Date Due

MAY 8 2000		
8-29-04		
SEP 2 4 2010		

BRODART, CO.   Cat. No. 23-233-003   Printed in U.S.A.

Textbook of Fetal and Perinatal Pathology

SECOND EDITION

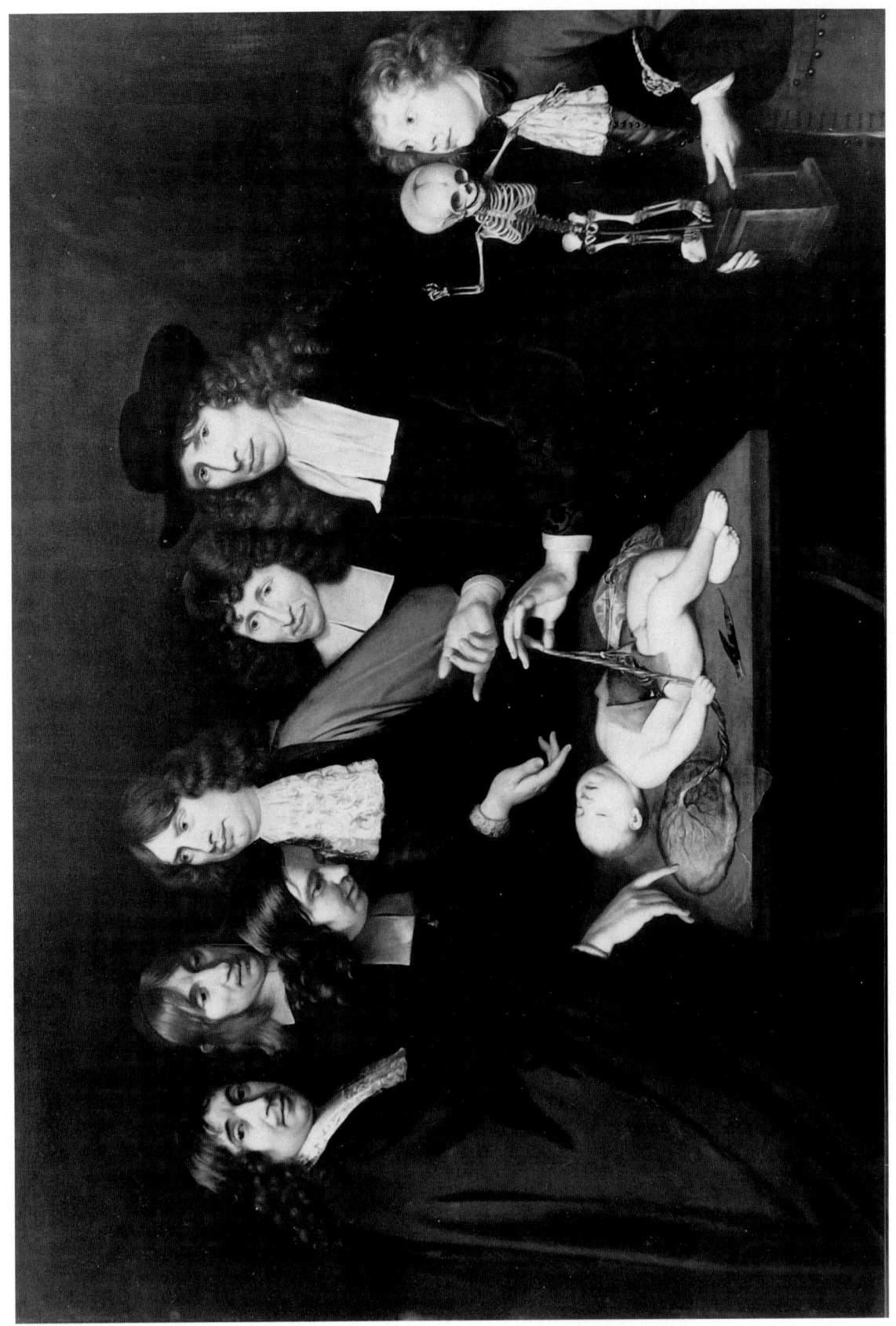

Textbook of Fetal and Perinatal Pathology

SECOND EDITION

Edited by

JONATHAN S. WIGGLESWORTH, MD, FRCPATH
Professor of Perinatal Pathology
Department of Histopathology
Division of Investigative Science
Imperial College School of Medicine
Hammersmith Hospital
London, England

DON B. SINGER, MD
Developmental and Pediatric Pathology Program
Brown University School of Medicine
Women and Infants' Hospital
Providence, Rhode Island

b

**Blackwell
Science**

FEB 3 '99

© 1998 by Jonathan S. Wigglesworth and Don B. Singer
Blackwell Science
Editorial Offices:
Commerce Place, 350 Main Street, Malden, Massachusetts 02148,
    USA
Osney Mead, Oxford OX2 0EL, England
25 John Street, London WC1N 2BL, England
23 Ainslie Place, Edinburgh EH3 6AJ, Scotland
54 University Street, Carlton, Victoria 3053, Australia

Other Editorial Offices:
Blackwell Wissenschafts-Verlag GmbH
Kurfürstendamm 57
10707 Berlin, Germany

Blackwell Science KK
MG Kodenmacho Building
7-10 Kodenmacho Nihombashi
Chuo-ku, Tokyo 104, Japan

Acquisitions: Christopher Davis
Production: Irene Herlihy
Manufacturing: Lisa Flanagan
Cover Design: Meral Dabcovich, Visual Perspectives
Typeset by Best-set Typesetter Ltd., Hong Kong
Printed and bound by Braun-Brumfield, Inc.

The Blackwell Science logo is a trade mark of Blackwell Science
Ltd., registered at the United Kingdom Trade Marks Registry

Distributors:

USA

Blackwell Science, Inc.
Commerce Place
350 Main Street
Malden, Massachusetts 02148
    (Telephone orders: 800-215-1000 or 781-388-8250;
    fax orders: 781-388-8270)

CANADA

Login Brothers Book Company
324 Saulteaux Crescent
Winnipeg, Manitoba, R3J 3T2
    (Telephone orders: 204-224-4068)

AUSTRALIA

Blackwell Science Pty, Ltd.
54 University Street
Carlton, Victoria 3053
    (Telephone orders: 03-9347-0300; fax orders: 03-9349-3016)

OUTSIDE NORTH AMERICA AND AUSTRALIA

Blackwell Science, Ltd.
c/o Marston Book Services, Ltd.
P.O. Box 269
Abingdon
Oxon OX14 4YN
England
    (Telephone orders: 44-01235-465500;
    fax orders: 44-01235-465555)

Printed in the United States of America
98 99 00 01 5 4 3 2 1

Library of Congress Cataloging-in-Publication Data

Textbook of fetal and perinatal pathology / [edited by] Jonathan
    S. Wigglesworth, Don B. Singer.—2nd ed.
        p.   cm.
        Includes bibliographical references and index.
        ISBN 0-86542-396-2
        1. Fetus—Diseases.   2. Infants (Newborn)—Diseases.
    I. Wigglesworth, Jonathan S.   II. Singer, Don B.
        [DNLM: 1. Fetal Diseases—pathology.
    2. Infant, Newborn, Diseases—pathology.
    WQ 211 T355 1997]
    RG626.T47   1998
    618.3'3207—dc21
    DNLM/DLC
    for Library of Congress   97-21930
                                                        CIP

CONTENTS

Derek A. Applegarth, PhD, FRCMG
Head, Biochemical Diseases Laboratory
Department of Pathology
Children's and Women's Health Centre of British Columbia;
Professor of Pediatrics, Pathology and Medical Genetics
University of British Columbia
Vancouver, British Columbia
Canada

Frederic B. Askin, MD
Professor of Pathology
Director, Surgical Pathology
Department of Pathology
Johns Hopkins Medical Institutions
Baltimore, Maryland

Virginia J. Baldwin, BSc, MD, FRCP(C)
Pediatric Pathologist
Children's and Women's Health Centre of British Columbia;
Associate Professor of Pathology
University of British Columbia
Vancouver, British Columbia
Canada

J. Patrick Barbet
Service d'Anatomie Pathologique
Hôpital Saint Vincent de Paul
Paris, France

M. Michael Cohen, Jr., DMD, PhD
Professor of Oral and Maxillofacial Pathology
Faculty of Dentistry
Professor of Pediatrics
Faculty of Medicine
Dalhousie University
Halifax, Nova Scotia
Canada

Derek J. deSa, MBBS, DPhil(Oxon), FRCPath, FRCP(C)
Department of Pathology
Children's and Women's Health Centre of British Columbia;
Professor of Pathology
University of British Columbia
Vancouver, British Columbia
Canada

James E. Dimmick, MD, FRCP(C)
Director
Department of Pathology
Children's and Women's Health Centre of British Columbia;
Professor of Pathology and Laboratory Medicine
University of British Columbia
Vancouver, British Columbia
Canada

William H. Donnelly, MD
Professor of Pathology and Pediatrics
Department of Pathology
University of Florida College of Medicine
Gainesville, Florida

Ferechte Encha-Razavi, MD
Laboratoire de Neuropathologie
C.H.V. Henri Mondor
Creteil, France

Alec Garner, MD, PhD, FRCP, FRCPath, FRCOphth
Emeritus Professor of Pathology
Institute of Ophthalmology
University of London
London, England

Enid F. Gilbert-Barness, MD
Professor of Pathology and Laboratory
  Medicine, Pediatrics, and Obstetrics and
  Gynecology
University of South Florida;
Director of Pediatric Pathology
Tampa General Hospital
Tampa, Florida

Frank Gonzalez-Crussi, MD
Head of Laboratories
Children's Memorial Hospital;
Professor of Pathology
Northwestern University School of Medicine
Chicago, Illinois

**Robert J. Gorlin, DDS, MS, DSc (Athens,
  Thessaloniki)**
Regents' Professor, Oral Pathology and Genetics
Division of Oral Pathology and Genetics
Department of Oral Science
University of Minnesota Schools of Dentistry and
  Medicine
Minneapolis, Minnesota

Ronald Jaffe, MB, BCh
Pathologist-in-Chief
Children's Hospital of Pittsburgh;
Professor of Pathology and Pediatrics
University of Pittsburgh School of Medicine
Pittsburgh, Pennsylvania

Gareth P. Jevon, MB, ChB
Department of Pathology
Children's and Women's Health Centre of British
  Columbia
The University of British Columbia
Vancouver, British Columbia
Canada

Dagmar K. Kalousek, MD, FRCP(C), FCCMG
Department of Pathology
Children's and Women's Health Centre of British
  Columbia;
Professor of Pathology
The University of British Columbia
Vancouver, British Columbia
Canada

**Jean W. Keeling, MB, BS, FRCPath, FRCP(Edin.),
  FRCPCH**
Head of Pathology and Cytogenetics
Department of Paediatric Pathology
Royal Hospital for Sick Children
Edinburgh, Scotland

Brian D. Lake, BSc, PhD, FRCPath
Professor of Histochemistry
Department of Histopathology
Great Ormond Street Hospital for Children
London, England

Jeanne-Claudie Larroche, MD
Institut National de la Santé et de la Recherche Médicale
Paris, France

Stuart C. Lauchlan, MB, ChB, FRCP(C)
Director of Surgical Pathology and Cytopathology
Women and Infants' Hospital
Providence, Rhode Island

Geoffrey A. Machin, MD, PhD, FRCP(C)
Fetal/Genetic Pathologist
Department of Pathology
The Permanente Medical Group
Oakland, California

Trevor A. Macpherson, MB, ChB, MRCOG
Associate Professor of Pathology
University of Pittsburgh School of Medicine;
Chief of Pathology and Director of Research
Magee-Womens Hospital
Pittsburgh, Pennsylvania

John M. Opitz, MD, DSci(HC), MD(HC) SAAP
Professor of Pediatrics and Human Genetics and
  Obstetrics/Gynecology
University of Utah
Salt Lake City, Utah

Calvin E. Oyer, MD
Developmental and Pediatric Pathology Program
Brown University School of Medicine
Women and Infants' Hospital
Providence, Rhode Island

Halit Pinar, MD
Assistant Professor of Pathology and Pediatrics
Brown University School of Medicine;
Director, Division of Perinatal Pathology
Women and Infants' Hospital
Providence, Rhode Island

Juhani Rapola, MD
Pathology Unit
Children's Hospital
University of Helsinki
Helsinki, Finland

Harvey S. Rosenberg, MD
Professor of Pathology and Pediatrics
University of Texas Medical School
Houston, Texas

D. Ian Rushton, MB, ChB, FRCPath, FRCPCH
Senior Lecturer in Pathology
University of Birmingham;
Honorary Consultant Perinatal Pathologist
The Birmingham Maternity Hospital
Birmingham, England

Don B. Singer, MD
Developmental and Pediatric Pathology Program
Brown University School of Medicine
Women and Infants' Hospital
Providence, Rhode Island

Cirilo Sotelo-Avila, MD
Cardinal Glennon Children's Hospital
St. Louis University School of Medicine
St. Louis, Missouri

Chien-Ren Sung, MD
Developmental and Pediatric Pathology Program
Brown University School of Medicine
Women and Infants' Hospital
Providence, Rhode Island

Marie Valdes-Dapena, MD
Professor Emerita of Pathology and Pediatrics
Department of Pathology
University of Miami School of Medicine
Miami, Florida

Hilary D. Vallance, MD, FRCP(C)
Head, Newborn Screening Program
Department of Pathology and Laboratory Medicine
Children's and Women's Health Centre of Britis Columbia
Vancouver, British Columbia
Canada

Jonathan S. Wigglesworth, MD, FRCPath
Professor of Perinatal Pathology
Department of Histopathology
Division of Investigative Science
Imperial College School of Medicine
Hammersmith Hospital
London, England

R. Douglas Wilson, MSc, MD, FRCS(C)
Department of Medical Genetics/Obstetrics and
    Gynecology
Children's and Women's Health Centre of British
    Columbia;
Associate Professor
The University of British Columbia
Vancouver, British Columbia
Canada

S. Samuel Yang, MD
Former Attending Pathologist
William Beaumont Hospital
Royal Oak, Michigan

One of the purposes of science is to analyze phenomena, and then to reanalyze them as new techniques are developed. In less than a decade since the first edition, our knowledge of basic human biology has grown enormously. The new diagnostic methods, particularly in molecular biology, provide for the recognition of expanded or altered categories of disease. Furthermore, the definition of subtle differences in conditions that were formerly considered single entities has caused "splitters" to rejoice and "lumpers" to reconsider. We have encouraged contributors to this second edition to respond to the challenges implicit in our evolving specialty by retaining pertinent information from the first edition while incorporating advances in a concise and relevant manner. We are aware the publications on molecular and genetic sciences are outdated as soon as they appear in print, but we hope that the chapters herein may lead readers to appropriate journals and investigators to obtain more current data. Our intention is to provide a timely and comprehensive textbook of pathology of the embryo, placenta, fetus, and newborn infant.

We welcome new contributors J. P. Barbet, MD, M. Michael Cohen, Jr., DMD, PhD, Jevon Gareth, MB, ChB, Robert Gorlin, DDS, DDc, Calvin Oyer, MD, Halit M. Pinar, MD, Hilary D. Vallance, MD, and R. Douglas Wilson, MD.

Many of the errors that appeared in the first edition have been corrected. We thank our readers who have detected these errors and notified us of them and we encourage them to repeat the effort with this edition. We especially thank Christopher Davis, Irene Herlihy, and the editors at Blackwell Science, Inc. who have provided immeasurable help and stewardship as we moved to the completion of this edition. Our heartfelt thanks go to Joan Wigglesworth and Estelle Singer for their continued patience, encouragement, support, understanding, and love.

J.S.W.
D.B.S.
November 1997

There is a steadily increasing popular and medical interest in embryonic, fetal, and neonatal well-being. Popular interest reflects recent cultural changes in developed countries where there is a prevalence of small families and older mothers. Each pregnancy is now a major event and is embarked on with high expectations of a successful outcome. The demand to explain the occasional death, or handicapped surviving infant, becomes ever more insistent. Medical interest is stimulated by advances in obstetric, prenatal, perinatal, and neonatal medicine. New imaging techniques allow the obstetrician to study and relate to his unborn patient. New methods in laboratory diagnosis have expanded our knowledge of genetic and nongenetic abnormalities. New diseases have been described and old ones more completely understood. These factors combine to make clinical assessments of individual cases more critical and in some respects more complex. The foundations of knowledge of developmental pathology on which clinical decisions in perinatal medicine need to be based have become ever wider.

A number of texts on fetal and neonatal pathology have been published in the last 5 years and the need for a new one demands explanation. An earlier, smaller book written by one of us (J.S.W.) was intended to provide a practical working knowledge of the subject of perinatal pathology and to serve as the starting point for academic study. In planning a more comprehensive text we have been concerned to fulfill the needs of perinatal and pediatric pathologists for a relatively detailed reference work. In addition we hope that such a work would find a place on the shelves of perina-tologists, neonatologists, and geneticists as well as the libraries consulted by general pathologists, obstetricians, pediatricians, and others who are involved with the care of the fetus and newborn infant.

In planning the text for our own use we have tried to select an important range of topics for special consideration, in addition to the major organ systems, and to incorporate the data and tables to which rapid access would be most helpful. We have been fortunate in persuading many distinguished colleagues from both sides of the Atlantic to contribute chapters on areas where they have particular expertise and which cover the field from embryogenesis through to term and beyond to the first months of life. The editors are most appreciative of these experts' efforts: without them our task would have been impossible. The extensive references to most chapters are intended to fill many of the gaps of information unavoidably omitted, even in a work of this size. Although we have included slightly unusual topics such as the pathology of facial development, we are conscious that a number of other equally relevant subjects have been left out.

We are confident that readers and reviewers will inform us of the extent to which we have succeeded in our aims and what faults of omission or commission may require correction in any subsequent edition.

J.S.W.
D.B.S.
July 1990

Part

I

Principles and Major Problems

Role of Pathology in Modern Perinatal Medicine

JONATHAN S. WIGGLESWORTH

Fetal and perinatal pathology is largely a postmortem specialty concerned with causes and mechanisms of reproductive loss. Increasing interest in this field has come at a time when the adult postmortem is in decline and when numbers of deaths in the strict perinatal period have decreased to 10 per 1000 births or less in most developed countries. The role of the perinatal pathologist at such a time requires some explanation, both for the benefit of those who are commencing this work and for those who may be concerned with the organization and funding of services in perinatal medicine.

VALUE OF EXAMINATION OF EMBRYO, FETUS, AND NEONATE

The Embryo

The major part of total pregnancy loss occurs in the first half of pregnancy, before the stage of viability [1–5]. Causes of such loss vary according to the developmental age of the conceptus. Deaths associated with gross chromosomal and genetic defects are most frequent in the earlier weeks, representing 60% in aborted embryos, and decrease as pregnancy proceeds [2, 6–9]. Deaths at a later stage include an increasing proportion due to problems that have arisen during pregnancy, such as infections, premature rupture of the membranes, and a range of problems resulting in impairment of uteroplacental transfer.

Much of this loss can be regarded as a necessary deletion of reproductive failures. Examination of the products of abortion in every case is not currently achievable and could be regarded as an uneconomic use of scarce professional skills. Such examination is of importance in the individual case, either where a particular cause for the loss is suspected

or in an attempt to determine the mechanisms in cases of repeated abortions. Reasons for requiring examination in the individual case might include investigation of possible effects of potentially toxic or teratogenic agents, such as drugs administered to the mother, or maternal viral infections, such as rubella. Periodic surveys of types and causes of abortion are of scientific importance in establishing current patterns of pregnancy loss, particularly as a range of chromosomal anomalies, including triploidy and XO fetuses, is so heavily represented in this group [2, 8].

In addition, the trends in prenatal diagnosis are for methods that can be utilized earlier in gestation. The chorion villous sampling procedure can now allow diagnosis of a large range of genetic disorders in the first trimester [10], either by means of enzyme assay on cell cultures or by DNA analysis [11], enhanced if necessary by the polymerase chain reaction technique [12]. The rapidly expanding knowledge of specific gene loci for disease, including malformations and inborn errors of metabolism [13–19], will undoubtedly increase prenatal diagnosis by molecular techniques. These methods are leading to earlier termination of pregnancy for medical reasons, with consequent demand for accurate diagnostic confirmation by the pathologist to provide validation of the technique [20].

The Fetus and Neonate

As pregnancy proceeds toward and past the stage of viability, the frequency of loss decreases and the concerns over an individual loss may be expected to increase. In late first and early second trimester, diagnosis of fetal anomaly by ultrasound becomes a major factor leading to termination, while legally permissible, at up to 20 weeks' gestational age. Even in centers with a high rate of accurate prenatal ultrasound diagnosis, 37% of fetuses with correctly diagnosed anomalies may have additional defects that were not recognized prenatally [21]. Abnormalities that may require pathological confirmation include those of the brain, cardiovascular system, respiratory system, alimentary system, and urinary tract. The need for pathological examination of fetus and placenta is not confined to cases with a prenatally diagnosed abnormality. It may be demanded equally by clinical concern to exclude the presence of a recurrent problem and by the need to provide an explanation of the pregnancy loss to the parents.

Parental concern over a fetal death does not fall into a neat pattern related to gestation length, and significant grief reactions may be experienced in 70% of cases following termination for fetal anomaly [22]. Explanation of the pathology related to a fetal or neonatal death may not be of immediate help in determining the course of the grief reaction, but it is important in providing a positive focus for planning a subsequent pregnancy. Pathology cannot answer the bereaved parents' question, "Why did this happen to us?" It can, however, be an important aid to answering the questions, "Will the same thing happen next time?" and, "How can it be prevented?"

Paradoxically, the level of sophistication in the questions that parents ask about fetal and perinatal deaths has increased as the frequency of death has declined. Twenty or thirty years ago the loss of a baby was regarded as a largely unpredictable event, prompting recommendation to the parents to "go home and try again." Detailed questioning as to why or how the baby had died was neither expected nor welcomed by the medical profession. Parents planning a modern small family in the late 1990s expect to receive a baby in perfect order. In the event of perinatal death or handicap, the providers of perinatal care may be asked searching questions and, if answers are inadequate, may be called to answer for their actions in court. Adequate investigation of perinatal death in such a critical environment must involve an informed postmortem examination, even if clinicians feel confident of the premortem diagnosis made on the basis of imaging or other forms of assessment. The author has been involved in more than one case where the quality of a postmortem examination of a macerated fetus was a significant factor in determining the outcome of litigation relating to a handicapped surviving twin.

The value of a postmortem examination to the clinicians responsible for managing the index pregnancy, and for planning the management of a likely future pregnancy in the same family, is not readily separable from the value to the parents. If the clinician is confident of his or her strategy to detect potential recurrence in a subsequent pregnancy, this can only be to the parents' benefit. Improved management of other similar cases as a result of knowledge gained in the one case will be to the benefit of other parents in the future. Discussion of postmortem findings at regular perinatal mortality meetings, or indeed fetal pathology meetings, is a

further means of providing valuable training to medical personnel.

It must be stressed here, as previously [18, 23], that both positive and negative findings are equally important to parents and clinicians. It may be impossible to pinpoint a cause of death in the well-grown baby who dies unexpectedly in labor. This must at least mean that most of the conditions described in the one thousand two hundred-odd pages of this text have been excluded! The apparently healthy nutritional status of such an infant also suggests that, whatever the precise mechanism leading to death, the process must have operated briefly during, or near to, the time of labor. The message for the obstetrician may well be to induce labor in a succeeding pregnancy at a slightly earlier gestation in order to avoid recurrence. The role of the pathologist thus includes the ability to recognize and to report clearly all those features that are normal in such a way that logical conclusions may be drawn. This is often a problem in that pathologists are primarily concerned with diagnosis of disease rather than with description of nondisease. Poor perinatal postmortem reports often may be due to the loss of enthusiasm by the pathologist on failing to find evidence of a gross pathological process that can explain death.

PERINATAL PATHOLOGY AND RESEARCH

The perinatal postmortem can subserve a range of research purposes. At the simplest level will be the local hospital or district perinatal mortality audit. Assessment of postmortem findings is of considerable assistance in clarifying the patterns of mortality and locating areas where improvements in perinatal care should be sought. Postmortem observations are important for many clinicopathological studies on the development of disease processes (e.g., cerebral pathology in the perinatal period) or on the influence (beneficial or otherwise) of new methods of management (e.g., methods of mechanical ventilation and the lung).

In addition, the material studied at the postmortem examination may be critical for basic studies on normal human development (e.g., studies on normal lung development) as well as for gaining an understanding of the pathogenesis of pathological processes not readily seen in animals (e.g., intraventricular hemorrhage). Observations made on the human fetus or neonate can prompt questions that can be investigated further by the performance of an appropriate experiment. Experiments set up in this way by the author included the influence of uterine ischemia on fetal growth and the effect of spinal cord transection on fetal lung growth [24, 25].

EXPERIENCE AND SKILLS
NEEDED FOR PERINATAL PATHOLOGY

In the recent past, the examination of fetuses and neonates was regarded as the least demanding of pathological skills and was often delegated to the most junior pathologists in training. It is now realized that special skills and knowledge are required for this area of pathology, but there is a shortage of centers where appropriate expertise can be gained, and it may be difficult to recruit trained staff when specialist posts are advertised.

Macroscopic observational skills remain of particular importance in fetal and perinatal pathology, although training in adult histopathology now tends to be concerned more with utilization of microscopic and ultrastructural methods of diagnosis, a difference emphasized by the decline in adult postmortem rates. Development of the necessary observational skills requires experience of a considerable number of cases, but the decline in perinatal mortality means that such experience can be gained only in a regional center with a large number of referred cases or specimens. The essential skills needed are the ability to carry out an appropriate dissection; to recognize, analyze, and describe the information available from macroscopic examination; and to set in motion any further investigations needed to establish or refute putative diagnoses. Some of these can be achieved by following a standard protocol as described in Chapter 5, but there will always be situations that require individual decisions on appropriate further studies. How comprehensive a postmortem protocol may be, whether for instance photography, radiography, or microbiology are performed in every case, will inevitably depend on local considerations of cost or expediency. There have been many publications detailing the rationale for performing good fetal and perinatal postmortem examinations and the techniques for carrying them out [26–37]. They reiterate many of the points covered in this chapter, with varying emphasis on genetic or non-genetic aspects of perinatal pathology according to the persuasion and interests of the authors. However, there is no protocol that absolves the pathologist from the need to make his or her own observations on minor deviations from the normal, which may suggest the need for some additional diagnostic procedure that is not in any standard scheme. There is, in fact, no way that a protocol can substitute for a skilled dissector and observer.

RELATIVE ROLES OF INDIVIDUALS CONCERNED IN DIAGNOSIS IN FETAL AND PERINATAL CASES

The pathologist is only one of a team of individuals concerned with diagnosis in the fetal and perinatal period. The first and central clinician is now usually the obstetrician who, particularly in the modern role as a practitioner in fetal medicine, may make definitive or presumptive diagnoses with the powerful medium of ultrasound [21, 38, 39]. Recognition of a fetal abnormality, such as hydrocephalus, may lead directly to termination and referral to the pathologist for elucidation of the underlying pathogenetic mechanism.

In many cases, an abnormal ultrasound scan may prompt consultation with a second major specialist, the clinical geneticist, either before or after termination or spontaneous delivery. Many clinical geneticists now specialize in dysmorphology, and excel in recognizing characteristic dysmorphic syndromes from their external appearances and radiographs [40]. In addition, they may have links with, or control of, cytogenetic laboratories and will be able to analyze the chromosomal constitution of the fetus or neonate. Some genetic centers have laboratories where scientists carry out their own dissections of abnormal fetuses [2].

In the event of an ill liveborn infant, the diagnostic effort will be initiated or maintained by the neonatologist using neonatal ultrasound, radiology, biochemistry, hematology, and microbiology as adjuncts.

The pathologist may receive a fetus or neonate for examination at any stage of this process, with any degree of sophistication of diagnosis already made by other specialists. The pathologist's role may be merely to confirm a substantive diagnosis and to check that no subsidiary (e.g., iatrogenic) pathology is present. Often, there is only a partial diagnosis: An abnormality such as hydrocephalus or a renal cystic disorder has been recognized but not categorized further. Sometimes there has been no diagnosis, or an erroneous diagnosis has been made. It is important that the various specialists concerned recognize their own limitations and the value of other members of the team. The pathologist needs the help of the clinical geneticist in unravelling complex problems in dysmorphology. The dysmorphologist requires the pathologist to analyze the interactions between disease processes in the fetus and normal development, e.g., in the fetus with arthrogryposis.

Further scientific advances in perinatal medicine require an orderly combined approach, with preservation of tissues for future DNA analysis in cases where current knowledge fails to provide the answer.

ORGANIZATION OF PERINATAL PATHOLOGY SERVICES

Combined pressures from parents, obstetricians, and neonatologists have prompted a more constructive approach to the establishment and organization of services in fetal and perinatal pathology.

Reports from the British House of Commons and the Royal College of Pathologists some years ago stressed the importance of increased training, and an increased number of posts, in perinatal pathology [41–43]. It was recommended that specialist departments should be located within the regional tertiary neonatal intensive care facility [43], preferably at a teaching hospital and in close association with a university pathology department, and linked to regional centers for pediatric surgery and prenatal diagnosis. It was envisioned that each department would be staffed by two full time specialist perinatal/pediatric pathologists.

The work of such a department includes the performance of perinatal and neonatal postmortem examinations on babies dying in the associated obstetric and neonatal units, and examination of second trimester fetuses following spontaneous or therapeutic abortion. In addition, the regional department can undertake postmortem examinations on fetal, perinatal, and neonatal deaths referred from other hospitals in the region. All histopathologists in district general hospitals with maternity units should be able to perform a competent perinatal postmortem examination and handle routine cases, but might wish to refer more complex cases to the regional center. Advice on handling such cases should be available from the regional center by phone, and fixed organs (e.g., brains and malformed hearts), as well as histological sections, can be referred for specialist opinion. The regional center should be involved in any epidemiological studies carried out on fetal and perinatal deaths. The regional perinatal pathology department should have a major commitment to teaching junior pathologists and often may be involved in undergraduate teaching also. Often, the department will be concerned with pediatric surgical pathology and the investigation of postperinatal deaths, such as cases of sudden infant death syndrome, in addition to strictly fetal and perinatal pathology.

The need for such a center to produce reports rapidly and to liaise over local disposal requirements for a number of referring hospitals demands good secretarial and technical support. Other ancillary needs for the practice of perinatal pathology are discussed in Chapter 5.

Regional centers for perinatal pathology as outlined above have developed, or acquired increased staffing, over the last 6 years within the United Kingdom and they are an established feature of other jurisdictions, particularly in the United States and Canada. However, the distribution of such centers remains uneven and provision for perinatal pathology varies considerably from one region or state to the next.

TIME-SCALE OF EVENTS IN FETAL AND PERINATAL MEDICINE

Fetal and perinatal pathology represents a deviation from the normal at some time in development. Failure of development of the vascular system in the embryo and placenta is seen in a high proportion of early abortuses [44]. An extremely high proportion of early embryonic failure is related to gross chromosomal abnormality, as described in Chapter 6. Other fetuses with chromosomal anomalies are destined to be aborted or die in utero at later stages of the first and early second trimester. Single gene abnormalities may exert their effects in an obvious way from relatively early in development, as in a number of the chondrodysplasias. Others have a less gross influence, recognizable only in the late second or early third trimester, or indeed may involve the lack of an enzyme, such as one of the urea-cycle enzymes, that becomes essential for life only after birth,

causing rapid neonatal demise of an apparently normally developed infant. All such abnormalities may be regarded as inevitable disasters, programmed, like time bombs, to wreck development at some predetermined stage. Accurate diagnosis is essential to prevent a second disaster in the family.

More subtle are those disorders interfering with development in a quantitative way. Inadequacy of the transfer of oxygen or nutrients across the placenta may result in a similar outcome of a growth-retarded or hypoxic fetus, irrespective of whether the primary abnormality involves the maternal cardiorespiratory system, the development of the spiral artery supply to the intervillous space, or a problem of multiple placentation (see Chap. 2).

Secondary interference with fetal development occurs through sudden stresses, which may be purely physical, such as acute interference with the uteroplacental circulation by a motor accident affecting the pregnant mother (see Chap. 21), or may be infective, such as transplacental infection with *Listeria monocytogenes* or ascending infection with group B β-hemolytic streptococcus (see Chap. 17).

Further complexity is provided by the effects of an anomaly on later development of functionally related tissues. Thus, the lack of amniotic fluid consequent to renal agenesis results in external distortion and impairment of lung growth. The lack of urine production in such a case is associated with the failure of normal bladder development. Damage to muscle development, due either to a primary abnormality of muscle or central nervous system development or to anoxic destruction of spinal neurons, will result in muscle contractures, the picture of arthrogryposis.

Failure of function during the phase of rapid prenatal growth thus may be expressed rapidly in terms of structural alteration in a way that is not seen in the slower growth phases of later childhood or in the stable adult state.

The role of fetal and perinatal pathology is to disentangle these structural and functional interactions in order to determine the primary and secondary events that underlie a particular set of abnormal structural findings. For this purpose, an adequate understanding of the dynamic background processes of growth and development is essential. It is also essential to have access to ranges of appropriate normal measurements for all stages and areas of normal development. This is the subject of Chapter 2.

REFERENCES

1. Edmonds DK, Lindsay KS, Miller JF, Williamson E, Wood PJ. Early embryonic mortality in women. *Fertil Steril* 1982; 38:447–53.
2. Opitz JM. Prenatal and perinatal death: the future of developmental pathology. *Pediatr Pathol* 1987; 7:363–94.
3. Stein Z. Early fetal loss. *Birth Defects, Orig Artic Ser* 1981; 17(1):95–111.
4. Warburton D, Fraser FC. Spontaneous abortion risk in man: data from reproductive histories collected in a medical genetics unit. *Am J Hum Genet* 1964; 16:1–25.
5. Wilcox AJ, Weinberg CR, Wehmann RE, Armstrong EG, Canfield RE, Nisula BC. Measuring early pregnancy loss: laboratory and field methods. *Fertil Steril* 1985; 44:366–74.
6. Bauld R, Sutherland GR, Bain AD. Chromosomal studies in investigations of stillbirths and neonatal deaths. *Arch Dis Child* 1974; 49:782–8.

7. Boué A, Boué J, Gropp A. Cytogenetics of pregnancy wastage. *Adv Hum Genet* 1985; 14:1–57.

8. Boué J, Boué A, Lazar P. Retrospective and prospective epidemiological studies of 1500 karyotyped spontaneous human abortions. *Teratology* 1975; 12:11–26.

9. Gilbert EF, Opitz JM. Developmental and other pathologic changes in syndromes caused by chromosome abnormalities. *Perspect Pediatr Pathol* 1982; 7:1–63.

10. Daffos F. Access to the other patient. *Semin Perinatol* 1989; 13:252–9.

11. Holzgreve W, Miny P. Genetic aspects of fetal disease. *Semin Perinatol* 1989; 13:260–77.

12. Crisan D, Diven WF, Hartle K, Osborne PT, Mason L. Prenatal diagnosis of haemoglobinopathies by using polymerase chain reaction and allele-specific oligonucleotide probes. *Clin Chem* 1989; 35:1854.

13. Kerem B, Rommens JM, Buchanan JA, Markiewicz D, et al. Identification of the cystic fibrosis gene: genetic analysis. *Science* 1989; 245:1073–80.

14. McKusick VA, Amberger JS. The morbid anatomy of the human genome: chromosomal location of mutations causing disease. *J Med Genet* 1993; 30:1–26.

15. McKusick VA, Amberger JS. The morbid anatomy of the human genome: chromosomal location of mutations causing disease (update 1 December 1993). *J Med Genet* 1994; 31:265–79.

16. Riordan JR, Rommens JM, Kerem B, et al. Identification of the cystic fibrosis gene: cloning and characterisation of complementary DNA. *Science* 1989; 245:1066–73.

17. Rommens JM, Ianuzzi MC, Kerem B, et al. Identification of the cystic fibrosis gene: chromosome walking and jumping. *Science* 1989; 245:1059–65.

18. Wigglesworth JS. *Perinatal Pathology*. Philadelphia: Saunders, 1984, p. 1.

19. Wilkie AO, Amberger JS, McKusick VA. A gene map of congenital malformations. *J Med Genet* 1994; 31:507–17.

20. Joint Study Group on Fetal Abnormalities. Recognition and management of fetal abnormalities. *Arch Dis Child* 1989; 64:971–6.

21. Manchester DK, Pretorius DH, Avery C, et al. Accuracy of ultrasound diagnoses in pregnancies complicated by suspected fetal anomalies. *Prenat Diagn* 1988; 8:109–17.

22. Lloyd J, Laurence KM. Sequelae and support after termination of pregnancy for fetal malformation. *Br Med J* 1985; 290:907–9.

23. Keeling JW. The perinatal necropsy. In: Keeling JW, ed. *Fetal and Neonatal Pathology*, 2nd ed. London: Springer-Verlag, 1993, pp. 1–46.

24. Wigglesworth JS. Experimental growth retardation in the foetal rat. *J Pathol Bacteriol* 1964; 88:1–13.

25. Wigglesworth JS, Desai R. Effects on lung growth of cervical cord section in the rabbit fetus. *Early Hum Dev* 1979; 3:51–65.

26. Baldwin VJ, Kalousek DK, Dimmick JE, Applegarth DA, Hardwick DF. Diagnostic/pathologic investigation of the malformed conceptus. *Perspect Pediatr Pathol* 1982; 7:65–108.

27. Barson AJ. The perinatal postmortem. In: Barson AJ, ed. *Laboratory Investigation of Fetal Disease*. Bristol: John Wright, 1981, pp. 476–97.

28. Bruyere HJ Jr, Arya S, Kozel JS, et al. The value of examining spontaneously aborted human embryos and placentas. *Birth Defects, Orig Artic Ser*, 1987; 23:169–78.

29. Carey JC. Diagnostic evaluation of the stillborn infant. *Clin Obstet Gynecol* 1987; 30:342–51.

30. Driscoll SG. Autopsy following stillbirth: a challenge neglected. In: Ryder OA, Byrd ML, eds. *One Medicine*. Berlin: Springer-Verlag, 1984, pp. 20–31.

31. Gau G. The ultimate audit. *Br Med J* 1977; 1:1580–82.

32. Langley FA. The perinatal postmortem examination. *J Clin Pathol* 1971; 24:159–69.

33. Manchester DK, Shikes RH. The perinatal autopsy: special considerations. *Clin Obstet Gynecol* 1983; 23:1125–34.

34. Meir PR, Manchester DK, Shikes RH, Clewell WH, Stewart M. Perinatal autopsy: its clinical value. *Obstet Gynecol* 1986; 67:349–51.

35. Mueller RF, Sybert VP, Johnson J, Brown ZA, Chen WJ. Evaluation of a protocol for postmortem examination of stillbirths. *N Engl J Med* 1983; 309:586–90.

36. Naeye RL. The investigation of perinatal death. *N Engl J Med* 1983; 309:611–12.

37. Tyson W, Manchester D. Pathologic aspects of fetal death. *Clin Obstet Gynecol* 1987; 30:331–41.

38. Chervenak FA, Isaacson G, Mahoney MJ. Advances in the diagnosis of fetal defects. *N Engl J Med* 1986; 315:305–7.

39. Persson P-H, Kullander S. Long-term experience of general ultrasound screening in pregnancy. *Am J Obstet Gynecol* 1983; 146:942–7.

40. Clayton-Smith J, Farndon PA, McKeown C, Donnai D. Examination of fetuses after induced abortion for fetal abnormality. *Br Med J* 1990; 300:295–7.

41. Great Britain Parliament House of Commons Social Services Committee. First report on perinatal, neonatal and infant mortality (HC 54). HMSO, London, 1988.

42. Great Britain Department of Health. Perinatal, neonatal and infant mortality. Government reply to the 1st report from the Social Services Committee, Session 1988–89 (Cm. 741). HMSO, London, 1989.

43. Royal College of Pathologists Working Party. Report of the RCPath Working Party on paediatric and perinatal pathology. *Bull RCPathol* 1990; 69:10–13.

44. Rushton DI. Simplified classification of spontaneous abortions. *J Med Genet* 1978; 15:1–9.

Fetal Growth and Maturation: With Standards for Body and Organ Development

Don B. Singer   Chien-Ren Sung   Jonathan S. Wigglesworth

The first essential when examining the embryo, fetus, or infant is to determine where the case fits in the scale of human development. Typically, human form, function, and size change in a normal and predictable manner from conception through adolescence. If pathologic processes are to be understood, the changes during normal growth and development must have reference either to the age of the subject or to the stage of gestation. The most obvious change with time is an increase in size or mass, and the simplest view of human fetal and infant development would regard weight as the main criterion needed for the assessment of fetal maturity. Small newborns have more significant morbidity and mortality than individuals in any other comparable time of life [1–3], and the smaller the baby, the greater the risk. Survival with birth weight less than 1000 grams was a condition worthy of publication a few decades ago [4]. Now, however, such reports are commonplace and are evidence of the mounting interest received by these tiny patients [5–9].

The simple determination that a baby weighs either more than or less than 2500 grams is the most telling epidemiologic fact for predicting outcome, so it is not surprising that this figure was chosen years ago to define the limit between "prematurity" and "maturity" [10–12]. Fatality among babies with low birth weight (LBW; <2500 g) is some 200 times that of babies with normal birth weight [10, 13–16]. In the past two decades, improvements in care have resulted in survival of 95% of neonates with birth weights between 1250 and 1500 grams. Increased survival is also noted in babies as small as 500 grams at birth, although morbidity remains a significant factor in these fragile patients [10, 17–20]. The effect on mortality and morbidity of the severity of neonatal illness can be estimated through clinical scoring systems (e.g., Score for Neonatal Acute Physiology [SNAP]), which provide refined estimates to predict outcome in sick neonates. Birth weight is only one of the items considered in the SNAP scores [21]. While the data are not universally accepted, some studies suggest that babies with LBW may have continued morbidity and retarded growth through 14 years of age [22].

GESTATIONAL AGE

Weight alone is not a suitable criterion for inquiry in perinatal pathology [23]. Linear growth can also aid with assessments but the duration of gestation is most important [24, 25]. The recognition of specific morphological, functional, and pathological features of the mature, but growth-impaired, fetus or infant emphasizes the need to use time from conception as the independent variable against which all changes in form or function should be measured [26].

Of the three determinants, weight, length, and gestational age, the last is the most difficult to assess. It cannot be measured in a simple objective manner, and practical problems often result in a lack of cogent data for important epidemiological studies, such as those on perinatal mortality. Nevertheless, several ways exist to estimate gestational age while the fetus is in utero, and others are appropriate to the neonate or for use by the pathologist.

Menstrual and Obstetrical Estimates

Using Naegele's rule, we reckon a conceptus' menstrual age, taking the first day of the gravida's last menstrual period as the starting point. By counting ahead 7 days, subtracting 3 months, and adding 1 year, the expected date of birth is determined. In simpler terms, a full-term pregnancy should extend forward for 280 to 282 days, or 40 weeks, or 10 lunar months after the last menstrual period. In this chapter it is understood, unless stated otherwise, that the duration of gestation begins with the first day of the gravida's last menstrual period; i.e., we reckon gestation on the basis of menstrual age. In the embryological literature, gestation is usually reckoned from the time of fertilization. By convention, this is assumed to be on the same day as human ovulation and, also by convention, this is 14 days or 2 weeks after the first day of the last menstrual period. The ovulation age or fertilization age is always 14 days shorter than the menstrual age. The duration of embryogenesis is 56 days or 8 full weeks, but it extends to the end of the 10th week after the last menstrual period. The fetal period begins with the 9th week of development, but begins with the 11th week after the last menstrual period. Similarly, term gestation calculated from the time of ovulation or fertilization is 266 to 268 days or 38 weeks, and is 280 to 282 days or 40 weeks after the last menstrual period.

Using menstrual dates entails a significant chance for error due to biologic variation or misinterpretations of vaginal bleeding or lack thereof. Only 4–5% of babies are born on the expected day of delivery and only 35% within 5 days of the calculated date [27, 28]. One reason for the error is found in the variable duration of the preovulatory portion of the menstrual cycle. Many women have successive cycles that vary from 25 to 35 days. Nishimura and colleagues [29] demonstrated that both developmental stage and crown–rump length vary widely for embryos at a single gestational age. Conversely, at any single developmental stage

or at any crown–rump measurement, the gestational age can vary by as much as 20 days (Fig. 2.1).

Occasional breakthrough bleeding in early pregnancy occurs in as many as 20% of primigravidas and 38% of multigravidas, erroneously shortening the pregnancy [28, 30, 31]. Another biological variable is the true duration of pregnancy from one gravida to another, and from one pregnancy to the next in a particular gravida. Guerrero and Florez [32] found a standard deviation of 16 days in the length of pregnancy measured prospectively from the date of rise of maternal basal body temperature in more than 1300 women (Fig. 2.2). Kirkpatrick et al [33] found that by 16 weeks' gestation, 43.6% of gravidas had menstrual histories compatible with 16 weeks, while 32% had gestations by menstrual histories of less than 15 weeks or more than 17 weeks. Gestations extending beyond 295 days (43 weeks) are designated postterm and often have associated abnormalities of fetal growth and well-being; mortality among babies born after 44 weeks may be as much as 10% [27, 34].

Dating by last menstrual period (LMP) only overestimates the prevalence of prematurity and postmaturity. Obstetric estimates (using LMP corrected by ultrasound data) correlate better with observations at birth. Data for birth weights from 24 to 43 weeks of gestation by obstetric estimates are given in Table 2.1 [35].

The current standard method for timing a gestation is the gravida's recollection of the first day of the last menstrual period, combined where possible with an ultrasound assessment [36–38].

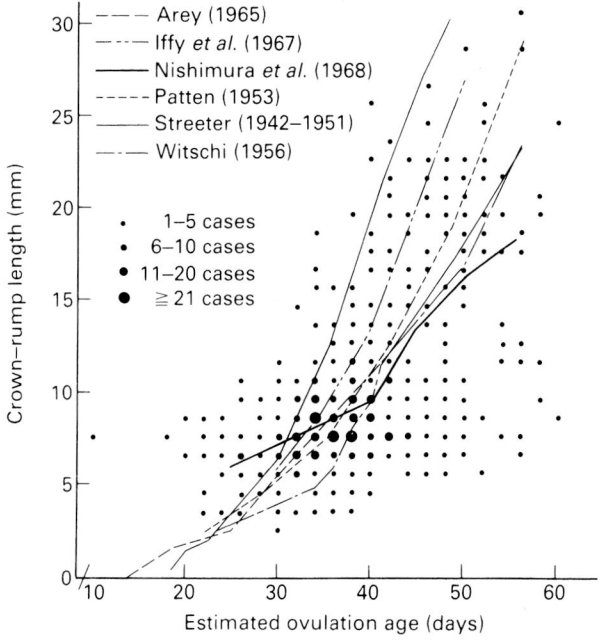

FIGURE 2.1. *Relation between estimated ovulation age and crown–rump length (675 embryos from mothers with regular cycles). (Courtesy of Nishimura et al [29].)*

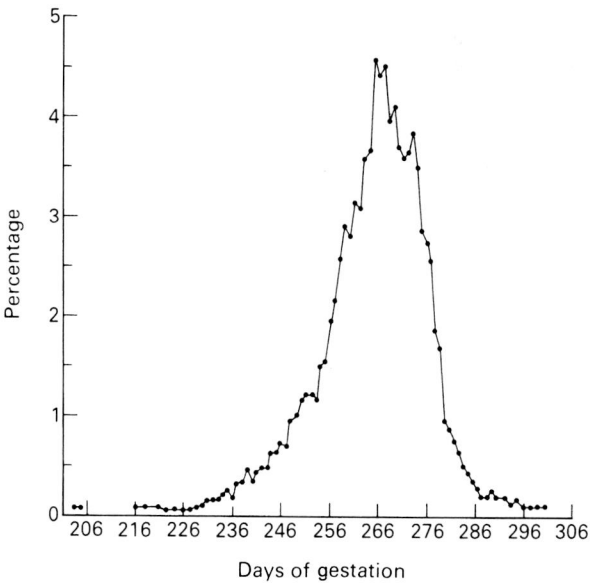

FIGURE 2.2. *Distribution of days of gestation from day of rise in basal body temperature in 1336 spontaneous full-term deliveries. Mean = 264.79 days; SD = 11.87. (From Ref. 32, with permission.)*

Table 2.1. Measurements of babies born at gestations determined by last menstrual period and corrected by fetal ultrasound examinations

Gestation (weeks)	Body weight (gm)	SD	Length (cm)	SD	Head circumference (cm)	SD
24	598	108	31.0	2.1	21.6	1.6
25	693	118	33.0	3.2	22.7	1.8
26	812	150	33.6	2.2	24.0	1.9
27	910	172	35.0	3.0	25.0	1.9
28	1037	199	36.1	2.8	25.3	1.8
29	1192	250	38.0	3.6	26.3	1.8
30	1371	248	39.1	2.8	27.7	1.5
31	1542	226	40.5	2.5	28.9	1.9
32	1683	273	42.1	2.5	29.5	1.8
33	1860	293	43.1	2.5	30.1	1.6
34	2061	347	43.9	2.4	30.9	1.6
35	2272	353	45.0	2.7	31.7	1.6
36	2493	336	45.9	2.4	32.2	1.5
37	2809	417	47.2	2.4	33.0	1.5
38	3050	428	48.3	2.5	33.6	1.4
39	3225	446	49.0	2.5	34.0	1.4
40	3364	445	49.5	2.6	34.3	1.4
41	3501	447	50.2	2.4	34.7	1.4
42	3598	494	50.5	2.5	34.9	1.4
43	3734	506	50.7	2.6	35.0	1.6

SD = standard deviation.
From Dombrowski et al [35].

Radiologic and Sonargraphic Assessment

Campbell [37] endorses the use of sonargraphy in making corrections to menstrual age, as he claims that one-third of pregnant women are uncertain of their menstrual dates. If the menstrual age does not agree with the sonargraphic age, serial sonargrams should be obtained to establish either accurate dating or a diagnosis of retardation of fetal growth [39]. In assessing fetal age in the 12- to 40-week range, two measurements are most often used: the biparietal diameter (BPD) and the femur length [39].

The usefulness of the BPD derives from the sagittal falx, which enables accurate alignment of the head and allows measurement precisely in the correct plane. Extra care is warranted toward the end of fetal gestation because the incremental growth of the BPD (and all other linear measurements) slows appreciably, leading to small differences over several weeks' time [39]. Femoral length is a valuable adjunct to BPD in assessing fetal age. Undermeasurement can be a problem if a tangential section of the calcified portion of the femur is obtained. Artifactual bowing may appear, depending on the angle of "view" of the bone. Poor lateral resolution and variation in beam width can increase the measurement [39].

Other structures used to determine fetal age include the kidney, the outer orbital diameter, head circumference, abdominal circumference, lengths of several long bones other than the femur, and crown–rump length. Of these, the BPD and femoral length are the most thoroughly studied and standardized [39]. The sonargraphic measurements of BPD, femoral length, and the corresponding gestational ages are shown in Table 2.2.

Estimates of gestation can be established within ± 1 week in at least 70% of pregnancies by measuring the amniotic sac sonargraphically between the 6th and 14th week of pregnancy. The sac is round until the 7th week when it becomes elongated in the cranio-caudad axis and ovoid in the transverse axis [39–41]. Gestational age is proportional to sac volume and linear dimensions from 6 to 12 weeks (Table 2.3).

Were it not for the hazard of radiation injury, the gestational age of the living conceptus could be determined by radiographic examination of various gestational age ossification "centers" [42]. This method is certainly available to the pathologist, and the data provided in Table 2.4 may be useful. Early gestations can be evaluated by this means, as the clavicle and mandible (the first two bones to ossify) are sufficiently mineralized to be detected in radiograms during the 9th week of gestation (7th week of development) [42, 43]. This is followed in 1 to 2 weeks by ossification of the humerus, the radius, and the femur. The fibula, then the distal phalanges of the fingers, the vomer, and the tympanic ring are ossified by the 12th week of gestation. The distal femoral epiphysis is not ossified until about the 36th week of gestation [43, 44]. As with other methods of establishing gestational age, considerable variation is observed in the

Table 2.2. Ultrasonic measurements and gestational age

Biparietal diameter (cm)	Femur length (cm)	Gestation (weeks)
2.0	0.8	11.6
2.2	1.0	12.6
2.4	1.2	13.1
2.6	1.3	13.6
2.8	1.6	14.6
3.0	1.8	15.0
3.2	1.9	15.5
3.4	2.2	16.5
3.6	2.4	17.0
3.8	2.7	17.9
4.0	2.9	18.4
4.5	3.3	19.9
5.0	3.6	21.3
5.5	4.2	23.3
6.0	4.7	24.7
6.5	4.9	26.2
7.0	5.4	28.6
7.5	5.8	30.6
8.0	6.5	33.0
8.5	6.8	35.0
9.0	7.2	36.9
9.5	7.5	39.0
9.7	7.6	39.8

Data extracted from Sanders and James [39].

Table 2.4. Gestational ages at which various ossification centers appear

7 weeks	Mandible; clavicle
8 weeks	Occipital bone (squamous portion); superior maxilla; scapula; ribs 5,6,7; humerus; radius and ulna; femur; tibia
9 weeks	Occipital bone (lateral and basal portion); temporal bone; sphenoid (inner lamellae and pterygoid process); frontal bone; ribs 2,3,4,8,9,10,11; fingers (terminal phalanges), fingers (basal phalanges) 2,3; metacarpals 2,3; vertebral arches C1–7, D1,2; ilium; fibula; metatarsals 2,3; toe (distal phalanx) 1
10 weeks	Sphenoid (greater wings); nasal bone; ribs 1,12; fingers (basal phalanges) 1,4; metacarpals 1,4,5; vertebral arches D3–12, L1,2; vertebral bodies D2–L5; metatarsals 1,4,5; toes (terminal phalanges) 2–4
11 weeks	Fingers (basal phalanx) 5; vertebral arches L3–5; vertebral bodies, upper cervical and sacral
12–14 weeks	Sphenoid (lesser wings and anterior body); finger (middle phalanx) 5 m; vertebral arches, upper S; vertebral bodies, upper C to lower S; toe (terminal phalanx) 5; basal phalanges 1–5
15–20 weeks	Bony labyrinth; deciduous teeth rudiments; vertebral arch S4; odontoid process of axis, ischium
21–30 weeks	Hyoid bone, greater cornu; sternum; vertebral costal processes C6,7; vertebral transverse processes C–L; os pubis; astragalus; cuboid; toes (middle phalanges) 2–4
32–34 weeks	Vertebral costal process C5; toe (middle phalanx) 5
35–40 weeks	Vertebral body, coccygeal 1; vertebral costal processes C2–4; femoral distal epiphysis

C = cervical; D = dorsal thoracic; L = lumbar; S = sacral.
After Potter and Craig [42].

Table 2.3. Gestational sac volume and measurements by ultrasound

Gestation (weeks)	Volume (mL)		Diameters (cm) Transverse × A-P × Longitudinal
	Sanders & James	Reinold	Hellman et al
5	<2.0		
6	<2.0	2.98	0.49 × 0.35 × 0.50
7	2.5	8.06	1.09 × 0.80 × 1.15
8	10–35	16.43	1.77 × 1.29 × 1.83
9	20–50	31.13	2.65 × 1.88 × 2.61
10	40	54.00	3.43 × 2.51 × 3.51
11	50	85.32	4.48 × 3.06 × 4.49
12	75–125	100+	

A-P = anteroposterior.
Data estimated from published curve and extrapolated from tables in Sanders & James [39], Reinold [40], and Hellman et al [41].

times of ossification of various bones. Diseases that cause intrauterine growth retardation can delay ossification [45, 46].

Clinical Assessment

Gestational age can be assessed by a combination of neurological responses and physical characteristics, the latter including breast development, genital development (especially scrotal rugae), facial features, skin turgor, skin color, etc. [47, 48]. By assigning numerical scores to each factor, this system of determining gestational age (the Dubowitz score) is reliable for infants with gestations of 28 weeks or more. Ballard et al [49] evaluated seven physical features: the skin, lanugo, plantar creases, breast tissue, ear, and genitals, and correlated them with six of Dubowitz's neurological tests. Few infants whose gestations are less than 28 weeks have been evaluated by either the Dubowitz or the Ballard system, so these methods at younger gestational ages are not considered accurate. Furthermore, neither the Dubowitz nor the Ballard scoring system for estimating gestational age is concordant with the obstetric age (LMP with adjustments indicated by sonargraphic data) [50]. Nevertheless, for the latter stages of gestation, Dubowitz and Ballard scores are of direct use to clinicians, and they may be of use later to pathologists who can evaluate some of the physical features, such as breast and scrotal development.

Pathologic Assessment

Pathologists may best assess gestational age by a combination of measurements and qualitative assessments of organ maturation [51]. The total body weight, the total body length (crown–heel length; CH), the sitting height (crown–rump length; CR), and the length of the foot (FL) are the most useful measurements of the fetus or neonate [42, 46, 52–59]. Gestational age is said to correlate better with linear measurement than with weight [60], but either is useful and both should always be determined. Such measurements can be compared with the corresponding measurements from large series of fetuses and newborns. Average measurements from necropsy series, that is from large groups of fetuses and infants who die, are usually less than average measurements from surviving infants [36, 58, 61]. According to Gruenwald [36], up to one-third of babies who die and who have birth weights less than 2500 grams have gestations greater than 36 weeks. Conversely, fewer than 10% of surviving babies have such low birth weights. The tables derived from either necropsies or from surviving patients are useful for evaluating individual patients. Several tables and charts are presented in this chapter; most have gestational age as the independent variable because this is considered of utmost importance when evaluating fetuses and neonates [24].

Assessment of organ maturation aids in the establishment of gestational age [62, 63]. The gyral pattern of the brain [58, 64], the myelination pattern of the brain and spinal cord [65, 66], the number of generations of glomeruli in the cortex and the thickness of the nephrogenic zone [64, 67, 68], the quantity of extramedullary erythropoiesis in the liver [69], the pulmonary vascular development [43, 63, 70], the parenchymal development of the lung [71, 72], and the ratio of stroma to parenchyma in the pancreas, the thickness of the fetal skin, and the development of fat deposits in the subcutaneous tissues [45] can all be used to assess gestational age. In a particular patient, all of these measurements and qualitative evaluations should be assessed. In practice, the gestational age is based on the greatest concordance of all the measurements and qualitative assessments.

GROWTH

Growth in biological terms is more than "getting larger" [53]. An integral part of the process is the functional developmental maturation of organs and tissues, which involves subtle changes in their composition and size relative to the body as a whole [55].

Human growth has been viewed as a continuous process with changing velocity as the individual ages. In fact, as much as 95% of infancy is growth-free! Using serial length measurements in normal infants during the first 21 months of life, Lampl et al [73] determined that linear growth is discontinuous, with bursts of 0.5 to 2.5 centimeters separated by intervals of absent growth lasting as long as 63 days.

At the cellular level, growth is the result of two processes: increase in numbers of cells and increase in size of cells [74]. Winick and colleagues [75] elaborated these two principal types of growth in fetuses, neonates, and children. The earliest growth in an organism is in numbers of cells (i.e., hyperplasia). In the first few divisions of the zygote, the size of cells actually decreases. At the 16+ to 32+ to 64+ cell stages, the developing conceptus increases little in total mass [76]. From the stage of the morula onward, the conceptus grows dramatically as the number of cells increases. The rate of growth in the early embryonic period is much more rapid than later. Based on the propositions that the conceptus weighs between 6×10^{-7} and 15×10^{-7} grams at the one-cell stage, that the doubling time of cells in the first week of gestation is about 24 to 36 hours, and that this rate is maintained until adulthood, the fully grown 20-year-old would weigh 437 logs of times greater than the planet Earth, which weighs 25×10^{29} kilograms [55, 76]. However, deceleration of hyperplastic growth begins in the first week after fertilization and extends to the end of adolescence, when linear growth stops completely and the healthy individual simply replaces lost cells or cytoplasmic content.

Neither the rate of hyperplastic growth nor absolute growth is consistent from week to week [77]. The most notable example of the variable rate of growth is the acceleration (reversal of deceleration) of growth at the time of adolescence. Similar but less dramatic spurts are observed during intrauterine growth and in infancy and childhood

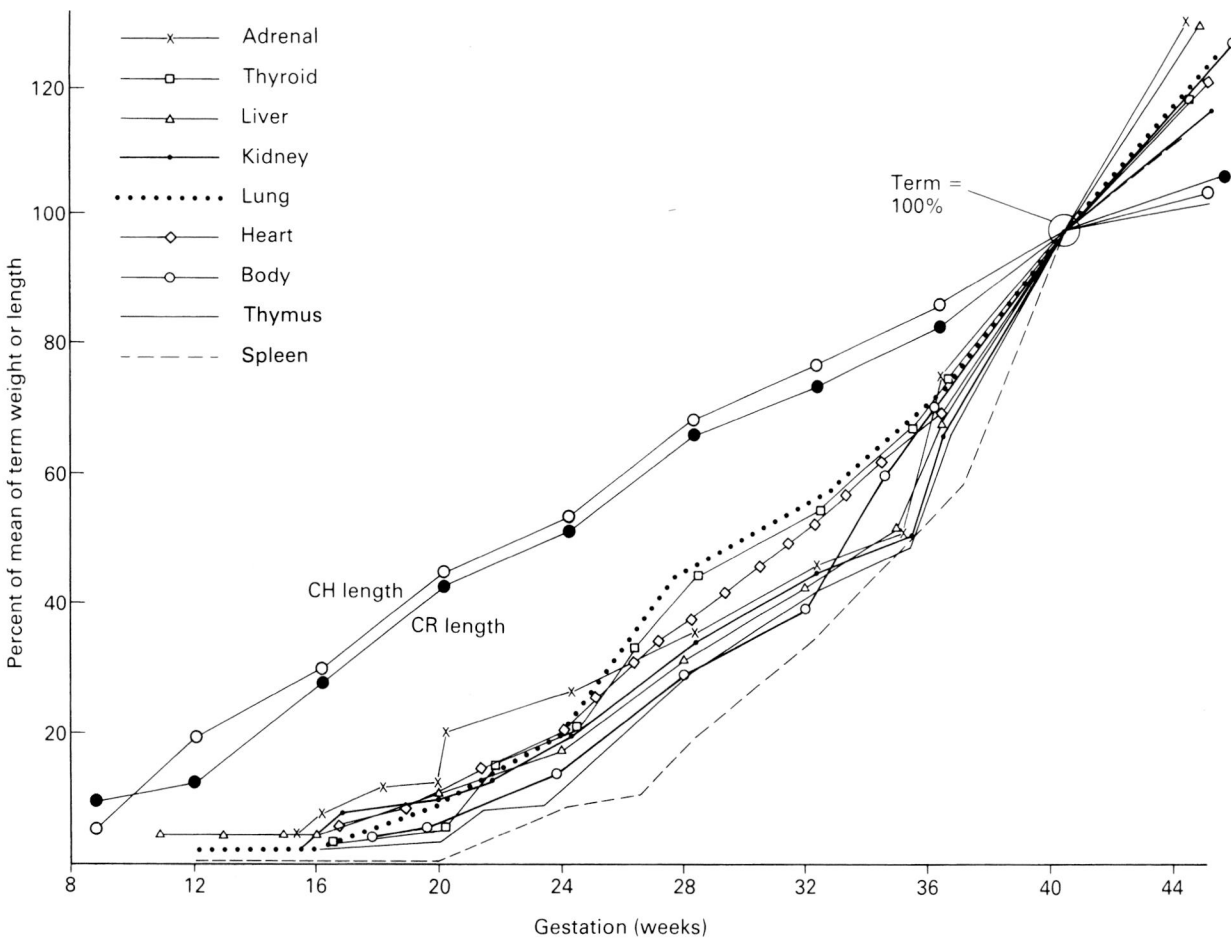

FIGURE 2.3.   *Growth of fetal body length compared with body and organ weights. Linear growth tends to be arithmetic, while weights of the body and internal organs tend to increase geometrically.*

[45, 53]. The accelerated growth of skin and subcutaneous fat in the last 8 to 10 weeks of fetal life and that of the lymphoid tissue in infancy and early childhood are examples of variable growth rates among organs and tissues [45]. The relative rates of growth of several organs and the total body weight throughout gestation are presented in Figure 2.3 and Table 2.5.

In mid-gestation, both cellular hyperplasia and cellular hypertrophy participate in growth of the total organism [75]. As the end of gestation approaches, hypertrophy plays a larger role and hyperplasia becomes less prominent in the overall growth of the fetus.

It is obvious from a cursory examination of developing organ structure that different organs develop over quite separate time courses and that within each organ, various tissues develop and mature at different rates. Thus in the human brain, the neurons within the cerebrum proliferate primarily in the period of 12- to 18-weeks' gestation, while the cerebellar neurons proliferate over the first year of postnatal life [78]. Proliferation of glial elements persists well into the second postnatal year.

The quantitative measurements of DNA content within whole organs, on which the Winick growth model is based, take no account of the process of cell death (e.g., apoptosis). Cell losses varying in the range of 20–70%, according to site and species, have been demonstrated in many areas of the developing mammalian central nervous system [79]. The process may be important in organs such as the brain, both for structural remodeling and to allow for elimination during development of errors in connectivity. This process of concomitant loss and accretion of cells undoubtedly would influence the results of growth patterns derived only from quantitative DNA measurements.

Nevertheless, the Winick model, though it does not take into account detailed growth processes, does agree with the observation that pathologic processes in early fetal life will reduce the number of cells, having hampered hyperplasia, which is the prominent factor in cell growth at that particular stage. In chronic insults, the recovery of the number of cells is never complete. The effect on the fetus, as it may be observed several months or years later, is quite different from the same insult at a later stage of gestation when the number

Table 2.5.   Growth of placenta and fetus

Gestation (weeks)	Placental weight (gm)	Percent of expected term weight	Fetal weight (gm)	Percent of expected term weight
24	195	41	680	21
26	220	47	880	27
28	280	58	1070	33
30	290	60	1330	41
32	320	68	1690	52
34	370	77	2090	62
36	420	87	2500	77
38	450	93	2960	91
40	480	100	3250	100
42	495	103	3410	105

From Hendricks [216].

of cells is fairly well established. Naeye and Blanc [80] have proposed that fetal viral infections such as rubella retard cell hyperplasia; starvation and other insults may do the same [81]. The timing of the insult and its intensity are important in determining the extent of the growth retardation due to low cell population and may limit later catch-up growth within an organ or tissue (Fig. 2.4).

During the first months of postnatal life, cellular hypertrophy becomes more prominent, while hyperplasia is limited in almost every organ and tissue.

CONTROL OF FETAL GROWTH

Control of cell multiplication and differentiation within different organs is a complex process involving many different genetically determined stimuli from endocrine and paracrine factors and so on. The sum of individual effects is the *genetic growth potential* of the fetus. The optimal expression of this growth potential is dependent on substrate availability via the placenta. Unlike growth in infancy and childhood, there is no essential requirement for pituitary growth hormone or thyroid hormones to modulate overall body growth in the fetus [82]. The fetus need not attain a predetermined size to allow organs to mature or to be born alive. For any particular genetic growth potential, the size actually attained by the fetus will vary widely according to available nutrients and other external constraints on or allowances for growth. If nutrient supply is suboptimal, genetic factors may account for only 40% of the variation in birth weight [83]. Within quite wide limits, this may be regarded as a highly effective means of adaptation, allowing the birth of healthy infants, with a wide range of birth

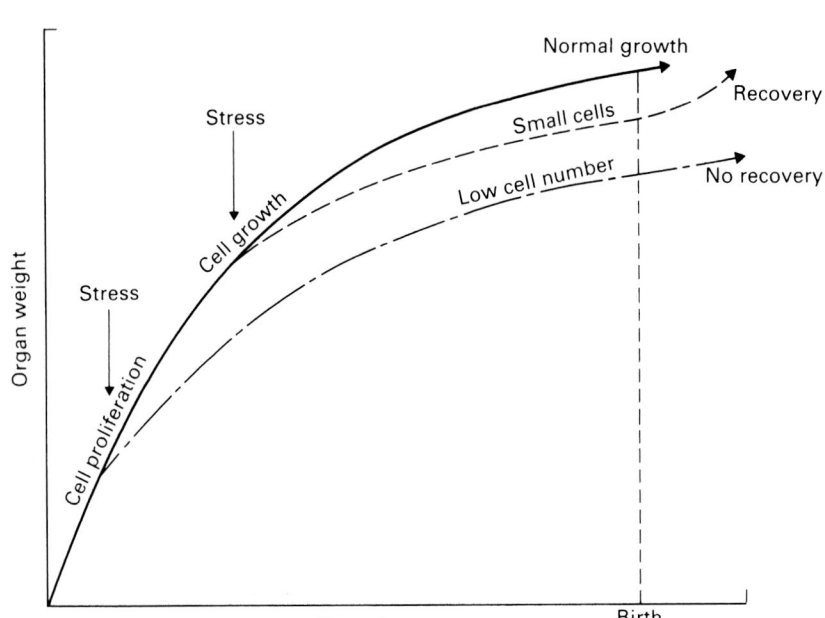

FIGURE 2.4.   *Diagrammatic illustration of the concept that a growth-retarding stress during the phase of cell proliferation in an organ will cause permanent restriction of cell population, while a similar stress during the later growth phase may cause a reversible impairment in cell size.*

weights, without interfering with their potential eventual adult size. How one defines the limits of normality within this spectrum of biological adaptation is largely a matter of personal philosophy [84].

Hormones

Most of the hormones known to control growth of differentiated tissues and organs are polypeptide hormones, and these are believed to be incapable of crossing the placenta from the mother to the conceptus. Presumably, the conceptus is responsible for its own production of growth hormone. The polypeptide growth factors act through specific plasma membrane receptors to regulate both components of growth: cell division and hypertrophy. The receptors for insulin, insulin-like growth factor (IGF-I), platelet-derived growth factor (PDGF), epidermal growth factor (EGF), and other such factors have much in common; conversely cells of epithelial, mesenchymal, neural, lymphoid, and hematopoietic lineage respond to different sets of growth factors.

We are just beginning to understand the influence of hormones on fetal growth. Various influences other than hormones (i.e., nervous elements, cell-cell contacts, and extracellular matrix) also act to modify growth. The embryo apparently does not produce growth hormone, insulin, or insulin-like growth factors. Studies in humans have not been adequate to show whether embryonic growth is augmented by EGF or alpha-transforming growth factor (α-TGF) [85]. Neither has it been proved conclusively whether maternal growth factors cross the placenta early in embryogenesis. Insulin, at least, does not seem to cross the placenta after the 10th to 11th week of gestation [86].

A number of hormones have been excluded as having a major role in fetal growth control [87]. Growth hormone can be excluded, as Laron dwarfs who lack receptors for growth hormone are of normal weight at birth. Rarely, pregnancies are associated with a lack of placental lactogen; in these, also, birth weight is normal, thereby effectively excluding another popular contender for an essential role in fetal growth control.

Insulin appears to have a powerful influence on fetal somatic growth. Fetal insulin production begins in the pancreatic islets at about 9 to 10 weeks of gestational age [88]. Insulin-like growth factors (IGF-I, IGF-II), the somatomedins, may also play an important role in fetal growth. Insulin, IGF-I, and IGF-II belong to a family that includes relaxin and possibly nerve growth factor (NGF). IGF-I shares 62% homology with IGF-II and 47% homology with insulin. Both IGF-I and IGF-II are potent mitogens for mesenchymal cells. IGF-I and IGF-II are synthesized in the liver and kidneys and likely in the mesenchyme itself. Deficiency of IGF-I is considered the cause for short stature in pygmies. IGF-II is the fetal analogue of IGF-I and is under the control of human placental lactogen. IGF-II production continues in the adult liver, kidney,

colon, and brain. In the latter two organs, its function is unknown [85]. Maternal levels of IGF-I show a direct correlation with birth weight, and a similar correlation has been shown for fetal umbilical IGF-I levels. A role for the IGFs in fetal growth control has not been proven conclusively yet, but neither has it been excluded [87].

Among premature neonates, body weights correlate directly with plasma levels of arachidonic acid. The effect may be related to the role of arachidonic acid as a precursor of certain fats or to its structural function in membrane lipids [89].

By measuring the soluble carboxypropeptide of type I procollagen, one may be able to monitor growth rates in infants and children. This procollagen has not been measured in infants less than 3 weeks of age, so its usefulness in neonates has not yet been determined [90].

Maternal Factors

Mothers with growth-retarded infants themselves have lower-than-average birth weights [91–93]. Mothers who as adults weigh less than 90% of average for their height have slightly smaller babies than mothers with weights closer to average for height [94]. Maternal height correlates better with fetal weight than does maternal pre-pregnancy weight. Tall mothers have heavier babies than short mothers [93]. In humans and other species, either maternal stature or weight has more influence than does the paternal stature or weight on a baby's weight and length [83, 84]. These observations do not conflict with the view of an overall genetic influence on fetal growth potential. Rather, they emphasize the wide range of the adaptation of fetal growth to the environment or to the maternal regulation previously mentioned [94, 95].

Environmental Factors

Altitudes more than 3000 meters above sea level are enormously effective in reducing fetal weight. Babies born in Lake County, Colorado (alt. 3100 m), weigh 200 to 300 grams less than babies born at sea level; the rate of low birth weight (<2500 gm) in Lake County is three times that of the rest of Colorado, which is 1500–2000 meters above sea level [56, 96].

Other Factors

Premature birth is a factor with significant effect on postnatal growth. Most very-low-birth-weight infants have some catch-up during the first year and more during the succeeding 2 years. However, at 3 years of age, the mean length is at the 5th percentile, weight at the 10th percentile, and head circumference at the 5th percentile. This is a sort of extrauterine growth retardation (EUGR) [97].

Normal male babies gain approximately 30 grams per day in the first month of life, only approximately 15 grams per day at 6 months of age, and only 10 grams per day at 12 months of age. Normal female babies gain about 1 to 2 grams less per day than males. As for length, males and females both grow slightly more than 1 millimeter per day in the first 2 months. This rate slows to approximately 0.6 millimeters per day by 6 months of age and to approximately 0.4 millimeters per day by 12 months of age [98]. Growth is not uniform from day to day, or even from month to month, in the first 2 years of life [73].

CHANGES IN FORM AND FUNCTION IN THE FETAL PERIOD

The details of embryonic development and previable development up to 20 weeks of gestational age are summarized in Chapter 7 and will not be given here. Some major structural features of the fetus at various stages of the second half of pregnancy are outlined below as an introduction to the consideration of problems of abnormal growth and the methods of growth assessment.

20–26 Weeks

During this period, the face and body of the fetus gradually assume an appearance more like that of the newborn infant. The eyelids and eyebrows are well developed, but the eyelids are fused. The fingernails are present. The skin is thin and may appear wrinkled due to faster growth than that of underlying tissues. The thin epidermis renders the underlying capillary bed visible, so that the skin appears red in the live fetus. Lanugo hair develops, and vernix caseosa appears. There is little subcutaneous fat.

During this period, the lung matures from the canalicular stage to the saccular stage, and with the appearance of surfactant, the infant achieves viability. The primary sulci of the brain appear.

27–30 Weeks

The eyes open, and the pupillary membrane disappears. The eyebrows and eyelashes are well developed, and scalp hair lengthens. Increasing subcutaneous fat results in rounding of the body contours. There is an increasing complexity of the cerebral convolutional pattern but a persistence of prominent subependymal matrix.

31–35 Weeks

Muscle mass and fat progressively increase and the skin becomes thicker, changing from red to pink. The fingernails reach to the tips of the fingers; the toenails are present and the testes descend into the scrotum. The lung changes from saccular to an early alveolar form. The brain shows a further complexity in convolutional pattern but a decrease in the quantity of subependymal matrix.

36–40 Weeks

Skeletal muscle and subcutaneous fat increase. Toenails have reached the tips of the toes. Almost all of the lanugo hair is shed and the skin is covered with vernix caseosa. The insula of the brain is covered by the enlarging frontal and temporal lobes (the opercula), and myelination is more pronounced. The formation of new renal glomeruli ceases.

PROBLEMS OF PRETERM BIRTH

The problems of preterm birth reflect the degree of structural and functional immaturity of various organs and tissues at the time of birth. As there is a continuous process of maturation, the patterns of illness will vary with the precise gestational age at which the infant is born. As stated earlier, infants of very low birth weight have the highest mortality and morbidity to which the problems of preterm birth are the greatest contributors. The pathology of preterm birth, therefore, is discussed in nearly every chapter of this book and so has not been given a major section on its own. A recent overview is given by Batcup [99]. A summary of the more commonly encountered pathologic changes follows.

Problems of Management

Intensive care of infants of very low birth weight at the limits of viability inevitably leads to a wide range of management-related or iatrogenic problems. These are discussed in Chapter 3.

Infection

Preterm infants have an increased susceptibility to infection. This is due both to an immature immune system and to a greater ease with which structural barriers to infection, such as the skin, can be breached. (See Chap. 16.)

Respiratory System

The state of maturity of the lungs is the most critical feature in determining viability of the preterm infant. Few infants survive at gestations below 24 weeks, the time at which the critical maturation to the saccular phase normally occurs. Above that gestation, the preterm infant is at a gradually decreasing risk of developing hyaline membrane disease until about 35 weeks' gestation. An associated risk is that of bronchopulmonary dysplasia. (See Chap. 19.)

Central Nervous System

Problems of the immature brain include subependymal and intraventricular hemorrhage and periventricular leukomalacia. The former is most frequent up to 30 to 32 weeks' gestation when the subependymal matrix commences to regress, while the latter may develop in any hypotensive preterm infant, as well as in some asphyxiated full-term infants. Late problems include posthemorrhagic hydrocephalus, severe cerebral palsy, and neurodevelopmental handicap. Kernicterus is a complication of hepatic immaturity with unconjugated hyperbilirubinemia. The condition can occur in preterm infants with hypoxia or sepsis at relatively low levels of serum bilirubin. (See Chap. 21.)

Alimentary System

Necrotizing enterocolitis (NEC) affects preterm infants, although a small proportion of cases occur in full-term infants. (See Chap. 24.)

Retrolental Fibroplasia

Most cases of retrolental fibroplasia occur in preterm infants. (See Chap. 23.)

Other Problems

These include structural problems such as increased incidence of patent ductus arteriosus due to hypoxia and inadequate development of ductal media and intima; and metabolic problems such as hypothermia, hypoglycemia, and hyperkalemia. Late complications include an increased risk of sudden infant death, in addition to respiratory and neurodevelopmental handicaps.

PROBLEMS OF FETAL GROWTH

Ethnic Variations in Frequency of Low Birth Weight

On a worldwide basis low birth weight (<2500 gm) is most prevalent in middle South Asia, with a rate of 31.1% [100]. Asia as a whole has a rate of low birth weight of 19.7%, followed by Africa with 14%, Latin America with 10.1%, North America with 6.8%, and Europe with 6.5% [100]. In Table 2.6, data from six centers worldwide are presented. The 50th percentile of birth weights ranged from 1000 grams to 1250 grams in preterm neonates at 28 weeks' gestation; from 1700 grams to 1900 grams at 32 weeks' gestational age; from 2600 grams to 2900 grams at 36 weeks' gestational age; and from 3300 grams to 3600 grams at 40 weeks' gestational age [61, 101].

In countries where maternal nutrition is thought to be optimal throughout pregnancy and where health is maximally maintained, fetal growth continues to accelerate through the 41st week of gestation [27]. Conversely, in undernourished mothers and those from poor socioeconomic circumstances, the curve of fetal growth seems to flatten at an earlier stage of gestation [75, 102, 103]. In Israel, a country with disparate genetic and ethnic origins of its population, the average birth weights vary depending on the group under study (Table 2.7).

Data on birth weights from several other countries around the world are indicated in Table 2.8. Whites of European background, wherever they currently live, have the largest babies, both in weight and length. Babies of Asian and African descent are smaller [45, 104, 105].

Table 2.6.   Average birth weights at gestations of 28–42 weeks in seven locations throughout the world

Nearest week of gestation	Denver	Baltimore	Montreal	Portland	Britain	Amsterdam	Lagos*
28	1150	1050 ± 310	1113 ± 150	1172 ± 344	—	1249	1300 ± 116
29	1268	1200 ± 350	1228 ± 165	1322 ± 339	1165 ± 540	1336	1163 ± 133
30	1392	1380 ± 370	1373 ± 175	1529 ± 474	1250 ± 450	1419	1556 ± 190
31	1537	1560 ± 400	1540 ± 200	1757 ± 495	1575 ± 445	1604	1630 ± 320
32	1661	1750 ± 410	1727 ± 225	1881 ± 427	1870 ± 550	1808	2008 ± 635
33	1844	1950 ± 420	1900 ± 250	2158 ± 511	2015 ± 640	1989	2066 ± 110
34	2117	2170 ± 430	2113 ± 280	2340 ± 552	2200 ± 670	2203	2231 ± 235
35	2385	2390 ± 440	2347 ± 315	2518 ± 468	2410 ± 675	2389	2472 ± 310
36	2618	2610 ± 440	2589 ± 350	2749 ± 490	2680 ± 640	2642	2780 ± 373
37	2809	2830 ± 440	2868 ± 385	2989 ± 466	2895 ± 560	2909	2870 ± 223
38	2946	3050 ± 450	3133 ± 400	3185 ± 450	3070 ± 500	3163	3084 ± 325
39	3076	3210 ± 450	3360 ± 430	3333 ± 444	3225 ± 465	3298	3246 ± 366
40	3178	3280 ± 450	3480 ± 460	3462 ± 456	3360 ± 455	3444	3380 ± 368
41	3266	3350 ± 450	3567 ± 475	3569 ± 468	3450 ± 460	3539	3583 ± 381
42	3307	3400 ± 460	3513 ± 480	3637 ± 482	3510 ± 480	3619	3604 ± 273

From Gruenwald [103].
* Data from Olowe [101].

Table 2.7.   Birth weights among various ethnic groups in Israel

Ethnic group of mother	Birth weight (gm)
Arab, Moslem	3250
Arab, Druse	3240
Arab, Christian	3340
Asian Jewish	3220
Israeli Jewish	3310
Western European Jewish	3300

From Eveleth and Tanner [106].

Table 2.8.   Birth weights and lengths for males and females at term for various populations*

Geographic and ethnic group	Birth weight (M/F)	Length (CH) (M/F)
Indomediterranean		
Beirut (poor)	3400/3300	50.1/49.5
Beirut (well-off)	3500/3300	50.2/49.7
Delhi (poor)	2800/2750	49.0/48.1
Delhi (well-off)	3300/3100	50.0/50.0
Iran	3370/3280	50.2/49.8
Asiatic		
Manila (poor)	3070/2940	
Bangkok	3120/3010	
Taipei	3210/3100	
Jakarta	3090/3010	
Eskimo	3370/3260	
Sioux Indian	3440/3370	
African		
Nigeria	2900/2800	
Senegal	3200/3100	
Dominican Republic	3400/3400	
Jamaica (urban)	3100/3100	
Jamaica (rural)	3500/3300	
Washington, DC	3200/3300	
European		
Brazil	3250/3090	50.1/49.2
Argentina	3470/3200	50.8/49.5
Denver	3200/3200	49.6/49.0
Ohio	3430/3350	
Stockholm	3570/3450	51.0/–
Zurich	3500/3500	50.0/–
The Netherlands	3500/3400	51.8/–
London	3440/3230	
Dublin	3480/3360	50.8/–
Naples	3500/3350	51.5/51.0
Sofia	3390/3250	51.4/–
Australia and Pacific Islands		
Western New Guinea	2900/2800	
Chimba, New Guinea	3400/2950	
Australian aborigines	2890/2860	
Australian aborigines (north)	3100/2900	
Pitjant-Jatjara	3100/3000	

CH = crown–heel length.
*   Weight is given in gm, length in cm.
Data derived from Eveleth and Tanner [106].

The populations with the lowest average birth weights are found in Guatemala and among the Ngaya pygmies of equatorial Africa. In Guatemala, the average birth weight at term is 2560 grams, both sexes combined [106]. One must question whether nutrition among these mothers is adequate. Among the Ngaya pygmies in whom the average height of adults is less than 150 centimeters, the average weight at birth is 2610 grams, both sexes combined [106]. Low levels of IGF-I in pygmies may have a negative effect on fetal growth, although insulin and IGF-II are the potent fetal growth hormones, not IGF-I [85].

Despite considerable genetic differences in postnatal growth and the ultimate adult stature and configuration, genetic underpinning has less to do with fetal growth than does environment [106]. To emphasize this point, consider multiple births; beyond the 28th to 32nd week of gestation, growth in either of twins is markedly reduced relative to singletons born to the same mother [23, 107]. In a low socioeconomic group in the Netherlands, children of Mediterranean parents gained significantly more weight than children of Dutch parents by 2 years of age. Length at 2 years of age was not related to ethnic background [108].

CAUSES OF FETAL GROWTH IMPAIRMENT

Causes of fetal growth impairment may operate at the maternal, placental, or fetal level, as illustrated in the diagram in Figure 2.5.

Maternal Undernutrition

The relationship of fetal growth to maternal health and adequate maternal nutrition has been widely studied throughout the world [109–111]. With acute maternal starvation in previously well-nourished gravidas, the average size of newborn infants is reduced by as much as 300 to 400 grams [109] (Table 2.9).

Chronic maternal undernutrition may also be associated with impaired fetal growth. Moghissi and colleagues [102] have shown that women who consume less than 50 grams of protein in their daily diets have babies who weigh almost 400 grams less than babies born to mothers who consume 70 or more grams of protein daily. On the other hand, in the study reported by Rush and colleagues [112] similar high protein supplements produced increased prematurity and reduced growth among the prematurely born infants. Pubescent and adolescent gravidas (ages 10–16 years) who are themselves still growing were thought to compete with their fetuses for growth-sustaining nutrients. Unless these mothers are afforded the figurative cushion of obesity, babies

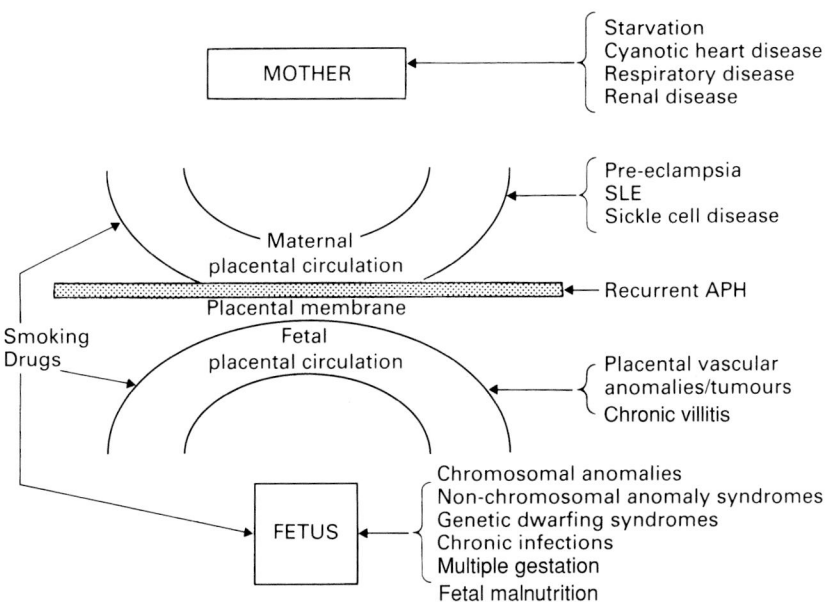

FIGURE 2.5. *Diagrammatic representation of causes of fetal growth impairment and their postulated sites of action. APH = antepartum hemorrhage.*

Table 2.9.   Various factors that influence birth weight

Characteristic	Effect = deviation from average weight or length at birth of white males in the US	
	Weight (gm)	Length (cm)
Positive effect		
Maternal diabetes	+300–1000	+1.0–4.0
Gestation of >42 weeks	+230–250	+0.7–1.0
Tall mother	+100–150	+1.0–2.0
Multiparous mother	+50–70	
Negative effect		
Female sex	−70–100	−0.1–0.3
Black parents	−150–170	−0.2–0.5
Mothers of low birth weight	−170	
Alcoholic mother	−165–200	−0.3–1.0
Mother who smokes	−175–220	−1.2–1.3
Altitude	−200–300	−1.2–1.5
Maternal hypertension	−200–500	−0.2–1.5
Malnutrition	−300–500	−0.1–3.0
Fetal diseases and malformations	−500–800	
Multiple births	−600–1000	−0.5–2.0

Starvation affects the total number of cells and the size of cells, depending on the stage of gestation during which the gravida is undernourished [81]. The period of greatest absolute fetal growth is in the last 6 to 7 weeks of gestation. A fetus may add 800 to 2000 grams during this interval [102]. Therefore, the effects of undernutrition are most dramatic during this time when much of the retarded growth is due to lack of increased cytoplasmic mass in adipose tissue and muscle. Visceral organs respond variably to maternal malnutrition. The liver is depleted most severely while the brain is relatively spared. The spleen and thymus are small unless fetal infection is superimposed in which case the mass of the spleen is increased. Placental growth retardation is usually parallel to total growth retardation in humans and other mammals [75, 116, 117].

Maternal Addictions

The adverse effect of maternal smoking on fetal growth has been demonstrated repeatedly over the last 30 years. Nieberg and colleagues have applied the term "fetal tobacco syndrome" to the condition affecting offspring of mothers who smoke [118]. Maternal cigarette smoking reduces fetal weights by 170 grams to 220 grams and fetal lengths by 1.2 centimeters to 1.3 centimeters [119–121]. These effects are not due to blunted maternal appetites. In fact, smoking gravidas may have more robust appetites than non-smokers [121]. The normal body proportions of small infants at birth and the poor growth and educational attainment in long-term follow-up studies suggest that the effects are due to impaired fetal growth potential rather than impaired fetal nutrition [122, 123]. The ways in which the effect may be produced are numerous. Injection of nicotine into pregnant monkeys causes uterine vasoconstriction with reduced

born to them may be growth-retarded due to a sort of starvation [113]. However, Stevens-Simon et al [114] refute the notion that growing adolescents compete with their fetuses for nutrients. In fact, in their study pregnant adolescents less than 16 years of age transferred more of their weight gain to their fetuses than did older gravidas. Hard physical work by an undernourished gravida may produce reduced uteroplacental blood flow, and this may account for much of the reduced birth weights in developing countries [115].

perfusion of the intervillous space [124]. Carbon monoxide in cigarette smoke destroys the oxygen-combining power of hemoglobin and myoglobin, effectively causing hypoxia that may compromise fetal growth. The low concentration of hydrocyanic acid within tobacco smoke is partly detoxified by combination with thiosulfate to form thiocyanate, a hypotensive agent. The cyanide may cause cellular anoxia by inactivating cytochrome oxidase. Either or both of these mechanisms could impair fetal growth. Finally carbonic anhydrase activity may be decreased in red blood cells of both mother and fetus owing to inhibition by cyanide, thiocyanate, and carbon monoxide. This may in turn interfere with cellular respiration in the fetus, with resultant tissue hypoxia, acidosis, and retarded growth. Aside from the effects on growth, smoking results in increased fetal mortality. Among gravidas who consume more than 20 cigarettes per day, the risk of fetal death is 1.75 times that of non-smokers [125]. Increased prematurity is 20% more common among mothers who smoke at least one pack of cigarettes per day [126]. A small but statistically significant catch-up growth was noted among infants born to mothers who smoked during pregnancy [108].

Illicit substances also seem to produce impaired fetal growth retardation [125]. Marijuana smoking results in reduced birth weights by an average of 79 grams. Cocaine use results in a 93-gram reduction in birth weight and a 0.43-centimeter smaller head circumference [127]. At birth, babies born to mothers addicted to amphetamines have lower mean birth weight, length, and head circumferences. This smaller size persists for all three measurements through 4 years of age [128].

The fetal alcohol syndrome was first recognized among babies with small heads and shortened palpebral fissures [129]. Growth retardation in such babies is now well established and may be dose related. Fetal weights are reduced by 165 to 200 grams among mothers who drink more than 50 milliliters of absolute alcohol or more than three to five alcoholic drinks per day [130, 131]. Mothers who drink pulque, a mild alcoholic beverage, may have babies with only slightly reduced birth weights compared with offspring of non–pulque-drinking mothers [132]. Head circumference, body length, and weight are all lower than normal at birth among infants of alcoholic mothers. Iosub et al [131] found that more than half of drinking mothers have fetuses who are growth retarded and these children are still small when measured at 3 years of age. By contrast, Sampson et al [133] found that by 8 months of age and thereafter through 14 years, growth of these offspring was normal, and the same is true of offspring born to mothers who drink pulque [132].

Mothers who take anticonvulsants and steroids have fetuses with impaired growth. Coffee drinking, when controlled for smoking and other maternal factors related to fetal growth, seems to have no effect on fetal weight or length [134].

Maternal Hypertension

Early onset or severe pre-eclampsia is associated with fetal growth impairment, while late onset or mild pre-eclampsia has no such association [135, 136]. Essential hypertension may pose no increased risk of fetal growth retardation [135], and placental growth is normal unless there is superimposed proteinuria, when the effects are similar to those of pre-eclampsia [137]. Reduced uteroplacental blood flow owing to failure of adaptation of the uteroplacental circulation to the demands of pregnancy is considered to be responsible for the growth failure. In animals, a similar effect on fetal growth can be produced by ligating uterine vessels [138] and if the placenta is bilobed, as it is in the rhesus monkey, by ligating the placental vascular pedicle between the primary and secondary lobes [117].

In humans, the weights of babies born to hypertensive mothers may be reduced by 200 to 500 grams and lengths by 1 to 3 centimeters. Simple therapeutic measures may reverse these effects. In the study by Uzan et al [139], small doses of aspirin given to pregnant women who had a previous pregnancy with reduced fetal growth halved the rate of subsequent impaired fetal growth.

Other Maternal Illnesses

Fetal growth impairment occurs frequently in cases of maternal cyanotic heart disease and was reported in 52% of pregnancies in this group as compared with 9% of pregnancies in the acyanotic group [140].

Chronic respiratory disease such as maternal asthma has been associated with reduced fetal growth in older studies, but with modern therapy it may be a complication only of occasional cases where control is poor [141]. In cystic fibrosis, the severity of maternal hypoxemia and hypercapnea may determine the adequacy of fetal growth, although the severity of pancreatic involvement and intestinal malabsorption also may be relevant [142]. Bronchiectasis and kyphoscoliosis have also been associated with reduced fetal growth [143, 144].

Chronic renal disease of moderate severity is associated with impaired fetal growth in up to 24% of cases [145], although it may be difficult to distinguish between any direct effect of the renal impairment and that of associated hypertension [146].

Systemic lupus erythematosus (SLE) is associated with retarded fetal growth [147]. It may be difficult to differentiate the influence of renal lesions and treatment with immunosuppressive drugs from those of the decidual bed vasculopathy associated with SLE [148].

Anemia is often associated with nutritional problems, making the assessment of anemia per se difficult in cases of fetal growth impairment. Some have cast doubt on the role of maternal anemia when reduced fetal growth is present [135, 147]. Women with sickle cell disease have an increased incidence of growth-impaired infants, as may those with sickle-thalassemia and sickle-hemoglobin C disease [149]. The basis of reduced fetal growth in sickle cell disease is almost certainly impaired uteroplacental circulation due to obstruction by sickled cells, with resultant placental microinfarcts.

Placental Factors

Circumvallate placenta is the only abnormality of placental development accepted by Fox [150] as being associated with reduced fetal growth. In fact, few primary placental conditions affect fetal growth, and the term "placental insufficiency" is regarded as obsolete now that the secondary nature of this organ's role is more clearly understood.

Ratios of placental to fetal weights fall as normal gestations progress (see Table 2.5). In the Perinatal Collaborative Project in the United States, Naeye [151] found that only 84 fetal deaths per 100,000 births were associated with very small placentas. Most growth-impaired fetuses have a lower placental/fetal weight ratio than that seen in normally grown fetuses. In the case of multiple births, placental mass increases at a slower rate than the total mass of all the fetuses, so placental insufficiency can be invoked in this situation.

In gestations at high altitudes, the placental/fetal ratio is increased relative to gestations at sea level, suggesting an adaptive mechanism to compensate for the relative maternal hypoxia [152]. Maternal smoking in pregnancy may similarly cause an increase in placental/fetal weight despite a lower birth weight [153]. Vascular anomalies of the fetal side of the placenta, including single umbilical artery and large chorioangiomas, are significantly associated with fetal growth reduction [150, 154, 155], as are chronic villitis of unknown etiology and chronic chorioamnionitis [156–158].

Recurrent antepartum hemorrhage in the first and second trimesters is strongly associated with fetal growth impairment [135]. This may be due to impaired development of the uteroplacental circulation, but placenta previa shows no such association [159]. Hypoxia and undernutrition may induce changes in placental growth by still-to-be-defined mechanisms [84].

Fetal Factors

Multiple Pregnancy

Beyond the 28th to 32nd week of gestation, growth in either of twins is markedly reduced relative to singletons born to the same mother [107, 160, 161]. Multiple births produce the greatest deviations of fetal growth from recorded norms for singletons [42, 107, 160–162] (see Table 2.9). McKeown and Record [160] studied birth weights and gestational ages of 688 sets of twins, 284 sets of triplets, and 27 sets of quadruplets. With this large series of cases, they were able to develop statistics for the inverse relationship of "the number of fetuses" to birth weight of each fetus and lengths of gestations. For twins, the average birth weight was

2400 grams, and the average duration of gestation was 261.6 days; for triplets the corresponding average values were 1800 grams and 246.8 days, and for quadruplets 1400 grams and 236.8 days, respectively. Lubchenco and colleagues [56] showed that each member of a twin pair plotted on the 50th percentile line for singletons until about 34 weeks, at which time the curve for twins' weights flattened, falling to the 10th percentile by 42 weeks' gestation. As the number of fetuses increases, the sex ratio shifts in favor of females [160]. This sex difference may slightly influence the lower birth weights in triplets, quadruplets, and so on. Conversely, as maternal parity increases, the sum of fetal weights increases, just as singletons born to multiparous mothers tend to be larger than those born to primiparas.

At term, the difference in weight between two members of a twin pair is 521 grams, on average [42]. The twin-twin transfusion syndrome causes even more variation in weight and length [107]. Both cell number and sizes of individual cells are reduced in twins [161]. Compared with normal singletons, the number of cells can be reduced by 25% in monozygous twins with monochorionic placentas [161]. In long-term follow-up studies of twins, if the difference in birth weights is more than 300 grams, the larger twins have IQ scores that are on average 5 points higher than the smaller twins [163].

Dizygous twins tend to be larger than monozygous ones [107, 162]. While monozygous twinning occurs at a constant rate in populations throughout the world, dizygous twins occur with greater frequency among certain ethnic groups and in certain families indicating definite genetic influences [162]. Increased parity also increases the number of dizygous twins but not the number of monozygous twins.

Data for the mid-1980s showed marked reduction in mortality for triplets and higher-order multiple births compared with the early 1960s. At birth weights greater than 999 grams, triplets and higher-order multiple births actually had mortality rates better than for singletons at the same birth weights. From 500 grams through 999 grams, the mortality rates were equal among triplets and higher-order multiple births and for singletons at the same birth weights [164].

Other Fetal Factors

Fetal malnutrition is encountered in every culture and every socioeconomic class. About 2–3% of babies born in the United States have fetal malnutrition. Its pathogenesis is extremely complex, involving not only genetic factors and noxious environmental factors, but also the proportions of various nutrients which, even though present in adequate quantities, may interfere with each other's transfer mechanisms [165]. Malnourished fetuses, should, with appropriate prenatal treatment, be able to start life with healthy organs [166].

Fetal infection, particularly viral infections such as rubella and cytomegalovirus infection, may reduce fetal weight and length to 80–85% of control values [167, 168]. Among rubella babies who survive the neonatal period, retarded growth continues for months to years [169]. Much of the growth retardation in fatal cases of congential rubella is associated with severely reduced cell populations in the fetal tissues [80]. Growth impairment as a result of other congenital viral infections is rather poorly documented [170], although it has been reported in herpes simplex and varicella zoster. Among bacterial infections, listeriosis is sometimes associated with reduced growth. Congenital syphilis and toxoplasmosis may also cause growth impairment.

Low birth weight is significantly associated with malformations of all types. For liveborn infants with birth weights less than 1500 grams, the risk for a major malformation is about five times greater than for infants with normal birth weights; infants weighing 1500 to 1999 grams have a risk four times greater, and infants weighing 2001 to 2499 grams have a risk two times greater. Infants with birth weights equal to or greater than 4000 grams have a slightly reduced risk of major malformation compared with infants having birth weights between 2500 and 3999 grams [171].

While some genetic abnormalities may be associated with fetal growth acceleration, most chromosomal and genetic abnormalities cause reduced fetal growth. The severity of undergrowth varies with the abnormality. Birth weights were 141 grams less than reference values among Dutch infants with the subsequent diagnosis of phenylketonuria. Postnatal growth through 3 years showed further decline in length from the reference values despite treatment, but head circumferences reached reference values after 1 year of age [172]. In Turner syndrome, the average birth weight at term is 84% of the normal; and in trisomy 13 the average birth weight is 80% of the normal, whereas in trisomy 21 the birth weight is 80–90% of the normal [83]. More severe growth retardation is seen in fetuses with trisomy 18, with an average birth weight of only 62% of the normal. Unbalanced autosomal anomalies, such as deletions, are also associated with reduced birth weight [83], and severe reduced growth is a feature of fetuses with triploidy [173]. Other malformation syndromes associated with reduced growth include anencephaly, osteogenesis imperfecta, renal agenesis, and renal dysplasia [174, 175].

A number of infants with hyperplastic and enlarged pancreatic islets show intrauterine growth impairment rather than accelerated fetal growth [176]. Somatostatin-producing cells may be responsible for the enlarged islets; their hormone(s) can suppress insulin and perhaps other growth hormones, which may explain part of this apparent paradox. The insulin receptor gene, the code for which has been localized to chromosome 19, may be defective in Donohue syndrome (leprechaunism), thereby providing a geneticmolecular basis for the etiology and pathogenesis of reduced fetal growth in this condition with hyperplastic islets [177].

We have seen a severely undergrown baby with triploidy syndrome (69 XXX) whose somatostatin-producing cells in the pancreas were markedly enlarged; individual cells mea-

sured up to 70 microns in diameter. We inferred from this case that somatostatin suppressed insulin production by paracrine action. Preliminary studies in rats show that fetal weight is inversely related to the volume proportion of somatostatin-producing cells in their pancreatic islets [178].

Wit and van Unen [179] studied growth in 15 infants with deficiency of neonatal growth hormone. Five of the 15 infants had a length at birth more than two standard deviations below the mean. Eight infants had an immediate deviation from the normal growth curve as measured through 9 months of age. Four of the infants had complete growth hormone deficiency, while two others had poor response to provocation tests.

ACCELERATED FETAL GROWTH

Babies of above-average birth weight are most frequently born to women of increased height and weight. Familial tall stature is a normal feature among some babies who are born weighing 4000 grams or more [180]. Among obese mothers, the weights of the fetuses are usually increased but not the lengths or head circumferences. Babies born to obese mothers weigh, on average, 220 grams more and as much as 700 grams more than babies born to mothers of normal weight [181–183].

PATHOLOGY OF ABNORMAL FETAL GROWTH

Reduced Fetal Growth

Major contributions to our knowledge of the pathology of fetal growth impairment were made by Gruenwald [36], Naeye [81], and Naeye and Blanc [80].

Gruenwald conducted extensive analyses of postmortem data to show that severely growth-impaired infants (i.e., infants of at least two standard deviations in weight below the mean in surviving infants for the gestation) had relatively large brains but small livers, lungs, and thymuses. They also tended to have increased length relative to their weight. These changes were similar to those in fetuses of starved animals (e.g., fetal lambs of ewes maintained on a low plane of nutrition) [184]. A second group of infants had long thin bodies with little subcutaneous fat and loose, often meconium-stained, wrinkled skin, but had weights within normal range for gestation. These fetuses were considered to have subacute intrauterine distress of a few days' duration at or after term gestation. Clifford [185] had similar descriptions of infants, who he declared had "post-maturity with placental dysfunction." Gruenwald described a continuum between those infants with obvious evidence of malnutrition suffered in late gestation and those who suffered prolonged stress causing more subtle impairment of growth [36] (Fig. 2.6).

Markers of maturation, such as brain convolutions, and histological development of the internal organs, such as the

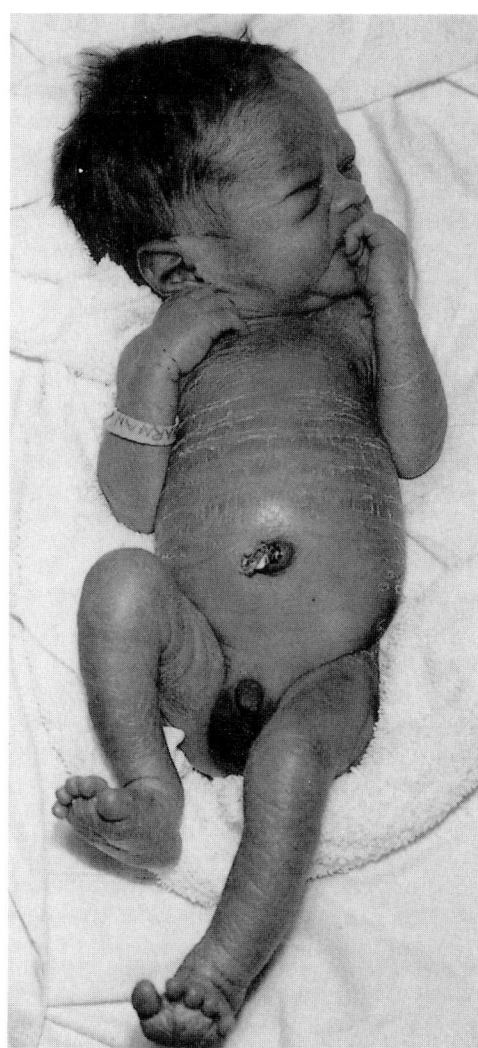

FIGURE 2.6. *A growth-impaired full-term infant weighing 2400 grams and showing cracked peeling skin over the trunk, indicative of late intrauterine stress.*

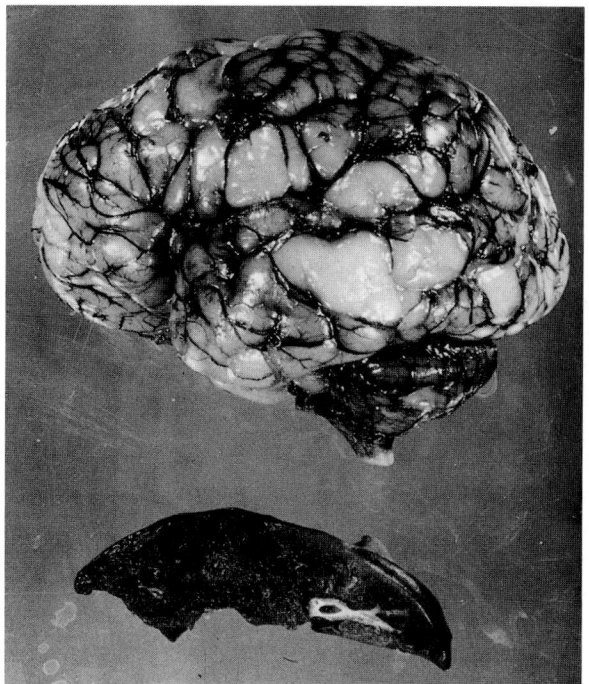

FIGURE 2.7. *Brain and coronal liver slice from an infant weighing 1100 grams at 34 weeks' gestation. Brain/liver weight ratio is 6:1.*

kidney, lung, and liver, are appropriate for gestational age in these growth-impaired fetuses and infants. Because the brain is relatively large and liver relatively small, the ratio of the brain weight to liver weight (usually about 2.8:1 over the last 3 months of gestation) is increased to 5:1 or more in many severely growth-impaired infants [186] (Fig. 2.7). Changes of acute terminal asphyxia are noted, such as amniotic or meconium aspiration, and lymphocytic depletion in the thymus may be seen. Placentas frequently have extensive infarcts in cases of maternal pre-eclampsia, and a variety of other placental lesions have been described (e.g., poorly vascularized or avascular villi) [36]. This is of interest in view of reports of reduced villous arterial counts in cases with abnormal Doppler measurements of umbilical blood flow [187, 188]. At the time when Gruenwald was investigating the pathology of these infants, they frequently died in the

early neonatal period owing to problems such as acute hypoglycemia, resulting in low glycogen stores within their small livers, or hypothermia due to lack of fat stores. A terminal feature in some cases was massive pulmonary hemorrhage. Growth-impaired infants are now more likely to present to the pathologist in developed countries following preterm death in utero or after emergency preterm delivery with neonatal death following intensive care. Problems of maceration, immaturity, or iatrogenic lesions may be superimposed on the basic features of growth retardation.

Following delineation of the most frequent "malnutrition" form of reduced fetal growth, it became apparent that a separate group exists with a different pattern of organ weights and clinical associations. The most typical example of this group is the infant with congenital rubella whose organs may retain the approximate proportions seen in the normally grown infant, but whose maturation is appropriate to gestational age. These infants appear "symmetrically" growth impaired. As mentioned, the organs of this group of infants have a predominant reduction in cell population, whereas those of the "malnutrition" or "asymmetrical" growth-impaired infants have a predominant reduction in size of cells. Symmetrical growth reduction is characteristic of forms of growth impairment induced early in pregnancy, such as those associated with chromosomal or other anomalies originating at or near organogenesis. The timing may be as important as the mechanism in determining the growth pattern characteristic of a particular form of prenatal stress (see Fig. 2.4).

The Pathologically Large Infant

The growth-accelerated infant of the tall, heavy multiparous mother has normal bodily proportions and is large in all respects. In contrast, the infant of the diabetic mother (IDM) is heavy and obese with a characteristic pattern of organomegaly. Adipose tissue, the liver, heart, and adrenals are disproportionately increased in mass [189–191]. The facial appearance has been described as cherubic. The liver may be twice the expected weight for the body size and has steatosis as well as increased erythropoiesis [69]. Naeye [191] found that liver cells were increased in both size and number. Despite the large liver, Petry et al [192] have demonstrated that the iron stores in this organ and in other tissues are reduced, presumably to provide this mineral for the increased production of red blood cells. The heart may be enlarged even in IDMs who do not have other signs of organomegaly. Ventricular hypertrophy may be asymmetrical [193]. Histological examination of the septum may show whorling and disarray of muscle fibers and foci of necrosis. Cardiac failure sometimes develops. Pancreatic findings include increased size and number of islet cells. Beta cells are enlarged and hyperchromatic. Eosinophils sometimes infiltrate the islets and peri-insular connective tissues. The brain is often relatively small compared with other organs and the body as a whole and may be small for the gestational age [194]. The brain is generally of normal size when compared with brains from babies born to non-diabetic mothers at a given stage of gestation. In any case, the brain/liver weight ratio is markedly reduced, and indeed the brain sometimes may be smaller than the liver [61]. The size of the head will reflect that of the enclosed brain, and the resultant discrepancy between size of head and shoulders may predispose to shoulder dystocia in some of these infants. Not all infants of diabetic mothers are overgrown; those mothers with vascular disease may have growth-impaired infants [194].

Susa and colleagues [195] demonstrated insulin's trophic effect by implanting insulin-secreting pumps in the subcutaneous tissue of rhesus fetuses 2 weeks prior to delivery; these fetuses had significant increases in body mass relative to untreated fetuses. It is clear that hyperinsulinemia occurs in fetuses of diabetic mothers and that growth is usually excessive in such fetuses.

Conditions other than maternal diabetes can produce hyperinsulinemia, islet cell hyperplasia, and excessive fetal growth (e.g., the infant giant in whom islet hyperplasia and hyperinsulinemia are features but whose mother is not diabetic). In Sotos syndrome or cerebral gigantism, the mean birth weight is 3400 grams, but the mean length is proportionately greater, 55.2 centimeters, and osseous maturation is accelerated [180]. "Sotosoid" (Cohen's term) conditions

are sometimes associated with remarkable overgrowth of fibrous tissue [180, 196].

Trisomy for the IGF-II has been implicated in the Beckwith-Wiedemann syndrome in which there may be additional genetic material in the p-15 band of chromosome 11 [85]. This is the region where the genes for both insulin and IGF-II reside. High levels of IGF-II, similar to those in the developing fetus, have been demonstrated in Wilms' tumor, a condition which in some patients is associated with mutation of chromosome 11 at the p-13 locus [85].

Marked acceleration of osseous maturation with relative failure to thrive and unusual facial features are described in both the Marshall-Smith and Weaver syndromes. Psychomotor delay, frontal bossing, micrognathia and a long philtrum, respiratory distress, upturned nares, proptosis, hypertrichosis, failure to thrive, and early death are features of the Marshall-Smith syndrome [197]. Accelerated postnatal growth, large ears, camptodactyly, loose skin, hypertelorism, thin hair, and survival to adult life characterize the Weaver syndrome [198]. Some feel that these two syndromes are one-and-the-same [199]. Head size and weight are the most accelerated features, as well as with carpal bone maturation. Other conditions said to have accelerated carpal development are the Marshall-Smith syndrome, Beckwith-Wiedemann syndrome, and acrodysostosis [200].

MEASUREMENT AND ASSESSMENT OF EMBRYOS, FETUSES, NEONATES

Total Body and Selected Organs

Surprisingly few studies relate organ weights to gestational ages. For embryos and early fetuses, the most useful data are provided by Nishimura and colleagues [201], Tanimura and colleagues [202], and Potter and Craig [42] (Tables 2.10–2.12; see also Fig. 2.1). Several authors have published

Table 2.10.   Embryonic stages, gestational ages, crown–rump (CR) lengths and weights

Stage	Days	CR length (mm)	Weight (mg)
12	30	3.9	—
13	32	5.1	16
14	34	6.8	47
15	36	8.0	80
16	38	9.2	125
17	40	11.5	211
18	42	13.5	339
19	44	15.9	521
20	46	19.2	790
21	48	21.1	1020
22	50	22.8	1346
23	52	28	2098

From Nishimura et al [201].

Table 2.11. Weights and measurements of early-stage fetuses

Body wt. (gm)	Gestation (weeks)	CR length (cm)	Brain (gm)	Lungs (gm)	Liver (gm)	Kidneys (gm)	Heart (gm)	Adrenals (gm)	Spleen (gm)	Thymus (gm)	Thyroid (gm)
20	12	4.0	3.0	0.7	1.2	0.1	0.1	0.1	0.01	0.01	0.01
50	15	7.5	7.5	1.8	2.6	0.3	0.4	0.2	0.02	0.04	0.02
100	17	10.0	15.0	3.8	5.0	0.8	0.7	0.4	0.06	0.09	0.04
			±4.0	±1.4	±2.2	±0.3	±0.3	±0.2	±0.03	±0.08	±0.03
200	19	13.0	30.0	6.8	10.0	1.6	1.4	0.9	0.18	0.27	0.08
			±9.0	±1.1	±4.0	±0.7	±0.6	±0.4	±0.12	±0.13	±0.06
300	20	16.0	45.0	9.0	16.0	2.5	2.1	1.3	0.32	0.50	0.13
			±12.0	±4.0	±7.0	±1.0	±0.9	±0.7	±0.20	±0.23	±0.11
400	22	18.0	58.0	10.5	21.0	3.3	2.8	1.7	0.50	0.80	0.17
			±17.0	±5.5	±8.0	±1.3	±1.2	±0.9	±0.28	±0.32	±0.14
500	23	20.0	70.0	11.2	26.0	4.1	3.5	1.8	0.61	1.15	0.20
			±22.0	±7.1	±11.0	±1.8	±1.6	±1.0	±0.35	±0.40	±0.17

Data visually estimated from graphs in Tanimura et al [202].

data for fetuses and neonates born after 23 weeks' gestation [42, 58, 203, 204]. The values presented by Gruenwald and Minh [203], Potter and Craig [42], and Larroche [58] correspond relatively closely. The values presented by Schulz et al [204], while they include separate tables for males and females, vary from those of the other investigators. In this chapter, the data of Gruenwald and Minh are selected for presentation. These tables are in wide use, the authors specifically excluded cases that might alter the statistics, and the data are arranged by gestational age in increments of 2 weeks. The latter points are considered important (Table 2.13). Larroche's data are also presented because they show 10th, 25th, 50th, 75th, and 90th percentiles for weights of various organs at gestational ages from 26 to 40 weeks [58] (Table 2.14). Our own data are presented for liveborn infants and macerated stillborn infants (Tables 2.15 and 2.16).

The ponderal index equals the weight in grams ×100 divided by the cube of the length in centimeters, but it should be used with caution because concurrent abnormalities in weight and length will produce normal values. The

Table 2.12. Weights and measurements of fetuses of 8–26 weeks' gestation (mean values ± 1 SD)

Gestation (weeks)	Weight (gm)[a]	CH length (cm)[a]	CR length (cm)[a]	Foot length (cm)[b]
8	10 ± 2	2 ± 2		
9	11 ± 11	3 ± 3		
10	14 ± 20	4 ± 3	0.8 ± 0.5	
11	14 ± 16	6 ± 3	4 ± 3	0.9 ± 0.7
12	25 ± 20	7 ± 3	6 ± 2	1.1 ± 0.8
13	27 ± 24	9 ± 3	7 ± 2	1.4 ± 0.9
14	38 ± 17	10 ± 3	8 ± 2	1.7 ± 0.8
15	53 ± 22	13 ± 3	9 ± 2	2.1 ± 0.8
16	73 ± 46	14 ± 4	10 ± 2	2.2 ± 0.7
17	122 ± 59	17 ± 3	12 ± 2	2.4 ± 0.7
18	161 ± 91	19 ± 4	13 ± 3	2.6 ± 0.8
19	188 ± 87	20 ± 4	14 ± 3	2.9 ± 0.6
20	227 ± 99	21 ± 4	15 ± 3	3.2 ± 0.6
21	303 ± 75	24 ± 2	16 ± 2	3.4 ± 0.8
22	384 ± 111	26 ± 3	18 ± 2	3.8 ± 0.8
24	379 ± 142	27 ± 3	19 ± 2	4.1 ± 0.8
26	394 ± 140	27 ± 6	18 ± 4	

[a] Measurements from Potter and Craig [42].
[b] From Hern [57].

Table 2.13.   Fetal lengths and organ weights (mean values ± 1 SD)

Gestation (weeks)	N	Body wt. (gm)	Heart (gm)	Lungs (gm)	Spleen (gm)	Liver (gm)	Adrenals (gm)	Kidneys (gm)	Thymus (gm)	Brain (gm)	CH length[a] (cm)	Foot length[b] (cm)
24	108	638	4.9	17	1.7	32	2.9	6.4	2.7	92	31.3	5.0
		±240	±1.6	±6	±1.1	±15	±1.4	±2.6	±1.4	±31	±3.0	±0.3
26	143	845	6.4	18	2.2	39	3.4	7.9	3.0	111	33.3	5.3
		±246	±2.0	±6	±1.5	±15	±1.5	±2.9	±2.3	±39	±3.6	±0.3
28	139	1020	7.6	23	2.6	46	3.7	10.4	3.8	139	36.0	5.7
		±340	±2.3	±7	±1.4	± 16	±1.7	±3.6	±2.1	±48	±4.2	±0.2
30	148	1230	9.3	28	3.4	53	4.2	12.3	4.6	166	37.6	5.8
		±340	±3.3	±11	±2.0	±19	±2.2	±3.9	±2.3	±55	±3.6	±0.2
32	150	1488	11.0	34	4.1	65	4.3	14.5	5.5	209	40.5	6.3
		±335	±3.7	±11	±2.1	±22	±2.3	±4.8	±2.3	±44	±4.5	±0.3
34	104	1838	13.4	40	5.2	74	5.5	17.7	7.5	246	42.8	7.0
		±530	±3.9	±13	±2.1	±27	±2.3	±5.3	±3.8	±58	±4.5	±0.4
36	87	2465	15.1	46	6.7	87	6.4	21.6	8.1	288	45.0	7.3
		±600	±4.8	±16	±3.0	±33	±3.0	±6.7	±4.2	±62	±4.6	±0.4
38	102	2678	18.5	53	8.8	111	8.4	23.8	9.7	349	47.2	7.8
		±758	±5.5	±15	±4.2	±40	±3.5	±7.0	±4.8	±56	±4.6	±0.4
40	220	3163	20.4	56	10.0	130	8.6	25.6	9.5	362	49.8	7.8
		±595	±5.3	±15	±3.9	±45	±3.4	±6.5	±4.4	±55	±3.9	±0.3
42	112	3263	21.9	56	10.2	139	9.1	25.8	10.4	405	50.3	7.9
		±573	±6.2	±18	±4.3	±45	±4.0	±7.5	±4.4	±54	±3.6	±0.5
44	42	3600	25.8	60	11.2	149	9.3	28.4	10.3	417	52.8	7.8
		±800	±4.5	±17	±4.1	±35	±4.4	±7.6	±4.7	±55	±2.8	±0.4

N = number of cases in each group.
[a] Data from Gruenwald and Minh [203].
[b] Data from Usher RL, McLean F. Intrauterine growth of live-born Caucasian infants at sea level: standards obtained from measurements in 7 dimensions of infants born between 25 and 44 weeks of gestation. *J Pediatr* 1969; 74:901–10.

mean ponderal index at 27 weeks' gestation is about 2.2 ± 0.4; at term the mean ponderal index is about 2.4 ± 0.4 [205].

The rates of growth of the total body and various organs are graphically represented in Figure 2.3. The linear measurements progress in an arithmetic fashion throughout most of gestation, while the weights that are directly proportional to volume progress geometrically. The rates of change and the stages of gestation at which growth spurts take place vary minimally. One exception is the adrenal, which shows an early growth spurt between 18 and 24 weeks and which thereafter slows; another is the spleen, which lags behind the other organs until 26 to 28 weeks when its growth accelerates to "catch up" with the rest of the body (see Fig. 2.3). The ratio of sizes of several major organs to total body size also varies throughout development. For example, the brain and liver are prominent throughout the first half of gestation but gradually occupy a smaller proportion of the total body as the limbs and soft tissues become more prominent. (Fig. 2.8).

Weight loss in the first days after birth is inversely proportional to the gestational age and birth weight. The time to recovery of the initial birth weight is likewise inversely proportional to birth weight and gestational age (Fig. 2.9).

Between 1987 and 1991, Wright et al [206] developed growth curves for hospitalized preterm infants whose birth weights were 1500 grams or less. These infants regained birth weight more quickly and had larger average daily weight gains than babies reported previously [207]. The dip in weight in the first few days of life is now less pronounced, perhaps due to improved methods of supplying nutrients to these tiny infants and equally due to the more effective general care given to them [206]. However, for infants with birth weights of 1250 grams and less, catch-up growth may take several years [208].

Upper and Lower Extremities

Dimensions of the extremities of newborns have not received the attention accorded birth weights and total lengths, even though data have been accumulating for the past century [55]. The extensive studies by Streeter published in 1920 [52], and by Scammon and Calkins published in 1929 [53], contain data that are still valid according to recent measurements [31, 46, 57, 59, 209–211]. The foot length, measured from the calcaneus to the end of the longest toe, usually the second toe [57, 211], is especially useful in evaluating material from therapeutic abortions in which curet-

Table 2.14. Percentiles of organ weight (gm) in relation to gestational age

Gestation (weeks)	Brain 10	25	50	75	90	Liver 10	25	50	75	90	Kidneys 10	25	50	75	90	Lung 10	25	50	75	90
26		102	120				31.5	42.5				7	9.6				17.5	23.2		
27	94		110		120	29		37		47	6.1		8		10.9	15.5		19.2		26.1
28		135	160				42	54.5				10.5	13.7				24	31		
29	125		147		170	38		46.7		60	9.5		11.4		15	20.8		26.8		34.2
30		180	203				47.5	61				12	15				30	36.7		
31	170		190		217	43		54		67	10.5		13.3		17	26.5		31.6		39.8
32		201	234				57	72.5				16.1	20				33.4	42.9		
33	190		210		252	52.2		63.5		79	14.5		17.8		22.5	31		38.4		48.7
34		240	280				65	86				19	24				41.2	49.6		
35	226		251		287	61.1		75		99.6	17		21.6		27.2	37.9		45.8		54.4
36		295	328				90	107				20.3	26.3				50.1	60		
37	280		311		346	77.2		103		114.9	16.8		21.7		32.1	42.5		54		71.7
38		332	328				120	130				23	30.1				45.1	77.3		
39	317		356		346	100		123		141	20.3		25		33	41		53.8		81.3
40		400	440				130.5	156				30	37				53.5	81		
	370		420		463	124.2		142		165.6	27		34.7		44	47.2		63.4		86.6

Gestation (weeks)	Heart 10	25	50	75	90	Thymus 10	25	50	75	90	Spleen 10	25	50	75	90	Adrenals 10	25	50	75	90
26		6.3	8.7				1.5	2.5				1.4	2.5				2.2	3.5		
27	5.2		7		10	1.4		2		3.3	1		1.5		3.5	1.9		2.8		4
28		8.8	12				3	5				1.9	3.3				2.8	4.1		
29	8		10		13.2	2.6		4		6.8	1.6		2.5		4.1	2.3		3.3		4.7
30		10	14				4.2	6.5				2.5	4				3.3	4.5		
31	9		12		16	3.3		5.5		7	2		3.3		4.6	2.5		4		5.4
32		12.5	15.6				4.9	8				4	6				4	5.7		
33	11		14		17	4.1		6.3		9.3	3.2		4.4		7.2	3.5		4.7		6.9
34		14	21.5				7	12.7				5.2	7.7				4.5	5.5		
35	13.1		18		25.2	5.8		8.5		13.7	4.7		6.1		8.9	4.3		4.8		6.1
36		19	24				7	12				5.6	9.5				5.5	6.4		
37	16.5		20.8		26.5	5.8		8.7		13.3	5		7		10	4.8		6		7.9
38		20.2	24.5				10.7	13.8				8.3	12.3				7.5	9.6		
39	14		22.4		28	8.8		13		14.4	6.8		10.5		13.3	6.5		8.2		11.3
40		24.3	30.5				9.2	14.7				9.1	13				8.3	11.8		
	20		27		33	8.8		11		17.6	8		10.9		13.6	7.6		10		12

From Larroche [58].

tage is employed. Tables 2.17 and 2.18 show foot lengths, hand lengths, and measurements of segments of the upper extremities, each related to either the gestational age, crown–rump length, or crown–heel length (see Tables 2.14–2.18).

Yau and Chang [212] reported measurements of arm area, arm muscle, and arm fat area in preterm small-for-gestational-age (SGA) infants. By the post-conceptional age of 37 to 40 weeks, the SGA babies had accumulated as much or more fat but less muscle mass, body weight, body length, and head circumference than appropriate-for-gestational-age (AGA) infants.

Merlob and Sivan [205] correlated thigh circumference with head circumference, body length, birth weight, and gestational age in 87 term and 111 preterm infants. A thigh-to-head ratio of 0.38 and a ponderal index of 2.3 were considered the lower limits of normal in term infants. At 27 weeks' gestation the mean thigh-to-head ratio is 0.38, and at term it is about 0.44.

Placental Weight

Placental growth is almost entirely by hyperplasia. Amounts of DNA and RNA in the human placenta are parallel and

T a b l e 2 . 1 5 .   Means and standard deviations of weight and measurements of liveborn infants

Gestation (weeks)	Body weight (gm)	Crown–rump (cm)	Crown–heel (cm)	Toe–heel (cm)	Brain (gm)	Thymus (gm)	Heart (gm)	Lungs (gm)	Spleen (gm)	Liver (gm)	Kidneys (gm)	Adrenals (gm)	Pancreas (gm)
20	381	18.3	25.6	3.6	49	0.8	2.8	11.5	0.7	22.4	3.7	1.8	0.5
	±104	±2.2	±2.2	±0.7	±15	±2.3	±1.0	±2.9	±0.3	±8.0	±1.3	±1.0	±0.5
21	426	19.1	26.7	3.8	57	1	3.2	12.9	0.7	24.1	4.2	2	0.5
	±66	±1.2	±1.7	±0.1	±8	±0.3	±0.4	±2.8	±0.2	±4.2	±0.7	±0.5	
22	473	20	27.8	4	65	1.2	3.5	14.4	0.8	25.4	4.7	2	0.6
	±63	±1.3	±1.6	±0.4	±13	±0.3	±0.6	±4.3	±0.4	±5.2	±1.5	±0.6	±0.3
23	524	20.8	28.9	4.2	74	1.4	3.9	15.9	0.8	26.6	5.3	2.1	0.7
	±116	±1.9	±3.0	±0.5	±11	±0.7	±1.3	±4.9	±0.4	±8.0	±1.8	±0.8	±0.4
24	584	21.6	30	4.4	83	1.5	4.2	17.4	0.9	28	6	2.2	0.8
	±92	±1.4	±1.7	±0.3	±15	±0.7	±1.0	±5.9	±0.5	±7.1	±1.8	±0.8	±0.5
25	655	22.5	31.1	4.6	94	1.8	4.7	19	1.1	29.7	6.8	2.2	0.9
	±106	±1.6	±2.0	±0.4	±25	±1.2	±1.2	±5.3	±1.6	±9.8	±1.9	±1.4	±0.3
26	739	23.3	32.2	4.8	105	2	5.2	20.6	1.3	32.1	7.6	2.4	1
	±181	±1.9	±2.4	±0.7	±21	±1.1	±1.3	±6.3	±0.7	±10.9	±2.5	±1.1	±0.5
27	836	24.2	33.4	5	118	2.3	5.8	22.1	1.7	35.1	8.6	2.5	1.2
	±197	±2.5	±3.5	±0.5	±21	±1.2	±1.9	±9.7	±1.0	±13.3	±3.0	±1.1	±0.5
28	949	25	34.5	5.2	132	2.6	6.5	23.7	2.1	38.9	9.7	2.7	1.4
	±190	±1.7	±2.3	±0.6	±29	±1.5	±1.9	±10.0	±0.8	±12.6	±12.0	±1.2	±0.5
29	1077	25.9	35.6	5.4	147	3	7.2	25.3	2.6	43.5	10.9	3	1.5
	±449	±2.8	±4.4	±0.8	±49	±1.9	±2.7	±12.6	±0.9	±15.8	±4.4	±1.2	±1.0
30	1219	26.7	36.7	5.7	163	3.5	8.1	26.9	3.3	49.1	12.3	3.3	1.7
	±431	±3.3	±4.2	±0.7	±38	±2.6	±2.6	±20.3	±2.0	±18.8	±8.5	±2.7	±1.0
31	1375	27.6	37.8	5.9	180	4	9	28.5	4	55.4	13.7	3.7	1.8
	±281	±3.8	±3.1	±0.7	±34	±3.4	±2.8	±13.2	±1.2	±17.3	±5.2	±1.3	±0.6
32	1543	28.4	38.9	6.1	198	4.7	10.1	30.2	4.7	62.5	15.2	4.1	2
	±519	±9.5	±5.7	±1.1	±48	±3.6	±4.4	±19.0	±5.4	±30.0	±7.4	±1.7	±0.8
33	1720	29.3	40	6.3	217	5.4	11.2	31.8	5.5	70.3	16.8	4.6	2.1
	±580	±3.3	±3.5	±0.7	±49	±3.2	±4.0	±13.5	±3.5	±25.4	±7.7	±1.5	±0.8
34	1905	30.1	41.1	6.5	237	6.1	12.4	33.5	6.4	78.7	18.5	5.1	2.3
	±625	±4.3	±4.0	±0.6	±53	±3.8	±2.8	±16.5	±3.0	±30.2	±9.3	±2.2	±1.1
35	2093	30.9	42.3	6.7	257	6.9	13.7	35.2	7.2	87.4	20.1	5.6	2.5
	±309	±2.0	±2.9	±0.4	±45	±4.5	±3.6	±20.5	±5.2	±30.6	±10.9	±2.8	±0.6
36	2280	31.8	43.4	6.9	278	7.7	15	36.9	8.1	96.3	21.7	6.1	2.6
	±615	±3.9	±5.9	±1.1	±96	±5.0	±5.1	±17.5	±3.1	±33.7	±6.8	±3.1	±0.7
37	2462	32.6	44.5	7.1	298	8.4	16.4	38.7	8.8	105.1	23.3	6.6	2.8
	±821	±5.0	±7.0	±1.2	±70	±5.6	±5.7	±22.9	±6.4	±33.7	±9.9	±3.3	±0.9
38	2634	33.5	45.6	7.3	318	9	17.7	40.6	9.5	113.5	24.8	7.1	3
	±534	±3.2	±5.1	±0.8	±106	±2.8	±5.4	±17.1	±3.5	±34.7	±7.2	±2.9	±1.1
39	2789	34.3	46.7	7.5	337	9.4	19.1	42.6	10.1	121.3	26.1	7.4	3.3
	±520	±1.9	±4.4	±0.5	±91	±2.5	±2.8	±14.9	±3.5	±39.2	±4.9	±2.5	±0.5
40	2922	35.2	47.8	7.7	356	9.5	20.4	44.6	10.4	127.9	27.3	7.7	3.6
	±450	±2.8	±4.2	±0.8	±79	±5.0	±5.6	±22.7	±3.3	±35.8	±11.5	±3.0	±1.3
41	3025	36	48.9	7.9	372	9.1	21.7	46.8	10.5	133.1	28.1	7.8	3.9
	±600	±3.1	±5.4	±0.8	±65	±4.8	±10.9	±26.2	±4.5	±55.7	±12.7	±2.8	±1.5
42	3091	36.9	50	8.1	387	8.1	22.9	49.1	10.3	136.4	28.7	7.8	4.3
	±617	±2.4	±3.8	±1.1	±61	±3.8	±6.2	±14.6	±3.6	±38.9	±9.7	±3.2	±1.9

Data from Women & Infants Hospital, Providence, Rhode Island.

equal until about the 34th to 36th week of gestation when the DNA RNA ratio becomes less than 1. According to some authors, by the middle of the 38th week of gestation, the growth of the placenta ceases altogether, and its mass may actually regress [213, 214]. Teasdale [215] describes the interval from the beginning of gestation until 36 weeks as the phase of growth, while the last 4 to 5 weeks of gestation compose the phase of placental maturation. According

to Hendricks [216], the placenta continues to grow, albeit slowly, through the 40th week of gestation. In any case, after embryonic life, the fetal weight increases more rapidly than does the placental weight (Table 2.19; see also Table 2.5).

All elements of growth are not completely reflected in the placental weight. As Teasdale and others have shown, the villous and microvillous surface areas for exchange and the configuration and numbers of syncytiovascular membranes

Table 2.16. Means and standard deviations of weights and measurements of stillborn infants

Gestation (weeks)	Body weight (gm)	Crown–rump (cm)	Crown–heel (cm)	Toe–heel (cm)	Brain (gm)	Thymus (gm)	Heart (gm)	Lungs (gm)	Spleen (gm)	Liver (gm)	Kidneys (gm)	Adrenals (gm)	Pancreas (gm)
20	313	18.0	24.9	3.3	41	0.4	2.4	7.1	0.3	17	2.7	1.3	0.5
	±139	±2.0	±2.3	±0.6	±24	±0.3	±1.0	±3.0	±1.0	±9	±2.9	±0.6	±0.1
21	353	18.9	26.2	3.5	48	0.5	2.6	7.9	0.4	18	3.1	1.4	0.5
	±125	±4.8	±3.6	±0.6	±18	±0.3	±0.9	±3.8	±0.6	±7	±1.3	±0.7	±0.4
22	398	19.8	27.4	3.8	55	0.6	2.8	8.7	0.5	19	3.5	1.4	0.6
	±117	±9.6	±2.5	±0.4	±15	±0.4	±0.9	±3.1	±0.4	±10	±0.8	±0.6	±0.5
23	450	20.6	28.7	4	64	0.8	3	9.5	0.7	21	4.1	1.5	0.7
	±118	±2.3	±3.3	±0.5	±18	±0.5	±1.4	±5.7	±0.5	±7	±1.7	±0.8	±0.3
24	510	21.5	29.9	4.2	74	0.9	3.3	10.5	0.9	22	4.6	1.5	0.7
	±179	±3.1	±4.3	±0.8	±25	±0.7	±1.8	±5.6	±0.7	±8	±2.4	±0.8	±0.3
25	581	22.3	31.1	4.4	85	1.1	3.7	11.6	1.2	24	5.3	1.6	0.8
	±178	±4.0	±6.5	±0.8	±31	±0.8	±1.3	±4.9	±0.4	±35	±2.4	±0.8	±0.7
26	663	23.2	32.4	4.7	98	1.4	4.2	12.9	1.5	26	6.1	1.7	0.8
	±227	±4.1	±5.3	±0.9	±37	±1.4	±2.2	±8.7	±1.1	±16	±3.6	±0.9	±0.7
27	758	24.1	33.6	4.9	112	1.7	4.8	14.4	1.9	29	7	1.9	0.9
	±227	±2.9	±3.2	±1.4	±37	±1.1	±3.6	±9.7	±1.0	±24	±3.1	±1.5	±0.3
28	864	24.9	34.9	5.1	127	2	5.4	16.1	2.3	32	7.9	2.1	1
	±247	±2.2	±5.6	±1.2	±39	±2.1	±2.6	±7.0	±1.1	±32	±2.5	±1.6	±0.3
29	984	25.8	36.1	5.3	143	2.4	6.2	18	2.7	36	9	2.4	1.1
	±511	±4.1	±5.9	±1.2	±57	±2.6	±2.4	±13.6	±2.0	±23	±4.5	±1.2	±1.2
30	1115	26.6	37.3	5.6	160	2.8	7	20.1	3.1	40	10.1	2.7	1.2
	±329	±2.4	±3.6	±0.7	±72	±4.1	±2.8	±8.6	±1.5	±22	±6.0	±1.3	±0.2
31	1259	27.5	38.6	5.8	178	3.2	8	22.5	3.6	46	11.3	3	1.4
	±588	±3.0	±2.7	±0.7	±32	±1.9	±3.1	±10.1	±4.0	±38	±4.1	±1.8	±1.4
32	1413	28.4	39.8	6	196	3.7	9.1	25	4.2	52	12.6	3.5	1.6
	±623	±2.8	±5.4	±0.6	±92	±2.2	±4.1	±10.7	±2.4	±32	±8.0	±1.8	±0.6
33	1578	29.2	41.1	6.2	216	4.3	10.2	27.8	4.7	58	13.9	3.9	1.8
	±254	±3.5	±3.1	±0.4	±51	±1.5	±2.0	±5.8	±2.3	±17	±3.5	±1.4	±0.8
34	1750	30.1	42.3	6.5	236	4.8	11.4	30.7	5.3	66	15.3	4.4	2
	±494	±3.5	±4.3	±0.8	±42	±5.6	±3.2	±15.2	±2.5	±22	±5.1	±1.3	±0.5
35	1930	30.9	43.5	6.7	256	5.4	12.6	33.7	5.9	74	16.7	4.9	2.3
	±865	±3.9	±5.8	±0.9	±70	±3.4	±5.3	±14.3	±6.8	±46	±7.1	±1.9	±0.7
36	2114	31.8	44.8	6.9	277	6.1	13.9	36.7	6.5	82	18.1	5.4	2.6
	±616	±4.0	±7.2	±0.8	±94	±4.1	±5.8	±16.8	±2.9	±36	±6.3	±2.4	±2.6
37	2300	32.7	46	7.2	297	6.7	15.1	39.8	7.2	91	19.4	5.8	2.9
	±647	±5.1	±7.9	±0.9	±69	±3.9	±9.9	±11.1	±6.3	±57	±9.7	±6.2	±3.1
38	2485	33.5	47.3	7.4	317	7.4	16.4	42.9	7.8	100	20.8	6.3	3.2
	±579	±2.6	±3.9	±0.8	±83	±6.1	±4.4	±15.7	±5.9	±44	±6.0	±2.1	±1.6
39	2667	34.4	48.5	7.6	337	8.1	17.5	45.8	8.5	109	22	6.7	3.5
	±596	±3.7	±4.9	±0.5	±132	±4.7	±3.9	±15.2	±4.5	±53	±5.8	±5.3	±1.9
40	2842	35.2	49.7	7.8	355	8.9	18.6	48.6	9.2	118	23.1	7	3.9
	±482	±6.4	±3.2	±0.7	±57	±4.3	±12.9	±19.4	±4.1	±49	±8.6	±2.9	±1.7
41	3006	36.1	51	8.1	373	9.6	19.5	51.1	9.9	126	24.1	7.1	4.2
	±761	±3.7	±5.4	±0.8	±141	±5.6	±4.9	±17.0	±4.5	±53	±10.5	±3.0	
42	3156	36.9	52.2	8.3	389	10.4	20.3	53.2	10.6	135	24.9	7.2	4.5
	±678	±2.0	±3.0	±0.5	±36	±5.0	±4.5	±10.1	±3.7	±54	±8.1	±2.9	±2.3

Data from Women & Infants Hospital, Providence, Rhode Island.

tend to increase throughout gestation. Large placentas (e.g., from cases of maternal diabetes mellitus) have increased numbers of cells, but individual cells are of normal size [215, 217, 218]. Small placentas, as determined by weight alone, account for few cases of reduced growth. Naeye [151] found that in the collaborative perinatal project in the US, only 84 of 100,000 births were associated with placentas more than two standard deviations below the mean.

Singleton placentas gain weight uniformly, throughout gestation but twin placentas accelerate in weight between 24 and 36 weeks' gestation, reaching a plateau at 37 to 38 weeks. Singleton placentas in our hospital are heavier than those previously reported in the literature. Twin placentas do not weigh twice that of a singleton placenta of the same gestational age [219] (Tables 2.20 and 2.21).

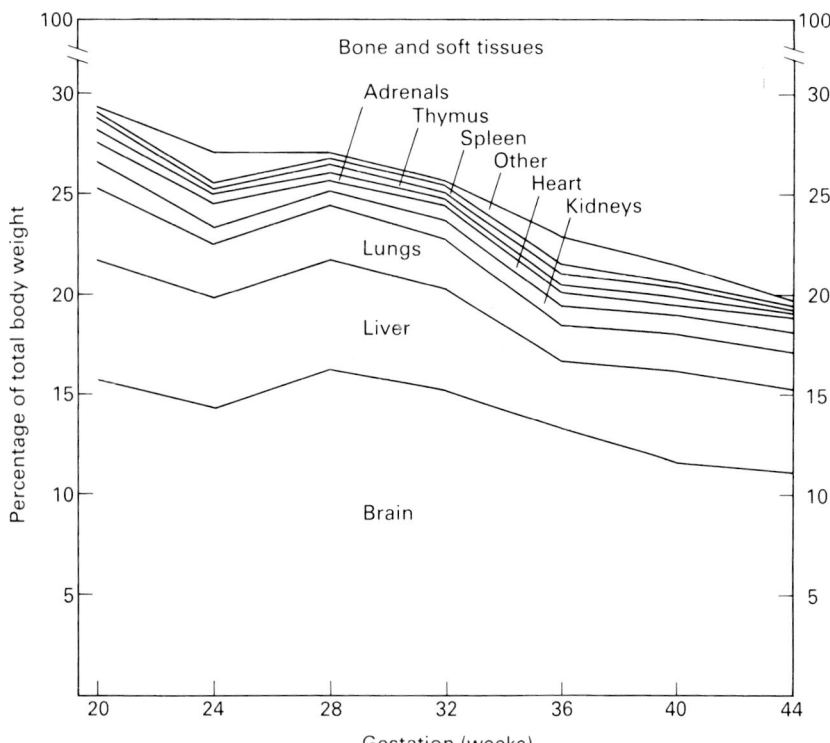

FIGURE 2.8. *Percentage of total body weight contributed by various organs and tissues at different gestational ages.*

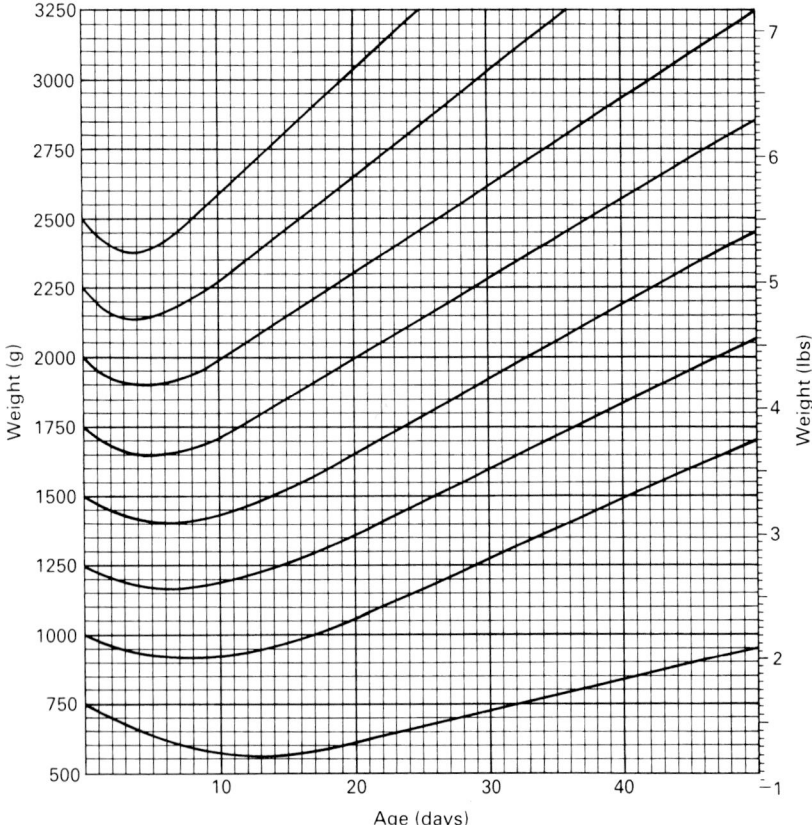

FIGURE 2.9. *Weight curves for liveborn infants at various gestational ages and birth weights. Note that babies with low birth weights maintain weight loss for long periods of time. (From Ref 207.)*

Table 2.17. Lengths of hand, foot, crown–heel (CH), and crown–rump (CR) at various gestational ages

Gestation (weeks)	Hand (cm)	Foot (cm)	CH (cm)	CR (cm)
12	0.55	0.48	7.08	5.17
16	1.56	1.84	15.54	10.76
20	2.43	3.00	22.79	15.54
24	3.20	4.02	29.20	19.77
28	3.91	4.96	35.05	23.63
32	4.55	5.82	40.43	27.18
36	5.16	6.63	45.47	30.51
40	5.72	7.38	50.20	33.63

Data compiled from several tables in Scammon and Calkins [53].

Table 2.18. Upper extremity measurements*

Gestation (weeks)	Arm length	Upper arm	Forearm	Hand	Middle finger
27	14.26 ± 0.66	6.23 ± 0.36	5.54 ± 0.35	4.12 ± 0.31	1.73 ± 0.10
30	15.70 ± 0.69	6.91 ± 0.44	6.00 ± 0.36	4.60 ± 0.28	1.99 ± 0.13
35	18.57 ± 0.87	8.07 ± 0.46	6.95 ± 0.52	5.53 ± 0.35	2.34 ± 0.14
38	20.17 ± 0.76	8.64 ± 0.36	7.68 ± 0.45	6.05 ± 0.31	2.55 ± 0.13
40	20.61 ± 0.86	8.88 ± 0.32	7.81 ± 0.42	6.14 ± 0.31	2.65 ± 0.16

* The arm is measured from the acromion to the tip of the middle finger, with the arm in full extension and parallel to the body; the upper arm is measured from the acromion to the olecranon, with the elbow bent at 90 degrees; the forearm is measured from the olecranon process to the distal end of the styloid process of the radius, with the elbow bent at 90 degrees; hand length is measured from the distal wrist crease to the tip of the middle finger, and the middle finger length is obtained by measuring the distance from the proximal flexion crease of the middle finger to the tip of the middle finger.
Adapted from Sivan et al [210].

Maturation of the Central Nervous System

The fetal and neonatal brain is the largest of the organs usually listed in tables of organ weights (e.g., brain, heart, lungs, liver, kidneys). Between 20 weeks' and 40 weeks' gestation, the human fetal brain accounts for from 15.6% to about 11.5% of the total body weight (see Fig. 2.8). Its rate of growth parallels that of the total body from the 8th through the 40th week of development (see Fig. 2.3). Some of the morphologic milestones in early brain development (from approximately 4 weeks to 24 weeks) are listed in Table 2.22. The actual weights range from 92 grams (standard deviation, 31 grams) at 24 weeks' to 362 grams (standard deviation, 55 grams) at 40 weeks' gestational age [42, 54, 58, 204, 220] (see Tables 2.12–2.14). As for head circumference, the measurements are shown at various gestations in Table 2.1. Postnatal growth of the head circumference in premature babies, when corrected for post-conceptional age, shows catch-up at 18 months compared with babies born at term. However, when the premature infant weighs less than 1000 grams and has a gestation pre-sumed to be less than 27 weeks, catch-up growth takes more time [221].

By 10 to 12 weeks of gestation, all the cellular anlage of the brain can be discerned. Hippocampal folds and the anterior part of the corpus callosum are visible by 15 weeks. Between 20 and 28 weeks, waves of migrating cells travel from the periventricular germinal matrix to the cortex. Subsequent waves of neurons leapfrog over the first waves, which come to rest in the deepest layers of the cortex. The migration depletes the germinal matrix so that by 34 to 36 weeks, remnants are seen mainly in the anterior portion. By 40 weeks, the germinal matrix area is almost completely devoid of primitive cells. Migration in the cerebellum is not as uniform as that of the cerebrum. Cells in the cerebellum are said to arrive at their destinations after "a very complicated ballet" of movement [58].

The gyral pattern is of particular value in assessing gestational age in the middle of fetal development from about the 20th to the 36th week. At 20 weeks, the surface of the brain is essentially smooth, while by 34 weeks, most of the secondary gyri have formed. This phase of gyral and sulcal

Table 2.19.   Placental weights and body weights from postmortem babies and survivors for each gestational age (mean values in grams ± 1 SD)

Gestation (weeks)	Placental weights		Body weights	
	Postmortem (n)	Survivor (n)	Postmortem (n)	Survivor (n)
24	225 (108) ±69	—	638 (108) ±240	—
26	256 (143) ±74	—	845 (143) ±246	—
28	277 (139) ±62	256 (9) ±71	1020 (139) ±340	1333 (9) ±405
30	303 (148) ±69	310 (13) ±71	1230 (148) ±340	1625 (13) ±550
32	362 (150) ±79	375 (11) ±80	1488 (150) ±335	1928 (11) ±438
34	410 (104) ±92	389 (23) ±80	1838 (104) ±530	2380 (23) ±483
36	453 (87) ±76	407 (63) ±93	2165 (87) ±600	2705 (63) ±500
38	465 (102) ±74	469 (225) ±88	2678 (102) ±758	2990 (225) ±383
40	469 (220) ±82	483 (555) ±88	3163 (220) ±595	3318 (555) ±438
42	508 (112) ±80	507 (296) ±96	3263 (112) ±573	3508 (296) ±360
44	518 (42) ±111	497 (112) ±100	3690 (42) ±800	3513 (112) ±360

Data from Gruenwald and Minh [54].

Table 2.20.   Percentiles of singleton placenta weight (gm) in relation to gestational age

Gestation (Weeks)	90	75	Mean	25	10	N
21	3	114	128	143	158	172
22	6	122	138	157	175	191
23	7	133	151	172	193	211
24	9	145	166	189	212	233
25	19	159	182	208	233	256
26	14	175	200	227	255	280
27	9	192	219	248	278	305
28	16	210	238	270	302	331
29	11	229	259	293	327	357
30	12	249	281	316	352	384
31	14	269	303	340	377	411
32	24	290	325	364	403	438
33	30	311	347	387	428	464
34	32	331	369	411	453	491
35	44	352	391	434	477	516
36	36	372	412	457	501	542
37	32	391	432	478	524	566
38	62	409	452	499	547	589
39	103	426	470	519	567	611
40	193	442	487	537	587	632
41	87	456	502	553	605	651

N = number of cases in each group.
From Pinar et al [219].

Table 2.21. Percentiles of twin placenta weight (gm) in relation to gestational age

Gestation (Weeks)	N	10	25	Mean	75	90
19	2	161	185	212	239	263
20	3	166	190	218	245	270
21	2	176	202	231	260	286
22	5	191	219	251	282	310
23	2	210	241	276	311	343
24	3	232	267	307	346	382
25	5	257	297	341	386	426
26	4	284	330	380	430	475
27	8	314	365	421	478	528
28	7	345	401	464	527	584
29	12	377	439	509	579	641
30	17	409	478	554	631	700
31	13	441	516	600	683	758
32	29	472	554	644	734	815
33	27	503	590	687	783	870
34	53	531	624	727	830	923
35	52	558	656	764	873	971
36	66	582	684	798	912	1014
37	58	602	708	827	945	1051
38	54	619	728	850	972	1082
39	38	631	743	868	993	1105
40	47	639	753	879	1005	1118
41	12	642	756	882	1009	1123

N = number of cases in each group.
From Pinar et al [219].

Table 2.22. Milestones in the development of the central nervous system

Event	CR length (mm)	Gestation (weeks)
Neural tube closes	3	3–4
Olfactory bulb appears	12	6
Spinal cord fills neural canal	30	9
Vertebral arches close	34	11
Chorioid plexus appears, 3rd V	77	12
Sylvian fossae appear	77	12
Corpus callosum appears	80–150	12–20
Cord ends at 1st sacral ganglion	111	14
Primary fissure of cerebellum appears	132	16
Nerve roots myelinate	132	16
Spinal cord ends at L3–L4 interspace	221	23
Central, parieto-occipital, and calcarine fissures appear	150–230	20–24

Fom Minckler J. *Pathology of the Nervous System*, vol. 2. New York: McGraw-Hill, 1971, p. 1856.

Table 2.23. Brain surface structure during gestation

Gestation (weeks)	
22	Calcarine fissure and parieto-occipital fissure appear
24	Rolandic fissure begins, cingulate sulcus visible
26	Frontal and parietal sulci appear
28	Superior temporal sulcus present
30	Growth and more finished appearance
32–34	No striking changes, except for growth
36	Operculum closes over insula
40	Tertiary sulci appear

Adapted from descriptions in Dorovini-Zis and Dolman [64].

development, while very active, is at the same time fairly predictable and provides the pathologist with a major tool to determine gestational age [64, 65] (Table 2.23). Gyral and sulcal development are not usually affected by most of the conditions that produce intrauterine growth impairment. Indeed in so-called symmetrical growth retardation, a small brain may have a mass similar to that of a fetus (e.g., of 24 weeks' gestational age) but can have the gyral pattern of a fetus at 30 to 32 weeks' gestation, establishing the true length of gestation at the higher figure. On the other hand, the brain's gyral development may not be totally immune to the effects of diseases; one report describes acceleration of gyral pattern by about 2 weeks in fetuses whose mothers have pre-eclampsia [222].

Myelinization first occurs in the spinal cord at 22 weeks. The medial longitudinal fasciculus of the pons myelinates next. By 30 weeks, medial and lateral lemnisci myelinate; then at 34 weeks, the process begins in the cerebral structures. In general, the pattern of myelination proceeds from proximal to distal structures in long tracts, from the phylogenetically older to newer structures (i.e., in a caudocephalad direction) in the cerebral white matter. By 40 weeks' gestation, cranial nerves are myelinated as are all the spinal cord tracts, except the anterior and lateral corticospinal tracts. Limbic and some extrapyramidal and reticular formations myelinate late, mostly during the first 12 to 18 months of postnatal life [58, 65, 66].

Kidney Development

In tissue culture, early nephrogenic blastema can form glomerular structures without the benefit of vascular participation [223, 224]. The mature elements consist of epithelial derivatives, including epithelial basal laminae. Elements such as endothelial basal laminae, mesangial cells, and juxtaglomerular apparatus require the participation of vessels. Renin-producing cells appear in the fetal renal vascular pole as early as the 5th week of gestation [225].

In fetal development, the ratio of width of the glomerulogenic zone to the width of the definitive glomerular zone (gz:dz) correlates well with birth weight [68]. The glomerulogenic zone extends from the undersurface of the capsular connective tissue through the S-shaped and densely cellular tubular structures, to the definitive glomerulus closest to the capsular surface. The definitive glomerular zone extends from the top of the superficial-most definitive glomerulus to the bottom of the deepest glomerulus at the junction with the medulla. At 500 grams, the gz:dz ratio is 0.208;

the ratio decreases in a linear fashion as the birth weight increases (Fig. 2.10). In babies with birth weights of 2500 grams, the ratio is 0.008. This system of evaluating organ (renal) maturation in relation to birth weight is useful in detecting infants with reduced intrauterine growth in whom the gz:dz ratio is less than expected for the birth weight.

Gestational age can be estimated by counting the number of rows of glomeruli between two well-oriented columns of Bertin from the arcuate artery to the nephrogenic zone. This system works well between gestations of 23 weeks to 33 weeks [64]. Three rows ("generations") of glomeruli are present at 16 to 17 weeks' gestation. The nephrogenic zone is quiescent until about 23 weeks when glomeruli start to form at the rate of one row per week and continue for the next 10 to 11 weeks. When glomerulogenesis ceases, there are 10 to 14 rows or "generations" of glomeruli from the arcuate artery to the capsule of the kidney, the oldest and largest glomeruli in the deepest part of the cortex (Table 2.24). In practical use, estimates are usually within ±1 week of the actual gestational ages, as may be determined by a variety of other means. Certain chromosomal abnormalities, such as Down syndrome, can retard renal maturation. The system is useless in Potter syndrome and in infants or fetuses with dysplastic kidneys, but cases of autosomal recessive polycystic kidney disease can be evaluated in this way.

The kidney's major functions correlate well with anatomic maturation. Proximal convoluted tubules increase in volume throughout childhood [226]. Even in the early days and weeks of life, functional maturation is measurable with increased glomerular filtration rates and clearance rates for creatinine. Fractional excretions of sodium, alpha amino

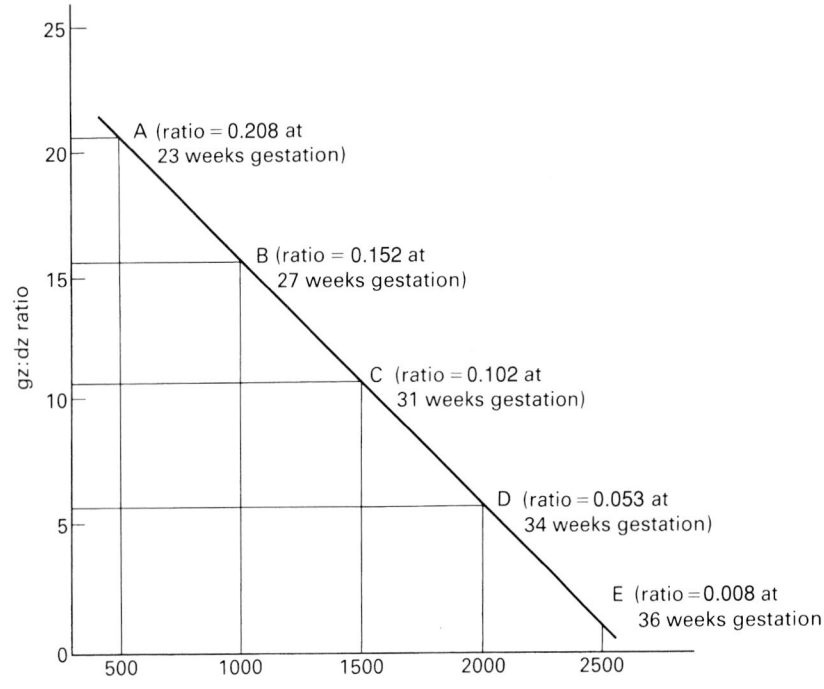

FIGURE 2.10.   *The ratio of the renal glomerulogenic zone to the definitive glomerular zone (gz:dz) is represented on the Y-axis. Birth weights in normally grown babies are represented on the X-axis.*

Table 2.24.   Development of glomeruli in gestations of 16–40 weeks

Gestation (weeks)	Rows of glomeruli between columns of Bertin
16–23	3
24	4 ± 1
25	5 ± 1
26	6 ± 1
27	7 ± 1
28	8 ± 1
29	9 ± 1
30	10 ± 1
31	11 ± 1
32	12 ± 1
33	12–13
34	12–14
35–42	12–14
Newborn to adult	12–14

From Dorovini-Zis and Dolman [64].

Table 2.25.   Hepatic erythropoiesis and gestational age

Gestation (weeks)	n	Ratio of erythroids to hepatocytes + sinusoids × 100 (± 1 SD)
22–25	8	10.39 (4.56)
26–29	8	8.85 (2.69)
30–33	7	6.11 (3.16)
34–37	5	5.36 (3.26)
38–40	5	1.38 (0.30)
41–43	5	1.26 (0.54)

Data from Singer [69].

Table 2.26.   Radial alveolar counts at various gestational ages

Gestation (weeks)	Alveoli intersected[b] (± 1 SD)
24–27	2.2 (0.6)
28–31	2.6 (0.8)
32–35	3.2 (0.9)
36–39	3.6 (0.9)
40	4.4 (0.9)
1–4.5[a]	5.5 (1.4)

[a] Postnatal age, weeks.
[b] The radial alveolar count is measured by extending an imaginary straight line from the center of terminal bronchioles or respiratory bronchioles to their nearest pleural surface or the nearest interlobular septum of fibrous tissue; the number of alveoli crossed represents the count.
From Emery and Mithal [71].

acids, and glucose decrease as the kidney matures during the first months of life [227].

Liver Erythropoiesis

In newborn mice at term, erythroids make up a large proportion of total hepatic mass, but in human fetuses the amount of hepatic erythropoiesis decreases progressively through the last half of gestation and is quite sparse at term. This decline is measurable and therefore can be correlated with gestational age. Many factors commonly associated with perinatal mortality are responsible for persistent hepatic erythropoiesis (e.g., hypoxia and anemia). Since there is a lag of about 3 to 4 days between such events and the appearance of hyperplastic erythroid tissue, cases with sudden fatal insults can be used to establish the expected curve of decline. The ratio of volume-proportion of erythroids to volume-proportion of hepatocytes plus sinusoids is inversely proportional to gestational age [69] (Table 2.25).

Lung Growth and Maturation

The development of air spaces beyond 20 weeks' gestation is a useful morphologic feature to estimate gestational age. Qualitative changes include the flattening of pneumocytes beginning at about 23 weeks and the gradual enlargment of air spaces at the expense of the extensive interstitial tissues. Vessels become more numerous and move closer to the epithelial cells. Between 28 and 40 weeks, further flattening of epithelium and enlargement of air spaces with apposed capillaries characterize the mature fetal lung. Functionally, of course, the development of surface-active phospholipids is of major significance but their morphologic identification is not practical [70, 228].

Morphometric evaluations are best done with special injection techniques, but morphometry is possible in material collected with standard autopsy techniques [229]. One such evaluation is the radial alveolar count described by Emery and Mithal [71]. By extending an imaginary straight line from the center of a terminal bronchiole or respiratory bronchiole to the nearest pleural surface or the nearest interlobular septum of fibrous tissue, the number of alveoli crossed can be determined and is proportional to gestational age (Table 2.26). Radial alveolar counts are most useful in evaluating cases of pulmonary hypoplasia.

In terms of functional pulmonary maturation, ethnic background and environment both play a role. Assuming that hyaline membrane disease is a sign of relative pulmonary immaturity, Ross and Naeye [230] demonstrated more mature lungs (less hyaline membrane disease) among babies of cigarette-smoking mothers and among babies born to Ethiopian mothers, many of whom were poorly nourished, than among white babies or South African black babies whose mothers had prenatal care. In the United States, black babies of low birth weight have less hyaline membrane disease than do white babies of the same weight [231].

Table 2.27. Palpebral fissure size and gestational age

Gestation (weeks)	Palpebral fissure length ± 1 SD (cm)
32	1.48 ± 0.2
34	1.5 ± 0.2
36	1.6 ± 0.2
38	1.7 ± 0.2
40	1.7 ± 0.2

From Jones et al [232].

Head, Eyes, and Ears

Scammon and Calkins [53] measured 21 different features of the face and head, only three or four of which are still widely used. Streeter [52] developed an index, the head modulus, with which he hoped to standardize head measurements. The head modulus consisted of the largest horizontal circumference plus the biauricular diameter, the sum of which is divided by two. These examples may have been useful in attempting to discriminate normal from abnormal development, but they are not appropriate for establishing gestational age. The most useful head measurement is the biparietal diameter (see Table 2.2). Other measurements, such as the circumference of the head, suboccipital-mental diameter, and bregmatic-occipital diameter, are less useful, mostly due to differences in interpretation of fetal and neonatal anatomy.

At term, the distance from left outer canthus to right outer canthus is 6.3 centimeters (range, 5.3–7.4 c); the inter-pupillary distance, measured to the center of each pupil, is 3.8 centimeters (range, 3.3–4.5 c); the distance from left inner canthus to right inner canthus is 2.6 centimeters (range, 1.5–3.6 c) [232]. The lengths of the palpebral fissure at various gestations are shown in Table 2.27. No differences in these lengths are due to the sex of the baby, but blacks have slightly longer fissures than Hispanics (+0.5 mm) and whites (+1.5 mm) [233]. Ear lengths have also been measured. At term, the 50th percentile of lengths of pinnae is 3.6 centimeters (10th–90th percentile, 2.9–4.3 cm) [234].

Sex Organs and Gestational Age

Phalluses have been measured in formalin-fixed fetuses of both sexes from the 10th through the 24th week of gestation [235]. At 10 weeks, the lengths of the phalluses are essentially equal in males and females; the mean for both sexes is approximately 2.5 millimeters. Thereafter, the length of the penis outstrips that of the clitoris (Table 2.28). Measurements after about 18 weeks' gestation were made only in males.

Gastrointestinal Growth

The gut length is quite variable depending on the methods used to measure the intestine, the nutritional status of the

Table 2.28. Length of phalluses related to gestational age*

Gestation (weeks)	Penile length (mm)	Clitoral length (mm)
10	2.5	2.5
14	3–7	1.5–4
18	3.5–10	2–4.5
20	4–12	
24	6–13+	
28	15–25	
32	18–32	
36	20–34	
40	22–42	

* Phalluses were measured from the pubic bone to the tip of the glans. Clitoral lengths were not measured beyond 18 weeks' gestation. The ranges of values were determined by visual estimates from the published curves, there being no tabulated data. The mean length of the penis at 40 weeks' gestation was 35 mm (± 7 = 2 SD).
Data from Feldman and Smith [235].

Table 2.29. Length of small and large intestines at various gestational ages

Body length (cm)	Gestation (weeks)	Small intestine (cm)	Large intestine (cm)
12.5	14	6	5
18.3	16	50	9
22.0	20	80	14
30.0	24	129	25
36.0	28	184	51
42.0	32	200	60
46.2	36	250	40
50.0	40	310	45

From data in Bryant [236].

fetus or neonate at the time of death, and the presence or absence of inflammation in the gut or the serosal tissues. Measurements are presented in Table 2.29 [236, 237]. The mean length of small intestine from the ileocecal valve to the ligament of Treitz is related to the crown–heel length. Shanklin and Cooke [237] fixed the intestines in formalin solution before removing them from the mesentery and mesocolon. The lengths they recorded are somewhat less than those of Bryant [236] whose data are shown in Table 2.29. In the range of premature and newborn babies, the length of the small intestine is approximately four to five times that of the total body length (one standard deviation being roughly equal to the body length). For example, in the study reported by Siebert [238], when the body length is 40 centimeters, the length of the small intestine is 164 ± 54 centimeters; when the body length is 50 centimeters, the length of the small intestine is 239 ± 67 centimeters.

The diameter of the anus in the newborn has a linear relationship with fetal weight [239]. The anal diameter, best measured with graded sounds, is equal in millimeters to

Table 2.30. Anal diameters relative to fetal weight

Weight (kg)	Mean anal diameter (mm)
1.0–1.5	8.6
1.5–2.0	9.1
2.0–2.5	9.7
2.5–3.0	10.4
3.0–3.5	11.1
3.5–4.0	12.0
4.0–4.5	12.8

After El Haddad and Corkery [238].

$7 + (1.3 \times \text{weight in kg})$. Values for normal anal diameters relative to body weight are shown in Table 2.30.

REFERENCES

1. Little WJ. On the influence of abnormal parturition, difficult labor, premature birth, and asphyxia neonatorum on the mental and physical condition of the child, especially in relation to deformities. *Lancet* 1861; 2:378–80.
2. Schwarz H, Kohn JL. The infant of low birth weight: its growth and development. *Am J Dis Child* 1921; 21:296–306.
3. Simpson JW, Geppert LJ. The responsibility of the obstetrician to the fetus. 1. An analysis of fetal and neonatal mortality in 10,000 deliveries. *Am J Obstet Gynecol* 1951; 62:1062–70.
4. Dale ML. Report on a premature infant weighing 820 grams. *J Pediatr* 1947; 30:199–200.
5. Saigal S, Rosenbaum P, Stoskopf B, Milner R. Follow up of infants 501 to 1500 gm birth weight delivered to residents of a geographically defined region with perinatal intensive care facilities. *J Pediatr* 1982; 100:606–13.
6. Cohen RS, Stevenson DK, Malachowski N, et al. Favorable results of neonatal intensive care for very-low-birth-weight infants. *Pediatrics* 1982; 69:621–5.
7. Driscoll JM Jr, Driscoll YT, Steir ME, et al. Mortality and morbidity in infants less than 1001 grams birth weight. *Pediatrics* 1982; 69:21–6.
8. Hack M, Fanaroff AA, Merkatz IR. The low-birth-weight infant—evolution of a changing outlook. *N Engl J Med* 1979; 301:1162–1166.
9. Kimble KJ, Ariagno RL, Stevenson DK, Sunshine P. Growth to age 3 years among very-low-birth-weight sequelae-free survivors of modern neonatal intensive care. *J Pediatr* 1982; 100:622–4.
10. McCormick MC. The contribution of low birth weight to infant mortality and childhood morbidity. *N Engl J Med* 1985; 312:82–90.
11. Herron MA, Katz M, Creasy RK. Evaluation of a preterm birth prevention program: preliminary report. *Obstet Gynecol* 1982; 59:452–6.
12. Horwood SP, Boyle MH, Torrance GW, Sinclair JC. Mortality and morbidity of 500 to 1499 gram birth weight infants live-born to residents of a defined geographic region before and after neonatal intensive care. *Pediatrics* 1982; 69:613–20.
13. Joshi VV. Primary causes of perinatal mortality: autopsy study of 100 cases. *Arch Pathol Lab Med* 1976; 100:106–111.
14. Valdes-Dapena M, Arey JB. The causes of neonatal mortality: an analysis of 501 autopsies on newborn infants. *J Pediatr* 1970; 77:366–75.
15. Nesbitt REL, Anderson GW. Perinatal mortality: clinical and pathologic aspects. *Obstet Gynecol* 1956; 8:50–86.
16. Karlberg P, Ericson A. Perinatal mortality in Sweden: analyses with international aspects. *Acta Paediatr Scand* 1979; 275:28–34.
17. Roth J, Resnick MB, Ariet M, et al. Changes in survival patterns of very low-birth-weight infants from 1980 to 1993. *Arch Pediatr Adolesc Med* 1995; 149:1311–17.
18. Allen MC, Donohue PK, Dusman AE. The limit of viability—neonatal outcome of infants born at 22–25 weeks' gestation. *N Engl J Med* 1993; 329:1649–50.
19. Hack M, Fanaroff AA. Outcomes of extremely-low-birth-weight infants between 1982 and 1988. *N Engl J Med* 1989; 321:1642–7.
20. Ross G, Lipper EG, Auld PAM. Physical growth and developmental outcome in very low birth weight premature infants at 3 years of age. *J Pediatr* 1985; 107:284–6.
21. Richardson DK, Phibbs CS, Gray JE, et al. Birth weight and illness severity: independent predictors of neonatal mortality. *Pediatrics* 1993; 91:969–75.
22. Rantakallio P. A 14-year follow-up of children with normal and abnormal birth weight for their gestational age. *Acta Pediatr Scand* 1985; 74:62–9.
23. McKeown T, Gibson JR. Observations on all births (23970) in Birmingham, 1947 IV "Premature Birth." *Brit Med J* 1951; 2:513–23.
24. Philip AGS, Little GA, Polivy DR, Lucey JF. Neonatal mortality risk for the eighties: the importance of birth weight/gestational age groups. *Pediatrics* 1981; 68:122–30.
25. Vohr BR, Oh W, Rosenfield AG, Cowett RM, Berstein J. The preterm small-for-gestational age infant: a two-year follow-up study. *Am J Obstet Gynecol* 1979; 133:425–31.
26. Wilcox A, Skjaerven R, Buekens P, Kiely J. Birth weight and perinatal mortality. *JAMA* 1995; 273:709–11.
27. Lindell A. Prolonged pregnancy. *Acta Obstet Gynecol Scand* 1956; 35:135–63.
28. Eastman NJ. *Williams Obstetrics*, 11th ed. New York: Appleton-Century-Crofts, 1956, p. 216.
29. Nishimura H, Takano K, Tanimura T, Yasuda M. Normal and abnormal development of human embryo: first report of the analysis of 1213 intact embryos. *Teratology* 1968; 1:281–90.
30. Gruenwald P. Growth of the human fetus. 1. Normal growth and its variation. *Am J Obstet Gynecol* 1966; 94:1112–9.
31. Golbus MS, Berry LC Jr. Human fetal development between 90 and 170 days postmenses. *Teratology* 1977; 15:103–8.
32. Guerrero R, Florez PE. The duration of pregnancy. *Lancet* 1969; ii:268–9.
33. Kirkpatrick A, Cohen M, Prescott GH, et al. The importantce of accurate gestational age estimation in screening for fetal neural tube defects using maternal serum alpha-fetoprotein levels. In: Crandall BR, Brazier MAB, eds. *Prevention of Neural Tube Defects*. New York: Academic Press, 1978, pp. 199–205.
34. Daichman I, Gold EM. Postdate labor: effects on mother and fetus. *Am J Obstet Gynecol* 1954; 68:1129–35.
35. Dombrowski MP, Wolfe HM, Brans YW, Saleh AAA, Sokol RJ. Neonatal morphometry: relation to obstetric, pediatric, and menstrual estimates of gestational age. *Am J Dis Child* 1992; 146:852–6.
36. Gruenwald P. Chronic fetal distress and placental insufficiency. *Biol Neonate* 1963; 5:215–65.
37. Campbell S. The antenatal assessment of fetal growth and development: the contribution of ultrasonic measurement. In: Roberts DF, Thomson AM, eds. *The Biology of Human Fetal Growth*. London: Taylor and Francis, 1976, pp. 15–38.
38. Robinson JS. Growth of the fetus. *Br Med Bull* 1979; 35:137–44.
39. Sanders RC, James AE Jr. *The Principles and Practice of Ultrasonography in Obstetrics and Gynecology*, 3rd ed. Norwalk, CT: Appleton-Century-Crofts, 1985.
40. Reinold E. *Ultrasonics in Early Pregnancy: Diagnostic Scanning and Fetal Motor Activity*. Basel: S Karger, 1976, pp. 56ff.
41. Hellman LM, Kobayashi M, Fillisti L, Lavenhar M, Cromb E. Growth and development of the human fetus prior to the twentieth week of gestation. *Am J Obstet Gynecol* 1969; 103:789–98.
42. Potter EL, Craig JM, *Pathology of the Fetus and the Infant*, 3rd ed. Chicago: Year Book Medical, 1975, pp. 15–24.
43. O'Rahilly R, Gardner E. The initial appearance of ossification in staged human embryos. *Am J Anat* 1972; 134:291–304.
44. O'Rahilly R, Meyer DB. Roentgenographic investigation of the human skeleton during early life. *Am J Roentgenol Radium Ther Nucl Med* 1956; 76:455–68.
45. Silverman WA. *Dunham's Premature Infants*, 3rd ed. New York: Paul B Hoeber, Inc, 1961.
46. Usher RL, McLean F. Intrauterine growth of live-born caucasian infants at sea level: standards obtained from measurements in 7 dimensions of infants born between 25 and 44 weeks of gestation. *J Pediatr* 1969; 74:901–10.
47. Dubowitz L, Dubowitz V, Goldberg C. Clinical assessment of gestational age in the newborn. *J Pediatr* 1970; 77:1–10.
48. Koenigsberger MR. Judgment of fetal age. 1. Neurologic development. *Pediatr Clin North Am* 1966; 13:823–33.
49. Ballard JL, Novak KK, Driver M. A simplified score of fetal maturation of newly born infants. *J Pediatr* 1979; 95:769–74.
50. Sanders M, Allen M, Alexander GR, et al. Gestational age assessment in preterm neonates weighing less than 1500 grams. *Pediatrics* 1991; 88:542–6.
51. Nacye RL, Kelly JA. Judgement of fetal age. *Pediatr Clin North Am* 1966; 13:849–62.
52. Streeter GL. Weight, sitting height, head size, foot length, and menstrual age of the human embryo. Carnegie Institute of Washington, Publication 274. *Contrib Embryol* 1920; 11:143–90.

53. Scammon RE, Calkins LA. *The Development and Growth of the External Dimensions of the Human Body in the Fetal Period.* Minneapolis: University of Minnesota Press, 1929.

54. Gruenwald P, Minh HN. Evaluation of body and organ weights in perinatal pathology. 1. Normal standards derived from autopsies. *Am J Clin Pathol* 1960; 34:247–53.

55. Boyd E. Origins of the study of human growth. In: Savara BS, Schilke JF, eds. Portland: University of Oregon Health Sciences Center, 1980.

56. Lubchenco LO, Hansman C, Dressler M, Boyd E. Intrauterine growth as estimated from liveborn birth-weight data at 24 to 42 weeks of gestation. *Pediatrics* 1963; 32:793–800.

57. Hern WM. Correlations of fetal age and measurements between 10 and 26 weeks gestation. *Obstet Gynecol* 1984; 63:26–32.

58. Larroche J-C. *Developmental Pathology of the Neonate.* Amsterdam: Excerpta Medica, 1977, pp. 5–21.

59. Merlob P, Sivan Y, Reisner SH. Lower limb standards in newborns. *Am J Dis Child* 1984; 138:140–2.

60. Naeye RL, Simms EA, Welsh GW III, Gray MJ. Newborn organ abnormalities: a guide to abnormal maternal glucose metabolism. *Arch Pathol* 1966; 81:552–60.

61. Wigglesworth JS. *Perinatal Pathology.* Philadelphia: Saunders, 1984, pp. 1–18.

62. Valdes-Dapena MA. *Histology of the Fetus and Newborn.* Philadelphia: Saunders, 1979.

63. Nishimura H. *Atlas of Human Prenatal Histology.* Tokyo: Igaku Shoin, 1983.

64. Dorovini-Zis K, Dolman CL. Gestational development of brain. *Arch Pathol Lab Med* 1977; 101:192–5.

65. Rorke LB, Riggs HE. *Myelination of the Brain in the Newborn.* Philadelphia: Lippincott, 1969.

66. Brody BA, Kinney HC, Kloman AS, Gilles FH. Sequence of central nervous system myelination in human infancy. I. An autopsy study of myelination. *J Neuropathol Exp Neurol* 1987; 46:283–301.

67. Potter EL, Craig JM. *Pathology of the Fetus and the Infant,* 3rd ed. Chicago: Year Book Medical, 1975, pp. 15, 18, 19, 72, 434–8.

68. Singer DB, Klish W. Morphometric studies of the renal glomerulogenic zone. *Am J Pathol* 1970; 59:32a.

69. Singer DB. Hepatic erythropoiesis in infants of diabetic mothers: a morphometric study. *Pediatr Pathol* 1986; 5:471–9.

70. Haworth SG, Hislop AA. Normal structural and functional adaptation to extrauterine life. *J Pediatr* 1981; 98:915–7.

71. Emery JL, Mithal A. The number of alveoli in the terminal respiratory unit of man during late intrauterine life and childhood. *Arch Dis Child* 1960; 35:544–7.

72. Emery JL. The postnatal development of the human lung and its implications for lung pathology. *Respiration* 1970; 27(suppl):41–50.

73. Lampl M, Veldhuis JD, Johnson ML. Saltation and stasis: a model of human growth. *Science* 1992; 258:801–3.

74. Goss RJ. Adaptive mechanisms of growth control. In: Falkner F, Tanner JM, eds. *Human Growth,* vol. 1: *Principles and Prenatal Growth.* New York: Plenum, 1978, p. 3.

75. Winick M. *Nutrition and Fetal Development.* New York: John Wiley & Sons, 1974.

76. Corner GW. *Ourselves Unborn.* New Haven, CT: Yale University Press, 1944, pp. 1–6.

77. Snow MHL, Tam PP. Timing in embryological development. *Nature* 1980; 286:107.

78. Dobbing J, Sands J. Timing of neuroblast multiplication in developing human brain. *Nature* 1970; 226:639–40.

79. Wigglesworth JS. Plasticity in the developing brain. In: Pape K, Wigglesworth JS, eds. *Perinatal Brain Lesions.* Boston: Blackwell Scientific, 1989, pp. 253–69.

80. Naeye RL, Blanc WA. Pathogenesis of congenital rubella. *JAMA* 1965; 194:1277–83.

81. Naeye RL. Malnutrition: probable cause of fetal growth retardation. *Arch Pathol* 1965; 79:284–91.

82. Parkes MJ. Endocrine factors in fetal growth. In: Cockburn F, ed. *Fetal and Neonatal Growth.* Chichester: Wiley, 1988, pp. 33–48.

83. Polani PE. Chromosomal and other genetic influences on birth weight variation. In: *Size at Birth, Ciba Foundation Symposium 27 (New Series).* Amsterdam: Elsevier, 1974, pp. 127–59.

84. Warshaw JB. Intrauterine growth retardation: adaptation or pathology? *Pediatrics* 1985; 76:998–9.

85. Anon. Polypeptide growth factors: a clinical perspective. *Lancet* 1985; 2:251–3.

86. Adam PA, Teramo K, Raika N, Gitlin D, Schwartz R. Human fetal insulin metabolism early in gestation: Response to acute elevation of the fetal glucose concentration and placental transfer of human insulin I-131. *Diabetes* 1969; 18:409–20.

87. Chard T. Hormonal control of growth in the human fetus. *J Endocrinol* 1989; 123:3–9.

88. Like AA, Orci L. Embryogenesis of the human pancreatic islets: a light and electron microscopic study. *Diabetes* 1972; 21(suppl 2):511–32.

89. Koletzko B, Braun M. Arachidonic acid and early human growth: is there a relation? *Ann Nutr Metab* 1991; 35:128–31.

90. Trivedi P, Risteli J, Risteli L, et al. Serum concentrations of the type I and III procollagen propeptides as biochemical markers of growth velocity in healthy infants and children and in children with growth disorders. *Pediatr Res* 1991; 30:276–80.

91. Ounsted MK. Unconstrained foetal growth in man. *Dev Med Child Neurol* 1966; 8:3–8.

92. Ounsted MK. Maternal constraint of foetal growth in man. *Dev Med Child Neurol* 1965; 7:479–91.

93. Miller HC, Merritt TA. *Fetal Growth in Humans.* Chicago: Year Book Medical, 1979.

94. Haworth JC, Ellestad Sayed JJ, King J, Dilling LA. Relation of maternal cigarette smoking, obesity and energy consumption to infant size. *Am J Obstet Gynecol* 1980; 138:1185–9.

95. Yates JRW. The genetics of fetal and postnatal growth. In: Cockburn F, ed. *Fetal and Neonatal Growth.* Chichester: Wiley, 1988, pp. 1–10.

96. Lichty JA, Ting RY, Bruns PD, Dyar E. Studies of babies born at high altitude: relation of altitude to birth weight. *Am J Dis Child* 1957; 93:666–9.

97. Daily DK, Kilbride HW, Wheeler R, Hassanein R. Growth patterns for infants weighing less than 801 grams at birth to 3 years of age. *J Perinatol* 1994; XIV:454–60.

98. Guo S, Roche AF, Fomon SJ, et al. Reference data on gains in weight and length during the first two years of life. *J Pediatr* 1991; 119:355–62.

99. Batcup G. Prematurity. In: Keeling JW, ed. *Fetal and Neonatal Pathology,* 2nd ed. London: Springer-Verlag, 1993, pp. 199–222.

100. *WHO Weekly Epidemiological Record* 1981; 59:205–12.

101. Olowe SA. Standards of intrauterine growth for an African population at sea level. *J Pediatr* 1981; 99:489–95.

102. Moghissi KS, Churchill JA, Brown K, Kurrie D. In: Moghissi KS, ed. *Birth Defects and Fetal Development: Endocrine and Metabolic Factors.* Relationship of maternal nutrition to fetal development. Springfield, IL: Charles C Thomas, 1974, pp. 23–32.

103. Gruenwald P. Pathology of the deprived fetus and its supply line. In: *Size at Birth Ciba Foundation Symposium 27 (New Series).* Amsterdam: Elsevier, 1974, pp. 3–19.

104. Verhoestrate LJ, Puffer RR. Challenge of fetal loss, prematurity, and infant mortality: a world vision. *JAMA* 1958; 167:950.

105. Baldwin W. Half empty, half full: what we know about low birth weight among blacks. *JAMA* 1986; 255:86–8.

106. Eveleth PB, Tanner JM. *Worldwide Variation in Human Growth.* Cambridge: Cambridge University Press, 1976.

107. Benirschke K, Kim S. Multiple pregnancy. *N Engl J Med* 1973; 288:1277–84.

108. Herngreen WP, van Buuren S, van Wieringen JC, et al. Growth in length and weight from birth to 2 years of a representative sample of Netherlands children (born in 1988–89) related to socioeconomic status and other background characteristics. *Ann Hum Biol* 1994; 21:449–63.

109. Stein Z, Susser M, Saenger G, Marolla F. *Famine and Human Development: The Dutch Hunger Winter of 1944–5.* New York: Oxford University Press, 1975.

110. Smith CA. Effects of maternal undernutrition upon the newborn infant in Holland (1944–1945). *J Pediatr* 1947; 30:229–43.

111. Antonov AN. Children born during the siege of Leningrad in 1942. *J Pediatr* 1947; 30:250–9.

112. Rush O, Stein Z, Susser M. Diet in pregnancy: a randomized controlled trial of prenatal nutritional supplements. *Birth Defects* 1980; 16:1–197.

113. Naeye RL. Teenaged and pre-teenaged pregnancies: consequences of the fetal-maternal competition for nutrients. *Pediatrics* 1981; 67:146–50.

114. Stevens-Simon C, McAnarney ER, Roghmann KJ. Adolescent gestational weight gain and birth weight. *Pediatrics* 1993; 92:805–9.

115. Hytten FE. Nutrition in relation to fetal growth. In: Van Assche FA, Robertson WB, eds. *Fetal Growth Retardation.* Edinburgh: Churchill Livingstone, 1981, pp. 57–62.

116. Barry LW. The effects of inanition in the pregnant albino rat, with special reference to the changes in the relative weights of various parts, systems, and organs of the offspring. Carnegie Institute of Washington, Publication 53. *Contrib Embryol* 1920; XI:91–136.

117. Myers RE, Hill DE, Holt AB, et al. Fetal growth retardation produced by experimental placental insufficiency in the rhesus monkey. 1. Body weight, organ size. *Biol Neonate* 1971; 18:379–94.

118. Nieberg P, Marks JS, McLaren NM, Remington PL. The fetal tobacco syndrome. *JAMA* 1985; 253:2998–9.

119. Fielding JE. Smoking and pregnancy. *N Engl J Med* 1978; 298:337–9.

120. Pirani BBK. Smoking during pregnancy. *Obstet Gynecol Surv* 1978; 33:1–13.

121. Haworth JC, Ellestad-Sayed JJ, King J, Dilling LA. Fetal growth retardation in cigarette-smoking mothers is not due to decreased maternal food intake. *Am J Obstet Gynecol* 1980; 137:719–23.

122. Butler NR, Goldstein H. Smoking in pregnancy and subsequent child development. *Br Med J* 1973; 4:573–5.

123. Miller HC, Hassanein K. Maternal smoking and fetal growth of full term infants. *Pediatr Res* 1964; 8:960–3.

124. Suzuki K, Horiguchi T, Comas-Urrutia AC, et al. Pharmacologic effects of nicotine upon the fetus and mother in the Rhesus monkey. *Am J Obstet Gynecol* 1971; 111:1092–1101.

125. Hill RM, Stern L. Drugs in pregnancy: effects on the fetus and newborn. *Drugs* 1979; 17:182–197.

126. Shiono PH, Klebanoff MA, Rhoads GG. Smoking and drinking during pregnancy: their effects on preterm birth. *JAMA* 1986; 255:82–4.

127. Zuckerman B, Frank DA, Hingson R, et al. Effects of maternal marijuana and cocaine use on fetal growth. *N Engl J Med* 1989; 320:762–8.

128. Eriksson M, Jonsson B, Steneroth G, Zetterstrom R. Cross-sectional growth of children whose mothers abused amphetamines during pregnancy. *Acta Paediatr* 1994; 83:612–7.

129. Lemoine P, Harousseau H, Borteyru J. Children of alcoholic parents. Observed anomalies (127 cases). *Ouest Medical* 1968; 21:476–82.

130. Ouellette EM, Rosett HL, Rosman NP, Werner L. Adverse effects on offspring of maternal alcohol abuse during pregnancy. *N Engl J Med* 1977; 197:528–30.

131. Iosub S, Fuchs M, Bingol N, Gromisch DS. Fetal alcohol syndrome revisited. *Pediatrics* 1981; 68:475–9.

132. Flores-Huerta S, Hernandez-Montes H, Argote RM, Villapando S. Effects of ethanol consumption during pregnancy and lactation on the outcome and postnatal growth of the offspring. *Ann Nutr Metab* 1992; 36:121–8.

133. Sampson PD, Bookstein FL, Barr HM, Streissguth AP. Prenatal alcohol exposure, birthweight, and measures of child size from birth to age 14 years. *Am J Public Health* 1994; 84:1421–8.

134. Linn S, Schoenbaum SC, Monson RR, et al. No association between coffee consumption and adverse outcomes of pregnancy. *N Engl J Med* 1982; 306:141–5.

135. Fedrick J, Adelstein P. Factors associated with low birth weight of infants delivered at term. *Br J Obstet Gynaecol* 1978; 85:1–7.

136. Long PA, Abell DA, Beischer NA. Fetal growth retardation and pre-eclampsia. *Br J Obstet Gynaecol* 1980; 87:13–8.

137. Boyd PA, Scott A. Quantitative structural studies on human placentas associated with pre-eclampsia, essential hypertension and intrauterine growth retardation. *Br J Obstet Gynaecol* 1985; 92:714–21.

138. Wigglesworth JS. Experimental growth retardation in the foetal rat. *J Pathol Bacteriol* 1964; 88:1–13.

139. Uzan S, Beaufils M, Breart G, et al. Prevention of fetal growth retardation with low-dose aspirin: findings of the EPREDA trial. *Lancet* 1991; 337:1427–31.

140. Shime J, Mocarski EJM, Hastings D, Webb GD, McLaughlin PR. Congenital heart disease in pregnancy: short and long-term implications. *Am J Obstet Gynecol* 1987; 156:313–22.

141. Greenberger PA, Patterson R. Beclomethasone dipropionate for severe asthma during pregnancy. *Ann Intern Med* 1983; 98:478–80.

142. Palmer J, Dillon-Baker C, Tecklin JS, et al. Pregnancy in patients with cystic fibrosis. *Ann Intern Med* 1983; 99:596–600.

143. Thaler I, Bronstein M, Rubin AE. The course of pregnancy associated with bronchiectasis. *Br J Obstet Gynaecol* 1986; 93:1006–8.

144. Kopenhager T. A review of 50 pregnant patients with kyphoscoliosis. *Br J Obstet Gynaecol* 1977; 84:585–7.

145. Katz AI, Davison JM, Hayslett JP, Singson E, Lindheimer MD. Pregnancy in women with kidney disease. *Kidney Int* 1980; 18:192–206.

146. Brem AS, Singer D, Anderson L, Lester B, Abuelo JG. Infants of azotemic mothers: a report of three live births. *Am J Kidney Dis* 1988; 12:299–303.

147. Carlson DE. Maternal diseases associated with intrauterine growth retardation. *Semin Perinatol* 1988; 12:17–22.

148. Abramowsky CR, Vegas ME, Swinehart G, Gyves MT. Decidual vasculopathy of the placenta in lupus erythematosus. *N Engl J Med* 1980; 303:668–72.

149. Powars DR, Sandhu M, Niland-Weiss J, et al. Pregnancy in sickle cell disease. *Obstet Gynecol* 1986; 67:217–28.

150. Fox H. Placental malfunction as a factor in intrauterine growth retardation. In: Van Assche FA, Robertson WB, eds. *Fetal Growth Retardation*. Edinburgh: Churchill Livingstone, 1981, pp. 117–25.

151. Naeye R. Causes and consequences of placental growth retardation. *JAMA* 1978; 239:1145–7.

152. Kruger H, Arias-Stella J. The placenta and the newborn infant at high altitudes. *Am J Obstet Gynecol* 1970; 106:586–91.

153. Naeye RL. Effect of maternal cigarette smoking on the fetus and placenta. *Br J Obstet Gynaecol* 1978; 85:146–50.

154. Bryan EM, Kohler HG. The missing umbilical artery. *Arch Dis Child* 1974; 49:844–52.

155. Froehlich LA, Fujukura MD. Significance of a single umbilical artery. *Am J Obstet Gynecol* 1966; 94:274–9.

156. Altemani AM, Fassoni A, Marba S. Cord IgM levels in placentas with villitis of unknown etiology. *J Perinat Med* 1989; 17:465–8.

157. Nordenvall M, Sandstedt B. Placental villitis and intrauterine growth retardation in a Swedish population. *APMIS* 1990; 98:19–24.

158. Gersell DJ, Phillips NJ, Beckerman K. Chronic chorioamnionitis: a clinicopathologic study of 17 cases. *Int J Gynecol Pathol* 1991; 10:217–29.

159. Gabert HA. Placenta praevia and fetal growth. *Obstet Gynecol* 1971; 38:403–6.

160. McKeown T, Record RG. Observations on foetal growth in multiple pregnancy in man. *J Endocrinol* 1952; 8:386–401.

161. Naeye RL. Organ abnormalities in the human parabiotic syndrome. *Am J Pathol* 1965; 46:829–38.

162. Bulmer MG. *The Biology of Twinning in Man.* Oxford: Clarendon Press, 1970.

163. Hardy J. Birth weight and subsequent physical and intellectual development. *N Engl J Med* 1973; 289:973–4.

164. Kiely JL, Kleinman JC, Kiely M. Triplets and higher-order multiple births: time trends and infant mortality. *Am J Dis Child* 1992; 146:862–8.

165. Metcoff J, Cole TJ, Luff R. Fetal growth retardation induced by dietary imbalance of threonine and dispensable amino acids with adequate energy and protein-equivalent intakes in pregnant rats. *J Nutr* 1981; 111:1411–24.

166. Crosby WM. Studies in fetal malnutrition. *Am J Dis Child* 1991; 145:871–6.

167. Miller HC. Intrauterine growth retardation: an unmet challenge. *Am J Dis Child* 1981; 135:944–8.

168. Naeye RL. Cytomegalic inclusion disease: the fetal disorder. *Am J Clin Pathol* 1967; 47:738–44.

169. Singer DB, Rudolph AJ, Rosenberg HS, Rawls WE. Pathology of the congenital rubella syndrome. *J Pediatr* 1967; 71:665–75.

170. Waterston AP. Virus infections (other than rubella) during pregnancy. *Br Med J* 1979; 2:564–6.

171. Mili F, Edmonds LD, Khoury MJ, McClearn AB. Prevalence of birth defects among low-birth-weight infants: a population study. *Am J Dis Child* 1991; 145:1313–8.

172. Verkerk PH, van Spronsen FJ, Smit GP, Sengers RC. Impaired prenatal and postnatal growth in Dutch patients with phenylketonuria. The National PKU Steering Committee. *Arch Dis Child* 1994; 71:114–8.

173. Doshi N, Surti U, Szulman AE. Morphologic anomalies in triploid liveborn fetuses. *Hum Pathol* 1983; 14:716–23.

174. Honnebier WJ, Swaab DF. The influence of anencephaly upon intrauterine growth of fetus and placenta and upon gestation length. *J Obstet Gynaecol Br Commonw* 1973; 80:577–88.

175. Elias S, Simpson JL, Griffin LP. Intrauterine growth retardation in osteogenesis imperfecta. *JAMA* 1978; 239:23.

176. Oh W, Coustan D. Intrauterine fetal growth retardation: perinatal diagnosis and management. *Ann Nestlé* 1982; 40:17–29.

177. Elsas LJ, Endo F, Strumlauf E, Elders J, Priest JH. Leprechaunism: an inherited defect in a high affinity insulin receptor. *Am J Hum Genet* 1985; 37:73–88.

178. Lipsey L, Singer S, Singer DB. Relation of fetal growth to pancreatic insulin and somatostatin [unpublished data].

179. Wit JM, van Unen H. Growth of infants with neonatal growth hormone deficiency. *Arch Dis Child* 1992; 67:920–4.

180. Cohen MM Jr. The large-for-gestation-age (LGA) infant in dysmorphic perspective. In: Willey AM, Carter TP, Kelly S, Porter IM, eds. *Clinical Genetics: Problems in Diagnosis and Counseling.* New York: Academic Press, 1982, pp. 153ff.

181. Kliegman R, Gross T, Morton S, Dunnington R. Intrauterine growth and postnatal fasting metabolism in infants of obese mothers. *J Pediatr* 1984; 104:601–7.

182. Calandra C, Abell DA, Beischer NA. Maternal obesity in pregnancy. *Obstet Gynecol* 1981; 57:8–12.

183. Hickey RJ, Clelland RC, Bowers EJ. Maternal smoking, birth weight, infant death, and the self-selection problems. *Am J Obstet Gynecol* 1978; 131:805–11.

184. Wallace LR. The effect of diet on foetal development. *J Physiol* 1946; 104:34P–5P

185. Clifford SH. Postmaturity with placental dysfunction. *J Pediatr* 1954; 44:1–13.

186. Gruenwald P. Growth and maturation of the foetus and its relationship to perinatal mortality. In: Butler NR, Alberman ED, eds. *Perinatal Problems*. Edinburgh: Livingstone, 1969, pp. 141–62.

187. Bracero LA, Beneck D, Kirshenbaum N, et al. Doppler velocity and placental disease. *Am J Obstet Gynecol* 1989; 161:388–93.

188. Giles WB, Trudinger BJ, Baird PJ. Fetal umbilical artery flow velocity waveforms and placental resistance: pathological correlation. *Br J Obstet Gynaecol* 1985; 92:31–8.

189. Fee BA, Weil WB Jr. Body composition of infants of diabetic mothers by direct analysis. *Ann NY Acad Sci* 1963; 110:869–97.

190. Morriss FH Jr. Infants of diabetic mothers: fetal and neonatal pathophysiology. *Perspect Pediatr Pathol* 1984; 8:223–34.

191. Naeye RL. Infants of diabetic mothers: a quantitative morphologic study. *Pediatrics* 1965; 35:980–8.

192. Petry CD, Eaton MA, Wobken JD, et al. Iron deficiency of liver, heart, and brain in newborn infants of diabetic mothers. *J Pediatr* 1992; 121: 109–14.

193. Gutgesell HP, Speer ME, Rosenberg HS. Characterization of the cardiomyopathy in infants of diabetic mothers. *Circulation* 1980; 61:441–7.

194. Gruenwald P. Growth of the human fetus. II. Abnormal growth in twins and infants of mothers with diabetes, hypertension, or isoimmunization. *Am J Obstet Gynecol* 1966; 94:1120–32.

195. Susa JB, Neave C, Sehgal P, et al. Chronic hyperinsulinemia in the fetal rhesus monkey: effects of physiologic hyperinsulinemia on fetal growth and composition. *Diabetes* 1984; 33:656–60.

196. Elejalde BR, Giraldo C, Jiminez R, Gilbert EF. Acrocephalopolydactylous dysplasia. *Birth Defects* 1977; 13(suppl 3B):53–67.

197. Marshall RE, Graham CB, Scott CR, Smith DW. Syndrome of accelerated skeletal maturation and relative failure to thrive: a newly recognised clinical growth disorder. *J Pediatr* 1971; 78:95–101.

198. Weaver DD, Graham CB, Thomas IT, Smith DW. A new overgrowth syndrome with accelerated skeletal maturation, unusual facies and camptodactyly. *J Pediatr* 1974; 84:547–62.

199. Smyth RL, Gould JDM, Baraitser M. A case of Marshall-Smith or Weaver syndrome. *J R Soc Med* 1989; 82:682–3.

200. Ramos-Arroyo MA, Weaver DD, Banks ER. Weaver syndrome: a case without early overgrowth and review of the literature. *Pediatrics* 1991; 88: 1106–11.

201. Nishimura H, Tanimura T, Semba R, Uwabe C. Normal development of early human embryos: observation of 90 specimens at Carnegie stages 7 to 13. *Teratology* 1974; 10:1–8.

202. Tanimura T, Nelson T, Hollingsworth RR, Shepard TH. Weight standards for organs from early human fetuses. *Anat Rec* 1971; 171:227–36.

203. Gruenwald P, Minh HN. Evaluation of body and organ weights in perinatal pathology. II. Weight of body and placenta in surviving and in autopsied infants. *Am J Obstet Gynecol* 1961; 82:312–9.

204. Schulz DM, Giordano DA, Schulz DH. Weights of organs of fetuses and infants. *Arch Pathol* 1962; 74:244–50.

205. Merlob P, Sivan Y. Thigh circumference and thigh-to-head ratio in preterm and term infants. *J Perinatol* 1994; xiv:479–82.

206. Wright K, Dawson JP, Fallis D, Vogt E, Lorch V. New postnatal growth grids for very low birth weight infants. *Pediatrics* 1993; 91:922–6.

207. Avery MA, Taeusch W Jr. *Schaffer's Diseases of the Newborn*, 5th ed. Philadelphia: Saunders, 1984.

208. Casey PH, Kraemer HC, Bernbaum J, Yogman MW, Sells JC. Growth status and growth rates of a varied sample of low birth weight, preterm infants: a longitudinal cohort from birth to three years of age. *J Pediatr* 1991; 119:599–605.

209. Munsick RA. Human fetal extremity lengths in the interval from 9 to 21 menstrual weeks of pregnancy. *Am J Obstet Gynecol* 1984; 149:883–7.

210. Sivan Y, Merlob P, Reisner SH. Upper limb standards in newborns. *Am J Dis Child* 1983; 137:829–32.

211. Meredith HV. Human foot length from embryo to adult. *Human Biol* 1944; 16:207–82.

212. Yau KI, Chang MH. Growth and body composition of preterm, small-for-gestational-age infants at a postmenstrual age of 37–40 weeks. *Early Hum Dev* 1993; 33:117–31.

213. Brasel J, Winick M. Regulation of nucleic acid synthesis in fetus and placenta during normal growth and malnutrition. In: Moghissi KS, ed. *Birth Defects and Fetal Development: Endocrine and Metabolic Factors*. Springfield, IL: Charles C Thomas, 1974, pp. 10ff.

214. Aherne W, Dunnill MS. Quantitative aspects of placental structure. *J Pathol Bacteriol* 1966; 91:123–39.

215. Teasdale F. Gestational changes in the functional structure of the human placenta in relation to fetal growth: a morphometric study. *Am J Obstet Gynecol* 1980; 137:560–8.

216. Hendricks CH. Pattern of fetal and placental growth: the second half of normal pregnancy. *Obstet Gynecol* 1964; 24:357–68.

217. Winick M, Coscia A, Noble A. Cellular growth in human placenta. *Pediatrics* 1967; 39:248–51.

218. Singer DB. The placenta in pregnancies complicated by diabetes mellitus. *Perspect Pediatr Pathol* 1984; 8:199–212.

219. Pinar H, Sung CJ, Oyer CE, Singer DB. Reference values for singleton and twin placental weights. *Pediatr Pathol Lab Med* 1996; 16:901–7.

220. Gilles F, Leviton A, Dooling EC. *The Developing Human Brain: Growth and Epidemiologic Neuropathology*. Boston: John Wright PSG, 1983, p. 50.

221. Sheth RD, Mullett MD, Bodensteiner JB, Hobbs GR. Longitudinal head growth in developmentally normal preterm infants. *Arch Pediatr Adolesc Med* 1995; 149:1358–61.

222. Hadi HA. Fetal cerebral maturation in hypertensive disorders of pregnancy. *Obstet Gynecol* 1984; 63:214–7.

223. Bernstein J, Cheng F, Roszka J. Glomerular differentiation in metanephric culture. *Lab Invest* 1981; 45:183–90.

224. Winick M, McCrory WW. Renal differentiation: a model for the study of development. *Birth Defects, Orig Art Ser* 1968; IV: no 5.

225. Phat VN, Camilleri JP, Bariety J, et al. Immunohistochemical characterization of renin-containing cells in the human juxtaglomerular apparatus during embryonal and fetal development. *Lab Invest* 1981; 45:387–90.

226. Fetterman G, Shuplock NA, Philipp FJ, Gregg HS. The growth and maturation of human glomeruli and proximal convolutions from term to adulthood: studies by microdissection. *Pediatrics* 1965; 35:601–9.

227. Arant BS Jr. Developmental patterns of renal functional maturation compared in the human neonate. *J Pediatr* 1978; 92:705–12.

228. Inselman LS, Mellins RB. Growth and development of the lung. *J Pediatr* 1981; 98:1–15.

229. Langston C, Thurlbeck WM. Lung growth and development in late gestation and early postnatal life. *Perspect Pediatr Pathol* 1982; 7:203–35.

230. Ross S, Naeye RL. Racial and environmental influences on fetal lung maturation. *Pediatrics* 1981; 68:790–5.

231. Binkin NJ, Williams RL, Hogue CJR, Chen PM. Reducing black neonatal mortality: will improvement in birth weight be enough? *JAMA* 1985; 253:372–5.

232. Jones KL Jr, Hanson JW, Smith DW. Palpebral fissure size in newborn infants. *J Pediatr* 1978; 92:787–90.

233. Fuchs M, Iosub S, Bingol N, Gromisch DS. Palpebral fissure size revisited. *J Pediatr* 1980; 96:77–8.

234. Feingold M, Bossert WH. Normal values for selected physical parameters: an aid to syndrome delineation. *Birth Defects* 1974; 10: no 13.

235. Feldman KW, Smith DW. Fetal phallic growth and penile standards for newborn male infants. *J Pediatr* 1975; 86:395–8.

236. Bryant J. Length and growth of the human intestine. *Am J Med Sci* 1924; 167:499–519.

237. Shanklin DR, Cooke RJ. Effects of intrauterine growth on intestinal length in the human fetus. *Biol Neonate* 1993; 64:76–81.

238. Siebert JR. Small-intestine length in infants and children. *Am J Dis Child* 1980; 134:593–5.

239. El Haddad M, Corkery JJ. The anus in the newborn. *Pediatrics* 1985; 76:927–8.

Pathology of Perinatal and Neonatal Care

Halit Pinar

INTRODUCTION

Almost any ministration to the human body for the purpose of diagnosis or therapy has some unwanted side effects. While we no longer see some of the lesions that were described in the early days of high-risk obstetric and neonatal care, with advances in technology and improvements in patient care we started seeing others. Some new treatments described in this chapter are still being evaluated. In some instances, human applications were initiated before proper animal studies were performed. The pathologist is the expert in investigating possible pathology that may be associated with these new techniques. As pathologists, we should alert our clinician-colleagues about unexpected lesions that come to our attention even with established and time-proven methods of diagnosis and treatment. In a litigious society, it is imperative to correctly diagnose and document any disorder that is related to diagnostic and management procedures.

PRENATAL PERIOD

Effects of Maternal Drugs on the Fetus and Neonate

During pregnancy, drugs affect not only the mother but also her unborn offspring. In most instances, the risk of adverse fetal effects from drugs taken by the mother is not known. The maternal dose usually is not predictive of an adverse outcome. Because these risks cannot be experimentally analyzed, our knowledge is based on retrospective analyses, cohort studies, and case reports.

The timing of the drug exposure is extremely important. The developing embryo is most susceptible from 15 to 60 days after conception. Some drugs are lethal to the developing embryo, and some taken after organogenesis can affect the growth and development of the fetus. Some drugs may have longer lasting damaging effects on the central nervous system of the fetus and neonate. A drug taken during pregnancy can also act as a transplacental carcinogen. For a given pregnancy, published risk may not accurately reflect the risk to that particular fetus. Genetic factors have a strong influence on susceptibility to certain teratogens. Table 3.1 summarizes the effects on the fetus and neonate of the most commonly used maternal drugs [1, 2].

Amniocentesis

Amniocentesis is the oldest and, when performed after 16 weeks' gestation, the most commonly performed invasive procedure for prenatal diagnosis. In experienced hands, the procedure-related pregnancy loss rate is 0.2–0.5% above the spontaneous loss rate at 16 weeks' gestation, which is estimated at 2–3% [3]. Pregnancy loss rates seem to be associated with the number of failed needle insertions during one session and with vaginal bleeding after amniocentesis. Leakage of amniotic fluid through the cervix is a relatively frequent complication, affecting approximately 1–2% of patients, but it usually is of minor long-term consequence; in most patients, it resolves after bed-rest. On the other hand, prolonged amniotic fluid leakage, although rare, may lead to severe oligohydramnios, with lung hypoplasia in the fetus [4, 5]. The risk of severe amnionitis endangering maternal health is very low, around 0.1%. Likewise, fetal injury by the needle is rare with ultrasound guidance, but injuries to the brain and viscera still occur. The risk of Rh isosensitization after amniocentesis in Rh-negative women with Rh-positive fetuses has been estimated to increase by 1% above the background risk [6, 7].

Table 3.1.   Effects of maternal drugs on the fetus and neonate

Drug	Side effects
Acetaminophen	Neonatal renal failure
Acetylsalicylic acid	Depresses maternal urinary estriol secretion. Birth defects: skeletal and heart defects, especially patent ductus arteriosus if taken during the third trimester, cleft lip and palate, hypospadias, cyclopia, and intrauterine growth retardation. High-dose maternal aspirin intake may cause pulmonary hypertension in the newborn.
Alcohol (ethyl)	Fetal alcohol syndrome: prenatal and postnatal growth retardation, microcephaly, mental deficiency, short palpebral fissures, midface hypoplasia, ptosis, short nose, cleft palate, cardiac septal defects, fused cervical vertebrae, hemangiomas, malformed ears
Amantadine	Congenital heart disease: single ventricle with pulmonary atresia
Aminogylcosides	Eighth nerve toxicity in the neonate
Amitryptyline	Fetal malformations; urinary retention in the fetus
Ammonium chloride	Inguinal hernia, cataracts, benign tumors
Anisindione	Birth defects: stippled epiphyses; chondrodysplasia punctata; hypoplastic nasal bridge, resulting in upper airway obstruction; growth retardation; hypoplastic extremities; microphthalmia; mental retardation
Antineoplastic agents	Almost all are associated with multiple and different congenital defects; aminopterin, methotrexate, cyclophosphamide, and 5-fluorouracil cause distinct anomalies.
Antithyroid agents	Intrauterine growth retardation, goiter, hypo- or hyperthyroidism, and focal scalp defects (methimazole).
Azathioprine	Leukopenia, thrombocytopenia, immunosuppression, transient chromosomal aberrations
Bromides	Polydactyly, gastrointestinal malformations, clubfoot, and congenital dislocation of hip; may also cause neonatal bromism (poor suck, decreased Moro's reflex, and hypotonia)
Calcifediol	Increases calcium levels; may be associated with supravalvular aortic stenosis syndrome
Captopril	Angiotensin-converting enzyme (ACE); intrauterine growth retardation, neonatal respiratory distress, renal failure; embryopathic in animals
Carbamazepine	Microcephaly, spina bifida, and encephalocele
Carbimazole	Cutis aplasia
Clomiphene	Neural tube defects
Chloroquine	Congenital deafness, motor delay, chorioretinitis, and hemihypertrophy
D-Amphetamine	Congenital heart disease, biliary atresia, eye defects
D-Penicillamine	Cutaneous hyperextensibility, joint hyperflexibility, contractures (similar to Ehler-Danlos syndrome), low set ears, and micrognathia
Digoxin	Fetal death with maternal overdose
Diethylstilbesterol	Females: vaginal adenosis, cervical eversion, cervical ridges, abnormal uteri. Males: epididymal cysts, hypoplastic testes, cryptorchidism, quantitative and qualitative sperm abnormalities, urethral stenosis, and seminal anomalies. Incidence of mesoblastic nephroma is mildly increased.
Disulfiram	Fetal malformations and spontaneous abortions
Glucose-6-phosphate dehydrogenase (G-6-PD) deficiency	Drugs that will affect the neonate with G-6-PD deficiency when maternally taken: antimalarials, ascorbic acid, aspirin, chloramphenicol, methylene blue, nitrofurantoin, phenacetin, quinidine, sulfonamides, vitamin K
Glucocorticoids	Neonatal and maternal leukocytosis and neonatal lymphocytopenia; in some studies: cataracts, cyclopia, ventricular septal defect, gastroschisis
Guaifenesin	Inguinal hernias with first-trimester use
Indomethacin	Premature closure of the ductus, persistent pulmonary hypertension, renal failure, intestinal perforation, and death
Levothyroxine	Cardiovascular anomalies and polydactyly
Lindane (Kwell)	Neurotoxicity and aplastic anemia
Minoxidil (Rogaine)	Neonatal hypertrichosis
Menadione	Hyperbilirubinemia, with increased risk of kernicterus if given at term
Nicotine	Dose-related low-birth-weight infants; increased risk of stillborn or neonatal death and sudden infant death
Non-steroidal anti-inflammatory agents	Oligohydramnios, premature or partial closure of the ductus arteriosus, persistent pulmonary hypertension, and neonatal oliguria
Oral contraceptives	Progestational activity: clitoral hypertrophy, labioscrotal fusion, penile urethra in females; phallic enlargement in males; hyperbilirubinemia in the newborn
Phenobarbital	Birth defects: wide-set eyes, depressed nasal bridge, ptosis, and growth retardation Neonatal withdrawal syndrome, hypocalcemia, coagulation defects
Phenytoin (Dilantin)	Birth defects: fetal hydantoin syndrome [FHS], i.e., broad, low nasal bridge; epicanthal folds; short, upturned nose; ptosis, strabismus; hypertelorism; malformed ears; wide mouth with prominent lips; hypoplasia of the distal phalanges; intrauterine growth retardation; microcephaly; mental or motor retardation Neuroblastoma, cataracts, and vascular anomalies with congenital heart disease Neonatal hemorrhage due to the competitive inhibition of clotting factor synthesis
Povidone-iodine (betadine)	Fetal exposure by means of scalp electrode sites. Elevated iodine and thyroid-stimulating hormone and decreased levels of thyroxin concentrations are seen in the neonate.
Quinidine	Neonatal thrombocytopenia
Quinine	Congenital deafness, thrombocytopenia, limb anomalies, esophageal atresia, hydrocephaly, and mental retardation
Retinoids (Accutane)	Low set, small, or absent external ears and canals, microcephaly, hydrocephaly, facial palsy, thymic hypoplasia, congenital heart disease
Valproic acid	Spina bifida, intrauterine growth retardation, diastasis recti abdominis, inguinal hernia, hemangiomas, telangiectasia, supernumerary nipples, abnormal ears, hypertelorism, groove under the eyes, flat nasal bridge, congenital heart disease, hyperglycinemia, hyperbilirubinemia
Warfarin (Coumadin)	Same as anisindione

Data from Briggs et al [1] and Gilstrap and Little [2].

With improved ultrasound technology and increasing experience with ultrasound-guided manipulations, early amniocentesis has become an attractive alternative to chorionic villous sampling late in the first trimester [8, 9]. *Early amniocentesis* refers to aspiration of amniotic fluid for analysis before 15 weeks' gestation. Complications with early amniocentesis include bleeding, uterine cramping, leakage of fluid, and infection. Rupture of membranes after early amniocentesis is observed in 2.5% of patients. The total unintentional fetal loss after early amniocentesis ranges between 1.4% and 4.2% [10, 11]. In all series, slightly increased fetal loss rates occur after amniocentesis performed at 11 or 12 weeks' gestation [12, 13]. In comparison with CVS, however, early amniocentesis has a lower rate of pseudomosaicism and maternal cell contamination.

Chorionic Villous Sampling

Chorionic villous sampling (CVS) procedures, whether transcervical, transabdominal, or transvaginal, are most commonly performed between 9 and 12 weeks of gestation. After 13 weeks, the procedure usually is best done transabdominally. The likelihood of spontaneous abortion in women at 8 to 11 weeks is 3–5%, and this rate increases with maternal age [14, 15]. Both Canadian and American collaborative studies documented a loss rate in the CVS group of 0.6–0.8% in excess of background loss, which is not significantly different from the loss rate in the early amniocentesis group [16].

Concerns over the safety of CVS have been raised by Firth et al [17] and Burton et al [18]. In two small series in which procedures were done by relatively inexperienced physicians, they claimed a 1% increased risk of limb reduction defects. In contrast, evaluation of over 125,000 cases from experienced centers worldwide reveals that the incidence of limb reduction or any other defects is identical to that of the background population [19]. Froster and Jackson [20] recently reported the experience from 139,000 CVS procedures. In this series, the incidence of limb defects was similar to the incidence in the control population. A slightly increased risk exists with CVS procedures done at 6 to 7 weeks' gestation as opposed to the usual time of 9 to 12 weeks' gestation or done by inexperienced personnel, but the data suggest that CVS is otherwise safe and effective.

Internal Fetal Monitoring

Scalp electrodes for fetal heart monitoring can cause abscesses [21]. These usually develop by about 5 days postpartum. The incidence of such abscesses is 0.1–4.5%. Multiple aerobic and anaerobic organisms have been implicated. These include streptococci groups A, B, D, *Escherichia coli*, *Klebsiella pneumoniae*, *Peptococcus*, and *Bacterioides*. Osteomyelitis after application of scalp electrodes has also been described [22]. Herpes simplex I and II have been inoculated

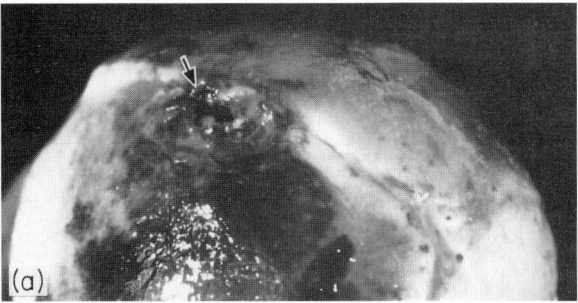

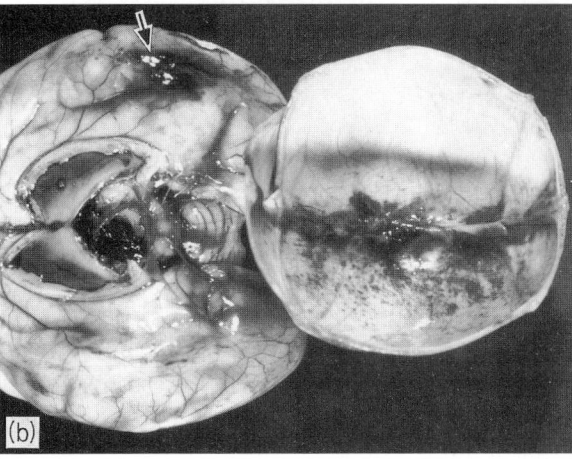

FIGURE 3.1. *Injury due to hook from scalp monitor.* (a) *Damage to sagittal suture* (arrow). (b) *Meningeal laceration* (arrow). *(Courtesy of Dr. DB Singer.)*

by fetal scalp electrodes in cases where the mother has no overt clinical signs of infection [23, 24].

Other complications that are associated with scalp electrodes include local trauma, ranging from minor abrasions and skin puncture to more extensive scalp lacerations and significant hemorrhage [25] (Fig. 3.1).

Cordocentesis

Percutaneous Umbilical Blood Sampling

Introduced by Daffos and associates in 1983 for the diagnosis of fetal infections [26], percutaneous umbilical blood sampling (PUBS) rapidly gained wide acceptance. Indications for PUBS are diagnosis of infections such as toxoplasmosis or rubella, karyotyping, detection of coagulation disorders such as hemophilia and factor deficiencies, diagnosis of platelet disorders, rhesus isoimmunization, hemoglobinopathies, and general assessment of fetal well-being. In experienced hands, the risk of fetal loss is relatively small, approximately 1% [27–29]. Other complications, typically associated with excessive needle manipulations, include hematoma of the umbilical cord and placental abruption. If one of the umbilical vessels tears, hematoma results; such hemorrhages can be fatal. Maternal complications are generally negligible, although one case of life-threatening amnionitis has been reported [30]. The risks are higher when the mother is obese, the placenta is posterior, and when the sampling is performed relatively early in gestation (i.e., before 19 weeks).

Fetal Transfusions

In cases of isoimmunization with hydrops fetalis, fetal transfusion is the therapy of choice but may be associated with a traumatic death rate of up to 5%. In years past, fetal intra-abdominal transfusions were given for severe anemia. Hazards included ruptured or punctured abdominal viscera and circulatory overload with heart failure and graft-versus-host disease (see Graft-Versus-Host Disease under Invasive Procedures) [31].

Infectious complications are the same as for any transfusion. The current bloodbank screening methods have increased the safety of fetal transfusions.

Fetal Surgery

Fetal surgery was first attempted in the early 1960s. With increasing sophistication of ultrasound and surgical methods, results improved somewhat over the years [32, 33].

Two methods are used. The first is percutaneous surgery. This includes shunt placement for congenital hydrocephalus, obstructive uropathy, or pleural effusions. The success rates with these procedures are low. The second method is open surgery, and the success rates with this method are even lower than with percutaneous methods.

The results achieved with ventriculoamniotic shunts are disappointing [34]. As of March 1993, 45 cases of fetal ventriculomegaly treated in utero by ventriculoamniotic shunts had been reported to the International Fetal Surgery Registry [34]; 41 fetuses with hydrocephalus were treated by ventriculoamniotic shunting, and 34 of these fetuses survived. Of the 7 deaths, 4 could be attributed directly to trauma at the time of catheter placement. The 34 surviving infants have been followed, and most of them have profound central nervous system handicaps. Data on shunting of obstructive uropathy are similar. Of 98 cases collected until 1992, the mortality rate after catheter placement was 40.8% [34]. A sodium level greater than 100 mmol/L in fetal urine was an indicator of poor outcome [35, 36]. Iatrogenic abdominal wall defects were described as complications of urinary shunts [34].

Although the percutaneous approach under ultrasonographic guidance is preferred for placing a shunt in a hollow enlarged organ, the correction of more complex fetal anomalies requires extensive surgery on both mother and fetus. Throughout the 1980s and early 1990s, the San Francisco fetal therapy group has performed approximately 70 open fetal surgeries for obstructive uropathies, congenital diaphragmatic hernias, congenital cystic adenomatoid malformations of the lung, and sacrococcygeal teratomas. Complications include amniotic leakage, infection, premature labor, and fetal death [37]. Creating vesicostomies for obstructive uropathy and pulmonary lobectomies for cystic adenomatoid malformations have been successful in saving most of these severely affected fetuses. Repair of congenital diaphragmatic hernias has been almost impossible [38].

Fetal surgery may have a role in preventing irreversible organ damage in selected congenital anomalies. Its widespread application is unlikely, however, unless or until some fundamental obstacles such as premature labor and difficulties of operating on tiny fetuses are overcome.

Embryo Reduction

With an increasing number of pregnancies achieved through assisted reproduction, the number of multiple gestations has increased dramatically. Many of these are triplets, quadruplets, quintuplets, and more. The hazards of these larger multiple gestations are significant, and many such patients undergo therapeutic embryo-reduction procedures [39–42].

The pathologic evaluation of these specimens is entirely similar to that of the "vanished twin." The placental membranes contain plaques and flattened mounds of fibrotic material measuring a few centimeters in diameter. Often, a dark blue-black pigmented spot, 1 to 2 mm in diameter is identified at one end of the thickened mass. This represents the retina of an ablated embryo. Radiographs may disclose well-preserved skeletal structures if the ablation is performed after 10 to 12 weeks. The ablated embryonic remnant may rest in the free membranes or be firmly encased in membranes on the fetal surface of the placenta (Fig. 3.2). Hazards to the surviving embryos are rare, but inadvertent transfer of high concentrations of potassium to another sibling can occur, presumably though vascular anastomosis.

Artifacts Associated with Therapeutic Termination of Pregnancies

Therapeutic abortions can be performed using different techniques. The most common procedures are dilatation and extraction (D&E) and use of prostaglandin and urea. Characteristic artifacts are seen in these procedures.

In D&E, extraction can be performed by vacuum or curettage. When curettage is used, the fetus is fragmented and difficult to examine. Depending on the size of the fragments, certain malformations—mainly involving the extremities, palate, spinal cord, or internal organs—can be identified.

Urea is used as a hypertonic solution for termination. Following the application of urea, prostaglandin is used usually as a suppository to initiate the labor process [43]. In this procedure, the fetus is delivered intact but shows marked congestion and autolysis. The skin is red and friable and may disintegrate upon handling. The internal organs are also congested and fragile. Samples for cytogenetic studies may not yield viable tissue for successful harvesting. In this situation, multiple samples from different sites should be submitted.

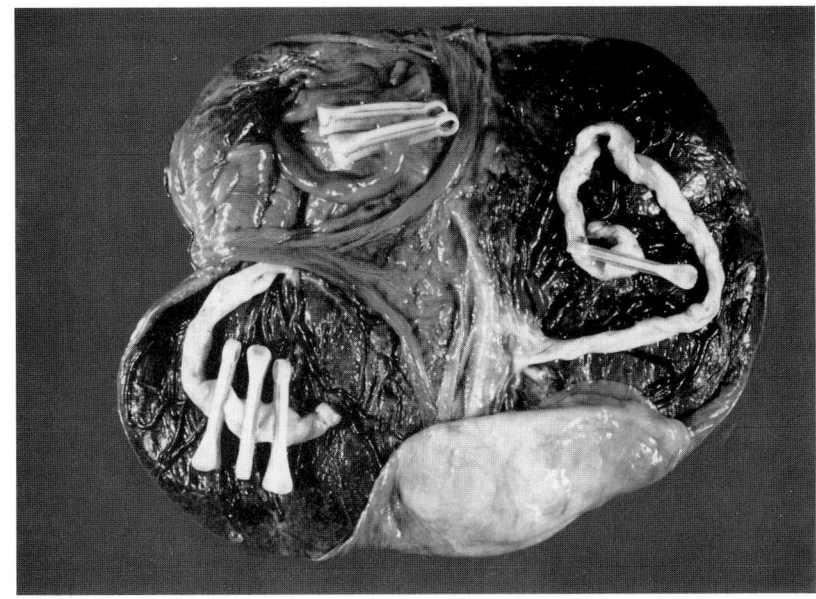

FIGURE 3.2. *A quadruplet placenta from a pregnancy after in vitro fertilization (IVF). There were four embryos at the beginning of the pregnancy. One was reduced (fetus papyraceous) (arrow); another died in utero (two cord clamps). Two healthy babies survived.*

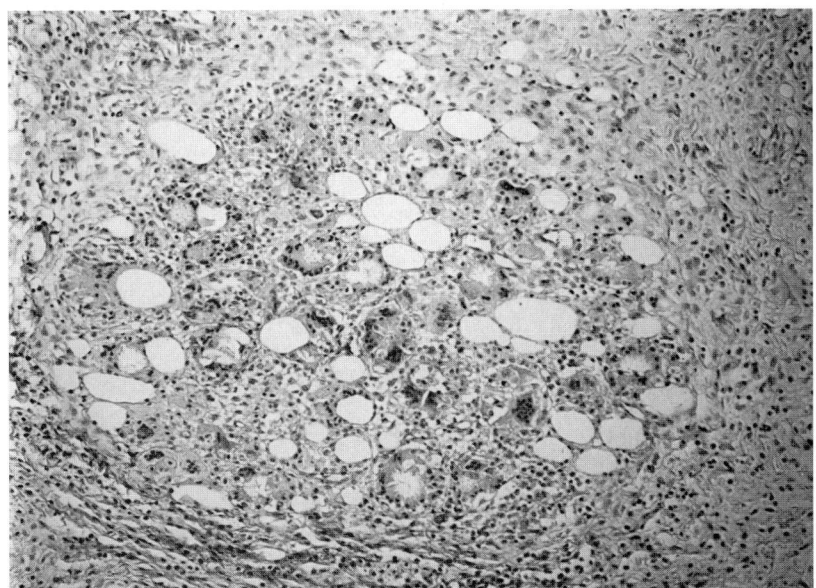

FIGURE 3.3. *Fat necrosis with lipogranulomas consisting of multinucleated giant cells with a lymphohistiocytic cell infiltrate. Asteroid bodies (arrows) are present. H&E stain. ×40.*

INTRAPARTUM CONDITIONS

Birth Trauma

Birth trauma, sustained during labor and delivery, accounts for fewer than 2% of the neonatal deaths and stillbirths in this country and up to 8 injuries per 1000 live births [44]. It is most often observed in large-for-gestational-age babies, where the labor is protracted, and when the delivery is precipitous, breech, or otherwise complicated.

Superficial Lesions

Abrasions, ulcerations, ecchymoses, lacerations, or areas of pressure necrosis of the presenting part may be seen after prolonged labor, vacuum extraction [45], application of forceps [46] or scalp electrodes [47], fetal blood sampling, or cesarean section. Breech delivery can be associated with marked bruising of the buttocks and legs. Testicular injury can also occur [48].

Fat Necrosis

Fat necrosis is an uncommon, sharply circumscribed, indurated subcutaneous nodule or plaque appearing on the extremities, trunk, or buttocks during the first weeks of life and has been attributed to trauma, shock, cold, and asphyxia. Microscopically, there are foci of necrosis of the adipose tissue with a lymphohistiocytic infiltrate. Lipogranulomas with multinucleated giant cells are formed. Typical asteroid bodies may be present [49] (Fig. 3.3).

Table 3.2.   Types of traumatic hemorrhage in the neonate

Occult hemorrhage before birth
Feto-maternal
   Traumatic amniocentesis
   Spontaneous during delivery
   After external cephalic version
Obstetric accidents, malformations of the placenta and the cord
Rupture of a normal umbilical cord
   Precipitous delivery
   Entanglement
Hematoma of the cord and placenta
Rupture of a malformed umbilical cord
   Varices
   Aneurysm
Rupture of anomalous vessels
   Aberrant vessel
   Velamentous insertion
   Communicating vessels in a multilobed placenta
Incision of the placenta during cesarean section
Internal hemorrhages
Intracranial
Cephalhematoma
Subgaleal
Retroperitoneal
Laceration of the liver
Ruptured spleen

Caput Succedaneum

Caput succedaneum is a diffuse, edematous, occasionally hemorrhagic swelling of the scalp that occurs secondary to compression of local vessels associated with prolonged labor. Since it involves the scalp, it is not limited by periosteal seams and crosses the cranial suture lines. Similar lesions may develop with other presenting parts (e.g., scrotum, labia majora, extremities). Edema recedes in a few days; ecchymoses, if present, clear in several weeks.

Hemorrhages

Hemorrhages associated with birth trauma can occur in different organs and tissues. Some congenital malformations complicate the normal delivery process and cause hemorrhage (Table 3.2).

Cephalhematoma   Cephalhematoma is rarely present at birth. It occurs in up to 20% of vacuum-assisted deliveries [50], develops after delivery, and expands during the first day as blood accumulates under the periosteum of a calvarial bone. Usually the parietal bones are involved. The cephalhematoma is rounded and discrete, with boundaries limited by cranial suture lines. The blood contained in a cephalhematoma may take several weeks to resorb and prolongs neonatal jaundice. In very-low-birth-weight newborns, the degree of hyperbilirubinemia secondary to a cephalhematoma may be severe enough to warrant exchange transfusion.

Subgaleal Hemorrhage   Subgaleal hemorrhages are less common than cephalhematomas. Hemorrhage occurs under the epicranial aponeurosis. It feels crepitant with less pitting than the edema of the caput succedaneum. Because there is little anatomic restriction to subgaleal fluid accumulation, large volumes may redistribute and deplete total blood volume. This lesion has been associated with vacuum extraction, and death occurs in 22.8% of the reported cases [51, 52].

Other Hemorrhages   Bleeding from internal organs such as liver [53, 54], spleen, and kidneys [55] can occur in traumatic deliveries. Significant bleeding can occur in skeletal muscle. Rupture of a subcapsular hematoma of the liver can cause hemoperitoneum, which may be life-threatening. This may complicate a breech or a difficult cesarean section delivery, but most cases occur in premature infants, especially those with pneumothorax, pulmonary interstitial emphysema, or sepsis.

Hemorrhages in the skeletal muscles are easily overlooked [55]. Extensive bruising of muscle tissues may be a major hazard to low-birth-weight premature babies when they are delivered vaginally. The hemorrhage is particularly severe over the buttocks.

Ruptures of spleen or liver have been described in newborns with severe erythroblastosis fetalis.

Retinal hemorrhages are present in up to 50% of all neonates [56] and are more common after vacuum-assisted delivery [57, 58]. The exact significance of neonatal retinal hemorrhage is uncertain. Most such hemorrhages resolve within several weeks after birth, and little long-term morbidity has been documented [56].

Intracranial hemorrhage [59, 60] and tentorial tears [61, 62] have been reported as complications of vacuum-assisted delivery.

Fractures and Dislocations

Long, difficult labor, particularly with the breech position, a large infant, or fetal distress requiring rapid extraction, makes birth injuries more likely. Birth fractures almost always involve the clavicle, humerus, or femur [63]. Rarely do birth fractures occur below the elbow or below the knee. On occasion, the fractures are not diagnosed because the extremity is minimally deformed.

A fracture through the proximal epiphyseal plate of the humerus is one of the most common skeletal injuries associated with a difficult delivery. A fracture separation of the distal humeral epiphysis is rare. Fractures of the proximal or distal femoral epiphysis are uncommon. Fracture of the proximal femoral epiphysis can be confused with congenital hip dislocation or acute pyarthrosis.

Clavicular fractures most often occur following shoulder dystocia. Fetuses or neonates with cleidocranial dysplasia may present with pseudofractures of the clavicle. In any newborn with fractures, skeletal dysplasias such as osteogenesis imperfecta should be ruled out.

Skull fractures are rare in the newborn [64]. They are usually linear fractures of the parietal bones, extending radially from the suture lines, and may cause epidural hemorrhages. They occur during difficult breech extraction or forceps delivery [46]. Depressed or indentation fractures usually occur in the parietal bone [65]. The most severe complication of any skull fracture is a torn underlying dural sinus leading to obstruction, vasocongestion, or hemorrhage. Brain emboli have been described with massive skull fractures. Some of these cases may go unrecognized clinically, being instead considered complicated forceps deliveries. Frequent use of cesarean sections and careful monitoring in high-risk deliveries decrease the incidence of these lesions.

Occipital Osteodiastasis Traumatic separation of the squamous and lateral parts of the occipital bone is called *occipital osteodiastasis* [66]. After splitting, the sharp edge of the bone may rupture the dura and cause subdural hemorrhage into the posterior fossa or sometimes may even lacerate the cerebellum. The overriding calvarial bones in a macerated fetus should not be mistaken for occipital osteodiastasis.

Traumatic Nerve Injuries

Traumatic neuropathy of the brachial plexus is one of the more common birth injuries. It is caused by traction and lateral flexion of the neck. There are three types of obstetric brachial plexus palsy, each with characteristic clinical findings [67]. The upper plexus type is called *Erb-Duchenne's palsy*, and in this lesion spinal cord roots C5 and C6 are affected; C7 is less involved. The lower plexus type is called *Klumpke's palsy*, and in this lesion C8 and T1 roots are involved. The third type is the involvement of all the roots of the plexus. In Erb-Duchenne's palsy the shoulder is internally rotated, with the forearm supinated and elbow extended and the wrist and fingers flexed. In Klumpke's palsy the hand is totally flaccid, with little or no control. When the entire plexus is involved, the total extremity is flaccid.

Facial paralysis occurs with difficult deliveries, especially when forceps are forcefully or inappropriately used. It may be associated with intracranial hemorrhages with or without fractures. The incidence of facial paralysis varies from 0.05–1.8% [68]. This condition should be differentiated from congenital absence of the seventh cranial nerve nuclei, a rare condition.

In an early report from the Children's National Medical Center of 135 infants born with a difficult delivery, different types of birth traumas were summarized [67]. In this series, torticollis, facial palsies, subluxations of the shoulder, fractures of the humerus and clavicle, slippage of the radial head, subluxation of the cervical spine with evidence of traction injury of the cervical cord, ipsilateral diaphragmatic paralysis, and adrenal hemorrhage were described. Horner syndrome was seen in 8 infants. Phrenic nerve paralysis accounted for some of the infants' respiratory distress.

Spinal Cord Injuries

Neonates born with evidence of severe hypoxic ischemia may have ischemic necrosis of the spinal cord gray matter. Spinal cord injury can occur after difficult breech extraction [69]. Persistent intrauterine hyperextension of the head can result in impingement of the cervical and upper thoracic spine [70]. High cervical injuries result from complications caused by rotational forceps.

Umbilical artery catheterization has caused spinal cord infarction as well as other major organ infarctions [71]. In such cases, the tips of the intra-aortic catheters were located high in relation to the thoracic spinal cord and produced thrombotic or embolic occlusion of the arterial supply to the anterior spinal cord.

In macerated stillborn fetuses, the spine may rupture internally, depositing portions of the semisolid autolyzed spinal cord into the chest, simulating soft, gray neoplasms.

Resuscitation

Complications related to cardiopulmonary resuscitation (CPR) are numerous and involve nearly every organ system. Some complications are related to the performance of chest compressions; others are related to equipment, such as endotracheal tubes, needles, or bag-valve-mask devices.

Trauma to the neck is associated primarily with attempts to intubate the newborn. Hyoid bone and thyroid cartilage can be damaged during positioning of the baby for ventilation [72]. Injury to the esophagus can occur during attempts to pass a nasogastric tube to decompress the stomach. Esophageal rupture has been reported as a complication of chest compressions [73, 74].

Most of the complications during CPR involve the thorax. Rib and sternal fractures are common, especially in small, premature infants. Hemopericardium can occur during attempts at intracardiac injection. Use of excessive force may result in ventricular contusion and rupture or laceration with pericardial tamponade secondary to hemopericardium [75]. Another common problem is pneumothorax.

Gastric contents are commonly aspirated. Pulmonary edema may develop during or after CPR. The etiology of this is not known.

Another frequent site of complication during CPR is the abdomen. Gastric rupture may result from an overdistended viscus. Overly strong chest compressions may cause laceration of stomach, liver, or spleen [75]. Pneumoperitoneum may result secondary to a perforated viscus or dissection of air from the thorax.

Fat or bone marrow emboli after CPR have been described [76]. Electrolyte abnormalities such as hyperkalemia or hypokalemia have also been reported [77].

Birth Asphyxia

Fetal asphyxia is primarily due to dysfunction of the fetoplacental unit. It is a major cause of morbidity and mortality among fetuses and newborns [78]. Although the original cause of fetoplacental compromise is not iatrogenic, failure to detect the condition and to take the necessary precautions can be iatrogenic. Asphyxia is detected by the biophysical profile of the fetus [79]. Five ultrasound-monitored fetal biophysical variables (i.e., fetal breathing movements, tone, heart rate, reactivity, and semiquantitative amniotic fluid volume determination) are used to assess fetal risk of asphyxia. Repeatedly evaluating the biophysical profile in compromised fetuses is imperative.

Acute fetal asphyxia is relatively uncommon except in obstetric emergencies such as a cord prolapse or major abruption of the placenta. Therefore, most asphyxiated fetuses exhibit both subacute and chronic signs of the disease process (see Chap. 10).

Meconium-stained Amniotic Fluid and Meconium Aspiration Syndrome

Meconium first appears in the fetal ileum between 10 and 16 weeks of gestation as a viscous, green liquid composed of gastrointestinal secretions, cellular debris, bile and pancreatic juice, mucus, blood, lanugo, and vernix. Meconium-stained amniotic fluid (MSAF) is seen in approximately 12% of live births [80, 81]. MSAF usually occurs after 38 weeks' gestation. The incidence of MSAF increases thereafter, and approximately 30% of newborns have MSAF after 42 weeks' gestation. An association between MSAF, fetal compromise, and perinatal morbidity has been clearly demonstrated. In infants with a normal fetal heart rate pattern, MSAF generally carries a low risk of perinatal mortality. The gasping respiratory efforts accompanying fetal asphyxia are thought to contribute to the entry of meconium into the respiratory tract, causing meconium aspiration syndrome (MAS). Problems with MSAF include failure to recognize the condition and to proceed with the emergency delivery or to inadequately aspirate the oropharynx and nasopharynx or trachea when the baby's head is delivered.

Lungs from infants with severe MAS contain meconium, vernix, fetal squamous cells, and cellular debris in the air spaces [82]. Grossly, lungs are green, and meconium can be seen in the airways. An inflammatory response with polymorphonuclear leukocytes, macrophages, and alveolar edema may be observed only if the aspirated material is infected [83]. Large quantities of sterile meconium may be present without an inflammatory response. Hyaline membranes, pulmonary hemorrhage, and necrosis of the pulmonary vasculature and epithelium can occur. Platelet-rich microthrombi in small arterioles and thickening of the muscular layer of the distal arterioles have been described [84].

INVASIVE PROCEDURES

Venipuncture and Peripheral Access

In addition to the traditional venous sites, heelstick is used to obtain blood samples when only a small amount of blood is needed or when there is difficulty obtaining samples by venipuncture. Capillary blood gas sampling and blood cultures when venous access is not possible can also be done by heelstick [85]. Complications are usually infectious. Cellulitis and osteomyelitis by direct inoculation of bacteria have been described [86–88]. Osteomyelitis usually involves the calcaneous bone, and *Staphylococcus aureus* is the most common organism responsible for such cases. This complication can be prevented if the center of the heel is avoided during the procedure [89]. Other complications are scarring of the heel and calcified nodules at old heelstick sites [90].

The following veins can be used for venipuncture in the newborn: supratrochlear, superficial temporal, posterior auricular, external jugular, cephalic, accessory cephalic, basilic, cubital, dorsal arch of the hands and feet, femoral, and greater saphenous veins. Complications are usually related to hemorrhage or hematoma formation. Venous thrombosis is often unavoidable. In premature neonates, veins thrombose after a very short time period and are devastating if they occur in the external jugular and femoral veins. Meningitis and encephalitis have been described when the external jugular vein was used for repeated venipunctures [91]. Thrombosis of the femoral vein may adversely affect the femoral head. Osteomyelitis and abscess formation involving the femoral head and the joint space have been reported with femoral vein punctures [92, 93]. For these reasons, the jugular and femoral veins are avoided.

If there are no indications for central venous or arterial access, peripheral venous cannulation is used; it is the easiest form of access. Basilic, cephalic, and median cubital veins in the antecubital fossa are the most frequently used veins. Interdigital veins of the hand, scalp veins, and the saphenous veins are especially used in preterm infants. Complications of peripheral venous access include local infection, bacteremia, septicemia, phlebitis, infiltration with or without necrosis, thrombosis, and embolism.

Venous Cutdown

Venous cutdown is considered when attempts at vascular cannulation have been unsuccessful. The saphenous vein or the basilic vein are usually used. The risk of infection with cutdowns is significantly higher than with percutaneous cannulation.

Central Venous Access

Central venous catheters are used for hemodynamic monitoring and administration of fluids, drugs, blood products, and parenteral hyperalimentation. The most common sites for central venous cannulation are the subclavian, internal jugular, and femoral veins. Antecubital and external jugular veins are used less frequently. In the newborn age group, the femoral vein is sparingly used [94]. Bleeding, venous thrombosis, arterial puncture, pneumothorax, air embolus, pulmonary thrombus, caval thrombosis, intracardiac catheter-tip

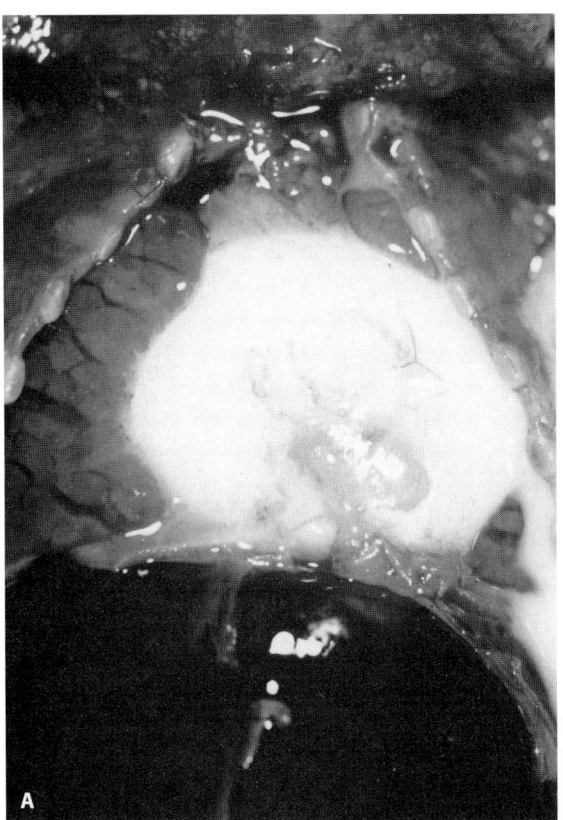

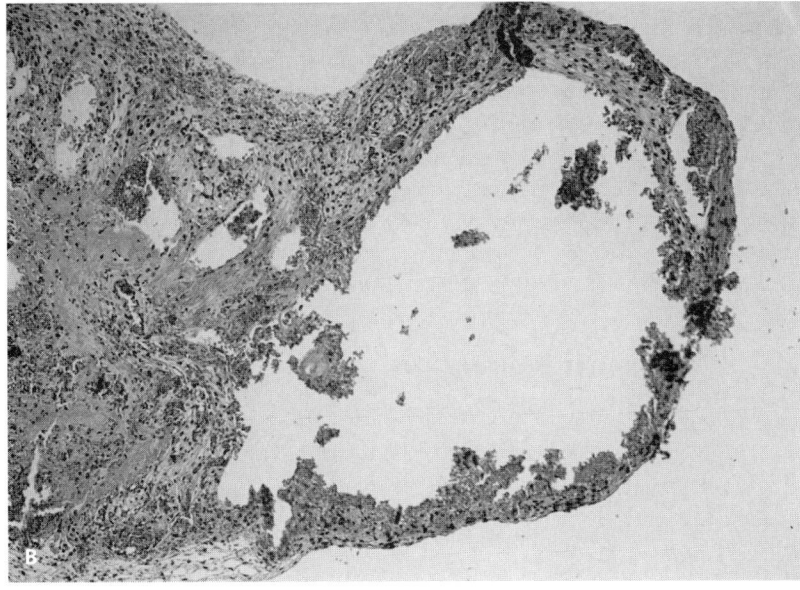

FIGURE 3.4. *Complications of central venous catheters used for total parenteral nutrition (TPN). A. Pericardial tamponade with intralipid solution secondary to rupture of right atrial appendage with a central venous catheter. B. Low-power view of the right atrium showing the perforation site. H&E stain. ×40.*

thrombus formation, sepsis, hydrothorax, vessel perforation, catheter discontinuity, infection, and dysrhythmias are complications [95]. The tip of the central venous catheter may be misplaced and hyperalimentation solutions infused to unwanted spaces. Mah et al [96] described a case where the tip of the catheter was in the subarachnoid space; the cerebrospinal fluid was contaminated with the intralipid solution. Two cases were documented in which venous catheters perforated the superior vena cava or the right atrium and

fluid entered the pericardial cavity. In both cases there was significant intralipid tamponade [97] (Fig. 3.4).

Pulmonary Artery Access

Pulmonary artery catheters are used to measure pressures in the right atrium, pulmonary artery, or the pulmonary arterial wedge pressure, and to sample pulmonary artery and pulmonary arterial wedge blood for blood gas determination. Through this access, cardiac output can be determined by thermodilution. The most common indications for pulmonary artery catheterization are cardiogenic shock, respiratory failure, shock unresponsive to volume infusion, and when routine monitoring proves inadequate and additional information is required. Pulmonary artery rupture, pulmonary embolus, pulmonary infarction, catheter knotting, balloon rupture, dysrhythmia during insertion, and valve damage are possible risks when using pulmonary artery catheters.

Arterial Puncture and Peripheral Arterial Access

Peripheral arterial punctures are performed to measure arterial blood gases when there is no indwelling arterial catheter. The radial artery is the site of choice. The presence of an ulnar artery is checked before the radial artery is punctured. The brachial artery is avoided because compromise to its circulation will have a devastating effect. When there is suspicion of significant ductal shunting, right radial artery blood gases (preductal) are measured simultaneously with umbilical artery samples (postductal). The most common complication of arterial punctures is vasospasm, which is usually transient. Thrombosis and infection can also occur.

Indwelling arterial catheters are used for continuous blood pressure monitoring, frequent arterial blood gas sampling, and as withdrawal ports for exchange transfusion. Arterial catheter blood pressure readings may be more accurate than cuff measurements in the hypotensive neonate with elevated systemic vascular resistance. Newborns receiving vasopressors or vasodilators usually require continuous intra-arterial blood pressure monitoring. The most commonly used sites are radial, posterior tibial, dorsalis pedis, femoral, and axillary arteries. Brachial and superficial temporal arteries are not used because of poor collateral flow. Complications are rare but include thrombosis and infection.

Umbilical Vessel Access

The umbilical vessels are accessible during the first several days of life, and in some infants they can be cannulated after 2 weeks of age, either directly or by infraumbilical cutdown. At skin level, the umbilical vein is usually at the 12 o'clock position. The umbilical artery is used for blood pressure measurement, blood sampling, and infusion of drugs and fluids. The umbilical vein is used for central venous pressure measurement, blood sampling, and infusion of drugs and fluids.

The tips of umbilical artery catheters should lie below the ductus arteriosus but above the celiac axis, or between the inferior mesenteric artery and the aortic bifurcation. The umbilical venous catheter tip should lie a few centimeters into the umbilical vein or in the inferior vena cava; it should not lie within the liver.

The most common complications are thrombosis of varying degrees (<90%), bacterial colonization (57%), sepsis (5%), and vasospasm (<20%) [98]. Blood loss and vascular perforation are also significant and are seen relatively commonly. Perforation occurs just deep to the umbilicus or at the junction with the internal iliac artery.

A long list of rare complications has been described in the literature [99]. These are mainly procedural errors or exaggerated thrombotic complications. For umbilical artery catheters, complications include: erroneous insertion of the catheter into the umbilical vein, iliac vein, or subarachnoid space and paraplegia [100]; perforation of the aorta and false aneurysm formation [101, 102]; perforation of the bladder; urinary ascites; and blockage of different arteries at their origins, resulting in ischemic necroses in the kidneys, gastrointestinal tract, or soft tissue. Thrombotic complications include infarcts in the liver, kidneys, adrenals, intestines, and spleen (Fig. 3.5). Renal artery embolism and hypertension have also been described [103]. Infectious complications include osteomyelitis [104], pyarthrosis [105], peritonitis secondary to perforation of the gastrointestinal tract [106], and endocarditis [107].

Umbilical vein catheters have been associated with portal vein thrombosis, with embolization leading to portal hypertension [108], thrombophlebitis and necrosis, and abscesses of the liver [109, 110] (Fig. 3.6). Sepsis, bacteremia, and endocarditis can also occur. Infusion of hypertonic and acidic solutions through umbilical venous catheters can cause necrosis and abscess formation [111].

The use of umbilical venous catheters has decreased in recent years due to the relatively high rate of complications. Peripheral and central venous catheters are more widely used in the care of the sick or preterm neonate. Although umbilical arterial catheters are still widely used, monitoring devices such as transcutaneous Po_2 monitors ($TcPo_2$) and pulse oximeters have diminished their use.

Intraosseous Access

Intraosseous infusion (IOI) remains largely a resuscitative measure, used until other access is secured. Short-term IOI is safe [112]. The preferred site for IOI is the flat, anteromedial surface of the proximal tibia. Infusion is given into the medullary cavity, which is a non-collapsible venous network with rapid drainage into the central circulation. Complications include extravasation, compartment syndromes, bone fractures, osteomyelitis, and fat and bone marrow emboli [113]. This technique is rarely used in low-birth-weight infants.

Exchange Transfusion

The primary aim of exchange transfusion is to prevent the toxic effects of bilirubin by removing it from the body. Other indications include sepsis; disseminated intravascular coagulation; metabolic disorders causing severe acidosis, such

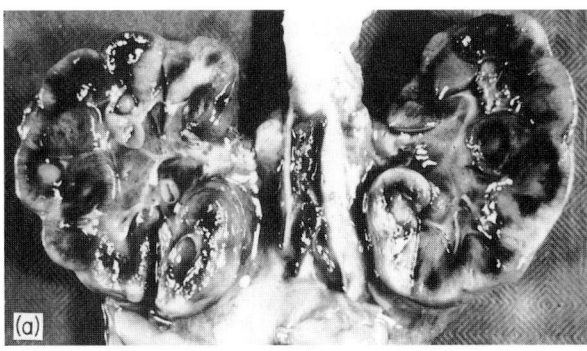

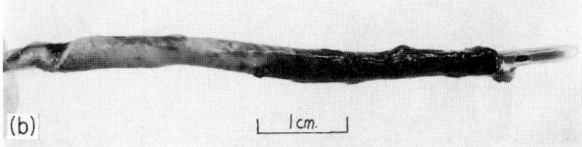

1 cm.

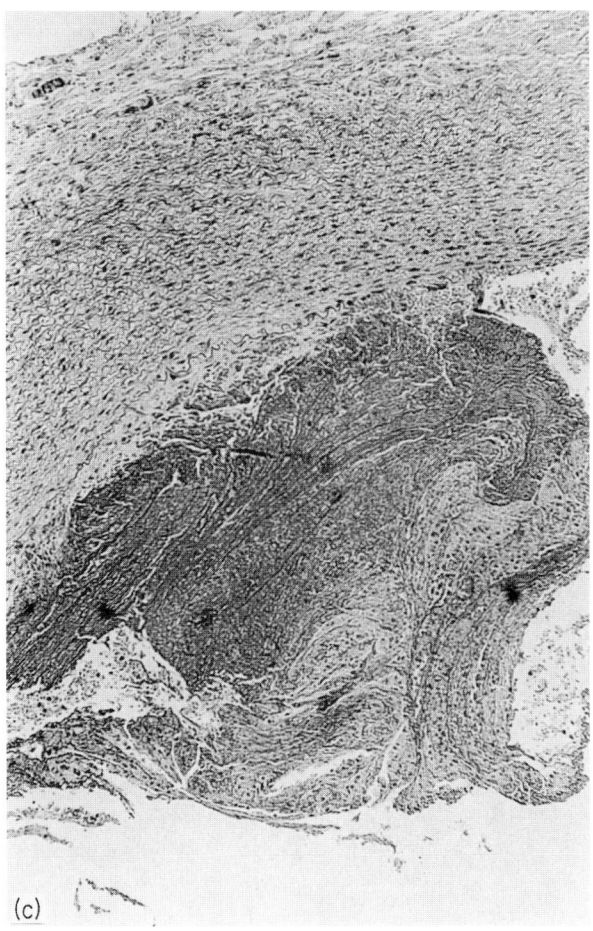

FIGURE 3.5. *Thrombosis due to umbilical artery catheterization. (a) Mural thrombus of aorta with renal artery spread and renal infarction. (b) Thrombus forming a sheath around an umbilical artery catheter. (From Gupta et al [99]). (c) Low-power microscopic view of aortic thrombus in 5-day-old infant with an umbilical artery catheter.*

as aminoaciduria with associated hyperammonemia; severe fluid or electrolyte imbalances such as hyperkalemia or hypernatremia; fluid overload; polycythemia; and severe anemia. Three types of exchange transfusions are commonly used: 2-volume exchange, isovolumetric 2-volume exchange, and partial exchange. Simple 2-volume exchange transfusion is used for uncomplicated hyperbilirubinemia. Isovolumetric 2-volume exchange transfusion is used when volume shifts during a simple exchange might cause or aggravate cardiac insufficiency; it is performed using a double setup with two operators. Partial exchange transfusion is used mainly in the treatment of polycythemia.

Complications with exchange transfusions can be metabolic, catheter-induced, or related to the exchange procedure itself.

The anticoagulant citrate in citrate phosphate dextrose (CPD) blood binds ionic calcium and magnesium and produces a significant depression in these divalent cations. The temporary hypomagnesemia has not been associated with clinically recognizable problems, but hypocalcemia is a hazard [114]. Potassium levels increase rapidly in stored blood. Hyperkalemia can occur with the use of old red blood cells [115]. This complication is avoided by washing the red blood cell units.

All the catheter induced complications that were discussed in the previous sections can occur with exchange transfusions. Other significant complications are necrotizing enterocolitis, graft-versus-host disease, and blood-borne infections.

Necrotizing Enterocolitis
Necrotizing enterocolitis (NEC) with intestinal perforation has been reported following exchange transfusion [116–119] in both full-term and preterm infants and after both single and multiple exchanges. The cause remains obscure, but malposition of the umbilical venous catheter in the portal system, with its close relation to the mesenteric veins, may produce retrograde obstruction with hemorrhage and thrombosis at the microcirculatory level. The pathology of NEC is well described [120]. (See Chap. 24.)

Graft-Versus-Host Disease
Graft-versus-host disease (GVHD) has occurred in infants who received intrauterine transfusions and who subsequently received postnatal exchange transfusions [121]. A clinical syndrome of transient maculopapular rash with associated eosinophilia, thrombocytopenia, and mild lymphopenia was described in 21 of 35 neonates who received both intrauterine transfusions and postnatal exchange transfusions, and in 6 of 17 neonates who received multiple exchange transfusions for erythroblastosis fetalis [122].

Pathological examination of biopsies and postmortem tissue samples with GVHD show infiltrates of lymphocytes, plasma cells, and eosinophils in the skin, spleen, bone marrow, esophagus, stomach, and intestines. Great numbers of histiocytes infiltrate lymphoid tissues and bone marrow.

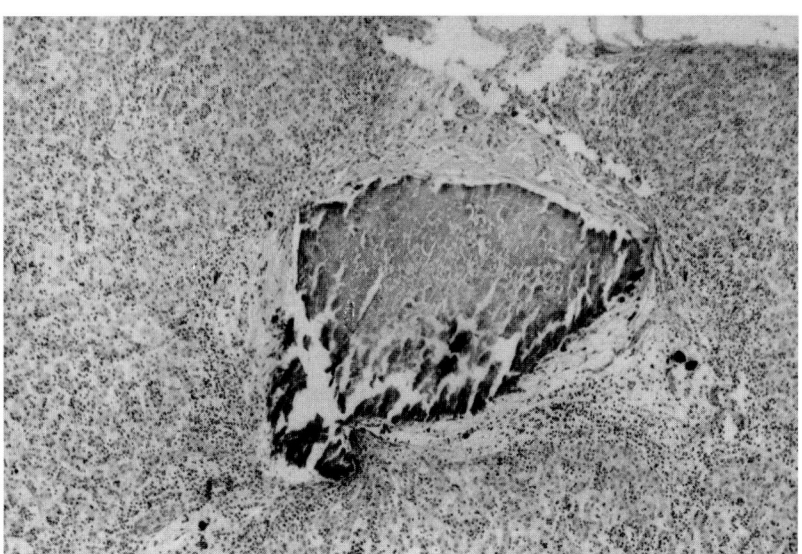

FIGURE 3.6. *Hepatic venous thrombus with calcification secondary to umbilical venous catheterization, ×47. (Courtesy of Dr. DB Singer.)*

Dyskeratosis in the skin, periportal necrosis in the liver, generalized depletion of lymphocytes, and hypoplasia of the bone marrow have been described [121, 123].

Exchange transfusion also carries the usual risk of any blood product. With the newer screening techniques for blood donors the risk of acquired immunodeficiency syndrome, hepatitis, and cytomegalovirus infection is low [124, 125].

Diagnostic and Therapeutic Centeses

Pericardiocentesis

The indications for pericardiocentesis are treatment of cardiac tamponade caused by pneumopericardium or pericardial effusion and to obtain pericardial fluid for diagnostic studies.

The complications of pericardiocentesis are multiple. The most serious complications are myocardial and coronary artery lacerations [126, 127]. Pneumothorax, hemothorax, pulmonary edema after evacuation of pericardial effusions [128], and acute right ventricular volume overload [129] have been reported. Dysrhythmias and infectious complications also can occur.

Thoracentesis

Thoracentesis is performed either to relieve dyspnea or to improve ventilation and gas exchange in the newborn with a significant pleural effusion and to determine the nature of the effusion when its cause is not known.

Complications of thoracentesis include vasovagal reactions, hemothorax from laceration of an intercostal artery, pneumothorax, infection of the pleural space, and puncture of the lung, liver, spleen, or kidney [130]. Additional complications during or after therapeutic thoracentesis are related to the removal of large volumes of pleural fluid. These are hypoxemia and unilateral pulmonary edema [131, 132].

Abdominal Paracentesis

Indications for abdominal paracentesis are to obtain peritoneal fluid for diagnostic tests and as a therapeutic procedure to aid in ventilation.

The complications associated with paracentesis are few and usually not serious. Intestinal perforation may occur more frequently than suspected [133]; however, it is seldom of any consequence because the perforation rapidly seals upon withdrawal of the needle. Perforation of a blood vessel, either intraperitoneally or extraperitoneally, usually closes rapidly, although hematomas may form. Bacterial contamination and peritonitis may result from a break in the sterile technique or from soiling by intestinal contents if an intestinal perforation failed to seal. Rapid removal of a large volume of ascitic fluid can result in a reflexive decrease in the intravascular volume and subsequent hypotension. Perforation of the bladder has been reported [134]. If the "Z-track" technique is not used, persistent ascitic fluid leak can occur.

Chest Tubes

Indications for placement of chest tubes are the presence of a tension pneumothorax causing respiratory compromise or decreased venous return to the heart, with decreased cardiac output and hypotension; pneumothorax compromising ventilation and causing increased work of breathing, hypoxia, and increased Pco_2; and to drain a pleural effusion.

The most common complication is perforation of the lung(s) [135] (Fig. 3.7). This may cause persistent pneumothorax, significant hemorrhage, and hemothorax. Bleeding may also be caused by perforation of one of the major vessels (intercostal, axillary, pulmonary, or mammary). Chylothorax has been reported [136]. Phrenic or intercostal nerve damage can occur [137]. Like all the other invasive procedures, local infection of the pleural cavity or sepsis can be seen with chest tube placement. This author has seen as many as six chest tubes, four on one side, two on the other disorders such as meningitis or subarachnoid hemorrhage, administration of intrathecal medications, and monitoring the efficacy of antibiotics used to treat CNS infections. Until recently, serial LPs were used to drain the cerebrospinal fluid in communicating hydrocephalus associated with intraventricular hemorrhages. Intraventricular catheters draining cerebrospinal fluid to the outside are now utilized in most centers.

Complications from this essential procedure are especially prone to develop in small preterm neonates. Positioning the baby (i.e., left side with hips flexed at 90 degrees) may cause transient hypoxemia or cardiac compromise. Apnea and bradycardia significant enough to warrant resuscitative measures have occurred. Spinal cord and nerve injuries have been described but are rare. Herniation of cerebral tissue through the foramen magnum is not a common problem in the intensive care nursery because of the open fontanelles, but meningitis, bacteremia, and sepsis can be seen. Osteomyelitis and abscess formation in the epidural space, secondary to direct inoculation of the vertebrae during the procedure, have been reported [138]. Delayed development of an intraspinal epidermoid tumor or epidermoid cyst can result from performing a LP with a needle without stylet (e.g., butterfly needles) [139]; the cause is thought to be a "plug" of epithelial tissue displaced into the dura.

Urinary Bladder Catheterization and Aspiration

In the newborn, the urinary bladder is catheterized for accurate measurement of urinary output. Urine specimens obtained by catheters are often contaminated, so suprapubic bladder tap is preferred for cultures.

The incidence of infection is high in newborns with urinary catheters [140]. The risk of infection increases with duration of catheterization; it is estimated to increase at 5–10% per day of catheterization. In very-low-birth-weight preterm infants, the rate is even higher. Hematuria, urethral trauma, and strictures can also occur.

Infectious complications are much lower in bladder taps. The main complications of bladder taps are bowel perforation and microscopic hematuria. Bowel perforations spontaneously seal and usually do not cause major problems.

Circumcision

Circumcision is probably one of the oldest of all surgical procedures. Especially in the United States, it is performed in the neonatal age group. Although it is a relatively safe procedure, the complication rate ranges from 2–10% [141–142]. The common complications are hemorrhage and sepsis. In the majority of cases, bleeding is minor. Excessive bleeding may be due to anomalous vessels or a bleeding disorder. Infection occurs after circumcision in up to 10% of patients. In the majority of cases, this is usually mild with local inflammatory changes, but septic death, necrotizing

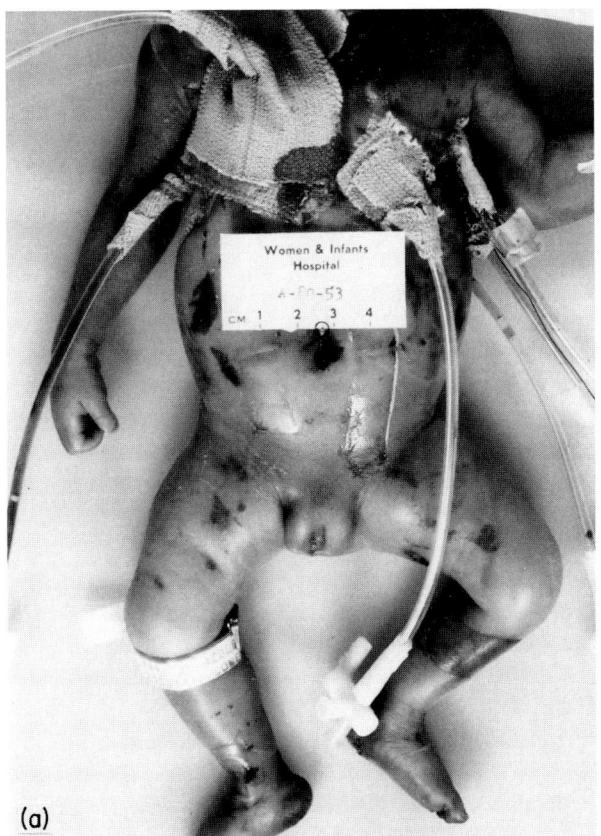
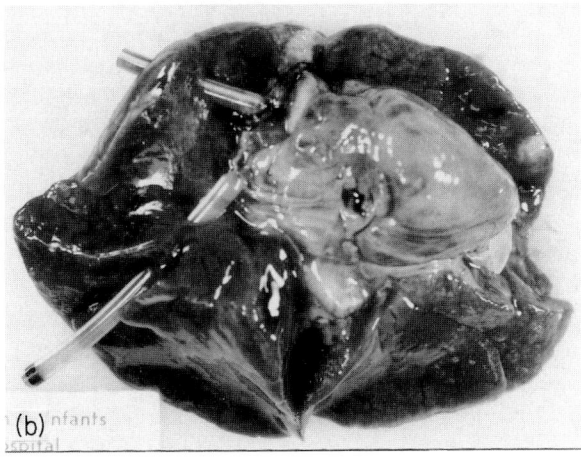

FIGURE 3.7. (a) *Infant at postmortem examination with multiple drainage tubes in situ.* (b) *Heart and lungs showing drainage tubes penetrating right lung.*

side, in one infant whose lungs were ruptured by several of the tubes. Softer plastic in newer tubes has reduced this complication.

Lumbar Puncture

Indications for lumbar puncture (LP) are to obtain cerebrospinal fluid for the diagnosis of central nervous system fasciitis, gangrene, scalded skin syndrome, and osteomyelitis have been described. Rare complications include amputation of the glans [143], total ablation of the penis secondary to diathermy injury [141], urethrocutaneous fistula [141], and meatal stenosis [141].

COMPLICATIONS OF
THERAPEUTIC MODALITIES

Chemical Blepharoconjunctivitis

Chemical blepharoconjunctivitis is caused by silver nitrate that is used for neonatal eye prophylaxis. It peaks on the second day of life with copious secretions and edema, but it is self-limited. Brown-gray pigmentation of the eye can also occur with silver nitrate. This disappears after 7 to 10 days. Tearing or persistent eye crusting after the first 2 days requires further evaluation. Erythromycin ointment has replaced silver nitrate for eye prophylaxis in many institutions [144].

Vaccinations

In the newborn age group, vaccination with hepatitis B vaccine is recommended. Pain at the injection site and fever are the most common reported complications. Allergic reactions have been described. Postvaccination surveillance for 3 years after the licensure of the plasma-derived vaccine suggested an association of borderline significance between Guillain-Barré syndrome and receipt of the first vaccine dose. No association has been demonstrated in postvaccination surveillance for the recombinant hepatitis B vaccines [145].

Bacille Calmette-Guérin (BCG) vaccination is still used in some countries in the neonatal age group. This vaccine has more reported complications than the hepatitis B vaccine. Granulomatous abscess formation [146], osteomyelitis [147], and non-caseating granulomatous hepatitis have been reported. The hepatitis is believed to be caused by a hypersensitivity reaction related to the vaccine [148].

Oxygen Therapy

Hypoxic infants who are able to maintain an adequate minute ventilation are assisted with free-flow of oxygen or air-oxygen mixtures.

Oxygen hoods provide an enclosure for blended air-oxygen supply, humidification, and continuous oxygen concentration monitoring. Hoods are easy to use and provide access and visibility to the infant.

Mask oxygen is not suitable for infants because of poor control and lack of monitoring the oxygen supply.

Nasal cannulae are used for infants needing low concentrations of oxygen. Delivery can be controlled by flow meters.

Table 3.3.   Complications of hyperoxia

Retinopathy of prematurity
Pulmonary complications
   Proliferation of pulmonary capillaries
   Hyperplasia of type II pneumocytes
   Alveolar and interstitial hemorrhage
   Pulmonary edema
RBC hemolysis
Decreased myocardial metabolism
CNS damage
Seizures

Complications of Hyperoxia

Under normal conditions, a delicate balance exists between the production of free radicals and the antioxidant defenses that protect cells in vivo. Free radicals are molecules with extra electrons, and they are toxic to living tissues. Oxygen has a unique structure and is abundant within cells. It readily accepts free electrons generated by oxidative metabolism within the cell, producing free radicals. The balance may be disturbed by increased free-radical production under conditions of hyperoxia, reperfusion, or inflammation. The complications of hyperoxia are summarized in Table 3.3 [149].

Retinopathy of Prematurity   Retinopathy of prematurity (ROP) is a disorder of the developing retinal vasculature due to interruption of normal progression of newly forming retinal vessels [150, 151]. Vasoconstriction and obliteration of the advancing capillary bed is followed in succession by neovascularization extending into the vitreous, retinal edema, retinal hemorrhages, fibrosis, and traction on and eventual detachment of the retina. In most cases, the process is reversed before fibrosis occurs.

In the United States, approximately 400 to 600 children per year may be blinded by ROP, representing 20% of blindness in preschool children.

In the normally developing retina, there are no retinal vessels until about 16 weeks' gestation. Until then, oxygen diffuses to the retina from the underlying choroidal circulation. At 16 weeks, in response to an unknown stimulus (relative hypoxia as the retina thickens has been suggested), cells derived from mesenchyme traveling in the nerve fiber layer emanate from the optic nerve head. These cells, called *spindle cells*, are the precursors of the retinal vasculature system. A fine capillary network advances through the retina to the ora serrata; more mature vessels form behind this advancing network. Vascularization on the nasal side of the ora serrata is complete at about 8 months' gestation, whereas that on the temporal side is ordinarily complete at term. Once completely vascularized, the retinal vasculature is no longer susceptible to the insult of hyperoxia. The classification of ROP is summarized in Table 3.4 [152].

Respiratory Complications   Pulmonary complications of hyperoxia include proliferation of pulmonary capillaries,

Table 3.4.   Classification of retinopathy of prematurity (ROP)

Stage	
1	Demarcation line (thin non-elevated white line at the junction between vascularized and avascular retina)
2	Ridge (elevated demarcation line)
3	Ridge with extraretinal fibrovascular proliferation (ERP), mild (A), moderate (B), severe (C)
4	Subtotal retinal detachment Extrafoveal (A), foveal (B)
5	Total retinal detachment
Zone	
1	Distal to 2% disc to foveal distance
2	Disc to nasal ora and temporal equator
3	Disc to ora nasally and temporally

Plus disease: Retinal vascular tortuosity and dilatation; iris vascular engorgement; pupillary rigidity; vitreous haze or hemorrhage. From [152].

Table 3.5.   Complications of endotracheal tubes

Local trauma to nose, larynx, and trachea [157]
Perforation of bronchi, trachea [158, 159]
Perforation of the esophagus [160]
Kinking and blockage leading to hypoxia
Infections
Pneumothorax
Raised intracranial pressure
Squamous metaplasia and necrosis of trachea
Postextubation atelectasis
Palatal groove
Midfacial hypoplasia
Vocal cord damage
Subglottic tracheal stenosis [161, 162]
Persistent stridor or hoarseness
Stricture of nasal vestibule
Abnormal dentition
Foreign bodies

Data from Gould and Graham [156].

hyperplasia of type II pneumocytes, alveolar and interstitial hemorrhage, patchy atelectasis, pulmonary edema, fibroproliferative bronchiolitis, and bronchopulmonary dysplasia [153].

Iatrogenic Respiratory Distress Syndrome   Neonatal respiratory distress syndrome (RDS) continues to be an important complication of elective repeat cesarean section. This point was made and examined in detail by Bowers et al [154]. Fifteen years later, the problem still exists. Among 1207 repeat cesarean births without labor, 18 neonates of gestational age of at least 37 weeks or birth weights of at least 2500 grams were admitted to the neonatal intensive care unit (NICU); 5 of the 18 neonates admitted met the criteria of RDS. This represented an incidence of 0.41%. These 5 neonates had complications such as pneumothorax and pulmonary hemorrhage [155]. While this shows a decrease in incidence from 4.3% described in the report by Bowers et al, RDS still occurs in infants born by cesarean section, presumably at term gestations.

Endotracheal Intubation and Suctioning

Endotracheal intubation is used to mechanically ventilate the sick newborn. It is mostly used in the form of an oropharyngeal tube, but in some centers nasotracheal tubes are preferred. Complications associated with endotracheal tubes are summarized in Table 3.5.

Mechanical Ventilation

Respiratory distress and failure may be defined as either apnea, hypercarbia, or hypoxia. Mechanical ventilation reestablishes the normal ventilatory balance by removing the CO_2 and restores oxygenation. Techniques range from simple

Table 3.6.   Complications of continuous positive airway pressure (CPAP)

Local and nasal erosion from nasal prongs
Nasal edema and stenosis
Facial trauma from face masks
Neck ulceration from head box
Gastric distention
Gastric perforation
Pneumothorax, pneumomediastinum
Water intoxication from nebulizer
Paradoxical hypoxemia
Increased work of breathing from nasal prongs
Wide swings in oxygen concentration
Inadequacy in maintaining seals
Hydrocephalus from head box
Cerebral hemorrhage
Noise trauma

bag-and-mask ventilation to microprocessor-controlled and extremely complicated instruments.

Continuous Positive Airway Pressure

Mask, nasal prongs, or endotracheal tubes can be used to apply continuous positive airway pressure (CPAP), which improves PaO_2 by stabilizing the airway and allowing alveolar recruitment. Retention of CO_2 may result from excessive distending airway pressure. Nasal deformities secondary to nasal CPAP have been reported [163]. Complications associated with CPAP are summarized in Table 3.6.

Bag-and-Mask or Bag-to-Endotracheal Tube Ventilation

These handheld assemblies allow for emergency or temporary ventilatory support. All handheld units must have pop-off valves to avoid excessive pressures to the infant's airway. Because these are all manual units, the main complication is application of excessive peak inspiratory pressure (PIP), which causes air leaks such as pneumothorax and pneumomediastinum. Sometimes the practice of manually closing the pop-off valve is employed, especially during vigorous resuscitation of a poorly responding infant. This practice can be particularly detrimental to the airway of the infant.

Pressure Control Ventilators

These are the standard, classic ventilators. They are the most commonly used ventilators in the NICU. They are time-cycled and the pressure can be adjusted.

Volume Control Ventilators

Previously, these ventilators were not used for newborns because measurement, adjustment, and monitoring of tidal volumes were not possible in this age group. With improvements in equipment, however, this is now possible, and volume control respirators are more widely used in neonatal care.

High-Frequency Ventilators

Infants who are 2 or 3 weeks old, ventilator-dependent, and in need of supplemental oxygen require high frequency ventilators (HFVs). HFV refers to a variety of strategies and devices designed to provide ventilation at rapid rates and very low tidal volumes. This decreases the barotrauma. Rates in HFV are often expressed in Hertz (Hz). A rate of 1 Hz (1 cycle/sec) is equivalent to 60 bpm (breaths per minute). Definite indications for HFV are pulmonary interstitial emphysema, severe bronchopleural fistula, and clinical deterioration necessitating extracorporeal membrane oxygenation (ECMO) (see Extracorporeal Membrane Oxygenation below). Possible indications are pulmonary hypertension, severe hyaline membrane disease, meconium aspiration syndrome, and diaphragmatic hernia with pulmonary hypoplasia. Two types of HFV instruments are in common use.

High-Frequency Jet Ventilators   The high-frequency jet ventilator (HFJV) injects a high-velocity stream of gas into the endotracheal tube, usually at frequencies between 240 and 600 bpm, and tidal volumes are equal to or slightly greater than dead space. Indications are the same as for HFV.

High-Frequency Oscillatory Ventilators   The high-frequency oscillatory ventilator (HFOV) generates tidal volume less than or equal to dead space by means of an oscillating piston or diaphragm. This mechanism creates active expiration as well as inspiration. Indications are the same as for HFV.

Surfactant Replacement Therapy

In 1959, Avery and Mead [164] demonstrated that saline extracts from the lungs of preterm infants who died from RDS were deficient in pulmonary surfactant. Successful

Table 3.7.   Lung surfactant preparations

Active substance	Trade name
Phospholipids with additives	Exosurf, ALEC
Animal lung minces, extracted and modified	Curosurf, Survanta, Surfacten, Surfactant TA
Animal lung lavage surfactant extract	Infrasurf, Alveofact
Human surfactant in amniotic fluid	

exogenous surfactant replacement therapy was first described by Fujiwara et al [165], who demonstrated improvement of lung function and decreased morbidity in infants treated with a surfactant prepared from an organic solvent extract of bovine lung. Between 1985 and 1993, more than 35 controlled trials evaluating different preparations of lung surfactants were reported [166]. There are four groups of surfactant preparations; these are summarized in Table 3.7. Desaturation, bradycardia, and apnea are frequent adverse effects, unless the dose is administered slowly. During the clinical trials, pulmonary hemorrhage emerged as one possible complication of surfactant replacement therapy [167, 168]. A recent meta-analysis of surfactant clinical trials confirmed the increased risk of pulmonary hemorrhage [169]. Most of the pathologic studies in surfactant-treated neonates did not reveal significant pulmonary findings [170–172], but one study suggested a slight increase in pulmonary hemorrhage when compared with a control group [173].

Nitric Oxide

Nitric oxide (NO) is an endogenous endothelium-derived relaxing factor that contributes to the regulation of vascular tone in many circulations, including the perinatal lung [174]. Because NO is a gas, inhalational NO therapy has been studied for its potential efficacy in causing selective pulmonary vasodilation in experimental and clinical settings [175, 176]. NO produces marked improvement in oxygenation in term newborns with severe persistent pulmonary hypertension who meet the criteria for ECMO therapy. The usual dose is 20 ppm, and multiple doses are given. Although clinical trials are just starting, premature infants with problems ranging from prolonged rupture of membranes, oligohydramnios, suspected hypoplastic lungs, and group B streptococcus sepsis have been treated with NO with reasonably good results [177, 178].

The complications associated with NO therapy are multiple and potentially serious. Increases in bleeding time have been noted in normal adult subjects who have received inhaled NO [179, 180]. Peliowski et al [177] reported two deaths associated with massive intracranial hemorrhage in eight preterm neonates treated with NO for respiratory problems associated with prolonged rupture of membranes. Increased bleeding time has been noted in rabbits receiving as little as 3 ppm of inhaled NO [181]. In other studies, methemoglobinemia is described [177]. Moreover, at concentrations of 50 ppm, impaired memory and delayed brainstem nerve conduction have been observed in rats [182]. Finally, there is recent evidence that peroxynitrites, which form when NO combines with superoxide, can inhibit surfactant function [183].

Liquid Ventilation

Fluids such as saline, silicones, and fluorocarbons to facilitate or support respiration have been under study for several decades. Researchers studying the effects of war gas poisoning in the 1920s found that the lungs could tolerate lavage procedures with large quantities of saline solution. The concept of land mammals breathing liquids was first introduced into the medical literature with Kylstra's experiments on fluid-breathing mice [184]. In the early 1960s, it was discovered that fluorocarbon, a substance first produced during World War II as part of the Manhattan Project, is an excellent carrier of oxygen.

Perfluorocarbons are derived from common organic compounds such as benzene. They are clear, colorless, odorless liquids. They are stable, can be stored indefinitely at room temperature, and can be autoclaved without change. They are not soluble in water or lipids, nor are lipids and water soluble in them [185]. They are excellent solvents for oxygen, carbon dioxide, and most gases, but very poor solvents for almost everything else that exists in biological systems. Perfluorocarbons are chemically and biologically inert, scavenged by macrophages, are not catabolized, and leave the body by volatilization through the lung and transpiration through the skin [186, 187]. Whether perfluorocarbons are injected or breathed, very small quantities are absorbed and distributed. The highest tissue concentration has been found in the adipose tissue. In primates, small amounts of the liquid persisted in the lungs as long as 3 years following fluorocarbon ventilation. Marked pulmonary damage was demonstrated in the lungs of adult rabbits, but, in a more recent study, the newborn rabbit lung had no ultrastructural lesions [188]. Because perfluorocarbons can accumulate in the adipose tissue, the effect on the developing brain is unknown.

Despite advances in mechanical ventilation of the sick newborn and use of artificial surfactant, barotrauma is still a major problem that causes further lung damage in these already compromised infants. Such infants are candidates for liquid ventilation. Numerous animal studies have shown that barotrauma can be markedly reduced and that ventilation can be accomplished with perfluorocarbon ventilation [189]. The perfluorocarbon solution (Liquivent) is circulated to and from the lungs via an endotracheal tube in a tidal fashion, and through an extracorporeal membrane "lung" to continuously add oxygen and remove carbon dioxide. Greenspan et al [190] in 1990 ventilated two terminally ill preterm neonates with perfluorocarbon. Although the

neonates died within 19 hours of liquid ventilation, the gas exchange prior to death had improved. There was no evidence of retained perfluorocarbon in the lungs or pleural space. More recently, Hirschl et al [191] reported satisfactory gas exchange in nineteen patients with this technique. This series included ten adults, five children, and four neonates with severe respiratory failure. The liquid ventilation was alternated with extracorporeal life support. All the patients survived and tolerated the procedure well. Their ventilatory status showed marked improvement during the liquid ventilation phase of their treatment. Complications were pneumothoraces (9 patients) and pulmonary hemorrhage (1 patient).

Complications of Respiratory Therapy

Airway Injury
Necrotizing tracheobronchitis (NT) has been described as a specific complication with high-frequency ventilatory therapy [192]. Some investigators suggested that inadequate humidification was the cause of this necrotizing lesion [193]. Further studies reveal no statistically significant difference in the incidence of NT between conventional versus high-frequency ventilators [194].

Histologically, NT consists of mucosal and submucosal necrosis, acute inflammatory infiltrates, and, in severe cases, chondritis. Chronic lesions include squamous metaplasia of the surface epithelium, fibrosis, and glandular proliferation.

Air Leak Syndromes
The pulmonary leak syndromes (pneumothorax, pneumomediastinum, pneumopericardium, pulmonary interstitial emphysema [PIE], persistent interstitial pulmonary emphysema [PIPE], and air embolism) comprise a spectrum of diseases with the same underlying pathophysiology. Overdistention of alveolar sacs or terminal airways leads to disruption of tissues and dissection of air into surrounding tissues and spaces. The common etiologic factor in all air leak syndromes is barotrauma.

Pathology of air leak syndromes has been described in detail [195]. In PIE, gross examination of the lungs shows small elliptical or spherical spaces in the septa and under the pleura. The pleural surface appears coarse. Intraparenchymal blood vessels appear to "hang" with small attachments to septal connective tissues because of air or gas dissecting into the tissue and forming a space surrounding them. Hemorrhage is frequently present in the same areas.

Blebs of interstitial air may sometimes be trapped in the lung for a long period of time and can trigger a foreign body reaction with multinucleated giant cells; this is called *persistent interstitial pulmonary emphysema* (PIPE) [196].

Air embolism is a rare but serious complication [195, 197] (Fig. 3.8). It can occur as a complication of vigorous resuscitation or accidentally during a procedure involving venous or arterial access. If the diagnosis is suspected as a contributing cause of death, the pathologist should take

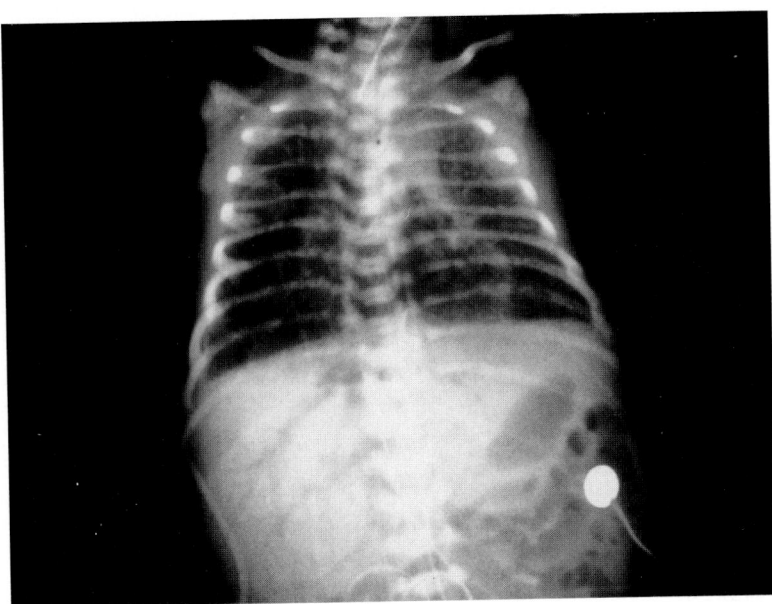

FIGURE 3.8.   *Gas emboli involving the heart and major blood vessels. (Courtesy of Dr. B Waters.)*

postmortem x-rays prior to the autopsy to further document the process.

Bronchopulmonary Dysplasia

Bronchopulmonary dysplasia (BPD) has become a general term for a variety of chronic lung diseases developing in preterm infants who are treated with mechanical ventilation for RDS [198]. The term *bronchopulmonary dysplasia* was coined by Northway et al [199] in 1967. The infants in their study were more mature and larger at birth than many survivors of RDS today. Two recent clinical definitions of BPD have been suggested. In the first, the diagnosis of BPD is made in an infant who requires positive-pressure ventilation in the first week of life and has clinical signs of chronic respiratory disease, an oxygen requirement, and an abnormal chest x-ray film at 28 days of age [200]. In the second, BPD is diagnosed by a persistent requirement of oxygen at 36 weeks' postconceptual age [201].

The microscopic features of BPD evolve from an early exudative/reparative stage, to a subacute and fibroproliferative stage, and a final chronic stage characterized by marked interstitial fibrosis with smooth muscle proliferation and vascular wall thickening. The lung with end-stage BPD reveals a cobbled-appearing pleural surface. Alternating areas of atelectasis and emphysema are striking. The cut surface is firm and has a honeycomb appearance. Large and small dilated air spaces can be intermixed. Fibrous bands are felt and seen.

Atrophy of the Diaphragmatic Muscle

Babies who require prolonged mechanical ventilation develop a form of disuse atrophy of the muscles of respiration, especially the diaphragm. This may contribute to difficulties in weaning infants from mechanical ventilators [202].

Extracorporeal Membrane Oxygenation

Extracorporeal membrane oxygenation (ECMO) is used in infants with respiratory failure complicated by pulmonary hypertension and significant extrapulmonary right-to-left shunting of blood. These infants have severe hypoxemia that persists despite conventional medical therapy.

ECMO is similar to cardiovascular-pulmonary bypass procedures used in adults. Surgical access to the circulation is established through the internal jugular vein (Fig. 3.9). The infant's venous blood is pumped through a membrane oxygenator where oxygen is added and carbon dioxide is removed. The blood is then pumped back into the patient's venous (venovenous ECMO) or arterial circulation (venoarterial ECMO) [203]. In venoarterial ECMO, during removal of the cannula, the internal carotid artery is ligated. For this reason, venovenous ECMO is becoming more widely used. The procedure allows the lungs to rest and averts continuous high-pressure mechanical ventilation in severe respiratory failure. During ECMO, the lungs continue to function at a low volume and pressure to prevent atelectasis and to maintain minimal alveolar ventilation, but the baby is entirely dependent on the membrane for oxygenation and removal of carbon dioxide.

ECMO is currently used primarily for critically ill full-term newborns with reversible respiratory failure who have failed maximal medical management. The selection criteria for ECMO entry are summarized in Table 3.8.

Diseases that have been treated by ECMO include meconium aspiration syndrome, congenital diaphragmatic hernia, persistent pulmonary hypertension (usually secondary to meconium aspiration, severe asphyxia, or severe hyaline membrane disease), cardiac failure after open heart surgery, intractable respiratory distress syndrome, and sepsis/pneumonia. The results have been encouraging. In larger babies with meconium aspiration syndrome, the mortality

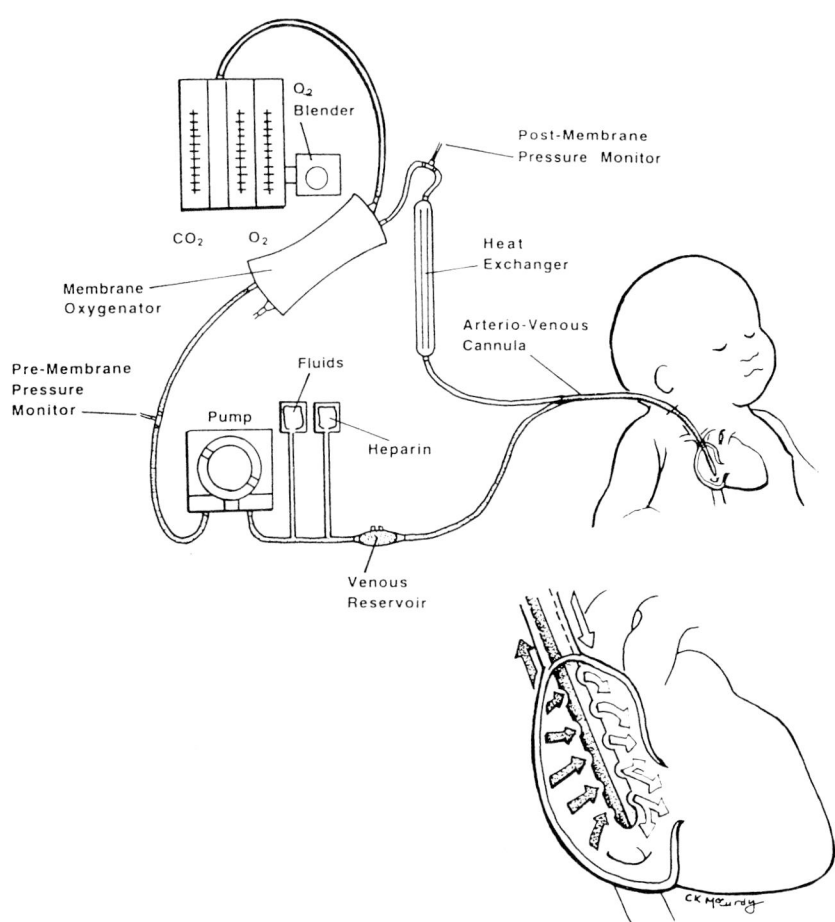

FIGURE 3.9. *Components of the veno-venous extracorporeal membrane oxygenation (ECMO) circuit. (Modified from Short [203]).*

Table 3.8. Selection criteria for neonatal ECMO

Gestational age >34 weeks
Birth weight >2000 grams
Ventilated for <10 days
No intraventricular hemorrhage
Oxygenation index (mean arterial pressure $\times$ FiO$_2$ [%]/postductal oxygen tension [mm Hg]) >40 or intractable CO$_2$ retention
Treatable primary diagnosis

Table 3.9. Mortality with ECMO treatment

Diseases	%
Meconium aspiration syndrome	5
RDS/HMD with PPHN	20
Pneumonia/sepsis	23
Diaphragmatic hernia	48

RDS = respiratory distress syndrome; HMD = hyaline membrane disease; PPHN = persistent pulmonary hypertension of the newborn.
Data from Kanto [204].

significantly dropped with ECMO treatment. The mortality rates in different diseases are summarized in Table 3.9 [204].

Complications are multiple and mainly related to hemorrhage [205]. Data from 7600 neonates entered into the Neonatal ECMO Registry are summarized in Table 3.10 [204]. Evans et al [206] described pathological complications of non-survivors of neonatal ECMO. Hemorrhagic complications were common, and sepsis occurred in 6 of the 12 cases (Table 3.11). Vogler et al [207] described thromboemboli in 22 of 23 infants who died after ECMO. Aluminum emboli were seen in 12 infants and involved multiple organs except the lungs. They suggested that this was a complication of the aluminum heat-exchanger units used in the

process, and the manufacturer subsequently corrected the problem.

Phototherapy and Transillumination

Phototherapy is used in mildly or moderately jaundiced infants. It is an effective means of lowering serum bilirubin concentration, and its use reduces the risks of exchange transfusions [208, 209]. Although considered one of the safest therapeutic techniques used in the NICU, certain issues need to be discussed.

Table 3.10.   Complications associated with neonatal ECMO

Complications	%*
Mechanical problems	
Clots in circuit	19
Problems with cannulae	9
Air in circuit	5
Oxygenator failure	4
Cracks in connectors	3
Other mechanical failures	6
Patient-related problems	
Hemorrhage from different sites	23
Cranial infarct and/or hemorrhage	17
Seizures	14
Dialysis	13
Hypertension	11
Blood creatinine >1.5 mg/dL	10
Hemolysis	9
Hyperbilirubinemia	6
Infection/sepsis	6
Other	6

* More than one complication occurred in the same patient.
Data from Kanto [204].

Table 3.11.   Autopsy findings in neonates who died during or after ECMO (n = 12)

Findings	Neonates*
Hemorrhage	
Lungs	6
Cerebellum	4
Cerebrum	3
Kidneys	1
Stomach	1
Pericardium (occurred before ECMO)	1
Sepsis	6
Periventricular leukomalacia	5
Myocardial ischemia	3
Thrombi	2
Endothelial damage at the site of cannulation	2
Necrotizing enterocolitis (occurred before ECMO)	1

* More than one lesion seen in the same neonate.
Data from Evans et al [206].

Exposure of cells to light intensities similar to those used in phototherapy can produce DNA strand breaks [210], sister chromatid exchanges, and mutations [211]. Bilirubin acts as a photosensitizing agent, enhancing DNA damage in cells exposed to phototherapy in vitro. However, bilirubin is a weak photosensitizer, and there is no evidence of photodynamic damage in babies receiving phototherapy. If abnormal levels of endogenous or exogenous photosensitizing pigments are present, as in some porphyrias, phototherapy is contraindicated [212].

Phototherapy has significant effects on hyperalimentation. The exposure of amino acid solutions to blue light produces reductions in tryptophan. In addition, when a multivitamin solution is added to the amino acids, a reduction in methionine and histidine occurs in association with decreased levels of riboflavin [213, 214]. Studies with several animal species have demonstrated potential toxic effects of light on the retina. In monkeys, all the experimentally exposed retinas showed some loss of rod and cone cells when compared with the controls. These changes represent a form of premature aging of the retina [215].

Infants with cholestatic jaundice who receive phototherapy may develop a dark gray-brown discoloration of the skin, serum, and urine [216, 217]. This is called the "bronze baby syndrome." The brown color probably results from the phototransformation of copper porphyrins subsequent to an electron transfer between photoexcited bilirubin and copper ion [218].

Other complications of phototherapy include watery diarrhea [219], poor weight gain, decrease in the luteinizing hormone [220], burns [221], late closure of the ductus arteriosus [222], and hypocalcemia.

Human, animal, and in vitro studies suggest that the products of photodecomposition have no direct neurotoxic effects [223].

Transillumination

Transillumination is used for non-invasive detection of air- or space-occupying lesions in semitransparent, hollow locations. Most commonly, it is used to diagnose pneumothorax, pneumoperitoneum, pneumopericardium, hydrocephaly, and hydranencephaly. Cases of focal burns have been described with transillumination light sources [224].

Hypothermia and Hyperthermia

The newborn infant must be kept warm and dry to prevent heat loss and its consequences. In a neutral thermal environment, the least amount of oxygen consumption and metabolic expenditure is needed for the infant to maintain a normal body temperature. Preterm infants are predisposed to heat loss because they have less subcutaneous fat, an increased ratio of surface area to body weight, and reduced glycogen and brown fat stores. Mechanisms of heat loss in the newborn include radiation, conduction, convection, and evaporation. Hypothermia causes grave consequences. Hypoglycemia develops secondary to depletion of glycogen stores. Metabolic acidosis occurs by peripheral vasoconstriction with anaerobic metabolism and acidosis. Hypoxia with increasing oxygen demand and decreased growth is seen with increased metabolic rate. Clotting disorders and pulmonary hemorrhage have been described in protracted hypothermia. Shock, apnea, bradycardia, and intraventricular hemorrhage have been reported.

Acrocyanosis, Cutis Marmorata, Sclerema Neonatorum

Other well-described entities are associated with a cold environment. These are acrocyanosis, cutis marmorata, and sclerema neonatorum. *Acrocyanosis,* blue hands and feet, is usually transient, but severe circulatory compromise can occur in the extremities after prolonged exposure. Mottling or a lacy red pattern may be seen in a normal infant or with cold stress, hypovolemia, or sepsis. If the mottling persists, it is called *cutis marmorata* [224a]. Persistent cutis marmorata can occur in other conditions such as trisomies 21 and 18 and de Lange syndromes. Sclerema neonatorum more commonly affects the preterm or severely debilitated infant. It has a similar etiology and adipose tissue findings as in fat necrosis. Cold stress alone can produce this injury.

Hyperthermia can cause several problems in the neonate including tachycardia, tachypnea, irritability, apnea, periodic breathing, dehydration, acidosis, brain damage, and death.

Traumatic and Other Skin Lesions

The skin of preterm infants is fragile and is vulnerable to mishandling (Fig. 3.10). Adhesive tapes and probe and electrode patches easily damage the skin. Local and systemic infections such as scalded skin syndrome and sepsis have

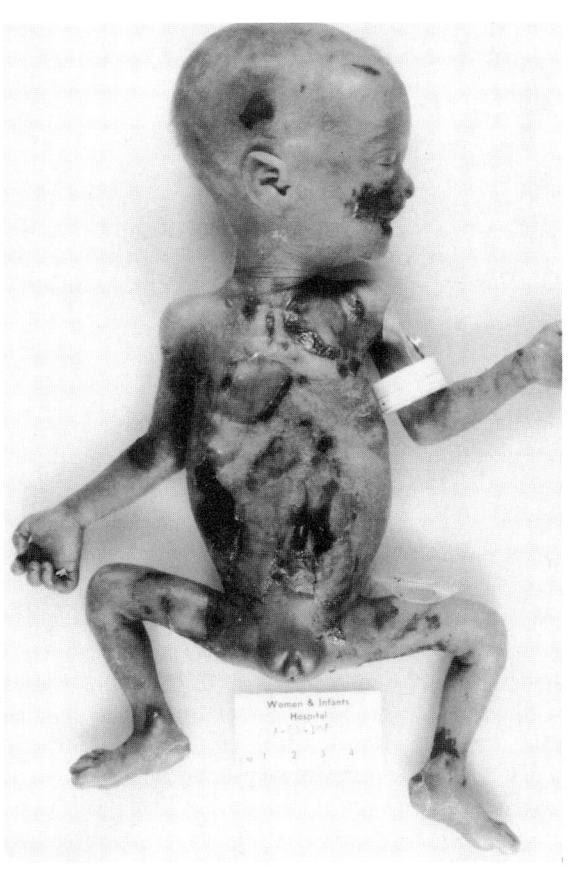

FIGURE 3.10.   *Multiple areas of skin excoriation in a preterm infant after 7 days of intensive care. (Courtesy of Dr. DB Singer.)*

been described [225]. Large areas of denudation cause loss of fluid, protein, and blood. Now available are sheet skin barriers that cover large surface areas or hydrogel adhesive, which can be removed easily with water.

Scalded Skin Syndrome

Scalded skin syndrome (Ritter disease, staphylococcal toxic epidermal necrolysis) is a bullous and exfoliative disorder caused by phage group II *S. aureus,* which may be a nosocomial infection. Tenderness, erythema, Nikolsky's sign, and shedding of the skin are clinical findings. Bullae develop through the granular layer where desmosomes are destroyed. Minimal inflammatory changes develop initially in the epidermis and dermis. Healing occurs without scarring [225].

PHARMACOLOGICAL AGENTS USED IN THE NEWBORN

Many and various medications are used in the NICU. Since the pharmacodynamics and metabolism of the commonly used medications are different in the neonatal age group, the side effects also may be different. The adverse effects of some of the most commonly used medications are listed in Table 3.12.

FLUID, ELECTROLYTE THERAPY, AND NUTRITION

Protein-Calorie Undernutrition

Although protein-calorie undernutrition or protein-energy malnutrition (PEM) is a major problem in the developing world, in this age of careful and scientific enteral and total parenteral nutrition (TPN), it is rarely seen in the intensive care nursery [228, 229]. Most cases of PEM are subtle and rapidly corrected. Full-term newborns' caloric requirements are approximately 120 kcal/kg/day. Low-birth-weight and very-low-birth-weight infants' caloric requirements are even higher. When the babies are sick, it may be difficult to provide these requirements, and low-level PEM can be seen.

Although the morphological features of PEM have been described in studies performed in the developing world, the pathologic changes are similar in the infants who die after a protracted course in the nursery.

The liver may have fatty change. Atrophy of the villi and the microvilli develops in the small intestine. Mitoses are absent in the epithelium of the crypts. The bone marrow is often hypoplastic with decreased erythroid precursors. Cerebral atrophy and impaired myelinization of the white matter develop in the central nervous system. Thymic and lymph node atrophy are noted [229].

Hypovitaminoses

Since nutritional demands of the preterm infants are significant, failure to provide the essential nutrients is a significant cause of morbidity. One of the most common problems

Table 3.12.   Adverse reactions of commonly used medications in the NICU

Drugs	Adverse reactions
Acetaminophen	Hepatic necrosis with overdosage; rash, fever, blood dyscrasias (neutropenia, pancytopenia, leukopenia, thrombocytopenia); may be hepatotoxic with chronic use
Acyclovir	Transient elevation of serum creatinine, thrombocytosis, jitters, rash, and hives
Albumin (human)	Rapid infusion may cause vascular overload and congestive heart failure; hypersensitivity reactions include chills, fever, nausea, and urticaria
Aminoglycosides	Ototoxicity and nephrotoxicity
Amphotericin B	Fever, chills, vomiting; thrombophlebitis at injection sites; renal tubular acidosis, renal failure; hypomagnesemia, hypokalemia; bone marrow suppression with reversible decline in hematocrit; hypotension, hypertension, wheezing, and hypoxemia
Ampicillin	Rubella-like rash and eosinophilia
Atropine sulfate	Xerostomia, blurred vision, mydriasis, tachycardia, palpitations, constipation, urinary retention, ataxia, tremor, and hyperthermia
Caffeine citrate	Nausea, vomiting, gastric irritation, agitation, tachycardia, diuresis, tonic-clonic seizures, and arrhythmias
Calcium chloride and calcium gluconate	Arrhythmias and deterioration of cardiovascular function; extravasation causes skin sloughing
Cephalosporins	Allergic reactions including fever, rash, urticaria; may also cause leukopenia, thrombocytopenia, eosinophilia, positive Coombs' test, renal failure, cholelithiasis, and hepatic toxicity
Cimetidine	Diarrhea, rash, myalgia, confusion, neutropenia, gynecomastia, and elevated liver function tests
Clindamycin	Pseudomembranous colitis, Stevens-Johnson syndrome, granulocytopenia, thrombocytopenia, and sterile abscess at the injection site
Cortisone acetate	Glucose intolerance, Cushing's syndrome, pituitary-adrenal suppression, edema, hypertension, cataracts, hypokalemia, and skin atrophy
Ergocalciferol	Hypercalcemia, weakness, diarrhea, polyuria, metastatic calcification, and nephrocalcinosis
Furosemide (Lasix)	Ototoxicity, hypokalemia, alkalosis, dehydration, hyperuricemia, and nephrocalcinosis
Ganciclovir	Antiviral medication against cytomegalovirus; causes retinal detachment, neutropenia, and thrombocytopenia
Heparin sodium	Bleeding, allergic reactions, thrombocytopenia, alopecia
Indomethacin	Decreased platelet aggregation, gastrointestinal ulcers, necrotizing enterocolitis, nausea, diarrhea, and blood dyscrasias; nephrotoxic
Phenobarbital	Sedation, lethargy, gastrointestinal distress, ataxia, and rash
Phenytoin	Gingival hyperplasia, hirsutism, dermatitis, blood dyscrasias, ataxia, systemic lupus erythematosus, and Stevens-Johnson–like syndromes, lymphadenopathy, liver damage, and nystagmus
Prostaglandin E$_1$	Cutaneous vasodilatation, seizure-like activity, jitteriness, hyperthermia, hypocalcemia, apnea, thrombocytopenia, hypotension
Ribavirin	Rash, conjunctivitis, hypotension, and anemia
Sodium polystyrene sulfonate	Used as an enema for treatment of hyperkalemia; may cause fecal impaction and rectal ulcerations
Surfactant (Beractant)	Most frequent adverse effects are associated with administration of the surfactant to the infant and include transient bradycardia, oxygen desaturation, and apnea; may be associated with increased incidence of intraventricular and pulmonary hemorrhage
Theophylline	Hyperglycemia, diuresis, dehydration, feeding intolerance, tachyarrhythmias, hyperreflexia, and seizures
Tolazoline	Used for treatment of persistent pulmonary hypertension; causes tachycardia, nausea, vomiting, gastrointestinal bleeding, hypotension, thrombocytopenia, and agranulocytosis
Tromethamine (Tham)	Used for refractory acidosis; causes respiratory depression, thrombophlebitis, venospasm, and electrolyte disturbances; extravasation causes sloughing of the skin
Vancomycin	Ototoxicity, nephrotoxicity, and allergic reactions. "Red man syndrome" (i.e., rash, chills, and fever) can occur.

Data from Marx and Cronin [226] and Roberts [227].

encountered in this age group is hypovitaminoses. This is reviewed in detailed by several authors [230–232].

Vitamin A
Multiple compounds have vitamin A activity; the most important and active is retinol. Its derivatives, such as retinal and retinoic acid, also have some vitamin A activity. Carotenoids, which are vitamin A precursors, also have important metabolic roles. Among these, beta carotene is the most well known [233].

Functions of vitamin A include maintenance of specialized, mainly mucus-secreting epithelia, providing critical prosthetic groups in the retinal pigment, enhancing immunity to infections, and acting as an antioxidant.

Preterm infants, particularly those who are critically ill, have low vitamin A levels. This is a result of their missing the last trimester of placental transfer and is compounded by the fact that vitamin A adheres to plastic tubing when added to the TPN solution [234].

Vitamin A deficiency is characterized by reduced wound healing, increased squamous metaplasia in the respiratory tract, increased incidence of infection, night blindness, and xerophthalmia [235] (Fig. 3.11). In 1985, Shenai et al [236] showed that infants with bronchopulmonary dysplasia (BPD) had lower plasma vitamin A levels than those with no lung disease. Giving vitamin A supplements decreased the incidence of BPD [237].

Vitamin D
Dietary vitamin D is derived from plants as ergosterol (D$_2$) and from animals as cholecalciferol (D$_3$). In animals and humans, D$_3$ can be synthesized endogenously in the skin

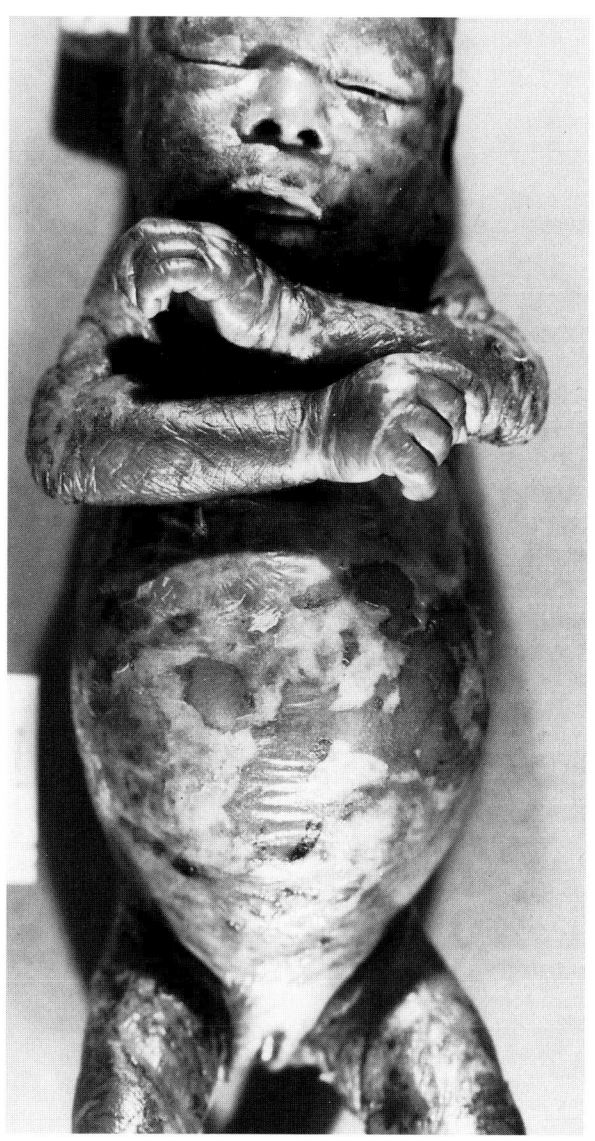

FIGURE 3.11. *Infant with skin changes of vitamin A deficiency following total parenteral nutrition for 3 weeks. (Courtesy of Dr. DB Singer.)*

after exposure to ultraviolet (UV) light. In the liver, vitamin D is 25 hydroxylated to 25-hydroxyvitamin D (25 OHD). In the proximal tubular cells of the kidney, 25 OHD is hydroxylated further to $1,25(OH)_2D$, which is the most active vitamin D metabolite. It exerts its action through modulation of the cellular genome by binding to specific nuclear receptors in numerous cell types. Through this mechanism $1,25(OH)_2D$ affects cell growth, differentiation, and immune and endocrine functions. Calcium homeostasis and bone mineralization are maintained by $1,25(OH)_2D$ primarily by increasing vitamin D–dependent calcium absorption through the gut.

Deficiency of vitamin D causes rickets and hypocalcemia in the newborn [238, 239]. Clinical findings in neonatal rickets include rachitic rosaries; enlargement of the wrists, knees, and ankles; and frontal bossing. Fractures may be the presenting symptom [240]. The soft rib cage, fractures, and respiratory muscle weakness may result in late respiratory distress [241].

The most important radiological finding of the skeletal system is cupping of the ends of tubular bones, which is especially noticeable at the lower end of the ulna. Similar cupping occurs much later in the radius and other bones.

Physeal growth zones are widened and thickened with irregular vascular invasion, poor removal of cartilage, and persistent hypertrophic chondrocytes in the zone of provisional ossification (metaphysis). The abnormal large cellular metaphyseal cartilage columns are surrounded by broad osteoid seams. This abnormal zone is the widened rachitic metaphysis. The cortex and the cancellous bone of the shaft also show abnormal remodeling with poor mineralization.

Vitamin E

Vitamin E refers to several chemically related compounds classified generically as tocopherols. Alpha-tocopherol is the primary, naturally occurring member of this group. Vitamin E functions as an antioxidant, and this is the rationale for clinical administration to premature neonates. Vitamin E concentrations in many preterm neonates are significantly low at birth. Animal studies suggest that vitamin E protects against oxidant injury to the lung and eye [242]. Initial favorable effects of vitamin E on BPD and retinopathy of prematurity (ROP) were not confirmed in subsequent studies. In one study, not only was there no significant change in the incidence of ROP but an increased incidence of necrotizing enterocolitis and retinal hemorrhages was found [243].

Vitamin E deficiency was first described in 1967 by Oski [244], who found preterm infants with an anemia unresponsive to iron, high reticulocyte counts, increased hydrogen peroxide hemolysis, and puffy feet. With the advent of balanced TPN and supplementation, vitamin E deficiency became extremely rare. The main problem with vitamin E is the tragedy that occurred in the early years of 1980s. After preliminary data suggested that the antioxidant effect of vitamin E might be useful in BPD and ROP, it became fashionable to supplement the preterm infants with vitamin E. In addition to oral supplements, some centers empirically started to use a parenteral version of vitamin E. In 1984 and 1985, a new symptom complex emerged and included pulmonary deterioration, thrombocytopenia, liver failure, ascites, and renal failure leading to death in some cases [245–248]. These symptoms were attributed to a specific brand of alpha-tocopherol acetate, E-Ferol (distributed by O'Neill, Jones and Feldman Pharmaceuticals, St. Louis, MO), which was administered intravenously. This syndrome disappeared after the use of E-Ferol was discontinued. It was never completely clear whether the toxicity was due to alpha-tocopherol, the polysorbate emulsifiers, or an unknown contaminant [249, 250]. Sepsis, necrotizing enterocolitis, and intraventricular hemorrhage also have been attributed to treatment of neonates with vitamin E [251]. The Committee on Fetus and Newborn concluded that pharmacologic doses of vitamin E should be regarded as experimental and not routinely indicated for infants weighing less than 1500 grams [252].

Vitamin K

Vitamin K is a cofactor necessary for the gamma-carboxylation of a prothrombin precursor to active prothrombin [253, 254]. In the absence of vitamin K, this precursor (proteins induced by vitamin K absence [PIVKA]) can be detected in the plasma. Relative to adults, normal newborns are vitamin K deficient [255]. Significant vitamin K deficiency causes late hemorrhagic disease of the newborn.

Babies born to mothers who are on anticonvulsant medications (recall the mnemonic "3 Ps": phenytoin, phenobarbital, primidone) are at particularly high risk of having vitamin K deficiency [256] or *early hemorrhagic disease of the newborn.*

Other Deficiencies

Iron Deficiency

Iron deficiency has remained one of the most common causes of anemia in infancy and childhood despite widespread availability of iron-fortified formulas, hyperalimentation solutions, supplements, and cereals. Although a full-term infant is born with adequate iron reserves, these stores begin to be depleted at about 4 months of age and "physiologic iron deficiency" appears at 6 to 9 months [257].

Low-birth-weight neonates are born with inadequate iron stores. Excessive blood sampling of these infants further depletes their iron stores and speeds the development of iron-deficiency anemia. Iron supplements are important in this groups of infants. The American Academy of Pediatrics currently recommends that iron supplements of 2 mg/kg/day be started in all preterm infants by the age of 2 months [258]. Although iron supplementation does not affect the development of early physiologic anemia, meta-analysis of controlled studies shows significant reductions in the incidence of iron-deficiency anemia at 6 and 11 months of age [259]. Recent studies suggest that iron supplementation for the extremely preterm infant should be started at 2 weeks of age [260]. Higher doses up to 4 mg/kg/day should be given. Neonates who are on recombinant human erythropoietin should also be on higher doses of iron supplementation [261].

In progressive iron deficiency, a series of events occurs. First, the stainable iron in the bone marrow disappears. Next, serum iron decreases and serum iron-binding capacity increases; percent saturation falls below normal. If iron is still not available, free erythrocyte protoporphyrins increase. During these changes, peripheral smears are characteristic of iron-deficiency anemia. Microcytosis, hypochromia, poikilocytosis, and, in some cases, thrombocytosis occurs. Bone marrow findings are also typical. Bone marrow is markedly hypocellular and is composed of empty marrow spaces filled with fat, fibrous stroma, and clusters of lymphocytes and plasma cells. In less extreme cases, occasional red cell precursors are seen. Iron stains are negative.

Essential Fatty Acid Deficiency

Dietary polyunsaturated fatty acids (PUFA) have long been considered a necessary component of dietary lipids. In addition to providing energy for growth, cellular metabolism, and muscle activity, some PUFAs also are regarded as essential fatty acids (EFAs) because they serve as precursors of eicosanoids, such as prostaglandins, prostacyclins, thromboxanes, and leukotrienes. During the past two decades, attention has focused on the role of omega-3 PUFAs in the prevention of cardiovascular disease, regulation of blood pressure, and modulation of platelet function and immunologic status. The role of dietary omega-3 fatty acids during the perinatal period was recently recognized. Several studies have shown that these key nutrients are essential for the promotion of fetal growth, reactivity of uterine and placental vascular tone, initiation of labor and delivery, and development of neonatal brain and visual function [262–265].

In 1929, the first EFA deficiency was described in rats on a fat-free diet. When given fat, symptoms of skin rash and growth delay disappeared [266]. It was not until the introduction of fat-free parenteral nutrition that typical symptoms in neonates were seen. It is now apparent that two PUFAs, linoleic acid (omega-6 18:2) and alpha-linolenic acid (omega-3 18:3), are essential for the preterm infant and that deficiency of the latter is subtle. Linoleic acid elongates and saturates to become the precursor of arachidonic acid; linolenic acid is metabolized to eicosapentaenoic acid (EPA) and docohexaenoic acid (DHA) by the same mechanism. In addition to the roles that were described above, EPA and DHA may provide structure to the phospholipid layer, influencing important membrane functions [267]. DHA and EPA are present in breast milk; formula-fed infants' levels slowly decrease with time [268]. The American Academy of Pediatrics suggests that 3% of energy intake should be linoleic acid [269]. Intralipid solutions that supplement the parenteral hyperalimentation and new formulas and formula additives meet this requirement.

Clinical EFA deficiency commonly is related to a combined deficiency of linolenic and linoleic acids. The clinical signs of this syndrome include poor growth, dermatitis, hypopigmentation, hypotonia, increased metabolic rate, impaired water balance, increased fragility and permeability of cell membranes, electroencephalographic and electrocardiographic changes, and increased susceptibility to infections [270].

Linoleic acid deficiency in rats causes scaling of the skin, alopecia, and injury to renal and testicular tubular epithelium. Newborns fed on a formula containing less than 0.1%

of calories as linoleic acid failed to grow and developed scaly skin changes [229].

Trace Elements

Zinc Zinc is an essential nutrient for growth and development, and it plays a major role in bone structure and as a metalloenzyme [271]. Over 200 zinc metalloenzymes have been identified and are associated with carbohydrate and energy metabolism, protein catabolism and synthesis, nucleic acid synthesis, heme biosynthesis, and many other vital reactions. Under normal circumstances, zinc homeostasis appears to be maintained primarily by changes in the fecal excretion of endogenous zinc through bile, pancreatic secretions, mucosal sloughing of epithelial cells, and dietary factors that influence the fractional absorption of zinc. The primary route of excretion of endogenous zinc is via feces, with smaller quantities being excreted in the urine. Parenterally fed infants excrete zinc via the kidneys.

Zinc deficiency in formula-fed newborns is very rare. Very-low-birth-weight infants on parenteral hyperalimentation deficient in zinc develop zinc deficiency. Therapeutic use of dexamethasone impairs normal zinc absorption and storage, thus causing zinc deficiency [272].

Acute zinc deficiency causes growth failure, diminished food intake, skin lesions, poor wound healing, hair loss, decreased protein synthesis, and depressed immune function. Severe zinc deficiency is relatively easy to diagnose because of the severity of the clinical and biochemical presentation. In addition to the findings described, plasma zinc levels and alkaline phosphatase activity are usually below normal. Zinc deficiency in rats causes corneal vascularization, alopecia, keratinization of the skin and esophagus, and finally death in a few weeks.

Copper Copper, like zinc, is an essential constituent of many enzymes. Of special importance are the copper-dependent oxidative enzymes, including cytochrome oxidase, the terminal oxidase in the electron transport chain. The most abundant copper-containing enzymes are the superoxide dismutase enzymes, which are involved in protection of cell membranes against oxidative damage. Ceruloplasmin, a weak oxidase, comprises about 60% of the copper in plasma and interstitial fluids; its main function is copper transport. Copper deficiency can lead to anemia because ceruloplasmin also plays a role in iron transport from hepatic storage sites to transferrin and may be necessary for the seroconversion of ferric to ferrous iron prior to attachment of iron to transferrin.

Copper deficiency has been reported in infants fed primarily cows' milk–based formula [273] and in infants fed copper-free parenteral formulation [274]. Several cases of neonatal copper deficiency were reported in the 1980s [274, 275]. The principal features of copper deficiency are hypochromic, microcytic anemia unresponsive to iron therapy, neutropenia, osteoporosis of the metaphysis, and retarded bone age.

Selenium Although selenium deficiency has been described infrequently in infants, selenium is recognized as a nutritionally essential trace element [276]. Its only established physiologic function is an integral part of the selenium-dependent enzyme glutathione peroxidase. The type I iodothyronine 5′-deiodinase enzyme is a recently identified selenozyme [277]. Selenium and vitamin E have overlapping functions. Selenium, through glutathione peroxidase, is involved in cell membrane protection from peroxidase damage through detoxification of peroxides and free radicals.

Selenium deficiency has been described in infants and adults receiving selenium-free parenteral nutrition [278]. Clinical manifestations of selenium deficiency include color changes in skin and hair (pseudoalbinism) [279], macrocytosis [279], and biochemical and functional abnormalities of red cells and granulocytes [278]. Myositis, characterized by pain, tenderness, and increasing weakness, has been reported to improve in one child and three adults upon selenium supplementation [279]. Severe, often fatal, cardiomyopathy has been described in a few adults and children [280].

Other Trace Elements Although other trace elements [281], such as chromium, molybdenum, and manganese have important metabolic and biochemical roles, their deficiency states have not been well defined in the newborn. In one study, magnesium deficiency has been associated with spasms of umbilical vessels in the newborn [282]. Molybdenum deficiency was described by Arnold et al [283], and neonatal convulsions were attributed to this deficiency by Slot et al [284].

Tube Feedings

Tube feedings can be administered with nasogastric, orogastric, transpyloric, or gastrostomy tubes. Hazards of nasogastric and orogastric tubes include partial airway obstruction, increased airway resistance, and incompetence of the esophagocardiac sphincter when the tubes are in place. Additional complications are excessive nasal secretions, bacterial and fungal colonization with indwelling tubes, ulceration or perforation of the nasal septum, malplacement into the trachea, and perforation of the esophagus and stomach. Nasogastric tubes are more stable in position, but orogastric tubes cause less airway obstruction.

Transpyloric continuous feedings have been introduced to improve the tolerance of the very-low-birth-weight infants to enteral feedings. Although better growth in these infants has been reported, impaired assimilation of fat and potassium [285] and increased bacterial contamination of the jejunum have been documented [286]. A few cases of duodenal and jejunal perforations, midgut volvulus, and necrotizing enterocolitis have occurred [287].

Gastrostomy

The rate of major complications of gastrostomy in infants is between 2.5% and 5.8% [288]. Complications include intra-abdominal leaks with peritonitis, leaks around the tube requiring surgical closure, and bleeding. Minor complications occur at a rate of 4.3–10.8% and include leaks not requiring surgery, delayed closure, and displacement of tube. The mortality rates directly attributed to gastrostomy reported in old studies were between 0.4% and 4.7% [288, 289]. The current incidence is probably lower.

Total Parenteral Nutrition

Parenteral nutrition of the critically ill newborn has been in use for over 20 years. It is indicated for preterm or term infants who cannot receive enteral feedings in acute or chronic disease. In its most recent form, it is composed of 2–4% protein and 15–20% glucose, lipid, trace elements, and multivitamin solutions [290]. Complications of TPN include infections, catheter-related complications, metabolic complications, nutritional deficiencies, hepatobiliary lesions, and fat emulsion–related complications (Table 3.13).

Infection

Sepsis can occur in infants receiving central TPN. The most common organisms include coagulase-positive and coagulase-negative *Staphylococcus*, *Streptococcus viridans*, *Escherichia coli*, *Pseudomonas* spp, *Klebsiella* spp, and *Candida albicans*. Contamination of the central line can occur as a result of infection at the insertion site or of use of the line for blood sampling or administration of blood or blood products.

Catheter-Related Complications

Complications associated with placement of central catheters (especially the subclavian vein) occur in 4–9% of patients. Complications include pneumothorax, pneumomediastinum, hemorrhage, and chylothorax. Thrombosis of the vein adjacent to the catheter tip, resulting in "superior vena cava syndrome" (edema of the face, neck, and eyes), may be seen. Pulmonary embolism can occur secondary to thrombosis. Malpositioned catheters may result in collection of fluid in the pleural cavity causing hydrothorax, or in the pericardial space causing pericardial tamponade. (See Central Venous Access under Invasive Procedures above.)

Metabolic Complications

Hyperglycemia resulting from excessive intake or change in metabolic rate such as infections can occur. Hypoglycemia from sudden cessation of infusion can be seen. Azotemia from excessive intake of protein solutions, hyperammonemia, abnormal serum and tissue amino acid pattern, and metabolic alkalosis are some of the metabolic complications that can be seen with TPN.

Nutritional Deficiencies

If TPN is administered without fat emulsions, deficiency of essential fatty acids occurs. This deficiency is associated with

decreased platelet aggregation (thromboxane A_2 deficiency), thrombocytopenia, poor weight gain, scaly rash, and sparse hair growth [291].

Since most of the minerals are normally transferred to the fetus during the last trimester of pregnancy, if the

Table 3.13. Complications of total parenteral nutrition (TPN)

Infection
  Sepsis
  Infection at the insertion site
Placement-related complications
  Pneumothorax
  Pneumomediastinum
  Hemorrhage
  Chylothorax
  Thrombosis
  Pulmonary embolism
  Hydrothorax
  Pericardial tamponade
Metabolic complications
  Hyperglycemia
  Hypoglycemia
  Azotemia
  Hyperammonemia
  Abnormal serum and tissue amino acid pattern
  Metabolic alkalosis
Nutritional deficiencies
  Essential fatty acid deficiency
    Decreased platelet aggregation
    Thrombocytopenia
    Poor weight gain
    Scaly rash
    Sparse hair growth
  Osteopenia
  Rickets
  Pathologic fractures
  Zinc deficiency
    Poor growth
    Diarrhea
    Alopecia
    Increased susceptibility to infections
    Acrodermatitis enteropathica
Hepatobiliary lesions
  Cholestatic hepatitis
  Hepatic steatosis
  Bile duct proliferation
  Hepatocellular damage
  Cirrhosis
  Hepatocellular carcinoma
  Gallbladder distention and cholelithiasis
Fat emulsion–related complications
  Elevation of serum triglycerides and free fatty acids
  Displacement of albumin-bound bilirubin by free fatty acids
  Decrease in pulmonary function
  Decrease in reticuloendothelial function
  Infection with *Malassezia furfur*

preterm neonate is not given mineral supplements, severe deficiencies can occur. Osteopenia, rickets, and pathologic fractures are common. Zinc deficiency may occur if zinc is not added to the TPN after 4 weeks. Infants with zinc deficiency present with poor growth, diarrhea, alopecia, increased susceptibility to infection, and skin desquamation around the mouth and anus (acrodermatitis enteropathica). Zinc losses increase in the presence of ileostomy or colostomy. Infants with copper deficiency present with osteoporosis, hemolytic anemia, neutropenia, and depigmentation of the skin.

Hepatobiliary Lesions

Continuous use of total parenteral nutrition causes significant hepatobiliary morbidity. This is reviewed by Goplerud and Quigley in detail [292, 293].

Cholestatic Hepatitis   Evidence of cholestasis develops in 30% of neonates on TPN. In most cases, this is transient but in some cases it progresses to hepatocellular damage, fibrosis, and finally cirrhosis. Liver histology reveals marked structural disorganization and hepatocellular and canalicular cholestasis. There may be mild fibrosis. The hepatocytes are often arranged in acinar fashion.

Hepatic Steatosis   TPN enhances hepatic fatty acid synthesis and decreases triglyceride secretion. This causes steatosis in the hepatocytes. This change is usually diffuse and reversible.

Bile Duct Proliferation   Prolonged TPN may cause marked bile duct proliferation. Bile plugs in these bile ducts can be seen. When this lesion occurs with fibrosis, an erroneous diagnosis of extrahepatic biliary atresia may be made.

Hepatocellular Damage   Long-term TPN administration may cause hepatocellular damage. The hepatocytes show ballooning degeneration with disorganization of liver cell plates and pseudoacinar transformation (Fig. 3.12). Sometimes giant cells can be seen.

Cirrhosis   In the lesions associated with TPN, varying degrees of fibrosis are seen. The fibrosis can form bridges between the portal tracts and can be marked. In final stages, cirrhosis can occur.

These hepatic lesions can occur separately, but frequently a mixture of all the described patterns is seen [294]. Histological features change with the duration of treatment. In early stages, canalicular cholestasis, periportal inflammation with occasional eosinophilic leukocytes, steatosis, and extramedullary hematopoiesis are seen. Later, fibrosis and cirrhosis are described (Table 3.14). Ultrastructural studies reveal increased collagen in the spaces of Disse, hypertrophy of the smooth endoplasmic reticulum, and dilatation of the bile canaliculi by plugs of inspissated bile.

Hepatocellular Carcinoma   Hepatocellular carcinoma has been described in a non-cirrhotic infant after prolonged parenteral nutrition [295].

Gallbladder Distention and Cholelithiasis   Distention of the gallbladder has been reported in infants on TPN (Fig. 3.13).

Table 3.14.   Histopathologic liver findings in infants according to duration of TPN

Duration of TPN (wks)	Histopathology
<2	Cholestasis
	Aggregates of macrophages
2–6	Marked cholestasis (zone 3 > zone 1)
8–12	Fibrosis
>12	Cirrhosis

Data from Mullick et al [294].

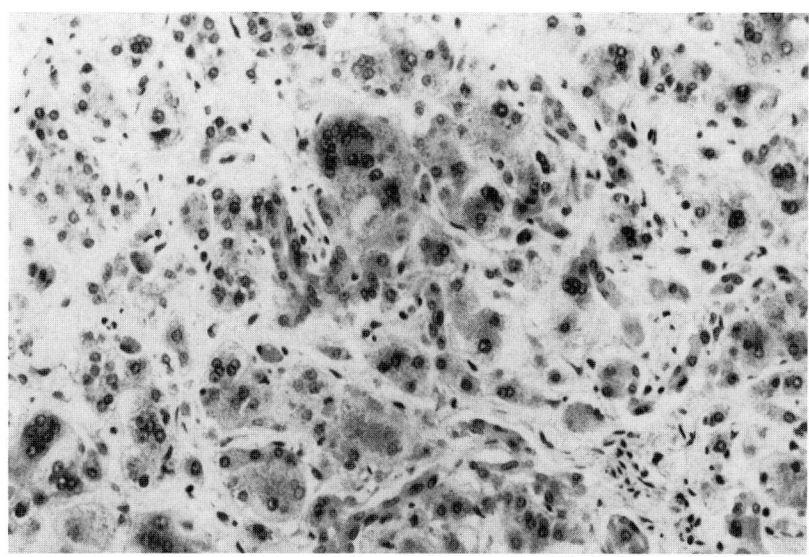

FIGURE 3.12.   *Distortion of architecture and hepatic fibrosis following total parenteral nutrition for 5 weeks, ×190. (Courtesy of Dr. DB Singer.)*

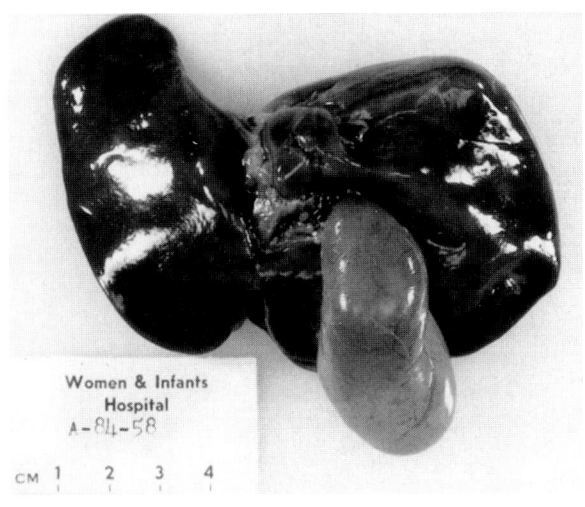

FIGURE 3.13.   *Gallbladder distention in an infant following 6 weeks of total parenteral nutrition.*

A predisposing factor in addition to TPN is lack of enteral feedings and consequent failure in the release of cholecystokinin [296]. Cholelithiasis has been described in infants on prolonged TPN. Risk factors include prolonged fasting, ileal disease, ileal resection, and exposure to opiates or anticholinergic drugs.

Fat Emulsion–related Complications

Fat emulsions are usually added to the parenteral nutrition of the newborns in the neonatal intensive care unit [297]. Usually 10% or 20% concentrations are used.

Elevation of triglycerides and free fatty acids occurs if an infant's ability to metabolize fat is exceeded. This may be due to developmental insufficiency of lipoprotein lipase or its activator.

Lipid emulsions have little effect on bilirubin binding to albumin, but the free fatty acids generated during hydrolysis of triglycerides compete for albumin. This creates problems when the infant who requires TPN also is icteric.

Lipid emulsions have deleterious effects on pulmonary function. Arterial Po_2 values decrease if lipid solution is infused during the first week of life. This drop in Po_2 may be due to changes in erythrocyte membrane structure or coating of the erythrocytes with lipid. Pulmonary blood flow can be reduced, possibly related to deposition of lipid in arterioles and capillaries or to release of prostaglandins. Fat embolism has occurred with high infusion rates.

Lipid-emulsion usage is associated with decreased reticuloendothelial function. Chylomicrons are taken up by the reticuloendothelial system of the liver, lung, and other organs, and may interfere with fighting infection, particularly in an immunocompromised infant. *Malassezia furfur* (*Pityrosporum orbiculare*) colonization evolves to pneumonia and sepsis in neonates with lipid emulsions and indwelling central catheters.

NOSOCOMIAL INFECTIONS

The nosocomial infections are mostly those associated with intensive care, e.g., liberal use of antimicrobial drugs and invasive therapies such as catheters in vessels, nasogastric and chest tubes, and surgical operations, among others.

Group B streptococcus, *E. coli*, *S. viridans*, *Proteus* spp, *Pseudomonas* spp, *Listeria monocytogenes*, *Serratia marcescens*, *Klebsiella pneumoniae*, *Streptococcus faecalis*, *Candida albicans*, *Hansenula anomala*, *Aspergillus*, *Malassezia furfur*, and a large variety of other infectious organisms have been isolated from typical cases [298–304].

The clinical features of nosocomial sepsis may be subtle. They include poor feeding, circumoral cyanosis, lethargy, hypotonia, and either fever or hypothermia. Meningitis is a common clinical manifestation; pneumonia and septicemia may also be noted.

Pneumonias in nosocomial sepsis may be due to a variety of organisms, each with its particular pattern of inflammation and repair. Thus, coagulase-positive *Staphylococcus* infection can produce abscesses and an intense pleural reaction or empyema. *Malassezia furfur* produces a localized indolent chronic infection in which lipid deposits are found in capillary and arterial endothelium [301, 302]. Organisms that invade and destroy blood vessel walls (e.g., *Pseudomonas* or *Aspergillus*) result in pulmonary infarcts, with hemorrhage and marginating inflammation. Lobar or bronchopneumonia may be clearly seen in nosocomial pneumonia due to any of the same infectious agents that produce a diffuse pneumonia or an extended aspiration pattern in early onset pneumonia [305, 306].

Other features of neonatal nosocomial sepsis include hepatic abscesses [307], otitis, facial cellulitis, and septic arthritis. Osteomyelitis has been reported in babies whose heels were traumatized by lancets during blood-drawing procedures [308]. Urinary tract infections, though rare in young infants, may occur in males up to 3 months of age, and are more apt to occur in females beyond that age [309]. Necrotizing enterocolitis, often associated with, if not the result of, infection, is commonly described as a nosocomial event [310–312]. Endocarditis may also be a nosocomial disease [313].

Table 3.15 summarizes selected outbreaks of nosocomial infections.

Table 3.15.   Selected outbreaks of nosocomial infections in newborn nurseries

Organism	Diseases	Mode of transmission
Bacteria		
Salmonella newport	Diarrhea	Infected nurse
Listeria monocytogenes	Sepsis, meningitis	Unknown
Proteus mirabilis	Sepsis, meningitis	Infected nurse
Pseudomonas aeruginosa	Eye infections	Resuscitation equipment
	Sepsis, pneumonia	? Hand carriage
Pseudomonas pickettii	Bacteremia	"Sterile" water for injection
Escherichia coli	Diarrhea	? Hand carriage
Serratia marcescens	Sepsis, meningitis, abscesses	Hand carriage, scalp needles
	Sepsis, meningitis	Scrub brushes
Enterobacteriaceae	Sepsis, meningitis, conjunctivitis	Unknown
Enterobacter cloacae	Bacteremia, pneumonia	Unknown
	Sepsis	Unknown
	Bacteremia	Enteral solutions
Enterobacter cloacae and *agglomerans*	Sepsis	Intravenous fluids
Klebsiella pneumoniae	Unspecified	Hand carriage
Staphylococcus epidermidis	Sepsis	Central venous catheters
Staphylococcus aureus	Sepsis, pneumonia, conjunctivitis	Hand carriage
	Impetigo, sepsis	Hand carriage
	Pneumonia, bacteremia, conjunctivitis, soft tissue abscesses	? Hand carriage
	Conjunctivitis	? Hand carriage
	Bacteremia, meningitis, osteomyelitis, abscesses	Unknown
Citrobacter diversus	Meningitis	Monitoring equipment
Enterococcus faecalis	Sepsis	Unknown
	Bacteremia, meningitis	Hand carriage
Campylobacter jejuni	Meningitis	Unknown
Group B streptococcus	Sepsis	Colonized personnel
Acinetobacter calcoaceticus	Bacteremia	Warm-air humidifiers
Viruses		
Influenza type A	Apnea, lethargy, pneumonia	Ill visitors and staff
Respiratory syncytial virus	Pneumonia, apnea	Ill visitors and staff
Rotavirus	Gastroenteritis	Hand carriage
Echovirus 11	Sepsis-like syndrome	Hospital personnel
Parainfluenza, type 3	Respiratory tract infection	Nursery personnel
Adenovirus, type 8	Upper respiratory infection, conjunctivitis	Unknown
Hepatitis A	Asymptomatic	Nursery personnel
Herpes simplex	Disseminated infection	Scalp electrodes
Fungi		
Malassezia furfur	Pneumonia	Infant-to-infant by personnel, and colonization of central catheters used in infusing intralipid solutions
Candida albicans	Fungemia	Contaminated syringes
Microsporum canis	Tinea capitis, tinea corporis	Infected nurse
Other		
Ureaplasma urealyticum	Pneumonia, osteomyelitis	Unknown

Data from Peter and Cashore [314].

REFERENCES

1. Briggs GG, Freeman RK, Yaffe SJ. *Drugs in Pregnancy and Lactation*, 3rd ed. Baltimore: Williams & Wilkins, 1990.
2. Gilstrap LC, Little BB. *Drugs and Pregnancy*. New York: Elsevier, 1992.
3. National Institute of Child Health and Human Development (NICHD) National Registry for Amniocentesis Study Group. Midtrimester amniocentesis for prenatal diagnosis: safety and accuracy. *JAMA* 1976; 236:1471–6.
4. Nimrod C, Varela-Gittings F, Machin G, et al. The effect of very prolonged membrane rupture on fetal development. *Am J Obstet Gynecol* 1984; 148:540–3.
5. Crane JP, Rohland BM. Clinical significance of persistent amniotic fluid leakage after genetic amniocentesis. *Prenat Diagn* 1986; 6:25–31.
6. Golbus MS, Stephens JD, Cann HM, et al. Rh isoimmunization following genetic amniocentesis. *Prenat Diagn* 1982; 2:149–56.
7. Murray JC, Karp LE, Williamson RA, et al. Rh isoimmunization as related to amniocentesis. *Am J Hum Genet* 1983; 16:527–34.

8. Hanson FW, Zorn EM, Tennant FR, et al. Amniocentesis before 15 weeks gestation: outcome, risks and technical problems. *Am J Obstet Gynecol* 1987; 156:1524–31.

9. Penso CA, Frigoletto FD. Early amniocentesis. *Semin Perinatol* 1990; 14:465–70.

10. Stripparo I, Buscaglia M, Longatii L, et al. Genetic amniocentesis: 505 cases performed before the sixteenth week of gestation. *Prenat Diagn* 1990; 10:359–64.

11. Nevin J, Nevin NC, Dornan JC, et al. Early amniocentesis: experience of 222 consecutive patients from 1987–1988. *Prenat Diagn* 1990; 10:79–83.

12. Dunn LK, Godmilow L. A comparison of loss rates for first trimester chorionic villous sampling, early amniocentesis and midtrimester amniocentesis in a population of women of advanced maternal age. *Am J Hum Genet* 1990; 47(suppl):A273. Abstract.

13. Elejalde BR, de Elejalde MM, Acuna JM, et al. Prospective study of amniocentesis performed between weeks 9 and 16 of gestation: its feasibility, risks, complications and use in early genetic amniocentesis. *Am J Med Genet* 1990; 35:188–96.

14. Williams J 3rd, Wang BB, Rubin CH, Aiken-Hunting D. Chorionic villous sampling: experience with 3016 cases performed by a single operator. *Obstet Gynecol* 1992; 80:1023–9.

15. Wass DM, Brown GA, Warren PS, Saville TA. Completed follow-up of 1,000 consecutive transcervical chorionic villous samplings performed by a single operator. *Aust N Z J Obstet Gynaecol* 1991; 31:240–5.

16. Simpson JL. Incidence and timing of pregnancy losses: relevance to evaluating safety of early prenatal diagnosis. *Am J Med Genet* 1990; 35:165–73.

17. Firth HV, Boyd PA, Chamberlain P, et al. Severe limb abnormalities after chorionic villous sampling at 56–66 days' gestation. *Lancet* 1991; 337:762–3.

18. Burton BK, Schulz CJ, Burd LI. Limb anomalies associated with chorionic villous sampling. *Obstet Gynecol* 1992; 79:726–30.

19. Drugan A, Isada NB, Johnson MP, Hallak M, Evans MI. Prenatal diagnosis: procedures and trends. In: Avery GB, Fletcher MA, MacDonald MG, eds. *Neonatology: Pathophysiology and Management of the Newborn*, 4th ed. Philadelphia: JB Lippincott, 1994; 144–53.

20. Froster UG, Jackson L. Limb defects and chorionic sampling: results from an international registry, 1992–94. *Lancet* 1996; 347:489–94.

21. Ashkenazi S, Metzker A, Merlob P, Ovadia J, Reisener SH. Scalp changes after fetal monitoring. *Arch Dis Child* 1985; 60:267–9.

22. McGregor JA, McFarren T. Neonatal cranial osteomyelitis: a complication of fetal monitoring. *Obstet Gynecol* 1989; 73:490–2.

23. Kaye EM, Dooling EC. Neonatal herpes simplex meningoencephalitis with fetal scalp monitor scalp electrodes. *Neurology* 1981; 31:1045–7.

24. Goldkrand JW. Intrapartum inoculation of herpes simplex virus by fetal scalp electrode. *Obstet Gynecol* 1982; 59:263–5.

25. Scanlon JW, Walkley EI. Neonatal blood loss as a complication of fetal monitoring. *Pediatrics* 1972; 50:934–6.

26. Daffos F, Capella-Pavlovsky M, Forestier F. Fetal blood sampling via the umbilical cord using a needle guided by ultrasound: report of 66 cases. *Prenat Diagn* 1983; 3:271–7.

27. Ward RHT, Modell B, Fairweather DVI. Obstetric outcome and problems of midtrimester fetal blood sampling for antenatal diagnosis. *Br J Obstet Gynaecol* 1981; 88:1073–80.

28. Hoskins IA. Cordocentesis in isoimmunization and fetal physiologic measurement, infection and karyotyping. *Curr Opin Obstet Gynecol* 1991; 3:266–71.

29. Duchatel F, Oury JF, Mennesson B, Murray JM. Complications of diagnostic ultrasound-guided percutaneous umbilical blood sampling: analysis of a series of 341 cases and review of literature. *Eur J Obstet Gynecol Reprod Biol* 1993; 52:95–104.

30. Wilkins I, Mezrow G, Lynch L, et al. Amnionitis and life threatening respiratory distress after percutaneous umbilical blood sampling. *Am J Obstet Gynecol* 1989; 160:427–8.

31. Valdes-Dapena M. Iatrogenic disease in the perinatal period as seen by the pathologist. In: Naeye RL, Kissane JM, Kaufman N, eds. *Perinatal Diseases*. Baltimore: Williams & Wilkins, 1981, pp. 382–418.

32. Adzick NS, Harrison MR. Fetal surgical therapy. *Lancet* 1994; 343:897–902.

33. Luks F. Fetal surgery. In: Steegers EAP, Eskes TKAB, Symonds EM, eds. *Baillière's Clinical Obstetrics and Surgery: International Practice and Research*, vol. 9. Philadelphia: Ballière Tindall, 1995; 571–7.

34. Evans MI, Harrison MR, Johnson MP, Holzgreve W. Fetal therapy. In: Avery GB, Fletcher MA, MacDonald MG eds. *Neonatology: Pathophysiology and Management of the Newborn*, 4th ed. Philadelphia: Lippincott. 1994, pp. 171–83.

35. Crombleholme TM, Harrison MR, Golbus MS, et al. Fetal intervention in obstructive uropathy: prognostic indicators and efficacy of intervention. *Am J Obstet Gynecol* 1990; 162:1239–44.

36. Nicolini U, Fisk NM, Beacham J, Rodeck CH, et al. Urine biochemistry: an index of renal maturation and dysfunction. *Br J Obstet Gynaecol* 1992; 99:46–50.

37. Longaker MT, Golbus MS, Filly RA, et al. Maternal outcome after open fetal surgery: a review of the first 17 human cases. *JAMA* 1991; 265:737–41.

38. Harrison MR, Adzick NS, Flake AW. Correction of diaphragmatic hernia in utero: hard earned lessons. *J Pediatr Surg* 1993; 28:1411–8.

39. Jauniaux E, Leroy F, Wilkin P, Oodesch F, Hustin J. Clinical and morphologic aspects of the vanishing twin phenomenon. *Obstet Gynecol* 1988; 72:577–81.

40. Benirschke K. Intrauterine death of a twin: mechanisms, implications for surviving twin, and placental pathology. *Semin Diagn Pathol* 1993; 10:222–31.

41. Goldman GA, Dicker D, Feldberg D, et al. The vanishing fetus: a report of 17 cases of triplets and quadruplets. *J Perinat Med* 1989; 17:157–62.

42. Benirschke K, Kaufmann P. *Pathology of the Human Placenta*, 2nd ed. New York: Springer-Verlag, 1990, pp. 680–4.

43. Hannah ME, Hannah WJ, Hellman J, et al. Induction of labor as compared with serial antenatal monitoring in post-term pregnancy. *N Engl J Med* 1992; 326:1587–9.

44. Schullinger JN. Birth trauma. *Pediatr Clin North Am* 1993; 40:1352–8.

45. Williams MC. Vacuum assisted delivery. *Clin Perinatol* 1995; 22:933–49.

46. Thompson JP. Forcep deliveries. *Clin Perinatol* 1995; 22:953–72.

47. Scanlon JW, Walkley EI. Neonatal blood loss as a complication of fetal monitoring. *Pediatrics* 1972; 50:934–6.

48. Dunn PM. Testicular birth trauma. *Arch Dis Child* 1975; 50:744–5.

49. Friedman SJ, Winkelmann RK. Subcutaneous fat necrosis of the newborn: light, ultrastructural and histochemical microscopic studies. *J Cutan Pathol* 1989; 16:99–105.

50. Johanson RB, Rice C, Doyle M, et al. A randomized prospective study comparing the new vacuum extractor policy with forceps delivery. *Br J Obstet Gynaecol* 1993; 100:524–30.

51. Plauche WC. Subgaleal hematoma: a complication of instrumental delivery. *JAMA* 1980; 244:1597–8.

52. Florentino-Pineda I, Ezhuthachan SG, Sineniu LG, Kumar SP. Subgaleal hemorrhage in the newborn infant associated with silicone elastomer vacuum extractor. *J Perinatol* 1994; 14:95–100.

53. Brown JM. Hepatic hemorrhage in the newborn. *Arch Dis Child* 1957; 32:480–3.

54. French CE, Waldstein G. Subcapsular hemorrhage of the liver in the newborn. *Pediatrics* 1982; 2:374–80.

55. Wigglesworth JS. Pathology of intrapartum and early neonatal death in the normally formed infant. In: Wigglesworth JS, Singer DB, eds. *Textbook of Fetal and Perinatal Pathology*, vol. 1. Boston: Blackwell, 1991, pp. 300–1.

56. Levin S, Janive J, Mintz M, et al. Diagnostic and prognostic value of retinal hemorrhages in the neonate. *Obstet Gynecol* 1980; 55:309–14.

57. Egge K, Lying G, Maltau JM. Effect of instrumental delivery on the frequency and severity of retinal hemorrhages in the newborn. *Acta Obstet Gynecol Scand* 1982; 60:153–15.

58. Ehlers N, Jensen IK, Hansen KB. Retinal hemorrhages in the newborn: comparison of delivery by forceps and by vacuum extractor. *Acta Ophthalmol* 1974; 52:73–81.

59. Ferrari B, Tonni G, Luzietti R, et al. Neonatal complications and risk of intraventricular-periventricular hemorrhage. *Clin Exp Obstet Gynecol* 1992; 19:253–8.

60. Aguero O, Alvarez H. Fetal injury due to vacuum extractor. *Obstet Gynecol* 1962; 19:212–7.

61. Hanigan WC, Morgan AM, Stahlberg LK, et al. Tentorial hemorrhage associated with vacuum extraction. *Pediatrics* 1990; 85:534–9.

62. Huang CC, Shen ET. Tentorial subdural hemorrhage in term newborns: ultrasonographic diagnosis and clinical correlates. *Pediatr Neurol* 1991; 7:171–7.

63. Griffin PP. Orthopedics. In: Avery GB, Fletcher MA, MacDonald MG, eds. *Neonatology: Pathophysiology and Management of the Newborn*, 4th ed. Philadelphia: Lippincott, 1994, pp. 1190–1.

64. Gresham EL. Birth trauma. *Pediatr Clin North Am* 1975; 22:317–28.

65. Leestma JE. Forensic neuropathology. In: Duckett S, ed. *Pediatric Neuropathology*. Philadelphia: Williams & Wilkins, 1995, pp. 243–83.

66. Wigglesworth JS, Husemeyer RP. Intracranial birth trauma in vaginal breech delivery: the continued importance of injury to the occipital bone. *Br J Obstet Gynaecol* 1977; 84:684–91.

67. Eng GD, Koch B, Smokvina MD. Brachial plexus palsy in neonates and children. *Arch Phys Med Rehabil* 1978; 59:458–64.

68. Falco NA, Eriksson E. Facial nerve palsy in the newborn: incidence and outcome. *Plast Reconstr Surg* 1990; 85:1–4.

69. Koch BM, Eng GD. Neonatal spinal cord injury. *Arch Phys Med Rehabil* 1979; 60:378–81.

70. Fotter R, Sorantin E, Schneider U, et al. Ultrasound diagnosis of birth-related spinal cord trauma: neonatal diagnosis and follow-up and correlation with MRI. *Pediatr Radiol* 1994; 24:241–4.

71. Brown MS, Phibbs RH. Spinal cord injury in newborns from use of umbilical artery catheters: report of two cases and review of the literature. *J Perinatol* 1988; 8:105–10.

72. Gregersen M, Vesterby A. Iatrogenic fractures of the hyoid bone and the thyroid cartilage: a case report. *Forensic Sci Int* 1981; 17:41–3.

73. McGrath RB. Gastroesophageal lacerations: a fatal complication of closed chest cardiopulmonary resuscitation. *Chest* 1983; 83:571–2.

74. Topsis J, Kinas HY, Kandall SR. Esophageal perforation: a complication of neonatal resuscitation. *Anesth Analg* 1989; 69:532–4.

75. Brill JE. The performance of CPR in infants and children. In: Fuhrman BP, Zimmerman JJ, eds. *Pediatric Critical Care.* St. Louis Mosby, 1992, pp. 1315–29.

76. Powner DJ, Holcombe PA, Mello LA. Cardiopulmonary resuscitation-related injuries. *Crit Care Med* 1984; 12:54–5.

77. Eisenberg MJ. Electrolytes measurements during in-hospital cardiopulmonary resuscitation. *Crit Care Med* 1990; 18:25–6.

78. Low JA, Panagiotopoulos C, Derrick EJ. Newborn complications after intrapartum asphyxia with metabolic acidosis in the term fetus. *Am J Obstet Gynecol* 1994; 170:1081–7.

79. Manning FA, Platt LD, Sipos L. Antepartum fetal evaluation: development of a fetal biophysical profile. *Am J Obstet Gynecol* 1980; 136:787–95.

80. Bacsik RD. Meconium aspiration syndrome. *Pediatr Clin North Am* 1977; 24:463–79.

81. Katz VL, Barnes WA. Meconium aspiration syndrome: reflections on a murky subject. *Am J Obstet Gynecol* 1992; 166:171–4.

82. Ohlsson A, Cumming WA, Najjar H. Neonatal aspiration syndrome due to vernix caseosa. *Pediatr Radiol* 1985; 15:193–5.

83. Lauweryns J, Bernat R, Lerut A, Detournay G. Intrauterine pneumonia: an experimental study. *Biol Neonate* 1973; 22:301–18.

84. Murphy JD, Vawter GF, Reid LM. Pulmonary vascular disease in fatal meconium aspiration. *J Pediatr* 1984; 104:758–62.

85. Knudson RP, Alden ER. Neonatal heelstick blood culture. *Pediatrics* 1980; 65:505–7.

86. Goldber I, Shauer L, Klier I, Seelenfreund M. Neonatal osteomyelitis of the calcaneus following a heel pad puncture: a case report. *Clin Orthop* 1981; 158:195–7.

87. Canale ST, Manugian AH. Neonatal osteomyelitis of the os calcis: a complication of repeated heel punctures. *Clin Orthop* 1981; 156:178–82.

88. Lilien LD, Harris VJ, Ramamurthy RS, Pildes RS. Neonatal osteomyelitis of the calcaneus: complication of heel puncture. *J Pediatr* 1976; 88:478–80.

89. Blumenfeld TA, Turi GK, Blanc WA. Recommended site and depth of newborn heel skin puncture based on anatomical measurements and histopathology. *Lancet* 1979; 1:230–3.

90. Sell EJ, Hansen RC, Struck-Pierce S. Calcified nodules on the heel: a complication of neonatal intensive care. *J Pediatr* 1980; 96:473–5.

91. Klein JO, Marcy M. Bacterial sepsis and meningitis. In: Remington JS, Klein JO, eds. *Infectious Diseases of the Fetus and Newborn Infant,* 4th ed. Philadelphia: Saunders, 1995, pp. 835–90.

92. Zych GA, McCollough NC. Acute psoas abscess in a newborn infant. *J Pediatr Orthoped* 1985; 5:89–91.

93. Asnes RS, Arendar GM. Septic arthritis of the hip: a complication of femoral venipuncture. *Pediatrics* 1966; 38:837–41.

94. Stenzel JP, Green TP. Percutaneous femoral venous catheterization: a prospective study of complications. *J Pediatr* 1989; 114:411–5.

95. Chathas MK, Paton JB, Fisher DE. Percutaneous central venous catheterization: three years experience in a neonatal intensive care unit. *Am J Dis Child* 1990; 144:1246–50.

96. Mah MP, Fain JS, Hall SL. Radiological case of the month. *Am J Dis Child* 1991; 145:1439–40.

97. Rogers BB, Berns SD, Maynard EC, Hansen TWR. Pericardial tamponade secondary to central venous catheterization and hyperalimentation in a very low birth weight infant. *Pediatr Pathol* 1990; 10:819–23.

98. Hodson WA, Truog WE. Principles of management of respiratory problems. In: Avery GB, Fletcher MA, MacDonald MG, eds. *Neonatology: Pathophysiology and Management of the Newborn,* 4th ed. Philadelphia: Lippincott, 1994, pp. 478–503.

99. Gupta JM, Robertson NRC, Wigglesworth JS. Umbilical artery catheterization in the newborn. *Arch Dis Child* 1967; 43:382–7.

100. White LE, Montes JE, Chaves-Carballo E, et al. Radiological case of the month. *Am J Dis Child* 1987; 141:903–4.

101. Shandall AA, Leopold PW, Shan DM, et al. Visceral aortic aneurysm in a $4\frac{1}{2}$ year old child: an unusual complication of umbilical artery. *Surgery* 1986; 100:928–31.

102. Wynn ML, Rowen M, Rucker RW, Sperling DR, Gazzaniga AB. Pseudoaneurysm of the thoracic aorta: a late complication of umbilical artery catheterization. *Ann Thoracic Surg* 1982; 34:186–91.

103. Ford KT, Teplick SK, Clark RE. Renal artery embolism causing neonatal hypertension: a complication of umbilical artery catheterization. *Radiology* 1974; 113:169–70.

104. Lim MO, Gresham EL, Franken EA Jr, et al. Osteomyelitis as a complication of umbilical artery catheterization. *Am J Dis Child* 1977; 131:142–4.

105. Pittard WB, Thullen JD, Fanaroff AA. Neonatal septic arthritis. *J Pediatr* 1976; 88:621–4.

106. Barson AJ. A postmortem study of infection in the newborn from 1976 to 1988. In: deLouvois J, Harvey D, eds. *Infection in the Newborn.* New York: John Wiley & Sons, 1990, pp. 13–34.

107. McGuiness GA, Schieken RM, Maguire GF. Endocarditis in the newborn. *Am J Dis Child* 1980; 134:577–80.

108. Oski FA, Allen DM, Diamond LK. Portal hypertension: a complication of umbilical vein catheterization. *Pediatrics* 1963; 31:297–302.

109. Brans YW, Ceballos R, Cassady G. Umbilical catheters and hepatic abscess. *Pediatrics* 1974; 53:264–6.

110. Fraga JR, Javate BA, Venkatessan S. Liver abscess and sepsis due to *Klebsiella pneumoniae* in a newborn: a complication of umbilical vein catheterization. *Clin Pediatr* 1974; 13:1081–2.

111. Scott J. Iatrogenic lesions in babies following umbilical vein catheterization. *Arch Dis Child* 1965; 40:426–8.

112. Rosetti VA. Intraosseous infusion: an alternative route of pediatric intravascular access. *Ann Emerg Med* 1985; 14:885–8.

113. Strauss RH. The performance of CPR in infants and children. In: Fuhrman BP, Zimmerman JJ, eds. *Pediatric Critical Care.* St. Louis: Mosby, 1992, pp. 1315–25.

114. Maisels MJ, Li TK, Peichocki JT. The effect of exchange transfusion on serum ionized calcium. *Pediatrics* 1974; 53:683–6.

115. Blanchette VS, Gray E, Hardie MJ. Hyperkalemia after neonatal exchange transfusion: risk eliminated by washing red cell concentrates. *J Pediatr* 1984; 105:321–4.

116. Orme RL, Eades SM. Perforation of the bowel in the newborn as a complication of exchange transfusion. *Br Med J* 1968; 4:349–51.

117. Shapiro N, Stein H, Olinsky A. Necrotizing enterocolitis and exchange transfusion. *S Afr Med J* 1973; 47:1236–8.

118. Kliegman RM, Fanaroff AA. Neonatal necrotizing enterocolitis: a nine year experience. I. Epidemiology and uncommon observations. *Am J Dis Child* 1981; 135:603–7.

119. Kliegman RM, Fanaroff AA. Necrotizing enterocolitis. *N Engl J Med* 1981; 310:1093–1103.

120. deSa DJ. The spectrum of ischemic bowel disease in the newborn. *Perspect Pediatr Pathol* 1976; 3:273–309.

121. Parkman R, Mosier D, Umansky I, Cochran W, Carpenter C. Graft-versus-host disease after intrauterine and exchange transfusions for hemolytic disease of the newborn. *N Engl J Med* 1974; 290:359–63.

122. Chudwin DS, Ammann AJ, Wara DW. Post-transfusion syndrome: rash, eosinophilia, and thrombocytopenia following intrauterine and exchange transfusions. *Am J Dis Child* 1982; 136:612–4.

123. Wigger HJ. Influence of perinatal management. In: Wigglesworth JS, Singer DB, eds. *Textbook of Fetal and Perinatal Pathology,* vol. 1. Boston: Blackwell, 1991, pp. 49–76.

124. Walker RH. Special report: transfusion risks. *Am J Clin Pathol* 1987; 88:374–8.

125. Dodd RY. The risk of transfusion-transmitted infection *N Engl J Med* 1992; 327:419–21.

126. Rutsky EA, Rostand SG. Treatment of uremic pericarditis and pericardial effusion. *Am J Kidney Dis* 1987; 10:2–8.

127. Sobol SM, Thomas HM Jr, Evans RW. Myocardial laceration not demonstrated by continuous electrocardiographic monitoring occurring during pericardiocentesis. *N Engl J Med* 1975; 292:1222–3.

128. Van Dyke WH, Cure J, Chakko CS. Pulmonary edema after pericardiocentesis for cardiac tamponade. *N Engl J Med* 1983; 309:595–6.

129. Armstrong WF, Feigenbaum H, Dillon JC. Acute right ventricular dilation and echocardiographic volume overload following pericardiocentesis for relief of cardiac tamponade. *Am Heart J* 1984; 107:1266–70.

130. Rice TB, Pontus SP Jr. Diagnostic and therapeutic centesis. In: Fuhrman BP, Zimmerman JJ, eds. *Pediatric Critical Care.* St. Louis: Mosby, 1992, pp. 144–7.

131. Brown NE, Zamel N, Aberman A. Changes in pulmonary mechanics and gas exchange following thoracentesis. *Chest* 1978; 74:540–2.

132. Brandstetter RD, Cohen RP. Hypoxemia after thoracentesis: a predictable and treatable condition. *JAMA* 1979; 242:1060–1.

133. Wyllie R, Arasu MB, Fitzgerald JF. Ascites: pathophysiology and management. *J Pediatr* 1980; 97:167–76.

134. Gomella TL, Cunningham MD, Eyal FG. *Neonatology*, 3rd ed. Norwalk, CT: Appleton-Lange, 1994, pp. 159–60.

135. Banagale RC, Outerbridge EW, Aranda JV. Lung perforation: a complication of chest tube insertion in neonatal pneumothorax. *J Pediatr* 1979; 94:973–5.

136. van Straaten HL, Gerards LJ, Krediet TG. Chylothorax in the neonatal period. *Eur J Pediatr* 1993; 152:2–5.

137. Odita JC, Khan AS, Dinçsoy M, et al. Neonatal phrenic nerve paralysis resulting from intercostal drainage of pneumothorax. *Pediatr Radiol* 1992; 22:379–81.

138. Bergman I, Wald ER, Meyer JD. Epidural abscess and vertebral osteomyelitis following serial lumbar punctures. *Pediatrics* 1983; 72:476–80.

139. Shaywitz B. Spinal taps and epidermoid tumors. *Hosp Pract* 1973; 8:79–84.

140. Lohr JA, Donowitz LG, Sadler JE. Hospital acquired urinary tract infection. *Pediatrics* 1989; 82:193–9.

141. Williams N, Kapila L. Complications of circumcision. *Br J Surg* 1993; 80:1231–6.

142. Niku SD, Stock JA, Kaplan GW. Neonatal circumcision. *Urol Clin North Am* 1995; 22:57–65.

143. Gluckman GR, Stoller ML, Jacobs MM, Kogan BA. Newborn penile glans amputation during circumcision and successful reattachment. *J Urol* 1995; 153:778–9.

144. Chen JY. Prophylaxis of ophthalmia neonatorum: comparison of silver nitrate, tetracycline, erythromycin and no prophylaxis. *Pediatr Infect Dis J* 1991; 11:1026–30.

145. American Academy of Pediatrics. *1997 Red Book*. Report of the Committee on Infectious Diseases. Elk Grove, IL: AAP, 1997, pp. 250–60.

146. Hengster P, Schnapka J, Fille M, Menardi G. Occurrence of suppurative lymphadenitis after a change in BCG vaccine. *Arch Dis Child* 1992; 67:952–5.

147. Kroger L, Brander E, Korppi M, et al. Osteitis after newborn vaccination with three different Bacillus Calmette-Guérin vaccines: twenty-nine years of experience. *Pediatr Infect Dis J* 1994; 13:113–6.

148. Simma B, Dietze O, Vogel W. Bacille Calmette-Guérin associated hepatitis. *Eur J Pediatr* 1991; 150:423–4.

149. Rao HKM, Elhassani SB. Iatrogenic complications of procedures performed on the newborn: Part 2. Respiratory procedures. *Perinatal Neonatol* 1980; 4:43–52.

150. Phelps DL. Retinopathy of prematurity. *Pediatr Rev* 1995; 16:50–6.

151. Bossi E, Koerner F. Retinopathy of prematurity. *Intensive Care Med* 1995; 21:241–6.

152. Committee members. An international classification of retinopathy of prematurity. *Pediatrics* 1984; 74:127–33.

153. Anderson WR, Strickland MB, Tsai SH. Light microscopic and ultrastructural study of the adverse effects of oxygen therapy on the neonate lung. *Am J Pathol* 1973; 73:327–31.

154. Bowers SK, MacDonald HM, Shapiro ED. Prevention of iatrogenic neonatal respiratory distress syndrome: elective repeat cesarean section and spontaneous labor. *Am J Obstet Gynecol* 1982; 142:186–9.

155. Parilla BV, Dooley SL, Jansen RD, Socol M. Iatrogenic respiratory distress syndrome following elective repeat cesarean delivery. *Obstet Gynecol* 1993; 81:392–5.

156. Gould SJ, Graham J. Long term pathological sequelae of neonatal endotracheal intubation. *J Laryngol Otol* 1989; 103:622–5.

157. Joshi VV, Mandavia SG, Stern L. Acute lesions induced by endotracheal intubation. *Am J Dis Child* 1972; 124:646–9.

158. Holcomb GW 3d, Templeton JM Jr. Iatrogenic perforation of the bronchus intermedius in a 1100g neonate. *J Pediatr Surg* 1989; 24:1132–4.

159. McLeod BJ, Sumner E. Neonatal tracheal perforation: a complication of tracheal intubation. *Anesthesia* 1986; 41:67–70.

160. Grunebaum M, Horodniceanu C, Wilunsky E, Reisner S. Iatrogenic transmural perforation of the esophagus in the preterm infant. *Clin Radiol* 1980; 31:257–61.

161. Dankle SK, Schuller DE, McClead RE. Risk factors for neonatal acquired subglottic stenosis. *Ann Otol Rhinol Laryngol* 1986; 95:626–30.

162. Marcovich M, Pollauf F, Burian K. Subglottic stenosis in newborns after mechanical ventilation. *Prog Pediatr Surg* 1987; 21:8–19.

163. Loftus BC, Ahn J, Haddad J Jr. Neonatal nasal deformities secondary to nasal continuous positive airway pressure. *Laryngoscope* 1994; 104:1019–22.

164. Avery ME, Mead J. Surface properties in relation to atelectasis and hyaline membrane disease. *Am J Dis Child* 1959; 97:517–23.

165. Fujiwara T, Chida S, Watanabe Y, et al. Artificial surfactant therapy in hyaline membrane disease. *Lancet* 1980; 1:55–9.

166. Jobe AH. Pulmonary surfactant therapy. *N Engl J Med* 1993; 328:861–8.

167. Valencia GB, Allen L, Claude S, et al. Pulmonary hemorrhage: a severe complication in preterm infants administered surfactant replacement therapy. *Pediatr Res* 1992; 31:226A. Abstract.

168. Russell L, White A, Andrews E, et al. Observational study of synthetic surfactant in 11,455 infants. *Pediatr Res* 1992; 31:100A. Abstract.

169. Raju TNK, Langenberg P. Pulmonary hemorrhage and exogenous surfactant therapy: a metaanalysis. *J Pediatr* 1993; 123:603–10.

170. Pinar H, Makarova N, Rubin LP, Singer DB. Pathology of the lung in surfactant-treated neonates. *Pediatr Pathol* 1994; 14:627–36.

171. deMello DE, Noguchi A, Gunkel H. Absence of Survanta-related lung histologic changes at autopsy in infants with hyaline membrane disease. *Pediatr Res* 1993; 33:323A. Abstract.

172. Thornton CM, Halliday HL, O'Hara MD. Surfactant replacement therapy in preterm neonates: a comparison of postmortem pulmonary histology in treated and untreated infants. *Pediatr Pathol* 1994; 14:945–53.

173. Pappin A, Shenker N, Hack M, Redline RW. Extensive intraalveolar pulmonary hemorrhage in infants dying after surfactant therapy. *J Pediatr* 1994; 124:621–6.

174. Moncada S, Higgs A. The L-arginine-nitric oxide pathway. *N Engl J Med* 1993; 329:2002–12.

175. Zayek M, Wild L, Roberts JD, Morin FC. Effect of nitric acid oxide on the survival rate and incidence of lung injury in newborn lambs with persistent pulmonary hypertension. *J Pediatr* 1993; 123:947–52.

176. Geggel RL. Inhalational nitric oxide: a selective pulmonary vasodilator for treatment of persistent pulmonary hypertension of the newborn. *J Pediatr* 1993; 123:76–9.

177. Peliowski A, Finer NN, Etches PC, Tierney AJ, Ryan CA. Inhaled nitric oxide for premature infants after prolonged rupture of the membranes. *J Pediatr* 1995; 126:450–3.

178. Abman SH, Kinsella JP, Schaffer MS, Wilkening RB. Inhaled nitric oxide in the management of a premature newborn with severe respiratory distress and pulmonary hypertension. *Pediatrics* 1993; 92:606–9.

179. Gaston B, Keith JF. Nitric oxide and bleeding time. *Pediatrics* 1994; 94:134–5.

180. Högman M, Frostell C, Arnberg H, Hedenstierna G. Bleeding time prolongation and NO inhalation. *Lancet* 1993; 341:1664–5.

181. Högman M, Frostell C, Arnberg H, Sandhagen B, Hedenstierna G. Prolonged bleeding time during nitric oxide inhalation in the rabbit. *Acta Physiol Scand* 1994; 151:125–9.

182. Groll-Knapp E, Haider M, Kienzl K, Handler A, Trimmel M. Changes in discrimination learning and brain activity (ERP's) due to combined exposure to NO and CO in rats. *Toxicology* 1988; 49:441–7.

183. Haddad IY, Ischiropoulos H, Holm BA, et al. Mechanisms of peroxynitrite-induced injury to pulmonary surfactants. *Am J Physiol* 1993; 265:L555–64.

184. Kylstra JA, Tissing MO, Van der Maen A. Of mice and fish. *Trans Am Soc Artif Intern Organs* 1962; 8:378–83.

185. Wolfson MR, Clark LC, Hoffman RE, et al. Liquid ventilation of neonates; uptake, distribution, and elimination of the liquid. *Pediatr Res* 1990; 27:37A. Abstract.

186. Deoras KS, Coppola D, Wolfson MR, et al. Liquid ventilation of neonates: tissue histology and morphometry. *Pediatr Res* 1990; 27:29A. Abstract.

187. Fuhrman BP, Paczan PR, DeFrancisi M. Perfluorocarbon-associated gas exchange. *Crit Care Med* 1991; 19:712–22.

188. Forman D, Bhutani BK, Hilfer SF, Shaffer TH. A fine structure study of the liquid-ventilated newborn rabbit. *Fed Proc* 1984; 43:647A. Abstract.

189. Shaffer TH, Wolfson MR, Clark LC. Liquid ventilation. *Pediatr Pulmonol* 1992; 14:102–9.

190. Greenspan JS, Wolfson MR, Rubenstein D, Shaffer TH. Liquid ventilation of human preterm neonates. *J Pediatr* 1990; 117:106–11.

191. Hirschl R, Pranikoff T, Gauger P, et al. Liquid ventilation in adults, children, and full-term neonates. *Lancet* 1995; 346:1201–2.

192. Hanson JB, Waldstein G, Hernandez JA, Fan LL. Necrotizing tracheobronchitis. *Am J Dis Child* 1988; 142:1094–8.

193. Circeo LE, Heard SO, Griffiths E, Nash G. Overwhelming necrotizing tracheobronchitis due to inadequate humidification during high frequency jet ventilation. *Chest* 1991; 100:268–9.

194. Polak MJ, Donnelly WH, Bucciarelli RL. Comparison of airway pathologic lesions after high frequency jet or conventional ventilation. *Am J Dis Child* 1989; 143:228–32.

195. Valdes-Dapena M. Iatrogenic disease in the perinatal period. *Pediatr Clin N Am* 1989; 36:67–93.

196. Stocker JT, Madewell JE. Persistent interstitial pulmonary emphysema: another complication of the respiratory distress syndrome. *Pediatrics* 1977; 59:847–57.

197. Brown ZA, Clark JM, Jung AL. Systemic gas embolus: a discussion of its pathogenesis in the neonate, with a review of the literature. *Am J Dis Child* 1977; 131:984–5.

198. Zimmerman JJ, Farrell PM. Advances and issues in bronchopulmonary dysplasia. *Curr Probl Pediatr* 1994; 24:159–70.

199. Northway WH Jr, Rosan C, Porter DY. Pulmonary disease following respiratory therapy of hyaline membrane disease. *N Engl J Med* 1967; 76:357–68.

200. Bancalari E, Abdenour GE, Feller R. Bronchopulmonary dysplasia: clinical presentation. *J Pediatr* 1979; 95:819–23.

201. Shennan AT, Dunn MS, Ohlsson A, Lennox K, Hoskins EM. Abnormal pulmonary outcomes in premature infants: prediction from oxygen requirement in the neonatal period. *Pediatrics* 1988; 82:527–32.

202. Knisely AS, Leal SM, Singer DB. Abnormalities of diaphragmatic muscle in neonates with ventilated lungs. *J Pediatr* 1988; 113:1074–7.

203. Short BL. Physiology of extracorporeal membrane oxygenation (ECMO). In: Polin RA, Fox WW, eds. *Fetal and Neonatal Physiology.* Philadelphia: Saunders, 1992, pp. 932–8.

204. Kanto WP. A decade of experience with neonatal extracorporeal membrane oxygenation. *J Pediatr* 1994; 124:335–47.

205. Zwischenberger JB, Nguyen TT, Upp JR Jr, et al. Complications of neonatal extracorporeal membrane oxygenation: collective experience from the Extracorporeal Life Support Organization. *J Thorac Cardiovasc Surg* 1994; 107:838–48.

206. Evans MJ, McKeever PA, Pearson GA, Field D, Firmin RK. Pathological complications of non-survivors of newborn extracorporeal membrane oxygenation. *Arch Dis Child* 1994; 71:88–92.

207. Vogler C, Sotelo-Avila C, Lagunoff D, et al. Aluminum-containing emboli in infants treated with extracorporeal membrane oxygenation. *N Engl J Med* 1988; 319:75–9.

208. Cashore WJ, Stern L. The management of hyperbilirubinemia. *Clin Perinatol* 1984; 11:339–57.

209. Cashore WJ. The neurotoxicity of bilirubin. *Clin Perinatol* 1990; 17:437–47.

210. Speck WT, Rosenkranz HS. Intracellular deoxyribonucleic acid—modifying activity of phototherapy lights. *Pediatr Res* 1976; 10:553–5.

211. McGinty LD, Fowler RG. Visible light mutagenesis in *Escherichia coli. Mutat Res* 1982; 95:171–81.

212. Brown AK, McDonagh AF. Phototherapy for neonatal hyperbilirubinemia: efficacy, mechanism and toxicity. In: Barness LA, eds. *Advances in Pediatrics.* Chicago: Year Book, 1980, p. 341.

213. Ennever JF, Carr HS, Speck WT. Potential for genetic damage from multivitamin solutions exposed to phototherapy illumination. *Pediatr Res* 1983; 17:192–4.

214. Amin HJ, Shukla AK, Snyder F, et al. Significance of phototherapy-induced riboflavin deficiency in the full-term neonate. *Biol Neonate* 1992; 61:76–81.

215. Messner KH. Light toxicity to newborn retina. *Pediatr Res* 1978; 12:530–2.

216. Purcell SM, Wians FH Jr, Ackerman NB Jr, Davis BM. Hyperbiliverdinemia in the bronze baby syndrome. *J Am Acad Dermatol* 1987; 16:172–7.

217. Ashley JR, Little CM, Burgdof WH, Brann BS. Bronze baby syndrome: report of a case. *J Am Acad Dermatol* 1985; 12:325–8.

218. Jori G, Reddi E, Rubaltelli FF. Bronze-baby syndrome: an animal model. *Pediatr Res* 1990; 27:22–5.

219. Berant M, Diamond E, Brik R, Yurman S. Phototherapy-associated diarrhea: the role of bile salts. *Acta Paediatr Scand* 1983; 72:853–5.

220. Dacou-Voutetakis C, Anagnostakis D, Matsaniotis N. Effect of prolonged illumination (phototherapy) on concentrations of luteinizing hormone in human infants. *Science* 1978; 199:1229–31.

221. Siegfried EC, Stone MS, Madison KC. Ultraviolet light burn: a cutaneous complication of visible light phototherapy of neonatal jaundice. *Pediatr Dermatol* 1992; 9:278–82.

222. Rosenfeld W, Sadhev S, Brunot V, et al. Phototherapy effect on the incidence of patent ductus arteriosus in premature infants: prevention with chest shielding. *Pediatrics* 1986; 78:10–4.

223. Silberberg DH, Johnson L, Schutta H. Effects of photodegradation products of bilirubin on myelinating cerebellum cultures. *J Pediatr* 1970; 77:613–8.

224. Church S, Adamkin DH. Transillumination in neonatal intensive care: a possible iatrogenic complication. *South Med J* 1981; 74:76–7.

224a. Picascia D, Esterly NB. Cutis marmorata telangiectasia congenita: report of 22 cases. *J Am Acad Dermatol* 1989; 20:1098–1100.

225. Itani O, Crump R, Mimouni F, Tunnessen WW. Ritter's disease: staphylococcal scalded skin syndrome. *Am J Dis Child* 1992; 146:425–6.

226. Marx CM, Cronin JH. Medications used in the newborn. In: Cloherty JP, Stark AR, eds. *Manual of Neonatal Care,* 3rd ed. Boston: Little, Brown, 1991, pp. 619–33.

227. Roberts RJ. *Drug Therapy in Infants.* Philadelphia: Saunders, 1984.

228. van Beek RH, Carnielli VP, Sauer PJ. Nutrition in the neonate. *Curr Opin Pediatr* 1995; 7:146–51.

229. Pinkerton H. Vitamins and deficiency diseases. In: Anderson WAD, Kissane JM, eds. *Pathology,* 7th ed, Vol. 1. St. Louis: Mosby, 1977, pp. 623–39.

230. Argao EA, Heubi JE. Fat-soluble vitamin deficiency in infants and children. *Curr Opin Pediatr* 1993; 5:562–6.

231. Powers HJ. Micronutrient deficiencies in the preterm neonate. *Proc Nutr Soc* 1993; 52:285–91.

232. Rucker RB, Stites T. New perspectives on function of vitamins. *Nutrition* 1994; 10:507–13.

233. Tee ES. Carotenoids and retinoids in human nutrition. *Crit Rev Food Sci Nutr* 1992; 31:103–5.

234. Hartline JV, Zachman RD. Vitamin A delivery in total parenteral nutrition solution. *Pediatrics* 1976; 58:448–51.

235. Zachman RD. Role of vitamin A in lung development. *J Nutr* 1995; 125:1634S–8S.

236. Shenai JP, Chytil F, Stahlman MT. Vitamin A status of neonates with bronchopulmonary dysplasia. *Pediatr Res* 1985; 19:185–8.

237. Robbins ST, Fletcher AB. Early vs delayed vitamin A supplementation in very low birth weight infants. *J Parenter Enteral Nutr* 1993; 17:220–5.

238. Reichel H, Koeffler HP, Norman AW. The role of vitamin D endocrine system in health and disease. *N Eng J Med* 1989; 320:980–91.

239. DeLuca HF, Krisinger J, Darwish H. The vitamin D system. *Kidney Int* 1990; 38(suppl 29):S2.

240. Gefter WB, Epstein DM, Anday EK, Dalinka MK. Rickets presenting as multiple fractures in premature infants on hyperalimentation. *Radiology* 1982; 142:371–4.

241. Glasgow JFT, Thomas PS. Rachitic respiratory distress in small preterm infants. *Arch Dis Child* 1977; 52:268–73.

242. Johnson L, Schaffer D, Boggs TR. The premature infant, vitamin E deficiency and retrolental fibroplasia. *Am J Clin Nutr* 1974; 27:1158–73.

243. Phelps DL, Rosenbaum AI, Isenberg SJ, et al. Tocopherol efficacy and safety for preventing retinopathy of prematurity: a randomized, controlled, double-masked trial. *Pediatrics* 1987; 79:489–500.

244. Oski FA, Barness LA. Vitamin E deficiency: a previously unrecognized cause of hemolytic anemia in the premature. *J Pediatr* 1967; 70:211–20.

245. Phelps DL. Local and systemic reactions to the parenteral administration of vitamin E. *Dev Pharmacol Ther* 1981; 2:156–71.

246. Center for Disease Control. Unusual syndrome with fatalities among premature infants: association with a new intravenous vitamin E product. *MMWR* 1984; 33:198–9.

247. Bodenstein CJ. Intravenous vitamin E and deaths in the intensive care unit [Letter]. *Pediatrics* 1984; 73:387.

248. Lorch V, Murphy D, Hoersten LR, et al. Unusual syndrome among premature infants: association with a new intravenous vitamin E product. *Pediatrics* 1985; 75:598–602.

249. Balistreri WF, Farrell MK, Bove KE. Lessons from the E-Ferol tragedy. *Pediatrics* 1986; 78:503–6.

250. Martone WJ, Williams WW, Mortensen ML. Illness with fatalities in premature infants: association with an intravenous vitamin E preparation, E-Ferol. *Pediatrics* 1986; 78:591–600.

251. Johnson L, Bowen FW, Abbasi S, et al. Relationship of prolonged pharmacologic serum levels of vitamin E to incidence of sepsis and necrotizing enterocolitis in infants with birth weights of 1500 grams or less. *Pediatrics* 1985; 75:619–38.

252. American Academy of Pediatrics. Committee on Fetus and Newborn. Vitamin E and the prevention of retinopathy of prematurity. *Pediatrics* 1985; 76:315.

253. Thorpe JA, Gaston L, Caspers DR, Pal ML. Current concepts and controversies in the use of vitamin K. *Drugs* 1995; 49:376–87.

254. Shearer MJ. Vitamin K. *Lancet* 1995; 345:229–34.

255. von Kries R, Greer FR, Suttie JW. Assessment of vitamin K status of the newborn infant. *J Pediatr Gastroenterol Nutr* 1993; 16:231–4.

256. Blayer WA, Skinner AL. Fetal neonatal hemorrhage after maternal anticonvulsant therapy. *JAMA* 1976; 235:626–8.

257. Milman N, Agger AO, Nielsen OJ. Iron status markers and serum erythropoietin in 120 mothers and newborn infants: effect of iron supplementation in normal pregnancy. *Acta Obstet Gynecol Scand* 1994; 73:200–4.

258. American Academy of Pediatrics Committee on Nutrition. Nutritional need of low-birth-weight infants. *Pediatrics* 1985; 75:976–86.

259. Doyle JJ, Zipursky A. Neonatal blood disorders. In: Sinclair JC, Bracken MB, eds. *Effective Care of the Newborn Infant.* Oxford: Oxford University Press, 1992, pp. 426–53.

260. Lundström U, Siimes MA, Dallman PR. At what age does iron supplementation become necessary in low birth weight infants? *J Pediatr* 1991; 91:878–83.

261. Maier RF, Obladen M, Scigalla P, et al. The effect of epoietin beta on the need for transfusion in very low birth weight infants. *N Engl J Med* 1994; 330:1173–8.

262. Innis SM. Essential fatty acids in growth and development. *Prog Lipid Res* 1991: 30:39–103.

263. Simopoulos AP. Ω-3 fatty acids in health and disease and in growth and development. *Am J Clin Nutr* 1991; 54:438–63.

264. Sardesai VM. The essential fatty acids. *Nutr Clin Pract* 1992; 7:179–86.

265. Uauy-Dagach R, Mena P, Hoffman DR, Essential fatty acid metabolism and requirements for LBW infants. *Acta Paediatr* 1994; 405:78–85.

266. Burr GO, Burr MM, A new deficiency disease produced by rigid exclusion of fat from the diet. *J Biol Chem* 1929; 82:345–7.

267. Uauy R, Treen M, Hoffman DR. Essential fatty acid metabolism and requirements during development. *Semin Perinatol* 1989; 13:118–30.

268. Carlson SE, Rhodes PG, Ferguson MG. Docohexaenoic acid status of preterm infants at birth and following feeding with human milk or formula. *Am J Clin Nutr* 1986; 44:798–804.

269. American Academy of Pediatrics, Committee on Nutrition. Nutritional needs of low birth weight infants. *Pediatrics* 1985; 75:976–86.

270. Uauy R, Hoffman DR. Essential fatty acid requirements for normal eye and brain development. *Semin Perinatol* 1991; 15:449–55.

271. Simmer K, Thompson PH. Zinc in the fetus and newborn. *Acta Paediatr Scand* 1985; 319:158–63.

272. Wang Z, Atkinson SA, Bertolo RF, et al. Alterations in intestinal uptake and compartmentalization of zinc in response to short term dexamethasone therapy or excess dietary zinc in piglets. *Pediatr Res* 1992; 33:118–24.

273. Seely JR, Humphrey GB, Matter BJ. Copper deficiency in a premature infant fed on iron fortified formula. *N Eng J Med* 1972; 286:109–10.

274. Tokuda Y, Yokoyama, S, Tsuji M, et al. Copper deficiency in an infant on prolonged total parenteral nutrition. *J Parenter Enteral Nutr* 1986; 19:242–4.

275. Goel R, Misra PK. Plasma copper in fetal malnutrition. *Acta Paediatr Scand* 1982; 71:421–3.

276. Litov RE, Combs GF. Selenium in pediatric nutrition. *Pediatrics* 1991: 87:339–51.

277. Arthur JR. The role of selenium in thyroid hormone metabolism. *Can J Physiol Pharmacol* 1991; 69:1648–52.

278. Baker SS, Lerman RH, Krey SH. Selenium deficiency with total parenteral nutrition: reversal of biochemical and functional abnormalities by selenium supplementation: a case report. *Am J Clin Nutr* 1983; 38:769–74.

279. Vinton NE, Dahlstrom KA. Macrocytosis and pseudoalbinism: manifestations of selenium deficiency. *J Pediatr* 1987; 111:711–7.

280. Collip PJ, Chen SY. Cardiomyopathy and selenium deficiency in a 2-year-old girl. *N Engl J Med* 1981; 304:1304–5.

281. Koo WW, Tsang RC, Mineral requirements of low-birth-weight infants. *J Am Coll Nutr* 1991; 10:474–86.

282. Altura BM, Altura BT, Carella A. Magnesium deficiency-induced spasms of umbilical vessels: relation to pre-eclampsia, hypertension, growth retardation. *Science* 1983; 221:376–8.

283. Arnold GL, Greene CL, Stout JP, Goodman SI. Molybdenum cofactor deficiency. *J Pediatr* 1993; 123:595–8.

284. Slot HM, Overweg-Plandsoen WC, Bakker HD, et al. Molybdenum-cofactor deficiency: an easily missed cause of neonatal convulsions. *Neuropediatr* 1993; 24:139–42.

285. Roy RN, Pillnitz RP, Hamilton JR, Chance GW. Impaired assimilation of nasojejunal feeds in healthy low-birth-weight newborn infants. *J Pediatr* 1977; 90:431–4.

286. Challacombe D. Bacterial microflora in infants receiving nasojejunal tube feeding. *J Pediatr* 1974; 85:113.

287. Sun SC, Samuels S, Lee J, Marquis JR. Duodenal perforation: a rare complication of neonatal nasojejunal tube feeding. *Pediatrics* 1975; 55:371–5.

288. Haws EB, Sieber WK, Kiesewetter WB. Complications of tube gastrostomy in infants and children. *Ann Surg* 1966; 164:284–90.

289. Holder TM. Gastrostomy: its uses and dangers in pediatric patients. *N Eng J Med* 1972; 286:1345–7.

290. Lipsky CL, Spear ML. Recent advances in parenteral nutrition. *Clin Perinatol* 1995; 22:141–55.

291. Okada A, Takagi Y, Nezu R, Sando K, Shenkin A. Trace element metabolism in parenteral and enteral nutrition. *Nutrition* 1995; 11:106–13.

292. Goplerud JM. Hyperalimentation associated hepatotoxicity in the newborn. *Ann Clin Lab Med* 1992; 22:79–84.

293. Quigley EM, Marsh MN, Shaffer JL, Markin RS. Hepatobiliary complications of total parenteral nutrition. *Gastroenterology* 1993; 104:286–301.

294. Mullick FG, Moran CA, Ishak KG. Total parenteral nutrition: a histo-pathologic analysis of the liver changes in 20 children. *Mod Pathol* 1994; 7: 190–4.

295. Patterson K, Kapur SP, Chandra RS. Hepatocellular carcinoma in a non-cirrhotic infant after prolonged parenteral nutrition. *J Pediatr* 1985; 106:797–9.

296. Saldanha RL. Stein CA, Kopelman AE. Gall-bladder distension in ill preterm infants. *Am J Dis Child* 1983; 137:1179–80.

297. Crouch JB, Rubin LP. Nutrition. In: Cloherty JP, Stark AR, eds. *Manual of Neonatal Care*, 3rd ed. Boston: Little, Brown, 1991; pp. 526–58.

298. Baker CJ. Group B streptococcal infection in newborns: prevention at last? *N Engl J Med* 1986; 314:1702–4.

299. LaGamma EF, Drusin LM, Macles AW, Machalek S, Auld PAM. Neonatal infections: an important determination of late NICU mortality in infants less than 1000 g at birth. *Am J Dis Child* 1983; 137:838–41.

300. Murphy N, Buchanan CR, Damjanovic V, et al. Infection and colonization of neonates by *Hansuela anomala*. *Lancet* 1986; i:291–3.

301. Powell DA, Aungst J, Snedden S, Hansen N, Brady M. Broviac catheter-related *Malassezia furfur* sepsis in five infants receiving intravenous fat emulsions. *J Pediatr* 1984; 105:987–90.

302. Redline RW, Redline SS, Boxerbaum B, Dahms BB. Systemic *Malassezia furfur* infections in patients receiving intralipid therapy. *Hum Pathol* 1985; 16:815–22.

303. Vawter GF. Listeria monocytogenes: the perinatal infection. *Perspect Pediatr Pathol* 1981; 6:153–66.

304. Walsh MC, Simpser EF, Kliegman RM. Late onset of sepsis in infants with bowel resection in the neonatal period. *J Pediatr* 1988; 112:468–71.

305. MacGregor AP. Pneumonia in the newborn. *Arch Dis Child* 1939; 14:323–31.

306. Morison JE. *Foetal and Neonatal Pathology*. London: Butterworth, 1963, pp. 474ff.

307. Moss TJ, Pysher TJ. Hepatic abscess in neonates. *Am J Dis Child* 1981; 135:726–8.

308. Lilien LD, Harris VJ, Ramamurthy RS, Pildes RS. Neonatal osteomyelitis of the calcaneus: complication of heel puncture. *J Pediatr* 1976; 88:478–80.

309. Ginsburg CM, McCracken GH Jr. Urinary tract infection in young infants. *Pediatrics* 1982; 69:409–12.

310. Book LS, Overall JC Jr, Herbst JJ, et al. Interruption of necrotizing enterocolitis clustering by infection control measures. *N Engl J Med* 1977; 197:984–5.

311. Han VKM, Sayed H, Chance GW, Brabyn DG, Shaheed WA. An outbreak of *Clostridium difficile* necrotizing enterocolitis: a case for oral vancomycin therapy. *Pediatrics* 1983; 71:935–41.

312. McCracken GH Jr, Eitzman DV. Necrotizing enterocolitis. *Am J Dis Child* 1972; 132:1167–8.

313. McGuinness GA, Schieken RM, Maguire GF. Endocarditis in the newborn. *Am J Dis Child* 1980; 134:577–80.

314. Peter G, Cashore WJ. Infections acquired in the nursery: epidemiology and control. In: Remington JS, Klein JO, eds. *Infectious Diseases of the Fetus and Newborn Infant*, 4th ed. Philadelphia: Saunders, 1995, pp. 1264–86.

Causes and Classification of Fetal and Perinatal Death

Jonathan S. Wigglesworth

INTRODUCTION

The causes and classification of fetal and perinatal deaths can be considered at several levels and from a variety of viewpoints. National perinatal mortality statistics are used for political purposes in making claims as to how good or bad the maternity services are. Local figures, if bad, similarly may be used to bolster claims for improved services or, if improving, to show that the expensive services provided are fulfilling their role. Classifications of death by cause or disease process provide further material for epidemiologists to utilize in studying patterns of death in relation to age, place, time, or social status. National figures form a yardstick against which the significance of local figures can be assessed. Changes in some area of mortality (such as hypoxic perinatal deaths) in a hospital population can be assessed against national figures to provide some form of quality control for local perinatal care.

The validity of all such uses of the statistical data related to perinatal death is dependent on the consistency of definition and recording of the original information. There is considerable variation in practice between different countries with respect to definitions and recording practice. Pathologists are inevitably involved in this process, as they have to provide an assessment of cause or mode of death in the individual case, even if they do not become concerned with surveys of local perinatal mortality.

DEFINITIONS OF PERINATAL MORTALITY

Fetal Death

Fetal death is defined by the World Health Organization (WHO) as "death prior to the complete expulsion or extraction from its mother of a product of conception, irre-

spective of the duration of pregnancy; the death is indicated by the fact that after such separation the fetus does not breathe or show any other evidence of life such as beating of the heart, pulsation of the umbilical cord, or definite movement of voluntary muscles" [1, 2]. Most analyses of fetal death relate to late fetal death, i.e., fetal deaths after 28 weeks' gestation. Late fetal death or stillbirth rates are normally quoted per 1000 total births.

Neonatal Death

Neonatal deaths are deaths of liveborn infants in the first 4 weeks after birth. The neonatal death rate is normally quoted as deaths per 1000 livebirths.

Perinatal Death

Perinatal deaths comprise late fetal deaths and neonatal deaths in the first week after birth. The perinatal death rate is the late fetal deaths plus the first-week neonatal deaths per 1000 total births.

Viability

Definitions of fetal death, neonatal death, and perinatal death are affected significantly by the point selected for the lower limit of viability. In the United Kingdom, an act of parliament in 1925 determined that it was reasonable to assume viability in any fetus of 28 completed weeks of gestation. As a result, any fetus that died in utero before this time was regarded as an abortus and was excluded from perinatal mortality figures. Since many fetuses born at an earlier gestation now survive, it was possible for one of a pair of twins born at 24 weeks' gestation, for example, to be registered as a livebirth while a stillborn co-twin of similar size was excluded from consideration. The decrease in the upper time limit for abortion to 24 weeks' gestation in 1990 has caused this to be recognized as the lower limit for presumption of viability in the United Kingdom. Termination for severe malformation is allowed at any gestational age. A missed abortion, where fetal death has occurred many weeks before birth but the mother has delivered more than 24 weeks after commencement of her last menstrual period, should be registered as a stillbirth in the United Kingdom as should a fetus papyraceus born as one of a pair of twins. In Japan, all pregnancies lasting 13 weeks have to be registered [3]. In the United States, the lower limit for registering births is set at 20 weeks of age, and separate figures are quoted for fetal deaths (from 20 weeks) and late fetal deaths (from 28 weeks).

The World Health Organization, recognizing the difficulties in some countries of assessing gestational age, recommends that domestic perinatal figures should be quoted for infants of at least 500 grams' birth weight or 25 cm crown–heel length (equivalent to 22 weeks' gestational age), whereas "standard perinatal statistics" for international comparisons should be based on deaths of infants of at least 1000 grams' birth weight or 35 cm crown–heel length.

Registration

Irrespective of the definitions of viability and of fetal death and neonatal death adopted in different countries, there are considerable variations in registration practice, which influences the official figures. In the United Kingdom, for example, not all doctors would register an extremely small macerated fetus born at 24 weeks' gestation as a stillbirth if it was apparent that death had occurred in utero several weeks previously. This might apply particularly to the example given above of a fetus papyraceus as unexpected co-twin to a healthy infant.

There are also problems in deciding whether to register an extremely immature fetus as a livebirth. Livebirth is defined by the World Health Organization as "the complete expulsion or extraction from its mother of a product of conception, irrespective of the duration of pregnancy, which after such separation, breathes or shows any other evidence of life such as beating of the heart, pulsation of the umbilical cord, or definite movement of voluntary muscles" [54]. If the presence of a heartbeat alone is accepted as evidence of livebirth, then many aborted fetuses of less than 20 weeks' gestation could be recorded as livebirths. There are likely to be considerable variations in the diligence with which such signs are sought and in the efforts made to resuscitate extremely immature fetuses, according to gestational age, which is perceived as being compatible with viability in a particular institution [4]. A minor difference in management may shift a significant number of fetuses from the non-registered group to the neonatal deaths. This is less of a problem in those jurisdictions where all fetuses beyond 20 weeks' gestational age have to be registered.

Other pressures or local procedures may influence whether a dead infant is registered as a late fetal death or a neonatal death, as pointed out by Golding [5]. In some countries, an infant that dies before registration as a livebirth is counted as a fetal death. In others, the rules relating to entitlement to a maternity grant may influence the pattern of registration. Administrative failures also may lead to lack of registration of 10–31% of perinatal deaths in different cities or states [5–10]. The largest group of non-registrations are those fetuses with birth weights below 1000 grams who die soon after birth. Failure of registration is particularly likely in such infants born to ethnic minorities of low socioeconomic status or with language problems.

COMPONENTS OF PERINATAL MORTALITY

Comparisons of perinatal mortality between two different populations, or within the same population at two different times, require that similar definitions and accuracy of registration have been established for each population or time period under review. Even if these factors are comparable, interpretation of the mortality figures requires an understanding of the birth population from which they have been drawn. Many perinatal surveys are still carried out without an understanding of the rather basic point that the number and pattern of perinatal deaths may be altered significantly by a minor change in the proportions of the population most at risk to perinatal death. The frequency of perinatal death is inversely related to gestational age and thus also to birth weight (Fig. 4.1). However, most babies are born at term and have a low risk of death (Fig. 4.2). The net effect of the combination of large numbers of large mature infants at low risk of death with progressively smaller numbers of births of less-well-grown, less mature infants at progressively higher risk of death is a wide spread of birth weight and gestational age in those infants who die (Fig. 4.3).

In most birth populations, about one-third of perinatal deaths are in relatively well-grown infants of 2.5 kilograms

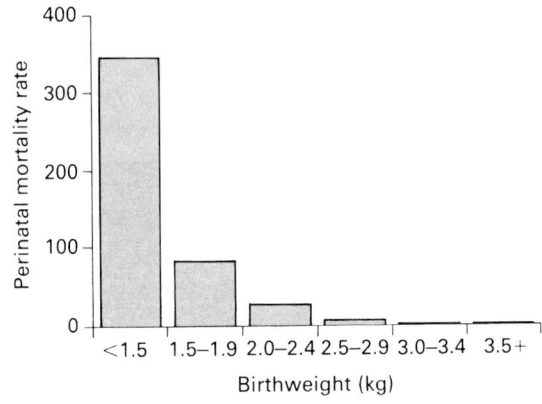

FIGURE 4.1.   *Perinatal mortality rate for different birthweight groups, England and Wales, 1986. (Data from the OPCS [16].)*

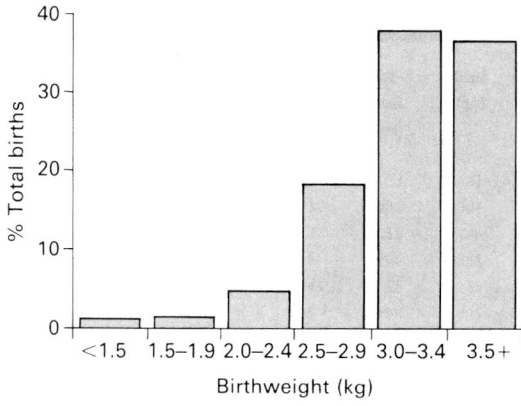

FIGURE 4.2. *Birth-weight distribution of liveborn and stillborn infants (known birth weights only), England and Wales, 1986. (Data from the OPCS [16].)*

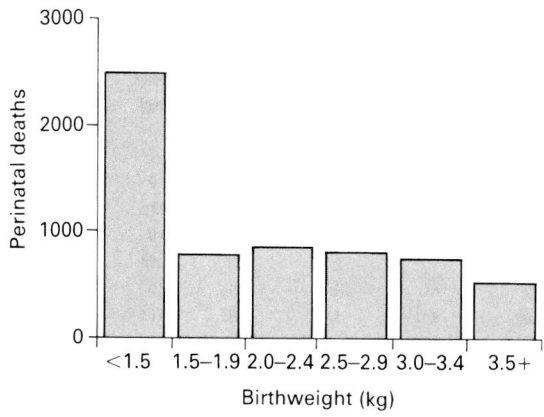

FIGURE 4.3. *Birth-weight distribution of perinatal deaths, England and Wales, 1986. (Data from the OPCS [16].)*

of birth weight or more, while two-thirds are in infants of low birth weight (see Fig. 4.3). However, a rather slight difference in the proportion of markedly preterm births in a population would be expected to have a marked effect on the overall perinatal mortality. Many terminations are now performed for congenital anomaly before the start of the recognized perinatal period. This may account for up to one-third of the decline in perinatal mortality noted in the period 1985–1990 [11].

As the perinatal mortality period only includes the first week after birth, any increase in the rate of resuscitation of very small ("previable") fetuses will increase the perinatal mortality rate if they die within 7 days but will decrease it if they survive beyond that period. Neonatal care that leads to prolonged survival of sick or malformed neonates may decrease the perinatal mortality rate but increase the late neonatal death rate or the infant mortality rate according to whether the infant dies within the first month after birth or later in the first year. It has been suggested that the perinatal mortality rate would form a more useful measure of the effectiveness of perinatal care if it included late neonatal deaths [12, 13].

Comparison of the United Kingdom perinatal mortality rates for 1978 with those for Sweden for the same year indicated that the United Kingdom was lagging behind Sweden in perinatal care. However, the United Kingdom perinatal mortality figures differed little from those for Sweden for most birth-weight subgroups. The higher crude British perinatal mortality rate was due to a larger proportion of infants of low birth weight [14]. This might suggest that background social factors responsible for birth weight and maturity were more important than purely medical ones.

The proportions of late fetal deaths show a similar inverse relationship with gestational age, to that of perinatal deaths as a whole. It may be assumed readily that there is a higher risk of the fetus dying in utero in the early third trimester than near term. However, the correct denominator for still-

births at a particular gestation is the total number of unborn infants rather than the number of births [15]. Thus, the risk of an unborn fetus dying in utero increases steadily toward term and rises rapidly past 41 weeks' gestation when there are few fetuses remaining undelivered.

CURRENT PATTERNS OF PERINATAL MORTALITY

In the United Kingdom in 1986 the stillbirth rate was 5.0, the neonatal death rate was 4.7, and the perinatal death rate was 8.8 [16]. These figures represent a continuing fall by some 50% over 10 years from 1975. The United Kingdom comes only thirteenth in a World League, but the change in rates is virtually a universal phenomenon [17]. Further decreases in perinatal mortality since the late 1980s are less pronounced than in earlier years. In 1995 (after the inclusion of deaths at 24 to 27 weeks' gestation) the perinatal death rate for the United Kingdom was 8.8 and the stillbirth rate 5.5, but the neonatal death rate had declined to 4.2 [18].

A study in Finland [19] showed a decline in perinatal mortality from 17.9 in 1968 to 7.0 in 1982, or from 14.8 to 4.6 when infants of less than 1000 grams were excluded. All cases underwent postmortem examination in this series. Neonatal deaths declined more markedly than fetal deaths and accounted for two-thirds of the mortality at the start of the study period and one-third at the end. The greatest decline occurred in the neonatal deaths of infants of low birth weight. Significant declines occurred also in perinatal mortality due to maternal illness, placental and umbilical cord complications, other forms of asphyxia, and respiratory distress syndrome.

In Western Australia, the stillbirth rate fell from 12.24 in 1971 to 8.65 in 1981, and the neonatal death rate from 12.19 to 5.91 over the same period [20]. As in the Finnish study, the fall in neonatal mortality was the greater. In 1981 the major causes of perinatal and infant death were congenital malformations, stillbirths of unknown cause, preterm births, and crib deaths.

Both Australian and Finnish authors concluded that the improvements were due to better obstetric and pediatric services and to the introduction of neonatal intensive care rather than to changes in social factors.

FACTORS ASSOCIATED WITH PERINATAL DEATH

Epidemiological studies reveal that a large number of factors are associated with high or low perinatal mortality. It is often claimed loosely that these associated factors "cause" perinatal death, whereas in fact the causative factors responsible for the association are often obscure and inaccessible to the epidemiological approach.

Maternal Factors

Maternal Disease
Perinatal mortality is well recognized to be higher in major forms of maternal disease, including diabetes, heart disease, chronic renal disease, liver disease, and respiratory disease [21].

Maternal Age
There is increased perinatal mortality at both ends of the age scale, in mothers younger than 20 years and steadily increasing in those older than 30 [22, 23]. The association may be explicable in terms of the development of the uterus and its blood supply, with poor development in very young mothers and an inadequate response of the uterine vascular system in older mothers. A study in Jamaica showed that advanced maternal age was mainly associated with antepartum fetal deaths and that teenage pregnancy carried an increased risk of neonatal death associated with immaturity [5].

Parity
Second and third pregnancies have the lowest risk of perinatal death, but there is a steadily increasing risk for higher parities [22].

Maternal Height
There is an increased risk of perinatal death in short rather than tall mothers [22].

Maternal Smoking
Maternal smoking is associated with a decrease in birth weight and an increase in premature birth and perinatal mortality [24, 25].

Disorders of Pregnancy

Severe pre-eclampsia (a maximum diastolic blood pressure of 110 mmHg or more) is associated with a considerably increased risk of perinatal mortality, but the British perina-

tal mortality survey showed that mild pre-eclampsia (a maximum diastolic blood pressure of 99 mmHg or less) was not associated with increased risk of death [22]. Antepartum hemorrhage of all types is associated with high perinatal mortality rates. In several classifications of perinatal mortality, antepartum hemorrhage constitutes a major category [26, 27].

Influence of Obstetric Care

Surveys such as the Finnish and Australian ones cited above have suggested that improvements in obstetric care have played a significant role in recent years in lowering perinatal mortality rates, particularly in relation to intrapartum fetal deaths. Some studies have claimed that intrapartum fetal deaths have declined with increased electronic monitoring [28, 29]. A study of all singleton births in New York City during 1976–1978 showed that, compared with Level 3 maternity units (perinatal intensive care), births in Level 1 units (community hospitals) had a 61% excess risk of intrapartum fetal death, and births in Level 2 units (intermediate level of care) had a 35% excess risk of intrapartum deaths [30]. There was little difference in the relative risk of antepartum fetal death according to the level of care. The authors emphasize that fetal deaths in labor are especially sensitive to the level of obstetric care. Although the frequency of electronic fetal monitoring was higher with the increased level of maternity unit, it was not certain whether this was the major factor involved.

Influence of Neonatal Care

A number of the studies previously discussed have found a more rapid fall in neonatal deaths than in fetal deaths. Similar findings were demonstrated in a study of perinatal deaths in Manitoba from 1977 to 1983 [31]. In 1977 neonatal deaths represented 53% of all perinatal deaths, but by 1981 neonatal deaths accounted for only 40% of perinatal deaths. This change was attributed to the introduction of neonatal intensive care. Other investigators have specifically considered neonatal mortality in infants of low birth weight and have been able to demonstrate a major beneficial effect of neonatal intensive care [32–34].

A concern has been the possible effect of neonatal intensive care in shifting early neonatal deaths to late neonatal or infant deaths as a result of maintaining small infants on ventilators, or by palliative management of severe congenital anomalies. Recent figures give no indication that this is occurring with sufficient frequency to distort the overall pattern of neonatal and infant mortality [33, 35]. It may, however, blunt the original relatively sharp distinction between first-week neonatal deaths as being due to obstetric factors and later deaths as being due largely to factors arising de novo. In fact, most late neonatal and some postneonatal deaths represent late deaths from congenital anomalies or late deaths from problems of prematurity.

Influence of Ethnic Factors

The influence of ethnic factors on perinatal mortality is shown starkly by the British Office of Population Censuses and Surveys figures for perinatal death rates by country of birth of the mother [16]. For mothers born in the United Kingdom, the perinatal mortality rate for 1986 was 9.4, for mothers born in the Caribbean the rate was 12.1, and for mothers born in Pakistan the rate was 16.9. These differences are despite the availability of the same National Health Service maternity facilities to all groups (private maternity care being utilized only by a minute fraction of the population). Of the two immigrant communities, the Caribbean group has been in the United Kingdom for more than 30 years. More recent arrivals have entered an established community; they speak English and can make full use of medical facilities. There is a high unemployment rate and poor housing, which will be accentuated for first-generation immigrants, although there is no evidence that these factors increase perinatal mortality [5]. Extensive immigration to the United Kingdom from Pakistan is a more recent phenomenon. The immigrant women do not speak English and in the Muslim tradition live relatively secluded lives. Language and cultural differences make it difficult for this group to obtain maximum benefit from the health care available. There are nutritional inadequacies, particularly among vegetarian groups, and a high rate of intermarriage. The major part of the increased mortality rate is reported as being due to congenital anomalies [36]; any effect of possible differences in quality of health care received remains to be determined.

Socioeconomic Status

There are marked differences in perinatal mortality according to social class differences.

From the figures for England and Wales shown in Table 4.1, it can be seen that there is an inverse relationship between social class as defined by the Registrar General and stillbirth, neonatal death, and perinatal mortality rates. The stillbirth rate is 78% higher in social class V than in social class I; the perinatal mortality rate is 58% higher and the neonatal death rate 50% higher. The causal factors responsible for such differences are likely to be complex and not amenable to simple forms of analysis.

APPROACHES TO CLASSIFICATION

Problem of Perinatal Death Classification

The basic problem in the classification of perinatal deaths is the complexity of the clinical situation within which the fetus or newborn infant dies. The previous discussion of definitions already indicates the difficulty of determining limits of the proportion of total reproductive loss that we may wish to classify. In any form of comprehensive classification, the major difficulty is the need to consider both the mother

Table 4.1. Stillbirth, perinatal mortality, and neonatal death rates in England and Wales in 1986 by social class: legitimate births only

Social class*	Stillbirth rate	Perinatal mortality rate	Neonatal death rate
I	3.7	7.2	4.1
II	4.0	7.2	4.1
IIIN	4.8	8.4	4.3
IIIM	5.2	8.9	4.7
IV	5.7	9.9	5.4
V	6.6	11.4	6.0

* Classified by husband's occupation: I—professional, e.g., lawyers, doctors; II—intermediates, e.g., teachers and managers; IIIN—skilled non-manual, e.g., clerks, shop assistants; IIIM—skilled manual, e.g., bricklayers, underground miners; IV—semiskilled, e.g., postmen, bus conductors; V—unskilled and others, e.g., porters, laborers.
Data from the OPCS [16].

and the fetus as separate individuals, as well as interactions between the two through the placenta.

If we take into account prepregnancy influences on the mother, problems arising in pregnancy, complications of birth, genetic factors affecting the fetus, neonatal disorders, and complications of management, the analysis of perinatal death may appear to defy any logical form of classification. There are, however, insistent and justifiable demands for classification and determination of causation on medical, political, and sociological grounds. If the factors all acted in sequence so that, for instance, a poor maternal nutritional background resulted in poor placental and fetal growth, which in turn resulted in fetal death in utero, the analysis might not be too difficult. Unfortunately, the varying factors may act in parallel so that unfavorable maternal pregnancy factors occur with genetically determined fetal abnormalities.

Although it might be possible to design a classification that would take all influences into consideration, the practical problem would arise of the quantity of information available in any one case. Thus, pathological data are not available for all cases and cannot, therefore, be used as a basis for classification in institutions, much less at a national or international level. Classification systems need to be designed in terms of the data that are available or can be obtained, and in a form that will allow subsequent analysis in terms of the questions most likely to be posed [37].

Classification Systems Currently Used or Suggested

WHO Classification System

The method of classification recommended by the WHO for the purpose of international comparisons is by use of

BIRTHS AND DEATHS REGISTRATION ACT 1953

(Form prescribed by the Registration of Births, Deaths and Marriages (Amendment) (No. 2) Regulations 1985)

MEDICAL CERTIFICATE OF CAUSE OF DEATH OF A LIVE-BORN CHILD
DYING WITHIN THE FIRST TWENTY-EIGHT DAYS OF LIFE

For use only by a Registered Medical Practitioner WHO HAS BEEN IN ATTENDANCE during the deceased's last illness,
and to be delivered by him forthwith to the Registrar of Births and Deaths.

Registrar to enter
No. of Death Entry

Name of child ....

Date of death .... day of .... 19 .... Sex ....

Age at death .... days (complete period of 24 hours) .... hours

Place of death ....

Place of birth ....

Last seen alive by me .... day of .... 19 ....

1 The certified cause of death has been confirmed by post-mortem.
2 Information from post-mortem may be available later.
3 Post-mortem not being held.
4 I have reported this death to the Coroner for further action.
[See overleaf]

Please ring appropriate digit and letter.

a Seen after death by me.
b Seen after death by another medical practitioner but not by me.
c Not seen after death by a medical practitioner.

CAUSE OF DEATH

a. Main diseases or conditions in infant ....

b. Other diseases or conditions in infant ....

c. Main maternal diseases or conditions affecting infant ....

d. Other maternal diseases or conditions affecting infant ....

e. Other relevant causes ....

I hereby certify that I was in medical attendance during the above named deceased's last illness, and that the particulars and cause of death above written are true to the best of my knowledge and belief.

Signature ....

Address ....

Qualifications as registered by General Medical Council ....

Date ....

For deaths in hospital: Please give the name of the consultant responsible for the above-named as a patient ....

FIGURE 4.4. *Current neonatal death certificate used in the United Kingdom. This provides space for information on both maternal and infant disorders relevant to the death.*

the detailed list of three-digit categories (with or without fourth-digit subcategories) in the *International Classification of Diseases*. If this is not possible, the basic tabulation list of 307 causes [38] may be used. The use of the WHO perinatal death certificate would, in theory, allow this information, as well as birth weight and gestation data and a considerable quantity of further information, to be collected routinely for statistical analysis. Although this certificate is in use in a number of European countries, it has not been introduced to the United Kingdom or North America. In the United Kingdom and in the United States, new perinatal death certificates giving some of the required basic information have been introduced (Fig. 4.4).

Aberdeen Classification

This classification, originally introduced by Baird et al in Aberdeen [26] and expanded for use in relation to the

British Perinatal Mortality Survey of 1958 [39], classifies perinatal death purely from an obstetric point of view in terms of maternal conditions. The results of pathological studies on the dead infant are not taken into account. Baird and Thomson [39] stated that the "chief purpose of a classification of deaths is to assist prevention." They stated further that postmortem findings may be inconclusive from this point of view because they indicate how but not why the baby died; and that the aim of their classification was to identify "the factor that probably initiated the train of events leading to death." The classification thus makes the assumption that there is such a simple sequence, although, as was pointed out earlier, this often is not valid. Although the approach may be adequate for considering maternal aspects of perinatal death, it does not provide a fully acceptable way for neonatologists or pathologists to analyze perinatal death. Thus, the category "prematurity cause unknown" is clearly

Table 4.2. Modified Aberdeen classification of Cole et al [40]

Baird and Thomson [4]	Cole et al [17]	Cole et al subclassification
Malformation	Congenital anomaly	Neural tube defects Other anomalies
Serological incompatibility	Isoimmunization	Due to the rhesus (D) antigen Due to other antigens
Toxemia	Pre-eclampsia	Without APH Complicated by APH
APH (without toxemia)	APH	With placenta previa With placental abruption APH of uncertain origin

Mechanical	Mechanical	Cord prolapse or compression in vertex
		    or face presentation
		Other vertex or face presentation
		Breech presentation
		Oblique or compound presentation,
		    uterine rupture, etc.

Maternal disease	Maternal disorder	Maternal hypertensive disease Other maternal disease Maternal infection
Infection of the fetus or infant	Miscellaneous	Neonatal infection
Miscellaneous		Other neonatal disease Specific fetal conditions

Uncertain
  Mature
  Premature
	
	Unexplained ≥2.5 kg
	Unexplained <2.5 kg	

Unclassified	Unclassifiable	

APH = antepartum hemorrhage.

an inadequate way to describe all deaths in infants weighing less than 2500 grams, although in 1969 it may have seemed reasonable to obstetricians.

An updating of this obstetric approach has been carried out, with alteration of the terminology and definitions to agree with current international practice [40] (Table 4.2). The current working definitions are as follows:

Congenital anomaly: Any genetic or structural defect arising at conception or during embryogenesis incompatible with life or potentially treatable but causing death.

Isoimmunization: Death ascribable to blood group incompatibility.

Pre-eclampsia: Only significant pre-eclampsia, i.e., a diastolic blood pressure of 90 mmHg or more on two separate days after 20 weeks' gestation (140 days) with significant proteinuria in the absence of existing hypertensive disease before pregnancy. The full definition of pre-eclampsia is the same as that given by the International Federation of Gynaecology and Obstetrics to the terms pre-eclampsia and eclampsia in the 9th Edition of the *International Classification of Diseases* (ICD Codes 642.4–642.6).

Antepartum hemorrhage: Vaginal bleeding after 20 weeks' gestation (140 days), whether revealed or not, excluding antepartum hemorrhage secondary to pre-eclampsia (which is classified under pre-eclampsia). Minor degrees of hemorrhage at the start of labor (a "show") and hemorrhage due to a cervical erosion or polyp should be ignored, but significant or recurrent bleeding of uncertain origin that is followed fairly closely by preterm labor should not be ignored.

Mechanical: Any death from uterine rupture and those deaths from birth trauma or intrapartum asphyxia that are associated with problems in labor, such as disproportion, malpresentation, cord prolapse, cord compression, or breech delivery in babies weighing 1000 grams or more. If there is no evidence of difficulty in labor, deaths from asphyxia or trauma should be classified as "unexplained." Antepartum deaths associated with cord entanglement in the absence of strong circumstantial evidence that cord compression caused death (e.g., fetal death soon after external version) also should be classified as "unexplained."

Maternal disorder: Includes maternal trauma (such as automobile accident), diabetes, appendicitis, and cardiac disease, etc., if severe enough to jeopardize the baby. It includes significant renal disease or essential hypertension known to be present before pregnancy and includes also symptomatic and asymptomatic maternal infection when this results in the death of the baby.

Miscellaneous: Specific fetal and neonatal conditions only; does not include conditions directly ascribable to prematurity or asphyxia before birth, because these deaths are attributable to the relevant underlying obstetric disorder; includes, however, specific fetal conditions (e.g., twin-to-twin transfusion) or neonatal conditions (e.g., inhalation of milk) where these are not ascribable directly to intrapartum anoxia or preterm delivery; includes also postnatally acquired infection, except in babies weighing less than 1000 grams (here, the reason for the low birth weight is the codable factor).

Unexplained: Deaths with no obstetric explanation, including unexplained antepartum stillbirths, deaths resulting from unexplained preterm delivery (including hyaline membrane disease, intraventricular hemorrhage, etc.) and cases of intrapartum asphyxia or trauma if the baby weighed less than 1000 grams at birth or delivery was unassociated with any obvious mechanical problem. Cases should be subclassified into those babies weighing 2500 grams or more and those of less than 2500 grams at birth.

Unclassifiable: Cases where little or nothing is known about pregnancy or delivery. Use this category as sparingly as possible.

Classification by Pathological Findings

A classification by primary postmortem findings was introduced by Bound et al [41] and later used in reporting the results of the 1958 British Perinatal Mortality Survey [22]. This was also used in a survey of perinatal deaths in southeast London [42]. The coding was designed to give cause of death rather than to detail all pathological lesions present. The problem was determining which condition represented the primary cause of death, e.g., in an immature infant with hyaline membrane disease and intraventricular hemorrhage. This approach to classification has been reconsidered by Hey et al [43], who have suggested modifications (Table 4.3) and have provided a flow chart for perinatal death coding. These authors claim that the use of modern diagnostic procedures, such as the range of imaging techniques applicable in perinatal and infant periods, allows quite sophisticated pathological diagnoses, even in infants who never undergo postmortem examination.

Naeye's Classification   Richard Naeye designed a classification involving placental and fetal pathological findings, which was used for analysis of data from the US Collaborative Perinatal Project [27].

Potter's Classification   Edith Potter devised her own pathological classification that would fit on a standard punch card [44]. This is mainly organized on a standard organ system

design, but allows recording also of relevant maternal disorders.

Other Classifications

Hovatta et al [45] and Autio-Harmainen et al [35] have produced classifications for stillbirths and neonatal deaths, respectively.

SNOMED System   Classification using Systemized Nomenclature for Medicine (SNOMED) can be achieved using the Microglossary for Pediatrics, Pediatric Pathology, and Perinatal Medicine [46]. SNOMED has six fields or axes for classification: topography, morphology, etiology, function, disease, and procedure, designated by code letters T, M, E, F, D, and P, respectively. Of these, topography is the base to which all other fields must be linked. Any medical event coded must be linked either to a specific site within the body or to the body as a whole (T-00010). The use of the code letters is critical, as there are identical code numbers in different fields. Within fields, particularly within the morphology field, the classification has a hierarchical structure, allowing retrieval of cases with inclusive diagnoses as well as those with specific diagnoses. Thus, M29000 (placenta, abnormal, not otherwise specified) can be used to retrieve all abnormally formed placentae, whereas the different forms of twin placenta are coded as M29040-twin monochorionic diamniotic, M29050-twin monochorionic monoamniotic, and M29060-twin dichorionic diamniotic. The fifth digit modifiers for more accurate definition are obtained where needed from the main SNOMED. There is a perinatal section of the microglossary that includes codes for clinical details relating to maternal problems, gestation, and mode of delivery, which allows considerable detail to be coded in an individual case.

Analysis by Temporal Relationship of Death to Birth, External Appearances, and Birth Weight

Some years ago, it was pointed out that a small number of major subgroups of perinatal deaths could be defined using a combination of the known timing of death (before commencement of labor, during labor or delivery, or in the neonatal period), external appearances, and any information obtained in life [14]. These subgroups comprised:

1. Normally formed macerated stillborn infants.
2. Congenital malformations (stillbirth or neonatal death).
3. Conditions associated with immaturity (neonatal death).
4. Asphyxial conditions developing in labor (fresh stillbirth or neonatal death).
5. Other specific conditions (e.g., known beta-hemolytic streptococcal infection).

To the embarrassment of the author, this grouping has become known as the "Wigglesworth classification," although it was originally presented as an illustration of how

Table 4.3.   Classification by fetal and neonatal factors of Hey et al [43]

Butler and Bonham [22]	Hey et al [43]	Hey et al subclassification*	Category
Congenital malformation	Congenital anomaly	Chromosomal defect	1
		Inborn error of metabolism	2
		Neural tube defect	3
		Congenital heart disease	4
		Renal abnormality	5
		Other anomaly	6
Isoimmunization	Isoimmunization		7
Antepartum death with:	Antepartum asphyxia		8
(a) postmortem evidence of anoxia			
(b) no postmortem evidence of anoxia			
Intrapartum death with postmortem evidence of:	Intrapartum asphyxia		9
(a) anoxia			
(b) anoxia + trauma			
(c) neither			
Cerebral birth trauma	Birth trauma		10
Neonatal death (no postmortem abnormality)	Pulmonary immaturity		11
Hyaline membrane	HMD	HMD	12
		HMD with IVH	13
		HMD with infection	14
IVH	Intracerebral hemorrhage	IVH	15
		Other intracerebral bleeding	16
Pulmonary infection	Infection	Necrotizing enterocolitis	17
		Antepartum infection	18
		Intrapartum infection	19
		Postpartum infection	20
Massive pulmonary hemorrhage	Miscellaneous		21
Miscellaneous	Miscellaneous		
No postmortem examination	—	—	—
—	Unclassified or unknown	Crib death	22
		Unattended delivery	23
		Undocumented or unclassified	24

HMD = hyaline membrane disease; IVF = intraventricular hemorrhage.
* Further detailed subclassification obtainable by use of *International Classification of Diseases* codes for each abnormality or factor.

perinatal deaths could be investigated rather than as an established classification.

The groups require less sophistication to define than those of the more detailed breakdown of Bound et al [41], as redefined by Hey et al [43], but do present some problems. There may, for instance, be inadequate information on the precise time of fetal death in a case where a woman presents in early labor with an absent fetal heart. In such a case, the presence or absence of maceration may be used to decide which category the death comes into. If this information is not available, then at least it indicates the need for improved documentation. Many preterm infants who die soon after birth do so apparently as a result of an asphyxial event relating to the birth, such as antepartum hemorrhage or a vaginal breech delivery. It may be necessary to specify that neonatal death in a normally formed infant below a

certain weight or gestation (e.g., 800 gm or 26 weeks) is always regarded as being due to conditions associated with immaturity, whereas a similar infant above such a weight may be coded as dying from asphyxia if death occurs within a certain time after birth (e.g., 4 hours). There are also problems in determining how severe a malformation should be to justify coding it as a cause of death, and how to code death due to a deformation such as pulmonary hypoplasia secondary to prolonged leakage of amniotic fluid.

Hey et al [43] suggest the following approach to coding anomalies: If the defect is one that would inevitably cause death if the infant were born alive (such as bilateral renal agenesis), classification is easy, although it may not be possible to explain why the infant died in utero. In the case of a severe, but potentially treatable, malformation such as exomphalos, it may be reasonable also to code death as being "due" to the anomaly, as there is known to be an increased incidence of fetal death in such cases. In the case of less severe malformations, such as localized intestinal atresia, death is only ascribed to the malformation if it occurred as a direct or indirect consequence of it. This might be due to some complication of corrective surgery or due to a complication of preterm birth induced by polyhydramnios. Infants in whom the only "anomaly" is pulmonary hypoplasia are coded as "other specific condition" if there is reasonable evidence that the lung growth impairment was due to oligohydramnios following prolonged membrane rupture, but are coded as "congenital anomaly" if the cause of lung hypoplasia is obscure. Stillborn infants with three or more minor anomalies (e.g., extra digits, low-set ears, small cardiac septal defects) are coded as deaths due to anomaly. This is important in such cases where there is no consent to postmortem examination. Single-gene defects, such as cystic fibrosis or galactosemia, are coded with the congenital anomalies. A further objection is to the use of the term "asphyxial" to describe non-malformed deaths related to birth events. This may be a reasonable term to use scientifically to encompass the range of anoxic and ischemic events that can cause death at this time. To the legal mind, the term may suggest a preventable cause and thus a fit subject for litigation, an attitude that does not require further encouragement at present.

These various problems and objections are considered by Hey et al [43], who have provided a revised "short classification of perinatal death."

The purpose of having a simple basic classification is for epidemiological use in the study of perinatal death in populations where postmortem examinations will have been performed only in a proportion of the deaths. The subgroups selected can provide useful information on quality of perinatal care if they are related to the birth weight and/or gestational age grouping of the deaths and back-

ground birth population, as originally suggested [14]. Thus, the mortality rate of babies of different weights or gestations from "conditions arising in labor" can give some indication of the quality of obstetric care, while the mortality related to "problems of preterm birth," particularly weight or gestation groups, may relate more to the quality of neonatal management.

This approach has proved to be of practical help in a number of epidemiological and hospital studies [47–51], although there has been some lack of consistency in use [5]. An attempt to refine this classification has been published [52].

CURRENT MAJOR CONTRIBUTORS TO PERINATAL MORTALITY

In the first edition I stated that the rapid fall in perinatal mortality rates in the developed countries caused published figures rapidly to become out-of-date and quoted figures from Scotland [53] as providing useful up-to-date analyses. Since that time there has been a less dramatic fall in perinatal mortality rates with the added complication in the United Kingdom of a change in the definition of stillbirth to include deaths with a lower limit of 24 weeks' completed gestation rather than 28 weeks.

However, the 1987 Scottish figures can usefully be compared with those for Wales published in 1995 in the All Wales Perinatal Survey [54] in that both reports contain tables for breakdown of perinatal mortality by the Aberdeen classification of Baird and Thomson [39] (as modified by Cole et al [40]) as is shown in Table 4.4. The crude perinatal mortality rate is the same in both surveys despite the inclusion of the additional early stillbirths in the more recent study. Breakdown of the more recent figures by the "extended Wigglesworth" classification is shown in Table 4.5. The obstetric classification indicates the continuing fall

Table 4.4. Modified obstetric classification of deaths

	Perinatal mortality		Neonatal mortality	
	Scotland	Wales	Scotland	Wales
Total	8.1	8.1	4.0	3.9
Congenital anomaly	1.6	1.0	1.3	0.8
Isoimmunization	0.0	0.1	0.0	0.0
Hypertension of pregnancy	0.3	0.6	0.2	0.4
Antepartum hemorrhage	1.0	1.5	0.4	0.7
Trauma/mechanical	0.3	0.3	0.2	0.2
Maternal disorder	0.4	0.7	0.2	0.4
Other	0.3	0.4	0.2	0.2
Unknown (body wt <2.5 kg)	2.7	2.5	1.2	0.9
Unknown (body wt >2.5 kg)	1.4	1.0	0.2	0.3
Postnatal cause only	0.0	0.0	0.2	0.0

Comparison of figures for Scotland 1987 [53] with those for Wales 1995 [54].

Table 4.5.   Stillbirth and neonatal mortality rates by "Extended Wigglesworth" Classification

	Stillbirth	Early neonatal rate	Late neonatal rate
Total	5.1	3.0	0.9
Congenital anomaly	0.4	0.7	0.1
Unexplained before labor	3.1	—	—
Placental abruption before labor	0.7	—	—
Intrapartum event (asphyxia, trauma)	0.4	0.4	0.1
Immaturity (liveborn)	—	1.6	0.6
Infection	0.2	0.1	0.05
Other specific causes*	0.3	0.1	0.05
Accidental (nonintrapartum)	0.0	0.0	0.0
Sudden infant death of unknown cause	—	0.1	0.03
Unclassifiable	0.0	0.0	0.0

Wales 1995 [54].
*   Includes twin-twin transfusion, nonimmune hydrops, tumurs, inborn metabolic errors, etc.

in deaths from congenital anomaly in cases included within the perinatal period. This is undoubtedly due mainly to increased availability of early prenatal diagnosis and termination of affected fetuses. The report for Wales includes information that the number of terminations for congenital anomaly in the late second trimester was equal to the number of infants with anomalies who died in the perinatal period. The extended Wigglesworth classification shows that normally formed antepartum stillbirths constitute the largest proportion of perinatal deaths, with problems related to immature birth constituting the largest group of both early and late neonatal deaths.

A similar analysis of other populations at other times might give a very different breakdown. The prevention of known causes of late stillbirth leaves an increasing proportion of unexplained antepartum deaths in normally formed infants.

The effects of increasing attempts to maintain very small fetuses alive by means of neonatal intensive care may be to increase the proportion, or even the numbers, of deaths due to conditions associated with preterm birth. A fall in asphyxial deaths may result from improved obstetric care. A fall in frequency of congenital anomalies may sometimes reflect an improvement in general health impinging on the multifactorial causes of most anomalies, but as shown above is now mainly due to prenatal diagnosis and termination which shifts such cases out of the registrable period.

SELECTION OF A CLASSIFICATION SYSTEM

The selection of a classification system in a particular set of circumstances is dependent on the purpose to which the classification is to be put. The pathologist wishing to retrieve various types of cases from his hospital files will need to use a pathological system such as SNOMED or a simple local system such as Potter's.

The hospital or local region with a consistent approach to pathology may wish to undertake an analysis of more broadly based pathological groups using a system such as that described by Hey et al [43]. Some regions may wish to use a combined maternal and fetal approach, with dual classification of maternal and fetal factors, as suggested by Cole et al [40]. For study, at an epidemiological level, of large groups of cases with variable pathological input, a simple basic classification such as the modified Wigglesworth classification described above is most likely to be applicable.

A problem with any classification of perinatal death is the need to assume a single ultimate cause in order to simplify analysis. In reality, it may be quite obvious that a number of different factors have contributed to death in a way that cannot be explained in terms of a single sequence.

USE OF DEATH CERTIFICATES

In the absence of the availability of any coded classification of the cause of death or pathological findings, it is customary to perform epidemiological studies using the causes obtained from the death certificate. A number of studies have shown that these are frequently in error [55–57]. Thus, Fedrick and Butler [57] found that even for such a clearly recognizable condition as anencephalus only 90% of cases had the anomaly recorded on the death certificate. Problems that arise are the completion of death certificates before postmortem examination and the variety of "causes" of death that may be recorded. Recent improvement in the format of the certificate may allow improved reporting [55, 58].

REFERENCES

1. Chiswick ML. Commentary on current World Health Organization definitions used in perinatal statistics. *Br J Obstet Gynaecol* 1986; 93:1236–8.

2. World Health Organization. *Manual of the International Statistical Classification of Diseases, Injuries and Causes of Death*, 9th Revision, Vol. 1. Geneva: WHO, 1977.

3. Kamimura K. Epidemiology of twin births from a climatic point of view. *Br J Prev Soc Med* 1976; 30:175–9.

4. Goldenberg RL, Nelson KG, Dyer RL, Wayne J. The variability of viability: the effect of physicians' perceptions of viability on the survival of very low-birth-weight infants. *Am J Obstet Gynecol* 1982; 143:678–84.

5. Golding J. Epidemiology of fetal and neonatal death. In: Keeling J, ed. *Fetal and Neonatal Pathology*, 2nd ed. London: Springer Verlag, 1993, pp. 165–81.

6. Alley J, Terry J. Under-reporting of neonatal deaths—Georgia 1974–77. *CDC Morbid Mortal Weekly Rep* 1979; 28:253–4.

7. Doornbos JPR, Nordbeck HJ, Treffers PE. The reliability of perinatal mortality statistics in The Netherlands. *Am J Obstet Gynecol* 1987; 156:1183–7.

8. McCarthy BJ, Terry J, Rochat RW, Quave S, Tyler CW Jr. The under-registration of neonatal deaths: Georgia 1974–77. *Am J Public Health* 1980; 70:977–82.

9. Scott MJ, Ritchie JW, McClure BG, Reid MM, Halliday HL. Perinatal death recording: time for a change? *Br Med J* 1981; 282:707–10.

10. Tzoumaka-Bakoula C. Assessment of the incidence of perinatal deaths in Greece using two separate sources. In: Golding J, ed. *The Third Report of the WHO Study of Social and Biological Effects on Perinatal Mortality*. Geneva: WHO, 1987.

11. Gissler M, Ollila E, Teperi J, Hemminki E. Impact of induced abortions and statistical definitions on perinatal mortality figures. *Paediatr Perinat Epidemiol* 1994; 8:391–400.

12. Campbell MK, Webster KM. Age at neonatal death in Ontario, 1979–1987: implications for the interpretation of mortality markers. *Paediatr Perinat Epidemiol* 1993; 7:426–33.

13. Cartlidge PH, Stewart JH. Effect of changing the stillbirth definition on evaluation of perinatal mortality rates. *Lancet* 1995; 346:486–8.

14. Wigglesworth JS. Monitoring perinatal mortality: a pathophysiological approach. *Lancet* 1980; 2:684–6.

15. Yudkin PL, Wood L, Redman CWG. Risk of unexplained stillbirth at different gestational ages. *Lancet* 1987; i:1192–4.

16. Office of Population Censuses and Surveys Series DHS no. 20. 1986 *Mortality Statistics, Perinatal and Infant: Social and Biological Factors*. London: HMSO, 1988.

17. National Center for Health Statistics: Health United States, 1987. DHHS Publ. No. (PHS) 88–1232, Public Health Service. US Government Printing Office, Washington, 1988.

18. *Infant and Perinatal Mortality 1995*. ONS Population and Health Monitor, DHS 96/1. London: Office of National Statistics Publications Unit, 1996, p. 4.

19. Piekkala P, Erkkola R, Kero P, Tenovuo A, Sillanpaa M. Declining perinatal mortality in a region of Finland, 1978–82. *Am J Public Health* 1985; 75:156–60.

20. Stanley FJ, Waddell VP. Changing patterns of perinatal and infant mortality in Western Australia: implications for prevention. *Med J Aust* 1985; 143:379–81.

21. Naeye RL, Tafari N, eds. *Risk Factors in Pregnancy and Diseases of the Fetus and Newborn*. Baltimore: Williams & Wilkins, 1983.

22. Butler NR, Bonham DG, eds. *Perinatal Mortality*. Edinburgh: Churchill Livingstone, 1963, pp. 278–9.

23. Pharoah POD, Alberman ED. Annual statistical review. *Arch Dis Child* 1988; 63:1511–5.

24. Butler NR, Goldstein H, Ross EM. Cigarette smoking in pregnancy: its influence on birth weight and perinatal mortality. *Br Med J* 1972; 2:127–30.

25. Pirani BBK. Smoking during pregnancy. *Obstet Gynecol Surv* 1978; 33:1–13.

26. Baird D, Walker J, Thomson AM. The causes and prevention of stillbirths and first week deaths. Part III. A classification of deaths by clinical cause. *J Obstet Gynaecol Br Emp* 1954; 61:433–48.

27. Naeye RL. Causes of perinatal mortality in the US Collaborative Perinatal Project. *J Am Med Assoc* 1977; 238:228–9.

28. Erkolla R, Gronoos M, Punnonen R, Kilkku P. Analysis of intrapartum fetal deaths: their decline with increasing electronic fetal monitoring. *Acta Obstet Gynecol Scand* 1984; 63:459–63.

29. Parer JT. Fetal heart-rate monitoring. *Lancet* 1979; 2:632–3.

30. Kiely JL, Paneth N, Susser M. Fetal death during labor: an epidemiologic indicator of level of obstetric care. *Am J Obstet Gynecol* 1985; 153:721–7.

31. Morrison I. Perinatal mortality: basic considerations. *Semin Perinatol* 1985; 9:144–50.

32. Cohen RS, Stevenson DK, Malachowski N, et al. Favorable results of neonatal intensive care for very low-birth-weight infants. *Pediatrics* 1982; 69:621–5.

33. Horwood SP, Boyle MH, Torrance GW, Sinclair JC. Mortality and morbidity of 500- to 1499-gram birth weight infants live-born to residents of a defined geographic region before and after neonatal intensive care. *Pediatrics* 1982; 69:613–20.

34. Paneth N, Kiely JL, Wallenstein S, et al. Newborn intensive care and neonatal mortality in low-birth-weight infants: a population study. *N Engl J Med* 1982; 307:149–55.

35. Autio-Harmainen H, Rapola J, Hoppu K, Osterlund K. Causes of death in a paediatric hospital neonatal unit. *Acta Paediatr Scand* 1983; 72:333–7.

36. Gillies DRN, Lealman GT, Lumb KM, Congdon P. Analysis of ethnic influence on stillbirths and infant mortality in Bradford 1975–81. *J Epidemiol Community Health* 1984; 38:214–17.

37. Wigglesworth JS. Classification of perinatal deaths. *Soz Praventivmed* 1994; 39:11–4.

38. FIGO Standing Committee on Perinatal Mortality and Morbidity. *Report of the Committee following a Workshop on Monitoring and Reporting Perinatal Mortality and Morbidity*. London: Chameleon, 1982.

39. Baird D, Thomson AM. The effects of obstetric and environmental factors on perinatal mortality by clinicopathological causes. In: Butler NR, Alberman ED, eds. *Perinatal Problems*. Edinburgh: Churchill Livingstone, 1969, pp. 211–26.

40. Cole SK, Hey EN, Thomson AM. Classifying perinatal death: an obstetric approach. *Br J Obstet Gynaecol* 1986; 93:1204–12.

41. Bound JP, Butler NR, Spector WG. Classification and causes of perinatal mortality. *Br Med J* 1956; ii:1191–6.

42. Machin GA. A perinatal mortality survey in South East London 1970–73: the pathological findings in 726 necropsies. *J Clin Pathol* 1975; 28:428–34.

43. Hey EN, Lloyd DJ, Wigglesworth JS. Classifying perinatal death: fetal and neonatal factors. *Br J Obstet Gynaecol* 1986; 93:1213–23.

44. Potter EL, Craig JM. Causes of fetal and infant death. In: *Pathology of the Fetus and the Infant*, 3rd ed. London: Lloyd Luke, 1976, pp. 72–82.

45. Hovatta O, Lipasti A, Rapola J, Karjalainen O. Causes of stillbirth: a clinico-pathological study of 243 patients. *Br J Obstet Gynaecol* 1983; 90:691–6.

46. Donelly WH, Buchholz C, eds. Systematized nomenclature of medicine. *Microglossary for Pediatrics, Pediatric Pathology and Perinatal Medicine*. Skokie, IL: College of American Pathologists, 1984.

47. Ashley D, McCaw-Binns A, Foster-Williams K. The perinatal morbidity and mortality study of Jamaica. *Paediatr Perinat Epidemiol* 1988; 2:138–47.

48. Barson AJ, Tasker M, Lieberman BA, Hillier VF. Impact of improved perinatal care on the causes of death. *Arch Dis Child* 1984; 59:199–207.

49. Clarke M. Perinatal audit: a tried and tested epidemiological method. *Community Med* 1982; 4:104–7.

50. Clarke M, Clayton DG. Quality of obstetric care provided for Asian immigrants in Leicestershire. *Br Med J* 1983; 286:621–3.

51. Raghuveer G. Relevance of Wigglesworth's classification. *Paediatr Perinat Epidemiol* 1992; 6:45–50.

52. Keeling JW, MacGillivray I, Golding J, et al. Classification of perinatal death. *Arch Dis Child* 1989; 64:1345–51.

53. *Scottish Stillbirth and Neonatal Death Report, 1987*. Information and Statistics Division Common Services Agency for the Scottish Health Services, Edinburgh, 1988.

54. Cartlidge PHT, Stewart JH, Hopkins JM. All Wales Perinatal Survey and Confidential Enquiry into Stillbirths and Deaths in Infancy. Annual Report 1995. Cardiff, University of Wales College of Medicine, 1996.

55. Duley LMM. A validation of underlying cause of death as recorded by clinicians on stillbirth and neonatal death certificates. *Br J Obstet Gynaecol* 1986; 93:1233–5.

56. Edouard L. Validation of the registered underlying causes of stillbirth. *J Epidemiol Community Health* 1982; 36:231–4.

57. Fedrick J, butler NR. Accuracy of registered causes of neonatal deaths. *Br J Prev Soc Med* 1972; 26:101–5.

58. Chalmers I. Enquiry into perinatal death. *Br J Obstet Gynaecol* 1985; 92:545–9.

The Perinatal Autopsy

Trevor A. Macpherson Marie Valdes-Dapena

INTRODUCTION

What is required of the perinatal postmortem is guidance in the management of the next case. (Barson [1])

The information sought at the perinatal autopsy differs in many respects from that in the adult. In addition to documenting disease and, if possible, establishing the cause of death, the performance of the perinatal autopsy requires the consideration of disorders that are unique to the maternal–fetal–placental unit, the evaluation of anatomical maturity, growth, and development of the infant and the infant's individual organs, and assessment of the possibility of recurrence in future pregnancies. An additional concern is the recognition of unsuspected complications of medical care, particularly in the neonate in whom such observations at autopsy may contribute to evaluation of new diagnostic and therapeutic modalities [2–4].

The perinatal autopsy will fulfill these roles only when performed by a pathologist interested in perinatal events and when its components include an acceptable clinical review, external examination, adequate dissection procedure, methods for determining weights and measures, adequate tissue sampling, special studies (including radiography and photography), placental examination, microscopic examination of tissue sections, a protocol for data recording, appropriate charts for evaluating maturity and growth, and a good commentary. Interpretation of the information thus gathered is facilitated when the pathologist knows obstetric and neonatal practice in his/her hospital, as well as the current background frequency of the conditions that may be encountered.

To date, the autopsy rate for the perinatal period has not suffered the decline that has occurred in adults. At the Magee-Womens Hospital in Pittsburgh the perinatal autopsy rate for 1985 was 68%, while that at an affiliated adult hospital was about 30%. The perinatal autopsy rate for stillborns was 83% and for neonatal deaths 62%, the lowest rate being for those of ≤750 g birth weight and dying in the first 4 hours after birth [5]. One reason for the decline in the adult hospital's autopsy rate is considered to be the delegation of the autopsy to junior staff, trainees, or pathologist's assistants without close supervision, reflecting the fact that pathologists themselves consider the autopsy to have low priority [6, 7]. The more favorable perinatal autopsy rate, probably the result of the greater desire for families and clinicians to have explanations for perinatal events, is best maintained and enhanced by commitment on the part of the pathologist to the quality of the perinatal autopsy [5, 8]. Apart from the essential components listed above, improvement in this area requires close supervision of the autopsy by pathologists experienced in and interested in perinatal pathology. This supervision should include, at a minimum, participation in the clinical review and external examination, inspection of the organs in situ, review of the microscopic sections, and review of the commentary.

We have found that the use of ultrasound during pregnancy has resulted in an increase in the perinatal autopsy rate and has also placed new demands on the pathologist to make correlations between autopsy and ultrasound findings. Since many of the lesions seen by ultrasound are complex, the involvement of an interested and experienced pathologist is essential. The purpose of the perinatal autopsy, the value of a standardized protocol, and the essential components of a high-quality perinatal autopsy have been presented elsewhere [9]. The dissection procedure has been described [10–14], as have methods and charts for anthropometric measurements [15] and methods for evaluation of the first-trimester fetus [16].

The aim of this chapter is to provide information that will help the prosector and pathologist to perform an autopsy of high quality on the fetus/infant of ≥20 weeks' gestation or ≥250 g birth weight.

AUTOPSY FACILITIES

The performance of the perinatal autopsy is enhanced by adequate facilities, including work space, storage space, lighting, photographic and other equipment, access to imaging techniques, and good instruments. Moderately comprehensive lists of these are included in the autopsy manual of Valdes-Dapena and Huff [13]. In certain cases, such as patients with hepatitis or AIDS, the autopsy must be performed with infectious disease precautions [17].

BACKGROUND INFORMATION

Clinical Information

Close scrutiny of the maternal and infant history is an essential component of the perinatal autopsy. Pathologists are in the fortunate position of having information on the complete life history of the infant; they have the responsibility of arranging it as an accurate sequence of events. Beyond the review of the physician's case records, pathologists will find invaluable information in the nurse's notes, particularly when the times of certain clinical events, treatments, or diagnostic procedures are important. Completing a clinical information sheet (Table 5.1) is a useful means of recording important clinical data. Such a sheet should preferably be completed by the physician requesting the autopsy, particularly if the case notes are bulky. Finally, we find, as does Wigglesworth [14], that discussion with the clinician(s) before beginning the dissection is invaluable for providing important information that may not be in the case notes (as indicated in Table 5.2). Prior to undertaking the autopsy, the pathologist should check the permission papers and adhere to any restrictions. Accurate identification of the body must be maintained at all times; this is most easily done by leaving the hospital wrist or ankle tag attached throughout the autopsy.

WEIGHTS AND MEASURES

Weights and measures are essential to evaluate maturity (anatomical age), growth, and development. They are of most value when performed carefully and according to standard procedure, which for measurements should follow that recommended by Merlob et al [15] and Valdes-Dapena and Huff [13]. All weights and measures must be interpreted as normal or abnormal by comparing them with the standard tables. These tables are most convenient when space is provided below each body weight or gestational age for data entry from a particular autopsy, thereby facilitating comparison with expected normal values. Certain body parameters

are best interpreted when plotted on percentile charts (see Merlob et al [15]), which permits growth to be categorized as appropriate (AGA), small (SGA), or large (LGA) for gestational age. In addition to weights and measures, the gyral pattern of the brain and histological evaluation of some organs (e.g., kidney and lung) are valuable for assessing anatomical maturity [18]. Reference charts for other measurements on infants of low gestational age have been published by Roberts and Thompson [19]. The size and weight of the body and organs vary primarily with gestational age, and secondarily by events that cause disorders of growth or development.

Weights

Weights should be determined using scales accurate to 5 g for body weight and placental weight, 0.5 g for most organ weights, and 0.1 g for smaller organs. We have found that the newer digital scales (Mettler PE 3600—Analytical Instruments Company Inc.) are reliable and convenient for organ weights in that they permit zeroing of the scale without the need for cleaning the weighing surface between weighings. Routine weights include body weight, placental weight, and organ weights (brain, heart, lungs, liver, spleen, thymus, kidneys, adrenals, thyroid, gonads, and pancreas).

Measurements

The method for determining various external body measurements has been described elsewhere [13] and is illustrated in Figures 5.1 through 5.3. The crown to heel (CH) and crown to rump (CR) lengths should be measured in all cases and to the nearest 0.5 cm. Since the CR length is normally two-thirds of CH, if there should be lower limb abnormalities the CH length can be calculated in infants who do not have collapsed heads. The occipitofrontal circumference (OFC) should be measured to the nearest 1 to 2 mm. There is a built-in check on the accuracy of some measurements; for example, if the CR and OFC differ by more than 1 cm, the measurements should be verified. If a difference is confirmed, some explanation for the unusual head size should be sought (i.e., a large OFC suggests hydrocephalus or fetal malnutrition, while a small OFC suggests microcephaly or cranial distortion by face mask or molding during delivery) [14]. When the head is abnormal, as in anencephaly or hydrocephalus, one can correct for that by multiplying the CH to CR difference by three [20].

Other useful, but not essential, measurements are shown in Figure 5.1 and include chest circumference (CC) at the nipple level, abdominal circumference (AC) at the umbilicus, foot length (FL), facial measurements for dysmorphology (Fig. 5.2), size of fontanelles, inter-nipple distance (IND), and length of the umbilical cord. The three circumference measurements (OFC, CC, AC) normally diminish as one proceeds caudally; a failure to diminish indicates that

Table 5.1. Clinical history information sheet

Institution: _____ Autopsy #: _____

Name: Last _____ Race: _____ B _____ W _____ O _____ Other _____

    First (Mother) _____ Hosp #: _____ Sex: _____ F _____ M _____ ? _____

    First (Baby) _____ Hosp #: _____ Birth weight: _____ g

Gestational age: _____ by LMP _____ by sonar _____ by clinical evaluation _____ by other: _____

Birth sequence: _____ Singleton _____ Twin A _____ Twin B _____ Other: _____

Birth: _____ d _____ m _____ y _____ am/pm Type of death: _____ NND

Death: _____ d _____ m _____ y _____ am/pm   _____ Non-macerated SB

Age: _____ y _____ d _____ h _____ m   _____ Macerated SB

(at death)

Transfer: Maternal _____ yes _____ no   Neonatal _____ yes _____ no

        (before birth)   (after delivery)

        From: _____ When: _____ d _____ m _____ y _____ am/pm

            (name of hospital)

Attending: Obstetrician: _____

         Neonatologist: _____

         Other: _____ _____

        _____ _____

            (specialty)   (name)

Paternal history: Age: _____ y   Other: _____

Maternal history:

    Age: _____ y Para: _____ Grava: _____ Blood Group: _____ BP: _____ / _____ Smoking: _____ no _____ yes _____ # packs/day

    Previous pregnancy: # Ab's 6–2 w _____ Spont _____ Ind   Hospital #'s: _____

                   13–20 w _____ Spont _____ Ind   Hospital #'s _____

                # Deaths >20 w _____   Hospital #'s _____

    Diagnoses for above: _____

    Maternal complications in previous pregnancy: _____

    Present pregnancy:

        Clinical problem list: 1 _____   2 _____

                   3 _____   4 _____

        Treatment/diagnostic modalities: 1 _____   2 _____

                   3 _____   4 _____

Labor: _____ spontaneous _____ augmented _____ induced

    Duration: 1st stage _____ h   2nd stage _____ h _____ min

    Rupture of membranes _____ h _____ min

Fetal monitoring: Late decelerations _____ yes _____ no Scalp pH _____ yes _____ no value: _____

Presentation: _____ vertex _____ breech _____ transverse _____ other: _____

Delivery: _____ spontaneous

    _____ assisted: _____ forceps _____ vac _____ C/S _____ elective _____ repeat _____ stat

                _____ other: _____

Neonatal history:

    Apgar: _____ 1 min _____ 5 min _____ 10 min

    Cord gases: pH _____ pO$_2$ _____ pCO$_2$ _____ BE _____ HCO$_3$ _____

    First ABG: pH _____ pO$_2$ _____ pCO$_2$ _____ BE _____ HCO$_3$ _____

        Clinical problem list: 1 _____   2 _____

                   3 _____   4 _____

                   5 _____   6 _____

                   7 _____   8 _____

        Diagnostic/treatment modalities: 1 _____   2 _____

                   3 _____   4 _____

                   5 _____   6 _____

                   7 _____   8 _____

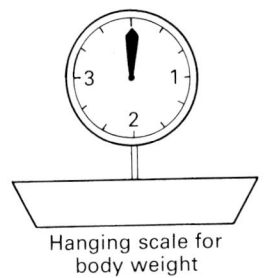

Hanging scale for
body weight

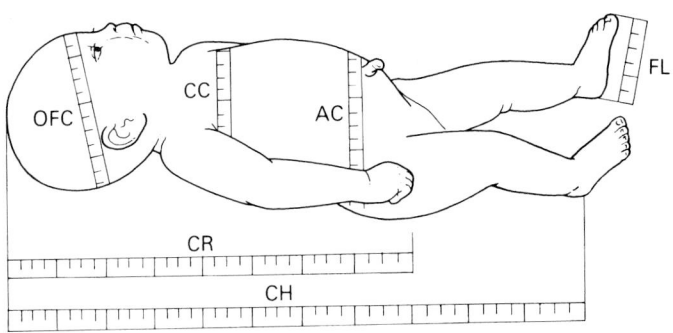

FIGURE 5.1. *Body measurements: CR = crown–rump length; CH = crown–heel length; OFC = occipitofrontal circumference; CC = chest circumference; AC = abdominal circumference; FL = foot length.*

T a b l e 5 . 2 . Clinician–pathologist pre-autopsy discussion

Clinical events or findings that require pathological correlation
The best estimate of gestational age established by the clinician
Laboratory tests required that were not performed premortem
Laboratory results that are pending (i.e., cytogenetics, viral cultures)
Unusual diagnoses suspected but not confirmed premortem (i.e., metabolic disease)
Potential "iatrogenic" events

(Adapted from Wigglesworth [14].)

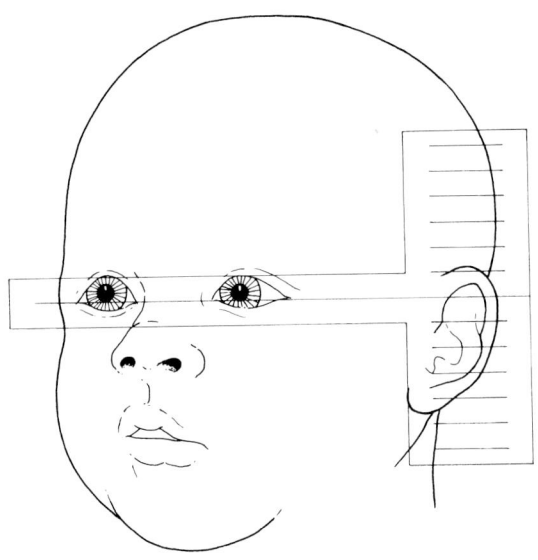

FIGURE 5.3. *Evaluation for low-set ears. Ear length = maximum distance from the superior aspect to the inferior aspect of the ear (pinna). Ear above eyeline = distance from the superior aspect of the ear to the inner canthi level.*

$$Percent\ of\ ear\ above\ eyeline = \frac{Ear\ above\ eyeline}{Total\ ear\ length}$$

(Adapted from Merlob et al [15].)

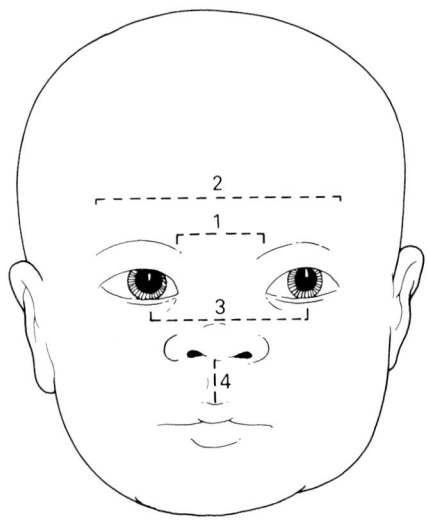

FIGURE 5.2. *Facial measurements: 1 = inner canthus; 2 = outer canthus; 3 = interpupillary distance; 4 = philtrum length.*

something is wrong. The FL is particularly useful in fetuses of early gestational age [21], in severely macerated fetuses, and in infants with major head or spinal column abnormalities such as anencephaly or amniotic band syndrome. The IND is increased in some chromosomal syndromes

(18+, 4p+, etc.), in facial defects, and in fetal hydantoin syndrome, while it is decreased in Jeune syndrome [15]. Facial measurements (Fig. 5.2) and evaluation of the size and location of the ears (Fig. 5.3) are of value in documenting the dysmorphology and abnormalities associated with numerous malformation syndromes [15]. The publication of Merlob et al [15] includes useful charts for plotting most of the body measurements, including the hands and portions of limbs, thus facilitating recognition of abnormal values [15]. Measurements of the fontanelles are best performed after reflection of the scalp, and their regular measurement will ensure examination of sutures for defects and for evidence of hydrocephalus. Umbilical cord length is discussed in further detail in Chapter 7.

Apart from measurements to evaluate growth and development of the body and organs, it is important to measure volumes when abnormal fluid collections are noted, such as effusions, extravascular blood, and distended bladder. In specialized centers, lung volumes after perfusion are sometimes recorded.

EXTERNAL EXAMINATION

After external measurements the remaining external examination is done to detect abnormalities of the surface and subcutaneous tissues, and to evaluate development of structures such as the face, mouth, ears, eyes, limbs, and body orifices. We concur with Barson that "it is necessary for the pathologist to be as thorough in his external examination of the infant as the pediatrician" [1]. This is best achieved in an orderly manner, starting with the head and proceeding caudally to ensure external abnormalities are recognized and photographed; the body will not be available for further review after it has been removed from the hospital for burial or cremation, so such lesions will be unavailable for further evaluation. In stillborn infants, apart from the recognition of abnormalities, the external evaluation of color and peeling are part of the assessment of the degree of maceration. In all infants, the external surface is examined for cyanosis, edema, jaundice, petechial hemorrhage, meconium staining, bruising (which, in many instances, is an indication of a presenting part being "constricted" by the cervix), vernix, ischemia (i.e., gangrene), and skin lesions suggestive of infection. Evidence of trauma due to mechanical devices such as tape, monitoring equipment, needles, tubes, and lines are noted. Trauma to the mouth and gums is often noted when there has been prolonged intubation, and meconium already cleaned from the skin may still be detected in the external auditory meatus. Dehydration is present if skin turgor is reduced, as evidenced by its remaining "tented" when pinched; excess tissue folds, due to loss of subcutaneous tissue, suggest intrauterine growth retardation. The flexibility of the ear lobe, appearance of the skin, extent of plantar creases, size of the breast bud, amount of lanugo, descent of the testes, characteristics of scrotal rugae, appearance of the external female genitalia, and the length of the

toe and fingernails contribute to the evaluation of fetal maturity [22]. Post-term infants often have nails that extend beyond the ends of the digits.

The morphology and development of several structures are checked as part of the external examination. The ears are examined with reference to shape and structure, and the method illustrated in Figure 5.3 is used to determine if they are set low. The hard and soft palate are carefully examined for any clefts or abnormally high arching, and one can check for choanal atresia by passing a probe through each naris, first backward toward the occiput 1 cm and then abruptly caudally into the nasopharynx. If there is no choanal atresia, membranous or bony, the probe will slide in easily for more than 2 cm [13]. Patency of the anus and vagina are checked using a probe. Limb changes, such as distortion or unusual positioning of the hands and feet, suggest intrauterine compression due to prolonged oligohydramnios or a congenital neuromuscular abnormality. Dermatoglyphics, including occipital hair pattern, are an important part of certain syndromes [15, 23] and are best recorded using an ink pad. We have found that recording the findings on diagrams such as those displayed in Figure 5.4 are a useful way to capture the myriad of external lesions that might be present. In addition, photographs are essential for accurate documentation of all important lesions noted externally. The multiplicity of external and internal developmental abnormalities that are possible require that the pathologist refer frequently to good reference books [23–25].

Postmortem radiology is a simple yet informative procedure that should be a part of many perinatal autopsies. Some pathologists use radiology routinely [26], while we recommend it only for certain indications as proposed by Griscom and Driscoll [27]. It is essential for an accurate diagnosis of skeletal dysplasias, and for recognition of skeletal abnormalities in malformation syndromes such as VATER association, amniotic band "syndrome," and radial dysplasia [28]. We also consider it to be essential for the exclusion of skeletal anomalies in infants at high risk for such lesions as those with an abnormal karyotype or in the infant of a diabetic mother. An x-ray is useful in evaluating fetal maturity via examination of ossification centers, and some suggest that it also has value in recognizing intrauterine growth retardation [29, 30]. Occasionally, soft-tissue calcification can be recognized on an x-ray suggesting intrauterine infection or meconium peritonitis, although there may be calcification of intraluminal meconium in infants with anorectal malformations [31]. Radiography is also an excellent method of documenting pneumothorax and pneumopericardium. When vascular anomalies are suspected, postmortem angiography provides useful information more readily than does dissection [32]. We take anteroposterior and lateral views of individual limbs when indicated. The films are available to the pathologist before dissection begins; after completion of the autopsy, a written report, which is included in the final autopsy protocol, is issued by the radiologist.

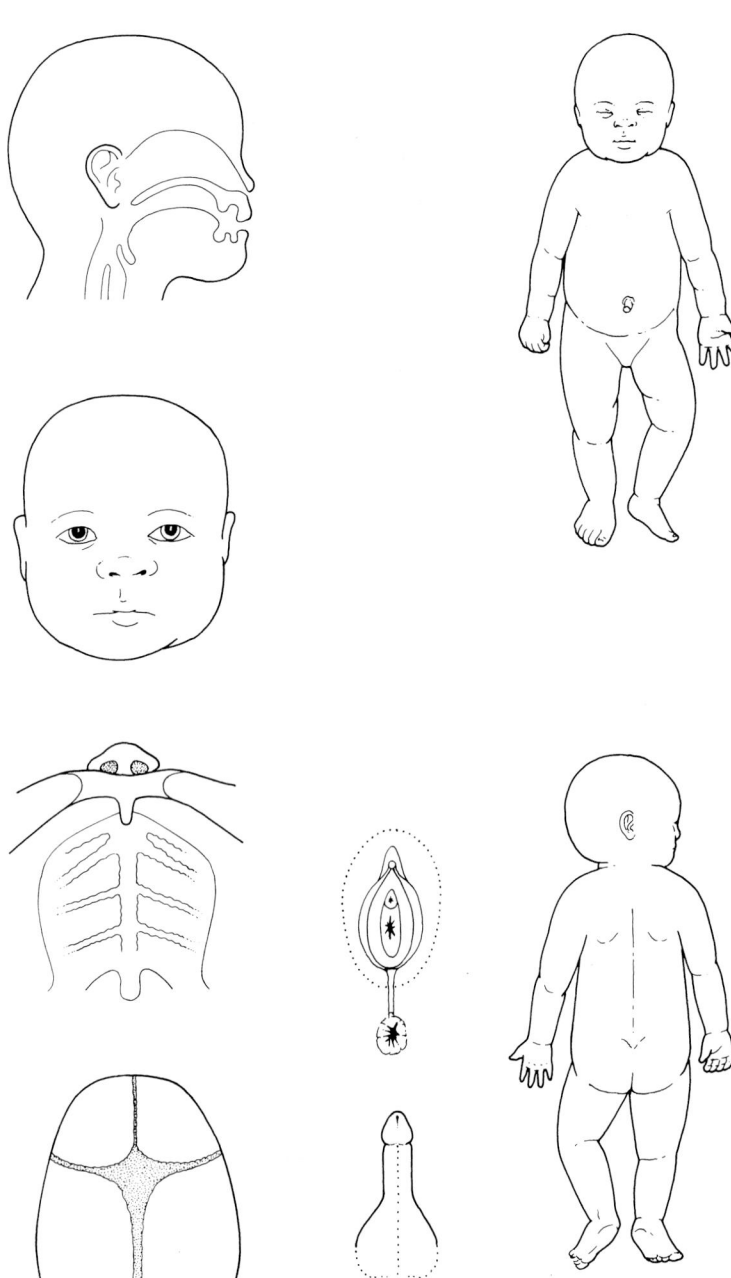

FIGURE 5.4.   *External body diagrams from Magee-Womens Hospital autopsy protocol.*

At the conclusion of the external examination, the pathologist should have determined whether dysmorphic lesions, abnormal dermatoglyphics, or any congenital abnormalities are evident; if they are, karyotyping is indicated. Evidence of abnormal nutrition, trauma, dehydration, infection, and asphyxia may also be apparent. This information, combined with weights and measures, will give the pathologist an initial impression as to growth and development and whether these are consistent with the clinical conclusions of the obstetrician and neonatologist [33]. This impression will be reevaluated at completion of the autopsy when additional information is available on internal organs.

INCISIONS

Skin Invasion

A variety of skin incisions have been described, including a straight simple midline cut from the level of the larynx to the symphysis pubis, a T-shaped variant of the former with the horizontal component extending from one shoulder top to the other, and an inverted Y-shape with the two lower extremities overlying the umbilical arteries [14]. We have found that the most advantageous is an upright Y-shaped cut extending cranially to the top of each acromioclavicular junction, or above that point (Rokitansky procedure).

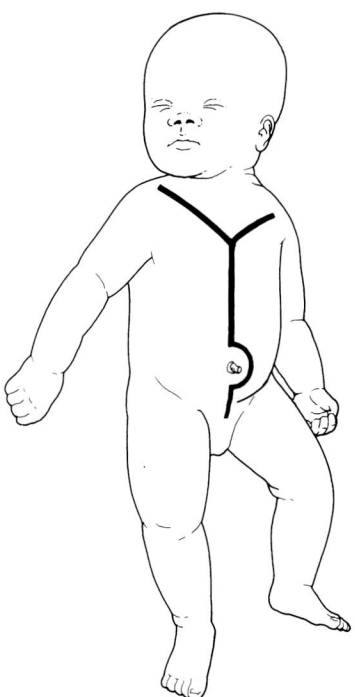

FIGURE 5.5. *Y-shaped skin incision.*

These two arms of the Y are joined over the xiphoid process. The single vertical leg passes just to the left of the umbilicus (making a little arc around it) and then proceeds to the symphysis pubis (Fig. 5.5). There are two advantages of this incision: 1) the uppermost flap facilitates removal of the tongue and all of the neck organs without any incision in the skin of the neck, and 2) as the Rokitansky procedure is accomplished the little leftward arciform deflection to the side of the umbilicus becomes the first step in routine removal of the base of the umbilical cord in continuity with the umbilical arteries and urachus.

Thorax

After the Y-shaped skin incision has been made, one can proceed to mobilize the triangular flap of skin over the upper chest, taking special care over the anterior aspect of the neck to avoid accidentally cutting the overlying skin. Dissection by repeatedly spreading the blades of a Metzenbaum scissors is a useful technique. The skin flap is mobilized all the way up to the lower border of the mandible and from one angle of the jaw to the other. At this time, reduced subcutaneous fat suggests intrauterine growth retardation, while pale or poorly developed muscle together with a narrow chest may indicate neurogenic atrophy.

Next, the flaps of skin on the two sides of the chest are dissected away from the external aspects of the rib cage. It is important to expose the ribs clearly in this procedure for two reasons: 1) to identify the costochondral junctions for

a definitive incision through the cartilages in removal of the plastron and for sampling those junctions for microscopic sections; and 2) to be able to count the ribs.

At this point in the autopsy on a neonate, it is advisable to check each side of the chest for pneumothorax. Several techniques have been described, but probably the best one is to use a sterile needle and a syringe partly filled with sterile saline. Using a lateral point of entry, any air under pressure within the chest will enter the needle and the bubbles will then rise through the saline within the barrel of the syringe. This method prevents any fluid from entering the chest and thus maintains the original microbiological state of the thoracic cavity. Finally, if a radiograph was taken at autopsy it should be examined for evidence of pneumothorax.

Removal of the sternocleidomastoid allows exposure of the deeper structures of the neck and removal of the submandibular glands. These present as small, firm, lobulated structures tucked up under the angle of the jaw.

Abdomen

The umbilical vein can be explored by opening it with a scissors from below. In the perinatal period, the lumen is patent and often contains a little liquid blood. After it has been examined thoroughly, the vessel can be ligated and transected. The internal aspect of the umbilicus may be explored for possible omphalomesenteric or vascular remnants.

One can now incise the skin and subcutaneous tissue around the right side of the umbilicus, thereby freeing the umbilicus itself and the attached stump of cord, maintaining their continuity with the two umbilical arteries and the urachal remnant. Then the cord, the umbilicus, the umbilical arteries, and the urachus, as a block, can be laid down caudally to overlie the symphysis pubis while the remaining abdominal contents are explored in detail.

At this point it is important to reflect the skin and subcutaneous tissue flaps completely away from the lower chest, clearing entirely the lower margins of the rib cage on each side so that the lower edge of each caudal rib is clean and well exposed.

IN SITU EXAMINATION AND DISSECTION

We concur with Barson that "the precise order and manner of dissection of the organs is of secondary importance to its thoroughness and the clarity with which it demonstrates" any pathological lesions of the case [1]. However, it is helpful to follow a routine that reduces the likelihood of missing important changes.

Abdomen and Pelvis

As soon as the abdomen has been opened, all the peritoneal surfaces should be scanned from the diaphragm to the pelvis and from one flank to the other in search of organomegaly, ascites, hemorrhage, peritonitis, or pneumoperitoneum, as well as areas of infarction or necrotizing enterocolitis. When these are noted, the mesentery should be left attached at these sites for the evaluation of mesenteric vessels. Some sharply demarcated shiny surfaces, discolored green, brown, or black, are readily recognized as being so because of postmortem (probably) sulfur or bile staining originating in the content of the small or large bowel; frequently, the process affects two loops abutted against each other. This phenomenon is not to be confused with the discoloration of necrotic bowel, the surface of which, by contrast, is usually dull and friable.

If "puddles" or patches of yellow or green fibrinopurulent exudate are seen, aerobic and anaerobic cultures should be taken and, after establishing relationships in the immediate vicinity, the structures involved should be separated gingerly in an attempt to determine the site of perforation or other source of the localized inflammatory reaction.

If any clear fluid is present in the peritoneal cavity, it should be suctioned out carefully, and the volume determined. If the content is abundant, liquid, and puriform, it should be cultured when first observed.

The site of any fibrinous or fibrous adhesions must be noted: the former may be teased apart carefully in search of any underlying acute pathological process; the latter require transection with scalpel blade or scissors, which may be a challenging task if damage to related structures is to be avoided.

It is generally best to examine the abdominal structures systematically, moving from the diaphragm itself in a caudal direction. The height and integrity of each leaf of the diaphragm can be determined by sliding a moistened right index finger high into its dome and then counting downward with the left forefinger to ascertain the number of the rib or interspace overlying the exploring fingertip. In the perinatal period, the right leaf is the more cranial and both are unexpectedly high compared to adults or older infants.

The liver is observed for symmetry and for focal lesions, such as subcapsular hemorrhage, abscesses, and so on. The distance to which the lower border of the liver extends below the costal margin on each side may be measured in the anterior axillary line.

The presence, size, and position of the gallbladder can be determined at this time, lifting the right hepatic lobe if necessary, and the falciform and triangular ligaments may be cut.

Next, the spleen should be examined. Normally, the spleen is hidden high in the left upper quadrant of the abdomen, well above the costal margin, with its hilus directed medially toward the greater curvature of the stomach. If it extends below the costal margin, the distance by which it does so should be recorded. A careful search should be made for accessory spleens. It is our impression that at least one is almost universal. Most accessory spleens are tiny, about 2 to 3 mm in diameter, spherical, and purple. They are ordinarily in the vicinity of the hilus of the spleen and in clear associ-

ation with the dorsal mesogastrium; a few are to be found rather deeply embedded in the tail of the pancreas. They can always be differentiated from lymph nodes by their typically spherical shape, if not by their purple color.

The position, shape, and size of the stomach can be noted, including the diameter of its midportion (from the lesser to the greater curvature) and the sheen of its ordinarily light-pink or tan serosa.

The state of the greater omentum should be noted. It is a delicate structure during the perinatal period, containing almost no adipose tissue and resembling layers of moist cobwebs lying like a transparent veil suspended above from the greater curvature of the stomach and draped over the loops of bowel below.

The small bowel is normally clustered together in many small loops, with a shiny, pale pink serosa and a diameter of 0.5 to 0.8 cm in the center of the abdomen. Color, diameter, and anomalies such as constrictions, atresias, ectopic tissue, or annular pancreas should be noted while tracing the course of the small bowel from the ligament of Treitz to the cecum. Malrotation and/or malfixation can be detected also at this time. The positions of the cecum and of the appendix can be observed. The colon may then be followed from the cecum to the rectum to determine its orientation, color and diameter.

The root of the mesentery of the small intestine can be examined by sweeping all of the small bowel to the right and slightly cephalically, and holding it there gently while inspecting its linear attachment to the posterior abdominal wall. Intestinal malrotations often have a narrow mesenteric root. The foramen of Winslow can be seen close to the origin of the superior mesenteric artery. The nature and integrity of the mesentery and the lymph nodes embedded within it can be observed at this stage, followed by inspection of the mesocolon and the pancreas.

Moving in a caudal direction thereafter, it is a good idea to check on the state of the adrenal glands, the kidneys, the ureters (these may be lifted up through the peritoneum to ascertain that there is only one on each side), the urinary bladder, the internal inguinal rings, the testis, epididymis and vas on each side (by opening the inguinal canal), or, if the body is that of a female infant, the uterus, fallopian tubes, and ovaries.

The presence of normal kidneys, ureters, and bladder confirms the patency of the urinary tract. Urethral obstruction (posterior valves, stricture, or agenesis) causes bladder distension, with hypertrophy, hydronephrosis, or renal dysplasia. Other renal conditions observed grossly include organomegaly, agenesis, infarcts, abscesses, and congestion. The adrenal glands are normally one-third of the size of the kidney in the term newborn.

Neck and Thorax

The plastron should be removed by incising the cartilage on both sides medial to the costochondral junction using the tip of the scalpel blade. Removal of the plastron and the strap muscles covering the anterior surface of the neck organs exposes the thymus, thyroid, and trachea. If mediastinal emphysema is present, it will be seen at this point. We often reflect the clavicle on each side by cutting through the cartilage between it and the 2nd rib and the sternum.

The thymus is removed next, taking care to avoid damage to the innominate vein lying deep to it. Any nick in the vein wall allows a large amount of blood to escape, which obscures the field and reduces the amount of blood available for culture via right atrial puncture. The thymus is usually quite large and fills the anterior mediastinum. Significant atrophy indicates prolonged stress, and hemorrhage is noted in asphyxia. Mediastinal emphysema may involve the perithymic tissues. If the thymus is absent from its normal location, the neck and superior chest must be examined carefully for thymic tissue. (Absence of thymic tissue is part of the DiGeorge syndrome.)

This having been accomplished, one can proceed to identify the phrenic nerve on each side and to culture the lungs. This we do ordinarily by pulling the lower lobe forward and medially with a hemostat; with the lobe stabilized over the mediastium, one can cut out a little (3-mm) wedge from an angle which has not yet been touched, using two opposing No. 22 sterile scalpel blades. The wedge is then dropped into liquid medium in a test tube. We find that we obtain better results with less contamination by this method. If there are any focal lesions, such as areas of consolidation or pleural exudate, these must be cultured. Inspect the lungs, making a note of their size, color, the sheen of the pleural surfaces, and the number of lobes. Gross pulmonary diagnoses include petechial hemorrhage, subpleural emphysema, bronchopulmonary dysplasia, and abscesses impinging on the pleural surface. If interstitial emphysema is present, it will be seen as a delicate network of tiny subpleural bubbles of about 1 mm or less in diameter, highlighting "the outlines of pulmonary lobules." If any chest tubes are in place, the course of each within the pleural space must be ascertained and special attention paid to the possibility that one or more may have penetrated a lobe of the lung.

If there is any fluid present in either pleural cavity, the amount, color, and clarity must be noted. If the fluid is turbid, it should be cultured separately. As part of the investigation of the thorax, it is necessary to inspect both the azygos and hemiazygos veins—especially with regard to their size and course. At the same time, one can inspect the sympathetic chain bilaterally.

The logical next structure to approach is the *pericardial sac*. We are accustomed to removing the anterior portion of the parietal pericardium in one sheet, cutting it with scissors as close as possible to the hilus of the lung on each side, to the great vessels cranially and the diaphragm caudally. The sheet can then be saved in a commonly used fixative. Before proceeding further one should obtain blood samples (2.0–3.0 mL) from the right atrium for aerobic and anaerobic cultures using a No. 18 needle. If any difficulty is encountered in obtaining the required amount, it is possible to increase the yield by elevating the head and/or the lower extremities for a few moments. More reliable culture results are obtained by changing needles between withdrawal of the blood and its injection into the culture medium. The visceral pericardium should be inspected, especially for fibrin deposition. Any blood, excess of fluid, or adhesions within the sac must be noted.

Following inspection of the heart, the aortic arch and great vessels should be explored, with clearance of the surrounding loose connective tissues. At this stage, we tie the major branches of the aortic arch about 1.0 cm above the arch. The distal portion of the aortic arch should then be examined for coarctation. It will usually be seen as a sharp indentation at least 1 to 2 mm deep, directly opposite the entrance of the ductus arteriosus.

External features of the heart should be assessed, including the size and position of the atria, the distribution pattern of the coronary arteries, the size, position, and form of each ventricle, the relative size and orientation of the two great arteries, the positions of the superior and inferior venae cavae, and the locations of the pulmonary veins and the major branches of the pulmonary artery. Special care must be given to recognizing venous anomalies because relationships of these structures may be lost once the organs have been removed from the body.

If the gross appearance of the heart is normal, it is best opened in situ at this stage. Opening the heart in situ can be accomplished in six easy steps, three incisions on the right and three on the left (Fig. 5.6). The first connects the two venae cavae, proceeding from a nick in the lateral aspect of the superior, down along the right side of the right atrium and running into the inferior vena cava. The second originates, like the stem of a letter T, in the middle of the first cut and then proceeds down the back of the heart, immediately to the right of the descending coronary artery, to the apex.

These incisions expose the inflow tract of the entire right heart. At this point one must assess the state of the foramen ovale, since it is easily torn and is not as accurately examined when the heart has been removed from the body. Because liquid blood is still present in the left atrium, the normal valve flap for the foramen ovale is, at this point, stretched over the blood, holding it back. A little pressure applied on the interatrial septum will cause the flap to bulge toward the right without blood draining through. Then, on touching the flap itself near its normal opening with the rounded tip of a probe, blood leaks to the right thus demonstrating that the valve flap is anatomically patent but adequate for functional closure.

The third incision on the right side begins at the apex and goes straight up the front of the heart, again immediately to the right of the septum and the descending coronary artery, to end within the pulmonary artery. At this point, all features of the interior of the right heart are

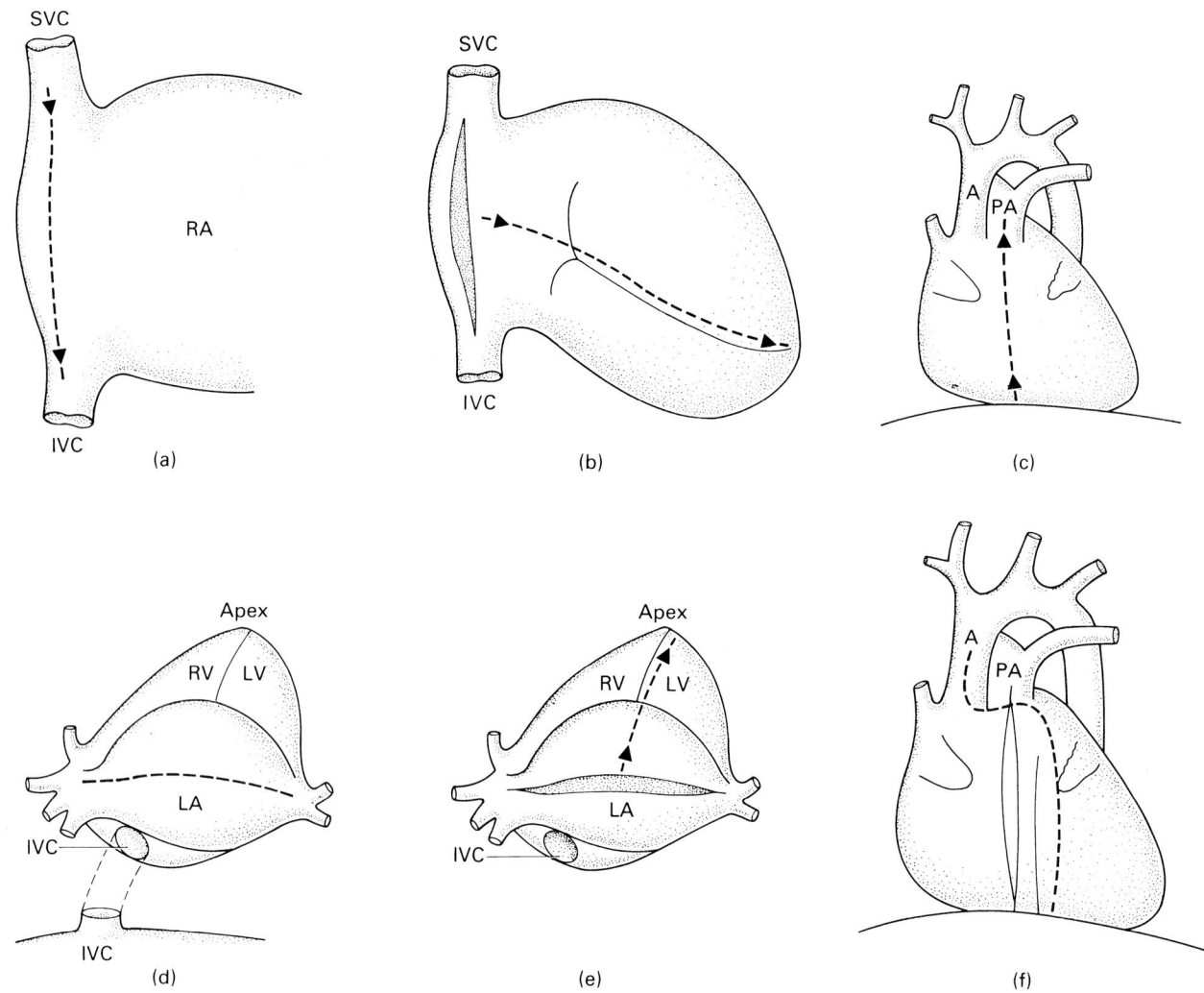

FIGURE 5.6.   *Opening the heart in situ. (a) 1st cut (right atrium exposed); (b) 2nd cut (right inflow tract exposed); (c) 3rd cut (right outflow tract exposed); (d) 4th cut (left atrium exposed); (e) 5th cut (left inflow tract exposed); (f) 6th cut (left outflow tract exposed). A = aorta; PA = pulmonary artery; SVC = superior vena cava; IVC = inferior vena cava; RA = right atrium; LA = left atrium; RV = right ventricle; LV = left ventricle.*

exposed for examination. The cut should be extended into the ductus arteriosus, the patency of which is determined at this stage. Probing the pulmonary arteries is useful at this point.

The fourth cut connects the entering pulmonary veins on the two sides of the left atrium. In order to expose the atrium, however, it is necessary to transect the inferior vena cava first and then "flip" the heart upward. In this way, all four pulmonary veins can be visualized and then connected on each side with a single transverse incision.

The fifth cut, like the second, extends "down" the middle of the back of the heart (but now that the heart is upside-down, the actual incision is made in an upward direction) to the apex, just to the left of the septum, with the "inside" blade of the scissors against the septum.

The sixth and final cut is made after the heart has been returned to its original position, from the apex up the front

of the organ to the aorta. This task, however, cannot be accomplished on the left as easily and directly as it is on the right because, near the top, it is necessary to bend to the right (your left) and to transect the pulmonary artery just above that valve in order to open the ascending aorta while leaving the pulmonic valve intact. If one prefers not to cut the pulmonary artery, it will be necessary to separate the aorta and pulmonary artery near their origins by using the spreading technique.

At the time of making the various cardiac incisions the ventricles should be evaluated for dilatation and the walls and septum for hypertrophy, particularly septal hypertrophy sufficient to compromise left ventricular outflow, as is sometimes noted in infants of diabetic mothers.

In congenital heart lesions, it is critical to identify carefully each chamber as right or left according to established morphological criteria [34]. If the heart is separated from the abdominal organ block, it is useful to leave a portion of the liver attached to the inferior vena cava. In anomalous pulmonary venous return, which involves thoracic and abdominal vessels, the organ block should be left intact to retain accurate anatomical relationships. A text on congenital heart disease should be consulted when cardiovascular anomalies are encountered [35]. A history of congenital heart block, a condition associated with maternal systemic lupus erythematosus, or significant cardiac arrhythmia may indicate the need for dissection of the conduction system [36].

At this stage, one should inspect the neck organs. The thyroid should be examined carefully to confirm that both lateral lobes are present and of equal size and that there is not a persistent midline "pyramidal" lobe arising from the isthmus. Any abnormally prominent cervical lymph nodes should be noted, as well as any laterally placed ectopic nodules of thymic tissue.

EVISCERATION

General Organs

In common with most North American pediatric pathologists, we consider that removal of the thoracic and abdominal organs en bloc in the Rokitansky procedure is the most effective autopsy procedure because it maintains intact most of the interrelationships of the organs until they can be dissected individually. Some authors [11, 12, 14, 37] recommend alternative methods of removal of the organs in several blocks.

In general, evisceration proceeds from the neck caudally. The neck organs are freed from their posterior attachments by incising the connective tissues on each side from the top of the pleural space medial to the carotid arteries to the angle of the mandible bilaterally, and then making an incision from below upward all the way around the inside of the mandible—with the blade of the scalpel held flat against the bone—separating the tongue and floor of the mouth from the lower jaw. This same cut is extended up to form an arch between the soft and hard palate, leaving the soft palate and tonsillar pillars attached to the tongue. Thereafter, by slipping a moistened, gloved, index fingertip upward between the tongue and the mandible, one can hook the tongue and pull it and the neck organs downward.

As the tongue is being delivered caudally, the connective tissue attachments between the nasopharynx and the bony spine and angles of the mandible embracing it are severed. Using the tongue as a handle one can continue to eviscerate, pulling gently but firmly the block of neck and thoracic organs caudally toward the diaphragm.

The leaves of the diaphragm and crurae are then detached peripherally. At this junction, one must incise the peritoneum in each gutter vertically, lateral to the kidneys, all the way down to the inguinal region without cutting the iliac vessels; then reflect the united kidneys and adrenal glands medially. The "pull" is continued in the direction of

the pelvis, with posterior and lateral attachments being severed all the while, down to the pelvic brim, leaving the psoas muscle intact on each side. The iliac vessels can either be carried along with this block or, if one cuts and ties the aorta above the bifurcation, left in place.

At this time it is best to lay the block of organs back in place in order to separate the pelvic organs from the pubis; this is accomplished by cutting into the space of Retzius and then dividing the connecting tissues, again by blunt dissection, down to the pelvic floor and sweeping laterally to the inguinal area on each side. Any remaining attachments can then be severed laterally and the urethra transected below the prostate (in the male), the vagina (in the female) and the anus as far distally as possible.

When congenital anomalies of the genitourinary tract and/or anorectal region are suspected it is important to remove them en bloc, including the perineal and anal regions, thereby maintaining complete continuity of these organ systems to the exterior. The first step is to bisect the symphysis pubis and carefully clear the connecting tissues all around the pelvis. In the male, the spreading technique is then used to separate the muscular component of the penis from the overlying skin by working along the length of the penis. The skin of the tip is cut where it attaches to the glans penis. The penis is then extracted from its skin sheath. In the female, the skin of the perineum is cut where the vaginal wall and perineum meet. Using the spreading dissection technique, the vagina is cleared laterally so that it can be delivered into the pelvic cavity. In both the male and the female, the anorectal region is freed by cutting around the anus where the anal canal and perineal skin meet. The anal canal is freed and delivered into the pelvic cavity. The organ block is then removed as described previously.

Once the organ block has been removed, systematic exploration of the nasopharynx should include examination of the eustachian tubes and posterior choanae. The adenoids may be removed for histological examination. The neck, thoracic cavity, abdominal cavity, and pelvic cavity should then be inspected for changes that might have been missed when the organs were in place.

Brain

In Figure 5.7 we illustrate our method for opening the scalp and skull. The initial incision in the scalp is made as a straight line from just behind one pinna to just behind the other, crossing over the top of the head in the vicinity of the posterior fontanelle. Combined skin and galea of both the anterior and posterior flaps are then reflected, the anterior to the level of the eyebrows and the posterior to the base of the skull.

To visualize the posterior aspect of the pons, medulla, and upper cervical cord in continuity with the brain, a second incision needs to be made in the midline posteriorly down through the posterior flaps and over the atlas, axis, and upper cervical spinous processes. Following

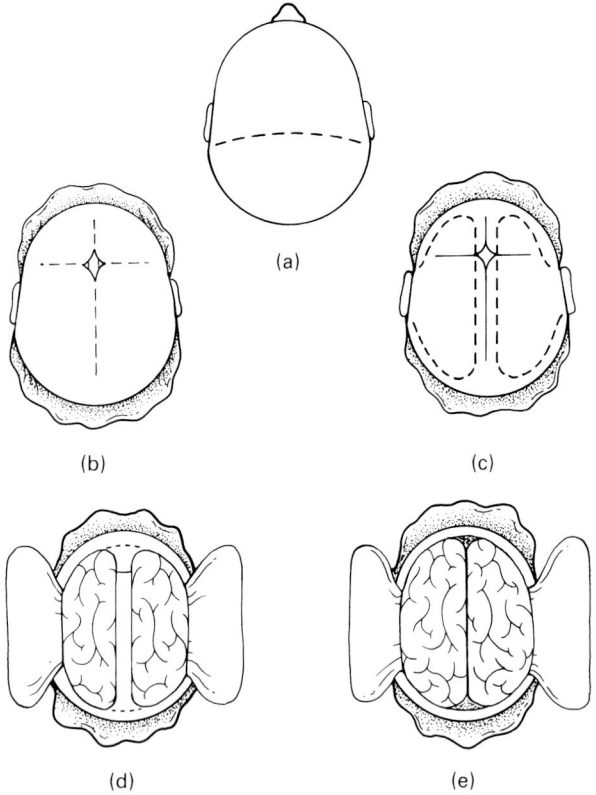

FIGURE 5.7. *Method for opening the scalp and skull: (a) incision of the scalp; (b) scalp reflected with two incisions in the dura; (c) definite cuts through bone and dura; (d) skull flaps laid back to reveal leptomeninges and brain; (e) leptomeninges and brain following removal of bone strip with midline sagittal sinus. (Courtesy of Valdes-Dapena and Huff [13].)*

exposure of the calvarium one measures the greatest dimensions, length and width, of the anterior and posterior fontanelles, and examines all of the sutures carefully for their orientation and movability.

In the fetus and newborn we are accustomed to exposing the brain by creating and bending down large lateral flaps of the calvarium bilaterally (as does Potter [20]), beginning with a longitudinal nick in the dura at the lateral extremities of the anterior fontanelle and completing the cuts, as illustrated in Figure 5.7, using stout bone scissors. There remains, at the bottom of each flap, an intact thin strip of bony calvarium only 1 to 2 cm in length, which serves as a hinge for its ready replacement (for cosmetic purposes) following completion of the autopsy. Be warned that the edges of this bony flap are surprisingly sharp and can easily cut one's gloves or hands; once the flap is replaced, they may also cut the leptomeninges. To prevent tearing of the delicate leptomeninges, which are important for keeping the friable infant brain intact during removal, we drape each bony flap with a wet paper towel as soon as possible. In addition to their value in reconstruction of the head, the

two paper-wrapped flaps may also serve as handles with which to stabilize the skull during some of the procedures.

At this point one must remember, particularly in the case of a liveborn neonate, to inspect the tentorium bilaterally for tears or fraying due to cranial birth trauma at the junction of the falx cerebri and tentorium cerebelli. To see the angle clearly, one can tilt the head, forehead down, and then slide a wet scalpel handle between each occipital pole and the calvarium—pushing the hemisphere slightly forward—just far enough to bring the junction of the falx cerebri and tentorium cerebelli into clear view.

After the tentorium has been inspected one can move on to the falx cerebri, which is seen readily with the help of a wet scalpel handle. Once more, gravity can be of assistance as one tilts the head to the appropriate side, to drop the hemisphere away from the falx cerebri while pushing the hemisphere delicately with the scalpel handles. Any tears or bleeding in the area are documented. The next logical step in the procedure is removal of the long, slender remaining strip of bone, together with the underlying sagittal sinus, which can be opened later and examined.

There are two important elements in the technique from this point forward: 1) gloved hands (and everything else that comes in contact with this fragile organ) must be wet, or they will adhere to and tear the leptomeninges; and 2) gravity is a great ally in this process—as much as possible one ought to permit the head to lie on the table top by its own weight, then one can tilt the head this way and that to permit the brain to fall in the desired direction. Ultimately, after all important connections have been severed, the base of the skull is delivered caudally and up, permitting the free brain to remain lying on the moistened surface of the table. In general, we prefer not to hold the head while working, because this inactivates one hand—gravity and the table top will suffice. Furthermore, the less one touches the brain during this process, the better the results.

Freeing the Attachments of the Brain

At the beginning of this stage, the head lies on the occipital bone (or face up) with the vertex directed to the operator and both lateral flaps deflected. As the cranium is tilted gently to one side and then the other, all of the cranial nerves and large vessels should be identified and transected (as close to the bone as possible), proceeding from front to back, and the anterior portion of the falx cerebri cut loose. As the posterior fossa is approached, the tentorium is cut away from the interior of the skull, around its entire perimeter, then the falx cerebri is transected just above the tentorium.

As the attachments on both sides of the posterior fossa are severed, the brain stem and cord come into view. When the upper cervical cord can be seen clearly, it should be transected as far caudally as possible. With that, the entire brain will slide out easily on to the moistened table top. The technique described by Langley [11] is a useful means of achieving this (Fig. 5.8). It should be weighed and then fixed in

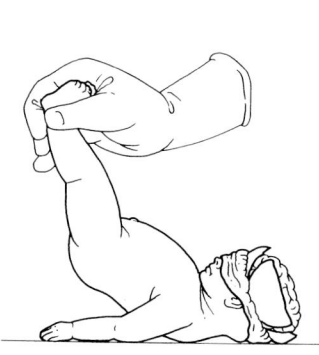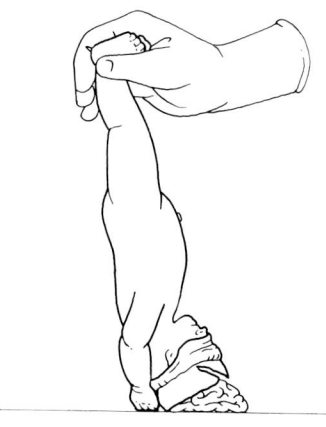

FIGURE 5.8. *Removal of the brain by gravity.
(Courtesy of Langley [11].)*

10 times its volume of 10% buffered formalin. Any abnormalities of the base of the skull are best documented by photography at this stage.

All of the dural sinuses are then opened in search of thrombi as is the Great Vein of Galen. The fragile pituitary is probably best removed within the cartilagenous sella by using a sharp scalpel, and is fixed as it is—attached to the sella.

In all perinatal autopsies the middle ears ought to be inspected and, if necessary, cultured. Even in infants of this size, the petrous portion of the temporal bone is extremely hard. Using strong bone shears, one can make two straight cuts angling down through the temporal bone from above to join each other in the main cavity of the middle ear. The more lateral incision is flat against the inner table of the skull, just inside the pinna; the opposing incision is at about a 30° angle to the first coming down, front to back, through the petrous portion of the temporal bone to meet the bottom end of the first cut inside the middle ear. The wedge of bone between the two incisions is removed and the middle ear explored. Any puriform fluid is cultured. The ossicles are inspected, as is the inner aspect of the drum. By sliding a blunt-ended probe into the external canal and touching the outside of the drum with it, one can demonstrate readily the normal translucency of that delicate structure. In certain malformation syndromes, anomalies of the middle and inner ear may be present. These are best looked for by using the technique described by Sando for the removal and examination of these structures [38].

The eyes—their size, orientation, lids, and appendages—are studied carefully in every perinatal autopsy. However, in many malformation syndromes and in a variety of other circumstances (i.e., prolonged oxygen exposure) it is desirable to remove the globes for further detailed measurements and examination. The procedure is, in fact, easier than it would seem. After the brain has been removed, the thin, orbital roof, an almost translucent plate of bone on top of each globe is seen readily in each anterior fossa. Using bone-cutting medium-sized scissors, one can cut readily all the way around and then remove the bony plate. At first glance, what one sees within is pure adipose tissue; however, deeper than that is the globe itself, with its voluntary muscles attached. By pushing gently with one's finger on the globe itself, from outside, through the closed eyelids while tugging from above with forceps on the various attached muscles, one can deliver the intact eye upward and out. The eyes can also be removed from the front with dissection facilitated by use of a small ophthalmology retractor. Even though there is written permission to remove the eyes, we recommend discussing the matter with the funeral director beforehand. The best sections of the eye are obtained using plastic embedding after formalin fixation.

Spinal Cord

There are two standard approaches for removal of the spinal cord: anterior and posterior. The anterior approach is simple in fetuses and neonates. Initially, it is necessary to stabilize the body on a firm surface in a sort of opisthotonic supine position, so that the now-bared thoracolumbar spine arches forward prominently. One first removes approximately two lumbar vertebrae, which are then at least halved and fixed in formalin.

Into the opening thus created, a single blade or small bone-cutting scissors can be inserted, in a cranial direction, blades tilted toward one side or the other. Then two parallel cuts are made upward through the two pedicles of all of the thoracic and lower cervical vertebrae to facilitate removal of the corresponding vertebral bodies and visualization of the entire spinal cord.

The status of the cord is then documented and an incision made, with fine scissors, through the entire length of the dura, anterior to the cord, in the midline, this incision permits removal of the cord without inadvertent crushing, as it is bent necessarily during removal.

By making a transverse cut through the filum terminale (near its caudal end), together with the dura, one can then remove the cord by grasping the opened dura caudally (which now forms a kind of cradle to support the cord) and lifting it up progressively from below, toward the cervical region with the cord resting safely in its embrace. A portion of the filum terminale is included with the cord.

The posterior approach commences with a midline skin incision extending from the nape of the neck to the lumbosacral region (this procedure is almost required if the case involves an Arnold-Chiari malformation; in such an instance, the aforementioned posterior midline scalp incision is simply continued caudally, in the midline as described above, down to the lumbosacral region). If there is a lumbar myelomeningocele or a related lesion at that level, the skin incision may be brought completely around it in an elongated oval so that the entire lesion—with affected vertebral bodies—can be removed in continuity with the spinal cord. A similar en bloc technique can be used for lesions involving the spine or vertebral column that project forward into the body cavity.

In a non-complicated case, the dorsal skin and subcutaneous tissues are then reflected to the two sides of the body, thus exposing the spinous processes and laminae of the bony vertebrae. The backs of the thoracic and lumbar vertebrae are removed by cutting through the laminae on each side of the midline with small bone-cutting scissors—creating one continuous strip—and then lifting it steadily upward from below. Then one proceeds to remove the exposed spinal cord and dura in virtually the same fashion as is described above for the anterior approach.

Special techniques are important to consider for achondroplasia. In infants with osteochondrodysplasia the dissection technique described by Knisely and Singer permits more accurate assessment of both spinal cord stenosis and spinal cord injury [39]. This is important since spinal cord stenosis is a well-recognized cause of respiratory dysfunction, paralysis, and death in achondroplasia [40].

Bones

In a routine case, we remove two segments of rib and two vertebral bodies for histological sections. Arbitrarily, we use the 6th and 7th ribs and take from each a 1.0-cm segment, including the costochondral junction. In cases that involve a disease of the bones, other samples are also selected; the bones chosen would depend, of course, upon the nature and extent of the disease. When an entire long bone is to be removed (e.g., the tibia), we often consult with the funeral director beforehand; he or she frequently will agree to the procedure provided that we perfuse the extremity with formalin (via the major arteries) before removing the bone. This is especially important in older infants. Further, to facilitate the work of the funeral director, we usually attempt to reconstruct the limb by replacing the bone with a piece of wood or plastic of approximately the same size and shape.

Muscle and Nerve

It is our custom, in routine cases, to remove two skeletal muscle samples, namely, one leaf of the diaphragm and one psoas muscle. In cases of primary or secondary muscle disease, appropriate individually labeled samples of both normal (if possible) and affected muscles are also removed for further study, as indicated. It is important to sample tissues both for longitudinal and cross-sectional study. Samples should also be taken for electron microscopy and frozen tissue for enzyme studies. Proximal and distal muscles of both limbs should be sampled.

If sections of nerve are desired, we usually sample the sciatic nerve; the phrenic nerve and the left recurrent laryngeal nerve are also readily available for sampling.

Lymph Nodes

Customarily, we remove a pie-shaped segment of the mesentery of the small bowel, about 1.0 cm length, at its perimeter. A longitudinal histological section of the sample will ordinarily include an adequate number of lymph nodes, two or three, for routine microscopic examination. If, on the other hand, the case is one that involves primary or secondary disease of the lymph nodes, appropriate individually labeled nodes should also be removed; very thin sections should be taken from larger nodes and touch preparations or special fixatives may be employed. The hilar region of the lung is also a ready source of lymph nodes.

Dissection of Organs

After the block of organs has been removed from the body, it is dissected further in a systematic manner beginning at the tongue and then proceeding stepwise in a generally caudal direction.

We find that a readily available and inexpensive commercial plastic sponge or block greatly facilitates this operation. We prefer to use a sponge roughly the size and shape of an ordinary building brick. This must be kept moist from the outset and may be cleansed with water once or twice during the dissection.

The major visceral block of organs, from tongue to rectum, is first stretched longitudinally over the sponge with the posterior aspect displayed for dissection. Usually, the tongue will be left hanging over one end of the sponge and the pelvic organs over the other.

Dissection begins with examination of the tongue, especially the dorsal surface posteriorly, for any remnants of the thyroglossal duct. At the same time, the tonsillar pillars, soft palate, and the uvula are inspected for either congenital or acquired lesions, as are the hyoid bone, the pharynx, larynx, and trachea. We usually open the pharynx first, then proceed caudally, incising the esophagus longitudinally in the midline, down the posterior aspect, to the level of the diaphragm, which takes the incision close to the esophagogastric junction to permit examination of the entire length of the mucosa. Disorders such as ectopic gastric mucosa (a sharply demarcated, slightly velvety, slightly elevated, ovoid, pink island, which is a different shade of pink from that of the surrounding esophageal mucosa) and tracheo-esophageal fistula are detected at this time. If a tracheo-esophageal fistula is suspected, the trachea should be opened anteriorly rather than posteriorly, as described later. Following its examination, the normal esophagus, together with the pharynx, is separated from the upper airway and then laid down caudally over the stomach. This exposes the posterior wall of the pericardium and the posterior aspect of the airway. The latter can then be opened with scissors, by cutting the midline posterior membranous portion of the trachea and bronchi in a craniocaudal direction. The interior of the larynx and trachea can then be examined, taking particular care to look for endotracheal tube trauma, necrosis, and plugging with meconium, mucus, or other aspirated material. If an endotracheal tube has been left in situ its level in the tracheobronchial tree should be recorded.

The neck organs are then cut away en bloc from the main unit, with transection at a point just below the isthmus of the thyroid and the bifurcation of the trachea.

The tonsils are removed next, each with a small cuff of surrounding mucosa. The tongue is detached from the larynx with the hyoid bone, and fixed as a whole. The larynx, trachea, and thyroid are also fixed as one unit.

The abdominal aorta is dissected next and opened longitudinally in the midline posteriorly, from the level of the diaphragm to its bifurcation. The location of catheter tips should be documented and thrombus formation excluded. The two renal arteries are opened and the celiac and superior mesenteric arteries are inspected. The thoracic aorta is then reflected cranially up to the level of the left main bronchus. After removal of the posterior wall of the pericardial sac, the thoracic organs can be separated from the abdominal organs by simply cutting across the inferior vena cava as close to the diaphragm as possible. (This should not be done when anomalous pulmonary venous return involves infradiaphragmatic structures.)

The heart is separated from the lungs, if there are no congenital cardiac anomalies, by isolating and then transecting each of the following vessels separately: 1) the right lower pulmonary vein, 2) the right middle and upper pulmonary veins, 3) the right pulmonary artery, 4) the left lower pulmonary vein, 5) the left upper pulmonary vein, 6) the left pulmonary artery, 7) the right and left cardiac mesenteries from the right and left bronchi, and 8) the aorta at the level of the diaphragm, leaving the descending part of the aortic arch and the ductus arteriosus intact and separating the caudal portion of the trachea from the aorta.

The lungs are inspected for lobation, pleural lesions, and for correct situs by observing the anatomy of the major bronchial branches. At this juncture, some pathologists prefer to make serial thin slices through each lung horizontally—usually with a Durham knife—and to take representative sections for fixation from each lobe and from any gross lesions. Others, instead, perfuse formalin through the main bronchus of each lung (or one lung) and then fix the organ

as a whole by total immersion prior to sectioning. Perfusion is best performed via a closed-circuit pump system for 24 hours at a pressure of 25 cm H_2O [41]. If a pump is not available, an intravenous set can be used, again at a pressure of 25 cm H_2O. If pulmonary hypoplasia is a consideration, perfusion is the best method of fixation since it fixes the lung in what approximates to its inflated state.

The inferior vena cava is then opened cranio-caudally from the level of the diaphragm to the bifurcation, and both renal veins are also opened. The diaphragm is removed with the crurae—in one piece—and fixed spread out flat (on a paper towel) in its entirety. Each adrenal gland is now removed very carefully to avoid crushing them, because they are extremely fragile in the newborn. One method of removal begins with grasping firmly a bit of attached loose connective tissue near one pole of the gland, which allows one to lift the organ upward while cutting under it and separating it from the kidney. At this time, the periadrenal autonomic neural tissue can be inspected.

In preparation for removal of the spleen, one should first open and inspect the splenic and portal veins. Then only should the pedicle of the spleen be transected and the organ examined, weighed, cut in thin serial sections, and selected sections fixed.

Before dissecting the stomach and liver, the gastrohepatic ligament can be cut, leaving the common bile duct intact. In addition, one should sever all attachments of the pancreas to the stomach and to retroperitoneal tissue.

At this point, the genito-urinary tract is dissected. First, each kidney is freed in turn and hemisected in the coronal plane (with a Durham knife) by holding it up with one hand while it is still attached to its hilar structures, to provide stability. The capsule can then be stripped from one half, but should be left attached to the portion chosen for microscopic study to avoid damage to the outer cortex. The cut surface is examined with particular attention to the number and color of the pyramids and the size and shape of the pelvis. The normal number of pyramids is 8 to 12 per kidney. The ureter is opened from the pelvis to the bladder. One should open the bladder then from the outlet to the dome and inspect the trigone (including the ureteral orifices). The kidneys, ureters, and urinary bladder are now removed in continuity with one another—together with attached testes and vasa (or ovaries, tubes, uterus, and vagina—thus separating them from the rectum and anus.

The next step is to remove the entire intestinal tract. Some pathologists commence this process at the rectum and, using scissors to sever its attachments, work upward to the cecum and then to the small bowel. It is our custom to begin at the ligament of Treitz, after transecting the duodenum. Proceeding distally, the attachment of the mesentery to the small bowel is cut with scissors throughout its length, leaving behind any tags of mesentery, which may cause the bowel to kink or curl during opening. The large bowel is then removed from its attachments. As soon as the bowel is removed, the length of each portion (i.e., small and large intestine) should be measured. Opinions differ as to the best method of taking samples of intestine for microscopic sections; some prefer to open the bowel first, empty it, and then examine the mucosa before taking sections—which they usually mount, serosa down, on pieces of dry paper towel. It is probably preferable to remove small unopened cross-sectional segments prior to opening the gut, and to fix them intact together with their content; this method provides better preservation of the mucosa, which is easily damaged during emptying of the lumen.

Exploration of the biliary tree is commenced by removing the gallbladder from its bed, without transecting the cystic duct. The first part of the duodenum is then opened to display the ampulla of Vater. One can then press upon the gallbladder to force bile through the common duct into the duodenum, thus demonstrating the patency of the extrahepatic biliary duct system. Alternatively, water or saline can be injected via a large-bore needle into the gallbladder. The duodenohepatic ligament is then severed to separate the liver from the upper gastrointestinal block.

Once the liver is free, it should be turned upside down and placed on its diaphragmatic surface; this exposes the veins embedded in the underside of the organ, which can then be investigated. The umbilical vein is opened from below upward, commencing from the severed free end and then continuing, with a turn to the prosector's right, to open the left portal vein (formerly the sinus intermedius), the portal vein, and then, if possible, the ductus venosus. The liver is then weighed and sectioned serially in the sagittal plane, and representative sections are taken for fixation. Possible differences in the color of the right and left lobes are noted.

The pancreas must first be cleaned of the loose connective tissue that surrounds it and then the duodenum should be removed from its attachment to the head. The organ can be sectioned serially, in the sagittal plane, and fixed in its entirety. An alternative method is to leave the duodenum attached to the head of the pancreas.

The linear incision made earlier through the length of the esophagus should now be extended distally along the greater curvature of the stomach so that the two organs, in continuity, can be laid cut flat, serosa down, on a dry paper towel. The stomach contents are noted. In this fashion, the mucosa is thoroughly exposed for inspection, following which the two organs together can be fixed in toto.

Dissection of the genito-urinary block differs in the male and the female. In the female, the first step in the procedure is to separate the internal genital organs en bloc from the urinary bladder. Next, one excises the umbilical arteries, separating them from the ureters and sides of the bladder up to the umbilicus. The urachal remnant should be severed as close to the umbilicus as possible. One then fixes the umbilicus with the attached arteries. In the male, the genital organs sectioned include the testis and prostate. The male gonads are often congested in breech presentation. In the female, one

ovary and tube are submitted and a sagittal section of the uterus, cervix, and vagina. Small cysts are sometimes noted in the ovary and are probably not significant.

MICROSCOPIC EXAMINATION

Apart from the recognition of pathological processes, microscopy is also part of the evaluation of organ growth and development. This requires knowledge of the normal histology and development of fetal tissues [42].

SPECIAL STUDIES

In many autopsies, the clinical and/or gross findings indicate that special studies are necessary for accurate diagnosis of certain disorders. Apart from bacteriology studies, the studies discussed below need not be repeated if adequate samples have been taken premortem.

Microbiology Studies

Except for severely macerated stillbirths, we routinely culture heart's blood, one lung, and the liver for aerobic and anaerobic organisms. Other sites are sampled via swabs, fluid, or tissue based on clinical or gross findings (i.e., exudates, chorioamnionitis, etc.). Viral cultures are done when indicated, usually by the clinical history and signs of sepsis, with negative bacterial cultures. In systemic viral infections, heart muscle has been suggested as a source of tissue for viral cultures [1].

Immunopathology Studies

These are useful in the diagnosis of infection and hydrops fetalis. In the case of a specific infection, TORCH titers or general serum electrophoresis may be indicated. In a newborn infant, an elevated IgM level indicates intrauterine infection; this is particularly useful in the differential diagnosis of non-immune hydrops fetalis. IgG levels are less valuable, but need to be compared with the mother's IgG titers since these immunoglobulins cross the placenta. These samples should be collected within 12 to 24 hours of death [14]. Immunohistochemistry or in situ DNA hybridization can be used for identifying certain organisms in tissue sections. It is useful to freeze portions of tissue and excess serum in some cases.

Hematology Studies

We do not do hematocrit and hemoglobin analyses routinely, since these studies are generally unreliable when performed after death.

Biochemistry

These are performed primarily to diagnose inborn errors of metabolism. One uses fluids (urine and blood) and tissue samples for enzyme assays and the latter for morphology, including electron microscopy. Time is of the essence if accurate quantitative and qualitative estimations of lipids, carbohydrates, and mucopolysaccharides are to be performed on samples of liver, spleen, kidney, heart, and muscle tissues. Enzymes can also be evaluated on fibroblast cultures taken at autopsy [14]. Barson has found the vitreous humor to be the least labile fluid biochemically [1]. Haan and Danks have reviewed the clinical investigation of suspected metabolic disease [43] and Wigglesworth has compiled a useful list of those inborn errors likely to cause perinatal death [14].

Histochemistry/Immunohistochemistry

Frozen tissue is required to characterize skeletal muscle fibers by enzyme analysis and for the evaluation of cholinesterase for the diagnosis of Hirschsprung disease. Many other immunohistochemical procedures, such as the evaluation of infection, pancreatic polypeptides, and liver alpha-1-antitrypsin, can be performed on formalin-fixed paraffin-embedded tissues.

Frozen Tissues

It is useful to freeze tissue when viral infection and metabolic disease (inborn errors of metabolism) are suspected. In addition, when resources and policy permit, a frozen tissue bank is an invaluable resource for future molecular investigation of development.

Photographs

Photographs are an essential part of the perinatal autopsy. External, in situ, and gross organ abnormalities are best documented in this manner, particularly in the macerated infant where descriptions may be difficult. Whole-body (front and back), close-up of the full face, and right and left profiles are invaluable for the future review of dysmorphology and congenital anomalies. They are also essential for good communication among pathologists and clinicians in teaching conferences. We also receive requests from patients for photographs of their infants.

Tissue Culture for Cytogenetic and Other Studies

Tissues taken for cytogenetic studies will grow in tissue culture even when derived from a macerated fetus (up to grade I, and up to several days after death) [44]. The indications for cytogenetic studies include fetuses or neonates known, suspected, or likely to have congenital malformations or tumors. Suspicious features include nuchal edema, ambiguous genitalia, and dysgenetic gonads [13]. Other indications for tissue culture include molecular studies for the diagnosis of osteogenesis imperfecta, cystic renal disease, cystic fibrosis, and Duchenne muscular dystrophy [45].

A METHOD FOR EXAMINING THE BRAIN AFTER FIXATION

Brain Fixation

The brain should be maintained in 10% formalin for 2 weeks, and then in 80% alcohol for 2 days before sectioning. It is then cut as described below; the cassettes bearing tissue samples are placed in 80% alcohol for 2 more days. Tissue processing in a Technicon includes 4 hours in 95% alcohol, 4 hours in 100% alcohol, and 2 hours in Parasol rather than xylene. Sections are then cut and stained routinely. Special stains of tissue sections may be used for the evaluation of myelin.

Sectioning the Fixed Brain

The fixed brain is washed in running water overnight and its weight recorded. The dura, falx cerebri, and tentorium cerebelli are examined and the dural sinuses opened. The leptomeninges are inspected. The 12 pairs of cranial nerves and the branches of the circle of Willis are identified. The general appearance and symmetry of the cerebral hemispheres are noted. The degree of development of the cerebral convolutions is compared with the normal for gestational age (Fig. 5.9) and the maturity by gyral pattern determined.

The size and general appearance of the cerebellum are noted. The components of the brain stem are identified.

The cerebrum is separated from the cerebellum and brain stem by cutting through the cerebral peduncles as far rostrally as possible using a No. 22 scalpel. The cerebrum is placed upside down (base up) on the cutting board. It is sliced in serial coronal sections using a brain knife, beginning at the frontal pole and ending at the occipital pole. The thickness of the slices is determined by the consistency of the brain. Firm brains can be sliced at 1-cm intervals and soft friable ones at greater intervals. The location of the cuts can be varied according to the position of observed or suspected lesions. Each slice is laid on a flat tray, in sequence, with the anterior surface on the board, convex edge pointing "north" and right side on the right. Anatomical landmarks are identified. The size and shape of the ventricles and appearance of the ependyma are noted.

The brain stem is separated from the cerebellum by cutting through the cerebellar peduncles with a No. 22 scalpel. Each is weighed separately if their growth appears arrested. Using a Durham knife, the cerebellum is sectioned serially in the horizontal plane beginning at the superior surface. The slices are laid out sequentially with the inferior surface of each slice on the tray, the dorsal edge pointing "north" and the right side on the right. Anatomical landmarks are identified.

Using a Durham knife again, the brain stem is sectioned serially at 2-mm intervals from the rostral to the caudal ends. The slices are laid out with the caudal surface of each on the tray, the dorsal surface up and the right side on the

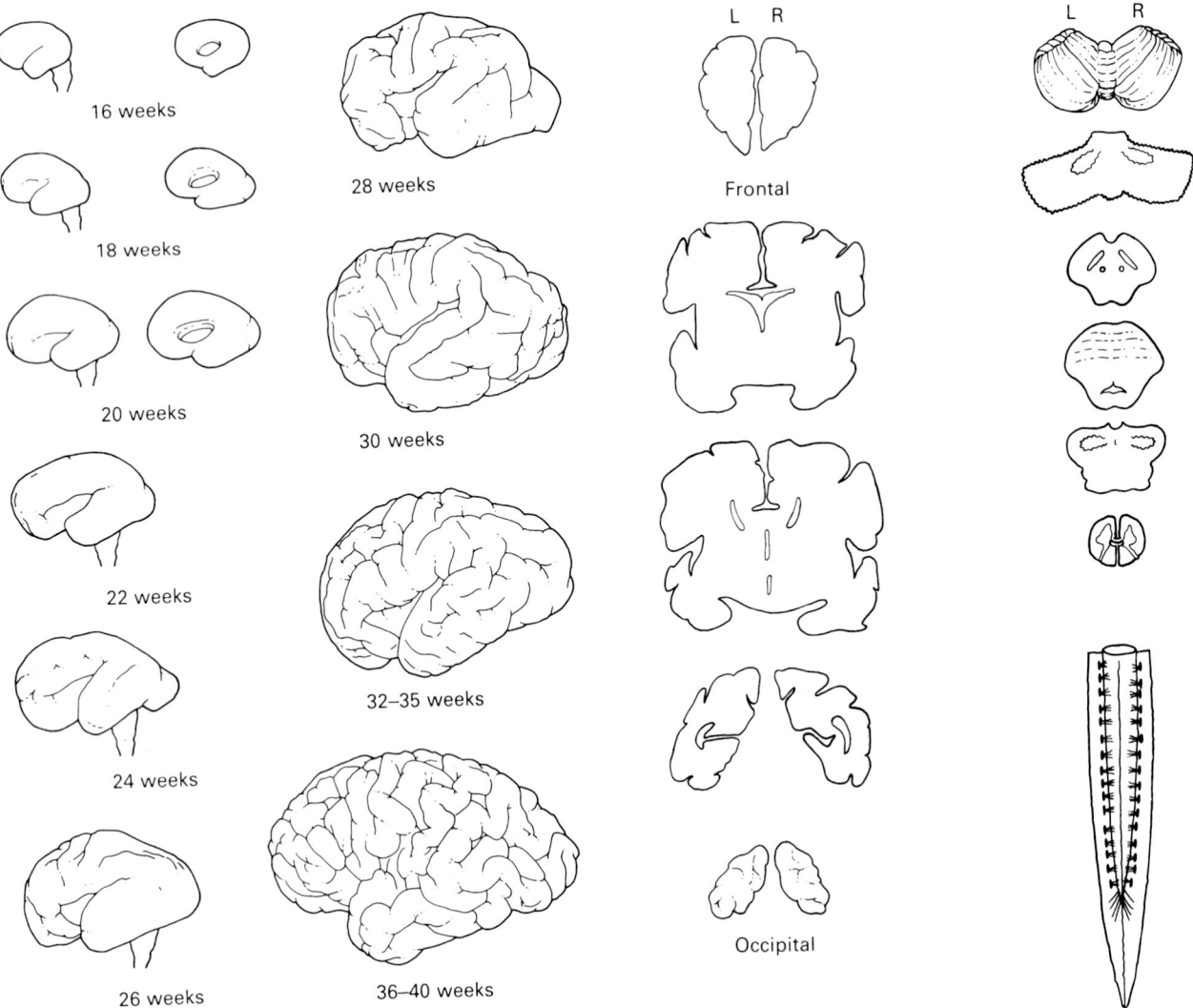

FIGURE 5.9. *Development of the fetal brain. The degree of gyral development is a crude measure of gestational age—accurate at best within two or more weeks of gestation. The rate of development varies among individuals. The right and left hemispheres may develop asynchronously. The ability to detect the earliest evidence of a sulcus or gyrus varies with the state of preservation of the specimen and the method of examination. (Courtesy of Valdes-Dapena and Huff [13].)*

FIGURE 5.10. *Sectioned brain and cord. The posterior surfaces of the cerebrum and spinal cord face the prosector, as do the superior surfaces of the cerebellum and brain stem. The brain is ready for final inspection and selection of sections. (Courtesy of Valdes-Dapena and Huff [13].)*

right. The size of the aqueduct of Sylvius and of the 4th ventricle is noted. Normal landmarks are identified.

If it has not been cut already (during removal), the dorsal dura of the spinal cord is incised longitudinally in the midline. The anterior and posterior surfaces of the dura can then be opened like double doors and the surfaces of the cord examined. The cord is cut transversely at several levels, without cutting the dura, leaving the cord attached to the dura. The cut surfaces can be examined without losing the anatomical orientation of the cord.

At this point the entire cerebrum, cerebellum, brain stem, and cord are all laid out in sequential slices, all uniformly oriented (Fig. 5.10). Sections can be selected. These should

be no more than 2.5 × 1.5 cm. The exact location of any sections taken should be recorded on a cut-down sheet (Table 5.3), and lesions recorded on the diagram presented in Figure 5.10.

A METHOD FOR EXAMINATION OF THE PLACENTA

The placenta is examined, maternal surface down, on a flat surface. The membranes are spread out and the point of rupture determined.

The cord length and average diameter are measured and the number of vessels determined (this may require a fresh cut of the cord). Any constrictions, fusiform enlargements, and abnormalities of Wharton's jelly are noted. The cord is

Table 5.3. Neuropathology cut-down sheet (courtesy of Hanna Kinney)

Autopsy number . . . .
Cut by . . . .
Autopsy date . . . .   Autopsy time . . . . .a.m.☐ p.m.☐
Tissue cut date . . . .   Autopsy time . . . . .a.m.☐ p.m.☐

Cassette	Site	Section	
		Yes	No
Cerebral hemispheres			
1*	Orbital frontal cortex and white matter	☐	☐
2*	Superior frontal gyrus, cingulate gyrus, corpus callosum, and white matter to include corona radiata and deep centrum ovale at level of anterior horn	☐	☐
3	Posterior frontal cortex and white matter with germinal matrix at thalamostriate junction at level of foramen of Monroe	☐	☐
4	Lenticular nucleus with insular cortex at level of genu of capsule; includes optic tract and hypothalamus	☐	☐
5*	Hippocampus, cingulum, and optic tract	☐	☐
6	Internal capsule, posterior limb and thalamus	☐	☐
7	Proximal optic radiation, just lateral to làteral geniculate body; includes hippocampus and adjacent temporal lobe	☐	☐
8*	Pulvinar with rostral midbrain	☐	☐
9*	Parietal cortex and periventricular white matter with splenium corpus callosum	☐	☐
10	Parietal cortex and periventricular white matter with distal optic radiation and choroid plexus	☐	☐
11	Occipital cortex to include calcarine cortex and periventricular white matter	☐	☐
Cerebellum/midbrain/pons/medulla			
12 A	Lateral hemisphere with dentate nucleus	☐	☐
B	Vermis	☐	☐
13	Midbrain—rostral	☐	☐
	or		
	Midbrain—caudal	☐	☐
14*	Pons—rostral; pons—mid (exit of cranial V)	☐	☐
15	Medulla	☐	☐
Spinal cord			
16	Cervical spinal cord	☐	☐
17*	Thoracic spinal cord	☐	☐
18	Lumbar spinal cord	☐	☐
Dura/sinus			
19*	Dura with superior sagittal sinus	☐	☐

* Sections are optional but useful. All other sections are considered to be essential.

examined with regard to color and the surface examined for any changes in translucency. Insertion of the cord is determined and findings such as velamentous insertion and vasa previa are recorded. A cross-section of the cord is taken about 10 cm from the placental end and any other focal lesions should be sampled. The cord is then trimmed close to its placental insertion.

The membranes not covering the placental disc are examined with regard to their translucency, color, completeness (complete or incomplete), insertion at the placental edge (to look for placenta extrachorialis), and presence of any vessels (i.e., possible vasa praevia). A strip of membranes is then cut from the estimated point of rupture to the placental edge (i.e., a strip up to 3 × 4 cm), rolled,

pinned, and fixed for section after fixation. The membranes are then trimmed from the placental disc.

The placental disc is now measured (average diameter and average thickness) and weighed. The fetal surface is examined with regard to shape (normally round), color, surface, translucency, surface lesions (i.e., amnion nodosum), and state of fetal vessels in the chorionic plate (i.e., thrombosis, rupture, etc.). If cultures are indicated, they are taken from this surface after sterilizing the amnion, stripping it from the chorion by aseptic technique and sampling chorion and/or villous tissue. Scrapings for Gram and other stains can also be made from the amnion and chorion.

The maternal surface of the placental disc is now examined with regard to color, completeness, and appearance of the uncut surface (blood clots, focal lesions, etc.). Before cutting the placenta at 1-cm intervals, it is important to palpate the placenta through its full thickness because focal lesions, such as infarcts or chorangiomas, may be identified readily in that manner. The placenta is then cut at 1-cm intervals.

The following sections of the placenta are taken:

1. One centrally near the midpoint of the placenta.
2. One from a midzone section (i.e., between the midpoint of the placenta and its edge).
3. Sections of any focal lesions of the placenta.
4. One section of cord and rolled membranes.

All sections of the placenta should be no more than 3 mm thick and should be full thickness—that is, include both the decidual and amniotic surfaces in each section.

A METHOD FOR TRIMMING TISSUE FOR MICROSCOPIC SECTIONS

General

It is very helpful to place the trimmed tissue in plastic cassettes for processing. Each cassette can be labeled with the autopsy number followed by the cassette number. The type and number of tissue blocks placed in each numbered cassette can be recorded on a "cut-down" sheet, which becomes a permanent part of the autopsy report. The histotechnologist labels each slide with the autopsy number and cassette number. This makes retrieval of specific slides and blocks very easy. Furthermore, using cassettes forces one to trim the tissue to the appropriate thickness of 3 to 4 mm, since the cassettes are only 4 mm deep. This enhances the quality of microscopic sections.

Table 5.4.   General autopsy—cut-down sheet

Autopsy number . . . .
Cut by . . . .
Autopsy date . . . .   Time . . . . ☐ a.m. ☐ p.m.
Tissue cut date . . . .   Time . . . . ☐ a.m. ☐ p.m.

Cassette	Organ	No. of Pieces in Cassette
1	*Left heart* ☐ *Right heart* ☐ Interventricular septum ☐	—
2	*Larynx* ☐ *Trachea* ☐ *Esophagus* ☐ *Thyroid* ☐	—
3	Lower trachea ☐ Bronchi ☐	—
4	*Right lung* ☐	—
5	*Left lung* ☐	—
6	Submaxillary gland ☐ *Pancreas head* ☐ tail ☐	—
7	Liver ☐	—
8	*Esogastric* ☐ Pyloduodenal ☐ Ileocecal ☐ Anorectal ☐	—
9	*Small bowel* ☐ *Colon* ☐	—
10	*Kidney right* ☐ left ☐	—
11	Bladder ☐ *Female genitalia* ☐ *Male genitalia* ☐	—
12	*Adrenal* ☐ Pituitary ☐ Testis/epididymis ☐ Ovary/tube ☐	—
13	*Thymus* ☐ Spleen ☐ Mesentery ☐ Tonsil ☐ Adenoid ☐	—
14	Tongue ☐ Diaphragm ☐ Psoas ☐ +Nerve ☐	—
15	Costochondral junction ☐ Vertebra ☐	—
16	Skin ☐ +Nipple ☐ *Umbilicus* ☐	—
17	Umbilical vein ☐ *Umbilical cord* ☐	—
18, 19	*Placenta central* ☐ *margin* ☐ *lesion* ☐	—

Note: Sections in italic are considered to be essential; the others are very useful.
(Adapted from the Perinatal Autopsy Manual [13].)

The quality of microscopic sections is best if the tissue is trimmed within 24 hours of the autopsy and then processed immediately. Sections taken are recorded on a cut-down sheet (Table 5.4).

Heart

Two longitudinal sections of the heart are taken: one through the right and one through the left posterior free atrioventricular junction. Each should include the full thickness of the atrial and ventricular walls, the atrioventricular valve, a papillary muscle, and a chorda tendinea. These sections can be up to 2.5 cm long, 1.5 cm wide, and 3 mm thick. A section of the interventricular septum is useful in some circumstances. They are placed in cassette no. 1.

Neck Organs

The larynx, trachea, upper esophagus, and thyroid are serially cross-sectioned at 3 mm intervals. A representative complete cross-section at the level of the isthmus is submitted in cassette no. 2. This block will include a complete cross-section of the thyroid, trachea, and esophagus, and will often contain ectopic lobules of thymus and both parathyroids IV. In the case of small fetuses, two or more of these cross-sections may fit in this cassette.

Lungs, Trachea, and Bronchi

Sections of lower trachea and bronchi are placed in cassette no. 3. One section of the periphery and one of the hilum are taken from each lung. Each rectangular section can be 2.0 × 1.5 cm. The two from the right are placed in cassette no. 4 and those from the left in cassette no. 5.

Accessory Digestive Organs

Cassette no. 6 contains a complete section of one submaxillary gland and a complete coronal section of the head of the pancreas, including the attached duodenal wall and papilla of Vater. With smaller specimens, a cross-section of the other submaxillary gland and a complete coronal section of the tail of the pancreas may fit into this cassette.

Liver

In larger fetuses, a complete coronal section of the tail of the pancreas and a rectangular section of liver are put in cassette no. 7. These should be no more than 2 × 1.5 cm.

Digestive Tract

Longitudinal sections 2 cm long and 3 mm wide are cut through the full thickness of the esophagogastric junction, pyloric-duodenal junction, ileocecal junction, including the valve, and the anorectal canal. These are all put in cassette no. 8. Cross-sections of the small bowel and colon are placed in cassette no. 9.

Kidney

One section from each kidney is included in cassette no. 10. Each should include an entire lobule from the renal capsule to the tip of the pyramid, with attached calyceal walls. These can be up to 2 × 1.5 cm.

Bladder and Genital Organs

Cassette no. 11 contains a strip of the full thickness of the bladder wall and a longitudinal section of the full thickness of the uterus, cervix, and vagina. These can be up to 3 cm long and 4 mm wide. The section of cervix and vagina should include as much of the uterus as the 3-cm length will allow. In smaller preterm babies, a complete mid-sagittal section of the intact uterus, cervix, and upper vagina may fit into this cassette. For males, one or more complete cross-sections of the prostate and attached seminal vesicles, and the ampoules of the vasa replace the section of uterus and vagina.

Endocrine Glands

Usually one or two longitudinal sections of testis and attached epididymis, a cross-section of adrenal gland, and a mid-sagittal section of pituitary will all fit into cassette no. 12. For females, several cross-sections of ovary and attached tubes will fit, in place of the sections of testis.

Lymphoid Tissue

Cassette no. 13 contains one square of thymus and one of spleen, measuring 1.5 × 1.5 cm, and a 2-cm section of the full thickness of the mesentery containing lymph nodes. Sections of tonsils and adenoids should be included when indicated.

Skeletal Muscle

A mid-sagittal section of posterior tongue measuring 1.5 × 1.5 cm, including mucosa, foramen cecum, and skeletal muscle; a strip of diaphragm 2 cm long; and a portion of psoas, including underlying nerve, make up the contents of cassette no. 14.

Bone

Cassette no. 15 contains a longitudinal section of one costochondral junction and a mid-sagittal section through one or two vertebrae (depending on the size of the fetus), including an intervertebral disc, if possible. These are submitted for decalcification (after trimming to the correct size and thickness to reduce the time required for decalcification). Fetal and neonatal bones can usually be trimmed with a scalpel.

Skin

Cassette no. 16 is for a section through the breast bud, including the nipple, overlying skin, surrounding fat, and underlying pectoralis muscle. A section of the full thickness of the umbilicus and surrounding skin and abdominal wall is also included, measuring approximately 2 × 1.5 cm.

Umbilical Cord and Placenta

A 3-mm-thick section of umbilical cord and a 3-mm-thick cross-section of a roll of chorioamniotic membrane are placed in cassette no. 17.

Table 5.5.   Guidelines for perinatal death review committee

Have representatives from those specialties involved in perinatal care, i.e.,
    obstetrics, neonatology, pathology, and anesthesiology
Establish criteria for review of perinatal deaths, i.e., review of all deaths ⩾20
    weeks' gestation or ⩾500 g birth weight
Evaluate appropriateness of care
Maintain an adequate autopsy rate
Establish guidelines for placental examination
Use a system for categorization/classification of perinatal deaths
Prepare a comprehensive annual report of perinatal deaths
Maintain confidentiality

(From Macpherson et al [5].)

Table 5.6.   Items for inclusion in annual report on review of perinatal deaths

Summary of major conclusions of the report
Recommendations for changes in clinical practice
Identification of areas requiring clinical research
Overall perinatal mortality review (PMR) for current year
Comparison of current PMR with PMR of previous years
Annual report (%) overall, for stillbirths and for neonatal deaths
Placental evaluation rate (%)
PMR by birth weight and gestational age
PMR by maternal age, parity, presentation, and route of delivery
PMR by maternal diagnosis
PMR by perinatal cause of death
List of congenital anomalies
PMR by race and obstetric service (clinic/private/referral)
Miscellaneous (items that require emphasis for a particular year)

(From Macpherson et al [5].)

Cassette nos. 18 and 19 contain a section of the placenta, one from the central portion and the other from the midzone. Each of these should be approximately 2 × 1.5 cm.

Central Nervous System

Sections of specific lesions and normal structures are taken as indicated in Table 5.3. The specific sites of the lesions should be recorded on a cutdown sheet, while the nature of the lesions can be recorded on the diagrams presented in Figure 5.10.

The above instructions are artificially specific and only suggest an appropriate set of routine sections. The number, site, and size of sections should be tailored to the individual case. Sections of lesions can replace or be added to the suggested list of routine sections. In any case, the general principles concerning size and thickness of sections should be followed. Sections should be no more than 3 to 4 mm thick and should not be crowded into the cassettes.

CONCLUSION

"The pathologist's role in perinatal mortality and morbidity is to provide the accurate diagnostic support necessary to ensure his contribution to education, research and the quality of care in perinatology" [5]. This begins with the pathologist's commitment to the perinatal autopsy as demonstrated by his or her close supervision of the work, a good protocol, issue of timely and informative reports, communication of autopsy findings to health care providers, and participation in the review of perinatal deaths. There have been several recent reports on the clinical value of [3, 17, 45–49] and concerns about the perinatal and neonatal autopsy [50, 51]. The worth of the perinatal autopsy is realized fully when epidemiological and pathological data regarding individual deaths are used in formal reviews of perinatal mortality. A uniform system for categorizing perinatal deaths will facilitate the work of review committees and if widely accepted will permit collection of accurate perinatal mortality statistics on regional, national, and international levels [14]. When there are set standards for

perinatal mortality review committees (Table 5.5) and appropriate items are included in their annual reports (Table 5.6), then their recommendations are taken seriously by colleagues, hospital administrators, and those responsible for perinatal health care policy.

In this regard, we have found the sorting process developed by Wigglesworth to be most valuable (Fig. 5.11). The degree of sophistication of final decisions in this process is determined by the completeness, skill, experience, and resources available.

At the conclusion of an autopsy, the pathologist should be able to make a statement on the sequence of events, fetal growth (AGA, SGA, LGA), nutrition, severity of stress, occurrence of trauma, complications of medical care, prenatal organ failure, and obvious pathological changes such as dysmorphology, congenital anomalies, hemorrhage, or infection [14]. This set is best presented with the final autopsy diagnoses. The commentary should include the following discussions:

1. A review of important features concerning father, mother, pregnancy, labor, and delivery.
2. A presentation of the clinical sequence of events.
3. A clinical-pathological correlation.
4. An interpretation of congenital abnormalities.
5. An interpretation of abnormalities in intrauterine growth.
6. Conclusions as to major factors contributing to death.
7. A categorization of the death.

Finally, and most importantly, the significance of the case for subsequent pregnancies should be addressed.

Perinatology needs the support of pathologists with special interests, training, and expertise in perinatal pathology. When this support is provided, the accurate perinatal

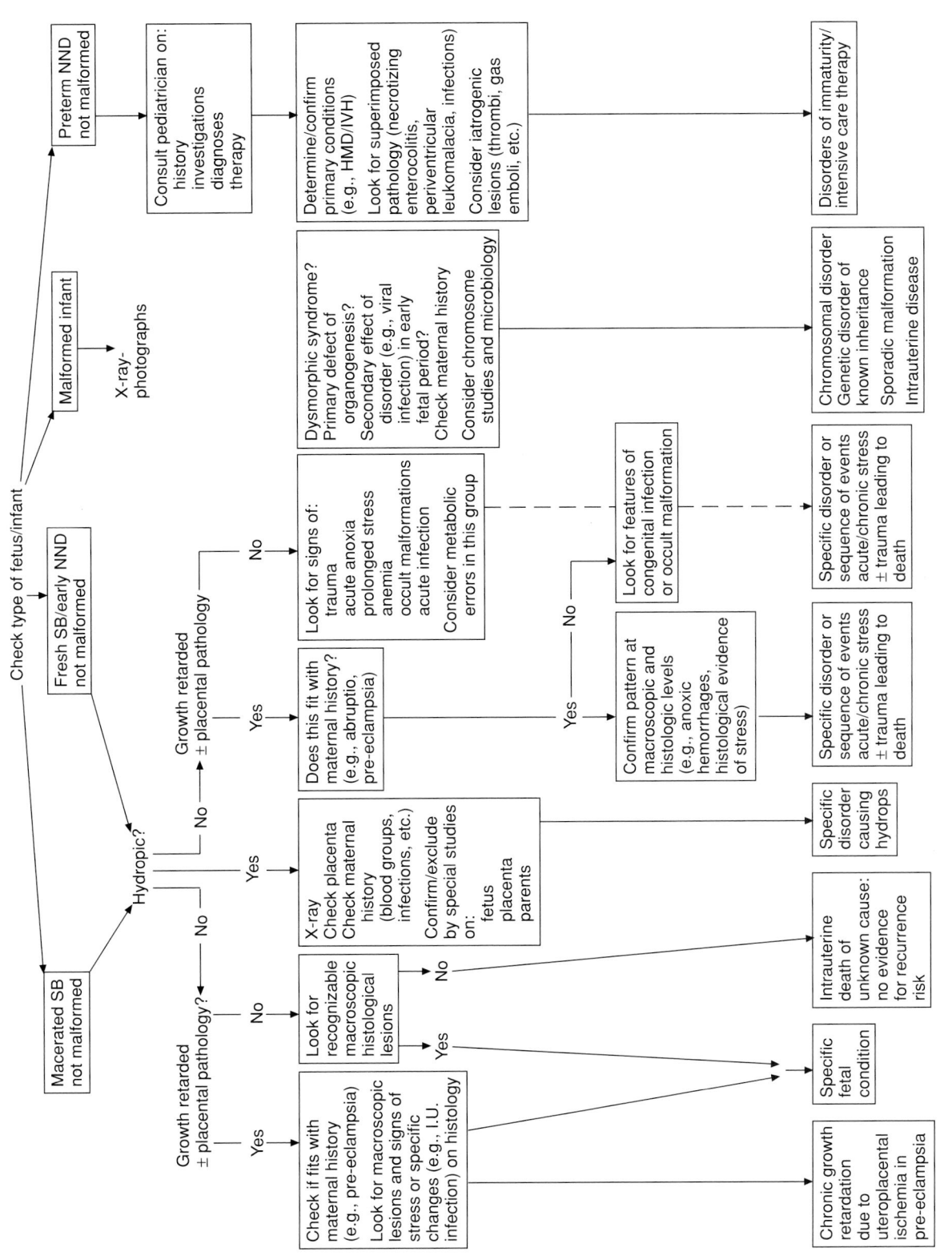

FIGURE 5.11. *A representation of the perinatal autopsy as a sorting process. (Courtesy of Wigglesworth [14].)*

pathology data gathered will benefit individual families, institutions, communities, and the general population [5].

REFERENCES

1. Barson AJ. The perinatal postmortem. In: Barson AJ, ed. *Laboratory Investigation of Fetal Disease*. Bristol, John Wright & Sons, 1981, pp. 476–97.

2. Kassner EG, Haller JO. Iatrogenic disorders of the fetus. In: Kassner EG, ed. *Iatrogenic Disorders of the Fetus, Infant and Child*, Vol. 1. New York: Springer-Verlag, 1985, pp. 81–123.

3. Macpherson TA, Valdes-Dapena M, Shen SS. Preventing and reducing iatrogenic disorders in the newborn. In: Guthrie R, ed. *Clinics in Critical Care Medicine: Recent Advances in Neonatal Intensive Care*. New York: Churchill Livingstone, 1988, 271–312.

4. Valdes-Dapena M. Iatrogenic disease in the perinatal period as seen by the pathologist. In: Naeye RL, Kissane JM, Kaufman N, eds. *Perinatal Diseases*. Baltimore: Williams & Wilkins, 1981, pp. 382–418.

5. Macpherson TA, Valdes-Dapena M, Kanbour A. Perinatal mortality and morbidity: the role of the anatomic pathologist. *Semin Perinatol* 1986; 10:179–86.

6. Lowbeer L. The inadequacy of autopsy examinations. *Hum Pathol* 1983; 14:94.

7. Robinson MJ. The autopsy 1983: can it be revived? *Hum Pathol* 1983; 14:566–8.

8. Macpherson TA. The role of the anatomical pathologist in perinatology. *Semin Perinatol* 1985; 9:257–62.

9. Macpherson TA. *A Model Perinatal Autopsy Protocol*. Washington, DC: American Registry of Pathology, AFIP: 1994.

10. Attwood HD. *The Perinatal Necropsy*. Broadsheet No. 3. Australia: College of Pathologists, 1969, pp. 1–12.

11. Langley FA. The perinatal post mortem examination. *J Clin Pathol* 1971; 24:159–69.

12. Pryse-Davies J. The perinatal autopsy. In: Anthony PP, MacSween RWM, eds. *Recent Advances in Histopathology*. Vol. II. London: Churchill Livingstone, 1981, pp. 65–82.

13. Valdes-Dapena M, Huff D. *Perinatal Autopsy Manual*. Washington, DC: AFIP, 1983.

14. Wigglesworth JS. Performance of the perinatal autopsy. In: Wigglesworth JS, ed. *Perinatal Pathology*. Philadelphia: W.B. Saunders, 1984, pp. 27–47.

15. Merlob P, Sivan Y, Reisner SH. Anthropometric measurements of the newborn infant (27 to 41 gestational weeks). *Birth Defects* 1984; 202(7).

16. Byrne JM. *Fetal Pathology Laboratory Manual*. Birth Defects Original Article Series, Vol. 19, No. 2. March of Dimes Birth Defects Foundation, 1983.

17. Maas AE. AIDS autopsy precautions. *Pathologist* 1985; 39:20–1.

18. Chi JG, Dooling EC, Gilles FH. Gyral development of the human brain. *Ann Neurol* 1977; 1:86–93.

19. Roberts DF, Thompson AM. *The Biology of Human Fetal Growth*. New York: Halsted, 1976.

20. Potter EL, Craig JM. *Pathology of the Fetus and the Infant*, 3rd ed. Chicago: Year Book Medical, 1976.

21. Berry CL. The examination of embryonic and fetal material in diagnostic histopathology laboratories. *J Clin Pathol* 1980; 33:317–26.

22. Ballard JL, Novak KK, Driver M. A simplified score for assessment of fetal maturation of newly born infants. *J Pediatr* 1979; 95:769–74.

23. Graham JM Jr. *Smith's Recognizable Patterns of Human Deformation*. 2nd ed. Philadelphia: W.B. Saunders, 1986.

24. Friede RL. *Developmental Neuropathology*. New York, Springer-Verlag, 1975.

25. Jones KL. *Smith's Recognizable Patterns of Human Malformation*. 4th ed. Philadelphia: W.B. Saunders, 1988.

26. Foote GA, Wilson AJ, Stewart JH. Perinatal postmortem radiography—experience with 2500 cases. *Br J Radiol* 1978; 51:351–6.

27. Griscom NT, Driscoll SG. Radiography of stillborn fetuses and infants dying at birth. *Am J Roentgenol* 1980; 134:485–9.

28. Lachman R. Radiology of pediatric syndromes. *Curr Probl Pediatr* 1979; 9:1–52.

29. Emery JL, Kalpaktsoglou KP. The costochondral junction during later stages of intrauterine life and abnormal growth patterns in association with perinatal death. *Arch Dis Child* 1967; 42:1–13.

30. Russel JGB. Radiologic assessment of age, retardation and death. In: Barson AJ, ed. *Laboratory Investigation of Fetal Disease*. Bristol: John Wright & Sons, 1981, pp. 3–16.

31. Silverman FN. The gastrointestinal tract. In: Silverman FN, ed. *Caffry's Pediatric X-ray Diagnosis*. Chicago: Year Book Medical 1985; 1863–73.

32. Talamo TS, Macpherson TA, Dominquez R. Sirenomelia, angiographic demonstration of vascular anomalies. *Arch Pathol Lab Med* 1982; 106:347–8.

33. Dubowitz LMS, Dubowitz V, Goldberg C. Clinical assessment of gestational age in the newborn infant. *J Pediat* 1970; 77:1.

34. Shinebourne EA, Macartney FJ, Anderson RH. Sequential chamber localization—logical approach to diagnosis in congenital heart disease. *Br Heart J* 1976; 38:327–40.

35. Arey JB. *Cardiovascular Pathology in Infants and Children*. Philadelphia: W.B. Saunders, 1984.

36. Roberts NK, Pepin DWJ. The atrioventricular node, His bundle and bundle branches. *Stain Technol* 1977; 52:131–5.

37. Keeling JW. *Fetal and Neonatal Pathology*. London: Springer-Verlag, 1987, pp. 1–43.

38. Sando I, Doyle WJ, Okuno H, et al. A method for the histopathological analysis of the temporal bone and the eustachian tube and its accessory structures. *Ann Otol Rhinol Laryngol* 1986; 95:267–74.

39. Knisely AS, Singer DB. A technique for necropsy evaluation of stenosis of the foramen magnum and rostral spinal cord in osteochondrodysplasia.

40. Reid CS, Pyeritz RE, Kopits SE, et al. Cervicomedullary compression in young patients with achondroplasia: value of comprehensive neurologic and respiratory evaluation. *J Pediatr* 1987; 110:522.

41. Langston C, Thurlbeck WM. Lung growth and development in late gestation and early postnatal life. *Perspect Pediatr Pathol* 1982; 7:203–35.

42. Valdes-Dapena M. *Histology of the Fetus and Newborn*. Philadelphia: W.B. Saunders, 1979.

43. Haan EA, Danks DM. Clinical investigation of suspected metabolic disease. In: Barson AJ, ed. *Laboratory Investigation of Fetal Disease*. Bristol: John Wright & Sons, 1981, pp. 410–28.

44. Macpherson TA, Garver KL, Turner JH, et al. Predicting *in vitro* tissue culture growth for cytogenetic evaluation of stillborn fetuses. *Eur J Obstet Gynecol Reprod Biol* 1985; 19:167–74.

45. Meier PR, et al. Perinatal autopsy: its clinical value. *Obstet Gynecol* 1986; 67:349–51.

46. Craft H, et al. Autopsy. High yield in neonatal population. *Am J Dis Child* 1986; 140:1260–62.

47. Dahms B. The autopsy in pediatrics. *Am J Dis Child* 1986; 140:445.

48. Manchester DK, et al. The perinatal autopsy: special considerations. *Clin Obstet Gynecol* 1980; 23:1125–34.

49. Maniscalco WM, et al. Factors influencing neonatal autopsy rate. *Am J Dis Child* 1982; 136:781–4.

50. Problems with perinatal pathology [letter]. *Br Med J (Clin Res)* 1982; 284:1475–1576.

51. Rushton DI. Problems with perinatal pathology [letter]. *Br Med J (Clin Res)* 1982; 284:1266.

Pathology of Abortion: The Embryo and the Previable Fetus

DAGMAR K. KALOUSEK   R. DOUGLAS WILSON

INTRODUCTION

Spontaneous abortion represents a large and incompletely quantified source of pregnancy loss, with estimates of some 40% of conceptions lost by 20 weeks' gestation [1]. Over half of all spontaneous deaths of the conceptus are associated with defective genes and chromosomal abnormalities. These deaths are more frequent in the earlier than in the middle and later weeks of pregnancy [2]. The remaining spontaneous previable pregnancy losses, often multifactorial or unknown in etiology, are due to a wide range of maternal, placental, and embryonic/fetal conditions in which infections are prominent in the second trimester. In addition to spontaneous abortions, many conceptions are terminated following diagnosis of fetal abnormality or disease. The adequate investigation of spontaneous abortions and medical terminations often is neglected, although this area of pathology deserves as much attention as fetal or infant death in the perinatal period.

Methods of Studying the Conceptus During Intrauterine Life

An understanding of many non-invasive and invasive techniques available for assessment of the in utero embryo or fetus (Table 6.1) is helpful when considering the pathological evaluation of abortion.

Initial prenatal diagnosis reports can be traced to the 1960s, with the first diagnosis of in utero Down syndrome and biochemical disorders being reported [3–5]. In the 1970s, technology allowed an increasing number of fetal conditions to be evaluated. Congenital malformations, such as neural tube defects, were identified by increased intra-amniotic alpha-fetoprotein. This was followed by non-invasive screening, recognizing that increased levels of maternal serum alpha-fetoprotein could also predict certain con-

genital anomalies, such as neural tube defects, abdominal wall defects, as well as twins [6, 7]. The availability of ultrasound allowed specific malformations such as central nervous system and cardiac abnormalities to be diagnosed visually [8, 9]. Initial Doppler assessments of blood flow [10] and direct access to the fetus with fetoscopic techniques were also reported [11]. In the 1980s, changes in ultrasound technology allowed an explosion of invasive techniques to be used, such as amniocentesis, chorionic villus sampling, and cordocentesis [12–14]. Combination of these techniques and molecular DNA technology provided the identification of increasing numbers of genetic conditions. The report of Cooper and Schmidtke [15] on a registry of molecular diagnosis listed more than 300 conditions. The genetic inheritance of these conditions showed 152 being dominant, 82 recessive conditions, and 70 X-linked conditions. The recognition that maternal serum screening could identify, in addition to developmental defects, certain fetal chromosome abnormalities increased the usefulness of such screening in pregnancy [16]. Identification of fetal cells in the maternal circulation and their utilization for obtaining information about the fetus with no risk for pregnancy loss [17, 18] represented a further advance for assessment of the in utero embryo or fetus.

A catalog of prenatally diagnosed conditions [19] reported a listing of 601 conditions. Recognized entities included 84 chromosomal abnormalities, 265 congenital malformations, 12 dermatological conditions, 11 fetal infections, 25 hematological abnormalities, 96 inborn errors of metabolism, 50 tumors and cysts, and 58 other prenatal conditions.

Non-invasive Techniques

Real-time ultrasound allows the identification of a large number of congenital malformations [9] (Table 6.2). Major

Table 6.1. Non-invasive and invasive assessment of the in utero embryo or fetus

	Embryo (<10 weeks' gestation)	Fetus (previable) (≥10–23 weeks' gestation)
Non-invasive		
Ultrasound	Vaginal	Vaginal
	Abdominal	Abdominal
	Doppler—uterine blood flow	Detail—cardiac
		Doppler—uterine blood flow
		—fetal blood flow
Biochemical screening	PAPP-A	AFP
	Free beta subunit	hCG
		Unconjugated estriol
Fetal cells/maternal circulation	Nucleated erythrocytes	Trophoblast
	Lymphocytes	
	Trophoblast	
Invasive		
Chorionic villus (placenta)	Minimal risk of fetal vascular disruption defects	Transcervical (10–12 weeks)
		Transabdominal (10–23 weeks)
Amniocentesis (fluid)	No procedure	Mid-trimester (>14 weeks)
		Early (11–13 weeks)
Cordocentesis (fetal blood)	No procedure	Transabdominal (>16 weeks)
Fetoscopy (flexible, small gauge)	Transabdominal (outside amniotic cavity)	Transabdominal (intra-amniotic)
Embryoscopy	Transcervical (outside amniotic cavity)	

AFP = alpha-fetoprotein; hCG = human chorionic gonadotropin; PAPP-A = pregnancy-associated plasma protein A.

anatomical fetal anomalies can be evaluated in a systematic approach and may indicate increased chromosomal or genetic risks [20] (Table 6.3).

In the first trimester with transvaginal scanning [21], ultrasound allows improved embryo/fetal detail unless conditions are optimal for transabdominal ultrasound evaluation [22]. First trimester ultrasounds are usually limited to: 1) screening pregnancy viability when bleeding is present; 2) pregnancy-dating when obstetric procedures (e.g., chorionic villus sampling, early amniocentesis) are required prior to 16 weeks' gestation; 3) maternal history of recurrent spontaneous abortion; and 4) evaluation of possible ectopic pregnancies. Optimal gestational age for fetal ultrasound assessment is between 18 and 20 weeks, as fetal size will generally allow accurate detail to be seen.

Maternal serum biochemical screening for malformations and chromosome abnormalities is routinely offered in both low- and high-risk pregnancies. The most common screening methods are maternal serum alpha-fetoprotein alone or in combination as a double or triple screening, using serum measurements of alpha-fetoprotein (AFP), human chorionic gonadotropin (hCG), and unconjugated estriol (UE3) between 15 and 20 weeks of pregnancy. These measurements are used, combined with the woman's age, gestational age, racial background, maternal weight, and presence or absence of insulin-dependent diabetes, to provide an estimate of the risk of the fetus having a neural tube defect, abdominal wall defect, or chromosomal abnormality (trisomy 21, trisomy

18). This form of serum screening will identify approximately 90–95% of neural tube defects and 70–90% of in utero Down syndrome (depending on maternal age of the patient). Maternal serum screening is a *screening test* only, and a positive result requires confirmation by invasive prenatal diagnosis, either chorionic villus sampling, amniocentesis, or cordocentesis [23].

Recent research indicates that other biochemical markers, such as PappA (pregnancy-associated plasma protein), free beta subunit of hCG, and inhibin may give similar screening potentials [24].

The identification and analysis of fetal-nucleated erythrocytes in maternal blood may allow prenatal cytogenetic or molecular diagnosis and eliminate some of the concerns of long-term fetal lymphocyte survival from previous pregnancies. Published studies [25] indicate sensitivities varying from 50–100% with positive predictive values of 82–100%. Further work in the area of fetal/maternal physiology is required to define optimal fetal cell type, cell separation technique, gestational age, and genetic evaluation (polymerase chain reaction, fluorescence in situ hybridization, biochemical, and cell culture) before this non-invasive form of prenatal diagnosis can be used routinely.

Invasive Techniques

Chorionic villus sampling (CVS) is an ultrasound-guided invasive prenatal diagnosis technique using either a transcervical or transabdominal approach. The transcervical approach

Table 6.2.   Ultrasound diagnosis and congenital malformations

Central nervous system
  Hydrocephalus
    Aqueductal stenosis
    Dandy-Walker malformation
    Choroid plexus papilloma
  Neural tube defects
    Spina bifida
    Anencephaly
  Cephalocele
  Porencephaly
  Hydranencephaly
  Microcephaly
  Holoprosencephaly
  Iniencephaly
  Intracranial arachnoid cysts
  Intracranial tumors

Neck
  Cystic hygroma
  Teratoma of the neck

Lungs
  Chylothorax
  Congenital cystic adenomatoid malformation of the
    lung
  Lung sequestration
  Bronchogenic cysts

Abdominal wall
  Diaphragmatic hernia
  Omphalocele
  Gastroschisis
  Body stalk anomaly
  Bladder exstrophy and cloacal exstrophy

Gastrointestinal tract and intra-abdominal organs
  Esophageal atresia with and without
    tracheo-esophageal fistula
  Duodenal atresia
  Bowel obstruction
  Meconium peritonitis
  Splenomegaly/polysplenia/asplenia
  Hepatomegaly

Heart
  Structure:
    Atrial septal defects
    Ventricular septal defects
    Atrioventricular septal defects
    Univentricle heart
    Ebstein's anomaly
    Hypoplastic left heart syndrome
    Hypoplastic right ventricle
    Tetralogy of Fallot
    Complete transposition of the great vessels
    Double outlet right ventricle
    Truncus arteriosus
    Coarctation and tubular hypoplasia of the aortic arch
    Pulmonic stenosis
    Aortic stenosis
    Cardiomyopathies
    Total anomalous pulmonary venous return
    Tumors of the heart
    Cardiosplenic syndrome
  Rhythm:
    Premature atrial and ventricular contractions
    Supraventricular tachyarrhythmias
    Atrioventricular blocks

Genital tract
  Fetal gender

Umbilical cord
  Single umbilical artery
  Cystic lesions of the umbilical cord
  Vascular lesions of the umbilical cord

Urinary tract and adrenal glands
  Bilateral renal agenesis
  Infantile polycystic kidney disease
  Adult polycystic kidney disease
  Multicystic kidney disease
  Ureteropelvic junction obstruction
  Megaureter
  Posterior urethral valves
  Prune-belly syndrome

Skeletal limb defects
  Achondroplasia
  Achondrogenesis
  Thanatophoric dysplasia
  Skeletal dysplasias associated with a small thorax
  Skeletal dysplasias characterized by bone
    demineralization:
    Osteogenesis imperfecta
    Hypophosphatasia
    Limb reduction abnormalities

Other anomalies
  Twin pregnancies
  Conjoined twins
  Twin-reversed arterial perfusion
  Non-immune hydrops fetalis (see conditions
    associated with non-immune fetal hydrops)
  Sacrococcygeal teratoma

Table 6.3.   Frequency of chromosomal abnormalities identified in fetuses with isolated or multiple malformations identified by ultrasound

Ultrasound abnormality	Frequency of chromosomal abnormality
Isolated malformation alone	8.8%
Associated with oligoamnios or hydramnios	10.2%
Associated with IUGR	20.4%
Associated with oligoamnios or hydramnios plus IUGR	21.4%
Multiple malformations alone	28.7%
Associated with oligoamnios or hydramnios	35.6%
Associated with IUGR	50.0%
Associated with oligoamnios or hydramnios plus IUGR	41.1%
Oligoamnios or hydramnios	2.9%
IUGR	6.9%
IUGR and oligoamnios or hydramnios	8.7%

IUGR = intrauterine growth retardation.
From Boué [20].

using a flexible catheter is limited to a gestational age of 10 to 20 weeks, while the transabdominal approach using a 19- or 20-gauge spinal needle can be done from 10 to 40 weeks of gestation. Indications for CVS are increased risks for chromosomal, metabolic, and DNA disorders. The major advantage of CVS is the availability of a first trimester diagnostic result. Three large collaborative studies [26–28] have indicated that CVS, when performed by expert operators, is a relatively safe procedure and may be considered an acceptable alternative to mid-trimester genetic amniocentesis. Limb defects are not increased when CVS is performed by experts (see Chap. 3). The procedure-related risk of spontaneous loss for CVS is estimated at 1–2% above the background rate, in comparison to a 0.5–1.0% risk for amniocentesis. The background risk for spontaneous abortion in the advanced maternal age population is estimated at 4–6% when the pregnancy has been shown to be viable by ultrasound at 10 weeks' gestation [29–31].

The disadvantage of utilizing CVS is the presence of confined placental mosaicism in 1–2% of pregnancies from women with advanced maternal age (greater than 35 years of age at estimated date of delivery). When such mosaicism is diagnosed, it is important to distinguish it from generalized mosaicism, and additional invasive techniques are required, such as amniocentesis or cordocentesis, to prove the chromosome abnormality is confined to the placenta and does not involve the fetus itself.

Amniocentesis is an ultrasound-guided second trimester prenatal diagnosis procedure, usually performed after 14 weeks' gestation. Indications for amniocentesis include advanced maternal age, history of previous stillborn or liveborn child with a chromosome abnormality, parental chromosome translocations, history of specific congenital anomalies (neural tube defects), and other biochemical or molecular genetic diseases where diagnosis can be obtained from amniocytes or amniotic fluid. The technique is performed with a 20- or 22-gauge spinal needle with removal of 15 to 30 milliliters of amniotic fluid. The main advantage of amniocentesis is an accurate analysis of fetal karyotype, as the cells of extra-embryonic origin are not present. Other genetic diseases can also be diagnosed from the cultured amniocytes or by measurement of specific substances in the amniotic fluid. The major risk of amniocentesis includes fetal loss due to fluid leakage, infection, or bleeding.

Table 6.4 compares and summarizes the procedures of amniocentesis and CVS. The disadvantage of amniocentesis is the lack of availability of results before 17 to 20 weeks' gestational age. Due to this drawback, early amniocentesis is being evaluated in research protocols. Early amniocentesis is done at 11 to 13 weeks' gestation. The long-term risks of this procedure are not known, and randomized trials are under way to compare early amniocentesis with mid-trimester amniocentesis.

Invasive prenatal diagnosis by *cordocentesis* allows vascular (umbilical vein) access to the fetus. The common fetal indications for cordocentesis involve chromosome analysis, blood disorders (autoimmune, alloimmune), infection, and metabolic, biochemical, and blood gas status. Reported success rates for cordocentesis range from 93.7–98.5%. Cordocentesis is an ultrasound-guided technique usually using a 22-gauge needle. It is usually performed at a gestational age of 16 weeks or greater, but blood sampling has been done between 12 and 16 weeks. Fetal losses are higher (5–6%) if the technique is done prior to 16 weeks compared with 2.5% at 19 to 21 weeks [32]. Fetal blood sampling after 18 weeks has a 0.5–1.0% risk of associated miscarriage [33]. The risk of fetal loss is greater if fetal anomalies or intrauterine growth restrictions are present and is estimated at 3.25% [34]. Cordocentesis can be useful for determining the fetal status for factors such as complete blood count, platelets, electrolytes, glucose, lactate, antibody (titers, presence), blood gases, and other components of fetal blood [34].

A small flexible fetoscope allowing direct visualization or access to the fetus for prenatal diagnosis or treatment has

Table 6.4.   Summary and comparison of amniocentesis and chorionic villus sampling

Parameter	Amniocentesis	Chorionic villus sampling (transcervical/transabdominal)
Procedure	Amniotic fluid removed by needle and syringe	Chorionic villi removed by transcervical catheter and syringe or transabdominal needle insertion
Timing	15 to 17 weeks	10 to 11 weeks plus 6 days (>12 weeks, transabdominal CVS only)
Added risk of miscarriage due to procedure	0.5%	0.5–1.0%
Fetal malformation risks	Possible respiratory effects or limb deformation	Perhaps increased vascular limb malformation in inexperienced hands
Chance of successful sampling	Approximately 99%	Approximately 99%; if unsuccessful, can follow with amniocentesis
Time required for cytogenetic diagnosis	2 to 3 weeks	2 weeks
Accuracy (chromosomes)	Highly accurate	Highly accurate
Confined placental mosaicism	Very low	1–2%
NTDs	AFP in amniotic fluid detects approximately 95% of NTDs	Ultrasound and AFP in maternal serum (16–18 weeks) detects approximately 90–95% of NTDs

AFP = alpha-fetoprotein; NTD = neural tube defect.

been developed. This is presently a research tool and is not commonly available. The technique allows a flexible optical system to be inserted down an 18- to 19-gauge needle into the amniotic cavity. Multiple congenital anomaly syndromes, such as Meckel-Gruber syndrome, have been diagnosed by this technique [35].

Definitions Used in the Study of Abortions

Basic Terms

The *conceptus* (or products of conception) includes all the structures that develop from the zygote: the embryo or fetus and the placenta. The developing human is considered to be an embryo until the end of the 8th week following conception (10th week of gestation measured from the last menstrual period) by which time all major organ systems have been formed. Some reserve the term *embryo* for that period between the formation of the embryonic disc (2nd week) and the end of the 8th week [8]. From the beginning of the 9th week until birth, the developing human is called a *fetus*.

Developmental (or fertilization) *age* is the term used most by embryologists, teratologists, and anatomists; it extends from the presumed day of ovulation/fertilization (or 14 days after the first day of the last menstrual period [LMP]) to the death of the embryo/fetus within the mother or to live-birth. In contrast, clinicians, epidemiologists, and statisticians usually use *gestational* (or menstrual) *age*, which extends from the LMP to the expulsion or removal of the conceptus. Gestational age is often cited in completed weeks and is 2 weeks more than the developmental age. *Retention* refers to the time period between the death of the embryo/fetus and its expulsion or removal (Fig. 6.1).

Abortion (the lay term being *miscarriage*) has many meanings. *Spontaneous abortion* refers to the unassisted premature expulsion of the dead or living conceptus from the uterus before the fetus is "viable," or before it is able to sustain life after it has been born. In some jurisdictions, the legal lower limit of viability is defined solely in terms of gestational age; 28, 24, or 20 weeks are the most common, the differences reflecting changes in neonatal care. In this chapter, 20 weeks is considered the lower limit of viability. Other measures of

viability are sometimes used in conjunction with gestational age and include weight [36] and length. Practicing pathologists should learn the current definitions used in their jurisdiction and be prepared for inconsistencies.

A number of clinical definitions related to abortion are commonly used. A *threatened abortion* is characterized by bloody discharge from the pregnant uterus without cervical dilatation, whereas *inevitable abortion* is associated with profuse or prolonged bleeding with cervical dilatation or effacement. An *incomplete abortion* means that all of the presumably dead conceptus has not yet passed; if a dead conceptus is retained for at least 4 weeks, it is called a *missed abortion*. The *habitual aborter* refers to a woman who has had at least three consecutive spontaneous abortions. An *induced abortion* or termination of pregnancy (as opposed to a spontaneous abortion) may be performed because the mother's health is threatened (*therapeutic abortion*) or for a wide variety of social reasons, including removal of a defective fetus.

In this chapter, we divide spontaneous abortion into early and late. The *early spontaneous abortion* is that occurring in the embryonic period (up to the end of the 8th developmental week); the *late spontaneous abortion* will refer to death in the 9th to 18th week of the fetal period.

Terms Related to Embryonic and Fetal Abnormalities

These terms are defined in the report of an International Working Group [37], and the definitions are given in Chapter 13. They include *malformation, disruption, deformation, dysplasia, polytopic field defect, sequence, syndrome*, and *association*.

Failure to distinguish between etiology and pathogenesis has retarded the understanding of developmental pathology. *Potter's sequence*, for example, refers to a phenotype of abnormalities that includes fetal deformities (altered facies, clubbed feet or hands), pulmonary hypoplasia, and amnion nodosum. Its pathogenesis (or the process by which the phenotype is produced) is thought to be oligohydramnios. Its etiology (or the initiator[s] of the pathogenesis) is heterogeneous and includes renal agenesis, urinary tract obstruction, or chronic leakage of amniotic fluid.

Understanding pathogenetic mechanisms in embryopathology relies heavily on knowledge of the sequence of

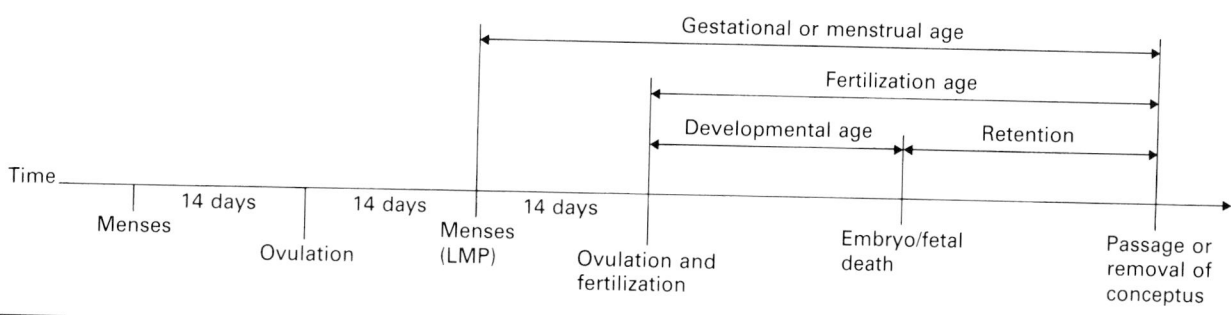

FIGURE 6.1.   *Time relationships used in embryo/fetal pathology. LMP-last menstrual period.*

tissue and organ development and on the timing of each step relative to the next. For decades, experimental teratologists have used the concept of "termination period" as meaning the last possible time in the developmental sequence at which an etiologic agent could bring about specific abnormalities. The actual time at which the agent initiates the injury ("determination period" or "teratogenic window") always precedes the termination period.

Current knowledge of etiology and pathogenesis of specific conditions varies widely. By definition, we know the pathogeneses of deformations and disruptions but usually not the etiologies; the same applies to constellations of anomalies defined as polytopic field defects and many sequences. In contrast, etiology is better understood than pathogenesis in some malformations and dysplasias and in syndromes. There are numerous situations (including associations), in which neither pathogenesis nor etiology is clear.

Examination and Classification of Products of Conception

The diagnosis of products of conception is based on identifying placental villi, trophoblast, or embryonic/fetal parts. Trophoblastic tissue can be detected, if need be, with immunoperoxidase staining for hCG or human placental lactogen (hPL). Often the pathologist cannot tell if the entire conceptus has passed, and if only fragments of placental tissue are seen, intrauterine fetal demise cannot be assumed. The diagnosis of products of conception in material from the uterine cavity removes the possibility of ectopic pregnancy, except for the very rare occurrence of one twin being intrauterine and the other ectopic [38].

Every spontaneous abortus should be examined in the pathology laboratory not only to confirm that it is, in fact, a product of conception, but also to determine the presence or absence of an embryonic/fetal developmental defect and to gain knowledge of benefit to the parents.

If a pregnancy is to be terminated because of an alleged fetal defect, it is mandatory to try to confirm that defect in the conceptus. The obstetrician should favor the method of termination that will optimize that confirmation. Thus, a procedure that will remove the conceptus quickly (such as suction curettage) is preferable to a slower procedure (such as saline injection) when confirming a chromosomal abnormality originally diagnosed by genetic amniocentesis or CVS. Whenever possible, the tissue used to confirm a fetal chromosomal abnormality should come from the fetus itself or its amnion. When confined placental mosaicism [39, 40] is to be confirmed, the sampling must involve both the chorion and the fetus. Conversely, an anatomic defect (such as meningomyelocele) is best confirmed on an intact fetus, thus favoring prostaglandin induction.

On making the final diagnosis on a spontaneously aborted conceptus, the pathologist may classify it in order to facilitate data analysis. Of the many anatomic and pathologic classifications, we mention three different types,

although none of them utilizes correlations with cytogenetic analysis.

1. The classification of Fujikura et al [41] was based on gross examination of 353 early and late abortuses excluding hydatidiform moles and ectopic pregnancies.
2. The classification of Poland et al [42] focused on early spontaneous abortions and was based on the gross examination of over 1000 complete embryonic specimens. These specimens were divided into three categories:
   I   Normal embryos
   II Embryos with focal defects
   III Embryos with generalized abnormal development (growth disorganization)
3. Rushton's classification [43], based on microscopic placental morphology, is particularly useful in classifying curettage specimens and abortuses without a grossly evident embryo or fetus. It was derived from the examination of some 814 abortuses including hydatidiform moles. These specimens were divided into three groups:
   Group 1 Chorionic sacs and placentas associated with early conceptuses (mean fertilization age, 9.4 weeks)
   Group 2 Placentas associated with macerated embryos or fetuses (mean fertilization age, 14.1 weeks)
   Group 3 Placentas associated with non-macerated fetuses (mean fertilization age, 18.6 weeks)

EPIDEMIOLOGICAL ASPECTS OF SPONTANEOUS ABORTION

All epidemiological inferences that relate to the developing human are conditioned by three features of intrauterine life: 1) conceptus death is very frequent; 2) the conceptus is totally dependent on the mother; and 3) the conceptus is maturing and growing at non-uniform but very rapid rates. Unlike the neonate, the conceptus is still difficult to examine during its development, and most of our knowledge is based on morphologic abnormalities found in abortuses. Thus, the processes that result in embryonic or fetal abnormality and death are often inferred at the end rather than observed during their development.

The Frequency of Early and Late Spontaneous Abortion

It is not yet known how frequently spontaneous abortion occurs throughout the entire course of pregnancy; that is, after the zygote has formed. Some 15% of clinically recognized pregnancies spontaneously abort in the first trimester [44]; and, of these, mothers can recall the event in no more than three-fourths of cases [45]. Prospective studies of discrete populations have been reported, in which women were enrolled as soon as they were known to be pregnant and were observed until the end of pregnancy [46–50]. A prospective study of more than 30,000 pregnant women in the Kaiser Health Plan, Northern California, used life-table methods and showed an estimated probability of spontaneous abortion of 14.4% between 5 and 28 weeks of gestation [47].

Stimulated by the need to assess the risk of CVS, a number of studies report spontaneous embryonic/fetal deaths as detected by ultrasound [30, 31, 51–54]. These are generally comparable with each other (about 10% loss by the 10th week) but are much higher than corresponding life-table estimates [47, 55]. Ultrasonically detected loss rates increase with maternal age.

It has long been recognized that the highest conceptus mortality exists in the earliest weeks of pregnancy, usually before mothers realize that they are pregnant [56, 57]. In-vitro fertilization studies show that only 12–50% of embryos have the capacity to implant; up to 21–32% of the implantation failures can be attributed to embryonic non-viability and some 31–64% to uterine factors [58, 59]. Other studies have been based on repetitive pregnancy testing of women who might conceive. One such study reports that 43% of the conceptions aborted before 20 weeks and that 33% of these conceptions had been diagnosed only with beta-subunit hCG pregnancy testing [1]; another found that 61.9% of the conceptuses were lost prior to 12 weeks, most occurring subclinically [60]. It is likely that even these estimates are low since the beta-subunit hCG pregnancy test may not become positive until the blastocyst implants at about 7 days' postfertilization.

Our current inability to measure all loss of conceptuses (particularly in the earliest weeks) and to assess embryonic injury before death has two important implications as noted years ago by Roberts and Lowe [61]. First, we cannot assume that spontaneous abortion of clinically recognized pregnancies is a valid index of teratogenicity. The effect of a potential teratogen, such as dioxin, might be expressed by lethal preimplantation injury, chromosomal aberration, or faulty implantation occurring before the mother realizes that she is pregnant and before the currently available pregnancy test becomes positive. Second, we cannot yet compare rates of conceptus death as they occur in groups of women who differ in such obvious ways as age, race, ethnicity, occupation, or exposure to a specific environmental toxin. Most of the studies done in these areas [47, 48, 62–65] are inconclusive because they can measure only the outcome of clinically evident pregnancies and lack data on early conception losses where the bulk of mortality occurs.

Types of Embryonic and Fetal Illness in Spontaneous Abortion

General statements to the effect that spontaneous abortion in the first trimester is often associated with chromosomal abnormalities and in the second trimester with infections

[66], or that the disease process starts in the embryo (or fetus), in the placenta or in the mother [67], are oversimplifications. Taken together, they do emphasize the diversity of disease processes affecting the conceptus and the close relationship between mother and conceptus.

Chromosomal Abnormalities
Conceptuses that spontaneously abort before the end of the 2nd week of development have a 78.3% rate of chromosomal abnormalities, while those aborting between the first missed menstrual period and the 20th week have a 62.1% rate [2]. About half of the abnormal karyotypes that occur in the first trimester are various forms of autosomal trisomy, of which trisomy 16 is the most frequent; sex chromosome monosomy is detected in about 20% and chromosomal polyploidy in 25% [68]. Thus, chromosomal abnormalities are closely associated with obviously defective early development and with lethal outcomes. The frequency of chromosomal abnormalities declines steadily during middle and late fetal periods such that 5–10% of previable fetuses, 6% of stillbirths, and only 0.5% of liveborns have chromosomal aberrations [2].

Infections
The major effects of infection on a conceptus of any age are embryonic or fetal death, developmental disruptions, intrauterine growth retardation, low birth weight, premature birth, and persisting postnatal disease [69]. Infections of the conceptus during the embryonic and early fetal periods are usually acquired by hematogenous spread of the organism from the mother; the fetus is rarely infected in the absence of placentitis. Transcervical infection is commonly associated with premature rupture of membranes and becomes increasingly frequent after the first trimester. The specific organisms causing intrauterine infections vary with environmental and cultural factors in the general population. Even in a single hospital, studies over a 5-year period showed marked alterations in the relative frequencies of specific infection [70].

Immunovascular Diseases
The condition and integrity of maternal blood vessels that communicate with the placental intervillous space are important determinants of fetal mortality. After implantation, the walls of uterine spiral arterioles are normally invaded by trophoblast, causing the vessel diameters to increase. This vascular dilatation is absent in some cases of chronic and gestational maternal hypertension, in which spiral arteriole morphology resembles that seen in rejected renal transplants [71]. Intramural immunoglobulin deposits with vasculopathy have been described in the spiral arterioles of women with pre-eclampsia [72], lupus erythematosus, and lupus anticoagulant [73], all conditions associated with spontaneous abortion or placental infarction and fetal growth retardation. Lupus anticoagulant represents a heterogeneous group of antibodies that react with negatively charged phospholipids.

These antibodies may exist in immunoglobulin G and M forms. The association of antiphospholipid antibodies with systemic lupus erythematosus is reported [74] but has been less well studied in the absence of the systemic disease [75]. There appears to be a close relationship between the consequences of these conditions and less specific graft-versus-host immunopathies that may account for substantial spontaneous abortion [76]. Decidual sloughing found in the placentae of many abortuses [77] may be an expression of the maternal rejection of the placental allograft. Lack of integrity of fetal vessels within the placenta can result in numerous pathological states and fetal death. These include maternal sensitization to fetal blood-group incompatibilities, maternal-fetal lymphocyte engraftment, and chronic feto-maternal [78] and maternofetal [79] hemorrhage.

Repeated spontaneous abortions may be related to sharing human leukocyte antigen (HLA) maternal and paternal loci and have been observed in women who fail to develop antibodies against paternal T and B lymphocytes; immunization with paternal lymphocytes appears to increase the chances of the next pregnancy being successful, particularly if the immunization is received before or within the first 40 days of pregnancy [80]. Recently the class I antigen HLA-G expressed in human trophoblast has been found to be of great importance in pregnancy maintenance [81].

Effects of Maternal Nutrition

Maternal undernutrition affects both fetal growth and development depending on when it started relative to the development of the conceptus, how long it lasted, and on its type and severity. Preterm birth and small-for-dates newborns are more frequent in acutely undernourished populations [82], but in chronic situations it remains unclear how much to attribute to undernutrition and how much to other environmental factors such as endemic malaria. The continuum of cellular growth and differentiation in most tissues, including brain, appears to be deranged by deficient maternal dietary intake, by reduced nutrient availability to the conceptus, and by hypoxia [83]. Only limited data are available on the effects of absolute or relative lack of specific nutrients. Preconceptual folic acid supplementation of the maternal diet may be responsible for decreasing recurrence of neural tube defects and may prevent first occurrence of neural tube defects [84–86]. Additional benefits of preconceptual folic acid supplementation may be the reduction of other congenital defects such as cardiovascular malformations. The prevalence of cleft lip with or without cleft palate was not affected by this supplementation. Deficiency of maternal dietary zinc decreases antimicrobial activity of amniotic fluid [87].

Effects of Maternal Medication

Shepard [88] has edited a compendium, listing references to the proved and alleged teratogenicity of specific drugs. Thalidomide is now off the market, but its study illustrates many principles of assessing the effect of maternal medication. The problem with thalidomide might not have come to light 1) if the drug had been more lethal, therefore producing only early embryonic death, or 2) if its manifestations had not been both dramatically unusual and externally visible [89]. There are undoubtedly drugs and environmental toxins not yet identified as teratogenic because they do not share these properties. Further study of thalidomide showed that not all fetuses were affected and that the high risk of teratogenic effect was related to the developmental age at which the fetus was exposed to the drug [89]. The concept of a particular time during which the embryo or fetus is vulnerable to developmental disruption assumes that the developmental sequence in that fetus is "normal." Extraordinary efforts are needed to obtain complete drug histories with dates and dosages [90, 91]. Ideally, such histories should start before the woman conceives. Non-prescription drugs are a particular problem since they are easy to obtain, taken in an unscheduled way, and easily forgotten. A single substance, perhaps teratogenic, may be an ingredient of many medications and in varying amounts. For example, agenesis of the cloacal membrane has been related to maternal ingestion of doxylamine succinate; this substance is contained in at least fourteen prescription and non-prescription drugs [92]. As in the investigation of other possible teratogens, prospective studies are required in which preconceptual or pregnant women who take the drug(s) are observed throughout their pregnancies and their offspring examined after birth [93].

Four common medical conditions require chronic medical treatment and may complicate pregnancy. These are insulin-dependent non-gestational diabetes mellitus [94], epilepsy [95], chronic hypertension [96], and psychiatric illness [97] (i.e., bipolar affective disorder).

Insulin-dependent non-gestational diabetes increases the risks of congenital anomalies of the central nervous system, heart, renal and urinary tract; lower limb reduction defects; and axial skeleton and caudal dysgenesis. The risk of birth defects increases with the lack of diabetic control (normoglycemia) [94].

Infants of epileptic women are at an increased of birth defects with specific defects related to valproic acid (spina bifida), phenytoin and carbamazepine (congenital heart disease, distal digital hypoplasia, dysmorphic facial features), and trimethadione (congenital heart disease). Women with epilepsy are recommended to use folic acid periconceptually. The risk of birth defects is present whether or not the fetus is exposed to an anticonvulsant but increases with anticonvulsant use [95].

The majority of common antihypertensive medications are safe in pregnancy such as adrenoreceptor blocking agents (alpha, beta), methyldopa, hydralazine, and calcium channel blockers. Angiotensin-converting enzyme (ACE)-inhibitors are contraindicated in pregnancy [96].

Psychiatric medications such as lithium carbonate increase the risk of a specific fetal cardiac anomaly (Ebstein's anomaly—tricuspid valve). Among the tranquilizers, chlordiazepoxide, meprobamate, and diazepam in general are felt to be safe during pregnancy.

Medication use in pregnancy is common, with estimates that 60–75% of pregnant women use from three to ten medications. These estimates do not include illicit or recreational drugs (alcohol, marijuana, cocaine, LSD), use of which may range from 5–30% [98].

It is now generally accepted that alcohol drinking during pregnancy is associated with developmental defects in the infant and predisposes to spontaneous abortion [99]. The effect of smoking on the risk of abortion is difficult to evaluate and appears to be less dose-dependent than that of alcohol. None of the other socially used drugs (LSD, cannabis, crack) has been shown unequivocally to increase the risk of spontaneous abortion, but cocaine has been shown to cause abruptio placenta and fetal vascular disruptive defects.

EARLY SPONTANEOUS ABORTION

Review of Normal Embryonic Development

The major anatomic contributions to early human development have been made during the 20th century. One of the best classic descriptions of human organogenesis can be found in the *Manual of Human Embryology*, edited by Keibel and Mall in 1910 and 1912 [100]. The first formal classification of human embryos was published in 1917 [101]. Embryonic development, that is from fertilization until the embryo has attained a crown–rump (CR) length of some 30 millimeters, is conventionally categorized into 23 stages [102, 103], each characterized by either somite development during early stages or by specific size of the embryo during later stages and by specific embryonic external features (Table 6.5). This classification allows an easy and accurate evaluation of human embryonic specimens.

A brief summary of normal embryonic development with reference to developmental stages is given below.

Fertilization and Implantation (Stages 1–3)

Embryonic development commences with fertilization. Normal fertilization is a sequence of events that begins with contact between a sperm and a secondary oocyte and ends with the fusion of the nuclei of the sperm and ovum, each carrying a reduced number of chromosomes. The fertilization process requires about 24 hours and results in formation of a *zygote*, a diploid cell with 46 chromosomes containing genetic material from both parents. The usual site of fertilization is the ampulla of the uterine tube.

The embryo's sex is determined at fertilization by the type of sperm that fertilizes the ovum. An X-bearing sperm produces an XX zygote, which normally develops into a female; whereas fertilization by a Y-bearing sperm produces an XY zygote, which normally develops into a male.

Table 6.5. Embryonic development

Crown–rump length (mm)	Days after ovulation	Stage	Main external features
	0–2	1	Fertilized oocyte
	2–4	2	Morula
	4–6	3	Blastocyst
0.1		4	Bilaminar embryo
0.2–0.4	6–15	5	Bilaminar embryo with primary yolk sac
		6	Trilaminar embryo
0.4–1.0	15–17	7	Trilaminar embryo with primitive streak
1.0–1.5	18–20	8	Primitive pit and notochordal canal formed
1.5–2.0	20–22	9	Deep neural groove; first somites present
2.0–3.0	22–24	10	Neural folds begin to fuse; embryo straight
3.0–4.0	24–26	11	Rostral neuropore closing; embryo curved
4.0–5.0	26–30	12	Upper-limb buds appear; caudal neuropore closed; tail appearing
5.0–6.0	28–32	13	Four pairs of branchial arches; lower-limb buds appear; tail present
6.0–7.0	31–35	14	Lens pits and nasal pits visible; optic cups present
7.0–10.0	35–38	15	Hand plates formed; lens vesicles and nasal pits prominent
10.0–12.0	37–42	16	Foot plates formed; nasal pits face ventrally; pigment visible in retina
12.0–14.0	42–44	17	Finger rays appear; auricular hillocks developed
14.0–17.0	44–48	18	Toe rays and elbow regions appear; eyelids are forming
16.0–20.0	48–51	19	Trunk elongating and straightening; midgut herniation to umbilical cord
20.0–22.0	51–53	20	Fingers distinct but webbed; scalp vascular plexus appears
22.0–24.0	53–54	21	Fingers free and longer; toes still webbed
24.0–28.0	54–56	22	Toes free and longer; eyelids and external ear more developed
28.0–30.0	56–60	23	Head more rounded; fusing eyelids

Data from Moore [144], O'Rahilly [102], Streeter [103], and Jirasek JE. *Atlas of Human Prenatal Morphogenesis*. Martinus Nijhoff, 1983.

As the zygote passes down the uterine tube, it undergoes a series of rapid mitotic cell divisions known as *cleavage*. These divisions produce progressively smaller cells, *blastomeres*. On entering the uterine cavity 3 to 4 days later, the developing conceptus is made of a solid ball of 12 to 16 cells resembling a mulberry and therefore called the *morula*.

At about 4 days, hollow spaces appear inside the compact morula, and fluid soon passes into these cavities from the surrounding uterine mucosa, allowing one large space to form and converting the morula into the *blastocyst*. The blastocyst cavity separates the embryonic cells into an outer cell layer, the *trophoblast*, which gives rise to the epithelial lining of the placenta, and a group of centrally located cells known as the *inner cell mass*, which gives rise to both the embryo proper and extra-embryonic tissue of the placenta. It has been shown that only a small number of cells (3–5) of the whole inner cell mass will become involved in the formation of an embryo proper [104]. A disproportionate distribution of progenitor cells for embryo proper and extra-embryonic tissues at the blastocyst stage is important in the development of different types of chromosomal mosaicism among conceptuses [39, 40, 105, 106].

The zona pellucida disappears at about 4 to 5 days, and the blastocyst attaches to the endometrial epithelium. The trophoblastic cells then start to invade the epithelium and its underlying stroma.

The implantation of the blastocyst usually takes place in the mid-portion of the body of the uterus, slightly more frequently on the posterior than the anterior wall. Implantations in the lower segment of the uterus near the internal os of the cervix may result in *placenta previa*, a placenta that covers or adjoins the internal ostium and may cause severe bleeding during pregnancy or at delivery. Cervical pregnancy, where implantation occurs in the true cervical canal, is rare. It is likely that some of these pregnancies are not recognized because the conceptus is expelled early in gestation. Implantation occurring outside the cavity of the uterus is referred to as an *ectopic pregnancy*. The majority of ectopic implantations occur in the uterine tube, frequently resulting in rupture of the uterine tube and hemorrhage during the first 8 weeks, followed by death of the conceptus. The tubal rupture and subsequent hemorrhage obviously constitute a threat to the mother's life. Ectopic pregnancies occurring on the surface of the ovary, on the peritoneum of the broad ligament, on the mesentery of the intestine, or in the recto-uterine pouch are rare.

Many conceptuses unable to implant due to their abnormal genetic make-up are lost during the first week of development.

Second Week of Development (Stages 4–5)

Implantation of the blastocyst continues during the second week while significant morphological changes occur in the inner cell mass. The second week of development is sometimes referred to as "the period of twos" [107] because a bilaminar embryonic disc forms, amniotic and primary yolk sac cavities develop, and two layers of trophoblast, cytotrophoblast and syncytiotrophoblast, differentiate (Fig. 6.2).

The two-layered disc arrangement of the embryo separates the blastocyst cavity into two unequal parts (smaller amniotic cavity and larger primary yolk cavity) during the early part of the second week. The thick layer of embryonic cells bordering the amniotic cavity is called the *epiblast* (ectoderm), and a thin layer bordering the primary yolk cavity is called the *hypoblast* (endoderm).

Rapid proliferation of the trophoblast and its differentiation into two layers, an inner cytotrophoblast and an outer syncytiotrophoblast, are important features of this period. While the trophoblast continues to penetrate deeper into the endometrium, the differentiating inner cell mass never lies deeper than a few millimeters from the surface of the endometrium. At the end of the second week, the site of implantation may be recognized as a small elevated area of endometrium having a central pore filled with a blood clot.

Third Week of Development (Stages 6–9)

The third week is characterized by the formation of the primitive streak and three germ layers (ectoderm, mesoderm, and endoderm), from which all tissues and organs of the embryo develop.

The primitive streak (Fig. 6.3) is represented by the opacity caused by a proliferation of ectodermal cells at the caudal end of the embryonal disc. The cells of the primitive streak undergo extensive proliferation and expand laterally, cephalically, and caudally between the ectoderm and endoderm of the embryonic disc to form the embryonic mesoderm.

While the primitive streak is giving rise to the embryonic mesoderm, a solid cord of cells grows cephalically from the primitive knot, which is the cephalic end of the primitive streak, and becomes attached to the endoderm below the point of fused ectoderm and endoderm in the region of the future buccopharyngeal membrane. This cord of cells is the *notochord* (see Fig. 6.3). It not only represents a base around which the vertebral column and the caudal part of the base of the skull develop but also a craniocaudal axis of embryonic development.

Thickening of ectodermal cells lying in close proximity to the developing notochord gives rise to the neural plate. The neural plate is the first appearance of the nervous system. Shortly after its appearance, the neural plate becomes depressed below the surface along the long axis of the embryo to form the neural groove. As the neural groove deepens, its margins fuse in the mid-line to form the neural fold (see Fig. 6.3). The process of fusion begins in the region of the future embryonic neck and extends toward the cephalic and caudal ends of the embryo. The fusion is completed during the fourth week of development. The neural tube ultimately will give rise to the central nervous system. The cephalic end will dilate to form the forebrain, midbrain, and hind-brain. The remainder of the tube will become the spinal cord.

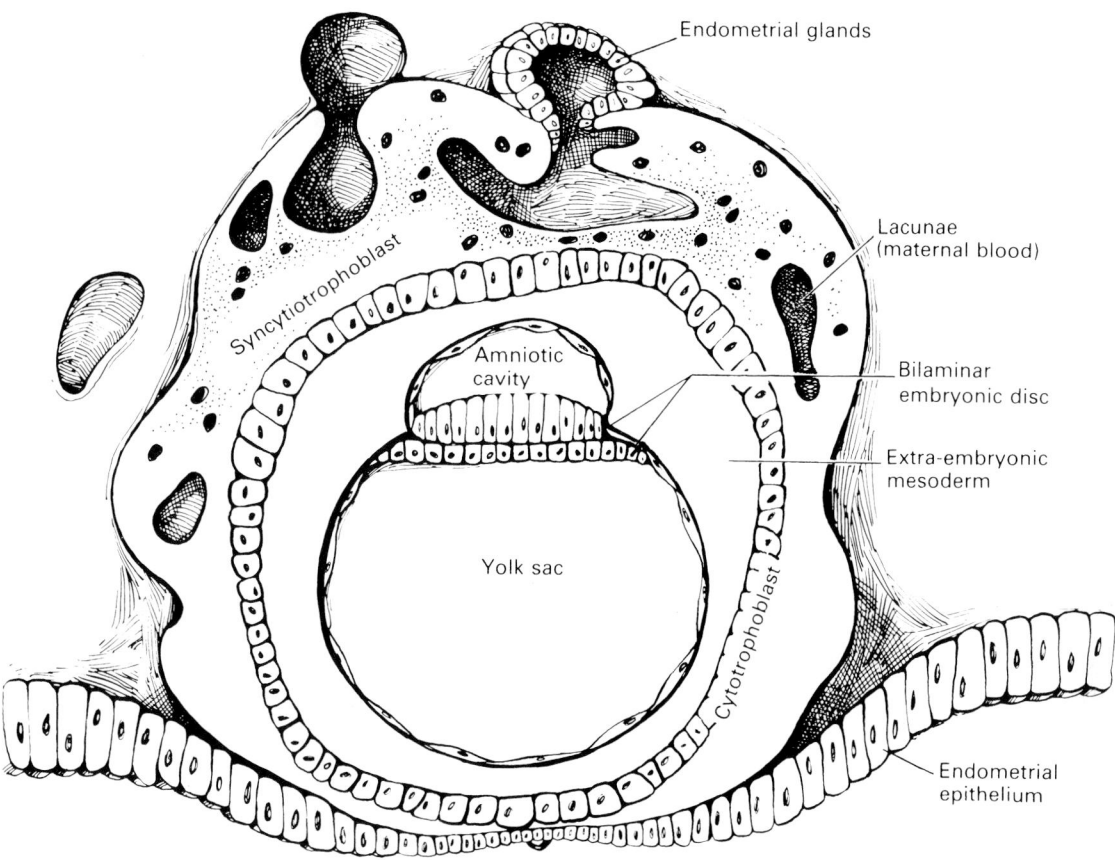

FIGURE 6.2.   *The bilaminar embryonic disc with amniotic and primary yolk sac cavities, surrounded by extra-embryonic mesoderm and differentiating trophoblast. Note positioning of the conceptus in the endometrium.*

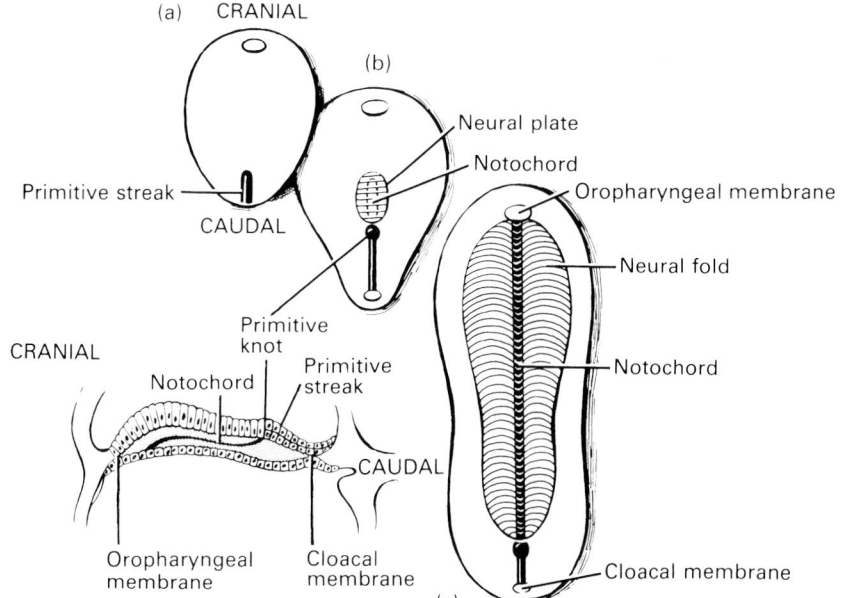

FIGURE 6.3.   *The development of primitive streak* (a), *notochord* (b), *and neural folds* (c), *in trilaminar embryo.*

While the neural tube is developing, mesoderm situated on either side of the mid-line of the embryo, also known as *paraxial mesoderm*, undergoes segmentation by which it becomes divided into segmental blocks or somites. There are eventually approximately 43 pairs of somites. Each somite later differentiates into bones, cartilage, and ligaments of the vertebral column and part of the base of the skull, as well as into skeletal voluntary muscles, dermis, and subcutaneous tissue of the skin. The intermediate mesoderm, the mesodermal tissue present on both sides of the embryo between the paraxial mesoderm and the lateral mesoderm, gives rise to portions of the urogenital system. The lateral mesoderm is involved in the development of pericardial, pleural, and peritoneal cavities, as well as the muscle of the diaphragm.

Mesoderm also gives rise to a primitive cardiovascular system during the third week of development. Blood vessel formation begins in the extraembryonic mesoderm of the yolk sac, the connecting stalk, and the chorion. It is followed by development of embryonic vessels 2 days later. The primitive heart forms from mesenchymal cells differentiating into muscular and connective tissue in the cardiogenic area. The linkage of the primitive heart tube with blood vessels takes place toward the end of the third week, after which the circulation of the embryo's blood begins.

As the embryo progressively changes shape from a disc to a tube, exhibiting cranial and caudal ends with head and tail, endoderm, the third germ layer, becomes incorporated into the interior of the embryo where it contributes to the formation of the epithelial components of most internal organs.

Further development of the placenta, specifically formation of chorionic villi, takes place in the third week. Primary chorionic villi acquire cores of mesenchyme and become secondary chorionic villi. Before the end of the third week, capillaries develop in the villi, transforming them into tertiary chorionic villi. At the same time, the cytotrophoblast cells of the chorionic villi penetrate the layer of syncytiotrophoblast to form a cytotrophoblastic shell, which attaches the chorionic sac to the endometrial tissues [108].

Fourth Week of Development (Stages 10–12)

During the fourth week of development, the embryo measuring 2 to 5 millimeters becomes easily recognizable by the naked eye. At Stage 10, the embryo (22–24 days) is almost straight, and between four and twelve somites produce conspicuous surface elevations (Fig. 6.4). The neural tube is closed opposite the somites but is widely open at the rostral and caudal neuropore. The first and second pair of branchial arches become visible.

During Stage 11, a slight curve is produced in the embryo by folding the head and tail. The heart produces a large ventral prominence. The rostral neuropore continues to close, and optic vesicles are formed (Fig. 6.5).

Stage 12 is characterized by three pairs of branchial arches, complete closure of the rostral hemisphere, and the presence of recognizable upper limb buds on the ventral lateral body wall. The otic pits, the primordia of the inner

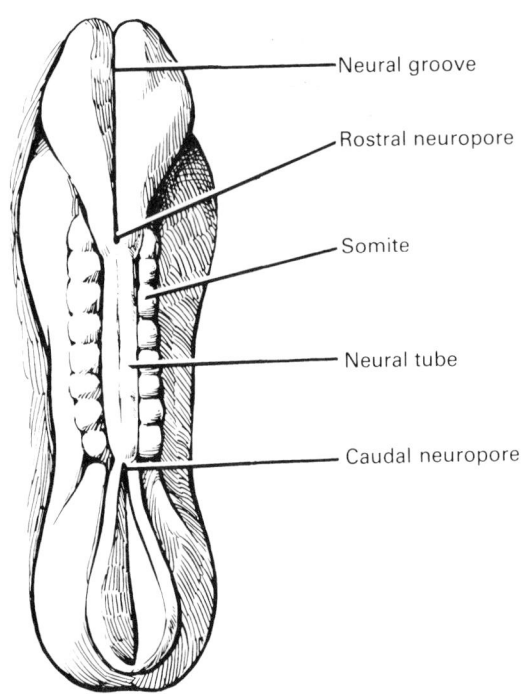

FIGURE 6.4.   *Human embryo Stage 10, showing partial fusion of neural folds, resulting in formation of neural tube with rostral and caudal neuropores.*

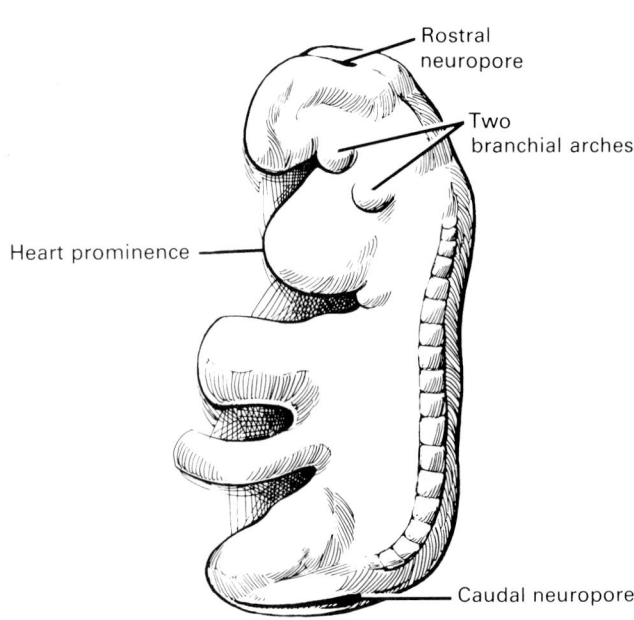

FIGURE 6.5.   *Human embryo Stage 11, with closing rostral neuropore, two pairs of branchial arches, heart prominence, and widely open caudal neuropore.*

ears, are also clearly visible (Fig. 6.6). The growth of the forebrain produces prominent elevation of the head, and further folding of the embryo in the longitudinal plane gives the embryo a characteristic C-shape curvature. Narrowing of the connection between the embryo and the yolk sac produces a body stalk containing one umbilical vein and two umbilical arteries.

Fifth Week of Development (Stages 13–15)
The embryo measures 5 to 10 millimeters in length. Changes in body form seen during this week are minor compared to those that occurred during the 4th week and are characterized by rapid head growth. This extensive head

growth is caused mainly by the rapid development of the brain and leads to further increase in embryonic curvature. As a result, the face lies in close contact to the heart prominence. The upper limbs begin to show regional differentiation as the hand plates develop toward the end of this week. The fourth pair of branchial arches and the lower limb bud are present by 28 to 32 days of development. Lens placodes indicating the future lenses of the eyes are visible on the sides of the head. The attenuated tail with its somites is a characteristic feature at the beginning of the fifth week (Fig. 6.7).

Sixth Week of Development (Stages 16–17)
The CR length of the embryo in this time period is approximately 10 to 14 millimeters. The main external features of Stage 16 can be summarized as follows: nasal pits face ventrally, retinal pigment becomes visible, auricular hillocks appear, and the foot plate is formed. During Stage 17 the C shape of the embryo is still present, even though the trunk begins to straighten. Development of finger rays is one of the main hallmarks of this stage. Basic facial structure formation advances dramatically. The upper lip appears when medial nasal prominences and maxillary prominences merge. Nostrils become clearly defined, and eyes are directed more anteriorly (Fig. 6.8).

Seventh Week of Development (Stages 18–19)
At the end of the 7th week, embryos attain a CR length of 20 millimeters. During this week, the head continues to enlarge rapidly, and the trunk straightens. Elbow regions can be recognized on upper limbs, and toe rays appear on lower limbs. Eyelids are formed, and nipples become visible. The physiological herniation of the intestinal tract into the umbilical cord occurs. The intestinal loops normally "return" to the abdomen by the end of the 10th week.

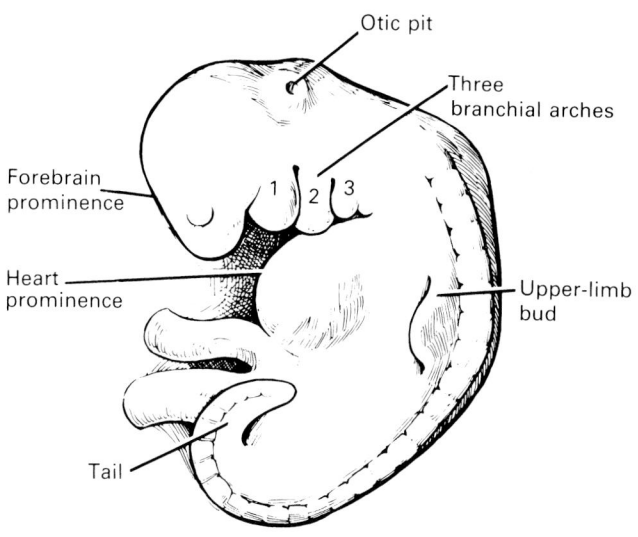

FIGURE 6.6. *Human embryo Stage 12, with forebrain prominence, three pairs of branchial arches, upper-limb buds, and developing tail.*

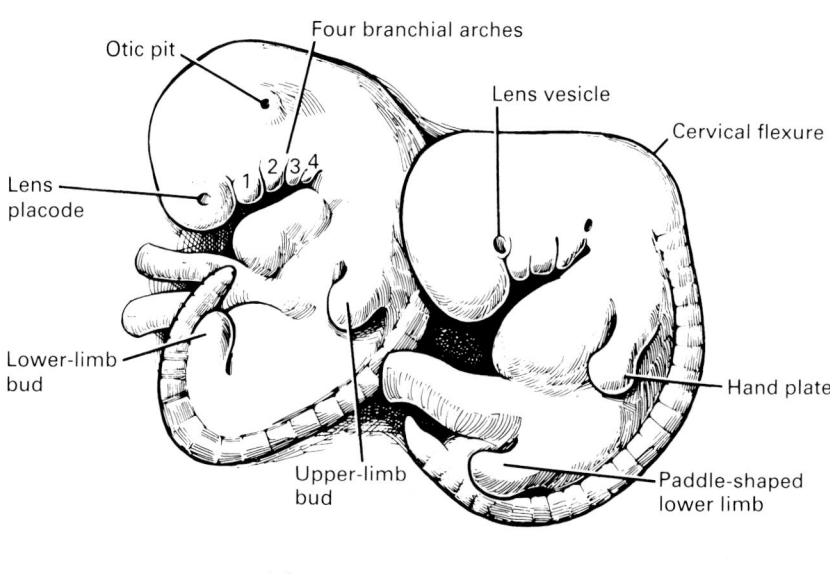

(a) (b)

FIGURE 6.7. *(a) Human embryo Stage 13, showing the presence of all four branchial arches, lens placode, and otic pit. Note that lower-limb bud is recognizable. (b) Lens vesicle and hand plate formation are prominent features of Stage 15 human embryo.*

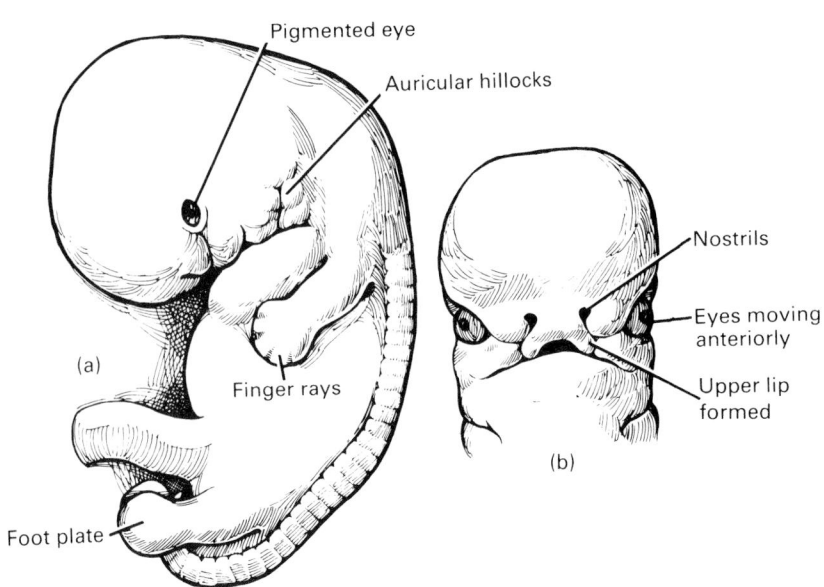

FIGURE 6.8. *Stage 17 human embryo, with pigmented eye and auricular hillocks shown on lateral view (a); nostril and upper lip formation on front view (b). The presence of finger rays and foot plate represents other hallmarks of this stage.*

Eighth Week of Development (Stages 20–23)

At the beginning of the 8th week, the fingers are distinct but still webbed. There are notches between toe rays, and a scalp vascular plexus appears. Toward the end of the week, fingers become free and longer, and the development of hands and feet approach each other. The head becomes more rounded and shows typical human characteristics. The embryo measures 20 millimeters from crown to rump at the beginning of the week and 30 millimeters at the end (Fig. 6.9). All major organ systems are formed by now, and the fetal period begins.

For more detailed description of human embryology, the reader is referred to comprehensive textbooks such as Hamilton et al's *Human Embryology* [108].

Morphological Studies

Principles of Examination

Accurate pathological evaluation of the aborted products of conception requires that all aborted tissues be submitted for examination and be accompanied by a complete obstetrical, medical, and family history. The need for full information, the obstetrical and medical history, and details of the current pregnancy up to the time of abortion, is similar to that required for other types of intrauterine death. Menstrual dates are a valuable help for dating of the gestational sac and embryo. The information about drug ingestion (e.g., anticonvulsive medication) or about exposure to infection during the pregnancy (e.g., rubella) is essential for proper handling of the specimen. The history of previous reproductive failures or family history of congenital morphological and metabolic defect will significantly influence the investigative approach.

The aborted tissue should be submitted fresh, not fixed in formalin, in a sterile or at least clean plastic, tightly closed

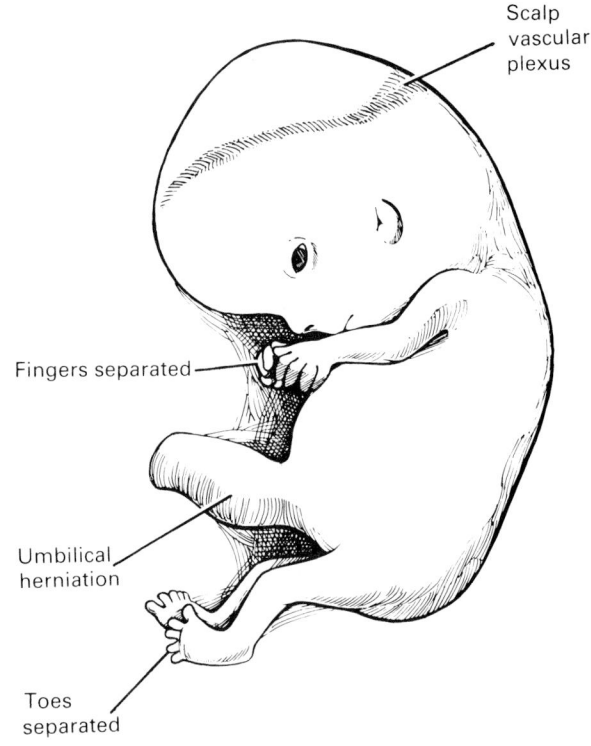

FIGURE 6.9. *Human embryo Stage 23, emphasizing the completed development of face, hands, and feet. Note persistence of umbilical herniation of some loops of the small bowel.*

container or bag, to avoid drying. The small specimens should be kept moist with gauze soaked in sterile saline.

The specimen of early spontaneous abortion is best examined in a large sterile Petri dish with sterile instruments under a dissecting microscope, which is essential for the

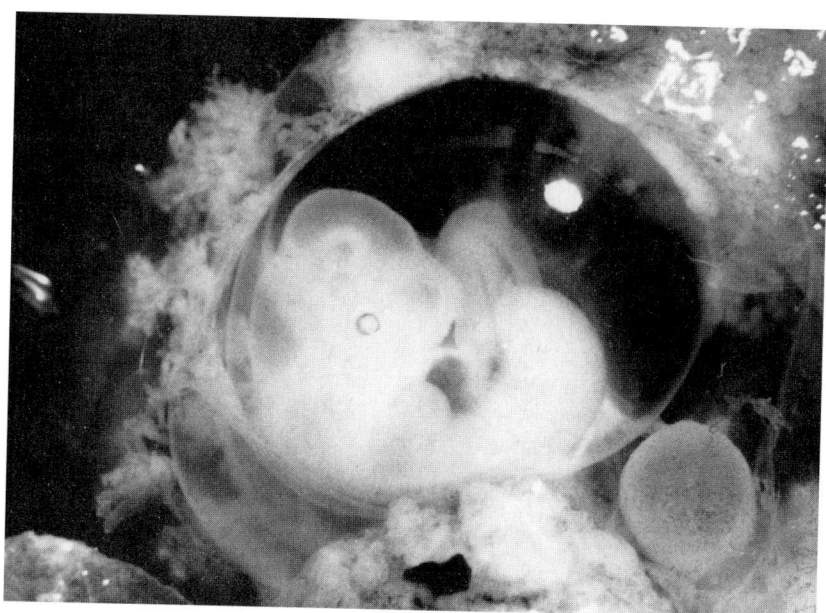

FIGURE 6.10. *Opened chorionic sac with an intact amniotic sac containing normal human embryo Stage 17 is shown. Note degenerating yolk sac outside amniotic sac (right lower corner).*

evaluation of both embryo and chorionic villi. Sterile technique allows samples to be taken for tissue culture and chromosome analysis if such sampling is indicated after examination under the dissecting microscope. The dissecting microscope should have a camera attachment allowing for color photographic documentation as a useful supplement to the gross description. When a small embryo is identified after recording its position in the sac and taking a picture, it is best transferred to a smaller sterile dish for further examination. As embryonic specimens are generally fragile, it is recommended to examine them floating in saline or after fixation.

Types of Specimens

A complete specimen of early abortion consists of an intact chorionic sac, which may be empty or may contain various embryonic or extra-embryonic tissues (see Examination of Chorionic Sacs). Some decidual tissue and blood clots are usually present. Often the chorionic sac is ruptured or, following uterine curettage, it is fragmented. Careful examination of all submitted material for the presence of an embryo is essential, as an embryo may be present outside the ruptured chorionic sac or among curettings. When the embryo is not found, a damaged chorionic sac is categorized as an incomplete specimen. In many instances only decidua and blood clots, with or without chorionic villi, are available for pathological examination.

Examination of Chorionic Sacs

The intact chorionic sac is commonly found as a fluctuant globular structure in a pear-shaped specimen, representing a decidual cast of the uterine cavity. Such specimens should be carefully opened from the narrow end to release the intact chorionic sac. Smaller intact chorionic sacs may be received free, surrounded only by some blood clots. The

dimensions of the chorionic sac vary from 10 to 80 millimeters, and in diameter the surface is usually completely covered by abundant chorionic villi. These villi are of uniform diameter with a symmetrical branching appearance and multiple buds along their length. A sparse development and abnormal morphology (swelling, clubbing, and hypoplasia) of chorionic villi are common in specimens of early abortion and may be best observed with the dissecting microscope. Villi with swollen tips are decribed as *clubbed*, villi with clear vesicles at their ends are referred to as *cystic*, and villi that have few buds or thin irregular branches are described as *hypoplastic*. Histologically, clubbed and cystic villi are usually hydropic and avascular. Hypoplastic villi show fibrosis and vascular obliteration.

After opening the intact chorionic sac, the presence or absence of amniotic sac, yolk sac, body stalk/cord, and embryo should be noted. When an amniotic sac is present, its size and relationship to the chorionic sac should be recorded (Fig. 6.10). An abnormal sized amniotic sac and premature fusion with chorion are the most frequent abnormalities. Aberrant amniotic sac development in the form of cysts has also been reported [109]. The record of an abnormal size and position of the yolk sac allows further insight into the sequence and timing of early embryogenesis insults. A ruptured chorionic sac has a collapsed corrugated appearance due to a loss of amniotic fluid. An embryo is frequently missing from such a sac. Even in the absence of the embryo, the evaluation of the presence or absence of the amniotic sac, its size and relationship to chorion, presence of body stalk, and yolk sac, together with histological examination of the villi allows categorization of the specimen as a normally or abnormally developing gestational sac.

Even a fragmented chorionic sac without a detectable embryo can yield information about embryonic development if the villi are histologically examined. The histological abnormalities in the chorionic villi relate to the time at which embryogenesis has been disturbed. If embryonic death occurred before establishment of the embryonic circulation in the placental villi, then the villi will be avascular, hydropic, and will have attenuated trophoblast layers. On the other hand, if the embryonic circulation was established, increased villous stromal cellularity, fibrosis, and vascular obliteration occur as a result of cessation of blood flow [110].

Examination of Embryos

Early experience of pathological examination of aborted human embryos was summarized by Mall in several publications [111–113]. Based on his extensive knowledge of morphologic findings in early spontaneous abortions, Mall made two important observations: He recognized that embryonic developmental anomalies are more common than congenital defects at birth [113], and he observed that many embryonic defects are difficult to identify as specific malformations. He referred to the embryos with ill-defined abnormal development as *stunted* or *cylindrical embryos* [112]. The high incidence of abnormal embryos in abortion specimens has been confirmed by many other investigators [42, 114–116]. In the study of Poland et al [42], which is one of the largest morphologic studies of early spontaneous abortion, normal embryos were detected in only 16% of 1126 specimens, whereas abnormal embryos were seen in 84%. Among abnormal embryos, a specific systemic or localized defect(s) in otherwise normally developing embryos occurred in only 5%, while generalized abnormal embryonic development was reported in 79%.

For determination of the developmental stage, embryonic length and characteristic facial, limb, and body features are evaluated with the dissecting microscope. The developmental age is established by correlating the embryonic CR length and the developmental stage (see Table 6.5). The difference between the developmental age derived from morphology of embryos and calculated age from the last menstrual period reflects the length of time of retention in utero after embryonic death.

The CR length of the embryo is obviously the most important single measurement. It should be taken without attempting to straighten out normal flexures. As embryos of the 3rd and early 4th week are nearly straight, their linear measurement indicates the greatest length. In those with greatly flexed heads (5th and 6th week of development), the CR length is actually a neck–rump measurement. The true CR length is measured in older embryos. As the length of an embryo is not the only criterion for establishing age, the pathologist should not refer to "the 5-millimeter stage" but should evaluate the developmental characteristics of the embryo of that length and judge the embryo on both its length and its developmental status.

Any discrepancy between the embryonic length and a specific developmental hallmark points to the existence of developmental defect. For example, if a well-preserved fresh embryo measures 5 millimeters and there is an incomplete closure of the rostral neuropore, this is diagnostic of an open neural tube defect. For an accurate evaluation of embryonic development, it is essential to have a set of pictures of normal human embryos from anterior, posterior, and lateral views, as well as a set of actual fixed embryonic specimens, both illustrating the normal development of each stage.

Although the CR length is important for staging normally developing embryos and embryos with focal defects, it is meaningless for embryos with growth disorganization (see Growth Disorganized Embryos) as these do not follow the normal pattern.

Normal Embryos A human embryo classified as "normal" is an embryo harmoniously developed at a certain stage. For example, at Stage 15 a normal embryo measures 7.0 to 10.0 millimeters in CR length and shows a prominent embryonic curvature, regional differentiation of the upper limbs, the presence of lower limb buds, and all four branchial arches. Lens vesicles and nasal pits are prominent features in facial development. Such an embryo is usually found in well-developed amniotic and chorionic sacs, the latter being covered by plentiful secondary and tertiary villi.

Embryos with Specific Developmental Defect(s) Specific defects in an otherwise well-developed embryo (5 to 30 mm CR length) are seen much less frequently than generalized growth disorganization. It should be remembered that most of the defects routinely recognized in embryos are external, as internal dissection or serial histological sectioning is impractical for routine pathological examination. Neural tube defects, cleft lip and palate, and defects of limb development are the most commonly detected specific defects in embryos. Due to incomplete morphogenesis during the embryonic period, the diagnosis of a specific defect present in an embryo depends on the correct evaluation of the developmental stage. Anomalies cannot be diagnosed at a stage that precedes normal structural development. For example, agenesis of the upper limbs cannot be diagnosed before the 26th to 27th day of developmental age, polydactyly of hands before finger digital rays appear (41 to 43 days), cleft lip before the 47th to 50th day (Fig. 6.11), or cleft palate before 61 days of developmental age.

The etiology of the specific embryonic defect should be established as precisely as possible to place genetic counseling and management of further pregnancy on a sound basis. A chromosomal analysis should be routine on all conceptuses with an isolated embryonic defect to allow distinction between polygenic (multifactorial) or monogenic and chromosomal etiology of the defect. For example, an embryonic neural tube defect is commonly seen in chromosomal triploidy or trisomy. Therefore, chromosomal etiology should always be excluded before making a diagnosis of multifactorial causation of a neural tube defect in an embryo. Genetic counseling differs significantly in each of the three conditions.

Growth Disorganized Embryos Based on the degree of abnormal embryonic development, four categories of growth disorganization (GD), GD1 to GD4, can be distinguished [42].

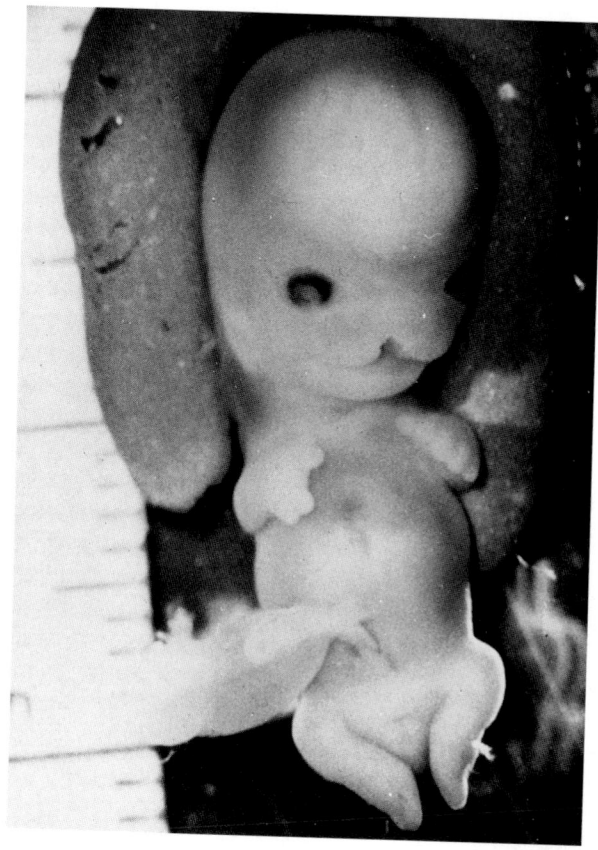

FIGURE 6.11. *Human embryo Stage 19, showing mid-line cleft lip.*

The first category, *GD1* (empty intact sac or unembryonic sac), represents complete or very early failure of development of the embryo proper. The intact sac contains slightly mucoid fluid with no evidence of an embryo or body stalk (Fig. 6.12). The amnion, if present, is usually closely applied to the chorion (fusion of amnion and chorion prior to 10 weeks of gestation represents an abnormal finding) and is structurally abnormal. Chorionic villi are generally sparse, clubbed, and cystic. Microscopically they are avascular, hydropic, and have an attenuated trophoblast.

GD2 (a nodular embryo) consists of chorionic sac containing solid embryonic tissue 1 to 4 millimeters in length, with no recognizable external features and no retinal pigment (Fig. 6.13). Thus, it is impossible to differentiate between caudal and cephalic poles of the embryo. The embryo can be firmly attached to the chorionic plate, or a short body stalk may be identified. A yolk sac is often present and can be macroscopically distinguished from the embryo proper by its position between amnion and chorionic plate. An intact sac containing a yolk sac with no other solid embryonic tissue is also classified as GD2. Abnormal development of amnion is a common finding in these gestations. The amniotic sac is usually too large and adheres to the chorion. Villi show similar abnormalities as in GD1.

GD3 (a cylindrical embryo) in Mall's classification [112] represents elongated smooth embryos up to 10 millimeters without any morphological hallmarks but with retinal pigment (Fig. 6.14). The presence of retinal pigment allows the recognition of caudal and cephalic poles. Limb buds are absent, but a body stalk is present. The size of both the chorionic sac and amniotic sac is usually large and out of proportion to the size of the embryo. Chorionic villi are sparse and hypoplastic, showing hydropic degeneration.

GD4 (a stunted embryo) is usually 10 millimeters in CR length, with a major distortion of body shape. These embryos have a recognizable head, trunk, and limb buds.

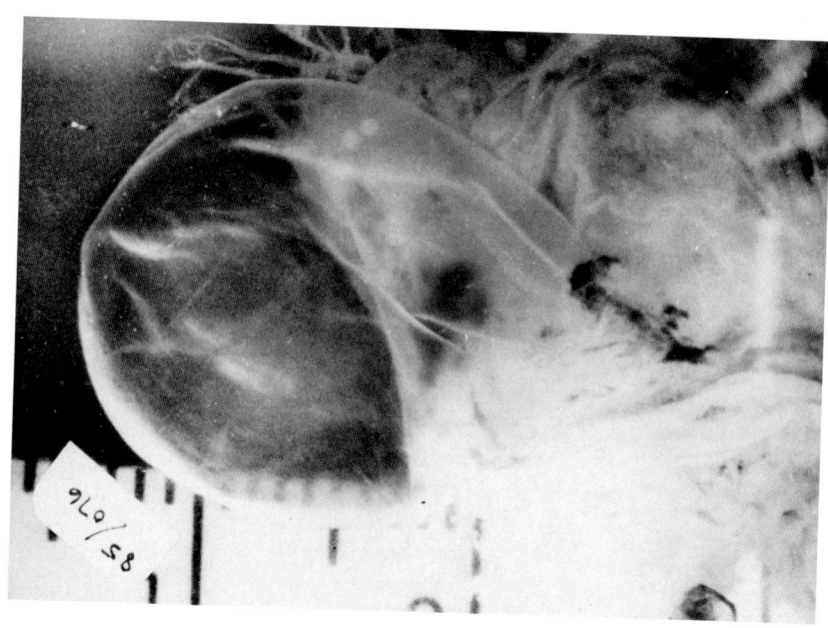

FIGURE 6.12. *Empty intact sac with sparse hypoplastic villi (right upper and lower corner).*

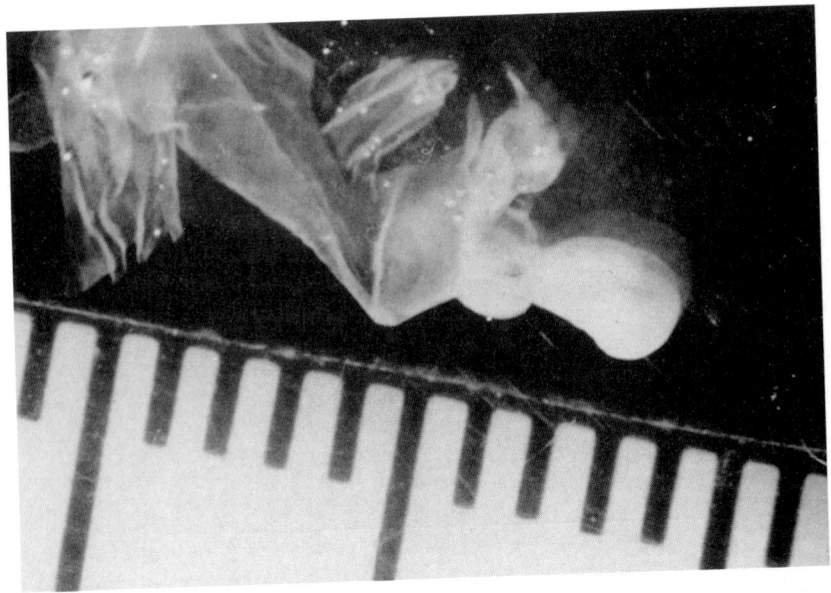

FIGURE 6.13. *Opened chorionic and amniotic sac with a nodular embryo (GD2) measuring 2 millimeters in length.*

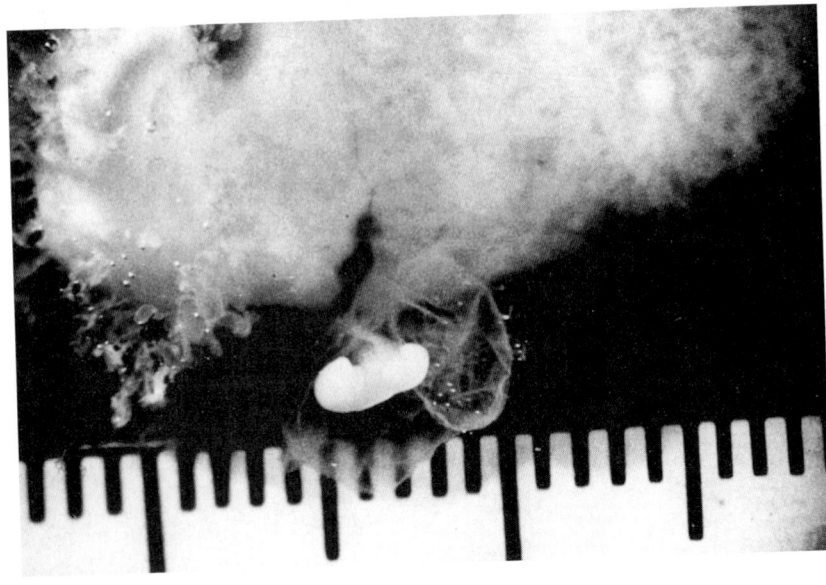

FIGURE 6.14. *Cylindrical embryo (GD3) with retinal pigment at cranial end and no limb buds in an intact amniotic sac. Chorionic sac is opened and sparse; villi at the edge can be seen.*

However, when developmental age is established based on CR length and retinal pigment development, the size of the head is too small and limb buds are profoundly retarded in their development (Fig. 6.15). The face is also abnormal, and there is often fusion of mouth or chin to chest. The cervical flexure is either absent or abnormal.

An intact sac containing a well-developed body stalk (5 mm in length) and either no embryonic tissue or a 2- to 3-millimeter nubbin of tissue attached to the free end of the stalk, usually represents a conceptus in the GD3 or GD4 category. On careful inspection, a necrotic area sealed with fibrin can be identified in the wall of such a chorionic sac, and occasionally a GD3 or GD4 embryo can be found outside a seemingly intact chorionic sac.

Molar Pregnancies

Complete hydatidiform moles have an incidence on the North American continent of approximately 1:2000 and

represent abnormal pregnancies, with a rapidly progressing hydatidiform change affecting chorion in the absence of an embryo and amnion [117]. Histology of complete hydatidiform moles has been well defined [118–120]. The majority of complete moles have a 46,XX karyotype, resulting either from *dispermy*, the fertilization of anuclear ovum by two spermatozoa, or duplication of haploid sperm in an anuclear ovum (diploid androgenesis [121]). XY moles, which represent only some 4% of complete moles, originate from dispermy [122]. No significant difference has been noted in the gross and microscopic findings between the XY and XX complete moles [118]. Studies of invasive moles and choriocarcinomas have led to the suggestion that heterozygous complete moles (caused by dispermy) may have a more malignant potential than their homozygous counterparts arising through diploid androgenesis [123, 124].

Partial moles differ from complete moles in three respects:

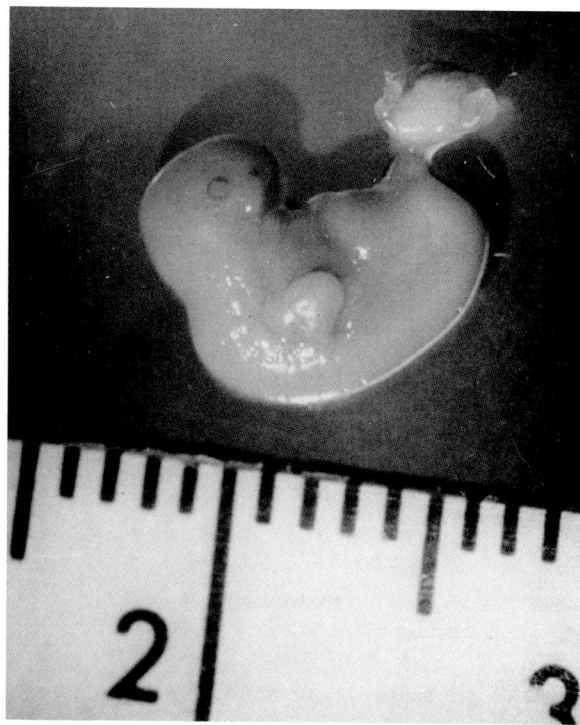

FIGURE 6.15. *Stunted embryo (GD4) showing disproportionate development of head, trunk, and limbs for its crown–rump length of 9 millimeters.*

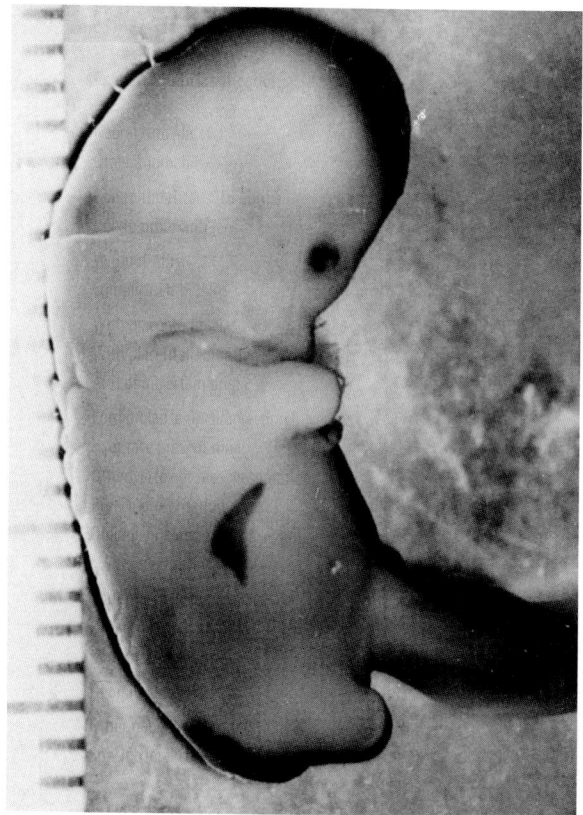

FIGURE 6.16. *Typical phenotype of embryo with chromosomal triploidy (69,XXY) characterized by presence of facial dysplasia, retardation of limb development, presence of symmetrical subectodermal hemorrhages (opposite hemorrhage not seen), and open neural tube defect of lower spine.*

1. An embryo/fetus is commonly present.
2. The microcystic pattern may be diffuse or focal and is not as prominent as in a complete mole.
3. Histologically, trophoblastic hyperplasia is less prominent and sometimes strikingly focal.

Genetically, partial moles are usually triploid with two paternal and one maternal haploid complement [125, 126]. Occasionally, trisomic conceptuses with partial mole morphology have been described [120]. It is important to distinguish between partial and complete moles, as the malignant transformation rate in partial hydatidiform mole is the same as in any non-molar pregnancy [127].

Cytogenetic Studies

The cytogenetic approach to early spontaneous abortion is different from the morphologic one. Each specimen containing at least some villi can be evaluated cytogenetically and categorized as normal or abnormal. Study of several thousand early abortion specimens showed that 50–60% have chromosomal abnormalities resulting mainly from meiotic non-disjunction, abnormal fertilization, or abnormal cleavage [2, 63, 68]. The proportion of chromosomally abnormal conception is even higher in morphologically abnormal embryos [42].

There does not seem to be any consistent correlation between the specific chromosomal defect and morphological abnormality in complete specimens of early spontaneous

abortions. The majority of chromosomally abnormal conceptuses abort as growth-disorganized embryos. Although some chromosomal defects, such as trisomy 13–15, monosomy X, and triploidy, may show specific embryonic phenotypes, these are not consistent findings. Trisomy 13–15 embryos may abort showing advanced embryonic development (Stages 20–23) and focal defects such as holoprosencephaly with or without cyclopia or cebocephaly, severe facial clefting, post-axial polydactyly or retarded limb development, or abnormal heart development. Apparently normal embryonic morphogenesis may be seen in monosomy X embryos. Despite their normal external appearance, monosomy X embryos show uniform degeneration due to prolonged intrauterine retention after embryonic demise. The presence of encephalocele is a common finding in morphologically abnormal 45,X embryos [128]. Conceptuses with chromosomal triploidy may abort as typical GD1–GD3, or show a phenotype similar but not identical to GD4 (Fig. 6.16). This phenotype is characterized by limb retardation in relation to developmental age, facial dysplasia, symmetrical or mid-line subectodermal hemorrhages, and cystic changes in the placenta microscopically characterized by irregular outline and hydropic alteration of secondary and tertiary villi. These cystic changes in placenta seen only in some types of triploidy are frequently the basis for classifying such conceptions as partial hydatidiform moles.

Cell cultures for cytogenetic studies from early abortion specimens are most easily initiated from the amnion and the chorionic villi. The embryo proper is frequently degenerated due to long periods of intrauterine retention following embryonic death, thus providing a poor source of viable cells. The chorionic villi selected for culture must be freed from decidual contamination under the dissecting microscope, to avoid overgrowth of maternal cells, and repeatedly washed in balanced salt solution containing both antibacterial and antifungal agents to prevent infection. The amnion represents the ideal source of dividing cells in culture, as it is of ectodermal origin and no maternal contamination needs to be feared. However, it degenerates relatively easily and becomes non-viable in conceptions retained in utero for long periods of time. Therefore, to ensure the success of the cultures, both amnion and chorion should be set up from early abortion specimens.

Traditional cytogenetic methodologies are enhanced and augmented by using fluorescence in situ hybridization (FISH), applied to nondividing *interphase nuclei* [129]. Classical cytogenetic analysis reveals information about the entire karyotypic complement of an individual but is reliant on availability of mitotically active fresh tissue. Interphase FISH eliminates artifacts such as culturally induced biases and low number of dividing cells. Its application to studies of human spontaneous abortions is promising [130]. FISH not only detects numerical chromosomal abnormalities in non-dividing nuclei, but it also can be used for accurate diagnosis of microdeletion syndromes and for localization of oncogenes or translocation breakpoints, which are not assessable by traditional cytogenetics [131].

FISH involves hybridization of chromosome-specific biotin or digoxigenin-labeled nucleic acid probes to interphase nuclei. The site of hybridization is detected using antibodies, and the signals are currently analyzed using a standard light microscope adapted for fluorescence. FISH is a rapid alternative method for cytogenetic analysis useful in the studies of chromosomal mosaicism [132]. FISH can be applied to tissues that have been frozen, fixed, or embedded in paraffin [133]. In addition to detection of chromosome defects, FISH can be used for detection of foreign DNA (e.g., viral particles) [134].

Microbiology Studies

The incidence of embryonic bacterial and viral infections and their effects on very early stages of human pregnancy development (Stages 1–4) are generally unknown [135]. The effect of viral infections during later embryonic development depends more on the embryonic developmental stage at the time of viral penetration than on the specific virus. This was demonstrated in both chicken and human embryos for several viruses (rubeola, poliovirus, influenza) [135]. Only

a small percentage of embryos from mothers infected during the first trimester show evidence of embryopathy.

Colonization of the female genital tract by *Chlamydia* is commonly described. However no significant evidence of chlamydial involvement in the causation of an early pregnancy loss has been reported [136].

Genital mycoplasmas have become implicated in the etiology of repeated spontaneous abortion when it has been shown that the organisms were isolated more often from the endometrium of habitual aborters than from controls. The rates of isolation of genital mycoplasma from the lower genital tract of habitual aborters did not differ from normal [137]. Eradication of genital mycoplasma infection by antibiotic therapy has also been reported to result in an increased number of successful pregnancies, but controlled studies with a placebo are lacking [138, 139].

Microbiologic studies, specifically ureaplasma and mycoplasma cultures, are, therefore, indicated in cases of repeated, unexplained early spontaneous abortions. To initiate such studies, the gestational tissue must be not only fresh but also received as soon as possible after curettage or spontaneous passage. Samples should be taken from the inside of the gestational sac and not from areas contaminated by vaginal environment. They should be promptly delivered in special media to a laboratory equipped to culture and identify genital mycoplasma organisms [140].

Clinical Significance of Pathological Evaluation

Following spontaneous abortion, the questions of "cause" and "risk of recurrence" are likely to arise. The examination of early spontaneous abortion specimens by the pathologist provides important information relating to the developmental age and morphology of the conceptus. It also allows for conclusions regarding the cause of spontaneous pregnancy loss or failure of normal embryonic development and provides the basis for counseling the parents.

Examination of embryos is as important as performing perinatal postmortem examinations. This can be clearly illustrated in the case of specific developmental defects. A higher incidence of developmental defects such as limb defects, cleft lip, and neural tube defects exists in embryos as compared to liveborn infants [116, 141, 142]. The probability of recurrence of these defects if they are multifactorial in origin is approximately 3–5%. It may be much higher in the case of autosomal dominant or recessive genes or significantly lower if these defects are part of a chromosomal syndrome, such as neural tube defect in triploidy. Therefore, valuable information for genetic counseling and specific prenatal investigation in a future pregnancy is lost if pathological investigation of early spontaneous abortion specimens is omitted.

The morphological diagnosis of embryonic growth disorganization is less informative. It points to a high possibility of several types of de novo chromosomal abnormalities such as trisomy, monosomy, triploidy, and tetraploidy. These chromosomal mutations, either de novo in parental gametes (trisomy) or the result of failure of normal fertilization (triploidy) and cleavage (tetraploidy), are not hereditary. A small proportion of structural chromosomal abnormalities and rare numerical defects may be inherited from a carrier parent, but cytogenetic studies of early spontaneous abortions are fully justified and necessary when there is a history of repeated early spontaneous abortions [143].

Understanding the relationship between karyotype and phenotype of the conceptus in habitual abortions is important. A normal karyotype in a specimen with embryonic growth disorganization suggests either a teratogenic effect interfering with normal embryogenesis or submicroscopic lethal genetic defects. The detection of triploidy or tetraploidy indicates the sporadic nature of the embryonic maldevelopment. An unbalanced chromosomal rearrangement indicates a high probability of one parent being a carrier of a balanced form of the rearrangement. The identification of a well-developed, non-degenerated, normal embryo in an early spontaneous abortion specimen suggests abnormal hormonal function of the corpus luteum or an endometrial disorder.

Incomplete specimens are difficult to evaluate meaningfully on morphological examination. Decidua is not a product of conception, and specimens consisting of decidua only should not be used for definitive confirmation of pregnancy loss. Hormone treatment, ectopic pregnancy, and premenstrual endometrium can confuse the issue. In a fragmented or ruptured empty chorionic sac, the existence of an embryo can be established following histologic examination of villous vascularization. Avascular hydropic villi allow a specific diagnosis of an unembryonic sac with its high risk of de novo chromosomal error. However, if there is appropriate vascularization or villous fibrosis with vascular obliteration, any questions about the specific phenotype of a lost embryo from that sac will remain without an answer.

LATE SPONTANEOUS ABORTION

Review of Normal Fetal and Placental Development

Previable Fetal Development

There is no formal system of fetal staging as exists for the embryonic period. Development during the fetal period (9 weeks to term) is primarily concerned with growth and further differentiation of organs and tissues. There are no dramatic changes in external appearance and, therefore, greater emphasis is placed on CR, toe-heel (TH), and crown-heel (CH) measurements in establishing fetal developmental age. Between the 9th and 20th weeks of pregnancy, the CR length of the fetus increases from 30 to 180 millimeters (Table 6.6). The weight of the fetus in the previable weeks (9–20) is variable and unreliable as a measure of developmental age [36]. Changes in the external appearance of the fetus and in the relationship of head and limbs is subtle but progressive during the previable fetal period.

Table 6.6.   Crown–rump length and developmental age (previable fetuses)

Crown–rump length (mm)	Days after ovulation	Crown–rump length (mm)	Days after ovulation
30–31	53	107–108	94
32–34	54	109–110	95
35–36	55	111–112	96
37	56	113–114	97
38–39	57	115–116	98
40–41	58	117–118	99
42	59	119–120	100
43–44	60	121–122	101
45–46	61	123–124	102
47–48	62	125–126	103
49	63	127–128	104
50–51	64	129	105
52–53	65	130–131	106
54	66	132–134	107
55–56	67	135–136	108
57–58	68	137–138	109
59–60	69	139	110
61–62	70	140–141	111
63–64	71	142–143	112
65	72	144–145	113
66–67	73	146–147	114
68–69	74	148–149	115
70–71	75	150	116
72–73	76	151–152	117
74	77	153	118
75	78	154–155	119
76–78	79	156–157	120
79–80	80	158	121
81	81	159–160	122
82	82	161–162	123
83–86	83	163–164	124
87–89	84	165	125
90–91	85	166	128
92–93	86	167	130
94	87	168	131
95–97	88	169	132
98–99	89	170–172	133
100–101	90	173–174	134
102–103	91	175–177	135
104	92	178–179	136
105–106	93	180	137

The head is about one-third the size of the fetal body at 12 weeks and approximately one-fourth at the 16th week. The CH length increases more rapidly than the CR length due to increased rate of growth of the lower limbs compared to the upper limbs which, during the embryonic period, were advanced in development. The marked cervical flexure present in the embryo is lost by the 12th week and is replaced by a dorsal flexure. The flexure of arms and legs increases so that at 16 weeks forearms and legs are crossed, and the fingers are also flexed.

A summary of the most obvious hallmarks of fetal development follows: During the 9th week, eyes are closing or closed. External genitalia are still not distinguishable as male or female. Intestines are still herniated into umbilical cord. The 10th week is characterized by return of the intestine into the abdomen. During the 11th and 12th weeks, the external genitalia of male and female fetuses can be reasonably easily distinguished from one another provided magnification is used. Fingernails are clearly developed in the 13th week. Lower limb development is finalized by the 14th week. Eyebrows and head hair become visible at the end of 20th week.

Functional maturation of individual organs begins in the fetal stage and approaches completion at about the 36th week of pregnancy. More information on the development and maturation of the individual systems can be found in embryology textbooks [108, 144, 145] and in Chapter 2.

Placental Development

The placenta develops into a circumscribed and discrete organ from about the 10th gestational week of pregnancy. There is no clear demarcation between the embryonic and fetal stages of placental development, but rather a gradual merging with loss of function of those villi not involved in the formation of the mature organ.

Up to about the 8th week, villi cover the entire surface of the chorionic sac. As the sac grows, the villi facing the uterine cavity (decidua capsularis) lose their blood supply and degenerate, giving rise to the chorion laeve. At the same time, the villi associated with the decidua basalis proliferate and branch rapidly, giving rise to the chorionic plate and the chorionic villi of the placenta. The placental shape is usually discoid. As a result of villous invasion into maternal decidua, the surface of the placenta is divided into ten to thirty irregular convex areas or lobules, not cotyledons. Technically, each cotyledon represents the villous tree served by the fetal vessels in a stem villus. Lobules may have two or more main stem villi and their many vascular branches. The separation between lobules is provided by maternal, wedge-shaped, decidual tissue.

The placental membranes are formed by fusion of the chorion laeve and the amniotic sac at about 9 weeks of development; their fusion before 9 weeks is abnormal and characteristic of embryonic growth disorganization (see Growth Disorganized Embryos under Early Spontaneous Abortion above). Delayed fusion or lack of it may be seen in amniotic band syndrome when extra-embryonic coelom between chorion and amnion persists.

The umbilical cord develops from the connecting stalk, which is extra-embryonic mesoderm joining the caudal end of the embryonic disc and primary yolk sac to the internal surface of the chorion. As the tail fold of the embryo is formed and the embryo grows, the connecting stalk becomes attached to the ventral surface of the embryo and contains the vitelline duct (communication between the yolk sac and the midgut of the embryo) and the allantoic diverticulum, accompanied by the allantoic vessels (two umbilical arteries and two umbilical veins, only one of the latter persisting). The mature umbilical cord consists of two umbilical arteries and one vein within the mesodermal core of loose mesenchyme (Wharton's jelly). The cord is covered by amniotic epithelium and may contain remnants of the allantois as a microscopic and usually discontinuous epithelial strand. The umbilical cord is at first very short, but, as the amnion and chorion grow, its length increases rapidly. At the third month, the average length of the umbilical cord is 60 millimeters. At full term, it is normally about 54 centimeters [108].

Morphologic Studies of Fetuses and Placentas

Principles of Examination

Late-abortion specimens usually consist of fetus and placenta, and each can be examined separately. As in the examination of early abortuses, it is essential that the obstetrical history be available to the pathologist. Both fetus and placenta should be submitted fresh without fixation, so that cytogenetic, microbiologic, or biochemical studies can be done. It is most important that the aborted fetus and placenta be taken as quickly as possible to the pathology department. If immediate transport is not possible, the fetus and placenta should be refrigerated in a sterile, dry, tightly closed container.

Examination of the Fetus

The fetus should be weighed and CR length, CH length, and head circumference should be recorded. CR length is the principal value used for establishing the fetal developmental age as illustrated in Table 6.6. Tables are also available for determining developmental age from the foot and hand lengths (Table 6.7). These can be used instead of CR length when the specimen is incomplete or fragmented or for verification of the accuracy of CR measurement. Careful inspection of the face, eyes, nose, mouth, palate, and ears should take place, remembering that features of common syndromes, such as trisomy 21 or trisomy 18, may be poorly developed or even absent in previable fetuses [146]. The examination of limbs with a record of their length, the number of digits, and their position, and the presence or absence of flexion deformities is important. The external genitalia are well formed and gender can be easily distinguished from the 12th week of development. Macerated and damaged fetuses should not be disregarded, even though they may appear to be grossly distorted. Despite molding and distortion, major external malformations such as neural tube defect, cleft lip and palate, syndactyly, polydactyly, amputations, and constrictions can be easily diagnosed (Fig. 6.17). Amputations of digits and constrictions of limbs and umbilical cord represent common findings in the amniotic band syndrome and should be sought in macerated fetuses. This condition is one hundred times more common in previable fetuses than in newborns [147, 148].

Table 6.7.   Hand and foot lengths correlated with developmental age (previable fetuses)

Developmental age (weeks)	Hand length (mm)	Foot length (mm)
11	10 ± 2	12 ± 2
12	15 ± 2	17 ± 3
13	18 ± 1	19 ± 1
14	19 ± 1	22 ± 2
15	20 ± 3	25 ± 3
16	26 ± 2	28 ± 2
17	27 ± 3	29 ± 4
18	29 ± 2	33 ± 2
19	32 ± 2	36 ± 1

Modified from McBride ML, Baillie J, Poland BJ. Growth parameters in normal fetuses. *Teratology* 1984; 29:185–101; supplemented with unpublished data.

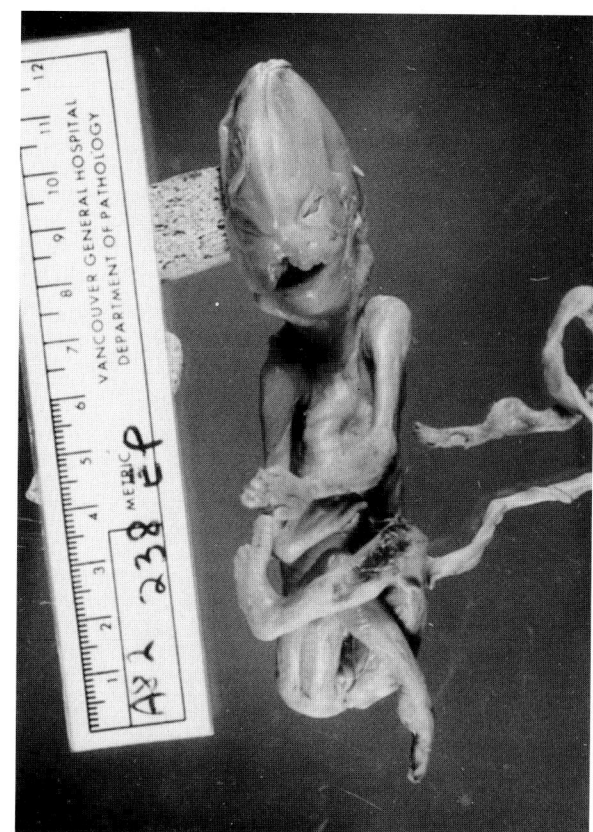

FIGURE 6.17.   *Severely macerated male fetus of 14 developmental weeks with amniotic band syndrome. Note the irregular bilateral right-sided cleft lip and palate, as well as amputation of bilateral distal phalanges with attached amniotic bands and partial amputation of left third toe.*

Both external and internal examination of the non-macerated fetuses is usually done in a fresh state. However, macerated fetuses can sometimes be better examined when fixation precedes internal dissection. It may be helpful to secure the fetal limbs on a cork board. Smaller fetuses (9–11 weeks) can also be examined with the dissecting microscope after slicing the trunk at 0.5- to 1-centimeter intervals [149]. The internal examination should not be directed only toward the diagnosis of obvious abnormalities such as renal agenesis, diaphragmatic hernia, or malrotation of the intestine. Meticulous dissection, identical to that of perinatal autopsy technique, should identify all internal malformations, including congenital heart defects. Detailed dissection using a magnifying lens or a dissecting microscope is especially important in cases with abnormal external morphogenesis. If no external malformations are present, Rushton [110] estimates that the likelihood of finding major internal malformation is only 2%. All internal organs should be weighed and the weight compared to normal values for developmental age [150]; this is particularly important whenever organ hypoplasia is suspected.

Examination of the brain is feasible only in a fresh, spontaneously aborted fetus. In a macerated fetus the brain is usually partially or completely liquefied. The removal of brain tissue should be done after ample fixation in situ in 10% formaldehyde with a widely open skull. All precautions to avoid the damage of immature brain tissue must be used [151]. The examination of the brain not only allows diagnosis of specific developmental defects such as hydrocephalus, but it is particularly important in any case of suspected symmetrical intrauterine growth retardation. A significant discrepancy between the developmental age established by CR length and brain maturation confirms the diagnosis of intrauterine growth retardation.

Morphological assessment of the abnormal fetus should routinely include radiographic examination for the purpose of determining bone developmental age and documenting skeletal anomalies. This is best done prior to evisceration. An antero posterior (A-P) projection of the whole fetus can be conveniently accommodated on an 18 × 24 centimeter film and is sufficient in most circumstances. If skeletal abnormalities are demonstrated in the A-P projection, then appropriate lateral views and detailed views of the abnormalities should be obtained. Fetal radiography is most useful for the examination of fetal dwarfism or of a fetus with skeletal dysplasia. However, even when a skeletal defect is not suspected, radiographic examination permits detection of anomalies that are difficult to demonstrate by dissection, such as abnormal vertebrae or hypoplasia of the phalanges (see Fig. 6.19b).

Photographic documentation of all detected developmental defects is mandatory. Anterior and lateral photographs of the whole fetus are a useful minimum record, but detailed photographs of all detected malformations should also be taken. Photographs of internal malformations are usually taken under a dissecting microscope to allow a magnified view. The importance of photographic recording of fetal abnormalities cannot be stressed enough. It enables identification of the range of abnormalities within a particular syndrome, allows comparisons to be made, and makes re-evaluation of the case possible.

Common Abnormal Morphological Findings

Neural Tube Defects

Central nervous system defects are among the most devastating human developmental defects. Current estimates indicate that 5% of all newborns have some type of congenital anomaly. Neural tube defects, including spina bifida, anencephaly, and congenital hydrocephalus, are the most common and second only to congenital heart defects in causing infant mortality [152]. Researchers believe that neural tube defects in humans are caused by a combination of multiple genes and environmental factors [153, 154]. Heritability has been estimated to account for approximately 60% of all anencephaly and spina bifida cases [155–157]. Diet also seems to play a significant role, because folic acid supplementation beginning at conception reduces the incidence in women at high risk [84, 85, 158, 159]. Drugs such as valproic acid, when taken during the first few weeks of pregnancy, can increase the incidence of neural tube defects [157].

Anencephaly

Anencephaly is the commonest open neural tube defect seen among previable fetuses. It is diagnosed in the second trimester either on ultrasound examination or because of a raised maternal alpha-fetoprotein level, but it is rarely seen among spontaneously aborted fetuses. For a detailed discussion of anencephaly, see Chapter 21.

Encephalocele

Encephalocele is usually occipital. Frequently it is accompanied by hydrocephalus or microcephaly. Encephalocele may be covered by normal scalp skin but more commonly by membranes only. Although encephalocele usually represents an isolated neural tube defect, it may be a manifestation of amniotic band syndrome or a recessive gene mutation such as occurs in Meckel syndrome. Encephalocele is a rare finding among spontaneously aborted fetuses. For a detailed discussion of encephalocele, see Chapter 21.

Meningomyelocele

Meningomyelocele is a form of an open neural tube defect along the spinal canal, which occasionally may be completely covered by skin. It is usually diagnosed by raised maternal alpha-fetoprotein if open, or by ultrasound examination when closed. Meningomyelocele is commonly associated with chromosomal trisomies and triploidy. When a spontaneously aborted fetus shows the defect, cytogenetic examination of cultured fetal fibroblasts must be requested. A detailed discussion of meningomyelocele is found in Chapter 21.

Amnion Rupture Sequence

Amnion rupture sequence (ARS) is defined as a disruption complex characterized by rupture of the amnion with secondary effects on the fetus, producing (1) malformations due to interruption of normal morphogenesis, (2) deformations due to distortion of established structures, or (3) mutilations of structures already formed. It is considered an uncommon, sporadic condition among liveborn infants. Its incidence among previable fetuses is about one hundred times higher than it is after 23 to 24 weeks of gestation. Constrictions of the umbilical cord by amniotic bands are a common cause of intrauterine death [148].

Posterior Cervical Hygroma

Posterior cervical hygroma, once considered diagnostic of fetal Turner syndrome, is now recognized as a non-specific malformation [160]. It consists of fluid accumulation in lymphatic channels of the neck and surrounding connective tissue, reflecting failure or delay in the development of the connection between the jugular lymph sac and the internal jugular vein. Significance and fetal outcomes of first trimester nuchal anomalies detected by ultrasound have been reported [161, 162]. Physiological fluid collections in the nuchal area are found in 40% of embryos before 10 weeks of gestation. However, at 17 weeks of gestation, increasing amounts of nuchal fluid are suggestive of chromosomal anomalies [163]. Because ultrasound diagnosis of posterior cervical hygroma is a frequent indication for termination of pregnancy, it is of utmost importance for genetic counseling of the parents that the correct fetal condition associated with the cervical hygroma be established [148].

Omphalocele

Omphalocele is the result of failure of reduction of the physiological midgut herniation, when abdominal contents remain in a membranous sac composed of amnion and peritoneum beyond 7 to 8 weeks of development. Associated developmental anomalies are frequent. Chromosomal defects were found in two-thirds of fetuses karyotyped because of prenatal diagnosis of omphalocele [148, 164].

Omphalocele must be clearly distinguished from other abdominal wall defects, such as gastroschisis and body stalk defect, to allow for accurate genetic counseling.

Renal Anomalies and Urethral Obstruction

Oligohydramnios is the most common presenting symptom of renal anomalies, which range from renal agenesis, cystic renal dysplasia, infantile polycystic disease, to Meckel syndrome. Pathological examination should distinguish between the different types of renal disease so that accurate risks of recurrence are given to parents and appropriate investigation initiated in subsequent pregnancies [165]. Urethral obstruction producing prune belly syndrome is also commonly associated with variable renal anomalies (hydronephrosis, renal cystic dysplasia, renal hypoplasia, and isolated medullary hypoplasia) and requires a detailed pathological examination [166–168]. Megacystis-microcolon-intestinal hypoperistalsis syndrome needs to be differentiated from less lethal conditions characterized by bladder obstruction [169]. Renal anomalies are discussed in detail in Chapter 29.

Heart Defects

Heart defects are common findings among both spontaneously aborted and terminated fetuses. A cardiac anomaly may represent an isolated defect or be a part of a syndrome such as a chromosomal trisomy. For a detailed discussion of congenital heart defects, see Chapter 20.

Artifacts due to Trauma or Autolysis

Artifactual abnormalities are present frequently in both terminated and spontaneously aborted fetuses. Traumatic defects are commonly seen in the neck and abdominal wall. The confusion with developmental defects can be avoided by careful microscopic examination of the margins of the defect. In traumatic defects, the edges are irregular and show all different layers of the abdominal wall or neck. Disruption of developmental defects, such as the sac of an omphalocele or encephalocele, is a common finding. The presence of cerebral tissue in the retroperitoneal space can be confused with primitive neuroectodermal tumor in macerated fetuses. This finding is common (1 in 4 macerated fetuses). Brain tissue can be also found under the pleura, in the neck, and inguinal areas.

Fixation of the fetus in formaldehyde prior to examination makes the evaluation of facial dysmorphology and limb contractures very difficult.

Examination of the Placenta

A well-formed placenta of a previable fetus consists of umbilical cord, membranes, and chorionic plate with villi. The process of its examination is identical to that of the placenta in the perinatal period; the reader is therefore referred to Chapter 7.

Cytogenetic Studies

The incidence of cytogenetic abnormalities among late abortions is significantly lower (5–10%) than among early abortions [68, 170]. The most frequently detected chromosomal abnormalities are trisomies, sex chromosome monosomy, and triploidy. Because the majority of chromosomal defects are found among morphologically abnormal fetuses, all fetuses with developmental defects should have chromosomal studies.

In contrast to chromosomal defects in embryos, many of the chromosomally abnormal fetuses show a characteristic

phenotype. A classical fetal phenotype for sex chromosomal monosomy (45,X) consists of generalized subcutaneous edema, posterior cervical cystic hygroma, and intrauterine retention following fetal death [171]. Fetal posterior cervical hygroma is not limited to 45,X, it is also present in Noonan syndrome, chromosomal trisomies (21, 18, 13), congenital heart disease, familial pterygium colli, fetal alcohol syndrome, and idiopathic posterior cervical hygroma [172, 173]. As sex chromosome monosomy is one of the most common abnormalities among second trimester spontaneous abortions, its accurate diagnosis has an important value in genetic counseling of parents. A reliable diagnostic morphological finding other than karyotype, which may not be possible due to frequent non-viability of aborted tissues, is necessary. An aortic preductal coarctation fulfills this requirement. It is consistently found among spontaneously aborted previable fetuses with sex chromosome monosomy [160]. Other developmental anomalies such as an abnormal bicuspid aortic valve, horseshoe kidney, ventricular septal defect, and single umbilical artery are commonly but not consistently seen. These findings indicate the importance of a complete internal examination of any fetus with posterior cervical hygroma. The cytogenetic analysis of cultured fetal tissues remains essential for differential diagnosis of posterior cervical hygroma whenever aortic preductal coarctation is not identified.

Fetal triploidy (Fig. 6.18) should be suspected in fetuses showing severe intrauterine growth retardation, syndactyly of digits (usually between the third and fourth finger), abnormal development of brain (microcephaly, hydrocephalus, neural tube defect), and severe adrenal hypoplasia [174]. Placental cystic changes in triploid conceptuses are observed only when triploidy arises from one maternal and two paternal haploid complements [125].

Contrary to the situation among early abortuses, only a few specific autosomal trisomies, represented by trisomies 9, 13, 18, and 21, are usually found among late abortions. Trisomies 9, 13, or 18 are relatively easily diagnosed or suspected on the basis of morphologic examination alone. Even during early fetal development many classic features of the affected term infant are present (microcephaly, heart and limb malformations in trisomy 9; polydactyly, cleft lip and palate, abnormal brain and eye development in trisomy 13; severe intrauterine growth retardation, abnormal positioning of second and fifth finger, overlapping of third and fourth finger, congenital heart disease in trisomy 18). In trisomy 21, the fetal phenotype is frequently normal. Only a careful search for subtle features such as midphalangeal hypoplasia of the fifth finger (Fig. 6.19), simian crease, flat occiput bone, and presence of congenital heart disease (typically arterioventricular defect) may prompt the pathologist to think of trisomy 21 and to culture tissue for cytogenetic analysis.

Sampling of the tissue for culturing and cytogenetic analysis of late abortions is simple. A small piece of chorion and amnion is sufficient in most cases when the fetus itself

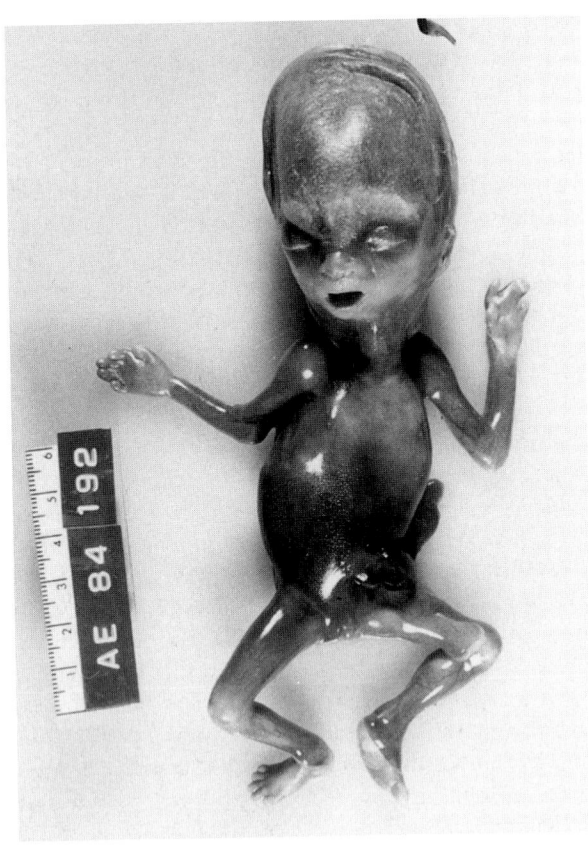

FIGURE 6.18.   *Fetus of 15 developmental weeks with chromosomal triploidy (69,XXY), showing hydrocephaly, bilateral syndactyly (third and fourth fingers), ambiguous genitalia, and marked intrauterine growth retardation.*

is macerated. When a large fresh fetus is available, short-term lymphocyte culture from cord or heart blood should be attempted, as the results are obtained much faster. Fibroblast cultures initiated from chorion and amnion can be set up as a backup for lymphocyte cultures. Short-term thymocyte cultures also may provide an effective and quick method of providing a karyotype analysis compared to fibroblast culture [175]. Chondrocyte culture from fetal cartilage can often be successfully initiated when only a macerated fetus is available [176].

Confined Placental Mosaicism and Uniparental Disomy

Even when the chromosomal preparation derived from fetal tissues is of an excellent quality, the detection of a diploid karyotype in the cells of fetal origin does not necessarily mean a normal complement, because *uniparental disomy* (UPD), the derivation of a pair of homologues from one parent, cannot be detected cytogenetically. UPD most often results from chromosome loss in a preimplantation trisomic embryo [177, 178]. Postzygotic mitotic errors during embryonic development lead to a discrepancy between the

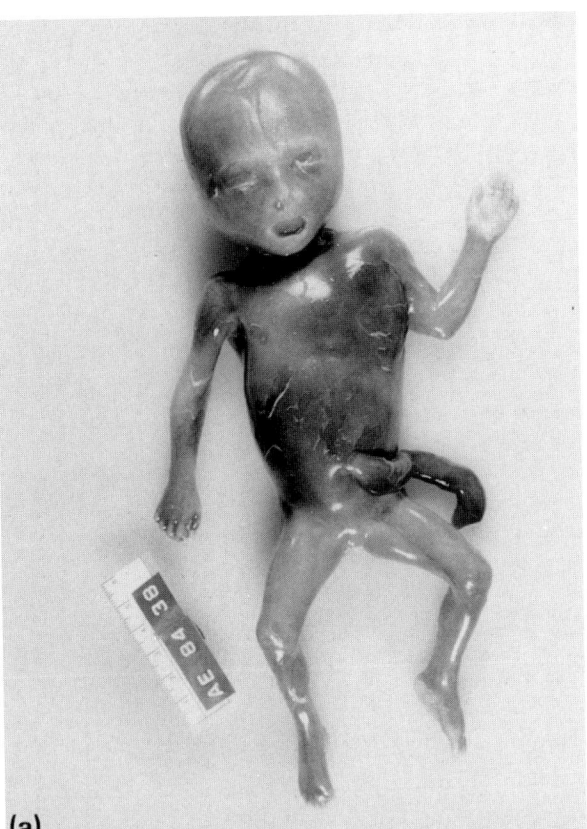

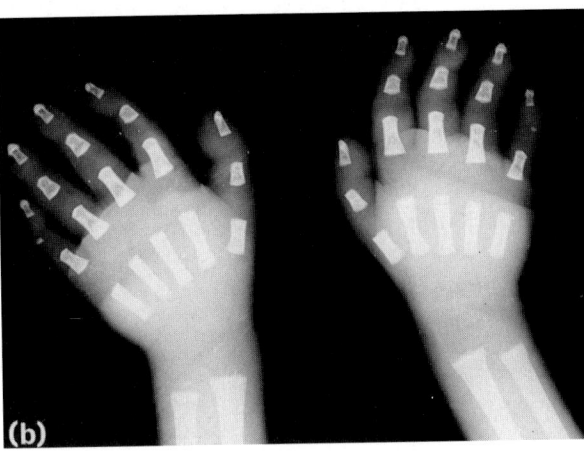

FIGURE 6.19.   (a) *Female fetus of 19 developmental weeks with trisomy 21. Note the lack of any diagnostic phenotypic features.* (b) *X-ray of hands of fetus with trisomy 21, showing hypoplasia (left) and nearly aplasia (right) of mid-phalanx of fifth finger.*

chromosomal complement of the fetus and its placenta, known as *confined placental mosaicism* (CPM). CPM can be detected prenatally in about 2% of viable human pregnancies at 10 to 12 weeks of gestation [179]. One of several pathways producing CPM is the trisomic zygote rescue. Such rescue may result in either a liveborn trisomic fetus or a diploid fetus. Whether the fetus will be trisomic or diploid depends on the cell lineage involved in the somatic loss of the extratrisomic chromosome. A diploid cell line, the product of the random loss of a trisomic chromosome, is expected to have UPD for the chromosome pair involved in the original trisomy in one-third of these cases [177, 180]. In humans, this mechanism appears to be the most common source of heterodisomy where the pair is made up of two non-recombinant homologous chromosomes. In isodisomy, the uniparental pair is a duplicate of a same chromosome. UPD may affect the prenatal or postnatal development of an individual either if the involved chromosomal pair carries imprinted DNA segment(s) or recessive disease genes. The effect of genomic imprinting will be observed in both heterodisomy or isodisomy. In cases of isodisomy, the likelihood of inheriting a severe or lethal form of recessive disease is significantly increased.

The main effect of UPD on prenatal or postnatal development is dependent on the presence of "imprinted" genes carried by the involved chromosomal pair. The term *genomic imprinting* refers to the phenomena that induce genetic marking of genes before fertilization so that they are transcriptionally silenced at one of the parental alleles in the offspring. Among the first and most general indicators of the effect of genomic imprinting were observations that both complete maternal and paternal sets of chromosomes are essential for undisturbed embryonic and fetal development in mice [181]. Neither androgenic (diploid paternal) nor gynogenic (diploid maternal) embryos could complete normal intrauterine development. Gynogenic embryos constructed by replacement of male pronucleus with female pronucleus were found to grow normally only to early somite stages with unusually small quantities of extra-embryonic placental tissue. An inverse situation was observed in androgenic embryos induced by transplantation of a male pronucleus into a zygote from which the female pronucleus had been removed. These gave rise to predominantly extra-embryonic placental tissues with severely stunted embryos.

From these experiments it was concluded that certain genes that are essential for growth of trophoblastic tissue are expressed preferentially from the paternally transmitted genome, while the maternally transmitted genome can provide all the essential genes needed for early development of the embryo proper. More specific evidence for the non-equivalence of maternal and paternal genomes came from breeding experiments using lines of mice that carried various chromosomal translocations. In appropriate crosses, it was possible to produce uniparental disomies for particular chromosomes or chromosomal regions [182]: for example, one type of cross generated fetus containing two copies of a large portion of the maternal chromosome 7 but no copies of the corresponding portion of the paternal chromosome 7. These fetuses were developmentally retarded, showed small placentas, and died in utero at mid-gestation. The converse cross, resulting in two paternal and no maternal chromosome 7 homologues, produced conceptuses that died at a much earlier stage [183]. By this approach, several differ-

ent chromosomes and subchromosomal regions were scored for their ability to produce an abnormal phenotype when they were inherited as uniparental disomies. Because only a subset of chromosomal regions showed evidence of harboring imprinted genes by this assay, these observations have allowed the assignment of "imprinted" and "non-imprinted" regions in the mouse genome [184].

Similar effects of genomic imprinting have been described in humans for the whole maternal and paternal sets of chromosomes as well as for specific chromosomal regions [180]. Complete moles, which are composed mostly of trophoblastic tissue, were found to contain solely a reduplicated paternal complement of chromosomes [185], while ovarian dermoids, which differentiate into a broad spectrum of somatic tissues but which never show placental elements, invariably contain a reduplicated complement of maternal chromosomes derived from an unfertilized oocyte [186]. The differential effect of the paternal versus the maternal genetic contribution on development has also been noted in studies of human triploidy. Human triploidy, which occurs in 1% of recognized pregnancies, is associated with two distinct placental phenotypes: partial mole and non-molar morphology [119, 120]. The development of a partial hydatidiform mole correlates highly with the paternal origin of the extra chromosome set, and non-molar morphology with the maternal one [187]. The parental origin of the extra haploid set has also been shown to have a detectable effect on the fetal phenotype. Two fetal phenotypes have been delineated: type I fetuses, associated with a large cystic placenta, have relatively normal fetal growth and microcephaly; type II fetuses, associated with small non-cystic placentas, are markedly growth retarded and have a disproportionately large head [188].

Among the clearest and best studied examples of human genetic diseases due to imprinted genes are Prader-Willi syndrome (PWS) and Angelman syndrome (AS) [106], although other genetic syndromes have also been recognized (Beckwith-Wiedemann syndrome due to segmental UPD for chromosome 11) [189, 190]. Both syndromes, PWS and AS, include mental retardation, but the associated features are entirely distinct and even to some degree opposite: individuals with PWS are overweight and slow moving, while individuals with AS are thin and hyperactive, with a characteristic "happy puppet" appearance and inappropriate laughter. Pathogenetically both syndromes often result from chromosomal deletions in bands 15q11–13, which are cytogenetically indistinguishable.

A possible role for genomic imprinting in producing the distinct phenotypes was raised when it was found that the deleted DNA in the two syndromes was of opposite parental origin: In each case of PWS the deletion had occurred on the paternal chromosome 15, while for each case of AS it had occurred on the maternal homologue. Recent high-resolution mapping of the minimal deleted regions supports a hypothesis that PWS and AS are caused by two very closely linked but distinct genes (or gene clusters which are oppositely imprinted). Additional evidence for genomic imprinting in the two syndromes was produced by the detection of PWS cases with maternal disomy for the entire chromosome 15 and AS cases with paternal disomy 15 [106].

Uniparental disomy often results from trisomic zygote rescue. The concept of trisomic zygote rescue involves the postzygotic mutation, and the end result is dependent on the cell lineage involved. When the trisomic chromosome is lost in the trophoblast, a viable non-mosaic trisomic infant is delivered [191]. When a similar mutation occurs in the embryonic progenitor cell, a diploid fetus/newborn develops supported by a trisomic placenta. One-third of these diploid fetuses/newborns, resulting from the random loss of a trisomic chromosome, are expected to have UPD for the chromosomal pair involved in the original trisomy [177, 180, 192].

In pregnancies resulting from trisomic zygote rescue, an increased rate of pregnancy complications is observed, including intrauterine fetal growth restriction, pregnancy-associated hypertension, and intrauterine fetal death [193–195]. It remains to be established whether these complications in pregnancies with a diploid fetus are due to placental trisomy or whether some of the complications are related to the presence of UPD in the fetus itself [192]. In pregnancies with a trisomic fetus, the effect of UPD in a diploid trophoblast on placental function has not yet been studied.

Microbiology Studies

Among late abortions, infections are more common than cytogenetic abnormalities or fetal morphologic defects. The infections of previable second trimester pregnancies are predominantly caused by bacteria and fungi. The most common manifestation is inflammation of the placental membranes and chorionic plate resulting from ascending vaginal organisms. Whether the infection occurs prior to rupture of the membranes or is secondary to it is not clear. Once bacteria or fungi are in the amniotic sac, they cause maternal leukocyte migration from the intervillous space toward the amniotic cavity. This leads to the loss of translucency of the membrane, which becomes creamy yellow in color. Most bacteria or fungi affect the membranes diffusely. However, candidiasis produces a characteristic nodular eruption on the umbilical cord and membranes.

Infection of the fetus from the mother by the hematogenous route requires transfer of organisms across the placental villi, that is, from the maternal intervillous space, across the trophoblast layer, and into the lumen of fetal capillaries. The villi appear to form an effective barrier to transfer of most bacteria but do not seem to hinder passage of a number of viruses. Hematogenously acquired infections are less commonly associated with pregnancy loss and/or intrauterine fetal death than ascending infections. *Chlamydia trachomatis* infections have been recorded in several preterm infants and stillbirths [196] but not in previable fetuses. On the other hand, the isolation of genital mycoplasmas in conceptuses spontaneously lost prior to 20 weeks of gestation has been described many times [197–199]. It has been illustrated on second trimester amniocentesis specimens that during pregnancy genital mycoplasmas may colonize the endometrium, fetal membranes, and amniotic fluid [200]. Also, amniotic fluids collected from patients with clinical intra-amniotic infection showed a high association with *Mycoplasma hominis* [201].

Bacteriological and viral cultures should be initiated only from selected aborted fetuses. The indication should be either fetal/placental phenotype (intrauterine growth retardation, placental lesions or fetal specific malformations, and focal lesions typical for a particular infection) or a maternal history of repeated pregnancy loss or exposure to a particular infection. The specimen must be fresh and the cultures taken into a specific media, dependent on the type of suspected infection. Viral culture samples of different tissues (brain, liver, placenta, etc.) taken under sterile conditions should be submitted and the suspected viral agent indicated.

Clinical Significance of Pathological Evaluation

Single anatomical malformations are more frequent among spontaneously aborted previable fetuses than in stillbirths or liveborn infants [42]. Their identification and accurate diagnosis provide assistance in prenatal care of future pregnancies. Six times more congenital heart defects are detected in previable fetuses than in later stillbirths and thirteen times more than in liveborn infants. Similar rates have been derived for other developmental defects (gastrointestinal, genitourinary, and musculoskeletal).

Because most single anatomical malformations are inherited in multifactorial fashion, this finding demonstrates the importance of complete examination of aborted previable fetuses for genetic counseling and for prenatal care during future pregnancies. For example, isolated cleft palate carries a recurrence risk of 4%, while cleft lip encompassing both cleft palate and lip pits is inherited in autosomal dominant fashion. Congenital heart disease of multifactorial inheritance has a recurrence risk in future pregnancies of 2–5% depending on the type of defect, but the recurrence risk for heart defect is not increased in cases of congenital heart disease associated with chromosomal defect (e.g., trisomy 13). Neural tube defects are even more heterogeneous, as these can be of multifactorial origin, caused by single gene defect (Meckel syndrome), chromosome defect (trisomy 13, 18, triploidy), or non-genetic mechanism (amniotic bands). The recurrence risk for each of these pathogenetic mechanisms significantly differs. The quality of pathological investigation determines the quality of future medical and preventive care for the couple and their relatives. When a normal fetus is aborted, the cause of the abortion may be related to uterine and/or placental abnormalities or ascending infection, not to a genetic factor. In these cases, the identification of the normally developed fetus and the determination of the non-genetic cause is important.

PREGNANCY TERMINATION FOLLOWING PRENATAL DIAGNOSIS OF FETAL ABNORMALITY

The different methods of diagnosis, varying accuracy of diagnostic techniques, and varying stages at which termination is performed may present the pathologist with specific problems or requirements.

Chorionic Villus Sampling

Pregnancy termination during the first trimester following chorion villus biopsy is done by curettage or suction, so that a mixture of fragments of embryo/fetus, chorionic sac, and decidua is received by the pathologist. A careful separation of maternal and embryonic tissues is necessary. The morphological external and internal examination of embryo/fetus is usually hampered severely because of fragmentation (Fig. 6.20). Confirmatory cytogenetic, biochemical, or DNA testing is necessary in most cases.

Amniotic Fluid Testing

The confirmation of an open neural tube defect after elevated levels of alpha-fetoprotein and acetylcholinesterase is a simple task, usually requiring only photographic and x-ray documentation plus a routine morphologic examination. A problem arises only when there is no detectable fetal neural tube defect. The most likely explanation in such cases is the presence of ultrasound-undetected twin pregnancy with fetus papyraceus. A careful examination of placentas and membranes, and a search for a partially resorbed twin fetus is necessary in such cases [202].

Pregnancy terminations of cytogenetically abnormal conceptuses can be divided into three main categories from the point of view of how much confirmatory effort they require. In the first category, no cytogenetic confirmation is required, as the morphology of the fetus is diagnostic. Into this category belong the majority of autosomal trisomies (Fig. 6.21), triploidy, sex chromosome monosomy, and some unbalanced chromosomal rearrangements. Trisomy 21 needs no confirmatory cytogenetics if dermatoglyphic abnormalities or a typical congenital heart defect (atrioventricular canal) is present. When no morphologic features allowing the diagnosis of trisomy 21 are present, such a fetus should be moved into a second category. In this category, typical cases would be sex chromosome aneuploidies, such as 47,XXY, 47,XYY, or 47,XXX. A sampling of a single tissue (amniotic membrane, chorionic villi, or muscle tendon) for initiation of culture and cytogenetic analysis of three cells is sufficient in this category for confirmation of prenatal diagnosis. The third category is represented by cases with prenatal cytogenetic diagnosis of chromosomal mosaicism. The confirmation requires a sampling of different tissues of both fetal and placental origin to establish accurately the type of the mosaicism [39, 203]. The tissues must be submitted in separate well-labeled containers to allow accurate cytogenetic evaluation of the individual tissues.

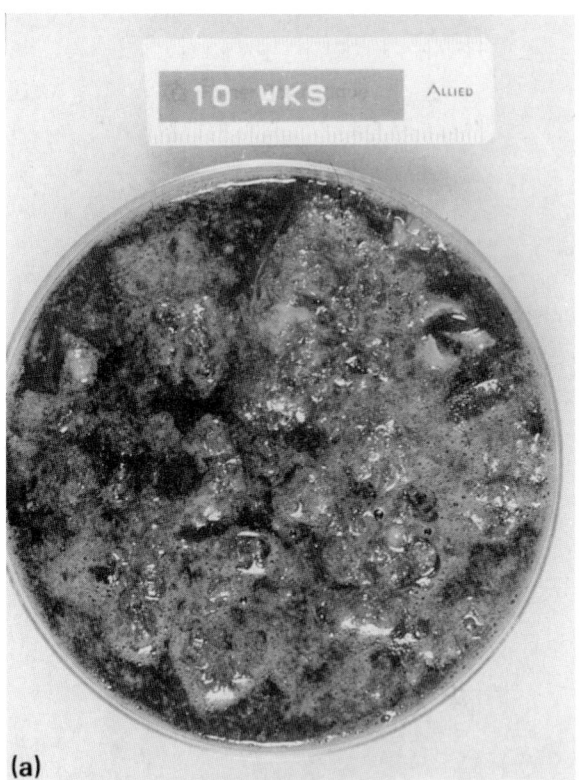

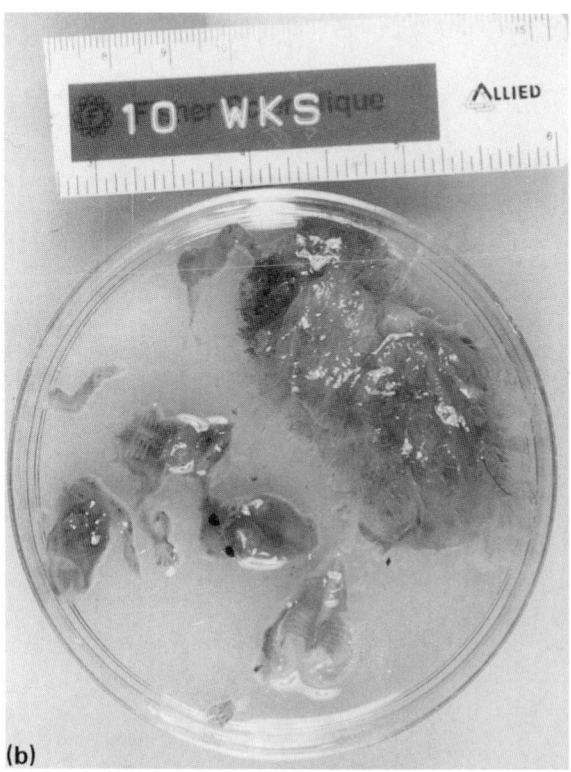

FIGURE 6.20. (a) *Pregnancy termination specimen obtained by suction. Note large amount of decidua and blood clots completely obscuring fetal parts and chorionic sac fragments.* (b) *The same specimen after removal of decidua and blood clots. Fragmented but nearly complete fetus is identified.*

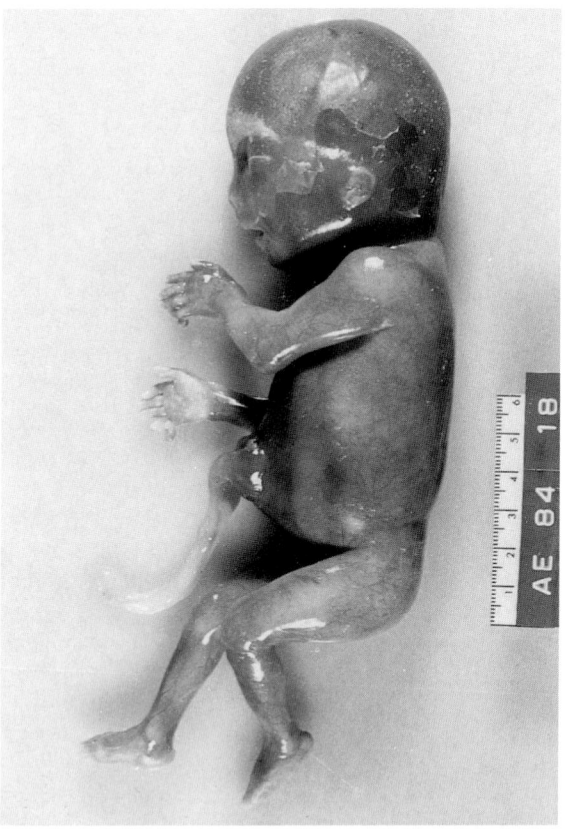

FIGURE 6.21. *Male fetus of 17 developmental weeks with trisomy 13, showing microcephaly, abnormal positioning of eyes, and bilateral postaxial polydactyly.*

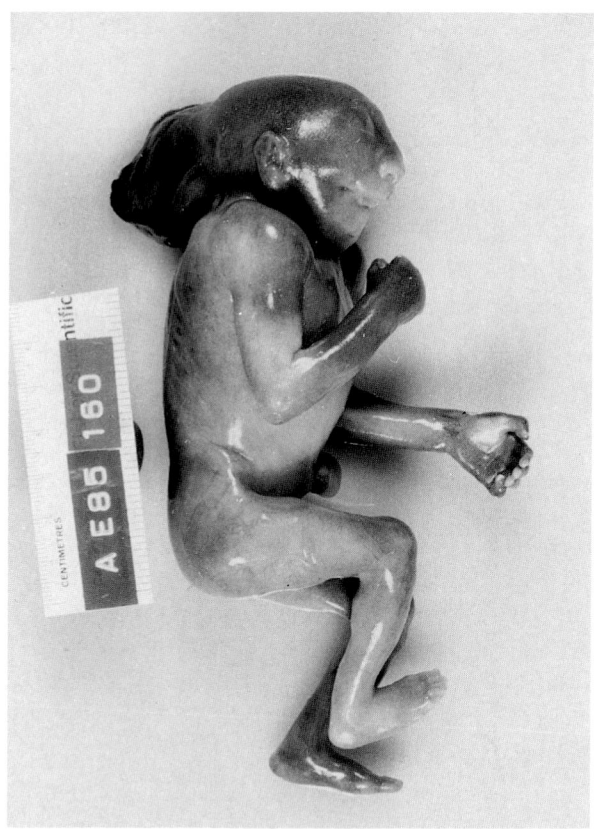

FIGURE 6.22. *Female fetus of 16 1/2 developmental weeks, with a large occipital encephalocele.*

When pregnancies are terminated because of inherited metabolic defects, it is essential that the pathologist has been informed of both the nature of the defect and the identity of the laboratory where diagnosis was made. In most cases, there is no anatomical abnormality of the fetus and confirmation of the diagnosis depends on confirmatory assays done on collected fetal tissues. Biochemical analysis of specific fetal organs or histochemical demonstration of abnormal accumulation of metabolites in tissues (e.g., Tay-Sachs disease) are helpful in some circumstances. Individual laboratories often have preferences with respect to the types of tissue, the method of freezing, and subsequent storage; therefore a consultation between the pathologist and referral biochemical laboratory should take place prior to beginning the examination. Generally, in all biochemical disorders diagnosed prenatally, repeat biochemical testing should be initiated regardless of whether the morphology contributes to the confirmation.

Some hematologic disorders such as alpha-thalassemia already have severe phenotypic presentation at 20 weeks of gestation when termination is done following direct gene analysis [204]. In such a case, morphologic diagnosis alone

is sufficient. On the other hand, in cases of sickle cell anemia or beta-thalassemia, there are no morphologic defects in second trimester fetuses, and confirmatory testing must be initiated [205].

Ultrasound Examination

Abnormalities commonly detected by this technology include defects of central nervous system (Fig. 6.22), heart, genitourinary tract, abdominal wall, bowel, and skeleton. Abnormal quantities of amniotic fluid—polyhydramnios and oligohydramnios—frequently associated with congenital abnormalities can also be detected.

In cases where pregnancy is terminated on the basis of an ultrasound-detected defect, the pathologist should be familiar with the ultrasound report and perform the examination with the aim of confirming the prenatal diagnosis. In case of any discordance, careful documentation (photo, x-ray, drawing) is necessary as well as contact and communication between the pathologist and clinician responsible for the ultrasound examination (Fig. 6.23). Apart from documenting and reporting the findings, it is also important to

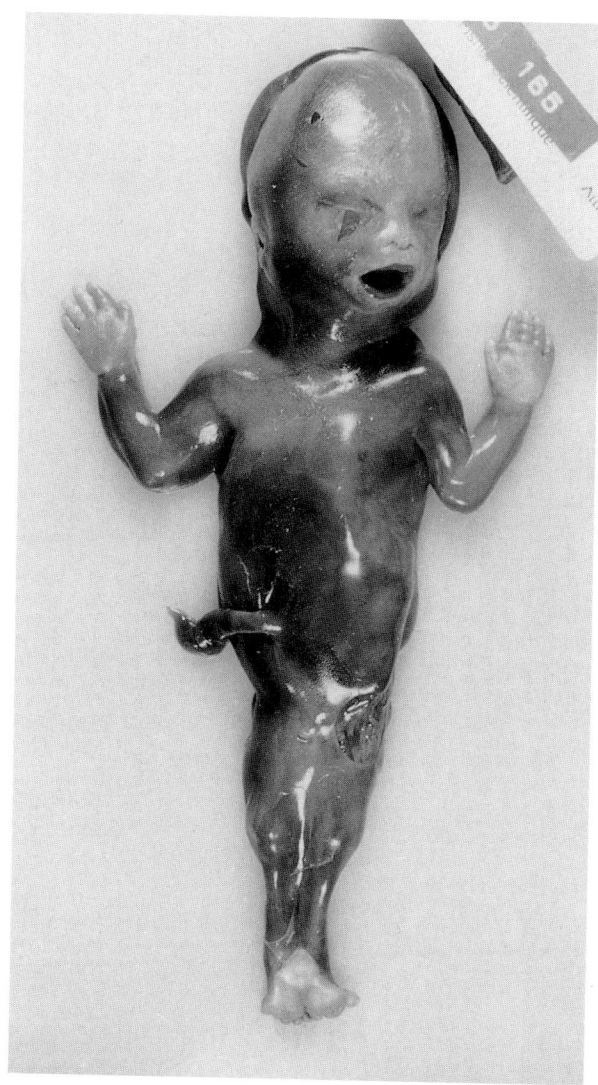

FIGURE 6.23. *Male fetus of 19 developmental weeks, with caudal regression syndrome diagnosed on ultrasound as renal agenesis.*

organize regular sessions aimed at evaluation of the results of prenatal diagnosis. These sessions should be attended by all physicians involved in prenatal diagnosis.

REFERENCES

1. Miller JF, Williamson E, Glue J, et al. Fetal loss after implantation: a prospective study. *Lancet* 1980; 2:554–6.
2. Gilbert EF, Opitz JM. Developmental and other pathologic changes in syndromes caused by chromosome abnormalities. *Perspect Pediatr Pathol* 1982; 7:1–63.
3. Jeffecote TNA, Fliegner JRH, Russell SH, Davis JC, Wade AP. Diagnosis of the adrenogenital syndrome before birth. *Lancet* 1965; 2:553.
4. Nadler HL. Antenatal detection of hereditary disorders. *Pediatrics* 1968; 42:912.
5. Valenti C, Schutta EJ, Kehaty T. Prenatal diagnosis of Down's syndrome. *Lancet* 1968; 2:220.
6. Brock DJH, Bolton AE, Monaghan JM. Prenatal diagnosis of anencephaly through maternal serum-alpha fetoprotein measurement. *Lancet* 1973; 2:923.
7. Brock DJH, Sutcliffe RG. Alpha-fetoprotein in the antenatal diagnosis of anencephaly and spina bifida. *Lancet* 1972; 2:197.
8. Garrett WJ, Robinson DE. Fetal heart size measured in vivo by ultrasound. *Pediatrics* 1970; 46:25.
9. Romero R, Pilu G, Jeanty P, Ghidini A, Hobbins JC. *Prenatal Diagnosis of Congenital Anomalies.* Norwalk, CT: Appleton & Lange, 1988.
10. Wolfson RN, Zador IE, Pillay SK, Timor-Tritsch IE, Hertz RH. Antenatal investigation of human fetal systolic time intervals. *Am J Obstet Gynecol* 1977; 129:203–9.
11. Valenti C. Endoamnioscopy and fetal biopsy: a new technique. *Am J Obstet Gynecol* 1972; 114:561–9.
12. Daffos F, Capella-Pavlovsky M, Forestier F. Fetal blood sampling via the umbilical cord using a needle guided by ultrasound. *Prenat Diagn* 1983A; 3:271.
13. Kazy Z, Rozovsky IS, Bakharev VA. Chorion biopsy in early pregnancy: a method of early prenatal diagnosis for inherited disorders. *Prenat Diagn* 1982; 2:39.
14. Smidt-Jensen S, Hahnemann N. Transabdominal fine needle biopsy from chorionic villi in the first trimester. *Prenat Diagn* 1984; 4:163.
15. Cooper DN, Schmidtke J. Diagnosis of genetic disease using recombinant DNA. *Hum Genet* 1991; 87:519–60.
16. Merkatz IR, Nitowsky HM, Macri JN, Johnson WE. An association between low maternal serum alpha-fetoprotein and fetal chromosomal abnormalities. *Am J Obstet Gynecol* 1984; 148:886.
17. Bianchi DW, Flint AF, Pizzimenti MF, Latt SA. Demonstration of fetal gene sequences in nucleated erythrocytes isolated from maternal blood. *Am J Hum Genet* 1989; 45:A252. Abstract.
18. Gray J, Pinkel D, Yu L-C, et al. Fluorescence in situ hybridization (FISH) applied to prenatal diagnosis. *Am J Hum Genet* 1988; 43:A235. Abstract.
19. Weaver DD. *Catalog of Prenatal Diagnosed Conditions,* 2nd ed. Baltimore: Johns Hopkins University Press, 1992.
20. Boué A. Le risque d'anomalies est imprévisible. In: *Médicine Prénatale: Biologie Clinique du Foetus.* Flammarion: Médicine-Sciences, 1989, pp. 212–40.
21. Bronshtein M, Blumenfeld Z. Transvaginal sonography—detection of findings suggestive of fetal chromosomal anomalies in the first and early second trimesters. *Prenat Diagn* 1992; 12:587–93.
22. Green JJ, Hobbins JC. Abdominal ultrasound examination of the first-trimester fetus. *Am J Obstet Gynecol* 1988; 159:165.
23. Report of the RCOG Working Party on Biochemical Markers and the Detection of Down's Syndrome. Royal College of Obstetricians and Gynaecologists, July 1993.
24. Wald NJ, Kennard A, Hackshaw AK. First trimester screening for Down's syndrome. *Prenat Diagn* 1995; 15:1227–40.
25. Langlois S, Wilson RD. Non-invasive prenatal fetal testing by analysis of maternal blood. *Clin Invest Med* 1993; 16:333–8.
26. Canadian Collaborative CVS-Amniocentesis Clinical Trial Group. Multicentre randomized clinical trial of chorion villus sampling and amniocentesis. *Lancet* 1989; 1:1–7.
27. Medical Research Council European Trial of Chorion Villus Sampling. *Lancet* 1991; 337:1491–9.
28. Rhoades GG, Jackson LG, Schlesselman SE, et al. The safety and efficacy of chorionic villus sampling for early prenatal diagnosis of cytogenetic abnormalities. *N Eng J Med* 1989; 320:611–7.
29. Cashner KA, Christopher CR, Dysert GA. Spontaneous fetal loss after demonstration of a live fetus in the first trimester. *Obstet Gynecol* 1987; 70:827–30.
30. Gilmore DH, McNay MB. Spontaneous fetal loss rate in early pregnancy. *Lancet* 1985; 1:107.
31. Wilson RD, Kendrick V, Wittmann BK, McGillivray BC. Risk of spontaneous abortion in ultrasonically normal pregnancies. Lancet 1984; 2:920–1.
32. Orlandi F, Damiani G, Jakil C, et al. The risks of early cordocentesis (12–21 weeks): analysis of 500 procedures. *Prenat Diagn* 1990; 10:425–8.
33. Daffos F. Access to the fetus. *Nouv Rev Fr Hematol* 1990; 32:431.
34. Wilson RD, Farquharson DF, Wittmann BK, Shaw D. Cordocentesis: overall pregnancy loss rate as important as procedure loss rate. *Fetal Diagn Ther* 1994; 9:142–8.
35. Quintero RA, Abuhamad A, Hobbins JC, Mahoney MJ. Transabdominal thin-gauge embryofetoscopy: a technique for early prenatal diagnosis and its use in the diagnosis of a case of Meckel-Gruber syndrome. *Am J Obstet Gynecol* 1993; 168:1552–7.
36. Golbus MS, Berry LC Jr. Human fetal development between 90 and 170 days post menses. *Teratology* 1977; 15:103–8.

37. Spranger J, Benirschke K, Hall JG, et al. Errors in morphogenesis: concepts and terms. Recommendations of an International Working Group. *J Pediatr* 1982; 100:160–5.

38. Rubin GL, Peterson HB, Dorfman SF, et al. Ectopic pregnancy in the United States, 1970 through 1978. *JAMA* 1983; 249:1725–9.

39. Kalousek DK, Barrett IJ. Placental mosaicism and stillbirth. *Pediatr Pathol* 1994; 14:151–9.

40. Kalousek DK, Dill FJ. Chromosome mosaicism confined to the placenta in human conceptions. *Science* 1982; 221:665–7.

41. Fujikura T, Froehlich LA, Driscoll SG. A simplified anatomic classification of abortions. *Am J Obstet Gynecol* 1966; 95:902–5.

42. Poland BJ, Miller JR, Harris M, Livingston J. Spontaneous abortion: a study of 1961 women and their conceptuses. *Acta Obstet Gynecol Scand* 1981; 102(suppl):5–32.

43. Rushton DI. The classification and mechanisms of spontaneous abortion. *Perspect Pediatr Pathol* 1984; 8:269–86.

44. Glass RH, Golbus MS. Pregnancy wastage: habitual abortion. In: Creasy RK, Resnik R, eds. *Maternal-Fetal Medicine: Principles and Practice*. Philadelphia: Saunders, 1984, pp. 385–94.

45. Wilcox AJ, Horney LF. Accuracy of spontaneous abortion recall. *Am J Epidemiol* 1984; 120:727–33.

46. French FE, Bierman JM. Probabilities of fetal mortality. *Public Health Rep* 1962; 77:835–47.

47. Shapiro S, Bross D. Risk factors for fetal death in studies of vital statistics data: inference and limitations. In Porter IH, Hook EB, eds. *Human Embryonic and Fetal Death*. New York: Academic Press, 1980, pp. 89–105.

48. Shapiro S, Levin HS, Abramovicz M. Factors associated with early and late fetal loss. In: *Advances in Planned Parenthood*, vol. 6th ed. Amsterdam: Excerpta Medica, 1970, pp. 45–63.

49. Wilcox AJ, Weinberg CR, Wehmann RE, et al. Measuring early pregnancy loss: laboratory and field methods. *Fertil Steril.* 1985; 44:336–74.

50. Yerushalmy J, Bierman JM, Kemp D, Connor A, French FE. Longitudinal studies of pregnancy on the island of Kauai: analysis of previous reproductive

51. Alpin JD. Implantation, trophoblast differentiation and hemochorial placentation: mechanistic evidence in vivo and in vitro. *J Cell Sci* 1991; 99:681–99.

52. Christiaens GCML, Stoutenbeek P. Spontaneous abortion in proven intact pregnancies. *Lancet* 1984; 2:571–2.

53. Gustavii B. Chorionic biopsy and miscarriage in the first trimester. *Lancet* 1984; 2:562.

54. Lind T, McFadyen JR. Human pregnancy failure. *Lancet* 1986; 1:91–2.

55. Harlap S, Shiono PH, Ramcharan S. A life table of spontaneous abortions and the effects of age, parity and other variables. In: Porter IH, Hook EB, eds. *Human Embryonic and Fetal Death*. New York: Academic Press, 1980, pp. 145–58.

56. Hertig AT, Rock J, Adams EC, Menkin MC. Thirty-four fertilized human ova, good, bad and indifferent, recovered from 210 women of known fertility. *Pediatrics* 1952; 23:202–11.

57. Kline J, Stein Z. Very early pregnancy. In: Dixon RL, ed. *Reproductive Toxicology*. New York: Raven, 1985, pp. 251–65.

58. Edwards RG, Craft I. Development of assisted conception. In: Edwards RG, ed. Assisted human conception. *Br Med Bull* 1990; 46:565–79.

59. Yovich JL. Embryo quality and pregnancy rates in in-vitro fertilization. *Lancet* 1985; 1:283–4.

60. Edmonds DK, Lindsay KS, Miller JF, Williamson E, Wood PJ. Early embryonic mortality in women. *Fertil Steril* 1982; 38:447–53.

61. Roberts CJ, Lowe CR. Where have all the conceptions gone? *Lancet* 1975; 1:498–9.

62. Curran WJ. Dangers for pregnant women in the work place. *N Engl J Med* 1985; 312:164–5.

63. Hook EB. Human chromosomal abnormalities. In: Bracken MB, ed. *Perinatal Epidemiology*. New York: Oxford University Press, 1984, pp. 10–22.

64. Kline J, Stein Z. Spontaneous abortion (miscarriage). In: Bracken MB, ed. *Perinatal Epidemiology*. New York: Oxford University Press, 1984, pp. 23–51.

65. Stein Z, Kline J, Susser E, et al. Maternal age and spontaneous abortion. In: Porter IH, Hook EB, eds. *Human Embryonic and Fetal Death*. New York: Academic Press, 1980, pp. 107–27.

66. Driscoll SG. Early reproductive wastage. Course on Gynecological and Obstetric Pathology, Harvard Medical School, 1983.

67. Gruenwald P. Fetal deprivation and placental pathology: concepts and relationships. *Perspect Pediatr Pathol* 1975; 2:101–49.

68. Jacobs P, Hassold T. Chromosome abnormalities: origin and etiology in abortions and livebirths. In: Vogel F, Sperling K, eds. *Human Genetics*. Berlin: Springer-Verlag, 1987, pp. 233–44.

69. Klein JO, Remington JS, Marcy SM. Current concepts of infections of the fetus and newborn infant. In: Remington JS, Klein JO, eds. *Infectious Diseases of the Fetus and Newborn Infant*. Philadelphia: Saunders, 1983, pp. 1–26.

70. Campognone P, Singer DB. Neonatal sepsis due to nontypable *Haemophilus influenzae*. *Am J Dis Child* 1986; 140:117–21.

71. Robertson WB, Brosens I, Dixon HG. The pathological response of the vessels of the placental bed to hypertensive pregnancy. *J Pathol Bacteriol* 1967; 93:581–92.

72. Kitzmiller JL, Benirschke K. Immunofluorescent study of placental bed vessels in pre-eclampsia of pregnancy. *Am J Obstet Gynecol* 1973; 115:248–51.

73. DeWolf F, Carreras LO, Moerman P, et al. Decidual vasculopathy and extensive placental infarction in a patient with repeated thromboembolic accidents, recurrent fetal loss, and a lupus anticoagulant. *Am J Obstet Gynecol* 1982; 142:829–34.

74. Scott JR, Rote WS, Branch DW. Immunologic aspects of recurrent abortion and fetal death. *Obstet Gynecol* 1987; 70:645–56.

75. Harris EN, Spinnato JA. Should anticardio-lipidin tests be performed in otherwise health pregnant women. *Am J Obstet Gynecol* 1991; 165:1272–7.

76. Fox H. *Pathology of the Placenta*. Philadelphia: Saunders, 1979, pp. 337–8.

77. Gruenwald P. Decidual sloughing in abortion, premature birth, and abruptio placentae. *Bull Johns Hopkins Hosp* 1965; 116:363.

78. Hutchison AA, Drew JH, Yu VYH, et al. Nonimmunologic hydrops fetalis: a review of 61 cases. *Obstet Gynecol* 1982; 59:347–52.

79. Bowman JM, Lewis M, deSa DJ. Hydrops fetalis caused by massive maternofetal transplacental hemorrhage. *J Pediatr* 1984; 104:769–72.

80. Mowbray JF, Underwood JL, Michel M, et al. Immunisation with paternal lymphocytes in women with recurrent miscarriage. *Lancet* 1987; 2:679–80.

81. Kovats S, Main EK, Librach C, et al: A class I antigen HLA-G expressed in human trophoblasts. *Science* 1990; 735:220–5.

82. Stein Z, Susser M, Saenger G, Marolla F. *Famine and Human Development: The Dutch Hunger Winter of 1944–45*. New York: Oxford University Press, 1975.

83. Brasel JA. Cellular changes in intrauterine malnutrition. In: Winick M, ed. *Nutrition and Fetal Development*. New York: John Wiley & Sons, 1974, pp. 13–25.

84. Czeizel AE, Dudas I. Prevention of the first occurrence of neural tube defects by periconceptual vitamin supplementation. *N Eng J Med* 1992; 327:1832–5.

85. MRC Vitamin Study Research Group. Prevention of neural tube defects: results of the Medical Research Council Vitamin Study. *Lancet* 1991; 338:131–7.

86. Smithells RW, Sheppard S, Schorah CJ, et al. Apparent prevention of neural tube defects by periconceptional vitamin supplementation. *Arch Dis Child* 1981; 56:911–8.

87. Naeye RL. Disorders of the placenta, fetus and neonate. In: *Diagnosis and Clinical Significance*. Mosby St. Louis Mosby-Year Book, 1992.

88. Shepard TH. *Catalog of Teratogenic Agents*, 7th ed. Baltimore: The Johns Hopkins University Press, 1992.

89. Taussig HB. A study of the German outbreak of phocomelia: the thalidomide syndrome. *JAMA* 1962; 180:1106–14.

90. Heinonen OP, Shone D, Shapiro S. *Birth Defects and Drugs in Pregnancy*. Littleton, MA: John Wright-PSG, 1983.

91. Quirk JG. Use and misuse of drugs in pregnancy. In: Fabro S, Scialli A, eds. *Drug and Chemical Action in Pregnancy: Pharmacologic and Toxicologic Principles*. New York: Marcel Dekker, 1986, pp. 477–510.

92. Robinson HB, Tross K. Agenesis of the cloacal membrane: a probable teratogenic anomaly. *Perspect Pediatr Pathol*. 1984; 8:79–96.

93. Koren G. *Maternal-Fetal Toxicology: A Clinicians Guide*. New York: Marcel Dekker, 1990.

94. Martinez-Frias ML. Epidemiological analysis of outcomes of pregnancy in diabetic mothers: identification of the most characteristic and most frequent congenital anomalies. *Am J Med Genet* 1994; 51:108–13.

95. Donaldson JO. Neurologic disorders of pregnancy. In: Reece AE, Hobbins JC, Mahoney MJ, Petrie RH eds. *Medicine of the Fetus and Mother*. Philadelphia: Lippincott, 1992, pp. 1097–1102.

96. Fairlie FM, Sibai BM. Hypertensive diseases in pregnancy. In: Reece AE, Hobbins JC, Mahoney MJ, Petrie RH, eds. *Medicine of the Fetus and Mother*. Philadelphia: Lippincott, 1992, pp. 925–42.

97. Mattison DR, Jelovsek FR. Risk assessment for developmental toxicity: effects of drugs and chemicals on the fetus. In: Reece AE, Hobbins JC, Mahoney MJ, Petrie PH, eds. *Medicine of the Fetus and Mother*. Philadelphia: Lippincott, 1992, pp. 328–41.

98. Chasnoff IJ, Landress HJ, Barrett ME. The prevalence of illicit-drug or alcohol use during pregnancy and discrepancies in mandatory reporting in Pinellas County, Florida. *N Engl J Med* 1990; 322:1202–10.

99. Harlap S, Shiono PH. Alcohol, smoking, and incidence of spontaneous abortions in the first and second trimesters. *Lancet* 1980; ii:173–6.

100. Keibel F, Mall FP, eds. *Manual of Human Embryology*, Vol. I, II. Philadelphia/London: Lippincott, 1910–1912.

101. Mall FP. On stages in the development of human embryos from 2 to 25 mm long. *Anat Anz* 1914; 46:78–84.

102. O'Rahilly R, Muller F. Developmental stages in human embryos. Washington, DC: Carnegie Institution of Washington, 1987.

103. Streeter GL. *Developmental Horizons in Human Embryos*. Washington: Carnegie Institute of Embryology, 1951.

104. Markert CL, Petters RM. Manufactured hexaparental mice show that adults are derived from three embryonic cells. *Science* 1978; 202:56–8.

105. Kalousek DK. Confined chorionic mosaicism in human gestations. In: Fraccaro M, Simoni B, Brambati B, eds. *First Trimester Fetal Diagnosis*. Berlin: Springer, 1985, pp. 130–6.

106. Kalousek DK, Barrett I. Genomic imprinting related to prenatal diagnosis. *Prenat Diagn* 1995; 14:1191–201.

107. Crowley LV. *An Introduction to Clinical Embryology*. Chicago: Year Book Medical Publishers, 1974.

108. Hamilton WJ, Boyd JD, Mossman MW. *Human Embryology*, 4th ed. Baltimore: Williams & Wilkins, 1978.

109. Shepard TM, Fantel AG. Embryonic and early fetal loss. In: Warshaw JB, ed. *Clinics in Perinatology*. Philadelphia: Saunders, 1979, pp. 219–43.

110. Rushton DI. Examination of products of conception from previable human pregnancies. *J Clin Pathol* 1981; 34:819–35.

111. Mall FP. On measuring human embryos. *Anat Rec* 1907; 6:129–40.

112. Mall FP. A study of the causes underlying the origin of human monsters. *J Morphol* 1908; 19:3–368.

113. Mall FP. On the frequency of localized anomalies in human embryos and infants at birth. *Am J Anat* 1917; 22:49–72.

114. Hertig AT, Rock J. A series of potentially abortive ova recovered from fertile women prior to the first missed menstrual period. *Am J Obstet Gynecol* 1949; 58:968–93.

115. Kajii T, Ferrier A, Niikawa N, et al. Anatomic and chromosomal anomalies in 639 spontaneous abortuses. *Hum Genet* 1980; 55:87–98.

116. Nishimura M, Takano K, Tanimura T, Yasuda M. Normal and abnormal development of human embryos. *Teratology* 1968; 1:281–90.

117. Bracken MB, Brinton LA, Hayashi K. Epidemiology of hydatidiform mole and choriocarcinoma. *Epidemiol Rev* 1984; 6:52–75.

118. Kajii T, Kurashige M, Ohama K, Uchino F. XY and XX complete moles: clinical and morphological correlation. *Am J Obstet Gynecol* 1984; 150:57–64.

119. Szulman AE, Surti U. The syndromes of hydatidiform mole. II. Morphologic evolution of the complete and partial mole. *Am J Obstet Gynecol* 1978; 132:20–7.

120. Szulman AE, Surti U. The clinicopathologic profile of the partial hydatidiform mole. *Obstet Gynecol* 1982; 59:597–602.

121. Kajii T, Ohama K. Androgenetic origin of hydatidiform mole. *Nature* 1977; 268:633–4.

122. Ohama K, Kajii T, Okamoto E: Dispermic origin of XY hydatidiform moles. *Nature* 1981; 292:551–2.

123. Davis JR, Surwit EA, Garay JP, Fortier KJ. Sex assignment in gestational trophoblastic neoplasia. *Am J Obstet Gynecol* 1984; 148:722–5.

124. Fisher AR, Lawler SD. Heterozygous complete hydatidiform moles: do they have a worse prognosis than homozygous complete moles? *Lancet* 1984; 2:51.

125. Hunt PA, Jacobs PA, Szulman AE. Molar pregnancies and nonmolar triploids: results of a 7-year cytogenetic study. *Am J Hum Genet* 1983; 35:135A. Abstract.

126. Lawler SD, Fisher A, Pickthall JV, Povey S, Evans WM. Genetic studies on hydatidiform moles: the origin of partial moles. *Cancer Genet Cytogenet* 1982; 5:309–20.

127. Stone M, Bagshawe KD. Hydatidiform mole: two entities. *Lancet* 1976; 1:535–6.

128. Warburton D, Byrne J, Caulir N. *Chromosome anomalies and prenatal development: An Atlas*. Oxford: Oxford Monographies on Medical Genetics, Oxford University Press, 1991.

129. Herrington CS, McGee J O'D. Interphase cytogenetics. *Neurochem Res* 1990; 15:467–74.

130. Phillips C, Meadows L, Hebert M, et al. Screening for chromosome abnormalities by fluorescent in situ hybridization: application to human spontaneous abortions. *Am J Hum Genet* 1992; 51:A11. Abstract.

131. Alvarado M, Harold NB, Caldwell S, et al. Miller-Dieker syndrome: detection of a cryptic chromosome translocation using in situ hybridization in a family with multiple affected offspring. *Am J Dis Child* 1993; 147:1291–4.

132. Harrison KJ, Barrett IJ, Lomas BL, Kuchinka BD, Kalousek DK. Detection of confined placental mosaicism in trisomy 18 conceptions using interphase cytogenetic analysis. *Hum Genet* 1993; 92:353–8.

133. Lomax B, Kalousek D, Kuchinka B, et al. The utilization of interphase cytogenetic analysis for the detection of mosaicism. *Hum Genet* 1994; 93:243–7.

134. Rogers BB, Singer DB, Mak SK, et al. Detection of human parvovirus B19 in early spontaneous abortuses using serology, histology, electron microscopy, in situ hybridization, and the polymerase chain reaction. *Obstet Gynecol* 1993; 81:402–8.

135. Grumbach A, ed. *Pranatale Infektionen in Bibliotheca Microbiologica*, Fasc. I. Basel/New York: Karger, 1960.

136. Schachter J. Chlamydial infection. *N Engl J Med* 1978; 298:490–5.

137. Stray-Pedersen B, Eng J, Reikvam TM. Uterine T-mycoplasma colonization in reproductive failure. *Am J Obstet Gynecol* 1978; 130:307–11.

138. Quim PA, Shewchuk AB, Shuber J, et al. Efficacy of antibiotic therapy in preventing spontaneous pregnancy loss among couples colonized with genital mycoplasma. *Am J Obstet Gynecol* 1983; 145:239–44.

139. Taylor-Robinson D, McCormack MW. The genital mycoplasmas. *N Eng J Med* 1980; 302:1003–10, 1063–7.

140. Clyde WA Jr. Mycoplasma species identification based upon growth inhibition by specific antisera. *J Immunol* 1964; 9:958–64.

141. Nishimura H. Prenatal versus postnatal malformations based on the Japanese experience on induced abortions in the human being. In: Blandon RJ, eds. *Ageing Gametes, Their Biology and Pathology*. Basel: Karger, 1975, pp. 349–68.

142. Nishimura H, Takano K, Tamimura T. High incidence of several malformations in the early human embryo as compared with infants. *Biol Neonate* 1966; 10:93–105.

143. Hassold JT. Cytogenetic study of repeated spontaneous abortion. *Am J Hum Genet* 1980; 32:723–30.

144. Moore KL, Persaud TVN. *The Developing Human: Clinically Oriented Embryology*, 5th ed. Philadelphia: Saunders, 1993.

145. Moore KL, Persaud TVN, Shiota K. *Color Atlas of Clinical Embryology*. Philadelphia: Saunders, 1994.

146. Fantel AG, Shepard TH, Vadheim-Roth C, Stephens TD, Coleman C. Embryonic and fetal phenotypes: prevalence and other associated factors in a large study of spontaneous abortion. In: Porter IH, Hook EB, eds. *Human Embryonic and Fetal Death*. New York: Academic Press, 1980, pp. 71–86.

147. Kalousek DK, Bamforth S. Amniotic bands and ADAM sequence in previable fetuses. *Am J Med Genet* 1988; 31:63–73.

148. Kalousek DK, Fitch N, Paradice B. *Pathology of the Human Embryo and Previable Fetus*. New York: Springer Verlag, 1990.

149. Berry CL. The examination of embryonic and fetal material in diagnostic histopathology laboratories. *J Clin Pathol* 1980; 33:317–26.

150. Tanimura T, Nelson T, Hollingsworth RR, Shepard TH. Weight standards for organs from early human fetuses. *Anat Rec* 1971;171:226–36.

151. Isaacson G. Postmortem examination of infant brains: techniques for removal, fixation and sectioning. *Arch Pathol Lab Med* 1984; 108:80–1.

152. Marin-Padilla M. Cephalic axial skeletal neural dysraphic disorders: embryology and pathology. *Can J Neurol Sci* 1991; 18:153–95.

153. Campbell LR, DH Dayton, Sohal GS. Neural tube defects: a review of human and animal studies on the etiology of neural tube defects. *Teratology* 1986; 34:171–87.

154. Laurence KM. The genetics and prevention of neural tube defects and "uncomplicated" hydrocephalus. In: Emery AEH, Rimoin DL, eds. *Principles and Practice of Medical Genetics*, 2nd ed. Edinburgh: Churchill Livingstone, 1990, pp. 323–46.

155. Copp AJ. Genetic models of mammalian neural tube defects. In: *Neural Tube Defects*. Ciba Foundation Symposium, Vol. 181. Chichester: John Wiley & Sons, pp. 118–35.

156. Emery AEH. Multifactorial inheritance. In: *Methodology in Medical Genetics*, 2nd ed. Edinburgh: Churchill Livingstone, pp. 55–66.

157. Thompson MW, McInnes RR, Willard HR. *Thompson & Thompson, Genetics in Medicine*, 5th ed. Philadelphia: Saunders, 1991.

158. Milunsky A, Jick H, Jick SS, et al. Multivitamin/folic acid supplementation in early pregnancy reduces the prevalence of neural tube defects. *JAMA* 1989; 262:2847–52.

159. Wald N, Sneddon J, Densem J, et al. MRC Vitamin Study Research Group. Prevention of neural tube defects: results of the medical research council vitamin study. *Lancet* 1991; 338:131–7.

160. Kalousek DK, Seller MJ. A characteristic and constant phenotype of 45,X previable fetuses. *Am J Med Genet* 1987; 3:(suppl)83–92.

161. Ville Y, Lalondrelle C, Doumerc S, et al. First-trimester diagnosis of nuchal anomalies: significance and fetal outcome. *Ultrasound Obstet Gynecol* 1992; 2:314–6.

162. van Zalen-Sprock RM, van Vugt JMG, van Geijn HP. First trimester diagnosis of cystic hygroma—course and outcome. *Am J Obstet Gynecol* 1992; 167:94–8.

163. Wilson RD, Venir N, Farquharson DF. Fetal nuchal fluid—physiological or pathological?—in pregnancies less than 17 menstrual weeks. *Prenat Diagn* 1992; 12:755–63.

164. Nicolaides KH, Rodeck CH, Gosden CM. Rapid karyotyping in non-lethal fetal malformations. *Lancet* 1986; i:283–7.

165. Johnson MP, Bukowski TP, Reitleman C, et al. In utero surgical treatment of fetal obstructive uropathy: a new comprehensive approach to identify appropriate candidates for vesicoamniotic shunt therapy. *Am J Obstet Gynecol* 1994; 170:1770–9.

166. Harrison MR, Filly RA. The fetus with obstructive uropathy: pathophysiology, natural history, selection, and treatment. In: Harrison MR, Golbus MS, Filly RA, eds. *The Unborn Patient*, 2nd ed. Philadelphia: Saunders, 1990, pp. 329–44.

167. Nicolaides KH, Cheng HH, Snijders RJM, Moriz CF. Fetal urine biochemistry in the assessment of obstructive uropathy. *Am J Obstet Gynecol* 1992; 166:932–7.

168. Nicolini U, Tannirandorn Y, Vaughan J, et al. Further predictors of renal dysplasia in fetal obstructive uropathy: bladder pressure and biochemistry of "fresh" urine. *Prenat Diagn* 1991; 11:159–66.

169. Vintzileos AM, Eisenfeld LI, Herson VC, et al. Megacystis-microcolon-intestinal hypoperistalsis syndrome—prenatal sonographic findings and review of the literature. *Am J Perinatol* 1986; 3:297–315.

170. Carr DH, Gedeon M. Population cytogenetics of human abortuses. In Hook EB, Porter IH eds. *Population Cytogenetics*. New York: Academic Press, 1977, pp. 1–9.

170. Singh RP, Carr DM. The anatomy and histology of human XO fetuses. *Anat Rec* 1996; 155:869–83.

172. Chervenak FA, Isaacson G, Blackmore K, et al. Fetal cystic hygroma: cause and natural history. *New Engl J Med* 1983; 309:822–5.

173. Shulman LP, Emerson DS, Felker RE, et al. High frequency of cytogenetic abnormalities in fetuses with cystic hygroma diagnosed in the first trimester. *Obstet Gynecol* 1992; 80:80–2.

174. Niebuhr E. Triploidy in man: cytogenetical and clinical aspects. *Hum Genet* 1974; 21:103–25.

175. Stanley WS, Khan T. Use of short-term thymocyte suspension culture for chromosome analysis following fetal, neonatal and childhood death. *Am J Hum Genet* 1985; 38:119A. Abstract.

176. Chen M, Yu CW, Mulhern R, Fowler M, Al Saadi A. Chromosome preparations of chondrocytes cultured from human cartilages. *Am J Med Genet* 1980; 6:179–81.

177. Engel E, De Lozier-Blanchet CD. Uniparental disomy, isodisomy and imprinting: probable effects in man and strategies for their detection. *Am J Med Genet* 1991; 40:432–9.

178. Spence EJ, Perciaceante RG, Greig GM, et al. Uniparental disomy as a mechanism for human genetic disease. *Am J Hum Genet* 1988; 42:217–26.

179. Ledbetter DH, Zachary JM, Simpson JL, et al. Cytogenetic results from the U.S. collaborative study on CVS. *Prenat Diagn* 1992; 12:317–54.

180. Hall JG. Genomic imprinting: review and relevance to human diseases. *Am J Hum Genet* 1990; 46:857–73.

181. Surani MAH, Barton SC, Norris ML. Development of reconstituted mouse eggs suggests imprinting of the genome during gametogenesis. *Nature* 1984; 308:548–50.

182. Searle AG, Beechey CV. Genome imprinting phenomena on mouse chromosome 7. *Genet Res* 1990; 56:237–44.

183. Ferguson-Smith AC, Cattanach BM, Barton SC, et al. Embryological and molecular investigations of parental imprinting on mouse chromosome 7. *Nature* 1991; 351:667–70.

184. Searle AG, Peters J, Lyon MF, et al. Chromosome maps of men and mouse. *Am Hum Genet* 1989; 53:89–140.

185. Lawler SD, Povey S, Fisher RA, et al. Genetic studies on hydatidiform moles. II. The origin of complete moles. *Ann Hum Genet* 1982; 46:209–22.

186. Linder D, McCaw BK, Hecht F. Parthenogenic origin of benign ovarian teratomas. *N Engl J Med* 1975; 292:63–6.

187. Jacobs PA, Szulman AE, Funkhouser J. Human triploidy: relationship between parental origin of the additional haploid complement and development of partial hydatidiform mole. *Ann Hum Genet* 1982; 46:223–31.

188. McFadden DE, Kalousek DK. Two different phenotypes of fetuses with chromosomal triploidy: correlation with parental origin of the extra haploid set. *Am J Med Genet* 1991; 38:535–8.

189. Henry I, Puech A, Rieswijk A, et al. Somatic mosaicism for partial paternal isodisomy in Wiedemann-Beckwith syndrome: a poststerilization event. *Eur J Hum Genet* 1993; 1:19–29.

190. Henry I, Bonaiti-Pellie C, Chehensse V, et al. Uniparental paternal disomy in a genetic cancer-predisposing syndrome. *Nature* 1991; 351:665–67.

191. Kalousek DK, Barrett IJ, McGillivray BC. Placental mosaicism and intrauterine survival of trisomies 13 and 18. *Am J Hum Genet* 1989; 44:338–43.

192. Kalousek DK, Langlois S, Barrett I, et al. Uniparental disomy for chromosome 16 in humans. *Am J Hum Genet* 1993; 52:8–16.

193. Johnson A, Wagner RJ, Davis GH, Jackson LG. Mosaicism in chorionic villus sampling: an association with poor perinatal outcome. *Obstet Gynecol* 1990; 75:573–7.

194. Langlois S, Wilson RD, Yong SL, Kalousek DK. Prenatal and postnatal growth failure associated with maternal heterodisomy for chromosome 7. Presented at the seventh International Conference on Early Prenatal Diagnosis, Jerusalem, Israel, 1994, A19.

195. Leschot NJ, Wolf H. Is placental mosaicism associated with poor perinatal outcome? *Prenat Diagn* 1991; 11:403–4.

196. Martin DH, Koutsky L, Eschenbach DA, et al. Prematurity and perinatal mortality in pregnancies complicated by maternal chlamydia trachomatis infections. *JAMA* 1982; 247:1585–8.

197. Dische RM, Quinn PA, Czegledy-Nagy E, Sturgess JM. Genital mycoplasma infection. *Am J Clin Pathol* 1972; 72:167–74.

198. Friberg J. Mycoplasmas and ureaplasmas in infertility and abortion. *Fertil Steril* 1980; 33:351–9.

199. Sompolinsky D, Solomon F, Elkina L, et al. Infections with mycoplasma and bacteria in induced midtrimester abortion and fetal loss. *Am J Obstet Gynecol* 1975; 121:610–6.

200. Cassell GM, Davis OR, Waites KB, et al. Isolation of *Mycoplasma hominis* and *Ureaplasma urealyticum* from amniotic fluid at 16–20 weeks of gestation. *Sex Transm Dis* 1983; 10:294–302.

201. Blanco JD, Gibbs RS, Malherbe H, et al. A controlled study of genital mycoplasmas in amniotic fluid from patients with intra-amniotic infection. *J Infect Dis* 1983; 147:650–3.

202. Baldwin VJ. *Pathology of Multiple Pregnancies*. New York: Springer-Verlag, 1994.

203. Kalousek DK, Dill FS, Pantzar T, et al. Confined chorionic mosaicisms in prenatal diagnosis. *Hum Genet* 1987; 77:163–7.

204. Kan YW, Lee KY, Forbetta M, Angus A, Coa A. Polymorphism of DNA sequence in globlin gene region: application to prenatal diagnosis of thalassaemia in Sardinia. *N Engl J Med* 1980; 302:185–8.

205. Blanche P. Advances in the prenatal diagnosis of hematologic diseases. *Blood* 1984; 64:329–49.

Pathology of Placenta

D. Ian Rushton

INTRODUCTION

The role of the placenta in the causation of perinatal mortality and morbidity remains uncertain in the majority of compromised babies. While increasingly sophisticated techniques are being used by the obstetrician to assess fetal well-being in utero at all stages of pregnancy, including labor, correlating the results of these investigations with morphological variations in the placenta has been difficult if not impossible. Immunohistochemical techniques, while often of theoretical interest, have yet to find a role in the routine examination of the placenta. The range of these clinical investigations is subject to continuous review, and as some are discarded others appear.

Fetal scalp blood sampling, the biochemistry of amniotic fluid, ultrasonic visualization of the fetus and placenta, the assessment of fetal and placental blood flow using Doppler methods, and the biochemical assessment of the status of the fetoplacental unit are or have been commonplace in the management of pregnancy in modern maternity units, though not without hazard [1, 2]. The introduction of these investigative procedures has necessitated a reappraisal of the importance of the placenta by clinician and pathologist alike. The placenta is no longer the universal scapegoat for unexplained perinatal death. This benefits both clinician and pathologist. For the former, it is a stimulus to use modern technology to study normal as well as abnormal pregnancies in an attempt to determine the events that precede fetal distress or intrauterine death. For the latter, it provides the basis for a more honest approach to perinatal death and, in particular, emphasizes that a significant proportion of perinatal deaths remain mysterious even after full clinical and pathological assessment. The availability of accurate methods of dating pregnancies has yet to be fully reflected in the pathological assessment of the placenta. The reader will recall that virtually all the foundation studies of placental pathology were performed when the most accurate method of dating was the last menstrual period.

It must be emphasized that it may be positively detrimental to provide unsubstantiated placental causes for perinatal deaths simply to satisfy the obstetrician or to bolster the pathologist's ego. This change in attitude is nowhere more apparent than in the area of so-called placental insufficiency, a term still used in clinical practice, which has neither reliable diagnostic parameters nor specific or characteristic pathological features. Indeed, it has been argued that the term should be discarded [3]. Certainly, as will become apparent, there is no evidence that the vast majority of clinical cases of placental insufficiency are the result of a primary failure in placental function.

It has become common practice to attempt to condense placental development and pathology into a single chapter in texts on pediatric and perinatal pathology, with little consideration of the relevance of much of the data to perinatal morbidity and mortality. Much of the information is of little interest to the obstetrician or neonatologist and is frequently given undue importance by the pathologist. Those readers requiring a more detailed description of the placenta and its diseases should consult one or more of the monographs included in the reference section.

PLACENTAL MATURATION AND ADAPTATION

Because the placenta appears to show little or no change in its gross appearance (apart from an increase in size) as pregnancy progresses, it is frequently visualized by both clinician and pathologist as a structurally static organ, the structure at any particular gestation being a reflection of a predetermined and fixed pattern of development that is independent of its local environment. Yet, it would be surprising if an organ with such diverse functions as the placenta were unable to adapt to a hostile environment. As will become apparent, the ability to adapt should be considered an additional essential function of the placenta and one of paramount importance. This stems from understanding that there is no clear line of demarcation between the processes of physiological adaptation to changes in the normal placental environment and those occurring in a pathological environment. It follows that there is a continuous spectrum of adaptation both functionally and structurally. However, current histopathological techniques do not allow us to differentiate between the normal and the abnormal, except at the extremes of these spectra. While the identification of these changes may permit an explanation of some fetal disorders, the reverse is not true, and we are unable to predict with certainty either the gestation or the condition of the fetus from examination of the placenta, except perhaps where the fetus has been dead for some days. It is only when these processes of adaptation fail to compensate for the hostile environment that the fetus begins to suffer. Current histopathological techniques do not allow us to distinguish between physiological and pathophysiological adaptive failure. However, this ability of the placenta to adapt underlies the concept of a *placental reserve*. This reserve has two basic components:

1. An inherent functional reserve in that, like any normal organ, the placenta will not normally be operating at full capacity.
2. An ability to adapt to changes in its environment by modifying both its structure and function.

Because fetal growth outstrips placental growth from about the 16th week of pregnancy, it is self-evident that the placenta must increase its functional efficiency by some means other than by a simple increase in size. This increased efficiency is explained on the basis of structural changes in the villous architecture, which result in a progressive reduction in the thickness of the placental tissue between the maternal and fetal circulations, combined with an increase in surface area [4, 5]. How these changes are controlled is unknown, as are the relative importance of maternal, placental, and fetal factors in this process, though some clues are beginning to appear [6, 7]. There is, however, considerable evidence to suggest that in certain pathological states, the rate of progress of these structural changes may be modified (*vide infra*). If they are accelerated, it follows that the placenta will appear more mature than the clinical data might suggest, the opposite being true if the changes are retarded. The failure of placental morphology to coincide with that predicted for a particular gestation in the presence of a normally grown fetus is frequently interpreted as evidence that the often similar appearances demonstrated in the presence of an abnormally grown fetus are of no significance. If, however, they are, as is suggested, indications that the placenta is adapting to a hostile environment, then it is not only their presence but also their extent and possibly their timing that must be considered. It is, therefore, essential to have a dynamic image of the placenta as an organ continually responding to its environment by modifying both its metabolic activity and its structure. The structural and probably the metabolic changes that occur in pathological situations are, for the most part, brought about by variations in the rate of normal maturation of villous architecture combined, in many instances, with the more specific effects of hypoxia and/or ischemia. In the vast majority of cases, the placenta must be successful in compensating for variations in its environment, but in a small proportion the response is inadequate and is associated with both perinatal morbidity and mortality.

Because the pathology of the placenta in early pregnancy and in multiple pregnancies is discussed elsewhere, only those maternal and fetal disorders that are associated with placental lesions, together with a small number of primary placental lesions of clinical significance, will be discussed here. It must be emphasized that primary disorders of the placenta are extremely rare and indeed, where present, are usually associated with fetal abnormalities (e.g., placental sulfatase deficiency [8]), an entirely predictable situation since the placenta and fetus both originate from the same fertilized ovum. The vast majority of significant placental pathology stems from disturbances in the environment provided by the mother [9]: in particular, the quality and quantity of the maternal circulation through the intervillous space. In order that the importance of the maternal circulation is understood, it is first necessary to detail two fundamental aspects of placental development:

1. The acquisition of the maternal intervillous circulation and its relationship to the basic anatomical structure of the placenta.
2. The adaptive changes that occur within the villi that allow the efficiency of transfer to increase progressively with gestation.

DEVELOPMENT OF THE MATERNAL CIRCULATION WITHIN THE PLACENTA

The survival of the human race is dependent on the fertilized ovum obtaining and maintaining adequate nutrition and oxygenation during its 9-month period of intrauterine life. Because, to all intents and purposes, the environment in which exchange between mother and fetus occurs is the maternal blood that bathes the placental villi, the development of an adequate maternal circulatory system is essential for the growth and development of both the placenta and embryo or fetus. By the end of a normal pregnancy, the blood flow through the placenta is some hundred times greater than that of the non-pregnant endometrium [10]. Such a dramatic increase cannot and does not result from simple dilatation of the normal endometrial vessels but follows profound structural changes in the spiral arteries lying beneath the placenta (i.e., in the placental bed).

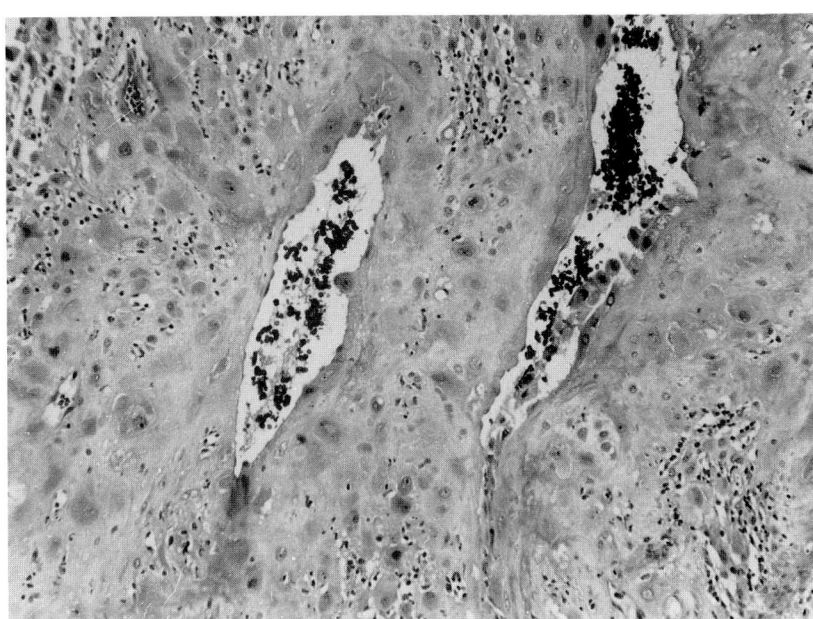

FIGURE 7.1. *Adaptive changes in spiral arteries in the decidua. The vessel wall is replaced by fibrinoid material and the lumen contains trophoblastic cells. H&E, ×105.*

The spiral arteries, which in the non-pregnant state are hormone sensitive, supply the functional endometrium; the basal endometrium and adjacent myometrium are supplied by the basal arteries. It is from the relatively small number of spiral arteries in the future placental bed that the entire intervillous blood flow is derived. While the presence of pathological changes in these vessels in certain abnormal pregnancies has been recognized for many years [11, 12], the detailed description of the normal physiological response of these arteries to pregnancy, on which current concepts of placentation are based, can be attributed to Brosens et al [13], though in early pregnancy Hamilton and Boyd [14] clarified what was until then a somewhat confused picture. The essential features may be listed as follows:

1. The process of adaptation is biphasic, the initial phase beginning at the time of implantation and continuing until about the fourth month of pregnancy, involving primarily the decidual portion of the spiral artery (Fig. 7.1). The second phase modifies much of that part of the spiral artery lying within the myometrium. It may be pertinent that the transition between these two phases roughly corresponds with the period when the relative autonomy of the trophoblast (with respect to the embryo or fetus) is lost. In the early stages of development, placental function, as determined endocrinologically [15], and possibly uterine vascular adaptation may progress normally in the absence of an embryo, but in later pregnancy an established embryonic or fetal circulation appears essential for trophoblastic survival and thus for the progression of uterine vascular adaptation [16].

2. The key to the adaptive process is the endovascular extension of cytotrophoblast into the arteries beneath the implanting ovum and developing placenta. Though tro-

phoblast cells are found outside the arteries within the decidua, the importance of the endovascular trophoblast is emphasized by the failure of the basal arteries, which do not communicate with the intervillous space, to undergo adaptive changes, even though they may be surrounded by decidua-containing trophoblastic cells. This may be correlated with the expression of adhesion molecules by the interacting endovascular trophoblast and decidual vascular endothelial cells [17]. However, it is not clear why similar changes do not occur in the veins draining the intervillous space.

3. The endovascular trophoblast invades the vessel wall, with the destruction of its constituents being associated with fibrinoid necrosis, and the fibrinoid material giving the vessels a blurred indistinct outline with routine hematoxylin and eosin (H&E) preparations (see Fig. 7.1). The muscular and elastic elements of the vessel wall are destroyed, and the vessels dilate and increase in tortuosity. Because their contractile elements are destroyed, these portions of the spiral arteries will no longer be responsive to humoral and neural stimuli. This may provide an important protective mechanism in that maternal stresses that lead to vasoconstriction of the peripheral circulation will not significantly affect blood flow to the placenta.

Concurrently with these adaptive changes within the uterine vasculature, the intervillous space, which begins with the formation of lacunae within syncytial trophoblast cells, undergoes remodeling and organization as the cotyledonary structure of the mature placenta develops. The lobular or cotyledonary structure of the placenta, which becomes increasingly apparent from the middle of the second trimester, was demonstrated clearly by the elegant injection studies of Wigglesworth [18] (Fig. 7.2). In the normal

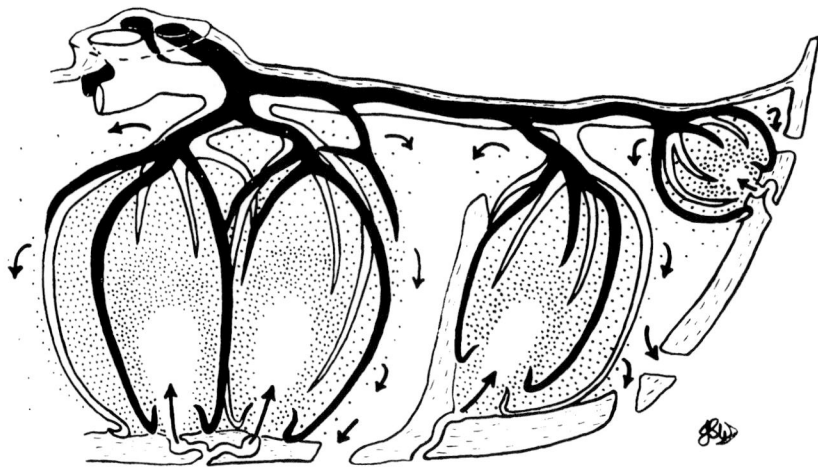

FIGURE 7.2. *Diagrammatic representation of the normal placental circulations. (From Wigglesworth [18].)*

human full-term placenta, the fetal cotyledons are bell-shaped structures that arise from a single-stem villus and number approximately 100, each being supplied by the terminal branch or branches of a single spiral artery. The cotyledonary structure described above is not always evident on examination of the intact placenta, as the lobules visible to the naked eye frequently consist of two or more fetal cotyledons. Because the survival of the conceptus depends on the maternal blood supply and because there is little or no collateral circulation between fetal cotyledons, these terminal branches of the spiral arteries are, in effect, *end arteries*, a factor of great importance in the understanding of the most significant lesions associated with perinatal morbidity and mortality.

As a result of the cotyledonary structure, the intervillous space is not uniform either structurally or functionally. Blood entering the intervillous space in the center of the cotyledons is arterial, yet by the time it has reached the periphery of the cotyledon it is of venous composition. The presence of this metabolic gradient across the cotyledons necessarily means that the normal environment of the villus at the periphery of the cotyledon is substantially different from a centrally sited villus. Because the environment of the villus appears to influence its structure [19], consideration of the morphology and maturation of villi requires knowledge of the location of the villus in relation to the architecture of the cotyledon. Indeed, each cotyledon may be considered to be a miniature representation of the entire placenta. It is customary when maturation of the placenta is discussed to infer a mean level of maturation for the entire villous population. However, within individual cotyledons variations around this mean are to be found, the least mature villi being centrally placed while the most mature are sited at the periphery. Since the trophoblast, weight for weight, has at least twice the oxygen consumption of the fetus [20], any decline in the oxygen supply to the placenta will affect the fetus to a greater degree than the placenta, because the trophoblast has first call on the available oxygen. Furthermore, the peripheral zones of the cotyledons will be affected

earlier and more severely than the central areas. It is therefore of paramount importance that microscopic examination of placental tissue be performed in the knowledge of these architectural features, as comparison of lesions in different placentae is only valid if the areas sectioned are from similar zones within cotyledons. Indeed, histological blocks of placental tissue should, wherever possible, include entire cotyledons.

It also follows from the cotyledonary structure that some mechanism must exist to ensure that the blood emerging from adjacent cotyledons does so at similar pressure, since gross differences could result in turbulence and the risk of thrombosis. It is estimated that there is a pressure gradient of approximately 20 mmHg across a cotyledon and that flow velocities of 300 millimeters per second in the spiral artery fall to 0.1 millimeters per second at the periphery [21]. It is probable that the control of pressure is mediated through the density of the villi within the cotyledons, those with the best arterial supply being the largest and most efficient, though the exact mechanisms involved are unknown. In addition to the graduated environment within cotyledons, there are differences in placental function and anatomy between areas adjacent to the basal plate and those beneath the chorion where villi are relatively sparse, the blood forming subchorionic lakes [22].

ADAPTIVE CHANGES OF STRUCTURE AND FUNCTION WITHIN VILLI

The first primitive villi develop at about 12 days, and during the next week the trophoblast becomes organized radially around the chorion. The cytotrophoblast proliferates on the chorionic surface of the trabeculae to produce a cellular core forming the true primary villus. The development of a mesodermal core converts the primary villus into a secondary villus, and vascularization of the latter gives rise to the tertiary or true functional villus. A basement membrane forms between the villous stromal core and the cytotrophoblast, which stains with periodic acid–Schiff (PAS) and

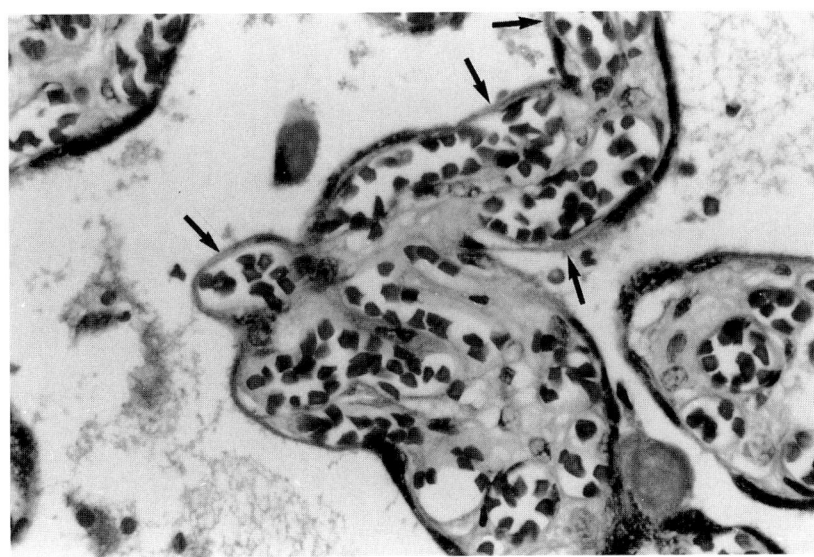

FIGURE 7.3.   *Vasculosyncytial membranes (arrows) in 36-week placenta. H&E, ×430.*

silver stains. Both the cytotrophoblast and syncytial trophoblast come into direct contact with the basement membrane on the outer surface, while on the inner surface there may be fusion of the trophoblastic and fetal capillary basement membranes to form the vasculosyncytial membranes (Fig. 7.3). There is some dispute as to the constancy of thickness of the basement membrane, but it would appear that it gradually increases in thickness with the duration of pregnancy, although there may be local variations in thickness in different parts of individual villi. Thus, Burgos and Rodriguez [23] found that the basement membrane was 200 Å thick at the site of the vasculosyncytial membranes—the so-called alpha zone—and 600 Å thick in the beta zone. These zones are believed to be sites of specialized trophoblastic activity, the former being a site for optimum transfer of metabolites and the latter for synthetic activity. Thus, in the early placenta, fetal blood may be separated from maternal blood by fetal vascular endothelial cells, fetal vascular basement membrane, villous stroma, trophoblastic basement membrane, cytotrophoblast, and syncytial trophoblast, whereas in the mature villus the vasculosyncytial membrane consists of an attenuated extension of the fetal vascular endothelial cell, the fused fetal vascular and trophoblastic basement membranes, and an attenuated syncytial cell. Concurrently, the villous diameter decreases from 618 microns on the 100th day of pregnancy to 268 microns at term [5], thus increasing the surface area per unit volume [4]. These modifications in structure clearly permit increased transfer across the placental "membrane." It cannot be overemphasized that the structure varies both within cotyledons and individual villi, and thus the assessment of placental maturity is fraught with difficulties [24]. Under normal circumstances, these modifications of villous architecture adequately compensate for the relative decrease in the rate of placental growth as compared with that of the fetus after the 16th week of pregnancy. Thus, recent studies have shown

that there is a relationship between these increasing abilities to transfer oxygen and fetal weight gain [25].

DEVELOPMENTAL VARIATIONS AND ABNORMALITIES

The characteristic discoid placenta with a centrally inserted umbilical cord is subject to numerous variations both in shape and in the site of insertion of the umbilical cord. The vast majority of these variations are of no clinical significance. Ovoid, cardioid, and reniform placentae are common variants. Multilobate placentae are found in 1–4% of pregnancies, the majority being bilobed and approximately 0.1% being trilobed or multilobate [26]. Bilobed placentae are reported to be more frequent in elderly women, in women suffering from prolonged infertility [27], and in grand multipara. Apart from an increased incidence of bleeding in early pregnancy, multilobate placentae do not endanger the fetus.

Accessory or succenturiate lobes occur in up to 10% of pregnancies. They may be connected to the body of the placenta by an isthmus of placental tissue or by the chorion alone, the former being much more frequent. In some instances, a small accessory lobe may be difficult to differentiate from a normal cotyledon with a deep septal fissure, and this may in part account for the differences in reported incidence of these variants. Accessory lobes not attached to the body of the placenta may become detached at delivery and result in postpartum hemorrhage associated with a placental "polyp." If the lobe is large, the compression of the vessels in the intervening chorion or their rupture may result in fetal distress or, rarely, fetal exsanguination.

Placenta Extrachorialis

In the normal placenta, the chorionic plate and the basal plate are of roughly equal dimensions, so that they fuse at the margins of the placenta. The *extrachorial placenta* results

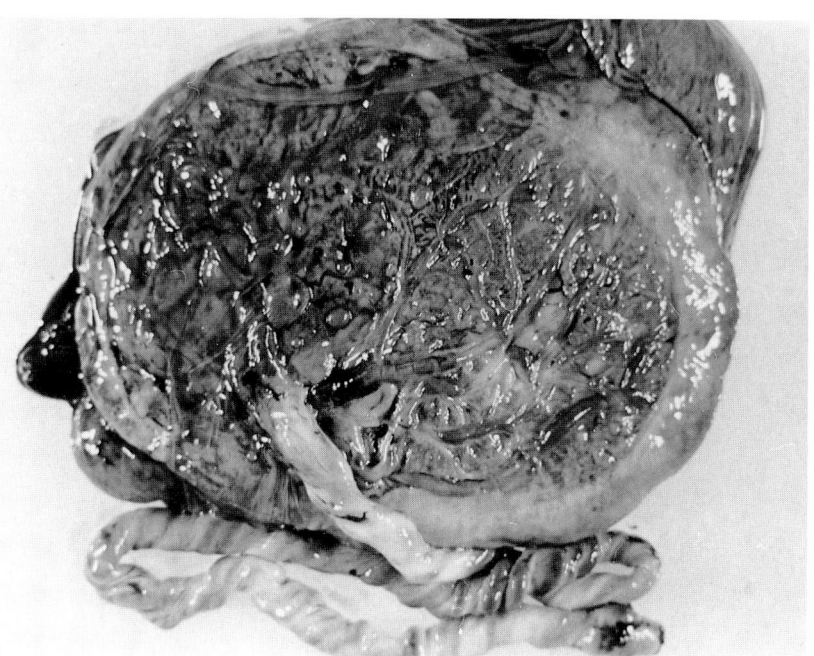

FIGURE 7.4.   *Circummarginate placenta. The opaque extrachorionic extension forms a crescent on the right of the placenta.*

when the chorionic plate is smaller than the villous portion, so the latter projects beyond the periphery of the attachment of the membranes. The junctional zone may be smooth, the *circummarginate placenta* (Fig. 7.4), or elevated, the *circumvallate placenta* (Fig. 7.5), the former being the much commoner variant. The overall incidence of these conditions is variously reported as 15–30%, with 1–7% showing the circumvallate form. The extrachorionic villous tissue may involve the entire circumference, though partial involvement is considerably more frequent. Both circummarginate and circumvallate forms may be observed in a single placenta. Personal experience indicates that extrachorial placentae are more frequently associated with an ovoid form. Circumvallate placentae frequently show very numerous and extensive subchorionic fibrin plaques.

Examination of extrachorial placentae reveals that the large fetal vessels appear to end abruptly at the edge of the ring, but Scott [28] demonstrated by injection and radiography that the vessels continue into the extrachorial villi at a deeper level. In the marginate placenta, the chorion may be stripped from the underlying extrachorial placenta without disruption of the vessels. The circumvallate placenta is associated with the formation of folds or plicae in the chorion. These plicae may contain amnion, chorion, ghost villi, fibrin, blood clot, and, very rarely, active villi [28]. The clinical significance and etiology of extrachorial placentation remain controversial. This is further complicated by the failure of many surveys to distinguish between circummarginate and circumvallate placentae, since the former has no clinical significance [29, 30].

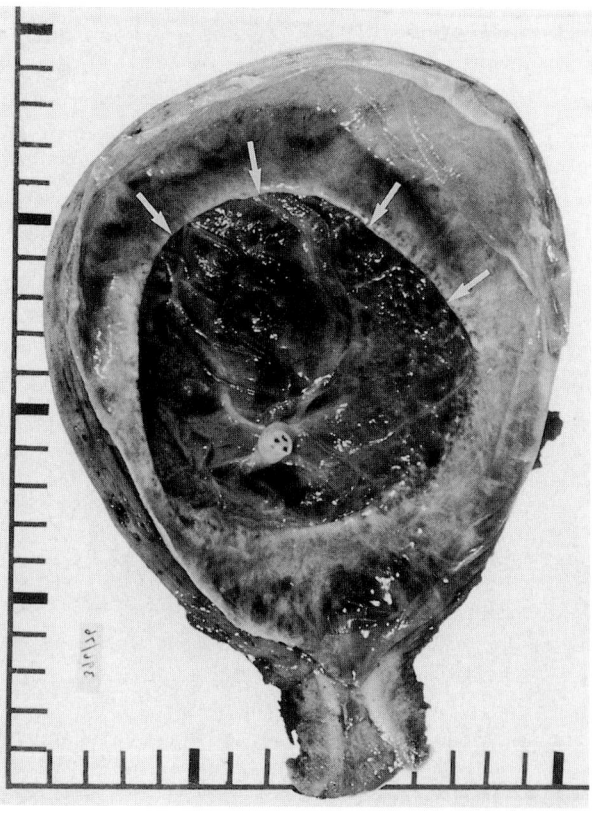

FIGURE 7.5.   *Circumvallate placenta in situ in 22-week pregnancy. The overlapping fold of membranes and decidua (arrows) is as yet not adherent to the placenta.*

The clinical complications reported in association with extrachorial placentation include second trimester abortion (McKay and Hertig, quoted by Scott [28]), premature labor [31, 32], antepartum and postpartum hemorrhage—the latter being associated with placental retention and manual removal [28, 33, 34]—and vaginal loss of amniotic fluid [28, 35, 36]. There is general agreement that the incidence of antepartum hemorrhage is increased, but that this is not of major clinical significance and does not materially affect the fetal outcome.

The pathogenesis of the extrachorial placenta is obscure; thus Benirschke and Driscoll [37] described it as the "placental anomaly of hypotheses." Any adequate hypothesis must explain the spectrum of anomalies and their coexistence in one placenta, their relative rarity before the 20th week of pregnancy, and the increased incidence of circummarginate placentae, but not circumvallate placentae, in multiple pregnancies [28]. Benirschke and Driscoll [37] consider endometritis, cornual implantation, an initially excessively small chorionic plate, and abnormalities in the depth of implantation as unproven, while Fox [38] considers the most plausible hypothesis to be that of Torpin [39], who suggests that abnormally deep implantation of the ovum is the primary factor.

Several *in-situ* specimens have been reported, and a further example is illustrated in Figure 7.5. In this specimen, obtained at 18 weeks' gestation, a fold in the membranes and decidua is clearly evident, involving only part of the circumference. At the time of hysterectomy, it was not adherent to the placental surface. Such folds might develop as a result of unequal growth rates in the decidua, particularly along the axis of the fold, which in association with normal uterine growth might result in a "line of stress" in the chorionic plate and lead to infolding of the membranes. As further growth of the placenta occurred, it would extend

beneath these folds, which would then become applied to the marginal surface.

Placenta Membranacea

Placenta membranacea is a rare anomaly [40] in which the entire chorion is covered by villi and, while an incidence of 1 in 3300 deliveries has been reported by Aguero [41], only two cases in more than 65,000 placentae has been encountered in pregnancies over 28 weeks' gestation at Birmingham Maternity Hospital, a figure comparable to that of Hurley and Beischer [42] who found an incidence of 1 in 21,500 deliveries. All these placentae must, by definition, also be previa, and the latter authors found an incidence of membranous placenta of 1 in 184 placenta previa. Premature labor and antepartum hemorrhage are frequent complications. The placenta is usually very thin (Fig. 7.6). The etiology of placenta membranacea is uncertain, but the frequent association with placenta accreta would seem to indicate that endometrial hypoplasia may be important.

Placenta Accreta, Increta, and Percreta

Normal placental separation is facilitated by the presence of a layer of decidua between the villi and uterine wall. Morbidly adherent placenta (MAP), of which there are three forms—placenta accreta, increta, and percreta—is defined as "the abnormal adherence either in whole or in part of the afterbirth to the underlying uterine wall" [43]. The incidence of MAP is uncertain, since minor degrees of accreta are not uncommon and must be underdiagnosed. Overall estimates vary from 1 in 540 [44] to 1 in 93,000 [45]. In our experience, the incidence is approximately 1 in 4500 deliveries [46], a figure comparable with that of Hill and Beischer [47]. About one in five cases involve the lower

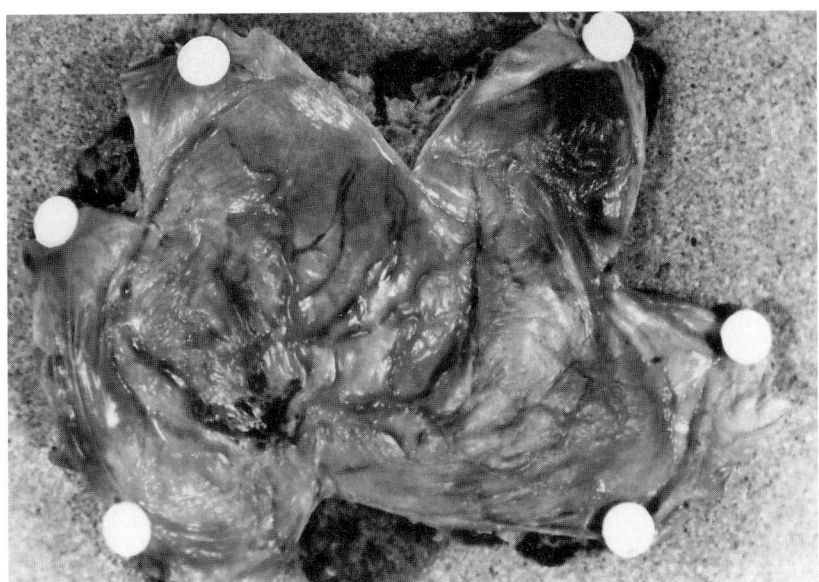

FIGURE 7.6. *Placenta membranacea. The entire surface of the chorion is covered by villous tissue.*

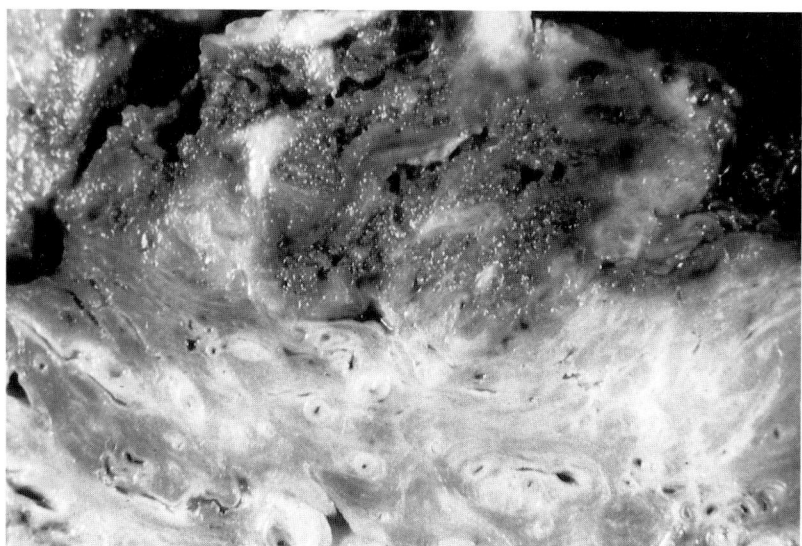

FIGURE 7.7.   *Placenta accreta. Villous tissue interdigitates with the myometrium.*

segment [48], this being particularly hazardous to the mother, frequently necessitating an emergency hysterectomy [46]. The majority of cases are accreta, and the least common form is percreta, where the placenta penetrates the entire thickness of the uterine wall.

The cause of MAP is generally accepted to be a failure of decidualization, which in most instances is probably secondary to endometrial hypoplasia [49]. The latter may be secondary to uterine disease or surgery or, rarely, a primary disorder [50]. Thus MAP is very uncommon in primigravidae. An endemic form has been reported from Papua New Guinea [51], and there may be an association with myotonic dystrophy [52].

Macroscopic examination of MAP in situ reveals various degrees of penetration and interdigitation of the placenta into the uterine (or cervical) wall (Fig. 7.7). Microscopically, villi are directly apposed to the myometrium or cervical connective tissue, with either an incomplete or absent layer of decidua (Fig. 7.8).

A recent study of the placental bed in MAP [53] demonstrated a diminution of placental bed giant cells, the trophoblast being either mononuclear or binuclear. The trophoblastic penetration of the myometrium was reduced in density. Curiously, large radial or arcuate arteries showed physiological adaptation, while some spiral arteries retained their non-pregnant appearance. They suggest that MAP may be due to a defective interaction between decidua and the migrating trophoblast.

Placenta Previa

Macroscopic examination of the placenta in isolation will not enable the diagnosis of placenta previa to be made with any degree of certainty, though it is not infrequent for

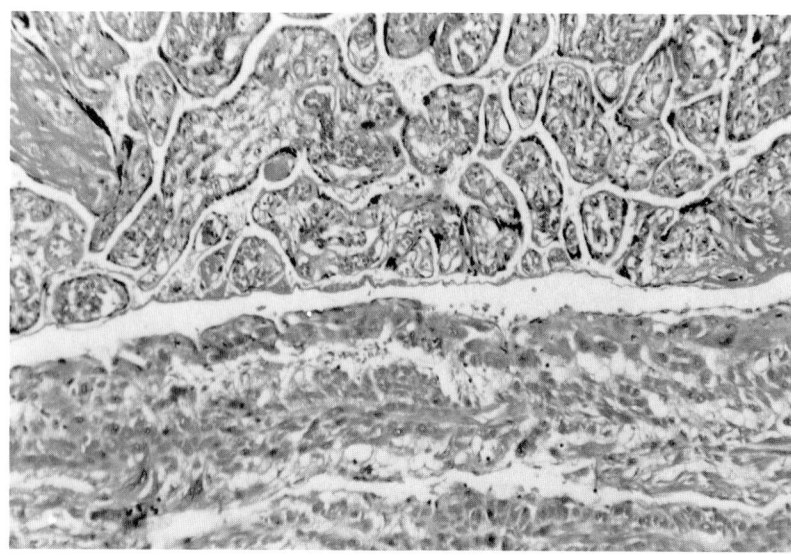

FIGURE 7.8.   *Placenta accreta. Villous tissue is in direct apposition with the myometrium with no intervening decidua. H&E, ×106.*

known clinical cases to deliver placentae in which an irregular thinned projection from the margin is identifiable. The clinical grading and classification of placenta previa is discussed in current textbooks of obstetrics. The associated complication of placenta accreta has been discussed previously, but a further complication, which may result in life-threatening postpartum hemorrhage, may be important to the pathologist. It was indicated earlier that among the physiological changes involved in uterine adaptation to pregnancy, the superficial portions of the uterine vessels are modified, with destruction of the muscle and elastic tissues in their walls. The author has observed three cases in which these modified vessels in the lower segment of the uterus were identified as the cause of torrential postpartum hemorrhage, necessitating an emergency hysterectomy.

MICROSCOPIC LESIONS OF THE PLACENTA

Prior to consideration of maternal and fetal disorders affecting the placenta, the limited microscopic responses will be discussed. As emphasized already, microscopic examination of the placenta is dependent on the knowledge of the normal anatomy, and preparation of blocks of tissue to include an entire cotyledon is of critical importance. As will become apparent, it is not so much the individual lesion but the constellation of lesions that may be indicative of a specific clinical disorder. Examination should proceed in a standard manner, which, provided it is consistent for each observer, can be adapted to individual preferences. The author examines villous tissue from the syncytial surface inward, finishing with the luminal surface of the fetal vasculature; thus, the microscopic lesions will be described in this order. Certain lesions, including calcification and some inherited metabolic disorders, may affect several villous components and will be discussed under separate headings.

Trophoblastic Lesions

Primary lesions of the trophoblast in clinically confirmed pregnancies are extremely rare, with the exception of hyperplasia and malignant change. This may be surprising in view of the diverse functions of the trophoblast, although it should be readily apparent that any major abnormality will almost certainly result in failure of implantation or early embryonic death. There are, however, rare examples of inherited metabolic disorders, which may be manifest in the trophoblast (*vide infra*). Two major factors are responsible for trophoblastic lesions—disturbances of the maternal circulation (*vide supra*) and of the fetal circulation. Both may lead to similar lesions, though presumably by different mechanisms.

Syncytial Knots
The interrelationship between disturbances in the maternal and fetal circulations and syncytial knots is discussed below, as is their structure, and they will not be considered further here. Among the many functions of the trophoblast is that of a vascular endothelial cell. The syncytium on the surface of villi is permanently bathed in maternal blood. Damage to the surface will result in the deposition of fibrin and adherence of platelets. Such fibrin deposits are a feature of all placentae, and it must be assumed that in the vast majority of instances they are rapidly removed and the surface repaired by a combination of fibrinolysis, phagocytosis, and cell growth. In this respect, the trophoblast may have a distinct advantage over the vascular endothelial cell, in that it has the capability of destroying and ingesting cells and other tissue constituents, a function essential in the process of implantation.

Fibrin Deposition
The deposition of fibrin and other constituents of the maternal blood on the surface of and between villi occurs in several differing patterns.

Focal Perivillous Fibrin Deposition Focal deposition of fibrin occurs most commonly at the placental margin, in the junctional zones between cotyledons, and beneath the chorionic plate to form subchorionic plaques [54]. Deposits visible to the naked eye are evident in at least one-third of all full-term placentae, and microscopic deposits are seen at all gestations. Macroscopic deposits are typically yellow-white, slightly opalescent lesions with an irregular but sharp line of demarcation from the adjacent normal placenta (Fig. 7.9).

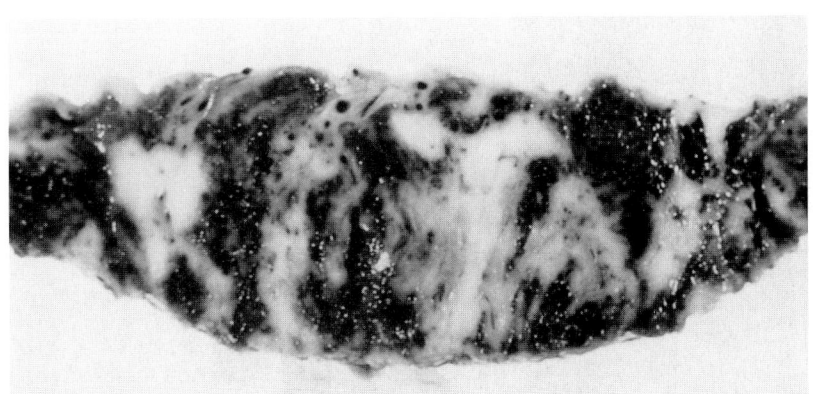

FIGURE 7.9.   *Fibrin deposition. The fibrin (pale areas) is largely sited in the intercotyledonary zones.*

Well-established deposits easily can be mistaken for infarcts, particularly in the unsliced placenta, and may require histological confirmation.

Histological examination reveals the villi to be partially or completely encased in fibrin, the latter being associated with obliteration of the intervillous space. Remnants of syncytium may be evident in recent deposits, but as the lesion ages these disappear. The cytotrophoblast frequently proliferates and may appear unduly prominent. The trophoblastic basement membrane thickens and the villous vessels collapse and are eventually obliterated, while the villous stroma undergoes sclerotic changes. The final result is a group of avascular collagenized villi embedded in a relatively homogeneous matrix of fibrin. Occasional irregular channels may persist within the fibrin and communicate with the intervillous space; these are sometimes lined with attenuated syncytial cells. In the past, there has been considerable debate as to the nature of the material surrounding the villi, but immunofluorescent techniques have demonstrated conclusively that the material is predominantly fibrin derived from maternal blood [55].

Subchorionic Fibrin Deposition   Subchorionic fibrin plaques occur in 15–20% of full-term placentae and are evident as irregular yellow-white plaques visible through the membranes on the fetal surface of the placenta. Slicing reveals these to be discoid or wedge-shaped, yellowish, often slightly gelatinous deposits that, on close examination, frequently have a clearly laminated structure. They may vary from a few millimeters to several centimeters in diameter. Histological examination shows them to consist almost entirely of a fine laminar meshwork of fibrin, in which are embedded platelets and occasional red cells and rarely villi. Subchorionic plaques may fuse and become very extensive, which, in the author's experience, is particularly common in circumvallate placentae. Occasionally, there may be numerous smaller deposits of 2 to 5 millimeters in diameter, giving a miliary pattern.

The etiology of both perivillous and subchorionic fibrin deposition is now accepted as being the result of local disturbances in the maternal circulation within the placenta. Fox [38, 54] has emphasized that the former lesion is associated with a very good maternal blood supply. It is believed that the lesions are not of any clinical significance, even if 20–30% of the villi are involved.

Massive Perivillous Fibrin Deposition (MPFD)   Rarely, the deposition of fibrin extends to involve the majority of the cotyledons, with obliteration of much of the intervillous space in a remarkably uniform manner. In the author's experience, this type of fibrin deposition is more common in the late second and early third trimester of pregnancy and has been associated with recurrent pregnancy wastage and fetal growth retardation. The uniformity of the process suggests that there may be diffuse trophoblastic damage, resulting in either a failure of the normal antithrombogenic properties of the syncytium or destruction of the syncytium at a rate in excess of the ability of the cytotrophoblast to replace the lost trophoblast. The placenta is typically of a firm or rigid consistency, often being relatively thick (in comparison with the diameter) and having a pale yellowish cut surface in which dark-red areas consisting of surviving functional villi are scattered (Fig. 7.10).

Microscopy reveals that the villi are embedded in the fibrin deposits, the individual villi frequently having prominent cytotrophoblastic shells between the stroma and surrounding fibrin (Fig. 7.11). The stroma of the villi may show an increased fibrous tissue component and obliteration of the fetal vasculature, although these vessels frequently remain patent. These lesions are *not* associated with infarction of the villi. Within the deposits of fibrin, there are irregular vascular channels, often without identifiable lining cells, although occasionally small islands of syncytial cells may be identified. In some instances, these channels may contain large numbers of mononuclear cells, both macrophages and lymphocytes, raising the possibility that the trophoblastic injury

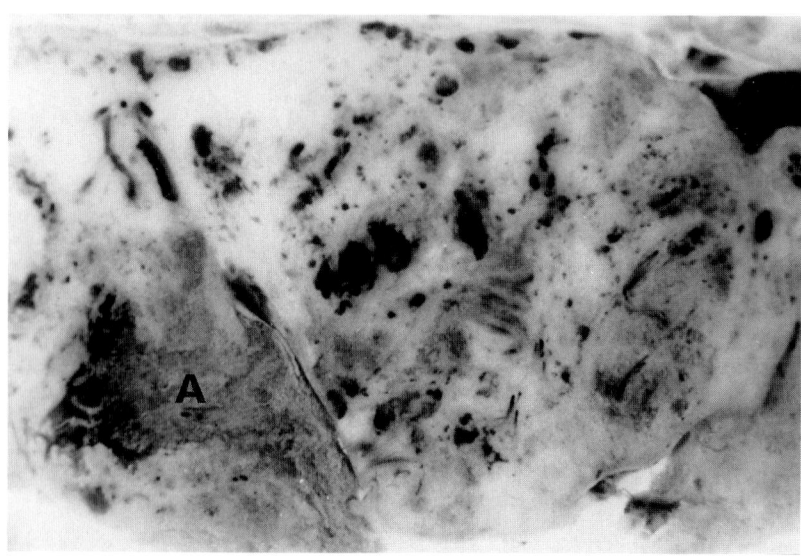

FIGURE 7.10.   *Massive perivillous fibrin deposition. There are groups of unaffected villi (A), but the vast majority are embedded in homogeneous fibrin traversed by vascular channels.*

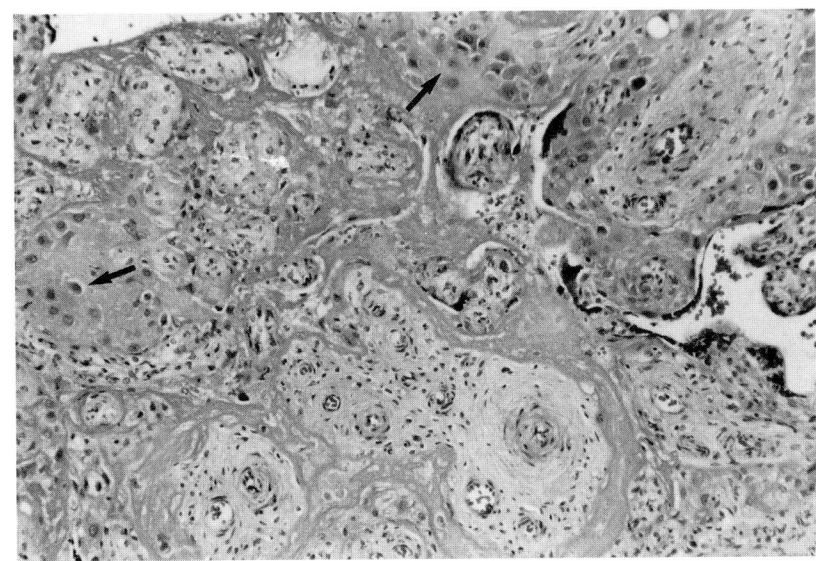

FIGURE 7.11. *Massive perivillous fibrin deposition. Viable villi are encased in fibrin, which contains collections of cytotrophoblastic cells (or X cells, arrows). H&E, ×106.*

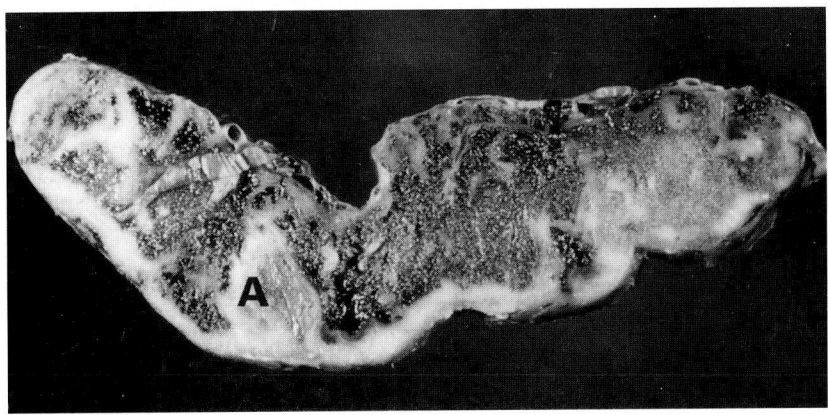

FIGURE 7.12. *Early maternal floor infarction. A layer of fibrin deposition is present on the maternal surface. There is an old infarct (A).*

is immunologically mediated. Whether this condition is related to massive chronic intervillousitis, which has also been associated with recurrent early pregnancy loss, remains uncertain. The surviving villi are generally normal or show accelerated maturation. Though MPFD can be interpreted as an extreme example of focal deposition, in the author's opinion this seems unlikely. The lesion is remarkably uniform, and it does not show any predilection for sites where disturbances of flow within the maternal component of the placental circulation might occur (e.g., focal and sub-chorionic fibrin deposition).

As has been indicated, the pathogenesis of MPFD is obscure, but the possibility that it represents the outcome of an "immunological" insult cannot be ignored. There would appear to be some confusion between MPFD and maternal floor infarction (MFI) of the placenta, a lesion first described by Benirschke and Driscoll [37] in macerated twins. This lesion, which is not an infarctive process, is common in macerated abortions [56] and differs from MPFD in that the fibrin deposition begins at the maternoplacental interface, gradually extending toward the chorionic plate until the entire villous population is involved and the intervillous

space is largely obliterated (Fig. 7.12). It is invariably associated with villous fibrosis and vascular obliteration, and cytotrophoblastic proliferation does not occur. Islands of normal surviving villi are absent, the free villi also showing stromal fibrosis and vascular obliteration, often in association with syncytial knot formation and trophoblastic basement membrane thickening and/or mineralization.

Fibrinoid Necrosis Fibrinoid necrosis occurs in about 3% of villi in normal full-term placentae [57] but is much more common in diabetic and rhesus placentae, with a less striking increase in pre-eclamptic toxemia [58, 59]. The lesion begins with the accumulation of acidophilic PAS-positive material between the trophoblast and basement membrane (Fig. 7.13). The deposits may increase in size until they appear to completely separate the trophoblast from the villous core. There are similarities between this lesion and fibrinoid necrosis of blood vessels in diseases unrelated to pregnancy, in particular to some autoimmune disorders, though there is no evidence to suggest a similar etiology for the placental lesion. Indeed, the distinction between fibrinoid necrosis and small healing lesions of fibrin deposition is far from clear-cut, and it is possible that the two lesions

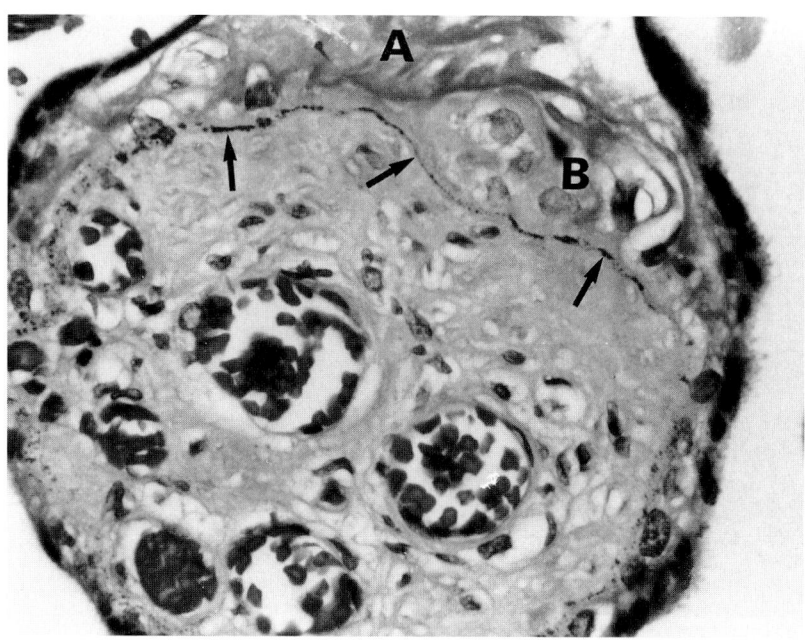

FIGURE 7.13.   *Fibrinoid necrosis. Fibrin (A) is deposited beneath the syncytium but outside the trophoblastic basement membrane (arrows), to which is attached a small group of cytotrophoblastic cells (B). H&E, ×476.*

represent part of a spectrum of trophoblastic damage and repair associated with fibrin deposition.

Trophoblastic Necrosis

Necrosis of the trophoblast (syncytial and cytotrophoblast) is typical of placental infarction, though small foci of full thickness or of syncytial necrosis may occur in otherwise normal placentae, in placentae of pre-eclamptic patients, and in association with villitis.

Maturation Acceleration and Delay

The problems in assessing disturbances of maturation have been discussed earlier, and their identification necessarily demands accurate knowledge of the duration of the pregnancy.

Becker [24] has termed the mature placenta found with the premature infant as *maturitas praecox*, while the reverse combination is termed *maturitas retarda placentae*. It is estimated that the former occurs in 1–2% of premature deliveries, although incidences as high as 25% have been reported [60]. The latter is commoner, being found both in term and postmature pregnancies. Personal experience suggests that accelerated maturation is frequently seen in mid-trimester abortions, particularly in those with other evidence of uteroplacental ischemia. Immaturity is particularly notable in diabetic pregnancies and may account for the high rate of late stillbirths in diabetic mothers. Becker [24] has emphasized the possible role of immaturity of the placenta in fetal distress and fetal growth retardation. Decreased formation of vasculosyncytial membranes is associated with a high risk of fetal hypoxia [38].

Postmaturity and the Placenta   It is estimated that approximately 5% of pregnancies have a duration in excess of 43 weeks and a further 5–10% in excess of 42 weeks but less than 43 weeks [61]. Approximately three-fourths of these

fetuses are delivered without evidence of pathology, although there is an excess of infants over 4 kilograms, as might be anticipated. The remainder show features of the postmaturity syndrome, the clinical features of which have been described by Vorherr [62].

There is disputed evidence that fetal [63] and placental function either levels off or declines from approximately 36–38 weeks of pregnancy. The following factors are pertinent to this argument:

1. The mean birth weight levels off at 42 weeks and may then show a slight decline [64].
2. Amniotic fluid volume falls rapidly from about the 38th week of pregnancy [65].
3. Uteroplacental blood flow falls after 40 weeks [66–68], although Magnin and Gabriel [69] found no abnormality in the uteroplacental vessels.
4. Placental and fetal growth rates decline at about term, although it must be emphasized that they do not cease [38, 70–72].

Many of these features may also be associated with uteroplacental ischemia earlier in pregnancy, and it has therefore been argued that "placental insufficiency" is the cause of the complications and hazards associated with postmaturity, although there is little or no firm evidence to support this concept. There is a rise in the perinatal mortality rate from the 42nd to the 44th weeks to between ten and twenty times that at term [73–75], but this may be more closely related to the problems associated with the delivery of large babies than to placental insufficiency. Thus, Vorherr [62] in an analysis of perinatal mortality found that 9–30% of deaths occurred before the onset of labor and 45–93% during labor, emphasizing the risks of delivery, particularly the increased risk of birth trauma due to the high percentage of large babies. The reduced uteroplacental blood flow may explain the findings of Walker [75], who demon-strated that the umbilical venous blood oxygen content was reduced by one-third at 43 weeks' gestation. This reduction resulted in the umbilical venous blood oxygen level approaching the normal arteriovenous difference of the fetus, thus significantly diminishing the reserve capacity to supply oxygen to the fetus. Because these measurements were made in the resting state, it is readily apparent that the stress of labor could, under these circumstances, precipitate severe fetal hypoxia. Fox [38], on reviewing the placental changes associated with postmaturity, emphasizes the absence of characteristic macroscopic lesions. He subdivides the histological lesions into four categories:

1. Those with normal histology for a full-term placenta—25–35% of specimens—probably from pregnancies of shorter duration than the dates suggest.
2. Those with normal villous vessels but with mild ischemic lesions (i.e., cytotrophoblastic proliferation and thickening of the trophoblastic basement membrane, due to reduced intervillous blood flow)—10–15% of specimens.
3. Those with inadequately vascularized villi due to collapse of the peripheral villous vessels—15–20% of specimens. However, it is debatable whether the vascular collapse is a secondary phenomenon and not an indication of significant vascular pathology.
4. Those with both inadequately vascularized villi and mild ischemic lesions—40% of cases. Fox believes that this group is the only one of clinical significance and that the combination of mild ischemia with reduced fetal villous blood flow results in impaired maternofetal transfer.

Because postmaturity may be considered a manifestation of a failure of the normal mechanism, which leads to the spontaneous onset of labor at term, the clarification of the pathology of postmaturity will require a better understanding of the relative importance of maternal, placental, and fetal factors in this process. Some of the observed changes may be secondary lesions attributable to this failure and, while they may be characteristic of postmaturity, as Fox [38] has suggested, they do not give us a clear insight into their origin. They do, however, provide at least a partial explanation of the apparent "placental insufficiency" of postmaturity.

Prematurity and the Placenta   Because the causes of premature delivery are varied or unknown, there are no specific pathological changes in the placentae of premature babies. Obstetric complications, such as pre-eclampsia, placental abruption, and premature rupture of the membranes, are frequently associated with premature labor. A proportion of cases of prematurity are totally unexplained. The villous tissue of the majority of placentae from premature deliveries appears to be normal for the gestation. This is also true of many mid-trimester abortions, in which the fetus is apparently normal until the time of expulsion, although a significant proportion do show accelerated maturation of the placenta [56]. However, evidence of inflammatory changes in the placental membranes is very common (*vide infra*).

Placental infarction, perivillous fibrin deposition, subchorionic fibrin plaques, and calcification are less common than at term [5, 76]. Wigglesworth [77] described considerable variation in villous structure in premature placentae, but this is almost certainly a reflection of villous growth, which is active at this stage of pregnancy. The two common pathological findings are chorioamnionitis and undue maturity of the placenta. Approximately one-half of premature placentae show chorioamnionitis [78] and, while this may simply be a reflection of ascending infection through prematurely ruptured membranes, there is an increasing suspicion that infection is in fact causal in a proportion of premature deliveries. The possible significance of early maturation of the placenta (Fig. 7.14) has been previously

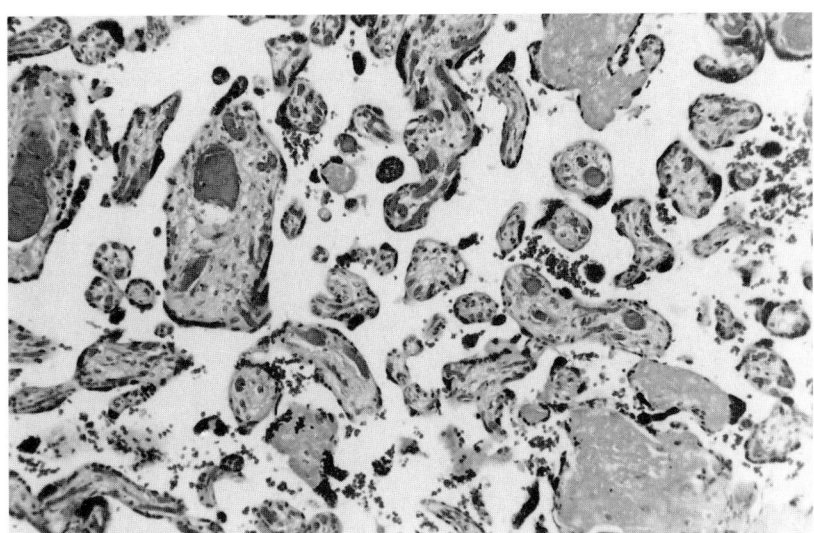

FIGURE 7.14.   *A 28-week gestation placenta from mother with pre-eclamptic toxemia with growth-retarded fetus. The villi are small and poorly vascularized with numerous syncytial knots and an overall reduction of density within the cotyledon. H&E, ×105.*

discussed, although the etiology remains obscure. It is possible that the attainment of maturity is inextricably linked with the physiological processes concerned in the initiation of normal labor, thus accounting for some premature deliveries. Because prematurity is the greatest single factor contributing to perinatal mortality, with approximately 6% of pregnancies ending prematurely, a better understanding of the mechanisms involved would undoubtedly have a significant effect on perinatal mortality and morbidity.

Routine histological methods can only detect relatively major disturbances in maturation, although it may safely be assumed that less obvious variations are much more frequent, involving either the entire placenta or individual cotyledons. However, it must be remembered that current concepts of placental maturity are relatively simplistic; thus "immaturity" is frequently used to describe a paucity of terminal villi due to failure of maturation of the villous tree. Attempts have been made to subclassify disturbed maturation and to relate disturbances to the timing of their onset in pregnancy [79], but the value of such classifications has yet to be proven, either clinically or pathologically.

Trophoblastic Basement Membrane

Only two lesions are worthy of discussion: thickening and mineralization of the basement membrane.

Thickening of Basement Membrane

As has been stated, the trophoblastic basement membrane varies in thickness, depending on the function of the particular area of the villous surface and on the gestation. It is difficult, therefore, to assess minor increases in thickness, although major increases are usually apparent even on routine staining of villi with H&E (Fig. 7.15). Little is understood about the mechanisms that lead to thickening or the effects that thickening has on the fetus [80].

Mineralization of Basement Membrane

See Placental Calcification under Miscellaneous Placental Lesions.

Villous Stroma

Probably the most important stromal lesions are those associated with infection, and these are discussed elsewhere.

Stromal Fibrosis

Stromal fibrosis is the most common pathological change and inevitably follows fetal death; the placenta is retained in utero either in part or in toto for several days after cessation of the fetal circulation. The end result of local occlusion of the fetal circulation within a cotyledon will be stromal fibrosis and, in such cases, normal and fibrotic villi may be seen side by side (Fig. 7.16). Fibrosis is also associated with obliteration of the vascular tree within the villus, the two changes occurring concurrently after fetal death. Initially, an increase of stromal reticulin precedes the formation of collagen and, therefore, in equivocal cases a reticulin stain may be helpful. It may also be of value in the identification of stromal edema.

Stromal edema (villous hydrops) is also common. There is some confusion in the literature between the terms "hydatidiform change" and "hydrops," particularly in early abortions. It is the author's contention that the term *hydrops* should be retained for changes that occur in vascularized villi and the term *microscopic hydatidiform change* be used for the avascular enlarged villi seen in blighted ova. Thus, hydropic villi are an indication of fetal diseases, such as intrauterine cardiac failure, anemia, and hypoproteinemia. It should be noted that immature villi frequently appear mildly hydropic. If fetal death occurs in the presence of a hydropic placenta (as opposed to a placenta with microscopic hydatidiform change), stromal fibrosis will ensue and, although

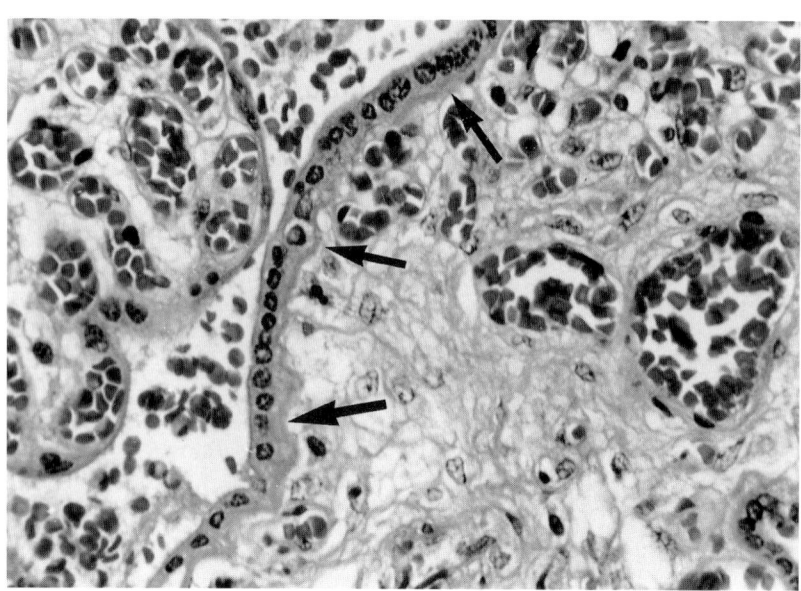

FIGURE 7.15. *Thickened trophoblastic basement membrane (arrows) from diabetic mother of 37 weeks' gestation. H&E, ×448.*

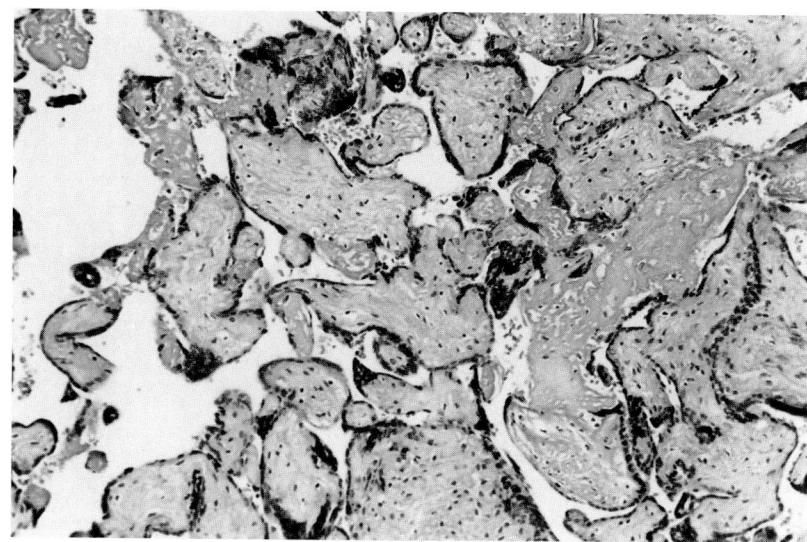

FIGURE 7.16. *Fibrotic villi. The vessels are obliterated and the stroma collagenized. There are syncytial knots on the surface. H&E, ×105.*

the macerated fetus may still appear hydropic, all evidence of placental hydrops may be obliterated.

Hofbauer Cells

The number of Hofbauer cells within the villous stroma varies with gestation. They are relatively more numerous in the earlier months of pregnancy. Increases in numbers are associated with inflammatory disorders, usually of an infective origin, and are discussed elsewhere.

Villous Vessels

Obliteration

The vessels within villi may become obliterated by a process of contraction and intimal proliferation after cessation of the circulation within them. This process is frequently termed *obliterative arteritis*, an erroneous description, as there is no evidence of an arteritis. The lesion may be diffuse, involving all villi, as occurs after fetal death, or focal, as occurs after interruption of the blood supply to a part or the whole of a cotyledon.

Medial Hypertrophy

Thickening of the media is frequently a subjective diagnosis and, as with all assessments of vascular wall lesions, may be influenced greatly by the contents of the vessels and the extent to which contraction or relaxation of the musculature occurs after cessation of the circulation. Thus, while it is possible to argue that an elevated maternal blood pressure raises the pressure in the intervillous space and thus necessitates a rise in the fetal blood pressure to overcome the increased pressure transmitted to the villous core, it should also be remembered that the increased intervillous pressure will provide support for the villous vessel. Unlike the systemic circulation, the forces within and without the vessel will be balanced and no additional stress will be put on the vessel wall. Under such circumstances, the stimulus to hypertrophy will be removed. It is the author's view that the

diagnosis of medial hypertrophy is best avoided unless morphometry under standardized conditions is performed.

Intimal Thickening and Fibrosis

Intimal thickening is subject to the same limitations as medial hypertrophy. Intimal fibrosis may be circumferential or crescentic in distribution (Fig. 7.17). It is most commonly seen in the chorionic vessels but also follows partial or total thrombosis. Its significance depends on the size and number of vessels involved.

Hemorrhagic Vasculosis

This term has been coined by Sander and Stevens [81] for a lesion in which villous vessels are partially obliterated by intimal proliferation, which divides the lumen into numerous minute vascular channels (Fig. 7.18). The histological appearances have much in common with those that occur after fetal death and that lead to obliteration of the lumen. The villus with no fetal circulation but with an intact maternal circulation can be considered as an in vivo tissue culture, and it is not yet certain whether the lesions described in such villi precede the cessation of the circulation or are secondary events. Sander and Stevens [81] favor the view that hemorrhagic vasculosis is a primary phenomenon and a cause of fetal death, but the author remains unconvinced, as lesions occurring in this unique environment cannot necessarily be interpreted in the same manner as those in which there is only a single circulation. Furthermore, similar lesions may be seen in the remnants of umbilical vessels in perinatal deaths in the absence of any vascular lesions in the placenta. Be that as it may, the lesions described by Sander and Stevens [81] are by no means rare.

Vascular Thrombosis

Thrombosis of chorionic and villous vessels is a common incidental finding and usually involves a single vessel and a small group of villi (Fig. 7.19). It is not easy to distinguish arteries and veins within the placenta without injection

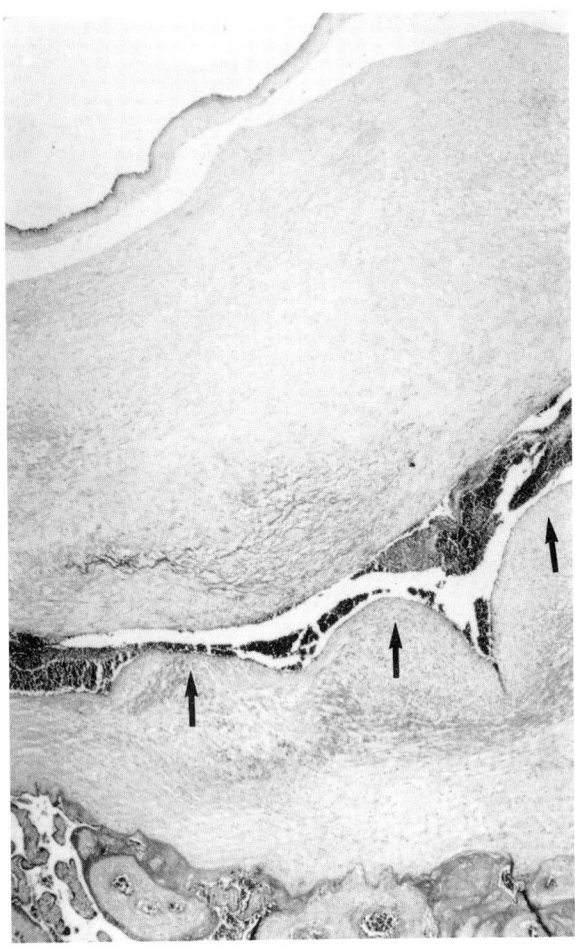

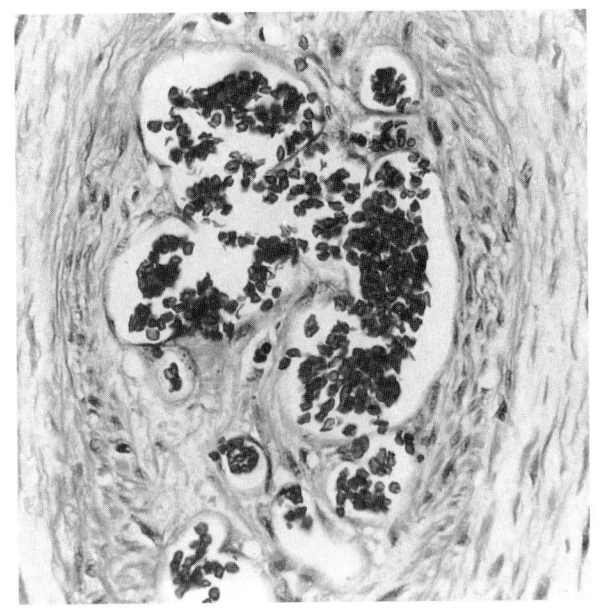

FIGURE 7.18.   *Hemorrhagic vasculosis. Early lesion. The vessel lumen is divided into multiple small channels by fibrous tissue from the intima. H&E, ×287.*

FIGURE 7.17.   *Chorionic vessel. There are irregular fibrous intimal cushions (arrows) with extension of fibrous tissue into the media. H&E, ×117.*

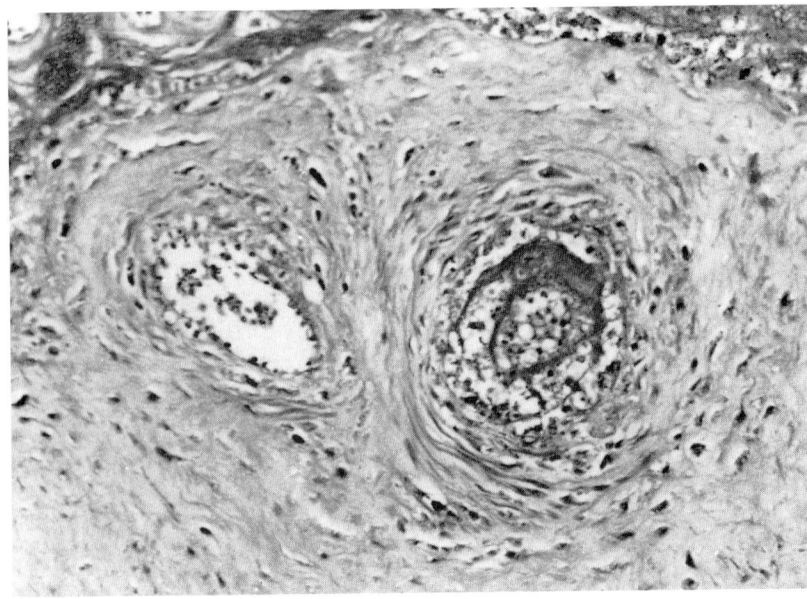

FIGURE 7.19.   *Thrombosed vessel in stem villus draining an infarcted cotyledon. H&E, ×263.*

studies, but it is probable that the majority of thrombi form in the venous side of the fetal circulation. When a large vessel is occluded, the lesion may result in a visible abnormality of the placenta, the affected villi forming an irregular pale area that initially retains the normal spongy appearance of the adjacent unaffected villi, unlike an infarct due to maternal vascular disease. Partial or complete occlusion of villous vessels by thrombus or fibrin is frequently seen in association with villitis, and chorionic vessels may be affected in the presence of inflammation of the membranes. Theoretically, such thrombi might be the source of emboli to the fetus, although, even in the presence of ischemic lesions in fetal organs, this is virtually impossible to confirm.

MATERNAL DISEASE AND THE PLACENTA

Armed with an understanding of the development and maturation of the placenta and the likely response to changes in its environment, it is possible to consider the effects of maternal diseases on the placenta. The most important of these disorders are those that affect the quantitative or qualitative status of the maternal blood supply to the placenta. Those that affect the quality of the blood supply are almost entirely the result of preexisting maternal diseases affecting organs other than the reproductive tract and are not specifically related to the pregnant state, although it is not uncommon for pregnancy to modify the severity of these diseases. Quantitative disturbances of the maternal blood supply may result from maternal cardiac disease, but the majority of those associated with fetal or perinatal morbidity and mortality are due to uterine vascular pathology.

The major maternal diseases that affect the placenta are listed in Table 7.1. Clinically, the most important of these in developed countries are pre-eclamptic toxemia (and eclampsia) and maternal diabetes mellitus. Not only do they affect the fetus, but the former is the most important cause of

Table 7.1.   Maternal disease and placental pathology

Qualitative disturbances in maternal blood flow
Anemia
Hypoxia—cyanotic heart disease, altitude, respiratory disease
Metabolic—diabetes mellitus, renal disease, starvation, endocrine disorder, phenylketonuria, drugs
Infection

Quantitative disturbances in maternal blood flow
Uterine vascular disease—gestational hypertension, pre-eclampsia, eclampsia, essential hypertension, diabetes mellitus, maternal collagen diseases

Abnormalities of placentation
Morbidly adherent placenta
Placenta previa
Placenta membranacea

Malignancy
Metastatic disease

pregnancy-related maternal death. In developing countries, malnutrition and anemia are clearly of major significance.

Primary placental disease is only rarely a cause of fetal or perinatal morbidity and mortality.

Trophoblastic Response to Hypoxia

Prior to the consideration of specific pathological lesions of the placenta, one further aspect of placental adaptation pertinent to maternal disorders must be mentioned, i.e., the response of the trophoblast to hypoxia and ischemia.

Because placental growth and survival is inextricably linked with the maternal blood supply, which in turn is dependent on the activities of the trophoblast within and around the uterine spiral arteries, any disease process that compromises this blood supply after the initiation of the vascular adaptive changes should, on teleological grounds, result in a compensatory response. This will be directed toward either halting or reversing the decline in blood flow, while increasing the physiological efficiency of the functional placental tissue.

After the establishment of an embryonic circulation within the villi, villous growth normally proceeds by the formation of syncytial buds or sprouts, which sequentially develop cytotrophoblastic and then stromal cores into which capillaries grow from the established intravillous circulation [82]. In the earlier stages of placental growth, the cytotrophoblast is a prominent feature of villous architecture, but as the rate of placental growth declines it becomes relatively inconspicuous. As the cytotrophoblast is the source of the syncytiotrophoblast, it must, however, persist to allow for continued growth and to replace syncytial cells, which may be lost or damaged on the villous surface. Under adverse conditions, the cytotrophoblast may remain conspicuous or return to prominence. Thus, in rhesus isoimmunization, it may be stimulated by increased turnover of syncytial cells, while in the diabetic placenta the immaturity of the villi may be a reflection of disturbances in growth. However, both clinical and pathological evidence indicate that one of the most important stimuli to cytotrophoblastic proliferation is uteroplacental ischemia, which is classically associated with pre-eclamptic toxemia and, to a lesser extent, with other maternal hypertensive disorders. There must also be mechanisms by which the fetus can influence placental growth, although as yet they are unknown.

Experimental evidence from cultured villi indicates that one important stimulus to cytotrophoblastic proliferation is reduced oxygen tension in the environment [83, 84]. During pregnancy the oxygen tension may be reduced either as a result of a decline in the maternal blood supply or a reduction in the oxygen content of the maternal blood. In the former situation, not only the supply of oxygen but also the supply of nutrients and removal of fetal metabolites will be compromised, whereas in the latter the blood flow may be maintained, with only oxygenation being reduced. This distinction is important in that a reduced blood supply, although stimulating a compensatory response, may, by preventing the supply of adequate nutrients, obtund that response, whereas a simple reduction in oxygen tension, providing that it is not extreme, will result in an appropriate cytotrophoblastic response leading to villous growth. In such circumstances, e.g., maternal anemia [85–87], maternal cyanotic heart disease [88], and pregnancy at high altitude [89], the size of the placenta (relative to the fetus) may be increased, though this increase may in part be explained by reduced fetal growth secondary to chronic hypoxia. More recent studies on placentae from populations living at high altitude would seem to indicate that, while the villous tree is reduced in size, there is a compensatory increase in maturity of the villi, in that the length of capillaries per fixed length of villus is greater than in lowland placentae [90]. This suggests that the increased placental/fetal weight ratio reflects fetal growth retardation rather than increased placental size.

A second type of syncytial sprout or bud has been described by Hamilton and Boyd [91]; these initially appear similar to those destined to form new villi but fail to develop a central core. They gradually become isolated from the villi to which they are attached by narrow stalks, which become attenuated and eventually separate to form trophoblastic emboli that are deported to the lungs. As many as 100,000 of these emboli may enter the maternal circulation each day [92]. Their role, if any, is uncertain, but they may be concerned in the control of the immunological interrelationships between mother and fetus. Currently, they are under investigation as a possible source of cells for prenatal diagnosis [93]. The numbers of emboli are very much larger in eclamptic patients, and clumps of trophoblastic cells may be found in the small pulmonary vessels (Fig. 7.20) of mothers dying of eclampsia [92]. This second type of syncytial sprout or bud has much in common with the syncy-

tial knot, a collection of syncytial cell nuclei found on the surface of villi in several pathological states, among which uteroplacental ischemia is prominent.

Several mechanisms may be implicated in the trophoblastic response to hypoxia or ischemia:

1. There may be a direct effect on the cytotrophoblast, as suggested by the experimental evidence.

2. Since the syncytial trophoblast has an extremely high oxygen requirement to enable it to carry out its many metabolic activities (e.g., hormone synthesis, transport of metabolites, etc.), it is very sensitive to a fall in the oxygen tension of its local environment and, as a result, the turnover of cells may be increased, requiring compensatory cytotrophoblastic proliferation to replace them. In pre-eclampsia, the archetypal complication of pregnancy associated with decreased perfusion of the maternal component of the placental circulation—focal syncytial necrosis—is prominent; these areas of necrosis appear as small superficial ulcer-like craters on the surface of the villi when examined by scanning electron microscopy [94]. These almost certainly heal fairly rapidly because their persistence would provide a suitable nidus for fibrin and platelet deposition, which, though often present in such placentae, is not a major feature of the pre-eclamptic placenta. If hypoxic stimulation of the cytotrophoblast is combined with an increased turnover of syncytial cells and the two processes remain in balance, the only histological abnormality will be persistently active cytotrophoblast. In these circumstances, the trophoblast will retain a bilaminar structure, and the villi may appear immature for the gestation. If the syncytial damage exceeds the ability of the cytotrophoblast to replace lost cells, fibrin and platelet deposition may become widespread. When the cytotrophoblastic prolif-

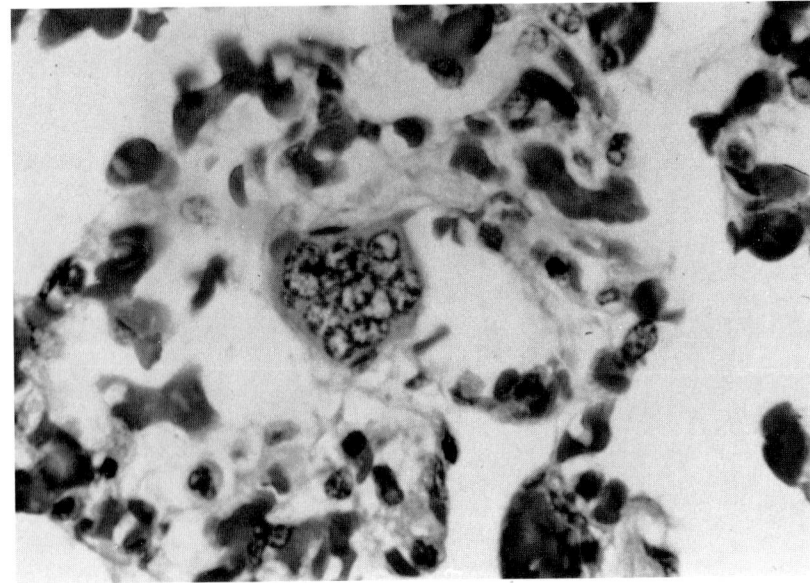

FIGURE 7.20. *Trophoblastic embolus in lung of mother dying of cerebral hemorrhage associated with pre-eclamptic toxemia. H&E, ×460.*

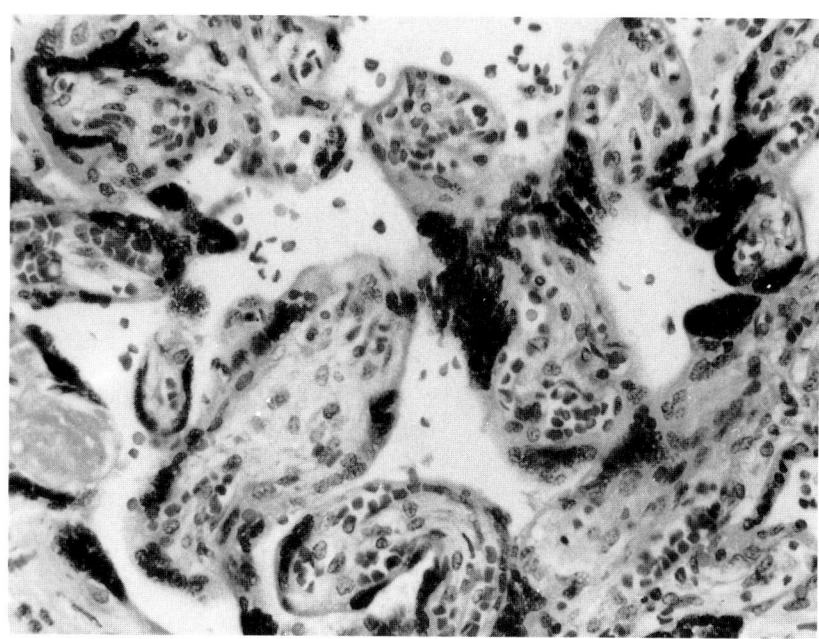

FIGURE 7.21. *Syncytial knots in 32-week placenta from pre-eclamptic mother. H&E, ×263.*

eration exceeds the loss of syncytial cells, then excess syncytial nuclei will accumulate, resulting in the formation of syncytial knots (Fig. 7.21). It is not surprising, therefore, that there are conflicting reports in the literature about the effects of pre-eclampsia on the trophoblast [95–98], with descriptions of both syncytial hyperplasia and syncytial degeneration with premature aging. These differences possibly reflect different stages in the evolution of the pathological manifestations of the disease. Syncytial knots may represent abortive attempts at new growth, in that original buds or sprouts, which under normal conditions would have developed into villi, fail to acquire stromal and vascular cores, possibly because their environment has become too hostile to support stromal and vascular proliferation. Other authors, notably Jones and Fox [99], have argued that they represent sequestrated groups of surplus or senescent syncytial nuclei.

3. Alterations in the hormonal milieu resulting from hypoxia or ischemia may stimulate trophoblastic growth either directly or possibly via the fetus. The role of the fetus is unknown, but ligation of fetal arteries in the monkey placenta results in increased syncytial knot formation on the villous surface [100]. Syncytial knots are also prominent in the placentae of intrauterine deaths. It is possible that the secondary vascular proliferation necessary for villous growth does not occur in the absence of a fetal circulation and thus syncytial sprouts again fail to mature into villi, the excess syncytial cells persisting as knots.

In summary, it is clear that hypoxia and ischemia modify the function and structure of the trophoblast. Initially, there may be a hyperplastic response, a concept supported by the demonstration that patients destined to develop pre-eclampsia have a larger placental mass in early pregnancy, as judged by biochemical parameters [101], than those who remain normotensive. A similar mechanism may account for the elevated levels of serum alphafetoprotein in early pregnancy of women destined to develop pre-eclampsia [102]. This should also be true of those pregnancies with qualitative deficiencies in the oxygen content of the maternal blood. In later pregnancy, if the process is primarily ischemic, the hyperplastic response will be obtunded and placental growth inhibited, with morphometric studies confirming that villous tissue is reduced in pre-eclampsia and some other hypertensive disorders of pregnancy [103, 104]. The final stage occurs when the circulation through the spiral arteries is insufficient to maintain the trophoblast, and infarction results.

One of the major histological manifestations of an obtunded hyperplastic or proliferative response is the syncytial knot. (See item 2 above.) Syncytial knots occur in 10–30% of villi at term [105], and they are more common at the periphery of the cotyledons, in the subchorionic space and in marginal cotyledons. Their frequency increases in pre-eclampsia, essential hypertension, severe maternal diabetes, prolonged pregnancy, in villi adjacent to infarcts, in retained placental tissue either following delivery or intrauterine death, and distal to fetal arterial occlusions. They are said to be distinctly uncommon under 32 weeks' gestation, although they may be found in 10–15% of mid-trimester abortions [56]. Routine histological studies will only detect relatively large increases in their numbers, although morphometric techniques are more sensitive. However, major increases are unlikely to be missed, even with low-power microscopy, since they will involve villi from all areas of the cotyledon. Studies on trophoblastic specializations [106] have suggested that while syncytial sprouts in early pregnancy and in diabetic pregnancies represent the early stages of villous growth, syncytial knots, sprouts, and bridges in later pregnancy are predominantly artifacts due to tangential sectioning of the villi. It is not clear, however, why tangential sectioning should be influenced by the gestation at which the placenta is delivered. In a small proportion where the authors considered there to be genuine lesions, they were considered to be degenerative changes.

It must be clear from the foregoing discussion that hypertensive disease affecting the mother during pregnancy is the most important clinical factor associated with placental hypoxia and ischemia. The effects of hypertensive disease are mediated through damage to the spiral arteries, and thus placental insufficiency and placental ischemia are more appropriately termed *uteroplacental insufficiency* and *ischemia*. The importance of uterine vascular disease cannot be overestimated, and it is probable that over one-third of all small-for-dates babies are attributable to uterine vascular disease [107]. Unfortunately for the pathologist, though fortunately for the mother, uterine vessels are rarely available for histological examination in routine practice; although, as Wigglesworth [18] demonstrated, the terminal portions of the spiral arteries may be identified on the maternal surface of the freshly delivered placenta. Techniques for measuring uterine blood flow during pregnancy by non-invasive methods may at least partly resolve this problem [108].

Uterine Vascular Pathology

In general terms, uterine vascular disease resulting in fetal compromise may arise as the result of:

1. Preexisting maternal vascular disease, e.g., essential hypertension, systemic lupus erythematosus, diabetes mellitus.
2. Failure of the normal processes of physiological adaptation of vessels in the placental bed.
3. Development of lesions within the uterine vessels, whether physiological adaptation has proceeded normally or abnormally, e.g., acute atherosis, fibrinoid necrosis, thrombosis.

Workers from three European centers [109] have reviewed the techniques and problems associated with obtaining and interpreting placental bed biopsies. In order to assess fully the status of the uteroplacental circulation, a biopsy must include both decidua and myometrium from the placental site. The criterion for identifying the latter is the presence of extra-villous trophoblast—both mononuclear cytotrophoblast and syncytial giant cells—in the decidua and myometrium. Additional confirmatory evidence includes the presence of remnants of anchoring villi and vessels showing physiological modification. While, as discussed earlier, physiological adaptation extends to the myometrial segments of the spiral arteries after the first trimester, the extent of the changes is diminished at the margins of the placenta, a

feature that may result in the inexperienced misinterpreting the biopsy as showing a failure of adaptation.

In summarizing the pathology, these authors emphasize that, despite a growing consensus concerning the lesions associated with proteinuric and non-proteinuric hypertension, and intrauterine growth retardation in the absence of hypertension, the current data largely apply to these disorders as studied in the third trimester. Data relating to earlier pregnancy are scanty, though undoubtedly of crucial importance, as the lesions seen in the third trimester stem from events occurring in the first and second trimesters.

Two groups of lesions are currently described:

1. In pre-eclampsia and eclampsia, physiological adaptation is confined to the decidual portions of the spiral arteries, although some spiral arteries fail to show any adaptive changes [110]. In the absence of proteinuria and in intrauterine growth retardation (IUGR) without hypertension, the extent of physiological adaptation is less certain but is almost certainly restricted.
2. Lesions within the arteries, which in proteinuric hypertension of pregnancy are best demonstrated in the decidua vera and include fibrinoid necrosis and acute atherosclerosis (Figs 7.22 and 7.23). These may lead to thrombosis, placental ischemia and infarction, retroplacental hemorrhage, and abruption. The first description of vascular lesions in the placental bed is that of Williams [111]. Hertig [11] detailed the changes that Zeek and Assali [12] subsequently called *acute atherosis*, which was demonstrated in 30% of the decidual specimens from beneath infarcted placentae and in almost 50% from cases of clinical toxemia.

The lesion of acute atherosis typically develops in small muscular arteries in the placental bed and decidua vera at the margin of the placenta. The evolution of acute atherosis has been studied by De Wolf et al [112]. Initially, there is accumulation of lipid in the muscle of the media and within the intima. Whether this is the result of primary abnormalities within the muscle cells or due to disturbance of the lipid transport across vessel walls is uncertain. The lipid-laden cells necrose and release fat, which is taken up by macrophages. Because these changes occur in vessels in the placental bed, it would suggest that a local factor, possibly of placental origin, may play a role in their pathogenesis. Although the mechanism that initiates these lesions is unknown, their similarity to the lesions found in rejected renal transplants [113] has led to speculation that in pre-eclampsia they may be immunological in nature. If this is the case, the immunological mechanisms are yet to be identified. The accumulation of foamy lipid-laden macrophages (lipophages) on the intimal surface and in the walls of these vessels with transmural fibrinoid necrosis is characteristic. Essential hypertension in pregnancy does not appear to modify the adaptive processes in the spiral arteries, although they may show arteriosclerotic changes. If pre-eclampsia develops in a patient with essential hypertension, then vas-

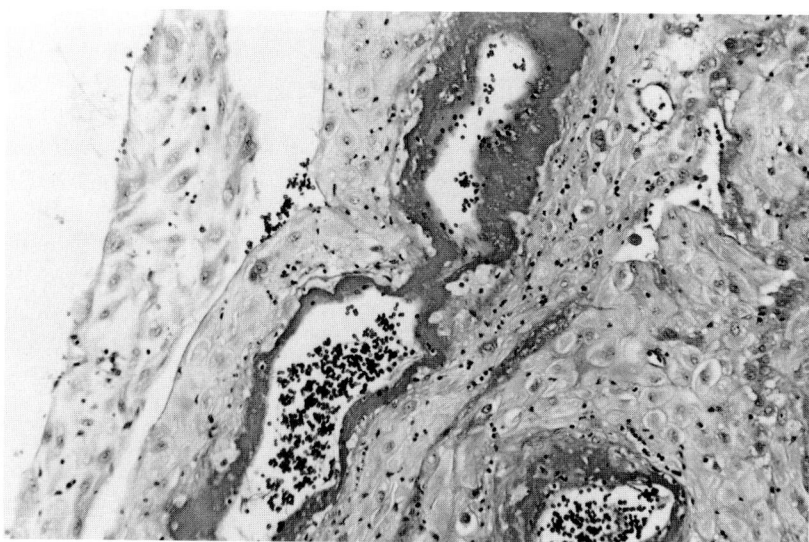

FIGURE 7.22. *Fibrinoid necrosis of decidual vessels. Fulminating pre-eclampsia at 28 weeks' gestation. H&E, ×105.*

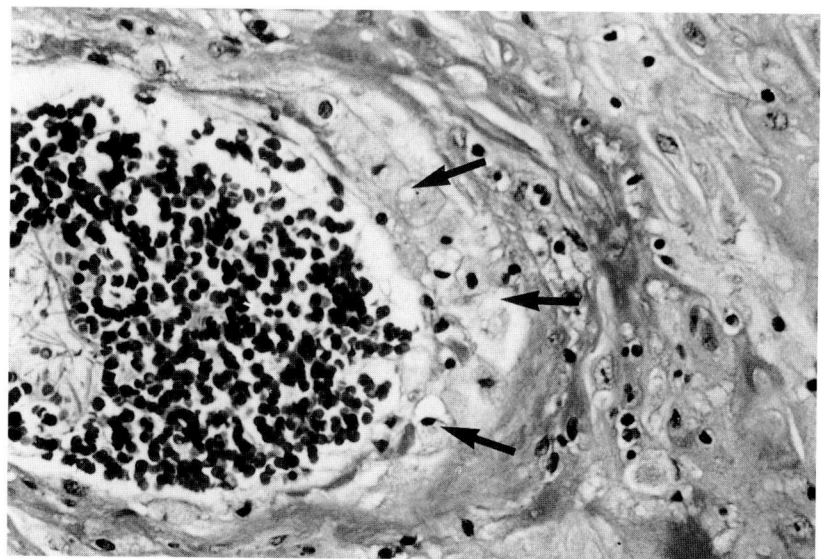

FIGURE 7.23. *Acute atherosis. There are numerous lipid-laden macrophages in the intima (arrows). H&E, ×263.*

cular adaptation is modified as it is in pre-eclampsia. The spiral arteries in the myometrium and basal decidua in such cases may show a profound hyperplastic arteriosclerosis in their unadapted segments.

It should be noted that while a properly obtained placental bed biopsy is necessary to assess the degree of physiological adaptation, lesions in the spiral arteries can be demonstrated in decidua and in the remnants of vessels attached to the maternal surface of the placenta [114].

Many fundamental problems remain unresolved. Why does the endovascular trophoblast not extend along uterine veins in the same manner as it does along arteries? How is trophoblastic invasion controlled? Why do the destructive changes associated with vascular adaptation not result in thrombosis? Finally, and of crucial importance, what is the pathogenesis of the vasculopathies of pregnancy? Until these questions are answered, the major factors responsible for perinatal wastage (i.e., prematurity, hypertensive disease

of pregnancy, and intrauterine growth retardation) will continue to concern obstetricians and neonatologists and bedevil perinatal pathologists.

Placental Pathology Associated with Uterine Vascular Disease

The response of the placenta to maternal vascular disease depends on both the extent and rate of progression of the vascular damage. Involvement of isolated vessels, as may typically occur at the margin of the placenta or in relation to preexisting uterine pathology (e.g., fibroids), is likely to affect only a small number of cotyledons and is unlikely to lead to fetal compromise. Diffuse vascular disease, though not necessarily affecting all uterine vessels equally, will affect the entire placenta and therefore may well be followed by fetal morbidity or mortality. Equally, a slowly progressive disease may be compensated for by the adaptive processes enumerated earlier, whereas acute lesions, particularly super-imposed on diffuse vascular disease, may have a catastrophic effect on the fetus.

At a macroscopic level, there are few lesions associated with uterine vascular disease, of which the most important is the placental infarct. However, on light microscopy, the interpretation of suspected abnormalities is far from straight-forward, in that the placenta appears to have a relatively simple structure (that belies its complex metabolic func-tions), which in turn is capable of only a limited number of recognizable pathological responses, as discussed previ-ously. These are, in general, relatively non-specific and form a continuum from the normal, through adaptations to a hostile environment that may permit normal fetal growth and survival, to those that are associated with growth retar-dation and fetal or perinatal death.

Furthermore, the correlation of placental pathology with fetal or neonatal disease is fraught with difficulties, in that the fetal end-points are imprecise. Though death may be seen as a clear-cut end-point, such deaths are often either inexplicable or inadequately explained. IUGR and fetal dis-tress are two examples of clinical end-points where attempts to correlate placental pathology are often made, yet both are of multifactorial origin and both suffer from lack of clarity of definition. If, in addition, there is doubt about the dura-tion of the pregnancy, clinicopathological correlation of fetal disease with placental pathology will be particularly poor, except in the most severe examples of maternal, fetal, and placental disease. Furthermore, there is growing evidence that the interpretation of histopathological changes in the placenta is not consistent even among those pathologists with special knowledge of the organ [115, 116].

This apparent lack of correlation is used as an argument for the abandonment of placental examination. Such exam-inations are indeed of limited value, not least because they are retrospective in nature and rarely influence postnatal management. Even acute obstetric emergencies, such as placental abruption (see below) and massive retroplacental hemorrhage, may leave no mark on the placenta if delivery ensues rapidly after their onset. However, placental exami-nation may still provide explanations or clues to particular fetal disorders or, alternatively, exclude suspected clinical causes. As methods of intrauterine assessment become increasingly precise, the range of placental "lesions" previ-ously described may well be reassessed. The increasing shift of obstetrics from an art (when most of the descriptive pathology of the placenta was recorded) to a science pro-vides the pathologist with almost unlimited scope for research into the human placenta and for the revision of past misconceptions.

Pre-eclamptic Toxemia and Eclampsia

The adoption of a universally acceptable definition of pre-eclamptic toxemia is far from agreed [117]. From the pathol-ogist's point of view, pre-eclamptic toxemia is a clinical syndrome associated with maternal hypertension and pro-teinuria peculiar to the pregnant state and, as a syndrome, it does not necessarily follow that all cases have an identi-cal etiology, any more than respiratory distress in the neonate is always due to hyaline membrane formation. The complexities of the problem of pre-eclampsia have been reviewed thoroughly by MacGillivray [117]. Although the etiology remains unknown, there is increasing evidence that the pathogenesis of the disorder relates to events that occur several weeks, if not months, prior to the disease becoming clinically manifest; i.e., in effect there is an "incubation" period. The pathological evidence and, to a lesser extent, the clinical evidence would seem to indicate that this "incuba-tion" period is variable in duration, and it is probable that in some cases delivery ensues before maternal symptoms are manifest. In such circumstances there are fertile grounds for argument about the specificity or otherwise of lesions demonstrated in the placental bed, placenta, and fetus. However, while opinion on the specificity of spiral artery lesions in pre-eclampsia remains divided, it is clear that the placental and fetal responses to a reduced maternal blood flow to the placenta are non-specific. Thus, none of the diseases associated with uteroplacental ischemia can be diagnosed unequivocally by examination of the placenta, although certain groups of lesions occurring together may induce in high index of suspicion that the mother has one of these disorders.

However, the lack of specificity of pathology should not deter the pathologist from examining the placenta, as positive findings may, for example, explain IUGR while negative findings may stimulate the search for alternative explanations for poor fetal growth.

Placental Infarction

The lesion most commonly associated with toxemia of preg-nancy is the placental infarct. Placental infarcts are frequently erroneously identified, particularly by obstetricians. They should *never* be diagnosed without slicing of the placenta, because many so-called infarcts, identified as pale, roughly circular lesions on the maternal surface of the placenta, will, on slicing, be shown to be local collections of fibrin or decidua attached to the base of otherwise normal cotyle-dons. A placental infarct can be defined as an area of ischemic necrosis within the territory or territories of one or more spiral arteries, the occlusion of which deprives the affected area of the placenta of a maternal blood supply.

As with infarcts in other organs, placental infarcts vary in color depending on the duration of the ischemia; thus, the most recent are dark red, while old lesions are yellowish white (Fig. 7.24). It is, however, generally impossible to judge the age of the infarct with any degree of accuracy from these color changes.

The effects of ischemia on the placenta are very rapid in onset due to the high metabolic activity and oxygen con-sumption of the trophoblast. Initially, the intervillous space may contain maternal blood, which forms a central throm-bus in the cotyledon, and the villous vessels are dilated and

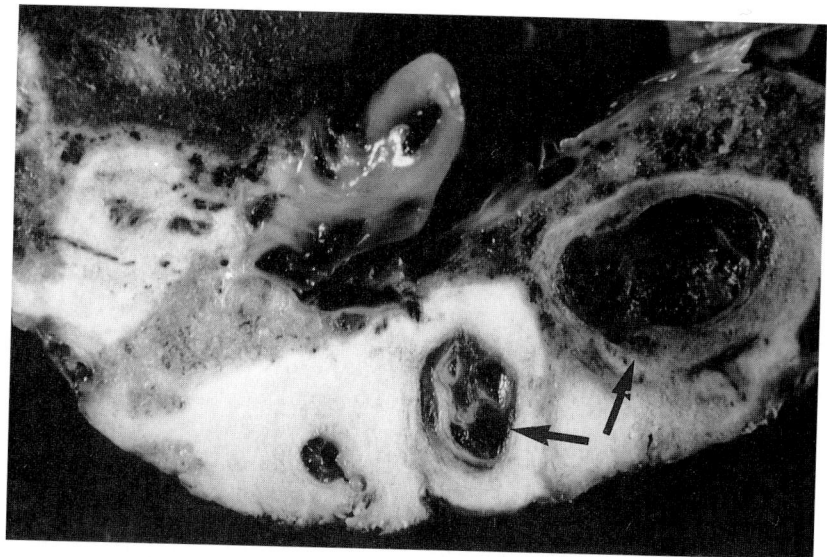

FIGURE 7.24. *Multiple placental infarcts, of which two contain hematomas (arrows). (From Rushton DI. Placenta as a reflection of maternal disease. In: Perrin EVKD, ed.* Pathology of the Placenta. *New York: Churchill Livingstone, 1984, pp. 57–87.)*

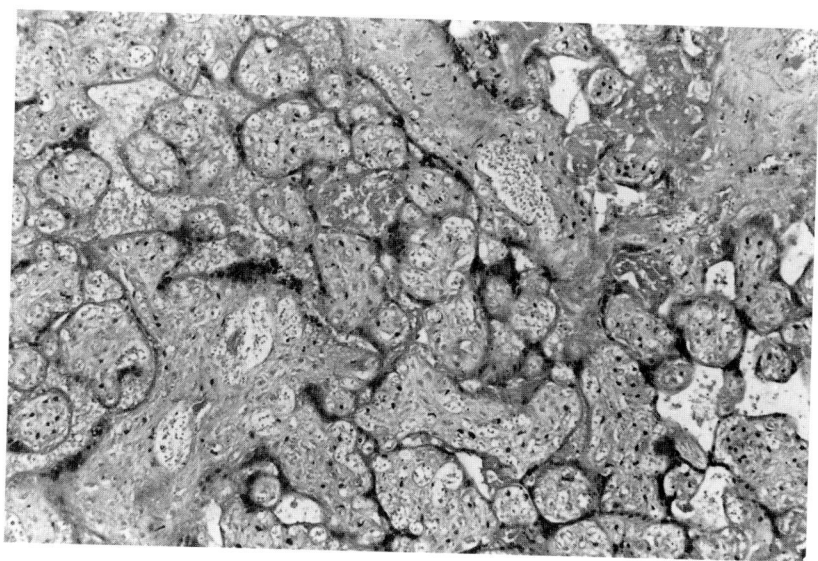

FIGURE 7.25. *Early infarct. The trophoblast is necrotic and the vessels within the villi are dilated. H&E, ×105.*

intensely congested, thus accounting for the dark-red color and the early lesion. Congestion of the vessels is commonly seen in villi overlying a retroplacental hemorrhage. This may be accentuated by villous hemorrhage associated with retroplacental hemorrhage [118]. The syncytial trophoblast undergoes rapid necrosis with loss of the brush border, loss of cytoplasmic basophilia, and eventually nuclear staining to form a faintly granular or amorphous eosinophilic layer of the surface of the villus (Fig. 7.25). With the loss of the distensive action of the maternal circulation, the intervillous space collapses and the villi become apposed, except where fibrin is deposited or a thrombus forms as the result of the release of thromboplastic substances from the necrotic tissues. The dilated fetal vessels collapse, though the mechanism involved is obscure. Though thrombi may be identified in some villous vessels, in infarcts they are by no means frequent, and it would seem probable that local release of vasoactive substances results in contraction of the vessels

with expulsion of the fetal blood into the functional circulation. Once the fetal circulation has ceased, the process of necrosis extends to involve the entire villus, which in old infarcts is only visible as a ghost-like remnant. Unlike infarcts elsewhere, placental infarcts do not undergo fibrosis and scarring, nor do they induce any significant inflammatory or histiocytic response in adjacent tissues. However, they may be infiltrated focally by maternal polymorphs, particularly at their margins where non-specific villitis is common. This should not be interpreted as evidence of an infective process.

While infarcts may occur in any cotyledon, they are most frequently seen at the placental margins, where they are usually of no clinical importance to the fetus. Central infarction may result from local uterine pathology, such as a submucous fibroid. However, central infarction, particularly where more than one cotyledon is affected, may reflect generalized uterine vascular disease and ischemia; thus, the adjacent non-infarcted cotyledons may also be underperfused, a pattern frequently associated with maternal hypertension and fetal growth retardation.

The extent of the placental infarction consistent with fetal survival will depend on the functional capacity of the surviving tissue and, to a lesser extent, on the degree of shunting of the fetal blood through the infarcted villi in the early stages of the evolution of the lesion. Thus, some fetuses may survive loss of one-third of the placenta, while a growth-retarded fetus with generalized disease of the uterine vessels may succumb after the loss of one or two cotyledons.

After 28 weeks' gestation, infarction involving in excess of 10–15% of the placenta is almost invariably confined to the hypertensive mother [119, 120], though in the second trimester there may be both extensive infarction and IUGR in the absence of maternal hypertension [56]. In mothers with pre-eclampsia, infarcts were found in one-third of placentae where the disease was classified as mild [119] and in almost two-thirds where the disease was classified as severe. In both groups there was a high fetal morbidity and mortality. These findings are emphasized by data derived from the British Perinatal Mortality Survey [121, 122]. Approximately 44% of perinatal deaths in the survey were attributed to obstetric factors, of which 65% were related to "placental insufficiency" or pre-eclamptic toxemia, particularly when severe. Mild pre-eclampsia, particularly of late onset, may not be associated with any identifiable placental pathology and has led some authors to speculate as to whether severe early-onset disease is a separate entity [123]. The effects of uteroplacental ischemia on the fetus depend not only on the extent of the lesions in the placental bed but also on the functional reserve of the placenta (*vide supra*). Since the effects of diminution of the maternal blood flow through the placenta may not result in an immediate parallel reduction in the fetal blood flow through the affected villi, shunting of deoxygenated blood is likely to occur. This may result in either temporary arrest or retardation of growth, which may return to normal after shunting ceases, providing that there is adequate remaining functional placenta. Emery and Kalpaktsoglou [124] showed that such periods of growth arrest may be detected by examination of the costochondral junctions of the ribs (see Chap. 2).

In those fetuses that survive the effects of uteroplacental ischemia, a significant number show serious sequelae, which in some instances may be fatal. In a series of just under 100 children with cerebral palsy under 1 year of age, Brown [125] found that perinatal asphyxia was implicated in one-fourth. In almost 40% of asphyxiated babies, placental problems (insufficiency, separation, and antepartum hemorrhage) were present.

Retroplacental Hematoma, Placental Hematoma, Intervillous Thrombus, and Subchorionic Hematoma

Thrombosis and hemorrhage into the maternal component of the placental circulation occur in several sites. Although only the retroplacental and placental hematomas have been related to pre-eclampsia and maternal hypertensive disease, they will be considered together.

Retroplacental Hematoma Separation of the placenta is an essential component of the process of parturition and, of necessity, deprives the placenta of its maternal blood supply; however, under normal conditions this is of little consequence to the fetus. Still, partial separation prior to the onset of labor or delivery may result in severe fetal distress or an acute hypoxic death. Such separations are usually associated with retroplacental hemorrhage and frequently with vaginal hemorrhage. The accumulation of blood beneath the placenta results in the formation of a retroplacental hematoma (Fig. 7.26). If localized, such hematomas result in ischemia of the overlying placenta, and if delivery does not follow rapidly evidence of infarction will appear. However, in the

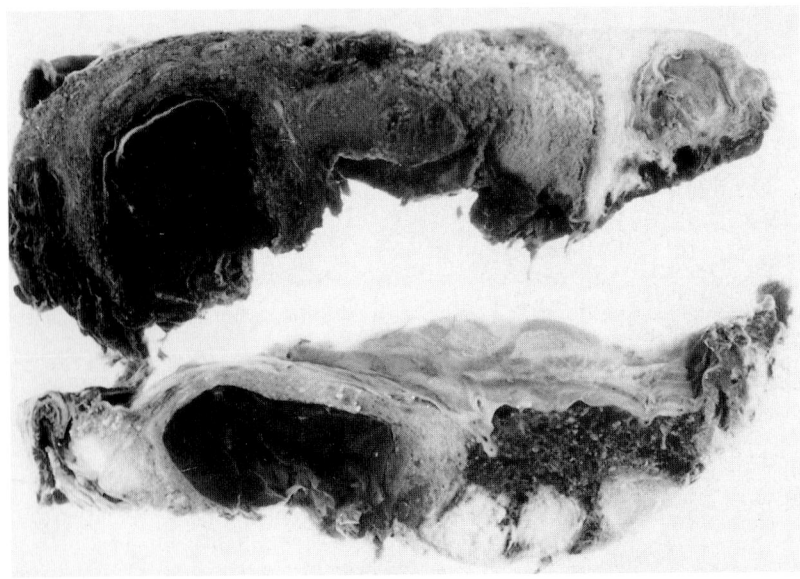

FIGURE 7.26. *Excavating retroplacental hemorrhages.*

majority of cases, the hemorrhages occur immediately prior to delivery, or concurrent acute fetal distress leads to emergency delivery; thus, macroscopic evidence of infarction is absent. Yet, there may be microscopic evidence in that the fetal vessels of the affected area will be intensely congested and dilated. In addition there may be intravillous hemorrhage, which is considered to be a possible marker of placental abruption [118].

Retroplacental hematoma is discussed frequently in the context of hypertensive disease, although the relationship between high blood pressure and these hemorrhages is tenuous, with the vast majority occurring in normotensive women. However, in the severe pre-eclamptic or eclamptic woman with low platelet count and disseminated intravascular coagulation, such hemorrhages may be anticipated.

The hemorrhages probably arise from basal vessels in the decidua, though larger acute lesions might arise from spiral arteries. It is not certain whether they are due to primary vascular pathology [18] or are preceded by local decidual necrosis; indeed, both mechanisms may be important. The bleeding is primarily intradecidual (i.e., in effect, they are dissecting hemorrhages of the decidua, there being a layer of decidua beneath the hemorrhage attached to the uterus and a layer above attached to the placenta). There is a continuous spectrum of lesions, from the acute hemorrhage with no obvious lesion in the placenta, through the recent lesion with adherent clot on the maternal surface of the placenta without any excavation, to the older excavating lesion with overlying infarction. As a result, the true incidence of such lesions is uncertain, since early lesions cannot be identified reliably. However, both Wilkin [5] and Fox [38] showed an incidence of approximately 5%. Fox [38] also demonstrated that women with pre-eclampsia had a three-fold increase in incidence, while there was no increase in women with essential hypertension. In the former, there is some evidence that decidual arteriolar disease may be an important factor [126]. While the hazards of such lesions to the fetus are readily apparent, it must also be remembered

that larger lesions may be associated with a consumptive coagulopathy in the mother, which on occasion may be fatal.

Allied to the retroplacental hemorrhage is the marginal hematoma, which occurs in about 1% of placentae and is of no clinical importance to the fetus providing that it is not in continuity with a retroplacental lesion. Marginal hematomas occur beneath the marginal cotyledons and adjacent membranes and probably arise as a result of rupture of decidual veins [5] during the early phases of placental separation. They may occur in both early and late pregnancy.

Placental Hematoma The placental hematoma is closely allied to the placental infarct, and the two lesions are frequently associated. The hematoma is a non-laminated thrombus situated in the center of a cotyledon, frequently an infarcted cotyledon, and is invariably associated with uteroplacental ischemia (Fig. 7.24). It has been suggested that the lesion is due to slow aneurysmal dilatation of a spiral artery proximal to a thrombosed segment, with subsequent rupture into the overlying infarcted cotyledon [18]. This mechanism, however, remains speculative. Alternatively, the peripheral villous infarction may initiate the lesion by leading to impaired blood flow through the more peripheral zones of the cotyledon, which, in the presence of continued but decreased flow into the central zones, may distend the central cavity of the cotyledon. Subsequent release of thromboplastic substances from the infarcted villi would induce clotting of this blood. It is important to distinguish the hematoma from the intervillous thrombus, as the latter is not considered to be of major clinical significance. Peripheral villous infarction is absent and the intervillous thrombus is generally laminated.

Intervillous Thrombosis Intervillous thrombi consist of clotted blood lying free within the intervillous space. Such thrombi may occur as isolated lesions, or there may be numerous thrombi within a single placenta. Characteristically, they are situated near or within the center of a cotyledon (Fig. 7.27) and tend to expand the intervillous space

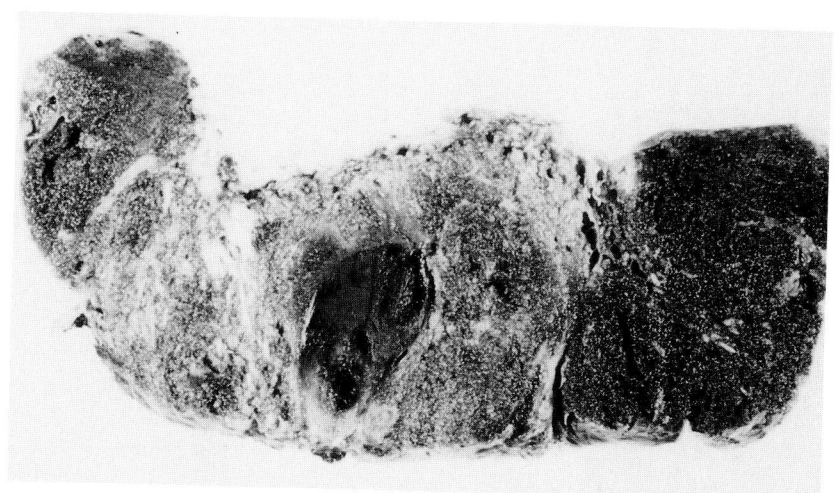

FIGURE 7.27. *Intervillous thrombus. The darker villi at the right-hand margin are intensely congested due to partial separation of the placenta prior to delivery.*

(the divergent villous lesions of Carter et al [127]). The incidence has been reported variously from 28% [5] to 48% [128].

Recent thrombi are dark red in color and may have a clearly visible laminated pattern on the cut surface. The older thrombus is yellow-brown or white, and the laminar pattern is often more readily apparent. Intervillous thrombi vary from several millimeters to several centimeters in diameter, the average size being between 0.5 and 2.5 centimeters.

Aging of these thrombi results in lysis of red cells, the invasion of macrophages—which eventually contain much hemosiderin—focal invasion with polymorphs, and not infrequently further thrombosis on the surface of the lesion. However, true organization of intervillous thrombi does not occur, because the placenta appears incapable of forming granulation tissue [129]. The adjacent villi may become encased in fibrin, but villous infarction does not occur. The stroma of these villi frequently contains numerous mononuclear cells resembling plasma cells, although the significance of these cells remains uncertain. It would seem that they are not an indication of a response of the fetus following the exposure of the fetal tissue to maternal antigens [37].

The genesis of central intervillous thrombi remains uncertain. Fetal hemorrhage has been incriminated, particularly because these lesions are said to be more common in cases of rhesus isoimmunization [130, 131], although this view is not supported by Wilkin [5]. It is clear that the majority of the blood in these thrombi is of maternal origin [132]. Some thrombi, if not all, undoubtedly contain a proportion of fetal red cells. It has been argued that a fetomaternal bleed may precipitate local thrombosis in the intervillous space [131]. The cause of the fetal hemorrhages is also uncertain, although it is probably due to rupture of the vasculosyncytial membranes because it is at this site that healing of defects in the trophoblast by fibrin deposits is most frequently observed [119]. If the underlying etiology of intervillous thrombi is not fetal bleeding or the release of thromboplastic material into the intervillous space from the villi, then the only likely alternative mechanism is a disturbed pattern of maternal blood flow through the intervillous space. In this respect, the intervillous space is likely to be modified significantly by villous hydrops, and this might be the cause of the increased frequency of intervillous thrombi in Rhesus placentae.

Subchorionic Hematoma   The accumulation of thrombus in the subchorionic intervillous lake results in the formation of a subchorionic hematoma. Small lesions are common, but massive collections of thrombus occur in about 1 in 2000 births [133]. Although commoner in association with fetal death, they occur in live births and have been detected ultrasonically in utero [134, 135]. In early pregnancy, a similar lesion is described as the so-called Breus' mole. Large lesions may be several centimeters in thickness and are traversed by the stem vessels of the individual cotyledons. The hematomas may project into the amniotic cavity, particularly in those cases associated with fetal death. The mechanisms of pathogenesis are obscure [136].

Summary

Maternal hypertensive disease mediates its effects on the placenta through lesions in the spiral arteries, these being primarily ischemic and their extent depending on the type of hypertension and its severity. The microscopic lesions are summarized in Table 7.2.

Table 7.2.   Microscopic lesions of the placenta and their effect on maternal diseases

	Syncytial knots	Fibrinoid necrosis	Maturation acceleration	Maturation delay	Thickened basement membrane	Mineralized basement membrane	Stromal fibrosis	Stromal edema	Hofbauer cells	Obliterated fetal vessels	Hemorrhagic vasculosis	Cytotrophoblast	Vasculosyncytial membranes
Essential hypertension	↑	–	↑	–	+	–	–	–	–	–	–	↑	–
Gestational hypertension	↑	–	↑	–	+	–	–	–	–	–	–	↑	–
Pre-eclampsia/eclampsia	↑	↑	↑	–	+	+	±	–	–	–	–	↑	±↑
Diabetes mellitus	↑±	↑	–	↓	+	–	–	+	–	–	–	↑	↓
Maternal collagen disease	↑	–	↑	–	+	–	–	–	–	–	–	↑	–↓
Fetal hydrops	–	↑	±↓	±↓	+	–	–	+	+	–	–	↑	↓
Metabolic disorders	–	–	–	–	–	–	–	+	+	–	–	↑	–
Intrauterine death	↑	–	–	–	+	+	–	–	–	+	+	–	–

↑ Increased; ↓ decreased; + present.

Maternal Diabetes Mellitus

Modern intensive management of the pregnant diabetic female has radically altered the perinatal outcome. Thus, in the latter part of the first half of this century, a perinatal mortality of 40–50% [137] was not uncommon, while today the outcome is comparable with the non-diabetic mother, although the high incidence of congenital malformations has not been reduced significantly [138–142]. White [143] and, more recently, West [144] classified diabetic patients into four major groups and demonstrated that the outcome of pregnancy was closely related to the severity of the disease and to treatment. In overtly diabetic patients, much has been and can be achieved, but there is a growing suspicion that occult diabetes may contribute to a significant number of late unexplained stillbirths in perinatal mortality statistics.

The four groups of diabetic mothers are:

1. Those with insulin-dependent diabetes that precedes conception. These patients may derive benefit from pre- or periconceptional care [145, 146].
2. Those with early disease, in whom hyperglycemia is detected in pregnancy and persists after delivery.
3. The gestational diabetic patient in whom disturbances of glucose metabolism are only found during pregnancy.
4. The prediabetic or one with occult diabetes with no clinical evidence of diabetes either during or after pregnancy who subsequently develops diabetes in later life. Such women may, in addition to unexplained late stillbirths, also deliver typical diabetic cherubs.

While the large cherubic baby with abundant subcutaneous fat, visceromegaly, and microscopic abnormalities of the internal organs—particularly in the liver and pancreas—typifies the effect of diabetes on the conceptus, it must be remembered that, prior to modern management (and even

occasionally in spite of it), IUGR may occur [147] in the absence of any manifest additional disorder, such as pre-eclampsia. In the presence of such a wide range of maternal and fetal manifestations, the lack of any consistent placental pathology is unsurprising, although the typical case may show a constellation of characteristic lesions [148].

Macroscopically, the placenta is bulky and edematous [149], often with a thick edematous umbilical cord. Though amnion nodosum has been described in association with maternal diabetes [150], this is probably a secondary phenomenon and not a specific feature of diabetes. However, fetal vascular thrombosis occurs both in fetal organs and the placenta [151], with an incidence of up to 10% in the latter. The so-called fetal infarct differs from the commoner infarct due to uterine vascular disease, in that the pathological changes do not affect the viability of the tissues that are dependent on the maternal blood supply. Macroscopically, the affected villi become pale (Fig. 7.28) but without any significant change in the consistency or texture of the placenta, providing that the circulation in the intervillous space is maintained. The microscopic changes were described earlier (see Vascular Thrombosis).

Microscopically, the villi of the diabetic placenta are typically large and immature (Fig. 7.29), a change best seen at the center of cotyledons. The vascular component is prominent, but vasculosyncytial membranes are underrepresented. The stroma stains poorly with H&E due to the presence of increased glycosamino-glycans [152], and there are increased numbers of Hofbauer cells. Other features include cytotrophoblastic hyperplasia, stromal and subtrophoblastic edema, increased syncytial knots and bridges, thickened trophoblastic basement membrane, and fibrinoid necrosis. These changes are only seen in about one-third of all diabetic placentae, and while there does appear to be a relationship between the severity of the diabetes and their development, in that they are less common in placentae from gestational diabetic patients [153, 154], the effects of better diabetic

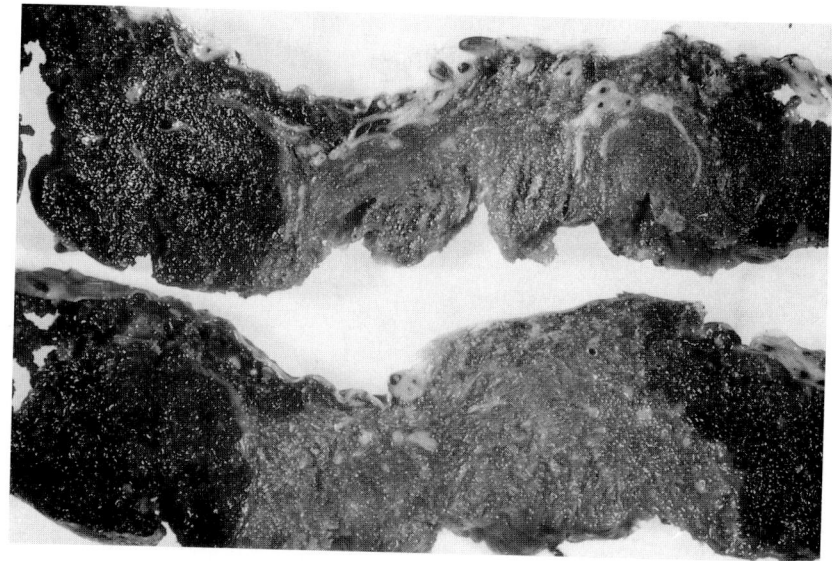

FIGURE 7.28.   *Fetal infarct. The villi in the central portion of the placenta are pale, but they retain the normal spongy appearance of the normal villi on either side.*

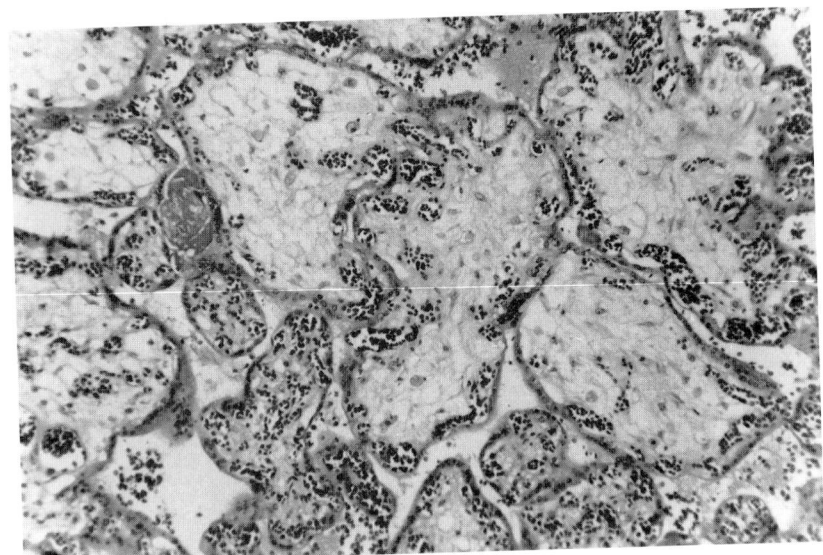

FIGURE 7.29.   *Diabetic placenta of 38 weeks' gestation. The villi are large with abundant stroma, deeply placed vessels without vasculosyncytial membranes, and a bilaminar trophoblast. H&E, ×105.*

control in ameliorating them are uncertain. A recent morphometric study in highly controlled diabetics has shown that the incidence and severity of changes in these placentae are not influenced by either the duration or the severity of the diabetes [155]. It has also raised fundamental questions about current thinking on the pathological changes in the placenta associated with maternal diabetes by casting doubt on the concept of villous immaturity, suggesting that the villi of the diabetic placentae were more mature than controls. However, these patients had neither significantly larger babies nor placentae compared to the control group, and the relevance of the findings to the poorly controlled mother having a diabetic cherub must be questioned.

The placental bed has been studied [69, 156], but the results are contradictory, with no consistent abnormality being demonstrated in the absence of other complications of pregnancy, such as hypertension.

Maternal Collagen Diseases

Many of the collagen diseases result in widespread vascular pathology and, therefore, it may be anticipated that where the uterine vasculature is involved, placental lesions will ensue. Unfortunately, while there has been considerable clinical interest in the effects of these diseases on the mother and fetus and the effects of pregnancy on the course of these diseases, there are few data on the placenta [157]. Abortion and premature delivery rates are increased in mothers with systemic lupus erythematosus (SLE), but placentae have been reported variously as normal [38, 158] and as infarcted with necrotizing decidual arteriolitis [37]. Personal experience has revealed no consistent pattern in such cases and, since pre-eclamptic toxemia is not uncommon in patients with SLE [159], some cases are likely to show lesions described in association with pre-eclamptic toxemia. There are no characteristic lesions in rheumatoid arthritis, scleroderma, or polyarteritis nodosa [160].

Qualitative Disturbances of Maternal Blood Flow

These have been discussed earlier in relation to maternal cardiac disease and altitude. Anemias have also been considered, as they affect oxygenation of the conceptus. Sickle cell disease is not only associated with anemia but also with the risk of sickling, which may occlude the uterine vasculature, resulting in placental infarction. Sickle cells may be readily identifiable in the intervillous space.

FETAL DISEASE AND THE PLACENTA

The vast majority of fetal anomalies are not associated with identifiable placental lesions. Where present, placental lesions are generally non-specific, although they may give a clue to the etiology of the fetal disorders (e.g., villitis and infection). Of the non-specific disorders related to fetal abnormalities and acquired disease, hydrops is one of the commonest.

Placental Hydrops

The distinction between hydropic degeneration of the placenta and hydatidiform degeneration has been discussed earlier. Hydrops fetalis is almost invariably associated with some degree of placental hydrops. The most common etiological factors are hemolytic disease due to rhesus isoimmunization or other blood group incompatibilities between the mother and fetus; and, in certain areas of the world, due to hemoglobinopathies, in particular alpha-thalassemia. Other suspect or proven maternal disorders include diabetes mellitus and fetomaternal hemorrhage. Fetal disorders include twin transfusion syndrome (in the recipient twin), achondroplasia, cystic adenomatoid malformation of the lung, mongolism and other trisomies, pulmonary lymphangiectasia, multiple congenital malformations, congenital nephrosis, chorionic or umbilical vein thrombosis, fetal neuroblastomatosis, and certain infections (i.e., parvovirus and cytomegalovirus infection, toxoplasmosis, syphilis, leptospirosis, Chagas disease, and congenital hepatitis). A proportion of cases (5–10%) remain unexplained or idiopathic [37, 161–163]. The majority of fetal abnormalities are readily diagnosed during life or at postmortem examination but, in the absence of information about the fetus, no case should be classified as idiopathic.

The hydropic placenta is characteristically pale, bulky, and friable, and transudation of fluid occurs freely after delivery so that storage of these placentae will result in progressive loss of weight. Fresh placentae from severely affected full-term infants frequently weigh between 1 and 2 kilograms. There is edema of the spongy layer of the chorion and of the umbilical cord. The membranes and cord may be pale yellow-green or orange-yellow. In mildly affected fetuses with rhesus isoimmunization, there may be little macroscopic abnormality. In those cases in which the etiology of the hydrops is not apparent from the clinical history or examination of the fetus, histological examination of the placenta is essential, although all placentae with hydrops should be examined microscopically.

The histological features in hemolytic disease include stromal edema, with increased cellularity and prominent Hofbauer cells; retention of a bilaminar trophoblast, with easily identifiable cytotrophoblast even at term; and prominent peripherally situated capillaries filled with nucleated red cells and their precursors (Fig. 7.30).

True hemopoiesis occurring in the villous stroma is extremely rare, if it occurs at all. The presence of mitotic activity in the cytotrophoblast and in stroma cells indicates that placental growth continues into the last trimester of pregnancy. Other histological features include thickening of the trophoblastic basement membrane, fibrinoid necrosis, and possibly increased syncytial knotting. Swelling of the endothelial cells of the villous vessels is frequently prominent. In addition to the edema of the membranes and cord, there are often numerous pigment-filled macrophages in the chorion, much of this pigment being hemosiderin. Iron-laden cells may also be identified in the villi, and iron may be deposited on the trophoblastic and fetal capillary basement membranes and within the villous stroma. Many of these histological abnormalities are found in other non-immunological cases of hydrops, although evidence of hemopoietic activity may be absent, and there may be additional lesions (e.g., evidence of villitis in infections).

The mechanisms concerned in the genesis of the placental lesions in immunological hydrops are obscure and, equally, there is doubt as to the pathogenesis of the hydrops. Fetal anemia, hypoproteinemia, and cardiac and renal factors may be implicated, although their respective roles are far from clear. Thus, anemia per se in prenatally exsanguinated fetal lambs does not lead to hydrops [164]. Low serum protein levels may be significant [165], although Macafee et al [163] found little evidence to support this in their earlier study. The possible mechanisms involved in the pathogenesis of the histological lesions in the placenta are reviewed by Fox [38].

Metabolic Disorders

Placental lesions identifiable by light microscopy occur in certain inherited metabolic disorders associated with storage of mucopolysaccharides and lipids [166–170]. These disorders are now diagnosed antenatally [171, 172], but they may present as fetal ascites [166]. While biochemical and electron microscopic studies are required for confirmation of the type of disorder present, examination of the placenta may provide the first clue that a metabolic disease is present. If the fetus is macerated, it may be the only evidence available.

The characteristic lesions are found in the Hofbauer cells, which are large and vacuolated, and in the syncytial trophoblast, which shows similar vacuolation (Fig. 7.31). Further delineation of the disease may be possible by

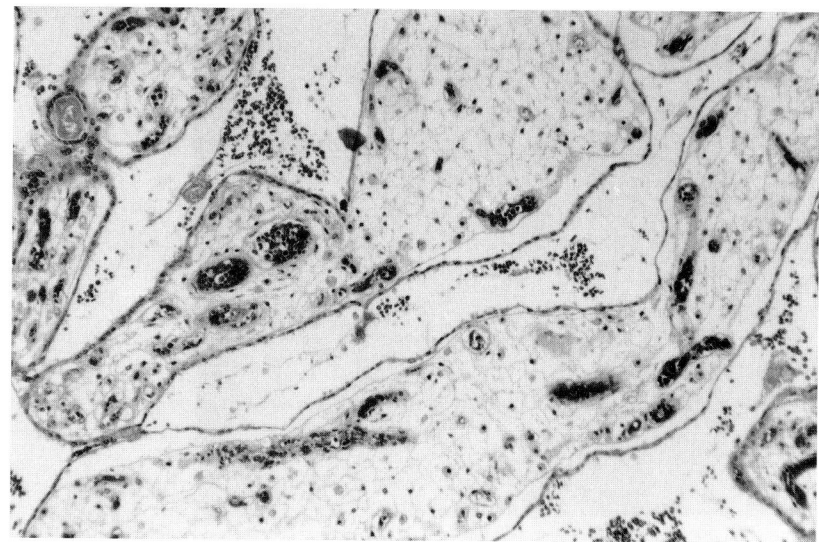

FIGURE 7.30. *Rhesus isoimmunization. Hydropic villi. H&E, ×105.*

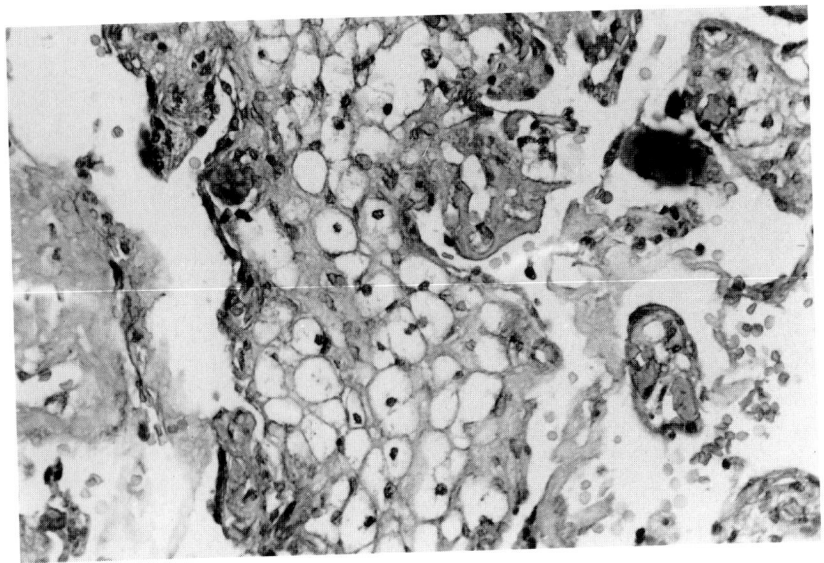

FIGURE 7.31.   *I cell disease. The villous stroma contains numerous storage cells with clear cytoplasm and small eccentrically placed nuclei. H&E, ×263.*

histochemical means [167]. Sialic acid storage disease, mucolipidosis II (I cell disease), and GM1 gangliosidosis may be differentiated in part by electron microscopy, on the basis of the distribution of membrane-bound inclusions within placental cells [170].

Miscellaneous Fetal Disorders

Small placentae may be found in certain karyotypic abnormalities (see below). Ehlers-Danlos syndrome (type 1)—an autosomal dominant disorder of collagen production—is associated with premature rupture of the fetal membranes, thought to be due to deficient collagen in the placental membranes [173]. Amniotic bands have been reported in association with Ehlers-Danlos type IV and the severe lethal form of osteogenesis imperfecta [174].

MISCELLANEOUS PLACENTAL LESIONS

Small and Large Placentae

The size and weight of the placenta in isolation are of little value and require additional data, including gestation, fetal weight, and the macroscopic and microscopic status of the organ, before interpreting the significance of these parameters. The normal fetal placental weight ratio for differing gestations has been documented fully by Boyd and Hamilton [82] but rarely is used in either clinical or pathological practice. Attempts have been made to relate placental size to its functional capacity, and placental weight to birth weight [175–177], but such data are of little value to the perinatal pathologist.

Small placentae, while frequently found attached to small babies, do not necessarily imply a causal relationship; indeed, in many cases there is likely to be a common factor for both, be it uteroplacental ischemia or a malformation syndrome such as trisomy 18.

Large placentae (i.e., those weighing over 1 kg at term in the absence of obvious pathology [e.g., hydrops]) are rare and usually remain unexplained. In the author's experience, they frequently show villous immaturity, and in the presence of a large baby (>4.5 kg), they should alert the pathologist to the possibility of a prediabetic state in the mother.

In the last few years, it has become apparent that there may be differences in the karyotype of the placenta and the fetus and that these differences may affect fetal survival and/or growth. Placental mosaicism has been implicated in fetal growth retardation, but as more studies are completed its significance, if any, is becoming less clear. In particular, karyotypic studies on the placentae of small-for-dates babies have given conflicting results, and their relevance to the growth disturbances remains uncertain [178–180].

Placental Calcification

The calcium content of the placenta rises rapidly in the last month of pregnancy, doubling between 37 weeks and term [181], and is increased between 28 and 36 weeks' gestation in placentae from toxemic mothers when compared with controls, although there is no difference at term. It is higher in stillbirths born before 37 weeks' gestation, being equal to that in placentae in live births at term. Calcium deposition in the placenta occurs in two distinct patterns, each having a different etiology and significance. Extravillous calcification is a common finding in full-term pregnancies. Intravillous calcification is associated with embryonic or fetal death and with fetal intrauterine cardiac failure.

Extensive extravillous calcification is readily recognizable as irregular yellow-white gritty deposits on the maternal surface of the placenta (Fig. 7.32). Slicing reveals that these deposits extend along the edges of the placental septa and in the intercotyledonary zones. The calcium is deposited entirely in relation to fibrin deposits in the basal plate and septa and on the surface of villi.

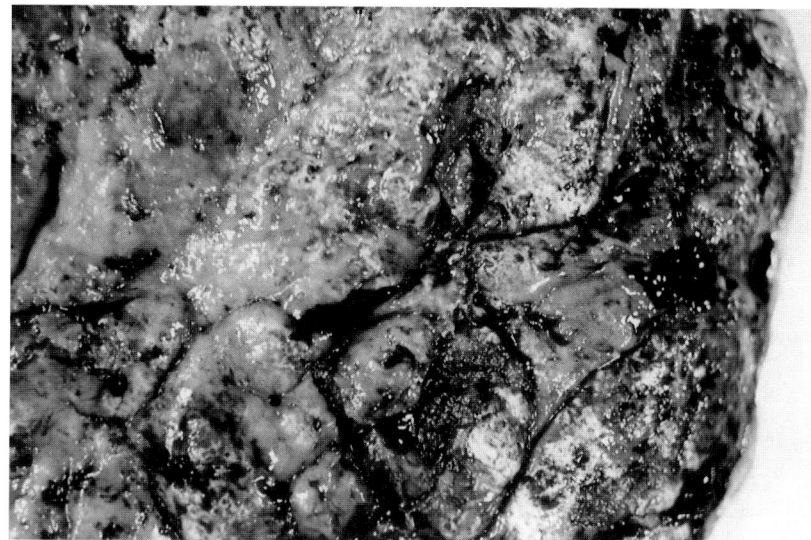

FIGURE 7.32. *Placental calcification. Abundant white deposits on the maternal surface.*

Tindall and Scott [182], using x-ray techniques, demonstrated a uniform reticular pattern of calcification that gradually increased in extent as pregnancy continued. Fox [183] found that almost one-fourth of full-term placentae were calcified; Fujikura [27, 184] found that the incidence of calcified placentae was related to the season, being more frequent in the summer months. It was also more common in primigravid mothers. The evidence suggests that the principal controlling factor is the maternal serum calcium level and that calcification of the extravillous areas of the placenta is normal rather than pathological. The concept of the unhealthy gritty placenta, beloved of midwives and obstetricians, is a myth. Calcification is influenced by maternal dietary intake of calcium and vitamin D and exposure to ultraviolet light. It is usually stated that calcification is more common in postmature pregnancies, but the evidence is conflicting.

Mineralization of the basement membrane is identified readily on routine staining, the deposits containing both iron and calcium (Fig. 7.33). It is most typically seen after fetal death if the placenta is retained in utero for about 1 week or more, but it may be seen in association with live births, particularly those where there is evidence of major circulatory disturbance in the fetus or where the demand for iron and/or calcium is reduced due to fetal disease. The author has observed basement membrane mineralization in association with congenital heart disease, osteogenesis imperfecta, and dyserythropoietic anemia.

The deposition is likely to reflect an imbalance between the iron and calcium transferred across the trophoblastic barrier and fetal demand. In some cases, deposition may also involve the stroma of the villus and the basement membrane of the fetal capillaries. Rarely, iron and calcium deposits may occur in larger vessel walls, notably in the media, and in

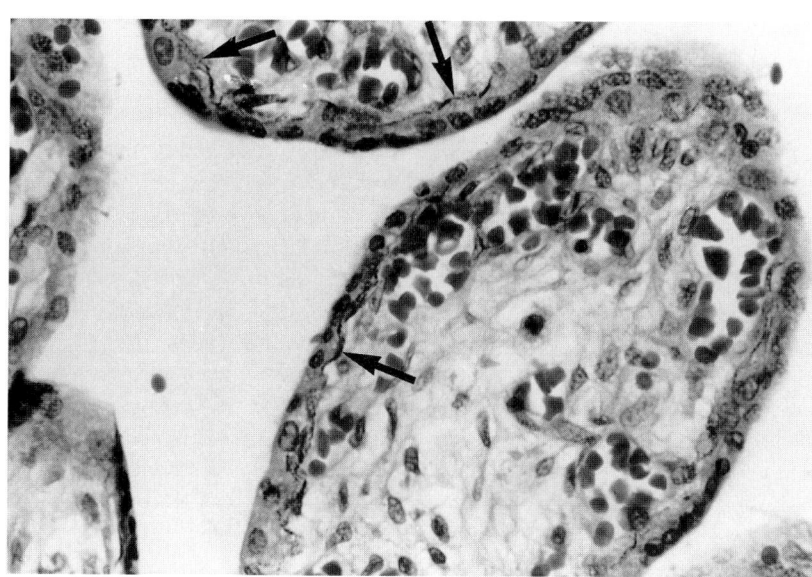

FIGURE 7.33. *Mineralization of the trophoblastic basement membrane* (arrows). *H&E, ×420.*

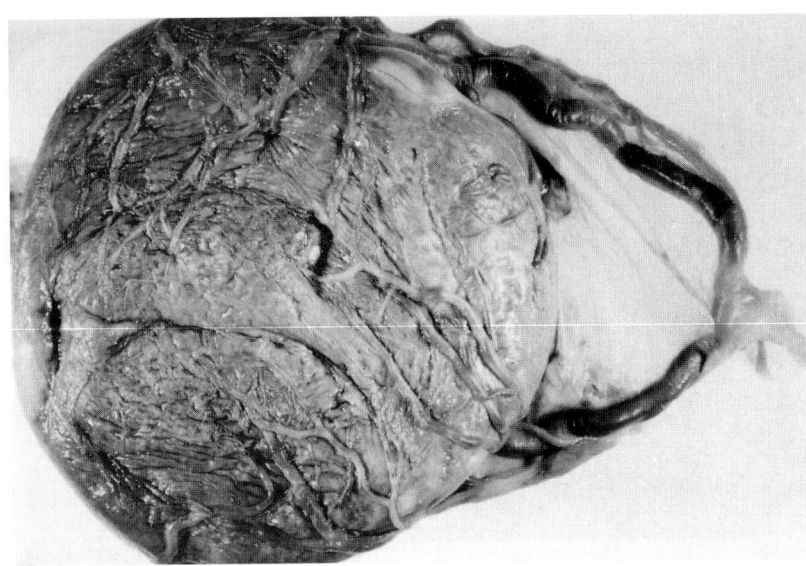

FIGURE 7.34.   *Velamentous insertion of the cord. The vessels cross the membranes unprotected by Wharton's jelly for up to 7 cm.*

these circumstances may be associated with similar lesions in the vessels of the umbilical cord and the fetus [185, 186].

THE UMBILICAL CORD

Variations in Insertion of the Umbilical Cord

Approximately 85–90% of umbilical cords are inserted into the placenta within the limits of the chorionic plate. A further 5–10% are inserted into the margin, and approximately 1% are inserted into the membranes (Fig. 7.34). It is possible that the major determinant of the site of insertion is the relationship of the embryonic disc of the early conceptus to the developing chorion frondosum and the degenerating chorion laeve. An alternative explanation is the concept of trophotropism (Strassmann, quoted by Benirschke and Driscoll [37]), in which the placenta grows differentially in a specific direction toward a better site of implantation. This hypothesis is particularly attractive in explaining the high incidence of velamentous insertion associated with twin pregnancy (approximately seven times as great as in singleton placentae). Velamentous insertion, where the umbilical vessels run for variable distances in the membranes unprotected by Wharton's jelly, is also associated with a high incidence of an absent umbilical artery (one in eight, according to Little [187]). It is difficult to be certain if the velamentous insertion and the absence of an umbilical artery are separately acquired abnormalities or whether they represent part of a general response to a teratological insult to the early conceptus, as both are associated with an increased incidence of malformation in the embryo or fetus.

Apart from the increased incidence of malformations, velamentous insertion is associated with an increased risk of fetal mortality and morbidity during labor, because the unprotected vessels may be compressed or torn by the presenting part or, on occasion, by the obstetrician during arti-

ficial rupture of the membranes. Marginal insertion of the umbilical cord has also been associated with an increased risk of fetal abnormality, but considerable doubt has been cast on this view [188, 189].

Absence of an Umbilical Artery

A single umbilical artery has been reported variously as occurring in between 0.2% [190] and 12.0% [191] of placentae. This wide variation in incidence is a reflection of the population studied; thus, Molz [191] examined only postmortem material, where the range extends from 2.7% [192] to 12.0%. The largest postmortem series of 1554 cases [193] recorded an incidence of 2.9%. In consecutive obstetrical patients, the highest incidence (1.22%) was found among 11,371 white singleton pregnancies [194] in a total series of 26,539 consecutive single births where the overall incidence was 0.76%. This is in close agreement with Bryan and Kohler [195], who demonstrated 0.72% in 20,000 placentae. This is approximately three times the incidence in our own series, which is in agreement with the lowest figure (0.2%) recorded above.

Kristoffersen [196] noted that the observed incidence in fixed material was higher than in unfixed specimens, both macroscopically and microscopically. He recommends treatment of a segment of cord with glacial acetic acid, which makes the cord translucent. There is a tendency to overdiagnose an absent vessel in unfixed material, particularly if there is a gross discrepancy in the size of the arteries; thus, histological confirmation should be sought in every case.

A high incidence has been noted by some authors in twin pregnancies [197, 198]; Benirschke [197] reported a series of 250 successive twin pregnancies containing 3.6% of cords with a single artery. This was not observed by Kristoffersen [196], who found one affected cord in 106 pairs of twins.

The proportion of malformed fetuses among conceptions with a single umbilical artery varies in the range 0–100% [196], although these extremes only occur in very small series. As would be anticipated, the postmortem series showed a consistently high proportion of malformed infants; Seki and Strauss [193] found that 73.3% were abnormal, while Molz [191] found that 93% were abnormal. Froehlich and Fujikura [194], in their very large series, demonstrated that 23% of the fetuses were malformed. The incidence of malformations in those series comprising consecutive pregnancies and which include over 20 examples of a single umbilical artery varies from 10% [199] to 48% [187]. Our own experience suggests an incidence of between 10% and 20%, as found by Bryan and Kohler [195]; although this is influenced clearly by the effectiveness of follow-up because certain malformations, particularly those of paired organs, may not become apparent until well beyond the perinatal period. It must be emphasized, however, that the majority of malformations associated with a single umbilical artery are very gross.

The pathogenesis of a single umbilical artery is uncertain, although there are two possible explanations. The artery may never have developed (agenesis), or two arteries may have been present initially, one later undergoing atrophy. Among 48 cases studied by Altshuler and Russell [200], atrophic vascular remnants were found in 19 cases, the remainder considered to be examples of agenesis. In order to establish the origin of the lesion, it is necessary to examine multiple sections of affected cords. In some instances, the single artery is thought to be a vitelline artery [201, 202], a feature of some interest, in that the very rare examples of supernumerary vessels [203, 204] have been considered to be due to persistence of vitelline vessels. Rarely, angiomatous lesions of the cord are identified and, while these may arise from the normal vascular components, it is also possible that some originate from vitelline vessels (see Chorangioma under Lesions of the Amnion and Chorion).

It will be clear from the preceding discussion that the true incidence and significance of a single umbilical artery in relation to fetal malformations is uncertain and requires further investigation. While it is not difficult to examine large numbers of cords in a maternity unit, it is more difficult to obtain a large enough series of cases with single umbilical arteries to assess its relationship to other fetal, placental, or maternal abnormalities. Thus, the largest series published to date only includes 203 cases [194]. In twin pregnancies, the difficulty is even greater.

The perinatal mortality associated with a single umbilical artery shows an equally wide variation; thus Benirschke and Driscoll [37] in their review of published series noted a range of 7.2–76.0%. The high mortality is primarily the result of lethal malformations, but it appears that there is also an increased mortality in morphologically normal infants [187, 194, 195, 205, 206]. Bryan and Kohler [195] found a perinatal mortality among 118 normal infants of 4.2% compared with a 2.66% mortality in normal infants with normal umbilical arteries. The incidence of a single umbilical artery in non-malformed stillbirths and neonatal deaths was 1.1% compared with 0.72% in all newborn infants. Thus, it does appear that perinatal mortality is increased in the absence of an umbilical artery in otherwise anatomically normal fetuses.

In several series, it has been observed that there is an association between a single umbilical artery and small-for-dates infants [194, 195, 207–209], this being true even in those infants without anatomical malformations.

Benirschke and Brown [207], Seki and Strauss [193], Kristoffersen [196], and Bryan and Kohler [195] all noted that, where a single umbilical artery was present in one of a pair of twins, the twin with the abnormal cord was commonly smaller than its normal sibling. It is not clear whether the increased number of small-for-dates infants is sufficient to account for the high perinatal mortality in anatomically normal fetuses.

Among the clinical features found in the mothers of children with a single umbilical artery are an increased incidence of diabetes mellitus, from 6.4% [194] to 14% [193], and an increased incidence of pre-eclampsia and polyhydramnios [207]. Associated placental abnormalities include circumvallate placentae and velamentous insertions, Seki and Strauss [193] finding the latter lesion in 5% of cases.

The incidence of a single umbilical artery appears to be higher in spontaneous abortions; thus, Javert and Barton [131] and Thomas [209] recorded 2.4% and 2.7%, respectively. In my own series, the incidence is 3.1% but this may, in part, be accounted for by the high incidence of gross malformations in abortions. The gender ratio reported in cases with single umbilical arteries varies from all male [210] to a preponderance of females, thus Bryan and Kohler [195] recorded a ratio of 1.4:1.0 in favor of females. While male predominance is most commonly found in postmortem series, where more males would be expected, the excess of females may be due to the high proportion of anencephalic patients. It therefore seems probable that the gender ratio is not significantly disturbed in fetuses with single umbilical arteries, if allowance is made for the effect of malformations with gender ratios that vary from the norm.

In summary, it may be stated that there is an association between malformations; increased perinatal mortality; small-for-dates infants, particularly in twins; maternal diabetes; spontaneous abortion; and single umbilical artery. However, in the absence of gross malformations in the fetus, the presence of a single umbilical artery should not be considered an indication for intensive investigation of an apparently normal infant to exclude minor abnormalities.

Abnormal Length of the Umbilical Cord

The normal full-term umbilical cord measures between 45 and 75 centimeters, with a mean of approximately 60 centimeters [26], and has a diameter of 1 to 2 centimeters.

Gross abnormalities of cord length are rare and of doubtful significance, although Naeye [150] has related short cords to poor fetal mobility, often due to neuromuscular disease. Occasionally, a very long cord may become entangled with the fetal limbs or wound around the neck, a nuchal cord being found in between 15% and 33% of pregnancies [211–213]. However, the majority of such cases are associated with a cord of normal length. Earn [32] found that 87% of cases with unusually long cords had loops around the neck. The longest cord encountered by the author measured 122 centimeters and was associated with a macerated stillbirth, the cause of death being thrombosis of the umbilical vein. Similar cases have been reported by Benirschke and Driscoll [37].

Very short cords are less common, and Browne [214] found that they are associated with placental abruption, uterine inversion, and fetal hemorrhage into the cord. Rupture of the cord may occur during delivery.

Compression of the Cord

Compression of the umbilical cord of sufficient degree to obstruct the fetal circulation [215–218] may result from entanglement with the fetal limbs or by encirclement of the neck, prolapse of the cord with entrapment by the presenting part in labor, constriction by amniotic bands [219–221], and velamentous insertion. In monoamniotic twins, there may be entanglement of both cords, which may result in both fetuses succumbing. Occasionally, true knots may be implicated in the death of singleton fetuses. It is clear from the etiological factors that only a few will be apparent to the pathologist examining the placenta.

Prolapse of the umbilical cord is an obstetric emergency and occurs in about 0.3% of pregnancies [222]. These authors found a perinatal mortality rate of 11.4% among 70 potentially salvageable babies. Histological study of such placentae may show intense congestion of the fetal vessels, although this may be indistinguishable from a very early placental infarct. Occasional stillbirths may be received with the cord wound around the neck, but it is not always clear that this is the cause of intrauterine death. It is also difficult to be certain if these deaths are due to compression of the umbilical vessels or, possibly, due to compression of the vessels in the neck of the fetus. A tight nuchal cord may be associated with neonatal hypovolemic shock [223].

Knots of the Cord

Knots of the umbilical cord are of two categories. *True knots*, as the term implies, involve entanglement of the cord. *False knots* are due to inequalities in the lengths of the umbilical vein and umbilical arteries, the latter being longer. This results in the formation of loops in the arteries (Fig. 7.35). These loops may become twisted and tortuous as a result of spiraling of the afferent and efferent limbs around each other; they are of little clinical significance, although rarely an umbilical artery may thrombose. Occasionally, a large false knot with varicose vessels may be compressed by the presenting part during labor and cause severe fetal distress. Whether these are simply minor malformations of the umbilical cord or have a hemodynamic significance is unknown, but they are commoner in early pregnancy than at term.

True knots should be diagnosed at delivery because the pathologist can never be certain that knots in the delivered cord and placenta have not been tied by a tidy-minded obstetrician or midwife. True knots occur in approximately 0.5% of deliveries [32, 214]. The presence of a knot in an otherwise normal umbilical cord is unlikely to be a direct cause of fetal death and, in the absence of thrombus in the

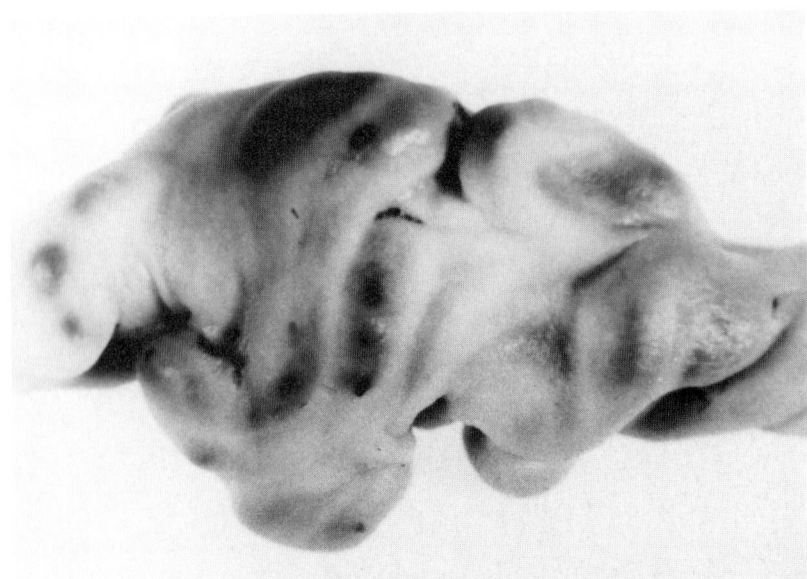

FIGURE 7.35. *False knot in cord due to unequal growth of the constituent vessels.*

vessels, the pathologist should be wary of accepting the obstetrician's word that it was the cause of fetal demise. Long-standing knots may be confirmed by histological examination, in some instances, by the presence of adhesions between the amniotic surfaces of the loops.

It is pertinent to note that any lesion impeding flow in the umbilical vein will result in dilatation of the vein proximal to the obstruction and extreme congestion of the fetal vessels within the placenta. Compression of an umbilical artery will result in edema of the cord and little or no abnormality of the placenta.

Edema of the Cord

Edema of the umbilical cord (Fig. 7.36) is largely ignored, although unusual cases with very gross edema appear periodically in the literature [224–226]. Javert and Barton [227] draw attention to edema of the cord in spontaneous abortions. The definition of edema of the umbilical cord is critical, and Coulter et al [228] have accepted an arbitrary cross-sectional area of 1.3 cm² or more as an indication of significant edema. Edema may be generalized or segmental, and edematous blebs are not uncommon in otherwise normal cords. Coulter et al [228] found edema to be associated with placental abruption, maternal diabetes, macerated intrauterine deaths, Rhesus isoimmunization, prematurity, respiratory distress, and infants delivered by caesarean section, but *not* with fetal distress, neonatal asphyxia, maternal hypertension, or edema. The significance of these findings is uncertain, since it is clear that many of the negative correlations are themselves associated with positive associations (i.e., fetal distress and caesarean section). They suggest that edema of the cord may be of value as a prognostic indicator of respiratory distress in the fetus. The etiology of edema of the cord is also uncertain. Arterial obstruction, low plasma proteins, and changes in intraplacental vascular resistance may be implicated, but in most cases adequate clinical information is not available to determine the etiology.

Torsion of the Umbilical Cord

The vessels in the cord normally show a varying degree of spiraling around the long axis. This spiraling may become accentuated, particularly after fetal death in utero, and should not be interpreted as the cause of death unless there is further evidence of vascular occlusion, such as thrombosis or congestion of the fetus or placenta [37]. Cases of fetal death due to torsion have been reported by Weber [218], Wilkin [5], Benirschke and Driscoll [37], and Phillipe [26].

Hemorrhage into and from the Umbilical Cord

Bleeding from the vessels of the cord is usually the result of obstetric trauma either at the time of delivery or occasionally as a result of puncture during diagnostic amniocentesis. The unprotected vessels of a velamentous insertion are at particular risk during delivery. A very short umbilical cord may be torn or avulsed during the second stage of labor. Hemorrhage into the substance of the cord is usually venous in origin, although if extensive it may surround all three vessels and result in compression, the most severe effects being on the vein [229]. It is difficult to be certain that cord hemorrhages (Fig. 7.37) found on routine examination of the placenta are significant, since the majority will be the result of handling during labor. The incidence of true antepartum hematomas is low (1 in 5505 according to Dippel [230]). The lesions are usually segmental, measuring up to 10 centimeters in length, although up to 42 centimeters of cord have been involved. Other than trauma, etiological factors that have been implicated include inflammation, abnormal vessels, varicosities, syphilis, and idiopathic calcification [37]. The mortality associated with this lesion is high, and Schreier and Brown [231] in a review of 36 cases in the literature found that almost one-half succumbed. Calcification of the umbilical vessels has been reported by Ivemark et al [232] and is associated with calcification of vessels in the fetus. The etiology is obscure.

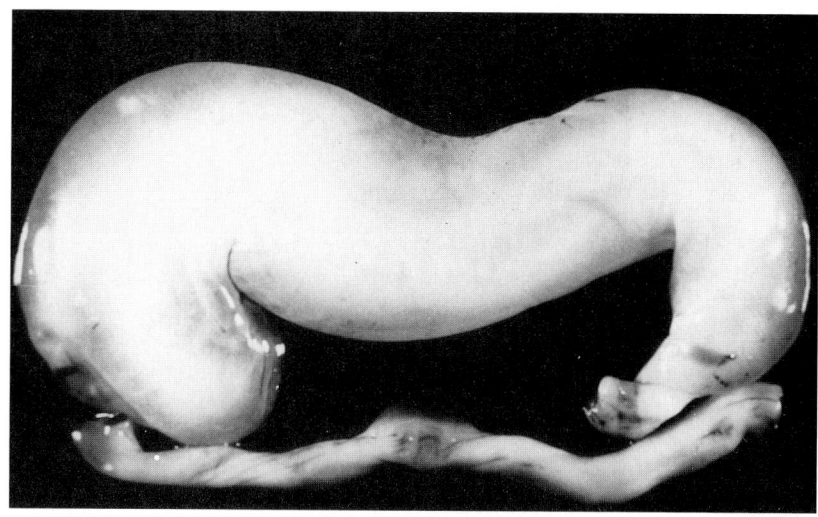

FIGURE 7.36.   *Segmental edema of umbilical cord.*

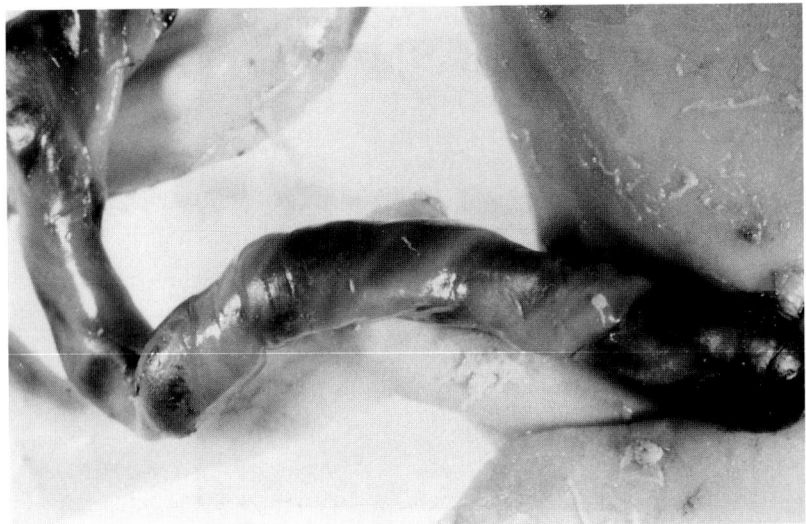

FIGURE 7.37. *Hemorrhage and thrombosis of umbilical cord associated with amniotic bands.*

Puncture of the umbilical cord should always be sought carefully when unexplained intrauterine death occurs following amniocentesis.

Embryological Vestiges

Two embryological vestiges may be related to cyst formation in the umbilical cord—the omphalomesenteric duct and the allantoic diverticulum—although in most instances these structures can be identified only by microscopic examination.

The omphalomesenteric or vitelline duct in the early conceptus connects the developing embryo to the yolk sac. As growth occurs, the duct becomes elongated and discontinuous, and the yolk sac degenerates. Structures derived from this duct include Meckel's diverticuli, umbilical polyps, and cysts in the cord [233] that may contain structures found in Meckel's diverticuli, i.e., pancreas, small intestinal mucosa [234], and gastric mucosa [229]. In the latter instance, the mucosa ulcerated and led to rupture of the vein, with fetal exsanguination.

The allantoic diverticulum or duct is frequently identified if the umbilical cord is sectioned close to its fetal attachment. It may or may not have an identifiable lumen and is lined by flattened cuboidal or transitional epithelium without any associated muscle. Cysts have been reported in the remnants of the duct [214] and patent urachus has been associated with giant umbilical cord, which some believe to be due to leakage of urine into Wharton's jelly [224, 235–238]. Rarely, remnants of the omphalomesenteric blood vessels are identified.

Thrombosis of the Umbilical Cord

Thrombosis of the cord is a rare complication of pregnancy, occurring in about 1 in 1500 placentae [239], while in high-risk pregnancies the risk may be as high as 1 in 250 pla-

centae. The vein is more commonly affected than the arteries, thus venous thrombosis occurred alone in approximately 70% of cases, venous and arterial thrombosis in approximately 20% of cases, and arterial thrombosis alone in 10%. As with a single umbilical artery, there is apparently a strong association with perinatal mortality and morbidity as the result of a selection of cases retrospectively, but prospective data [239] do not reveal such an association.

Thrombosis is frequently associated with umbilical cord abnormalities, such as prolapse, knotting, nuchal entanglement, stricture, short cord, and inflammation. Arterial thrombosis is associated with a greater morbidity and mortality, and thrombosis of both arteries was associated with a stillbirth rate of 90%. There is also an association with obstetric problems and complications such as maternal diabetes mellitus, multiple pregnancy, hemolytic disease, and fetomaternal hemorrhage.

Hemangioma of the Umbilical Cord

See Chorangioma under Lesions of the Amnion and Chorion.

LESIONS OF THE AMNION AND CHORION

Discoloration of the Amnion

The amniotic surface of a normal placenta is smooth, translucent, and dark-red-blue. The vessels within the chorionic plate are readily visible, with the arteries running over the surface of the veins. Following delivery, the membranes and cord may take on a greenish tinge if they are stored for any length of time, and, if there is significant bacterial contamination, there may be red or red-brown staining by breakdown products derived from hemoglobin.

Discoloration of the cord or membranes in freshly delivered placentae may be due to meconium staining, intrauterine death, bacterial infection, intra-amniotic hemorrhage, or hemolytic disease. Hemolytic disease, bacterial infection, and intra-amniotic hemorrhage are discussed elsewhere.

Meconium staining of the placenta varies from dark green to olive green and bronze, the meconium being passed by the distressed fetus. There is little evidence of cellular damage on exposure to meconium for less than 6 hours. Subsequently, the amniotic epithelium becomes swollen and pseudostratified, many of the cells being club-shaped. Some of the epithelial cells become stained by the pigment and, between 12 and 24 hours after passage of meconium, macrophages containing greenish-yellow pigment may be identified within the compact layer of the amnion. According to Miller et al [240], the meconium-laden macrophage may migrate to the chorion in as little as 3 hours. In cases of prolonged exposure, the amniotic epithelium may be lost entirely and, where this involves the chorion laeve, there may be necrosis of the underlying decidua. Eventually, a sterile chorioamnionitis may develop.

Intrauterine death, if recent, may have little effect on the membranes, although there may be meconium staining if death was due to hypoxia. Prolonged retention of the dead fetus results in red-brown and then green-brown or khaki membranes and cord. The amniotic fluid contains much brown particulate matter derived from the fetal skin, which may become adherent to the amnion. The amniotic epithelium eventually degenerates and is also shed into the fluid. There is usually no significant inflammatory response to this necrotic debris.

Chorionic Edema, Cysts, and Hemorrhage

The spongy layer of the amnion, like Wharton's jelly in the umbilical cord, is derived from the magma reticulare within the extracoelomic cavity and contains a thixotropic gel [241] that liquefies on compression and is hydrophilic. This is the site at which edema fluid accumulates [242], and it is the site at which cleavage occurs between the amnion and chorion; it is also the site at which blood from ruptured chorionic vessels may accumulate. Rarely, amniotic fluid may dissect this potential space, and it has been suggested that this is a possible route by which amniotic fluid embolism might reach the maternal circulation [243]. The causes of edema of the membranes are similar to those associated with placental hydrops. Cysts on the fetal surface of the placenta are usually subchorionic and are found in 3–5% of placentae. They may be single or multiple and can measure several centimeters in diameter. They contain thin, slightly mucinous blood-stained or yellow-green fluid, and they are most frequent in the central regions of the placenta, particularly at the root of the cord. Marginal lesions are also common. Similar cysts may be identified in the placental septa, and it would appear that both varieties are of similar origin. In many cases, there is continuity between the subchorionic cyst and a placental septum. Benirschke and Driscoll [37] have noted numerous cysts of this type in association with maternal floor infarction of the

placenta, but my own experience is that this is not a common association.

The cysts have no definite lining cell and are surrounded by X cells, which are the major constituents of placental septa. The pathogenesis of the cysts is disputed but appears not to be due to infarction. Paddock and Greer [244] consider that they may be formed by trophoblastic dissolution within decidual septa. Septal cysts occur more frequently than subchorionic cysts and reported incidences vary from 0.15–56.0%, but our own experience suggests that approximately 10% of full-term placentae contain macroscopically identifiable cysts in the septa.

Subamniotic hemorrhage occurs in approximately 5% of placentae and may vary from small local extravasations of blood to massive fetal hemorrhage covering the entire surface of the placenta and extending into the extrachorial membranes. Such hemorrhages may be associated with fetal anemia and, very rarely, fetal death. The lesions in the chorionic vessels associated with these hemorrhages have been investigated by deSa [245, 246], who found that the hemorrhages arise from varices of the surface veins. deSa is of the opinion that these vessels have been subject to raised pressures for some time prior to rupture and has demonstrated intimal cushions, which he believes are derived from organizing thrombi. However, only six placentae were studied, and further cases must be investigated prior to acceptance of these findings. In the author's experience, the most common cause of subamniotic hemorrhage has been tearing of the vein at the site of insertion of the umbilical cord, presumably as a result of undue traction during delivery.

Squamous Metaplasia and Amnion Nodosum

The surface of the amnion is normally smooth. Occasionally, a single, opaque, yellow-white nodule of approximately 5 millimeters in diameter may be observed in the amnion. This is the yolk sac remnant, and histological examination shows an amorphous, sometimes coarsely granular, lipid- and mineral-containing debris. The amniotic epithelium may show microscopic changes when exposed to meconium, with columnar change and vacuolation [247]. A curious and possibly specific pattern of vacuolation in association with gastroschisis but not omphalocele has been described [248]. Less frequently, there may be diffuse nodularity of the amnion. Excluding infections of the membranes with herpes and pox viruses and *Candida albicans*, these nodules are of two types: squamous metaplasia and amnion nodosum.

Squamous Metaplasia

The first and more common type of diffuse nodularity of the amnion squamous metaplasia, appears to have no clinical significance. The normal amnion is covered by cuboidal or flattened columnar cells arranged as a monolayer on a basement membrane. As pregnancy progresses, the cells tend to become increasingly columnar, with the nuclei migrating to the surface of the cells, giving them a peg-like

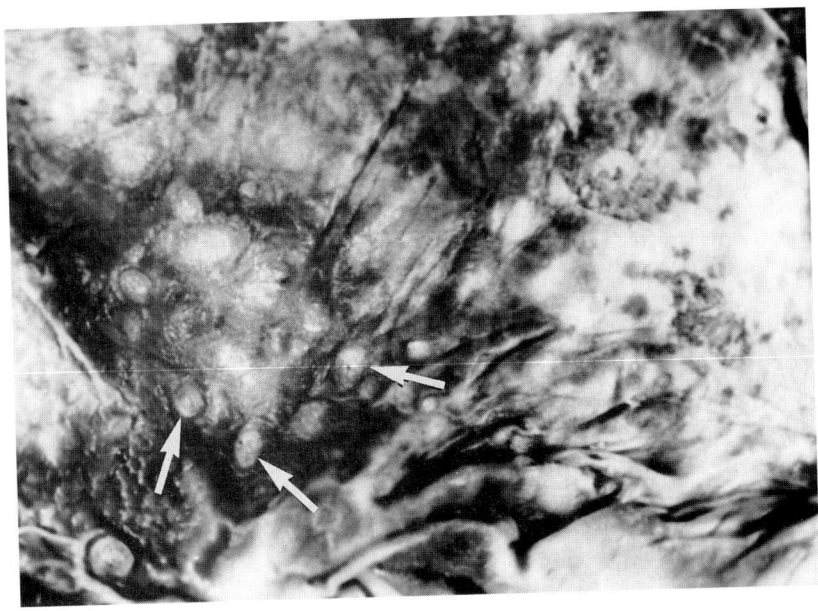

FIGURE 7.38.   *Amnion. Squamous metaplasia. Multiple rounded plaques (arrows) of squamous cells derived from the amniotic epithelium.*

appearance. Increasing numbers of these cells are shed into the amniotic fluid as pregnancy progresses and their lipid content rises.

In postmature pregnancies, there may be areas of amnion denuded of surface cells. These changes in the amniotic surface cells have been used as an indicator of the duration of pregnancy, but such techniques are relatively inaccurate. Squamous metaplasia, as the term implies, results from the normal amniotic cells taking on the appearances of squamous cells. This is considered to be due to metaplasia rather than seeding from the squamous epithelium on the surface of the fetus. The nodules are usually opaque, yellow-white or silvery-gray (Fig. 7.38) and sometimes have concentric lamination visible to the naked eye. They usually measure 2 to 3 millimeters in diameter, though occasionally they may be larger. Squamous metaplasia frequently involves the umbilical cord. Bourne [242] found the lesion in 4% of placentae.

Amnion Nodosum

The second type of nodularity is amnion nodosum, which is of major clinical importance since it is almost invariably associated with oligohydramnios. It occurs classically in association with renal agenesis (Potter sequence) but may also be found in association with other abnormalities of the urinary tract in which there is decreased or absent urine excretion, following prolonged rupture of the membranes with vaginal loss of amniotic fluid, and less frequently with prolonged retention of a dead fetus [243, 249, 250].

The lesions of amnion nodosum are usually smaller than those of squamous metaplasia (measuring 1–2 mm in diameter), more numerous, and frequently only semiopaque or translucent (Fig. 7.39). They tend to occur in depressions in the amnion between blood vessels and around the insertion of the cord. The nodules consist of desquamated fetal cells and vernix covered by a layer of amniotic cells

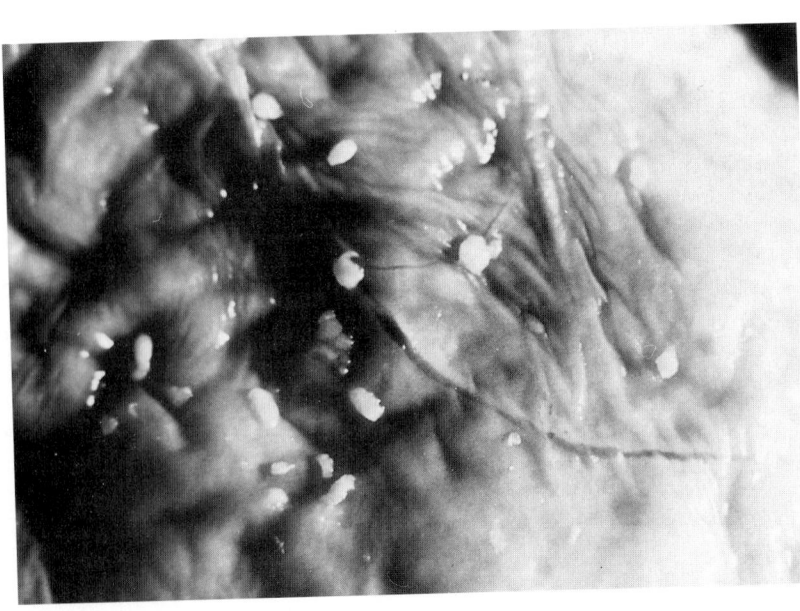

FIGURE 7.39.   *Amnion nodosum of fetus with renal agenesis. Small clumps of fetal squames "stuck on" the surface of the amnion.*

(Fig. 7.40). They arise as cellular debris, in the amniotic fluid, adheres to the surface of the amnion and is subsequently incorporated by overgrowth of the amniotic epithelium [251, 252].

Amniotic Bands

Amniotic bands occur in between 1 in 1200 and 1 in 15,000 births [253] and are significantly more common in early pregnancy [56, 254]. Clusters of cases have been reported [255].

They arise as the result of adhesions between the amnion and embryonic or fetal parts and frequently are associated with fetal malformations, which include limb, craniofacial, and visceral defects. They may occur between the fetus and the umbilical cord and between one part of the fetus and another; in most instances, the site of the attachment of the band is deformed [256].

Classically, amniotic bands have been associated with intrauterine amputations and constriction rings. These are widely believed to result from tears in the amnion in the first trimester [257], with part of the fetus coming to lie in a false cavity outside the amniotic sac. Strips or fronds of the amnion and chorionic connective tissue become attached to the limbs, often encircling them and leading to constriction or amputation (Fig. 7.41). It is not clear whether the amnion is physically torn or whether it develops as a fenestrated membrane. If the latter, it would form part of a spectrum of which the most severe form is the anamniotic blighted ovum of the first trimester. Other limb malformations include pseudosyndactyly, clubbed feet, and abnormal dermatoglyphics.

Craniofacial lesions are frequently asymmetrical and do not conform to the anatomy of the normal facial clefts. They include cleft lip, cleft palate, microphthalmia, abnormal skull calcification, as well as anencephaly, encephalocele, and decapitation [258]. Visceral defects most frequently involve the ventral body wall (omphalocele, gastroschisis) and abdominal constriction ring [259]. Constriction of the umbilical cord has been reported by several authors [221, 260, 261].

In humans, amniotic bands are not believed to be inherited abnormalities, although similar malformations of the limbs in rabbits, in the absence of bands, may be inherited [262]. Similar anomalies are found in mice [263] and may be induced in rabbits and chickens by vasopressor substances and selenium, respectively [264].

Amniotic bands are probably not the only causes of intrauterine amputation in humans; thus, Warkany [265] has documented examples of recessively inherited reduction malformations, and Hoyme et al [266] have reported amputations following occlusion of the brachial artery by emboli arising in the placenta.

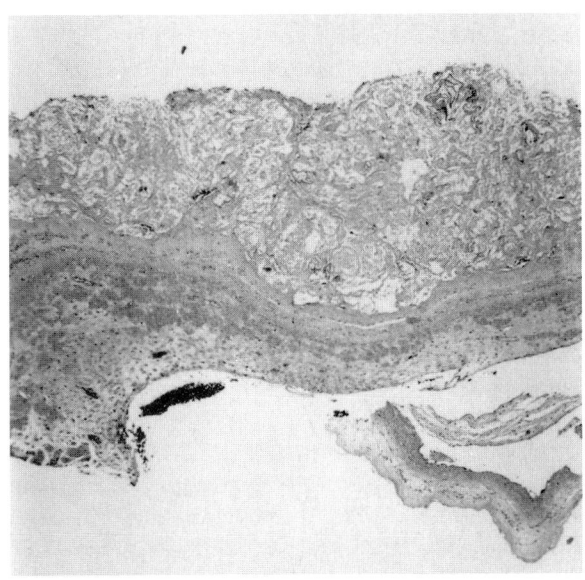

FIGURE 7.40. *Amnion nodosum. Cell debris adherent to the amniotic surface. H&E, ×99.*

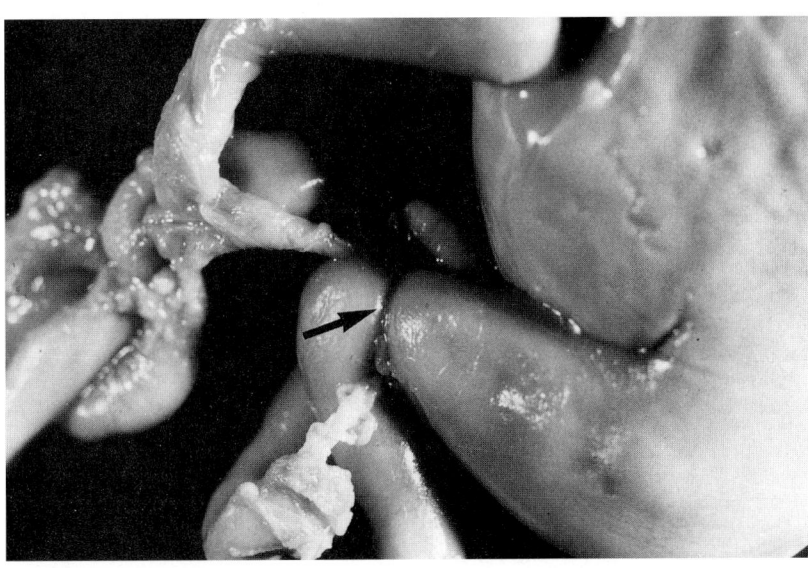

FIGURE 7.41. *Amniotic bands involving umbilical cord and limbs. There is a constriction ring around the thigh (arrows).*

Amniotic bands may arise following amniocentesis in rats [267] and have been reported as a complication in humans [268, 269]. It must be emphasized, however, that none of the malformations associated with bands is unique, and even asymmetrical facial lesions have been described in their absence in primates [270].

Extramembranous Pregnancy

This is a rare complication in which the membranes rupture, usually during the second trimester, and the fetus continues to develop outside the gestation sac. The fetus may be partly or completely extramembranous. Inevitably, this condition is associated with continuous loss of liquor. This subject has been reviewed by Torpin [271], and several further examples have been recorded since [272, 273]. The placentae associated with extramembranous pregnancies are, without exception, circumvallate, but it remains uncertain whether this is the cause or the result of the condition. The amniotic cavity is small, and it is readily apparent that the fetus is too large to be contained within it. The defect in the sac has a thickened, opaque, rolled edge, and the remaining membranes of the sac are usually thick and opaque, although this may be a reflection of the presence of chorioamnionitis. Amnion nodosum may be found in this situation, particularly if the breech is extramembranous.

Extra-amniotic pregnancy is even less frequent [257, 274]. The fetus is contained within the chorion, and thus liquor is retained. The amnion shrinks and may only be visible around the attachment of the cord to the placenta.

Placental Tumors

Choriocarcinoma will not be discussed in this text, and the reader is referred to one of the many texts in the gyneco-logical literature for specific information. Very rarely choriocarcinoma in full-term placentae may be associated with massive fetomaternal hemorrhage [275]. Hydatidiform degeneration and hydatidiform mole will be considered in relation to spontaneous abortion, to which they are closely allied. There have been occasional reports of teratomas arising in the placenta [276], in one instance with an ovarian teratoma [277], but the only common tumor of the placenta is the chorangioma.

Chorangioma and Hemangioma of the Placenta and Umbilical Cord

Angiomatous malformations of the placenta are the most common "tumor"-like lesions of the placenta, although it is probable that they should be classified properly as hamartomas rather than neoplasms. The incidence of chorangiomas is uncertain, as they may vary in size from a few millimeters to 22 centimeters in diameter [278]. Undoubtedly, many small lesions are missed, but it is probable that they occur in approximately 1% of full-term placentae [129, 279–281].

Macroscopically, chorangiomas vary considerably in appearance, largely as a result of variations in the proportions of vascular and stromal tissue. Small lesions may be indistinguishable from infarcts, particularly if the stromal component predominates. Larger lesions form lobular masses, which may project into the amniotic cavity (Fig. 7.42). Vascular lesions are dark red and of firm or spongy consistency, while others may be white, myxomatous, or even cartilaginous in appearance. Rarely, the tumors appear to arise from the umbilical cord to which they are attached by a vascular pedicle. Areas of necrosis, calcification, and mucinous degeneration may occur.

Histological examination reveals a varying admixture of capillaries and fibrous and myxomatous stroma. Occasion-

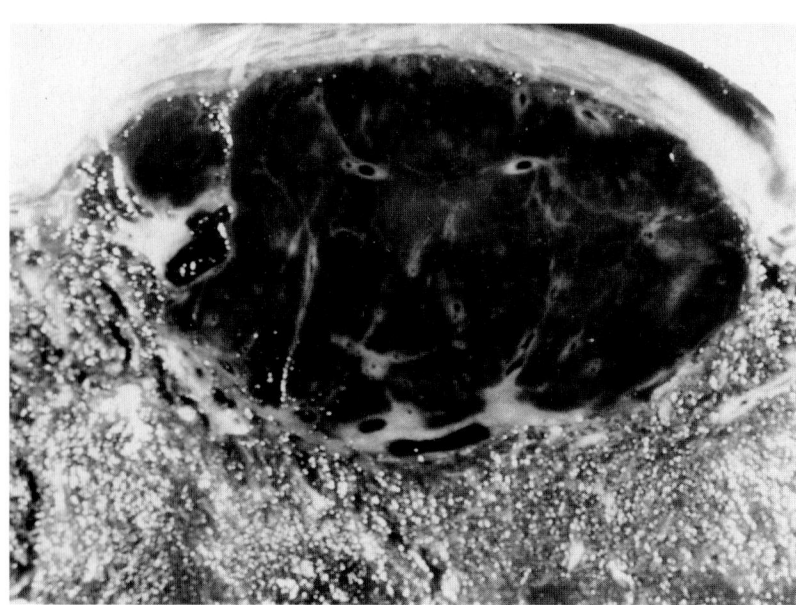

FIGURE 7.42. *Chorangioma. A solid vascular tumor lying immediately beneath the membranes.*

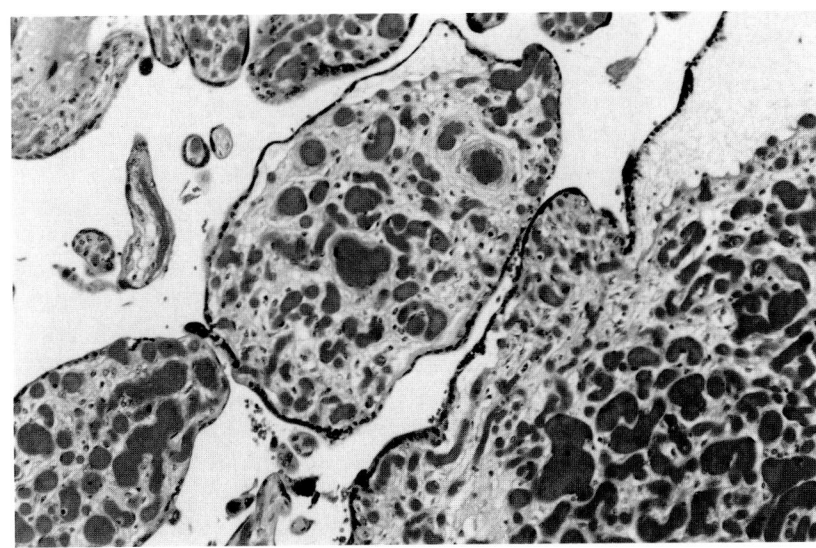

FIGURE 7.43. *Chorangioma. The main body of the lesion is in the bottom right-hand corner. Note the adjacent villi with increased numbers of vascular channels (chorangiosis). H&E, ×105.*

ally, there may be large numbers of extravascular cells with clear cytoplasm and rounded nuclei, the origin of which is uncertain. The vascular components may be distributed focally or diffusely within the stroma. Adjacent villi frequently show chorangiosis (Fig. 7.43). There may be considerable quantities of hemosiderin in the stroma and, in cases occurring in association with rhesus isoimmunization, evidence of hemopoietic activity. Lesions within the placenta usually have a trophoblastic covering, but those arising from the cord do not. Recurrence of hemangiomas in successive pregnancies is extremely rare, although the author has encountered a family in which there were chorangiomas in three successive pregnancies.

Chorangiomas may be associated with polyhydramnios, this being particularly true of large subamniotic lesions, although the cause of the hydramnios is uncertain [279, 282]. Cardiac failure in utero may be precipitated by the extra load on the fetal circulation, and cardiomegaly has been noted in some instances where the fetus has succumbed soon after delivery [283]. Cardiac failure coupled with transudation from large subamniotic lesions may be the major factors in the production of polyhydramnios. Large lesions, particularly those in which thrombosis occurs, may lead to intrauterine or postpartum thrombocytopenia and disseminated intravascular coagulation.

Some chorangiomas are associated with pre-eclamptic toxemia [281], although it is not clear how these two conditions are correlated. Hemangiomas may be found in the fetus [57, 284], and other cardiovascular anomalies appear to be more frequent.

Rarely, there may be diffuse involvement of the placenta with all the villi showing excess vascular channels. The placenta with chorangiomatosis or chorangiosis is generally enlarged, weighing in excess of 1 kilogram. Such a case is described and illustrated by Potter and Craig [285]. It is uncertain whether this is part of a spectrum of vascular anomalies that includes the chorangioma, or whether it should be considered as a separate entity.

Hemangiomas in the umbilical cord have similar variability in structure to those in the placenta [286, 287]. They may be associated with elevation of maternal serum and amniotic fluid alpha-fetoprotein [288]. They do not appear to be associated with hydramnios, nor have they been associated with vascular lesions in the babies.

Metastatic Tumors of the Placenta

Potter and Schoenemann [289] reviewed the world literature on placental metastases and found 24 reported cases, of which almost one-half were secondary melanomas and one-sixth breast carcinomas. These authors analyzed the incidence of malignant disease in pregnancy and concluded that approximately 1 in 61,000 pregnant women had cancer. Only 7 cases of metastatic carcinoma were reported in over 61 million pregnancies, indicating that the conceptus is not a common site of metastasis. One-quarter of the fetuses in their analysis died of metastases, but 2 infants with metastatic melanoma survived and the tumors regressed. The 8 cases of metastasis to the fetus consisted of 7 with melanoma and 1 with lymphosarcoma.

Invasion of villi was evident in 7 of 16 cases, and of these only 1 fetus survived. They suggest that the trophoblast may play a protective role in preventing villous invasion and fetal metastasis.

In the Birmingham Maternity Hospital there have been two cases of carcinoma of the cervix, two of carcinoma of the breast, and one reticulum cell carcinoma diagnosed either prior to or during pregnancy (this excludes hemopoietic malignancies) in over 40,000 pregnancies, and in none of these was there evidence of placental metastasis. One referred case of secondary gastric carcinoma is illustrated (Fig. 7.44) from a 42-year-old mother who died of metastatic disease 2 weeks after delivery of an unaffected

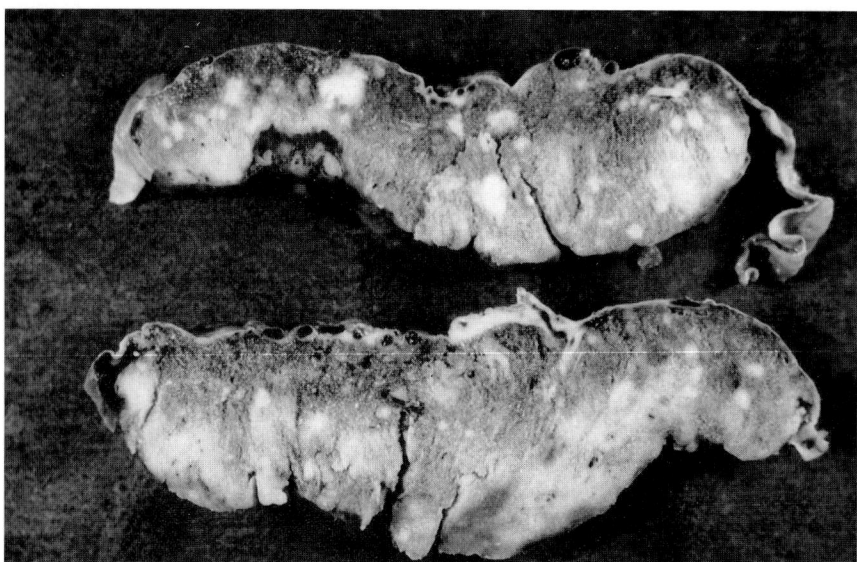

FIGURE 7.44. *Secondary gastric carcinomas in the placenta manifest as multiple white deposits within the parenchyma.*

infant. A metastatic tumor was identified in the uterus at postmortem examination.

Rarely, the fetus may be the source of the placental tumor, the most common malignancy being congenital leukemia [290], a condition that may result in intrauterine death and stillbirth.

EXAMINATION OF THE PLACENTA

Because the vast majority of human placentae are macroscopically normal, the placenta is neglected by both clinician and pathologist. However, many macroscopically normal placentae do show histological abnormalities, such as chorioamnionitis, hypoxic-ischemic lesions, or disturbances in maturation. Though these findings may not be of immediate clinical importance, they may add to the totality of the clinical assessment of an individual case, particularly where there is associated morbidity or mortality.

There are two reasons for examination of the placenta:

1. To identify lesions that may be of significance to the mother (e.g., completeness of the membranes and parenchyma, infection).
2. To identify lesions that are related to the pathology in the fetus.

Ideally, all placentae should be examined both macroscopically and microscopically, so as to retain familiarity with both the normal and the abnormal. However, such an approach is usually precluded for logistical reasons, and case selection is essential. Such selection should be agreed between the pathologist and clinicians and a formal protocol established that is familiar to both midwifery and medical staff. In the author's department, all placentae falling into the categories in Table 7.3 are examined both macroscopically and microscopically. Using these categories, the placentae of over 95% of all neonatal deaths are examined fully, as well as those from all stillbirths. As with other sur-

Table 7.3. Indications for histological examination of the placenta

Diabetes mellitus
Essential hypertension
Gestational hypertension, pre-eclampsia, eclampsia
Rhesus isoimmunization (and other types of isoimmunization)
Pyrexia immediately prior to, or during, labor
Prolonged rupture of membranes (>24 hours)
Premature rupture of the membranes (<36 weeks' gestation)
Babies under 2.5 kg birth weight
Malformed babies
Stillborn babies
Two vessels in umbilical cord
Unusual or equivocal macroscopic placental pathology
Miscellaneous (e.g., history of maternal infection in pregnancy, or history of diagnostic procedure involving placenta)

gical pathology specimens, certain clinical data are required with the placenta (Table 7.4). This may be incorporated easily on a standard request form.

Following assessment of the completeness of the organ, the cord and membranes should be trimmed from the parenchyma and the organ weighed. Some authors, notably Fox [38], argue that weighing the placenta is of no value, as the quantity of both maternal and fetal blood within the delivered organ is variable, although this may be overcome partly by allowing the organ to drain prior to weighing. It is also impossible to correlate the functional capacity of the organ with the weight. There is, however, a broad correlation of fetal and placental weight [82], and major deviations from these parameters are generally significant. The size of the placenta may also be recorded.

The fetal surface of the membranes should be examined for translucency, discoloration, and nodularity, which may indicate inflammation, meconium passage, fetal distress, and

Table 7.4. Data required with placentae sent for pathological examination

Date and time of delivery
Estimated date of delivery or gestation
Date and time of rupture of membranes
Parity
Antenatal complications
    Maternal diabetes
    Pre-eclamptic toxemia
    Other maternal hypertension
    Presence of maternal antibodies
    Antepartum hemorrhage
    Diagnostic procedures (e.g., amniocentesis, chorionic villus biopsy)
    Other maternal disease (e.g., pyrexia in labor)
    Mode of delivery and presentation
Outcome
    Live birth, stillbirth, birth weight, malformations

oligohydramnios. The maternal surface may reveal evidence of calcification, retroplacental hemorrhage, or infarction, although the latter should not be diagnosed without slicing the organ.

The organ should be sliced in strips of approximately 0.5 centimeters in width and all macroscopic lesions noted.

The cord should be examined for knots, torsion, adhesions, thrombosis and the number of vessels.

Microscopic examination should include non-placental and placental membranes, the umbilical cord, and at least one block of central placental tissue that appears macroscopically normal, in addition to any gross lesions. The blocks should be taken in the knowledge of the cotyledonary structure and should be full thickness so as to include both the chorionic and basal plates. It may be possible to identify remnants of maternal vessels on the maternal surface, which may also be examined microscopically.

Staining techniques are a matter of individual preference, the most useful techniques beyond H&E being PAS, trichrome, fibrin and calcium, and/or iron stains.

CONCLUSION

There is no special mystique about the placenta, the rewards from its examination being commensurate with the diligence of the observer. The ancient Egyptians considered the placenta to be of major importance [82], depicting it on their sculptures. Today, interest is again increasing, as obstetrics, neonatology, and in particular immunology press back the frontiers of medical science. The pathologist should be aware that there is yet much to be learned from this essential component of human reproduction.

REFERENCES

1. Nuttal ID. Perforation of a placental fetal vessel by an intrauterine catheter. *Br J Obstet Gynaecol* 1978; 85:573–4.
2. Trudinger BJ, Pryse-Davies J. Fetal hazards of the intrauterine pressure catheter: five case reports. *Br J Obstet Gynaecol* 1978; 85:567–72.
3. Fox H. The histopathology of placental insufficiency. *J Clin Pathol* 1976; 29:1–8.
4. Aherne W. Morphometry. In: Gruenwald P, ed. *The Placenta and its Maternal Supply Line*. Baltimore: University Park Press, 1975, pp. 80–98.
5. Wilkin P. *Pathologie due Placenta*. Paris: Masson et Cie, 1965.
6. Roby KF, Soares MJ. Trophoblast cell differentiation and organisation: role of fetal and ovarian signals. *Placenta* 1993; 14:529–45.
7. Shurtz-Swirski R, Simon RJ, Cohen Y, Barnea ER. Human embryo modulates placental function in the first trimester: effects of neural tissues upon chorionic gonadotropin and progesterone secretion. *Placenta* 1991; 12:521–31.
8. Attenburrow AA, Heslip M, Henderson MJ, et al. Placental steroid sulphatase deficiency. *Arch Dis Child* 1984; 59:1187–9.
9. Rushton DI. The placenta—an environmental problem. *Br Med J* 1973; 1:344–8.
10. Browne JC McC, Veall N. The maternal placental blood flow in normotensive and hypertensive women. *J Obstet Gynaecol Br Emp* 1953; 60:141–7.
11. Hertig AT. Vascular pathology in the hypertensive albuminuric toxaemias of pregnancy. *Clinics* 1945; 4:602–14.
12. Zeek PM, Assali NS. Vascular changes in the decidua associated with eclamptogenic toxaemia of pregnancy. *Am J Clin Pathol* 1950h; 20:1099–109.
13. Brosens I, Robertson WB, Dixon HG. The physiological response of the vessels of the placental bed to normal pregnancy. *J Pathol Bacteriol* 1967; 93:569–79.
14. Hamilton WJ, Boyd JD. Development of the human placenta in the first three months of gestation. *J Anat* 1960; 94:297–328.
15. Aspillaga MO, Whittaker PG, Grey CE, Lind T. Endocrinological events in early pregnancy failure. *Am J Obstet Gynecol* 1983; 147:903–8.
16. Rushton DI. The classification and mechanisms of spontaneous abortions. *Perspect Pediatr Pathol* 1984; 8:269–87.
17. Burrows TD, King A, Loke YW. Expression of adhesion molecules by endovascular trophoblast and decidual endothelial cells: implications for vascular invasion during implantation. *Placenta* 1994; 15:21–33.
18. Wigglesworth JS. Vascular anatomy of the human placenta and its significance for placental pathology. *J Obstet Gynaecol Br Commonw* 1969; 76:979–89.
19. Critchley GR, Burton GJ. Intralobular variation in barrier thickness in the mature human placenta. *Placenta* 1987; 8:185–94.
20. Campbell AGH, Dawes GS, Fishman AP, Hyman AI, James GB. The oxygen consumption of the placenta and foetal membranes in the sheep. *J Physiol* (London) 1966; 182:439–64.
21. Adamson K, Myers RE. Circulation in the intervillous space: obstetrical considerations in fetal deprivation. In: Gruenwald P, ed. *The Placenta and its Maternal Supply Line*. Baltimore: University Park Press, 1975, pp. 158–77.
22. Teasdale F. Functional significance of the zonal morphologic differences in the normal human placenta. *Am J Obstet Gynecol* 1978; 30:773–81.
23. Burgos MH, Rodriguez EM. Specialised zones in the trophoblast of the human term placenta. *Am J Obstet Gynecol* 1966; 96:342–56.
24. Becker V. Abnormal maturation of the villi. In: Gruenwald P, ed. *The Placenta and its Maternal Supply Line*. Baltimore: University Park Press, 1975, pp. 232–43.
25. Mayhew TM, Jackson MR, Boyd PA. Changes in oxygen diffusive conductances of human placentae during gestation (10–41 weeks) are commensurate with the gain in fetal weight. *Placenta* 1993; 14:51–61.
26. Philippe E. *Histopathologie Placentaire*. Paris: Masson et Cie, 1974.
27. Fujikura T. Placental calcification and seasonal difference. *Am J Obstet Gynecol* 1963; 87:46–7.
28. Scott JS. Placenta extrachorialis (placenta marginata and placenta circumvallata): a factor in antepartum haemorrhage. *J Obstet Gynaecol Br Emp* 1960; 67:904–18.
29. Benson RC, Fujikura T. Circumvallate and circum-marginate placenta: unimportant clinical entities. *Obstet Gynecol* 1969; 34:799–804.
30. Fox H, Sen DK. Placenta extrachorialis: a clinico-pathological study. *J Obstet Gynaecol Br Commonw* 1972; 79:32–5.
31. Earn AA. Placental anomalies. *Can Med Assoc J* 1951; 64:118–20.
32. Earn AA. The effect of congenital abnormalities of the umbilical cord and placenta on the newborn and mother: a survey of 5676 consecutive deliveries. *J Obstet Gynaecol Br Emp* 1951; 58:456–9.
33. Morgan J. Circumvallate placenta. *J Obstet Gynaecol Br Emp* 1955; 62:899–900.
34. Pinkerton JHM. Placenta circumvallata, its aetiology and clinical significance. *J Obstet Gynaecol Br Emp* 1956; 63:743–7.
35. Paalman RJ, Van der Veer CG. Circumvallate placenta. *Am J Obstet Gynecol* 1953; 65:491–7.
36. Ziel HA. Circumvallate placenta, a cause of antepartum bleeding, premature delivery and perinatal mortality. *Obstet Gynecol* 1963; 22:798–802.

37. Benirschke K, Driscoll SG. *The Pathology of the Human Placenta*. Berlin: Springer-Verlag, 1967.

38. Fox H. *Pathology of the Placenta (Major Problems in Pathology)*. London: Saunders, 1978.

39. Torpin R. Evolution of a placenta circumvallata. *Obstet Gynaecol* 1966; 27:99–101.

40. Pryse-Davies J, Dewhurst CJ, Campbell S. Placenta membranacea. *J Obstet Gynaecol Br Commonw* 1973; 80:1106–10.

41. Aguero O. *Anomalias Morphologicas de la Placenta y su Significado Clinico*. Caracas, Venezuela: Artegrafia. 1957.

42. Hurley VA, Beischer NA. Placenta membranacea: case reports. *Br J Obstet Gynaecol* 1987; 94:798–802.

43. Irving C, Hertig AT. A study of placenta accreta. *Surg Gynecol Obstet* 1937; 64:178–200.

44. Sumawong V, Nondasatu A, Thanapath S, Budthmimedhee V. Placenta accreta: a review of the literature and a survey of 10 cases. *Obstet Gynecol* 1966; 27:511–16.

45. Althabe O, Althabe O. Placenta accreta. *Sem Med* 1963; 123:118–25.

46. Sturdee DW, Rushton DI. Caesarean and post partum hysterectomy 1968–1983. *Br J Obstet Gynaecol* 1986; 93:270–4.

47. Hill DJ, Beischer NA. Hysterectomy in obstetric practice. *Aust N Z J Obstet Gynaecol* 1980; 20:151–3.

48. Millar WG. A clinical and pathological study of placenta accreta. *J Obstet Gynaecol Br Emp* 1959; 66:353–64.

49. Fox H. Placenta accreta 1945–1969. *Obstet Gynecol Surv* 1972; 27:475–90.

50. Sturdee DW, Rushton DI. Caesarean and post partum hysterectomy. In: Studd J, ed. *Progress in Obstetrics and Gynaecology*, Vol. 6. Edinburgh: Churchill Livingstone, 1987, pp. 195–209.

51. Barss P, Misch KA. Endemic placenta accreta in a population of remote villagers in Papua New Guinea. *Br J Obstet Gynaecol* 1990; 97:167–74.

52. Freeman RM. Placenta accreta and myotonic dystrophy: two case reports. *Br J Obstet Gynaecol* 1991; 98:594–5.

53. Khong TY, Robertson WB. Placenta creta and placenta praevia creta. *Placenta* 1987; 8:399–409.

54. Fox H. Perivillous fibrin deposition in the human placenta. *Am J Obstet Gynecol* 1967; 98:245–51.

55. Moe N. Deposits of fibrin and plasma proteins in the normal human placenta: an immunofluorescence study. *Acta Pathol Microbiol Scand* 1969; 76:74–88.

56. Rushton DI. Placental pathology in spontaneous miscarriage. In: Beard RW, Sharp F, eds. *Early Pregnancy Loss. Mechanisms and Treatment*. London: Royal College of Obstetricians and Gynaecologists, 1988, pp. 149–57.

57. Fox H. Fibrinoid necrosis of placental villi. *J Obstet Gynaecol Br Commonw* 1968; 75:448–52.

58. Anderson WR, McKay DG. Electron microscopic study of the trophoblast in normal and toxemic placentas. *Am J Obstet Gynecol* 1966; 95:1134–48.

59. Sen DK, Langley FA. Villous basement membrane thickening and fibrinoid necrosis and normal and abnormal placentas. *Am J Obstet Gynecol* 1974; 118:276–81.

60. Aladjem S. Placenta of the premature infant. *Am J Obstet Gynecol* 1968; 102:311–12.

61. Perkins RP. Antenatal assessment of fetal maturity: a review. *Obstet Gynaecol Surv* 1974; 29:369–84.

62. Vorherr H. Placental insufficiency and postmaturity. *Eur J Obstet Gynecol Reprod Biol* 1975; 5:109–22.

63. Chard T, Yoong A, MacIntosh M. The myth of fetal growth retardation at term. *Br J Obstet Gynaecol* 1993; 100:1076–81.

64. Hoffman HJ, Stark CR, Lundin FE Jr Ashbrook JD. Analysis of birth weight, gestational age and fetal viability, US births 1968. *Obstet Gynecol Surv* 1974; 29:651–81.

65. Elliot PM, Inman WHW. Volume of liquor amnii in normal and abnormal pregnancy. *Lancet* 1961; 2:835–40.

66. Browne JC McC. Placental insufficiency. *Scott Med J* 1963; 8:459–65.

67. Dixon HG, Browne JC McC, Davey DA. Choriodecidual and myometrial blood flow. *Lancet* 1963; 2:369–73.

68. Robertson WB, Dixon HG. Uteroplacental pathology. In: Klopper A, Diczfalusy E, eds. *Foetus and Placenta*. Oxford: Blackwell Scientific, 1969, pp. 33–60.

69. Magnin P, Gabriel H. Les scléroses vasculaires de la cadaque profonde. *Gynecol Obstet* 1966; 65:37–56.

70. Boyd PA. Quantitative structure studies of the normal human placenta from 10 weeks of gestation to term. *Early Hum Dev* 1984; 9:297–307.

71. Geier G, Schumann R, Kraus H. Regional unterschiedliche zellproliferation innerhalb der plazentone reifer menschlicher plazenten: autoradiograische untersuchungen. *Arch Gynakol* 1975; 218:31–7.

72. Sands J, Dobbing J. Continuing growth and development of the third trimester human placenta. *Placenta* 1985; 6:13–22.

73. Kloosterman GJ. Prolonged pregnancy. *Gynaecologia* 1956; 142:373–88.

74. Sinnathuray TA. A study of uncomplicated prolongation of pregnancy. *Aust N Z J Obstet Gynaecol* 1972; 12:225–7.

75. Walker J. Foetal anoxia. *J Obstet Gynaecol Br Commonw* 1954; 61:162–80.

76. Fox H. The placenta in premature onset of labour. *J Obstet Gynaecol Br Commonw* 1969; 76:240–44.

77. Wigglesworth JS. The gross and microscopic pathology of the prematurely delivered placenta. *J Obstet Gynaecol Br Commonw* 1962; 69:934–43.

78. Chellam VG, Rushton DI. Chorioamnionitis and funiculitis in the placentas of 200 births weighing less than 2.5 kg. *Br J Obstet Gynaecol* 1985; 92:808–14.

79. Hopker WW, Ohlendorf B. Placental insufficiency: histomorphologic diagnosis and classification. In: Grundmann E, ed. *Current Topics in Pathology No. 66 Perinatal Pathology*. Berlin: Springer-Verlag, 1979, pp. 57–81.

80. Fox H. Basement membrane changes in the villi of the human placenta. *J Obstet Gynaecol Br Commonw* 1968; 75:302–6.

81. Sander CH, Stevens NG. Hemorrhagic endovasculitis of the placenta: an in depth morphologic appraisal with initial clinical and epidemiological observations. *Pathol Annu* 1984; 19:37–79.

82. Boyd JD, Hamilton WJ. *The Human Placenta*. Cambridge: W. Heffer, 1970.

83. Fox H. Effect of hypoxia on trophoblast in organ culture: a morphologic and autoradiographic study. *Am J Obstet Gynecol* 1970; 107:1058–64.

84. MacLennan AH, Sharp F, Shaw-Dunn J. The ultrastructure of human trophoblast in spontaneous and induced hypoxia using a system of organ culture: a comparison with ultrastructural changes in preeclampsia and placental insufficiency. *J Obstet Gynaecol Br Commonw* 1972; 79:113–21.

85. Agboola A. Placental changes in patients with a low haematocrit. *Br J Obstet Gynaecol* 1975; 82:225–7.

86. Beischer NA, Holsman M, Kitchen WH. Relations of various forms of anaemia to placental weight. *Am J Obstet Gynecol* 1968; 101:801–9.

87. Beischer NA, Sivabamboo R, Vohra S, Silpisornkosal S, Reid S. Placental hypertrophy in severe pregnancy anaemia. *J Obstet Gynaecol Br Commonw* 1970; 77:398–409.

88. Clavero JA, Botella Llusia J. Measurement of villus surface in normal and pathologic placentas. *Am J Obstet Gynecol* 1963; 86:234–40.

89. McClung J. Effects of high altitude on human birth. In: *Observations on Mothers, Placentas and the Newborn in Two Peruvian Populations*. Cambridge, MA: Harvard University Press, 1969.

90. Jackson MR, Mayhew JM, Haas JD. Morphometric studies on villi in human term placentae and the effects of altitude, ethnic grouping and sex of the newborn. *Placenta* 1987; 8:487–96.

91. Hamilton WJ, Boyd JD. Specialisations of the syncytium of the human chorion. *Br Med J* 1966; 1:1501–6.

92. Attwood HD, Park WW. Embolism to the lungs by trophoblast. *J Obstet Gynaecol Br Commonw* 1961; 68:611–17.

93. Covone AE, Mutton D, Johnson PM, Adinolfi M. Trophoblast cells in peripheral blood from pregnant women. *Lancet* 1984; II:841–3.

94. Fox H, Agrafojo-Blanco A. Scanning electron microscopy of the human placenta in normal and abnormal pregnancies. *Eur J Obstet Gynecol Reprod Biol* 1974; 4:45–50.

95. Alvarez H. Prolifération du trophoblaste et sa relation avec l'hypertension artérielle de la toxémie gravidique. *Gynecol Obstet* 1970; 69:581–8.

96. Cibils LA. The placenta and newborn infant in hypertensive conditions. *Am J Obstet Gynecol* 1974; 118:256–40.

97. Paine CG. Observations on placental histology in normal and abnormal pregnancies. *J Obstet Gynaecol Br Emp* 1957; 64:668–72.

98. Sauramo H. Histology of the placenta in normal, premature and overterm cases and in gestosis. *Ann Chir Gynaecol Fenn* 1951; 40:164–88.

99. Jones CPJ, Fox H. Syncytial knots and intervillous bridges in the human placenta: an ultrastructural study. *J Anat* 1977; 124:275–86.

100. Myers RE, Fujikura T. Placental changes after experimental abruptio placentae and fetal vessel ligation of rhesus monkey placenta. Am J Obstet Gynecol 1968; 100:846–51.

101. Gant NF, Hutchinson HT, Siiteri PK, MacDonald PC. Study of the metabolic clearance rate of dehydroisoandrosterone sulfate in pregnancy. *Am J Obstet Gynecol* 1971; 111:555–61.

102. Boyd PA, Keeling JW. Raised maternal serum alpha-fetoprotein in the absence of fetal abnormality—placental findings: a quantitative morphometric study. *Prenat Diagn* 1986; 6:369–14.

103. Boyd PA, Scott A. Quantitative structural studies on human placentas associated with pre-eclampsia, essential hypertension and intrauterine growth retardation. *Br J Obstet Gynaecol* 1985; 92:714–21.

104. Teasdale F. Histomorphometry of the human placenta in pre-eclampsia associated with severe intrauterine growth retardation. *Placenta* 1987; 8:119–28.

105. Fox H. The significance of villous syncytial knots in the human placenta. *J Obstet Gynaecol Br Commonw* 1965; 72:347–55.

106. Cantle SJ, Kaufman P, Luckhardt M, Schweikhart G. Interpretation of syncytial sprouts and bridges in the human placenta. *Placenta* 1987; 8:221–34.

107. Dawes GS. General discussion. In: Elliott KM, Knight J, eds. *Size at Birth.* Ciba Foundation Symp No. 27. Amsterdam: Excerpta Medica, 1974.

108. Trudinger BJ, Giles WB, Cook CM. Uteroplacental blood flow velocity–time waveforms in normal and complicated pregnancy. *Br J Obstet Gynaecol* 1985; 92:39–45.

109. Robertson WB, Khong TY, Brosens I, et al. The placental bed biopsy: review from three European centres. *Am J Obstet Gynecol* 1986; 155:401–12.

110. Khong TY, Liddell HS, Robertson WB. Defective haemochorial placentation as a cause of miscarriage: a preliminary study. *Br J Obstet Gynaecol* 1987; 94:649–55.

111. Williams JW. Premature separation of the normally implanted placenta. *Surg Gynecol Obstet* 1915; 21:541–54.

112. De Wolf F, Robertson WB, Brosens I. The ultrastructure of acute atherosis in hypertensive pregnancy. *Am J Obstet Gynecol* 1975; 123:164–74.

113. Goodwin WE, Kaufman JJ, Minas MM, et al. Human renal transplantation. I. Clinical experiences with six cases of renal homotransplantation. *J Urol* 1963; 89:13–24.

114. Khong TY, Chambers HM. Alternative method of sampling placentas for the assessment of uteroplacental vasculature. *J Clin Pathol* 1992; 45:925–7.

115. Khong TY, Staples A, Moore L, Stewart RW. Observer reliability in assessing villitis of unknown aetiology. *J Clin Pathol* 1993; 46:208–10.

116. Khong TY, Staples A, Bendon RW, et al. Observer reliability in assessing placental maturity by histology. *J. Clin Pathol* 1995; 48:420–3.

117. MacGillivray J. *Pre-eclampsia. The Hypertensive Disease of Pregnancy.* London: Saunders, 1983.

118. Mooney EE, Al Shunnar A, O'Regan M, Gillan JE. Chorionic villous haemorrhage is associated with retroplacental haemorrhage. *Br J Obstet Gynaecol* 1994; 101:965–9.

119. Fox H. The significance of placental infarction in perinatal morbidity and mortality. *Biol Neonat* 1967; 11:87–105.

120. Wentworth P. Placental infarction and toxaemia of pregnancy. *Am J Obstet Gynecol* 1967; 99:318–26.

121. Butler RN, Alberman ED. *Perinatal Problems.* The second report of the 1958 British Perinatal Mortality Survey. Edinburgh: Livingstone, 1969.

122. Butler NR, Bonham DG. *Perinatal Mortality.* The first report of the 1958 British Perinatal Mortality Survey. Edinburgh: Livingstone, 1963.

123. Moore MP, Redman CWG. Case control study of severe pre-eclampsia of early onset. Br Med J 1983; II:580–3.

124. Emery JL, Kalpaktsoglou PK. The costochondral junction during later stages of intrauterine life, and abnormal growth patterns found in association with perinatal death. *Arch Dis Child* 1967; 42:1–13.

125. Brown JK. Infants damaged during birth: pathology. In: Hull D, ed. *Recent Advances in Paediatrics.* Edinburgh: Churchill Livingstone, 1976, p. 37.

126. Brosens I, Renaer M. On the pathogenesis of placental infarcts in pre-eclampsia. *J Obstet Gynaecol Br Commonw* 1972; 79:794–9.

127. Carter JE, Vellios F, Huber CP. Histologic classification and incidence of circulatory lesions of the human placenta with a review of the literature. *Am J Clin Pathol* 1963; 40:374–8.

128. Wentworth P. The incidence and significance of intervillous thrombi in the human placenta. *J Obstet Gynaecol Br Commonw* 1964; 71:894–8.

129. Dunn RIS. Haemangioma of placenta (chorio-angioma): report of 9 cases. *J Obstet Gynaecol Br Emp* 1959; 66:51–7.

130. Benirschke K. A review of the pathologic anatomy of the human placenta. *Am J Obstet Gynecol* 1962; 84:1595–1622.

131. Javert CT, Reiss C. The origin and significance of macroscopic intervillous coagulation hematomas (red infarcts) of the human placenta. *Surg Gynecol Obstet* 1952; 94:257–69.

132. Potter EL. Intervillous thrombi in the placenta and their possible relation to erythroblastosis fetalis. *Am J Obstet Gynecol* 1948; 56:959–61.

133. Shanklin DR, Scott JS. Massive subchorial thrombohaematoma (Breus' mole). *Br J Obstet Gynaecol* 1975; 82:476–87.

134. Almond DC, Fenton DW, Kennedy A, Pryce WIJ. Ultrasonic evidence that massive subchorial haematoma is an antemortem event. *J Clin Ultrasound* 1983; 11:49–53.

135. Olah KS, Gee H, Rushton I, Fowlie A. Massive subchorionic thrombohaematoma presenting as a placental tumour: case report. *Br J Obstet Gynaecol* 1987; 94:995–7.

136. Torpin R. Subchorial haematoma mole: hypothetical aetiology. *J Obstet Gynaecol Br Emp* 1960; 67:990.

137. Hagbard L. Pregnancy and diabetes mellitus: a clinical study. *Acta Obstet Gynecol Scand* 1956; 35:1–180.

138. Adashi EY, Pinto H, Tysen JE. Impact of maternal euglycaemia on fetal outcome in diabetic pregnancy. *Am J Obstet Gynecol* 1979; 133:268–74.

139. Day RE, Insley J. Maternal diabetes mellitus and congenital malformation: survey of 205 cases. *Arch Dis Child* 1976; 51:935–8.

140. Editorial. Diabetes and malformation. *Lancet* 1982; II:587–8.

141. Editorial. Congenital abnormalities in infants of diabetic mothers. *Lancet* 1988; I:1313–15.

142. Kitzmiller JL, Cloherty JP, Younger MD, et al. Diabetic pregnancy and perinatal morbidity. *Am J Obstet Gynecol* 1978; 131:560–80.

143. White P. Pregnancy complicating diabetes. *Am J Med* 1949; 7:609–16.

144. West KM. Epidemiology of diabetes and its vascular lesions. In: *Current Concepts, Natural History Classifications and Definitions.* New York: Elsevier, 1978.

145. Steel JM, Johnstone FD, Smith AF. Five years experience of a pregnancy clinic for insulin dependent diabetics. *Br Med J* 1982; 2:353–6.

146. Watkins PJ. Congenital malformations and blood glucose control in diabetic pregnancy (Leading article). *Br Med J* 1982; I:1357–8.

147. Pedersen J. *The Pregnant Diabetic and Her Newborn: Problems and Management,* 2nd ed. Copenhagen: E. Munksgaard, 1977.

148. Haust MD. Maternal diabetes mellitus—effects on the fetus and placenta. In: Naeye RL, Kissane JM, Kaufman N, eds. *Perinatal Diseases.* Baltimore: Williams & Wilkins, 1981, pp. 201–85.

149. Nummi S. Relative weight of the placenta and perinatal mortality: a retrospective clinical and statistical analysis. *Acta Obstet Gynaecol Scand* 1972; 17:1–69.

150. Naeye RL. The outcome of diabetic pregnancies: a prospective study. In: *Pregnancy Metabolism, Diabetes and the Fetus.* Ciba Foundation Symp No. 63. Amsterdam: Excerpta Medica, 1978, pp. 227–41.

151. Fox H. Thrombosis of foetal arteries in the human placenta. *Am J Obstet Gynecol* 1966; 73:961–5.

152. Wasserman L, Shlesinger H, Abramovici A, Goldman JA, Allalouf D. Glycosaminoglycan patterns in diabetic and toxaemic term placentas. *Am J Obstet Gynecol* 1980; 138:769–73.

153. Fox H. Pathology of the placenta in maternal diabetes mellitus. *Obstet Gynecol* 1969; 34:792–8.

154. Jones CJP, Fox H. An ultrastructural and ultrahistochemical study of the placenta of diabetic women. *J Pathol* 1976; 119:91–9.

155. Mayhew TM, Sorensen FB, Klebe JG, Jackson MR. Growth and maturation of villi in placentae from well-controlled diabetic women. *Placenta* 1994; 15:57–65.

156. Pinkerton JHM. The placental bed arterioles in diabetes. *Proc R Soc Med* 1963; 56:1021–2.

157. Denman AM. Pregnancy and immunological disorders. *Br Med J* 1982; I:999–1000.

158. Haustein UF. Electron mikroscopische untersuchungen der plazenta bei lupus erythematodes visceralis. *Z Gynakol* 1973; 95:1818–23.

159. Houser MT, Fisher AJ, Tagatz FE. Pregnancy and systemic lupus erythematosus. *Am J Obstet Gynecol* 1980; 138:409–13.

160. Reed NR, Smith MT. Periarteritis nodosa in pregnancy: report of a case and review of the literature. *Obstet Gynecol* 1980; 55:381–4.

161. Beischer NA, Fortune DW, Macafee J. Non-immunologic hydrops fetalis and congenital abnormalities. *Obstet Gynecol* 1971; 38:86–95.

162. Keeling JW, Gough DJ, Iliff P. The pathology of non rhesus hydrops. *Diagn Histopathol* 1983; 6:89–111.

163. Macafee CAJ, Fortune DW, Beischer, NA. Non immunological hydrops fetalis. *J Obstet Gynaecol Br Commonw* 1970; 77:226–37.

164. Hutchinson DL, Horger EO. Hydrops fetalis. Antenatal diagnosis and treatment. *Am J Obstet Gynecol* 1969; 103:967–71.

165. Baum JD, Harris D. Colloid osmotic pressure in erythroblastosis fetalis. *Br Med J* 1972; 1:601–3.

166. Gillan JE, Lowden JA, Gaskin K, Coty E. Congenital ascites as a presenting sign of lysosomal storage disease. *J Pediatr* 1984; 104:225–31.

167. Jauniaux E, Vamos E, Libert J, Elkhazen N, Wilkin P, Hustin J. Placental electron microscopy and histochemistry in a case of sialic acid storage disorder. *Placenta* 1987; 8:433–42.

168. Powell HC, Benirschke K, Favara BE, Plweger OH. Foamy changes of placenta in fetal storage disorder. *Virch Arch A* 1976; 369:191–6.

169. Rapola J, Aula P. Morphology of the placenta in fetal I cell disease. *Clin Genet* 1977; 11:107–13.

170. Sekelis K, Ornoy A, Cohen R, Kohn G. Mucolipidosis IV: fetal and placental

pathology. A report on two subsequent interruptions of pregnancy. *Monogr Hum Genet* 1978; 10:47–53.

171. Poenaru L, Castelnau L, Dumez Y, Thepot F. First trimester prenatal diagnosis of mucolipidosis II (I cell disease) by chorionic biopsy. *Am J Hum Genet* 1984; 36:1379–85.

172. Vamos E, Elkhazen N, Jauniaux E, et al. Prenatal diagnosis and confirmation of infantile sialic acid storage disease. *Prenat Diagn* 1986; 6:437–46.

173. Barabas AP. Ehlers-Danlos syndrome associated with prematurity and premature rupture of the foetal membranes. *Br Med J* 1966; 2:682–4.

174. Young ID, Lindenbaum RH, Thompson EM, Pembrey ME. Amniotic bands in connective tissue disorders. *Arch Dis Child* 1985; 60:1061–3.

175. Garrow JS, Hawes SF. The relationship of size and composition of the human placenta to its functional capacity. *J Obstet Gynaecol Br Commonw* 1971; 98:22–8.

176. Girmes DH, Hamilton WJ. Tolerance limits of fetal and placental growth relationships. *J Obstet Gynaecol Br Commonw* 1971; 78:620–3.

177. Thomson AM, Billewicz WZ, Hytton FE. The weight of the placenta in relation to birthweight. *J Obstet Gynaecol Br Commonw* 1969; 76:865–71.

178. Kalousek DK, Howard-Peebles PN, Olson SB, et al. Confirmation of CVS mosaicism in term placentae and high frequency of intrauterine growth retardation: association with confined placental mosaicism. *Prenat Diagn* 1991; 11:743–50.

179. Kennerknecht I, Kramer S, Grab D, Terinde R, Vogel W. No association of intrauterine growth retardation and confined placental mosaicism: a prospective study. *Prenat Diagn* 1992; 12(suppl):S104.

180. Wapner RJ, Simpson JL, Golbus MS, et al. Chorionic mosaicism: association with fetal loss but not with adverse perinatal outcome. *Prenat Diagn* 1992; 12:347–55.

181. Jeacock MK, Scott J, Plester JA. Calcium content of the human placenta. *Am J Obstet Gynecol* 1963; 87:34–40.

182. Tindall VR, Scott JS. Placental calcification: a study of 3025 singleton and multiple pregnancies. *J Obstet Gynaecol Br Commonw* 1965; 72:356–73.

183. Fox H. Calcification of the placenta. *J Obstet Gynaecol Br Emp* 1964; 71:759–65.

184. Fujikura T. Placental calcification and maternal age. *Am J Obstet Gynecol* 1963; 87:41–5.

185. Blanc WA. The future of antepartum morphological studies. In: Adamsons, K, ed. *Diagnosis and Treatment of Fetal Disorders.* New York: Springer-Verlag, 1968, p. 20.

186. deSa DJ. Disease of the umbilical cord. In: Perrin, EVDK, ed. *Pathology of the Placenta.* New York: Churchill Livingstone, 1984, pp. 121–39.

187. Little WA. Umbilical artery aplasia. *Obstet Gynecol* 1961; 17:695–700.

188. Uyanwah-Akpom PO, Fox H. The clinical significance of marginal and velamentous insertion of the cord. *Br J Obstet Gynaecol* 1977; 84:941–3.

189. Woods DL, Malan AF. The site of umbilical cord insertion and birthweight. *Br J Obstet Gynaecol* 1978; 85:332–33.

190. Lenoski EF, Medovy H. Single umbilical artery: incidence clinical significance and relation to autosomal trisomy. *Can Med Assoc J* 1962; 87:1229–31.

191. Molz G. Aplasie einer nabelartorie und angeborene fehlbildungen. *Helv Paediatr Acta* 1965; 20:403–14.

192. Faierman E. The significance of one umbilical artery. *Arch Dis Child* 1960; 35:285–8.

193. Seki M, Strauss L. Absence of one umbilical artery. Analaysis of 60 cases with emphasis on associated developmental aberrations. *Arch Pathol* 1964; 78:446–55.

194. Froelich LA, Fujikura T. Significance of single umbilical artery. Report from the collaborative study of cerebral palsy. *Am J Obstet Gynecol* 1966; 94:274–9.

195. Bryan EM, Kohler HG. The missing umbilical artery 1. Prospective study based on a maternity unit. *Arch Dis Child* 1974; 49:844–52.

196. Kristoffersen K. The significance of absence of one umbilical artery. *Acta Obstet Gynecol Scand* 1969; 48:195–223.

197. Benirschke K. Major pathologic features of the placenta, cord and membranes. *Proc Symp on the Placenta National Foundation, New York.* 1965; 1:52–77.

198. Benirschke K, Bourne GL. The incidence and prognostic implication of congenital absence of one umbilical artery. *Am J Obstet Gynecol* 1960; 79:251–4.

199. Cairns JD, McKee J. Single umbilical artery: a prospective study of 2000 consecutive deliveries. *Can Med Assoc J* 1964; 91:1071–3.

200. Altshuler G, Russell P. The human placental villitides: a review of chronic intrauterine infection. *Curr Top Pathol* 1975; 60:64–112.

201. Kampmeier OF. On sireniform monsters with a consideration of the causation and the predominance of male sex among them. *Anat Rec* 1927; 34:365–89.

202. MacPherson TA. Angiographic evaluation of vascular anomalies at autopsy in the fetus and neonate. *Lab Invest* 1982; 46:10A. Abstract.

203. Meyer WW, Lind J, Moinian M. An accessory fourth vessel of the umbilical cord: a preliminary study. *Am J Obstet Gynecol* 1969; 105:1063–8.

204. Nadkarni BG. Congenital anomalies of the umbilical cord: a light and electron microscope study. *Indian J Med Res* 1969; 57:1018–27.

205. Fujikura T. Single umbilical artery and congenital malformations. *Am J Obstet Gynecol* 1964; 88:829–30.

206. Peckham CH, Yerushalmy J. Aplasia of one umbilical artery. Incidence by race and certain obstetric factors. *Obstet Gynecol* 1965; 26:359–66.

207. Benirschke K, Brown WH. A vascular anomaly of the umbilical cord. *Obstet Gynecol* 1955; 6:399–404.

208. Fischer A. Fetal atrophie bei fehlerhafer anlabe der nabelarterien und kleinheit der placenta (Ein beitrag zur frage nichterblicher missbildungen). *Frankf Z Pathol* 1957; 68:497–506.

209. Thomas J. Untersuchungsergebnisse uber die aplasie einer nabelartorie unter besonderer berucksichtigung der zwillingsschwagerschaft. *Geburtshilfe Frauenheilk* 1961; 21:984–92.

210. Hyrtl J. Die blutgefasse der menschlichen nachgeburt in normalen und abnormen. Wein: Verhaltnissen Braumuller, 1870.

211. Crawford JS. Cord round neck: incidence and sequelae. *Acta Paediatr Scand* 1962; 51:594–603.

212. Crawford JS. Cord round neck: further analysis of incidence. *Acta Paediatr Scand* 1964; 53:553–7

213. Walker CW, Pye BG. The length of the umbilical cord: a statistical report. *Br Med J* 1960; i:546–8.

214. Browne FJ. On abnormalities of the umbilical cord which may cause antenatal death. *J Obstet Gynaecol Br Emp* 1925; 32:17–48.

215. Daly JW, Gibbs CE. Cord prolapse. *Am J Obstet Gynecol* 1968; 100:264–6.

216. Niswander KR, Friedman EA, Hoover DB, Pietrowski H, Wesphal M. Fetal morbidity following potentially anoxigenic obstetric conditions. III. Prolapse of the umbilical cord. *Am J Obstet Gynecol* 1966; 95:853–9.

217. Pathak UN. Presentation and prolapse of the umbilical cord. *Am J Obstet Gynecol* 1968; 101:401–5.

218. Weber J. Constriction of the umbilical cord as a cause of fetal death. *Acta Obstet Gynecol Scand* 1963; 42:259–68.

219. Heifetz SA. Strangulation of the umbilical cord by amniotic bands: report of six cases and review of the literature. *Pediatr Pathol* 1984; 2:285–304.

220. Hong CY, Simon MA. Amniotic bands knotted about umbilical cord: a rare cause of fetal death. *Obstet Gynecol* 1963; 22:667–70.

221. Kohler HG, Collins ML. Ligation of the umbilical cord by torn amniotic membranes. *J Obstet Gynaecol Br Commonw* 1972; 79:183–4.

222. Brant HA, Lewis BV. Umbilical cord prolapse. *Lancet* 1966; 2:1443–5.

223. Vanhaesebrouck P, Vanneste K, De Praeter C, Van Trappen Y, Thiery M. Tight nuchal cord and neonatal hypovolaemic shock. *Arch Dis Child* 1987; 62:1276–7.

224. Chantler C, Baum JD, Wigglesworth JS, Scopes JW. Giant umbilical cord associated with a patent urachus and fused umbilical arteries. *J Obstet Gynaecol Br Commonw* 1969; 76:273–4.

225. Howorka E, Kapczynski W. Unusual thickness of the fetal end of the umbilical cord. *J Obstet Gynaecol Br Commonw* 1971; 78:283.

226. Walz W. Uber das odem der nabelschnur. *Zentralbl Gynakol* 1947; 69:144–8.

227. Javert CT, Barton B. Congenital and acquired lesions of the umbilical cord and spontaneous abortions. *Am J Obstet Gynecol* 1952; 63:1056–77.

228. Coulter JBS, Scott JM, Jordan MM. Oedema of the umbilical cord and respiratory distress in the newborn. *Br J Obstet Gynaecol* 1975; 82:453–9.

229. Blanc WA, Allan GW. Intrafunicular ulceration of persistent omphalomesenteric duct with intra-amniotic hemorrhage and fetal death. *Am J Obstet Gynecol* 1961; 82:1392–6.

230. Dippel AL. Hematomas of the umbilical cord. *Surg Gynecol Obstet* 1940; 70:51–7.

231. Schreier R, Brown S. Hematoma of the umbilical cord. *Obstet Gynecol* 1962; 20:798–800.

232. Ivemark BI, Lagergren C, Ljungqvist A. Generalised arterial calcification associated with hydramnios in two stillborn infants. *Acta Paediatr Scand* 1962; 135:103–10.

233. Heifetz SA, Rueda-Pedraza ME. Omphalomesenteric duct cysts of the umbilical cord. *Pediatr Pathol* 1983; 1:325–36.

234. Harris LE, Wenzl JE. Heterotopic pancreatic tissue and intestinal mucosa in the umbilical cord: report of a case. *N Engl J Med* 1963; 268:721–2.

235. Benton BF, Lanford HG, Hardy JD. Patent urachus. *Am J Surg* 1954; 88:513–15.

236. Ente G, Penzer PH, Kenigsberg K. Giant umbilical cord associated with patent urachus: an external anomaly due to an internal anomaly. *Am J Dis Child* 1970; 120:82–3.

237. McCauley RT, Lichtenheld FR. Congenital patent urachus. *South Med J* 1960; 53:1138–41.

238. Tsuchida Y, Ishida M. Osmolar relationship between enlarged umbilical cord and patent urachus. *J Pediatr Surg* 1969; 4:465–7.

239. Heifetz SA. Thrombosis of the umbilical cord: analysis of 52 cases and literature review. *Pediatr Pathol* 1988; 8:37–54.

240. Miller PW, Coen RW, Benirschke K. Dating the time interval from meconium passage to birth. *Obstet Gynecol* 1985; 66:459–62.

241. McKay DG, Roby CC, Hertig AT, Richardson MV. Studies of the function of early human trophoblast. II. Preliminary observations on certain chemical constituents of chorionic and early amniotic fluid. *Am J Obstet Gynecol* 1955; 69:735–41.

242. Bourne GL. *The Human Amnion and Chorion*. London: Lloyds-Luke, 1962.

243. Landing BH. Amnion nodosum: a lesion of the placenta apparently associated with deficient secretion of fetal urine. *Am J Obstet Gynecol* 1950; 60:1339–42.

244. Paddock R, Greer ED. Origin of common cystic structures of human placenta. *Am J Obstet Gynecol* 1927; 13:164–73.

245. deSa DJ. Rupture of fetal vessels on placental surface. *Arch Dis Child* 1971; 46:495–501.

246. deSa DJ. Intimal cushions in foetal placental veins. *J Pathol* 1973; 110:347–52.

247. Bartman J, Blanc WA. Ultrastructure of human fetal placental membranes in chorioamnionitis and meconium exposure. *Obstet Gynecol* 1970; 35:554–61.

248. Ariel IB, Landing BH. A possibly distinctive vacuolar change of amniotic epithelium associated with gastroschisis. *Pediatr Pathol* 1985; 3:283–9.

249. Blanc WA. Vernix granulomatosis of amnion (amnion nodosum) in oligohydramnios: lesion associated with urinary anomalies, retention of dead fetuses and prolonged leakage of amniotic fluid. *NY State J Med* 1961; 61:1492–5.

250. Scott JS, Bain AD. Amnion nodosum. *Proc R Soc Med* 1958; 51:512–13.

251. Bartman J, Driscoll SG. Amnion nodosum and hypoplastic cystic kidneys: an electron microscopic and microdissection study. *Obstet Gynecol* 1968; 32:700–5.

252. Salazar H, Kanhour AI. Amnion nodosum ultrastructure and histopathogenesis. *Arch Pathol* 1974; 98:39–46.

253. Seeds JW, Cefalo RC, Herbert WNP. Amniotic band syndrome. *Am J Obstet Gynecol* 1982; 144:243–8.

254. Patterson TJS. Amniotic bands. In: Bourne G, ed. *The Human Amnion and Chorion*. London: Lloyd-Luke 1962, pp. 250–64.

255. Herva R, Rapola J, Rosti J, Karlson H. Cluster of severe amniotic adhesion malformations in Finland. *Lancet* 1980; I:818–9.

256. Ballantyne JW. *Manual of Antenatal Pathology and Hygiene: The Foetus*.

257. Torpin R. *Fetal Malformations Caused by Amnion Rupture during Gestation*. Springfield, IL: Charles C. Thomas, 1968.

258. Swinburne LM. Spontaneous intrauterine decapitation. *Arch Dis Child* 1967; 42:636–41.

259. Imber G, Guthrie RH, Goulian D. Congenital band of the abdomen and the amniotic aetiology of bands. *Am J Surg* 1974; 127:753–4.

260. James PD, Beilby JOW, Steele SJ. An unusual cause of intrauterine death. *J Obstet Gynecol Br Commonw* 1969; 76:752–4.

261. Burrows S, Phillips N. Strangulation of umbilical cord by amniotic band. *Am J Obstet Gynecol* 1976; 124:697–8.

262. Greene HSN, Saxton JA. Hereditary brachdactylia and allied abnormalities in the rabbit. *J Exp Med* 1939; 69:301–14.

263. Bagg HJ, Little CC. Hereditary structural defects in the descendants of mice exposed to roentgen ray irradiation. *Am J Anat* 1924; 33:119–38.

264. Rushton DI. Amniotic band syndrome: leading article. *Br Med J* 1983; 1:919–20.

265. Warkany J. *Congenital Malformations: Notes and Comments*. Chicago: Year Book Medical Publishers, 1971, pp. 946–7.

266. Hoyme HE, Jones KL, Vanall-Saunders BG, Benirschke K. The vascular pathogenesis of transverse limb reduction defects. *Clin Res* 1982; 30:134A. Abstract.

267. Demyer W, Baird I. Mortality and skeletal malformations from amniocentesis and oligohydramnios in rats: cleft palate, club foot, microstomia and adactyly. *Teratology* 1969; 2:33–8.

268. Firth HV, Boyd PA, Chamberlain PF, et al. Analysis of limb reduction defects in babies exposed to chorionic villus sampling. *Lancet* 1994; 343:1069–71.

269. Kohn G. The amniotic band syndrome: a possible complication of amniocentesis. *Prenat Diagn* 1987; 7:303–5.

270. Tingpalapong M, Chapple FE, Andrews WK. Unilateral hypoplasia of the palate and associated structures in a white handed gibbon (*Hylobates* Lar). *J Med Primatol* 1981; 10:274–8.

271. Torpin R. Extramembranous pregnancy. *J Med Assoc Ga* 1966; 55:174–9.

272. Gregersen E. Extramembranous pregnancy with amniorrhoea. *Acta Obstet Gynecol Scand* 1976; 55:69–71.

273. Kohler HG, Peel KR, Hoar RA. Extramembranous pregnancy and amniorrhoea. *J Obstet Gynaecol Br Commonw* 1970; 77:809–12.

274. Kohler HG, Jenkins DM. Extra-amniotic pregnancy: a case report. *Br J Obstet Gynaecol* 1976; 83:251–3.

275. Santamaria M, Benirschke K, Carpenter PM, Baldwin VJ, Pritchard JA. Transplacental haemorrhage associated with placental neoplasms. *Pediatr Pathol* 1987; 7:601–15.

276. Nickell KA, Stocker JT. Placental teratoma: a case report. *Pediatr Pathol* 1987; 7:645–50.

277. Gayer N, Blumenthal N, Ruhen L. Placental teratoma: simultaneous occurrence with ovarian teratoma complicating pregnancy. *Br J Obstet Gynaecol* 1994; 101:720–2.

278. Marchetti AA. Consideration of certain types of benign tumours of the placenta. *Surg Gynecol Obstet* 1939; 68:733–43.

279. Fox H. Vascular tumours of the placenta. *Obstet Gynaecol Surv* 1967; 22:697–711.

280. Siddall RS. The occurrence of chorioangiofibroma (chorangioma): a study of six hundred placentas. *Johns Hopkins Hosp Bull Baltimore* 1926; 38:355–7.

281. Wentworth P. The incidence and significance of haemangioma of the placenta. *J Obstet Gynaecol Br Commonw* 1965; 72:81–8.

282. McInroy RA, Kelsey HA. Chorangioma (haemangioma of placenta) associated with acute hydramnios. *J Pathol Bacteriol* 1954; 68:519–23.

283. Benson PF, Joseph MC. Cardiomegaly in a newborn due to placental chorangioma. *Br Med J* 1961; 1:102–5.

284. DeCosta EJ, Gerbie AB, Andersen RH, Gallanis TC. Placental tumours: hemangiomas with special reference to an associated clinical syndrome. *Obstet Gynecol* 1956; 7:249–59.

285. Potter EL, Craig JM. *Pathology of the Fetus and the Infant*, 3rd ed. Chicago: Year Book Medical Publishers, 1976.

286. Heifetz SA, Rueda-Pedraza ME. Hemangiomas of the umbilical cord. *Pediatr Pathol* 1983; 1:385–98.

287. Mishriki YY, Vanyshelbaum Y, Epstein H, Blanc W. Hemangioma of the umbilical cord. *Pediatr Pathol* 1987; 7:43–9.

288. Barson AJ, Donnai P, Ferguson A, Donnai D, Read AP. Haemangioma of the cord: further cause of raised maternal serum and liquor alpha fetoprotein. *Br Med J* 1980; II:1252–3.

289. Potter JF, Schoenemann M. Metastasis of maternal cancer to the placenta and fetus. *Cancer* 1970; 25:380–8.

290. Gray ES, Balch NJ, Kohler H, Thompson VD, Simpson JG. Congenital leukaemia: an unusual cause of stillbirth. *Arch Dis Child* 1986; 61:1001–6.

APPENDIX: PLACENTAL INFECTION AND INFLAMMATION

The commonest pathological lesion of the placenta encountered in routine practice is evidence of inflammation, usually of the placental membranes. In the majority of instances, the cause of the inflammation is either unknown or conjectural, as routine microbiological sampling of the placenta is rarely carried out. Indeed, because, with the exception of transabdominal deliveries, the placenta passes through a non-sterile environment that may contain potential if not actual pathogens, the value of routine placental culture is questionable. Gibbs [1] notes that between 18% and 49% of placentas with histological chorioamnionitis are sterile on culture, while 15–45% of those membranes with positive cultures do not show histological evidence of inflammation. Thus, not all mothers who carry group B hemolytic streptococci in their vaginal flora will develop either placental or fetal infection, yet the organism might well be isolated from a vaginally delivered placenta in such cases [2, 3]. The lack of correlation between inflammatory changes and isolation of infecting organisms is particularly true where villous tissue is involved (*vide infra*).

There is, however, no doubt that infection is a major cause of reproductive wastage both in humans and in animals [4]. The most common placental pathology in spontaneously occurring human, anatomically normal, fresh midtrimester abortions [5] and premature viable deliveries [6] is chorioamnionitis occurring in association with amniotic cavity infection. It is still debated as to whether chorioamnionitis is the cause or effect of membrane rupture [7]. Obstetric risk factors that are associated with amniotic cavity infection include low parity, increased numbers of vaginal examinations in labor, prolonged labor, prolonged membrane rupture and internal fetal monitoring, and bacterial vaginosis [8–10].

Indeed, there is evidence that asymptomatic non-pregnant women may carry potential pathogens in their uterine cavities prior to conception [11]. Coitus in pregnancy has been implicated, though this is disputed [12, 13]. There is also a relationship between the presence of certain organisms and/or their antigens or antibodies in the urine of pregnant women and premature labor [14]. There is little doubt that the prevention of amniotic cavity infections would result in a significant decrease in the number of premature deliveries and thus in the perinatal mortality rates, especially where these rates are already low.

ROUTES OF INFECTION

There are two major and two lesser routes by which infection may reach the placenta that reflect its anatomical relationship with the mother. These have been comprehensively reviewed by Remington and Klein 1995 [15].

1. The most important both numerically and in terms of fetal wastage is the *ascending route via the vagina*. There is evidence that some, if not all, women have commensal organisms in the uterine cavity as well as the vagina [11]. Whatever the source of infection, involvement of the amniotic cavity may result in chorioamnionitis, with or without funisitis, and in a proportion of cases of fetal infection. Such infections are usually bacterial and are usually caused by organisms normally carried in the vagina or on the perineum.
2. The second major route is via the *maternal blood-stream*, and though very much less common than ascending infection it is a significant cause of fetal morbidity and mortality. This route is typically followed by viral infections such as rubella, but any organism infecting the mother that enters her blood-stream has the potential to cause placental and/or fetal infection. It is characterized by inflammation of placental villi (villitis) and/or aggregation of inflammatory cells in the intervillous space (intervillositis).

Table 7A.1. Organisms isolated from amniotic fluid in cases with amniotic cavity infection

Organism	Percent (%)
Aerobes and anaerobes	48
Aerobes only	38
Anaerobes only	8
No organisms	6
Ureaplasma	47–50
Mycoplasma	31–35
Anaerobes	
Bacteroides	11–29[a]
Peptostreptococcus	7–33
Fusobacterium	6–7[a]
Aerobes	
Group B streptococcus	12–19[b]
Enterococci	5–11
Escherichia coli	8–12[b]
Other gram-negative rods	5–10
Gardnerella	24

[a] Organisms more commonly isolated among premature babies.
[b] Most common cause of neonatal infections.
Note: In addition to these bacterial and mycoplasma infections, certain fungi, chlamydia, viruses, and protozoa may cause ascending infections. These include *Candida* species, *Aspergillus, Actinomyces, Torulopsis*, ovine chlamydia, herpes simplex, and possibly cytomegalovirus [46].
Modified from Gibbs [1].

3. In a few instances, there may be transmission of infection as a result of *contiguous spread from the uterus or cervix*. This route may be more important as a cause of fetal infection because early delivery obtunds the development of an inflammatory response in the placenta.
4. A small number of cases follow *obstetric interventions* such as chorionic villous sampling, amniocentesis and cordocentesis, intrauterine transfusion, and cervical cerclage.

CAUSE OF AMNIOTIC CAVITY INFECTION

The organisms that have been identified as causing infection of amniotic fluid are both numerous and diverse. A complete listing of responsible organisms is of little value other than to those wishing to record a new addition. It is likely that most pathogenic organisms are capable of infecting the amniotic cavity. The majority of infections are due to mixed organisms, both aerobes and anaerobes being isolated. In a proportion of cases, no organisms are identified (Table 7A.1).

RESPONSE TO INFECTION

The role of amniotic fluid in preventing or obtunding infection is uncertain, and the inflammatory response in the placenta is unique in that it involves the immune systems of two individuals. Furthermore, the potential to respond differs between these individuals both with the gestation and the site of response. These cellular and immunological responses and their development have been reviewed by Lewis and Wilson [16]. The response in the membranes of chorion laeve (that part of the chorionic plate not covered by villous tissue) will be maternal and in the umbilical cord will be fetal, while the response in the membranes of the chorion frondosum (that part of the chorionic plate covered by villous tissue) may be both fetal and/or maternal. In villous tissue, the major component of the response will be fetal, and the role of maternal contribution remains uncertain. Likewise, the response in the intervillous space will be predominantly maternal.

The evolution of the response to infection within the amniotic cavity follows basic pathological principles. The presence of pathogenic organisms and/or toxins produced by organisms adjacent to the gestation sac results initially in the margination of polymorphs from the maternal bloodstream on and in the trophoblast of the maternal side of the chorionic plate and at the junction of the decidua (Fig. 7A.1) and the trophoblast of the chorion laeve. Margination in fetal vessels in the chorionic plate and the umbilical cord may occur concurrently or may be delayed. The marginated cells from these sites then invade the chorion and amnion (Fig. 7A.2) (or the vessel wall and eventually Wharton's jelly in the umbilical cord), finally congregating in their largest numbers immediately below the amniotic epithelium or within Wharton's jelly in the cord where the response may organize concentrically around the blood vessels (Fig. 7A.3). In florid infections, pus may form on the surface of the membranes, and the membranes become creamy and opaque obscuring the superficial chorionic vessels (Fig. 7A.4). The amnion may remain intact or become ulcerated

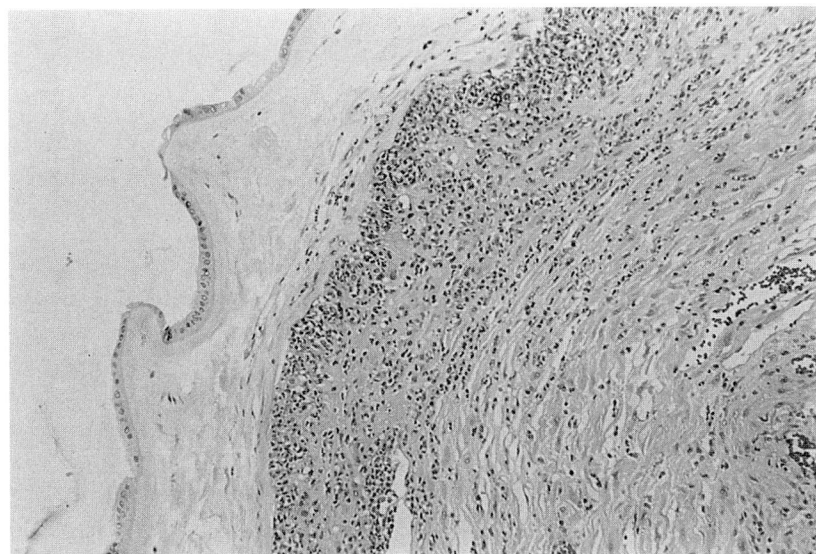

FIGURE 7A.1. *Early acute chorioamnionitis. Polymorphs are aggregated at the junction between the chorion and decidua. H&E, ×30.*

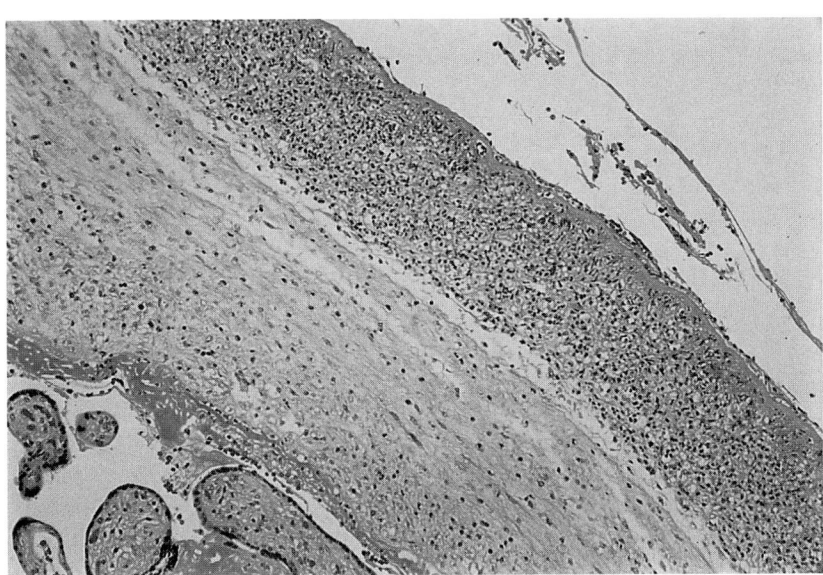

FIGURE 7A.2. *Acute chorioamnionitis. The inflammatory infiltrate is concentrated below the amniotic epithelium. H&E, ×30.*

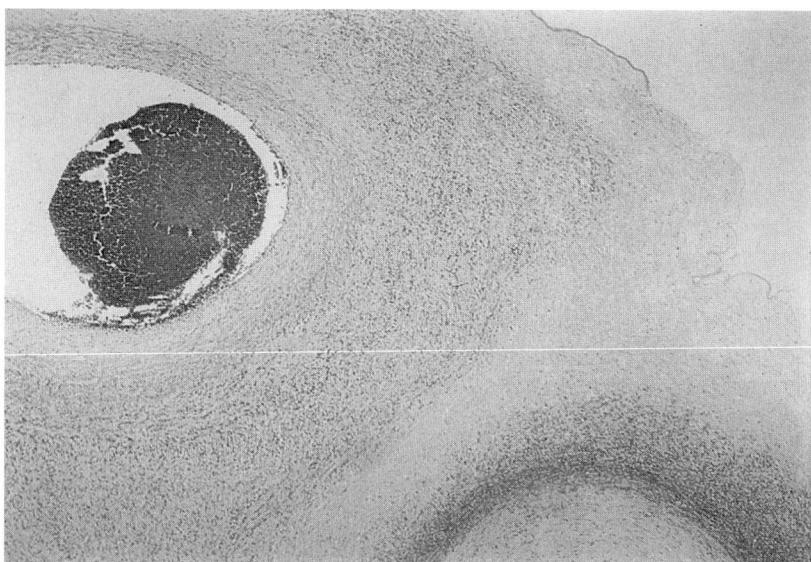

FIGURE 7A.3. *Acute funisitis. Inflammatory cells are arranged concentrically around blood vessels in the umbilical cord. H&E, ×30.*

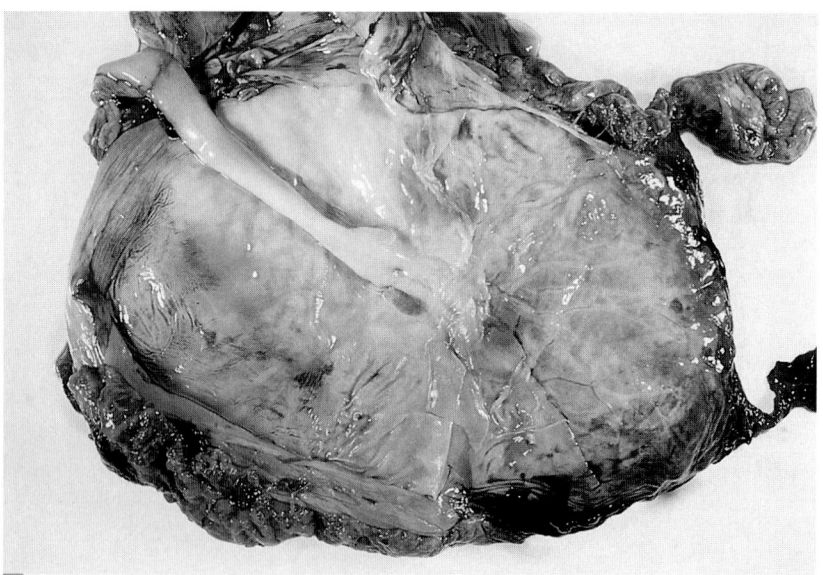

FIGURE 7A.4. *Acute chorioamnionitis. The placental membranes are opaque and creamy. (Group B streptococcal infection).*

depending on the nature and virulence of the infecting organism. Where the cord is involved, this may result in necrotizing funisitis. Polymorphs may also enter the amniotic cavity and thus be aspirated or swallowed by the fetus. It has been shown that in the fetal lung many of the polymorphs seen in so-called congenital pneumonia are of fetal origin [17, 18]; however, the origin of these cells may vary. Thus, where there is amniotic cavity infection and the fetal lungs contain large numbers of aspirated squames as well as polymorphs, it is likely that a significant number of the latter will be of maternal origin. Where the infection resolves, the cellular response first abates on the maternal or fetal aspects (i.e., on the maternal surface of the chorionic plate and intimal surface of the fetal vessels). Thus, the deeper aspects of the chorionic plate will show clearing of the inflammatory response before the fetal aspects. Where the acute reaction resolves completely, there may be a residual population

of macrophages and mononuclear cells that may contain iron and, on occasion, meconium-derived pigments. In most instances, bacterial infections produce diffuse though sometimes patchy lesions. Other organisms, notably fungal and yeast infections, may produce focal or spotty lesions on both the membranes and umbilical cord.

VILLITIS AND INTERVILLOSITIS

Inflammation of the villi and intervillous space is, as has been indicated, far less frequent than involvement of the placental membranes, mainly because these parts of the placenta are far less accessible to invading organisms. Villitis is the result of an inflammatory response mounted by the fetus against an external antigenic stimulus within the villous component of the placenta [19]. The etiology of such inflammation can be broadly divided into those cases

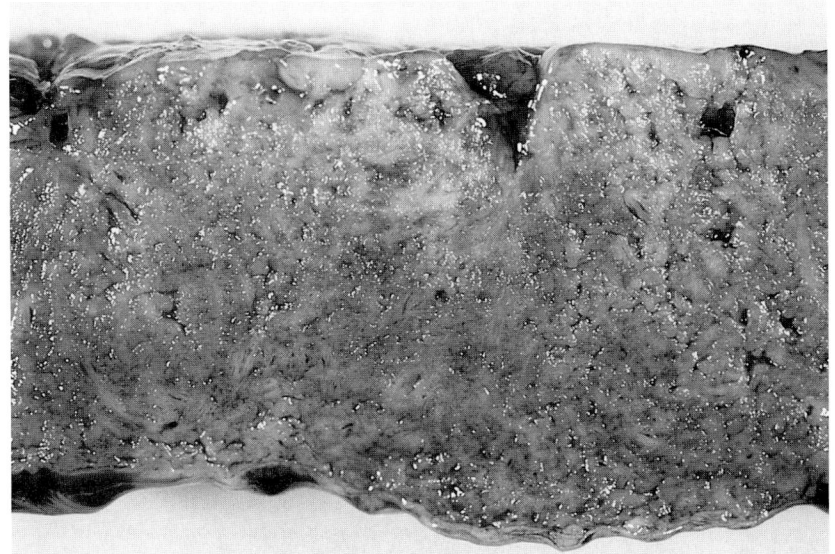

FIGURE 7A.5. *"Consolidated" placenta. There is loss of texture with a homogeneous cut surface. Ovine chlamydial infection.*

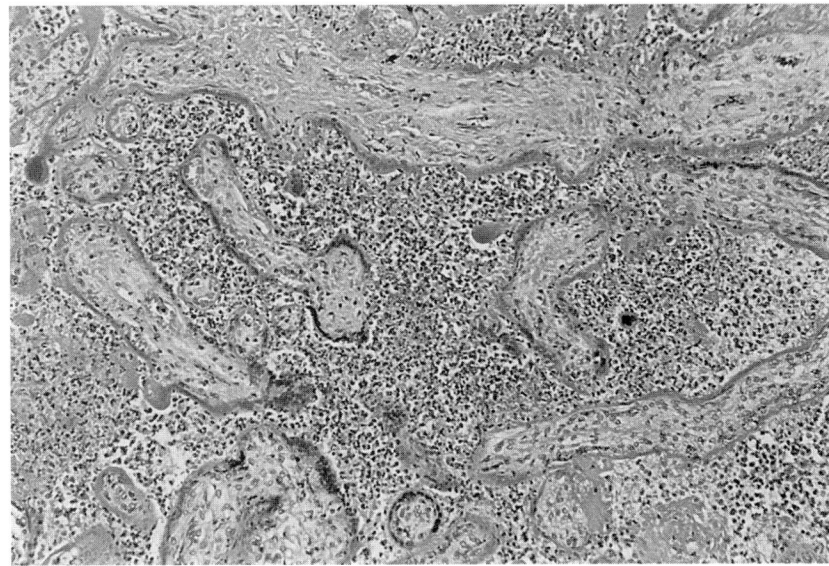

FIGURE 7A.6. *Listeriosis. An acute intervillositis with little villous involvement. H&E, ×78.*

where a specific organism has or can be identified and those where the cause is unknown, often termed non-specific villitis or villitis of unknown etiology (VUE). The latter is seen in twin pregnancies [20] and in association with small-for-dates babies [21], and the possibility that it represents an immunological disorder has been suggested [22, 23]. While the clinical significance of villitis due to infection is self-evident, in that it is a possible marker of fetal infection, the significance is unclear as might be anticipated with a disorder of unknown and possibly multiple causes [24].

Macroscopically, placentae with villous inflammation may appear normal, while in other instances they may appear unusually solid ("placental consolidation") (Fig. 7A.5), the latter being found in very florid infections. Where the inflammation is categorized as nonspecific, there are usually no macroscopic abnormalities, though in those cases associ-

ated with uteroplacental ischemia, pre-eclampsia, and/or eclampsia, there may be infarcts or hematomas.

In bacterial diseases such as listeriosis (Fig. 7A.6) or group B streptococcal infection, the microscopic features are those of acute inflammation, with a polymorphonuclear cellular response both in the villous stroma and often in the intervillous space. In cytomegalovirus (Fig. 7A.7) and many other viral infections, a more chronic response with mononuclear cells, probably derived from the Hofbauer cells and resembling plasma cells and lymphocytes, is typically seen. In some infections, it may appear granulomatous [25]. Where the villitis is non-specific, the inflammatory infiltrate may be mixed, but it is usually less intense (Fig. 7A.8) and often predominantly lymphocytic. The most common form is very similar in appearance to the villitis seen in chicken pox [26].

Villitis associated with specific infections is usually more

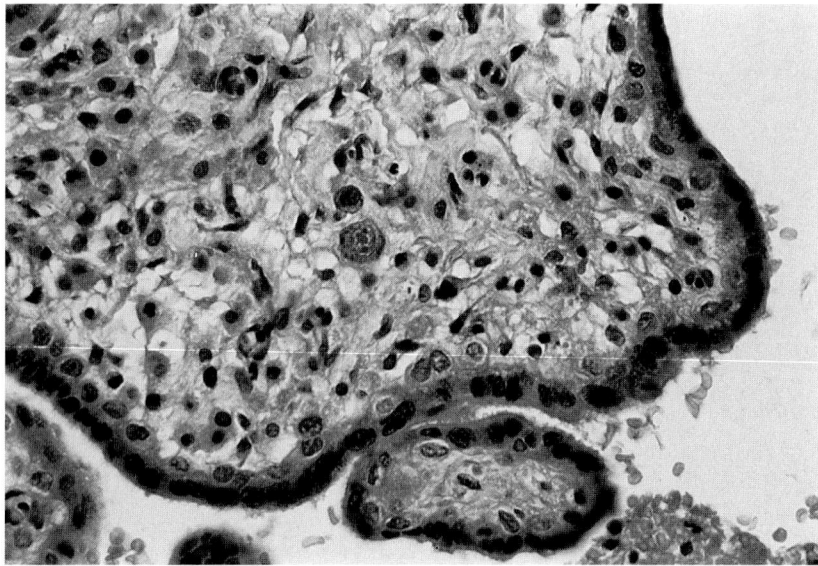

FIGURE 7A.7.   *Cytomegalovirus villitis. Occasional viral inclusions are evident (arrows) H&E, ×125.*

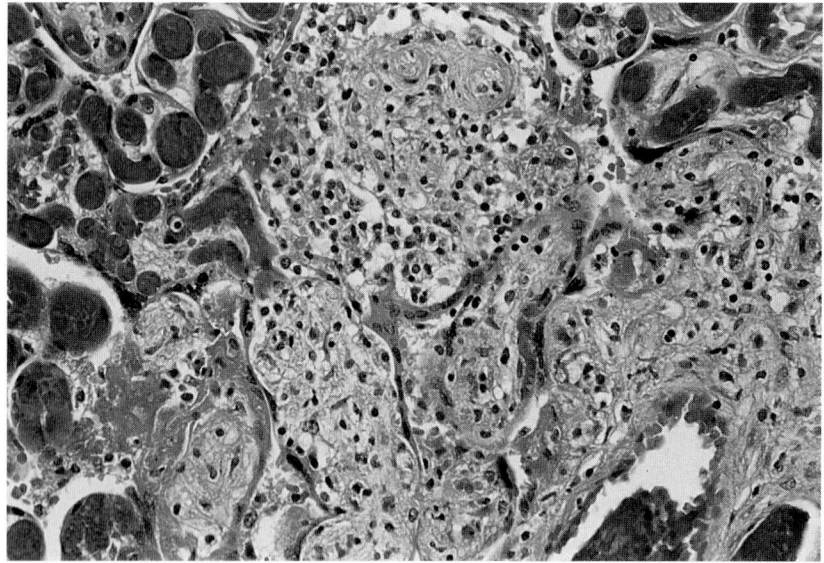

FIGURE 7A.8.   *Non-specific villitis. Low-grade focal villitis associated with maternal pre eclampsia. H&E, ×125.*

diffuse, whereas non-specific villitis is frequently focal and may involve very small numbers of villi. The evolution of the inflammatory response in villous tissue is more variable than in the membranes, in that some viruses such as that causing rubella may pass to the fetus with minimal evidence of placental involvement, while others such as cytomegalovirus may produce a florid though often focal villitis, with or without the characteristic viral inclusion bodies. Bacterial infections tend to produce an acute polymorphonuclear response in both the intervillous space and villous tissue, with or without chorioamnionitis. However, there are no absolute criteria for identifying the type of villitis, unless the causative organism is isolated, produces pathognomonic lesions, or can be demonstrated by specific tinctorial or immunological techniques [27–32]. Many organisms may infect and/or cross the placenta to infect the fetus, and some are associated with villitis and/or intervillositis (Table 7A.2). The list in Table 7A.2, however, is not exhaustive. It is not intended to describe the placental lesions in each individual infection, as these are often quite similar and definitive diagnosis depends on identification of the causative organism.

Intervillositis is usually associated with villositis and is most commonly an acute response. A massive chronic form of intervillositis has been described [33, 34], which, at least in some instances, is associated with recurrent early pregnancy loss or toxemia of pregnancy. The chronic inflammatory infiltrate consists largely of monocytic macrophage cells with occasional T lymphocytes (Fig. 7A.9) and again suggests that this lesion may represent an immunological attack on the conceptus (see Massive Perivillous Fibrin Deposition).

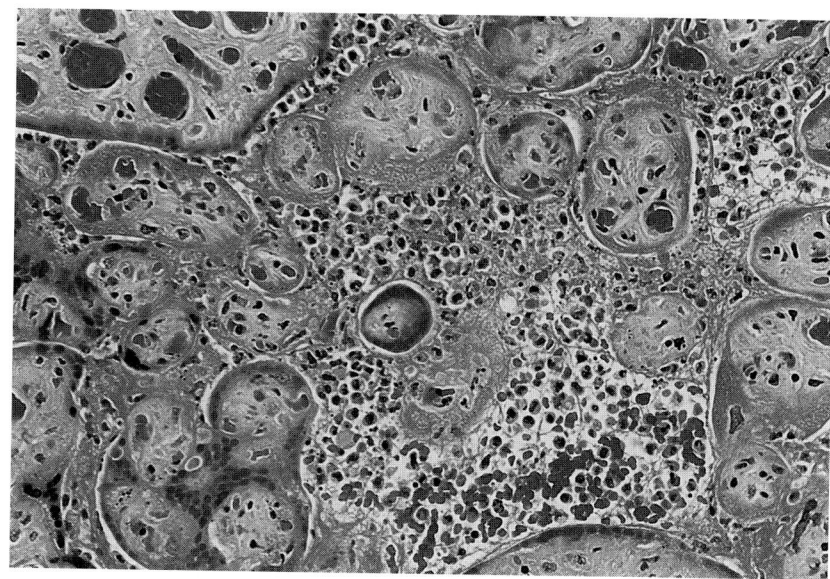

FIGURE 7A.9. *Chronic intervillositis. The intervillous space is filled with mononuclear cells. The trophoblast is degenerate with focal fibrin deposition. H&E, ×125.*

Table 7A.2. Organisms infecting the placenta via the hematogenous route

Bacteria	Viruses	Miscellaneous
Staphylococcus	Cytomegalovirus	*Treponema pallidum*
Streptococcus	Rubella	*Vibrio cholerae*
Pneumococcus	Hepatitis	*Chlamydia*
Enteric bacteria	Herpes simplex	*Mycoplasma*
Listeria	Varicella zoster	*Rickettsia*
Campylobacter fetus	Variola alastrim	Coccidiodomycosis
Salmonella	Vaccinia	*Toxoplasma*
Brucella	Mumps	*Plasmodium malariae*
Borrelia	Measles	*Trypansoma*
Mycobacteria	Coxsackie	*Schistosoma*
Francisella tularensis	Poliomyelitis	*Leptospira*
	Parvovirus	
	Epstein-Barr virus	
	ECHO	
	HIV	
	Western equine encephalitis	

HIV = human immunodeficiency virus.
Note: While all these organisms may infect the placenta and/or the fetus, they are not all invariably associated with either villitis or intervillositis.

SIGNIFICANCE OF PLACENTAL INFLAMMATION

There are, as has been suggested, two broad categories of placental inflammation, those with an identifiable or conjectural etiology based on direct or indirect methods of identification of the infecting organism and those where no cause has been identified. The latter category is almost entirely made up of cases of so-called VUE.

Clinically, the importance of amniotic cavity infections and, thus, the pathological finding of chorioamnionitis is threefold and lies in:

1. Their relationship with the premature onset of labor.
2. Their relationship with infection of the infant.
3. Their relationship with the risk of serious maternal infection.

Of these, undoubtedly the most important in developed countries in terms of morbidity and mortality is the contribution of these infections to premature delivery or infection of the fetus, with all the incumbent risks and financial consequences that stem therefrom. However, in developing countries, their contribution to maternal mortality may be of equal or greater importance.

The clinical management of the infected fetus or mother will depend on the isolation of the organism concerned, and while placental microbiology may be positive it does not obviate the need for fetal and maternal sampling, if only for the reason that the placenta may have been contaminated during delivery by irrelevant though potential pathogens.

The investigation of the role of infection in the etiology of premature rupture of the membranes and of premature labor in an individual case is more problematic, as in nearly all cases the infection is only identified after delivery. In the majority of cases, there is no recurrence in further pregnancies. In the few women who have recurrent midtrimester losses or premature labors associated with chorioamnionitis, there is no certainty that each loss will be caused by the same organism, even if it is identified (not infrequently there is either no evidence of placental examination or the examination is so cursory that it is not clear whether evidence of infection has been sought). However, some of these women do suffer repeated infections with a single organism, most commonly in our experience due to *Gardnerella*, an infection that may not be clinically apparent [35].

The role of amniotic cavity infections in the etiology of premature labor is still controversial [36]. While the majority of identified cases of infection are associated with premature rupture of the membranes, there is no doubt such infections may precede rupture [37]. What is not clear is the relative importance of the physical effects of rupture of the membranes with loss of amniotic fluid and of the infection in the onset of labor. Recent evidence suggests that attempts to suppress labor in women with premature rupture of the membranes with tocolytic drugs are much less likely to succeed if infection is present [38]. There are also good theoretical grounds to suggest infection may lead to the premature onset of labor through the effect of inflammatory mediators on prostaglandin synthesis in the decidua [39–41].

Currently, the relationship between premature and prolonged rupture of the membranes, chorioamnionitis and neurological damage in the fetus, and cerebral palsy and neurodevelopmental outcome in the infant are under investigation [42–44]. The significance of villitis is more difficult to assess. In those cases where a pathogen is identified, there is frequently also fetal infection, and it is uncertain whether any of the non-specific fetal abnormalities such as intrauterine growth retardation are due to the effects of the infection on the fetus or are mediated through effects on the placenta.

Where no pathogen is isolated, the problem is even more confusing. VUE is a diagnosis made by exclusion, yet even this definition is not without problems [45]. The finding of an isolated inflamed villus or group of inflamed villi is not uncommon. There is no generally accepted guidance as to whether the finding of a single inflamed villus is acceptable for a diagnosis of non-specific villitis to be made. If it is not, then how many affected villi are necessary to make the diagnosis? It is almost certainly true that if every placenta were subjected to complete microscopic examination, all would contain at least one inflamed villus. It is also true that inflamed villi are frequently found in relation to other placental lesions, such as infarcts, where they are viewed as a secondary consequence of the underlying uteroplacental ischemia. However, as Khong et al [45] have indicated, there is no guidance as to how far away from an ischemic lesion an inflamed villus must be sited to be classified as being of unknown cause. These authors compared inter-observer variation among experienced placental pathologists and found significant differences in their assessment of villitis of unknown etiology. In that it has been related to clinical disorders such as intrauterine growth retardation, pre-eclampsia, and stillbirth, one must question whether it is an epiphenomenon or a true etiological factor in these disorders. Suggestions that it may be an indication of an underlying immunological assault on the conceptus by the maternal immune system, while interesting, would seem as yet to have no greater standing than suggestions that pre-eclampsia is an immunological disorder.

The frequency of the disorder varies widely from 6% in North America to 33.8% in South America [46]. If these differences are real, epidemiological studies may provide clues as to the nature of the disease process. It does, however, seem unlikely that there would be major differences in the immunological response to pregnancy in these populations that are racially heterogeneous. It is also not clear whether this is a true indication of a genuine difference or a reflection of differences in sampling techniques, the degree to which specific causes are sought and excluded, and observer variation. Blanc [47] has pointed out that the incidence of viral infections or illnesses typical of viral infection and often classified as flu-like illnesses have an incidence similar to that of VUE in North America and does not discount the possibility that a significant number of VUE cases are due to undiagnosed viral infections. The advent of polymerase chain reaction (PCR) techniques for the detection of very small quantities of infective material may allow clarification of this conundrum.

The clinical significance of the finding of villitis remains uncertain. Salafia [48] has linked the condition with preterm delivery. In a few instances, it has been reported to recur in subsequent pregnancies where the severity of the lesions is remarkably similar in successive pregnancies [46].

Thus, while placental inflammatory lesions are extremely common, their significance in influencing the outcome of pregnancy is not always straightforward. The pathologist confronted with morphological evidence of inflammation, be it macroscopic or microscopic, would be wise not to overinterpret the significance of these findings, particularly if there are no clinical data available, because, in the author's experience, many an inflamed placenta is associated with a normal baby and a fit mother.

REFERENCES

1. Gibbs RS. Obstetric factors associated with infections of the fetus and newborn infant. In: Remington JS, Klein JO, eds. *Infectious Diseases of the Fetus and Newborn Infant*, 4th ed. Philadelphia: Saunders, 1995, p. 1248.
2. Islam AKMS. Primary carrier sites of group B streptococci in pregnant women correlated with serotype distributions and maternal parity. *J Clin Pathol* 1981; 34:84–6.
3. Sanderson PJ, Ross J, Stringer J. Source of group B streptococci in the female genital tract. *J Clin Pathol* 1981; 34:78–81.
4. Lessing JB, Auster R, Berger SA, Peyser MR. Bacterial infection and human fetal wastage. *J Reprod Med* 1989; 34:975–6.
5. Rushton DI. Placental pathology in spontaneous miscarriage. In: Beard RW, Sharp F, eds. *Early Pregnancy Loss Mechanisms and Treatment. Proceedings of the Eighteenth Study Group of the Royal College of Obstetricians and Gynaecologists.* London: Royal College of Obstetricians and Gynaecologists, 1987, p. 153.
6. Chellam VG, Rushton DI. Chorioamnionitis and funiculitis in the placentas of 200 births weighing less than 2.5 kgs. *Br J Obstet Gynaecol* 1985; 92:808–14.
7. Annotation. Chorioamnionitis: cause or effect. *Lancet* 1989; 1:362.
8. Hay PE, Lamont RF, Taylor-Robinson D, et al. Abnormal bacterial colonisation of the genital tract and subsequent preterm delivery and late miscarriage. BMJ 1994; 308:295–8.
9. MacDermott RIJ. Bacterial vaginosis: a review. *Br J Obstet Gynaecol* 1995; 102:92–4.
10. Soper DE, Mayhall CG, Dalton HP. Risk factors for intraamniotic infection: a prospective epidemiological study. *Am J Obstet Gynecol* 1989; 161:562–5.
11. Hemsell DL, Obregon VL, Heard MC, Nobles BJ. Endometrial bacteria in asymptomatic non pregnant women. *J Reprod Med* 1989; 34:872–4.
12. Klebanoff MA, Nugent RP, Rhoads GG. Coitus during pregnancy: is it safe? *Lancet* 1984; 2:914.
13. Naeye RL. Coitus and associated amniotic fluid infections. *N Engl J Med* 1979; 301:1198–9.
14. McKenzie H, Donnet ML, Howie PW, Patel NB, Genvie DT. Risk of preterm delivery in pregnant women with group B streptococcal urinary infections or

urinary antibodies to group B streptococcal and *E. coli* antigens. *Br J Obstet Gynaecol* 1994; 101:107–13.

15. Remington JS, Klein JO. Current concepts of infection of the fetus and newborn infant. In: Remington JS, Klein JO, eds. *Infectious Diseases of the Fetus and Newborn Infant*, 4th ed. Philadelphia: Saunders, 1995, Chap. 1.

16. Lewis DB, Wilson CB. Developmental immunology and role of host defenses in neonatal susceptibility to infection. In: Remington JS, Klein JO, eds. *Infectious Diseases of the Fetus and Newborn Infant*, 4th ed. Philadelphia: Saunders, 1995, pp. 20–98.

17. Schuring-Blom GH, Keijzer M, Jakobs ME, et al. Investigation of the fetal pulmonary inflammatory reaction in chorioamnionitis using an in situ Y chromosome marker. *Pediatr Pathol* 1994; 14:997–1003.

18. Scott RJ, Peat D, Rhodes CA. Investigation of the fetal pulmonary inflammatory reaction in chorioamnionitis using an in situ Y chromosome marker. *Pediatr Pathol* 1994; 14:997–1003.

19. Altshuler G, Russell P. The human placental villitides: a review of chronic intrauterine infection. *Curr Top Pathol* 1975; 60:63–112.

20. Jacques SM, Qureshi F. Chronic villitis of unknown etiology in twin gestations. *Pediatr Pathol* 1994; 14:575–84.

21. Labarrere C, Althabe O, Telenta M. Chronic villitis of unknown aetiology in placentae of idiopathic small for gestational age infants. *Placenta* 1982; 3:309–18.

22. Labarrere C, Althabe O, Caletti E, Muscolo D. Deficiency of blocking factors in intrauterine growth retardation and its relationship with chronic villitis. *Am J Reprod Immunol Microbiol* 1986; 10:9–14.

23. Laberrere CA, McIntyre JA, Faulk WP. Immunohistologic evidence that villitis in human normal term placentas is an immunologic lesion. *Am J Obstet Gynecol* 1990; 162:515–22.

24. Knox WF, Fox H. Villitis of unknown aetiology: its incidence and significance in placentae from a British population. *Placenta* 1984; 5:395–402.

25. Popek EJ. Granulomatous villitis due to *Toxoplasma gondii*. *Pediat Pathol* 1992; 12:281–8.

26. Robertson NJ, McKeever PA. Fetal and placental pathology in two cases of maternal varicella infection. *Pediatr Pathol* 1992; 12:545–50.

27. Backe E, Jimenez E, Unger M, et al. Demonstration of HIV-1 infected cells in human placenta by in-situ hybridisation and immunostaining. *J Clin Pathol* 1992; 45:871–4.

28. Fleming KA. Analysis of viral pathogenesis by in-situ hybridisation. *J Pathol* 1992; 166:95–6.

29. Garcia AGP, Basso NG, Da S, Ferreira-Fonseca ME, Outani HN. Congenital ECHO virus infection: morphological and virological study of fetal and placental tissue. *J Pathol* 1990; 160:123–7.

30. Garcia AGP, Basso NG, Da S, et al. Enterovirus associated placental morphology: a light, virological, electron microscopic and immunohistologic study. *Placenta* 1991; 12:533–47.

31. Morey AL, O'Neill HJ, Coyle PV, Fleming KA. Immunohistological detection of human parvovirus B19 in formalin-fixed paraffin embedded tissues. *J Pathol* 1992; 166:105–8.

32. Sachden R, Nuovo GJ, Kaplan C, Greco MA. In-situ hybridisation analysis for cytomegalovirus in chronic villitis. *Pediatr Pathol* 1990; 10:909–17.

33. Doss BJ, Greene MF, Hill J, et al. Massive chronic intervillositis associated with recurrent abortions. *Hum Pathol* 1995; 26:1245–61.

34. Labarrere CA, Mullen E. Fibrinoid and trophoblastic necrosis with massive chronic intervillositis: an extreme variant of villitis of unknown etiology. *Am J Reprod Immunol Microbiol* 1987; 15:85–91.

35. Rosevear SK, Hope PL. Subclinical intraamniotic infection with *Gardnerella vaginalis* with preterm labour: case report. *Br J Obstet Gynaecol* 1989; 96:491–3.

36. Minkoff H, Grunebaum AN, Schwarz RH, et al. Risk factors for prematurity: a prospective study of vaginal flora in pregnancy. *Am J Obstet Gynecol* 1984; 150:965–72.

37. Mazor M, Chaim W, Bar-David J, et al. Prenatal diagnosis of microbial infection of the amniotic cavity with *Campylobacter coli* in preterm labour. *Br J Obstet Gynaecol* 1995; 102:71–2.

38. Carroll SG, Ville Y, Greenough A, et al. Preterm labour amniorrhexis: intrauterine infection and interval between membrane rupture and delivery. *Arch Dis Child* 1995; 72:F43–6.

39. Bejar R, Curbelo V, Davis C, Giuck L. Premature labour. II. Bacterial sources of phospholipase. *Obstet Gynecol* 1981; 57:479–82.

40. Lopez Bernal A, Hansell DJ, Khong TY, Keeling JW, Turnbull AC. Prostaglandin E production by fetal membranes in unexplained preterm labour and preterm labour associated with chorioamnionitis. *Br J Obstet Gynaecol* 1989; 96:1133–9.

41. Lundin-Schiller S, Mitchell MD. Prostaglandin production by human chorion laeve cells in response to inflammatory mediators. *Placenta* 1991; 12:353–63.

42. Morales WJ. The effects of chorioamnionitis on the developmental outcome of preterm infants at one year. *Obstet Gynecol* 1987; 70:183–7.

43. Nelson KB, Ellenberg JH. Antecedents of cerebral palsy: multivariate analysis of risk. *N Engl J Med* 1986; 315:81–6.

44. Spinillo A, Capuzzo E, Stronati M, et al. Effect of preterm premature rupture of the membranes on neurodevelopmental outcome: follow-up at two years of age. *Br J Obstet Gyaecol* 1995; 102:882–7.

45. Khong TY, Staples A, Moore L, Byard RW. Observer reliability in assessing villitis of unknown aetiology. *J Clin Pathol* 1993; 46:208–10.

46. Russell P. Infections of the placental villi (villitis). In: Fox H, Wells M, eds. *Haines and Taylor Obstetrical and Gynaecological Pathology*, 4th ed. New York: Churchill Livingstone, 1995, pp. 1553–5.

47. Blanc WA. Pathology of the placenta, membranes and umbilical cord in bacterial, fungal and viral infections in man. In: Naeye RL, Kissane JM, Kaufman N, eds. *Perinatal Diseases*. Baltimore: Williams & Wilkins 1981, p. 72.

48. Salafia CM, Vogel CA, Vintzileos AM, et al. Placental pathologic findings in preterm birth. *Am J Obstet Gynecol* 1991; 165:934–8.

Pathology of Multiple Pregnancy

Virginia J. Baldwin

INTRODUCTION

The scientific interest in twins and higher multiples has been concerned with two areas in particular: the relative rates of genetic and environmental influences on human development and disease as revealed by twin studies; and the pathology of multiple pregnancy, especially the aberrations of monozygous twinning. The pathologist has a critical role in both areas of interest, because complete and accurate descriptions of the placentae and infants from multiple gestations are essential to the validity of any study. Aspects of single gestations, including perinatal pathology, embryology, and placentology, are part of the consideration of multiple gestation, and they are detailed elsewhere in this volume. This chapter considers those aspects of perinatal pathology that are unique to multiple gestations.

TWINNING MECHANISMS, RATES, AND INFLUENCES; TWIN STUDIES; ZYGOSITY DETERMINATION

Twinning Mechanisms, Rates, and Influences

These aspects of twinning must now take into account new information about early intragestational loss of twins, the results of hormonal stimulation of ova, and the effects of extracorporeal manipulation of egg, sperm, and embryo. However, all multiple births can still usefully be considered to have arisen from one egg or from several eggs, and these two categories of twinning can be discussed separately.

Polyovular twinning occurs when two or more individual eggs are each fertilized by individual sperm to create separate, genetically distinct embryos. This can occur naturally and is subject to endogenous hormone levels that are affected by genetic and environmental influences [1]. Exogenous hormones may produce polyovulation by direct action on the ovary or through the pituitary, occasionally producing very high multiples [2]. Differences in twinning

rates among such drugs may be due to differences in early resorptions [3].

The eggs may come from single or separate follicles maturing in the same cycle, or possibly in sequential cycles (superfetation), although the latter phenomenon has yet to be documented unequivocally [4]. They may be fertilized by sperm from one source, either by coitus, artificial insemination, or in vitro fertilization [5]; or by sperm from separate sources by coitus (superfecundation) [6] or, theoretically, from pooled donor semen used for artificial insemination.

There are three possible mechanisms of single egg twinning: fertilization of the oocyte and its first polar body by separate sperm [7]; "splitting" of the developing embryo with the two halves developing as separate individuals [8], the degree of separateness depending on when this occurs [9]; and development of separate organizing loci leading to two individuals that are more or less separate depending on timing and other factors [10]. The polar body theory may explain some of the anomalies of monozygous twinning, particularly the chorangiopagus parasiticus (CAPP) twin (see below). The splitting hypothesis has been used to explain mirror-image structural and functional variations in single egg twins, such as handedness and facial clefts [11]. The concept of codominant axes has been used to explain the excess of monozygous twins in ectopic gestations [12], the excess of females in aberrations of single egg twinning, and the generation of asymmetric monozygous twins [13].

The implication that single egg twinning is itself an anomaly is reinforced by the greater frequency of all malformations in single egg twins and particular increases in some malformations that may have implications for both the mechanism of twinning and the malformations in question. These specific associations include chromosomal loss [14, 15], anterior neural tube defects [16], sirenomelia [17], caudal duplication [18], esophageal atresia [19], and the Duhamel anomalad [13].

The occurrence of single egg twinning is related to genetic factors [20], use of oral contraceptives [21], X-bearing sperm [22], and in vitro fertilization [23].

Reported overall rates of multiple gestation as well as rates of specific types of plural births need to be reassessed to include knowledge of fetal death during pregnancy [24], accurate prospective determination of zygosity [25], and recognition of racial influences on the different types of twinning [26–28].

Twin Studies

Twin studies are based on the premise that by comparing a feature in monozygous and dizygous twins, the different degrees of genetic and environmental influences on that feature can be determined. Interpretation of the conclusions of the studies does, however, require consideration of at least six inherent problems [29].

Without adequate zygosity determination, concordant dizygous twins and discordant monozygous twins may be mislabeled, leading to erroneous interpretations of pathophysiology [1]. The excess of perinatal mortality among members of monozygous multiple gestations is not often considered, creating a bias against more lethal conditions [30]. Also, usually it is not appreciated that "environmental" influences may be exerted even prior to conception, and certainly in utero, so that some observations are mislabeled as "genetic" [31]. Reporting requirements and definitions of what constitutes fetal death or neonatal death vary widely, so that twin studies from different populations may not be comparable [32]. Other biases of ascertainment are legion and may be as simple as the observation that female pairs are more likely to volunteer for twin studies than male pairs [22]. Twin studies have yet to consider the apparent magnitude of early pregnancy loss and its significance regarding genetic or environmental influences on multiple gestation.

Part of the difficulty in assessing twins, clinically or pathologically, is that the sources of variability are nearly infinite. There may be characters in the cytoplasmic mass of the egg that are not represented equally in the zygotes. The sperm/egg combinations at fertilization lead to variations in zygote chromosomal composition, which may be complicated further by differences in postzygotic mitotic chromosomal migrations. The basic genetic makeup of the zygote affects fetal growth and responses. Implantation may be asymmetric, and asymmetric chorion development can be reflected in twin growth. Intertwin vascular connections can create strikingly dissimilar twins. Even the consequences of labor and delivery may lead to markedly dissimilar fetal outcomes and characteristics completely unrelated to events up to that point.

Zygosity Determination

Zygosity studies are best initiated at the time of delivery using cord blood and placenta [1, 25]. However, blood tests and chromosomal studies can be performed long after birth and even by a reference laboratory at some distance from the patient. Zygosity determination after intragestational fetal death remains a problem if chromosome culture is not possible, although DNA probes may be considered in some cases. Concordance is no certain indicator of monozygosity, although the probability increases with each similarity; detailed tables are available [33–35]. Discordance is evidence of dizygosity except in very rare cases of polar body twinning.

Concordance of physical features is quite variable and may be misleading. Discordant sex indicates dizygosity except for rare events, such as postzygotic mitotic errors.

Macroscopic and histologic delineation of placental structure is an important aid to zygosity determination: monochorionicity is a virtually certain indicator of monovular origin. There are three allelic autosomal genes for placental alkaline phosphatase, from which six phenotypes can be determined, and up to 60% of dizygotic twins can be identified with this assessment.

Blood components of the infants can be analyzed, particularly red cell blood groups (ABO, Rh, Kell, MNS, Duffy), red cell isoenzymes (acid phosphatase, phosphoglucomutase, adenylate kinase, peptidase A and B), and HLA haplotypes.

Chromosome polymorphism is identified with banding techniques [36], and minisatellite DNA probes may be used [37].

Additional methods may be used in unusual situations [6, 38, 39], such as secretor status, hepatic or other isoenzymes, karyotypes of several tissues, assays for specific markers, and mixed lymphocyte cultures. Reciprocal skin grafts may not be totally reliable, as complete acceptance may require that there was vascular sharing during gestation, not just monozygosity [40].

THE PLACENTA IN MULTIPLE PREGNANCY

Introduction

Some aspects of the pathology of the placenta in multiple pregnancy have received attention for years, and particularly outstanding is the contribution of Schatz to the study of vascular communications (cited in Kloosterman [41] and in Strong and Corney [40]). Systematic approaches to all aspects of the placenta in multiple gestation have been contributed by Strong and Corney [40], Benirschke and Driscoll [9], Potter and Craig [42], Fox [43], Shanklin and Perrin [12], Benirschke and Kaufmann [44], and Baldwin [45], and these excellent references should be consulted for expansion of the following discussion. The pathologist's analysis of multiple pregnancy includes documentation of placental morphology, with two aspects to be considered.

The first aspect is the examination for those lesions encountered in singleton gestations, as outlined in Chapter 7. The second aspect of placental morphology includes those features due to the multiple nature of the gestation, specifically the pattern of the disc and membrane relationships and the pattern and degree of anastomoses of the body stalk and chorionic vasculature. While the membrane relationships do not always identify the zygosity of the infants, the patterns of placentation may have other significance for fetal development, particularly overall growth [46, 47]. The consequences of the various patterns of vascularization in monochorial placentae can be bizarre and can influence the co-twin from early gestation to the neonatal period. If placental examination is not adequate in these cases, an erroneous attribution of causation may be made, with inaccurate conclusions drawn and inappropriate counseling given.

Patterns of Discs and Membranes

The patterns of placentation in multiple pregnancy depend on the type of twinning, polyovular (dizygous) or monovular (monozygous); the timing of the twinning event in monozygous twins; and the geography of implantation in the uterus for all dizygous and some monozygous twins. Variations in rates of the different patterns depend on the differing rates of dizygous twinning, and the population of origin must be considered when reviewing such data [1, 48].

When the conceptuses arise from separate ova, each embryo has the full complement of membranes, both amnion and chorion. The proximity of implantation in the uterine wall determines whether the gestational sacs are completely separate, share membranes, or actually fuse into an apparent single mass with a dividing septum. Although Cameron stated in 1968 [49], and it has been emphasized before and since, that the degree of fusion of the chorionic discs is not a reliable indication of zygosity, this misinterpretation is still made. In one series [50], dichorial monozygous twin placentae were fused six times more frequently than they were separate, but other series reported that monozygous dichorial placentae were fused or separate with equal frequency [9, 33]. Thus, it is very unreliable to assume that twins of the same sex with a single placenta are monozygotic, and it is far from true that separate placentae are a good indication of dizygosity. Also, when the developing embryos are each invested with a layer of chorion, any conjunction of membranes between them virtually always will contain chorionic tissue, which may or may not be separable visually into two layers, either grossly or microscopically.

There are three possible patterns of placentation of monovular twins: separate complete gestational sacs (dichorionic diamniotic) with separate or fused discs (as with dizygous twins), a single chorion with separate amniotic sacs inside (monochorionic diamniotic), or a single cavity and placental disc (monochorionic monoamniotic). The pattern is considered to be related to the timing of the twinning event, which is thought to be distributed randomly [9] over the first 14 days of development, leading to decreasing barriers between the twins as the separation occurs later

in development, and culminating in the conjoined twins with a single cord and a single sac. Definition of the pattern of placentation of monozygous twins is aided by delineations of zygosity in sets of like-sex dichorionic twins, which obviously represent the group for which placental morphology is not helpful in determining dizygous or monozygous origin [51]. The pattern of attachment of the separating membranes to a fused disc is variable. Usually, when there is chorion between the amnions, the attachment parallels the vascular equator of the chorionic plate vessels for each twin, and hence the border of the chorionic tissue between twins [40, 48]. When the layers are only amnion, such attachment often bears no relation to the vascular equator and in fact may even be at 90° to it.

Virtually all twin placentations with separate discs are dichorial, whether the membranes are shared or not. Virtually all monochorial placentae are single discs. However, a number of dichorial placentae will be fused to a single disc, and differentiation of the nature of the separating membranes will separate these placentae from the monochorial diamniotic placentae.

A summary flow chart using Cameron's data [49] is shown in Figure 8.1, and a pictorial representation of the possible patterns is shown in Figure 8.2.

There are a number of reports in the literature giving the distribution frequencies of the various membrane patterns in twin placentations. The results of some of these reports are presented in Table 8.1, and a graphic representation of one study is shown in Figure 8.3.

Although Corney [48] suggested that differentiation of dichorial placentae into "separate" and "fused" was of doubtful biologic significance, more recent studies [46, 47] suggest that whether the discs are fused or separate is in fact an appropriate distinction to be recorded, because it is significant in regard to fetal growth.

Vascular Patterns

Anomalies of the insertion of the umbilical cord are more frequent in multiple gestation. They may occur as a function of the intrauterine crowding with two or more embryos, and they may have clinical significance in the outcome of the affected pregnancy. In our cases (1016 twins), anomalous cord insertions were present in 16.25% of all twins, 25.4% of monochorial twins, and 11.8% of dichorial twins. Marginal cord insertions occurred in 14% of monochorial twins compared with 4.3% of dichorial twins, and 8.9% of monochorial twins had velamentous cord insertions compared with 5.2% of dichorial twins. Cord anomalies were more common with dichorial fused than dichorial separate placentae. Intrauterine position did not seem important, as twins A and B were equally affected. Patterns of cord insertion from three studies are presented in Table 8.2.

Differential rates in the dichorial group may be associated with irregular expansion of the fused placenta [49]. An

Table 8.1.   Statistical reports of membrane patterns (in percent)

Source	DCDA-S	DCDA-F	DCDA-US (i.e., DZ)	DCDA-LS DZ	DCDA-LS MZ	MC MCDA	MC MCMA	?
Baldwin (508 twin placentae)	31.8	28.0				←32.8→		7.4
			23.4	←49.2→				27.4
Benirschke [9] (USA)	35.2	34.0				29.6	1.2	
Cameron [49] (Birmingham)			35.0	37.0	8.0	←20.0→		
Pauls [181]							0.83	
Myrianthopoulos [71] (USA)			33.0	15.0	7.8	16.6	1.5	25.8
Benirschke [1] (USA)			35.0	37.0	8.0	←20.0→		
Soma [138] (Japan)	20.3	18.5	14.8					
Sekiya [53] (Japan)						56.5	4.6	
Segreti [51]					25.0		1.0	
Cameron [25] (Birmingham, Ghent)						52.5	7.5	14.7
Robertson [61] (USA)	37.0	39.0	34.0	35.0	9.0	19.5	2.4	
Shanklin [12] (Chicago and Florida)	34.4	36.6	40.0	20.0	11.3	25.5	0	
			←————71.0————→			20.4	3.2	

DC = dichorionic; DA = diamniotic; S = separate; F = fused; US = unlike sex; LS = like sex; MC = monochorionic; MA = monoamniotic; ? = unknown; DZ = dizygotic; MZ = monozygotic.

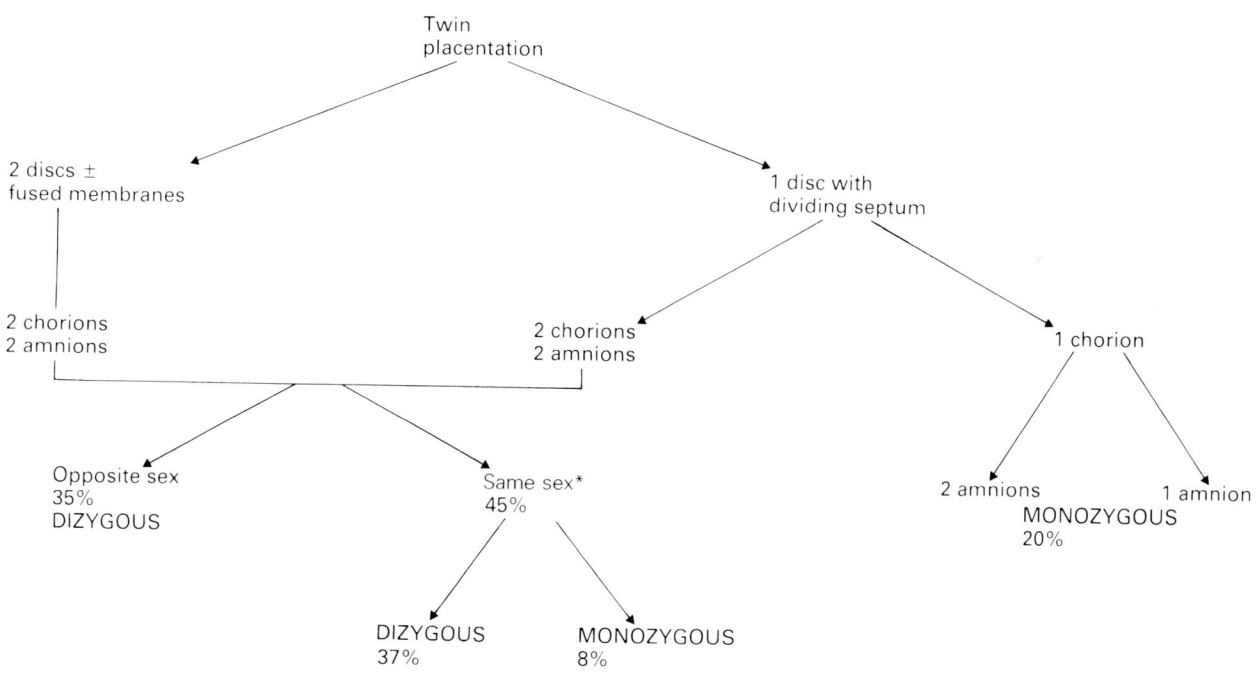

FIGURE 8.1.   *Placentation in twin pregnancy. (*Differentiation requires additional zygosity tests.)*

extensive review of velamentous cord insertions recorded a frequency of velamentous cords that was nine times higher for twins than for singletons and four times higher in monochorial than in dichorial placentae, and velamentous cords were almost the rule in triplets [52]. A number of abnormalities have been ascribed to velamentous insertions, including fetal anomalies, a greater rate of abortions, prematurity, polyhydramnios, abnormal presentation, premature rupture of membranes, postpartum hemorrhages, and decreased fetal weight. An increased association of fetal malformations has been reported with marginal cord insertions (5.3%) and velamentous insertions (8.5%). The presence of only one umbilical artery is also more frequent, ranging from 3.6% [1] to 35% of the twins studied [53].

The subject of vascular anastomosis is reviewed in a later section on the pathology of monozygosity.

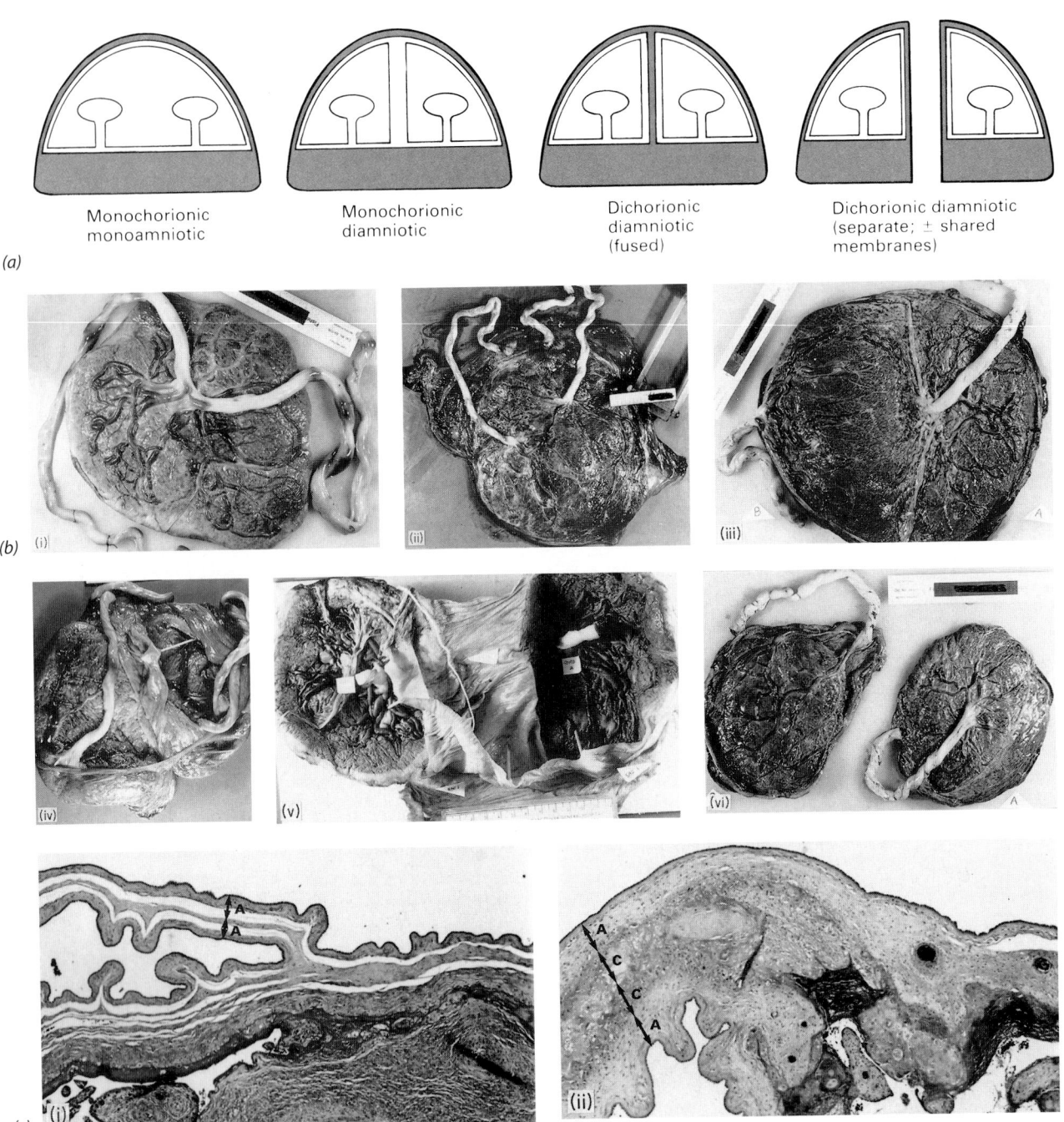

FIGURE 8.2.   *Possible patterns of placentation of twins. (a) Diagrammatic representation of patterns: shaded zone represents chorion, fine line, amnion. (b) Examples: (i) monochorionic monoamniotic, cords very closely inserted; (ii) monochorionic monoamniotic, cords farther apart; (iii) monochorionic diamniotic—note very delicate membrane layer across middle of disc (one cord inserts at separating membranes); (iv) dichorionic diamniotic, fused disc with thick separating membrane across middle; (v) dichorionic diamniotic, separate discs but shared overlapping membranes—white cord outlines edge of one disc; (vi) dichorionic diamniotic, separate discs (note velamentous cord insertion of one twin). (c) Separating membranes: (i) amnion only, from monochorionic placentation—only two layers of amnion (A) (tissue in middle is part of amnion connective tissue); (ii) amnion and chorion, from dichorionic placentation—two layers of amnion (A) and two layers of chorion (C), which may be fused variably to look like one (note atrophic villi in chorion layer).*

Molar Disease

One aspect of placental pathology in multiple gestation is the occurrence of gestational trophoblastic disease. There are three relationships to be considered: Twins may develop ges-

tational trophoblastic disease [54]; hydatidiform moles have been reported to occur in other pregnancies of mothers of twins at 6.7 times the expected incidence [55]; and it has been suggested that a coexistent hydatidiform mole and a normal fetus may represent dizygous twinning. Five patterns

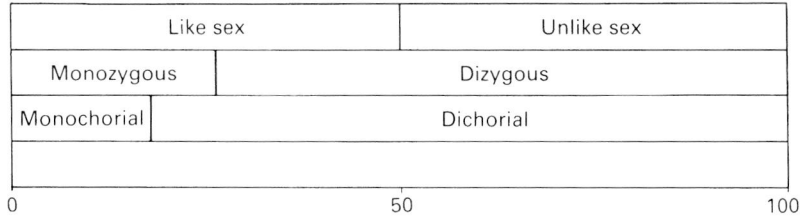

	Like sex		Unlike sex

Monozygous		Dizygous	

Monochorial	Dichorial		

0   50   100%

FIGURE 8.3. *Comparison of zygosity, chorionicity, and sex in twins. (Data from Cameron [49], after Hafez [262].)*

Table 8.2. Cord insertion patterns: percent of infants with anomalous insertions in twin pregnancies

	MM	MD	DD-F	DD-S
Velamentous patterns				
Cameron [49]	0.0	23.3	12.6	2.7
Benirschke [1]	—	11.4	7.0	3.4
Shanklin [12]	—	10.0	10.0	0.0
Other patterns				
Shanklin [12]				
marginal	—	27.0	6.0	1.0
lateral	—	0.0	42.0	60.0
central	—	—	27.0	39.0
Benirschke [9]				
marginal	16.6	19.5	10.0	6.2
marginal or velamentous	16.6	31.0	17.0	9.6

MM = monochorial monoamniotic; MD = monochorial diamniotic; DD-F = dichorial diamniotic fused; DD-S = dichorial diamniotic separate.

of pathology of coexistent hydatidiform mole and normal fetus have been described [56]. Very focal vesicular degeneration in a single placenta, such as a single cotyledon, is probably not a multiple gestation. Multifocal vesicular degeneration throughout a single placenta and complete hydatidiform degeneration of a single placenta are often called "partial" moles and are often triploid, and thus possibly are not indicative of multiple gestation either. Extensive but quite distinct molar change in a portion of a single placenta may represent an origin in multiple gestation. The most convincing pattern, however, is that of two separate placentae, one normal and one molar, sometimes quite separately attached to the uterus [57]. This pattern may well represent a dizygous conception, with molar change of one conceptus. Further support for the dizygous nature of this pattern comes from an analysis of chromosome polymorphism in a 46,XX mole and coexistent 46,XY fetus [36], and from an analysis of DNA fingerprints of three placentae, molar tissue, and parents using a minisatellite probe in a quadruplet conception [58].

A review of cases of normal fetuses with distinct molar masses identified 46 twin, one triplet [36], and one quadruplet gestation [58]. Among the cases where the fetal sex was reported, there were 15 males and 12 females as the coexisting fetuses. However, most of these cases were not confirmed with chromosomal polymorphism, so triploidy with minimal manifestations cannot be ruled out. A further aspect of these dizygous molar pregnancies is the outcome of the associated fetus. Usually the pregnancies terminate sponta-

neously in the second trimester and the infants do not survive, but survivals have been reported [56, 59, 60]. The data are incomplete, but there appear to be no greater risks for the normal twin beyond that of prematurity in those pregnancies that terminate beyond 31 weeks. This may be a reflection of the fact that over half of these cases had distinct molar and normal placentae.

Examination

The references cited at the beginning of this section contain systematic approaches to examination of the twin placenta and can be consulted for details. All placentae from multiple gestation should be examined grossly and microscopically, and fresh tissues are easier to examine than fixed tissues. Speculation as to birth order can sometimes be made on the basis of patterns of membrane rupture, thickness of umbilical cords correlated with stated fetal weights, evidence of ascending infection in one sac, or maceration changes associated with a dead twin. However, there is no guaranteed method of reconstruction of the gestational order unless the cords are identified adequately in the delivery room. Adequate clinical information is also critical, including general and obstetric maternal history; family history; details of the current pregnancy, labor, and delivery; and details of infant weight, sex, condition, and course. Correlation with ultrasound or cytogenetic findings is also important.

The approach to a singleton placenta is described in Chapter 7 of this volume and should be consulted.

It is valuable to take the time to orient the twin placentae, perhaps with the first delivered twin's portion to the right, determining the degree of separateness of the discs/membranes, the orientations of the cords, and the relative sizes of the twins' portions. If the discs are separate or share membranes only, complete descriptions of each can be done in sequence. When the parenchyma is shared, it is useful to combine the descriptions: cord and membranes of each twin in turn (noting how far apart the cords are), the pattern of the separating membranes, the nature of the chorionic circulations, and, finally, the disc as a whole.

A dividing septum that contains chorion will be fixed firmly to the placental surface, while one of amnion only will come away readily. An apparent single sac due to separation of the amnion is more common than a truly monoamniotic sac, and care is required to be certain in the latter case that there is no remnant of a septum.

There are two concerns regarding the chorionic surface vascularization—relative proportions and anastomoses. The relative proportions of the chorionic surface occupied by vessels from each twin are important, because asymmetry of this pattern can be significant in regard to overall fetal development in both monochorial and dichorial placentae.

Vascular anastomoses are frequent in monochorial placentae and are often very significant in asymmetric fetal development, so every effort should be made toward demonstration and detailed description in these cases. Direct artery-to-artery and vein-to-vein anastomoses usually are readily identifiable on the surface, both visually and by shunting blood back and forth by compressing the vessels. The arteries are superficial to the veins on the chorionic surface [9, 12].

"Third circulation" anastomoses, which are arterial-capillary-venous anastomoses, can be suspected grossly by identifying unaccompanied vessels from each twin that terminate close to each other on the chorionic surface. Ordinarily, the members of an artery-vein pair penetrate the chorionic plate within millimeters of each other, but an artery from one twin that penetrates the chorionic surface adjacent to a vein from the other twin is a potential site of a shared cotyledon and requires injection for confirmation. Vessels involved in this clinically important pattern of sharing may be of quite small caliber. A number of complex perfusion techniques have been described [25, 61], but India ink or air using a 50-cm^3 syringe with needle and forceps also works well. The volume of the shared cotyledon can be assessed occasionally when the parenchyma is sectioned.

Details of any anastomosis identified should be recorded, including the sizes and types of vessels involved and the twin from which each vessel came. A diagram of complex patterns of cord insertions, membrane relationships, and/or vascular anastomoses is often more helpful than a photograph, although both are valuable.

Asymmetries of the chorionic development for each twin—area, volume, and quality—are of critical importance in some cases and are to be assessed and recorded in each case.

The approach to triplets and higher multiples is simply a methodical expansion of the techniques used for twins, with careful attention to precise documentation of membrane relationships and vascular patterns.

MORTALITY AND MORBIDITY IN MULTIPLE PREGNANCY

Introduction

The risks of disease and death are greater for all members of a plural gestation from the moment of conception to the end of their life span [62], but while there seems to be universal agreement on this concept, the statistical magnitude and details reported vary widely. There are three major trends. First, there are distinct risks at different times in the life of a twin, and discoveries as to cause and decisions in connection with care are made more readily when these patterns are appreciated. Secondly, increased awareness, particularly of the perinatal problems that twins face, has led to significant improvements in this period [63–65]. Thirdly, the importance of intrauterine fetal death of twins is better appreciated [66].

The mortality of twins is recorded as being, overall, four to 11 times the rate of single infants [27, 32, 63, 67–69]. The excess mortality occurs both antenatally and neonatally. Twins are stillborn 3 [1] to 13 [70] times more frequently than singletons. Actual rates of stillbirth are 8.1% of all twins [28, 71], or 25.3–39.6% of all twin deaths in any one series [63, 72, 73]. In one series, 25.3% of the stillborn twins died antepartum and 14.3% intrapartum [72]. In another series, 16% of the stillborn twins were fresh stillbirths, 18% were macerated, and 2% were fetus papyraceus [63]. Neonatal death occurs six to seven times [1, 74] more frequently among twins than among singletons. Actual rates of neonatal death are 9.2% of all twins [28, 71] or 60.3–70.3% of all twin deaths [63, 72, 73].

Combining stillbirth and neonatal deaths to measure overall perinatal mortality in twins gives rates of 14.2% [1] to 17.3% [28, 71]. The perinatal mortality of 16.81% for twins compares with one report of 7.15% for singletons [75]. The perinatal mortality of twins has been reported as high as 11 times the rate of singletons, peaking between 2 and 48 hours of life [74]. Both twins of a pair died in 5.7% [63] to 37% [70] of cases.

Changes in patterns of care have affected disease frequencies in twins over the years, and definitions of causes of death vary in the different reports so that it becomes difficult to compare frequencies of causes from series to series. For example, deaths attributed to hyaline membrane disease range from 8% [72] to 52% [68], and "immaturity" is listed as the cause in 17.4% [76] to 24.5% [77].

Discussions of causes of death of twins all emphasize the importance of prematurity and its complications as contributing factors to neonatal mortality [28, 42, 71–73, 76, 77]. Anoxia and causes unknown are recorded most often as leading to stillbirths of twins [42].

Of the 280 twin postmortems in our series, the main cause of death was recorded as complications of prematurity in 30.3%, asphyxia alone in 9.2%, asphyxial insult with prematurity in 7.1%, fetal anomalies in 10.7%, "immaturity" in 5.7%, lesions of monozygosity in 20%, miscellaneous other diseases/disorders in 7.1%, and cause not determined in 12.5%. When the cause of death in our cases is related to the age of the infant at death, it is seen that prematurity and its complications are responsible for deaths not only early but over a long time span, as shown in Table 8.3.

The Collaborative Perinatal Study in the United States has been a source of much information on twin gestations [28, 71, 78]. Monozygous twins died more often from anoxia/asphyxia, malformations, or unknown causes, while dizygous twins died more often from early fetal death and "other" causes. The rates for the idiopathic respiratory distress syndrome and trauma were about equal for monozygous and dizygous twins. Male twins died more often as

Table 8.3. Cause of death related to duration of survival

Cause	Stillbirth	1 day	2–7 days	8–28 days	1–12 months	1 year
Prematurity	—	37.2	46.6	41.3	43.7	11.1
Asphyxia	19.4	6.3	6.6	6.9	—	—
Prematurity/ asphyxia	—	5.4	17.7	6.9	12.5	—
Anomalies	4.2	9.0	8.8	27.5	12.5	22.2
Cause not determined	45.8	0.9	4.4	—	—	—
Immaturity	—	13.6	—	—	—	—
Monochorial monozygosity	27.7	23.6	8.8	13.8	12.5	11.1
Other	2.9	1.8	4.4	3.4	12.5	55.5

Figures represent percentage of deaths from each cause for the duration of survival shown.

immature fetuses or from asphyxia/anoxia, while female twins died more often from the idiopathic respiratory distress syndrome, malformations, or the effects of trauma or hemorrhage. However, in all the statistics in this monumental study there remained large groups of "other" or "unknown," which might have affected the distributions reported if they could have been clarified.

One report considered that 26.6% of twin deaths were unavoidable and 59.4% were probably unavoidable, but causes of death in these cases were not specified [67]. Causes of death in the 13.9% of deaths considered to be avoidable were largely obstetric complications, such as prolapsed cord or vessels, interlocking of twins, and abruptio placenta, but also included the idiopathic respiratory distress syndrome. Late diagnosis of twin gestation will profoundly influence perinatal outcome, and in this report one-third of the pregnancies were not diagnosed as being twins until the onset of labor. A bimodal risk for fetal loss related to maternal age and parity is described, with the lowest risk in mothers in their 30s and in the third or fourth pregnancy, respectively [67].

Death rates correlated with placental membrane patterns are presented in Table 8.4. It has been noted that it was more common for both of the monochorial twins to die: both twins died in 13.6% of cases with monochorial pla-

centae, but there were no double deaths with dichorial placentae [53]. Up to 25.3% of perinatal twin deaths have been attributed to problems associated with monozygosity [76]. Higher mortality rates of monozygous twins as compared with dizygous twins were reported by Potter [73] (11.2% and 3.5%, respectively) and by the Collaborative Perinatal Project [28, 71] (14.8% and 7.6%, respectively). The monochorionic placenta of monozygous twins seems to be most important, as perinatal twin death rates of 7.1% of monochorial twins, 4.6% of dichorial twins of the same sex, and 3.6% of dichorial twins of opposite sex have been reported from a study of perinatal deaths of twins who both weighed more than 1000 grams at birth [79]. There were no common causes in the perinatal deaths of dichorial twins [80], although both died slightly more often if they had dichorial diamniotic separate placentae than if they had dichorial diamniotic fused placentae [49].

Many authors record a sex differential in perinatal deaths, although the reports are sometimes conflicting [67, 75]. The rates generally are reported higher for male twins (11.7%) than for female twins (9.4%) [42]. Also, like-sex twins are at greater risk than unlike-sex pairs: 12.2% and 7.3%, respectively [42]. This excess is largely in the fetal and early neonatal period, and often both twins die [32]—probably owing to a greater number of monozygous pairs among these peri-

Table 8.4. Percentage of twin deaths compared with patterns of placentation

Source	MC total	MCMA	MCDA	DCDA total	DCDA-S	DCDA-F
Benirschke [80]	24.6	50.0	23.3	7.3	9.4	4.7
Potter [73]	13.2	—	—	9.3	10.0	8.3
Benirschke [1, 184]	25.9	50.0	26.0	9.0	9.6	8.2
Myrianthopoulos [28, 71]	—	28.0	22.0	10.9	—	—
Potter [42]	13.2	—	—	9.6	—	—
Sekiya [53]	—	67.0	18.0	6.0	—	—

MC = monochorial; MA = monoamniotic; DC = dichorial; DA = diamniotic; S = separate; F = fused.

natal deaths. Like-sex male twins are especially at risk [1, 50]. After the neonatal period, rates are more nearly equal for like-sex and unlike-sex pairs.

Opinions vary as to whether birth order is related to chance of survival. It has been suggested that the second twin is less subject to trauma because it does not dilate the birth passage but, on the other hand, is more subject to anoxia because of possible placental ischemia or even separation after the reduction in uterine size following the birth of the first twin. Several authors have reported no difference in perinatal mortality for the second twin as compared with the first [33, 63, 75], while others state that the neonatal death rates are greater for twin B, although stillbirth rates are equivalent [65, 72]. The Collaborative Perinatal Project suggested that the mortality for B twins was greater antenatally, whereas the rates were equal neonatally [28, 71]. When measures more sensitive than perinatal death were used, it was found that there were statistically significant differences favoring twin A in 1-minute Apgar scores; umbilical venous pH, PCO_2, and PO_2; and umbilical artery PO_2 [81, 82]. When these results were examined with respect to route of delivery, chorionicity, interval between the delivery of the twins, and vertex-only deliveries (to eliminate the possible effects of malpresentation), the comparisons persistently favored the firstborn twin. These results suggest that the second twin is definitely at greater risk, although the consequences may not always be fatal. On the other hand, active intervention to deliver twin B may add to its risks of adverse consequences [1]. A different measure of the greater risk for twin B than for twin A noted that A twins survived an average of 62.8 hours while B twins survived an average of 34.2 hours [50].

Twins die of different causes at different gestational ages. Of twins of 29 to 38 weeks' gestation, 17% died antepartum of unstated causes, 15% died intrapartum with low birth weight and/or malformations, and 68% died as neonates from complications of prematurity. Those twins delivered after 38 weeks were stillborn for unstated reasons in 58%, succumbed to intrapartum obstetric complications in 19%, and died neonatally of a mixture of causes unrelated to prematurity in 23% [83]. More than 70% of the perinatal mortality of twins has been reported to occur at less than 30 weeks of gestation and could be attributed almost entirely to complications of prematurity [84]. Perinatal mortality after 34 weeks of gestation has been associated with intrauterine growth retardation, the twin-to-twin transfusion syndrome, fetal anomalies, or unknown causes. Another study reported 80% mortality of infants of fewer than 31 weeks of gestational age, 20% mortality between 31 and 33 weeks, and 6.7% mortality at 34 to 36 weeks [77].

Selected Aspects of Mortality and Morbidity

Obstetric Aspects

The obstetric aspects of perinatal pathology in twins include the influence of maternal disorders, those pregnancy complications that are increased in twin gestations, and problems with labor and delivery leading to traumatic and asphyxial damage of the infants. Maternal mortality related to twin pregnancy is rarely described; fulminant intrapartum eclampsia is one cause that has been recorded [63].

It appears that maternal disorders affect twins the same as they do singletons [74]. Discordant fetal response to an apparently homogeneous maternal state has been identified in erythroblastosis fetalis due to rhesus isoimmunization [1, 85, 86], fetal macrosomia with maternal diabetes [87], and malformations and malignancy due to maternal therapy with cyclophosphamide [88], and is usually attributed to fetal genetic heterozygosity.

Some of the problems that twins face in utero are the obstetric complications of having two or more fetuses growing in a space meant ideally for one [27, 65]. Disorders of glucose intolerance do not appear to be increased with multiple pregnancy until there are three or more fetuses [89, 90]. Hypertensive syndromes of pregnancy are reported to occur up to 13 times as often as in singleton gestations, with conflicting reports as to their frequency in monozygous as opposed to dizygous twins. There was no greater mortality of the affected twins, but there were an increase in intrauterine growth retardation, a decrease in total fetal weights, and greater interfetal weight differences, and adverse perinatal outcome was more likely to be associated with severe pre-eclampsia [91]. Although maternal anemia is more common in multiple gestation and there is also a greater increase in plasma volume due to hemodilution, no effect on fetal outcome has been reported. There is apparently no increase in antepartum hemorrhage due to either placenta previa or abruptio placenta in twin pregnancies, although abruptio placenta is listed as a cause in 4.5% of perinatal deaths [92]. Apparently there is no increase in threatened abortion as manifested by first- or second-trimester bleeding.

Hydramnios is a very subjective finding, but it seems to be more common in twin pregnancies [63]. Fetal mortality in these cases is high, 23–87% [1], but is likely to be related to the underlying cause of the hydramnios, such as fetal malformation or twin-to-twin transfusion, or to the fact that hydramnios leads to premature delivery [63]. Acute hydramnios, occurring within a few days, has been reported [93] in 2% of twin pregnancies and occurs in the second trimester. Acute hydramnios is associated with monochorial development of normal twins, but its precipitate course usually terminates the pregnancy in a few days. The twin-to-twin transfusion syndrome is important in cases of acute hydramnios whereas chronic hydramnios is usually associated with fetal anomalies.

Intrauterine fetal death with retention of the dead fetus may be complicated by a maternal defibrination syndrome. Defibrination is also a risk when one infant of a multiple pregnancy dies, due to either a natural process or iatrogenic intervention, and the pregnancy continues. Such a situation can be handled clinically so that a mature infant can be delivered without threat to the mother [94]. In the case of a retained singleton death, this situation is attributed to thromboplastin entering the maternal circulation from the dead conceptus. However, it happens so rarely in situations of intrauterine fetal death of one of a multiple gestation, where the dead infant is retained and where the pregnancy continues, that this appears to be an incomplete explanation for this complication.

A malpositioned or undiagnosed twin may lead to problems during delivery, such as obstructed labor, leading to birth asphyxia or actual birth trauma [95]. Up to 58% of twins may have abnormal presentations [64], more frequently twin B [77]. Interlocking of twins is rare (0.1%) but has a perinatal mortality rate of 31% [1]. A survey of 362 pairs of twins [96] suggested that neither position nor presentation was a significant factor in perinatal mortality or morbidity, and that after delivery of twin A there was no urgency to deliver twin B if electronic monitoring of fetal heart rate showed no abnormality, thus avoiding trauma associated with mechanically assisted delivery, including caesarean section. In one study [97], birth injuries were listed as the cause of death in 11.5% of all perinatal twin deaths—14.3% of twin A and 4.1% of twin B deaths—but in another study [74] an increased perinatal death rate due to trauma was not observed.

Complications of labor and delivery that contribute to perinatal asphyxia have been implicated in low Apgar scores in both monochorial (2% in twin A, 4% in twin B) and dichorial twins (5% in twin A, 10% in twin B) [53]. Perinatal asphyxia was listed as a cause of death for 15% of A twins and 25% of B twins in one study [92] and for 27% of singletons, 34% of A twins, and 42% of B twins in another study [74], although in the latter report aspiration syndromes occurred with equal frequency. Perinatal asphyxia/hypoxia caused 30% of twin deaths in one study and was associated with antepartum hemorrhage in one-third of cases (intrapartum premature separation in the majority); cord accidents (prolapse of cords, entangled monoamniotic cords) in 16.6%; maternal toxemia and fetal intrauterine growth retardation in 11% each; and prolonged second stage due to dystocia and an undiagnosed second twin in cases where ergotrate had been administered after the first twin, in 5.5% each. No cause for asphyxia was identified in 16.6% of the cases. Although uterine distention has been blamed for the increase of pre-eclamptic toxemia and premature labor in twins, hypotonia of the uterus was not reported as a problem [63].

In a review of patterns and mechanisms of brain damage in twins, anoxic lesions due to perinatal asphyxia were identified in 16.6% of cases [98]. Differences in brain size identified in three of five pairs of twins on postmortem examination were attributed to unequal blood supply during intrauterine growth. A third group of lesions consisted of cavitated and destructive lesions with or without abnormal neuronal migration. These were associated with cerebral ischemia and resulted from inequalities in perfusion that could be due to a variety of vascular insults, such as abruptio placenta, placenta previa, or other cord or placental catastrophes, as well as inequalities of monochorial shunting.

Factors of placentation, particularly vascular aspects contributing to asphyxia in twins, were described by Benirschke and Gille in 1977 [99]. They noted a sevenfold increase in vasa previa in twins with an increased risk of rupture and fetal shock. Cord entanglements were the major source of perinatal mortality or severe neurologic sequelae in monoamniotic twins. Vascular anastomoses between twins could be associated with chronic or acute intertwin transfusions, with effects on intrauterine development and perinatal survival.

Prematurity and Sequelae
Although there have been marked improvements in perinatal care, prematurity and its sequelae are still a major source of mortality and morbidity in multiple gestations [96]. Prematurity has been listed as the cause of up to 90% of neonatal deaths and 54% of fetal deaths [69], although it is not clear how fetal (intrauterine) death can be attributed to prematurity. Premature delivery occurred in 12% of singletons and 39% of twins in one study [74], while another study suggested that only 57% of twins delivered at term compared with 93% singletons [100]. Death rates have been related directly to gestational age, with 100% perinatal mortality at 21 to 24 weeks, 67% at 25 to 28 weeks, 27.7% at 29 to 32 weeks, 9% at 33 to 36 weeks, and 3.5% at over 37 weeks [67].

Problems can be encountered in defining prematurity [27], as twins tend to be underweight for dates, although their length may be equivalent to that of a singleton of the same age [101]. The reasons for premature delivery of a multiple pregnancy have not been clarified completely, although uterine distention is usually quoted as being important [100], and preterm premature rupture of membranes occurs more frequently in twin than in singleton gestations (7.4% vs. 3.7%) [102]. A total weight of 5450 grams has been stated as the limit that a uterus could accommodate [53], although our data would not support this, as combinations totaling over 8 kg have been carried easily to term, and twins can be contained until term, one each in a horn of a bicornuate uterus [103]. A factor contributing to premature delivery of twins may be that an incompetent cervix is encountered two to three times more often with twins than with singletons [104].

Gestational age at delivery has been correlated with patterns of placentation [12], and greater prematurity was identified with monochorial gestations. About 48% of twins with dichorial fused placentae had been delivered by 38 weeks, 52% of dichorial twins with separate placentas by 37 weeks, but 67% of monochorial twins by 37 weeks. Fourteen percent of monochorial twins were born at fewer than 28 weeks of gestation, compared with 4% of dichorial like-sex twins and 2% of dichorial unlike-sex twins [79].

The problem that twins face after premature delivery is the increased risk of complications, particularly hyaline membrane disease (HMD) and its sequelae, including intracranial hemorrhage. HMD was diagnosed in 8% of A twins and 12% of B twins, was the stated cause of perinatal death in 34%, and was complicated by intracranial hemorrhage in 11.9% [92].

Infants in the group with HMD were more premature, had lower birth weights, had lower Apgar scores, were more often monozygous, had been delivered by caesarean section more frequently, and had a higher mortality than the non-HMD group [105]. In 63% of twin pairs, both twins were affected; these infants had a lower gestational age and birth weight and were more often monozygous. In 32% of the pairs, only twin B was affected and usually had lower Apgar scores and higher birth weight than the corresponding twin A. In only one pair was twin A alone affected. In the pairs where both twins were affected, they were equally affected in just over half of the cases, and twin B was more severely affected in the remainder. Thus, HMD occurs in twins for reasons of pulmonary immaturity, just as it occurs in singletons, but monozygous twins may be predisposed to HMD because they are more likely to be premature, and twin B has a greater risk of the disease because of birth asphyxia [105]. The incidence of HMD has been related to birth order and presence or absence of premature rupture of membranes, although no comment was made as to whether or not chorioamnionitis was present pathologically [106]. The highest rate of HMD was 77% of B twins without premature ruptured membranes; 69% of B twins with premature ruptured membranes, 54% of A twins without premature ruptured membranes, and 13% of A twins with premature ruptured membranes developed HMD. Male gender is also a factor contributing to the increased risk of pulmonary complications of prematurity, including bronchopulmonary dysplasia [107].

In Norman's series of brain-damaged twins [98], periventricular infarction—a lesion of prematurity—was found in 22% of the cases. Subependymal cell plate hemorrhage was present in 61%, and it had ruptured into the ventricles in just under half of the cases.

Low Birth Weight

Both low birth weight and intrauterine growth retardation are important problems with twins. One series reported that 55% of twins weighed less than 2500 grams at birth and 23.5% were small for gestational age. Twenty percent of A twins and 27% of B twins were growth retarded [77]. The majority (86%) of twins who died of unspecified causes weighed less than 2000 grams at birth [72], and 83% of neonatal deaths were of twins who weighed less than 1500 grams at birth. One-third of twins born after 32 weeks of gestational age are growth retarded [84].

The causes of low birth weight in twins are the same as for singletons, with additional factors related to the infants' sex and placentation pattern [77]. Unlike-sex pairs tend to be heavier than male pairs, who in turn are heavier than female pairs [32]. These differences may be related in part to patterns of placentation, because dichorionic dizygous twins are heavier than dichorionic monozygous twins, who in turn are heavier than monochorionic monozygous pairs

[53, 108]. It has been suggested that the maternal circulatory adaptation to a twin-bearing uterus may be less than adequate since some twin pairs have elevated hemoglobins and red cell mass, which may be a response to low-grade hypoxia [33, 76, 109]. The more striking examples of low birth weight, however, are associated with marked intrapair discrepancies (see below).

While low birth weight is an important problem in multiple gestation, any discussion of it requires careful distinction between low birth weight due to prematurity and true intrauterine growth retardation, because the consequent risks are different [27]. One study that maintained this distinction [53] reported perinatal death rates of 36% for small-for-gestational-age preterm twins, 11% for small-for-gestational-age twins at term, 6% for appropriate-for-gestational-age preterm twins, and 0% for appropriate-for-gestational-age twins at term. The factors that contribute to perinatal death of intrauterine growth-retarded singletons are thought to be operative in the case of growth-retarded twins as well, and low birth weight is reported to be a factor in 50% [76] to 85% [75] of the overall perinatal mortality of twins.

The question has been raised, however, whether it is valid to use singleton growth standards for twins, that possibly twins and singletons with the same apparent degree of growth retardation are not equivalent in either cause or consequences [27]. Also, weight alone as a standard for intrauterine growth retardation in macerated twins [68] is not valid, so the criteria used in studies of intrauterine growth retardation with fetal death [64] must be examined carefully. Singleton standards for measurements of fetal linear growth and head size may be useful for assessing twins, but twins can be expected to weigh less at birth without apparent detrimental effect [101]. Naeye has collected organ weight data differentiated for monozygous and dizygous twins [110, 111].

Twin A has been reported to weigh more than twin B [32], the same [92], or less [74]. In this last report, 29% of singletons weighted less than 1500 grams at birth, compared with 54% of B twins and 66% of A twins. Another group stated that 31% of A twins were growth retarded compared with 40% of B twins. An intrapair weight discrepancy greater than 500 grams is reported to occur with the same frequency in like-sex as in unlike-sex pairs [32]. When twins are discordant in size, the smaller twin has an equal chance to be A or B [105]. Intrauterine growth retardation and discordant weights have a disproportionately greater incidence in monochorial monozygous twins than in dichorial monozygous twins [79], which suggests that monochorionicity contributes to growth retardation. Of twins weighing less than 1000 grams at birth, 15% were monochorial, 4% were like-sex dichorial, and 3% were unlike-sex dichorial.

In a study of intrapair weight differences of over 25% and of 20–24%, the frequency was virtually the same (8.9% and 8.7%, respectively) for 460 twin pairs, but the risk of fetal death was 6.5 times greater, and the risk of perinatal death was 2.5 times greater, for the over 25% group than for the 20–24% group [112]. However, causes of death, placental data, and zygosity were not described in that study.

Determining the cause of intrapair weight variation is just as important as determining the cause of low birth weight. Discordant placental pathology, such as chronic villitis of unknown etiology, may be a factor in asymmetric fetal growth [113]. A number of studies [46, 47] suggest that some of the inequalities in both monozygous and dizygous twin birth weights may be related to placental proximity and hence placental growth, perhaps representing differences in adequacy of implantation sites in the uterus. This asymmetry may be grossly evident as early as the 37th day of gestation [114]. Thus, when the pathologist is assessing twin birth weights and intrapair variations, the chorionicity, degree of separation, and degree of symmetry of volume of the respective chorionic tissues are all relevant. There are obviously other causes of intrapair weight variations, such as fetal malformations, discordant responses to intrauterine insults (e.g., blood group incompatibility, infection, ischemia), and all the lesions possible with monozygous twinning, but asymmetries of placentation are probably just as important. In our material, intrapair weight variations greater than 25% were associated with chorion asymmetries, as well as discordant anomalies and villus pathology (Fig. 8.4).

Abnormal growth patterns of twins during pregnancy have been correlated with possible causes and three patterns have been identified [101, 115]. A first-trimester growth discordant twin is at increased risk for congenital anomalies. The onset of growth discrepancy in the second trimester reflected twin transfusion syndrome and other potentially severe problems, while onset in the third trimester was related to intrauterine nutrition and these twins were less severely affected. The growth-retarded twins were small in all three measures of growth—head circumference, length, and weight—when compared with well-grown twins who matched singletons in head circumference and length.

The long-term significance of low birth weight in twins is not certain. It has been noted that when one twin dies in utero, the other fetus attains normal singleton standard growth, including weight, if there are no anomalies or other problems [27]. This might suggest that each twin has a full potential for growth that is inhibited only by the intrauterine environment. However, postnatal growth may still be impaired, as even apparently normal twins can retain their growth differences for many years [116].

Other Disorders/Diseases in Twins

Infants of multiple gestation are subject to all the diseases that occur in singletons, with five additional categories of disorders. There are diseases that may be more frequent in twins because they *are* twins. These include complications of prematurity because these infants are more often premature, growth dissimilarities for the reasons described above, and the problems of labor and delivery already discussed. There are those disorders that are unique to twins, such as

the twin transfusion syndrome described below. Some diseases may be modified in their expression because of the twin situation, such as discordance in the manifestation of rhesus blood group incompatibility already described in dizygous twins, or possible variations in the manifestations of metabolic or infectious disease through vascular anastomoses. Some studies suggest that the twinning stimulus may affect the potential for neoplasms, and concordance for leukemia in monozygous twins is described below. Finally, social aspects, such as fear of twins or the extra burden of caring for twins, may contribute to abuse or neglect [27, 75]. The pathologist will do well to keep these considerations in mind when assessing disease processes in twins.

Twins are reported to die as a consequence of infection in the newborn period at a rate equivalent to that of singletons [74]. Twin B may succumb four times as often as twin A, although twin A was described as being septicemic more often than twin B [92]. Congenital infection is said to be discordant more often when ascending and concordant when hematogenously acquired [1]. However, infections that must have been acquired in utero can have very different manifestations in twins (or triplets, etc.) that do not fit with the usual concepts of pathophysiology. Genetically based differences in fetal resistance or the placental barrier to infection could explain discordant fetal response to infection, and this would seem to be borne out by the case reports. Concordant infection (as evidenced by immunologic methods) with clinically discordant disease has been reported for rubella [116], toxoplasmosis [116, 117], cytomegalovirus [69], and echovirus 11 [118]. Discordant infection and disease leaving one twin ill or dead and the other twin normal have been reported for cytomegalovirus [119]. Maternal and fetal death with systemic coccidioidomycosis without apparent infection of the uterus or placenta has been reported [120]. Ascending infection may be concordant, even in high multiples, without apparent explanation [121]. A reported increased risk of listeriosis during multiple gestation is unexplained [122].

While neoplasia seems to have a lower prevalence in twins than in singletons [1, 16], there are several relationships between twinning and tumors. A variety of tumors are associated with some malformation syndromes, congenital functional defects (particularly immunologic), or chromosomal errors (especially trisomy 21) [123]. Therefore, it is conceivable that there could be tumors in this group if the associated disease was present in one or both twins. However, this relationship has not been addressed specifically in reference to cancer and twins. Sacrococcygeal teratomas have been related to twinning [124]: 7.5% of those affected were one of twins, and twinning occurred in the families of 50% of those responding to a follow-up questionnaire. Some congenital tumors have a strong genetic component and may be a special class of malformation, which could therefore be expected to appear simultaneously in monozygous twins [125]. A report of concordant bilateral congenital retinoblastoma without family history, in

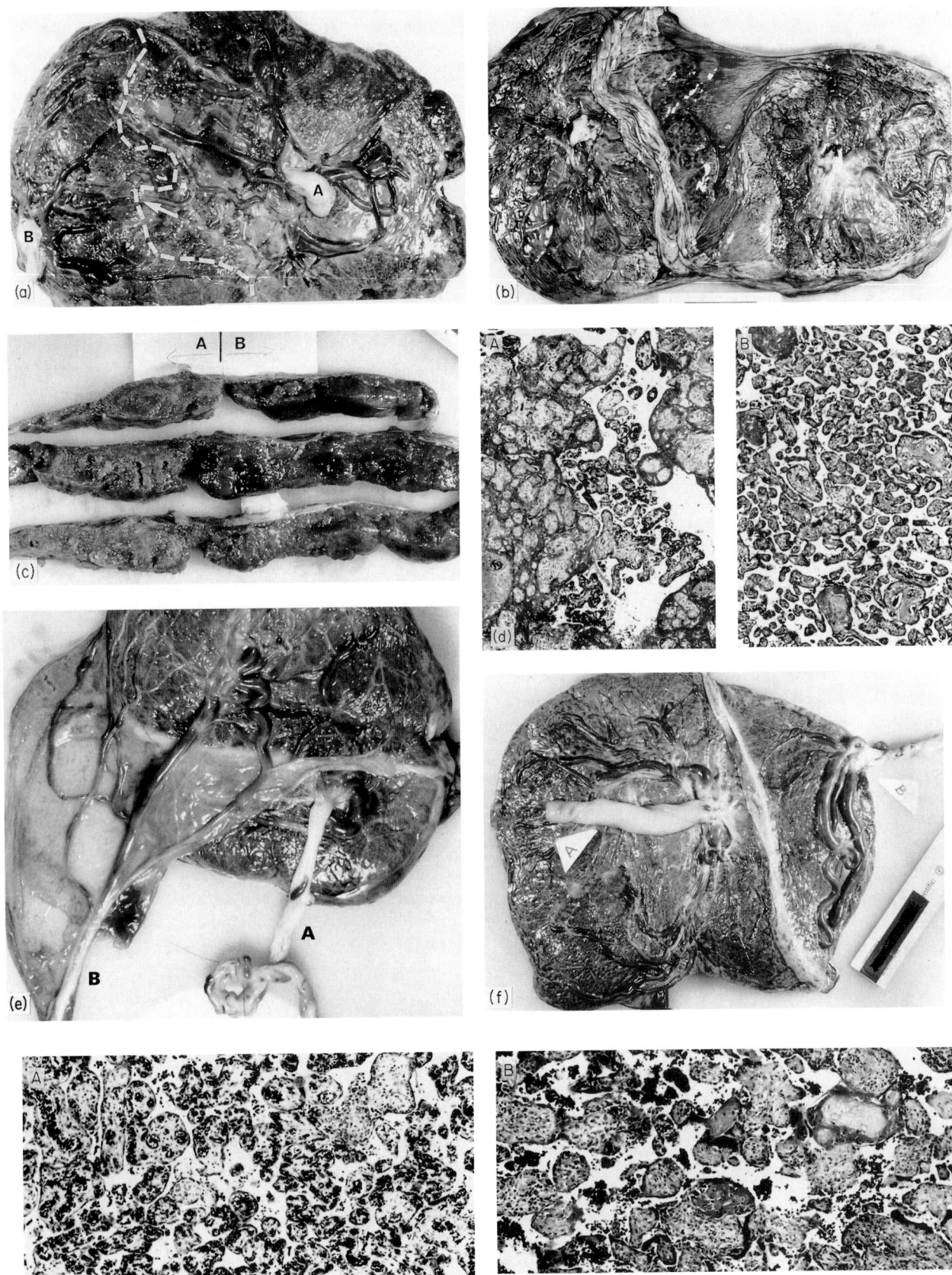

twins stated to be dizygotic, suggested unspecified intrauterine factors in tumorigenesis [126]. Otherwise, broad-based population studies [127, 128] suggest that aside from leukemia and renal cancer there does not seem to be an increased risk for concordance of tumors in twins. Also, in many of the case reports, the basis of statements of monozygosity is not given.

Wilms' tumors have been reported to occur at four times the expected rate in twins, and 80% of such tumors occurred in concordant monozygous pairs [127]. The subject of leukemia in twins has received considerable attention, and it has been suggested [127] that if leukemia is diagnosed in one twin under 1 year of age, the other twin should also be examined. Concordance for leukemia may be as high as 10:1 in monozygous pairs, and leukemia in the concordant twin may be diagnosed within a month in 75% of such twin pairs. Concordance has also been identified in early childhood leukemia, late childhood leukemia, and adult onset leukemia in monozygous twins, but the greatest concordance was in the perinatal-congenital period.

Twins are vulnerable to the same diseases as singletons, but the numbers of cases of concordant or discordant disease described are few and thus biases of ascertainment and reporting must be kept in mind when reviewing these discussions. Also, zygosity assignment is rarely detailed, so that the significance of concordance or discordance cannot be developed.

The incidence of twins in any group of individuals afflicted with cerebral palsy is greater than in the normal population. Twin pregnancies produce a child with cerebral palsy 8 to 12 times more often than singleton pregnancies, and triplets 47 times more often [129, 130]. In such twin sets, the firstborn has cerebral palsy twice as often as the secondborn, but there is greater mortality among the secondborn. In a detailed correlation of the type of cerebral palsy with birth order [131], there was discordance in all types. It was concluded that the first twin suffered trauma as it dilated the cervix leading to spastic diplegia, while the second twin was anoxic and either died or survived with spastic or athetoid tetraplegia. Detrimental consequences of intertwin placental vascular anastomoses have been suggested as mechanisms for some types of brain damage in twins [132]. Unfortunately, the review of cerebral palsy in twins does not describe the anatomy of the placenta of the affected twins; therefore, this concept of transvascular etiology for the lesions of cerebral palsy cannot be assessed further.

Sudden infant death syndrome has been reported to be increased in twins [133], with rates in all infants of 1.81 per 1000 births compared with 3.56 per 1000 for all twins. Firstborn twins have a rate of 1.53 per 1000, while secondborn twins have a risk nearly four times as great, with a rate of 5.6 per 1000. No mention is made of concordance or zygosity, but the differential raises the question of the significance of the second-twin syndrome, particularly in relation to perinatal asphyxia.

In some societies, twins inspire fear, and for some families twins may simply be too much of a burden to care for [27], so that neglect and abuse may be encountered [75]. The Munchausen syndrome [134] has been reported in a set of dizygous twins.

Anomalies

It should be kept in mind that reports concerning anomalies in twins are susceptible to a number of biases [135], including biases of ascertainment, probable underreporting of discordancy, tyranny of small numbers, exclusion of stillbirth data, lack of pathologic confirmation, and poor to non-existent placental morphology and documentation of zygosity.

Infants of multiple pregnancies have anomalies that fall into one of two categories: malformations of the type that occur in single infants and malformations associated with the twinning process. The first category is of interest because of what the pattern of occurrence (concordant or discordant) may indicate about the pathogenesis of the anomaly, but the pathologic examination of these malformations is no different when they occur in a twin. The second category includes those anomalies that are seen more often in twins or are associated with twinning in the family, and those anomalies that occur only in twins.

General reviews of anomalies in twins are numerous [1, 25, 28, 30, 53, 70, 72, 75, 92, 97, 116, 136–138], but many suffer from one or more of the biases referred to above.

Using thorough zygosity studies, malformation rates of 2.5% of all dizygous individuals and 3.7% of all monozygous

FIGURE 8.4. *(facing page) Placental variations associated with asymmetric fetal growth. (a) Monochorionic diamniotic twin girls at 32 weeks. A = 2080 gm, B = 1525 gm. Chorionic asymmetry: 3/4 of surface vascularization associated with cord A (dotted line); note that fetal asymmetry is opposite to that of A-to-B arteriovenous shunt (arrow). (Separating membranes have been removed for easier demonstration of shunts.) (b) Dichorionic diamniotic separate discs with shared membranes of twin girls at 39 weeks. Infant/placenta weights are: A, 3080 gm/435 gm; B, 2320 gm/280 gm. No other lesions to explain growth asymmetry, except asymmetric placentae. (c) Dichorionic diamniotic fused placenta of twin boys at 28 weeks. A = 1080 gm, B = 2310 gm. Twin A drained 2/5 of chorionic surface and had markedly increased perivillus fibrin on section; note different textural quality of parenchyma between A and B due to greater fibrin in A (d). (e) Dichorionic diamniotic twin boys at 35 weeks. A = 1860 gm, B = 1250 gm. Chorion disc asymmetry is opposite to twin size—twin A has 1/3 of surface with fewer vessels, but twin B has a very abnormal cord insertion (long intramembranous). This suggests influence of abnormal cord insertion on fetal growth. (f) Dichorionic diamniotic twin girls at 30 weeks from in vitro fertilization conception. A = 3100 gm, B = 1720 gm. Surface area asymmetry: A = 3/4, B = 1/4. Villi of B also ischemic. (g) Monochorionic diamniotic twins at 38 weeks. A = 2381 gm, B = 1790 gm. No vascular anastomoses but marked asymmetry of placental involvement by villitis, suggesting significance of asymmetric villus disorder on relative twin growth.*

individuals have been reported [25]. One-third of the anomalies in the monozygous individuals were concordant, and the remainder were discordant. It should be noted, however, that while concordance in proven monozygous twins is suggestive of genetic origin, nongenetic teratogenic factors, such as infection, drugs, disease during pregnancy, and intrauterine position should also be considered as likely to affect both embryos, leading to an acquired concordance. Similarly, discordance cannot be taken to exclude genetic factors, since genetically determined predispositions may not be manifest and a discordant response to common environmental factors may be due to genetic factors. Newer techniques of genetic investigation are providing explanations for puzzling patterns of discordance in monozygotic twins [139]. For example, nonrandom inactivation of the X chromosome was identified as the reason for discordant Hunter disease (mucopolysaccharidosis type II) in proven monozygotic twin girls [140]. Even something as basic as pattern of placentation may provide a threshold effect for anomalous development for one of twins who both have a predisposition.

One of the most exhaustive analyses of malformations in twins was that undertaken by the Collaborative Perinatal Project in the United States [28]. There was a statistically significant increase of twins with malformations compared with singletons but not of multiple malformation complexes or multiply malformed individuals. This increased rate was due to monozygous individuals. The difference was highly significant and applied to both major and minor malformations. Compared with rates in singletons, twins had twice the rate of cardiovascular and gastrointestinal anomalies. Central nervous system and related skeletal anomalies were also of greater frequency in twins, but they were less significant. The cardiovascular system, gastrointestinal tract, and central nervous system anomalies were virtually all major ones, however. Also significantly greater in twins were mixtures of minor and major anomalies of the ear, upper respiratory tract, and mouth. When specific malformations were considered, almost all were increased in twins, although for some the numbers were small, and meaningful comparisons with singletons could not be made. Major malformations that were significantly increased in twins were macrocephaly, encephalocele, cleft lip and palate, diaphragmatic anomalies, tracheoesophageal fistula, intestinal malrotation, inguinal and umbilical hernias, and cystic kidneys. Significantly increased minor malformations were deformed pinnae, preauricular skin tags, and accessory spleens. Hypospadias was not identified in twins. While malformations were reportedly associated with 6.6% of all twin deaths in the study, twins who died in the neonatal period died of causes other than the consequences of malformations.

Blacks had a slightly but significantly higher incidence of malformations, consisting mainly of polydactyly and branchial cleft anomalies. There were more males with major malformations and male twins had a higher rate of malformations than male singletons, while female twins and singletons had the same rate. Monozygous white twins had both major and minor anomalies, while black monozygous twins had mostly minor anomalies. The malformation rate in monoamniotic twins was high; 16.7% had major anomalies and another 16.7% had minor anomalies. When malformations were correlated with birth order—an association that might reflect influence of intrauterine position or placentation—no differences were noted.

In a significant number of cases where one twin had a malformation, the co-twin also had a malformation, although not necessarily the same type as the first twin. All dizygous concordant pairs were concordant for at least one similar malformation. Of the concordant monozygous pairs, 69% had at least one similar malformation and 31% had different malformations. With reference to specific anomalies, the concordance rate for monozygous twins was consistently greater than for dizygous twins, but only in musculoskeletal malformations was it statistically significant (60% and 10%, respectively). Concordance of central nervous system defects in twins was low. The majority of musculoskeletal malformations comprised the three types of clubfoot, and in all concordant twins the clubfoot was bilateral in both twins, whereas in discordant pairs it was bilateral in half of the cases. Major and minor hand anomalies and anomalies of the hip joint were not identified in monozygous twins. Concordance rates for cardiovascular anomalies were low, with the exception of fused hearts in conjoined twins, which is obviously a very special situation. Gastrointestinal anomalies were generally discordant. More than 50% of all skin malformations were hemangiomas, for which all twin pairs were discordant.

A monumental review of single umbilical artery [141] recorded a 3 to 4 times greater incidence of single umbilical artery among members of multiple gestation, but the affected infants had associated malformations at the same rate as singletons and there was no consistent pattern to these malformations. Most twins were discordant for single umbilical artery, and the infant with the single umbilical artery was the smaller of the two in 82.4% of the cases where the weights of both were known. Concordance was greater in monozygous twins than in dizygous twins, but 37% of the twins with single umbilical artery were monozygous and 63% were dizygous. Cases of chorangiopagus twins (acardia) were excluded. The presence of only a single umbilical artery connoted a greater risk of perinatal mortality beyond that due to any associated malformation.

Series of cardiovascular malformations have been reported [70, 142]. Lesions occurring in greater than 5% of twins were ventricular septal defect in 21%, tetralogy of Fallot in 15%, pulmonary stenosis in 11%, patent ductus arteriosus in 10%, and aortic stenosis and atrial septal defects in 7% each. There are conflicting reports in these reviews on concordance. Malformations of the central nervous system are reported [70], but the varied occurrence in twin pairs, including concordant dizygous twins and discordant conjoined twins, proves neither genetic nor environmental hypotheses [116]. Unfavorable local conditions, such as those associated with the twinning process itself, may be important. Visceral transposition and mirror imaging in twins have been discussed [11,

125]. It appears that visceral inversion may be due to factors having no particular relation to factors in twinning, except possibly with conjoined twins (see below). It has been suggested, however, that there may be some degree of "mirror imagery" in up to 25% of monozygous pairs, in features such as hair patterns and finger-print patterns [143]. Phenotypically discordant responses to exogenous teratogens have been attributed to dizygosity and hence to genetic makeup in the fetal hydantoin syndrome [144], in the fetal alcohol syndrome [145], and with thalidomide [146]. The amniotic band syndrome, a disruption complex, has been reported to be both discordant and concordant in twins [147, 148], and an inter-twin vascular etiopathogenesis has been proposed for cases of clefts/constrictions/amputations in the presence of normally intact amnion [149]. Falsely elevated alphafetoprotein (AFP) levels in twins have been reported [150].

It has been suggested, concerning relative survival rates of concordantly or discordantly malformed twins, that the presence of the normal twin might allow the pregnancy to continue, whereas a concordant pregnancy may abort [151].

Both numerical and structural chromosomal anomalies have been described [14, 15, 152, 153], with discordant manifestations in some sets of monozygous twins. These are referred to as monozygotic heterokaryotic twins (MZHT). The commonest abnormality is discordance for phenotypic sex due to a variety of chromosomal errors. In a review of 14 cases of discordant chromosomal and phenotypic sex [154], the normal member was a male in four cases and a female in 10, and the abnormal member usually phenotypically had the Turner syndrome. The chromosomal makeup of the abnormal twin varied with at least some 45,X, but it was usually a mosaic with cell lines identical to the normal twin (46,XX or 46,XY) and occasionally some 47,XXX lines.

Other numerical chromosomal discordances have been limited largely to chromosome 21, and monozygous twins are generally concordant and dizygous twins discordant for trisomy 21. Discordance in monozygous twins has been associated with mosaics [154], and concordance in truly dizygous infants is uncommon but reported [152]. A 22:22 translocation discordant in twins has been reported [154]. A number of karyotypic discordances in chorangiopagus twins (acardiacs) are described below. In a review of triploid fetuses [15], the frequency of twins was the same as that among spontaneous abortions overall. Structural rearrangement has also been reported to be discordant in twins [155].

In twins there are components of the twinning phenomenon itself that provide influences in addition to those of genetic and environmental origin [20]. Crowding of two infants in a uterus that is ideally meant for only one may result in fetal deformities. Crowding can also affect placentation and thus have potential secondary vascular consequences to the infants. The actual process that leads to monozygotic twinning itself may influence the further development of such twins. The evidence for this is the greater frequency of anomalies in monozygous twins than can be explained by hereditary influences alone, and the fact that the rates of malformation increase with increasing proximity of monozygous twins. An excess of midline malformations, such as symmelia, cloacal extrophy, tracheo-esophageal fistula, and neural tube defect, have been associated with monozygous twins [7, 16, 19].

Mortality During Gestation

Introduction

A pregnancy that starts as a multiple gestation may not continue or terminate as such, and fetal loss between conception and delivery can take several forms. Such intragestational fetal loss has different causes and consequences at different times during the pregnancy, although the distinctions become blurred when the dead fetus is retained for a prolonged period of time.

Third-trimester loss is the most familiar pattern of twin mortality. If all fetuses die, the pregnancy will terminate with delivery of stillborn infants who are more or less macerated. If only one fetus dies, it may be delivered and the pregnancy may continue for a variable period of time until delivery of the remaining fetus or fetuses. Alternatively, the dead fetus may be retained and be delivered as a macerated co-twin at the time of delivery of the surviving fetus or fetuses.

Second-trimester loss also has been recognized for some time. If all fetuses die, they are usually "aborted" or "stillborn" depending on the timing of delivery and the regional legal definition of point of viability. If only one fetus dies, it may be delivered with persistence of the pregnancy, or it may be retained to become a fetus papyraceus. Selective iatrogenic termination of one or more infants in the second trimester may be undertaken to allow normal infants to be delivered at maturity [9, 156].

Finally, a much higher early reproduction loss is being identified than had been recognized formerly [157, 158]. These early embryo deaths may be aborted and available for embryopathologic evaluation or they may be resorbed with little or no pathologic evidence of their previous existence on the placenta of the surviving infant delivered later in pregnancy. Elective embryo/fetal reductions are being performed more frequently in cases of higher multiple conceptions, both spontaneous and induced, and documentation of the residues is often possible [159, 160].

Early Pregnancy Loss

Ultrasound studies have reported overall rates of early pregnancy loss that have ranged from 50% [3] to 70% [161]. Losses from spontaneous multiple gestations have ranged from 63% [3] to 100% [161]. Losses from induced multiple gestations have averaged 28–29% [3, 161], with the greatest loss 64%, associated with clomiphene induction [3]. Comparing rates of fetal loss with the time during pregnancy that twins were diagnosed has shown that the loss occurs in the first and early second trimester [162]. Twin gestations identified at less than 10 weeks' gestational age ended with delivery of singletons in 71% of cases. Twins still present at 10 to 15 weeks of gestation were reduced to singletons at delivery in 62% of cases. When twins were both still present after 15 weeks of gestation, all were delivered.

Fetal loss may consist of death of either or both of the embryos. If both embryos are lost, they may be blighted ova or they may be aborted as larger embryos; the latter group accounts for 17–29% of the wastage [24, 163]. In 37–49% of the cases of fetal loss, only one embryo is a blighted ovum and the normal co-twin survives [24, 163]. The only sign of fetal loss in this group may be an episode of slight vaginal bleeding, and the process of fetal death of the co-twin does not seem to affect the development of the survivor. Pathologic evaluation of these cases consists of documentation of the embryopathology of the aborted material or identification of the embryonic residue on the placenta of the surviving twin.

Detailed reviews of the pathology of spontaneously aborted embryos (less than 8 weeks) and fetuses (8–18 weeks) identified three times more twins among aborted pregnancies when compared with the ratios at term [164, 165]. They were largely monochorial twins (17.5:1) and most were lost as embryos. The exact cause of the gestational loss was not identified in all cases, but anomaly rates were similar to those identified among all abortions, including growth disorganizations of 88% of the embryos and a variety of malformations in 21% of the fetuses, often with chromosomal errors. There was a preponderance of females.

The dead twin's residue that the pathologist may identify on the delivered placenta of the survivor has different forms (Fig. 8.5). It may be simply a flattened mass of sclerotic placental tissue, which is present as part of the healthy disc of a cotwin, or it may be a variably separate mass accessory in position in the membranes. The only clue to the true nature of these zones may be the presence of a collapsed but definite sac of membranes on the surface, distinct from the membranes of the surviving co-twin. Very occasionally, a tiny fragile clump of amorphous tissue can be recognized in this space, and even more rarely a recognizable embryo that can be dated and examined is found. Occasionally, the pathologist is called on to document the results of selective iatrogenic interventions in multiple pregnancies. In the first trimester, some of the embryos of an induced multiple gestation may be "treated" to allow fewer fetuses to grow [166].

The causes of fetal wastage in this period are not established, aside from those factors encountered in embryo singleton abortuses for which a very high rate of chromosomal abnormalities is responsible. The high proportion of monozygous conceptions suggests that there may be a basic problem secondary to the monozygous twinning process, although the nature of this problem is not known. Additionally, there may be implantation asymmetries that are lethal to one of the embryos.

Midpregnancy Loss

Fetal wastage in the second trimester may result in abortion of the entire contents of the uterus, or the dead fetus may be retained, becoming compressed to a fetus papyraceus or

fetus compressus by the growing sac of the surviving twin as the fluid in its own sac is resorbed.

The term "fetus papyraceus" is usually considered to mean a fetus who dies in the second trimester but who is delivered with the co-twin in the third trimester. This category can become blurred at both ends of the time frame. A fetus who dies in the 12-to-20-week period but is not delivered until after 20 weeks may be classed as a fetus papyraceus. In later third trimester, a fetal death may merge with the "retained macerated" stillbirth group depending on the gross description of the fetus. Careful definitions are required in order to be able to estimate the date of fetal death. The overall rate of fetus papyraceus is 0.54% of twin pregnancies and is reportedly higher in triplets [52], sometimes with two papyraceous fetuses and a normal survivor [167].

The survivor is generally normal, although complications have been reported and include ileal atresia [52, 168], congenital skin defects [76], limb amputations [169], and gastroschisis [170]. The mechanism of these complications is not clear, except in the case where the cord of the papyraceous fetus was wound around the leg of its monoamniotic co-twin, leading to amputation of the leg. It has been suggested that transanastomotic vascular complications, such as disseminated intravascular coagulopathy or transient sublethal blood loss, following the death of the co-twin may be important [171, 172]. Of greatest concern are the nonlethal but handicapping neurologic deficits identified in one of a twin pair following the intrauterine death of a co-twin [173]. These deficits are discussed further in the section on twin-to-twin transfusion syndrome.

Unless there are extensive intertwin vascular communications, cessation of the fetal circulation in that portion of the placenta associated with the dead twin leads to gradual reduction of maternal circulation to that villous territory. This leads to ischemic damage and eventual collapse of the villi. This compaction is associated with deposition of increased fibrin around the villi. The dead twin's portion of the placenta in the delivered placenta of the survivor is thus represented by a firm, pale, and sclerotic mass with avascular villi embedded in fibrin. It may be present as a separate mass or a residual portion of a single disc, depending on the original pattern of placentation [42].

The twin itself is variably compacted, usually gray tan, with extensive tissue autolysis. Anomalies aside from cord lesions are rarely identified. There may be problems determining the time of death of the papyraceous fetus. The size may suggest a growth arrest or possibly death at a certain date, but the clinical data may suggest a different date [168]. Therefore, in some cases it is possible that growth was initially impaired or arrested by the process that eventually led to the fetal death.

The cause of death of these fetuses that will become papyraceous is not known in the majority of cases. Anomalous insertions of the cord, particularly velamentous insertions, have been implicated [52, 170, 174]. Monochorial

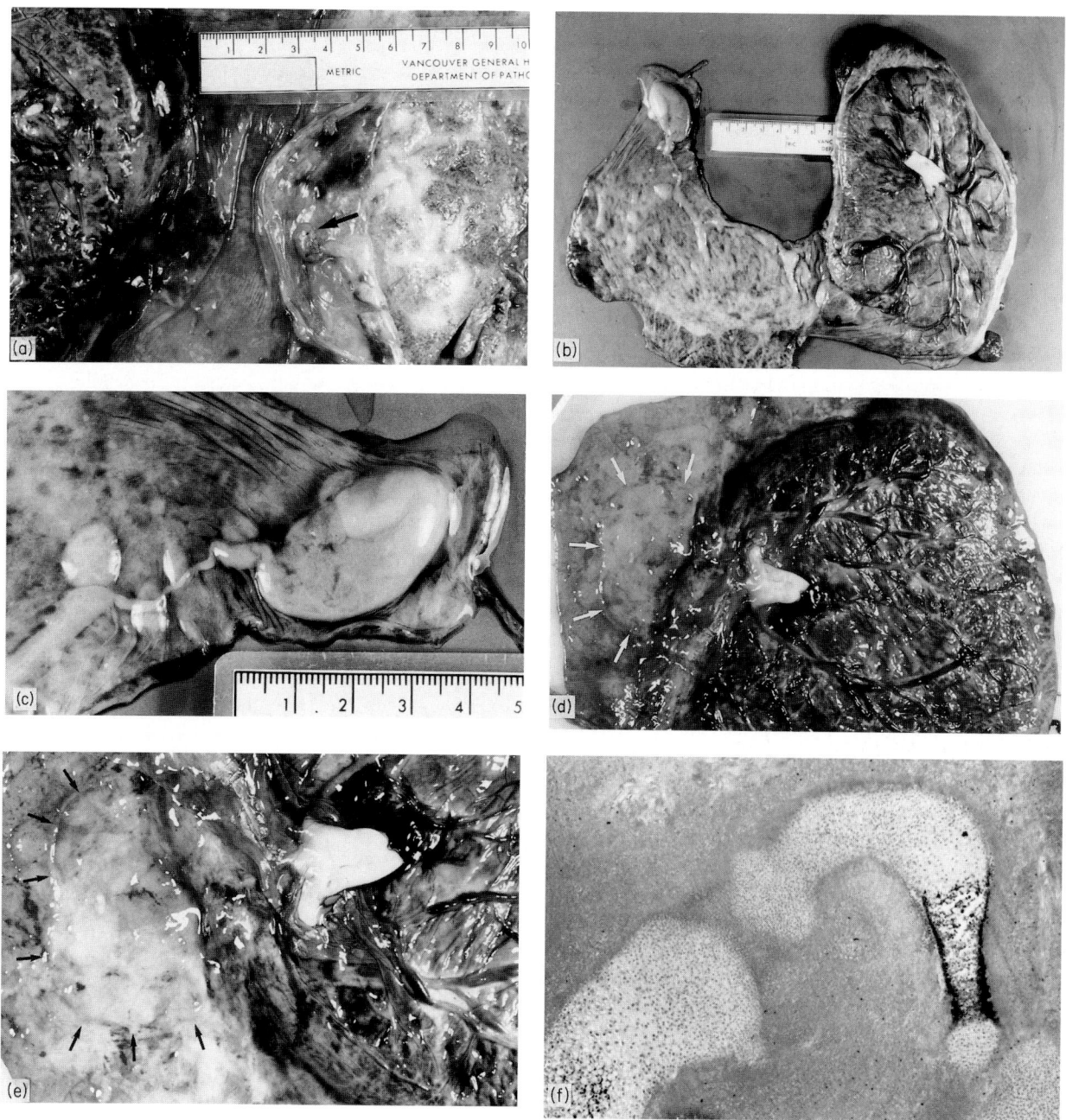

FIGURE 8.5.   *Twin residues after fetal death during gestation. (a) Clinically unsuspected dichorionic diamniotic twin pregnancy with death of one twin at about 6 weeks' gestation by size. The residue consists of a plaque in the membranes with a collapsed sac and macerated but identifiable gray-green embryo (arrow) with retinal pigment. Cause of embryonic death not known. (b) and (c) Clinically unsuspected dichorionic diamniotic twin pregnancy with death of one twin at about 9 weeks' gestation by size. The residue is present as a plaque in the membranes, with definable sac and grayish embryo still with amnion. Note umbilical cord. Delivered at 26 weeks, co-twin normal. Cause of embryonic death not known. (d), (e), and (f) Documented growth retardation of one twin with death between 12 and 14 weeks' gestation. No sign on ultrasound thereafter and thought to have been passed. Spontaneous delivery at 41 weeks of 4366-gm, normal boy. The residue is present as plaque in membranes (arrow). Fetal bones identified histologically. Dichorionic gestation. Cause of fetal death not known.*

twins may succumb due to a severe twin transfusion syndrome [7, 75, 175]. Cord entanglements of monoamniotic twins can lead to fetal death [169]. As many as 50% of papyraceous fetuses are said to have been growth retarded at the time of intrauterine fetal death [64], but the criteria

of failure of fetal growth are unclear. Males may be affected more often than females [174].

Intrauterine fetal death of one twin may also be induced in the second trimester [159, 176] for reasons of discordant metabolic/structural/cytogenetic disorders, or to allow survival of at least one twin in a twin-to-twin transfusion situation [9, 156]. It is the pathologist's responsibility in these cases to confirm the diagnosis of the abnormality if possible, although, since the pregnancies may continue for several months, such confirmation is often difficult.

Late Pregnancy Loss

Late pregnancy loss may involve delayed delivery or stillbirth [177]. Occasionally, the fetuses of twin or higher multiple pregnancy are delivered at intervals of days to months apart [178]. The pathophysiology is not understood, and reported fetal pathology is nonspecific. The placentations are usually described as having involuted or sclerotic but otherwise unremarkable portions or discs corresponding to the earlier delivered fetus, and a normal portion that may have evidence of premature separation or ascending infection.

Twins are at greater risk of stillbirth than singletons [68, 70, 92, 100], and rates of stillbirth in twins range from 3% [69] to 14% [179]. The stillborn twins are more likely to have died antepartum (75% compared with less than half of stillborn singletons) than intrapartum [34]. Of all twin deaths in one series, 16% were fresh stillbirths and 18% were macerated stillbirths [63].

THE PATHOLOGY OF MONOCHORIAL MONOZYGOSITY

Monoamniotic Twins

Except for genetic considerations, monozygous twins with dichorial placentae have similar developmental and gestational risks as dizygotic twins. Monochorial monozygous twins, however, have two additional sources of problems—vascular anastomoses between the fetuses and/or abnormalities of duplication [20]. Monochorial placentae represent 5% (Africa [52]) to 71% (Japan [138]) of all twin placentae, depending on the rate of monozygous twinning in the population, and they represent up to nearly three-quarters [49] of all monozygous twins. Monoamniotic placentae represent 6–12% of monochorial gestations and require special consideration.

Monoamniotic pregnancy was first described in 1612, and several comprehensive reviews of regional and worldwide experience are availabe [179–181]. Care is required to avoid overdiagnosis. The amnion tends to separate from the chorion in a mature placenta, and the absence of a diamniotic septum must be documented carefully unless the cords are unequivocally tangled. Monoamniotic placentae usually arise when the twinning event occurs after the ectodermal plate and amniotic sac have developed—i.e., 7 to 13 days after fertilization [9].

In monoamniotic pregnancies, fetal mortality is high (60%), due almost entirely to cord entanglements and knots that may be quite complex [182]. However, asymmetry of chorionic development is also described and has been associated with 39% of monoamniotic stillbirths [179]. The sex of the twins is not always reported, but females are described

twice as often as males, which is consistent with the previous comments on the greater rate of female embryos as proximity of the embryos to one another increases. Interlocking of twins would seem to be a distinct possibility in monoamniotic sacs, but apparently it is rarely encountered. Anomalies have been described in 10% of these infants, including discordant lesions [28, 181]. Vascular anastomoses have been identified in nearly all cases in which they were sought. Remarkably, however, the twin-to-twin transfusion syndrome is uncommon [9], identified in 4.6% of one series [180] and in none of 16 cases in another series [179].

Intertwin Vascular Anastomoses

Description and Significance

With rare exceptions, vascular communications between twins are present only in monochorial placentae. Nearly 100% of such placentae have been reported to have vascular anastomoses, but there is marked variation in the number, size, and direction of these haphazardly formed connections [183]. In any series, the demonstrable anastomoses may vary depending on their suitability for injection, since demonstration may be difficult if there is placental fragmentation or previous formalin fixation. Also, it is possible that some of the anastomotic vessels may regress in later pregnancy and therefore not be demonstrable by injection of the delivered placenta. Reported instances of demonstrable anastomoses have ranged from 76% [100] through 85% [9] to 98% [61].

The pattern of anastomosis is variable [76, 183]. Artery-to-artery connections on the chorionic surface are the most common pattern and have been identified in up to 75% of injected monochorial placentae. Vein-to-vein anastomoses on the chorionic surface have been identified in up to 46% of such placentae. Anastomoses that involve the capillary bed of the villous tissue create a so-called "common villous district" or "third circulation." These anastomoses involve the connection of an artery of one twin to the vein of the other twin through the intervening capillaries, and have been identified in up to 58% of injected placentae. Isolated shunts and combinations are identified with the following frequencies: an artery-to-artery connection plus an artery-to-vein connection is the most common combination and is reported in 28% of cases, an artery-to-artery alone in 21%, artery-to-vein alone in 19%, and the remaining possible combinations in 3–5% each. One vessel may be demonstrated to have several connections, occasionally in both directions.

Although the relaxed size of surface vessels may bear little relation to their diameter in vivo, a rough approximation of the potential direction and volume of flow occasionally can be made by measuring midpoint diameters of the vessels involved [12]. The vessels involved can vary greatly in diameter from less than 1 mm to 5–6 mm, and occasionally vessels of different sizes anastomose. Generally, the farther apart the cord insertions are, the smaller will be the anastomotic channels. The actual number of anastomoses in any one placenta is quite variable, and there can be numerous connections. Occasionally, the volume of the shared villous territory can be demonstrated with injection techniques.

While anatomic vascular anastomoses in dichorial placentae are extremely rarely documented pathologically [49, 52], they occasionally must be inferred to have been present, at least transiently, because of the demonstration of rare cases of blood chimerism in dichorial twins [9, 184].

Static analysis of the vascular anatomy of the delivered placenta is an indication only of potential hemodynamic flow patterns. The functional effect must be ascertained from the condition of the fetuses [41, 79].

Potentially balanced shunt situations are those in which there is a surface artery-to-artery or vein-to-vein anastomosis, or in which an arteriovenous shunt is present with either a surface anastomosis or a second reversed arteriovenous shunt. Flow might vary in these shunts depending on the respective hemodynamic status of each twin at any one time, but twin mortality is considerably less in cases with these patterns of vessels [80]. These balanced anastomoses may have nonhemodynamic significance because they may allow intermingling of blood components sufficient to enhance intertwin skin grafts [1], create blood chimeras in heterokaryotic twins [39], or allow transchorionic disseminated intravascular coagulation (DIC) when one twin dies in utero (see below).

There are three patterns of hemodynamically imbalanced anastomotic circulations: chorangiopagus asymmetric twin (acardius) (see below) and acute and chronic twin-to-twin transfusion syndrome (TTS). The percentage of placentae with demonstrable vascular anastomoses that are associated with clinically recognizable TTS is variable, ranging from 5.5% [61] to 33% [114]. In 132 liveborn twin pairs [185], there were 42 with monochorial placentae, 75% of which had vascular anastomoses. Thirty-four percent of these had clinical evidence of TTS, and of these 18% had an acute syndrome and 82% a chronic syndrome. The same study noted that one-third of stillborn pairs had vascular anastomoses with a diagnosis of TTS made because of differential plethora and pallor of the twins without other cause. Occasional instances of bidirectional intraparenchymal anastomoses with one artery connected to veins of both twins may provide a possible explanation for spontaneous clinical correction of TTS during pregnancy.

Twin-to-Twin Transfusion Syndrome

The twin-to-twin transfusion syndrome (TTS) generally is considered possible only if there is a monochorial placenta with vascular anastomoses.

The acute transfusion syndrome results from a rapid loss of blood from one twin across the vascular anastomoses (usually superficial) into the circulation of the other twin. This most often occurs during labor and delivery, and the loss may be out of the severed cord of the already delivered twin. Twins with this syndrome are the same length and weight, but one will be paler than the other [186] (Fig. 8.6). Hemoglobin levels assessed at birth will be equal, as there will have

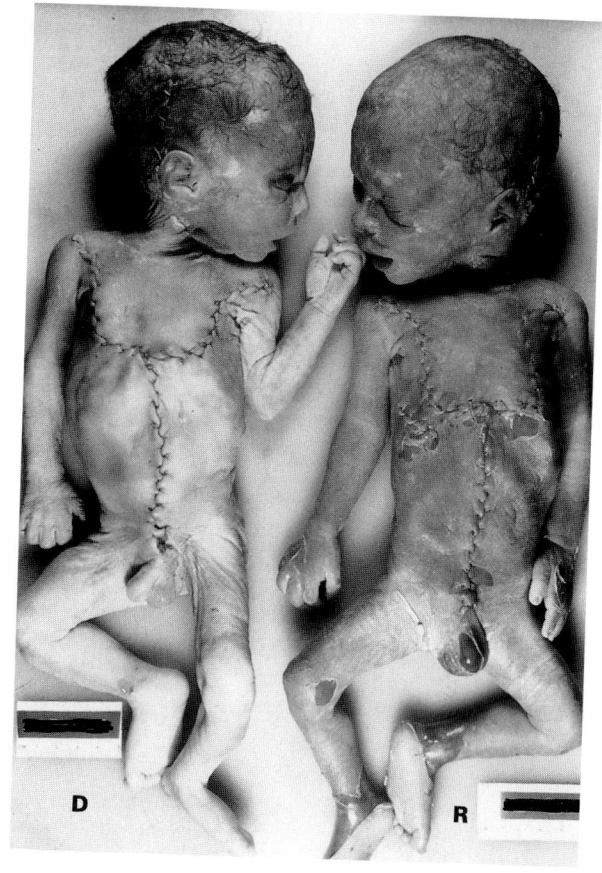

FIGURE 8.6. *Acute twin-to-twin transfusion syndrome. Note the nearly equal development but marked plethora of the recipient (R). There were a number of superficial and third circulation anastomoses.*

been no time for adaptation to have occurred [187]. It should be noted, however, that not all pale members of a twin pair are necessarily donor twins of an acute TTS. Fetal maternal hemorrhage from one monochorial twin may be responsible [188]. It is noteworthy that simple acute TTS is relatively rare, clinically, compared with the frequency of demonstrable surface anastomoses in monochorial placentae [49].

Much more frequent is acute transfusion as a complication of chronic transfusion. In one series, 45% of the autopsy cases of chronic transfusion were interpreted as having been complicated by an acute transfusion just prior to fetal death [183]. Acute-on-chronic transfusion has been implicated as the cause of brain damage noted in some survivors after fetal death of one monochorionic twin [189].

The chronic transfusion syndrome is seen more frequently and is usually associated with asymmetric third circulation anastomoses [80]. These shunts do not have to be very large, and the actual amount of blood being lost by the donor need not be great [1, 41, 76, 190]. The effect on these infant pairs is a composite of anemic growth retardation and polycythemic plethora, possibly compounded by osmotic effects due to induced differences in serum protein concentrations [41, 188, 190].

The more severe examples of chronic transfusion can be identified as early as the 10th week of development embryopathologically [1] and by 12 to 14 weeks ultrasonographically [101], manifested by developmental asymmetry in both general growth and size of specific viscera, particularly the heart. The plethoric recipient may produce more urine because of enhanced release of atrial natriuretic factor from the overloaded heart [191], creating hydramnios in over half the cases [192], and contributing to premature delivery. Twin mortality associated with TTS is high, up to 70% [1], although in some cases the complications of prematurity associated with the syndrome may be the greater risk. The donor sac will often have reduced fluid with secondary effects on fetal development, but occasionally it may also contain excessive amounts [1], and hydropic donor twins have been described [193].

The features found in chronically affected twin pairs include monochorial placentation with demonstrable appropriate anastomoses, plethora of one twin with pallor of the other, size and weight discrepancies that rarely may exceed 1000 grams [1, 109, 192] and red cell hematologic discrepancy that may reach 19 gm/dL of hemoglobin and 60% of hematocrit, although the differential is usually on the order of 5 gm/dL [186].

The placental pathology of chronic TTS includes details of the vascular connections and morphology of the villus tissues. It is worth emphasizing that some of the apparently less significant shunts anatomically may be quite important pathophysiologically, and may be present even though the cords are inserted quite far apart on the chorionic surface (up to 25 cm in our material). The donor villus tissue may look relatively immature with villus edema [190], possibly due to hypoproteinemia. This change reduces the intervillous space [194] and affects fetal capillary resistance [109], both of which would influence placental exchange and fetal nutrition. Occasionally, the donor placenta may have an ischemic appearance [1], either as a different pattern of placental response or as a later stage of the more edematous reaction pattern. The recipient's placental tissue is relatively normal developmentally, but the capillaries are markedly dilated and congested.

The lesions identified pathologically in the infants with chronic TTS include effects on development and complications of prematurity [109, 192]. Donor twins manifest changes due to chronic malnutrition, including marked reduction in weight but less reduction in length compared with that expected for gestational age, and reduced organ weights due to reduced cytoplasmic mass, particularly liver, spleen, thymus, and fetal adrenal cortex. The heart is particularly small, often only half the expected weight, due to decreased number and mass of cardiac fibers. These findings become more striking when donor and recipient are compared (Fig. 8.7). The recipient is of normal length and weight or may be slightly heavier than expected. The organs that are reduced in weight in the donor are heavier than expected in the recipient. The recipient's heart may weigh four times that of the donor and have signs of right-sided cardiomyopathy [195]. Parallel changes in pulmonary and systemic vessel muscle and elastic tissues also occur [196], and pulmonary artery calcification has been correlated with vascular overload [197]. Cutaneous hematopoiesis has been identified in the donor twins [198], but recipient twins tend to have more hepatic hematopoiesis [40]. The risk to the donor seems less than to the recipient for consequences of abnormal blood volume and composition [185, 198]. The donor may be at risk for ischemic/anoxic lesions due to the anemia, while the recipient may suffer from complications of plethora and hemoconcentration. The classic appearances of intertwin discrepancies are shown in Figure 8.7. Both the donor and the recipient appear to be equally susceptible to the complications of prematurity, which are important causes of death in these infants.

It is worth reemphasizing that not all growth discordancy in monochorial twins can be attributed to the twin-to-twin transfusion syndrome. Although simply documenting anastomoses is not necessarily confirmation that there actually was an asymmetry of flow, lack of appropriate anastomosis might indicate a search for other causes of asymmetry, such as asymmetric chorion development or fetomaternal hemorrhage from one twin. However, there may be cases of discordant twin development where anastomoses cannot be identified because of technical problems or because the shunts have become obliterated late in pregnancy.

Since Benirschke's description in 1961 [80], a number of cases have been reported that attribute apparently ischemic visceral lesions in the surviving twin who has a macerated co-twin to transchorionic disseminated intravascular coagulopathy [199]. The suggested mechanism is that thromboplastin-rich macerating blood from the dead twin crosses to the live twin, initiating a coagulopathy and leading to the consequences reported. The lesions described have included hydrancephaly and porencephaly [132], intestinal atresia [200, 201], renal cortical necrosis [202–204], multicystic encephalomalacia with cerebral palsy [132], and aplasia cutis [205]. However, monozygosity is proven in only a few instances [204], and even fewer reports refer to the placenta as actually being monochorionic or describe any vascular communications [202]. The lack of such corroborating evidence raises serious doubts about the explanations proposed in many of these reports. One Doppler study of blood flow patterns in the umbilical cord artery of the surviving twin failed to identify any abnormal flow patterns in the 24 hours between the death of the co-twin and the delivery of the survivor, although vascular anastomosis between the twins was confirmed pathologically [206]. Hypoxic/ischemic lesions could also be explained on the basis of an episode of shock or altered perfusion that could affect one twin or both twins such that one twin dies and one survives but is damaged [98].

There is no question that intrauterine vascular accidents occur in twins and that the presence of scarring and secondary anomalies attests to their occurrence some time before delivery [201, 202, 207]. The type of defect may vary with the approximate time in gestation that the perfusion insult occurred [207]. Early insults cause tissue damage that may be resorbed, leading to absence or atresia of structures. Such a mechanism may explain intestinal atresia, first and second branchial arch syndromes, and some terminal limb reduction defects. Later lesions leave residues of tissue necrosis and are exemplified by destructive lesions in the central nervous system and kidney. However, consumptive coagulopathy has not been well documented in surviving twins at delivery nor has thromboplastin been identified in their circulation. One investigation demonstrated that such twins had normal platelets and bleeding times and no problems with clinical hemostasis, although they were anemic [203].

Other causes of impaired intrauterine vascular supply or perfusional abnormalities in twins could be abruptio placenta, cord compression, fetomaternal hemorrhage [208], suddenly altered TTS hemodynamics across larger vessels [202, 209], vascular damage due to infection, vascular toxins, or premature ablation of transient vessels [207]. While transchorionic DIC may not be the cause in any one case, it is important to identify a potential vascular cause for an abnormality, because such a mechanism is unlikely to have genetic considerations and interpretative counseling can be given accordingly [207].

Because of the high mortality and morbidity in severe chronic twin transfusion syndrome, a number of therapeutic approaches have been tried. Selective feticide is fraught with unforseeable complications for the survivor [210]. Repeated amniocenteses of the hydramniotic sac have been more successful, but the outcome is still often unpredictable [211]. The most direct approach is interruption of the anastomotic vessels, but there are few centers with the appropriate procedural skills [212]. The pathologist may be required to assess the intertwin vasculature in some detail in these cases in order to explain unanticipated outcomes and complications.

Asymmetric Duplication

Endoparasitic and Ectoparasitic Twins

Although monozygous twins are often called "identical," implying symmetric duplication, some of the most bizarre anomalies of reproduction occur in this group of twins. These anomalies consist of various asymmetric duplications, including acardius/acephalus monsters, parasitic partial duplications, fetus-in-fetu, and the varieties of conjoined twins. When one developing embryo has an advantage over the other, the one suffering the disadvantage will be reduced in size and may be very abnormal in form. In fact, the abnormal embryo may not survive unless it is able to parasitize the more normal co-twin, either by anastomoses of chorionic circulations (chorangiopagus parasiticus or acardius/acephalus) or by actually attaching to the co-twin, externally (ectoparasite or heteroparasite) or internally

(endoparasite or fetus-in-fetu). This parasitism would allow the smaller member of a twin pair to survive with pronounced disturbances in structure, even if it has been reduced to a poorly differentiated mass of tissue more closely resembling a tumor and bearing no resemblance to its twin. Sometimes it can be very difficult to differentiate between abnormalities that result from twinning and those caused by primary neoplasia or by abnormal development of an isolated portion of a body [42]. The possible factors and forces leading to such asymmetries are reviewed in depth by Stockard [213]. Concepts of monozygotic duplication can be summarized as shown in Figure 8.8. The boundaries among these three patterns of asymmetric parasitic twins are far from distinct, and individual examples sometimes are not readily differentiated from teratomas or some of the cases described as conjoined twins.

The pathologic differentiation of a teratoma from an amorphous fetus, whether internal or external, remains to be defined [214]. One extensive review of over 100 reported cases of amorphous or variably fetiform masses failed to support the value of presence or absence of an umbilical cord and/or skeletal organization to differentiate a fetus amorphous from a teratoma [215]. These cases are rare, so as much should be learned from each case as possible.

Endoparasitic twins (fetus-in-fetu) are usually located in the upper abdominal retroperitoneum, with close anastomoses to the vitelline circulation [216]. Sex ratios are equal. Some are a single mass, others are subdivided into apparently nonduplicated parts [217]. Common tissues represented are vertebra, dermal structures, extremities, intestines, and neural tissues. Less common are gonads, adrenals, heart, and lungs. Pancreas and spleen are rare. The resemblance to the chorangiopagus parasitic twin can be striking. Detailed molecular studies have not yet settled whether these internal masses are unequally divided included twins or complex teratomas of premiotic stem cell origin [218].

The ectoparasitic partial duplications consist of various portions of duplicated parts, usually extremities, which are most often attached at the caudal end of the spine [219]. The degree of duplication may vary, and when there is more complete representation of the abnormal twin, this class of asymmetric duplication is indistinct from the class of conjoined twins [220]. Some of these anomalous duplications may be associated with an individual normal twin in the same conception, but, unfortunately, details of zygosity are usually lacking [221]. Chromosomal aneuploidy has been reported [222].

Chorangiopagus Parasiticus Twins

This classification of the asymmetric abnormality of monozygous twinning, referred to as "external" in the scheme in Figure 8.8, has gone through several phases. Although there are basic similarities, no two examples of this anomaly are identical, so the purely descriptive nosology based on external appearance has become quite complex. This is particularly so when classifications are modified, stating features of

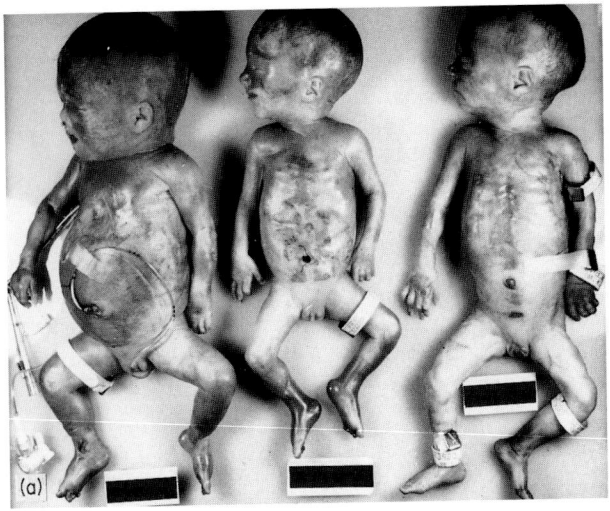

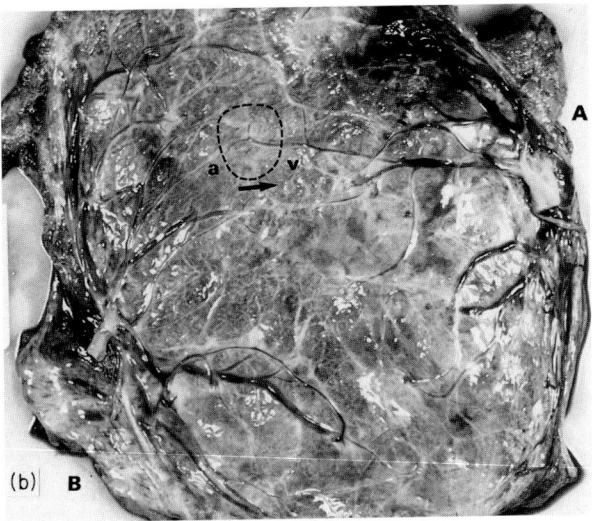

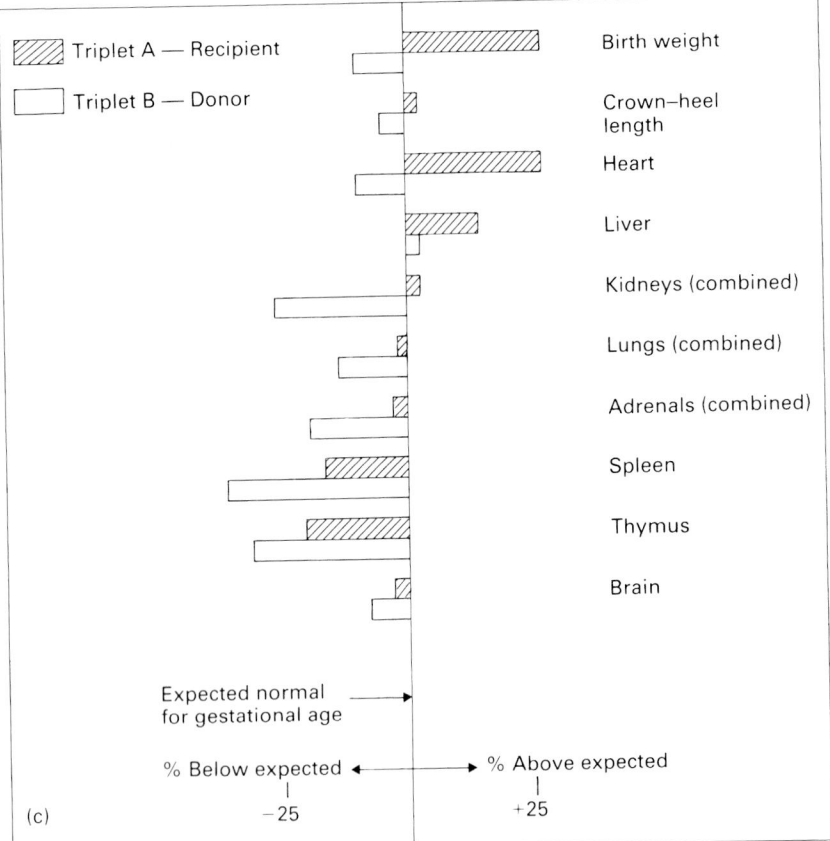

- Triplet A — Recipient
- Triplet B — Donor

Birth weight

Crown–heel length

Heart

Liver

Kidneys (combined)

Lungs (combined)

Adrenals (combined)

Spleen

Thymus

Brain

Expected normal for gestational age →

% Below expected ← → % Above expected

−25   +25

(c)

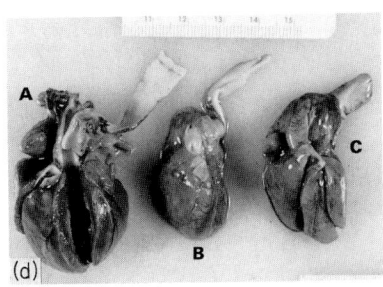

(d)

FIGURE 8.7. *(facing page and above) Chronic twin-to-twin transfusion syndrome. These triplets were delivered by caesarean section at 26 weeks after 4 weeks of repeated amniocentesis because of hydramnios. Triplets A and B were monochorionic diamniotic with intertwin anastomoses and twin-to-twin transfusion syndrome. Triplet C was a dizygous (by blood group) normal triplet for gestational age, used here as a standard for the other two. (a) Triplets—note the plethoric, edematous, and largest triplet A (1100 gm), the recipient of the twin-to-twin transfusion syndrome; the smallest triplet B (580 gm), the donor of the twin-to-twin transfusion syndrome; and the normally grown triplet C (840 gm). (b) Placenta of twin-to-twin transfusion syndrome pair. The disc is 660 gm and the cords are 18 cm apart. The surface is symmetrically vascularized with equal numbers of chorionic vessels. An arteriovenous shunt is located in the circled area with the artery (a) of triplet B to the vein (v) of triplet A. (c) Comparative growth and organ weights of the twin transfusion pair. Note particularly the disparity in weight and heart size. Even in those cases where the viscera weigh less than expected in both twins, the donor's organs weighed less than those of the recipient. (d) Hearts of all the triplets—note the relative sizes of the hearts. Triplet C's heart is the expected size for age. Triplet A's heart (recipient) is twice the expected weight and triplet B's heart (donor) is less than the expected weight by 27%. (e) Placental histology of triplets. Note the well-vascularized and normally cellular villi of the normal triplet (N), the sparser and poorly vascularized villi of the donor (D), and the bulkier, edematous villi of the recipient (R). (f) Placental histology at 24 weeks' gestation in another case of twin-to-twin transfusion syndrome to demonstrate the degree to which donor (D) and recipient (R) villous territories may differ. Taken in midzone of the placenta at the same magnification in each case. The donor tissue has a distinctly hypermature and ischemic appearance.*

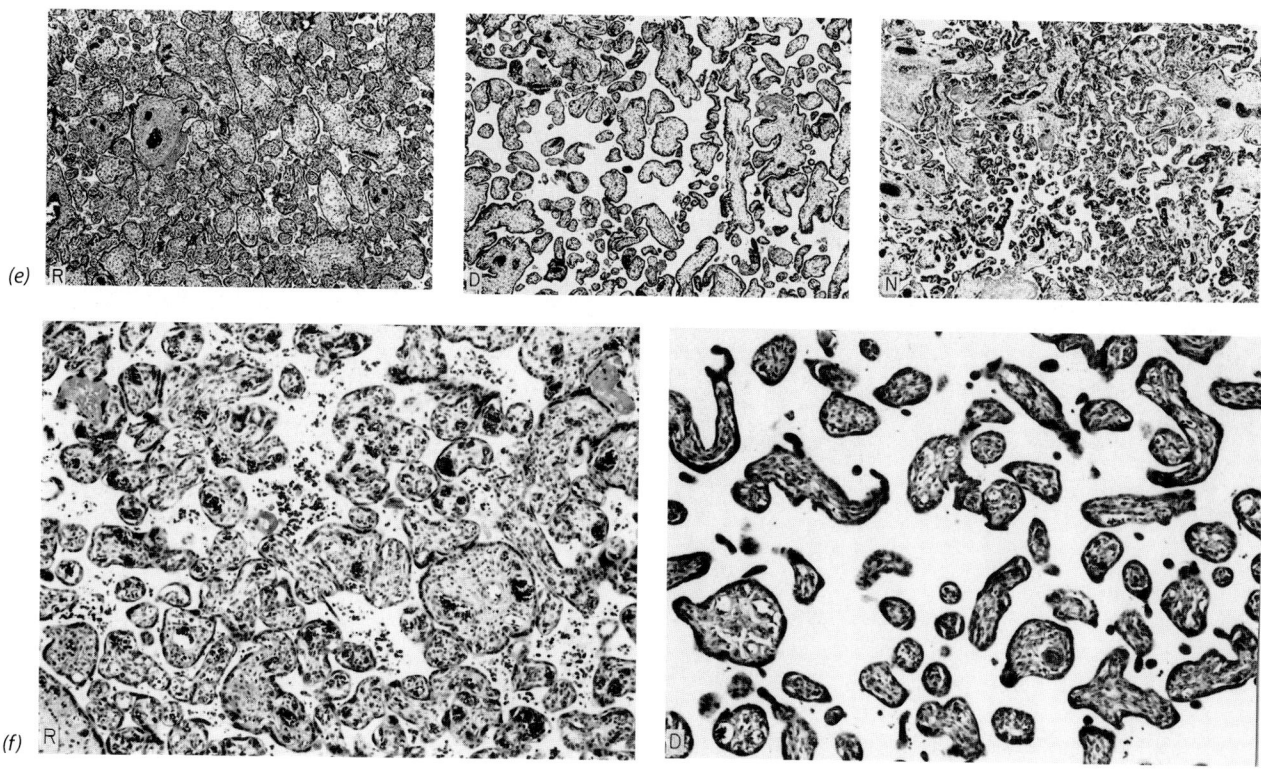

(e)

(f)

FIGURE 8.7. *Continued.*

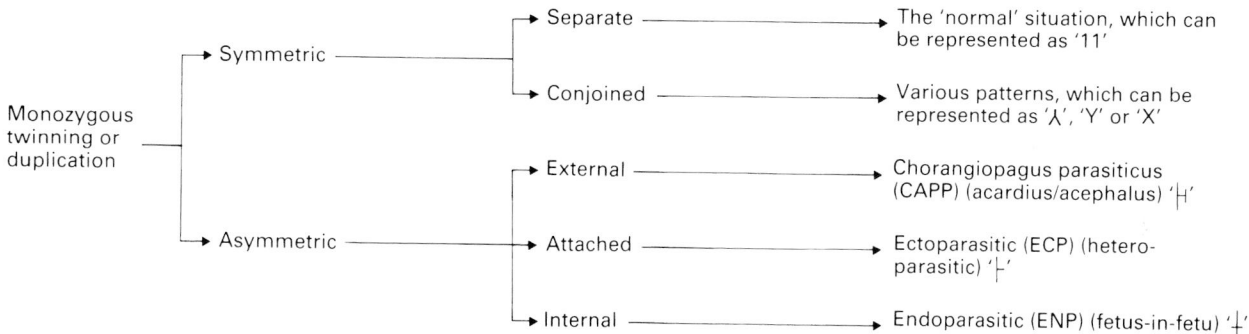

FIGURE 8.8. *Concepts of monozygotic duplication.*

Table 8.5. Classification and distribution of chorangiopagus parasiticus (CAPP) twins

Expanded classification with distribution [223]		Percent	Simplified classification [224]
Acardius holosomus (14.7%)	—holocranius	12.5 ⎤	Acardius anceps
	—hemicranius	2.3 ⎦	
Acardius hemisomus (68%)	—acephalus	10.2 ⎤	
	—holocranius	3.4	
	—hemicranius	6.8	
	—acranius	35.2	Acardius acephalus
	—athorax	6.8	
	—arrhachis	3.4 ⎦	
	—acormus—incompletus	1.1 ⎤	Acardius acormus
	—completus	1.1 ⎦	
Acardius amorphus (17%)	—externus	8.0	Acardius myelocephalus
	—totalis	9.1	Acardius amorphus

radiographic and dissection findings. Up to 12 different classes of the anomaly have been described, some of which have several names that are dissimilar [223, 224]. As can be seen from Table 8.5, the word "acardius" is common to all and often has been used to refer to the group as a whole. Auerback and Wigglesworth [225] recommended that the description of the placental-umbilical circulation findings be included and the term "twin reversed arterial perfusion" or TRAP sequence was suggested [226], because not all these abnormal twins are actually acardiac.

This anomaly represents the most common form of asymmetric twinning, occurring in 1% of monozygous twin pairs or 1 in 35,000 births [227]. It can be identified by ultrasound as early as 12 weeks [228]. The asymmetric twin survives only by parasitizing the more normally developed co-twin by way of circulatory conjunction of one form or another. The anomaly could thus be considered a form of conjoined twin in which the conjunction is at the chorionic circulation, hence chorangiopagus parasiticus [229]. It is suggested that this term represents the most uniform aspect of these cases because it indicates where these twins are joined without implications as to the shape of the abnormal twin or the presence or absence of other contributing abnormalities, such as chromosomal errors. Even the acronym, CAPP, is to an extent descriptive of the gross form.

The form of all CAPP twins consists of a gradient of malformations and reduction anomalies of virtually all tissues [229]. The form ranges from a fetus weighing several thousand grams who has a partially developed head, a deformed face, trunk, and arms, and virtually complete internal viscera, to an amorphous mass that might be confused with a teratoma [43, 125]. Even conjoined CAPP fetuses with a normal fetus in a triplet gestation have been described [227], as has a CAPP fetus conjoined to a normal twin through the gastrointestinal tract analogous to the endoparasitic asymmetric twin [230].

The most common pattern consists of a markedly edematous fetoform mass with relatively well-developed legs, incomplete pelvis and lower spine, and a central body cavity containing some incomplete abdominal viscera but usually no thoracic organs. The upper portion of the twin is usually a rounded dome that may have a barely visible suggestion of upper extremities or head and neck structures. Edematous tissues may be quite cystic in the "neck" region. This parasitic perfused twin has no placental vascular connections, and its cord vessels are conjoined with those of the supporting or parasitized pump twin on the surface of the placenta or somewhere along the cord in direct artery-to-artery and vein-to-vein anastomoses.

All of the pump twins available for analysis in one study had evidence of cardiovascular overload with cardiac failure but had no structural malformations or evidence of embolic phenomena [229]. In another study, however [20], 10% of the pump twins had malformations, and the anomalies were of the same type as in the CAPP twins that they nourished. Discordant diffuse visceral arterial medial calcification has been described in a pump twin [231], and pulmonary calcification

in the pump twin has been related to volume overload [197]. The heart of the pump twin is enlarged, with right ventricular hypertrophy and relative pulmonary stenosis. There is also hepatosplenomegaly with ascites and hypoalbuminemia due to impaired synthesis [232]. There may be edema severe enough to be considered hydrops [233].

Requirements for the CAPP situation are twofold [229]. First, there must be close proximity of the developing vessels of the two embryos on a common placenta so that direct vascular anastomoses can occur at the 18-to-21-day stage when the vascular network of the placenta connects with the umbilical allantoic vessels of the embryo. Second, there must be discordant development between the embryos, allowing the larger twin to assume the circulation of the delayed twin. The source of the initial delay or asymmetry could be a variety of influences, such as chromosomal anomalies [154], polar body twinning [40], a single umbilical artery cord [234], primary cardiac defects [42], or other structural malformations [226]. The blighted conceptus that results is able to survive only because of the vascular anastomoses to the co-twin, but there is a reversal of blood flow in the abnormal twin and the perfused twin receives poorly oxygenated "used" blood flowing in a reverse direction [76]. It is this hypoxic, abnormally flowing blood that is supposedly responsible for the resorption and reduction of previously formed tissues [235], with the caudal end of the embryo slightly better perfused and therefore more complete. In this situation the pump twin is also receiving an increased load of deoxygenated used blood as the flow from the CAPP returns directly to the co-twin without going through the placenta. It is possible that the severity of this abnormal perfusion is what determines the size, completeness, and organization of the CAPP. While the presence of only one umbilical artery in the cord is thought to be a prerequisite for this syndrome, enough cases with three-vessel cords have been described [223, 229] to suggest that the fact of vascular anastomoses is more important than the number of arteries in the cord.

There are extensive reviews available [116, 223, 226, 235, 236]. These reviews suggest that there is no sex differential, but two-thirds of our cases were males. There is a higher proportion of monoamniotic pairs and three times the frequency of CAPP twin pairs as part of a triplet set. The reported form of the CAPP twin spans the possibilities alluded to and is represented by some of our cases (Fig. 8.9). Perinatal mortality of the pump twin is 35% in twins and 45% in triplets overall [237], but improves if delivery can be delayed beyond 37 weeks. In our cases where pump twins survived, their co-twins were the most rudimentary of CAPP twins.

The recurrence risk seems not to be increased in subsequent pregnancies, as this abnormality has not been reported to recur.

Conjoined Twins

Conjoined twins are an abnormality of twinning in which two individuals of equal size are incompletely separated but

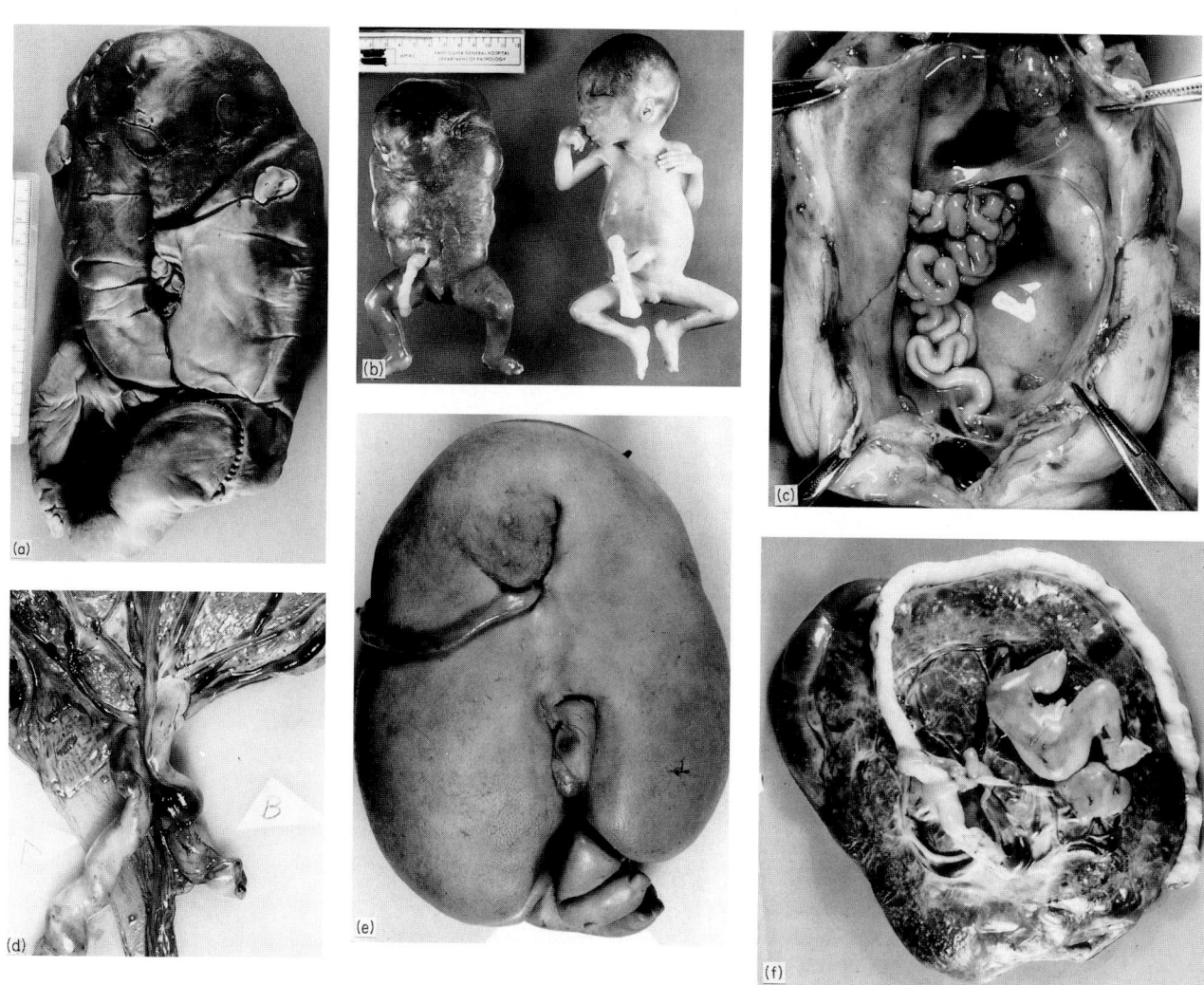

FIGURE 8.9.   *Chorangiopagus parasiticus (CAPP) twins. (a) A relatively large (1220 g) and moderately well-formed CAPP male of 32 weeks' gestation had a small disorganized multichambered, but thrombosed, heart. Pump twin died just before delivery. (b) Polyhydramnios led to premature delivery at about 20 weeks' gestation. The pump twin died in the newborn period due to immaturity and had no malformations but enlarged heart and liver. The CAPP twin was missing arms and most internal viscera but had a remarkable amount of brain tissue. It died just before delivery, with numerous thromboses of internal vessels. (c) This CAPP twin had a simple tubular "heart" in the upper part of the body cavity and some indeterminate bowel which ended in a rectum. Also, there was an allantois with cystic dysplastic kidneys, and normal testes were present internally. Note the very edematous subcutaneous tissues. There were extensive areas of ischemic brain damage with scarring. The pump twin had heart failure in utero but survived after spontaneous delivery at 32 weeks. (d) This represents the conjunction of the CAPP twin in (c)—a direct artery-to-artery and vein-to-vein anastomosis at the level of the cord of the pump twin (B). The membranes between the cords are the diamniotic separating membranes. (e) One of the more rudimentary but large (1780 gm) CAPP twins with a direct artery-to-artery and vein-to-vein anastomosis at the placental margin. The pump twin was normal and did well. Internal viscera consisted of a length of bowel, a gonad, and a kidney in a space about 3 cm in diameter. (f) Unsuspected CAPP twin parts with a normal male full-term pump twin. By foot length, 15 weeks' development. "Legs" unattached at time specimen received. Amorphous mass attached to long two-vessel "cord." Monoamniotic.*

have an overall symmetry no matter what the pattern of conjunction. The unity or duality of conjoined twins is an interesting philosophical and ethical consideration, particularly when a process of surgical separation is being considered that may require sacrifice of one twin. Even the pathologist may be faced with the mundane question as to whether to assign one postmortem number or two to a set of conjoined twins.

The incidence of conjoined twins quoted is 1 in 33,000 to 1 in 165,000 Caucasian deliveries [1, 28, 238, 239], 1 in 58,000 in Singapore [240], and a much higher rate of 1 in 6454 reported by the Taipei collaborative study [30]. Six

percent of conjoined twins are part of triplets [20]. There is a striking female preponderance of up to 95% of the reported cases [42], although females usually represent around 70% in any series [28, 238]. This excess of females may be related to the pathogenesis of the anomaly analogous to the previous discussion of the mechanisms of monozygous twinning and its relation to delay factors and the XX zygote.

Conjoined twinning does not appear to be related to factors of maternal age or gravidity. The relationship to a family history of twins is less certain. Apparently, more than 1000 descendants of Chang and Eng Bunker have been

Table 8.6.   Classification and terminology of conjoined twins. (From Guttmacher and Nichols [243].)

Terata catydidymus

Single in the lower body and double above, or a pair of twins joined by some portion of the lower body.

Variants

Diprosopus—2 faces with 1 head and 1 body.

Dicephalus—2 heads and necks with one body.

Ischiopagus—joined by the inferior margins of the coccyx and sacrum, the two completely separate spinal columns lying in the same axis.

Pyopagus—joined by the lateral and posterior surfaces of the coccyx and sacrum, which are single, the rest of the two bodies being normally duplicated; these twins are almost back to back.

Terata anadidyma

Single in the upper portion of the body and double below, or a pair of twins joined by some region of the upper part of the body.

Variants

Dipygus—1 head, thorax, and abdomen with 2 pelves with or without two sets of external genitalia and up to 4 legs.

Syncephalus—joined by the face. The faces are turned laterally and are each made up of the right side of one and the left side of the other. The twins may be separate except for this or further joined by the thorax, but are separate from the umbilicus down.

Craniopagus—joined at some homologous portion of the cranial vault, being separate at all other points.

Terata anacatadidyma

Twins joined by the midportion of the body and being separate and double above and below the shared region.

Variants

Thoracopagus—part of the thoracic wall and contained viscera is common to both twins.

Omphalopagus—these twins are joined from the umbilicus to the xiphoid.

Rachipagus—twins united at the vertebral column at any point above the sacrum.

traced with only one set of twins identified [240]. However, a family history of monozygous twins was identified in a group of Arab conjoined twins [241].

The patterns of conjoined twins are infinitely varied. If the twins are more separate than fused, they are usually joined anteriorly, posteriorly, cranially, or caudally. If they are more fused than separate, they are usually joined laterally [42]. The degrees of conjunction in any of these alignments can be considered as part of a continuum from the single individual to the separate pair of twin individuals. Whole systems of conjoined twins are possible [242]. As might be imagined, the classification of these twins is complicated and tends to be descriptive of the site and extent of the union, sometimes including details of head and extremity numbers and orientation. Also, there does not seem to be agreement on whether to emphasize the zone that is conjoined or to describe the portions that are duplicated. Basically, the conjunction can be of upper body portions, lower body components, or middle zone regions, as indicated by the symbols in Table 8.6. The classification used by Guttmacher and Nichols [243] is etymologically accurate and straightforward and is useful as a broad scheme of categorization into which most cases could be placed, with further descriptive modifiers as needed (see Table 8.6).

In addition to the terms in Table 8.6, some additional terms have become accepted. Syncephalus twins may also be known as janiceps or cephalothoracopagus twins, depending on the degree of fusion [244]. The diprosopus twins have also

been termed lateral cephalothoracopagus anomalies [245]. The lateral rostral duplications have been described in some of the most complex terms, with combinations of words used to specify the number of heads, arms, and legs in each case—e.g., dicephalus tribrachius dipus. Omphalopagus twins are also referred to as xiphopagus [246].

When the frequencies of the different patterns of conjunction are analyzed (Table 8.7), centrally conjoined twins

Table 8.7.   Frequencies of different patterns of conjoined twins

		Edmonds [238]	Rudolph [263]
Catadidyma 6.2	Dicephalus	3.7	—
	Pyopagus	2.5	18.8
	Ischiopagus	—	5.9
Anadidyma 8.6	Syncephalus	2.4	—
	Craniopagus	6.2	1.7
Anacatadidyma 59.3	Thoracopagus	18.5	73.4
	Omphalopagus	9.9	
	Xiphopagus	2.5	
	Thoraco-omphalopagus	28.4	
Other 25.9	Parasitic	9.9	
	Combination	12.3	
	Not stated	3.7	

Numbers refer to percentages of each type in the individual series.

Table 8.8. References for conjoined twins

Conjoined twins generally	Bergsma [87], Tan [240], Potter [42], Edmonds [238]
Diprosopus	Barr [251], Chervenak—31 cases [252]
Dicephalus	Konstantinova [222]
Cephalothoracopagus	Herring [244], Merwin [245]
Thoracopagus	Nichols—42 cases [247]
Xiphopagus	Harper—36 cases [246]
Pyopagus	Gupta [264]

are considerably more common than all of the others combined. Since somite development begins centrally and spreads caudally and cranially, the extremities of the embryo may be able to duplicate later than the central portions. This may account for the preponderance of thoracopagus twins.

Conjoined twins have a high mortality rate [238]. Nearly 40% are stillborn and an additional one-third die in less than 24 hours. The cases that die soon after birth are usually extensively joined with serious abnormalities of internal organs, which are often fused. Why the individuals in some sets of minimally conjoined twins die very close together in time is still not understood (e.g., Chang and Eng Bunker), although some form of disseminated intravascular coagulopathy or exsanguination across the shared circulation into the dead twin is possible.

Because the pathology of these twins is infinitely variable, only a brief review of the more common basic patterns is presented here, and the references given should be consulted for further details if one is faced with the examination of one of these cases (Table 8.8). One of the most extensive photographic catalogues is provided by Potter and Craig in their text [42].

The placentae are always monochorionic monoamniotic, and there may be a single cord from the surface of the placenta, or two cords that originate separately may fuse closer to the infant(s). The numbers of cord vessels range from one artery and one vein to four arteries and two veins.

There are two types of malformations in the affected infants [230]: those malformations of the conjoined organs that probably are related to the process of impaired twinning itself, and those malformations in nonconjoined organs that may or may not be related to the twinning process. These two types of malformations may be termed secondary and primary, respectively, and either can be concordant or discordant.

The most common pattern of conjoined twins is face-to-face fusion of the thorax and variable portions of the abdomen—thoracopagus. There is extensive literature concerning the anatomy of such twins, with particular reference to the possibility of surgical separation [87].

Although thoracopagus twins are basically symmetric, there is often a degree of disparity of size and hardiness [247]. One of the most critical factors in survival or sepa-

ration of these twins is the degree of cardiac fusion. Although cardiac fusion is present in 75% of cases [248], the degree of fusion cannot be predicted by the degree of thoracic fusion [249]. Atrial fusion is almost always present if any fusion exists at all, and a common pericardium is observed in 90% of cases. The conjoined heart is in the frontal plane, although the bodies are in the lateral plane. Detailed analyses of the cardiovascular defects are available [247, 248, 250].

The degree of fusion of other viscera varies. The liver is shared in all cases, but the intestinal tract is shared in only about half of the cases. Pleural spaces are usually separate. There may be an omphalocele at the site of a conjoined umbilicus. One of the limiting factors in the survival of these infants is that there is often a lethal degree of pulmonary hypoplasia due to loss of thoracic volume secondary to the conjunction.

Many of the anomalies in these twins seem to be manifestations of alterations in body symmetry [249]. The normally asymmetric structures (heart and great vessels, lungs, liver, spleen, and gastrointestinal tract) are rendered more symmetric. The normally symmetric structures (brain, upper respiratory tract, urogenital system, and skeleton) are less severely affected or not affected at all.

The most readily separable conjoined twins are the omphalopagus twins, since their union may involve only skin and portions of liver, as in Chang and Eng Bunker, occasionally including portions of the sternum [247]. The reported distribution of conjoined tissue in xiphopagus twins is as follows: liver in 81% of cases, cartilage in 56%, diaphragm in 17%, genitourinary tract in 3%, and skin only in 6.0% [246]. In 53% of the cases, both twins survived. Twenty-five percent had concordant cardiac malformations and 33% had concordant gastrointestinal anomalies.

Neural tube defects are frequently associated with craniofacial duplications [244, 251]. While there is a spectrum of facial duplication from isolated nasal duplication to the complete doubling of all facial structures, as in the diprosopus [252], it might be questioned whether this type of anomaly is truly a conjoined twin or merely a regional duplication for some other reason. Is there in fact a class of so-called conjoined twins who are not the result of incomplete fission or codominant axes, but who are the result of forces leading to the variable duplications of localized parts, analogous to other regional duplications, such as polydactyly? The varieties of facial duplications are to be considered separately from the median cleft face syndromes, however [251].

In the lateral conjunctions of the lower body, there is duplication of the viscera roughly proportional to that of the cerebrospinal axis.

In the cephalothoracopagus twins [244], the cranial fusions may be lateral or janiceps type. The thoracic or abdominal organs are usually duplicated. The heart and anterior intestinal derivatives tend to be oriented anteroposteriorly and to be shared by the twins rather than belonging to the right or left individual. The posterior organs tend to maintain a right and left orientation.

Nine cases of conjoined twins as parts of triplet sets have been described [253]. Two-thirds were thoracopagus twins and the normal triplet was of the same sex in all but one case, although zygosity was not stated. Conjoined CAPP twins have also been described in a monochorionic triplet pregnancy [227].

TRIPLETS AND HIGHER MULTIPLES

Triplet gestations represent 1 in 1014 deliveries in Eastern Nigeria [26], 1 in 1300 in the southeastern United States [12], 1 in 3687 in Taipei [30], and 1 in 10,000 in Chicago [12] and in the Collaborative Perinatal Project in the United States [71]. All the aspects of multiple gestation that have so far been discussed also apply to triplets and any higher multiples [254, 255]. It has been suggested that as many as one-third of the pregnancies that begin as triplets deliver as singletons [167, 256]. There are well-described cases where one or two members of a triplet gestation were papyraceous fetuses at the time of delivery of the survivor [167], and other examples of delayed delivery of surviving triplets after earlier death and/or delivery of one or two members [178]. In one survey [26], one-third of the infants died around the time of birth and the mortality rate varied with birth order: 22% for triplet 1 and 38.9% each for triplets 2 and 3. The death rates were equal for both sexes. Patterns and concordance of malformations in triplets have the same considerations as those in twins. Heterokaryotic triplets with anomalies of sex chromosomes or trisomy 21 are described [152, 154]. A triplet pregnancy may also include a set of conjoined twins [221, 227, 253] or CAPP twins [20]. The placentation in triplets ranges from monochorionic monoamniotic [179] to trichorionic triamniotic separate discs [12]. The commonest pattern is two discs, one of which is monochorionic diamniotic or dichorionic diamniotic. Fox [43] recorded the chorionicity in triplets as 42% trichorionic, 42% dichorionic, and 16% monochorionic. In one series [26], 44% of the triplet sets were of the same sex, of which 58% were male and 42% female. Of the mixed sets, 70% consisted of two females with one male, and 30% consisted of two males with one female.

The higher multiples of human conceptions are sufficiently rare that they are often the subject of single case reports. Mayer [257] gave a delightful review of probable, possible, and pretentious reports of six to 365 "infants" at a single parturition. He described some reasonably well-documented and truly phenomenal examples of fertility, which occurred long before the so-called "fertility drugs." The unfortunate features of some of these reports are that details of the placental relationships are incomplete and zygosity is often assessed inaccurately. The zygosity combinations in natural multiples [258] probably represent a random distribution, whereas drug-induced multiples are usually polyovulatory [259]. All the considerations that have been discussed regarding twins apply just as well to these grand multiples. Fortunate indeed is the pathologist who has the opportunity of examining the placentae and infants from such a gestation.

EXTRAUTERINE MULTIPLE PREGNANCY

Extrauterine multiple pregnancies are rare, although it has been suggested that combined pregnancies (one intrauterine and one tubal or intrauterine multiples plus tubal) may become more common with drug-induced ovulation [260].

Bilateral tubal ectopic pregnancies, tubal twins, and tubal triplets have been reported with a greater ratio of monochorial gestations than usual. Tubal lesions that lead to delay in transport of the fertilized egg may predispose to monozygous twinning, or monochorial embryos may be more prone to implantation in the tubes [12]. Ovarian twin pregnancies have also been reported [261].

CONCLUSION

The pathology of multiple pregnancy includes considerations of basic processes in reproduction and embryology, normal development and teratology, genetic and environmental influences on development, as well as all the concepts of disease and developmental disorders encountered in single infants. Similarly, the placentology of multiple conceptions adds several dimensions to the interpretations required in singletons. It is no wonder that this is an area that has attracted medical attention over the years. The quality and usefulness of much of the material that has been written concerning multiple gestations are in direct proportion to the thoughtful precision and completeness of the pathologic components of the descriptions and interpretations.

REFERENCES

1. Benirschke K, Kim CK. Multiple pregnancy. *N Engl J Med* 1973; 288:1276–84, 1329–36.
2. Wyshak G. Statistical findings on the effects of fertility drugs in plural births. Twin Research: Biology & Epidemiology. In: Nance W, ed. *Progress in Clinical & Biological Research* 1978; 24B:17–33.
3. Schneider L, Bessis R, Simonnet T. The frequency of ovular resorption during the first trimester of twin pregnancy. *Acta Genet Med Gemellol* 1979; 28:271–2.
4. Zeilmaker GH, Alberda AT, van Gent I. Fertilization and cleavage of oocytes from a binovular human ovarian follicle: a possible cause of dizygotic twinning and chimerism. *Fertil Steril* 1983; 40:841–3.
5. Yovich JL, Stanger JD, Grauaug A, et al. Monozygotic twins from *in vitro* fertilization. *Fertil Steril* 1984; 41:833–7.
6. Terasaki PI, Gjertson D, Bernoco D, et al. Twins with two different fathers identified by HLA. *N Engl J Med* 1978; 299:590–92.
7. Nance WE. Malformations unique to the twinning process. Twin Research 3: Twin Biology and Multiple Pregnancy. In: Gedda L, Parisi P, Nance WE, eds. *Progress in Clinical & Biological Research* 1981; 69A:123–33.
8. Golan A, Amit A, Baram A, David MP. Unusual cord intertwining in monoamniotic twins. *Aust NZ J Obstet Gynecol* 1982; 22:165–7.
9. Benirschke K, Driscoll SG. *The Pathology of the Human Placenta*. New York: Springer-Verlag, 1967, pp. 91–179.
10. Boklage CE. On the timing of monozygotic twinning events. Twin Research 3: Twin Biology and Multiple Pregnancy. In: Gedda L, Parisi P, Nance WE, eds. *Progress in Clinical & Biological Research* 1981; 69A:155–65.
11. Gedda L, Brenci G, Franceschetti A, Talone C, Ziparo R. A study of mirror imaging in twins. Twin research 3: Twin biology and multiple pregnancy. In: Gedda L, Parisi P, Nance WE, eds. *Progress in Clinical & Biological Research* 1981; 69A:167–8.

12. Shanklin DR, Perrin EVDK. Multiple gestation. In: Perrin EVDK, ed. *Pathology of the Placenta, Contemporary Issues in Surgical Pathology*, Vol. 5. New York: Churchill Livingstone, 1984, Ch. 7, pp. 165–82.

13. Smith DW, Bartlett C, Harrah LM. Monozygotic twinning and the Duhamel anomalad (inperforate anus to sirenomelia): a nonrandom association between two aberrations in morphogenesis. *Birth Defects Orig Artic Ser* 1976; 12(5):53–63.

14. Flannery DB, Brown JA, Redwine FO, Winter P, Nance WE. Antenatally detected Klinefelter's syndrome in twins. *Acta Genet Med Gemellol* 1984; 33:51–6.

15. Uchida IA, deSA DJ, Whelan DT. 45,X/46,XX mosaicism in discordant monozygotic twins. *Pediatrics* 1983; 71:413–17.

16. Windham GC, Sever LE. Neural tube defects among twin births. *Am J Hum Genet* 1982; 34:988–98.

17. Wright JCY, Christopher CR. Sirenomelia, Potter's syndrome and their relationship to monozygotic twinning (a case report and discussion). *J Reprod Med* 1982; 27:291–4.

18. Rowe MI, Ravitch MM, Ranniger K. Operative correction of caudal duplication (dipygus). *Surgery* 1968; 63:840–48.

19. German JC, Mahour GH, Wooley MM. The twin with esophageal atresia. *J Pediatr Surg* 1979; 14:432–5.

20. Schinzel AAGL, Smith DW, Miller JR. Monozygotic twinning and structural defects. *J Pediatr* 1979; 95:921–30.

21. Macourt DC, Stewart P, Zaki M. Multiple pregnancy and fetal abnormalities in association with oral contraceptive use. *Aust NZ J Obstet Gynecol* 1982; 22:25–8.

22. James WH. Sex ratio and placentation in twins. *Ann Hum Biol* 1980; 7:273–6.

23. Mettler L, Riedel H-H, Grillo M, et al. Schwangerschaft und Geburt monozygoter weiblicher Zwillinge nach In-Vitro-Fertilisation und Embryotransfer (IVF-ET). *Geburtshilfe Frauenheikd* 1984; 44:670–76.

24. Robinson HP, Caines JS. Sonar evidence of early pregnancy failure in patients with twin conceptions. *Br J Obstet Gynaecol* 1977; 84:22–5.

25. Cameron AH, Edwards JH, Derom R, Thiery M, Boelaert R. The value of twin surveys in the study of malformation. *Eur J Obstet Gynecol Reprod Biol* 1983; 14:347–56.

26. Eqwuatu VE. Triplet pregnancy: a review of 27 cases. *Int J Gynecol Obstet* 1980; 18:460–64.

27. Marivate M, Norman RJ. Twins. *Clin Obstet Gynecol* 1982; 9(B):723–43.

28. Myrianthopoulos NC. Congenital malformation in twins: epidemiologic survey. *Birth Defects Orig Artic Ser* 1975; X1(8):1–39.

29. Allen G. Errors of Weinberg's difference method. Twin Research 3: Twin Biology and Multiple Pregnancy. In: Gedda L, Parisi P, Nance WE, eds. *Progress in Clinical & Biological Research* 1981;69A:71–4.

30. Emanuel I, Huang S-W, Gutman LT, Yu F-C, Lin C-C. The incidence of congenital malformations in a Chinese population: the Taipei collaborative study. *Teratology* 1972; 5:159–69.

31. Phillips DIW. Twin studies in medical research: can they tell us whether diseases are genetically determined? *Lancet* 1993; 341:1008–9.

32. Hoffman HJ, Bakketeig LS, Stark CR. Twins and perinatal mortality: a comparison between single and twin births in Minnesota and in Norway, 1967–1973. Twin Research: Biology & Epidemiology. In: Nance W, eds. *Progress in Clinical & Biological Research* 1978; 24B:133–42.

33. Bulmer MG. *The Biology of Twinning in Man*. Oxford: Clarendon, 1970.

34. Corney G, Robson EB. Types of twinning and determination of zygosity. In: MacGillivray I, Nylander PPS, Corney G, eds. *Human Multiple Reproduction*. Philadelphia: W.B. Saunders, Ch. 2, pp. 16–39.

35. Smith SM, Penrose LS. Monozygotic and dizygotic twin diagnosis. *Ann Hum Genet* 1955; 19:273–89.

36. Fisher RA, Sheppard DM, Lawler SD. Twin pregnancy with complete hydatidiform mole (46,XX) and fetus (46,XY): genetic origin proved by analysis of chromosome polymorphism. *Br Med J* 1982; 284(6324):1218–20.

37. Hill AVS, Jeffreys AJ. Use of minisatellite DNA probes for determination of twin zygosity at birth. *Lancet* 1985; 21/28:1394–5.

38. Bieber FR, Nance WE, Morton CC, et al. Genetic studies of an acardiac monster: evidence of polar body twinning in man. *Science* 1981; 213:775–7.

39. Gilgenkrantz S, Marchal C, Wendremaire P, Seger M. Cytogenetic and antigenic studies in a pair of twins: a normal boy and a trisomic 21 girl with chimera. Twin Research 3: Twin Biology and Multiple Pregnancy. In: Gedda L, Parisi P, Nance WE, eds. *Progress in Clinical & Biological Research* 1981; 69A:141–53.

40. Strong SJ, Corney G. *The Placenta in Twin Pregnancy*. Norwich, UK: Pergamon, 1967.

41. Kloosterman GJ. The "Third Circulation" in identical twins. *Ned Tijdschr Verloskd Gynaecol* 1963; 63:395–412.

42. Potter EL, Craig JM. *Pathology of the Fetus and the Infant*. 3rd ed. Chicago: Year Book Medical Publishing, 1975, pp. 180–97, 207–37.

43. Fox H. Pathology of the placenta. In: Benninger JL, ed. *Major Problems in Pathology*, Vol. II. Philadelphia: W.B. Saunders, 1978.

44. Benirschke K, Kaufmann P. *Pathology of the Human Placenta*. 2nd ed. New York: Springer-Verlag, 1990, pp. 638–43.

45. Baldwin VJ. *Pathology of Multiple Pregnancy*. New York: Springer-Verlag, 1994, pp. 29–56, 227–8.

46. Buzzard IM, Uchida IA, Norton JA, Christian JC. Birth weight and placental proximity in like sex twins. *Am J Hum Genet* 1983; 35:318–23.

47. Corey LA, Nance WE, Kang KW, Christian JC. Effects of type of placentation on birthweight and its variability in monozygous and dizygous twins. *Acta Genet Med Gemollol* 1979; 28:41–50.

48. Corney G. Placentation. In: MacGillivray I, Nylander PPS, Corney G, eds. *Human Multiple Reproduction*. Philadelphia: W.B. Saunders, 1975, Ch. 3, pp. 40–76.

49. Cameron AM. The Birmingham twin survey. *R Soc Med Proc* 1968; 61:229–34.

50. Fujikura T, Froehlich LA. Twin placentation and zygosity. *Obstet Gynecol* 1971; 37:34–43.

51. Segreti WO, Winter PM, Nance WE. Familial studies of monozygotic twinning. Twin Research: Biology & Epidemiology. In: Nance W, ed. *Progress in Clinical & Biological Research*, Vol. 24B. 1978, pp. 55–60.

52. Ottolenghi-Pretti GF. Sopra un rarissimo caso di gravidanza gemellare con un feto papiraceo e con inserzione velamentosa del funicolo del feto vivo. *Ann Ostet Ginecol Med Perinat* 1972; 93:173–99.

53. Sekiya S, Hafez ESE. Physiomorphology of twin transfusion syndrome: a study of 86 twin gestations. *Obstet Gynecol* 1977; 50:288–92.

54. La Vecchia C, Franceschi S, Fasoli M, Mangioni C. Gestational trophoblastic neoplasms in homozygous twins. *Obstet Gynecol* 1982; 60:250–52.

55. De George FV. Hydatidiform moles in other pregnancies of mothers of twins. *Am J Obstet Gynecol* 1970; 108:369–71.

56. Beischer NA. Hydatidiform mole with coexistent foetus. *Aust NZ J Obstet Gynecol* 1966; 6:127–41.

57. Yee B, Tu B, Platt LD. Coexisting hydatidiform mole with a live fetus presenting as a placenta previa on ultrasound. *Am J Obstet Gynecol* 1982; 144:726–8.

58. Hoshi K, Morimura Y, Azuma C, et al. A case of quadruplet pregnancy containing complete mole and three fetuses. *Am J Obstet Gynecol* 1994; 170:1372–3.

59. Hohe PT, Cochrane CR, Gmelich JT, Austin JA. Coexistent trophoblastic tumor and viable pregnancy. *Obstet Gynecol* 1971; 38:899–904.

60. Suzuki M, Matsunobu A, Wakita K, Nishijima M, Osanai K. Hydatidiform mole with a surviving coexisting fetus. *Obstet Gynecol* 1980; 56:384–8.

61. Robertson EG, Neer KJ. Placental injection studies in twin gestations. *Am J Obstet Gynecol* 1983; 147:170–4.

62. Farr V. Prognoses for the babies, early and late. In: MacGillivray I, Nylander PPS, Corney G, eds. *Human Multiple Reproduction*. Philadelphia: W.B. Saunders, 1975, Ch. 14, pp. 188–211.

63. Bender S. Twin pregnancy (a review of 472 cases). *J Obstet Gynecol Br Common* 1952; 59:510–17.

64. Desgranges M-F, de Muylder X, Moutquin J-M, Lazaro-Lopez F, Leduc B. Perinatal profile of twin pregnancies: a retrospective view of 11 years (1969–1979) at Hopital Notre-Dame, Montreal, Canada. *Acta Genet Med Gemellol* 1982; 31:157–63.

65. MacGillivray I. Twins and other multiple deliveries. *Clin Obstet Gynecol* 1980; 7:581–600.

66. Knuppel RA, Rattan PK, Scerbo JC, O'Brien WF. Intrauterine fetal death in twins after 32 weeks of gestation. *Obstet Gynecol* 1985; 65:172–5.

67. Keith L, Ellis R, Berger GS, Depp R. The Northwestern University multihospital twin study. I. A description of 588 twin pregnancies and associated pregnancy loss, 1971 to 1975. *Am J Obstet Gynecol* 1980; 138:781–9.

68. Manlan G, Scott KE. Contribution of twin pregnancy to perinatal mortality and fetal growth retardation: reversal of growth retardation after birth. *Can Med Assoc J* 1978; 118:365–8.

69. Sehgal NN. Perinatal mortality in twin pregnancies (implications for clinical management). *Postgrad Med* 1980; 68:231–4.

70. Layde PM, Erickson JD, Falek A, McCarthy BJ. Congenital malformations in twins. *Am J Hum Genet* 1980; 32:69–78.

71. Myrianthopoulos NC. An epidemiologic survey of twins in a large, prospectively studied population. *Am J Hum Genet* 1970; 22:611–29.

72. Ferguson WF. Perinatal mortality in multiple gestations (a review of perinatal deaths from 1609 multiple gestations). *Obstet Gynecol* 1963; 23:861–70.

73. Potter EL. Twin zygosity and placental form in relation to the outcome of pregnancy. *Am J Obstet Gynecol* 1963; 87:566–77.

74. Zahalkova M. Perinatal and infant mortality in twins. Twin Research: Biology & Epidemiology. In: Nance W, ed. *Progress in Clinical & Biological Research*, 1978; 24B:115–20.

75. Chandra P, Harilal KT. Plural births—mortality and morbidity. Twin Research: Biology & Epidemiology. In: Nance W, ed. *Progress in Clinical & Biological Research* 1978; 24B:109–14.

76. Leroy F. Major fetal hazards in multiple pregnancy. *Acta Genet Med Gemellol* 1976; 25:299–306.

77. Ho SK, Wu PYK, Perinatal factors and neonatal morbidity in twin pregnancy. *Am J Obstet Gynecol* 1975; 122:979–87.

78. Naeye RL. *Disorders of the Placenta, Fetus, and Neonate: Diagnosis and Clinical Significance*. St. Louis: Mosby Year Book, 1992, pp. 277–92.

79. Gruenwald P. Environmental influences on twins apparent at birth (a preliminary study). *Biol Neonat* 1970; 15:79–93.

80. Benirschke K. Twin placenta in perinatal mortality. *NY State J Med* 1961; 61:1499–1508.

81. Ordorica SA, Hoskins IA, Young BK. Acid-base differences in preterm and term twin pregnancy. *Acta Genet Med Gemellol* 1991;40:345–51.

82. Young BK, Suidan J, Antoine C, et al. Differences in twins: the importance of birth order. *Am J Obstet Gynecol* 1985; 151:915–21.

83. Puissant F, Leroy F. A reappraisal of perinatal mortality factors in twins. *Acta Genet Med Gemellol* 1982; 31:213–19.

84. Hawrylyshyn PA, Barkin M, Bernstein A, Papsin PR. Twin pregnancies—a continuing perinatal challenge. *Obstet Gynecol* 1982; 59:463–6.

85. Knuppel RA, Shah DM, Rattan PK, O'Brien WF, Lerner A. Rhesus isoimmunization in twin gestation. *Am J Obstet Gynecol* 1984; 150:136–41.

86. Manning FA, Bowman JM, Lange IR, Chamberlain PF. Intrauterine transfusion in an Rh-immunized twin pregnancy: a case report of successful outcome and a review of the literature. *Obstet Gynecol* 1985; 65:25–55.

87. Bergsma D, Blattner RJ, Nichols BL, Rudolph AJ. Conjoined twins. *Birth Defects Orig Artic Ser* 1967; 3(1):1–147.

88. Zemlickis D, Lishner M, Erlich R, Koren G. Teratogenicity and carcinogenicity in a twin exposed in utero to cyclophosphamide. *Teratogenesis Carcinog Mutagen* 1993; 13(3):139–43.

89. Elliott J, Radin T. Glucose tolerance testing in high order multiple gestations. *Am J Obstet Gynecol* 1993; 168(1, part2):331.

90. Henderson CE, Scarpelli S, Divon MY. The prevalence of gestational diabetes is similar for twin and singleton gestations. *Am J Obstet Gynecol* 1993; 168(1, part 2):406. Abstract.

91. Blickstein I, Ben-Hur H, Borenstein R. Perinatal outcome of twin pregnancies complicated with preeclampsia. *Am J Perinatol* 1992; 9(4):258–60.

92. Koivisto M, Jouppila P, Kauppila A, Moilanen I, Ylikorkala O. Twin pregnancy, neonatal morbidity and mortality. *Acta Obstet Gynecol* 1975; 44:21–9.

93. Weir PE, Ratten GL, Beischer NA. Acute polyhydramnios—a complication of monozygous twin pregnancy. *Br J Obstet Gynaecol* 1979; 86:849–53.

94. Romero R, Duffy TP, Berkowitz RL, Chang E, Hobbins JC. Prolongation of a preterm pregnancy complicated by death of a single twin in utero and disseminated intravascular coagulation. *N Engl J Med* 1984; 10:772–4.

95. Jakobovits AA. The abnormalities of the presentation in twin pregnancy and perinatal mortality. *Eur J Obstet Gynecol Reprod Biol* 1993; 52(3):181–5.

96. Chervenak FA, Johnson RE, Youcha S, Hobbins JC, Berkowitz RL. Intrapartum management of twin gestation. *Obstet Gynecol* 1985; 65:119–24.

97. Pettersson F, Smedby B, Lindmark G. Outcome of twin birth (review of 1636 children born in twin birth). *Acta Pediatr Scand* 1976; 65:473–9.

98. Norman MG. Mechanisms of brain damage in twins. *Can J Neurol Sci* 1982; 9:339–44.

99. Benirschke K, Gille J. Placental pathology and asphyxia. In: Gluck L, ed. *Intrauterine Asphyxia and the Developing Fetal Brain*. Chicago: Year Book Medical Publishers, 1977, Ch. 7, pp. 117–36.

100. Gedda L. Why can the study of twins be called gemellology? Twin Research: Biology & Epidemiology. In: Nance W, ed. *Progress in Clinical & Biological Research* 1978; 24B:1–8.

101. Crane JP, Tomich PG, Kopta M. Ultrasonic growth patterns in normal and discordant twins. *Obstet Gynecol* 1980; 55:678–83.

102. Mercer BM, Crocker LG, Pierce F, Sibai BM. Clinical characteristics and outcome of twin gestation complicated by preterm premature rupture of the membranes. *Am J Obstet Gynecol* 1993; 168:1467–73.

103. Nhan VQ, Huisjes HJ. Double uterus with a pregnancy in each half. *Obstet Gynecol* 1983; 61:115–17.

104. Farquharson DF. Personal communication, 1985.

105. de la Torre Verduzco R, Rosario R, Rigatto H. Hyaline membrane disease in twins—a 7 year review with a study in zygosity. *Am J Obstet Gynecol* 1976; 125:668–71.

106. Yeung CY. Effects of prolonged rupture of membranes on the development of respiratory distress syndrome in twin pregnancy. *Aust Pediatr J* 1982; 18:197–9.

107. Chen SJ, Vohr BR, Oh W. Effects of birth order, gender, and intrauterine growth retardation on the outcome of very low birth weight in twins. *J Pediatr* 1993; 123(1):132–6.

108. Hrubec Z, Rubinette CD. The study of human twins in medical research. *N Engl J Med* 1984; 310(7):435–41.

109. Naeye RL. Organ abnormalities in a human parabiotic syndrome. *Am J Pathol* 1965; 46:829–42.

110. Naeye RL. The fetal and neonatal development of twins. *Pediatrics* 1964; 38:546–53.

111. Naeye RL, Letts HW. Body measurements of fetal and neonatal twins. *Arch Pathol* 1964; 77:393–6.

112. Erkkola R, Ala-Mello S, Piiroinen O, Kero P, Sillanpaa M. Growth discordancy in twin pregnancies: a risk factor not detected by measurements of biparietal diameter. *Obstet Gynecol* 1985; 66:203–6.

113. Jacques SM, Qureshi F. Chronic villitis of unknown etiology in twin gestations. *Pediatr Pathol* 1994; 14:575–84.

114. Boyd JD, Hamilton WJ. The placenta in multiple pregnancy. In: *The Human Placenta*. Cambridge: W. Heffer & Sons, 1970, pp. 313–34.

115. Weissman A, Achiron R, Lipitz S, Blickstein I. The first-trimester growth-discordant twin: an ominous prenatal finding. *Obstet Gynecol* 1994; 84:110–14.

116. Warkany J. *Congenital Malformations*. Chicago: Year Book Medical Publishers, 1971, p. 151.

117. Wiswell TE, Fajardo JE, Bass JW, Brien JH, Forstein SH. Congenital toxoplasmosis in triplets. *J Pediatr* 1984; 105:59–60.

118. Bose CL, Gooch WM, Sanders GO, Bucciarelli RL. Dissimilar manifestation of intrauterine infection with Echovirus 11 in premature twins. *Arch Pathol Lab Med* 1983; 107:361–3.

119. Morton R, Mitchell I. Neonatal cytomegalic inclusion disease in a set of twins, one member of whom was a hydropic stillbirth, the other completely uninfected. Case report. *Br J Obstet Gynaecol* 1983; 90:276–9.

120. Shafai T. Neonatal coccidioidomycosis in premature twins. *Am J Dis Child* 1978; 132:634.

121. Neri A, Wielunsky E, Henig E, Friedman S, Ovadia J. Group B streptococcus amnionitis with intact membranes associated with quintuplet delivery. *Eur J Obstet Gynecol Reprod Biol* 1984; 17:29–32.

122. Mascola L, Ewert DP, Eller A. Listeriosis: a previously unreported medical complication in women with multiple gestations. *Am J Obstet Gynecol* 1994; 170:1328–32.

123. Miller RW. Relation between cancer and congenital defects: an epidemiologic evaluation. *J Nat Cancer Inst* 1968; 40:1079–85.

124. Gross RE, Clatworthy HW, Meeker IA. Sacrococcygeal teratomas in infants and children (a report of 40 cases). *Surg Gynecol Obstet* 1951; 92:341–54.

125. Willis RA. *The Borderland of Embryology and Pathology*. 2nd ed. London: Butterworth, 1962, pp. 135–47, 442–62.

126. Amino K, Ichioka H, Matsubara K, Lin YW, Ohta S. Retinoblastoma in dizygotic twins born as extremely low birth weight infants. *Jpn J Ophthalmol* 1992; 36(3):310–14.

127. Keith L, Brown E. Epidemiologic study of leukemia in twins (1928–1969). *Acta Genet Med Gemellol* 1971; 20:9–22.

128. Windham GC, Bjerkedal T, Langmark F. A population-based study of cancer incidence in twins and in children with congenital malformations or low birth weight, Norway, 1967–1980. *Am J Epidemiol* 1985; 121:49–56.

129. Grether JK, Nelson KB, Cummins SK. Twinning and cerebral palsy: experience in four northern California counties, births 1983 through 1985. *Pediatrics* 1993; 92:854–8.

130. Petterson B, Nelson KB, Watson L, Stanley F. Twins, triplets, and cerebral palsy in births in Western Australia in the 1980s. *Br Med J* 1993; 307:1239–43.

131. Griffiths M. Cerebral palsy in multiple pregnancy. *Dev Med Child Neurol* 1967; 9:713–31.

132. Jung JH, Graham JM, Schultz N, Smith DW. Congenital hydrancephaly/porencephaly due to vascular disruption in monozygotic twins. *Pediatrics* 1984; 73:467–9.

133. Getts A. SIDS: increased risk to secondborn twins. *Am J Public Health* 1981; 71:317–18.

134. Lee DA. Munchausen syndrome by proxy in twins. *Arch Dis Child* 1979; 54:646–7.

135. Hay S, Wehrung DA. Congenital malformations in twins. *Am J Hum Genet* 1970; 22:662–78.

136. Bonney GE, Walker M, Gbedeman K, Konotey-Ahulu FID. Multiple births and visible birth defects in 13,000 consecutive deliveries in one Ghanaian

hospital. Twin Research: Biology & Epidemiology. In: Nance W, ed. *Progress in Clinical & Biological Research* 1978; 24B:105–8.

137. Little J, Bryan E. Congenital anomalies in twins. *Semin Perinat* 1986; 10(1):50–64.

138. Soma H, Yoshida K, Tada M, Mukaida T, Kikuchi T. Fetal abnormalities associated with twin placentation. *Teratology* 1975; 12:211. Abstract.

139. Baldwin VJ. *Pathology of Multiple Pregnancy*. New York: Springer-Verlag, 1994, pp. 170–2.

140. Winchester B, Young E, Geddes S, et al. Female twin with Hunter disease due to nonrandom inactivation of the X-chromosome: a consequence of twinning. *Am J Med Genet* 1992; 44:834–8.

141. Heifetz SA. Single umbilical artery. A statistical analysis of 237 autopsy cases and review of the literature. *Perspect Pediatr Pathol* 1984; 8(4):345–78.

142. Anderson RC. Congenital cardiac malformations in 109 sets of twins and triplets. *Am J Cardiol* 1977; 39:1045–50.

143. Wilkinson JL, Holt PA, Dickinson DF, Jivani SK. Asplenia syndrome in one of monozygotic twins. *Eur J Cardiol* 1979; 10:301–4.

144. Bustamante SA, Stumpff LC. Fetal hydantoin syndrome in triplets (a unique experiment of nature). *Am J Dis Child* 1978; 132:978–9.

145. Christoffel KK, Salafsky I. Fetal alcohol syndrome in dizygotic twins. *J Pediatr* 1975; 87:963–7.

146. Mellin GW, Katzenstein M. The saga of thalidomide (neuropathy to embryopathy, with case reports of congenital anomalies). *N Engl J Med* 1962; 267:1184–93, 1238–44.

147. Bieber FR, Moustoufi-Zadeh M, Birnholz JC, Driscoll SG. Amniotic band sequence associated with ectopia cordis in one twin. *J Pediatr* 1984; 105:817–19.

148. Pysher TJ. Discordant congenital malformations in monozygous twins: the amniotic band disruption complex. *Diagn Gynecol Obstet* 1980; 2:221–5.

149. van Allen MI, Siegel-Bartelt J, Dixon J, et al. Constriction bands and limb reduction defects in two newborns with fetal ultrasound evidence for vascular disruption. *Am J Med Genet* 1992; 44:598–604.

150. Huber J, Wagenbichler P, Bartsch F. Biaminal alpha fetoprotein concentration in twins, one with multiple malformations. *J Med Genet* 1984; 21:377–9.

151. Hall JG, Reed SD, McGillivray BC, et al. Part II. Amyoplasia: twinning in amyoplasia—a specific type of arthrogryposis with an apparent excess of discordantly affected identical twins. *Am J Med Genet* 1983; 15:591–9.

152. Avni A, Amir J, Wilunsky E, Katznelson MBM, Reisner SH. Down's syndrome in twins of unlike sex. *J Med Genet* 1983; 20:94–6.

153. Ratcliffe CG, Melville MM, Stewart AL, Jacobs PA, Keay AJ. Chromosome studies on 3500 newborn male infants. *Lancet* 1970; 1:121–2.

154. Dallapiccola B, Stomeo C, Ferranti G, Di Lecce A, Purpura M. Discordant sex in one of three monozygotic triplets. *J Med Genet* 1985; 22:6–11.

155. Juberg RC, Stallard R, Straughen WJ, Avotri KJ, Washington JW. Clinicopathologic conference: a newborn monozygotic twin with abnormal facial appearance and respiratory insufficiency. *Am J Med Genet* 1981; 10:193–200.

156. Wittmann BK, Farquharson DF, Thomas WDS, Baldwin VJ, Wadsworth LD. The role of feticide in the management of severe twin transfusion syndrome. *Am J Obstet Gynecol* 1986; 155:1023–6.

157. Benson CB, Doubilet PM, David V. Prognosis of first-trimester twin pregnancies: polychotomous logistic regression analysis. *Radiology* 1994; 192:765–8.

158. Spirtos NJ, Hayes MF, Magyar DM, Cossler NJ. Spontaneous abortion following ovulation induction. In: Hafez ESE, ed. *Spontaneous Abortion*. Wingham, MD: MTP, 1984, pp. 81–98.

159. Baldwin VJ. *Pathology of Multiple Pregnancy*. New York: Springer-Verlag, 1994, pp. 89–118.

160. Evans MI, Dommergues M, Timor-Tritsch I, et al. Transabdominal versus transcervical and transvaginal multifetal pregnancy reduction: international collaborative experience of more than one thousand cases. *Am J Obstet Gynecol* 1994; 170:902–9.

161. Hellman LM, Kobayashi M, Cromb E. Ultrasonic diagnosis of embryonic malformation. *Am J Obstet Gynecol* 1973; 115:615–23.

162. Levi S. Ultrasonic assessment of the high rate of human multiple pregnancy in the first trimester. *J Clin Ultrasound* 1976; 4:3–5.

163. Kurjak A, Latin V. Ultrasound diagnosis of fetal abnormalities in multiple pregnancy. *Acta Obstet Gynecol Scand* 1979; 58:153–61.

164. Livingston JE, Poland BJ. A study of spontaneously aborted twins. *Teratology* 1980; 21:139–48.

165. Uchida IA, Freeman VCP, Gedeon M, Goldmaker J. Twinning rate in spontaneous abortions. *J Hum Genet* 1983; 35:987–93.

166. Farquharson DF, Wittmann BK, Hansmann M, et al. Management of quintuplet pregnancy by selective embryocide. *Am J Obstet Gynecol* 1988; 158:413–16.

167. Hommel H, Festge B. Drillingsschwangerschaft mit fetus papyraceus. *Zentralbl Gynaekol* 1979; 101:845–7.

168. Saier F, Burden L, Cavanagh D. Fetus papyraceus (an unusual case with congenital anomaly of the surviving fetus). *Obstet Gynecol* 1975; 45:217–20.

169. Balfour RP. Fetus papyraceus. *Obstet Gynecol* 1976; 47:507.

170. Baker VV, Doering MC. Fetus papyraceus: an unreported congenital anomaly of the surviving infant. *Am J Obstet Gynecol* 1982; 143:234–235.

171. Benirschke K. Intrauterine death of a twin: mechanisms, implications for surviving twin, and placental pathology. *Semin Diagn Pathol* 1993; 10(3):222–31.

172. Clark DA. Hydrops fetalis attributable to intrauterine disseminated intravascular coagulation. *Clin Pediatr* 1981; 20:61–2.

173. Rydhstrom H, Ingemarsson I. Prognosis and follow-up of a twin after antenatal death of the co-twin. *J Reprod Med* 1993; 38(2):142–6.

174. Kindred JE. Twin pregnancies with one twin blighted (report of two cases with comparative study of cases in the literature). *Am J Obstet Gynecol* 1944; 48:642–82.

175. Gilardi G, Giannone E. Osservazioni cliniche, morfologiche e patogenetiche su un caso di gravidanza gemellare con trasformazione papiracea di uno dei feti. *Arch Ostet Ginecol* 1972; 77:256–63.

176. Redwine FO, Hays PM. Selective birth. *Semin Perinat* 1986; 10(1):73–81.

177. Dudley DKL, D'Alton ME. Single fetal death in twin gestation. *Semin Perinat* 1986; 10(1):65–72.

178. Wittmann BK, Farquharson D, Wong GP, et al. Delayed delivery of second twin: report of four cases and review of the literature. *Obstet Gynecol* 1992; 79:260–3.

179. Wharton B, Edwards JH, Cameron AM. Monoamniotic twins. *J Obstet Gynecol Br Common* 1968; 75:158–63.

180. Colburn DW, Pasquale SA. Monoamniotic twin pregnancy. *J Reprod Med* 1982; 27:165–8.

181. Pauls F. Monoamniotic twin pregnancy. A review of the world literature and a report of two new cases. *Can Med Assoc J* 1969; 100:254–6.

182. Decker J. Monoamniotic twins with true knot between cords. *Cent Afr J Med* 1976; 22:137–8.

183. Baldwin VJ. *Pathology of Multiple Pregnancy*. New York: Springer-Verlag, 1994, pp. 215–75.

184. Benirschke K. Origin and clinical significance of twinning. *Clin Obstet Gynecol* 1972; 15:220–35.

185. Galea P, Scott JM, Goel KM. Feto-fetal transfusion syndrome. *Arch Dis Child* 1982; 57:781–94.

186. Rausen AR, Seki M, Strauss L. Twin transfusion syndrome. *J Pediatr* 1965; 66:613–28.

187. Tan KL, Tan R, Tan SH, Tan AM. The twin transfusion syndrome: clinical observations on 35 affected pairs. *Clin Pediatr* 1979; 18:111–14.

188. Bryan EM. IgG deficiency in association with placental edema. *Early Hum Dev* 1977; 1/2:133–43.

189. Fusi L, McParland P, Fisk N, Nicolini U, Wigglesworth J. Acute twin-twin transfusion: a possible mechanism for brain-damaged survivors after intrauterine death of a monochorionic twin. *Obstet Gynecol* 1991; 78:517–20.

190. Aherne W, Strong SJ, Corney G. The structure of the placenta in the twin transfusion syndrome. *Biol Neonat* 1968;12:121–35.

191. Wieacker P, Wilhelm C, Prömpeler H, et al. Pathophysiology of polyhydramnios in twin transfusion syndrome. *Fetal Diagn Ther* 1992; 7:87–92.

192. Naeye RL. Human intrauterine parabiotic syndrome and its complications. *N Engl J Med* 1963; 268:804–9.

193. Lubinsky M, Rapoport P. Transient fetal hydrops and "prune belly" in one identical female twin. *N Engl J Med* 1983; 308:256–7.

194. Abraham JM. Intrauterine feto-fetal transfusion syndrome. *Clin Pediatr* 1967;6:405–10.

195. Zosmer N, Bajoria R, Weiner E, Rigby M, Vaughan J, Fisk NM. Clinical and echographic features of in utero cardiac dysfunction in the recipient twin in twin-twin transfusion syndrome. *Br Heart J* 1994; 72:74–9.

196. Nicosia RF, Krouse TB, Mobini J. Congenital aortic intimal thickening (its occurrence in a case of twin-transfusion syndrome). *Arch Pathol Lab Med* 1981; 105:247–9.

197. Popek EJ, Strain JD, Neumann A, Wilson H. In utero development of pulmonary artery calcification in monochorionic twins: a report of three cases and discussion of the possible etiology. *Pediatr Pathol* 1993; 13:597–611.

198. Schwartz JL, Maniscalco WM, Lane AT, Currao WJ. Twin transfusion syndrome causing cutaneous erythropoiesis. *Pediatrics* 1984; 74:527–9.

199. Szymonowicz W, Preston H, Yu VYH. The surviving monozygotic twin. *Arch Dis Child* 1986; 61:454–8.

200. David TJ, Vascular basis for malformations in a twin. *Arch Dis Child* 1985; 60:166–7.

201. Hoyme HE, Higginbottom MC, Jones KL. Vascular etiology of disruptive structural defects in monozygotic twins. *Pediatrics* 1981; 67:288–91.

202. Dimmick JE, Hardwick DF, Ho-Yuen B. A case of renal necrosis and fibrosis in the immediate newborn period—association with the twin to twin transfusion syndrome. *Am J Dis Child* 1971; 122:345–7.

203. Moore CM, McAdams AJ, Sutherland J. Intrauterine disseminated intravascular coagulation: a syndrome of multiple pregnancy with a dead twin fetus. *J Pediatr* 1969; 74:523–8.

204. Shah NB, Jenkins ME, Jones GW. Renal cortical necrosis in a homozygous twin neonate. *J Urol* 1972; 108:146–8.

205. Mannino FL, Jones KL, Benirschke K. Congenital skin defects and fetus papyraceus. *J Pediatr* 1977; 91:559–64.

206. Erskine RLA, Ritchie JWK, Murnaghan GA. Antenatal diagnosis of placental anastomosis in a twin pregnancy using Doppler ultrasound. *Br J Obstet Gynaecol* 1986; 93:955–9.

207. Jones KL, Benirschke K. The developmental pathogenesis of structural defects: the contribution of monozygotic twins. *Semin Perinat* 1983; 7:239–43.

208. Reisman LE, Pathak A. Bilateral renal cortical necrosis in the newborn—associated with fetomaternal transfusion and hypermagnesemia. *Am J Dis Child* 1966; 111:541–3.

209. Grafe MR. Antenatal cerebral necrosis in monochorionic twins. *Pediatr Pathol* 1993; 13:15–19.

210. Baldwin VJ, Wittmann BK. Pathology of intragestational intervention in twin to twin transfusion syndrome. *Pediatr Pathol* 1990; 10:79–93.

211. Pinette MG, Pan Y, Pinette SG, Stubblefield PG. Treatment of twin-twin transfusion syndrome. *Obstet Gynecol* 1993; 82:841–6.

212. De Lia JE, Cruikshank DP, Keye WR Jr. Fetoscopic neodymium:yag laser occlusion of placental vessels in severe twin-twin transfusion syndrome. *Obstet Gynecol* 1990; 75:1046–53.

213. Stockard CR. Developmental rate and structural expression: an experimental study of twins, "double monsters" and single deformities, and the interaction among embryonic organs during their origin and development. *Am J Anat* 1921; 28:115–277.

214. Baldwin VJ. *Pathology of Multiple Pregnancy*. New York: Springer-Verlag, 1994, pp. 279–85.

215. Stephens TD, Spall R, Urfer AG, Martin R. Fetus amorphus or placental teratoma? *Teratology* 1989; 40:1–10.

216. Chi JG, Lee YS, Park YS, Chang KY. Fetus-in-fetu: report of a case. *Am J Clin Pathol* 1984; 82:115–19.

217. Gonzalez-Crussi F. The "included-twin" hypothesis. In: *Extra-gonadal Teratomas, Atlas of Tumor Pathology*, 2nd Series, Fascicle 18. Washington: Armed Forces Institute of Pathology, 1982, pp. 20–24.

218. Hing A, Corteville J, Foglia RP, et al. Fetus in fetu: molecular analysis of a fetiform mass. *Am J Med Genet* 1993; 47:333–41.

219. Silbermann M, Bar-Maur JA, Auslander L. Craniofacial microsomia in a parasite of a heteropagus conjoined twin; a clinical and histopathologic evaluation. *Head Neck Surg* 1984; 6:792–800.

220. Yasuda Y, Ohtsuki H, Torii S, Tomoyoshi E, Clark CF. Epigastrius with oomphalocele—report of a case. *Teratology* 1984; 30:297–309.

221. Vestergaard P. Triplets pregnancy with a normal fetus and a dicephalus dibrachius sirenomelius. *Acta Obstet Gynecol Scand* 1972; 51:93–4.

222. Konstantinova B. Morphologic and cytogenetic studies on conjoined twins. *Acta Genet Med Gemellol* 1976; 25:55–8.

223. Sato T, Kaneko K, Konuma S, Sati I, Tamada T. Acardiac anomalies: review of 88 cases in Japan. *Asia-Oceana J Obstet Gynecol* 1984; 10:45–52.

224. Simonds JP, Gowen GA. Fetus amorphus (report of a case). *Surg Gynecol Obstet* 1925; 41:171–9.

225. Auerback P, Wigglesworth FW. Congenital absence of the heart: observation of a human funiculopagus twinning with insertio funiculi furcata, fusion, forking and interposito velamentosa. *Teratology* 1978; 17:143–50.

226. Stephens TD. Muscle abnormalities associated with the twin reverse-arterial-perfusion (TRAP) sequence (acardia). *Teratology* 1984; 30:311–18.

227. Amatuzio JC, Gorlin RJ. Conjoined acardiac monsters. *Arch Pathol Lab Med* 1981;105:253–5.

228. Lindahl SA, Baldwin VJ, Wakeford J, Wittmann BK. Early diagnosis of an acardiac acephalus twin by ultrasound. *Med Ultrasound* 1984; 8:105–7.

229. van Allen MI, Smith DW, Shepard TH. Twin reversed arterial perfusion (TRAP) sequence: a study of 14 twin pregnancies with acardius. *Semin Perinat* 1983; 7:285–93.

230. Ornoy A, Navot D, Menashi M, Laufer N, Chemke J. Asymmetry and discordance for congenital anomalies in conjoined twins: a report of six cases. *Teratology* 1980; 22:145–54.

231. Royston D, Geoghegan F. Disseminated arterial calcification associated with acardius acephalus. *Arch Dis Child* 1983; 58:641–3.

232. Harkavy KL, Scanlon JW. Hydrops fetalis in a parabiotic acardiac twin. *Am J Dis Child* 1978; 132:638–9.

233. van Allen MI. Fetal vascular disruptions: mechanisms and some resulting birth defects. *Pediatr Ann* 1981; 10:219–33.

234. Benirschke K, des Roches Harper V. The acardiac anomaly. *Teratology* 1977; 15:311–16.

235. Kaplan C, Benirschke K. The acardiac anomaly. New case reports and current status. *Acta Genet Med Gemellol* 1979; 28:51–9.

236. James WH. A note on the epidemiology of acardiac monsters. *Teratology* 1977; 16:211–16.

237. Healey MG. Acardia: predictive risk factors for the co-twin's survival. *Teratology* 1994; 50:205–13.

238. Edmonds LD, Layde PM. Conjoined twins in the United States, 1970–1977. *Teratology* 1982; 25:301–8.

239. Källén B. Conjoined twins—an epidemiological study based on 312 cases. The International Clearinghouse for Birth Defects Monitoring Systems. *Acta Genet Med Gemellol* 1991; 40:325–35.

240. Tan KL, Goon SM, Salmon Y, Wee JH. Conjoined twins. *Acta Obstet Gynecol Scand* 1971; 50:373–80.

241. Jachevatzky OE, Goldman B, Kampf D, Wexler H, Grunstein S. Etiologic aspects of double monsters. *Eur J Obstet Gynecol Reprod Biol* 1980; 10:343–9.

242. Ingalls TH, Bazemore MK. Prenatal events antedating the birth of thoracopagus twins. *Arch Environ Health* 1969; 19:358–64.

243. Guttmacher AF, Nichols BL. Teratology of conjoined twins. In: Bergsma D, ed. *Birth Defects Orig Artic Ser* 1967; 3(1):3–4.

244. Herring SW, Rowlatt UF. Anatomy and embryology in cephalothoracopagus twins. *Teratology* 1981; 23:159–73.

245. Merwin MC, Wright J. Lateral cephalothoracopagus: a case report. *Teratology* 1984; 29:181–4.

246. Harper RG, Kenigsberg K, Sia CG, et al. Xiphopagus conjoined twins: a 300 year review of the obstetric, morphopathologic, neonatal and surgical parameters. *Am J Obstet Gynecol* 1980; 137:617–29.

247. Nichols BL, Blattner RJ, Rudolph AJ. General clinical management of thoracopagus twins. *Birth Defects Orig Artic Ser* 1967; 3(1):38–51.

248. Marin-Padilla M, Chin AJ, Marin-Padilla TM. Cardiovascular anomalies in thoracopagus twins. *Teratology* 1981; 23:101–13.

249. Singer DB, Rosenberg HS. Pathologic studies of thoracopagus conjoined twins. *Birth Defects Orig Artic Ser* 1967; 3(1):97–105.

250. Gerlis LM, Seo J-W, Ho SY, Chi JG. Morphology of the cardiovascular system in conjoined twins: spatial and sequential segmental arrangements in 36 cases. *Teratology* 1993; 47:91–108.

251. Barr M. Facial duplication: case, review, and embryogenesis. *Teratology* 1982; 25:153–9.

252. Chervenak FA, Pinto MM, Heller CI, Norooz H. Obstetric significance of fetal craniofacial duplication. *J Reprod Med* 1985; 30(1):74–6.

253. Tan K-L, Tock EPC, Dawood MY, Ratnam SS. Conjoined twins in a triplet pregnancy. *Am J Dis Child* 1971; 122:455–8.

254. Deale CJC, Cronje HS. A review of 367 triplet pregnancies. *S Afr Med J* 1984; 66:92–4.

255. Loucopoulos A, Jewelewicz R. Management of multifetal pregnancies: sixteen years' experience at the Sloan Hospital for Women. *Am J Obstet Gynecol* 1982; 143:902–5.

256. Sulak LE, Dodson MG. The vanishing twin: pathologic confirmation of an ultrasonographic phenomenon. *Obstet Gynecol* 1986; 68:811–15.

257. Mayer CF. Sextuplets and higher multiparous births: a critical review of history and legend from Aristotle to the 20th century. *Acta Genet Med Gemellol* 1952; 1:118–35, 242–75.

258. Neubecker RD, Blumberg JM, Townsend FM. A human monozygotic quintuplet placenta. *J Obstet Gynecol Br Commun* 1962; 69:137–9.

259. Cameron AH, Robson EB, Wade-Evans T, Wingham J. Septuplet conception: placental and zygosity studies. *J Obstet Gynecol Br Commun* 1969; 76:692–8.

260. Reece EA, Petrie RH, Sirmans MF, Finster M, Todd WD. Combined intrauterine and extrauterine gestations: a review. *Am J Obstet Gynecol* 1983; 146:323–30.

261. Stanley JR, Harris AA, Gilbert CF, Lennon YA, Dellinger EH. Magnetic resonance imaging in evaluation of a second-trimester ovarian twin pregnancy. *Obstet Gynecol* 1994; 84:648–52.

262. Hafez ESE. Physiology of multiple pregnancy. *J Reprod Med* 1974; 12:88–98.

263. Rudolph AJ, Michaels JP, Nichols BL. Obstetric management of conjoined twins. *Birth Defects Orig Artic Ser* 1967; 3(1):28–37.

264. Gupta JM. Pyopagus conjoined twins. *Br Med J* 1966; 2:868–71.

Fetal Death and the Macerated Stillborn Fetus

DON B. SINGER   TREVOR A. MACPHERSON

INTRODUCTION

Human development is a continuum not significantly altered by birth. The diseases that affect the conceptus preceding birth are part of that continuum. Asphyxia, infection, hematologic and circulatory abnormalities, malformations, tumors, trauma, and iatrogenic conditions all occur in the fetus as they do in the liveborn infant. The effects of these lesions and diseases are similar in both cases, but may be more difficult to ascertain in the fetus due to its relative inaccessibility. Amnioscopy, ultrasound, electronic monitors, and other techniques for fetal examination have improved prenatal diagnosis, but confirmation at autopsy is still required in instances of fetal death. Autolysis and maceration increase the difficulty of examining dead fetuses. Nevertheless, we concur with Ballantyne, who stated "the custom of saying that because the foetus was macerated, there was no use in examining it microscopically or bacteriologically must be abandoned" [1]. Placentae must be carefully examined, but the autopsy is the essential tool for complete evaluation of stillborn fetuses [2]. It is the most thorough procedure available and the standard against which all other techniques should be measured.

INCIDENCE OF FETAL DEATH

Throughout the world some 5 million deaths occur each year among fetuses between 24 weeks and term gestation [3, 4]. For the last 35 to 50 years in the United States and other developed countries, fetal deaths have been roughly equal in number to neonatal deaths, and all perinatal deaths have accounted for three-fourths of infant mortality [5]. Fetal death rates range between 4 and 40 per 1000 total births, with developing countries having the higher rates [6].

When considered by international comparisons—that is, gestations of at least 28 weeks or birth weights greater than 1000 grams—fetal deaths account for 45–55% of all perinatal deaths in developed countries. In some populations, such as South African blacks, the fetal death rate accounts for 70% of all perinatal deaths [4, 7]. When evaluating fetal deaths in one region, state, or county, definitions and social factors must be considered [8–10]. Including all stillborn fetuses and liveborn infants with birth weights of 500 grams or more in Women and Infants Hospital, Rhode Island, the fetal death rate in 1994 was 4.5 per 1000 while the neonatal death rate was 2.8 per 1000. The socially disadvantaged have higher rates than the general population [11, 12]. Political factors have an effect. In New York State, after elective abortions became legal, fetal death rates dropped from about 15 per 1000 to 9.6 per 1000 total births [11]. These rates compare with those in other highly developed areas. The definition of perinatal death was recently altered in England and Wales to include all fetal deaths at 24–27 completed weeks of gestation in addition to those after 28 weeks. In a cohort analysis of this very premature group (<28 weeks) in 1993, there were 221 stillbirths and 92 early neonatal deaths (313 perinatal deaths). The neonatal mortality rate among those born alive between 24 and 28 weeks gestation was only 37.8% (36 deaths/95 livebirths.) Another 52 fetuses were stillborn, and five babies died after 28 days of age. The total perinatal mortality rate was 60% in this very premature group [13].

Low fetal death rates may be attributable simply to the provision of prenatal care without consideration of scientific advances in the type of care [9, 14, 15]. In 1921, Ballantyne noted that among healthy women who received prenatal care, the fetal death rate was 5.9 per 1000, a rate as low as that reported today [1]. On the contrary, a contemporary religious group whose members eschew obstetric care have a fetal death rate three times (and a maternal death rate 100 times) that of the surrounding general population [10].

DURATION AND CONDITIONS OF PREGNANCY AT THE TIME OF FETAL DEATH

Without considering losses before 20 weeks of gestation [16], the distribution of fetal deaths is skewed toward the later weeks. About 35% occur after 37 weeks, about 30% between 34 and 37 weeks, and the remainder prior to 34 weeks [17–19]. At Magee-Womens Hospital during the five years 1982–1986, the percentages of stillbirths by birth weight and gestational age are presented in Table 9.1. The rate of fetal death, when expressed as the total number of fetuses in utero of the same gestational age, is fourfold greater after 39 weeks than between 32 and 36 weeks [20] (Fig. 9.1).

Maternal hypertension, diabetes mellitus, and post-term pregnancies account for much of the fetal mortality around 40 weeks gestation. About half of these term fetal deaths are due to inadequate prenatal care and are therefore deemed preventable [18]. Infections, placental and umbilical cord catastrophic lesions, and acute maternal diseases account for most of the fetal deaths in midgestation. Anomalies and chromosomal abnormalities are responsible for most of the early fetal deaths [21].

Maternal age less than 20 years or greater than 29 years and increased parity at any maternal age are associated with increased fetal death [22], but particularly intrapartum fetal death [23]. Maternal diseases that antedate the onset of pregnancy are associated with as few as 6% to as many as 40% of the fetal deaths [24, 25].

Pregnancy induced hypertension (PIH) is associated in 3.2–19.9% of fetal deaths [4, 6, 19, 24, 26]. The incidence of fetal deaths rises to 3 to 4 times that of normal mothers as the degree of hypertension and proteinuria increases [27]. Abruptio placentae is often associated with PIH and can be an immediate cause of death in such cases [19, 28]. Among 24 stillborn fetuses reported long ago by Strachan, 14 of the mothers had PIH and another four had extensive placental infarcts [29]. In the mid-twentieth century, preexisting hypertensive cardiovascular disease accounted for about one-third of stillbirths that were attributed to maternal hypertensive disorders [30], but this is no longer the case.

Maternal diabetes mellitus is reported in 0–17% of fetal deaths in various series [2, 4, 6, 19]. Maternal cardiovascular disease is another significant risk factor for fetal death. In the study by Whittemore et al [31], 55% of the mothers with cyanotic heart disease had stillborn fetuses and most of the remaining 45% had infants with growth retardation. On the other hand, palliative surgery in the mothers resulted in 72% live births and normal size in about three-fourths of the liveborn infants. In the past, maternal renal disease has prevented successful completion of pregnancy, but several babies have been born to mothers on chronic hemodialysis [32, 33]. Maternal connective tissue and autoimmune diseases are not often directly associated with increased fetal death, but the incidence of stillbirth is higher among such mothers than among mothers with no chronic illness [34]. Maternal thromboembolic diseases can be treated successfully with anticoagulants such as coumadin and heparin, but fetal deaths may occur in as many as 2% of such cases and the fetopathy of coumadin remains a hazard [35].

Maternal infection, especially acute sepsis, is responsible for small numbers of fetal deaths. We have observed two cases associated with maternal acute appendicitis. Simpson and Geppert found maternal infections of all kinds in 5.2% of their series of fetal deaths [17]. Mothers with urinary tract infections reportedly have more premature deliveries, fetuses with growth retardation, and a risk of fetal death 2.4 times that of normal pregnancies [36], but these observations are not universally accepted as true or accurate [37].

Certain maternal occupations are associated with 1.5 to 2 times the general population's risk for fetal death. Those

Table 9.1.   Perinatal mortality by gestational age and birth weight: 834 deaths

Birth weight in grams		Gestational age in weeks	
<751	29%	<26	23%
751–1000	11%	26–28	13%
1001–2500	31%	29–36	34%
>2500	28%	>36	30%

Data from Magee-Womens Hospital Perinatal Mortality and Morbidity Report, 1982–1986. Includes perinatal deaths at gestational age of 20 weeks or more or at a weight of 500 mg or more.

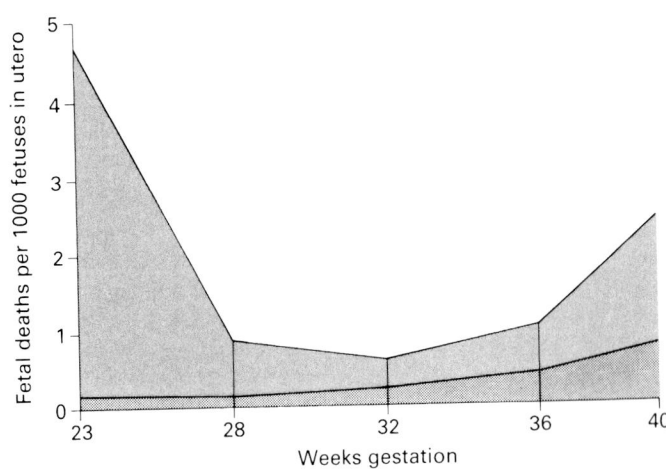

FIGURE 9.1.   *The number of cases of fetal death of unknown cause (dark shaded area) increases markedly as term approaches, as Yudkin et al have shown [20]. This graph shows that all fetal deaths also increase as full-term gestation approaches. (Data from Women and Infants Hospital of Rhode Island Perinatal Mortality Committee statistics.)*

pregnant women at increased risk work in farming, in the metal, wood, textile, and chemical industries, and as flight attendants, pet shop workers, veterinarians or their assistants, hairdressers, x-ray technicians, and medical laboratory technicians [22].

Maternal drug abuse, even to the point of addiction, may be unassociated with increased stillbirth [38]. However, most reports show that habitual use of tobacco, drugs, and alcohol is implicated in fetal deaths [39–41]. Fetal deaths, especially late in gestation, are increased by as much as 50% if mothers smoke three or more cigarettes per day compared with non-smoking mothers [42, 43]. Naeye found that abruptio placentae and placenta previa were more common among smoking mothers [44]. Cocaine, particularly its more active base form ("crack"), has been assigned a causal role in instances of acute and sometimes massive placental separations [45–47]. With cocaine, vasoconstriction results in reduced uterine blood flow, and decidual ischemia is followed by necrosis, hemorrhage, and placental separation [48]. Some therapeutic drugs, such as salicylates, are associated with an increased rate of fetal deaths, while others, such as anticonvulsants, are associated with increased anomalies but apparently not with fetal deaths [49, 50].

Lupus anticoagulant is associated with a high incidence of spontaneous abortions and with fetal deaths in the second and third trimesters of gestation. Lupus anticoagulant is a double misnomer. It is occasionally found in healthy pregnant women, and clot formation is unimpeded. In fact, thrombotic phenomena predominate, particularly in the decidua and basal layers of the placenta, often resulting in infarcts [34, 51]. Lupus anticoagulants are either IgG or IgM antibodies that interfere with phospholipid-dependent coagulation assays, particularly those related to factors Va and Xa and calcium-dependent reactions [51–53]. The diagnosis of lupus anticoagulant is suggested when prothrombin time and partial thromboplastin time are prolonged, and is confirmed by prolonged snake venom clotting time. Other laboratory tests include demonstration of antibodies to phosphatidylserine or cardiolipin [51, 54]. In mothers with untreated lupus anticoagulant, the rate of pregnancy loss is nearly 100% [55, 56]. In a population of women with normal pregnancies, lupus anticoagulant can be detected in less than one per thousand [57]. In a population of pregnant women whose fetuses died in utero, the incidence of lupus anticoagulant is 4%, and 10% have elevated antiphospholipid antibodies [58]. In the case reported by Grimmer et al, IgM antitrophoblast antibodies were present along with lupus anticoagulant [59]. In many cases, subsequent pregnancies can be successfully carried to term if aspirin or corticosteroids are taken [55, 56, 58, 60].

Multiple births, especially among those with monochorial placentae, are associated with an increased rate of fetal death [61]. In Driscoll's study of 100 fetal deaths, 10% of the cases were associated with either twins or triplets [2].

Siblings of infants and children with congenital malformations have a high rate of fetal death. If a previous pregnancy ended in fetal or neonatal death, subsequent fetal death is threefold more likely to occur compared with prior normal births [15, 23, 62].

Table 9.2.   Stillbirths according to degree of maceration according to criteria of Langley [66].

Degree of maceration	Number
Fresh stillbirth	13
Grade 0	8
Grade I	17
Grade II	21
Grade III	40

Data from Magee-Womens Hospital autopsy series, 1986. Autopsy rate for stillbirths, 77%.

PREPARTUM VERSUS INTRAPARTUM FETAL DEATH

Until the past few years, fully one-third of fetal deaths were intrapartum and produced fetuses with little or no maceration, the so-called "fresh stillborn" [63]. In Machin's series (1974), the fresh and macerated stillborns were almost equal in number [64]. These ratios are changing [65]. In Women and Infants Hospital's autopsy series, the ratio of macerated to nonmacerated fetuses is 12:1. Ratios ranging from 4:1 to 8:1 are reported by others [18, 23, 24]. Driscoll's 1984 series of 100 cases had 71 macerated and autolyzed fetuses while 29 were "fresh stillbirths" approaching the 2:1 ratio of old [2]. At Magee-Womens Hospital, Langley's criteria were used to classify maceration in 99 stillborn fetuses examined at autopsy in 1986 [66]. They were distributed as shown in Table 9.2.

PATHOGENESIS OF FETAL DEATH

Some of the conditions commonly associated with neonatal death have no bearing on fetal death [67]. Neither immaturity nor prematurity is ever a cause of fetal death [2]. No matter how striking they are, pulmonary, cardiac, gastrointestinal, hepatic, and renal lesions and malformations are rarely the primary cause of fetal death, since the exchange with the mother through the placenta facilitates the processes of respiration, nutrition, excretion, and detoxification. On the other hand, general conditions such as sepsis, severe anemia, thromboses, trauma, exogenous toxic substances, and local lesions of metabolic nature or of the cardiovascular and nervous systems may lead to fetal death [24].

About one-quarter to one-half of all cases of fetal death have an identified direct cause [2, 67–70]. On the other hand, associated major disorders of known pathogenesis may be found at autopsy in about 85–90% [2, 71].

Causes and associations with fetal death should, in the first instance, be classified broadly [67] (see Chap. 4).

Significant associated conditions that may or may not be directly responsible for death might include, for example, asphyxia and major malformations.

Of all fetal deaths, 20–60% are attributed to fetal asphyxia [2, 17, 19, 68, 69, 72, 73]. In most studies, figures are in the higher range. The causes of fetal asphyxia are not all clearly understood. Among those with clear pathogeneses, abruptio placentae is the leading single cause of fetal asphyxia and is also the leading single cause of fetal death [26]. Abruptio placentae accounts for one-tenth [6, 19, 44, 69] to one-half of all cases of fetal death [2, 4, 17, 26, 28, 74]. The causes of abruptio placentae are not entirely understood. Maternal vascular disease is one factor. Lack of a placental platelet inhibitor has been assigned an important role in its pathogenesis [75].

Cord accidents (nuchal cord, true knots, and prolapse) comprise 5–18% of all cases of fatal fetal asphyxia, although such accidents are not often substantiated by pathologic examination [2, 19, 26]. In Morrison's study of full term asphyxiated infants, 48% had cord accidents [19]. Nuchal cord with one loop around the neck occurs in at least 20% of all deliveries. When there are two loops or more around the neck, this is considered sufficient evidence for fetal asphyxial episode [19]. At autopsy, a pale groove in the neck or plethora of the face and scalp are further evidence for such a causal role. True knots occur in about 1% of all pregnancies but account for fetal death in a tiny proportion of such cases (Fig. 9.2). Twisting of the cord at the fetal umbilical skin is commonly observed in fetal death and is usually considered a postmortem artifact due to unrestrained twisting of the dead fetus for several revolutions in one direction. Whether or not this is always the case is a matter of continued debate [76].

Between 10% and 30% of fetal deaths are associated with poor uteroplacental blood flow leading to numerous or large and acutely acquired placental infarcts [2, 26, 69, 77]. Probably most of these occur in mothers with PIH or lupus anticoagulant [77].

Unexplained asphyxia is fairly commonly invoked as a cause of fetal death, accounting for rates of 50 to 360 fetal deaths per 1000 births in selected groups such as postdate deliveries or in fetuses of diabetic mothers [20, 26, 78]. One should use this designation only with the positive pathologic evidence or with ultrasonic or electronic evidence before death occurs. Pathologic signs of asphyxia can be detected in fetuses, even when severely macerated, and include thoracic visceral and serosal petechiae; aspirated squames in distal air spaces; adrenal hemorrhagic necrosis; renal, splenic, and hepatic infarcts or necroses; and cerebral subependymal and intraventricular hemorrhages.

Brain damage is commonly found in stillborn fetuses. After 27 weeks' gestation, nearly half of the stillborn fetuses in one study had damaged brains that were thought to have been caused by asphyxia or circulatory disorders. The lesions were ischemic injury in the white matter with reactive astrocytosis and macrophagic infiltration, karyorrhexis, and

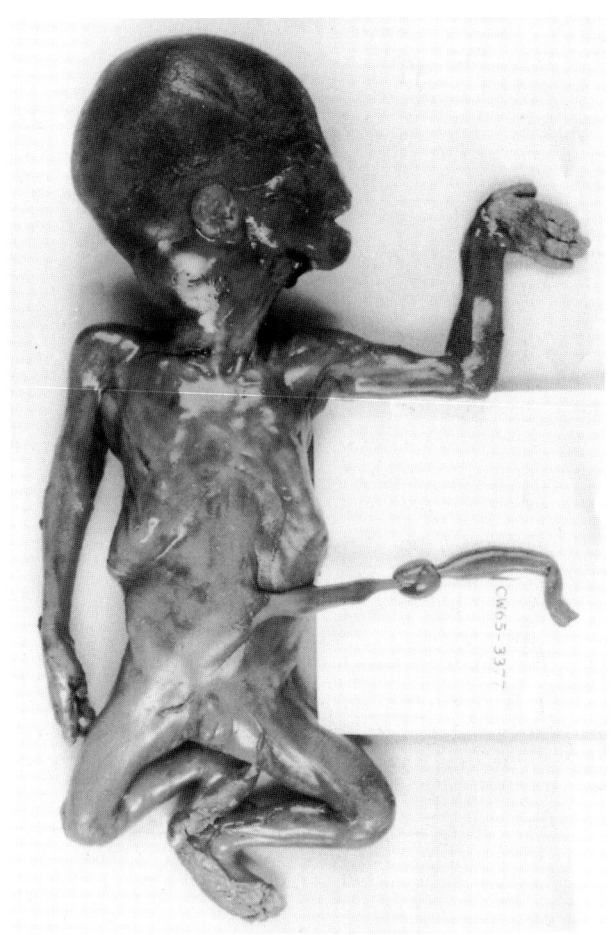

FIGURE 9.2.   *Macerated fetus with tight true knot in umbilical cord.*

endothelial swelling. Approximately 30% also had hemorrhages [79]. Another rare cause of severe hypoxic damage is diffuse meningocerebral angiomatosis. This affects the whole cortex with necrosis of both gray and white matter and may present in stillborn fetuses with extensive subarachnoid hemorrhage [80]. Brain damage was found in more than 80% of stillborn fetuses with nonimmune hydrops fetalis. The lesions included microcalcifications, cerebral and cerebellar hypoplasia, microcephaly, encephalomalacia, cavitary lesions, astrocytosis, polymicrogyria, and severe neuronal loss. Cranial ultrasonography failed to detect many of these lesions. Furthermore, six of the 10 survivors of nonimmune hydrops fetalis had neurologic abnormalities [81]. Burke and Tannenberg correlated placental lesions with those of the brain among 175 stillborn fetuses [82]. By using glial fibrillary acidic protein and H&E stains, they detected microscopic evidence of ischemic cerebral injury in 70 of 175 brains (40%). Most often, these lesions were in the periventricular white matter. More than half of these cases had macroscopic or microscopic infarcts in the placenta.

The rate of malformations among stillborns is higher than in the general population; major malformations occur in 4–26% of stillborn fetuses in several reported series of cases [3, 6, 19, 24, 68, 71, 83]. Renal and skeletal anomalies are more frequent than those of other organs. In Driscoll's series of 100 cases, 17 had malformations: five were multiple and 12 were isolated defects [2]. Manning et al found major anomalies in 56% of their fetal deaths, but all of their cases were from a high-risk maternity service [15]. In some instances, fetal death can be attributed to the malformation, but many such lesions are not considered lethal [4, 17]. Of the major lethal fetal anomalies, those of the central nervous system predominate [24].

A variety of structural and nonstructural cardiovascular diseases occur in the fetus. Dysrhythmias are usually transient and are rarely fatal. Common among these are supraventricular tachycardia and bradycardia due to complete atrioventricular block [53]. Cardiac conduction tissues were hemorrhagic in one of our cases of intrapartum fetal death [84]. Rare vascular malformations may also be detected in stillborn fetuses [85].

Minor anomalies are more common in cases of fetal death compared with the general population [17, 86, 87]. Among singleton fetal deaths, single umbilical artery was observed in 3.1%, versus 0.5% in the general population [88]. Single umbilical artery is observed in 10% of stillborn twins whereas the incidence is about 3.6% in the general population of twins [17]. Velamentous cord and marginal insertion of the cord are 3 to 4 times more frequent among those with fetal deaths compared with the general population [17].

About 60% of embryonic or early fetal deaths are associated with chromosomal abnormalities. This rate drops to 5–12% by the end of the 6th month of gestation [89, 90]. Monosomy X and trisomy 21 are particularly apt to be associated with fetal hydrops. The phenotypic features of the chromosomal abnormality may be partially obscured by anasarca, but are detectable if carefully sought (Fig. 9.3). Szulman found triploidy in three fetuses of gestations greater than 19 weeks [91]. Machin found chromosome abnormalities in 9% of macerated stillborns (using amnion as the source of cells) and in 4.1% of fresh stillborns (using amnion and gonad as sources of cells) [64]. Ellis and Bain successfully obtained karyotypes in 77% of their macerated fetuses by using amnion as the source of cells [90]. Among the cases of fetal deaths, 6.8% had abnormal chromosomes: six had 45 monosomy X (Turner syndrome), two had 47 + 21, one had 47 + 13, and one had 47 + 18 [90]. Saal et al reported successful chromosome analysis with the use of amniotic fluid obtained as soon as possible after fetal death occurs— i.e., before significant maceration sets in [92]. Macpherson et al predicted the likelihood of tissue growth from stillborn fetuses as graded by Langley's criteria [93] (Table 9.3). Provided the fetus is refrigerated after birth, cells remain viable for several days even in cases with grade 1 maceration.

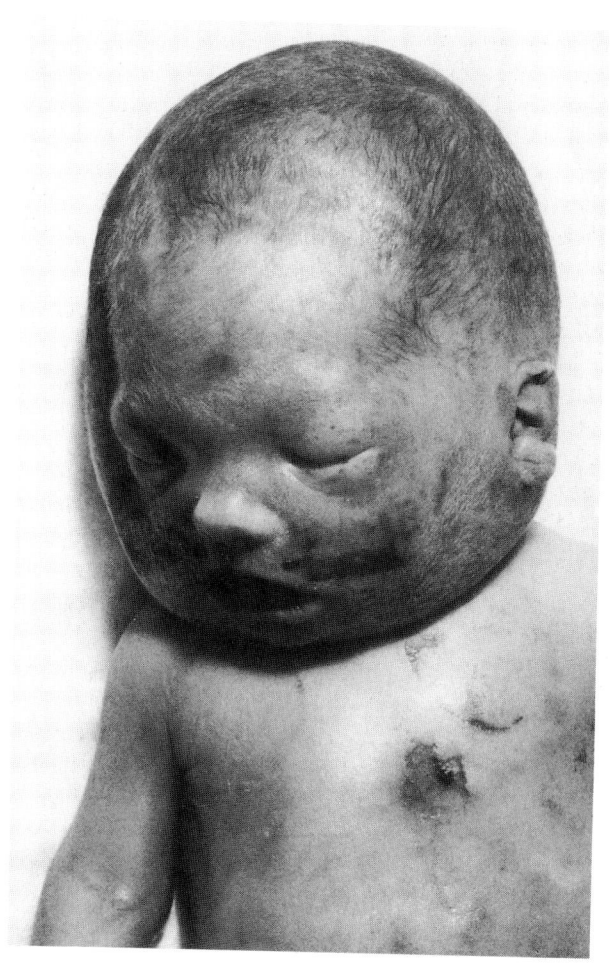

FIGURE 9.3. *Minimal maceration in a fetus with Down syndrome. The facial features and small ear are characteristic. The fetus also had single palmar creases, an endocardial cushion defect, and characteristic pelvic radiographs. Chromosome studies of pericardial tissue were successful, showing trisomy 21.*

Fetal infection is often responsible for intrauterine deaths, especially in gestations of less than 36 weeks [77]. Inflamed placental membranes may be found in 10–67% of all cases of fetal death [2, 68, 77]. The inflammation associated with carriage of a dead fetus—e.g., cases in which mater-

Table 9.3. Successful growth of tissues in culture samples from stillborn fetal autopsies

Maceration grade	Growth frequency
Fresh stillbirth	69%
Grade 0	61%
Grade I	45%
Grade II	00%
Grade III	00%

Maceration grade according to Langley's criteria [66, 93].

nal leukocytes are attracted by the dead tissues to the sub-chorionic layers of the placental disc—must be distinguished from the fetus' own inflammatory response, which is best identified in the umbilical vein, the umbilical arteries, or the fetal vessels in the chorionic plate. While 67% of Driscoll's cases had chorioamnionitis, she found that only 20% of the fetuses had infection [2]. At that, the 20% rate is higher than those in most series of fetal deaths. Intrauterine pneumonia was found in 14%, and all of these had associated chorioamnionitis.

Causative organisms are usually identified with difficulty. The bacteria can propagate in the chorionic and decidual layers, sites where most of the inflammatory cells are found [94]. Infection and abruptio placentae often occur together. In some cases, infection seems to play the primary role by damaging decidual blood vessels; in others, repeated episodes of maternal vaginal bleeding may precede the infection by several weeks [77]. In about one-third of cases, premature rupture of membranes occurs, and it is assumed that the infection precedes rupture in most such cases.

Viral, spirochetal, and protozoal agents cause fetal death. None of these is frequent, but the more common ones are parvovirus, cytomegalovirus, syphilis, and toxoplasmosis [4]. The characteristic pathologic features, despite extensive tissue autolysis and maceration, may still be clearly visible. Spirochetes are usually detected in macerated stillborn fetuses with Warthin-Starry or other silver stains. Acute villitis with neutrophils migrating to the subtrophoblast area, nucleated red blood cells in the villous capillaries, and enlarged placentae and livers are helpful clues to the diagnosis in these cases [95]. *Listeria monocytogenes*, uncommon in the United States except in epidemics, may produce fetal death. Acute villitis with microabscesses is highly characteristic of this infection. Gas-producing anaerobes, such as *Clostridium* species, produce rapid fetal death and a devastating tissue autolysis and maceration. Gas can also be demonstrated radiologically in cases of aerobic gas formers such as *E. coli*. This should not be confused with small amounts of carbon monoxide, a by-product of hemoglobin breakdown, demonstrable in the cardiac atria of stillborn fetuses (Fig. 9.4).

Prior to the use of Rh immune globulin prophylaxis, blood group incompatibility with severe anemia accounted for 5–6% of fetal deaths. By 1983, this figure had been reduced to 3.3% [26], and it is still lower today. About 2–11% of fetal deaths are attributable to other causes of erythroblastotic anemia—e.g., alpha thalassemia, atypical blood group incompatibility, parvovirus, and other causes of red-cell destruction [2, 6]. Most of these now fall under the rubric of nonimmune hydrops [21].

Hemorrhages, usually located in the cerebrum, developed in 9% of fetal deaths in Huff's series [68]. Harcke and colleagues noted that 6% of well-preserved stillborn fetuses have intraventricular hemorrhage [96]. Among our own cases of perinatal cerebral hemorrhage, 10% occur in still-

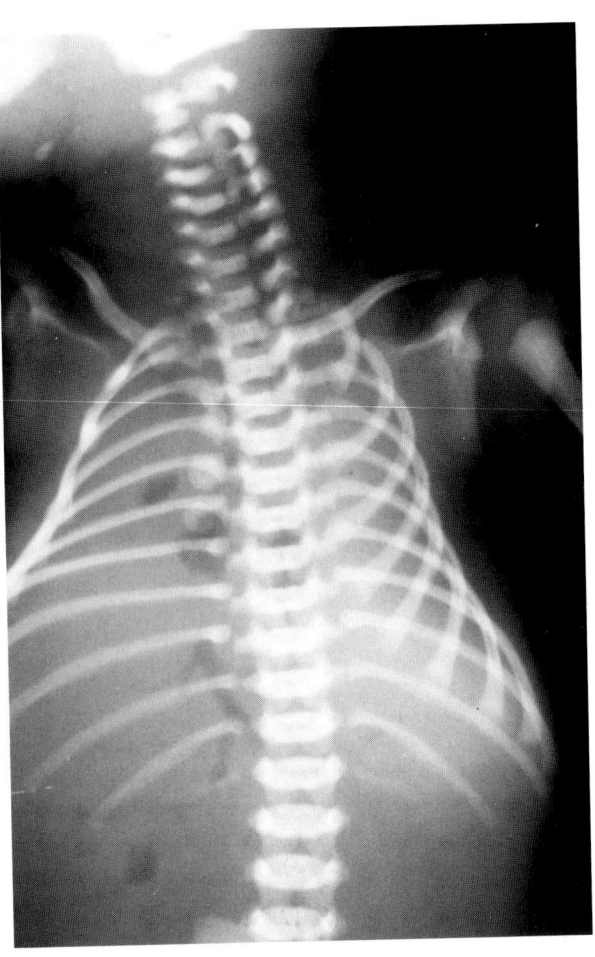

FIGURE 9.4.   *Radiograph of stillborn fetus showing gas in atria and vena cavae. This is probably carbon monoxide derived from breakdown of hemoglobin.*

born fetuses, and most of these are in macerated and autolyzed brains. These features and others of similar nature are observed by other investigators [79, 80].

Fetal bleeding (fetal-maternal, fetal-fetal, and intrafetal) caused 2.9% of the fetal deaths in the series reported by Simpson and Geppert [17]. In one case of fetal-maternal hemorrhage at Magee-Womens Hospital, an estimated 150 mL of fetal blood loss was demonstrated; the Kleihauer-Betke test disclosed that 3.5% of the red blood cells in the mother's circulation were of fetal origin.

Thrombi are rarely found in fetuses. They usually occur in the renal veins or branches of the portal veins. In six of Driscoll's 100 cases, three had thrombi in placental chorionic veins and one each in renal vein, splenic vein, and umbilical artery [2].

In the 1951 study by Simpson and Geppert, traumatic lesions accounted for 10.4% of fetal deaths, and most of these were located intracranially [17]. Trauma accounted for only one case of fetal death in Huff's series of 56 cases and three in Driscoll's study of 100 cases [2, 68].

Leukemia, tumors, and in situ tumors have been recognized in cases of fetal death, although they may have been only indirectly related to the demise [68, 97]. Umbilical cord hemangiomas are occasionally associated with fetal death [98].

Unknown Cause of Fetal Death

Using only data from death certificates, up to 50% of all fetal deaths are unexplained [20, 99]. Even with autopsies, maceration causes difficulty in establishing correct diagnoses, and the unknown rate, while less, is not reduced to satisfactorily low levels [19, 24, 43, 100]. In Driscoll's autopsy series of 100 cases, 13% had disorders that could not be identified [2]. The rate of fetal death due to unknown causes is higher in those gestations of 37 or more weeks [18, 20]. This is illustrated in our own series at Women and Infants Hospital (see Fig. 9.1). Among the clinical harbingers, vaginal bleeding, oligohydramnios, and reduced fetal activity are often associated with unexplained fetal death [101]. With careful prepartum fetal monitoring, fetal deaths due to unknown causes can be reduced to as few as 8% of cases [15].

DIAGNOSIS OF FETAL DEATH

The diagnosis of fetal death may first be made by the mother who notices reduced or absent fetal movement. This sign is not totally reliable, since some women will interpret shifts in the floating dead fetus as movement [73]. After a week or more, the mother fails to gain weight or may even lose weight [102]. The physician can usually detect fetal death by observing absence of fetal heart tones. Fetal skull radiographs show overriding skull sutures (Spalding's sign). This is due to softening of the brain and dissolution of the collagen in the sutures and occurs about 4 or 5 days after fetal death [102, 103]. Abnormal curvature of the spine and gas in the abdomen are two other radiologic signs used to establish fetal death [102]. Laboratory tests to confirm fetal demise have not been used, although, long ago, Rezek promoted use of a modified Aschheim-Zondek rabbit ovary reaction [103].

Electronic fetal monitoring is now commonly used to diagnose fetal well-being and also to confirm intrauterine fetal death. Ultrasound in real time has been used to demonstrate the lack of true fetal movement or cardiac action. This is now considered the definitive sign of fetal death.

In an effort to detect warning signs of potentially lethal fetal distress, particularly in pregnancies that progress beyond 40 weeks, obstetricians have adopted a protocol that includes the mother's daily documentation of the number of fetal movements, twice weekly nonstress tests, and weekly ultrasound examinations [104]. The frequency of the electronic and ultrasonic monitoring is increased if there is evidence of fetal compromise.

THE PATHOLOGY OF FETAL DEATH

When fetal death occurs, the tissues quickly lose all tone. Autolysis and maceration have begun. One of the earliest macroscopic manifestations is in the umbilical cord and the skin [105, 106]. After 4 to 8 hours, vascular permeability increases and imparts a "parboiled" appearance. Minimal shearing force causes the epidermis to slip away from the underlying dermis, exposing a shiny, moist, red surface. Even without shearing and slippage, fluid soon collects under the epidermis, producing small vesicles and blisters. These must not be confused with congenital bullous dermatoses or vesicles of herpes infections. The bullae may coalesce to form larger bullae, which can reach diameters of 8 to 10 cm before rupture occurs (Fig. 9.5). Later, hemolysis and leaking of blood and plasma from the damaged capillaries and venules produce a red-brown discoloration of soft tissues. Joints become lax, and joint tissues soon dissolve. Rigor mortis is lost by lysis of muscle tone and of joint tissues.

The brain becomes semiliquid and the sutures of the skull dissolve. Even so, if the brain is carefully dissected in

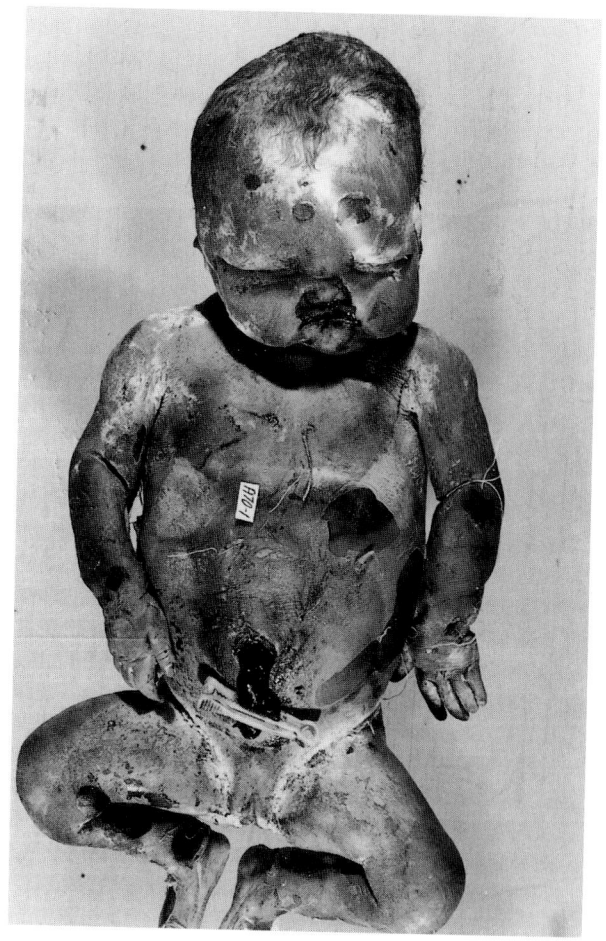

FIGURE 9.5. *Grade II maceration. The peeling skin is autolyzed extensively (see Table 9.4).*

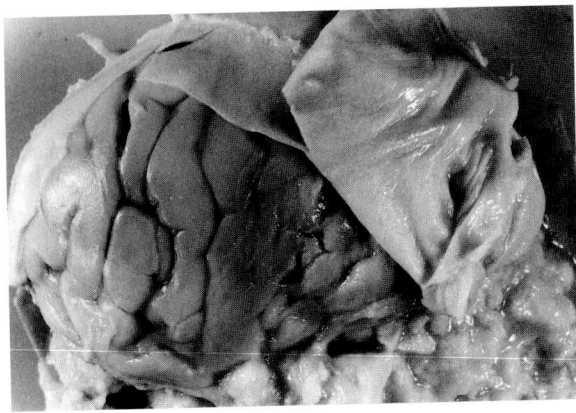

FIGURE 9.6.   *The cerebral gyral pattern is preserved although the brain tissue is autolyzed. Careful dissection from the skull, keeping the brain within the dura, facilitates this observation. Estimates of gestational age are possible from such examinations.*

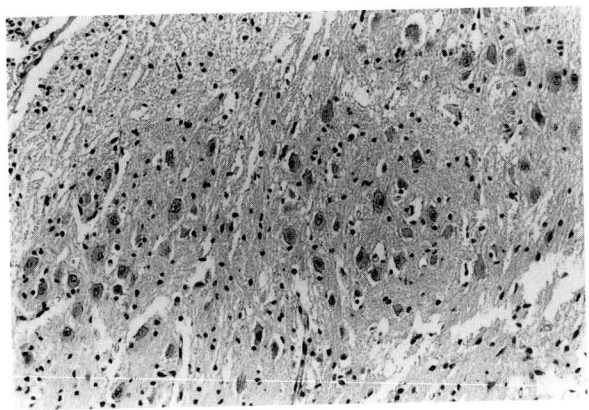

FIGURE 9.7.   *Neurons and glia in the brainstem are remarkably well preserved, despite extensive autolysis of the brain, rendering it grossly semisolid. H&E, ×175.*

an intact dura, the pattern of cerebral convolutions can be studied (Fig. 9.6). After 4 or 5 days, the skull bones overlap [103]. Forensic pathologists have noted that acidosis produces more rapid liquefaction in the brain [107]. After a few days the scalp becomes a fluctuant bag containing the bony plates of the skull and semisolid brain. This change is sometimes mistaken for hydrocephalus. Rupture of soft tissues in the spinal column allows pasty nervous system tissue to ooze into the chest; this material may be mistaken for a necrotic neurogenic tumor [107a]. Despite the loss of integrity of nervous system tissue, microscopy shows remarkably clear cellular detail (Fig. 9.7). This is more characteristic of the brain and spinal cord than of any other tissue in the body.

The fetal bone marrow turns a muddy brown and is easily expressed from the ribs by moderate pressure. In spite of this, cytologic detail of hematopoietic elements may be well preserved.

The abdominal contents become green due to seeping of bile pigments from the gall bladder or the meconium into the devitalized tissues. If the fetus is retained for longer than a week or two, the bowel wall may dissolve, releasing meconium into the peritoneal cavity. The meconium itself is enzymatically degraded and becomes less tenacious the longer the fetus is retained.

The liver undergoes autolysis quickly with loss of cohesion and loss of histologic detail in 48 to 72 hours. Hepatic erythropoietic tissue is more resistant to autolysis than is hepatocellular tissue.

When the fetus is retained for more than a week or 10 days, the color of the skin gradually fades and changes to a light olive brown [73]. The younger the fetus, the more rapid is this change, because of the lower concentration of red blood cells and the paucity of fetal fat [73, 108]. In younger or older fetuses with extensive edema—e.g., fetuses with cystic hygroma, fetal hydrops, etc.—the red-maroon discoloration may develop quickly and persist for several

weeks after death [73]. In small fetuses, abdominal wall disruption may occur and should not be confused with omphalocele or gastroschisis.

Weights of most organs progressively decrease from those of liveborn infants due to loss of tissue water [108]. Standard weights for macerated fetuses have recently become available.

Histology should be done on all organs in every case. Although hepatic, intestinal, and pancreatic tissues undergo autolysis within 1 to 3 days, cross striations in muscle fibers are clearly seen and lung structure is well preserved for several days. One can detect aspirated meconium and debris from the amniotic sac in cases of asphyxia. While renal histologic features may deteriorate within a few hours, renal maturity can still be assessed by counting the number of ranks of glomeruli beneath the nephrogenic zone [109] (Fig. 9.8). Effects of chronic stress can be detected in the thymus where cortical lymphocytes have abandoned the condensed stroma. Medullary corpuscles can be detected, even in the most severely macerated tissues (Fig. 9.9). Despite autolysis, tumors such as cardiac rhabdomyomas and sacrococcygeal teratomas can be diagnosed with fair accuracy. Congenital leukemia has also been diagnosed [73]. The collagenous skeleton of the spleen may be accentuated in autolyzed fetuses (Fig. 9.10).

Special stains are usually useful. Elastic tissue stains and trichrome stains can accentuate elastic and collagen fibers (Fig. 9.11). Using oil red-O and Sudan stains, Becker and Becker found that the distribution of adrenal cortical lipid could be correlated with duration of fetal distress preceding death in utero and the associated causative conditions [110]. They showed that when lipid was diffusely depleted, acute asphyxia was the associated feature, whereas when the deep fetal cortical cells retained lipid and the superficial fetal cortex was depleted, chronic distress was indicated. Fat was always identified in the definitive adult adrenal cortex, however macerated and autolyzed the tissue became.

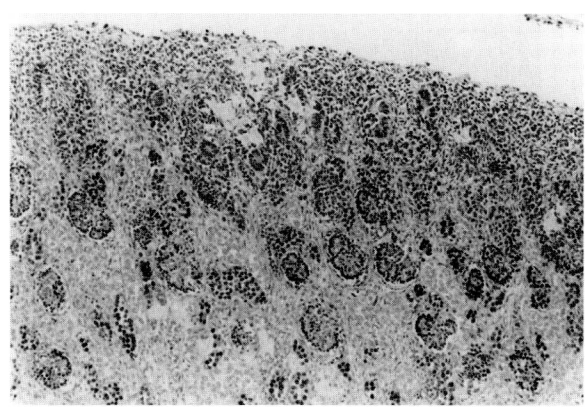

FIGURE 9.8. *Columns of renal glomeruli, the nephrogenic zone, and remnants of tubules are readily visible in this autolyzed kidney. Estimates of gestational age are possible from such examinations. H&E, ×85.*

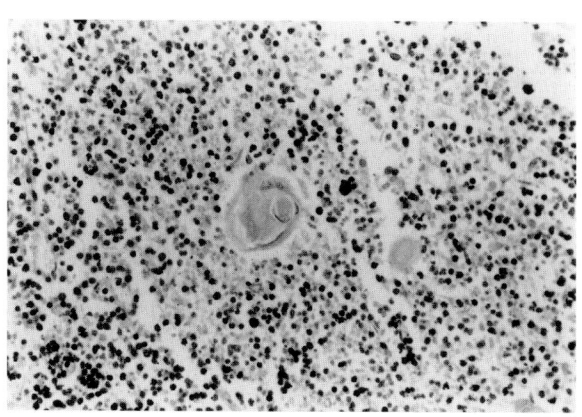

FIGURE 9.9. *Thymic involution is shown by loss of lymphocytes, indicating intrauterine stress. A thymic (Hassall's) corpuscle is clearly shown. H&E, ×175.*

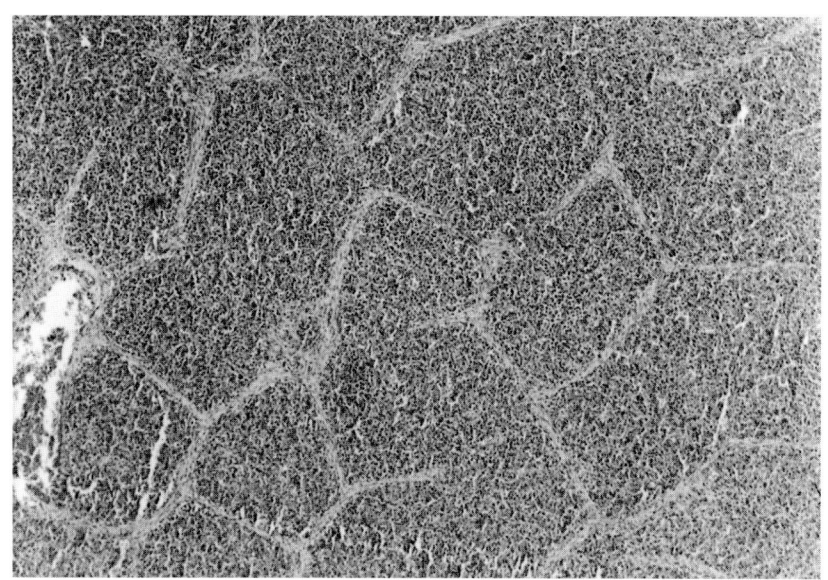

FIGURE 9.10. *Autolysis sometimes accentuates architecture, as in this spleen with the prominent fibrous skeleton. H&E, ×45.*

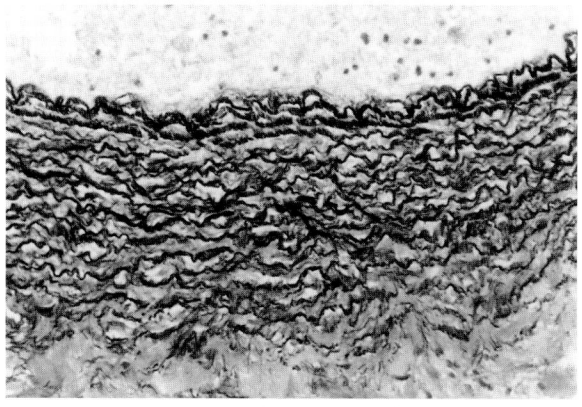

FIGURE 9.11. *Elastic tissue staining of the aorta shows elastic fibers as clearly as in a nonautolyzed specimen. H&E, ×175.*

Fetus Compressus, Fetus Papyraceus, Adipocere, and Lithopedions

Fetus compressus and fetus papyraceus are almost always the result of multiple gestation wherein a sibling survives [111] (Fig. 9.12). In the affected fetus, the thorax is often flattened tangentially so that most of the ventral or anterior aspect of the body is on the concave surface. The whole surface of the body has a gray-yellow, slightly dry character, and there is usually no bloating or swelling. The epidermis shrinks to a thin layer, which might represent the remnants of the basement membrane. Striations of muscle fibers are readily visible and nuclei along muscle fibers may be preserved in outline although the chromatin does not usually stain with hematoxylin. The liver often is evident only as a mass of yellow material inferior to the diaphragm. The heart may or may not be flattened, depending on the state of the

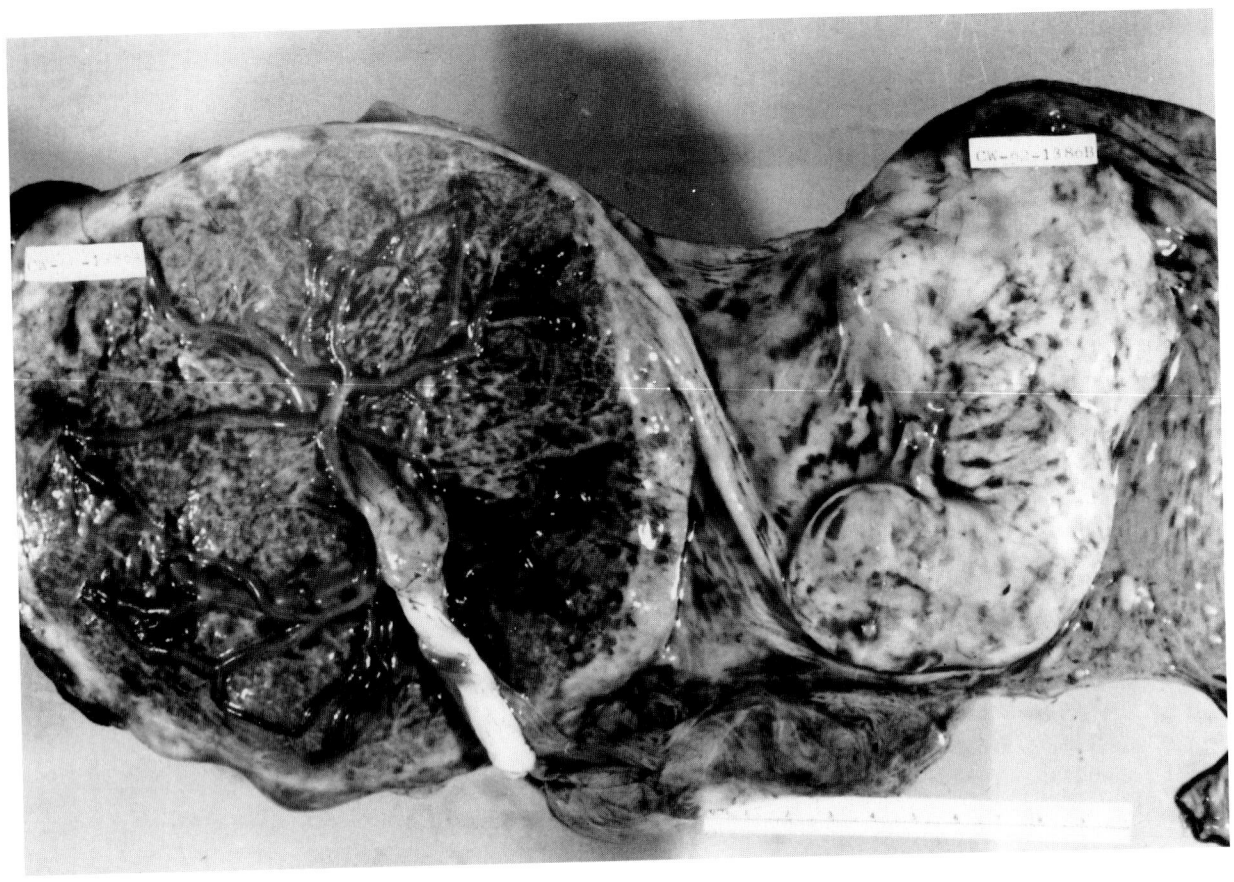

FIGURE 9.12.   *Fetus papyraceus and fetus compressus in a twin gestation. The other twin was healthy.*

overlying rib cage, which can form a protective arch over it. Most flattened fetuses are drier than those not flattened, and more of them are monochorial [111]. Saier et al stated that fetus papyraceus occurs once in every 180 to 190 twin pregnancies [112]. When the fetus dies, the mother may have amniotic fluid leaks, sudden lower abdominal pain, and vaginal bleeding.

"Adipocere" is the term applied to the peculiar waxy substance formed during decomposition of bodies buried in moist places, hence the term "grave wax." Fatty acids and their salts form the waxlike materials. In adults, this process requires at least 2 to 4 months of interment [107]. The condition occurs in fetuses retained in utero for lengthy periods of time following death. Dehner described such a fetus in an extrauterine pregnancy that was surgically removed a full 10 months after the due date and 8 months after the mother noted cessation of fetal movement [113]. The fetus, a female weighing 2000 grams, was mummified and waxy, developed to term proportions, and had subcutaneous tissues that were firm and woody. Deep, broad grooves coursed over the surface of the face and head and the placental remnants were hyalinized. Gill described an intrauterine pregnancy in which the large 8-lb fetus was "adherent" to the endometrium [114]. The cranium contained fluid but very little brain substance, and the hands were clubbed. The fetal

tissue was mottled brown and had a firm, almost brittle texture. In a macabre circumstance during the examination of this fetus, one hand snapped off at the wrist and one leg at the knee without bleeding from these broken surfaces.

"Lithopedion" ("stone baby") is the term applied to calcified fetuses that have been carried, usually intra-abdominally, for years or even decades. Some remarkable cases have been described in which subsequent pregnancies were successfully carried to term while the calcified or ossified fetus was still in situ. In one instance, the fetus was extracted 31 years after conception and was reported to have six teeth; in another, twins were carried in the mother's abdomen for 6 years [115]. Lithopedions of different ages have been reported in mothers' abdomens. In another set of twins, one developed intra-abdominally and the other in the uterus, terminating with a liveborn infant whose intra-abdominal twin became a lithopedion [116].

The Dead Fetus Syndromes

The death of a monozygotic twin shortly before birth may result in ordinary maceration and autolysis in the dead fetus, but produces extensive infarcts in many organs of the surviving twin. Studies with in utero ultrasound have disclosed severe brain lesions in the surviving twin [117, 118], and

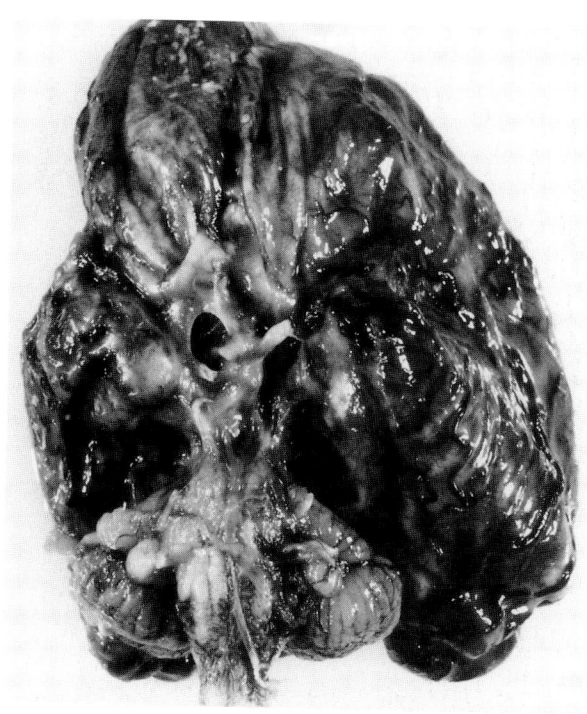

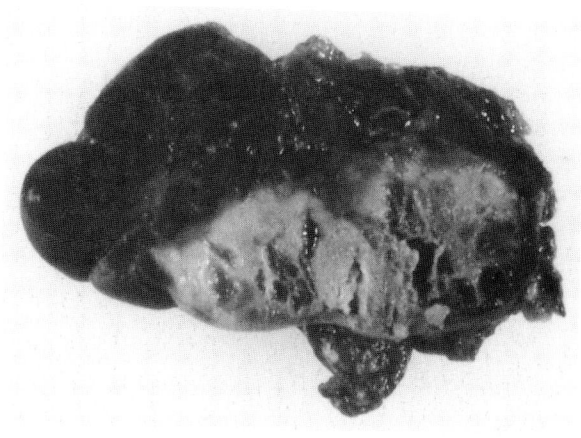

FIGURE 9.14. *Atrophy of the spleen with a large infarct from a liveborn twin whose partner in utero died several weeks before delivery. (Same case as in Figs. 9.13 and 9.15.)*

FIGURE 9.13. *Extensive necrosis and atrophy in the brain of a liveborn twin whose partner in utero died several weeks before delivery. (Same case as in Figs. 9.14 and 9.15.)*

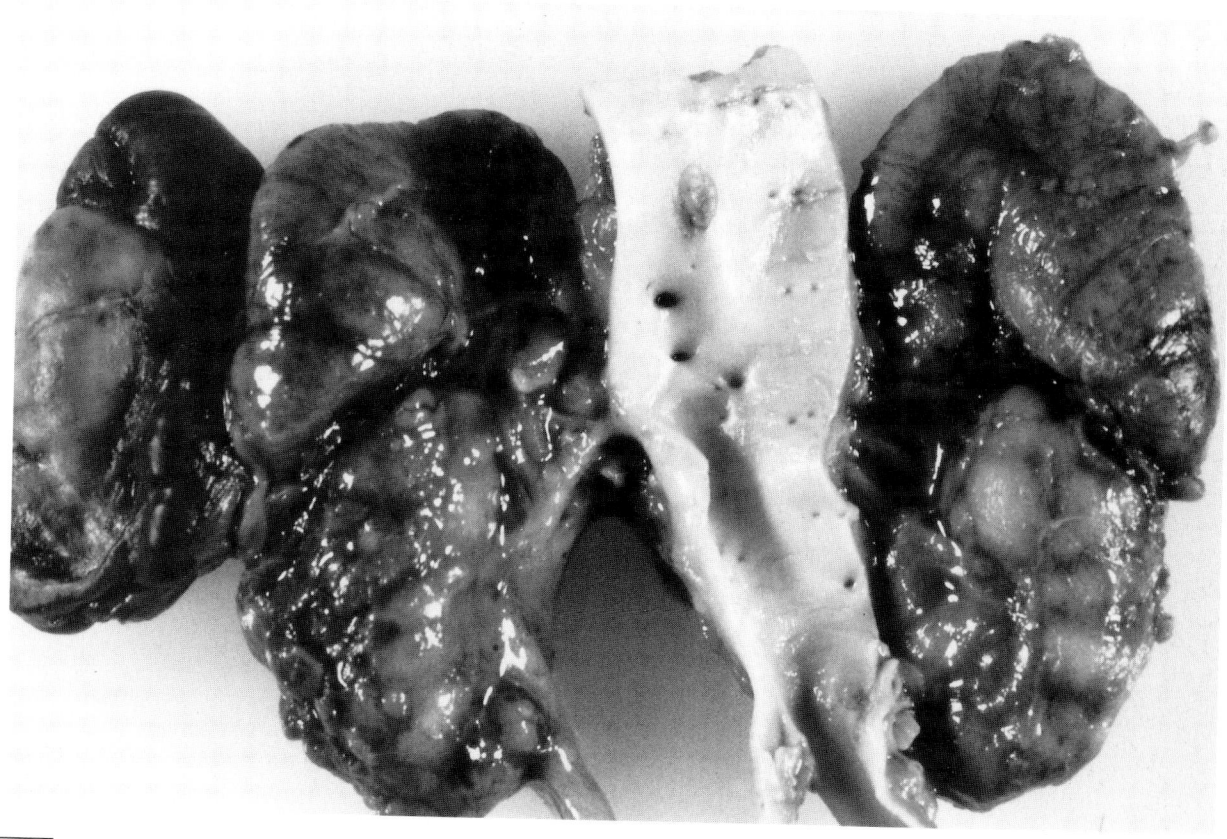

FIGURE 9.15. *Atrophy and infarcts of the spleen and the kidneys, and hemorrhagic infarct of the left adrenal from a liveborn twin whose partner in utero died several weeks before delivery. (En bloc specimen, posterior view; same case as in Figs. 9.13 and 9.14.)*

other frequent lesions are infarcts in the spleen and kidney [48, 61] (Figs. 9.13–9.15). Cases have been described with cardiac and hepatic infarcts [119], with intestinal atresia [112], and with necrosis of an extremity in the surviving twin [120]. Mannino and colleagues have shown that skin defects (aplasia cutis congenita) involving the trunk and limbs often occur in the liveborn monozygotic twin whose stillborn twin sibling is a fetus papyraceus [121]. Yet Kindred, in a review of 150 cases of fetus papyraceus, did not describe skin defects or other ischemic lesions in the survivors [111]. Triplets, quadruplets, and higher multiples are also susceptible to this complication, but only if the circulation seems to communicate with that of the dead sibling [74]. The postulated mechanisms are circulatory and vascular insults with ischemia of the affected tissues, lethal in one twin but sublethal in the other. Thrombosis due to passage of thromboplastic material through the placenta from the dead twin to the live twin is another theory that was recanted in favor of shock caused by hemorrhage from the survivor into the relaxed vessels of the deceased sibling [61, 122].

Maternal coagulation defects develop, but rarely unless the dead fetus has been carried in utero for a month or more. Almost all dead fetuses are delivered spontaneously within 2 weeks after their demise, so this syndrome is not often seen. If the pregnancy continues, about 25% of such mothers develop hypofibrinogenemia, elevated fibrin degradation products, and moderate thrombocytopenia [74]. Extrauterine pregnancy with fetal death has also been associated with maternal coagulopathy [113].

PLACENTAL CHANGES AFTER FETAL DEATH

The placental changes after fetal death are quite dissimilar to those in the fetus itself, because the integrity of placental tissues depends on maternal circulation more than on fetal circulation. Nearly all placentae associated with fetal death have either gross or microscopic abnormalities [123].

Grossly, placental infarcts may be found. When infarcts occupy more than 10% of the placental parenchyma, a cause-effect relationship may be invoked for the fetal death [124]. The basement membranes of trophoblast become thickened and may become mineralized within as few as 5 days [73]. The surface trophoblast is attenuated, and syncytial knots become numerous. These changes can obscure villous edema and acute inflammatory changes that may have been directly responsible for the fetal death. Conversely, infarcts and variations in placental size may be reflections of preceding disease rather than the changes associated with the stillbirth itself [73].

Syncytial knots are not increased in number until after 7 days [125]. Villous collagen, intervillous fibrin, fetal endothelial cell proliferation, calcium deposits, and villous edema increase negligibly in the first week but then became abundant. This is followed by increasing fibrosis of villi with obliteration of villous capillaries (Fig. 9.16). Fetal stem arteries become thickened and sclerotic as villous fibrosis

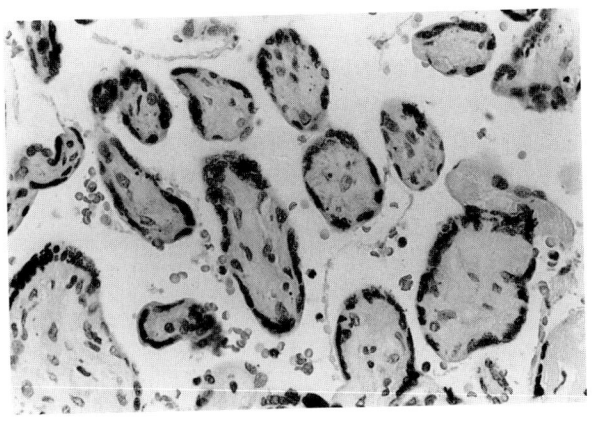

FIGURE 9.16.   *Fibrosis of the placental villi in a case with fetal death 16 days prior to delivery. H&E, ×175.*

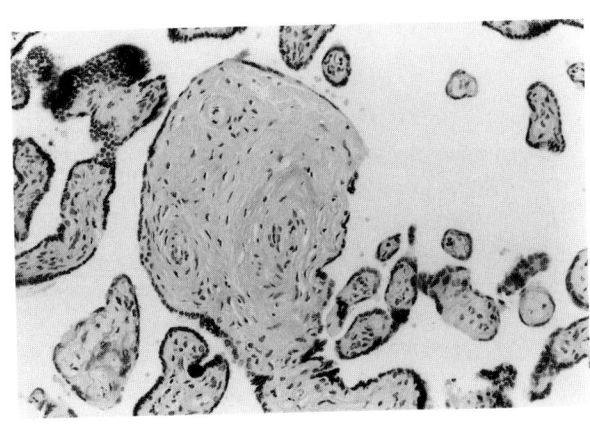

FIGURE 9.17.   *Obliteration of vessels in stem villi in a case with fetal death 16 days prior to delivery. H&E, ×40. (Same case as in Fig. 9.16.)*

increases and trophoblast basement membranes thicken in a corresponding time frame (Fig. 9.17). Proliferation of cytotrophoblast is intense in the first few days following fetal demise and slackens after 7 days.

Among grossly observed changes in placental form in fetal death, Liban and Salzberger found a fourfold increase of velamentous cord insertion and marginal cord insertion and a sevenfold increase in the incidence of single umbilical artery in their series of 1108 stillbirths [6]. Heifetz noted that nearly 60% of single umbilical arteries occur in stillborn fetuses [88]. Rayburn et al found gross abnormalities of placental form in 12% of the fetal deaths [123].

Fetal deaths that occur in gestations beyond 18 weeks have inflammatory changes in as many as 60% of placentae [69, 126]. Chorioamnionitis is the predominant inflammatory lesion and is attributed to attraction of maternal inflammatory cells by chemotactic substances elaborated from the dead fetus inside the amniotic sac.

In mothers with recurrent fetal deaths, placentae are pale and have friable villous tissue. Intervillous fibrin deposits

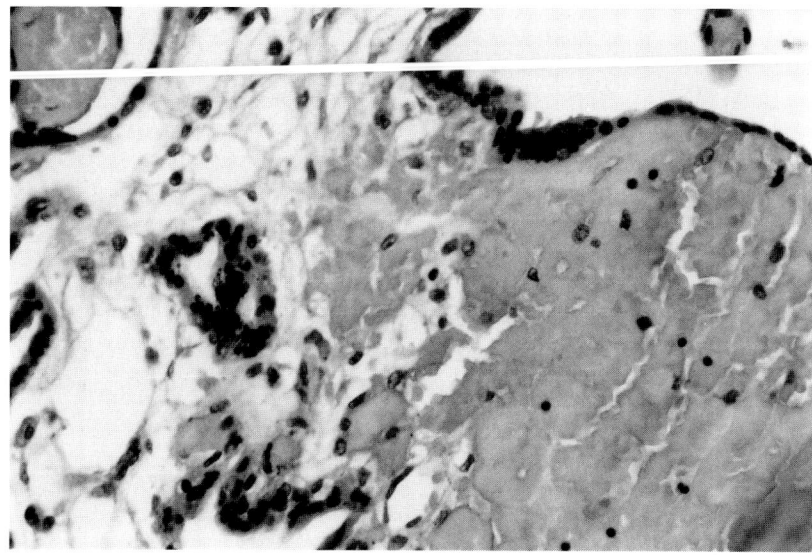

FIGURE 9.18. *Hemorrhagic endovasculitis. In this case, the baby was liveborn at 30 weeks' gestation and had multiple malformations. H&E, ×215.*

surround and choke the chorionic villi. Idiopathic villitis, sometimes with microabscesses but more often of chronic type, widespread necroses, villous vasculitis involving large vessels in the stem-villi, and lymphocytic deciduitis are also described in such cases [127–129].

With lupus anticoagulant and anticardiolipin antibodies, the placenta may be massively infarcted with necrotizing decidual vasculopathy and thromboses. In some cases, subtle nonspecific alterations are found in the placenta [34, 55, 130].

In fetal hydrops, the placentas are enlarged, boggy, and pale. Microscopically, nucleated red blood cells in fetal vessels indicate severe anemia due to maternal-fetal blood group incompatibility, fetal-maternal hemorrhage, fetal hemoglobin dyscrasias such as alpha thalassemia, or parvovirus infection.

Sander and Stevens have observed a microangiopathic process affecting chorionic vessels with thrombi, microthrombi, fragmented and extravasated red blood cells, and nucleated red blood cells [129]. These changes are designated hemorrhagic endovasculitis and are found in up to 17% of the placentae in fetal deaths. Liveborn infants, especially if born before 30 weeks' gestation, may also have placentae with these lesions [123] (Fig. 9.18). The incidences in Sander's series are from a regional placenta registry and are probably artificially high, and the clinical significance may have been overemphasized. In a series of routine placental evaluations, Shen-Schwarz et al found hemorrhagic endovasculitis in only 0.6% of cases and considered the changes as consequences of thrombosis or vascular occlusion with the morphologic features dependent on whether venous or arterial obstruction occurred [131].

A word should be said about the term "placental insufficiency." This term has been regarded by most pathologists as a "dustbin diagnosis" [99]. On the other hand, in the British survey of perinatal mortality, fairly precise criteria are used in the definition—i.e., meconium stained amniotic fluid without obvious cause (and with no clear logic), or a fetal-placental weight ratio greater than 7:1, or placental infarcts involving more than 25% of the placental mass [19]. Using one or another of these criteria, "placental insufficiency" occurs in 17% of all fetal deaths and in 50% of all full-term fetal deaths [19]. So-called immature or dysmature placentae are not generally associated with fetal deaths except as they are correlated with maternal diabetes, erythroblastosis, and other such conditions. Mercer and Brown have reported a large number of fetal deaths of unknown pathogenesis associated with oligohydramnios [101].

DURATION OF FETAL DEATH BEFORE DELIVERY

Some 57% of fetal deaths occur within 24 hours of delivery. Fewer than 20% of stillborn fetuses are carried for more than 1 week after intrauterine death, and the great majority of deliveries occurs within 2 weeks of fetal demise [17, 74]. The duration of carriage in utero after fetal death is extremely difficult to establish by either macroscopic or microscopic examination. Only crude estimates are possible. Potter mentions that skin slippage occurs after only a few hours of intrauterine carriage following fetal death [106]. After 8 to 10 days, the skin changes to a dry olive brown [108]. Langley described four grades of maceration [66], Bain used three [83], and both temporally correlated them as shown in Table 9.4.

Langley noted that in some cases of severe neonatal edema, living babies may have blistering and skin slippage but this is uncommon [66]. Bain graded maceration as "slight" with intrauterine carriage up to 48 hours after death, "moderate" from 2 to 7 days characterized by blood-stained, watery serous effusions, and "severe" from 8 days onward characterized by absence of bloody fluid in serous cavities and extensive autolysis of tissues [83]. Attempts to

Table 9.4.   Temporal correlation of grade of maceration

Grade of maceration		Physical features	Duration of fetal demise before delivery	
Langley [66]	**Bain [83]**		**Langley [66]**	**Bain [83]**
0	Slight	"Parboiled" reddened skin	<8 hours	0–48 hours
I	Slight	Skin slippage and peeling	>8 hours	0–48 hours
II	Moderate	Extensive skin peeling, red serous effusions in chest and abdomen	"Later still"	2–7 days
III	Severe	Yellow-brown liver, turbid effusions, may be mummified	"Prolonged"	≥8 days

Table 9.5.   Time of fetal death as determined by placental examination [132]

1. Villous intravascular karyorrhexis—6 or more hours
2. Vascular lumen abnormalities of stem villi, including fibroblast septation and total obliteration of lumen—multifocal 2 or more days; extensive 2 or more weeks
3. Extensive fibrosis of terminal villi—2 or more weeks.

Table 9.6.   Time of fetal death as determined by external examination of the fetus [105]

1. Desquamation at least 1 cm and brown-red discoloration of umbilical cord stump—6 or more hours
2. Desquamation involving face, abdomen, or back—12 or more hours
3. Desquamation involving 5% or more of the body surface—18 or more hours
4. Brown skin discoloration—24 or more hours
5. Mummification—2 or more weeks

Table 9.7.   Time of fetal death as determined by histologic examination of fetal tissues [133]

1. Loss of nuclear basophilia in isolated cells in renal cortical tubules—4 hours
2. Loss of nuclear basophilia in isolated cells in liver—24 hours
3. Loss of nuclear basophilia in isolated cells in inner half of myocardium—24 hours
4. Loss of nuclear basophilia in isolated cells in outer half of myocardium—48 hours
5. Loss of nuclear basophilia in isolated cells in bronchial epithelium—96 hours
6. Loss of nuclear basophilia in isolated cells in tracheal cartilage—1 week
7. Loss of nuclear basophilia in all cells in liver—96 hours
8. Loss of nuclear basophilia in all cells in GI tract—1 week
9. Loss of nuclear basophilia in all cells in adrenal—1 week
10. Loss of nuclear basophilia in all cells in kidney—4 weeks

Above changes accelerated by hydrops and delivery to autopsy interval greater than 24 hours.
Above changes decelerated by fetal gestational age less than 25 weeks.

refine the estimates of duration of fetal death have met with difficulty because of the tremendous variation in conditions—viz., maternal temperature, the presence or absence of infection (especially putrefactive infections), the presence or absence of oligohydramnios, fetal edema or dehydration, etc. The placenta may provide additional information in the first week following fetal death. Fox found that if cytotrophoblasts are increased in number but other changes have not been very prominent, the likely duration of fetal death is less than 7 days, but that if fibrosis, fibrin, calcium deposits, increased syncytial knots, thick basement membranes, and sclerotic fetal stem arteries predominate, the fetus has probably been dead for more than 7 days [125] (see Figs. 9.16 and 9.17).

Genest and his colleagues have produced valuable data regarding the pathologist's role in determining the duration of fetal death before delivery [105, 132, 133]. The results of their studies are summarized in Tables 9.5–9.7.

Even under the controlled conditions of animal experiments, investigators have encountered widely variable results in correlating autolysis and maceration with duration of intrauterine carriage after fetal death.

MACERATION AND AUTOLYSIS

Maceration (from the Latin *macerare*, to soften) is defined as the process by which tissues waste away or are softened by steeping or soaking so as to separate the parts. More simply, it is the softening of a solid by soaking [134] and is the term usually applied to the degenerative changes that take place in the dead fetus retained in utero [135]. Much of the softening of tissues occurs not just by soaking but by way of autolysis—i.e., the spontaneous disintegration of tissues or of cells by the action of autogenous enzymes. Autolysis occurs after death in a manner similar to the way it does in many nonfatal pathologic conditions.

The processes of maceration and autolysis occur in a moist environment at 37°C or higher temperatures, but are of relatively short duration—hours, days, or weeks. Exceptions are usually encountered only for fetus papyraceus and lithopedions [111].

Maceration is both associated with and confused with the process of autolysis. When tissues from liveborn infants (heart, lung, stomach, intestine containing abundant coliform bacteria, skin, kidney, pancreas, liver, muscle, and brain) are steeped in amniotic or ascitic fluids, in their intrinsic tissue fluids, or in plasma at 37°C for up to 15 days, negligible change can be detected. Vesicle formation fails to form in skin, and histology is well preserved. Other factors must be necessary for the changes observed in naturally macerated and autolyzed fetuses.

The autolytic process is one in which endogenous lytic enzymes play a role. The protease kallikrein is one such enzyme [7]. All the kallikreins are proteolytic and esterolytic and share with trypsin the ability to hydrolyze peptide bonds. Tissue kallikreins are located in salivary glands and pancreas, hence the rapid autolysis of these glands in devitalizing or ischemic processes. Kallikreins are also abundant in the liver and intestine, and this may account for the extensive autolysis seen in these organs in stillborn fetuses. Kallikrein also plays a role in the permeability of vessels. During life, this promotes exudation; after death, vascular permeability and hemolysis lead to the peculiar red-brown exudate of the macerated fetus. The suffusion of the umbilical cord with its peculiar cloudy purple-maroon discoloration is probably due to a combination of hemolysis and the effect of kallikrein in the umbilical vessels [7]. Serotonin and 5-hydroxytryptamine are also potent in producing vascular permeability and may be activated in autolysis and maceration.

In cases of infection, particularly with gas-forming bacilli such as *Clostridium perfringens*, the process of autolysis may be greatly accelerated, with virtual complete dissolution of the soft tissues in as little as 12 to 24 hours.

Experimental Fetal Death

Rat fetuses incubated at 37°C in salt solutions have changes of maceration distinct from putrefaction [136–138]. Just as in the human, rat fetuses become macerated before the placentae. Autolysis begins in the liver after about 12 hours. If the fetuses are incubated at 24°C, the process of autolysis is much slower, reaching a comparable level only after 72 hours [138]. In rat fetuses retained in utero after death, most of the maceration and autolytic changes occur within 12 to 24 hours [136, 139]. Desquamation of skin begins at 24 hours, and by 72 hours skin adheres in only a few areas to the underlying dermis. Internal organs change as early as 12 hours after fetal death, with cartilage or fibrous tissue retaining form and preservation for several days. Cartilage from large joints, fascia lata, or abdominal fascia are often used for attempted tissue culture for cytogenetic and other studies. Variation is the rule with these animal experiments. Corey noted astonishingly good preservation of some animals retained in utero as long as 10 days after death, while others were severely autolyzed in 48 to 72 hours [139]. The order of dissolution of tissues in the mouse model in general is as follows: capillaries, epidermis, ear, lens, retina, brain, esophagus, stomach, gonads, anterior spinal cord, metanephros, posterior spinal cord, intestines, liver, sclerotome, heart, and finally precartilage. A different order has been observed in other experiments and in humans [139]. Human kidney, liver, and intestines are among the first tissues to undergo severe autolysis.

Shanklin et al examined fetuses of NZ white rabbits by ligating umbilical cords between days 23 and 30 [135]. At 72 hours, specimens had maximimum liquefaction, and by 96 hours fetuses appeared compressed. Changes in various tissues are described below.

Skin: Gross slippage began at 12 hours and peaked at 96 hours. Microscopically, perinuclear halos formed in the epidermal cells within 90 minutes; these disappeared after 12 hours. Leaking of red blood cells from vessels and laking of them in the dermis occurred after 90 minutes. Blebs appeared at the epidermal-dermal junction in 9 hours. By 48 hours, the vesicles sloughed and staining with hematoxylin was more difficult. After 150 hours, minimal basophilia could be detected in stained preparations of skin. *Kidney:* After 90 minutes of interrupted umbilical cord blood flow, the nuclei in the ducts of Bellini became irregular. Between 6 and 12 hours, ribbons of these cells detached from their basement membranes and sloughed into the ductal lumina. Endothelial cells in renal vessels sloughed in ribbons into the vascular lumina after 30 hours. Basophilia persisted in the nephrogenic zone cells for 48 hours after cessation of blood flow, but by 150 hours this had faded virtually completely. *Liver:* Loss of hepatocytic cohesiveness developed within 90 minutes. Bile duct epithelium sloughed at 15 hours. Basophilia was lost by 30 hours and was complete by 120 hours. This is in contrast to observations in human liver tissue in which loss of cytoarchitecture and basophilia occurs more quickly, within 24 to 48 hours. *Lung:* The pattern of sloughing of epithelium of bronchi and vessels is similar to those described for other organs. Proteinaceous fluid fills air spaces and becomes stained with hemoglobin from laked red blood cells. This imparts a purple color in the gross examination of lungs. Pulmonary cytologic detail is preserved long after disappearance in other viscera—e.g., liver and kidney. Overall, the earliest changes observed in this experiment were laking of red blood cells and pyknosis of nuclei, particularly those of

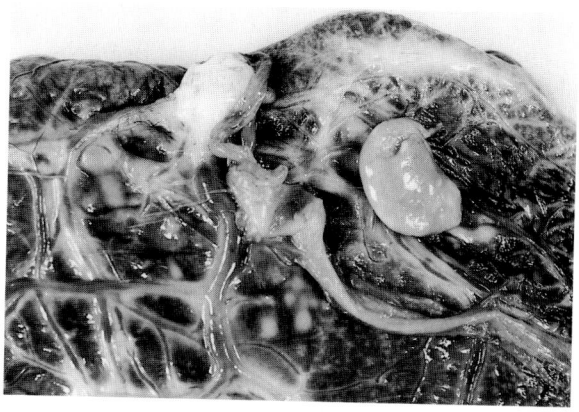

FIGURE 9.19. *Dead embryo, incorporated into amniotic membrane of placenta. The twin was liveborn at term.*

extramedullary hematopoiesis in the liver and protein fluid leaks into air spaces in the lungs [135].

Comparisons of these experimental results with changes observed in humans should be made with caution, particularly in view of the variations in the experimental data and the known differences between intrauterine temperatures in rabbits (about 40.5°C, or 105°F) and humans (37°C, or 98.6°F).

While resorption of fetuses is commonly observed among small animals, particularly rodents, its occurrence in human intrauterine pregnancies is doubted [108]. In cases of blighted ova, the embryo is either expelled or is never formed. In some instances of twins, triplets, and other multiple gestations, early loss of one or more of the conceptuses may be obscured by compression of the embryos or fetuses into a scarcely recognizable fibrous mat or plaque on the surface of the placenta or in the free membranes (Fig. 9.19).

REFERENCES

1. Ballantyne JW. Ante-natal, intra-natal, and neo-natal death: causes, pathology and prevention, with special reference to ante-natal death. *Brit Med J* 1992; 2:583–8.
2. Driscoll SG. Autopsy following stillbirth: a challenge neglected. In: Ryder OA, Byrd ML, eds. *One Medicine*. Berlin: Springer-Verlag, 1984, pp. 19–31.
3. Shepard TH, Fantel AG. Embryonic and early fetal loss. *Clin Perinatol* 1979; 6:219–43.
4. Woods DL, Draper RR. A clinical assessment of stillborn infants. *S Afr Med J* 1980; 57:441–3.
5. Anonymous. *Vital Statistics Annual Report*. Rhode Island Department of Health, 1986.
6. Liban E, Salzberger M. A prospective clinicopathological study of 1108 cases of antenatal fetal death. *Israel J Med Sci* 1976; 12:34–44.
7. Wilhelm DL. Inflammation and healing. In: Anderson WAD, Kissave J, eds. *Pathology*. 7th ed. St. Louis: Mosby, 1977, pp. 25–37.
8. Crawford MD, Gardner MJ, Sedgwick PA. Infant mortality and hardness of water supplies. *Lancet* 1972; 1:918–922.
9. Hein HA, Lathrop SS, Papke KP. Comparing perinatal mortality. *Obstet Gynecol* 1985; 66:346–9.
10. Kaunitz AM, Spence C, Danielson TS, Rochat RW, Grimes DA. Perinatal and maternal mortality in a religious group avoiding obstetric care. *Am J Obstet Gynecol* 1984; 150:826–31.
11. Hook EB, Porter IH. Terminologic conventions, methodological considerations, temporal trends, specific genes, environmental hazards, and some other factors pertaining to embryonic and fetal death. In: Porter I, Hook E, eds. *Human Embryonic and Fetal Death*. New York: Academic Press, 1980, pp. 1ff.
12. Teller CH, Clyburn S. Trends in infant mortality. *Texas Business Review* 1974; October:240–6.
13. Cartlidge PH, Stewart JH. Effect of changing the stillbirth definition on evaluation of perinatal mortality rates. *Lancet* 1995; 346:486–8.
14. Hussey HH. Neonatal mortality. *JAMA* 1976; 235:944.
15. Manning FA, Morrison I, Lange IR, Harman CR, Chamberlain PF. Fetal assessment based on fetal biophysical profile scoring: experience in 12,620 referral high-risk pregnancies. I. Perinatal mortality by frequency and etiology. *Am J Obstet Gynecol* 1985; 151:343–50.
16. Bierman JM, Siegel E, French FE, Simonian K. Analysis of the outcome of all pregnancies in a community. Kauai pregnancy study. *Am J Obstet Gynecol* 1965; 91:37–45.
17. Simpson JW, Geppert LJ. The responsibility of the obstetrician to the fetus. 1. An analysis of fetal and neonatal mortality in 10,000 deliveries. *Am J Obstet Gynecol* 1951; 62:1062–70.
18. Cruikshank DP, Linyear AS. Term stillbirth: causes and potential for prevention in Virginia. *Obstet Gynecol* 1987; 69:841–44.
19. Morrison I, Olsen J. Weight specific stillbirth and associated causes of death: an analysis of 765 stillbirths. *Am J Obstet Gynecol* 1985; 152:975–80.
20. Yudkin PL, Wood L, Redman CWG. Risk of unexplained stillbirth at different gestational ages. *Lancet* 1987; 1:1192–4.
21. Becker MJ, Becker AE. *Pathology of Late Fetal Stillbirth*. Edinburgh: Churchill Livingstone, 1989, p. 128.
22. Vaughan TL, Daling JR, Starzyk PM. Fetal death and maternal occupation. An analysis of birth records in the state of Washington. *J Occup Med* 1984; 26:676–8.
23. Kiely JL, Paneth N, Susser M. An assessment of the effects of maternal age and parity in different components of perinatal mortality. *Am J Epidemiol* 1986; 123:444–54.
24. Mcllwaine GM, Howat RCL, Dunn F, MacNaughton MC. The Scottish Perinatal Mortality Survey. *Brit Med J* 1979; 2:1103–6.
25. Turkel SB. Perinatal autopsy. *N Engl J Med* 1984; 310:394.
26. Hovatta O, Lipasti A, Rapola J, Karjalainen O. Causes of stillbirth: a clinicopathological study of 243 patients. *Br J Obstet Gynaecol* 1983; 90:691–6.
27. Friedman E. *Hypertension in Pregnancy*. New York: Wiley, 1976.
28. Abdella TN, Sibai BM, Hays JM Jr, Anderson GD. Relationship of hypertensive disease to abruptio placentae. *Obstet Gynecol* 1984; 63:365–8.
29. Strachan G. The pathology of foetal maceration. *Br Med J* 1922; 2:80–2.
30. Eastman NJ. *The Toxemias of Pregnancy*. In: Williams Obstetrics, 11th ed. New York: Appleton-Century-Crofts, 1951, p. 691.
31. Whittemore R, Hobbins JC, Engle MA. Pregnancy and its outcome in women with and without surgical treatment of congenital heart disease. *Am J Cardiol* 1982; 50:641–5.
32. Rotellar C, Ferragui A, Borrull J. Pregnancy in a patient on regular hemodialysis. *Nephron* 1983; 35:66–7.
33. Brem A, Singer DB, Lester B, Abuelo JG. Infants of azotemic mothers: a report of three live births. *Am J Kidney Dis* 1988; 12:299–303.
34. Scott JR, Rote NS, Branch DW. Immunologic aspects of recurrent abortion and fetal death. *Obstet Gynecol* 1987; 70:645–56.
35. Hall J, Pauli R, Wilson K. Maternal and fetal sequelae of anticoagulation during pregnancy. *Am J Med* 1980; 68:122–38.
36. McGrady GA, Daling JR, Peterson DR. Maternal urinary tract infection and adverse outcomes. *Am J Epidemiol* 1985; 121:377–81.
37. Anonymous. Urinary tract infection during pregnancy. *Lancet* 1985; 2:190–2.
38. Anonymous. Maternal drug addiction and the neonate. *Lancet* 1973; 1:527.
39. Kuhnert BR, Kuhnert PM. Placental transfer of drugs, alcohol, and components of cigarette smoke and their effects on the human fetus. In: Chang CN, Lee CC, eds. *Prenatal Drug Exposure, Kinetics and Dynamics*. Rockville, MD: National Institute of Drug Abuse, 1985.
40. Kahn EL, Neumann LL, Polk G-A. The course of heroin withdrawal syndrome in newborn infants treated with phenobarbital and chlorpromazine. *J Pediatr* 1969; 75:495–500.
41. Clarren SK, Smith DW. The fetal alcohol syndrome. *N Engl J Med* 1978; 298:1063–7.
42. Butler NR, Goldstein H, Ross EM. Cigarette smoking in pregnancy. Its influence on birth weight and perinatal mortality. *Br Med J* 1972; 2:127–30.
43. Niswander NR, Gordon M. *National Institute of Neurological Disease and Stroke: The Women and Their Pregnancies*. Bethesda: DHEW Publication (NIH), 1972, pp. 73–379.
44. Naeye RL. Abruptio placentae and placenta praevia. Frequency, perinatal mortality and cigarette smoking. *Obstet Gynecol* 1980; 55:701–4.
45. Chasnoff IR, Burns WJ, Schnoll SH, Burns KA. Cocaine use in pregnancy. *N Engl J Med* 1985; 313:666–9.
46. Bingol N, Fuchs M, Diaz V, Stone RK, Gromisch DS. Teratogenicity of cocaine in humans. *J Pediatr* 1987; 110:93–6.
47. Oro AS, Dixon SD. Perinatal cocaine and methamphetamine exposure: maternal and neonatal correlates. *J Pediatr* 1987; 111:571–8.
48. Moore TR, Sorg J, Miller L, Key TC, Resnik R. Hemodynamic effects of intravenous cocaine on the pregnant ewe and fetus. *Am J Obstet Gynecol* 1986; 155:883–8.
49. Turner G, Collins E. Fetal effects of regular salicylate ingestion in pregnancy. *Lancet* 1975; 2:338–9.
50. American Academy of Pediatrics, Committee on Drugs. Anticonvulsants and pregnancy. *Pediatrics* 1979; 63:331–2.
51. Woodhouse S. The lupus anticoagulant and the dilute Russell viper venom test. *Pathologist* 1984; 38:432–3.
52. Lockshin MD, Druzin ML, Goei S, et al. Antibody to cardiolipin as a predictor of fetal distress or death in pregnant patients with systemic lupus erythematosus. *N Engl J Med* 1985; 313:152–4.
53. Gleicher N, Friberg N. IgM gammopathy and the lupus anticoagulant syndrome in habitual aborters. *JAMA* 1985; 253:3278–81.
54. Triplett DA, Brandt JT, Musgrave KA, Orr CA. The relationship between lupus anticoagulants and antibodies to phospholipids. *JAMA* 1988; 259:550–4.

55. Lubbe WF, Butler WS, Palmer SJ, Liggins GC. Fetal survival after prednisone suppression of maternal lupus-anticoagulant. *Lancet* 1983; i:1361–3.
56. Branch DW, Scott JR, Kochenour NK, Hershgold E. Obstetric complications associated with the lupus anti-coagulant. *N Engl J Med* 1985; 313:1322–6.
57. Rix P, Stentoft J, Aunsholt NA, et al. Lupus anticoagulant and anticardiolipin antibodies in an obstetric population. *Acta Obstet Gynecol Scand* 1992; 71:605–9.
58. Bocciolone L, Meroni P, Parazzini F, et al. Antiphospholipid antibodies and risk of intrauterine fetal death. *Acta Obstet Gynecol Scand* 1994; 73:389–92.
59. Grimmer D, Landas S, Kemp JD. IgM antitrophoblast antibodies in a patient with pregnancy-associated lupuslike disorder, vasculitis and recurrent fetal demise. *Arch Pathol Lab Med* 1988; 112:191–3.
60. Feinstein DI. Lupus anticoagulant, thrombosis, and fetal loss. *N Engl J Med* 1985; 313:1348–50.
61. Benirschke K. Twin placenta in perinatal mortality. *NY J Med* 1961; 61:1499–1508.
62. Fedrick J, Adelstein P. Preceding pregnancy loss as an index of risk of stillbirth or neonatal death in the present pregnancy. *Biol Neonate* 1977; 31:84–93.
63. Fujikura T, Froehlich LA, Driscoll SG. A simplified classification of abortions. *Am J Obstet Gynecol* 1966; 95:902–5.
64. Machin GA. Chromosome abnormality and perinatal death. *Lancet* 1974; i:549–51.
65. Löfgren O, Polberger S. Perinatal mortality: changes in the diagnostic panorama 1974–1980. *Acta Paediatr Scand* 1983; 72:327–32.
66. Langley FA. The perinatal postmortem examination. *J Clin Pathol* 1971; 24:159–69.
67. Wigglesworth JS. Monitoring perinatal mortality. A pathophysiological approach. *Lancet* 1980; 2:684–6.
68. Huff DS. Which stillborn fetus should have an autopsy. *Lab Invest* 1983; 48:6p.
69. Keeling J. Macerated stillbirth. In: Keeling JW, ed. *Fetal and Neonatal Pathology*. London: Springer-Verlag, 1987, pp. 167–77.
70. Saller DN Jr, Lesser KB, Harrel U, Rogers BB, Oyer CE. The clinical utility of the perinatal autopsy. *JAMA* 1995; 273:663–5.
71. Rushton DI. Prognostic role of the perinatal postmortem. *Br J Hosp Med* 1994; 52:450–4.
72. Huidi C, Dixian J. Analysis of 645 autopsy findings in fetuses and newborn infants from the clinical obstetric viewpoint. *Chinese Med J* 1980; 93:474–6.
73. Wigglesworth JS. *Perinatal Pathology*. Philadelphia: WB Saunders, 1984, pp. 84–92.
74. Pritchard JA, MacDonald PC, Gant NF. *Williams Obstetrics*. 17th ed. Norwalk: Appleton-Century Crofts, 1984, pp. 218–20.
75. O'Brien WF, Knuppel RA, Saba HI, et al. Platelet inhibitory activity in placentas from normal and abnormal pregnancies. *Obstet Gynecol* 1987; 70:597–600.
76. Glanfield PA, Watson R. Intrauterine fetal death due to umbilical cord torsion. *Arch Pathol Lab Med* 1986; 110:357–8.
77. Naeye RL. The investigation of perinatal deaths. *N Engl J Med* 1983; 309:611–12.
78. Rosenthal AH, Smith JH, Gold EM, Jacobziner H. Postmaturity as a factor in fetal wastage. *NY State J Med* 1956; 56:691–704.
79. Squier M, Keeling JW. The incidence of prenatal brain injury. *Neuropath Appl Neurobiol* 1991; 17:29–38.
80. Bloxham CA. Angiodysgenetic necrotising encephalopathy: presentation as an intrauterine death. *Acta Neuropathologica* 1992; 84:221–4.
81. Laneri GG, Claassen DL, Scher MS. Brain lesions of fetal onset in encephalopathic infants with nonimmune hydrops fetalis. *Pediatr Neurol* 1994; 11:18–22.
82. Burke CJ, Tannenberg AE. Prenatal brain damage and placental infarction. An autopsy study. *Dev Med Child Neurol* 1995; 37:555–62.
83. Bain AD. The perinatal autopsy. In: Cockburn F, Drillien CM, eds. *Neonatal Medicine*. Oxford: Blackwell Scientific, 1974, pp. 820–34.
84. Singer DB. Hemorrhage in cardiac conduction tissue in premature infants. *Arch Pathol Lab Med* 1985; 109:1093–6.
85. Kasznica J, Nisar N. Congenital vascular malformation of the uterus in a stillborn: a case report. *Hum Pathol* 1995; 26:240–1.
86. Reece EA, Lockwood CJ, Rizzo N, et al. Intrinsic intrathoracic malformations of the fetus: sonographic detection and clinical presentation. *Obstet Gynecol* 1987; 70:627–33.
87. Gilbert WM, Nicolaides KH. Fetal omphalocele: associated malformations and chromosomal defects. *Obstet Gynecol* 1987; 70:633–5.
88. Heifetz S. Single umbilical artery: a statistical analysis of 237 autopsy cases. *Lab Invest* 1983; 48:6p.
89. Alberman ED, Creasy MR. Frequency of chromosomal abnormalities in miscarriages and perinatal deaths. *J Med Genet* 1977; 143:13–315.
90. Ellis PM, Bain AD. Cytogenetics in the evaluation of perinatal death. *Lancet* 1984; 1:630–1.
91. Szulman AE. Chromosomal aberrations in spontaneous human abortions. *N Engl J Med* 1965; 272:811–18.
92. Saal HM, Rodis J, Weinbaum PJ, DiMaggio R, Landrey TM. Cytogenetic evaluation of fetal death. The role of amniocentesis. *Obstet Gynecol* 1987; 70:601–3.
93. Macpherson TA, Garver KL, Turner JH, et al. Predicting in vitro tissue culture growth for cytogenetic evaluation of stillborn fetuses. *Eur J Obstet Gynecol Reprod Biol* 1985; 19:167–74.
94. Evaldson GR, Malmborg A-S, Nord CE. Premature rupture of the membranes and ascending infection. *Br J Obstet Gynaecol* 1982; 89:793–801.
95. Young SA, Crocker DW. Occult congenital syphilis in macerated stillborn fetuses. *Arch Pathol Lab Med* 1994; 118:44–7.
96. Harcke HT, Naeye RL, Storch A, Blanc WA. Perinatal cerebral intraventricular hemorrhage. *J Pediatr* 1972; 80:37–42.
97. Shanklin DR, Sotelo-Avila C. In situ tumors in fetuses, newborns and young infants. *Biol Neonat* 1969; 14:286–316.
98. Heifetz S, Rueda-Pedroza ME. Hemangiomas of the umbilical cord. *Pediatr Pathol* 1983; 1:385–98.
99. Anonymous. Unexplained stillbirth. *Lancet* 1987; 1:22–3.
100. Cordier MP, Sournies G, Domenichini Y, et al. Bilan de 100 autopsies practiquées dans le service de Maternité de L'Hotel Dieu de Lyon sur un période de 18 mois. *J Genet Hum* 1985; 33:295–300.
101. Mercer LJ, Brown LG. Fetal outcome with oligohydramnios in the second trimester. *Obstet Gynecol* 1986; 67:840–2.
102. Pritchard JA, MacDonald PC, Gant NF. *Williams Obstetrics*. 17th ed. Norwalk: Appleton-Century-Crofts, 1984, pp. 404–43.
103. Rezek GH. A biologic test for the diagnosis of intrauterine fetal death. *Am J Obstet Gynecol* 1936; 32:976–81.
104. Small ML, Phelan JP, Smith CV, Paul RH. An active management approach to the postdate fetus with a reactive nonstress test and fetal heart rate decelerations. *Obstet Gynecol* 1987; 70:636–40.
105. Genest DR, Singer DB. Estimating the time of death in stillborn fetuses: III. External fetal examination: a study of 86 stillborns. *Obstet Gynecol* 1992; 80:593–600.
106. Potter EL. *Pathology of the Fetus and Infant*. Chicago: Year Book Medical Publishers Inc, 1961.
107. Janssen W. *Forensic Histopathology*. Berlin: Springer-Verlag, 1984.
107a. Kalousek DK, Pantzar T, Craver R. So-called primitive neuroectodermal tumor in aborted previable fetuses. *Pediatr Pathol* 1988; 8:503–11.
108. Potter EL, Craig JM. *Pathology of the Fetus and Infant*. 2 ed. Chicago: Year Book Medical Publishers, 1975, p. 595.
109. Dorovini-Zis K, Dolman CL. Gestational development of brain. *Arch Pathol Lab Med* 1977; 101:192–5.
110. Becker MJ, Becker AE. Fat distribution in the adrenal cortex as an indication of the mode of intrauterine death. *Hum Pathol* 1976; 7:495–504.
111. Kindred JE. Twin pregnancies with one twin blighted. Report of two cases with comparative study of cases in the literature. *Am J Obstet Gynecol* 1944; 48:642–82.
112. Saier FS, Burden L, Cavanagh D. Fetus papyraceus: an unusual case with congenital anomaly of the surviving fetus. *Obstet Gynecol* 1975; 45:217–18.
113. Dehner LP. Advanced extrauterine pregnancy and the fetal death syndrome. Report of a case with clinicopathologic considerations. *Obstet Gynecol* 1972; 40:525–34.
114. Gill JJ. Fetus adipocere monster. *Am J Obstet Gynecol* 1945; 49:440–1.
115. Gould GM, Pyle WL. *Anomalies and Curiosities of Medicine*. New York: Bell, 1956, pp. 50–64.
116. Mathieu A. Lithopedion developed from extrauterine gestation in intrauterine and extrauterine pregnancy. *Am J Obstet Gynecol* 1939; 37:297–302.
117. Yoshioka H, Kadomoto Y, Mino M, et al. Multicystic encephalomalacia in liveborn twin with a stillborn macerated co-twin. *J Pediatr* 1979; 95:798–800.
118. Dudley DKL, D'Alton ME. Single fetal death in twin gestation. *Semin Perinatol* 1986; 10:65–72.
119. Moore CM, McAdams AJ, Sutherland J. Intrauterine disseminated intravascular coagulation: a syndrome of multiple pregnancy with a dead twin fetus. *J Pediatr* 1969; 74:523–7.
120. Balfour RP. Fetus papyraceus. *Obstet Gynecol* 1976; 47:507.
121. Mannino FL, Jones KL, Benirschke K. Congenital skin defects and fetus papyraceus. *J Pediatr* 1977; 91:559–64.

122. Benirschke K. Intrauterine death of a twin: mechanisms, implications for surviving twin, and placental pathology. *Semin Diag Pathol* 1993; 10:222–31.

123. Rayburn W, Sander C, Barr M Jr, Rygiel R. The stillborn fetus: placental histologic examination in determining a cause. *Obstet Gynecol* 1985; 65: 637–41.

124. Fox H. *Pathology of the Placenta*. London: WB Saunders, 1978, pp. 115–23.

125. Fox H. Morphological changes in the human placenta following fetal death. *J Obstet Gynaecol Br Commonw* 1968; 75:839–43.

126. Ornoy A, Salamon-Arnon J, Ben-Zur Z, Kohn G. Placental findings in spontaneous abortions and stillbirths. *Teratology* 1981; 24:243–52.

127. Russell P, Atkinson K, Krishnan L. Recurrent reproductive failure due to severe placental villitis of unknown etiology. *J Reprod Med* 1980; 24:93–8.

128. Redline RW, Abramowsky CR. Clinical and pathologic aspects of recurrent placental villitis. *Hum Pathol* 1985; 16:727–31.

129. Sander CH, Stevens NG. Hemorrhagic endovasculitis of the placenta: an in depth morphologic appraisal with initial epidemiological observations. *Pathol Annu* 1984; 19:37–79.

130. DeWolf F, Carreras LO, Moerman P, et al. Decidual vasculopathy and extensive placental infarction in a patient with repeated thromboembolic accidents, recurrent fetal loss and lupus anticoagulant. *Am J Obstet Gynecol* 1982; 142:829–31.

131. Shen-Schwarz S, Macpherson TA, Mueller-Heubach E. The clinical significance of hemorrhagic endovasculitis of the placenta. *Am J Obstet Gynecol* 1988; 159:48–51.

132. Genest DR. Estimating the time of death in stillborn fetuses: II. Histologic evaluation of the placenta: a study of 71 stillborns. *Obstet Gynecol* 1992; 80:585–92.

133. Genest DR, Williams MA, Greene MF. Estimating the time of death in stillborn fetuses: I. Histologic evaluation of fetal organs: an autopsy study of 150 stillborns. *Obstet Gynecol* 1992; 80:575–84.

134. Dorland WAN. *The American Illustrated Medical Dictionary*. Philadelphia: WB Saunders Co, 1951.

135. Shanklin DR, Cimino DA, Lamb TH. Fetal maceration. 1. An experimental sequence in the rabbit. *Am J Obstet Gynecol* 1964; 88:213–23.

136. Crosman AM. An experimental study of dissolution and absorption of retained dead fetuses. *Am J Obstet Gynecol* 1936; 32:964–75.

137. Long CNH, Parkes AS. On the nature of foetal reabsorption. *Biochem J* 1924; 18:800–6.

138. Nicholas JS. Embryonic rat tissue survival. *Proc Soc Exp Biol Med 2* 1931; 19:188–90.

139. Corey EL. The maceration and resorption of fetuses in the rat. *Anat Rec* 1933; 56:195–209.

Pathology of Intrapartum and Early Neonatal Death in the Normally Formed Infant

Jonathan S. Wigglesworth

INTRODUCTION

Intrapartum and early neonatal deaths of normally formed infants constitute a group of perinatal deaths that cause continuing concern in developed countries. This concern stems from the unexpected occurrence of most such deaths and the theoretically preventable nature of many of them.

The problem of birth asphyxia commands particular attention in view of the high frequency, in developed countries, of medicolegal claims alleging birth asphyxia as the cause of permanent neurologic handicap. Although there can be no doubt that sometimes this may be the case, recent studies indicate that prenatal brain damage may account for a major proportion of such handicaps [1–3].

The second group of conditions that may cause death in normally developed infants—those associated with mechanical trauma—are equally unacceptable in developed countries and equally likely to provoke medicolegal actions on behalf of handicapped survivors. Trauma is linked closely with asphyxia and needs to be discussed along with it rather than under the separate heading of iatrogenic disorders.

The third problem relevant to this chapter, that of unexplained death during or soon after birth, is a practical one that is linked with asphyxia and trauma, but touches also on infection and metabolic abnormalities, which are the subjects of Chapters 17 and 18, respectively.

BIRTH ASPHYXIA

Mechanisms of Birth Asphyxia

Normal Fetal Cardiorespiratory State

Some 30–40% of the fetal cardiac output perfuses the placenta by the middle of human pregnancy [4], whereas 15% perfuses the brain, 10% the intestine, 3% the kidneys, and 2% the heart. Similar figures are obtained in species such as the rhesus monkey and the lamb, although the proportion of cardiac output to the brain is lower in these species [5, 6]. Work on the fetal lamb indicates that the fetus maintains cardiac output near maximum through a high mean systemic pressure modulated through a relatively high blood volume and low systemic vascular resistance [7]. Although a further increase in blood volume causes a limited further increase in cardiac output, any decrease in volume causes both right atrial pressure and cardiac output to decline [7]. The oxygen tension in the umbilical vein is about 28 mm Hg and that in the umbilical artery is 15 mm Hg [8]. The fetal heart rate ranges from 120 to 160 beats per minute but shows considerable beat-to-beat variation. The fetus undertakes periodic respiratory movements in the form of low-amplitude/high-frequency excursions of the diaphragm, with lesser, largely paradoxical movements of the thoracic wall. In addition, the fetus shows considerable general activity, making a wide range of active body movements, as well as swallowing.

Influence of Labor

Normal labor has significant effects on fetal cardiorespiratory function. Amniotomy may cause transient changes in fetal heart rate [9]. Uterine contractions inevitably cause a decrease in uteroplacental blood flow, as shown many years ago in the rhesus monkey by Ramsey et al [10]. Maternal posture during late pregnancy and labor may influence placental perfusion. When the mother is supine there is a risk of compression of the aorta and vena cava by the gravid uterus [11, 12]. In normal human labor, there may be a fall of capillary pH during the first and second stages of labor [13].

Most information about the effects of normal and abnormal labor on fetal well-being in the human infant comes from studies of fetal heart rate, uterine contractions, and fetal scalp pH [14–17]. These studies, although helpful and scientifically interesting, cannot of course give a complete picture of fetal response during pregnancy and labor. The lack of ability to measure fetal blood pressure in particular must strictly limit the value of the information that can be derived from fetal monitoring studies. The fetal heart rate normally shows accelerations of up to 15 beats per minute (bpm) with fetal movement; decelerations of a similar magnitude coincident with uterine contractions (type 1 dips) may also be normal. An increase in baseline fetal heart rate may occur in both normal and abnormal labor but is more common in abnormal labor and may be the first sign of fetal hypoxic stress [16].

Maternal levels of circulating catecholamines are lower during pregnancy than in the nonpregnant state. Jones and Greiss [18] found that levels of both adrenaline and noradrenaline rise during the course of labor, and adrenaline levels exceed those in the nonpregnant state. The same authors found high levels of catecholamines in the umbilical artery at birth, indicating significant fetal output during labor. Since it has been shown that increased fetal catecholamine levels cause a switch in the fetal lung from a phase of liquid secretion to liquid resorption [19], one effect of this process may be partly to "dry up" the fetal lungs before birth. Caesarean section before the onset of labor is not associated with increased catecholamine output, and the lungs at birth may retain most of the fetal lung liquid with consequent increased delay in full gaseous expansion after birth (transient tachypnea of the newborn). Thus, the "stress" of labor may be a normal and beneficial process aiding physiologic adaptation to birth.

The Fetal Response to Hypoxia

In the classic acute asphyxial experiments on fetal animals delivered into a warm saline environment after umbilical cord occlusion [20], the initial effect was a short period of respiratory efforts, which ended abruptly and was followed by a phase of apnea (primary apnea). There was then a period of repeated gasps, which became more frequent and weaker before ceasing. During the final phase of secondary or terminal apnea, the blood pressure and heart rate fell rapidly and the fetus would die unless revived by mechanical ventilation with oxygen. This type of experiment may be similar to the effect of umbilical occlusion due to prolapsed umbilical cord in the human fetus or the terminal phases of any fatal asphyxial process, but does not relate closely to the early stages of slowly progressive fetal or intrapartum asphyxia.

Detailed studies of the effects of prolonged hypoxia on the fetus have been performed mainly in the lamb. During hypoxemia in unanesthetized fetal lambs in utero, fetal arterial pressure increases and fetal heart rate decreases with a fall in cardiac output [21]. There is maintenance of blood flow to the placenta, an increased flow to brain, heart, and adrenals, but decreased flow to lungs, kidneys, spleen, gut, and carcass. Blood flow to the central nervous system

(CNS), heart, and adrenals in this species increases in inverse relation to the fetal arterial O_2 content between 6 and 1 mmol/L [6]. The relatively much greater size of the human fetal brain (12% rather than 2% of body mass) must inevitably limit the extent to which cerebral flow can be increased in the hypoxic human fetus. Studies in the fetal primate [22] showed effects on blood flow similar to those in the lamb. The increased proportion of cardiac output supplying the brain in asphyxia was distributed to preserve greater blood flow in noncortical areas, with a relatively greater increase (per gram of tissue) going to the brainstem.

During hypoxia, the fetus has to engage in anaerobic metabolism and utilize alternative energy sources, such as lactate. There is inevitably an increasing metabolic acidosis, accentuated by the reduced circulation to many tissues. The increasing carbon dioxide tension within the fetal blood has its own effects on the circulation, such as enhancing cerebral vasodilatation. In the clinical situation there is never a pure hypoxia but always a condition of asphyxia—i.e., a combination of hypoxia and acidosis. Fetal survival in asphyxia depends on the maintenance of myocardial function, which in turn may depend on factors such as the level of myocardial glycogen stores available for anaerobic glycolysis [23].

Study of human fetal respiratory activity in utero shows cessation of normal fetal respiratory movements in response to hypoxia [24], as observed in the early stages of acute experimental asphyxia.

In the late stages of asphyxia, the human fetus also may undertake gasping respirations and inhale amniotic fluid with squames and meconium if meconium has been passed. The passage of meconium is a frequent occurrence in acute fetal or intrapartum asphyxia, but a small amount of meconium staining of the amniotic fluid is common and may be seen in a high proportion of pregnancies at term.

Modern diagnosis and assessment of human fetal hypoxia depends on the interpretation of fetal heart rate tracings and scalp pH records in relation to uterine contractions. During metabolic acidosis there is often a loss of the normal beat-to-beat variation in fetal heart rate. This has been found to be a useful sign of depression of fetal reflex activity, such as that due to asphyxia, prior to labor [25]. However, the interpretation of fetal heart traces before the onset of labor poses considerable problems. More than 90% of growth-retarded fetuses have been reported to show some impairment of fetal heart activity or reactivity [26, 27].

A number of other significant fetal heart rate patterns may be observed. The early decelerations, coincident with the uterine contraction phase (type 1 dips) already mentioned, may occur in response to fetal head compression and are associated with normal fetal acid-base status [15, 17]. In contrast, the pattern of decelerations commencing late in the uterine contraction phase (type 2 dips) is considered ominous and is associated with fetal hypoxia and acidosis. A pattern of decelerations varying in shape and timing of onset from one contraction cycle to the next (variable decelerations) may be due to umbilical cord compression and can also be of serious significance, particularly if associated with reduced or absent beat-to-beat variability [28, 29]. Although most maternity units in developed countries perform electronic fetal monitoring (EFM), it has not been proved to be more effective than intermittent auscultation (IA) for preventing death from asphyxia, and widespread use of the technique has not been associated with a significant reduction in the population of permanently handicapped infants [28]. The Dublin trial of fetal monitoring did show a halving of the risk of neonatal seizures in low-risk labors monitored by EFM rather than by IA, but there was no difference in the frequency of neurologic handicap at follow-up [30].

Factors Associated with Perinatal Asphyxia

Factors associated with or causing perinatal asphyxia may relate to the mother, the placenta, or the fetus.

Maternal Factors

Several medical disorders of the mother are associated with a risk of fetal asphyxia, including diabetes [31], renal disease, essential hypertension, malnutrition, and anemia of any cause. Disorders related to pregnancy that are associated with an increased risk of fetal asphyxia include pre-eclampsia, prolonged gestation, and grand multiparity. In addition, pelvic pathology, such as fibroids or ovarian cysts, may predispose to breech delivery with consequent risk of asphyxia.

Drugs administered to the mother may act on the uteroplacental vessels to cause asphyxia or may cross the placenta to cause fetal CNS depression. Drugs involved include anesthetics, barbiturates, and hypotensive narcotic and oxytocic agents. However, the effects are complex, and a review of the evidence indicated favorable as well as deleterious actions [32].

Placental Factors

The most striking examples are abruption and placenta previa, where there is physical separation of the uteroplacental connections. The presence and rupture of velamentous vessels and obstruction of umbilical cord vessels by prolapse, entanglement, or the tightening of true knots are further examples. Other placental factors include alterations in villous structure that impair placental exchange, such as the edematous villi of fetal hydrops, and the destruction of the villous integrity of placental infarction. The latter is the result of obstruction of uteroplacental arteries and equally may be considered to be a maternal condition.

Fetal Factors

The extremes of fetal size are associated with increased risk of perinatal asphyxia [33]. Unduly large fetuses predispose to prolonged and difficult labor and specific asphyxial events, such as shoulder impaction. Unduly small fetuses are also associated with asphyxia, whether the small size is due to short gestation or to fetal growth retardation. The importance of birth asphyxia may well be underestimated in preterm infants where pathology that is more obviously associated with immaturity (hyaline membrane disease and intraventricular hemorrhage) may command the attention of clinicians and pathologists [34].

Incomplete flexion of the head may predispose to asphyxia, as may some forms of fetal anomaly (e.g., Klippel-Feil) and fetal malpresentations such as breech, persistent occipitoposterior position, face, and brow.

The association of breech presentation with birth asphyxia is accounted for largely by the conditions that predispose to the breech presentation [35]. Of these, one of the most important is preterm birth. The large volume of amniotic fluid relative to fetal size in early pregnancy allows the fetus to move around freely until about 34 weeks, when a cephalic presentation is normally adopted. Conditions that impede fetal movement, including oligohydramnios, multiple pregnancy, and fetal neuromuscular abnormalities, predispose to breech presentation, as, conversely, do those that allow excessive fetal movement, such as polyhydramnios and the lax uterus of the multipara. Factors such as placenta previa, fibroids in the lower uterine segment, or fetal anomalies—e.g., hydrocephalus—which impede engagement of the fetal head, also encourage breech presentation.

After allowing for the morbidity and mortality associated with these factors, vaginal breech delivery carries obvious asphyxial hazards for the infant, including cord prolapse and delay in delivery of the head due to descent through an incompletely dilated cervix. In addition, there is a risk of trauma resulting from manipulations performed to expedite delivery (see below).

Frequency of Fresh Stillbirth and Early Neonatal Death in Normally Formed Infants

There are no large, recently published surveys based on postmortem studies to show the proportion either of births or of perinatal deaths represented by this group. The figures for fresh stillbirths merely give an indication of such deaths.

Recent figures show considerable variations in both the frequency of fresh stillbirths and the proportion of perinatal deaths that they represent. Scandinavian studies have shown that intrapartum deaths comprised only 9.1% of stillbirths in Helsinki [36] and 8.3% of stillbirths in Malmo [37]. In contrast, a study in a socially disadvantaged area of the United States found that 66% of stillbirths occurred prior to the onset of labor [38]. This would leave 34% of stillbirths occurring intrapartum, representing 3.5 deaths per 1000 births. A comparison of perinatal deaths to Asian and European women in Leicester showed perinatal mortality rates of 15.7% and 7.9% per 1000 births, respectively, in 1983–1985 [39]. There was, however, little difference between them in respect to the proportion of perinatal deaths represented by fresh stillbirths (8.1% as compared with 8.8%).

Pathology of Birth Asphyxia

A number of descriptions of the pathology of infants who have died from birth asphyxia have been published within recent years [40–43]. These reports were written mainly from first-hand observation by the authors, as is the following description.

External Features

The fetus or neonate who has died as result of birth asphyxia most likely will show features of the condition that predisposed to the asphyxial injury. There may be evidence of fetal malnutrition with a low body weight for length, lack of subcutaneous tissue, and a relatively large head circumference. There is often evidence of meconium staining of skin, fingernails, and the fetal surface of the placenta and membranes. Traces of meconium may be recognizable in skin creases or ears, even if the infant has been cleaned before being shown to the parents. Petechial hemorrhages are sometimes visible in areas of the skin subjected to increased capillary pressure, including the legs and lower trunk in breech delivery, the head in cases where the cord is tightly wound around the neck during cephalic delivery, or a single limb that has prolapsed through the cervix—e.g., in preterm birth. Excessive molding of the head may be recognizable if labor was prolonged, and abnormal flattening or excessive mobility of the occiput may suggest associated trauma (Fig. 10.1).

If the infant has been maintained on a ventilator for several days, there will be signs of therapy and the fontanelle may be tense, indicating brain swelling.

Internal Macroscopic Features

Hemorrhages   The main internal features of acute asphyxia are congestion, with petechial hemorrhages into internal organs.

Small hemorrhages are seen over the lungs in most cases and are often visible also on the parietal pleura. Over the heart, the hemorrhages tend to be distributed along the line of the coronary arteries and sometimes within the adventitia at the bases of the great arteries. Similar hemorrhages frequently are present over the thymus, where they involve the cortex rather than the medulla. Subcapsular hemorrhages may be seen over the congested liver, and the cerebral veins frequently are engorged. The adrenals may appear hemorrhagic, and there is sometimes acute necrotizing enterocolitis in infants who survive for several days.

Infants who die as a result of placental abruption have an accentuation of the hemorrhagic changes throughout the body, but particularly over the heart and lungs (Fig. 10.2). There may be large ecchymoses or streaky hemorrhages into the lungs and prominent hemorrhages over the heart and thymus. It has been postulated that the florid hemorrhages are the result of sudden augmentation of the fetal blood volume due to placental compression by a retroplacental clot [44] (Fig. 10.3).

Other Findings   Meconium may stain the tongue and may be recognized within major airways. It is sometimes possible to recognize a greenish tinge to the lungs in cases of massive meconium inhalation, and swallowed meconium

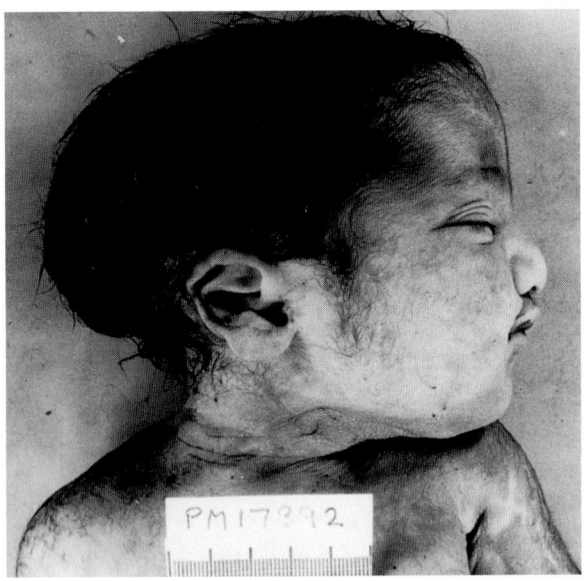

FIGURE 10.1.   *Head of stillborn infant at term showing abnormal shape of occiput due to occipital osteodiastasis.*

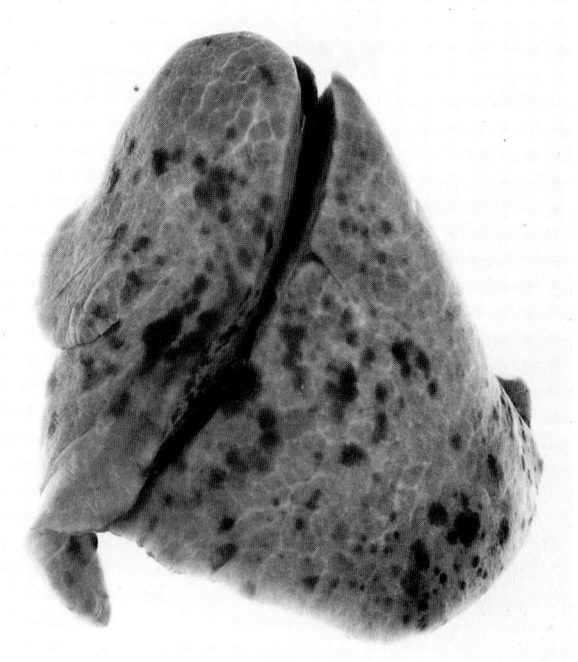

FIGURE 10.2.   *Hemorrhages over the lung in a case of abruptio placentae. (From Ref. 43.)*

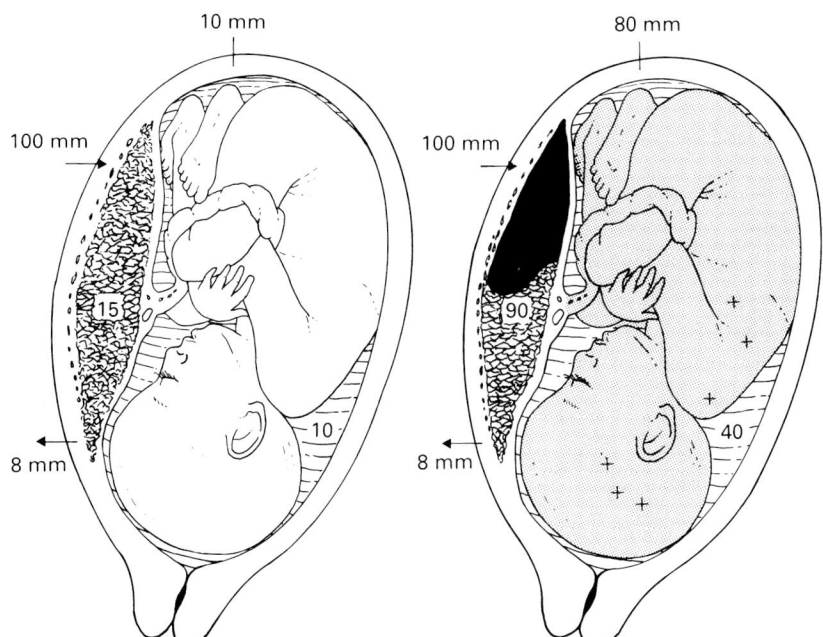

FIGURE 10.3.   *Diagram illustrating how pressure changes associated with retroplacental hemorrhage may cause overloading of the fetal circulation with accentuation of petechial hemorrhages in viscera. (From Ref. 44.)*

often can be seen in the esophagus and stomach. The lungs may be expanded partly by the inhaled material, but more frequently are collapsed and of small volume.

Interstitial emphysema or pneumothorax are seen frequently in infants who die soon after an asphyxial birth. The condition may be caused by overenthusiastic resuscitation attempts by staff unused to handling newborn infants and occurs most often in cases of meconium aspiration. A large infant at term may make sufficiently vigorous respiratory efforts to create a pneumothorax in cases where impacted mucus or meconium causes a ball-valve obstruction in the small airways. This subject is handled in more detail in Chapter 19.

Another form of lung pathology that may be observed in association with birth asphyxia is a massive pulmonary hemorrhage. This sometimes presents almost immediately after birth, with blood appearing within the endotracheal tube during resuscitation in the delivery room. Alternatively, the condition may develop at several hours of age. The bleeding may be a manifestation of a consumption coagulopathy due to disseminated intravascular coagulation, or related to some primary coagulation defect. A further possibility is that the condition is analogous to the "shock lung" seen in adults [43].

Brain changes vary both with the pattern of asphyxia and with the time at which the infant dies. In infants who are stillborn or die within a few hours after birth following a brief period of acute asphyxia, the changes are usually relatively nonspecific, comprising little more than a generalized congestion without apparent brain swelling. In infants who die after being maintained for some days on a ventilator, the brain is usually pale and swollen, with flattening

of the convolutions, obliterations of sulci, and a pale cortex on section. There is often herniation of the uncus through the tentorial incisura into the posterior fossa, or tonsillar herniation through the foramen magnum into the cervical canal. In addition, there may be localized infarction within the territory of one of the cerebral arteries. On section, there may be a pale cortical ribbon with acute congestion of white matter, thalamus, midbrain, cerebellum, and brainstem if the infant has lived only 2 to 3 days (Fig. 10.4). With longer survival there may appear to be just mild edema and cerebral softening without focal lesions.

Macroscopic changes in the kidney comprise acute congestion, often generalized or affecting the medulla (Fig. 10.5). There is sometimes an obvious accentuation of congestion at the corticomedullary junction.

The placenta may show changes of infarction or abruption.

Histologic Features

Lungs   Lung histology in cases of acute perinatal asphyxia confirms the acute congestion and hemorrhages seen at gross level with capillary engorgement and bleeding into interstitial tissue and alveoli. Airspaces show a variable degree of expansion, and there are often masses of inhaled epithelial squames and granular debris within bronchi, bronchioles, and down to saccular or alveolar level in some lobules (Fig. 10.6). Fresh meconium appears on histology as yellow granules. Staining with Alcian blue, or Alcian green in Attwood's stain [45], reveals the presence of inspissated mucus.

The pathologic findings may be modified considerably in infants who die after being maintained for days or weeks on

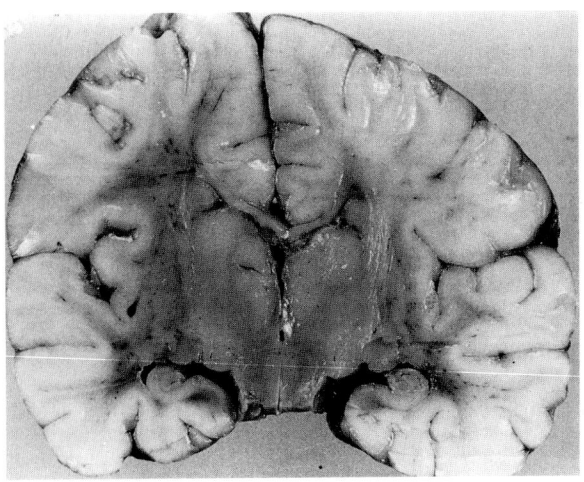

FIGURE 10.4. *Coronal section through an infant brain at term, showing compression of the ventricles and congestion of basal ganglia and white matter due to intrapartum asphyxia. (From Ref. 58.)*

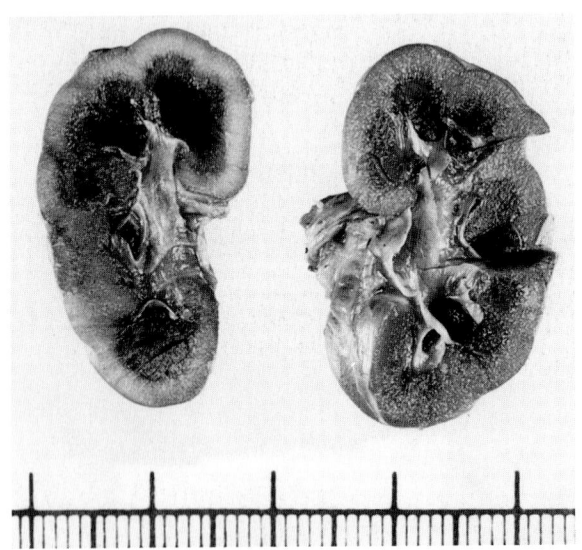

FIGURE 10.5. *Kidneys from an infant at term who died at 5 days of age following asphyxia. Pallor of the renal cortex and congestion of the medulla were associated with necrosis of the proximal renal tubules. See Figure 10.9. (From Ref. 43.)*

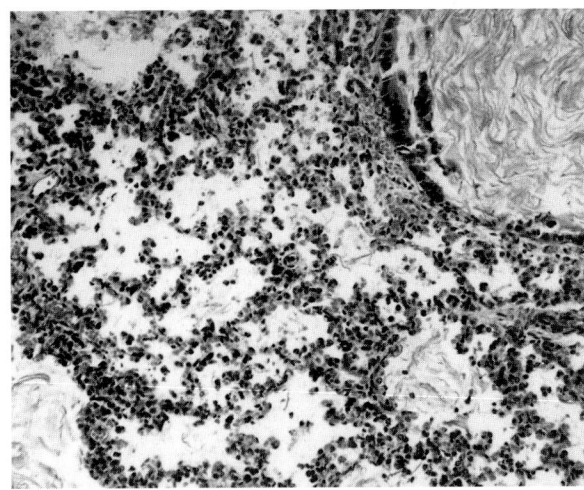

FIGURE 10.6. *Lung from a fresh stillborn infant at term, showing masses of epithelial squames plugging bronchioles and air spaces. H&E, ×100.*

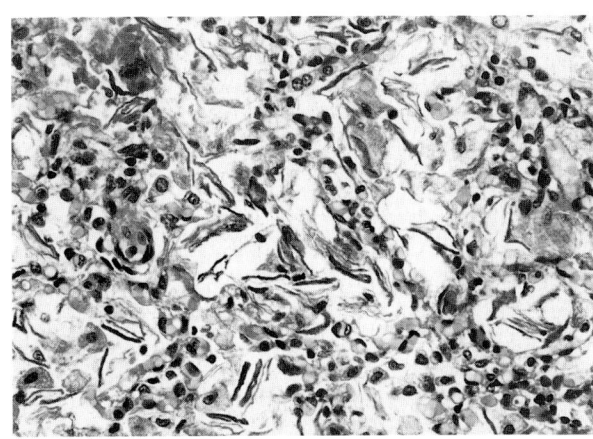

FIGURE 10.7. *Lung from an infant born at 42 weeks' gestation who appeared healthy for the first 4 days of life but died after 18 days following apneic attacks and convulsions. Air spaces are packed with epithelial squames, evidently inhaled during an asphyxial episode in utero. H&E, ×300.*

ventilators. The congestion and hemorrhages may resolve, but inhaled epithelial squames often persist for many weeks (Fig. 10.7). Superimposed changes occurring in the first few days include development of hyaline membranes, presence of milk inhalation, or pneumonia. Pulmonary artery branches may show evidence of persistent fetal circulation, with thick muscular and adventitial layers due to maintenance of a fetal-type high pulmonary vascular resistance.

Brain   Changes of anoxic-ischemic damage are seen in all infants who die at 2 days of age or later following clinical evidence of neurologic injury, irrespective of the macroscopic appearance of the brain. If damage has been sustained prenatally, lesions may be recognized in those who die earlier. Areas of the brain that are most likely to show anoxic-ischemic change include the thalamus, midbrain, pons, and dentate nucleus (Fig. 10.8). Astrocytic hypertrophy often may be recognized within the edematous white matter of the centrum semiovale, and there is sometimes leukomalacia affecting periventricular or subcortical regions. Prenatal damage may present as periventricular leukomalacia with cyst formation or calcification, or as neuronal necrosis affecting the sites listed above and associated with

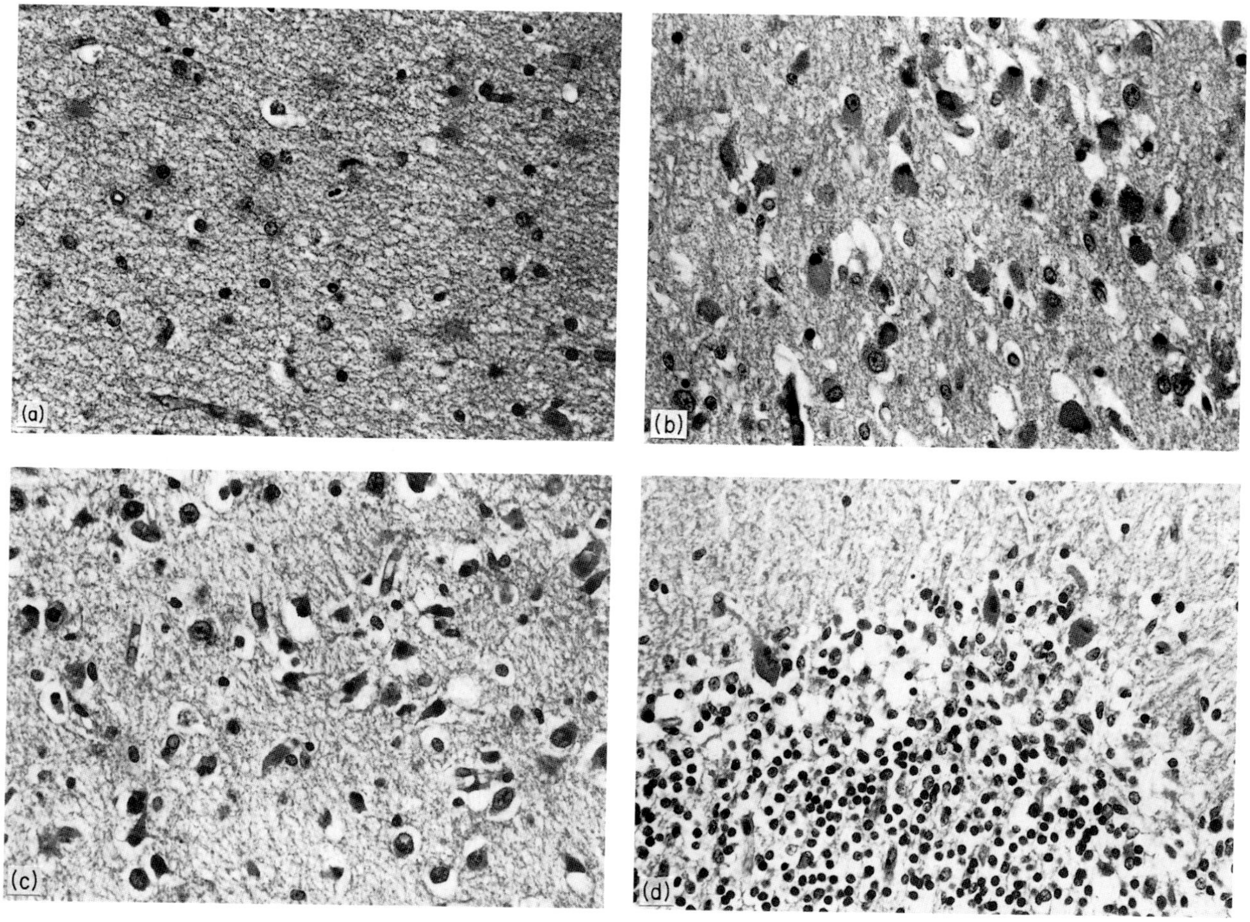

FIGURE 10.8.   *Sections of brain from an infant at term who died at 3 days of age following severe intrapartum asphyxia. H&E, ×300. (a) Cerebral white matter showing edema with early hypertrophy of astrocytes. (b) Thalamus showing necrosing neurons with pyknotic nuclei. (c) Ventral pons with shrunken necrotic neurons. (d) Cerebellum at junction of molecular and internal granular layers, showing three necrotic Purkinje's cells.*

extensive gliosis. The topic of anoxic–ischemic brain damage is dealt with more fully in Chapter 21.

Heart   There are seldom any recognizable cardiac lesions other than the acute epicardial hemorrhages mentioned above. Acute myocardial necrosis is seen occasionally, and foci of established ischemic necrosis are recognized in a few infants who survive for days or weeks on ventilators.

Kidney   Histology characteristically shows acute tubular necrosis in the cortex of cases of placental abruption. Other infants with birth asphyxia may have tubular necrosis affecting either cortex or medulla, or there may be necrosis of the renal papillae (Fig. 10.9). The lesions indicate that the infant suffered an episode of acute shock and hypotension some time before death.

Thymus   Evidence of acute stress may also be manifest in the thymus in the form of a "starry sky" appearance on histology.

Other organs that sometimes show evidence of stress include:

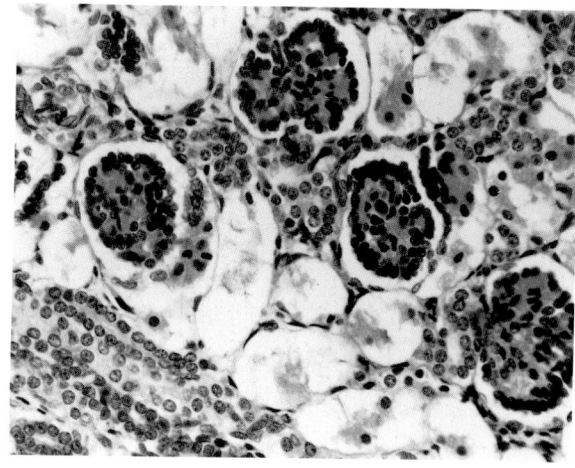

FIGURE 10.9.   *Kidney from an infant of 34 weeks' gestation who died at 2 hours old. H&E, ×300. Proximal tubules show acute epithelial necrosis indicative of an episode of acute renal ischemia due to prenatal asphyxia.*

Liver   Foci of necrosis or fatty infiltration may be seen.

Pancreas   Acute necrosis of islet tissue is occasionally observed.

Adrenal   The hemorrhagic appearance observed macroscopically may be seen to represent hemorrhagic infarction; ischemic infarction may also develop.

Intestine   Necrotizing enterocolitis sometimes develops.

Costochondral Junction   Irregularity of cartilage formation and ossification may indicate prenatal stress.

Placenta   Histology may show changes of chronic hypoxia or ischemia in addition to those of infarction (see Chapter 7).

BIRTH TRAUMA

Birth trauma is an even more emotive subject than birth asphyxia, as it would seem that traumatic delivery always should be avoidable in modern obstetric practice. In reality, the subject is more complex than it might appear, and some degree of mechanical trauma may be quite unavoidable in certain circumstances, such as a fetus with the lethal form of osteogenesis imperfecta (Sillence type 11A).

Frequency of Fatal Mechanical Trauma at Birth

Although the frequency of mechanical trauma at birth has fallen dramatically with greater recourse to caesarean section in cases of potential dystocia, cases of trauma still present with sufficient frequency to merit detailed consideration. In recent studies, the incidence of death due to mechanical birth injury has varied from 0.2 to 0.7 per 1000 births [46–48]. An analysis of the postmortem records of 515 infants who died intrapartum or in the first week of life over the 10 years 1976–1985, and were referred to Hammersmith Hospital for postmortem examination, revealed significant cranial or intracranial trauma in 47, an incidence of 9.1% [49]. Trauma was considered to be a major factor leading to death in 13 cases. Over the period 1980–1991, the frequency of cranial birth trauma in autopsies on term infants at Hammersmith was 4.2% [50].

A recent series of 25 live cases of traumatic intracranial hemorrhage recognized by computerized tomography was estimated to have been derived from a population of about 130,000 births [51]. These were nearly all well-grown mature infants who presented with signs referable to the CNS.

Trauma is not limited to infants at term. Larroche [52] found subdural bleeds in 11% of preterm infants who died. Of the Hammersmith Hospital series [49], 33 of the 47 were below 2.5 kg in weight and 28 were of less than 36 weeks' gestation, a distribution similar to that of perinatal deaths in general.

Relation between Trauma and Asphyxia

The diagnosis of primary birth trauma is seldom made in life. Most infants who are found to have traumatic lesions at postmortem examination come from the group of infants diagnosed as suffering from asphyxia and managed in neonatal intensive care units. During the course of treatment, the traumatic nature of some features may have been noted, but there is often considerable delay in diagnosis of the true nature of rather obvious and potentially fatal traumatic lesions, such as spinal cord transection. Serious traumatic lesions, such as occipital osteodiastasis, are very seldom recognized in life. Structural lesions of the CNS that many cause apnea at birth have been reviewed by Brazy et al [53].

Asphyxia and mechanical trauma are related in several ways. The recognition of fetal distress in labor may prompt efforts to expedite delivery by potentially traumatic means, such as the application of forceps. An asphyxiated infant may be at increased risk of trauma due to lack of fetal tone and possibly engorgement of the cerebral vessels with blood. Infants who are susceptible to asphyxia may, for different but associated reasons, be equally susceptible to trauma. Thus, a growth-retarded infant at risk of asphyxia due to impaired placental exchange is likely to present as a breech and has a relatively large head and thin cranium, factors that make it susceptible to cranial trauma. The infant with congenital muscular dystrophy and hypoplastic lungs that result in asphyxia at birth also has long, thin bones and stiff unyielding limbs, which increase the risk of trauma.

In addition, the cranial distortion associated with trauma, the occurrence of intracranial bleeding, or secondary cerebral swelling may each cause cerebral ischemia, leading to a depressed neurologic state similar to that of asphyxial encephalopathy.

Traumatic Lesions

Extracranial and Extradural Hemorrhage

The range of sites of lesions is shown in Figure 10.10.

Caput Succedaneum   A degree of edema with a minor hemorrhagic component over the presenting part is extremely frequent and of little significance. The hemorrhagic edema involves the skin and superficial fascia and is due to circulatory stasis caused by compression of the presenting part by the uterus or cervix.

Subaponeurotic Hemorrhage   This form of bleeding, also known as subgaleal hemorrhage or "severe" caput succedaneum, originates deep to the epicranial aponeurosis—the thin tendinous sheet uniting the frontal and occipital parts of the occipitofrontalis muscle. The aponeurosis is attached laterally to the zygomatic arch, the auricular muscles, and the tissues of the posterior triangle. If bleeding into this site occurs, it may spread over the entire scalp and dissect between the muscle fibers into the subcutaneous tissue of the posterior triangle and suboccipital regions (Fig. 10.11). Massive hemorrhage may occur into this site, particularly after delivery by vacuum extractor [54], and has resulted in death in 22.8% of reported cases [55].

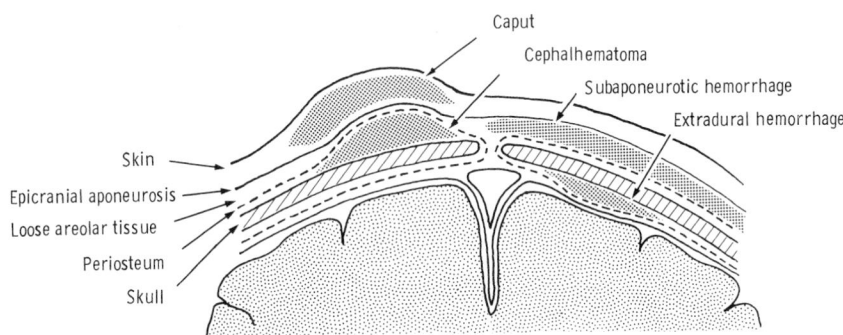

FIGURE 10.10. *Sites of extracranial and extradural hemorrhage in the newborn. (From Ref. 58.)*

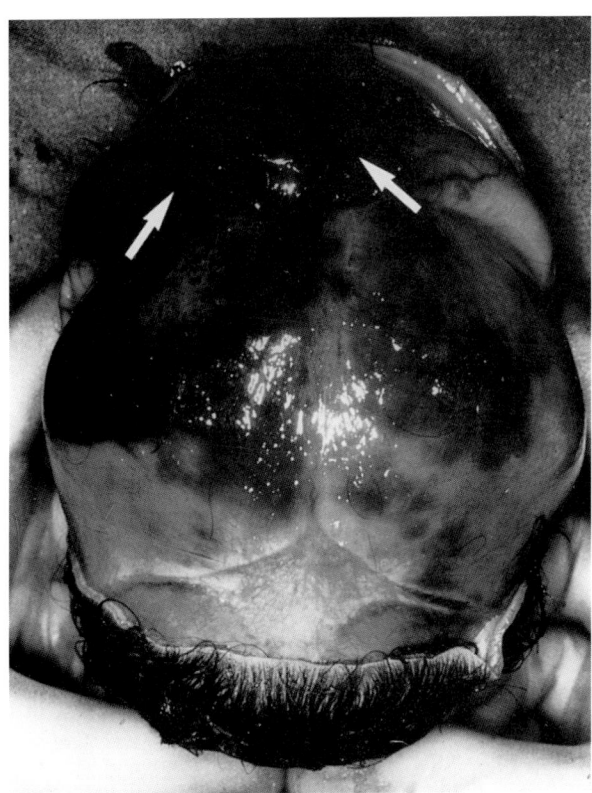

FIGURE 10.11. *Subaponeurotic hemorrhage (arrows) and bilateral cephalohematomas at postmortem examination. (From Ref. 58.)*

Hemostatic abnormalities may predispose to this form of hemorrhage.

Cephalohematoma Although in the strict sense all bleeds over the head may be called "cephalohematoma," the term is usually restricted to the subperiosteal variety. The most frequent site is over one of the parietal bones. In this site, the bleeding is limited by the periosteal attachments to the bone margins. The bleeding is seldom of clinical significance and resolves slowly in the weeks after birth, although the prominent swelling may cause parental concern.

Extradural Hemorrhage This form of hemorrhage involves the plane between the inner table of the skull and the internal periosteum, and is an internal variety of cephalohematoma. It is usually associated with skull fracture, is of minor extent, and is seldom seen at postmortem examination [56].

Skull Fracture

The anatomy of the newborn infant skull, comprising poorly mineralized bones separated by membranous sutures, allows considerable distortion to occur during birth without risk of fracture. The fractures that are most frequent are linear fractures of the parietal bones extending radially along the lines of cleavage. These fractures are seen in infants who die following difficult breech extraction or cephalic forceps delivery. Less often, a depressed fracture may occur as a result of localized trauma in the newborn period. In either case, the fracture itself is unlikely to be significant, and the clinical course depends on the extent of injury to the underlying brain.

Separation of the Squamous and Lateral Parts of the Occipital Bone: Occipital Osteodiastasis

The one area of the fetal cranium that is disrupted readily is the syndesmosis between the squamous and lateral parts of the occipital bone (Fig. 10.12). The mobility of this cartilaginous joint is an important factor, which allows molding of the cranium during labor. In the normal infant, the joint undergoes bony fusion during the second year of life.

The lower margin of the squamous occipital bone forms the posterior boundary of the foramen magnum, centrally, and is closely related to the occipital sinuses, on each side, near their junction with the lateral parts.

Traumatic separation of the cartilaginous joints on one or both sides is caused readily by excessive pressure on the suboccipital region during birth [57, 58]. This results in displacement and forward rotation of the lower edge of the squamous occipital bone (Fig. 10.13). The sharp edge of the bone, freed from the cartilage, may shear through the dura and occipital sinuses, causing gross subdural hemorrhage in the posterior fossa and sometimes laceration of the cerebellum. In preterm infants, the joint displacement causes

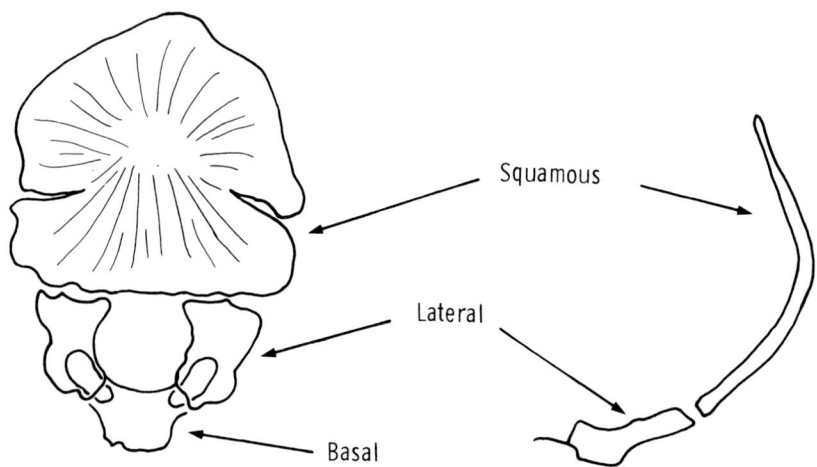

FIGURE 10.12.   *Diagram of the occipital bone at term. (From Ref. 58.)*

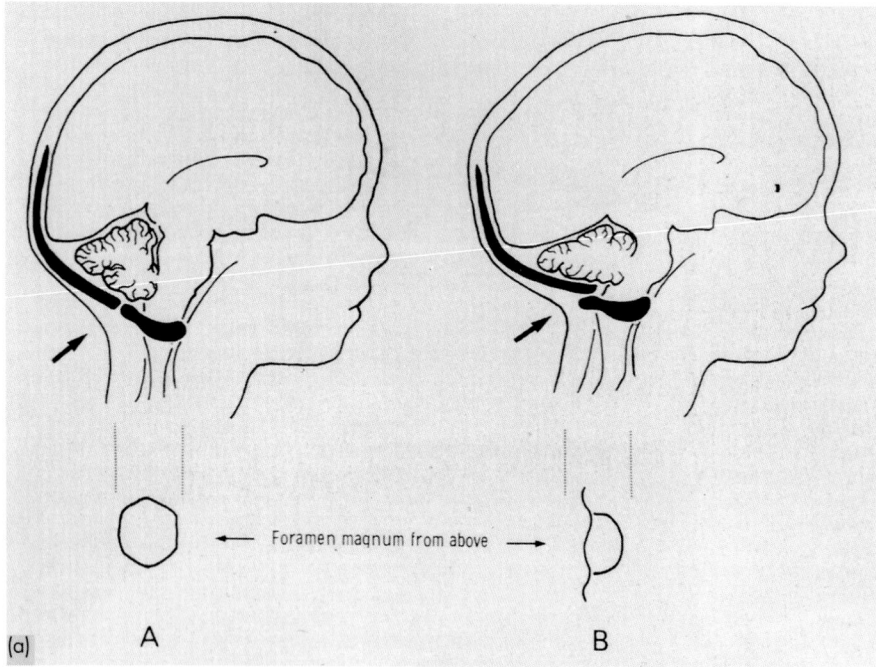

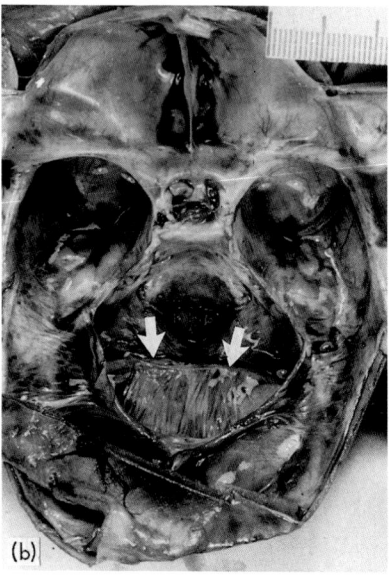

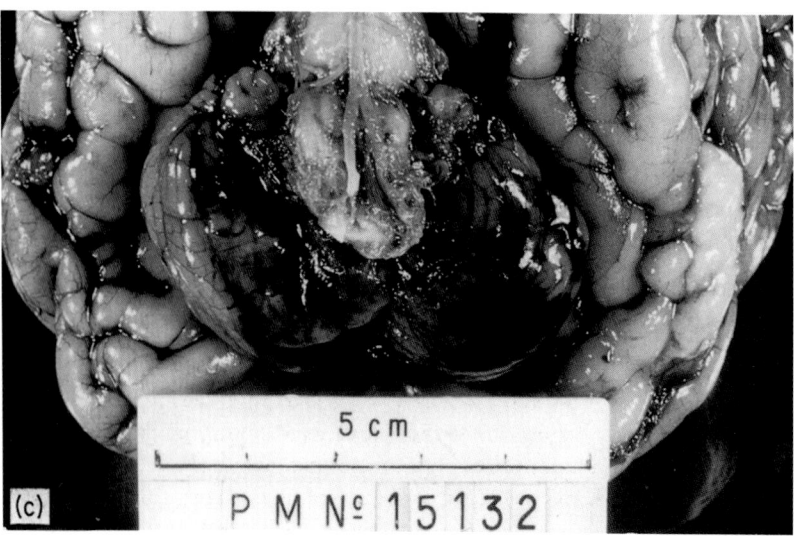

FIGURE 10.13.   *Occipital osteodiastasis. (a) Mechanism of injury. (From Ref. 58.) (b) Base of the skull after dissection, showing the ridge produced in the posterior fossa (arrows). (From Ref. 43.) (c) Inferior surface of hindbrain, showing laceration of cerebellum. (From Ref. 57.)*

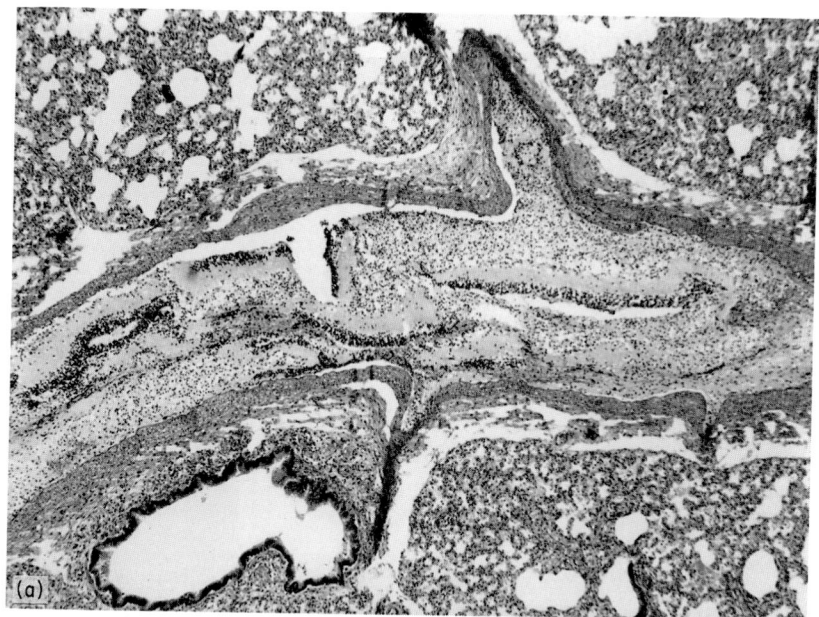

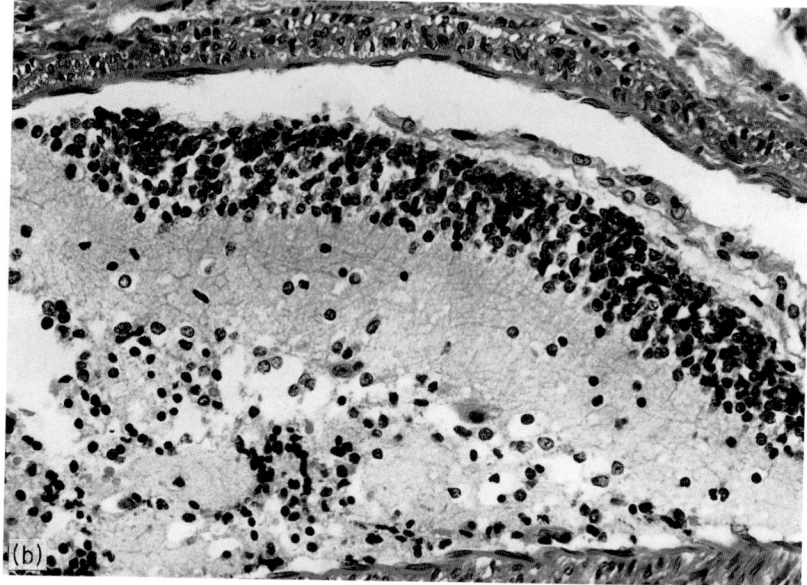

FIGURE 10.14.   *Section of lung from an infant who died 20 minutes after a forceps delivery. No abnormality of cranium or brain recognized at postmortem examination. (a) Masses of fetal cerebellar cortex plugging a pulmonary artery branch. H&E, ×42. (b) Details of cerebellar histology, including external granular layer, molecular layer, and several Purkinje's cells. H&E, ×280. (From Ref. 43.)*

compression of the posterior fossa without massive subdural bleeding [59].

The injury occurs most readily during manipulations to deliver the aftercoming head in breech delivery, but may be seen also following delivery of the head in the occipitoposterior position or via rotational forceps delivery for transverse arrest or delay in spontaneous cephalic rotation.

Occipital osteodiastasis occurs at all gestational ages from 27 weeks up to term. The pathologic significance of the lesion depends on the extent of displacement: separation of the occipital bone with minor displacement is entirely benign and can be recognized on lateral skull x-rays in surviving infants. Major displacement results in distortion and obstruction of venous sinuses in the posterior fossa or direct pressure on the cerebellum and brainstem, with a rapidly fatal outcome. Occipital osteodiastasis is almost certainly the most frequent cause of the rare but bizarre occurrence of multiple cerebral emboli within pulmonary and other vessels following delivery, as most of the reported cases involved fragments of cerebellum [43, 60, 61] (Fig. 10.14). Damage to both dural sinus and cerebellum would allow the cerebellar tissue to be squeezed or sucked into the sinus.

Subdural Hemorrhage: Tears of Tentorium and Falx

Subdural hemorrhage associated with tentorial tears represents the most classic form of cranial birth trauma. The subdural bleeding, however, is usually derived from tears of the unsupported bridging veins passing between the brain and

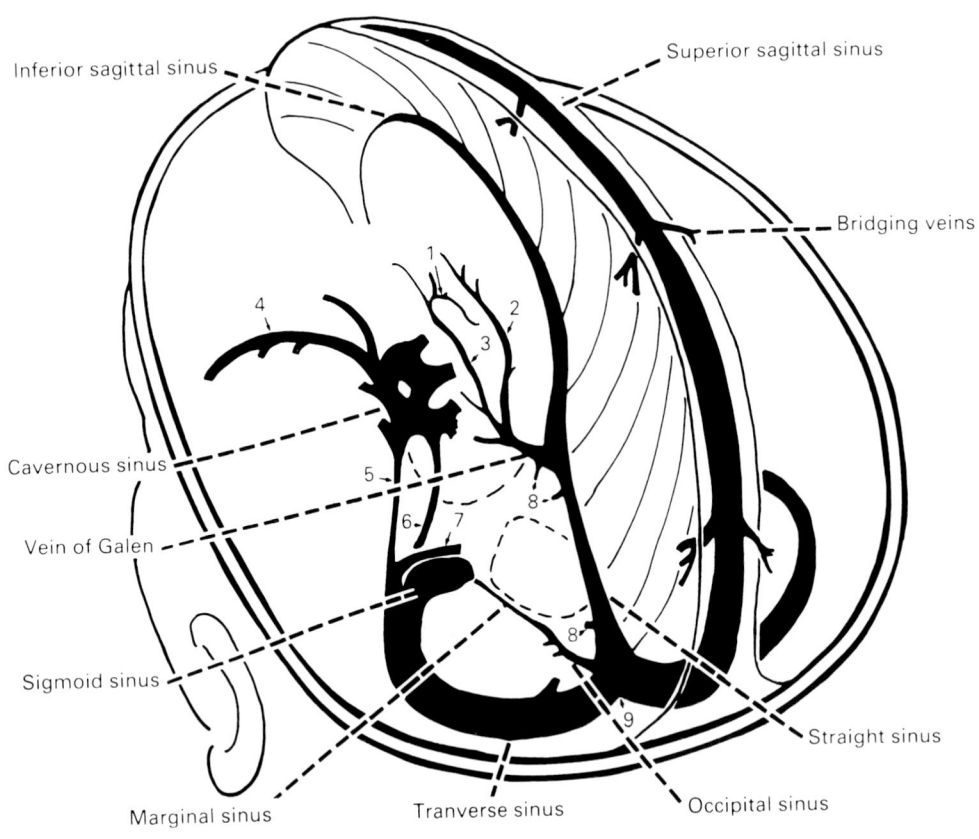

FIGURE 10.15.   *Venous sinuses in the newborn. 1, terminal vein; 2, basal vein; 3, internal cerebral vein; 4, sphenoparietal sinus; 5, superior petrosal sinus; 6, inferior petrosal sinus; 7, petrosal vein of Dandy; 8, superior cerebellar veins; 9, torcular Herophili. (From Ref. 58.)*

the dural sinuses, rather than from the torn tentorium. Only occasionally does a tear of the tentorium extend into one of the venous sinuses to cause massive subdural hemorrhage. An alternative source is from laceration of a cerebral vein or sinus by the margin of a fractured or separated skull bone.

Anatomy of the Dural Folds   The falx cerebri and the leaves of the tentorium cerebelli are two-layered structures with a radiating pattern of fibers that indicate the normal lines of stress. The dural folds are strengthened with additional bands of fibers at the free margins. The falx is usually thinner than the tentorium and often has fenestrations anteriorly, which should not be confused with traumatic lacerations. The relationships of the cerebral veins and venous sinuses to the dural folds are shown in Figure 10.15. The superior cerebral veins cross the subdural space to enter the superior sagittal sinus, and the vein of Galen crosses the space to enter the straight sinus.

Mechanisms of Injury to Veins and Subdural Folds   Evenly applied compression seldom causes damage to the fetal head. Damage to bridging veins or dural folds usually results either from excessive fronto-occipital compression or from oblique distortion. Fronto-occipital compression may cause kinking, obstruction, and tears of the vein of Galen or the closely related superior cerebellar veins. Oblique compression, such

as may be caused by an incorrect application of forceps, places one tentorial leaf under tension while relaxing the opposite one. Similar uneven pressures are exerted on the bridging veins.

Subdural hemorrhage usually originates from one or more of the groups of superior cerebral bridging veins. The subdural bleed presents at postmortem examination as a film of blood or clot over one or both cerebral hemispheres (Fig. 10.16). There may be an associated subarachnoid hemorrhage if the bridging vein has been avulsed at its origin from a cerebral vein. The ruptured veins often cannot be demonstrated at postmortem examination. Sometimes it has been shown that a particular group of veins was intact over an unaffected hemisphere but was missing from the corresponding site over the hemisphere involved in the hemorrhage.

Tears of the tentorium almost invariably involve the free margin close to the junction with the falx. They may be full thickness or may affect only one of the layers of fibers. Extension of such tears medially into the straight sinus or laterally into the lateral sinus is, in this author's experience, very rare, although such extensions have been stressed as important occurrences by several authors [44, 62]. Oval tears of the falx may be seen in association with tentorial tears

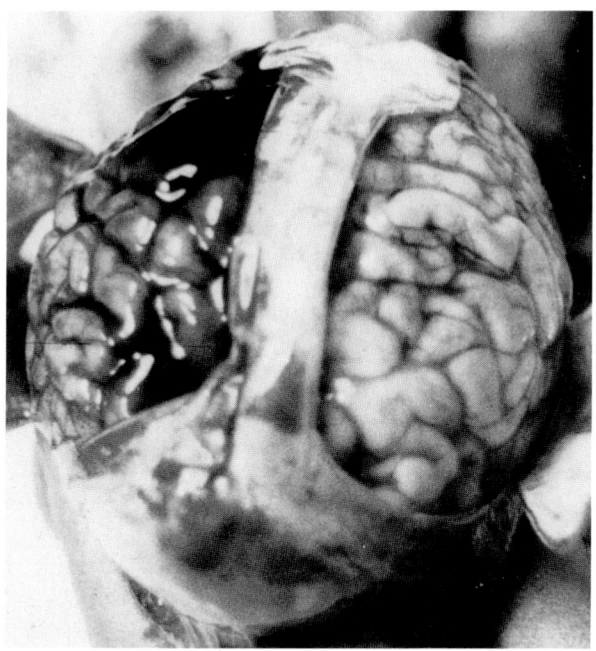

FIGURE 10.16.   *Subdural and subarachnoid hemorrhage over the left hemisphere of a growth-retarded infant at term.*

or occasionally as the sole lesion. In cases of vaginal breech delivery, it is not unusual to find tentorial tears as an accompaniment to occipital osteodiastasis.

Posterior fossa hemorrhage has been recorded as an important cause of death following cranial birth trauma. Sources of bleeding into this site include the superior cerebellar veins, which drain into the vein of Galen and straight sinus (see Fig. 10.15), and the occipital sinuses. The latter are at risk in severe cases of occipital osteodiastasis.

Govaert and colleagues have provided evidence that focal cerebral infarcts may develop in association with cranial birth trauma and have suggested that this may be due to stretching of branches of the middle or posterior cerebral arteries or to spasm resulting from basal subdural hemorrhage [63].

Relationships Among Tears of Dural Folds, Subdural Hemorrhage, and Cerebral Damage   Subdural hemorrhage (from torn bridging veins) and tears of the dural folds are commonly found together because they result from the same type of injury. In some cases, the massive nature of the subdural hemorrhage may be considered an adequate cause of death. A more frequent finding is the association of tears of one or both leaves of the tentorium with a trivial subdural bleed. It may be questioned reasonably whether the cranial trauma is of any significance in such cases. The older writers considered that a baby might be born in a state of concussion because of cranial trauma (see discussion in Ref. 59). In recent years it has become customary to ascribe any shocklike state in a newborn baby to birth asphyxia rather than trauma, unless massive subdural hemorrhage develops in life or is revealed at postmortem examination. Tears of

the dural folds can occur only as a result of gross distortion of the cranium. The basic question that the pathologist has to consider is whether the stresses that caused the tears were likely also to have caused damage to the brain in the absence of massive hemorrhage. It seems probable that any cranial deformation that was severe enough to damage the dural folds might be expected to have caused direct damage to the brain also, by a mechanism such as acute brainstem ischemia. It seems justifiable for the pathologist to regard any evidence of cranial trauma in a case of intrapartum or neonatal death as being of possible major significance.

Extracranial Lesions

Soft-tissue Injuries   These injuries comprise bleeding from internal organs, including liver, spleen, and kidneys, and hemorrhage into skeletal muscles.

Rupture of a subcapsular hematoma of the liver, with resultant peritoneal hemorrhage, is one of the most frequently recognized forms of soft-tissue trauma in the newborn infant (Fig. 10.17). The risk of this lesion is enhanced by hepatic congestion or by an operative delivery, such as breech extraction. Similar considerations apply to hemorrhage from spleen or kidneys. A major peritoneal hemorrhage is recognized readily at postmortem examination: in most cases, the extent of bleeding is such as to suggest that it was a contributory rather than a primary cause of death. Hemorrhage into the muscles is overlooked more readily at postmortem examination, unless the pathologist remembers the possibility. Extensive bruising into muscle tissues may be a major hazard of small preterm infants subjected to vaginal delivery. Massive hemorrhage

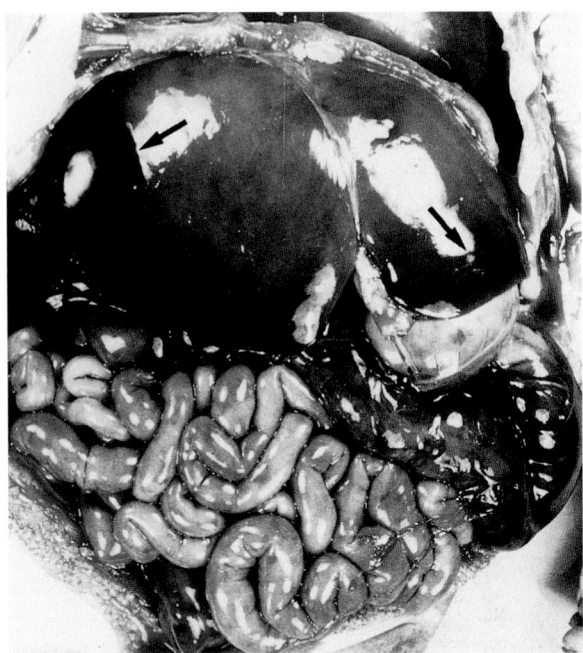

FIGURE 10.17. *Unruptured subcapsular hematomas of the liver (arrows) in an infant at term who died following severe birth asphyxia. (From Ref. 43.)*

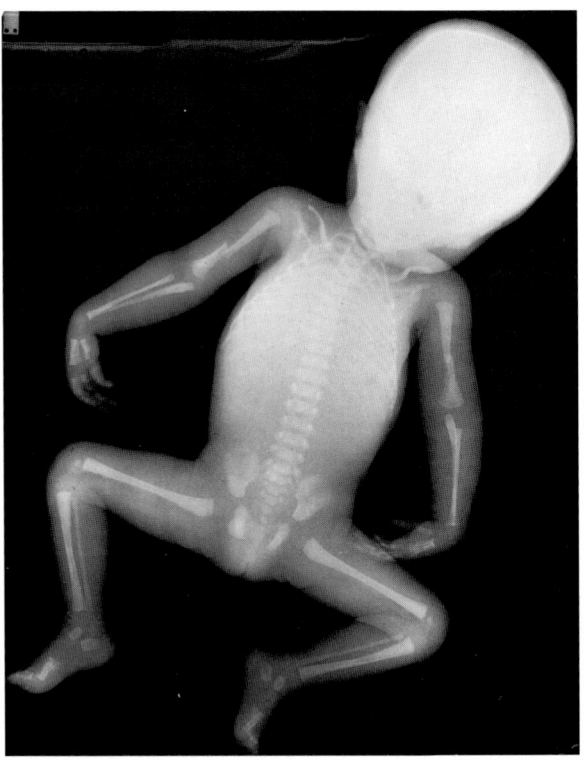

FIGURE 10.18. *Bilateral fractures of the humeri recognized at postmortem examination in an infant with congenital muscular dystrophy, delivered by the breech, in whom it proved difficult to bring down the arms. (From Ref. 43.)*

into the muscles, with little or no superficial bruising, can be seen in infants delivered in the breech position. The hemorrhage is particularly severe over the buttocks and may be accentuated in preterm infants. This form of hemorrhage has been reported to cause the renal picture of crush syndrome [64].

Peripheral Nerve Injuries   These injuries are more likely to be recognized in life than at postmortem examination. They tend to occur in large infants, particularly those subjected to obstetric manipulations for shoulder dystocia [65, 66]. If there has been a traumatic delivery or history of an Erb's palsy, diaphragmatic paralysis, or Klumpke's paralysis, the nerve roots should be examined with particular care at postmortem examination.

Bony Injuries   Fractures of long bones are found quite frequently in infants who die following birth trauma. Long bone fractures, like nerve injuries, usually result from obstetric manipulations [66] (Fig. 10.18). Common minor lesions, such as midshaft fractures of the clavicle, can be overlooked readily unless postmortem x-rays are made routinely.

Spinal Injuries   The chief mechanisms postulated as causes of spinal injury in the past have been most likely to operate during breech delivery. They include excessive longitudinal stretching, hyperextension of the head, excessive traction via the brachial plexus, and ischemic injury due to narrowing or occlusion of the vertebral arteries. However, severe spinal injuries in association with breech delivery have become relatively infrequent with the use of caesarean section to avoid the need for difficult breech extractions. The most frequent

site of transection in cases of breech delivery is the lower cervical cord. Separation of the vertebrae should be apparent readily on x-ray or dissection, and the cord injury is seen easily on opening of the spinal canal at postmortem examination. No such case has been observed in a normally formed infant at Hammersmith Hospital over the past 30 years.

Far more difficult to recognize are cases in which cord transection occurs during a cephalic delivery, because in these cases the injury is at the upper end of the cervical cord (C3 or higher) or within the medulla, where it is almost certain to be missed by the standard dissection technique. High cervical transection invariably occurs during rotational forceps delivery and may be associated with little or no evidence of injury to the bony spine or ligaments. Because the infant is unable to breathe at birth, the lesion has been recognized regularly only since the advent of life-support systems. This condition has been regarded as extremely uncommon, and published reports all relate to single cases [67–69]. Having personally dissected three cases from our own neonatal unit (each referred from a different maternity hospital) over the last 18 years, and being aware of a number of others, this author believes that this must now be the most important form of cord transection (Fig. 10.19). Two of our own cases were associated with occipi-

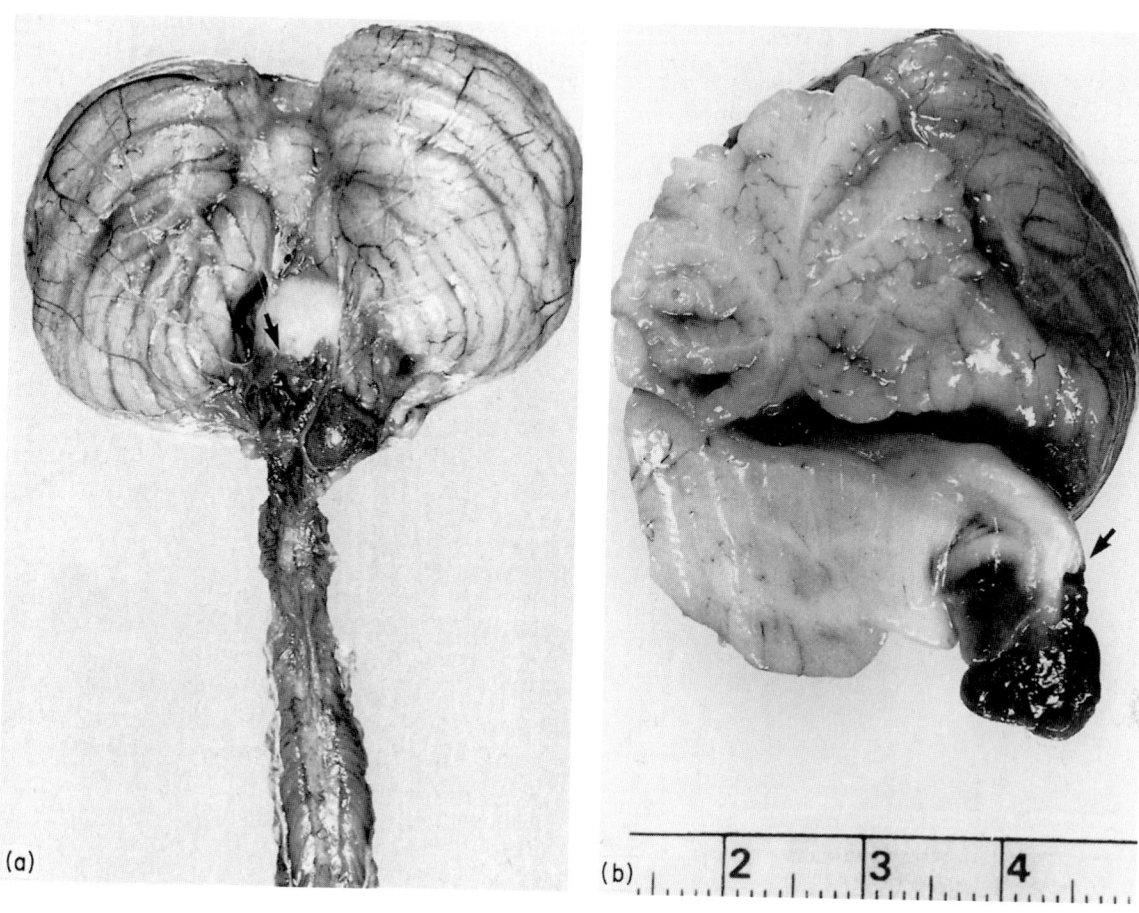

FIGURE 10.19.   *Traumatic transection of the medulla (arrows): (a) posterior view; (b) sagittal section. (From Ref. 58.)*

tal osteodiastasis and tentorial tears [49]. Examination of the site of transection in these cases suggested that the displaced lower margin of the occipital bone may have sheared the lower medulla. In the third case, there was infarction of the ventral cord below the site of transection, indicating damage to the arterial supply via the vertebral arteries. It is important that obstetricians who favor the use of rotational forceps should remain aware of the ease with which the medulla and spinal cord can be damaged by this procedure. Imaging techniques can now detect such lesions in life [70, 71]. Use of rotational forceps has been associated with other forms of trauma, notably tentorial tears [72], although other authors have defended their use [73, 74].

PROBLEM OF THE UNEXPLAINED EARLY NEONATAL DEATH

Intrapartum death in normally developed infants nearly always can be explained on the basis of asphyxia and/or trauma. Rarely, an infant who dies during labor may show evidence of infection as the major or contributory factor.

Infants who appear well at birth but develop a rapidly progressive fatal illness, or die unexpectedly in the first few days after birth, present a far greater diagnostic problem for the clinician and pathologist.

Signs preceding death may include tachypnea and grunting (with or without gross disturbances of acid–base status), hypotonia, convulsions, hypoglycemia, and jaundice. From the pattern of appearance and progression of signs, the neonatologist may be able to make an accurate differential diagnosis and instigate appropriate investigations to provide the definitive diagnosis. In some cases, death supervenes before full investigations can be set in motion, or the infant may die unexpectedly with no prior recognizable signs. Inevitably, the pathologist may have to supplement the investigations commenced before death or attempt to make a diagnosis from scratch.

Postmortem examination in such cases may yield a fairly obvious structural cause of death, such as cardiovascular anomaly. Examples seen at Hammersmith Hospital in recent years have included total anomalous pulmonary venous drainage (diagnosis considered but rejected on ultrasound) and arteriovenous aneurysm of the vein of Galen. Such anomalies should be revealed readily at a competent perinatal postmortem examination and will not be considered further here.

Table 10.1. Some inborn errors that may prove fatal in the perinatal period

Type of defect	Clinical presentation	Examples	Postmortem findings	Tissue for biochemical diagnosis
Urea cycle defect	Vomiting, CNS signs, and acute respiratory failure with hyperammonemia	Ornithine transcarbamylase deficiency, citrullinemia, and argininosuccinic aciduria	None specific	Liver, kidney, brain, or fibroblast culture
Disorders of amino acid metabolism	Vomiting, CNS signs, and acute respiratory failure with hypoglycemia and acidosis	Maple syrup urine disease, propionic acidemia, and methylmalonic acidemia	None specific	Liver, kidney, brain, or fibroblast culture
Disorders of carbohydrate metabolism	Vomiting, jaundice, hepatomegaly, hypoglycemia, and acute liver failure	Galactosemia and hereditary fructose intolerance	Jaundice, hemostatic failure, and typical liver pathology	Liver or fibroblast culture
Glycogen storage disease	Cardiac failure hypotonia, CNS signs, and hepatosplenomegaly	Type II (Pompe disease)	Cardiomegaly and excess glycogen storage in liver, heart, and muscles	Liver, heart, or fibroblast culture
Deficiencies of mitochondrial enzymes involved in lipid metabolism	Hypoglycemia, metabolic acidosis, and sudden death. Some have dysmorphic features	Long-chain acyl coenzyme A dehydrogenase deficiency and multiple coenzyme A dehydrogenase deficiency	Lipid infiltration of liver, heart, kidney, and skeletal muscle	Heart, liver, or fibroblast culture
Lipid storage diseases	Hepatosplenomegaly	GM, gangliosidosis type 1; Niemann-Pick disease type A; Gaucher disease; mucopolysaccharidosis VII; mucolipidosis II	Storage cells in spleen, liver, bone marrow, and placental villi	Spleen, liver, brain, or fibroblast culture
Mucopolysaccharide storage disease and mucolipid storage diseases	Some present with hydrops; some have facial features and x-rays characteristic of Hurler syndrome			Spleen, liver, brain, or fibroblast culture plasma or other body fluids

Investigation of Infective or Biochemical Abnormalities

The two groups of cases that are most likely to require appropriate, nonhistologic studies are infective and biochemical abnormalities.

Infection

Bacterial and virologic cultures should always be taken in unexpected deaths at any age: in this age group, the most likely bacterial infections are those due to group B β hemolytic streptococcus or *Haemophilus influenzae*, although a wide range of common gram-positive and gram-negative bacterial pathogens can present as rapidly progressive early-onset sepsis in the newborn. A less common organism is *Listeria monocytogenes*. Viral infections to consider include the coxsackie group and herpes viruses. Further details of these various infections are given in Chapter 17.

Inborn Errors of Metabolism

The range of inborn errors of metabolism that can present with rapidly progressive fatal illness in the immediate newborn period is considerable. Moreover, if the infant dies without any evidence as to the type of error present, sub-

sequent attempts at postmortem diagnosis may be doomed to failure. A useful clinical pointer to an inborn error as the underlying cause is a history of a period of normality immediately after birth. The subsequent pattern of deterioration may provide a clue to the underlying type of defect.

Table 10.1 shows some inborn errors that may need to be considered in the infant who dies unexpectedly in the newborn period, along with their clinical presentation and techniques for postmortem diagnosis. Among these are the recently recognized group of congenital abnormalities of mitochondrial enzymes involved in fatty acid metabolism, which may present with rapidly fatal hypoglycemia and acidosis in the first few weeks or months of life (Fig. 10.20). For further information, see Chapter 18.

Interpretation of Minimal Pathology

This group of infants may not show convincing evidence of any type of inborn error, and the pathologist may have to attempt to interpret minimal pathologic changes. One pattern seen occasionally is the infant who was thought to be well at birth, with a good Apgar score, but who collapses and dies after a feed within the first day or two of life. Postmortem examination may reveal changes suggestive of birth asphyxia, including evidence of inhaled amniotic debris and

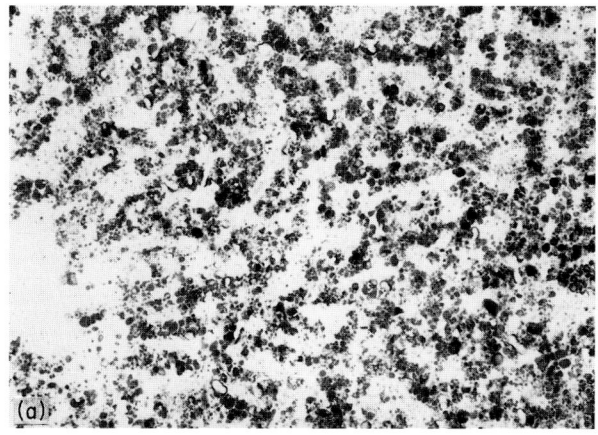

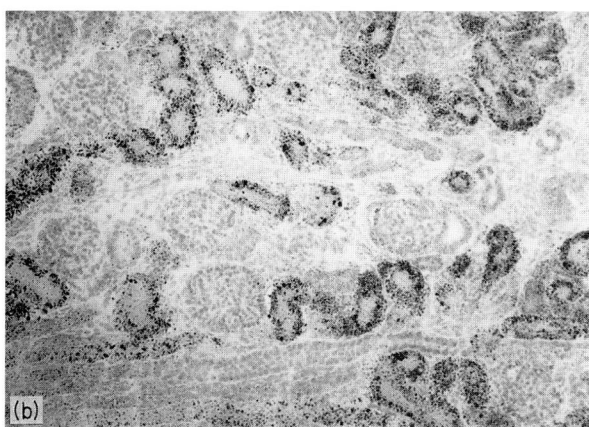

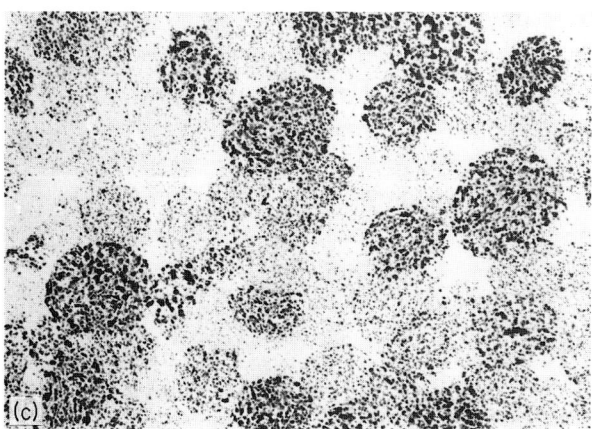

FIGURE 10.20. *Sections from an infant at term who was found dead unexpectedly at 30 hours old. Biochemical investigations revealed a defect in the oxidation of long-chain fatty acids, subsequently shown to be due to mitochondrial carnitine-acylcarnitine translocase deficiency. (a) Liver, showing microvesicular lipid infiltration. (b) Renal cortex, showing lipid within proximal tubules. (c) Skeletal muscle fibers, showing extensive lipid infiltration. All sections stained for neutral lipid by oil red O. (a) and (b) ×100, (c) ×300.*

epithelial squames, with superimposed aspirated feed. A reasonable explanation for such a case would be that a prenatal asphyxial episode had resolved sufficiently by the time of birth to allow the infant to appear normal, but that persistent depression of the swallowing reflex allowed subsequent inhalation of feed. In newborn monkeys subject to prenatal asphyxia, an excellent initial response to resuscitation might be followed some hours later by the onset of irreversible cardiogenic shock [75]. A similar occurrence in the human neonate may explain some unexpected, early neonatal deaths.

There are often subtle signs that tend to confirm the occurrence of prenatal asphyxia or other forms of prenatal stress. These signs include the cerebral, renal, hepatic, skeletal, and thymic changes previously listed for asphyxia. Evidence of myocardial injury should be looked for with particular care.

There remains a small group of cases for which no explanation is forthcoming after detailed study. This raises the question as to the point at which overlap may occur between perinatal death and the sudden infant death syndrome.

REFERENCES

1. Bejar R, Wozniak P, Allard M, et al. Antenatal origin of neurologic damage in newborn infants. 1. Preterm infants. *Am J Obstet Gynecol* 1988; 159:357–63.
2. Blair E, Stanley F. Intrapartum asphyxia: a rare cause of cerebral palsy. *J Pediatr* 1988; 112:515–19.
3. Nelson KB. What proportion of cerebral palsy is related to birth asphyxia? *J Pediatr* 1988; 112:572–4.
4. Rudolph AM, Heymann MA, Teramo KAW, Barrett CT, Raiha NCR. Studies on the circulation of the previable human fetus. *Pediatr Res* 1971; 5:452–65.
5. Paton JB, Fisher DE, Peterson EN, deLannoy CW, Behrman RE. Cardiac output and organ blood flows in the baboon fetus. *Biol Neonate* 1973; 22:50–7.
6. Peeters LLH, Sheldon RE, Jones MD, Makowski EL, Meschia G. Blood flow to fetal organs as a function of arterial oxygen content. *Am J Obstet Gynecol* 1979; 135:637–46.
7. Gilbert RD. Control of the fetal cardiac output during changes in blood volume. *Am J Physiol* 1980; 238:H80–6.
8. Low JA. Maternal and fetal blood gas and acid–base metabolism. In: Philipp E, Barnes J, Newton M, eds. *Scientific Foundations of Obstetrics and Gynaecology*. 3rd ed. London: Heinemann Medical Books, 1986, pp. 376–89.
9. Smis B, Thiery M. Fetal heart rate pattern before, during and after amniotomy. *Eur J Obstet Gynecol Reprod Biol* 1980; 11:163–71.
10. Ramsey EM, Corner GW, Donner MW. Serial and cineangioradiographic visualization of maternal circulation in the primate (hemochorial) placenta. *Am J Obstet Gynecol* 1963; 86:213–25.
11. Atkins AJF, Watt JM, Milan P, Davies P, Crawford S. The influence of posture upon cardiovascular dynamics throughout pregnancy. *Eur J Obstet Gynecol Reprod Biol* 1981; 12:357–72.
12. Crawford JS, Burton M, Davies P. Time and lateral tilt at Caesarean section. *Br J Anaesth* 1972; 44:477–84.
13. Beard RW, Morris ED, Clayton SG. pH of foetal capillary blood as an indicator of the condition of the foetus. *J Obstet Gynaecol Br Commonw* 1967; 74:812–22.
14. Hon EH. The fetal heart rate patterns preceding death *in utero. Am J Obstet Gynecol* 1959; 78:47–56.
15. Kubli FW, Hon EH, Khazin AF, Takamura H. Observations on heart rate and pH in the human fetus during labor. *Am J Obstet Gynecol* 1969; 104:1190–206.
16. Low JA, Cox MJ, Karchmar EJ, et al. The effect of maternal, labor, and fetal factors upon fetal heart rate during the intrapartum period. *Am J Obstet Gynecol* 1981; 139:306–10.
17. Mendez-Bauer C, Arnt IC, Gulin L, Escarcena LA, Caldeyro-Barcia R. Relationship between blood pH and heart rate in the human fetus during labour. *Am J Obstet Gynecol* 1967; 97:530–45.

18. Jones CM, Greiss FC. The effect of labor on maternal and fetal circulating catecholamines. *Am J Obstet Gynecol* 1982; 144:149–53.

19. Olver RE. Of labour and the lungs. *Arch Dis Child* 1981; 56:659–62.

20. Dawes GS. *Foetal and Neonatal Physiology.* Chicago: Year Book Medical Publishers, 1968, p. 149.

21. Cohn HE, Sacks EJ, Heymann MA, Rudolph AM. Cardiovascular responses to hypoxemia and acidemia in fetal lambs. *Am J Obstet Gynecol* 1974; 120:817–24.

22. Behrman RE, Lees MH, Peterson EN, De Lannoy CW, Seeds AE. Distribution of the circulation in the normal and asphyxiated fetal primate. *Am J Obstet Gynecol* 1970; 108:956–69.

23. Friedman WF, Kirkpatrick SE. Fetal cardiovascular adaptation to asphyxia. In: Gluck L, ed. *Intrauterine Asphyxia and the Developing Fetal Brain.* Chicago: Year Book Medical Publishers, 1977, pp. 149–65.

24. Ritchie K. The fetal response to changes in the composition of maternal inspired air in human pregnancy. *Semin Perinatol* 1980; 4:295–9.

25. Schifrin BS. Antepartum fetal heart rate monitoring. In: Gluck L, ed. *Intrauterine Asphyxia and the Developing Fetal Brain.* Chicago: Year Book Medical Publishers, 1977, pp. 205–24.

26. Flynn AM, Kelly J, O'Connor M. Unstressed antepartum cardiotocography in the management of the fetus suspected of growth retardation. *Br J Obstet Gynaecol* 1979; 86:106–10.

27. Visser GMA, Redman CWG, Huisjes HJ, Turnbull AC. Non-stressed antepartum heart rate monitoring: implication of decelerations after spontaneous contractions. *Am J Obstet Gynecol* 1980; 138:429–35.

28. Boylan P. Intrapartum fetal monitoring. *Bailliere's Clin Obstet Gynaecol* 1987; 1:73–95.

29. Hon EH. Detection of asphyxia *in utero.* In: Gluck L, ed. *Intrauterine Asphyxia and the Developing Fetal Brain.* Chicago: Year Book Medical Publishers, 1977, pp. 167–77.

30. MacDonald D, Grant A, Sheridan-Pereira M, Boylan P, Chalmers I. The Dublin randomized controlled trial of intrapartum fetal heart rate monitoring. *Am J Obstet Gynecol* 1985; 152:425–539.

31. Brudenell J. Delivery of the baby of the diabetic mother. *JR Soc Med* 1978; 71:207–11.

32. Myers RE, Myers SE. Use of sedative, analgesic, and anesthetic drugs during labor: bane or boon? *Am J Obstet Gynecol* 1979; 133:83–104.

33. Fedrick J. Comparison of birth weight/gestation distribution in cases of stillbirth and neonatal death according to lesions found at necropsy. *Br Med J* 1969; 3:745–8.

34. Barson AJ, Tasker M, Lieberman BA, Hillier VF. Impact of improved perinatal care on the causes of death. *Arch Dis Child* 1984; 59:199–207.

35. Faber-Nijholt R, Huisjes HJ, Touwen BCL, Fidler VJ. Neurological follow-up of 281 children born in breech presentation: a controlled study. *Br Med J* 1983; 286:9–12.

36. Hovatta O, Lipasti A, Rapola J, Karjalainen O. Causes of stillbirth: a clinicopathological study of 243 patients. *Br J Obstet Gynaecol* 1983; 90:691–6.

37. Lofgren O, Polberger S. Perinatal mortality: changes in the diagnostic panorama 1974–1980. *Acta Paediatr Scand* 1983; 72:327–32.

38. Brans YB, Escobedo MB, Hayashi RH, et al. Perinatal mortality in a large perinatal center: five year review of 31,000 births. *Am J Obstet Gynecol* 1984; 148:284–9.

39. Clarke M, Clayton DG, Mason ES, MacVicar J. Asian mothers risk factors for perinatal death—the same or different? A 10 year review of Leicestershire perinatal deaths. *Br Med J* 1988; 297:384–7.

40. Claireaux AE. Pathology of perinatal hypoxia. *J Clin Pathol* 1977; 30(11):142–8.

41. Gillan JE. Intrapartum events. In: Reed GB, Claireaux AE, Cockburn F, eds. *Disorders of the Newborn.* 2nd ed. London: Chapman and Hall, 1995, pp. 284–317.

42. Keeling JW. Intrapartum asphyxia and birth trauma. In: Keeling JW, ed. *Fetal and Neonatal Pathology.* 2nd ed. London: Springer-Verlag, 1993, pp. 237–52.

43. Wigglesworth JS. *Perinatal Pathology.* 2nd ed. Philadelphia: WB Saunders, 1996, pp. 87–103.

44. Morison JE. *Foetal and Neonatal Pathology.* 3rd ed. London: Butterworth, 1970, p. 294.

45. Attwood HD. The histological diagnosis of amniotic fluid embolism. *J Pathol Bacteriol* 1958; 76:211–5.

46. Geirson RT. Birth trauma and brain damage. *Bailliere's Clin Obstet Gynaecol* 1988; 2:195–212.

47. O'Driscoll K, Meagher D, MacDonald, D, Geoghegan F. Traumatic intracranial haemorrhage in first-born infants and delivery with obstetric forceps. *Br J Obstet Gynaecol* 1981; 88:577–81.

48. Walker CHM. Birth trauma. In: Crawford JW, ed. *Risks of Labour.* Chichester: Wiley, 1985, pp. 71–93.

49. Wigglesworth JS. Trauma and the developing brain. In: Kubli F, Patel N, Schmidt W, Lindekamp O, eds. *Perinatal Events and Brain Damage in Surviving Children.* Berlin: Springer-Verlag, 1988, pp. 64–9.

50. Govaert P. *Cranial Haemorrhage in the Term Newborn Infant.* London: MacKeith, 1993, pp. 5–8.

51. Welch K, Strand R. Traumatic parturitional intracranial haemorrhage. *Dev Med Child Neurol* 1986; 28:156–64.

52. Larroche JC. *Developmental Pathology of the Neonate.* Amsterdam: Excerpta Medica, 1977, p. 358.

53. Brazy JE, Kinney HC, Oakes WJ. Central nervous system structural lesions causing apnoea at birth. *J Pediatr* 1987; 111:163–75.

54. Plauche WC. Fetal cranial injuries related to delivery with the Malmstrom vacuum extractor. *Obstet Gynecol* 1979; 53:750–7.

55. Plauche WC. Subgaleal hematoma. A complication of instrumental delivery. *J Am Med Assoc* 1980; 244:1597–8.

56. Gresham EL. Birth trauma. *Pediatr Clin North Am* 1975; 22:317–28.

57. Hemsath FA. Birth injury of the occipital bone with a report of thirty-two cases. *Am J Obstet Gynecol* 1934; 27:194–203.

58. Wigglesworth JS, Husemeyer RP. Intracranial birth trauma in vaginal breech delivery: the continued importance of injury to the occipital bone. *Br J Obstet Gynaecol* 1977; 84:684–91.

59. Pape KE, Wigglesworth JS. *Haemorrhage, Ischaemia and the Perinatal Brain.* London: Heinemann, 1979, p. 68.

60. Gardiner WR. Massive pulmonary embolization of cerebral cortical tissue: an unusual fetal birth injury. *Stanford Med Bull* 1956; 14:226–9.

61. Hauck AJ, Bambara JF, Edwards WD. Embolism of brain tissue to the lung in a neonate. Report of a case and review of the literature. *Arch Path Lab Med* 1990; 114:217–18.

62. Potter EL, Craig JM. *Pathology of the Fetus and the Infant.* 3rd ed. Chicago: Year Book Medical Publishers, 1976, p. 107.

63. Govaert P, Vanhaesebrouck P, de Praeter C. Traumatic neonatal intracranial bleeding and stroke. *Arch Dis Child* 1992; 67:840–5.

64. Ralis ZA. Birth trauma to muscles in babies born by breech delivery and its possible fatal consequences. *Arch Dis Child* 1975; 50:4–13.

65. Sjoberg I, Erichs K, Bjerre I. Cause and effect of obstetric (neonatal) brachial plexus palsy. *Acta Paediatr Scand* 1988; 77:357–64.

66. Wikstrom I, Axelsson O, Bergstrom R, Meirik O. Traumatic injury in large-for-date infants. *Acta Obstet Gynecol Scand* 1988; 67:259–64.

67. Gould SJ, Smith JF. Spinal cord transection, cerebral ischaemic and brain-stem injury in a baby following a Kielland's forceps rotation. *Neuropathol Appl Neurobiol* 1984; 10:151–8.

68. Pridmore BR, Hey EN, Aherne WA. Spinal cord injury of the fetus during delivery with Kielland's forceps. *J Obstet Gynaecol Br Commonw* 1974; 81:168–72.

69. Shulman ST, Madden JD, Esterly JR, Shanklin DR. Transection of spinal cord: a rare complication of cephalic delivery. *Arch Dis Child* 1971; 46:291–4.

70. Babyn PS, Chuang SH, Daneman A, Davidson GS. Sonographic evaluation of spinal cord birth trauma with pathologic correlation. *Am J Roentgenol* 1988; 151:763–6.

71. Lamska MJ, Roessman U, Wiznitzer M. Magnetic resonance imaging in cervical cord birth injury. *Pediatrics* 1990; 85:760–4.

72. Chiswick ML, James DK. Kielland's forceps: association with neonatal morbidity and mortality. *Br Med J* 1979; 1:7–9.

73. Cardozo LD, Gibb DMF, Studd JWW, Cooper DJ. Should we abandon Kielland's forceps? *Br Med J* 1983; 287:315–7.

74. Healey DL, Quinn MA, Pepperall RJ. Rotational delivery of the fetus: Kielland's forceps and two other methods compared. *Br J Obstet Gynaecol* 1982; 89:501–6.

75. Myers RE. Experimental models of perinatal brain damage: relevance to human pathology. In: Gluck L, ed. *Intrauterine Asphyxia and the Developing Fetal Brain.* Chicago: Year Book Medical Publishers, 1977, pp. 37–97.

Causes of Human Maldevelopment

GEOFFREY A. MACHIN

INTRODUCTION

Many developmental diseases continue to need clarification in terms of anatomic description and classification; however, standard pathologic methods are now often a starting point, giving clues as to the choice of definitive methods of genetic diagnosis. There are numerous examples of developmental diseases that have long been familiar to perinatal pathologists as anatomic entities but that now can be precisely defined in cytogenetic and/or molecular terms; this leads to specific diagnosis in pedigrees (e.g., carrier status) and in the prenatal period. Close collaboration among clinicians, pathologists, and specialized diagnostic laboratories (e.g., cytogenetic and DNA laboratories) yields a harvest of definitive information on the etiologies and pathogeneses of these diseases. Correlations between genotypes of humans and mice are useful, as are mouse "knock-out" models.

Such are the power and simplicity of molecular genetics that there are no clear distinctions among the mechanisms that produce diseases of metabolism (mutations are known in the genes coding for Gaucher disease, Wilson disease, Tay-Sachs disease, hemophilia, cystic fibrosis, and Duchenne muscular dystrophy), neuronal migration/differentiation (familial Hirschsprung disease and lissencephaly), important malformation syndromes (Williams, Beckwith-Wiedemann, and Noonan syndromes), osteochondrodysplasias, genodermatoses (ichthyoses and epidermolysis bullosa), syndromal synostoses (Crouzon, Saethre-Chotzen, Pfeiffer, and Boston types), dominant polycystic kidney disease, Marfan syndrome, and early onset neoplasms (Wilms' tumor, Ewing's tumor, desmoplastic small cell carcinoma, and acute myelogenous leukemia). The alliance of cytogenetics with molecular genetics [via fluorescent in situ hybridization (FISH) and small structural chromosome abnormalities] has been fruitful. The identification of loci on chromosomes involved

in common aneuploidies (13, 18, 21, X) allows analysis of the components of these syndromes that have large-scale genetic disturbances. The intersex conditions and related disorders such as azoospermia can be analyzed according to several gene loci on the Y chromosome that are syntenic with X-chromosome loci and not subject to X-chromosome inactivation. The mechanisms whereby small numbers of progenitor cells of the inner cell mass give rise to the 200 types of differentiated cells are now being investigated. They probably involve "default" or ground states that are moved to new states by the actions of transcription factors. The fanning out of cell types in the adenohypophysis and bone marrow are good examples, as is sex determination. An understanding of pattern formation in the early embryo is being gained by analysis of the heterotaxy conditions. Genes involved in early patterning and segmentation are widely conserved in all species studied, most notably the HOX and PAX genes.

Unusual, apparently non-mendelian mechanisms, including gonadal and somatic mosaicism, postzygotic mutations, uniparental disomy, X-inactivation, and imprinting, may go some way toward explaining disorders previously regarded as "multifactorial" and/or "polygenic."

These increments in diagnostic power have profound effects on the specificity and simplicity of counseling and prenatal diagnosis. A working knowledge of cytogenetic and molecular mechanisms of maldevelopment aids the pediatric pathologist in selecting diagnostic tests on tissue samples such that naked-eye, light microscopic, and electron microscopic pathology will form a system of triage. However, it is clear that different mutations in different regions of a given gene confer differences in phenotypic severity. For example, mutations in the cystic fibrosis transmembrane regulator (CFTR) gene may cause mild, late onset chronic obstructive pulmonary disease or severe early liver disease;

collagen gene mutations may cause precocious osteoarthritis or lethal osteochondrodysplasias; and mutations in the neurofibromatosis, fibrillin, and dominant polycystic kidney disease genes may give standard presentations in adult life and also (often as yet unexplained) severe or lethal perinatal phenotypes. Perinatal pathologists should therefore be original, vigilant, and diligent in finding new manifestations of known diseases as well as identifying new diseases.

This chapter reviews many of the known mechanisms of maldevelopment. These mechanisms involve at least three major categories: malformation, disruption, and deformation. It has to be admitted that the present understanding of these categories is incomplete and provisional, with many overlaps. The number of malformations that can be diagnosed at the level of gene mutations and cytogenetic abnormality is increasing dramatically. There is considerable discussion on the concept of disruption, whereas mechanical deformation is rather more readily understood. These three entities of congenital anomaly can often be linked by cascades or sequences whereby multiple congenital anomalies in a given clinical case may actually be linked as consequences of one primary malformational or disruptional event. In addition, final disease states, such as hydrops fetalis, can be shown to arise from complex networks of mechanisms and primary causes, which are frequently genetic.

CAUSES AND DISTRIBUTION OF CYTOGENETIC ABNORMALITIES

Abnormal prezygotic meiotic and postzygotic mitotic events lead to frequent and varied chromosome abnormalities, which can be detected in studies of sperm and eggs, in abnormally developed in vitro fertilization (IVF) embryos, in spontaneous miscarriages, and in malformed fetuses and infants in the perinatal period. These abnormalities include aneuploidy for many chromosomes (trisomy and monosomy), abnormal ploidy (haploidy, triploidy, tetraploidy), structural abnormalities (deletions, insertions, inversions, translocations, and ring chromosomes), and mosaicism (which may be gonadal, somatic, placental, and within pairs of monozygotic twins). Considerations of uniparental disomy and imprinting apply to many of these anomalies.

Aneuploidy most commonly results from abnormal allocation of chromosomes (nondisjunction) in gametogenesis. The effects may be modified by postzygotic events that lead to mosaicism. The principal mechanisms are as follows. (1) Parents who are aneuploid (e.g., 21-trisomic) produce aneuploid gametes; 21-trisomic women produce disomic gametes if the secondary oocyte contains two copies of chromosome 21. (2) Parents who carry balanced robertsonian (centric fusion) nonhomologous translocations may produce unbalanced or balanced gametes (Fig. 11.1). In studies of spermatogenesis in balanced robertsonian translocation carriers, the frequency of unbalanced sperm varied from 3–26% (Table 11.1) [1–4]. The origins of robertsonian translocations can be traced. In a series of 30 de novo nonhomologous cases,

Table 11.1.   Frequency of chromosomally unbalanced sperm produced by robertsonian translocation carriers [1–4]

Translocation	Unbalanced product, %
t(13q;14q)	8
t(13q;15q)	10
t(14q;21q)	27
t(21q;22q)	3
t(15q;22q)	10
t(13q;14q)	26

Table 11.2.   Parental origin of free autosomal trisomies: informative cases [8–13]

	Maternal		Paternal		Author
	No.	%	No.	%	
Trisomy 16	62	100	0	0	Hassold et al [8]
Trisomy 13	16	100	0	0	Bugge et al [9]
Trisomy 18	48	89	6	11	Nöthen et al [10]; Kupke and Muller [11]; Babu and Verma [12]
Trisomy 21	184	95	9	5	Antonarakis [13]
TOTAL	310	95.4	15	4.6	

26 were maternally derived and four were paternally derived [5]. Similar considerations apply to other structural abnormalities, which may frequently be found in parents who have recurrent pregnancy losses. Again, the parents may show these structural chromosomal abnormalities in somatic cells or be presumed to have gonadal mosaicism. (3) The most common cause of trisomy is de novo nondisjunction during oogenesis, often linked to advanced maternal age (Table 11.2). Although nondisjunction is common in oogenesis, it should also be noted that errors in second meiosis (M2) result in abnormal ova, and that the aneuploid ovum is probably the only available one in that cycle. M2 nondisjunction affects only half of the spermatozoa derived from one spermatogonium, and there may be selection against aneuploid sperm in a given ejaculate.

FREE ANEUPLOIDY CAUSED BY NONDISJUNCTION

Details of the frequency and types of nondisjunction in oocytes are given in the publications of Plachot [6, 7]. The extent of maternal contribution to autosomal trisomic fetuses has been examined by molecular techniques and is summarized in Table 11.2 [8–13]. In 45,X̊ fetuses, the majority have one normal maternal X, and it is thought that a structurally abnormal paternal sex chromosome (X or Y)

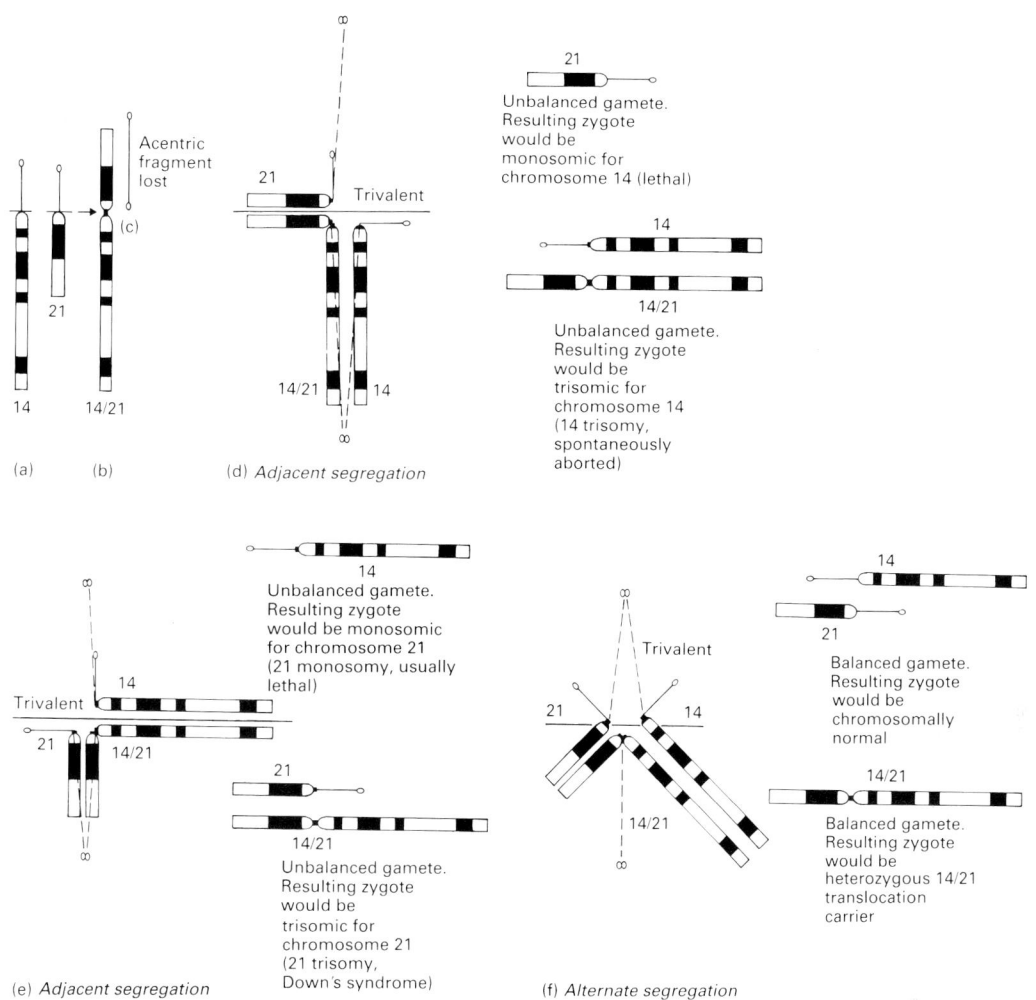

FIGURE 11.1. *Robertsonian (centric fusion) translocation. Breaks occur in the short arms very close to the centromeres of acrocentric chromosomes (a). The fused chromosome is dicentric, and the acentric fragment is usually lost (b, c). Carriers have a normal phenotype. At meiosis I synapsis, a trivalent is formed. Adjacent segregations (d, e) result in trisomy or monosomy for whole acrocentric chromosomes. Alternate segregation results in balanced gametes and zygotes (f). The monosomies are thought to be lethal. 14/21 translocation is the most common cause of translocation trisomy 21, and it may arise from unbalanced meiosis in the germ cells of a translocation carrier parent, or as a de novo event in the germ cells of a chromosomally normal parent.*

is preferentially lost during postzygotic nondisjunction. Common structural X-chromosome abnormalities include iso-X, partially deleted, and large ring X chromosomes, and these are preferentially inactivated [14]. In the case of X-autosomal translocations, X-inactivation may spread to involve autosomal genes.

Using DNA restriction fragment length polymorphisms (RFLPs), it has been shown for trisomy 16 that there are fewer than expected numbers of recombination events in maternal M1 prophase. This suggests that there may often be a failure of synapsis; homologous chromosome pairs may wander at random, with incorporation into daughter nuclei occurring by happenstance [8].

Nondisjunction in early postzygotic mitosis is the source of fetal mosaicism for aneuploidy. Depending on where and when this occurs, mosaic cell lines may be present in all

components of the zygote; alternatively, they may be limited to trophoectoderm or inner cell mass, limited to one of a pair of MZ twins, or unequally distributed in the inner cell mass so as to produce gonadal mosaicism or pigmentary dysplasias (see Chap. 33). Most commonly, a trisomic chromosome set reverts to disomy because one of the trisomic chromosomes fails to participate normally in mitotic disjunction. A diploid cell line may lose one sex chromosome to produce 46,XX or 46,XY/45,X mosaicism; as mentioned, this frequently results in the loss of a structurally abnormal X or Y chromosome. Two successive nondisjunction events may occur in one chromosome group, resulting in three cell lines (e.g., 47,XXY/46,XX/45,X); such events may affect more than one chromosome group (e.g., 47,XY,+8/45,X mosaicism, with presumed intermediate 46,XY or 46,X,+8 cell lines) [15]. When trisomy reverts

Table 11.3.   Patterns of mosaicism involving chorionic villus sampling [16, 17]

	Type I	Type II	Type III	Type IV
Cytotrophoblast (direct analysis)	Aneuploid or aneuploid/euploid mosaic	Euploid	Aneuploid or aneuploid/euploid mosaic	Euploid
Villous mesenchyme (culture analysis)	Euploid	Aneuploid or aneuploid/euploid mosaic	Aneuploid or aneuploid/euploid mosaic	Euploid
Fetal blood or tissue	Euploid	Euploid	Euploid	Aneuploid
Comment	"False positive" by direct analysis	"False positive" by culture analysis.	"False positive" by direct and culture analysis	"False negative"
	Normal fetal outcome	Aneuploid mesenchyme may cause fetal growth retardation.	Aneuploid chorion causes fetal growth failure or demise.	A necessary condition for survival to term of 13- and 18-trisomic fetuses

Table 11.4.   U.S. Collaborative study on chorionic villus sampling [18]

Chorionic trophoblast mosaicism	Chorionic mesenchyme mosaicism	Fetal tissue	
36	0	21/21 (60%) euploid	Type I
0	45	7/33 (21%) true mosaicism	
		26/33 (79%) euploid	Type II
10	10	3/8 (37.5%) true mosaicism	
		5/8 (62.5%) euploid	Type III

11,436 cytogenetic results, 91 (0.8%) mosaicism. True mosaicism accounts for 10 of 62 cases (16%). Confined placental mosaicism accounts for 52 of 62 cases (84%). Of 52 confined cases, 40%, 50%, and 10% were type I, II, and III, respectively.

Table 11.5.   Chromosome mosaicism in four monozygotic twin pairs

Author	Chromosome mosaicism
Perlman et al [19]	45,X and 46,XY
Deacon et al [20]	45,X and 46,XX
Rogers et al [21]	47,XX, +21 and 46,XY
Heydanus et al [22], case No. 2	47,XX, +13 and 46,XX

Rare patients show mosaic aneuploidy for different chromosomes in different tissue—i.e., mosaic variegated aneuploidy [23–25].

to disomy, there is the possibility of uniparental disomy (see below). Ratios of mosaic cell lines may vary from tissue to tissue. For instance, the lymphocyte mosaicism ratios may not faithfully represent the degree of aneuploidy in the brain.

Confined mosaicism poses problems in prenatal diagnosis and also explains some phenotypic variability and severity of chromosome abnormality syndromes [16, 17]. Confined placental/fetal mosaicism occurs in four patterns (Table 11.3). It should be noted that chorionic mesenchymal mosaicism may not be confined but may truly represent the fetal status, as assessed by amniocentesis and/or analysis of fetal cells. The types of mosaicism have been numerically analyzed in a large collaborative study of chorionic villous sampling results (Table 11.4) [18].

Amniotic fluid cell mosaicism generally reflects fetal mosaicism.

Mosaicism may also be confined in monozygotic twin pairs (heterokaryotypia), as summarized in Table 11.5 [19–22].

ABNORMALITIES OF PLOIDY

Abnormal syngamy causes abnormal ploidy. Although haploid IVF embryos have been identified, no such embryos have been found among spontaneous miscarriages. Triploidy and tetraploidy may be found in pure or mosaic form.

Abnormal syngamy can take the form of exclusion of the female pronucleus, resulting in an androgenic diploid zygote (true hydatidiform mole), or of inclusion of more than two haploid chromosome sets in the zygote. Diandric triploidy can result from fertilization of a normal haploid ovum by two normal haploid sperm or one diploid sperm. Digynic triploidy results from fertilization of a diploid ovum by a haploid sperm. Classic cytogenetic analysis suggested that diandry led to partial hydatidiform moles (PHMs), while most of the digynic triploids could survive to term with the typical clinical syndrome of triploidy [26]. DNA RFLP analysis has confirmed this [27]. Two phenotypes are found: in type I (diandry) there is PHM in a relatively well-grown fetus, while in type II (digyny) the fetus has head-sparing growth retardation and a normal placenta.

Tetraploidy can arise from triandry [28, 29] or failure of cytokinesis in early postzygotic mitosis [30]. The phenotype is PHM, which may progress to trophoblastic neoplasia.

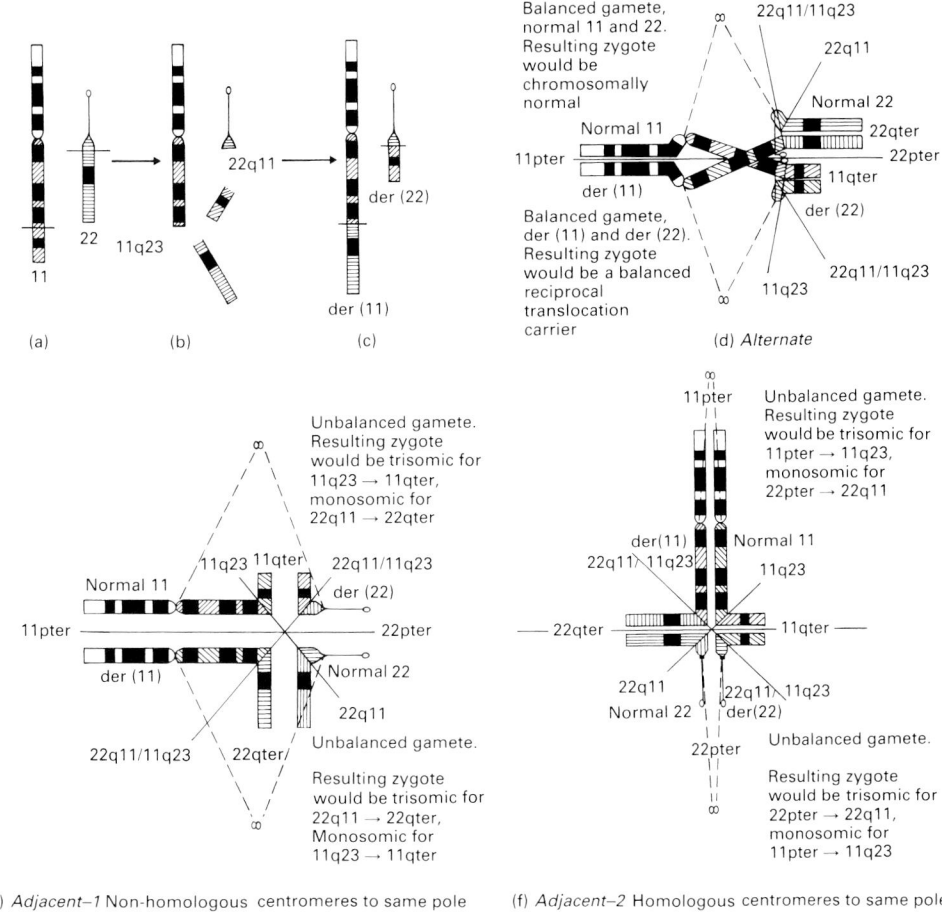

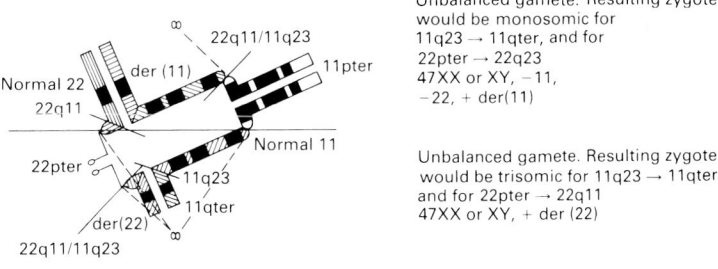

FIGURE 11.2. *Reciprocal translocation (a, b, c). Breaks at chromosome 11q23 and chromosome 22q11 result in the most common reciprocal translocation in humans. At meiosis I synapsis, quadrivalents are formed, and the mode of segregation determines the karyotype of the resulting gametes and zygotes. In alternate segregation (d), alternate centromeres of the quadrivalent pass to the same daughter cell pole; this is the only mechanism whereby chromosomally balanced gametes and zygotes can be formed. (e) Adjacent-1 segregation results in nonhomologous centromeres of the quadrivalent passing to the same pole, whereas in adjacent-2 segregation (f), homologous adjacent centromeres pass to the same pole. In both cases, zygotes will be partially monosomic and partially trisomic for the four affected chromosome segments. In discordantly oriented segregation (g), the centromeres of the normal nonhomologous chromosomes are both free to pass at random to either pole, and 2:2 and 3:1 segregations therefore occur. The figure shows the two known types of gametes from 3:1 discordant segregation. Of these, the segregation 46,XX or XY, +der(22) is the most frequent. It results in trisomy for part of chromosome 22 and part of chromosome 11. This is not apparent from inspection of the karyotype of the propositus, and parental carrier status needs to be established.*

STRUCTURAL CHROMOSOME ANOMALIES

Structural chromosome abnormalities are important because pairing of homologous chromosomes is disturbed at M1 of gametogenesis; this can lead to a variety of unbalanced karyotypes, with trisomy or monosomy for entire chromosomes or significant lengths of chromosomes. In addition, reciprocal translocations vary in their effects according to the sites of breakpoints in relation to exonic, intronic, and intergenic DNA; such translocations may also yield very small chromosome fragments that are easily lost in meiotic and mitotic cell divisions, leading to monosomy for groups of genes (so-called cryptic translocation). Such mechanisms can give rise to the "contiguous gene syndromes" (see below). In fact, the structural chromosome abnormalities have been fruitful as a bridge between classic cytogenetics and single gene diseases, often through the medium of FISH methods that can paint entire chromosomes, chromosomal centromeres, or single genes on chromosomes.

For simplicity, this section considers only the two main types of translocations—i.e., centric fusion and reciprocal. Special texts can be consulted for the consequences of insertions/deletions, inversions, and ring chromosomes.

Centric fusion (robertsonian) translocation eliminates the very short short-arms of two acrocentric chromosomes (in groups D and/or G), the new chromosome having the long arms of two chromosomes. Some cases of homologous translocation (e.g., 13;13q,21q;21q) are actually isochromosomes [31]; this applies to the chromosomes of zygotes with unbalanced translocations. Balanced translocation zygotes may have homologous robertsonian translocations to which both parents have contributed [32, 33]. Centric fusion translocations per se do not result in loss of genetic material; however, isochromosomes may well cause uniparental disomy (see below).

Reciprocal translocations arise from breakpoints in chromatids of nonhomologous chromosomes, with exchange of chromosomal segments. Such translocations may have four effects:

1. Even if the breakpoints are outside genomic DNA, misassortment at M1 gametogenesis yields partially trisomic or monosomic gametes and zygotes (Fig. 11.2).
2. Likewise, there may be loss of small products of translocation, including important genes for which the patient could be nullisomic (Fig. 11.3).
3. One breakpoint may occur within a gene, which cannot be transcribed because it is distributed on two chromosomes after translocation (Fig. 11.4).
4. Both breakpoints may occur within genes; following translocation, hybrid or chimeric genes are produced, giving rise to fusion transcripts. For example, the 5′-part of an actively expressed gene (e.g., a housekeeping gene, including its promoter region) may be fused to any part of a gene that should be suppressed. The second gene is inappropriately switched on, and may act as an oncogene (e.g., Philadelphia chromosome, Burkitt's lymphoma, Ewing's tumor, desmoplastic small round cell tumor; Fig. 11.5).

UNIPARENTAL DISOMY (UPD) AND IMPRINTING

These phenomena can arise through several mechanisms, including:

1. Isochromosomes, including isochromosomes resembling homologous robertsonian translocations (Table 11.6) [31]
2. Trisomy with the postzygotic loss of the single chromosome derived from one parent, leaving a chromosome pair derived from the other parent
3. Gamete complementation, with ovum and sperm disomic and nullisomic, respectively, for a given chromosome
4. Gamete complementation with ovum and sperm nullisomic and disomic, respectively, for a given chromosome
5. Postzygotic mitotic nondisjunction, yielding a monosomic line that undergoes duplication for that chromosome

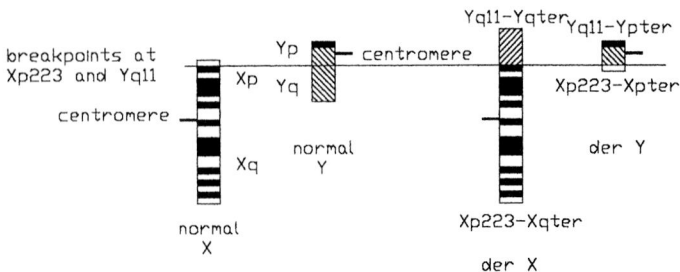

FIGURE 11.3. *X-linked ichthyosis is a component of a contiguous gene syndrome. The genes are situated very near the telomeric end of Xp. In a reciprocal translocation between Xp223 and Yq11, a small derY chromosome fragment is produced which may be lost during meiosis. The breakpoints occur in intergenic DNA.*

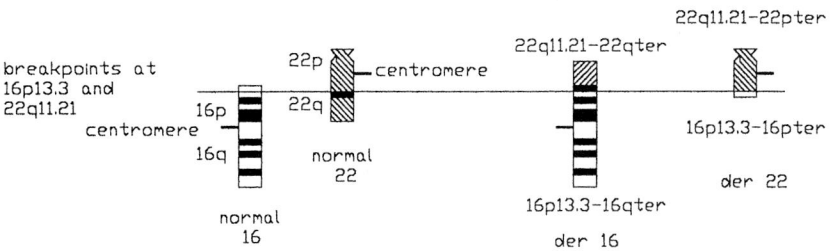

FIGURE 11.4.   *The gene for autosomal dominant polycystic kidney disease (PKD1) was mapped to chromosome 16p13.3. In a particular family, affected individuals have a reciprocal translocation in which one breakpoint is within the PKD1 gene; as a result, the gene is disrupted, one part being present in the der16 chromosome and the other in the der22 chromosome. The disrupted gene cannot be transcribed. The other breakpoint, at 22q11.21, apparently does not pass through a gene.*

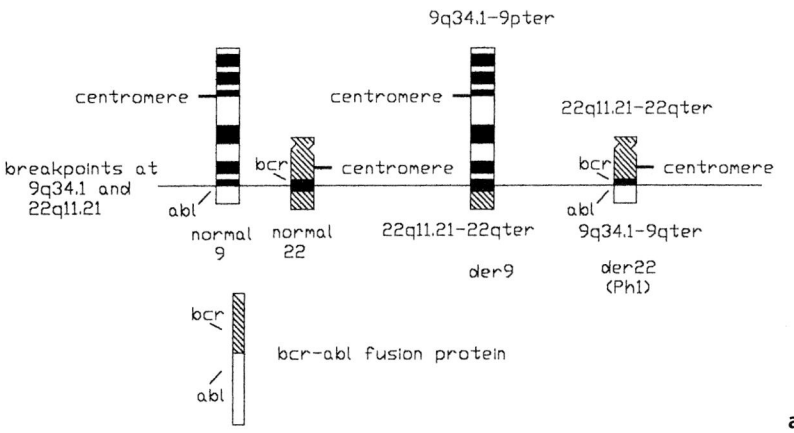

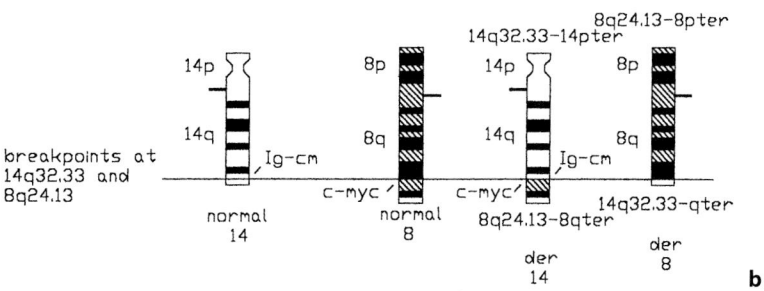

FIGURE 11.5.   *Reciprocal translocations causing neoplasia by producing chimeric genes. (a) The t(9;22) translocation of chronic myelogenous leukemia produces the der22 Philadelphia chromosome. Both breakpoints disrupt genes. At 9q34.1 is the c-ab1 oncogene; this codes for transmembrane tyrosine kinase receptor and was isolated from the Abelson murine leukemia virus. There is a breakpoint cluster region (bcr) at 22q11.21. As a result of the translocation, a bcr-ab1 fusion protein is produced, and this acts as an oncogene. (b) In Burkitt's lymphoma, the most common reciprocal translocation affects the c-myc proto-oncogene at 8q24.13 and an immunoglobulin gene at 14q32.33, allowing malignant transformation. (c) The most common translocation in Ewing's tumor produces a chimeric gene composed of the first exons of the EWS gene at 22q12 and the last four exons of the FLI1 gene at 11q24. The FLI1 gene codes for a transcription factor. Hence, there is activation of inappropriate transcription. (d) In desmoplastic small round cell tumor, the EWS gene is disrupted in the same region, between exons 7 and 8. A chimeric gene is made with the last three exons of the WT1 gene. This is a transcription factor with zinc finger motifs coded by exons 7–10. Again, there is activation of inappropriate transcription.*

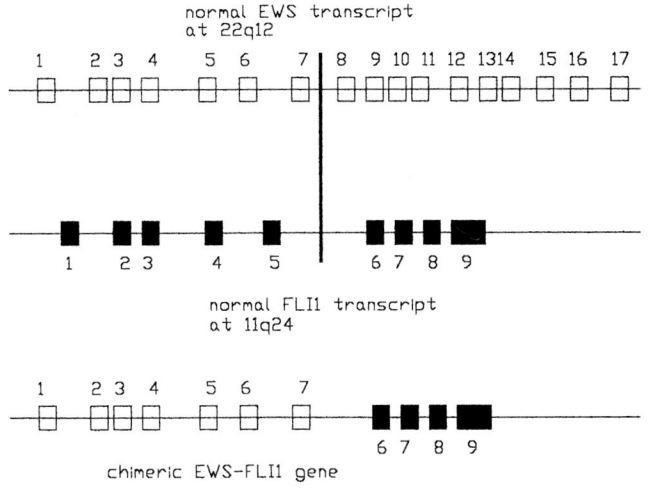

Ewing's tumor results from a
t(11;22)(q24;q12) translocation,
producing a chimeric EWS-FlI1 gene

normal EWS transcript
at 22q12

normal FLI1 transcript
at 11q24

c   chimeric EWS-FLI1 gene

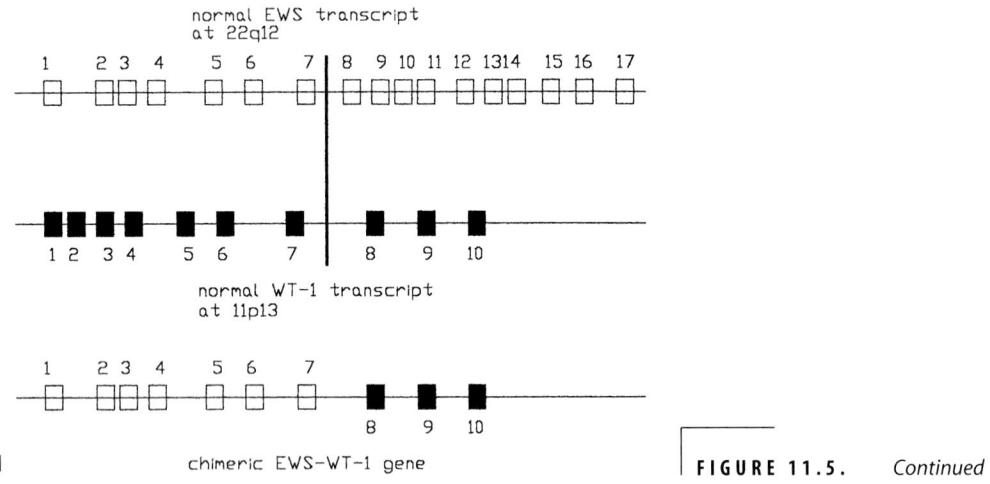

Desmoplastic small round cell tumor (DSCRT)
results from a t(11;22)(p13;q12) translocation,
producing a chimeric EWS-WT1 gene

normal EWS transcript
at 22q12

normal WT-1 transcript
at 11p13

d   chimeric EWS-WT-1 gene

FIGURE 11.5.   *Continued*

Table 11.6. Consequences of homologous robertsonian translocations and isochromosomes [31]

Karyotype	Phenotype	Other	Homologous status
t(15q15q)	Normal	Multiple early loss	Biparental
t(15q15q)	Angelman syndrome	—	Paternal uniparental disomy (UPD)
t(15q15q)	Prader-Willi syndrome	—	Maternal uniparental disomy (UPD)
t(21q21q)	Normal	21-trisomic	Biparental
t(21q21q)	Normal	Multiple early loss	Paternal UPD 21
t(22q22q)	Normal	Multiple early loss	Biparental
t(14q14q)	Mild mental retardation	—	Maternal UPD 14

The main consequences of disomy are:

1. The possibility of inheriting two copies of a deleterious mutant gene from a single heterozygous parent—e.g., cystic fibrosis [34] or hemophilia A [35].
2. Growth retardation and early embryonic failure [36–38].
3. Considerations of imprinting. The classic instance of isodisomy and imprinting effects is the relationship between Prader-Willi syndrome (PWS) and Angelman syndrome (AS). Both involve abnormalities of chromosome 15, region 15q11.2-q12 [39]. PWS is caused by paternal deficiency of this region, through either paternal chromosome 15 deletion (74%) or maternal UPD (26%). In AS, 72% have maternal chromosome 15 deletion, and 5% have paternal UPD. Some cases of AS may have single maternal gene mutations. It is likely that the two defects are caused by abnormal expression of two imprinted genes that are closely linked in the q11.2-12 region of chromosome 15. Confined placental trisomy 15 mosaicism has been found in some cases of PWS [40, 41]; presumptive evidence of such a mechanism has been observed in two interesting cases. In one, a diagnosis of 46,XX/47,XX,+15 mosaicism was made at amniocentesis and confined in the infant. There were combined phenotypic effects of maternal UPD and trisomy 15 [42]. In the other case, there were combined features of PWS and Bloom syndrome. There was maternal UPD for chromosome 15; the (recessive) gene for Bloom syndrome is at 15q26.1, and the newborn was presumably homozygous for the maternally inherited gene [43].

Another example of imprinting is the inheritance of a severe congenital form of myotonic dystrophy when the mutant gene is maternal rather than paternal in origin [44, 45].

Imprinting of chromosome regions is thought to take place by a process of methylation similar to that occurring in X-chromosome inactivation. Like mosaicism, it may help to explain unusual, apparently non-mendelian genetic effects.

FREQUENCY AND TYPES OF CYTOGENETIC ABNORMALITIES

1. IVF embryos have been studied in two ways:
   (a) A wide range of unusual and severe chromosome abnormalities has been seen in morphologically abnormal embryos unsuitable for implantation [6, 46]. Given the difficulties and the limitations of the IVF techniques, these results imply that the majority of such embryos are chromosomally abnormal, with high rates of polyploidy and mosaicism.
   (b) In spontaneous losses after IVF [47], 62% of cases were chromosomally abnormal, most commonly with 45,X and trisomy 14 karyotypes. These results are quite similar to those for spontaneously conceived early losses.
2. Spontaneous miscarriage. Results from several large series are summarized in Tables 11.7 and 11.8 [48]. Rates of chromosome abnormality are highest in early losses; early active removal and karyotyping of spontaneous losses yields an abnormality rate of 76% [49].

Table 11.7.   Principal types of chromosomal abnormalities found in spontaneous abortions (modified from Creasy [48])

Chromosome anomaly	Chromosomally abnormal cases, %
Autosomal trisomy	50
45,X	18
Triploid, euploid and aneuploid	15
Tetraploid, euploid and aneuploid	5
Structural abnormalities	4
Mosaic, various	4
Trisomy, double and triple	2
Other	2
TOTAL	100

Table 11.8.   Specific autosomal trisomies in spontaneous abortions (modified from Creasy [48])

Trisomic autosome	%
1	0
2	5
3	1
4	2
5	<1
6	<1
7	4
8	3
9	3
10	2
11	<1
12	<1
13	6
14	4
15	7
16	30
17	<1
18	5
19	<1
20	3
21	12
22	9
TOTAL	100

3. Perinatal deaths. Chromosome abnormalities are found in 3.6% of fetuses and newborn infants dying in the perinatal period (Table 11.9) [50–52].

4. Prenatal diagnosis for selected fetal anomalies. The situation is complicated by variations in expertise in obstetric ultrasound; also, the types and combinations of anomalies may be reported singly or in combination. General patterns are summarized in Table 11.10 [53–61]. The highest frequency of chromosome abnormality is seen in fetal omphalocele and cystic hygroma.

SINGLE GENE DEFECTS

Until a few years ago, the only well-known human single gene mutation was that causing sickle cell disease. Many genes have now been identified and sequenced that code for diseases regularly diagnosed by pediatric pathologists (Table 11.11), including genes for genetic metabolic diseases, tissue dysplasias, malformation syndromes, and pediatric neoplasms. A few genes have been identified that are clearly

involved in the early development of normal structure and function of tissues and organs (e.g., PAX genes, Wilms' tumor gene-1, and retinoblastoma gene-1); it seems likely that genes will soon be found for major regional malformations such as neural tube defects, holoprosencephaly, and bilateral renal agenesis. Several genes have been found that are implicated in some of the classic pediatric neoplasms (see Fig. 11.5). Contiguous gene deletion syndromes form a link between classic cytogenetics and molecular genetics (see Fig. 11.3) [62, 63].

The typical structure and function of a gene are summarized in Figure 11.6. The effects of mutations depend on three main factors:

1. The type and extent of the mutation—e.g., point mutation, deletion mutation, splice site mutation
2. The effect of a mis-sense point mutation on change of amino acid residue function
3. The situation of the mutation in the gene—i.e., whether at the proximal (5'-) or distal (-3') end

Point mutations substitute one base for another in a codon (triplet code for one amino acid residue). Such substitutions are synonymous when the amino acid does not change, although its codon does. For instance, there are six codons for arginine (Arg), and a series of point mutations could merely change the code for Arg: AGC → AGA → CGA → CGG → CGC → CGT.

Mis-sense mutations do change the coded amino acid residue. The severity of the effect of these mutations depends on the size and charge of the old and new amino acid residues, and whether they have any critical role in the three-dimensional structure and function of the protein. For instance, Arg has a basic side chain, and is frequently involved in DNA-binding sites of transcription factor proteins (see below). Glycine (Gly) has the smallest side chain,

Table 11.9. Chromosomal abnormalities among 2832 fetuses and infants dying in the perinatal period [50–52]

Chromosomal abnormality	% of Abnormalities
Autosomal trisomy	55
45,X	15
Triploidy	15
Structural	9
Gonosomal trisomy	7
Unbalanced translocation	3
Other	2

Table 11.10. Karyotypic analysis of anatomically abnormal fetuses diagnosed by obstetric ultrasound

Anomaly	Chromosomally abnormal	Authors
Symmetric growth retardation	9/50 (18%)	Gagnon et al [53]
Moderate/severe hydramnios	29/356 (8%)	Damato et al [54]
		Brady et al [55]
		Hendricks et al [56]*
		Eydoux et al [57]
		Stoll et al [58]*
Single malformation	29/239 (12%)	Eydoux et al [57]
Multiple malformations	19/65 (29%)	Eydoux et al [57]
All malformations	122/936 (13%)	Eydoux et al [57]
Cystic hygroma	21/29 (72%)	Gagnon et al [53]
Cardiovascular malformation	19/52 (37%)	Paladini et al [59]
Omphalocele	19/35 (54%)	Gilbert and Nicolaides [60]*
Diaphragmatic hernia	4/18 (22%)	Gagnon et al [53]*
		Sharland et al [61]*

Table 11.11.   Some common developmental diseases and their genes

Disease Groups	Genes and Mutations
1. Collagenopathies	*COL1A1*—osteogenesis imperfecta—numerous mutations, usually involving mis-sense mutations from Gly; Ehlers-Danlos syndrome (EDS) type V11A [64–67] *COL1A2*—osteogenesis imperfecta, EDS type VIIB [64, 65] *COL2A1*—achondrogenesis type II, hypochondrogenesis, Stickler syndrome, spondylo-epiphyseal dysplasia, Kniest syndrome [64, 65] *COL3A1*—EDS type IV [64] *COL4A5*—Alport syndrome [64, 68] *COL5A1*—EDS1/hypomelanosis of Ito [69, 70] *COL7A1*—Dystrophic epidermolysis bullosa [71, 72] *COL9A2*—multiple epiphyseal dysplasia [73] *COL10A1*—Schmid metaphyseal chondrodysplasia [74]
2. Cystic fibrosis and related disorders	*CFTR*—numerous mutations throughout the large gene cause phenotypic variability in severity of disease of lungs, liver, pancreas, vas deferens [75–80]
3. Myopathies	*DMD* Duchenne and Becker muscular dystrophy are caused by large and smaller deletions respectively [81–83] *LAM* Congenital muscular dystrophy [84] *LGMD2F* autosomal recessive limb-girdle muscular dystrophy AR sarcoglycan [85] *STA* Emery-Dreifus [86] *MTM1* X-linked myotubular myopathy [87] *DM* myotonic dystrophy [88, 89] adhalin protein in autosomal recessive muscular dystrophy [90] calpain gene in limb girdle muscular dystrophy type 2A [91] plectin gene in muscular dystrophy/epidermolysis bullosa [92]
4. Marfan syndrome and related disorders	*FBN1* [93–96] *FBN2* [97]
5. Williams syndrome	*LIMK* [98, 99] elastin [100]
6. Hirschsprung	*RET* receptor tyrosine kinase mutations [101] *GDNF* (?ligand of RET) mutations not sufficient, but may contribute [102, 103] *EDNRB*, a G-protein coupled endothelin-B receptor *EDN3*, endothelin 3 causes a Hirschsprung/Waardenburg phenotype [104]
7. CNS malformations	Lissencephaly *LIS1* [105] Schizencephaly *EMX2* [106] *PAX3 Waardenburg* [107] *MITF* Waardenburg type II [108] L1CAM X-linked hydrocephalus [109] *SMN, NAIP, p44* spinal muscular atrophy [110–112] *PAX6* aniridia [113] *SHH* autosomal dominant holoprosencephaly (114) *UBE3A* Angelman syndrome [115]
8. Osteochondrodsyplasias	*COL2A1*—achondrogenesis type II, hypochondrogenesis—see collagenopathies *COL9A2*—multiple epiphyseal dysplasia—see collagenopathies FGFR3—achondroplasia, hypochondroplasia, thanatophoric dysplasia [116] *DTDST*—diastrophic dysplasia, atelosteogenesis II and achondrogenesis type IB [117–119] *SOX9*—campomelic dysplasia [120] *CDMP-1*—in acromesomelic, Hunter-Thompson type [121]; Grebe type [122] *OSF2/CBFA1* cleidocranial dysostosis [123]
9. Overgrowth syndromes	$p57^{KIP2}$ (cyclin-cdk inhibitor) mutations in 5 of 52 cases of Beckwith-Wiedemann syndrome [124–126] *SGBS* Simpson-Golabi-Behmel syndrome [127]
10. Treacher-Collins syndrome	*TCOF1* [128]
11. EDS	*COL5A1* Type I/hypomelanosis of Ito [69, 70] Type IV *COL3A1* [64] Type VI *lysyl hydroxylase* [129, 130] *COL1A1* Type VIIA [64] *COL1A2* Type VIIB [64]

Table 11.11. *Continued*

Disease Groups	Genes and Mutations
12. BOR	*EYA1* [131]
13. Hypogammaglobulinemia	BtK X-linked hypo/agammaglobulinemia [132, 133]
	hyperIgM hypogammaglobulinemia [134]
14. Pallister Hall	*GLI3* [135]
15. Alagille	*BJAG1* [136]
16. Cardiovascular	*TBX5* Holt-Oram syndrome [137]
	NODAL, HTX1 mutations in heterotaxy [138–142]
17. Wilson	*ATP7B* [143–145]
18. Batten	*CLN3* [146]
19. Rieger	*RIEG* is a bicoid-related homeobox gene. The syndrome has oculodental anomalies and failure of involution of umbilical skin [147]
20. Genodermatoses	hair cortex keratin monilethrix [148]
	integrin beta4 junctional epidermolysis bullosa (EB) with pyloric atresia [149]
	laminin 5 junctional EB [150]
	KTN9 epidermolytic palmoplanatar keratoderma [151]
	EDA X-linked anhidrotic ectodermal dysplasia [152]
	Sjogren-Larsson ichthyosis [153]
	COL17A1 atrophic benign EB [154]
	X-linked ichthyosis steroid sulfatase [155]
	transglutaminase 1 lamellar ichthyosis [156]
	K5, K14 EB simplex [157]
	K16, 17 pachyonychia congenita [158]
	epidermolytic hyperkeratosis *K1, K10* [157]
	plectrin mutations in muscular dystrophy/EB [92]
	XPB/ERCC3 trichothiodystrophy [159]
21. Storage disorders	Gaucher disease [160]
	Lysosomal sialidase sialidosis [161]
	Hunter disease [162]
	mucopolysaccharidosis type VII [163]
22. Hemophilia A	flip tip mutation [164]
23. Tuberous sclerosis	*TS1* [165]
24. Autosomal dominant polycystic kidney disease	*PKD1* [166]
25. FGFR disorders	*FGFR1–3* mutations cause several dyschondroplasias and craniosynostoses [167–171]
26. Craniosynostoses	Numerous *FGFR1–3 mutations*—see FGFR section
	TWIST mutations in Saethre-Chotzen [172]
	MSX mutation in Boston type [173, 174]
	FBNI mutation in Shprintzen-Goldberg syndrome [93]
27. Peroxisomal disorders	*PEX7* rhizomelic chondrodysplasia punctata [175]
	PEX12 group 3 disorders (Zellweger) [176]
	PAF-2 group C peroxisomal disorders [177]
	X-linked adrenoleukodystrophy [178]
28. Developmental gene mutation summary	*HOXD13* sympolydactyly [179]
	MSX1 tooth agenesis [180]
	PTC Gorlin syndrome *(basal cell nevus syndrome)* [181]
	HOXA13 hand-foot-genital syndrome [182]
	EYA1 BOR syndrome [131]
	PAX6 aniridia [112]
	PAX3 Waardenburg [107]
	TBX5 Holt-Oram syndrome [137]
	TBX3 ulnar-mammary syndrome [183]
	PAX2 renal coloboma syndrome [184]
	SRY gonadal dysgenesis [185]
	SOX9 campomelic dysplasia [120]
	SHH autosomal dominant holoprosencephaly [137]
	WT1 Denys-Drash syndrome [186]

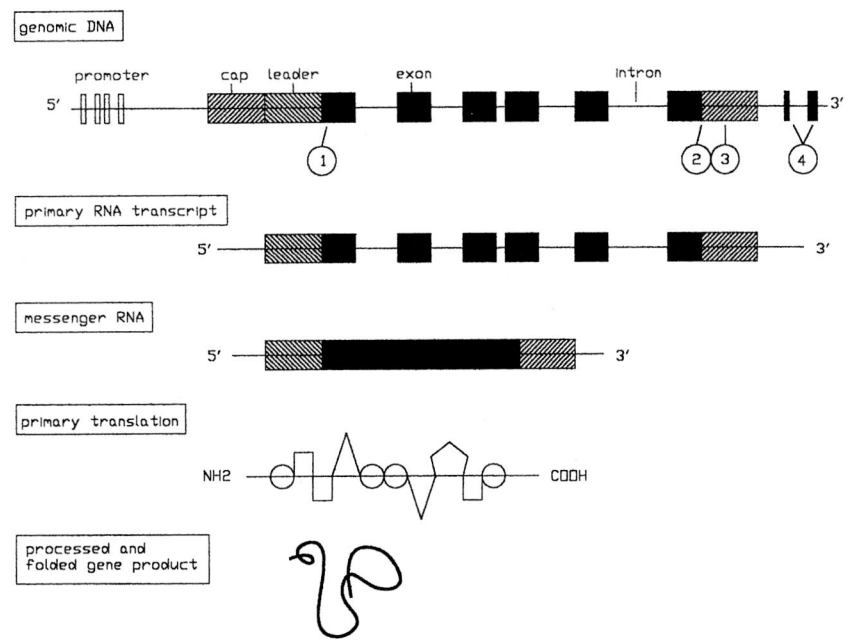

FIGURE 11.6. *Typical structure of a gene and its relation to the gene product. The upstream promoter region is the site of action of transcription factors that modify expression of the gene. The initiator codon (1) is the same as that for methionine (AUG), but the methionine residue is subsequently removed from the protein gene product. At the end of the last exon there is a STOP or termination code (2), followed by a trailer segment (3). There are often downstream enhancer regions (4). Sequences in DNA that are translated into segments of protein gene product are termed exons. Intervening intronic sequences are spliced out of the primary RNA transcript in the production of messenger RNA. Abnormal splicing can result from mutation in the 5′-splice site (usually -gt-) or the 3′-splice site (usually -ag-), causing loss or gain of exons in the translation to protein. Alternate splicing is a normal mechanism that allows the production of more than one gene product from a given gene. The primary, linear translated protein adopts its functional form by folding that is dictated by the properties of the side chains of the amino acid residues. This process occurs rapidly; in part the process is spontaneous, but chaperone molecules are also involved.*

and is involved in tight packing of fibrillar proteins—e.g., in the triple helical structures of collagen. Most of the point mutations in the collagenopathies cause mutation from Gly to a bulkier amino acid, whose size disrupts the triple helical structure of collagen. Mutations in the fibrillin gene (Marfan syndrome) frequently abolish cysteine-S-S-cysteine bridges or create new ones in the many epidermal growth-factor-like regions of the protein. Hence, many mis-sense mutations in Marfan patients substitute other amino acids for cysteine or introduce new cysteine residues.

Nonsense mutations substitute one of the three STOP codons for an amino acid, or vice versa. A premature STOP codon usually results in the production of a truncated protein translation; mutation from a normal termination point of transcription results in an elongated protein.

CpG pairs readily undergo mutation to TpG, such that there are fewer than expected CpG pairs in exonic DNA. C → T mutations in the CpG pairs at the template (non-coding strand) result in a CpG → CpA mutation in the coding strand. Up to 40% of all point mutations involve C → T mutations in the coding or template strands. Arg is involved again, since four of its six codes contain CpG pairs; a common nonsense point mutation is CGA → TGA, Arg → STOP.

Mutations involving changes in DNA length are insertions and deletions. They may affect small numbers of bases or large segments of genes. Where deletions and insertions involve small numbers of bases, three bases or multiples of three bases deleted or inserted will maintain transcription in-frame. For instance, the ΔF508 mutation in the CFTR gene (cystic fibrosis gene) does not cause frame shift. However, insertions and deletions of three bases or multiples of three bases may not occur in-frame; hence, nonsense and mis-sense mutations may take place. Deletions and insertions of other than three bases or multiples do cause frame shift and this usually results in a new STOP triplet downstream, with premature termination of transcription.

Deletional mutations are frequent (about 5% of all mutations) and are found particularly in the larger genes, such as the dystrophin gene. Large deletions are thought to be caused by misalignment of coding and template strands during mitosis, usually because similar regions are repeated along the gene, leading to misrecognition.

Splice site mutations at either end of the introns result in loss or gain of translated exons. In some mis-sense mutations, it is difficult to know whether the base change causes the disease or if it is only a harmless polymorphism. If the mutation affects an amino acid that is highly conserved across several species, it is reasonable to assume that the mutation has had a significant effect on protein conformation and function.

SOME EXAMPLES OF RECENTLY ASCERTAINED GENES AND THEIR MUTATIONS

There is rapid accumulation of data on mutations in many genes that cause developmental diseases such as those listed in Table 11.11 [64–185]. On-line catalogues are used to archive this information and to make it accessible. For instance, it is estimated that two new mutations are found every week in the CFTR gene. For many of the classic genetic diseases, the responsible genes and their various mutations have been found. This section highlights a small selection of these reports as listed in Table 11.11. It also draws attention to some correlations between genotype and phenotype.

The Collagenopathies

The collagen genes code for very long proteins that consist largely of rodlike domains but with specialized sequences at the NH_2- and -COOH ends that are probably important in assembling the triple helices of pro-α chains (64–74). The linear part of the collagen molecule is coded by about 50 exons, each having a length of 54 codons or multiples of 54. The exon thus codes for a length of 18 amino acids, consisting of six repeats of a sequence of the form (-Gly-X-Y-) in which X and Y residues are frequently proline and hydroxyproline, respectively. The pro-α chains are arranged in β-helices, and the triple helix is arranged as an α-helix. There are many different pro-α collagen chains, and the different types of collagen molecules are made up of different combinations of pro-α chains in the triple helix. In building the triple helix, glycine residues are found at the center, while the proline and hydroxyproline residues face outward. The center of the triple helix is tightly packed. Glycine residues have no side chains; hence, mis-sense mutations from glycine to any other amino acid disturb the tight packing. Such mutations are frequently found in the collagenopathies.

The formation of the triple helix from the three pro-α chains begins at the -COOH end of the polypeptide. Therefore, mutations affecting that end of the fibrillar part of the protein (i.e., those in higher-numbered exons and codons) can produce more severe phenotypic effects (e.g., lethal perinatal osteogenesis imperfecta) than mutations in the midsection of the gene (type III, progressive bone deforming osteogenesis imperfecta) [65, 66]. However, several other types of mutations have been described, including 5′-splice site mutations and frame shift mutations leading to premature termination in various parts of the gene [66].

Clearly, mutations at the −COOH, nonrod end of the gene are likely to interfere with the formation of the triple helix. This has been found in mutations of the α1(X) chain of the collagen type X that occur in metaphyseal chondrodysplasia type Schmid [74].

It is notable that there are quite wide variations in the phenotypic effects of mutations in the COL2A1 gene; these range through achondrogenesis/hypochondrogenesis, Stickler syndrome, Kniest dysplasia, and spondyloepiphyseal dysplasia with premature osteoarthropathy. Data on the collagen type 7 mutations in dystrophic epidermolysis bullosa are given in Chapter 33.

Cystic Fibrosis and Mutations in the CFTR Gene

The cystic fibrosis transmembrane conductance regulator (CFTR) gene codes for a chloride channel regulated by cyclic AMP [75–80]. It has 27 exons; the complete gene product has 1480 peptides arranged in five functional domains. Two membrane-spanning domains contribute to the physical structure of the chloride channel, two nucleotide-binding domains (NBD) interact with cytosolic nucleotides, and a single R domain, coded by exon 13, controls channel activity and must be phosphorylated by a protein kinase for the channel to open.

Some early analyses of mutation effects have shown severely defective protein production by a variety of mutations toward the 5′- end of the gene. Other mutations, including the most frequent one in Caucasians (ΔF508), prevent protein processing, so that the protein does not arrive at the cellular apical membrane. Defective regulation occurs with mutations in the NBDs. Mutations in the membrane-spanning domains permit the channel to open for an abnormally short time period. Attempts are now being made to correlate specific mutations with stronger or weaker expressions of some of the clinical components of cystic fibrosis, such as pulmonary and pancreatic disease, congenital absence of the vas deferens, etc. [79, 80].

Mutations in the Dystrophin Gene

The dystrophin gene is very large, with 74 exons spread over 2300 kb [81–83]. The upstream, NH_2- portion of the protein is an actin-binding domain, while there are 24 homologous α-helical repeats in the rod region of the molecule. There is a cysteine-rich zone followed by a region that is unique to dystrophin, having no known homology in any other cytoskeletal proteins. Sixty percent of patients with Duchenne muscular dystrophy have out-of-frame deletional mutations causing severely truncated proteins. By contrast, patients with Becker-type dystrophy have semifunctional dystrophin molecules caused by in-frame internal deletions. Because of the size of the gene and its product, genotype/phenotype correlations are relatively crude. However, it is clear that these two major groups of deletional mutations occur at two different "hot spots."

Mutations in the Fibrillin Gene

Marfan syndrome is caused by mutations in the gene for fibrillin (FBN1). Fibrillin is a major component of microfibrils in the extracellular matrix. The protein structure is highly repetitive, with 65 exons having many motifs resembling epidermal growth factor (EGF). These EGF motifs have six cysteine residues in a 12 amino acid sequence; these residues form 3 -S-S- cross-linking pairs [93–97]. Almost all fibrillin mutations are "private," de novo mutations found only in one family. Despite this, there is phenotypic diversity among affected members of a given family. However, a severe neonatal phenotype has been noted, in which the following mutations have been found: skipping of a complete EGF-like exon because of frame shift mutations at or about exon 32, an in-frame insertion mutation of an extra cysteine residue at position 160, and mis-sense point mutations involving cysteine residues in the same region. In general, mis-sense mutations that substitute for cysteine residues cause severe phenotypes.

Williams Syndrome

The majority of cases have deletions in the gene for elastin, and there may be a contiguous gene syndrome effect to account for hypercalcemia by involvement of the adjacent calcitonin receptor gene [96–100].

Hirschsprung Disease

About 20% of cases of Hirschsprung disease are familial, with autosomal dominant inheritance. The responsible RET gene codes for a tyrosine kinase proto-oncogene that is expressed in cells derived from neural crest [101–104]. Mutations have been found in the extracellular liganding portion of the protein.

Lissencephaly Gene

A gene for lissencephaly (LIS1) has recently been isolated. Large deletions at the 5′- end of the gene have been detected in patients with Miller-Dieker syndrome [105]. The gene product is involved in cell-signalling pathways whereby neuroblasts migrate out of the subependymal germinal zone to the cerebral cortex.

Achondroplasia Mutation

The gene mutated in achondroplasia has recently been identified [116]. The ACH gene codes for fibroblast growth factor 3 (FGFR3), which is a transmembrane tyrosine kinase receptor protein that is expressed in pre-bone cartilage rudiments. Of 16 cases investigated, 15 had the same mutation, Gly 380 Arg, in the single transmembrane domain. This is a typical CpG to TpG mutation on the template strand (Fig. 11.7).

-380- 5′-TAC-GGG-GTG-3′ -Tyr-Gly-Val-	coding strand	normal allele
3′-ATG-CCC-CAC-5′	template strand	normal allele
3′-ATG-TCC-CAC-5′	template strand	mutant allele
-380- 5′-TAC-AGG-GTG-3′ -Tyr-Arg-Val-	coding strand	mutant allele

FIGURE 11.7. *A typical example of a C → T mutation in a CpG pair. In this case, the CpG pair is present on the template strand. It results in a CG → CA mutation in the coding strand at codon 380 of the fibroblast growth factor receptor 3 gene. This is the most common point mutation causing achondroplasia.*

Diastrophic Dysplasia

Diastrophic dysplasia (DTD) combines osteochondrodysplasia with spinal deformity and joint pathology. The DTD gene is a sulfate transporter, malfunction of which probably affects sulfation in cartilage matrix [117]. Three mutations have been found, two being single base deletions leading to premature STOP codons, and the other a 3′-splice acceptor site mutation.

Mutations in Bruton Tyrosine Kinase Gene

Mutations in the gene for Bruton's tyrosine kinase (BtK) gene cause agammaglobulinemia. The protein is involved in signal transduction in B cells. Point mutations are found in the kinase domain [132, 133].

Wilson Disease

Wilson disease results from a failure to export copper from hepatocytes into the bile. The Wilson disease gene (WND) is a P-type ATPase [143–145]. Many different mutations have been described; there is a special SEHP motif that may be essential for copper binding. Forty-two percent of cases have a mis-sense mutation involving the SEHP motif.

X-Linked Ichthyosis

Many patients with X-linked ichthyosis have a contiguous gene syndrome caused by a breakpoint at Xp223 (see Fig. 11.3). However, point mutations are also described [155], and these mutations occur at amino acid residues that are highly conserved across species.

Mutations in the Keratin 5 Gene

Mutations in the Keratin 5 gene cause epidermolysis bullosa simplex [157] (see Chapter 33).

Mutations in the Glucocerebrosidase Gene

The glucocerebrosidase gene codes for 11 exons and has been completely sequenced [160]. At least 30 different mutations have been found so far in Gaucher cases. Genotype/phenotype correlations are not yet clear; patients with a Leu $\rightarrow$ Pro mutation at amino acid residue 444 have severe (type II) disease, often with ichthyosis, renal hypoplasia, and hydrops fetalis.

Hemophilia A

One of the more unusual mutations commonly occurs in hemophilia A, whereby the factor VIII gene splits into two halves that face in opposite directions and cannot therefore be transcribed in continuity. This "flip-tip" mutation is found in half of all cases with severe hemophilia A [164].

Tuberous Sclerosis

The locus for tuberous sclerosis on chromosome 16 (TSC2) is close to the gene for dominant polycystic kidney disease (PKD1). Patients have constitutional heterozygosity for loss of 16p alleles, while there is loss of heterozygosity in hamartomas of these patients. The gene has been characterized as a transcription factor of leucine-zipper type. Mutations include very large deletions possibly also involving extragenic DNA, as well as intragenic mutations [165].

Polycystic Kidney Disease

The gene for dominant polycystic kidney disease (PKD1) has been found close to the TSC2 gene on chromosome 16p13.3 [166]. One remarkable Portuguese family has a translocation at this site (see Fig. 11.4) such that both diseases are transmitted; dominant polycystic kidney disease is transmitted from the maternal translocation carrier to a daughter. A son has tuberous sclerosis because of loss of the der22 chromosome fragment (see Fig. 11.4). The TSC2 gene is situated just distal to the breakpoint on chromosome 16. There are some cases of tuberous sclerosis who have significant renal cystic disease. It is not clear whether the PKD1 gene is implicated in these cases.

Crouzon Craniosynostosis

Crouzon craniosynostosis is caused by mutations in the FGFR2 gene [167–171]. Point mutations are found in one of the immunoglobulin-like domains (the B exon), most commonly affecting the cysteine residue at position 342.

The mutations listed above and in Table 11.11 occur in genes coding for structure and function in differentiated cells as well as in genes that control early development in embryogenesis. It is perhaps surprising that holoprosencephaly is the only large, regional anomaly that has, at the time of writing, been ascribed to a mutation in a developmental gene [114]. This may be because other major developmental genes show overlapping spheres of functional

Table 11.12.   Syndromes and anomaly complexes in which renal agenesis/dysplasia may occur

DiGeorge syndrome [188]
Familial unilateral agenesis with segmental glomerulosclerosis [189]
Familial or "recurrent" (hereditary renal adysplasia) [190]
Bilateral agenesis with cystic adenomatoid malformation of lung and left heart hypoplasia [191]
Penile agenesis [192]
Sirenomelia (recurrent) [193]
Brachio-oto-renal syndrome [194]
Unilateral agenesis in "cat eye syndrome" [195]
Mayer-Rokitansky-Kuster-Hauser syndrome [196]
MURCS association [197]
Cerebro-reno-digital syndrome [198]
Holzgreve syndrome [199]
Trisomy 22 [200], other trisomies (13, 18)
45,X/46,XY mosaicism [201]
Turner syndrome [202]
Kallman syndrome [203]
Bartsocas-Papas syndrome [204]
Fraser syndrome (syndromal cryptophthalmos) [205]
Branchio-oculo-facial syndrome [206]
Goldenhar syndrome [207]
Short rib polydactyly syndromes [208]
Omphalocele-exstrophy-imperforate-anus-spina bifida (OEIS) complex [209]
Meckel syndrome [210]
Roberts syndrome [211]
Zellweger syndrome [212]
Renal-hepatic-pancreatic dysplasia [213]

Table 11.13.   Syndromes and anomaly complexes in which diaphragmatic hernia may occur (72% of prenatally diagnosed cases have other anomalies)

Ectrodactyly, congenital heart defect, agenesis of corpus callosum association [214]
Cystic adenomatoid malformation, extralobar sequestration, laryngotracheoesophageal cleft association [215]
Denys-Drash syndrome [216]
Trisomy 18 [217]
Trisomy 22 [218]
C-trigonocephaly syndrome [219]
Chromosome 1; 15 translocation [220]
Fryns syndrome [221]
Brachmann-de Lange syndrome [222]
"Familial" [223]
Pallister-Killiam syndrome [224]
Simpson-Golabi-Behemel syndrome [225]

influence, such that mutations in any one gene are not as severe as might be expected.

Further clues to the effects of mutations in developmental genes will probably result from several other approaches:

1. The realization that well-known anomalies, such as renal agenesis [188–213] and diaphragmatic hernia [214–225], can occur as isolated malformations and also as components of syndromes and associations, the genetic basis for which is understood in some instances (Tables 11.12 and 11.13).

2. The realization from serial prenatal fetal ultrasound that anomalies that were previously thought to be distinct may in fact develop one from the other (e.g., renal agenesis from multicystic renal dysplasia) [226, 227]. The histologic subtypes of congenital cystic adenomatoid lung are well known. But it is now clear that prenatal lung masses may grow or disappear, the latter suggesting progressive maturation of zones of lungs that lagged behind the normal rate of lung development [228].

3. The elucidation of phenotypes of mouse knockout models of developmental disease. For instance, several knockouts cause renal agenesis. It is not surprising that the null *WT1* mouse does so [229]; but it is interesting to find that knockouts for *RET* [230] and *GDNF* [231] also result in renal agenesis, implying that there may be a significant role for neural crest cells in nephrogenesis.

4. In groups of congenital diseases for which the mutational basis is now being elucidated, advocates of "lumping" and "splitting" classifications are both simultaneously vindicated and invalidated. In the chondrodysplasias, quite a variety of genes are involved, despite the fact that the phenotypes are closely similar. On the other hand, achondroplasia, hypochondroplasia, and thanatophoric dysplasia are phenotypically delineated fairly rigorously in most cases, yet have very similar mutational origins. The complexities of genotype-phenotype correlations are nowhere illustrated more graphically that in the *FGFR* gene mutations (Table 11.14; Fig 11.8).

5. The mutational basis for a number of familiar pediatric neoplasms is now becoming clear. Not surprisingly, some of these involve translocations that disrupt the function of developmental genes: Ewing's tumor [232], retinoblastoma [233], Wilms' tumor [186], and desmoplastic small round cell tumor [234]. This helps to explain the fact that mutations in a single gene (*WT1*) can cause the following overlapping phenotypes that include neoplasia, malformation, and chronic structural change in later life (Table 11.15): 1) predisposition to Wilms' tumor [186], 2) other genitourinary maldevelopment, with (Denys-Drash syndrome) [186, 187] or without

Table 11.14. Genotype-phenotype correlations of point mutations in the genes *FGFR1–3*

GENE	POINT MUTATION	PHENOTYPE
FGFR1	P252R	Apert[a]
FGFR2	S252W	Apert
	P253R	Apert[a]
	S267P; W290G,R; Y328C,R; G338R; Y340H; C342W,F; A344G; S347C; S354C; V359F	Crouzon
	C278F	Pfeiffer, Crouzon
	Q289P	J-W,[b] Crouzon
	A314S; D321A; T341P; A344P; V349F	Pfeiffer
	C342S,Y	Crouzon, Pfeiffer
	C342R	Crouzon, Pfeiffer, JW
	S372C; Y375C	B-S[cd]
FGFR3	R248C; S249C	TDI[e]
	P250R	NSC[a,f]
	G346E	ACH[g]
	G370C; Y373C	TDI[d]
	S371C	TDI
	G375C; G380R	ACH
	N540K	HYP[h]
	K650E	TDII[i]
	X807G,R,C,[j] L	TDI

[a] Mutations in analogous sites in the -ERSPHR- sequence of the three genes cause two different phenotypes, Apert in *FGFR1* and *2*, but nonsyndromal craniosynostosis in *FGFR3*.
[b] J-W Jackson-Weiss craniosynostosis.
[c] B-S Beare-Stevenson syndrome.
[d] Mutations in analogous sites of *FGFR2* and *FGFR3* cause B-S and TDI, respectively.
[e] TDI thanatophoric dysplasia, type I.
[f] NSC non-syndromic craniosynostosis.
[g] ACH achondroplasia.
[h] HYP hypochondroplasia.
[i] TDII thanatophoric dysplasia, type II.
[j] Two mutations, A2421C and A2421T both result in X807C.

There is a mutation "hot spot" in *FGFR2* at position C342, with six mutations to five other amino acids:

TGC → AGC,TCC	C342S	Crouzon, Pfeiffer
TGC → TTC	C342F	Crouzon
TGC → TAC	C342Y	Crouzon, Pfeiffer
TGC → CGC	C342R	Crouzon, JW, Pfeiffer
TGC → TGG	C342W	Crouzon

This indicates that the mutational basis for these related disorders is a set of alleles; it is presumably the modifying actions of other genes that cause the phenotypic variability in expression of, for instance, the single mutation C342R.

All the mis-sense mutations causing TDI and both the mutations causing B-S result in the substitution of a cysteine for another amino acid residue. This raises the likelihood that dimerization may occur via -S-S- bridges.

Only one mutation, P252R causing Apert, has so far been found in *FGFR1*. The NSC mutation in FGFR3 is the only craniosynostosis expressed on that gene, whereas the chondrodysplasias are not coded on *FGFR1* or *FGFR2*. TDII, ACH, HYP, B-S, NSC, J-W and Apert craniosynostoses have limited mutational repertoires in comparison with Crouzon and Pfeiffer craniosynostoses and TDI.

Only one set of nonsense mutations (X807G,R,C,L) is seen in the group discussed here, causing TDI. Five of the eight possible point nonsense mutations have now been found at this site.

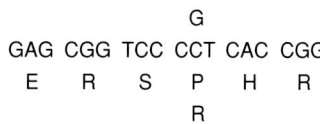

Pro252Arg in FGFR1 causing Pfeiffer Syndrome
Pro253Arg in FGFR2 causing Apert Syndrome
Pro250Arg in FGFR3 causing non-syndromal craniosynostosis

FIGURE 11.8. *Mutations at the same site in FGFR1–3 cause different but similar diseases. The conserved amino acid sequence - ERSPHR- occurs in the linker region between the second and third Ig-like domains of FGFR1–3. Identical point mutations (CCT → CGT) from proline (P) to arginine (R) cause different phenotypes according to the gene in which they occur.*

Table 11.15. Phenotype-genotype correlations in *WT1* gene mutations

Disease	Site of WT1 mutation
Denys-Drash syndrome (mesangial sclerosis, male pseudohermaphroditism, predisposition to Wilms' tumor)	exons 8,9
Pure mesangial sclerosis	exon 9, intron 9
Frasier syndrome (mesangial sclerosis, male pseudohermaphroditism)	intron 9

(Frasier syndrome) [235] Wilms' tumor; and 3) mesangial sclerosis without any of the above [236].

Perhaps it will not be long before we have a full "genetic theory of everything" to account for the large majority of congenital disorders with which pediatric pathologists are so familiar.

REFERENCES

1. Martin RH. Chromosomal analysis of human spermatozoa. In: Verlinsky Y, Kuliev A, eds. *Preimplantation Genetics.* New York: Plenum, 1991, pp. 91–102.
2. Symie RM, Martin RH. Meiotic segregation of a 21;22 robertsonian translocation. *Hum Reprod* 1992; 7:825–9.
3. Martin RH, Ko E, Hildebrand K. Analysis of sperm chromosome complement from a man heterozygous for a robertsonian translocation 45,XY,t(15q;22q). *Am J Med Genet* 1992; 43:855–7.
4. Martin RH. Cytogenetic analysis of sperm from a male heterozygous for a 13;14 robertsonian translocation. *Hum Genet* 1988; 30:357–61.
5. Shaffer LG, Jackson-Cook CK, Stasiowski BA, Spence JE, Brown JA. Parental origin determination in thirty de novo robertsonian translocations. *Am J Med Genet* 1992; 43:957–63.
6. Plachot M. Chromosome analysis of oocytes and embryos. In: Verlinsky Y, Kuliev A, eds. *Preimplantation Genetics,* New York: Plenum, 1991, pp. 103–12.
7. Plachot M, Veiga A, Montagut J, et al. Are clinical and biological parameters correlated with chromosomal disorders in early life: a multicenter study. *Hum Reprod* 1988; 3:627–35.
8. Hassold T, Merrill M, Adkins K. Recombination and nondisjunction: molecular studies of trisomy 16. *Am J Hum Genet* 1995; 57:867–74.
9. Bugge M, Petersen MB, Hertz JM, et al. Nondisjunction studies in trisomy 13. *Am J Hum Genet* 1994; 55(suppl):Abstract No. 566.
10. Nothen MM, Eggermann T, Endmann J, et al. Retrospective study of the parental origin of the extra chromosome in trisomy 18 (Edwards syndrome). *Hum Genet* 1993; 92:347–9.
11. Kupke KG, Muller V. Parental origin of the extra chromosome in trisomy 18. *Am J Hum Genet* 1989; 45:599–605.
12. Babu A, Verma RS. The heteromorphic marker on chromosome 18 using restriction endonuclease *Alu* I. *N Engl J Med* 1986; 38:549–54.
13. Antonarakis SE and the Down's syndrome collaborative group. Parental origin of the extra chromosome in trisomy 21 as indicated by analysis of DNA polymorphisms. *N Engl J Med* 1991; 324:872–6.
14. Jacobs PA, Betts PR, Cockwell AE, et al. A cytogenetic and molecular reappraisal of a series of patients with Turner's syndrome. *Ann Hum Genet* 1990; 54:204–23.
15. Schofield B, Babu A, Punales-Morejon D. et al. Double mosaic aneuploidy: 45,X/47,XY,+8 in a male infant. *Am J Med Genet* 1992; 44:7–10.
16. Simoni G, Fraccaro M. Does confined placental mosaicism affect the fetus? Editorial. *Hum Reprod* 1992; 7:139–40.
17. Kalousek DK, Barnet IJ, McGillivray BC. Placental mosaicism and intrauterine survival of trisomies 13 and 18. *Am J Hum Genet* 1989; 44:338–43.
18. Ledbetter DH, Zachary JM, Simpson JL, et al. Cytogenetic results from the U.S. collaborative study on CVS. *Prenat Diagn* 1992; 12:317–45.
19. Perlman E, Stetten G, Tuck-Miller CM, et al. Sexual discordance in monozygotic twins. *Am J Med Genet* 1990; 37:551–7.
20. Deacon JS, Machin GA, Martin JM, et al. Investigation of acephalus. *Am J Med Genet* 1980; 5:85–99.
21. Rogers JG, Voullaire L, Gold H. Monozygotic twins discordant for trisomy 21. *Am J Med Genet* 1982; 11:143–6.
22. Heydanus R, Santema JG, Stewart PA, Mulder PGM, Wladimiroff JW. Preterm delivery rate and fetal outcome in structurally affected twin pregnancies: a retrospective matched control study. *Prenat Diagn* 1993; 13:155–162.
23. Meck JM, Kozma C, Stratakis C, et al. Mosaic variegated aneuploidy with microencephaly. A rare cytogenetic syndrome. *Am J Hum Genet* 1994; 55(suppl):Abstract No. 631.
24. Mehta L, Babu A, Willner J, Hirschhorn K. Mosaic variegated aneuploidy associated with a dysmorphic syndrome and mental handicap. *Am J Hum Genet* 1994; 55(suppl):Abstract No. 632.
25. Warburton D, Anyane-Yeboa K, Taterka P, Yu CY, Olsen D. Mosaic variegated aneuploidy with microencephaly; a new human mitotic mutant? *Am Genet* 1991; 34:287–92.
26. Jacobs PA, Szulman AE, Funkhouser J, Matsuura JS, Wilson CC. Human triploidy: relationship between parental origin of the additional haploid complement and development of partial hydatidiform mole. *Ann Hum Genet* 1982; 46:223–31.
27. McFadden DE, Kwong LC, Yam IYL, Langlois S. Parental origin of triploidy in human fetuses: evidence for genomic imprinting. *Hum Genet* 1993; 92:465–9.
28. Sheppard DM, Fisher RA, Lawler SD, Povey S. Tetraploid conceptus with three paternal contributions. *Hum Genet* 1982; 62:371–4.
29. Surti V, Szulman, Wagner K, Leppert M, O'Brien SJ. Tetraploid partial hydatidiform moles: two cases with a triple paternal contribution and a 92,XXXY karyotype. *Hum Genet* 1986; 72:15–21.
30. Lange JM, Weinberg DS, Yavner DL, Bieber FR. The biology of tetraploid hydatidiform moles. Histopathology, cytogenetics and flow cytometry. *Hum Pathol* 1989; 20:419–25.
31. Robinson WP, Bernasconi F, Basaran S, et al. A somatic origin of homologous robertsonian translocations and isochromosomes. *Am J Hum Genet* 1994; 54:290–302.
32. Robinson WP, Bernasconi F, Lefort G, Binkert F, Schinzel AA. Molecular studies of free and translocation trisomy 13. *Am J Hum Genet* 1994; 55(suppl):Abstract No. 661.
33. Tomkins DJ, Maye JS, Whelan DT, Cox DW. Maternal uniparental disomy of chromosome 14 in a boy with t(14q14q) associated with a paternal t(13q14q). *Am J Hum Genet* 1994; 55(suppl):Abstract No. 685.
34. Spence JE, Perciaccante RG, Greig GM, et al. Uniparental disomy as a mechanism for human genetic disease. *Am J Hum Genet* 1988; 42:217–26.
35. Lusher JM, Zuelzer WW, Evans RK. Hemophilia A in chromosomal female subjects. *J Pediatr* 1969; 74:265–71.
36. Schnizel AA, Robinson WP, Binkert F, et al. Exclusively paternal X chromosomes in a girl with short stature. *Hum Genet* 1993; 92:175–8.
37. Harrison KB, Eisenger K, Yeboa K-A, Brown S. Maternal uniparental disomy of chromosome 2 in a baby with trisomy 2 mosaicism in amniotic fluid culture. *Am J Hum Genet* 1995; 55(suppl):Abstract No. 603.
38. Sherman LS, Bennett PR, Moore GE. Early embryonic failure: expression and imprinted status of candidate genes in human chromosome 21. *Am J Hum Genet* 1994; 44(suppl):Abstract No. 1681.

39. Roberts E, Stevenson K, Cole T, et al. Prospective prenatal diagnosis of Prader-Willi syndrome due to maternal disomy for chromosome 15 following trisomic zygote rescue. *Prenat Diagn* 1997; 17:780–3.

40. Purvis-Smith SG, Saville T, Manass S, et al. Uniparental disomy 15 resulting from "correction" of an initial trisomy 15. *Am J Hum Genet* 1992; 50:1348–50.

41. Cassidy SB, Lai L-W, Erickson RP, Magnuson L. Trisomy 15 with loss of the paternal 15 as a cause of Prader-Willi syndrome due to maternal disomy. *Am J Hum Genet* 1992; 51:701–8.

42. Milunsky JM, Wyaudt HE, Amos JA, Kang Z, Huang SL, Milunsky A. Trisomy 15 mosaicism and uniparental disomy (UPD) in a liveborn infant. *Am J Hum Genet* 1994; 55(suppl):Abstract No. 636.

43. Woodage T, Prasad M, Dixon JW, et al. Bloom syndrome and maternal uniparental disomy for chromosome 15. *Am J Hum Genet* 1994; 55:74–80.

44. Harper PS. Congenital myotonic dystrophy in Britain. II. Genetic basis. *Arch Dis Child* 1975; 50:514–8.

45. Lavenden C, Hoffmann-Radvanyi H, Shelbourne P, et al. Myotonic dystrophy. Size- and sex-dependent dynamics of CTG meiotic instability, and somatic mosaicism. *Am J Hum Genet* 1993; 52:875–83.

46. Munne S, Grifo J, Cohen J, Weier H-VG. Chromosome abnormalities in human arrested preimplantation embryos: a multiple-probe FISH study. *Am J Hum Genet* 1994; 55:150–9.

47. Plachot M. Chromosome analysis of spontaneous abortions after IVF. A European survey. *Hum Reprod* 1989; 4:425–9.

48. Creasy MR. The cytogenetics of spontaneous abortion in humans. In: Beard RW, Sharp IF, eds. *Early pregnancy loss. Mechanisms and treatment.* Berlin: Springer-Verlag, 1988.

49. Guerneri S, Beltio D, Simoni G, et al. Prevalence and distribution of chromosome abnormalities in a sample of first trimester interval abortions. *Hum Reprod* 1987; 2:735–9.

50. Machin GA. Chromosome abnormality and perinatal death. *Lancet* 1974; i:549–51.

51. Kuleschov NP. Chromosome anomalies of infants dying during the perinatal period and premature newborn. *Hum Genet* 1986; 81:151–60.

52. Dimmick JE, Kalousek DK. *Developmental pathology of the embryo and fetus.* Philadelphia: Lippincott, 1992, Ch. 4, Table 4-1.

53. Gagnon S, Fraser W, Fouquette B, et al. Nature and frequency of chromosomal abnormalities in pregnancies with abnormal ultrasound findings: analysis of 117 cases with review of the literature. *Prenat Diagn* 1992; 12:9–18.

54. Damato N, Filly RA, Goldstein RB, et al. Frequency of fetal anomalies in sonographically detected polyhydramnios. *J Ultrasound Med* 1993; 12:11–14.

55. Brady K, Polzin WJ, Kopelman JN, Read JA. Risk of chromosomal abnormalities in patients with idiopathic polyhydramnios. *Obstet Gynecol* 1992; 79:234–8.

56. Hendricks SK, Conway L, Wang K, et al. Diagnosis of polyhydramnios in early gestation: indication for prenatal diagnosis? *Prenat Diagn* 1991; 11:49–54.

57. Eydoux P, Choiset A, Porrier N, et al. Chromosomal prenatal diagnosis: study of 936 cases of intrauterine abnormalities after ultrasound assessment. *Prenat Diagn* 1989; 9:255–68.

58. Stoll CG, Alembik Y, Dott B. Study of 156 cases of polyhydramnios and congenital malformations in a series of 118,265 births. *Am J Obstet Gynecol* 1991; 165:586–90.

59. Paladini D, Calabro R, Palmeri S, D'Andria T. Prenatal diagnosis of congenital heart disease and fetal karyotyping. *Obstet Gynecol* 1993; 81:679–82.

60. Gilbert WM, Nicolaides KH. Fetal omphalocele: associated malformations and chromosomal defects. *Obstet Gynecol* 1987; 70:633–5.

61. Sharland GK, Lockhart SM, Heward AJ, Allan LD. Prognosis in fetal diaphragmatic hernia. *Am J Obstet Gynecol* 1992; 166:9–13.

62. Ross JB, Allerdice PW, Shapiro LJ, et al. Familial X-linked ichthyosis, steroid sulphatase deficiency, mental retardation and nullisomy for Xp 223-pter. *Arch Dermatol* 1985; 121:1524–8.

63. Emanuel BS. Molecular cytogenetics: toward dissection of the contiguous gene syndromes. *Am J Hum Genet* 1988; 43:575–8.

64. Beighton P, De Paepe A, Hall JG, et al. Molecular nosology of the heritable disorders of connective tissue. *Am J Hum Genet* 1992; 42:431–48.

65. Byers PH, Wallis GA, Willing MC. Osteogenesis imperfecta: translation of mutation to phenotype. *J Med Genet* 1991; 28:433–42.

66. Willing MC, Deschenes SP, Scott DA, et al. Osteogenesis type I: molecular heterogeneity for COL1A1 null alleles of type I collagen. *Am J Hum Genet* 1994: 55:638–47.

67. Willing MC, Dechennes SP, Slayton RL, Roberts EJ. Premature chain termination is a unifying mechanism for COL1A1 null alleles in osteogenesis imperfecta type I cell strains. *Am J Hum Genet* 1996; 59:799–809.

68. Knebelman B, Breillat C, Forestier L, et al. Spectrum of mutations in the COL4A5 collagen gene in X-linked Alport syndrome. *Am J Hum Genet* 1996; 59:1221–32.

69. Toriello HV, Glover TW, Takahar K, et al. A translocation interrupts the COL5A1 gene in a patient with Ehlers-Danlos syndrome and hypomelanosis of Ito. *Nat Genet* 1996; 13:361–5.

70. DePaepe A, Nuytinck L, Ubagai I, et al. Mutations in the COL5A1 gene are causal of the Ehlers-Danlos syndromes I and II. *Am J Hum Genet* 1997; 60:547–54.

71. Gardella R, Belletti L, Zoppi N, et al. Identification of two splicing mutations in the collagen type VII gene (COL7A1) of a patient affected by the *localisata* variant of recessive dystrophic epidermolysis bullosa. *Am J Hum Genet* 1996; 59:292–300.

72. Schumann H, Hammami-Hauasli N, Pulkkinen L, et al. Three novel homozygous point mutations and a new polymorphism in the COL17A1 gene: relation to biological and clinical phenotypes of junctional epidermolysis bullosa. *Am J Hum Genet* 1997; 60:1344–53.

73. Muragaki Y, Mariman ECM, van Beersum SEC, et al. A mutation in the gene encoding the alpha2 chain of the fibril-associated collagen IX, COL9A2, causes multiple epiphyseal dysplasia (EDM2). *Nat Genet* 1996; 12:103–5.

74. Wallis GA, Rash B, Sweetman WA, et al. Amino acid substitutions in conserved residues in the carboxyl-terminal domain of the a1(X) chain of type X collagen occur in two unrelated families with metaphyseal chondrodysplasia type Schmid. *Am J Hum Genet* 1994; 54:169–78.

75. Kerem B, Rommens JM, Buchanan JA, et al. Identification of the cystic fibrosis gene: genetic analysis. *Science* 1989; 245:1073–80.

76. Welsh MJ, Smith AE. Molecular mechanisms of CFTR chloride channel dysfunction in cystic fibrosis. *Cell* 1993; 73:1251–4.

77. Collins FS. Cystic fibrosis: molecular biology and therapeutic implications. *Science* 1992; 256:774–9.

78. Cystic Fibrosis Genotype-Phenotype Consortium. Correlation between genotype and phenotype in patients with cystic fibrosis. *N Engl J Med* 1993; 329:1308–13.

79. Highsmith WE, Burch LH, Zhon Z, et al. A novel mutation in the cystic fibrosis gene in patients with pulmonary disease but normal sweat chloride concentration. *N Engl J Med* 1994; 331:974–80.

80. Miller PW, Hamosh A, Macek M, et al. Cystic fibrosis transmembrane conductance receptor regulator (CFTR) gene mutations in bronchopulmonary aspergillosis. *Am J Hum Genet* 1996; 59:45–51.

81. Koenig M, Beggs AH, Moyer M, et al. The molecular basis for Duchenne versus Becker muscular dystrophy: correlation of severity with type of deletion. *Am J Hum Genet* 1989; 45:498–506.

82. Ahn AN, Kunkel LM. The structural and functional diversity of dystrophin. *Nature Genet* 1993; 3:283–91.

83. Lindlof M, Kiuru A, Kaariainen H, et al. Gene deletions in X-linked muscular dystrophy. *Am J Hum Genet* 1989; 44:496–503.

84. Nissinen M, Helbling-Leclerc A, Zhang Z, et al. Substitution of a conserved cysteine-996 in a cysteine-rich motif of the laminin alpha2-chain in congenital muscular dystrophy with partial deficiency of protein. *Am J Hum Genet* 1996; 58:1177–84.

85. Nigro V, Moreira E, Piluso G, et al. Autosomal recessive limb-girdle muscular dystrophy, LGMD2F, is caused by a mutation in the delta-sarcoglycan gene. *Nat Genet* 1996; 14:195–8.

86. Nagano A, Koga R, Ogawa M, et al. Emerin deficiency at the nuclear membrane in patients with Emery-Dreifuss muscular dystrophy. *Nat Genet* 1996; 12:254–9.

87. Laporte J, Hu LJ, Kretz C, et al. A gene mutated in X-linked myotubular myopathy defines a new putative tyrosine phosphatase family conserved in yeast. *Nat Genet* 1996; 13:175–82.

88. Harley HG, Brook JD, Rundle SA. Expansion of an unstable DNA region and phenotypic variation in myotonic dystrophy. *Nature* 1992; 355:345–6.

89. McNally EM, Passso-Bueno MR, Bennemann CG, et al. Mild and severe muscular dystrophy caused by single gamma-sarcoglycan mutation. *Am J Hum Genet* 1996; 59:1040–7.

90. Roberds SL, Leturcq F, Allamand V, et al. Missense mutations in the adhalin gene linked to autosomal recessive muscular dystrophy. *Cell* 1994; 78:625–33.

91. Richard I, Broux O, Allamand V, et al. Mutations in the proteolytic enzyme calpain 3 cause limb-girdle muscular dystrophy type 2A. *Cell* 1995; 81:27–40.

92. Smith FJD, Eady RAJ, Leigh IM, et al. Plectin deficiency results in muscular dystrophy with epidermolysis bullosa. *Nat Gene,* 1996; 13:450–7.

93. Kairulainen K, Karttunen L, Puhakka L, Sakai L, Peltonen L. Mutations in the fibrillin gene responsible for dominant ectopia lentis and neonatal Marfan syndrome. *Nature Genet* 1994; 6:64–9.

94. Price CE, Wang M, Wang J, Godfrey M. Fibrillin mutations in the Marfan syndrome. *Am J Hum Genet* 1994; 55(suppl):Abstract No. 1378.

95. Milewicz DM, Duvic M. Severe neonatal Marfan syndrome resulting from a de novo 3-bp insertion into the fibrillin gene on chromosome 15. *Am J Hum Genet* 1994; 54:447–53.

96. Sood S, Eldadah ZA, Krause WL, et al. Mutations in fibrillin-1 and the Marfanoid-craniosynostosis (Shprintzen-Goldberg) syndrome. *Nat Genet* 1996; 12:209–11.

97. Wang M, Clericuzio CL, Godfrey M. Familial occurrence of typical and severe lethal congenital contractural arachnodactyly caused by missplicing of exon 34 of fibrillin-2. *Am J Hum Genet* 1996; 59:1027–34.

98. Perez Jurado LA, Peoples R, Kaplan P, et al. Molecular definition of the chromosome 7 deletion in Williams syndrome and parent-of-origin effects on growth. *Am J Hum Genet* 1995; 59:781–92.

99. Tassabehji M, Metcalfe K, Fergusson WD, et al. LIM-kinase deleted in Williams syndrome. *Nat Genet* 1996; 13:272–4.

100. Nickerson E, Greenberg F, Keating MT, et al. Deletions of the elastin gene at 7q11.23 occur in approximately 90% of patients with Williams syndrome. *Am J Hum Genet* 1995; 56:1156–61.

101. Edery P, Lyonnet S, Mulligan LM, et al. Mutations of the RET proto-oncogene in Hirschsprung's disease. *Nature* 1994; 367:378–80.

102. Angrist M, Bolk S, Halushka M, et al. Germline mutations in glial cell-line derived neurotropic factor (*GDNF*) and RET in a Hirschsprung disease patient. *Nat Genet* 1996; 14:341–4.

103. Salomon R, Attie T, Pelet A, et al. Germline mutations of the RET ligand GDNF are not sufficient to cause Hirschsprung disease. *Nat Genet* 1996; 14:345–7.

104. Edery P, Attie T, Amiel J, et al. Mutation of the endothelin-3 gene in the Waardenburg-Hirschsprung disease (Shah-Waardenburg) syndrome. *Nat Genet* 1996; 12:422–4.

105. Corrozzo R, Kabota T, McKinney MJ, et al. Frequent deletions of the LIS1 gene in classical lissencephaly. *Am J Hum Genet* 1994; 55:(suppl):Abstract No. 568.

106. Brunelli S, Faielle A, Capra V, et al. Germline mutations in the homeobox gene *EMX2* in patients with severe schizencephaly. *Nat Genet* 1996; 12:94–6.

107. Baldwin CT, Hoth CT, Macina RA, Milunsky A. Mutations in PAX3 that cause Waardenburg syndrome type I: ten new mutations and review of the literature. *Am J Med Genet* 1995; 58:115–22.

108. Nobokuni Y, Watanabe A, Takeda K, et al. Analyses of loss-of-function mutations of the *MITF* gene suggest that haploinsufficiency is a cause of Waardenburg syndrome type 2A. *Am J Hum Genet* 1996; 59:76–83.

109. Gu S-M, Orth U, Zankl M, et al. Molecular analysis of the L1CAM gene in patients with X-linked hydrocephalus demonstrates eight novel mutations and suggests non-allelic heterogeneity of the trait. *Am J Med Genet* 1997; 71:336–40.

110. Lefebvre S, Burglen L, Reboullet S, et al. Identification and characterization of a spinal muscular atrophy-determining gene. *Cell* 1995; 80:155–65.

111. Bussaglia E, Clement O, Tizzano E, et al. A frame-shift deletion in the survival motor neuron gene in Spanish spinal muscular atrophy patients. *Nat Genet* 1995; 11:335–7.

112. Burglen L, Seroz T, Miniou P, et al. The gene encoding p44, a subunit of the transcription factor TFIH, is involved in large-scale deletions associated with Werdnig-Hoffmann disease. *Am J Hum Genet* 1997; 60:72–9.

113. Martha A, Strong LC, Ferrell RE, Saunders GF. Three novel aniridia mutations in the human PAX6 gene. *Hum Mutat* 1995; 6:44–9.

114. Ressler E, Belloni E, Gaudenz K, et al. Mutations in the human *Sonic Hedgehog* gene cause holoprosencephaly. *Nat Genet* 1996; 14:357–60.

115. Vu TH, Hoffman AR. Imprinting of the Angelman syndrome gene, *UBE3A*, is restricted to brain. *Nat Genet* 1997; 17:12–13.

116. Shiang R, Thompson LM, Zhy Y-Z, et al. Mutations in the transmembrane domain of FGFR3 cause the most common genetic form of dwarfism, achondroplasia. *Cell* 1994; 78:355–42.

117. Hastbacka J, de la Chapelle A, Mahtani MM, et al. The diastrophic dysplasia gene encodes a novel sulfate transporter: positional cloning by fine-structure linkage disequilibrium mapping. *Cell* 1994; 78:1073–87.

118. Superti-Fuerga A, Hastbacka J, Wilcox WR, et al. Achondrogenesis type IB is caused by mutations in the diastrophic dysplasia sulphate transporter gene. *Nat Genet* 1996; 12:100–2.

119. Hastbacka J, Superti-Furga A, Wilcox WR, et al. Atelosteogenesis type II is caused by mutations in the diastrophic dysplasia sulfate-transported gene (DTDST): evidence of a phenotypic series involving three chondrodysplasias. *Am J Hum Genet* 1996; 58:255–62.

120. Cameron FJ, Hageman RM, Cooke-Yarborough C, et al. A novel germ line mutation in *SOX9* causes familial campomelic dysplasia and sex reversal. *Hum Molec Genet* 1996; 5:1625–30.

121. Thomas JT, Lin K, Nadedkar M, et al. A human dyschondroplasia due to a mutation in a TGF-beta superfamily gene. *Nat Genet* 1996; 12:315–7.

122. Thomas JT, Kilpatrick MW, Lin K, et al. Disruption of human limb morphogenesis by a dominant negative mutation in *CDMP1*. *Net Genet* 1997; 17:58–64.

123. Lee B, Thirunavukkarasu K, Zhou L, et al. Missense mutations abolishing DNA binding of the osteoblast-specific transcription factor *OSF2/CBFA1* in cleidocranial dysostosis. *Nat Genet* 1997; 16:307–10.

124. O'Keefe D, Dao D, Zhao L, et al. Coding mutations in p57^{KIP2} are present in some cases of Beckwith-Wiedemann syndrome but are rare or absent in Wilms tumors. *Am J Hum Genet* 1997; 61:295–303.

125. Hatada I, Ohashi H, Fukushima Y, et al. An imprinted gene p57^{KIP2} is mutated in Beckwith-Wiedemann syndrome. *Nat Genet* 1996; 14:171–3.

126. Lee MP, DeBraun M, Randhawa G, et al. Low frequency of p57^{KIP2} mutation in Beckwith-Wiedemann syndrome. *Am J Hum Genet* 1997; 61:304–9.

127. Pilia G, Hughes-Benzie RM, MacKenzie A, et al. Mutations in *GPC3*, a glypican gene, cause the Simpson-Golabi-Behmel overgrowth syndrome. *Nat Genet* 1996; 12:241–7.

128. Edwards S, Gladwin AJ, Dixon MJ. The mutational spectrum in Treacher Collins syndrome reveals a predominance of mutations that create a premature termination codon. *Am J Hum Genet* 1997; 60:515–24.

129. Hyland J, Ala-Kobbo L, Royce P, et al. A homozygous stop codon in lysyl hydroxylase gene in two siblings with Ehlers-Danlos syndrome type VI. *Nat Genet* 1992; 2:228–31.

130. Heikkinen J, Toppinen T, Yeowell H, et al. Duplication of seven exons in the lysyl hydroxylase gene is associated with longer forms of a repetitive sequence within the gene and is a common cause for the type VI variant of Ehlers-Danlos syndrome. *Am J Hum Genet* 1997; 60:48–56.

131. Abdelhak S, Kalatzis V, Heilig R, et al. A human homologue of the *Drosophila eyes absent* gene underlies Branchio-Oto-Renal (BOR) syndrome and identifies a novel gene family. *Nat Genet* 1997; 15:157–64.

132. Saffran DC, Parolini O, Fitch-Hilgenberg ME, et al. Brief report: a point mutation in the 5H2 domain of Bruton's tyrosine kinase in atypical X-linked agammaglobulinemia. *N Engl J Med* 1994; 330:1488–91.

133. Vetrie D, Vorechovsky I, Sideras P, et al. The gene involved in X-linked agammaglobulinemia is a member of the src family of protein-tyrosine kinases. *Nature* 1993; 361:226–33.

134. Macchi P, Villa A, Strina D, et al. Characterization of nine novel mutations in the CD40 ligand gene in patients with X-linked hyper IgM syndrome of various ancestry. *Am J Hum Genet* 1994; 56:898–906.

135. Kang S, Graham JM, Olney AH, Bieseker LG. *GLI3* frameshift mutations cause autosomal dominant Pallister-Hall syndrome. *Nat Genet* 1997; 15: 266–8.

136. Oda T, Elkahoun AG, Pike B, et al. Mutations in the human *Jagged1* gene are responsible for Alagille syndrome. *Nat Genet* 1997; 16:235–42.

137. Li QY, Newbury-Ecob RA, Terrett JA, et al. Holt-Oram syndrome is caused by mutations in *TBX5*, a member of the *Brachyury* (*T*) gene family. *Nat Genet* 1997; 15:21–9.

138. Casey R, Devoto M, Jones KL, Ballabio A. Mapping a gene for familial situs abnormalities to human chromosome Xq24-q27.1. *Nature Genet* 1993; 5:403–7.

139. Gebbia M, Ferrero GB, Pilia G, et al. X-linked *situs* abnormalities result from mutations in ZIC3. *Nat Genet* 1997; 17:305–8.

140. Brown NA, Lander A. On the other hand. . . . *Nature* 1993; 363:303–4.

141. Horwich A, Brueckner M. Left, right and without a cue. *Nature Genet* 1993; 5:321–2.

142. Yokoyama T, Copeland NG, Jenkins NA, et al. Reversal of left-right asymmetry: a situs inversus mutation. *Science* 1993; 260:679–82.

143. Thomas GR, Ball PC, Roberta EA, Walshe JM, Cox DW. Haplotype studies in Wilson disease. *Am J Hum Genet* 1994; 54:71–8.

144. Thomas GR, Forbes JR, Roberts EA, et al. The Wilson disease gene: spectrum of mutations and their consequences. *Nat Genet* 1995; 9:250–7.

145. Shah AB, Chernov I, Zhang HT, et al. Identification and analysis of mutations in the Wilson disease gene (*ATP7B*): population frequencies, genotype-phenotype correlation, and functional analysis. *Am J Hum Genet* 1997; 61:317–28.

146. Munroe PB, Mitchison HM, O'Rawe AM, et al. Spectrum of mutations in Batten disease gene, *CLN3*. *Am J Hum Genet* 1997; 61:310–6.

147. Semina EV, Reiter R, Leysens NJ, et al. Cloning and charcterization of a novel *bicoid*-related homeobox transcription factor gene, *RIEG*, involved in Rieger syndrome. *Nat Genet* 1966; 14:392–9.

148. Winter H, Rogers MA, Langbein L, et al. Mutations in the hair cortex keratin hHb6 cause the inherited hair disease monilethrix. *Nat Genet* 1997; 16:372–4.

149. Vidal F, Aberdam D, Miquel C, et al. Integrin beta 4 mutations associated with junctional epidermolysis bullosa with pyloric atresia. *Nat Genet* 1995; 10:229–34.

150. Kivirkko S, McGrath JA, Baudoin C, et al. A homozygous nonsense mutation in the alpha 3 chain gene of laminin 5 (LAMA3) in lethal (Herlitz) junctional epidermolysis bullosa. *Hum Mol Genet* 1995; 4:959–62.

151. Rothnagel JA, Wojcik S, Liefer KM, et al. Mutations in the 1A domain of keratin 9 in patients with epidermolytic palmoplantar keratoderma. *J Invest Dermatol* 1995; 104:430–3.

152. Kere J, Srivastava AK, Montonen O, et al. X-linked anhidrotic (hypohidrotic) ectodermal dysplasia is caused by mutation in a novel transmembrane protein. *Nat Genet* 1996; 13:409–16.

153. De Laurenzi V, Rogers GR, Hamrock DJ, et al. Sjogren-Larsson syndrome is caused by mutations in the fatty aldehyde dehydrogenase gene. *Nat Genet* 1996; 12:52–7.

154. Gatalica B, Pulkkinen L, Li K, et al. Cloning of the human type XVII collagen gene (COL17A1), and detection of novel mutations in atrophic benign epidermolysis bullosa. *Am J Hum Genet* 1997; 60:352–65.

155. Alperin ES, Shapiro LJ. Characterization of point mutations in patients with X-linked ichthyosis (XLI). *Am J Hum Genet* 1994; 55(suppl):Abstract No. 1217.

156. Russell LJ, Di Giovanna JJ, Rogers GR, et al. Mutations in the gene for transglutaminase 1 in autosomal recessive lamellar ichthyosis. *Nat Genet* 1995; 9:279–83.

157. Fuchs E, Coulombe P, Cheng J, et al. Genetic bases for epidermolsis bullosa simplex and epidermolytic hyperkeratosis. *J Invest Dermatol* 1994; 103:255–305.

158. McLean WH, Rugg EL, Lunny DP, et al. Keratin 16 and keratin 17 mutations cause pachyonychia congenita. *Nat Genet* 1995; 9:273–8.

159. Weeda G, Eveno E, Donker I, et al. A mutation in the *XPB/ERCC3* DNA repair transcription gene, associated with trichothiodystrophy. *Am J Hum Genet* 1997; 60:320–9.

160. Buetler E. Gaucher disease: new molecular approaches to diagnosis and treatment. *Science* 1992; 256:794–9.

161. Pshezhetsky AV, Richard C, Michaud L, et al. Cloning, expression and chromosomal mapping of human lysosomal sialidase and characterization of mutations in silalidosis. *Nat Genet* 1997; 15:316–20.

162. Rathmann M, Bunge S, Beck M, et al. Mucopolysaccharidosis type II (Hunter syndrome): mutation "hot spots" in the iduronate-2-sulfatase gene. *Am J Hum Genet* 1996; 59:1202–9.

163. Vervoort R, Islam MR, Sly WS, et al. Molecular analysis of patients with beta-glucuronidase deficiency presenting as hydrops fetalis or as early mucopolysaccharidosis VII. *Am J Hum Genet* 1996; 58:457–71.

164. Tuddenham EGD. Flip tip inversion and hemophilia A. *Lancet* 1994; 343:307–8.

165. The European Chromosome 16 Tuberous Sclerosis Consortium. Identification and characterization of the tuberous sclerosis gene on chromosome 16. *Cell* 1993; 75:1305–15.

166. The European Polycystic Kidney Disease Consortium. The polycystic kidney disease 1 gene encodes a 14 Kb transcript and lies within a duplicated region on chromosome 16. *Cell* 1994; 77:881–94.

167. Reardon W, Winter RM, Rutland P, et al. Mutations in the fibroblast growth factor receptor 2 gene cause Crouzon syndrome. *Nature Genet* 1994; 8:98–103.

168. Bellus GA, Gaudenz K, Zackai EH, et al. Identical mutations in three different fibroblast growth factor receptor genes in autosomal recessive craniosynostosis syndromes. *Nat Genet* 1996; 15:174–6.

169. Muenke M, Gripp KW, McDonald-McGinn DM, et al. A unique point mutation in the fibroblast growth factor receptor 3 gene (*FGFR3*) defines a new craniosynostosis syndrome. *Am H Hum Genet* 1997; 60:555–64.

170. Park W-J, Bellus GA, Jabs EW. Mutations in fibroblast growth factor receptors: Phenotypic consequences during eukaryotic development. *Am J Hum Genet* 1995; 57:748–54.

171. Przylepa KA, Paznekas W, Zhang M, et al. Fibroblast growth factor receptor 2 mutations in Beare-Stevenson cutis gyrata syndrome. *Nat Genet* 1996; 13:492–4.

172. Howard TD, Paznekas WA, Green ED, et al. Mutations in *TWIST*, a basic helix-loop-helix transcription factor, in Saethre-Chotzen syndrome. *Nat Genet* 1997; 15:36–41.

173. Jabs EW, Muller V, Li X, et al. A mutation in the homeodomain of the human MSX2 gene in a family affected with autosomal dominant craniosynostosis. *Cell* 1993; 75:443–50.

174. Ma L, Golden S, Wu L, Maxson R. The molecular basis of Boston-type craniosynostosis. *Hum Molec Genet* 1996; 5:1915–20.

175. Braverman N, Steel G, Obie C, et al. Human *PEX7* encodes the peroxisomal PTS2 receptor and is responsible for rhizomelic chondrodysplasia punctata. *Nat Genet* 1997; 15:369–71.

176. Chang C-C, Lee W-H, Moser H, et al. Isolation of the human *PEX12* gene, mutated in group 3 of the peroxisomal biogenesis disorders. *Nat Genet* 1997; 15:385–8.

177. Fukuda S, Shimozawa N, Suzuki Y, et al. Human peroxisomal assembly factor-2 (PAF-2): a gene responsible for group C peroxisomal biogenesis disorder in humans. *Am J Hum Genet* 1996; 59:1210–20.

178. Fiegelbaum V, Lombard-Platet G, Guidoux S, et al. Mutational and protein analysis of patients and heterozygous women with X-linked adrenoleukodystrophy. *Am J Hum Genet* 1996; 58:1135–44.

179. Muragaki Y, Mundlos S, Upton J, Olsen BR. Altered growth and branching patterns in sympolydactyly caused by mutations in HOXD13. *Science* 1996; 272:548–51.

180. Vastardis H, Karimbux N, Gythua SW, et al. A human *MSX1* homeodomain missense mutation causes selective tooth agenesis. *Nat Genet* 1996; 13:417–21.

181. Johnson RL, Rothman AL, Xie J, et al. Human homologue of *patched*, a candidate gene for the basal cell nevus syndrome. *Science* 1996; 272:1668–71.

182. Mortlock DP, Innis JW. Mutation of HOXA13 in hand-foot-genital syndrome. *Nat Genet* 1997; 15:179–80.

183. Bamshad M, Lin RC, Law DJ, et al. Mutations in human *TBX3* alter limb, apocrine and genital development in ulnar-mammary syndrome. *Nat Genet* 1997; 16:311–5.

184. Schimmenti LA, Cunliffe HE, McNoe LA, et al. Further delineation of renal-coloboma syndrome in patients with extreme variability of phenotype and identical *PAX2* mutations. *Am J Hum Genet* 1997; 60:869–78.

185. Nordqvist K, Lovell-Badge R. Setbacks on the road to sexual fulfillment. *Nature* 1994; 7:7–9.

186. Bruening W, Bardeesy N, Silverman BL, et al. Germline intronic and exonic mutations of the Wilms' tumor gene (WT1) affecting urogenital development. *Nat Genet* 1992; 1:114–8.

187. Ogawa O, Eccles MR, Yun L, et al. A novel insertion mutation in the third zinc finger coding region of the WT1 gene in the Denys-Drash syndrome. *Hum Molec Genet* 1993; 2:203–4.

188. Wilson TA, Blethen SL, Vallone A, et al. DiGeorge anomaly with renal agenesis in infants of mothers with diabetes. *Am J Med Genet* 1993; 47:1078–82.

189. Arfeen S, Roseborough D, Luger AM, Nolph KD. Familial unilateral renal agenesis and focal and segmental glomerulosclerosis. *Am J Kidney Disease* 1993; 21:663–8.

190. Sherer DM, McAndrew JA, Liberto L, Woods JR. Recurring bilateral renal agenesis diagnosed by ultrasound with the aid of amnioinfusion at 18 weeks' gestation. *Am J Perinatol* 1992; 9:49–51.

191. Carles D, Dallay D, Serville F, et al. Cystic adenomatoid malformation of the lung, bilateral renal agenesis and left heart hypoplasia. An unusual association in Potter's syndrome. *Ann Pathol* 1992; 12:367–70.

192. O'Connor TA, La Cour ML, Friedlander ER, Thomas R. Penile agenesis associated with urethral and bilateral renal agenesis. *Urology* 1994; 43:130–1.

193. Selig AM, Bennacerraf B, Greene MF, et al. Renal dysplasia, megalocystis, and sirenomelia in siblings. *Teratology* 1993; 47:65–71.

194. Chitayat D, Hodgkinson KA, Chen MF, et al. Branchio-oto-renal syndrome: further delineation of an underdiagnosed syndrome. *Am J Med Genet* 1992; 43:970–5.

195. Legros y Carrenard JR, Martinez Cortes F, Martin Sanchez J. "Cat eye syndrome" with right renal agenesis. Report of a case and review of the literature. *An Esp Pediatr* 1992; 36:317–9.

196. Strubbe EH, Willemsen WN, Lemmeus JA, et al. Mayer-Rokitansky-Kuster-Hauser syndrome: distinction between two forms based on excretory urographic, sonographic, and laparoscopic findings. *AJR* 1993; 160:331–4.

197. Fernandez CO, McFarland RD, Timmons C, et al. MURCS association: ultrasonographic findings and pathologic correlation. *J Ultrasound Med* 1996; 15:867–70.

198. Piantanida M, Tiberti A, Plebani A, et al. Cerebro-reno-digital syndrome in two sibs. *Am J Med Genet* 1993; 47:420–2.

199. Thomas IT, Honore GM, Jewett T, et al. Holzgreve syndrome: recurrence in sibs. *Am J Med Genet* 1993; 45:767–9.

200. Van Buggenhout GJ, Verbruggen J, Fryns JP. Renal agenesis and trisomy 22: case report and review. *Ann Genet* 1995; 38:44–8.

201. Wax JR, Probhakar G, Giraldez RA, et al. Unilateral renal hypoplasia and contralateral renal agenesis: a new association with 45,X/46,XY mosaicism. *Am J Perinatol* 1994; 11:184–6.

202. Benjamin B, al-Harbi N. Renal agenesis and uretropelvic junction obstruction in an infant with Turner syndrome. *An Trop Paediatr* 1997; 17:101–3.

203. Kirk JM, Grant DB, Besser GM, et al. Unilateral renal aplasia in X-linked Kallman syndrome. *Clin Genet* 1994; 46:260–2.

204. Hennekam RC, Huber J, Variend D. Bartsocas-Papas syndrome with internal anomalies: evidence for a more generalized epithelial defect or new syndrome? *Am J Med Genet* 1994; 53:102–7.

205. Fryns JP, van Schoubroeck D, Vandenberghe K, et al. Diagnostic echographic findings in cryptophthalmos syndrome (Fraser syndrome). *Prenat Diagn* 1997; 17:582–4.

206. McCool M, Weaver DD. Branchio-oculo-facial syndrome: broadening the spectrum. *Am J Med Genet* 1994; 49:414–21.

207. Ritchey ML, Norbeck J, Huang C, et al. Urologic manifestations of Goldenhar syndrome. *Urology* 1994; 43:88–91.

208. Yang SS, Langer LO Jr, Cacciarelli A, et al. Three conditions with neonatal asphyxiating thoracic dysplasia (Jeune) and short rib-polydactyly syndrome spectrum. *Am J Med Genet* 1987; (suppl 3):191–207.

209. Lizcano-Gil LA, Garcia-Cruz D, Sanchez-Corona J. Omphalocele-exstrophy-imperforate-anus-spina-bifida (OEIS) complex in a male prenatally exposed to diazepam. *Arch Med Res* 1995; 26:95–6.

210. Wright C, Healicon R, English C, Brun J. Meckel syndrome: what are the minimum diagnostic criteria? *J Med Genet* 1994; 31:482–5.

211. Van Den Berg DJ, Francke U. Roberts syndrome: a review of 100 cases and a new rating system for severity. *Am J Med Genet* 1993; 47:1104–23.

212. Wright C, Healicon R, English C, Burn J. Meckel syndrome: what are the minimum diagnostic criteria? *J Med Genet* 1994; 31:482–5.

213. Torra R, Alos L, Ramos J, Estevill X. Renal-hepatic-pancreatic dysplasia: an autosomal recessive malformation. *J Med Genet* 1996; 33:409–12.

214. Saal HM, Bulas DI. Ectrodactyly, diaphragmatic hernia, congenital heart defect, and agenesis of the corpus callosum. *Clin Dysmorphol* 1995; 4:246–50.

215. Ryan CA, Finer NN, Etches PC, et al. Congenital diaphragmatic hernia: associated malformations—cystic adenomatoid malformation, extralobar sequestration, and laryngotracheal cleft: two case reports. *J Pediatr Surg* 1995; 30:883–5.

216. Devriendt K, Deloof E, Moerman P, et al. Diaphragmatic hernia in Denys-Drash syndrome. *Am J Med Genet* 1995; 57:97–101.

217. Bollmann R, Kalache K, Mau H, et al. Associated malformations and chromosomal defects in congenital diaphragmatic hernia. *Fetal Diagn Ther* 1995; 10:52–9.

218. Kim EH, Cohen RS, Ramachandran P, et al. Trisomy 22 with congenital diaphragmatic hernia and absence of corpus callosum in a liveborn premature infant. *Am J Med Genet* 1992; 44:437–8.

219. Addor C, et al. "C" trigonocephaly syndrome with diaphragmatic hernia. *Genet Couns* 1995; 6:113–120.

220. Smith SA, Martin KE, Dodd KL, Young ID. Severe microphthalmia, diaphragmatic hernia and Fallot's tetralogy associated with chromosome 1;15 translocation. *Clin Dysmorphol* 1994; 3:287–91.

221. Langer JC, Winthrop AL, Whelan D. Fryns syndrome: a rare familial case of congenital diaphragmatic hernia. *J Pediatr Surg* 1994; 29:1266–7.

222. Cunniff C, Cwry CJ, Covey JC, et al. Congenital diaphragmatic hernia in Brachmann-de Lange syndrome. *Am J Med Genet* 1993; 47:1018–21.

223. Narayan H, De Chazal R, Barrow M, et al. Familial congenital diaphragmatic hernia: prenatal diagnosis, management and outcome. *Prenat Diagn* 1993; 13:893–901.

224. McPherson EW, Ketterer DM, Salsburey DJ. Pallister-Killiam and Fryns syndromes: nosology. *Am J Med Genet* 1993; 47:241–5.

225. Chen E, Johnson JP, Cox VA, Golabi M. Simpson-Golabi-Behmel syndrome: congenital diaphragmatic hernia and radiologic findings in two patients and follow-up of a previously reported case. *Am J Med Genet* 1993; 46: 574–8.

226. Mesrobian HG, Rushton HG, Bulas D. Unilateral renal agenesis may result from in utero regression of multicystic renal dysplasia. *J Urol* 1993; 150: 793–4.

227. Hitchcock R, Burge DM. Renal agenesis: an acquired condition? *J Pediatr Surg* 1994; 29:454–5.

228. Winters WD, Effmann EL, Nghiem HV, Nyberg DA. Disappearing fetal lung masses: importance of postnatal imaging studies. *Pediatr Radiol* 1997; 27:535–7.

229. Kreidberg JA, Sariola H, Loring JM, et al. WT-1 is required for early kidney development. *Cell* 1993; 74:679–91.

230. Schuchardt A, D'Agati V, Lorsson-Blomberg L, et al. RET-deficient mice: an animal model for Hirschsprung's disease and renal agenesis. *Ann Intern Med* 1995; 238:327–32.

231. Sanchez MP, Silos-Santiago I, Frisen J, et al. Renal agenesis and the absence of enteric neurons in mice lacking GDNF. *Nature* 1996; 382:70–3.

232. Delattre O, Zucman J, Melot T, et al. The Ewing family of tumors—a subgroup of small round cell tumors defined by specific chimeric transcripts. *N Engl J Med* 1994; 331:194–299.

233. Yandell DW, Campbell TA, Dayton SH, et al. Oncogenic point mutations in the human retinoblastoma gene: their application to genetic counseling. *N Engl J Med* 1989; 321:1689–95.

234. Ladanyi M, Gerald W. Fusion of the EWS and WT1 genes in the desmoplastic small round cell tumors. *Cancer Res* 1994; 54:2837–40.

235. Barbaux S, Niaudet P, Gubler M-C, et al. Donor splice-site mutations in WT1 are responsible for Frasier syndrome. *Nat Genet* 1997; 17: 467–70.

236. Jeanpierre C, et al. Isolated mesangial sclerosis: identification of constitutional WT1 mutations and analysis of genotype-phenotype correlations using a computerized mutation database. *Am J Hum Genet* 1997; 61(Suppl). Abstract No. 885.

Chromosome Abnormalities

ENID F. GILBERT-BARNESS   JOHN M. OPITZ

INTRODUCTION

An International Standing Committee on Human Cytogenetic Nomenclature [1] has standardized technical terminology referring to normal primate chromosomes and to structural and numerical chromosome abnormalities (Table 12.1). High-resolution methods have increased the number of recognizable human chromosome regions and bands to almost 1000 [2, 3], resulting in more precise and accurate determinations of chromosome abnormalities.

Chromosome abnormalities represent the largest category of causes of death in humans. Abortuses that have reached a 2-week stage of development have a 78.3% rate of chromosome abnormalities [4, 5]. However, this rate declines to 62.1% for abortions occurring after the first missed period, but before the 20th week [4, 5]. The proportion of fetuses with chromosome defects drops continuously, with only 5.8% of stillborn infants having chromosome defects [6–8]. In liveborn infants, the rate of chromosome defects is 5.9 per 1000 [9]. Chromosomal imbalance may also be the major cause of failure of development of 31% of ova lost before implantation. Witschi [10] in 1969 and Boué et al [11] in 1975 estimated that from the time of conception at least one-half of all human ova have chromosome abnormalities. The incidence of the types of chromosome abnormalities in spontaneous abortions is shown in Table 12.2. Maternal age has long been known as a predisposing factor for chromosome abnormalities.

More than one-third of cytogenetically abnormal liveborn infants have an extra sex chromosome (47, XXX; 47, XXY; 47, XYY); these infants do not seem to suffer excessive prenatal mortality. About one-quarter have autosomal trisomy, and about two-fifths (40%) have structural chromosome defects. Those with balanced structural chromosome defects are phenotypically normal, but have 15% fewer liveborn offspring than their chromosomally normal siblings [12]. Thus, about 99% of all conceptuses with chromosome abnormalities die prenatally, including almost all 45, X, polyploid, and autosomal trisomy cases; even trisomy 21 is a "sublethal" condition, and more than one-half die prenatally [13]. Forty percent of liveborn Down syndrome children are dead by the end of the first year of life [14, 15]. Machin and Crolla [8] found chromosome abnormalities in 13.4% of infants and fetuses with lethal malformations. It is apparent that nondisjunction appears to be a nonrandom event, with women who have had chromosomally unbalanced fetuses being more likely to have other aneuploid fetuses if they miscarry again than women whose first miscarried fetuses were chromosomally normal.

SIGNIFICANCE OF MINOR ANOMALIES AND MILD MALFORMATIONS

It has become evident that most congenital anomalies in conditions attributable to chromosome imbalance are minor anomalies or mild malformations that can no longer be ignored as trivial. Minor anomalies should be regarded as defects of phenogenesis, and mild malformations as defects of organogenesis. Minor anomalies include all those human developmental variants seen more or less frequently in various normal populations, including epicanthic and mongolian folds, variants of scalp-hair patterns, auricular configuration, height of bridge of nose, variant dermatoglyphics, broad thumbs, clinodactyly, "trigger" thumbs, hairy ears, synophrys, long or short upper lip, micrognathia, thin vermilion border of upper lip, and other anomalies. Anomalies of facial appearance or configuration of the auricles should be documented photographically; dermatoglyphics should be described and/or printed, and minor skeletal variants should be recorded by x-ray examination.

Table 12.1.   Glossary of terminology and cytogenetic nomenclature

Aneuploid
An unbalanced state that arises through loss or addition of either whole chromosomes or pieces of chromosomes, always considered deleterious.

Chromosome
The location of hereditary (genetic) material within the cell.

Deletion
Pieces of chromosomes that are missing, in persons having 46 chromosomes.

Diploid (2n)
The double set of chromosomes in a somatic cell.

Duplications
Extra pieces of chromosomes that are present in individuals with 46 chromosomes.

Genotype
The total of the genetic information contained in the chromosomes.

Haploid (n)
The half-set of chromosomes of a gamete.

Homologues
The individual members of a pair of chromosomes.

Inversion
Inversions require two breaks; both breaks on one side of the centromere result in a pericentric inversion; breaks in both arms result in a pericentric inversion.

Isochromosomes
Arise from several different mechanisms, principally transverse rather than longitudinal division of the centromere during mitosis or meiosis.

Monosomy
Lack of one whole chromosome.

Mosaicism
The presence of two or more chromosomally different cell lines in the same person.

Nondisjunction
Failure of paired chromosomes or sister chromatids to disjoin at anaphase either in a mitotic division or in the first or second meiotic division.

Polyploidy
The presence of more than two complete sets of chromosomes (i.e., 69 is triploidy, 92 is tetraploidy).

Ring chromosomes
At least two breaks are required and can be mitotically unstable; they rarely survive meiosis to be transmitted from one generation to the next.

Tetrasomy
Two extra chromosomes (of one pair); if they belong to two different pairs, the state is called *double trisomy.*

Translocation
A reciprocal exchange of material between two chromosomes in which the unbalanced state of one or the other altered chromosome in offspring represents a duplication/deficiency, which can also arise through crossing-over in a pericentric inversion.

Triploidy
Three copies of a haploid set (69,XXX, 69,XXY, or 69,XYY).

Trisomy
One whole extra chromosome.

A mild malformation is a morphologic anomaly and should be interpreted as reduced expressivity (severity) of a major anomaly under the following circumstances:

1. If a laterally paired organ has a more severe defect of the same developmental type (e.g., right pretragal tag, left microtia).

Table 12.2.   Incidence of the types of chromosome abnormalities in 1500 spontaneous abortions [11]

Abnormality	Incidence, %
Autosomal trisomies	52.00
Triploidy	19.86
45,X	15.30
Tetraploidy	6.18
Double trisomy	1.73
Translocations	3.80
Mosaicism	1.08

2. When anomalies are known to be associated with the defect as part of a developmental field defect (bifid distal phalanx of thumb with ipsilateral renal agenesis as an acrorenal field defect, or presence of single umbilical artery with unilateral renal agenesis).

3. When the defect is present in more severe form in a twin or other first-degree relative.

4. When associated functional or structural defects indicate aneuploidy (e.g., in a slightly short 4th metacarpal in the Ullrich-Turner syndrome; or absence of the palmaris longus muscles in the trisomy 18 syndrome).

It has been suggested that the retention of genes that code for phylogenetically older structures that are usually repressed may explain the production of atavisms, such as the presence of the pectoralis minimus and latissimocondyloideus muscles in the trisomy 18 syndrome [16].

The chromosome defects causing the most damage are autosomal trisomy, polyploidy, and monosomy X, which carries a 98–99% prenatal lethality. Autosomal trisomy is associated with increased maternal age, but the contrary is true of monosomy X. The occurrence of chromosome abnormalities is nonrandom; radiation and other environmental factors (viruses?) can increase the risk of nondisjunction. Generally, the effect of autosomal aneuploidy is worse than that of gonosomal aneuploidy. The exception to this rule is the unusual lethality of 45, X, which raises the suspicion that most surviving Ullrich-Turner syndrome patients are mosaics with a normal cell line, a hypothesis supported by the documented fertility in a considerable number of such women. In the case of structural chromosome defects, deletions generally are more deleterious than duplications.

The discovery of the fragile site of the tip of the long arm of the X chromosome, Fra(X)(q28), in the macroorchidism-X-linked mental retardation (Fra(X)) syndrome represents a great advance in its diagnosis, nosology, carrier detection, and genetic counseling. Fra (X) syndrome has a prevalence of 2 per 1000 males [17]. Special culture conditions are required to demonstrate the marker. Prenatal diagnosis is possible with karyotype or DNA analysis.

Chromosome abnormalities may be symptomatic manifestations of known or presumed underlying defects of

DNA repair, as seen in Bloom syndrome, ataxia telangiectasia, xeroderma pigmentosum, and Fanconi's aplastic anemia. In these disorders, the chromosome abnormalities are results, not causes, of the conditions.

DEVELOPMENTAL EFFECTS OF ANEUPLOIDY

Aneuploidy is usually associated with disturbances of growth, beginning prenatally as intrauterine growth retardation.

All unbalanced chromosome abnormalities are associated with multiple congenital anomalies (MCAs), syndromes consisting of various permutations of minor and major anomalies. Most cases of chromosome imbalance affect CNS function, and most autosomal defects are associated with mental retardation (MR).

All gross aneuploidy has more or less severely deleterious developmental effects on gonads. The Ullrich-Turner syndrome is associated with gonadal dysgenesis or late fetal ovarian degeneration, and Klinefelter syndrome with congenital micro-orchidism.

All well-studied aneuploidy syndromes have increased numbers of dysplasias, which probably are responsible for their increased risk of cancer—e.g.: associations of 13q⁻ and retinoblastoma; 11p⁻ and Wilms' tumor; trisomy 21 and leukemia, retinoblastoma and perhaps CNS and testicular tumors; Klinefelter syndrome and breast cancer; trisomy 13 syndrome and retinoblastoma and leukemia; and trisomy 18 syndrome and Wilms' tumor.

The most common aneuploidy syndromes are discussed in this chapter; for more extensive and detailed reviews, the reader is referred to the works by Yunis [18], Zellweger and Simpson [19], de Grouchy and Turleau [20], and Schinzel [21], to the many sections and volumes on new chromosomal syndromes from the Annual Birth Defects Meetings published in the Birth Defects Original Articles Series, and to a catalogue of chromosomal variants and anomalies [22].

TRISOMY 21: DOWN SYNDROME (DS)

Approximately 95% of all cases of DS have primary trisomy 21; about 4% have a translocation, and 1% are mosaics. The most frequent translocation is between chromosome 21 and a chromosome of the D (usually 14) or G (usually 22) group. More than 50% of the D/G and 90% of the G/G translocations occur de novo, both parents having normal karyotypes. The remaining cases with D/G or G/G translocation have a parent with the same translocation in a balanced form; a balanced translocation can be found in several members of such families. The risk to offspring of D/G translocation is 11% in the mother and 2.4% in the father. In the very rare instance of (21q; 21q) translocation, the risk is 100% [23]. Trisomy 21 resulting from nondisjunction is maternal-age-dependent (Table 12.3). An increased paternal age also contributes slightly to an increased incidence of Down syndrome; the effect becomes evident beyond the age of 55 [24–26]. The chromosome aberration corresponding

to trisomy 21 is also found in the chimpanzee [27], gorilla [28], and orangutan [29].

Infants with DS have intrauterine growth retardation (IUGR). They are hypotonic, with hyperextensibility of joints, and have diminished sucking and swallowing reflexes. There are 10 cardinal signs of trisomy 21 in the newborn infant [30] (Table 12.4). The phenotype of Down syndrome can be recognized easily in the fetus as early as 24 weeks' gestation (Fig. 12.1). The dermatoglyphic patterns in DS include an increased number of ulnar loops, third interdigital distal loops, radial loops on digits IV and V, a decreased number of whorls and arches, a single palmar crease (simian line) or an extended proximal transverse crease (Sydney line), and a distal axial triradius [31–33] (Fig. 12.2).

Mental retardation is the most consistent manifestation of DS; the IQ score is usually in the range of 35–55 [19]. Anatomic studies at the University of Wisconsin have confirmed the inferences of developmental delay in DS [34]. Major anomalies are found in 50% of affected infants. The most common anomalies, in order of frequency, are cardiac defects, duodenal obstruction, talipes equinovarus, cataracts, imperforate anus, cleft lip and/or palate, congenital megacolon, and meningomyelocele [35]. Congenital cardiac defects (Table 12.5) have an incidence of about 50% [36]

Table 12.3. Down syndrome and maternal age [251]

Age of mother (years)	Risk of Down syndrome
20	1:1000
25	1:1524
30	1:1163
32	1:610
35	1:324
38	1:322
40	1:95
43	1:64
45	1:30

Table 12.4. Clinical features of trisomy 21 in the newborn infant [30]

Sign	Frequency, %, in Down syndrome
Flat face (hypoplastic maxilla)	90
Slanting palpebral fissures	80
Abundant nuchal skin	80
Hyperextensibility of joints	80
Muscular hypotonia	80
Absent Moro's reflex	80
Dysplastic pelvis	70
Dysplastic ears	60
Dysplastic middle phalanx of 5th finger	60
Simian crease (at least of one hand)	50

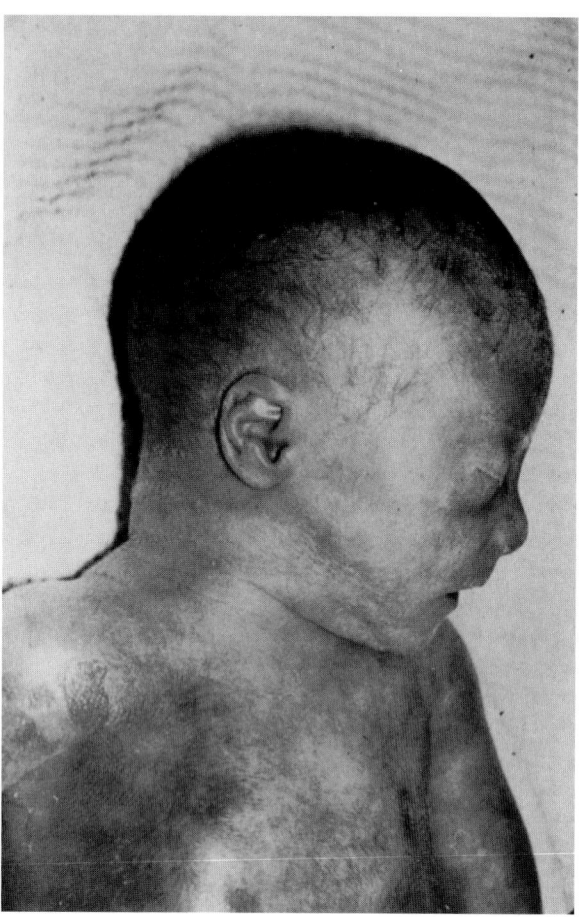

FIGURE 12.1. *A 24-week fetus with typical features of Down syndrome.*

Table 12.5. Congenital cardiovascular defects in Down syndrome [36]

Defect	Incidence, %
Endocardial cushion defect	50
Ventricular septal defect	25
Tetralogy of Fallot	8
Patent ductus arteriosus	7
Atrial septal defect (secundum type)	3
Other heart lesions	7

the glomeruli near the capsule as characteristic of fetal and early postnatal life. Hemangiomas of the kidney have been present in several cases [43]. Retardation in maturation of the nephrogenic zone of the cortex and persistent fetal lobulation were the only consistent findings in our cases with DS.

Hematologic abnormalities include a transient myeloproliferative syndrome that can be seen early in infancy in DS patients; this syndrome usually disappears after some weeks or months. One percent of all patients with DS develop leukemia [19]; acute myeloblastic leukemia is the most common congenital type. Leukemia in older children with DS is predominantly of acute lymphocytic type. Polycythemia unassociated with cyanotic heart disease can occur. Miller and Todaro [44] have shown an increased oncogenic effect of SV40 virus on trisomy 21 cells compared with euploid cells, which could explain the high leukemia incidence in DS. Other malignant tumors that occur with greater frequency in DS include retinoblastoma, testicular tumors, and brain tumors [19, 45].

Endocrine disorders also have been reported in DS. Hypothyroidism [46] has occasionally been associated with precocious puberty or diabetes mellitus [47–49]. It has been hypothesized that the hypofunctioning thyroid gland may enhance the release of not only thyroid stimulating hormone (TSH), but follicle stimulating hormone (FSH) as well. A gonadotropic effect of TSH would account for the precocious puberty. Hyperthyroidism may rarely be present.

Hypogenitalism is frequently present in DS in the male; although the penis and testes are usually small and cryptorchidism may be present, it is rare to find macrogenitosomia praecox with adrenal hyperplasia [50]. Postpubertal testes on microscopic examination have revealed interstitial fibrosis and hypoplasia of the seminiferous tubules, with few tubules showing normal spermatogenesis [51, 52]. These changes are frequently indistinguishable from those seen in Klinefelter syndrome. In females, the ovaries are usually small [43] and there is hypoplasia with persistence of atretic corpora lutea and little follicular activity. About one-half of female patients with DS do not ovulate [51]. The development of axillary and pubic hair and breasts is usually deficient.

and occur about 40 times more frequently in patients with DS than in the general population. They account for more than 5% of all cases of congenital heart malformations. Pulmonary hypertension and pulmonary vascular sclerosis [37] occur with higher frequency in DS. We have also observed periarteritis nodosa involving the coronary vessels in DS [35].

Gastrointestinal obstruction is the second most frequent group of major malformations in DS. Esophageal atresia occurs in approximately 1%, duodenal atresia in 30%, annular pancreas in 24%, congenital intestinal aganglionosis in 2%, and anorectal malformations in 2% of cases of DS [19]. Almost one-third of all cases of congenital duodenal obstruction occur in association with DS [38]. Diastasis recti and umbilical hernia occur in about 10% of cases.

Developmental disorders of the kidney in DS are uncommon and have been reviewed [39]. Stricture at the ureteropelvic junction, hydronephrosis, and focal cystic malformation of the collecting tubules with immature glomeruli have been reported [40, 41]. Renal dysplasia and nodular renal blastema were described by Kissane [42]. Benda [43] considered the kidneys to be small and described

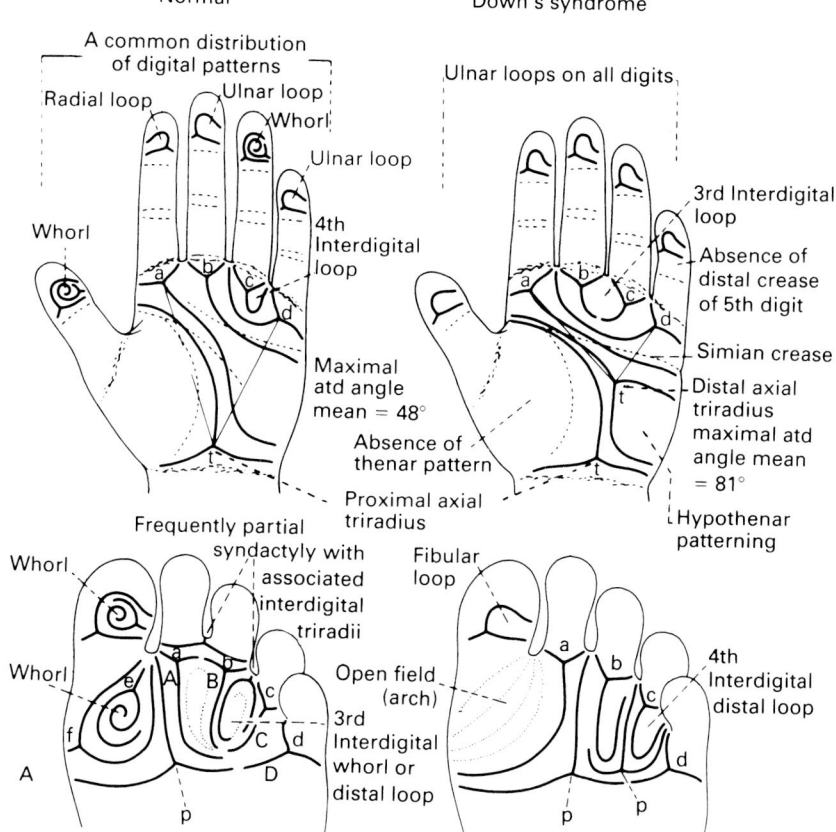

Normal
Down's syndrome

A common distribution of digital patterns
Radial loop
Ulnar loop
Whorl
Ulnar loop
Whorl
4th Interdigital loop
Maximal atd angle mean = 48°
Absence of thenar pattern
Proximal axial triradius

Ulnar loops on all digits
3rd Interdigital loop
Absence of distal crease of 5th digit
Simian crease
Distal axial triradius maximal atd angle mean = 81°
Hypothenar patterning

Frequently partial syndactyly with associated interdigital triradii
Whorl
Whorl
A
Fibular loop
Open field (arch)
3rd Interdigital whorl or distal loop
4th Interdigital distal loop

FIGURE 12.2. *Dermatoglyphic patterns of hands and feet in Down syndrome (right) compared with normal patterns (left). (Courtesy of Dr. M. Bat-Miriam; prepared by Mr. R. Lee of the Kennedy-Galton Centre near St Albans, UK; reprinted with permission of W.B. Saunders, Philadelphia, PA.)*

There is well-documented evidence for immunodeficiency in DS (Table 12.6). Children with DS may have T-cell deficiency [53]. The thymus is usually small and may be dysplastic, with lymphocytic depletion, a small contracted cortex, and loss of corticomedullary demarcation in a histologic pattern resembling thymic involution. Large Hassall's corpuscles with calcification and cystic changes (Fig. 12.3) appear to be characteristic of the thymus in DS, and these corpuscles have been suggested as markers for DS [54]. The spleen has marked lymphocyte depletion in the thymic-dependent periarteriolar sheaths, and the germinal follicles may be diminished in number. Lymph nodes also have depleted T-dependent zones [53]. There is a high incidence of hepatitis B surface (HbS) antigenemia [55]. The significance of this finding is not clearly understood.

The morphology of the brain may be variable, but certain features appear to be quite consistent. The weight of the brain is usually less than normal; the brain is delayed in maturity for gestational age and the convolutions are small. Myelination is retarded. The cerebral convolutions are flat and the frontal and temporal poles are compressed. The brain is brachycephalic; the gyri are flattened. The frontal poles are markedly flattened. Hypoplasia of the superior temporal gyrus and open operculum are characteristic of the DS brain (Fig. 12.4). A short corpus callosum, hypoplasia of

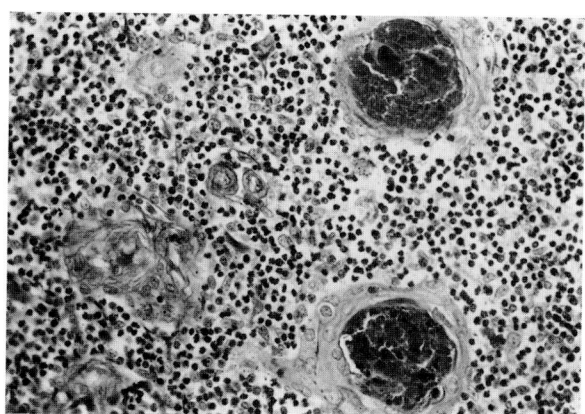

FIGURE 12.3. *Microscopic section of thymus in Down syndrome. Hassall's corpuscles are large, cystic, and calcified. H&E, ×100. (From Gilbert and Opitz [35]; reprinted with permission of Masson Publishing USA, New York.)*

the brainstem and medulla, and hypoplasia of the cerebellar hemispheres are other fairly constant features.

The spinal cord changes include enlargement of the central canal with irregular ependymal proliferation, hypoplasia of the gray matter, and lack of separation of

Table 12.6.   Immunodeficiency in Down syndrome [35]

Clinical findings
Increased incidence of infections, particularly respiratory
Increased incidence of lymphatic leukemia
High incidence of hepatitis B surface antigenemia
High incidence of thyroid autoantibodies
Immunologic findings
Diminished number of blood lymphocytes
Diminished phagocytic activity
B cells:
  normal number
  immunoglobulin production, no consistent abnormality
T cells:
  diminished number
  diminished blast transformation with phytohemagglutinin (PHA)
  diminished delayed skin hypersensitivity to PHA
  diminished leucocyte migration inhibition factor with PHA
  deficient interferon production
  respond in vivo and in vitro to thymic humoral factor
Pathologic findings
Thymus:
  small with marked lymphocyte depletion
  contracted, depleted cortex
  giant and cystic Hassall's corpuscles
  increased cellularity around some Hassall's corpuscles
Spleen:
  depleted T-zone lymphocytes
Lymph nodes:
  depleted T-dependent zones

found a paucity of neuronal elements, although the existing neurons had an increase of nucleoplasm. Typical Alzheimer lesions (Fig. 12.5) may appear early in DS, as may senile plaques and neurofibrillary tangles. In DS, these changes occur earlier than in non-DS Alzheimer's disease and can be found in the brains of adolescent and young adult patients [58–61]. Granulovacuolar degeneration of neurons may be present by 30 years [62].

The cerebellum may show asymmetric development with the presence of tuber flocculus (Fig. 12.6), which is a focus of undifferentiated cell piles found in the earliest differentiation of the cerebellum at about 5 weeks' gestation; this persists in the cerebellum in more than 60% of the brains of DS patients.

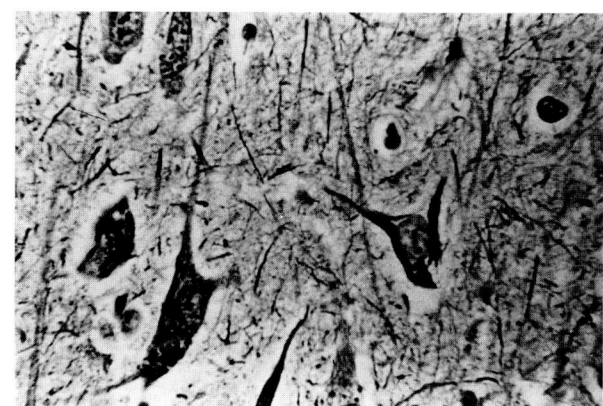

FIGURE 12.5.   *Microscopic section of brain in Down syndrome, showing neurofibrillary tangles. H&E, ×100.*

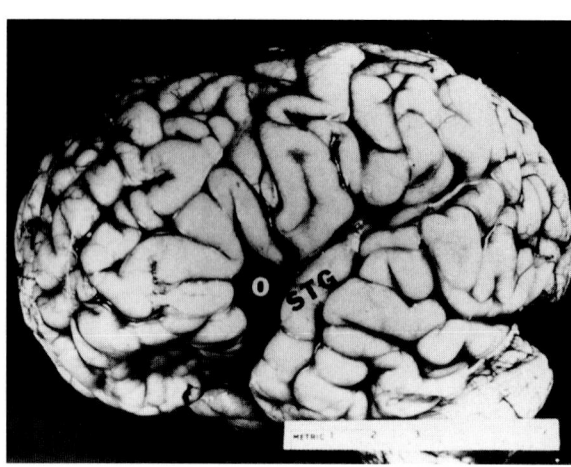

FIGURE 12.4.   *Gross appearance of the brain in Down syndrome. The brain is brachycephalic, the operculum is open, and the superior temporal gyrus is hypoplastic.*

Clarke's columns [56]. Atlanto-occipital or atlantoaxial instability is common in DS and may potentiate spinal cord injury.

On microscopic examination, the architecture of the cortex of the cerebrum and cerebellum is irregular, with alternating zones of dense and scanty neurons. Colon [57]

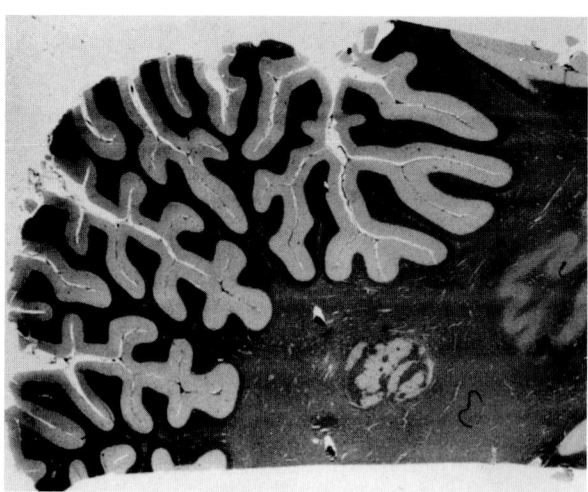

FIGURE 12.6.   *Microscopic section of brain, showing tuber flocculus within the cerebellum. H&E, ×40. (From Gilbert and Opitz [35]; reprinted with permission of Masson Publishing USA, New York.)*

The cerebral cortex shows arrested differentiation and myelination. The U fibers are not developed, and demyelination often is associated with deposits of calcium and secondary sclerosis.

The liver in DS tends to be increased in size and shows moderate to severe fatty metamorphosis [63]. This does not appear to be related to malnutrition, but possibly to a defect in the mobilization and transport of lipids.

TRISOMY 13

Trisomy 13 was first cytogenetically defined by Patau et al [64], and the clinical phenotype was first described by Patau et al [64]. Trisomy 13 due to nondisjunction is found in the majority of cases. Translocation is found in about 20%, and trisomy 13 mosaicism is found in less than 10% [19]. Abnormalities are listed in Table 12.7.

Table 12.7.   Abnormalities observed in trisomy 13

Craniofacial abnormalities	Micromulticystic kidneys
Microcephaly	Double kidney
Receding forehead	Double ureter
Epicanthal folds	Hydronephrosis and hydroureters
Deep-set eyes	Male:
Sparse curled eyelashes	cryptorchidism
Midline scalp defect at vertex of head	anomalies of scrotum
Horizontal palpebral fissures	hypoplasia of Leydig's cells
Broad and flat nose	agenesis of testes
Low-set ears, flat and poorly defined	Female:
Midline facial defect, cleft lip/palate	bicornuate uterus
Abnormal ears	hypertrophy of clitoris
Incisor teeth present at birth	double vagina
Hypotelorism	**Cardiovascular malformations**
External malformations	Ventricular septal defect
Prominent calcaneus	Patent ductus arteriosus
Rocker-bottom feet	Atrial septal defect
Talipes equinovarus	Dextrocardia/dextroposition
Talipes calcaneovalgus	Patent foramen ovale
Hexadactyly of hands and/or feet	Valvular, pulmonic stenosis
Flexed fingers, retroflexed thumbs	Bicuspid aortic valve
Clinodactyly of little fingers	Transposition, great arteries
Camptodactyly	Truncus arteriosus
Narrow and hyperconvex nails	Double outlet right ventricle
Hemangiomas—face, forehead, nape of neck	Valvular, pulmonic atresia
Hypoplastic or absent 12th ribs	Aortic coarctation
Hypoplastic pelvis with flattened acetabular angle	Left superior vena cava
Kyphoscoliosis	**Central nervous system malformations**
Dermatoglyphics	Arrhinencephaly-holoprosencephaly
Distal axial triradius	Cerebellar anomalies
Single palmar crease (simian line)	Corpus callosum defects
Arch fibular or arch fibular S pattern	Heterotopias
Ocular malformations	Arnold-Chiari malformation
Microphthalmia-anophthalmia	Vascular malformations
Cataract	Anencephaly
Corneal opacities	Migration defects
Retinoschisis	**Visceral malformations**
Hypoplasia of optic nerve	Abnormal lobation of lungs
Persistent hyperplastic primary vitreous	Abnormal lobation of liver
Coloboma of iris or retina	Elongation, hypoplasia, or malrotation of
Aniridia	gallbladder
Retinal dysplasia	Ectopic pancreas in spleen
Retinoblastoma	Abnormally large fetal cortex of adrenals
Hematologic abnormalities	Accessory spleens
Multiple projections in neutrophil nuclei	Meckel's diverticulum
Increased fetal and Gower-2 hemoglobin	Absent mesentery
Genitourinary malformations	Inguinal and/or umbilical hernia

At least 85% of translocation cases involve two D chromosomes. Trisomy 13 has an estimated incidence of 1 per 5000 livebirths [65] and is associated with advanced maternal age. Prenatal wastage is high; most trisomy 13 conceptuses are spontaneously aborted.

In the series by Warkany et al [66] of 200 liveborn infants with trisomy 13, 28% died within the first week, 44% within the first month, and 73% within the first 4 months of life. The oldest reported living children with this disorder were 10, 11 and 19 years of age [67, 68].

The infant with trisomy 13 is small for gestational age and may have a spectrum of midline facial defects that includes premaxillary agenesis, cebocephaly, ethmocephaly, and cyclopia (Fig. 12.7). Other classic external phenotypic abnormalities include micrognathia, malformed ears, and polydactyly (Fig. 12.8). About one-third of trisomy 13 infants have scalp defects in the region of the vertex (Fig. 12.9). Two-thirds of cases have capillary hemangiomas. Omphalocele, large umbilical hernias, retroflexed thumb, hyperconvex nails, and anomalies of the feet, such as talipes equinovarus and talipes calcaneovalgus, are frequent. The calcaneus is often prominent, and rocker-bottom feet, although less frequent than in trisomy 18, may be seen.

Dermatoglyphic patterns include a high incidence of a single palmar crease, distal axial triradius, and increased numbers of arches on the fingertips. An S-shaped fibular arch pattern in the hallucal areas of the soles is a valuable diagnostic sign of trisomy 13 [35].

Pettersen et al [69] have made extensive anatomic studies in trisomy 13. The six most frequent and consistent muscle variations are the absence of palmaris longus, peroneus tertius, palmaris brevis, plantaris, pectorodorsalis, and extensor indicis muscles.

Congenital cardiovascular malformations are found in 80% of cases [66, 70]. Respiratory tract defects include abnormal lobation of the lungs, tracheoesophageal fistula, and bifid uvula.

Abdominal malformations include omphalocele, malrotation of the gut, and, less often, Meckel's diverticulum, heterotopia of the pancreas, and accessory spleens.

The adrenal glands may be enlarged and morphologically abnormal [71], and the association of adrenocortical carcinoma and neuroblastoma has been described [72].

The genital system shows a fairly regular pattern of abnormalities. In the female, bicornuate uterus occurs in 80% of cases. The fallopian tubes may insert abnormally; anomalies of the external genitalia, such as clitoral hypertrophy and duplication of the labia, are rare [71]. The ovaries may be agenetic, normal, hypoplastic, or enlarged [73]. In the male, cryptorchidism and hypoplasia of the external genitalia are common.

Urogenital abnormalities include micromulticystic kidneys (Fig. 12.10), hydronephrosis, hydroureter, duplication of kidneys and ureters, dysplastic kidneys [74], unilateral renal agenesis [75], and nodular renal blastema [76].

Horseshoe kidneys are less common than in trisomy 18. Megacystis and persistent urachus have been seen infrequently.

Cryptorchidism is an almost constant finding in males with trisomy 13. The penis and scrotum are small, and hypospadias is sometimes present. Scrotal skin may extend to the penis. The female may have bicornuate uterus, biseptate uterus, or uterus duplex. These anomalies are much more frequent in trisomy 13 than in other chromosome defects and suggest that the extra chromosome 13 affects fusion at the caudal end of the müllerian duct.

Fatal hemoglobin is present in greater than normal amounts in newborn infants with trisomy 13 and tends to decrease at a slower rate than in normal infants. Hematologic abnormalities include neutrophilic nuclear projections [77–79]. Hemoglobin Gower-2 persists throughout the gestational period and after birth into the early neonatal period. Acute myeloblastic leukemia has been reported in trisomy 13 [80, 81].

Central Nervous System

The central nervous system (CNS) abnormalities in trisomy 13 include the spectrum of arrhinencephaly-holoprosencephaly (Fig. 12.11). DeMyer et al [82] relate the facial defects to the malformation of the brain. Mesoderm migrates anterior to the notochord and is responsible for the induction of the differentiation of the forebrain and the midline facial structures. Failure of this migration results in a defect encompassing this developmental field.

The optic chiasm and optic nerves are usually hypoplastic. Arnold-Chiari malformation and myelomeningocele may be present. Heterotopias are frequent within the cortex, particularly in the dentate nucleus of the cerebellum. We have observed [83] herniation of the cochlear nuclei into the eighth cranial nerve, the presence of gray matter in the 11th cranial nerve, arteriovenous malformations of leptomeningeal and intracerebral vessels, arachnoid cyst of the cauda equina, and retinal pigment epithelium within the optic nerve. Heterotopic neuroblasts may be present within the external granular layer of the cerebellum, and the external granular layer may persist on the outer surface of the pons and extend along the lateral surface of the brainstem around the origins of the seventh and eighth cranial nerves with glia extending into the eighth nerve. The corticospinal tracts of the spinal cord may lack myelination.

Formation of the ocular vesicle may be defective. Colobomas resulting in various ocular malformations, including anophthalmia, microphthalmia (Fig. 12.12), and cyclopia [73, 84], lead to intrusion of extraorbital mesenchyme into the optic vesicle and abnormal differentiation of intraocular mesoderm. Dysplastic changes of the cornea, iris, and anterior chamber can lead to corneal opacity, hypoplasia of iris stroma, and immature chamber angle. Partial absence of Descemet's membrane and corneal epithelium is seen in some cases [85]. Retinal dysplasia appears to

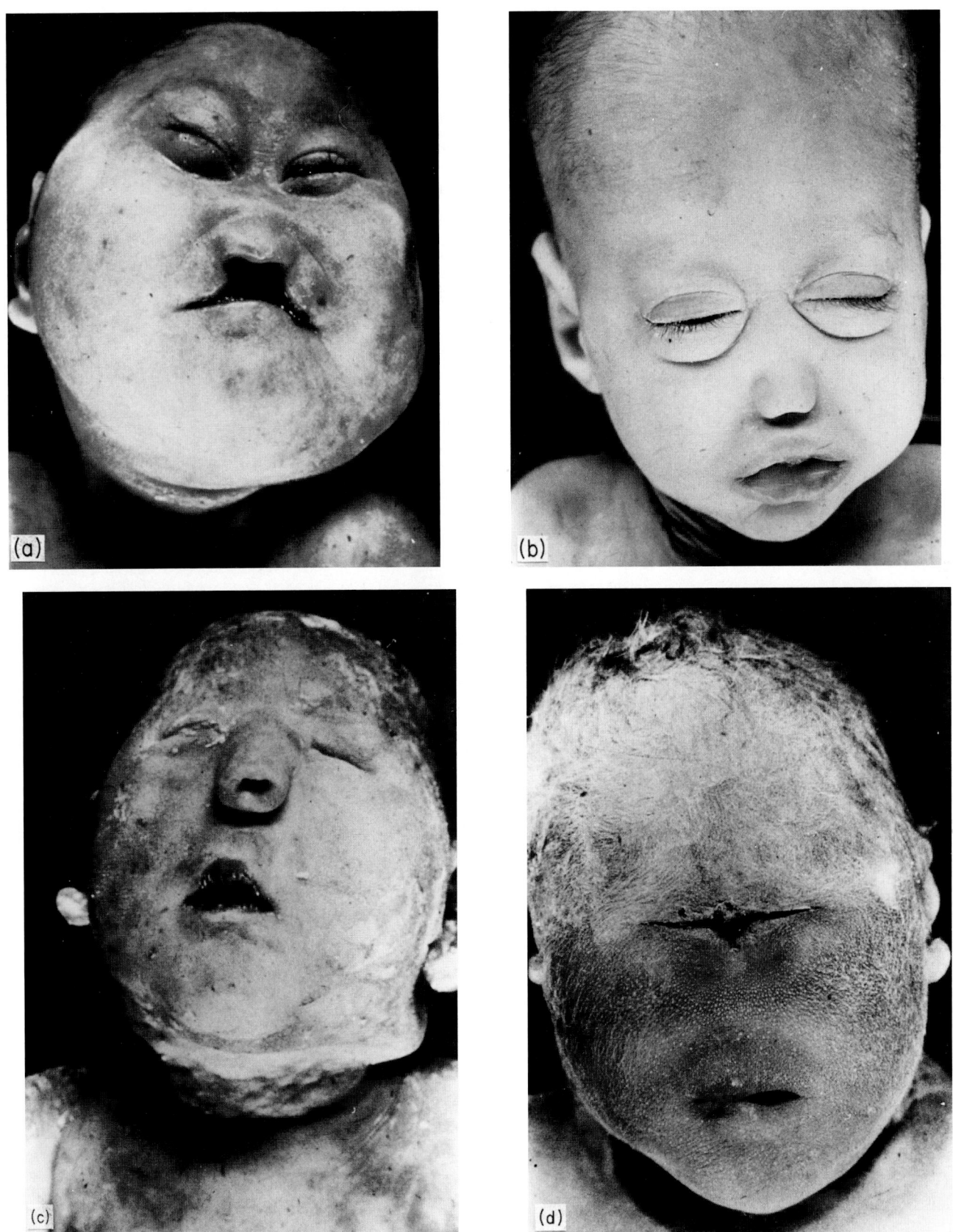

FIGURE 12.7.   *Midline facial defects in trisomy 13: (a) bilateral cleft lip, premaxillary aplasia, and hypotelorism; (b) cebocephaly; (c) ethmocephaly; (d) cyclopia. (From Gilbert and Opitz [35]; reprinted with permission of Masson Publishing USA, New York.)*

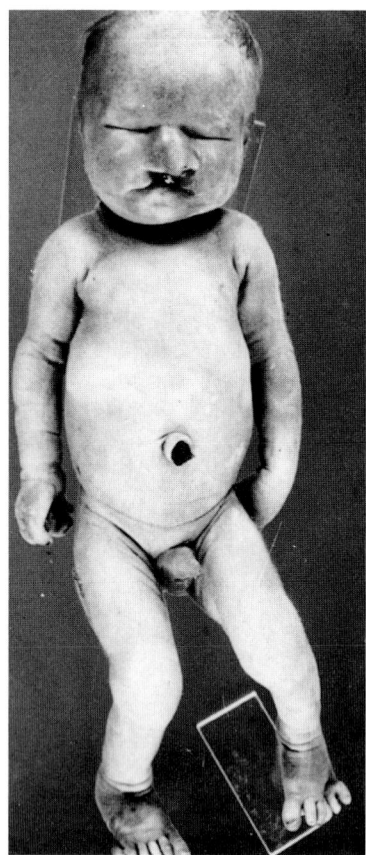

FIGURE 12.8.   *Newborn full-term infant showing typical phenotype of trisomy 13, with midline facial defect, hypotelorism, and polydactyly.*

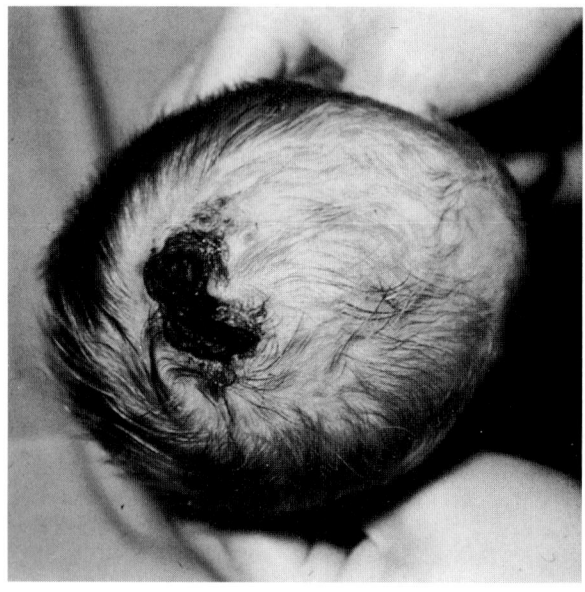

FIGURE 12.9.   *Midline defect over the vertex of the scalp in trisomy 13.*

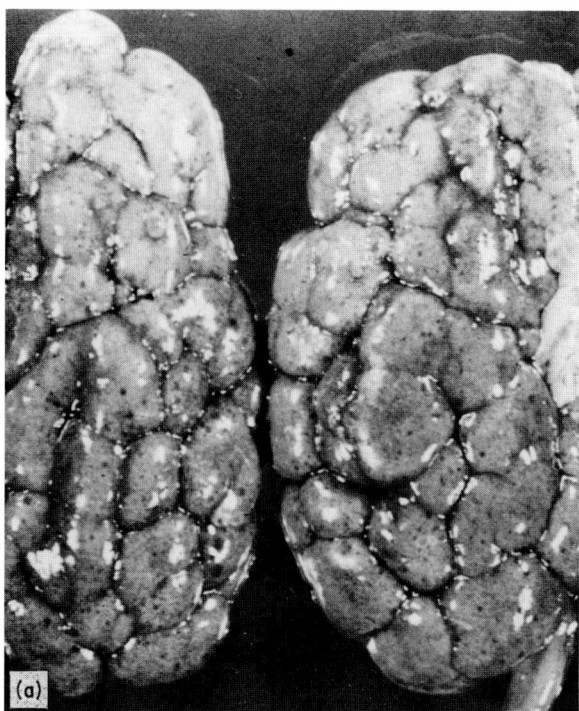

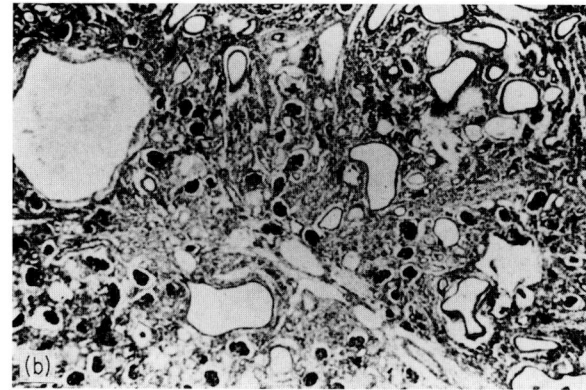

FIGURE 12.10.   *Kidney in trisomy 13: (a) excessive fetal lobulations with multiple small cortical cysts; (b) micromulticystic kidney with small glomerular and tubular cysts. H&E, ×100.*

be a constant feature. We have also observed retinoblastoma in trisomy 13 (Fig. 12.13).

DUPLICATIONS, DELETIONS, AND MOSAICISM OF CHROMOSOME 13

As a result of banding techniques, duplications can be subdivided into two groups trisomic for, respectively, the proximal $1/3$–$1/2$ and the distal $2/3$–$1/2$ portions of the long arm of chromosome 13 [86]. Excess for the distal segment [87, 88] and for the proximal segment [89] is associated with specific malformations.

Duplication of the proximal segment of the long arm of chromosome 13 is associated with rather nonspecific clinical features: psychomotor retardation, microcephaly, low-set

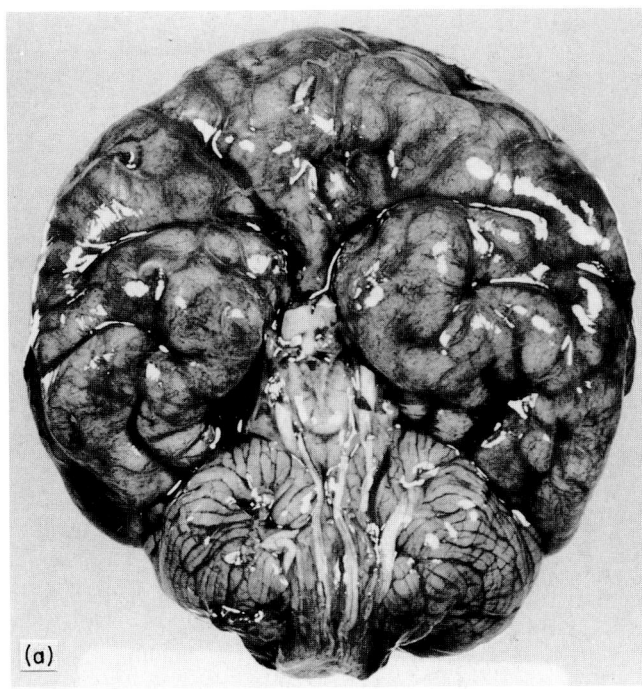
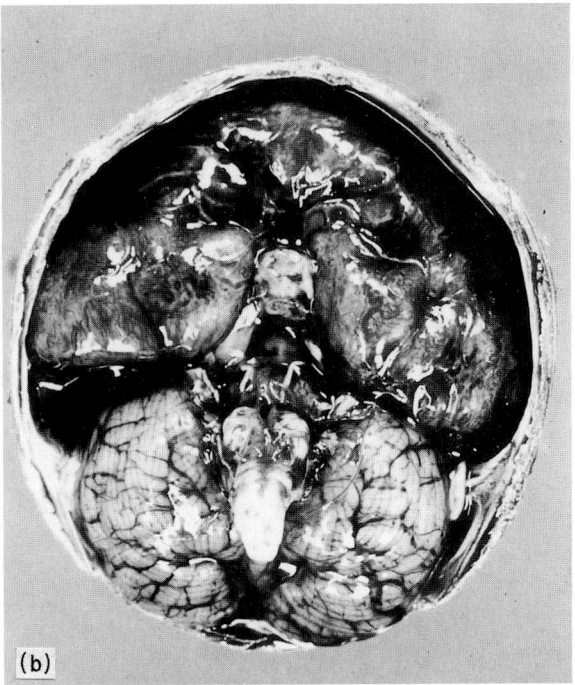

FIGURE 12.11. *Brain in trisomy 13: (a) arrhinencephaly with absence of olfactory bulbs and tracts and semilobar holoprosencephaly; (b) alobar holoprosencephaly with failure of cleavage of forebrain.*

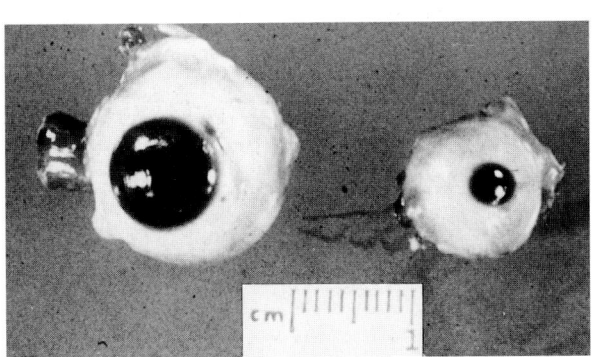

FIGURE 12.12. *Eyes in trisomy 13. Extreme microphthalmia on the right. (From Gilbert and Opitz [35]; reprinted with permission of Masson Publishing USA, New York.)*

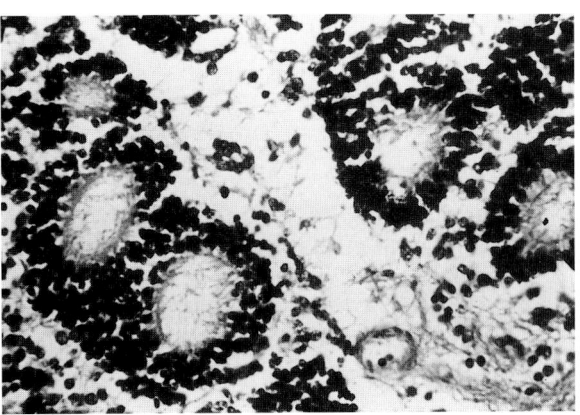

FIGURE 12.13. *Microscopic section of retina in trisomy 13, showing typical rosettes of retinoblastoma.*

ears, microstomia, micrognathia, distal triradius, and incurved fifth fingers. A few patients also have exhibited microphthalmia, hemangioma, cleft palate, and epicanthic folds.

Duplication of the distal $^2/_3–^1/_2$ of the long arm is associated with features that are not very different from those seen in complete trisomy 13 syndrome, although deafness, eye malformations, cleft palate, cleft lip, and cardiac defects are observed less frequently. However, duplication of the distal $^1/_3–^1/_2$ of the long arm of chromosome 13 seems to be critical for polydactyly, hemangioma, frontal bossing, and narrow temples [87]. Receding forehead with midbrain defects, harelip, eye malformations, and increased number of

nuclear projections of neutrophils are probably dependent on trisomy for most of the long arm. Fetal hemoglobin concentration has been normal in patients with trisomy for the distal $^1/_3$ of the long arm. Two patients, trisomic for the distal portion, have had a hallucal fibular arch. Simple arches on all 10 fingers, a finding more characteristic of trisomy 18, has been observed [86].

Chromosome 13 Deletion Syndrome

Approximately 60% are associated with a ring chromosome formation. About one-quarter of patients present with a 13q chromosome constitution, with a terminal or interstitial deletion. A prosencephalic brain defect may be observed in del(13q). Ventricular and atrial septal defects, aplasia of the gallbladder, and hypoplastic kidneys are frequent malformations. Unilateral renal agenesis and hydronephrosis may be present. Prominent nasofrontal bones, large ears with deep sulci and large overdeveloped lobules, hypoplasia or agenesis of the thumbs, and imperforate anus are conspicuous features. On the basis of specific clinical traits, Niebuhr [86] delineated four separate categories of patients with chromosome 13 deletions (Fig. 12.14).

Category 1 may reflect a peculiar behavior of the ring in early embryonic life. Loss of the telomere and the most distal band of 13q34 are essential for the development of these abnormalities. Microcephaly with hypertelorism, ears with large deep sulci and overdeveloped lobules, ocular abnormalities, and anogenital malformations are occasional features.

In category 2, patients have absent or hypoplastic thumbs. Craniofacial abnormalities include a triangular shape of the calvarium, frontal bossing, hypertelorism, epicanthic folds, and a protruding maxilla. Microphthalmia, coloboma, and genital malformations are frequent. Thumb defects range from a unilateral, boneless, rudimentary fold to bilateral absence of the thumbs without rudiments. Bilateral fusion of the fourth and fifth toes and absent fifth toes with only four metatarsals have been observed. On the other hand, only mild psychomotor retardation associated with very few

congenital malformations has been reported. Deletion of the 13q31 segment is necessary for the development of category 2 features [86].

Category 3 involves deletion of 13q14 and is associated with the development of retinoblastoma [90–93]. On the basis of concordance data, Matsunaga [94] has shown that the retinoblastoma of 13q⁻ cases is biologically different from that due to autosomal dominant mutations, and therefore suggests that this locus probably does not map to 13q.

Category 4 is associated with deletion of 13q21 [86]. Psychomotor retardation, microcephaly, hypertelorism, large but well-formed ears, and cardiac defects characterize this defect; thumbs are normal and the patients do not have retinoblastoma. Microstomia and mongoloid slant of the palpebral fissures may be present.

Mosaicism for trisomy 13 has a readily recognizable phenotype of trisomy 13; however, patients with relatively fewer trisomic cells have a less diagnostic clinical appearance.

TRISOMY 18

Trisomy 18 is due to nondisjunction in approximately 80% of cases, mosaicism in 10%, translocation in 5%, and trisomy 18 plus sex chromosome aneuploidy in 5% of cases [19]. The incidence of trisomy 18 has been estimated to be between 1 in 3000 in 1 in 10,000 livebirths; most are spontaneously aborted. Of those who are liveborn, more than

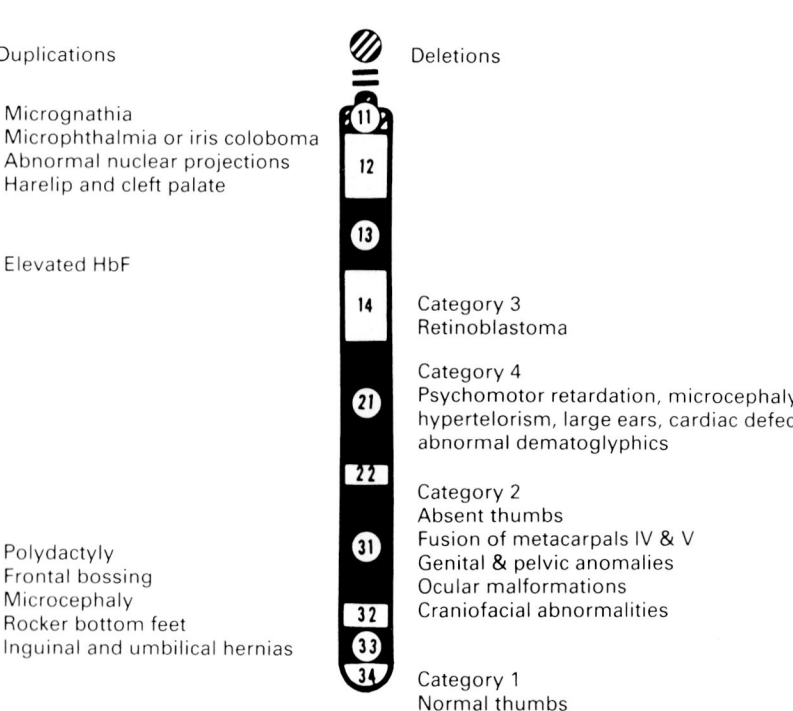

FIGURE 12.14. *Diagrammatic representation of chromosome 13, showing effects of deletions and duplications of specific segments. (From Gilbert and Opitz [35]; reprinted with permission of Masson Publishing USA, New York.)*

one-half die by 2 months, and survival beyond 1 year is rare. The female/male ratio is approximately 3:1 [95]. As in other trisomic states, there is a relationship to advanced maternal age. The spectrum of clinical and postmortem findings in trisomy 18 has been reviewed by Moerman et al [96].

A list of abnormalities noted in the trisomy 18 syndrome is shown in Table 12.8. The typical phenotype of trisomy 18 can be recognized in the second-trimester fetus (Fig. 12.15).

Prenatal growth failure is frequent. More than one-half of the cases are associated with polyhydramnios; this may be related to defective sucking and swallowing reflexes in utero. The placenta is frequently disproportionately small and may have a single umbilical artery. Some anomalies occur with equal frequency in trisomy 13 and trisomy 18. Delayed psychomotor development and severe mental retardation are constant findings. The classic phenotype is an infant with hypertonia, limited hip abduction, and flexion deformities. The head is dolichocephalic with a prominent occiput. The low-set ears have a pointed upper helix. Small palpebral fissures, small mouth, micrognathia, barrel chest with short sternum, frequently a single umbilical artery, small pelvis and camptodactyly with the index finger overlapping the middle and ring fingers, short thumb and short hallux, and rocker-bottom feet occur with high frequency. Clefts of the lip and palate are not as common as in trisomy 13. Abnormal retinal pigmentation has been described [97]. Diastasis recti, umbilical hernia, omphalocele, short and dorsiflexed hallux, and partial syndactyly between the second and third toes may be present. Dermatoglyphics show a high number of arches in the fingers.

In extensive anatomic dissections of the head and neck in the trisomy 18 syndrome, Ramirez-Castro and Bersu [98] have described hypoplasia of the muscles of facial expression, fusion of the muscles around the corners of the mouth, and a supernumerary muscle band that extends from the corner of the mouth to the occipital attachment of the trapezius. The otomandibular region shows a variable spectrum of muscular, skeletal, arterial, and salivary gland variations.

A congenital cardiac defect is an almost constant feature of trisomy 18 [99]. The atrioventricular and semilunar valves of the heart are dysplastic, with vacuolar and lacunar degeneration of the spongiosa and a lack of elastic tissue in the proximalis and the spongiosa layers. The valves have a gelatinous nodular appearance with obliterated interchordal spaces and hyperplastic papillary muscles (Fig. 12.16). This has been a consistent finding in our cases [100]. These valvular lesions are reminiscent of the normal fetal appearance of valves at about 4 months of gestation and suggest failure of maturation of the loose myxoid mesenchyme of the valvular anlagen. Endocardial fibroelastosis [101] and diffuse myocardial fibrosis [102] have also been described.

CNS abnormalities have not been consistent but have included abnormal gyri, parietal lobe defects, absent corpus

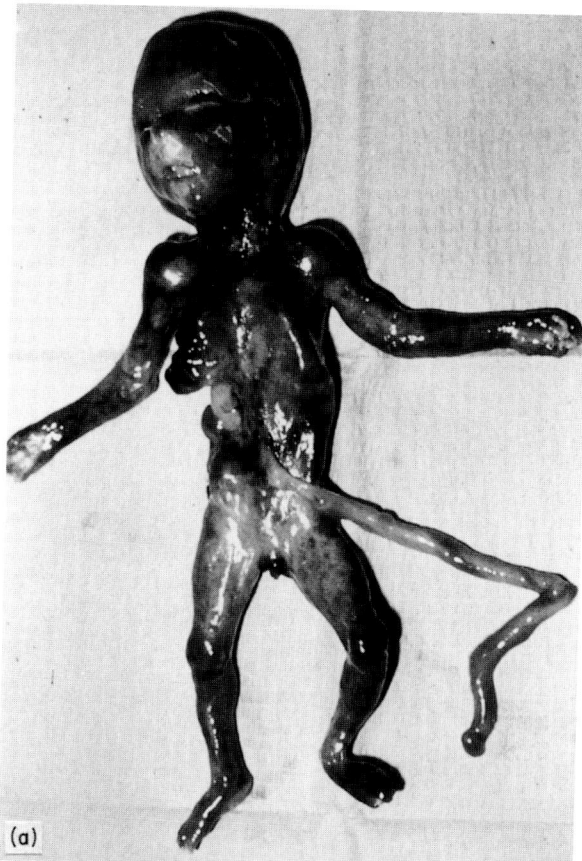

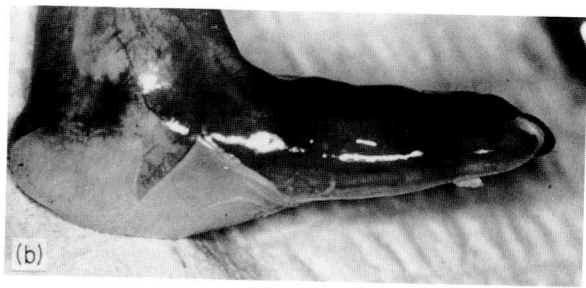

FIGURE 12.15. *(a) Fourteen-week fetus, showing typical phenotype of trisomy 18. (b) Rocker-bottom feet.*

callosum, cerebellar abnormalities, hydrocephalus, and meningomyelocele [20]. Holoprosencephaly and anencephaly [103] have been observed.

Malformations of the genitourinary tract are frequent and are found in approximately 75% of cases; horseshoe kidneys are present in 25%. Duplication of ureters and/or kidney, hydroureters, hydronephrosis, cystic dysplastic kidneys and renal hypoplasia, unilateral aplasia, or agenesis may be present. Cryptorchidism and hypospadias are frequent in males. Nests of undifferentiated metanephric blastema resembling minute foci of Wilms' tumor and overt Wilms' tumor have been reported [104].

Table 12.8.   Abnormalities observed in trisomy 18

Craniofacial abnormalities	Syndactyly of 2nd and 3rd digits
Dolichocephaly	Postaxial hexadactyly
Protuberant occiput	Lobster-claw anomaly
Small bitemporal diameter	Phocomelia
Microencephaly	Partial cutaneous syndactyly of toes
Wide fontanelles	Arthrogryposis
Slender bridge of nose	**Dermatoglyphics**
Nares upturned	Low arch pattern on fingers
Palpebral fissures horizontal	Absent distal flexion crease of fingers
Epicanthal folds	Single transverse palmar crease (simian line)
Hypertelorism	Distal axial triradius
Microstomia	Tetralogy of Fallot
Micrognathia	Eisenmenger's complex
Cleft lip/cleft palate (rare)	Dextrocardia
Ears low set and "fawnlike"—pinna flat—upper	Dextroversion
portions pointed	Hypoplastic left atrium
Atresia of external auditory canal (rare)	Parachute mitral valve
Patent metopic suture	Abnormal coronary arteries
Thorax and abdomen malformations	Diffuse myocardial fibrosis
Short webbed neck	Endocardial fibroelastosis
Short sternum	Double inferior vena cava
Small nipples	**Central nervous system malformations**
Umbilical and inguinal herniae	Meningomyelocele
Diastasis recti	Cerebellar anomalies
Narrow pelvis	Abnormal gyri
Marked lanugo at birth	Hydrocephalus
Pilonidal sinus	Arnold-Chiari malformation
Limb malformations	**Visceral malformations**
Hyperflexed position	Abnormal lobation of lung
Clenched fists	Tracheoesophageal fistula
Index finger overlaps 3rd finger and 5th finger	Esophageal atresia
overlaps 4th finger	Meckel's diverticulum
Camptodactyly	Heterotopic pancreas or spleen
Clinodactyly	Pyloric stenosis
Hypoplastic hyperconvex nails	Omphalocele
Limitation of thigh abduction	Malrotation of intestine
Congenital dislocation of hips	Common mesentery
Radial hypoplasia or aplasia	Hypoplasia of diaphragm
Thumb aplasia	Extrophy of cloaca
Thumb duplication	Anomalies of pancreas
Rocker-bottom feet	Adrenal hypoplasia
Big toe short and dorsiflexed	Thymic hypoplasia
Absent 12th ribs	Thyroid hypoplasia

THE 18Q–(DUP(18Q)) SYNDROME

Most cases of dup(18q) have a specific duplicated chromosome segment, 18q21, and most of these cases have had the major features of full trisomy 18. This suggests that the 18q21 segment is responsible for the major stigmata of the trisomy 18 phenotype.

The phenotype includes a carp-shaped mouth, maxillary hypoplasia, hypoplastic ears, upper epicanthic folds, short palpebral fissures, congenital cataracts, maleruption and malocclusion of the teeth, micrognathia, camptodactyly,

abnormal dermatoglyphics, rocker-bottom feet, crowding of toes, and congenital cardiac defects including double outlet right ventricle, ventricular septal defect, patent foramen ovale, and pulmonary artery stenosis. The brain may have a striking resemblance to that seen in Down syndrome (Fig. 12.17).

THE 18Q–(DEL(18Q)) SYNDROME

This syndrome is associated with severe mental and somatic growth retardation and multiple congenital anomalies.

Table 12.8.   *Continued*

Diaphragmatic hernia	Patent ductus arteriosus
Ectopic pancreas in duodenal wall	Pulmonic stenosis/bicuspid valve
Imperforate anus	Bicuspid aortic valve
Accessory spleens	Atrial septal defect
Umbilical and inguinal herniae	Dysplastic valves
Genitourinary malformations	Coarctation of aorta
Horseshoe kidney	Double outlet right ventricle
Ectopic kidney	Hypoplastic left heart
Hydronephrosis	Abnormal coronary artery
Megaloureter or double ureter	Persistent left superior vena cava
Micromulticystic kidneys	Absent right superior vena cava
Severe hypoplasia of kidneys	Transposition, great arteries
Bilateral duplication of ureters and pelvis	Corpus callosum defects
Urethral atresia	Holoprosencephaly
Megacystis	Frontal lobe defect
Patent urachus	Migration defect
Male:	Anencephaly
cryptorchidism	**Ocular malformations (rare)**
Female:	Abnormal retinal pigmentation
vaginal agenesis (rare)	Cataract
hypotrophy of clitoris	Coloboma
hypoplasia of labia majora	Clouding of corneae
bifid uterus	Microphthalmia
ovarian hypoplasia	**Placental abnormalities**
streak ovaries (rare)	Polyhydramnios
Cardiovascular malformations	Small placenta with multiple infarcts (postmature)
Ventricular septal defect (with or without	Single umbilical artery
overriding aorta)	

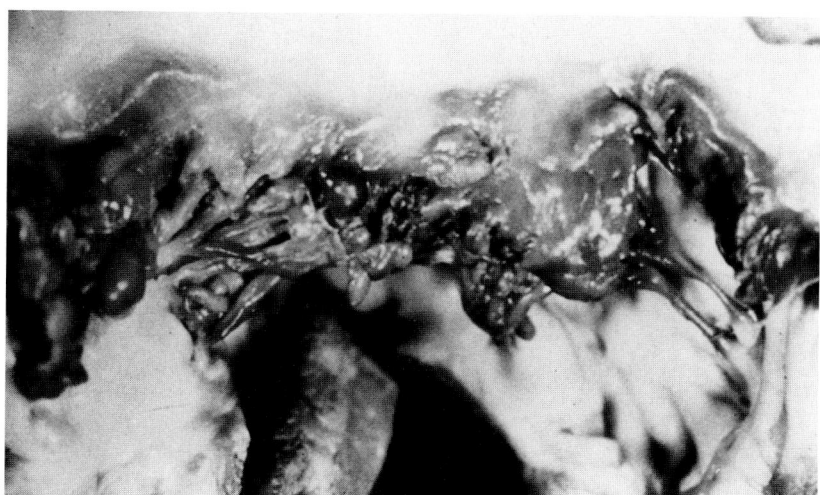

FIGURE 12.16.   *Appearance of heart valves in trisomy 18. The mitral valve is thickened and gelatinous. (From Gilbert and Opitz [35]; reprinted with permission of Masson Publishing USA, New York.)*

Hypotonia and seizures are frequent. Skin dimples may be present over the subacromion and epitrochlear areas, lateral to the patellae, and over the metacarpophalangeal joints. Subcutaneous nodules may be present on the cheeks at the usual site of the dimples. The fingers are long and tapering, and supernumerary ribs may be present. Cardiovascular anomalies, principally ventricular septal defects, are frequent.

Hypogenitalism is usually present in both sexes. Craniofacial anomalies include midfacial hypoplasia and microcephaly with deep-set eyes, often with ophthalmologic defects, carp-shaped mouth, short nose, and abnormal ears, and frequently with atresia of external auditory canals. Cleft lip and/or cleft palate is present in 40% of cases [20]. Low serum levels of immunoglobulin A have been reported

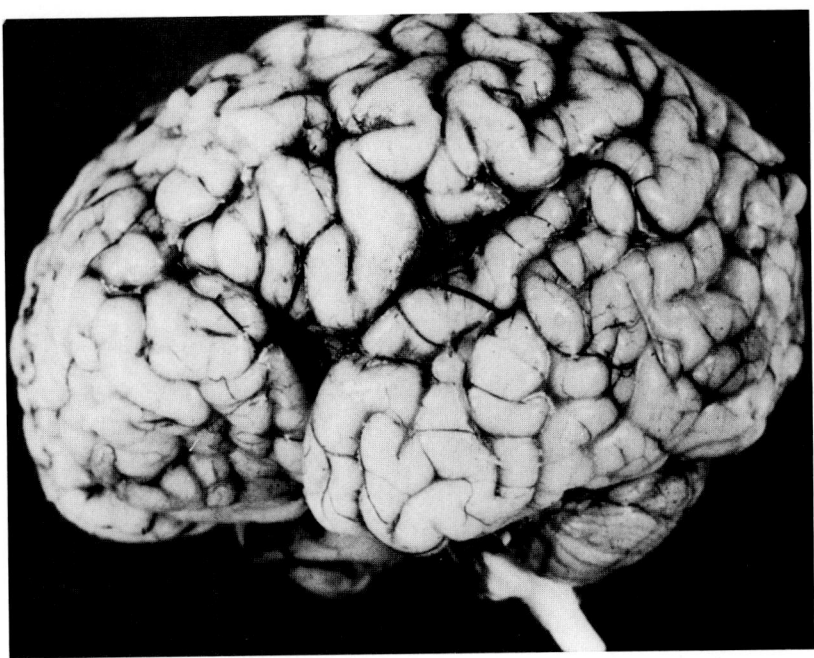

FIGURE 12.17. *Brain in dup(18q). Note similarity to Down syndrome—brachycephaly with open operculum and hypoplastic superior temporal gyrus. (From Gilbert and Opitz [35]; reprinted with permission of Masson Publishing USA, New York.)*

[105]. Dermatoglyphic characteristics include fingerprint whorls exceeding five in number and a high frequency of large composite patterns [106].

Cryptorchidism and hypospadias may be present in the male, and horseshoe kidney has been reported [105] as well as bilateral cortical nephrogenic rests [35] (Fig. 12.18). This has also been noted in partial dup(20p) [107, 108]. Additional abnormalities that we have observed in four cases have included intrauterine growth retardation, micrognathia, depressed nasal bridge, macrostomia, highly arched palate, puffy lower eyelids with semilunar-shaped palpebral fissures, minimal mongoloid slant of the palpebral fissures, extremely well-developed dermal ridges, rocker-bottom feet, umbilical hernia, and a very short perineal body [35]. One of our cases had papillary thyroid carcinoma with lymph node metastases at 9 years.

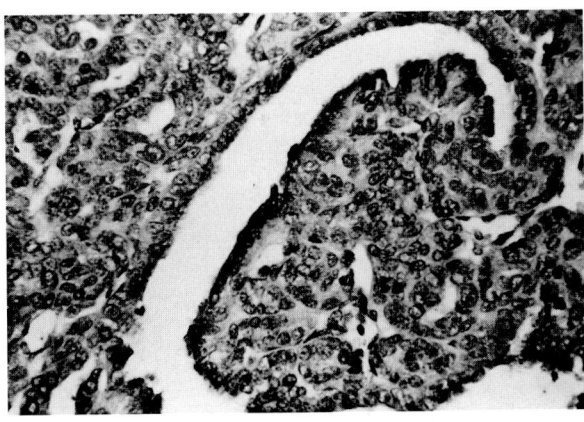

FIGURE 12.18. *Microscopic section of kidney in dup(18q), showing cortical nephroblastomatosis. H&E, ×100.*

THE 18P–(DEL(18P)) SYNDROME

Deletion of the short arm of chromosome 18 is associated with mental retardation of variable degree. It has a 2:1 male/female sex ratio. Birth weight is low, somatic growth is retarded, and the ears are apparently low-set, large, floppy, and poorly formed. Hypotonia, hypertelorism, short neck, ptosis, micrognathia, epicanthic folds, pterygium colli, and microcephaly are frequent, and there may be striking resemblance to Ullrich-Turner and Noonan syndromes [19]. Short fingers and alopecia are observed less frequently. Variable degrees of holoprosencephaly, including cyclopia and agenesis of the corpus callosum, have been described [109–112]. We have observed early onset of extremely severe rheumatoid arthritis in one patient.

THE 4P–(DEL(4P)) SYNDROME (WOLF-HIRSCHHORN SYNDROME)

This syndrome is characterized by severe psychomotor and growth retardation, low birth weight, diminished fetal activity, hypotonia, and seizures. One-third die during the first year of life [21]. The oldest reported cases have been 24 years of age [113, 114]. The clinical features (Fig. 12.19) include microcephaly, cleft lip and/or cleft palate, and micrognathia, and large low-set ears are noted frequently [115]. Abnormalities that have been described are listed in Table 12.9. Hemangioma on the brow, prominent glabella, ocular hypertelorism, divergent strabismus, eyelid ptosis, antimongoloid

Table 12.9. Abnormalities observed in the 4p⁻ (Wolf-Hirschhorn) syndrome

Craniofacial abnormalities
Frontal bossing
High frontal hairline
Hemangioma over forehead or glabella
Proptosis due to hypoplasia of orbital ridges
Hypertelorism
Upslanting palpebral fissures
Ptosis
Exotropia and ectopic pupils
Broad and beaked nose
Prominent bridge of nose and shallow septum
Stenosis or atresia of nasolacrimal ducts
Short, prominent philtrum
Downturned corners of mouth
Small mandible
Large, floppy, misshapen ears
Scalp defect with or without underlying bone defect
Long, slender fingers with additional flexion creases
Trunk and skeletal malformations
Long, narrow chest
Hypoplastic and widely shaped nipples
Diastasis recti
Sacral sinus
Umbilical or inguinal herniae
Hypoplasia or duplication of thumbs
Hypoplasia or duplication of big toes
Hypoplasia of pubic bones
Abnormalities of vertebrae and ribs
Defective calcification of calvaria
Osteoporosis
Delay in bone maturation
Genitourinary malformations
Hypoplastic kidneys
Cystic dysplastic kidneys
Unilateral agenesis of kidney
Hydronephrosis
Extrophy of bladder
Large clitoris in females

Hypoplastic external genitalia in males
Uterine hypoplasia
Bicornuate or unicornuate uterus
Agenesis of vagina, cervix, or uterus
Ovarian streaks
Cryptorchidism and hypospadias
Cardiovascular malformations
Persistent left superior vena cava
Abnormalities of valves
Complex defects
Central nervous system malformations
Hypoplasia of cerebellum
Cavum septi pellucidi
Hypoplasia or aplasia of corpus callosum
Hypoplasia or absence of olfactory bulbs and tracts
Microgyria
Migration defects
Hydrocephalus
Ocular malformations
Colobomata
Microphthalmia
Megalo- or sclerocornea
Cataract
Hypoplastic anterior chamber
Hypoplastic ciliary body of iris
Persistence of lenticular membrane
Hypoplastic retina with formation of rosettes
Cup-shaped optic discs
Congenital nystagmus
Rieger's anomaly
Dermatoglyphics
Hypoplastic dermal ridges ("laundress hands")
Internal malformations
Accessory spleens
Abnormal shape of pancreas
Absence of gallbladder
Abnormal lung lobations

obliquity of the palpebral fissures, and iris coloboma are seen occasionally. Cryptorchidism and hypospadias may occur in males, and absent uterus and streak gonads may occur in females [116]. Congenital heart malformations [117], simian palmar creases, dermal ridges, and hypoplastic fingers are frequently present [118]. If deletion occurs in both arms of the chromosome, a ring chromosome is produced. Advanced parental age has been observed [19].

THE 5P–(DEL(5P)) SYNDROME (CRI DU CHAT OR CAT-CRY SYNDROME)

This is probably the most frequent autosomal deletion syndrome in humans and has an estimated incidence of 1 in 50,000 and a prevalence among mentally retarded of 1.5 in

1000. The syndrome was reviewed thoroughly by Schinzel [21, 119]. Table 12.10 lists the abnormalities that may be noted.

The cat-cry syndrome is characterized by a kitten-like, weak cry in infancy caused by hypoplasia of the larynx. Balanced translocation in a parent accounts for 10–15% of cases [120]. The characteristic cry usually disappears with time, even within a few weeks of age. There is usually severe growth and mental retardation (IQ less than 35), failure to thrive, and hypotonia in infancy. The head is microcephalic and the face is round; hypertelorism, antimongoloid obliquity of palpebral fissures, epicanthal folds, bilateral alternating strabismus, broad nasal bones, and low-set ears comprise the typical phenotype (Fig. 12.20). Preauricular tags are occasionally noted. Most patients have mild micrognathia. In

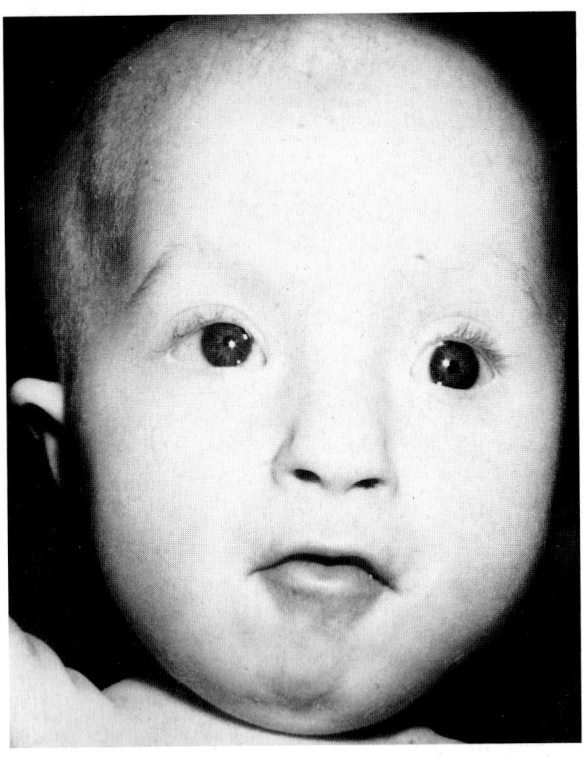

FIGURE 12.19.   *Wolf-Hirschhorn syndrome—del(4p). Typical facial appearance with hypertelorism. (From Gilbert and Opitz [35]; reprinted with permission of Masson Publishing USA, New York.)*

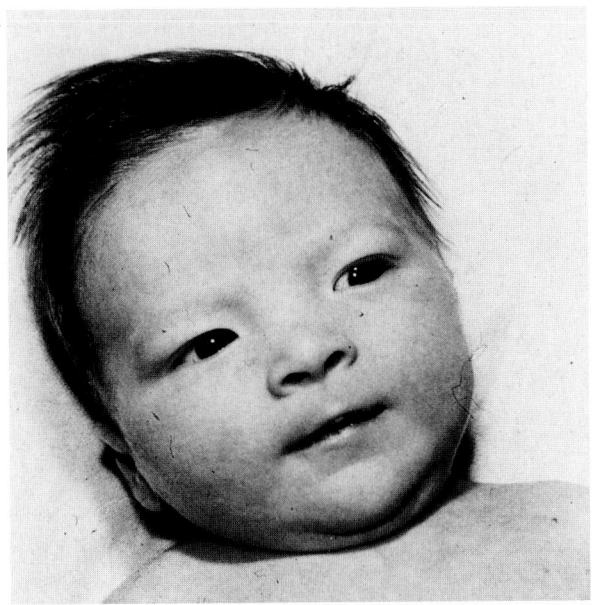

FIGURE 12.20.   *Cri du chat syndrome—del(5p). Typical oval face with hypertelorism and antimongoloid slant of palpebral fissures. (From Gilbert and Opitz [35]; reprinted with permission of Masson Publishing USA, New York.)*

Table 12.10.   Abnormalities observed in the 5p⁻ (cat-cry) syndrome

At birth
Growth retardation
Microcephaly
Mewing cry
Full cheeks, round face
Depressed nasal bridge
Inner epicanthal folds
Downward slant of palpebral fissures
Short fingers
Clinodactyly of little fingers
Talipes equinovarus
Cleft palate
Preauricular fistulas
Hypospadias
Cryptorchidism
Syndactyly of 2/3 toes and fingers
Oligosyndactyly
Malrotation of gut
Thymic dysplasia
Childhood
Small, narrow, often asymmetric face
Malocclusion
Scoliosis
Graying of hair
Muscle tone normal or increased
Shortness of metacarpals 3–5

time, the roundness of the face and the ocular hypertelorism disappear and the face becomes thin and the philtrum short. Premature graying of the hair has been noted in about 30% of cases. Oligosyndactyly malrotation and thymic dysplasia have been noted in more severe cases [121]. Although females menstruate and develop normal secondary sex characteristics, none have so far reproduced. Dental malocclusion is commonly present. Musculoskeletal anomalies include flat feet, mild scoliosis, large frontal sinuses, small ilia, syndactyly, and short metacarpals and metatarsals [122, 123]. Simian creases occur in 35%, 50% have thenar patterns, and distal axial triradii and deficiency of ulnar loops are frequent [124].

TRISOMY 8

Complete trisomy 8 (Fig. 12.21) is usually lethal; normal/trisomy 8 mosaicism is more common. Trisomy 8 mosaicism may vary from a phenotypically normal individual to a severe malformation syndrome (Warkany syndrome). Mental retardation is frequent and varies from mild to severe, although some have normal intelligence [125–129]. Abnormalities that have been noted are listed in Table 12.11.

The phenotype of trisomy 8 mosaicism includes an abnormally shaped skull, reduced joint mobility, various vertebral anomalies, supernumerary ribs, strabismus, absent patellae, short neck, long slender trunk, cleft palate, and deep palmar and plantar creases. Plantar creases are highly characteristic of the syndrome. However, it should be noted that deep palmar and plantar creases also have been seen in a

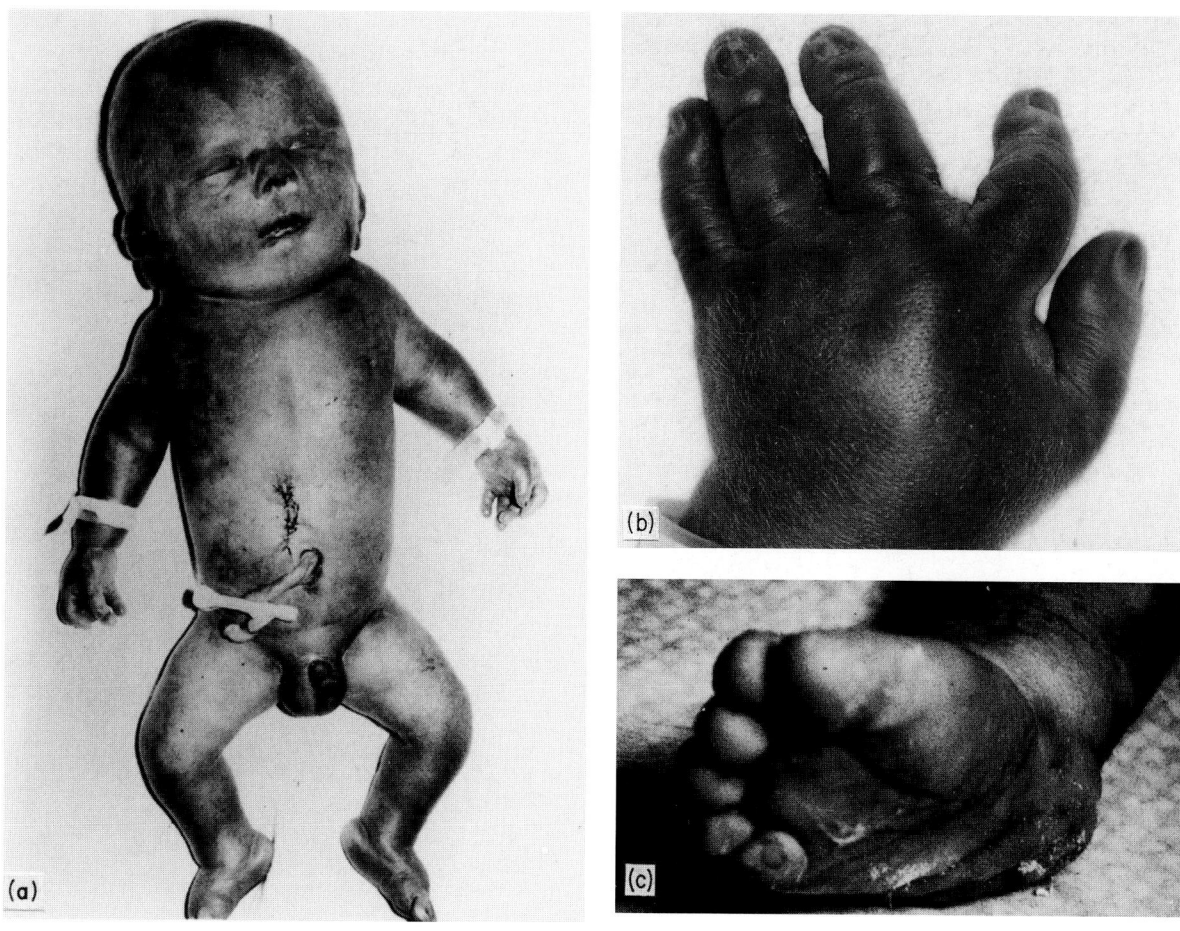

FIGURE 12.21. *Complete trisomy 8 in liveborn infant who died shortly after birth: (a) phenotypic appearance with lymphedema and multiple anomalies; (b) hand is broad, with short and malformed fingers; (c) foot with deep plantar furrow and malpositioned toes. (From Gilbert and Opitz [35]; reprinted with permission of Masson Publishing USA, New York.)*

patient with 6p− syndrome [130] and in two with duplication of the long arm of chromosome 10 [131]. A few have exhibited agenesis of the corpus callosum.

Cardiac defects include ventricular septal defect, patent ductus arteriosus, and cor triatriatum; digital abnormalities of both feet also have been observed [35].

In 75% of these cases, severe ureteral and renal anomalies occurred, predominantly obstructive uropathy with hydronephrosis and secondary chronic pyelonephritis [132, 133].

Dermatoglyphic patterns include a low total ridge count and increased number of arches, distal palmar triradius, and a single palmar crease. Partial factor 7 deficiency has been reported [134]. Skeletal malformations may include supernumerary skeletal and lumbar vertebrae, supernumerary ribs, small pelvic bones, absent patellae, vertebral dysplasia, "locked" vertebrae, hemivertebrae, and spina bifida.

Localization of the gene for glutathione reductase on chromosome 8 bears diagnostic importance in patients with trisomy 8 in whom high levels of the enzyme have been

detected [135]. Apparently complete trisomy 8 demonstrated in all cultures from skin fibroblasts, bone marrow, and peripheral lymphocytes rarely occurs [35]. We have observed an infant with complete trisomy 8. Abnormalities included generalized lymphedema, brachycephalic skull, antimongoloid slant of eyes, flat nasal bridge, ankylosis of the tongue, hypertelorism, epicanthic folds, cleft palate micrognathia, abnormally shaped ears, bilateral camptodactyly, shield chest, shortened neck, sacral dimple, hypospadias, deep furrows on the soles of the feet, truncus arteriosus with a supracristal ventricular septal defect, aplasia of the left diaphragm, hypoplasia of the left lung, and posterior urethral valves causing urinary obstruction with bilateral hydronephrosis and hydroureters.

Trisomy 8 cell lines have been found in the bone marrow of patients with various hematologic disorders, such as acute and chronic myeloid leukemia, myelosclerosis, and sideroachrestic anemia with polycythemia [136–138]. Trisomy 8 is not found in blood lymphocytes and cultured skin fibroblasts under these conditions, and disappears from

Table 12.11. Trisomy 8 mosaicism

Skeletal malformations	Downslanting palpebral fissures
Hemivertebrae	**Trunk malformations**
Extra vertebrae	Narrow pelvis
"Butterfly" vertebrae	Trunk long and slender
Spina bifida occulta	**Limb malformations**
Broad dorsal ribs	Clinodactyly
Narrow and hypoplastic iliac wings	Deep skin furrows on soles and/or palms
Absent patellae	Camptodactyly
Kyphoscoliosis	Syndactyly of toes
Pectus carinatum	**Genitourinary malformations**
Radioulnar synostosis	Hydronephrosis
Growth normal or advanced	Ureteral obstruction
Ocular malformations	Horseshoe kidney
Microphthalmia	Unilateral agenesis of kidney
Iridal coloboma	Cryptorchidism
Glaucoma	Testicular hypoplasia
Corneal or lenticular opacities	Hypospadias
Craniofacial anomalies	**Cardiovascular malformations**
Scaphocephaly	Interrupted aortic arch
Abnormal ears	**Gastrointestinal malformations**
Hypertelorism	Diaphragmatic hernia
Strabismus	Esophageal atresia
Broad-bridged, upturned nose	Malrotation or absence of gallbladder
Thick, everted lower lip	**Central nervous system malformations**
Micrognathia	Hydrocephalus
High-arched palate	Agenesis of corpus callosum
Coarse, pear-shaped nose	Large sella turcica

the marrow cells during remission of these hematologic disorders.

RECOMBINANT CHROMOSOME 8 SYNDROME (RC8S)

RC8S is an inherited chromosome abnormality associated with multiple congenital anomalies and has been described in 33 large kindreds in several western states [139]. All the kindreds have been of Hispanic origin. It has also been described in an Argentinian child [140]. The partial trisomy is caused by a recombinant chromosome 8 with duplication of the long arm and, probably, deletion of a very small portion of the distal end of the short arm: rec(8), dur q, inv(8) (p23q22). The abnormal chromosome results from the unequal meiotic recombination in the gamete cells of a parent who is heterozygous for a specific pericentric inversion of chromosome 8: inv(8) (p23q22).

Developmental delay and mental retardation become evident soon after birth. Facial abnormalities include hypertelorism, short prominent philtrum, hirsutism, broad square face, low frontal hairline, brachycephaly, short thick neck, long palpebral fissures, anteverted nostrils, high nasal bridge, square ear lobules, camptodactyly of fifth fingers, arch dermal pattern on five or more digits, and deep plantar furrows. Internal malformations include a high incidence of

congenital cardiac and genitourinary defects. Cardiac anomalies include ventricular septal defect, atrial septal defect, patent ductus arteriosus, tetralogy of Fallot, pulmonary atresia and stenosis, and persistent left superior vena cava. Genitourinary abnormalities include bilateral ureterovesical obstruction, double collecting system, cystic kidneys, hypoplastic ureters, hydronephrosis, dysplastic kidneys, and cryptorchidism in males.

TRISOMY 9

The first living infant with probable full trisomy 9 was reported by Juberg et al [141]; the infant had craniofacial anomalies, microcephaly, flat nasal bridge, epicanthal folds, micrognathia, apparently low-set ears, and a cleft palate. Bilateral cystic dysplastic kidneys were observed with atresia of the proximal ureters and a rudimentary atretic urinary bladder. A similar case reported by Blair [142] shared a number of external and visceral anomalies and, in addition, had hepatic and pancreatic dysplasia as well as cystic dysplastic kidneys and atretic ureters. These cases were recorded before Giemsa banding studies were available, but the phenotype of these cases is consistent with trisomy 9. Additional cases have been reported [143–148]. Table 12.12 lists the abnormalities that have been noted in trisomy 9.

Complex congenital cardiac defects occur in two-thirds of the cases, renal malformations in about one-half, and brain defects, particularly cystic dilatation of the fourth ventricle with lack of midline fusion of the cerebellum, in two-thirds of cases. Less frequent anomalies include microphthalmia, corneal opacities, coloboma of the iris, absence of corpus callosum, cleft lip and/or palate, abnormal lobation of lungs, malrotation of the large bowel, imperforate anus, and vertebral anomalies.

Trisomy 9 Mosaicism Syndrome

This syndrome was first reported by Haslam et al [147]. It is associated with joint contractures, congenital cardiac defects, apparently low-set malformed ears, sloping forehead, deeply set eyes, and micrognathia. Genitourinary abnormalities have included micropenis, cryptorchidism, bladder diverticulum, double ureters, and microscopic renal cysts [149].

THE 11P–(DEL(11P)) SYNDROME

The triad of aniridia, ambiguous genitalia, and mental retardation (AGR triad) comprises the clinical characteristics of interstitial 11 short-arm deletion, del(11p) (Fig. 12.22), which has been delineated clearly by Riccardi et al [150]. One-third of these patients have Wilms' tumor. There is phenotypic variability. Facial characteristics include prominent nasal bridge, eversion of the lower lip, prominent forehead, cranial asymmetry, highly arched narrow palate, short neck, simplified pinnae, and ptosis. Additional eye abnormalities

Table 12.12.   Phenotype of trisomy 9 (12 cases)

Frequent anomalies	Deeply furrowed or simian crease
Microcephaly	Hypoplastic/hyperconvex nails
Low-set and malformed ears	Hypoplastic/absent phalanges or metacarpal bones
Micrognathia	Rocker-bottom feet
Broad nose with bulbous tip	Talipes calcaneovalgus
Abnormal brain	Longitudinal sole crease
Congenital heart disease	Short humerus and femur
Abnormal hands/feet	Folded helix, prominent antihelix, posterior rotation
Dislocation of joints: elbow/knee/hip	Brachycephaly
Cryptorchidism	Hydrocephalus
Micropenis	Pouched cheek
Growth failure, psychomotor retardation, and/or early death	Low-pitched cry
Less frequent anomalies	Long philtrum
Dolichocephaly	Long trunk
Third fontanelle present	Narrow chest
Narrow temples	13 ribs
Occipital bossing	S-shaped upper lip
Facial asymmetry	Short xiphoid
Enophthalmos	Hyposegmented lungs
Small palpebral fissure	Malrotation of large bowel
Hypotonia	Posterior urethral valves
Epicanthic folds	Cholestasis
Mongoloid slant	Absent 5th sacral segment
Hypertelorism	Absent tarsal/calcaneal bone
Hypotelorism	Inguinal hernia
High-arched palate	Ectopic adrenal tissue on testis
Cleft lip/palate	Single umbilical artery
Small mouth	**Central nervous system defects**
Thin upper lip	Large 4th ventricle
Prominent maxilla	Nonfusion of cerebellum
Low hairline	Hypoplastic temporal lobes
Loose, webbed, or short neck	Wide cranial sutures
Shield chest	Leucomalacia
Widely spaced nipples	**Cardiac defects**
Umbilical hernia	Dextroposition
Kyphosis/scoliosis	Aorta from right ventricle
Renal cysts	Persistent left superior vena cava
Hydronephrosis	Ventricular septal defect
Absent pubic bone	Atrial septal defect
Absent/hypoplastic tibia/fibula	Patent ductus arteriosus
Abnormal/absent toes	Coarctation
Hypoplastic scrotum	Pulmonic/tricuspid valve dysplasia or atresia
Rare anomalies	
Malformed/overlapping fingers	

include poor vision, nystagmus, glaucoma, pale fundus or optic disc, and cataracts. Dermatoglyphic findings have included helical open field patterns and digital radial loops. When this syndrome is associated with Wilms' tumor, the age of appearance of the tumor has averaged 18 months, whereas isolated Wilms' tumor occurs between 3 and 5 years.

In the United Kingdom, aniridia was found in 1 in 43 cases of Wilms' tumor patients; bilateral tumors were present in 36% (in Wilms' tumor without aniridia, only one had bilateral tumors). The presence of a del(11)(p13) indicates a high risk for the development of Wilms' tumor [151]. Recently, Riccardi et al [152] reported on Wilms' tumor with sporadic aniridia and normal chromosomes. The evaluation, follow-up, and ultimate prognosis of del(11p) patients remains to be clarified. We have observed disorganization of the renal parenchyma in the del(11p) syndrome with a Wilms' tumor that occupied the medulla of the kidney in contradistinction to the usual cortical origin of Wilms' tumor.

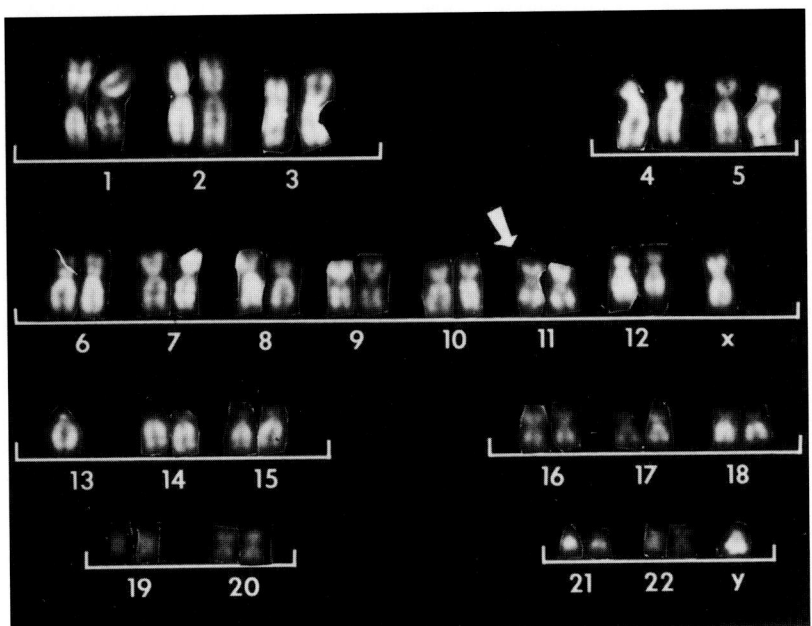

FIGURE 12.22.   *Karyotype of del(11p).*

Yunis and Ramsey [153] have contributed considerably to the expanding knowledge of the aniridia–Wilms' tumor association. In their study, a woman had a balanced interstitial translocation from the short arm of chromosome 11 to the long arm of chromosome 2; familial Wilms' tumor–aniridia syndrome occurred in three first-degree relatives.

Two patients with Wilms' tumor and iris dysplasia, with normal chromosomes and no gene loss demonstrable by enzyme markers and direct DNA analyses, have been reported [152]; these findings have suggested that aniridia defines a risk for Wilms' tumor even in the absence of del(11)(p13). It has not yet been determined whether patients with Wilms' tumor and aniridia exhibit subcapsular nephroblastomatosis, as found in children with the hereditary form of Wilms' tumor [154].

THE 17P–(DEL(17P))
MILLER-DIEKER SYNDROME

Miller-Dieker syndrome (MDS, lissencephaly type I) [155] is characterized by minor facial anomalies, occasional hirsutism, clouding of corneae, polydactyly, variable malformations of other organs, and severe brain anomalies, including lissencephaly with only four instead of six cortical layers [156–167].

Congenital heart disease, agenesis of one kidney [163], fetal lobulation, and cystic kidneys [157, 162] have been described in MDS. In two of four cases reported by Van Allen and Clarren [167], renal abnormalities were noted that included bilateral double collecting systems, hydronephrosis, and abnormal calyceal patterns.

By high-resolution chromosome analyses, Dobyns et al [155] have found abnormalities of chromosome 17 in two of three unrelated patients with MDS, one with a ring chromosome 17 and the other with an unbalanced translocation resulting in partial monosomy of 17p13. In addition, abnormalities of chromosome 17 have been found in all previously reported families in which two or more children had MDS. The abnormality is restricted to chromosome 17 (rings or deletions) or unbalanced translocations resulting in partial deletion of 17p in addition to duplication of some other autosomal segment. Two patients reported by Dobyns et al [158] had normal chromosomes. He has suspected that there may be submicroscopic deletions of 17p in these cases. A second aneuploidy syndrome involving deletion of 17p is being recognized, this one involving an interstitial deletion closer to the centromere. Clinically, however, this is quite a different syndrome. The diagnosis can be made in cases with deletions by fluorescent in situ hybridization (FISH) microscopy.

ISODICENTRIC 22(PTER-Q11)
CAT-EYE SYNDROME
(SCHMID-FRACCARO SYNDROME)

More than 30 cases of this syndrome have been recorded [168]. The extra chromosome probably is an isodicentric (22) (pter-q11).

Clinical features vary greatly (Table 12.13). Mild cases of trisomy 22 may have almost normal intelligence. Familial occurrence is more frequent in trisomy 22 than in other trisomies. In milder forms of this disorder, reproduction has occurred, allowing for a dominant mode of inheritance

Table 12.13. Clinical features of trisomy 22 (Schmid-Fraccaro or cat-eye syndrome)

Mental retardation
Antimongoloid slant of palpebral fissures
Cleft palate
Anal atresia
Iris coloboma
Microphthalmia
Preauricular appendages and fistulae
Congenital heart defects
Congenital hip dislocation
Deafness
Renal aplasia
Hydronephrosis
Anal atresia with fistula
Finger-like thumb
Rare malformations:
malrotation of gut
biliary atresia
microphthalmia
reduction of external ear
atresia of external auditory canal

[169]. An extra-small G-like chromosome that appears to be an isochromosome for the juxtacentromeric region of an acrocentric chromosome has been found [168].

Characteristic features are ocular coloboma, which can involve the iris, choroid, and/or optic nerve; preauricular skin tags and/or pits, which are probably the most consistent abnormality; congenital heart defects; anal atresia with a fistula; renal malformations, such as unilateral absence, unilateral or bilateral hypoplasia, and cystic dysplasia; and antimongoloid slant of palpebral fissures. Intelligence is usually low to normal, although moderate retardation is also reported. There is great variability in the clinical findings, ranging from near-normal to lethal malformations. Less frequent, but also characteristic, findings are microphthalmia, microtia with atresia of the external auditory canal, intrahepatic or extrahepatic biliary atresia and malrotation of the gut, cerebellar hypoplasia, and cyanotic heart defect.

G DELETION SYNDROMES

The 21q–(del(21q)) Syndrome

In patients with 21q– syndrome, there is hypertonia, antimongoloid slant, prominent nasal bridge, wide external ear canals, highly arched or cleft lip/palate, and micrognathia; mental retardation is usually severe. Other malformations include nail and skeletal anomalies, cryptorchidism, hypospadias, inguinal hernia, pyloric stenosis, thrombocytopenia, eosinophilia, and hypogammaglobulinemia [170, 171]. Dermatoglyphic analyses have shown a marked increase in radial loops [172].

The 22q–(del(22q)) Syndrome

The features of the 22q– syndrome are not distinctive and consist of severe mental retardation, muscular hypotonia, microcephaly, epicanthic folds, ptosis, flat nasal bridge, large apparently low-set ears, highly arched palate, syndactyly of toes, and bifid uvula. Dermatoglyphic analyses have shown a marked increase in furrows, a decrease in ulnar and radial loops, a distal axial triradius, and hypothenar patterns and increased leucocyte alkaline phosphatase [173].

TRIPLOIDY

Triploidy is one of the most frequent chromosome aberrations in first-trimester abortions [174].

Table 12.14. Clinical features of triploidy

Maternal
Midtrimester pre-eclampsia
Polyhydramnios
Proteinuria, hypertension
Infant
Prenatal growth failure
Large posterior fontanelle
Hydrocephalus
Arnold-Chiari malformation
Meningomyelocele
Holoprosencephaly
Hypoplasia of basal ganglia, cerebellum, and occipital lobe
Iris coloboma, microphthalmia
Malformed ears
Large, bulbous nose
Incomplete ossification of calvarium
Congenital heart lesions
Abnormal lobation of lungs
Adrenal hypoplasia
Aplasia of gallbladder
Renal hypoplasia and cysts
Hypospadias
Cryptorchidism, Leydig's cell hyperplasia
Syndactyly between 3rd and 4th fingers
Simian crease
Talipes equinovarus
Aplasia of corpus callosum
Lumbosacral myelomeningocele
Cleft lip and cleft palate
Malrotation of colon
Hydronephrosis
Micropenis, bifid scrotum
Hypoplasia of ovaries
Proximal displacement of thumbs
Placenta
Partial hydatidiform mole
Mild trophoblastic proliferation
Large villi with scalloping
Large cisternae within villi
Trophoblastic inclusions

The extra haploid set of chromosomes is the result of double fertilization of the ovum (diandry) or failure of the ovum to extrude a polar body (digyny). By studying fetal and parental heteromorphisms, Jacobs and Morton [175] and Jacobs et al [12] have concluded that 66% of triploids are the result of dispermy, 24% the result of fertilization of a haploid ovum by a diploid sperm resulting from failure of the first meiotic division in the male, and 10% the result of a diploid egg resulting from failure of the first maternal meiotic division. Most triploidies are aborted. If liveborn, death occurs within a few hours after birth; however, one XXX triploidy infant lived for 26 days [19].

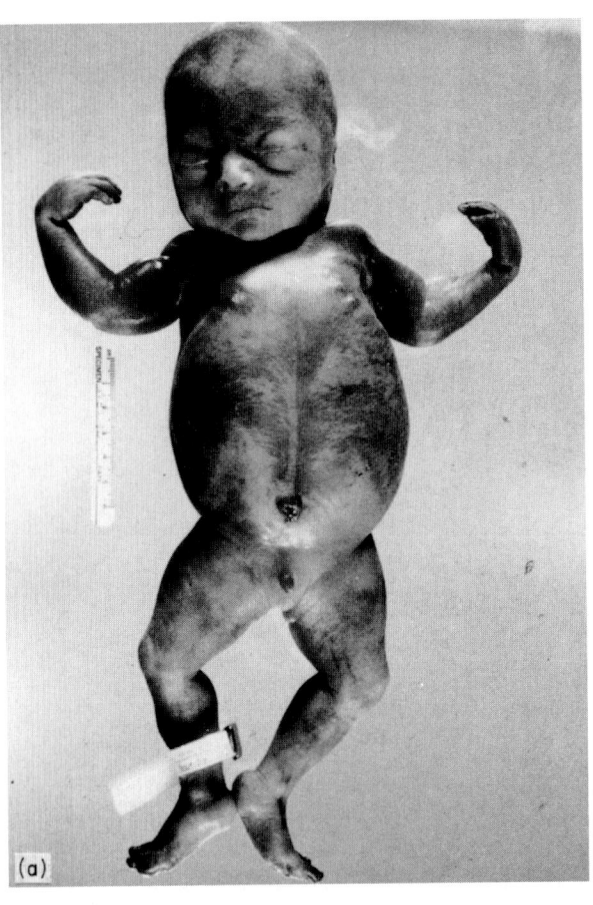

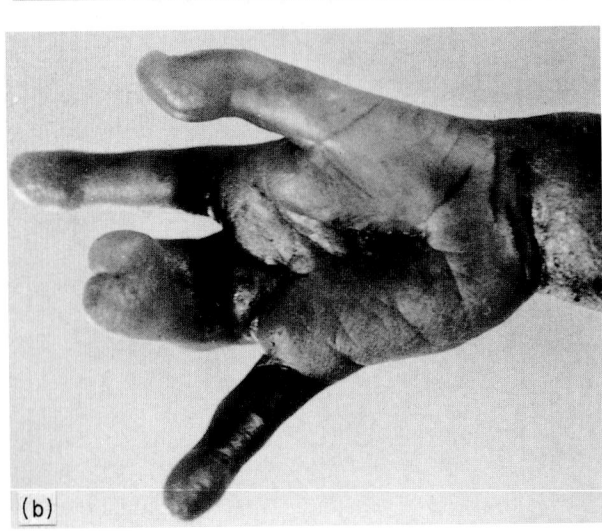

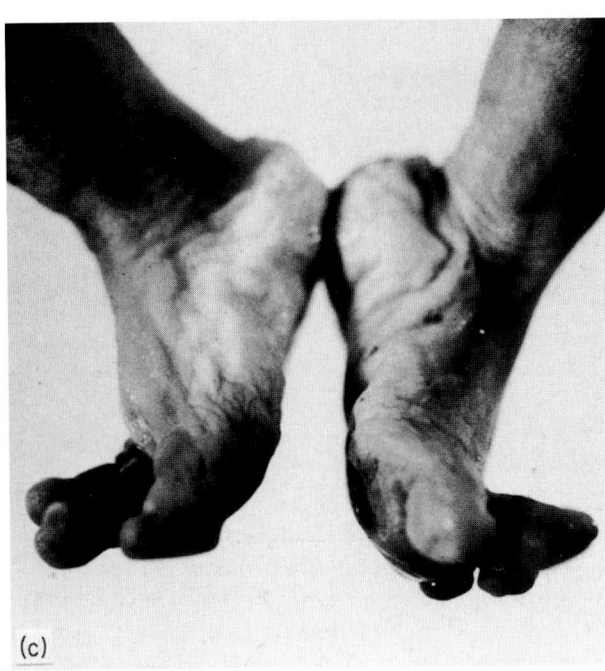

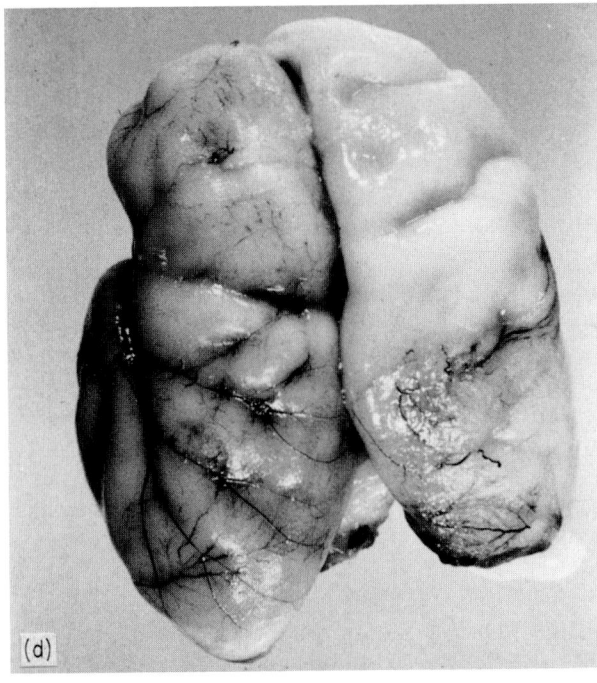

FIGURE 12.23.   *(a) A 26-week liveborn infant with triploidy who died 2 hours after birth. (b) Hands and (c) feet, showing syndactyly and bizarre appearance of fingers and toes. (d) Brain with lissencephaly, most striking on right.*

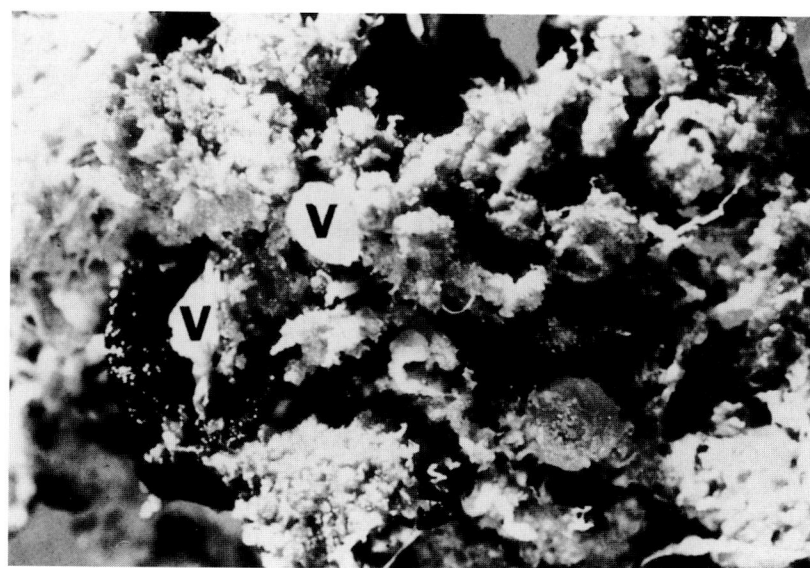

FIGURE 12.24. *Partial hydatidiform molar placenta in triploidy. Many chorionic villi (v) are large and edematous.*

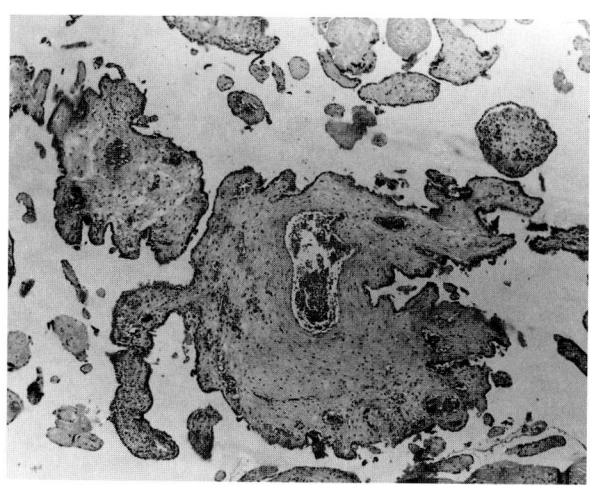

FIGURE 12.25. *Microscopic section of the placenta in a partial mole of triploidy. The chorionic villi are large, with scalloping at the margins and an edematous stroma. H&E, ×100.*

Diploid/triploid mosaic infants may survive with moderate to severe mental retardation. About two-thirds of the cases of triploidy have been XXY and about one-third XXX, rarely XYY [176]. We have observed one case of triploidy with XXYY. Triploidies usually have female internal and external sex organs, with hypoplastic gonads with poorly developed primordial follicles [177]. Table 12.14 lists the abnormalities reported in triploidy.

Microphthalmia, coloboma, ovoid cornea, hypertelorism, and abnormal ears are frequent [19], while syndactyly and bizarre abnormalities of fingers and toes and talipes equinovarus may be present (Fig. 12.23). Congenital cardiac lesions occur in two-thirds of the cases and include

atrial and ventricular septal defects, endocardial cushion defects, pulmonary valvular stenosis, and valvular anomalies. Adrenal aplasia has been described. Simian creases are not infrequent.

Rarer anomalies include Dandy-Walker malformation, eccentric pupils, hypoplasia of the iris and retina [177], choanal atresia [178], hypoplasia of the thyroid, thymus and pancreas [179], tracheoesophageal fistula [178], omphalocele, diaphragmatic hernia, chondrodysplasia punctata [180], and thumb duplication.

Triploid pregnancy is associated with polyhydramnios, proteinuria, hypertension, edema, and midtrimester pre-eclampsia [181]. The placenta of triploidy is usually a partial hydatidiform mole (Fig. 12.24) (85%); in fact, triploidy should be suspected in all partial moles [182–184]. The microscopic appearance of the chorionic villi (Fig. 12.25) is distinctive.

Histologically, the partial mole of triploidy is characterized by molar changes interdigitating with seemingly unaffected placental villi [185]. Hydatidiform changes include large villi with scalloping of their margins and mild trophoblastic hyperplasia with vacuolization, similar to that seen in young placentae up to 6 to 7 weeks' menstrual age. Large cisternae are present within the edematous villi. Trophoblastic inclusions are seen in 70% of cases [186–188]. These are deep and narrow invaginations of trophoblasts into the villous stroma.

Extremely rarely do triploid gestations reach term [186, 189–191].

We have observed a triploid stillborn 70,XXYY infant with an elevated maternal serum level and a borderline elevated amniotic alphafetoprotein level. This may be related to the partial hydatidiform molar placenta that may pass more alphafetoprotein back from the amniotic fluid to the maternal serum [192].

KLINEFELTER SYNDROME

Klinefelter syndrome comprises about 0.2% of live male births and includes XXY, XXYY, XY/XXY mosaicism, and other rarer forms. Eighty per cent are XXY, 10% are mosaic, and the remainder are XXYY and the less frequent types. About 10% of male sterility is due to Klinefelter syndrome [193]. Some cases have associated trisomy 21. Tallness, borderline intelligence, and aggressive behavior problems are present in some cases.

Postpubertal males have small, firm testes with tubular hyalinization and usually a normal number of Leydig cells, aspermia, gynecomastia, elevated urinary gonadotropins, and low concentrations of urinary 17-ketosteroids. Before puberty, the testis may be of normal size and microscopic appearance. During adolescence, however, the testes fail to enlarge; the seminiferous tubules become shrunken, hyalinized, and irregularly arranged and are lined solely by Sertoli cells; elastic fibers are absent around the tunica propria of the tubules; Leydig cells are clumped; and spermatogenesis is inconspicuous or absent. The penis is usually of normal circumference, but can be shorter than normal.

The kidneys have been described as symmetrically enlarged, with small cysts 0.1 to 0.8 cm in diameter throughout the parenchyma [194]. Histologically, these cysts are lined with undifferentiated epithelium, and some of them may contain several glomerular loops and connective tissue between the cysts. The ureters may be very thin but not atretic, the bladder small and cylindrical. Calyces and papillae may not be recognized. Kidney cysts, hydronephrosis, hydroureters, and ureterocele have been noted on rare occasions [70].

Gynecomastia develops after puberty in about 50% of patients; facial hair is sparse, axillary hair may be deficient, and 50% have a female pubic escutcheon. Mosaic individuals may be affected less severely. An increased incidence of diabetes mellitus [195] and chronic pulmonary diseases, chronic bronchitis, bronchiectasis, asthma and emphysema [196, 197] has been reported. Endocrine studies by Hsueh et al [198] documented a low concentration of plasma testosterone and an elevated plasma concentration of luteinizing hormone (LH) and FSH. Patients with Klinefelter syndrome have decreased radioactive iodine uptake and diminished response to TSH; however, growth hormone and glucocorticoid secretion are normal.

ULLRICH-TURNER SYNDROME (UTS)

Approximately 60% of patients with the UTS phenotype have a monosomy-X (45,X) chromosome constitution. Mosaicism of various types, and short- and long-arm deletions of an X chromosome, account for the remainder of the cases. UTS has been estimated to occur in 1 per 2500 female births [199]. Fetal mortality is high; 95–98% of the 45,X conceptuses are spontaneously aborted.

The UTS phenotype (Table 12.15) includes short stature, broad chest with wide spacing of nipples, ovarian dysgene-

sis with hypoplasia to absence of germinal elements, primary amenorrhea, sexual infantilism and sterility, congenital lymphoedema with residual puffiness of the dorsum of the fingers and toes (80%), anomalous ears, webbed posterior neck (50%), cubitus valgus, excessive number of pigmented nevi (50%), and cardiac defects (20%).

In older patients, the histologic appearance of the dysgenetic gonad of UTS consists of long streaks of white, wavy connective tissue stroma without follicles, although follicles are usually present in fetal and infantile ovaries. Skeletal anomalies include cubitus valgus, short fourth metacarpals, deformity of the medial tibial condyle, osteoporosis with hypoplasia of the first cervical vertebra, and a small carpal angle [200–202]. Neck blebs or cystic hygromas (Fig. 12.26) are common prenatally [203, 204]. It has been suggested that the lymphedema results from the generalized hypoplasia and partial agenesis of the lymphatic system that ceases to extend peripherally at an early embryonic stage [205].

The renal anomalies that occur in 76% of cases are most commonly horseshoe kidney, double or clubbed renal pelvis, hypoplasia or hydronephrosis and bifid ureters, duplication of kidneys and/or ureters, unilateral renal agenesis with

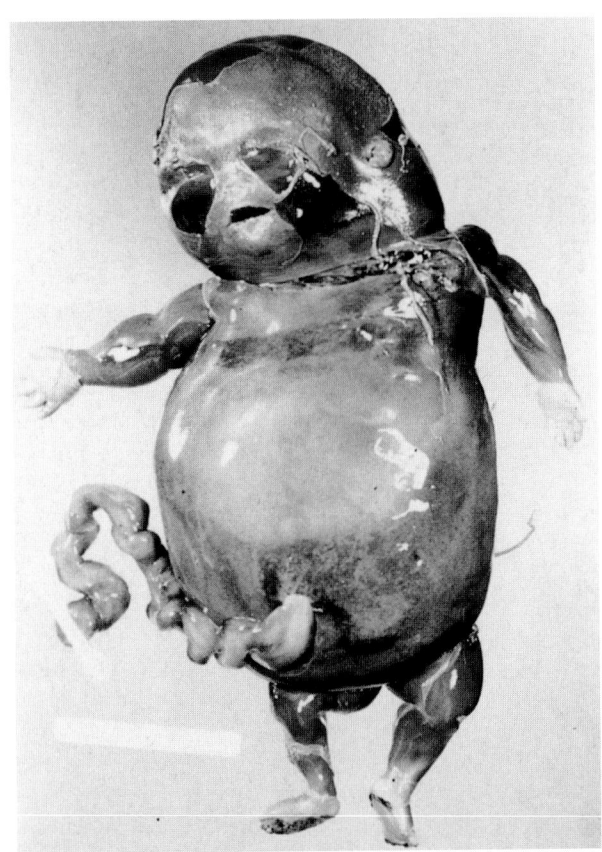

FIGURE 12.26.   *Ullrich-Turner syndrome. Fourteen-week fetus with massive lymphedema and cystic hygromas.*

Table 12.15. Abnormalities observed in Ullrich-Turner syndrome

Infant	Membranoproliferative glomerulonephritis
Small for gestational age	Gonadal malignancy if Y chromosomal component present
Lymphedema of dorsum of hands and feet	**Cardiovascular malformations**
Deep-set nails	Coarctation of the aorta
Excess skin on nape of neck (becomes pterygium colli later in life)	Cystic medial necrosis of aorta
	Dissecting aneurysm
Cystic hygroma	Floppy mitral or aortic valves (myxoid degeneration)
At puberty	Aortic valvular stenosis
Small stature	**Central nervous system malformations**
Neck short and webbed	Slight cortical dysplasia
Low posterior hairline	Gray matter heterotopia
Cubitus valgus	Hydrocephalus
Shortness of 4th and 5th metacarpals (brachymetacarpia)	**Sense organ malformations**
	Severe myopia
Multiple nevi	Congenital cataracts
Nails hypoplastic and hyperconvex	Congenital deafness
Tendency to keloid scars	**Skeletal malformations**
Craniofacial anomalies	Inner tibial plate low, slightly slanted downward and inward, and projects beyond metaphysis (Kosowicz' sign)
Triangular face	
Antimongoloid slant of palpebral fissures	
Epicanthus	Shortness of 4th and 5th metacarpals
Ptosis	Raised semilunar carpal bones
Highly arched palate	**Endocrine abnormalities**
Hypoplasia of mandible, retrognathia	Low serum levels of estrogens and pregnanediol; increased FSH
Low-set ears	
Thorax malformations	17-ketosteroids, low levels in urine
Broad, shield-shaped	Hashimoto's thyroiditis (autoimmune)
Widely spaced hypoplastic nipples	**Nongonadal neoplasms**
Gastrointestinal malformations	Ganglioneuroblastoma of adrenal
Intestinal hemorrhage due to hemangiomas or telangiectasia	Carcinoid tumor of cecum and appendix
	Multiple granular cell myoblastomas
Genitourinary malformations	Medulloblastoma
Infantile female external genitalia	Cerebellar glioma
Pubic hair scanty or absent	Meningioma
Axillary hair absent	Melanoma
Clitoral hypertrophy	Pituitary chromophobe adenoma
Streak gonads	Retroperitoneal mesenchymoma
Uterus hypoplastic, sometimes bifid or absent	Thyroid carcinoma
Failure of development of secondary sex characteristics	Anaplastic lung tumor
	Pituitary adenoma
Horseshoe kidney	Hibernoma
Double or clubbed renal pelvis	Adenocarcinoma of endometrium
Anomalies of renal rotation	Gastrointestinal adenocarcinoma (stomach and large bowel)
Hypoplasia or renal agenesis	
Hydronephrosis	Adenocanthoma of uterus
Bifid ureters	Squamous cell carcinoma of vulva
Micromulticystic kidneys	Acute myelogenous leukemia

abnormalities of the contralateral kidney, and renal hypoplasia [70, 206–213]. A retrocaval ureter with massive hydronephrosis was reported in one case by Cleeve et al [214]. Goodyer et al [215] have reported persistent complement activation and membranoproliferative glomerulonephritis in UTS with 46,X, del(X)(p11). Micromulticystic renal disease has also been observed [35].

Intestinal hemorrhage due to congenital hemangiomas, venous ectasia, or telangiectasia occurs in about 7% of cases [216]. Multiple telangiectasias of the intestinal wall may lead to anemia as a result of repeated gastrointestinal bleeding [217].

Cardiovascular malformations are found in approximately 40% of cases with apparently monoclonal 45,X constitution.

The most frequent cardiovascular malformations are atrial septal defect, patent ductus arteriosus, transposition of the great arteries, and retroesophageal subclavian artery [218, 219]. Coarctation of the aorta, congenital aortic valvular stenosis, dilatation of the proximal aorta, and cystic medial necrosis of the aortic wall may occur with aortic rupture [220]. Dermatoglyphic ridge counts are high.

NEOPLASIA ASSOCIATED WITH CHROMOSOME ABERRATIONS

Certain chromosome defects are consistently associated with specific types of human cancer [221]. Chromosome defects are present in most neoplasms [90, 222–228]. It has also been shown that active oncogenes occur in various types of human cancer, and when taken up by certain viruses can be used to induce neoplasia in experimental animals or to transform cells in culture [229].

The most common chromosome defect in neoplasia is either a band deletion or a reciprocal translocation between two chromosomes. In a few instances, trisomy is present. In acute nonlymphocytic leukemia (ANLL) and in acute lymphocytic leukemia (ALL), most patients have chromosome defects, with two-thirds demonstrating one of several distinctive abnormalities [222, 227]. Ninety-eight percent of patients with non-Hodgkin, non-Burkitt lymphomas show chromosome abnormalities.

The fact that virtually every cancer contains at least one chromosome abnormality suggests that the *c-onc* and *onc*-like genes may be responsible for tumorigenesis and tumor progression in most, if not all, cancers [230].

A translocation involving chromosomes 9 and 22 or a variant translocation of chromosome 22 is present in 95% of adults with chronic myelogenous leukemia (CML) [221, 231] and translocation of chromosomes 15 and 17 in 41% of patients with ANLL of the M3 type [232].

Trisomy of chromosome 12 has been observed in about one-third of patients with either chronic lymphocytic leukemia (CLL) or its lymphomatous counterpart, small lymphocytic lymphoma (SLL) [222, 228, 233, 234]. Trisomy of chromosome 8 has been found in 5–10% of patients with ANLL, and inversion of chromosome 16 is present in acute myelomonocytic leukemia (M4).

In Burkitt's lymphoma, the human cellular oncogene *myc* (*c-myc*), located on chromosome 8, appears to become activated when rearranged with either the immunoglobulin heavy-chain genes of chromosome 14 or the immunoglobulin light-chain genes of chromosomes 2 and 22 [235–239].

A translocation of chromosomes 8 and 14 or a variant form of this defect is present in 100% of cases of Burkitt's lymphoma [223, 225, 240].

Solid tumors that most consistently show a chromosome aberration include disseminated neuroblastoma, retinoblastoma, and cancers of the lung, cervix, vulva, retina, kidney, colon, ovary, bladder, and breast [220, 224, 226]. A significant proportion (>60%) of neuroblastomas have been reported to contain deletions or other rearrangements of the short arm of chromosome 1, resulting in the loss of structural material distal to band 1p31 [241].

In cells from Ewing's sarcoma, two- and three-way reciprocal translocations have been identified recently, always involving a break at band 22q12 (most commonly resulting in the exchange of material between chromosomes 11 and 22): t(11; 22) (q24; q12) [242, 243].

The karyotypes from rhabdomyosarcomas have shown a reciprocal translocation between chromosomes 2 and 13: t(2; 13) (q37; q14) [244].

Cytogenetic analysis of retinoblastoma cells has demonstrated deletions and rearrangements resulting in the loss of structural material from the long arm (q) of chromosome 13, at band 13q14 [245]. This has been reported in cases with tumor in one or both eyes—the former is usually sporadic, the latter is always heritable—and in patients who carry deletions of 13q14 in somatic, as well as tumor, cells (constitutional 13q deletion syndrome) [245]. This deletion of 13q14 is associated with a 50% loss of esterase D activity (the loci for retinoblastoma and esterase D are linked), whereas individuals with duplication of this site show no tumor and an increased level of esterase D [246, 247].

Wilms' tumor has been seen in association with aniridia in individuals who also carry constitutional deletions of the short arm of chromosome 11, always including band 11–13, [248]. These patients also show a 50% loss of catalase activity since the catalase gene is located in 11p(13) [249]. Duplication of this segment is associated with increased activity of catalase and no development of tumor.

Cytogenetic studies of meningiomas have described the loss of one chromosome 22 in 70% of cases. In nearly half of these cases of monosomy 22, other chromosomes were also missing [250].

REFERENCES

1. ISCN. An international system for human cytogenetic nomenclature. *Cytogenet Cell Genet* 1978; 21:309.
2. Francke U, Oliver N. Quantitative analysis of high-resolution trypsin-Giemsa bands of human prometaphase chromosomes. *Hum Genet* 1978; 45:137.
3. Yunis JJ. Nomenclature for high resolution human chromosomes. *Cancer Genet Cytogenet* 1980; 2:221.
4. Boué J, Boué A. Anomalies chromosomiques dans les avortements spontanes. In: Boué A, Thibault CD, eds. *Les Accidents Chromosomiques de la Reproduction.* Paris: INSERM, 1973, p. 29.
5. Boué J, Philippe E, Giroud A, et al. Phenotypic expression of lethal chromosome anomalies in human abortuses. *Teratology* 1976; 14:3.
6. Bauld R, Sutherland GR, Bain AD. Chromosome studies in investigations of stillbirths and antenatal deaths. *Arch Dis Child* 1974; 49:782.
7. Kuleshov NP, Alekhin VI, Egolina NA, et al. Frequency of chromosomal anomalies in children dying in the perinatal period (Plenum translation). *Genetika* 1975; 11:107.
8. Machin GA, Crolla JA. Chromosome constitution of 500 infants dying during the perinatal period. *Humangenetik* 1974; 23:183.
9. Jacobs PA. Epidemiology of chromosome abnormalities in man. *Am J Epidemiol* 1977; 105:180.

10. Witschi E. Teratogenic effects from overripeness of the egg. In: Fraser FC, McKusick VA, eds. *Congenital Malformations*. New York: Excerpta Medica, 1970, p. 157.

11. Boué J, Boué A, Lazar P. Retrospective and prospective epidemiological studies of 1500 karyotyped spontaneous human abortions. *Teratology* 1975; 12:11.

12. Jacobs PA, Aitken J, Frackiewicz A, et al. The inheritance of translocations in man: data from families ascertained through a balanced heterozygote. *Ann Hum Genet* 1970; 34:119.

13. Greasy MR, Crolla JA. Prenatal mortality of trisomy 21 (Down syndrome). *Lancet* 1974; i:473.

14. Gustavson KH, Hagberg B, Hagberg G, et al. Severe mental retardation in a Swedish county. I. Epidemiology, gestational age, birth weight, and associated CNS handicaps in children born 1959–1970. *Acta Paediatr Scand* 1977; 66:373.

15. Gustavson KH, Hagberg G, Sars K. Severe mental retardation in a Swedish county. II. Etiologic and pathogenetic aspects of children born 1959–1970. *Neuropaediatrie* 1977; 8:293.

16. Barash BA, Freedman L, Opitz JM. Anatomic studies in the 18-trisomy syndrome. *Birth Defects, Orig Artic Ser* 1970; VI(4):3.

17. Opitz JM, Sutherland GR. Editorial comment. X-linked mental retardation. *Am J Med Genet* 1980; 7:407.

18. Yunis JJ. *New Chromosomal Syndromes*. New York: Academic Press, 1977.

19. Zellweger H, Simpson J. *Chromosomes of Man*. Philadelphia: JB Lippincott, 1977.

20. de Grouchy JD, Turleau C. *Clinical Atlas of Human Chromosomes*. New York: Wiley, 1984.

21. Schinzel A. *Catalogue of Unbalanced Chromosome Aberrations in Man*. New York: Walter de Gruyter, 1984.

22. Borgaonkar DS. Chromosomal variation in man. *A Catalog of Chromosomal Variants and Anomalies*. 3rd ed. New York: AR Liss, 1980.

23. Hamerton JL. Fetal sex. *Lancet* 1970; i:516.

24. Erickson JD, Bjerkedal T. Down syndrome associated with father's age in Norway. *J Med Genet* 1981; 18:22.

25. Hook EB. Unbalanced robertsonian translocations associated with Down's syndrome or Patau's syndrome: chromosome subtype, proportion inherited, mutation rates, and sex ratio. *Hum Genet* 1981; 59:235.

26. Stene J, Stene E, Stengel-Rutkowski S, et al. Paternal age and Down's syndrome. Data from prenatal diagnoses (DFG). *Hum Genet* 1981; 59:119.

27. McClure HM. Features of Down's-like syndrome in a chimpanzee. *Am J Pathol* 1972; 67:413.

28. Turleau C, de Grouchy J, Klein M. Phylogénie chromosomique de l'homme et des primates hominiens (*Pan troglodytes, Gorilla gorilla, et Pongo pygmaeus*): essai de reconstitution du caryotype de l'ancêtre commun. *Ann Genet* 1972; 15:225.

29. Andrle M, Fiedler W, Rett A, et al. A case of trisomy 22 in *Pongo pygmaeus*. *Cytogenet Cell Genet* 1979; 24:1.

30. Hall B. Mongolism in newborn infants. An examination of the criteria for recognition and some speculations on the pathogenetic activity of the chromosomal abnormality. *Clin Pediatr* 1966; 5:4.

31. Bergsin D. Memorandum on dermatoglyphic nomenclature. *Birth Defects, Orig Artic Ser* 1968; IV:1.

32. Reed T, Christian JC. A comparison of the dermatogram with other indices for the diagnosis of Down's syndrome. *Clin Genet* 1976; 10:139.

33. Zellweger H, Schochet S Jr, Simpson J, et al. Chromosomal aneuploidies excluding Down's syndrome. In: Vinken PJ, Bruyn GW, eds. *Handbook of Clinical Neurology*. Ch. 31. Amsterdam: North-Holland, 1977.

34. Bersu ET. Anatomical analysis of the developmental effects of aneuploidy in man: the Down syndrome. *Am J Med Genet* 1980; 5:399.

35. Gilbert EF, Opitz JM. Developmental and other pathologic changes in syndromes caused by chromosome abnormalities. In: Rosenberg HS, Bernstein J, eds. *Perspectives in Pediatric Pathology*. vol. 7. New York: Masson, 1982, pp. 1–63.

36. Greenwood RD, Nadas AS. The clinical course of cardiac disease in Down's syndrome. *Pediatrics* 1976; 58:893.

37. Chi TPL, Krovetz LJ. The pulmonary vascular bed in children with Down syndrome. *J Pediatr* 1975; 86:533.

38. Fonkalsrud EW, deLorimier AA, Hays DM. Congenital atresia and stenosis of the duodenum. *Pediatrics* 1969; 43:79.

39. Friedmann AL, Gilbert EF, Opitz JM. Genetic aspects of renal disease. In: Holiday M, Barratt M, Nesices R, eds. *Pediatric Nephrology*. 2nd ed. Baltimore: Williams & Wilkins, 1985, pp. 183–92.

40. Ariel I, Wells TR, Landing BH, Singer DB. The urinary system in Down syndrome: a study of 124 autopsy cases. *Pediatr Pathol* 1991; 11:879–88.

41. Özer FL. Kidney malformations in mongolism. *Birth Defects, Orig Artic Ser* 1974; 10:189.

42. Kissane JM. Congenital anomalies. In: *Pathology of Infancy and Childhood*. 2nd ed. St. Louis: CV Mosby, 1975, p. 577.

43. Benda CA. *The Child With Mongolism (Congenital Acromicria)*. New York: Grune & Stratton, 1960.

44. Miller RS, Todaro GJ. Viral transformation of cells from persons at high risk of cancer. *Lancet* 1969; i:81.

45. Herrmann J, Gilbert EF, Opitz JM. Dysplasia, malformations and cancer, especially with respect to the Wiedemann–Beckwith syndrome. In: Nichols WW, Murphy DG, eds. *Regulation of Cell Proliferation and Differentiation*. New York: Plenum, 1977, pp. 1–64.

46. Aarskog D. Autoimmune thyroid disease in children with mongolism. *Arch Dis Child* 1969; 44:454.

47. Farquhar JW. Down's syndrome with diabetes mellitus and hypothyroidism. *Arch Dis Child* 1974; 49:750.

48. Lawrence RD. Three diabetic mongol idiots. *Br Med J* 1942; 1:695.

49. Litman NN. Down's syndrome, hypothyroidism and diabetes mellitus. *J Pediatr* 1968; 73:798.

50. Schachter M. L'arrieration mongolienne. *An Port Psiquiatr* 1958; 10:97.

51. Benda CE. *Down's Syndrome*. 2nd ed. New York: Grune & Stratton, 1969.

52. Engler M, *Mongolism (Peristatic Amentia)*. Bristol: Wright, 1949.

53. Levin S, Schlesinger M, Handzel Z, et al. Thymic deficiency in Down's syndrome. *Pediatrics* 1979; 63:80.

54. Hubbard JD. Down's syndrome—dilated Hassall's corpuscles as a histopathologic marker. Pediatric Pathology Club Interim Meeting, Providence, RI, 11–13 October, 1979.

55. Sutnick AI, London WT, Blumberg BS. Persistent anicteric hepatitis with Australia antigen in patients with Down's syndrome. *Am J Clin Pathol* 1972; 57:2.

56. Solitare GB. The spinal cord of the mongol. *J Ment Defic Res* 1968; 13:1.

57. Colon EJ. The structure of the cerebral cortex in Down syndrome. *Neuropaediatrie* 1972; 3:362.

58. Burger PC, Vogen SF. The development of the pathologic changes of Alzheimer's disease and senile dementia in patients with Down's syndrome. *Am J Pathol* 1973; 73:457.

59. Haberland C. Alzheimer's disease in Down's syndrome. *Acta Neurol Belg* 1969; 69:369.

60. Olson MJ, Shaw C. Presenile dementia and Alzheimer's disease in mongolism. *Brain* 1969; 92:146.

61. Owen SD, Dawson JD, Losin S. Alzheimer's disease in Down's syndrome. *Am J Ment Defic* 1971; 75:606.

62. Schochet SS, Lampert PW, McCormick WF. Neurofibrillary tangles in patients with Down's syndrome. *Acta Neuropathol* 1973; 23:342.

63. Gilbert EF, Opitz JM. Personal observations.

64. Patau K, Smith DW, Therman E, Inhorn SL, Wagner HP. Multiple congenital anomaly caused by an extra chromosome. *Lancet* 1960; i:790.

65. Nielsen J, Sillesen J. Incidence of chromosome aberrations arising in 11,148 newborn children. *Humangenetik* 1975; 30:1.

66. Warkany J, Passarge E, Smith LD. Congenital malformations in autosomal trisomy syndromes. *Am J Dis Child* 1966; 112:502.

67. Marden PM, Yunis JJ. Trisomy D_1 in a 10-year-old girl: normal neutrophils and fetal hemoglobin. *Am J Dis Child* 1967; 114:662.

68. Redheendran R, Neu RL, Bannerman RM. Long survival in trisomy-13-syndrome: 21 cases including prolonged survival in two patients 11 and 19 years old. *Am J Med Genet* 1981; 8:167.

69. Pettersen JC, Koltis GG, White MF. An examination of the spectrum of anatomic defects and variations found in eight cases of trisomy 13. *Am J Med Genet* 1979; 3:183.

70. Egli F, Stalder G. Malformations of kidney and urinary tract in common chromosomal aberrations. *Humangenetik* 1973; 18:1.

71. Marin-Padilla M, Hoefnagel D, Benirschke K. Anatomic and histopathologic study of two cases of D_1 (13–15) trisomy. *Cytogenetics* 1964; 3:258.

72. Nevin NC, Dodge JA, Allen IV. Two cases of trisomy D associated with adrenal tumors. *J Med Genet* 1972; 9:119.

73. Towns H, Jones HW. Cyclopia in association with D trisomy and gonadal agenesis. *Am J Obstet Gynecol* 1968; 102:53.

74. Gilbert E, Opitz J. Renal involvement in genetic-hereditary malformation syndromes. In: Hamburger J, Crosnier J, Grunfeld JP, eds. *Nephrology*. vol. 64. New York: Wiley, 1979, pp. 909–94.

75. Townes PL, Dehart GK Jr, Hecht F, Manning JA. Trisomy 13–15 in a male infant. *J Pediatr* 1962; 60:528.

76. Keshgegian AA, Chatten J. Nodular renal blastema in trisomy 13. *Arch Pathol Lab Med* 1979; 103:73.

77. Huehns ER, Lutzner M, Hecht F. Nuclear abnormalities of the neutrophils in D_1 (13–15) trisomy syndrome. *Lancet* 1964; i:589.

78. Powars D, Rhode R, Graves D. Foetal hemoglobin and neutrophil anomaly in the D₁ trisomy syndrome. *Lancet* 1964; i:1363.

79. Walzer S, Gerald PS, Breau G, et al. Hematologic changes in the D₁ trisomy syndrome. *Pediatrics* 1966; 34:419.

80. Schade H, Scholler L, Schultze KW. D-Trisomie (Patau-Syndrom), mit kongenitaler myeloider Leukaemie. *Med Welt* 1962; 2:2690.

81. Zuelzer WW, Thompson RI, Mastrangelo R. Evidence for a genetic factor related to leukemogenesis and congenital anomalies: chromosomal aberrations in pedigree of an infant with partial D trisomy and leukemia. *J Pediatr* 1968; 72:367.

82. DeMyer W, Zeman W, Palmer CG. The face predicts the brain: diagnostic significance of median facial anomalies for holoprosencephaly (arrhinencephaly). *Pediatrics* 1964; 34:256.

83. Gilbert LA, Dudley AW, Meisner L, et al. New neuropathological findings in trisomy 13. *Arch Pathol Lab Med* 1977; 101:540.

84. Taysi K, Tinaztepe K. Trisomy D and the cyclops malformation. *Am J Dis Child* 1972; 124:710.

85. Hoepner J, Yanoff M. Ocular anomalies in trisomy 13–15. *Am J Ophthalmol* 1972; 74:729.

86. Niebuhr E. Partial trisomies and deletions of chromosome 13. In: Yunis JJ, ed. *New Chromosomal Syndromes.* New York: Academic, 1977, p. 273.

87. Escobar JI, Sanchez O, Yunis JJ. Trisomy for the distal segment of chromosome 13. *Am J Dis Child* 1974; 128:217.

88. Pettersen JC. Anatomical studies of a boy trisomic for the distal portion of 13q. *Am J Med Genet* 1979; 4:383.

89. Escobar JI, Yunis JJ. Trisomy for the proximal segment of the long arm of chromosome 13. A new entity? *Am J Dis Child* 1974; 128:221.

90. Knudson AG, Meadows AT, Nichols WW, et al. Chromosomal deletion and retinoblastoma. *N Engl J Med* 1976; 29:1120.

91. Lele KP, Penrose LS, Stallard HB. Chromosome deletion in a case of retinoblastoma. *Ann Hum Genet* 1963; 27:171.

92. Orye E, Delbeke MH, Vandenabeele B. Retinoblastoma and long arm deletion of chromosome 13. Attempts to define the deleted segment. *Clin Genet* 1974; 5:457.

93. Wilson MG, Melnyk J, Towner JW. Retinoblastoma and deletion D (14) syndrome. *J Med Genet* 1969; 6:322.

94. Matsunaga E. Host resistance and 13q deletion. *Hum Genet* 1980; 56:53.

95. LeMarec B, Senecal J. Sex ratio et age maternal dans la trisomie 18. *J Genet Hum* 1975; 23:119.

96. Moerman P, Fryns JP, Goddeeris P, Lauweryns JM. Spectrum of clinical and autopsy findings in trisomy 18 syndrome. *J Genet Hum* 1982; 30:17.

97. Rodrigues MM, Punnet HH, Valdes-Dapena M, et al. Retinal pigment epithelium in a case of trisomy 18. *Am J Ophthalmol* 1973; 76:265.

98. Ramirez-Castro JL, Bersu ET. Anatomical analysis of the developmental effects of aneuploidy in man—the trisomy 18 syndrome. II. Anomalies of the upper and lower limbs. *Am J Med Genet* 1978; 2:285.

99. Schinzel A. Cardiovascular defects associated with chromosome aberrations and malformation syndromes. *Prog Med Genet* 1983; 5:303.

100. Matsuoka R, Matsuyama S, Yamamoto Y, et al. Trisomy 18q: a case report and review on karyotype-phenotype correlations. *Hum Genet* 1981; 57:78.

101. Lewis AJ. The pathology of trisomy 18. *J Pediatr* 1964; 65:92.

102. Kurien VA, Duke M. Trisomy 17–18 syndrome: report of a case with diffuse myocardial fibrosis and review of cardiovascular abnormalities. *Am J Cardiol* 1968; 21:431.

103. Merrild U, Schioler V, Christensen F, et al. Anencephaly in trisomy 18 associated with elevated alpha-1-fetoprotein in amniotic fluid. *Hum Genet* 1978; 45:85.

104. Karayalcin G, Shanske A, Honigman R. Wilms' tumor in a 13-year-old girl with trisomy 18. *Am J Dis Child* 1981; 135:665.

105. Wertelecki W, Gerald PS. Clinical and chromosomal studies on the 18q– syndrome. *J Pediatr* 1971; 78:44.

106. Mavalwala J, Wilson MG, Parker CD. The dermatoglyphics of the 18q– syndrome. *Am J Phys Anthropol* 1970; 32:443.

107. Francke U. Partial duplication 20p. In: Yunis JJ, ed. *New Chromosomal Syndromes.* New York: Academic, 1977, p. 262.

108. Schinzel A. Trisomy 20pter-q11 in a malformed boy from at (13; 20) (p11; q11) translocation-carrier mother. *Hum Genet* 1980; 53:169.

109. Gorlin RJ, Yunis J, Anderson VE. Short arm deletion of chromosome 18. *Am J Dis Child* 1968; 115:453.

110. Nitowsky HM, Sindhavanada N, Konigsberg U, et al. Partial 18 monosomy in the cyclops malformation. *Pediatrics* 1966; 37:260.

111. Sabater J, Antich J, Lluch M, et al. Deletion of short arm of chromosome 18 with normal levels of IgA. *J Ment Defic Res* 1972; 16:103.

112. Uchida IA, McRae KN, Wang HC, et al. Familial short arm deficiency of chromosome 18 concomitant with arrhinencephaly and alopecia congenita. *Am J Hum Genet* 1965; 17:410.

113. Fryns JP, de Muelenaere A, van den Berghe H. The 4p– syndrome in a 24-year-old female. *Ann Genet* 1981; 24:110.

114. Wilson MG, Towner JW, Coffin GS, et al. Genetic and clinical studies in 13 patients with the Wolf-Hirschhorn syndrome [del(4p)]. *Hum Genet* 1981; 59:297.

115. Arias D, Passarge E, Engle MA, et al. Human chromosomal deletion—two patients with the 4P–syndrome. *J Pediatr* 1970; 76:82.

116. Wilcock MG, Adams FG, Cooke P, et al. Deletion of short arm of No. 4 (4p–). A detailed case report. *J Med Genet* 1970; 7:171.

117. Judge CG, Garson OM, Pitt DB, et al. A girl with Wolf-Hirschhorn syndrome and mosaicism 46, XX/46, XX4p. *J Ment Defic Res* 1974; 18:79.

118. Nicolas H, Ravise N, Boue J, Boue A. Etude comparative du developpement des conceptions trisomiques 21 et de la croissance in vitro de leurs cellules. *Arch Fr Pediatr* 1977; 34:101.

119. Schinzel A. Autosomale Chromosomenaberrationen. *Arch Genet* 1979; 52:1.

120. de Capoa A, Warburton D, Breg WR, et al. Translocation heterozygosis: a cause of five cases of the cri du chat syndrome and two cases with a duplication of chromosome number five in three families. *Am J Hum Genet* 1967; 19:586.

121. Taylor MJ, Josifek K. Multiple congenital anomalies, thymic dysplasia, severe congenital heart disease, and oligosyndactyly with a deletion of the short arm of chromosome 5. *Am J Med Genet* 1981; 9:5.

122. Mennicken Y, Pfeiffer RA, Puyn U, et al. Klinische und cytogenetische Befunde von 7 Patienten mit Cri-du-chat Syndrom. *Z Kinderheilkd* 1968; 104:230.

123. Neuhauser G, Lother K. Das Katzenschrei-Syndrom. *Monatsschr Kinderheilkd* 1966; 114:278.

124. Warburton D, Miller OJ. Dermatoglyphic features of patients with a partial short arm deletion of a B-group chromosome. *Ann Hum Genet* 1967; 31:189.

125. Bishun P. Normal trisomy C mosaicism in the mother of a "mongoloid" child. *Acta Paediatr Scand* 1958; 57:243.

126. Caspersson T, Lindsten J, Zech L, et al. Four patients with trisomy 8 identified by the fluorescence and Giemsa banding techniques. *J Med Genet* 1972; 9:1.

127. Giraud F, Mattei JF, Blanc-Pardigon M, et al. Trisomie 8 en mosaique. *Arch Fr Pediatr* 1975; 32:177.

128. Stenbjerg S, Husted S, Bernsen A, et al. Coagulation studies in patients with trisomy 8 syndrome. *Ann Genet* 1975; 19:241.

129. Stolte L, Evers J, Blankenborg G. Possible trisomy in chromosome 6–12 in a normal woman. *Lancet* 1964; ii:480.

130. de Grouchy J, Veslot J, Bonnette J, et al. A case of ? 6p–chromosomal aberration. *Am J Dis Child* 1968; 115:93.

131. Yunis J, Sanchez O. A new syndrome resulting from partial trisomy for the distal third of the long arm of chromosome 10. *J Pediatr* 1974; 84:567.

132. Kosztolanyi G, Buhler EM, Elmiger P, Stalder GR. Trisomy 8 mosaicism. A case report and a proposed list of clinical features. *Eur J Pediatr* 1976; 123:293.

133. Riccardi V, Atkins L, Holmes LB. Absent patellae, mild mental retardation, skeletal and genitourinary anomalies, and group C autosomal mosaicism. *J Pediatr* 1970; 77:664.

134. de Grouchy J, Josso F, Beguin S, et al. Deficit en facteur VII de la coagulation chez trois sujets trisomiques 8. *Ann Genet* 1974; 17:105.

135. de la Chapelle A, Vunopio P, Icen A. Trisomy 8 in the bone marrow associated with high red cell glutathione reductase activity. *Blood* 1976; 47:815.

136. Jonasson J, Gahrton G, Lindsten J, et al. Trisomy 8 in acute myeloblastic leukemia and sideroachrestic anemia. *Blood* 1974; 43:557.

137. Niss R, Passarge E. Trisomy 8 restricted to cultured fibroblasts. *J Med Genet* 1976; 13:229.

138. Rowley JL. Nonrandom chromosomal abnormalities in hematologic disorders of man. *Proc Natl Acad Sci USA* 1975; 72:152.

139. Williams TM, McConnell TS, Martinez F Jr, Smith ACM, Suhansky E. Clinicopathologic and dysmorphic findings in recombinant chromosome 8 syndrome. *Hum Pathol* 1984; 15:1080.

140. Lovell M, Herrera J, Coco R. A child with recombinant of chromosome 8 inherited from a carrier mother with a pericentric inversion. *Medicina (Buenos Aires)* 1982; 42:359.

141. Juberg RC, Gilbert EF, Salisbury RS. Trisomy C in an infant with polycystic kidneys and other malformations. *J Pediatr* 1970; 76:598.

142. Blair JD. Trisomy C and cystic dysplasia of kidneys, liver and pancreas. *Birth Defects, Orig Artic Ser* 1976; 12:139.

143. Anneren G, Sedin G. Trisomy 9 syndrome. *Acta Paediatr Scand* 1981; 70:125.
144. Feingold M, Atkins L. A case of trisomy 9. *J Med Genet* 1973; 10:184.
145. Francke U, Benirschke K, Jones OW. Prenatal diagnosis of trisomy 9. *Humangenetik* 1975; 29:243.
146. Frohlich GS. Delineation of trisomy 9. *J Med Genet* 1982; 19:316.
147. Haslam RHA, Broske SP, Moore CM, Thomas GH, Neill CA. Trisomy 9 mosaicism with multiple congenital anomalies. *J Med Genet* 1973; 10:180.
148. Mantagos S, McReynolds JW, Seashore MR, et al. Complete trisomy 9 in two liveborn infants. *J Med Genet* 1981; 18:377.
149. Bowen P, Ying KL, Chung GSH. Trisomy 9 mosaicism in a newborn infant with multiple malformations. *J Pediatr* 1974; 85:95.
150. Riccardi VM, Hittner HM, Francke U, et al. The aniridia–Wilms' tumor association: the critical role of chromosome band 11p13. *Cancer Genet Cytogenet* 1980; 2:131.
151. Shannon RS, Mann JR, Harper E, et al. Wilm's tumour and aniridia: clinical and cytogenetic features. *Arch Dis Child* 1982; 57:685.
152. Riccardi VM, Hittner HM, Strong LI, et al. Wilms' tumor with aniridia/iris dysplasia and apparently normal chromosomes. *J Pediatr* 1982; 100:574.
153. Yunis JJ, Ramsey NK. Familial occurrence of the aniridia–Wilms' tumor syndrome with deletion 11p13–14.1. *J Pediatr* 1980; 96:1027.
154. Bove KE, McAdams AJ. The nephroblastomatosis complex and its relationship to Wilms' tumor: a clinicopathological treatise. *Perspect Pediatr Pathol* 1976; 3:185.
155. Dobyns WB, Stratton RF, Parke JT, et al. Miller–Dieker syndrome: lissencephaly and monosomy 17p. *J Pediatr* 1983; 102:552.
156. Daube JR, Chou SM. Lissencephaly: two cases. *Neurology* 1966; 16:179.
157. Dieker H, Edwards RH, ZuRhein G, et al. The lissencephaly syndrome. *Birth Defects, Orig Artic Ser* 1969; 5:53.
158. Dobyns WB, Stratton RF, Greenberg F. Syndromes with lissencephaly: I. Miller–Dieker and Norman–Roberts syndromes and isolated lissencephaly. *Am J Med Genet* 1985; 22:157.
159. Garcia CA, Dunn D, Trevor R. The lissencephaly (agyria) syndrome in siblings: computerized tomographic and neuropathologic findings. *Arch Neurol* 1978; 35:608.
160. Hanaway J, Lee SI, Netsky MG. Pachygyria: relation of findings to modern embryologic concepts. *Neurology* 1968; 18:791.
161. Jellinger K, Rett A. Agyria-pachygyria (lissencephaly syndrome). *Neuropediatrics* 1976; 7:66.
162. Jones KL, Gilbert EF, Kaveggia EG, Opitz JM. The Miller-Dieker syndrome. *Pediatrics* 1980; 66:277.
163. Miller JQ. Lissencephaly in 2 siblings. *Neurology* 1963; 13:841.
164. Norman MG, Roberts M, Sirois J, Tremblay LJM. Lissencephaly. *J Can Sci Neurol* 1976; 3:39.
165. Stewart RM, Richman DP, Caviness VS Jr. Lissencephaly and pachygyria, an architectonic and topographical analysis. *Acta Neuropathol* 1975; 31:1.
166. Toro-Sola MA, Rivera de Quinones H. Lissencephaly: a clinicopathologic study in a Puerto Rican female. Birth Defects Conference, Memphis, TN, 1977.
167. Van Allen M, Clarren SK. A spectrum of gyral anomalies in Miller-Dieker (lissencephaly) syndrome. *J Pediatr* 1983; 102:559.
168. Schinzel A, Schmid W, Fraccaro M, et al. The "Cat Eye syndrome": dicentric small marker chromosome probably derived from a No. 22 (tetrasomy 22pter-7q11) associated with a characteristic phenotype. Report of 11 patients and delineation of the clinical picture. *Hum Genet* 1981; 57:148.
169. Smith DW. *Recognizable Patterns of Human Malformations*. 2nd ed. Philadelphia: WB Saunders, 1976.
170. Embinger JM, Rey J, Rieu D, et al. Trisomie du groupe (47, XX, C8). *Arch Fr Pediatr* 1970; 27:1081.
171. Kelch RP, Franklin M, Schmickel RD. Group G deletion syndromes. *J Med Genet* 1971; 8:341.
172. Schindeler JD, Warren RJ. Dermatoglyphics in the G deletion syndromes. *J Ment Defic Res* 1973; 17:149.
173. De Cicco F, Stelle MW, Pan S, et al. Monosomy of chromosome No. 22. A case report. *J Pediatr* 1973; 83:836.
174. Boué JG, Boué A. Les aberrations chromosomiques dans les avortements spontanes humains. *Presse Med* 1970; 78:635.
175. Jacobs PA, Morton NE. Origin of human trisomies and polyploids. *Hum Hered* 1977; 27:59.
176. Niebuhr E. Triploidy in man. *Humangenetik* 1974; 21:103.
177. Butler LJ, Chantler C, France H, et al. A liveborn infant with complete triploidy (69, XXX). *J Med Genet* 1969; 6:413.
178. Niebuhr E, Sparrevohn S, Henningsen K, et al. A case of liveborn triploidy (69, XXX). *Acta Paediatr Scand* 1972; 61:203.
179. Al Saadi A, Juliar JF, Harm J, et al. Triploidy syndrome. A report of two live-born (69, XXY) and one still-born (69, XXX) infants. *Clin Genet* 1976; 9:43.
180. Prats J, Sarret E, Moragas A. Triploid live full-term infant. *Helv Paediatr Acta* 1971; 26:164.
181. Toaff R, Toaff ME, Peyser MR. Mid-trimester pre-eclamptic toxemia in triploid pregnancies. *Isr J Med Sci* 1976; 12:234.
182. Jacobs PA, Hunt PA, Matsuura JS, Wilson CC. Complete and partial hydatidiform mole in Hawaii: cytogenetics, morphology and epidemiology. *Br J Obstet Gynaecol* 1982; 89:258.
183. Jacobs PA, Szulman AE, Funkhouser J, Matsuura JS, Wilson CC. Human triploidy: relationship between parental origin of the additional haploid complement and development of partial hydatidiform mole. *Ann Hum Genet* 1982; 46:223.
184. Szulman AE, Philippe E, Boué JG, Boué A. Human triploidy: association with partial hydatidiform moles and nonmolar conceptuses. *Hum Pathol* 1981; 12:1016.
185. Szulman AE, Surti U. The syndromes of hydatidiform mole. II. Morphologic evolution of the complete and partial mole. *Am J Obstet Gynecol* 1978; 132:20.
186. Jacobs PA, Angell RR, Buchanan IM, et al. The origin of human triploids. *Ann Hum Genet* 1978; 42:49.
187. Philippe E. *Histopathologie Placentaire*. Paris: Masson et Cie, 1974.
188. Philippe E, Boué JG. Le placenta des aberrations chromosomiques letales. *Ann Anat Pathol* 1969; 14:249.
189. Beisher NA, Fortune DW, Fitzgerald MG. Hydatidiform mole and coexistent foetus, both with triploid chromosome constitution. *Br Med J* 1967; 3:476.
190. Jones WB, Lauersen NH. Hydatidiform mole with coexistent fetus. *Am J Obstet Gynecol* 1975; 122:267.
191. Szulman AE, Surti U. The clinico-pathological profile of the triploid partial mole. (Cited in Ref. 216).
192. Louie RR, Arya S, Gilbert EF, Meisner L. Triploidy (70, XXYY) with an extra sex chromosome and elevated alpha-fetoprotein levels. In: Gilbert EF, Opitz JM, eds. *Genetic Aspects of Developmental Pathology*, Vol. 23. New York: Alan R. Liss, pp. 333–9.
193. Williams DL, Runyan JW Jr. Sex chromatin and chromosome analysis in the diagnosis of sex anomalies. *Ann Intern Med* 1966; 64:422.
194. Côté GB, Tsomi K, Papadakou-Lagoyanni S, Petmezaki S. Oligohydramnios syndrome and XYY karyotype. *Ann Genet* 1978; 121:226.
195. Rimoin DL, Schimke RN. *Genetic Disorders of the Endocrine Glands*. St. Louis: CV Mosby, 1971.
196. Daly JJ, Hunter H, Rickards DF. Klinefelter syndrome and pulmonary disease. *Am Rev Respir Dis* 1968; 98:717.
197. Domm BM, Vassallo CL. Klinefelter syndrome, obesity and respiratory failure. *Am Rev Respir Dis* 1973; 107:123.
198. Hsueh WA, Hsu TH, Federman DD. Endocrine features of Klinefelter's syndrome. *Medicine (Baltimore)* 1978; 57:447.
199. MacLean N, Court-Brown WM, Jacobs P, et al. A survey of sex chromosome abnormalities in mental hospitals. *J Med Genet* 1968; 6:165.
200. Finby N, Archibald RM. Skeletal abnormalities associated with gonadal dysgenesis. *Am J Roentgenol* 1963; 89:1222.
201. Koswicz J. The roentgen appearance of the hand and wrist in gonadal dysgenesis. *Am J Roentgenol* 1965; 93:354.
202. Lemli L, Smith DW. The XO syndrome. A study of the differential phenotype in 25 patients. *J Pediatr* 1963; 63:577.
203. Rushton DI, Faed M, Richards S, et al. The fetal manifestations of the 45, XO karyotype. *J Obstet Gynaecol Br Commonw* 1969; 76:266.
204. Singh RP, Carr DH. The anatomy and histology of XO human embryos and fetuses. *Anat Rec* 1966; 155:369.
205. Vander Putte SCJ. Lymphatic malformation in human fetuses. A study of fetuses with Turner's syndrome or status Bonnevie-Ullrich. *Virchows Arch A* 1977; 376:233.
206. Brook CGD, Murset G, Zachmann M, Prader A. Growth in children with 45, XO Turner syndrome. *Arch Dis Child* 1974; 49:789.
207. de la Chapelle A. Cytogenetical and clinical observations in female gonadal dysgenesis. *Acta Endocrinol Suppl* 1962; 65:1.
208. Gilbert E, Opitz J. Renal abnormalities in malformation syndromes. Ch. 45. In: Edelman CM, Bernstein J, eds. *Pediatric Kidney Disease*. 2nd ed. Boston: Little, Brown & Co. (in press).
209. Lindsten J. *The Nature and Origin of X Chromosome Aberrations in Turner's Syndrome*. Stockholm: Almqvist & Wiksell, 1963.
210. Rossle R. Hypertrophie und atrophie. *Jahreskurse Aerztl Fortbild* 1922; XIII:13.
211. Smith DW. *Recognizable Patterns of Human Malformation*. 3rd ed. Philadelphia: WB Saunders, 1982.

212. Turner HH. A syndrome of infantilism, congenital webbed neck, and cubitus valgus. *Endocrinology* 1938; 23:566.

213. Weiss L. Additional evidence of gradual loss of germ cells in the pathogenesis of streak ovaries in Turner's syndrome. *J Med Genet* 1971; 8:540.

214. Cleeve DM, Older RA, Cleeve LK, Bredael JJ. Retrocaval ureter in Turner syndrome. *Urology* 1979; 13:544.

215. Goodyer PR, Fong JSC, Kaplan BS. Turner's syndrome, 46X, del(X)(p11), persistent complement activation and membranoproliferative glomerulonephritis. *Am J Nephrol* 1982; 2:272.

216. Burge DM, Middleton AW, Kamath R, et al. Intestinal haemorrhage in Turner's syndrome. *Arch Dis Child* 1981; 56:557.

217. Schultz LS, Assimacopoulos CA, Lillihei RC. Turner's syndrome with associated gastrointestinal hemorrhage: a case report. *Surgery* 1970; 68:485.

218. Engle MA, Ehlers KH. Cardiovascular malformations in the syndrome of Turner phenotype with normal karyotype. *Birth Defects, Orig Artic Ser* 1972; 8:104.

219. Siggers DC, Polani PE. Congenital heart disease in male and female subjects with somatic features of Turner's syndrome and normal sex chromosomes. *Br Heart J* 1972; 34:41.

220. Kostich ND, Opitz JM. Ullrich-Turner syndrome associated with cystic medial necrosis of the aorta and great vessels. *Am J Med* 1965; 38:943.

221. Sandberg AA. *The Chromosomes in Human Cancer and Leukemia*. Amsterdam: Elsevier/North-Holland, 1980.

222. Yunis JJ. *Cancer Genet Cytogenet*. (Cited in Ref. 247.)

223. Yunis JJ. Chromosomes and cancer: new nomenclature and future directions. *Hum Pathol* 1981; 12:494.

224. Yunis JJ. New chromosome techniques in the study of human neoplasia. *Hum Pathol* 1981; 12:540.

225. Yunis JJ. Specific fine chromosomal defects in cancer: an overview. *Hum Pathol* 1981; 12:503.

226. Yunis JJ. Unpublished data, cited in Ref. 246.

227. Yunis JJ, Bloomfield CD, Ensrud K. All patients with acute nonlymphocytic leukemia may have a chromosomal defect. *N Engl J Med* 1981; 305:135.

228. Yunis JJ, Oken MM, Kaplan ME, et al. Distinctive chromosomal abnormalities in histologic subtypes of non-Hodgkin's lymphoma. *N Engl J Med* 1982; 307:1231.

229. Temin HM. Viral oncogenes. *Cold Spring Harbor Symp Quant Biol* 1980; 44:1.

230. Yunis JJ. The chromosomal basis of human neoplasia. *Science* 1983; 221:227.

231. Mitelman F, Levan G. Clustering of aberrations to specific chromosomes in human neoplasms. IV. A survey of 1871 cases. *Hereditas* 1981; 95:79.

232. Second International Workshop on Chromosomes in Leukemia (1979). *Cancer Genet Cytogenet* 1980; 2:89.

233. Autio K, Turuner O, Penttila O, et al. Human chronic lymphocytic leukemia: karyotypes in different lymphocyte populations. *Cancer Genet Cytogenet* 1979; 1:147.

234. Gharton G, Robert KH, Friberg K, Zech L, Bird AG. Extra chromosome 12 in chronic lymphocytic leukemia. *Lancet* 1980; i:146.

235. Dalla-Favera R, Bregni M, Erikson J, et al. Human *c-myc onc* gene is located on the region of chromosome 8 that is translocated in Burkitt lymphoma cells. *Proc Natl Acad Sci USA* 1982; 79:7824.

236. Dalla-Favera R, Martinotti S, Gallo RC, Erikson J, Croce CM. Translocation and rearrangements of the *c-myc* oncogene locus in human undifferentiated B-cell lymphoma. *Science* 1983; 219:963.

237. Marcu KB, Harris LJ, Stanton LW, et al. Transcriptionally active *c-myc* oncogene is contained within NIARD, a DNA sequence associated with chromosome translocations in B-cell neoplasia. *Proc Natl Acad Sci USA* 1983; 80:519.

238. Shen-Ong GLC, Keath EJ, Piccoli SP, Cole MD. Novel *myc* oncogene RNA from abortive immunoglobulin-gene recombination in mouse plasmacytomas. *Cell* 1982; 31:443.

239. Taub R, Kirsch L, et al. Translocation of the *c-myc* gene into the immunoglobulin heavy chain locus in human Burkitt lymphoma and murine plasmacytoma cells. *Proc Natl Acad Sci USA* 1982; 79:7837.

240. Rowley JD. Identification of the constant chromosome regions involved in human hematologic malignant disease. *Science* 1982; 216:749.

241. Gilbert F, Balaban G, Moorhead P, Branchi D, Schlesenger H. Abnormalities of chromosome 1p on human neuroblastoma tumour cell lines. *Cancer Genet Cytogenet* 1982; 7:33.

242. Aurias A, Rimabaut C, Buffe D, Dubousset J, Mazabraud A. Chromosomal translocations in Ewing sarcoma. *N Engl J Med* 1983; 309:496.

243. Turc-Carel C, Philip I, Berger MP, Philip T, Lenoir GM. Chromosomal translocation in Ewing sarcoma. *N Engl J Med* 1983; 309:497.

244. Seidal T, Mark J, Hagman B, Angervall L. Alveolar rhabdomyosarcoma. *Acta Pathol Microbiol Immunol Scand, Sect A*: 1982; 90:345.

245. Balaban G, Gilbert F, Nichols W, Meadows A, Shields J. Abnormalities of chromosome 13 in retinoblastomas from individuals with normal constitutional karyotypes. *Cancer Genet Cytogenet* 1982; 6:213.

246. Rivera H, Turleau C, de Grouchy J, et al. Retinoblastoma—del(13q14): report of two patients, one with a trisomy sib due to maternal insertion. Gene-dosage effect for esterase D. *Hum Genet* 1981; 59:211.

247. Sparkes RS. Regional assignment of genes for human esterase D and retinoblastoma to chromosome band 13q14. *Science* 1980; 208:1042.

248. Riccardi VM, Sujansky E, Smith AC, Francke U. Chromosomal imbalance in the aniridia–Wilms' tumor association: 11p interstitial deletion. *Pediatrics* 1978; 61:604.

249. Junien C, Turleau C, et al. Regional assignment of catalase (CAT) gene to band 11p13. Association with the aniridia–Wilms' tumor–gonadoblastoma (WAGR) complex. *Ann Genet* 1980; 23:165.

250. Zankl H, Zang KD. Correlations between clinical and cytogenetical data in 180 human meningiomas. *Cancer Genet Cytogenet* 1980; 1:351.

251. Trimble BK, Baird PA. Maternal age and Down syndrome: age-specific incidence rates by single-year intervals. *Am J Med Genet* 1978; 2:1.

Congenital Anomalies: Malformation Syndromes

Enid F. Gilbert-Barness   John M. Opitz

DEFINITION OF TERMS

The International Working Group (IWG) [1] has recommended a terminology of developmental and other congenital abnormalities. These terms are pertinent to the conditions discussed in this chapter.

General Terminology

Hypoplasia refers to underdevelopment and hyperplasia to overdevelopment of an organism, organ, or tissue resulting from a decrease or an increase in the number of cells, respectively. Hypotrophy and hypertrophy refer to a decrease and an increase in the size of an organ, of tissue, or of cells, respectively. Agenesis is the absence of a part of the body caused by a presumed absence of the anlage (primordium). Aplasia refers to a rudimentary structure that results from a failure of the anlage to develop (completely); it can be regarded as an extreme degree of hypoplasia. Atrophy is used when a normally developed mass of tissue(s) or organ(s) shrinks because of a decrease in cell size or cell number.

Developmental fields are those morphogenetic units of the embryo in which the development of the complex structure appropriate to them is determined and controlled inductively in a spatially coordinated, temporally synchronous, and epimorphically hierarchical manner.

Development of fields may be abnormal due to intrinsic (i.e., genetic) or extrinsic causes: the former lead to primary developmental field defects (malformations), and the latter to secondary developmental field defects (disruptions, secondary malformations). Developmental field defects may be monotopic or polytopic.

A monotopic field defect includes contiguous anomalies (e.g., cyclopia and holoprosencephaly, cleft lip, and cleft palate).

In a polytopic field defect, there are disturbed inductive processes that result in more distantly located defects—e.g., acrorenal field defect (lack of or interference with the inductive effect of the mesonephros results in a defect of limb-bud cartilage proliferation and differentiation) or DiGeorge anomaly (failure of neural crest cells to cause normal development of derivatives of pharyngeal pouches III and IV and their branchial arch arteries and of normal development of conotruncal septation).

All malformations are causally heterogeneous and represent either anomalies of incomplete differentiation or defects of abnormal differentiation, in mild or severe form.

The six periods in human development are pregenesis, embryogenesis, blastogenesis, organogenesis, metamorphosis (the transition from the 8th week to the fetal period), and phenogenesis (Table 13.1).

The Midline as a Developmental Field

The midline is a special kind of "field." It seems to be a developmentally weakly knit part of the "fabric of the human body." It represents not only the plane of cleavage in monozygotic twinning but also the plane around which the symmetry of visceral position is determined. Morphogenetic midline events include, among others, fusions, segmentation, programmed cell death with morphogenetic "necroses" or resorptions, rotations, and other morphogenetic movements. In some anomalies involving the midline, there is an increased incidence of monozygotic twinning (including VATER association and caudal "regression" sequence). Midline anomalies (mostly defects of incomplete differentiation) include such defects as the holoprosencephaly complex, agenesis of corpus callosum, cleft lip, cleft palate, the midface cleft complex, spina bifida, omphalocele, congenital heart defects, hypospadias, and

Table 13.1.   Six periods in human development

Period	Description
Pregenesis	All stages of development from the separation of the germline early in embryogenesis to the moment of fertilization
Embryogenesis	Development from fertilization to the end of the 8th week (10th gestational week)
Blastogenesis	All stages of development from the time of fertilization until the end of gastrulation (day 28)
Organogenesis	Development from day 28 to the 8th week (day 55–56) postconception. Morphogenesis (formation of organs) and hindogenesis (formation of cells and tissues) occur during organogenesis
Metamorphosis	Transition from the end of the 8th week to the fetal period
Phenogenesis	Developmental period from the end of metamorphosis to birth (38 weeks postconception)

imperforate anus. A generalized weakness of midline development increases the chance of having several midline defects, as has been demonstrated by Czeizel [2] in data from the Hungarian Congenital Malformations Registry in so-called schisis associations.

Lubinsky developed a theory pertaining to dysmorphogenetic vulnerability of the mammalian midline by proposing a model relying on positional information for the control of the process of embryonic determination. According to Lubinsky [3], the topologic properties of the midline as an early plane of symmetry imply positional informational weaknesses that should decrease developmental stability in this area for two reasons. First, the unique location on a cusp between two mirror-image fields is conceived as a "null" position for differentiation. Second, this location between two presumably equal positional values eliminates a lateral gradient that aids in regaining information after disruptions. Under Lubinsky's model, midline malformations would be expected to be primarily determinative defects with a particular disturbance of pattern and tissue abnormalities (i.e., dysplasia). Lubinsky has presented initial evidence in support of this hypothesis, which makes midline anomalies consequences of developmental field properties even though, technically speaking, the midline is not itself a field. Rather, the midline must be regarded as the morphogenetically most important landmark of the primary field—i.e., of the embryo until the end of blastogenesis.

Mild Malformations Versus Minor Anomalies

Mild Malformations
All malformations, including their least severe forms, are all-or-none traits; even when least severe, none "shades" into

normality. Mild malformations should not be viewed as normal variants in the population, regardless of how mild or common. Some examples of mild malformations are bipartite uvula, abnormal lobation of lungs, enterohepatic gallbladder, annular pancreas, accessory spleens, renal microcysts, and Meckel's diverticulum, Mild malformations usually are autosomal dominant traits and are frequently present in aneuploidy syndromes.

Minor Anomalies
Anatomically, minor anomalies and normal developmental variants are indistinguishable and constitute, respectively, abnormal and normal variations of final structure. They arise during phenogenesis (i.e., all of those morphogenetic events that occur after organogenesis) and are the traits that constitute our morphologic uniqueness, and are also the heritage of ethnic group and family inheritance. The final results of end-stage "fine-tuning" of development do not involve major threshold decisions of morphogenesis (organogenesis) and are controlled polygenically. To our knowledge, no mendelian minor anomalies are known. All normal development variants can occur as minor anomalies and vice versa, but, while developmentally identical, they have different causal implications. In Down syndrome, there usually are a sufficient number of minor anomalies characteristic enough to be diagnostic. Aneuploidy disturbs preeminently end-stage fine-tuning of development, as is evident from the well-known fact that most anomalies in such conditions are minor anomalies and that such individuals lack family resemblance. Normal variants are familial; syndromic minor anomalies usually are not.

Syndrome

A syndrome is a causally defined entity in the sense formalized at the VIIth International Congress on Human Genetics [4]: "A syndrome is a recognizable pattern of anomalies that are known or thought to be causally related." This is a genetic definition. However, in medical usage, the older understanding of syndrome as a set of pathogenetically related manifestations persists and is used to this day, but with the now explicit understanding that in every case where an entity is spoken of in such terms, causal heterogeneity is not excluded, and indeed must be presumed to be present until proven otherwise. In clinical genetics it is becoming common practice to speak of a set of causally heterogeneous entities as a phenotype—e.g., the Sanfilippo phenotype—and of the individual causally defined entities of Sanfilippo syndrome type A, B, C, D, etc. [4]. No structural component anomaly of any malformation syndrome is obligatory, and none is pathognomonic of any syndrome. Malformation syndromes consist of two or more developmental field defects, or a single (major) field defect and several minor anomalies.

Disruptions (Secondary Malformations)

"A disruption is a morphological defect of an organ, part of an organ or larger region of the body resulting from an extrinsic breakdown of, or an interference with, an originally normal developmental process" (IWG). Disruptions are causally heterogeneous and may be anatomically identical to malformations. In a given case, the distinction may be made on the basis of the associated malformations or the history of gestational exposure to a teratogenic cause or event.

Types of Disruptions

1. Radiation disruption
2. Teratogenic disruption (e.g., thalidomide, 13-*cis*-retinoic acid, fetal alcohol syndrome)
3. Metabolic disruption (maternal diabetes, maternal PKU)
4. Infectious disruption (rubella syndrome)
5. Immunologic/autoimmune disruption (congenital graft-versus-host reaction)
6. Chorion–yolk sac rupture with ectopia cordis and other anomalies
7. Amnion rupture–oligohydramnios disruption sequence (early) (cyllosomus, pleurosomus)
8. Amniotic deformities-adhesions-mutilation (ADAM) complex (late)
9. Maternal myoma uteri and uterine malformations as a cause of fetal disruption and defect of implantation, placentation, and body stalk formation
10. Ischemic disruption
11. Dysplastic disruptions
12. Twinning disruption
13. Thermodisruptive anomalies
14. Circumvallate placenta disruptions

Sequence

"A sequence is a pattern of multiple anomalies derived from a single known or presumed prior anomaly or mechanical factor" (IWG).

In the Potter sequence, the initiating event is oligohydramnios of genetic or nongenetic cause, and due to malformation (renal agenesis or dysplasia—e.g., polycystic kidney) or a mechanical factor (amniotic fluid leakage). Lack of amniotic fluid leads to restriction of fetal movement and fetal compression, with resultant typical changes of the Potter sequence (Fig. 13.1).

Deformation

"A deformation is an abnormal form, shape or position of part of the body caused by mechanical forces" (IWG). This may be extrinsic due to intrauterine constraint (e.g., lack of amniotic fluid) or intrinsic due to a defect of the nervous system resulting in hypomobility. Examples of deformities

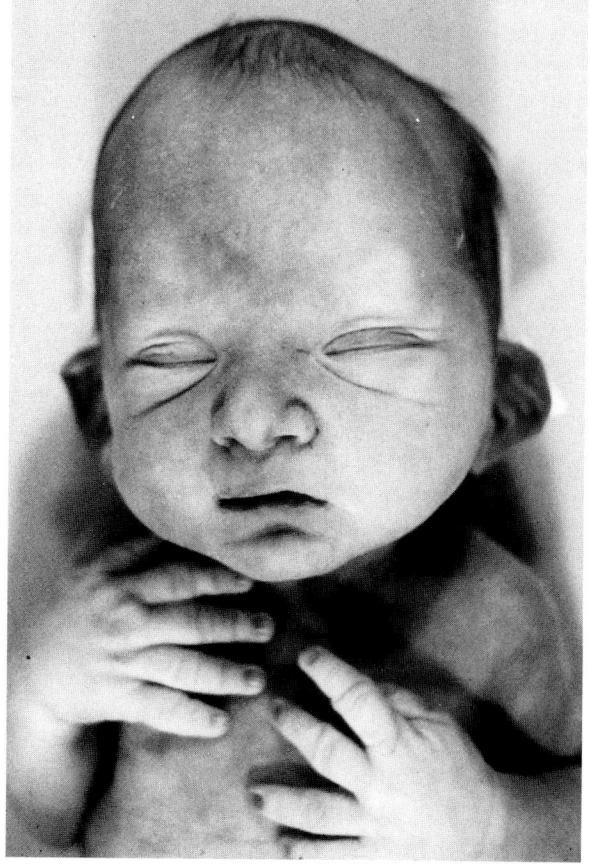

FIGURE 13.1.   *Infant with Potter sequence, illustrating the facial appearance. Courtesy of Prof. J. S. Wigglesworth.*

are talipes equinovarus and arthrogryposis. About 1–2% of newborn infants have deformations.

Dysplasia

"A dysplasia is an abnormal organization of cells into tissue(s) and its morphological result(s). In other words: a dysplasia is the process (and the consequence) of dyshistogenesis" (IWG). A dysplasia is abnormal differentiation of tissue structure. Dysplasias also are causally nonspecific. Dysplasias may or may not be metabolically induced. They may involve one or several germ layers, may be generalized or localized, and tend to be sporadic in occurrence.

Dysplasias represent defects of tissue differentiation—i.e., dyshistogenesis (in contradistinction to malformations, which are defects of morphogenesis of organ structure—a "dysmorphogenesis"). Many dysplasias can be viewed as developmental fine-tuning defects of histogenesis. Small, minor dysplasias are exceedingly common in the normal population and include freckling, capillary hemangioma over the glabella and metopic suture area of the forehead, café-au-lait spots, moles, and nevi. Most dysplasias occur sporadically. If they are mendelian traits, they usually represent autosomal dominant mutations. Dysplasias are components of every aneuploidy syndrome and probably are one of the reasons for the increased incidence of cancers in such syndromes. Dysplasias may be induced environmentally through a variety of influences, including radiation, viruses, and carcinogens.

Association

"Associations represent the idiopathic occurrence of multiple anomalies during blastogenesis" (IWG) [1, 5, 6]. At the 1984 Birth Defects Conference, Lubinsky [7] proposed a definition and suggested that: "associations are derivatives of causally non-specific disruptive events acting in developmental fields." The presumption is that the disruptive exogenous agents or events acted essentially simultaneously, affecting all primordia sensitive or vulnerable and capable of reacting dysmorphogenetically at that time in organogenesis. This is a noncausal understanding of the entity association; but, in contradistinction to the medical understanding of the concept of syndrome, the implication of pleiotropy is lacking in this view of the term "association." Thus, in addition to clinical methods, associations are evaluated in terms of biologic or teratologic modeling and by epidemiologic methods. The clinician attempts to delineate the VATER association and its numerous variants and to understand it pathogenetically, and the epidemiologist attempts to find associated factors that might have a predisposing relationship to the association, such as monozygotic twinning or maternal diabetes [7].

MONOTOPIC DEVELOPMENTAL FIELD DEFECTS

Under this heading we include only a few examples. The large number of monotopic developmental field defects that involve single organ systems are discussed in the relevant chapters elsewhere in the book and will not be considered here.

Sirenomelia

This severe developmental field defect is probably due to an early defect of the posterior axis caudal blastema, resulting in fusion of the lower limb buds (Fig. 13.2). It dates to the primitive streak stage during the 3rd week of gestation, prior to development of the allantois, for there usually is an absence of allantoic vessels [8–10]. Sirenomelia appears to involve a wedge-shaped defect of the caudal midline such that the lower limb is fused. It has been claimed recently that sirenomelia is the result of a vascular steal phenomenon, as all cases dissected show an abnormal single large artery arising from the abdominal aorta, with malformation or absence of tissues arising caudal to it [11]. This sporadic defect occurs in about 1 in 60,000 newborn infants; it has

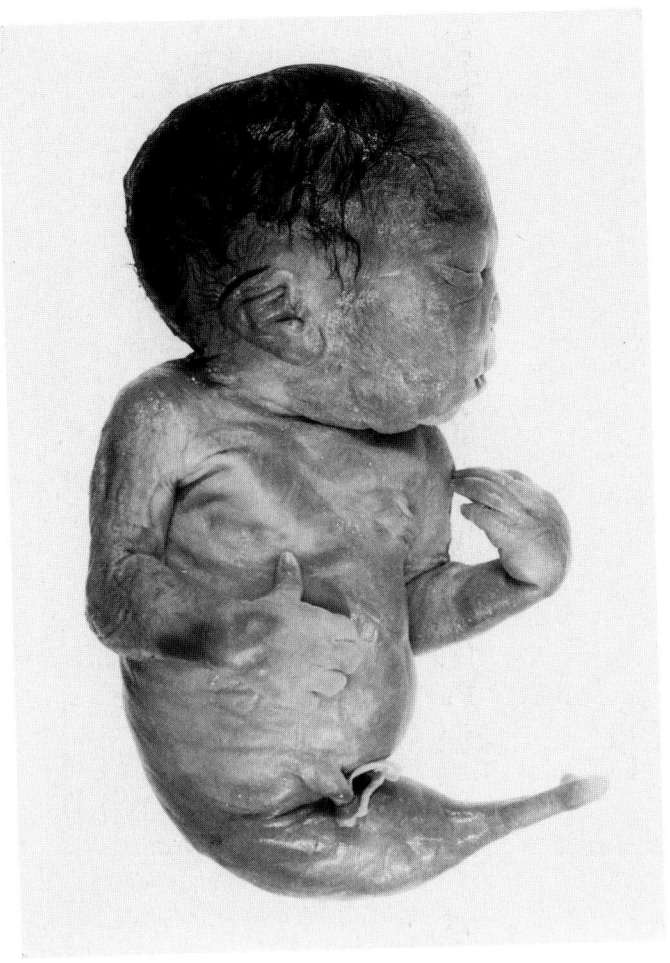

FIGURE 13.2.   *Sirenomelia with normal upper limbs and fused lower limbs ending in single digit. Courtesy of Dr. D. I. Rushton.*

a male sex preponderance and is more common in one of identical twins. Other defects of the caudal axis include malformations of the coccygeal vertebrae, sacral defects, chordomas from notochordal rests at the coccygeal site, imperforate anus, lower vertebral defects, and genitourinary defects. The presence of radial aplasia, esophageal atresia, and tracheoesophageal fistula in some cases suggests that the VATER association may represent a lesser degree of the caudal regression sequence. The latter malformation may occur in infants of diabetic mothers. Opitz and Gilbert [12] hypothesized a generalized developmental midline weakness to explain this defect. We have observed ectopic renal tissue within the gastrointestinal tracts of sirenomelic fetuses. Renal agenesis and cystic renal dysplasia have occurred [8].

Robinson Defect

Agenesis of the cloacal membrane results in a persistent cloaca with absence of external genitalia and urinary, genital, and anal orifices [13]; the bladder may be massively distended (and ruptured) with hydroureters, hydronephrosis, and cystic renal dysplasia. Bilateral renal agenesis has been described. Abdominal wall distension with marked distension of the bladder may result in the wrinkled appearance of the abdominal wall seen in the prune belly sequence.

Otocephaly

Otocephaly is a causally heterogeneous single developmental field defect affecting structures in the face and upper neck, with absence of the mandible and approximation of the ears in the midline region normally occupied by the mandible (Fig. 13.3). It has been related to defects in neural crest cells of cranial origin and/or to underlying mesodermal support elements of these cells [14]. Cardiac defects and renal anomalies have been observed [15]. It may be associated with microphthalmia and/or cyclopia and its association with cyclopia is well known. Most cases have been sporadic [14, 16, 17] although familial occurrence in siblings has been noted, suggesting autosomal recessive inheritance [15].

Otocephaly is different from agnathia/holoprosencephaly, which is an autosomal recessive trait [15]. In humans, otocephaly is rarely associated with holoprosencephaly as it frequently is in guinea pigs [18, 19].

POLYTOPIC DEVELOPMENTAL FIELD DEFECTS

Microtia-Auriculo-Facio-Vertebral Complex (First and Second Branchial Arch Syndrome, Oculoauriculo-Vertebral Dysplasia, Hemifacial Microsomia, Goldenhar Syndrome)

This condition is usually sporadic and represents defects in morphogenesis of the first and second branchial arches [20–25]. Facial anomalies include hypoplasia of the malar, the maxillary, and/or the mandibular region, especially the ramus and condyle of the mandible and temporomandibular joint, macrostomia, and hypoplasia of facial muscles (Fig. 13.4). Microtia, accessory preauricular tags and/or pits, middle-ear anomaly with variable deafness, diminished-to-absent parotid secretion, anomalies of the tongue and soft palate, and hemivertebrae are frequent.

Less frequent manifestations include epibulbar dermoid, strabismus, microphthalmia, deafness, cleft lip, cleft palate, and cardiac defects. Branchial cleft remnants in the anterior-lateral neck, laryngeal anomaly, hypoplasia or aplasia of lung, occipital encephalocele, renal anomalies, and psychomotor and growth retardation may be seen.

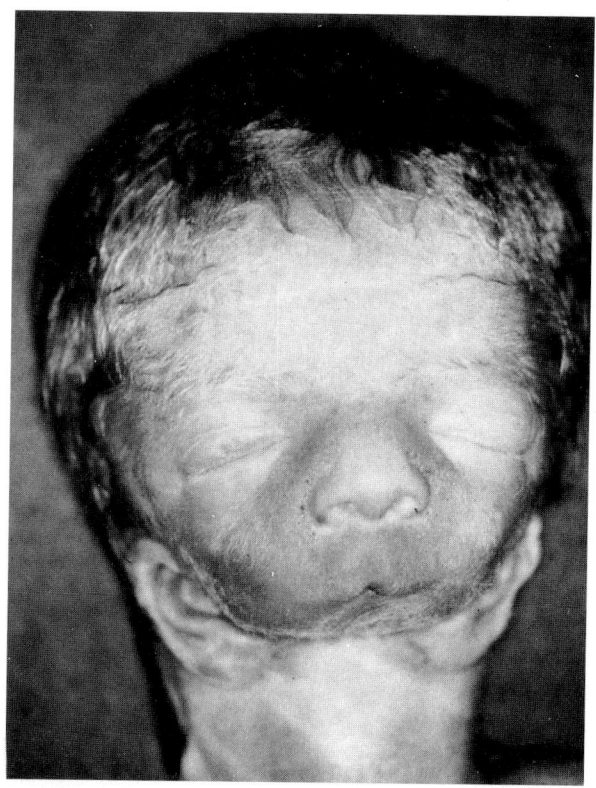

FIGURE 13.3. *Otocephaly. The ears are displaced downward and approximate the midline; there is virtual agnathia.*

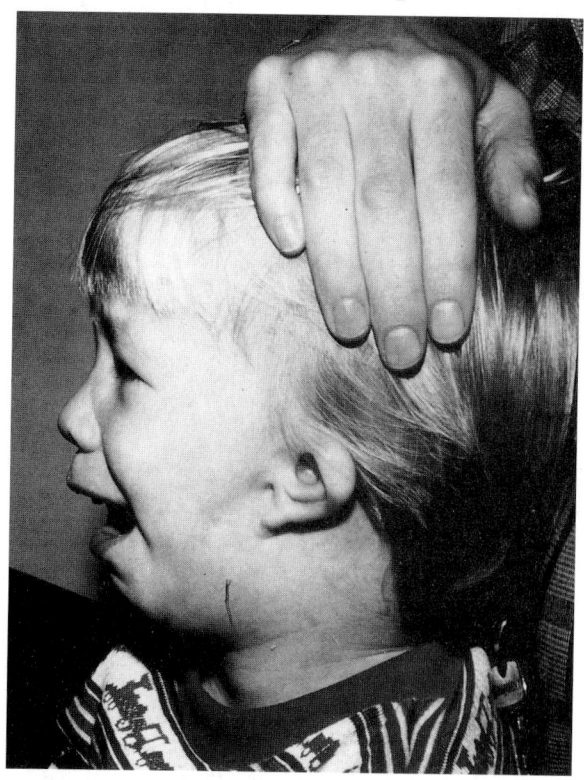

FIGURE 13.4. *Goldenhar syndrome, with mandibular hypoplasia, microtia, and mild hemifacial microsomia.*

Hanhart and Poland-Möbius Complexes

These conditions were studied extensively and redefined by Herrmann et al [26]. The Hanhart anomaly usually includes severe limb defects of at least one hand or foot (Fig. 13.5), frequently associated with severe oral abnormalities. The condition associated with cranial nerve palsies is called the Hanhart-Möbius complex. Most cases are reported as aglossia-adactylia syndrome, aglossia-hypomelia syndrome, or oromandibular limb hypogenesis spectrum, and some cases may be reported as glossopalatine ankylosis or ankyloglossia superior-Möbius syndrome. The condition should be separated from the Poland-Möbius syndrome. The Poland-Möbius syndrome involves the Poland anomaly (i.e., chest defect and/or symbrachydactyly) and cranial nerve palsies.

Both of these conditions are malformation complexes, which implies that they are etiologically nonspecific developmental field complexes. In the Hanhart complex, Bersu et al [27] postulated a common ectodermal pathogenetic disturbance for oral and limb defects, thus suggesting that the manifestations represent a single anomaly rather than a syndrome. Pauli and Greenlaw [28] have related splenogonadal fusion to limb deficiency and complex ectromelia conditions, such as the Hanhart complex. The Hanhart complex should be considered as an example of "ectoderm ring" developmental disturbance.

DISRUPTIONS

Radiation Disruption

Fetal radiation damage was well defined by Murphy [29] and Goldstein and Murphy [30], who documented microcephaly, skull defects, spina bifida, microphthalmia, cleft palate, micromelia, clubfoot, and other abnormalities after heavy maternal X-irradiation. Atomic bomb casualty studies have also documented microcephaly and mental retardation related to the distance from the hypocenter [31, 32].

Teratogenic Disruptions

Aminopterin and Folic Acid Deficiency
Aminopterin, a folic acid antagonist, administered during the first trimester of pregnancy along with methotrexate, the methyl derivative [33–35], may result in a pattern of malformations consisting of cranial and foot anomalies, growth deficiency, and microcephaly. Craniofacial anomalies include severe hypoplasia of frontal, parietal, temporal, or occipital bones, wide fontanelles, upsweep of frontal scalp hair, broad nasal bridge, shallow supraorbital ridges, prominent eyes, micrognathia, cleft palate, apparently low-set ears, maxillary hypoplasia, and epicanthal folds. The limbs are relatively short. Dislocation of hips, short thumbs, partial syndactyly of third and fourth fingers, dextroposition of the heart, and hypotonia may be present occasionally.

Folic acid deficiency has been observed in a high percentage of women who have had infants with neural tube defects (NTDs). Deficiency appears to result in up to 70% of infants with NTDs—particularly anencephaly [36]. It has been recommended that there be a periconceptional intake of 0.4 mg of folic acid daily; such a regimen is estimated to reduce significantly the risk of NTDs [37].

Fetal Iodine Deficiency
Fetal iodine deficiency results in mental deficiency, spastic diplegia, deafness, and strabismus [38, 39]. It requires severe maternal iodine deficiency (less than 20 μg per day) during the first half of gestation, as may occur in northern Italy and in some mountainous areas of New Guinea, the Himalayas, and the Andes.

Thalidomide
Thalidomide was first recognized as a teratogen by Lenz [40] and McBride [41]. Maternal administration during the critical period (23rd to 28th day of gestation) may result in a number of defects (Table 13.2), most notable of which are limb defects ranging from triphalangeal thumb to tetra-amelia or phocomelia of upper and lower limbs, at times with preaxial polydactyly of six or seven toes per foot. Congenital heart defects, urinary tract anomalies, genital defects,

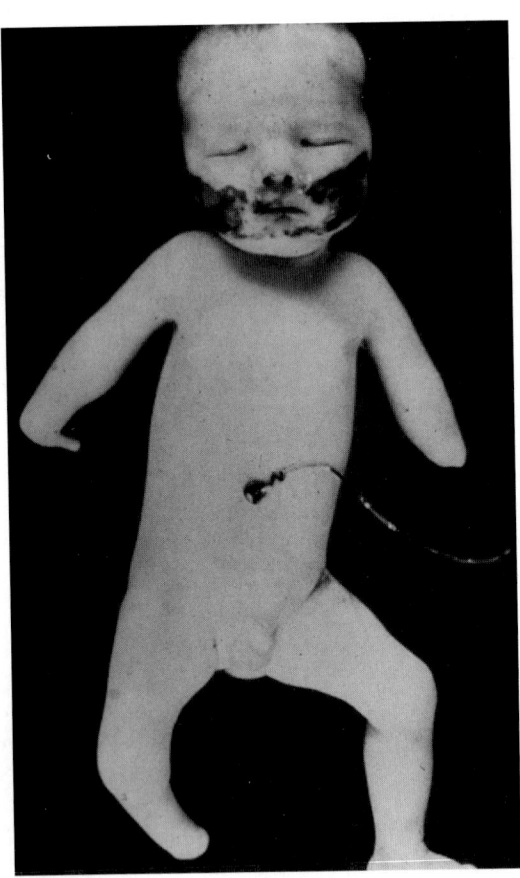

FIGURE 13.5. *Hanhart complex with severe limb defects (marks on face result from tape).*

Table 13.2. Abnormalities reported in thalidomide embryopathy

Skeletal defects
Absent radii
Hand
  Limited extension
  Clubhand
  Hypoplastic or fused phalanges
  Finger syndactyly
  Carpal hypoplasia or fusion
  Radial deviation
Ulna
  Short and malformed
  Unilaterally absent
  Bilaterally absent
Humerus
  Hypoplastic
  Absent
Shoulder girdle (abnormally formed with absent glenoid fossa and acromion
    process, and hypoplastic scapula and clavicle)
Hips
  Unilaterally or bilaterally dislocated
Legs
  Coxa valga
  Femoral torsion
  Tibial torsion
    bilateral
    unilateral
  Stiff knee
  Abnormal tibiofibular joint
  Dislocated patella(e)
Feet
  Overriding 5th toe
  Calcaneovalgus deformity
  Other foot deformity
Ribs
  Asymmetric 1st rib
  Cervical rib
Spine
  Cervical spina bifida
  Fused cervical spine
Mandibular hypoplasia
Maxillary hypoplasia
Cardiac anomalies
Tetralogy of Fallot
Atrial septal defect
Patent foramen ovale
Dextrocardia
Congestive heart failure leading to death
Systolic murmur
Cardiomegaly
Suspected congenital heart disease
Apparently low-set ears and malformations extending to microtia
Urogenital anomalies
Micrognathia
Meckel's diverticulum
Uterine anomalies

gastrointestinal anomalies, eye defects, ear malformations, and dental anomalies may be observed. McCredie has postulated an interference with neural-crest-based sclerotomal organization as a pathogenetic basis of the limb malformations [42–48]. Recently, North and McCredie [49] expanded this conception by studying retrospectively the visceral anomalies in infants who died of multiple congenital anomalies with longitudinal limb defects, to determine if neural crest injury would impair the development of structures supplied by the sensory and autonomic nerves derived from the injured zone of the neural crest. Sclerotome maps of the segmental sensory innervation of the skeleton were used to analyze the limb defects in terms of their nerve supply. Anatomic resources provided data on the presumed contribution of neural crest to the autonomic innervation of internal organs, and "viscerotome" diagrams were constructed. Application of sclerotomal and viscerotomal maps to the postmortem data showed a neuroanatomic correlation in 89% of cases. North and McCredie [49] propose the challenging concept of a developmental correlation within multiple congenital anomaly syndromes on the basis of neurotomes or (embryonic) developmental fields with common regional innervation.

Trimethadione

Infants affected with the trimethadione syndrome have a quite characteristic facial appearance, with unusual eyebrows and apparently low-set ears with anteriorly folded helix, highly arched palate, and irregular teeth. They may also be short and mentally retarded and have a cleft palate and cardiac anomalies.

Warfarin

Warfarin [50–52] may cause a syndrome—warfarin embryopathy—of shortness of stature and characteristic facial appearance with hypoplastic nose and chondrodysplasia punctata [53]. When warfarin is given in the later part of pregnancy, brain damage with mental retardation due to CNS bleeding may occur [54].

Teratogenic Effects of Hormonal Drugs

Synthetic progestins, such as 17-ethinyl-19-nortestosterone, can induce enlargement of the clitoris in female fetuses [55] and hypospadias in males [56]. Diethylstilbestrol may cause vaginal adenosis in prenatally exposed females [57] and reproductive anomalies in similarly exposed males [58].

Rarer types of teratogenic drugs in humans include congenital exposure of the fetus to mercury, which may cause severe brain damage called Minamata disease. It occurred in epidemic proportions on a Japanese island following the maternal ingestion by humans and cats of shellfish contaminated with an organic mercury compound (methyl mercury) [54]. Folic acid antagonists—methotrexate, cyclophosphamide, busulphan, and quinine—are teratogenic [54], while meclizine, ACTH, and cortisone (Fig. 13.6) are suspected of causing cleft lip and cleft palate [54].

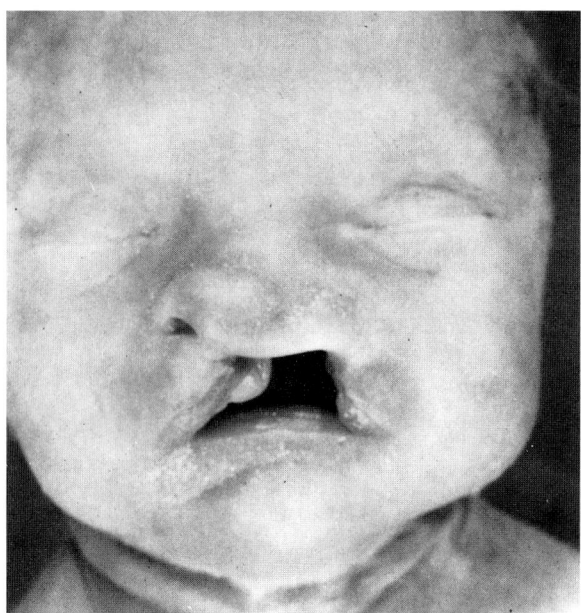

FIGURE 13.6.   *Stillborn infant with cleft lip and cleft palate following maternal cortisone treatment during pregnancy.*

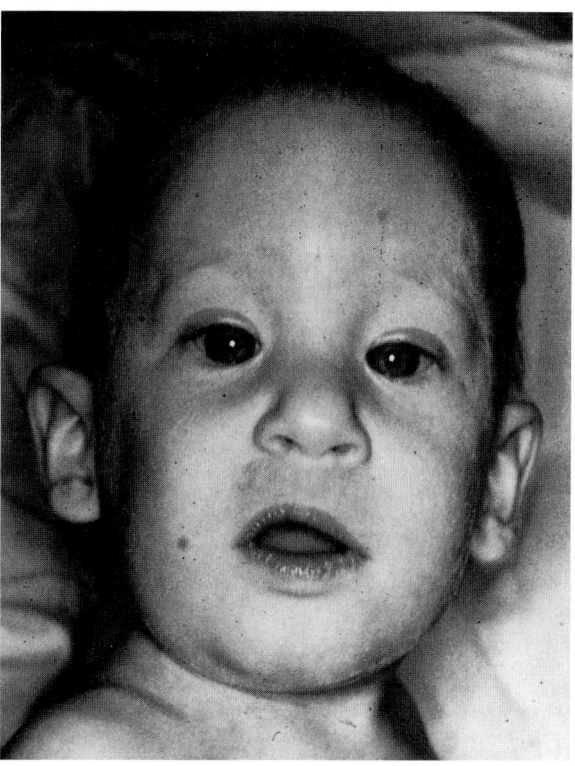

FIGURE 13.7.   *Fetal alcohol syndrome with typical facial appearance. There is a long upper lip, thin upper lip vermilion, short and upward slanted palpebral fissures, epicanthal folds, and mild hirsutism.*

Vitamin A Analogue: Retinoic Acid

Isotretinoin (Accutane), a vitamin A analogue, is 13-*cis*-retinoic acid and is one of the most potent teratogenic agents known. It inhibits sebaceous gland function and is used in the treatment of cystic acne [59]. Exposure to this drug during the first trimester of pregnancy has resulted in a high incidence of spontaneous abortion and malformations in the fetus, including craniofacial anomalies, hypertelorism, downward slant of palpebral fissures, cleft palate and hypoplasia of the midface and mandible, the DiGeorge sequence, and brain malformations.

Microtia with or without agenesis of the external ear canal, CNS abnormalities, and congenital heart defects have been described [60, 61].

Alcohol

Alcohol is probably the most common and important teratogen in humans [62, 63]. For a diagnosis of fetal alcohol syndrome (FAS) to be made, the patient must have three characteristics: pre- and postnatal growth retardation (greater than or equal to 2 SD for length and weight), facial anomalies, and CNS dysfunction. Patients with FAS usually weigh less than 2500 grams at birth. Among the distinctive facial anomalies are absent-to-indistinct philtrum, epicanthal folds, short palpebral fissures, thin vermilion border of the upper lip, and short upturned nose (Fig. 13.7). Joint, limb, and cardiac anomalies are also often present. CNS dysfunction includes mental retardation, hyperactivity, sleep disorders, spastic tetraplegia, seizures, and miscellaneous behavior difficulties. Limb defects include shortness of metatarsals

and/or metacarpals or severe ectrodactyly [64]. Unusual hirsutism is present at birth but disappears with age in many infants; it may be retained in North American Indians. Cystic hygromas may occur and should be distinguished from other conditions associated with them (Table 13.3). In spite of a small head circumference and initially slow psychomotor maturation, some infants with FAS may progress to a normal range of intelligence. FAS is also a carcinogenic syndrome with tumors virtually identical to those seen in the fetal hydantoin syndrome.

Diphenylhydantion

Diphenylhydantoin (Dilantin) may be associated with a syndrome of microcephaly and mental retardation, cleft palate, and congenital heart defect, with a characteristic facial appearance (Fig. 13.8) [65]. Fetal exposure to diphenylhydantoin is now also known to be carcinogenic. Neuroblastoma has been observed in three infants with the fetal hydantoin syndrome. Ganglioneuroblastoma has been observed in a child with both fetal hydantoin and alcohol syndromes. Malignant mesenchymoma has been recorded in a young adult exposed to diphenylhydantoin in utero. A newborn infant has been described with fetal hydantoin syndrome and extrarenal Wilms' tumor [66].

Table 13.3. Conditions associated with cystic nuchal hygromas

Single gene disorders
    Familial neck webbing (autosomal dominant)
    Lymphedema distichiasis syndrome (autosomal dominant)
    Roberts-SC syndrome (autosomal recessive)
    Cowchock syndrome (autosomal recessive?)
Chromosome disorders
    45, X Ullrich-Turner syndrome
    X-chromosome polysomy
    13q– syndrome
    18p– syndrome
    Trisomy 18 syndrome
    Trisomy 21 syndrome
    Trisomy 22 mosaicism syndrome
Teratogenic disorders
    Fetal alcohol syndrome
    Fetal aminopterin syndrome
    Fetal trimethadione syndrome
Disorders of unknown cause
    Noonan syndrome (autosomal dominant?)

Metabolic Disruptions

Maternal diabetes may be associated with fetal anomalies (Fig. 13.9). In diabetic embryopathy, defects include congenital heart defect, spina bifida, the so-called "caudal regression anomaly," sirenomelia, imperforate anus, radius aplasia, and renal abnormalities including renal agenesis and dysplasia. Frequently, anomalies present may constitute the VATER association [67–73].

Malformations (Table 13.4) emerge as the most important cause of mortality in infants of diabetic mothers [74, 75]. The overall incidence of major malformations is 6–9% in large studies [74–76]—about twice that found in a general neonatal population—the "normal" incidence being about 5% [77].

Recently it has been found that there is a close correlation between hemoglobin A_{1c} (HbA_{1c}) and the incidence of major congenital anomalies in infants of diabetic mothers [78]. HbA_{1c} is a normal minor hemoglobin that is distinguished from hemoglobin A by the addition of a glucose moiety to the amino-terminal valine of the beta chain. Glycosylation of hemoglobin A occurs during circulation of the red cell and depends on the average concentration of

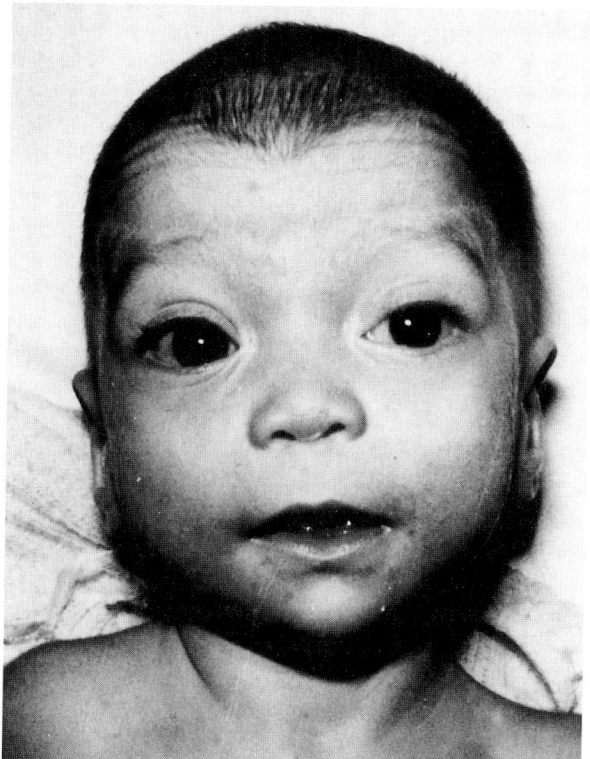

FIGURE 13.8. *Diphenylhydantoin embryopathy. The infant has hypertelorism, prominent eyes, micrognathia, and microcephaly.*

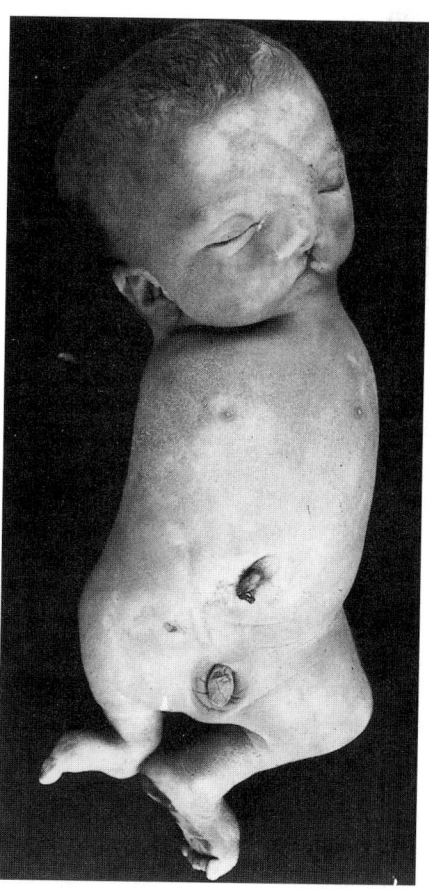

FIGURE 13.9. *Diabetic embryopathy with amelia, cleft lip, micrognathia, and caudal regression.*

Table 13.4.   Major congenital anomalies in offspring of diabetic mothers

CNS
   Anencephaly
   Holoprosencephaly
   Arhinencephaly
   Occipital encephalocele
Cardiovascular
   Transposition of the great arteries
   Ventricular septal defect
   Atrial septal defect
   Tetralogy of Fallot
   Single ventricle
   Mitral valve atresia
   Pulmonary stenosis
   Hypoplastic left heart, Ebstein malformation
Other
   Bilateral auricular atresia
   Cleft lip
   Omphalocele
   Unilateral renal agenesis
   Hypoplastic lungs
   Caudal regression
   Amelia of upper limbs

glucose to which the red cell has been exposed during its life cycle [79]. Measurement of HbA_{1c} provides an index of glucose, hence of diabetes control [80]. There is a higher incidence of major congenital anomalies in the offspring of women with elevated HbA_{1c}. Inadequately controlled diabetes is associated with an increased risk of such anomalies.

Uncontrolled diabetes mellitus in early pregnancy is associated with an increased risk of major structural malformations in offspring. HbA_{1c} values should be useful in the individual assessment of risk of the major congenital malformations.

In a study by Key et al [81] of HbA_{1c} levels during pregnancy, values that exceeded 11.5% were associated with congenital abnormalities in 66% of the offspring, whereas levels less than 9.5% were not associated with an increased frequency of anomalies in the infant. Subsequently it has been found that major fetal anomalies do not increase significantly until the first trimester HbA_{1c} are 14.4% more [82].

Maternal Phenylketonuria (PKU)

Maternal PKU leads to defects in all fetuses conceived, including intrauterine and postnatal growth retardation, microcephaly and mental retardation, cardiovascular defects, dislocated hips, and other anomalies [83]. All infants of phenylketonuric mothers are heterozygous, and since PKU heterozygotes are generally normal, the defect in the fetus must be attributed to the maternal metabolic disturbance.

Infectious Disruptions

Infections, particularly those of the toxoplasmosis, rubella cytomegalovirus infection, herpes and syphilis group, may cause fetal disruptions. The earlier in pregnancy the infection occurs, the greater the likelihood of embryonic death and of fetal anomalies. Most frequent are intrauterine growth retardation, microcephaly and mental retardation, deafness, cataracts, retinopathy, microphthalmia, glaucoma, myopia, and congenital heart defects.

Periventricular calcifications and chorioretinitis are frequent in toxoplasmosis. Other organisms that may be implicated in human congenital anomalies are *Herpesvirus hominis* type 2 (severe congenital brain defect), varicella, Venezuelan equine encephalitis, coxsackievirus, and syphilis [84].

Immunologic Autoimmune Disruptions

In graft-versus-host disease, immunologic mechanisms have been invoked in endocardial fibroelastosis [85], following paternal leukocyte injections received by the mother [86] and in congenital lupus.

Rupture of Chorion or Yolk Sac Sequence: Ectopia Cordis and Cleft Sternum

Kaplan et al [87] have suggested that rupture of the chorion or yolk sac around 3 weeks of gestation with subsequent mechanical compression may interfere with normal cardiac descent, resulting in ectopia cordis with cephalic-pointing cardiac apex and cleft sternum, and thoracic and pulmonary hypoplasia. Congenital heart defects associated with ectopia cordis may represent deformations secondary to mechanical distortions of the developing heart. Thoracoabdominal ectopia cordis results from tethering of the heart to periumbilical structures by bands.

Early Amnion Rupture: Oligohydramnios Disruption

Early amnion rupture may interfere with fetal development, resulting in severe defects of body wall with extrusion of viscera and absence of an ipsilateral or contralateral limb, neural tube defects with scoliosis, postural deformations, growth deficiency, and a short umbilical cord [88]. These complex groups of defects have been designated "pleurosomus" and "cyllosomus." Oligohydramnios and uterine compression appear to be the underlying pathogenetic mechanisms.

The ADAM Complex (Amniotic Deformities, Adhesions, Mutilations)

The ADAM defect is due to adhering, constricting, and swallowed amniotic bands. It is common and may affect one in every 1200 live- and stillborn fetuses. In the ADAM complex, amniotic bands frequently adhere to the head. Swallowing of amniotic bands may produce bizarre orofacial clefts (Fig. 13.10) as well as distortions and disruptions of craniofacial structures, widely separated eyes, nose displaced onto the forehead, and exencephaloceles. Limbs or parts of limbs may be amputated. Exomphalocele may be present. Strands of amnion may still be present at birth. The least severe end of the spectrum of amniotic band disruption is a constriction groove on a limb (Streeter band).

The result of early amnion rupture is external compression and/or disruption; there are rarely any internal anomalies. The etiology is unknown. Generally, it is a sporadic event. Anecdotally, a few cases have been associated with trauma; we have observed an association with maternal exposure to radiation. Two families with amniotic bands in relatives were reported recently [89]; generally, however, the recurrence risk is negligible. The temporal relationship of abnormalities in early amnion rupture—ADAM complex—is shown in Table 13.5.

Myoma Uteri and Uterine Malformation

In particular, a bicornuate uterus may cause fetal compression and constraint and result in a malformed fetus. Also, such uterine malformations seem to predispose to abnormalities in implantation, placentation and body stalk formation, late fetal cord complications, and increased risk of stillbirth.

Ischemic and Vascular Disruptions

Interference with blood supply may result in ischemic disruptions. The acardia/acephalus anomaly is due to artery/artery transfusion (see Chap. 8) With diversion of arterial blood from a donor twin, the perfusion of blood is greater to the lower part of the body of the recipient twin. This results in disruption of existing tissue as well as incomplete morphogenesis of tissues that are differentiating. The result may be an amorphous twin, acardia/acephalus, or variable absence of the head, heart, upper limbs, lungs, pancreas, and upper intestine [90].

Cutis marmorata telangiectatica congenita (CMTC) [91] is a vascular disruption characterized by atypical capillaries, venules, and veins in different cutaneous layers. Clinically, the lesions are manifested as telangiectasis, capillary hemangioma, cutis marmorata, venous hemangiomas, and varicose veins, depending on the type of vessels involved in the layer of skin affected. Secondary thrombosis with subsequent localized atrophy and ulceration may occur. It occurs sporadically with female preponderance, with occasional minor manifestations in close relatives.

Nosologically, the Klippel-Trénaunay-Weber dysplasia and capillary hemangiomatosis must be considered. In CMTC, bona fide toe malformations (oligodactyly, syndactyly) and gigantism of digits have been observed.

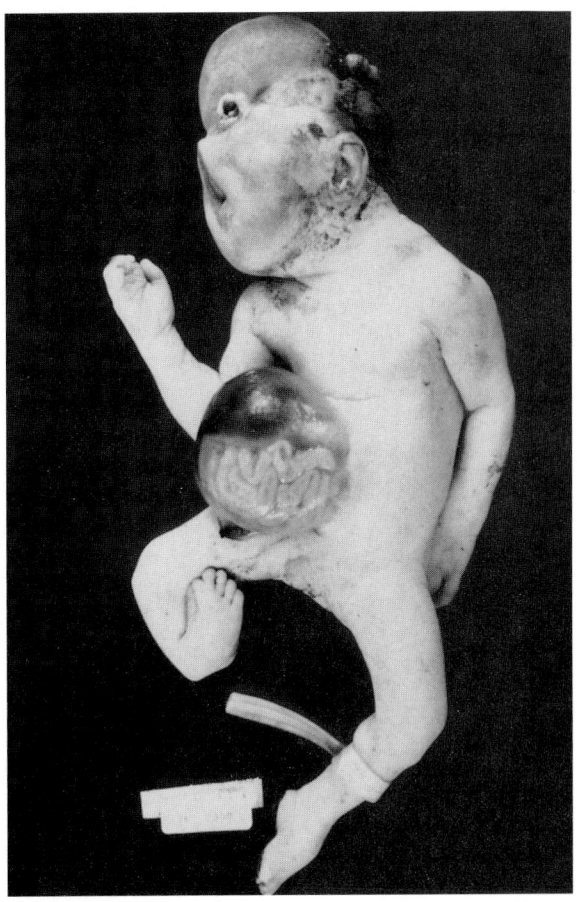

FIGURE 13.10. *ADAM complex with multiple developmental disruptions, omphalocele, pseudosyndactyly, and distortion of craniofacial structures due to swallowed bands of amnion.*

Dysplastic Disruptions

Dysplastic disruptions most commonly involve presacral teratomas, which may be associated with anencephaly; spina bifida; meningocele; imperforate anus; duplication of the lower intestinal tract, uterus, vagina, and of a ureter and renal pelvis; patent urachus; cleft palate; and esophageal and duodenal atresia. A rare form of presacral teratoma, imperforate anus, and sacral defect may be inherited dominantly.

Twinning Disruptions

Twinning disruptions involve mostly vascular defects [92]. The "Swiss cheese" brain defect is an example in a surviving monozygotic twin (see Chap. 8 and 21). Acardia/acephalus, "caudal regression"/sirenomelia, and VATER association may also be disruptive sequences of the twinning process.

Thermodisruptive Anomalies

Hyperthermia is an antimitotic teratogen that interferes mostly with CNS development, producing usually micro-

Table 13.5. Temporal relationship of abnormalities in early amnion rupture—ADAM complex

Fetal timing	Craniofacial	Limbs	Other
3 weeks	Anencephaly Facial distortion, proboscis Unusual facial clefting Eye defects Encephalocele, meningocele		Placenta attached to head and/or abdomen Short umbilical cord
5 weeks	Cleft lip Choanal atresia	Limb deficiency Polydactyly Syndactyly	Abdominal wall defects Thoracic wall defects Scoliosis
7 weeks and onward	Cleft palate Micrognathia Ear deformities Craniostenosis	Amniotic bands Amputation Hypoplasia Pseudosyndactyly Distal lymphoedema Foot deformities Dislocation of hip	Short umbilical cord Omphalocele
Later	Oligohydramnios deformation sequence		

From Jones KL. *Smith's Recognisable Patterns of Human Malformation.* 4th ed. Philadelphia: WB Saunders, 1988, p. 596, with permission.

cephaly with or without microphthalmia and mild distal limb deficiencies. Smith et al [283] found severe mental deficiency, seizures in infancy, microphthalmia, midface hypoplasia, and mild distal limb abnormalities. Hyperthermia at 7 to 16 weeks may be associated with hypotonia, neurogenic arthrogryposis (Fig. 13.11), and/or CNS dysgenesis [93]. Shiota [94] studied 100 embryos with CNS defects and found that 18% of the mothers of anencephalics had hyperthermia at the critical embryonic stage.

The defects relate to the timing of the hyperthermia. Most of the cases relate to febrile illness with a temperature of 38.9°C or higher [95–101], most commonly 40°C or above. Two cases of severe hyperthermia were induced by sauna bathing. Retrospective human studies suggest that possibly 10% of neural tube defects, including anencephaly, meningomyelocele, and occipital encephalocele, may be related to hyperthermia [90]. Microcephaly, neuronal heterotopias, and/or polymicrogyria have been described. Other anomalies include microphthalmia, small midface, micrognathia, cleft lip and palate and defects in ear morphogenesis, and, less frequently, minor limb defects, including syndactyly and arthrogryposis.

Circumvallate Placenta Disruption

Circumvallate placenta is associated with an increase in perinatal death, prematurity, and congenital malformations. We have postulated a possible genetic origin in some cases, as exemplified by three sisters who died neonatally with a syndrome of bleeding and vascular fragility and a skeletal dys-

plasia manifested by blue sclerae and thin fragile bones associated with a circumvallate placenta [102]. Recently, a similar case was brought to our attention (R. J. Rowlatt).

DEFORMATIONS

CNS defects, weakness, and/or congenital hypotonia may result in deformations. Congenital limb deformities most commonly are tibial bowing, mild metatarsus varus, talipes equinovalgus and varus, and flexural contractures of arthrogryposis (Fig. 13.12). Twins and multiple fetuses may "interlock" and, with additional lack of space, may have considerable deformities. Skeletal dysplasias may be associated with deformities of pre- and/or postnatal onset. Deformations frequently are the result of mechanical pressure on the fetus, as may be present in oligohydramnios. The head may be misshappen if it resides in the horn of a bicornuate uterus.

NONMETABOLIC DYSPLASIA SYNDROMES

Beckwith-Wiedemann (EMG) Syndrome

Wiedemann [103] and Beckwith [104] reported on a syndrome of exomphalos, macroglossia, and gigantism (EMG).

Craniofacial abnormalities (Fig. 13.13a) include macroglossia, prominent eyes with relative infraorbital hypoplasia, capillary nevus flammeus of the central forehead and eyelids, metopic ridge in the central forehead, large fontanelles, prominent occiput, and malocclusion with tendency toward

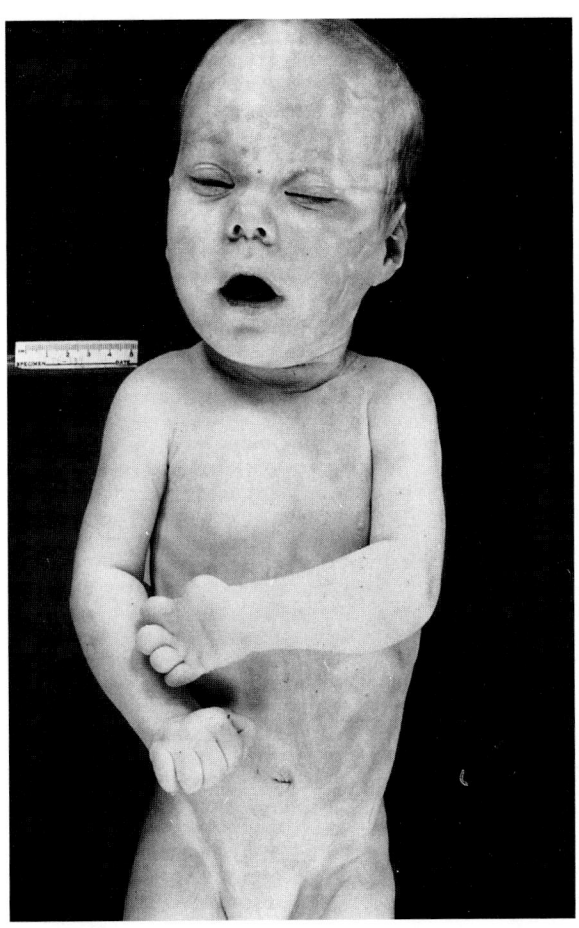

FIGURE 13.11. *Neurogenic arthrogryposis due to maternal hyperthermia.*

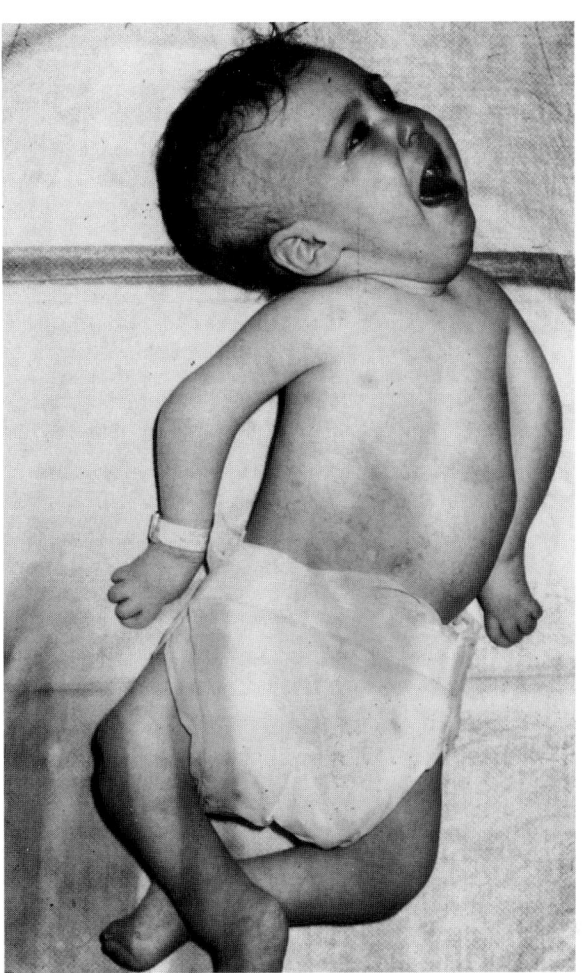

FIGURE 13.12. *Neurogenic arthrogryposis due to CNS dysfunction.*

mandibular prognathism. The unusual linear fissures in the lobule of the external ear (Fig. 13.13b) appear to be a marker for this syndrome, as well as semilunar indentations of the posterior rim of the helix. Mild microcephaly, hemihypertrophy, clitoromegaly, large ovaries, hyperplastic uterus and bladder, bicornuate uterus, hypospadias, and immunodeficiency may also be present.

Most cases have been sporadic, although occasional familial cases have been reported. A delayed mutation of an unstable premutated gene has been postulated [105]. In other families, this is a dominant mutation with variable expression.

There is a relatively high incidence of polyhydramnios and prematurity. This syndrome accounted for at least 11.7% of the cases of omphalocele reviewed by Irving [106]. The large tongue may partially occlude the respiratory tract and lead to feeding difficulties.

This syndrome also includes neonatal hypoglycemia, organomegaly, cytomegaly of the adrenal cortex (Fig. 13.13c) and islet cells of the pancreas, and a predisposition to the development of malignant tumors, including Wilms'

tumor (Fig. 13.13d), adrenocortical carcinoma, hepatoblastoma, gonadoblastoma, and brainstem glioma [105].

The kidneys may be strikingly enlarged, and their surfaces are traversed by numerous irregularly disposed shallow fissures, markedly increasing the number of lobulations [104]. The parenchyma is disorganized, with minute lobulations crowding one another, each with a distinctly demarcated cortex and medulla.

Other renal changes include persistent glomerulogenesis, medullary dysplasia, diffuse bilateral nephroblastomatosis, metanephric hamartomas, hydronephrosis and hydroureters, and duplications [105]. Wilms' tumor associated with this syndrome may be bilateral.

Interstitial cell hyperplasia of the testes, pituitary hyperplasia, neonatal polycythemia, diastasis recti, posterior diaphragmatic eventration, and cryptorchidism may occur.

Perlman Syndrome

Perlman syndrome is an autosomal recessive syndrome of renal dysplasia, Wilms' tumor, hyperplasia of the endocrine

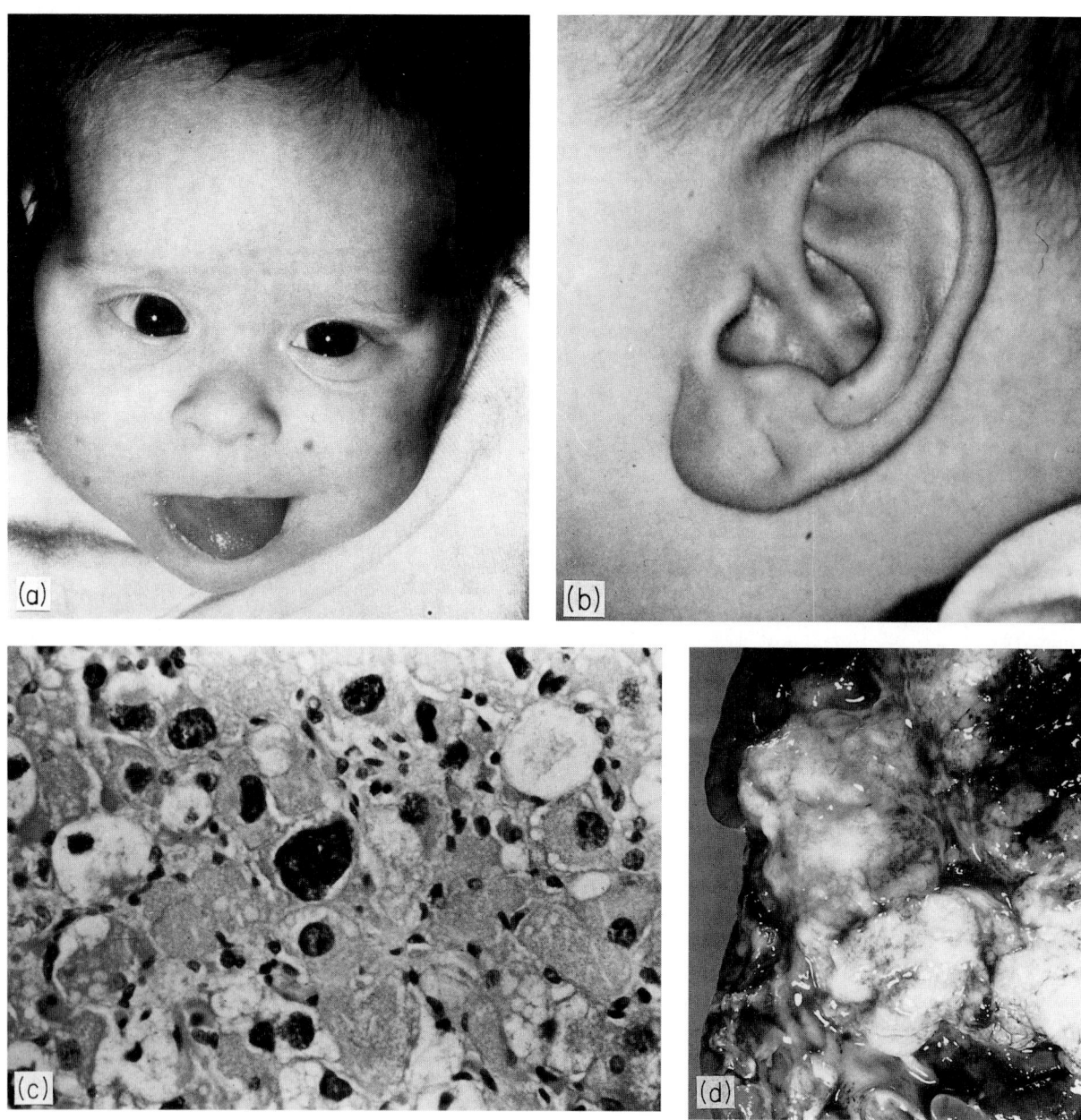

FIGURE 13.13.   *Wiedemann-Beckwith syndrome: (a) macroglossia, prominent eyes, and infraorbital hypoplasia; (b) ears show pits and grooves on the lobule; (c) cytomegaly of the adrenal cortex; (d) Wilms' tumor of the kidney.*

pancreas, fetal gigantism, multiple congenital anomalies, and mental retardation. This condition was described by Perlman et al [107, 108] and later by Neri et al [109].

The kidneys show persistence of fetal lobation, nodular renal blastema, immature glomeruli, sclerotic glomeruli, and primitive tubular structures, as well as medullary hamartomatous dysplasia. The pancreas shows an increase in the number of islets. The frequent occurrence of Wilms' tumor has led to the speculation that persistence of foci of renal blastema or nephroblastomatosis is a lesion predisposing to the development of Wilms' tumor. The condition has some similarity to the Wiedemann-Beckwith (or EMG) syn-

drome, and is easily differentiated from it on the basis of inheritance (EMG syndrome being an autosomal dominant trait), strikingly different minor facial anomalies and appearance, different natural history, and different constellations of associated malformations.

METABOLIC DYSPLASIA SYNDROMES

Williams Syndrome

Williams syndrome represents a maternal gestational derangement of vitamin D or calcium metabolism. Infantile hypercalcemia occurred in epidemic proportions in England and West Germany when increased amounts of vitamin D were added to pasteurized milk ingested by pregnant women. It has been suggested that populations of English and German origin may carry genes that predispose to fetal hypercalcemic reactions to vitamin D. The syndromal characteristics include growth and mental retardation, microcephaly and congenital hypotonia, and "elfin face" with short palpebral fissures, depressed nasal bridge, epicanthal folds, and anteverted nares. Neonatally, many infants have a symptom complex of "irritable failure to thrive"; in more severely affected infants, manifestations of hypercalcemia may be life-threatening or lethal. Cardiovascular defects include supravalvular aortic stenosis, peripheral pulmonary artery stenosis, pulmonic valvular stenosis, and ventricular and atrial septal defects. Renal artery stenosis with hypertension, hypoplasia of the aorta, and other arterial anomalies have been noted. Recently, Culler et al [110] have studied the hormonal control of calcium metabolism in patients with Williams syndrome. Intravenous calcium and parathyroid hormone infusions as provocative stimuli showed delayed clearance of calcium after intravenous calcium loading and blunted calcitonin responses after calcium infusion, as compared with a group of seven normal children. No abnormalities of vitamin D metabolism were found either before or after parathyroid hormone stimulation. The studies of Culler et al suggested that Williams syndrome patients may have a defect in the synthesis or release of immunoreactive calcitonin.

Zellweger (Cerebrohepatorenal) Syndrome (ZS)

An autosomal recessive trait, this disorder is lethal in infancy and dominated clinically by severe CNS dysfunction [111]. Generally, affected infants are born at term and do not manifest intrauterine growth retardation. The component anomalies are listed in Table 13.6 and include pear or light-bulb shape of head, large fontanelles, flat occiput, high forehead with shallow supraorbital ridges and flat face (Fig. 13.14a), minor ear anomalies, inner epicanthic folds, Brushfield's spots, mild micrognathia, and redundant skin of neck. Because of the hypotonia and "mongoloid" appearance, these infants are sometimes thought to have Down syndrome. The infant with ZS usually has a paucity of spontaneous movements, weakness and severe hypotonia with inability to suck, reduced deep tendon reflexes, and a total lack of psychomotor development [112–114]. Death before 1 year of age usually results from respiratory complications. Some atypical cases of ZS (Versmold variant) have hypertonia [115, 116] and may live longer. Other manifestations include congenital heart defects (anomalies of aortic arch, patent ductus arteriosus, and ventricular septal defect), stippled calcification of the epiphyses, and hepatomegaly with signs of hepatic dysfunction and occasional jaundice. Increased serum iron content and evidence of tissue siderosis can be established

Table 13.6. Clinical findings in Zellweger syndrome

Craniofacial anomalies
  Macrocephaly, high forehead, dolichocephaly
  Large anterior fontanelle, open metopic suture
  Mongoloid slant of palpebral fissures, hypertelorism, shallow supraorbital ridges, epicanthal folds
  Highly arched palate, posterior cleft of palate
  Minor anomalies of ears
Limbs
  Talipes equinovarus
  Camptodactyly
  Contractures
Eyes
  Cataracts, prominent Y-suture
  Glaucoma
  Corneal clouding
  Brushfield's spots
  Pigmentary retinopathy
  Optic nerve "dysplasia," hypoplasia
CNS
  Hypotonia, rarely hypertonia
  Severe mental retardation
  Seizures
  Nystagmus, oculogyric fits
  Absent neonatal reflexes
Other
  Cardiac defects
  Jaundice with hepatomegaly
  Cryptorchidism, clitoromegaly
  Simian creases
  DiGeorge developmental field defect
Radiologic abnormalities
  Chondrodysplasia calcificans (especially patellae)
  Delayed skeletal maturation
  Bell-shaped thorax
  Large fontanelles

in most cases before death and is helpful diagnostically [117].

Postmortem findings are shown in Table 13.7 and include focal lissencephaly (Fig. 13.14b) and other cerebral gyral abnormalities, heterotopic cerebral cortex, olivary nuclear dysplasia, defects of the corpus callosum, numerous lipid-laden macrophages and histiocytes in cortical and periventricular areas, and dysmyelination [118]. The liver is characterized by hepatic lobular disarray (micronodular cirrhosis), biliary dysgenesis, and siderosis. The kidneys show persistence of fetal lobulations with cortical cysts (Fig. 13.14c). Albuminaria and aminoaciduria may be observed. Biochemical abnormalities that have been found include hypoglycemia, elevated serum iron, siderosis, hyperpipecolic acidemia, hepatic and cerebral glycogen storage, elevated very-long-chain fatty acids, abnormal bile acids, dicarboxylic aciduria, and hypocarnitinemia.

Renal cysts (Fig. 13.14d) have been a consistent finding and may be a pathologic marker for this condition. They

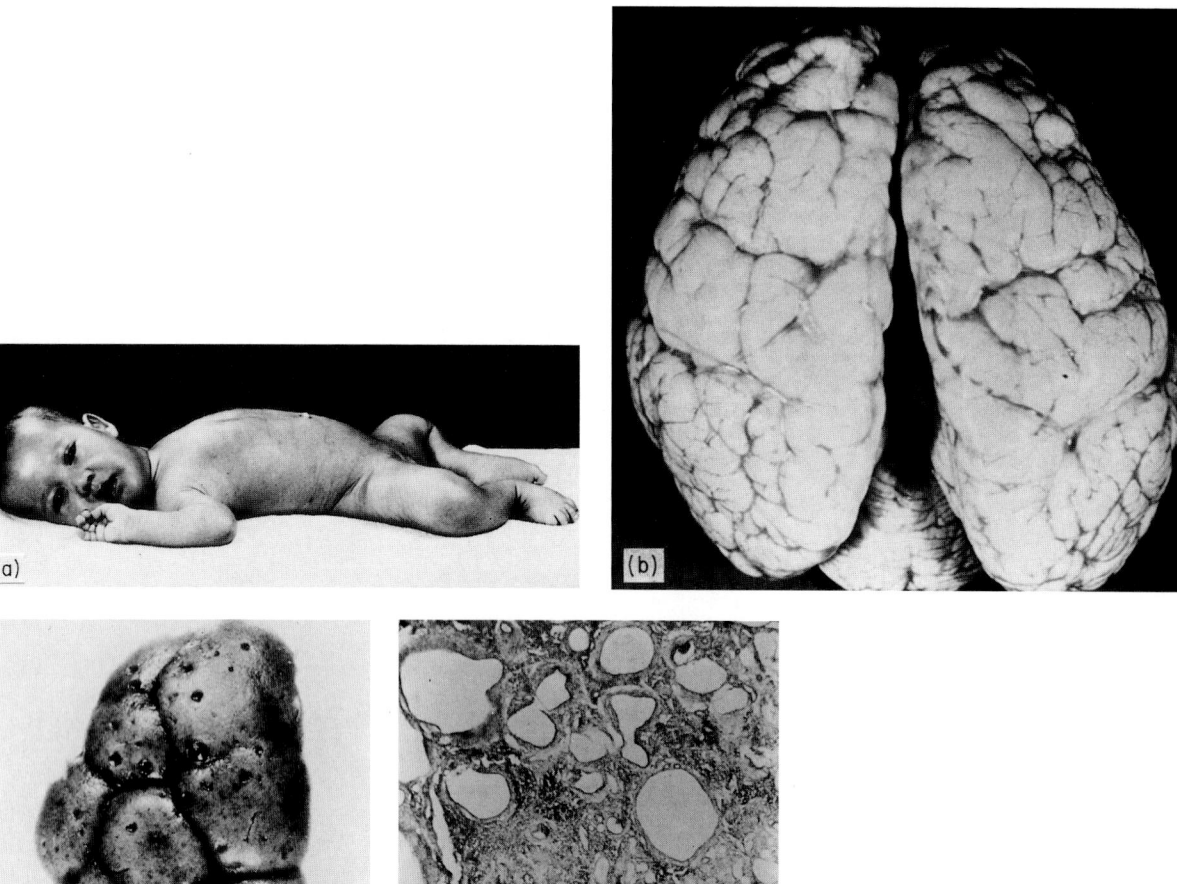

FIGURE 13.14. *Zellweger syndrome: (a) infant with hypotonia and characteristic facial appearance; (b) brain showing pachygyria and partial lissencephaly; (c) gross appearance of kidney with multiple small cortical cysts; (d) microscopic section of kidney with multiple small tubular cysts.*

have been more commonly glomerular in origin and occasionally have appeared to connect directly to terminal ends of collecting tubules without an intervening tubular segment, suggesting focally deficient metanephric differentiation. Cystic dysplastic changes may also be observed [119]. Horseshoe kidneys and ureteral duplication have been noted [115]. The DiGeorge sequence has been seen in several infants with the Zellweger syndrome [120].

This inborn error appears to be a defective production of a peroxisomal membrane protein or of a cytochrome b oxidase enzyme required for import of peroxisomal proteins into this organelle [121]. Absence of peroxisomes in the liver was first recognized by Goldfischer et al [122]. It is pre-

sumed that all congenital anomalies and subsequent pre- and postnatal organ and cellular structural changes represent a metabolic dysplasia sequence. In ZS there are no morphologically demonstrable peroxisomes. Adrenocortical cells in the inner portion of the adrenal cortex identified by ultrastructural examination contain lamellae and lamellar-lipid profiles of very-long-chain fatty acids and cholesterol esters that are also characteristic of adrenoleukodystrophy. This morphologic observation further emphasizes the common pathogenetic manifestation of ZS and adrenoleukodystrophy.

Zellweger syndrome is one of several peroxisomal disorders in which there appears to be an impairment of more than one peroxisomal function. It has been postulated that

Table 13.7. Pathologic and radiologic abnormalities in Zellweger syndrome

Brain
    Cerebellar, olivary hypoplasia
    Abnormal cerebral convolutions (microgyria, pachygyria)
    Partial lissencephaly
    Agenesis/hypoplasia of corpus callosum
    Cerebral/cerebellar heterotopias
    Enlarged lateral ventricles
    Sudanophilic leukoencephalomyelopathy
    Gliosis
Liver
    Biliary dysgenesis
    Cirrhosis
    Siderosis
    Ultrastructural: absent peroxisomes
    Abnormal mitochondria
    Diminished smooth endoplasmic reticulum
Kidneys
    Multiple cortical microcysts: glomerular and tubular cystic dysplasia
    Hydronephrosis
    Horseshoe kidney
Heart
    VSD, PDA, patent foramen ovale
Pancreas
    Islet cell hyperplasia
Thymus
    Thymic hypoplasia

in these disorders the primary biochemical lesion is at the level of the peroxisomal membrane protein, which is essential for the transport of peroxisomal enzymes from the cytoplasm to the inside of the peroxisome.

Prenatal diagnosis of ZS has been established by the observation of increases in very-long-chain fatty acids, particularly hexacosanoic acids (C26:0 and C26:1); in plasma, cultured skin fibroblasts, and amniotic cells [123]; and in chorionic villus biopsy obtained by transcervical catheter aspiration during the first trimester of pregnancy [124, 125].

Cultured skin fibroblasts or leukocytes from patients with ZS show the activity of acyl-CoA-dihydroxyacetone phosphate (DHAP) acyltransferase to be deficient [126, 127]. This enzyme is required for plasmalogen synthesis and is located in peroxisomes [128, 129].

Smith-Lemli-Opitz (SLO) Syndrome

SLO has recently been found to be due to a deficiency of 7 dehydrocholesterol reductase whereby the immediate precursor of cholesterol-7 dehydrocholesterol is several thousand times greater than in controls and results in greatly reduced plasma cholesterol concentrations [130, 131]. Anteverted nostrils and/or distinct craniofacial appearance

with microcephaly, ptosis of eyelids, inner epicanthal folds, strabismus, micrognathia, syndactyly of second and third toes, hypospadias, cryptorchidism in males, and mental deficiency are the main characteristics of this common, autosomal recessive condition [132–135]. Serious defects in brain morphogenesis include microencephaly, hypoplasia of the frontal lobes, hypoplasia of cerebellum and brainstem, dilated ventricles, irregular gyral patterns, and irregular neuronal organization.

Atypical mononuclear giant cells in pancreatic islets have been described (Fig. 13.15a) [136]. Less frequent anomalies are rudimentary postaxial hexadactyly, congenital heart defect, and multiple anomalies of renal and spinal cord development. Cystic renal disease (Fig. 13.15b), hypoplasia, hydronephrosis, and abnormalities of the ureters are frequent. Rare patients have severe perineoscrotal hypospadias. The reported higher frequency of affected males versus females may be related to the ascertainment bias of the genital anomaly.

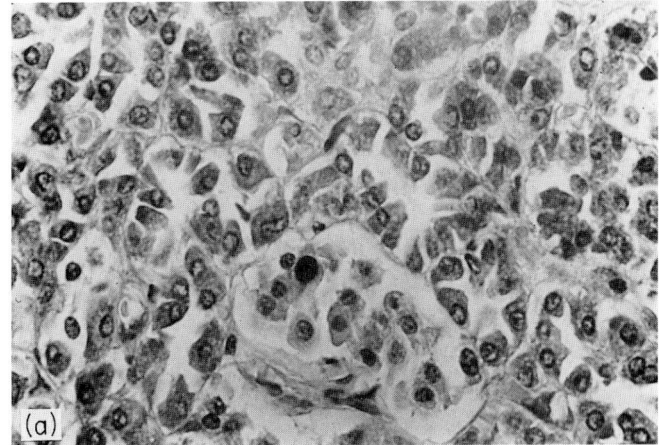

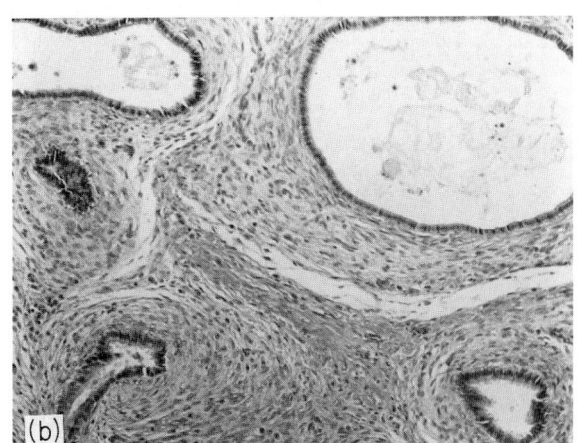

FIGURE 13.15. *Smith-Lemli-Opitz syndrome: (a) microscopic section of pancreas showing large mononuclear giant cells in pancreatic islets. ×100; (b) microscopic appearance of kidney.*

SEQUENCES

DiGeorge Sequence

The primary defect is in the development of the fourth branchial arch and derivatives of the third and fourth pharyngeal pouches. The condition was first described by DiGeorge [137] and later by others [138–141]. It includes defects of the thymus, parathyroids, and great vessels. Facial anomalies include hypertelorism, short philtrum, downslanting palpebral fissures, and ear anomalies. Thymic hypoplasia or aplasia results in a deficit of cellular immunity. Hypoplasia or absence of parathyroids results in hypocalcemia and tetany in early infancy. Cardiovasular defects include aortic arch anomalies (such as right aortic arch), interrupted aorta, conotruncal anomalies (truncus arteriosus and ventricular septal defect), patent ducts arteriosus, and tetralogy of Fallot. Esophageal atresia, choanal atresia, imperforate anus, and diaphragmatic hernia may be accompanying abnormalities. Death usually occurs in early infancy due to the cardiovascular defects, tetany, or infection related to the defect of cellular immunity. It has now become apparent that the DiGeorge "syndrome" is causally heterogeneous and is a polytopic developmental field defect [142, 143]. Experimental studies [144–146] have shown that impairment of the inductive and morphogenetic functions of the neural crest cells is responsible for the defects of the epithelial organ derivatives of the third and fourth pharyngeal pouches and of the corresponding branchial arteries. Because of the role played by cephalic neural crest in morphogenesis of the heart, conotruncal heart defects are commonly seen in children with the DiGeorge anomaly. Because of the neural crest–midline pathogenetic origin of the DiGeorge anomaly, this condition is associated frequently with other midline anomalies, schisis associations, and arrhinencephaly. It may be related causally to the fetal alcohol [147, 148] and fetal accutane [61, 149–151] disruptions, as well as to the effects of maternal diabetes [152]. It has been related to partial monosomy of the proximal long arm of chromosome 22 and partial 8q trisomy (see Chap. 16).

Robin Sequence

The defects in this condition include micrognathia, glossoptosis, and cleft soft palate. Hypoplasia of the mandibular area before 9 weeks of gestation allows the tongue to be posteriorly located and is presumed to prevent the closure of the posterior palatal shelves [153, 154]. Posterior airway obstruction in the Robin sequence is most commonly noted; the prognosis is good if survival occurs beyond the early period of respiratory obstruction. It may also be a result of early mechanical constraint in utero, with limitation of growth prior to palatine closure. The Pierre Robin sequence should alert the clinician to the possible presence of Stickler syndrome in order to assist in prevention of blindness due to high myopia and prevention of recurrence through correct genetic counseling.

Prune Belly Sequence and Related Defects

Prune belly sequence occurs sporadically and is a triad of apparent absence of abdominal muscles, urinary tract defects, and cryptorchidism [155, 156]. There is cephalad displacement of the umbilicus, flaring of rib margins, Harrison's groove, and pectus deformities, all apparently secondary to the muscle defect. There is a frequent association with talipes equinovarus [157, 158].

A presumed early mesenchymal maldevelopment between the 6th and 10th weeks of development [159], resulting in a developmental field defect, has been discussed by Opitz [160] and postulated by Straub and Spranger [161]. Burton and Dillard [162] have reported a case of prune belly sequence in which they speculate that splitting of the abdominal wall occurred due to massive bladder dilatation. This hypothesis is supported by the demonstration of attenuation of smooth muscle elements, with lack of differentiation into circular and longitudinal orientation of smooth muscle fibers within the bladder with replacement by collagen [163]. Renal dysplasia may be present. The urinary tract is greatly dilated, usually with urethral or bladder neck obstruction. Neonatal death occurs in 20% of infants; however, long-term survival without significant renal impairment may occur. Megalourethra [164], megacystis, megaureters, renal hypoplasia, and hydronephrosis have been described. Decreased spermatogenesis, absence of spermatogonia [165], and salt-losing nephritis have also been observed [166].

ASSOCIATIONS

VATER Association

The nonrandom association of vertebral defects, imperforate anus, and esophageal atresia with tracheoesophageal fistula was noted by Quan and Smith [167], who coined the acronym to include Vertebral defects, Anal atresia, T-E fistula with esophageal atresia, and Radial (and Renal) abnormalities. Cardiac defects and a single umbilical artery, as well as prenatal growth deficiency, were included by Temtamy and Miller [168], who used the acronym VATERS association. Other less frequent defects include prenatal growth deficiency, ear anomalies, large fontanelles, defects of the lower limbs, and rib anomalies. This pattern of malformations occurs sporadically. The concept of an expanded VATER association (Fig. 13.16) has been introduced recently, and the suggestion has been made that the VATER association may represent a less severe degree of the sirenomelia malformation sequence [7, 169].

VACTERL is one of many expansions used to include cardiac and limb defects. Likewise, there is an overlap caudally with MURCS association [170] and cephalically with tracheal agenesis and hemifacial microsomia and other facial asymmetry syndromes [171, 172]. The genitourinary defects include renal dysplasia or agenesis, renal ectopia, persistent urachus, hypospadias, and caudally displaced hypoplastic

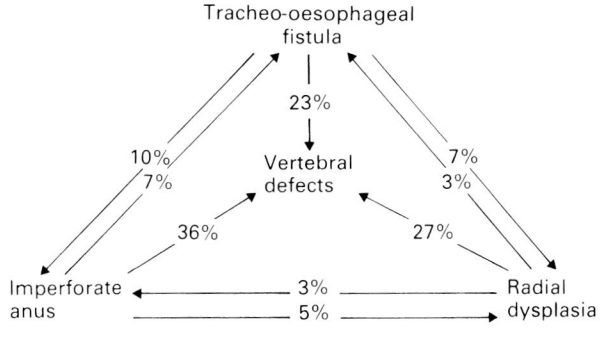

(a)

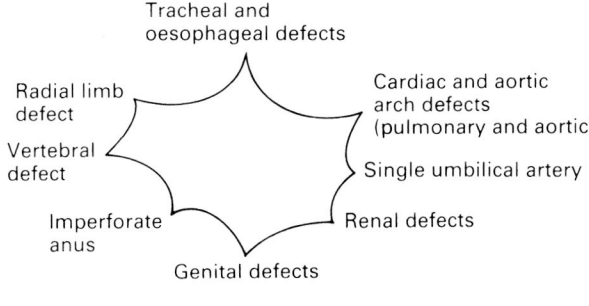

(b)

FIGURE 13.16.   *(a) The VATER association. (b) The expanded VATER association.*

penis. Embryologically, the VATER association seems to originate in a disturbance occurring before the 35th day of gestation [173].

This nonrandom association appears to be related to a common developmental pathogenesis due to a defect in mesoderm in early development before 35 days of gestation. All of the following occur prior to 35 days:

1. The rectum and anus are formed by a mesodermal urorectal shelf, which divides the cloaca into the urogenital sinus and rectum and anus.
2. A mesodermal septum separates the trachea from the esophagus.
3. The radius is formed by a condensation of mesenchymal tissue in the limb bud.
4. The vertebrae are formed by migration and organization of somite mesoderm.

Lubinsky et al [174] have suggested that all of the VATER associations represent disruption sequences, as exemplified in the common metabolic disruptive condition of maternal diabetes in infants with the VATER association.

MURCS Association

MURCS is an acronym for *M*üllerian duct aplasia, *R*enal aplasia, and *C*ervicothoracic *S*omite malformation resulting in cervicothoracic vertebral defects, especially from C5 to T1

[175, 176]. Absence of the vagina [177], absence or hypoplasia of the uterus, and renal abnormalities occur. The latter include renal agenesis and ectopy. This condition is sporadic.

CHARGE Association

CHARGE is an acronym for *C*oloboma, *H*eart disease, *A*tresia choanae, and *R*etarded *G*rowth and development. Associated anomalies include genital and ear anomalies, tracheoesophageal fistula, facial palsy, micrognathia, cleft lip, cleft palate, omphalocele, congenital cardiac defects, and holoprosencephaly. The CHARGE association shows some phenotypic overlap with the VATER association. Familial cases have been observed; since these may be genetic, the designation of CHARGE syndrome may be more appropriate.

Heart defects include tetralogy of Fallot, patent ductus arteriosus, double outlet right ventricle with a common atrioventricular canal, ventricular septal defect, atrial septal defect, and right-sided aortic arch. Ear anomalies and/or deafness may be present. Many of the anomalies may be related to altered morphogenesis during the 2nd month of gestation. The choanae are formed between days 35 and 38 of gestation. Colobomas result from failure of the fetal

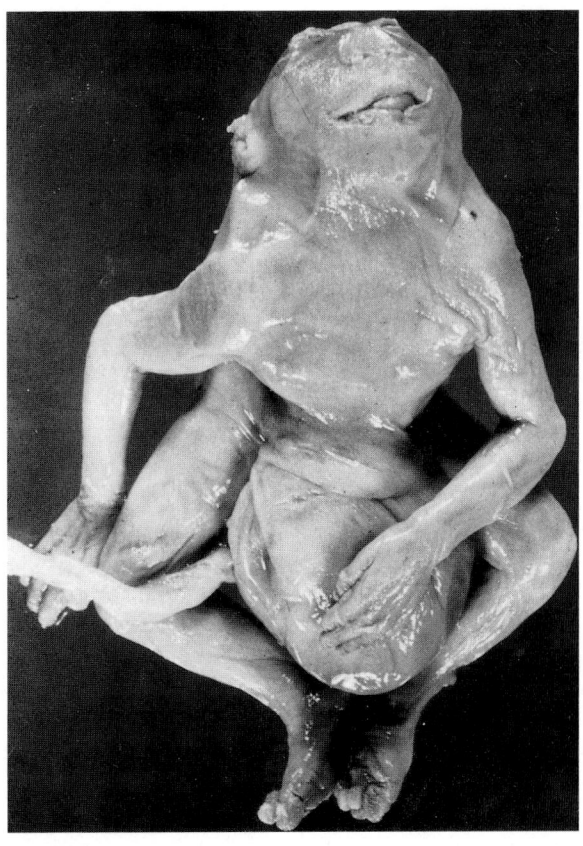

FIGURE 13.17.   *Schisis association in a stillborn infant with anencephaly and omphalocele.*

choroid fissure to close during the 5th week of gestation. Cardiac septation occurs on day 38 and is reasonably complete by day 45. Holoprosencephaly may reflect altered morphogenesis during the 4th to 5th week of gestation.

There have been instances in which familial occurrence of some of the associated anomalies has suggested a genetic cause [178]. With normal parents of an affected child, there appears to be a low but not negligible risk of recurrence [90].

Schisis Association and Its Variants

Czeizel [2] has shown that schisis (midline) defects, including neural tube defects (anencephaly, encephalocele, and meningomyelocele), oral clefts (cleft lip and palate and posterior cleft palate), omphalocele (Fig. 13.17), and diaphragmatic hernia, associate with one another far more frequently than at the expected random combination rates. The schisis association is frequently a lethal abnormality. It occurs more often in girls, in twins (4.6%), in breech presentations (13.7%), and in association with lower mean birth weight and with a shorter gestational period. Congenital cardiac defects, limb deficiencies, and defects of the urinary tract, mainly renal agenesis, are defects that have a high association [2]. Schisis-type abnormalities therefore appear to be the manifestations of nonrandom occurrences.

AUTOSOMAL DOMINANT MUTATIONS

Nail-patella (Hereditary Onycho-Osteodysplasia) Syndrome (NPS)

Onychodysplasia of fingers and toes includes hypoplasia, longitudinal ridging, and hemiatrophy. The nails of the thumbs and great toes are most severely involved. The patellae are small and sometimes absent. Iliac osseous spurs, described as "horns," are usually present. A peculiar heterochromia may be seen in the iris. Proteinuria may be associated with a nephrosis-like renal disease.

Light microscopy and electron microscopy show thickening of the glomerular basement membrane, which contains focal collections of collagen fibers within the lamina densa [179]. This appears to be specific for NPS and has been observed by us in a spontaneously aborted affected fetus (Fig. 13.18). Immunofluorescence shows a nonspecific focal distribution of IgM or complement.

The nail-patella and the ABO blood group loci are linked [180, 181] on chromosome 9.

Branchio-Otorenal (BOR) Syndrome

The BOR syndrome is an autosomal dominant trait characterized by branchial arch anomalies (preauricular pits and branchial fistulas), hearing loss, and renal hypoplasia and dysplasia [90, 182]. A preauricular pit at birth is a marker for this syndrome and suggests one chance in 200 of severe hearing loss [183]. The renal anomalies range from minor defects to marked hypoplasia with renal failure.

Townes-Brocks Syndrome (Thumb, Auricular, Anal, and Renal Anomalies)

This autosomal dominant disorder includes thumb, auricular, anal, and renal anomalies [184–186], congenital heart defects, and anomalies of other internal organs [187]. It encompasses many of the anomalies of both the VATER association and the Treacher Collins complex [90].

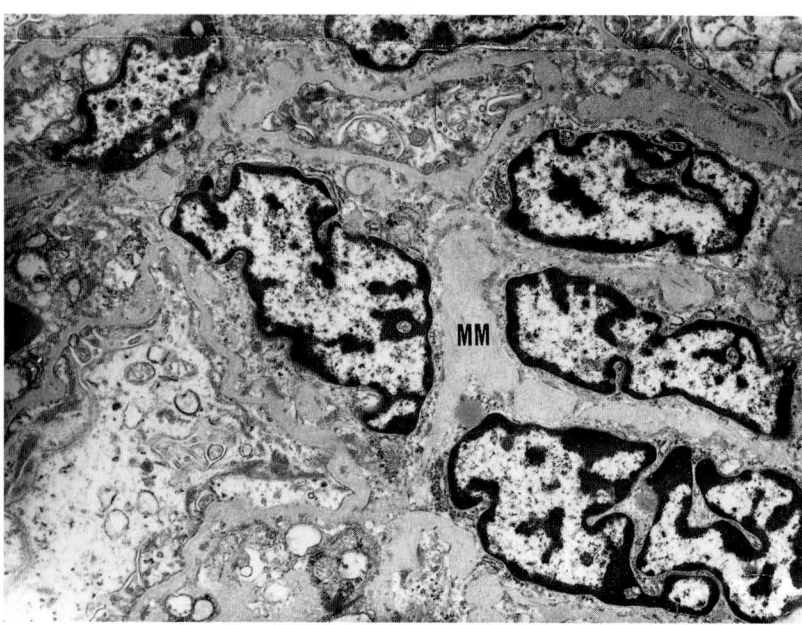

FIGURE 13.18.   *Nail-patella syndrome. Electron micrograph shows thickened capillary walls with intramembranous (MM) and subendothelial electron-dense deposits.*

Opitz Syndrome
(G Syndrome; Opitz-Frias Syndrome)

This condition was initially reported by Opitz et al in 1969 and named the G syndrome using the initial of the surname of the first family studied having this syndrome. The clinical manifestations include maxillary hypoplasia, hypertelorism, epicanthic folds and micrognathia (Fig. 13.19a), stridor, swallowing difficulties, hypospadias, and wheezing and hoarseness [188, 189]. Pathologic studies have documented a laryngotracheal cleft (Fig. 13.19b), malformations of the larynx, tracheoesophageal fistula, high carina, pulmonary hypoplasia, cardiac defects, renal defects, imperforate anus, cryptorchidism, agenesis of the gallbladder, and duodenal stricture. Males are usually affected more severely than females. The condition is autosomal dominant, with partial sex limitation [190–193].

Mandibulofacial Dysostosis
(Treacher Collins Syndrome) or
Franceschetti-Klein-Zwahlen Syndrome

This is not a syndrome but a causally nonspecific developmental field defect that may be inherited as an autosomal dominant defect. The main characteristics of this defect include malar hypoplasia with downslanting palpebral fissures, defects of the lower lid, mandibular hypoplasia, and malformations of the external ear (Fig. 13.20) [194–198]. Analysis of affected families shows that some cases appear to be autosomal dominant mutations. An excess of affected offspring from affected females and of normal offspring from affected males has been found. There is wide variability in expression but moderate similarity with a given sibship. Other abnormalities include partial to total absence of the lower eyelashes, external ear canal defects, conductive deafness, cleft palate, incompetent soft palate, and a projection of scalp hair onto the lateral cheek. Pharyngeal hypoplasia, microphthalmia, macrostomia, microstomia, choanal atresia, blind fistulas and skin tags between the auricle and the angle of the mouth, absence of the parotid gland, congenital heart defects, and cryptorchidism are rarely reported.

Holt-Oram or Cardiac-Limb Syndrome

This syndrome of skeletal and cardiovascular abnormalities was first described by Holt and Oram [199] in 1960. In

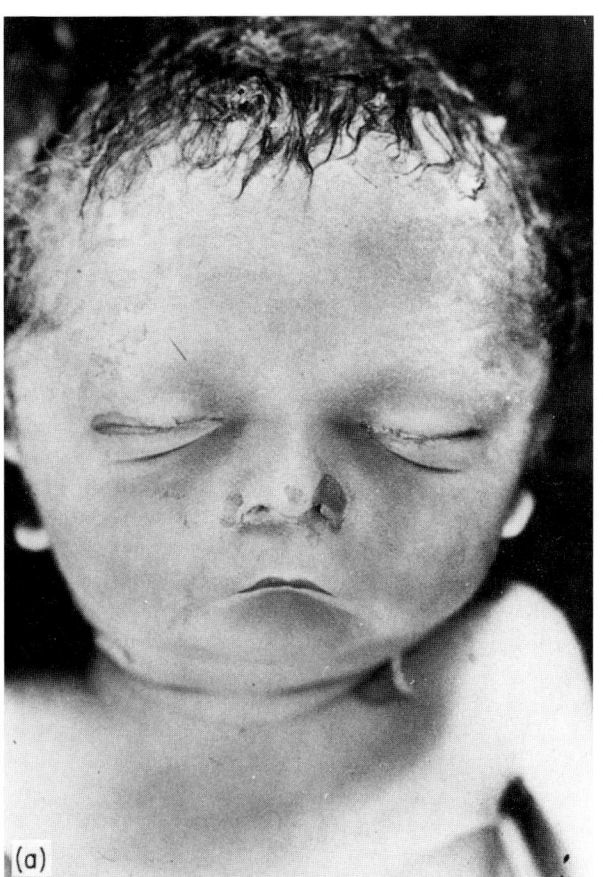
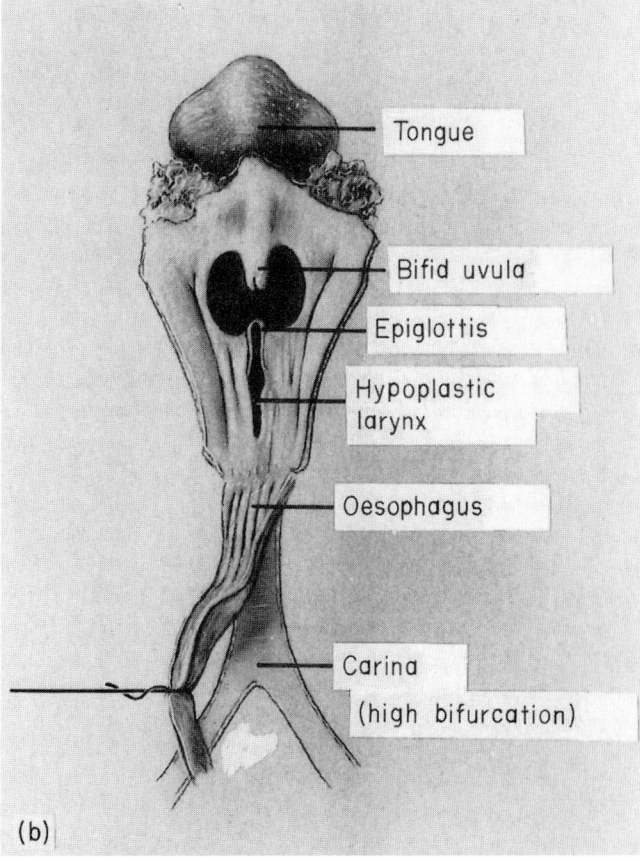

FIGURE 13.19. *Opitz syndrome (G syndrome; Opitz-Frias syndrome): (a) hypertelorism with midface hypoplasia; (b) diagram of laryngotracheal cleft.*

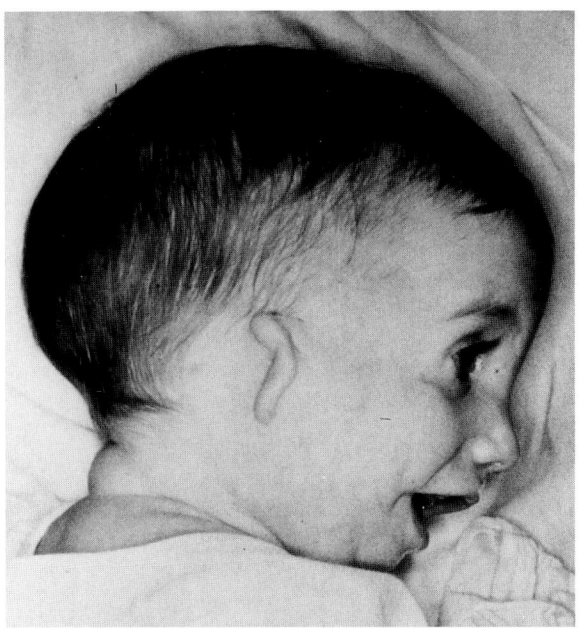

FIGURE 13.20.   *Mandibulofacial dysostosis. Mandibular and zygomatic hypoplasia, macrostomia, and microtia.*

families with Holt-Oram syndrome (HOS), an autosomal dominant mode of inheritance with variable expressivity has been demonstrated [196, 199–204].

Skeletal abnormalities in the upper limb range from thumb hypoplasia to phocomelia. There is a preponderance of left-sided involvement. Hypoplasia or absence of the first metacarpal and radius and defects of the ulna, humerus, clavicle, scapula, and sternum may be present.

The most frequently described cardiac lesion is a secundum-type atrial septal defect. Numerous reports have described a variety of cardiac anomalies. Ventricular septal defects, transposition of great vessels, subclavian artery malformations, common atrioventricular canal, pulmonary stenosis, patent ductus arteriosus, right aortic arch, electrocardiographic abnormalities (some with arrhythmias), tetralogy of Fallot, persistent left superior vena cava, truncus arteriosus, total anomalous pulmonary venous return, and hypoplasia of peripheral vessels are the cardiovascular defects that have been described so far [199–207]. Infrequent abnormalities of the coronary artery have been described. Lewis et al [203] described a patient with a single coronary artery arising from the aorta with no other cardiac lesion present. We have observed a single anomalous left coronary artery arising from the pulmonary artery with an associated patent ductus arteriosus (PDA), ventricular septal defect (VSD) and myocardial infarction [208].

BBB Syndrome (Hypertelorism-Hypospadias or Opitz Syndrome)

This dominantly inherited condition was described in three families by Opitz et al [209], using the initials of the surnames of these three families. Affected males usually have ocular hypertelorism and hypospadias, whereas affected females have only hypertelorism. Cardiac anomalies, cleft lip or palate, cranial asymmetry, strabismus, and downslanting palpebral fissures may be present [210]. There is considerable overlap between G and BBB syndrome manifestations, and some investigators have suggested that the entities are one and the same and should be called the Opitz syndrome [211]. Neonatally, infants with the BBB syndrome can be recognized by their hypertelorism, hypospadias, and occasional additional anomalies, such as cleft lip and/or congenital heart defects. Most are less severely affected.

Apert Syndrome (Acrocephalosyndactyly Type I)

This autosomal dominant mutation includes irregular craniosynostosis, especially of coronal sutures, midface hypoplasia, syndactyly, and a broad distal phalanx of the thumb and big toe [212–214]. Mental retardation may be present as well as normal intelligence. Craniofacial anomalies include a short anterior-posterior skull diameter with a high, full forehead and flat occiput, flat face, supraorbital horizontal groove, shallow orbits, hypertelorism, downslant of palpebral fissures, small nose, and maxillary hypoplasia. Cutaneous syndactyly of all toes, with or without osseous syndactyly, is present. Synostosis of the radius and humerus, pyloric stenosis, ectopic anus, pulmonary aplasia, anomalous tracheal cartilages, pulmonary stenosis and other cardiac malformations, cystic kidneys, hydronephrosis, and bicornuate uterus may occur. The condition is easily diagnosed at birth, but the possibility has been raised that Apert infants with (webbed) polydactyly—especially of the toes—represent a nosogically different entity.

The designation of Apert syndrome includes what used to be called acrocephalosyndactyly type II, or Vogt cephalodactyly, or Apert-Crouzon disease. It has been suggested that this entity is probably a variant of Apert syndrome [215].

Saethre-Chotzen Syndrome (Acrocephalosyndactyly Type III)

A dominant disorder with variability in expression, Saethre-Chotzen syndrome is characterized by brachycephaly with a high forehead, synostosis of coronal suture, maxillary hypoplasia, facial asymmetry, shallow orbits, hypertelorism, ptosis of eyelids, small ears, large fontanelles, cutaneous syndactyly (most commonly of the second and third fingers and/or the third and fourth toes), brachydactyly, a single palmar crease, and broad thumbs and great toes. These anomalies are clearly visible neonatally. Occasionally, mental deficiency, small stature, deafness, vertebral anomalies, cryptorchidism, and renal anomalies may be present [216–219].

Pfeiffer Syndrome (Acrocephalosyndactyly Type V)

The numeric designations of these entities are relics of earlier classifications from which type IV has disappeared. Similarly, Noack syndrome has disappeared as a nosologically distinct entity, being considered a variant of Pfeiffer syndrome [215]. Pfeiffer syndrome is an autosomal dominant mutation, with most cases representing new mutations [220–222]. Craniosynostosis of coronal and/or sagittal sutures, ocular hypertelorism, antimongoloid palpebral fissures, small nose and sometimes cloverleaf skull (kleeblattschädel), broad distal phalanges of thumb and big toe, partial syndactyly of fingers and toes, and sometimes radiohumeral synostosis characterize this syndrome. Craniofacial abnormalities tend to improve with age. Intelligence is usually normal, although severe (secondary) brain defects

have been seen with the kleeblattschädel anomaly (Fig. 13.21) [220].

Crouzon Craniofacial Dysostosis

Inherited as an autosomal dominant trait, Crouzon craniofacial dysostosis [223–226] is a relatively common disorder that includes craniofacial anomalies with shallow orbits and ocular proptosis, hypertelorism, frontal bossing, and maxillary hypoplasia with a curved parrot-like nose. Craniosynostosis may involve coronal, lambdoid, and sagittal sutures. The teeth are peg-shaped and widely spaced with a large tongue and deviation of the nasal septum, atresia of the auditory meatus, and deafness. Surgical procedures may allow for more normal brain development in the presence of increased intracranial pressure; facial operations may be required to correct extreme midface hypoplasia and proptosis.

Robinow Syndrome (Fetal Face Syndrome)

The infant with Robinow syndrome has a facial appearance resembling a fetal face [227, 228]. This includes macrocephaly, large anterior fontanelle, frontal bossing, hypertelorism, small upturned nose, long philtrum, and triangular mouth with downturned angles and micrognathia (Fig. 13.22). The forearms are short with brachydactyly. Hemivertebrae can be seen on roentgenograms. A small penis, clitoris and labia majora, cryptorchidism, pectus excavatum,

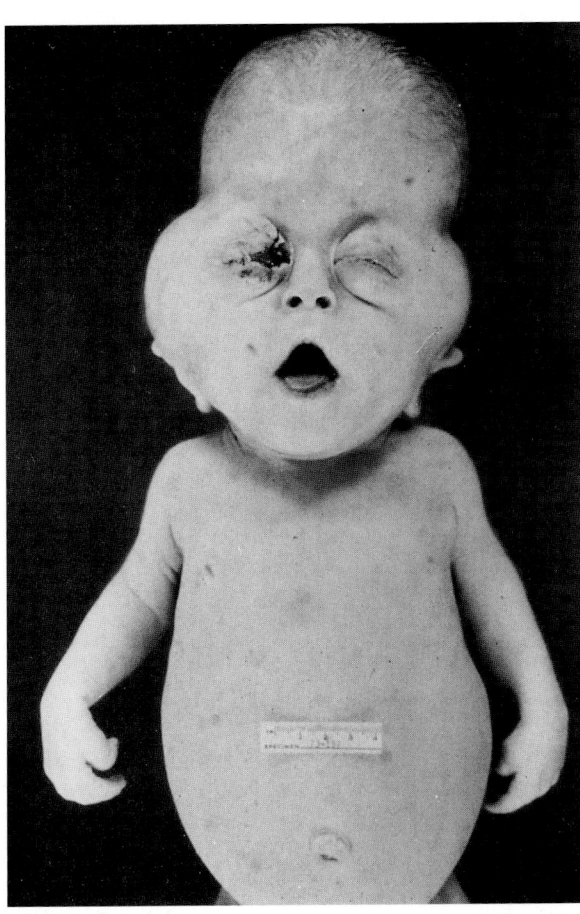

FIGURE 13.21.   *Pfeiffer syndrome with cloverleaf skull.*

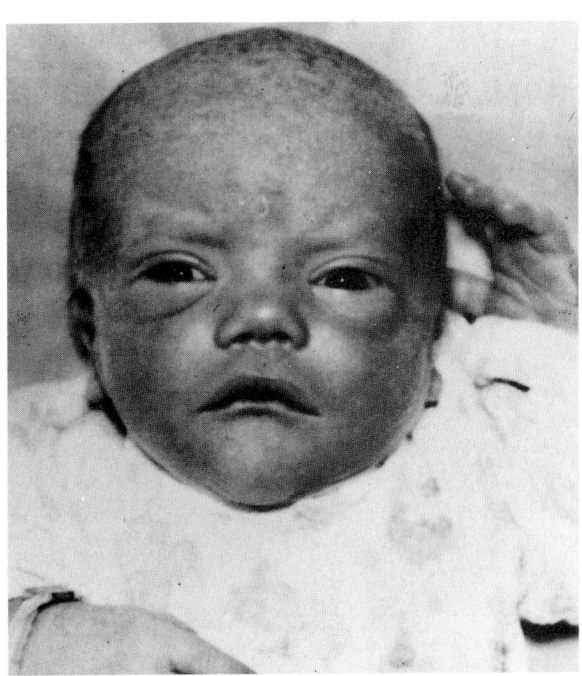

FIGURE 13.22.   *Robinow syndrome with typical "fetal face" appearance.*

rib anomaly, inguinal hernia, and cardiac anomalies may be present.

Stickler Syndrome (Hereditary Arthro-Ophthalmopathy)

First described by Stickler et al [229, 230] and later documented by Spranger [231] and by Herrmann et al [232], this condition includes facial anomalies with depressed nasal bridge, epicanthal folds, midface hypoplasia (Fig. 13.23), cleft of hard palate, micrognathia, deafness, and myopia with frequent retinal detachment and/or cataracts. Musculoskeletal abnormalities include hypotonia, marfanoid habitus, prominence of large joints, and spondyloepiphyseal dysplasia. Stickler syndrome should be considered in every newborn infant with the Pierre Robin sequence. It is an autosomal dominant trait with highly variable expression.

Noonan Syndrome

Webbing of the neck, pectus excavatum, cryptorchidism, and pulmonic stenosis characterize this syndrome, which was first clearly differentiated from the Ullrich-Turner syndrome by Dr. Jacqueline Noonan [233]. Short stature, mental retardation, epicanthal folds, ptosis of eyelids, hypertelorism, myopia, apparently low-set and/or abnormal auricles, and abnormalities of vertebrae are usually seen. Edema

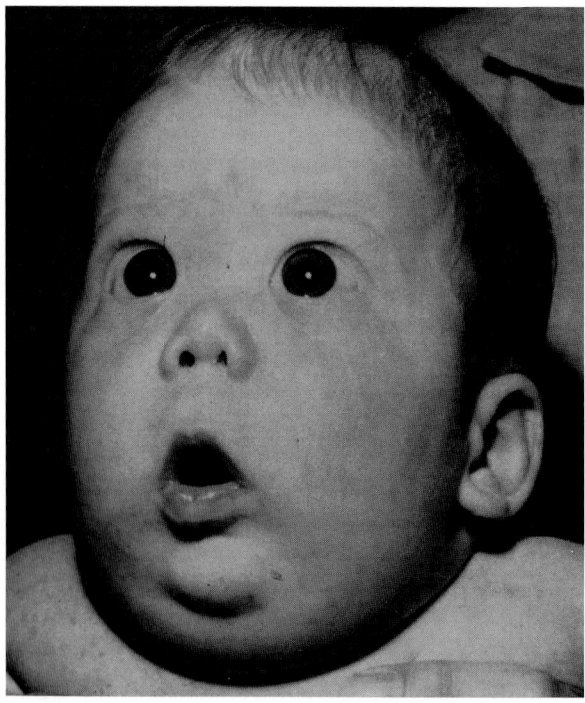

FIGURE 13.23. *Stickler syndrome. Abnormal facial appearance with extreme myopia, flat face, depressed nasal bridge, anteverted nostrils, epicanthal folds, and micrognathia.*

of the dorsum of the hands and feet may also simulate that observed in the Ullrich-Turner infant.

Brachmann-De Lange Syndrome

The Brachmann-de Lange syndrome (BDLS) has been reviewed by Kousseff et al [234, 235]. It is a syndrome of growth and mental retardation, microbrachycephaly, and hirsutism. There is extreme variability in expression. The major manifestations include mental retardation (100%), synophrys (94%), hirsutism (84%) and thin downturned vermilion borders (80%). Other common anomalies include dental abnormalities with late eruption of widely spaced teeth (93%), and male genital abnormalities such as cryptorchidism and hypospadias (94% of males) [236]. A recurrence risk of 2–5% has been reported [237] and there have been case reports of concordance in monozygotic twins [238, 239]. Several cases of familial occurrence in mildly affected individuals confirm dominant inheritance. Although there is some phenyotypic overlap of BDLS and the dup(3q) syndrome [240, 241], these entities are distinct [242, 243] and distinguishable. BDLS appears now to be due to a ring q chromosome that is related to deficiency of pregnancy-associated plasma protein (PAPPA)—a large zinc glycoprotein of placental origin that has been mapped to chromosome q [244].

Occasional anomalies include myopia, microcornea, astigmatism, optic atrophy, coloboma of the optic nerve, strabismus, proptosis, choanal atresia, low-set ears, cleft palate, congenital heart defects (most commonly ventricular septal defect), hiatus hernia, duplication of the gut, malrotation of the colon, brachyesophagus, pyloric stenosis, inguinal hernia, small labia majora, radial hypoplasia, short first metacarpal, absent second to third interdigital triradius, and diaphragmatic hernia.

AUTOSOMAL RECESSIVE MUTATIONS

Meckel Syndrome (MS)

This condition was first described by Meckel in 1822. Gruber coined the term dysencephalia splanchnocystica in 1934. The condition was reviewed by Opitz and Howe [245] in 1969, who suggested the eponym "Meckel's syndrome."

MS is recessively inherited and leads to death perinatally or in early infancy; prolonged survival to 28 months has been reported [246]. In Finland, the incidence of MS was found to be 1 in 9000 births, with an equal sex ratio [247]; in other parts of the world, the incidence varies from 1 in 140,000 [248] to 1 in 13,250 [249]. The classic diagnostic triad is polydactyly, occipital encephalocele (Fig. 13.24a), and cystic kidneys. Other central nervous system malformations may occur, including cranial rachischisis, Arnold-Chiari malformation, hydrocephalus, and polymicrogyria. Ocular anomalies, cleft palate, congenital heart defects, hypoplasia of the adrenal glands, pseudohermaphroditism in males, and other malformations may be present. Large cystic dysplastic kidneys (Fig. 13.24b) may cause marked abdominal distension. This appears to be a fairly constant defect [250].

On average, there is a 10-to-20-fold increase in the size of the kidneys in MS. It should be possible to distinguish between MS and infantile polycystic kidney disease (IPCD). In MS the cysts are spherical, glomeruli are absent, and interstitial fibrosis is prominent. In IPCD the cysts are huge, tubules are linearly arranged, normal glomeruli are present, and stromal connective tissue is not prominent. The cysts display an orderly, progressive increment in cyst size from capsule to calyx [251].

Sometimes there are also cysts of the liver and pancreas. Other genitourinary anomalies include agenesis, atresia, hypoplasia and duplication of ureters, and absence or hypoplasia of the urinary bladder. The maternal and fetal alphafetoprotein levels may be elevated due to the presence of an encephalocele, and ultrasonography may disclose the presence of large cystic kidneys. These studies may provide prenatal diagnosis [252]. Difficulty may be encountered in differentiating very mild MS from rather severe Smith-Lemli-Opitz syndrome cases, the hydrolethalus syndrome, trisomy 13, and Ivemark syndrome.

The morphologically heterogeneous CNS anomalies also included hydrocephalus and micropolygyria.

Fibrosis and proliferation of the bile ducts in the hepatic portal tracts, severe hypoplasia of male genitalia with cryptorchidism, epididymal cysts and ductal dilatation, as well as fibrosis of the pancreas, are common anomalies [253].

Cryptophthalmos (Fraser) Syndrome

The association of cryptophthalmos with a specific range of other anomalies was initially reported by Fraser, and there have been many subsequent reports [254–256].

Facial findings of this autosomal recessive condition include cryptophthalmos with eye defects, hypoplastic and notched nares, and dysplastic, usually cupped, ears. Partial midfacial clefts may be present. The hands and feet often show cutaneous syndactyly, and males may show hypospadias and cryptorchidism. Internal anomalies commonly include laryngeal stenosis or atresia, renal agenesis, and abnormalities of the female genital tract, including bicornuate uterus and absent vagina.

Leprechaunism (Donohue-Uchida Syndrome)

This autosomal recessive disorder is characterized by adipose tissue deficiency and pre- and postnatal growth deficiency. Children with leprechaunism have a strikingly characteristic facial appearance, mental retardation, hirsutism, excessive skin folding, more or less pronounced skeletal involvement, hyperinsulinemia, and failure to thrive and grow rivaling that seen in severe aneuploidy syndromes. Much recent research in the USA and Japan has

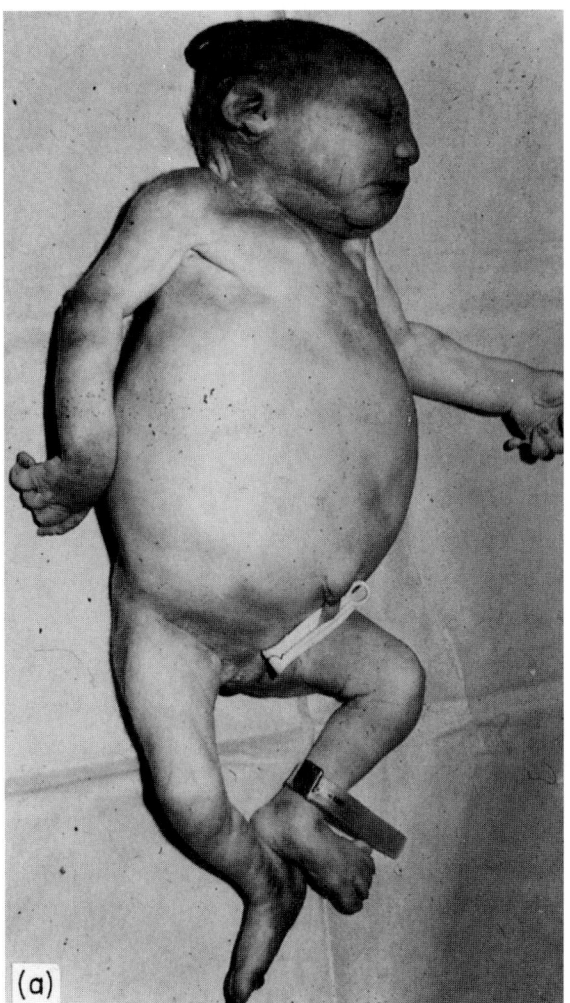

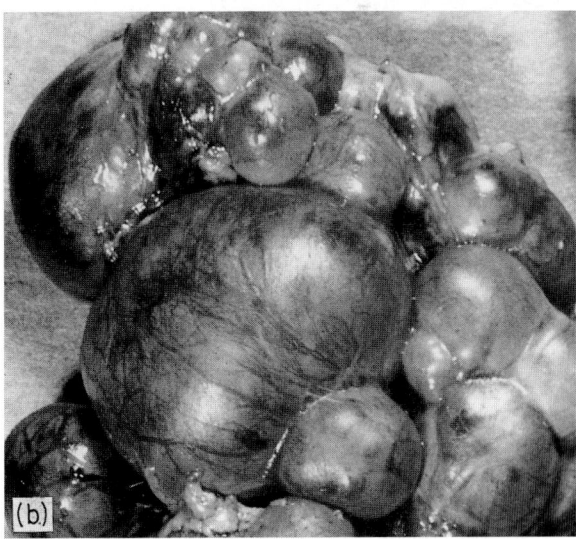

FIGURE 13.24. *Meckel syndrome: (a) characteristic facial appearance with encephalocele and polydactyly; (b) large cystic kidney.*

demonstrated that leprechaunism is an autosomal recessive congenital disorder of extreme insulin resistance, occasionally demonstrable in heterozygous carriers. Grigorescue et al [257] found a one-third to one-half reduction of insulin binding to intact erythrocytes and monocytes due to a decrease in receptor number. However, in transformed lymphocytes and monocytes, Vesely et al [258] found insulin receptor binding to be normal. These investigators demonstrated a postreceptor defect or reduction in guanylate cyclase activity and in transcellular messenger cyclic GMP concentration without ruling out a receptor defect in some cases. Genetic studies by Taylor et al [259] suggested the existence of at least two types of mutations in leprechaunism—namely, decreased in vivo receptor binding and a qualitative abnormality of insulin receptors on EB virus-transformed lymphocytes. Thus, leprechaunism has emerged as a fascinating and complex prototype entity demonstrating the pre- and postnatal developmental effects of defective insulin binding.

Cockayne Syndrome (CS)

Cockayne syndrome is an autosomal recessive disorder leading to retarded growth and development and multiple organ failures, including progressive neurologic impairment (ataxia, spasticity) and dementia [260–265]. It generally becomes manifest in early infancy and leads to death from intercurrent infection before adulthood.

There appears to be more than one possible nonallelic form of CS.

CS is characterized by a progeria-like syndrome with dwarfism, severe mental retardation, chorioretinitis, and intracranial calcification. Hypertension and renal disease are early complications, and death from early atherosclerosis may occur.

The pathogenesis of this condition is unexplained. However, CS is regularly associated with impairment in cellular DNA repair and RNA synthesis after ultraviolet light irradiation (as tested with cell cultures) [266]. It seems likely that these basic cytologic defects lead to the widespread changes that characterize the disease. Prenatal diagnosis has been made on the basis of sensitivity of amniocytes to ultraviolet light [267].

The brain in CS is characterized by microcephaly, hydrocephalus, patchy irregular loss of myelin and axons in a tigroid pattern, focal calcification (especially in basal ganglia), cerebellar atrophy, peripheral neuropathy, bizarre astrocytosis, and oligodendroglial dysplasia.

OFD (Orofaciodigital) Syndrome Type II (Mohr Syndrome)

OFD syndrome type II [268–270] is characterized by cleft tongue, conductive deafness, and partial duplication of the hallux. This is an autosomal recessive disorder; the X-linked OFD syndrome type I is described separately. Syndromal anomalies include low nasal bridge with lateral displacement of inner canthi, broad nasal tip, midline partial cleft of lip, hypertrophy of frenulum, midline cleft of the tongue and nodules on the tongue, and hypoplasia of the maxilla and mandible. The hands are short, with clinodactyly of the fifth finger. Occasionally, there may be wormian cranial bones, missing central incisors, cleft palate, pectus excavatum, and scoliosis. OFD syndrome is not associated with mental retardation.

Seckel Syndrome (Bird-Headed Dwarfism)

Seckel syndrome is associated with severe prenatal growth and mental deficiency, with microcephaly and premature synostosis, hypoplasia of maxilla with prominent nose, malformed ears, sparse hair, clinodactyly of fifth finger, hypoplasia of proximal radius, dislocation of hip and hypoplasia of proximal fibula, and 11 pairs of ribs and cryptorchidism in males [271–274]. It is inherited as an autosomal recessive trait.

Dubowitz Syndrome

Unusual facial appearance, infantile eczema, small stature, and mild microcephaly characterize this autosomal recessive disorder [275]. Infants with this syndrome are small for gestational age, with an average birth weight of 2.3 kg and variably retarded osseous maturation. The clinical manifestations include mild mental deficiency, mild microcephaly, small face, shallow supraorbital ridges with the nasal bridge at about the same level as the forehead, hypertelorism, and micrognathia. The facial characteristics bear some resemblance to those seen in the fetal alcohol syndrome. Other abnormalities include submucous cleft palate, pes planus, metatarsus adductus, hypospadias, cryptorchidism, clinodactyly of the fifth finger, and pilonidal dimple [276, 277].

Pena-Shokeir Phenotype (Pena-Shokeir I Syndrome)

Pena and Shokeir [278] first described this early lethal disorder of neurogenic arthrogryposis, pulmonary hypoplasia, and hypertelorism. It has an estimated frequency of one in 12,000 births, with a heterozygote frequency of 1:55. It has been postulated that the phenotypic manifestations are nonspecific and may be caused by decreased or absent in utero movements, thus resulting in the fetal akinesia deformation sequence [279]. There is genetic heterogeneity. Half of the cases are sporadic and half are familial and appear to be autosomal recessive or, in some cases, possibly X-linked. Therefore, Hall [280] proposed the term Pena-Shokeir "phenotype," since it is now recognized that this is not a specific syndrome but rather a description of a phenotype produced by fetal akinesia (see also Chap. 32).

Polyhydramnios, a small placenta, and a relatively short umbilical cord are frequently found. Infants are small for gestational age. Approximately 30% are stillborn. Most die of the complications of pulmonary hypoplasia within the first few weeks. Death occurs before 6 months of life.

Facial abnormalities include prominent eyes, hypertelorism, telecanthus, epicanthal folds, malformed ears, depressed tip of the nose, small mouth, highly arched palate, and micrognathia [278, 281–283].

Failure of normal deglutition results in polyhydramnios. Neuromuscular deficiency in the function of the diaphragm and intercostal muscles results in pulmonary hypoplasia. Multiple ankyloses at elbows, knees, hips, and ankles, rocker-bottom feet, talipes equinovarus, and camptodactyly are present. Absence of the flexion creases on the fingers and palms and sparse dermatoglyphic ridges are frequent. The phenotype resembles that of trisomy 18, from which it should be distinguished.

Neuropathologic findings include thin cerebral and cerebellar cortices, polymicrogyria, and multiple foci of encephalomalacia, with loss of neurons and gliosis. There is usually spinal cord involvement, with reduction in the anterior motor horn cells. Skeletal muscles show diffuse and group atrophy, consistent with neurogenic atrophy.

Pterygium formation is one of the manifestations of the Pena-Shokeir phenotype. The lethal form of the recessively inherited multiple pterygium syndrome [284–286] may represent a severe form of the Pena-Shokeir phenotype [287].

Prenatal diagnosis may be possible with prior occurrence and a high index of suspicion. Pulmonary hypoplasia may be detected by prenatal ultrasonography [288].

Cerebro-Oculofascioskeletal (COFS) Syndrome

This syndrome, characterized by neurogenic arthrogryposis, microcephaly, microphthalmia, and/or cataracts, is an autosomal recessive disorder. Death is due to pulmonary infections and spinal cord degenerative changes [289–293]. Anomalies are microcephaly, prominent root of nose, large pinnae, upper lip overlapping lower lip, mild micrognathia, and hirsutism. The eyes are deep set, with microphthalmia, cataracts, and nystagmus. Contractural deformities of the limbs, elbows, and knees; rocker-bottom feet with vertical talus; and posteriorly placed second metatarsal and longitudinal grooves in the soles along the second metatarsal are frequent.

Roberts-SC Syndrome

This condition has been described under the names pseudothalidomide or SC syndrome [22, 294–296], SC-phocomelia syndrome [215, 297], total phocomelia [298], hypomelia–hypotrichosis–facial hemangioma syndrome [299], and others [300]; the acronym SC refers to the initials of the surnames of the first two families described with the syndrome.

Roberts-SC syndrome is a malformation syndrome that includes as the most prominent characteristics a nearly symmetric phocomelia-like limb deficiency; prenatal and postnatal growth retardation; microbrachycephaly; eye abnormalities, including shallow orbits, prominent eyeballs, and cloudy corneae; cleft lip with or without cleft palate; and prominent premaxilla. Minor craniofacial abnormalities include sparse silvery blond hair, extensive hemangiomas, micrognathia, hypoplastic nasal cartilages, and malformed ears with hypoplastic lobules [301]. Nuchal cystic hygromas have been described [302]. The condition is inherited as an autosomal recessive trait, and infants have been stillborn or have died in early infancy. Premature centromere separation with puffing and splitting is a valuable laboratory diagnostic marker for this syndrome [303].

Postmortem studies have shown cystic dysplastic kidney, horseshoe kidney, and ureterostenosis with hydronephrosis [22].

TAR (Thrombocytopenia–Absent Radius) Syndrome

Gross et al [304] first described this entity in siblings; many other cases have been reported subsequently. It is inherited as an autosomal recessive trait. Almost half of the patients with this condition die during early infancy.

Hematologic abnormalities include thrombocytopenia with absence or hypoplasia of megakaryocytes; leukemoid granulocytosis, especially during bleeding episodes; and frequently eosinophilia and anemia. The limb defects include absence or hypoplasia of the radius with the presence of thumbs. It is usually bilateral with associated ulnar hypoplasia and defects of the hands, legs, and feet. Mental retardation is present in 7% of cases.

Other abnormalities may be a congenital heart defect, spina bifida, brachycephaly, strabismus, micrognathia, syndactyly, short humerus, and dislocation of the hips. A genitourinary anomaly occurred in 1 of 40 cases reviewed by Hall et al [305]; this patient had a unilateral agenesis of the kidney with hypospadias and transposition of the penis and scrotum.

Prenatal diagnosis can be accomplished by demonstration of the defects of the upper limbs by ultrasonography.

Leukemoid granulocytosis is present in two-thirds of the patients, particularly during bleeding episodes. About 40% of the patients have died during early infancy. The babies are liable to have eosinophilia and seem more prone to developing an allergy to cow's milk.

Hydrolethalus Syndrome

Hydrolethalus syndrome [306] includes hydrocephalus, micrognathia, polydactyly and abnormal lobation of the lungs, and frequently microphthalmia, cleft lip/palate, small tongue, anomalous nose, and low-set malformed ears. Bilateral pulmonary agenesis may be an associated manifestation [307]. Renal anomalies include unilateral renal agenesis and hypoplasia or tubular cysts [308]. We have observed a

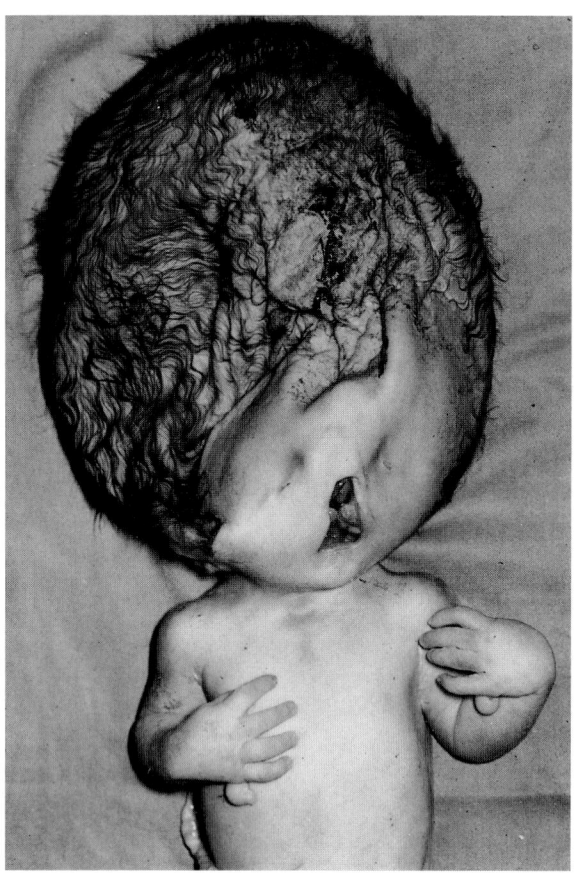

FIGURE 13.25. *Hydrolethalus syndrome.*

hydrolethalus case delivered after withdrawal of 3000 mL of cerebrospinal fluid to decompress the huge cranium (Fig. 13.25).

X-LINKED MUTATIONS

Lowe Syndrome (Oculocerebrorenal Syndrome)

Hypotonia, cataracts, renal tubular dysfunction, and mental retardation as an X-linked disorder were first described by Lowe et al [309]. The renal tubular defect results in limited ammonium production, hyperchloremic acidosis, phosphaturia, hypophosphatemia, generalized aminoaciduria, albuminuria, osteoporosis, sometimes rickets, and organic aciduria [310, 311]. Death is usually due to renal failure. Lowe syndrome is inherited as an X-linked mutation.

Menkes Syndrome (Menkes Kinky-Hair Syndrome)

Menkes et al [312] described this disorder of progressive cerebral deterioration with seizures and twisted and fractured hair in five related male infants. Danks et al [313, 314] subsequently related the disorder to copper deficiency due to a defect in intestinal copper absorption with low levels

of serum copper and ceruloplasmin. The cheeks are pudgy and the hair is sparse, stubby, coarse, and brittle, with a steel-wool appearance (Fig. 13.26a). It is lightly pigmented and shows twisting with partial breakage by magnified inspection (Fig. 13.26b). The skeletal changes include wormian bones and metaphyseal widening, particularly of ribs and femora, with lateral spurs. Arteriograms show widespread arterial elongation and tortuosity due to deficiency of copper-dependent cross-linking in the internal elastic membrane of the arterial wall. Progressive deterioration, with death in infancy, usually occurs.

By histofluorescence for the identification of catecholamines, peculiar torpedo-like swellings of catecholamine-containing axons are seen in the peripheral nerve tracts [315], as well as reduced numbers of nonadrenergic fibers in the midforebrain. The adrenergic nerve fibers and vascular regulatory disturbance may contribute to the progressive deterioration of various organs [315]. The gene has been localized to chromosome Xq13.3.

OFD (Orofaciodigital) Syndrome Type I

The clinical manifestations of OFD type I syndrome include hypertelorism, hypoplasia of alar cartilages, and milia of ears and upper face in infancy, sometimes with frontal bossing, malar hypoplasia and micrognathia, webbing between buccal mucous membrane and the alveolar ridge, partial clefts in mid-upper lip and tongue with irregular complete cleft of soft palate, anomalous teeth and absent lateral incisors, enamel hypoplasia, supernumerary teeth, hamartomas of the tongue, and fistulas in the lower lip. This X-linked form is more common and better known than the autosomal recessive type II OFD syndrome.

Clinodactyly, syndactyly, and asymmetric shortness of digits occur. The scalp is dry and rough, with sparse hair. Mental deficiency occurs in about 50% of cases. Brain malformations include absence of corpus callosum and heterotopia of gray matter in about 20% of patients.

This condition [316–321] is due to an X-linked dominant mutant gene with a lethal effect in the male. The ratio of female to male offspring of affected women has been 2:1; no affected woman has had a son with the OFD syndrome. Therefore, the risk of the OFD mother having an affected daughter is one in three.

SPORADIC DISORDERS

Klippel-Trénaunay-Weber Vascular Malformation Dysplasia

Hypertropy of usually one but occasionally more than one limb, hemangiomas that may be capillary or cavernous, phlebectasias, and varicosities characterize this disorder [322–325]. The legs, buttocks, abdomen, and lower trunk are the usual sites of the vascular lesions. Less common abnormalities include arteriovenous fistulae, lymphangiomas,

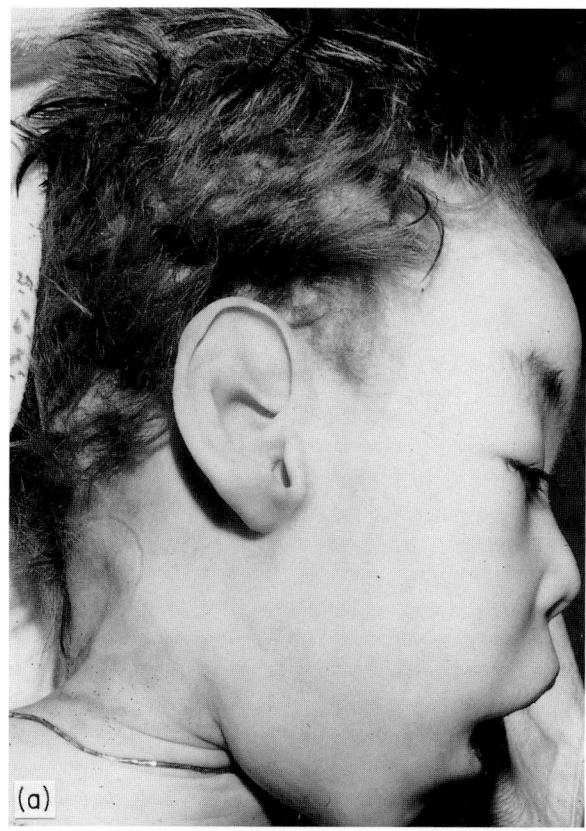

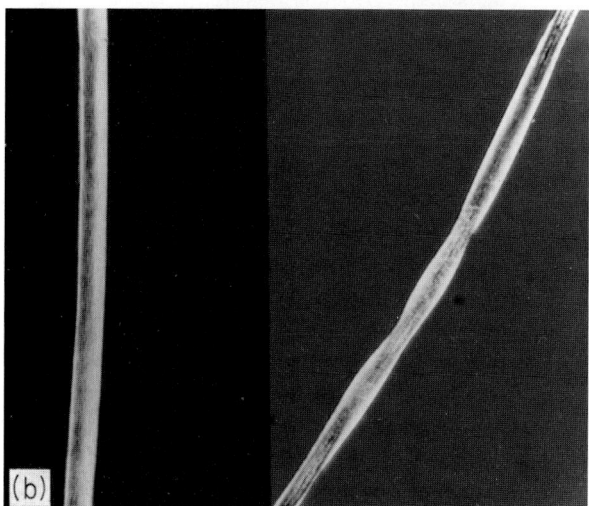

FIGURE 13.26. *(a) Menkes kinky-hair syndrome. (b) Hair under polarized light, showing kinking and twisting (right) compared with normal hair (left).*

macrodactyly, syndactyly, polydactyly, hyperpigmented nevi, and telangiectasia. Craniofacial abnormalities include asymmetric facial hypertrophy, hemangiomas, intracranial calcifications, and eye abnormalities. Visceromegaly and hemangiomas of the intestinal tract, urinary system, and mesentery may be present. Mental deficiency and seizures may occur with facial hemangiomatosis. This condition is sporadic.

Sturge-Weber Dysplasia

The association of hemangiomas in the facial skin, eyes, and meninges appears to be related to an early localized defect in vascular morphogenesis. Hemangiomas most commonly occur in a trigeminal facial distribution [326, 327]. Meningeal hemangiomas occur in the occipital and temporal areas. Cerebral cortical atrophy, sclerosis, and calcification, with seizures and mental deficiency, occur. This condition is sporadic.

Hallermann-Streiff Syndrome (Oculomandibulodyscephaly with Hypotrichosis)

This condition was first reported by Audry [328] in 1983; Hallermann and Streiff independently described three cases at a later time. It is characterized by microphthalmia, a small pinched nose, and hypotrichosis [329–333]. Infants with this syndrome have proportionate small stature, brachycephaly with frontal and parietal bossing, thin calvaria, malar hypoplasia, micrognathia, and anterior displacement of the temporomandibular joint. Bilateral microphthalmia (80%) and cataracts (94%), which may resorb spontaneously, are frequent. Facial anomalies include a thin, small, pointed nose, with hypoplasia of the cartilage and becoming parrot-like; microstomia; and a narrow, high-arched palate. There is atrophy of the skin, most prominent over the nose and suture areas of the scalp; thin hair; and hypotrichosis, especially of the scalp, eyebrows, and eyelashes. Ocular manifestations may include cataracts, spherophakia, blue sclerae, nystagmus, strabismus, colobomata, glaucoma, and various chorioretinal pigment alterations.

Rubinstein-Taybi Syndrome

This mental retardation syndrome of broad thumbs and toes, slanted palpebral fissures, and hypoplastic maxilla was first described by Rubinstein and Taybi in 1963 [334]. More than 200 cases have been reported. Other abnormalities include short stature and small cranium, mental retardation, beaked nose with nasal septum extending below nasal alae, epicanthal folds, strabismus, apparently low-set and/or malformed auricles, excess dermal ridge patterning in thenar and first interdigital areas of the palm, cryptorchidism, and cardiac defects (ventricular septal defect and patent ductus arteriosus are most common). Cataracts, colobomata, ptosis of eyelids, long eyelashes and hypertrichosis, polydactyly, simian crease, distal axial triradius, cardiac anomalies, and renal anomalies have been described. The condition is sporadic.

Hypomelanosis of Ito Syndrome (Incontinentia Pigmenti Achromians)

First described by Ito [335] in 1952, this disorder has been reviewed by Schwartz et al [336]. The triad of streaked, whorled, or mottled areas of hypopigmentation that fluoresce under Wood's lamp, mental deficiency, and severe intractable seizures that are difficult to control are present from birth and help to diagnose this condition. Strabismus, iridal heterochromia, asymmetry in leg length, macrocephaly, and hirsutism may be components of this condition [337]. The skin manifestations bear a resemblance to those of incontinentia pigmenti and the ash leaf lesion of tuberous sclerosis. This condition is sporadic. The neuropathologic changes are similar to those of tuberous sclerosis without glial proliferation and nodules. Many Ito syndrome cases probably have the Pallister [338] mosaic aneuploidy syndrome, and all infants with the diagnosis of Ito syndrome should undergo fibroblast chromosome analysis to detect the aneuploid cell line (47, +i (12p)) (see also Chap. 33).

REFERENCES

1. Spranger JW, Benirschke K, Hall JG, et al. Errors in morphogenesis: concepts and terms. Recommendations of an International Working Group. *J Pediatr* 1982; 100:160.
2. Czeizel A. Schisis associations. *Am J Med Genet* 1981; 10:25.
3. Lubinsky MS. Midline developmental "weakness" as a consequence of determinative field properties. The Enid Gilbert–Barness Festschrift. *Am J Med Genet Suppl* 1987; 3:23.
4. Opitz JM, Czeizel A, Evans JA, et al. Nosologic groupings in birth defects. In Vogel F, Sperling K, eds. *Human Genetics. Proceedings of VII International Congress on Human Genetics, Berlin.* Heidelburg: Springer-Verlag, 1987, pp. 382–5.
5. Opitz JM. Blastogenesis and the "primary field" in human development. *Birth Defects Orig Artic Ser* 1993; 29:3.
6. Van Allen M. Vascular disruptions. In: Gilbert-Barness E, ed. *Potter's Pathology of the Fetus and Infant.* Philadelphia: Mosby, 1997.
7. Lubinsky M. Invited editorial comment—associations in clinical genetics with a comment on the paper by Evans et al on tracheal agenesis. *Am J Med Genet* 1986; 21:35.
8. Chappard D, Lauras B, Fargier P, Knopf JF. Sirenomélie et dysplasie rénale multicystique. *J Genet Hum* 1983; 31:403.
9. Crawfurd MDA, Ismail SR, Wigglesworth JS. A monopodal sireniform monster with dermatoglyphic and cytogenetic studies. *J Med Genet* 1966; 3:212.
10. Duhamel B. From the mermaid to anal imperforation: the syndrome of caudal regression. *Arch Dis Child* 1961; 36:152.
11. Stevenson RE, Jones KL, Phelan MC, et al. Vascular steal: the pathogenetic mechanism producing sirenomelia and associated defects of the viscera and soft tissues. *Pediatrics* 1986; 78:451.
12. Opitz JM, Gilbert EF. Pathogenetic analysis of congenital anomalies in humans. In: Ioachim HL, ed. *Pathobiology Annual.* New York: Raven, 1982.
13. Robinson HB, Tross K. Agenesis of the cloacal membrane: a probable teratogenic anomaly. In: Rosenberg HS, Bernstein J, eds. *Perspectives in Pediatric Pathology.* vol. 8. New York: Masson, 1984, p. 79.
14. Pauli RM, Graham JM, Barr M. Agnathia, situs inversus and associated malformations. *Teratology* 1981; 23:85.
15. Pauli RM, Pettersen JC, Arya S, Gilbert EF. Familial agnathia-holoprosencephaly. *Am J Med Genet* 1983; 14:677.
16. Gaba AR, Andersen GJ, Van Dyke DL, Chason JL. Alobar holoprosencephaly and otocephaly in a female infant with a normal karyotype and placental villitis. *J Med Genet* 1982; 19:78.
17. Mollica F, Pavone L, Nuciforo G, Sorge G. A case of cyclopia. Role of environmental factors. *Clin Genet* 1979; 16:69.
18. Wright S. On the genetics of subnormal development of the head (otocephaly) in the guinea pig. *Genetics* 1934; 19:471.
19. Wright S. The genetics of vital characteristics of the guinea pig. *J Cell Comp Physiol* 1960; 56(suppl):123.
20. Converse JM, Coccaro PJ, Becker M, Wood-Smith D. On hemifacial microsomia. The first and second branchial arch syndrome. *Plast Reconstr Surg* 1973; 51:268.
21. Goldenhar M. Associations malformatives de l'oeil et de l'oreille. *J Genet Hum* 1952; 1:243.
22. Gorlin RJ, Pindborg JJ, Cohen MM Jr. *Syndromes of the Head and Neck.* New York: McGraw-Hill, 1976, pp. 125–7, 630–3.
23. Mellow DH, Richardson JE, Douglas DM. Goldenhar's syndrome—oculoauriculo-vertebral dysplasia. *Arch Dis Child* 1973; 48:537.
24. Pashayan H, Pinsky L, Fraser FC. Hemifacial microsomia-oculo-auriculo-vertebral dysplasia. A patient with overlapping features. *J Med Genet* 1970; 7:185.
25. Summitt RL. Familial Goldenhar syndrome. *Birth Defects Orig Artic Ser* 1969; V(2):106.
26. Herrmann J, Pallister PD, Gilbert EF, et al. Studies of malformation syndromes of man XXXXIB: nosologic studies in the Hanhart and the Möbius syndrome. *Eur J Pediatr* 1976; 122:19.
27. Bersu ET, Pettersen JC, Charboneau WJ, Opitz JM. Studies of malformation syndromes of man XXXXIA: anatomical studies in the "Hanhart syndrome"—a pathogenetic hypothesis. *Eur J Pediatr* 1976; 121:1.
28. Pauli RM, Greenlaw A. Limb deficiency and splenogonadal fusion. *Am J Med Genet* 1982; 13:81.
29. Murphy DP. The outcome of 625 pregnancies in women subjected to pelvic radium or roentgen irradiation. *Am J Obstet Gynecol* 1929; 18:179.
30. Goldstein L, Murphy DP. Microcephalic idiocy following radium therapy for uterine cancer during pregnancy. *Am J Obstet Gynecol* 1929; 18:189.
31. Miller RW. Effects of ionizing radiation from the atomic bomb on Japanese children. *Pediatrics* 1968; 41:257.
32. Plummer G. Anomalies occurring in children exposed *in utero* to atomic bomb in Hiroshima. *Pediatrics* 1952; 10:687.
33. Milunsky A, Graef JW, Gaynor MF Jr. Methotrexate induced congenital malformations with a review of the literature. *J Pediatr* 1968; 72:790.
34. Shaw EB, Steinbach HL. Aminopterin-induced fetal malformation. *Am J Dis Child* 1968; 115:477.
35. Thiersch JB. Therapeutic abortions with a folic acid antagonist, 4-aminopteroylglutamic acid (4-amino P.G.A.) administered by the oral route. *Am J Obstet Gynecol* 1952; 63:1298.
36. Werler MM, Shapiro S, Mitchell AA. Periconceptional folic acid exposure and risk of occurrent neural tube defects. *JAMA* 1993; 269:1257–61.
37. Lin-Fu JS, Anthony M. *Folic acid and neural tube defects. A fact sheet for health care providers.* Maternal and Child Health Bureau, Health Resources and Services Administration, Public Health Service, May, 1993.
38. Connolly KJ, Pharoah POD, Hetzel BS. Fetal iodine deficiency and motor performance during childhood. *Lancet* 1979; 2:1149.
39. Hetzel BS, Hay ID. Thyroid function, iodine nutrition, and fetal brain development. *Clin Endocrinol* 1979; 11:445.
40. Lenz W. Kindliche Missbildungen nach Medikament während der Gravidität? *Dtsch Med Wochenschr* 1961; 86:2555.
41. McBride WG. Thalidomide and congenital abnormalities. *Lancet* 1961; 2:1358.
42. McCredie J. The action of thalidomide on the peripheral nervous system of the embryo. *Proc Aust Assoc Neurol* 1975; 12:135.
43. McCredie J. Congenital fusion of bones: radiology, embryology and pathogenesis. *Clin Radiol* 1975; 26:47.
44. McCredie J. Embryonic neuropathy. A hypothesis of neural crest injury as the pathogenesis of congenital malformations. *Med J Aust* 1974; 1:159.
45. McCredie J. Neural crest defects. A neuroanatomic basis for classification of multiple malformations related to phocomelia. *J Neurol Sci* 1976; 28:373.
46. McCredie J. Segmental embryonic peripheral neuropathy. *Pediatr Radiol* 1975; 3:162.
47. McCredie J. Thalidomide and congenital Charcot joints. *Lancet* 1973; 2:1058.
48. McCredie J, McBride WG. Some congenital abnormalities: possibly due to embryonic peripheral neuropathy. *Clin Radiol* 1973; 24:204.
49. North K, KcCredie J. Neurotomes and birth defects: a neuroanatomic method of interpretation of multiple congenital malformations. Enid Gilbert–Barness Festschrift. *Am J Med Genet Suppl* 1987; 3:29.
50. Barr M, Burdi AR. Warfarin-associated embryopathy in a 17-week abortus. *Teratology* 1976; 14:129.
51. Hall JG, Pauli RM, Wilson KM. Maternal and fetal sequelae of anticoagulation during pregnancy. *Am J Med* 1980; 68:122.
52. Shane WL, Emery H, Hall JG. Chondrodysplasia punctata and maternal warfarin during pregnancy. *Am J Dis Child* 1975; 129:360.
53. Warkany J. Warfarin embryopathy. *Teratology* 1976; 14:205.
54. Shepard TH. *Catalog of Teratogenic Agents.* 3rd ed. Baltimore: John Hopkins University, 1980.
55. Wilkins L, Jones HW Jr, Holman GH, Stempfel RS Jr. Masculinization of the female fetus associated with administration of oral and intramuscular progestins during gestation: non-adrenal female pseudohermaphrodism. *J Clin Endocrinol Metabol* 1958; 18:559.

56. Aarskog D. Maternal progestins as a possible cause of hypospadias. *N Engl J Med* 1979; 300:75.

57. Heinonen OP. Diethylstilbestrol in pregnancy. Frequency of exposure and usage patterns. *Cancer* 1973; 31:573.

58. Whitehead ED, Leiter E. Genital abnormalities and abnormal semen analysis in male patients exposed to diethylstilbestrol *in utero*. *J Urol* 1981; 125:47.

59. Peck GL, Olson TG, Yoder FW, et al. Prolonged remission of cystic and conglobate acne with 13-*cis*-retinoic acid. *N Engl J Med* 1979; 300:329.

60. Rosa FW. Isotretinoin: a newly recognized human teratogen. *MMWR* 1984; 33:171.

61. Rosa FW. Teratogenicity of isotretinoin. *Lancet* 1983; 2:513.

62. Jones KL, Smith DW, Streissguth AP, Myrianthopoulos NC. Outcome in offspring of chronic alcoholic women. *Lancet* 1974; 1:1076.

63. Lemoine P, Harousseau H, Borteyru JP, Menuet JC. Les enfants de parents alcoöliques: anomalies observées, a propos de 127 cas. *Arch Fr Pediatr* 1968; 25:830.

64. Herrmann J, Pallister PD, Opitz JM. Tetraectrodactyly and other skeletal manifestations in the fetal alcohol syndrome. *Eur J Pediatr* 1980; 133:221.

65. Hanson JW, Myrianthopoulos NC, Harvey MAS, Smith DW. Risks to the offspring of women treated with hydantoin anticonvulsants, with emphasis on the fetal hydantoin syndrome. *J Pediatr* 1976; 89:662.

66. Taylor WF, Myers M, Taylor WR. Extrarenal Wilms' tumour in an infant exposed to intrauterine phenytoin. *Lancet* 1980; 2(8192):481.

67. Comess LJ, Bennett PH, Man MB, Burch TA, Miller M. Congenital anomalies and diabetes in the Pima Indians of Arizona. *Diabetes* 1967; 18:471.

68. Haust MD. Maternal diabetes mellitus—effects on the fetus and placenta in perinatal disease. In: Naeye RL, Kissane JM, Kaufman N, eds. *International Academy of Pathology Monograph*. Baltimore: Williams & Wilkins, 1981, p. 201.

69. Krous HF, Richie JP, Sellers B. Glomerulocystic kidney: a hypothesis of origin and pathogenesis. *Arch Pathol Lab Med* 1977; 101:462.

70. Kučera J, Lenz W, Maier W. Missbildungen der Beine und der kaudalen Wirbelsäule bei Kindern diabetischer Mütter. *Dtsch Med Wochenschr* 1965; 90:901.

71. Passarge E. Congenital malformations and maternal diabetes. *Lancet* 1965; 1:324.

72. Rusnak SL, Driscoll SG. Congenital spinal anomalies in infants of diabetic mothers. *Pediatrics* 1965; 35:989.

73. Stehbens JA, Baker GL, Kitchell M. Outcome at ages 1, 3, and 5 years of children born to diabetic women. *Am J Obstet Gynecol* 1977; 127:408.

74. Gabbe SG, Mestman JH, Freeman RK, et al. Management and outcome of pregnancy in diabetes mellitus, classes B to R. *Am J Obstet Gynecol* 1977; 129:723.

75. Kitzmiller JL, Cloherty JP, Younger MD, et al. Diabetic pregnancy and perinatal morbidity. *Am J Obstet Gynecol* 1978; 131: 560.

76. Pedersen J. *The Pregnant Diabetic and Her Newborn: Problems and Management*. 2nd ed. Baltimore: Williams & Wilkins, 1977, p. 123.

77. Holmes LB. Congenital malformations. In: Cloherty JP, Stark AR, eds. *Manual of Neonatal Care*. Boston: Little Brown, 1980, p. 91.

78. Miller E, Hare JW, Cloherty JP, et al. Elevated maternal hemoglobin A_{1c} in early pregnancy and major congenital anomalies in infants of diabetic mothers. *N Engl J Med* 1981; 304:1331.

79. Bunn HF, Haney DN, Kamin S, Gabbay KH, Gallop PM. The biosynthesis of human hemoglobin A_{1c}: slow glycosylation of hemoglobin *in vivo*. *J Clin Invest* 1976; 57:1652.

80. Dunn PJ, Cole RA, Soeldner JS, et al. Temporal relationship of glycosylated haemoglobin concentrations to glucose control in diabetics. *Diabetologia* 1979; 17:213.

81. Key TC, Giuffrida RG, Moore TR, Resnik R. Early pregnancy glycosylated hemoglobin as a predictor of pregnancy outcome. Society of Perinatal Obstetricians. Annual Meeting, Las Vegas, NV, 1985.

82. Greene MF, Hare JW, Clohertz JB, Benacerraf BR, Soeldner JS. First trimester hemoglobin A_1 risk for major malformations and spontaneous abortion in diabetic pregnancy. *Teratology* 1989; 39:225–31.

83. Yu JS, O'Halloran MT. Children of mothers with phenylketonuria. *Lancet* 1970; 1:210.

84. Sever JL, Fuccillo DA, Bowes WA. Environmental factors: infections and immunizations. In: Brent RL, Harris MI, eds. *Prevention of Embryonic, Fetal and Perinatal Diseases*. Washington: U.S. Government Printing Office, 1976, p. 199.

85. Rosenquist GC, Glass LE, Simpson E. Familial incidence of endocardial fibroelastosis: circulating maternal antiheart antibody as a possible etiology. *Birth Defects Orig Artic Ser* 1972; VIII(5):30.

86. Scott JR. Immunology of pregnancy loss. 1987 ACOG Update. A clinical continuum. *Obstet Gynecol*. vol. 13, no. 4.

87. Kaplan LC, Matsuoka R, Gilbert EF, Opitz JM, Kamil DM. Ectopia cordis and cleft sternum: evidence for mechanical teratogenesis following rupture of the chorion or yolk sac. *Am J Med Genet* 1985; 21:187.

88. Miller ME, Graham JM Jr, Higginbottom MC, Smith DW. Compression-related defects from early amnion rupture: evidence for mechanical teratogenesis. *J Pediatr* 1981; 98:292.

89. Lubinsky M, Sujansky E, Sanger W, Salyards P, Severn C. Familial amniotic bands. *Am J Med Genet* 1983; 14:81.

90. Smith DW. *Recognizable Patterns of Human Malformation*. 3rd ed. Philadelphia: WB Saunders, 1982.

91. Way BH, Herrmann J, Gilbert EF, Johnson SAM, Opitz JM. Cutis marmorata telangiactatica congenita. *J Cutaneous Pathol* 1974; 1:10.

92. Myrianthopoulos NC. Congenital malformations in twins: epidemiologic survey. *Birth Defects Orig Artic Ser* 1975; XI(8).

93. Plect H, Graham JM, Smith DW. Central nervous system and facial defects associated with maternal hyperthermia at 4 to 14 weeks' gestation. *Pediatrics* 1981; 67:785.

94. Shiota K. Neural tube defects and maternal hyperthermia in early pregnancy: epidemiology in a human embryonic population. *Am J Med Genet* 1982; 12:281.

95. Chance PI, Smith DW. Hyperthermia and meningomyelocele and anencephaly. *Lancet* 1978; 1:769.

96. Clarren SK, Smith DW, Harvey MAS, Ward RH. Hyperthermia—a prospective evaluation of a possible teratogenic agent in man. *J Pediatr* 1979; 95:81.

97. Edwards MJ. Clinical disorders of fetal brain development: defects due to hyperthermia. In: Hetzel BS, Smith RM, eds. *Fetal Brain Disorders*. Amsterdam: Elsevier/North-Holland, 1981, p. 335.

98. Fisher NL, Smith DW. Hyperthermia as a possible cause for occipital encephalocele. *Clin Res* 1980; 28:116A.

99. Halperin LR, Wilroy RS. Maternal hyperthermia and neural tube defects. *Lancet* 1978; 2:212.

100. Miller P, Smith DW, Shepard T. Maternal hyperthermia as a possible cause of anencephaly. *Lancet* 1978; 1:519.

101. Smith DW, Clarren SK, Harvey MAS. Hyperthermia as a teratogenic agent. *J Pediatr* 1978; 92:877.

102. Deacon JSR, Gilbert EF, Viseskul C, Herrmann JRR, Opitz JM. Polyhydramnios and neonatal hemorrhage in three sisters—a circumvallate placenta syndrome? *Birth Defects Orig Artic Ser* 1974; X(7):41.

103. Wiedemann HR. Complexe malformatif familial avec hernie ombilicale et macroglossie—un "syndrome nouveau"? *J Genet Hum* 1964; 13:223.

104. Beckwith JB. Macroglossia, omphalocele, adrenal cytomegaly, gigantism, and hyperplastic visceromegaly. *Birth Defects Orig Artic Ser* 1969; 5(2):188.

105. Kosseff AL, Herrmann J, Gilbert EF, et al. Studies of malformation syndromes of man XXIX: the Wiedemann-Beckwith syndrome. Clinical, genetic and pathogenetic studies of 12 cases. *Eur J Pediatr* 1976; 123:139.

106. Irving I. Exomphalos with macroglossia: a study of 11 cases. *J Pediatr Surg* 1967; 2:499.

107. Perlman M, Goldberg GM, Bar-Ziu J, Danovitch G. Renal hamartomas and neuroblastomatosis with fetal gigantism: a familial syndrome. *J Pediatr* 1973; 83:414.

108. Perlman M, Levin M, Wittels B. Syndrome of fetal gigantism, renal hamartomas, and neuroblastomatosis with Wilms' tumor. *Cancer* 1975; 35:1212.

109. Neri G, Martini-Neri ME, Katz BE, Opitz JM. The Perlman syndrome: familial renal dysplasia with Wilms tumor, fetal gigantism and multiple congenital anomalies. *Am J Med Genet* 1984; 19:195.

110. Culler FL, Jones KL, Deftos LJ. Impaired calcitonin secretion in patients with Williams syndrome. *J Pediatr* 1985; 107(5):720.

111. Smith DW, Opitz JM, Inhorn SL. A syndrome of multiple developmental defects including polycystic kidneys and intrahepatic biliary dysgenesis. *J Pediatr* 1965; 67:617.

112. Bowen P, Lee CSN, Zellweger H, Lindenberg R. A familial syndrome of multiple congenital defects. *Bull Johns Hopkins Hosp* 1964; 114:402.

113. Opitz JM, ZuRhein GM, Vitale L, et al. The Zellweger syndrome (cerebro-hepato-renal syndrome). *Birth Defects Orig Artic Ser* 1969; V(2):144.

114. Taylor JC, Zellweger H, Hanson JW. A new case of the Zellweger syndrome. *Birth Defects Orig Artic Ser* 1969; V(2):159.

115. Friedman A, Betzhold J, Hong R, et al. Clinicopathologic conference: a three-month-old infant with failure to thrive, hepatomegaly and neurological impairment. *Am J Med Genet* 1980; 7:171.

116. Versmold HT, Bremer HJ, Herzog V, et al. A metabolic disorder similar to Zellweger syndrome with hepatic acatalasia and absence of peroxisomes,

altered content and redox state of cytochromes, and infantile cirrhosis with hemosiderosis. *Eur J Pediatr* 1977; 124:261.

117. Vitale L, Opitz JM, Shahidi NT. Congenital and familial iron overload. *N Engl J Med* 1969; 280:642.

118. Volpe JJ, Adams RD. Cerebro-hepato-renal syndrome of Zellweger: an inherited disorder of neuronal migration. *Acta Neuropathol (Berlin)* 1972; 20:175.

119. Bernstein J, Brough AJ, McAdams AJ. The renal lesion in syndromes of multiple congenital malformations. *Birth Defects Orig Artic Ser* 1973; X(16):35.

120. Hong R, Horowitz SD, Borzy MF, et al. The cerebrohepato-renal syndrome of Zellweger: similarity to and differentiation from the DiGeorge syndrome. *Thymus* 1981; 3:97.

121. Heymans HSA, Schutgens RBH, Tan R, van den Bosch H, Borst P. Severe plasmalogen deficiency in tissues of infants without peroxisomes (Zellweger syndrome). *Nature* 1983; 306:69.

122. Goldfischer S, Moore CL, Johnson AB, et al. Peroxisomal and mitochondrial defects in the cerebro-hepato-renal syndrome. *Science* 1973; 182:62.

123. Moser AE, Singh I, Brown FR, et al. The cerebrohepatorenal (Zellweger) syndrome: increased levels and impaired degradation of very-long-chain fatty acids and their use in prenatal diagnosis. *N Engl J Med* 1984; 310:1141.

124. Hajra AK, Datta NS, Jackson LG, et al. Prenatal diagnosis of Zellweger cerebrohepatorenal syndrome. *N Engl J Med* 1985; 312:445.

125. Jackson L, Wapner R, Grebner E, Barr M. Fetal diagnosis by chorionic villus sampling. In: Filkins K, ed. *Prenatal Diagnosis*. New York: Marcel Dekker, in press.

126. Datta NS, Wilson GN, Hajra AK. Deficiency of enzymes catalyzing the biosynthesis of glycerol-ether lipids in Zellweger syndrome: a new category of metabolic disease involving the absence of peroxisomes. *N Engl J Med* 1984; 311:1080.

127. Schutgens RBH, Romeyn GJ, Wanders RJA, et al. Deficiency of acyl-CoA: dihydroxyacetone phosphate acyltransferase in patients with Zellweger (cerebro-hepato-renal) syndrome. *Biochem Biophys Res Commun* 1984; 120:179.

128. Hajra AK, Bishop JE. Glycerolipid biosynthesis in peroxisomes via the acyl dihydroxyacetone phosphate pathway. *Ann NY Acad Sci* 1982; 386:170.

129. Hajra AK, Burke CL, Jones CL. Subcellular localization of acyl coenzyme A:dihydroxyacetone phosphate acyltransferase in rat liver peroxisomes (microbodies). *J Biol Chem* 1979; 254:10896.

130. Irons M, Elias ER, Salen G, Tint GS, Batten AK. Defective cholesterol biosynthesis in Smith-Lemli-Opitz syndrome. *Lancet* 1993; 341:1414.

131. Tent GS, Irons M, Elias E, et al. Defective cholesterol biosynthesis associated with Smith-Lemli-Opitz syndrome. *N Engl J Med* 1994; 330:107–13.

132. Dallaire L, Fraser FC. The syndrome of retardation with urogenital and skeletal anomalies in siblings. *J Pediatr* 1966; 69:459.

133. Garcia CA, McGarry PA, Boirol M, Duncan C. Neurological involvement in the Smith-Lemli-Opitz syndrome. *Dev Med Child Neurol* 1973; 15:48.

134. Nevo S, Benderly A, Levy J, Katznelson MB. Smith-Lemli-Opitz syndrome in an inbred family. *Am J Dis Child* 1972; 124:431.

135. Smith DW, Lemli L, Opitz JM. A newly recognized syndrome of multiple congenital anomalies. *J Pediatr* 1964; 64:210.

136. Kohler HG. Brief clinical report: familial neonatally lethal syndrome of hypoplastic left heart, absent pulmonary lobation, polydactyly, and talipes, probably Smith-Lemli-Opitz (RSH) syndrome. *Am J Med Genet* 1983; 14:423.

137. DiGeorge AM. Congenital absence of the thymus and its immunologic consequences: concurrence with congenital hypoparathyroidism. In: Good RA, ed. *Immunologic Deficiency Diseases*. vol. IV/1. New York: National Foundation, 1968, p. 116.

138. Conley ME, Beckwith JB, Mancer KFK, Tenkoff L. The spectrum of the DiGeorge syndrome. *J Pediatr* 1979; 94:883.

139. Freedom RM, Rosen FS, Nadas AS. Congenital cardiovascular disease and anomalies of the third and fourth pharyngeal pouches. *Circulation* 1972; 46:165.

140. Kretschmer R, Say B, Brown D, Rosen FS. Congenital aplasia of the thymus gland (DiGeorge's syndrome). *N Engl J Med* 1968; 279:1295.

141. Lobdell DH. Congenital absence of the parathyroid glands. *Arch Pathol* 1959; 67:412.

142. Carey JC. Spectrum of the DiGeorge "syndrome." *J Pediatr* 1980; 96:955.

143. Lammer EJ, Opitz JM. The DiGeorge anomaly as a developmental field defect. *Am J Med Genet Suppl* 1986; 2:113.

144. Bockman DE, Kirby ML. Dependence of thymus development on derivatives of the neural crest. *Science* 1984; 223:498.

145. Kirby ML, Bockman DE. Neural crest and normal development: a new perspective. *Anat Rec* 1984; 209:1.

146. Kirby ML, Gale TF, Stewart DE. Neural crest cells contribute to normal aorticopulmonary septation. *Science* 1983; 220:1059.

147. Amman AJ, Wara DW, Cowan MJ, Barrett DJ, Stiehm ER. The DiGeorge syndrome and the fetal alcohol syndrome. *Am J Dis Child* 1982; 136:906.

148. Johnson S, Knight R, Marmer DW, Steele RW. Immune deficiency in fetal alcohol syndrome. *Pediatr Res* 1981; 15:908.

149. De la Cruz E, Sun S, Vangvanichyakorn K, Desposito F. Multiple congenital malformations associated with maternal isotretinoin therapy. *Pediatrics* 1984; 74:428.

150. Lammer EJ. Retinoic acid embryopathy: a neural crest migrational abnormality. *Am J Hum Genet* 1984; 36(4):61S. Abstract 177.

151. Lott IT, Bocian M, Pribram HW, Leitner M. Fetal hydrocephalus and ear anomalies with maternal use of isotretinoin. *J Pediatr* 1984; 105:597.

152. Gosseye S, Golaire MC, Verellen G, Van Lierde M, Claus D. Association of bilateral renal agenesis and DiGeorge syndrome in an infant of a diabetic mother. *Helv Paediatr Acta* 1982; 37:471.

153. Hanson JW, Smith DW. U-shaped palatal defect in the Robin anomaly: developmental and clinical relevance. *J Pediatr* 1975; 87:30.

154. Latham RA. The pathogenesis of cleft palate associated with the Pierre Robin syndrome. *Br J Plast Surg* 1966; 19:205.

155. Eagle JF, Barrett GS. Congenital deficiency of abdominal musculature with associated genitourinary abnormalities: a syndrome; report of nine cases. *Pediatrics* 1950; 6:721.

156. Parkes RW. Absence of abdominal muscles in an infant. *Lancet* 1895; 1:1252.

157. Tuch BA, Smith TK. Prune-belly syndrome: a report of twelve cases and review of the literature. *J Bone Joint Surg* 1978; 60A:109.

158. Wigger JH, Blanc WA. The prune belly syndrome. In: Sommers S, Rosen P, eds. *Pathology Annual*. New York: Appleton-Century-Crofts, 1977, p. 17.

159. Harley LM, Chen Y, Rattner WH. Prune belly syndrome. *J Urol (Baltimore)* 1972; 108:174.

160. Opitz JM. The developmental field concept in clinical genetics. *J Pediatr* 1982; 101:805.

161. Straub E, Spranger J. Etiology and pathogenesis of the prune belly syndrome. *Kidney Int* 1981; 20:695.

162. Burton BK, Dillard RG. Brief clinical report: prune belly syndrome: observations supporting the hypothesis of abdominal overdistention. *Am J Med Genet* 1984; 17:669.

163. Palmer JM, Tesluk H. Ureteral pathology in the prune belly syndrome. *J Urol (Baltimore)* 1974; 111:701.

164. Cremin BJ. The urinary tract anomalies associated with agenesis of the abdominal wall. *Br J Radiol* 1971; 44:767.

165. Uehling DT, Gilbert EF, Chesney RW. Urologic implications of the VATER association. *J Urol* 1983; 129:352.

166. McLoughlin TG, Shanklin DR. Pathology of Laurence-Moon-Bardet-Biedl syndrome. *J Path Bacteriol* 1967; 93:65.

167. Quan L, Smith DW. The VATER association, vertebral defects, anal atresia, T-E fistula with esophageal atresia, radial and renal dysplasia: a spectrum of associated defects. *J Pediatr* 1973; 82:104.

168. Temtamy SA, Miller JD. Extending the scope of the VATER association: definition of VATER syndrome. *J Pediatr* 1974; 85:345.

169. Evans JA, Reggin J, Greenberg C. Tracheal agenesis and associated malformations: a comparison with tracheoesophageal fistula and the VACTERL association. *Am J Med Genet* 1986; 21:21.

170. Duncan PA, Shapiro LR. MURCS and VATER associations: vertebral and genitourinary malformations with distinct embryologic pathogenetic mechanisms. *Teratology* 1979; 19:24A.

171. Duncan PA, Shapiro LR. Sirenomelia, the VATER association and facial asymmetry: interrelated disorders. *Teratology* 1981; 23:33A.

172. Evans JA. Numerical taxonomy in the study of birth defects. In: Persaud TVN, ed. *Advances in the Study of Birth Defects Volume 5. Genetic Disorders, Syndromology and Prenatal Diagnosis*. Lancaster: MTP, 1982.

173. Quan L, Smith DW. The VATER association: vertebral defects and atresia, tracheoesophageal fistula with esophageal atresia, radial dysplasia. *Birth Defects Orig Artic Ser* 1972; VIII(2):75.

174. Lubinsky M, Severn C, Rapoport JM. Fryns syndrome: a new variable multiple congenital anomaly (MCA) syndrome. *Am J Med Genet* 1983; 14:461.

175. Duncan PA. Embryologic pathogenesis of renal agenesis associated with cervical vertebral anomalies (Klippel-Feil phenotype). *Birth Defects Orig Artic Ser* 1977; XIII(3D):91.

176. Duncan PA, Shapiro LR, Stangel JJ, Klein RM, Addonizio JD. The MURCS association: müllerian duct aplasia, renal aplasia, and cervicothoracic somite dysplasia. *J Pediatr* 1979; 95:399.

177. Griffin JE, Edwards C, Madden JD, Harrod MJ, Wilson JD. Congenital absence of the vagina. *Ann Intern Med* 1976; 85:224.

178. Pagon RA, Graham JM Jr, Zonana J, Yong S. CHARGE association: coloboma, congenital heart disease, and choanal atresia with multiple anomalies. *J Pediatr* 1981; 99:223.

179. Gubler MC, Levy M, Naizot C, Habib R. Glomerular basement membrane changes in hereditary glomerular disease. *Renal Physiol* 1980; 3:405.

180. Schleutermann DA, Bias WB, Murdoch JL, McKusick VA. Linkage of the loci for the nail-patella syndrome and adenylate kinase. *Am J Hum Genet* 1969; 21(6):606.

181. Westerveld A, Jongsma APM, Meera Khan P, van Someren H, Bootsma D. Assignment of the AK1:Np:ABO linkage group to human chromosome 9. *Proc Natl Acad Sci USA* 1976; 73(3):895.

182. Melnick M, Bixler D, Silk K, Yune H, Nance W. Autosomal dominant branchio-oto-renal dysplasia. *Birth Defects Orig Artic Ser* 1975; XI(5):121.

183. Fraser FC, Sproule JR, Halal F. Frequency of the branchio-oto-renal (BOR) syndrome in children with profound hearing loss. *Am J Med Genet* 1980; 7:341.

184. Kurnit DM, Steele MW, Pinsky L, Dibbins A. Autosomal dominant transmission of a syndrome of anal, ear, renal and radial congenital malformations. *J Pediatr* 1978; 93:270.

185. Reid IS, Turner G. Familial anal abnormality. *J Pediatr* 1976; 88:992.

186. Townes PL, Brocks ER. Hereditary syndrome of imperforate anus with hand, foot, and ear anomalies. *J Pediatr* 1972; 81:321.

187. Monteiro de Pina-Neto JM. Phenotypic variability in Townes-Brocks syndrome. *Am J Med Genet* 1984; 18:147.

188. Little JR, Opitz JM. The G syndrome. *Am J Dis Child* 1971; 121:505.

189. Opitz JM, Frias JL, Gutenberger JE, Pellett JR. The G syndrome of multiple congenital anomalies. *Birth Defects Orig Artic Ser* 1969; 5(2):95.

190. Arya S, Viseskul C, Gilbert EF. Letter to the editor: the G syndrome—additional observations. *Am J Med Genet* 1980; 5:321.

191. Gilbert EF, Viseskul C, Mossman HW, Opitz JM. The pathologic anatomy of the G syndrome. *Z Kinderheilk* 1972; 111:290.

192. Kasner J, Gilbert EF, Viseskul C, et al. Studies of malformation syndromes VID: the G syndrome. Further observations. *Z Kinderheilk* 1974; 118:81.

193. Opitz JM. Editorial comment: G syndrome (hypertelorism with esophageal abnormality and hypospadias, or hypospadias-dysphagia, or "Opitz-Frias" or "Opitz-G" syndrome—perspective in 1987 and bibliography. *Am J Med Genet* 1987; 28(2):275.

194. Franceschetti A, Klein D. *The Mandibulofacial Dysostosis—A New Hereditary Syndrome.* Copenhagen: E Munksgaard, 1949.

195. Peterson-Falzone S, Pruzansky S. Cleft palate and congenital palatopharyngeal incompetency in mandibulofacial dysostosis. *Cleft Palate J* 1976; 13:354.

196. Shprintzen RJ, Berkman MD. Pharyngeal hypoplasia in Treacher Collins syndrome. *Arch Otolaryngol* 1979; 105:127.

197. Thomson A. Notice of several cases of malformation of the external ear, together with experiments on the state of hearing in such persons. *Month J Med Sci* 1946; 7:420.

198. Treacher Collins E. Case with symmetrical congenital notches in the outer part of each lower lid and defective development of the malar bones. *Trans Ophthalmol Soc UK* 1900; 20:90.

199. Holt M, Oram S. Familial heart disease with skeletal malformations. *Br Heart J* 1960; 22:236.

200. Gall JC, Stein AM, Cohen MM, Adams MS, Davidson RT. Holt Oram syndrome: clinical and genetic study of a large family. *Am J Hum Genet* 1966; 18:187.

201. Kaufman RL, Rimoin DC, McAlister WH, Hartmann AF. Variable expression of the Holt Oram syndrome. *Am J Dis Child* 1974; 127:21.

202. Letts RM, Chudley AE, Cumming G, Skokin MD. The upper limb–cardiovascular syndrome. *Clin Orthop Relat Res* 1976; 116:149.

203. Lewis KB, Bruce RA, Baum D, Motulsky AG. The upper limb–cardiovascular syndrome. *J Am Med Assoc* 1965; 193:98.

204. Sanz G, Nadal-Girard B, Mata LA, Buertello L. The upper limb–cardiovascular syndrome (Holt-Oram syndrome). *Clin Pediatr* 1973; 12:687.

205. Smith AT, Sack GH, Taylor GJ. Holt Oram syndrome. *J Pediatr* 1979; 95:538.

206. Brans YW, Lintermans JP. The upper limb—cardiovascular syndrome. *Am J Dis Child* 1972; 124:779.

207. Poznanski AK, Garn SM, Gall JC, Stern AM. Objective evaluation of the hands in the Holt Oram syndrome. *Birth Defects Orig Artic Ser* 1972; VII(5):125.

208. Hoganson G, McPherson E, Piper P, Gilbert EF. Single coronary artery arising anomalously from the pulmonary trunk. *Arch Pathol Lab Med* 1983; 107:199.

209. Opitz JM, Smith DW, Summitt RL. Hypertelorism and hypospadias. *J Pediatr* 1965; 67:968. Abstract.

210. Gonzalez CH, Hernmann J, Opitz JM. The hypertelorism-hypospadias BBB syndrome: case report and review. *Eur J Pediatr* 1977; 125:1.

211. Cappa M, Borrelli P, Morini R, Neri G. The Opitz syndrome: a new designation for the clinically indistinguishable BBB and G syndromes. *Am J Med Genet* 1987; 28:303.

212. Apert E. De l'acrocéphalosyndacylie. *Bull Soc Med* 1906; 23:1310.

213. Blank CE. Apert's syndrome (a type of acrocephalosyndactyly) observations on British series of thirty-nine cases. *Ann Hum Genet* 1960; 24:151.

214. Park EA, Powers GF. Acrocephaly and scaphocephaly with symmetrically distributed malformations of the extremities. A study of the so-called "Acrocephalosyndactylism." *Am J Dis Child* 1920; 20:235.

215. McKusick VA. *Mendelian Inheritance in Man; Catalogs of Autosomal Dominant, Autosomal Recessive and X-linked Phenotypes.* 7th ed. Baltimore: Johns Hopkins University, 1986.

216. Bartsocas CS, Weber AL, Crawford JD. Acrocephalosyndactyly type III: Chotzen's syndrome. *J Pediatr* 1970; 77:267.

217. Chotzen F. Eine Eigenartige familiäre Entwicklungsstörung (Akrocephalosyndaktylie, Dysostosis craniofacialis und Hypertelorismus). *Monatsschr Kinderheilkd* 1932; 55:97.

218. Friedman JM, Hanson JW, Graham CB, Smith DW. Saethre-Chotzen syndrome: a broad and variable pattern of skeletal malformations. *J Pediatr* 1977; 91:929.

219. Saethre H. Ein Beitrag zum Turmschädelproblem (Pathogenese, Erblichkeit und Symptomatologie). *Dtsch Z Nervenheilkd* 1931; 117:533.

220. Hodach RJ, Viseskul C, Gilbert EF, et al. Studies of malformation syndromes in man XXXVI: the Pfeiffer syndrome, association with Kleeblattschädel and multiple visceral anomalies. *Z Kinderheilkd* 1975; 119:87.

221. Martsolf JT, Cracco JB, Carpenter GG, O'Hara AE. Pfeiffer syndrome. An usual type of acrocephalosyndactyly with broad thumbs and great toes. *Am J Dis Child* 1971; 121:257.

222. Pfeiffer RA. Dominant erbliche Akrocephalosyndactylie. *Z Kinderheilkd* 1964; 90:301.

223. Bertelsen TI. The premature synostosis of the cranial sutures. *Acta Ophthalmol Suppl* 1988; 51:1–1016.

224. Crouzon O. Dysostose cranio-faciale héréditaire. *Bull Mem Soc Med Hop (Paris)* 1912; 33:545.

225. Dodge HW Jr, Wood MW, Kenned RL. Craniofacial dysostosis: Crouzon's disease. *Pediatrics* 1959; 23:98.

226. Vulliamy DG, Normandale PA. Craniofacial dysostosis in a Dorset family. *Arch Dis Child* 1966; 41:375.

227. Robinow M, Silverman FN, Smith HD. A newly recognized dwarfing syndrome. *Am J Dis Child* 1969; 117:645.

228. Wadlington WB, Tucker VL, Schimke RN. Mesomelic dwarfism with hemivertebrae and small genitalia (the Robinow syndrome). *Am J Dis Child* 1973; 126:202.

229. Stickler GB, Pugh DG. Hereditary progressive arthro-ophthalmopathy. II. Additional observations on vertebral abnormalities, a hearing defect, and a report of a similar case. *Mayo Clin Proc* 1967; 42:495.

230. Stickler GB, Belau PG, Farrell FJ, et al. Hereditary progressive arthro-ophthalmopathy. *Mayo Clin Proc* 1965; 40:433.

231. Spranger J. Arthro-ophthalmopathia hereditaria. *Ann Radiol (Paris)* 1968; 11:359.

232. Herrmann J, France TD, Spranger JW, Opitz JM, Wiffler C. The Stickler syndrome (hereditary arthroophthalmopathy). *Birth Defects Orig Artic Ser* 1975; XI(2):76.

233. Noonan J. Noonan syndrome (comments). *Birth Defects Orig Artic Ser* 1972; VIII:122.

234. Kousseff BJ, Newkirk P, Root AW. Brachmann-de Lange syndrome. 1994 update. *Arch Pediatr Adolesc Med* 1994; 148:749–55. (See editorial by JM Opitz).

235. Van Allen MI, Filippi G, Siegel-Bartelt J, et al. Clinical variability within Brachmann-de Lange syndrome: a proposed classification system. *Am J Med Genet* 1993; 47:947–58.

236. Hawley PP, Jackson LG, Kurnit DM. Sixty-four patients with Brachmann-de Lange syndrome: a survey. *Am J Med Genet* 1985; 20:453.

237. Pashayan H, Whelan D, Guttman C, Fraser FC. Variability of the de Lange syndrome: report of 3 cases and genetic analysis of 54 families. *J Pediatr* 1969; 75:853.

238. Choo PB, Bianchi GN. Brachmann-de Lange syndrome. *Aust Paediatr* 1965; 1:236.

239. Motl M, Opitz JM. Phenotypic and genetic studies of the Brachmann-de Lange syndrome. *Hum Hered* 1971; 24:1.

240. Beck B, Mikkelson M. Chromosomes in the Cornelia de Lange syndrome. *Hum Genet* 1981; 59:271.

241. Wilson G, Hicher VC, Schmickel RD. The association of chromosome 3 duplication and the Cornelia de Lange syndrome. *J Pediatr* 1978; 93:783.

242. Breslau EJ, Disteche C, Hall JG, Thuline H, Cooper P. Prometaphase chromosomes in five patients with Brachmann-de Lange syndrome. *Am J Med Genet* 1981; 10:170.

243. Francke U, Opitz JM. Chromosome 3q duplication and the Brachmann-de Lange syndrome (BDLS). *J Pediatr* 1979; 95:161.

244. Westergaard JG, Chemnitz J, Teisner B, et al. Pregnancy-associated plasma protein A: a possible marker in the classification and prenatal diagnosis of syndrome. *Prenat Diagn* 1983; 3:225–32.

245. Opitz JM, Howe JJ. The Meckel syndrome (dysencephalia splanchnocystica, the Gruber syndrome). *Birth Defects Orig Artic Ser* 1969; V(2):167.

246. Lowry RB, Hill RH, Tischler B. Survival and spectrum of anomalies in the Meckel syndrome. *Am J Med Genet* 1983; 14:417.

247. Salonen R, Norio R. The Meckel syndrome in Finland; epidemiologic and genetic aspects. *Am J Med Genet* 1984; 18:691.

248. Seller MJ. Meckel syndrome and the prenatal diagnosis of neural tube defects. *J Med Genet* 1978; 15:462.

249. Holmes LB, Driscoll SG, Atkins L. Etiologic heterogeneity of neural-tube defects. *N Engl J Med* 1976; 294:365.

250. Salonen R. The Meckel syndrome: clinicopathological findings in 67 patients. *Am J Med Genet* 1984; 18:671.

251. Anderson VM. Meckel syndrome: morphologic considerations. *Birth Defects Orig Artic Ser* 1982; 18(3B):145.

252. Scully RE, Mark EJ, McNeely BU. Case records of the Massachusetts General Hospital: Case 11–1983. *N Engl J Med* 1983; 308:642.

253. Rapola J, Salonen R. Visceral anomalies in the Meckel syndrome. *Teratology* 1985; 31:193.

254. Codère F, Brownstein S, Chen MF. Cryptophthalmos syndrome with bilateral renal agenesis. *Am J Ophthalmol* 1981; 91:737.

255. Fraser CR. Our genetical "load." A review of some aspects of genetical variation. *Ann Hum Genet* 1962; 25:387.

256. Lurie IW, Cherstvoy ED. Renal agenesis as a diagnostic feature of the cryptophthalmos-syndactyly syndrome. *Clin Genet* 1984; 25:528.

257. Grigorescue F, Herzberg V, King G, et al. Defect in insulin binding and autophosphorylation of erythrocyte insulin receptor in patients with syndromes of severe insulin resistance and their parents. *J Clin Endocrinol Metab* 1987; 64(3):549.

258. Vesely DL, Schedecoie HK, Kemp SF, Frinaik JP, Elders MJ. Decreased cyclic guanosine-3′,5′-monophosphate and guanylate cyclase activity in leprechaunism: evidence for a post receptor defect. *Pediatr Res* 1986; 20(4):329.

259. Taylor SI, Marcus-Samuels B, Ryan-Young J, Levenskol S, Elders MJ. Genetics of insulin receptor defect in a patient with extreme insulin resistance. *J Clin Endocrinol Metab* 1986; 62(6):1130.

260. Cockayne EA. Dwarfism with retinal atrophy and deafness. *Arch Dis Child* 1936; 11:1.

261. Gandolfi A, Horoupian D, Rapin I, DeTeresa R, Hyams V. Deafness in Cockayne's syndrome: morphological, morphometric, and quantitative study of the auditory pathway. *Ann Neurol* 1984; 15: 135.

262. Grunnet ML, Zimmerman AW, Lewis RA. Ultrastructure and electrodiagnosis of peripheral neuropathy in Cockayne syndrome. *Neurology* 1983; 33:1606.

263. Guzzetta F. Cockayne-Neill-Dingwall syndrome. In: Vinken PJ, Bruyn GW, eds. *Handbook of Clinical Neurology.* vol. 13. Amsterdam: North-Holland, 1972, p. 431.

264. Moossy J. The neuropathology of Cockayne's syndrome. *J Neuropathol Exp Neurol* 1967; 26:654.

265. Smits MG, Garbreëls FJM, Renier WO, et al. Peripheral and central myelinopathy in Cockayne's syndrome. Report of 3 siblings. *Neuropediatrics* 1982; 13:161.

266. Robbins JH. Hypersensitivity to DNA-damaging agents in primary degenerations of excitable tissue. In: Friedberg EC, Bridges BR, eds. *Cellular Responses to DNA Damage.* New York: Alan R. Liss, 1983, p. 671.

267. Lehmann AH, Francis AJ, Giannelli F. Prenatal diagnosis of Cockayne's syndrome. *Lancet* 1985; 1:486.

268. Mohr OL. A hereditary sublethal syndrome in man. *Skr Nor Vidensk Akad Oslo 1* 1941; 14:3.

269. Pfeiffer RA, Majewski F, Mannkopf H. Das Syndrom von Mohr und Claussen. *Klin Paediatr* 1972; 184:224.

270. Rimoin DL, Edgerton MT. Genetic and clinical heterogeneity in the oral-facial-digital syndromes. *J Pediatr* 1967; 71:94.

271. Harper RG, Orti E, Baker RK. Birdheaded dwarfs (Seckel's syndrome). A familial pattern of developmental, dental, skeletal, genital, and central nervous system anomalies. *J Pediatr* 1967; 70:799.

272. Mann TP, Russell A. Study of a microcephalic midget of extreme type. *Proc R Soc Med* 1959; 52:1024.

273. McKusick VA, Mahloudji M, Abbott MH, Lindenberg R, Kepan D. Seckel's bird-headed dwarfism. *N Engl J Med* 1967; 277:279.

274. Seckel HPG. *Bird-Headed Dwarfs.* Springfield, IL: Charles C Thomas, 1960, p. 241.

275. Dubowitz V. Familial low birth weight dwarfism with an unusual facies and a skin eruption. *J Med Genet* 1965; 2:12.

276. Opitz JM, Pfeiffer RA, Herrmann JPR, Kushnick T. The Dubowitz syndrome. Further observations. *Z Kinderheilkd* 1973; 116:1.

277. Wilroy RS Jr, Tipton RE, Summitt RL. The Dubowitz syndrome. *Am J Med Genet* 1978; 2:275.

278. Pena SDJ, Shokeir MHK. Syndrome of camptodactyly, multiple ankyloses, facial anomalies and pulmonary hypoplasia: a lethal condition. *J Pediatr* 1974; 85:373.

279. Moessinger AC. Fetal akinesia deformation sequence: an animal model. *Pediatrics* 1983; 72:875.

280. Hall J. Analysis of the Pena-Shokeir syndrome. *Am J Med Genet* 1986; 25:99.

281. Dimmick JE, Berry K, MacLeod PM, Hardwick DF. Syndrome of ankylosis, facial anomalies and pulmonary hypoplasia: a pathologic analysis of one infant. In: Bergsma D, Lowry RB, eds. *Embryology and Pathogenesis and Prenatal Diagnosis.* Birth Defects Original Article Series. vol. XIII (3D). New York: Alan R. Liss, 1977, p. 133.

282. Mease AD, Yeatman GW, Pettett G, Merenstein GB. A syndrome of ankylosis, facial anomalies and pulmonary hypoplasia secondary to fetal neuromuscular dysfunction. In: Bergsma D, Schimke RD, eds. *Cytogenetics, Environment and Malformation Syndromes.* Birth Defects Orig Artic Ser. vol. XII/5. New York: Alan R. Liss, 1976, p. 193.

283. Pena SDJ, Shokeir MHK. Syndrome of camptodactyly, multiple ankyloses, facial anomalies and pulmonary hypoplasia: further delineation and evidence of autosomal recessive inheritance. In: Bergsma D, Schimke RM, eds. *Cytogenetics, Environment and Malformation Syndromes.* Birth Defects Original Article Series. vol. XII. New York: Alan R. Liss, 1976, p. 201.

284. Chen H, Chang CH, Misra RP, et al. Multiple pterygium syndrome. *Am J Med Genet* 1980; 7:91.

285. Chen H, Immken L, Blumberg B, et al. Lethal form of multiple pterygium syndrome: a prenatally diagnosable entity. *Am J Med Genet* 1984; 17:809.

286. Chen H, Immken L, Lachman R, et al. Syndrome of multiple pterygia, camptodactyly, facial anomalies, hypoplastic lungs and heart, cystic hygroma and skeletal anomalies: delineation of a new entity and review of lethal forms of multiple pterygium syndrome. *Am J Med Genet* 1984; 17:809.

287. Chen H, Blumberg B, Immken L, et al. The Pena-Shokeir syndrome: report of five cases and further delineation of the syndrome. *Am J Med Genet* 1983; 16:213.

288. Bovicelli L, Rizzo N, Orsini LF, Calderoni P. Ultrasonic real-time diagnosis of fetal hydrothorax and lung hypoplasia. *J Clin Ultrasound* 1981; 9:253.

289. Pena SDJ, Shokeir MHK. Autosomal recessive cerebro-oculo-facio-skeletal (COFS) syndrome. *Clin Genet* 1974; 5:285.

290. Preus M, Fraser FC. The cerebro-oculo-facio-skeletal syndrome. *Clin Genet* 1974; 5:294.

291. Scott-Emuakpor A, Heffelfinger J, Higgins JV. A syndrome of microcephaly and cataracts in four siblings. A new genetic syndrome? *Am J Dis Child* 1977; 131:167.

292. Shokeir MHK. Pena-Shokeir II syndrome: cerebro-oculo-facio-skeletal (COFS) syndrome. In: Myrianthopoulos N, ed. *Handbook of Clinical Neurology: Neurogenetic Directory.* part II, vol. 45. Amsterdam: North-Holland, 1982, p. 341.

293. Surana RB, Fraga JR, Sinkford SM. The cerebro-oculo-facio-skeletal syndrome. *Clin Genet* 1978; 13:486.

294. Herrmann J, Opitz JM. Dermatoglyphic studies in a Rubinstein-Taybi patient, her unaffected dizygous twin sister and other relatives. *Birth Defects Orig Artic Ser* 1969; 5(2):22.

295. Judge C. A sibship with the pseudothalidomide syndrome and an association with Rh incompatibility. *Med J Aust* 1973; 2:280.

296. Lenz WD, Marquardt E, Weicker H. Pseudothalidomide syndrome. *Birth Defects Orig Artic Ser* 1974; 10(5):97.

297. Herrmann J, Opitz JM. The SC phocomelia and the Roberts syndrome: nosologic aspects. *Eur J Pediatr* 1977; 125:117.

298. O'Brien HR, Mustard HS. An adult living case of total phocomelia. *J Am Med Assoc* 1921; 77:1964.

299. Hall BD, Greenberg MH. Hypomelia–hypotrichosis–facial hemangioma syndrome. *Am J Dis Child* 1972; 123:602.

300. Levy M, Sacrez R, Luckel JC, et al. Malformations graves des membres et oligophrénie dans une famille (avec études chromosomiques). *Ann Pediatr* 1972; 19:313.

301. Herrmann J, Feingold M, Tuffli GA, Opitz JM. A familial dysmorphogenetic syndrome of limb deformities, characteristic facial appearance and associated anomalies: the "pseudothalidomide" or "SC-Syndrome." *Birth Defects Orig Artic Ser* 1969; 5(3):81.

302. Graham JM Jr, Stephens TD, Shepard TH. Letter to the Editor: Nuchal cystic hygroma in a fetus with presumed Roberts syndrome. *Am J Med Genet* 1983; 15:163.

303. Tomkins D, Hunter A, Roberts M. Cytogenetic findings in Roberts–SC phocomelia syndrome(s). *Am J Med Genet* 1979; 4:17.

304. Gross H, Groh CH, Weippl G. Kongenitale hypoplastische Thrombopenie mit Radialaplasie. Ein Syndrom multipler Abartungen. *Neue Oesterr Z Kinderheilkd* 1956; 1:574.

305. Hall JG, Levin J, Kuhn JP, et al. Thrombocytopenia with absent radius (TAR). *Medicine* 1969; 48:411.

306. Salonen R, Herva R, Norio R. The hydrolethalus syndrome: delineation of a "new," lethal malformation syndrome based on 28 patients. *Clin Genet* 1981; 19:321.

307. Toriello HV, Bauserman SC. Bilateral pulmonary agenesis: association with the hydrolethalus syndrome and review of the literature from a developmental field perspective. *Am J Med Genet* 1985; 21:93.

308. DeBuse PJ, Morris G. Bilateral pulmonary agenesis, esophageal atresia, and the first arch syndrome. *Thorax* 1973; 28:526.

309. Lowe CU, Terrey M, MacLachland EA. Organic-aciduria, decreased renal ammonia production, hydrophthalmos, and mental retardation. *Am J Dis Child* 1952; 83:164.

310. Illig R, Dumermuth G, Prader A. Das oculocerebro-renale Syndrom (Lowe). *Helv Paediatr Acta* 1963; 18:173.

311. Richards W, Donnell GN, Wilson WA, Stowens D, Perry T. The oculo-cerebro-renal syndrome of Lowe. *Am J Dis Child* 1965; 109:185.

312. Menkes JH, Alter M, Steigler GK, Weakley DR, Snug JH. A sex-linked recessive disorder with retardation of growth, peculiar hair, and focal cerebral and cerebellar degeneration. *Pediatrics* 1962; 29:764.

313. Danks DM, Campbell PE, Stevens BJ, et al. Menkes' kinky hair syndrome. An inherited defect in copper absorption with widespread effects. *Pediatrics* 1972; 50:188.

314. Danks DM, Stevens BJ, Campbell PE, et al. Menkes' kinky hair syndrome. *Lancet* 1972; 1:1100.

315. Uno H, Arya S, Laxova R, Gilbert EF. Menkes' syndrome with vascular and adrenergic nerve abnormalities. *Arch Pathol Lab Med* 1983; 107:286.

316. Doege TC, Thuline HC, Priest JH, Norby DE, Bryant JS. Studies of a family with the oral-facial-digital syndrome. *N Engl J Med* 1964; 271:1073.

317. Gorlin RJ, Psaume J. Orodigitofacial dysostosis—a new syndrome. *J Pediatr* 1962; 61:520.

318. Jacquemart CJ, Trotter TL, Kaplan AH, Beauchamp RF. The oral-facial-digital syndromes reviewed: the role of computerized axial tomography in management. *Arizona Med* 1980; 37:261.

319. Majewski F, Lenz W, Pfeiffer RA, Tünte W. Das oro-facio-digitale Syndrom. Symptome und Prognose. *Z Kinderheilkd* 1972; 112:89.

320. Papillon-Léage M, Psaume J. Une malformation héréditaire de la muqueuse buccale: brides et freins anormaux. *Rev Stomatol (Paris)* 1954; 55:209.

321. Whelan DT, Feldman W, Dost I. The oro-facial–digital syndrome. *Clin Genet* 1975; 8:205.

322. Klippel M, Trenaunay P. Du naevus variqueux ostéo-hypertrophique. *Arch Gen Med* 1900; 185:641.

323. Kuffer FR, Starzynski TE, Girolami A, Murphy L, Grabstald H. Klippel-Trenaunay syndrome, visceral angiomatosis, and thrombocytopenia. *J Pediatr Surg* 1968; 3:65.

324. Lindenauer SM. Congenital arteriovenous fistula and the Klippel-Trenaunay syndrome. *Ann Surg* 1971; 174:248.

325. Parkes-Weber F. Angioma formation in connection with hypertrophy of limbs and hemi-hypertrophy. *Br J Dermatol* 1907; 19:231.

326. Butterworth T, Strean LP. *Clinical Genodermatology.* Baltimore: Williams & Wilkins, 1962.

327. Chao DH-C. Congenital neurocutaneous syndromes of childhood. III. Sturge-Weber disease. *J Pediatr* 1959; 55:635.

328. Audry C. Variété d'alopecia congénitale; alopécie suturale. *Ann Dermatol Syphiligr* 1893; 4:899.

329. François J. A new syndrome: dyscephalia with bird face and dental anomalies, nanism, hypotrichosis, cutaneous atrophy, microphthalmia and congenital cataract. *Arch Ophthalmol* 1958; 60:842.

330. Golomb RS, Porter PS. A distinct hair shaft abnormality in the Hallermann-Streiff syndrome. *Cutis* 1975; 16:122.

331. Guyard M, Perdriel G, Ceruti F. Sur deux cas de syndrome dyscéphalique a tête d'oiseau. *Bull Soc Ophtalmol Fr* 1962; 62:443.

332. Hoefnagel D, Benirschke K. Dyscephalia mandibulo-oculo-facialis (Hallermann-Streiff syndrome). *Arch Dis Child* 1965; 40:57.

333. Judge C, Chalcanovskis JF. The Hallermann-Streiff syndrome. *J Ment Defic Res* 1971; 15:115.

334. Rubinstein JH, Taybi H. Broad thumbs and toes and facial abnormalities. A possible mental retardation syndrome. *Am J Dis Child* 1963; 105:588.

335. Ito M. Studies on melanin XI. Incontinentia pigmenti achromians. *Tohoku J Exp Med* 1952; 55(suppl):57.

336. Schwartz MF, Esterly NB, Fretzin DF, Pergament E, Rozenfeld IH. Hypomelanosis of Ito. *J Pediatr* 1977; 90:236.

337. Ross DL, Liwnicz BH, Chun RWM, Gilbert E. Hypomelanosis of Ito (incontinentia pigmenti achromians)—a clinicopathologic study: macrocephaly and gray matter heterotopias. *Neurology* 1982; 32:1013.

338. Pallister PD, Herrmann J, Spranger JW, et al. The W syndrome. *Birth Defects Orig Artic Ser* 1974; X(7):51.

Hydrops Fetalis and Other Forms of Excess Fluid Collection in the Fetus

JEAN W. KEELING

INTRODUCTION

Water is the major constituent of the human body. Its contribution to body mass changes with maturity, comprising 88% of fetal mass at 18 to 20 weeks' gestation, 73% at term, and falling to 60% of body mass in the mature adult [1]. Excessive fluid accumulation (edema) can be localized within the tissues of a restricted anatomical region in response to inflammation or obstruction to lymphatic or venous drainage. It can be localized within a single body cavity, such as pleural effusion or ascites. Edema may be generalized; in the fetus, this is often designated "hydrops." In the hydropic fetus, there is both an increase in total body water and an imbalance of fluid distribution between body compartments. Even when edema is generalized, local differences in the extent of edema are common and are probably related to the composition and structure of subcutaneous tissues.

The incidence of generalized edema in the fetus is difficult to quantify. Minor fetal hydrops is very common, particularly among preterm neonates, and is often unexplained [2]. Major or severe fetal hydrops, defined as generalized edema of >5-mm subcutaneous edema in a third-trimester fetus and accompanied by an effusion in at least one body cavity, was identified in 1:1400 pregnancies when cases caused by rhesus incompatibility had been excluded [3]. Severe hydrops is more likely to be diagnosed prenatally and its cause identified. In the third trimester, generalized fetal edema is often accompanied by polyhydramnios and edema of the placenta, but these features are not always present. Second-trimester fetal hydrops is rarely accompanied by polyhydramnios; this probably reflects the changing relationship between fetus and amniotic fluid as pregnancy progresses.

While there may be differences in both pathogenesis and etiology between localized and generalized fluid accumula-tion and polyhydramnios, it should not be forgotten that, in the fetus, neither is a static condition and that any one may progress to another [153]. We should also remember that even major degrees of generalized hydrops can disappear over a period of several weeks, both with [4, 5] and without [6, 7] medical treatment.

DISTRIBUTION AND CONTROL OF FLUID IN THE FETUS AND AMNIOTIC SAC

Fluid distribution in the fetus will be considered first, and then the relationship between fetal fluid and fluid within the amniotic cavity will be discussed.

Water within the fetus may be intracellular or extracellular, the latter comprising both the intravascular compartment and the interstitial space. The volume of water within the intracellular compartment depends on the relationship between osmotic forces both within the cell and in the local interstitial space, and on a functional sodium pump within cell membranes.

The distribution of extracellular water between interstitial and intravascular compartments is dependent on, and affected by, a variety of mechanisms. Its control is clearly more complex than that postulated by Starling: that the difference between the colloid osmotic pressure of the interstitial space and the hydrostatic pressure of the intravascular compartment effected loss of intravascular water at the arterial end of the capillary bed while a change in the balance of these forces promoted return of fluid to the intravascular space at the venous end of the capillary network, any excess interstitial fluid being returned to the venous circulation via lymphatics [8].

The work of Mayerson et al [9] suggests that bulk flow of water accompanies protein molecules across capillaries in the lung and liver, where pores in capillary walls are large enough to permit the passage of protein molecules. In other sites, it is more likely that water escapes from the intravascular compartment by a process of simple diffusion through intercellular clefts in the capillary wall.

The stability of the relationship between interstitial and intravascular fluid seems to depend on the structure and components of the interstitial space. This comprises a gel of mucopolysaccharide molecules, much of this being hyaluronic acid, lying in the spaces of a collagen network. The gel contains protein and salts, particularly sodium ions, and is only partially saturated with water. Under normal circumstances, no free fluid is present within the interstitial space. Water is attracted into the interstitial space by the partially saturated gel, and removed by the small, negative hydrostatic force exerted by the pumping action of the lymphatics. Small changes in interstitial water content produce large changes in interstitial fluid pressure until saturation of the gel occurs, when a large increase in water content has little effect on interstitial fluid pressure [10]. At this point, any more water entering the interstitial space results in pooling of free fluid and edema. This free interstitial fluid can move under the influence of gravity.

The volume of amniotic fluid increases as pregnancy progresses towards term, although not at a constant rate. Its chemical composition alters as the fetus matures. The relationship between fetal size, weight, and amniotic fluid volume also changes with increasing fetal maturity.

During embryogenesis, amniotic fluid volume is greatly in excess of embryo volume. A fluid-filled amniotic cavity is recognizable around the time of implantation, before the embryo is distinguishable [11]. At this stage, amniotic fluid is not dependent on the embryo, as it continues to accumulate in the amniotic sac when the fetus fails to develop or is resorbed; presumably, it is secreted by the amnion.

In the early fetal period, amniotic fluid volume is closely related to fetal size [12–14], increasing from 25 mL at 10 weeks' gestation to about 400 mL at 20 weeks. During this time, the composition of amniotic fluid closely resembles fetal plasma [14] and there is rapid diffusion of water between fetus and amniotic fluid at a rate of 400 to 500 mL per hour. This rate is grossly in excess of the net increase in amniotic fluid volume, which is calculated at about 0.5 mL per hour, derived from a steady increase in amniotic fluid volume of about 100 mL per week. In the first half of pregnancy, both fetal skin and umbilical cord amnion are freely permeable to water and solutes [15, 16]. Work in rhesus monkeys [17] shows that amniotic fluid volume may change in order to maintain the tonicity of fetal extracellular fluid. Before mid-pregnancy, it is unlikely that fetal swallowing or micturition exerts any influence on either the volume or composition of amniotic fluid.

In the second half of pregnancy, the relationship between fetal size and amniotic fluid volume is no longer linear. Although the latter increases to around 800 mL at term, the rate of increase is outstripped by the rate of increase of fetal size and weight. Keratinization of fetal skin begins at 19 to 20 weeks' gestation and is well developed by 25 weeks, so that free diffusion of water and solutes through the skin is no longer possible. Thus, the amniotic fluid changes from having both physical and physiological buffer functions as an extension of the fetal extracellular compartment into an externalized fluid with an entirely physical protective role. Its volume is increased continually by voiding of urine by the fetus, and a similar volume is removed by fetal swallowing [13]. The fetal lung secretes fluid at the rate of 4 to 6 mL per hour per kg body weight in a variety of animal species. There is no reason to suppose that the human fetal lung behaves differently [18] and at this rate, would produce about 500 mL per day at term. At least some of this enters the amniotic fluid to account for the presence of surfactant in amniotic fluid toward the end of pregnancy.

During the last trimester of pregnancy, fetal anomalies that interfere with swallowing are often accompanied by polyhydramnios and reduced voiding of urine with oligohydramnios. Water can cross both umbilical cord amnion and the chorionic plate of the placenta at term [19]. However, there is no evidence to suggest that fluid exchange at either site modifies amniotic fluid volume in the presence of a healthy fetus, but such routes might be important when this is not the case.

The volume of amniotic fluid falls rapidly after 40 weeks' gestation to around 400 mL at 42 weeks and then to 200 mL at 44 weeks [20, 21].

MECHANISMS OF FETAL HYDROPS

Consideration of the factors involved in the maintenance of fetal fluid balance suggests that there are a number of pathological states which might adversely affect the maintenance of homeostatic mechanisms. The most important of these are chronic, severe fetal anemia, leading to hypoxic capillary damage; hypoproteinemia, reducing colloid osmotic pressure; and fetal heart failure, leading to reduction of arterial hydrostatic pressure [22]. To these must be added interference with the fetoplacental circulation, usually impedance to venous return from the placenta, leading to placental villous edema, and reduced efficiency of gas and solute exchange between maternal and fetal circulations [23]. Fetal hydrops has been precipitated by in utero closure of the ductus arteriosus brought about by maternal prostaglandin inhibitor administration in the presence of critical aortic stenosis [24].

When we consider the role of particular mechanisms in the development of fetal hydrops, it becomes apparent that the extent of underlying abnormality observed, such as a low hemoglobin or reduced serum albumin level, often does not correlate well with the extent of hydrops present. There are three factors that appear to modify the effect of the primary abnormality:

1. The stage of gestation when the disorder is first manifest. If this occurs during early fetal life, then

the fetus appears to be able to compensate for gross degrees of abnormality, such as the very low hemoglobin level in erythrogenesis imperfecta or the extremely low serum protein level in analbuminemia. When onset of the causative process occurs later in pregnancy, fetal tolerance seems to be much reduced.

2. The rate of progression of the primary mechanism. This may be accelerated effectively in the second half of pregnancy by rapid fetal growth, with consequent expansion of both intravascular and interstitial compartments.

3. Development of villous edema within the placenta, consequent on fetal hydrops, will impair oxygen transfer to the fetus and may reduce transport of proteins as well.

By the time that the fetal hydropic state is apparent, additional mechanisms usually have been brought into play. Phibbs et al [25] observed that the degree of hydrops in rhesus incompatibility was related more closely to serum albumin level than to packed cell volume. Moerman [26] found that the extent of generalized edema in nonimmunological hydrops correlated better with serum albumin than hemoglobin level. Impairment of the fetoplacental circulation can occur as a complication of the primary mechanism. Moise et al [27] demonstrated lower hematocrit and colloid osmotic pressure in gestation-matched hydropic, compared with non-hydropic, fetuses who were also anemic. There was also minor umbilical venous pressure elevation in the hydropic fetuses. The authors concluded that minor abnormalities of intravascular Starling forces could have a role in the development of hydrops when anemia was present. This may be effected either at villous capillary level—for example, by extramedullary hemopoiesis within the placenta—or as impedance to venous return by increased intrathoracic or intra-abdominal pressure following rapid enlargement of viscera or fluid accumulation within body cavities.

The fetus responds appropriately to both anemia and hydrops by increasing its secretion of atrial natiuretic factor to stimulate urine production [28]. Plasma aldosterone level is also increased in anemic and hydropic states [29].

LOCALIZED FLUID ACCUMULATION

Polyhydramnios

Polyhydramnios, an excess of amniotic fluid, has been defined either in terms of a fixed upper limit of normal amniotic fluid volume (both 1500 mL and 2000 mL have been suggested), or the volume of fluid has been related to gestational age [30]. Precise volumes are of little use in practice, however, as polyhydramnios is usually a clinical diagnosis; currently, it is often diagnosed by ultrasound. Measurement of amniotic fluid volume is not undertaken as part of patient management in these circumstances and the

perceived and actual amniotic fluid volume bear little relationship to each other [31].

A diagnosis of polyhydramnios is made in between 0.3% [32] and 1% of pregnancies, irrespective of whether this is made on clinical grounds or by ultrasound examination [33]. A relationship between amniotic fluid volume and fetal size has been demonstrated in late pregnancy [34]. The association between polyhydramnios and both gestational diabetes and diabetes mellitus is largely the result of this relationship rather than an increased incidence of malformation in the offspring of women with diabetes. The frequency of polyhydramnios increases with the severity of the diabetic state [35, 36].

Polyhydramnios is observed more frequently in multiple than in single pregnancy. It was present in 4% of Law's [37] cases and observed in 3.9% of twin pregnancies in the British Perinatal Mortality Survey [32]. An excess of fluid may be present in only one gestation sac and in some cases the disparity is seen in association with twin–twin transfusion and generalized hydrops of one twin.

Polyhydramnios occurs more frequently in pregnancies where the fetus is malformed. Jeffcoate and Scott [34] described fetal anomalies of a type that might be expected to interfere with fetal swallowing in 32% of 169 consecutive pregnancies that were complicated by polyhydramnios. The most frequently observed anomaly was anencephaly. Esophageal atresia and small intestinal obstruction due to atresia or volvulus are also associated with polyhydramnios. Butler and Alberman [32] found polyhydramnios in 59.5% of pregnancies where the fetus was anencephalic, in 10% of cases with spina bifida, and 33% of other CNS malformations. They also found an association between esophageal atresia (38%) and duodenal atresia (54%) and polyhydramnios.

Polyhydramnios was more common in Down syndrome, even when those babies with upper intestinal obstruction had been excluded. The overall incidence of polyhydramnios in babies with major malformations was 28%. Butler and Claireaux [38] found that polyhydramnios complicated the pregnancy of 19 babies with diaphragmatic hernia; two-thirds of these babies had other major defects, but six had diaphragmatic hernia alone. None of the babies were hydropic. In one American institution [36], unspecified malformations were present in 19.8% of pregnancies complicated by polyhydramnios.

Polyhydramnios was described in 25% to 30% of pregnancies where there was a large angioma in the placenta [39]. In some cases, generalized fetal hydrops, due to high-output cardiac failure because of arteriovenous anastomosis within the tumor, was also present. A decrease in amniotic fluid volume to normal has been observed over a period of several weeks, and thrombosis of the angioma observed after delivery [40, 41].

Recurrent polyhydramnios in the following or subsequent pregnancies is not common. Beischer et al [42] found an incidence of 1:1720 of their pregnant patients. Fetal macrosomia, maternal diabetes mellitus, and major malformations were common predisposing factors. Perinatal mortality was increased because of malformations and, since polyhydramnios causes premature onset of labor, deaths due to diseases of prematurity also increased.

There is an increased incidence of cord prolapse and malpresentation in pregnancies complicated by polyhydramnios, and postpartum hemorrhage is also encountered more often [5, 36]. In the third trimester of pregnancy, it is usual for generalized fetal hydrops to be accompanied by polyhydramnios [40, 43]. The increase in amniotic fluid volume may be very rapid and is often accompanied by preeclampsia [5]. Fetal hydrops in the second trimester of pregnancy is not usually accompanied by an increase in amniotic fluid volume.

Pleural Effusions

Pleural effusions are commonly observed in sick neonates as a manifestation of heart failure, but are unusual in the fetus. When they do occur, they are usually seen in the fetus with severe, generalized hydrops [40, 44] and are rarely present in isolation.

Pleural effusions are present at birth in the fetus with primary pulmonary lymphangiectasis [45–47] (Fig. 14.1). The effusions often appear serous at birth, although the lymphocyte content is usually elevated; they appear opalescent or frankly chylous after milk feeding is initiated. Pleural effusions are uncommon when pulmonary lymphangiectasis is secondary to cardiovascular malformations, such as total anomalous pulmonary venous drainage [48, 49]. In this situation, lymphatic distention occurs after lung expansion, and the accompanying interstitial edema serves to splint the lung, reduce the degree of collapse on expiration, and

increase lung volume so that the lungs eventually fill the thoracic cavities.

Brus et al [50] argue that lymphatic obstruction within and on the surface of an extrapulmonary sequestration, giving rise to a massive unilateral pleural effusion, is the mechanism for pulmonary hypoplasia and generalized hydrops, rather than the increasing size of the sequestration acting directly by increasing intrathoracic pressure. I would be more convinced if they had found disproportionate ipsilateral pulmonary hypoplasia as encountered in diaphragmatic hernia.

Dark red or brownish fluid is frequently found in the pleural cavities of macerated stillbirths at postmortem examination. The fluid accumulates after fetal death. Its volume is usually small, but larger amounts may raise the possibility of premortem accumulation. Long-standing pleural effusions in the fetus result in loss of the sharp borders of lung lobes and the concave inferior surface of both lower lobes.

Fetal Ascites

Ascites as an isolated pathological fluid accumulation in the fetus is less commonly detected than is ascites as part of generalized hydrops with fluid excess in other body cavities as well. Fetal ascites is reported in infants of diabetic mothers and in fetal anemia without blood group incompatibility [4]. It is described in association with maternal polyhydramnios, without serious sequelae [51]. Transitory fetal ascites is documented by Platt et al [7] and Mueller-Heubach and Mazer [52].

The associations of fetal ascites are similar to those malformations that may be accompanied sometimes by generalized edema, suggesting a progression from one to the other. Although examination of the associations of fetal

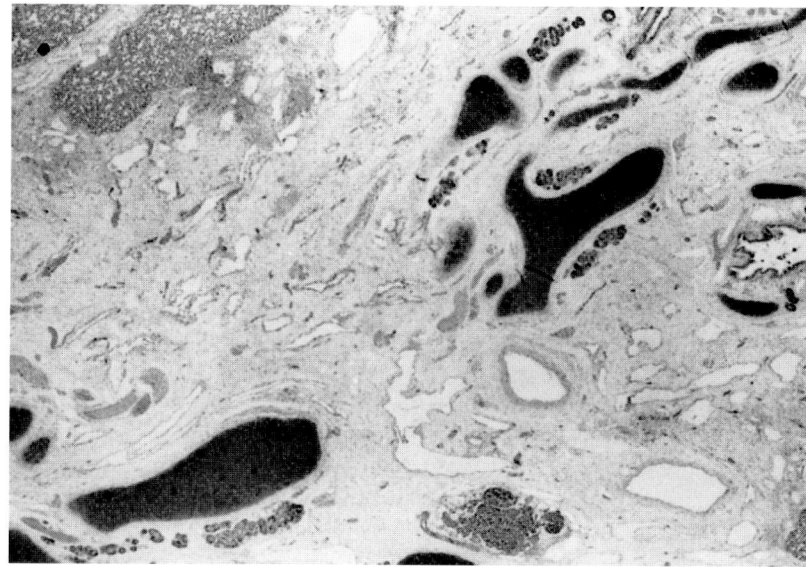

FIGURE 14.1. *Pulmonary lymphangiectasis. Section through the hilum of the lung; cartilage bars are irregular. There is an excess of connective tissue within which an excess of dilated branching lymphatic channels is present.*

ascites [53] reveals proportionally more babies with local intra-abdominal abnormalities, particularly lower urinary tract obstruction, liver disease, both hepatitis and extrahepatic biliary atresia have been described and intestinal perforation. Prenatal intussusception [54] and multiple intestinal atresias [55] can also provoke fetal ascites.

Fetal ascites has been described in the fetus with major cardiovascular malformations, such as hypoplastic left heart syndrome and bilateral pulmonary sequestration [56] and sacral agenesis [4]. The author has seen massive accumulation of ascites in a fetus with disordered bronchial branching and atresias of intrapulmonary airways. The lungs were massively overdistended by secreted lung fluid, similar to the situation in laryngeal atresia (Fig. 14.2a,b). Isolated ascites have also been seen in a fetus with high-output cardiac failure resulting from diffuse leptomeningeal angiomatosis. Other reported associations are premature closure of the foramen ovale [57], ruptured ovarian cyst [58], and genetic metabolic disease, such as sialidosis, Salla disease, GM_1 gangliosidosis, and Gaucher disease [53, 59–61].

When ascites is long-standing, the intestines are compressed into the central part of the abdominal cavity and the liver loses its normal contour with a sharp lower margin and becomes more symmetrical and rounded in outline.

Pericardial Effusion

Significant pericardial effusion is rarely seen at birth in the non-hydropic infant. When present, it is usually associated with a local structural abnormality, such as an intrapericardial teratoma (Fig. 14.3) [62, 63] or visceral herniation into the pericardial sac as a consequence of absence of the central tendon of the diaphragm [3, 64]. The effusion associated with a teratoma is characteristically large, serous, and symp-

tomatic, leading to cardiac tamponade. It usually reaccumulates rapidly after pericardiocentesis [62].

The pathogenesis of isolated pericardial effusion in the fetus is unclear (Fig. 14.4). It may result from mechanical irritation of the sac lining [3]. The increased surface area of the sac may permit more rapid transudation of fluid into its cavity.

Postnuchal Fluid Accumulation (Cystic Hygroma)

Postnuchal fluid accumulation (usually, albeit incorrectly, called "cystic hygroma" in the obstetrical and ultrasound literature) is a frequent finding in the second-trimester fetus, becoming less common as pregnancy advances. It may be an isolated finding, seen in association with a structural defect or as part of generalized fetal hydrops. The presence of a small fluid-filled bleb overlying the neck and occiput (Fig. 14.5) is now distinguished from massive fluid accumulation extending upward to the vertex, down to the shoulders, and easily seen from the front (Fig. 14.6). The thickness of the nuchal pad increases slightly as gestation advances; the upper limit of normal varies slightly in different publications. A bleb of <10 mm can be described as small, and >10 mm is large [65]. The presence or absence of septae giving rise to a multilocular lesion is also important [66].

A fluid bleb of ≥5 m carries an increased risk of chromosome anomaly (23% in one study) [67, 68]. Several different chromosome abnormalities, particularly trisomy 21 and a wide variety of other disorders including skeletal dysplasias, cardiac anomalies, and genetic metabolic disease are described with postnuchal fluid bleb. Structural abnormalities were seen in 91% and chromosome abnormalities in 37% of cases referred to one fetal medicine unit [66]. The

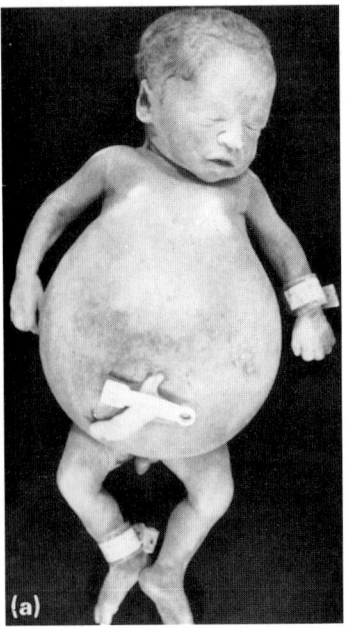

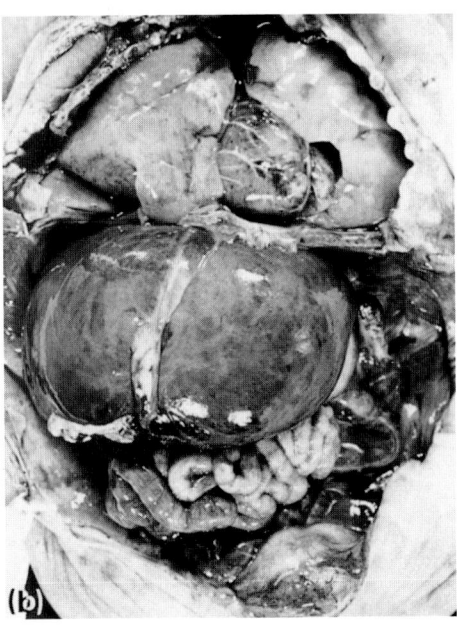

FIGURE 14.2.   *(a) Preterm neonate with massive abdominal distension due to ascites. There is no associated subcutaneous edema. (b) Same fetus. Inspection of the body cavities reveals bulky lungs filling the chest and impeding venous return to the heart. Within the large abdominal cavity the liver has rounded borders and the intestine is crowded into the central part of the cavity as a result of long-standing ascites.*

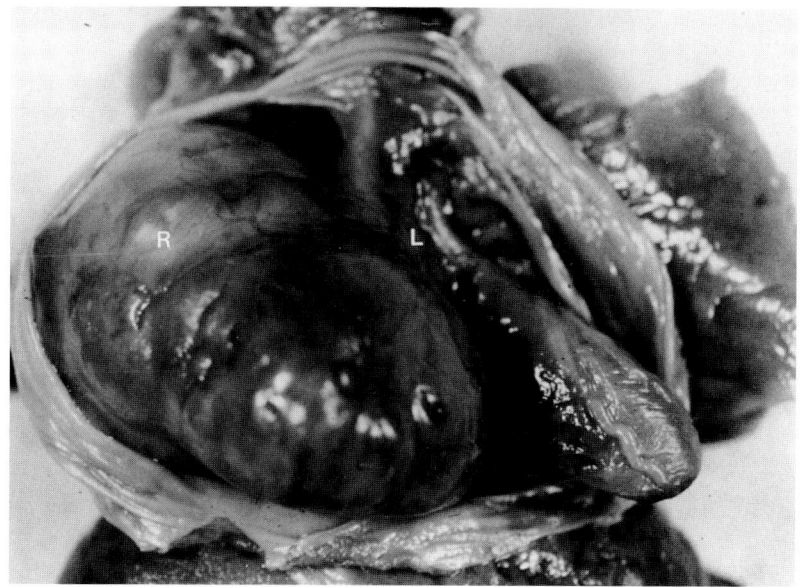

FIGURE 14.3.   *The reflected pericardial sac gives an indication of the volume of a pericardial effusion which distorted intrathoracic anatomy. A teratoma (R) arises from the base of the heart (L).*

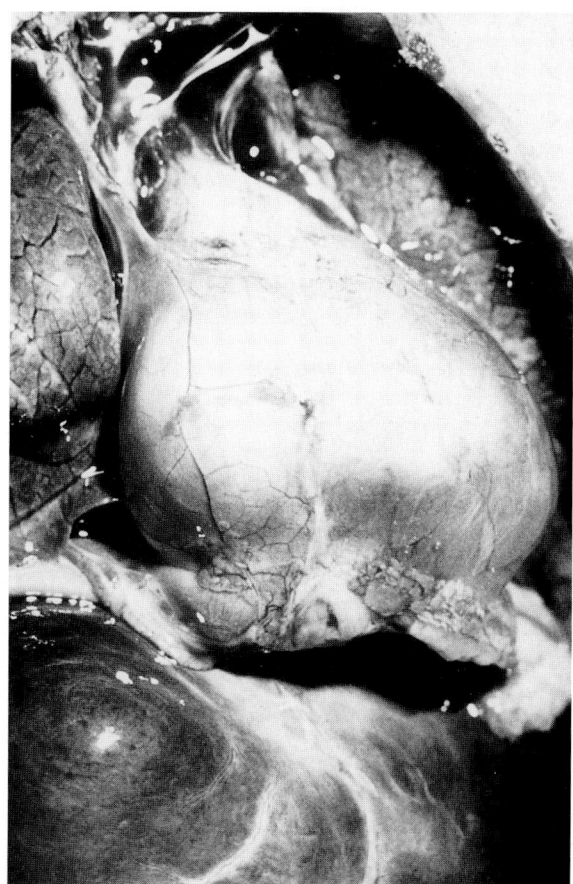

FIGURE 14.4.   *Isolated pericardial effusion in a neonate at term. The pericardial sac is tense and distended by a serous effusion.*

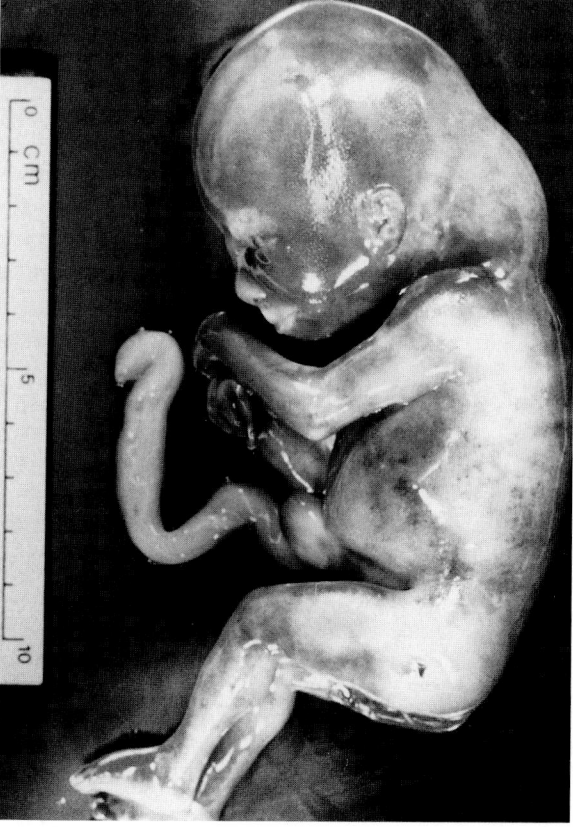

FIGURE 14.5.   *Trisomy 18. There is a small postnuchal fluid-filled bleb; typical dysmorphic features and visceral anomalies associated with this karyotype were present.*

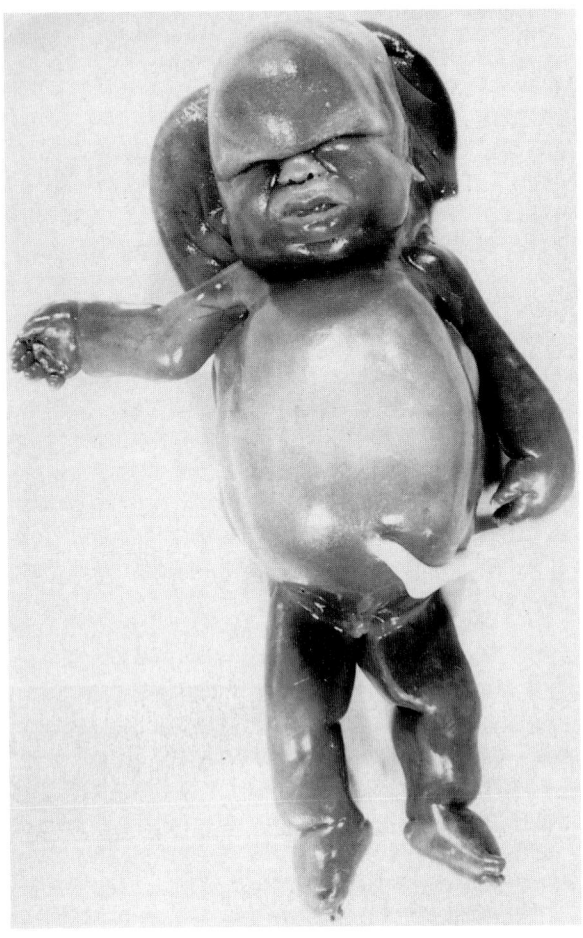

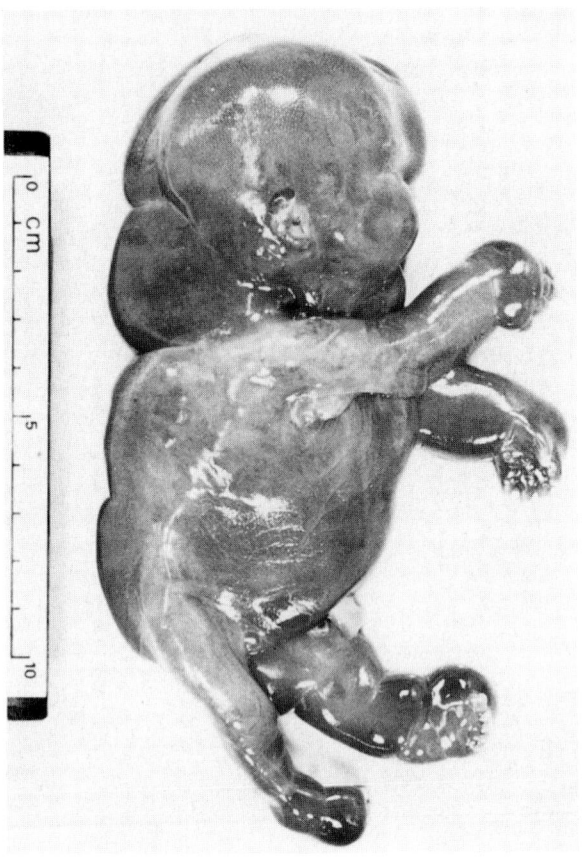

FIGURE 14.7.   *Fetus with postnuchal fluid accumulation and generalized hydrops, a combination designated Turner-like phenotype, but this fetus had trisomy 18 karyotype.*

FIGURE 14.6.   *45,XO karyotype. Fetus with massive postnuchal fluid-filled sac. There is generalized edema and effusions in body cavities. The distal aortic arch was hypoplastic.*

same group found enhanced prediction of fetal trisomy in older women using a combination of maternal age and deliberate search for fetal nuchal bleb, rather than using maternal age and biochemical screening [69]. Another study found much less predictive effect—only 8 of 14 fetuses with trisomy 21 had a nuchal bleb ≥6 mm, and no association was found with other chromosome abnormalities [70].

Boyd et al [65] followed up 92 pregnancies where postnuchal fluid accumulation had been discovered prenatally. Of 42 of these cases with an abnormal karyotype, 34 pregnancies were terminated and there were four fetal deaths and four live births. Twenty-five conceptuses had a normal karyotype, although on additional scan abnormality was present. Ten of the 25 were liveborn, seven had significant abnormalities, but two, both diaphragmatic hernias, were successfully treated. Seventeen of 24 fetuses with an isolated postnuchal bleb were liveborn and are normal, but two died in utero.

Gross postnuchal fluid accumulation in the second-trimester abortus is most commonly a manifestation of the

45,XO (Turner) karyotype (Fig. 14.6). Additionally, generalized hydrops is usually present in those fetuses that abort spontaneously [71, 72], but is not always present when pregnancy is terminated after identification of the fluid-filled sac by ultrasound examination. This appearance has been designated "Turner-like phenotype" [73], but this designation is disputed by Byrne et al [71] who stress the importance of chromosome culture or Barr body counts in such fetuses. We have seen similar fetuses with trisomy 18 (Fig. 14.7), trisomy 21, and normal karyotype; Marchese et al [74] report a similar experience.

Most fetuses with Turner karyotype and post-nuchal fluid have hypoplasia of the third part of the aortic arch and may also have anomalous origin of the aortic arch branches (Fig. 14.8a,b) and cardiac septal defects. Kalousek and Seller [75] suggest that tubular hypoplasia of the aortic arch, together with a postnuchal-fluid-filled sac, is pathognomonic of the 45,XO karyotype. Furthermore, they suggested that those fetuses with aortic arch hypoplasia who developed postnuchal fluid accumulation, went on to develop generalized hydrops, and died in utero constitute the "worst end" of the phenotype. Even this is not always the case, and an appar-

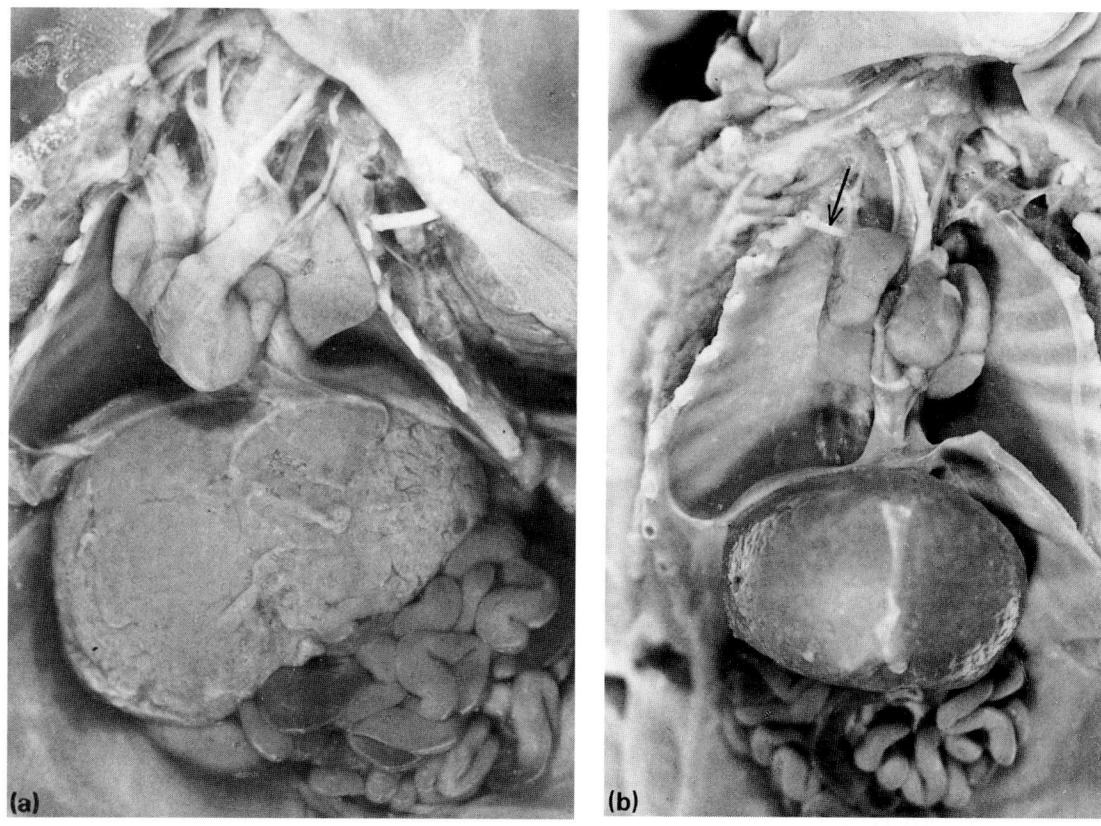

FIGURE 14.8. *Aortic arch anomaly in 45,XO karyotype. (a) Tubular hypoplasia of aortic isthmus. The pulmonary trunk is larger than the ascending aorta. (b) The right subclavian artery arises from the descending aorta and emerges behind the apex of the right lung (arrow).*

ent Turner phenotype with aortic arch hypoplasia examined recently in my department was subsequently found to have the 47,XX + 18 karyotype.

Byrne et al [71] described postnuchal fluid in a fetus with cardiac septal defects, situs inversus abdominis, intestinal malrotation, and polysplenia. The fetus also appeared to have ambiguous cardiac situs. Similar cardiac anomalies have been reported in fetuses with generalized hydrops [40, 76]. Cowchock et al [77] reported the familial occurrence of postnuchal blebs in fetuses with cleft palate and normal chromosomes.

Byrne et al [71] found the incidence of a nuchal-filled sac to be 1 in 875 of spontaneous aborted fetuses, rising to 1 in 200 in those fetuses whose crown–rump length is <3 cm. Occasionally, occipital encephaloceles or cervical teratoma are mistaken on ultrasound examination for postnuchal fluid accumulation. Neither should present the pathologist with a serious diagnostic problem.

When incised, free fluid is released from tissue spaces of differing size, which have poorly defined margins. The "cystic hygroma" is poorly circumscribed and overlying skin cannot be dissected easily off it. Histological examination shows irregular spaces divided by poorly cellular connective tissue. The spaces do not have an endothelial lining, although

dilated lymphatics are sometimes identified within the lesion. This lack of endothelium has often been explained as a result of autolysis or poor fixation, as many fetuses die in utero or are placed whole in formalin. This, however, is not a spurious finding. The fluid is lying free in connective tissue and not in distended lymphatics. Van der Putte [78] describes failure of cervical lymphatic primordia to connect with the jugular vein in the second-trimester fetus with Turner's syndrome. Dilatation and irregularity of the main lymph trunk occurs secondarily. He also found local or generalized hypoplasia of peripheral lymphatics in the trunk or limbs of some fetuses. The degree and distribution of peripheral lymphatic abnormalities was not related to the extent of subcutaneous edema, which was gross in every case. The lesion differs both in macroscopic and microscopic features from cystic hygroma, which is identified occasionally in the second-trimester fetus [79] (Fig. 14.9). This is a localized hamartoma, and comprises an overgrowth of endothelial-lined spaces of widely differing size; it contains thick-walled vessels which have smooth muscle in their wall and lymphoid aggregates within the connective tissue component (Fig. 14.10). The appearances are very similar to those lesions encountered in neonates and infants, in the anterior cervical region or upper limbs.

HYDROPS FETALIS

Fetal hydrops is generalized fetal edema which, when severe, is usually accompanied by effusions in body cavities. The reported associations of fetal hydrops are numerous (Table 14.1). With some, a causal relation is clear (rhesus disease,

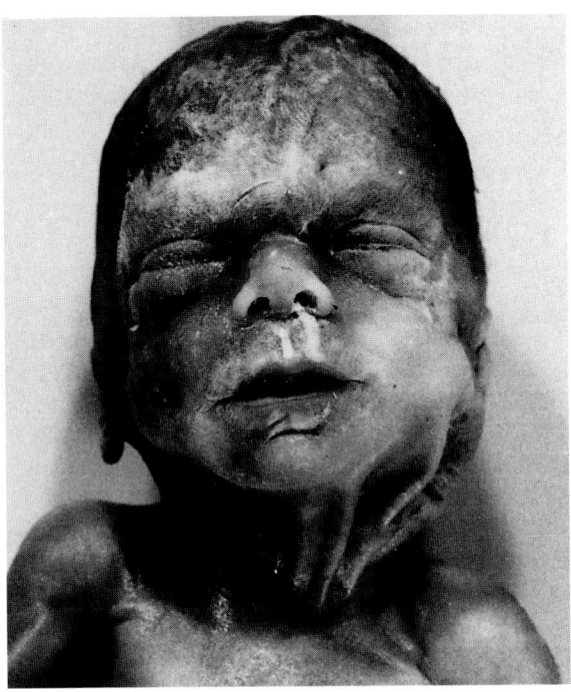

FIGURE 14.9.   *Second-trimester fetus with left-sided cervical cystic hygroma. Formalin fixation has reduced the size of the neck and redundant skin folds are present on the left side.*

alpha-thalassemia, adenomatoid malformation of lung), whereas in others identifying the mechanism taxes the imagination; but careful in utero investigation or postmortem examination yields results that suggest the underlying mechanism. One example is the demonstration of a transient myeloproliferative disorder accompanied by severe anemia in trisomy 21 [80]. Some associations of fetal hydrops showed marked geographic variation, either because of the high prevalence of an inherited disorder within a population, such as alpha-thalassemia in the eastern Mediterranean countries and Southeast Asia, or infection, such as syphilis, which is common in the childbearing population, as observed in South Korea [81]. The successful prevention of rhesus disease in Australia, Europe, and North America (Table 14.2) has resulted in a marked change of emphasis in the investigation and management of pregnancy complicated by fetal hydrops.

Examination of the associations of nonimmunological hydrops in a reported series of 10 or more cases gives an idea of their relative importance (Tables 14.3 and 14.4). Caution must be exercised in the interpretation of the lack of diversity of findings in some series, which reflect interests of particular units [82]. Others more truly represent the associations of hydrops within a local population [26, 40, 43]. More than one-quarter of cases from combined series are associated with structural anomalies (Fig. 14.11a,b) or hamartomata in the fetus (Fig. 14.12) or placenta (Fig. 14.13a,b), and a further 16% exhibit stigmata of chromosome anomaly or inherited metabolic disease. About 10% of cases of nonimmunological hydrops appear to be complications of monozygous twin pregnancy. Most are the result of twin–twin transfusion (Fig. 14.14a,b,c) through deep anastomoses within the placenta between the two circulations; a few are due to major structural anomalies, such as acardia,

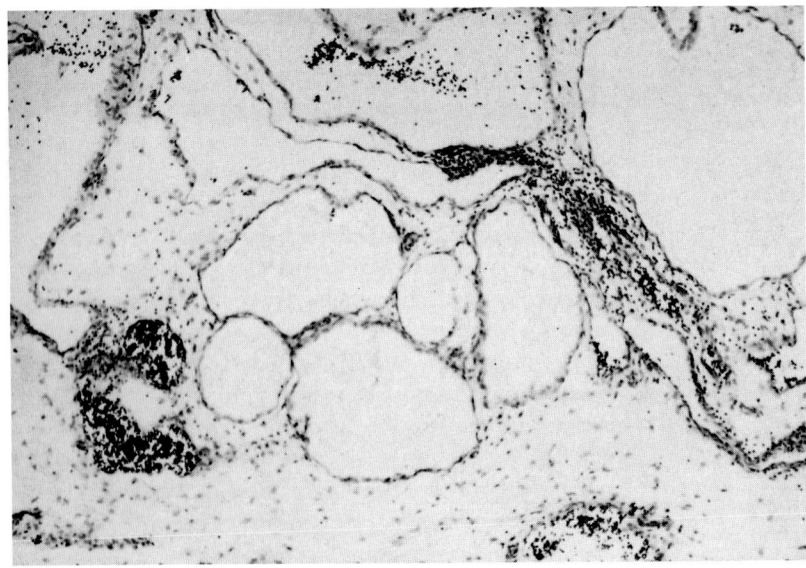

FIGURE 14.10.   *Same fetus as in Figure 14.7. Histological section through the circumscribed cervical mass. It is composed of endothelial-lined spaces filled with fluid and lymphocytes which lie in a connective tissue stroma. Lymphoid aggregates are present within the stroma.*

Table 14.1. Conditions described in association with fetal hydrops

Hematological disorders

Inherited:

Rhesus incompatibility [83]

ABO incompatibility [84–86]

Kell incompatibility [87, 88]

Alpha-thalassemia [89–91]

Hemoglobin Bart's [92, 93]

Glucose-6-phosphate dehydrogenase deficiency [94, 95]

Hemoglobin Bart's +H [96]

Hemophilia A [97]

Diamond-Blackfan syndrome [98]

Absent thumb, immune disorder, anemia [99]

Diserythropoetic anemia [100, 101]

Acquired:

Chronic feto-maternal hemorrhage [44, 97, 102]

Feto-fetal hemorrhage (twin transfusion syndrome) [40, 97, 100]

Hemorrhage into fetal organs

Intracranial associated with ischemia [104–105]

Intracranial associated with tumor [105]

Intra-abdominal [106]

Structural cardiac anomalies

Complex with ambiguous cardiac situs [40, 76]

Transposition of great arteries [40, 89]

Tetralogy of Fallot [76, 107]

Truncus arteriosus [89, 108]

Atrial septal defect [89]

Atrioventricular canal defect [76, 82, 109]

Large ventricular septal defect [89, 104, 110]

Single ventricle [89]

Aortic valve atresia [111]

Aortic valve stenosis [26, 82]

Hypoplastic left heart syndrome [43, 82, 89]

Mitral atresia + EFE [112]

Pulmonary valve atresia [82, 113]

Absent pulmonary valve + EFE [76, 111]

Tricuspid valve atresia [40, 89]

Tricuspid valve atresia and ectopia cordis [82]

Ebstein's anomaly [82, 111]

Acardia (twin pregnancy) [76, 105]

Double outlet right ventricle [114, 115]

Other cardiac pathology

Myocarditis [17, 40, 44, 116]

Myocardial infarction (coronary artery embolus) [76]

Cardiomyopathy [82, 89]

Premature closure foramen ovale [117–119]

Premature closure ductus arteriosus [120–122]

Premature closure ductus arteriosis (iatrogenic) [24]

EFE ± hepatitis [40, 110]

Cardiac tumors

Rhabdomyoma [40, 76]

Rhabdomyoma and tuberous sclerosis [123]

Cardiac teratoma [97]

Atrial angioma [124]

Cardiac arrhythmias

Paroxysmal atrial tachycardia [108, 125, 126]

Supraventricular tachycardia [76, 125]

Bundle branch block [127]

Complete heart block [89, 104]

Complete heart block and maternal connective tissue disease [59, 96, 128–130]

Arrhythmia + EFE [131]

Arrhythmia and conduction system anomaly [132, 133]

Familial heart block [134]

Bradycardia [108]

Wolff-Parkinson-White syndrome [135]

Intrathoracic abnormalities

Adenomatoid malformation [40, 76, 136]

Pulmonary sequestration [76, 104]

Tracheal atresia [40, 44, 109]

Tracheobronchomalacia [137]

Diaphragmatic hernia [40, 76, 109]

Laryngeal atresia/stenosis (Fraser's syndrome) [40, 105, 138]

Congenital mesenchymal malformation [139, 140]

Vascular abnormalities

Hemangioma

fetus [40, 141, 142]

fetus multiple [143]

placenta [40, 144, 145]

Calcific arteriopathy [40, 43, 146, 147]

Pulmonary lymphangiectasia [43, 148]

Diffuse lymphangiectasia [46, 149]

Cystic hygroma [40, 104]

Acardiac monozygous twin pregnancy [76, 105]

Vena caval thrombus [150]

Coronary artery embolus [76]

Fetal entanglement umbilical cord [40]

Meningeal angiodysplasia [105, 131]

Musculoskeletal

Achondrogenesis I [44]

Achondrogenesis II [26, 53, 62, 89, 152]

Chondroectodermal dysplasia [97]

Saldino-Noonan [153]

Osteogenesis imperfecta [43, 44]

Jeune's asphyxiating thoracic dystrophy [43, 154]

Thanatophoric dysplasia [4]

Multiple pterygium syndrome [89]

Popliteal pterygium syndrome [97]

Neu-Laxova [89]

Pena Shokeir [89]

Myotonic dystrophy [97]

Hydrocephaly, arthrogryposis [89]

Holoprosencephaly [44]

Amniotic bands [89]

Achondrogenesis III [154]

Noonan's syndrome [155]

Greenberg dysplasia [156]

Oral-facial-digital (Mohr's) syndrome [154]

Urogenital abnormalities

Cystic renal dysplasia [157]

Renal hypoplasia [40, 104]

Urethral obstruction: valves [89]

Urethral obstruction: atresia [40]

Congenital nephrotic syndrome [44, 158]

Meckel syndrome [105]

Cystic kidneys/tracheal atresia [40, 109]

Vaginal atresia, hydrometrocolopos syndrome [26, 43]

Mesoblastic nephroma [142]

Autosomal recessive kidney disorder [154]

Gastrointestinal

Esophageal atresia [156]

Jejunal atresia [110]

Table 14.1. *Continued*

Small intestinal volvulus [106]
Meconium ileus ± peritonitis [43, 104]
Intestinal infarction [89]
Intestinal obstruction [97]
Hepatitis [40, 43, 159]
Hepatic necrosis [43]
Cirrhosis [40, 110]

Tumors
Neuroblastoma [26, 160–163]
Teratoma
    sacrococcygeal [43, 164]
    mediastinal [4, 159]
    intrapericardial [89, 97]
Mesoblastic nephroma [142]
Cardiac rhabdomyoma [40, 123]
Atrial angioma [124]
Glioblastoma multiforme [165]
Primitive neurectodermal tumor [105]

Genetic metabolic disease
Infantile Gaucher [44, 108, 166]
Mucopolysaccharidosis [97]
Neonatal hemochromatosis [167]
Günther's disease [168]
Niemann-Pick [169]
? GM$_1$ gangliosidosis [104]
Hypoalbuminemia [170]

Chromosome anomalies
45, XO [40, 76, 97]
Trisomy 21 [26, 40, 89, 108, 171]
Trisomy 18 [40, 86]
Trisomy 13 [97, 172]
Triploidy [43]
Cystic hygroma and hypoplastic aortic arch [40]
Unbalanced translocation 3/11 [173]

Infection
Cytomegalovirus (CMV) [43, 89, 104]
Herpesvirus I [108, 174]
Rubella virus [110]
Toxoplasmosis [110, 175–177]
Syphilis [178–179]
Coxsackievirus [116]
Myocarditis NOS [40, 44]
Parvovirus [180–182]
Listeriosis [114]
Ureaplasma ureolyticum [183]
Adenovirus [184]

Maternal disorders
Connective tissue disorders [128, 129]
Diabetes mellitus [185]
Maternal anemia with two hydropic pregnancies [86, 157]
Choriocarcinoma [186]

EFE = subendocardial fibroelastosis.

Table 14.2. Changing importance of causes of fetal hydrops over two decades

	Macafee [86] Melbourne 1958–69		Kanbour & Klionsky [187] Pittsburgh 1965–76		Machin [188] Calgary 1967–80		Wright & Dimmick [in Ref. 188] Vancouver 1972–77		Andersen et al [189] Melbourne 1970–79	
Isoimmunization	149	82%	30	65%	7	25%	7	41%	130	64%
Alpha-thalassemia	—				3					
Twins	6				6				73	
Cardiac malformation	2				2		1		(61 of these	
Cardiac tumor	—				1		1		cases are	
High-output failure	1		9		—		1		reported by	
Obstructed venous return	3				3		—		Hutchison	
Congenital infection	—				—		1		et al [43]) (see	
Miscellaneous	8				—		2		Table 14.3)	
Idiopathic	13		7		6		4			
Total	182	100%	46	100%	28	100%	17	100%	203	100%

in one fetus. Other groups of associations, such as fetal infection or tumor, are found in <5% of cases.

Examination of the associations of hydrops and the stage of gestation at which hydrops was diagnosed show gestation-related differences [40, 105]. In the second trimester, chromosome anomalies, alpha-thalassemia, and parvovirus infection are important associations; in the third trimester major structural anomalies, cardiac dysrhythmias, and multiple pregnancy are important and chronic fetal infection and tumors are more likely to be found.

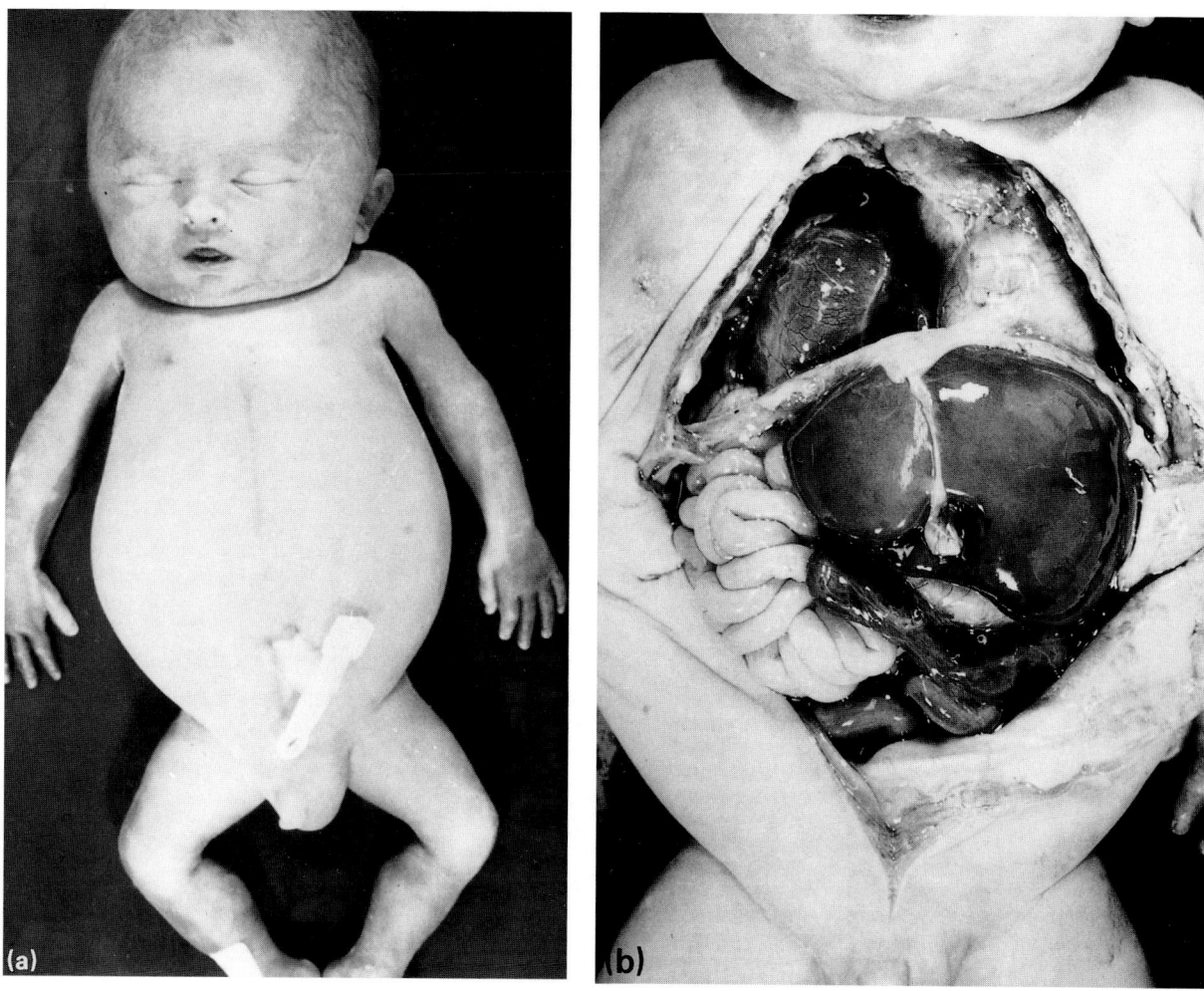

FIGURE 14.11.   *(a) Fetus with edema of trunk, head, and neck and massive ascites. (b) Same fetus. A right diaphragmatic hernia is present. Most of the right lobe of the liver lies within the right hemithorax. The mediastinum is displaced to the left [40].*

Pathological Findings

Generalized edema is often accompanied by pallor because of anemia. Soft-tissue edema will tend to obscure dysmorphic features, which would be expected, for example, with chromosome abnormality. At the same time, the edema may introduce a deformity that can mimic specific dysmorphic features, such as the ears in Apert syndrome. Edema of the limbs is often less marked than that affecting the head and trunk (see Fig. 14.11a), but may be gross (Fig. 14.15).

Cardiomegaly and hepatomegaly are commonly found in the hydropic fetus, even when specific abnormalities that may be related causally to the hydropic state are not present in those organs. When generalized edema is due to high-output cardiac failure, the heart and liver are often spectacularly enlarged (Fig. 14.16).

In rhesus disease and other causes of chronic anemia, hepatosplenomegaly will be present and is often gross (Fig.

14.17). Hepatosplenomegaly is usually present in the hydropic fetus with congenital infection. Other macroscopic abnormalities related to the infection, such as periventricular necrosis and calcification, may suggest the likely diagnosis. Histological examination (Fig. 14.18a), more specific techniques (Fig. 14.18b), or culture may enable precise diagnoses to be made. Cardiovascular (Fig. 14.19) and pulmonary anomalies (Fig. 14.20) are relatively common associations of fetal hydrops and should be sought with care. When the heart is anatomically normal and no other structural abnormality is present, the heart should be retained so that the conduction system can be examined if there is no histological evidence of infection (including myocarditis) or endocardial fibroelastosis. The last condition is often not as readily apparent in the fetus as in the neonate in unfixed organs, and often requires histological examination for diagnosis (Fig. 14.21a,b). Malformations in other organ systems can sometimes present with generalized edema (Fig.

Table 14.3.   Associations of fetal hydrops in published series of 10 or more cases

	Potter [109] Chicago	Beischer et al [159] Melbourne 1951–70	Etches and Lemons [104] Denver 1975–78	Spahr et al [110] Pittsburgh 1969–78	Machin [188] Calgary 1967–80	Hutchison et al [43] Melbourne 1970–79	Kleinman et al [76] Yale	Moerman et al [26] Leuven 1960–81	Keeling et al [40] Oxford 1976–82
Cardiac malformations	1	5	1	2	2	1	4	1	6
Arrhythmias	—	—	—	1	—	1	3	—	2
Cardiac, other	—	—	—	—	1	1	1	—	1
Arterial pathology	—	2	—	—	—	1	1	—	6
Pulmonary malformation	—	2	2	—	—	3	2	2	1
Diaphragmatic hernia	1	1	—	—	—	1	1	—	3
Renal anomaly	1	1	1	1	—	2	—	—	5
Skeletal anomaly	—	—	—	—	—	2	—	2	—
Other malformation	—	—	—	1	4	—	—	1	—
Chromosome abnormality	—	1	—	—	—	3	—	2	5
Cystic hygroma	—	—	1	—	—	—	—	—	3
Monochorionic twin pregnancy	2	8	1	2	6	3	1	—	1
Infection	—	—	2	2	—	1	—	—	6
Fetal anemia	—	—	2	—	3	4	—	—	—
Tumors	—	1	—	1	2	3	—	2	—
Gastrointestinal pathology	—	2	1	1	—	4	—	—	2
Genetic metabolic disorder	—	—	1	—	—	—	—	—	—
Obstructed venous return	—	—	—	—	1	—	—	—	1
Unexplained	12	22	8	8	6	27	—	—	8
Total	17	44	22	19	21	61	13	10	50
Incidence		1:3538	1.4:1000	1:3975		1:3748		1:466	1:1400

	Graves et al [185] Halifax	Holzgreve et al [89] San Francisco 1978–83	Im et al [108] Toronto	Mahoney et al [97] San Francisco 1978–82	Mostoufi-Zadeh et al [44] Boston 1975–83	Allan et al [82] London 4 yrs	Nakamura et al [190] Kurume 14 yrs	Boyd and Keeling [105] Oxford 1983–88
Cardiac malformations	5	5	1	4	—	10	6	3
Arrhythmias	4	2	3	2	1	8	—	—
Cardiac, other	—	1	—	1	—	3	—	—
Arterial pathology	1	—	1	—	—	—	2	2
Pulmonary malformation	—	1	—	—	—	—	4	2
Diaphragmatic hernia	—	2	—	—	—	—	—	—
Renal anomaly	—	1	—	—	2	2	—	1
Skeletal anomaly	—	7	—	2	2	—	4	—
Other malformation	6	—	—	1	2	3	—	1
Chromosome abnormality	1	7	2	3	4	3	5	22
Cystic hygroma	—	—	—	—	—	—	3	17
Monochorionic twin pregnancy	4	4	4	1	3	9	6	6
Infection	2	2	1	—	3	—	2	11
Fetal anemia	1	5	—	6	4	—	—	—
Tumors	—	2	—	1	2	1	1	1
Gastrointestinal pathology	—	1	—	1	—	—	2	—
Genetic metabolic disorder	—	—	3	1	1	—	—	—
Obstructed venous return	—	—	—	—	—	—	—	—
Unexplained	2	10	5	4	16	13	14	6
Total	26	50	20	27	40	52	50	72
Incidence	1:1469		1:2029		1:1510			

Table 14.3. *Continued*

	Bagozzi et al [138] Milan 1980–87	Schmid et al [114] Bonn 1984–87	Shimokawa et al [191] Fukuoka 1983–86	Hansmann et al [192] Bonn 1979–88	Villaespesa et al [115] Madrid 1967–87	van Maldergem et al [154] Loverval 1976–78
Cardiac malformations	4	1	3	—	8	2
Arrhythmias	3	2	2	71	—	—
Cardiac other	3	2	2	—	5	—
Arterial pathology	—	—	1	—	1	2
Pulmonary malformations	—	1	2	23	2	—
Diaphragmatic hernia	—	—	1	—	8	—
Renal anomaly	5	—	—	9	2	2
Skeletal anomaly	1	—	—	—	3	3
Other malformations	—	—	1	18	1	3
Chromosome abnormality	1	3	2	54	3	18
Cystic hygroma	—	1	1	48	3	—
Monochorionic twin pregnancy	—	—	2	2	7	5
Infection	1	2	—	11	2	3
Fetal anemia	2	1	—	37	—	—
Tumors	—	1	1	—	2	—
Gastrointestinal pathology	5	—	1	8	2	—
Genetic metabolic disorder	—	—	—	—	—	1
Obstructed venous return	—	—	—	—	—	—
Unexplained	6	18	14	121	10	19
Total	31	31	33	402	59	58

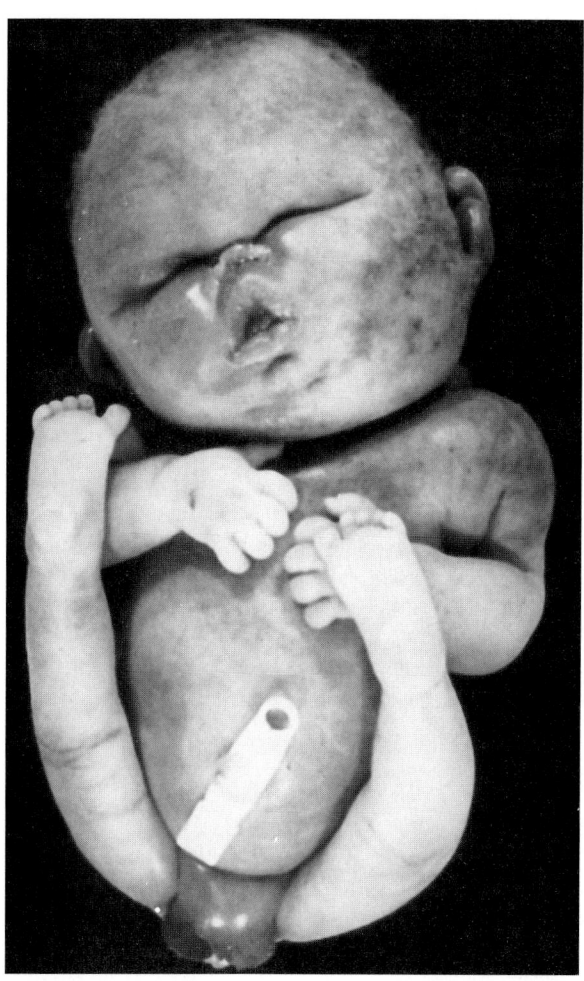

FIGURE 14.12. *Hydropic stillbirth at term. A large angioma is seen over the left face, head, and shoulder. The angioma has involved underlying soft tissue and muscle, the upper airway and thymus. (From Keeling JW (Ed.) Fetal and Neonatal Pathology. Springer-Verlag, London, Heidelberg, 1987, with permission.)*

Table 14.4.   Associations of nonimmunological fetal hydrops

	Number of Associations	Percentage Association
Cardiovascular abnormalities	221	18.3
Non-cardiovascular anomalies	168	13.9
Chromosome anomaly	216	17.9
Monochorionic twin pregnancy	77	6.4
Infection	51	4.2
Fetal anemia	65	5.3
Tumors	21	1.7
Hepatic pathology	16	1.7
Genetic metabolic disease	7	0.6
Meconium peritonitis	14	1.2
Obstructed venous return from placenta	2	0.2
Unexplained	349	28.9
Total	1207	100%

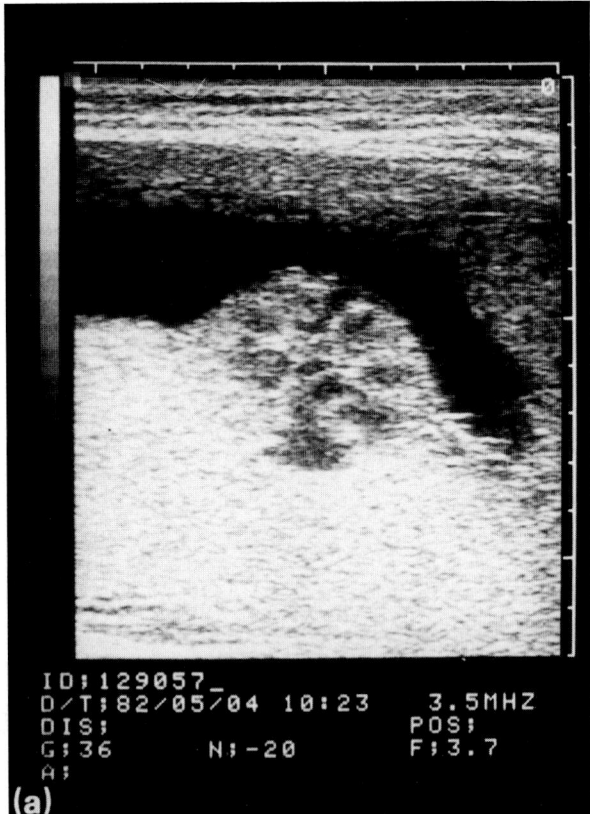

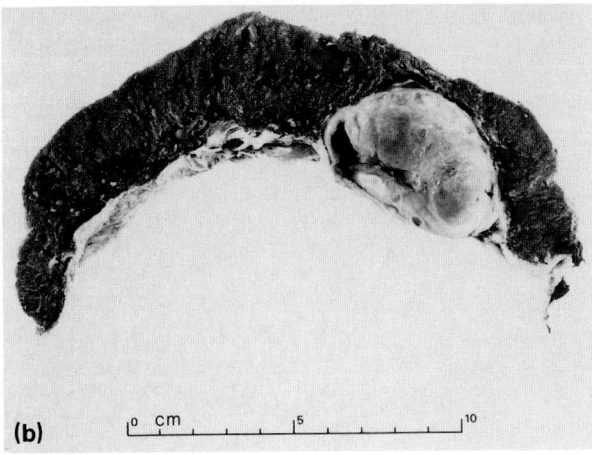

FIGURE 14.13.   *Placental angioma. (a) An echogenic mass beneath the chorionic plate protrudes into the amniotic cavity. (b) A slice through fixed placenta 4 weeks later. A large, localized angioma is present* [40].

14.22a,b), so a thorough postmortem examination of every hydropic fetus should be undertaken.

Cerebral pathology identified in the hydropic fetus may be present when TORCH infection is the primary abnormality. Intracranial tumor [105, 165] is reported in a few hydropic fetuses (Fig. 14.23). The chronicity of hemorrhage accompanying such lesions may be supported by the finding of obstructive hydrocephaly secondary to obstruction of aqueduct or foramina caused by hemorrhage within glial tissue. Evidence of fetal cerebral ischemia, with or without secondary hemorrhage, is sometimes found in the hydropic fetus which, from its gross and histological appearance has been present for days or weeks before birth [193, 194].

Interpretation of Pathological Findings in the Hydropic Fetus

Interpretation of the status of any pathological abnormality requires some care so that an etiological role is not assigned inappropriately. Inappropriate interpretation may result in failure to initiate particular investigations or in incorrect advice to parents about recurrence risks. The latter is particularly important as fetal hydrops is recognized as the presenting feature of many different genetic metabolic disorders and malformation syndromes [80, 154, 173].

Edema-induced deformity and loss of dysmorphic features have been mentioned, making karyotype analysis a mandatory investigation. Some pathological features, such as subendocardial fibroelastosis (EFE) and cerebral ischemia/hemorrhage, may be the result of reduced vascular perfusion because of heart failure or reduced arterial PO₂ from placental edema in some cases. However, hepatic fibrosis and EFE resulting from fetal (viral) infection early in gestation

may also have an etiological role. The description of a prenatal form of infantile cortical hyperostoses (Caffey disease), which restricts normal pulmonary development and can be complicated by fetal hydrops [195], would seem to be another example.

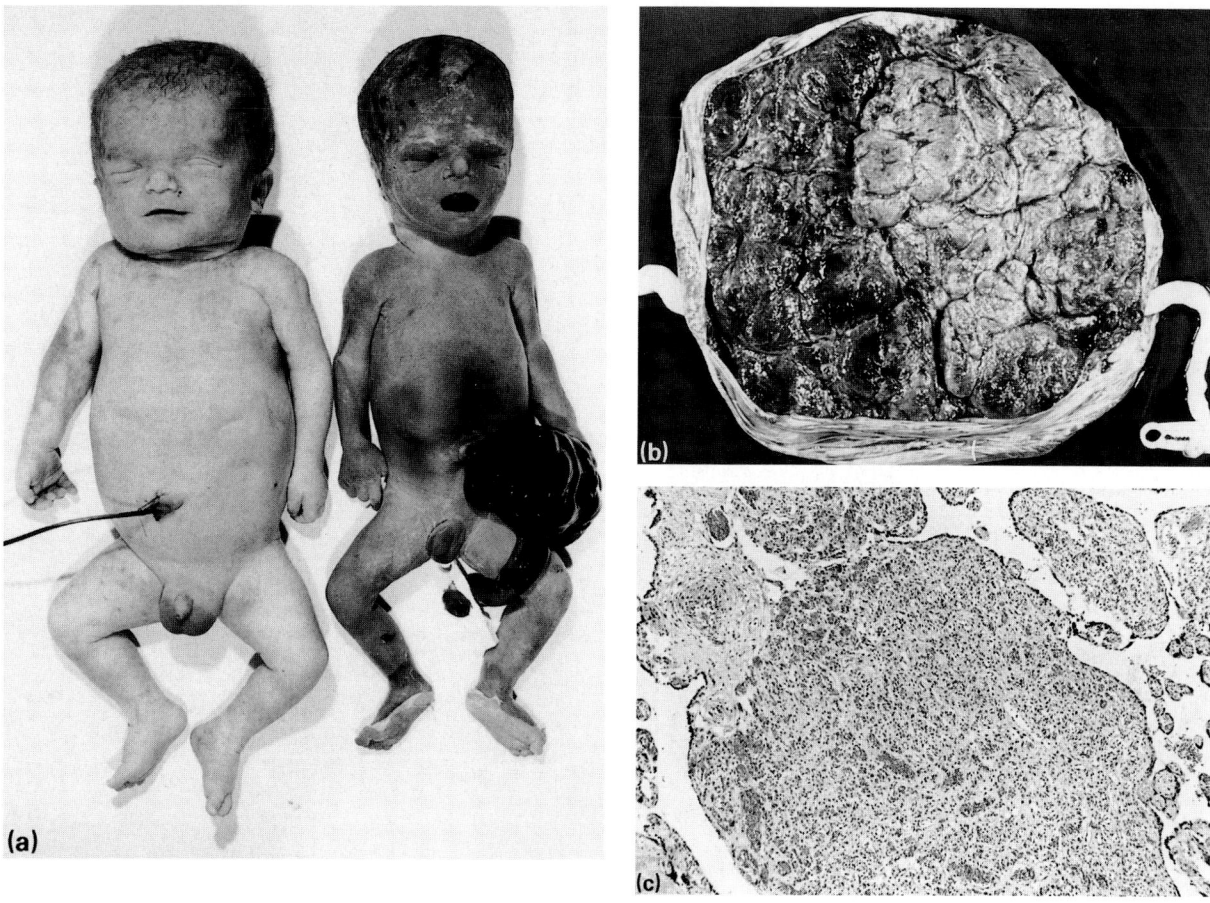

FIGURE 14.14. *Twin–twin transfusion syndrome. (a) Monozygotic twins. Liveborn pale hydropic twin contrasts with stillborn plethoric sibling. (b) Monochorionic twin placenta. Left congested placenta of recipient contrasts with bulky pale placenta of donor twin. (From Keeling JW (Ed.) Fetal and Neonatal Pathology. Springer-Verlag, London, Heidelberg, 1987, with permission.) (c) Chorangiosis of villi within monochorionic placenta. Such lesions permit shunting between the two fetal circulations.*

The Placenta

In many pregnancies complicated by fetal hydrops, the placenta is bulky (weight >1000g), pale, and friable and the umbilical cord is edematous. Histological examination reveals edema of the villous cores, Hofbauer cells are easily seen, villi appear immature for gestational age, and the cytotrophoblast may persist. The immature trophoblast demonstrates excess human chorionic gonadotrophin (hCG) immunostaining [196]. This is probably the origin of elevated maternal serum hCG levels which can cause confusion in the interpretation of Down syndrome screening scores. Knowles and Flett [197] point out the cause of this confusion and stress the need to karyotype all cases so identified.

When rhesus disease (or any other blood group incompatibility) is the cause of the hydropic state, nucleated red cells are identified easily in villous capillaries, and focal hemopoiesis may be present. In rhesus disease, villous hydrops is often patchy; plugging of capillaries by hemopoietic foci protects against hydropic change (Fig. 14.24). Examination of the placenta from the hydropic fetus with neuroblastoma may reveal clumps of tumor cells within villous capillaries (Fig. 14.25). Invasion of villous stroma by tumor is not usual. Angiomatoid structures effecting arteriovenous connection between the two circulations in a monochorionic twin pregnancy may be demonstrated histologically (see Fig. 14.14c). Accumulation of metabolites within a placental trophoblast producing cytoplasmic vacuolation and increased thickness of the trophoblast layer is apparent in some genetic metabolic disorders such as sialidosis (Fig. 14.6). In others, enlargement and cytoplasmic vacuolation is present in macrophages. This is described in beta-glucuronidase deficiency [198].

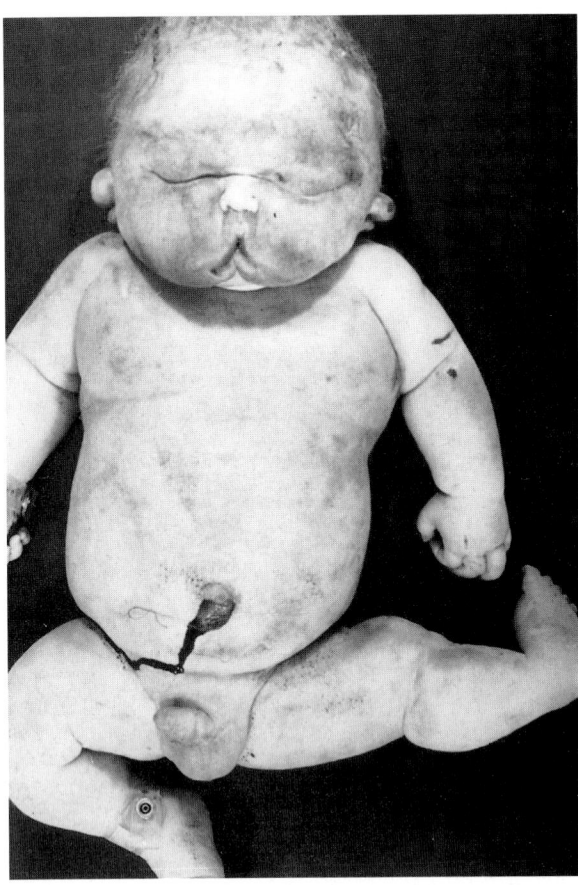

FIGURE 14.15. *Generalized fetal hydrops affecting limbs as well as trunk and head. Effusions are present in thorax and abdomen [40].*

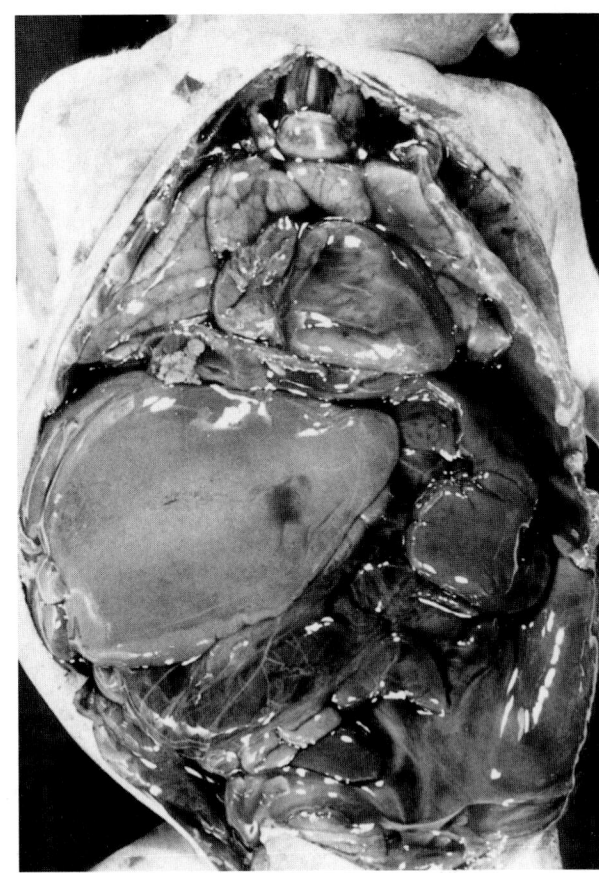

FIGURE 14.17. *Rhesus hydrops. There is massive hepatosplenomegaly. (From Keeling JW (Ed.)* Fetal and Neonatal Pathology. *Springer-Verlag, London, Heidelberg, 1987, with permission.)*

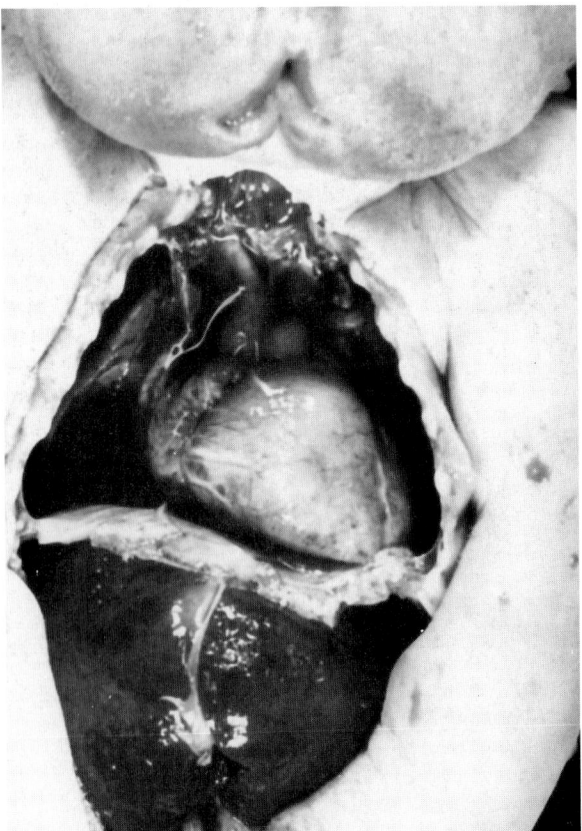

FIGURE 14.16. *Same baby as in Figure 14.15. There is cardiomegaly with biventricular hypertrophy and hepatomegaly. In this baby, hydrops complicated the familial arterial calcification.*

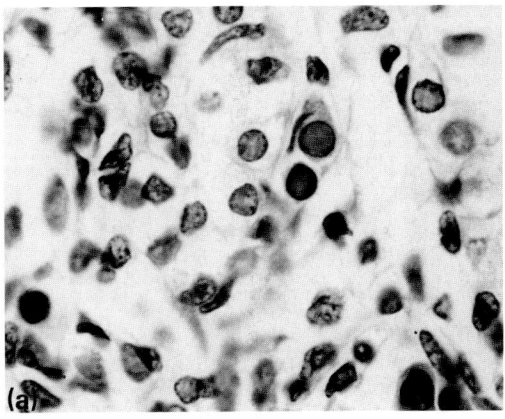
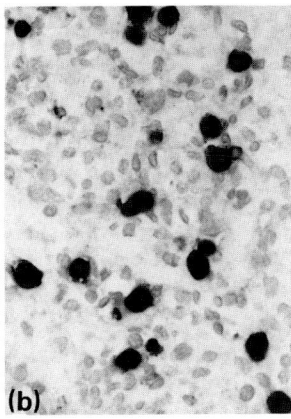

FIGURE 14.18.   *Parvovirus infection. (a) Histological section of lung. Intranuclear inclusions are present at center field, lower left, and right. (Courtesy of Dr P.A. Burton, Bristol.) (b) In situ hybridization technique demonstrates many more intranuclear inclusions than are apparent by H&E staining [182].*

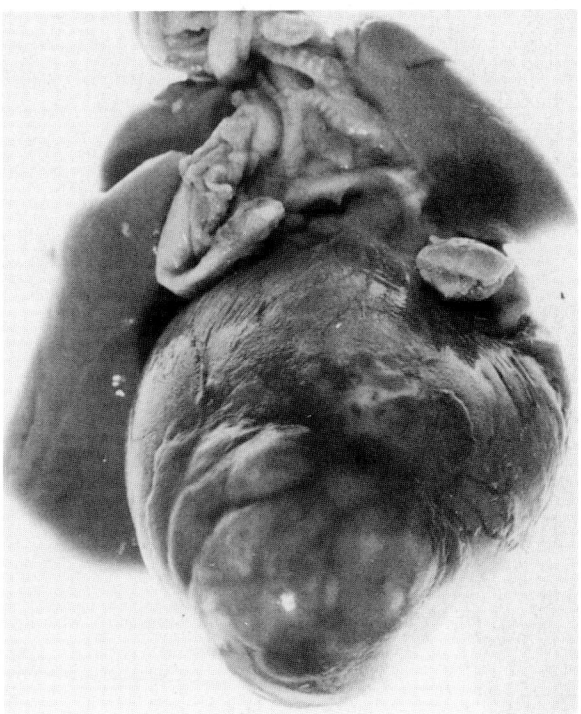

FIGURE 14.19.   *Stillbirth at 32 weeks. Cardiomegaly and hydrops identified prenatally. A mass arises from the ventricular myocardium. Histologically this was a rhabdomyoma.*

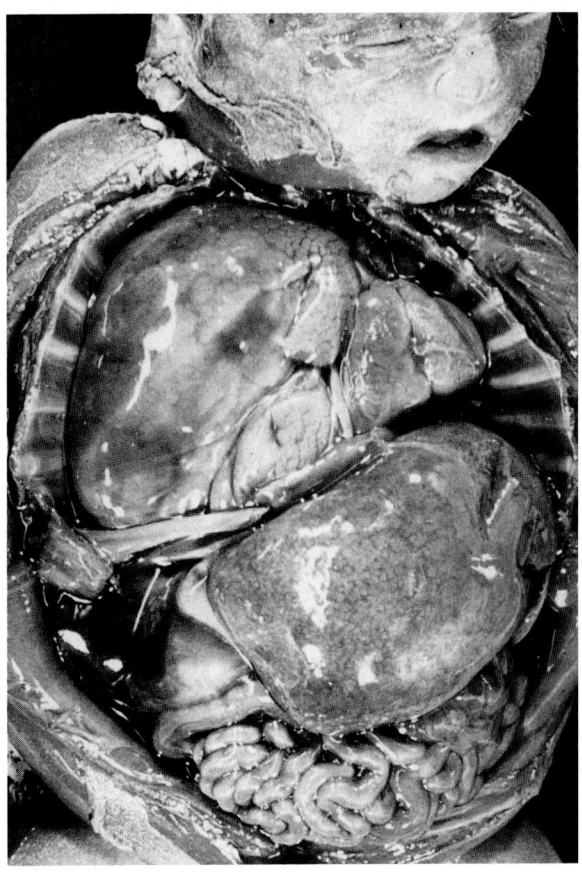

FIGURE 14.20.   *Hydropic stillbirth. There is expansion of the right upper lobe of the lung, with displacement of mediastinum and liver to the left. An adenomatoid malformation was confined to a single lung lobe [40].*

When hydrops results from fetal viral infection, placental involvement is usual. In cytomegalovirus infection, villitis is a common finding. A dense but patchy round cell infiltration of the villus stroma is seen. Viral inclusions are often present in capillary endothelium. When infection is well established, villus fibrosis with loss of capillaries is apparent. When there is parvoviral infection, viral inclusions are readily apparent in circulating erythrocyte precursors and macrophages. Endothelial injury in villus capillaries may be evident [199] with karyorrhexis and perivascular inflammatory cell infiltration. Villous capillary damage with consequent loss of a substantial part of the capillary bed may be an important factor in the development of hydrops in these cases.

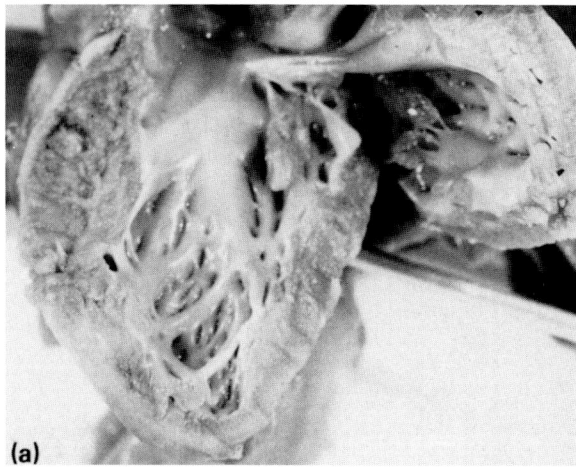

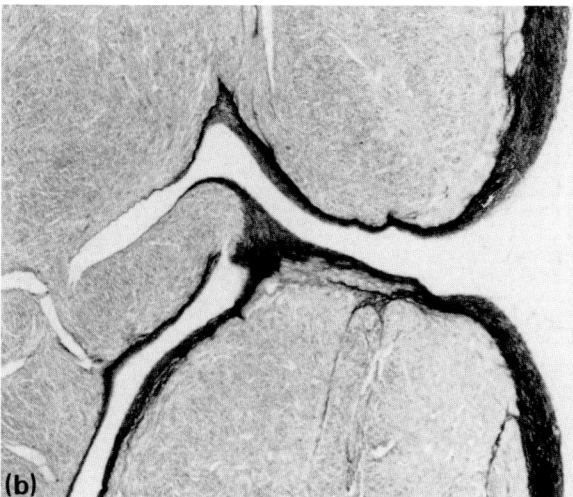

FIGURE 14.21. *Neonatal death at 36 weeks. (a) Left ventricular endocardial fibroelastosis accentuates the trabecular pattern. (b) A dense band of fibroelastic tissue is present beneath the endocardium (Weigert's elastic van Gieson's method). (From Keeling, JW (Ed.)* Fetal and Neonatal Pathology. *Springer-Verlag, London, Heidelberg, 1987, with permission.)*

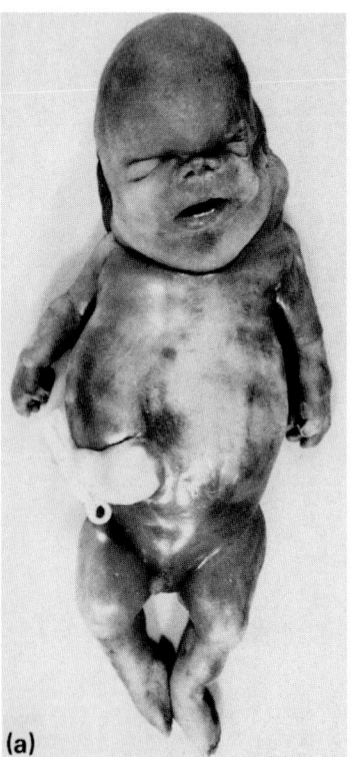

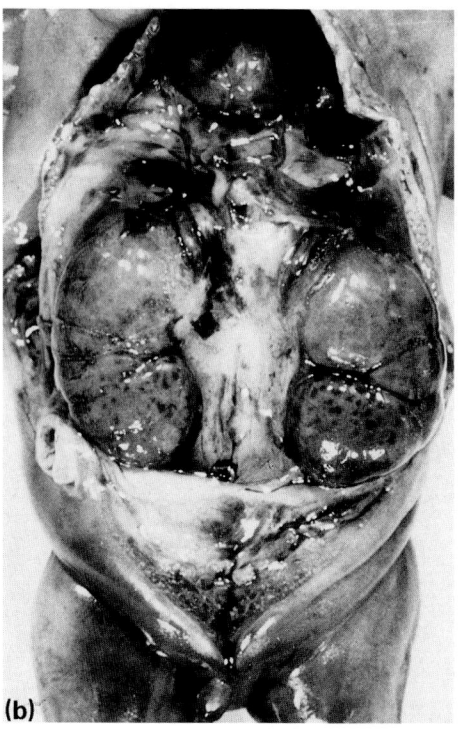

FIGURE 14.22. *Meckel syndrome. Fetus at 22 weeks' gestation. (a) Massive ascites, shortening of all limbs, and abdominal distension. (b) Massive renomegaly.*

Investigation of Fetal Hydrops

The aims of the investigation of mother and fetus following the recognition of generalized fetal edema or localized fluid accumulation are to document the severity and site of fluid accumulation, to elucidate the cause or associated abnormality, and to evaluate fetal well-being. The combina-

tion of umbilical venous pressure and heart-size monitoring may be a useful measure of cardiac function [200]. When hydrops is discovered prenatally, the investigations listed in Tables 14.5 and 14.6 should be undertaken urgently. Cardiac arrhythmias, a cause of hydrops treatable in utero, may be intermittent. Repeated scanning or continuous cardiotocographic recording may be required for diagnosis [201]. Thor-

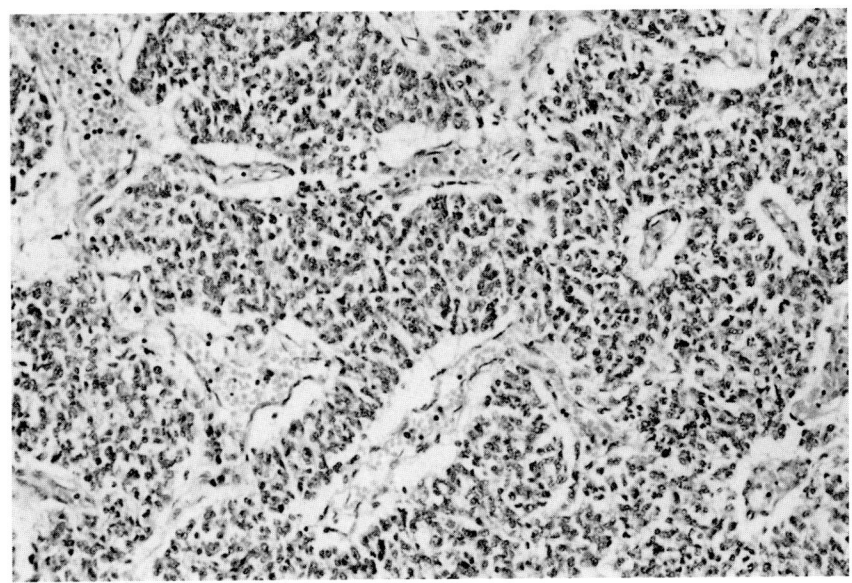

FIGURE 14.23. *Hydropic stillbirth with hydrocephaly. Intraventricular hemorrhage and a hemorrhagic temporal lobe mass. Histological section shows a cellular, extremely vascular, primitive neuroectodermal tumor.*

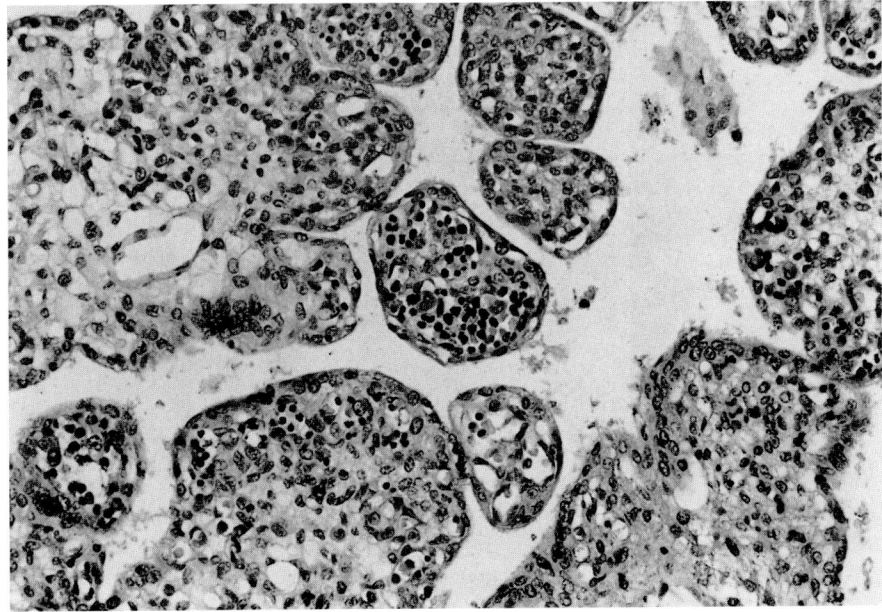

FIGURE 14.24. *The placenta in rhesus hydrops. Hydropic change is non-uniform. Capillaries of non-hydropic villi are plugged by erythropoietic foci. (From Keeling JW (Ed.)* Fetal and Neonatal Pathology. *Springer-Verlag, London, Heidelberg, 1987, with permission.)*

ough investigation of both mother and fetus are essential so that fetal therapy can be initiated or delivery expedited should either be appropriate. Urgent investigations of the hydropic neonate are set out in Table 14.7. Table 14.8 lists postmorterm investigations that are essential should the fetus or neonate die.

Management of Fetal Hydrops

Elucidation of the underlying cause of fetal hydrops is essential before appropriate in utero treatment can be initiated in those cases where it is likely to be effective. A combination of specific and palliative measures is now pursued in some

centers once karyotypic normality has been established. Palliative measures include infusion of albumin or packed red cells into the fetal peritoneal cavity. This results in increased fetal urine production and often in reduction of the edema [191]. This method has the advantage of repeatability without concern about umbilical vein thrombosis. Specific measures include blood transfusions through the umbilical vein to increase osmolality and improve anemia [202]. Repeated blood transfusion has been successful in treating anemia due to parvovirus B$_{19}$ infection and feto-maternal hemorrhage [203] and "other" hematological abnormalities [192], as well as improving survival in severe rhesus disease. Oepkes et al [204] found a relationship between the degree

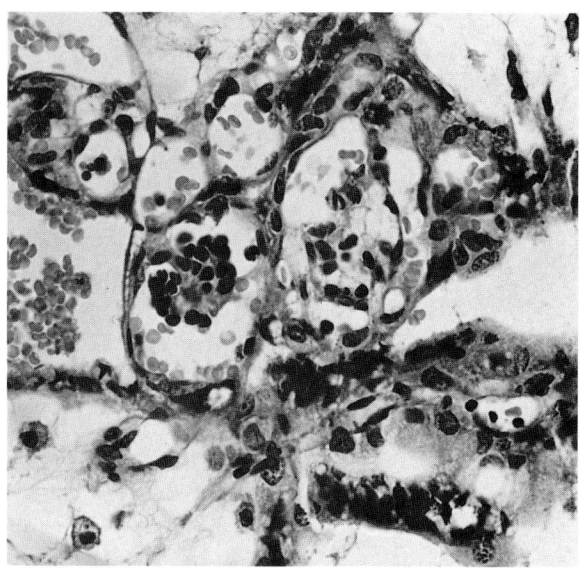

FIGURE 14.25.   *Hydropic fetus with neuroblastoma. Tumor emboli are present within villous capillaries in the placenta.*

Table 14.5.   Investigation of the mother when fetal hydrops is diagnosed

Hemoglobin, Kleihauer
ABO and rhesus group
Minor blood group antigens
Hemolysins, hemagglutinins
Hemoglobin-electrophoresis
G-6-PD screen
Serological tests for syphilis
Glucose tolerance test
Antinuclear factor
Autoantibodies
TORCH/parvovirus titers
Alpha-fetoprotein

G-6-PD = Glucose-6-phosphate dehydrogenase.

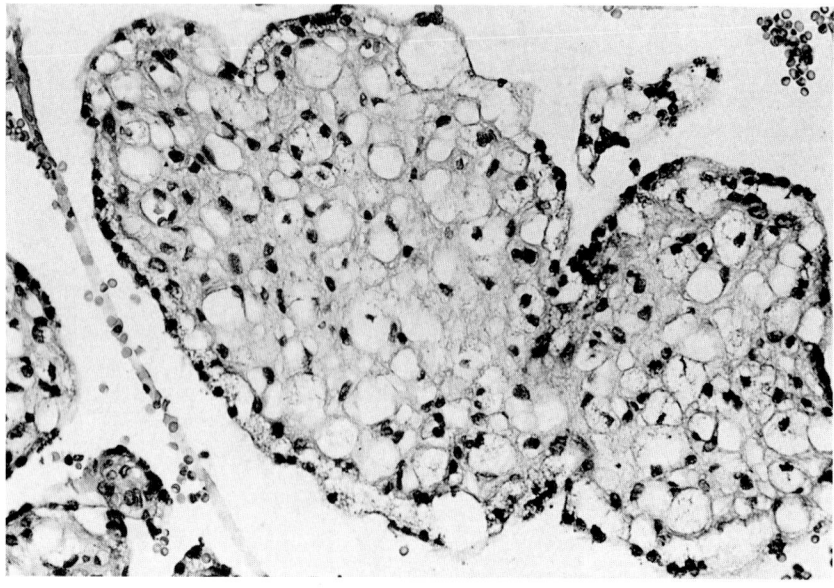

FIGURE 14.26.   *Fetal hydrops in lysosomal storage disease (sialidosis). The trophoblast is cuboidal and vacuolated.*

of anemia and splenic size on sonograms and suggest that serial splenic measurement is useful for assessment of the need for further intervention. Tachyarrhythmia may be more effectively treated by administering antiarrhythmic drugs directly to the fetus rather than via the mother when the dosage delivered is less precise.

Drainage of hydrothorax to permit lung growth is an attractive idea. These effusions reaccumulate rapidly [192], although removal of fluid just before delivery makes postpartum resuscitation easier [191].

Treatment of twin transfusion has apparently been successfully achieved by obliteration of the connecting vessels, but isolation of these is difficult [205] and may result in fetal demise. Feticide of the hydropic twin has resulted in the development of hydrops in the co-twin [206]. When hydrops results from high output failure from shunting through an acardiac co-twin, ligation of the umbilical cord of the acardiac twin has been successful.

Fetal surgery to remove a cystic adenomatoid malformation (CAM) when the fetus has become hydropic may be

Table 14.6. Investigation of the fetus when hydrops is diagnosed

Ultrasonography
    Severity of hydrops and polyhydramnios
    Multiple pregnancy
    Fetal heart rate/rhythm
    Cardio-thoracic ratio
    Umbilical venous pressure
    Major fetal anomaly
        Heart
        Other systems
Dysmorphic features suggestive of a syndrome
    Placenta
        Thickness
        Angioma, other abnormality
    Placental biopsy
        Rapid karyotype
        Fibroblast culture for GMD
        DNA for molecular genetic analysis
        Virus culture
    Cord blood
        Full blood count
        Hematocrit
        Hemolysins
        Rapid karyotype
        Viral antibodies

Table 14.7. Investigation of the hydropic neonate at birth

Full blood count, PCV
Blood sugar
Blood group and antibodies
Hemoglobin electrophoresis
Clotting screen
Red cell enzymes
Liver function tests
TORCH screen
Viral antibodies
WR, karyotype
Electrocardiograph
Radiological examination
Ultrasound examination
    Heart
    Abdomen
    Brain
Effusions
    Culture
    Biochemical analysis
Urine
    Protein
    GMD screening
Examination of placenta

GMD = genetic metabolic disease.

Table 14.8. Postmortem examination of the hydropic fetus or neonate

Photographic record
Radiograph
Weight and measurements
Malformations
    Cardiac
    Other
Lung weight
Virus culture and antibodies
Blood group and antibodies
Urine
    Protein
    GMD screen
Effusions
    Virus culture
    Biochemistry
Tissue for DNA extraction
Tissue for fibroblast culture (GMD)
Histological examination of all organs

GMD = genetic metabolic disease.

lifesaving [207]. Successful outcome is also recorded following neonatal surgery and extracorporeal membrane oxygenation support [208]. However, the prognosis with CAM type 3 remains poor [209], especially when hydrops is established [210]. Where specific in utero treatment is not currently an option, palliative measures and a clear plan of management for the duration of pregnancy, delivery, and the immediate neonatal period are important. Such measures have produced some increase in survival and have reduced morbidity, although the mortality of both rhesus and nonimmune hydrops remains high even when these are carried out [211, 212]. Emergency caesarean section is only appropriate in a few circumstances, such as feto-maternal hemorrhage, but in other situations often results in neonatal death despite active resuscitation because of the combined problems of hydrops and prematurity [213]. The associated maternal morbidity should not be forgotten.

REFERENCES

1. Friis-Hansen B. Body composition during growth. In vivo measurements and biochemical data correlated to differential anatomical growth. *Pediatrics* 1971; 47(2):264–74.
2. Cartlidge PHT, Rutter N. Serum albumin concentrations and oedema in the newborn. *Arch Dis Child* 1986; 61:657–60.
3. Iliff PJ, Eyre JA, Westaby S, de Leval M, de Sousa C. Neonatal pericardial effusion associated with central eventration of the diaphragm. *Arch Dis Child* 1983; 58:147–9.
4. Fleischer AC, Killam AP, Boehm FH, et al. Hydrops fetalis: sonographic evaluation and clinical implications. *Radiology* 1981; 141:163–8.
5. Gough JD, Keeling JW, Castle B, Iliff PJ. The obstetric management of nonimmunological hydrops. *Br J Obstet Gynaecol* 1986; 93:111–19.
6. Iliff PJ, Nicholls JM, Keeling JW, Gough JD. Non-immunologic hydrops fetalis: a review of 27 cases. *Arch Dis Child* 1983; 58:979–82.
7. Platt LD, Collea JV, Joseph DM. Transitory fetal ascites: an ultrasound diagnosis. *Am J Obstet Gynecol* 1978; 132:905–6.

8. Guyton AC. Capillary dynamics, and exchange of fluid between the blood and interstitial fluid. In: *Textbook of Medical Physiology*. Philadelphia: W.B. Saunders, 1986, pp. 348–60.

9. Mayerson HS, Wolfram CG, Shirley HH Jr, Wasserman K. Regional differences in capillary permeability. *Am J Physiol* 1960; 198:155–60.

10. Guyton AC. A concept of negative interstitial pressure based on pressures in implanted perforated capsule. *Circ Res* 1963; 12:399–414.

11. Boyd JD, Hamilton WJ. *The Human Placenta*. Cambridge: Heffer, 1970, p. 22.

12. Abramovich DR. The volume of amniotic fluid in early pregnancy. *J Obstet Gynaecol Br Commonw* 1968; 75:728–31.

13. Abramovich DR. Fetal factors influencing the volume and composition of liquor amnii. *J Obstet Gynaecol Br Commonw* 1970; 77:865–77.

14. Lind T, Kendall A, Hytten FE. The role of the fetus in the formation of amniotic fluid. *J Obstet Gynaecol Br Commonw* 1972; 79:289–98.

15. Abramovich DR, Heaton B, Page KR. Transfer of labelled urea, creatinine and electrolytes between liquor amnii and the fetoplacental unit in midpregnancy. *Eur J Obstet Gynecol Reprod Biol* 1974; 4(4):143–6.

16. Page KR, Abramovich DR, Garden AS, Jandial L. Solute levels in uterine fluids of patients with normal values of amniotic fluid and with hydramnios. *Eur J Obstet Gynecol Reprod Biol* 1978; 8(5):287–93.

17. Schruefer JJ, Seeds AE, Behrman RE, Hellegers AE, Bruns PD. Changes in amniotic fluid volume and total solute concentration in the rhesus monkey following replacement with distilled water. *Am J Obstet Gynecol* 1972; 112:807–15.

18. Walters DV. Fetal lung fluid. In: Hanson MA, Spencer JAD, Rodeck CH, Walters DV, eds. *Breathing*. New York: Cambridge Univ Press, 1994, pp. 42–62.

19. Abramovich DR, Page KP. Pathways of water transfer between liquor amnii and the fetoplacental unit at term. *Eur J Obstet Gynecol Reprod Biol* 1973; 3(5):155–8.

20. Elliott PM, Inman WHW. Volume of liquor amnii in normal and abnormal pregnancy. *Lancet* 1961; ii:835–40.

21. Queenan JT, Thompson W, Whitfield CR, Shah SI. Amniotic fluid volumes in normal pregnancies. *Am J Obstet Gynecol* 1972; 114:34–8.

22. Barnes E, Bryan EM, Harris DA, Baum JD. Oedema in the newborn. *Mol Aspects Med* 1977; 1:187–282.

23. Bryan EM, Chaimongkol B, Harris D. Alpha-thalassaemic hydrops fetalis. *Arch Dis Child* 1981; 56:476–8.

24. Saenger JS, Mayer DC, D'Angelo LJ, Manci EA. Ductus-dependent fetal cardiac defects contraindicate indomethacin tocolysis. *J Perinatol* 1992; 12:41–7.

25. Phibbs RH, Johnson P, Tooley WH. Cardiorespiratory status of erythroblastotic newborn infants: II. Blood volume, hematocrit, and serum albumin concentration in relation to hydrops fetalis. *Pediatrics* 1974; 53:13–23.

26. Moerman P. Nonimmunological hydrops fetalis. *Arch Pathol Lab Med* 1982; 106:635–40.

27. Moise KJ Jr, Carpenter RJ Jr, Hesketh DE. Do abnormal Starling forces cause fetal hydrops in red blood cell alloimmunization? *Am J Obstet Gynecol* 1992; 4:907–12.

28. Ville Y, Proudler A, Abbas A, Nicolaides K. Atrial natriuretic factor concentration in normal, growth-retarded, anemic, and hydropic fetuses. *Am J Obstet Gynecol* 1994; 171:777–83.

29. Ville Y, Proudler A, Kuhn P, Nicolaides KH. Aldosterone concentration in normal, growth-retarded, anemic and hydropic fetuses. *Obstet Gynecol* 1994; 84:511–14.

30. Gadd RL. The volume of the liquor amnii in normal and abnormal pregnancies. *J Obstet Gynaecol Br Commonw* 1966; 73:11–22.

31. Hytten FE. The physiology and pathology of amniotic fluid formation. In: Fox H, ed. *Obstetrical and Gynaecological Pathology*. Edinburgh: Haines & Taylor, Churchill Livingstone, 1987, pp. 1177–87.

32. Butler NR, Alberman ED. *Perinatal Problems. The Second Report of the 1958 British Perinatal Mortality Survey*. Edinburgh: E & S Livingstone, 1969, pp. 128,290–91.

33. Zameh NM, Gillieson MS, Walters JH, Hall PF. Sonographic detection of polyhydramnios. A five-year experience. *Am J Obstet Gynecol* 1982; 143:523–7.

34. Jeffcoate TNA, Scott JS. Polyhydramnios and oligohydramnios. *Can Med Assoc J* 1959; 80:77–86.

35. Peel J. Diabetes in pregnancy. Foetal macrosomia and increased perinatal mortality. *Proc R Soc Med* 1963; 56:1009–11.

36. Queenan JT, Gadow EC. Polyhydramnios: chronic vs acute. *Am J Obstet Gynecol* 1970; 108:349–55.

37. Law RG. *Standards of Obstetric Care: The Report of the North West Metropolitan Regional Obstetric Survey*. Edinburgh: E & S Livingstone, 1967.

38. Butler N, Claireaux AE. Congenital diaphragmatic hernia as a cause of perinatal mortality. *Lancet* 1962; i:659–65.

39. Siddall RS. Chorioangiofibroma (chorioangioma). *Am J Obstet Gynecol* 1924; 8:430–56.

40. Keeling JW, Gough DJ, Iliff P. The pathology of non-Rhesus hydrops. *Diagn Histopathol* 1983; 6:89–111.

41. MacIntosh AM, Osborn RA. Chorangioma of the placenta. *Med J Aust* 1968; 2:313–4.

42. Beischer N, Desmedt E, Ratten G, Sheedy M. The significance of recurrent polyhydramnios. *Aust & NZ J Obstet Gynecol* 1993; 33:25–30.

43. Hutchison AA, Drew JH, Yu VYH, Williams ML, Fortune DW, Beischer NA. Nonimmunologic hydrops fetalis: a review of 61 cases. *Obstet Gynecol* 1982; 59:347–52.

44. Mostoufi-Zadeh M, Weiss LM, Driscoll SG. Non-immune hydrops fetalis: a challenge in perinatal pathology. *Hum Pathol* 1985; 16:785–9.

45. Giammalvo JT. Congenital lymphangiomatosis of the lung: a form of cystic disease. *Lab Invest* 1955; 4:450–56.

46. Laurence KM. Congenital pulmonary cystic lymphangiectasis. *J Pathol Bacteriol* 1955; 70:325–33.

47. Laurence KM. Congenital pulmonary lymphangiectasis. *J Clin Pathol* 1959; 12:62–9.

48. Felman AH, Rhatigan RM, Pierson KK. Pulmonary lymphangiectasia. Observation in 17 patients and proposed classification. *Am J Roentgenol Radium Ther Nucl Med* 1972; 116:548–58.

49. Noonan JA, Walters LR, Reeves JT. Congenital pulmonary lymphangiectasis. *Am J Dis Child* 1970; 120:314–19.

50. Brus F, Nikkels PGJ, van Loon AJ, Okken A. Non-immune hydrops fetalis and bilateral pulmonary hypoplasia in a newborn infant with extralobar pulmonary sequestration. *Acta Pædiatr* 1993; 82:416–18.

51. Bryan EM. Benign fetal ascites associated with maternal polyhydramnios. A report of transitory ascites in two newborn infants. *Clin Pediatr* 1975; 14:88–91.

52. Mueller-Heubach E, Mazer J. Sonographically documented disappearance of fetal ascites. *Obstet Gynecol* 1983; 61:253–7.

53. Machin GA. Diseases causing fetal and neonatal ascites. *Pediatr Pathol* 1985; 4:195–211.

54. Woodall DL, Birken GA, Williamson K, Lobe TE. Isolated fetal-neonatal abdominal ascites: a sign of intrauterine intussusception. *J Pediatr Surg* 1987; 22:506–7.

55. Skoll MA, Marquette GP, Hamilton EF. Prenatal ultrasonic diagnosis of multiple bowel atresias. *Am J Obstet Gynecol* 1987; 156:472–3.

56. Cederqvist LL, Williams LR, Symchych PS, Saary ZI. Prenatal diagnosis of fetal ascites by ultrasound. *Am J Obstet Gynecol* 1977; 128:229–38.

57. Arger PH, Morantz J, Mennuti M, et al. Premature closure of the foramen ovale as a cause of intrauterine ascites. *Rev Interam Radiol* 1979; 4:93–4.

58. Vyas ID, Variend S, Dickson JAS. Ruptured ovarian cyst as a cause of ascites in a newborn infant. *Z Kinderchir* 1984; 39:143–4.

59. Abu-Dalu KI, Tamary H, Livri N, et al. GM₁ gangliosidosis presenting as neonatal ascites. *J Pediatr* 1982; 100:940–3.

60. Aylsworth AS, Thomas GH, Hood JL, et al. A severe infantile sialidosis. Clinical, biochemical and microscopic features. *J Pediatr* 1980; 96:662–8.

61. Gillan JE, Lowden JA, Gaskin K, Cutz E. Congenital ascites as a presenting sign of lysosomal storage disease. *J Pediatr* 1984; 104:225–31.

62. Reynolds JL, Donahue JK, Pearce CW. Intrapericardial teratoma: a cause of acute pericardial effusion in infancy. *Pediatrics* 1969; 43:71–8.

63. Zerella JT, Halpe DCE. Intrapericardial teratoma—neonatal cardiorespiratory distress amenable to surgery. *J Pediatr Surg* 1980; 15:961–3.

64. Einzig S, Munson DP, Singh S, Castaneda-Zuniga W, Amplatz K. Intrapericardial herniation of the liver: uncommon cause of massive pericardial effusion in neonates. *Am J Roentgenol* 1981; 137:1075–7.

65. Boyd PA, Anthony MY, Manning N, et al. Antenatal diagnosis of cystic hygroma or nuchal pad—report of 92 cases with follow up of survivors. 1996; 74:F38–F42.

66. Nicolaides KH, Azar G, Snijders RJ, Gosden CM. Fetal nuchal oedema: associated malformations and chromosomal defects. *Fetal Diagn Ther* 1992; 7:123–31.

67. Wilson RD, Venir N, Farquharson DF. Fetal nuchal fluid—physiological or pathological?—in pregnancies less than 17 menstrual weeks. *Prenat Diagn* 1992; 12:755–63.

68. Nadel A, Bromley B, Benacerraf BR. Nuchal thickening or cystic hygromas in first- and early second-trimester fetuses: prognosis and outcome. *Obstet Gynecol* 1998; 82:43–8.

69. Nicolaides KH, Brizot ML, Snijders RJ. Fetal nuchal translucency: ultrasound screening for fetal trisomy in the first trimester of pregnancy. *Br J Obstet Gynaecol* 1994; 101:782–6.

70. Watson WJ, Miller RC, Menard MK, et al. Ultrasonographic measurement of fetal nuchal skin to screen for chromosomal abnormalities. *Am J Obstet Gynecol* 1994; 170:583–6.

71. Byrne J, Blanc WA, Warburton D, Wigger J. The significance of cystic hygroma in fetuses. *Hum Pathol* 1984; 15:61–7.

72. Chervenak FA, Isaacson G, Blakemore KJ, et al. Fetal cystic hygroma: cause and natural history. *N Eng J Med* 1983; 309:822–5.

73. Poland BJ, Dill F, Paradice B. A Turner-like phenotype in the aborted fetus. *Teratology* 1980; 21:361–5.

74. Marchese C, Savin E, Dragone E, et al. Cystic hygroma: prenatal diagnosis and genetic counselling. *Prenat Diagn* 1985; 5:221–7.

75. Kalousek DK, Seller MJ. Differential diagnosis of posterior cervical hygroma in previable fetuses. *Am J Med Genet Suppl* 1987; 3:83–92.

76. Kleinman CS, Donnerstein RL, DeVore AR, et al. Fetal echocardiography for evaluation of in utero congestive heart failure: a technique for study of nonimmune fetal hydrops. *N Eng J Med* 1982; 306:568–75.

77. Cowchock FS, Wapner RJ, Kurtz A, Chatzkel S, Barnhart JS Jr, Lesnick DC. Brief clinical report: not all cystic hygromas occur in the Ullrich-Turner syndrome. *Am J Med Genet* 1982; 12:327–31.

78. van der Putte SCJ. Lymphatic malformation in human fetuses: a study of fetuses with Turner's syndrome or Status Bonnevie-Ullrich. *Virchows Arch Pathol Anat Histol* 1977; 376:233–46.

79. Adam AH, Robinson HP, Pont M, Hood VD, Gibson AAM. Prenatal diagnosis of fetal lymphatic system abnormalities by ultrasound. *J Clin Ultrasound* 1985; 7:361–4.

80. Hendricks SK, Sorensen TK, Baker ER. Trisomy 21, fetal hydrops, and anemia: prenatal diagnosis of transient myeloproliferative disorder? *Obstet Gynecol* 1993; 82:703–5.

81. Bryan EM, Nicholson E. Hydrops fetalis in South Korea. *Ann Trop Paediatr* 1981; 1:181–7.

82. Allan LD, Crawford DC, Sheridan R, Chapman MG. Aetiology of nonimmune hydrops: the value of echocardiography. *Br J Obstet Gynaecol* 1986; 93:223–5.

83. Whitfield CR. Prediction of Rhesus haemolytic disease. In: Barson AJ, ed. *Laboratory Investigation of Fetal Disease*. Bristol: John Wright & Sons, 1981, pp. 299–319.

84. Gauthier E. *Anasarque fœto-placentaire en dehors des incompatibilités de groupes. A propos de 29 cas.* Thèse doctorat en médecine, Paris 1978.

85. Huchet J, Soulié JC. Anasarque fœto-placentaire et incompatibilité ABO. *Rev Fr Transfus Immuno-hémat* 1979; 22:191–3.

86. Macafee CAJ, Fortune DW, Beischer NA. Non-immunological hydrops fetalis. *J Obstet Gynaecol Br Commonw* 1970; 77:226–37.

87. Miser A, Geraci TK, Wennberg RP. Fetal erythroblastosis fetalis due to anti-Kell isoimmune disease. *J Pediatr* 1975; 86:567–9.

88. Scanton JW, Muirhead DM. Hydrops fetalis due to anti-Kell isoimmune disease: survival with optimal long-term outcome. *J Pediatr* 1976; 88:484–5.

89. Holzgreve W, Curry CJR, Golbus MS, Callen PW, Filly RA, Smith JC. Investigation of nonimmune hydrops fetalis. *Am J Obstet Gynecol* 1984; 150:805–12.

90. Pearson HA, Shanklin DR, Brodine CR. Alpha-thalassemia as a cause of nonimmunologic hydrops fetalis. *Am J Dis Child* 1965; 109:168–72.

91. Thumasathit B, Nondasuta A, Silpisornkosol S, Lousuebsakul B, Unchalipongse P, Mangkornkanok M. Hydrops fetalis associated with Bart's haemoglobin in Northern Thailand. *J Pediatr* 1968; 73:132–8.

92. Boer HR, Anido G. Hydrops fetalis caused by Bart's haemoglobin. *South Med J* 1979; 72:1623–4.

93. Weatherall DJ, Clegg JB, Wong Hock Boon. The haemoglobin constitution of infants with the haemoglobin Bart's hydrops fetalis syndrome. *Br J Haematol* 1970; 18:357–67.

94. Mentzer WC, Collier E. Hydrops fetalis associated with erythrocyte G-6-P.D. deficiency and maternal ingestion of fava beans and ascorbic acid. *J Pediatr* 1975; 86:565–9.

95. Perkins RP. Hydrops fetalis and stillbirth in a male glucose-6-phosphate dehydrogenase deficient fetus possibly due to maternal ingestion of sulfisoxazole. *Am J Obstet Gynecol* 1971; 111:379–81.

96. Lie Injo Luan Eng, Lie Hong Gie. Abnormal haemoglobin production as a probable cause of erythroblastosis and hydrops foetalis in uniovular twins. *Acta Hematol* 1961; 25:192–9.

97. Mahony BS, Filly RA, Callen PW, Chinn DH, Golbus MS. Severe nonimmune hydrops fetalis: sonographic evaluation. *Radiology* 1984; 151:757–61.

98. Scimeca PG, Weinblatt ME, Slepowitz G, Harper RG, Kochen JA. Diamond-Blackfan syndrome: an unusual cause of hydrops fetalis. *Am J Pediatr Hematol/Oncol* 1988; 10:241–3.

99. Semmekrot BA, Haraldsson A, Weemaes CM, et al. Absent thumb, immune disorder, and congenital anemia presenting with hydrops fetalis. *Am J Med Genet* 1992; 42:736–40.

100. Carter C, Darbyshire PJ, Wickramasinghe SN. A congenital dyserythropoietic anaemia variant presenting as hydrops foetalis. *Br J Haematol* 1989; 72:289–90.

101. Roberts DJ, Nadel A, Lage J, Rutherford CJ. An unusual variant of congenital dyserythropoietic anaemia with mild maternal and lethal fetal disease. *Br J Haematol* 1993; 84:549–51.

102. Debelle GD, Gillam GL, Tauro GP. A case of hydrops foetalis due to foeto-maternal haemorrhage. *Aust Paediat J* 1977; 13:131–3.

103. Bose C. Hydrops fetalis and in utero intracranial haemorrhage. *J Pediatr* 1978; 93:1023–4.

104. Etches PC, Lemons JA. Nonimmune hydrops fetalis: report of 22 cases including three siblings. *Pediatrics* 1979; 64:326–32.

105. Boyd PA, Keeling JW. Fetal hydrops. *J Med Genet* 1992; 29:91–7.

106. Seward JF, Zusman J. Hydrops fetalis associated with small bowel volvulus. *Lancet* 1978; ii:52–3.

107. Sameshima H, Nishibatake M, Ninomiya Y, Tokudome T. Antenatal diagnosis of tetralogy of Fallot with absent pulmonary valve accompanied by hydrops fetalis and polyhydramnios. *Fetal Diagn Ther* 1993; 8:305–8.

108. Im SS, Rizos N, Joutsi P, Shime J, Benzie RJ. Non-immunologic hydrops fetalis. *Am J Obstet Gynecol* 1984; 148:566–9.

109. Potter EL. Universal edema of the fetus unassociated with erythroblastosis. *Am J Obstet Gynecol* 1943; 46:130–34.

110. Spahr RC, Botti JJ, MacDonald HM, Holzman IR. Non-immunologic hydrops fetalis: a review of 19 cases. *Int J Gynaecol Obstet* 1980; 18:303–7.

111. Moller JH, Lynch RP, Edwards JE. Fetal cardiac failure resulting from congenital anomalies of the heart. *J Pediatr* 1966; 68:699–703.

112. Wilkin P, Parmentier R. Hydrops foeto-placentaire et fibroelastose sousendocardique. *Bull Soc R Belge Gynec Obstet* 1961; 31:35–44.

113. Ito T, Engle MA, Holswade GR. Congenital insufficiency of the pulmonic valve. *Pediatrics* 1961; 28:712.

114. Schmid G, Fahnenstich H, Redel D, et al. Nicht-immunologischer Hydrops fetalis—eine übersicht über 31 fälle. *Klin Padiatr* 1988; 200:287–93.

115. Villaespesa AR, Mier MPS, Ferrer PL, Baleriola IA, Gonzalez JIR. Nonimmunologic hydrops fetalis: an etiopathogenetic approach through the postmortem study of 59 patients. *Am J Med Genet* 1990; 35:274–9.

116. Bates HR. Coxsackie virus B3 calcific pancarditis and hydrops fetalis. *Am J Obstet Gynecol* 1970; 106:629–30.

117. Benner MC. Premature closure of the foramen ovale. Report of two cases. *Am Heart J* 1939; 17:437.

118. Naeye RL, Blanc WA. Prenatal narrowing or closure of the foramen ovale. *Circulation* 1964; 30:736–42.

119. Pesonen E, Haavistu H, Anumala P, Teramu IC. Intrauterine hydrops caused by premature closure of the foramen ovale. *Arch Dis Child* 1983; 58:1015–16.

120. Arcilla RA, Thilenius OG, Ranniger K. Congestive heart failure from suspected ductal closure in utero. *J Pediatr* 1969; 75:74–8.

121. Becker AE, Becker MJ, Wagenvoort CA. Premature contraction of the ductus arteriosus: a cause of fetal death. *J Pathol* 1977; 121:187–91.

122. Kohler HG. Premature closure of the ductus arteriosus (P.C.D.A.): a possible cause of intrauterine circulatory failure. *Early Hum Dev* 1978; 2(1):15–23.

123. Ostor AG, Fortune DW. Tuberous sclerosis initially seen as hydrops fetalis: report of a case and review of the literature. *Arch Pathol Lab Med* 1978; 102:34–9.

124. Platt LD, Geirmann CA, Turkel SB, Young G, Keegan KA. Atrial hemangioma and hydrops fetalis. *Am J Obstet Gynecol* 1981; 141:107–9.

125. Radford DJ, Izukawa T, Rowe RD. Congenital paroxysmal atrial tachycardia. *Arch Dis Child* 1976; 51:613–17.

126. Silber DL, Durnin RE. Intrauterine atrial tachycardia associated with massive edema in a newborn. *Am J Dis Child* 1969; 117:722–6.

127. Cowan RH, Waldo HB, Harris G, et al. Neonatal paroxysmal supraventricular tachycardia with hydrops. *Pediatrics* 1975; 55:248–50.

128. Altenberger KM, Jedziniak M, Roper WL, et al. Congenital complete heart block associated with hydrops fetalis. *J Pediatr* 1977; 91:618–20.

129. Hardy JD, Solomon S, Banwell GS, Beach R, Wright V, Howard FM. Congenital complete heart block in the newborn associated with maternal systemic lupus erythematosus and other connective tissue disorders. *Arch Dis Child* 1979; 54:7–13.

130. McCue CM, Mantakes ME, Tingelstad JB, Ruddy S. Congenital heart block in newborns of mothers with connective tissue disease. *Circulation* 1977; 56:82–90.

131. Hull D, Binns BAO, Joyce D. Congenital heart block and widespread fibrosis due to maternal lupus erythematosus. *Arch Dis Child* 1966; 41:688–90.

132. Esscher E, Scott JS. Congenital heart block and maternal systemic lupus erythematosus. *Br Med J* 1979; i:1235–8.

133. Ho SY, Mortimer G, Anderson RH, Pomerance A, Keeling JW. Conduction system defects in three perinatal patients with arrhythmia. *Br Heart J* 1985; 53:158–63.

134. Cooke RWI, Mettau JW, Van Ceppelle AW, de Villeneuve VH. Familial congenital heart block and hydrops fetalis. *Arch Dis Child* 1980; 55:479–80.

135. Lauener, P-A, Payot M, Micheli J-L. Congenital hydrops and WPW syndrome. *Pediatr Cardiol* 1985; 6:113–16.

136. Gottschalk W, Abramson D. Placental edema and fetal hydrops: a case of congenital cystic and adenomatoid malformation of the lung. *Obstet Gynaecol* 1957; 10:626–31.

137. Phillips RR, Batcup G, Vinall PS. Non-immunologic hydrops fetalis. *Arch Dis Child* 1985; 60:84.

138. Bagozzi DC, Tagliabue P, Salmoiraghi MG, et al. Neonatal evaluation of non-immunologic hydrops fetalis. Report of 31 cases. *Pathologica* 1988; 80:677–86.

139. Khong TY, Keeling JW. Massive congenital mesenchymal malformation of the lung: another cause of non-immune hydrops. *Histopathology* 1990; 16:609–11.

140. McGinnis M, Jacobs G, El-Naggar A, Redline RW. Congenital peribronchial myofibroblastic tumor (so-called "congenital leiomyosarcoma"). A distinct neonatal lung lesion associated with nonimmune hydrops fetalis. *Mod Pathol* 1993; 6:487–92.

141. Daniel SJ, Cassady G. Non-immunological hydrops fetalis associated with a large hemangio-endothelioma. *Pediatrics* 1968; 42:829–33.

142. Larroche J-Cl. Nonimmunologic hydrops fetalis. In: *Developmental Pathology of the Neonate*. Amsterdam: Excerpta Medica, 1977, pp. 179–81.

143. Shturman-Ellstein R, Greco MA, Myrie C, Goldman EK. Hydrops fetalis, hydramnios and hepatic vascular malformation associated with cutaneous haemangioma and chorioangioma. *Acta Paediatr Scand* 1978; 67:239–43.

144. Jones CE, Rivers RPA, Taghizadeh A. Disseminated intravascular coagulation and fetal hydrops in a newborn infant in association with a chorioangioma of placenta. *Pediatrics* 1973; 50:901–7.

145. Sweet L, Reid WD, Roberton NRC. Hydrops fetalis in association with chorangioma of the placenta. *J Pediatr* 1973; 82:91–4.

146. Ivemark BI, Lagergren C, Ljungqvist A. Generalised arterial calcification associated with hydramnios in two stillborn infants. *Acta Paediatr (Stockholm) Suppl* 1962; 135:103–10.

147. Jones DED, Pritchard KI, Gioannini CA, Moore DT, Bradford WD. Hydrops fetalis associated with idiopathic arterial calcification. *Obstet Gynecol* 1972; 39:435–40.

148. Moerman P, Vandenberghe K, Delieger H, et al. Congenital pulmonary lymphangiectasis with chylothorax: a heterogeneous lymphatic vessel abnormality. *Am J Med Genet* 1993; 47:54–8.

149. Windebank KP, Bridges NA, Ostman-Smith I, Stevens JE. Hydrops fetalis due to abnormal lymphatics. *Arch Dis Child* 1987; 62:198–200.

150. Rudolph N, Levin EJ. Hydrops fetalis with vena caval thrombosis in utero. *NY State J Med* 1977; 77:421–3.

151. Drut R, Sapia S, Gril D, Velasco JC, Drut RM. Nonimmune hydrops fetalis, hydramnios, microcephaly, and intracranial meningeal hemangioendothelioma. *Pediatr Pathol* 1993; 13:9–13.

152. Golbus MS, Hall BD, Filly RA, Poskaizer LR. Prenatal diagnosis of achondrogenesis. *J Pediatr* 1977; 91:464–6.

153. Richardson MM, Wagner ML, Malini S, Rosenberg HS, Lucci JA. Prenatal diagnosis of recurrence of Saldino-Noonan dwarfism. *J Pediatr* 1977; 91:467–71.

154. Van Maldergem L, Jauniaux E, Fourneau C, Gillerot Y. Genetic causes of hydrops fetalis. *Pediatrics* 1992; 89:81–6.

155. Katz VL, Kort B, Watson WJ. Progression of nonimmune hydrops in a fetus with Noonan syndrome. *Am J Perinatol* 1993; 10:417–18.

156. Chitayat D, Gruber H, Mullen BJ, et al. Hydrops-ectopic calcification—moth-eaten skeletal dysplasia (Greenberg dysplasia): prenatal diagnosis and further delineation of a rare genetic disorder. *Am J Med Gene* 1993; 47:272–7.

157. Larroche J-Cl. Anasarque foeto-placentaire (hydrops) sans immunisation. *Med Hyg* 1982; 40:2061–73.

158. Worthen HG, Vernier RL, Good RA. Infantile nephrosis. *Am J Dis Child* 1959; 98:731–48.

159. Beischer NA, Fortune DW, Macafee J. Nonimmunologic hydrops fetalis and congenital abnormalities. *Obstet Gynecol* 1971; 38:86–95.

160. Anders D, Kindermann G, Pfeifer U. Metastasing fetal neuroblastema with involvement of the placenta simulating fetal erythroblastosis. *J Pediatr* 1973; 82:50–3.

161. Johnson AT, Halbert D. Congenital neuroblastoma presenting as hydrops fetalis. *NC Med J* 1974; 35:289–91.

162. Moss TJ, Kaplan L. Association of hydrops fetalis with congenital neuroblastoma. *Am J Obstet Gynecol* 1978; 132:905–6.

163. van der Slikke JW, Balk AG. Hydramnios with hydrops fetalis and disseminated fetal neuroblastoma. *Obstet Gynecol* 1980; 55:250–3.

164. Kohler H. Sacrococcygeal teratoma and "non-immunological" hydrops fetalis. *Br Med J* 1976; ii:422–3.

165. Sabet LM. Congenital glioblastoma multiforme associated with congestive heart failure. *Arch Pathol Lab Med* 1982; 106:31–4.

166. Ginsburg SJ, Groll M. Hydrops fetalis due to infantile Gaucher's disease. *J Pediatr* 1973; 82:1046–8.

167. Wisser J, Schreiner M, Diem H, Roithmeier A. Neonatal hemochromatosis: a rare cause of nonimmune hydrops fetalis and fetal anemia. *Fetal Diagn Ther* 1993; 8:272–8.

168. Verstraeten L, van Regemorter N, Pardou A, et al. Biochemical diagnosis of a fatal case of Gunther's disease in a newborn with hydrops fœtalis. *Eur J Clin Chem Clin Biochem* 1993; 31:121–8.

169. Rossier A, Caldera R, Sarrut S. Sur un cas de maladie de Niemann-Pick chez un nouveau-né. *Presse Med* 1958; 66:535–7.

170. Turski DM, Shahidi N, Viseskul C, Gilbert E. Non-immunologic hydrops fetalis. *Am J Obstet Gynecol* 1978; 131:586–7.

171. Fujimoto A, Ebbin AJ, Wilson MG. Down's syndrome and nonimmunological hydrops fetalis. *Lancet* 1973; i:329.

172. Sahn DJ, Shenker L, Reed KL, Valdes-Cruz LM, Sobonya R, Anderson C. Prenatal ultrasound diagnosis of hypoplastic left heart syndrome in utero associated with hydrops fetalis. *Am Heart J* 1982; 104:1368–72.

173. Willekes C, Roumen FJME, van Elsacker-Niele A-MW, et al. Human parvovirus B19 infection and unbalanced translocation in a case of hydrops fetalis. *Prenat Diagn* 1994; 14:181–5.

174. Greene D, Watson WJ, Wirtz PS. Non-immune hydrops associated with congenital herpes simplex infection. *S Dakota J Med* 1993; 46:219–20.

175. Bain AD, Bowie JH, Flint WF, Beverley JKA, Beattie CP. Congenital toxoplasmosis simulating haemolytic disease of the newborn. *J Obstet Gynaecol Br Commonw* 1956; 63:826–32.

176. Kettler L. Kongentale toxoplasmose und erythroblastose. *Zentralbl Allg Pathol* 1954; 91:92.

177. Zuelzer WW. Infantile toxoplasmosis. *Arch Pathol* 1944; 38:1–19.

178. Bulova SI, Schwartz E, Harrer WV. Hydrops fetalis and congenital syphilis. *Pediatrics* 1972; 49:285–7.

179. Henderson JL. Erythroblastosis or congenital syphilis. *J Obstet Gynaecol Br Emp* 1942; 49:499–511.

180. Anand A, Gray ES, Brown T, Clewley JP, Cohen BJ. Human parvovirus infection in pregnancy and hydrops fetalis. *N Engl J Med* 1987; 4:183–6.

181. Burton PA. Intranuclear inclusions in marrow of hydropic fetus due to parvovirus infection. *Lancet* 1976; ii:1155.

182. Porter HJ, Khong TY, Evans MF, Chan VT-W, Fleming KA. Parvovirus as a cause of hydrops fetalis; detection by in situ hybridisation. *J Clin Pathol* 1988; 41:381–3.

183. Ollikainen J, Hiekkaniemi H, Korppi M, Katila ML, Heinonen K. Hydrops fetalis associated with ureaplasma urealyticum. *Acta Pædiatr* 1992; 81:851–2.

184. Towbin JA, Griffin LD, Martin AB, et al. Intrauterine adenoviral myocarditis presenting as non-immune hydrops fetalis: diagnosis by polymerase chain reaction. *Pediatr Infect Dis J* 1994; 13:144–50.

185. Graves GR, Baskett TF. Nonimmune hydrops fetalis: antenatal diagnosis and management. *Am J Obstet Gynaecol* 1984; 148:563–5.

186. Zarafu IW, Tseng PI, Chuachingco J. Hydrops fetalis, fetal maternal transfusion and choriocarcinoma of the placenta. *Pediatr Res* 1978; 12:537.

187. Kanbour AI, Klionsky BL. Idiopathic fetal hydrops. *Lab Invest* 1978; 38:390.

188. Machin GA. Differential diagnosis of hydrops fetalis. *Am J Med Genet* 1982; 12:341–50.

189. Andersen HM, Drew JH, Beischer NA, Hutchison AA, Fortune DW. Nonimmune hydrops fetalis: changing contribution to perinatal mortality. *Br J Obstet Gynaecol* 1983; 90:636–9.

190. Nakamura Y, Komatsu Y, Yano H, et al. Non-immunologic hydrops fetalis: a clinicopathological study of 50 autopsy cases. *Pediatr Pathol* 1987; 7:19–30.

191. Shimokawa H, Hara K, Maeda H, et al. Intrauterine treatment of idiopathic hydrops fetalis. *J Perinat Med* 1989; 16:133–8.

192. Hansmann M, Gembruch U, Bald R. New therapeutic aspects of nonimmune hydrops fetalis based on four hundred and two prenatally diagnosed cases. *Fetal Ther* 1989; 4:29–36.

193. Squier MV, Keeling JW. The incidence of prenatal brain injury. *Neuropath Appl Neurobiol* 1991; 17:29–38.

194. Larroche JC, Aubry MC, Narcy F. Intrauterine brain damage in non-immune hydrops fetalis. *Biol Neonate* 1992; 61:273–80.

195. Lécolier B, Bercau G, Gonzalès M, Afriat R, et al. Radiographic, haematological, and biochemical findings in a fetus with Caffey disease. *Prenat Diagn* 1992; 12:637–41.

196. Kamat BR, Greco MA, Demopoulos RI. Immunocytochemical staining patterns of placentas associated with hydrops fetalis. *Int J Gynecol Pathol* 1989; 8:246–54.

197. Knowles S, Flett P. Multiple marker screen positivity in the presence of hydrops fetalis. *Prenat Diagn* 1994; 14:403–5.

198. Nelson J, Kenny B, O'Hara D, Harper A, Broadhead D. Foamy changes of placental cells in probable β glucuronidase deficiency associated with hydrops fetalis. *J Clin Pathol* 1993; 46:370–1.

199. Morey AL, Keeling JW, Porter JH, Fleming KA. Clinical and histopathological features of parvovirus B19 infection in the human fetus. *Br J Obstet Gynaecol* 1992; 99:566–74.

200. Johnson P, Sharland G, Allan LD, Tynan MJ, Maxwell DJ. Umbilical venous pressure in non-immune hydrops fetalis: correlation with cardiac size. *Am J Obstet Gynecol* 1992; 167:1309–13.

201. Stephenson T, Zuccollo J, Mohajer M. Diagnosis and management of non-immune hydrops in the newborn. *Arch Dis Child* 1994; 70:F151–4.

202. Rejjal AL, Nazer H. Resolution of cystic hydroma, hydrops fetalis, and fetal anemia. *Am J Perinatol* 1993; 10:455–9.

203. Downing CG, Vandenboom E, Thorp JA. Antepartum fetomaternal hemorrhage. Report of a case with the use of cordocentesis in diagnosis and management. *J Reprod Med* 1992; 37:566–8.

204. Oepkes D, Meerman RH, Vandenbussche FP, et al. Ultrasonographic fetal spleen measurements in red blood cell-alloimmunized pregnancies. *Am J Obstet Gynecol* 1993; 169:121–8.

205. Burke MS, Heyborne K, Bruno A, Porreco RP. Selective feticide in the second trimester: percutaneous ultrasound guided intracardiac placement of a thrombogenic coil. *Am J Obstet Gynecol* 1991; 164:337. Abstract.

206. Mahone PR, Sherer DM, Abramowicz JS, Woods JR Jr. Twin-twin transfusion syndrome: rapid development of severe hydrops of the donor following selective feticide of the hydropic recipient. *Am J Obstet Gynecol* 1993; 169:166–8.

207. Adzick NS, Harrison MR, Flake AW, et al. Fetal surgery for cystic adenomatoid malformation of the lung. *J Pediatr Surg* 1993; 28:806–12.

208. Etches PC, Tierney AJ, Demianczuk NN. Successful outcome in a case of cystic adenomatoid malformation of the lung complicated by fetal hydrops, using extracorporeal membrane oxygenation. *Fetal Diagn Ther* 1994; 9:88–91.

209. Revillon Y, Jan D, Plattner V, et al. Congenital cystic adenomatoid malformation of the lung: prenatal management and prognosis. *J Pediatr Surg* 1993; 28:1009–11.

210. Pinson CW, Harrison MW, Thornburg KL, Campbell JR. Importance of fetal fluid imbalance in congenital cystic adenomatoid malformation of the lung. *Am J Surg* 1992; 163:510–14.

211. Harris JP, Alexson CG, Manning JA, Thompson HO. Medical therapy for the hydropic fetus with congenital complete atrioventricular block. *Am J Perinat* 1993; 10:217–9.

212. Thompson PJ, Greenough A, Brooker R, Nicolaides KH, Gamsu HR. Antenatal diagnosis and outcome in hydrops fetalis. *J Perinat Med* 1993; 21:63–7.

213. Walton JM, Rubin SZ, Soucy P, Benzie R, Ash K, Nimrod C. Fetal tumors associated with hydrops: the role of the pediatric surgeon. *J Pediatr Surg* 1993; 28:1151–3.

Congenital Tumors

FRANK GONZALEZ-CRUSSI   CIRILO SOTELO-AVILA

GENERAL CONSIDERATIONS

Although malignant neoplasms are rare in children, they account for significant morbidity and mortality, being the second leading cause of death in the first 14 years of life, after accidents.

It is difficult to obtain reliable data and information on the incidence of childhood neoplasms; however, some extremely useful generalizations for understanding the problem of childhood neoplasia can be made from surveys in the literature [1–9]. Among these generalizations are the following:

1. The major histological types of malignant congenital tumors occurring in children of all ethnic groups are leukemia, neuroblastomas, and soft-tissue sarcomas [1].
2. In the first month of life, leukemia is the most frequent cause of death attributable to cancer [1]. Beyond the neonatal period, leukemia is the most common malignancy observed in white children, accounting for approximately one-third of all malignant tumors. Leukemia in black children is comparatively less frequent than in white children (percentage distribution for white children was 33.1, in contrast to 22.1 for non-whites in the Greater Delaware Valley Pediatric Tumor Registry, which was based on a population of 2 million) [5].
3. Congenital acute non-lymphocytic leukemia is nine times more frequent than acute lymphocytic leukemia [10]. This is exactly the opposite ratio of what occurs in later years. Congenital acute leukemia has a rapid and frequently fatal outcome.
4. Lymphoma is exceedingly rare in early life [11] and Hodgkin's disease has not been observed in children under 2 years of age.

The frequencies of various tumor types compiled by the Paediatric Pathology Society in Great Britain [2] for infants under 1 month of age were as follows: teratomas, 23.5%; neuroblastomas, 22.5%; soft-tissue sarcomas, 8.1%; kidney tumors, 7.1%; central nervous system tumors, 5.9%; leukemia, 5.9%; and others, 2.7% (Table 15.1). It is evident that the figures reported in different studies vary not only with the population studied and the methods used to collect the data, but also with the criteria that are used to select the cases. For instance, when mortality under 29 days of age is used as an indicator of frequency, leukemia emerges as the most common type of tumor. Neuroblastomas, soft-tissue sarcomas, and renal, liver, and central nervous system tumors follow in frequency [1]. However, in terms of strict incidence, not considering the ability to cause death, neuroblastomas are more prevalent than leukemia. Of 130 malignant tumors diagnosed annually in newborn infants in the United States, one-half are found on the first day of life, and two-thirds in the first week [1]. Table 15.1 summarizes seven congenital and neonatal tumor series from different sources [1, 2, 12–16].

ETIOLOGY AND CARCINOGENETIC MECHANISMS

It has been the hope, overtly expressed or implicit in epidemiological studies, to identify the cause or causes of malignancies that occur in early life. In particular, the limited temporal nature of intrauterine development, and its distinct spatial confinement, provide a unique opportunity to identify carcinogenic stimuli. Fetal and/or maternal exposure to exogenous factors, including ionizing irradiation, drugs, and viruses, may set in motion the biological mechanisms responsible for tumor formation. Unfortunately, the quest for specific carcinogenic factors has produced few concrete

Table 15.1. Incidence* of congenital and neonatal tumors (benign and malignant)

	O'Brien et al [15]	Fraumeni and Miller [12]	Wells [16]	Bader and Miller [1]		Barson [2]	Issacs [14]	Gale et al [13]
		Mortality		Incidence rate	Mortality rate			
Neuroblastomas all sites	49 (43.0)	27 (20.8)	23 (34.9)	21	70	64 (23.0)	14 (12.3)	11 (50.0)
Renal neoplasms, all types	4 (3.5)	9 (6.9)	5 (7.6)	5	21	† (7.0)	6 (5.4)	1 (4.5)
Liver neoplasms, all types	5 (4.4)	10 (7.7)		0	15		4 (3.6)	
Teratomas, all sites	1 (0.9)	9 (6.9)	1 (1.5)	0	11	67 (24.0)	40 (36.4)	3 (14.0)
Soft tissue tumors	14 (12.3)	12 (9.2)	33 (50.0)	4	29	† (8.0)	24 (21.8)	3 (14.0)
Central nervous system tumors	9 (7.9)	7 (5.4)	1 (1.5)	1	12	† (6.0)	5 (4.6)	
Unclassified			3 (4.5)					
Retinoblastomas	17 (14.9)				1		2 (1.8)	
Leukemia, all types	8 (7.0)	44 (33.9)		5	101	† (6.0)	11 (10.0)	3 (14.0)
Lymphomas				1	2			
Carcinomas				1	6		2 (1.8)	1 (4.5)
Other	7 (6.1)	12 (9.2)		1	27	† (26.0)	2 (1.8)	
Total	114	130	66	39	295	285	110	22

* Numbers in parentheses are percentages.
† Not stated.

results of practical benefit, but the importance of discoveries in this area is unquestionable. Administration of diethylstilbestrol to mothers may result in the development of vaginal adenosis, dysplastic changes of several types, and clear cell adenocarcinomas of the vagina in their daughters [17]. Hydantoin exposure in utero is associated with the development of neuroblastomas [18], and possibly with a wide spectrum of tumors of neural crest origin. A positive association between irradiation in utero and childhood cancer has been reported [19]; in particular, the risk has been considered higher for infants of mothers who undergo roentgenographic studies during the first trimester, and the incidence of exposure to radiation is thought to be higher in cases of children who develop leukemia early in life [20]. On the other hand, there are studies [6] that show no effect of carcinogenic factors on the progeny of mothers exposed to the potential carcinogen. Salonen [6], in a study conducted in Finland, found no significant correlation between maternal pelvic roentgenograms and the development of malignancy in the young.

Developmental errors during embryonal and fetal neruration may result in embryonic tumors. Durante's [21, 22] and Cohnheim's [23] "cell rest" theory, long discarded for the majority of human tumors, may well be pertinent to embryonic neoplasms. These authors believed that more cells are produced than are required for the formation of an organ or tissue and the origins of embryonic tumors rest in developmental errors in these surplus embryonic rudiments. The cellular and architectural features of embryonic tumors, as well as their presentation at or shortly after birth, suggest an origin in faulty embryogenesis (dysontogenesis). Embryonic tumors developing after infancy are explained by the

persistence of cell rests or developmental vestiges [24]. Developmentally anomalous tissue—choristomas, hamartomas, and dysgenetic gonads—is a source of neoplasms in older children and adults. When any of this developmentally abnormal tissue is present at birth, it is inferred that the cells failed to mature, migrate, or differentiate properly during intrauterine life.

Neoplastic transformation of cells in tissue culture and in vivo carcinogenesis are dynamic, multistep, and complex processes that can be separated artificially in three phases: initiation, promotion, and progression [25, 26]. Although not every tumor exhibits the entire chain of events shown in Figure 15.1, these phases may be applied to the natural history of virtually all human neoplasms, including embryonic tumors.

Initiation is the result of exposure of cells or tissues to an appropriate dose of a carcinogen; an initiated cell is permanently damaged and has a malignant potential. Initiation alone is not sufficient for tumor formation, but resultant daughter cells have a selective advantage over the surrounding unaffected cells. The initiated cells can persist for months or years before becoming malignant. During the *promotion* phase, initiated cells clonally expand [26]. Promotion may be modulated or reversed by a variety of environmental conditions [25]. In the last phase, *progression*, the transformed cell develops into a tumor, ultimately with metastasis. Fundamental carcinogenic mechanisms are virtually the same, regardless of age, and embryonic tumors can also be considered as defects in the integrated control of cell differentiation and proliferation.

A useful conceptual scheme was proposed more than 20 years ago by Knudson and colleagues [27, 28] to explain the

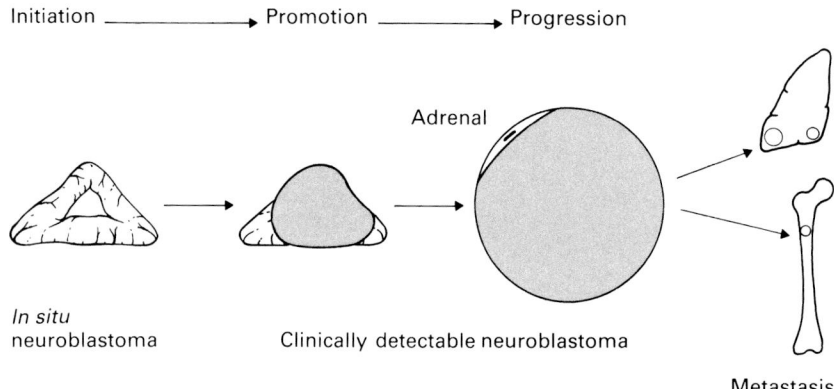

FIGURE 15.1.   *Natural history of neoplasia.* Initiation *is the interval during which a carcinogenic agent can induce a change in a cell which predisposes it to a malignant transformation.* Promotion *is the interval during which repeated exposures to an active (promoting) agent can induce the initiated cell to express the transformed phenotype.* Progression *is the interval in which the transformed cell develops into a tumor.*

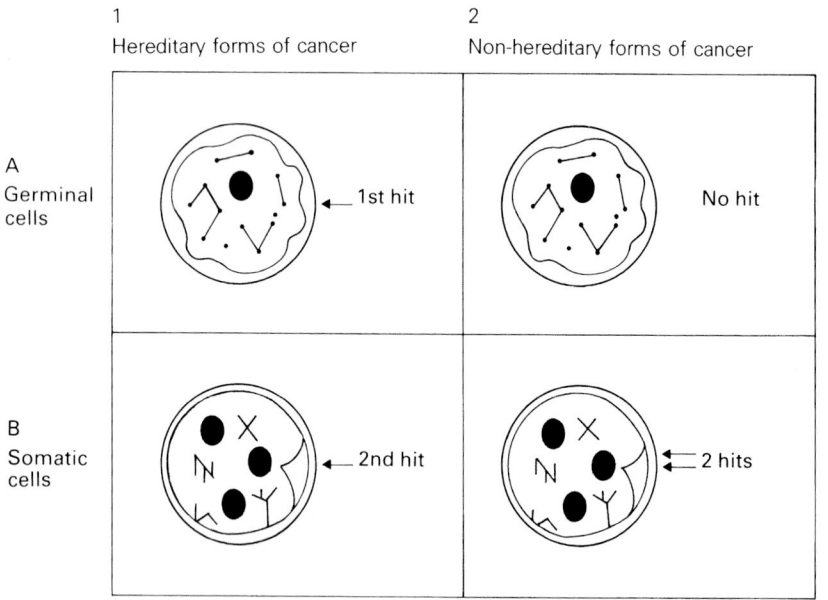

FIGURE 15.2.   *Mutation model for cancer.*

origin of retinoblastoma. Although recent advances have superseded some of its premises, it continues to be a helpful model to understand the inception of embryonal tumors. Knudson proposed that two events or "hits" in sequence must occur and are the rate-limiting step in the development of the tumor. The nature of the first hit was generally understood to be a mutation. The occurrence of two events results in the inactivation of both copies of a single *tumor suppressor gene* (see below). Inactivation of only one copy is insufficient to cause a tumor: both alleles of the gene must be destroyed or made functionally inadequate. If the first event is a constitutional mutation that the patient inherited from the sex cells of one of the parents, then all the patient's cells carry the abnormality in one of the alleles. The second event could be a new mutation or a chromosomal mishap during mitosis, such as mitotic nondisjunction, or mitotic recombination involving the wild type allele (Fig. 15.2).

The "two hit" hypothesis is not meant to give a full account of the origin of childhood tumors, but it introduced the concept of sequential insults to the genome as fundamental to neoplastic inception. Interestingly, whereas malignant tumors of breast and colon in adults usually associate with loss of heterozygosity (LOH) at multiple chromosomes, the LOH in "blastomas" of childhood seems restricted to few chromosomes, among which the short arm of chromosome 11 figures prominently. This may be because "blastomas" are embryonic tumors, in which the target cells are not fully differentiated, and thus may require fewer mutational events to become neoplastic.

The concept of tumor suppressor genes is especially relevant to the origin of childhood tumors. It is appropriate to recapitulate on how this concept was established. In the 1950s and 1960s, virologists had been able to obtain tumor transformation by injecting viruses into cells [29]. Because this injection causes a gain of genetic information (the viral genome is added), the thought that dominated thinking among oncologists early on was that cancer was due to the addition of genetic information, not the loss of the same. Moreover, because this addition of genetic material prevailed functionally over the normal set of genes, causing the malignant transformation of the phenotype, it was firmly believed that the gain of genetic information acted in a *dominant* fashion. A few years later it became possible to fuse two different cells into a single, composite unit or "hybrid." When a normal cell and a malignant cell were fused together, the resulting cell was malignant. Therefore, for some time it was believed that a gain, not a loss, of genes causes cancer, and this gain was thought to act upon the cell in a dominant fashion (i.e., a single added gene was sufficient for malignant transformation).

However, two researchers from Oxford, Sir Henry Harris and John Watson [30], refused to accept this conclusion. They noted that cells from tumors produced by injecting hybrid cells in animals always contained fewer chromosomes than the cells originally injected [31]. This suggested that the loss of genetic information was important. Moreover, there was also a long lag period between injection of hybrid cells and the development of malignancy. This suggested that the hybrid cells initially grew very poorly, and the malignant phenotype did not appear until certain chromosomes, presumably from the normal parent cell, were lost ("segregated"). A series of painstaking experiments with hybrid cells injected into suitable F_1 genetically compatible, hybrid animals confirmed these suspicions [32]. It took many years to convince the scientific community, but in the end the weight of the evidence could not be ignored: a loss, not a gain, of genetic material was crucial for the development of certain tumors. Moreover, the mutations taking place in crosses between normal and malignant cells behaved genetically in a *recessive*, not in a dominant, fashion.

Additional work firmly established the new concept. Serially cultivated "hybrid" cells were repeatedly inoculated into suitable experimental animals (nude mice). After a certain number of inoculations, malignant tumors did appear. Comparison of the karyotypes of the nontumorigenic hybrids and the tumorigenic "segregants" allowed one to examine the differences. It turned out that loss of chromosome 11 was implicated, with a high degree of statistical probability, in the development of malignancy. One of the two number 11 chromosomes was lost. It must be recalled that in "hybrid" cells each of the two chromosomes of a set comes from a cell of different kind: for instance, fusing a HeLa epithelial cell with a fibroblast. It was logical to think that the chromosome 11 of the HeLa cell was driving the cell toward malignancy, whereas the corresponding chromosome of the normal fibroblast was suppressing this drive in the nontumorigenic hybrids. With the techniques available in these early investigations it was not possible to determine which of the two members of the set was lost, either the one coming from the HeLa cell or the one from the fibroblast. Techniques such as RFLP (restric-

tion fragment length polymorphisms) then became available that permit identification of the lost one. Because loss of the normal gene accompanied transformation, it became apparent that something is present in chromosomes that "restricts" or "puts the brake" on the process of malignant transformation; when lost, a malignant neoplasm develops. This "something" consists of tumor-suppressor genes [33]. Refinements in technique presently allow selective transfer of a "tagged" individual chromosome into the cancer cell line investigated, thus helping to ascertain the role of specific chromosomes in the etiology of embryonal tumors of infancy and childhood [34, 35].

BENIGNITY OF NEONATAL AND INFANTILE TUMORS

Some neonatal and infantile tumors have a benign clinical behavior despite malignant histological features. Well-documented examples include congenital neuroblastomas, sacrococcygeal teratomas in infants under 4 months of age, hepatoblastomas below 1 year of age, congenital and infantile fibromatosis, and yolk sac carcinomas of the infantile testis in boys under 2 years of age [36]. Spontaneous regression of retinoblastomas, although rare, has also been documented [37]. The regressive tendency or cytodifferentiative capacity of these tumors and the rarity of other malignancies, such as Wilms' tumors and rhabdomyosarcomas, during the neonatal period led Bolande [38] to postulate an "oncogenic period of grace" which begins in utero and extends through the first few months of extrauterine life. The mechanisms responsible for this phenomenon are unknown.

RELATION BETWEEN CANCER AND CONGENITAL DEFECTS

In the last several decades, numerous examples of childhood tumors associated with congenital malformations have been documented [39–45], supporting the concept that oncogenesis and teratogenesis have shared mechanisms during embryonic development. Bolande [46–48] postulates that teratogenesis and oncogenesis are simultaneous or sequential cellular and tissue reactions to certain injurious agents. The degree of cytodifferentiation, the metabolic or immunological state of the embryo or fetus, and the length and time of exposure to the agent will determine whether the effect is teratogenic, oncogenic, both, or neither. Teratogenesis may be the more primitive expression of an injury, and oncogenesis the result of late gestational or postnatal exposure. Many biological, chemical, and physical agents known to be teratogenic to the fetus or embryo are carcinogenic postnatally [39]. Alternatively, a teratogenic event during intrauterine life may predispose the fetus to an oncogenic event later in life. This would explain neoplastic transformation occurring in hamartomas, developmental vestiges, heterotopias, and dysgenetic tissues. It is possible that the anomalous tissues harbor latent oncogenes which, under appropriate environmental conditions, are activated resulting in malignant transformation of a tumor. For instance, the transplacental effects of diethylstilbestrol on the fetus that leave the vestiges of anomalous tissue such as vaginal adenosis, and the hormonal stimulation that accompanies puberty may be responsible for the development of clear cell adenocarcinoma of the adolescent vagina [49].

Systemic study of embryonal tumors in large and relatively unselected populations, based on death certificates and hospital charts of patients with childhood tumors [41–45] and data from multi-institutional studies of children with specific tumors (e.g., the National Wilms' Tumor Study [50]), have made it apparent that some childhood neoplasms are associated with specific congenital defects and syndromes (Table 15.2). Of all the embryonic tumors, none demonstrates more strikingly than Wilms' tumor the relationship between teratogenesis and oncogenesis, both as a general phenomenon and in specific associations.

Aniridia–Wilms' Tumor Association

The aniridia–Wilms' tumor association was detected during a multihospital survey of Wilms' tumor, when aniridia was found in 6 out of 440 children with this tumor [51]. Conversely, of 27 children with aniridia, six developed Wilms' tumor [52]. Aniridia, genitourinary anomalies, and mental retardation are the major components of a malformation association that also affects other organs and systems, including the musculoskeletal and central nervous system, and the external ear. Growth retardation, microcephaly, craniofacial dysmorphism, hamartomas, lipomas, and inguinal and umbilical hernias have also been described [53]. About two-thirds of all cases of aniridia are familial, with an autosomal dominant inheritance; the rest are sporadic, presumably representing new mutations [54]. The anomaly affects about 1 in 64,000 persons in the United States [54]. Aniridia is present in one in 75 [51] to one in 127 cases of Wilms' tumor [50], a frequency that is 500 times greater than that of aniridia in the general population. Wilms' tumor occurs almost exclusively in patients with sporadic aniridia. The average age of patients with the aniridia–Wilms' tumor association is significantly lower than that of other cases of Wilms' tumor [50]. High-resolution chromosomal studies of both familial and sporadic cases of Wilms' tumor have shown 11p interstitial deletion of the p13 band [55–57]. However, this is not a consistent finding [58], indicating that Wilms' tumor may arise from a variety of pathogenetic mechanisms [59].

Hemihypertrophy and Intra-abdominal Malignancy

Patients with hemihypertrophy are at risk from the development of intra-abdominal malignancy, particularly Wilms' tumor, adrenal cortical carcinomas, and hepatoblastomas [42, 50, 60–62]. Neuroblastomas [63], myeloblastic leukemia [64], sarcomas of the lung [65], and benign mesenchymomas [66], although rare, are well documented. Four of 129 patients (ratio 1:32) with hemihypertrophy and segmental hemihypertrophy reviewed by Ringrose et al [67] had tumors (Wilms' tumor, "sarcoma" of the lung, adrenal carcinoma, and lipoma). Conversely, the hemihypertrophy to Wilms' tumor ratio is 1:41 [50], 1:31 in children with adrenal cortical carcinomas [61], and 1:35 for hepatoblastomas [68]. In a study of 27 patients with coexisting hemihypertrophy and intra-abdominal malignancy (nephroblastoma, adrenal cortical carcinoma, and hepatoblastoma), 19 tumors developed on the hypertrophied side of the body and the rest developed contralaterally [42]. In another study, there was no predilection of Wilms' tumor to the hypertrophied side [50].

The hemihypertrophy–Wilms' tumor constellation is distinct from the aniridia–Wilms' tumor association. Aniridia and hemihypertrophy rarely occur together [50]. Patients with hemihypertrophy frequently have malignancies other than Wilms' tumor, whereas aniridia is rarely associated with other malignancies [69]. Both aniridia and hemihypertrophy, as well as Wilms' tumor, are associated with genitourinary tract anomalies and hamartomas [42, 62, 67, 70].

Since a number of kidney anomalies coexist with Wilms' tumor, one might expect to see congenital defects instead of Wilms' tumor as the renal expression of hemihypertrophy. Indeed, a number of cases of hemihypertrophy in asso-

Table 15.2.   Pediatric neoplasms associated with specific teratogenic disorders or anomalies

Wilms' tumor
Sporadic aniridia
Hemihypertrophy
Beckwith-Wiedemann syndrome
Genitourinary tract anomalies and pseudohermaphroditism
Pigmented nevi

Leukemia
Down syndrome
Ataxia telangiectasia
Bloom's syndrome
Fanconi's anemia
Poland's syndrome

Adrenal cortical carcinoma and hepatoblastoma
Beckwith-Wiedemann syndrome
Hemihypertrophy

Sacrococcygeal teratoma
Lower vertebra anomalies
Genitourinary tract and anorectal anomalies

Lymphoma
Ataxia telangiectasia
Wiskott-Aldrich syndrome
Agammaglobulinemia
Chediak-Higashi syndrome

Basal cell carcinoma, medulloblastoma, rhabdomyosarcoma
Basal cell nevus syndrome

ciation with medullary sponge kidney [71–73] and anomalies of the urinary tract [74] have been described in the literature. Meadows et al [75] described a family in which certain elements of the hemihypertrophy–Wilms' tumor association were distributed among several members of the family rather than being concentrated in a single individual. Three children had Wilms' tumor and a fourth had duplication of the left renal collecting system; the mother had congenital hemihypertrophy.

Beckwith-Wiedemann Syndrome and Neoplasia Complex

The Beckwith-Wiedemann syndrome is a constellation of clinical abnormalities which includes varying combinations of macroglossia, nephromegaly, defects of closure of the abdominal wall (omphalocele, umbilical hernia, diastasis recti), natal and/or postnatal gigantism, facial flame nevus, hepatomegaly, ear-lobe anomalies, neonatal polycythemia and hypoglycemia, microcephaly, advanced bone age, hemihypertrophy, mental retardation, and clitoral enlargement. Pathological abnormalities are commonly seen in the adrenal glands (cortical cytomegaly and cysts), pancreas (hypertrophy and hyperplasia of the islets of Langerhans and ducts, and nesidioblastosis), and kidneys (nephromegaly with prominent lobulations, persistent nephrogenesis, medullary dysplasia, and medullary sponge kidney disease).

Patients with the Beckwith-Wiedemann syndrome have a substantially increased risk for the development of tumors [76]. Of over 200 reported cases, 26 patients had 22 malignant and 7 benign neoplasms (Table 15.3) [76–81]. A recent review of reports of children with hemihypertrophy disclosed 18 patients who might have Beckwith-Wiedemann syndrome, either incompletely manifested (forme fruste) or insufficiently described [82]. As a group, these patients had 19 malignant and 4 benign tumors (Table 15.4) [76, 80, 83–84].

It is not known whether cases of intra-abdominal malignancy associated with a single manifestation of Beckwith-Wiedemann syndrome represent incomplete forms of the latter, but the two malformations, Beckwith-Wiedemann syndrome and hemihypertrophy, are associated with each other. Of 174 patients with Beckwith-Wiedemann syndrome [76], 22 had hemihypertrophy (1:8); and of 26 children with Beckwith-Wiedemann syndrome in whom a tumor had arisen, hemihypertrophy was present in eight (1:3.1) [76–81]. All but two of the 18 patients with incomplete forms of Beckwith-Wiedemann syndrome had hemihypertrophy [76, 80, 82–84].

Genitourinary Tract Malformations and Wilms' Tumor

Congenital malformations of all types were identified in 262 of 1905 patients with Wilms' tumor registered in the National Wilms' Tumor Study between 1968 and 1981 [50].

Table 15.3. Tumors associated with Beckwith-Wiedemann syndrome: review of 26 patients*

Malignant		Benign	
11	Wilms' tumor	1	Adrenal cortical tumor (bilateral)
5	Adrenal cortical carcinomas	1	Hemangioma, liver
1	Neuroblastoma	1	Fibrous hamartoma, heart
1	Hepatoblastoma	1	Myxoma, umbilicus
1	Glioblastoma	1	Ganglioneuroma, retroperitoneal
1	Rhabdomyosarcoma, retro-orbital	1	Carcinoid tumor, appendix
1	Pancreatoblastoma	1	Extra-adrenal cortical adenoma
1	Lymphoma		
Total: 22		Total: 7	

* Three patients had two tumors each: Wilms' tumor and cardiac hamartoma; adrenal carcinoma and extracapsular adrenal adenoma; and bilateral adrenal cortical tumor and liver hemangioma.

Table 15.4. Tumors associated with forme fruste of Beckwith-Wiedemann syndrome: review of 18 patients*

Malignant		Benign	
9	Wilms' tumor	1	Congenital mesoblastic nephroma
4	Hepatoblastomas	1	Lumbar lipoma
3	Adrenal cortical carcinomas	1	Breast fibroadenoma
1	Hepatocellular carcinoma	1	Adrenal adenoma
1	Soft-tissue sarcoma		
1	Pancreatic adenocarcinoma		
Total: 19		Total: 4	

* Four patients had two or more tumors: Wilms' tumor with adrenal adenoma; bilateral adrenal cortical carcinoma and lipoma; Wilms' tumor and soft-tissue sarcoma; and Wilms' tumor, adrenal cortical carcinoma, and fibroadenoma.

Anomalies of the genitourinary tract were the most frequent, accounting for 28% of all malformations. Of the 89 patients with genitourinary tract malformations, there were 29 children with double collecting systems and 7 with fused kidneys. Other anomalies included lobulated kidney (4), renal ectopia (2), hydronephrosis (2), cystic kidney (2), "malformed" kidney (1), ureteral "obstruction" (1) and female hypospadias (1), cryptorchidism (25), and hypospadias (16). Two males and one female were pseudohermaphrodites and one male had an extra testicular sac.

NEOPLASTIC AND PRENEOPLASTIC LESIONS OF THE INFANTILE KIDNEY

Congenital Mesoblastic Nephroma of Infancy

In 1967, Bolande and associates [85] first recognized this tumor as a distinctive clinicopathological entity, adopting the term congenital mesoblastic nephroma of infancy, and emphasizing its congenital nature, preponderant mesenchymal components, renal location, and possible relationship to Wilms' tumor. Polyhydramnios and premature delivery have complicated the pregnancies of women whose infants had congenital mesoblastic nephromas [52, 86, 87]. Most congenital mesoblastic nephromas are detected at birth or in the neonatal period, usually up to 3 months of age and seldom later in childhood [88]. The oldest patient reported is 9 years [89]. There is a slight male predilection (M:F ratio, 1.8:1) [89]. A palpable abdominal mass is the predominant clinical presentation in about 94% of patients [89].

The benign behavior of this tumor has been emphasized in numerous publications. With a few exceptions [89–94], the majority of infants do well after complete removal of the tumor. In two [90, 92] of five patients [89, 92–94] with recurrence, the initial resected tumor extended to the surgical margin. In the third child, tumor recurrence was fatal [94]. In the fourth child, the tumor recurred 6 months after removal, despite chemotherapy [89]. In the fifth infant, pulmonary metastases developed simultaneously with local recurrence 2 months afte removal of the congenital mesoblastic nephroma [93]. Pulmonary metastases had been noted in only one previous instance [91]. Other complications observed in congenital mesoblastic nephromas relate to associated surgery, chemotherapy, or radiotherapy [89].

A congenital mesoblastic nephroma is the most common renal neoplasm in the first 3 months of life [88, 89], but its actual frequency is unknown. In a series of 57 Wilms' tumor cases reported by Bolande and associates [85], six were congenital mesoblastic nephromas. Favara and associates [52] combined their experience in three pediatric hospitals and identified three cases of congenital mesoblastic nephroma in over 300 renal tumors. Fifty-one (2.7%) congenital mesoblastic nephromas were identified among 1905 pediatric renal tumors submitted to the National Wilms' Tumor

Study Center [89]. More than 100 cases with congenital mesoblastic nephromas have been reported to date [88, 89]. Seven of the 51 patients studied by Howell et al [89] had associated anomalies, including genitourinary malformations (3), polydactyly (1), and hydrocephalus (1). This high association with congenital anomalies is similar to that reported for Wilms' tumor [50].

All congenital mesoblastic nephromas reported have been unilateral. The involved tumor is grossly enlarged, with the renal capsule stretched over the surface of the tumor (Fig. 15.3a). The tumor weight varies from 35 to 550 g and occupies 50% to 90% of the renal parenchyma [88]. Congenital mesoblastic nephromas are unencapsulated, with finger-like projections of the tumor extending into the adjacent normal kidney and even penetrating the perirenal soft tissue. The cut surface is yellow-grey, firm, rubbery, whorled, and trabeculated, resembling a leiomyoma (Fig. 15.3b). Hemorrhage and necrosis are not features of congenital mesoblastic nephromas, but small or large smooth-walled cysts may be present [88, 95].

Tight interlaced bundles of fibroblasts and myofibroblasts, with eosinophilic and fibrillar cytoplasm and round-to-oval nuclei with 1 to 3 small nucleoli surrounded by fine granular chromatin, are characteristically present [52, 88, 96]. Mitoses are infrequent, except in highly cellular areas. Normal glomeruli and tubules are often trapped by the tumor. At the junction with a normal kidney, the tumor infiltrates the renal parenchyma, blending imperceptibly with the kidney stroma (Fig. 15.4). Sometimes, a loose myxoid stroma predominates. Prominent lymphocytic infiltrate at the periphery of the tumor has been reported [88]. In focal areas, large tortuous vascular spaces surrounded by thick fibromuscular walls or thin-walled channels lined by endothelium give the tumor an angiomatous pattern. Hemopoiesis, immature cartilage, and dysplastic glomeruli

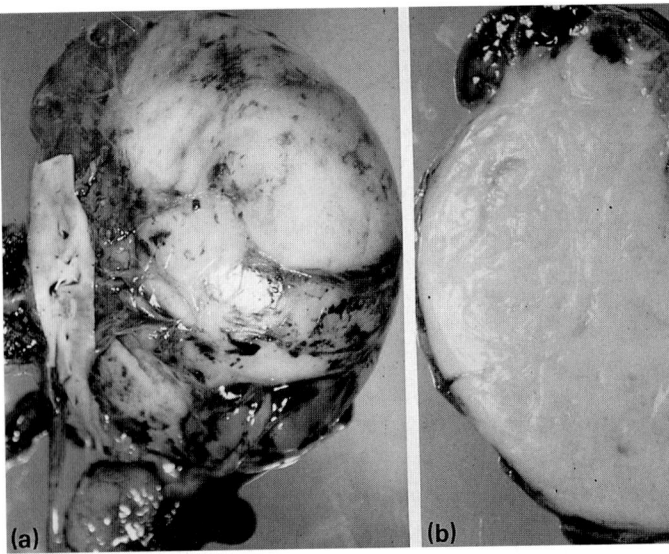

FIGURE 15.3. (a) External surface of mesoblastic nephroma. A small portion of normal kidney can be seen in the upper and lower poles. (b) Section surface of the same kidney showing the infiltrative character of the tumor.

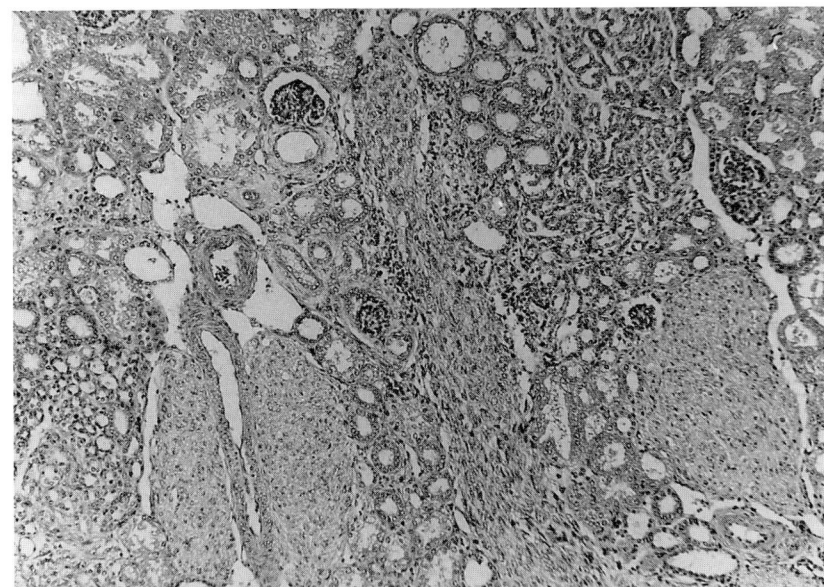

FIGURE 15.4. *Congenital mesoblastic nephroma. Normal kidney interface demonstrating bundles of spindle cells projecting into the kidney.*

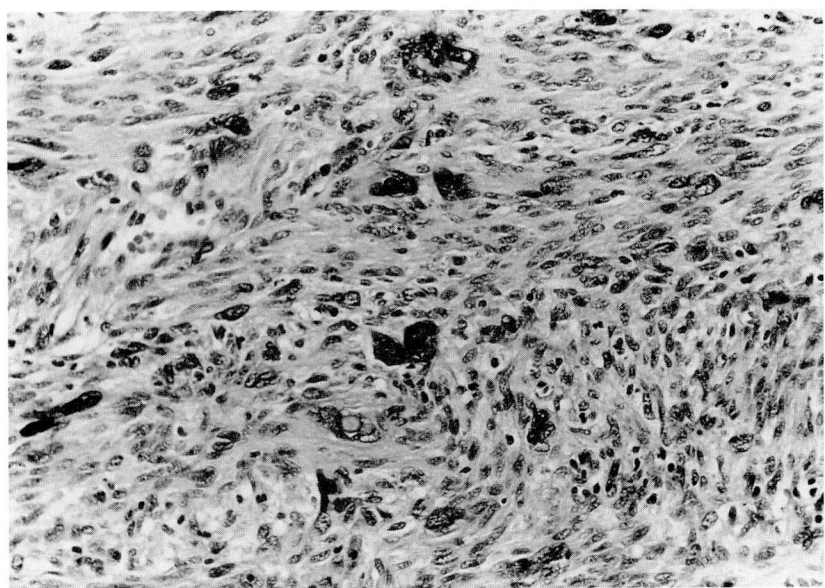

FIGURE 15.5. *Anaplasia in congenital mesoblastic nephroma is marked by nuclear enlargement and hyperchromasia.*

and tubules may be present. Argyle and Beckwith [97] reported anaplastic changes, including marked cellular pleomorphism, numerous giant cells and hyperchromatic bizarre nuclei in congenital mesoblastic nephromas of four children aged 3 to 7 years (Fig. 15.5). One of the patients died; the other three were well for 1 to 10 years after diagnosis. Although the authors concluded that these anaplastic changes have no prognostic significance, no statements were made regarding chemotherapy and radiotherapy administered to these children.

The nature and histogenesis of the tumor remain controversial. Bolande [88] and Beckwith [98] consider it to be a cytodifferentiated form of Wilms' tumor. Wigger [99]

believes that Wilms' tumor originates from primary mesenchyme or mesoblast, and that a congenital mesoblastic nephroma originates from secondary mesenchyme or more mature mesoblastic derivatives. In the chick embryo, two distinctive lines of mesenchyme have been described. The primary mesenchymal cells are derived directly from the primitive streak and aggregate to form the epithelia of somite and nephrogenic and lateral mesoderm. The secondary mesenchyme arises subsequently and forms most of the somatic connective tissue, but does not give rise to epithelia. If this avian model is applicable to the human kidney, Wilms' tumor with its epithelial and mesenchymal components is derived from the primary mesenchyme (mesoblast) and represents a mesoblastoma. Since a congenital mesoblastic nephroma is composed of cells with features of secondary mesenchyme and its differentiating derivatives, including fibroblasts, myofibroblasts, and cartilage, this tumor may derive from secondary mesenchyme; the lack of epithelial differentiation supports this view. Wigger [99] and Favara et al [52] prefer the term fetal mesenchymal hamartoma rather than congenital mesoblastic nephroma because of the exclusive mesenchymal character, frequent immature appearance, and absence of destructive invasiveness. Because of an occasional superficial histological resemblance to clear cell sarcoma of the kidney, Beckwith and Yokomori [100] propose that clear cell renal sarcomas originate by malignant transformation of congenital mesoblastic nephromas.

Nephroblastomatosis

Nephroblastomatosis or persistent renal blastema, as defined by Machin [101], is the persistence of renal blastema after 36 weeks of gestation (the stage at which nephrogenesis is completed) or the presence of renal blastema in abnormal quantities or distribution prior to 36 weeks of gestation. Morphologically, nephroblastomatosis may be classified as [102]:

1. Multifocal superficial (juvenile)
    (a) Nodular renal blastema
    (b) Metanephric hamartoma
        (i)   sclerosing metanephric hamartoma
        (ii)   tubular metanephric hamartoma
        (iii) sclerosing metanephric hamartoma with central adenoma
        (iv)   sclerosing metanephric hamartoma with incipient Wilms' tumor
    (c) Wilms' tumorlet

2. Diffuse pancortical (infantile)
3. Diffuse superficial (late infantile)

Multifocal Superficial Nephroblastomatosis

Multifocal superficial nephroblastomas are a closely related family of lesions and are the most common type of nephroblastomatosis. They do not cause nephromegaly, but may be associated with Wilms' tumor or malformation syndromes predisposing to Wilms' tumor [101], such as the Beckwith-Wiedemann syndrome [76].

Nodular Renal Blastema   Nodular renal blastema—variously referred to in the literature as incipient nephroblastomas [103], undifferentiated or abnormal metanephric blastomas [104], micronodules of blastematous tissue [105, 106], and in situ nephroblastomas [107]—is a well-circumscribed non-encapsulated renal lesion of fetuses, newborns, and young infants, cytologically indistinguishable from the blastemal component of Wilms' tumor. It is characterized by multiple, isolated subcapsular 50 to 250 μm nodules of primitive metanephric tissue (Fig. 15.6). Nodular renal blastema may also be found along the nodular septae or in the center of the columns of Bertin. Nodular renal blastema is considered to be the result of abnormal maturation or growth of nephrogenic precursors occurring at or shortly after birth [102].

Nodular renal blastema has been described in association with multiple congenital malformations [106–108], chromosomal anomalies [106–111], and Wilms' tumor [102, 109]. Of the 23 cases of nodular renal blastema studied by Bennington and Beckwith [108], 15 had associated congenital malformations, eight of which involved the urinary tract. A high incidence of multiple major anomalies was also observed by Bove et al [109] in postmortem examinations of infants with nodular renal blastema: five had trisomy 18

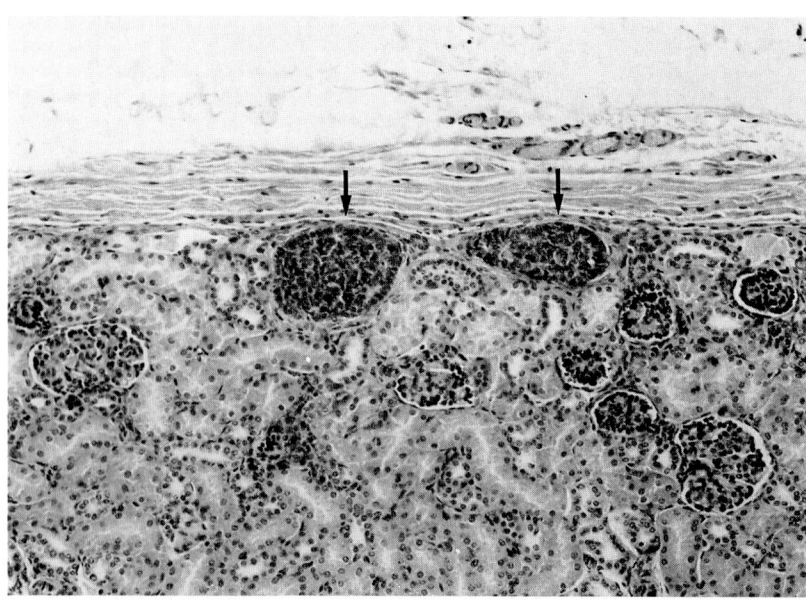

FIGURE 15.6.   *Subcapsular renal blastema nodules (arrow). Nephrogenesis is complete.*

and three had ventricular septal defects. Potter [103] identified nodular renal blastema in seven infants with normal kidneys and in five with type II cystic kidney disease. Four of the infants with normal kidneys had other anomalies, including anterior abdominal wall agenesis, eventration of the viscera, spinal column anomalies, and ventricular septal defect. Other congenital malformations accompanying nodular renal blastema include anencephaly and rachischisis [107], trisomy 18 [107, 109, 110], trisomy 13 [105, 111], and thanatophoric dwarfism [112].

Because of its anaplastic and primitive histological appearance, nodular renal blastema was considered to be a premalignant lesion by Potter [103, 104]. The term "in situ nephroblastoma" [107] implies that a certain proportion of these microscopic lesions will progress to Wilms' tumor. Although the microscopic anatomy of nodular renal blastema is not conclusive of its neoplastic nature, there is growing evidence which suggests that it may be a precursor of Wilms' tumor [113–117]. In nodular renal blastema, differentiation and proliferation occur long before the development of Wilms' tumor. During this process of cytodifferentiation, other renal lesions may evolve—tubular or sclerosing metanephric hamartoma (with or without adenoma and with or without incipient Wilms' tumor) and Wilms' tumorlet [101, 102]. This helps, in part, to account for the disparity between the postmortem frequency of nodular renal blastema (one in 115 postmortems in infants under 3 months of age) [108] and the expected incidence of Wilms' tumor (1.7 in 100,000 children under 12 months) [1]. The frequency with which nodular renal blastema progresses into Wilms' tumor is unknown. Nodular renal blastema probably represents a hyperplastic nodule of initiated cells awaiting a second hit [36, 107, 117, 118] before transforming to Wilms' tumor.

Metanephric Hamartoma This lesion can be subclassified morphologically as 1) sclerosing metanephric hamartoma, 2) tubular metanephric hamartoma, 3) sclerosing metanephric hamartoma with central adenoma, and 4) sclerosing metanephric hamartoma with incipient Wilms' tumor [102]. Typically, these lesions range from 1 mm to 3 cm in diameter, are made of epithelial elements and collagenized stroma, and are usually superficial and clearly demarcated from the adjacent cortex.

The sclerosing metanephric hamartomas consist grossly of either diffuse, broad subcapsular plaques of collagen up to several millimeters thick or focal clefts extending into the deep renal cortex producing abnormal kidney lobulations. Histologically, the lesion may contain plump mesenchymal cells or rare tubular structures with nuclear hyperchromatism, and may be in continuity with the margin of Wilms' tumor. They probably represent end-stage regression of tubular metanephric hamartomas.

The tubular metanephric hamartoma is characterized by poorly circumscribed collections of tubules lined by hyperchromatic cuboidal epithelium. Psammoma bodies may be found within the lumen of these tubules. The stroma is composed of sclerotic collagen.

The sclerosing metanephric hamartoma with central adenoma is histologically similar to the tubular hamartoma, but is larger and contains one or more benign papillary or tubular adenomas (Figs. 15.7 and 15.8).

The sclerosing metanephric hamartoma with incipient Wilms' tumor is, in part, indistinguishable from tubular hamartoma and may also contain adenomas; in addition, they contain fairly well-circumscribed tubules of embryonic and partially differentiated tubular epithelium identical to that seen in Wilms' tumor. The epithelium exhibits a high mitotic rate and the supporting stroma is well

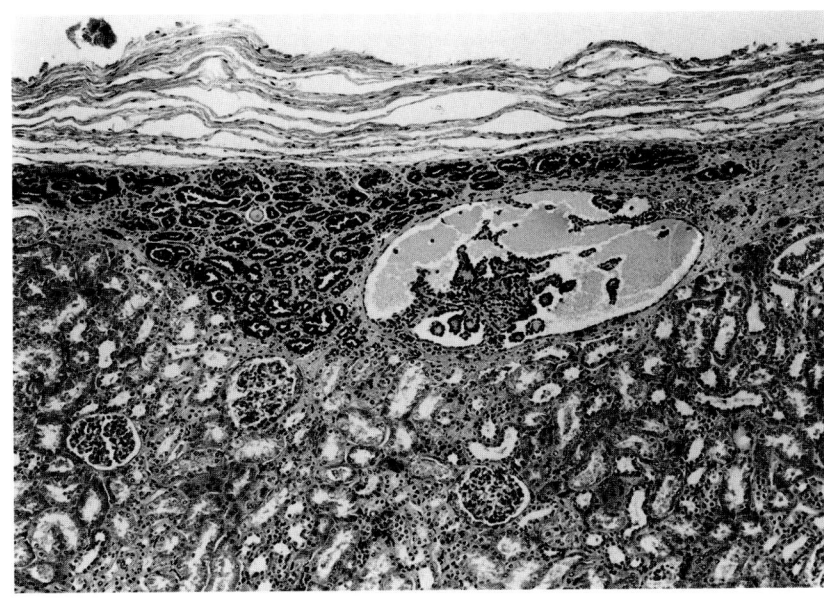

FIGURE 15.7. *Tubular metanephric hamartoma with an incipient papillary adenoma.*

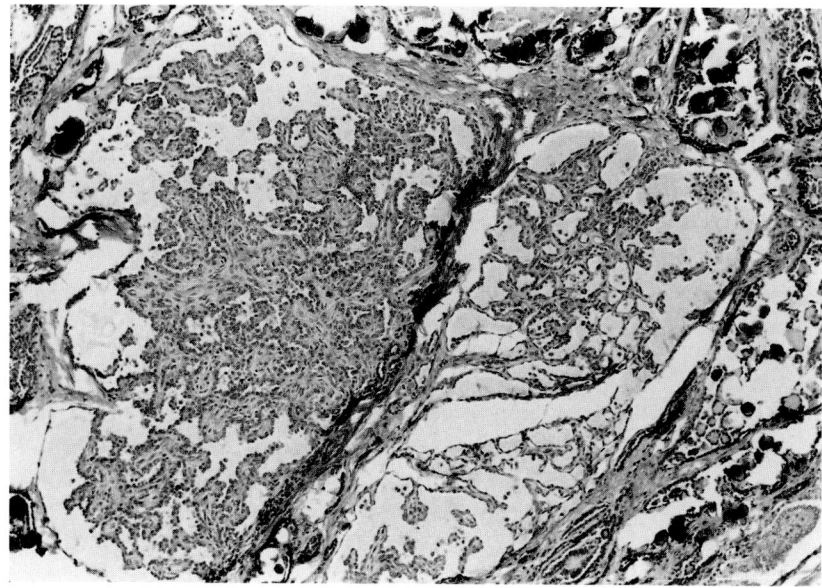

FIGURE 15.8.   *Well-developed papillary metanephric adenoma. A sclerosing tubular metanephric hamartoma surrounds the lesion.*

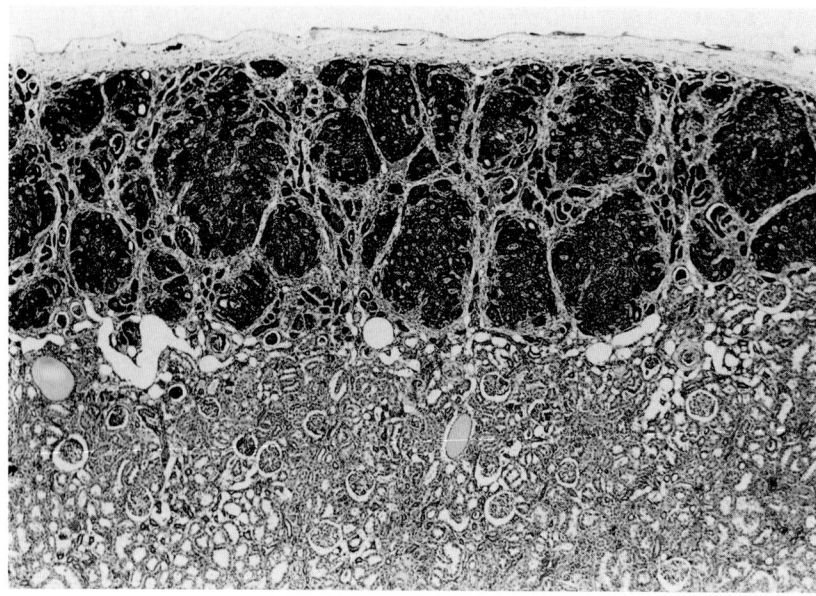

FIGURE 15.9.   *Multifocal superficial nephroblastomatosis. This photograph shows entire superficial cortical involvement; other areas of the same kidney were not involved by the nephroblastomatosis. This lesion was associated with a predominantly blastemal Wilms' tumor.*

vascularized. This lesion has been considered by Bove and McAdams [102] to be the progenitor of Wilms' tumor (Fig. 15.9).

Wilms' Tumorlets   Wilms' tumorlets are circumscribed neoplastic nodules of embryonic monomorphous epithelium identical to that seen in Wilms' tumor (Figs. 15.10 and 15.11). Wilms' tumorlets are distinguished from Wilms' tumor by size (1.0–3.5 cm in diameter) and lack of infiltration into the adjacent tissue. Wilms' tumorlets are invariably surrounded by metanephric hamartomas in varying degrees of involution. Although rare, Wilms' tumorlets have been described in an adult [119].

Diffuse Pancortical Nephroblastomatosis

Diffuse pancortical nephroblastomatosis is the rarest form of nephroblastomatosis; it is characterized by diffuse, symmetrical, and massive enlargement of both kidneys. Microscopically, the entire renal cortex is replaced by a mantle of primitive metanephric tissue composed of collecting tubules, blastema, and dysplastic nephrogenesis. This lesion, described by Hou and Holman [120] in a premature infant who died of respiratory failure after 13 hours, is considered to be both a malformation and a neoplasm. According to Machin [101], diffuse pancortical nephroblastomatosis represents a failure of interaction between the ureteric bud and the metanephric blastema, followed by proliferation of blastema and minimal epithelial differentiation.

Diffuse Superficial Nephroblastomatosis

As the name indicates, diffuse superficial nephroblastomatosis is a complete or nearly complete layer of persistent metanephric tissue in the superficial cortex of the kidney (Figs. 15.12 and 15.13). This lesion may produce bilateral but not necessarily symmetrical nephromegaly. It is probably related to multifocal superficial (juvenile) nephroblastomatosis and is intermediate in usual age of discovery between pancortical (infantile) and multifocal (juvenile) nephroblastomatosis. Like multifocal superficial nephroblastomatosis, the diffuse superficial type is also associated with Wilms' tumor or malformation syndromes, such as Klippel-Trenaunay syndrome [121].

Beckwith and colleagues [121a] proposed a new classification for precursor lesions of Wilms' tumor. The generic term *nephrogenic rest* was used in two major categories, perilobar and intralobar. The nephrogenic rest (NR) was defined as a focus of abnormally persistent nephrogenic cells retaining cells that can be induced to form a Wilms' tumor. Nephroblastomatosis was defined as diffuse or multifocal nephrogenic rests or their derivatives. Perilobar NRs are positioned at the periphery of a renal lobule or reniculus and have smooth borders, whereas intralobar NRs are randomly positioned in the renal lobule and have indistinct, irregular borders. Perilobar NRs have predominantly blastemal components early, and epithelial and sclerosing components late, in development. Intralobar NRs have predominantly primitive stroma along with blastema and epithelial components. Perilobar NRs are numerous and may form a diffuse rim at the perimeter of a renal lobule; intralobar NRs are usually single and rarely numerous. These authors described apparent progressive changes in the NRs from nascent to hyperplastic to neoplastic rests.

Wilms' Tumor

Wilms' tumor rarely presents at or shortly after birth (Fig. 15.14). A review of the literature by Giangiacomo and Kissane [122] disclosed only five cases of congenital Wilms' tumor, and two of these five cases [123, 124] were subsequently reclassified by Palmer [125] as malignant rhabdoid tumors of the kidney. Wells [16], in 1940, accepted only five

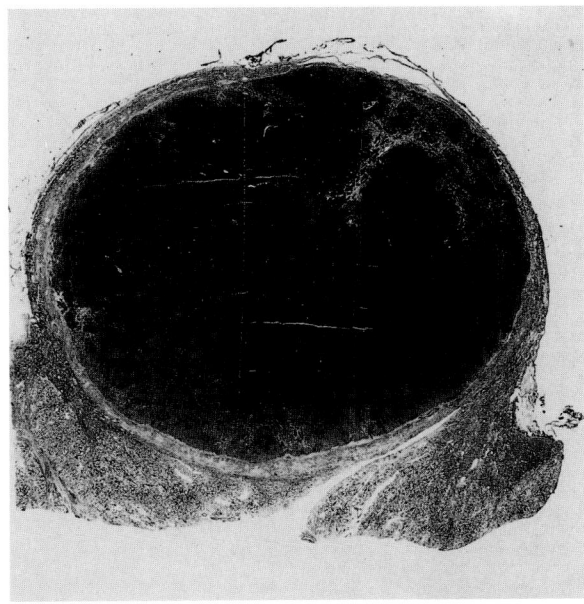

FIGURE 15.10. *Wilms' tumorlet. Notice the expansile and non-infiltrative nature of the tumor.*

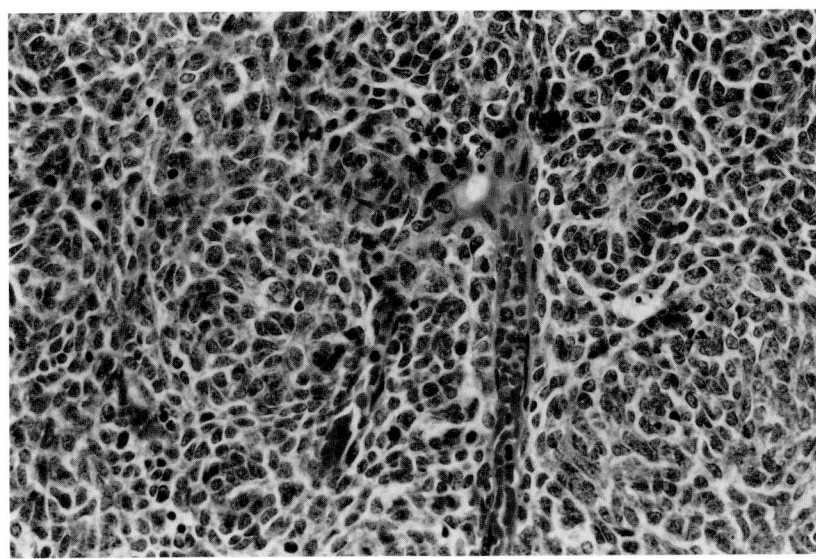

FIGURE 15.11. *Histological section of kidney shown in Figure 15.10, demonstrating the monomorphous blastemal pattern and occasional rosettes.*

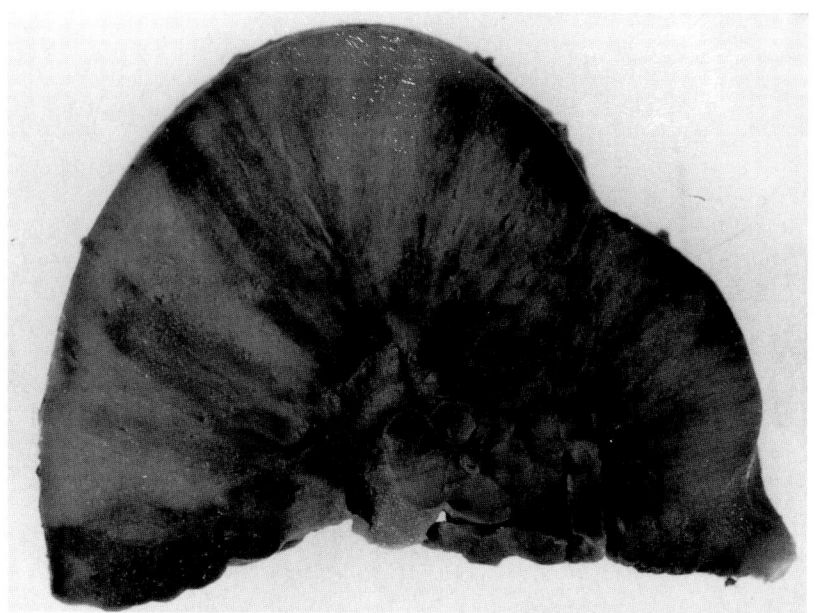

FIGURE 15.12. *Upper pole of kidney with diffuse superficial (late infantile) nephroblastomatosis. A small portion of medulla is seen in the center of the specimen.*

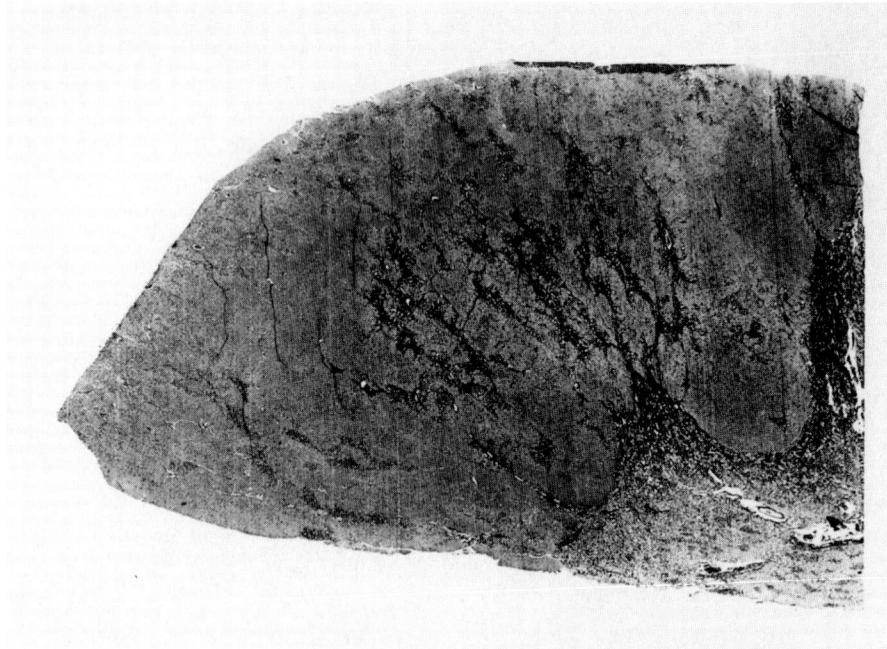

FIGURE 15.13. *Histological section of kidney shown in Figure 15.12.*

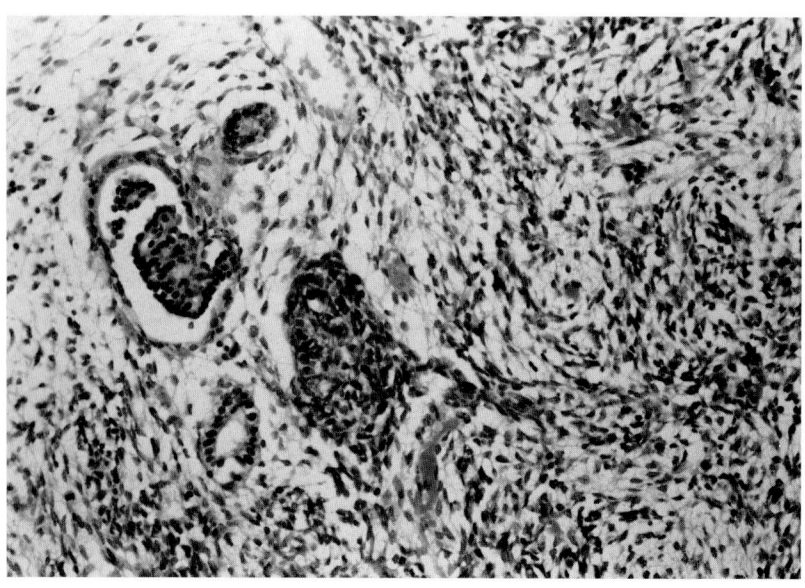

FIGURE 15.14. *Congenital Wilms' tumor in a patient with B–C translocation. The epithelial, blastemal, and stromal components are shown.*

cases in the world's literature as authentic examples of congenital malignant renal tumors. However, some of these may represent instances of congenital mesoblastic nephroma rather than Wilms' tumor. In a review of 205 consecutive primary renal tumors at the Children's Memorial Hospital in Chicago, no cases of Wilms' tumor were seen in patients under 6 months of age [126]. Of the 77 children with nephroblastomas reported by Sullivan et al [127], only one occurred in a newborn. A similar incidence was reported by Isaacs [14]: 3 newborns among 170 children with nephroblastomas (1.8%).

The peak incidence of Wilms' tumor is during the second year of life, with 48% of cases diagnosed in patients under 3 years of age and 75% in patients under 5 years [128]. Thus, a solid renal tumor during the first 3 months of life will most likely be a congenital mesoblastic nephroma rather than Wilms' tumor.

Typically, Wilms' tumor consists of a mixture of blastemal, epithelial, and stromal tissues (Fig. 15.15). However, the diagnosis should not be restricted to those neoplasms in which all three cell lines are present. A number of monomorphous blastemal (Fig. 15.16) or epithelial variants (Fig. 15.17) often can be identified. Primary renal rhabdomyosarcoma may represent a monomorphous variant of Wilms' tumor. The distinction is important since therapy may be determined, at least in part, by the histopathology of the tumor. Most, if not all, cells in the metanephros probably ultimately derive from the metanephric blastema, so

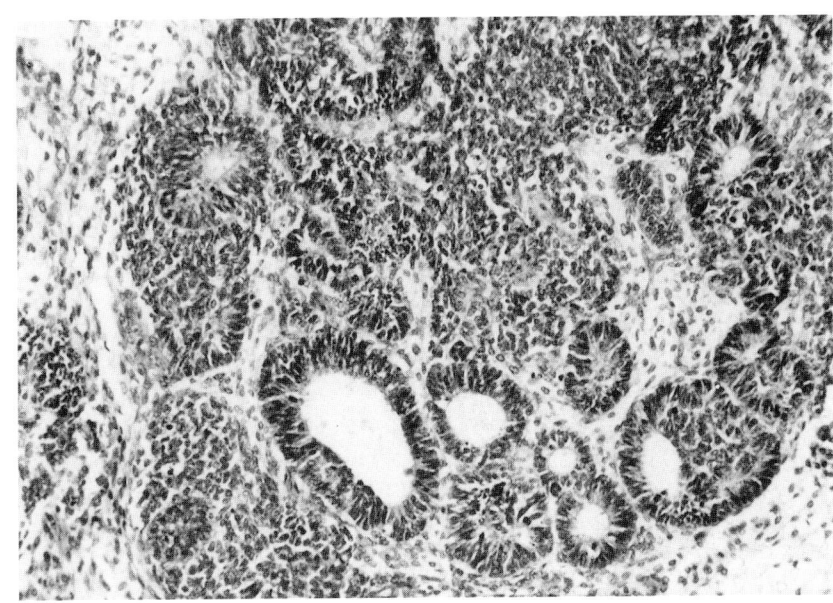

FIGURE 15.15. *Typical triphasic Wilms' tumor showing epithelial, blastemal, and stromal components.*

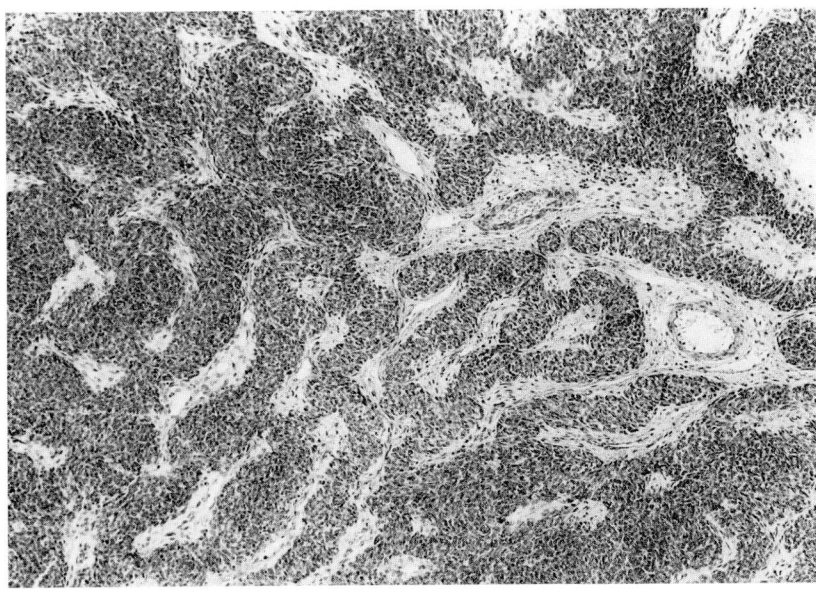

FIGURE 15.16. *Monomorphous blastemal Wilms' tumor manifested as ribbons of cells embedded in loose connective stroma.*

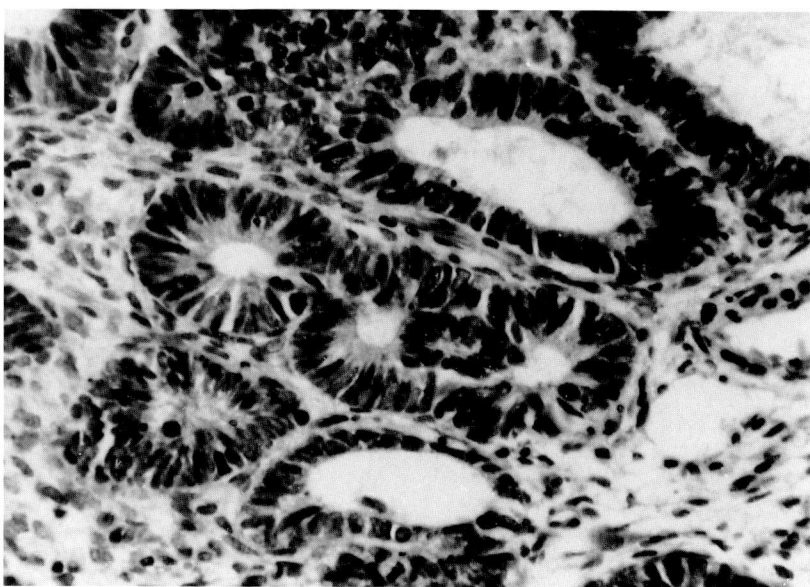

FIGURE 15.17.   *Monomorphous epithelial Wilms' tumor demonstrating back-to-back tubules.*

that Beckwith [129] may well be correct in proposing that virtually all renal tumors are related to nephroblastomas.

WT-1 was presumably the first "tumor suppressor gene" implicated in the etiology of nephroblastoma, but abnormalities in this gene do not contain the key to all Wilms' tumors. Wilms' tumor develops in 59% of patients with the Beckwith-Wiedemann syndrome (BWS). It is currently thought that the chromosomal region 11p15.5 is associated with this syndrome. Molecular studies have shown duplication of 11p15 in many cases. Interestingly, the duplication has been of the chromosome of paternal origin; the mother's genetic material is lost. It appears that the phenomenon of *genomic imprinting* manifests in BWS [130]. Increased expression of IGF2 has been reported in tumors that occur at higher incidence in BWS, including Wilms' tumor [131]. IGF2 is parentally imprinted during normal embryogenesis and is overexpressed in 95% of Wilms' tumor, from 10- to 100-fold compared to normal adult kidney tissue; blastema cells of the tumors seem to be mainly implicated in this overexpression. Chromosome 1p3 shows abnormalities, in keeping with other pediatric tumors such as neuroblastoma, retinoblastoma, and rhabdomyosarcoma. In summary, changes in chromosome 11 are abundantly confirmed, but are believed to be insufficient to cause Wilms' tumor, and other genetic tumor loci must be affected.

At the molecular level, the catalase (CAT) gene, encoding the erythrocytic enzyme catalase, produces reduced blood levels of this enzyme, because of a deletion at 11p13. Patients with aniridia and Wilms' tumor but with normal karyotype may have normal levels of catalase; this means that the linkage of the Wilms' tumor gene and those of catalase and aniridia is close but not absolute. Some patients were reported with 11p13 deletion and Wilms' tumor, but without aniridia or mental retardation; this indicates that the

loci for Wilms' tumor and aniridia are genetically distinct. Further work led to the identification of two genes, transcribed in opposite directions, named WT and WT-1, whose transcripts are most abundant in RNA from fetal kidneys, and are found at much lower levels in renal tissue from children and adults. By the occurrence of different combinations of alternative splicing, four different WT-1 mRNAs are produced [132].

Familial Wilms' tumor is well documented: some cases present as autosomal dominant inheritable disease with incomplete penetrance. Familial Wilms' tumor comprises less than 2% of all cases but this is far less than the 30% predicted by the two-hit hypothesis. Also, the incidence of Wilms' tumor in the offspring of parents with Wilms' tumor is not as high as the two-hit hypothesis would predict. Multicentric Wilms' tumor is uncommon, and patients bearing this form of tumor do not differ in age of presentation from the sporadic, unilateral, and unicentric form of the disease [132]. The two-hit hypothesis may be applicable to specific events occurring during Wilms' tumor formation, though not accounting for tumorigenesis entirely. The most common karyotypic abnormality of Wilms' tumor is structural change of the short arm of chromosome 11, which occurs in about 25% of cases, but may be subtle cytogenetically [133]. Bands 11p13 and 11p15 are preferentially affected. In addition, there is loss of heterozygosity (LOH) for markers in 16q.

Patients with the Denys-Drash syndrome (DDS) manifest three phenotypes simultaneously: ambiguous genitalia, nephrotic syndrome (usually as a result of mesangial sclerosis), and nephroblastoma. DDS is believed to comprise an abnormality of growth (hypertrophy) and differentiation of glomerular tissue structures. The nephropathy is the central feature of the syndrome. Variants may consist of nephropathy and Wilms' tumor, or nephropathy and ambiguous genitalia, or other genitourinary malformations. Germline mutations of WT-1 are also thought to be responsible for the genitourinary malformations of DDS. In almost all cases examined, LOH in the WT-1 gene has been found in the tumors of these individuals [132].

There is nonuniform expression of WT-1 in the cells of nephroblastoma. Tumors that remain highly undifferentiated, such as those made predominantly of blastema cells, do not express the gene, whereas those that show evidence of epithelial differentiation in the form of vesicles or "proglomeruli" express it strongly. The expression of WT-1 in Wilms' tumor seems to recapitulate the expression in the embryonic kidney.

Clear Cell Sarcoma of the Kidney

A clear cell sarcoma of the kidney is an uncommon but distinctive renal tumor of childhood, with a characteristic histological pattern and a marked proclivity to metastasize to bone. It deserves mention here because of its occurrence, albeit rare, in the neonatal period [134]. No association with congenital anomalies has been noted for this tumor. The term "clear cell sarcoma" was proposed by Beckwith and Palmer [135] to distinguish it from the renal rhabdoid tumor whose neoplastic cells have a characteristic and abundant eosinophilic cytoplasm. Its recognition is of practical importance because of its malignant clinical behavior; it requires more aggressive therapy than Wilms' tumor. Its overall frequency among primary renal tumors seen in the U.S. pediatric population varies from 2.5% [129] to 5.6% [136]; in the U.K., the frequency is slightly lower at 1.6% [137].

Histologically, a clear cell sarcoma of the kidney is characterized by its cellularity: haphazardly arranged cells with clear, vesicular, round-to-oval nuclei, indistinct nucleoli, and poorly stained cytoplasm with discrete projections from the cell surface. The stroma is uniform and delicate, containing fine capillaries throughout (Fig. 15.18). With hematoxylin and eosin, the cytoplasm of many cells fails to stain altogether, hence the name "clear cell" sarcoma. Microscopic foci of necrosis and randomly distributed myxoid areas are commonly seen throughout the tumor. A highly characteristic feature of clear cell sarcoma of the kidney is a net of arborizing fascicles of spindle fibroblasts and myofibroblasts dividing the tumor into cords (Fig. 15.19). A clear cell sarcoma of the kidney is not the only sarcoma of the kidney, but it is the most common renal sarcoma of childhood [136]. Its histogenesis is unknown.

Malignant Rhabdoid Tumor

A rhabdoid tumor is another distinctive renal neoplasm that occurs in newborn and young infants. Malignant rhabdoid tumors of the kidney represent about 2% of all tumors entered in the National Wilms' Tumor Study 1 and 2 [125]. These 21 children ranged in age from 3 to 42 months, with a mean age of 18 months; 16 children were diagnosed before their second birthday and 10 were less than 1 year old. Malignant rhabdoid tumors of the kidney have been reported in the newborn period in at least three patients [123, 124, 138]. The rapid appearance of metastasis, often to multiple sites, and the short subsequent survival make this tumor one of the most malignant childhood neoplasms. Hypercalcemia observed in infants with malignant rhabdoid tumors of the kidney has been ascribed to elevated serum parathormone produced by the tumor [139–141]. This neoplasm is characterized by sheets, cords, and nests of cells containing a large hyaline, globular, PAS-positive cytoplasmic inclusion, a prominent nucleolus, and an eccentric nucleus (Fig. 15.20). The most distinctive ultrastructural feature is the presence of parallel cytoplasmic intermediate filaments

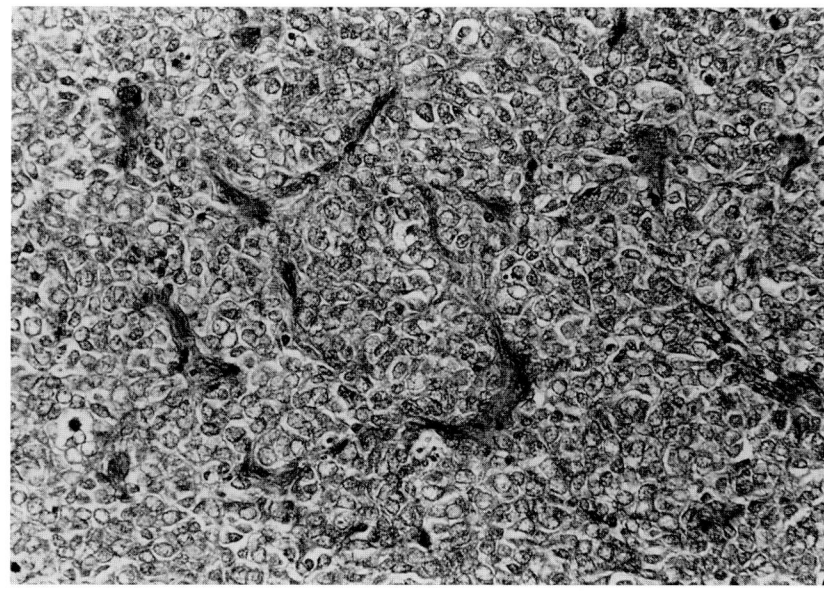

FIGURE 15.18. *Clear cell sarcoma of the kidney. Fine capillary network and cells with vesicular nuclei and indistinctive cytoplasm characterize this tumor.*

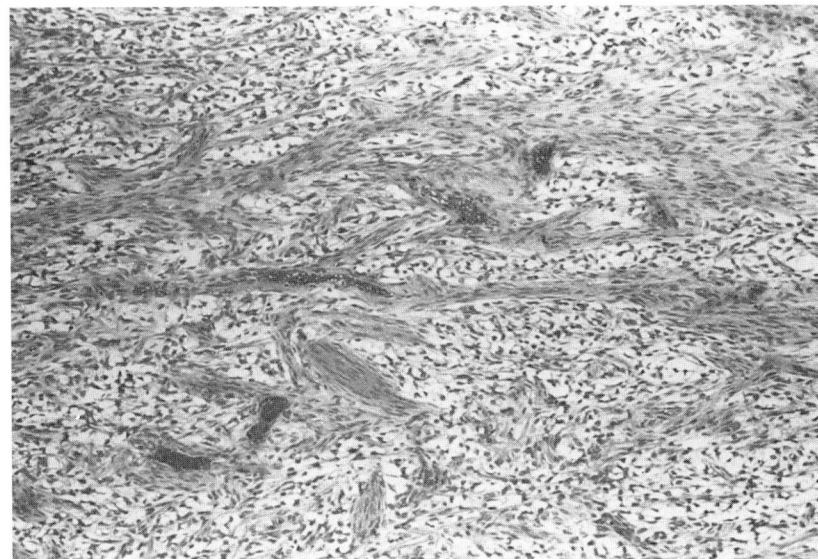

FIGURE 15.19.   *Clear cell sarcoma of the kidney. Notice the haphazardly arranged tumor cells and the arborizing fascicles of fibroblasts and myofibroblasts.*

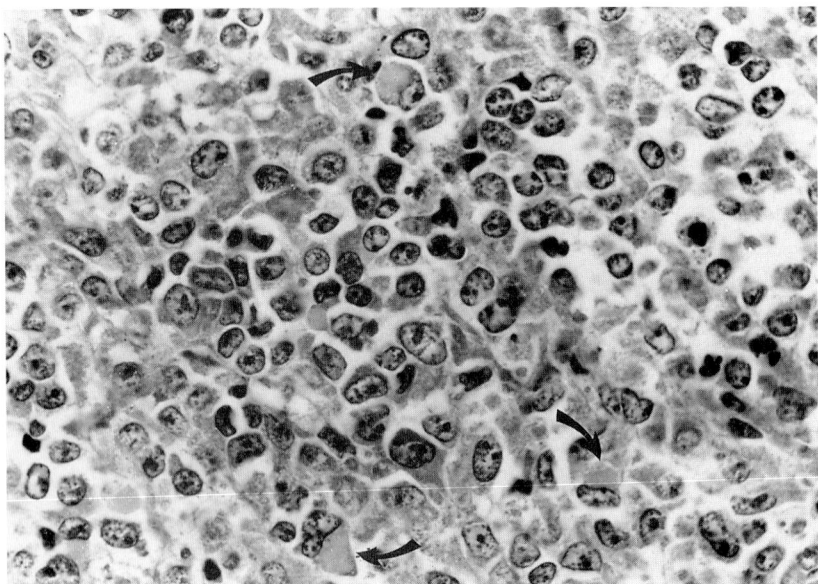

FIGURE 15.20.   *Rhabdoid tumor of the kidney. Loosely arranged tumor cells contain large cytoplasmic inclusions (arrow).*

packed in concentric whorls (Fig. 15.21) [142]. The presence of vimentin and 54-kDa cytokeratin suggest both epithelial and mesenchymal differentiation of these tumors [15]. Malignant rhabdoid tumors of the kidney have been associated with metastatic and primary central nervous system tumors, including cerebellar medulloblastoma and medulloepithelioma, pinealoblastoma, primitive neuroepithelial tumor, and malignant subependymal giant cell astrocytoma of the cerebellum [138]. Because of this association and the observation of similar intracytoplasmic intermediate filaments in a number of tumors of the APUD system, Haas et al [142] suggest a neural crest histogenetic origin for this tumor.

Extrarenal rhabdoid tumors have been identified as primary neoplasms in the prostate [143], thymus [144], par-

avertebral [145], pelvis [146], heart [147], chest-wall soft tissue, liver and dorsum of foot [148], central nervous system [149], and shoulder [150].

NEOPLASMS OF THE LIVER

Benign Tumors and Tumor-like Lesions

Perinatal hepatic tumors may be benign or malignant. The most frequent primary neoplasm is the hemangioendothelioma (Fig. 15.22), although pathologists do not encounter this tumor in the laboratory as frequently as it is encountered in the clinic. See the discussion of angiomas later in this chapter.

Also distinctive of infants, although not exclusive to this age group, is the mesenchymal hamartoma of the liver, a

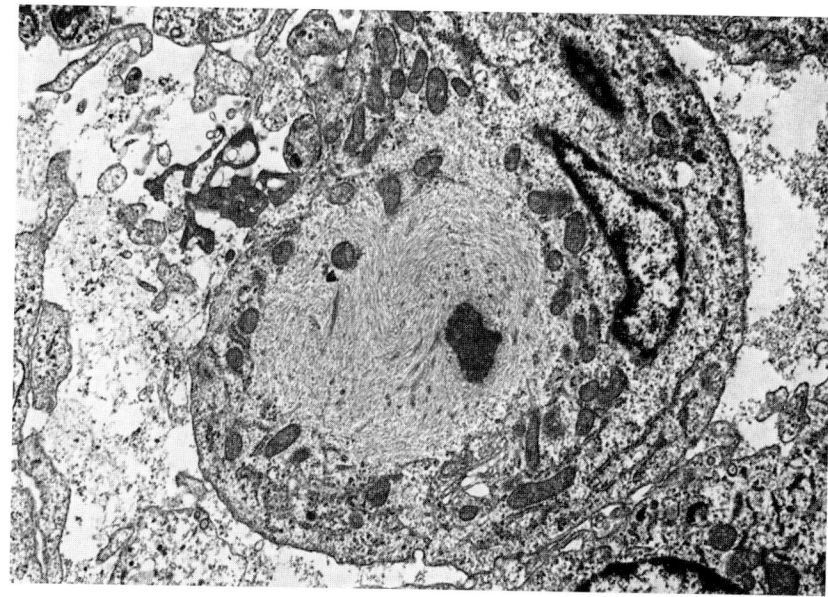

FIGURE 15.21. *Rhabdoid tumor cell shows tightly packed intermediate filaments in paranuclear position. (×10,200.)*

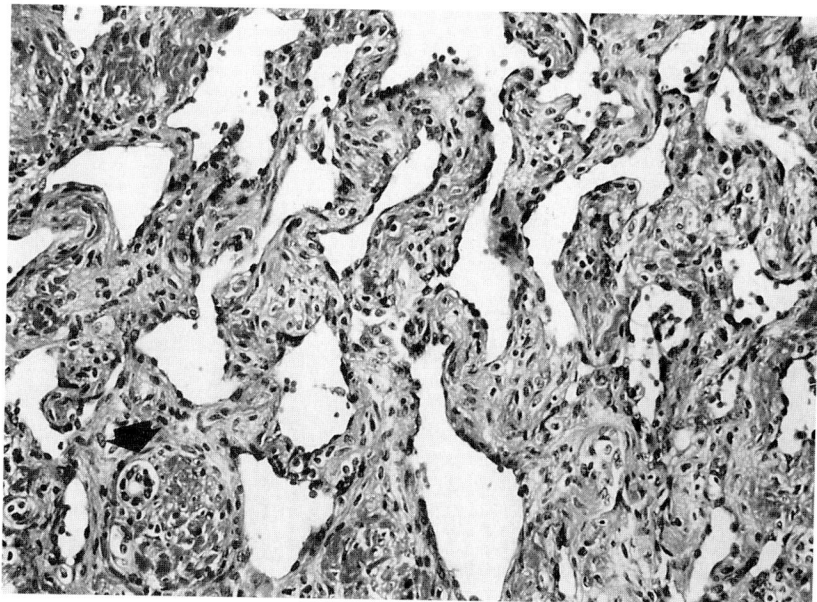

FIGURE 15.22. *Hemangioma of the liver in a newborn. The area illustrated here is no different from cavernous hemangiomas of the soft tissues, but cellularity varies greatly, ranging from "solid"-appearing zones to areas of marked cavitation. Note residual portal tract with bile duct (arrow).*

benign neoplasm that consists of a mixture of myxoid, embryonal-appearing mesenchyme, proliferating bile ducts, and blood vessels (Fig. 15.23a,b). "Cystification" may occur, leading to confusion with lymphangioma (Fig. 15.23c), the most common misidentification of this lesion. The cavities are pseudocysts formed by seepage of tissue fluid with no discernible lining. This hamartoma seems to reflect abnormal development of the portal tracts [151]. True cysts, most often asymptomatic and discovered incidentally, do occur in the infantile liver. Cysts may develop during embryonic development, probably as a result of inclusion of celomic epithelium in the liver parenchyma, and are sometimes called "nonparasitic" cysts to distinguish them from echinococcal cysts. They are perfectly encapsulated, usually single, uncon-

nected to the biliary system, and lined by a uniform small, cuboidal or attenuated layer of cells of probable mesothelial derivation (Fig. 15.24). Hepatic *adenoma* is rare in the pediatric age before adolescence, and almost unheard of in infancy. Nonetheless, a recent study shows that adenomas, albeit exceptionally, may be congenital, and associated with metabolic inheritable diseases [152]. *Focal nodular hyperplasia* is a tumor-like lesion that may be seen in infants, although its peak incidence is in adults and in children between the ages of 6 and 10 years. It may be a regenerative proliferation following a hypothetical vascular accident, because large vessels with fibrotic intimal changes are regularly seen in or near the center of this lesion, within scar tissue of more or less "stellate" shape. Fibrous tracts

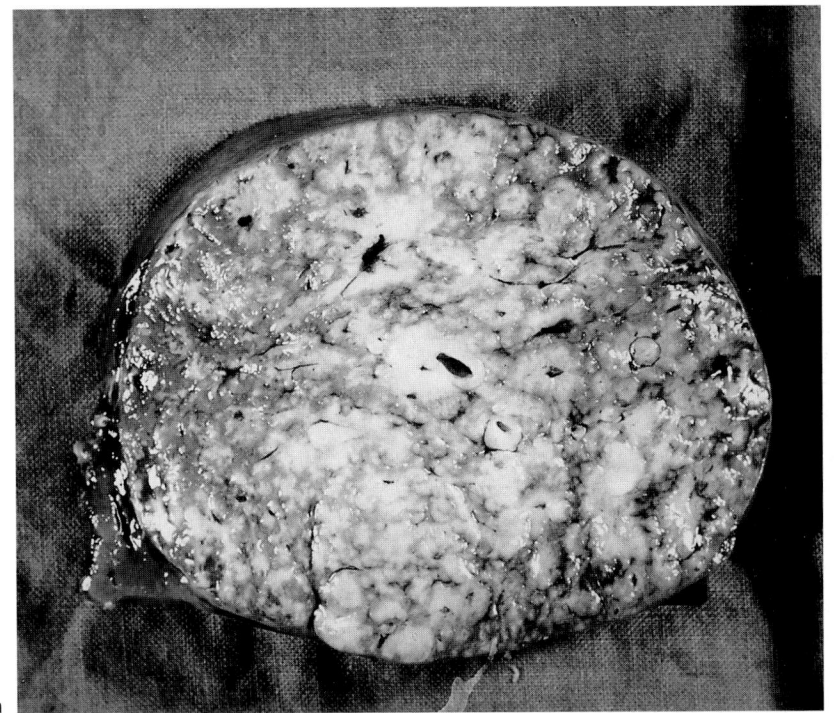

a

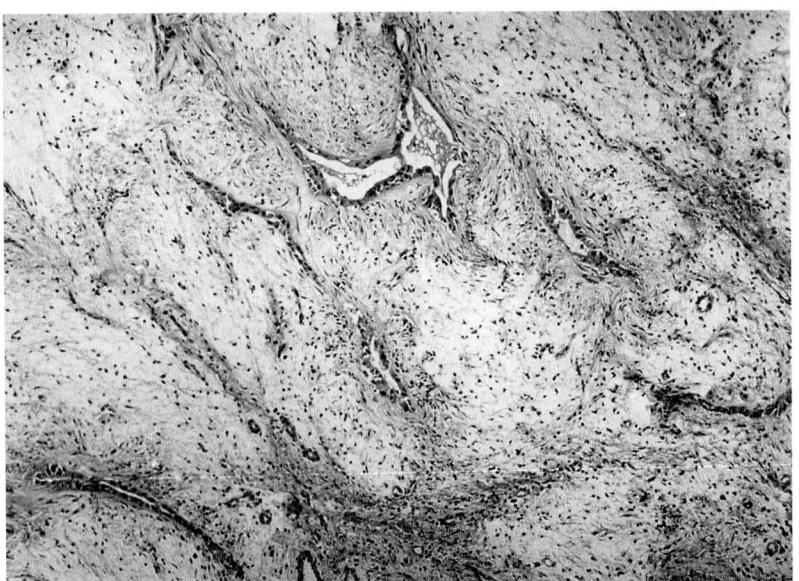

b

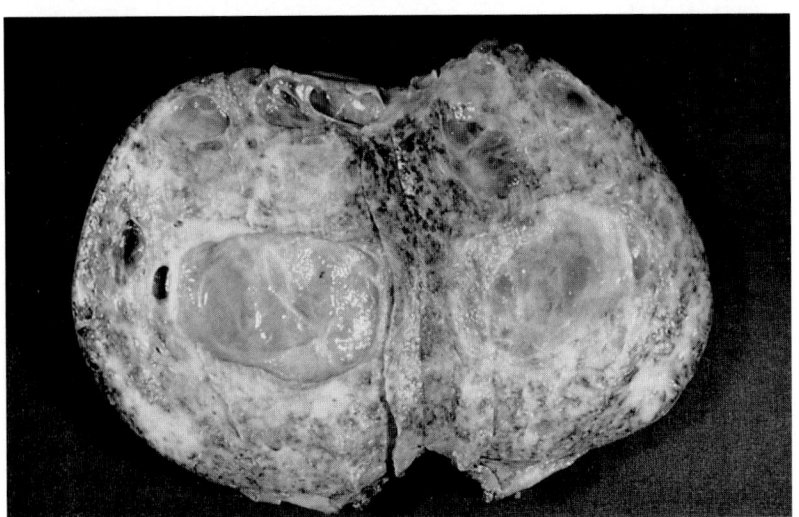

c

FIGURE 15.23. *(a) Typical gross appearance of mesenchymal hamartoma of the liver in an infant. The tumor is well demarcated, although not encapsulated, and could be removed in its entirety. The tumor parenchyma shows nacreous, whitish nodules interspersed with, and largely replacing, the normal brownish liver tissue. (b) Representative microscopic appearance of the whitish nodules of the hepatic mesenchymal hamartoma. The tumor tissue consists of loose mesenchyme, which may be more or less collagenized, in which are set bile ducts and blood vessels. (c) In this example of congenital mesenchymal hamartoma of the liver, pseudocysts have formed by fluid infiltration of the tumor. When this change occurs, the fluid-containing mass grossly resembles a lymphangioma.*

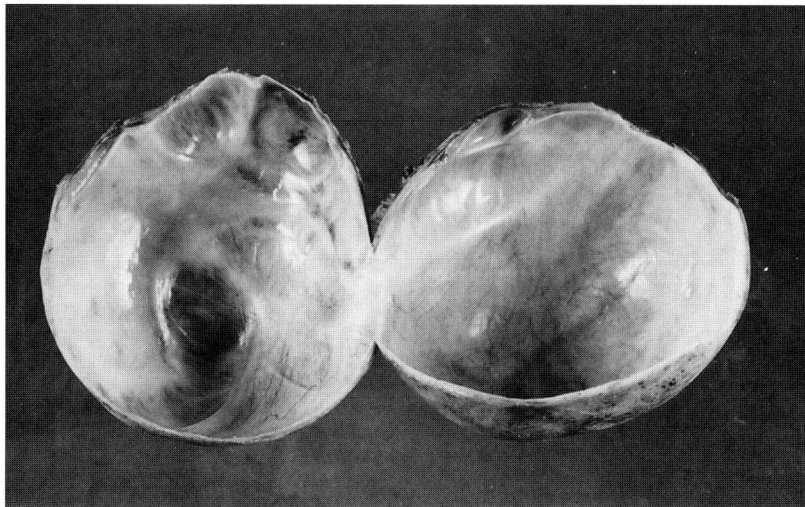

FIGURE 15.24. *Intrahepatic "simple" cyst of an asymptomatic infant. The lesion was discovered when hepatomegaly was detected on a routine check-up. Note smooth contour and lining.*

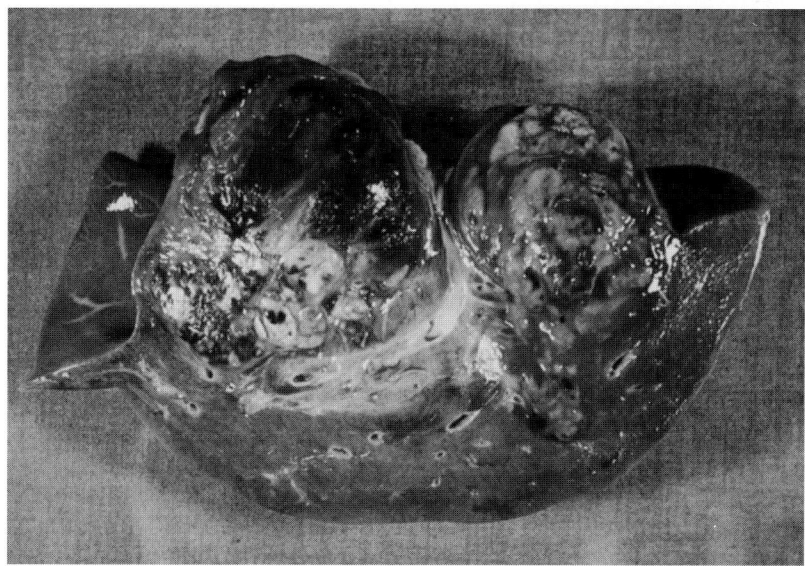

FIGURE 15.25. *Gross appearance of hepatoblastoma discovered in an infant who died before 1 year of age. Although the liver is characteristically non-cirrhotic, two large masses are present in close proximity, suggesting rapid growth of "satellite" nodule.*

carrying blood vessels irradiate from the central scar and partition the parenchyma of this lesion into irregular lobules.

Hepatoblastoma

Hepatoblastomas are the embryonic tumors of the liver and, although rare (their frequency is only a fraction of that of other solid malignancies, such as neuroblastomas or Wilms' tumor), they are the most common primary hepatic malignancies in infants under 3 years of age [68]. They may be congenital, and usually arise in a non-cirrhotic liver [14]. Hepatoblastomas often present as single palpable masses. We have seen large satellite nodules (Fig. 15.25) which, when present, make complete surgical excision more difficult to perform. Hepatoblastomas may be distinguished from hepatocarcinomas both histologically and clinically. Hepatic carcinomas are rarely seen in patients under 6 years of age. The

histological appearance of hepatoblastomas may be exclusively epithelial or mixed epithelial and mesenchymal. The epithelial component is made up of primitive hepatocytes that are reminiscent of the parenchymal liver cells of the fetus or embryo. These cells occur in different arrangements, depending on maturation of the tumor, from cord-like arrays that are virtually identical to normal liver, to nodules, rosettes, or diffuse masses without a specific architectural pattern (Fig. 15.26). Hemopoietic cell clusters are common between liver cell cords in the well-differentiated areas. Thus, the well-differentiated forms of hepatoblastomas have a histological appearance similar to normal fetal liver. Poorly differentiated tumors show no histological similarity to the normal liver (Fig. 15.27). It would be tempting to propose a better prognosis for the cytodifferentiated types, but there is no evidence at present in favor of this contention. The prognosis is a function of adequacy of surgical resection. The

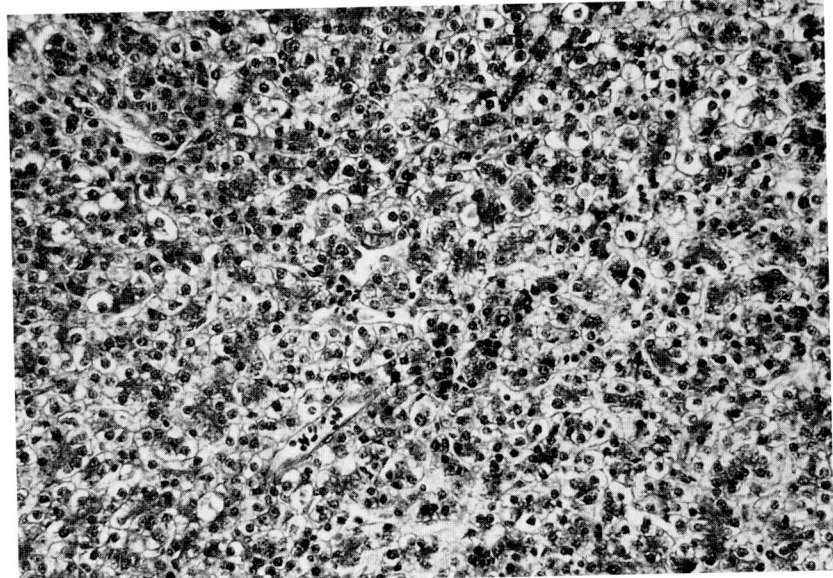

FIGURE 15.26. *Microscopic appearance of well-differentiated hepatoblastoma. The tumor closely reproduces the histology of normal liver, including the formation of liver cell plates, sinusoids, and central veins. No portal tracts are formed by hepatoblastomas, however, and cell size is smaller than in the normal, non-neoplastic liver.*

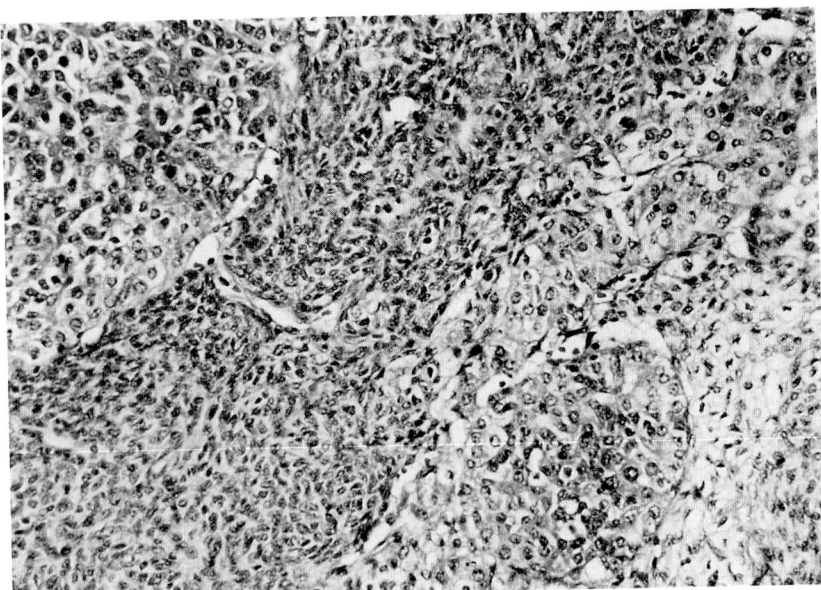

FIGURE 15.27. *Poorly differentiated area in a hepatoblastoma of "mixed" type, probably representing immature mesenchymal elements in close aggregation. Areas of undifferentiation do not reproduce the normal liver architecture.*

chances of survival are increased greatly when the tumor is resected entirely, before metastases appear. Chemotherapy is capable of bestowing some benefit, and sometimes impressive remissions.

The most malignant, and fortunately the rarest, form of hepatoblastoma is the anaplastic, small cell hepatoblastoma. It is entirely composed of small cells similar to neuroblasts or lymphoma cells. However, their hepatocytic lineage may be established by immunostaining or ultrastructural study [153]. To our knowledge, no long-term survivors have been reported with this highly aggressive tumor.

Embryonal Sarcoma

The liver sarcomas are extremely rare tumors, but may arise in newborn infants [154]. Rhabdomyosarcoma primary of the bile duct apparatus is similar to rhabdomyosarcoma botryoides of other sites, especially of the genitourinary tract. Undifferentiated (embryonal) sarcomas of the liver, apparently unrelated to the bile duct system, arise from primitive mesenchymal elements, without the features of cytodifferentiation apparent with conventional histological techniques [154]. With immunological and electron micro-

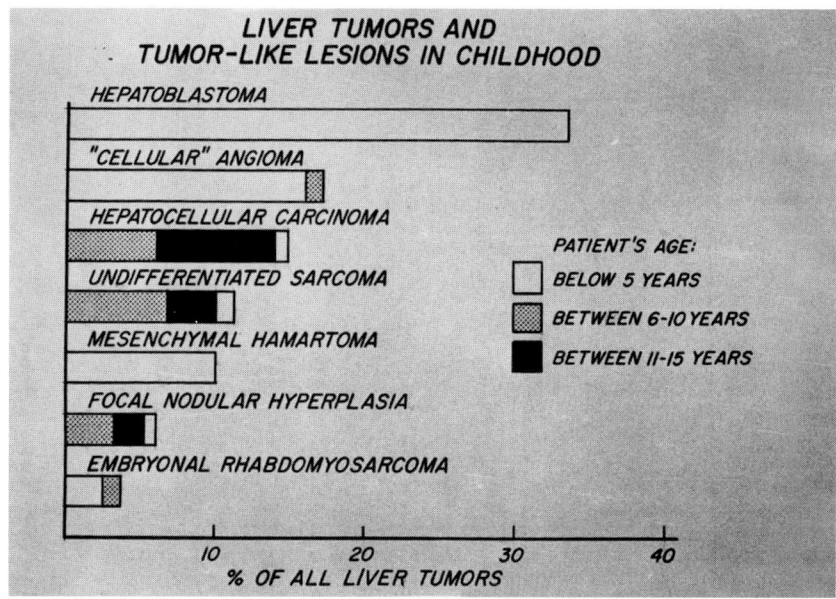

FIGURE 15.28. *Distribution of the major pathologic categories of hepatic tumor and tumor-like masses, according to age.*

scopic techniques it may be possible to detect evidence of rhabdomyoblastic or leiomyoblastic differentiation of the sarcoma cells. The differential diagnosis must include the mesenchymal component of a hepatoblastoma since, as previously noted, some hepatoblastomas have both hepatocytic and mesenchymal components ("mixed" hepatoblastoma). The distinction rests on the presence of an epithelial or hepatocellular component, which is not seen in primary sarcomas of the liver.

It should be emphasized that malignant primary hepatic tumors in the neonate or young infant are extremely uncommon, and the majority are hepatoblastomas. The rare liver sarcomas when found in the neonate are almost always rhabdomyosarcomas of bile duct origin. Undifferentiated (embryonal) hepatic sarcomas may occur in infants, but the greatest incidence is in older children and adolescents. Other primary liver tumors reported in newborns include mesenchymal hamartomas [14] and teratomas [155]. A hepatocellular carcinoma associated with macronodular cirrhosis in a 5-day-old infant has been reported [156] (Fig. 15.28).

NEUROBLASTOMA

Neuroblastomas are enigmatic and fundamentally different childhood tumors whose wide variety of biological vagaries sets them apart from any other human neoplasms. These vagaries, excellently summarized by Jaffe [157], include a high rate of spontaneous remission, regression, or maturation, variable prognosis, possible susceptibility to immune mechanisms, secretion of specific biochemical markers, familial occurrence, peculiar syndromes, consumptive coagulopathies, and occasional coexistence with other diseases or tumors of neural crest origin.

Neuroblastomas—tumors derived from the neural crest—are the fourth most common malignant tumors of childhood (after leukemia, central nervous system tumors, and lymphomas). It is estimated that 1 in 100,000 children under 15 years of age develops neuroblastomas [8]. In the newborn period, neuroblastomas are the most frequent malignant neoplasms, accounting for 30% to 50% of all malignancies in this age group [13, 14].

Tumors derived from neuroblasts present a wide spectrum of histological variations, ranging from poorly differentiated malignancies to fully mature neoplasms. Accordingly, they can be classified into five types, as follows:

1. *Undifferentiated* or *poorly differentiated neuroblastomas*—malignant tumors composed of diffuse sheets of uniformly small, dark neuroblasts considerably larger than lymphocytes. The neoplastic cells have little cytoplasm and a relatively large round nucleus, no visible nucleolus, and fine evenly dispersed chromatin. The neuroblasts have minimal fibrils, variable pseudo-rosette formation, and poor compartmentalization.
2. *Differentiated neuroblastomas*—where the neuroblasts have a tendency to aggregate, clump or form Homer-Wright pseudo-rosettes. The latter lack a central lumen but contain abundant eosinophilic fibrillar material. A delicate fibrovascular stroma divides the tumor cells into compartments or nests (Fig. 15.29).
3. *Ganglioneuroblastomas*—which consist of a not necessarily equal mixture of both neuroblasts and ganglion cells against a background of neurofibrils and nerve fibers.

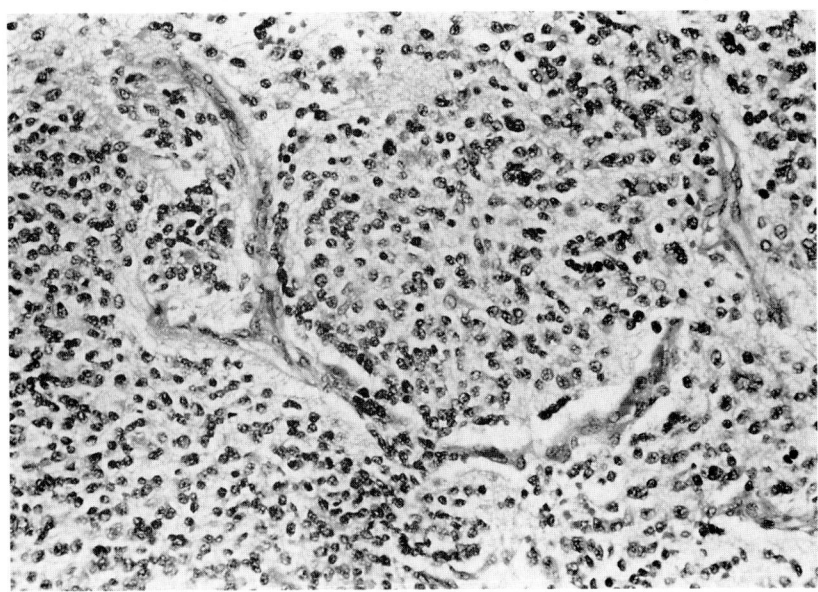

FIGURE 15.29. *Classic histopathology of a differentiating neuroblastoma. Note the compartmentalization of tumor cells by a fine fibrovascular network.*

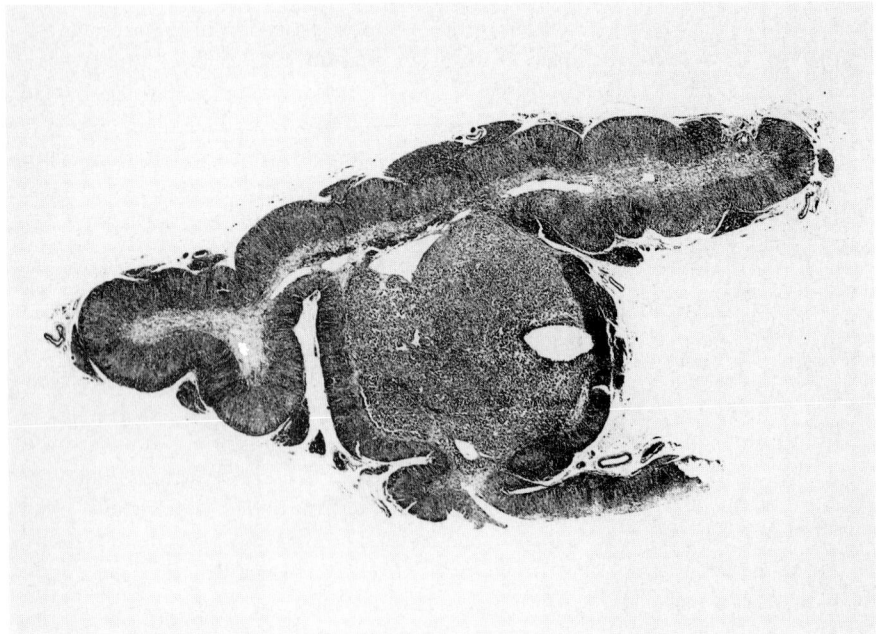

FIGURE 15.30. *In situ neuroblastoma. Notice the expansile nature of the nodule.*

4. *Ganglioneuromas*—benign neoplasms composed of mature ganglion cells in a background of Schwann cells, neurofibrils arranged in coarse interlacing fascicles, and fibrous tissue.
5. *Composite ganglioneuroblastomas*—subsets of ganglioneuromas which contain foci of poorly or partially differentiated neuroblasts that retain the capacity to metastasize. The ganglion cells are surrounded by mature neuromatous stroma similar to that of ganglioneuromas.

In Situ Neuroblastoma

One of the most intriguing phenomena in a neuroblastoma is its evolution from an in situ lesion to a fully developed and metastatic malignant tumor. An in situ neuroblastoma was defined by Beckwith and Perrin [158] as a minute, incidentally encountered, adrenal tumor of newborns and young infants, composed of neuroblasts indistinguishable from cells of a typical neuroblastoma (Figs. 15.30 and 15.31). These authors proposed that the in situ lesion represents an early stage in the development of a neuroblastoma. In normal fetal and newborn adrenal glands, primitive sympathetic cells migrate to and locate in the central medullary regions, where cell division and differentiation occur (Fig. 15.32) [159]. A certain proportion of the sympathetic cells differentiate into neuroblasts and ganglion cells, whereas others differentiate into pheochromoblasts and chromaffin cells (Fig. 15.33). This requires a precise equilibrium between cell proliferation and differentiation. In an in situ neuroblastoma, dividing and proliferating neuroblasts can be seen in the central adrenal region but differentiation into ganglion cells has been documented rarely (Fig. 15.34). Neuroblasts of an in situ neuroblastoma do not express a distinct phenotype; they are histologically and ultrastructurally identical to normal neural crest aggregates of the fetal adrenal glands

[160]. It has been suggested that an in situ neuroblastoma is not a tumor, but rather a hyperplastic nodule of initiated preneoplastic cells lacking a second "hit" [161].

In situ neuroblastomas have been identified in about one in 150 to 300 pediatric postmortems in infants under the age of 3 months [107, 158], which is 50- to 70-fold greater than the incidence of neuroblastomas. This suggests that the great majority of these lesions cytodifferentiate into normal constituents of the adrenal medulla or undergo necrosis and calcification (Figs. 15.35 and 15.36).

Although a variety of malformations have been found in association with in situ neuroblastomas [107, 158, 162], a statistically probable relationship has not been established yet. Infants with pathologically diagnosed neuroblastomas in situ are drawn from postmortem populations heavily

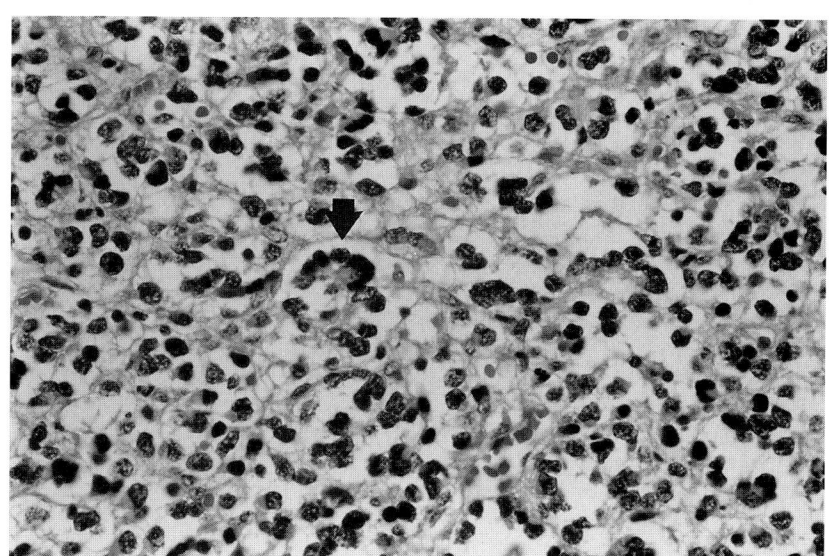

FIGURE 15.31. *In situ neuroblastoma demonstrating cellularity and poor pseudorosette formation* (arrow).

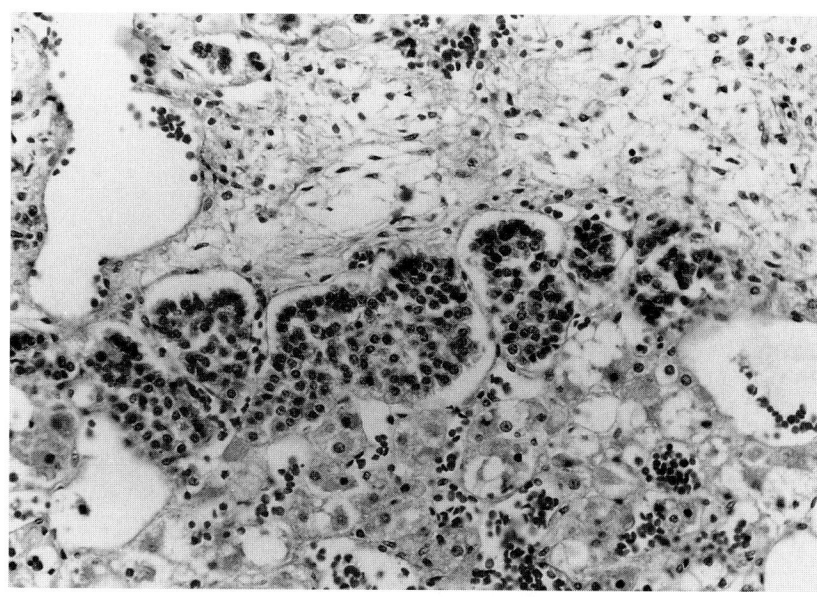

FIGURE 15.32. *Neuroblastic rests are shown in the center of this photograph.*

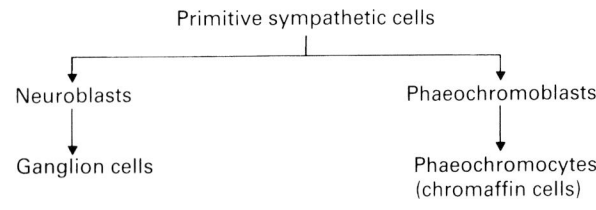

Primitive sympathetic cells

Neuroblasts   Phaeochromoblasts

Ganglion cells   Phaeochromocytes
                     (chromaffin cells)

FIGURE 15.33.   *Histogenesis of ganglion cells and chromaffin cells.*

weighted by malformations [107]. Similarly, a putative association between neuroblastomas and specific congenital anomalies has not been established and, when identified, they follow no regular pattern [163–165].

Remission, Regression, and Maturation

Neuroblastomas may spontaneously remit and mature into ganglioneuromas [166]. Most cases of histological maturation are associated with extra-adrenal neuroblastomas, and

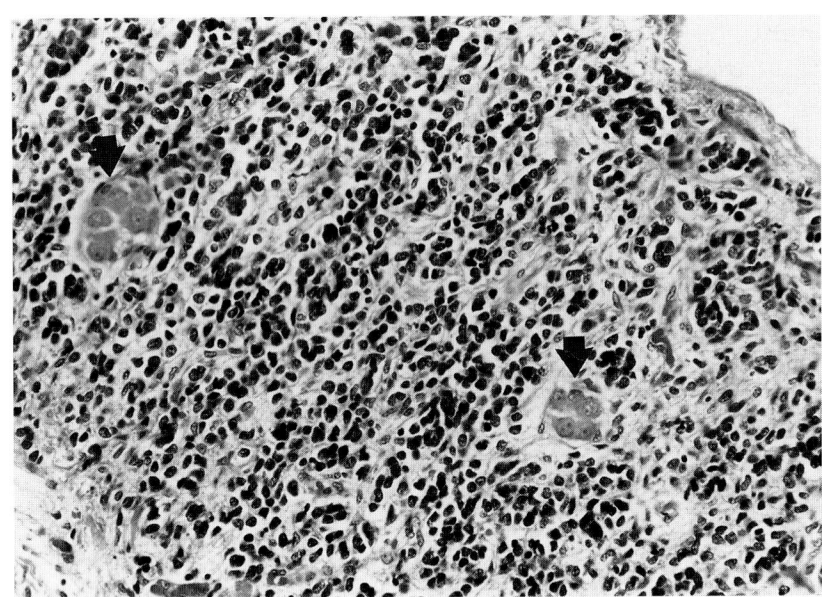

FIGURE 15.34.   *In situ neuroblastoma showing focal collections of ganglion cells (arrow). The central adrenal vein is seen in the upper right corner.*

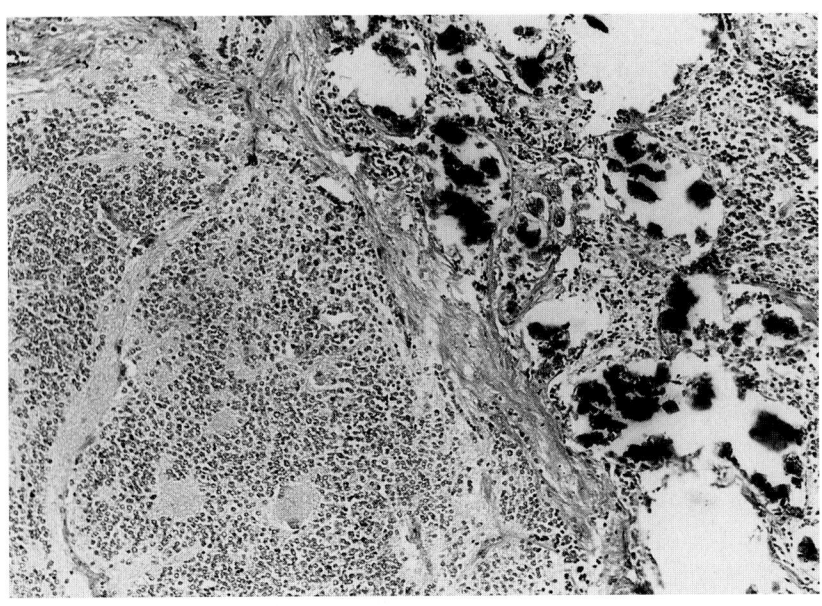

FIGURE 15.35.   *In situ neuroblastoma showing extensive necrosis and calcification.*

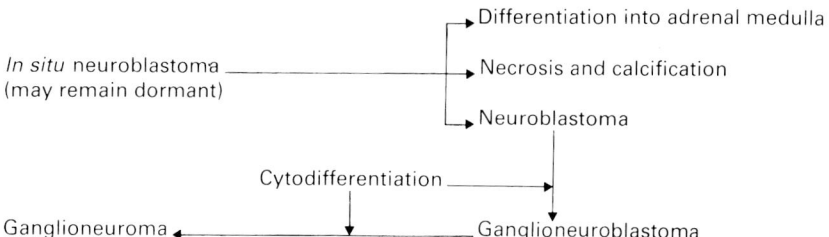

FIGURE 15.36. *Histogenesis and possible fates of neuroblastoma.*

Table 15.5. Clinical staging of a neuroblastoma

Stage I	Tumor confined to the organ or structure of origin
Stage II	Tumor extending in continuity beyond the organ or structure of origin but not crossing the midline. Regional lymph nodes on the ipsilateral side may be involved*
Stage III	Tumor extending in continuity beyond the midline. Regional lymph nodes may be involved bilaterally
Stage IV	Remote disease involving the skeleton, organs, soft tissue, or distant lymph nodes
Stage IV-S	Patients who would otherwise be stage I or II, but who have remote disease confined to the liver, skin, or bone marrow, and who have no radiographic evidence of bone metastases on complete skeletal survey

* For tumors arising in midline structures, e.g., the organ of Zuckerkandl, penetration beyond the capsule and lymph node involvement are considered to be stage II. Bilateral extensions of any sort are considered to be stage III.

are seen in older children without bone metastases [157]. The factors responsible for maturation are unknown, but nerve growth factor [167] and chemotherapy [157] have been implicated. The most dramatic spontaneous regression of neuroblastomas occurs in stage IV-S (Table 15.5). This special form of disseminated neuroblastoma, predominantly occurring in patients in the first year of life, makes up to 11% of the total number of patients with neuroblastomas [168].

Knudson and Meadows [161] believe that the multiple lesions observed in a IV-S neuroblastoma are neither metastases nor multiple primary tumors, but are nodules of hyperplastic neural crest elements with a germinal one-hit mutation. Delayed maturation may transform these nodules into ganglioneuromas or neurofibromas. A second hit may transform the hyperplastic nodules or the ganglioneuromas–neurofibromas into neuroblastomas or neurofibrosarcomas, respectively.

Prognostic Factors

The prognosis of children with neuroblastomas is influenced by two independent variables: the age of the patient at time of diagnosis, and the clinical stage [169].

Age and Stage

The age of the patient in which this tumor is diagnosed is one of the major prognostic determinants [157]. Stage for stage, children less than 1 year of age fare better than do older children. Cure is most often seen in children under the age of 1 year (about 60%) as compared to those over 2 years (13%) [166]. The staging system proposed by Evans et al [170] is useful for estimating prognosis and for planning therapy (Table 15.5). Children under the age of 1 year with a stage IV neuroblastoma have a significantly better prognosis than older children in the same stage, but their prognosis is still poor (18% survival) [171]. Children less than 1 year old with a stage I or IV-S neuroblastoma have an extremely good prognosis (90% survival) [171].

Miscellaneous Prognostic Factors

Site of Origin and Metastases Another factor known to influence the outcome of children with neuroblastomas is the site of origin. Patients with primary tumors in the cervical and thoracic areas have a better prognosis than those with retroperitoneal tumors [172, 173]. The site of the metastases also influences the outcome of the disease. Spinal cord metastases are usually associated with relatively high survival rates, whereas bone metastases accompanied by roentgenographic evidence of bone involvement are associated with an unfavorable outcome.

Oncogenes It has been found that amplification of the *N-myc* gene in a primary untreated neuroblastoma correlates with an advanced disease state [174]. Seeger et al [175] have demonstrated an association between genomic amplification and tumor growth, and suggest that genomic amplification plays a key role in determining the aggressiveness of the neuroblastoma.

Histopathology Various systems for the histological grading of neuroblastomas have been devised [176, 177]. One of the simplest classifications is that of Beckwith and Martin [176], who divided neuroblastomas into four grades according to the quality and quantity of the neoplastic cells:

Grade I Predominantly differentiated: over 50% differentiating cells.

Grade II Predominantly undifferentiated: 5% to 50% differentiating cells.

Grade III Slightly differentiated: under 5% differentiating cells.

Grade IV Undifferentiated: no recognizable neurogenesis.

Beckwith and Martin [176] analyzed these grades with age and site of primary tumor. Their data showed a clear maturation–survival relationship, but no statistically significant correlation was found between grade and age of the patient at diagnosis. Neuroblastomas arising in the adrenal glands tended to be undifferentiated.

Following the widely used classification developed by Shimada et al [177], a primitive neuroblastoma in which more than 5% of the cells show morphologic evidence of differentiation (enlargement of the nucleus and the cytoplasm, conspicuous appearance of nucleolus, cytoplasmic eosinophilia) is called "differentiating." With still greater maturation, Schwannian stromal cells increase in number, and the neuroblastic cells progress toward ganglion cells; when only a few, scattered neuroblasts are present, the stage is designated an *intermixed, stroma rich* neuroblastoma. Joshi [178] has discussed the criteria used in the histologic grading of neuroblastoma, and recognized that there is a blurred demarcation between a well-differentiated, "stroma rich" neuroblastoma and what many pathologists call ganglioneuroblastoma. *Ganglioneuroma* is the final stage of maturation, in which the stromal elements dominate the morphology, with only mature ganglion cells surrounded by satellite cells in the stroma.

It seems established that, biologically, neuroblastomas are of two kinds: one may show a tendency to regress or to mature, and is associated with good prognosis, and the other follows an aggressive course and responds poorly to therapy. Multidisciplinary research has been geared to understand the basis underlying these "favorable" and "unfavorable" tumor forms. Substrate-adherent growth in tissue culture is a feature of neuroblastoma cells, supported by chemical compounds and growth factors (cyclic AMP, papaverine, prostaglandin E1, nerve growth factor, cytosine arabinoside, etc.). The ability to establish a permanent cell line correlates with "unfavorable" biologic behavior. Chromosome 1 deletions, at the critical area 1p36, are the most characteristic karyotypic abnormality of neuroblastoma, and are thought to be associated with damage to a neuroblastoma suppressor gene, as they correlate with malignant transformation [179]. Loss of heterozygosity at the distal short arm of chromosome 1 was recently demonstrated in about 20% of primary neuroblastomas [180]; cloning of the putative gene at 1p36.2–1p36.3 is now awaited. Amplification of the MYCN (N-*myc*) oncogene is associated with rapid progression and worse outcome than tumors without this feature, even in the presence of low clinical stage [179]. Ploidy is another important parameter. Paradoxically, abnormally high DNA content is correlated with better prognosis; in infants with localized disease, the tumor is usually hyperdiploid [181]. Expression of the nerve growth factor receptor encoded by the TRK proto-oncogene (also known as TRKA), a transmembrane glycoprotein with tyrosine kinase activity, is associated with "favorable" neuroblastoma [182].

Numerous laboratory tests and clinical observations have been developed to predict with considerable accuracy the prognosis of an individual case. Basic understanding of the biologic substratum of the behavior of the tumor has progressed considerably. Many of these evaluative measures are applied to the resected tumor tissue, but much needs to be learned before the prognostic assessment can be done preoperatively.

Ultrastructure and Biochemical Markers

Ultrastructural features common to neuroblastomas, ganglioneuroblastomas, and ganglioneuromas are cytoplasmic neuritic processes and dense-core neurosecretory granules (Fig. 15.37) [183]. The cytoplasmic neuritic processes increase in number with advancing cytodifferentiation from neuroblastoma to ganglioneuroma [184]. Neurosecretory granules are most commonly found within neuritic processes and occasionally in the perinuclear cytoplasm. Microtubules, desmosomes, and microfilaments are relatively common in neuroblastomas, but they are neither consistently present nor sufficiently distinctive in separating neuroblastomas from other small round-cell tumors [134].

A positive correlation between increased numbers of neurosecretory granules and prognostically favorable biochemical excretory patterns has been reported by Romansky et al [184]. Conversely, low numbers of neurosecretory granules are associated with an unfavorable biochemical pattern and fatal clinical course [184]. Urine catecholamine metabolites are elevated in about 75% to 80% of patients with neuroblastomas [185]. For patients with a stage IV neuroblastoma, the higher the urinary vanillic acid to homovanillmandelic acid ratio, the better the prognosis. Absolute amounts of urinary homovanillic acid do not have a predictive value, whereas the higher the vanillmandelic acid, the better the prognosis [186]. Other biochemical markers used to monitor tumor activity include dopamine, adrenaline, noradrenaline, 3-methoxy-4-hydroxyphenylethylene glycol, dopamine beta-hydroxylase, cystathionine, and carcinoembryonic antigen.

Immunohistochemistry

Neurone-specific enolase has been immunohistochemically demonstrated in neuroblastomas, ganglioneuromas, and paragangliomas, but it is not restricted to nervous system neoplasms or APUD-derived tumors [187, 188]. Glycoxylic acid-induced catecholamine fluorescence of the cytoplasm of neoplastic cells and tissue culture morphology are also helpful diagnostic tools in the identification of neuroblastomas [189].

Miscellaneous peculiarities described in the neuroblastoma include consumptive coagulopathy [190], nesidioblastosis [191], opsoclonus–myoclonus syndrome [192], and Horner syndrome [193]. Familial neuroblastomas have been described in the literature. In one report [13], four out of five children in a family had neuroblastomas; their mother had persistently elevated urinary catecholamines and a posterior mediastinal mass, presumably a ganglioneuroma [194].

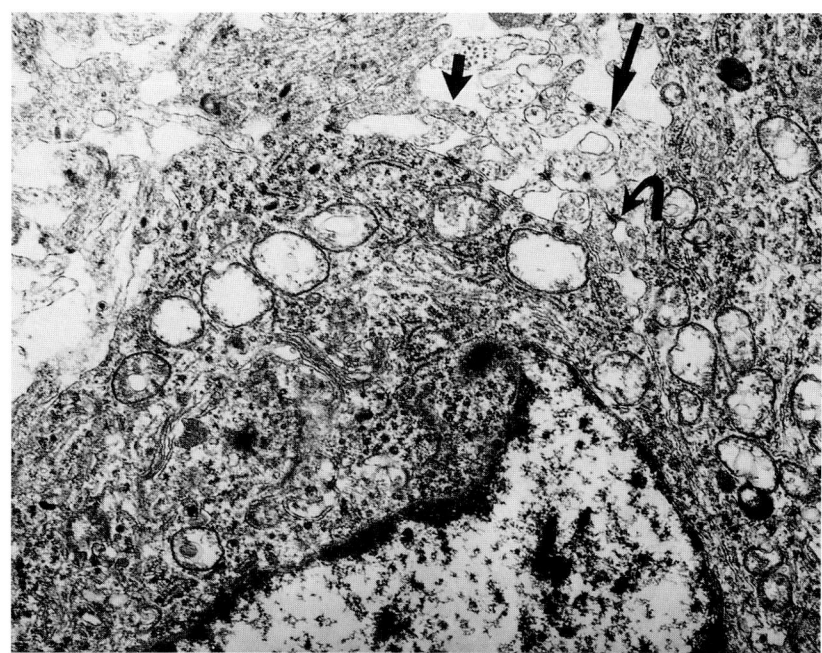

FIGURE 15.37. *Typical ultrastructural features of a neuroblastoma include cytoplasmic neuritic processes* (short arrow) *and dense core neurosecretory granules* (long arrow). *A poorly developed cytoplasmic junction is present* (curved arrow). *(×21,900.)*

Neuroblastomas have been linked to a constellation of genetically related diseases, generically termed neurocristopathies [195]. Pheochromocytoma, neurofibromatosis, medullary carcinoma of the thyroid, carcinoid tumors, Hirschsprung disease, and non-chromaffin paragangliomas are some of the related disorders whose origin has been linked to abnormal migration, growth, and differentiation of neural crest elements. We have seen megakaryocytic leukemia (M7) in the liver that simulated metastatic neuroblastoma. Thus, combined immunohistochemistry and electron microscopy may be necessary to arrive at a correct diagnosis in poorly differentiated tumors.

TERATOMA

A teratoma is generally defined as a tumor arising from pluripotent cells, and it is precisely the heterogeneity of tissues present in such a tumor that best characterizes it; it is also commonly accepted that a teratoma must contain derivatives of more than one blastodermic layer, according to traditional concepts of embryonic ontogenesis. An important characteristic of teratomas of the newborn is their surprising capacity to form structures that "simulate" or "reproduce" organ development, as observed in the embryo and fetus. In general, this ability correlates with the degree of differentiation of the teratoma, and the resulting tissues are called "organoid" structures. There is virtually no tissue in the body that cannot find its simile in teratomas: pancreatic acini, myocardium, endocrine tissues, glia, neurones, skin, bowel, and others have been identified in teratomas at one time or another. Even the ocular lens is a structure

reported to occur, though rarely, in teratomas. The capacity for differentiation of teratoma cells is so great that it is rash to state that one or other type of tissue "is never found" in these tumors. Whenever such a statement has been made, subsequent reports have disproved the validity of this generalization [196].

Teratomas, unlike most human neoplasms, are classified into benign, malignant, and immature. They are, by definition, composed of a wide variety of tissues haphazardly arranged, usually representing derivatives of the three germ layers (although this is not indispensable for diagnosis), and of a nature that is alien to the site where they originate. Immature teratomas may be defined as teratomas composed of tissues whose maturity lags behind with respect to the tissues of the host. Thus, restricted foci of neuroblasts are not unusual in the periventricular region of the brain in a newborn, and may be expected in a teratoma of a neonate, but would be discrepant in a child several years old. In general, a large amount of immature tissues bespeaks potential aggressiveness, although this statement must be qualified according to the site of origin and other clinical characteristics of the neoplasm. The caveat must be reiterated that in discussing germ cell tumors of infancy it is difficult to generalize; cases must be evaluated individually. For instance, testicular teratomas in infants and young children may contain abundant immature somatic tissues, but no case has been known to pursue an aggressive, metastasizing course in the absence of germ cell malignant tumor as part of the teratoma. Nonetheless, various histologic grading systems have been developed that use the amount of immature tissues present in a teratoma as a criterion to

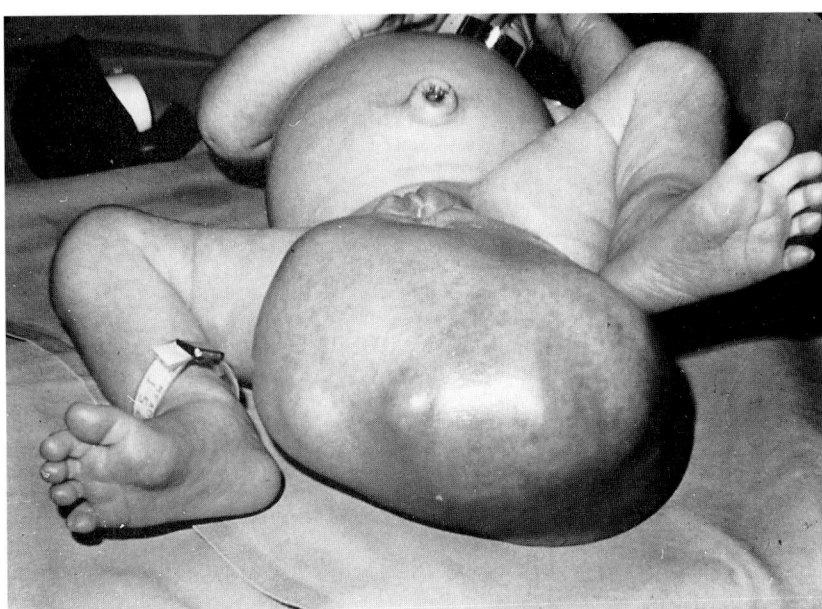

FIGURE 15.38. *Common appearance of a congenital sacrococcygeal teratoma. Although the dimensions of these tumors may be massive, surgical excision is usually well tolerated by newborn patients.*

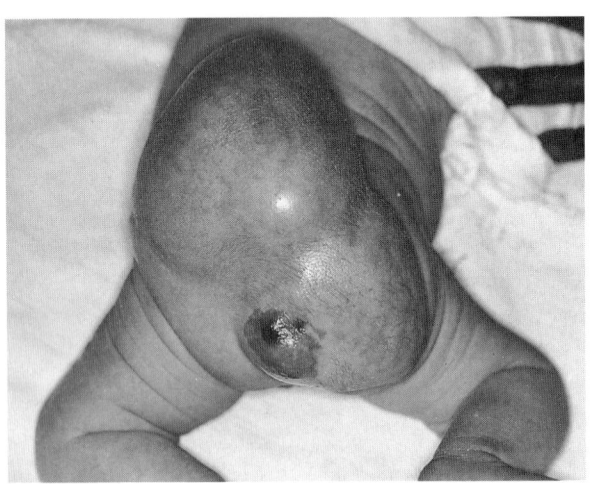

FIGURE 15.39. *Asymmetrical growth of sacrococcygeal mass in this patient is due to the simultaneous presence of a sacrococcygeal teratoma and myelomeningocele. Myelomeningocele may simulate teratoma clinically, and constitutes an important differential diagnosis.*

gauge prognosis [196]; this approach has been validated by experience.

Sacrococcygeal teratoma appears typically as a mass attached by a broad pedicle to the sacrococcygeal region of term infants, predominantly of the female sex. It may also be hidden in the hollow of the sacrum, retroperitoneally. As all teratomas, it may be cystic or solid. The majority are benign, but tend to recur when they are not surgically excised en bloc with the coccyx. Occasionally, a sacrococ-

cygeal teratoma that was diagnosed as benign after thorough sampling of the resected primary may recur as an undifferentiated tumor. Although the reasonable assumption is that in such cases a focus of malignancy went undetected, the true explanation is not always clear. Regardless of the cause, a practical corollary is that oncofetal markers of high sensitivity, such as alpha-fetoprotein, should be investigated in the serum of patients with teratomas, regardless of their histologic appearance. A persistent rise after surgery is prima facie evidence of recurrence, and a stronger indication of the probable malignancy of the tumor than the histologic assessment of the primary.

Teratoma was the most frequent tumor at the Children's Hospital of Los Angeles, with 40 examples among 110 neonatal tumors [14]. Of all teratomas, sacrococcygeal tumors are the most prevalent in newborns (Figs. 15.38 and 15.39) [14, 196, 197]. Since the advent of ultrasonography, diagnosis is frequently made prenatally. With modern imaging techniques, complications such as severe dystocia caused by the teratoma, nonimmunological fetal hydrops, polyhydramnios, or bleeding of the tumor from tears during parturition are preventable [198, 199]. The affected infant is female in over three-quarters of the cases [196, 197, 200], and the tumor is, in most cases, unaccompanied by any other life-threatening anomalies [196]. Surgical correction is therefore the dominating concern, and this should be undertaken as soon as possible. In the present state of surgical and medical advance, it is often possible and important to excise the tumor completely, even when massive, on the first day of life. The chances for malignancy to manifest in the tumor are greater the longer it is allowed to remain in the patient. Up to the fourth month of life, most teratomas are benign and composed of mature tissues (Figs. 15.40 and 15.41); but

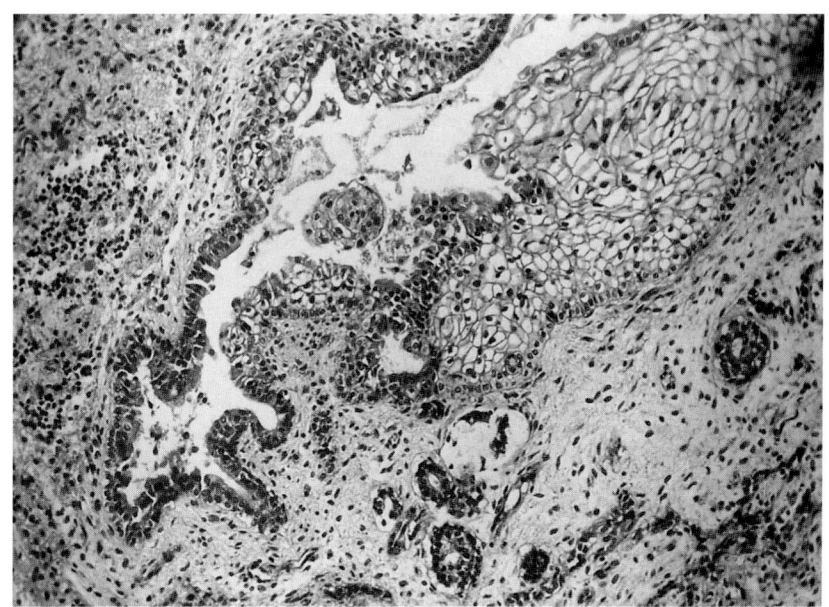

FIGURE 15.40. *Histological area from a benign sacrococcygeal teratoma. In these tumors, cysts are very common, and appear lined by different types of epithelium. In the area illustrated, a cyst is lined partly by squamous epithelium and partly by columnar, ciliated epithelium. Glia is present around the cyst.*

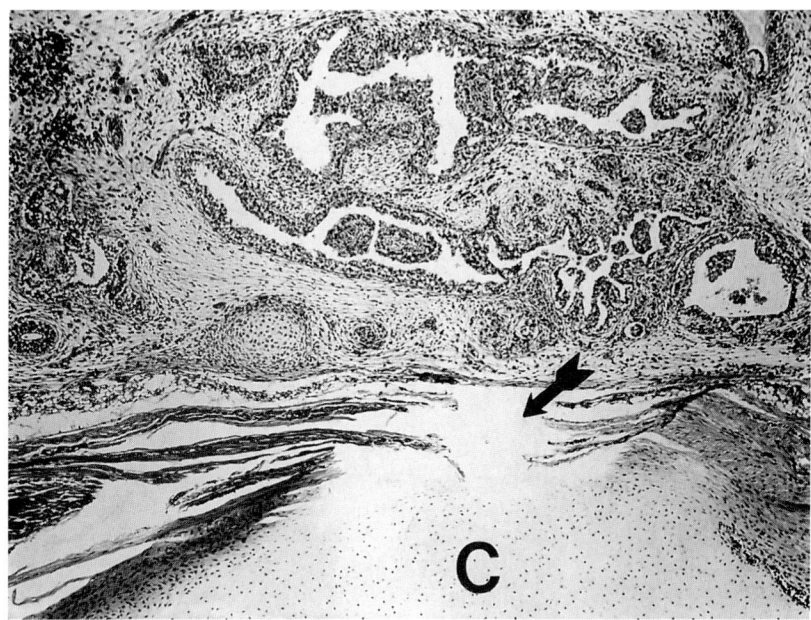

FIGURE 15.41. *Teratomatous tissues in close proximity to the patient's coccyx (C) illustrate the need to surgically remove the coccyx en bloc with the tumor, in order to avoid recurrence. Break in the perichondrial fibrous tissue (arrow) may be artefactual in nature.*

the majority of those removed in older children, especially over 2 years of age, are malignant. It is not well understood why this should be the case, since malignancy probably does not develop de novo in a preexistent tumor. It may be that primitive germ cells remain dormant for a time but embark on a differentiation pathway of germ cell malignancy if the tumor remains undisturbed in its host [196].

In most cases, when the teratoma is malignant it owes its malignant character to tissue having the morphology of a yolk sac carcinoma or endodermal sinus tumor. Accordingly, the detection of alpha-fetoprotein in the serum of these

patients is a useful clinical tool. This type of malignancy is observed generally in teratomas of childhood. Rarely do the malignant tissues of a teratoma adopt a different form (Fig. 15.42). On occasion, probably no more than in 2% of teratomas, it is the immature neuroectodermal component that behaves aggressively, including the development of metastases [196]. The rarity with which this occurs justifies a cautiously conservative attitude vis-à-vis the teratomas that contain no germ cell malignancy; however, teratomas that contain a very large amount (half or more of the total bulk of the tumor) of primitive neuroectodermal tissue should be

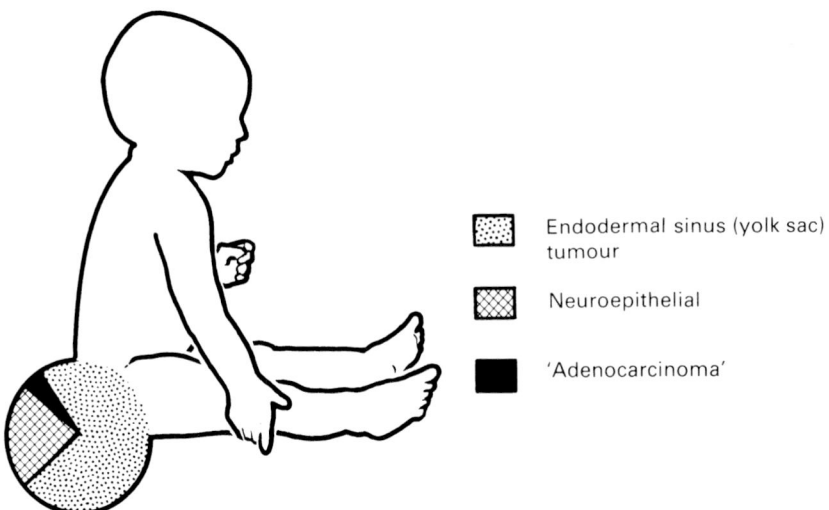

FIGURE 15.42.   *Malignancy in sacrococcygeal teratomas is due, in more than three-quarters of the cases, to endodermal sinus (yolk sac) tumor; metastases are frequent. Less than one-quarter of these tumors have inordinate amounts of primitive neuroectodermal tumor; metastases in such cases are possible, but quite rare. An "adenocarcinoma" pattern is uncommonly reported, but its histogenesis is unclear; some of these cases may correspond to neuroectodermal tubule-forming tissue, incorrectly interpreted as secretory gland formation.*

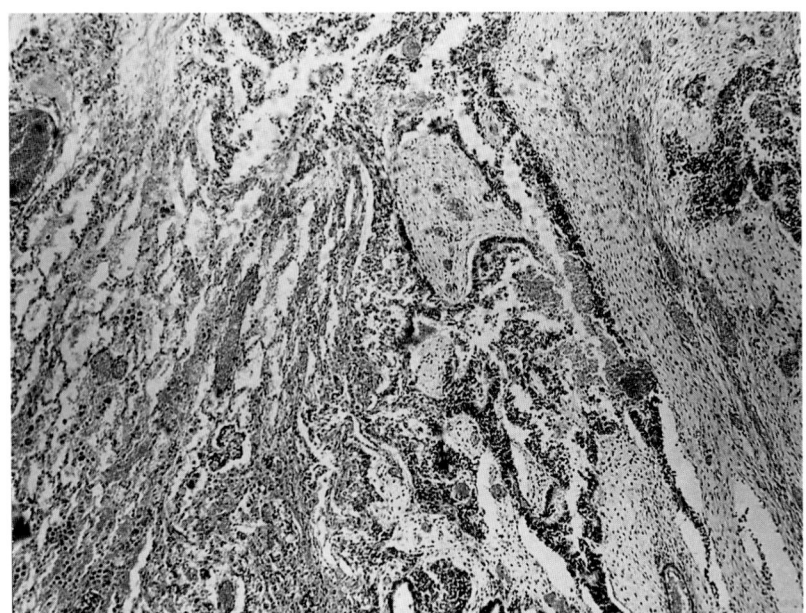

FIGURE 15.43.   *Primitive neuroectodermal tissue metastatic to lung from a sacrococcygeal teratoma. Although exceptional, this occurrence demonstrates the malignant potential of neuroectodermal tissue.*

viewed as potentially malignant (Figs. 15.43 and 15.44). In our experience, widely metastasizing neuroectodermal tissue in teratomas often contains tubular structures reminiscent of the primitive embryonic neural tube. The tubular histological appearance often misleads the pathologist into diagnosing "adenocarcinomas" of various histogeneses, an error that may be avoided today by performing immunohistological procedures that reveal the presence of neural antigens.

Teratomas occur in other sites of the body, generally along the midline; the biology of this tumor seems to depend to some extent on the anatomical location in which they arise and on the age of the patient. Teratomas of the testis in infants have a good prognosis (Fig. 15.45). We know of no well-authenticated case of a testicular teratoma with metastases at presentation in individuals below the age of 4 years. This is in striking contrast to testicular teratomas of adolescents or young adults. By the same token, testicular teratomas of young children or infants appear to be composed of somatic tissues of various degrees of differentiation and maturation, but usually do not contain areas of germ

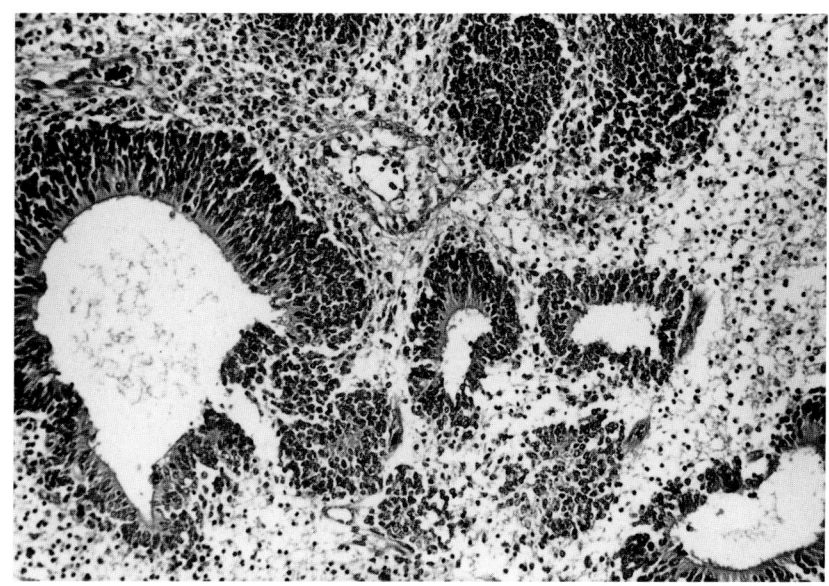

FIGURE 15.44.   *Primitive neuroectodermal tissue forming tubular structures. When neuroepithelium vastly predominates, the resulting histological appearance is often called an "adenocarcinoma."*

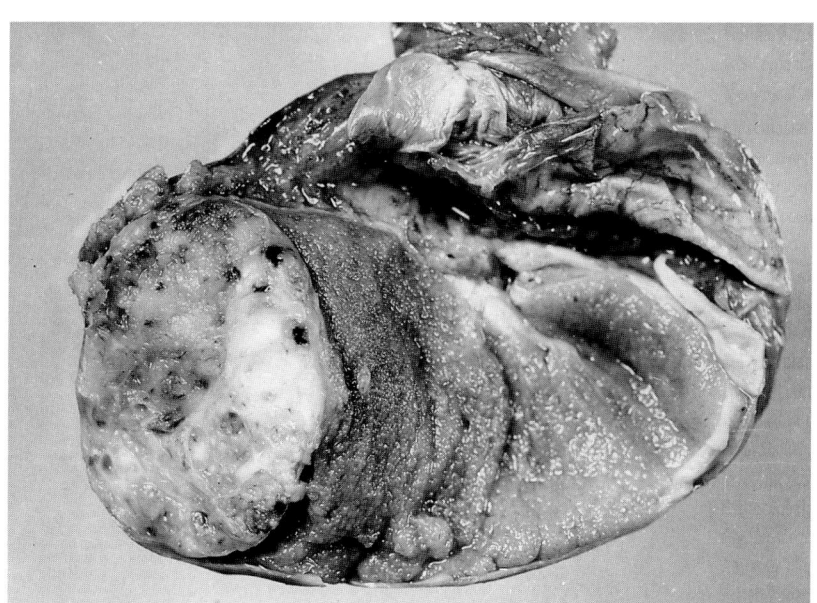

FIGURE 15.45.   *Testicular teratoma appearing as a firm, light-colored, well-circumscribed mass within the testicular parenchyma. Teratomas of this location have never been known to be malignant in young children less than 4 years of age.*

cell malignancy; teratomas of the testis in older patients may harbor zones of embryonal carcinoma or variants thereof. Endodermal sinus tumors may be present in the testis of young children, but usually not in the infantile period, and when present they manifest in a "pure" form, that is, without any other histological pattern being present. This is in contrast to adult patients, in whom endodermal sinus tumors rarely occur by themselves, and are usually seen in combination with other histological types of tumor, such as teratomas, embryonal carcinomas, choriocarcinomas, or seminomas [196].

Other sites at which teratomas may be observed in newborns and young infants include the mediastinum, central nervous system, retroperitoneum, neck, palate and orophar-ynx, kidney, orbit, and stomach [14, 196, 199, 201–204]. The prognosis of teratomas of these anatomical sites is related to the critical regions in which they arise. For instance, mediastinal teratomas produce compression of cardiovascular structures, and intracranial teratomas may be fatal by disturbing central nervous system structures [14, 196, 204]. It is rare, however, that teratomas of these locations contain tissues capable of distant spread.

TUMORS OF THE CENTRAL NERVOUS SYSTEM

Central nervous system tumors figure prominently in surveys of neoplasia of childhood. These tumors are second only to leukemias; their annual incidence per million children, ages 0 to 14 years, is 26.44 for males and 25.74 for females [5]. However, in the newborn period, the frequency of neuroblastomas surpasses that of central nervous system tumors [205, 206]. Medulloblastomas and ependymomas are well documented in newborns [205–208] and are usually supratentorial, in contrast with the infratentorial location common in children over 2 years of age. Slightly over half of all the primary intracranial tumors of newborn infants are teratomas [204]. This tumor usually presents in the midline, frequently in the pineal region or third ventricle over the sella; we have seen a congenital teratoma of the posterior fossa originating in the cerebellum. Congenital intracranial teratomas may reach a massive size, lead to hydrocephalus and dystocia, and be fatal during the prenatal period. On occasion, an intracranial choriocarcinoma has been attributed to overgrowth of trophoblastic elements in a teratoma; this, however, is rare. In our experience, intracranial teratomas of the newborn period owe their lethal behavior more to size and critical location than to the inherently malignant quality of the tissues that comprise the tumor.

Warkani et al's [204] review of the literature includes examples of pineoblastomas, spongioblastomas, sarcomas, choroid plexus papillomas, craniopharyngiomas, and adamantinomas. Wells's classic review [16] includes a cerebral glioma in a newborn infant.

Clinical manifestations of intracranial hamartomas may be present at birth or may manifest themselves later in childhood. This tumor may cause increased intracranial pressure and neurological, metabolic, and endocrine manifestations, such as precocious puberty [204].

TUMORS OF SOFT TISSUE

Soft tissue includes all non-epithelial extraskeletal tissue of the human body, with the exception of the reticuloendothelial system, glia, and stroma of organs. By convention, it also includes the peripheral and autonomic nervous system because tumors arising in these structures present as soft-tissue masses and pose similar diagnostic and therapeutic problems [209].

Comprising approximately 10% of the congenital and neonatal tumors [210], tumors of fibroblastic and myofibroblastic composition are the most important category of soft tissue neoplasms [211]. Excellent reviews and treatises are available that describe the various clinico-pathologic entities occurring in this age group [212–214].

Congenital, or *infantile*, *myofibromatosis* designates nodular, proliferative lesions of myofibroblasts that may present as a single nodule in the subcutaneous tissue (solitary), or adopt a generalized, multifocal form, either with the lesions limited to the skin (multiple), or with involvement of viscera and skeleton (generalized). Thus the early classification of the cases into "solitary, multiple, and generalized" still seems useful, since it identifies cases in a scale of progressively

worse prognosis. The most important distinction has been thought to be between cases with and without visceral involvement; the two are morphologically indistinguishable from each other, but the former carry a more serious prognosis. Although the lesions are histologically benign, their multiplicity may determine a serious, even lethal, outcome. Numerous lytic bone lesions may cause hypercalcemia and bone fractures, visceral involvement may lead to intestinal obstruction, and rarely, the disease may directly affect critical sites, such as the central nervous system.

The participating cells are predominantly myofibroblasts, as implied in the name of this disease; many synonyms have been used (generalized hamartomatosis, congenital generalized fibromatosis, multiple leiomyomata, and others) for which there is currently little justification. The most frequent type is the solitary, subcutaneous form, which usually behaves as a self-limiting disease in which the nodules spontaneously regress. This intriguing phenomenon remains little understood [215]; apoptosis may contribute to it. About two-thirds of all the cases are identified in the neonatal period, but, as might be anticipated, single lesions are noted less frequently and later than generalized ones. After primary excision, 7% of single lesions may recur, but a new excision is usually curative. Microscopically, the appearance is characteristic, due to the phenomenon of "zonation"—that is, the central, intermediate, and peripheral portions of the lesion look different from each other. Zonation, however, is not perfect, as the lesions tend to be altered by the conditions proper to their anatomical location and by secondary changes. At the periphery, the cells aggregate in bundles which resemble smooth muscle fibers; true smooth muscle differentiation has been thought to occur [216]. Large parts of the lesion may show hyalinization or aggregation of spindle cells into criss-crossing fascicles, with variable amounts of collagen. The center is highly vascularized, and the vessels are arborizing and interanastomotic, so that the resulting pattern resembles a hemangiopericytoma. Necrosis is a frequent feature, especially in the central portion, a feature helpful to distinguish the lesion from musculo-aponeurotic fibromatosis. There is no encapsulation. Mitoses may be seen, but are not frequent; in rare cases their number may reach three or four per high power (400×) field, but always in very restricted foci throughout the lesion, and always of normal morphology. Estrogen receptors may be absent, and no gene amplification was found when several oncogenes (epidermal growth factor, *c-myc*, Neu, P53, *N-myc*) known to be important for fibroblast growth were investigated by molecular biology techniques [217].

Congenital myofibromatosis may be mistaken for a soft tissue sarcoma. This diagnostic error may be avoided by recalling that a diagnosis should not be made with a limited specimen, as with a needle biopsy. Mitotic activity in a newborn is not sufficient, by itself, to qualify a lesion as malignant. Furthermore, congenital myofibromatosis may show an "angiocentric" or perivascular pattern that likens the lesions to metastatic or vessel-invading neoplasms [217].

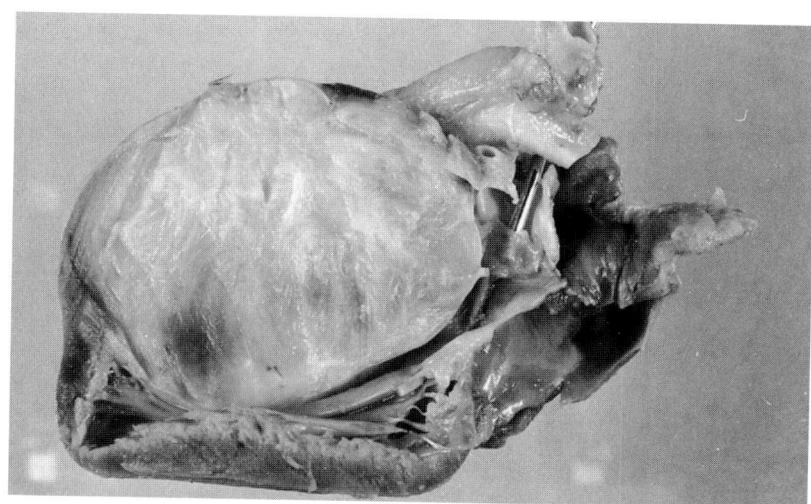

FIGURE 15.46. *Massive cardiac fibroma of the interventricular septum in an infant with multiple congenital anomalies.*

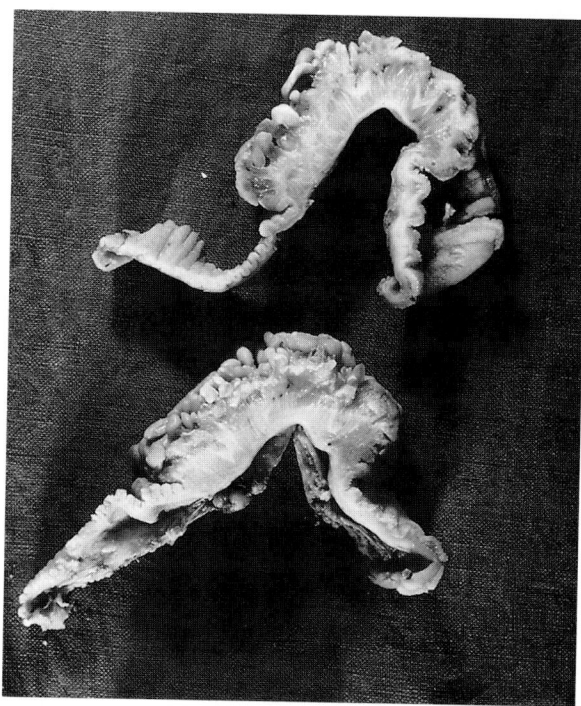

FIGURE 15.47. *Sections through a specimen of "solitary" intestinal fibromatosis that manifested as intestinal obstruction in the neonatal period. Note thickened area of the bowel wall.*

Awareness of the general features of the disease, by leading to the search for lesions that may have been initially unsuspected, such as skeletal deposits, should promote diagnostic accuracy. Some cases have shown a pattern of inheritance consistent with autosomal dominant transmission. Involvement of father and daughter, both with congenital tumors, has been described, as have brothers with multicentric disease [218, 219]. There is thus evidence for a genetic component in this disease.

Visceral myofibromatosis may adopt several forms, which are at present ill understood. *Cardiac fibromas* are known to manifest in infancy, either accompanying systemic diseases, or as isolated lesions (Fig. 15.46). *Solitary intestinal fibromatosis* is the name given to fibroblastic–myofibroblastic proliferations confined to the small intestine, rarely present in infants. Whether they represent the same entity as congenital myofibromatosis, in which the cutaneous involvement was inconspicuous and missed, is not clear (Fig. 15.47). The same may be said for diffuse myofibromatosis of the skin, a rare disease. In all these conditions, the basic proliferation is of fibroblasts and myofibroblasts of benign appearance.

Fibromatosis colli is a mass lesion usually detected in the sternocleidomastoid muscle of an infant between 2 and 4 weeks of age. It is composed of mature fibrous tissue that surrounds degenerating muscle fibers, and it is not clear whether it represents a true neoplasm or an inflammatory, reparative process. Often, but not always, there is a history of complicated delivery, and the lesion tends to regress spontaneously. There is no evidence that fibromatosis colli ever behaves aggressively or transforms into a malignant neoplasm. A conservative approach is favored, and the surgical pathologist encounters the lesion less frequently than formerly.

Digital fibromatosis is a distinctive form of fibromatosis of infants and young children that occurs almost exclusively in fingers and toes [219a]. It presents as a rounded, protruding mass arising from the lateral or dorsal surface of the involved phalanx, sometimes more than one, covered by erythematous skin. Histopathologically, intracytoplasmic inclusions are characteristic, which together with the digital localization permits the diagnosis. These are spheroidal, pale, eosinophilic, frequently paranuclear inclusions that vary in number from case to case, and at times may be so scanty that they are easily overlooked. They are PAS-negative, best demonstrated in sections stained with iron hematoxylin, which stains them black, but are adequately visualized by

Masson's trichrome stain or PTAH. The inclusions persist in tissue culture; however, it is well established that they do not represent viruses, and most probably are not viral-induced changes. The inclusions contain actin, and perhaps other constituents from the cytoskeleton, but their true significance and mechanism of formation remain unknown. Although typical of infantile fibromatosis, they are by no means specific to this disease, having been reported in tumors of other locations and in patients beyond infancy or childhood.

Fibrous hamartoma of infancy is a tumor characteristically occurring in the subcutaneous tissue of the trunk or extremities, less commonly in other sites, and often present at birth. On occasion the tumor may be quite large (10 cm or more), but it is usually small, and grossly has a nondescript appearance of fibrofatty tissue [220]. The diagnosis is easily established when the three characteristic histologic components are identified, namely, trabeculae of mature fibrous tissue, adipose tissue areas, and nest-like foci of immature mesenchymal tissue (Fig. 15.48). This lesion is benign, but recurrence may follow incomplete excision.

Calcifying aponeurotic fibroma is a tumor likely to arise in the hands and feet of children, but its anatomical distribution is wider and it is not exclusive of infants. Its histologic picture is characteristic, consisting of a fibrotic, ill-delimited nodule in whose central portion are discrete foci of calcification and/or chondrogenesis; the fibroblasts may show a tendency to palisade around these foci, and reactive giant cells are sometimes present. The fibroblasts are characteristically plump, with indistinct cell borders and round or ovoid, clear nuclei, and may be oriented in rows separated by dense, hyalinized collagen. These features, to which are added the focal calcifications and the primary location in the hand, usually allow the diagnosis. Contrary to digital fibromatosis, this lesion is uncommon in infants and new-

borns. It should be distinguished from *calcifying fibrous pseudotumor*, a lesion characterized by dense fibrous tissue containing calcified "psammoma bodies," first reported by Rosenthal and Abdul-Karim [220] in 1988 and thought to represent a healed stage of an inflammatory pseudotumor.

Musculoaponeurotic fibromatosis, the equivalent of "desmoid"-type fibromatosis of older patients, occurs in infants and newborns, affecting preferentially the shoulder region, neck, or extremities, and rarely other anatomical sites. This is a problematic entity, whose distinction from fibrosarcoma often represents a major diagnostic quandary. In its most typical form, it appears as an ill-delimited mass of fibrous tissue barely distinguishable from a scar. "Cellular" forms occur, simulating other sarcomas such as rhabdomyosarcoma by virtue of their greater cellularity and presence of myxoid, immature cellular components. Despite a bland histologic appearance, its tendency is to recur. The treatment of choice is surgical, but this may be technically impossible due to involvement of critical structures and widespread infiltration.

Fibrosarcoma is a tumor composed of densely aggregated, mitotically active fibroblasts, usually appearing as spindle-shaped cells that adopt a fascicular disposition and show a tendency to produce collagen and reticulin fibers. Other histopathologic patterns may be present. Stout [221] first noted that such a tumor may be congenital or manifest in the early infantile period—hence the name congenital-infantile fibrosarcoma (CIFS)—and that it tends to follow a clinical course more favorable than that of tumors of similar histology in adults. Pathologists have been prompted to question whether the term "fibrosarcoma" in CIFS is a misnomer [222], and whether the lesion exists at all [223], because CIFS rarely metastasizes and exceptional cases have been known to involute spontaneously [224]. The collective experience is that a few of these tumors, less than 10%,

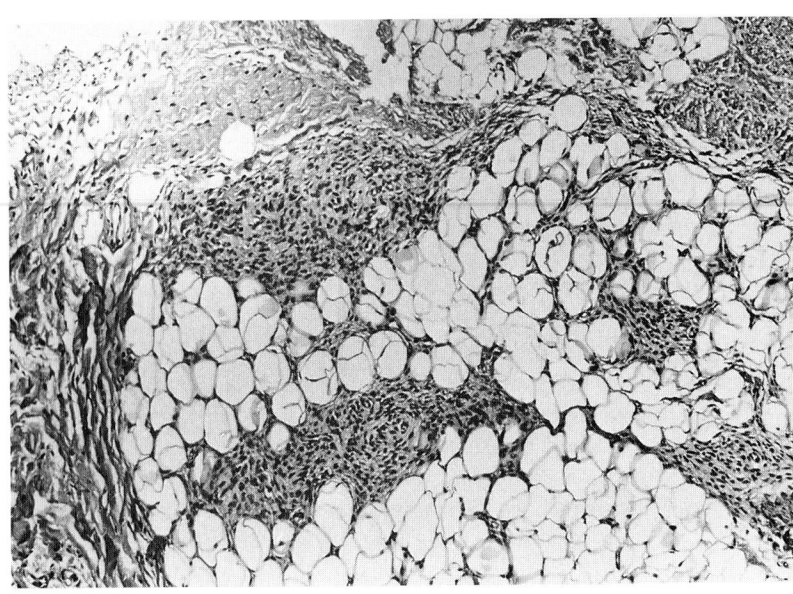

FIGURE 15.48.   *Histologic appearance of fibrous hamartoma of infancy showing adipose tissue, nests of highly cellular immature mesenchymal cells, and mature collagenous fibrous tissue.*

metastasize widely and follow a lethal course. The most common primary sites are the extremities. Second in frequency are the head and neck regions, followed by the chest wall, pelvis, and dorsum. Males are affected more commonly than females. Typically, the tumor presents at birth as a large mass that grossly distorts the shape of an extremity, although at times the size is very small. The overlying skin may be congested or ulcerated.

Grossly, the tumor is usually white or pink-white, its consistency depending on the amount of collagen present. Microscopically, the ovoid or spindle cells may be arranged in fascicular bundles, herringbone pattern, cords, bands, or sheets, with interspersed foci of necrosis, hematopoietic cell clusters, or myxoid matrix. Lymphocytic infiltration is common, and this feature is more characteristic of the infantile than the adult form of fibrosarcoma. Fibrosarcoma is one of several mesenchymal tumors that may exhibit focal areas of "hemangiopericytoma" pattern. The component cells express vimentin, but beyond this there appears to be no distinctive immunophenotype. According to Coffin et al [223], one-third of the cases react with antineuronal-specific enolase, muscle-specific and smooth muscle actin, and manifest estrogen receptors. However, cytokeratin, epithelial membrane antigen, and myelin basic protein are uniformly negative.

Congenital fibrosarcoma is usually diploid on DNA analysis. In most reports no correlation has been found between cellularity, anaplasia, mitotic index, necrosis, number of cells in S-phase, proliferative activity, and the ultimate outcome of the patient. Various chromosomal abnormalities, mainly nonrandom gains of chromosomes 8, 11, 17, and 20 have been reported [225]. It is possible to demonstrate this abnormality by fluorescent in situ hybridization (FISH) technique. This was recently done by Schofield and collaborators [226], who showed that the chromosomal abnormality is consistently present in congenital–infantile fibrosarcoma of patients up to 2 years of age, but only exceptionally in fibrosarcomas of older patients, and, interestingly, not at all in fibromatoses or congenital myofibromatoses.

Despite difficulties in characterization, the prognosis of congenital/infantile fibrosarcoma is predictable: most cases are effectively managed by complete surgical excision. In the experience of the Armed Forces Institute of Pathology, 84% of the patients were free of tumor 5 years after excision, and lethality due to metastases was less than 8%; other reported series have shown a comparable experience. Recurrences follow promptly after excision; only exceptional cases are on record in which the recurrence or metastasis took place years after the tumor was removed. Lundgren et al [227] have studied the differences between those infantile fibrosarcomas that tend to remain confined and those that metastasize. They identified three patients between 1 and 3 years of age bearing tumors that were similar in all respects to congenital–infantile fibrosarcoma, except that some cells showed ultrastructural and immunocytochemical evidence of rhabdomyoblastic differentiation. Two of these patients died from metastatic disease within 2 years of the operation, and the third had a recurrence at the time of the report. Cytogenetically, two tumors had a karyotype showing clones with monosomy 19; one had, in addition, monosomy 22. Lundgren and colleagues suggested that infantile fibrosarcomas that metastasize may constitute a different entity, for which the term "infantile rhabdomyofibrosarcoma" was proposed [227]. This intriguing proposal has yet to be confirmed.

For the pathologist, the main difficulty is perhaps the differential diagnosis. Cases initially presenting with the bland, paucicellular, and collagen-rich appearance of fibromatosis have been known to recur as highly cellular fibrosarcomas. The distinction between these two lesions is notoriously difficult and may be impossible. Differences have been pointed out, such as the greater number of nucleolar organizer regions (Ag NOR) in fibrosarcoma [228] or staining for nuclear activation antigens and p53 oncogene mutations [229], but there continues to be a pressing need for reliable, reproducible, and practical ways to establish this distinction in practice. The ability to detect chromosomal gains in fixed tumor samples, and the apparent differences in karyotype of fibrosarcoma and fibromatosis reported by Schofield et al [226] are reasons to hope that this traditionally vexing problem may soon be solved.

Another important distinction is with rhabdomyosarcoma, since the latter may adopt a thoroughly fascicular, herringbone architectural pattern; we have seen a pelvic tumor initially diagnosed and treated as fibrosarcoma that later metastasized with the appearance of embryonal rhabdomyosarcoma. Improvements in immunohistochemistry, including the greater sensitivity of antibodies to cellular antigens of muscle differentiation, may diminish the frequency of such misdiagnoses. Distinction from myofibroblastic proliferative processes that simulate malignancy, such as nodular fasciitis, is very important. Except in longstanding cases with much scarring, fasciitis tends to exhibit a myxoid character and displays a mixed cellular inflammatory infiltrate; its structure is less fascicular and more whorled in appearance; and it is sometimes possible to determine its origin from a fascia.

Fetal rhabdomyomas are rare tumors with a remarkable propensity to arise in the head and neck. At least half occur in patients 1 year of age or younger, and approximately 25% are present at birth; they are twice as common in boys as in girls. The face and preauricular region are favored primary sites, but the tumor may arise in the nasopharynx, tongue, larynx, palate, or buccal mucosa. They present as subcutaneous nodules; or, if present in the mucosa, they can present as polypoid masses that may reach a large size (over 10 cm) even when congenital. They are usually well circumscribed, but lack true encapsulation. Histologically, the so-called "classic" type is composed of benign-appearing spindle cells interspersed with striated muscle cells with the appearance of fetal myotubules set in a fibromyxoid stroma. The "classic" type corresponds to the least mature form. A higher number of well-differentiated rhabdomyoblasts gives rise to a type of fetal rhabdomyoma designated as "intermediate," but the appearance of fully mature striated muscle cells is not reproduced by these tumors.

Fetal rhabdomyomas are benign tumors. However, a problem exists concerning their distinction from the spindle-cell variant of rhabdomyosarcoma, a recently recognized morphologic type of embryonal rhabdomyosarcoma. To effect the distinction, we must recall that sarcomas are generally deeply situated, whereas fetal rhabdomyoma is usually subcutaneous. The degree of cellular pleomorphism and mitotic activity is greater in sarcomas than in benign tumors. Kapadia et al [230] deemed the absence of marked nuclear atypia the most reliable criterion, but fetal rhabdomyomas comprise a morphologic spectrum that includes examples with such degree of cellularity as would blur the distinction between rhabdomyoma and low-grade rhabdomyosarcoma. It is perhaps those problematic cases that account for reports of progression from benign to malignant.

Rhabdomyomatous mesenchymal hamartoma is a lesion of the skin of infants and newborns that also has a predilection for the face and neck. Fat, fibrous tissue, and disorderly grown nerves may enter into the composition of these subcutaneous masses, and some have been reported as "intraneural." Hamartomatous rhabdomyomas may accompany some systemic syndromes. Cardiac rhabdomyomas, questionably neoplastic growths, are well known to associate with tuberous sclerosis.

Rhabdomyosarcoma has a histopathologic variability. A recently proposed classification [231] includes the following types:

Embryonal—composed of undifferentiated mesenchymal cells that express rhabdomyogenesis, and thus may display great cytologic variation.

Botryoid—a subtype of the embryonal form that grows in polypoid fashion (Fig. 15.49) and displays a condensed layer of cells ("cambium" layer) at its surface.

Spindle cell—also a variant of embryonal, made of cellular bundles of elongated cells, as denoted in its name.

Alveolar—in which the cells arrange around spaces demarcated by fibrovascular connective tissue reminiscent of the alveoli of the lung, but which may also occur as a cytologically identical "solid" variant.

Undifferentiated sarcoma—a tumor with no specific features, negative to most immunostains used to characterize muscle-derived neoplasms, and only tentatively assimilated to the rhabdomyosarcoma group.

This classification was propounded based on its prognostic implications, with the best prognosis attached to botryoid and spindle-cell tumors, an intermediate prognosis associated with the embryonal type, and the worst clinical outcome correlating with alveolar and undifferentiated sar-

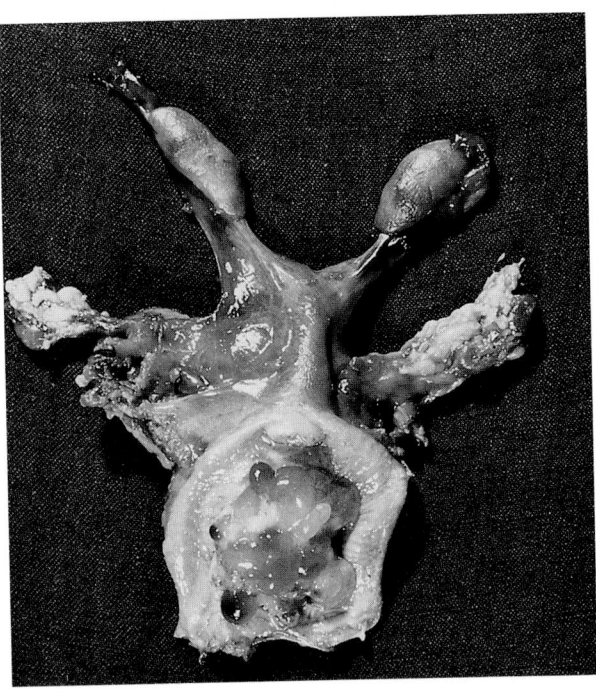

FIGURE 15.49. *Typical appearance of botryoid rhabdomyosarcoma of the infantile vagina. The tumor looks like a bunch of grapes filling the upper third of the vagina. The specimen includes uterus, tubes, and ovaries. Current therapy is conservative, and therefore surgical specimens such as this are no longer encountered.*

comas. Histopathology alone is not an entirely satisfactory prognostic index. Rhabdomyosarcoma poses special problems according to its anatomical localization. Accordingly, the following discussion will refer to the main primary sites observed.

In the head and neck, it is currently customary to classify the lesion into three main topographic types: parameningeal, orbital, and "other." This tripartite subdivision is fully justified by the different prognosis associated with each primary site. Orbital rhabdomyosarcomas—that is, those arising within the bony cavity that houses the eye globe, optic nerve, vessels, and extraocular muscles—tend to follow a less aggressive course. Only rarely do they actually involve the orbital bones (in which case they are classified as "parameningeal"); the majority remain confined to the site of origin, without extending to adjacent regions. Once the diagnosis is made by means of a biopsy, chemotherapy and radiotherapy often suffice to control the disease. Orbital exenteration is required only when there is a local relapse and no metastases are evident. Orbital rhabdomyosarcoma may have a better prognosis even in the presence of metastases, but this is still controversial.

Parameningeal rhabdomyosarcomas often arise medial to the tympanic membrane paranasal sinuses, nasopharynx, and the pterygopalatine and parapharyngeal areas. In all these locations, rhabdomyosarcomas are treated aggressively, on account of their tendency to infiltrate the base of the skull, with the consequent bad prognosis. In contrast, orbital RS rarely involves the bones of the base of the skull or seeds into the cerebrospinal fluid.

The scalp, the eyelid, the parotid gland, the cheek, the oral cavity including the soft tissues of the oropharyngeal wall, and the paraspinal neck muscles are other well-known sites from which a primary rhabdomyosarcoma may originate. Metastases to cervical lymph nodes are strikingly uncommon. This fact has rendered radical neck dissection unnecessary in the treatment of rhabdomyosarcoma of the head and neck. In contrast, childhood rhabdomyosarcoma of other locations, especially of the extremities, often disseminates to regional lymph nodes.

Pelvic rhabdomyosarcoma is particularly important in infants and newborns. In boys, the tumor may arise from the wall of the bladder, the prostate, or the loose connective tissue adjacent to these structures. Sometimes, the site of origin cannot be determined accurately. In girls, the vulva, vagina, and uterus, in addition to the bladder, are recognized sites of origin of rhabdomyosarcoma. It should be recalled that in infants and young children the vaginal primaries are much more common than the uterine; actual origin from the uterine body is very rare in infancy. Obstructive uropathy is a common manner of presentation. In the past, extensive initial surgery, including pelvic exenteration, was an accepted part of the therapeutic approach. Fortunately, the appalling morbidity and low quality of life associated with this approach have been alleviated by the introduction of nonoperative measures effective in tumor control. Bladder salvage is an important aim of current treatment, as is preservation of the uterus, ovaries, and vagina whenever possible. At present, a biopsy is first secured, sometimes by endoscopy. When obtained by laparotomy, iliac and paraaortic lymph node sampling is performed to determine the extent of disease, but a radical lymph node dissection is not indicated.

OTHER SOFT TISSUE TUMORS

Cranial fasciitis (Fig. 15.50), nodular fasciitis, calcifying aponeurotic fibromas, fibrohistiocytic tumors such as juvenile xanthogranulomas, and mesenchymomas are all examples of tumors that are rarely described in neonates.

Angiomas

Hemangiomas are the commonest tumors of the skin and soft tissues in infants. Attempts to establish criteria for distinguishing between malformations and tumors of blood vessels have been published [232, 233]. Capillary hemangioma is the most frequent type of angioma of the soft tissues. The overwhelming majority of these tumors arise in the skin and subcutaneous tissue and present as more or less raised nodules at birth, grow steadily for 6 to 8 months, then stabilize and eventually regress. Complete disappearance may take several years. They are composed of closely aggregated masses of capillary-sized vessels that form distinct lobules separated by stroma; hence the name *lobular hemangioma*, which adequately denotes the characteristic organization [234].

Capillary hemangiomas are part of a spectrum of lesions that originate from a more primitive form ("cellular angioma"), which would presumably transform into a better differentiated lesion ("cavernous" or other types of hemangioma made up of vessels of mature appearance). Certain clinical and pathologic features justify separating hemangiomas that may represent different phases of the same lesion.

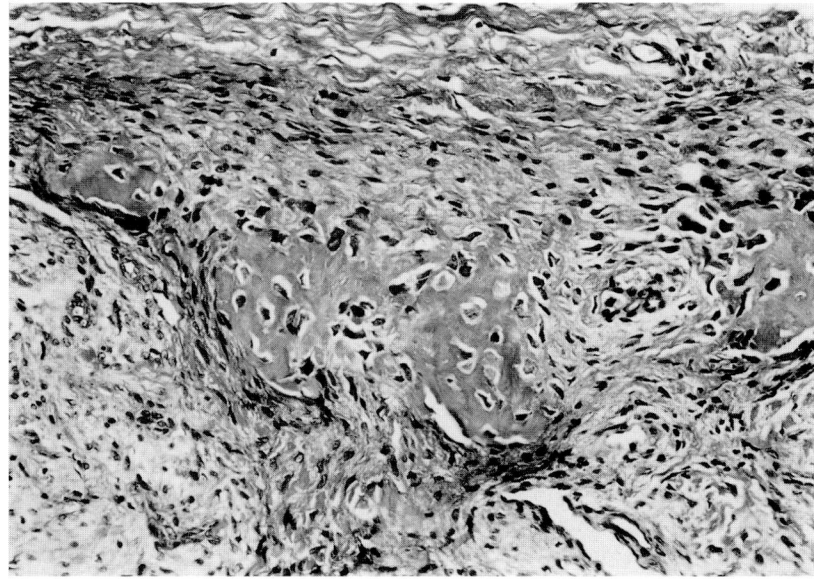

FIGURE 15.50. *Histological picture of cranial fasciitis demonstrating irregular fibroblastic proliferation, osseous metaplasia, and intimal attachment to fascia.*

"*Cavernous*" hemangiomas are constituted of vessels larger than capillary size. Presumably due to connections with larger feeding arteries, the blood vessels of a cavernous hemangioma become distended, engorged with blood, and form warm and pulsatile masses. These developments usually take place in more deeply located hemangiomas than do their capillary counterparts. Frequent complications are compression of thoracic or abdominal structures, thrombosis, stagnation of blood, calcification, sequestration of platelets within the tumor with severe thrombocytopenia (*Kasabach-Merritt syndrome* [234a]), or symptomatic arteriovenous shunts.

High intravascular pressure will eventually reproduce the appearance of arteries, and vessels with lesser pressure will resemble veins. Congeries of tortuous cavernous vessels are sometimes referred to as "*racemose*" hemangioma (from Latin *racemus*, a bunch of grapes) or "*cirsoid*" aneurysm (from Latin *cirrus*, plural *cirri*, "curl"), but these terms are descriptive and do not indicate well-defined pathologic entities. *Sinusoidal hemangioma* is another graphic term based on the microscopic resemblance of the tumoral vessels to sinusoids—that is, spaces larger than capillaries but lined by a tenuous single-layered endothelial coat. Adoption of such terminology does not yet serve any useful purpose. The terms "arteriovenous (A-V) fistula" or "A-V malformation" denote the existence of abnormal communication(s) between the arterial and venous sides of the circulation, and should not be used by the pathologist when the information supporting this abnormal shunting is lacking. Arteriovenous shunts include all the morphologic types of hemangioma. Furthermore, when a functional shunt exists, it may be superficial and asymptomatic, or be deeply situated and cause profound, sometimes life-threatening hemodynamic and oxygenation disturbances.

Cellular angioma of infancy (benign "infantile" or "juvenile" hemangioendothelioma) is a lesion of infancy, single or multiple, which may be defined as a capillary hemangioma in which the number of tumor cells greatly exceeds the vascular lumina present; in other words, there are more endothelial/pericytic cells than needed to line the vessels discernible by light microscopy, thereby resulting in so-called "solid" areas. On electron microscopy one sees tiny lumina below the resolving power of the light microscope, even in areas that seemed "solid" by conventional histologic means. The arrangement of the tumor cells in solid sheets, and the presence of mitoses (always, however, morphologically normal), joined to an infiltrative pattern of growth, may be the source of confusion with a soft tissue sarcoma, especially in deep-seated lesions. The latter sites include the mediastinum, the orbit, the parotid, or other sites with difficult access, including the central nervous system. In children, a tumor in the parotid is likelier to be a hemangioma than a neoplasm of salivary gland tissue. Clinically, the diagnosis of vascular tumor is suspected when the mass is fluctuant, cavitated, or fluid-filled but clinical identification may remain uncertain until excision. Cellular angiomas may

represent the most "immature" form of angiomas, but areas of typical capillary hemangioma are often seen at the periphery of the lobules. Immunostains with anti-actin antibodies enhance the vascular nature of the tumor better than stains for reticulin. Endothelial markers such as Factor VIII-related antigen, *Ulex europeus*, and CD34 fail to react consistently with the immature endothelial cells of cellular angiomas. These cells lack Weibel-Palade bodies, having instead crystalline formations with a multilamellar periodic substructure [235, 236].

The term "infantile hemangioendothelioma" arose from the belief that the tumor cells were exclusively endothelial, and grew *inside* the capillary (basement lamina) sheaths, in contrast to "pericytoma," in which the growth is *external* to this investment and, therefore, composed of pericytes. This nomenclature is well entrenched by protracted use, but is nonetheless ill advised. In the first place, the cellular composition of cellular angiomas is heterogeneous. Endothelium, pericytes, mast cells, and mesenchymal cells reactive to Factor XIIIa (probably "dendritic" connective tissue cells) are consistently present in these lesions [237]; accordingly, the demonstration of the mentioned cells is useful to establish the diagnosis in problematic cases. Secondly, the traditional use of reticulin stains to demonstrate the capillaries' framework of support, and to ascertain whether the cell growth is internal or external to this framework, is unreliable in practice, because the reticulin support is often imperfectly developed; immunostaining for actin may be helpful to accentuate the capillarization present in the tumor. Lastly, the term "hemangioendothelioma" has been applied to both benign and malignant lesions of adults, and its application to infantile lesions of proven benignity does little to dispel the ambiguities that may surround an individual case.

Deeply situated hemangiomas are more likely to be treated surgically. Those arising within the muscles do not differ fundamentally from the types discussed. However, certain secondary features, in part due to their location, confer to intramuscular hemangiomas characteristics deserving special consideration. They are more common in the trunk and lower extremities than in other sites. Growth of the component vessels along the surface of preexistent muscle fibers may determine the development of diagnostically helpful, "striated" patterns on angiography [238]. A high content of adipose tissue is frequently observed; it may greatly overshadow the vascular component, and may not represent the preexisting adipose tissue. This feature finds expression in the term "*infiltrating angiolipoma*," which denotes both the histologic composition and the locally infiltrating nature of the lesion [239]. Allen and Enzinger decried this designation [240], arguing that use of the word "angiolipoma" was preempted by its application to a subcutaneous lesion, and that distinction between angiomas and lipomas of muscle might be blurred by introduction of a compound name that implies both. Although neither objection is fully persuasive, there is much to be said for simplification of nomenclature. Other heterologous elements, such as smooth muscle or cartilage may be occasionally seen, but their frequency and extent fall far short of those of adipose tissue, and thus are reasonably explained as metaplastic foci. These tumors are benign, but a high frequency of local recurrence—variously reported between 9% and 50% [240, 241]—is attributable to difficulties attending complete excision. A problem of differential diagnosis with a primary angiosarcoma in muscle very rarely, if ever, poses itself. We know of no well-authenticated case of angiosarcoma of muscle in infants and newborns. Furthermore, the morphology of the proliferating vessels shows none of the features of atypia that would be expected in a malignant process.

"Tufted" hemangioma, also known as *angioblastoma*, resembles cellular angioma of infancy. Unlike the latter, the tendency to regress may not be apparent, and this leads to surgical excision—hence the name "acquired, progressive capillary hemangioma," [242, 243] which is a misnomer, since the lesion may be congenital. These are indurated, rapidly spreading, erythematous macules or papules between 1 and 10 cm in greatest diameter, which may be painful and are sometimes accompanied by local hyperhydrosis. Tufted hemangioma is subject to all the complications of hemangiomas, and thrombocytopenia may rarely be a component. The most common location is the skin and subcutaneous tissue of the neck and upper trunk, followed in frequency by the extremities, and, lastly, the head. Patients of any age may be affected, but clearly these tumors are most often seen in childhood: 60% are discovered in the first year of life, and 75% by the age of 10 years.

Histologically, these lesions may be confused with cellular angiomas of infancy. Both are "lobulated," but the architectural pattern of tufted hemangioma is less orderly: instead of being closely aggregated, the lobules exist far apart, reflecting a livelier pattern of spread. The tumor spread is said to follow the planes of least resistance, along the loose adventitial coats of preexisting vessels, the nerve sheaths (perhaps correlating with the dull soreness observed clinically), or the interstices between collagenous bundles, and into the subcutaneous adipose tissue. Solid masses of tumor cells sometimes appear partly surrounded by a crescentic sinusoidal space, giving the impression that the tumor protrudes into a thin vessel or a lymphatic. These subtle features, joined to the clinical manifestations, permit the diagnosis of the uncommon tufted hemangiomas.

Endovascular papillary angioendothelioma was described by Dabska [244] in 1969, and is sometimes referred to as "Dabska tumor." It is characterized by large vascular spaces, possibly lymphatic in origin, from whose endothelial lining arise papillary structures that project into the lumen. These endopapillary projections are lined by endothelial cells of variable appearance, some small, with dark nuclei and high nucleocytoplasmic ratio similar to lymphocytes. Other cells are epithelial-like, with abundant cytoplasm and nuclei oriented toward the luminal pole of the cell. Interest in this rare tumor was spurred by Dabska's documenting six children with this lesion, two of whom developed regional lymph node metastases [244]. However, no patient has been known to die from progression of the tumor or wide dissemination.

Infantile hemangiopericytoma is a controversial entity. In our experience, many cases have been called hemangiopericytomas that might be best classified as cellular angiomas (hemangioendotheliomas); this applies to some reported cases as well. However, some deep-seated cases have apparently behaved aggressively [245]. These two tumors may be related, as shown by the existence of apparent transition between peri- and endotheliomatous tumor morphology. When all this is taken into account, true hemangiopericytoma is a very uncommon neoplasm in infants and young children. In adults, tumors such as synovial sarcoma, meningioma, and others must be excluded; in infants, distinction must be made from "cellular" angioma and from congenital myofibromatosis, the latter of which characteristically shows hemangiopericytomatous areas. The diagnosis ought to be suspected when the tumor replicates the features attributed to hemangiopericytoma of adults and shows such a histomorphology consistently, throughout the entire extent of the tumor, not just focally. It is believed that the hemangiopericytoma of young children is biologically different from its adult counterpart, so the presence of mitoses and necrosis, which usually portend a poor outcome in adults, are not necessarily associated with bad prognosis in children. Accordingly, most cases can be treated adequately by surgical excision.

We found an extremely rare form of hemangioma of infants, *infiltrating, giant cell angioblastoma*, that must be added to vascular tumors of "borderline" prognosis. Its microscopic appearance appears to be distinctive, resembling granulomas with angiocentric arrangement (Fig. 15.51). Experience with this tumor is as yet very limited.

Pertinent to the present discussion are the hemangiomas that accompany various malformation syndromes. Their complete enumeration cannot be attempted here, but some of the best described will be listed.

Klippel-Trenaunay syndrome consists of cutaneous hemangiomas, varicose veins, and soft tissue and/or osseous hypertrophy of the extremities; the involvement is unilateral, but rarely are both limbs affected. Orofacial involvement may be present, with or without other features of Sturge-Weber syndrome.

Sturge-Weber syndrome, or encephalo-trigeminal angiomatosis, consists of congenital ("port wine stain") telangiectasis distributed over the branches of the trigeminal nerve. Intracranial, meningocerebral angiomas and telangiectatic vessels are part of the syndrome, accounting for the development of seizures in the first few years of life, as well as for mental retardation. Congenital glaucoma (buphthalmos) may give rise to enlargement of one eye; disparity in eye color may result from angiomatosis of the choroid.

Fabry disease is characterized by storage of glycosphingolipids (trihexosyl and digalactosyl ceramide) principally in

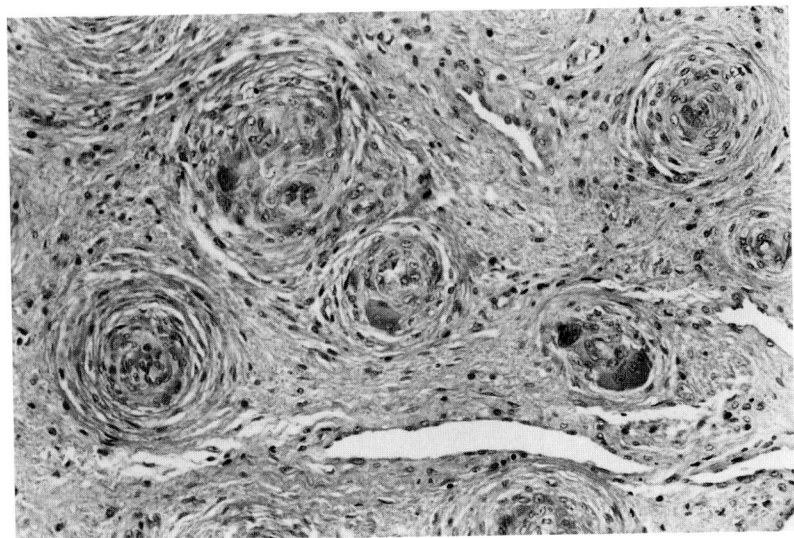

FIGURE 15.51.   *Infiltrating, giant cell angioblastoma, a recently reported vascular neoplasm, is characterized by angioblastic plump cells occurring in clusters around neoformed vessels. Plurinucleated cells are present, thus resembling granulomas. (Gonzalez-Crussi et al, Am J Surg Pathol 1991; 15:175.)*

the heart and kidneys as a result of absence or deficiency of the lysosomal enzyme alpha-galactosidase A, which hydrolyzes metabolic precursors of trihexosyl ceramide originating from senescent erythrocytes. The patients, predominantly of male sex, manifest skin angiokeratomas that appear in childhood, may be present at birth, and increase in size and number with age. There may also be telangiectasias of retinal and conjunctival vessels. The histopathology consists of cystically dilated capillaries that protrude into the upper dermis, flanked or entirely circumscribed by elongate rete ridges, and a thinned out overlying epidermis, which shows hyperkeratosis. The vessels are often filled with erythrocytes, but some of them contain only a proteinaceous fluid, suggesting that lymphatics participate in the formation of the lesions. Accordingly, it may be difficult to distinguish a small angiokeratoma from so-called "lymphangioma circumscriptum." As the dilated vessels do not aggregate into lobules, the appearance of incipient lesions is more that of a telangiectasia than a true tumor; however, lesions coalesce into larger, expanding plaques, may extend into the subcutaneous tissue, and their histopathology overlaps with cavernous hemangioma.

The association of hemangiomas of the skin and subcutaneous tissue with multiple hemangiomas of the liver forms a recognized syndrome known variously as *multicentric* or *multinodular hepatic hemangiomatosis*. This disease falls within the spectrum of hemangiomatosis, a continuum of disorders characterized by multiple (from a few to hundreds) hemangiomas of skin and viscera. Organs other than the liver may be the seat of hemangiomatosis, but it is interesting that more than half of children with cellular angiomas of the liver have associated cutaneous hemangiomas, whereas only 6% of children with nonhepatic hemangiomas have cutaneous lesions [246]. These children may manifest a clinical triad characterized by cutaneous hemangiomas, hepatomegaly, and cardiac failure (Fig. 15.52). The latter is

MULTINODULAR HEMANGIOMATOSIS

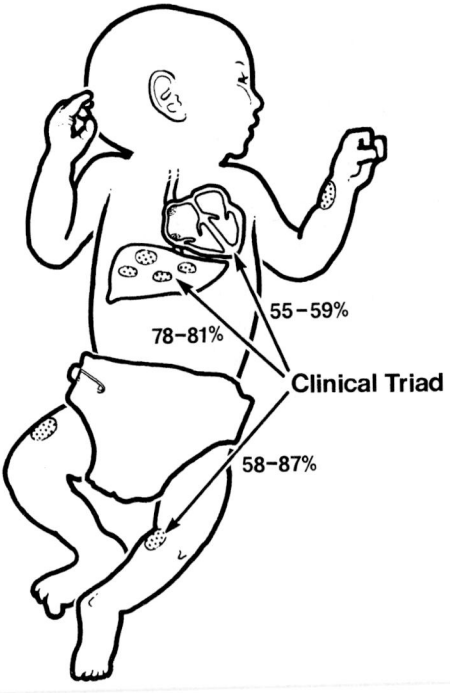

FIGURE 15.52.   *Diagram showing the reported proportions of the components of the clinical triad observed in multinodular hemangiomatosis of the liver.*

the result of perturbed hemodynamics: the blood is shunted from the arterial to the venous side of the circulation across multiple hemangiomas present in the liver. The cutaneous lesions are not invariably present. Hepatomegaly is out of proportion to the severity of heart failure; likewise, cardiac decompensation takes place in the absence of any specific congenital malformations. These two findings may lead an investigator to suspect the correct diagnosis. However, if cardiac failure is protracted it may obscure the diagnosis, because the right atrial pressure rise produced by increased venous return via the hepatic hemangiomas may force open a patent foramen ovale and produce a right-to-left shunt. Blood flow through the ductus arteriosus is usually reversed, due to low systemic arterial pressure, and this worsens the cyanosis. The hemangiomas in this condition are benign. *Hepatic angiosarcoma* is extremely rare in infants, but we have seen one case in which serial biopsies demonstrated an evolution of the tumors toward malignancy (Figs. 15.53a,b).

MISCELLANEOUS TUMORS

Histiocytosis-X, recently referred to as Langerhans' cell histiocytosis, is the only congenital tumor-like condition whose nosological position is still unclear. The clinical form of histiocytosis-X, designated Letterer-Siwe disease, may be congenital [247].

Melanocytic neuroectodermal tumor of infancy (melanotic progonoma) is a rare pigmented lesion that usually arises in the head and neck regions (92.8% of cases) [248]. This tumor has also been identified in the epididymis, mediastinum, scapular region, thigh, cerebellum, uterus, ovaries, femur, and temporal bone [249]. It is believed to be a tumor of neuroectodermal origin and usually has a benign clinical

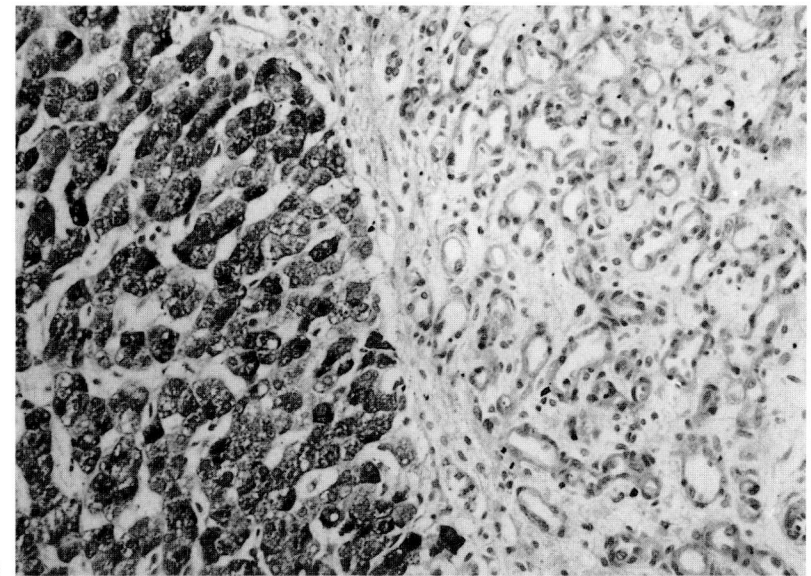

a

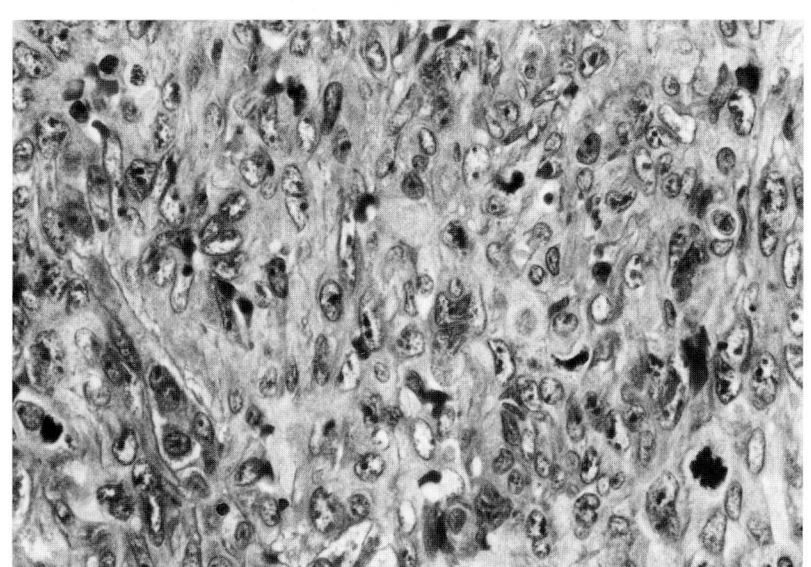

b

FIGURE 15.53. *(a) Hemangioma of the liver, in a case of multinodular hemangiomatosis. The microscopic appearance is that of a benign capillary hemangioma, shown here adjacent to the liver parenchyma. The tissue was stained with the PAS technique, which reveals abundant glycogen in the liver cells, but fails to stain basement membranes in the capillaries. (b) Biopsy specimen of hepatic hemangioma from the same patient a year after initial diagnosis. The histologic pattern is now solid, dense, and the cells show atypia and mitoses. The lesion is clearly sarcomatous.*

course. Of 166 cases reported, only six, including a maxillary tumor in a stillborn [250], were indisputably malignant [249]. This tumor has been identified in a 6-month-old child with the fetal hydantoid syndrome [251].

Pancreatic carcinomas in children are uncommon and have been classified as functioning (islet cell carcinomas) and non-functioning (adenocarcinomas) [252]. Pancreatic adenocarcinomas [252, 253], hamartomas [254], and islet cell adenomas have been reported in newborns.

Congenital leiomyosarcomas of the large intestine are extremely rare; no more than 10 examples have been reported in the literature [255]. Primary bronchopulmonary leiomyosarcoma in children is also extremely rare. Jimenez et al [256] uncovered 10 examples of this tumor in children under 15 years of age; two of these were newborns. Respiratory distress was the common denominator, especially in younger patients, whereas cough, anorexia, weight loss, hemoptysis, and pneumonia were more common in older children.

Retinoblastomas, although rare, are the most common intraocular tumors of childhood, accounting for about 1.2% of cancer deaths in children under 15 years of age in the United States [257]. Retinoblastomas are highly malignant tumors; if the tumor extends beyond the eye, mortality ranges between 90% and 100% [258]; but if confined to the eye, the 5-year survival rate is 92% [259]. About 25% to 30% of retinoblastomas are bilateral. Retinoblastomas occur in both heritable (autosomal dominant) and sporadic forms, as well as in association with an interstitial deletion on the long arm of chromosome 13 [260, 261]. Survivors of the heritable form of retinoblastoma subsequently developed second primary tumors (particularly osteosarcomas) at a substantially greater frequency than either the general population or survivors of the sporadic form [262]. Of 688 patients who survived radiation therapy for retinoblastoma, 89 developed second tumors—62 in the field of radiation and 27 out of the field. Of 23 patients who received no radiation, five developed second tumors. Sarcomas were the most common tumors in both, in and out of the field of radiation. The incidence of second tumors in patients treated with radiation increases with time: 20% of patients at 10 years, 50% at 20 years, and 90% of second primary tumors will have occurred by 30 years after initial treatment. In patients without radiation, the incidence is lower: 10% at 10 years, 30% at 20 years, and 68% at 32 years [263]. Histologically, the three basic cell patterns described in this tumor are undifferentiated retinoblast, rosettes, and fleurettes [261]. The cell of origin appears to be the photoreceptor cell of the retina.

Conclusions

It would not be wise for us to conclude that one or other histological type of tumor does not occur in neonates. We would rather cite selected and recent publications on benign and malignant congenital tumors. Benign mesenchymomas [264], papillary carcinomas of the thyroid [265], hemangiopericytomas of the tongue [266], fibrous hamartomas of the heart [267], melanoma [268], atypical chondroblastomas of the rib [269], sacrococcygeal chordoma [270], mesenchymal hamartomas of the chest [271], hepatocellular carcinomas [156], cystic choristoma of the head and neck [272], and liposarcomas of the back [273] are only some examples of the many histological forms of congenital tumors described in the literature.

MATERNAL OR PLACENTAL TUMOR METASTASIS TO THE FETUS

Although extremely rare, maternal tumors have been reported to metastasize to the fetus transplacentally. Fox [274] summarized 29 reported examples of placental metastases from maternal neoplasms, including melanomas (11), breast carcinomas (6), and bronchial carcinomas (3). Histologically, clusters or sheets of malignant cells were present in all cases in the intervillous space, and nine showed villous invasion. Of these nine, five were melanomas, three were carcinomas (breast, bronchus, and stomach), and one was a soft-tissue myxosarcoma. Two of the nine melanomas metastasized to the fetus. Both infants died, with a widespread metastatic melanoma [275, 276]. Documented fetal metastatic disease due to other carcinomas has not been identified.

Choriocarcinoma has been observed concurrently in mother and child in at least four instances [40, 277–279]. Both the maternal and infantile tumors are probably the result of metastases from a primary placental tumor.

REFERENCES

1. Bader JL, Miller RW. US cancer incidence and mortality in the first year of life. *Am J Dis Child* 1979; 133:157.
2. Barson AJ. Congenital neoplasia: the society's experience. *Arch Dis Child* 1978; 53:436. Abstract.
3. Davies JN. Some variations in childhood cancers throughout the world. In: Marsden HB, Stewart JK, eds. *Tumors in Children*. 2nd ed. New York: Springer-Verlag, 1976, pp. 28–58.
4. Ericsson JL, Karnstrom L, Mattson B, Childhood cancer in Sweden, 1958–1974. *Acta Paediatr Scand* 1978; 67:425.
5. Kramer S, Meadows AT, Jarrett P, Evans AE. Incidence of childhood cancer: experience of a decade in a population-based registry. *J Natl Cancer Inst* 1983; 70:49.
6. Salonen T. Prenatal and perinatal factors in childhood cancer. *Ann Clin Res* 1976; 7:27.
7. Williams AO. Tumors of childhood in Ibadan, Nigeria. *Cancer* 1975; 36:270.
8. Young JL Jr, Miller RW. Incidence of malignant tumors in US children. *J Pediatr* 1975; 86:254.
9. Young JL Jr, Percy CL, Asire AJ. Surveillance, epidemiology, and end results program: incidence and mortality data, 1973–77. *Natl Cancer Inst Monogr* 1981; 57:1.
10. Weinstein HJ. Congenital leukemia and the neonatal myeloproliferative disorders associated with Down's syndrome. *Clin Haematol* 1978; 7:147.
11. Valsamis MP, Levine PH, Rapin I, Santorineou M, Shulman K. Primary intracranial Burkitt's lymphoma in an infant. *Cancer* 1976; 37:1500.
12. Fraumeni JF Jr, Miller RW. Cancer deaths in the newborn. *Am J Dis Child* 1969; 117:186.
13. Gale GB, D'Angio GJ, Uri A, Chatten J, Koop CE. Cancer in neonates: the experience at the Children's Hospital of Philadelphia. *Pediatrics* 1982; 70:409.

14. Isaacs H Jr. Perinatal (congenital and neonatal) neoplasms: a report of 110 cases. *Pediatr Pathol* 1985; 3:165.

15. O'Brien A, Chan HSL, Campbell AN, Smith CR. Malignant neoplasms in the neonate. *Lab Invest* 1986; 54:6P.

16. Wells HG. Occurrence and significance of congenital malignant neoplasms. *Arch Pathol* 1940; 30:535.

17. Barnes AB, Colton T, Gundersen I, et al. Fertility and outcome of pregnancy in women exposed *in utero* to diethylstilbestrol. *N Engl J Med* 1980; 302: 609.

18. Pendergrass TW, Hanson JW. Fetal hydantoin syndrome and neuroblastoma. *Lancet* 1976; 2:150.

19. Berry CL. Aetiological factors in childhood neoplasia. *J Clin Pathol* 1976; 29:1032.

20. Court Brown WM, Doll R, Hill AB. Incidence of leukemia after exposure to diagnostic radiation *in utero*. *Br Med J* 1960; 2:1539.

21. Durante F. Nesso fisio-patologico tra la struttura dei nei materni e la genesi di alcuni tumori maligni. *Arch Memor Observ Chir Prat* 1874; 11:217.

22. Klavins JV. Letter to the Editor. *Lab Invest* 1984; 51:253.

23. Cohnheim J. *Lectures on General Pathology*. Vol. 2. London: The New Syndenham Society, 1889.

24. Bolande RB. *Cellular Aspects of Developmental Pathology*. Philadelphia: Lea & Febiger, 1967, pp. 88–143.

25. Pitot HC. The stability of events in the natural history of neoplasia. *Am J Pathol* 1977; 89:703.

26. Scott RE, Wille JJ Jr, Wier ML. Mechanisms for the initiation and promotion of carcinogenesis. A review and a new concept. *Mayo Clin Proc* 1984; 59:107.

27. Knudson AG. Mutation and cancer: statistical study of retinoblastoma. *Proc Natl Acad Sci USA* 1971; 68:820.

28. Knudson AG, Strong LC. Mutation and cancer: neuroblastoma and pheochromocytoma. *Am J Hum Genet* 1972; 24:514.

29. Barski G, Cornefert G. Characteristics of "hybrid"-type clonal cell lines obtained from mixed cultures in vitro. *J Natl Cancer Inst* 1962; 28:801.

30. Harris H. Cell fusion and the analysis of malignancy: the Croonian lecture. *Proc Roy Soc London Ser B* 1971; 179:1.

31. Harris H, Watkins JF. Hybrid cells derived from mouse and man: artificial heterokaryons of mammalian cells from different species. *Nature* 1965; 205:640.

32. Jonasson J, Povey S, Harris H. The analysis of malignancy by cell fusion. VII. Cytogenetic analysis of hybrids between malignant and diploid cells of tumours derived from them. *J Cell Sci* 1977; 24:217.

33. Klein G. The approaching era of the tumor suppressor genes. *Science* 1987; 238:1539.

34. Saxon PJ, Srivatsan ES, Leipzig GV, Sameshima JH, Stanbridge EJ. Selective transfer of individual human chromosomes to recipient cells. *Mol Cell Biol* 1985; 5:140.

35. Weissman BE, Saxon PJ, Pasquale SR, et al. Introduction of a normal human chromosome 11 into a Wilms' tumor cell line controls its tumorigenic expression. *Science* 1987; 236:175.

36. Bolande RP. Models and concepts derived from human teratogenesis and oncogenesis in early life. *J Histochem Cytochem* 1984; 32:878.

37. Nehen JH. Spontaneous regression of retinoblastoma. *Arch Ophthalmol* 1975; 53:647.

38. Bolande RP. Benignity of neonatal tumors and concept of cancer repression in early life. *Am J Dis Child* 1971; 122:12.

39. DiPaolo JA, Kotin P. Teratogenesis-oncogenesis: a study of possible relationships. *Arch Pathol* 1966; 81:3.

40. Mercer RD, Lammert AC, Anderson R, Hazard JB. Choriocarcinoma in mother and infant. *J Am Med Assoc* 1958; 166:482.

41. Miller RW. Down's syndrome (mongolism), other congenital malformations and cancers among the sibs of leukemic children. *N Engl J Med* 1963; 268:393.

42. Miller RW. Relation between cancer and congenital defects in man. *N Engl J Med* 1966; 275:87.

43. Miller RW. Relation between cancer and congenital defects: an epidemiologic evaluation. *J Natl Cancer Inst* 1968; 40:1079.

44. Miller RW. Peculiarities in the occurrence of adrenal cortical carcinoma. *Am J Dis Child* 1978; 132:235.

45. Miller RW, Fraumeni JF. Neuroblastoma: epidemiologic approach to its origin. *Am J Dis Child* 1968; 115:253.

46. Bolande RP. Relationships between teratogenesis and oncogenesis. In: Perrin EV, Finegold M, eds. *Pathology of Development—Or Ontogeny Revisited*. Baltimore: Williams & Wilkins, 1973, pp. 114–34.

47. Bolande RP. Congenital and infantile neoplasia of the kidney. *Lancet* 1974; 2:1497.

48. Bolande RP. Neoplasia of early life and its relationships to teratogenesis. *Perspect Pediatr Pathol* 1976; 3:145.

49. Herbst AL, Poskanzer DC, Robboy SJ, Friedlander L, Scully RE. Prenatal exposure to stilbestrol: a perspective comparison of exposed female offspring with unexposed controls. *N Engl J Med* 1975; 292:334.

50. Breslow NE, Beckwith JB. Epidemiological features of Wilms' tumor: results of the National Wilms' Tumor Study. *J Natl Cancer Inst* 1982; 68:429.

51. Miller RW, Fraumeni JF Jr, Manning MD. Association of Wilms' tumor with aniridia, hemihypertrophy, and other congenital malformations. *N Engl J Med* 1964; 270:922.

52. Favara BE, Johnson W, Ito J. Renal tumors in the neonatal period. *Cancer* 1968; 22:845.

53. Fraumeni JF. The aniridia–Wilms' tumor syndrome. *Birth Defects* 1969; 5:198.

54. Shaw MW, Falls HF, Neel JV. Congenital aniridia. *Am J Hum Genet* 1960; 12:289.

55. Fisher JH, Miller YE, Sparkes RS, et al. Wilms' tumor–aniridia association: segregation of affected chromosome in somatic cell hybrids, identification of cell surface antigen associated with deleted area, and regional mapping of *c*-Ha-*ras-l* oncogene, insulin gene and beta-globin gene. *Somat Cell Mol Genet* 1984; 10:455.

56. Nakagome Y, Ise T, Sakurai M, et al. High-resolution studies in patients with aniridia–Wilms tumor association, Wilms tumor or related congenital abnormalities. *Hum Genet* 1984; 67:245.

57. Yunis JJ, Ramsay NKC. Familial occurrence of the aniridia–Wilms' tumor syndrome with deletion 11p13–14.1. *J Pediatr* 1980; 96:1027.

58. Riccarde VM, Hittner HM, Strong LC, et al. Wilms' tumor with aniridia/iris dysplasia and apparently normal chromosomes. *J Pediatr* 1982; 100:574.

59. Riccardi VM, Sujansky E, Smith AC, Francke U. Chromosomal imbalance in the aniridia–Wilms' tumor association: 11p interstitial deletion. *Pediatrics* 1978; 61:604.

60. Benson PF, Vulliamy DG, Taubman JO. Congenital hemihypertrophy and malignancy. *Lancet* 1963; 1:468.

61. Fraumeni JF Jr, Miller RW. Adrenocortical neoplasms with hemihypertrophy, brain tumors, and other disorders. *J Pediatr* 1967; 70:129.

62. Muller S, Gadner H, Weber B, Vogel M, Riehm H. Wilms' tumor and adrenocortical carcinoma with hemihypertrophy and hamartomas. *Eur J Pediatr* 1978; 127:219.

63. Lewis D, Geschickter CF. Tumors of the sympathetic nervous system. *Arch Surg* 1934; 28:16.

64. Vergara B, Svarch E. Myeloblastic leukemia and congenital hemihypertrophy (letter to the editor). *J Pediatr* 1977; 90:1036.

65. Gorlin RJ, Meskin LH. Congenital hemihypertrophy. Review of the literature and report of a case with special emphasis on oral manifestations. *J Pediatr* 1962; 61:870.

66. Majeski JA, Paxton ES, Wirman JA, Schreiber JT. A thoracic benign mesenchymoma in association with hemihypertrophy. *Am J Clin Pathol* 1981; 76:827.

67. Ringrose RE, Jabbour JT, Keele DK. Hemihypertrophy. *Pediatrics* 1965; 36:434.

68. Ishak KG, Glunz PR. Hepatoblastoma and hepatocarcinoma in infancy and childhood. Report of 47 cases. *Cancer* 1967; 20:396.

69. Valdes-Dapena M, Arey JB. Multiple (4) primary neoplasms in a child with aniridia. *Am J Pathol* 1971; 62:22a. Abstract.

70. Fraumeni JF Jr, Geiser CF, Manning MD. Wilms' tumor and congenital hemihypertrophy: report of five new cases and review of the literature. *Pediatrics* 1967; 40:886.

71. Eisenberg RL, Pfister R. Medullary sponge kidney associated with congenital hemihypertrophy (asymmetry). *Am J Roentgenol* 1972; 116:773.

72. Levi M, MacKinnon KJ, Dossetor JB. Hemihypertrophy and medullary sponge kidney. *Can Med Assoc J* 1967; 96:1322.

73. Morris RC, Yamauchi H, Palubinska S, Howenstine J. Medullary sponge kidney. *Am J Med* 1965; 38:883.

74. Parker DA, Salko RG. Congenital asymmetry: report of 10 cases with associated developmental abnormalities. *Pediatrics* 1969; 44:584.

75. Meadows AT, Lichtenfeld JL, Koup CE. Wilms' tumor in three children of a woman with congenital hemihypertrophy. *N Engl J Med* 1974; 291:23.

76. Sotelo-Avila C, Gonzalez-Crussi F, Fowler JW. Complete and incomplete forms of Beckwith-Wiedemann syndrome: their oncogenic potential. *J Pediatr* 1980; 96:47.

77. Brown NJ, Goldie DJ. Beckwith's syndrome with renal neoplasia and alpha-feto-protein secretion. *Arch Dis Child* 1978; 53:435. Abstract.

78. Emery LG, Shields M, Shah NR, Garbes A. Neuroblastoma associated with Beckwith-Wiedemann syndrome. *Cancer* 1983; 52:176.

79. Odom LF. Written communication.

80. O'Hara D. Pancreatoblastoma—does it exist? *Pediatr Pathol* 1985; 3:118. Abstract.

81. Wiedemann HR. Tumours and hemihypertrophy associated with Wiedemann-Beckwith syndrome. *Eur J Pediatr* 1983; 141:129

82. Sotelo-Avila C, Gonzales-Crussi F, Starling KA. Wilms' tumor in a patient with an incomplete form of Beckwith-Wiedemann syndrome. *Pediatrics* 1980; 66:121.

83. Kelly DR, Buntain WL, Dearth JC. *Pancreatic Adenocarcinoma and Hepatoblastoma in a Child with Probable Beckwith-Wiedemann Syndrome.* Presented at the International Academy of Pathology meeting, Miami, FL, September 1984. Abstract.

84. Wockel W, Scheibner K, Lageman A. A variant of the Weidemann-Beckwith syndrome. *Eur J Pediatr* 1981; 135:319.

85. Bolande RP, Brough AJ, Izant RJ Jr. Congenital mesoblastic nephroma of infancy. *Pediatrics* 1967; 40:272.

86. Blank E, Neerhout RC, Burry KA. Congenital mesoblastic nephroma and polyhydramnios. *J Am Med Assoc* 1978; 240:1504.

87. Hartenstein H. Wilms' tumor in a newborn infant. Report of a case with autopsy studies. *J Pediatr* 1949; 35:381.

88. Bolande RP. Congenital mesoblastic nephroma of infancy. *Perspect Pediatr Pathol* 1973; 1:227.

89. Howell CG, Othersen HB, Kiviat NE, et al. Therapy and outcome in 51 children with mesoblastic nephroma: a report of the National Wilms' Tumor Study. *J Pediatr Surg* 1982; 17:826.

90. Fu Y-S, Kay S. Congenital mesoblastic nephroma and its recurrence. *Arch Pathol* 1973; 96:66.

91. Gonzalez-Crussi F, Sotelo-Avila C, Kidd JM. Malignant mesenchymal nephroma of infancy. Report of a case with pulmonary metastases. *Am J Surg Pathol* 1980; 4:185.

92. Joshi VV, Kay S, Milstein R. Congenital mesoblastic nephroma of infancy: report of a case with unusual clinical behavior. *Am J Clin Pathol* 1973; 60:811.

93. Steinfeild AD, Crowley CA, O'Shea PA, Tefft M. Recurrent and metastatic mesoblastic nephroma in infancy. *J Clin Oncol* 1984; 2:956.

94. Walker D, Richard GA. Fetal hamartoma of the kidney: recurrence and death of a patient. *J Urol* 1973; 110:352.

95. Ganick DJ, Gilbert EF, Beckwith JB, Kiviat N. Congenital cystic mesoblastic nephroma. *Hum Pathol* 1981; 12:1039.

96. Shen SC, Yunis EJ. A study of the cellularity and ultrastructure of congenital mesoblastic nephroma. *Cancer* 1980; 45:306.

97. Argyle JC, Beckwith JB. Significance of anaplasia in congenital mesoblastic nephromas. *Lab Invest* 1985; 52:1P. Abstract.

98. Beckwith JB. Mesenchymal renal neoplasms of infancy. *J Pediatr Surg* 1970; 5:405.

99. Wigger HJ. Fetal mesenchyma hamartoma of kidney. A tumor of secondary mesenchyme. *Cancer* 1975; 36:1002.

100. Beckwith JB, Yokomori K. *Clear Cell Sarcoma of the Kidney. Is It Derived from Mesoblastic Nephroma.* Presented at the Interim Meeting of the Pediatric Pathology Club, Vancouver, BC, Canada, October 1982.

101. Machin GA. Persistent renal blastema as a precursor of Wilms' tumor. In: Pochedly C, Baum ES, eds. *Wilms' Tumor.* New York: Elsevier, 1984, pp. 214–49.

102. Bove KE, McAdams AJ. The nephroblastomatosis complex and its relationship to Wilms' tumor: a clinicopathologic treatise. *Perspect Pediatr Pathol* 1976; 3:185–223.

103. Potter EL. *Normal and Abnormal Development of the Kidney.* Chicago: Year Book Medical, 1972, pp. 271–3.

104. Potter EL, Osathanondh V. Normal and abnormal development of the kidney. In: Mostofi FK, Smith DE, eds. *The Kidney.* Baltimore: Williams & Wilkins, 1966, pp. 1–16.

105. Feingold M, Cheradi GJ, Simmons C. Familial neuroblastoma and trisomy 13. *Am J Dis Child* 1971; 121:451.

106. Levert G, Gagne F. Micro-nodules d'aspect blastemateaux du cortex renal chez le jeune enfant. *Union Med Can* 1970; 99:1822.

107. Shanklin DR, Sotelo-Avila C. In situ tumors in fetuses, newborns, and young infants. *Biol Neonat* 1969; 14:286.

108. Bennington JL, Beckwith JB. Tumors of the kidney, renal pelvis, and ureter. *Atlas of Tumor Pathology*, 2nd Series, Fascicle 12. Washington, DC: Armed Forces Institute of Pathology, 1975.

109. Bove KE, Koffler H, McAdams AJ. Nodular renal blastema. Definition and possible significance. *Cancer* 1969; 24:323.

110. Hecht F, Bryant JS, Motulsky AG, Giblett ER. The No. 17–18 (E) trisomy syndrome. Studies on cytogenetics, dermatoglyphics, paternal age and linkage. *J Pediatr* 1963; 3:605.

111. Keshgegian AA, Chatten J. Nodular renal blastema in trisomy 13. *Arch Pathol* 1979; 103:73.

112. Coffin CM, Dehner LP. Nodular renal blastema and thanatophoric dwarfism: a newly reported association. *Am J Pediatr Hematol Oncol* 1982; 4:428.

113. Kulkarni R, Bailie MD, Bernstein J. Progression of nephroblastomatosis to Wilms' tumor (Letter to the Editor). *J Pediatr* 1980; 93:178.

114. Machin GA. Persistent renal blastema (nephroblastomatosis) as a frequent precursor of Wilms' tumor, a pathological and clinical review. Part 1. Nephroblastomatosis in context of embryogenesis and genetics. *Am J Pediatr Hematol Oncol* 1980; 2:165.

115. Machin GA. Persistent renal blastema (nephroblastomatosis) as a frequent precursor of Wilms' tumor, a pathological and clinical review. Part 2. Significance of nephroblastomatosis in the genesis of Wilms' tumor. *Am J Pediatr Hematol Oncol* 1980; 2:353.

116. Machin GA. Persistent renal blastema (nephroblastomatosis) as a frequent precursor of Wilms' tumor, a pathologial and clinical review. Part 3. Clinical aspects of nephroblastomatosis. *Am J Pediatr Hematol Oncol* 1980; 2:253.

117. Pochedly C. Persistent renal blastema: a seed of Wilms' tumor? *Hosp Pract* 1981; 16:83.

118. Bolande RP, Vekemans MJ-J. Genetic models of carcinogens. *Hum Pathol* 1983; 14:658.

119. Scharfenberg JC, Beckman EN. Persistent renal blastema in an adult. *Hum Pathol* 1984; 15:791.

120. Hou LT, Holman RL. Bilateral nephroblastomatosis in a premature infant. *J Pathol Bacteriol* 1961; 82:249.

121. Beckwith JB, Kiviat NB, Bonadio JF. Nephrogenic restis, nephroblastomatosis and the pathogenesis of Wilms' tumor. *Pediatr Pathol* 1990; 10:1–36.

121a. Mankad VN, Gray GF, Miller DR. Bilateral nephroblastomatosis and Klippel-Trenaunay syndrome. *Cancer* 1974; 33:1462.

122. Giangiacomo J, Kissane JM. Congenital Wilms' tumor. In: Pochedly C, Baum ES, eds. *Wilms' Tumor. Clinical and Biological Manifestations.* New York: Elsevier, 1984, pp. 103–10.

123. Kalousek DK, deChadarevian JP, Mackie GG, Bolande RP. Metastatic infantile Wilms' tumor and hydrocephalus. A case report with review of the literature. *Cancer* 1977; 39:1312.

124. Wexler HA, Poole CA, Fojaco RM. Metastatic neonatal Wilms' tumor: a case report with review of the literature *Pediatr Radiol* 1975; 3:179.

125. Palmer NF, Sutow W. Clinical aspects of the rhabdoid tumor of the kidney: a report of the National Wilms' Tumor Study Group. *Med Pediatr Oncol* 1983; 11:242.

126. Ugarte N, Gonzalez-Crussi F, Hsueh W. Wilms' tumor: its morphology in patients under one year of age. *Cancer* 1981; 48:346.

127. Sullivan MP, Hussey DH, Ayala AG. Wilm's tumor. In: Sutow WM, Vietti TJ, Fernbach DJ, eds. *Clinical Pediatric Oncology.* St. Louis: C.V. Mosby, 1973, p. 359.

128. Beckwith JB. Histopathologic aspects of renal tumors in children. In: *Renal Tumors: Proceedings of the First International Symposium on Kidney Tumors.* New York: Alan R. Liss, 1982, pp. 1–14.

129. Beckwith JB. Wilms' tumor and other renal tumors of childhood. A selective review from the National Wilms' Tumor Study Pathology Center. *Hum Pathol* 1983; 14:481.

130. Junien C. Beckwith-Wiedemann syndrome, tumorigenesis and imprinting. *Curr Opin Genet Dev* 1992; 2:431.

131. Rauscher FJ III. The Wilms' tumor gene product: a developmentally regulated transcription factor in the kidney that functions as a tumor suppressor. *FASEB J* 1993; 7:896.

132. Coppes MJ, Campbell CE, Williams BG. The role of WT1 in Wilms' tumorigenesis. *FASEB J* 1993; 7:886.

133. Wolman SR, Camuto PM, Eisenberg AJ, Feiner HD, Greco MA. Wilms' tumor: a search for the critical lesion. *Hum Pathol* 1990; 21:715.

134. Suzuki H, Honzumi M, Itoh Y, et al. Clear cell sarcoma of the kidney seen in a 3-day-old newborn. *Z Kinderchir* 1983; 38:422.

135. Beckwith JB, Palmer NF. Histopathology and prognosis of Wilms' tumor. Results from the first National Wilms' Tumor Study. *Cancer* 1978; 41:1937.

136. Sotelo-Avila C, Gonzales-Crussi F, Sadowinski S, Gooch WM III, Pena R. Clear cell sarcoma of the kidney. A clinicopathologic study of 21 patients with long term follow-up. *Hum Pathol* 1985; 16:1219.

137. Marsden HB, Lennox EL, Lawler W, Kinnier-Wilson LM. Bone metastases in childhood tumors. *Br J Cancer* 1980; 41:875.

138. Bonnin JM, Rubinstein LJ, Palmer NF, Beckwith JB. The association of embryonal tumors originating in the kidney and in the brain. A report of seven cases. *Cancer* 1984; 54:2137.

139. LaBlanc A, Caillaud JM, Hartmann O, et al. Hypercalcemia preferentially

occurs in unusual forms of childhood non-Hodgkin's lymphoma, rhab-domyosarcoma, and Wilms' tumor. *Cancer* 1984; 54:2132.

140. Mayes LC, Kasselberg AG, Roloff JS, Lukens JN. Hypercalcemia associated with immunoreactive parathyroid hormone in a malignant rhabdoid tumor of the kidney (rhabdoid Wilms' tumor). *Cancer* 1984; 54:882.

141. Rousseau-Merck MF, Boccon-Gibod L, Nogues C, et al. An original hypercalcemic infantile renal tumor without the bone metastases. Heterotransplantation to nude mice. Report of two cases. *Cancer* 1982; 50:85.

142. Haas JE, Palmer NF, Weinberg AG, Beckwith JB. Ultrastructure of malignant rhabdoid tumor of the kidney. A distinctive renal tumor of childhood. *Hum Pathol* 1981; 12:646.

143. Ekfors TO, Aho HJ, Kekomaki M. Malignant rhabdoid tumor of the prostatic region. Immunohistochemical and ultrastructural evidence for epithelial origin. *Virchows Arch A* 1985; 406:381.

144. Lemus LB, Hamoudi AB. Malignant thymic tumor in an infant (malignant histiocytoma). *Arch Pathol Lab Med* 1978; 102:84.

145. Lynch HT, Shurin SB, Dahms BB, et al. Paravertebral malignant rhabdoid tumor in infancy. *In vitro* studies of a familial tumor. *Cancer* 1983; 52:290.

146. Frierson HF, Mills SE, Innes DJ Jr. Malignant rhabdoid tumor of the pelvis. *Cancer* 1985; 55:1963.

147. Small EJ, Gordon GJ, Dahms BB. Malignant rhabdoid tumor of the heart in an infant. *Cancer* 1985; 55:2850.

148. Sotelo-Avila C, Gonzalez-Crussi F, deMello D, et al. Renal and extrarenal rhabdoid tumors in children: a clinicopathologic study of 14 patients. *Semin Diagn Pathol* 1986; 3:151–63.

149. Briner J, Bannwart F, Kleihues P, et al. Malignant small cell tumor of the brain with intermediate filaments—a case of a primary cerebral rhabdoid tumor. *Pediatr Pathol* 1985; 3:117–18. Abstract.

150. Tsuneyoshi M, Daimaru Y, Hashimoto H, Enjoji M. Malignant soft tissue neoplasms with the histologic features of renal rhabdoid tumors: an ultrastructural and immunohistochemical study. *Hum Pathol* 1985; 16:1235.

151. Stocker JT, Ishak KG. Mesenchymal hamartoma of the liver. Report of 30 cases and review of the literature. *Pediatr Pathol* 1983; 1:245.

152. Resnick MB, Kozakewich HPW, Perez-Atayde A. Hepatic adenoma in the pediatric age group. Clinicopathologic observations and assessment of cell proliferative activity. *Am J Surg Pathol* 1995; 19:1181.

153. Gonzalez-Crussi F. Undifferentiated small cell ("anaplastic") hepatoblastoma. *Pediatr Pathol* 1991; 11:155–61.

154. Stocker TA, Ishak KG. Undifferentiated (embryonal) sarcoma of the liver. Report of 31 cases. *Cancer* 1978; 42:336.

155. Dische MR, Gardner HA. Mixed teratoid tumors of the liver and neck in trisomy 13. *Am J Clin Pathol* 1978; 69:631.

156. McGoldrick JP, Boston VE, Glasgow JFT. Hepatocellular carcinoma associated with macronodular cirrhosis in a neonate. *J Pediatr Surg* 1986; 21:177.

157. Jaffe N. Biologic vagaries in neuroblastoma. In: Pochedly C, ed. *Neuroblastoma. Clinical and Biological Manifestations.* New York: Elsevier, 1982, pp. 293–309.

158. Beckwith JB, Perrin EV. *In situ* neuroblastomas: a contribution to the natural history of neural crest tumors. *Am J Pathol* 1963; 43:1089.

159. Coupland RE. *The Natural History of the Chromaffin Cell.* London: Longmans, Green, 1965, pp. 47–76.

160. Romansky SG. Neural crest aggregates in the human fetal adrenal gland. *Lab Invest* 1979; 40:9. Abstract.

161. Knudson AG Jr, Meadows AT. Regression of neuroblastoma IV–S: a genetic hypothesis. *N Engl J Med* 1980; 302:1254.

162. Sy WM, Edmonson JH. The developmental defects associated with neuroblastoma—etiologic implications. *Cancer* 1968; 22:234.

163. Knudson AG. Mutagenesis and embryonal carcinogenesis. *Natl Cancer Inst Monogr* 1979; 51:19.

164. Knudson AG Jr, Meadows AT. Developmental genetics of neuroblastoma. *J Natl Cancer Inst* 1976; 57:675.

165. Miller RW, Fraumeni JF, Hill JA. Neuroblastoma: epidemiologic approach to its origin. *Am J Dis Child* 1968; 115:253.

166. Jaffe N. Neuroblastoma: review of the literature and examination of its enigmatic character. *Cancer Treat Rev* 1976; 3:61.

167. Garvin JH Jr, Lack EE, Berenberg W, Frantz CN. Ganglioneuroma presenting with differentiated skeletal metastases. *Cancer* 1984; 54:357.

168. D'Angio GJ, Evans AE, Koop CE. Special pattern of widespread neuroblastoma with a favourable prognosis. *Lancet* 1971; 1:1046.

169. Breslow N, McCann B. Statistical estimation of prognosis of children with neuroblastoma. *Cancer Res* 1971; 31:2098.

170. Evans AE, D'Angio GJ, Randolph J. A proposed staging for children with neuroblastoma. Children's Cancer Study Group A. *Cancer* 1971; 27:374.

171. Jereb B, Bretsky SS, Vogel R, Helson L. Age and prognosis in neuroblastoma. Review of 112 patients younger than 2 years. *Am J Pediatr Hematol Oncol* 1984; 6:233.

172. Carachi R, Campbell PE, Kent M. Thoracic neural crest tumors. A clinical review. *Cancer* 1983; 51:949.

173. Filler RM, Traggis DG, Jaffe N, Vawter GF. Favorable outlook for children with mediastinal neuroblastoma. *J Pediatr Surg* 1972; 7:136.

174. Brodeur GM, Seeger RC, Schwab M, Varmus HE, Bishop JM. Amplification of *N-myc* in untreated human neuroblastomas correlates with advanced disease stage. *Science* 1984; 224:1121.

175. Seeger RC, Brodeur GM, Sather H, et al. Association of multiple copies of the *N-myc* oncogene with rapid progression of neuroblastomas. *N Engl J Med* 1985; 313:1111.

176. Beckwith JB, Martin RF. Observations on the histopathology of neuroblas-tomas. *J Pediatr Surg* 1968; 3:106.

177. Shimada H, Chatten J, Newton WA Jr, et al. Histopathologic prognostic factors in neuroblastic tumors: definition of subtypes of ganglioneuroblastoma and on age-linkd classification of neuroblastomas. *J Natl Cancer Inst* 1984; 73:405.

178. Joshi VJ. Small round cell tumors and related lesions of children. In: *Common Problems in Pediatric Pathology.* New York: Igaku-Shoin, 1994, p. 415.

179. Brodeur GM, Nakagawara A. Molecular basis of clinical heterogeneity in neuroblastoma. *Am J Pediatr Hematol Oncol* 1992; 14:111.

180. Maris JM, White PS, Beltinger CP, Sulman EP, et al. Significance of chromosome 1p loss of heterozygosity in neuroblastoma. *Cancer Res* 1995; 55:4664–9.

181. Look AT, Hayaes FA, Nitschke R, et al. Cellular DNA content as predictor of response to chemotherapy in infants with unresectable neuroblastoma. *New Engl J Med* 1984; 311:231.

182. Nakagawara A, Arima-Nakagawara M, Scavarda NJ, et al. Association between high levels of expression of the TRK gene and favorable outcome in human neuroblastoma. *New Engl J Med* 1993; 328:847.

183. Taxy JB. Electron microscopy in the diagnosis of neuroblastoma. *Arch Pathol Lab Med* 1980; 104:355.

184. Romansky SG, Crocker DW, Shaw KNF. Ultrastructural studies on neuroblastoma. Evaluation of cytodifferentiation and correlation of morphology and biochemical and survival data. *Cancer* 1978; 42:2392.

185. LaBrosse EH, Comoy E, Bohoun C, Zucker J-M, Schweisguth O. Catecholamine metabolism in neuroblastoma. *J Natl Cancer Inst* 1976; 57:633.

186. Laug WE, Siegel SE, Shaw KNF, Landing B, Baptista J, Gutenstein M. Initial urinary catecholamine metabolite concentrations and prognosis in neuroblastoma. *Pediatrics* 1978; 62:77.

187. Dranoff G, Bigner DD. A word of caution in the use of neuron-specific enolase expression in tumor diagnosis. *Arch Pathol Lab Med* 1984; 108:535.

188. Vinores SA, Bonnin JM, Rubistein LJ, Marangos PJ. Immunohistochemical demonstration of neuronspecific enolase in neoplasms of the CNS and other tissues. *Arch Pathol Lab Med* 1984; 108:536.

189. Reynolds CP, German DC, Weinburg AG, Smith RG. Catecholamine fluorescence and tissue culture morphology. Technics in the diagnosis of neuroblastoma. *Am J Clin Pathol* 1981; 75:275.

190. Scott JP, Morgan E. Coagulopathy of disseminated neuroblastoma. *J Pediatr* 1983; 103:219.

191. Grotting JC, Kassel S, Dehner LP. Nesidioblastosis and congenital neuroblas-toma. *Arch Pathol Lab Med* 1979; 103:642.

192. Senelick RC, Bray PF, Lahey MA, Van Dyk HJL, Johnson DG. Neuroblastoma and myoclonic encephalopathy: two cases and a review of the literature. *J Pediatr Surg* 1973; 8:623.

193. Jaffe N, Cassady JR, Filler RM, Petersen R, Traggis D. Heterochromia and Horner's syndrome associated with cervical and mediastinal neuroblastoma. *J Pediatr* 1975; 87:75.

194. Gerson JM, Chatten J, Eisman S. Familial neuroblastoma—a follow-up. (Letter to the Editor). *N Engl J Med* 1974; 290:1487.

195. Bolande RP. The neurocristopathies. A unifying concept of disease arising in neural crest maldevelopment. *Hum Pathol* 1974; 5:409.

196. Gonzalez-Crussi F. Extragonadal teratomas. *Atlas of Tumor Pathology.* 2nd Series, Fascicle 18. Washington, DC: Armed Forces Institute of Pathology, 1982.

197. Dehner LP. Neoplasms of the fetus and neonate. In: Naeye RL, Kissane JM, Kauffman N, eds. *Perinatal Diseases.* International Academy of Pathology Monograph. Baltimore: Williams & Wilkins, 1981, pp. 286–345.

198. Kohler HG. Sacrococcygeal teratoma and "nonimmunological" hydrops. *Br Med J* 1976; 2:422.

199. Rosenfeld CR, Coln CD, Duenhoelter JH. Fetal cervical teratoma as a cause of polyhydramnios. *Pediatrics* 1979; 64:176.
200. Billmire DF, Grosfeld JL. Teratomas in childhood: analysis of 142 cases. *J Pediatr Surg* 1986; 21:548.
201. Aubert J, Casamayou J, Denis P. Intrarenal teratoma in a newborn infant. *Eur Urol* 1978; 4:306.
202. Dehner LP. Intrarenal teratoma occurring in infancy: report of a case with discussion of extragonadal germ cell tumors in infancy. *J Pediatr Surg* 1973; 8:369.
203. Esposito G, Cigliano B, Paludetto R. Abdominothoracic gastric teratoma in a female newborn infant. *J Pediatr Surg* 1983; 18:304.
204. Warkani J, Lemire RJ, Cohen MM Jr. *Mental Retardation and Congenital Malformations of the Central Nervous System.* Chicago: Year Book Medical, 1981, p. 300.
205. Fessard C. Cerebral tumors in infancy. 66 clinicoanatomical case studies. *Am J Dis Child* 1968; 115:302.
206. Schoenberg BS, Schoenberg DG, Christine BW. The epidemiology of primary intracranial neoplasms of childhood. A population study. *Mayo Clin Proc* 1976; 51:51.
207. Amacher AL, Torres QU, Rittenhouse S. Congenital medulloblastoma: an inquiry into origins. *Child Nerv Syst* 1986; 2:262.
208. Heiskanen O. Intracranial tumors in children. *Child Brain* 1977; 3:69.
209. Enzinger FM, Lattes R, Torloni H. Histological typing of tissue tumours. *International Histological Classification of Tumours*, No. 3. WHO, Geneva, 1969, p. 13.
210. Keeling JW, ed. *Fetal and Neonatal Pathology.* 2nd ed. London: Springer-Verlag, 1993.
211. Kaufman SC, Stout AP. Congenital mesenchymal tumors. *Cancer* 1965; 18:460.
212. Allen PW. The fibromatoses: a clinicopathologic classification based on 140 cases. Part I. *Am J Surg Pathol* 1977; 1:255–270. Part II:305–321.
213. Enzinger FM, Weiss SW. Fibrous tumors of infancy and childhood. In: *Soft Tissue Tumors.* 3rd Ed. St. Louis: CV Mosby, 1995, p. 231.
214. Rosenberg HS, Stenback WA, Spjut HJ. The fibromatoses of infancy and childhood. *Perspect Pediatr Pathol* 1978; 4:269.
215. Fukasawa Y, Ishikura H, Takada A, et al. Massive apoptosis in infantile myofibromatosis. A putative mechanism of tumor regression. *Am J Pathol* 1993; 144:480.
216. Fletcher CDM, Achu P, Van Noorden S, McKee PH. Infantile myofibromatosis: a light microscopic, histochemical and immunohistochemical study suggesting true smooth muscle differentiation. *Histopathology* 1987; 11:245.
217. Kennedy S, Yunis E, Smith S, Locker J. Morphologic and molecular analysis of congenital myofibromatosis and fibromatosis. *Mod Pathol* 1990; 3:4P.
218. Bracko M, Cindro L, Golouh R. Familial occurrence of infantile myofibromatosis. *Cancer* 1991; 69:1294.
219. Venencie PY, Bigel P, Desgruelles C, Lortat-Jacob S, Dufier JL, Saurat JH. Infantile myofibromatosis: report of two cases in one family. *Br J Dermatol* 1987; 117:255.
219a. Reye RDK. Recurring digital fibrous tumors of childhood. *Arch Pathol* 1965; 80:228.
220. Rosenthal NS, Abdul-Karim FW. Childhood fibrous tumor with psammoma bodies: clinicopathologic features in two cases. *Arch Pathol Lab Med* 1988; 112:798.
221. Stout AP. Fibrosarcoma in infants and children. Cancer 1962; 15:1028.
222. Wilson MB, Stanley W, Sens D, et al. Infantile fibrosarcoma—a misnomer? *Pediatr Pathol* 1990; 10:901.
223. Coffin CM, Jaszcz W, O'Shea PA, Dehner LP. So-called congenital-infantile fibrosarcoma: does it exist and what is it? *Pediatr Pathol* 1994; 14:133.
224. Madden NP, Spicer RB, Allibore EB, et al. Spontaneous regression of neonatal fibrosarcoma. *Br J Cancer [Suppl]* 1992; 18:S72.
225. Mandahl N, Heim S, Rydholm A, Willen H, Mitelman F. Nonrandom numerical chromosome aberrations (+8, +11, +17, +20) in infantile fibrosarcoma [letter]. *Cancer Genet Cytogenet* 1989; 40:137.
226. Schofield DE, Fletcher JA, Grier HE, Yunis EJ. Fibrosarcoma in infants and children. Application of new techniques. *Am J Surg Pathol* 1994; 18:14.
227. Lundgren L, Angervall L, Stenman G, Kindblom LG. Infantile rhabdomyo-fibrosarcoma: a high-grade sarcoma indistinguishable from fibrosarcoma and rhabdomyosarcoma. *Hum Pathol* 1993; 24:785.
228. Egan MJ, Raafat F, Crocker J, Smith K. Nucleolar organizer regions in fibrous proliferations of childhood and infantile fibrosarcoma. *J Clin Pathol* 1988; 41:31.
229. Ohiro Y, Fukuda T, Tsuneyoshi M. Fibrosarcoma versus fibromatoses and nodular fasciitis. A comparative study of their proliferative activity using proliferating nuclear antigen, DNA flow cytometry, and p53. *Am J Surg Pathol* 1994; 18:712.
230. Kapadia SB, Meis JM, Frisman DM, Ellis GL, Heffner DK. Fetal rhabdomyoma of the head and neck: a clinicopathologic and immunophenotypic study of 24 cases. *Hum Pathol* 1993; 24:754.
231. Newton WA, Gehan EA, Webber BL, Marsden HB, van Unnik AJM, et al. Classification of rhabdomyosarcomas and related sarcomas. Pathologic aspects and proposal for a new classification—an Intergroup Rhabdomyosarcoma Study. *Cancer* 1995; 76:1073.
232. Mulliken JB, Glowacki J. Hemangiomas and vascular malformations in infants and children: a classification based on endothelial characteristics. *Plast Reconstruct Surg* 1982; 69:412–20. (See discussion by HG Thomson, *ibid*, pp. 421–42.)
233. Silverman RA. Hemangiomas and vascular malformations. *Pediatr Clin N Amer* 1991; 38:811.
234. Mills SE, Cooper PH, Fechner RE. Lobular capillary hemangioma: the underlying lesion of pyogenic granuloma: a study of 73 cases from the oral and nasal mucous membranes. *Am J Surg Pathol* 1980; 4:273.
234a. Kasabach HH, Merritt KK. Capillary hemangioma with extensive purpura. *Am J Dis Child* 1940; 69:1063.
235. Pasyk AK, Grabb WC, Cherry GW. Cellular hemangioma: light and electron microscopic studies of two cases. *Virchows Arch Pathol Anat* 1982; 396:103.
236. Pasyk KA, Grabb WC, Cherry GW. Crystalloid inclusions in endothelial cells of cellular and capillary hemangiomas. A possible sign of cellular immaturity. *Arch Dermatol* 1983; 119:134.
237. Gonzalez-Crussi F, Reyes-Mugica M. Cellular hemangiomas ("hemangio-endotheliomas") in infants. Light microscopic, immunohistochemical and ultrastructural observations. *Am J Surg Pathol* 1991; 15:769.
238. Angervall L, Nielsen JM, Stener B, et al. Concomitant arteriovenous malformation in skeletal muscle. *Cancer* 1979; 44:232.
239. Gonzalez-Crussi F, Enneking WF, Arean VM. Infiltrating angiolipoma. *J Bone Joint Surg* 1966; 48-A:1111.
240. Allen PW, Enzinger FM. Hemangioma of skeletal muscle. An analysis of 89 cases. *Cancer* 1972; 29:8.
241. Beham A, Fletcher CDM. Intramuscular angioma: a clinicopathologic analysis of 74 cases. *Histopathology* 1991; 18:53.
242. Alessi E, Bertani E, Sala F. Acquired tufted angioma. *Am J Dermatopathol* 1986; 8:426.
243. Padilla RS, Orkin M, Rosai J. Acquired "tufted" hemangioma (progressive capillary hemangioma). A distinctive clinicopathologic entity related to lobular capillary hemangioma. *Am J Dermatopathol* 1987; 9:292.
244. Dabska M. Malignant endovascular papillary angioendothelioma of the skin in childhood. Clinicopathologic study of 6 cases. *Cancer* 1969; 24: 503.
245. Jenkins JJ. Congenital malignant hemangiopericytoma. *Pediatr Pathol* 1987; 7:119.
246. Chabalko JJ, Fraumeni JF. Blood-vessel neoplasms in children: epidemiologic aspects. *Med Pediatr Oncol* 1975; 1:135.
247. Cohen DM, Mitchel CB, Alexander JW. Letterer–Siwe disease in a newborn. *Arch Pathol* 1966; 31:347.
248. Cutler LS, Chaudhry AP, Topazian R. Melanotic neuroectodermal tumor of infancy: an ultrastructural study, literature review, and reevaluation. *Cancer* 1981; 48:257.
249. Young S, Gonzalez-Crussi F. Melanocytic neuroectodermal tumor of the foot. Report of a case with multicentric origin. *Am J Clin Pathol* 1985; 84:371.
250. Lindahl F. Malignant melanocytic progonoma. One case. *Acta Pathol Microbiol Scand Sect A* 1970; 78:532.
251. Jimenez JF, Seibert RW, Char F, Brown RE, Seibert JJ. Melanotic neuroecto-dermal tumor of infancy and fetal hydantoin syndrome. *Am J Pediatr Hematol Oncol* 1981; 3:9.
252. Robey G, Daneman A, Martin DJ. Pancreatic carcinoma in a neonate. *Pediatr Radiol* 1983; 13:284.
253. Rich RH, Weber JL, Shandling B. Adenocarcinoma of the pancreas in a neonate managed by pancreatoduodenectomy. *J Pediatr Surg* 1986; 21:806.
254. Burt TB, Condon VR, Matlak ME. Fetal pancreatic hamartoma. *Pediatr Radiol* 1983; 13:287.
255. Posen JA, Bar-Maor JA. Leiomyosarcoma of the colon in an infant. A case report and review of the literature. *Cancer* 1983; 52:1458.
256. Jimenez JF, Uthman EO, Townsend JW, Gloster ES, Seibert JJ. Primary bronchopulmonary leiomyosarcoma in childhood. *Arch Pathol Lab Med* 1986; 110:348.
257. Miller RW. Fifty-two forms of childhood cancer: US mortality experience 1960–66. *J Pediatr* 1969; 75:685.
258. Kodilinye HC. Retinoblastoma in Nigeria: problems of treatment. *Am J Ophthalmol* 1967; 63:469.

259. Abramson DH, Ellsworth RM, Tretter P, Javitt J, Kitchin FD. Treatment of bilateral groups I through III retinoblastoma with bilateral radiation. *Arch Ophthalmol* 1981; 99:1761.

260. Potluri VR, Helson LL, Ellsworth RM, Reid T, Gilbert F. Chromosomal abnormalities in human retinoblastoma. A review. *Cancer* 1986; 58:663.

261. Rootman J, Carruthers JDA, Miller RR. Retinoblastoma. *Perspect Pediatr Pathol* 1987; 10:208.

262. Hansen MF, Koufos A, Gallie BI, et al. Osteosarcoma and retinoblastoma: a shared chromosomal mechanism revealing recessive predisposition. *Proc Natl Acad Sci* 1985; 82:6216.

263. Abramson DH, Ellsworth RM, Kitchin FD, Tung GT. Second nonocular tumors in retinoblastoma survivors: are they radiation induced? *Ophthalmology* 1984; 91:1351.

264. Bures C, Barnes L. Benign mesenchymomas of the head and neck. *Arch Pathol Lab Med* 1978; 102:237.

265. Mills SE, Allen MS Jr. Congenital occult papillary carcinoma of the thyroid gland. *Hum Pathol* 1986; 17:1179.

266. Alpers CE, Rosenau W, Finkbeiner WE, de Lorimier AA, Kronish D. Congenital (infantile) hemangiopericytoma of the tongue and sublingual region. *Am J Clin Pathol* 1984; 81:377.

267. Gonzalez-Crussi F, Eberts TJ, Mirkin D. Congenital fibrous hamartoma of the heart. *Arch Pathol* 1978; 102:491.

268. Naraysingh V, Busby GOD. Congenital malignant melanoma. *J Pediatr Surg* 1986; 21:81.

269. Kadell BM. Congenital atypical benign chondroblastoma of a rib. *J Pediatr Surg* 1970; 5:46.

270. Nix WL. Sacrococcygeal chordoma in a neonate with multiple anomalies. *J Pediatr* 1978; 93:995.

271. Brandt T, Hatch EL, Shaller RT, et al. Surgical management of the infant with mesenchymal hamartoma of the chest wall. *J Pediatr Surg* 1986; 21:556.

272. Tepas JJ, Deen HG, McArtor R, Southern TE. Giant cystic choristoma of the head and neck in a neonate: successful management of a life-threatening respiratory emergency. *J Pediatr Surg* 1982; 17:184.

273. Reddy DR, Mohan SR, Krishna RV. Congenital liposarcoma. *J Indian Med Assoc* 1982; 77:178.

274. Fox H. *Pathology of the Placenta*. Philadelphia: W. B. Saunders, 1978, pp. 357–60.

275. Brodsky I, Baren M, Kahn SB, Lewis G Jr, Tellem M. Metastatic malignant melanoma from mother to fetus. *Cancer* 1965; 18:1048.

276. Holland E. A case of transplacental metastases of malignant melanoma from mother to foetus. *J Obstet Gynaecol Br Emp* 1949; 56:529–36.

277. Daamen CBF, Bloem GWD, Westerbeek AJ. Chorionepithelioma in mother and child. *J Obstet Gynaecol Br Commonw* 1961; 68:144.

278. Kruseman ACN, Van Lent M, Blom AH, Lauw GP. Choriocarcinoma in mother and child, identified by immunoenzyme histochemistry. *Am J Clin Pathol* 1977; 67:279.

279. Witzleben CL, Bruninga G. Infantile choriocarcinoma: a characteristic syndrome. *J Pediatr* 1968; 73:374.

Disorders of the Lymphoid Tissues and the Immune System

Don B. Singer

The immune system is composed of a widely distributed and disparate set of elements. The immunologically specific components, also called the adaptive system, are the T and B lymphocytes. The nonspecific effector, also called the innate, components include the phagocytes, the dendritic cells of the spleen, the epidermal Langerhans' cells, specialized epithelial cells of the thymus, bone marrow, other lymphoid organs, the complement system, and similar substances [1, 2]. The cell products of the lymphocytes are cytokines and immunoglobulins (Ig). These interact with each other and with nonlymphoid elements as well. Receptors on T lymphocytes and B lymphocytes are similar in many respects. They are disulfide-linked heterodimers that can each react with only one antigenic determinant, a specificity predicted in the clonal selection theory [3]. B cells respond to free antigens directly and secrete their receptors as immunoglobulins while T cells, with their receptors for major histocompatibility complex (MHC) proteins, require presentation of the antigens by other cells, especially macrophages but also some endothelial and glial cells. The T cell receptors remain fixed to the cell membrane. In addition to B and T cells, the natural killer cells (NK cells) are characterized as one kind of large granular lymphocyte and seem to have some anti-tumor surveillance function. Antibody dependent cellular cytotoxic (ADCC) lymphocytes are not yet well characterized in fetuses and neonates [4].

FORMATION OF LYMPHOID TISSUES OF THE IMMUNE SYSTEM

Lymphatics

Angioblasts arise at the end of the second week to the middle of the third week of development [5]. Lymphatic vessels originate in discrete spaces in the mesenchyme. They develop independently of the blood vessels and of venous connections which develop a bit later. By progressive fusion, these spaces become continuous channels adjacent to the main primitive venous trunks. They form six main sacs: the paired jugular sacs, the unpaired retroperitoneal sac at the root of the mesentery, the unpaired cisterna chyli, and the paired posterior sacs adjacent to the sciatic veins. The thoracic duct develops from downgrowth of the jugular sacs which meet upgrowths from the cisterna chyli. The jugular sacs are the only ones that develop permanent connections to adjacent veins. Failure of these connections leads to cystic hygroma which commonly occurs in monosomy X (Turner syndrome) but may also be found in trisomy 21, trisomy 18, and trisomy 13 syndromes, and in other chromosomal and nonchromosomal conditions [6]. The thoracic duct is a rich source of T cells with few B cells. Thoracic duct disruption, as in cases of chylothorax, causes T cell depletion with immunosuppression [3]. Other forms of lymphatic maldevelopment include hypoplasia of pulmonary septal lymphatic vessels which produces pleural effusions, hypoplastic lungs, respiratory insufficiency, and fetal hydrops [7]. The surface lymphatics in the visceral pleura may be accentuated in congenital pulmonary lymphangiectasis (Chap. 21). Lymphatic aplasia and hypoplasia of other organs are described and are sometimes associated with abnormalities such as the double eyelash syndrome, gonadal dysgenesis, Milroy disease, and so on [8].

Lymph Nodes

During the third month of development, the lymph sacs begin to form plexuses of vessels, and primary lymph nodes appear in these areas. The plexus form in strands of mesenchymal tissue which proliferate to form nodules. Secondary nodes develop later along the course of the lymphatics which spread from these centers. The vessels are crowded to the periphery where the peripheral sinus appears. A connective tissue capsule condenses around the whole nodule. Nutrient blood vessels enter and leave the nodules via the hilus. Lymphocytic cells populate these nodules and form ill-defined follicles which become more discrete after 25 to 28 weeks of gestation (Figs. 16.1 and 16.2). Follicular centers (germinal centers) form normally only after 2 to 3 months of postnatal life [9]. They may develop precociously in fetal life if stimulated by certain antigens such as syphilis, cytomegalovirus, or rubella [10, 11] (Fig. 16.3).

Hemolymph nodes develop similarly to lymph nodes, but in relation to blood vessels rather than lymphatic vessels. The nutrient vessels arise independently of the sinuses although they eventually communicate [12]. The lymph nodes act as filters within the lymphatic vascular tree. Regional nodes respond to antigens introduced nearby and brought to them by afferent lymphatics [3].

Special Regional Lymphoid Tissues

Solvason and Kearney suggest that the omentum is a primary site for developing pre-B cells which are also thought to originate in the liver in late embryonic and early fetal life [13]. Gut-associated lymphoid tissue occurs in the intestines and liver. IgA production is important in this tissue which has a unique pattern of lymphocyte recirculation. Pre-B cells develop in Peyer's patches and, in the postnatal state, meet antigens in the lumen of the gut, then enter the general circulation only to home back to the gut. Bronchus-associated lymphoid tissues in the lower respiratory tract and hilar lymph nodes are also associated with IgA production to inhaled or aspirated antigens. Skin-associated lymphoid

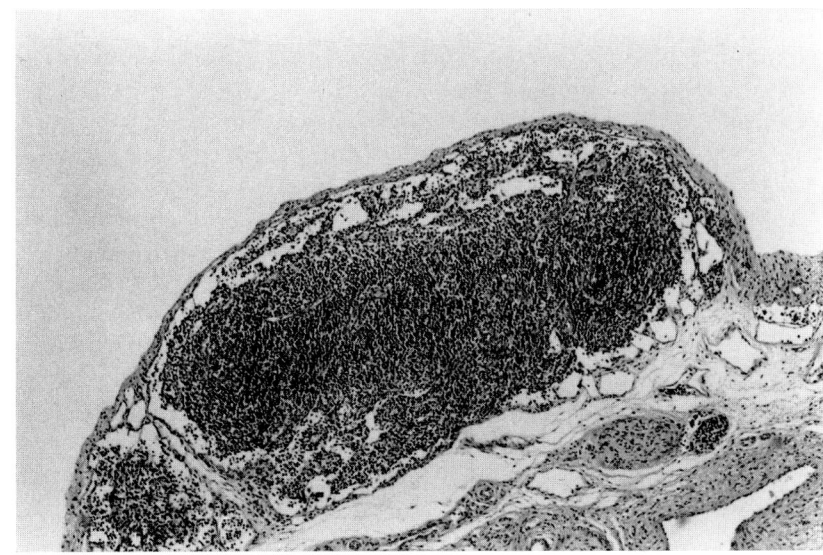

FIGURE 16.1.   *Lymph node from neonate of 21 weeks' gestation. The peripheral sinusoid is widely patent and lymphoid follicles are ill defined. (H&E, ×60.)*

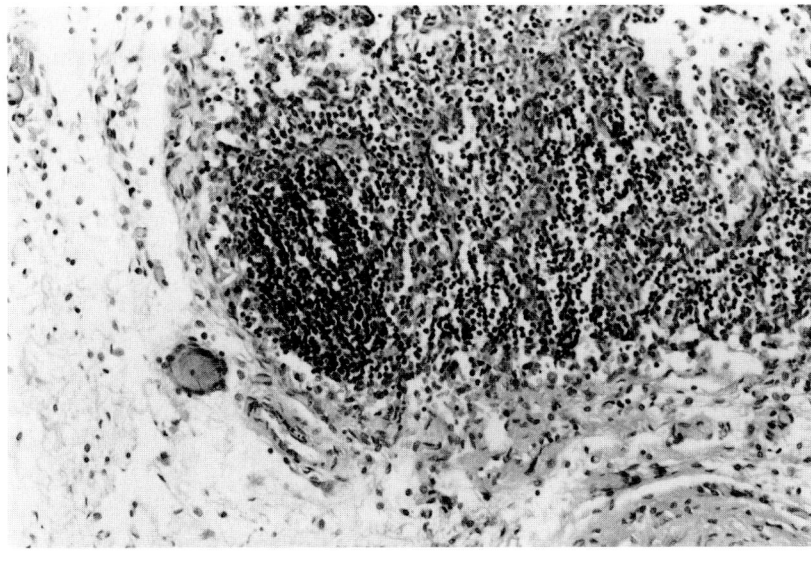

FIGURE 16.2.   *Lymph node from neonate of 26 weeks' gestation. The follicle is well defined but no germinal center has developed. (H&E, ×300.)*

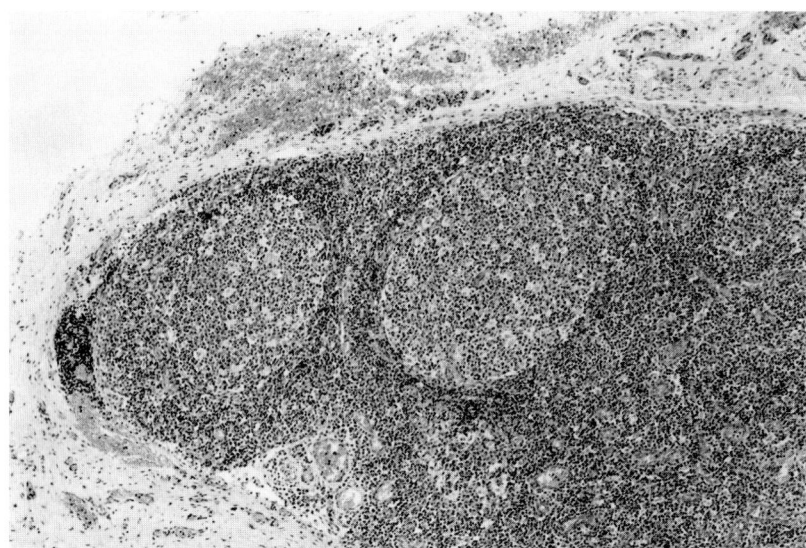

FIGURE 16.3.   *Lymph node from neonate of 28 weeks' gestation. A desquamating skin lesion was present at birth but an infectious agent was not identified. Note the large active germinal centers which indicate a strong antigenic stimulus in utero. (H&E, ×60.)*

tissue is stimulated by antigens presented via epidermal Langerhans' cells. Blood is an important immunoactive tissue with representatives of all the lymphoid and nonlymphoid cell lineages and substances [3].

Pathologic changes in the lymph nodes are to be described in the sections on various immune deficiency and hyperimmune disorder.

Spleen

The spleen is derived from small masses or hillocks of mesenchymal cells located between the layers of the dorsal mesogastrium and shaped by the stomach (foregut) during the 5th week of development [14]. The capsule, connective tissue, and parenchyma of the spleen all form from this mesenchyme. They soon become located on the dorsal body wall between the mesonephric and genital folds. By three months of development, the neonatal form is assumed by fusion of the two or several separate masses [15]. Specialization into red and white pulp seems to be dependent on the manner in which the vascular channels develop. Lymphoid tissue appears early, but splenic corpuscles or follicles which form around arteries are ill defined in normal circumstances until 6 months of gestation (Fig. 16.4). The red pulp develops subsequent to and outward from the white pulp. White pulp has a tight meshwork of reticulum whereas the red pulp has wider spaces forming venous sinusoids which are surrounded by smaller arterial sinusoids [16].

Erythropoiesis and myelopoiesis are both active in the fetal spleen, but this activity is less than that in the liver and it subsides in the last 8 to 10 weeks of prenatal life. Functionally, the spleen acts as a lymphoid filter within the blood vascular tree. It is an important site of antibody production in response to particulate antigens such as bacteria. It can clear the bloodstream of such particles and is especially

effective in this action when the particle is opsonized (coated with opsonizing antibodies). Particles other than bacteria, such as hematopoietic cells, may be similarly treated and cleared from the bloodstream [3]. Splenic function is evaluated by the number of pocked erythrocytes circulating in the blood. In term infants, 24% of the red blood cells have pocks; in premature infants 47% are pocked; and in very low birth weight infants of less than 1500 grams, 60% to 80% of the red blood cells are pocked, indicating that splenic function is more efficient with progressive fetal maturation [17, 18].

Accessory spleens are found incidently at autopsy or surgery in up to 19% of patients [19]. Their maximum dimensions are from 2 mm to 3.5 cm; about half are found in the hilum of the main spleen and the remainder are found in the spleno-renal ligament, the gastrosplenic ligament, the tail of the pancreas, the greater omentum, and in the connective tissue under the left leaf of the diaphragm. Rarely, accessory spleens form in the peritoneum and may be found in or adjacent to the gonads, even as distant as the scrotum. Splenic-gonadal fusion is seen occasionally in the left ovary or testicle [20]. It is more commonly found in males, and while it is often found in the scrotum, it may interfere with descent of the testis. Severe limb defects and micrognathia have been reported in cases of splenic-gonadal fusion [15, 20, 21]. Intestinal obstruction may be caused by a cord-like process consisting of splenic tissue that arises from the superior pole of the spleen and descends ventral to the intestine. In other cases the accessory splenic tissue is discontinuous in relation to the main spleen. Wandering spleen is associated with a stretched pedicle, frequently with torsion and splenic necrosis. It has not been reported in neonates [15].

Polysplenia and splenic agenesis are conditions with many similarities. Either may be an isolated defect or may

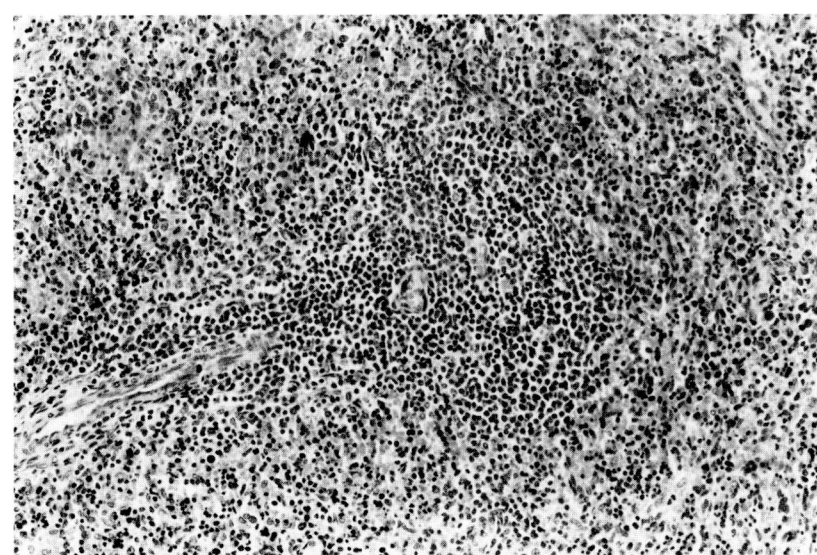

FIGURE 16.4. *Splenic follicle from neonate of 21 weeks' gestation. The arteriole has a sparsely cellular sheath of lymphocytes. (H&E, ×300.)*

have associated defects outside the embryonic field that are directly related to the splanchnic mesoderm. Males predominate among cases of splenic agenesis [15]. Polysplenia, the condition in which two, three, or more splenic masses of comparable size occupy the usual position of the spleen in the left upper quadrant, represents the failure of fusion of the embryonic hillocks in the dorsal mesogastrium. In a review of approximately 3000 autopsy records over a span of 16 years in a referral center, 23 examples of polysplenia (ratio of 1.3 female to 1.0 male); and 24 examples of splenic agenesis (ratio of 0.76 female to 1.0 male) were found. Both splenic agenesis and polysplenia were often associated with tracheobronchial anomalies, cardiac lesions, and disorders of visceral situs or heterotaxia [15, 22]. The splenic agenesis associated with Ivemark syndrome consists of complex congenital cardiac lesions of the conotruncal and endocardial cushion regions as well as tracheal abnormalities [22–24]. Congenital asplenia is also reported with congenital and neonatal infections although sepsis in these cases is usually a postneonatal event [25, 26].

Congenital hypoplasia of the spleen is rare. It was reported with severe infections in two sisters and their brother in one sibship [27]. One of the girls died at 10 months of age due to overwhelming infection with *Haemophilus influenzae*. Two other siblings were unaffected. These were children of a consanguineous union and an autosomal recessive inheritance pattern was suggested. No similar cases have been reported in the nearly 30 years since this report [27].

Thymus

The thymus is composed of both epithelial and lymphoid elements. It arises from the third and fourth branchial pouches, the same embryonic origin as the parathyroids,

about 4 to 6 weeks after conception [28]. This common origin occasionally results in thymic and parathyroid tissue sharing a common capsule. The cervical extensions of the mature thymus are found adjacent to the lower half of each lateral lobe of the thyroid. The thymus usually comes to rest in the anterior mediastinum with two main lobes lying anterior to the innominate vein. Occasionally, the thymus is found posterior to the innominate vein. The two lobes fuse in the midline about 50 days after conception. Soon thereafter, 53 to 58 days, the epithelial thymus is colonized by lymphoid stem cells from the embryonic or fetal liver [29]. Its volume increases 35-fold in 8 to 10 days [30]. Using monoclonal antibodies to a number of lymphoid and nonlymphoid elements, Haynes and his colleagues have found that T-cell development, dendritic cells, epithelial cells, macrophages, and stroma are all well developed by the end of the first trimester of pregnancy [28, 31, 32]. Select cytokines and adhesion molecules at discrete stages of T-cell maturation participate in and regulate the complex processes of T-cell development [33, 34]. The nonlymphoid components of the thymic microenvironment (epithelium, fibroblasts, macrophages) play critical roles in normal thymic development [28]. Epithelial-cell differentiation and fetal thymic lobulation are induced just prior to migration of lymphoid cells to the thymus. The epithelial cells are known to derive from the endodermal elements of the third pharyngeal pouch. The mesoderm-derived capsule penetrates the epithelial thymus and carries with it thymic vessels to form the separations between lobules. This occurs at about 10 weeks of gestation. Histologic distinction between cortex and medulla appears between 11 and 14 weeks and Hassall's corpuscles appear by 12 to 16 weeks of gestation. The thymus has dendritic epithelial cells in the cortex and interdigitating dendritic cells in the medulla. Some of the epithelial cells in the cortex are called "nurse" cells. Immature thymocytes occupy the cortex while mature thymocytes are found throughout but are concentrated in the medulla [28].

At term, the cortex comprises 85% of the total thymus while the medulla comprises 15% (Fig. 16.5). Most T cells never leave the thymus but die there by apoptosis [35]. This process is accelerated by stress in the fetus or neonate (Fig. 16.6). Thymic stress involution is "accidental" as differentiated from "age-related" involution. Stress-induced thymic involution consists of apoptosis of most and exodus of a few thymic lymphocytes with a quickly shrinking organ. The increase in cortical macrophages or uncovering of cortical nurse epithelial cells imparts a starry sky histologic pattern as the depletion of lymphocytes causes less intense blue staining in hematoxylin-stained section [36] (Fig. 16.7). The epithelial components of the medulla, including the thymic

(Hassall's) corpuscles, become conspicuous and tend to collapse upon each other. Van Baarlen et al [37] found a thymic involutional grading system useful in evaluating acute illness in fetuses and neonates: grade 1—some lymphophagocytosis in the cortex; grade 2—a starry sky pattern with some shrinking of the cortex and separation of the thymic lobules; grade 3—blurred corticomedullary demarcation, advanced lymphophagocytosis, narrowing of the cortex, and increased separation of thymic lobules; grade 4—pronounced lymphodepletion of cortex with reversed density, more lymphocytes in the medulla than in the cortex, prominent interstitium and vessels, advanced shrinking and separation of thymic lobules. Using this system, acute illness of less than 12 hours resulted in no changes in two-thirds of the cases, while grade 1 or grade 2 changes were found in the remaining one-third of cases. Illness of

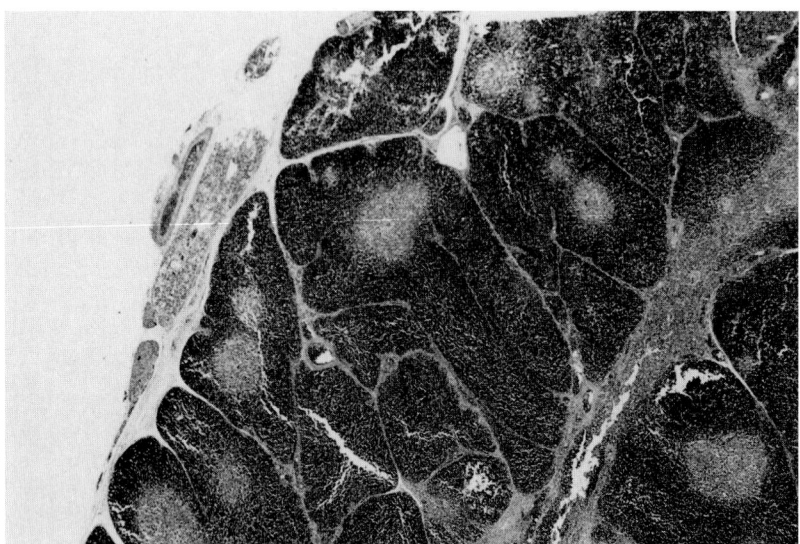

FIGURE 16.5.   *Thymus from neonate of 38 weeks' gestation. The densely cellular cortex and the medulla are clearly demarcated. The cortex occupies approximately 85% of the parenchyma. (H&E, ×15.)*

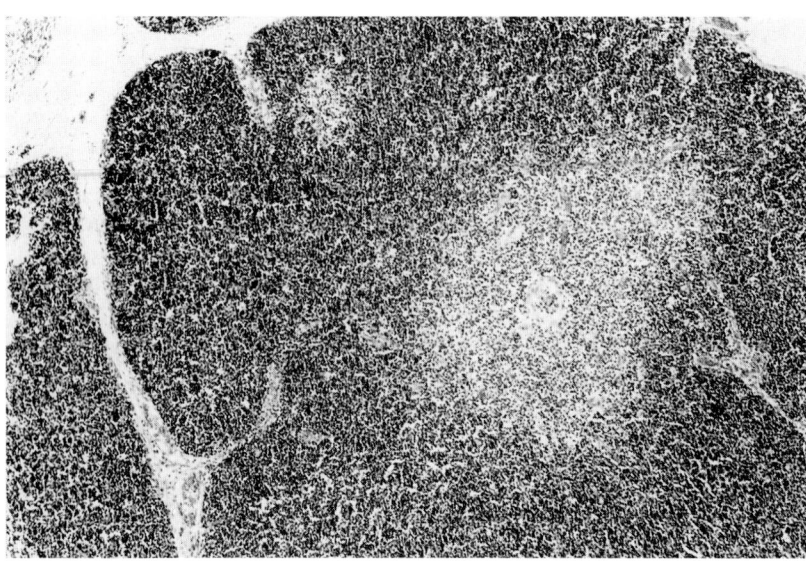

FIGURE 16.6.   *Thymus from neonate of 27 weeks' gestation who survived for 28 hours. Early stress involution is indicated by blurring of the corticomedullary junction and loss of cells from the cortex. A starry sky pattern is just beginning to form. (H&E, ×60.)*

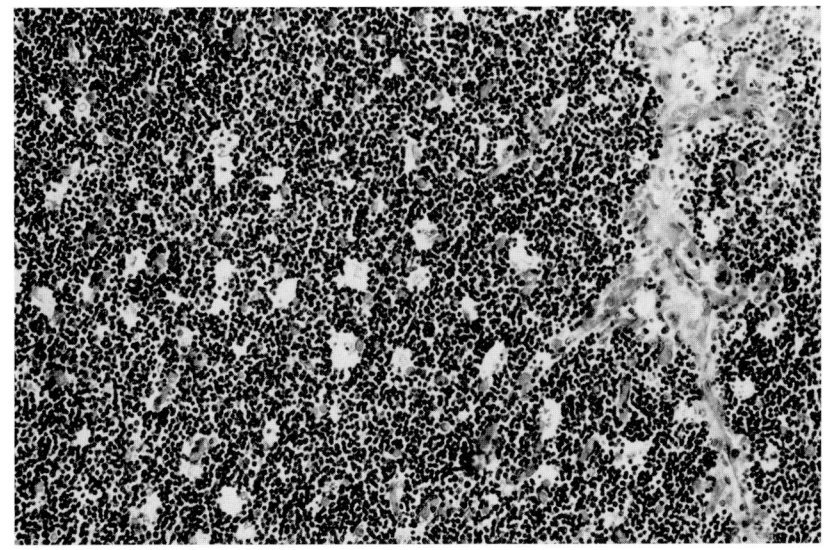

FIGURE 16.7. *Thymus from neonate who survived 22 hours. Note the starry sky pattern of stress involution due to loss of cortical lymphocytes and exposure of the epithelial "nurse" cells. (H&E, ×300.)*

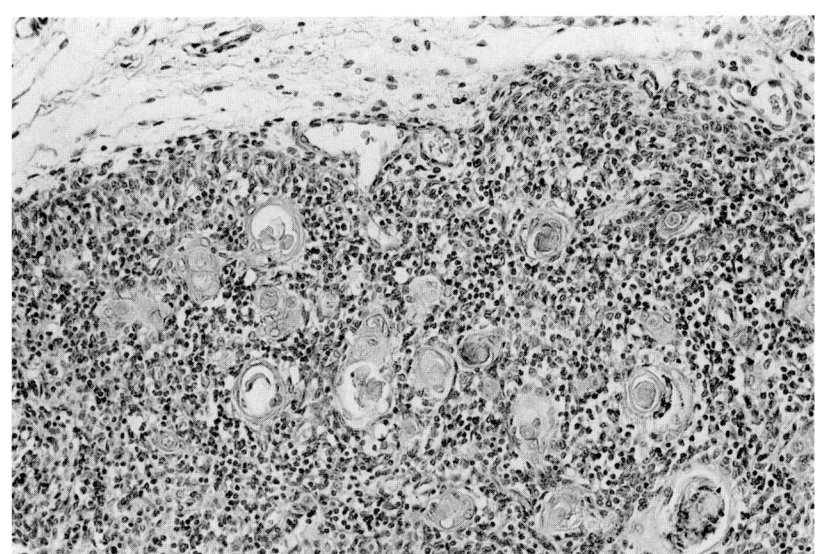

FIGURE 16.8. *Thymus from premature neonate who died at 29 days of age after several bouts of infection. The cortex is virtually completely depleted of lymphocytes and the Hassall's corpuscles have collapsed upon one another. (H&E, ×300.)*

12 to 24 hours' duration resulted in grade 1 changes in two-thirds of cases; illness of 24 to 48 hours resulted in grade 2 changes in three-fourths of cases; illness of 48 to 72 hours resulted in grade 3 changes in two-thirds of cases; and illness of >72 hours resulted in grade 4 changes in four-fifths of cases [37] (Fig. 16.8).

Structural and functional abnormalities of the thymus are discussed below in the sections on immunodeficiency diseases.

CELLS OF THE IMMUNE SYSTEM

The lymphoid and phagocytic cells originate in the pleuripotent hematopoietic islands of the yolk sac. They migrate through the body stalk to the embryonic liver and bone marrow and thence to the spleen, lymph nodes, lymphoid areas of the foregut, midgut, hindgut, and thymus.

Monocytes and Macrophages

The earliest phagocytes—the tissue macrophages and circulating monocytes—can be detected in the yolk sac and other foci of hematopoiesis in embryos of 4 to 5 weeks' gestation. Monocytes develop further in the bone marrow from monoblasts, themselves derivative of stem cells with granulocytic and monocytic potential. Maturation of the monoblast progresses through two stages in the bone marrow: promonocyte and monocyte. The monocyte enters the bloodstream within 24 hours and there it remains for a remarkably short time, 12 to 32 hours. Once the monocyte leaves the bloodstream, it does not return. In tissues, monocytes are transformed into macrophages without dividing, and there they may live for months, or perhaps years. The macrophage differs from the monocyte by its larger size (20 to 80 μm vs. 12 to 25 μm), large mitochondria, more prominent Golgi apparatus, and rough endoplasmic reticulum and numerous microvilli on the plasma membrane. Macrophages do not have primary azurophilic granules or peroxidase activity as do monocytes. At the molecular level, both monocytes and macrophages possess surface antigens directed by HLA-D genes. These are important in the class II MHC response of T cells. Macrophages also have receptors for the C3 component of complement and for the Fc element of immunoglobulins [38].

In spleen and lymph nodes, macrophages line the sinusoids. The so-called dendritic cells of the follicle are of mesenchymal origin and are unrelated to the monocyte/macrophage system although they are capable of phagocytosis. The bone marrow is also populated with macrophages and these again must be differentiated from the reticulum cells which also have phagocytic activity. The liver contains more macrophages, the Kupffer cells, than any other organ and these comprise the main phagocytic barrier of the body. Less numerous are the macrophages in the lung (alveolar macrophages), pleura, peritoneum, synovial fluid, and colostrum. Osteoclasts and Langerhans' cells in the epidermis are macrophages. Microglia are considered by some to be of monocytic origin. Formation of epithelioid cells and giant cells in particular inflammatory conditions is a feature of macrophages, but these responses are rarely prominent in fetuses and neonates [38].

Granulocytes

Granulocytes and macrophages evolve from a common progenitor cell, the colony-forming unit for granulocytes and macrophages (CFU-GM) after stimulation with colony-stimulating factor (CFS-GM). At about 7 to 8 weeks of development, granulocytes begin to circulate in the bloodstream [39]. Chemotaxis, phagocytosis, and bacterial killing are first detectable at 10 to 12 weeks' gestation. Thereafter, these functions develop quite gradually. Throughout gestation and the first months of extrauterine life, the occasionally sluggish chemotactic response does not always confer defense against invading microorganisms [39]. Even at term in normal newborns, indices of chemotaxis may be as low as 20% of adult values. Chemotactic responses reach adult status at about 8 to 12 months of postnatal age. The neonate's monocytes are less capable in these functions than are neutrophils [39]. Furthermore, in normal babies, that is, those with no stimulation from infectious agents, granulocyte-macrophage progenitor cells proliferate at a near maximal rate [40]. Similarly, in preterm infants the response to CSF-GM is nearly maximal and no further response is detectable when stimuli such as infection are added, although immature granulocytes are produced sufficiently in such instances to cause a left shift. The neonatal granulocytes fail to adhere to glass or nylon wool as do adult granulocytes. Chemotactic receptors are present in normal number on neonatal neutrophils, but cyclic AMP is reduced. Motility of neonatal granulocytes is related to the

cytoplasmic microtubule complex which orients the cells to the source of chemotaxis. Accurate orientation occurs in only 60% to 70% of neonatal granulocytes while 90% to 95% of adult cells properly orient [41]. Consequently, neonatal granulocytes migrate to sites of bacterial invasion slowly. Many neutrophils from newborn infants deform poorly after chemotactic stimulation. Receptors on the cell surface may fail to move to the side of the cell exposed to the stimulus or fail to change membrane potential after stimulation with chemotactic factors [42, 43]. The killing response, as reflected by the conversion of nitroblue tetrazolium dye (NBT) to a colored agent by the neutrophil granules, is increased in normal newborns compared with adults. But severely infected newborns may have a reduced oxidative metabolism in their neutrophils with reduced NBT response [44, 45].

Neonates, particularly preterm infants, commonly have a profound neutropenia in overwhelming infections. Noninfectious conditions such as low birth weight, respiratory distress, maternal pregnancy–induced hypertension, abruptio placentae, placenta praevia, postexchange transfusion, and postoperative state account for more than half the cases of neutropenia. Hypoxia rather than infection, may be the central abnormality in causing neutropenia. Perhaps the same conditions that result in neutropenia are also conducive to infection.

The several rare dysfunctions of granulocytes—such as lazy leukocyte syndrome, Job's syndrome, and variants, hyperactive IgE and IgA states, alpha-mannosidase deficiency, myeloperoxidase deficiency, lactoferrin deficiency, and membrane antigen deficiencies—are not usually recognized in fetuses and neonates [46].

Lymphocytes

Stem cell precursors of B cells originate in the blood islands of the yolk sac, migrate to the liver, and can be detected there by 8 to 9 weeks. They then migrate to the bone marrow where neighboring stromal cells promote their growth and differentiation. The microenvironment of the embryonic and fetal liver is favorable for the differentiation of pre-B cells. These are identified by the development of immunoglobulin IgM. Pre-B cells predominate over the more mature B cells while still in the liver. Production of pre-B cells and B cells is shifted from the liver to the bone marrow through the latter half of gestation. In postnatal life, the bone marrow is the only site where pre-B cells are normally found [47]. The fetus' immature B cells can be functionally inactivated by anti-IgM antibody or by any antigen introduced in proper concentration to crosslink their surface receptors. The resultant tolerance causes a marked inhibition of the cell's capacity to proliferate and differentiate, a phenomenon called *clonal anergy*. As the fetus matures, this vulnerable stage of development is passed by most, but not all, pre-B cells. In murine experiments, even pre-B cells in adults may become permanently anergic [47]. In those B cells that go on to proliferate and differentiate, it is assumed that by 6 months' gestation, human fetal lymphocytes can recognize and respond to virtually any antigenic determinant. Neonatal B cells respond much more readily to protein antigens than to polysaccharide antigens. While they have a full range of responsiveness to all antigens, they have had limited exposure and few of the memory cells have been activated. Therefore, humoral antibody response is sluggish with reduced IgG, and reduced type-specific antibody [48]. Fetal B lymphocytes produce IgG in amounts approximating 3% to 5% of average adult values. Relative to adult values, much more IgM is produced than is IgG [49].

T lymphocytes with cluster differentiation (CD) surface antigens CD7+ are found as early as 7 weeks' gestation in the yolk sac and by one week later they are concentrated in the mesenchymal areas of the upper fetal thorax. The CD7+ antigen is characteristic of early T cells [31]. By 15 to 16 weeks of development, differentiated T cells migrate widely throughout the body to lymph nodes, spleen, tonsils, and lower midgut (ileum, appendix, and colon). Most T cells, though, are destined to remain in the thymus until their death [50]. CD4+ and CD8+ cells are evident at about 10 weeks' gestation and mature T-cell antigens, CD3+ and p80, appear at 12 weeks [32]. T cells from embryonic liver at 7 weeks produce detectable responses in mixed lymphocyte cultures [51]. Rosettes form at 11 weeks from thymic lymphocytes and at 15 to 16 weeks from lymphocytes extracted from lymph nodes and spleen, albeit with reduced reaction [52]. Cytotoxic response to allografts is evident at 16 weeks' gestation, but inconsistently so. These observations suggest that the fetus of less than 20 weeks' gestation is immunologically active but is similar to the patient with AIDS or the infant with a syndrome of severe combined immunodeficiency. By the end of 40 weeks of development, graft rejection is intact in the newborn [53]. However, CD4+ helper cells are less numerous than in adults. T cells produce a variety of cytokines including IL-1, IL-2, IL-3, IL-4, IL-6, G-CSF, M-CSF, and GM-CSF [54] (Table 16.1).

Natural killer (NK) lymphocytes, morphologically characterized as large granular lymphocytes, are demonstrated as early as 9 weeks [55], and they are stimulated by interleukin-2, a lymphokine elaborated by T lymphocytes. Interferon [56] and interleukin-2 [57] induce NK cells in

Table 16.1.   Important interleukins and their actions

	Produced By	Activity
Interleukin 1 (IL-1)	Monocyte-macrophage and perhaps epidermis	Generated when antigen is presented to T lymphocyte and catalyzes T cell activity. The a,b types are also endogenous pyrogens, fibroblast stimulators, etc.
Interleukin 2 (IL-2)	T lymphocyte	Crucial for T-cell clonal expansion and has helper function for B cells, natural killer cells, etc.
Interleukin 3 (IL-3)	T lymphocyte	Promotes general cell growth during blastogenesis and thymic epithelium and is a colony-stimulating factor, especially for mast cells.
Interleukin 4 (IL-4)	T lymphocyte, mast cells	Promotes B cell proliferation and differentiation during blastogenesis. IgE induces class II MHC and FC receptors on B cells, granulocytes, megakaryocytes, and erythroids.
Interleukin 5 (IL-5)	T lymphocyte, mast cells	Eosinophil growth, proliferation, terminal differentiation of B cell idiotype.
Interleukin 6 (IL-6)	T lymphocytes, monocytes	Regulates immune processes, T and B growth, fibroblasts, and hemopoiesis.
Interleukin 7 (IL-7)	Marrow stromal cells	Regulates production of pre-B and pre-T cell co-mitogen with IL-2 for T-cell production.
Interleukin 8 (IL-8)	T lymphocytes, monocytes, firbroblasts, endothelium, keratinocytes	Aggregation of neutrophils, attracts T cells, related to platelet factor 4.
Interleukin 9 (IL-9)	T lymphocytes	Growth of erythroids, B cells, mast cells, megakaryocytes.
Interleukin 10 (IL-10)	T and B lymphocytes	Downregulates TNF-α and other T cell products, co-regulates mast cell growth, stimulates NK cells.
Interleukin 11 (IL-11)	Fibroblasts	Synergistic with IL-3,4 in hematopoiesis, modulates antibody response, potentiates megakaryocytes, regulates adipocytes in marrow.
Interleukin 12 (IL-12)	Dendritic cells, macrophages	Stimulates T helper cells and interferon gamma; initiates cell-mediated immunity.
Interleukin 13 (IL-13)	T lymphocytes	B lymphocyte growth; inhibits macrophage cytokine production; regulates inflammatory and immune response.
Interleukin 14 (IL-14)	B lymphocytes	B cell growth factor, autocrine or paracrine action [176].
Interleukin 15 (IL-15)	Many tissues, including skeletal muscle	Stimulates T lymphocytes to proliferate, shares properties with IL-2 [177].
Interleukin 16 (IL-16) initially	T lymphocytes	Previously known as lymphocyte chemoattractant factor, is a CD4+ T-cell competence growth factor described as a chemotactic factor for CD4+ cells.
Interleukin 17 (IL-17)	T helper lymphocytes	Induces IL-6 and IL-8 production and ICAM-1 in fibroblasts [178].

Source: [2, 179, 180].

neonates. In adults and older children, NK cells can be expected to function properly. Kohl et al found that neonatal NK cells, though increased in number, were unable to lyse herpes-infected cells when stimulated by interleukin-2 [58].

In fetuses of all gestational ages, fewer T cells (and relatively more B cells) are present than in older infants, children, and adults. Reduced thymic hormone levels in the serum of preterm and small-for-dates babies may play a role in the smaller numbers of T cells [59]. The concentration of T-helper cells (CD4 cells) is equivalent to that of adults but the T suppressor cells (CD8 cells) are less numerous than in adults through 19 to 28 weeks' gestation. The ratio of CD4 to CD8 cells may therefore be greater in fetuses and neonates than in adults.

In peripheral blood, the total number of lymphocytes at 12 to 20 weeks' gestation comprise 90% of circulating leukocytes [60]. These numbers decline about the third day of life only to reach steady-state values by 1 week of age. A reciprocal but earlier rise in neutrophils is noted during the first day of life. In Table 16.2, the proportional distribution of lymphocytes in various tissues is indicated.

IMMUNOLOGICALLY ACTIVE MOLECULES

Cytokines

Cytokines are soluble small molecules that act on the immune system and are made by a wide variety of cell types, including those of the immune system. Cytokines are nonspecific immunologically but their production may be antigen driven [3]. Those cytokines produced by lymphocytes are called lymphokines, and those that act between leukocytes are called interleukins.

Interleukin-1β (IL-1β) and cachectin, also known as tumor necrosis factor alpha (TNF-α), are products of macrophages stimulated by infections, especially gram-negative bacteria. The lipopolysaccharides of the bacterial cell walls, or endotoxins, or both stimulate the release of IL-1β and TNF-α. TNF-α can alter endothelial cells [61] and capillary basement membranes in the central nervous system, increasing the permeability. Serum levels of these two cytokines rise and fall quickly following challenge with

bacterial endotoxin. A constant recruitment of macrophages may result in a sustained increase. Amniotic fluid samples and placental and decidual tissues have abundant TNF [62, 63]. The placental villus plasma membrane has a specific receptor for TNF [64]. Preterm infants produce little TNF when compared with term infants and adults [65]. In a study of 55 infants and children, some as young as 1 month of age, TNF-α and IL-1 were elevated in 91% and 21%, respectively, in infants and children with severe gram-negative sepsis and purpura fulminans [66]. McCracken et al evaluated 41 neonates with gram-negative enteric bacillary meningitis and found that nearly all had IL-1β in the CSF as long as cultures were positive. There was no correlation between outcome and concentrations of TNF in the CSF [67]. The association of TNF-α with necrotizing enterocolitis has led to efforts to diminish the amount of TNF in the circulation and in the gut, perhaps enlisting interleukin-10 which is a natural regulator of TNF-α and other promoters of the inflammatory response [68].

Immunoglobulins

Immunoglobulins (Ig) are produced by B cells and are composed of polypeptide chains in various configurations. Five major classes (isotypes) are IgM, IgG, IgA, IgD, and IgE. Several subclasses also exist. Each Ig is composed of units with two heavy chains and two light chains. Two classes of light chains, kappa and lambda, exist. Chromosome 14 contains genes responsible for immunoglobulin heavy chains, chromosome 2 contains genes responsible for kappa light chains, and chromosome 22 contains genes responsible for lambda light chains. Both heavy and light chains have a constant region toward their C-terminal ends and a variable region toward their N-terminal ends. The variable regions impart antibody specificity. Each antigen will "fit" and be bound in a particular configuration (the *idiotope*) in the corresponding antibody [3].

IgM is composed of five subunits and does not cross the placenta so its presence in increased amounts or with particular antigen specificity is useful in the diagnosis of fetal and neonatal infections. The isotype IgG is the most abundant Ig in the serum of adults and has a half-life of approximately 3 weeks. Four subclasses of IgG are IgG1, IgG2, IgG3, and IgG4. The subclasses important to the fetus are IgG1 and IgG3 since they produce most of the anti-Rh antibodies in fetal maternal Rh-incompatibility. IgG3 may cross the placenta with greater facility than other IgG subclasses. Little IgA is produced in the fetus or neonate except in extraordinary circumstances and IgA does not cross the placenta. IgD is found on immature B cell surfaces; its biologic function is not well understood [3]. IgE is unique in that the Fc portion of the chain has high avidity to FcE receptors on mast cells and basophils, causing these leukocytes to degranulate with spectacular and sometimes devastating results [3]. Within a single fetal B cell, molecules can rearrange to form IgD and/or IgM; IgG 1, 2, 3, 4 and/or

Table 16.2.   Approximate percentages of T and B lymphocytes in various sites

Lymphoid Organ	T Lymphocytes (%)	B Lymphocytes (%)
Thymus	100	0
Bone marrow	10	90
Spleen	45	55
Lymph nodes	60	40
Blood	80	20

IgM; IgA 1, 2 and/or IgM; and IgE and/or IgM. In B cells from adults, only one immunoglobulin class usually occurs in a single cell [48].

The values of measurable immunoglobulins in preterm infants are: IgG at 7 g/L, IgA and IgM at 0; at age 10 days, IgG at 7 g/L, IgA at 50 mg/L, IgM at 250 mg/L; at age 30 days, IgG at 4 g/L, IgA at 50 to 75 mg/L, IgM at 400 to 500 mg/L [69]. In term infants, the values of IgG are the same as for preterm infants. IgA and IgM levels rise more quickly in term infants than in preterm infants.

The Complement System

All the components of complement have genetic deficiency states described in the literature but these are virtually never manifest in neonates [70]. Susceptibility to infection is especially characteristic of deficiencies of C3, C5, C6, and C7. Deficiency of C3 is associated with infections similar to those of antibody deficiency syndromes. Deficiency of the terminal components usually results in meningococcal or gonococcal disease in adults. A normal serum hemolytic complement is a test that will exclude all complement deficiencies.

Tuftsin

Tuftsin, a cytoactive tetrapeptide, Thr-Lys-Pro-Arg, is part of the heavy chain of gamma globulin and is highly specific in its action on the neutrophils and macrophages when cleaved from the carrier globulin. It acts by stimulating several phagocytic functions [71, 72]. A congenital deficiency of tuftsin with alteration or deletion of molecular structure has been reported but the symptoms were not present in fetal or neonatal life. Eczematous and seborrheic skin lesions with *Staphylococcus aureus* and monilia superinfection have been noted in infants. Acquired tuftsin deficiencies are reported in splenectomized older patients but such deficiencies have not been studied in cases of splenic agenesis.

ABNORMALITIES OF HUMORAL AND CELLULAR IMMUNITY

Humoral immune function can be detected in early fetal life at 7 to 8 weeks of development [51]. During the stage of tolerance or clonal anergy [51] noninflammatory lesions develop in some fetal viral infections, such as congenital rubella. Specific antibodies are generated well before 20 weeks' gestation. Germinal centers and plasma cells develop in lymphoid tissues of fetuses with syphilis, toxoplasmosis, and cytomegalovirus infection [10, 73] (see Fig. 16.3). Complement is produced in levels from one-half to two-thirds adult levels. IgM production is followed either by IgG, IgA, or IgD, depending on the lineage of the lymphocyte. Secretory IgA can be generated in significant quantities by infants 2 to 3 weeks of age when exposed to pathogenic bacteria [74]. Nevertheless, the formation of immunoglobulins in the

fetus and newborn is sluggish. For example, fetal and neonatal B cells are rarely infected with Epstein-Barr virus (EBV) [48]. If they become infected, the response to EBV, which is T-cell independent, is not fully developed until 2 to 3 years of age. By parallel logic, many immunizing vaccines for normal infants are withheld until several months of age when response will be salutory.

ACQUIRED IMMUNODEFICIENCY DISORDERS IN FETUSES AND NEONATES

Of disease states that are associated with acquired immunodeficiency in infants perhaps the most common is chronic malnutrition, with or without diarrhea [75]. This is rare in neonates. Intrauterine growth retardation, assumed in some cases to be a form of fetal malnutrition, has been studied in some babies with regard to immunocompetence. Delayed development of normal levels of immunoglobulins, complement, and poor responses to vaccines, particularly polio vaccine, have been noted [76, 77]. T lymphocytes respond either normally or poorly to in vitro stimulation with pokeweed mitogen [76, 77]. Cord blood lymphocytes from premature infants usually proliferate more readily when exposed to mitogens than do lymphocytes from term infants.

Maternal drug use may have a direct toxic effect on fetal immunologic development. Lymphocyte counts in cord blood are low, lymphocytic proliferation when exposed to phytohemagglutinin and pokeweed mitogen is blunted, and the CD4+/CD8+ ratio is decreased in infants born to mothers who use intravenous drugs. These changes are independent of fetal infection [78].

Of the fetal infections that impair immunity, rubella and AIDS have been most thoroughly studied. In some cases of rubella the restitution of adequate humoral immune status has taken more than a year following birth. Lymph nodes from rubella babies with diminished immune function have poorly formed lymphoid follicles and, in some cases, hypercellular T-dependent zones. Those with excessive immunoglobulin production have precocious germinal centers and cellular B cell zones [11].

Human immunodeficiency virus type 1 (HIV-1) is tropic for T-helper lymphocytes, macrophages, and possibly glial cells in children and adults [79]. The virus has been detected in embryonic tissue at as early as 8 weeks' gestation [80]. It has been cultured from thymic tissue from fetuses delivered at midgestation [81].

In a prospective study of pregnant women infected with HIV-1, 16 of 55 infants (29%) were infected with HIV-1 [82]. In follow-up studies, 9 of the 16 developed pediatric AIDS and 6 had less severe clinical manifestations of HIV-1 infection. One was symptom free but remained seropositive for HIV-1 beyond 15 months of age. HIV-1 infection was three times more likely to occur in preterm neonates than those delivered at 38 weeks' gestation or later. HIV-1 positive mothers who lacked antigen-band gp-120 on immunoblot were more apt to have infected babies than those with the band, irrespective of antibodies to this band. The route of delivery seemed to play no role in the transmission of HIV-1 to the baby. In yet another study of 20 infants born to HIV-1 infected mothers, Johnson et al found eight (40%) infected children [83]. Four of these were capable of synthesizing IgM against HIV-1. Five of the eight had p24 antigenemia. Opportunistic infections, lobar pneumonia, and failure to thrive were prevalent in the infected infants, but these problems arose after the first month of life. Four of the eight had pediatric AIDS by 1 year of age and another three had disease referable to HIV-1 infection [83].

Placentas from HIV-1 infected mothers have nonspecific chorioamnionitis more often than do control cases but villitis is not a feature [84]. Unusual infections may be transmitted to the fetus from symptomatic HIV-1 positive mothers. Cryptococcus organisms were colonized in the intervillous space of the placenta in one such case. The mother also had herpesvirus type 2. She died 2 days postpartum with disseminated cryptococcal infection. Neither the baby nor the infected placenta was undergrown and the baby was thriving at several months of age [85].

Marion et al described a malformation syndrome consisting of a box-shaped forehead, hypertelorism, blue sclerae, almond-shaped eyes, a flattened nasal bridge, triangular philtrum, and large patulous lips [86]. Qazi et al were unable to corroborate these malformations in a study of 30 children who were prenatally exposed to HIV-1 [87].

How do so many of the fetuses or the neonates become infected? Does the maternal HIV-1 laden macrophage or CD4+ lymphocyte cross the placenta, or is the free HIV-1 virus capable of invading syncytiotrophoblast? Perhaps the antibody-bound virus is carried into the chorionic villi. Despite the fact that the neonate is exposed to maternal blood and secretions at the time of birth, only 25% to 50% seem to become infected. Perhaps this figure will need to be revised upward since, in adults, silent HIV-1 infection can lie dormant for years [88]. A practical problem in the study of AIDS and care of the exposed neonates is the diagnosis of actual infection in neonates as differentiated from passive transfer of maternal antibody. Amplification of the HIV genome by polymerase chain reaction followed by hybridization with a specific probe appears to be a promising technique for detecting true HIV infection [88]. Most neonates with prenatal or perinatally acquired HIV-1 infection have a very poor prognosis and most become symptomatic before 1 year of age. Median survival in one study of 172 children was 38 months; mortality was highest in the first year of life when 17% of the total cohort died [89]. The use of anti-HIV therapy alters survival time.

The thymic histopathology in acquired immunodeficiency has been characterized as a precocious involution with severe lymphocytic depletion of the cortex and medulla with obscured corticomedullary demarcation. Microcystic change develops in remaining Hassall's corpuscles. The loss of Hassall's corpuscles may be variable with virtual total destruction in some cases. These changes are described in infants and children well beyond the neonatal period [90, 91]. Only 3 of 37 fetuses from HIV-seropositive mothers at 15 to 30 weeks' gestation had pathologic changes in the thymus. CD4+ macrophages were associated with epithelial stromal abnormalities in areas of some lymphocyte depletion in these three fetuses [92].

The transmission of HIV from mothers to fetuses and newborns is greatly reduced (from 25% to 8.3%) by administering zidovudine (AZT) to infected gravidas [93]. Provision of this drug (and medical care in general) to infected gravidas in developing countries is expensive, an issue that has yet to be resolved.

PRIMARY IMMUNODEFICIENCY DISORDERS

More than 50 primary immunodeficiency syndromes have been described [94]. Almost all the immunodeficiency states, genetic and acquired, manifest pathologically and clinically not in fetuses and neonates but in infants several months of age or in children [95]. Nevertheless, several of the more commonly recognized conditions are presented here since family histories may warrant study in fetuses or newborns [96]. Now, the molecular basis is known and the exact prenatal diagnosis is possible in at least three conditions: X-linked hyper-IgM syndrome, X-linked agammaglobulinemia and X-linked severe combined immunodeficiency [97]. Other immunodeficiency states that can be diagnosed prenatally include autosomal recessive severe combined immunodeficiency, Wiskott-Aldrich syndrome, the bald lymphocyte syndrome, MHC-II deficiency, leukocyte adhesion molecule deficiency, X-linked and autosomal recessive chronic granulomatous disease, adenosine deaminase deficiency, and purine nucleoside phosphorylase deficiency [94].

In rare instances with no preceding family history, the diagnosis of a primary immunodeficiency disease may be suspected in a neonate by finding a lymphocyte count less than 2.8 thousand per cubic milliliter. Signs of infection have been noted in the first day of life in such patients [98].

Many cases with severe immunodeficiency are associated with congenital anomalies that may result in early involvement by the perinatal pathologist. Vici et al described two brothers with agenesis of the corpus callosum, bilateral cataracts, hypopigmented skin, cleft lip and palate, and severe combined immunodeficiency [99]. Cases of DiGeorge anomaly present in the perinatal period, and many cases have microdeletions of chromosomal material in chromosome 22. Seemayer has pointed out the chromosomal and genetic aspects of selected immunodeficiencies that may have logical links to specific malformations [100]. Ratech et al have delineated the multisystemic changes in adenosine deaminase (ADA) deficiency, including those in the bones, kidneys, and liver [101]. The Nijmegen breakage syndrome has microcephaly as a component and cartilage-hair hypoplasia has bony and epidermal abnormalities [95, 102].

Table 16.3.   Immunodeficiency disorders involving lymphoid tissues

B Cell Immunodeficiency Disorders	
X-linked agammaglobulinemia (Bruton's)	Males, arrested development of B cells
Transient agammaglobulinemia	Males and females, often associated with defective helper T cell function
Common variable immunodeficiency (formerly acquired agammaglobulinemia)	Absence of or reduced numbers of B cells; or normal numbers with activation defect, failed helper T-cell function, or increased suppressor T-cell activity
IgG$_2$ or IgG$_3$ deficiency	IgG$_2$ deficiency associated with *H. influenzae*, pneumococcus, meningococcus infections [109]
Qualitative antibody deficiency syndrome	Abnormal response to carbohydrate antigens with recurrent infections and unresponsiveness to immunizations
Antibody deficiency associated with T cell dysfunction	Ig may be normal in amount but of poor quality as in T-cell signal transduction defect, T-cell activation signal defect, antibody deficiency secondary to lack of interleukin 2 secretion, severe combined immune deficiency with B cells but no T cells, HIV-1 infection
T Cell Immunodeficiency Disorders	
DiGeorge anomaly	Partial thymic aplasia, parathyroid function attenuated, hypocalcemia, abnormal facies, cardiovascular defects, T-cell deficiency and variable B cell deficiencies (CATCH-22), deletions in chromosome 22
Novel T-cell deficiency	Normal numbers of T cells but signal of transduction, activiation, or qualitative or quantitative interleukin 2 failure
Cellular immunodeficiency with normal or nearly normal immunoglobulins	Now consists of several known conditions which have in common B cells and immunoglobulins that are present but may be disordered. Thymus is devoid of Hassall's corpuscles. Subgroups with purine nucleoside phosphorylase deficiency or with absent MHC II molecules (bare lymphocyte syndrome) have Hassall's corpuscles [181]. Lumped under eponym "Nezelof syndrome"
Autosomal recessive SCID	Severe T and B cell deficiencies. Thymus dysplastic, without Hassall's corpuscles. Lymphoid tissues hypoplastic, no germinal centers
SCID with ADA deficiency	Multisystemic disorder with chondrodysplasia, adrenal and pituitary fibrosis; Hassall's corpuscles may be present
X-linked recessive SCID	Limited to males; similar to autosomal recessive SCID with some suggestion of slightly more lymphocytes in lymphoid organs
Reticular dysgenesis	Rare form of SCID with depleted bone marrow
Acquired immunodeficiency	Occurs with fetal and infantile malnutrition, certain infections such as HIV, rubella, infectious diarrhea. Lymphoid tissues hypoplastic; peripheral lymphocyte counts low; thymus severely involuted
Wiskott-Aldrich syndrome	X-linked, males with thrombocytopenia, eczema, reduced T cells, thymic dysplasia and involution. Treated with bone marrow transplants
Ataxia telangiectasia	Develops in early childhood with ataxic gait; oculocutaneous telangiectasia; absent Hassall's corpuscles; IgA, IgG, and IgE reduced
Nijmegen breakage syndrome	T cell and B cell deficiency with microcephaly, mental retardation or normal intelligence, radiation-sensitive cells with frequent breaks in chromosomes 7 and 14. Older children and adults develop lymphomas

SCID = severe combined immunodeficiency disease; ADA = adenosine deaminase.

Primary immunodeficiency syndromes (Table 16.3) are usually classified according to the type(s) of cells involved, that is B cells, T cells, and phagocytes and the immunoactive molecules such as complement, various cytokines, and adhesion molecules [94].

B Cell Immunodeficiency Disorders

B cell immunodeficiency disorders rarely manifest in fetuses or neonates since protective maternal IgG readily crosses the placenta.

X-Linked (Bruton's) Agammaglobulinemia

In X-linked agammaglobulinemia, infections in later infancy are caused by organisms such as pneumococci, streptococci, and haemophilus with resulting sinusitis, pneumonia, otitis, furuncles, meningitis, and septicemia. Fungal and viral infections are usually handled normally except for hepatitis, poliovirus, and other enteroviral infections such as echovirus, with particular susceptibility to prolonged bouts of enteroviral meningoencephalitis [1]. Serum levels of IgG, IgA, and IgM are well below the normal range as are specific antibodies to blood group substances and immunizing anti-

gens [103]. The number of T cells and their subsets are normal. Lymphocyte counts may be normal in the blood, but lymphoid tissues are depleted of follicles, and germinal centers and plasma cells are rare. The thymus is densely cellular and its Hassall's corpuscles are histologically normal. Pre-B cells are normal in number, but their maturation to B cells is impaired [95]. The defect is localized to the Xq21.3–Xq22 region of the X chromosome [100]. Mutations of the cytoplasmic tyrosine kinase gene *Btk* (Bruton's tyrosine kinase gene) are responsible for this condition [104]. The abnormal *Btk* gene in one report produced normal numbers of transcripts but the product had decreased stability, with a half-life of 4 hours, one-third that of normal [105]. Female carriers can be detected by mutation analysis for *Btk* [106].

Atypical X-linked agammaglobulinemia is characterized by fewer infections and slightly more circulating B lymphocytes (up to 2% of the total circulating leukocytes) than the classic syndrome (0.1%). Normal individuals have B lymphocytes comprising 5% to 15% of their circulating leukocytes. Growth hormone deficiency has been documented in some pedigrees with X-linked hypogammaglobulinemia [107].

Other Immunoglobulin Deficiencies

Common variable immunodeficiency, formerly called acquired hypogammaglobulinemia, is characterized by normal numbers of B lymphocytes in the blood but with decreased immunoglobulins. The faulty gene is on an autosome. Families with common variable immunodeficiency may have members with selective IgA deficiency. Older members tend to have autoimmune diseases [94].

With selective IgA deficiency, infections occur predominantly in the respiratory and intestinal tracts after 6 months of age. This is a common immunodeficiency disorder. A related rare defect is in the protein secretory piece which results in the lack of IgA in external secretions locally.

A selective IgM deficiency exists but has been reported in only a few cases. Deficiency of IgG and IgA with elevated polyclonal IgM is similar clinically to X-linked agammaglobulinemia except these patients have lymphoid hyperplasia [95]. The defect in X-linked immunodeficiency with hyper IgM, localized to Xq26–27, is thought to be a mutation in the T-cell ligand CD40L, the normal allele of which is bound by the B cell surface molecule CD40 to initiate various B cell idiotypes. When CD40L is abnormal, IgM is produced in excessive quantities [108].

Transient Hypogammaglobulinemia of Infancy

Transient hypogammaglobulinemia is likened to a prolonged accentuated physiologic decline in serum immunoglobulin, which usually ends at 3 to 6 months of life [95].

Immunoglobulin Subclass Deficiency

Any of the IgG subclasses may be subject to reduced serum levels in association with a wide range of diseases in older children and adults, such as various infections, food allergies, asthma, diabetes mellitus, Henoch-Schönlein purpura, Friedreich's ataxia, ataxia telangiectasia, and some autoimmune cytopenias [95]. A similar poor response occurs in individuals with selective IgA deficiency but with clinical symptoms most often limited to the respiratory and alimentary tracts [109].

Antibody Deficiency with Near-Normal Immunoglobulin Concentrations

Patients with normal T-cell function and normal concentrations of immunoglobulin may rarely have deficient functional antibody responses. Blood group antibodies are also absent. These patients are candidates for Ig replacement therapy [95].

X-Linked Lymphoproliferative Disease

X-linked lymphoproliferative disorder, also called Duncan disease, is a condition characterized by inadequate immune reaction to infection with Epstein-Barr virus (EBV). Fetal and neonatal infection with EBV is rare. In older children, death occurs during episodes of B cell proliferation in bouts of infectious mononucleosis. Antibody-dependent cell-mediated cytotoxicity and NK cell functions are both depressed. Lymphoid tissues are hyperplastic, and activated lymphocytes are sometimes prominent [95]. Restriction fragment length polymorphisms show linkage to the Xq24–27 region of the X chromosome [100].

T Cell and Combined Immunodeficiency Disorders

Cellular and combined immunodeficiency disorders occur with absolute or partial defects in T-cell function and are more severe than disorders of B cells. Though dysfunction can be detected in early stages of gestation, neither fetuses nor neonates are symptomatic in most of these disorders.

Thymic Hypoplasia (DiGeorge Anomaly)

The DiGeorge anomaly (formerly syndrome) results from failed formation of tissues derived from the third and fourth pharyngeal pouches. The thymus is hypoplastic or absent. Likewise, the parathyroid glands are hypoplastic or absent, leading to neonatal hypocalcemia. The aortic arch and conotruncal region of the heart may be malformed [110]. The most characteristic cardiac lesion is interrupted aortic arch, but septal defects and right aortic arch are fairly common as well. Other structures derived from this embryonic region may be malformed, thus patients may have a short philtrum of the upper lip, hypertelorism, receding chin, or low-set and notched ears. The anomaly is considered a developmental field defect and many variants are described [111].

Genetic transmission is uncertain in most patients with DiGeorge syndrome, although several cases have deletions of the long arm of chromosome 22(qll). These are now grouped with cases having cardiac and facial anomalies, hypoplastic thymuses, low serum levels of calcium, and the chromosomal deletion defect, together cleverly called CATCH-22. A few familial cases of the DiGeorge anomaly are reported. Some single gene defects and teratogenic exposures have been reported, and DiGeorge anomaly has been associated with other syndromes and anomalies such as Zellweger syndrome, cleft palate, Kallmann syndrome, and holoprosencephaly. The "complete" DiGeorge anomaly includes only those infants with thymic aplasia, parathyroid aplasia, and one of the usual conotruncal cardiovascular defects. The "partial" DiGeorge anomaly then refers to the disorder of an infant with less severe manifestations [112]. Both males and females are affected. Stillbirth is not uncommon.

The thymus is absent or markedly hypoplastic. Occasionally, small remnants of the cervical extensions of the thymus may be present with relatively normal histologic structure, including Hassall's corpuscles. Similarly, tiny parathyroid glands may be identified with careful search in the neck tissues. Paracortical areas of lymphoid structures show varying degrees of depletion [95]. The clinical features may be similar to severe combined immunodeficiency, for example, susceptibility to infection with fungi, viruses, and

Pneumocystis carinii. Total numbers of B cells are normal. T cells are decreased, but there is a normal proportion of CD4+ helper cells to CD8+ suppressor cells. Those with a persistently low number of CD4+ cells in early infancy are at greater risk for later infections [113]. Depending on the degree of thymic deficiency, the intradermal delayed hypersensitivity and T cell responses to mitogen stimulation may be slightly reduced to absent.

Cellular Immunodeficiency with Immunoglobulins (Nezelof Syndrome)

Lymphopenia, diminished paracortical (T-dependent) lymphoid tissue, abnormal thymic architecture, but normal or increased serum levels of all immunoglobulin classes characterize a group of distinct conditions which together were designated Nezelof syndrome [114]. Both autosomal recessive inheritance and X-linked inheritance have been proposed for various forms of this syndrome [94]. Thymuses are very small with poor corticomedullary distinction, a paucity of thymic lymphocytes, and virtually no Hassall's corpuscles. Yet thymic epithelium is present; it is sometimes prominent with structures resembling acini in the cortex. This is apparently dysplasia rather than the destructive involution that occurs in AIDS or in chronic diarrhea. Failure to thrive, oral or disseminated candidiasis, diarrhea, gram-negative sepsis, and recurrent skin infections may follow the development of Nezelof syndrome. Lymphopenia, neutropenia, and eosinophilia are also present [95]. Kurtzman et al have described a neonate with Nezelof syndrome who had giant pronormoblasts and depleted lymphoid cells and neutrophils. The baby was infected with parvovirus B19 [115]. IgE and IgD levels are elevated in some cases. T cells are reduced in number but with normal proportions of CD4+ helper to CD8+ suppressor subsets. This is in contrast to AIDS in which the ratio of CD4+ to CD8+ cells is reversed.

Progressive analysis of this syndrome results in definition of several disorders. Purine nucleoside phosphorylase (PNP) deficiency has an autosomal recessive inheritance pattern. In some cases the gene is thought to reside on chromosome 9, while in others the gene has been cloned and is located on chromosome 14q [116]. The abnormal gene is responsible in part for inhibiting cell division. PNP deficiency results in neurologic symptoms in about two-thirds of patients. Uric acid levels are low and guanosine triphosphate levels are high in the serum of these patients. The latter substance is thought to be toxic to T cells. Their thymuses have Hassall's corpuscles. As in idiopathic cases of Nezelof syndrome, T cells are reduced in number but with normal proportions of CD4+ helper to CD8+ suppressor subsets. However, NK cells are increased [95].

Another similar T-cell abnormality is the bare lymphocyte syndrome. In this condition, a defect in the formation of MHC II molecules prevents presentation of antigens (bacteria, fungi) to the CD4+ T helper cells and results in reduced antibody responses to those antigens, particularly viruses [1].

Severe Combined Immunodeficiency Disorders (SCID)

Severe combined immunodeficiency disorders (SCID) have nearly total absence of immune function and a diversity of features [95, 117]. They may have clinical onset in the neonatal period although death is usually delayed until several months or 1 to 2 years of age.

SCID with Leukopenia (Reticular Dysgenesis)

SCID with leukopenia is the most severe expression of SCID because not only lymphoid tissues but granulocytes and other marrow elements are profoundly depleted. Deaths from overwhelming infections have occurred in neonates. Thymuses are tiny and contain no Hassall's corpuscles. An autosomal mode of inheritance seems most likely [95].

Autosomal Recessive SCID

Autosomal recessive SCID, also called Swiss type SCID, was the first described SCID [118]. T cells are profoundly reduced in number, but like other T-cell deficiency states already mentioned, the ratio of CD4+ helper cells to CD8+ suppressor cells is normal. This is in contrast with acquired immunodeficiency due to HIV-1. Natural killer (NK) lymphocytes, the large granular lymphocytes, are essentially absent in most cases of SCID but a recently described phenotype of SCID has NK cells comprising virtually all the lymphocytes in the peripheral blood, illustrating the heterogeneity of these syndromes [95].

Lymph nodes are small, and both the cortical and paracortical populations are markedly reduced. Tonsils, adenoids, and Peyer's patches are depleted of lymphocytes. Thymuses are virtually always markedly diminished in size, usually weighing less than 1 gram, and they may fail to descend into the thorax. Few thymic lymphocytes are present (Fig. 16.9). Corticomedullary distinction is totally lost and Hassall's corpuscles are absent. Thymic epithelium is either normal or may appear to form clusters of small rosettes or acini (Figs. 16.10 and 16.11). This is in contrast to thymic architecture in AIDS wherein epithelial atrophy is severe and Hassall's corpuscles, if present, show destructive changes [90].

SCID with Adenosine Deaminase (ADA) Deficiency

The gene for adenosine deaminase (ADA) deficiency has been localized to 20q13-ter [94]. In the peripheral blood, the total leukocyte count is either markedly suppressed or moderately elevated. Lymphopenia is severe in most cases with a variable mild eosinophilia. The thymuses are uniformly small, weighing as little as 2% of the expected weight. Corticomedullary demarcation is absent in all the thymuses and intralobular sclerosis is variable. In older patients fatty infiltration is noted. Hassall's corpuscles are absent in most cases, but not in all of them. Weights of the spleen are variable; some are small and some are large, but all exhibit erythrophagocytosis. The large spleens are associated with infections due to

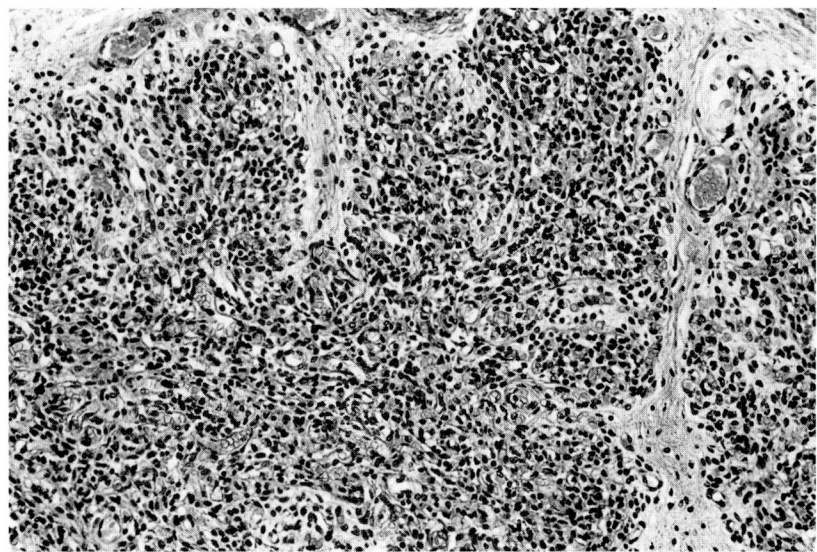

FIGURE 16.9. *Thymus from patient 8 months of age with autosomal recessive SCID. The cortical component is devoid of lymphocytes and the epithelium is dysplastic. No Hassall's corpuscles are present. (H&E, ×300.)*

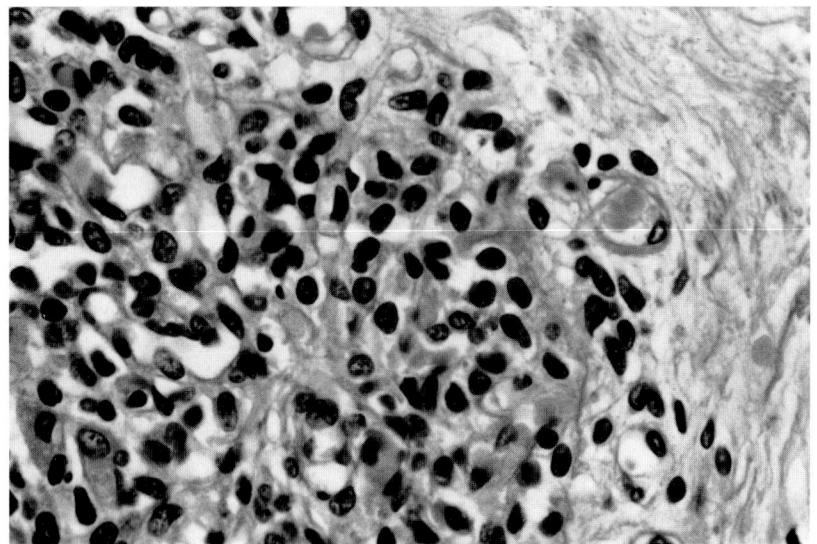

FIGURE 16.10. *Thymus from patient 8 months of age with autosomal recessive SCID. The cortex has a disordered epithelial structure with some poorly formed acini. (H&E, ×700.)*

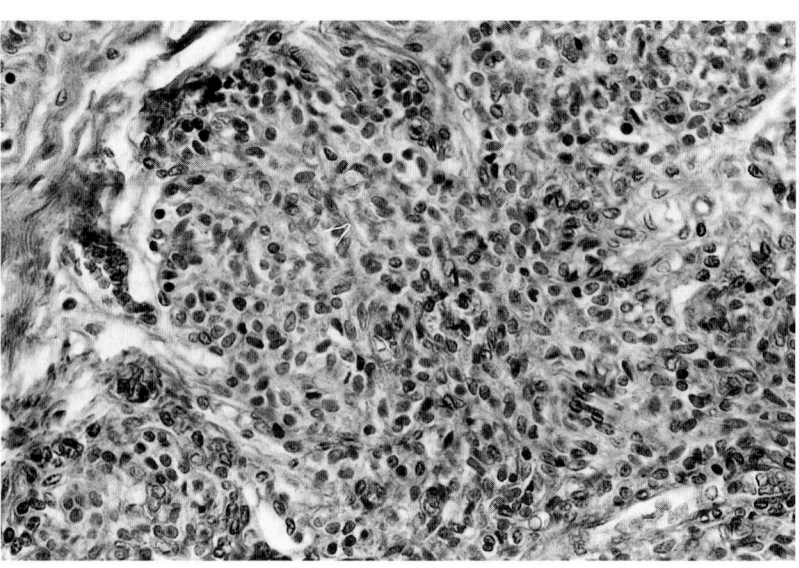

FIGURE 16.11. *Thymus from patient 5 months of age with autosomal recessive SCID. The cortex is dysplastic and has a more epithelioid cellular pattern than the example shown in Figures 16.9 and 16.10. (H&E, ×510.)*

encapsulated organisms. White pulp is variably reduced and rarely forms follicles. Eosinophils are not often found in the lymphoid tissues. Young patients have no lymphoid germinal centers and lymphoid cells are sparse in the gastrointestinal lymphoid tissue [119].

The multisystemic abnormalities for SCID with ADA deficiency include enlarged kidneys with glomerular mesangial sclerosis and sclerotic subcapsular adrenal cortex with fibrous tissue radiating into the cortex in long strands. The pituitary may have similar fibrotic strands. The skin has focal vacuolar degeneration of the basal layer with scattered necrotic epidermal cells. Rib abnormalities include bell-shaped costochondral junctions, and other bones have chondro-osseous dysplasia. The growth plates are short with few proliferating chondrocytes, some of which are hypertrophic with ballooned lacunae, and others of which are necrotic [101]. Hepatic fibrosis has been found in some autopsies of ADA-deficient babies. The damage may be due to the metabolic derangement attendant to the deaminase deficiency or, alternatively, the abnormal gene product may be deposited as aberrantly processed inclusions in hepatocytes, similar to the abnormality in alpha-1-antitrypsin deficiency. ADA-deficient patients do poorly with bone marrow transplants relative to patients with other forms of immunodeficiency, possibly because of the effects of abnormal metabolism in the liver and other tissues throughout the body [120]. Gene therapy holds some promise for these patients since Bodine et al demonstrated that the murine ADA gene can be successfully transferred to rhesus monkeys [121].

X-Linked Recessive Severe Combined Immunodeficiency Disease

X-linked recessive severe combined immunodeficiency disease is the most common form of SCID in the United States [95]. It is in most respects similar to the autosomal recessive form of SCID, but thymuses, lymph nodes, spleen, and gut-associated lymphoid areas tend to be less severely depleted of lymphocytes in the X-linked form than in the autosomal recessive form. The defect is localized to Xq13.1–13.3 [94] where it involves the gamma chain (gamma-C) of the receptor for several interleukins that promote T cell and B cell functions. In vitro correction with retroviral mediated insertion of the normal gene for gamma-C is considered a possible treatment for X-linked SCID [122]. Russell et al report a girl with Janus family tyrosine kinase deficiency (Jak3-deficiency) and features similar to X-linked SCID [123].

Defective Expression of Major Histocompatibility Complex (MHC) Antigens

Two conditions are characterized by the MHC class I antigen deficiency. These are the bare lymphocyte syndrome and the MHC class I deficiency with MHC class II antigen absence [124]. Both are autosomal recessive conditions with hypogammaglobulinemia, absent plasma cells, but only mod-

erate lymphopenia. The thymus is severely hypoplastic as are lymph nodes, tonsils, adenoids, and Peyer's patches [95].

Ataxia Telangiectasia

Ataxia telangiectasia has cutaneous and conjunctival telangiectasis which develops in childhood. Cerebellar ataxia is evident shortly after the infant begins to walk. Sinopulmonary infections occur in childhood and lymphoid and epithelial malignancies have been reported in adults. IgA deficiencies are most common but IgG and IgE may also be reduced. Among the T cells, CD4+ cells are reduced. The thymus is hypoplastic and lacks Hassall's corpuscles [95]. Chromosome breakage is demonstrated in irradiated specimens. The gene has been localized to chromosome 11 (11q22–23).

Nijmegen Breakage Syndrome

The Nijmegen breakage syndrome has T and B cell immunodeficiency with radiation-sensitive cells similar to but genetically distinct from ataxia telangiectasia [102]. This syndrome has associated microcephaly and either reduced or normal intelligence, but no ataxia and no telangiectasia. Most of the chromosomal breaks are found in chromosomes 7 and 14 [125]. Green et al established the diagnosis in a neonate whose sister had lack of involvement of chromosome 11 and the variant of the syndrome with normal intelligence [126]. In postmortem studies of two children, ages 4 years and 6.5 years, the brains had no degenerative changes of the type seen in ataxia telangiectasia, although they were approximately 40% of normal weights and one had hydrocephalus with stenosis of the aqueduct. Thymic tissue was suggestive of simple dysplasia; epithelium was present but Hassall's corpuscles were absent and lymphocytes were sparsely distributed. Lymphoid tissues in the intestine, spleen, and lymph nodes were slightly atrophic with sparse and small germinal centers but otherwise were structurally normal [127]. Seven lymphomas and one meningioma have been reported in longitudinal studies of 19 patients with this syndrome [128]. Other syndromes with microcephaly and immunodeficiency have been reported [129].

Wiskott–Aldrich Syndrome

Peacocke and Siminovitch [130] demonstrated that the locus of the gene for Wiskott-Aldrich syndrome was on the proximal end of the short arm of the X-chromosome (Xp11.22). Subsequent studies using linkage analysis showed a novel hypervariable genetic locus, DXS255, which was very closely linked to the disease gene for the Wiskott-Aldrich syndrome in five affected families [131]. Nonrandom inactivation of the X chromosome is found in the patients and in female carriers of the abnormal gene [132]. Two heavily glycosylated proteins are absent from platelets, lymphocytes, and phagocytes and these defects may account for some of the phenotypic features (small ineffective platelets and defective antibody production, especially low serum concentrations of IgM, and, because of adhesion molecule deficiency, poor inflammatory responses) [133]. Eczema, infection, and bleeding occur after several months of age. Bloody diarrhea is a common sign of illness in these patients. Lymphocyte depletion occurs in T-dependent zones. The thymus is usually severely involuted but has Hassall's corpuscles. Holmberg et al used the reduced platelet size and number in a sample of fetal blood to exclude the diagnosis in a fetus at risk for Wiskott-Aldrich syndrome [134].

Cartilage-Hair Hypoplasia

Short-limbed dwarfism and severe infections occur among Amish patients who also have redundant skin, hyperextensible joints of hands and feet but limited motion of elbows, and fine sparse light hair and eyebrows. Scalloped and sclerotic or cystic changes in the metaphyses and flared costochondral junctions are found in radiographs of the bones. Fatal varicella and vaccine-associated poliomyelitis may occur. Decreased T cells, defective antibody formation, or combinations have been variously described. Some patients have survived to old age [95].

Leukocyte Integrin Deficiency

Leukocyte integrins comprise a family of cell-surface glycoproteins responsible for chemotaxis and adhesion of leukocytes to matrix in areas of inflammation. One of these surface molecules, CR3, is the receptor for C3b, an opsonic fragment of the complement cascade which is fixed to the surface of microorganisms during complement activation [135]. Its absence or deficiency is characterized by a lack of infiltrates of leukocytes, including lymphocytes, granulocytes, and monocytes in areas of necrosis, infection, or other types of tissue damage usually attended by inflammatory infiltrates [136]. Neonates with deficient CR3 have delayed separation of umbilical cords, omphalitis, gingivitis, recurrent skin infections, otitis media, pneumonia, peritonitis, perianal abscesses, and impaired wound healing. Patients with this disorder may lack an intravascular marginated pool of neutrophils since there is a persistent neutrophilia even in the absence of infection [135]. The gene for leukocyte adhesion deficiency is localized to chromosome 21q and results in abnormal biosynthesis of CD18, a beta chain common to the C3b receptor [94]. Hawkins et al describe the autopsy findings in a baby 18 months of age with this disorder who died with pneumonia. Leukocytes were present in the air spaces of the lung suggesting an alternate means of sequestering leukocytes exists in this condition [137].

Other Adhesion Molecules

Several other adhesion molecules have been described. Some adhesion molecules are endothelial ligands and promote the homing activity of leukocytes, including lymphocytes as well as phagocytes. Examples of these are vascular cell adhesion molecule (VCAM), vascular adhesion protein (VAP), hyaluronate-binding cell adhesion molecule (HCAM), and several intercellular adhesion molecules (ICAM 1,2,3) [138]. Flow cytometric studies showed that levels of intercellular adhesion molecule 1 (ICAM-1; CD54) on cord blood dendritic cells were significantly lower than those on adult blood dendritic cells [5].

In the fetal intestine from 11 to 20 weeks' gestation, endothelial expression of ICAM-1 and diffuse staining of VCAM-1 are seen in the lamina propria. Intense expression of ICAM-1 and VCAM-1 in the developing Peyer's patches suggest that these molecules may be involved in the accumulation or organization of lymphoid tissue in the gut [139]. ICAM-1 can be upregulated on epithelial cells by various cytokines [140].

Phagocytic Cell Deficiencies

Chédiak-Higashi Syndrome

Gigantic lysomomes in white cells, melanocytes, and possibly other tissues characterize the morphologic feature of Chédiak-Higashi syndrome. Clinically, onset is in late infancy or in childhood with partial albinism and associated susceptibility to viral and enteric bacterial infections. Lymphadenopathy, anemia, and leukopenia are associated with hepatomegaly and neurologic symptoms including cerebral atrophy. Depressed chemotaxis is found in granulocytes and there is a marked deficiency of NK cells [95]. Prenatal diagnosis in humans and in cats has been accomplished by examining enlarged lysosomes in amniotic cells, chorionic villus cells, and neutrophils of fetuses [141–143].

Chronic Granulomatous Disease (CGD) of Childhood

Chronic granulomatous disease (CGD) is characterized by lack of lysis of phagocytosed catalase-positive bacteria such as *Staphylococcus aureus*, *Klebsiella*, *Proteus*, *Serratia marcescens*, and some fungi such as *Monilia* and *Aspergillus* [135]. Clinical onset of CGD is usually beyond the neonatal period. Normal lytic function in the cytoplasm of phagocytes can be tested in vitro by the reduction of the dye nitroblue tetrazolium (NBT) to a dark blue precipitate. This is the result of normal oxidation of glucose and hydrogen peroxide formation. The absence of these reactions fails to reduce NBT and is characteristic of CGD. The test may be misinterpreted in neonates since increased NBT reduction suggests exaggerated activity in phagocytes of normal babies while hypoxic babies may have depressed NBT reduction [95]. The more common X-linked form is localized to Xp21.1. Three of the less common autosomal recessive forms are localized to 16q24, 7q11.23, and 1q25 [94].

Histiocytosis

Familial Erythrophagocytic Lymphohistiocytosis

Familial erythrophagocytic lymphohistiocytosis is an uncommon disease of the lymphoid and reticuloendothelial system. The majority of the patients are diagnosed at less than 3 months of age. An autosomal recessive mode of inheritance is probable. Hepatosplenomegaly is a common finding but skin rash and lymphadenopathy are uncommon. There are no bone lesions. Anemia, thrombocytopenia, and absolute neutropenia are common. Erythrophagocytosis with increased histiocytes and lymphocytes is found in the bone marrow. Thrombocytopenia may result in severe bleeding. Granulocytes may demonstrate a maturation arrest. Erythroid hyperplasia is often present. Pulmonary infiltrates have been documented early in the course of disease. Lymphocytes infiltrate the portal tracts in the liver. Diffuse perivascular and parenchymal infiltration of lymphocytes and histiocytes occurs in the brain in almost one-third of the cases and may be the cause of death [144].

Histiocytosis X

Histiocytosis X rarely is found in neonates. In one large series of cases of all ages with histiocytosis X, only 2.4% occurred in neonates [145]. Nosologically, this condition is often included with tumors but the fit is uncomfortable. In Isaacs' series of 110 fetal and neonatal neoplasms, 2 cases of histiocytosis X were included [146]. Whether it is a tumor or not, it has a poor prognosis if the histiocytic lesions are widely disseminated in the body [147].

Spontaneously regressing histiocytosis limited to the skin has been described as a more benign congenital lesion [148–150]. The skin lesions are often raised, red-purple, ulcerated, and microscopically have dense infiltrates of cells. Most of the infiltrates are large pale histiocytes with indented nuclei and Birbeck granules in electron micrographs. Some eosinophils are associated with this neonatal lesion [148]. Caution is warranted when considering a good prognosis in babies with regression of skin lesions since some may later develop chronic or progressive disseminated lesions of histiocytosis X [147].

Graft-Versus-Host Disease

Graft-versus-host (GVH) disease is shown by chimerism of lymphocytes in the setting of eczematoid skin rashes, lymphopenia, thymic hypoplasia, and infections. The initial signs are fever, diffuse rash, and diarrhea. The rash can progress to bullae with widespread desquamation. Liver dysfunction may be expressed by jaundice. A chronic form of GVH may also occur with skin atrophy and ulcers, malabsorption, and pneumonitis [151]. Most neonatal cases have occurred in preterm or congenitally immunodeficient babies who have received un-irradiated blood transfusions [152]. GVH disease has also been reported in normal infants who have received exchange transfusions in utero for hemolytic disease of the newborn [153].

Omenn Syndrome

In 1965 Omenn described an infant with a familial reticuloendotheliosis, eosinophilia, disseminated skin eruptions, enlarged liver and spleen, recurrent infections, and general-

ized lymphadenopathy with prominent histiocytic cells infiltrating the lymphoid tissues. The patient history revealed that several other relatives had died with similar diseases [154]. Seven years later, Barth et al described clinical and pathologic features in two neonates with the syndrome who were cousins of Omenn's patient, thus confirming the familial nature of the disease [155]. The absence of Birbeck granules in the histiocytes of Omenn's disease helps to distinguish these cases from those of histiocytosis X [156]. Thymic hypoplasia and reduced proliferative responses to mitogens mark the disease. Onset may be in the first week of life and most patients have died before 12 months of age. It has been argued that the syndrome is caused by engraftment of maternal lymphocytes leading to GVH disease in infants who have a primary autosomal recessive immunodeficiency disease [156, 157], but no chimerism has yet been demonstrated in lymphocytes in these cases and the lack of maternal leukocytes (chimerism) rules out graft-versus-host disease [158]. Omenn syndrome may actually represent a range of defects in T-cell maturation with cytotoxic T-cell populations that mediate reactions resembling graft-versus-host disease [159]. In one such baby with non-consanguineous parents, the baby had hypoplastic ears, aplasia of the ossicles of the middle ear, communicating postauricular sinuses, flat nasal bridge and small nares, epicanthal folds, carp-like mouth, high arched palate, and coronal craniosynostosis. No thymic shadow may be seen at birth in chest X-rays. The thymic hypoplasia is further characterized by poorly developed or absent Hassall's corpuscles, with immature epithelial cells and macrophages making up the lobules. Peculiar stellate fibrinous deposits are found in the bone marrow. The skin lesion is characterized by hyperkeratosis, apoptotic cell death, CD4+ and CD8+ cells in the epidermis, and a progressive loss of the CD6+ positive Langerhans' cells. The basement membrane of the epidermis develops progressive destruction. The spleen has depleted lymphoid tissue although its overall size is increased. Lymph nodes are enlarged due to histiocytic infiltrates but lymphoid elements are depleted and follicles disappear [86]. Lymph nodes may have total effacement of the microscopic architecture resulting from a diffuse proliferation of interdigitating reticulum cells and a depletion of B lymphocytes, lacking a distinct cortex and with no follicle formation. Hyperplasia of S-100 protein positive nonphagocytic reticulum cells with large, pale Langerhans-like nuclei and ultrastructural features of interdigitating reticulum cells are described by Martin et al [160]. CD4CD8 double negative T lymphocytes have been reported and IL-5 production is said to be increased, accounting for the eosinophilia. Lack of interferon gamma, which inhibits IgE production, may account for some of the hematologic findings in Omenn syndrome [161].

Subsequent immunodeficiency may develop toward the end of the first year [159]. While treatment with interferon gamma may ameliorate some of the features of Omenn syndrome, bone marrow transplantation is as yet the lone successful therapy [155, 162].

HYPERIMMUNE DISORDERS
IN FETUSES AND NEONATES

Neonates with partial cellular and humoral immunodeficiencies are prone to develop a variety of autoimmune disorders, some with peculiar elevations of particular immunoglobulins. Most cases of hyperimmune disorders are of alloimmune type, with antibodies transferred from the mother to the fetus through the placenta. The most common historically is Rh incompatibility. Alloimmune thrombocytopenia is another such condition. These are both described in more detail in Chapter 34.

Transient neonatal myasthenia gravis occurs in about 20% of babies born to mothers with the disease. While the muscle paralysis is transient after birth, fetuses are at risk for arthrogryposis if movement in utero is sufficiently hampered [163, 164]. Both hyperthyroidism and hypothyroidism have been attributed to maternal TSH-binding inhibitor immunoglobulins [165, 166].

Neonatal lupus erythematosus is comprised of either a cutaneous disease or complete heart block, or in many cases both conditions. Autoantibodies anti-Ro or anti-La are found in the mother and these antibodies cross the placenta to react with antigens in fetal tissues such as the skin, heart, and liver [167]. The skin lesions are similar to those seen in adults. The heart lesion may include inflammation or, in healing stages, dystrophic calcification and endocardial fibrosis. Leukopenia, thrombocytopenia, and hemolytic anemia are also commonly found. In addition, the liver and spleen are frequently enlarged due apparently to congestive heart failure. Extramedullary hematopoiesis may also contribute to the hepatosplenomegaly. Laxer et al have recently reported substantial hepatocellular changes in neonatal lupus syndrome. Giant cell transformation, bile stasis, ductal obstruction, and excessive extramedullary hematopoiesis were seen in three survivors. Late healing stages include mild fibrosis and persistent lymphocytic infiltrates in portal zones [168].

AUGMENTATION OF IMMUNE
FUNCTION IN FETUSES AND NEONATES

Immunoglobulins of IgG classes can cross the placenta from the mother to the fetus. Subclasses IgG1 and IgG3 cross more readily than does IgG2 [169]. Antigen-specific antibodies produced by the mother may be concentrated by the fetus. For example, the ratio of cord serum to maternal serum for anti-tetanus. IgG is 1.77:1; for anti-*H. influenzae* IgG the ratio is 2.23:1; for anti-group A streptococci the ratio is 0.99:1. In addition to transplacental transfer of immunoglobulin, a major contribution is provided by mother's milk which has secretory IgA, lactoferrin, lysozyme, fatty acids, complement factors, T cells, and B cells [170]. Von Muralt and Sidiropoulos studied fetal and neonatal outcome among mothers who at 27 to 36 weeks' gestation had signs suggesting chorioamnionitis. Mothers in the

study group were given intravenous immunoglobulin. All of the babies received antibiotics. Among the newborn babies with birth weights greater than 1000 g, mortality was reduced from 44% (controls) to 8% (study group). Another group of mothers who received a fourfold increase in the immunoglobulin dose (24 g per day intravenously for 5 days) had no babies who died of sepsis [171].

Opsonization and phagocytosis are enhanced in neonatal serum in vitro by adding immunoglobulin [172]. Recent studies suggest that postnatal administration of intravenous immunoglobulins, especially in preterm infants shortly after birth, will reduce the incidence of sepsis but the data need to be confirmed [173].

Immunization with most of the routine vaccines results in an adequate response in babies born as prematurely as 26 to 28 weeks' gestation. Their chronologic postnatal age is the determining factor in the degree of response. The inference is that exposure to large numbers of external antigens, possible only outside the uterus, provides sufficient stimuli to the immune response [174, 175].

REFERENCES

1. Abbas AK, Lichtman AH, Pober JS. *Cellular and Molecular Immunology.* 2nd ed. Philadelphia: WB Saunders, 1994.
2. Janeway CA Jr, Travers P. *Immunobiology: The Immune System in Health and Disease.* London; New York: Current Biology; Garland, 1994.
3. Claman H. The biology of the immune response. *JAMA* 1987; 258:2834–40.
4. Paul W. *Fundamental Immunology.* 2nd ed. New York: Raven Press, 1989:pp. 3ff.
5. Hunt DW, Huppertz HI, Jiang HJ, Petty RE. Studies of human cord blood dendritic cells: evidence for functional immaturity. *Blood* 1994; 84:4333–43.
6. Jones K. *Smith's Recognizable Patterns of Human Malformation.* 4th ed. Philadelphia: WB Saunders, 1988:pp. 560–651.
7. Thibeault DW, Zalles C, Wickstrom E. Familial pulmonary lymphatic hypoplasia associated with fetal pleural effusions. *J Pediatr* 1995; 127:979–83.
8. Levine C. Primary disorders of the lymphatic vessels: a unified concept. *J Pediatr Surg* 1989; 24:233–40.
9. Arey L. *Developmental Anatomy.* Philadelphia: WB Saunders, 1965:p. 372.
10. Silverstein A, Lukes R. Fetal response to antigenic stimulus. *Lab Invest* 1962; 11:918–32.
11. Singer D, South M, Montgomery J, Rawls W. Congenital rubella syndrome, lymphoid tissue and immunologic status. *Am J Dis Child* 1969; 118:54–61.
12. Arey L. *Developmental Anatomy.* Philadelphia: WB Saunders: p. 347.
13. Solvason N, Kearney JF. The human fetal omentum: a site of B cell generation. *J Exper Med* 1992; 175:397–404.
14. Moore K. *The Developing Human. Clinically Oriented Embryology.* 4th ed. Philadelphia: WB Saunders, 1988.
15. Warkany J. *Congenital Malformations.* Chicago: Year Book Medical, 1971:pp. 745ff.
16. Blechschmidt E. *The Stages of Human Development before Birth.* Philadelphia: WB Saunders, 1961.
17. Freedman R, Johnston D, Mahoney M, Pearson H. Development of splenic reticuloendothelial function in neonates. *J Pediatr* 1980; 96:466–8.
18. Holroyde C, Oski F, Gardner F. The "pocked" erythrocyte. Red cell surface alterations in reticuloendothelial immaturity of the neonate. *N Engl J Med* 1969; 281:516–9.
19. Wadham B, Adams P, Johnson M. Incidence and location of accessory spleens. *N Engl J Med* 1981; 301:1111.
20. Putschar W, Manion W. Splenic-gonadal fusion. *Am J Path* 1956; 32:15–29.
21. Hines J, Eggum P. Splenic-gonadal fusion causing bowel obstruction. *Arch Surg* 1961; 83:887–90.
22. Landing B, Wells T. Tracheobronchial anomalies in children. *Perspect Pediatr Path* 1973; 1:1–32.
23. Ivemark B. Implications of agenesis of the spleen on the pathogenesis of conotruncus anomalies in childhood. *Acta Paediat Scandinav (suppl)* 1955; 104:1–56.

24. Putschar W, Manion W. Congenital absence of the spleen and associated anomalies. *Am J Clin Pathol* 1956; 26:429–70.

25. Nelson R, Venable D. Report of a case of congenital absence of the spleen and chronic amniotic fluid pneumonia. *J Lab Clin Med* 1941; 26:772–4.

26. Singer D. Postsplenectomy sepsis. *Perspect Pediatr Pathol* 1973; 1:285–311.

27. Kevy S, Tefft M, Vawter G, Rosen F. Hereditary splenic hypoplasia. *Pediatrics* 1968; 42:752–5.

28. Lobach D, Haynes B. Ontogeny of the human thymus during fetal development. *J Clin Immunol* 1987; 7:81–97.

29. Carlson B. *Patten's Foundations of Embryology*. 4th ed. New York: McGraw-Hill, 1981:pp. 437–9.

30. Haynes BF, Heinly CS. Early human T cell development: analysis of the human thymus at the time of initial entry of hematopoietic stem cells into the fetal thymic microenvironment. *J Exper Med* 1995; 181:1445–58.

31. Haynes B, Martin M, Kay H, Kurtzberg J. Early events in human T cell ontogeny. Phenotypic characterization and immunohistologic localization of T cell precursors in early human fetal tissues. *J Exp Med* 1988; 168:1061–80.

32. Lobach D, Hensley L, Ho W, Haynes B. Human T cell antigen expression during the early stages of fetal thymic maturation. *J Immunol* 1985; 135:1752–9.

33. Patel DD, Haynes BF. Cell adhesion molecules involved in intrathymic T cell development. *Semin Immunol* 1993; 5:282–92.

34. Uckun FM, Tuel Ahlgren L, Obuz V, et al. Interleukin 7 receptor engagement stimulates tyrosine phosphorylation, inositol phospholipid turnover, proliferation, and selective differentiation to the CD4 lineage by human fetal thymocytes. *Proc Natl Acad Sci* 1991; 88:6323–7.

35. Sprent J. T lymphocytes and the thymus. In: Paul WE, ed. *Fundamental Immunology*. 2nd ed. New York: Raven Press, 1989:pp. 69ff.

36. Butcher E, Weissman IL. Lymphoid tissues and organs. In: Paul WE, ed. *Fundamental Immunology*. 2nd ed. New York: Raven Press, 1989:pp. 117ff.

37. van Baarlen J, Schuurman H-J, Huber J. Acute thymus involution in infancy and childhood. A reliable marker for duration of acute illness. *Hum Pathol* 1988; 19:1155–60.

38. Lasser A. The mononuclear phagocytic system: a review. *Hum Pathol* 1983; 14:108–26.

39. Orlowski J, Sieger L, Anthony B. Bactericidal capacity of monocytes of newborn infants. *J Pediatr* 1976; 89:797–801.

40. Christensen R, Harper T, Rothstein G. Granulocyte-macrophage progenitor cells in term and preterm neonates. *J Pediatr* 1986; 109:1047–51.

41. Anderson D, Hughes B, Wible L, et al. Impaired motility of neonatal PMN leukocytes: relationship to abnormalities of cell orientation and assembly of microtubules in chemotactici gradients. *J Leukoc Biol* 1984; 36:1–15.

42. Hill H, Augustine N, Newton J, et al. Correction of a development defect in neutrophil activation and movement. *Am J Pathol* 1987; 128:307–14.

43. Repo H. Defects in phagocytic functions. *Ann Clin Res* 1987; 19:263–79.

44. Davies P. Bacterial infection in the fetus and newborn. *Arch Dis Child* 1971; 46:1–29.

45. Shigeoka A, Charette R, Wyman M, Hill H. Defective oxidative metabolic responses of neutrophils from stressed neonates. *J Pediatr* 1981; 98:392–8.

46. van der Valk P, Herman C. Biology of disease: leukocyte functions. *Lab Invest* 1987; 57:127–37.

47. Lawton A. Ontogeny of the immune system. In: Ogra PL, ed. *Neonatal Infections: Nutritional and Immunologic Interactions*. Orlando, FL: Grune and Stratton, 1984:pp. 3–20.

48. Cooper M. B lymphocytes. Normal development and function. *N Engl J Med* 1987; 317:1452–6.

49. Ferguson A, Cheung S-SC. Modulation of immunoglobulin M and G synthesis by monocytes and T lymphocytes in the newborn infant. *J Pediatr* 1981; 98:385–91.

50. Adkins B, Mueller C, Okada CY, et al. Early events in T-cell maturation. *Ann Rev Immunol* 1987; 5:325–65.

51. Ogra P. Ontogeny of the local immune system. *Pediatrics* 1979; 64:765–74.

52. Stites D, Pavia C. Ontogeny of human T cells. *Pediatrics* 1979; 64:795–802.

53. Cairo M, Worcester C, Rucker R, et al. Role of circulating complement and polymorphonuclear leukocyte transfusion in treatment and outcome in critically ill neonates with sepsis. *J Pediatr* 1987; 110:935–41.

54. Haynes BF, Denning SM, Le PT, Singer KH. Human intrathymic T cell differentiation. *Semin Immunol* 1990; 2:67–77.

55. Toivanen P, Uksile J, Leino A, et al. Development of mitogen responding T cells and natural killer cells in the human fetus. *Immunol Rev* 1983; 57:89–105.

56. Kohl S, Frazier J, Greenberg S, Pickering L, Loo L-S. Interferon induction of natural killer cytotoxicity in human neonates. *J Pediatr* 1981; 98:379–84.

57. Sancho L, Martinez A, Nogales A, de la Hera A, Mon M. Reconstitution of natural-killer-cell activity in the newborn by interleukin-1. *N Engl J Med* 1986; 314:57–8.

58. Kohl S, West S, Loo L. Defects in interleukin-2 stimulation of neonatal natural killer cytotoxicity to herpes simplex virus-infected cells. *J Pediatr* 1988; 112:976–81.

59. Chandra R. Serum thymic hormone activity and cell-mediated immunity in healthy neonates, preterm infants, and small-for-gestational age infants. *Pediatrics* 1981; 67:407–11.

60. Regelmann WE, Hill HR, Cates KL, Quie PG. Immunologic response and infection of the newborn. Immunology of the newborn. In: Feigen RD, Cherry JD, eds. *Textbook of Pediatric Infectious Diseases*. vol 1. 3rd ed. Philadelphia: WB Saunders, 1992:pp. 876–91.

61. Nawroth P, Bank I, Handley D, et al. Tumor necrosis factor/cachectin interacts with endothelial cell receptors to induce release of interleukin 1. *J Exp Med* 1986; 163:1363–75.

62. Casey M, Cox S, Beutler B, et al. Cachectin/tumor necrosis factor-alpha formation in human decidua. Potential role of cytokines in infection-induced preterm labor. *J Clin Invest* 1989; 83:430–6.

63. Jäättelä A, Kuusela P, Saksela E. Demonstration of tumor necrosis factor in human amniotic fluids and supernatants of placental and decidual tissues. *Lab Invest* 1988; 58:48–52.

64. Eades D, Cornelius P, Pekala P. Characterization of the tumour necrosis factor receptor in human placenta. *Placenta* 1988; 9:247–51.

65. Weatherstone K, Rich E. Tumor necrosis factor/cachectin and interleukin-1 secretion by cord blood monocytes from premature and term neonates. *Pediatr Res* 1989; 25:342–6.

66. Girardin E, Grau G, Dayer J, et al. Tumor necrosis factor and interleukin-1 in the serum of children with severe infectious purpura. *N Engl J Med* 1988; 319:397–400.

67. McCracken G, Mustafa M, Ramilo O, Olsen K, Risser R. Cerebrospinal fluid interleukin 1-beta and tumor necrosis factor concentrations and outcome from neonatal gram-negative enteric bacillary meningitis. *Pediatr Infect Dis J* 1989; 8:155–9.

68. Berg DJ, Kuhn R, Rajewsky K, et al. Interleukin-10 is a central regulator of the response to LPS in murine models of endotoxic shock and the Shwartzman reaction but not endotoxin tolerance. *J Clin Invest* 1995; 96:2339–47.

69. Kanakoudi-Tsakalidou F, Drossou-Agakidou V, Pratsidou P, et al. Prophylactic intravenous administration of immune globulin in preterm infants: effect on serum immunoglobulin concentrations during the first year of life. *J Pediatr* 1991; 119:624–9.

70. Frank M. Complement in the pathophysiology of human disease. *N Engl J Med* 1987; 316:1525–30.

71. Najjar V. The clinical and physiological aspects of tuftsin deficiency syndromes exhibiting defective phagocytosis. *Klin Wochenschr* 1979; 57:751–6.

72. Najjar V, Schmidt J. The chemistry and biology of tuftsin. *Lymphokine Rep* 1980; 1:157–79.

73. Hayward A, Lydyard P. B cell function in the newborn. *Pediatrics* 1979; 64s:758–64.

74. Mellander L, Carlsson B, Jalil F, Söderström T, Hanson L. Secretory IgA antibody response against *Escherichia coli* antigens in infants in relation to exposure. *J Pediatr* 1985; 107:430–2.

75. Girault D, Goulet O, LeDeist F, et al. Intractable infant diarrhea associated with phenotypic abnormalities and immunodeficiency. *J Pediatr* 1994; 125:36–42.

76. Chandra R. Fetal malnutrition and post-natal immunocompetence. *Am J Dis Child* 1975; 129:450–4.

77. Ferguson A. Prolonged impairment of cellular immunity in children with intrauterine growth retardation. *J Pediatr* 1978; 93:52–6.

78. Culver K, Ammann A, Partridge J, et al. Lymphocyte abnormalities in infants born to drug-abusing mothers. *J Pediatr* 1987; 111:230–5.

79. Ammann A. Human immunodeficiency virus infections in infants and children. *Adv Pediatr Infect Dis* 1988; 3:91–110.

80. Sprecher S, Soumenkoff G, Puissant F, Degueldre M. Vertical transmission of HIV in a 15 week old fetus. *Lancet* 1986; 2:288–9.

81. LaPointe N, Michaud J, Pekovic D, Chausseau J, Dupuy J. Transplacental transmission of HTLV III virus. *N Engl J Med* 1985; 312:1325–6.

82. Goedert JJ, Mendez G, Drummond JE, et al. Mother-to-infant transmission of human immunodeficiency virus type 1: association with prematurity or low anti-gp-120. *Lancet* 1989; 2:1351–4.

83. Johnson J, Nair P, Hines S, et al. Natural history and serologic diagnosis of infants born to human immunodeficiency virus-infected women. *Am J Dis Child* 1989; 143:1147–53.

84. Jauniaux E, Nessmann C, Imbert M, et al. Morphological aspects of the placenta in HIV pregnancies. *Placenta* 1988; 9:633–42.

85. Kida M, Abramowsky C, Santoscoy C. Cryptococcosis of the placenta in a woman with acquired immunodeficiency syndrome. *Hum Pathol* 1989; 20:920–1.

86. Marion R, Wiznia A, Hutcheon R, Rubinstein A. Human T-cell lymphotrophic virus type III (HTLV-III) embryopathy: a new dysmorphic syndrome associated with intrauterine HTLV-III infection. *Am J Dis Child* 1986; 140:638–40.

87. Qazi Q, Sheikh T, Fikrig S, Menikoff H. Lack of evidence for craniofacial dysmorphism in perinatal human immunodeficiency virus infection. *J Pediatr* 1988; 112:7–11.

88. Ochs H. The human immunodeficiency virus-infected infant. A diagnostic dilemma. *Am J Dis Child* 1989; 143:1138–9.

89. Scott G, Hutto C, Makuch R, et al. Survival in children with perinatally acquired human immunodeficiency virus type 1 infection. *N Engl J Med* 1989; 321:1791–6.

90. Joshi V, Oleske J, Saad S, et al. Thymus biopsy in children with acquired immunodeficiency syndrome. *Arch Pathol Lab Med* 1986; 110:837–42.

91. Schuurman H-J, Krone W, Broekhuizen R, Huber J, Goudsmit J. The thymus in acquired immune deficiency syndrome. Comparison with other types of immunodeficiency diseases, and presence of components of human immunodeficiency virus, type 1. *Am J Pathol* 1989; 134:1329–38.

92. Papiernik M, Brossard Y, Mulliez N, et al. Thymic abnormalities in fetuses aborted from human immunodeficiency virus type 1 seropositive women. *Pediatrics* 1992; 89:297–301.

93. Connor EM, Sperling RS, Gelber R, et al. Reduction of maternal-infant transmission of human immunodeficiency virus type 1 with zidovudine treatment. *N Engl J Med* 1994; 331:1173–80.

94. WHO Scientific Group. Primary immunodeficiency diseases—report of a WHO Scientific Group meeting. *Immunodeficiency Rev* 1992; 3:195–6.

95. Buckley R. Immunodeficiency diseases. *JAMA* 1987; 258:2841–50.

96. Durandy A, Dumez Y, Guy-Grand D, et al. Prenatal diagnosis of severe combined immunodeficiency. *J Pediatr* 1982; 101:995–7.

97. Puck JM. Molecular and genetic basis of X-linked immunodeficiency disorders. *J Clin Immunol* 1994; 14:81–9.

98. Hague RA, Rassam S, Morgan G, Cant AJ. Early diagnosis of severe combined immunodeficiency syndrome. *Arch Dis Child* 1994; 70:260–3.

99. Vici C, Sabetta G, Gambarara M, et al. Agenesis of the corpus callosum combined immunodeficiency, bilateral cataract and hypopigmentation in two brothers. *Am J Med Genet* 1988; 29:1–8.

100. Seemayer T. Molecular basis of selected primary immunodeficiency disorders. *Arch Pathol Lab Med* 1987; 111:1114–7.

101. Ratech H, Greco M, Gallo G, et al. Pathologic findings in adenosine-deaminase-deficient severe combined immunodeficiency. 1. Kidney, adrenal and chondro-osseious tissue alterations. *Am J Pathol* 1985; 120:157–69.

102. Weemaes CM, Hustinx TW, Scheres JM, et al. A new chromosomal instability disorder: the Nijmegen breakage syndrome. *Acta Paediatr Scand* 1981; 70:557–64.

103. Bruton O. Agammaglobulinemia. *Pediatrics* 1952; 9:722–7.

104. Vetrie D, Vorechovsky I, Sideras P, et al. The gene involved in X-linked agammaglobulinaemia is a member of the src family of protein-tyrosine kinases. *Nature* 1993; 361:226–33.

105. Saffran DC, Parolini O, Fitch-Hilgenberg ME, et al. Brief report: a point mutation in the SH2 domain of Bruton's tyrosine kinase in atypical X-linked agammaglobulinemia. *N Engl J Med* 1994; 300:1488–91.

106. Hagemann TL, Assa'ad AH, Kwan SP. Mutation analysis of the gene encoding Bruton's tyrosine kinase in a family with a sporadic case of X-linked agammaglobulinemia reveals three female carriers. *Am J Med Genet* 1995; 59:188–92.

107. Sitz K, Burks W, Williams L, Kemp S, Steele R. Confirmation of X-linked hypogammaglobulinemia with isolated growth hormone deficiency as a disease entity. *J Pediatr* 1990; 116:292–4.

108. DiSanto JP, Bonnefoy JY, Gauchat JF, et al. CD40 ligand mutations in X-linked immunodeficiency with hper IgM. *Nature* 1993; 361:541–3.

109. Hanson L, Söderström R, Avanzini A, et al. Immunoglobulin subclass deficiency. *Pediatr Infect Dis J* 1988; 7:S17–S21.

110. DiGeorge A. Discussion. In: Cooper MD, Peterson RDA, Good RA. A new concept of the cellular basis of immunity. *J Pediatr* 1965; 67(pt 2):907–8.

111. Lammer E, Opitz J. The DiGeorge anomaly as a developmental field defect. *Am J Med Genet* 1986; (suppl 2):113–27.

112. Greenberg F. What defines DiGeorge anomaly? *J Pediatr* 1989; 115:412–3.

113. Bastian J, Law S, Vogler L, et al. Prediction of persistent immunodeficiency in the DiGeorge anomaly. *J Pediatr* 1989; 115:391–6.

114. Lawlor G, Ammann A, Wright W, et al. The syndrome of cellular immunodeficiency with immunoglobulins. *J Pediatr* 1974; 84:183–92.

115. Kurtzman G, Ozawa K, Cohen B, et al. Chronic bone marrow failure due to persistent B19 parvovirus infection. *N Engl J Med* 1987; 317:287–94.

116. Markert ML. Purine nucleoside phosphorylase deficiency. *Immunodefic Rev* 1991; 3:45–81.

117. Rosen F, Cooper M, Wedgwood R. The primary immunodeficiencies. *N Engl J Med* 1984; 311:235–41,300–9.

118. Hitzig WH, Willi H. Hereditaire lymphoplasmocytase dysginesie. *Schweiz Med Wochenschri* 1961; 91:1625–33.

119. Ratech H, Hirschhorn R, Greco M. Pathologic findings in adenosine deaminase deficient-severe combined immunodeficiency. *Am J Pathol* 1989; 135:1145–56.

120. Bollinger ME, Arredondo-Vega FX, Santisteban I, et al. Brief report: hepatic dysfunction as a complication of adenosine deaminase deficiency. *N Engl J Med* 1996; 334:1367–71.

121. Bodine DM, Moritz T, Donahue RE, et al. Long-term in vivo expression of a murine adenosine deaminase gene in rhesus monkey hematopoietic cells of multiple lineages after retroviral mediated gene transfer into CD34+ bone marrow cells. *Blood* 1993; 82:1975–80.

122. Candotti F, Johnston JA, Puck JM, et al. Retroviral-mediated gene correction for X-linked severe combined immunodeficiency. *Blood* 1996; 87:3097–102.

123. Russell SM, Tayebi N, Nakajima H, et al. Mutation of Jak3 in a patient with SCIDF: essential role of Jak3 in lymphoid development. *Science* 1995; 270:797–800.

124. Touraine J, Betuel H, Souillet G, Jeune M. Combined immunodeficiency disease associated with absence of cell surface HLA-A and -B antigens. *J Pediatr* 1978; 93:47–51.

125. Taalman RD, Hustinx TW, Weemaes CM, et al. Further delineation of the Nijmegen breakage syndrome. *Am J Med Genet* 1989; 32:425–31.

126. Green AJ, Yates JR, Taylor AM, et al. Severe microcephaly with normal intellectual development: the Nijmegen breakage syndrome. *Arch Dis Child* 1995; 73:431–4.

127. Van de Kaa CA, Weemaes CM, Wesseling P, et al. Postmortem findings in the Nijmegen breakage syndrome. *Pediatr Pathol* 1994; 14:787–96.

128. Weemaes CM, Smeets DF, van der Burgt CJ. Nijmegen breakage syndrome: a progress report. *Int J Radiat Biol* 1994; 66:S185–S188.

129. Berthet F, Caduff R, Schaad UB, et al. A syndrome of primary combined immunodeficiency with microcephaly, cerebellar hypoplasia, growth failure and progressive pancytopenia. *Eur J Pediatr* 1994; 153:333–8.

130. Peacocke M, Siminovitch K. Linkage of the Wiskott-Aldrich syndrome with polymorphic DNA sequences from the X-chromosome. *Proc Natl Acad Sci* 1987; 84:3430–3.

131. de Saint Basile G, Arveiler B, Fraser NJ, et al. Close linkage of hypervariable marker DXS255 to disease locus of Wiskott-Aldrich Syndrome. *Lancet* 1989; ii:1319–21.

132. Wengler G, Gorlin JB, Williamson JM, et al. Nonrandom inactivation of the X chromosome in early lineage hematopoietic cells in carriers of Wiskott-Aldrich syndrome. *Blood* 1995; 85:2471–7.

133. Rosenstein Y, Park JK, Hahn WC, et al. CD43, a molecule defective in Wiskott-Aldrich syndrome, binds ICAM-1. *Nature* 1991; 354:233–5.

134. Holmberg L, Gustavii B, Jonsson A. A prenatal study of fetal platelet count and size with application to fetus at risk for Wiskott-Aldrich syndrome. *J Pediatr* 1983; 102:773–6.

135. Malech H, Gallin J. Neutrophils in human diseases. *N Engl J Med* 1987; 317:687–94.

136. Hawkins HK, Heffelfinger SC, Anderson DC. Leukocyte adhesion deficiency: clinical and postmortem observations. *Pediatr Pathol* 1992; 12:119–30.

137. Kishimoto T, Larson R, Corbi A, et al. The leukocyte integrins. *Adv Immunol* 1989; 46:149–82.

138. Butcher EC, Picker LJ. Lymphocyte homing and homeostasis. *Science* 1996; 272:60–6.

139. Dogan A, MacDonald TT, Spencer J. Ontogeny and induction of adhesion molecule expression in human fetal intestine. *Clin Exp Immunol* 1993; 91:532–7.

140. Brandtzaeg P, Halstensen TS, Huitfeldt HS, et al. Epithelial expression of HLA, secretory component (poly-Ig receptor), and adhesion molecules in the human alimentary tract. *Ann NY Acad Sci* 1992; 664:157–79.

141. Diukman R, Tanigawara S, Cowan MJ, Golbus MS. Prenatal diagnosis of Chediak-Higashi syndrome. *Prenat Diagn* 1992; 12:877–85.

142. Durandy A, Breton-Gorius J, Guy-Grand D, et al. Prenatal diagnosis of syndromes associating albinism and immune deficiencies (Chediak-Higashi syndrome and variant). *Prenat Diagn* 1993; 13:13–20.

143. Kahraman MM, Prieur DJ. Chediak-Higashi syndrome in the cat: prenatal diagnosis by evaluation of amniotic fluid cells. *Am J Med Genet* 1990; 36:321–7.

144. Shapiro D, Hutchinson R. Familial histiocytosis in offspring of two pregnancies after artificial insemination. *N Engl J Med* 1981; 304:757–9.

145. Greenberger J, Crocker A, Vawter G, et al. Results of treatment of 127 patients with systemic histiocytosis (Letterer-Siew syndrome, Schuller-Christian syndrome and multifocal eosinophilic granuloma). *Medicine* 1981; 60:311–38.

146. Isaacs H. Perinatal (congenital and neonatal) neoplasms: a report of 110 cases. *Pediatr Pathol* 1985; 3:165–216.

147. Cohen DM, Mitchell C, Alexander J. Letterer-Siwe disease in a newborn. *Arch Pathol* 1966; 81:347–51.

148. Dehner L, Bamford J, McDonald E. Spontaneous regression of congenital cutaneous histiocytosis X: report of a case with discussion of nosology and pathogenesis. *Pediatr Pathol* 1983; 1:99–106.

149. Jaffe R. Pathology of histiocytosis X. *Perspect Pediatr Pathol* 1987; 9:4–47.

150. Kapila P, Grant-Kels J, Allred C, Farouhar F, Capriglione A. Congenital spontaneously regressing histiocytosis: case report and review of the literature. *Pediatr Dermatol* 1985; 2:312–17.

151. Holland P. Prevention of transfusion-associated graft-vs-host disease. *Arch Pathol Lab Med* 1989; 113:285–91.

152. Seemayer T, Bolande R. Thymic involution mimicking thymic dysplasia: a consequence of transfusion-induced graft-versus-host disease in a premature infant. *Arch Pathol Lab Med* 1980; 104:141–4.

153. Parkman R, Mosier D, Umansky I, et al. Graft-versus-host disease after intrauterine and exchange transfusions for hemolytic disease of the newborn. *N Engl J Med* 1974; 290:359–63.

154. Omenn G. Familial reticuloendotheliosis with eosinophilia. *N Engl J Med* 1965; 273:427–32.

155. Barth R, Vergara G, Khurana S, Lowman J, Beckwith J. Rapidly fatal familial histiocytosis associated with eosinophilia and primary immunological deficiency. *Lancet* 1972; ii:503–9.

156. Junker A, Chan K, Massing B. Clinical and immune recovery from Omenn syndrome after bone marrow transplantation. *J Pediatr* 1989; 114:596–600.

157. Jouan H, Le Deist F, Nezelof C. Omenn's syndrome—pathologic arguments in favor of a graft versus host pathogenesis: a report of nine cases. *Hum Pathol* 1985; 18:1101–8.

158. Appleton AL, Curtis A, Wilkes J, Cant AJ. Differentiation of maternofetal GVHD from Omenn's syndrome in pre BMT patients with severe combined immunodeficiency. *Bone Marrow Transplant* 1994; 14:157–9.

159. Wirt D, Brooks E, Vacidya S, et al. Novel T-lymphocyte population in combined immunodeficiency with features of graft-versus-host disease. *N Engl J Med* 1989; 321:370–4.

160. Martin JV, Willoughby PB, Giusti V, Price G, Cerezo L. The lymph node pathology of Omenn's syndrome. *Am J Surg Pathol* 1995; 19:1082–7.

161. Melamed I, Cohen A, Roifman CM. Expansion of CD3+CD4 CD8 T cell population expressing high levels of IL 5 in Omenn's syndrome. *Clin Exp Immunol* 1994; 95:14–21.

162. Schandene L, Ferster A, Mascart Lemone F, et al. T helper type 2 like cells and therapeutic effects of interferon gamma in combined immunodeficiency with hypereosinophilia (Omenn's syndrome). *Eur J Immunol* 1993; 23:56–60.

163. Barlow C. Neonatal myasthenia gravis. *Am J Dis Child* 1981; 135:209.

164. Donaldson J, Penn A, Lisak R, et al. Antiacetylcholine receptor antibody in neonatal myasthenia gravis. *Am J Dis Child* 1981; 135:222–6.

165. Matsurira N, Yamada Y, Nohara Y, et al. Familial neonatal transient hypothyroidism due to maternal TSH-binding inhibitor immunoglobulin. *N Engl J Med* 1980; 303:738–41.

166. Yagi H, Takenchi M, Nagashuna K, et al. Neonatal transient thyrotoxicosis resulting from maternal TSH-binding inhibitor immunoglobulin. *J Pediatr* 1983; 103:591–3.

167. Lee L, Weston W. New findings in neonatal lupus syndrome. *Am J Dis Child* 1984; 138:233–6.

168. Laxer R, Roberts E, Gross K, et al. Liver disease in neonatal lupus erythematosus. *J Pediatr* 1990; 116:238–42.

169. Einhorn M, Granoff D, Nahm M, et al. Concentrations of antibodies in paired maternal and infants sera: relationship to IgG subclass. *J Pediatr* 1987; 111:783–8.

170. Goldman A, Ham Pong A, Goldblum R. Host defenses: development and maternal contributions. *Adv Pediatr* 1985; 32:71–100.

171. vonMuralt G, Sidiropoulos D. Prenatal and postnatal prophylaxis of infections in preterm neonates. *Pediatr Infect Dis J* 1988; 7:S72–S78.

172. Givner L, Edwards M, Anderson D, Baker C. Immune globulin for intravenous use: enhancement of in vitro opsonophagocytic activity of neonatal serum. *J Infect Dis* 1985; 151:217–22.

173. Noya F, Baker C. Intravenously administered immune globulin for premature infants: a time to wait. *J Pediatr* 1989; 115:969–70.

174. Conway S, James J, Smithells R, et al. Immunisation of the preterm baby. *Lancet* 1987; ii:1326.

175. Smolen P, Bland R, Heiligenstein E, et al. Antibody response to oral polio vaccine in premature infants. *J Pediatr* 1983; 103:917–9.

176. Ford R, Tamayo A, Martin B, et al. Identification of B-cell growth factors (interleukin-14; high molecular weight-B-cell growth factors) in effusion fluids from patients with aggressive B-cell lymphomas. *Blood* 1995; 86:283–93.

177. Grabstein KH, Eisenman J, Shanebeck K, et al. Cloning of a T cell growth factor that interacts with the beta chain of the interleukin-2 receptor. *Science* 1994; 264:965–8.

178. Yao Z, Painter SL, Fanslow WC, et al. Human IL-17: a novel cytokine derived from T cells. *J Immunol* 1995; 155:5483–6.

179. Fearon DT, Locksley RM. The instructive role of innate immunity in the acquired immune response. *Science* 1996; 272:50–4.

180. Richter GW, Solez K, Ryffel B. Cytokine-induced pathology. Part A: Interleukins and hemopoietic growth factors. Part B: Inflammatory cytokines, receptors and diseases. *Int Rev Exper Pathol* 34;1993.

181. Hauber I, Gulle H, Wolf HM, et al. Molecular characterization of major histocompatibility complex class II gene expression and demonstration of antigen-specific T cell response indicate a new phenotype in class II deficient patients. *J Exper Med* 1995; 181:1411–23.

Infections of Fetuses and Neonates

Don B. Singer

Infections in fetuses and neonates were considered rare through the first two decades of this century. The recognized conditions included pneumonia, endocarditis, ophthalmitis, scarlet fever, encephalitis, peritonitis, and otitis [1, 2]. Organisms identified in these conditions were common bacteria, such as *Staphylococcus*, *Streptococcus*, and of course *Treponema pallidum* [2]. In the 1920s and 1930s, other diseases were recognized such as toxoplasmosis, varicella, smallpox, diphtheria, typhoid, anthrax, and more rarely tuberculosis, malaria, leptospirosis, and disease due to gas bacillus [1].

As we approach the end of the twentieth century we know that infections account for as much as 20% of all fetal and neonatal diseases [3–5]. One large prospective study found infections were the most frequent cause of perinatal mortality, but in most studies infections rank third among cases of perinatal morbidity and mortality—only asphyxia and malformations are more numerous [6–9].

ROUTES OF INFECTION

Infectious agents reach the fetus either transplacentally from the mother's blood or ascend from the mother's vagina and cervix through the placental membranes into the amniotic fluid [10–12]. The ascending route is by far the more common. By a third route infectious organisms might ascend from the vagina and cervix, invade the endometrium, and propagate along the interface between decidua and chorion to reach the villous portion of the placenta, thereafter behaving in much the same manner as a maternal blood-borne infection (Table 17.1).

The transplacental route is the one taken by most of the viruses. Such infections usually occur long before birth [10, 11], but notable exceptions include most infections due to

herpes simplex viruses, hepatitis B virus, and human immunodeficiency virus. These agents usually infect the fetus at the time of birth by direct contact of the viruses to fetal skin and mucous membranes.

Most bacterial infections reach the fetus by way of the ascending route from the mother's colonized vagina and cervix, and the fetus is usually infected in the hours or days before birth. Indeed, bacterial infections of the amniotic sac may induce the onset of labor through prostaglandin production [13]. Rupture of the amniotic sac may thus be the result of ascending infection rather than preceding entry of the infectious agent [6]. Bacterial infections also are acquired during birth from the contact with colonized maternal birth canal.

In the normal course of pregnancy, the birth canal favors growth of certain organisms. In the first half of pregnancy, the majority of women in one study harbored coagulase-negative staphylococci and *Ureaplasma urealyticum* in the vagina. More than 15% of them also had *Corynebacterium* species, enterococci, *Mycoplasma hominis*, *Haemophilus vaginalis*, *Bacteroides* species, Enterobacteriaceae, and yeast. A smaller number, fewer than 15%, had trichomonads, group B streptococci, non-hemolytic streptococci, *Streptococcus viridans*, and chlamydia [14]. Normal intestinal flora frequently colonize the vagina and the external cervical os. These organisms are rarely sufficiently virulent to breach the cervix and cause fetal or neonatal infection, but some, such as group B streptococci and *Escherichia coli*, can cross the cervix and placental membranes to produce infections in utero. Colonization increases as pregnancy progresses with several organisms, including group B streptococci and *E. coli* [15, 16].

A small proportion of bacterial infections reach the fetus through the blood-borne transplacental route. *Listeria mono-*

Table 17.1. Diseases and their routes of infection in fetuses and neonatal infants

Diseases Associated with Transplacental Infection
  Cytomegalovirus infection
  Rubella infection
  Parvovirus infection
  Syphilis
  Listeriosis
  Toxoplasmosis
  Borrelia infection
  Chagas disease
  Malaria
Diseases Associated with Transcervical Infection and with Occasional
Transplacental Infection
  Group B streptococcus sepsis infection
  E. coli sepsis
  Unencapsulated H. influenzae sepsis
  Herpes simplex infection
  Hepatitis B virus infection (very rarely)
  Varicella virus infection (rarely)
  Human immunodeficiency virus infection
  Candidiasis

cytogenes frequently uses this route, while other organisms such as *E. coli* and *Streptococcus* do so uncommonly.

Infectious agents can invade the neonate after birth. The skin, respiratory tract, and gastrointestinal tract are bombarded by a variety of potential pathogens. Intensive care nurseries, with their inherent frequent handling of the babies, placement of intracorporeal catheters and tubes, and other maneuvers, provide several other sources of infections.

PROTECTIVE BARRIERS TO PERINATAL INFECTION

The natural physical barriers between infectious agents and the fetus are the mother's mucous membranes and their secretions, the placental villi, placental membranes, especially the amnion with its nearly impervious collagen layer, the amniotic fluid, and the fetal skin and mucous membranes.

Maternal Barriers to Perinatal Infection

Conditions that cause maternal protective barriers to break down may include coitus or pelvic examinations performed late in pregnancy [17, 18]. Foreign materials such as intrauterine devices and cervical sutures breach the maternal barriers and are associated with increased amniotic fluid infection and fetal infections.

The cervical mucus is generally an effective barrier to most infectious agents but the mucus and the unruptured membranes occasionally are invaded by bacteria with devastating, even lethal, fetal or neonatal infections [6]. The condition known as incompetent cervix, wherein a degree of

dilatation and some effacement occur early in pregnancy, is associated with infected membranes, but which event is the cause and which the effect remains unclear.

Amniotic fluid has increasing bacteriostatic properties after the 30th week of gestation [19, 20]. Before that time, the amniotic fluid provides a rich culture medium for most bacterial agents. After 40 weeks, bacteriostatic properties of the amniotic fluid may be variable [19]. A low-molecular-weight zinc-associated polypeptide with antibacterial properties has been described in the amniotic fluid. This protein is inhibited by phosphates which are present in high concentration in meconium [21]. Therefore, amniotic fluid contaminated by meconium may provide a better culture medium for bacteria than clear fluid [22]. This hypothesis may correct the erroneous impression that meconium itself induces either amniotic or pulmonary inflammation. Lauweryns et al demonstrated conclusively that sterile meconium does not induce pneumonia and that only infected meconium results in pulmonary inflammation [23]. Tafari et al found that in malnourished women zinc-deficient amniotic fluids were susceptible to bacterial invasion. By adding zinc to amniotic fluid in vitro, bacteriostatic properties were restored [20].

Fetal and Neonatal Barriers to Infection

Before the 30th week of gestation, the fetal skin has only one to three layers of squamous epithelium. The mucous membranes are similarly thin and relatively permeable to invading microorganisms. After infecting organisms breach these imperfect physical barriers, the fetal and neonatal responses are not optimal (Table 17.2).

The earliest phagocytes—that is, tissue macrophages and circulating monocytes—can be detected at 4 to 5 weeks. At 7 to 8 weeks of development, granulocytes form and begin to circulate in the bloodstream [24].

Chemotaxis, phagocytosis, and bacterial killing are first detectable at 10 to 12 weeks but these functions develop slowly and may fail against invading microorganisms. Adult activity levels are reached only after 8 to 12 months of postnatal age [24].

Table 17.2. Fetal and neonatal responses to infection

Humoral immunity	Present but attenuated
Cellular immunity	Present but attenuated
Phagocytosis	Present but slow
Bacterial killing	Present but attenuated
Febrile response	Poorly controlled, hypothermia common
White blood cells	Poorly controlled, neutropenia common
Red blood cells	Hemolysis and reduced production common
Platelets	Consumption and reduced production common
Hemodynamics	Shock common
Hemostasis	Accentuated, loss of clotting factors

The killing response, as reflected by the conversion of nitroblue tetrazolium dye (NBT) to a colored agent, is increased in normal newborns compared with adults but severely infected newborns may have a reduced NBT response [25, 26].

Neonates, particularly premature infants, may have a profound neutropenia in overwhelming infections. Myelopoiesis may be increased or reduced in spite of peripheral neutropenia in infected fetuses and neonates [27–29]. Noninfectious fetal and maternal conditions may be associated with neutropenia and may make the fetus susceptible to infections [30, 31].

Transfusion of neutrophils is useful in treating neonates infected with certain bacteria, particularly gram-negative organisms, but such transfusions are of limited value in rapidly progressive infections such as those due to group B streptococci and *Haemophilus influenzae* [32, 33]. Newer therapeutic measures include administration of granulocyte-stimulating factor [34, 35].

Perinatal Humoral and Cellular Immunity

Humoral immune function can be detected in late embryonic life at 7 to 8 weeks of development [36]. Histologic evidence consists of germinal centers and plasma cells in lymphoid tissues of fetuses with certain infections, such as syphilis, toxoplasmosis, and cytomegalovirus infections [37, 38]. Cells in the B lymphoid series are found in fetal liver, spleen, lymph nodes, and in blood. However, the formation of immunoglobulins in the fetus and newborn is sluggish. The humoral response to Epstein-Barr virus is not fully developed until 2 to 3 years of age [36]. Fortunately, maternal immunoglobulin-G crosses the placenta and antigen-specific antibodies may be concentrated by the fetus [39].

T cells are present at 3.5 weeks and natural killer lymphocytes and T cells with T4-T8 subtypes are detectable at about 9 weeks' gestational age [36]. Cytotoxic response to allografts is evident at 16 weeks' gestation but inconsistently so [36]. By the end of 40 weeks of development, graft rejection is intact in the newborn [40]. However, T4-helper cells are less numerous than in adults and are equal to or in an inverse ratio to T8-suppressor cells compared with normal adults [36].

Thymic and lymphoid tissues, like the immune cells and functions, mature gradually. Hassall's corpuscles are detected in about 60% to 70% of fetuses at 15 to 16 weeks' gestation and lymphoid tissue in the cortex is abundant by that time. Lymph nodes show a poorly cellular reticular and collagenous skeleton, with widely patent sinusoids but do not usually form distinct follicles until well past the 30th week of gestation. Follicular centers (germinal centers) are not visible until foreign antigens stimulate their formation. Normally, this occurs after 2 to 3 months of age. Only a few small collars of lymphocytes form around splenic arterioles before the 20th week of gestation. These gradually enlarge in the last weeks of intrauterine development.

The liver is the main source for white blood cells until after 30 weeks' gestation while the bone marrow gradually assumes its role as the primary producer of blood cells. Granulocyte precursors predominate in the portal connective tissue and are much less concentrated in hepatic sinusoids. But with infections, granulopoiesis is increased as much as 12-fold in the hepatic sinusoids [29].

In response to infection, some fetuses or newborn infants may develop transient abnormal myelopoiesis (TAM). This is a benign fetal and neonatal form of myeloproliferative disorder. Another label for this condition is acute leukemoid reaction and it must be differentiated from congenital leukemia [41]. In vitro assays for granulocyte macrophage-colony forming units (CFU-GM) are normal in TAM whereas with leukemia, abnormal maturation is found [42, 43]. In TAM, the peripheral blood may contain up to 90% blast forms. Tissues are not infiltrated by the immature leukocytes as they are in congenital leukemias.

The Placenta and Umbilical Cord as a Barrier to Fetal Infection

The placental membranes and the villi form the physical barriers which prevent or impede invasion of the fetus by infectious organisms. The most common histologic evidence of such invasion is chorioamnionitis and this is associated with true infection in most cases. Umbilical vasculitis is another feature and the mechanism of death in fetuses is related, at least in part, to the reduced flow of blood through inflamed umbilical vessels [44]. Acute or suppurative villitis may be caused by bacterial, viral, or fungal infections. Chronic villitis, on the other hand, is often noninfectious or is not currently amenable to demonstration of an infectious etiology.

INFECTION SYNDROMES OF FETUSES AND NEONATES

Transplacental Infections

Infections acquired by transplacental transmission are usually viral, but bacteria, fungi, and various protozoa may also reach the fetus by this route (see Table 17.1). Because these agents invade the fetal bloodstream from the chorionic villi, they become widely disseminated in the fetal organs and tissues. Growth retardation, depletion of or failure of development of fetal fat stores, and malformations or disruptions are common. Fetal anemia and heart failure are sometimes seen, resulting in infectious (nonimmune) hydrops fetalis. Postnatal jaundice is common with elevated serum levels of both unconjugated and conjugated bilirubin. Brain, eyes, and inner ears tend to be infected by hematogenous spread of the organisms. Precocious development of lymphoid tissues or direct infection of lymphoid structures with the opposite result—lymphoid depletion—may occur, sometimes in sequential fashion. Inflammatory reactions are mixed but tend to be chronic, with many lymphocytes, occasional eosinophils and plasma cells, macrophages, sometimes with ill-defined granulomas, and occasionally with a large fibrous tissue component.

Transcervical Infections: The Amniotic Sac Infection Syndrome

Amniotic sac infection was the most common cause of perinatal mortality with 6.17 deaths per 1000 births in the US national collaborative perinatal study [6]. The tendency for amniotic fluid infection to occur in mothers with poor obstetric histories has been well documented. In half of the cases the mothers had at least two previous pregnancy losses [45]. Although not specifically documented, many previous losses were probably also due to amniotic sac infection [46, 47].

Rupture of placental membranes is not necessary for the development of the amniotic sac infection syndrome [6]. In fact, logic suggests that the reason for the rupture, particularly in preterm cases, is that the membranes at the internal cervical os become infected. They rupture because of the associated inflammation and necrosis of tissue. When rupture occurs, the prospect for infection is much greater in a premature fetus than in a fetus or baby near term gestation. Of the 135 gravidas with ruptured membranes longer than 18 hours studied by Linder et al, 11 babies developed sepsis; 10 of these were premature. Neither maternal fever, neonatal leukocytosis, leukopenia, thrombocytopenia, nor positive gastric aspirate cultures were of use in predicting which babies would be infected. Among all the premature infants, fully 15% developed sepsis [48].

Infectious causes of perinatal mortality are especially prevalent during the second trimester of gestation [49–51] and in the last few weeks of gestation [6, 52, 53]. About 2% of all placentas in gestations greater than 37 weeks have severe acute chorioamnionitis and maternal fever and fetal tachycardia are frequently associated with this ominous sign. Neonatal pneumonia occurs in about one-third of such patients or about 4 per 1000 live births. Maternal fever, leukocytosis, and primiparous condition are all associated features [52, 54].

No matter when during gestation the syndrome of amniotic fluid infection occurs, one problem facing the pathologist is the interpretation of inflamed placental membranes. About half of all placentas which are carefully examined will have at least mild inflammation [55–57]. Conversely, among babies with proved infection, amniotic fluid can be sterile and similarly the placental membranes show no inflammation [58]. Gravett et al found that among amniotic fluid samples taken for evaluation of fetal lung maturity and presumably from unruptured sacs, 24% were positive for various bacteria, including *Mycoplasma hominis*, and/or *Candida albicans* [59]. Hillier et al recovered bacteria from 32% of all placentas with gestations of 35 weeks or less and in 19% of all placentas from gestations more than

35 weeks. Premature babies with positive placental cultures were at greatest risk for neonatal death [60]. Perkins et al found that inflammation precedes rupture of membranes in up to 30% of women who enter the hospital without labor; 22% of these women have babies with inflammation of the umbilical cord [61]. The onset of labor may be induced by polymorphonuclear leukocytes or by the organisms themselves, either of which may stimulate the production of significant levels of prostaglandin E [13]. In a case control study, Hillier et al found that inflammatory infiltrates in the membranes correlated with infection in premature deliveries [62]. Romero et al studied 92 patients with preterm labor and intact membranes. Amniotic fluid contained bacteria in 38% of the cases and these were associated with acute chorioamnionitis and funisitis in 96.6% of the specimens [63].

Severely inflamed membranes occur twice as often in fetuses and neonates with infection as in fetuses and neonates without infection and such placentas often have villous edema [64]. When the fetus is delivered prematurely (less than 34 weeks), and when the membranes are severely inflamed with confluent exudates and infiltrates in the amnion-chorion, and when at least two of three vessels in the umbilical cord are inflamed, the likelihood of clinical infection is about 85%. Lesser degrees of inflammation, especially in placentas near term, are less likely to be associated with infection [65]. Nevertheless, even mild degrees of membranitis can be found in fatal perinatal infections [47].

It must be admitted candidly that after decades of considering these processes, the interpretation of inflamed membranes and umbilical cords and positive bacterial cultures remains subjective as to which are causes, which are effects, and which have no relationship to clinical infection.

PATHOLOGY OF PLACENTAL INFECTION

Details of the placental pathology caused by specific infectious agents are given later in this chapter. In this section, general aspects only will be considered.

Macroscopic Appearances of Placental Infection

The appearance of the placenta with infected membranes is often indistinguishable from normal. The membranes usually appear cloudy or distinctly opaque in cases of severe chorioamnionitis (Fig. 17.1), although this may be partly masked by meconium staining. In addition, the placenta may have a foul odor. When examining placentas for possible infection, it is important to remember that any loss of translucency of the fetal surface of the preterm placenta is likely to be abnormal, whereas subchorial fibrin deposits may appear opaque on the fetal surface of the normal placenta at term.

Small yellow abscesses in the placental substance are characterisitic of listeriosis and small yellow/white spots on the umbilical cord are a feature of infection by *Candida albicans*.

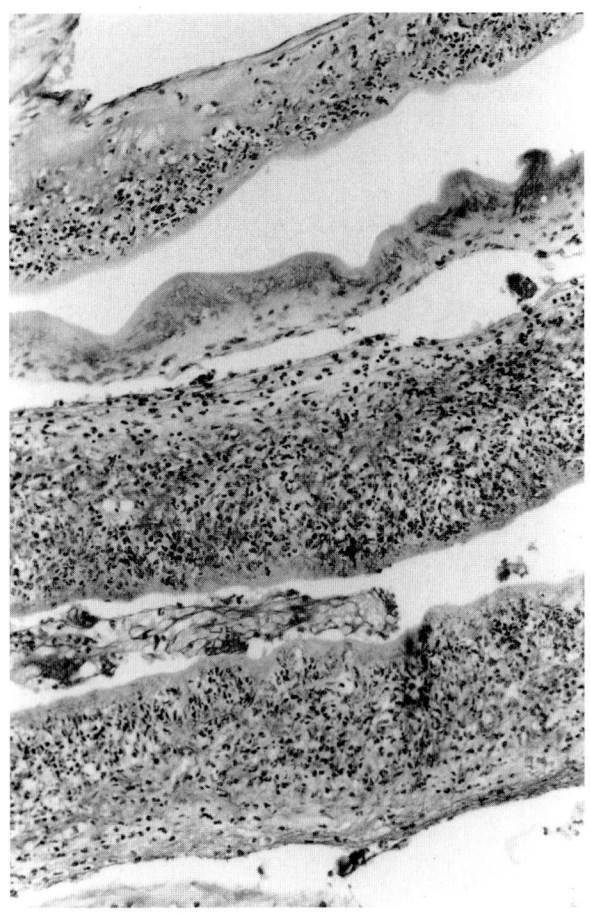

FIGURE 17.1.   *Acute and focally necrotizing chorioamnionitis. The membranes are from the placenta of a premature infant weighing 400 g, infected with group B streptococcus, and surviving only a few minutes. (H&E, ×60.)*

Pronounced subacute or necrotizing infection of the umbilical cord is recognizable in the form of a "barber pole" cord, in which the cord vessels are outlined by an opaque white or chalky exudate visible as spirals through the Wharton's jelly [66].

Microscopic Appearances of Placental Infection

Acute Chorioamnionitis

The earliest infiltration by maternal neutrophils occurs in placental membranes apposed to the internal cervical os [66]. The tissues stretch, the maternal blood flow diminishes, increasing the susceptibility to bacterial invasion at this site. Maternal leukocytes leave decidual vessels and invade the chorion and amnion, resulting in the classic appearances of established chorioamnionitis (see Fig. 17.1). Within the placenta, maternal leukocytes, mostly neutrophils, collect at the interface of the maternal sinusoids and the chorion. In the next phase, the maternal leukocytes infiltrate the chorion and migrate through the amnion to reach the amniotic

cavity, into which they pour. The maternal component of the infiltrate, either in the placenta or in the membranes, may be sparse or dense, varying with the intensity and duration of infection.

Fetal reaction to infection is leukocytic invasion of the chorionic and umbilical vessels; it commences later than the maternal reaction. It too may be sparse or dense, presumably depending on the intensity of the chemotactic stimulus and duration of the infection.

Villitis

Inflammation of placental villi is characteristic of infections reaching the placenta from the maternal bloodstream. Bacterial, viral, fungal, and protozoal infections cause villitis [67, 68]. The findings in specific infections such as cytomegalovirus, herpes simplex virus, syphilis, listeria, toxoplasmosis, and malaria are presented below. The general features include focal infiltration of the villi with maternal lymphocytes and histiocytes, necrosis, granulation tissue, and fibroblastic proliferation or fibrosis, according to the stage of evolution and organism involved [69, 70]. Granulomatous villitis has been described in toxoplasmosis [71]. There may be an associated vasculitis of villous stem arteries.

Once the diagnosis of chronic villitis is established, an effort must be made to identify the few known infectious causes. These include cytomegalovirus infection [72, 73], syphilis [67, 68, 74], toxoplasmosis [71, 75], and varicella [76, 77]. The specific diagnosis of these infectious agents can be enhanced with special techniques such as immunohistochemistry or in situ hybridization using molecular probes [73]. Greco et al found that cytomegalovirus (CMV) villitis has intense reactivity to macrophage markers [78]. Schwartz et al studied placentas known to be infected with CMV and found marked hyperplasia of Hofbauer cells and lymphocytic villitis [79].

Villitis of Unknown Etiology (VUE)

The significance of villitis remains controversial when it is an incidental finding in cases without recognizable infection elsewhere [80–88]. In villitis of unknown etiology (VUE), the inflammatory cells are mostly macrophages, T-helper lymphocytes, and some polymorphonuclear white blood cells, virtually all derived from the mother [70, 78, 82].

Since IgM concentrations are not elevated in the sera of mothers or babies, maternal and fetal infections, other than those already mentioned, are apparently unassociated with the lesions seen in VUE [88].

Chronic Chorioamnionitis

Chronic chorioamnionitis is an uncommon lesion. Chronic villitis and large intervillous fibrin deposits are found in many such cases but microorganisms are not usually present. Clinically, previous spontaneous abortions, small-for-dates babies, and preterm babies are associated with chronic chorioamnionitis [89, 90].

SYNDROME OF EARLY ONSET SEPSIS

Early onset sepsis affects liveborn infants within the first 4 or 5 days of life—usually within the first day, often at the time of birth. Bacteremia and pneumonia are the main clinical findings. Occasionally, meningitis is an added feature. Most such infections are acquired via the ascending route just before labor or during birth. The fetal counterpart is acute sepsis, usually with pneumonia, acute inflammatory infiltrates and exudates in various organs and tissues, and sometimes with acute meningitis. The pathogenesis includes asphyxia, apparently due to abnormal blood flow in the uteroplacental circulation [91]. With either fetal or neonatal sepsis, experiments have shown that endotoxins contribute to morbidity by inducing fibrin thrombi and hemorrhages with widespread endothelial damage [92]. Viruses, protozoa, and fungi may also produce their own forms of early onset sepsis (Table 17.3).

Early onset sepsis is associated with thrombocytopenia and neutrophilia or neutropenia [93]. Other lesions include those attributable to shock [94]. Liver damage is frequently severe and kernicterus is common [95, 96].

Localized forms of early sepsis (as differentiated from the generalized syndrome of neonatal sepsis) include neonatal appendicitis that, while rare, may be detected by cutaneous redness over the region encompassing McBurney's point [97]. Necrotizing enterocolitis, ocular infections, otitis media, and urinary tract infections may be found in neonates with early onset sepsis [98]. Ophthalmia neonatorum is a relatively minor infectious lesion seen in the first days following birth but rarely does this condition reach the attention of the pathologist. Examination of smears reveals intracellular gram-negative diplococci or cytoplasmic inclusions in conjunctival cells, indicative of the two most common causes of eye infections in the neonate, gonococcus and *Chlamydia trachomatis* [99, 100].

The Clinical Diagnosis of Early Onset Sepsis

One of the goals in neonatology is the rapid, accurate diagnosis of early onset sepsis so that treatment can be quickly started. Cultures are useful but require days for results in diseases that can be fatal in hours after the first signs appear.

Table 17.3. Infectious agents associated with early versus late onset disease

GBS	Early > Late
E. coli	Early > Late
Toxoplasmosis	Early = Late
Cytomegalovirus	Early = Late
HSV	Early = Late
Listeria	Early < Late
Candida	Early < Late

A clinical profile for the likelihood of neonatal sepsis includes the following features: premature rupture of the placental membranes (i.e., before labor commences), prolonged rupture of placental membranes for greater than 24 hours, gestation of less than 34 weeks, a male fetus, and maternal signs or symptoms of infection [101]. Maternal urinary tract infections may [102] or may not [103] qualify in this profile. A clinical feature sometimes overlooked is that the mothers have poor obstetric histories. Repeated losses, usually in the stages of gestation between 18 and 28 weeks, have already been mentioned. Maternal illicit drug use is also a risk factor for neonatal sepsis [104].

Many laboratory tests are used to diagnose fetal or neonatal sepsis. Amniotic fluid leukoattractants and cytokines are new analytes that may prove useful [105–108]. Simply measuring amniotic fluid glucose has proved a reasonably sensitive method of detecting fetal infection [109]. Neonatal tests include elevated white blood cell count, depressed white blood cell count, and acute phase reactants such as C-reactive protein, haptoglobin, sedimentation rate of red blood cells, and orosomucoid [101, 110]. A scoring system has been proposed wherein one point is assigned for each of seven abnormalities:

1. Abnormally elevated or depressed total leukocyte count
2. Abnormally elevated or depressed total polymorphonuclear leukocyte count
3. Elevated immature polymorphonuclear leukocyte count
4. Elevated ratio of immature to total polymorphonuclear leukocyte count
5. Ratio of 0.5 or greater of immature to mature polymorphonuclear leukocytes
6. Decreased platelet count (less than 150,000)
7. Morphologic evidence for degeneration of polymorphonuclear leukocytes

A score of 2 or less is almost never associated with infection (less than 1%) while a score of 3 or more is associated with a 30% likelihood of sepsis. Of course, high scores were more likely to be associated with sepsis than are relatively low scores such as 3 or 4 [111]. As with the fetus and the amniotic fluid, interleukins have been studied and show promise for aiding in the diagnosis of sepsis in the liveborn neonate [112]. Neonatal research groups in the United States are currently studying the efficacy of these analytes with the intent to find the most useful and timely tests for the diagnosis of early onset sepsis.

Physical signs in the neonate that indicate sepsis include lethargy, apnea, cyanosis, hemodynamic instability, respiratory distress, and temperature instability. Hypothermia is as common as hyperthermia [101, 113, 114].

Sepsis is diagnosed in the postmortem examination when one can demonstrate the appropriate inflammatory response and isolate the causative organism. One usually finds inflammation in the amniotic fluid, in the amnion and chorion of the placental disc or free membranes, and/or in the fetal airways and pulmonary air spaces or gastric mucus, with or without invasion of the mucosae of these organs (Figs. 17.2 and 17.3). An inflammatory response may be found, but a causative organism may not be isolated. Conversely, occasionally no inflammation is found when there are definite or highly suggestive clinical signs of infection and the appropriate organism is isolated. With regard to postmortem bacteriology, we have concluded that if sufficient care and judgment are exercised, valuable information can be obtained with the culture of blood, lung, and other organs at every postmortem examination.

Septicemia and Pneumonia

Neonatal septicemia and pneumonia most frequently occur together and form the syndrome of neonatal sepsis. This may be broadly considered bacterial infection during the first month of life, the primary site of invasion most often being the respiratory tract, the gastrointestinal tract, or the bloodstream, with spread to meninges in 25% to 30% of cases.

Septicemia can be defined as follows: a response in an infant who has two or more positive blood cultures with the same organism; or one positive blood culture and positive cultures from the cerebrospinal fluid, throat, or urine with the same organism as in the blood; or group B streptococcus, *E. coli*, or *Staphylococcus aureus* from any of these sites in an infant with symptoms of sepsis; or appropriate resolution of fever after antimicrobial treatment specific for the organism in question [115]. Specific pathologic lesions do not exist in septicemia, but hepatic sinusoids may have many more granulocytes and their precursors than normally found [29]. When septic shock is superimposed, the lesions include periventricular leukomalacia and intraventricular

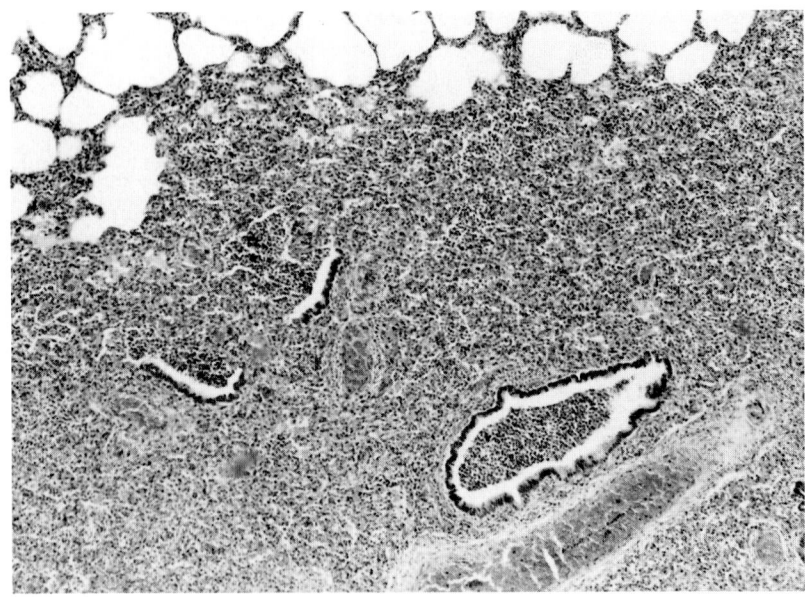

FIGURE 17.2.   *Intrauterine pneumonia is characterized by an aspiration pattern but it is more diffuse and has no foreign body reaction. (H&E, ×53.)*

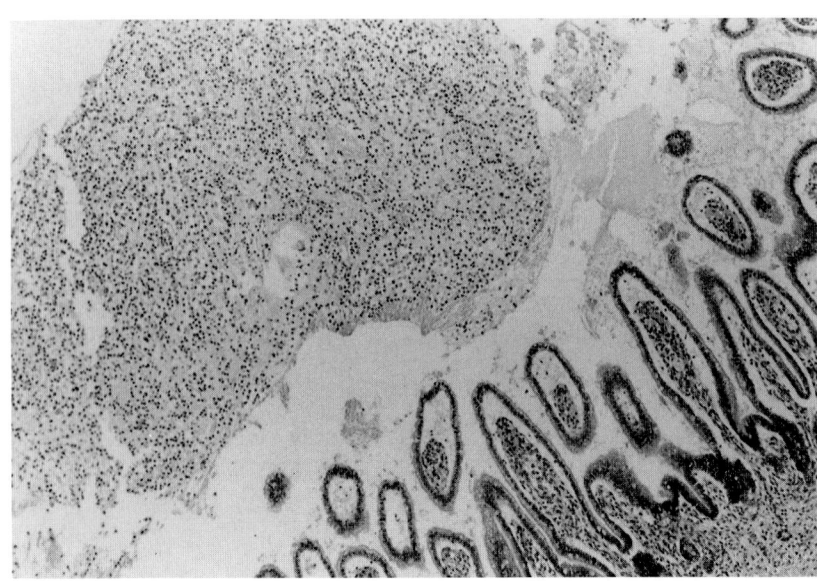

FIGURE 17.3.   *Proximal small intestine in a newborn infant. The lumen is filled with a purulent exudate, which was probably swallowed and undigested. (H&E, ×58.)*

hemorrhage; hepatic necrosis in a non-zonal irregular distribution; renal medullary hemorrhage, renal cortical necrosis, or acute renal tubular necrosis; and/or adrenal cortical and medullary hemorrhage and necrosis [116]. Lesions associated with coagulopathies may also be prevalent [117].

Pneumonia is the most common manifestation of neonatal sepsis. Despite the frequency with which it is observed clinically, pneumonia in the fetus and neonate is difficult, if not impossible, to recognize in the macroscopic inspection. The lungs are fleshy but not truly consolidated as they are in older infants or adults [118]. While closely resembling either hyaline membrane disease or hemorrhage, the lungs in neonatal pneumonia may be more voluminous than in the former condition and less moist than in the latter. In any case, one must depend upon microscopic examination to confirm the presence of pneumonia in cases with early onset. Rarely is a pleural reaction detected. When present, pleuritis usually consists of a delicate, stringy, clear, and mucoid substance rather than a yellow or tan fibrinous material.

In fetal or neonatal pneumonia the term "lobular" has been used but is not entirely accurate [5]. Lobar or bronchial patterns of pneumonia are almost never seen. These are aspiration pneumonias but in contrast to aspiration pneumonia in children and adults, the fetal or neonatal pattern is usually more widespread and has no associated foreign body response [118, 119] (Fig. 17.4). Polymorphonuclear leukocytes fill bronchioles and air sacs in an irregular distribution. There is no particular predilection for greater involvement of the right lung or the lower lobes compared with the left lung or other lobes. The inflammation is often diffuse, with all lobes of both lungs equally involved with exudate and infiltrate. This is particularly so with pneumonia in stillborn fetuses [120]. Bacteria may be demonstrated in the exudate or in the adjacent tissues, but this is frequently difficult to demonstrate in paraffin embedded tissues

[7]. When acquired in utero, pneumonia is classically described as an exudate without fibrin. One explanation for this phenomenon is that amniotic fluid inhibits the formation of fibrin or else dissolves it as it forms. Absence of air breathing is necessary for this phenomenon. When infants survive a few hours or days, fibrin is almost always found in the inflammatory reaction.

When the inflammatory reaction is limited to the lumens of air sacs and airways, it is possible that pneumonia does not truly exist but rather that the inflammatory cells were aspirated from a purulent exudate in the amniotic sac, in which instance many of the leukocytes are of maternal origin. Proof of the existence of pneumonia lies in the demonstration of infiltrate in the interstitium of the lung and evidence of an inflammatory reaction in blood vessels and lymphatics [119]. Even then, one could suppose that the maternal leukocytes which are aspirated from the amniotic fluid might migrate into fetal pulmonary interstitial tissues without a primary infection in the lung (Fig. 17.5). Demonstration of the y-antigen in the leukocytes of male fetuses or babies is proof of non-maternal origin in other cases [121].

Aspiration of amniotic fluid brings with it not only infectious agents but also amniotic debris. Squamous cells and other epithelial elements may be difficult to distinguish when pulmonary inflammation is intense. Meconium is frequently mixed with the amniotic debris, since the infection in utero is stressful and results in expulsion of meconium. Microscopically, meconium is recognized by green, yellow, or brown rounded globules (10 to 50 μm) or amorphous precipitate in aggregates (10 to 200 μm). The term "meconium pneumonia" is a misnomer, as aspirated meconium itself is not capable of inciting a pulmonary inflammatory response. Only when meconium is associated with bacteria or other infectious agents is pneumonia found [5, 23].

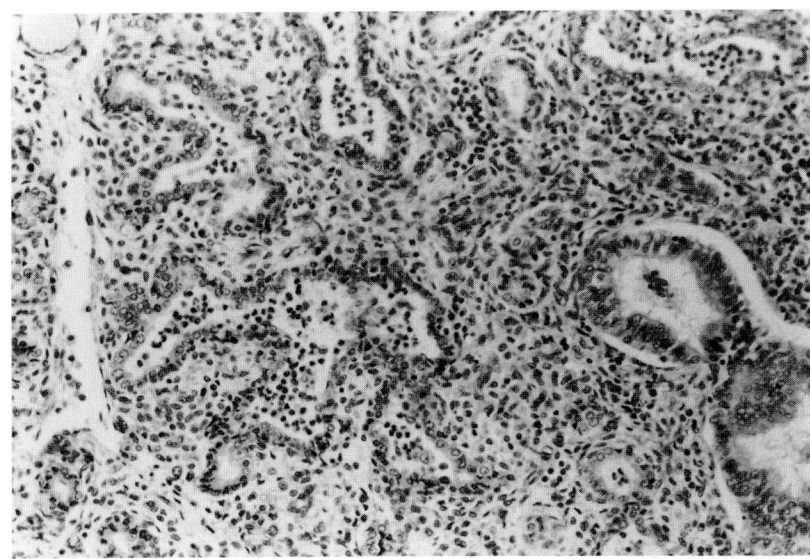

FIGURE 17.4. *Intrauterine pneumonia in a liveborn infant weighing 400 g at birth. The inflammatory cells occupy airspaces and also the interstitium. (H&E, ×280.)*

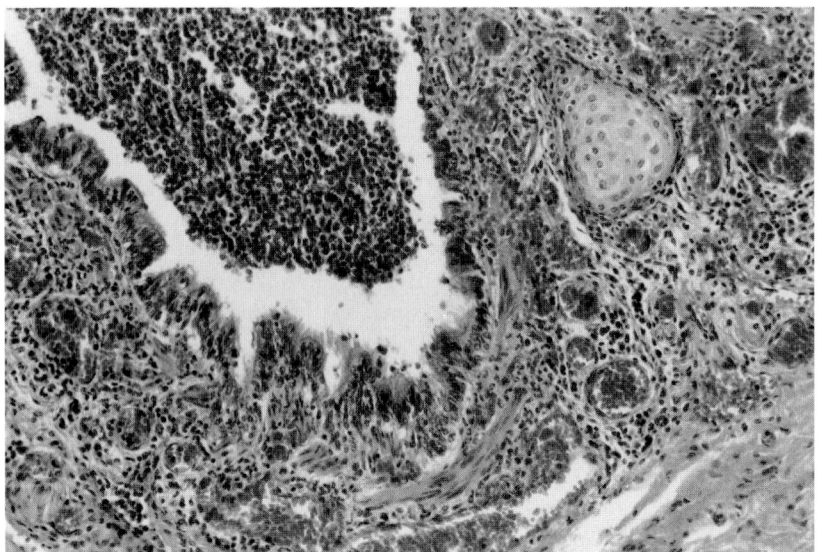

FIGURE 17.5.   *Intrauterine pneumonia in a liveborn infant weighing 3200 g at birth. The inflammation is in both the bronchial wall and in the bronchial lumen. It is also in the interstitium. (H&E, ×335.)*

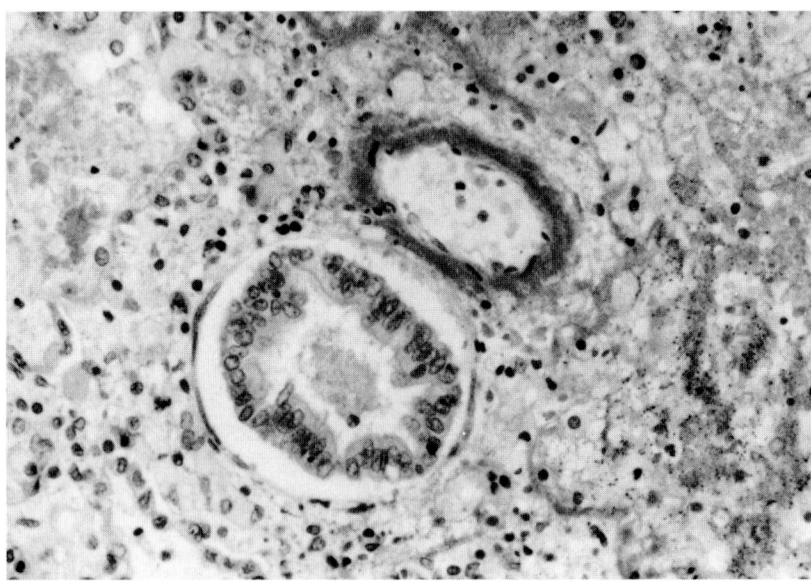

FIGURE 17.6.   *Infection of the neonatal lung with* Pseudomonas aeruginosa. *The arterial wall has a blue hazy appearance due to bacterial invasion. This is virtually pathognomonic of* Pseudomonas *infection [125]. (H&E, ×603.) (See Fig. 17.31 for the macroscopic lesion corresponding to this kind of infection.)*

Hemorrhage may accompany fetal or neonatal pneumonia and hyaline membrane formation is common. It is unclear whether the hyaline membranes are independent of or a consequence of the pneumonia [122, 123]. Clinically and radiologically, such cases are difficult to separate from respiratory distress due to surfactant deficiency [113, 122]. However, respiratory distress syndrome in an infant beyond 36 weeks' gestational age should at least raise the index of suspicion for pneumonia rather than surfactant deficiency [124].

Interstitial emphysema may also be a feature in neonatal pneumonia, but this is not common since pneumonia enhances lung compliance thereby reducing the likelihood of rupture of air sacs into the interstitium [113, 122].

Necrotic hemorrhagic pneumonia occurs when pseudomonad or proteus organisms or certain yeast or fungi are present. Leukocytes may be scanty. Fibrin and necrotic debris may predominate. In the case of *Pseudomonas*, yeast, or fungal infection, the organisms invade vessel walls. *Pseudomonas* imparts a hazy blue outline of the vessel. Usually small arteries and venules are involved, but occasionally larger vessels may have this pattern [125] (Fig. 17.6).

Meningitis

Meningitis, whether of early or late onset, is a diffuse process. Although rarely recognized, meningitis can occur in fetuses (Fig. 17.7). Diagnosis during life may be missed if

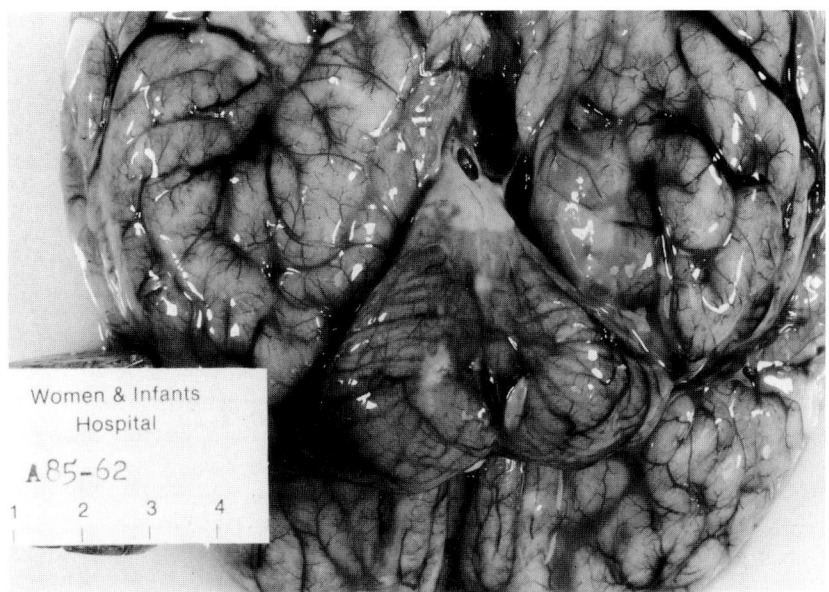

FIGURE 17.7.   *The basilar meninges are thickened in this case of fetal meningitis. The infecting organism was a hitherto unclassified* Pseudomonas, *according to the Centers for Disease Control, Atlanta.*

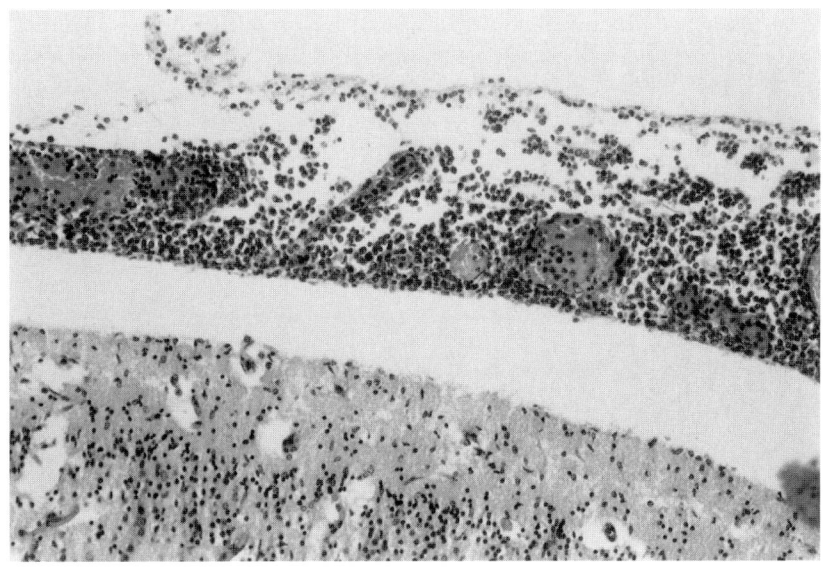

FIGURE 17.8.   *Purulent meningitis in a stillborn fetus. (H&E, ×335.)*

lumbar puncture is not performed [126]. Bacteria can gain access to the brain initially via the bloodstream to the choroid plexus and spread through the cerebral spinal fluid to the meninges [33]. Spread from the middle ears or through the cribriform plate probably plays a minor role [127]. In very small infants the inflammatory response may not be impressive macroscopically. Microscopically, one finds meningeal infiltrates of polymorphonuclear leukocytes and monocytes (Fig. 17.8). Lymphocytes are sparse in such cases. Extension is usually present along perivascular spaces around penetrating vessels in the cortex. Ventriculitis occurs in up to 90% of cases of neonatal meningitis [33]. Acute inflammatory cells infiltrate the ependyma and the subependymal tissues, destroying the surface epithelium. Hydrocephalus is a serious sequel of neonatal meningitis and

may be due either to destruction of absorptive granulations in the arachnoid meninges or to obstruction of narrow portions of the ventricular system such as the sylvian aqueduct. The association of cerebral palsy with peripartum sepsis has now been established by a case control study and probably represents the sequelae of meningoventriculitis [128]. Gram-positive organisms are twice as common as gram-negative ones in neonatal meningitis but mortality is higher with the gram-negative bacteria [129].

SYNDROME OF LATE ONSET SEPSIS

Late onset sepsis usually begins after 1 week of age but may occur as early as the third day or as late as 3 weeks to a few or several months after birth. The acquisition of the microorganism may have been in utero, during delivery, or after delivery. A long latent period is obviously necessary between the time that intrauterine or intrapartum inoculation takes place and the onset of symptoms and signs of infection. The supposition in such cases is that the baby is colonized in utero or at birth and then becomes infected when defenses are impaired; for example, surgery, shock, or some other untoward event allows the microorganisms to invade tissues or the bloodstream.

Group B streptococci, *E. coli*, *Streptococcus viridans*, *Proteus* species, *Pseudomonas* species, *Listeria monocytogenes*, *Serratia marcescens*, *Klebsiella pneumoniae*, *Streptococcus faecalis*, *Candida albicans*, *Hansenula anomala*, *Aspergillus*, *Malassezia furfur*, and a large variety of other infectious organsms have been isolated from typical cases [8, 130–135]. Herpes simplex viruses are also associated with syndromes of late onset sepsis [136].

The nosocomial infections can be associated with intensive care treatment, such as liberal use of antimicrobial drugs and invasive therapies such as catheters in vessels, nasogastric catheters, chest tubes, and surgical operations (Fig. 17.9) (Table 17.4).

The clinical features of late onset sepsis may be subtle. They include poor feeding, circumoral cyanosis, lethargy, hypotonia, and either fever or hypothermia. Meningitis is a common clinical manifestation; pneumonia and septicemia may also be noted.

Table 17.4.   Microbial agents in nosocomial infections associated with intensive care

Pseudomonas aeruginosa
Staphylococcus aureus
Serratia marcescens
Cytomegalovirus
Candida albicans
Hansenula anomala
Malassezia furfur

Pneumonias in late onset sepsis may be caused by any of several organisms, each with its particular pattern of inflammation and repair. Thus, coagulase-positive *Staphylococcus* infection can produce abscesses and an intense pleural reaction or empyema. *Malassezia furfur* produces a localized indolent chronic infection [133]. Organisms such as *Pseudomonas* or *Aspergillus* invade and destroy blood vessel walls resulting in pulmonary infarcts, with hemorrhage and marginating inflammation. Lobar or bronchopneumonia may be clearly seen in late onset pneumonia due to any of the same infectious agents that produce a diffuse pneumonia or an extended aspiration pattern in early onset pneumonia [5, 137].

Other features of late onset sepsis include hepatic abscesses [138], otitis, facial cellulitis, and septic arthritis (Fig.

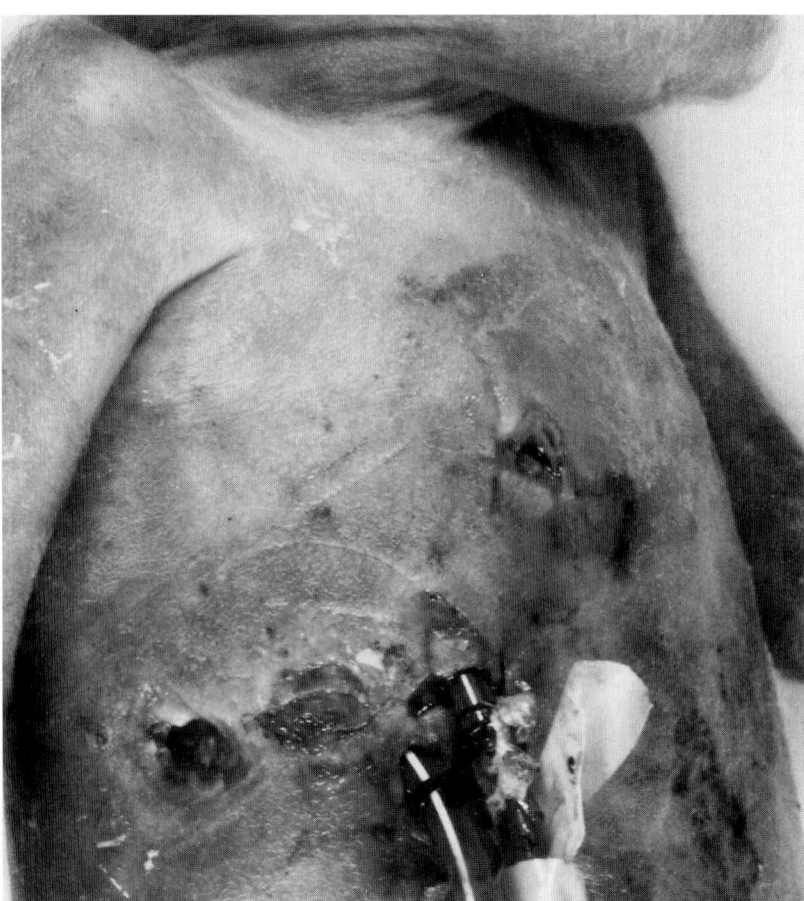

FIGURE 17.9.   *Cutaneous and subcutaneous necrosis is associated with* Pseudomonas *infection, complicating the prolonged use of several chest tubes. This premature baby survived for 2 weeks in the neonatal intensive-care unit.*

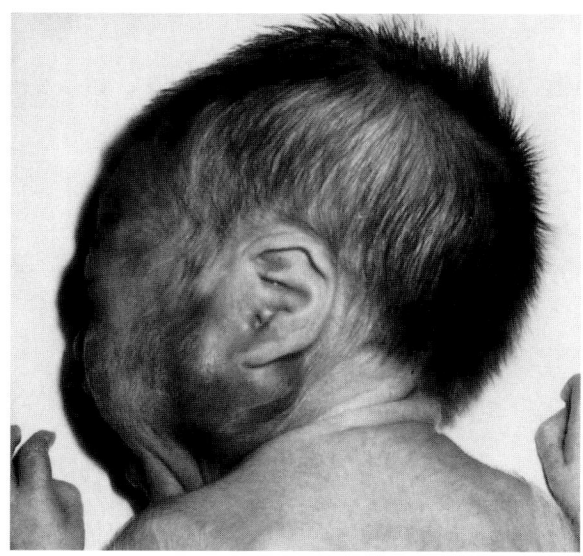

FIGURE 17.10. *Parotitis and facial cellulitis were due to* Staphylococcus *infection in this infant. Photograph generously provided by Dr. Murdina M. Desmond, Houston, Texas.*

17.10). Osteomyelitis has been reported in babies whose heels were traumatized by lancets during blood-drawing procedures [139]. Urinary tract infections, though rare in young infants, may occur in males up to 3 months of age. Females are usually older when they develop urinary tract infections [140]. Necrotizing enterocolitis, often associated with infection, if not actually the result of infection, is commonly described as an event of either early or late onset [141–143]. Endocarditis may also be either an early onset or late onset disease [144].

Reactive hemophagocytosis can occur in late onset sepsis due to viral, bacterial, fungal, or parasitic infections. This condition is characterised by pyrexia, wasting, lymphadenopathy, hepatosplenomegaly, and pancytopenia. The histologic hallmark is histiocytic proliferation, sometimes with atypia approaching malignant change and hemophagocytosis. The helper T cells may be markedly reduced and suppressor cells moderately elevated. Lymphoid tissues are atrophic while the stroma of lymph nodes and spleen are packed with histiocytes causing enlargement of these organs and structures [145].

VIRAL INFECTIONS

Most if not all viruses depend on cell surface receptors for particular tropism, and affect the internal cellular machinery of infected cells [146]. Several viruses can disrupt development during embryogenesis or early fetal life. Defective development of the central nervous system has been attributed to rubella virus, cytomegalovirus, herpes simplex viruses, coxsackie B viruses, Eastern equine encephalitis virus, mumps virus, and Western equine encephalitis virus [147–150]. In prospective studies, assignment of an infec-

tious cause to malformations has been more tenuous [151, 152]. Mumps has been associated with increased fetal mortality but not with malformations [152]. Some of the more carefully studied fetal and neonatal viral infections are described in detail below.

Rubella Virus Infection

N. McAlister Gregg is credited with recognizing the teratogenic effects of rubella. He observed a large number of infants and toddlers with cataracts in the months and years following an outbreak of rubella in Australia during the years 1939 to 1940 [153]. These children also had hearing deficits and heart murmurs, thus forming the classic triad of congenital rubella. During the 1964–65 epidemic in the United States, the rubella syndrome was expanded to include hepatitis, cholangitis, jaundice, failure to thrive superimposed on intrauterine growth retardation, purpuric skin rash, meningoencephalitis, osseous abnormalities, chorioretinitis, splenomegaly, thrombocytopenia, excessive extramedullary hematopoiesis, interstitial pneumonitis, lymphadenopathy, occasional pancreatic islet inflammation, and nephritis [154–157] (Figs. 17.11 and 17.12).

The various lesions develop along three pathways: 1) inhibition of cell growth, 2) cytolysis, and 3) interference with the blood supply. The lesions may be inflammatory, necrotic, or expressed as decreased growth or malformations [158–160].

Periconceptional maternal rubella is harmless if the rash appears before the 12th day following the last menstrual period [161]. All maternal infections noted between 3 weeks and 11 weeks of gestation result in infected fetuses [161, 162]. If maternal infection occurs during or after week 12, progressively fewer fetuses are infected [162].

Pathologic Findings in Congenital Rubella Syndrome
Placental lesions due to rubella are nonspecific but nevertheless characteristic. In gestations of less than 20 weeks, the villous vessels are damaged and sometimes are necrotic, with associated villous edema, increase in Hofbauer cells, and occasionally hemorrhage or necrosis [87, 158]. Necrosis of syncytial trophoblast is associated with encasement of the villi in fibrin. Lymphocytes, plasma cells, and neutrophils infiltrate the decidua. Umbilical cords are normal and there is no chorioamnionitis. When infection occurs in gestations close to term, villi are fibrotic and placentas are small [87]. Villitis is not described in congenital rubella infection. Villous vessels may have thin walls, atrophic media, and calcified thrombi [163].

Either precocious acceleration of lymphoid follicles with follicular (germinal) centers and increased humoral antibodies or depleted lymphoid tissues with depressed humoral and cellular immune function may be found [164, 165]. Beyond the neonatal period, lymphoid tissue has distorted structure with ill-defined follicles, changes that may take years to

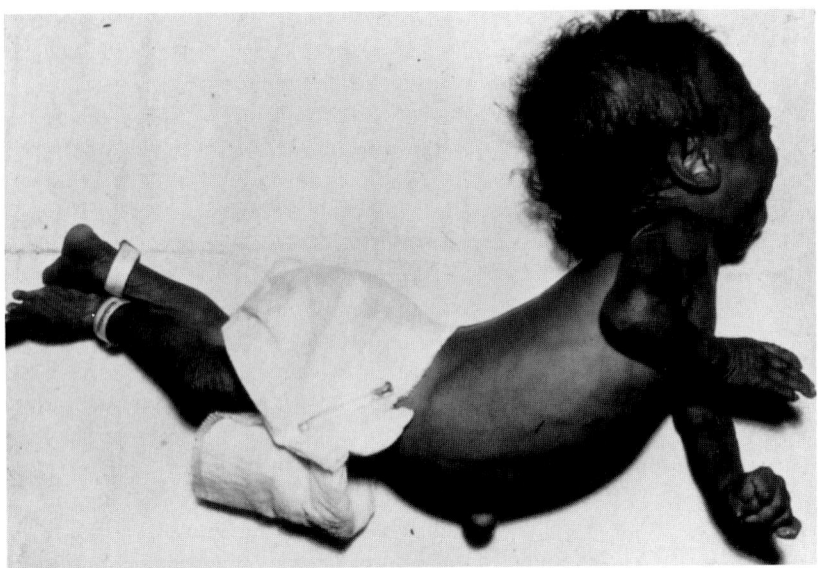

FIGURE 17.11. *Rubella meningitis causes a typical persistent opisthotonic posture in the affected baby. (From Desmond et al [171], used with permission from the publisher and Dr. Murdina M. Desmond, Houston, Texas.)*

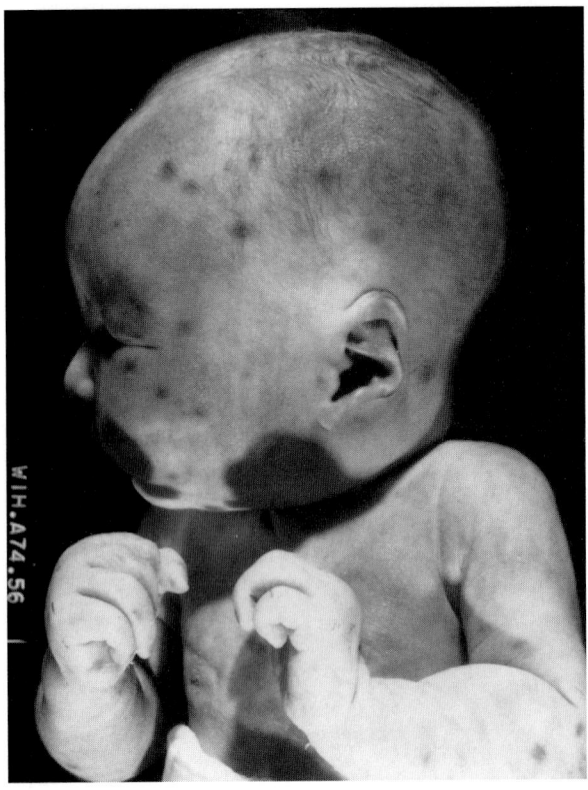

FIGURE 17.12. *Purpuric skin rash in congenital rubella.*

resolve [165]. Sinusoids of lymph nodes and spleen frequently have erythrophagocytosis and fibrin thrombi. Thymic involution is usual and bone marrow may be hyperplastic but usually is normally cellular [165, 166].

The incidence of fetal cardiovascular disease, other than patent ductus arteriosus, varies with the gestational age at onset of maternal rubella; incidence is highest in the first 4 weeks of development. Maternal infection after 16 weeks'

gestation is not associated with cardiovascular anomalies [160]. Patent ductus arteriosus affects about 80% of the infected neonates with collagenous replacement of ductal medias. Less common lesions are pulmonary artery branch stenosis, localized systemic arterial stenoses, myocarditis, and noninflammatory myocardial degeneration which is observed in stillborn fetuses. Aortic coarctations develop above and below the diaphragm [160, 166]. Fibromuscular proliferation without inflammation and without calcification characterizes these lesions. The aorta may show loose fibroblastic intimal proliferation with excess mucopolysaccharide in the stroma. The media may be fragmented with decreased elastic fibers. Vascular intimal sclerosis can also be found in the pulmonary arteries, renal arterial ostia, and iliac arteries. Branch stenoses are usually not detected until late in infancy [154]. Other lesions include malformations such as tetralogy of Fallot, truncus arteriosus, ventricular septal defects, atrioventricularis communis defects, tricuspid atresia, transpositions of the great arteries, supravalvular aortic stenosis, and nodular sclerosis of the valves. Chronic myocarditis is also described [154, 167].

Chronic pneumonia and interstitial pneumonitis are neonatal lesions that may persist for several weeks or months (Fig. 17.13). Alveolar septal metaplasia and fibrosis may evolve to chronic interstitial fibrosis [166]. Minimal residual fibrosis occurs in survivors and persistent pulmonary disease is rare [160].

Jaundice is a prominent clinical feature, partly as the result of a hemolytic anemia but largely due to liver damage [155, 166]. Hepatocellular swelling is followed by cholestasis, increased extramedullary hematopoiesis, portal phlebitis, giant cell transformation, and proliferation of bile ducts [154, 156]. Biliary atresia is rare [168]. Periportal fibrosis and extension of collagen into sinusoids occur later in a few cases, but overt cirrhosis has not been described [160].

Pancreatic involvement in rubella is uncommon but inflammation may occur in pancreatic ductal, acinar, and

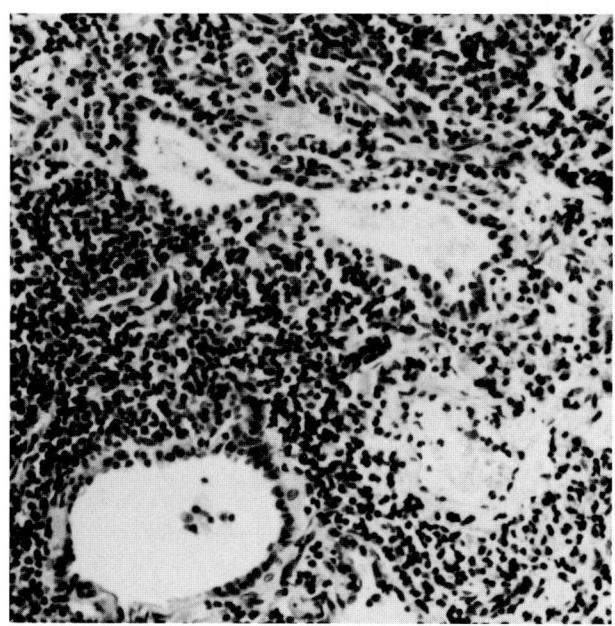

FIGURE 17.13. *Interstitial pneumonitis in congenital rubella. The inflammatory cells are almost exclusively lymphocytes. (H&E, ×360.)*

islet tissues. Juvenile-onset diabetes mellitus is increased in survivors of the congenital rubella syndrome [160].

The most characteristic bone lesion is reduced proliferative cartilage in the epiphyseal and metaphyseal growth zones. Osteoblasts and osteoclasts proliferate and ground substance contains increased myxoid connective tissue. Radiographs disclose longitudinal striations of alternating sclerosis and lucency in long bones. Spicules are thickened and maloriented in the metaphysis and diaphysis. Osteoid is decreased and cartilage extends into the diaphysis along spicules composed of poorly mineralized bone [154, 156, 157, 169]. Osteoporosis develops in survivors [160]. The epithelium of the enamel-forming organ in the teeth is destroyed in congenital rubella [166].

Cataractous lenses are spherical (spherophakia) with persistent nuclei in the central collagen. Microphthalmia is common. Iritis, pigmentary degeneration in the ciliary body, and degeneration of retinal ganglion cells are also noted [156, 166]. Neovascularization of the retina is one of the sequelae [160]. Glaucoma and fibrosis of conjunctiva also develop in later infancy [156].

The skin is purpuric with bland hemorrhages which are sometimes accompanied by clusters of extramedullary hematopoiesis (see Fig. 17.12). Seborrheic rashes develop in later infancy.

Lesions of the gastrointestinal and genito-urinary tracts have been infrequent. Jejunal atresia and distal urinary atresias are mentioned by Esterly and Oppenheimer [154]. Nephrocalcinosis occurs rarely as does chronic interstitial nephritis.

Deafness can be the only defect in congenital rubella, and tends to be the most common lesion in cases in which the mothers were infected later in gestation (beyond 12 to 14 weeks of pregnancy). However, deafness rarely occurs in infants infected after gestations of 16 weeks, although the virus can be isolated from 25% of such infants [162]. Pathologic changes are incompletely documented but include discontinuity of the cochlear duct and damage in Corti's organ. Inflammation of the striae vascularis is also described and collapse of the tectorial membrane is associated with adherence to the striae vascularis [166].

Fetuses and neonates have chronic lymphocytic/histiocytic meningitis. The most severe sequelae among survivors of congenital rubella infection are mental retardation and sensory and motor deficits [170]. Leukocytosis of the cerebrospinal fluid can be mild [166, 171, 172]. Encephalitis is characterized by glial proliferation, particularly in the basal ganglia, midbrain, and brain stem, but also in the cortex. These lesions are associated with perivascular cuffs of lymphocytes. Capillaries are disrupted and necrotic with mineralized deposits in vascular walls and in pericapillary tissues [171, 172].

In approximately 15% of neonatal deaths due to rubella, adrenal fetal cortical cytomegaly may be seen [156]. Lymphocytic thyroiditis is found in surviving patients with hypothyroidism. Hyperthyroidism and Addison's disease are also described in survivors but without pathologic data [160].

Swisher et al note that 50% of survivors show some form of regressive behavior and 12% are autistic [173]. Late infantile and early childhood death claim 20% in the first 18 months and another 5% die in the next several years [174]. Of the survivors, 92% have hearing loss, 65% have symptomatic congenital heart disease, 56% impaired vision, 32% behavioral disorders, 26% neurological residual, 19% combined hearing and visual difficulties, and 1% diabetes mellitus. Poor balance and muscle weakness persist in over half the survivors [170]. Growth retardation remains prominent. Of those survivors age 18 years and older with normal intelligence, 34% are below the 10th percentile for height, 29% below the 10th percentile for head circumference. Of those with subnormal intelligence 66% have growth retardation and 71% have small head circumferences [174].

In countries where the rubella vaccine is routinely available, the disease is all but extinguished as a cause of perinatal morbidity and mortality. The attenuated virus in the vaccine can cross the placenta but it is harmless. It has been isolated from fetuses and newborns whose mothers inadvertently receive vaccination while pregnant but has produced no disease [175], and among the 239 cases in which this was known to occur, demonstrable fetal or neonatal lesions or disease did not develop [176]. Although outbreaks among pregnant nurses have been reported as recently as 1980 where 12% of the female personnel at risk were not rubella immune [177], the situation has improved in the past several years. In 1986, only 12 congenital cases

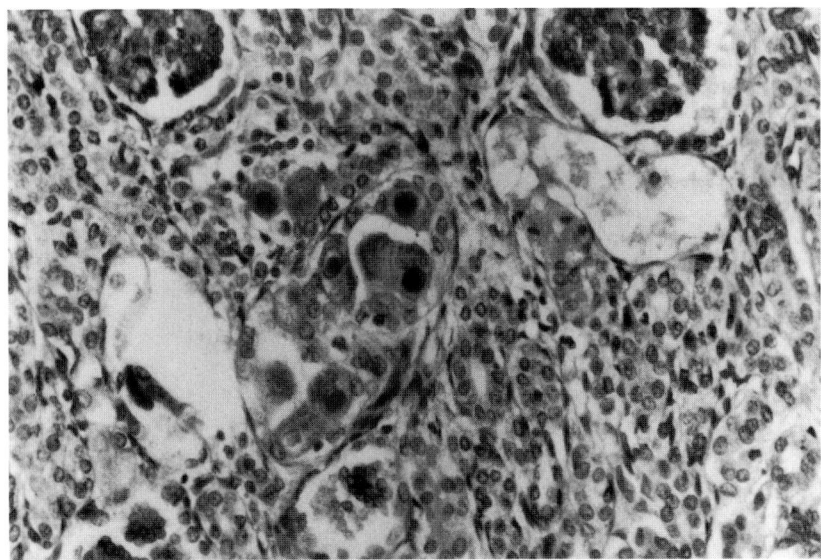

FIGURE 17.14. *Renal tubules infected with cytomegalovirus. The enlargement of cells, their nuclei, the intranuclear inclusions with halos, and the cytoplasmic inclusions forming an arc of darkly stained material are all characteristic of this infection. (H&E, ×603.)*

were reported among 551 total cases in the United States [178].

Cytomegalovirus Infection

Because of the unique features of the conspicuously enlarged cells, perinatal infection with cytomegalovirus (CMV) has been recognized (at least in retrospect) for the past 80 to 90 years [72] (Fig. 17.14). It is a relatively uncommon finding in autopsy material. Larroche mentions only 5 of 2000 perinatal autopsies in Paris with disseminated CMV infection [179]. Edith Potter saw no cases in the first 8000 perinatal autopsies she recorded at the Chicago Lying-In Hospital [180]. In the Aukland series, the rate of infection was one severe (fatal) perinatal case per 16,000 total births; 1 per 330 stillborn; and 1 per 200 neonatal deaths beyond 28 weeks' gestation [72]. In communities with low rates of immunity, fetal infections result in stillbirth in 2%, and a further 3% die as neonates. By 1 month of age, severe disease occurs in 15% of cases with primary maternal CMV infection but this figure rises to 50% if the infection occurs prior to the sixth month of gestation [181].

First identified as a human virus in salivary glands, the fatal generalized form of CMV disease was described in the 1950s and was called cytomegalic inclusion disease [182]. Fetterman was the first to report the diagnosis during life by examining urinary sediment. Thereafter, prospective study of the clinical course of the disease was possible [183]. Clinically inapparent infections can be tentatively diagnosed with elevated IgM in the cord blood correlated with positive cultures of urine or with anti-CMV specific IgM antibodies [184]. However, fetal IgM levels may be depressed in some congenital infections [185]. At least one case has been diagnosed by culture of amniotic fluid followed by elective abortion of the infected fetus [186].

The virus is found throughout the world with rates of seropositivity among pregnant women ranging from 10% in some countries to 100% in undeveloped areas including remote primitive populations [187]. About 50% of the adult population in the United States has antibodies against CMV [188]. From 0.25% to 3% of all pregnancies are complicated by primary maternal infection; 40% to 50% transmit CMV to the fetuses but these are not often symptomatic infections. In absolute numbers, an estimated 12,000 fetuses are infected every year in the United States and about 600 (5% to 10%) of these are symptomatic at birth [181, 187]. Early abortion may occur from an ascending CMV endometritis or hematogenous infection of the developing chorionic villi. The incidence of such events is unknown.

Reinfection or reactivation of latent infection occurs in many women. Viruria occurs in up to 5.9% of infected women in the third trimester and up to 28% of women may have positive cervical cultures in the latter part of pregnancy, particularly if they are young and of low parity. The source of the infection does not seem to be venereal, although semen may be infected and cervical infections may, like herpes simplex infections, be latent [189].

Severe symptomatic fetal infections result from maternal infections early in gestation (as contrasted with late infection) and are usually from mothers with primary infections [188]. Repeated or secondary maternal infections can also infect fetuses [188, 190, 191]. Huang et al have shown essentially identical viral genomes of isolates from mother-infant pairs [191].

Health care workers are not at particular risk from exposure to infected infants, but babies who remain in the intensive care nursery often acquire CMV [192, 193]. Blood transfusions are the common denominator for such cases and the resulting infection can prove fatal, especially in preterm infants [194, 195]. CMV-free blood is now available from blood banks. CMV may also be transmitted by mother's milk [188], although breast feeding is not associated with increased rates of infection [196]. A gray-baby syndrome with hepatosplenomegaly, atypical lymphocytes, and respiratory distress develops in some cases of postnatally acquired CMV [197].

The classic triad of congenital CMV infection consists of 1) chorioretinitis, 2) calcification of the cerebrum, and 3) microcephaly [181]. Jaundice, hemolytic anemia, pneumonitis, hepatosplenomegaly, thrombocytopenic purpura, and hydrocephaly are the other common features in symptomatic newborn babies.

The Cytomegalic Inclusion-Bearing Cell

Infected cells are characteristically enlarged to 20 to 35 μm and have intranuclear and cytoplasmic DNA inclusions. The cytoplasmic inclusions stain with PAS stains. The intranuclear inclusions are oval, round, or reniform and 5 to 10 μm in least diameter, separated from the nuclear membrane by a clear halo giving the "owl's-eye" appearance. This basic feature is recognizable even in autolyzed tissues of macerated stillborn fetuses in which the hematoxyphilia is completely lost (see Chap. 9). The intranuclear inclusion in plastic-embedded preparations may have lacunae or appear as a morula of fine granules. Cytoplasmic inclusions vary from minute dots to distinct rounded bodies 3 to 4 μm in diameter. The larger inclusions may show central vacuolation or lie within cytoplasmic vacuoles; they may be arranged in concentrically curved rows at a pole opposite the eccentric infected nucleus with its inclusion. In infected epithelial cells, a hobnail appearance is sometimes seen (Fig. 17.15). In early stages of infection, the intranuclear inclusion may resemble those of other viruses, particularly other herpesviruses. Nucleoli tend to be better preserved in cells infected with CMV compared with cells infected with other herpesviruses [72]. In later stages, the large size of the cytomegalovirus inclusion and its infected cell distinguish this disease from virtually all other viruses.

Fetal infection early in gestation results in widespread disease but with minimal inflammatory response in the placenta [198]. Later in gestation, the inflammation is intense with numerous plasma cells and thrombi in villous vessels. Placentas are pale, edematous, and have increased nucleated red blood cells. Inclusions may or may not be present in villous nuclei. Pigmented macrophages may contain hemosiderin deposits. Meconium-laden macrophages occur in the fetal membranes as a nonspecific sign of fetal distress. The early characteristic lesion is necrotizing villitis in terminal and stem villi. Villitis was noted in all eight CMV-infected placentas studied by Mostoufi-Zadeh and colleagues [199]. Trophoblast on the surfaces of such villi may or may not be preserved. Later, dense foci of plasmacytes infiltrate an avascular stroma. When plasma cells are present, inclusions can usually be found in the same cases [199]. In cases without characteristic lesions, immunoperoxidase stains and in situ hybridization techniques expose CMV organisms that otherwise go undetected [73]. Nonspecific changes in placentas include hydrops with weights sometimes exceeding 1000 g and chorioamnionitis with polymorphonuclear leukocytes [66]. Amniotic fluid often contains cells infected with CMV [200]. Hydrops fetalis and ascites are also described in several cases [199, 201, 202].

In tiny fetuses, inclusions are found in muscle, brain, skin, bile ductules, pulmonary interstitium, pancreas, and skin. Thrombi develop in pulmonary vessels. Myocarditis and microcephaly may be evident early. Fetal growth retardation is usual in fatal or severe neonatal CMV infection, especially when delivery is in the latter weeks of gestation.

Cytomegalovirus infection is thought to be the most common cause of perinatal brain damage, accounting for 0.1% to 0.3% of the total in the United States and United Kingdom [189]. The classic chronic lesion consists of periventricular calcification and necrosis. The acute lesions have multiple small necrotic foci with swollen eosinophilic microglial cells which are sparsely or diffusely distributed. Some cases have typical CMV inclusions, but in others the

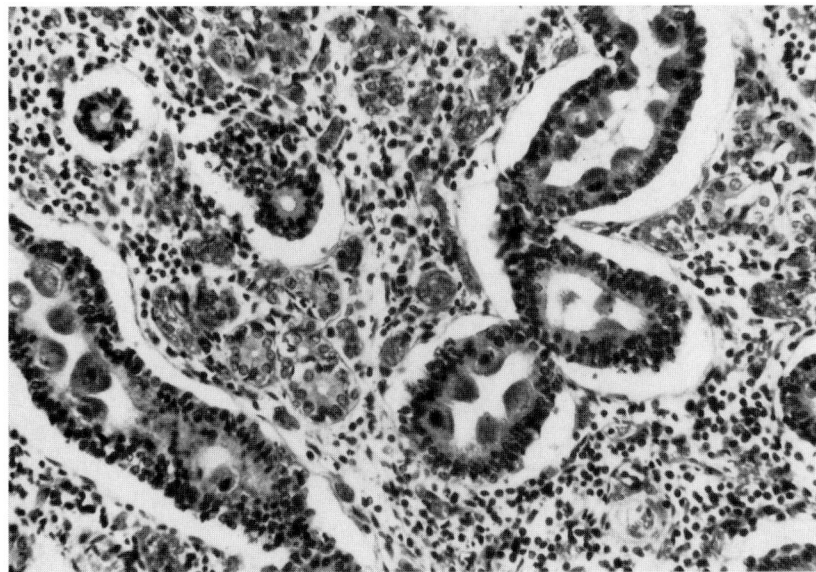

FIGURE 17.15. *Salivary gland infected with cytomegalovirus. The hobnail appearance and interstitial inflammation are characteristic of this infection. Demonstrable inclusions are sometimes limited to the salivary glands; in such cases, the fatal outcome is unrelated to the infection. (H&E, ×335.)*

lesion is simply an acute encephalitis. Inclusions are found in neurones, glia, ependyma, choroid plexus, meninges, and vascular endothelium and in cells lying free in ventricles. Cerebrospinal fluid may contain inclusion-bearing cells, but this is rare. Periependymitis may be present. Since many of these patients are preterm infants, the lesions of prematurity, such as intraventricular hemorrhage and periventricular leukomalacia, may also be present [72]. Microcephaly and hydrocephalus mark the destruction of brain tissue in the chronic brain lesions, although head size is a poor guide to brain pathology (Fig. 17.16). Old necrosis and various stages of resolution with hemosiderin or lipid-filled macrophages are present. The term granulomatous encephalomyelitis is used but the reaction is glial, not granulomatous [72]. Calcifications may involve individual cells of all types. In the periventricular location, calcium deposits are laminated and extracellular. Although the latter lesion is thought to be a classical one, in none of the 16 cases in the Aukland series did postmortem radiographs detect intracranial calcification [72].

Hearing loss is among the most common handicaps caused by congenital CMV infection. Virus has been isolated from Corti's organ and the spiral ganglia [181]. Inclusion-bearing epithelial cells are found in the vestibular (Reissner's) membranes and on the surfaces of the striae vascularis of the cochleae, the semicircular canals, saccules, and utricles and in the maculae and cristae. In routine histologic preparations the organs of Corti contain no inclusions nor are they edematous or infiltrated with lymphocytes [72]. Immunofluorescence has been used to demonstrate CMV antigens in Corti's organ in the absence of inclusions. Immune response and inflammation therefore play a major role in the damage to the ear in congenital CMV infection. We have detected CMV inclusions in the inner ear structures of a macerated fetus who died at 18 weeks' gestational age.

Chorioretinitis, optic neuritis, cataract, strabismus, microphthalmia, and colobomata are all described in congenital CMV infection. CMV has been isolated from anterior chamber fluid. In contrast to the chorioretinitis of toxoplasmosis, that of CMV infection apparently does not progress postnatally [72]. CMV inclusions have been described in areas of retinal necrosis and in retinal and chorioid vessels with associated retinal gliosis but without inflammation. Anophthalmia, optic atrophy, irregular retinal pigment, chorioretinitis, central corneal defect with adhesion to lens, and increased pressure in vitreous chamber have all been described with congenital CMV infection [203].

Lungs are the most favorable site for detecting inclusions in fetuses and neonatal infants. Inclusion-bearing cells may lie free in air spaces, their origin identified from the adjacent saccules. Bronchial and bronchiolar epithelia are rarely involved. Inflammation is often mild and consists of focal interstitial lymphocytic and plasmacytic infiltrates. Erythroid precursors may be numerous. Despite the lungs being the organ most often described as infected in postmortem material, symptomatic respiratory disease is not common in the newborn. On the other hand pneumonia is the most common manifestation of CMV infection beyond the perinatal period, as in neonates and young infants infected with contaminated transfused blood [72, 73].

Severe liver disease is not common, although inclusion-bearing cells are easily identified in small bile ducts and jaundice is a common finding. Hepatomegaly is noted in fewer than half the fatal neonatal cases. In severely infected neonates who survive for more than a few days, extensive neonatal hepatitis with giant cell transformation, cholangitis, and interstitial and portal fibrosis may be seen. Inclusions may be sparse in such cases. Progression to true cirrhosis has not been described. Hepatic calcifications are detected radiologically in infants with congenital CMV infection. The mineralized deposits are in periportal spaces and under the liver capsule with a fine marble-veined or network pattern [179]. The relationship of these calcium deposits to CMV is questionable. It is well known that dystrophic calcification commonly occurs in areas of necrosis [204]. We have observed similar calcifications in livers of fetuses without demonstrable CMV. Hepatic iron deposits have been confused with hemochromatosis in cases of fetal CMV infection [205]. Biliary epithelial infection with CMV may be responsible for the development of biliary atresia in older infants. Obliterative cholangitis with apparent paucity of intrahepatic bile ducts has also been described [206]. Pancreatic exocrine tissues and ducts are often infected [72].

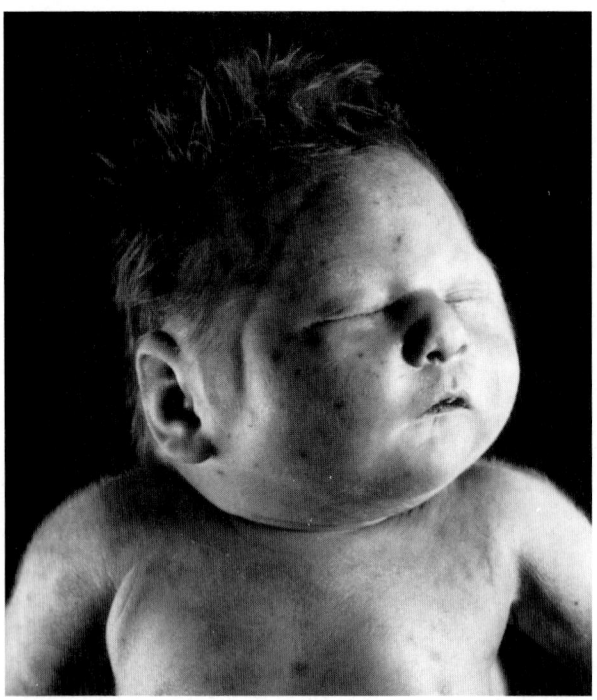

FIGURE 17.16. *Microcephaly in an infant with cytomegalovirus infection. Note also the purpuric skin rash sometimes seen in this infection as well as in rubella.*

Inclusion-bearing cells are easily found in distal convoluted tubules and collecting ducts of the kidneys (see Fig. 17.14). Bowman's capsules, proximal convoluted tubules, and Henle's loops are occasionally infected. The sloughed infected cells are excreted in the urine and can be detected there by simple microscopic examination [183]. Lymphocytes and plasma cells infiltrate infected areas, but renal function is rarely affected since the lesions are focal or at most multifocal [72].

Pancreatic islets, thyroid follicular cells, and parathyroid glands can be infected. Adrenal cortex is generally spared in neonates although it is a common site of infection in older infants and adults. The adrenal medulla may be infected in the fetus and neonate. CMV-infected cells should not be confused with adrenal cortical cytomegaly in the fetal adrenal cortex. The anterior hypophysis may have numerous inclusion-bearing cells but functional changes have not been documented, perhaps because of the lack of an inflammatory response [72].

Salivary glands are frequently infected (see Fig. 17.15). Inclusion-bearing cells have been described in the esophagus, stomach, and small intestinal mucosa and in vascular endothelium of ulcerating gastric lesions, especially in postnatal infections. CMV may infect the enteric ganglion cells resulting in hypoganglionosis, colonic dysmotility, and "pseudo-obstruction" [207, 208]. CMV in vascular endothelium within the intestine may result in classic short segment Hirschsprung disease and membranous colitis [208]. Pseudomeconium ileus has been described in neonates with CMV infection [209].

Eventration of the diaphragm with deficiency of the diaphragmatic muscle is reported in cases of CMV. Deficient abdominal muscles have also been described and CMV inclusions have been observed in sarcolemmal cells [72]. The radiographic "celery-stalk lesion," or longitudinal streaking in the metaphyses of long bones as found in congenital rubella, is also found in congenital CMV infection. The appearance is due to alternating sclerotic radiodense and demineralized radiolucent areas. Periosteal inflammation is a feature as is disordered growth at the cartilage-bone interface [72].

Thrombocytopenia is common among neonates with CMV and may persist for months [72]. The purpura noted in neonates is usually due to thrombocytopenia but some babies may also have circulating antithrombin [210] (Fig. 17.16). No inclusions were found in any marrow cells in the Aukland series of 16 cases. Inclusions are present but are uncommon in the spleen, thymus, and other lymphoid tissues. Splenomegaly develops in infants born close to term and is associated with hematopoiesis and diminished size of lymphoid follicles. Thymuses are small due to loss of lymphocytes. Precocious development of lymphoid follicles may be seen [72].

Altered immunity may be present in CMV-infected neonates. Increased numbers of bacterial infections are noted in small preterm infants with CMV [211]. Simultaneous infections with Epstein-Barr virus and herpes simplex virus have been described with congenital CMV infection [212, 213].

Malformations have been mentioned, but a true teratogenic effect of CMV infection is generally considered nonexistent. The phenotype of tyrosinemia is described in one case of CMV infection [214].

In milder or asymptomatic neonatal infections, 25% to 56% of survivors have such sequelae as sensorineural deafness and neurologic and mental deficits with a high incidence of school failure. Lowered intelligence can be expected at a rate 2.7 times that of uninfected babies [181, 215]. Virus may be excreted in the urine for as long as 3 years [215]. In neonates, symptoms that are considered high-risk features for later handicap are jaundice with increased conjugated bilirubin, hepatosplenomegaly, increased SGOT, petechiae, increased IgM, chorioretinitis, intracranial calcification, and atypical lymphocytes. Factors that impart little risk for long-term disability are small size for gestation, prematurity, minimal or questionable hepatosplenomegaly, and physiologic jaundice [215].

If symptoms are present at birth and are severe, fatal outcome occurs in almost one-third of cases before adolescence [215]; 70% have microcephaly, 53% to 60% are retarded, 30% to 65% have auditory problems, and 22% have microphthalmia with chorioretinitis [215, 216].

Herpes Simplex Viruses Infection

Herpes simplex virus (HSV) occasionally reaches the fetus through the placenta but most cases of congenital herpes infections are acquired by exposure to an infected birth canal [217]. At least one case has been attributed to application of a fetal scalp electrode to the buttocks, and postnatal acquisition can also occur [218, 219].

Mothers with primary HSV infection are the ones who have fetuses and neonates with serious perinatal morbidity. Of primary maternal infections in the second trimester, no fetal or neonatal infections may develop. When primary infection develops in the third trimester, growth retardation, prematurity, and fetal death are apt to occur, whether or not the fetus is infected with HSV [220]. In the study conducted by Prober et al, a population of 6904 pregnant women had an incidence of HSV infection of 0.2% [221]. All mothers were asymptomatic. Of the 14 infected mothers, 12 had secondary infections and none of their babies showed signs of disease. Of the two mothers with primary infections, one of their babies had significant clinical herpes infection.

In cases of maternal genital herpes in the latter stages of pregnancy, the practical aspects of care remain in a state of flux. Active lesions in the mother's cervix, vagina, or on the vulva or inner upper thighs have been considered sufficient reason for delivery by cesarean section [222]. To determine if the lesions are active, weekly cultures can be submitted. However, maternal genitalia and even the amniotic fluid can be infected without fetal infection [223]. On the other hand, asymptomatic mothers give birth to infected babies. Arvin et al found that among all mothers who have positive genital cultures at the time of delivery, none were positive one week earlier; conversely of 17 women with positive genital cultures one week prior to delivery, none were positive at delivery. This raises serious questions as to the validity of performing cultures in the last weeks of pregnancy [224].

Genital herpes infections increased ninefold in the years 1966 to 1984 with 140,000 to 150,000 new cases a year in the United States [225]. Similar increases were also noted in the United Kingdom [226]. The incidence of neonatal HSV infection ranges from 1 per 25,000 deliveries to 1 per 10,000 deliveries. More than 50% are prematurely born; at least 20% have no skin lesion. Antibodies to HSV-2 are not protective when HSV-1 is the infecting virus [227].

In the analysis by Whitley et al, localized HSV infection resulted in no deaths, whereas 57% of those with disseminated infection died. With encephalitis mortality was 15%; those with coma or who had disseminated coagulopathy had increased relative mortality risk of 5.2 and 3.8, respectively; preterm birth imparted a relative mortality risk of 3.7, and HSV pneumonia gave a risk of 3.6. Morbidity in survivors included encephalitis, coagulopathy, seizures, and was four times as likely with HSV-2 as with HSV-1. When lesions were limited to skin, eyes, or mouth, three or more recurrences of vesicles were associated with neurologic impairment compared with two or one or no recurrences of vesicles [228].

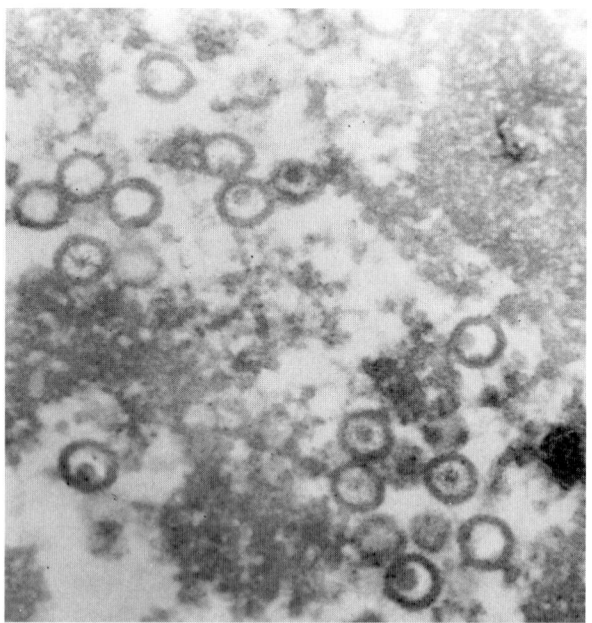

FIGURE 17.17. *Ultrastructure of herpesvirus particles. The bull's eye structures represent infectious viruses and measure about 70–90 nm in diameter. This is a postmortem preparation from adrenal tissue.*

Almost 80% of perinatal infections are due to HSV-2. The distinction is useful for epidemiological studies but may also be important for determining prognosis in survivors [229]. Corey et al found that CNS disease was more severe with HSV-2 than with HSV-1; pleocytosis, seizures, increased protein levels in cerebrospinal fluid, and cerebral damage were more intense in babies infected with HSV-2 than with HSV-1. However, mortality rates were equal in infants infected with HSV-1 and HSV-2. Recurrence in the maternal genital tract is eightfold more likely to be HSV-2 than HSV-1. Among women in venereal disease clinics, as many as 8% are infected with HSV-2, while fewer than 1.5% in private gynecologic practices have such infection [230].

In ultrastructural studies, all the herpesviruses are similar. The viral core is double-stranded DNA and measures about 20 to 30 nm; this is surrounded by a protein capsid with a diameter of about 70 to 90 nm and 162 capsomeres. The infectious particle has an envelope composed of lipid and glycoproteins. The whole viral particle has a characteristic bull's-eye appearance and a diameter of 120 to 150 nm (Fig. 17.17). The DNA codes 60 to 70 gene products [230]. The degree to which the virus becomes disseminated depends, in part, on the maturity of the infected host. In neonates the virus has wide-ranging tropism for many tissues, especially skin and mucous membranes, central nervous system, gastrointestinal tract, liver, and adrenal glands. In mice, the fetal adrenal is a target but not the liver [231]. Differences in cell receptors no doubt play a role in determining such tropism and such receptors may be exposed or activated in conditions with immune dysfunction. For example, in immunodeficient adults, the virus spreads as widely as it does in neonates, while in immunocompetent adults, the skin, central nervous system, and ganglia are usually the only targets. The virus invades ganglionic nerve cells within 2 days of mucosal inoculation. The lipid envelope is stripped as the virus travels centripetally but it reacquires an envelope in centrifugal travel out of the infected cell. The virus spreads to contiguous cells. Cell death is produced by two mechanisms: an inflammatory response and an inhibition of macromolecular synthesis which is upset by virions that may number up to 200,000 per cell [230]. Antibody-dependent cellular cytotoxicity with participation of neutrophils causes most of the damage in mature individuals. Lymphocytes destroy infected cells with HSV if antibody is present. Natural killer cells are stimulated by HSV and may be present in young infants, including neonates [232]. Phagocytes may carry viable virus to distant sites as they scavenge the debris [233].

Three types of lesions are encountered in humans: 1) intranuclear inclusion-bearing cells, 2) coagulative necrosis, and 3) intense inflammation [136]. Inclusions may be found in any type of cell but are particularly prominent in epidermis, esophagus, liver, adrenal, nerve ganglia, and central nervous system. Coagulative necrosis occurs in the liver, adrenal, lung, bone marrow, and ovary. Inflammation is prominent in the esophagus, skin, and brain.

Symptoms and signs of early fetal intrauterine HSV-2 infection are in some respects similar to infections with rubella, toxoplasmosis, and CMV syndromes—each disease has skin lesions, chorioretinitis, microphthalmia, microcephaly, and sometimes hydrocephaly. Congenital HSV differs from varicella in part by the absence of limb atrophy [234]. HSV is associated with a nonspecific increase in malformations, perhaps on the basis of chromosomal breakage [136, 149]. South et al reported the occurrence of severe brain "malformation" and atrophy in a fetus whose mother was infected with HSV-2 in midgestation [235]. In today's lexicon this lesion would be attributed to disruptive damage.

In newborn infants, the number of organs with herpetic lesions is inversely related to the age at which signs or symptoms first appear (Fig. 17.18). While there are many exceptions to the following generalizations, the liver and adrenal are almost always infected in disseminated fatal disease of early onset. The brain is involved more consistently in those babies whose onset was after day 10, with late onset disease [136]. Hemorrhagic diathesis and disseminated intravascular coagulopathy frequently precede death by a few hours or days. Purpuric skin lesions, mucosal hemorrhages in the gastrointestinal tract, pleural and peritoneal serosal hemorrhages, visceral hemorrhages in the liver, renal medulla, adrenal, heart, brain, and meninges are all described [136]. While the early onset form is widely disseminated, 70% of babies with either disseminated disease or encephalitis have no visible mucocutaneous lesion [236].

Microscopically, the inclusion-bearing cells are found in areas adjacent to necrotic zones. Such cells are sometimes slightly enlarged but are rarely smaller than normal. Cells are commonly multinucleated, particularly in epithelia, and in these cells all the nuclei may contain inclusions. Two types of inclusions are found; one is amphophilic and fills the nucleus, pushing the nuclear chromatin to the nuclear membrane. No halo surrounds this type of inclusion (Cowdry type B). It is rich in DNA, can be stained with Feulgen stain, immunofluorescent or immunoperoxidase reagents, and is considered infectious. The second type of inclusion is smaller, pale, eosinophilic, sometimes multiple, with a prominent halo separating the inclusion or inclusions from the peripherally displaced nuclear chromatin. This type (Cowdry type A) is considered effete, will not easily stain with Feulgen stain or immunoreagents, and is considered a noninfectious burned out remnant of the virus (Fig. 17.19).

Herpetic lesions have rarely been seen in the placenta even in cases in which maternal genital infection is severe. Localized necrosis of a villus or small clusters of villi with inclusion-like bodies in the syncytial trophoblast have been described in one case, suggesting hematogenous spread [217]. Herpetic chorioamnionitis and funisitis with inclusions and a necrotizing character have been seen in other cases, some with chronic inflammatory infiltrates, and these suggested ascending infection from the maternal genitalia [66]. HSV inclusion-bearing cells and HSV antigen, detected by immunohistologic techniques, have

Tissue	1	2	3	4	5	6	7	8	9	10	11	12	13	14	15	16	17	18	19	20	21	22
Liver	•	•	•	•	•		•	•	•	•	•	•	•	•	•	•	•	•	•			
Adrenal	•	•	•	•	•		•	•	•	•	•	•	•	•	•	•	•	•	•			
Oesophagus/tongue	•			o		•				•	•	o	•	•	•	•				•	•	•
Skin/eye	•			•	•				•	•			•	•				o		o	o	•
Lung	•		•		•	o		•	•		o		•	•								
Brain		o								o			o			o				•	o	o
Spleen	•							•		o		•	o			•						
Bone marrow	o	•	o					•					•					o				
Stomach/bowel	•							•								•						
Ovary			•					•														
Kidney	•					•																
Lymph node		•																				
Muscle	•																					
Pancreas																						

FIGURE 17.18. *Chart showing distribution of organs in 22 neonates with characteristic lesions due to perinatal herpes infection. The liver and adrenal were involved in all but four babies. (•) with inclusions, (o) without inclusions. (From Singer [213], used with permission from the publisher.)*

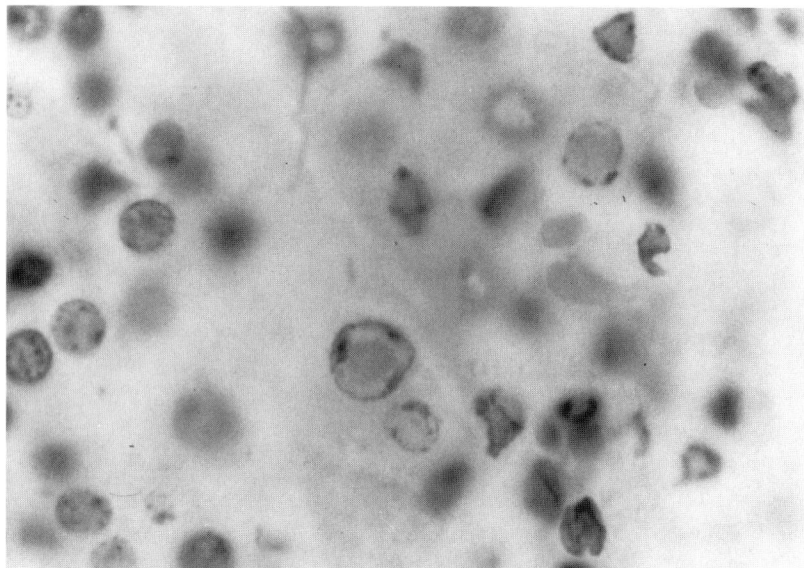

FIGURE 17.19.   *Liver tissue with extensive herpes infection. Prominent viral inclusions are noted. (H&E, ×1005.)*

(a)

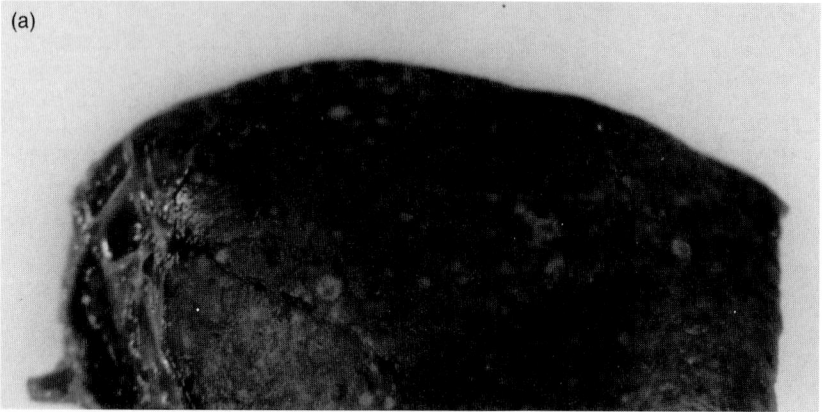

(b)

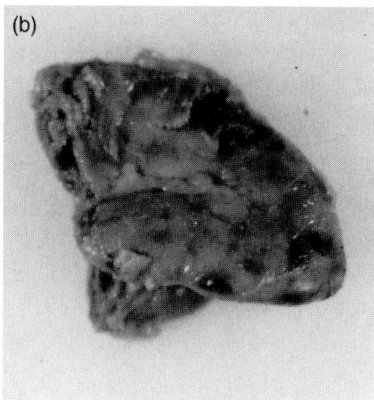

FIGURE 17.20.   *Capsular surfaces of the liver and adrenal are shown from a case of perinatal herpes infection. The hepatic lesions are yellow–white, some with focal hemorrhagic centers. The adrenal lesions are purple.*

been found in decidua, but while the virus may be present in the decidua, visual identification is not usually possible without special stains or techniques [237, 238]. Similar findings in a study of early spontaneous abortions suggested a relationship to HSV infection, but this latter work has not been verified [239]. Necrotizing funisitis and umbilical vasculitis are reported with herpes simplex infection [240].

HSV-infected lungs have small necrotic lesions scattered irregularly through the parenchyma. These usually are not detected grossly. In these lesions the interstitial cells and free alveolar macrophages have inclusions but pneumocytes seem to have none. Furthermore, respiratory epithelium in bronchioles, bronchi, and trachea rarely contain inclusions [136]. Localized hyaline membrane formation is sometimes found along with a chronic interstitial pneumonitis and localized

pleural inflammation. Disseminated disease is the rule when the lungs are infected, although in the case reported by Greene et al the esophagus was the only other involved tissue [241].

Herpes infection of the cardiovascular system is rare. In a case mentioned by Nahmias et al, the A-V bundle was infected and the infant had heart block [242]. Giant cell myocarditis was reported in a neonate with encephalopathy secondary to herpes simplex virus. The baby also had disseminated disease with involvement of the kidney, liver, and adrenal [243]. However the relationship of the myocardial lesion to HSV is questionable in this case. Thickened aortic intima with calcium and giant cells has been reported in neonatal herpes [244].

Hepatic herpetic lesions are grossly miliary (Fig. 17.20). They are yellow-white, measure from 0.5 to 3.0 mm, and are diffusely distributed throughout the parenchyma. A thin red rim surrounds each of the necrotic zones. The intervening tissue is often destroyed. As much as 80% of the hepatic parenchyma may thus be necrotic. There is no obvious collapse of parenchyma or wrinkling of the capsules and weights of the livers are neither increased nor decreased when compared with standard autopsy weights [136, 150]. Microscopically, the necrotic areas have no zonal distribution although central veins and portal tracts are often spared. All types of cells and tissues are necrotic in the zone of involvement, including hepatocytes, Kupffer cells, vessels, connective tissue, and hematopoietic cells. Reticular tissues are not collapsed (condensed) and bile ducts are not plugged with bile (Fig. 17.21). Inclusions are plentiful in the adjacent viable tissues, particularly in surviving hepatocytes and transitional bile ductules. Inflammatory cells tend not to infiltrate the areas of necrosis in the neonatal liver.

Grossly, necrotic lesions in the adrenal are opaque gray-white spots, 1 to 2 mm in diameter, or are larger hemorrhagic purple zones (see Fig. 17.20). Usually, no more than 20% to 30% of the adrenal is destroyed by herpesvirus infection. Inflammation and fibrin thrombi are sparse. The definitive or adult cortex is more severely involved than is the fetal cortex. Hemorrhage may or may not attend the infection. Accessory adrenal cortical tissue located in the inguinal region or scrotum may also be infected [136]. Mirra et al described cases of congenital HSV infection in which adrenals contained small nodules of necrosis, calcification, and giant cells [244].

The infant's esophagus and tongue are frequently infected with HSV. Vesicles occasionally form in a manner similar to that found in the skin but they apparently quickly rupture. Ulcers are much more commonly found than are vesicles. Inclusion-bearing cells are located at the edges of the

vesicles and ulcers. Inflammation may be intense at the bases of the ulcers. Inclusions may be seen in ganglion cells of the intermyenteric plexus and submucosal plexuses [136].

Cutaneous vesicles and ulcers are sometimes the only detectable lesions and when the disease is so limited, no untoward sequelae are expected in survivors. In some seriously infected babies (those with fatal outcome) the skin lesions tend to be more intense, but in the majority of such cases skin lesions are completely absent [236]. Hair follicles, sweat glands and ducts, and sebaceous glands have necrotic lesions and many inclusion-bearing cells. Acute and chronic inflammation are intense in the superficial dermis [136]. Vesicles can develop up to 87 days after birth in late onset disease [244]. The benign dermatologic condition known as herpes gestationis should not be confused with maternal herpes simplex infection. Herpes gestationis is uncommon, occurring in 1 out of 50,000 pregnant women in the second or third trimester. A pruritic rash around the mother's umbilicus spreads over trunk and extremities with urticarial papules and plaques followed by subepidermal vesicles and bullae. The rash persists until parturition but may wane late in pregnancy and exacerbate in the immediate postpartum period. The neonate is affected with preterm birth in about 20% of cases. Stillbirth occurs in 7% to 8%. About one in 10 babies will have skin papules which are transient and without sequelae [245].

Lymph nodes, spleen, and bone marrow cells may contain inclusions and may have areas of necrosis. In the spleen, lymphoid depletion is generally present during the first 2 weeks of life in babies with early onset HSV infection while in those with late onset infection, precocious lymphoid follicles with active follicular centers may be seen. Splenic veins have mononuclear infiltrates in the subintimal zones, a lesion

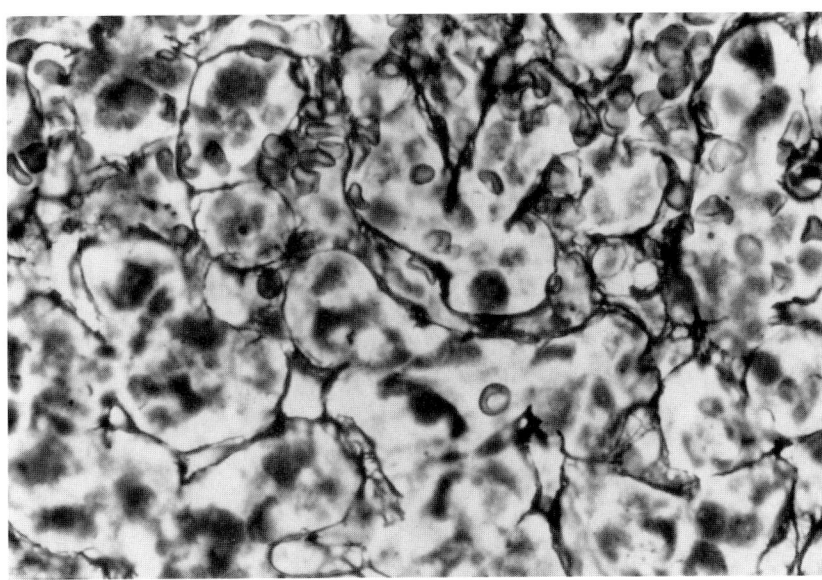

FIGURE 17.21. *Reticulum stain of liver tissue in a case of perinatal herpes infection. There is no collapse of the reticulum, despite extensive necrosis of cells. (Reticulum stain, ×1005.)*

reminiscent of Epstein–Barr virus infection of older children and a number of other lymphoproliferative disorders including leukemias [136].

Destructive lesions with intense inflammation may occur in any part of the central nervous system but tend to concentrate in the gray matter of the cerebral hemispheres, particularly the frontal and temporal poles. This is because the virus reaches the brain via the olfactory and trigeminal nerves or their sheaths [136]. Meningoencephalitis is common and perivascular cuffs consist of mixed acute and chronic inflammatory cells. Ventriculitis is also common. Porencephaly, hydranencephaly, and multicystic lesions have been described in survivors of neonatal CNS infection with HSV and some have persistent (chronic) virus infections [136, 244, 246]. Cerebral malacoplakia due to congenital HSV infection consists of parenchymal destruction of the cells with foamy histiocytes, plasma cells, lymphocytes, histiocytes with PAS-positive granules, and laminated calcospherules, the Michaelis–Gutmann bodies [244, 247]. No organisms are detected in these lesions by electron microscopy or fluorescence microscopy.

Inflammation of the conjunctivae can be noted clinically. Inside the ocular globe, a necrotizing iritis, uveitis, and retinitis occur with viral particles identified in these areas. Cataracts can develop, but this is uncommon [136].

Therapy with acyclovir or vidarabine has reduced perinatal mortality from 65% to 25% [230, 248]. Long-term studies, not yet performed, will be necessary to determine if morbidity is also reduced. Vidarabine has been used for cutaneous lesions but acyclovir is preferred in disseminated disease [249, 250]. Accumulation of acyclovir in babies with renal disease may result in hepatic toxicity [248].

Enterovirus Infections

Enteroviruses, which belong to the picornaviruses, are single-stranded RNA structures with diameters ranging from 24 to 30 nm and consist of naked protein capsids around a small dense RNA core. All enteroviruses are protected from nucleases by these protein coats that determine, among other things, antigenicity. The enteroviruses include the polioviruses 1-3, coxsackie A viruses 1-24, coxsackie B viruses 1-6, and echoviruses 1-34 [251]. Virtually all major enterovirus types have been reported in fetuses and newborn infants [252–255].

Enteroviruses as a group are four times more frequent than herpes simplex in causing perinatal infections. In adults, the gastrointestinal tract is the natural habitat for enteroviruses, but symptoms are not always referable to that tract. Aseptic meningitis and encephalitis, respiratory infections, and myocarditis occur in adults. Placental involvement is rarely seen. Extensive perivillous fibrin deposits and villous necrosis with inflammation were described by Baltcup et al in a rare case with intrauterine coxsackievirus A infection [256]. Garcia et al found villous necrosis, chronic villitis, and intervillositis in coxsackievirus B infections but

Table 17.5.   Perinatal infections characterized by encephalitis and hepatitis

Herpes simplex	(+ adrenal)
Echo	
Coxsackie	
Listeria	(+ adrenal)
Rubella	(+ adrenal, occasionally)
Cytomegalovirus	(+ adrenal, rarely)
Toxoplasmosis	(+ adrenal, rarely)
Chagas disease	

These infectious agents produce syndromes with both hepatitis and encephalitis; many also have associated infection of the adrenal.

Table 17.6.   Perinatal infections commonly associated with myocarditis

Coxsackie
Rubella
Toxoplasmosis
Chagas' disease

Benirschke claims that no meaningful lesions occur in placentas associated with enterovirus infections [257, 258]. The main target organs in fetuses and newborn infants are the liver, brain, heart, pancreas, and adrenal (Tables 17.5 and 17.6).

The exact diagnosis of viral species can be performed on viral isolates or, using molecular techniques, on tissue specimens. Bowles et al have established the diagnosis of coxsackievirus B from myocardial biopsy specimens [259]. Redline et al successfully diagnosed enteroviral infections using paraffin-embedded liver and cardiac tissues and polymerase chain reaction techniques [260]. Gauntt et al used coxsackieviral-specific antibodies on cells from the ventricular fluid of the brain [261], while Schlesinger et al used cerebrospinal fluid and polymerase chain reactions with appropriate molecular probes to establish the diagnosis in several cases of infantile enteroviral meningitis [262].

Intrauterine enteroviral infections develop rarely in early gestation while they are common in late pregnancy, especially during community outbreaks [256]. Such infections are usually not serious for mothers or their fetuses, but as many as 65% of mothers are symptomatic if their babies have positive cultures for enteroviruses.

Poliovirus Infection

Neonatal disease due to polioviruses has all but vanished in developed countries. In undeveloped countries, the disease was considered rare because most mothers were themselves exposed to the infection early in infancy, while still partially protected by maternal antibodies. However, studies of the causes of lameness in such countries suggest that poliomyelitis is still prevalent throughout the undeveloped world [263].

The placenta has no changes attributable to poliovirus infection [22]. The virus has a distinct tropism for tissue of the central nervous system. If the maternal infection occurs late in gestation, devastating fetal paralytic disease is apt to occur [264]. Fetal movements may cease and the neonate is limp, not stiff as in adults with acute poliovirus infections. Anterior horn cells in the spinal cord are destroyed and lateral horn cells are also affected. Lesions can be detected in the motor neurons of cranial nerves as high as the sixth and seventh nerves [265]. A chronic inflammatory infiltrate develops around vessels in the brain stem and spinal cord [5].

Coxsackievirus Infections

Coxsackie B infections are not associated with spontaneous abortions, but stillbirths late in pregnancy are described [252]. Between 30% to 50% of infected mothers will transmit the viruses through the placenta to their babies. Ascending infection from the vagina to the amniotic sac probably does not occur. The frequency of intrauterine transmission is unknown, but most neonatal infections are acquired during or after birth. Transmission to infants is usually by human-to-human contact, from the mother or other caretakers, especially those in the hospital or nursery where outbreaks are in progress [251]. The severity of neonatal illness ranges from asymptomatic to fatal disease [266].

Coxsackie B viruses are most often implicated in perinatal disease while coxsackie A viruses are rare in these patients [3]. Approximately 35% of neonatal coxsackie B infections occur in preterm infants. Those with the most severe disease have the onset before 10 days of age. Infections with coxsackieviruses, as those with polioviruses, occur most often in the summer and the fall. Maternal fever and headaches are described in nearly 60% of such cases. Several cases have been observed in nurseries with epidemics of neonatal myocarditis [267]. Among unselected children with severe neurological diseases such as hydrocephalus hydranencephaly, or hemimegencephaly, evidence of neonatal coxsackievirus B infection can be elicited in about 14%. Their cerebrospinal fluid contains antibodies against coxsackieviruses and more than one serotype can be found in some patients [261].

Babies may have exanthems, enanthems, pneumonia, gastroenteritis, necrotizing enterocolitis, hepatitis, pancreatitis, myocarditis, meningoencephalitis, generalized hemorrhage, shock, and sudden death. Severity of disease depends on several factors including the virus' strain, mode of transmission, and passive immunity from the mother's antibodies [252]. Intravenous immunoglobulin has been used therapeutically with success [266, 268].

The most seriously affected infants have involvement of the brain and the heart or both. The cardiac lesions are multiple myocardial necroses and lymphocytic infiltrates

and have been reported with coxsackie B1, B2, B3, and B4 viral infections. The left ventricle is more often involved than the right ventricle and pericarditis is often an associated lesion [269]. In experiments with mice, Gauntt et al produced sustained myocarditis without sustained virus replication and they suggest that antibodies to portions of the viral capsid mediate the inflammation in the heart [270]. RNA sequences of coxsackievirus can be demonstrated in digested tissues from healed stages of myocarditis [259].

Meningoencephalitis is associated with destruction of neurons and glia, lymphocytic and eosinophilic infiltrates in the meninges, and perivascular cuffs of lymphocytes. Such damage may lead to chronic brain disease [3].

The pancreas is often inflamed when infected with coxsackie B viruses [271]. Islets of Langerhans and interstitial tissues may have intense mononuclear infiltrates [272], leading to the speculation that these infectious agents are responsible for some cases of diabetes mellitus in infancy or childhood [271, 273, 274].

Overwhelming hepatitis syndrome is usually seen with echoviruses, but it has been reported with coxsackie B1 and B3 infection [253, 254]. Hepatitis associated with hemorrhagic pneumonia and lymphadenitis is described in rare cases of coxsackie B infection [3, 275].

An erythematous skin rash develops in nearly half the cases. Thrombocytopenia and enteritis are described in about 10% of the cases [276].

Echovirus Infections

Reports of fatal neonatal infections with echoviruses emerged in the early and mid-1970s [276–278] and continued into the subsequent decade [279–284]. Echovirus infections affect the fetus and infant in much the same way as infections with herpes simplex viruses. The route of entry in most cases is transplacental [277]. Postnatal infection is also possible. In two separate reports of fatal neonatal echovirus infection, neither of which was associated with maternal illness, the fathers were the source of infection. One father had headaches with probable aseptic meningitis and the other had gastroenteritis [280, 281].

Infected newborn infants may appear healthy at birth, but lethargy and poor feeding develop within a few days. If antibodies are present in the cord blood, overt neonatal disease is less apt to occur. Echovirus serotypes implicated in perinatal infections include 6, 7, 11 [279, 282–284], 14 [281], 19 [277], and 21 [280].

Although the virus can be isolated from brain, liver, spleen, lymph nodes, heart, adrenal, and other organs [279, 282], the main target organs for echoviruses are the liver and the brain [277, 283]. Hepatic necroses with little inflammatory reaction are characteristic [277, 284]. Up to 95% of the liver may be necrotic but the reticulum network and extramedullary hematopoietic tissue are preserved [281]. Giant cell transformation rarely occurs and iron deposits are not a feature [285]. Electron microscopy discloses virions 16 to 18nm in diameter, sometimes in crystalloid arrangements [281].

Encephalitis consists of collections of glial cells, neuronal necrosis, and perivascular lymphocytic infiltrates in the cortex and cerebellum [277]. Kernicterus has been described in at least one case [281].

Adrenal necrosis often develops with or without inflammation. Pancreatitis and sialadenitis are other lesions found in echovirus infections [281]. Hemorrhagic diathesis and disseminated intravascular coagulopathy frequently precede death by a few hours or days. Purpuric skin lesions, mucosal hemorrhages in the gastrointestinal tract, pleural and peritoneal serosal hemorrhages, and visceral hemorrhages in the renal medulla, adrenal, heart, brain, and meninges are all described [251, 277, 281, 284].

Rotavirus Infections

Rotavirus infection is a common cause of neonatal gastroenteritis but rarely is it fatal. Hemorrhagic diarrhea is the clinical feature of note. Stool contains characteristic virions; alternatively, the diagnosis can be made by enzyme-linked immunologic assay [286–289]. With either test the rate of error is about 5%.

Hepatitis Virus Infections

Trophoblast apparently has no receptors for the hepatitis virus B antigen structure and transplacental transmission is rare. The fetus is usually infected only during labor [290]. Such infections rarely cause clinical symptoms during the neonatal period but early infantile deaths due to fulminant hepatitis have been reported [291–293].

Maternal infection with hepatitis B virus during pregnancy can be fulminant with fetal death or preterm delivery [151, 294]. If the mother is a carrier for hepatitis B virus, there is little added risk for stillbirth, abortion, growth retardation, or malformation but the risk is increased for preterm birth [295]. The type of antigen carried by the mother determines the effect on the fetus. Maternal antigenemia with HBeAg is associated with a high rate of threatened abortion and with transmission of the virus to about 50% of the fetuses [296]. When mothers are carriers of HBsAg, this antigen is positive in the cord blood of 50% of their offspring, in the amniotic fluid of 33%, and in breast milk in 71%, but none of these factors seem to provide additional risk to the infant.

A major worldwide effort is under way to treat neonates exposed to mothers with hepatitis B virus antigenemia. Vaccine is effective in the neonatal period, even if passive immunization with hepatitis immune globulin is also used [291]. In Asia, 3% to 5% of all newborn infants are exposed and become chronic carriers. In Western countries, the incidence of the carrier state is much lower. Nevertheless, some 12,000 to 20,000 Americans become new carriers each year [297]. It is now common practice to screen all gravidas for

hepatitis antigens. The late sequelae of perinatal acquisition of hepatitis virus B infection are chronic carrier state in more than 80% with chronic hepatitis or hepatocellular carcinoma in 50% of the male carriers [295]. Most of these sequelae do not appear before adulthood but hepatoma has been reported in a child 7 years after perinatal infection [298]. Some ethnic groups have children, especially boys, who develop a carrier state by 6 weeks of age and cirrhosis in the first 2 years of life [296, 299]. Treatments with interferon gamma and other interferons have shown some promise in older patients with HVC and HVB infections [300].

Hepatitis A virus is rarely if ever transmitted to the fetus but neonates may acquire infection in the nursery, from blood transfusions, or at home [301–304]. Infection, even in premature infants, produces either no symptoms or only mild symptoms.

Hepatitis C virus has been transmitted from mothers to infants, probably at parturition, and is related to the viral load in the mother as well as with maternal intravenous drug use [305–307]. In one study, HCV infection in the offspring depended on concurrent HIV infection in the mother [308].

Another non-A, non-B hepatitis virus is known to exist and is water-borne. Infection is generally mild, with elevated hepatic enzymes persisting in the serum for 6 to 8 weeks [295]. In adults, the water-borne virus is more virulent than its counterpart, hepatitis virus A [304].

Reovirus Infection

Perinatal reovirus infection is not usually a significant problem with regard to mortality. However antibodies to reovirus type 3 have been demonstrated by some investigators in about 50% of cases of "neonatal" hepatitis, the onset of which is most often beyond the first month of life [309, 310]. The significance of this association has not gone unchallenged, and most authorities now believe that few cases of neonatal hepatitis are due to this infection [311].

Varicella–Zoster Infection

Varicella infection is fairly common among gravidas, yet fetal and neonatal infections are rarely seen. This is probably because the varicella-zoster virus has difficulty crossing the placental barrier during maternal viremia, particularly late in gestation. Even when the fetus is infected, maternal antibodies quickly develop and are protective when they cross to the fetal circulation. Varicella-zoster infection in earlier stages of gestation produces a syndrome that is characterized by cataracts, chorioretinitis, growth retardation, encephalitis, cortical brain atrophy, and cicatrices of skin, subcutaneous tissues, deep fascia, and even muscle. The lesions follow the dermatomes, a distribution similar to that seen in adult herpes zoster lesions [312–314]. Documented maternal infection prior to 20 weeks of gestation and the cicatricial lesions of the extremity are considered sine qua non for the diagnosis of early fetal varicella infection [315, 316]. A severe villitis may be found in the placenta with inclusion-bearing nuclei in villous stromal cells and trophoblast.

Significant danger to the older fetus or newborn exists when the mother is infected 5 days or less before delivery. This is before an adequate maternal antibody response can be mounted [317, 318]. Vesicles develop in fetal or neonatal skin and mucous membranes, just as in older children, but neonates can develop a severe and often fatal varicella pneumonia. Acute and chronic pulmonary inflammation with necrosis of the acinar epithelium leads to extensive hemorrhage. In disseminated varicella, visceral necrosis and hemorrhage occurs in virtually every organ in the body but especially the lung, liver, and brain. The placenta may also have such lesions. Viable infected cells have intranuclear inclusions similar to those seen in infections with herpes simplex virus. Varicella-zoster immune globulin (VZIG) is now available and can allay the more serious aspects of neonatal varicella infection [318].

Outcome for fetuses and neonates among 1739 cases complicated by varicella (chickenpox or herpes zoster) in the first 36 weeks of gestation was studied by Enders et al [319]. Congenital varicella syndrome was found in only 9 of the 1739 exposed fetuses, all 9 occurring in the first 20 weeks of gestation and all in mothers with chickenpox (i.e., none in the 366 mothers with herpes zoster). The abnormalities included hypoplasia and contractions of limbs, skin defects with scars, neurologic lesions such as dystrophies, and fetal and neonatal deaths [319].

Vaccinia Infection

Vaccinia can infect fetuses after primary vaccination of the mother. In a 14-week fetus described by Vorst and Galliard, hemorrhagic skin lesions were associated with Guarnieri-like bodies in fetal epidermis [320]. Miliary lesions formed in liver, lungs, kidneys, adrenal glands, and placenta. These were numerous white, sharply demarcated, 2 to 3 mm lesions with central necrosis, occasional calcification, and minimal peripheral leukocytic reaction. In the case described by Vorst and Galliard a necrotizing metaphyseal osteomyelitis with osteoporotic changes developed. Necrotic trabecular bone extended into the marrow while cartilage of the epiphyses appeared normal [320]. Necrotizing villitis may be seen in the placenta [320, 321].

Variola Infection

Since smallpox has been eradicated, fetal and neonatal variola infections are no longer a threat. The description by Garcia is included for historical interest [76]. A case of attenuated smallpox ("alastrim") occurred in a macerated fetus.

Guarnieri bodies were found in decidua and viral inclusions in the maternal floor of the placenta. Yellow crusted oval ulcers involved the fetal skin, along with "sinuous" necrosis of the thymus, heart, lungs, liver, pancreas, kidney, and adrenals. Gastric and intestinal ulcers were present. Pleural and peritoneal adhesions had formed and meninges had tortuous vessels.

Parvovirus Infection

Human parvovirus (B19) is a single-stranded DNA virus which in humans is cytopathic for nucleated red blood cell precursors. It is more commonly known as the etiologic agent for erythema infectiosum (fifth disease) in young children. It can also cause fleeting reticular rashes and mild arthritis in adults. Because the nucleated erythroblast is the primary target for this agent, parvovirus B19 is a dangerous pathogen in patients of any age with chronic anemia [322–324]. It causes an aplastic crisis when it attacks and destroys the erythropoietic cells which are constantly proliferating in these patients. In immunocompromised patients, transient neutropenia [325] and chronic anemia [326] have been attributed to parvovirus B19 infection. Resistance to infection has been demonstrated in those rare individuals (1 in 200,000) who do not have P antigen on their erythroids. The P antigen is the cellular receptor for parvovirus B19, and while the receptor is present on many cell types, the virus replicates only in erythroid precursors that have P antigen [327].

Human parvovirus (B 19) infection is now clearly associated with fetal deaths associated with hydrops fetalis [328]. Approximately 1% of all pregnant women in the United States will have primary parvovirus B19 infection during gestation [325]. This figure may rise to as much as 6% during community epidemics [329, 330]. Of those with primary infections, 33% will transmit the virus to their fetuses and an average of about 10% of these fetuses will have fatal disease. Another 25% will have symptoms of anemia. Immunoglobulins can be given to the mother [331] or directly to the fetus.

Most cases of fetal parvovirus B19 infection occur in early or midgestation, when nucleated erythroid precursors are most numerous. A few cases have also been reported in the latter weeks of pregnancy. Infants may be liveborn and some of these have residual lesions such as marked siderosis in the liver, portal fibrosis, and proliferation of portal bile ducts [332–334].

Fetal infections follow maternal infections by a few days to two weeks. Abundant viral particles are found in erythroid nuclei in the fetal liver, bone marrow, and in circulating blood (Fig. 17.22). The typical lesion is an intranuclear inclusion with moderate eosinophilic or amphophilic clearing of the normally dense, homogeneous nuclear chromatin. The residual chromatin is condensed at the nuclear membrane. Ultrastructurally, parvovirus particles are hexagonal, 20 to 26 nm in diameter, and may form crystalline arrays

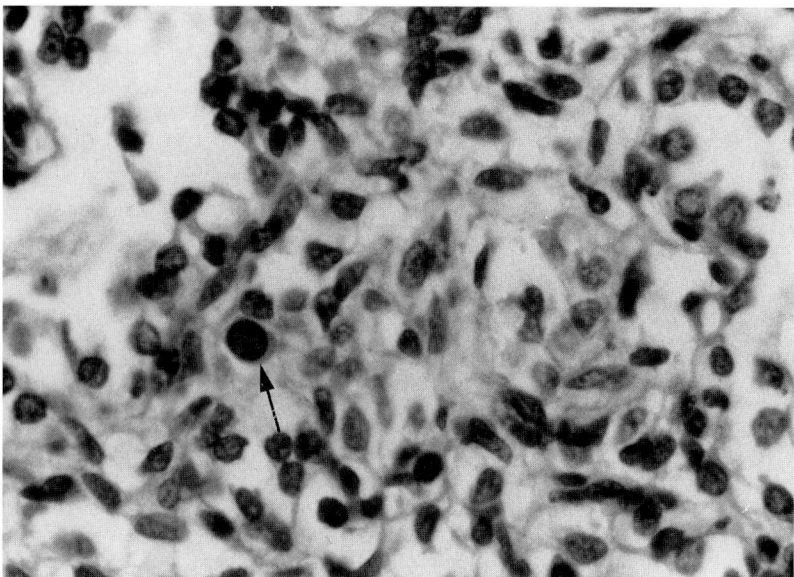

FIGURE 17.22.   *Parvovirus inclusion in a circulating nucleated erythroid cell (arrow). The tissue is lung from a macerated stillborn fetus. (H&E, ×792.)*

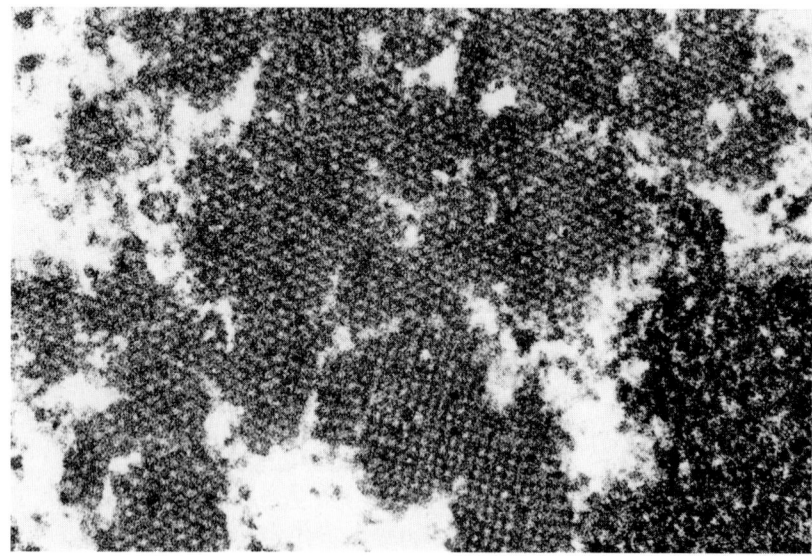

FIGURE 17.23.   *Ultrastructure of parvovirus in crystalline array within an erythroid nucleus. (×84,460.)*

[335, 336] (Fig. 17.23). The infected nucleus may be enlarged and ballooned. The majority of nucleated red blood cell precursors are infected. Anemia is profound, with hematocrits of 10 vol% and less in the cord blood. Other pathologic features are those common in hydrops fetalis based on destruction of red blood cells. Anasarca is prominent (Fig. 17.24). The placentas are greatly enlarged with pale boggy villous tissues. Hemosiderin deposits are dense in the liver and spleen, representing the residue of destroyed red blood cells. Secondary erythroblastosis, especially in the fetal liver, is prominent. Increased numbers of circulating nucleated red blood cells are detectable in other tissues and are frequently best preserved in the placental fetal circulation. While the hydropic appearance is due mainly to heart failure based on

severe anemia, there is some evidence that the myocardium may be infected directly [337].

Chromosomal defects have been associated with parvovirus B19 and hydrops fetalis [338] but these must be considered chance associations. Rogers et al examined autopsy materials retrospectively from 32 unselected cases of non-immune hydrops fetalis; 5 (15%) had parvovirus B19 infection as the cause of hydrops. Only 2 of 5 placentas had diagnostic inclusions [339]. In this same series of cases, routine histology with hematoxylin and eosin was as sensitive as molecular techniques in establishing the diagnosis. The molecular techniques, of course, add specificity not possible with routine histology [340].

In the 10 years or so since the first reported cases of fetal

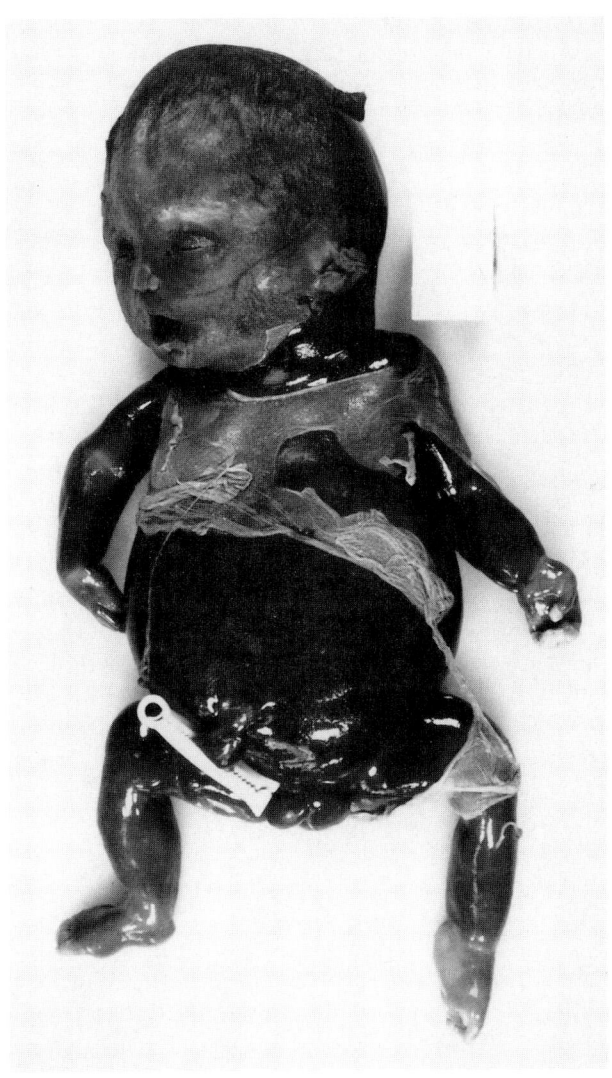

FIGURE 17.24.   *Macerated hydropic fetus infected with parvovirus.*

infection [328], convincing evidence for a teratogenic role for parvovirus B19 has not been reported. Periodically, a case with malformations is found in the literature [341], but the consensus is that the virus does not cause anomalies [330, 342, 343].

Rogers et al prospectively examined 80 spontaneously aborted embryos and fetuses in the first trimester of gestation in an attempt to determine the incidence and possible etiologic role of parvovirus B19. Maternal serology, routine histology, electron microscopy, in situ hybridization, and polymerase chain reaction (PCR) techniques were employed. Five mothers had seroconverted during pregnancy and two of their abortuses had parvovirus B19 demonstrated in the aborted tissues by PCR. Only one of the two had intranuclear inclusions in erythroid precursors. In five specimens from mothers who did not have serologic

evidence of infection (controls), false-positive inclusions were found in erythroid precursors in routine histologic preparations [344]. Isolated erythroids with presumed inclusions in abortuses should not prompt a diagnosis of parvovirus infection unless the majority of nucleated erythroids are involved. Proof lies with maternal serology or molecular diagnostic techniques.

The prenatal diagnosis of intrauterine infection can be established in several ways. Maternal serology has been used extensively with a rise in anti-parvovirus B19 antibodies indicating an infection. Amniotic fluid can be tested with molecular probes specific for parvovirus B19 [345, 346]. Elevated maternal serum alpha-fetoprotein (AFP) may be the first evidence of disease but by this time the fetus may be irreversibly damaged [347]. Air-dried smears of fetal or neonatal peripheral blood post-fixed in formalin and stained with hematoxylin and eosin will show the inclusions in nucleated red blood cells [348].

More than half of the adult population in the United States have had parvovirus B19 infections and have IgG antibodies specific to that agent [349]. Attempts to develop a vaccine have recently been reported [350]. Hall has suggested the following clinical protocol to use in potential primary infections in pregnancy. The mother at risk should be tested serologically for parvovirus B19-specific IgM, IgG, or DNA [351, 352]. Retesting after 4 weeks is recommended. Children and adults with typical rashes and arthralgias are no longer contagious, but HIV-positive patients or those with aplastic crisis may be regarded as infectious. The indications for treatment with intrauterine transfusions have not yet been defined [351]. Such transfusions have been used with varying success [330, 353, 354].

Human fetal parvovirus infection has been reported to produce vasculitis in placental villi [355]. In older children, necrotizing vasculitis has been associated with presumably chronic parvovirus B19 infection, but the virus may have been an opportunistic infection in these cases [356]. Active or recent parvovirus B19 infections were recently reported in children with Kawasaki disease [357]. Segmental proliferative glomerulonephritis has been reported in association with aplastic crisis and nephrotic syndrome in patients with sickle cell disease [358]. The rash of fifth disease may represent a vasculitis but this has yet to be shown histologically. In the many animal strains of parvovirus, which are distinct from the human B19 strain, the primary target cells and organs vary. The canine parvovirus is tropic for myocardium, especially in puppies. Now and then, human B19 infections are reported with myocarditis and fatal damage to the heart [337], but to date few of these cases are proved with in situ hybridization of parvovirus B19 in myocardial cells. Cases of premature closure of the ductus arteriosus and Ebstein malformation of the heart have been attributed to parvovirus infections [334, 359, 360]. Our own studies of six cases of Ebstein malformation showed no evidence of parvovirus infection. Most studies of parvovirus B19 have shown conclusive proof for direct infection only in nucleated erythroids [339, 361].

Human T-Cell Lymphotrophic Virus Infections

Human T-cell lymphotrophic viruses (HTLV) are transmitted through the placenta to the fetus. Data are most reliable for HTLV-I and HTLV-III (human immunodeficiency virus or HIV-1).

Fetal infection with HTLV-I, after delay to adulthood, results in T-cell lymphocytic leukemia/lymphoma or myelopathy [362, 363]. Some cases have occurred in early adolescence. Fetal infection with HTLV-II (HIV-2) has been reported in Uganda, often in patients also infected with HIV-1 [364]. Mother-to-child transmission occurs mostly with breast-feeding, but without signs or symptoms of neonatal disease [365].

Human Immunodeficiency Virus 1 Infection (HIV-1)

Human immunodeficiency virus 1 (HIV-1) has by the late 1990s infected millions of people throughout the world and produced its severe expression, acquired immunodeficiency syndrome (AIDS). Between 1978 and 1993, 14,920 infants with HIV were born in the United States. Through the year 1992, 4249 children under 13 years of age had developed AIDS in the United States, making it the eighth leading cause of death in children ages 1 to 4 years and the sixth leading cause of death in children in the United States [366]. More than 90% of these children received the virus from infected mothers. Each year since 1988, almost 7000 HIV-infected women have given birth to a live-born infant in the United States [367]. Based on a 25% vertical transmission rate, about 1750 infants are infected with HIV each year [368]. Pregnant women who have positive blood tests for HIV-1 are likely to have premature deliveries, infants with growth retardation, or premature rupture of placental membranes [369].

The most significant predictor of transmission is the severity of disease in the mother. CD4 cell counts below 400/µL were predictive of three times the transmission rate of higher CD4 counts. Rapidly proliferating virus in the mother is a similar risk factor. An additional risk factor is birth prior to 34 weeks' gestation. Prenatal transplacental infection is less of a factor than is transmission during labor and delivery by exposure to maternal blood.

Infection is established in infants and children at risk by any two of the following: positive culture, persistent antibody after 18 months of age, positive p24 antigen detection in serum, or the presence of an AIDS-defining illness. PCR alone on 3 mL of blood after 1 week and preferably before the end of 1 month is adequate for establishing the diagnosis. In this method, mononuclear cells are separated via Ficoll-Hypaque and DNA is amplified by PCR with primers and probes. Positive predictive value is 98.1% and negative predictive value 95.2%. Two concordant positive tests establish the diagnosis, while two consecutive negative

tests rule out infection to a greater than 99% degree of certainty. Infants with two negative tests should be retested at 12 to 24 months of age to document seroreversion [370]. Detection of the virus in the fetus or baby is the gold standard for determining the actual infection of the offspring [371].

The HIV-1 agent is tropic for T-helper lymphocytes and macrophages, possibly also for glial cells in the central nervous system [372]. The T-helper/T-suppressor ratio is lower than normal in infected infants, as it is in adults, and this test may serve as a means of presumptive diagnosis in neonates and young infants [373, 374]. Thymic lymphocytes with CD3+ and CD4+ antigens on their surface are infected and become severely depleted, probably in utero. An example of these features is illustrated in a 3-day-old baby reported by Rozenzweig et al. The baby was HIV seropositive. Replicating virus was demonstrated in thymocytes by in situ hybridization. CD3+ and CD4+ cells were decreased in number compared to 10 age-matched controls without HIV. CD3-CD4-CD8 cells remained in the thymus but no peripheral lymphopenia was detected and the baby had no symptoms [375].

Vertical transplacental transmission to fetuses is documented as early as the second trimester. Neonatal infection has been acquired from blood transfusions [376, 377] and breast milk or colostrum [378–380].

HIV-1 virus has been demonstrated in the brain, eye, and cord blood lymphocytes of aborted fetuses as early as 20 weeks' gestation [381] and in thymic tissue of a liveborn infant at 28 weeks' gestation [382]. HIV-1 infection in fetuses and neonates is either asymptomatic or enmeshed in the signs and symptoms of prematurity. Specific lesions and symptoms usually appear after several months have passed.

As for perinatal pathology, the placentas of infected fetuses have more chorioamnionitis than expected and placental villi which are hypercellular and hypovascularized. Villous cells are positive for p24 antigen but villitis is not reported in such cases. HIV has been cultured from amniotic fluid and HIV antigens have been demonstrated in amniotic cells and other tissues. Yet cultures of the placenta and cord blood have not been successful in growing HIV. The relatively low rate of transmission from mother to fetus and the lack of clear evidence (i.e., culture) for placental infection with HIV suggests that the virus is inactivated or attenuated in the placenta. Other fetal infections such as CMV, rubella, syphilis, and toxoplasmosis have a phase of placental infection which seems to be necessary before fetal infection takes hold. In HIV, there is a placental barrier. The barrier may be breached with the development of chorioamnionitis or syphilis [383].

While fetuses and neonates have no specific lesions due to infection with HIV, disease in later infancy can be devastating. Joshi has placed the lesions of pediatric AIDS into three categories: 1) primary lesions due to the HIV agent itself, including changes in the thymus, lymph nodes, and the brain; 2) secondary lesions due to direct and indirect sequelae of HIV infection, including opportunistic infections, lesions associated with Epstein-Barr virus, pulmonary lymphoid hyperplasia and lymphoid interstitial pneumonitis, lymphoproliferative disorders, lymphomas, inanition, maturation arrest of the testis, atrophy of intestinal villi, and iatrogenic lesions such as those due to parenteral nutrition, mechanical ventilators, etc.; 3) lesions due to undetermined factors including arteriopathy, cardiomyopathy, nephropathy, thrombocytopenia, and nonlymphomatous neoplasms [383]. Generalized lymphoid hyperplasia is followed by lymphoid depletion and superimposed infections, especially pneumonia with *Pneumocystis carinii*. Meningoencephalitis may be a primary HIV-1 infection [384] or can be caused by CMV or toxoplasmosis. HIV encephalopathy is common in children who acquired AIDS perinatally and is associated with severe morbidity and short survival [385]. Hepatosplenomegaly and myocarditis are also described [384, 386–389] (Table 17.7).

A clinical malformation syndrome due to AIDS was described early in the epidemic [390]. This consisted of box-shaped forehead, hypertelorism, blue sclerae, mild obliquity (almond-shape) of the eyes, flattened nasal bridge, triangular philtrum, and large patulous lips. Others have refuted the evidence for a malformation syndrome due to HIV-1 and no further reports of its existence have appeared in the literature [391].

Cholestasis within hepatocytes and canaliculi, giant cells, rare necrotic individual hepatocytes, occasional acinar configurations, and moderate lobular disarray were all described in a girl 9 months of age, born to a healthy mother with HIV antibodies [392]. Portal inflammation included mononuclear cells, eosinophils, and rare polymorphonuclear leukocytes, and portal fibrous tissue was moderately increased. Tubuloreticular inclusion structures were found in many endothelial cells while cylindrical conforming cisternae were found in both circular and "test-tube" forms in portal inflammatory cells. These latter changes are considered characteristic of HIV infection.

One of the most promising events in the HIV epidemic is the reduction of vertical transmission (mother to fetus or newborn infant) of fetal and neonatal infection from about 25% to 8% by giving zidovudine to infected asymptomatic or mildly symptomatic gravidas and to the infants for 6 weeks postnatally [393]. Another remarkable case report describes the apparent clearing of the HIV virus from the blood of an infected neonate. That baby was born to an HIV-positive mother at 36 weeks' gestation and had a positive HIV-1 culture of peripheral blood mononuclear cells at 19 and 51 days of age. The baby's plasma was also positive for HIV by polymerase chain reaction at 51 days of age. By 12 months of age, the serology was negative as were subsequent PCR analysis and culture. These tests remained consistently negative for the next 5 years [394]. The possibility remains, though, that the positive cultures may have been

from maternal cells circulating in and contaminating the infant's blood [395, 396].

To allay or delay the features of pediatric AIDS in babies known to have HIV infection, prophylaxis with zidovudine is given during the first month of life. This therapy may lead to superinfections, modifications of immunization schedules, monitoring of nutritional status, special education interventions, screen and treatment for tuberculosis, etc. [397, 398].

Epstein-Barr Virus Infection

Epstein-Barr virus (EBV) is the most prevalent of the herpesvirus infections, with over 90% of the U.S. population seroreactive [399]. Seroconversion in pregnancy occurs only rarely and then usually without adverse effects on the fetus. An infant 20 months of age with micrognathia, cryptorchidism, monocytosis, central cataract, metaphysitis, myotonia, and proteinuria provided a single instance of malformations following maternal EBV infection during gestation. The baby survived [400]. Prospective studies with viral isolation have been reported in only two neonates, both without disease. Joncas et al reported a baby with EBV but also with CMV [212]. Lymphocytes are the target cells for EBV but few can be found circulating even in cases of infectious mononucleosis. If HIV infection is also present, EBV may cause significant disease such as lymphocytic pneumonia, but this occurs in older infants, not neonates [398].

Respiratory Virus Infections

Adenovirus Infection

Fatal neonatal adenovirus pneumonia is rare [401]. One premature infant who died at 15 days of age (32 weeks postconception) had diffuse necrotizing bronchiolitis and pneumonia with rather indistinct intranuclear inclusions. Adenovirus type 30 was grown from the lung. Electron microscopy clearly showed evidence of the intranuclear virus in a crystalline array (Figs. 17.25 and 17.26). A second baby died at 2 weeks of age (35 weeks postconceptional age) and had multiple foci of gray-yellow pulmonary consolidation with some purulent material. Abscesses were present. Large basophilic intranuclear inclusions were found with typical ultrastructural features [401]. Meyer et al report a neonate with nonfatal pleural effusions due to adenovirus type 3 [402]. Kinney et al report a case treated successfully with extracorporeal membrane oxygenation (ECMO) [403]. Intussusception of the intestines is another hazard of adenovirus infection and has been reported in infants as young as 1 month of age [404].

Respiratory Syncytial Virus Infection

Respiratory syncytial virus (RSV) is a common cause of pneumonia in neonates, usually occurring in the winter [405]. In one nursery epidemic, 87% of the infected babies were less than 1 month of age [406]. Apnea is a common

Table 17.7.   Diagnosis of HIV infection in children

HIV Infected

1. Child <18 months of age known to be HIV seropositive or born to HIV-infected mother or whose mode of transmission is unknown and:

   a. has positive results on two separate determinations excluding cord blood by one or more of the following HIV detection tests:

      i.   HIV virus culture

      ii. HIV PCR

      iii. HIV antigen (p24)

   or

   b. meets diagnosis of AIDS based on the 1987 AIDS case definition

2. A child <18 months of age born to an HIV-infected mother or a child any age infected by blood, blood products, or other known mode of transmission such as sexual contact who is HIV antibody positive by repeatedly reactive enzyme immunoassay (EIA) and confirmatory test (e.g., Western blot or immunofluorescence assay)

   or

   meets any of the criteria in 1) above.

Perinatally Exposed (prefix E)

A child who does not meet the criteria above who:

1. Is HIV seropositive by EIA and confirmatory test (e.g., Western blot or IFA) and <18 months old at the time of test; or has unknown antibody status but was born to a mother known to be HIV infected.

Seroconverter (SR)

A child born to an HIV infected mother who:

has been documented to be HIV antibody negative (two or more negative EIA tests performed at age 6 to 18 months or one negative EIA test after age 18 months)

and

has no other lab evidence of infection (has not had two positive viral detections tests if performed)

and

has not had an AIDS defining condition.

CD4 Counts Vary with Age

0–11 months > 1500 > 25%	= no evidence of suppression	= IMMUNE CATEGORY 1
0–11 months 750–1499, 15% to 24%	= evidence of moderate suppression	= IMMUNE CATEGORY 2
0–11 months <750, <15%	= severe suppression	= IMMUNE CATEGORY 3

Clinical Categories

N = not symptomatic

A = mildly symptomatic; i.e., lymphadenopathy, hepatomegaly, splenomegaly, dermatitis, parotitis, recurrent/persistent URI or sinusitis or otitis

B = moderately symptomatic; i.e., anemia (hemoglobin <8 g/dL), neutropenia, <1000/fL, or thrombocytopenic < 100,000/fL persisting >30 days; bacterial meningitis, pneumonia, sepsis (single episode), candidiasis—thrush persistent >2 months in child >6 months of age; cardiomyopathy; CMV infection before 1 month of age; diarrhea, recurrent or chronic; failure to thrive; hepatitis; herpes stomatitis, recurrent >2 episodes in one year; HSV bronchitis, pneumonitis, esophagitis before 1 month of age; herpes zoster (shingles), two distinct episodes or more than one dermatome; leiomyosarcoma; lymphoid interstitial pneumonia or pulmonary lymphoid hyperplasia complex (LIP/PLH); nephropathy; nocardiosis; persistent varicella zoster; fever persisting >1 month; toxoplasmosis before 1 month of age; disseminated varicella.

C = severely symptomatic; any condition listed in 1987 case definition of AIDS except LIP, e.g., Pneumocystis carinii pneumonia, Mycobacterium avium intracellulare, Mycobacterium kansasii, progressive multifocal leukoencephalopathy, wasting, disseminated tuberculosis, lymphoma of non-cleaved Burkitt's type of immunoblastic or large cell of B cell or unknown immunologic phenotype; Kaposi's sarcoma, herpes simplex >1 month duration, encephalopathy, cryptosporidiosis, cryptococcosis.

Classification of Pediatric AIDS, 1987*

1. Virus in blood or tissue

2. HIV-positive antibody test in blood

3. Signs or symptoms of pediatric AIDS

   P-0   Indeterminant information

   P-1   Asymptomatic infection

      A   Normal immune function

      B   Abnormal immune function

      C   Immune function not tested

   P-2   Symptomatic infection

      A   Nonspecific symptoms

      B   Progressive neurologic disease

      C   Lymphocytic interstitial pneumonia

      D   Secondary infections

         1   Specific infectious agent

         2   Recurrent lesions

         3   Other

      E   Neoplasm

         1   Nonspecific

         2   Specific for AIDS

      F   Symptoms possibly due to AIDS

*   MMWR 1987; 36:91–96.

symptom in newborn infants infected with RSV, but the disease is not usually fatal unless pulmonary hypertension is also present [406–409].

The pathologic reaction in pulmonary tissues consists of acute endobronchiolitis and peribronchiolitis with bosselated bronchial mucosal cells at the surface [410–412]. Acinar (alveolar) epithelial cells may be necrotic or enlarged. Inflammatory infiltrates are composed of mixed neutrophils,

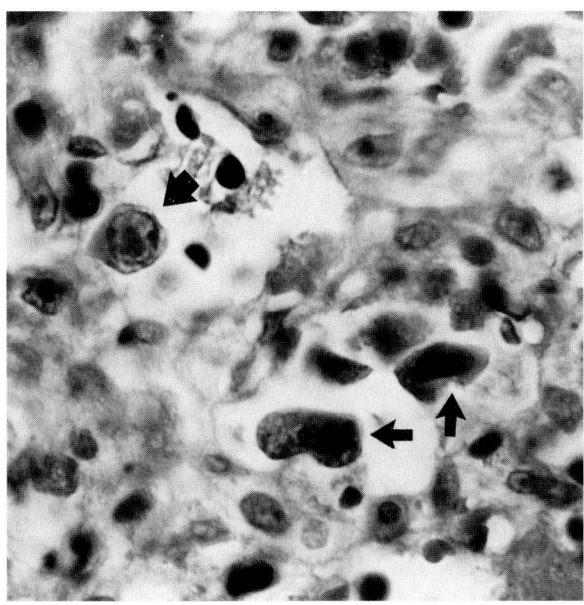

FIGURE 17.25.   *Pulmonary infection with adenovirus. Arrows point to inclusion-bearing cells. (From Shikes RH, Ryde JW. Adenovirus pneumonia in a newborn. Pediatr Pathol 1989; 9:199–202. Used with permission of the author and publisher.)*

lymphocytes, eosinophils, and macrophages. In many cases, large cytoplasmic inclusions are found; these are eosinophilic, rounded, 2 to 4 μm in diameter, and occupy the bronchiolar and acinar epithelial cells [408, 410, 411]. The diagnosis can be established by examining nasal and pharyngeal secretions for the antigen with immunofluorescent reagents [413]. Syncytial giant cells are rarely seen in vivo, the appellation for the disease being derived from observations of infected tissue cultures.

Treatment with maternal serum has had some salutary effect [414] as has treatment with ribavarin [405].

Rhinovirus Infection

Rhinovirus infections are most apt to occur in preterm infants who are ventilated mechanically. The illness is usually less severe than that caused by RSV. Viral deposits on plastic or metal fomites can remain infectious for several hours [415].

Human Papillomavirus Infection (HPV Infection)

The risk of developing laryngeal or tracheal papillomas is 1:500 to 1:1000 in vaginally delivered infants when the mother has condyloma acuminata. The rate among babies delivered by cesarean section is one-tenth that of babies delivered vaginally. These lesions develop in infants beyond the neonatal period [416]. In one such case, the virus type was among those associated with benignity in cervical lesions of adults [417].

Rubeola Virus Infection

Approximately 0.4 case of measles occurs per 10,000 pregnancies. The incidence is lower now that most of the women in developed countries are immunized in childhood. In susceptible pregnant women, the rubeola virus

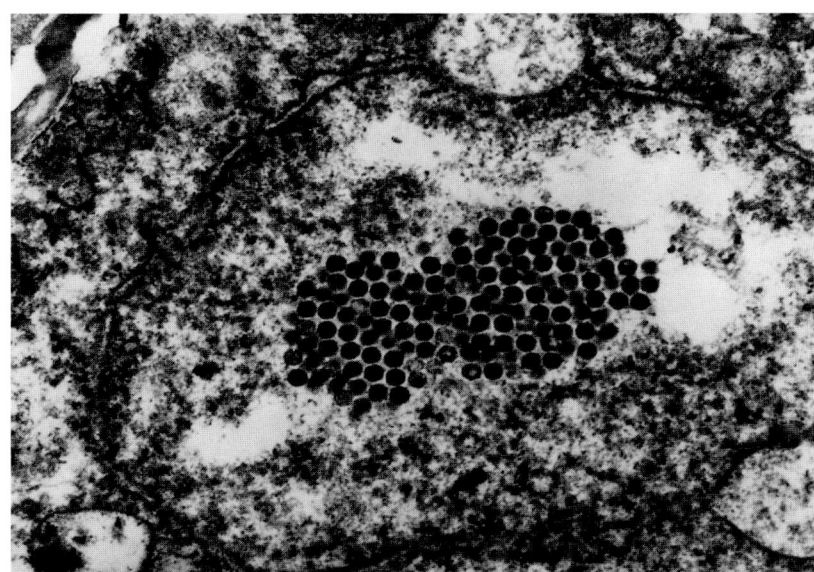

FIGURE 17.26.   *Ultrastructure of adenovirus in a case of neonatal pneumonia. (From Shikes RH, Ryder JW. Adenovirus pneumonia in a newborn. Pediatr Pathol 1989; 9:199–202. Used with permission of the author and publisher.)*

spreads through the bloodstream and, by the time an exanthem appears at around 12 to 14 days, is already well established in the mother's tissues. Measles during pregnancy is a more severe disease than in nonpregnant individuals. In the report by Atmar et al, 7 of 13 hospitalized women had respiratory complications and one died of measles pneumonia. Several of these patients also had clinical and laboratory evidence of hepatitis, premature delivery, and one had a stillborn fetus [418]. Similar findings have been reported by others [419, 420].

Malformations are reported in isolated cases but are most likely coincidental to the infection [421]. Normal fetal development is the rule, although increased rates of prematurity are reported and early spontaneous abortions are probably increased as well [151, 422, 423].

Congenital measles occurs when the interval between onset of exanthem in the mother and in the fetus or infant varies between 2 days and 10 days. The placenta is a moderately effective barrier to infection. One report suggests that the trophoblast may be the site of infection but histologic descriptions are lacking [424]. Up to 70% of babies born to mothers with active exanthems will have no evidence of disease. However, if the fetus or infant is infected, the disease is usually severe, with measles pneumonia apparently providing most of the morbidity and mortality. This is characterized by a chronic interstitial pneumonitis with many multinucleated giant cells formed from alveolar macrophages and pneumocytes. About 30% of infected newborn babies will die of the disease [421]. Postnatal death is said to be increased in survivors of congenital measles or in children born to mothers with gestational measles infection [425, 426].

Hemorrhagic Viral Infections

Of the many so-called hemorrhagic viral infections, the most information regarding fetuses and neonates has been collected for Lassa fever. Series of infections among pregnant women in Liberia and Sierra Leone have shown that Lassa fever is the most common cause of maternal mortality, especially when infection occurs in the third trimester [427, 428]. Fetal and neonatal loss was 87% among infected gravidas in the study from Sierra Leone [427]. The swollen baby syndrome is described as anasarca, pulmonary edema, swollen abdomen, and melena in fatal neonatal and infantile cases [428]. In autopsy studies, the necrotic lesions of liver, spleen, and adrenal and the cytoplasmic inclusions found in adrenal cells were not found in five fetuses who died after their mothers developed Lassa fever [429].

Puumala virus in Finland is one of the hantavirus strains, the reservoirs for which are rodents. Fetal infections have not been described in this mild form of hantavirus infection, though the more severe Korean hemorrhagic virus infection reportedly has produced lesions in fetal tissues [430].

Rickettsial Infection

Perinatal infections with *Rickettsia* organisms must be exceedingly rare. The only case of Rocky Mountain spotted fever in a pregnant woman recorded in the recent English literature resulted in a healthy baby born at term [431].

Chlamydia trachomatis Infection

In 1967 Schachter isolated chlamydial organisms from several aborted placentas [432]. Since then *Chlamydia trachomatis* has been repeatedly studied with inconsistent conclusions regarding its role in fetal disease [433, 434]. Up to 30% of women in prenatal clinics have cervical chlamydial colonization while women attending clinics for sexually transmitted diseases have higher colonization rates [434]. Transmission from colonized mothers to the neonate occurs at the time of parturition, although chorioamnionitis also occurs prepartum [435, 436]. Some 50% of the babies are infected and the major manifestations of disease are conjunctivitis and pneumonia [434, 437]. Conjunctivitis may consist of minimal erythema or the classic "sticky eye." Infection may be unilateral, but is usually bilateral. Follicular conjunctivitis doesn't develop because neonates lack sufficient lymphoid tissue in the eyelids or conjunctivae. Most cases heal without scars, with or without antimicrobial therapy; but corneal scarring occurs in a minority of cases. Those treated with systemic erythromycin or amoxicillin rather than topical therapy have the best long-term results [434, 438].

Chlamydial pneumonia is a distinctive neonatal pneumonia [439, 440]. Onset is usually after 4 weeks of age but many cases have been described as occurring early in the neonatal period. Pulmonary tissue is consolidated with mononuclear infiltrates of interstitium and peribronchial tissues. Eosinophils are also present. Pleural and septal congestion is prominent and bronchial necrosis has been described [434, 440].

BACTERIAL INFECTIONS

Spiral Organisms

Syphilis

Congenital syphilis is a transplacental infection passed from nonimmune infected mothers to the fetus. In developing countries, syphilis is still a significant cause of perinatal morbidity and mortality [441]. The same can be said for some regions and communities in the United States [442–445]. Pregnant women with primary or secondary syphilis are apt to deliver stillborn fetuses in 50% of the cases whereas women with tertiary syphilis have more variable results with their pregnancies. The overall perinatal mortality in recent years in the United States is 18% [74, 446].

Contrary to older theories of transmission, the spirochete crosses the placenta in all three trimesters of gestation [74, 446]. Spirochetes can be seen in first trimester placental villi, especially when immunofluorescent techniques are used [447]. Unlike adult syphilis which passes through stages, fetal or congenital syphilis has simultaneous development of lesions similar to all three classic stages [74]. In stillborn fetuses, which comprise the majority of cases born in the second trimester, maceration and hydrops were common features in the past but fewer cases of hydrops have occurred in recent decades [441]. In liveborn infants, snuffles, hemorrhagic rhinitis, enlarged livers and spleens, lymphadenopathy, lip fissures, and mucous patches of oral and anal mucosa are the main clinical features [446]. Preterm delivery is common. Marasmus in utero is described in cases born decades ago [74]. Apparently, intrauterine growth retardation is no longer such a common feature [441]. Among liveborn infants with severe disease, death usually occurs within a few days of birth. If the mother's infection occurs late in the third trimester, symptoms may be absent throughout the newborn period; failure to thrive with subsequent skin rash and snuffles develops after the first month of life [74].

Whether organs are enlarged, small, or of normal overall size, most have retarded development histologically [74]. Perhaps the most characteristic morphologic feature in congenital syphilis is increased fibrosis in many tissues and organs [74, 276]. Judge believes that the arteriopathy is the basic lesion and is mediated through a partially developed fetal immune response to the spirochete [441]. Oppenheimer and Dahms, citing infants who died four decades or more in the past [74], describe a triad consisting of gastrointestinal mucosal ulcers, pancreatic fibrosis, and pneumonia alba as characteristic for congenital syphilis. In more recent cases, the absence of pneumonia alba and the presence of hepatosplenomegaly and distinctive vascular inflammatory lesions are more characteristic. Fibrosis is less prominent or even absent in fetuses aborted in the second trimester [441, 446].

Spirochetemia occurs within hours of a primary exposure and presumably reaches the placenta during that time [74]. In some placentas, the organism is readily demonstrated [448], while in others, especially when the infection is several weeks or months old, few spirochetes can be found [74, 441]. Macerated fetuses from untreated mothers may be teeming with spirochetes [74]. When searching for the organisms, the liver and kidney provide positive results more often than the placenta or other organs [441]. In the liver, the spirochetes are mostly extracellular, as demonstrated by electron microscopy [449].

The spirochete of *Treponema pallidum* is about 15 μm long and has 13 to 15 turns in its spiral. It can be demonstrated with the Levaditi stain but the Warthin-Starry stain is equally useful and technically more easily applied.

Placentas are enlarged, sometimes massively, but without much edema. The placental-fetal weight ratios approach 0.5 [441]. Some placentas are pale and boggy [74]. A triad of changes consist of focal villitis, vascular changes including endothelial proliferation and perivascular inflammation, and

immature villi [448]. Knots of syncytial trophoblast are decreased in number [74]. Nucleated erythroid cells are sometimes present in vascular lumens. The decidua at the base of the placenta may have plasma cells and lymphocytes, particularly around maternal vessels. When the infection is more chronic, villous scarring may be seen [74]. Necrotizing funisitis is thought to be characteristic of syphilis, but Jacques and Qureshi found that only about 11% of these lesions were due to this infection [450]. Not every mother infected with syphilis will have placentas with the characteristic changes described above. In the study by Qureshi et al, fewer than 30% of mothers with proved gestational syphilis had chronic villitis, proliferative vascular changes, or villous edema [68]. In the study by Samson et al, the placentas from eight infants with congenital syphilis had IgM, C3, and rheumatoid factor demonstrated, suggesting that the reaction is immunologically mediated [67].

Pneumonia alba is a classic lesion but is waning in incidence [441]. White patches of firm parenchyma are grossly observed and acinar tissue has a fetal glandular pattern [74, 451]. Delicate strands of connective tissue with monocytic infiltrates are found in the interstitium in pneumonia alba.

Jaundice is a common clinical feature with congenital syphilis. The liver is enlarged and pale [74, 441, 449]. Minute gummata measuring up to 1 mm are scattered throughout the parenchyma [74, 449]. Increased fibrous tissue is found in the hepatic portal tracts and along the sinusoids. Liver cells are occasionally necrotic, and rarely, hepatocytic giant cells are seen [74].

In vessels throughout the body, perivascular lymphocytic and plasmacytic infiltrates are another classic feature. In the placenta, such lesions are usually seen in only one other condition, namely congenital CMV infection. The medias of small arteries are increased in thickness. Epicarditis and pericarditis are not uncommon, but the myocardium is infrequently inflamed [74].

The spleen is characteristically enlarged with increased hematopoiesis. Another classic lesion is laminated perivascular fibrosis forming "onion-skin" lesions around splenic arterioles. Small infarcts accompany some of these vascular lesions [74]. Lymphoid tissues may be hyperplastic with precocious development of follicles and follicular centers. Plasma cells infiltrate the sinusoids [38]. The thymus may be small due to loss of cortical lymphocytes. Dubois abscesses, consisting of mixed infiltrates in the medulla, are mentioned in the older literature [74] but seem to be less common in recent reports [441]. They may represent degenerating gummata. Hematopoiesis is increased in the liver, spleen, and many other organs [74,452]. Hydrops may develop in stillborn and liveborn infants on the basis of anemia, presumably due to destruction of red blood cells.

The skin has bullous lesions, characteristically extending to the palms and soles (Fig. 17.27). Cutaneous ulcers with gray, shaggy bases and borders with steep edges (rolled edges) have lymphocytic and plasmacytic infiltrates in the dermis. Cuffs of lymphoid cells surround skin appendages

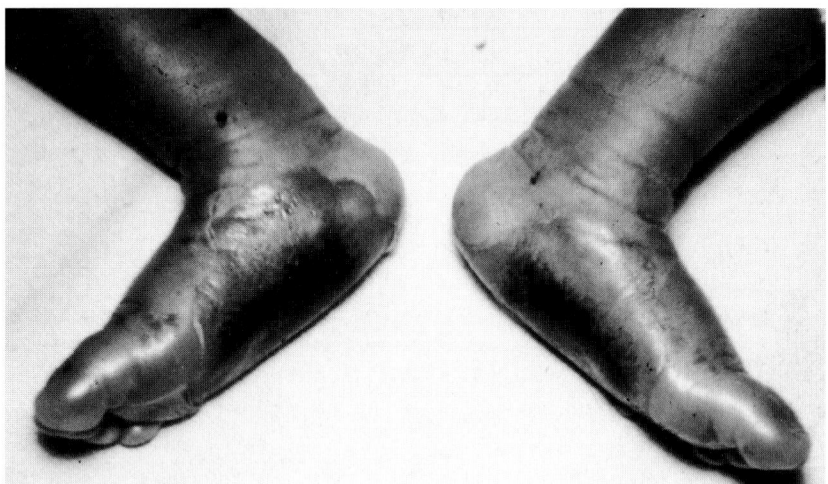

FIGURE 17.27.   *Feet from a baby with congenital syphilis. The lesions on the soles had been bullous originally; they ruptured and are now raw, weeping sores. (Photograph generously provided by Dr. Arnold J. Rudolph, Houston, Texas.)*

and vessels in the dermis and subcutaneous tissues. Dermal fibrosis is seen in more chronic stages. In older infants, fibrosis around the corners of the mouth leads to the wrinkles known as rhagades. Anal fissures may be present [74].

Bone lesions consist of focal destruction of bony tissue between the diaphysis and epiphysis. Periosteal inflammation and fibrosis produce a characteristic flared lesion. Granulation tissue may be exuberant, producing saber shin and bossing of the forehead in survivors. Irregular rarefactions of the metaphysis and diaphysis in long bones produce "celery-stalk" lesions, which occur in other congenital infections, most notably rubella and CMV infection. Epiphysitis results in irregular penetration of cartilage from the growth zone into the metaphysis, and osteoblasts are reduced in number [74].

Mononuclear inflammation of the pia-arachnoid is sometimes seen. Perivascular cuffing is commonly found deep within the tissues of the brain and spinal cord. The eyes occasionally have nonspecific uveitis [74].

In the endocrine glands, few lesions are described. Pituitary abscesses have occurred, and the adrenals may have scars in the cortex or nonspecific inflammation. Testes and epididymis are frequently infiltrated with chronic inflammatory cells, but the ovaries are usually normal. Thyroid pathology is not described in congenital syphilis [74].

Other Spiral Organisms and Their Infections

Yaws and pinta share many features with syphilis, but fetal and neonatal infections have not been described.

Abramowsky and colleagues described four fetuses of 17 to 23 weeks' gestation who had spirochetal microorganisms in their intestinal lumens and mucosa, but few in other organs. Chorioamnionitis and severe chronic villitis with villous vasculitis were noted along with chronic meningitis and mononuclear interstitial pneumonia. Bones, liver, and kidney had no detectable lesions. The mothers in these four cases had no clinical or laboratory evidence of syphilis, *Bor-*

relia infection, leptospiral disease, or *Campylobacter*. The conclusion was that these cases were infections with one or more species of gastrointestinal spirochetes [453]. *Leptospirosis canicola* has been cultured from the mother of a stillborn infant as reported by Coghlan and Bain [454]. *Borrelia recurrentis* and other *Borrelia* species have been associated with stillborn fetuses, and one liveborn infant had thrombocytopenia due to *Borrelia duttonii* with spirochetes demonstrated in the smears of cord blood [455]. Altschuler found fusobacteria in 18% of placentas with acute chorioamnionitis [456].

Lyme Disease   Lyme disease is caused by a tick-borne spirochete, *Borrelia burgdorferi* (Fig. 17.28). The organism undulates, unlike the tight spiral of *Treponema pallidum*. In older children and adults, the infection produces mild or severe symptoms that include arthritis and a characteristic annular skin rash, erythema chronicum migrans. The rash begins as a red papule and expands centrifugally with central clearing. Other lesions are meningoencephalitis and myocarditis. Lyme disease has occurred during all stages of pregnancy and about 25% of such cases have had poor outcome. Fetal deaths occur from 15 to 40 weeks' gestation. The organism is widely disseminated in the fetal tissues. Bacterial cultures of several organs taken at autopsy have been positive and have proved a useful means of diagnosis. However, no consistent fetal or placental lesions have been noted [457, 458]. In one series of five cases, three had dissimilar cardiovascular malformations. A skin rash was present at birth in a baby whose mother had meningoencephalitis 1 week prior to the term birth. The baby survived and the rash disappeared without sequelae [458]. In all the 46 cases of congenital Lyme borreliosis that have been reported, *Borrelia burgdorferi* has been demonstrated in liver, spleen, bone marrow, heart, brain, and kidney of fetuses and neonates. When maternal infection occurs during the first trimester, miscarriages tend to be delayed to 15 to 25 weeks of gestation and late fetal and neonatal deaths may show no signs of congenital infec-

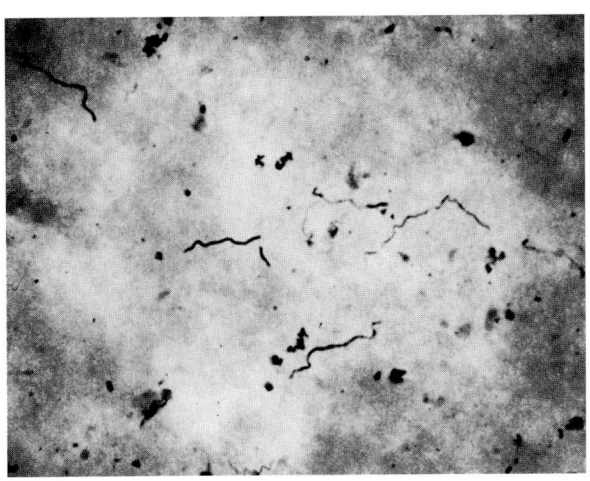

FIGURE 17.28. Borrelia burgdorferi *from a case of Lyme disease. The preparation is from the culture plate agar processed in a paraffin block. (Warthin-Starry stain, approximately ×1680.) (Photograph generously provided by Dr. A.B. MacDonald, Southampton, Long Island, New York.)*

tion. These clinical features are similar to those of congenital syphilis although pathologic lesions are not at all similar. As mentioned above, congenital heart lesions (ventricular septal defects, aortic stenosis, patent ductus arteriosus, atrial septal defects, coarctation, and endocardial fibroelastosis) are described in several cases of fetal and neonatal Lyme disease. Hydrocephalus unassociated with inflammation is also reported. Characteristically, fetal and neonatal tissues, even those with demonstrable spiral organisms, have no inflammation. Later manifestations of congenital infections consist of inflammatory multisystem disease of skin, synovia, lymph nodes, eyes, and central nervous system. The inflammatory cells are granulocytes, mast cells, and eosinophils, and tend to aggregate around vessels and in the meninges. Muscle atrophy is also described [459]. Placental pathology is variable, both as to type of lesions noted and the frequency with which lesions are found in cases of congenital Lyme disease. Focal chorioamnionitis, focal calcification, increased villous histiocytes, villous edema, villous fibrosis, and thrombosed vessels have been described. Spirochetes may be sparse or absent in such cases [459].

Gardner's review of congenital Lyme disease has shown that among cases with infection during gestation, the rate of fetal death is 11%, the rate of neonatal death is 3%, and of neonatal illness 15%. Normal outcomes are expected in about 70% [459].

Tuberculosis

Only 24 cases of congenital tuberculosis were recorded in the English literature in the 28 years following the introduction of isoniazid therapy [460, 461]. The congenital form

of the disease was never common. In past years, failure to thrive, jaundice, and central nervous system infection were prevalent. Now, liver and cutaneous involvement are the presenting features. In fatal cases, miliary lesions can be seen in omentum, spleen, liver, and lymph nodes, and in these organs and tissues one may find characteristic granulomas. Necrotic lesions occur in the lymph nodes [460]. The skin has deep dermal granulomas with giant cells and with caseous necrosis. Acid-fast bacilli can be demonstrated in these lesions. Intradermal antigen tests are rarely positive [460].

Leprosy

Perinatal leprosy is exceedingly rare. Morison refers to a report of transplacental infection but descriptions are not readily available [5]. Job et al describe fetal infections in 9-banded armadillos. The acid-fast bacilli of leprosy can be demonstrated in decidua, trophoblast, and fetal spleens of these mammals [462].

Common Bacterial Infections

Several bacterial agents produce a syndrome of early neonatal sepsis characterized chiefly by septicemia, pneumonia, meningitis/ventriculitis or combinations of these features. Other agents produce a variety of infections designated "late onset." Some bacteria can produce either early or late onset disease. The various bacterial agents predominating in perinatal infection have changed with each decade since the 1920s.

Group B Streptococcal Infection

Group B streptococcus (*Streptococcus agalactiae*) has become the most common cause of perinatal infection in many countries [4, 463–467]. It is found in the vagina or rectum of 10% to 50% of women in the United States [130, 465, 468]. Of babies born to colonized mothers, nearly 60% will be colonized [469]. Mothers with more heavily colonized genitalia are more apt to show peripartum symptoms and are more apt to produce fetuses and neonates with infections [470]. Maternal sepsis includes symptoms as mild as low-grade fever and as severe as septicemia, meningitis, and maternal endocarditis with mitral valve prolapse [15, 471]. Maternal symptoms tend to be more severe when labor begins before 32 weeks of gestation [472].

The rate of maternal carriage is 100 times that of fetal and neonatal infection [464]. The actual rate of perinatal sepsis due to GBS is approximately 2 per 1000 live births, but in some centers the rate seems to be dropping. Alternatively, the disease is becoming less fulminant. The number of stillborn fetuses with significant GBS sepsis is not known but several studies have had large numbers of fetal deaths among the cases of GBS sepsis [47, 465, 473]. Male offspring are more commonly infected than females, the ratio being about 3 to 2 [470, 474]. Before 1990, overall perinatal mortality was about 27% with much higher rates of mortality at gestations less than 28 weeks [464, 474, 475].

GBS have been serologically typed into five subgroups: Ia, Ib, Ic, II, III. Baker et al showed that of the group B streptococcus subtypes, Ia and Ib are usually found in the mothers during the third trimester but subtypes II and III predominate and are almost exclusively found late in gestation [468]. Subtype III is responsible for almost all of the cases of late onset disease, particularly meningitis [476]. In GBS sepsis of late onset, mothers often are not colonized with the organism but when they are, serologic typing shows concordance between the maternal organism and the neonatal organisms in 50% of the paired samples [464, 476]. These organisms may have properties that inhibit chemotaxis of polymorphonuclear leukocytes but histologic studies generally show adequate inflammatory responses [477].

Maternal prenatal treatment regimens have been a problem due to the high rate of colonization and the inability to routinely identify the women whose fetuses or babies are at great risk for GBS infection. Some early reports of perinatal sepsis due to GBS suggested that most cases occurred at or near term [474]. Oral antibiotics at 38 weeks were suggested as an appropriate treatment in such women but this regimen does not help the large number of fetuses and infants infected earlier in pregnancy [47, 466, 478, 479]. Indeed, septic abortions before 20 weeks' gestation are often due to GBS and were recorded in some of the earliest reports [466, 480]. There is some evidence that before 32 weeks, the rate of maternal colonization with GBS is three times that of mothers after 32 weeks [481].

Several investigators have administered intrapartum penicillin in colonized mothers or those at high risk for infection [482, 483]. Others have suggested treating all mothers whose urinary tract was infected with GBS [484]. Still others have given intramuscular penicillin to all mothers in labor greatly reducing the incidence of neonatal GBS sepsis; however, the overall morbidity and mortality were not changed with this regimen partly because of infections with organisms resistant to penicillin [485]. Intravenous immunoglobulin given to GBS-infected infants is of questionable benefit. The same may be said for other infections in neonates [486, 487].

Antibody levels in maternal serum have an effect on the incidence of and the severity of GBS sepsis in neonates. When the antibody titer is >1:40, approximately equivalent to 0.2 µg/mL, protection from GBS sepsis is achieved [168]. Baker and her colleagues have shown that pregnant women can be immunized at 32 weeks of gestation [486].

Both the American College of Obstetricians and Gynecologists and the American Academy of Pediatrics have developed treatment protocols for perinatal GBS infections (*Pediatrics* 1997; 99:489–496). In our own institution, both protocols have been used and we have seen a reduction in the number of infected fetuses and neonates. However, the reduction was evident prior to the use of these protocols,

suggesting another swing of the pendulum in the etiologies of neonatal and fetal sepsis [488, 489].

Perinatal GBS sepsis most often occurs in an early onset form with symptoms before 48 hours of age; death often occurs within 48 hours, sooner than with *E. coli* or most other infectious agents [475]. The late onset form has symptoms usually occurring around 5 to 15 days of age. The ratio of early onset sepsis to late onset sepsis is 6.6:1 while the rates are respectively 2 per 1000 live births vs. 0.3 per 1000 live births [488]. This can be compared with perinatal *E. coli* sepsis with a ratio of early to late onset of about 2:3 [488].

Acute chorioamnionitis, pneumonia, and septicemia are frequent features of GBS early onset sepsis [15, 47, 113, 122]. GBS pneumonia can mimic respiratory distress syndrome clinically and radiologically, although lung compliance is more nearly normal and pulmonary interstitial emphysema is less common when infection is present than when it is not [113]. Pressures required to insufflate the lung are not as high when infection with GBS is present [475]. Hyaline membranes develop in such cases and are infiltrated with gram-positive cocci, imparting a blue hazy hue to the ordinarily pink membranes [122]. In 1932, Farber and Wilson described this association in a baby with streptococcal pneumonia. The serotype of that streptococcus was not known since serotyping was not developed until 2 years later [123, 490]. Whether the hyaline membranes are due to the infection or whether they would have developed without the infection is still the subject of speculation. Pneumonia is more apt to occur in GBS sepsis than it is with *E. coli* or other infectious agents [475]. Extracorporeal membrane oxygenation has been employed in cases with severe pneumonia, and in some of these, bronchiolitis obliterans has developed [491].

About one-third of the cases of GBS sepsis occur in the second trimester of gestation, between 18 and 28 weeks [47]. Previous reproductive loss is a risk factor and maternal vaginal hemorrhage and premature rupture of membranes are common clinical warnings. Fetal deaths are as common as neonatal deaths, emphasizing the prepartum timing as well as the virulence of the infection in midgestation. Aside from the placenta and lung, inflammation rarely involves other tissues in these tiny premature fetuses and infants [47]. Otitis was a finding in one series [479].

Varying degrees of chorioamnionitis are seen, some with necrosis. Villitis is seen in some cases indicating longstanding infectious disease in the fetus or hematogenous spread from maternal bacteremia or endometritis [47]. According to Craig, chorioamnionitis is twice as prevalent and deciduitis three times as prevalent in GBS as these lesions are with other infectious agents [475]. Chorioamnionitis is not necessarily severe and umbilical cord inflammation may be mild [47].

While meningitis is one of the main characteristics of late onset sepsis, as few as one in four babies with late onset GBS sepsis has this lesion [129, 476]. GBS, more often than other organisms, is associated with periventricular leukomalacia [492]. Abnormal development, hydrocephalus, and other sequelae can be detected in about half of the babies who survive late onset sepsis due to GBS [493, 494].

Unusual features of late onset GBS sepsis include septic arthritis, which has been seen as late as 8 months after birth [476]. Right-sided diaphragmatic hernia, the explanation for which is not clear, is another unusual association [495–497]. Some have suggested that GBS is more apt to persist in such babies' lungs because of the lack of adequate movement of the right hemithorax during respiration [495]. Facial and submandibular cellulitis has also been reported in neonatal GBS sepsis of late onset and this may be the initial sign of the disease [498, 499].

Several methods have been suggested for early diagnosis of GBS in neonates. Rapid latex agglutination testing has not been uniformly successful [500].

Perinatal Infections with Other Streptococci (Non-GBS)

As a rule, non-group B streptococcal sepsis in neonates is not as virulent as group B streptococcal disease [501, 502]. Other streptococcal species that occasionally infect neonates include group D streptococci, both enterococci and non-enterococcal forms [503]. These organisms can produce meningitis, pneumonia with a typical respiratory distress syndrome, and fatal sepsis in neonates [504].

***Streptococcus pneumoniae* Infections** *Streptococcus pneumoniae* is responsible in some series for the majority of childhood bacteremias, but it is not a common cause of perinatal infection [505]. When it occurs, it may mimic sepsis caused by group B streptococcus and usually involves prematurely born infants [506, 507]. Meningitis and pneumonia with hyaline membranes have been the main features, but endophthalmitis has also been described [506, 508, 509].

Staphylococcal Infections

Coagulase-negative staphylococcus is now the main cause of neonatal nosocomial bacteremia in many neonatal intensive care units, surpassing infections with gram-negative organisms [510–514]. About 20 species of coagulase-negative staphylococci are involved, the majority of these being *Staphylococcus epidermidis* [515]. This is of particular concern because 75% of these staphylococci are resistant to antimicrobial agents including second generation beta-lactams. The infections tend to be more indolent and the organisms less virulent than infections with *Staphylococcus aureus*. Coagulase-negative staphylococci produce a slime that may impair antibiotic penetration and interfere with host defenses. The slime may also enhance bacterial adherence to infected cells [515]. The onset of disease usually ranges from 2 weeks to several months, and almost all are nosocomial. Most infected babies are preterm [516]. Intravenous immunoglobulin has been used to treat these patients with some success [517]. Few die, but among those who do the features resemble sepsis due to streptococci when the disease is of acute onset.

In patients who survive for long periods of time in neonatal intensive care units, coagulase-positive staphylococcal infections are apt to occur. Abscesses develop in the skin and in several organs or tissues if indwelling catheters become infected [518]. Use of lipid emulsions is associated with such infections [519]. Pulmonary infections with abscesses may be found [520]. Empyema is often a complicating feature. Treatment with vancomycin has been used in such cases with good effect [521].

Staphylococcal scalded skin syndrome (SSSS) occurs when infants or fetuses are infected with certain phage types of *Staphylococcus aureus*, specifically group 2 types 71, 55/71, 3A, and 3C/71 [522]. The same organisms are responsible for similar diseases in older infants and children (Lyell disease) and adults (Ritter disease). The earliest lesions in the skin are tender and have a sandpaper-like texture. Skin slippage (Nikolsky's sign) is quickly followed by the development of flaccid bullae. The skin then separates in sheets and within 48 hours, large areas are denuded, particularly around the mouth. Secondary desquamation persists for several days; purulent conjunctivitis and seborrhea may also be seen. Septicemia and bacterial endocarditis are complications. Microscopically, the skin develops intraepidermal bullae with degeneration and pyknosis of basal cell nuclei and hair follicles, often with no inflammatory reaction [522].

Escherichia coli Infections

Infections with *Escherichia coli* are only slightly less numerous and in some ways slightly less virulent than infections with group B streptococci. Geographic differences have been noted in time of onset of symptoms and also in rapidity of progression of disease [523]. The presence of the K1 antigen is important to the virulence of *E. coli*. McCracken et al found no fatalities among infants infected with K1-negative *E. coli* bacteria while several fatal cases occurred among infants infected with K1-positive *E. coli* [524]. The rate of infection in recent decades has been about 1 per 1000 live births or about half the rate of group B streptococcus, but these rates may change from location to location and from year to year within a center [488].

Neonates infected with *E. coli* are more apt to develop early jaundice than are those infected with other bacterial agents. Hepatocytic changes are not significant but cholestasis with canalicular bile plugs, occasional bile plugs in small ductules, and neutrophils in sinusoids are often found. Kupffer cells may be prominent. Pneumonia and meningitis are commonly found in fatal cases and premature infants are more apt to be infected than are those born at or near term. In meningitis the exudate is often more abundant than with other etiologic agents.

Neonates with galactosemia are prone to infection with *E. coli*. In addition to pneumonia and meningitis, some of these babies also have necrosis of the hepatic tissue [525]. Necrotizing enterocolitis is found in some cases of *E. coli* sepsis in which a heat labile enterotoxin is also present [526].

Haemophilus influenzae *Infections*

Haemophilus influenzae organisms are uncommon in the female genital tract. An estimated 0.8% to 1% of all pregnant women harbor *Haemophilus influenzae* [527–529]. Serotyping has disclosed that about 20% of perinatal *Haemophilus* infections are due to *H. influenzae* type B [528] and rarely type C [530]. The majority of the organisms are unencapsulated and therefore "non-typable" by serological tests. With biochemical reactions five generally accepted "biotypes" are identified (biotypes 1, 2, 3, 4, and 5), all of which are capable of producing perinatal infections. In one series, biotype 4 was the most prevalent agent colonizing the female genital tract [527]. In the Rhode Island series biotypes 3, 4, and 5 prevailed [531]. Fever appears in nearly half of the mothers and genitourinary infection in one-third. Occasionally, a mother will have septicemia [531].

Neonatal sepsis due to *H. influenzae* is emerging as a problem in several geographic centers. Recent series of cases have been reported from France and England but the largest series is reported from Rhode Island where 19 cases occurred in a period of 5 years [527, 531, 532]. In most infections with *H. influenzae* acute chorioamnionitis is found but it may be mild even in the fatal cases [531]. Funisitis and villitis are associated with fulminant and fatal cases.

Although other *Haemophilus* organisms are common causes of vaginitis, they are rarely found in fetuses or neonates. A cephalohematoma infected with *Haemophilus vaginalis* (so-called *Gardnerella vaginalis*) was successfully treated with no sequelae. Three mother-infant pairs are described with *Haemophilus pertussis* infections, none of which was fatal [533, 534].

Serratia marcescens *Infections*

Serratia marcescens infection is generally a nosocomial infection in the nursery. Early colonization but late onset of symptoms is the rule. Pneumonia occurs in about 15% and septicemia in about 10%; the latter is frequently fatal [535, 536]. Serratia meningitis can occur early in postnatal life and is almost uniformly fatal. Pneumonia may be absent in such cases [537]. *Serratia marcescens* can be associated with devastating necrosis and cavitation of the central nervous system. These changes are apparently due to compression and occlusion of cerebral vessels in the wake of the inflammatory process.

Citrobacter *Infections*

Citrobacter diversus produces meningitis in neonates, characteristically with intracerebral abscesses. Its occurrence may be endemic, and the neonatal fatality rate is one in three [538, 539].

Salmonellosis

Usually, salmonella infections develop after the first week of life. Two full-term neonates developed bloody stools within 24 hours of birth. Both had carrier mothers, one with diarrhea [540]. Stored human milk was responsible for one outbreak of neonatal salmonellosis [541]. No pathologic features have been reported from fetal or neonatal material.

Listeriosis

Adult cases of listeriosis were first recognized in the 1920s [179] and the first neonatal case was reported by Burn in 1935 [542]. Since then, fetal and neonatal infections have been recognized sporadically and in small epidemics, most of which are related to the mothers' ingestion of contaminated foodstuffs. Unpasteurized dairy products such as soft cheese have been the source of several outbreaks [134]. Incompletely pasteurized milk was blamed in one epidemic [543] and a bottle of contaminated mineral oil was involved in another [544]. Raw vegetables and coleslaw have also been the sources of outbreaks [269]. Of all cases of listeric infections in the United States, more than one-third are in fetuses or infants less than 1 month of age. Mortality occurs in about 20% of all cases of neonatal listeriosis [545, 546].

Neonatal infections are relatively common in France. Larroche states that 10 to 15 cases of listeriosis are treated each year in their neonatal intensive care unit [179]. In the United Kingdom, neonatal listeriosis occurs in 1 per 18,000 live births [547]. In absolute numbers, some 800 cases occur annually in pregnant women and fetuses in the United States. In our own institution, listeriosis accounted for only 3 cases among approximately 1300 perinatal autopsies in the 10 years from 1981 to 1990. Nevertheless, in febrile pregnant women, listeria infection should be on the list of possible causes [455]. Transabdominal amniocentesis with Gram's stain and culture has been used to establish the diagnosis [548, 549]. In unexplained fetal deaths, cultures should be performed specifically to search for listeria [550]. Virulent listeria organisms are small gram–positive bacilli, similar to cocci and especially pneumococci. The organisms form palisades in tissues with "X" and "Y" shaped aggregates. At 20°C in liquid media, the bacteria have a tumbling motility. Virulent strains accounting for 96% of cases in the U.S. have serotypes 1/2a, 1/2b, and 4b [551]. Avirulent strains may be filamentous. Silver stains or Giemsa stains are more useful than Gram's stain in demonstrating the organism in formalin-fixed tissues.

Some mothers may be asymptomatic, but maternal infections usually occur in prematurely interrupted gestation and are characterized by fever with leukocytosis and gastrointestinal, genitourinary, or upper respiratory symptoms. In other words, a flu-like illness often precedes delivery of an infected fetus or newborn infant [134, 179, 455, 546].

Clinically, perinatal or neonatal infections are divided into early onset infections and late onset infections [546, 552, 553]. In fetal and neonatal infections of early onset, widespread microabscesses in the villi and acute diffuse chorioamnionitis characterize placental infection with *Listeria monocytogenes* (Figs. 17.29 and 17.30). Such widespread involvement was at one time considered virtually pathognomonic for listeriosis [554, 555]. While *Listeria monocy-*

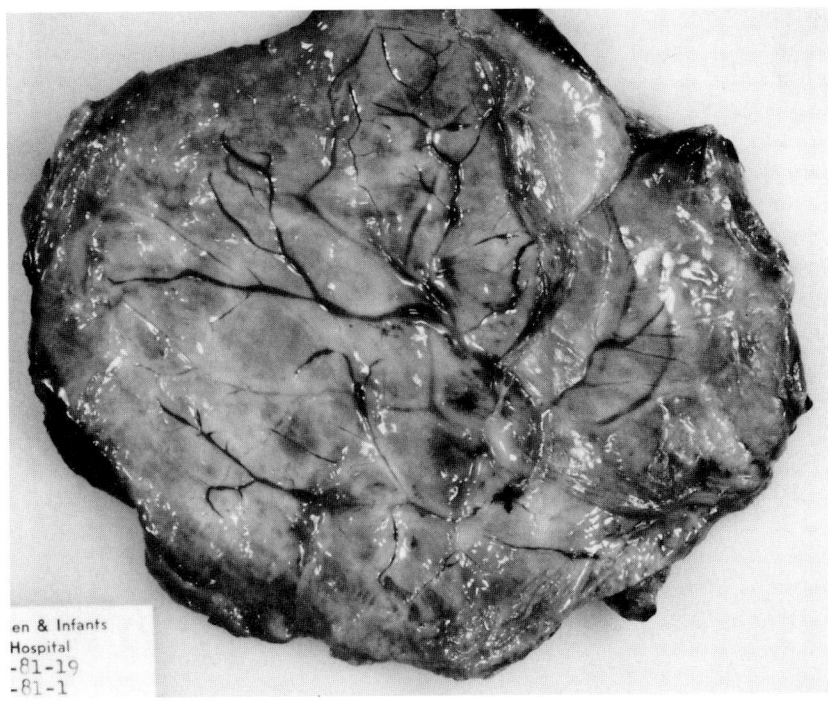

FIGURE 17.29.   *Fetal surface of the placenta with thick exudate. This was from a premature baby, 550 g, born at 23 weeks' gestation and fatally infected with* Listeria monocytogenes.

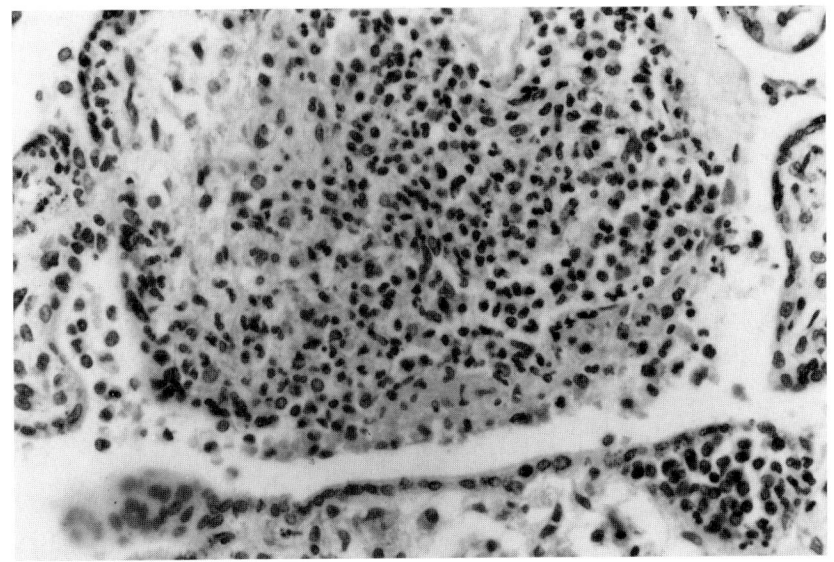

FIGURE 17.30.   *Placental villus with acute inflammation and microabscess formation. This was from a premature baby, 550 g, born at 23 weeks' gestation and fatally infected with* Listeria monocytogenes. *(H&E, ×600.)*

togenes remains the first consideration for an etiologic agent, we now know that other bacteria and viruses can produce similar placental lesions. Placental macroabscesses may measure up to 3 cm and are usually multiple. They may be mistaken for ischemic infarcts but larger ones have central cavitations [556].

In fetal infections, miliary abscesses develop in the skin, liver, adrenal, spleen, lung, and other organs. Mucosal necrosis is found in the gastrointestinal tract and listerial organisms may be found in the edges of the lesions. Nonspecific pneumonitis or hemorrhage may be present or the lungs

may be normal. Macroscopically, the lesions in the liver and adrenal mimic the necrotic lesions of congenital herpes simplex infection [134]. Listerial infection is yet another cause of hydrops fetalis [557].

Within the first week of life, jaundice, hemorrhages, disseminated intravascular coagulation, a pustular rash, tracheobronchitis, gastroenteritis, hepatitis, adrenalitis, and lymphorrhexis develop in the septic, early onset form. This is most apt to occur in preterm infants and in infants whose mothers are symptomatic [134, 179, 558]. Meningitis may be purulent although the onset may be delayed beyond 7 to 10 days [552]. Intraventricular hemorrhage and periventricular leukomalacia are described in some cases [134].

Late onset listeriosis is much more common than early onset disease and is most often found in term babies with asymptomatic mothers [558]. Late onset disease is characterized by meningitis. In long-standing cases the meningitis may be "granulomatous" but is better characterized as having a mononuclear inflammatory response. Neonates with listeriosis have higher circulating colony-stimulating factor-1 levels and subsequently higher monocyte counts than those of both noninfected newborns and newborns infected with non-listerial organisms [559]. The duration between birth and signs of illness is usually longer than for "late onset" neonatal infections with other organisms. Of the four common serotypes of *Listeria monocytogenes*, types I and IV account for 90% of the cases and type IV is most often implicated in neonatal meningitis [558].

With a concerted effort to educate health care workers and food producers regarding the dangers of listeriosis, the incidence of perinatal cases in the U.S. was decreased from 17.4 per 100,000 live births in 1989 to 8.6 per 100,000 live births in 1993 while the number of deaths was reduced from 481 in 1989 to 248 in 1993 [551].

Pseudomonas *Infections*

Pseudomonas infection usually occurs in infants who receive intensive care with the use of antibiotics. Respirator therapy is another predisposing factor, the source of infection being the humidifiers in the respirator equipment. The gastrointestinal tract is another portal of entry for *Pseudomonas* organisms. Of 265 neonatal infants studied by Somekh et al, 45 had *Pseudomonas* organisms in the stool. None of these had systemic illness and none died. The rate of diarrhea and abdominal distension was no higher in the babies with *Pseudomonas* colonization than in those without such organisms [560]. Occasionally, the infection can be acquired from the mother at the time of birth. Conjunctivitis may be an initial infection with dissemination to lungs, kidneys, and skin. Deep necrosis of the tongue, buccal mucosa, salivary gland, and extension to the middle ear are described [179]. Pneumonia is often necrotic and hemorrhagic. Macroscopically a typical bull's-eye lesion develops with a necrotic center, a reactive ring, and an outside hemorrhagic ring (Fig. 17.31). Systemic and pulmonary vascular lesions with bacterial growth in the media of blood vessels are characteristic [125] (see Fig. 17.6). Perichondritis of bronchial cartilage may be seen. Hemorrhagic plaques in the gastric or intestinal mucosa may also occur. Purulent meningitis is another feature of perinatal *Pseudomonas* infection [179]. Necrosis of skin with vasculitis and a green purulent discharge has been described in a case of intrauterine infection [561].

Campylobacter *Infections*

Campylobacter fetus or *C. jejuni* infections result in a bloody diarrhea in neonates. Few cases are fatal and histopathology has not been adequately described [562]. A nursery epidemic

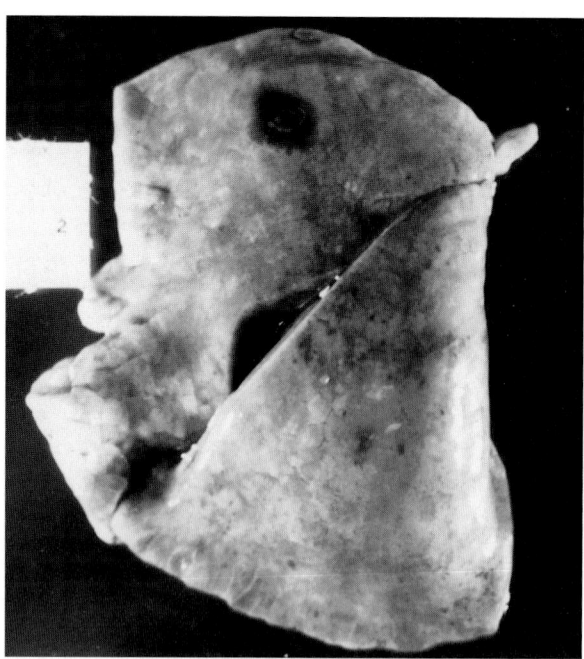

FIGURE 17.31. Pseudomonas aeruginosa *infection of the lung. Note the characteristic hemorrhagic lesion with the necrotic center. This was from a baby who required artificial ventilation for 9 days. (See Fig. 17.6, which shows the vascular necrosis responsible for this kind of lesion.)*

of *Campylobacter jejuni* meningitis affected 11 babies, all of whom were successfully treated with gentamicin and ampicillin [563].

Mycoplasma *and* Ureaplasma *Infections*

Mycoplasma hominis and *Ureaplasma urealyticum* are frequently cultured from the female genital tract, placentas, and tracheas of neonates [564, 565]. Pregnant women are more apt to harbor these organisms than are nonpregnant women [566]. Iwasaka and colleagues reported colonization rates up to 86% in a group of pregnant women, 40% of nonpregnant women, and 67% of sexually active nonpregnant women [567]. Infected sperm may carry the organism from males to females [568]. About half of the babies who are born to colonized mothers are themselves colonized [567].

In spite of the foregoing, the relationship of *Mycoplasma* organisms to perinatal disease remains a bit of a puzzle. Kundsin and colleagues believe that the probability of adverse outcome is greater in pregnancies complicated by infection with mycoplasmas than those with group B streptococci [569]. Acute chorioamnionitis is commonly associated with culture of ureaplasmas but the fetuses or neonates are not consistently affected [60, 568–570]. Abruptions of the placenta are described in conjunction with chorioamnionitis due to *Ureaplasma urealyticum* [568]. In prospective studies, premature labor (with or without rupture of membranes) is associated with *Ureaplasma urealyticum* but neither abortions nor stillbirths are increased, and cases of fetal or neonatal sepsis are not consistently increased [571–573]. Tumor necrosis factor is present in the amnion of such infected cases while uninfected placentas have no TNF [107]. Low-grade amniotic fluid infections can apparently persist for as long as 2 months [574].

In a study of two stillborn fetuses and one liveborn infant with *Mycoplasma* infection, Dische et al found acute chorioamnionitis and abscess formation [46]. Interstitial and bronchial inflammation were found in the lungs. Scanning electron micrographs were prepared to demonstrate a patchy loss of cilia in respiratory epithelium. Polymorphonuclear leukocytes in the airways and air spaces may have been aspirated from exudate in the amniotic fluid [46]. In a meta-analysis of several reports, the relative risk of chronic lung disease was increased (1.7) among children infected with *Ureaplasma* as neonates [575]. Meningitis and submandibular lymphadenitis are mentioned in neonates with *Mycoplasma hominis* infection [571, 576].

A significant proportion of neonatal sepsis (6%) and meningitis (13%) is due to ureaplasmas or mycoplasmas according to one study [573]. The retrospective studies of Maden and colleagues show that fetal growth is not affected but intra-alveolar polymorphonuclear leukocytes are increased in the lungs, the adrenals have pseudofollicular change with hemorrhage, and the placenta has villous edema and funisitis [577]. As with other infectious agents, preterm babies are more apt to be infected with these organisms than are full-term infants [578].

Neisseria *Infections*

Neisseria meningitis is rarely seen in the perinatal period and is less often fatal than it is when contracted later in infancy or childhood. Clegg et al described an infected infant 25 days of age with disseminated intravascular coagulation, acute renal tubular necrosis, and characteristic purpura of the skin along with congestive heart failure. The infant survived [579].

Neisseria gonorrhoeae produces a purulent conjunctivitis. Vaginitis, arthritis, and pharyngitis are other sequelae of gonococcal infections in neonates but sepsis is rare [580]. One case of infection in deep fetal tissues is recorded by Oppenheimer and Winn [581]. Minute abscesses were found in the pharyngeal and esophageal mucosa. Severe acute chorioamnionitis was also present.

Perinatal Infections with Anaerobes

Except for *Bacteroides* species and clostridia, infection with anaerobes is not commonly described in fetuses or neonates. Fusobacteria infection, while often demonstrated in inflamed placental membranes, is not usually associated with fetal or neonatal sepsis [456].

Clostridium tetani is still a common cause of neonatal death with infection beginning in the umbilical stump. In some developing countries, the severed umbilical stump is often treated with healing powders rich in tetanus organisms [582]. The onset of symptoms is usually 3 to 10 days following birth. In Colombia, neonatal tetanus is called the "disease of the seventh day" [583].

Gas-forming clostridia (*C. perfringens*, *C. welchii*, etc.) are responsible for a devastating necrotizing process in fetuses, with extensive tissue destruction and maceration. The process can virtually completely destroy a fetus in a matter of a few hours. Myriads of organisms may be found in the necrotic tissues. After birth several species of clostridia can quickly colonize the neonatal colon. Most of these are asymptomatic, despite the fact that toxin can be detected in stools or even in blood. *C. difficile*, *C. perfringens*, *C. paraputrificum*, or *C. sardiensis* have been implicated in several cases of neonatal necrotizing enterocolitis [584–586]. In adults, *C. difficile* has been associated with pseudomembranous colitis, and intense necrotizing colonic mucosal reaction secondary to the toxin. Neonates rarely have this condition, perhaps because they are unresponsive to the toxin. Two infants at ages 5 weeks and 12 weeks have been reported with pseudomembranous colitis. Both were premature infants who underwent intensive care and repeated treatments with antibiotics such as ampicillin [587, 588].

RICKETTSIAL INFECTIONS

Tularemia

Tularemia was reported in a stillborn of 5 days' duration. Villitis and intervillositis were noted and large bacilli could be seen in the inflammatory lesions. Fetal liver and spleen were enlarged with necrotic foci. Similar necroses were demonstrated in the kidney, adrenal, and thymus [589].

FUNGAL AND YEAST INFECTIONS

Fungal infections breach the maternal-fetal barriers with difficulty and therefore fetal infections with fungi are rare. Pulmonary blastomycosis occurs in neonates and is probably acquired from infected amniotic fluid. In perinatal blastomycosis, dissemination is not a feature and bone involvement has not been described [590]. Mortality is about 15% among neonates treated with amphotericin B [591]. Aspergillosis and mucormycosis may be encountered in neonates who are prolonged survivors of neonatal intensive care, as both are nosocomial infections. Molnar-Nadasdy et al reported a case of cryptococcal infection with abundant organisms in the placenta but no leukocytic reaction [86].

Candida albicans *Infections*

Although *Candida albicans* organisms are commonly isolated from the vaginas of pregnant women, fetal candidiasis is uncommon [179]. One of the first reports of placental and umbilical cord infection with *Candida* came in 1958 [592]. Most perinatal candidiasis occurs in preterm infants of very low birth weight, less than 1500 grams [593]. Most of these infections are nosocomial in babies surviving for several days or weeks. Many begin as the oral mucosal infection called thrush (Fig. 17.32). Antibiotics, intravascualr catheters, and other indwelling catheters are risk factors [594]. Repeated candida infections in successive infants born to the same mother have been reported [595]. Disseminated candida is also described in newborn infants who receive hydrocortisone for hypotension or other noninfectious conditions [596].

In fetal infections, multiple circumscribed miliary nodules, 0.2 to 2.0 mm, are present on the umbilical cord and on the skin and fetal surface of the placenta [597] (Fig. 17.33). Filaments and yeast invade Wharton's jelly and the amnion. Fetal vasculitis and funisitis are common, indicating the attempted fetal inflammatory response [179, 592]. In either the fetal or the postnatal disease, the gastrointestinal tract is commonly involved with ileitis, appendicitis, gastritis, and esophagitis. Gastric mucosa may show a mucoid felted mass with yeast and filaments superficially invading the glands [593] (Fig. 17.34). Vascular wall invasion occurs with secondary septicemia and pneumonia. In pulmonary infections, filaments invade the walls of air sacs. Cardiac involvement is not uncommon [179, 598]; we have seen a newborn infant in whose heart the His bundle had a discrete focus of yeast and filaments with clinically evident heart block. Renal involvement occurs in nearly two-thirds

of the cases and arthritis is noted in about 20% [594]. Meningitis occurs in many cases and seems to be growing in frequency. Some survivors have hydrocephalus [179]. Endophthalmitis due to candida produces a fluffy white lesion of the retina and vitreous [599].

PROTOZOAL INFECTIONS

Toxoplasmosis

In the United States and in the United Kingdom, one of every 1000 to 8000 livebirths may be infected with *Toxoplasma gondii* [75, 600]. The incidence of seropositive individuals is high in Paris (90%) and is moderately high in the United States (50%) [600]. High altitude and low humidity seem to be associated with fewer cases. *Toxoplasma* antibody in prenatal maternal sera is one-tenth as prevalent in Colorado as it is at sea level [601].

Toxoplasma organisms are found in cat feces and also in uncooked meat, unwashed fruit, and vegetables [600, 602]. The ingested cysts rupture, releasing sporozoites which enter intestinal lymphatics and disseminate through the vascular system. Adults and children may have suboccipital and submaxillary lymphadenopathy with characteristic giant cells [603]. Some may have a flu-like illness. In pregnant women the severity of symptoms is unrelated to fetal disease [75] but early fetal infection produces more severe fetal disease than does infection later in gestation [604]. Congenital toxoplasmosis has occurred together with HIV infection [605].

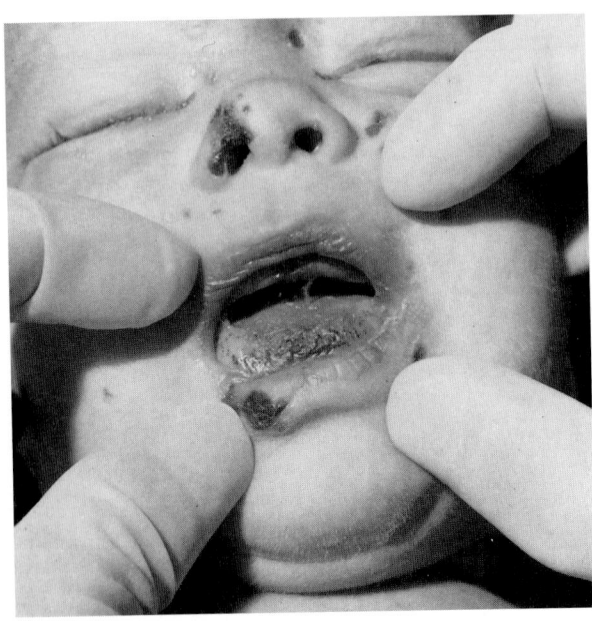

FIGURE 17.32.   *Candidiasis of the oral mucosa (thrush) in a newborn infant with a stormy course lasting 13 days. The cutaneous lesions and the lesion in the right naris are due to* Pseudomonas aeruginosa.

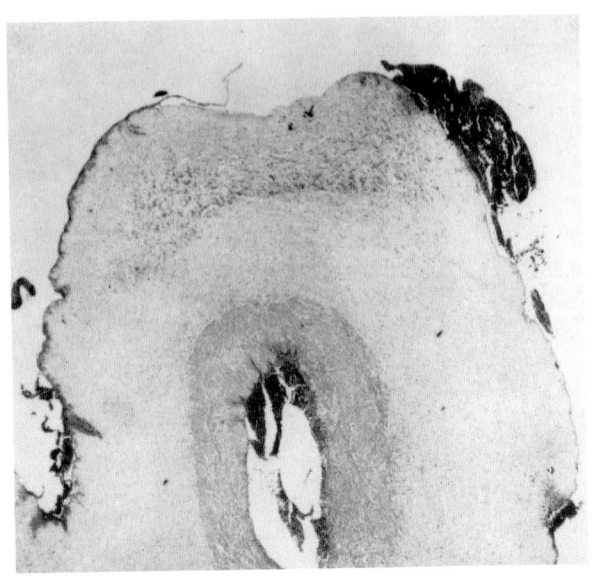

FIGURE 17.33.   *Funisitis due to fetal infection with* Candida albicans. *Note the necrotic and exudative lesion on the surface of the umbilical cord. (H&E, ×10.)*

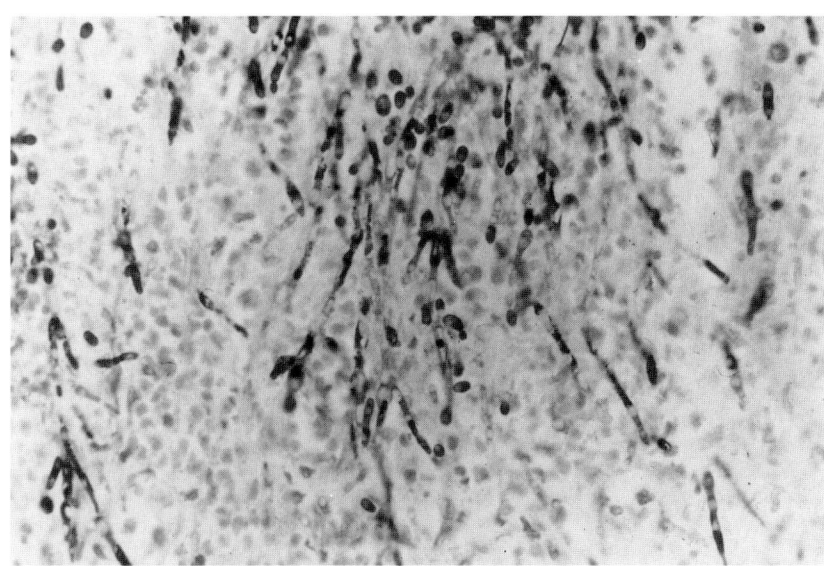

FIGURE 17.34. *Filaments and budding yeast forms from* Candida albicans *in the gastric mucosa. These formed a large felt-like mass covering the mucosal surface of the stomach and proximal duodenum. (H&E, ×490.)*

Daffos et al described a set of twins, only one of whom was infected with toxoplasmosis [603]. Maternal infections are transmitted to the fetus in 50% to 64% of cases [600, 603]. Mothers with previous toxoplasmosis infections are immune and usually do not transmit the disease to fetuses but treatment of the mother with corticosteroids may alter immunity sufficiently to result in repeated toxoplasmosis [606]. In Europe, treatment of primary infections with spiramycin has been effective but this drug is not available in the United States [600, 603].

Diagnosis is established by serological tests of the mother. The Sabin-Feldman dye test has been replaced by the immunofluorescent antibody titer test; specific tests for anti-toxoplasma IgM are available. Alternatively, homogenized infected tissues can be injected into mice or guinea pigs with demonstration of lesions and the organisms in inoculated animals. Freezing kills the organism [75]. A screening spot test of blood (serum) is now available and has been used to good advantage in the early detection and treatment of infants [607].

Toxoplasma gondii are arc-shaped or curved bow-shaped organisms which may appear round in cross section [608]. They are 4 to 7 μm long and 2 to 3 μm wide in smears; in fixed tissues these dimensions are 2 to 3 μm long and 0.5 to 1.5 μm wide. Organisms are Feulgen positive and with H&E they are pale blue with a conspicuous chromatin mass near the rounded end. Cysts are positively stained with periodic acid–Schiff stain but are perhaps better seen with Giemsa stains [75].

Intrauterine growth retardation is common. Cysts containing 50 to 60 trophozoites may be widespread in the body. They infect endothelial cells initially and produce a vasculitis. Toxoplasma cysts and trophozoites commonly aggregate in the brain and eyes. In fact, if they are not detected in these tissues, it is usually fruitless to search elsewhere. As long as the organisms remain encysted, little inflammatory reaction is observed but when trophozoites are released, the reaction may be intense. Central necrosis and marginal inflammation occur with organisms concentrated in the edges of the lesion. Miliary lesions can develop with granulomatous inflammation, usually around unruptured cysts. Chronic inflammatory reactions also occur with associated fibrosis in adjacent tissues or astrocytosis in the brain. All types of inflammation may develop in different sites in the same patient [75].

The septic form results in a petechial rash, jaundice, hepatosplenomegaly, convulsions and increased mortality [75]. Ascites and fetal hydrops have been observed and organisms have been found in amniotic fluid [75, 602, 603].

Placentas are pale, boggy, and edematous. The villous inflammation is commonly comprised of lymphocytes and occasional plasma cells but polymorphonuclear leukocytes may predominate and granulomatous inflammation is also described [71, 75]. Hofbauer cells are prominent and villous endarteritis may be observed [22]. The cysts and trophozoites are found with difficulty in the chorionic plate, syncytial trophoblast, or in villous stroma [22, 75, 600, 609]. They supposedly never infect the amnion but we have seen just such a case in our own material (Fig. 17.35).

Xanthochromic cerebrospinal fluid reflects the hemorrhage that often attends encephalitis due to toxoplasmosis [610]. Microcephaly, cerebral calcifications, hydrocephalus, chorioretinitis, and posterior uveitis were all recognized in some of the first cases described [611]. Convulsions are a common clinical feature [75] and new lesions can continue to develop in survivors [612]. Hydranencephaly and cysts in the brain stem and spinal cord can occur [613]. In fetuses less than 6 months of gestational age, toxoplasmosis produces liquefactive necrosis of the brain. The periventricular reaction is highly characteristic. The ependyma is destroyed

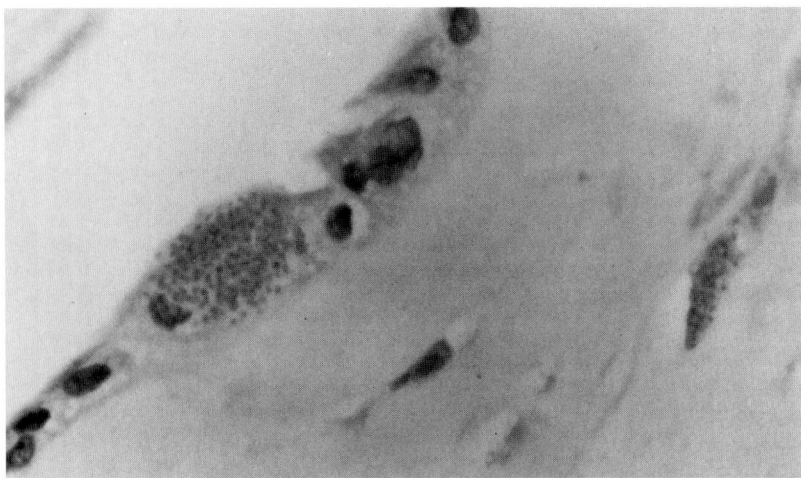

FIGURE 17.35.   Toxoplasma gondii *cysts in the amnion. Similar structures were present in the adrenal and in the brain from this macerated stillborn fetus. (H&E, ×1110.)*

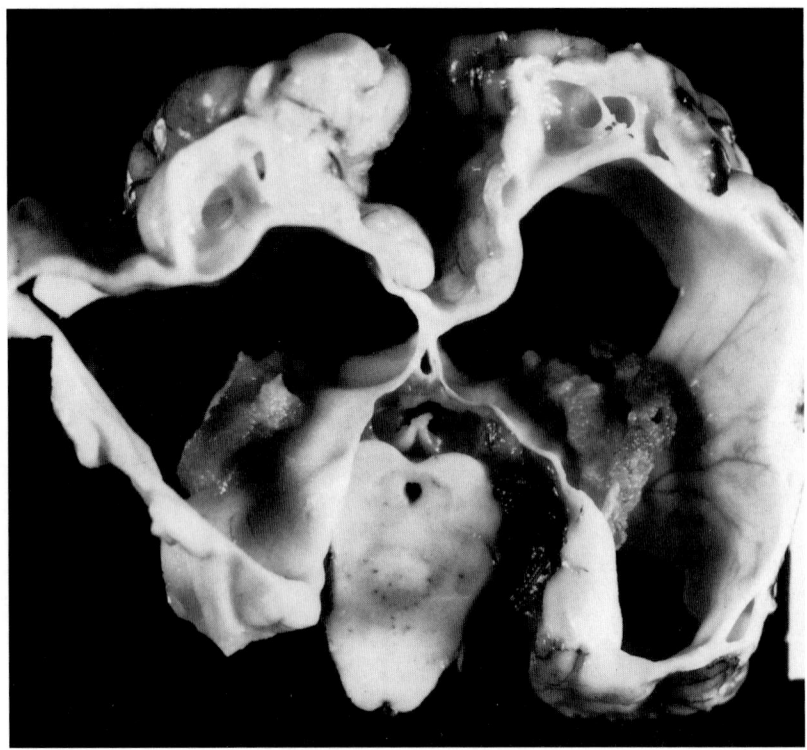

FIGURE 17.36.   *Coronal section of the cerebral hemispheres from a baby with congenital toxoplasmosis who died at 6 months of age. Periependymal calcification and cysts can be seen.*

and chorioid plexuses are edematous [75]. Dystrophic calcification in a periventricular distribution is a classic feature (Fig. 17.36). Zuelzer described granulomatous meningoencephalitis in cases characterized by lymphocytic, monocytic, and plasmacytic infiltrates in leptomeninges [608]. Porencephalic-like cysts may form and polymicrogyria can be seen through thickened, fibrotic, and inflamed meninges on cortical surfaces [75]. Trophozoites are found singly or in clusters; they may also occur in cysts within cells or lying free between cells or in the glia.

The eye is involved in the majority of cases of congenital toxoplasmosis [75, 614]. Melanin pigment in the uveal tract is irregularly dispersed; rods and cones are edematous; a yellow-white chorioretinitis develops [610]. Posterior chorioretinitis is particularly prominent with turbid vitreous fluid and disorganized retinal layers. Microphthalmia and optic nerve atrophy develop if the fetus is infected early in gestation. Optic vessels are often inflamed [75].

In 15% of survivors, hearing is deficient. Histologic

studies of the ear have shown ossification of the ligaments of the ossicles and granulation tissue [75].

Skeletal muscle fibers are also often infected with cysts and trophozoites [75, 608].

Myocardial infection with flabby ventricles and inflammation is relatively common. Myocardial necrosis may be present [608]. Cysts and free trophozoites may be demonstrated in myocardial fibers [75].

The lung is infrequently inflamed although mild interstitial pneumonitis may occur. It resembles viral pneumonitis if it is severe. Trophozoites can be found in vessels, septae, and pulmonary epithelium. Fibrosis does not usually occur [75].

The liver shows few changes although one case of giant cell transformation has been reported [608]. Hepatomegaly, bile stasis, bile duct proliferation, extramedullary hematopoiesis, and rarely, dystrophic calcification or portal fibrosis may also occur [75]. The pancreas is not usually involved but rarely may be necrotic with trophozoites and cysts [608].

Gastrointestinal and genitourinary tracts are not usually affected in congenital toxoplasmosis [75]. One case of necrotizing glomerulonephritis was described in an infant 11 days of age [608]. Renal petechiae, interstitial inflammation, and cysts in the bladder wall have all been seen in rare cases [75]. The testis may have necrotic seminiferous tubules but ovaries are spared [75, 608].

Unlike the lymphoid tissues of adults and children, fetal and neonatal lymph nodes and spleen show nonspecific changes such as precocious development of follicular centers [38]. Lymphadenopathy and splenomegaly are attended by karyorrhexis and extramedullary hematopoiesis [75, 608]. The bone marrow may show foci of necrosis with trophozoites [75].

Malaria

Malaria is uncommonly a cause of fetal or neonatal disease, probably because of the high incidence of maternal antibodies in the majority of females of childbearing age in endemic areas [120, 615, 616]. Intrauterine growth may be retarded in cases of maternal malaria [617]. Conversely, pregnancy may aggravate preexisting malaria in the gravida, particularly that due to *Plasmodium falciparum* [618].

Acute primary infection in the latter weeks of pregnancy can cause fetal disease [619]. While *P. falciparum* is the most common agent in such cases, all species of plasmodia have been recorded in neonates [620]. Measurement of antimalarial IgM in cord blood is diagnostic of intrauterine infection [621]. In some cases, smears of cord blood disclose the malaria parasites within red blood cells; in fatal cases, smears of organs, including brain, will disclose parasites [618, 622].

The placenta may show no gross abnormality [618, 623] but microscopically usually will have mild villitis or, in some instances, massive collections of maternal histiocytes in intervillous sinusoids. Malarial parasites can be seen in maternal red blood cells and malarial pigment can be found in villi [621, 624].

The fetal brain may show evidence of cerebral malaria, with ring hemorrhages around small cerebral arteries and veins. Similar hemorrhages occur in the fetal liver [625]. Splenomegaly is common and malarial pigment can be found in spleens [618].

Babesiosis

Transplacental infection with *Babesi microti* has been described in a full-term baby with parasites identified in 5% of fetal red blood cells. The infant recovered after treatment with clindamycin and quinine [626].

Trypanosomiasis

Trypanosoma brucei (subspecies *rhodesiense* or *gambiense*), transmitted by the tsetse fly, produces increased abortions, stillbirths, and preterm births with associated increased perinatal mortality. Pathologic features in these fetuses, infants, or their placentas have not been documented [627].

Trypanosma cruzi is the organism responsible for Chagas disease which is prevalent in all of South America, Central America, and occasionally extending into Texas. It is transmitted through the bite or the accidental ingestion of infected reduviid bugs. Armadillos, raccoons, and opossums can be infected; *T. cruzi* has been found in such animals as far to the northeast as Virginia [627].

Congenital infection has been described only in armadillos and humans [628, 629]. It is common in endemic areas and is transmitted either across the placenta or by aspiration or swallowing infected amniotic fluid. In humans, 2% of seropositive mothers will deliver infected fetuses or infants. Subsequent pregnancies are also at risk for infection [627]. About 30% of infected fetuses are stillborn; delivery rarely occurs at term and hydrops affects about 15% of the cases [628]. Target tissues are the placenta, cardiac muscle, gastrointestinal smooth muscle, lungs, central nervous system, and autonomic ganglia in contractile viscera [627–629]. Placentas are pale and boggy. Intracellular cysts with amastigote forms of the organism may be found in trophoblast, villous histiocytes (Hofbauer cells), and occasionally in the amnion. When the cysts rupture, free forms are released into adjacent tissues and into blood vessels to spread throughout the body. Severe necrotizing villitis may be seen in florid cases [628]. Hepatosplenomegaly, petechiae, anemia, jaundice with elevated unconjugated bilirubin in the serum, edema of myxedematous type, necrosis and hemorrhage in the skin, convulsions and tremors, megaesophagus, megaintestine, megaureters, and megacystis typify the infants infected with *T. cruzi* [628]. Myocardial disease affects fetuses and neonates with cardiac enlargement and a mononuclear inflammatory infiltrate in the interstitium [629] (Fig. 17.37). In the esophagus, intestines, ureters, and bladder, the ganglia are inflamed

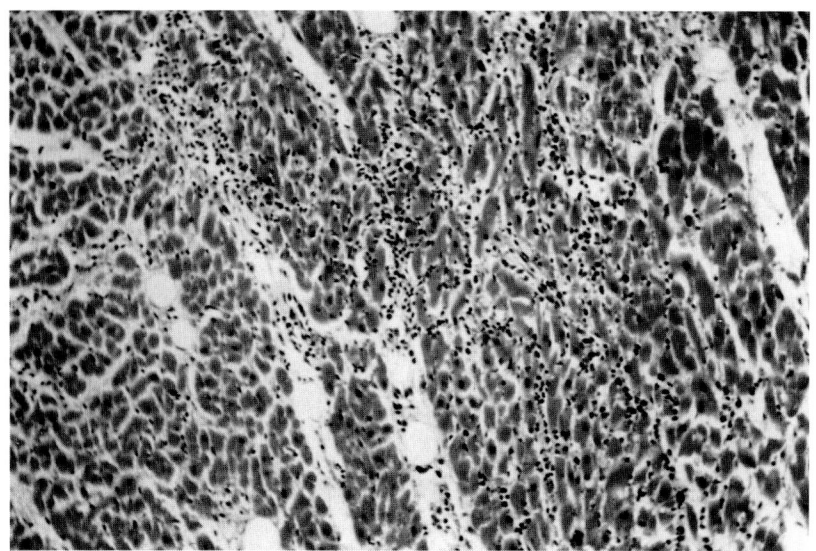

FIGURE 17.37. *Myocarditis in congenital Chagas disease. (H&E, approximately ×80.) (Photograph generously provided by Dr. B. DeGavaller, Newton, Massachusetts.)*

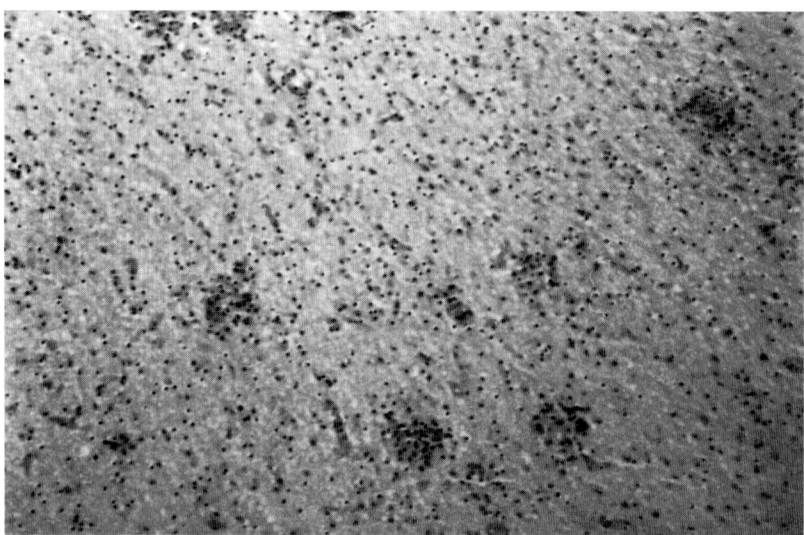

FIGURE 17.38. *Encephalitis in congenital Chagas disease. Note the punctate character of the lesions due to the perivascular distribution. (H&E, approximately ×80.) (Photograph generously provided by Dr. B. DeGavaller, Newton, Massachusetts.)*

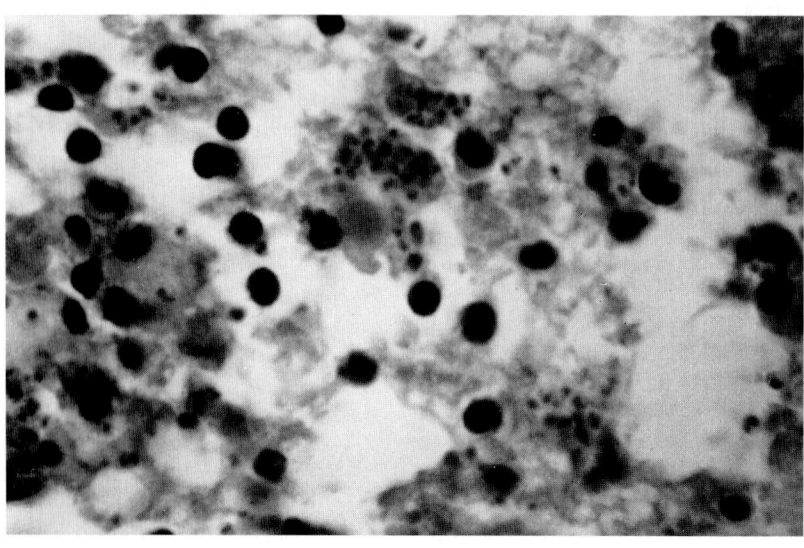

FIGURE 17.39. *Cysts and free forms (amastigotes) in the brain from a baby with congenital Chagas disease. (H&E, approximately ×490.) (Photograph generously provided by Dr. B. DeGavaller, Newton, Massachusetts.)*

with mononuclear inflammatory cells of all types, including plasma cells [628]. Visceral submucosal tissues and smooth muscle may also be inflamed with organisms demonstrable in the same areas. In the brain, perivascular cuffs of mononuclear inflammatory cells are found (Fig. 17.38). Parasitized cells may have either cyst forms or free amastigotes (Fig. 17.39). Subependymal granulomas with necroses may present as minute white nodules viewed en face in the ventricular lining. Precocious lymphoid follicles form, and fetal serum contains elevated levels of IgM antibodies specific for *T. cruzi* [628]. *T. cruzi* may be detected in the peripheral blood of infants. Skin may be inflamed with angiitis, fat necrosis, and subepidermal granulomas. Lungs are rarely involved but pneumonia has been described. Hepatic damage may be severe with extensive necrosis. Hepatic hematopoiesis is increased [628]. Some infected cells are gigantic, 100 to 200 μm in diameter.

Leishmaniasis

The visceral and cutaneous forms of leishmaniasis are transmitted by sandflies with wide distribution in temperate and tropical climates. Infants and young children are particularly susceptible to visceral leishmaniasis (kala azar). Congenital and neonatal infections have not been described [583].

REFERENCES

1. Crosby RMN, Mosberg WH Jr, GW S. Intrauterine meningitis as a cause of hydrocephalus. *J Pediatr* 1951; 39:94–101.
2. Duskes E, Dodge EF. Antenatal infection as a factor in fetal morbidity. *Am J Dis Child* 1928; 35:221–8.
3. Baker DA, Phillips CA. Maternal and neonatal infection with Coxsackie virus. *Obstet Gynecol* 1980; 55:12s–15s.
4. Christensen KK. Infection as a predominant cause of perinatal mortality. *Obstet Gynecol* 1982; 59:499–508.
5. Morison JE. *Foetal and neonatal pathology*. 2nd ed. London: Butterworth, 1963.
6. Naeye RL, Peters EC. Amniotic fluid infections with intact membranes leading to perinatal death: a prospective study. *Pediatrics* 1978; 61:171–7.
7. Davies PA, Gothefors LA. *Bacterial Infections in the Fetus and Newborn Infant*. Philadelphia: WB Saunders, 1984.
8. LaGamma EF, Drusin LM, Macles AW, Machalek S, Auld PAM. Neonatal infections. An important determination of late NICU mortality in infants less than 1000 g at birth. *Am J Dis Child* 1983; 137:838–41.
9. Becerra JE, Fry YW, Rowley DL. Morbidity estimates of conditions originating in the perinatal period: United States, 1986 through 1987. *Pediatrics* 1991; 88:553–9.
10. Benirschke K. Routes and types of infection in the fetus and newborn. *Am J Dis Child* 1960; 99:714–21.
11. Blanc WA. Pathways of fetal and early neonatal infection. Viral placentitis, bacterial and fungal chorioamnionitis. *J Pediatr* 1961; 59:473–96.
12. Slemons JM. Placental bacteremia. *J Am Med Assoc* 1915; 65:1265–8.
13. Lamont RF, Rose M, Elder MG. Effect of bacterial products on prostaglandin E production by amnion cells. *Lancet* 1985; ii:1331–3.
14. Minkoff H. Prematurity: infection as an etiologic factor. *Obstet Gynecol* 1983; 62:137–44.
15. Baker CJ, Barrett FF, Yow MD. The influence of advancing gestation on group B streptococcal colonization in pregnant women. *Am J Obstet Gynecol* 1975; 122:820–3.
16. Gibbs RS, Weinstein AJ. Puerperal infection in the antibiotic era. *Am J Obstet Gynecol* 1976; 124:769–87.
17. Naeye RL. Coitus and associated amniotic-fluid infections. *N Engl J Med* 1979; 301:1198–200.
18. Lenihan JP Jr. Relationship of antepartum pelvic examinations to premature rupture of the membranes. *Obstet Gynecol* 1984; 83:33–7.
19. Schlievert P, Larsen B, Johnson W, Galask R. Bacterial growth inhibition by amniotic fluid. *Am J Obstet Gynecol* 1975; 122:809–19.
20. Tafari N, Ross SM, Naeye RL, et al. Failure of bacterial growth inhibitor by amniotic fluid. *Am J Obstet Gynecol* 1977; 128:187–9.
21. Larsen B, Galask P. Host-parasite interactions during pregnancy. *Obstet Gynecol Surg* 1978; 33:297.
22. Fox H. *Pathology of the Placenta*. London: WB Saunders, 1978.
23. Lauweryns J, Bernat R, Lerut A, G D. Intrauterine pneumonia: an experimental study. *Biol Neonate* 1973; 22:301–18.
24. Orlowski JP, Sieger L, Anthony BF. Bactericidal capacity of monocytes of newborn infants. *J Pediatr* 1976; 89:797–801.
25. Davies PA. Bacterial infection in the fetus and new born. *Arch Dis Child* 1971; 46:1–29.
26. Shigeoka AO, Charette RP, Wyman ML, Hill HR. Defective oxidative metabolic responses of neutrophils from stressed neonates. *J Pediatr* 1981; 98:392–8.
27. Christensen RD, Rothstein G. Exhaustion of mature marrow neutrophils in neonates with sepsis. *J Pediatr* 1980; 96:316–18.
28. Squire E, Favara BE, Todd J. Diagnosis of neonatal bacterial infection: hematologic and pathologic findings in fatal and nonfatal cases. *Pediatrics* 1979; 64:60–4.
29. Stallmach T, Karolyi L. Augmentation of fetal granulopoiesis with chorioamnionitis during the second trimester of gestation. *Hum Pathol* 1994; 25:244–7.
30. Doron MW, Makhiouf RA, Katz VL, Lawson EE, Stiles AD. Increased incidence of sepsis at birth in neutropenic infants of mothers with preeclampsia. *J Pediatr* 1994; 125:452–8.
31. Engle WD, CR R. Neutropenia in high-risk neonates. *J Pediatr* 1984; 105:982–6.
32. Laurenti F, Feroo R, Isacchi G, et al. Polymorphonuclear leukocyte transfusion for the treatment of sepsis in the newborn infant. *J Pediatr* 1981; 98:118–23.
33. Hill HR. Phagocyte transfusion—ultimate therapy of neonatal disease. *J Pediatr* 1981; 98:59–61.
34. Murray JC, McClain KL, Wearden ME. Using granulocyte colony-stimulating factor for neutropenia during neonatal sepsis. *Arch Pediatr Adolesc Med* 1994; 148:764–6.
35. Givner LB, Nagaraj SK. Hyperimmune human IgG or recombinant human granulocyte-macrophage colony-stimulating factor as adjunctive therapy for group B streptococcal sepsis in newborn rats. *J Pediatr* 1993; 122:774–9.
36. Ogra PL. Ontogeny of the local immune system. *Pediatrics* 1979; 64:765–74.
37. Hayward AR, Lydyard PM. B-cell function in the newborn. *Pediatrics* 1979; 64(suppl):758–64.
38. Silverstein AM, Lukes RJ. Fetal response to antigenic stimulus. *Lab Invest* 1962; 11:918–32.
39. Einhorn MS, Granoff DM, Nahm MH, Quinn A, Shackelford PG. Concentrations of antibodies in paired maternal and infants sera: relationship to IgG subclass. *J Pediatr* 1987; 111:783–8.
40. Cairo MS, Worcester C, Rucker R, et al. Role of circulating complement and polymorphonuclear leukocyte transfusion in treatment and outcome in critically ill neonates with sepsis. *J Pediatr* 1987; 110:935–41.
41. Bain B. Down's syndrome. Transient abnormal myeloppoiesis and acute leukaemia. *Leuk Lymphoma* 1991; 3:309–17.
42. Jiang C-J, Liang D-C, Tien H-F. Neonatal transient leukaemoid proliferation followed by acute myeloid leukaemia in a phenotypically normal child. *Br J Haematol* 1991; 77:247–78.
43. Liang D-C, Ma S-W, Lu T-H, Lin S-T. Transient myeloproliferative disorder and acute myeloid leukemia: study of six neonatal cases with long-term follow-up. *Leukemia* 1993; 7:1521–4.
44. Fleming AD, Salafia CM, Vintzileos AM, et al. The relationships among umbilical artery velocimetry, fetal biophysical profile, and placental inflammation in preterm premature rupture of the membranes. *Am J Obstet Gynecol* 1991; 164:38–41.
45. Naeye RL BW. Unfavorable outcome of pregnancy: repeated losses. *Am J Obstet Gynecol* 1973; 116:1133–7.
46. Dische MR, Quinn PA, Czegledy-Nagy E, Sturgess JM. Genital mycoplasma infection. Intrauterine infection: pathologic study of the fetus and placenta. *Am J Clin Pathol* 1979; 72:167–74.
47. Singer DB, Campognone P. Perinatal group B streptococcal infection in midgestation. *Pediatr Pathol* 1986; 5:271–6.
48. Linder N, Ohel G, Gazit G, et al. Neonatal sepsis after prolonged premature rupture of membranes. *J Perinatol* 1995; 15:36–8.
49. Gaillard DA, Paradis P, Lallemand AV, et al. Spontaneous abortions during the second trimester of gestation. *Arch Pathol Lab Med* 1993; 117:1022–6.

50. Ariel I, Singer DB. *Streptococcus viridans* infections in midgestation. *Pediatr Pathol* 1991; 11:75–83.

51. Nadra L, Ariel I, Singer DB. Infections, preterm delivery, and perinatal death in midgestation. *Rhode Island Med J* 1991; 74:25–9.

52. Hauth JC, Gilstrap LC III, Hankins GDV, Connor KD. Term maternal and neonatal complications of acute chorioamnionitis. *Obstet Gynecol* 1985; 66:59–63.

53. Woods DL, Sinclair-Smith CC, Malan AF, Harrison A. Amniotic fluid infection at term. *S Afr Med J* 1978; 53:137–9.

54. Sperling RS, Ramamurthy RS, Gibbs RS. A comparison of intrapartum versus immediate postpartum treatment of intra-amniotic infection. *Obstet Gynecol* 1987; 70:861–5.

55. Driscoll SG. Genitourinary opportunists: mycoplasmas and chlamydiae. *Perspect Pediatr Pathol* 1981; 6:167–81.

56. Driscoll SG. Placental manifestations of malformation and infection. In: Greunwald P, ed. *The Placenta and Its Maternal Supply Line: Effects of Insufficiency on the Fetus*. Baltimore: University Park Press, 1975: pp. 244–59.

57. Woods DL, Edwards JNT, CC S-S. Amniotic fluid infection syndrome and abruptio placentae. *Pediatr Pathol* 1986; 6:81–5.

58. Svensson L, Ingemarsson I, Mårdh P-A. Chorioamnionitis and the isolation of microorganisms from the placenta. *Obstet Gynecol* 1986; 67:403–9.

59. Gravett MG, Hummel D, Eschenbach DA, Holmes KK. Preterm labor associated with subclinical amniotic fluid infection and with bacterial vaginosis. *Obstet Gynecol* 1986; 67:229–37.

60. Hillier SL, Krohn MA, Kiviat NB, Watts DH, Eschenbach DA. Microbiologic causes and neonatal outcomes associated with chorioamnion infection. *Am J Obstet Gynecol* 1991; 165:955–61.

61. Perkins RP, Zhou S-M, Butler C, Skipper BJ. Histologic chorioamnionitis in pregnancies of various gestational ages: implications in preterm rupture of membranes. *Obstet Gynecol* 1987; 70:856–60.

62. Hillier SL, Martius J, Krohng M, et al. A case-control study of chorioamnionic infection and histologic chorioamnionitis in prematurity. *N Engl J Med* 1988; 319:972–8.

63. Romero R, Salafia CM, Athanassiadis AP, et al. The relationship between acute inflammatory lesions of the preterm placenta and amniotic fluid microbiology. *Am J Obstet Gynecol* 1992; 166:1382–8.

64. Naeye RL, Maisels MJ, Lorenz RP, Botti JJ. The clinical significance of placental villous edema. *Pediatrics* 1983; 71:588–94.

65. Keenan WJ, Steichen JJ, Mahmood K, Altshuler G. Placental pathology compared with clinical outcome. A retrospective blind review. *Am J Dis Child* 1977; 131:1224–7.

66. Blanc WA. Pathology of the placenta, membranes and umbilical cord in bacterial, fungal, and viral infections in man. In: Naeye RL, Kissane JM, Kaufman N, eds. *Perinatal Diseases*. Baltimore: Williams & Wilkins, 1981, pp. 67–132.

67. Samson GR, Meyer MP, Blake DR, Cohen MC, Mouton SC. Syphilitic placentitis: an immunopathy. *Placenta* 1994; 15:67–77.

68. Qureshi F, Jacques SM, Reyes MP. Placental histopathology in syphilis. *Hum Pathol* 1993; 24:779–84.

69. Russell P. Inflammatory lesions of the human placenta. III. The histopathology of villitis of unknown aetiology. *Placenta* 1980; 1:227–44.

70. Redline RW, Patterson P. Villitis of unknown etiology is associated with major infiltration of fetal tissue by maternal inflammatory cells. *Am J Pathol* 1993; 143:473–9.

71. Popek EJ. Granulomatous villitis due to *Toxoplasma gondii*. *Pediatr Pathol* 1992; 12:281–8.

72. Becroft DMO. Prenatal cytomegalovirus infection: epidemiology, pathology, and pathogenesis. *Perspect Pediatr Pathol* 1981; 6:203–41.

73. Sachdev R, Nuovo GJ, Kaplan C, Greco MA. In situ hybridization analysis for cytomegalovirus in chronic villitis. *Pediatr Pathol* 1990; 10:909–17.

74. Oppenheimer EH, Dahms B. Congenital syphilis in the fetus and neonate. *Perspect Pediatr Pathol* 1981; 6:115–38.

75. Dische MR, Gooch WM III. Congenital toxoplasmosis. *Perspect Pediatr Pathol* 1981; 6:83–113.

76. Garcia AGP. Fetal infection in chickenpox and alastrim with histopathologic study of the placenta. *Pediatrics* 1963; 32:895–901.

77. Robertson NJ, McKeever PA. Fetal and placental pathology in two cases of maternal varicella infection. *Pediatr Pathol* 1992; 12:545–50.

78. Greco MA, Wieczorek R, Sachdev R, et al. Phenotype of villous stromal cells in placentas with cytomegalovirus, syphilis, and nonspecific villitis. *Am J Pathol* 1992; 141:835–42.

79. Schwartz DA, Khan R, Stoll B. Characterization of the fetal inflammatory response to cytomegalovirus placentitis. An immunohistochemical study. *Arch Path Lab Med* 1992; 116:21–7.

80. Altshuler G, Russell P. The human placental villitides: a review of chronic intrauterine infection. *Curr Top Pathol* 1975; 60:64–112.

81. Labarrere C, Altnabe O, Telenta M. Chorionic villitis of unknown aetiology in placentae of idiopathic small for gestational age infants. *Placenta* 1982; 3:309–18.

82. Altemani AM. Immunohistochemical study of the inflammatory infiltrate in villitis of unknown etiology. A qualitative and quantitative analysis. *Pathol Res Pract* 1992; 188:303–9.

83. Ilagan NB, Elias EG, Liang KC, et al. Perinatal and neonatal significance of bacteria-related placental villous edema. *Acta Obstet Gynecol Scand* 1990; 69:287–90.

84. Shen-Schwarz S, Ruchelli E, Brown D. Villous oedema of the placenta: a clinicopathological study. *Placenta* 1989; 10:297–307.

85. Martin AW, Smith SI, DeCoste D, et al. Immunohistochemical localization of human immunodeficiency virus p24 antigen in placental tissue. *Hum Pathol* 1992; 23:411–14.

86. Molnar-Nadasdy G, Haesly I, Reed J, Altshuler G. Placental cryptococcosis in a mother with systemic lupus erythematosus. *Arch Pathol Lab Med* 1994; 118:757–9.

87. Driscoll SG. Histopathology of gestational rubella. *Am J Dis Child* 1969; 118:49–53.

88. Altemani AM, Fassoni A, Marba S. Cord IgM levels in placentas with villitis of unknown etiology. *J Perinat Med* 1989; 17:465–8.

89. Gersell DJ, Phillips NJ, Beckerman K. Chronic chorioamnionitis: a clinicopathologic study of 17 cases. *Int J Gynecol Pathol* 1991; 10:217–29.

90. Gersell DJ. Chronic villitis, chronic chorioamnionitis, and maternal floor infarction. *Semin Diag Pathol* 1993; 10:251–66.

91. Christensen KK, Dahlander K, Ingemarsson I, et al. Relation between maternal urogenital carriage to group B streptococci and postmaturity and intrauterine asphyxia during delivery. *Scan J Infect Dis* 1978; 12:272–6.

92. Haesaert B, Ornoy A. Transplacental effects of endotoxemia on fetal mouse brain, bone, and placental tissue. *Pediatr Pathol* 1986; 5:167–81.

93. Tate DY, Carlton GT, Johnson D, et al. Immune thrombocytopenia in severe neonatal infections. *J Pediatr* 1981; 98:449–53.

94. Mardini MK. Septic shock in neonates, infants, and children. *King Faisal Specialist Hosp Med J* 1982; 2:47–53.

95. Ruebner BH, Bhagaran BS, Greenfield AJ, Campbell P, Danks DM. Neonatal hepatic necrosis. *Pediatrics* 1969; 43:963–70.

96. Pearlman MA, Gartner LM, Lee K-S, et al. The association of kernicterus with bacterial infection in the newborn. *Pediatrics* 1980; 65:26–9.

97. Shaul WL. Clues to the early diagnosis of neonatal appendicitis. *J Pediatr* 1981; 98:473–6.

98. Davies PA, Gothefors LA. *Bacterial Infections in the Fetus and Newborn Infant*. Philadelphia: WB Saunders, 1984.

99. Dillon HC Jr. Prevention of gonococcal ophthalmia neonatorum. *N Engl J Med* 1986; 315:1414–5.

100. Rowe DS, Aicardi EZ, Dawson CR, Schachter J. Purulent ocular discharge in neonates: significance of *Chlamydia trachomatis*. *Pediatrics* 1979; 63:628–32.

101. Philip AG. Acute-phase proteins in neonatal infection. *J Pediatr* 1984; 105:940–2.

102. Naeye RL. Causes of the excessive rates of perinatal mortality and prematurity in pregnancies complicated by maternal urinary tract infections. *N Engl J Med* 1979; 300:819–23.

103. Gleckman R. The controversy of treatment of asymptomatic bacteriuria in nonpregnant women—resolved. *J Urol* 1976; 116:776–7.

104. Beeram MR, Young M, Abedin M. Effect of maternal illicit drug use on the mortality of very low birth weight infants. *J Perinatol* 1995; 15:456–60.

105. Cherouny PH, Pankuch GA, Botti JJ, Appelbaum PC. The presence of amniotic fluid leukoattractants accurately identifies histologic chorioamnionitis and predicts tocolytic efficacy in patients with idiopathic preterm labor. *Am J Obstet Gynecol* 1992; 167:683–8.

106. Greig PC, Ernest JM, Teot L, Erikson M, Talley R. Amniotic fluid interleukin-6 levels correlate with histologic chorioamnionitis and amniotic fluid cultures in patients in premature labor with intact membranes. *Am J Obstet Gynecol* 1993; 169:1035–44.

107. Romero R, Mazor M, Sepulveda W, et al. Tumor necrosis factor in preterm and term labor. *Am J Obstet Gynecol* 1992; 166:1567–87.

108. Lencki SG, Maciulla MB, Eglinton GS. Maternal and umbilical cord serum interleukin levels in preterm labor with clinical chorioamnionitis. *Am J Obstet Gynecol* 1994; 170:1345–51.

109. Coultrip LL, Grossman JH. Evaluation of rapid diagnostic tests in the detection of microbial invasion of the amniotic cavity. *Am J Obstet Gynecol* 1992; 167:1231–42.

110. Manroe BL, Weinberg AG, Rosenfeld CR, Browne R. The neonatal blood count in health and disease. I. Reference values for neutrophilic cells. *J Pediatr* 1979; 95:89–98.

111. Rodwell RL, Leslie AL, Tudehope DI. Early diagnosis of neonatal sepsis using a hematologic scoring system. *J Pediatr* 1988; 112:761–7.

112. Shimoya K, Matsuzaki N, Taniguchi T, et al. Interleukin-8 in cord sera: a sensitive and specific marker for the detection of preterm chorioamnionitis. *J Infect Dis* 1992; 165:957–60.

113. Boyle RJ, Chandler BD, Stonestreet BS, Oh W. Early identification of sepsis in infants with respiratory distress. *Pediatrics* 1978; 62:744–50.

114. Voora S, Srinivasan G, Lilien LD, Yeh TF, Pildes RS. Fever in full-term newborns in the first four days of life. *Pediatrics* 1982; 69:40–4.

115. Todd JT, Roe MH. Rapid detection of bacteremia by an early subculture technique. *Am J Clin Pathol* 1975; 64:694–9.

116. Sáe-Llorens X, McCracken GH Jr. Sepsis syndrome and septic shock in pediatrics: current concepts of terminology, pathophysiology, and management. *J Pediatr* 1993; 123:497–508.

117. Levi M, tenCate H, van der Poll T, van Deventer SJH. Pathogenesis of disseminated intravascular coagulation in sepsis. *JAMA* 1993; 270:975–9.

118. Johnson WC, Meyer JR. A study of pneumonia in the stillborn and newborn. *Am J Obstet Gynecol* 1925; 9:151–67.

119. Bernstein J, Wang J. The pathology of neonatal pneumonia. *Am J Dis Child* 1961; 101:350–63.

120. Potter EL, Craig JM. *Pathology of the Fetus and the Infant*. 3rd ed. Chicago: Year Book Medical Publishers, 1975.

121. Scott RJ, Peat D, Rhodes CA. Investigation of the fetal pulmonary inflammatory reaction in chorioamnionitis using an in situ Y chromosome marker. *Pediatr Pathol* 1994; 14:997–1003.

122. Ablow RC, Driscoll SG, Effmann EL, et al. A comparison of early-onset group B streptococcal neonatal infection and the respiratory distress syndrome of the newborn. *N Engl J Med* 1976; 294:65–9.

123. Farber S, Wilson JL. The hyaline membrane in the lungs. I. A descriptive study. *Arch Pathol* 1932; 14:437–49.

124. Jacob J, Edwards D, Gluck L. Early-onset sepsis and pneumonia observed as respiratory distress syndrome. *Am J Dis Child* 1980; 134:766–8.

125. Teplitz C. Pathogenesis of pseudomonas vasculitis and septic lesions. *Arch Pathol* 1965; 80:297–307.

126. Wiswell TE, Baumgart S, Gannon CM, Spitzer AR. No lumbar puncture in the evaluation for early neonatal sepsis: will meningitis be missed? *Pediatrics* 1995; 95:803–6.

127. Ostrow PT, Moxon ER, Vernon N, Kapko R. Pathogenesis of bacterial meningitis. Studies on the route of meningeal invasion following *Haemophilus influenzae* inoculation of infant rats. *Lab Invest* 1979; 40:678–85.

128. Murphy DJ, Sellers S, MacKenzie IZ, Uudkin PL, Johnson AM. Case-control study of antenatal and intrapartum risk factors for cerebral palsy in very preterm singleton babies. *Lancet* 1995; 346:1449–54.

129. Franco SM, Cornelius VE, Andrews BF. Long-term outcome of neonatal meningitis. *Am J Dis Child* 1992; 146:567–71.

130. Baker CJ. Group B streptococcal infection in newborns. Prevention at last? *N Engl J Med* 1986; 314:1702–4.

131. Murphy N, Buchanan CR, Damjanovic V, et al. Infection and colonization of neonates by *Hansenula anomala*. *Lancet* 1986; i:291–3.

132. Powell DA, Aungst J, Snedden S, Hansen N, Brady M. Broviac catheter-related *Malassezia furfur* sepsis in five infants receiving intravenous fat emulsions. *J Pediatr* 1984; 105:987–90.

133. Redline RW, Redline SS, Boxerbaum B, Dahms BB. Systemic *Malassezia furfur* infections in patients receiving intralipid therapy. *Hum Pathol* 1985; 16:815–22.

134. Vawter GF. Listeria monocytogenes: the perinatal infection. *Perspect Pediatr Pathol* 1981; 6:153–66.

135. Walsh MC, Simpser EF, Kliegman RM. Late onset of sepsis in infants with bowel resection in the neonatal period. *J Pediatr* 1988; 112:468–71.

136. Singer DB. Pathology of neonatal herpes simplex virus infection. *Perspect Pediatr Pathol* 1981; 6:243–78.

137. MacGregor AP. Pneumonia in the newborn. *Arch Dis Child* 1939; 14:323–31.

138. Moss TJ, Pysher TJ. Hepatic abscess in neonates. *Am J Dis Child* 1981; 135:726–8.

139. Lilien LD, Harris VJ, Ramamurthy RS, Pildes RS. Neonatal osteomyelitis of the calcaneus: complication of heel puncture. *J Pediatr* 1976; 88:478–80.

140. Ginsburg CM, McCracken GH Jr. Urinary tract infection in young infants. *Pediatrics* 1982; 69:409–12.

141. Book LS, Overall JC Jr, Herbst JJ, et al. Interruption of necrotizing enterocolitis clustering by infection control measures. *N Engl J Med* 1977; 197:984–5.

142. Han VKM, Sayed H, Chance GW, Brabyn DG, Shaheed WA. An outbreak of *Clostridium difficile* necrotizing enterocolitis: a case for oral vancomycin therapy. *Pediatrics* 1983; 71:935–41.

143. McCracken GH Jr, Eitzman DV. Necrotizing enterocolitis. *Am J Dis Child* 1972; 132:1167–8.

144. McGuinness GA, Schieken RM, Maguire GF. Endocarditis in the newborn. *Am J Dis Child* 1980; 134:577–80.

145. Arya S, Hong R, Gilbert EF. Reactive hemophagocytic syndrome. *Pediatr Pathol* 1985; 3:129–41.

146. Southern P, Oldstone MBA. Medical consequences of persistent viral infection. *N Engl J Med* 1986; 314:359–67.

147. Fox MJ, Krumbiegel ER, Teresi JL. Maternal measles, mumps and chickenpox as a cause of congenital anomalies. *Lancet* 1948; i:746.

148. Johnson RT. Effects of viral infection on the developing nervous system. *N Engl J Med* 1972; 287:599–604.

149. Koskimies O, Lapinleimu K, Saxen L. Infections and other maternal factors as risk indicators for congenital malformations: a case control study with paired serum samples. *Pediatrics* 1978; 61:832–7.

150. Zuelzer WW, Stulberg CS. Herpes simplex virus as the cause of fulminating visceral disease and hepatitis in infancy. Report of eight cases and isolation of the virus in one case. *Am J Dis Child* 1952; 83:421–6.

151. Siegel M, Fuerst HT, Peress NS. Comparative fetal mortality in maternal virus diseases. A prospective study on rubella, measles, mumps, chickenpox, and hepatitis. *N Engl J Med* 1966; 274:768–71.

152. Siegel M. Congenital malformations following chickenpox, measles, mumps, and hepatitis. Results of a cohort study. *J Am Med Assoc* 1973; 226:1521–4.

153. Gregg NM. Congenital cataract following German measles in the mother. *Trans Ophthalmol Soc Aust* 1941; 3:35–46.

154. Esterly JR, Oppenheimer EH. Pathological lesions due to congenital rubella. *Arch Pathol* 1969; 87:380–91.

155. Rudolph AJ, Yow MD, Phillips CA, et al. Transplacental rubella in newly born infants. *J Am Med Assoc* 1965; 191:843–5.

156. Singer DB, Rudolph AJ, Rosenberg HS, Rawls WE. Pathology of the congenital rubella syndrome. *J Pediatr* 1967; 71:665–75.

157. Singleton EB, Rudolph AJ, Rosenberg HS, Singer DB. The roentgenographic manifestations of the rubella syndrome in newborn infants. *Am J Roentgenol Radium Ther Nucl Med* 1967; 97:82–91.

158. Naeye RL, Blanc WA. Pathogenesis of congenital rubella. *J Am Med Assoc* 1965; 194:1277–83.

159. Rawls WE, Melnick JL. Rubella virus carrier cultures derived from congenitally infected infants. *J Exp Med* 1966; 123:795–816.

160. Rosenberg HS, Oppenheimer EH, Esterly JR. Congenital rubella syndrome: the late effects and their relation to early lesions. *Perspect Pediatr Pathol* 1981; 6:183–202.

161. Enders G, Nickerl-Pacher U, Miller E, Cradock-Watson JE. Outcome of confirmed periconceptional maternal rubella. *Lancet* 1988; i:1445–6.

162. Miller E, Cradock-Watson JE, Pollock TM. Consequences of confirmed maternal rubella at successive stages of pregnancy. *Lancet* 1982; ii:781–4.

163. Blanc WA. Pathology of the placenta and cord in some viral infections. In: Hanshaw JB, JA Dudgeon, eds. *Viral Diseases of the Fetus and Newborn*. Philadelphia: WB Saunders, 1978, pp. 237–58.

164. Baublis JV, Brown GC. Specific response of the immunoglobulins to rubella infections. *Proc Soc Exp Biol Med* 1968; 128:206–10.

165. Singer DB, South MA, Montgomery JR, Rawls WE. Congenital rubella syndrome, lymphoid tissue and immunologic status. *Am J Dis Child* 1969; 118:54–61.

166. Esterly JR, Oppenheimer EH. Intrauterine rubella infection. *Perspect Pediatr Pathol* 1973; 1:313–8.

167. Simpson JW, Nora JJ, Singer DB, McNamara DG. Multiple valvular sclerosis in Turner phenotype and rubella syndrome. *Am J Cardiol* 1969; 23:94–7.

168. Strauss L, Bernstein J. Neonatal hepatitis in congenital rubella. *Arch Pathol* 1968; 86:317–27.

169. Reed G. Rubella bone lesions. *J Pediatr* 1969; 74:208–13.

170. Desmond MM, Fisher ES, Vorderman AL, et al. The longitudinal course of congenital rubella encephalitis in nonretarded children. *J Pediatr* 1978; 93:584–91.

171. Desmond MM, Wilson GS, Melnick JL, et al. Congenital rubella encephalitis. *J Pediatr* 1967; 71:311–31.

172. Rorke LB. Nervous system lesions in congenital rubella syndrome. *Arch Otolaryngol* 1973; 98:249–51.

173. Swisher CN, Swisher L. Congenital rubella and autistic behavior. *N Engl J Med* 1975; 293:198.

174. Desmond MM, Wilson GS, Melnick JL, et al. The health and educational status of adolescents with congenital rubella syndrome. *Dev Med Child Neurol* 1985; 27:721–9.

175. Preblud SR, Stetler HC, Frank JA Jr, et al. Fetal risk associated with rubella vaccine. *J Am Med Assoc* 1981; 246:1413–7.

176. Preblud SR. Some current issues relating to rubella vaccine. *J Am Med Assoc* 1985; 254:253–6.

177. Polk BF, White JA, DeGirolami PC, Modlin JF. An outbreak of rubella among hospital personnel. *N Engl J Med* 1980; 303:541–5.

178. *Morbidity and Mortality Weekly Report.* 1987; 36:91–6.

179. Larroche J-C. *Developmental Pathology of the Neonate.* Amsterdam: Excerpta Medica, 1977.

180. Potter EL. Placental transmission of viruses with especial reference to the intrauterine origin of cytomegalic inclusion body disease. *Am J Obstet Gynecol* 1957; 74:505–13.

181. Nankervis GA, Bhumbra NA. Cytomegalovirus infection of neonate and infant. *Adv Pediatr Infect Dis* 1986; 1:61–74.

182. Wyatt JP, Saxton J, Lee RS, Pinkerton H. Generalized cytomegalic inclusion disease. *J Pediatr* 1950; 36:271–93.

183. Fetterman GH. A new laboratory aid in the clinical diagnosis of inclusion disease of infancy. *Am J Clin Pathol* 1952; 22:424–7.

184. Reynolds DW, Stagno S, Stubbs KG, et al. Inapparent congenital cytomegalovirus with elevated cord IgM levels. *N Engl J Med* 1974; 290:291–6.

185. Cederqvist LL, Abdel-Latiff N, Meyer J, Doctor L. Fetal and maternal humoral immune response to cytomegalovirus infection. *Obstet Gynecol* 1986; 67:214–6.

186. Davis LE, Tweed GV, Chin TDY, Miller GL. Intrauterine diagnosis of cytomegalovirus infection: viral recovery from amniocentesis fluid. *Am J Obstet Gynecol* 1971; 109:1217–21.

187. Kinney JS, Onorato IM, Stewart JA, et al. Cytomegalovirus infection and disease. *J Infect Dis* 1985; 151:772–4.

188. Stagno S, Pass RF, Dworsky ME, et al. Congenital cytomegalovirus infection. The relative importance of primary and recurrent maternal infection. *N Engl J Med* 1982; 306:945–9.

189. Plotkin SA. Prevention of cytomegalovirus infection. *J R Soc Med* 1984; 77:94–5.

190. Ahlfors CE, Harris S, Ivarsson S, Svanberg L. Secondary maternal cytomegalovirus infection causing symptomatic congenital infection. *N Engl J Med* 1981; 305:284.

191. Huang ES, Alford CA, Reynods DW, Stagno S, Pass RF. Molecular epidemiology of cytomegalo-virus infection in women and their infants. *N Engl J Med* 1980; 303:958–62.

192. Dworsky ME, Stagno S. Occupational risk for primary CMV infection among pediatric health care workers. *N Engl J Med* 1983; 309:950–3.

193. Spector SA, Schmidt K, Ticknor W, Grossman M. Cytomegaloviruria in older infants in intensive care nurseries. *J Pediatr* 1979; 95:444–6.

194. Kalmin ND. Transfusion of cytomegalovirus: a review of the problem. *Lab Med* 1981; 12:489–91.

195. Sandler SG, Grumet FC. Posttransfusion cytomegalovirus infections. *Pediatrics* 1982; 59:650–2.

196. Hayes K, Danks DM, Gibas H, Jack I. Cytomegalovirus in human milk. *N Engl J Med* 1972; 287:177–8.

197. Ballard RA, Drew WL, Hufnagle KG, Riedel PA. Acquired cytomegalovirus in preterm infants. *Am J Dis Child* 1979; 133:482–5.

198. Benirschke K, Mendoza GR, Bazelay PL. Placental and fetal manifestations of cytomegalovirus infection. *Virchows Arch B* 1974; 16:121–39.

199. Mostoufi-Zadeh M, Driscoll SG, Biano SA, Kundsin RB. Placental evidence of cytomegalovirus infection of the fetus and neonate. *Arch Pathol Lab Med* 1984; 108:403–6.

200. Wilken H. Important clinical aspects of prenatal viral infections. *J Perinat Med* 1978; 6:257–74.

201. Morton R. Congenital cytomegalovirus infection presenting as massive ascites with secondary pulmonary hypoplasia. *Hum Pathol* 1986; 17:760.

202. Stocker JT. Congenital cytomegalovirus infection presenting as massive ascites with secondary pulmonary hypoplasia. *Hum Pathol* 1985; 16:1173–5.

203. Frenkel LD, Keys MP, Hefferen SJ, Rola-Pleszczynski M, Bellanti JA. Unusual eye abnormalities asociated with congenital cytomegalovirus infection. *Pediatrics* 1980; 66:763–6.

204. Rich AR. *The Pathogenesis of Tuberculosis.* 2nd ed. Springfield, IL: CC Thomas, 1951.

205. Kershisnik MM, Knisely AS, Sun C-CJ, Andrews JM, Wittwer CT. Cytomegalovirus infection, fetal liver disease, and neonatal hemochromatosis. *Hum Pathol* 1992; 23:1075–80.

206. Finegold MJ, Carpenter RJ. Obliterative cholangitis due to cytomegalovirus. A possible precursor of paucity of intrahepatic bile ducts. *Hum Pathol* 1982; 13:662–5.

207. Dimmick JE, Bove K. Cytomegalovirus infection of the bowel in infancy. Pathogenetic and diagnostic significance. *Pediatr Pathol* 1984; 2:95–102.

208. Sonsino E, Mony R, Foucand P, et al. Intestinal pseudoobstruction related to cytomegalovirus infection of myenteric plexus. *N Engl J Med* 1984; 311:196–7.

209. Déchelotte PJ MN, Bouvier RJ, Vanlieféringhen PC, Lémery DJ. Pseudo-meconium ileus due to cytomegalovirus infection: a report of three cases. *Pediat Pathol* 1992; 12:73–82.

210. Midulla M, Marzetti G, Bertolini L, et al. Generalized cytomegalic inclusion disease, hypergammaglobulinemia, and antithrombin activity in a newborn infant. *Helv Paediatr Acta* 1968; 23:205–10.

211. Kumar ML, Jenson HB, Dahms BB. Fatal *Staphylococcus epidermidis* infections in very-low-birth-weight infants with cytomegalovirus infection. *Pediatrics* 1985; 76:110–2.

212. Joncas JH, Alfieri C, Leyritz-Wills M, et al. Simultaneous congenital infection with Epstein-Barr virus and cytomegalovirus. *N Engl J Med* 1981; 304:1399–1403.

213. Singer DB. Pathology of neonatal herpes simplex virus infection. *Perspect Pediatr Pathol* 1981; 6:243–78.

214. Thoene J, Sweetman L, Shfai T, et al. Tyrosinemia associated with perinatal infections with cytomegalovirus. *J Pediatr* 1978; 92:108–12.

215. Pass RF, Stagno S, Myers GJ, Alford CA. Outcome of symptomatic congenital cytomegalovirus infection: results of long-term longitudinal follow-up. *Pediatrics* 1980; 66:758–62.

216. Williamson WD, Desmond MM, LeFevers N, et al. Symptomatic congenital cytomegalovirus. Disorders of language, learning, and hearing. *Am J Dis Child* 1982; 136:902–5.

217. Witzleben CL, Driscoll SG. Possible transplacental transmission of herpes simplex infection. *Pediatrics* 1965; 36:192–9.

218. Light IJ. Postnatal acquisition of herpes simplex virus by the newborn infant. A review of the literature. *Pediatrics* 1979; 163:480–2.

219. Parvey LS, Ch'ien LT. Neonatal herpes simplex virus infection introduced by fetal-monitor scalp electrodes. *Pediatrics* 1980; 65:1150–3.

220. Brown ZA, Vontver LA, Benedetti J, et al. Effects on infants of a first episode of genital herpes during pregnancy. *N Engl J Med* 1987; 317:1246–51.

221. Prober CG, Sullender WM, Yasukawa LL, et al. Low risk of herpes simplex virus infections in neonates exposed to the virus at the time of vaginal delivery to mothers with recurrent genital herpes simplex virus infections. *N Engl J Med* 1987; 316:240–4.

222. Randolph AG, Eugene Washington, Prober CG. Cesarean delivery for women presenting with genital herpes lesions. *JAMA* 1993; 270:77–82.

223. Zervoudakis IA, Silverman F, Senterfil LB, et al. Herpes simplex in the amniotic fluid of an unaffected fetus. *Obstet Gynecol* 1980; 55:16s–17s.

224. Arvin AM, Hensleigh PA, Prober CG, et al. Failure of antepartum maternal cultures to predict infants risk of exposure to herpes simplex virus at delivery. *N Engl J Med* 1986; 315:796–800.

225. JAMA. Leads from the MMWR. *JAMA* 1986; 256:575.

226. Woodman CBJ, Weaver JB. Virological screening for herpes simplex virus (HSV) in late pregnancy. *Lancet* 1986; i:744.

227. Brown ZA, Benedetti J, Ashley R, et al. Neonatal herpes simplex virus infection in relation to asymptomatic maternal infection at the time of labor. *N Engl J Med* 1991; 324:1247–52.

228. Whitley R, Arvin A, Prober C, et al. Predictors of morbidity and mortality in neonates with herpes simplex virus infections. *N Engl J Med* 1991; 324:450–4.

229. Halperin SA, Hendley JO, Nosal C, Roizman B. DNA fingerprinting in investigation of apparent nosocomial acquisition of neonatal herpes simplex. *J Pediatr* 1980; 97:91–3.

230. Corey L, Spear PG. Infections with herpes simplex viruses. *N Engl J Med* 1986; 314:686–91.

231. Nachtigal M, Caulfield JB. Early and late pathologic changes in the adrenal glands of mice after infection with herpes simplex virus type 1. *Am J Pathol* 1984; 115:175–85.

232. Kohl S, Frazier JJ, Greenberg SB, Pickering LK, Loo L-S. Interferon induction of natural killer cytotoxicity in human neonates. *J Pediatr* 1981; 98:379–84.

233. Daniels PA, Bodner S, Trofatter KF Jr. Scanning and transmission electron microscopic studies of complement-mediated lysis and antibody-dependent cell-mediated cytolysis of herpes simplex virus-infected human fibroblasts. *Am J Pathol* 1980; 100:663–82.

234. Hutto C, Arvin A, Jacobs R, et al. Intrauterine herpes simplex virus infections. *J Pediatr* 1987; 110:97–101.

235. South MA, Tompkins WAF, Morris CR, Rawls WE. Congenital malformation of the central nervous system associated with genital (type 2) herpesvirus. *J Pediatr* 1969; 75:13–7.

236. Arvin AM, Yeager AS, Bruhn FW, Grossman M. Neonatal herpes simplex infection in the absence of mucocutaneous lesions. *J Pediatr* 1982; 100:715–21.

237. Schwartz DA, Caldwell E. Herpes simplex virus infection of the placenta. The role of molecular pathology in the diagnosis of viral infection of placental-associated tissues. *Arch Pathol Lab Med* 1991; 115:1141–4.

238. Bendon RW, Perez F, Ray MB. Herpes simplex virus: fetal and decidual infection. *Pediatr Pathol* 1987; 7:63–70.

239. Robb JA, Benirschke K. Intrauterine herpes simplex virus infection in spontaneous abortions: chronic persistent infection detectd by glucose oxidase-avidin-biotin immunohistochemistry. *Lab Invest* 1984; 50:50a.

240. Heifetz SA BM. Necrotizing funisitis and herpes simplex infection of placental and decidual tissues: study of four cases. *Hum Pathol* 1994; 25:715–22.

241. Greene GR, King D, Romansky SG, Marble RD. Primary herpes simplex pneumonia in a neonate. *Am J Dis Child* 1983; 137:464–5.

242. Nahmias AJ, Alford CA, Korones SB. Infection of the newborn with *Herpesvirus hominis*. *Adv Pediatr* 1970; 17:285ff.

243. Drut RM, Drut R. Giant-cell myocarditis in a newborn with congenital herpes simplex virus (HSV) infection: an immunohistochemical study on the origin of the giant cells. *Pediatr Pathol* 1986; 6:431–7.

244. Mirra JM. Aortitis and malakoplakia-like lesions of the brain in association with neonatal herpes simplex. *Am J Clin Pathol* 1971; 56:104–10.

245. Karna P, Broecker AH. Neonatal herpes gestationis. *J Pediatr* 1991; 119:299–301.

246. Jay V, Becker LE, Blaser S, et al. Pathology of chronic herpes infection associated with seizure disorder: a report of two cases with tissue detection of herpes simplex virus by the polymerase chain reaction. *Pediatr Pathol Lab Med* 1995; 15:131–46.

247. Chang C-H, Nigro MA, Perrin EV. Cerebral malakoplakia and neonatal herpes simplex infection. *Arch Pathol Lab Med* 1980; 104:494–5.

248. Englund JA, Fletcher CV, Balfour HH J. Acyclovir therapy in neonates. *J Pediatr* 1991; 119:129–35.

249. Brunell PA. Prevention and treatment of neonatal herpes. *Pediatrics* 1980; 66:806–7.

250. Feder HM. Disseminated herpes simplex infection in a neonate during prophylaxis with vidarabine. *J Am Med Assoc* 1988; 259:1054–5.

251. Cherry JD. Enteroviruses. In: Remington JS, Klein JO, eds. *Infectious Diseases of the Fetus and Newborn Infant*. 4th ed. Philadelphia: WB Saunders, 1995: pp. 404–46.

252. Modlin JF. Perinatal echovirus and group B coxsackievirus infections. *Clin Perinatol* 1988; 15:233–47.

253. Kaplan MH, Klein SW, McPhee J, Harper RG. Group B coxsackievirus infections in infants younger than three months of age: a serious childhood illness. *Rev Infect Dis* 1983; 5:1019–32.

254. Krajden S, Middleton PJ. Enterovirus infections in the neonate. *Clin Pediatr* 1983; 22:87–92.

255. Haddad J, Gut JP, Wendling MJ, et al. Enterovirus infections in neonates. A retrospective study of 21 cases. *Eur J Med* 1993; 2:209–14.

256. Baltcup G, Holt P, Hambling MH, et al. Placental and fetal pathology in coxsackie virus A9 infection: a case report. *Histopathology* 1985; 9:1227.

257. Garcia AG, Basso NG, Fonseca ME, Zuardi JA, Outanni HN. Enterovirus associated placental morphology: a light, virological, electron microscopic and immunohistologic study. *Placenta* 1991; 12:533–47.

258. Benirschke K, Kaufmann P. *Pathology of the Human Placenta*. 2nd ed. New York: Springer-Verlag, 1990.

259. Bowles NE, Richardson PJ, Olsen EGJ, Archarel LC. Detection of coxsackie-B-virus-specific RNA sequences in myocardial biopsy samples from patients with myocarditis and dilated myocardiopathy. *Lancet* 1986; i:1120–3.

260. Redline RW GD, Tycko B. Detection of enteroviral infection in paraffin-embedded tissue by the RNA polymerase chain reaction technique. *Am J Clin Pathol* 1991; 96:568–71.

261. Gauntt CJ, Gudrangen RJ, Brans YW, Marlin AE. Coxsackievirus group B antibodies in the ventricular fluid of infants with severe anatomic defects in the central nervous system. *Pediatrics* 1985; 76:64–8.

262. Schlesinger Y, Sawyer JH, Storch GA. Enteroviral meningitis in infancy: potential role for polymerase chain reaction inpatient management. *Pediatrics* 1994; 94:157–62.

263. LaForce FM. Enteroviral infections. In: Hunter GW III, Swartzwelder JC, Clyde DF, eds. *Hunter's Tropical Medicine*. 6th ed. Philadelphia: WB Saunders, 1984: pp. 121–4.

264. Modlin JF, Kinney JS. Perinatal enterovirus infections. *Adv Pediatr Infect Dis* 1987; 2:57–78.

265. Elliott GB, McAllister JE. Fetal poliomyelitis. *Am J Obstet Gynecol* 1956; 72:896–902.

266. Isacsohn M, Eidelman AI, Kaplan M, et al. Neonatal coxsackievirus group B infections: experience of a single department of neonatology. *Israel J Med Sci* 1994; 30:371–4.

267. Avoiding the danger of enteroviruses to newborn infants. *Lancet* 1986; i:194–5.

268. Valduss D, Murray DL, Karna P, Lapour K, Dyke J. Use of intravenous immunoglobulin in twin neonates with disseminated coxsackie B1 infection. *Clin Pediatr* 1993; 32:561–3.

269. Singer DB. Infections of fetuses and neonates. In: Wigglesworth JS, Singer DB, eds. *Textbook of Fetal and Perinatal Pathology*. Boston: Blackwell Scientific, 1991: pp. 525–91.

270. Gauntt CJ, Arizpe HM, Higdon AL, et al. Molecular mimicry, anti-coxsackievirus B3 neutralizing monoclonal antibodies, and myocarditis. *J Immunol* 1995; 154:2983–95.

271. Rosenberg HS, Kohl S, Vogler C. Viral infections of the fetus and the neonate. In: Naeye RL, Kissane JM, Kaufman N, eds. *Perinatal Diseases*. Baltimore: Williams & Wilkins, 1981: pp. 133–200.

272. Ahmad N, Abraham AA. Pancreatic isleitis with Coxsackie virus B5 infection. *Hum Pathol* 1982; 13:661–2.

273. Jenson AB, Rosenberg HS, Notkins AL. Pancreatic islet-cell damage in children with fatal viral infections. *Lancet* 1980; ii:354–8.

274. Bolande RP. The pathology and pathogenesis of juvenile diabetes mellitus. *Perspect Pediatr Pathol* 1979; 5:269–91.

275. Castleman B, BU M. Case records of the Massachusetts General Hospital: case #20–1965. *N Engl J Med* 1965; 272:907–14.

276. Lake AM, Lauer BA, Clark JC, Wesenberg RL, McIntosh K. Enterovirus infections in neonates. *J Pediatr* 1976; 89:787–91.

277. Philip AG, Larson EJ. Overwhelming neonatal infection with ECHO 19 virus. *J Pediatr* 1973; 82:391–7.

278. Krous HF, Dietzman D, Ray CG. Fatal infection with echovirus types 6 and 11 in early infancy. *Am J Dis Child* 1973; 126:842–6.

279. Berry PJ, Nagington J. Fatal infection with echovirus 11. *Arch Dis Child* 1982; 57:22–9.

280. Georgieff MK, Belani K, Johnson DE, Thompson TR, Ferreieri P. Fulminant hepatic necrosis in an infant with perinatally acquired echovirus 21 infection. *Pediatr Infect Dis* 1987; 6:71–3.

281. Hughes JR, Wilfert CM, Moore M, Benirschke K, Hoyos-Guerara E. Echovirus 14 infection associated with fetal necrosis. *Am J Dis Child* 1972; 123:61–7.

282. Modlin JF. Fatal echovirus 11 disease in premature neonates. *Pediatrics* 1980; 66:775–80.

283. Halton N, Spector SA. Fatal echovirus type 11 infection. *Am J Dis Child* 1981; 135:1017–20.

284. Mostoufizadeh M, Lack EE, Gang DL, Perez-Atayde AR, Driscoll SG. Post-mortem manifestations of echovirus 11 sepsis in five newborn infants. *Hum Pathol* 1983; 14:818–23.

285. Dimmick JE. Liver disease in the perinatal infant. In: Wigglesworth JS, Singer DB, eds. *Textbook of Fetal and Perinatal Pathology*. Boston: Blackwell Scientific 1991: pp. 987–8.

286. Krause PJ, Hyam JS. Letter to the editor. *J Pediatr* 1984; 105:852.

287. Rand KH, Houck HJ, Swingle HM. Rotazyme assay in neonates without diarrhea. Am J Clin Pathol 1985; 84:748–51.

288. Rotbart HA, Nelson WL, Glode MP, et al. Neonatal rotavirus-associated necrotizing enterocolitis: case control study and prospective surveillance during an outbreak. *J Pediatr* 1988; 112:87–103.

289. Rubenstein AS, Miller MF. Comparison of an enzyme immunoassay with electron microscopic procedures for detecting rotavirus. *J Clin Microbiol* 1982; 15:938–44.

290. Lin H-H, Lee T-Y, Chen D-S, et al. Transplacental leakage of HBeAg-positive maternal blood as the most likely route in causing intrauterine infection with hepatitis B virus. *J Pediatr* 1987; 111:877–81.

291. Delaplane A, Yogev R, Crussi F, Shulman ST. Fatal hepatitis B in early infancy. *Pediatrics* 1983; 72:176–80.

292. Mosley JW. Vertical transmission of type B hepatitis. *J Am Med Assoc* 1972; 220:1128–9.

293. Schweitzer IL, Spears RL. Hepatitis associated antigen (Australia antigen) in mother and infant. *N Engl J Med* 1970; 283:570–2.

294. Banatvala JE. Acute hepatitis (HBsAG associated). In: Hanshaw JB, Dudgeon JA, eds. *Viral Diseases of the Fetus and Newborn*. Philadelphia: WB Saunders, 1978: pp. 222–6.

295. Snydman DR. Hepatitis in pregnancy. *N Engl J Med* 1985; 313:1398–401.

296. London WT, O'Connell AP. Transplacental transmission of hepatitis B virus. *Lancet* 1986; i:1037–8.

297. Arevalo JA, Washington AE. Cost-effectiveness of prenatal screening and immunization for hepatitis B virus. *J Am Med Assoc* 1988; 259:365–9.

298. Beasley RP, Shiao IS, Wu FC, Hwang L-Y. Hepatoma in an HBsAg carrier seven years after perinatal infection. *J Pediatr* 1982; 101:83–4.

299. Bartolotti F, Calzia R, Cadrobbi P, et al. Liver cirrhosis associated with chronic hepatitis B virus infection in childhood. *J Pediatr* 1986; 108:224–7.

300. Baron S, Tyring SK, Fleischmann WR Jr, et al. The interferons. Mechanisms of action and clinical applications. *JAMA* 1991; 266:1375–83.

301. Azimi PH, Roberto RR, Guralnik J, et al. Transfusion-acquired hepatitis A in a premature infant with secondary nosocomial spread in an intensive care nursery. *Am J Dis Child* 1986; 140:23–7.

302. Klein BS, Michaels JA, Rytel MW, Berg KG, Davis JP. Nosocomial hepatitis A. A multinursery outbreak in Wisconsin. *J Am Med Assoc* 1984; 252:2716–21.

303. Noble RC, Kane MA, Reeves SA, Roeckel I. Posttransfusion hepatitis A in a neonatal intensive care unit. *J Am Med Assoc* 1984; 252:2711–5.

304. Tabor E. Etiology, diagnosis and treatment of viral hepatitis in children. *Adv Pediatr Infect Dis* 1988; 3:19–46.

305. Weintrub PS, Veereman-Wauters G, Cowan MJ, Thaler MM. Hepatitis C virus infection in infants whose mothers took street drugs intravenously. *J Pediatr* 1991; 119:869–74.

306. Ohto H, Terazawa S, Sasaki N, et al. Transmission of hepatitis C virus from mothers to infants. *N Engl J Med* 1994; 330:744–50.

307. Degos F, Maisonneuve P, Thiers V, et al. Neonatal transmission of HCV from mother with chronic hepatitis. *Lancet* 1991; ii:338:758.

308. Zanetti AR, Tanzi E, Paccagnini S, et al. Mother-to-infant transmission of hepatitis C virus. *Lancet* 1995; 345:289–91.

309. Glaser JH, Balistreri WF, Morecki R. Role of reovirus type 3 in persistent infantile cholestasis. *J Pediatr* 1984; 105:912–5.

310. Morecki R, Glaser JH, Cho S, Balistreri WF, Horwitz MS. Biliary atresia and reovirus type 3 infection. *N Engl J Med* 1982; 307:481–4.

311. Brown WR, Sokol RJ, Levin MJ, et al. Lack of correlation between infection with reovirus 3 and extrahepatic biliary atresia or neonatal hepatitis. *J Pediatr* 1988; 113:670–6.

312. Gershon AA. Varicella in mother and infant: problems old and new. In: Krugman S, Gershon AA, eds. *Infections of the Fetus and Newborn Infant: Proceedings of a Symposium Held in New York City, March 1975*, New York: A. R. Liss, 1975: pp. 79–95.

313. Palmer CGS, Pauli RM. Intrauterine varicella infection. *J Pediatr* 1988; 112:506.

314. Srabstein JC, Morris N, Larke RPB, deSa DJ, Castelino BB, Sum E. Is there a congenital varicella syndrome? *J Pediatr* 1974; 84:239–43.

315. Alkalay AL, Pomerance JJ, Rimoin DL. Fetal varicella syndrome. *J Pediatr* 1987; 111:320–3.

316. Greenspoon JS, Masaki DI. Fetal varicella syndrome. *J Pediatr* 1988; 112:505–6.

317. Brunell PA. Placental transfer of varicella-zoster antibody. *Pediatrics* 1966; 38:1034–8.

318. Trompeter RS, Bradley JM, Griffiths PD. Varicella zoster in the newborn. *Lancet* 1986; i:744.

319. Enders G, Miller E, Cradock-Watson J, Bolley I, Ridehalgh M. Consequences of varicella and herpes zoster in pregnancy: prospective study of 1739 cases. *Lancet* 1994; 343:1548–51.

320. Vorst EJ, Gaillard JLJ. Vaccinial osteomyelitis in a case of generalized intrauterine virus infection. *Pediatr Pathol* 1983; 1:221–8.

321. Green DM, Reid SM, Rhoney K. Generalized vaccinia in the human foetus. *Lancet* 1986; i:1296–8.

322. Rao SP, Miller ST, Cohen BJ. Transient aplastic crisis in patients with sickle cell disease. B19 parvovirus studies during a 7-year period. *Am J Dis Child* 1992; 146:1328–30.

323. Mallouh AA, Qudah Ak. Acute splenic sequestration together with aplastic crisis caused by human parvovirus B19 in patients with sickle cell disease. *J Pediatr* 1993; 122:593–5.

324. Mallouh AA, Qudah A. An epidemic of aplastic crisis caused by human parvovirus B19. *Pediatr Infect Dis J* 1995; 14:31–4.

325. Koch WC. Human parvovirus B19 infections in women of childbearing age and within families. *Pediatr Infect Dis J* 1989; 8:83–7.

326. Griffin TC, Squires JE, Timmons CF, Buchanan GR. Chronic human parvovirus B19-induced erythroid hypoplasia as the initial manifestation of human immunodeficiency virus infection. *J Pediatr* 1991; 118:899–901.

327. Brown KE, Hibbs JR, Gallinella G, et al. Resistance to parvovirus B19 infection due to lack of virus receptor (erythrocyte P antigen). *N Engl J Med* 1994; 330:1192–6.

328. Anand A, Gray ES, Brown T, Clewley JP, Cohen BJ. Human parvovirus infection in pregnancy and hydrops fetalis. *N Engl J Med* 1987; 316:183–6.

329. Rodis JF, Hovick TJ Jr, Quinn DL, Rosengren SS, Tattersall P. Human parvovirus infection in pregnancy. *Obstet Gynecol* 1988; 72:733–8.

330. Török TJ. Human parvovirus B19 infections in pregnancy. *Pediatr Infect Dis J* 1990; 9:772–6.

331. Selbing A, Josefsson A, Dahle LO, Lindgren R. Parvovirus B19 infection during pregnancy treated with high-dose intravenous gammaglobulin. *Lancet* 1995; 345:660–1.

332. Berry PJ, Gray ES, Porter HJ, Burton PA. Parvovirus infection of the human fetus and newborn. *Semin Diag Pathol* 1992; 9:4–12.

333. Metzman R, Anand A, DeGjiulio PA, Knisely AS. Hepatic disease associated with intrauterine parvovirus B19 infection in a newborn premature infant. *J Pediatr Gastroent Nutr* 1989; 9:112–4.

334. White FV, Jordan J, Dickman PS, Knisely AS. Fetal parvovirus B19 infection and liver disease of antenatal onset in an infant with Ebstein's anomaly. *Pediatr Pathol Lab Med* 1995; 15:121–9.

335. Caul EW, Usher J, Burton PA. Intrauterine infection with human parvovirus B19: a light and electron microscopic study. *J Med Virol* 1988; 24:55–66.

336. Knisely AS, O'Shea PA, McMillan P, Singer DB, Magid MS. Electron microscopic identification of parvovirus virions in erythroid-line cells in fatal hydrops fetalis. *Pediatr Pathol* 1988; 8:163–70.

337. Porter HJ, Quantrill AM, Fleming KA. B19 parvovirus infection of myocardial cells. *Lancet* 1988; i:535–6.

338. Willekes C, Roumen FJME, Van Elsacker-Niele AMW, et al. Human parvovirus B19 infection and unbalanced translocation in a case of hydrops fetalis. *Prenatal Diagn* 1994; 14:181–6.

339. Rogers BB, Mark Y, Oyer CE. Diagnosis and incidence of fetal parvovirus infection in an autopsy series: I histology. *Pediatr Pathol* 1993; 13:371–9.

340. Mark Y, Rogers BB, Oyer CE. Diagnosis and incidence of fetal parvovirus infection in an autopsy series: II DNA amplification. *Pediatr Pathol* 1993; 13:381–6.

341. Van Elsacker-Niele A, Vermeij-Keers C, Oepkes D, Van Roosmalen J, Gorsira MCB. A fetus with a parvovirus B19 infection and congenital anomalies. *Prenat Diagn* 1994; 14:173–6.

342. Mortimer PP, Cohen BJ, Buckley MM. Human parvovirus and the fetus. *Lancet* 1985; 2:1102.

343. Guidozzi F, Ballot D, Rothberg AD. Human B-19 parvovirus infection in an obstetric population. *J Reprod Med* 1994; 39:36–8.

344. Rogers BB, Singer DB, Mak SK, et al. Detection of human parvovirus B19 in early spontaneous abortuses using serology, histology, electron microscopy, in situ hybridization, and the polymerase chain reaction. *Obstet Gynecol* 1993; 81:402–8.

345. Rogers BB, Mak SK, Dailey JV, Saller DN Jr, Buffone GJ. Detection of parvovirus B19 DNA in amniotic fluid by PCR DNA amplification. *Biotechniques* 1993; 15:406–8,410.

346. Török TJ, Wang Q-Y, Gary GW Jr, Yang C-F, Finch TM, Anderson LJ. Prenatal diagnosis of intrauterine infection with parvovirus B19 by the polymerase chain reaction technique. *Clin Infect Dis* 1992; 14:149–55.

347. Saller DN, Rogers BB, Canick JA. Maternal serum biochemical markers in pregnancies with fetal parvovirus B19 infection. *Prenat Diagn* 1993; 13:467–71.

348. Krause JR, Penchansky L, Knisely AS. Morphologic diagnosis of parvovirus B19 infection. A cytopathic effect easily recognized in air-dried, formalin-fixed bone marrow smears stained with hematoxylin-eosin or Wright-Giemsa. *Arch Pathol Lab Med* 1992; 116:178–80.

349. Gillespie SM, Cartter ML, Asch S, et al. Occupational risk of human parvovirus B19 infection for school and day-care personnel during an outbreak of erythema infectiosum. *JAMA* 1990; 263:2061–5.

350. Anderson S, Momoeda M, Kawase M, Kajigaya S, Young NS. Peptides derived from the unique region of B19 parvovirus minor capsid protein elicit neutralizing antibodies in rabbits. *Virology* 1995; 206:626–32.

351. Hall CJ. Parvovirus B19 infection in pregnancy. *Arch Dis Child* 1994; 71:F4–5.

352. Soderlund M, Brown CS, Cohen BJ, Wedman K. Accurate serodiagnosis of B19 parvovirus infections by measurement of IgG avidity. *J Infect Dis* 1995; 171:710–13.

353. Panero C, Azzi A, Carbone C, et al. Fetoneonatal hydrops from human parvovirus B19. Case report. *J Perinatal Med* 1994; 22:257–64.

354. Schwarz TF, Roggendorf M, Hottenträger B, et al. Human parvovirus B19 infection in pregnancy. *Lancet* 1988; ii:566–7.

355. Morey AL, Keeling JW, Porter HJ, Fleming KA. Clinical and histopathological features of parvovirus B19 infection in the human fetus. *Br J Obstet Gynaecol* 1992; 99:566–74.

356. Finkel TH, Török TJ, Ferguson PJ, et al. Chronic parvovirus B19 infection and systemic necrotising vasculitis: opportunistic infection or aetiological agent? *Lancet* 1994; 343:1255–8.

357. Nigro G, Zerbini M, Krzystofiak A, et al. Active or recent parvovirus B19 infection in children with Kawasaki disease. *Lancet* 1994; 343:1260–1.

358. Wierenga KJJ, Pattison JR, Brink N, et al. Glomerulonephritis after human parvovirus infection in homozygous sickle-cell disease. *Lancet* 1995; 346:475–6.

359. Silver MM, Zielenska M, Perrin D, MacDonald JK. Association of prenatal closure of the foramen ovale and fetal parvovirus B219 infection in hydrops fetalis. *Cardiovasc Pathol* 1995; 4:103–9.

360. Silver MM, Zielenska M, Perrin D, et al. Molecular evidence for an association of Ebstein anomaly with fetal parvovirus B19 infection. Society for Pediatric Pathology, Baltimore MD, Oct 26–27, 1995.

361. Schwarz TF, Nerlich A, Hottenträger B, et al. Parvovirus B19 infection of the fetus. Histology and in-situ hybridization. *Am J Clin Pathol* 1991; 96:121–6.

362. Hara T, Takahashi Y, Sonoda S, Kusuhara K, Ueda K. HTLV type I infection in neonates. *Am J Dis Child* 1987; 141:764–5.

363. Osame M, Igata A, Usuku K, Rosales RL. Mother-to-child transmission in HTLV-1 associated myelopathy. *Lancet* 1987; i:106.

364. Weiss SH, Lombardo J, Names MMc, et al. AIDS due to HIV-2 infection—New Jersey. *J Am Med Assoc* 1988; 259:969–72.

365. Van Dyke RB, Heneine W, Perrin M, et al. Mother-to-child transmission of human T-lymphotrophic virus type II. *J Pediatr* 1995; 127:924–8.

366. National Center for Health Statistics. Annual Summary of Births, Marriages, Divorces and Deaths: United States. 1993. Hyattsville, MD: US Department of Health and Human Services, Public Health Service, Centers for Disease Control and Prevention, 1994.

367. Rogers MF, Caldwell MB, Gwinn ML, Simonds RJ. Epidemiology of pediatric human immunodeficiency virus infection in the United States. *Ann NY Acad Sci* 1993; 693:4–8.

368. Davis SF, Byers RH Jr, Lindegren ML, et al. Prevalence and incidence of vertically acquired HIV infection in the United States. *JAMA* 1995; 247:952–5.

369. Minkoff H, Nanda D, Menez R, Fikrig S. Pregnancies resulting in infants with acquired immunodeficiency syndrome or AIDS-related complex. *Obstet Gynecol* 1987; 69:285–7.

370. Nelson RP Jr, Price LJ, Halsey AB, et al. Diagnosis of pediatric human immunodeficiency virus infection by means of a commercially available polymerase chain reaction gene amplification. *Arch Pediatr Adoles Med* 1996; 150:40–5.

371. Wara DW, Luzuriaga K, Martin NL, Sullivan JL, Bryson YJ. Maternal transmission and diagnosis of human immunodeficiency virus during infancy. *Ann NY Acad Sci* 1993; 693:14–9.

372. Ammann AJ. Human immunodeficiency virus infections in infants and children. *Adv Pediatr Infect Dis* 1988; 3:91–110.

373. Harnish DG, Hammerberg O, Walker IR, Rosenthal KL. Early detection HIV infection in a newborn. *N Engl J Med* 1987; 316:272–3.

374. Oleske J. Natural history of HIV infections. II. Report of the Surgeon General's Workshop on children with HIV infection and their families. DHHS Publ no. HRS-D-MC-87-1, 1987:24–6.

375. Rozenzweig M, Clark DP, Gaulton GN. Selective thymocyte depletion in neonatal HIV-1 thymic infection. *AIDS* 1993; 7:1601–5.

376. O'Duffy JF, Isles AF. Transfusion-induced AIDS in four premature babies. *Lancet* 1984; ii:1346.

377. Saulsbury FT, Wykoff RF, Boyle RJ. Transfusion-acquired human immunodeficiency virus infection in twelve neonates: epidemiologic, clinical and immunologic features. *Pediatr Infect Dis* 1987; 6:544–9.

378. Van de Perre P, Simonon A, Msellati P, et al. Postnatal transmission of human immunodeficiency virus type 1 from mother to infant. *N Engl J Med* 1991; 325:593–8.

379. Ziegler JB, Johnson RO, Cooper DA, Gold J. Postnatal transmission of AIDS: associated retrovirus from mother to infants. *Lancet* 1985; i:896–7.

380. Dunn DT, Newell ML, Ades AE, Peckham CS. Risk of human immunodeficiency virus type 1 transmission through breastfeeding. *Lancet* 1992; 340:585–8.

381. Jovaisas E, Koch MA, Schäfer A, Stauber M, Löwenthal D. LAV-HTLV-III in a 20 week fetus. *Lancet* 1985; ii:1129.

382. LaPointe N, Michaud J, Pekovic D, Chausseau JP, Dupuy JM. Transplacental transmission of HTLV III virus. *N Engl J Med* 1985; 312:1325–6.

383. Joshi VV. Pathology of Pediatric AIDS. Overview, update, and future direction. *Ann NY Acad Sci* 1993; 683:71–92.

384. Scott GB. Natural history of HIV infection in children. Report of the Surgeon General's workshop on children with HIV infection and their families. 1987:22–23.

385. Lobato MN, Caldwell B, Ng P, Oxtoby MJ. Encephalopathy in children with perinatally acquired human immunodeficiency virus infection. *J Pediatr* 1995; 126:710–5.

386. Joshi VV, Oleske JM, Minnefor AB, et al. Pathologic pulmonary findings in children with acquired immunodeficiency syndrome. A study of ten cases. *Hum Pathol* 1985; 16:241–6.

387. Joshi VV, Oleske JM. Pulmonary lesions in children with acquired immunodeficiency syndrome. A reappraisal based on data in additional cases and follow-up study of previously reported cases. *Hum Pathol* 1986; 17:641–2.

388. Joshi VV, Oleske JM, Connor EM. Morphologic findings in children with acquired immune deficiency syndrome: pathogenesis and clinical implications. *Pediatr Pathol* 1990; 10:155–66.

389. Rubinstein A, Sicklick M, Gupta A, et al. Acquired immunodeficiency with reversed T4/T8 ratios in infants born to promiscuous and drug addicted mothers. *J Am Med Assoc* 1983; 249:2350–6.

390. Marion RW, Wiznia AA, Hutcheon RG, Rubinstein A. Human T-cell lymphotropic virus type III (HTLV-III) embryopathy: a new dysmorphic syndrome associated with intrauterine HTLV-III infection. *Am J Dis Child* 1986; 140:638–40.

391. Qazi QH, Sheikh TM, Fikrig S, Menikoff H. Lack of evidence for craniofacial dysmorphism in perinatal human immunodeficiency virus infection. *J Pediatr* 1988; 112:7–11.

392. Witzleben CL, Marshall GS, Wenner W, Piccoli DA, Barbour SD. HIV as a cause of giant cell hepatitis. *Hum Pathol* 1988; 19:603–5.

393. Connor EM, Sperling RS, Gelber R, et al. Reduction of maternal-infant transmission of human immunodeficiency virus type 1 with zidovudine treatment. *N Engl J Med* 1994; 331:1173–80.

394. Bryson YJ, Pang S, Wei LS, et al. Clearance of HIV infection in a perinatally infected infant. *N Engl J Med* 1995; 332:833–8.

395. Gompels M, Spickett G, Curtis A. Clearance of HIV in an infant. *N Engl J Med* 1995; 333:319–20.

396. Krivine A, Lebon P. Clearance of HIV in an infant. *N Engl J Med* 1995; 333:319.

397. Perinatal human immunodeficiency virus testing. *Pediatrics* 1994; 95:303–6.

398. Peckham C, Gibb D. Mother-to-child transmission of the human immunodeficiency virus. *N Engl J Med* 1995; 333:298–302.

399. Stagno S, Whitley RJ. Herpes virus infections of pregnancy. *N Engl J Med* 1985; 313:1270–4,1327–30.

400. Goldberg GN, Fulginiti VA, Ray DG, et al. In utero Epstein-Barr virus (infectious mononucleosis) infection. *J Am Med Assoc* 1981; 246:1579–81.

401. Sun C-C, Duara S. Fatal adenovirus pneumonia in two newborn infants, one case caused by adenovirus type 30. *Pediatr Pathol* 1985; 4:247–55.

402. Meyer K, Girgis N, McGravey V. Adenovirus associated with congenital pleural effusion. *J Pediatr* 1985; 107:433–5.

403. Kinney JS, Hierholzer JC, Thibeault DW. Neonatal pulmonary insufficiency caused by adenovirus infection successfully treated with extracorporeal membrane oxygenation. *J Pediatr* 1994; 125:110–2.

404. Montgomery EA, Popek EJ. Intussusception, adenovirus, and children: a brief reaffirmation. *Hum Pathol* 1994; 25:169–74.

405. Update: Respiratory syncytial virus activity—United States, 1995–96 season. *JAMA* 1995; 275:29.

406. Hall CB, Kopelman AE, Douglas RG Jr, Greman JM, Meagher MP. Neonatal respiratory syncytial virus infection. *N Engl J Med* 1979; 300:393–6.

407. Anas N, Boettrick C, Hall CB, Brooks JG. The association of apnea and respiratory syncytial virus infection in infants. *J Pediatr* 1982; 101:65–8.

408. MacDonald NE, Hall CB, Suffin SC, et al. Respiratory syncytial virus infection in infants with congenital heart disease. *N Engl J Med* 1982; 307:397–400.

409. Wald ER. In re: ribavirin: a case of premature adjudication? *J Pediatr* 1988; 112:154–8.

410. Adams JM. Primary virus pneumonitis with cytoplasmic inclusion bodies. Study of an epidemic involving thirty-two infants with nine deaths. *J Am Med Assoc* 1941; 116:925–33.

411. Adams JM, Imagawa DT, Zike K. Epidemic bronchiolitis and pneumonitis related to respiratory syncytial virus. *J Am Med Assoc* 1961; 176:1037–9.

412. Shedden WIH, Emery JL. Immunofluorescent evidence of respiratory syncytial virus infection in cases of giant cell bronchiolitis in children. *J Pathol Bacteriol* 1965; 89:343–7.

413. Mintz L, Ballard RA, Sniderman SH, Roth RS, Drew WL. Nosocomial respiratory syncytial virus infections in an intensive care nursery. Rapid diagnosis by direct immunofluorescence. *Pediatrics* 1979; 64:149–53.

414. Murguia de Sierra T, Kumar ML, Wasser TE, Murphy BR, Subbarao EK. Respiratory syncytial virus-specific immunoglobulins in preterm infants. *J Pediatr* 1993; 122:787–91.

415. Valenti WM, Clarke TA, Hall CB, Menegus MA, Shapiro DL. Concurrent outbreaks of rhinovirus and respiratory syncytial virus in an intensive care nursery: epidemiology and associated risk factors. *J Pediatr* 1982; 100:722–6.

416. Shah K, Hashima H, Polk BF, et al. Rarity of cesarean delivery in cases of juvenile-onset respiratory papillomatosis. *Obstet Gynecol* 1986; 68:795–8.

417. Barnes L, Yunis EJ, Krebs FJ III, Sonmez-Alpan E. Verruca vulgaris of the larynx. Demonstration of human papillomavirus types 6/11 by in situ hybridization. *Arch Pathol Lab Med* 1991; 115:895–9.

418. Atmar RL, Englund JA, Hammill H. Complications of measles during pregnancy. *Clin Infect Dis* 1992; 14:217–26.

419. Stein SJ, Greenspoon JS. Rubeola during pregnancy. *Obstet Gynecol* 1991; 78:925–9.

420. Eberhart-Phillips JE, Frederick PD, Baron RC, Mascola L. Measles in pregnancy: a descriptive study of 58 cases. *Obstet Gynecol* 1993; 82:797–801.

421. Gershon AA. Chickenpox, measles and mumps. In: Remington JS, Klein JO, eds. *Infectious Diseases of the Fetus and Newborn Infant.* 4th ed. Philadelphia: WB Saunders, 1995: pp. 591–603.

422. Dyer I. Measles complicating pregnancy. Report of 24 cases with three instances of congenital measles. *South Med J* 1940; 33:601–4.

423. Packer AD. The influence of maternal measles (morbilli) on the newborn child. *Med J Austr* 1950; 1:835–8.

424. Moroi K, Saito S, Kurata T, Sata T, Yanagida M. Fetal death associated with measles virus infection of the placenta. *Am J Obstet Gynecol* 1991; 164:1107–8.

425. Susser M, Stein Z. Increased postperinatal child mortality among children of mothers exposed to measles during pregnancy. *Am J Epidemiol* 1991; 133:413.

426. Aaby P, Seim E, Knudsen K, et al. Increased postperinatal child mortality among children of mothers exposed to measles during pregnancy. *Am J Epidemiol* 1990; 132:531–9.

427. Price ME, Fisher-Hoch SP, Craven RB, McCormick JB. A prospective study of maternal and fetal outcome in acute Lassa fever infection during pregnancy. *Br Med J* 1988; 297:584–7.

428. Monson MH, Cole AK, Frame JD, et al. Pediatric Lassa fever: a review of 33 Liberian cases. *Am J Trop Med Hyg* 1987; 36:408–15.

429. Walker DH, McCormick JB, Johnson KM, et al. Pathologic and virologic study of fatal Lassa fever in man. *Am J Pathol* 1982; 107:349–56.

430. Partanen S, Kahanpää K, Peltola J, Lähdevirta J. Infection with the Puumala virus in pregnancy. Case report. *Br J Obstet Gynaecol* 1990; 97:274–5.

431. Gallis HA, Agner RC, Painter CJ. Rocky Mountain spotted fever in pregnancy. *N Carol Med J* 1984; 45:187–8.

432. Schachter J. Isolation of Bedsoniae from human arthritis and abortion tissues. *Am J Ophthalmol* 1967(1082–1086):390.

433. Frommel GT, Rotheberg R, Wang S, McIntosh K. Chlamydial infection of mothers and their infants. *J Pediatr* 1979; 95:28–32.

434. Hammerschlag MR, Anderka M, Semine DZ, McComb D, McCormack WM. Prospective studies of maternal and infantile infection with *Chlamydia trachomatis*. *Pediatrics* 1979; 64:142–8.

435. Donders GG, Moerman P, De Wet GH, Hooft P, Goubau P. The association between chlamydia cervicitis, chorioamnionitis, and neonatal complications. *Arch Gynecol Obstet* 1991; 249:79–85.

436. Abzug MJ, Hershey DW, Rotbart HA, Levin MJ. Incidence of nonbacterial intraamniotic infections in abnormal pregnancies. *J Reprod Med* 1991; 36:783–5.

437. Schachter J, Grossman M, Sweet RL, et al. Prospective study of perinatal transmission of *Chlamydia trachomatis*. *J Am Med Assoc* 1986; 255:3374–7.

438. Sandström KI, Bell TA, Chandler JW, et al. Microbial causes of neonatal conjunctivitis. *J Pediatr* 1984; 105:706–11.

439. Schachter J, Sweet RL, Grossman M, et al. Experience with the routine use of erythromycin for chlamydial infections in pregnancy. *N Engl J Med* 1985; 314:276–9.

440. Beem MO, Saxon EM. Respiratory tract colonization and a distinctive pneumonia syndrome in infants infected with *Chlamydia trachomatis*. *N Engl J Med* 1977; 296:305–10.

441. Judge DM. Congenital syphilis. In: Scarpelli DG, Migaki G, eds. *Transplacental Effects on Fetal Health: Proceedings of a Symposium Held in Bethesda, MD, November 5–6, 1987.* New York: A. R. Liss, 1988: pp. 87–106.

442. Sharrar RG, Goldberg M. Continuing increase in infectious syphilis—United States. *J Am Med Assoc* 1988; 259:975–6.

443. Donders GG, Desmyter J, DeWet DH, VanAssche FA. The association of gonorrhoea and syphilis with premature birth and low birthweight. *Genitourin Med* 1993; 69:98–101.

444. Rawstron SA, Jenkins S, Blanchard S, Li P-W, Bromberg K. Maternal and congenital syphilis in Brooklyn, NY. Epidemiology, transmission, and diagnosis. *Am J Dis Child* 1993; 147:727–31.

445. Zenker PN, Berman SM. Congenital syphilis: trends and recommendations for evaluation and management. *Pediatr Infect Dis J* 1991; 10:516–22.

446. Mascola L, Pelosi R, Blount JH, Alexander CE, Cates W Jr. Congenital syphilis revisited. *Am J Dis Child* 1985; 139:575–80.

447. Epstein H, King CR. Diagnosis of congenital syphilis by immunofluorescence following fetal death in utero. *Am J Obstet Gynecol* 1985; 152:689–90.

448. Russell P, Altshuler G. Placental abnormalities of congenital syphilis. A neglected aid to diagnosis. *Am J Dis Child* 1974; 128:160–3.

449. Brooks SEH, Audretsch JJ. Hepatic ultrastructure in congenital syphilis. *Arch Pathol Lab Med* 1978; 102:502–5.

450. Jacques SM, Qureshi F. Necrotizing funisitis: a study of 45 cases. *Hum Pathol* 1992; 23:1278–83.

451. McIntosh J. The occurrence and distribution of the *Spirochaeta pallida* in congenital syphilis. *J Pathol Bacteriol* 1909; 13:239–43.

452. Oppenheimer EH, Hardy JB. Congenital syphilis in the newborn infant. *J Hopkins Med J* 1971; 129:63–82.

453. Abramowsky C, Beyer-Patterson P, Cortinas E. Nonsyphilitic spirochetosis in second-trimester fetuses. *Pediatr Pathol* 1991; 11(6):827–38.

454. Coghlan JD, Bain AD. Leptospirosis in human pregnancy followed by death of the foetus. *Br Med J* 1969; 1:228–30.

455. Shirts SR, Brown MS, Bobbitt JR. Listeriosis and borreliosis as causes of antepartum fever. *Obstet Gynecol* 1983; 62:256–61.

456. Altshuler G. Fusobacteria. An important cause of chorioamnionitis. *Arch Pathol Lab Med* 1985; 109:739–43.

457. MacDonald AB. Human fetal borreliosis, toxemia of pregnancy and fetal death. Proceedings of the 2nd International Symposium on Lyme Disease, Vienna 1985.

458. Markowitz LE, Steere AC, Benach JL, Slade JD, Broome CV. Lyme disease during pregnancy. *J Am Med Assoc* 1986; 255:3394–6.

459. Gardner T, ed. Lyme disease. In: Remington JS, Klein JO, eds. *Infectious Diseases of the Fetus and Newborn Infant.* 4th ed. Philadelphia: WB Saunders, 1995: pp. 487–8.

460. Hageman J, Shulman S, Schreiber M, Luck S, Yogev R. Congenital tuberculosis: critical reappraisal of clinical findings and diagnostic procedures. *Pediatrics* 1980; 66:980–4.

461. Myers JP, Perlstein PH, Light IJ, et al. Tuberculosis in pregnancy with fatal congenital infection. *Pediatrics* 1981; 67:89–94.

462. Job CK, Sanchez RM, Hastings RC. Lepromatous placentitis and intrauterine fetal infection in lepromatous nine-banded armadillos (*Dasypus novemcinctus*). *Lab Invest* 1987; 56:44–8.

463. Becroft DMO, Farmer K, Mason GH, Morris MC, Stewart JH. Perinatal infection by group B beta-hemolytic streptococci. *Br J Obstet Gynaecol* 1976; 83:960–6.

464. Gotoff SP. Emergence of group B streptococci as major perinatal pathogens. *Hosp Pract* 1977; 12:85–97.

465. Hood M, Janney A, Dameron G. Beta hemolytic streptococcus group B associated with problems of the perinatal period. *Am J Obstet Gynecol* 1961; 82:809–18.

466. Hoogkamp-Korstanje JAA, Gerards LJ, Cats BP. Maternal carriage and neonatal acquisition of group B streptococci. *J Infect Dis* 1982; 145:800–3.

467. Reid TMS. Emergence of group B streptococci in obstetric and perinatal infections. *Br Med J* 1975; 2:533–6.

468. Baker CJ, Gotoff DK, Alpert S, et al. Vaginal colonization with group B streptococcus: a study in college women. *J Infect Dis* 1977; 135:392–7.

469. Anthony BF, Okada DM, Hobel CJ. Epidemiology of the group B streptococcus: maternal and nosocomial sources for infant acquisitions. *J Pediatr* 1979; 95:431–6.

470. Bobitt JR, Brown GL, Tull AH. Group B streptococcal neonatal infection: clinical review of plans for prevention and preliminary report of quantitative antepartum cultures. *Obstet Gynecol* 1980; 55:171s–177s.

471. Strasberg GD. Postpartum group B streptococcal endocarditis associated with mitral valve prolapse. *Obstet Gynecol* 1987; 70:485–7.

472. Pass MA, Gray BM, Santosh K, Dillon HC Jr. Prospective studies of group B streptococcal infections in infants. *J Pediatr* 1979; 95:437–43.

473. Bergqvist G, Holmberg G, Rydner T, Vaclavinkova V. Intrauterine death due to infection with group B streptococci. *Acta Obstet Gynecol Scand* 1978; 57:127–8.

474. Franciosi RA, Knostman JD, Zimmerman RA. Group B streptococcal neonatal and infant infections. *J Pediatr* 1973; 82:707–18.

475. Craig JM. Group B beta hemolytic streptococcal sepsis in the newborn. *Perspect Pediatr Pathol* 1981; 6:139–52.

476. Dillon HC Jr, Khare S, Gray BM. Group B streptococcal carriage and disease: a 6-year prospective study. *J Pediatr* 1987; 110:31–6.

477. McFail TL, Zimmerman GA, Augustine NH, Hill HR. Effect of group B streptococcal type-specific antigen polymorphonuclear leukocyte-endothelial cell interaction. *Pediatr Res* 1987; 21:517–23.

478. Merenstein GB, Todd WA, Brown G, Yost CC, Luzier T. Group B beta-hemolytic streptococcus. Randomized controlled treatment study at term. *Obstet Gynecol* 1980; 55:315–8.

479. deSa DJ, Trevenen CL. Intrauterine infections with group B beta-haemolytic streptococci. *Br J Obstet Gynaecol* 1984; 91:237–9.

480. Eickhoff TC, Klein JO, Daly AK, Ingall D, Finland M. Neonatal sepsis and other infections due to group B beta-hemolytic streptococci. *N Engl J Med* 1964; 271:1221–8.

481. Regan JA, Chao S, James LS. Premature rupture of membranes, preterm delivery, and group B streptococcal colonization of mothers. *Am J Obstet Gynecol* 1981; 141:184–6.

482. Boyer KM, Gotoff SP. Prevention of early-onset neonatal group B streptococcal disease with selective intrapartum chemoprophylaxis. *N Engl J Med* 1986; 314:1665–9.

483. Yow MD, Mason EO, Leeds LJ, et al. Ampicillin prevents intrapartum transmission of group B streptococcus. *J Am Med Assoc* 1979; 241:1245–7.

484. Thomsen AC, Mørup L, Brogaard Hansen K. Antibiotic elimination of group-B streptococci in urine in prevention of preterm labour. *Lancet* 1987; i:591–3.

485. Siegel JD, McCracken GH JR, Threlkeld N, Milvenen B, Rosenfeld CR. Single dose penicillin prophylaxis against neonatal group B streptococcal infections. A controlled trial in 18738 newborn infants. *N Engl J Med* 1980; 303:769–76.

486. Baker CJ, Rench MA, Edwards MS, et al. Immunization of pregnant women with a polysaccharide vaccine of group B streptococcus. *N Engl J Med* 1988; 319:1180–5.

487. Fanaroff AA KS, Wright LL, Wright EC, et al. A controlled trial of intravenous immune globulin to reduce nosocomial infections in very-low-birth-weight infants. *N Engl J Med* 1994; 330:1107–13.

488. Freedman RM, Ingram DL, Gross I, et al. A half century of neonatal sepsis at Yale. *Am J Dis Child* 1981; 135:140–4.

489. Gladstone IM, Ehrenkranz RA, Edberg SC, Baltimore RS. A ten-year review of neonatal sepsis and comparison with previous fifty-year experience. *Pediatr Infect Dis J* 1990; 9:819–5.

490. Lancefield RC. A serological differentiation of human and other groups of hemolytic streptococci. *J Exp Med* 1933; 57:571–95.

491. Mayock DE, O'Rourke FP, Kapur RP. Bronchiolitis obliterans: a complication of group B streptococcal disease treated with extracorporeal membrane oxygenation. *Pediatrics* 1993; 92:157–60.

492. Faix RG, Donn SM. Association of septic shock caused by early-onset group B streptococcal sepsis and periventricular leukomalacia in the preterm infant. *Pediatrics* 1985; 76:415–9.

493. Chin J. Current and future dimensions of the HIV/AIDS pandemic in women and children. *Lancet* 1990; 336:221–4.

494. Edwards MS, Rench MA, Haffar AAM, et al. Long-term sequelae of group B streptococcal meningitis in infants. *J Pediatr* 1985; 106:717–21.

495. Banagale RC, Watters JH. Delayed right-sided diaphragmatic hernia following group B streptococcal infection: a discussion of its pathogenesis, with a review of the literature. *Hum Pathol* 1983; 14:67–9.

496. Hall FK, Hall RT, Rising DR. Septicemia and hernia. *Am J Dis Child* 1982; 136:561–2.

497. Harris MC, Moskowitz WB, Engle WD, et al. Group B streptococcal septicemia and delayed-onset diaphragmatic hernia. *Am J Dis Child* 1981; 135:723–5.

498. Hauger SB. Facial cellulitis: an early indicator of group B streptococcal bacteremia. *Pediatrics* 1981; 67:376–7.

499. Patamasucon P, Siegel JD, McCracken GH Jr. Streptococcal submandibular cellulitis in young infants. *Pediatrics* 1981; 67:378–80.

500. Ascher DP, Wilson S, Mendiola J, Fischer GW. Group B streptococcal latex agglutination testing in neonates. *J Pediatr* 1991; 119:458–61.

501. Broughton RA, Krafka R, Baker CJ. Non-group D alpha-hemolytic streptococci: new neonatal pathogens. *J Pediatr* 1981; 99:450–4.

502. Buchino JJ, Ciambarella E, Light I. Systemic group D streptococcal infection in newborn infants. *Am J Dis Child* 1979; 133:270–3.

503. Bavikate K, Schreiner RL, Lemons JA, Gresham EL. Group D streptococcal septicemia in the neonate. *Am J Dis Child* 1979; 133:493–6.

504. Alexander JB, Giacoia GP. Early onset non-enterococcal group D streptococcal infection in the newborn infant. *J Pediatr* 1978; 93:489–90.

505. Roberts KB. Blood cultures in pediatric practice. *Am J Dis Child* 1979; 133:996–6.

506. Peter G, Singer DB. Respiratory distress and shock in a term neonate. *J Pediatr* 1980; 96:946–9.

507. Rhodes PG, Burry VF, Hall RT, Cox R. Pneumococcal septicemia and meningitis in the neonate. *J Pediatr* 1975; 86:593–5.

508. Weintraub MI, Otto RN. Pneumococcal meningitis and endophthalmitis in a newborn. *J Am Med Assoc* 1972; 219:1763–4.

509. Bortolussi R, Thompson TR, Ferrieri P. Early onset pneumococcal sepsis in newborn infants. *Pediatrics* 1977; 60:352–5.

510. Baumgart S, Hall SE, Campos JM, Polin RA. Sepsis with coagulase-negative staphylococci in critically ill newborns. *Am J Dis Child* 1983; 137:461–3.

511. Calonen G, Campognone P, Peter G. Coagulase-negative staphylococcal bacteremia in newborns. *Clin Pediatr* 1984; 23:542–4.

512. Freeman J, Platt R, Sidebottom DG, et al. Coagulase-negative staphylococcal bacteremia in the changing neonatal intensive care unit population. Is there an epidemic? *J Am Med Assoc* 1988; 258:2548–52.

513. Starr SE. Antimicrobial therapy of bacterial sepsis in the newborn infant. *J Pediatr* 1985; 106:1043–8.

514. Kacica MA, Horgan MJ, Ochoa L, et al. Prevention of gram-positive sepsis in neonates weighing less than 1500 grams. *J Pediatr* 1994; 125:253–8.

515. Hall SL. Coagulase negative staphylococcal infections in neonates. *Pediatr Infect Dis J* 1991; 10:57–67.

516. Noel GJ, Edelson PJ. *Staphylococcus epidermidis* bacteremia in neonates: further observations and the occurrence of focal infection. *Pediatrics* 1984; 74:832–7.

517. Baker CJ, Melish ME, Hall RT, et al. Intravenous immune globulin for the prevention of nosocomial infection in low-birth-weight neonates. *N Engl J Med* 1992; 327:213–9.

518. Spafford PS, Sinkin RA, Cox C, Reubens L, Powell KR. Prevention of central venous catheter—related coagulase-negative staphylococcal sepsis in neonates. *J Pediatr* 1994; 125:259–63.

519. Freeman J, Smith NE, Sidebottom DG, Epstein MF, Platt R. Association of intravenous lipid emulsion and coagulase-negative staphylococcal bacteremia in neonatal intensive care units. *N Engl J Med* 1990; 323:301–8.

520. Faden H, Neter E, McLaughlin S, Giacola G. Gentamicin-resistant *Staphylococcus aureus* in an intensive care nursery. *J Am Med Assoc* 1979; 241:143–5.

521. Barefield E, Phillips JB III. Vancomycin prophylaxis for coagulase-negative staphylococcal bacteremia. *J Pediatr* 1994; 125:230–2.

522. Melish ME, Glasgow LA. The staphylococcal scalded-skin syndrome. *N Engl J Med* 1970; 282:1114–9.

523. Mellander L, Carlsson B, Jalil F, Söderström T, Hanson LA. Secretory IgA antibody response against *Escherichia coli* antigens in infants in relation to exposure. *J Pediatr* 1985; 107:430–3.

524. McCracken GH Jr, Sarff LD, Glode MP, et al. Relation between *Escherichia coli* K 1 capsular polysaccharide antigen and clinical outcome in neonatal meningitis. *Lancet* 1974; ii:246–50.

525. Levy HL, Sepe SJ, Shih VE, Vawter GF, Klein JO. Sepsis due to *Escherichia coli* in neonates with galactosemia. *N Engl J Med* 1977; 297:823–5.

526. Cushing AH. Necrotizing enterocolitis with *Escherichia coli* heat labile enterotoxin. *Pediatrics* 1983; 71:626–30.

527. Quentin R, Goudeau A, Burfin E, et al. Infections materno-foetales à *Haemophilus influenzae*. *Presse Med* 1987; 16:1181–4.

528. Wallace RJ Jr, Baker CJ, Quinones FJ, et al. Nontypable haemophilus influenzae (Biotype 4) as a neonatal, maternal, and genital pathogen. *Rev Infect Dis* 1983; 5:123–36.

529. Schönheyder H, Grunnet N, Ejlertsen T. Non-encapsulated *Haemophilus influenzae* in the genital flora of pregnant and post-puerperal women. *Scan J Infect Dis* 1991; 23:183–7.

530. Barton LL, Dela Cruz R, Walentik C. Neonatal *Haemophilus influenzae* type C sepsis. *Am J Dis Child* 1982; 136:463–4.

531. Campognone P, Singer DB. Neonatal sepsis due to nontypable *Haemophilus influenzae*. *Am J Dis Child* 1986; 140:117–21.

532. Milne LM, Isaacs D, Crook PJ. Neonatal infections with *Haemophilus* species. *Arch Dis Child* 1988; 63:83–5.

533. McGregor J, Ogle JW, Curry-Kane G. Perinatal pertussis. *Obstet Gynecol* 1986; 68:582–6.

534. Nightingale LM, Eaton CB, Furehan AE, et al. Cephalohematoma complicated by osteomyelitis presumed due to *Gardnerella vaginalis*. *J Am Med Assoc* 1986; 256:1936–7.

535. Smith PJ, Brookfield DSK, Shaw DA, Gray J. *Serratia marcescens* infection in a neonatal unit. *Lancet* 1984; i:151–3.

536. Eisenfeld L ER, Wirtschafter D, Cassady G. Systemic bacterial infections in neonatal deaths. *Am J Dis Child* 1983; 137:645–9.

537. Nakamura Y, Nohara M, Nakashima T, et al. Meningoencephalitis due to *Serratia marcescens* infection in neonates. *Hum Pathol* 1984; 15:651–6.

538. Graham DR, Bard JD. *Citrobacter diversus* brain abscess and meningitis in neonates. *J Am Med Assoc* 1981; 245:1923–5.

539. Lin F-Y C, Devoe WF, Morrison C, et al. Outbreak of neonatal *Citrobacter diversus* meningitis in a suburban hospital. *Pediatr Infect Dis* 1987; 6:50–5.

540. Chhabra RS, Glaser JH. *Salmonella* infection presenting as hematochezia on the first day of life. *Pediatrics* 1995; 95:739–41.

541. Ryder RW, Crosby-Ritchie A, McDonough B, Hall WJ III. Human milk contaminated with *Salmonella kottbus*. A cause of nosocomial illness in infants. *J Am Med Assoc* 1977; 238:1533–4.

542. Burn CG. Clinical and pathologic features of an infection caused by a new pathogen of the genus listerella. *Am J Pathol* 1935; 12:341–50.

543. Fleming DW, Cochi SL, MacDonald KL, et al. Pasteurized milk as a vehicle of infection in an outbreak of listeriosis. *N Engl J Med* 1985; 312:404–7.

544. Schuchat A LC, Boome CV, Swaminathan B, Kim C, Winn K. Outbreak of neonatal listeriosis associated with mineral oil. *Pediatric Infect Dis J* 1991; 10:183–9.

545. Ahlfors CE, Goetzman BW HC, Sherman MP, Wennberg RP. Neonatal listeriosis. *Am J Dis Child* 1977; 131:405–8.

546. Boucher M, Yonekura ML. Perinatal listeriosis (early-onset): correlations of antenatal manifestations and neonatal outcome. *Obstet Gynecol* 1986; 68:593–7.

547. Listeriosis. *Lancet* 1985; ii:364–5.

548. Petrilli ES, d'Ablanig G, Ledger WJ. *Listeria monocytogenes* chorioamnionitis: diagnosis by transabdominal amniocentesis. *Obstet Gynecol* 1980; 55:5s.

549. Mazor M, Froimovich M, Lazer S, Maymon E, Glezerman M. Listeria monocytogenes. The role of transabdominal amniocentesis in febrile patients with preterm labor. *Arch Gynecol Obstet* 1992; 252:109–12.

550. Pitkin RM. Fetal death: diagnosis and management. *Am J Obstet Gynecol* 1987; 157:583–9.

551. Tappero JW, Schuchat A, Deaver KA, Mascola L, Wenger JD. Reduction in the incidence of human listeriosis in the United States. Effectiveness of prevention efforts? The listeriosis study group. *JAMA* 1995; 273:1118–22.

552. Visintine A, Oleske JM, Nahmias AJ. *Listeria monocytogens* infection in infants and children. *Am J Dis Child* 1977; 131:393–7.

553. Bortolussi R. Perinatal infection due to *Listeria monocytogenes*. *Clin Invest Med* 1984; 7:213–5.

554. Driscoll SG, Gorbach A, Feldman D. Congenital listeriosis: diagnosis from placental studies. *Obstet Gynecol* 1962; 20:216–22.

555. Yamazaki K, Price JT, Altshuler G. A placental view of the diagnosis and pathogenesis of congenital listeriosis. *Am J Obstet Gynecol* 1977; 129:703–5.

556. Topalovski M, Yang SS, Boonpasat Y. Listeriosis of the placenta: clinicopathologic study of seven cases. *Am J Obstet Gynecol* 1993; 169:616–20.

557. Gembruch U, Niesen M, Hansmann M, Knöpfle G. Listeriosis: a cause of non-immune hydrops fetalis. *Prenat Diag* 1987; 7:277–82.

558. Albritton WL, Wiggins GL, Feeley JC. Neonatal listeriosis: distribution of serotypes in relation to age of onset of disease. *J Pediatr* 1976; 88:481–3.

559. Grieg A, Roth P. Colony-stimulating factor 1 in the human response to neonatal listeriosis. *Infect Immun* 1995; 63:1595–7.

560. Somekh E, Abishai V, Hanani M, Gutman R, Mintz M. The clinical significance of *Pseudomonas aeruginosa* isolation from stool of neonates. *Arch Pediatr Adolesc Med* 1996; 150:108–9.

561. Ruvalo C, Bauer CR. Intrauterinely acquired pseudomonas infection in the neonate. *Clin Pediatr* 1982; 21:664–7.

562. Ander BJ, Lauer BA, Paisley JW. Campylobacter gastroenteritis in neonates. *Am J Dis Child* 1981; 135:900–2.

563. Goosens H, Henocque G, Kremp L, et al. Nosocomial outbreak of *Campylobacter jejuni* meningitis in newborn infants. *Lancet* 1988; ii:146–9.

564. Heggie AD, Jacobs MR, Butler VT, Baley JE, Boxerbaum B. Frequency and significance of isolation of *Ureaplasma urealyticum* and *Mycoplasma hominis* from cerebrospinal fluid and tracheal aspirate specimens from low birth weight infants. *J Pediatr* 1994; 124:956–61.

565. Embree JE, Krause VW, Embil JA, MacDonald S. Placental infection with *Mycoplasma hominis* and *Ureaplasma urealyticum*: clinical correlation. *Obstet Gynecol* 1980; 56:475–81.

566. McCormack WM, Braun P, Lee Y-H, Klein JO, Kass EH. The genital mycoplasmas. *N Engl J Med* 1973; 288:78–88.

567. Iwasaka T, Wada T, Kidera Y, Sugimori H. Hormonal status and mycoplasma colonization in the female genital tract. *Obstet Gynecol* 1986; 68:263–6.

568. Foulon W, Naessens A, DeWaele M, Lauwers S, Amy JJ. Chronic *Ureaplasma urealyticum* amnionitis associated with abruptio placentae. *Obstet Gynecol* 1986; 68:280–2.

569. Kundsin RB, Driscoll SG, Pelletier PA. *Ureaplasma urealyticum* incriminated in perinatal morbidity and mortality. *Science* 1981; 213:474–6.

570. Shurin PA, Alpert S, Rosner B, et al. Chorioamnionitis and colonization of the newborn infant with genital mycoplasmas. *N Engl J Med* 1975; 293:5–8.

571. Gewitz M, Dinwiddie R, Rees L, et al. *Mycoplasma hominis*. A cause of neonatal meningitis. *Arch Dis Child* 1979; 54:231–3.

572. Likitnukul S, Kusmiesz H, Nelson JD, McCracken GH Jr. Role of genital mycoplasmas in young infants with suspected sepsis. *J Pediatr* 1986; 109:971–4.

573. Waites KB, Crouse DT, Nelson KG, et al. Chronic *Ureaplasma urealyticum* and *Mycoplasma hominis* infections of central nervous system in preterm infants. *Lancet* 1988; i:17–21.

574. Cassell GH, Davis RO, Waites KB, et al. Isolation of *Mycoplasma hominis* and *Ureaplasma urealyticum* from amniotic fluid at 16–20 weeks gestation: potential effect on pregnancy outcome. *Sex Transmit Dis* 1983; 10:294–302.

575. Wang EEL, Ohlsson A, Kellner JD. Association of *Ureaplasma urealyticum* colonization with chronic lung disease of prematurity: results of a metaanalysis. *J Pediatr* 1995; 127:640–4.

576. Powell DA, Miller K, Clyde WA Jr. Submandibular adenitis in a newborn caused by *Mycoplasma hominis*. Pediatrics 1979; 63:798–9.

577. Madan E, Meyer MP, Amortegui AJ. Pathologic manifestations of perinatal genital mycoplasma infection. *Am J Clin Pathol* 1988; 90:512a.

578. Ollikainen J, Hiekkaniemi H, Korppi M, Sarkkinen H, Heinonen K. *Ureaplasma urealyticum* infection associated with acute respiratory insufficiency and death in premature infants. *J Pediatr* 1993; 122:756–60.

579. Clegg HW, Todres ID, Moylan FMB, Kevin DE, Shannon DC. Fulminant neonatal meningococcemia. *Am J Dis Child* 1980; 134:354–5.

580. Stark AR, Glode MP. Gonococcal vaginitis in a neonate. *J Pediatr* 1979; 94:298–9.

581. Oppenheimer EH, Winn KJ. Fetal gonorrhea with deep tissue infection occurring in utero. *Pediatrics* 1982; 69:74–6.

582. Neequaye J. Neonatal tetanus in Accra. *Lancet* 1984; ii:224–5.

583. Strickland GT, ed. *Hunter's Tropical Medicine.* 6th ed. Philadelphia: WB Saunders, 1984.

584. Cashore WJ, Peter G, Lauermann M, Stonestreet BS, Oh W. Clostridia colonization and clostridial toxin in neonatal necrotizing enterocolitis. *J Pediatr* 1981; 98:308–11.

585. Donta ST, Myers MG. *Clostridium difficile* toxin in asymptomatic neonates. *J Pediatr* 1981; 100:431–4.

586. Shereitz RJ, Sarubbi FA. The prevalence of *Clostridium difficile* and toxin in a nursery population: a comparison between patients with necrotizing enterocolitis and an asymptomatic group. *J Pediatr* 1982; 100:435–9.

587. Adler SP, Chandrika T, Berman WF. *Clostridium difficile* associated with pseudomembranous colitis. *Am J Dis Child* 1981; 135:820–22.

588. Singer DB, Cashore WJ, Widness JA, Campognone P, Hillemeier C. Pseudomembranous colitis in a preterm neonate. *J Pediatr Gastroenterol Nutr* 1986; 5:318–20.

589. Lide TN. Congenital tularemia. *Arch Pathol* 1947; 43:165–9.

590. Watts EA, Gard PD Jr, Tuthill SW. First reported case of intrauterine transmission of blastomycosis. *Pediatr Infect Dis* 1983; 2:308–10.

591. Cohen I. Absence of congenital infection and teratogenesis in three children born to mothers with blastomycosis and treated with amphotericin B during pregnancy. *Pediatr Infect Dis* 1987; 6:76–7.

592. Benirschke K, Raphael SI. Candida albicans infection of the amniotic sac. *Am J Obstet Gynecol* 1958; 75:200–2.

593. Whyte RK, Hussain Z, deSa DJ. Antenatal infections with *Candida*. *Arch Dis Child* 1982; 57:528–35.

594. Keller MA, Sellers BB JR, Melish ME, et al. Systemic candidiasis in infants. A case presentation and literature review. *Am J Dis Child* 1977; 131:1260–3.

595. Donders GG, Moerman P, Caudron J, Van Assche FA. Intra-uterine candida infection: a report of four infected fetuses from two mothers. *Europ J Obstet Gynecol Reprod Biol* 1991; 38:233–8.

596. Botas CM, Kurlat I, Yong SM, Sola A. Disseminated candidal infections and intravenous hydrocortisone in preterm infants. *Pediatrics* 1995; 95:883–7.

597. Dvorak AM, Gavaller B. Congenital systemic candidiasis. *N Engl J Med* 1966; 274:540–3.

598. Zenker PN, Rosenberg EM, Van Dyke RB, Rabalais GP, Daum RS. Successful medical treatment of presumed *Candida* endocarditis in critically ill infants. *J Pediatr* 1991; 119:472–7.

599. Baley JE, Annable WL, Kliegman RM. Candida endophthalmitis in the premature infant. *J Pediatr* 1981; 98:458–60.

600. McCabe R, Remington JS. Toxoplasmosis: the time has come. *N Engl J Med* 1988; 318:313–5.

601. Hershey DW, McGregor JA. Low prevalence of toxoplasma infection in a Rocky Mountain prenatal population. *Obstet Gynecol* 1987; 70:900–2.

602. Teutsch SM, Juranek DD, Sulzer A, Dubey JP, Sikes RK. Epidemic toxoplasmosis associated with infected cats. *N Engl J Med* 1979; 300:695–700.

603. Daffos F, Forestier F, Capella-Pavlovsky M, et al. Prenatal management of 746 pregnancies at risk for congenital toxoplasmosis. *N Engl J Med* 1988; 318:271–5.

604. Krogstad DJ, Juranek DD, Walls KW. Toxoplasmosis with comments on risk of infection from cats. *Ann Intern Med* 1972; 77:773–8.

605. Mitchell CD, Erlich SS, Mastrucci MT, et al. Congenital toxoplasmosis occurring in infants perinatally infected with human immunodeficiency virus. *Pediatr Inf Dis J* 1990; 9:512–8.

606. D'Ercole C, Boubli L, Franck J, et al. Recurrent congenital toxoplasmosis in a woman with lupus erythematosus. *Prenat Diagn* 1995; 15:1171–5.

607. Guerina NG, Hsu H-W, Meissner HC, et al. Neonatal serologic screening and early treatment for congenital *Toxoplasma gondii* infection. *N Engl J Med* 1994; 330:1858–63.

608. Zuelzer WW. Infantile toxoplasmosis. *Arch Pathol* 1944; 38:1–19.

609. Elliott WG. Placental toxoplasmosis. *Am J Clin Pathol* 1970; 53:413–7.

610. Wolf A, Cowen D, Paige BH. Toxoplasmic encephalomyelitis. III. A new case of granulomatous encephalomyelitis due to a protozoan. *Am J Pathol* 1939; 151:657–94.

611. Sabin AB, Feldman HA. Dyes as microchemical indicators of new immunity phenomena affecting protozoan parasite (toxoplasm). *Science* 1948; 108:660–3.

612. Koppe JG, Loewer-Sieger DH, deRoever-Bonnet H. Results of 20-year follow-up of congenital toxoplasmosis. *Lancet* 1986; i:254–6.

613. Altshuler G. Toxoplasmosis as a cause of hydranencephaly. *Am J Dis Child* 1973; 125:251–9.

614. Wilson CB, Remington JS, Stagno S, Reynolds DW. Development of adverse sequelae in children born with subclinical congenital toxoplasma infection. *Pediatrics* 1980; 66:767–74.

615. Harvey B, Remington JS, Sulzer AJ. IgM malaria antibodies in a case of congenital malaria in the United States. *Lancet* 1969; i:333–5.

616. Miglani N, Gupta BD, Gupta GL. Congenital and neonatal malaria. *Indian Pediatr* 1979; 16:637–8.

617. MacGregor JD, Avery JG. Malaria transmission and fetal growth. *Br Med J* 1974; 3:433–6.

618. Wickramasuriya GAW. Some observations on malaria occurring in association with pregnancy. *J Obstet Gynaecol Br Emp* 1935; 42:816–34.

619. Logie DE, McGregor IA. Acute malaria in newborn infants. *Br Med J* 1970; 2:404–5.

620. Woods WG, Mills E, Ferrieri P. Neonatal malaria due to *Plasmodium vivax*. *J Pediatr* 1974; 85:669–71.

621. Hindi RD, Azimi PH. Congenital malaria due to *Plasmodium falciparum*. *Pediatrics* 1980; 66:977–9.

622. Green JG. Three cases of subtertian malaria in the newborn. *Trop Dis Bull* 1939; 36:392–3.

623. Walter PR, Garin Y, Blot P. Placental pathologic changes in malaria: a histologic and ultrastructural study. *Am J Pathol* 1982; 109:330–42.

624. Galbraith RM, Faulk WP, Galbraith GMP, Holbrook TW, Bray RS. The human materno-foetal relationship in malaria: I. Identification of pigment and parasites in the placenta. *Trans R Soc Trop Med Hyg* 1980; 74:52–60.

625. Covell G. Congenital malaria. *Trop Dis Bull* 1950; 47:1147–67.

626. Esernio-Jenssen D, Scimeca PG, Benach JL, Tenenbaum MJ. Transplacental perinatal babesiosis. *J Pediatr* 1987; 110:570–2.

627. Wilcocks C, Manson-Bahr PEC, eds. *Manson's Tropical Diseases*. 17th ed. London: Ballière Tindall, 1972: pp. 109–16.

628. Bittencourt AL. Congenital Chagas' disease. *Am J Dis Child* 1976; 130:97–103.

629. DeGavaller B. Enfermedad de Chagas congènita. *Bol Maternidad 'Concepcion Palacios'* 1953; 4:59–64.

Chapter

18

Inborn Metabolic Diseases of the Perinatal Infant

James E. Dimmick   Derek A. Applegarth   Hilary D. Vallance

The scope of inherited metabolic disease in perinatal pathology includes the diagnosis of the ill newborn infant, prenatal diagnosis, newborn metabolic screening, and the study of disease evolution during intrauterine development. This discussion includes many metabolic diseases presenting to the perinatal pathologist (Table 18.1) and excludes those manifesting later in infancy. Some entities are discussed elsewhere within this volume under specific organ systems.

Many inborn metabolic disorders present in the neonatal period, others appear later in childhood, and a few do so before birth. There is great variation in the perinatal presentation of metabolic disease. Although storage diseases rarely produce severe illness in the fetus or neonate, they are an important albeit uncommon cause of hydrops fetalis. "Small-molecule," non-storage metabolic diseases (e.g., aminoacidopathies) often appear acutely in the newborn infant and rarely cause intrauterine clinical manifestations or pathology. Only a few of the inborn metabolic errors presently recognized cause abortion or intrauterine death of the infant.

The acute nature of many metabolic diseases in the newborn may be attributed to separation of the fetus from the presumed biochemical protection of the maternal-placental unit, exposure to substances from the gastrointestinal tract, and a metabolic shift from anabolism in the fetus to anabolism and catabolism in the newborn period. Since many inborn metabolic errors are in catabolic enzyme pathways, it is not surprising that the presentation of small-molecule metabolic diseases is in the newborn period.

Metabolic defects critical to anabolic pathways and embryogenesis are also now being elucidated, and the continued search for mechanisms whereby altered metabolism impacts embryogenesis promises interesting insights into dysmorphology. For example, some disorders of collagen, such as osteogenesis imperfecta, have been well characterized at the biochemical and molecular level, and a cholesterol synthesis defect underlies the Smith-Lemli-Opitz syndrome.

NEWBORN METABOLIC SCREENING

The purpose of a newborn screening program is to detect treatable disorders at an early or asymptomatic stage in order to effectively treat and avoid serious sequelae. Although this sounds admirable, screening programs have encountered problems, and so criteria and principles have been developed [1]. These principles state that 1) the condition sought should be an important health problem, 2) the natural history of the disease must be understood, 3) the screening test can detect the disease at an early or asymptomatic stage, 4) the test is reliable, sensitive, and acceptable to the population tested, 5) facilities for definitive diagnosis and treatment exist, 6) treatment at a presymptomatic or borderline stage should influence the course and prognosis of the disease favorably, 7) the cost of the case finding, including definitive diagnosis and treatment, should be balanced economically in relation to the total medical care cost, and 8) case findings should be continuous [1].

A screening test is, by nature, not diagnostic; a positive screen must be confirmed subsequently. Currently, there is a growing number of diseases included in newborn screening programs. Phenylketonuria, the first disease for which screening was instituted, was soon followed by tests for congenital hypothyroidism and galactosemia. Some centers screen for hemoglobinopathies, biotinidase deficiency, and congenital adrenal hyperplasia [2]. Screening for cystic fibrosis, Duchenne's muscular dystrophy, fatty acid oxidation disorders, and alpha-1-antitrypsin deficiency are controversial and presently are mostly done on a research basis.

Newborn metabolic screening programs may fall within the purview of the pathologist. For purposes of quality

Table 18.1.   Metabolic diseases of the neonate

Acute Metabolic Diseases of the Neonate	Subacute or Chronic Progressive Metabolic Diseases of the Neonate
Organic acidemia	Carbohydrate disorders
Propionic acidemia	Glycogen storage type I
Methylmalonic acidemia	Glycogen storage type II
Isovaleric acidemia	Glycogen storage type III
Multiple carboxylase deficiency	Glycogen storage type IV
Glutaric acidemia type II	Glycogen storage type VI
Pyruvate carboxylase deficiency	Lysosomal enzymopathies
Pyruvate dehydrogenase complex deficiency	GM1 gangliosidosis type I
Fatty acid oxidative disorders	Niemann-Pick disease
Urea cycle disorders	Gaucher disease
Carbamoyl phosphate synthetase deficiency	Farber disease
Ornithine transcarbamylase deficiency	Mucopolysaccharidoses I, II
Citrullinemia	Mucopolysaccharidosis VII
Argininosuccinic aciduria	Sialidosis
Aminoacidopathies	Mucolipidosis II
Tyrosinemia type I	Wolman disease
Maple syrup urine disease	Other
Non-ketotic hyperglycinemia	Peroxisomal diseases
Hypervalinemia	Cystic fibrosis
Hyper-beta-alaninemia	Alpha-1-antitrypsin deficiency
Lysinuric protein intolerance	Mitochondriopathies
Carbohydrate disorders	Smith-Lemli-Opitz syndrome
Hereditary fructose intolerance	Carbohydrate-deficient glycoprotein syndrome
Fructose-1,6-diphosphatase deficiency	
Classic galactosemia	
Glycogen storage disease type I	
Glycogen storage disease type II	
Lysosomal enzymopathies	
Those presenting with hydrops fetalis (Table 18.5) or ascites	
Wolman disease	
Niemann-Pick disease (type C)	
Other	
Peroxisomal diseases	
Neonatal iron storage syndrome	
Cystic fibrosis	
Alpha-1-antitrypsin deficiency	
Mitochondriopathies	

control, experience has shown that large centralized laboratories are the best way of handling tests for mass screening. Even in this setting, various technical and clerical errors occur [3]. Specifics regarding mass metabolic screening programs are addressed elsewhere [2].

INVESTIGATION AND DIAGNOSIS OF INBORN METABOLIC DISEASE IN THE NEONATE

Biochemical Investigation of Small-Molecule Diseases

Small-molecule diseases can, if not diagnosed and treated, lead to unexplained death or death mistakenly attributed to

some other cause. Diagnosis of a specific cause is essential because, even if treatment is unsuccessful, the diagnosis can often allow future prenatal diagnoses.

Table 18.2 lists signs and symptoms suspicious for metabolic disease in an infant. Table 18.3 shows biochemical findings that assist in reaching a diagnosis. The findings, like the signs and symptoms, are often nonspecific. Accordingly, Table 18.4 and the following discussion of biochemical tests help in the diagnosis of acute perinatal small-molecule metabolic diseases.

Plasma Amino Acids

Plasma amino acids are usually measured on a blood sample taken from the fasted infant. Some primary disorders of

Table 18.2. Clinical indicators of inborn metabolic disease

Neurological
Hypo- or hypertonicity
Lethargy
Coma, intermittent or constant
Convulsions
Deafness
Myopathic signs
Athetosis—ataxia
Progressive psychomotor degeneration
Cherry-red spot, macula
Cataract and corneal clouding

Gastrointestinal
Poor feeding
Vomiting (may mimic pyloric stenosis)
Diarrhea
Hepatomegaly
Ascites
Jaundice
Failure to thrive

Skeletal
Dysostosis multiplex
Arthropathy

Skin
Abnormal hair
Various skin abnormalities

Other
Hydrops fetalis
Dysmorphism
Severe or repeated infections; apparent sepsis
Peculiar odor (tomcat urine, maple syrup, mice, sweaty feet)
Family history of unexplained pediatric death or Reye syndrome
Leuko-, thrombo- or pancytopenia
Recurrent "ketoacidosis"

Table 18.3. Biochemical indicators of inborn metabolic disease

Increased anion gap (acidosis)
Unexplained hypoglycemia
Hyperammonemia
Respiratory alkalosis (often a sign of hyperammonemia)
Hyperglycinemia and/or hyperglycinuria
Lacticacidemia

amino acids, such as phenylketonuria and maple syrup urine disease, can be diagnosed immediately but there are secondary changes in amino acids indicating the presence of other disease. For instance, increased concentration of plasma glycine may suggest non-ketotic hyperglycinemia but can also be elevated in a disorder of organic acids, and increased concentration of tyrosine and/or methionine suggests liver disease. An increase in alanine may indicate lactic acidosis and suggests a defect in pyruvate metabolism or the mito-

Table 18.4. Tests needed to detect an acute metabolic disease

Blood	Urine
Blood glucose	Reducing substances by a nonspecific reducing sugar assay (alkaline copper method)
Plasma amino acids	Glucose (specific test for glucose only)
Blood ammonia	Organic acids
Blood gases	
Serum carnitine	
Plasma lactate	

chondrial electron transport chain. High concentration of glutamine may indicate hyperammonemia.

Blood Ammonia The major reason for measuring blood ammonia is to investigate a patient who is suspected of having a urea cycle defect. The finding of a high concentration of ammonia should always be followed by plasma amino acid analysis. Specific diseases of the urea cycle then may be recognized by characteristic amino acid patterns. Since hyperammonemia stimulates the respiratory center, the detection of an unexplained respiratory alkalosis should be followed by blood ammonia analysis.

Blood Gases and Electrolytes

Arterial blood gas analysis can provide evidence of a metabolic acidosis, and determination of plasma electrolytes can be used to determine the anion gap. The most common cause of metabolic acidosis in the acutely ill neonate is primary or secondary lactic acidemia. Determining the underlying defect in primary lactic acidosis remains one of the most difficult diagnostic problems in the field of metabolic disease. Secondary lactic acidosis due to liver failure or hypoxia may be easily identified. Urine organic acids, plasma amino acids and fasting glucose determinations will help to identify organic acid disorders that elevate lactate concentrations.

Urinary Organic Acids

If the metabolic acidosis is not due to a high lactate concentration, the urinary organic acid pattern should be examined. Some disorders of organic acids produce a distinct odor of the urine. However, one cause, trimethylamine, is probably innocuous [4]. Also, not all organic acid disorders are associated with metabolic acidosis. In this circumstance, clinical suspicion will determine whether urinary organic acids should be analyzed.

Urinary Reducing Substances

The ultimate aim of the urinary reducing substances test is to screen for galactosemia. Positive reducing substances and a urine test negative for glucose suggest galactosemia. However, galactosuria is not a diagnostic test because measurable amounts of galactose can be found in urine of normal newborns [237]. Diagnostic tests for galactosemia are discussed later (see the section on galactosemia). The child must be receiving galactose, usually as lactose, to diagnose galactosemia.

Biochemical Investigation of Storage Diseases

Storage disorders most often have an insidious, or subacute, clinical presentation and course. In general, the tests are presumptive or indicative and involve measuring the storage product as, for example, determination of mucopolysacchariduria. Definitive diagnoses are usually accomplished by enzyme assay. The laboratory approach summarizing presumptive and definitive diagnoses based on major organ or tissue manifestation is formulated in Table 18.5.

Morphological Investigation

Morphological techniques are valuable in the investigation and diagnosis of metabolic disease, especially in the neonate, and histopathologic findings may assist in directing the biochemical investigation. The role of histopathology in the prenatal diagnosis of metabolic disease is discussed later (see below). Histological investigation should begin with examination of the placenta, which provides easy access to tissues of the conceptus and an opportunity for rapid determination of the presence of storage disease (Fig. 18.1). An enlarging number of inborn errors of metabolism is associated with placental pathology [5–16] (Table 18.6).

Prominent microscopic vacuolation of Hofbauer and/or syncytiotrophoblast cells occurs. One must take care not to overdiagnose prominent Hofbauer cells or edema of the villus as storage cells. The foam cells of storage diseases are generally more significantly swollen and vacuolated. In Gaucher disease, stromal and trophoblast cells do not appear involved, but a few Gaucher cells may be found rarely in villous capillaries. Pompe disease, peroxisome deficiency disorders, and the infantile form of ceroid lipofuscinosis are identifiable by electron microscopy and are not associated with obvious vacuolation.

Given that the placenta may be unavailable, other tissues are used for screening purposes. Simplest is light microscopy of a peripheral blood film or bone marrow to search for vacuolated lymphocytes, bone marrow storage histiocytes, or inclusions in neutrophils, as seen in mucopolysaccharidosis (Alder-Reilly anomaly) [17] (Table 18.7).

Electron microscopy of peripheral blood lymphocytes is a focused, not a general, screening test and should be used only after rigorous clinical screening to reduce time-consuming and costly negative examinations. Ultrastructural presumptive diagnoses of some lysosomal storage diseases and definitive diagnoses of ceroid lipofuscinosis, glycogen storage disease type II, mucolipidosis type IV, and Niemann-Pick disease are possible (Fig. 18.2) [18]. Nonspecific cytoplasmic tubular, membranous, or vesicular structures, sometimes membrane-bound, occur commonly and must not be misinterpreted (Fig. 18.3).

In our opinion, electron microscopy of skin or conjunctival biopsies is more useful than peripheral lymphocytes. Skin and conjunctival biopsies provide tissue for initiation of fibroblast culture and allow for ultrastructural examination of epidermal and adnexal cells, fibrocytes, endothelial cells, pericytes, and myelinated and unmyelinated nerves (Figs. 18.4 and 18.5). Both biopsies require local anesthesia; neither requires suturing and, conveniently, conjuctival biopsy can be obtained in conjunction with ophthalmoscopic examination. The yield for ultrastructural pathology, including definitive diagnosis, may be high, particularly if patients are selected carefully by the pediatrician [19, 20]. Interpretation is based on the type of lysosomal inclusion and the cell type in which inclusions occur (see Table 18.7,

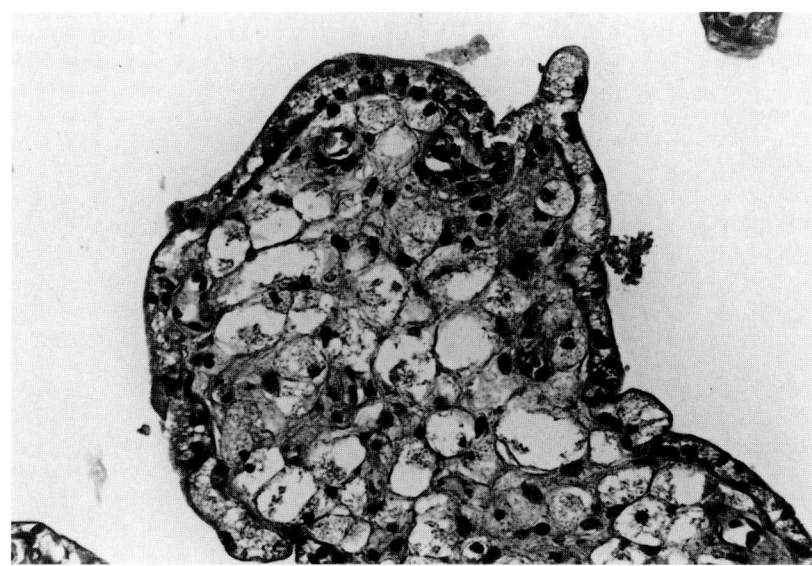

FIGURE 18.1. *Placental villus in sialidosis. Note vacuolated stromal and trophoblast cells. (×150.)*

T a b l e 18.5.   Storage diseases

Organ or Tissue	Manifestation	Disease to Be Considered	Presumptive Test	Diagnostic Test
Liver	Increased size; disordered liver function tests may be seen in some, but not all, patients with these diseases	Alpha-1-antitrypsin deficiency	Plasma alpha-1-antitrypsin	Electrophoresis and Pi typing; liver biopsy
		Mucopolysaccharidoses	Urine mucopolysaccharide quantitation; electron microscopy of conjunctiva	Specific enzyme analysis (Table 18.15)
		Glycoproteinoses	Urine oligosaccharides; electron microscopy of leukocytes, conjunctiva	Specific enzyme analysis (Table 18.4)
		Glycogen storage diseases	See Table 18.13; conjunctival biopsy (type 2); liver biopsy	See Table 18.13
		Gaucher disease	Gaucher cells in liver, bone marrow; increased serum total hexosaminidase or acid phosphatase	Leukocyte or fibroblast beta-glucosidase
		Niemann-Pick disease	Conjunctival, liver, or skin biopsy	Leukocyte or fibroblast sphingomyelinase
		Wolman disease	Liver biopsy	Fibroblast acid lipase
		Zellweger cerebrohepatorenal syndrome	Serum very-long-chain fatty acid; liver biopsy (peroxisomes)	Fibroblast or leukocyte very-long-chain fatty acid
Spleen	Increased size	Mucopolysaccharidoses	Urine mucopolysaccharide quantitation; electron microscopy of conjunctiva	Specific enzyme analysis (Table 18.15)
		Gaucher disease	Gaucher cells in bone marrow, liver	Leukocyte or fibroblast beta-glucosidase
		Niemann-Pick disease	Conjunctiva, bone marrow, or liver biopsy	Leukocyte or fibroblast sphingomyelinase
Bone	Dysostosis multiplex	Mucopolysaccharidoses	Urine mucopolysaccharide quantitations; electron microscopy of conjunctival biopsy	Specific enzyme analysis (Table 18.15)
		Glycoproteinoses	Urine oligosaccharide determination; electron microscopy of conjunctiva or leukocytes	Specific enzyme analysis (Table 18.16)
	Chondrodysplasia punctata	Chondrodysplasia punctata rhizomelic type	Serum phytanic acid	Fibroblast plasmalogen synthesis
Peripheral leukocytes; bone marrow	Cytoplasmic vacuolation		See Table 18.7	
Eye	Macular cherry-red spot	Tay-Sachs disease	Serum hexosaminidase A	Leukocyte or fibroblast hexosaminidase A
		Sandhoff disease	Serum total hexosaminidase	Leukocyte or fibroblast total hexosaminidase
		Niemann-Pick disease	Conjunctival, bone marrow, or liver biopsy	Leukocyte or fibroblast sphingomyelinase
		Generalized gangliosidosis	White cell beta-galactosidase; occasionally urine oligosaccharide increases can be seen by thin-layer chromatography; conjunctival, bone marrow biopsy	Leukocyte or fibroblast beta-galactosidase
		Sialidoses: myoclonus acid neuraminidase deficiency (mucolipidosis I)	Urinary oligosaccharide excretion; conjunctival biopsy	Fibroblast sialidase
	Corneal clouding	Mucopolysaccharidoses (Hurler, Scheie, Morquio, Maroteaux-Lamy diseases; beta-glucuronidase deficiency)	Urine mucopolysaccharides; conjunctival biopsy	Specific enzyme analysis (Table 18.15)
		Mucolipidoses II and III	Urinary oligosaccharide excretion; conjunctival biopsy	Fibroblast lysosomal enzymes
	Cataract	Galactosemia	Urinary galactose; red cell galactose or galactose-1-phosphate	Red cell galactose-1-phosphate uridyltransferase; galactokinase

Table 18.5.   *Continued*

Organ or Tissue	Manifestation	Disease to Be Considered	Presumptive Test	Diagnostic Test
Adrenal gland	Adrenal insufficiency on biochemical or clinical grounds	Adrenoleukodystrophy	Serum very-long-chain fatty acids; liver biopsy (peroxisomes)	Fibroblast or leukocyte very-long-chain fatty acids
	Bilateral adrenal calcification	Wolman disease	Liver biopsy	Fibroblast acid lipase
Cardiac muscle		Pompe disease	Electron microscopy of conjunctiva, lymphocytes, or skin	Lymphocyte or fibroblast alpha-glucosidase
		Glycogen storage disease—types III and IV	Liver biopsy—see Table 18.13	
Skeletal muscle	Myopathy involving skeletal muscle	Carnitine deficiency or carnitine palmitoyltransferase deficiency	Muscle biopsy	Measurement of muscle carnitine; measurement of carnitine palmityltransferase activity in muscle or fibroblast
Brain	Progressive mental and motor dysfunction; retardation	Krabbe disease	Conjunctival biopsy for electron microscopy; CSF protein (increased); sural nerve biopsy	Galactocerebroside beta-galactosidase, leukocytes, or fibroblast culture
		Metachromatic leukodystrophy	Conjunctival biopsy for electron microscopy; nerve biopsy; CSF protein (increased); sural nerve biopsy; nerve conduction studies	Arylsulfatase A, fibroblast culture
		Neuronal ceroid lipofuscinoses		Conjunctival biopsy for electron microscopy
		Farber disease	Tissue biopsy for electron microscopy	Fibroblast culture, lysosomal acid ceramidase
		Niemann-Pick disease	Conjunctiva, bone marrow or liver biopsy	Leukocyte or fibroblast sphingomyelinase
		Gaucher disease	Gaucher cells in bone marrow, liver	Leukocyte or fibroblast beta-glucosidase
		Mucopolysaccharidoses	Urine mucopolysaccharide quantitations; electron microscopy of conjunctival biopsy	Specific enzyme analysis (Table 18.15)
		Glycoproteinoses	Urine oligosaccharide determination; electron microscopy of conjunctiva or leukocytes	Specific enzyme analysis (Table 18.16)
		Tay-Sachs disease	Serum hexosaminidase A	Leukocyte or fibroblast hexosaminidase A
		Sandhoff disease	Serum total hexosaminidase	Leukocyte or fibroblast total hexosaminidase
		Generalized gangliosidosis GM1	White cell beta-galactosidase; occasionally urine oligosaccharide increases can be seen by thin-layer chromatography; conjunctival, bone marrow biopsy	Leukocyte or fibroblast beta-galactosidase
		Peroxisomal disorders	Serum very-long-chain fatty acid	Fibroblast very-long-chain fatty acid

Fig. 18.6). Sources of error in interpretation are artifacts created by the biopsy technique or fixation, or are due to misinterpretation of the normal morphology such as that of the mast cell or melanocyte.

Use of skin and conjunctival biopsy for investigation of lysosomal storage diseases has largely replaced biopsy of rectum and brain, but biopsy of specific organs is still required because of the limited expression of some diseases, such as mitochondriopathies, and there may be a need to obtain specific tissues for biochemical analysis.

The role for histopathology of cultured fibroblasts in the routine investigation of the newborn with possible disordered metabolism is limited but may be more significant in the setting of prenatal diagnosis using cultured amniotic fluid or chorionic villus cells. Histochemistry and electron microscopy are adjuncts to biochemical analysis [21]. Toluidine blue, PAS, Sudan black B, and histochemistry for acid phosphatase, to identify lysosomes, have greater usefulness than electron microscopy. Ultrastructural appearances of cultured cells may be confounded by tissue culture characteristics. Cells in alkaline pH media may mimic a lysosomal storage disease [22]. Ornoy et al caution that cultured fibroblasts of heterozygotes may have increased numbers of lysosomes compared to normals [23]. In all, morphological investigation of cultured fibroblasts appears to have minimal diagnostic value except in a research setting with carefully

Table 18.6.   Inherited metabolic diseases with placental involvement

Disease	Vacuolated Syncytiotrophoblast	Vacuolated Hofbauer Stromal Cells
GM1 gangliosidosis	+	?
Mucopolysaccharidosis I	–	+
Mucopolysaccharidosis III	+	+
Mucopolysaccharidosis IV	–	+
Mucopolysaccharidosis VII	–	+
Sialidosis	+	+
Mucolipidosis II	+	+
Mucolipidosis IV	–	+
Salla disease	+	+
Gaucher disease	–	–
Niemann-Pick disease	+	+
Wolman disease	?	?
Cholesterol ester storage disease	+	?
Pompe disease*	–	–
Ceroid lipofuscinosis*	–	–
Zellweger syndrome*	–	–

*   By electron microscopy.

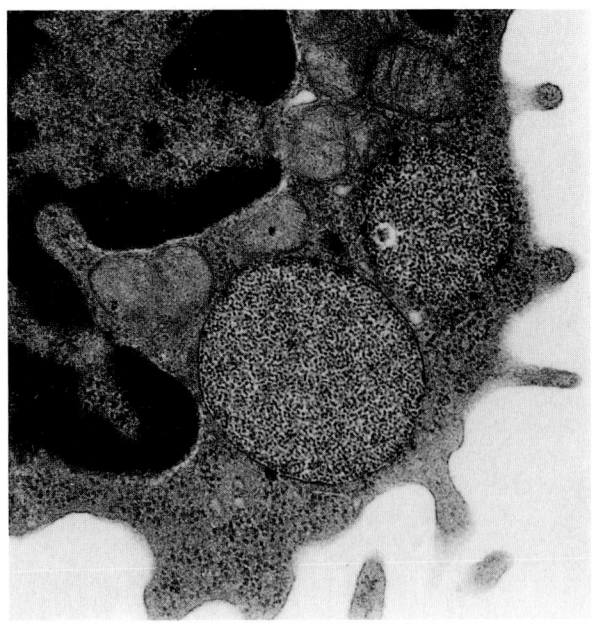

FIGURE 18.2.   *Lymphocyte in Pompe disease. Lysosomal glycogen is present. (×30,700.)*

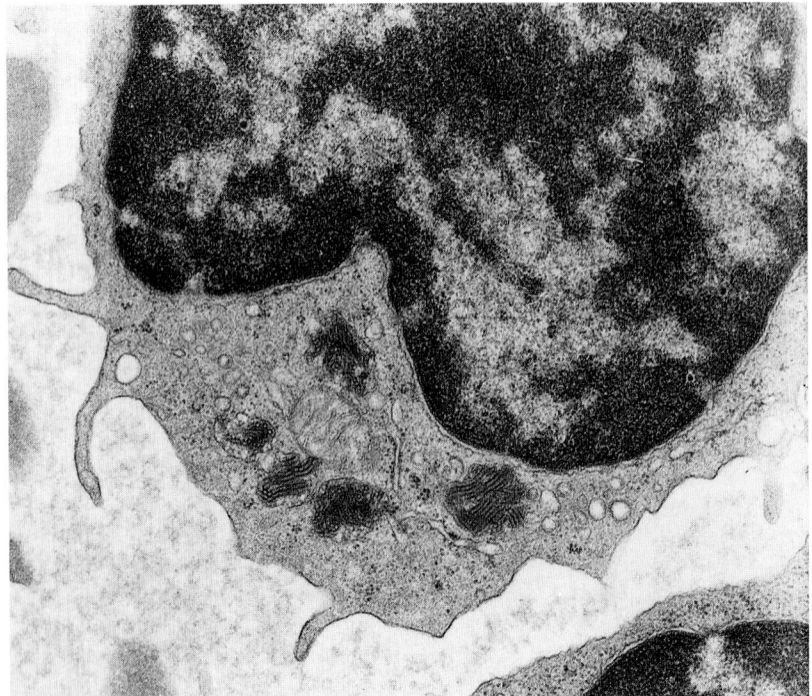

FIGURE 18.3.   *Lymphocyte showing nonspecific cytoplasmic tubular structures. (×20,000.)*

Table 18.7. Other tissues used for screening purposes

Disease	Peripheral Leukocytes*	Bone Marrow Foamy Histiocytes	Conjunctival/Skin Biopsy	
			Inclusion Type	**Site†**
Pompe disease	VL	–	Granular	EP,En,M,N
Niemann-Pick disease	VL	+	Pleomorphic, dense-lucent, lamellar	Ep,En,M,N
Gaucher disease	–	+	–	–
Krabbe disease	–	–	Crystal-like	N
Metachromatic leukodystrophy	–	–	Herringbone	N
Farber disease		+	Tubular "banana bodies," granular, membranous	M,En,N
Wolman disease	VL	+		
Mucopolysaccharidoses I,II,III	NG,VL	+	Fibrillogranular, membranous	Ep,M,N,En
GM1 gangliosidosis	VL	+	Fibrillogranular, membranous	Ep,En,M,N
Tay-Sachs disease	–	–	Membranous, granular	N,En,M
Sandhoff disease	–	–	Membranous, granular	N,En,M
Sialidosis	VL	+	Fibrillogranular, membranous	Ep,En,M,N
Mucolipidosis II	VL		Fibrillogranular, lamellar	M,En,N
Mucolipidosis III	VL		Fibrillogranular, lamellar	M,En,N
Mucolipidosis IV	VL		Fibrillogranular, lamellar	Ep,En,M,N
Fucosidosis	VL	+	Fine granular, sparse	Ep,En,M,N
Mannosidosis	VL	+	Fibrillogranular	M,En,N
Ceroid lipofuscinosis	VL (juvenile)	–	Granular, curvilinear, "fingerprint"	Ep,En,N

* VL = vacuolated lymphocyte; NG = neutrophil granules.
† EP = epithelial; En = endothelial; M = mesenchymal; N = neural.

controlled variables where the pathogenesis and therapy of metabolic diseases may be studied.

SPECIFIC INHERITED METABOLIC DISEASES
Disorders of Organic Acid Metabolism

Organic acidemias are rare metabolic disorders in which organic acids accumulate when there is a primary enzymopathy or secondary cofactor disturbance in the catabolism of amino acids, fatty acids, or pyruvate. The metabolites in these disorders are short-chain acids (up to 12 carbon atoms). They are non-reactive with ninhydrin and are not detected directly by amino acid assays. Gas-liquid chromatography and mass spectrometry are required for diagnosis. Some diseases, such as maple syrup urine disease, may be classified as either an aminoacidopathy or organic acidopathy. Organic acid diseases can affect amino acid concentrations and can produce lactic acidosis.

Organic acidemias may present in the newborn as an acute fulminant disorder, or later in infancy or childhood [24–26]. In the neonate, seizures, hypotonia, and coma occur with vomiting, sometimes to a degree suggesting the presence of pyloric stenosis. The disorders are exacerbated by infections or feeding changes. Older infants may fail to thrive. Odors are a feature of some organic acidemias, for example, isovaleric acidemia. Accumulated metabolites may suppress bone marrow precursor cells, resulting in neutropenia, thrombocytopenia, and sometimes anemia [27]. Organic acid disorders are broadly discussed elsewhere [28]. Diagnosis of organic acid diseases can be made by using the protocol for investigation of small-molecule disorders (see Table 18.4).

Propionic Acidemia and Methylmalonic Acidemia
Propionic acidemia (propionyl-CoA carboxylase deficiency) and methylmalonic acidemia (methylmalonyl-CoA mutase

deficiency) are clinically similar autosomal recessive disorders resulting from defects in the catabolism of isoleucine and odd-chain fatty acids. In the newborn, both disorders produce an acute fulminant disease with vomiting, hypotonia, respiratory distress, seizures, and coma leading to death. Modest hepatomegaly is often recorded. Infants are severely acidotic, usually ketotic, and have variably elevated levels of

ammonia, probably due to interference of N-acetyl glutamate synthetase, an activator of carbamoyl phosphate synthetase (see the discussion of urea cycle disorders), by propionyl CoA. Hypoglycemia also occurs and hyperglycinemia is usual. Urine organic acid excretion patterns include propionate, 3-hydroxypropionate, methylcitrate, and tiglylglycine. Methylmalonic acid is also elevated in methylmalonyl-CoA mutase deficiency. Ketone bodies are usually found in both disorders and may be long chain (butanone) or the conventional acetoacetate and acetone. Both diseases can be diagnosed by enzyme analysis using white cells or cultured fibroblasts [26]. Two complementation groups, pccA and pccBC, have been defined among propionyl-CoA carboxylase–deficient patients corresponding to mutations affecting genes coding for the alpha and the beta subunits of the carboxylase apoprotein.

Pathology of propionic acidemia and methylmalonic acidemia is poorly detailed. At autopsy hepatomegaly with hepatic macrovesicular steatosis is common [29–31]. Spongy change of the white matter, cerebellar hemorrhage, disruption or decrease in the external granular cell layer of cerebellum, and focal loss of Purkinje cells have been reported [29–31]. Alzheimer type II cells occur in some infants with marked hyperammonemia [30]. In one detailed study of a 12-day-old infant with propionic acidemia, there was moderate generalized hepatic steatosis [29]. Ultrastructurally, the lipid was located unbound within the cytoplasm; mitochondria were distended with a homogeneous amorphic substance and cristae appeared diminished. Hepatic siderosomes were increased. Isoleucine added to fibroblast cultures from the same infant with propionic acidemia caused an

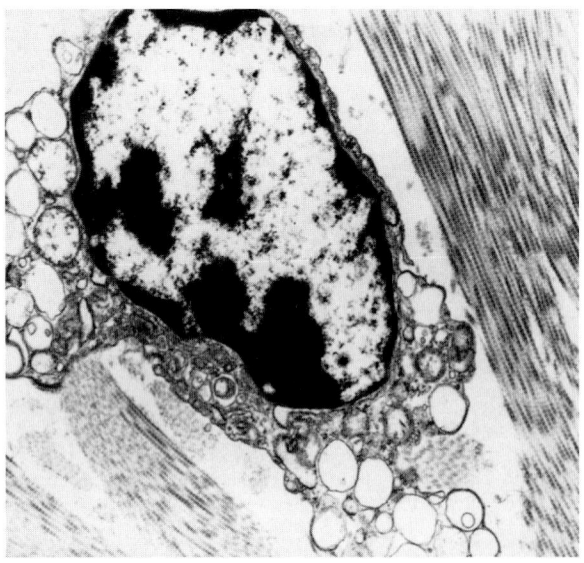

FIGURE 18.4. *Skin in sialidosis. Note the predominantly empty vacuoles. (×3100.)*

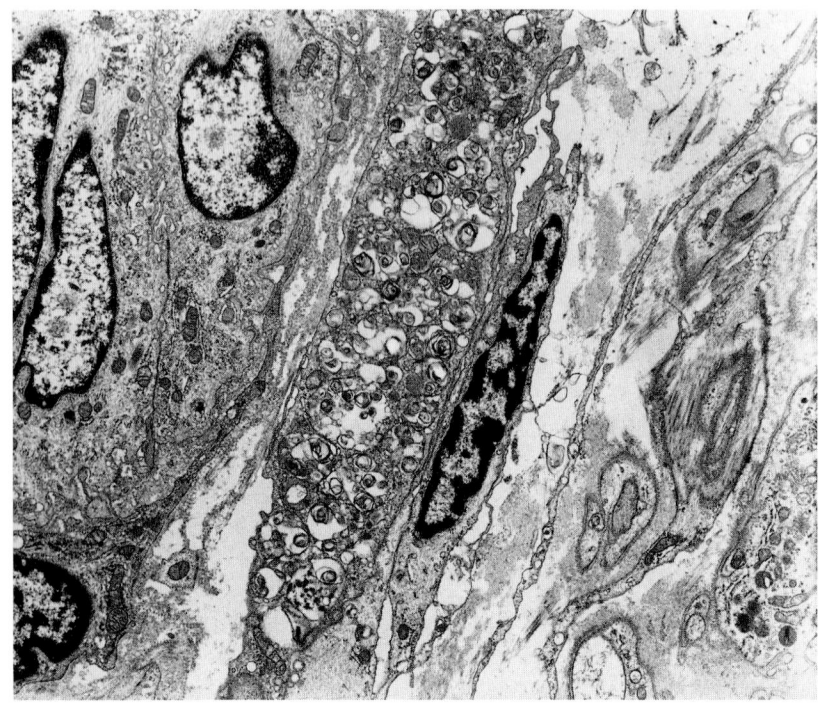

FIGURE 18.5. *Skin in Niemann-Pick disease. (×5670.)*

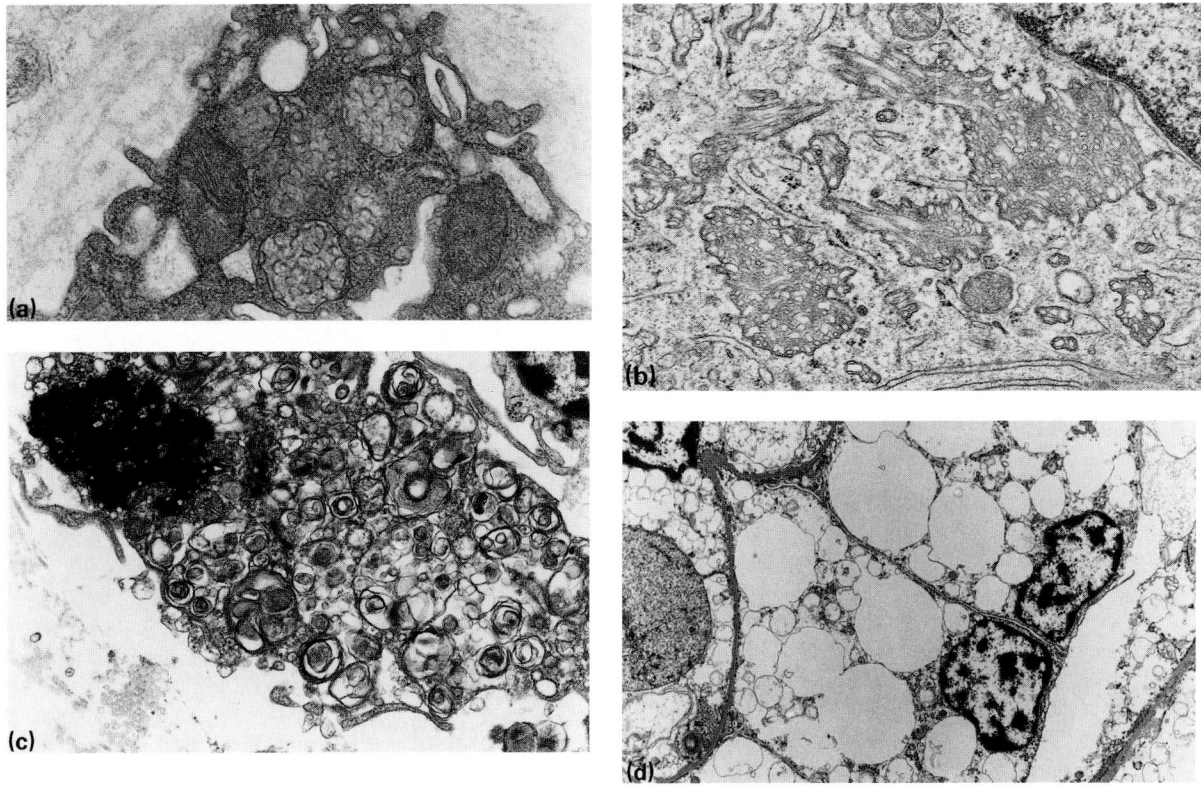

FIGURE 18.6.   *Inclusions seen in different forms of lysosomal disorder. (a) Ceroid lipofuscinosis. Curvilinear bodies in skin fibrocyte. (×41,750.) (b) Gaucher disease. Tubular inclusions in splenic histiocyte. (×25,000.) (c) Niemann-Pick disease. Membranous inclusions in bone marrow histiocyte. (×5250.) (d) Sialidosis. "Empty" lysosomes of renal tubule cell. (×5400.)*

increase in neutral lipid and lamellated osmophilic bodies but mitochondria remained normal, suggesting that lamellated bodies reflected lipid accumulation secondary to toxic injury of cell membranes [29].

Related Disorders   Propionic acid is also excreted in multiple carboxylase deficiency, caused by a defect in biotin metabolism which affects all four biotin-dependent carboxylases: propionyl-CoA carboxylase, acetyl-CoA carboxylase, pyruvate carboxylase, and 3-methylcrotonyl-CoA carboxylase. Most, if not all, of the respective organic acid metabolites are found in urine. In the neonatal form of multiple carboxylase deficiency, acidosis, ketosis, hyperammonemia, hypoglycemia, hyperglycinemia, coma, seizures, and an erythematous rash occur. A tomcat odor to the urine (due to methylcrotonoic acid) is noted. In fibroblast culture, low carboxylase enzyme activities are enhanced by the addition of biotin [32, 33].

Cobalamin, the cofactor of methylmalonyl CoA mutase, has a complex synthetic pathway and a number of defects in its synthesis have been described. Some of the cobalamin defects also affect homocysteine metabolism; therefore, it is worthwhile measuring total homocysteine in blood to look for this possibility [34]. Elucidation of the specific defect is essential for accurate diagnosis, treatment, and prenatal diagnosis.

Glutaric Acidemia Type I

Glutaric acidemia type I is caused by glutaryl-CoA dehydrogenase deficiency, an enzyme system present in mitochondria and peroxisomes [35, 36]. Macrocephaly at birth is common but dystonia and seizures rarely appear until after the neonatal period. Excretion of glutaric acid can be low or even absent. Therefore, a high index of clinical suspicion necessitates enzyme assay in leukocytes or fibroblasts. This disease is biochemically very different from glutaric acidemia type II (see below).

Isovaleric Acidemia

Isovaleric acidemia is caused by a deficiency of isovaleryl-CoA dehydrogenase, an enzyme in the catabolism of leucine. Clinical presentation, like that of propionic acidemia and methylmalonic acidemia, includes an acute fulminant form in the newborn with the additional finding of an odor of sweaty feet on the infant's breath or urine. In acute attacks, isovaleric acid concentration increases in the plasma and metabolites of isovaleryl-CoA accumulate. Isovaleric acid can be conjugated with glycine, forming isovaleryl glycine, or found free in plasma. Both can be detected using gas chromatography/mass spectrometry. Definitive diagnosis requires demonstration of the enzyme deficiency in fibroblast culture or leukocytes [37].

Pathology is as nonspecific as that of propionic acidemia and methylmalonic acidemia. Hemorrhages occur in the brain and other viscera, and the liver displays diffuse steatosis.

Fatty Acid Oxidation Defects

In recent years, our understanding of the clinical features and biochemical abnormalities of fatty acid beta-oxidation defects has greatly expanded [37]. Many fatty acid oxidation disorders are now known and it is likely that more are to be defined (Table 18.8). Clinical features include sudden metabolic decompensation with hypoketotic hypoglycemia and dysfunction of the organs (heart, skeletal muscle, and liver) dependent on fatty acid oxidation for energy. Crises are often triggered by viral illness or prolonged fasting. Misdiagnoses of sudden infant death syndrome or Reye syndrome may be made, or a similar illness may have occurred in a sibling [38, 39]. If detected early, many fatty acid oxidation defects are treatable, underlying the importance of early and accurate diagnosis.

Most fatty acid oxidation disorders have significant fatty infiltration of the liver (microvesicular or mixed micro- and macrovesicular) but steatosis may be mild and only observed after oil red O or similar staining techniques [40, 41]. When there is clinical suspicion, the liver, muscle, and other parenchymal organs should be stained specifically for lipids even if the gross appearance is normal. Abnormal metabolites are detected in urine, blood, and liver tissue (Table

18.9). Enzymatic diagnosis is often done using cultured skin fibroblasts. Most fatty acid metabolites are stable in fluids and tissues; therefore, tissue procurement during autopsy and storage at −70°C is worthwhile up to 72 hours postmortem [41].

Medium-Chain Acyl-CoA Dehydrogenase Deficiency Medium-chain acyl-CoA dehydrogenase deficiency (MCAD) is the most frequently diagnosed disorder of fatty acid beta-oxidation [42]. The most consistently abnormal metabolites during and between episodes of metabolic decompensation are *cis*-4-decenoic acid and hexanoylglycine which can be measured in the blood, urine, and liver [38, 40]. Molecular analysis has identified a common single point mutation (A985G) for which 80% of patients are homozygous and approximately 98% are heterozygous [43]. Although this mutation is common, its absence does not rule out a fatty acid oxidation defect.

Estimation by retrospective study of the incidence of MCAD among cases of sudden death in children suggests that it is not a common cause [44]. However, the incidence of fatty acid oxidation disorders among cases of sudden, unexpected death with a fatty liver identified on autopsy is significant. Boles et al suggest the incidence in such cases is as high as 10% [41]. MCAD appears to be most common in some regions of Great Britain or Northern Europe (1/10,000) [45] and is very rare among non-Caucasians, suggesting a founder effect of the A985G mutation.

Other Other fatty acid oxidative disorders occurring in the neonate and with hepatic involvement are discussed elsewhere (see Chapter 25).

Glutaric Aciduria Type II (Multiple acyl-CoA Dehydrogenase Deficiency) Glutaric aciduria type II or multiple acyl-CoA dehydrogenase deficiency is most often caused by deficiencies of electron transport flavoprotein (ETF). In some cases an undefined abnormality in flavin metabolism through which electrons from flavoprotein acyl-CoA dehydrogenases enter the respiratory chain appears responsible.

The severe form of glutaric aciduria type II is characterized by hypoketotic hypoglycemia, metabolic acidosis, an odor of "sweaty feet," hepatomegaly, hypotonia, and death in the neonatal period. Severe fatty change of the liver,

Table 18.8. Fatty acid oxidative defects

Defects of carnitine: acyl carnitine metabolism
  Plasma membrane carnitine uptake defect
  Carnitine palmitoyltransferase (CPT) deficiency
    CPT I—hepatic form
    CPT II—muscular form
      severe neonatal form
    Translocase deficiency
Acyl-CoA dehydrogenase defects
  Short-chain acyl-CoA dehydrogenase deficiency
  Short-chain 3-hydroxyacyl-CoA dehydrogenase deficiency
  Medium-chain acyl-CoA dehydrogenase deficiency
  Long-chain acyl-CoA dehydrogenase deficiency
  Very-long-chain acyl-CoA dehydrogenase deficiency
  Multiple acyl-CoA dehydrogenase defects
    Electron transfer flavoprotein (ETF) deficiency
    ETF-QC deficiency
2,4-dienoyl-CoA reductase deficiency
Trifunctional protein deficiency

Table 18.9. Investigation of fatty acid oxidative defects

Test	Sample
Glucose	Plasma, liver
Carnitine	Serum
Ketones	Serum or plasma, urine
Acylcarnitine analysis	Plasma, blood dot card preferred, urine if other specimens unavailable
Fatty acid analysis	Liver
Organic acid analysis	Urine
Molecular analysis (MCAD—A985G)	Blood dot card, whole blood, tissue

myocardium, and renal convoluted tubules, intraventricular hemorrhage of brain, and Alzheimer type II cells may be found [46, 47]. Infants with multiple acyl-CoA dehydrogenase deficiency may be dysmorphic; CNS anomalies, facial dysmorphism, cystic kidneys, cardiac defects, and intrahepatic biliary dysgenesis occur [48–51]. Urine organic acid analysis reveals glutaric acid; ethylmalonic acid 2-hydroxyglutaric, adipic, suberic, and sebacic acids; and other short-chain volatile acids. It can be difficult to diagnose this group of diseases by organic acid or enzyme assays.

For a thorough review of other fatty oxidation defects, see Roe et al [42].

Pyruvate Dehydrogenase Deficiency

Deficiency of the pyruvate dehydrogenase complex (PDHC) is a common cause of primary lactic acidemia. The severity tends to correlate with the degree of lactic acidemia. In the most severe form there is marked lactic acidosis at birth, and death occurs in the neonatal period. Some patients with PDHC deficiency have facial dysmorphism resembling fetal alcohol syndrome, microcephaly, and CNS anomalies which, like glutaric aciduria II, imply that disturbed metabolism has affected morphogenesis [52]. Pathology of the brain may resemble Leigh syndrome and agenesis of the corpus callosum is a feature in some cases. A milder phenotype presents with carbohydrate-induced episodic ataxia and mild developmental delay that may respond to a ketogenic diet.

PDHC may be due to a defect in any one of its components (E1-alpha, E2, E3, X-lipoate, or PDHC phosphatase proteins). The most common defect is in the E1-alpha component, which is on the X chromosome. This X-linked dominant form appears in equal numbers of female and male patients. Numerous point mutations and deletions have been described [53].

Diagnosis is achieved by PDHC assay in cultured fibroblasts. Due to X inactivation in females and the observation that the mutant allele may be inactivated to a greater extent than the normal allele in some patients, the assay is less reliable in females [54] and a normal result does not entirely rule out the diagnosis.

Pyruvate Carboxylase Deficiency

Pyruvate carboxylase (PC) deficiency, a rare autosomal recessive disorder, has acute neonatal and milder infantile forms. In the neonatal form there is no detectable enzyme protein and severe lactic acidosis occurs with citrullinemia, hyperammonemia, ketosis, and hyperlysinemia [52, 55, 56]. The fulminant neonatal form presents with respiratory distress, depressed central nervous system function, seizures, bleeding diathesis, and jaundice.

In one infant with the acute neonatal form, liver biopsy showed micro- and macrovesicular steatosis in all but the periportal hepatocytes, cholestasis, mild ductular proliferation with minimal portal septal fibrosis, and acinar rearrangement of hepatocytes [56] (Fig. 18.7). Hepatocytes were swollen with large nucleoli, and a few were mitotic, but none appeared necrotic. Ultrastructurally, mitochondria were slightly pleomorphic and had increased matrix density and prominent dilatation of the intracristal space. At autopsy the swollen brain contained bilateral symmetrical cavitated infarcts in the frontal lobes and diffuse gliosis between the cortex and central nuclei. Old cavitated hemorrhages were present in the germinal eminences.

Examination of one fetus confirmed to have pyruvate carboxylase deficiency and aborted at 20 weeks' gestation disclosed no gross or microscopic pathology of liver, brain, or other viscera [57].

PC deficiency can be confirmed in cultures of skin fibroblasts and lymphocytes. Multiple carboxylase deficiency

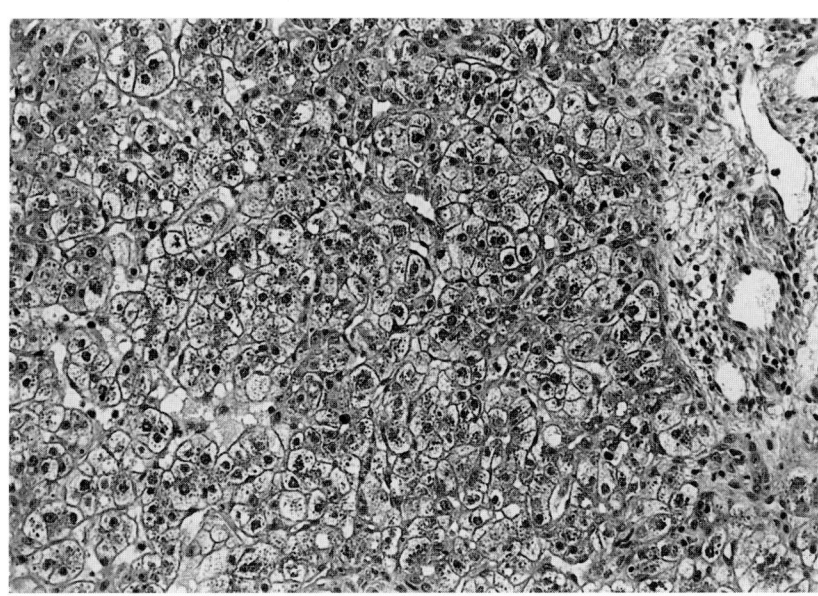

FIGURE 18.7. *Pyruvate carboxylase deficiency. Liver cells are swollen and have prominent nucleoli. There is steatosis and cholestasis. (×67.)*

should be ruled out by assay of one or more of the other carboxylase enzymes. Prenatal diagnosis is possible for both pyruvate dehydrogenase complex deficiency and pyruvate carboxylase deficiency using cultured chorionic villus tissue or amniocytes.

Mitochondrial Respiratory Chain Disorders

The mitochondrial respiratory chain is composed of electron carrier proteins that transfer reducing equivalents from NADH, succinate, and FADH2 to molecular oxygen in a series of oxidation-reduction steps which produce ATP. Situated in the mitochondrial membrane, each complex (I through V) is made up of multiple polypeptides, derived from a combination of mitochondrial (mtDNA) and nuclear DNA. Most human cells contain hundreds of mitochondria and thousands of mtDNAs. Since the mtDNA is predominantly transmitted through the oocyte cytoplasm, inheritance is maternal. Mutations are often heteroplasmic, meaning that there is a mixture of normal and mutant mitochondrial DNA in cells and tissues.

Tissues most dependent on oxidative metabolism, such as brain, skeletal and cardiac muscle, eye, and endocrine glands, are mostly affected (Fig. 18.8a and b). Primary lactic acidosis is virtually a universal finding in infantile forms, but may not occur with mitochondrial disorders presenting later.

In Table 18.10, specimens useful for investigation of mitochondriopathies are listed. The interpretation of an elevated lactate concentration can be difficult due to elevations that result from difficulties with infant venipuncture. It is, therefore, valuable to know that in mitochondriopathies a plasma amino acid assay may reveal an increased alanine concentration in the presence of lactic acidosis, and an elevated CSF lactate is very suggestive in the presence of neurological signs.

Biochemical assays of the respiratory chain complexes in skeletal muscle are often diagnostic, revealing isolated complex I, III, IV (cytochrome C oxidase), or V (ATPase) deficiency or a combined defect of more than one complex. There may be secondary disturbance of other enzymes such as pyruvate dehydrogenase complex activity [58]. The finding of normal respiratory chain enzyme activities in skeletal muscle does not rule out a mitochondrial defect in other tissues. Expression of defects may be more pronounced or only apparent in liver or brain [59, 60]. It is sometimes possible to demonstrate the biochemical defects in cultured fibroblasts.

Lethal Infantile Mitochondrial Disease (LIMD)

Infants with lethal infantile mitochondrial disease (LIMD) are often abnormal from birth and manifest hypotonia, respiratory distress, seizures, and severe lactic acidosis. Hepatic dysfunction and renal tubulopathy with generalized aminoaciduria are also common. Defects in complex I, complex III, complex IV, and combined defects (I and IV) have been described. Muscle often has lipid and glycogen accumulation but ragged red fibers are rarely seen. Electron microscopy may reveal abnormally shaped mitochondria with disordered cristae without paracrystalline inclusions.

Table 18.10. Specimens valuable for mitochondrial disorder investigations

Blood	Lactate; amino acids; carnitine; mtDNA analysis
Urine	Organic acids
CSF	Lactate
Muscle (or other tissue)	Histochemistry; electron microscopy; OXPHOS biochemistry; mtDNA analysis

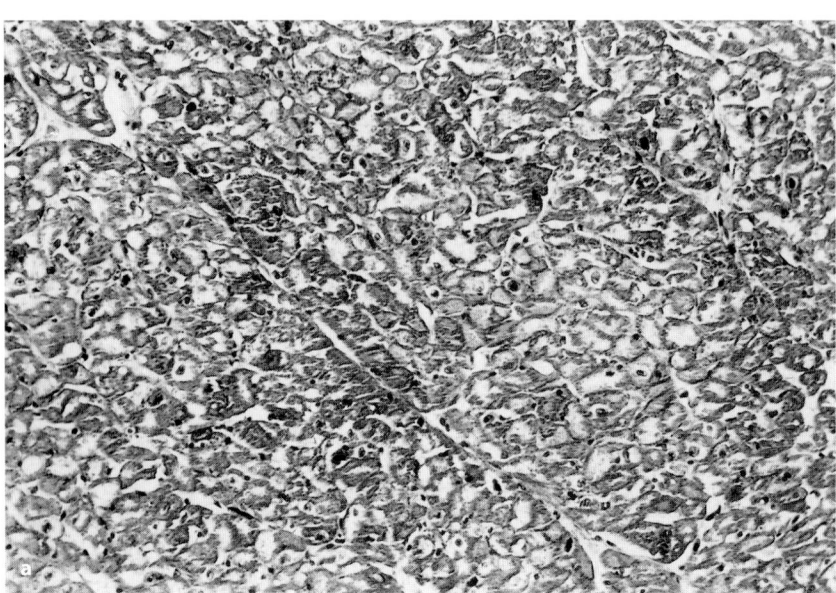

FIGURE 18.8. *Mitochondrial cardiomyopathy of an infant. (a) The myocardium has a vacuolated appearance, which is due to (b) an increased number of abnormal mitochondria. (a: H&E, ×40. b: ×9100.)*

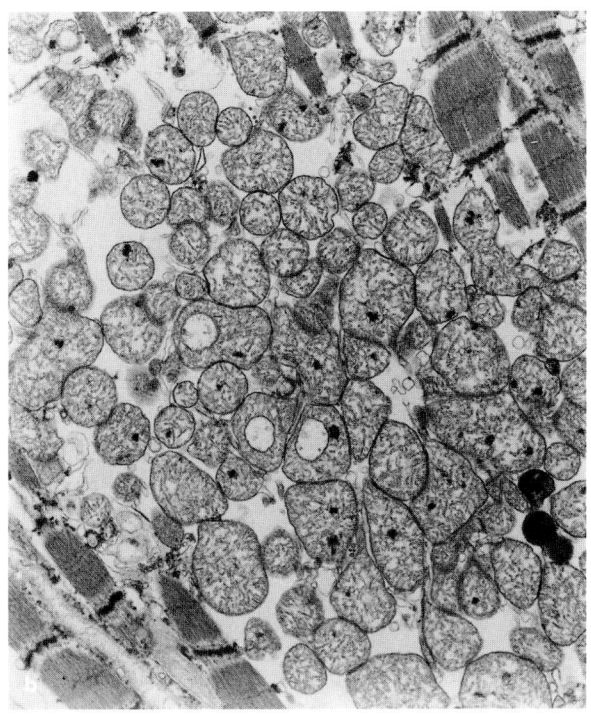

FIGURE 18.8. *Continued*

The pattern of inheritance is usually autosomal recessive but nuclear gene defects are uncommonly identified. Rare cases of LIMD are caused by depletion of mtDNA. Quantitative polymerase chain reaction (PCR) or Southern blot analysis shows that the ratio of mtDNA to nuclear DNA is greatly reduced.

A benign form of mitochondrial myopathy exists in which profound hypotonia, respiratory difficulties, and myopathy at birth abate and there is gradual improvement in the first year of life associated with normalization of oxidative phosphorylation (OXPHOS) activity in muscle [61]. The underlying defect is unknown but may be a fetal OXPHOS muscle isoform that diminishes with the switch to the adult isoform, allowing for clinical improvement.

Leigh Disease

Leigh disease (subacute necrotizing encephalopathy) is a neurodegenerative condition of the brain stem, cerebellum, and basal ganglia. There are well-demarcated symmetrical regions of necrosis, gliosis, and vascular proliferation [62]. Central nervous system dysgenesis and neuronal migrational defects are other frequent findings [63].

Complex I, IV, and V (ATPase) deficiencies have been described. A point mutation at 8993 of mtDNA in the ATPase 6 gene is responsible for many complex V deficiencies and can be tested for by a PCR-based assay [64]. The remainder of patients are likely to have nuclear genetic defects with presently an unknown molecular basis.

Hypertrophic Cardiomyopathy and Myopathy

A respiratory chain defect can sometimes be demonstrated in patients with hypertrophic cardiomyopathy and myopathy. Complex I and IV defects are found in cardiac muscle. Rarely, point mutations of mtDNA are described; an A to G mutation in the tRNA gene at bp 4269 of the mtDNA [65] and a mutation in the tRNA gene for isoleucine (A4317) have also been described [66]. A 4.5 kb deletion was found in another case [67].

Other Syndromes

An X-linked cardioskeletal myopathy has been described associated with growth retardation, neutropenia, endocardial fibroelastosis, and 3-methylglutaconic acid in the urine [68]. The gene was recently mapped to Xq28. Other neonatal mitochondriopathies with hepatic manifestations are described in Chapter 25.

Overall, the molecular basis of most of the mitochondrial disorders presenting in the perinatal period remain unknown.

Prenatal diagnosis of mitochondriopathies is generally not possible. Biochemical defects are often tissue specific, and those demonstrated in muscle or fibroblasts do not necessarily correlate with expression in other tissues or cultured cells.

Disorders of Amino Acid Metabolism

Urea Cycle Disorders

As with other inherited metabolic diseases, varying clinical expression of urea cycle disorders probably relates to the degree of enzyme deficiency. Inborn errors of all urea cycle enzymes, except arginase, cause severe illness in the newborn infant (Table 18.11). Without treatment, hypotonia, lethargy, and poor feeding are followed by seizures, coma, and death. Infants frequently vomit and have respiratory distress. Marked hyperammonemia is characteristic of all four inherited urea cycle disorders presenting in the neonatal period. Generally, the urea cycle disorders are not associated with hypoglycemia, ketosis, metabolic acidosis, or organic aciduria. In fact, hyperammonemia with respiratory alkalosis should suggest a urea cycle disorder.

Carbamyl Phosphate Synthetase Deficiency Carbamyl phosphate synthetase deficiency is an autosomal recessive disorder. Marked hyperammonemia is usually associated with diminished plasma citrulline and arginine. Orotic acid in urine is not elevated. There is no organic aciduria. Definitive diagnosis requires enzyme assay on liver tissue. Prenatal diagnosis was once only possible through fetal liver biopsy but now can be accomplished by linkage analysis with informative flanking markers [69–71].

In the brain, the most common findings are spongiosis, congestion, and Alzheimer type II astrocytic reaction [72]. Lesions attributable to anoxic-ischemic injury and hemorrhage may also occur. Pathology of liver includes mild steatosis and focal hepatocellular necrosis. Ultrastructurally,

Table 18.11.   Urea cycle diseases

Disorder*	Ammonia	Glutamine	Other Amino Acids†	Urine	Enzyme Deficiency	Assay Material
Carbamyl phosphate synthetase deficiency	↑↑↑	↑↑↑			Carbamoyl phosphate	Liver
Ornithine transcarbamoylase deficiency	↑↑↑	↑↑↑	Citrulline N or ↓ Arginine N or ↓	Orotic acid ↑↑	Ornithine transcarbamoylase (OTC)	Liver
Citrullinemia	↑↑	↑↑	Citrulline ↑↑ Arginine N or ↓	Citrulline ↑ Orotic acid ↑	Argininosuccinic acid synthetase	Liver, fibroblasts
Argininosuccinic acid lyase deficiency	↑	↑	ASA ↑↑↑ Citrulline ↑ Arginine N or ↓	ASA ↑↑↑ Orotic acid ↑	Argininosuccinic acid synthetase	Liver, fibroblasts, erythrocytes
Arginase deficiency	↑	↑	Arginine ↑↑↑ Ornithine N or ↓	Arginine ↑↑	Arginase	Liver, fibroblasts, erythrocytes

* With the exception of arginase deficiency, blood urea need not be strikingly low.
† N = normal.

mitochondria may be normal, swollen, increased in number but with normal cristae and matrix, or pleomorphic with increased matrix density [73]. Dense deposits in the mitochondrial matrix, short and forked cristae, and intercristal membranous whorls also occur [72]. The Golgi apparatus may appear increased, the smooth endoplasmic reticulum is vesicular, and the rough endoplasmic reticulum is concentrically configured [72, 73]. Loss of microvilli in dilated canaliculi also has been noted [73].

Ornithine Transcarbamylase Deficiency Ornithine transcarbamylase deficiency is an X-linked disorder in which hemizygous male infants suffer a fulminant neonatal disease. Beyond the neonatal period the disorder can mimic Reye syndrome. Heterozygous females have variable expression of the disease at a later age. Severe hyperammonemia and marked orotic aciduria occur, and there is often diminished plasma citrulline. Enzyme assay on liver biopsy may be done for confirmation. Prenatal diagnosis is similar to CPS deficiency: biochemical assay on fetal liver biopsy, linkage analysis, or if the mutation is known in the proband, direct mutation detection [74–76].

Alzheimer type II astrocytes and spongiosis of the brain occur, and hypomyelination and cerebellar heterotopias imply a possible prenatal insult by disturbed metabolism [77]. The liver of hemizygous male infants may be normal or enlarged with focal hepatocellular necrosis, and have mild steatosis. Hepatocellular necrosis, inflammation, steatosis, piecemeal necrosis, and fibrosis occur in heterozygous

females at an older age. Hepatic ultrastructure in male newborns suggests that the mitochondria are normal, unlike those of older infants in whom many mitochondrial abnormalities may occur [78]. Normal-sized peroxisomes may be decreased and small peroxisomes increased in number [79]. Hug et al noted varying-sized peroxisomes, some ballooned with flocculent matrices and disintegrating membranes [73]. A newborn male infant with ornithine transcarbamylase deficiency in our experience had normal mitochondria and swelling of peroxisomes with rarefaction of the matrix.

Argininosuccinate Synthetase Deficiency: Citrullinemia Citrullinemia due to deficient activity of argininosuccinate synthetase is an autosomal recessive disorder which, in its neonatal form, has a clinical behavior similar to the other urea cycle disorders. Marked hyperammonemia with low arginine and very high plasma citrulline levels occur. There is no argininosuccinic acid detectable in the urine or plasma. Orotic acid output may be increased mildly. Enzyme assays can be done on cultured fibroblasts, amniocytes, or chorionic villus samples [80, 81]. Citrulline is elevated in amniotic fluid of affected fetuses. Neuropathology of newborn infants dying with citrullinemia differs little from that of the other urea cycle disorders. Myelination may be normal or retarded and there may be myelin degeneration [82]. Lesions of hypoxic-ischemic injury are superimposed. The liver may be normal, or steatosis and focal hepatocellular necrosis may occur. Cholestasis is more common in citrullinemia than in the other neonatal urea cycle disorders [83]. Electron microscopic study of the liver from one newborn showed giant mitochondria with increased matrix density and widened intracristal spaces. The rough endoplasmic reticulum was arranged in a concentric fashion and circular or irregular cisternae were present. Peroxisomes and autolysosomes were increased [83].

Argininosuccinate Lyase Deficiency Argininosuccinic aciduria, which is autosomal recessive, is due to deficiency of argininosuccinate lyase. Neonatal, subacute, and delayed onset forms occur. Presentation in the newborn is similar to the other urea cycle disorders and usually occurs in the first week of life. Older infants may have abnormalities of the hair. In the newborn, hyperammonemia coexists with elevated argininosuccinic acid in plasma and urine; plasma citrulline is moderately elevated (see Table 18.8). Infants may have hepatomegaly and hypertransaminasemia. Enzyme assay is done on fibroblast culture, liver, or erythrocytes.

Pathologic changes are nonspecific. In the brain, spongy degeneration of the white matter, deficient myelination, and Alzheimer cells occur. In the liver, there is either no pathology or foci of hemorrhage and congestion. A less fulminant presentation in older infants may lead to clinical confusion with Reye syndrome, but the mitochondrial pathology of Reye syndrome is not present [84].

Other Disorders Argininemia due to arginase deficiency does not cause severe disease in the perinatal period. Transient hyperammonemia of the newborn is of unknown etiology and may or may not be symptomatic. Some preterm infants, often with respiratory distress, may have greatly elevated serum ammonia mimicking an inborn error of the urea cycle. Urea cycle enzyme activities are normal. Plasma amino acid determinations reveal normal to slightly elevated levels of citrulline, glutamine, and alanine. Urinary orotic acid is not elevated. Significantly, the onset of symptoms within 4 hours of birth is earlier than occurs with most urea cycle disorders. In the pathology of transient neonatal hyperammonemia, hepatic mitochondria may be pleomorphic with increased matrix density and decreased cristal profiles; autophagosomes may be increased; and rough endoplasmic reticulum and peroxisomes are normal [85]. The peribiliary dense zone may be broadened and canalicular microvilli focally decreased. This nonspecific pathology makes it impossible to distinguish transient neonatal hyperammonemia from inherited urea cycle disorders.

In one rare disorder, hyperornithinemia, hyperammonemia, and homocitrullinuria mitochondria are pleomorphic with giant forms, and have crystalloids and abnormalities of the mitochondrial outer membrane [86]. In a separate disease, deficiency of *N*-acetylglutamate synthetase is a cause of hyperammonemia in the newborn infant.

Tyrosinemia (Type I, Hepatorenal)

Tyrosinemia is an autosomal recessive error of fumarylacetoacetate hydrolase, the last enzyme in the degradative pathway of tyrosine [87]. Acute and chronic clinical forms exist; the former is more common and presents soon after birth. Infants fail to thrive and develop hepatomegaly with liver dysfunction, renal tubular dysfunction, renal failure, and acute porphyria-like episodes of peripheral neuropathy. Neurologic crises with respiratory insufficiency are a small but important cause of death [88]. In the past, most infants died of liver failure and bleeding or hepatocellular carcinoma. Tyrosinemia is uncommon in most populations (1 per 100,000 to 200,000) except in Quebec, where the incidence is 8 per 100,000 livebirths [89]. The presence of increased levels of succinylacetone in plasma or urine is diagnostic for this condition and can be detected by gas-liquid chromatography and mass spectrometry [90]. Detection of succinylacetone in amniotic fluid for prenatal diagnosis is available [89].

The pathogenesis of this disease is increasingly understood with the recognition that the metabolites maleyl- and fumarylacetoacetate are highly active compounds capable of producing cellular and DNA injury. Reducing these compounds by blocking the tyrosine degradative pathway proximally results in diminished clinical liver disease [91] and a possible, but yet to be demonstrated, reduction in liver cancer. Succinylacetoacetate and succinylacetone, byproducts of maleyl- and fumarylacetoacetate, react with glutathione, causing a deficiency of this compound which normally functions to reduce toxic injury [92]. Succinylacetone inhibits porphyrin metabolism, resulting in increased concentrations of delta-aminolevulinic acid which, as a neurotoxin, is implicated in acute episodes of peripheral neuropathy [93].

Major pathology involves the liver, kidney, pancreas, and peripheral nerve, but the liver is most seriously affected (Table 18.12) [94, 95]. Cirrhosis with acinar arrangement of hepatocytes and active formation of regenerative nodules is characteristic (Fig. 18.9). Cellular atypia is common in these nodules. Some contain aneuploid cells [96]. Increased pancreatic weight with islet cell hyperplasia occurs (Fig. 18.10). There is nephromegaly, sometimes profound, with cortical tubular ectasia and focal tubular calcification (Fig. 18.11). Portal hypertension with splenomegaly is common. In some infants, rickets and vascular mineralization occur. Central nervous system pathology includes hepatic encephalopathy and meningitis. Death from liver failure, usually accompanied by sepsis, is commonplace. Survival beyond 2 years of age for infants with chronic tyrosinemia imparts a high (37%) risk for hepatoma [97].

Little is known about the fetal pathology of tyrosinemia. No pathologic changes were found on examination of midgestation fetuses with biochemically confirmed tyrosinemia examined in our laboratory. Abnormally high concentrations of alpha-fetoprotein in the cord blood of newborn infants with tyrosinemia suggest that the liver pathology may be evolving, at least in late pregnancy [98].

Until recently, liver transplantation was the only effective treatment for type I tyrosinemia. Now clinical improvement has been demonstrated with use of a potent inhibitor of 4-hydroxyphenylpyruvate dioxygenase, an enzyme proximally

Table 18.12.   The pathology of acute tyrosinemia*

Patient	Age at Presentation (weeks)	Age at Death (weeks)	Liver Weight (grams)	Liver Nodules	Spleen Weight (grams)	Pancreas Weight (grams)	Islet Hyperplasia (area)	Kidney Weight (grams)	Renal Tubular Ectasia	Rickets	Vascular Mineralization
1	0	25	240 (240)	++	70 (18)	—	+ (80%)	260 (50)	+	−	+
2	0	7	174 (160)	+	8 (15)	17.5 (7)	+ (60%)	93 (36)	+	−	−
3	0	11	160 (180)	+	21 (15)	8.5 (8.5)	+ (50%)	84 (42)	+	+	−
4	2	12	116 (180)	+	21 (15)	—	+ (50%)	103 (42)	+	−	+
5	3	40	175 (260)	+++	70 (20)	18 (11)	+ (40%)	90 (62)	+	−	+
6	4	44	250 (300)	+++	NE	NE	NE	NE	NE	NE	NE
7	3	21	280 (240)	+++	80 (18)	23 (11)	+ (40%)	78 (58)	+	+	−
8	6	25	350 (240)	+++	80 (18)	16 (11)	+	66 (58)	+	−	−

* NE = not examined; figures in parentheses are expected normal weights.

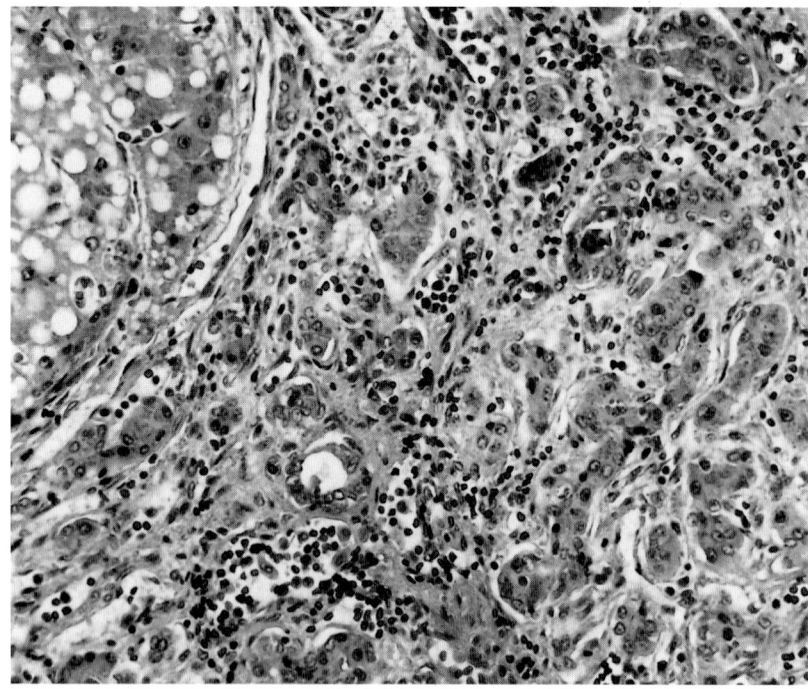

FIGURE 18.9.   *Hereditary tyrosinemia. The liver shows acinar hepatocellular transformation and lobular fibrosis. (×30.)*

located in the tyrosine catabolic pathway, that prevents the formation of the toxic metabolites, maleylacetoacetate and fumarylacetoacetate [91].

Maple Syrup Urine Disease (Branched-Chain Ketoaciduria)

Maple syrup urine disease, an autosomal recessive disorder of the branched amino acids leucine, isoleucine, and valine, is due to deficient activity of branched-chain keto acid decarboxylase. The incidence is 1 in 200,000 to 400,000 livebirths [99]. Most commonly, the disease presents as a severe disorder in the latter part of the first week of life, when the infant becomes irritable, fails to feed, vomits, develops alternating hypo- and hypertonicity, has a high-pitched cry, and develops seizures, ultimately leading to coma and death. Severe mental retardation follows if the infant survives. There is an odor of maple syrup from the urine or sweat. Diagnosis is easily made by plasma amino acid analysis. In Menkes' two cases, which came to autopsy at age 11 and 14 days, enlargement of the liver, kidneys, and brain was present in one infant [100]. The liver appeared to have increased glycogen. Dilatation of convoluted tubules in the kidneys was noted and the brain was edematous. Both infants had a failure of myelination in the pons and medulla. The second infant also had astrocytic swelling. Both infants had pneumonia. In older infants, the neuropathology is more profound and includes spongiosis, defective myelination, and gliosis. Disturbed myelination is absent if infants are treated [101].

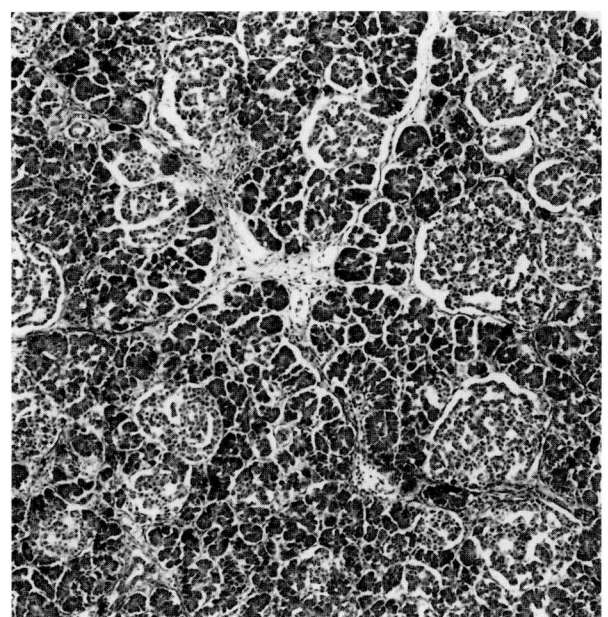

FIGURE 18.10. *Hereditary tyrosinemia. The pancreas shows islet-cell hyperplasia. (×84.)*

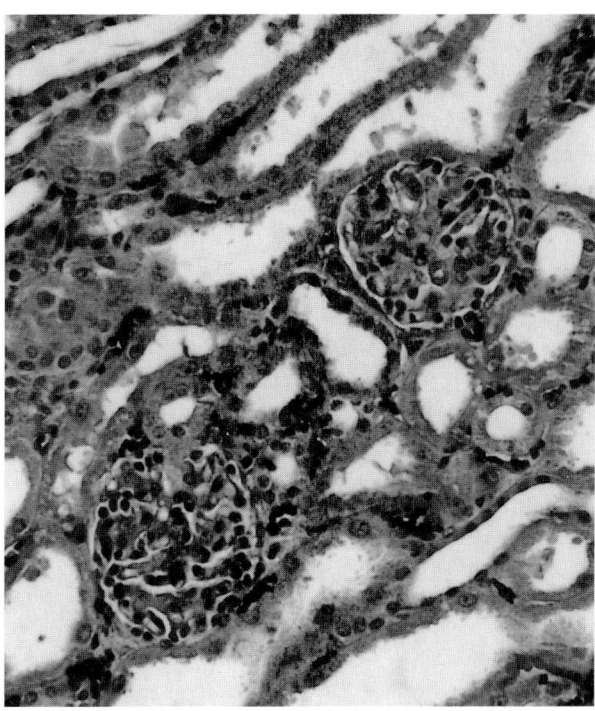

FIGURE 18.11. *Hereditary tyrosinemia. Renal cortical tubules are dilated. (×88.)*

Defective myelin synthesis is attributed to interference by the keto acids [102]. Other pathology is nonspecific. Bronchopneumonia is common; hepatomegaly with steatosis occurs and the kidneys, which may be enlarged, show tubular dilatation and vacuolation of epithelial cells [103]. In many organs, crystals within vacuoles may be seen on the frozen section [103]. Fetal pathology, if any, is unrecorded.

Non-Ketotic Hyperglycinemia

Non-ketotic hyperglycinemia (NKH) is an autosomal recessive condition in which glycine accumulates in the blood, cerebrospinal fluid (CSF), and brain. The incidence of this disease in British Columbia is 1 per 54,000 newborns over the period 1973 to 1988. This is the same incidence as that reported for Finland, so this is a relatively common disease. Presentation in the neonatal period is usual with hypotonia, respiratory distress, and seizures. Infants who survive the neonatal period have severe mental retardation and seizures. The disorder is caused by deficient activity of the glycine cleavage enzyme system, located in mitochondria, which splits glycine into carbon dioxide, ammonia, and methylene tetrahydrofolate, which then reacts with glycine to give serine.

NKH can be distinguished from other diseases with secondary hyperglycinemia (e.g., methylmalonic acidemia and propionic acidemia) by absence of ketosis and lack of abnormal organic acid excretion. Biochemical diagnosis of the disease is made initially by measurement of plasma glycine, which may be elevated only minimally, and then by measurement of CSF glycine, which is often 15 to 30 times elevated [104]. This greatly increased concentration of CSF

glycine is pathognomonic for the disease. Confirmation of the diagnosis is achieved by the measurement of glycine cleavage enzyme activity in liver or in cultures of Epstein-Barr–immortalized lymphoblasts [105]. Prenatal diagnosis is possible by enzyme assay in chorionic villus tissue [106].

Glycine has affinity for an *N*-methyl-D-aspartate receptor in the brain. Excessive stimulation is thought to be at least one factor that contributes to the intractable seizures and brain damage seen in this disorder [107]. Spongy myelinopathy, occurring in the central nervous system, in NKH is similar to other aminoacidopathies [108]. The liver may be normal or have nonspecific steatosis.

Phenylketonuria

Phenylketonuria is important in the perinatal period because of the availability of metabolic screening programs and the management of pregnancies of affected mothers who, if untreated, may give birth to children with mental retardation, microcephaly, and congenital heart disease [109].

Other Disorders

Other rare inherited aminoacidopathies occur in the newborn period. Hypervalinemia presents with vomiting and subsequently causes mental retardation. Hyper-beta-alaninemia manifests with polyhydramnios, reduced fetal movement, and lethargy and hyporeflexia in the neonate [110]. Lysinuric protein intolerance, more common in Finland, is an autosomal recessive disorder of cationic amino acid transport affecting the intestinal tract, kidney, and liver [111]. Because of the impaired absorption and renal loss, cationic amino acids are of low plasma concentration and the deficient transport at the hepatocyte level results in impairment of the urea cycle resulting in hyperammonemia. Poor feeding, vomiting, a large liver, and diarrhea may develop early in infancy. Pathology of the liver in neonatal cases consisted of only minimal fat deposition, whereas older patients developed peculiar clusters of pale hydropic-appearing hepatocytes with pyknotic nuclei. Ultrastructurally, little rough endoplasmic reticulum was found in the liver, and smooth endoplasmic reticulum was increased and had dilated cisternae. The mitochondria appeared normal.

Disorders of Carbohydrate Metabolism

Fructose Metabolism

Hereditary Fructose Intolerance   Hereditary fructose intolerance (HFI) is autosomal recessive and is caused by deficiency of fructose-1-phosphate aldolase in the liver, kidney, and intestinal mucosa. Clinical presentation and severity depend on the time of introduction of fructose in the diet. In the newborn the disease may be fulminant and lethal, whereas older infants may be difficult to wean from breast milk or be thriving poorly and have hepatomegaly. If the neonate is introduced to dietary fructose, vomiting, hepatomegaly and liver failure with ascites, jaundice, and coagulopathy may occur, often with sepsis. Some infants develop rickets [112]. Disseminated intravascular coagulopathy may also occur. Aminoaciduria and proteinuria are present. Infants are acidotic, hypokalemic, and hypophosphatemic; tyrosine,

methionine, and uric acid may be elevated. Hypoglycemia occurs in some but not in all. Diagnosis in early infancy may be difficult. The florid presentation mimics other acute metabolic diseases, such as galactosemia or tyrosinemia, and simulates sepsis, which may coexist.

ATP deficiency is implicated in the pathogenesis of HFI. Dietary fructose in the liver is phosphorylated using ATP to fructose-1-phosphate. In the normal liver, fructose-1-phosphate is converted to dihydroxyacetone phosphate and glyceraldehyde using fructose-1-phosphate aldolase, which is deficient in hereditary fructose intolerance. Because of the absent activity of this enzyme in HFI, the fructose-1-phosphate level increases and plasma phosphate levels diminish, as do cellular (liver) ATP concentrations [113]. Since the liver is the predominant site of fructose metabolism, it is most vulnerable to deficiency of fructose-1-phosphate aldolase. Following oral fructose intake, therefore, plasma phosphate and glucose levels fall. Decreased concentrations of potassium and increased plasma uric acid, lactate, methionine, and magnesium also occur.

As soon as 30 minutes after fructose administration to patients with HFI, electron microscopy of the liver reveals abnormalities attributable in part to diminished ATP [114]. Pathology of the liver in HFI is suggestive of the diagnosis. Steatosis with variable degrees of portal fibrosis, ductular proliferation, and cholestasis occurs in the acute disease of the young infant (Fig. 18.12). Hepatocellular necrosis and evolution to cirrhosis occurs rarely. Portal hypertension, ascites, congestive splenomegaly, islet cell hyperplasia of the pancreas, and cerebral edema have been noted at autopsy [115].

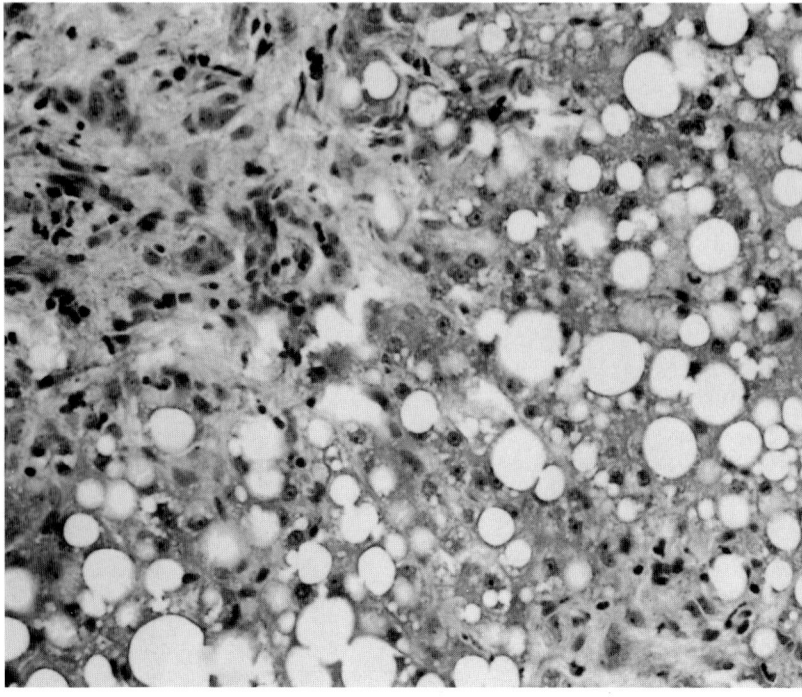

FIGURE 18.12.   *Hereditary fructose intolerance. Prominent steatosis is present in liver. There is minimal ductular proliferation. (×92.)*

Fructose-1,6-Bisphosphatase Deficiency   Hereditary fructose-1,6-bisphosphatase deficiency is characterized by episodic spells of hypoglycemia, ketosis, and lactic acidosis and can cause death in the neonatal period if not recognized early. A disorder of gluconeogenesis, episodes are precipitated by fasting. Fructose is not a precipitating factor [116]. Liver pathology consists of nonspecific steatosis. Diagnosis, therefore, is dependent upon biochemical investigations and definitive enzyme assay. Results from oral fructose testing are similar to hereditary fructose intolerance, implying a common pathogenesis.

Galactosemia

Classic galactosemia is an autosomal recessive disorder occurring with a frequency of 1 in 35,000 to 150,000 livebirths. Galactose-1-phosphate uridyltransferase (GALT) activity is deficient, causing accumulation of galactose, galactose-1-phosphate, and galactitol. These compounds are presumed to be responsible for most aspects of the disease. Non-enzymatic galactosylation may be responsible for cataract formation [117]. Galactokinase deficiency, in which no galactose-1-phosphate can be formed directly from galactose, causes no disease other than cataracts, so the pathogenesis may also relate to increased galactitol levels. Variants of galactosemia exist.

On exposure to lactose, galactosemic newborns fail to thrive, develop pronounced hyper-bilirubinemia, and show evidence of severe liver injury. Hepatomegaly and then splenomegaly, ascites, and death may occur. Sepsis, particularly with *Escherichia coli*, is common and is attributed to depressed neutrophil function by galactose [118]. Infants may also develop vomiting, diarrhea, hemorrhagic diathesis, hemolysis, acidosis, aminoaciduria, proteinuria, and, if still receiving lactose, will have galactosuria as indicated by positive reducing substances in the urine.

Comments on the diagnosis of galactosemia by using urine-reducing sugar tests are made in the first part of this chapter. Confirmatory diagnosis requires an assay for red cell galactose-1-phosphate uridyltransferase (GALT), which is not reliable if the child has recently received a blood transfusion. A presumptive diagnosis under these circumstances can be made by finding increased erythrocyte galactose-1-phosphate values in blood and by demonstrating that both parents have GALT values consistent with the carrier state.

Liver disease is characterized by marked steatosis with progressive acinar change of hepatocyte architecture, ductular proliferation, cholestasis, focal necrosis, and, ultimately, cirrhosis with regenerative nodule formation (Fig. 18.13) [94, 119, 120]. Pancreatic islet-cell hyperplasia, renal tubular dilatation, tubular epithelial vacuolation, and focal tubular necrosis have been found. Splenomegaly occurs with evolution of the liver disease and frequently evidence of the hemorrhagic diathesis is found at autopsy. In the brain, edema, neuronal injury attributed to hypoxic-ischemic damage, gliosis, and meningitis have been noted. Peritonitis, septicemia, cellulitis, and urinary tract infection occur.

Fetal pathology in galactosemia appears limited to incipient cataracts in the lens from a fetus of 20 weeks' gestation [121].

Glycogen Storage Diseases

Glycogen storage diseases (GSD) have an overall incidence of 1 in 50,000 to 100,000 livebirths; some become clinically apparent in the fetus or newborn (Table 18.13).

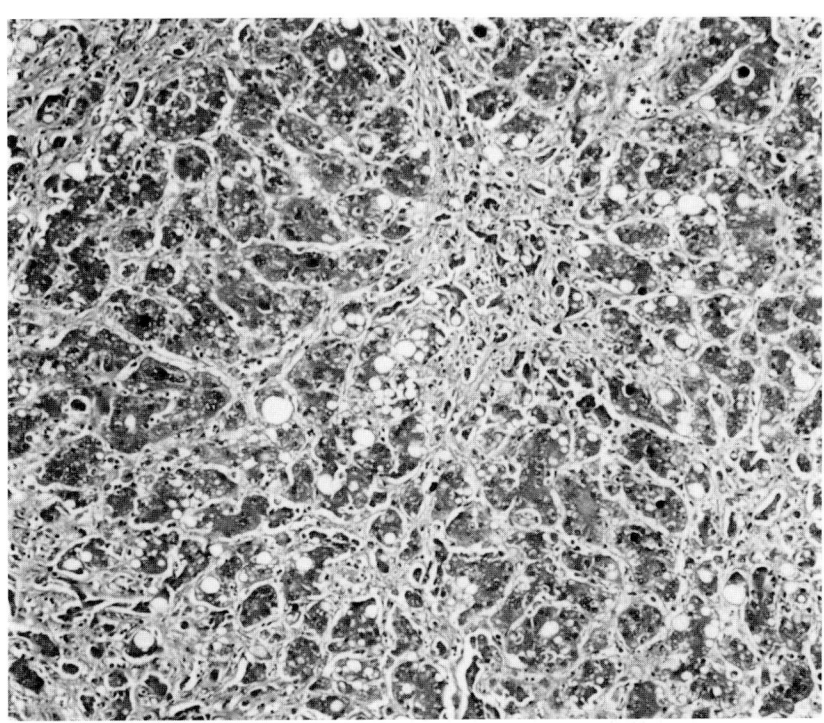

FIGURE 18.13.   *Classic galactosemia. The liver in the cirrhotic stage of the disease. (×32.)*

Table 18.13.   Summary of the chemical manifestations of the glycogen storage diseases

Types and Enzyme Defect	Fasting Blood Sugar	Glucose Tolerance Test	Response to Glucagon	Blood Lactate Pyruvate	Blood Lipids	Liver Function Tests	Organ	Pathology
Type I Glucose-6-phosphatase	↓	↑↑ Abnormal Delayed	No response ↑ Lactate	↑	↑↑	± Abnormal	Liver ++ Spleen o Kidney	Liver glycogen content ↑. Glycogen normal structure. Absent or low G-6-phosphatase.
Type II Glucose-1,4-glucosidase (acid maltase)	Normal	Normal	Normal	Normal	Normal	Normal	Liver + Spleen ± Heart ++	Multiple tissue infiltration by glycogen. Abnormal ECG. Liver enzyme ↓.
Type III Amylo-1,6-glucosidase (debrancher)	↓	Normal	No response, no rise in lactate	Normal	Normal	± Abnormal	Liver ++ Heart ++ Muscle	Glycogen content of liver and muscle ↑.
Type IV Amylo-1,4,1,6-transglucosidase (brancher)		Normal	+/− No response	Normal	Normal	++ Abnormal	Liver ++ Heart ++	Amylopectin infiltration in liver and heart. Abnormal glycogen structure.
Type VI Hepatic phosphorylase	↓ Mild–moderate	Normal	Variable; usually poor results	↑ (Mild)	↑ (Mild)	Normal	Liver ++ Leukocytes	Liver glycogen ↑. Liver phosphorylase ↓.

Glycogen Storage Disease Types Ia, b, c, and d   Glycogen storage disease type Ia is an autosomal recessive disorder caused by deficient glucose-6-phosphatase activity. Hydrolyzation of glucose-6-phosphate to glucose is the final step in gluconeogenesis and glycogenolysis. Deficiency results in profound hypoglycemia, lacticacidemia, hyperuricemia, hyperlipidemia, bleeding tendency, neutropenia, seizures, and hepatomegaly. Some infants thought to have sudden infant death syndrome have been reported to have GSD type I [122] but this is still in dispute. Glucose-6-phosphatase deficiency cannot be diagnosed prenatally by enzymatic methods in chorionic villous or amniotic fluid cells. Although the gene has recently been cloned [123], direct mutational analysis is not routinely available. Prenatal diagnosis may be possible by linkage analysis or as a last resort.

Types Ib, Ic, and Id are clinically similar to type Ia but are due to defects of specific glucose-6-phosphate translocases, which (respectively) transport glucose-6-phosphate, phosphate, and glucose across the microsomal membrane to the functional site of glucose-6-phosphatase [122, 124–126].

The liver and kidney contain excessive glycogen in type I glycogen storage disease and the liver has a mosaic pattern of bloated and steatotic hepatocytes. This liver pathology is sufficiently distinctive to allow a presumptive diagnosis while recognizing that biochemical confirmation is required (Fig. 18.14) [127].

Glycogen Storage Disease Type II   Glycogen storage disease type II (Pompe disease) is caused by deficient activity of lysosomal acid alpha-glucosidase. It can present in the

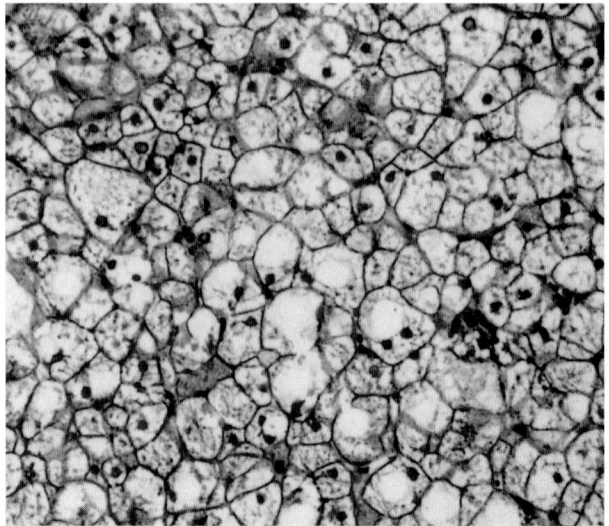

FIGURE 18.14.   *Glycogen storage disease type. I. Note the mosaic of swollen hepatocytes and nuclear hyperglycogenation. (×76.)*

neonatal period with hypotonia and cardiomegaly resulting from massive accumulation of glycogen in virtually all tissues [128]. Glucose homeostasis is normal and liver function only becomes abnormal when cardiac failure develops. Creatinine kinase in serum is usually elevated due to skeletal muscle involvement. In the severe form, infants usually succumb to heart failure in the first year of life.

The biochemical diagnosis of Pompe disease rests on demonstration of absent alpha-glucosidase (acid maltase) activity in peripheral blood lymphocytes (not a mixed leucocyte preparation), or in cultured skin fibroblasts [129]. In addition to the enzyme deficient in Pompe disease, there is an isoform in granulocytes and in kidney [130] that prevents the use of mixed leukocyte preparations for diagnosis. It has been our experience that carriers for the alpha-glucosidase deficiency of Pompe disease can have enzyme activities in lymphocytes that are close to zero. In such cases, enzyme activity in cultured fibroblasts must be assayed.

Diagnosis may also be made on tissue biopsies. Typical lysosomal-bound glycogen aggregates are found in many cell types in skin and conjunctival biopsies. Peripheral blood lymphocytes, vacuolated and containing PAS-positive diastase sensitive granules, suggest the disease and serve as a useful screening test.

Pompe disease is readily diagnosed prenatally [131, 132]. Intralysosomal glycogen, which occurs in uncultured amniocytes, permits rapid electron microscopic prenatal diagnosis in advance of the enzyme analysis which must be done on cultured cells (Fig. 18.15).

At autopsy, lysosomal glycogen storage is generalized and profound, although most heavily concentrated in skeletal and cardiac muscle and in the liver. Metachromatic material, sometimes seen in muscle, may be compacted and altered glycogen [133]. The heart is enlarged with generalized hypertrophy, pale myocardium, and sometimes endocardial fibroelastosis. Both myocardial cells and those of the conduction system share in glycogen storage (Fig. 18.16). The conduction system also may be malpositioned. Skeletal muscle has extreme vacuolation with both histochemical and electron microscopic presence of glycogen. Unexplained storage of neutral lipid in muscle may also occur [134]. Liver cells are enlarged and are finely vacuolated due to lysosomal glycogen storage.

The predominant expression of muscle disease in Pompe disease may be due to the mechanical effect of cell movement and myofibrillar trauma to lysosomes, which are fragile and when ruptured may cause enzymatic damage to other cell organelles. Low mitochondrial enzyme activity supports this hypothesis [135].

Glycogen Storage Disease Type III Glycogen storage disease type III, debrancher enzyme deficiency, is an autosomal recessive disorder similar to glycogen storage disease type I, although clinically usually more mild. Hepatomegaly may be noted in infancy and the consequences of hypoglycemia may occur. Glycogen storage in muscle is unlike glycogen storage disease type I, and may account for myopathic symptoms.

Assay of the debranching enzyme is surprisingly difficult, and although many groups have reported measurement in leukocytes [136], we have found the only satisfactory method to be that using cultured skin fibroblasts [Dr. BI Brown, personal communication]. Prenatal diagnosis by enzyme analysis may be done on cultured amniotic fluid cells and chorionic villus tissue.

Glycogen Storage Disease Type IV Glycogen storage disease Type IV is a very rare disorder caused by a recessively inherited deficiency of the brancher enzyme. There is a spectrum of age presentation, and a congenital form is known [137]. Variants with detectable activity of the enzyme in liver and cultured fibroblasts occur. The consequence of the deficient enzyme activity is an accumulation of structurally deranged glycogen with long outer chains and few branch points, which, presumably, produces cellular injury. Affected infants

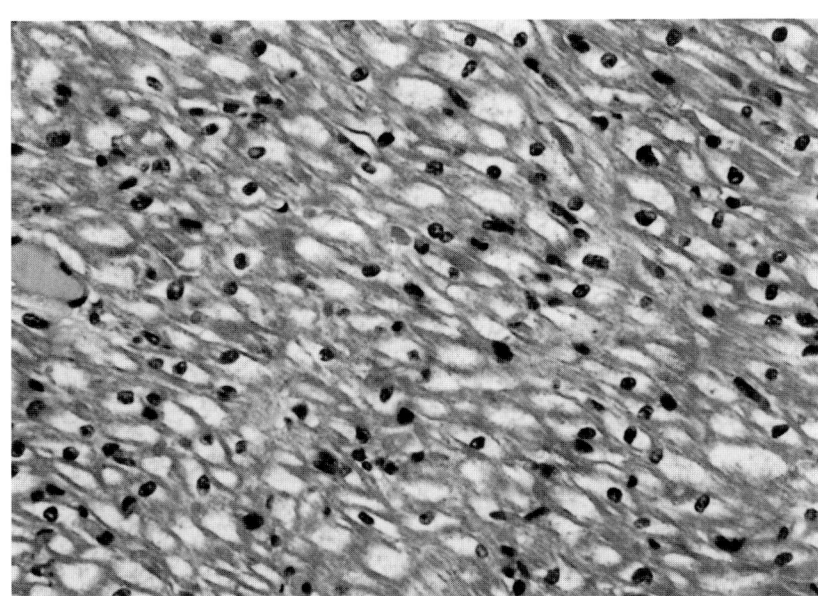

FIGURE 18.15. *Glycogen storage disease type II. Note the vacuolation of cardiac muscle. (×35.)*

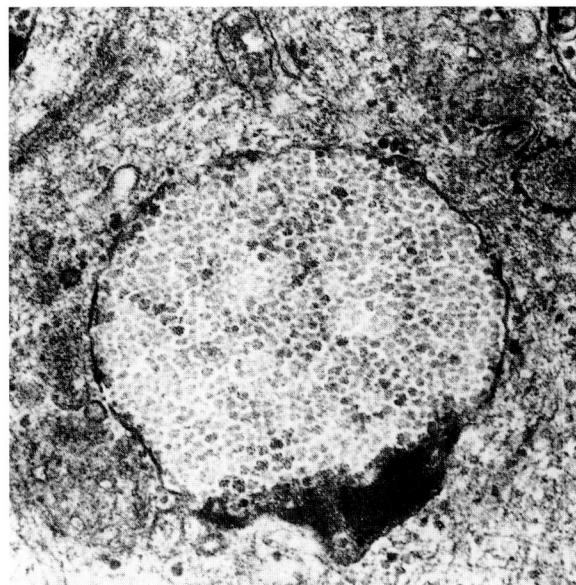

FIGURE 18.16. *Glycogen storage disease type II. An uncultured amniocyte contains membrane-bound glycogen. (×31,920.) (Reproduced with permission from Masson Publishing Company Inc.)*

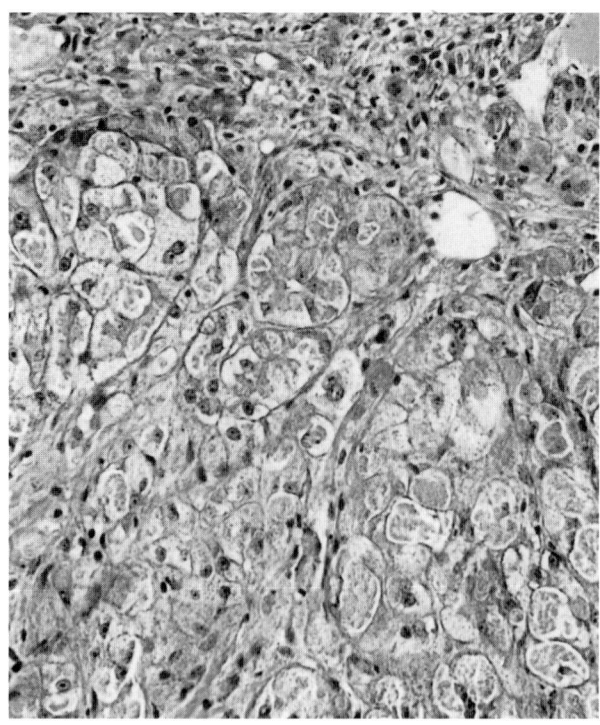

FIGURE 18.17. *Glycogen storage disease type IV. The liver is cirrhotic. Hepatocytes contain aggregates of abnormal glycogen. (×79.)*

may initially appear well but soon fail to thrive and develop hepatosplenomegaly and liver dysfunction, reflecting the aggressive liver disease. There may be neurological involvement manifested by hypotonia, muscle atrophy, and abnormal reflexes. Patients usually die within 2 years due to either cardiac or hepatic failure.

This disease is diagnosed by liver biopsy for histopathologic examination and enzyme assay. Liver disease evolves quickly into cirrhosis. Hepatocytes are enlarged by pale, slightly basophilic cytoplasmic masses which are PAS-positive and diastase-resistant (Fig. 18.17). Ultrastructurally, the inclusions are composed of fine fibrils, small granules, and some glycogen rosettes [138]. Diagnosis requires confirmation by enzyme assay [136].

Glycogen storage disease type IV is a generalized disorder. Therefore, at autopsy, many tissues, but particularly those of the heart and liver, contain the amylopectin-like inclusions. Both central and peripheral nervous systems are involved, and in the former the inclusions resemble Lafora bodies [139].

In one 19-week fetus examined in our laboratory, there was no light microscopic pathology and, by electron microscopy, fine fibrillar aggregates were found only in cardiac muscle.

Other Types of GSD   Other types of glycogen storage disease are uncommon in the fetus and neonate. There is a report of an infant with hypoglycemia who died of heart failure due to glycogen storage disease confined to the heart and

secondary to deficient cardiac phosphorylase kinase [140]. A cerebral glycogenosis, possibly owing to a defect in brain-specific glycogen phosphorylase, was identified in an infant of 38 weeks' gestation who presented with seizures and hypotonia in the neonatal period. Glycogen in the rosette form was stored in brain tissue [141].

Lysosomal Enzymopathies

Lysosomes are subcellular organelles responsible for hydrolyzing molecules as biochemically diverse as glycolipids, glycoproteins, and mucopolysaccharides (glycosaminoglycans). Lysosomal enzymes degrade large molecules in such a way that the terminal molecule is cleaved first and the remainder is degraded in sequence by separate enzymes. Deficiency of any one of the sequence of enzymes will fail to produce the correct substrate for the next enzyme, so degradation ceases and the product accumulates. The degradation pathway of glycolipids, with corresponding disorders, is shown in Figure 18.18.

Niemann-Pick Disease

Niemann-Pick disease type A, the acute neuronopathic form, commonly presents in early infancy. Types A and B, the latter being the chronic non-neuronopathic form, are due to an autosomal recessive inheritance of deficient sphin-

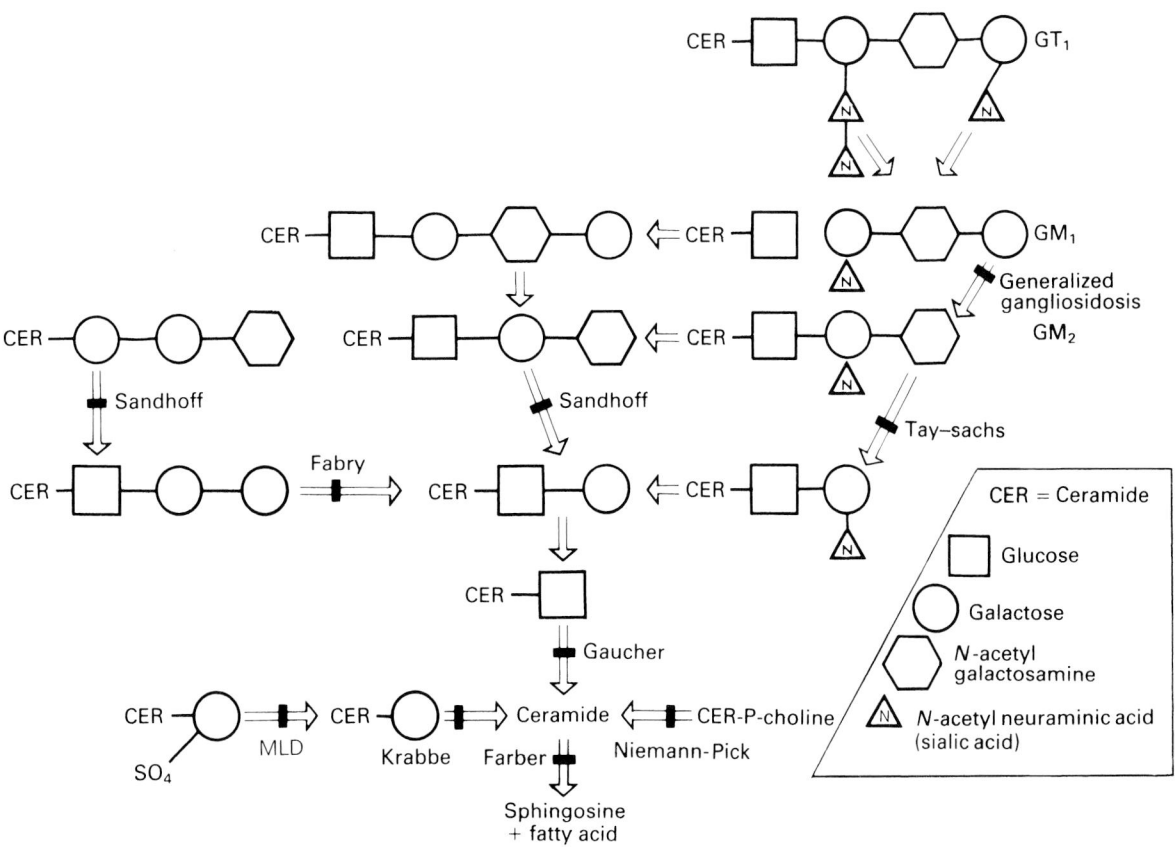

FIGURE 18.18.   *Glycolipid degradation pathway.*

gomyelinase. Acute neuronopathic Niemann-Pick disease presents in the first weeks of life with hepatosplenomegaly, failure to thrive, hypotonia, vomiting, diarrhea, and progressively worsening psychomotor retardation. An ocular cherry-red spot occurs in about 50% of patients. Respiratory symptoms are common and pneumonia is usual at death, which occurs by age 1 to 4 years. Type B Niemann-Pick disease may be detected in later infancy, often incidentally, due to the presence of hepatomegaly.

Niemann-Pick disease type C is an autosomal recessive disorder caused by an error in cellular trafficking of cholesterol that leads to the accumulation of unesterified cholesterol in lysosomes. Some infants have prolonged neonatal cholestasis and hepatomegaly with prominent liver involvement giving a histologic picture of neonatal hepatitis [142–144]. The gene was recently identified [144a].

The vacuolated foam cell, typical of Niemann-Pick disease, has a pale or clear cytoplasmic appearance, with tinges of yellow or brown reflecting lipofuscin content. Sphingomyelin, cholesterol, and ganglioside are also present. Ultrastructurally, membranous lamellar inclusions, pleomorphic bodies with dense and lucent zones, and dense gran-

ules, presumably lipofuscin, are present (Fig. 18.19). Niemann-Pick cells are found in the bone marrow, spleen, lymph nodes, lung, and kidney; Kupffer cells show the same histology. Hepatic parenchymal cells also are vacuolated. In the lung, foam cells in alveoli, septa, and vessels create a reticular radiological pattern and presumably influence the frequency of respiratory infections. Involvement of enteric ganglion cells and heavy infiltration of the intestinal lamina propria contribute to malabsorption, diarrhea, and malnutrition among these patients [145]. Cardiac involvement, including endocardial fibroelastosis, may occur [146]. The brain often is atrophic. Neurones are enlarged and stain positively with PAS, Sudan black B, oil red O, and Luxol fast blue. Ultrastructurally, membranous cytoplasmic bodies of concentric lamellae are present. Gliosis and secondary demyelination occur. In the peripheral nervous system, predominantly structureless electron-dense bodies can be found in Schwann cells [147].

The pathology of the fetus with Niemann-Pick disease is well established. As with other metabolic diseases involving storage in neurones, the most mature nerve cells are found, ultrastructurally, to be affected first. In Niemann-Pick

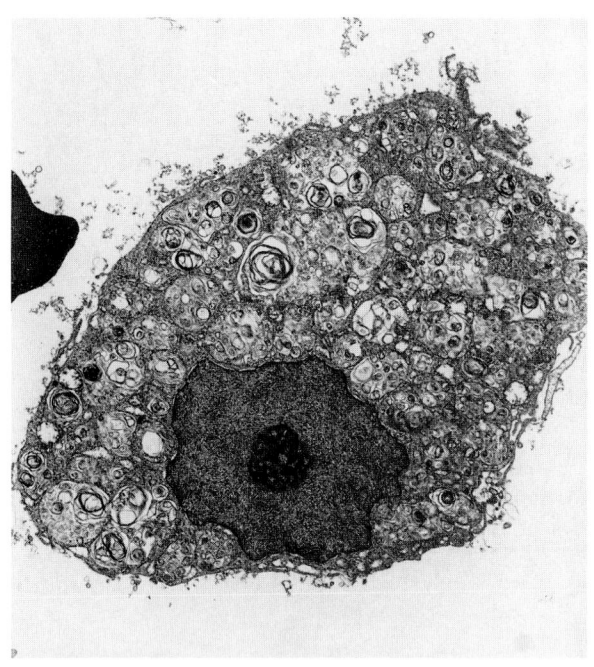

FIGURE 18.19. *Niemann-Pick cell. (×4900.)*

disease, neurones in the basal ganglia contain cytosomes and some neurones have a dilated endoplasmic reticulum containing dense granular material, a finding similar to that of Tay-Sachs disease in the fetus [148]. Vacuolated hepatocytes, splenic histiocytes and endothelial cells, but no typical Niemann-Pick foam cells, were observed. In these same cells, cytosomes bearing lipid lamellae could be seen ultrastructurally. In fetal life, Niemann-Pick disease predominates in viscera other than the nervous system; this pattern is paralleled in the newborn infant by the clinical presentation of hepatosplenomegaly, followed later by progressive neurological impairment [148, 149].

One may presumptively diagnose Niemann-Pick disease by demonstrating typical foamy histiocytes in bone marrow and by identifying electron-microscopically cytosomes in bone marrow histiocytes, conjunctival or skin biopsies (see Fig. 18.5), or liver and rectal biopsies. Peripheral blood lymphocyte preparations also may contain vacuolated lymphocytes with cytosomes. The definitive diagnosis of types A and B is made by demonstrating deficient activity of sphingomyelinase. In type C, sphingomyelinase activity varies from normal to half the control values [150]. For this type, diagnosis is made by demonstrating the cholesterol esterification defect in cultured fibroblasts. The same defect is sought for prenatal diagnosis, using cultured amniotic fluid cells or chorionic villus cells. The biochemical assay is supported by demonstrating with polyene antibiotic filipin staining abundant accumulation of cholesterol in the cultured cells [149].

Gaucher Disease

Acute neuronopathic Gaucher disease (type II) is the one form of this disorder presenting in early infancy. Due to deficient activity of glucocerebrosidase (lysosomal glucosylceramidase: beta-glucosidase), this autosomal recessive error is characterized by an accumulation of glucocerebroside (glucosylceramide) in large histiocytes or "Gaucher cells." Infants usually present in the first months of life with hepatosplenomegaly, feeding difficulty, and failure to thrive. Progressive neurological impairment then follows rapidly, and death occurs with respiratory infections usually by age 2 years. Newborn infants are less commonly affected, although they may present with neonatal ascites [8, 14].

Diagnosis of Gaucher disease in infancy is possible by demonstrating Gaucher cells in bone marrow or liver, either of which may be biopsied in the clinical setting of hepatomegaly. Gaucher cells in young infants may be less PAS-positive, and the striking "wrinkled silk" characteristic of cells from older patients may be developed incompletely. However, electron microscopic examination is diagnostic (Fig. 18.20). Confirmation requires assay of beta-glucosidase activity. There is often substantial residual enzyme activity when artificial substrates and detergents are used in the assay, which can make prenatal diagnosis more difficult than for other lysosomal enzyme diseases. There is also difficulty distinguishing between neuropathic and non-neuropathic Gaucher disease, both of which may have the same low level of residual beta-glucosidase activity [151]. Distinction between the three clinical subtypes of Gaucher disease has been reported using monoclonal antibodies directed against beta-glucosidase [152]. More recently, mutation analysis has been found to have considerable predictive value [153].

The pathology of acute neuronopathic Gaucher disease is characterized by storage cells throughout the reticuloendothelial system, but predominating in the spleen, liver, lymph nodes, and bone marrow. The brain contains perivascular collections of Gaucher cells and extensive loss of neurons. Neuronal storage and injury are probably due to accumulating cerebroside and toxic metabolites derived from cerebral ganglioside catabolism and not from hematogenous sources, which are the presumed origin of stored cerebroside in the liver [154].

Hydrops fetalis possibly is due to hypoproteinemia secondary to massive liver involvement, anemia, or vascular occlusion by Gaucher cells [8]. Gaucher cells can be found obstructing hepatic sinusoids and hepatic veins and in capillaries in placental villi. The fetal pathology of Gaucher disease is well known [155]. Morphological evidence of Gaucher disease has been found, particularly in the liver and spleen. In a fetus of 17 weeks' gestation, PAS-positive foam cells that lacked the typical striated appearance contained engulfed red blood cells as well as tubular cytosomes. No neuropathology was evident at that gestation or in a 20-week-old fetus. In contrast, a 26-weeks'-gestation infant

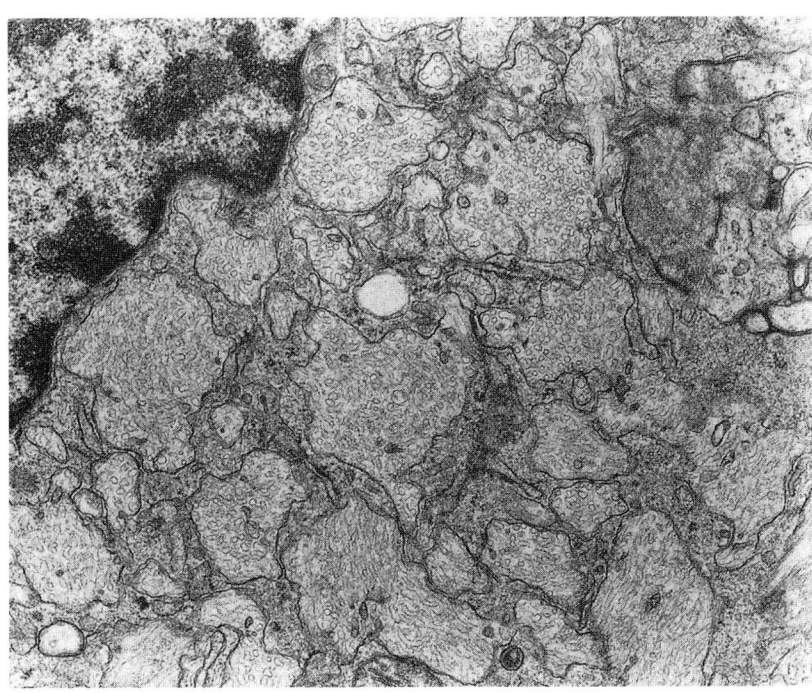

FIGURE 18.20.   *Gaucher cell. Note the tubular lysosomal inclusions. (×20,500.)*

examined in our laboratory had extensive neuronal loss and gliosis in brainstem, spinal cord, thalamus, and basal ganglia, those areas with the most mature neurons.

Krabbe Disease

Infants with Krabbe disease (globoid cell leukodystrophy) usually present between the third and sixth months of life and are not encountered clinically in the perinatal period. Only a few infants with earlier manifestations have been described [156]. The disease is autosomal recessive and is caused by deficient galactocerebroside beta-galactosidase. Enzyme assay with the use of the natural glycolipid substrate can establish the diagnosis in leukocytes or cultured fibroblasts. Prenatal diagnosis is possible with either amniotic fluid cells or via chorionic villus biopsy [157]. The pathology, confined to the nervous system, consists of lack of myelin, gliosis, and characteristic globoid cells and is attributed to increased concentration of psychosine, which is cytotoxic [158, 159]. Krabbe disease in therapeutically aborted fetuses, gestational age 18 to 23 weeks, manifests with leukodystrophy involving the most mature and earliest myelinating areas of the nervous system [160].

Metachromatic Leukodystrophy (MLD)

Metachromatic leukodystrophy (MLD) does not usually manifest in the perinatal period, although there are two incompletely documented cases of congenital MLD [161, 162, 42]. In one, the infant was full-term and died after 20 hours. In addition to the neuropathology of MLD, the infant had vacuolization of glomerular epithelial cells, tubular epithelium, and foam cells in the renal interstitium. In the liver, Kupffer cells but not hepatocytes were involved. Adrenal cortex and medullary cells and enteric plexus neurones were vacuolated. Foamy cells were found in lymph node sinuses. The pathology of the late infantile and other forms is described by Norman [158]. The disease is caused by a deficient activity of arylsulfatase A (ASA), which hydrolyzes galactocerebroside sulfate to galacto-cerebroside (see Fig. 18.18). A few patients have been described with MLD that have ASA activity in the normal or heterozygous range. These patients have been shown to have either a deficiency of cerebroside sulfatase activator protein or a Km mutant of ASA [162–164]. A low ASA activity does not necessarily establish the diagnosis of MLD because there is a deficiency of ASA activity found in some healthy individuals. This phenomenon, termed pseudodeficiency (PD), is caused by two mutations in a single allele, and is found in 7% to 15% of the general population [165]. Clinical and biochemical studies are reported to show that homozygosity for the PD allele is a benign condition.

A cerebroside sulfate loading test is used, in cultured fibroblasts, to establish the diagnosis of MLD and this may be needed for prenatal diagnosis [166]. Demonstration of an increased amount of sulfatide in urine will confirm the diagnosis but this may not be reliable in older patients [167]. Because of the variables, discussed above, the diagnosis of MLD requires extreme care.

Pathology in fetuses with MLD comprises metachromatic material and lysosomal inclusions in areas undergoing active myelination, namely spinal cord and peripheral nerves, at the time of therapeutic abortion. Demyelination is not evident. Laminated lysosomal material is found in fetal liver, and metachromatic material has been demonstrated in the kidney of an affected fetus aborted at 23-weeks' gestation [168].

Farber Disease

Farber disease is a very rare autosomal recessive disease caused by lysosomal acid ceramidase deficiency and accumulation of ceramide in tissues. Clinical manifestations begin as early as 2 weeks of age [169]. Hoarseness, respiratory difficulty, vomiting, and painful swollen joints develop. Ultimately, nodules emerge on the joints and in the subcutis. Infants fail to thrive, are febrile, and die usually with respiratory infections.

Lipogranulomata composed of foam cells with granulomatous reaction occur in respiratory tract, lungs, soft tissues, and joints. The neurons of the central nervous system and peripheral ganglion cells also are vacuolated. Foam cells may occur in the reticuloendothelial system, bone marrow, spleen, and liver [169, 170]. Ceramide, as well as mucopolysaccharides and gangliosides, accumulate in this disorder. Ultrastructurally, curvilinear tubular structures are found in foam cells. These typical ultrastructural inclusions are produced only with ceramide-containing non-hydroxylated fatty acids, which cause a granulomatous reaction when injected subcutaneously [171]. Other ultrastructural findings include membrane-bound reticulogranular material, presumably corresponding to mucopolysaccharide and zebra bodies of probable ganglioside origin in neurons, endothelial cells, and pericytes. So-called banana bodies have been found in Schwann cells [172].

One suspects the diagnosis of Farber disease from the clinical presentation. Biopsies of subcutaneous or articular and periarticular nodules should be examined by electron microscopy to search for the typical curvilinear inclusions. Confirmatory diagnosis requires tissue analysis for ceramide and determination of lysosomal acid ceramidase activity.

Wolman Disease (Acid Lipase Deficiency)

Deficiency of acid lipase activity causes Wolman disease or a milder phenotype, cholesteryl ester storage disease. Cholesteryl ester storage disease usually does not present in the immediate neonatal period, although hepatomegaly may be noted. In contrast, Wolman disease has an aggressive clinical course, leading to the death of an infant usually by 6 months of age. Infants become symptomatic shortly after birth, when they develop vomiting, diarrhea, abdominal disten-

tion, hepatosplenomegaly, and jaundice. Infants also have steatorrhea and fail to thrive. Liver function tests are abnormal and anemia is present. Bilateral adrenal calcification, a classic radiological sign of diagnostic import, begins in the fetus.

In Wolman disease, cholesteryl esters and triglycerides accumulate. The enlarged yellow liver is heavily lipid-laden and periportal fibrosis is progressive. Foam cells are present in the portal and periportal regions, and the hepatocytes and Kupffer cells are vacuolated. Ultrastructurally, lipid droplets are found within hepatocytes and macrophages, and cholesteryl ester clefts are seen in lysosomes [173]. In the adrenal, beginning in the fetus, the inner fasciculata, reticularis, and the fetal zone are transformed into foam cells which degenerate and become heavily calcified. Lipid foam cells also are present throughout the lymph nodes, spleen, lamina propria of the intestinal tract, and bone marrow; there also may be some in the lung. Lipid stains demonstrate deposition in vessel walls. In the brain, lipid vacuolation occurs in Schwann cells and oligodendroglia, and the ganglion cells of the enteric plexi also are involved [174].

Wolman disease is a rare disorder; diagnosis should be considered seriously if bilateral adrenal calcification is noted. Vacuolated peripheral lymphocytes and foamy histiocytes in the marrow are nonspecific, but they represent evidence of metabolic disease. Tissue biopsies should be stained for neutral lipid and cholesterol; unfixed frozen tissues should be examined for birefringent cholesterol crystals. Definitive diagnosis requires assay of lysosomal acid lipase (acid cholesteryl ester hydrolase) activity, and quantitation of tissue lipids may be carried out. Reduced acid lipase activity can be demonstrated by using natural as well as several synthetic substrates. Prenatal diagnosis is based on the absence of acid lipase activity in cultured chorionic villus cells.

Mucopolysaccharidoses

Mucopolysaccharidoses I (Hurler disease), II (Hunter syndrome), III, and VII appear clinically in infancy. Of these, type VII manifests especially in the neonatal period (Table 18.14). Infants with type I mucopolysaccharidosis are identified late in the first year of life when the coarse Hurler-type features begin to appear. An earlier appearance of the phenotype should lead one to consider infantile generalized GMI gangliosidosis, sialidosis, or mucolipidosis II (see Table 18.14).

The metabolic pathways involved in mucopolysaccharidoses are outlined in Figure 18.21, and in Table 18.15 the specimens necessary for enzyme assay are indicated. The investigation of a suspected case should include the collection of a randomly voided urine (frozen immediately after collection and stored frozen), plasma and white cell pellets for enzyme assays, and serum for N-acetylglucosaminidase and iduronate sulfatase assays. Light microscopy of peripheral white cells and electron microscopy of blood cells and skin conjunctival biopsies can provide indicative diagnostic information. It is necessary to confirm diagnoses by assays

Table 18.14. Disorders with Hurler phenotype in infants and children

Mucopolysaccharidosis I
Mucopolysaccharidosis II
Mucopolysaccharidosis VII*
Sialidosis*
Mucolipidosis II*
Mucolipidosis III
Mannosidosis
Fucosidosis
Aspartylglucosaminuria
Gangliosidosis, GM, generalized*
Sandhoff disease
Multiple sulfatase deficiency
Winchester syndrome
Kniest syndrome

* Manifests in early infancy.

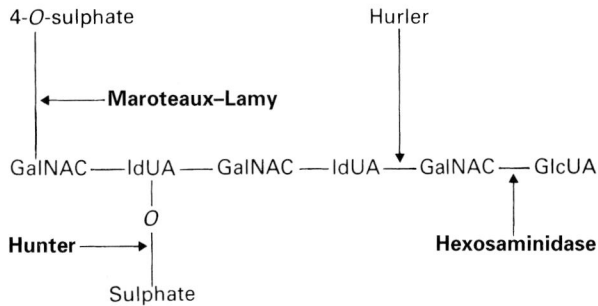

(a) Catabolism of dermatan sulphate

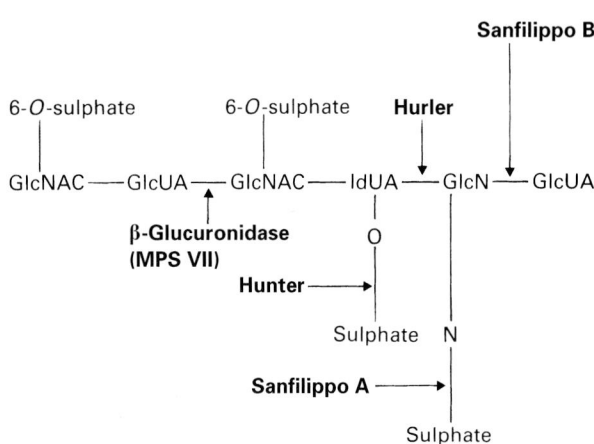

(b) Catabolism of heparin sulphate

FIGURE 18.21. *Mucopolysaccharidoses in the catabolic pathway.*
GalNAC = N-Acetylgalactosamine
GlcNAC = N-Acetylglucosamine
GlcN = Glucosamine
GlcUA = Glucuronic acid
IdUA = Iduronic acid

involving skin fibroblast cultures. The stored fibroblasts can be used for repeat investigations and family studies.

The method we use for quantitating urinary mucopolysaccharide output has been described [175]. Occasionally, it is difficult to decide whether a given output of mucopolysaccharide is abnormal. In this case, an increased ratio of high- to low-molecular-weight mucopolysaccharide is suggestive of mucopolysaccharidosis. Identification of excreted compounds by electrophoresis is usually helpful. If urinary mucopolysaccharides are not abnormal, the protocol for investigation of "pseudo-Hurler" diseases should be followed (Table 18.16).

Mucopolysaccharidosis type VII, an autosomal recessive disease caused by deficient beta-glucuronidase activity, has a variable onset from the perinatal age group to older children [176]. In addition to Hurler features, infants also present with hydrops fetalis [9, 12]. Pathology comprises cellular vacuolation in the brain, liver, heart, kidneys, and spleen. Endothelial vacuolation is also noted. The lungs may be hypoplastic, and there may be delayed maturation of the brain and kidneys [9]. In infants examined in our laboratory, cytoplasmic intralysosomal storage was found diffusely in epithelial, mesenchymal, and neural cells. The most prominent storage was in the reticuloendothelial system of the spleen, liver, and lymph nodes. Hepatocytes were involved, as were renal tubular epithelial cells, thyroid follicular cells, and endothelial cells (Fig. 18.22). Prominent involvement of placental Hofbauer cells but not trophoblastic cells was noted (Fig. 18.23). In addition, there was prominent islet cell hyperplasia of the pancreas, and the frontal lobes of the brain were foreshortened. Storage cell vacuoles were empty or contained a few lamellae, fibrils, or amorphous material. Endothelial cell involvement with resultant dysfunction may be important in the pathogenesis of hydrops in this condition.

Fetuses with mucopolysaccharidoses I, II, and III, ranging in gestational age from 18 to 23 weeks, have lysosomal storage in viscera, particularly the liver, and in mesenchymal cells [7, 177–179]. Neuronal involvement was not present in a fetus of 18 weeks' gestation but was found by electron microscopy in older fetuses. Ceuterick et al have also shown vacuolar involvement of placental stromal cells and syncytiotrophoblast in a fetus with Sanfilippo A disease [7]. In one fetus with Morquio disease we examined, no pathology other than unexplained pleural effusions and pulmonary hypoplasia could be found. Lack of evidence of storage in this fetus may reflect the later onset of clinical disease in Morquio disease.

Gangliosidoses

Gangliosides are glycosphingolipids bearing hydrophobic and hydrophilic components found in cell membranes,

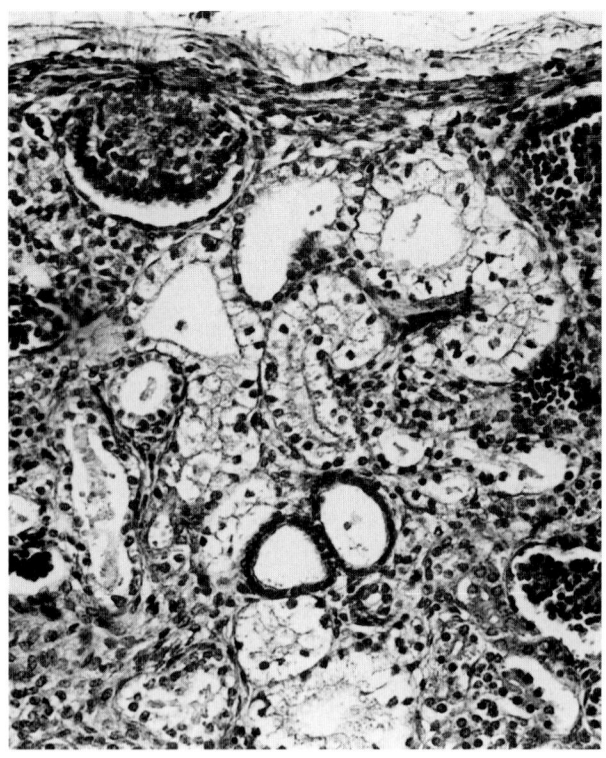

FIGURE 18.22. *Mucopolysaccharidosis type VII, kidney. Note the highly vacuolated tubular epithelium. (×100.)*

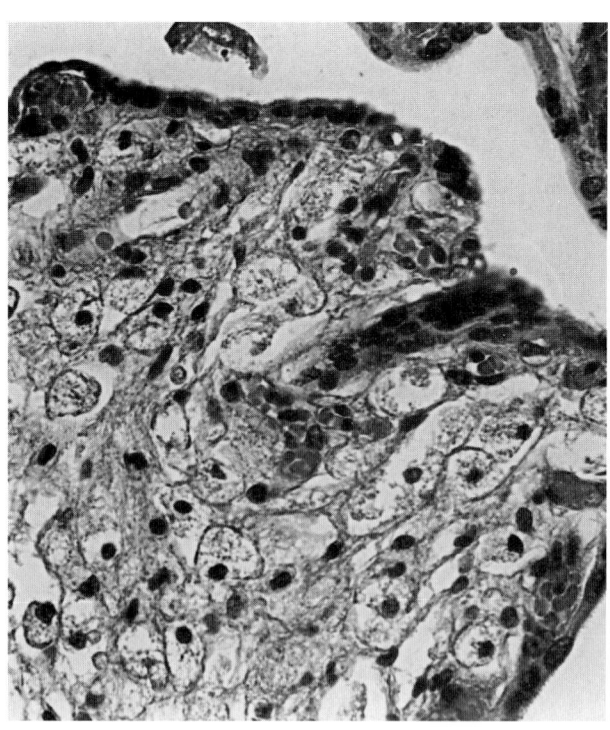

FIGURE 18.23. *Mucopolysaccharidosis type VII, placenta. Stromal cells are prominently vacuolated. Trophoblast is normal. (×190.)*

Table 18.15. Mucopolysaccharidoses

	Mucopolysaccharidosis	Major Storage	Enzymatic Defect	Biopsy Material Suggested*
I	Hurler	Dermatan sulfate and heparan sulfate	Alpha-L-iduronidase	Leukocytes
II	Hunter	Dermatan sulfate and heparan sulfate	Iduronate sulfatase	Serum
III A	Sanfilippo A	Heparan sulfate	Heparan sulfate sulfamidase	Leukocytes
III B	Sanfilippo B	Heparan sulfate	Alpha-N-acetylglucosaminidase	Plasma/serum
III C	Sanfilippo C	Heparan sulfate	Acetyl-CoA: aminodeoxyglucoside N-acetyltransferase	Leukocytes
III D	Sanfilippo D	Heparan sulfate	N-Acetylglucosamine-6-sulfatase	Leukocytes
IV	Morquio A	Keratan sulfate	N-Acetylgalactosamine-6-sulfatase	Leukocytes
	B	Keratan sulfate	β-galactosidase	Leukocytes
VI	Maroteaux–Lamy	Dermatan sulfate	N-Acetylgalactosamine-4-sulfatase (arylsulfatase B)	Leukocytes
VII	Beta-glucuronidase deficiency	Dermatan sulfate and heparan sulfate	Beta-glucuronidase	Leukocytes
Multiple sulfatase deficiency		Mucopolysaccharides and glycolipids	10 sulfatases, including aryl sulfatases A, B, and C	Leukocytes

* In all cases, the diagnosis can be confirmed using cultured fibroblasts, and prenatal diagnosis can be done by assay of cultured amniotic fluid cells, chorionic villus, or cultured chorionic villus.

especially in the nerve endings of neurons where they may be specific surface markers. Ganglioside degradation occurs in lysosomes by acid hydrolases, which also catabolize related substances. A consequence of degradative enzyme deficiencies is the accumulation of various lipid-rich substances. Refer to Figures 18.18 and 18.24 for the role of beta-galactosidase in glycolipid and catabolism. Of the gangliosidoses, only infantile GM1 gangliosidosis presents in the perinatal period. The GM2 gangliosidoses, Tay-Sachs and Sandhoff disease, appear at 3 to 6 months of age, although hypotonia may be present sooner. Infantile GM1 gangliosidosis is rare and autosomal recessive. Newborn infants may

Table 18.16. Investigation of pseudo-Hurler diseases

Sample Needed	Test to Be Done	Test Will Diagnose	Expected Result If Test Positive
Urine	Oligosaccharides by thin-layer chromatography	GM, gangliosidosis Mannosidosis Fucosidosis Mucolipidoses I, II, III	Increased amounts of oligosaccharides
	Amino acid chromatography	Aspartyl glucosaminuria	Aspartylglucosamine visible
Leukocytes	Beta-galactosidase Beta-mannosidase Beta-fucosidase	GM, gangliosidosis Mannosidosis Fucosidosis	Decreased or absent enzyme activity
Plasma	Hexosaminidase	Mucolipidoses II and III	Increased enzyme activity (at least a fivefold increase)
Fibroblasts	Sialidase	Mucolipidoses I, II, III Sialidoses I and II Confirmation of above diagnoses	Decreased or absent enzyme activity

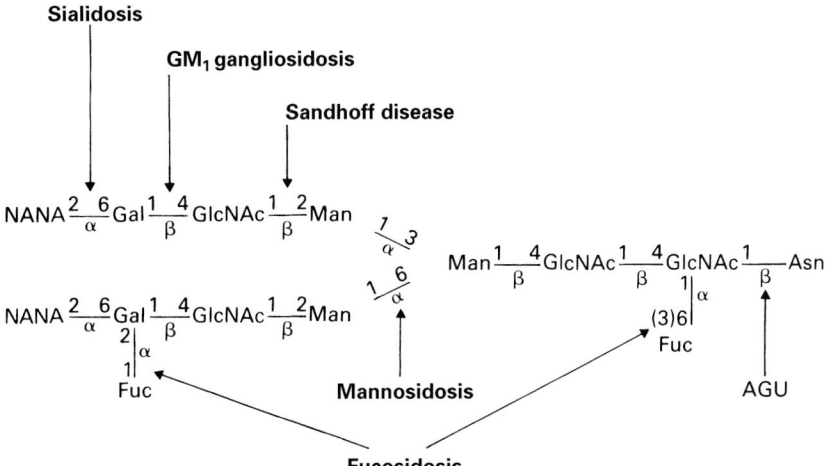

FIGURE 18.24. *Oligosaccharide pathway.*
NANA = N-acetylneuraminic acid (sialic acid), Gal = D-galactose, GlcNAc = N-acetyl-D-glucosamine, Man = D-Mannose, Fuc = L-Fucose, Asn = L-asparagine, AGU = Aspartylglucosaminuria.

be hydropic or may present with ascites [5, 8]. There is coarse facies with macroglossia, broad depressed nose, large ears, and frontal bossing of the head. The features resemble Hurler syndrome and, indeed, GM1 gangliosidosis is among the so-called pseudo-Hurler diseases (see Table 18.14). A cherry-red spot on the retina occurs in approximately 50% of patients. Infants also have hepatosplenomegaly and dysostosis multiplex. Psychomotor function is severely retarded and seizures often occur. Bronchopneumonia is common at the time of death, which usually occurs before the age of 2 years.

The widespread storage phenomenon permits presumptive diagnosis by tissue biopsy. In skin and conjuctival biopsies, fibrillogranular inclusions occur in fibroblasts and endothelial and epithelial cells, and membranous lysosomal inclusions occur in nerves. Bone marrow contains vacuolated histiocytes, and vacuolated lymphocytes are seen on a peripheral blood smear. Electron microscopy of a peripheral leukocyte preparation will show that most of the vacuoles are empty except for some sparse granular material. Definitive diagnosis of beta-galactosidase deficiency is readily made using leukocytes, cultured fibroblasts, or amniocytes. A variant of sialidosis has both sialidase and beta-galactosidase deficiency.

In infantile GM1 gangliosidosis, vacuolation of cells is found in all viscera, particularly the reticuloendothelial and nervous systems (Fig. 18.25). In the nervous system, lysosomal storage is predominantly sudanophilic, reflecting the storage of glycolipids; in other viscera, however, PAS-positive staining reflects polysaccharide storage. Electron microscopy of neuronal storage reveals membranous and lamellar intralysosomal structures, whereas in other viscera the lysosomes contain amorphous granular and a few lamellar structures [180, 181]. The pathology reflects the

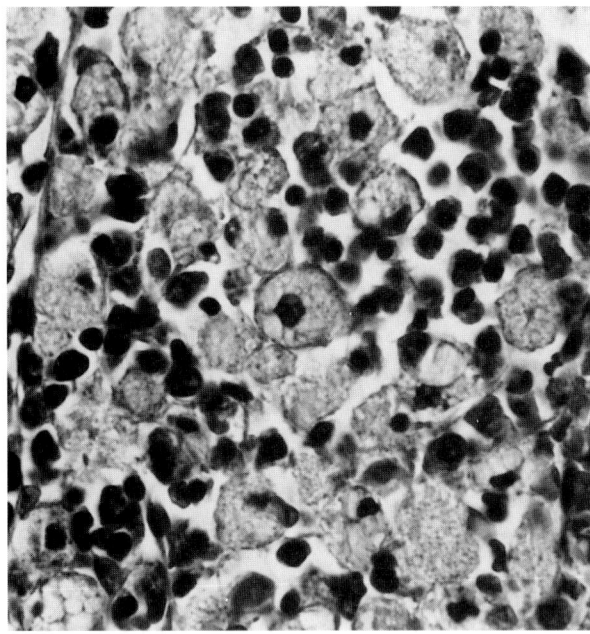

FIGURE 18.25. *GM₁ gangliosidosis. Many foam cells are present in bone marrow. (×344.)*

deficiency of beta-galactosidase which, in the neuron, is concerned predominantly with degradation of ganglioside; in other viscera it appears to have a role in the degradation of certain mucopolysaccharides.

Fetal pathology of the gangliosidoses has been examined extensively [11, 182–184]. Infantile GM1 generalized gangliosidosis is manifested by involvement of the most mature neurons and is thus seen most prominently in peripheral nervous system cells of the enteric plexus and with diminishing frequency in spinal cord neurons, Purkinje cells of the cerebellum, and maturing neurons in the deeper cerebral cortical plate. The earliest evidence of disease in the cerebral cortical cells is the presence of predominantly empty vacuoles with a few fine fibrils. In contrast, well-formed membranous cytoplasmic bodies were seen in cells of the peripheral nervous system [184]. Lowden et al noted a similar pattern in a 17-week fetus and also found vacuoles in the liver, renal tubules and glomeruli, lymphocytes, and the syncytiotrophoblast of the placenta [11]. In these cases, the pathology was subtle or even absent by light microscopy but was evident with electron microscopy even when the fetus was moderately macerated. Similarly, membranous cytoplasmic bodies in developing retinal ganglion cells and in the Purkinje cells of the cerebellum [183] have been demonstrated in Sandhoff disease in a fetus of 15 to 16 weeks' gestation. The earliest morphological expression of Tay-Sachs disease was in a fetus of 12 weeks' gestation in which membranous cytoplasmic bodies were found in spinal cord neurons [185]. The pattern of neuronal involvement is similar to generalized GMI gangliosidosis [182]. Morpho-

logical disease occurs first in the phylogenetically older parts of the nervous system (i.e., those areas that are first to mature).

Mucolipidoses

Mucolipidoses were conceived as a group of disorders having similarities to both mucopolysaccharidoses and sphingolipidoses. Subsequently, biochemical delineation showed that these are diverse: type I, now called sialidosis I (see below), is a disorder of degradation (sialidosis); types II and III are due to disordered targeting of lysosomal enzymes; and type IV is of unknown etiology. The pathology has been reviewed recently [186].

Sialidoses   The sialidoses are diverse. Most patients have increased amounts of sialic acid bound in glycopeptides but in one group, Salla disease, free sialic acid is stored. The defect in Salla disease is not known but in the other sialidoses a deficiency of sialidase is responsible for failure of hydrolysis of sialic acid from glycopeptides. Most classifications are based on that of Lowden and O'Brien, who divided sialidoses into normosomatic (type I) or dysmorphic (type II) [187]. The normosomatic type, usually presenting with a cherry-red spot (myoclonus phenotype), occurs either as sialidase deficiency alone or as part of a coexisting beta-galactosidase deficiency. The combined defect is caused by deficiency of a "protective protein," a serine protease that blocks beta-galactosidase and neuraminidase from degradation [188].

The dysmorphic type II sialidosis presents from neonatal to early adulthood ages, when it includes Goldberg syndrome and nephrosialidosis. Neonates with type II sialidosis present with hydrops fetalis, coarse facies, hepatosplenomegaly, corneal opacity, dysostosis multiplex, and sometimes cherry-red maculae. They fail to thrive and become mentally retarded; sepsis is frequent [6, 187, 189, 190]. Vacuolation of cells in the reticuloendothelial system, gastrointestinal tract, liver, kidney, and bone marrow predominate (Fig. 18.26). Peripheral lymphocytes also are vacuolated, as in all mucolipidoses, and both stromal and trophoblastic cells of placenta are vacuolated (see Fig. 18.1). Visceral and mesenchymal vacuoles tend to be populated sparsely by amorphous or fibrillogranular material. Membranous cytoplasmic bodies and pleomorphic bodies are noted in vacuoles of axons. Infants with sialidosis can, in theory, be diagnosed by identifying increased amounts of sialyl oligosaccharides in urine using thin-layer chromatography. In practice, this can be a difficult test to interpret unless the laboratory has available for comparison urine samples from patients with known oligosaccharide storage disease.

In addition to sialidosis, there are infants with storage and urinary excretion of free sialic acid associated with severe neonatal disease [191]. These patients are clinically similar to infantile sialidosis but lack dysostosis multiplex. Pathologically, many cell types, including epithelium, appear to be involved with lysosmal storage. Ultrastructurally, the vacuoles

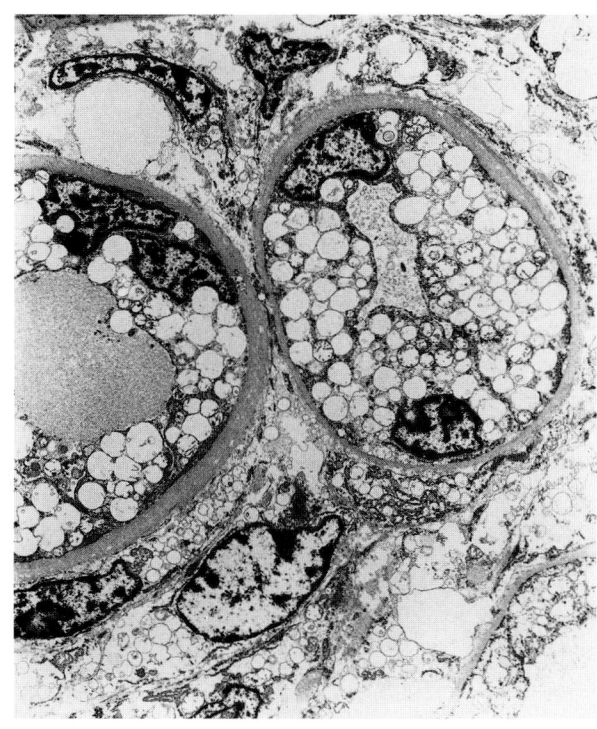

FIGURE 18.26.   *Sialidosis. Note the extensive, predominantly empty vacuoles of renal tubular epithelium. (×2750.)*

contain granular or floccular material and dense complex lamellae have been noted in axons.

Other Mucolipidoses Mucolipidoses II and III, or I-cell disease and pseudo-Hurler polydystrophy, respectively, are a group of autosomal recessive disorders of lysosomal protein processing and targeting caused by defective phosphorylation of mannose residues on newly synthesized lysosomal enzymes. Mannose-6-phosphate is a common marker for the proper targeting of these enzymes into lysosomes. The presence of at least three complementation groups suggests genetic heterogeneity of this disorder.

Type III mucolipidosis usually does not manifest in the perinatal period, whereas type II certainly does. Infants with I-cell disease (mucolipidosis II) are affected severely and have prominent Hurler features. Many viscera and cell types are involved by storage [192]. Cellular vacuolation and histiocytic accumulation are found in the heart, kidney, brain and meninges, liver, and bones. Lipid granulomata also occur. Cytoplasmic vacuoles are membrane-bound and contain variable material, including reticular, granular, and membranous lamellar bodies, reflecting the lack of localization of many lysosomal enzymes in the lysosome. The study by Martin et al emphasizes the predominantly mesenchymal involvement by vacuolar storage [193].

The diagnosis of mucolipidosis II and III is suggested by an at least seven or eightfold increase in plasma beta-hexosaminidase. In fetuses with mucolipidosis II, pathology

is already present by the 16th gestational week [194]. Vacuolation apparent in thin sections and by using electron microscopy predominates in mesenchymal cells and consists of membrane-bound aggregates of sparse fibrillogranular material and other vacuoles bearing polymorphic inclusions. Glomerular epithelial and mesangial cells are involved.

Mucolipidosis IV is not a disease of the perinatal period, although there may be clouding of the cornea in the first week of life [195]. The presence of cytoplasmic membrane-bound inclusions in cultured and uncultured amniotic fluid cells and in fetal tissues (predominantly epithelial) has been used both for intrauterine diagnosis and confirmation at autopsy [13, 196]. The placenta has vacuolation of the stromal cells. Vacuoles have nonspecific granular material, and lamellar structures are seen in endothelial cells of villous capillaries.

Three disorders—fucosidosis, mannosidosis, and aspartyl-glucosaminuria—are in the spectrum of metabolic disorders with Hurler-like features (see Table 18.14). These entities arise from defects in glycoprotein degradation (see Fig. 18.24), and although fucosidosis and mannosidosis have an infantile phenotype, none is clinically expressed in the neonatal period.

Peroxisomal Disorders

The peroxisome is an intracellular organelle found in all cells except mature red blood cells, and it is most prominent in liver and renal proximal tubular cells. They are the preferential site for oxidation of very-long-chain fatty acids and phytanic acid by metabolic pathways that generate hydrogen peroxide. The hydrogen peroxide generated is reduced to water by catalase contained within the organelle. Among the many functions of the peroxisome are plasmalogen and bile acid synthesis, glyoxylate transamination, and prostaglandin metabolism [197]. The organelle does not produce ATP.

In the past decade, genetically determined disorders have been identified in which there is peroxisomal dysfunction [198, 199]. These disorders can be classified into three groups: absence or paucity of the peroxisome organelle (group 1); or, in the presence of the organelle, deficiency of multiple enzymes (group 2); or, in the presence of the organelle, deficiency of a single enzyme (group 3) (Table 18.17). Clinical presentation often occurs in the neonatal period. The pathologic manifestations comprise dysmorphogenic abnormalities of as yet unidentified metabolic pathogenesis, storage phenomena presumably of very-long-chain fatty acid, and degenerative lesions with reparative responses [198, 199].

Group 1 peroxisomal disorders have in common an absence, or reduced number, of peroxisomes. The most common of this group is the cerebrohepatorenal (CHR) syndrome (Zellweger syndrome). This group of autosomal recessive disorders is characterized by hypotonia, dysmorphic features (prominent forehead, hypoplastic supraorbital

Table 18.17. Peroxisomal disorders

Group 1: Peroxisomes deficient
  Cerebrohepatorenal (Zellweger) syndrome (ZS)
  Neonatal adrenoleukodystrophy
  Infantile Refsum disease
  Hyperpipecolic acidemia
Group 2: Peroxisomes present, multiple enzymes deficient
  Rhizomelic chondrodysplasia punctata (RCDP)
  Zellweger-like syndrome
Group 3: Peroxisomes present, single enzyme deficient
  X-linked adrenoleukodystrophy
  Acyl-CoA oxidase deficiency (Pseudo-NALD)
  Bifunctional protein deficiency
  Peroxisomal thiolase deficiency (Pseudo-ZS)
  Dihydroxyacetone phosphate acyltransferase deficiency (DHAPAT-deficiency)
    (Pseudo-RCDP)
  Glutamyl-CoA oxidase deficiency
  Di- and trihydroxycholestanoic acidemia
  Hyperoxaluria type I
  Acatalasemia

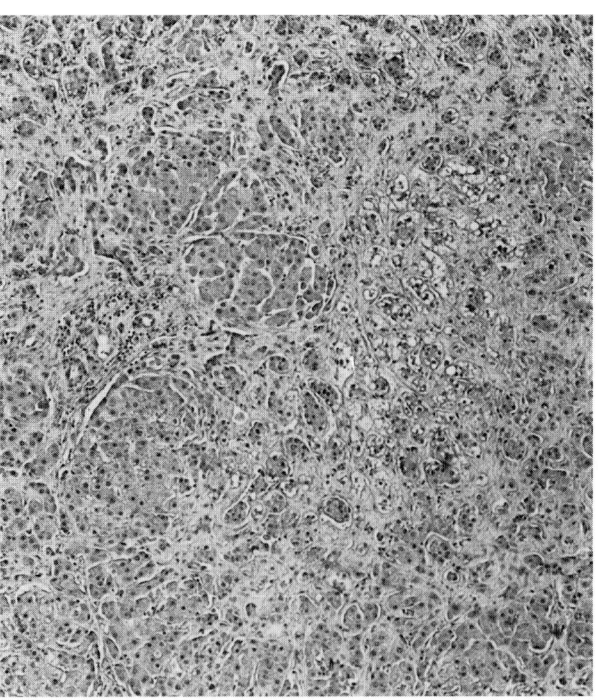

FIGURE 18.27. *Liver in Zellweger cerebrohepatorenal syndrome. The liver is cirrhotic with extensive lobular and portal fibrosis. (H&E, ×40.)*

ridges, anteverted nares, high arched palate), cryptorchidism, limb deformity, hepatomegaly with liver dysfunction, and cataracts and peripheral pigmentation of the retinas. Infants rarely survive beyond the first few months of life.

Neuronal heterotopias, polymicrogyria, and pachygyria, indicating disordered neuronal migration, are attributed to interferences by the abnormally high concentration of very-long-chain fatty acids. Dysmyelination and gliosis also occur. Stippled calcification of cartilage, tubular and glomerular renal cysts, and hepatic fibrosis progressing to cirrhosis are common (Fig. 18.27). Although mitochondria appear abnormal in the liver, the most striking ultrastructural pathology is the deficiency of peroxisomes [200–203].

Complementation studies have demonstrated that there are at least eight different genes responsible for the peroxisome-deficient syndromes. These genes are believed to be involved in the formation of normal peroxisomes and in the transport of peroxisomal enzymes [204]. There does not appear to be any obvious correlation between complementation groups and clinical phenotype. Two human peroxisomal proteins have been cloned: peroxisome assembly factor 1 (PAF-1) [205] and a transmembrane transporter gene PMP70 (3). Deleterious mutations have been described in both genes among patients with the cerebrohepatorenal syndrome phenotype [206].

In the group 2 disorder, rhizomelic chondrodysplasia punctata, there is much more chondrodysplasia and calcific stippling than in the Zellweger CHR syndrome, and neuronal migration defects are absent or minimal [198]. Phytanic acid may be elevated and deficient plasmalogen synthesis can be demonstrated in cultured fibroblasts. Group 3 disorders have defects of a single enzyme. X-linked

adrenoleukodystrophy (ALD), typical of this group, is by far the most common but does not present in the neonatal period. The affected fetus does have abnormal adrenal glands with enlarged fetal zone cells containing lamellar lipid profiles that are presumed to be very-long-chain fatty acids [207].

Identification of abnormally elevated concentrations of very-long-chain fatty acids and phytanic acid in plasma and/or cultured skin fibroblasts [208, 209] will diagnose group 1 disorders and most patients in groups 2 and 3. Plasmalogen synthesis can be assayed in cultured skin fibroblasts to investigate rhizomelic chondrodysplasia punctata [210, 211]. Peroxisomal disorders should be considered in the differential diagnosis of an infant with hypotonia and developmental delay, especially if there is facial dysmorphism, liver dysfunction, calcific stippling of cartilage, short limbs, or leukodystrophy in the central nervous system.

Miscellaneous Disorders

Alpha-1-Antitrypsin Deficiency

Alpha-1-antitrypsin (α_1AT) is a serine protease inhibitor (PI) which, by inhibiting primarily leukocyte elastase, has an important role in the control of tissue degradation. In the lung, α_1AT prevents elastase from degrading the elastin of the alveolar walls, the destruction of which would lead to emphysema. Idiopathic neonatal hepatitis syndrome and cirrhosis occur in some infants with the PI type ZZ. Neonatal liver dysfunction is not adequately explained but in part is thought to be due to aggregation of α_1AT in the endoplasmic reticulum. Hepatic pathology may be present by 20 weeks' gestation [212]. Diagnosis is achieved by measuring total plasma alpha-1-antitrypsin followed by PI typing (isoelectric-focusing). Prenatal diagnosis for the ZZ phenotype is readily available by direct DNA analysis using PCR-based methods [213].

Cystic Fibrosis

Cystic fibrosis can present in the perinatal period with meconium ileus, biliary tract obstruction, and neonatal hepatitis syndrome. Aborted fetuses have had a high incidence of meconium ileus [214]. Immunoreactive trypsin which is increased in the neonatal period [215] is often used for presumptive diagnosis until 4 to 6 weeks of age, at which time the sweat chloride test becomes reliable. Prenatal diagnosis of cystic fibrosis is now possible by direct DNA mutation analysis and linkage analysis. The major mutation, which accounts for 70% of alleles, is a 3-base-pair deletion causing loss of phenylalanine 508 [216].

Idiopathic Neonatal Iron Storage Syndrome (Neonatal Hemochromatosis)

A number of newborn infants have been described with excessive and predominantly parenchymal iron storage. These infants, both male and female, had serious liver disease and died usually within the first week of life, sometimes soon after birth [217]. The liver is extensively fibrotic with an acinar rearrangement of the remaining hepatocytes; lobular fibrosis, hepatic vein sclerosis, and hepatocytes are in varying stages of atrophy (Fig. 18.28). Cholestasis and bile ductule proliferation are also present. The iron content of the liver is almost exclusively limited to the hepatocytes. Hemosiderin is also present in myocardium, thyroid follicular cells, peribronchial glands, gastric mucosa, and renal cortical tubular epithelium. In the pancreas, iron is present in acinar and insular cells. The gland was moderately fibrosed and islets appeared hyperplastic relative to the atrophic acinar tissue. Little or no stainable iron is noted in lymph nodes, spleen, or bone marrow. Idiopathic neonatal iron storage syndrome is not now considered to be a specific entity but rather a manifestation of probably different injuries to the fetal liver, with secondary disturbances of iron metabolism. Although pathologic changes are similar to genetic hemochromatosis, there is no evidence of etiologic overlap [218, 219].

Smith-Lemli-Opitz Syndrome

The Smith-Lemli-Opitz (SLO) syndrome is an autosomal recessive disorder characterized by typical facial features, neurological and limb abnormalities, heart and kidney malformations, hypospadias, and endocrine disturbances [220]. Tint et al [221] recently found markedly elevated 7-

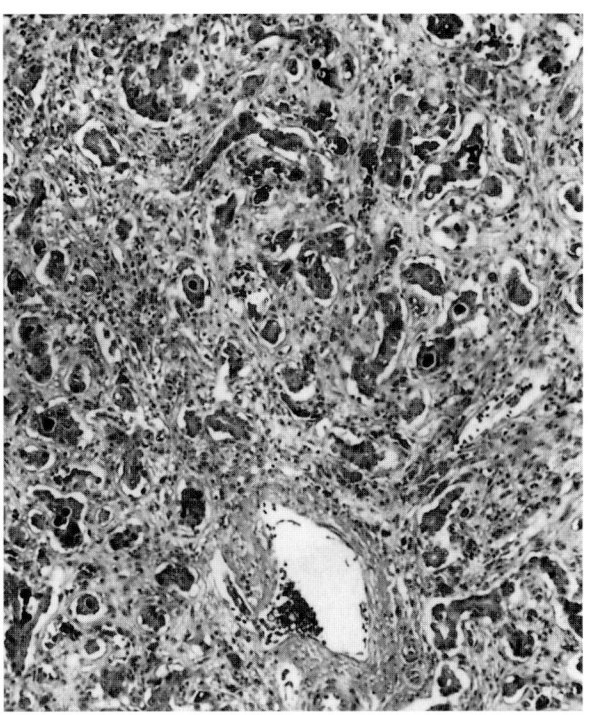

FIGURE 18.28. *Neonatal iron storage syndrome. Note the extensive lobular fibrosis of the liver. (×31.)*

dehydrocholesterol concentrations in SLO patients, suggesting that this disorder is in fact a metabolic disease. A defect in 7-dehydrocholesterol reductase, which catalyzes the final step in cholesterol biosynthesis, was demonstrated subsequently. As yet these biochemical abnormalities do not explain the dysmorphic phenotype. A case was recently detected prenatally in our hospital with an abnormally low material serum estriol level (abnormal triple marker screen). Prenatal diagnosis by both chorionic villus biopsy and amniocentesis is now available.

Carbohydrate-Deficient Glycoprotein Syndrome

The carbohydrate-deficient glycoprotein (CDG) syndrome is a recently recognized multisystem disease with autosomal recessive inheritance [222, 223]. Although the onset of disease is variable, the CDG syndrome may manifest in the neonatal period and can be life-threatening. There may be dysmorphic features (coarse facies, strabismus, inverted nipples, and abnormal gluteal fat pads). Liver dysfunction with steatosis progresses to portal fibrosis and cirrhosis. Severe neurological disturbances and olivopontocerebellar atrophy occur. Inclusions similar to membranous cytoplasmic bodies found in gangliosidosis are found in Purkinje cells. There are also renal tubular microcysts [224–227].

The most striking and consistent biochemical abnormality in the CDG syndrome is the presence of secretory glycoproteins that are deficient in some of their carbohydrate moieties. Isoelectric focusing of serum transferrin revealing missing terminal trisaccharides is the most commonly used diagnostic test [228]. This test has been used for prenatal diagnosis, but the abnormality is not consistently found in affected fetuses [229]. The underlying biochemical defect remains unknown.

PRENATAL DIAGNOSIS OF METABOLIC DISEASE

It is now possible to offer prenatal diagnosis for most inborn errors of metabolism, reinforcing the need to come to an accurate diagnosis in the proband. The devastating nature of many metabolic diseases and the recurrence risk in future pregnancies often discourage parents from having more children. Prenatal diagnosis addresses this concern by giving couples options in family planning.

Enzyme defects that can be demonstrated in cultured skin fibroblasts usually also can be identified in either cultured or uncultured chorionic villi or amniotic fluid cells. The advantage of a biopsy of chorionic villus is that the procedure is performed between 11 or 12 weeks' gestation and will provide results earlier than for amniocentesis. With use of these samples, the majority of enzyme defects can be investigated successfully if the laboratory offering prenatal testing has considerable experience with quality control and thorough familiarity with the diagnostic assays.

For enzymatic assays the disease being sought in the fetus must be confirmed biochemically in the family rather than relying on clinical or historical suspicion. It is especially important to determine the activity of the enzyme for het-

erozygotes and homozygotes within the family being investigated. Carriers with enzyme activity almost as low as in a homozygote sometimes occur and make it difficult to interpret low levels of enzyme activity in a fetus. Conversely some affected fetuses with disorders such as Hunter disease may have high residual enzyme activities that can complicate interpretation.

There has been a tremendous effort in recent years to clone genes and characterize mutations that result in inborn errors of metabolism. In some of these disorders identification of specific mutations occurring with relatively high frequency allows for direct screening of affected fetuses. If the mutation is identified, family studies can then be done. However, in the majority of disorders the frequency of individual mutations is small. Investigations then are aimed at the detection of novel mutations. Presently this work is laborious and mostly confined to research laboratories.

If the mutation or mutations are found in the proband and are clearly deleterious, prenatal diagnosis by direct mutational analysis on biopsied chorionic villi or amniotic fluid cells can be offered. The major advantage is that analyses can be done within days of the prenatal diagnostic procedure. For these assays, molecular testing to rule out maternal contamination of chorionic villi is essential.

In patients where the mutations have not been delineated, markers that flank the gene of interest can be used for linkage analysis as long as family members are available for testing and markers are informative. In recent years, highly informative markers throughout the human genome have been identified. In addition, the advent of the polymerase chain reaction (PCR) allows for rapid amplification of DNA, making results available quickly. Although markers can often be found very close to the gene of interest, recombination creates a small risk that can confuse results. Despite the potential of molecular testing, enzyme analyses are still the cornerstone for prenatal diagnosis of metabolic disorders. In the few biochemical disorders in which the defect is not expressed in chorionic villus tissue or amniocytes, such as ornithine transcarbamylase deficiency, linkage analysis or direct mutational analysis can be offered [230].

Role of Anatomic Pathology

Although the disorders that can be diagnosed prenatally by enzymatic or molecular methods are increasing, there are still some diseases in which neither is possible. In late infantile ceroid lipofuscinosis, a metabolic disease of unknown etiology, amniotic fluid cells from affected fetuses contain curvilinear bodies [16, 231, 232]. Mucolipidosis type IV, another disorder in which the biochemical defect is unknown, can also be diagnosed prenatally by electron microscopy of uncultured and cultured amniotic fluid cells because they contain membranous and granular cytosomes [233]. Rapid prenatal diagnosis can be obtained in Pompe disease (glycogen storage disease type II) by electron

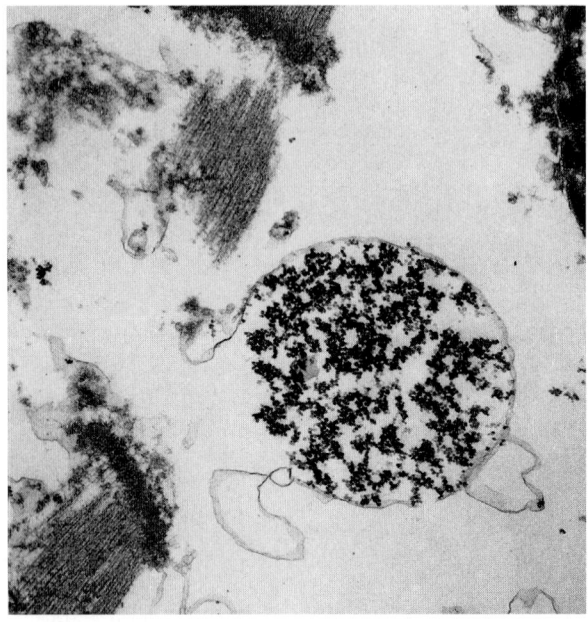

FIGURE 18.29. *Heart of macerated aborted fetus, Pompe disease. Note the lysosomal glycogen. (×26,220.)*

microscopy of uncultured amniocytes. Using enzyme histochemistry or immunohistochemistry for catalase, peroxisome deficiency may be investigated on chorionic villus tissue [132, 211] (see Fig. 18.16). For Niemann-Pick disease type C, filipin staining to identify excessive cholesterol in cultured amniocytes or chorionic villus cells is used to complement the biochemical assay [149]. Another productive use of histological techniques involves the prenatal diagnosis of genodermatoses, including some of a metabolic nature [234].

The "Emergency" or "Metabolic" Autopsy

The emergency or metabolic autopsy is so entitled to indicate the necessity of immediate involvement of the pathologist who has the expertise to match the broad etiological possibilities with types of specimens required for investigation. Such an autopsy, be it on an aborted fetus or a newborn infant with metabolic disease, should be conducted immediately upon receipt of permission and should be done with full clinical information and consultation with those who may be involved in special analyses of specimens. If parents are approached with sensitivity and if it is legally acceptable, autopsy permission may be obtained premortem when death is imminent or inevitable. When a delay in autopsy is expected or the autopsy has been refused, one should consider securing permission for needle biopsies of various viscera. In this way, the goal of the emergency autopsy will be met—to obtain a definitive diagnosis for the purposes of genetic counseling and possible future diagnoses or therapy, to ascertain that a prenatal diagnosis has been correct or in error, and to facilitate research on inborn metabolic diseases.

The approach to the emergency autopsy is discussed in detail elsewhere [131, 235, 236]. In most fetal cases, a metabolic disease will have been diagnosed prenatally and the autopsy protocol may then be quite specific. For a few fetal cases, and more commonly for newborn infants, metabolic disease may be only a possibility among differential diagnoses of chromosomal error, immunohemolytic disorders, or infectious disease. In the latter circumstances, biochemical analysis is required.

Biochemical Analysis

For biochemical analysis, as much tissue as is possible or reasonable should be obtained from the liver, kidney, brain, and skeletal muscle. The tissue is blocked into 0.5 cm cubes, snap-frozen in liquid nitrogen, wrapped in foil, and enclosed in a tight, labeled container for storage in a −70°C freezer until the biochemist chooses the tissue required for investigation. Special circumstances may require that other tissue specimens, blood, cerebrospinal fluid, and urine be sampled and stored similarly. If possible, plasma and cerebrospinal fluid should be collected in duplicate, with one sample deproteinized for amino acid analysis and the non-

deproteinized portion retained for organic acid determinations. With involvement of the central nervous system, one-half of the brain divided sagittally should be supported on stiff cardboard and frozen intact. In this way, samples from specific zones of the brain may be obtained for biochemical analysis.

Specimens for histochemistry are preferably rapid-frozen in chilled viscous isopentane immersed in liquid nitrogen.

Tissue Culture for Biochemistry and Cytogenetics

Fetuses delivered some time after induction of the abortion may be autolyzed, precluding standard biochemical analysis. Sterile samples of deep tissues, such as cartilage from the sternum, fascia, tendon, or placenta, may be taken for fibroblast culture. Specimens should be washed three times for 10 minutes in a 1% penicillin-streptomycin-fungizone solution and then placed in minimal essential media. The same procedure is followed for cytogenetic studies. In our experience for placenta the best tissue culture results are with samples of amnion taken near the insertion of the umbilical cord. Chromosomal analysis may also be initiated using peripheral blood samples if the postmortem interval is short.

DNA Analysis

For DNA analysis samples of the liver or spleen should be snap-frozen and retained deep-frozen for possible future analysis. Policies pertaining to DNA banking and special consent for doing so are currently being developed and likely will be required in addition to permission for autopsy examination.

Electron Microscopy

For electron microscopy specimens of the heart, brain, skeletal muscle, liver, kidney, and spleen are diced into 1.0 mm cubes in chilled 2.5% glutaraldehyde. Autolysis should not deter one from electron microscopy (see Fig. 18.28). Lysosomal storage products often survive cellular degeneration and can be identified. Even with a very macerated fetus, the placenta may be examined successfully by electron microscopy. When sampling the nervous system for electron microscopy, one should bear in mind that in fetal cases it is usually the most mature areas that will be involved by a storage disorder.

Other Procedures

Photography is invaluable for dysmorphic cases; similarly, radiological examination should be considered. If a hematological abnormality is entertained, blood and bone marrow specimens are required. For example, the hydropic newborn infant with hemoglobin Bart thalassemia may be diagnosed by hemoglobin electrophoresis done on postmortem blood samples. Finally, some infants and fetuses with suspected metabolic disease will have, instead, infectious diseases, and specimens for microbiological agents must be taken.

In our experience, the techniques most likely to lead to definitive diagnosis of inborn metabolic disease are histopathology; electron microscopy; routine special stains; and enzyme analysis of suitable tissues, when available, or of cultured fibroblasts. Chemical assay of tissues for storage material may be done but has not been as valuable in our practice. The pathologist should use the opportunity of an autopsy of non-metabolic cases to obtain tissues for the purposes of biochemistry controls.

CONCLUSION

Study of genetic metabolic disease has evolved from early attention to aminoacidopathies and lysosomal enzymopathies to organic acidemias and recent active interest in peroxisomal and mitochondrial disorders. Progress in biochemistry led to identification of more enzyme defects and better characterization of enzymes, with recognition of cofactor or activator protein anomalies. Better morphological definition of metabolic disease is due to histochemistry, electron microscopy, and immunotechnology. We now have rapidly evolving molecular technology to assist in diagnosis and, importantly, to further our understanding of pathogenesis, in particular the relationship of metabolic disease to dysmorphogenesis.

REFERENCES

1. Whitby LG. Screening for disease, definitions and criteria. *Lancet* 1974; ii:819.
2. Bickel H, Guthrie R, Hammersen G. *Neonatal Screening for Inborn Errors of Metabolism*. Berlin: Springer-Verlag, 1980.
3. Pitfalls in screening for neonatal hypothyroidism. Report of the New England Screening Program and the New England Congenital Hypothyroidism Collaborative. *Pediatrics* 1982; 70:16–20.
4. Todd WA. Psychosocial problems as the major complication of an adolescent with trimethylaminuria. *Pediatr* 1979; 94:936–7.
5. Abu-Dalu KI, Tamary H, Livni N, Rivkind AI, Yatziv S. GM1 Gangliosidosis presenting as neonatal ascites. *Pediatr* 1980; 100:940–3.
6. Beck M, Bender SW, Reiter HL, et al. Neuraminidase deficiency presenting as non-immune hydrops fetalis. *Eur J Pediatr* 1984; 143:135–9.
7. Ceuterick C, Martin JJ, Libert J, Farriaux JP. San-Filippo A disease in the fetus—comparison with pre- and post-natal cases. *Neuropaediatrie* 1980; 11:176–85.
8. Crocker AT, Vawter GF, Neuhauser EBD, Rosowsky A. Wolman's disease: three new patients with a recently described lipidosis. *Pediatrics* 1965; 35:770.
8. Gillan JE, Lowden JA, Gaskin K. Cutz E. Congenital ascites as a presenting sign of lysosomal storage disease. *J Pediatr* 1984; 104:225–31.
9. Irani D, Kim H-S, El-Hibri H, et al. Postmortem observations on beta glucuronidase deficiency presenting as hydrops fetalis. *Ann Neurol* 1983; 14:486–90.
10. Keeling JW, Gough DJ, Hiff P. The pathology of non-rhesus hydrops. *Diagn Histopathol* 1983; 6:89–111.
11. Lowden JA, Cutz E, Conen PE, Rudd N, Duran TA. Prenatal diagnosis of GM1 gangliosidosis. *N Engl J Med* 1973; 288:225–8.
12. Nelson A, Pederson L, Frampton B, Sly WS. Mucopoly-saccharidosis VII (beta glucuronidase deficiency) presenting as non-immune hydrops fetalis. *J Pediatr* 1982; 101:574–6.
13. Sekeles E, Ornoy A, Cohen R, Kohn G. Mucolipidosis IV: fetal and placental pathology. *Monogr Hum Genet* 1978; 10:47–50.
14. Sun CC, Panny S, Combs J, Gutberlett R. Hydrops fetalis associated with Gaucher's disease. *Pathol Res Pract* 1984; 179:101–4.
15. Roberts DJ, Ampola MG, Lage JM. Diagnosis of unsuspected fetal metabolic storage disease by routine placental examination. *Pediatr Pathol* 1991; 11:647–56.
16. Rapola J. Neuronal ceroid-lipofuscinoses in childhood. *Perspect Pediatr Pathol* 1993; 17:7–44.
17. Brunning RD. Morphologic alterations in nucleated blood and marrow cells in genetic disorders. *Hum Pathol* 1970; 1:99–124.
18. Dolman CL. Diagnosis of neurometabolic disorders by examination of skin biopsies and lymphocytes. *Semin Diagn Pathol* 1984; 1:82–97.
19. Ceuterick C, Martin JJ. Diagnostic role of skin or conjunctival biopsies in neurologic disorders. *J Neurol Sci* 1984; 65:179–91.
20. Libert J. Diagnosis of lysosomal storage diseases by the ultrastructural study of conjunctival biopsies. *Pathol Annu* 1980; 1:37–66.
21. Landing BH, Ng WG, Alfi O, Donnell GN. Fibroblast culture and the diagnosis of genetic metabolic diseases: comparative histochemical ultrastructure and biochemical studies. *Perspect Pediatr Pathol* 1979; 5:237–62.
22. Lie SO. Influence of cell culture medium on the metabolic behaviour of the fibroblast. In: Harkness RA, Cockburn F, eds. *The Cultured Cell and Inherited Metabolic Disease*. Baltimore: University Park Press, 1978, pp. 16–32.
23. Ornoy A, Sekeles E, Cohen R, Kohn G. Electron microscopy of cultured skin fibroblast and amniotic fluid cells and the diagnosis of hereditary storage diseases. *Monogr Hum Genet* 1978; 10:32–9.
24. Ampola MG. *Metabolic Diseases in Pediatric Practice*. Boston: Little, Brown, 1982, pp. 119–40.
25. Mahoney MJ. Organic acidemias. *Clin Perinatol* 1976; 3:61–78.
26. Rosenberg LE. Disorders of propionate and methyl malonate metabolism. In: Stanbury JB, Wyngaarden JB, Frederickson DS, Goldstein JL, Brown MS, eds. *The Metabolic Basis of Inherited Diseases*. 5th ed. New York: McGraw Hill, 1983, p. 474.
27. Hutchinson RJ, Bunnell K, Thoene JG. Suppression of granulopoietic progenitor cell proliferation by metabolites of the branched chain amino acids. *J Pediatr* 1985; 106:62–5.
28. Chalmers RA, Lawson AM. *Organic Acids in Man—the Analytical Chemistry, Biochemistry and Diagnosis of the Organic Acidurias*. London: Chapman & Hall, 1982.
29. Kott-Blumenkrantz R, Pappas CTE, Bensch KG. A study of the ultrastructure of the organs and of cultured fibroblasts incubated with isoleucine from a patient with propionic acidemia. *Hum: Pathol* 1981; 12:1141–8.
30. Shapiro LJ. Bocian ME, Raijman L, Cederbaum SD, Shaw KNF. Methylmalonyl CoA mutase deficiency associated with severe neonatal hyperammonemia: activity of urea cycle enzymes. *J Pediatr* 1978; 93:986–8.
31. Steinman L, Clancy RR, Cann H, Urich H. The neuropathology of propionic acidemia. *Dev Med Child Neurol* 1983; 25:87–94.
32. Ampola M. Multiple carboxylase deficiency: clinical and biochemical improvement following neonatal biotin treatment. *Pediatrics* 1981; 68:113–18.
33. Israels S, Haworth JC, Dunation, Applegarth DA. Lactic acidosis in childhood. *Adv Pediatr* 1975, 22:267–303.
34. Rosenblatt DS, Shevell MI. The neurology of cobalamin. *Can J Neurol Sci* 1992; 19:472–86.
35. Vamecq J, de Hoffmann E, Van Hoff F. Mitochondria and peroxisomal metabolism of glutaryl CoA. *Eur J Biochem* 1985; 146:663–9.
36. Vamecq J, Van Hoff F. Implication of a peroxisomal enzyme in the catabolism of glutaryl CoA. *Biochem J* 1985; 221:203–11.
37. Hale DE, Bennett MJ. Fatty acid oxidation disorders: a new class of metabolic diseases. *J Pediatr* 1992; 121:1–11.
37. Tanaka K, Rosenberg LE. Disorders of branched chain amino acid and organic acid metabolism. In: Stanbury JB, Wyngaarden JB, Frederickson DS, Goldstein JC, Brown MS, eds. *The Metabolic Basis of Inherited Disease*, 5th ed. New York: McGraw-Hill, 1983, pp. 440–73.
38. Bennett MJ, Pollitt RJ, Talz LS, et al. Medium chain acyl-CoA dehydrogenase deficiency: a useful diagnosis five years after death. *Clin Chem* 1990; 36:1695–97.
39. Bennett MJ, Powell S. Metabolic disease and sudden, unexpected death in infancy. *Hum Pathol* 1994; 25:742–6.
40. Losty HC, Lee P, Alfaham M, et al. Fatty infiltration in liver in medium chain acyl CoA dehydrogenase deficiency. *Arch Dis Child* 1991; 66: 727–8.
40. Farrell K, Dimmick JE, Applegarth DA, et al. Peroxisomal abnormality in neonatal adrenal leucodystrophy. *Ann Neurol* 1983; 14:379.

41. Boles RG, Spencer K, Martin MS, Blitzer MG, Rinaldo P. Biochemical diagnosis of fatty acid oxidation disorders by metabolite analysis of postmortem liver. *Hum Pathol* 1994; 25:735–41.

42. Roe CR, Coates PM. Mitochondrial fatty acid oxidation disorders. In: Scriver CR, Beaudet AL, Sly WS, Valle D, eds. *The Metabolic and Molecular Bases of Inherited Disease.* 7th ed. New York: McGraw-Hill, 1995; pp. 1501–33.

43. Yokota I, Coates PM, Hale DE, Rinaldo P, Tanaka K. Molecular survey of a prevalent mutation, A985 to G transition, and identification of five infrequent mutations in the medium-chain acyl-CoA dehydrogenase gene in 55 patients with medium chain acyl-CoA dehydrogenase deficiency. *Am J Hum Genet* 1991; 49:1280–91.

44. Arens R, Gozal D, Jain K, et al. Prevalence of medium-chain acyl-coenzyme A dehydrogenase deficiency in the sudden infant death syndrome. *J Pediatr* 1993; 122:715–18.

45. Seddon HR, Green A, Gray RGF, Leonard JV, Pollitt RJ, Regional variations in medium-chain acyl-CoA dehydrogenase deficiency. *Lancet* 1995; 345:135–6.

46. Goodman SI, Norenberg MD, Shikes RH, Breslich DJ, Moe PG. Glutaric aciduria: biochemical and morphologic considerations. *J Pediatr* 1977; 90:746–50.

47. Gregersen N. Riboflavin-responsive defects of beta oxidation. *J Inherited Metab Dis* 1985; 8:65–9.

48. Bernstein J. Hepatic and renal involvement in malformation syndromes. *Mt Sinai J Med* 1986; 53:421–8.

49. Harkin JC, Gill WL, Shapira E. Glutaric acidemia type II: phenotypic findings and ultrastructural studies of brain and kidney. *Arch Pathol Lab Med* 1986; 110:399–401.

50. Wilson GN, de Chadarevian J-P, Kaplan P, et al. Glutaric aciduria type II: review of the phenotype and report of an unusual glomerulopathy. *Am J Med Genet* 1989; 32: 395–401.

51. Kamiya M, Eimoto T, Kishimoto H, et al. Glutaric aciduria type II: autopsy study of a case with electron-transferring flavoprotein dehydrogenase deficiency. *Pediatr Pathol* 1990; 10:1007–19.

52. Robinson BH, Sherwood WG. Lactic acidemia. *J Inherited Metab Dis* 1984; 7:69–73.

53. Chun K, MacKay N, Petrova-Benedict R, Robinson BH. Mutations in the X-linked E1α subunit of pyruvate dehydrogenase leading to deficiency of the pyruvate dehydrogenase complex. *Hum Mol Genet* 1993; 2:449–54.

54. Brown GK. Pyruvate dehydrogenase E1α deficiency. *J Inher Metab Dis* 1992; 15:625–33.

55. Robinson BH, Oei J, Sherwood WG, et al. The molecular basis for the two different clinical presentations of classical pyruvate carboxylase deficiency. *Am J Hum Genet* 1984; 36:283–94.

56. Wong LTK, Davidson AGF, Applegarth DA, et al. Biochemical and histologic pathology in an infant with CRM (negative) pyruvate carboxylase deficiency. *Pediatr Res* 1986; 20:274–9.

57. Robinson BH, Toone JR, Benedict RP, et al. Prenatal diagnosis of pyruvate carboxylase deficiency. *Prenat Diagn* 1985; 5:67–71.

58. Sperl W, Ruitenbeek W, Sengers RCA, et al. Combined deficiencies of the pyruvate dehydrogenase complex and enzymes of the respiratory chain in mitochondrial myopathies. *Eur J Pediatr* 1992; 151:1922–95.

59. Edery P, Gerard B, Chretien D, et al. Liver cytochrome C oxidase deficiency in a case of neonatal-onset hepatic failure. *Eur J Pediatr* 1994; 153:190–4.

60. Morin C, Mitchell G, Larochelle J, et al. Clinical, metabolic, and genetic aspects of cytochrome C oxidase deficiency in Sagueray-Lac-Saint-Jean. *Am J Hum Genet* 1993; 53:488–96.

61. Tritschler HJ, Bonilla E, Lombes A, et al. Differential diagnosis of fatal and benign cytochrome C oxidase-deficient myopathies of infancy: an immunohistochemical approach. *Neurology* 1991; 41:300–5.

62. Van Erven PMM, Cillessen JPM, Eekhoff EMW, et al. Leigh syndrome, a mitochondrial encephalo(myo)pathy. *Clin Neurol Neurosurg* 1987; 89:217–30.

63. Chow CW, Anderson RMcD, Kenny GCT. Neuropathology in cerebral lactic acidosis. *Acta Neuropathol (Berl)* 1987; 74:393–6.

64. Tatuch Y, Pagon RA, Vlcek B, et al. The 8993 mtDNA mutation: heteroplasmy and clinical presentation in three families. *Eur J Hum Genet* 1994; 2:35–43.

65. Taniike M, Fukushima H, Yanagihara I, et al. Mitochondrial tRNA^{Ile} mutation in fatal cardiomyopathy. *Biochem Biophys Res Commun* 1992; 186:47–53.

66. Tanaka M, Ino H, Ohno K, et al. Mitochondrial mutation in fatal infantile cardiomyopathy. [Letter]. *Lancet* 1990; 336:1452.

67. Marin-Garcia J, Ananthakrishnan R, Carta M, et al. Mitochondrial dysfunction in a case of fatal infantile cardiomyopathy. *J Inher Metab Dis* 1994; 17:756–7.

68. Kelly RI, Clark BJ, Morton DH, Sherwood WG. X-linked cardiomyopathy, neutropenia, and increased urinary levels of 3-methylglutaconic and 2-ethylhydroacrylic acids. *Am J Hum Genet* 1989; 45(suppl 1):A7.

68. Yoshikatsu E, Takahiro T, Koda N, et al. Prenatal diagnosis of metachromatic leucodystrophy. *Arch Neurol* 1982; 39:29–32.

69. Fearon ER, Mallonee RL, Phillips III JA, et al. Genetic analysis of carbamyl phosphate I deficiency. *Hum Genet* 1985; 70:207–10.

70. Holzgreve W, Golbus MS. Prenatal diagnosis of ornithine transcarbamylase deficiency using fetal liver biopsy. *Am J Hum Genet* 1984; 36:320–8.

71. Fearon E, Mallonee R, Phillips J III, et al. Genetic analysis of carbamoyl phosphate synthesis I deficiency. *Hum Genet* 1985; 70:207–10.

72. Zimmermann A, Bachmann C, Colombo JP. Ultrastructural pathology in congenital defects of the urea cycle: ornithine transcarbamylase and carbamyl phosphate synthetase deficiency. *Virchows Arch A* 1981; 393:321–31.

73. Hug G, Kline J, Schubert W. Liver ultrastructure: dissimilarity between Reye's syndrome and heritable defect of carbamyl phosphate synthetase or ornithine transcarbamylase. *Pediatr Res* 1978; 12:437.

74. Horwich AL, Fenton WA, Williams KR, et al. Structure and expression of a complementary DNA for the nuclear coded precursor of human mitochondrial ornithine transcarbamylase. *Science* 1984; 224:1068–74.

75. Old JM, Briand PL, Purvis-Smith S, et al. Prenatal exclusion of ornithine transcarbamylase deficiency by direct gene analysis. *Lancet* 1985; i:73–5.

76. Grompe M, Muzny DM, Caskey CT. Scanning detection of mutations in human ornithine transcarbamylase by chemical mismatch cleavage. *Proc Natl Acad Sci USA* 1989; 86:5888–92.

77. Harding BN, Leonard JV, Erdohazi M. Ornithine carbamoyl transferase deficiency: a neuropathological study. *Eur J Pediatr* 1984; 141:215–20.

78. Capistrano-Estrada S, Marsden DL, Nyhan WL, et al. Histopathological findings in a male with late-onset ornithine transcarbamylase deficiency. *Pediatr Pathol* 1994; 14:235–43.

79. Landrieu P, Francois B, Leon G, van Hoof F. Liver peroxisome damage during acute hepatic failure in partial ornithine transcarbamylase deficiency. *Pediatr Res* 1982; 16:977–81.

80. Hill HZ, Goodman SI. Detection of inborn errors of metabolism. III. Defects in urea cycle metabolism. *Clin Genet* 1974; 6:70–81.

81. Schimke RT. Enzymes of arginine metabolism in cell culture. *J Biol Chem* 1964; 239:136–45.

82. Leibowitz J, Thoene J, Spector E, Nyhan W. Citrullinemia. *Virchows Arch A* 1978; 377:249–58.

83. Leibowitz J, Wick H, Mihatsch MJ, et al. Liver morphology in a case of citrullinemia [a light & electron microscopic study] *Beitr Pathol* 1974; 151:200–7.

84. Guertin SR, Levinsohn MW, Danms BB. Small droplet steatosis and intracranial hypertension in arginino-succinate lyase deficiency. *J Pediatr* 1983; 102:736–40.

86. Haust MD, Gatfield PD, Gordon BA. Ultrastructure of hepatic mitochondria in a child with hyperornithinemia, hyperammonemia and homocitrullinuria. *Hum Pathol* 1981; 12:212–22.

87. Kvittingen EA, Jellum E, Stokke O. Assay of fumaryl acetoacetate-fumaryl hydrolase in human liver—deficient activity in a case of hereditary tyrosinemia. *Clin Chim Acta* 1981; 115:311–9.

88. Mitchell G, Larochelle J, Lamber M, et al. Neurologic crises in hereditary tyrosinemia. *N Engl J Med* 1990; 322:432–7.

89. Gagne R, Lescault A, Grenier A, Laberge C, Melaneon SB, Dallaire L. Prenatal diagnosis of hereditary tyrosinemia: measurement in succinylacetone in amniotic fluid. *Prenat Diagn* 1982; 2:185–8.

90. Tuchman M, Whitley CB, Mramnaraine ML. Baower LD. Fregien KD. Krivit W. Detection of urinary succinyl acetone by capillary gas chromatography. *J Chromatog Sci* 1984; 22:211–15.

91. Lindstedt S, Holme E, Lock EA, et al. Treatment of hereditary tyrosinemia type I by inhibition of 4-hydroxyphenylpyruvate dioxygenase. *Lancet* 1992; 340:813–17.

92. Stoner E, Starkman H, Wellner D, et al. Biochemical studies of the patient with hereditary hepatorenal tyrosinemia, evidence of glutachicne deficiency. *Pediatr Res* 1984; 18:1332–6.

93. Sima AA, Kennedy JC, Blakeslee D, Robertson DM. Experimental porphyric neuropathy: a preliminary report. *Can J Neurol Sci* 1981; 8:105–13.

94. Hardwick DF, Dimmick JE. Metabolic cirrhosis of infancy and early childhood. *Perspect Pediatr Pathol* 1976; 3:103–44.

95. Russo P, O'Regan S. Visceral pathology of hereditary tyrosinemia type I. *Am J Hum Genet* 1990; 47:317–24.

96. Zerbini C, Weinberg DS, Hollister KA, Perez-Atayde AR. DNA ploidy abnormalities of the liver of children with hereditary tyrosinemia type I. Correlation with histopathologic features. *Am J Pathol* 1992; 140:11111–19.

97. Weinberg AG, Mize CE, Worthen HG. The occurrence of hepatoma in the chronic form of hereditary tyrosinemia. *J Pediatr* 1976; 88:434–8.

98. Hostetter MK, Levy HL, Winter HS, Knight GJ, Haddow JE. Evidence for liver disease preceding amino acid abnormalities in hereditary tyrosinemia. *N Engl J Med* 1983; 308:1265–7.

99. Naylor EW, Guthrie R. Newborn screening for maple syrup urine disease (branch chain ketoaciduria). *Pediatrics* 1978; 61:262–6.

100. Menkes JH, Hurst PL, Craig JM. A new syndrome: progressive familial infantile cerebral dysfunction associated with an unusual urinary substance. *Pediatrics* 1954; 14:462–7.

101. Silberman J, Dancis J, Feigin I. Neuropathological observations in maple syrup urine disease. *Arch Neurol* 1961; 5:351–63.

102. Prensky AL, Carr S, Moser HW. Development of myelin in inherited disorders of amino acid metabolism. *Arch Neurol* 1968; 19:552–8.

103. Roels H. Pathology of aminoacidurias. *Monogr Hum Genet* 1972; 6:79–98.

104. Perry TL, Urquhart N, MacLean J, et al. Nonketotic hyperglycinemia. Glycine accumulation due to absence of glycine cleavage in brain. *N Engl J Med* 1975; 292:1269–73.

105. Tada K, Kure S. Nonketotic hyperglycinemia: molecular lesion, diagnosis and pathophysiology. *J Inher Metab Dis* 1993; 16:691–703.

106. Toone JR, Applegarth DA, Levy HL. Prenatal diagnosis of non-ketotic hyperglycinemia: experience in 50 at-risk pregnancies. *J Inher Metab Dis* 1994; 17:342–4.

107. Johnson JW, Ascher P. Glycine potentiates the NMDA response in cultured mouse brain neurons. *Nature* 1987; 325:529–31.

108. Agamanolis DP, Potter JL, Herrick MK, Sternberger NH. The neuropathology of glycine encephalopathy: a report of five cases with immunohistochemical and ultrastructural observations. *Neurology* 1982; 32:975–85.

109. Levy HL. Maternal phenylketonuria. In: Scarpelli DG Miyaki G, eds. *Transplacental Effects in Fetal Health. Proceedings of a symposium held in Bethesda, Maryland, 1987.* New York: Alan R. Liss, 1988: pp. 227.

110. Scriver CR. Hyper-beta-alaninemia associated with beta-aminoaciduria and gamma-aminobutyricaciduria, somnolence and seizures. *N Engl J Med* 1966; 274:636.

111. Perheentupa J, Rapola J, Visakorpi JK, Eskelin L-E. Lysinuric protein intolerance. *Am J Med* 1975; 59:229–40.

112. Odievre M, Gentil C, Gautier M, Aiagille D. Hereditary fructose intolerance in childhood. *Am J Dis Child* 1978; 132:605–8.

113. Bode CL, Schumacher H, Goebell H, Zelder O, Pelzel H. Fructose induced depletion of liver adenine nucleotides in man. *Horm Metab Res* 1971; 3:289–90.

114. Froescn ER. Disorders of fructose metabolism. *Clin Endocrinol Metab* 1976; 5:606.

115. Dubois R, Loeb H, Malaisse-Lagae F, Toppet M. Etude clinique et anatomo-pathologique de deux cas d'intolerance congenitale au fructose. *Pediatrie* 1965; 20:5–14.

116. Rallison ML, Meikle AW, Zigrang WD. Hypoglycemia and lactic acidosis associated with fructose-1, 6-diphosphatase deficiency. *J Pediatr* 1979; 94:933–6.

117. Landing BH, Ang SM, Vallarreal-Engelhardt G, Donnell GN. Galactosemia: clinical and pathologic features, tissue staining patterns with labelled galactose- and galactosamine-binding lectins and possible loci of nonenzymatic galactosylation. *Perspect Pediatr Pathol* 1993; 17:99–124.

118. Kobayashi RH, Kettelbut BV, Kobayashi AL. Galactose inhibition of neonatal neutrophil function. *Pediatr Infect Dis* 1983; 2:442–5.

119. Dennehy PH, O'Shea PA, Abuelo DN. A newborn infant with bilious vomiting and jitteriness. *J Pediatr* 1985; 106:161–6.

120. Smetana HF, Olen E. Hereditary galactose disease. *Am J Clin Pathol* 1962; 38:3–25.

121. Vannas A, Hogan MJ, Golbus MS, Wood I. Lens changes in a galactosemic fetus. *Am J Ophthalmol* 1975; 80:726–33.

122. Burchell A, Bell J, Busuttil A, Hume R. The hepatic microsomal glucose-6-phosphatase and sudden infant death syndrome. *Lancet* 1989; 2:292–4.

123. Lei K-J, Shelly LL, Pan CJ, Sidbury JB, Chou JY. Mutations in the glucose-6-phosphatase gene that cause glycogen storage disease type 1a. *Science* 1993; 262:580–3.

124. Buchino JJ, Brown BI, Volk DM. Glycogen storage disease type 1b. *Arch Pathol Lab Med* 1983; 107:283–5.

125. Hawkins RA, Kamath KR, Dorney SFA, Adams A. Biochemical diagnosis of type Ib glycogen storage disease. *Aust Paediatr J* 1984; 20:217–20.

126. Narisawa K, Otoma H, Igarashi Y, et al. Glycogen storage disease type Ib due to a defect of glucose-6-phosphate translocase. *J Inherited Metab Dis* 1982; 5:227–8.

127. McAdams AJ, Hug G, Bove KE. Glycogen storage disease types 1-X. *Hum Pathol* 1974; 5:463–87.

128. Ninomiya N, Matsuda I, Matsuoka T, Iwamasa T, Nonakawa I. Demonstration of acid alpha glucosidase in different types of Pompe disease by use of an immunochemical method. *J Neurol Sci* 1984; 66:129–39.

129. Taniguchi N, Kato E, Yoshida H, et al. Alphaglucosidase activity in human leucocytes: choice of lymphocytes for the diagnosis of Pompe disease and the carrier state. *Clin Chim Acta* 1978; 89:293–9.

130. Broadhead D, Butterworth J. Pompe disease: diagnosis in kidney and leucocytes using 4-methylumbelliferyl-2-D-glycopyranoside. *Clin Genet* 1978; 13:504.

131. Baldwin VJ, Kalousek DK, Dimmick JE, Applegarth DA, Hardwick DF. Diagnostic pathologic investigation of a malformed conceptus. *Perspect Pediatr Pathol* 1982; 7:65–108.

132. Hug G, Soukup S, Ryan M, Chuck G. Rapid prenatal diagnosis of glycogen storage disease type II by electron microscopy of uncultured amniotic fluid cells. *N Engl J Med* 1984; 310:1018–22.

133. Griffin JL. Infantile acid maltase deficiency. *Virthows Arch B* 1984; 44:51–61.

134. Sarnat HB, Roth SI, Carroll JE, Brown BI, Dungan WT. Lipid storage myopathy in infantile Pompe disease. *Arch Neurol* 1982; 39:180–83.

135. Peters TJ, Jenkins W, Dubowitz V. Subcellular fractionation studies on hepatic tissue from a patient with Pompe's disease (type II glycogen storage disease). *Clin Sci* 1980; 59:7–12.

136. Huijing F. Glycogen and enzymes of glycogen metabolism. In: Curtius H, Roth M, eds. *Clinical Biochemistry*. Berlin: W. de Gruyter, 1974, pp. 1208–34.

137. Van Noort G, Straks W, Van Diggelen OP, Hennekam RCM. A congenital variant of glycogenosis type IV. *Pediatr Pathol* 1993; 13:685–98.

138. Reid GB, Dixon JFP, Neustein HB, Donnell GN. Type four glycogenosis. *Lab Invest* 1968; 19:546–57.

139. McMaster KR, Powers JM, Hennigar GR, Wohltmann HJ, Farr GH. Nervous system involvement in type 4 glycogenosis. *Arch Pathol Lab Med* 1979; 103:105–11.

140. Eishi Y, Takemura T, Sone R, et al. Glycogen storage disease confined to the heart with deficient activity of cardiac phosphorylase kinase: a new type of glycogen storage disease. *Hum Pathol* 1985; 16:193–7.

141. Towfighi J, Yoss BS, Wasiewski WW, et al. Cerebral glycogenosis, alpha particle type: morphologic and biochemical observations in an infant. *Hum Pathol* 1989; 20:1210–5.

142. Elleder M, Smid F, Hyniova H, et al. Liver findings in Niemann-Pick disease type C. *Histochem J* 1984; 16:1147–70.

143. Buchino JJ. Case 1. Niemann-Pick type C. *Pediatr Pathol* 1993; 13:841–5.

144. Kelly DA, Portmann B, Mowat AP, Sherlock S, Lake BD. Niemann-Pick disease type C: diagnosis and outcome in children with particular reference to liver disease. *J Pediatr* 1993; 123:242–7.

144a. Carstea ED, Morris JA, Coleman KG, et al. Niemann-Pick C1 disease gene—homology to mediators of cholesterol homeostasis. *Science* 1997; 277:228–31.

145. Dinari G, Rosenbach Y, Grunebaum M, Zahavi I, Alpert G, Nitzan M. Gastrointestinal manifestations of Niemann-Pick disease. *Enzyme* 1980; 25:407–12.

146. Westwood M. Endocardial fibroelastosis and Niemann-Pick disease. *Br Heart J* 1977; 39:1394–6.

147. Gumbinas M, Larsen M, Liu HM. Peripheral neuropathy and classic Niemann-Pick disease: ultra-structure of nerves and skeletal muscle. *Neurology* 1975; 25:107–13.

148. Schneider EL, Ellis WG, Brady RO, McCulloch JR, Epstein CJ. Prenatal Niemann-Pick disease: biochemical and histological examination of a 19 gestational week fetus. *Pediatr Res* 1972; 6:720–9.

149. Vanier MT, Rodriguez-Lafrasse C, Rousson R, et al. Prenatal diagnosis of Niemann-Pick type C disease: current strategy from an experience of 37 pregnancies at risk. *Am J Hum Genet* 1992; 51:111–22.

150. Poulos A, Hudson N, Ranieri E. Sphingomyelinase in cultured skin fibroblasts from normal and Niemann-Pick type C patients. *Clin Genet* 1983; 24:225–33.

151. Grabowski GA, Goldblatt J, Dinur T. et al. Genetic heterogeneity in Gaucher disease: physicokinetic and immunologic studies of the residual enzyme in cultured fibroblasts from non-neuronopathic and neuronopathic patients. *Am J Med Genet* 1985; 21:529–49.

152. Ginns EI, Tegelaers FPW, Barneveld R, et al. Determination of Gaucher disease phenotypes with monoclonal antibody. *Clin Chim Acta* 1983; 131:283–7.

153. Sidransky E, Tsuji S, Martin BM, Stubblefield B, Ginns EI. DNA mutation analysis of Gaucher patients. *Am J Med Genet* 1992; 42:331–6.

154. Suzuki K. Glucosyl ceramide and related compounds in normal tissues and in Gaucher's disease. In: Desnick RJ, Gatt S, Grabowski GA, eds. *Gaucher's Disease: A Century of Delineation and Research*. New York: Alan R. Liss, 1982, pp. 219–30.

155. Kamoshita S, Odawara M, Yoshida M. Fetal pathology and ultrastructure of neuropathic Gaucher's disease. *Adv Exp Med Biol* 1975; 68:63–75.

156. Clarke JGR, Ozere RL, Krause VW. Early infantile variant of Krabbe globoid leucodystrophy with lung involvement. *Arch Dis Child* 1981; 56:640–42.

157. Suzuki K. Enzymic diagnosis of sphingolipidoses. *Methods Enzymol* 1978; 50:468–71.

158. Norman MG. Leucodystrophy: diffuse cerebral sclerosis or Schilder's disease revisited. *Perspect Pediatr Pathol* 1975; 2:61–100.

159. Suzuki K. Biochemical pathogenesis of genetic leucodystrophies comprised of metachromatic dystrophy and globoid cell leucodystrophy (Krabbe's disease). *Neuropediatrics* 1984; 15:32–6.

160. Martin JJ, Leroy JG, Ceuterick C, Libert J, Dodinval P, Martin L. Fetal Krabbe leucodystrophy. *Acta Neuropathol* 1981; 53:87–91.

161. Bubis JJ, Adlesberg L. Congenital metachromatic leucodystrophy. *Acta Neuropathol* 1966; 6:298–302.

162. Fujibayashi S, Inui K, Wenger DA. Activator protein-deficient metachromatic leucodystrophy: diagnosis in leucocytes using immunologic methods. *J Pediatr* 1984; 104:739–42.

163. Harben AM, Krawiecki N, Marcus R, et al. A K_m mutant of arylsulfatase A. *Clin Chim Acta* 1982; 125:351–4.

164. Stevens RL, Fluharty AL, Kihars H, et al. Cerebroside sulfate activator deficiency induced metachromatic leucodystrophy. *Am J Hum Genet* 1981; 33:900–6.

165. Gieselmann V, Polten A, Kreysing J, von Figura K. Molecular genetics of metachromatic leukodystrophy. *J Inher Metab Dis* 1994; 17:500–9.

166. Kihara H, Ho C-K, Fluharty AL, et al. Prenatal diagnosis of metachromatic leucodystrophy in a family with pseudo arylsulfatase A deficiency by the cerebroside sulfate loading test. *Pediatr Res* 1980; 14:224–7.

167. Kolodny EH, Moser HW. Sulfatide lipidosis: metachromatic leucodystrophy. In: Stanbury JB, Wyngaarden JB, Fredrickson DS, eds. *The Metabolic Basis of Inherited Disease*. 5th ed. New York: McGraw-Hill, 1983, pp. 881–905.

168. Yoshikatsu E, Takahiro T, Koda N, et al. Prenatal diagnosis of metachromatic leucodystrophy. *Arch Neurol* 1982; 39:29–32.

169. Farber S, Cohen J, Uzman LL. Lipogranulomatosis. *J Mt Sinai Hosp* 1957; 24:816–37.

170. Tanaka T, Takahashi K, Hakozaki H, Kimoto H, Suziki Y. Farber's disease (disseminated granulomatosis). *Acta Pathol Jpn* 1979; 29:135–55.

171. Rutsaert J, Tondeur M, Vamos-Hurwitz E, Dustin P. The cellular lesions of Farber's disease and their experimental reproduction in tissue culture. *Lab Invest* 1977; 36:474–80.

172. Rauch HJ, Aubock L. "Banana Bodies" and disseminated lipogranulomatosis (Farber's disease). *Am J Dermatopathol* 1983; 5:263–6.

173. Miller R, Bialer MG, Rogers JF, Johnsson HT, Allen RV, Hennigar GR. Wolman's disease. *Arch Pathol Lab Med* 1982; 106:41–5.

174. Byrd JC, Powers JM. Wolman's disease: ultrastructural evidence of lipid accumulation in central nervous system. *Acta Neuropathol* 1979; 45:37.

175. Applegarth DA, Toone JR. In: Meiter S, ed. *Pediatric Clinical Chemistry*. 2nd ed. Washington: American Association of Clinical Chemistry, 1981, pp. 206–7, 320, 327–8, 482–4.

176. Lee JES, Falk RE, Ng WG, Donnell GN. Beta glucuronidase deficiency. *Am J Dis Child* 1985; 139:57–9.

177. Crawfurd M, Dean MF, Hunt DM, et al. Early prenatal diagnosis of Hurler syndrome with termination of pregnancy and confirmatory findings on the fetus. *J Med Genet* 1973; 10:144–53.

178. Lowden JA, Rudd N, Cutz E, Doran TA. Antenatal diagnosis of sphingolipid and mucopolysaccharide storage diseases. *Can Med Assoc J* 1975; 113:507–11.

179. Meier C, Wiesmann U, Herschkowitz N, Bischoff A. Morphological observations in the nervous system of prenatal mucopolysaccharidosis II. *Acta Neuropathol* 1979; 48:139–43.

180. Landing BH, Silverman FN, Craig JM, et al. Familial neurovisceral lipidosis. *Am J Dis Child* 1964; 108:503–22.

181. Severi F, Magrini U, Tettamanti G, Bianchi E, Lanzi G. Infantile GM1 gangliosidosis. Histochemical, ultrastructural and biochemical studies. *Helv Paediatr Acta* 1971; 26:192–209.

182. Cutz E, Lowden A, Conen PE. Ultrastructural demonstration of neuronal storage in fetal Tay-Sachs disease. *J Neurol Sci* 1974; 21:197–202.

183. Norby S, Jensen OA, Schwartz M. Retinal and cerebellar changes in early fetal Sandhoff's disease (GM2 gangliosidosis type II). *Metabol Pediatr Ophthalmol* 1980; 4:115–19.

184. Yamano T, Shimada M, Okada S, et al. Ultrastructural study on nervous system of fetus with GM1 gangliosidosis type 1. *Acta Neuropathol* 1983; 61:15–20.

185. Adachi M, Schneck L, Volk BW. Ultrastructural study of eight cases of fetal Tay-Sachs disease. *Lab Invest* 1974; 30:102–12.

186. Gilbert-Barness EF, Barness LA. The mucolipidoses. *Perspect Pediatr Pathol* 1993; 17:148–84.

187. Lowden JA, O'Brien JS. Sialidoses—a review of human neuraminidase deficiency. *Am J Hum Genet* 1979; 31:1–18.

188. Mueller OT, Henry W, Haley LL, et al. Sialidosis and galactosialidosis: chromosomal assignment of two genes associated with neuraminidase deficiency disorder. *Proc Natl Acad Sci USA* 1986; 83:1817–21.

189. Okada S, Sugino H, Kato T, et al. A severe infantile sialidosis (beta galactosidase-neuraminidase deficiency) mimicking GM1 gangliosidosis type I. *Eur J Pediatr* 1983; 140:295–8.

190. Yamano T, Shimada M, Sugino H, et al. Ultrastructural study on a severe infantile sialidosis (beta galactosidase-neuraminidase deficiency). *Neuropaediatrie* 1985; 16:109–12.

191. Tondeur M, Libert J, Vamos E, Van Hoof F, Thomas GH, Strecker G. Infantile form of sialic acid storage disorder: clinical ultrastructural and biochemical studies in two siblings. *Eur J Pediatr* 1982; 139:142–7.

192. Gilbert EF, Dawson G, Zu Rhein GM, Opitz JM, Spranger JW. I-cell disease, mucolipidosis II. Pathological, histochemical, ultrastructural and biochemical observations in four cases. *Z Kinderheilkd* 1973; 114:259–92.

193. Martin JJ, Leroy JG, van Eygen M, Ceuterick C. I-cell disease. *Acta Neuropathol* 1984; 64:34–242.

194. Aula P, Rapola J, Autio S, Raivio K, Karjalainen O. Prenatal diagnosis and fetal pathology of I-cell disease (mucolipidosis II). *J Pediatr* 1975; 87:221–6.

195. Crandall BF, Philipart M, Brown WJ, Bluestone DA. Review article: mucolipidosis IV. *Am J Med Genet* 1982; 12:301–8.

196. Kohn G, Livni N, Ornoy A, et al. Prenatal diagnosis of mucolipidosis IV by electromicroscopy. *J Pediatr* 1977; 90:62–6.

197. Van den Bosch H, Schutzens RBH, Wanders RJA, Tager JM. Biochemistry of peroxisomes. *Annu Rev Biochem* 1992; 61:157–97.

198. Dimmick JE, Applegarth DA. Pathology of peroxisomal disorders. *Perspect Pediatr Pathol* 1993; 17:45–98.

199. Fournier B, Smeitink JAM, Dorland L, et al. Peroxisomal disorders: a review. *J Inherit Metab Dis* 1994; 17:470–86.

200. Powers JM, Moser HW, Moser AB, et al. Fetal cerebrohepatorenal (Zellweger) syndrome: dysmorphic radiologic biochemical and pathologic findings in four affected fetuses. *Hum Pathol* 1985; 116:610–20.

201. Roels F, Espeel M, Poggi F, et al. Human liver pathology in peroxisomal diseases: a review including novel data. *Biochemie* 1993; 75:281–92.

202. Roels F, Espeel M, DeCraemer D. Liver pathology and immunocytochemistry in congenital peroxisomal diseases: a review. *J Inher Metab Dis* 1991; 14:873–5.

203. Hughes JL, Poulos A, Robertson E, et al. Pathology of hepatic peroxisomes and mitochondria in patients with peroxisomal disorders. *Virch Arch Path Anat Histopathol* 1990; 416:255–64.

204. Yajima S, Suzuki Y, Shimozawa N, et al. Complementation study of peroxisome-deficient disorders by immunofluorescence staining and characterization of fused cells. *Hum Genet* 1992; 88:491–9.

205. Shimozawa N, Tsukamoto T, Suzuki Y, et al. A human gene responsible for Zellweger syndrome that affects peroxisome assembly. *Science* 1991; 255:1132–4.

206. Gartner J, Moser H, Valle D. Mutations in the 70 K peroxisomal membrane protein gene in Zellweger syndrome. *Nature (Genetics)* 1992; 1:16–23.

207. Powers JM, Moser HW, Moser AB, Schaumburg HH. Fetal adrenoleukodystrophy. *Hum Pathol* 1982; 13:1013–9.

208. Moser HW, Moser AB. Measurement of saturated very long chain fatty acids in plasma. In: Hommes FA, ed. *Techniques in Diagnostic Human Biochemical Genetics: A Laboratory Manual*. New York: Wiley-Liss, 1991: Chapters 12, 13.

209. Vallance H, Applegarth D. An improved method for the quantification of very-long-chain fatty acids in plasma by GC-MS. *Clin Biochem* 1994; 27:183–6.

210. Wanders RJA, Schutgens RBH, Barth PG, Tager JM, van den Bosch II. Postnatal diagnosis of peroxisomal disorders: a biochemical approach. *Biochimie* 1993; 75:269–79.

211. Wanders RJA, Wiemer EAC, Brul S, et al. Prenatal diagnosis of Zellweger syndrome by direct visualization of peroxisomes in chorionic villus fibroblasts by immunofluoresence microscopy. J Inherited Metab Dis 1989; 12(suppl 2):301–304.

212. Roberts PF. P:ZZ Alpha-1-antitrypsin deficiency in a 20 week old fetus. *Hum Pathol* 1985; 16:188–90.

213. Kidd VJ, Wallace RB, Itakura K, Woo SLC. α1-Antitrypsin deficiency detection by direct analysis of the mutation in the gene. *Nature* 1983; 304:230.

214. Muller F, Aubry MC, Gasser B, et al. Prenatal diagnosis of cystic fibrosis. *Prenat Disgn* 1985; 5:109–17.

215. Davidson AGF, Wong LTK, Kirby LT, Applegarth DA. Immunoreactive trypsin in cystic fibrosis. *Pediatr Gastroenterol Nutr* 1984; 3:S79–88.

216. The cystic fibrosis genotype-phenotype consortium. Correlation between genotype and phenotype in patients with cystic fibrosis. *N Engl J Med* 1993; 329:1308–13.

217. Knisely AS, Magid MS, Dische RM, Cutz E. Neonatal hemochromatosis. In: Gilbert EF, Optiz JM, eds. *Genetic Aspects of Developmental Pathology*. Birth Defects Original Article Series 23. New York: Alan R. Liss, 1987, pp. 75–102.

218. Silver MM, Valberg L, Cutz E, Lines L, Phillips MJ. Hepatic morphology and iron quantitation in perinatal hemochromatosis. *Am J Pathol* 1993; 143:1312–25.

219. Knisely AS. Neonatal hemochromatosis. *Adv Pediatr* 1992; 39:383–403.

220. Smith DW, Lemli L, Opitz JM. A newly recognized syndrome of multiple congenital anomalies. *J Pediatr* 1964; 64:210–7.

221. Tint GS, Irons M, Elias ER, et al. Defective cholesterol biosynthesis associated with the Smith-Lemli-Opitz syndrome. *N Engl J Med* 1994; 330:107–13.

222. Jaeken J, Vancerschueren-Lodeweyck M, Casaer P, et al. Familial psychomotor retardation with markedly fluctuating serum prolactin, FS and GH levels, partial TBG deficiency, increased serum arylsulphatase A and increased CSF protein: a new syndrome. *Pediatr Res* 1980; 14:170–9.

223. Jaeken J, van Eijck HG, van der Heul C, et al. Sialic acid-deficient serum and cerebrospinal fluid transferrin in a newly recognized genetic syndrome. *Clin Chim Acta* 1984; 144:245–7.

224. Ramaekers VT, Stibler H, Kint J, Jaeken J. A new variant of the carbohydrate deficient glycoproteins syndrome. *J Inher Metab Dis* 1991; 14:385–8.

225. Condradi N, De Vos R, Jaeken J, et al. Liver pathology in the carbohydrate-deficient syndrome. *Acta Paediatr Scan (Supp)* 1991; 375:50–4.

226. Clayton PT, Winchester BG, Keir G. Hypertrophic obstructive cardiomyopathy in a neonate with the carbohydrate-deficient syndrome. *J Inher Metab Dis* 1992; 15:857–61.

227. Chang Y, Twiss J, Horoupian D, Caldwell S, Johnston K. Inherited syndrome of infantile olivopontocerebellar atrophy, micronodular cirrhosis and renal tubular microcysts: review of the literature and a report of an additional case. *Acta Neuropathol* 1993; 86:399–404.

228. Stibler H, Jaeken J. Carbohydrate deficient serum transferrin in a new systemic hereditary syndrome. *Arch Dis Child* 1990; 65:107–11.

229. Jaeken J, Carchon H. The carbohydrate-deficient syndromes: an overview. *J Inher Metab Dis* 1993; 16:813–20.

230. Matsuura T, Hoshide R, Fukushima M, et al. Prenatal monitoring of ornithine transcarbamoylase deficiency in two families by DNA analysis. *J Inher Metab Dis* 1993; 16:31–8.

231. MacLeod PM, Dolman CL, Nickel RE, Chang E, Zonana J, Silvey K. Prenatal diagnosis of neuronal ceroid-lipofuscinosis. *N Engl J Med* 1984; 310:595.

232. MacLeod PM, Nag S, Berry C. Ultrastructural studies as a method of prenatal diagnosis of neuronal ceroid-lipofuscinosis. *Am J Med Genet* 1988; 30(suppl 5):93–7.

233. Kohn G, Livni N, Ornoy A, et al. Prenatal diagnosis of mucolipidosis IV by electron microscopy. *J Pediatr* 1977; 90:62–6.

234. Anton-Lamprecht I. Genetically induced abnormalities of epidermal differentiation and ultrastructure in ichthyoses and epidermolyses: pathogenesis, heterogeneity, fetal manifestation and prenatal diagnosis. *J Invest Dermatol*, 1983; 81:149–56.

235. Wright VJ, Dimmick JE, Kalousek DK. The preliminary investigation (protocol) of the malformed fetus or neonate—or what to do until the pathologist comes. *Birth Defects Orig Artic Ser* 1979; 15:93–104.

236. Kalousek DK, Baldwin VJ, Dimmick JE, et al. Embryofetal-perinatal autopsy and placental examination In: Dimmick JE, Kalousek DK, eds. *Developmental Pathology of the Embryo and Fetus*. Philadelphia: Lippincott, 1992, pp. 799–824.

237. Hall WK, Cravey CE, Chen PT, et al. An evaluation of galactosuria. *J Pediatr* 1970; 77:625–30.

Pathology of Organ Systems

Respiratory Tract Disorders in the Fetus and Neonate

FREDERIC B. ASKIN

This chapter is devoted to a discussion of upper and lower respiratory tract disorders encountered in the perinatal patient. Congenital anomalies are studied in detail here, as are disorders of the transition between intra- and extra-uterine life. Iatrogenic problems and specific infections that affect the lungs of the fetus and neonate are considered as well. Rare congenital neoplasms may also be encountered in the respiratory tract [1–3].

LARYNX AND TRACHEA

The larynx arises from the respiratory diverticulum, a groove that forms at about the 20th day of development in the ventromedial aspect of the foregut [1, 4–8]. This diverticulum also gives rise to the trachea, bronchi, and, ultimately, the lungs. Indentations along the lateral aspect of the groove deepen and eventually separate the larynx and trachea from the esophagus. The septation is complete by the 5th gestational week. A definitive larynx is formed by approximately 40 days of intrauterine life and between the 8th and 10th weeks the epiglottis and then the true vocal cords develop, along with the appearance of the laryngeal ventricle [4, 5]. By the end of the 10th and 11th weeks of intrauterine life, the major laryngeal structures have appeared and the cartilagenous skeleton is beginning to develop.

At the end of the second trimester of pregnancy, the larynx has assumed the cone-shaped form and narrow sub-glottic lumen characteristic of the fetus [4, 5]. The neonate's larynx is, in comparison with the older child, located high in the neck (usually at the level of the 2nd or 3rd cervical vertebra), has more of a funnel shape, and has a distinct angle at the junction of the supra- and subglottic portions [4, 5].

The majority of pathological lesions in the neonate's larynx consist of congenital anomalies or iatrogenic injuries related to therapy of the respiratory distress syndrome (hyaline membrane disease) [1, 4–6, 9].

Laryngeal Atresia

Laryngeal atresia occurs in several patterns, involving the glottis, infraglottic area, or both the supra- and infraglottic areas [4, 5, 7, 10]. Three types were described in a study of nine cases [11]. In type 1, the vestibule was represented by a shallow cleft flanked by the apices of the arytenoid cartilages. Below this, the remainder of the vestibule and the laryngeal sinuses were replaced by a mass of muscle, the partly fused arytenoid cartilages, and the malformed cricoid cartilage. A persistent pharyngotracheal duct lined by respiratory epithelium and less than 1 mm in diameter passed behind the fused arytenoids and through the cricoid cartilage to open into the trachea. Type 2 differed from type 1 in having normally formed vestibule and laryngeal sinuses and separate arytenoid cartilages. The malformed cricoid cartilage was dome-shaped and the pharyngotracheal duct lay in a groove on the back of it. In type 3, seen in one case only, there was a mass of fibrous connective tissue and muscle with fused arytenoid cartilages occluding the glottis. The cricoid cartilage was normally formed. As in the other types, there was a persistent pharyngotracheal duct.

The condition appears to represent the arrest of laryngeal development, as each type of atresia resembles a stage of normal laryngeal formation [11]. Most cases present unexpectedly at birth, and die following unsuccessful attempts at intubation. Patients with laryngeal atresia have a high incidence of other congenital anomalies, including tracheal agenesis, tracheo-esophageal fistula, and components of the VATER syndrome [7, 12, 13].

Cases of laryngeal atresia without associated tracheal agenesis or tracheobronchial fistula have voluminous fluid-filled lungs [14]. Occasionally, the lungs are massive in size [15] but usually they are two to three times the expected weight and can be shown to have normal cell population but increased numbers of thin-walled alveoli of advanced maturation for the gestation [16]. The changes resemble those of experimental tracheal ligation in fetal rabbits or sheep.

Laryngeal Stenosis

Laryngeal stenosis, related to fibrous webs, is the most common congenital laryngeal anomaly [4, 12, 13, 17–21]. Most of the webs (75%) occur at the level of the glottis but similar supra- and infraglottic lesions occur [4, 13]. A small number of families with an autosomal dominant pattern of inheritance of webs has been reported. In contrast to atresia, there is no clearly demonstrated association of laryngeal stenosis with other organ system anomalies except in Fraser syndrome [7]. Subglottic stenosis associated with cartilage anomalies has also been described. Absence of the epiglottis is associated with recurrent aspiration and has been reported in association with a median mandibular cleft [22]. Bifid epiglottis may produce both aspiration and congenital stridor, due to abnormal mobility [23].

Laryngeal Clefts

Laryngeal clefts may be anterior and related to failure of fusion of the thyroid cartilage, but posterior laryngeal clefts are much more common [10, 24–26]. The defect represents faulty formation of the tracheo-esophageal septum and occurs in varying degrees of severity ranging from a small posterior laryngeal fissure (the most common form) to a complete cleft involving the trachea and extending to the level of the carina (esophagotrachea) (Fig. 19.1). Clinical problems include respiratory distress as well as recurrent aspiration. Polyhydramnios, the etiology unknown, often can be documented during the gestation of infants with these clefts. Posterior laryngeal cleft has been reported in families [25] and is also associated with a variety of other congenital anomalies and with anomaly syndromes such as VATER and the "G" syndrome.

Laryngeal, Epiglottic, and Pharyngeal Cysts

Laryngeal, epiglottic, and pharyngeal cysts may be present at birth and cause respiratory distress by virtue of obstruction of the upper airway [27]. Some of these cysts represent mucus retention, while others appear to be foregut duplication with a muscular wall [28]. Laryngoceles are very rare in infants [1, 7, 8]. These lesions are air-filled dilations of

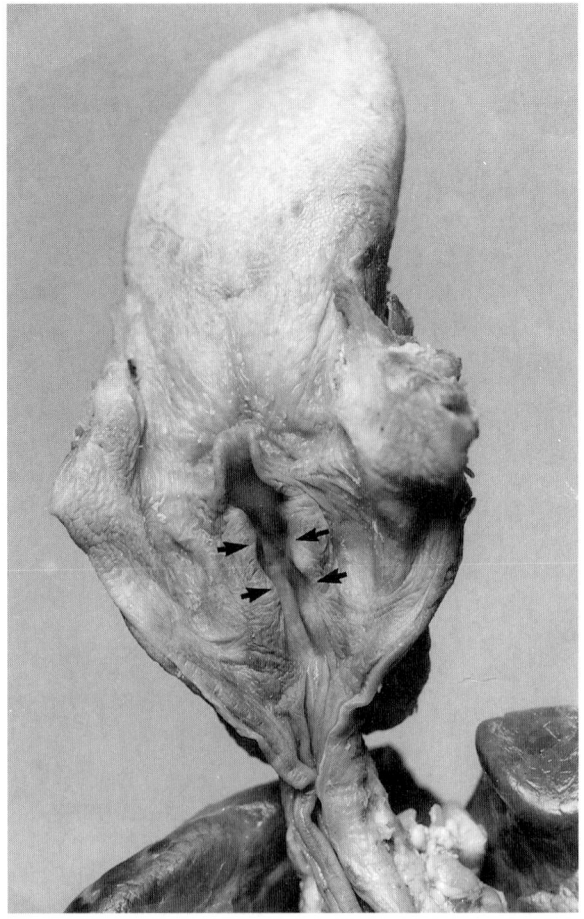

FIGURE 19.1.   *Large posterior laryngeal cleft (arrows). The esophagus is opened along the posterior aspect. (Courtesy of Kissane [6].)*

the ventricular saccule of the larynx and may present as extrinsic or intraluminal masses, or as both.

Laryngomalacia

Laryngomalacia is a clinical entity with very poorly described pathological findings [4, 8]. The basic problem is assumed to be relative flaccidity or instability of laryngeal and epiglottic cartilages, although specific morphological defects are not delineated [29]. The clinical problem is that of stridor and most infants will outgrow the problem as the larynx enlarges. A number of congenital anomaly syndromes are associated with functional laryngomalacia or with structural malformations of the larynx.

Congenital Paralysis of Vocal Cord

Congenital paralysis of the vocal cord may be unilateral or, more commonly, bilateral [4, 5, 30]. Unilateral lesions occur most frequently on the left and are usually associated with local (near the larynx) pressure on the vagus or recurrent laryngeal nerve. Delivery trauma or cardiovascular malformations may be associated. Isolated, idiopathic right vocal cord paralysis may also occur. Bilateral paralysis is most frequently associated with a central nervous system lesion, such as malformation or increased intracranial pressure and hydrocephalus.

Acquired Lesions of the Larynx

Acquired lesions of the larynx are rare in neonates; perhaps the most common is subglottic stenosis related to trauma from endotracheal tubes used in association with mechanical ventilation of severely ill neonates [31–33]. Mucosal necrosis and erosion are followed by granulation tissue and fibrosis in the subglottic larynx. There is some evidence that use of polyvinyl chloride plastics in the tracheal tubes has decreased the incidence of this disorder. Pharyngeal trauma may produce lesions that simulate intrinsic upper airway obstruction [34].

Infections of various types can involve the larynx; isolated laryngeal candidiasis has been reported in a neonate [35]. Tumors are discussed below.

Tracheal Atresia

Tracheal atresia has been reported in several different forms and may be an isolated finding [36–38]. In most instances, however, there is an associated tracheo-esophageal fistula [39], and associated cardiovascular, skeletal, pulmonary, and genitourinary tract anomalies are not uncommon [40]. Polyhydramnios may occur. In one form of tracheal atresia, the proximal trachea is affected but the distal trachea is present and usually connected to the esophagus. In two other types of atresia, the entire upper trachea is absent and the bronchi communicate with the esophagus either separately or through a common fistula. Unilateral bronchial communication with the esophagus may be a related entity but has been reported as "total sequestration of the lung."

Tracheal Stenosis

Tracheal stenosis may be diffuse, funnel-like, or segmental [41–45]. Cardiovascular and pulmonary anomalies may be associated with the lesion [41, 42]. Complete tracheal cartilaginous rings (Fig. 19.2) are usually found, although a muscular segmental stenosis, in which the affected portion of the trachea resembles the esophagus, has been reported as well [43]. Segmental stenosis appears to have an equal distribution in the upper and central trachea and in the area above the carina. In the lower trachea, anomalous tracheal bronchi are often associated with tracheal stenosis [46]. Funnel or "carrot"-like stenosis of the trachea is common in the left pulmonary artery sling syndrome. Clinically, infants with tracheal stenosis have stridor, dyspnea, wheezing, and feeding difficulties.

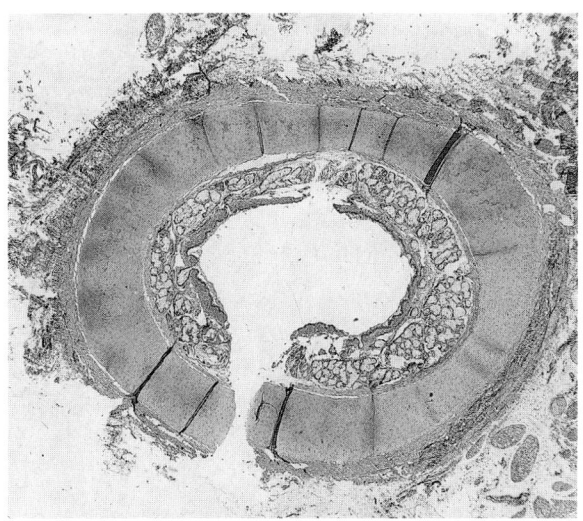

FIGURE 19.2. *Tracheal stenosis. This segmental lesion was caused by complete cartilaginous rings. (×40.) (Courtesy of Kissane [6].)*

A wide variety of tracheobronchial anomalies, especially cartilage patterns [7, 8], occur in the skeletal dysplasia syndromes and have been studied extensively by Landing and Wells [8]. Abnormal bronchial branching patterns also occur.

Tracheomalacia

Tracheomalacia, like bronchomalacia, may be diffuse or segmental, and congenital or acquired [29, 47]. The congenital diffuse lesion is a functional entity and the pathological features are poorly described, as in laryngomalacia. Segmental lesions may be acquired from external pressure (masses or anomalous vessels) but localized congenital absence of tracheal cartilage has also been described. Stridor, wheezing, and noisy respiration are clinical features of tracheomalacia and, as with the laryngeal lesion, the infant usually "outgrows" the problem.

Fibrous Tracheal Webs

Fibrous tracheal webs similar to those seen in the larynx have been reported [18, 48] and intraluminal tracheal cysts, possibly mucus retention cysts, may occur rarely [49].

Tracheal and Laryngeal Neoplasms

Tracheal and laryngeal neoplasms [50–53] are rare in infants, with the exception of subglottic capillary hemangioma. This potentially fatal lesion may extend into the larynx or down into the trachea as well [50]. Infantile fibromatosis [51] has been reported in the infant's larynx, as have so-called hamartomas [52]. These latter lesions merge into the spectrum of

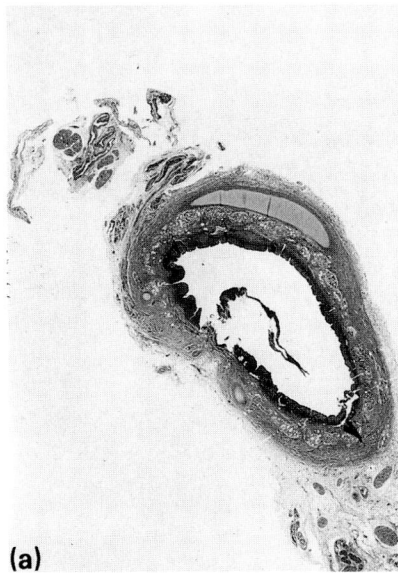

(a)

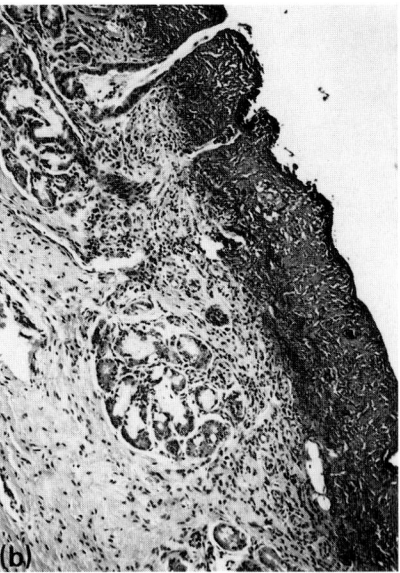

(b)

FIGURE 19.3. *Necrotizing tracheobronchitis in a neonate. This lesion was a complication of high-frequency jet ventilation in a patient with hyaline membrane disease. (a) Low-power view shows circumferential involvement of the trachea. (b) High-power view shows extensive necrosis of the tracheal mucosa with pseudomembrane formation. (Case courtesy of Dr. Jan Ophoven, St. Paul, MN [193].)*

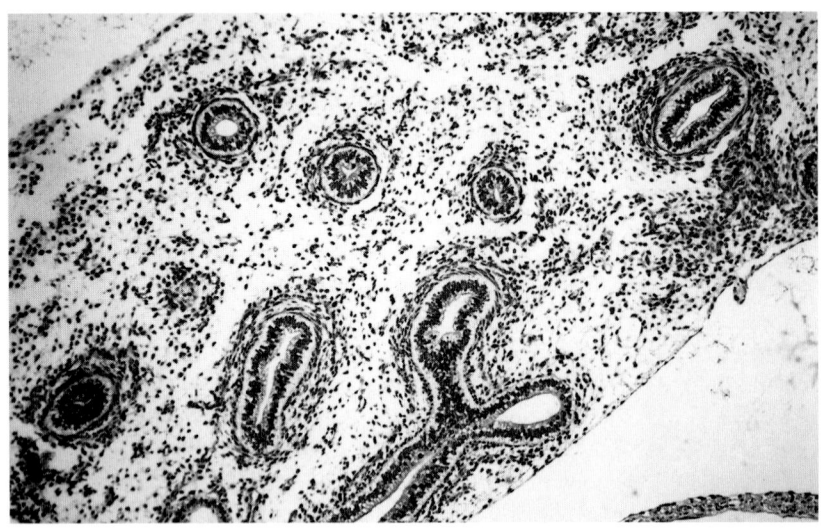

FIGURE 19.4. *Glandular phase of lung development. Branching channels lined by glycogen-rich epithelium are set in loose mesenchyme. (×200.)*

dermoid tumors or teratomas seen elsewhere in the head and neck region and on the tonsil. Lymphangiomas in the neck may involve the larynx as part of their local spread [53].

Tracheitis and tracheobronchitis in neonates is often iatrogenic and related to treatment of neonatal respiratory distress (Fig. 19.3) (see the discussion of bronchopulmonary dysplasia later in this chapter).

LUNG DEVELOPMENT

During the 4th week of gestation, the laryngotracheal groove forms in the esophageal portion of the endodermal tube. Development of the lung begins with evagination of two buds from the ventral surface of the groove and their subsequent invasion by dichotomous branching into the

thoracic mesenchyme [54–64]. The entire epithelial lining of the lung from bronchi to alveoli is of endodermal origin. The connective tissue and vessels are derived from the mesenchyme, which also appears to have a direct effect on the branching pattern of the lung [54]. By the end of the 6th week, the lobar and segmental branches of the bronchial tree are established and the conducting airway system is essentially complete by the end of the 16th week of intrauterine life [55, 56]. Pre-acinar pulmonary artery development parallels airway formation: during the early stages of lung development, pulmonary arteries develop from the 6th pair of aortic arches and invade the thoracic mesenchyme along with the bronchial buds [57]. These vessels are originally connected to systemic veins draining the trachea and foregut but subsequently develop connections to the pulmonary

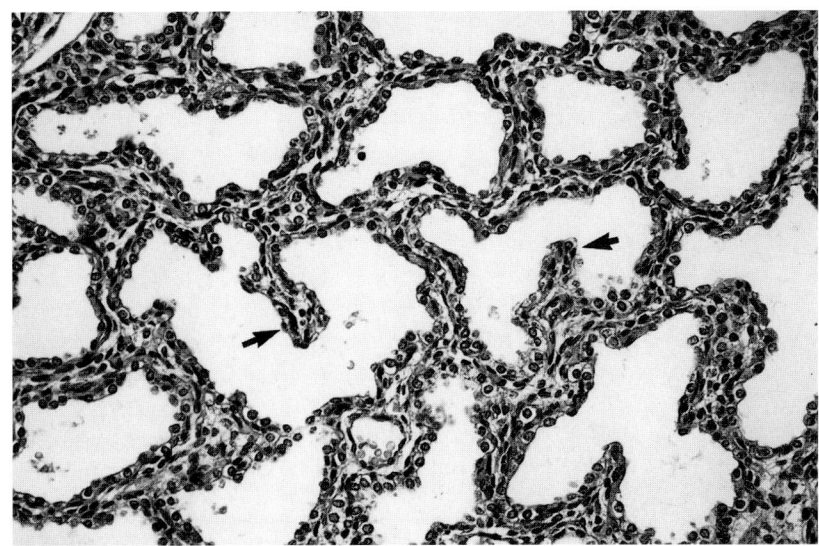

FIGURE 19.5.   *Saccular phase of lung development (approximately 28 weeks of gestation). Secondary crests (arrows) are seen. There is a separate capillary layer on each side of the septa. As primitive alveoli form, a single capillary will weave along both sides of the septum. (×400.)*

veins, which have grown out of the atrial portion of the heart.

The early stages of lung formation are termed the embryonic (up to 6 weeks of gestation) and the glandular phases (6–16 weeks) (Fig. 19.4) [55]. Subsequently, in the canalicular phase (16–28 weeks), acinar development begins with the formation of primitive airspaces and the apposition of capillaries to the wall of these structures with the first formation of blood–air barriers. Formation of acini appears to proceed from proximal to distal in the lung. From 28 to 36 weeks' gestation there is continued formation of potential airspaces as the primitive acinar saccules are subdivided by blunt mesenchymal protrusions called "secondary crests" [58, 59]. These crests have a capillary lining on both sides (Fig. 19.5). The existence of alveoli in the human lung prior to birth has been a subject of controversy, but recent studies by Langston et al suggest that alveoli may appear as early as of 32 weeks' gestation [58, 59]. They can be distinguished from spaces formed by secondary crests because alveoli have a single intertwining capillary in their septal wall and are polygonal rather than round. Alveoli continue to develop in the neonatal period and, in fact, increase by as much as tenfold in number between birth and late childhood [55, 58–61, 63].

Early branching of the pulmonary artery accompanies airway development, but "super-numerary" branches of the pulmonary artery exist and they supply distal airspaces directly without accompanying airways. These supernumerary vessels develop along with airspaces and continue to increase in number after birth, along with alveoli [55].

Changes in the cell lining of the lung also occur as pulmonary development proceeds [65, 66]. During the embryonic and early glandular stages, the lung is lined by a relatively homogeneous population of columnar cells. Differentiation into ciliated, goblet, and basal cells begins in the proximal airways and proceeds peripherally, along with development of smooth muscle and cartilage in the bronchi. Clusters of mucosal neuroendocrine cells also begin to appear. By the end of the 12th week, tracheal and then bronchial submucosal glands can be identified.

In the canalicular phase, distal airspaces are initially lined by a uniform layer of cuboidal epithelium. The cells are filled with glycogen but few organelles are apparent ultrastructurally. As the primitive acini are subdivided, the airspace-lining cells begin to differentiate so that two different types of cells are seen. Subsequently (by 20–24 weeks' gestation), alveolar type II cells with characteristic microvilli and intracytoplasmic osmiophilic lamellar bodies begin to appear, along with type I (squamous) lung cells [66–68]. These lamellar inclusions represent surface-active material required for lung stability during air-breathing [68, 69]. It seems that in human neonates, as has been demonstrated in animals, the proportion of type II cells present in alveoli is greater at birth than in adults or even in relatively young children. Exact morphometric data are not available.

Lung growth and cytological and functional maturity are affected and determined by a variety of physical, hormonal, chemical, and metabolic influences, many of which may be inferred from studies of pulmonary hypoplasia [69–73]. Glucocorticoids and thyroid hormone stimulate development of type II alveolar cells and surfactant synthesis. It is possible that corticoids also influence the development of beta-adrenergic receptors in alveolar lining cells, increasing their sensitivity to the endogenous catecholamines which appear to cause surfactant release into the alveolar lumen. Insulin may inhibit this maturational process. It has been suggested that prolactin and estradiol influence lung maturation, but clear-cut evidence of direct action of these hormones is not yet available.

Protein mediators, such as epidermal growth factor,

fibroblast pneumonocyte factor, and somatomedins, also appear to influence lung development [57–59, 63, 69, 70, 73]. Fibroblast pneumonocyte factor (FPF) represents an extension of the mesenchymal–epithelial interaction seen earlier in the embryonic lung, where thoracic mesenchyme influences the branching pattern of bronchial buds. The direct effect of FPF appears to be mediation of corticosteroid effects on lung epithelial cells.

CONGENITAL ANOMALIES OF THE LOWER RESPIRATORY TRACT

Pulmonary Agenesis

Congenital *absence* of the lung may be bilateral or unilateral [7, 74–82]. In either instance, the affected lung(s) may be absent completely or represented by a rudimentary bronchus. As part of this spectrum there may also be a dysplastic mass of pulmonary tissue, which occasionally may contain striated muscle (see "rhabdomyomatous dysplasia" in the section on heterotopia). Bilateral agenesis is quite rare and may be associated with an even wider spectrum of anomalies, involving tracheal and esophageal atresia [7, 41, 74]. Unilateral agenesis of the lung is a more common entity

and may be compatible with essentially normal life. Agenesis of the left lung appears to occur more frequently and in fact the prognosis is generally regarded as worse for patients with agenesis on the right [75, 76]. The excess morbidity in the latter case may be associated with tracheal or bronchial compression and distortion by a deviated aorta (Fig. 19.6); severe mediastinal shift may also occur. Unilateral pulmonary agenesis may also be associated with a variety of distal skeletal (thumb) and chest wall anomalies [77]. Morphometric analysis of the single lung in one case of unilateral agenesis revealed an increased volume, with an increased number of smaller-than-normal alveoli [78]. The number of bronchial branches was reduced.

Isolated absence of one or more lobes is a very rare occurrence [83] and should not be confused with the "bilateral left lungs" seen in association with cardiac defects (see below) [7, 8].

Bronchial Anomalies

Congenital bronchial anomalies include the bronchial isomerism syndromes ("bilateral" right or left lungs) associated with anisosplenia or polysplenia and various associated cardiac defects [7, 8, 84]. True supernumerary bronchi [7,

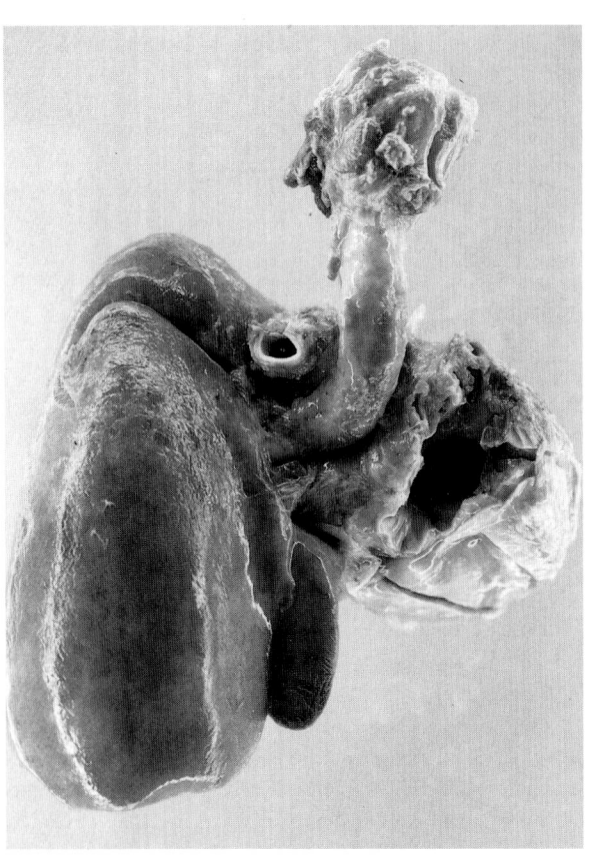

FIGURE 19.6.   *Agenesis of the right lung. The specimen is seen posteriorly. Note bronchial compression by the aorta.*

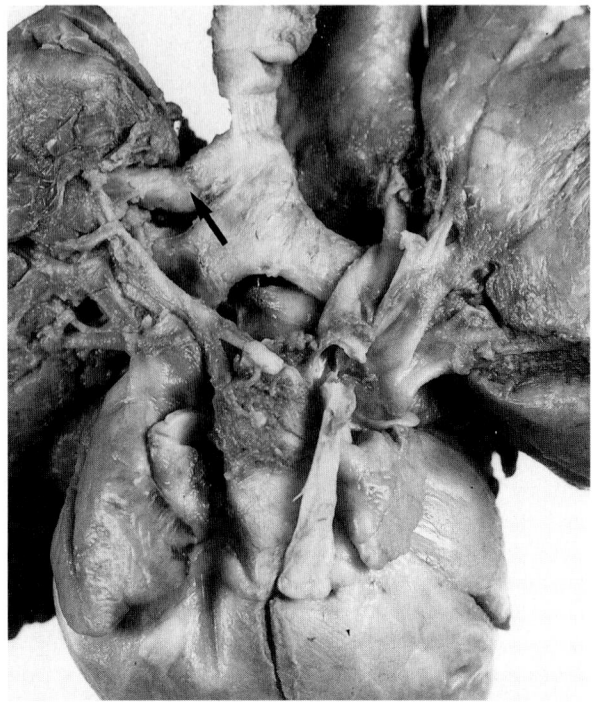

FIGURE 19.7.   *Tracheal bronchus (arrow). This displaced bronchus supplies a segment of the right upper lobe.*

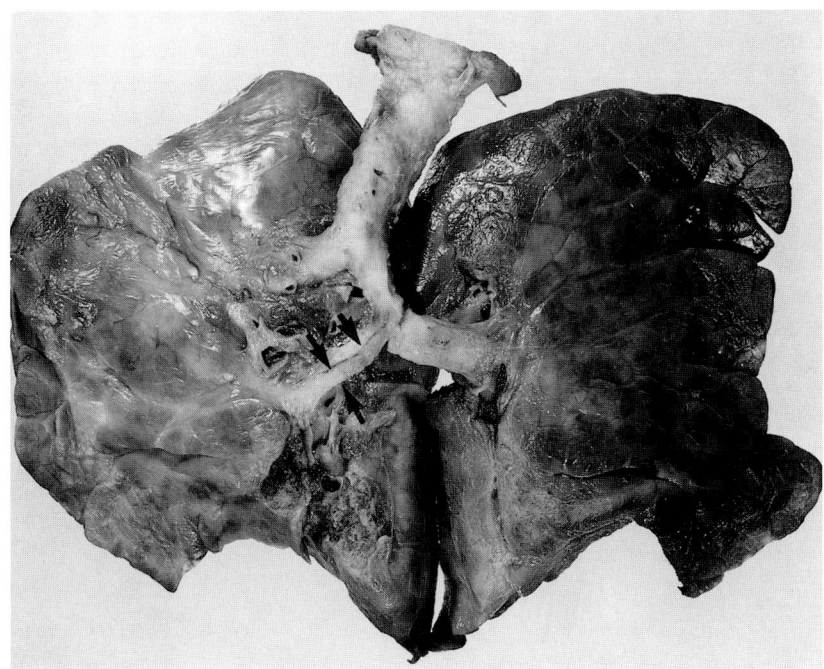

FIGURE 19.8.   *Bridging bronchus. The right lower lobe bronchus (arrows) arises from the left mainstem airway. (Courtesy of Dr. Frank Gonzalez-Crussi, used with permission of the Archives of Pathology and Laboratory Medicine and the American Medical Association.)*

85, 86] are rare and at least one reported case actually may be related more closely to another lung bud anomaly, such as extralobar sequestration or bronchogenic cyst [87]. Displaced bronchi are encountered, however, with some frequency [7, 8]. The tracheal bronchus [7, 85, 87–90] connects a segment of an upper lobe (usually, but not always, the right) to the trachea or (Fig. 19.7), less often, a mainstem bronchus. Both displaced and supernumerary bronchi have been described under this category. These lesions often produce no symptoms, but tracheal stenosis, recurrent infection, sublobar overinflation of the lung, or associated tracheo-esophageal anomalies may give rise to clinical problems. The so-called "bridging" bronchus connects the left lung to the right lower lobe by coursing across the mediastinum (Fig. 19.8) [91]. Other anomalous bronchi include the accessory cardiac bronchus which arises from the intermediate bronchus [7, 8], the origin of the anterior segmental upper lobe bronchus from the middle lobe bronchus ("postero-arterial bronchus") [92], and a variety of minor variations. Congenital intrinsic stenosis of a mainstem bronchus has been reported, associated with lobar atelectasis [93]. The lesion is vanishingly rare as compared to extrinsic compressive obstruction or with partial atresia associated with overinflation.

Bronchobiliary fistula is a rare anomaly which may be associated with the production of green sputum. A variety of biliary tract abnormalities have been reported in association with the lesion [94, 95]. Broncho-esophageal fistula is a rare lesion that may produce symptoms similar to those of the much more common tracheo-esophageal fistula [7].

Abnormal pulmonary fissures, usually absent or incomplete but also supernumerary, are probably the most common pulmonary anomalies [7, 85], and Landing and Dixon [7] stress that the number of external pulmonary lobes should not be taken as an indication of the number of lobar bronchi.

Horseshoe lung, fused behind the heart but anterior to the esophagus, is a rare entity [96, 97]; the lesion has been associated with anomalous pulmonary arteries and veins, including variants of the "scimitar syndrome" (p. 564).

Segmental bronchomalacia has been reported in the left mainstem bronchus. Functionally, there is narrowing and partial collapse of the airway on exhalation [47, 98]. The pathological features are poorly documented but include abnormal and abnormally spaced cartilaginous rings (Fig. 19.9). The etiology of the disorder is unknown [7], but familial cases have been reported [99].

Congenital bronchiectasis (Campbell-Williams syndrome) is an entity with a disputed pathogenesis originally described as a congenital disorder due to absence of bronchial cartilage; the entity now appears quite probably to be of postinfectious origin [7]. True congenital bronchiectasis on a structural basis may well exist but must be a very rare entity. Bronchiectasis associated with ultrastructurally abnormal cilia (with or without situs inversus) usually presents clinical problems in the older population but has been demonstrated in a neonate [100].

Pulmonary Hypoplasia

Pulmonary hypoplasia implies an abnormal reduction in the weight and/or volume of the lung without the absence of any of its lobes [64, 101–115]. A number of age-related standards have been proposed [101–103]. Page and Stocker [101] found that a lung weight/body weight of 0.010 identified pulmonary hypoplasia in most instances. Wigglesworth et al

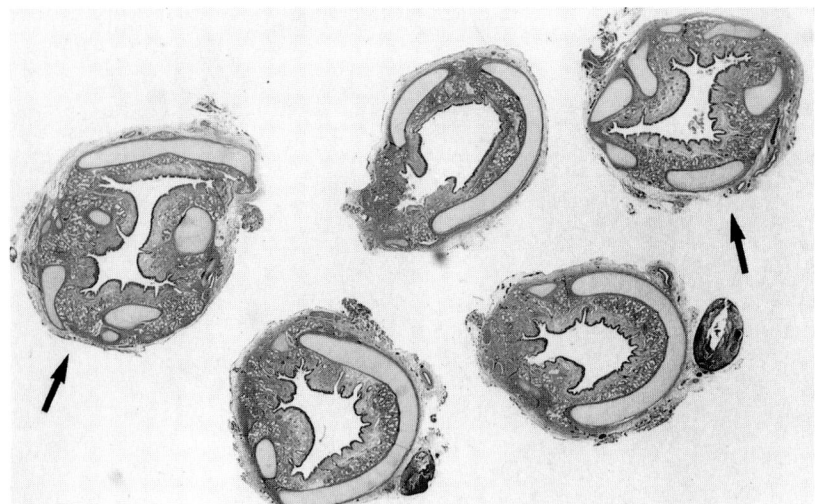

FIGURE 19.9. *Bronchomalacia. In this case, multiple abnormal cartilage segments were present in the affected segment* (arrows). *(×40.)*

[103, 116] indicated that a ratio of 0.015 was useful until 28 weeks' gestation but that after that time 0.012 was a more useful figure. Cooney and Thurlbeck [60, 61] employed the radial alveolar counting technique originally devised by Emery and Mithal and provided a set of normal standards for a gestational age of 18 weeks (1.5) through to the age of 18 years [102]. According to their figures, the count at term birth should be approximately 5. As another approach, the number of bronchial branches can be determined by bronchography and/or use of the dissecting microscope [55].

Hypoplasia represents the end result of many different and not necessarily related phenomena (Table 19.1). Structurally, decreased lung weight and volume could result from a decreased number of bronchial branches, reduced number of alveoli, decreased alveolar size, or from any combination of the three. Bilateral pulmonary hypoplasia is usually associated with conditions that can be grouped into several major categories (see Table 19.1), including oligohydramnios, thoracic wall abnormalities, lung compression by abdominal contents, abnormalities of the central nervous system, and a group of miscellaneous conditions [55, 58, 59, 103, 104, 107–113, 115]. The pathogenesis of lung hypoplasia under these conditions is often obscure. Experimentally, both distention of the lung with lung liquid and fetal respiratory movements are needed for normal fetal lung growth [115]. Oligohydramnios appears to cause compression of thoracic contents with a net loss of lung fluid into the amniotic cavity, resulting in reduced lung distension [111, 113, 114]. It is currently debated whether oligohydramnios also inhibits respiratory movements [117, 118]. Polyhydramnios, in contrast, may be associated with either small or large lungs [105]. Excess amniotic fluid in various forms of hydrops is often accompanied by pleural effusions, which could be expected to affect respiratory movements. Polyhydramnios may be due to fetal brainstem abnormality

Table 19.1. Conditions associated with bilateral pulmonary hypoplasia

Condition	Examples
Prolonged oligohydramnios	Renal agenesis
	Polycystic and dysplastic kidneys
	Urinary outlet obstruction
	Prolonged premature rupture of membranes
Thoracic wall anomalies or reduced intrathoracic space	Thanatophoric dwarfism
	Osteogenesis imperfecta
	Asphyxiating thoracic dysplasia
	Intrathoracic masses
Extrathoracic masses	Polycystic and dysplastic kidneys
	Large bladder in urinary outlet obstruction
	Other abdominal masses
Anomalies or damage to CNS or respiratory muscles	Anencephaly (involving brainstem)
	Intrauterine anoxic–ischemic damage to CNS (brainstem)
	Congenital muscular dystrophy
	Congenital amyoplasia of diaphragm
	Bilateral diaphragmatic hernia
Miscellaneous	Exomphalos
	Severe rhesus isoimmunization
	Extralobar sequestration of lung with pleural effusion
	Other forms of non-immunological hydrops
	Idiopathic

or neuromuscular abnormalities, which interfere both with fetal swallowing and respiratory movements.

In many of the disorders associated with impaired lung growth, multiple factors may operate. For instance, lower urinary tract obstruction causes oligohydramnios but the enlarged bladder and kidneys may form a mass that distorts the lower thoracic cage and compresses the lungs. Renal agenesis causes oligohydramnios but has been postulated also to interfere with collagen metabolism [55]. Primary or idiopathic lung hypoplasia may be sporadic or familial and has been reported in association with several malformation syndromes [7, 109, 112]. Diaphragmatic hernia is almost uniformly associated with hypoplasia of the ipsilateral and, to a lesser extent, contralateral lung. Unilateral hypoplasia of the lung is usually due to diaphragmatic hernia, but accessory diaphragm, pulmonary artery anomalies (usually absence), anomalous venous return, and idiopathic hypoplasia were causes of unilateral hypoplasia included in one recent series [119].

Heterotopia

Heterotopic tissues have been reported in the lung and include adrenal cortex [120], striated muscle "rhabdomyomatous dysplasia" [121, 122], and glial tissue [123]. Glial heterotopia is usually found in the lung parenchyma of anencephalic infants, probably on the basis of aspiration. Heterotopia must be separated from overt traumatic brain injury with emboli of central nervous system tissue to the pulmonary arteries [124].

Peripheral Dysplasias

Congenital alveolar capillary dysplasia (Fig. 19.10) is a rare developmental anomaly in which there is a profound absence of capillaries in the alveolar wall and there are anomalous veins in bronchovascular bundles. Extrauterine oxygenation of the lung is essentially too poor to support life [125]. Wagenvoort has described a similar entity as "misalignment of lung vessels" [126]. The disorder has been described in families and some infants have had phocomelia [127]. Rutledge and Jensen described an infant with "acinar dysplasia" of the lung [128]. This lesion is probably a form of adenomaterial malformation [129]. Airways were normally developed but alveoli and distal lung parenchyma, in general, were not well developed.

Pulmonary Vascular Anomalies

Arterial Anomalies

Arterial anomalies include origin of one or both pulmonary arteries from the aorta, its branches, or the ductus arteriosus [130–147]. Origin of the left pulmonary artery from the right (vascular sling) represents one of the multiple vascular anomalies, which can cause respiratory distress via compression of the trachea [131, 137].

The so-called *absent* or *occult pulmonary artery* actually represents interruption of the proximal portion of the vessel; the intrapulmonary branches of the vessel are usually present and complete [143]. Hislop et al reported three unusual cases of absent or hypoplastic pulmonary artery associated with mesenchymal dysplasia in the ipsilateral lung [139]. Diffuse hypoplasia of the pulmonary arterial system has been described as a consequence of intrauterine rubella [148]. Goldstein et al reported several other unusual cases in which the affected infant had hypoplastic pulmonary artery

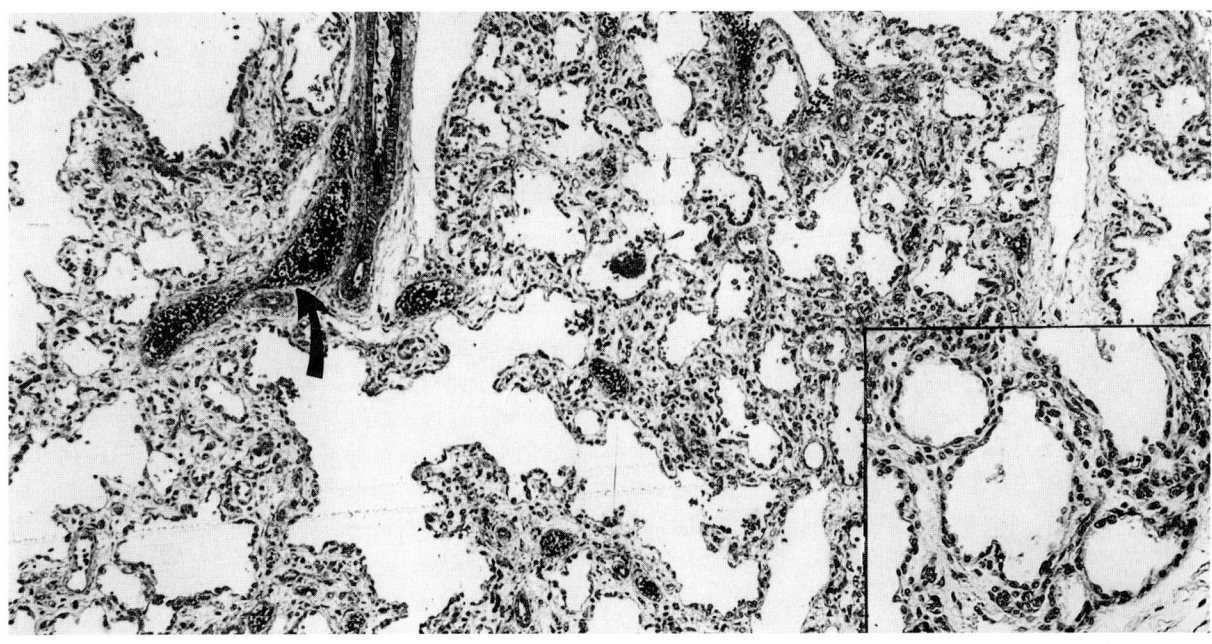

FIGURE 19.10. *Congenital alveolar capillary dysplasia. Alveoli (inset, ×400) are essentially devoid of capillaries. In addition, abnormal (? displaced) veins (arrow) are seen in the bronchovascular bundles. (×200.)*

branches in association with abnormal pulmonary venous connections and partial systemic arterial supply to both lungs [136].

Segmental stenosis in the pulmonary arterial system appears to represent a broad spectrum of disorders [140]. The stenosis may be single or multiple and may be peripheral or central in location. In some instances, cardiac anomalies may be present as well. Children with Alagille syndrome of cholestasis, paucity of intrahepatic bile ducts, and a peculiar facies often have peripheral stenotic lesions in the pulmonary arteries [7]. Peripheral stenosis has been described also in association with Down syndrome, in infants with Williams syndrome of supravalvular aortic stenosis and hypercalcemia [133], Ehlers-Danlos syndrome, cutis laxa, the "leopard" syndrome of multiple lentigenes and in association with café au lait spots, possibly representing a form of von Recklinghausen disease [7, 133, 140, 149].

Haworth and Reid studied the intrapulmonary vessels in cases of pulmonary valvular atresia and found a reduced number of intrapulmonary arteries [138]. The arteries that were present had thin muscular walls and an abnormally small diameter.

Arteriovenous Fistulas

Arteriovenous malformations (fistulas) occur in the lung either as an isolated entity or as part of the Rendu-Osler-Weber syndrome. The lesions can be acquired on the basis of trauma as well [134, 144, 146]. The blood supply of the fistula is usually derived from the pulmonary artery but may arise from systemic vessels. Abe et al reported direct connection of the right pulmonary artery to the left atrium [130]. We have seen a similar lesion in a neonate involving a segmental pulmonary artery. Rarely, an infant's lung may be infiltrated by a diffuse capillary hemangioma (Fig. 19.11) [147]. It is not clear whether or not this lesion is related to capillary hemangiomatosis as described in the adult. The lesion in infants seems to lack the prominent veno-

occlusion seen in the older patient. Complicated vascular malformations involving anastomosis of chest wall vessels to the lung have also been described [132].

Pulmonary Venous Abnormalities

Pulmonary venous abnormalities include anomalous venous return, either total or partial [150, 151]. In total anomalous return, all four main pulmonary veins converge and then drain into the innominate vein, coronary veins, or right atrium. They may also run below the diaphragm entering the inferior vena cava or portal vein. Lymphangiectasis may be prominent in the pulmonary parenchyma. Partial forms of anomalous venous return also occur; one such lesion is the so-called scimitar syndrome in which a large anomalous pulmonary vein drains in one lung, usually the right, into the inferior vena cava [152, 153]. The broad radiographic shadow of this vein forms the "scimitar." The affected lung is hypoplastic, has complete or at least partial systemic arterial blood supply, and may have abnormal lobation. This complicated syndrome may overlap with horseshoe lung or bronchopulmonary sequestration [7, 96, 154].

Isolated or multiple areas of stenosis or atresia may be found in the pulmonary veins [155–158]. These lesions are associated with diffuse or localized lymphangiectasis or hemorrhage and hemosiderin deposition in the lung (see veno-occlusive disease). Unilateral venous stenosis in association with ventricular septal defect may cause pulmonary hypertension very early in infancy [156]. Dilated, nonobstructed pulmonary veins (varices) are usually found in adults but have been described in children and even infants [159].

Bronchopulmonary Sequestration

Sequestration of pulmonary lobes or segments is generally defined as consisting of 1) absence of a normal connection to the airway system of the surrounding lung and 2) blood supply to the sequestered areas via systemic vessels arising

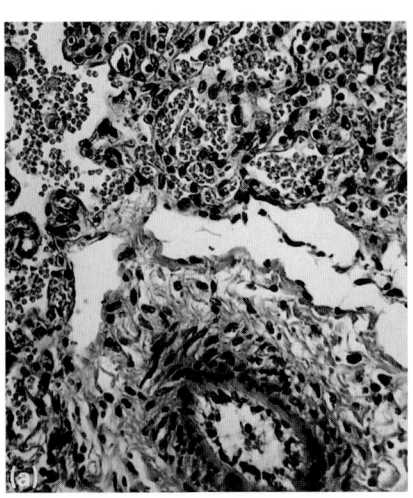 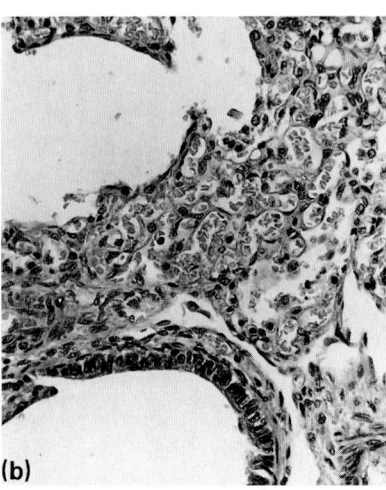

FIGURE 19.11. *Diffuse capillary hemangioma of the lung. Multiple capillary channels invade septa (a, ×200) and bronchovascular bundles (b, ×400). No septal veins were occluded and this lesion appears to differ from the angiomatous foci in pulmonary veno-occlusive disease. (Courtesy of Dr. B. Dahms, Cleveland, Ohio.)*

from the aorta or its branches either above or below the diaphragm [160–185]. Savic et al [176] and Stocker et al [177, 186] have produced extensive reviews of the subject. Two major types of sequestration occur: intralobar and extralobar. Rarely, both types of lesions occur in the same patient [7, 176].

Intralobar Sequestrations

Intralobar sequestrations (ILS) are incorporated within the pleural investment of a pulmonary lobe. The lesion occurs with almost equal frequency in children and adults [8, 176]. The usual, but not invariable, location is in the posterior segment of the left lower lobe [176], but upper lobe and even bilateral examples of ILS have been reported [166, 167]. One or more elastic arteries supply the area and the usual venous drainage is through the pulmonary system to the left atrium. The lesion is extremely rare in neonates in part because it is usually discovered during the investigation of recurrent localized pneumonia or as a mass lesion seen on a routine chest radiograph. Pathologically, the features are those of chronic pneumonitis and bronchiectasis. On gross examination the lesion may be solid or cystic, depending on the degree of inflammatory change and infection [7, 176].

Extralobar Sequestrations

Extralobar sequestrations (ELS, accessory lobes) are completely separate from the pleural covering of the normal lung [176, 178]. The usual location of the lesion is in the left lower hemithorax but ELS may be found in the mediastinum, near the esophagus or even within or below the diaphragm [7, 176]. Both the arterial supply and the venous drainage are usually of systemic origin. In contrast to ILS, the extralobar lesion is found predominantly in neonates and infants and may be associated with coexisting malformations, especially diaphragmatic hernia and pectus excavatum [7, 176–178]. In contrast to ILS, secondary infection and obstructive changes are not common features. On gross examination the lesion has a spongy character (Fig. 19.12) and the basic microscopic architecture (Fig. 19.13) often resembles that of immature lung or may resemble certain types of adenomatoid malformation. Striated muscle may be found within the parenchyma of an ELS [178]. Lymphatic dilation is common in ELS and several cases of massive pleural effusion and hypoplasia of the ipsilateral lung have been reported [170].

The origin of pulmonary sequestration has provided fertile ground for both debate and imagination [7, 64, 165, 186]. A practical classification is presented in Table 19.2. It seems certain that extralobar sequestration represents an accessory lung bud from the foregut. Some intralobar sequestrations may represent an accessory lung bud, presumably occurring later in embryogenesis than that associated with ELS. It has become increasingly clear that a portion of lesions classified as ILS are, in fact, acquired and represent recurrent localized inflammation [173, 179]. Aspi-

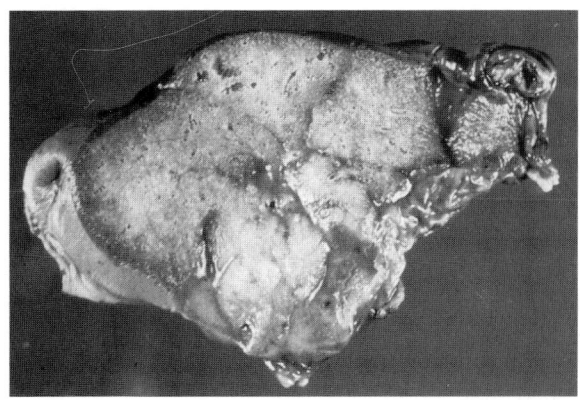

FIGURE 19.12. *Extralobar sequestration. This spongy mass of tissue was found incidentally during repair of a diaphragmatic hernia.*

Table 19.2. Practical classification of pulmonary sequestration

True sequestration
Intralobar
Extralobar
Bronchopulmonary foregut malformation
Intra- or extra-lobar sequestration with communication to esophagus or stomach
Pseudo-sequestration
Inflammatory intrabronchial mass and/or foreign body; recurrent infection with engorgement of normal pulmonary ligament arteries. This lesion represents an unknown proportion of lesions diagnosed as intralobar sequestration
Vascular anomalies
Systemic arterial supply to otherwise normal lung
Scimitar syndrome

rated foreign bodies, for example, could produce such a lesion [173]. With parenchymal inflammation there is enlargement of the small systemic arteries normally present in the pulmonary ligament [179]. Presumably, these recently demonstrated arteries play a role in the blood supply of ELS as well.

Reported complications of sequestration in neonates include clinically significant arteriovenous shunts and respiratory distress in a newborn related to a mediastinal mass [164, 183]. In some instances, with either ELS or ILS, the lung bud connection to the foregut may persist and connect the sequestered lobe or area to the esophagus or stomach "bronchopulmonary foregut malformation" [165, 168, 175]. Pancreatic tissue has been found in several intralobar sequestrations, presumably as part of this spectrum [161]. Not surprisingly, sequestration may occur in association with tracheo-esophageal fistula (also see total sequestration, below) and with duplication of portions of the gastrointestinal tract [160, 162, 169, 182, 187].

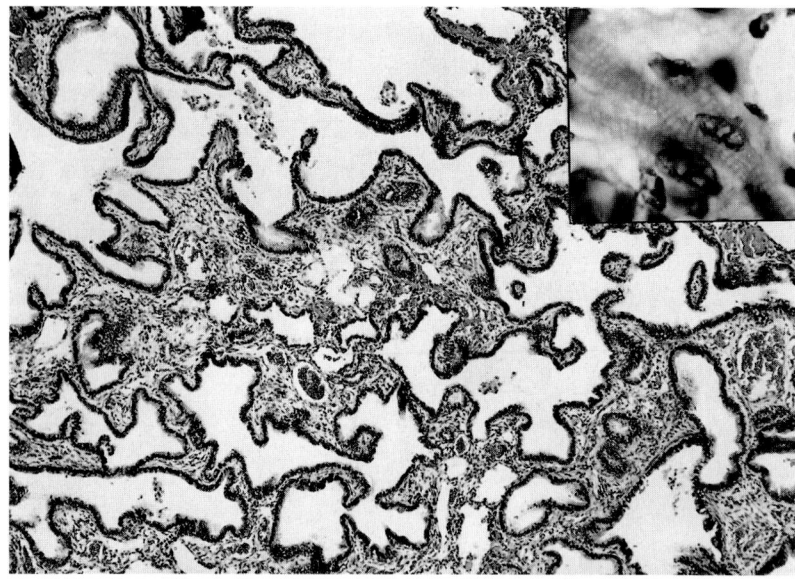

FIGURE 19.13. *Extralobar sequestration. In this case there are branching bronchiolar structures, which suggest adenomatoid malformation. (×200.) Striated muscle (inset, ×600) was also present.*

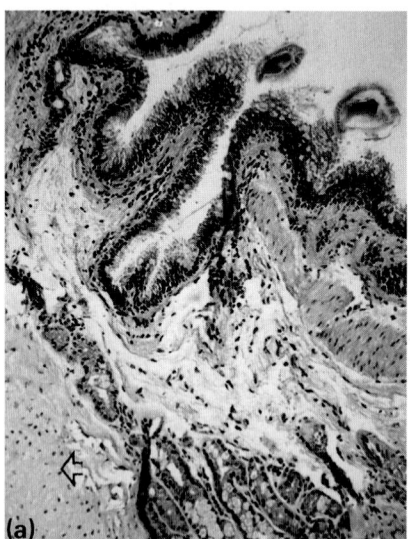 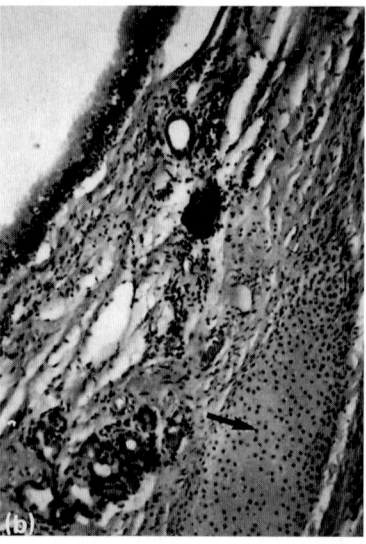

FIGURE 19.14. *Bronchogenic cyst. This paratracheal cyst has a ciliated columnar epithelial lining and (a) a wall composed of smooth muscle (arrow) and (b) fragments of cartilage (arrows). (×200.)*

Certain vascular anomalies may mimic or even belong in a broader spectrum of sequestion. Isolated systemic arterial supply of an otherwise normal lobe can occur and may produce a large shunt [163, 184]. In a very young infant without recurrent infection in the lung, it would be difficult to separate this lesion from ILS without a presurgical or specimen bronchogram. A variety of anomalous patterns of venous return have been noted in association with ELS or ILS [181] and the scimitar syndrome may, in fact, be related to sequestration. The term "total sequestration" (pulmonary ectoplasia) appears in the literature usually in reference to a malformed lung, with its main bronchial connection to the esophagus and a systemic arterial supply [171].

Bronchogenic and Other Cysts

Bronchogenic cysts also arise from accessory lung buds from the foregut [188–190]. In rare instances there may be a peripheral rim of poorly developed pulmonary tissue [165], but ordinarily these cysts are characterized by a muscular or fibrous wall with a lining of bronchial epithelium. Cartilage is present in the wall (Fig. 19.14) but may be difficult to find without multiple sections. Bronchogenic cysts are usually found in the anterior mediastinum but may appear within the lung substance as well [188]. Rare connections to the gut have been described, similar to those seen in sequestration [189]. A histologically similar lesion has been described in the skin of the neck or anterior chest wall

[191]. Bronchogenic cysts are unilocular and may contain mucus, watery fluid, or even pus. In the mediastinum they must be separated from enteric cysts, which are lined by gastric epithelium and usually occur in the posterior compartment [192, 193]. Within the lung, bronchogenic cysts may be confused with lung abscesses. The abscess, however, should have multiple bronchi communicating with the lesion, while the bronchogenic cyst will not. The nature of the epithelial lining may not be of help [194]. Bronchiectasis in infants has been described, mistakenly, in the past as a specific type of congenital cystic disease of the lung. Pneumatoceles are also cystic foci in the lung [7]. They probably result from areas of necrosis of bronchopulmonary tissue during infection, with subsequent escape of air into the interstitium. Staphylococcal pneumonia is the common antecedent but viral infection or, in older children, kerosene aspiration has also been implicated [195, 196].

Lymphangiectasis and pulmonary interstitial emphysema may also form grossly visible, but thin-walled, cysts in the lung parenchyma, as may the end stages of bronchopulmonary dysplasia. True congenital cysts of the lung are extremely rare and not well documented. Weinberg and Zumwalt described a patient with multiple lung cysts

and bilateral nephromegaly [197]. Postinfarction peripheral lung cysts are described in the section on pulmonary emboli.

Congenital Adenomatoid Malformation

The congenital adenomatoid malformation (CAM) is an unusual lesion combining features of dysplastic growth, hamartoma, or even neoplasia [198–210]. CAM is usually found in newborns or very young children, although cases have been described in adults [200]. Antenatal diagnosis has been reported [198, 206]. The lesion usually is restricted to a single lobe and presents as an expanding mass that causes respiratory distress and even death. The patient may have any of a variety of clinical presentations and the affected lung may have a gross appearance that ranges from solid to that of a large multiloculated cyst (Figs. 19.15–19.18). Fetal anasarca and stillbirth are not uncommon in infants with the solid variants of adenomatoid malformation [208, 209], and maternal polyhydramnios may be present [206]. Pneumothorax is a rare presenting feature [210]. Anomalous (systemic) arterial blood supply is distinctly rare but does occur [208].

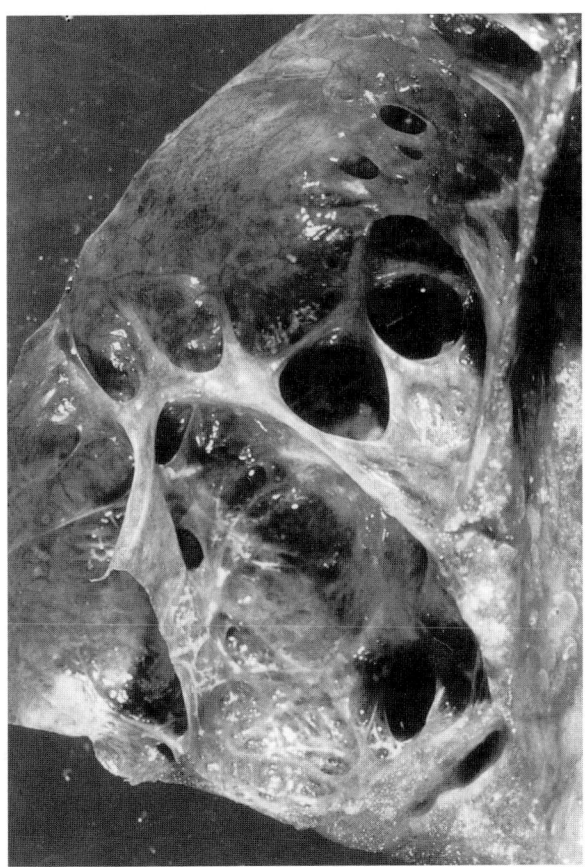

FIGURE 19.15.   *Adenomatoid malformation: a large cyst (Stocker type I) lesion.*

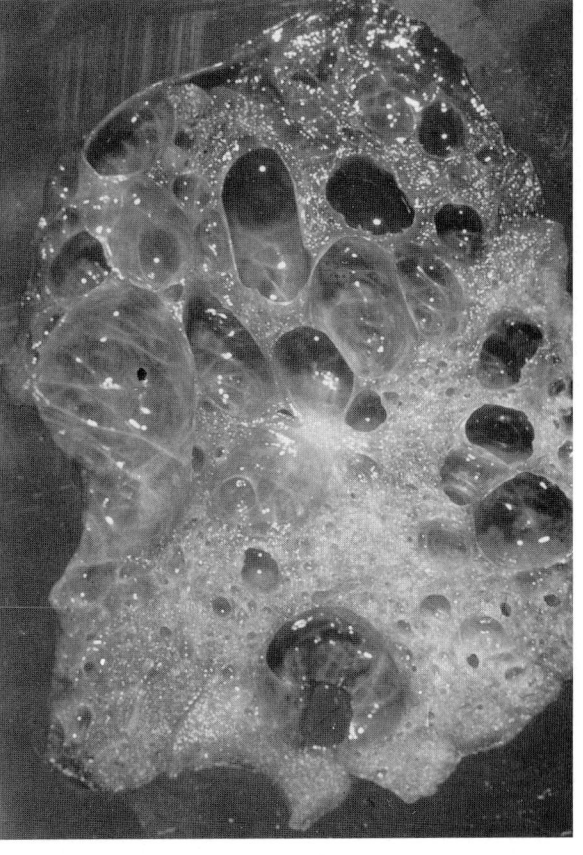

FIGURE 19.16.   *A small cyst (type II) adenomatoid malformation.*

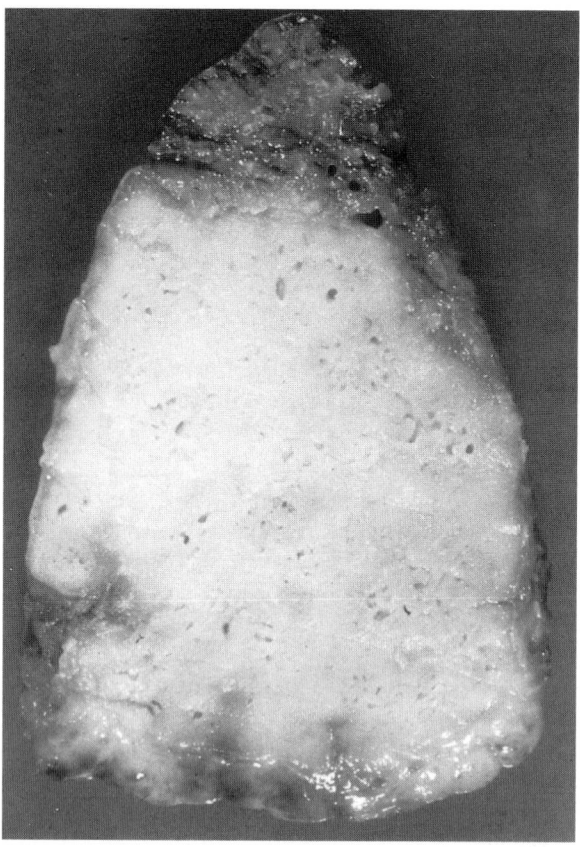

FIGURE 19.17.   *A solid (type III) adenomatoid malformation.*

In general, CAM lacks bronchi but does appear to communicate in many instances with the normal tracheobronchial tree, a feature that allows air-trapping and expansion to occur after birth. In a smaller number of cases, bronchial atresia has been found in association with the lesion [211]. In both solid and cystic forms, CAM is usually surrounded by a partial or complete peripheral rim of normal lung [202].

The microscopic appearance of CAM varies with that of the gross appearance [179]. Solid lesions are composed of multiple, curved, branched structures that resemble immature or dysplastic bronchioles (Fig. 19.19). Lesions with cysts of intermediate or large size contain similar areas of bronchiole-like structures interspersed between normal areas of lung (Fig. 19.20). Electron microscopic study of the cuboidal cells lining the bronchiolar areas in either solid or cystic lesions has suggested a resemblance to the cells of fetal airways [199]. All types of CAM, but especially the cystic lesions, may have prominent collections or tufts of mucigenic cells interspersed along thin septa (Fig. 19.21) [203]. Fischer et al reported a peculiar variant of CAM with papillary features [204], and we and others have seen a diffuse cartilaginous malformation (Fig. 19.22) that may be related to CAM [201].

The pathogenesis of the adenomatoid malformation is unknown. Overgrowth of bronchioles with suppression of alveolar differentiation has been suggested as the basic defect [208, 209]. The microscopic resemblance of some extralobar sequestrations to CAM is interesting but unexplained. A classification of CAM based on a combination of cyst size and microscopic features has been proposed and justified because of an apparent association of extrapulmonary anomalies with the small cyst lesion [209]. Stocker [129] has

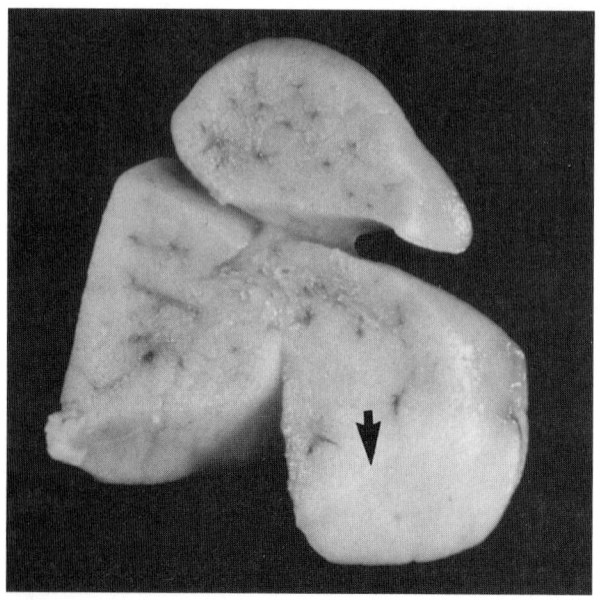

FIGURE 19.18.   *Adenomatoid malformation (arrow) in middle lobe of fetal lung (gestational age approximately 17 weeks). The lesion was diagnosed antenatally. Ultrasonic studies had been performed because of polyhydramnios.*

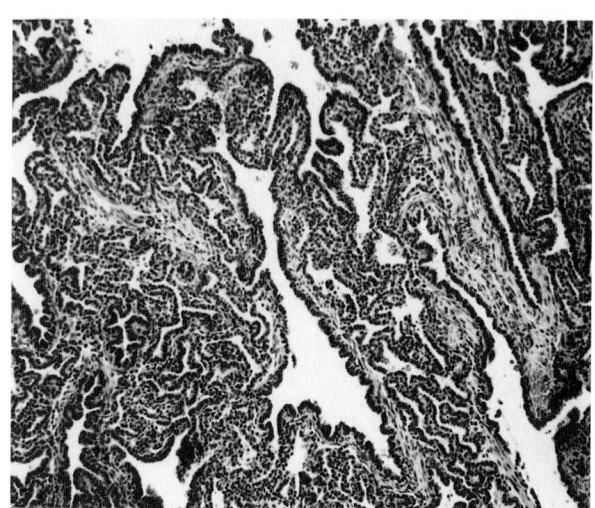

FIGURE 19.19.   *Solid adenomatoid malformation. The lesion is composed of multiple, curved, branching structures resembling bronchioles. (×200.)*

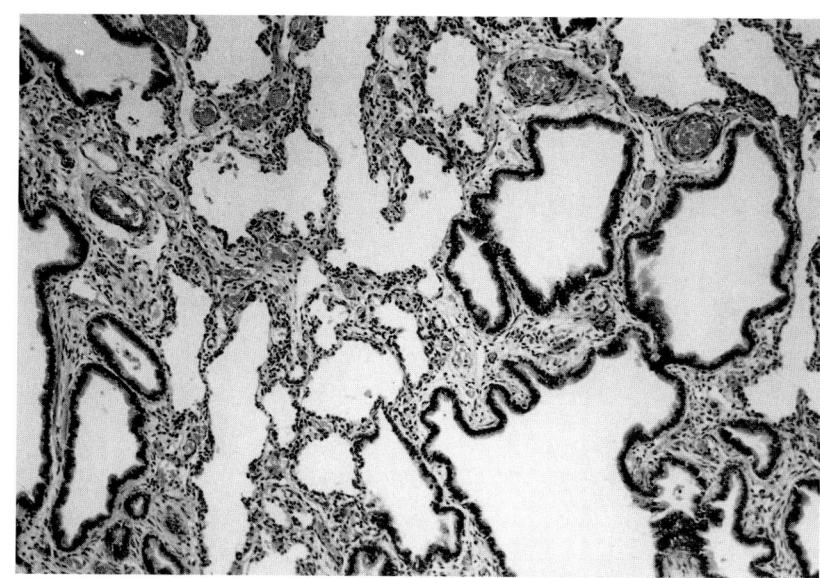

FIGURE 19.20. *Adenomatoid malformation, small cyst type. Dilated irregular bronchiolar structures are present. The lack of inflammation and fibrosis helps to separate this lesion from acquired bronchiectasis. (×400.)*

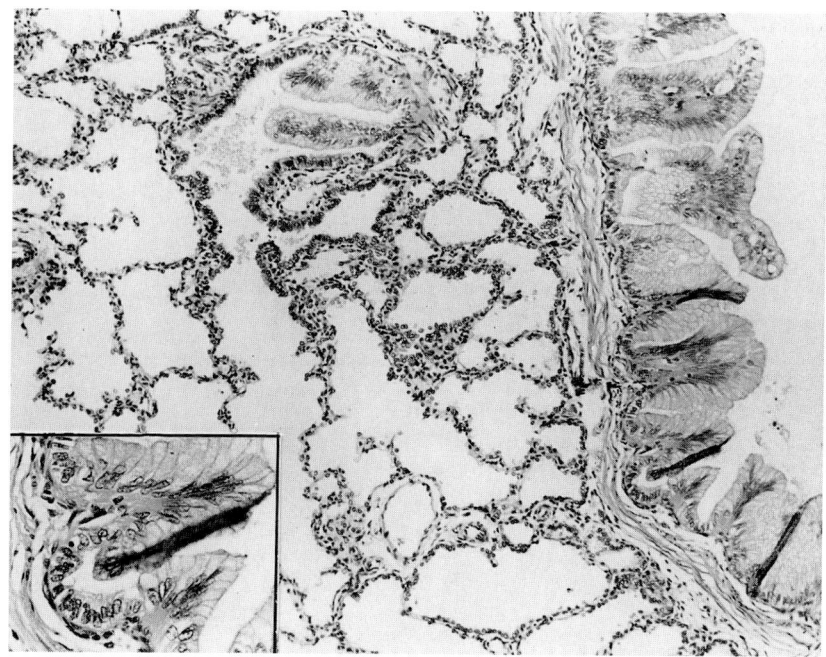

FIGURE 19.21. *Mucigenic cells (inset, ×600) line the cysts of a type I adenomatoid malformation. (×400.)*

prepared a recent update of the CAM classification (Table 19.3). Other investigators have not found a specific association of anomalies and prefer to separate only the cystic and the solid lesions [201, 208]. There does appear to be an association of CAM with all forms of renal dysgenesis [7, 208].

Embryonic malignant neoplasms, including pulmonary blastoma and embryonal rhabdomyosarcoma, have been reported to arise in congenital lung cysts; some of these were CAM and others were bronchogenic cysts [212, 213].

Congenital Pulmonary Lymphangiectasis

Congenital dilatation of pulmonary lymphatics is a rare lesion with a number of separate etiologies (Table 19.4) [214–219]. The disorder is characterized by a marked distension of the subpleural and septal lymphatics so that the lung has a cobblestone appearance. Lymphangiectasis most frequently occurs in the clinical setting of congenital heart disease with, and rarely without, pulmonary venous obstruction (total anomalous venous return, atresia of large pulmonary veins) [151, 155, 214, 218, 219]. Rarely, the disorder

Table 19.3. Characteristic features of congenital cystic adenomatoid malformations (CCAM)

	Type 0	Type I	Type II	Type III	Type IV
Origin	Tracheobronchial	Bronchial/bronchiolar	Bronchiolar	Bronchiolar/alveolar duct	Distal acinar
Clinical Features	Cyanosis at birth and survival for only few hours. Associated with CHD and dermal hypoplasia	Increasing respiratory distress shortly after birth. Older children present with cough, fever, or chest pain	Associated with other anomalies such as renal agenesis, dysgenesis, diaphragmatic hernia, and CHD	Occurs only in males. Associated with maternal polyhydramnios	Sudden respiratory distress from tension pneumothorax. May not have any symptoms
Macroscopic Features	Small and firm lungs. Diffusely granular surface	Cysts are limited to one lobe and rarely bilateral. Thin walled when distended	Lesions blend into normal parenchyma, multiple small cysts	Large bulky lesion involving entire lobe or even an entire lung producing mediastinal shift and compression of adjacent lung which is hypoplastic	Large thin-walled cysts located at the periphery of lobe
Frequency (%)	1–3	>85	20–25	8	2–4
Cyst Size (cm)	0.3–0.5	10	2.5	0.3–0.5	7
Epithelial Lining	Ciliated Pseudostratified Tall columnar with goblet cells	Ciliated Pseudostratified Tall columnar	Ciliated Cuboidal or columnar	Ciliated Cuboidal	Flattened Alveolar lining cells
Wall Thickness (μm)	100–500	100–300	50–100	0–50	25–100
Mucous Cells	Present in all cases	Present in 33%	Absent	Absent	Absent
Cartilage	Present in all cases	Present in 5% to 10%	Absent	Absent	Rare
Skeletal Muscle	Absent	Absent	Present in 5%	Absent	Absent

Source: Stocker [129].

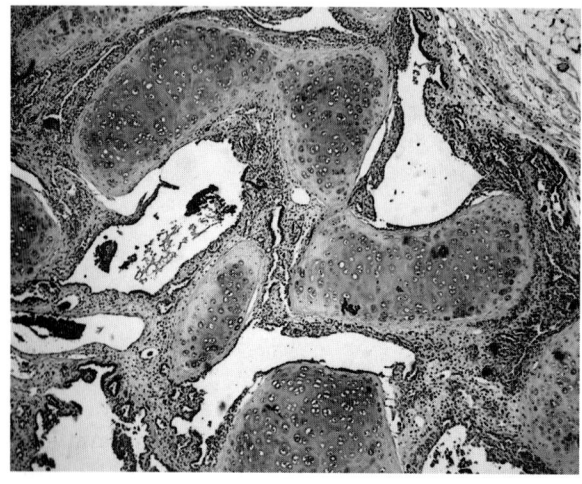

FIGURE 19.22. *Unusual adenomatoid malformation with abnormal cartilage. (×100.) (This case was published in* Chest *1987; 92:514–6.)*

may be primary in the lung or it may be part of a systemic disorder with chylous effusions, lymphangiectasis and lymphangiomas in many organs, and with "vanishing bones" [215].

Lymphangiectasis involves dilatation of normal structures (Fig. 19.23), a feature that helps to separate it from the destructive lesions seen with pulmonary interstitial air "emphysema."

Congenital Pulmonary Overinflation (Lobar or Segmental)

Congenital pulmonary overinflation occurs in several forms (Table 19.5). The term "emphysema" is inappropriate since there is no destruction of lung parenchyma [145, 220–229]. Congenital lobar overinflation occurs usually in neonates, although delayed onset of disease has been reported. A few familial cases have been described [228]. The expanding lung tissue, usually an upper or the middle lobe, compresses the

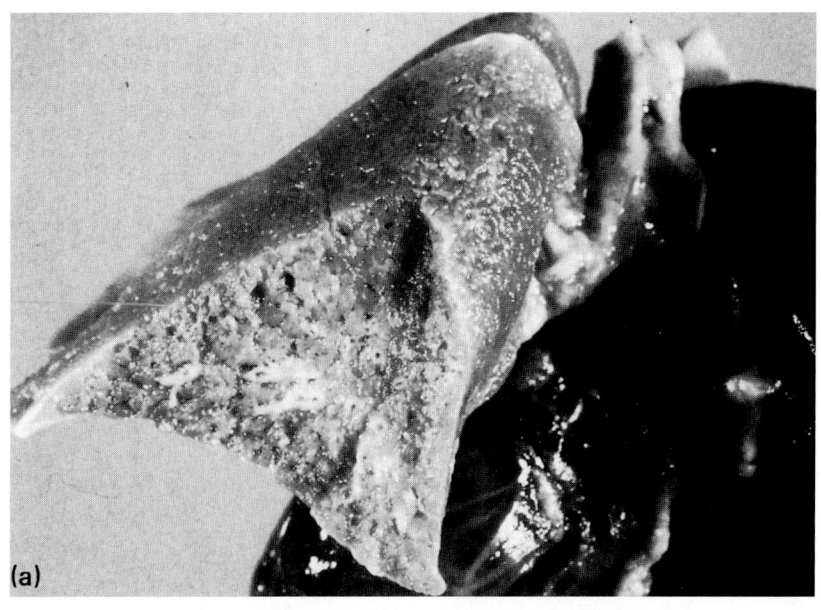

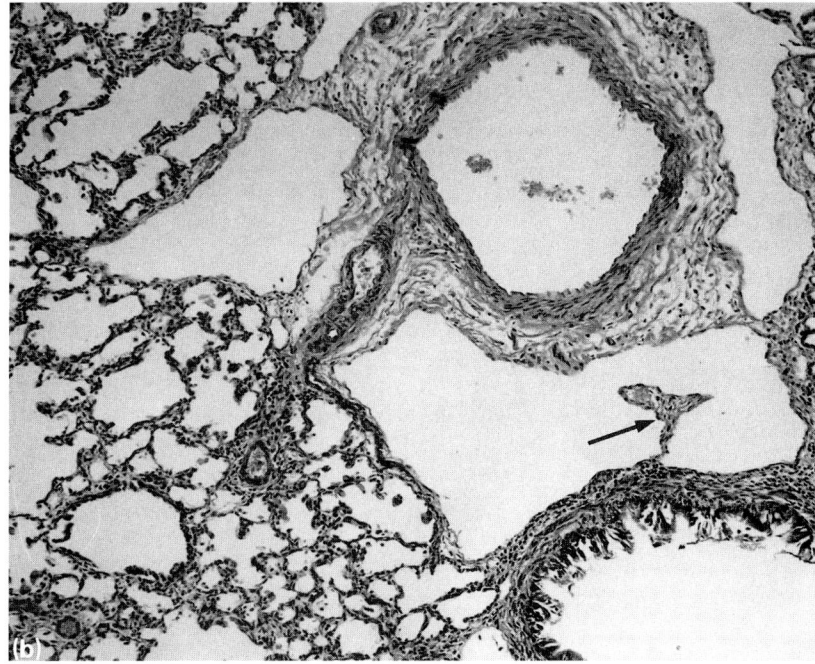

FIGURE 19.23. *Congenital pulmonary lymphangiectasis. (a) The lung has a coarse cobblestone appearance. (b) Microscopically dilated channels with lymphatic valves (arrow) are seen in septa and bronchovascular bundles. (×100.)*

Table 19.4. Classification of pulmonary lymphangiectasis

Cardiac
Mechanical or functional obstruction of large pulmonary veins
Noonan syndrome, asplenia, other cardiac defects without venous obstruction
Generalized
Multiple lymphangiomas, chylous effusions, "vanishing bones"
Primary
Isolated to the lung, no cardiac or venous anomalies demonstrable

remaining lung parenchyma and may cause fatal respiratory distress related to mediastinal shift (Fig. 19.24). In neonates, the lung initially may be radiographically opaque because of retained alveolar fluid [230]. The basic defect is partial obstruction of the lobar bronchus with resultant air-trapping. Complete obstruction will cause atelectasis. The immediate cause of obstruction may vary widely (see Table 19.5) but usually can be grouped under external compression (masses, engorged pulmonary arteries, aberrant vessels),

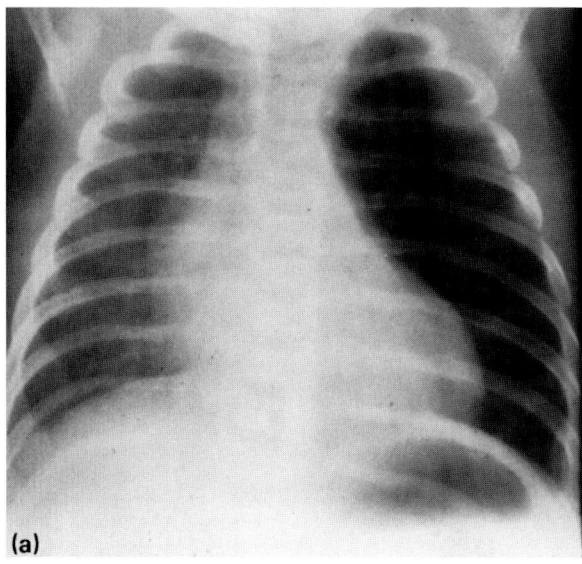

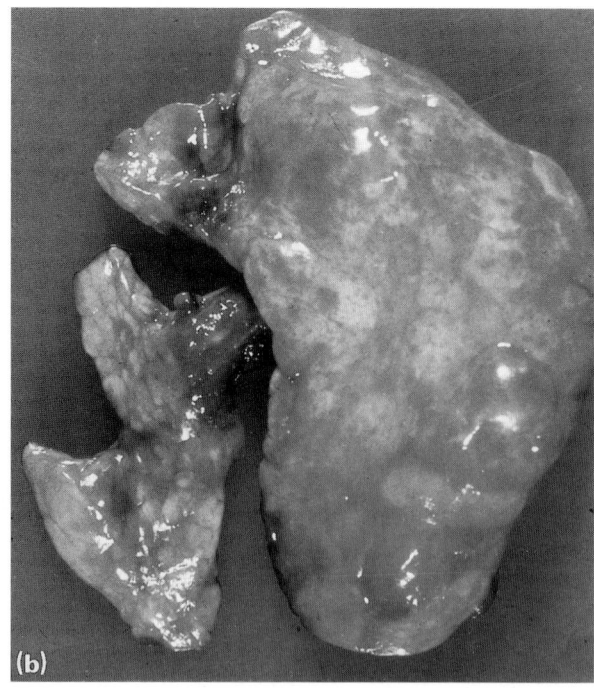

FIGURE 19.24. *Congenital lobar overinflation ("emphysema"). (a) The radiograph shows an overinflated left upper lobe with compression of the right lung. (b) The excised specimen shows overexpansion of the left upper lobe while the lingular is essentially normal. (Radiograph courtesy of Dr. William McAlister, St. Louis, MO.)*

Table 19.5. Pulmonary overinflation in neonates

Location	Cause	Patient Population
Congenital		
Lobar	External compression: vessels, masses ?torsion of lung pedicle Internal partial obstruction: physical—webs, masses, functional—absence of cartilage Polyalveolar lobe	Neonates
Segmental	Segmental bronchial atresia with mucocele	Older children or adults, rare cases in infants
Acquired		
Lobar	Bronchial granulation tissue with ball-valve effect—an iatrogenic lesion	Neonates

partial internal obstruction by webs, abnormal cartilage, or even apparent torsion of the lobe on its bronchial pedicle [221, 222, 225]. In this category, air-trapping can also result from defective or absent cartilage causing expiratory collapse of the lobar bronchus. Vascular compression of bronchi appears to account for the frequent association of lobar overinflation with congenital heart disease [145, 220, 226,

227]. Surgical removal of the affected lobe has been the usual form of therapy, although in a few cases the disorder has apparently resolved spontaneously [231]. Microscopically, the affected lobe has overinflated alveoli without destruction of septa. Rarely, a true structural anomaly of the lobar parenchyma, the so-called polyalveolar lobe, can be diagnosed by use of radial alveolar counts and is a rare cause of congenital overinflation of the lung [221, 223, 230]. The number of alveoli per acinus is increased.

An acquired form of lobar overinflation has been reported in infants with antecedent respiratory disease and described as related to partial bronchial obstruction by granulation tissue or polypoid areas of fibrosis. These lesions were apparently secondary to injury from repeated suctioning during the neonatal period [232]. Complete bronchial stenosis with lobar collapse has been described in the same population of infants [233].

Segmental bronchial atresia is associated with overinflation of the airspaces in the area distal to obstruction [234]. A mucus plug is usually found distal to the area of atresia in the bronchus. The disorder is usually diagnosed as an incidental finding on a chest radiograph taken for some unrelated ailment in an adult. We have, however, seen two cases in neonates; one with clinical features of lobar overinflation. The left upper lobe is the most frequent site of the lesion but other segments of the lung may be involved. Overinflation of the distal lung parenchyma is usually explained as related to collateral ventilation. Segmental overinflation may occur in the presence of a tracheal bronchus and that situation should not be confused with bronchial atresia as described above [221].

True destructive pulmonary emphysema has been reported in a neonate with Marfan syndrome [235].

DISORDERS OF THE TRANSITION TO EXTRAUTERINE LIFE

The lung in utero is distended by fluid secreted through the respiratory epithelium [57, 236–238]. Because of fetal respiratory movement this liquid has opportunity to mix, to a limited extent, with amniotic fluid and its particulates, and it is not uncommon to find fetal squames in the airspaces of any infant who is either stillborn or dies soon after birth.

The transition from intrauterine life to air-breathing requires removal of lung liquid, inflation of the lung with air, and development of sufficient lung stability to provide a pulmonary residual volume [56, 59, 116]. Forces from surface tension in the lung account for most of the collapsing pressure, and lung stability therefore depends to a great extent on the secretion of a surface-active material into the alveolar space and subsequent coating of alveolar and small airway walls. This "surfactant" is composed of a mixture of active ingredients, including phosphatidyl choline and phosphatidyl glycerol [56, 59, 69, 71–73, 236–238]. Protein moieties are present as well [239]. The presence of surfactant in alveolar lumens of the newborn depends on biochemical maturity of enzyme systems involved in phospholipid synthesis and on the release of adequate amounts of this material from the alveolar type 2 cells in which surfactant components are produced [68, 69]. Environmental and hormonal factors that accelerate or impede surfactant production are reviewed elsewhere, but include perinatal stress and steroid production [69, 72]. Insulin appears to impede functional maturation of type 2 cells, a phenomenon that partly explains the susceptibility of infants of diabetic mothers to the neonatal respiratory distress syndrome [69, 72]. Since fetal lung liquid exists in communication with the amniotic fluid, the surface-active material in amniotic fluid can be detected and used in a variety of methods as an index of the biochemical readiness of the fetal lung for extrauterine life [240]. Functional immaturity of the newborn lung may lead to a variety of complications, many iatrogenic, which result in further respiratory impairment. These disorders—hyaline membrane disease, bronchopulmonary dysplasia, and pulmonary interstitial air "emphysema"—constitute the major disorders of the "transition" period. Aspiration of meconium, pulmonary hemorrhage, and perinatal pneumonia are other life-threatening disorders seen in neonates. Disorders of lung structure such as hypoplasia, and also functional disorders such as persistent unexplained pulmonary hypertension in the newborn (per-

sistent fetal circulation), constitute the other major disorders of the immediate neonatal period.

Transient Tachypnea of the Newborn

Transient tachypnea of the newborn, or neonatal wet lung, is a mild disorder caused by delayed clearance of fetal lung liquid [230]. The infants characteristically exhibit mild tachypnea and have an alveolar filling pattern on chest radiographs. The disorder usually remits in 24 to 48 hours and no pathological description exists. Retention of lung liquid within cysts or other congenital lesions may, however, produce unusual and confusing radiographic pictures until the fluid is resolved.

Surfactant Protein-B Deficiency

Genetic disorders of surfactant protein production result in neonatal respiratory distress manifest histologically as an alveolar (air-space) filling disorder that mimics pulmonary alveolar proteinosis in the adult. Any infarct with congenital alveolar proteinosis should be evaluated for surfactant protein (usually SP-B) deficiency [241–244].

Hyaline Membrane Disease

Hyaline membrane disease (idiopathic neonatal respiratory distress syndrome) is a disorder related to deficiency of pulmonary surfactant [57, 63, 116, 237, 245–251]. The most usual cause of the deficit is biochemical immaturity of the lung, but it is clearly possible for multiple types of insult to inactivate surfactant and to damage the delicate enzyme systems involved in its production and secretion. The end result is high surface tension inside alveoli, with production of epithelial and endothelial permeability defects essentially comparable to diffuse alveolar damage in the adult. Hyaline membrane disease (HMD) occurs with increased frequency in a rather specific population of infants: premature white males, appropriate in size for their gestational age [237]. Other predisposing factors include maternal diabetes, twin gestation, and birth by caesarean section without a trial of labor. Although quantitative or qualitative deficiency of surfactant is a hallmark and probably the cause of HMD, biochemical surfactant deficiency in the lung may be a complication of many other neonatal lung problems and cannot be used as a sole diagnostic criterion of HMD [245].

Female and non-white infants appear to be relatively protected, as are infants with a variety of prenatal stresses including amniotic fluid infection and growth retardation [116, 247]. HMD has been described in infants at term but any deviation from occurrence in the usual population should cause intense consideration before a diagnosis is made.

Clinically, the affected infant develops respiratory distress at, or soon after, birth. The chest radiograph shows

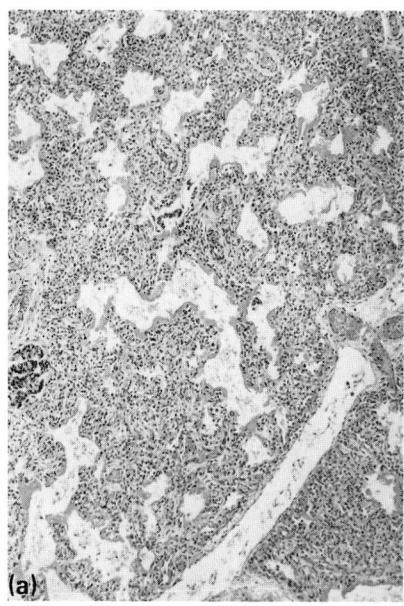

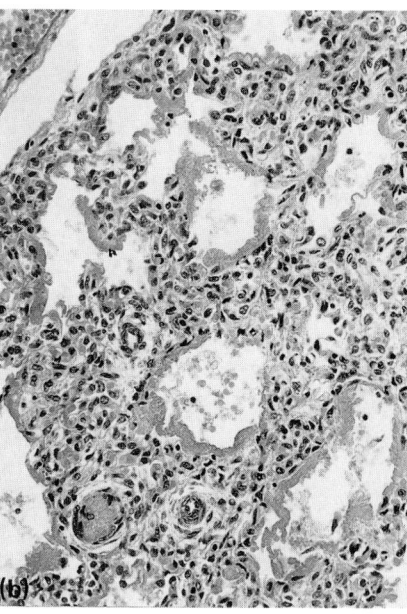

FIGURE 19.25.   *Hyaline membrane disease. (a) Low-power photomicrograph shows the characteristic collapse of airspaces. Septal lymphatics are markedly dilated as well. (×100.) (b) Higher magnification shows the characteristic hyaline membranes lining the distal airways. (×200.)*

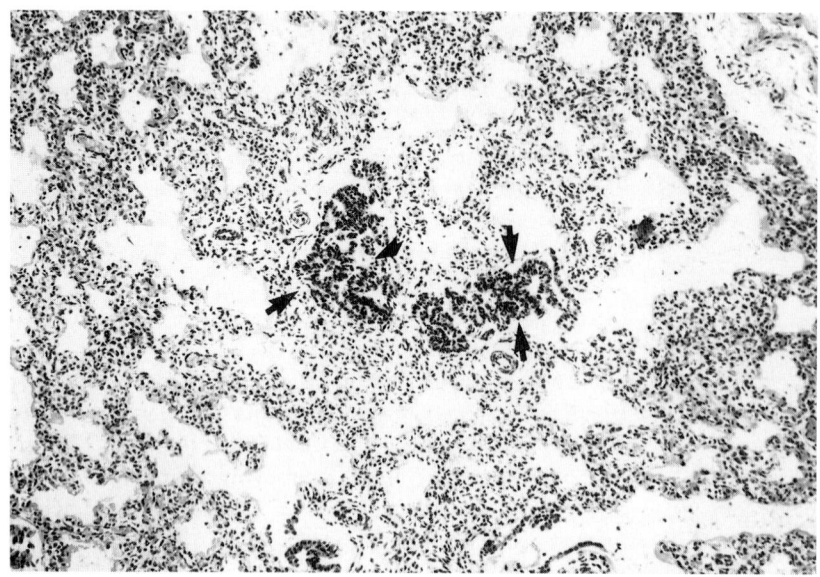

FIGURE 19.26.   *Hyaline membrane disease. Sloughing of bronchiolar epithelium has produced an artifact (arrows) which should not be misinterpreted as a congenital malformation. (×100.)*

ground-glass opacification of the lung fields and "air bronchograms" are seen [230, 249]. On gross inspection, the lungs have a solid or liver-like consistency. Microscopically, the most important feature is uniform airspace collapse [237, 246, 248–250]. The distal airways are dilated and lined by the characteristic eosinophilic membranes (Fig. 19.25). Septal lymphatics are often prominently dilated, and focal alveolar and interstitial hemorrhages and edema fluid may be seen. These features correlate with the radiographic appearance of the chest film in HMD and with physiological features of ventilation–perfusion inequity and decreased pulmonary compliance. The histological features may be altered by the fixative employed (mercury- or chromate-based solutions show the edema fluid more prominently)

[250], the time between death and autopsy [246], and the method of fixation of the lung. Fixation of the lung by perfusion of liquid through the airways removes the air–liquid interface and obscures the morphological effect of abnormally high surface tension on the lung. Under most circumstances, it is best to perfuse one lung with fixative through the bronchial tree and at least to sample the other lung without prior perfusion. In this way, both the expansion pattern and the interstitium of the lung can be examined. Hyaline membranes per se are not diagnostic of primary surfactant deficiency and the histological patterns seen in HMD can be mimicked by infection. In most other entities, however, the alveolar collapse pattern is neither as striking nor as diffuse as that seen in HMD.

Morphological variations of hyaline membrane disease include a peculiar rounded pattern of dilated airways alternating with collapsed alveoli and described by Gruenwald as exaggerated atelectasis [252], and sloughing of bronchial or alveolar epithelium to form a pseudoglandular pattern (Fig. 19.26). In infants dying after several days of disease, yellow-staining of the hyaline membranes, apparently by bilirubin, may be seen [253]. The diagnosis of HMD in very small preterm babies may be difficult histologically because the infants expire before membranes form or because the immature lung may not be able to collapse in the characteristic pattern.

Since most infants with HMD who die have been treated with oxygen, the histological features of resolving HMD are not clearly separable from bronchopulmonary dysplasia (see below) but it appears that an influx of macrophages, repair of alveolar walls, and proliferation of type 2 lining cells are major features [254]. The long-term prognosis of survivors of HMD is difficult to separate from that of preterm birth per se and from bronchopulmonary dysplasia. Prior to the advent of mechanical ventilation, most affected infants either died or recovered by 72 hours after birth. In the modern era, the majority of immediate fatalities from HMD occur in infants weighing less than 1 kg and the percentage of deaths attributable to HMD is greatest between 1 and 1.5 kg [255]. Among affected newborns, deaths secondary to HMD are consistently numerically greater in males [247].

The use of exogenous surfactant therapy has markedly reduced the morbidity and mortality from HMD. Pulmonary hemorrhage seems to be slightly more prevalent in babies who received this therapy but overall pulmonary pathologic change is reduced. This is especially so for pulmonary interstitial air and pneumothorax with its associated complications (see Chap. 3).

Complications of Hyaline Membrane Disease

Hyaline membrane disease in the neonate is associated with a variety of complications; these are often iatrogenic but related to therapeutic measures necessary to preserve life. Patent ductus arteriosus, bronchopulmonary dysplasia, and pulmonary interstitial air are the most common problems.

Patent Ductus Arteriosus   Persistent patency of the ductus arteriosus (PDA) as a complication of HMD has assumed an increasing role as a complication that parallels the increased survival of small neonates with HMD [256–262]. An overall 21% incidence of PDA in newborn babies weighing less than 2500 g was reported from one institution. Several studies have suggested that histological examination can identify a specific feature, the subendothelial elastic lamina, associated with those ducti likely to remain permanently patent [258].

Clinical and physiological symptoms related to the open ductus may vary from those seen in infants with minor problems to those associated with an acute and severe left-to-right vascular shunt. A third group of patients with predominant respiratory symptoms, such as bronchopulmonary

dysplasia (see below), have patent ductus arteriosus as part of their clinical and pathological picture. The exact role that the ductus plays in the production of pulmonary disease in neonates is not clear, although there is evidence that clinical HMD in very-low-weight newborn babies may be more a manifestation of ductal patency than of surfactant deficiency [260].

Factors promoting patency of the ductus are multiple and include hypoxia, E-type prostaglandins, and perhaps the naturally deficient musculature of large fetal pulmonary arteries [259]. In one study, infants treated with the diuretic furosemide had a higher risk of persistent ductal patency [120]. Both surgical and pharmacological methods for closure of the ductus have been effective [259].

Just as antenatal stress appears to reduce the incidence of HMD, there is morphological evidence that "maturation" and accelerated closure of the ductus may occur in preterm infants exposed to chronic intrauterine stress [261].

Other reported neonatal problems involving the ductus include necrosis [256] and aneurysm formation [262].

Bronchopulmonary Dysplasia   Bronchopulmonary dysplasia (BPD) is a complex, multistage, structural, and physiological alteration of the lungs that occurs as a prolonged response to acute injury in the neonatal period [116, 124, 230, 248, 263–282]. The acute insult was originally considered to be mechanical ventilation and high concentration of inspired oxygen in infants treated for HMD. Further studies have expanded the syndrome and it has been suggested that oxygen alone and mechanical ventilation without high oxygen concentration can also produce BPD [263, 264]. Furthermore, it appears that BPD can occur as a response to lung injury other than that associated with hyaline membrane disease [263, 264].

The typical infant with BPD is premature, has developed hyaline membrane disease, and has required prolonged ventilatory support [263, 264]. The incidence of BPD varies with the birthweight of the population studied, ranging from 10% in infants over 2500 g to 40% or even higher as birthweight decreases toward 1000 g [263, 264]. The original histological description of the evolution of BPD by Northway et al is still useful [248, 249] but has been refined somewhat in a classification proposed by Anderson and Engel (Table 19.6 [265]). All of the stages and histological features are based on infants studied at postmortem examinations, so it is difficult, if not impossible, to know whether one is actually observing an orderly progression of disease in these stages or whether different tissue responses or degrees of injury in individual patients account for the histological differences seen in patients dying early or late in the course of BPD. Furthermore, the relevance of lesions seen at postmortem examination to possible lung disease in survivors is not yet known. Diffuse alveolar damage and possibly reversible bronchiolar necrosis and obstruction characterize the early phase of the disease, while interstitial fibrosis is the predominant and probably irreversible feature of the late stage of the disease [263–266]. The histological changes

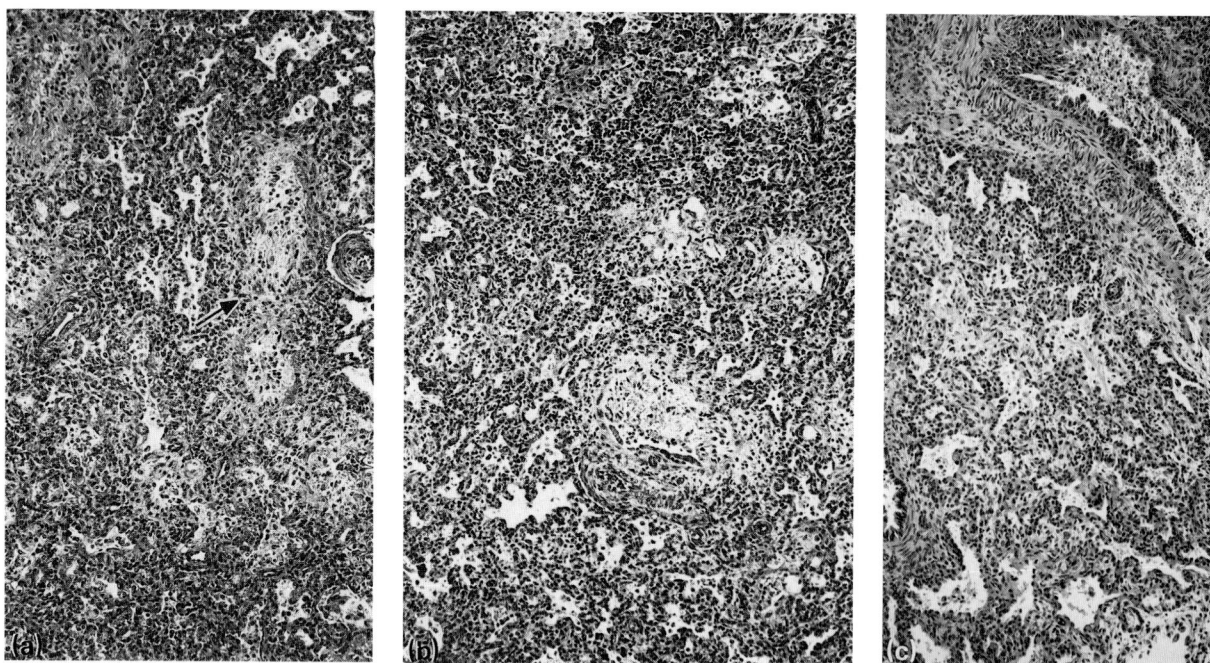

FIGURE 19.27. *Acute phase of bronchopulmonary dysplasia. (a) Acute bronchiolar necrosis, (b) fibroplasia in the lumen of bronchioles, (c) bronchiolitis obliterans. The bronchiolar muscle (arrow) remains identifiable. Elastic stains may be necessary to separate obliterated airways from vessels. (×200.)*

Table 19.6. Bronchopulmonary dysplasia: evolution

Stage	Pathological Features
Exudative, early reparative	Hyaline membranes, bronchial necrosis bronchiolitis obliterans, bronchiolectasis
	Early septal fibrosis
Subacute, fibroproliferative	Bronchiolitis obliterans, bronchiolectasis
	Rare residual hyaline membranes
	Type 2 cell hyperplasia/regeneration
	Perialveolar duct fibrosis,
	Increasing interstitial fibrosis, smooth-muscle proliferation
	Overexpanded/collapsed acini
Chronic, fibroproliferative	Interstitial fibrosis, smooth-muscle proliferation
	Honeycomb lung
	Vascular wall thickening
	No bronchiolitis obliterans or bronchiolectasis

(Modified from Anderson & Engel [265].)

seen in infants dying early in the course of BPD (1 to 2 weeks) are those of hyaline membrane disease upon which has been engrafted bronchiolar necrosis and obliterative, reparative bronchiolitis (Fig. 19.27). In some cases, fibrous obliteration of the bronchiolar lumen may lead to erroneous interpretation of the tubular structure as an artery. Elastic tissue stains showing the single submucosal fenestrated elastic lamina of the airway will resolve the question. Cystic dilatation of alveolar ducts and bronchioles may be a prominent feature (Fig. 19.28) [263, 264]. The ductus arteriosus is often patent at this stage.

Infants dying from 2 to 4 weeks after the onset of BPD show a subacute fibroproliferative stage of the disease [265]. Interstitial and perialveolar duct fibrosis becomes prominent. Reactive alveolar type II pneumocytes line the restructured airspaces and there is proliferation of interstitial capillaries. Small round cells in the alveolar wall interstitium may be interpreted as inflammatory cells but often can be identified as smooth muscle or as myofibroblasts by electron microscopy. The prominent restructuring of distal lung parenchyma is clearly analogous to the honeycombing and interstitial fibrosis which occur in the adult lung as a response to diffuse alveolar damage.

The chronic fibroproliferative stage of BPD is seen in infants dying several to many months after the onset of disease [263, 264, 267]. Hyaline membranes are no longer seen. Interstitial fibrosis is prominent and smooth-muscle hyperplasia may be seen in the septal wall (Fig. 19.29). Alternating areas of overexpanded and collapsed airspaces are present. The origin of this phenomenon is not clear. Air-trapping, true destructive emphysema, and honeycomb change may all play a role [263–266]. One might expect that loss of small airways may contribute to airtrapping, but

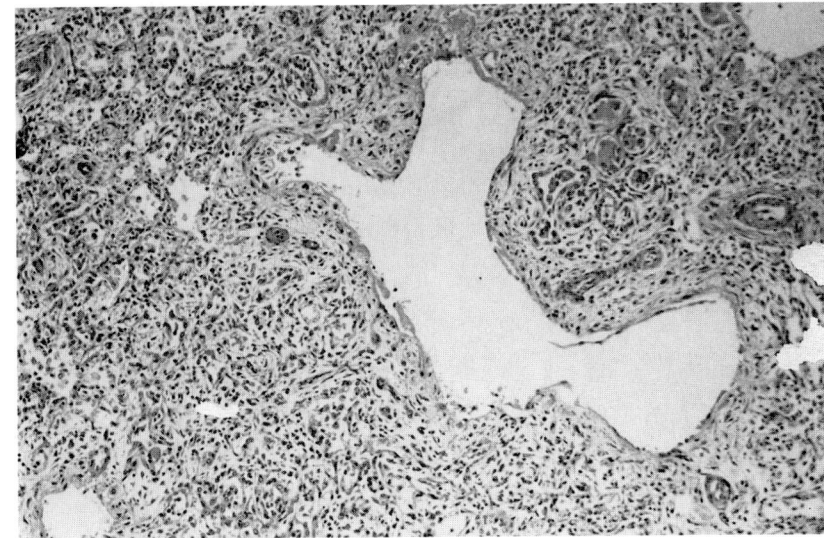

FIGURE 19.28.   *Bronchopulmonary dysplasia, subacute stage. Cystic bronchiolectasis and interstitial fibroplasia are seen. (×200.)*

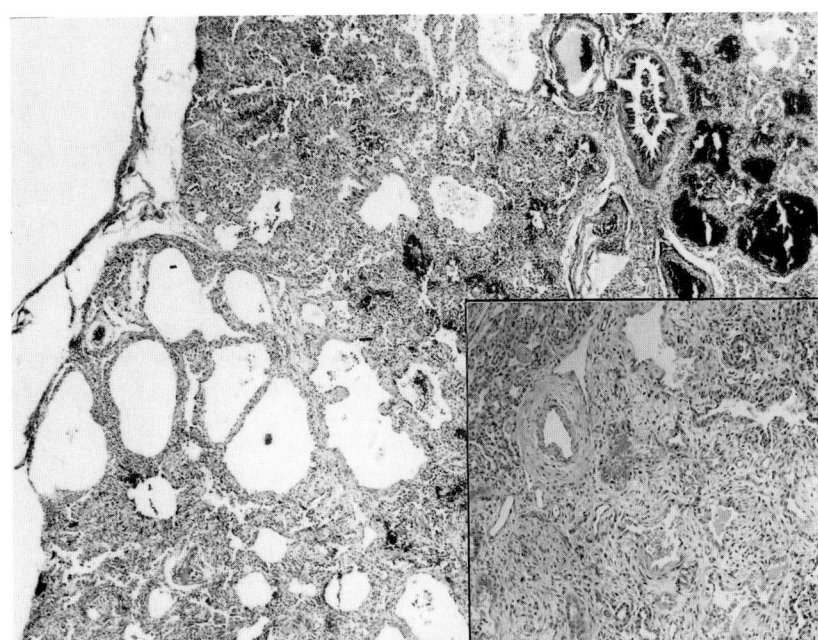

FIGURE 19.29.   *Late stage "healed" bronchopulmonary dysplasia. Interstitial fibrosis and honeycombing are characteristic features (inset, ×200). Bronchiolar lesions are not prominent. (×100.)*

in one morphometric study of a single case, this hypothesis could not be confirmed [268]. In contrast to the early stages of BPD, bronchiolitis obliterans is no longer seen, although squamous metaplasia may be found in the bronchial epithelium. Morphological evidence of pulmonary hypertension is often present (medial hyperplasia and intimal thickening of small arteries) and cor pulmonale may supervene.

There is, in general, only broad radiographic correlation with the pathological stage [263, 264, 269], and several studies have suggested a role for cytological evaluation of lung washings in the detection of early stages of BPD [270]. Early lung opacity is replaced by hyperinflation and a variety of radiographic "bubbles" in the lung parenchyma [230,

271]. In all stages of BPD, pulmonary interstitial air (see below) and pneumothorax and its complications may be an added clinical and pathological feature. Lobar overinflation or collapse may occur in relation to bronchial trauma, with resultant granulation of tissue and fibrosis causing either partial or complete luminal obstruction in large airways.

Postmortem studies and the availability of open-lung biopsy material have begun to show what is probably a variant or modified pattern of BPD in infants dying 3 or more months after birth [267, 272]. The patients are usually very small preterm infants who may have had either acute respiratory distress at birth (HMD) or the insidious onset of respiratory insufficiency during the first weeks of life. The chest radiograph shows both overexpanded and collapsed

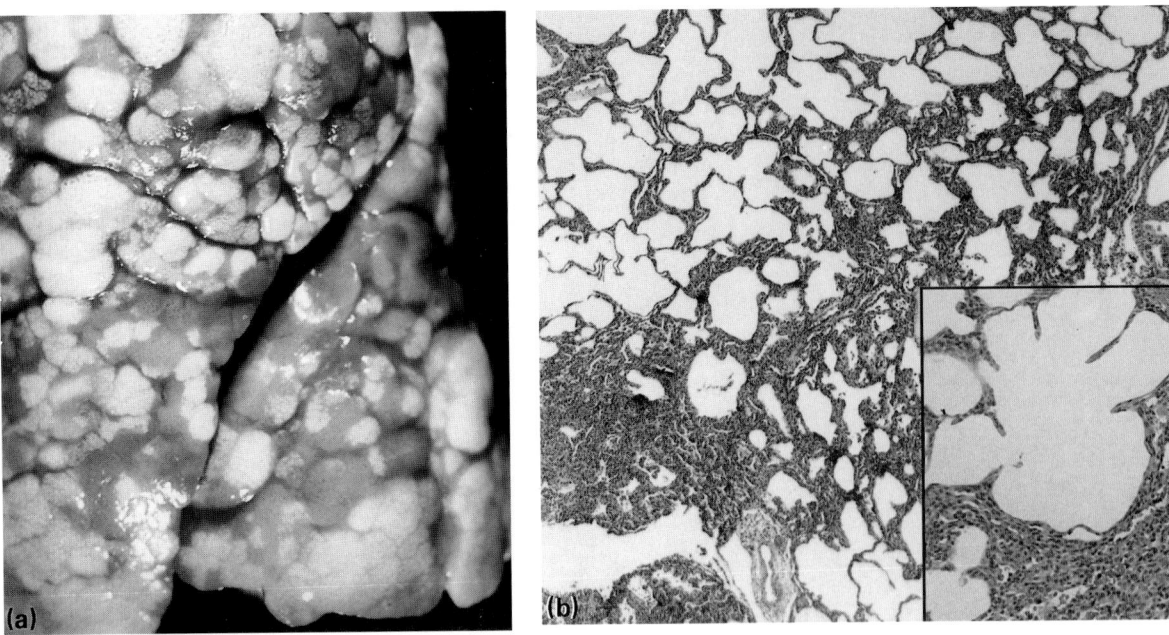

FIGURE 19.30.   *Variant BPD. (a) Gross photograph shows alternating areas of expansion and collapse. (b) Low-power (×200) photomicrograph shows characteristic areas of collapsed alveoli juxtaposed to dilated airspaces. This lesion is characteristically seen in premature infants with three or more months of respiratory symptoms and is probably the same as Wilson-Mikity disease.*

areas in the lung and the infants may have a prominent component of carbon dioxide retention. Microscopically, there are restructured, coalescent airspaces, and areas of over-expanded lung are juxtaposed to areas of collapse (Fig. 19.30). Fibrosis in the interstitium may be minimal in variant BPD. It is possible that this pattern may be an end stage of BPD related to honeycomb lung in the lung with ARDS, but the clinical course and microscopic features suggest that the evolution may be slower and the response less fibroblastic than seen in the acute disease described originally. Perhaps the more variant form is related to altered maturation and development of small premature infant lung than to direct tissue damage by oxygen and barotrauma. Histological similarity and the slow clinical evolution of disease suggest that this variant pattern is the same entity as that described earlier as the Wilson-Mikity syndrome [273].

The etiology of BPD is complex and unclear. Oxygen toxicity and barotrauma are clearly involved but antioxidant deficiency, increased pulmonary epithelial permeability, and blood flow through a patent ductus have also been implicated [263, 264]. Prematurity itself, with abnormal development of alveoli and small airways, may be a factor in the production of chronic effects of BPD [263, 274]. Furthermore, infants with a family history of asthma seem to have an increased susceptibility to bronchopulmonary dysplasia, a phenomenon that suggests a genetically predetermined decrease in tolerance to lung damage [263, 264].

Table 19.7.   Bronchopulmonary dysplasia: complications

Early	Pulmonary interstitial emphysema, pneumothorax
	Interstitial fibrosis
	Patent ductus
	Necrotizing enterocolitis
	Gastroesophageal reflux, aspiration
	Complications of hyperalimentation
	Growth failure, osteopenia
	Transient systemic hypertension
Late	Honeycomb lung
	Tracheal stenosis
	Apneic spells
	Respiratory failure during viral infection
	Small airway disease
	Bronchial hyper-reactivity

(From Nickerson [263] and O'Brodovich & Mellins [264].)

There is some experimental evidence that oxygen toxicity may be more responsible for bronchiolar necrosis than for fibrosis and restructuring of the distal lung parenchyma [275].

Pathophysiological alterations in BPD include hypoxia, CO_2 retention, decreased lung compliance, airflow obstruction, and ventilation perfusion inequity in varying combinations, depending upon the pathological stage of the disease [263, 264].

Many complications of BPD (Table 19.7) occur in relation to therapy but are not related directly to the lower respiratory tract [263, 264, 271, 275–279]. Tracheal scarring and stenosis may result from intubation. Necrotizing tracheobronchitis (see Fig. 19.3) has been reported as a complication of high-frequency jet ventilation [280]. Spells of apnea and of unexplained cyanosis are not uncommon. Feeding difficulties, including aspiration, gastroesophageal reflux and rumination occur frequently. Fat emboli may result from intravenous hyperalimentation [278]. Growth failure is common and osteopenia with multiple fractures may also occur. Long-term complications of BPD [276, 278, 279] include ramifications of psychosocial family trauma, recurrent respiratory problems with a distinct risk of respiratory failure during viral infection, and an apparent increased risk for the sudden infant death syndrome [279]. Central nervous system deficits may be demonstrable. Studies on 5- or 10-year survivors of BPD are not complete, but there is good evidence for small airway dysfunction and bronchial hyperreactivity [277]. There is some suggestion that children with BPD may be at risk of chronic airflow obstruction as adults [263, 264].

Pulmonary Interstitial Air   Pulmonary interstitial air or "pulmonary interstitial emphysema" (PIE), persistent interstitial pulmonary interstitial emphysema (PIPE), and resultant pneumothorax may occur spontaneously in neonates, but are usually a complication of hyaline membrane disease, BPD, or meconium aspiration in that population [283–292]. Infants with pulmonary hypoplasia are also at risk of PIE. Dissection of air into the connective tissue of bronchovascular bundles or interlobular septa may be followed by pneumothorax, pneumomediastinum, or pneumopericardium [285, 289].

In rare instances, pneumoperitoneum may occur, but that complication is much more likely to be a consequence of perforation of the stomach or of neonatal necrotizing enterocolitis. The radiographic appearance of PIE is that of coarse, linear cysts or bubbles which may coalesce to form large subpleural air collections (pseudocysts) [283].

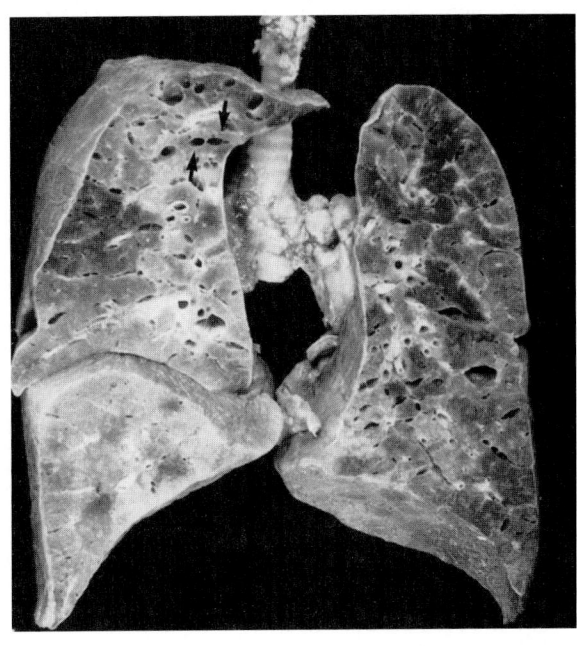

FIGURE 19.31.   *Acute diffuse pulmonary interstitial emphysema. Linear sausage-shaped spaces are seen* (arrows) *along interlobular septa and bronchovascular bundles.*

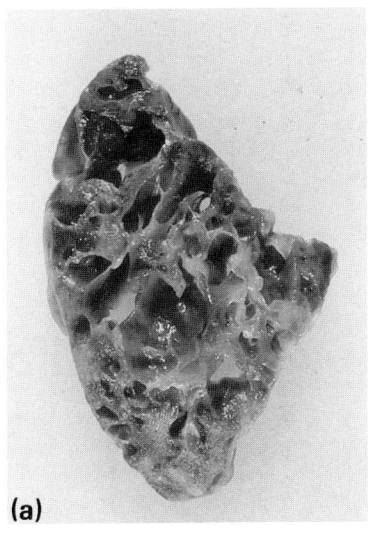

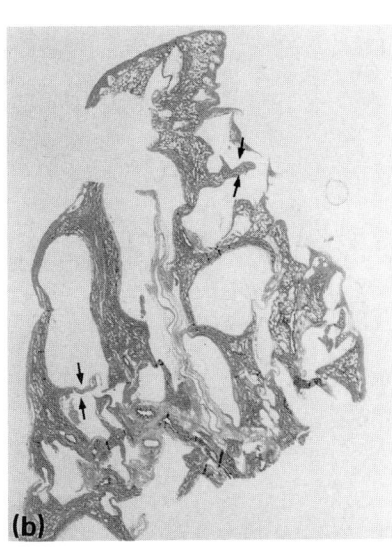

(a)   **(b)**

FIGURE 19.32.   *Lobar pulmonary interstitial emphysema. (a) Multiple cysts have replaced the parenchyma. This lesion presented as an expanding mass in the left upper lobe. (b) Low-power photomicrograph shows that air cysts have compressed the alveoli. The papillary structures* (arrows) *are residual bronchovascular bundles. (×40.)*

Several forms of persistent (present for several days) PIE are seen clinically [177]. The most common is that of diffuse multilobar involvement, but localized unilobar disease, or at least exaggerated involvement of a single lobe, may also occur [289–291]. In that instance, the major physiological problem is an expanding mass lesion in the thorax. Surgical therapy may be necessary. "Air block" is a rare phenomenon in which the hilar arteries and veins are compressed and occluded by the dissecting air [285, 288].

The pathogenesis of these pulmonary air-leak syndromes in the neonate is that of alveolar rupture, with escape of air into the interstitium [285, 288]. In contrast to older children and adults, neonatal air leakage is rather commonly associated with dissection of air into the septal lymphatics and even veins. Endolymphatic and intravenous air may then produce systemic emboli in the brain and other organs

[287]. Chest tube perforation of the lung may be an iatrogenic complication of therapy.

The characteristic gross pathological feature of diffuse pulmonary interstitial air is the presence of linear sausage-shaped spaces following septa and airways (Fig. 19.31). Subpleural blebs may also be seen. In lobar PIE, the spaces may be so large and round as to suggest a congenital cystic anomaly of the lung (Fig. 19.32). Microscopically, the air-filled spaces are variable in size and shape, and are often associated with destruction of adjacent lung parenchyma (Fig. 19.33). In persistent PIE, prominent giant cells forming a foreign-body reaction may be seen lining the wall of whatever tissue the air has invaded (Fig. 19.34).

The differential diagnosis of PIE includes pulmonary lymphangiectasis as the most common cause of confusion. Cystic forms of adenomatoid malformation may be suggested when interstitial air is localized. Post-infarction sub-

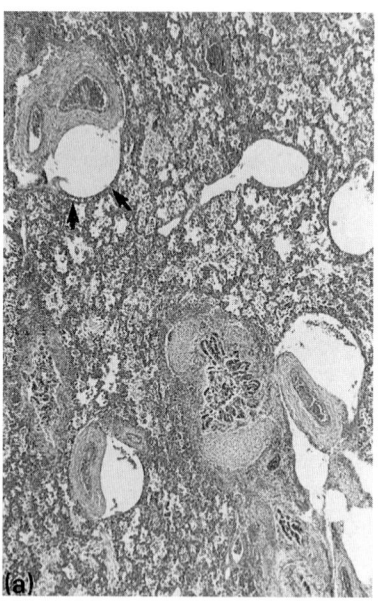
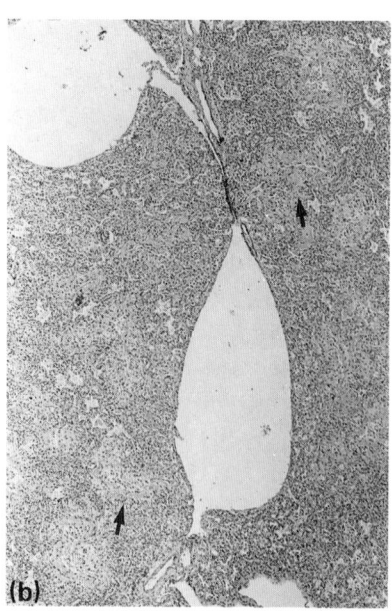

FIGURE 19.33.   *Acute pulmonary interstitial emphysema. (a) This patient aspirated meconium. Air has dissected into the septa and bronchovascular bundles (arrow). (b) Pulmonary interstitial emphysema in a patient with bronchopulmonary dysplasia. Air has dissected into the interlobular septa. Light areas (arrows) represent obliterative fibroplasia in bronchioles. (×100.)*

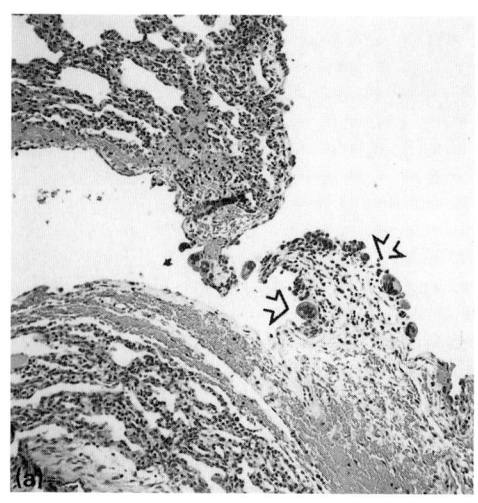
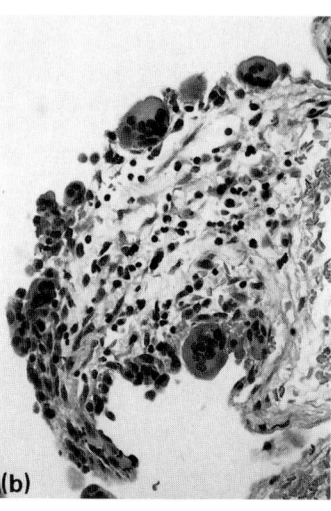

FIGURE 19.34.   *Persistent pulmonary interstitial emphysema. Dissection of air has produced a foreign-body reaction with giant cells. Arrows in (a) indicate area shown at higher power on the photomicrograph (b).*

pleural cysts are discussed in the section on pulmonary emboli.

Pulmonary Hemorrhage

Focal intra-alveolar or interstitial hemorrhage is not an unusual histological finding in the lungs of infants with hyaline membrane disease, BPD, or other neonatal lung disorders [293]. Massive bleeding into airways, airspaces, and, to some extent, the interstitium is a distinct clinical and pathological entity [293–297]. The affected infants are predominantly male, preterm, small for gestational age, or those who have suffered birth asphyxia or some other perinatal stress [295]. Both stillborn and liveborn infants manifest the lesion. Clinically, the affected infant collapses suddenly, usually in the first week of life, with blood-stained fluid pouring from the trachea and nose.

Microscopically, these are confluent areas of hemorrhage with blood filling the alveoli and dissecting into the interstitium [293, 294]. The presence of other pathological lesions, such as HMD or BPD, does not exclude the diagnosis of massive pulmonary hemorrhage.

The etiology of this disorder, other than a relationship to perinatal stress and asphyxia, is unknown. Multiple theories have been proposed, including a stress reaction to cold, to increased spinal fluid pressure, or to increased pulmonary blood flow and pressure. Capillary fragility and coagulation abnormalities have been suggested as well [294, 296, 297]. The occurrence of massive hemorrhage, predominantly in SGA preterm babies, suggests that the lesion is not an exaggerated form of hyaline membrane disease because intrauterine stress associated with growth retardation should stimulate the surfactant system.

Two clinical definitions are not particularly helpful to the pathologist. One defines BPD as present in a preterm infant who requires assisted respiration or oxygen therapy beyond 28 days of life. The other clinical definition is that BPD is present in infants who require continued oxygen therapy beyond 36 weeks' gestational age. Liquid ventilation with perfluorocarbon solution is another new method of treatment. Experience in neonates is limited, but patients subjected to barotrauma have benefited from liquid ventilation, sometimes alternated with extracorporeal membrane oxygenation (ECMO).

Meconium Aspiration

Acute intrauterine stress may cause the infant to pass meconium into the amniotic fluid and, concomitantly, to make deep respiratory movements [298–303]. Symptomatic aspiration of meconium is usually seen at delivery in term or posterm infants of appropriate gestational size.

Tenacious, mucoid, green meconium may coat the infant and placenta and can be seen in the larynx and trachea as well. Radiographically, patchy areas of infiltrate consistent with aspiration are seen, and there may be pulmonary interstitial air and pneumothorax. The latter two features are related to air-trapping distal to the airways that are partially obstructed by mucus and debris from the meconium [230].

The mortality of severe meconium aspiration is still high [298, 299]. At postmortem examination of infants dying soon after aspiration, the lungs often have a silvery green discoloration and sticky meconium can be seen in the bronchi. Microscopically, airways are obstructed not only by masses of fetal squamous cells but by aggregated mucus as well (Fig. 19.35). Bacterial infection and chemical pneumonitis associated with the components of meconium may supervene and, in infants dying later in the course of disease, mucus and even squames may not be obvious. At least one subset of infants with the meconium aspiration syndrome has morphological evidence of pulmonary hypertension, manifest microscopically by abnormally muscularized small pulmonary arteries [302]. This group may have had chronic intrauterine stress. Aspiration of vernix caseosa has been reported as a rare entity that may produce a similar clinical but not microscopic picture to that of meconium inhalation [303].

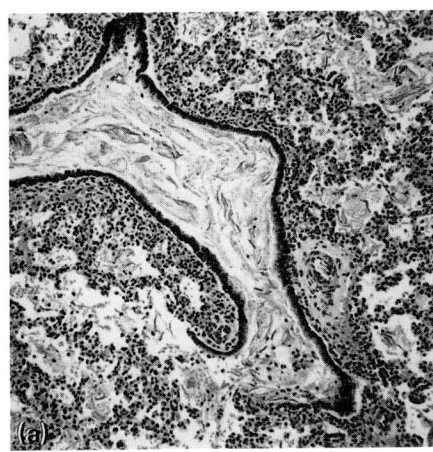
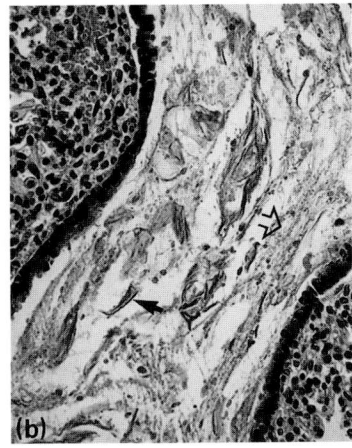

FIGURE 19.35.   *Meconium aspiration. (a) A bronchiole is filled with aspirated debris. (×100.) (b) At higher magnification not only squames (closed arrow) but, more importantly, mucin (open arrow) can be seen in the lumen. (×200.)*

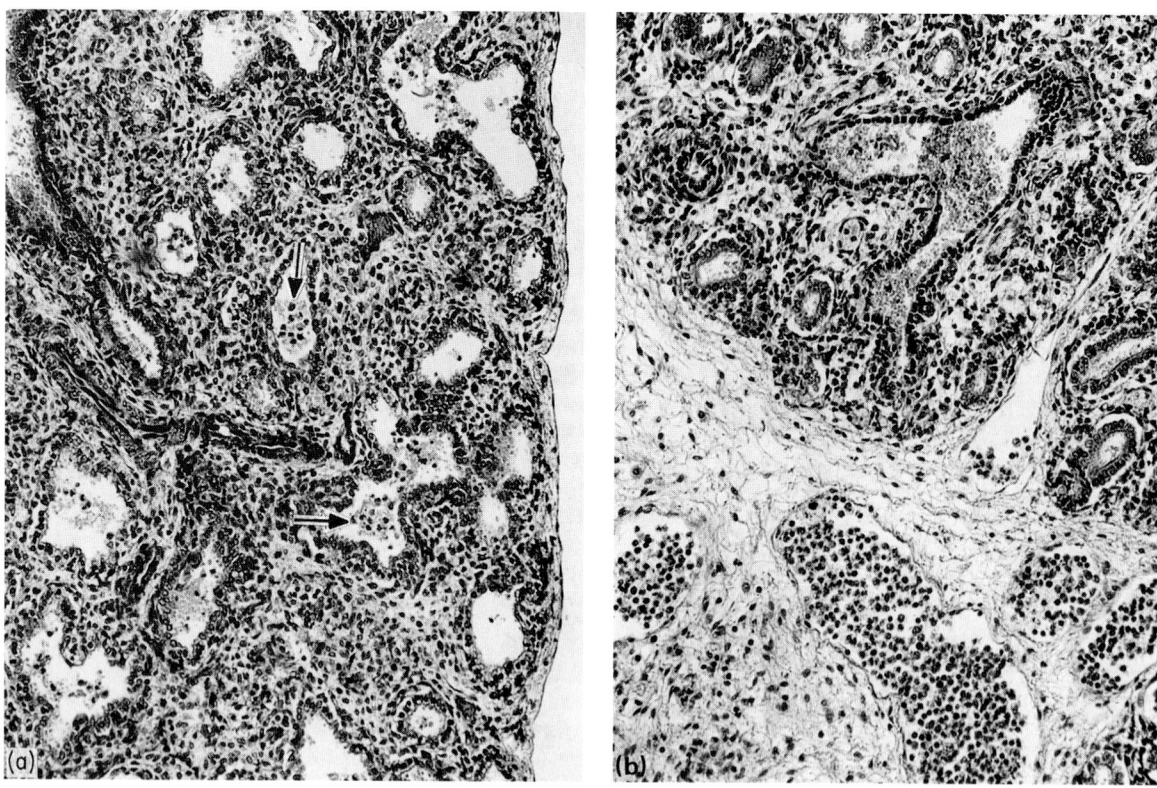

FIGURE 19.36.   *Intrauterine pneumonia. Preterm stillborn infants with amniotic fluid infection syndrome. (a) This infant has aspirated infected amniotic fluid. The intra-alveolar polys (arrows) are mostly of maternal origin. (×200.) (b) In this case, the lung vessels (bottom) are filled with polys as the fetus mounts a response to infection. (×200.)*

Table 19.8.   Perinatal pneumonia

Transplacental	Part of a systemic congenital infection, usually of maternal origin
Intrauterine	Present at birth; a form of aspiration pneumonia associated with infected amniotic fluid; usually due to organisms in the maternal vagina
Acquired during birth	Signs appear in the first week of life, usually associated with maternal vaginal infection
Acquired after birth	Appears in the first month of life; organisms acquired from the environment

The presence of isolated foci of fetal squames in alveoli is not unusual in any infant dying in the perinatal period, and squames alone do not prove that meconium aspiration has occurred.

Many babies with meconium aspiration syndrome (and diaphragmatic hernia with hypoplastic left lung) have been treated with extracorporeal membrane oxygenation therapy (ECMO). Early uses of this treatment had many problems with complications, mostly related to thromboembolic lesions and fluid balance. Refinements in techniques have improved the outcome with ECMO.

Perinatal Pneumonia

Certain general principles and a few specific disorders need to be considered in relation to infections in the lungs of the newborn.

Pulmonary infection is a common finding in neonatal postmortem examinations [116, 195, 196, 230, 304–310]. Pneumonia as a primary or complicating phenomenon was found in 36% of cases in the British Perinatal Mortality Survey and, including the "amniotic fluid infection syndrome," was thought to account for approximately 20% of neonatal deaths in the US Collaborative Perinatal Project [306]. The organisms and pathological manifestations vary with the clinical features. Pneumonias in the perinatal period can be classified on the basis of time of appearance of the lesion and how it was acquired (Table 19.8).

Congenital (Intrauterine) Pneumonia

Congenital intrauterine pneumonia is essentially a form of aspiration pneumonia and usually accompanies ascending infection of the amniotic fluid from a vaginal source. Both gram-positive and gram-negative organisms may be involved. Clusters of polymorphonuclear cells are found in bronchi and alveoli and concomitantly the placental membranes are inflamed. The membranes may have ruptured prematurely but it has been suggested that in many cases infection is the cause rather than the result of membrane rupture [116]. The presence of pulmonary vessels filled with polymorphonuclear cells has been used as a microscopic feature to differentiate infants with "true" pulmonary infection from those who drowned in pus from aspirated infected amniotic fluid. Basically, however, these lung findings represent different portions of the spectrum of the same disease (Fig. 19.36).

Pneumonia Acquired During Birth

Pneumonia acquired during birth usually represents a reaction to organisms acquired from the birth canal [116]. Group B streptococcal infection (GBS) has attracted major attention as an example of this phenomenon because of its rapidly fatal course and the histological feature, in some cases, of hyaline membranes, which may be interpreted as a manifestation of surfactant deficiency and thus obscure the true diagnosis of infection [304, 305, 307]. When present, the hyaline membranes often contain rows of gram-positive

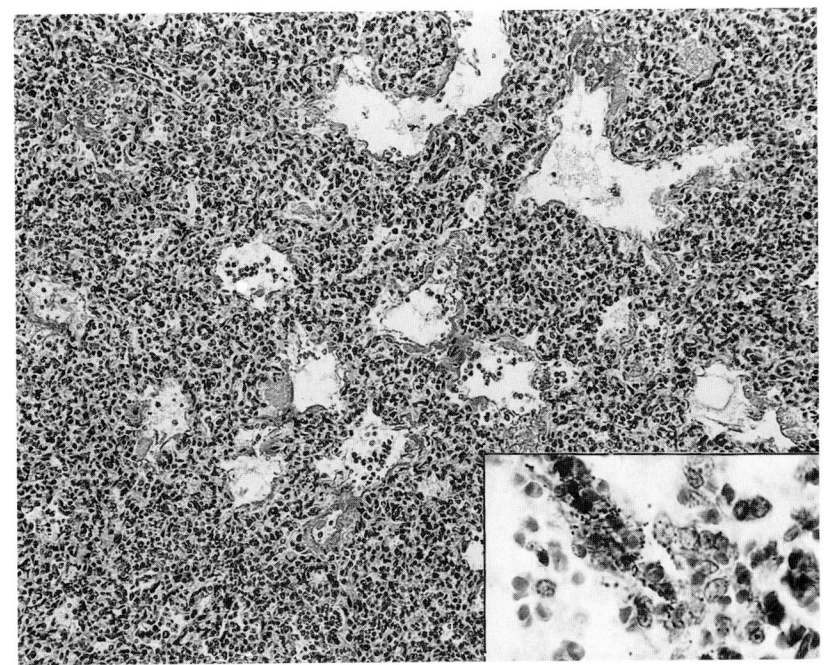

FIGURE 19.37. *Group B streptococcal pneumonia. Partial alveolar collapse and hyaline membranes may simulate hyaline membrane disease. The membranes in this case, however, are lined (inset, ×600) by cocci. Note the paucity of polymorphonuclear cells. (×100.)*

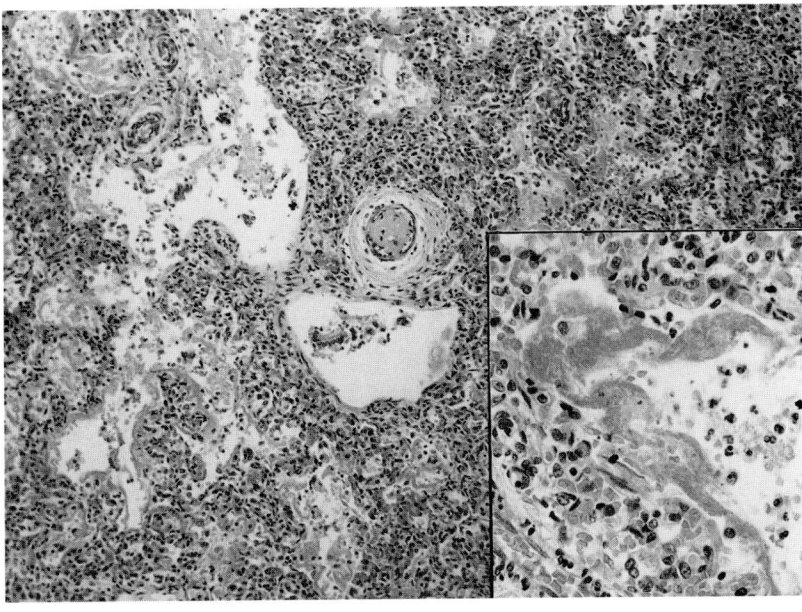

FIGURE 19.38. *Group B streptococcal pneumonia. Hyaline membranes and polymorphonuclear cells are seen in airways and airspaces. Alveolar collapse is not uniform. (×100.) (inset, ×400.)*

cocci (Figs 19.37 and 19.38) and there may, in fact, be an alveolar collapse pattern suggesting HMD. In other cases, cocci, polys, and edema fluid may fill the alveoli and in rare cases there may be a paucity of polymorphonuclear cells in the lung and in the circulating blood [304, 305]. A late-onset form of the disease with sepsis and meningitis may also be seen [307]. Group B streptococcal infection may also be acquired prior to delivery as a congenital pneumonia related to infected amniotic fluid [116]. Other causes of postnatal early-onset pneumonia are coliform organisms. *Haemophilus* infection may produce a clinical and pathological disease that mimics Group B streptococcal disease [116].

Although many viral pneumonias are acquired transplacentally, herpes infection may occur as a result of delivery of the infant through a vagina with active herpetic lesions [116, 307]. Adenovirus pneumonia is a rare cause of perinatal death [309]. Chlamydial pneumonitis is a distinctive pneumonitis in the neonate. The disease usually presents around 3 weeks of age with tachypnea and a staccato cough. Conjunctivitis may be seen in up to 50% of affected infants and an absolute blood eosinophilia is not uncommon [116, 307, 310]. Open-lung biopsy in one reported case showed bronchiolitis and an associated interstitial lymphocytic and plasma cell infiltrate in the pulmonary interstitium.

Late-Onset Pneumonia

Late-onset pneumonia represents a reaction to organisms acquired from human or environmental contacts and includes infection caused by staphylococci, coliform organisms, and pseudomonas, among others [116, 307]. Pulmonary infection with *Candida albicans* may occur as part of a systemic infection in neonates subjected to prolonged intravenous feeding [311]. Other forms of fungal pneumonia are extremely rare in neonates but pulmonary aspergillosis has been reported, usually also as part of a systemic infection [308].

Pulmonary Vascular Disorders in the Newborn

There appear to be marked histological differences in the clinicopathological grading of cardiac-shunt–associated pulmonary hypertension in children as opposed to adults [255, 312–318]. The normal anatomical differences in muscle distribution between the pulmonary arteries of infants and adults (see below) have led to studies that suggest that the classical Heath-Edwards grading system for cardiac-associated pulmonary hypertension may need to be replaced or at least supplemented, in infants, by a grading system that includes muscle distribution and loss of intra-acinar small arteries [313–315].

Persistent Pulmonary Hypertension

Persistent pulmonary hypertension of the newborn (PPHN, persistent "fetal" circulation) is an important cause of mortality in the neonate. The syndrome consists of many disorders that cause persistent high vascular resistance in the lung

Table 19.9.   Anatomical and functional causes of persistent pulmonary hypertension in the newborn (PPHN)

Failure of postnatal decrease in pulmonary vascular resistance (implies normal anatomical prenatal development)
  Increased blood viscosity
  Large unrestricted VSD
  ?Hypoxia
  Venous obstruction, structural or functional

Excessive prenatal muscularization of the distal pulmonary vasculature
  Idiopathic PPHN
  Meconium aspiration
  Congenital heart disease

Developmental decrease in cross-sectional area of the distal pulmonary vasculature
  Pulmonary hypoplasia
  Congenital diaphragmatic hernia
  Alveolar capillary dysplasia

(Modified from Geggel & Reid [313] and Rudolph [317].)

after birth, but the term "PPHN" is often used in reference to the idiopathic form of the disorder [255, 312–314, 317]. The classification proposed by Rudolph divides the etiologies of PPHN into several disparate categories (Table 19.9) [317]. The infants present with cyanosis, respiratory distress, and evidence of right-to-left shunt with elevated pulmonary artery pressure. By definition, cardiac anomalies causing pulmonary hypertension could be considered as part of the syndrome of PPHN, but most authors consider that etiology separately. Patients with pulmonary hypoplasia or diaphragmatic hernia (see below) commonly have PPHN, presumably as a consequence of reduced cross-sectional area of the pulmonary vascular bed [319]. In the idiopathic form a variety of perinatal stresses, such as fetal hypoxia and premature closure of the ductus arteriosus, have been postulated as responsible for increased pulmonary vascular smooth-muscle development [255, 314]. Leukotrienes have been suggested as a cause of pulmonary artery constriction [318]. Obstruction of an anatomically normal pulmonary arterial bed might occur in the presence of hyperviscosity of the neonate's blood or, as frequently seen in PPHN, in association with thrombi either in situ or as emboli from a pulmonary valve affected by non-bacterial endocarditis [320].

Microscopically, the idiopathic form of PPHN is characterized by a distinctive alteration of the normal muscular pattern of small pulmonary arteries [313, 314]. In the normal fetus at term and in the neonate, the intra-acinar pulmonary arteries distal to the level of the terminal bronchiole lack a muscular medial coat [313]. A muscular wall is ordinarily not well developed in these arteries until adolescence. In infants with idiopathic PPHN, there is abnormal extension of muscle into small intra-acinar arteries with resultant compromise of the lumen. In addition, there is proliferation of connective tissue in the adventitia of these vessels [313]. This remodeling is considered to represent the development of new muscle and not persistence of fetal musculature or constriction of normal arteries. The nature of the lesion suggests that it occurs before birth, probably in response to intrauterine stress. As noted above, intravascular thrombi and non-bacterial endocarditis are frequently associated with the other histological findings described for idiopathic PPHN.

Extracorporeal membrane oxygenation (ECMO) has been used to treat babies with PPHN. More recently nitric oxide, a potent pulmonary arterial vasodilator, has been successfully employed to improve oxygenation in these babies. Complications from nitric oxide therapy have included massive intracranial hemorrhage and methemoglobinemia. Ironically, nitric oxide may inhibit surfactant function.

Pulmonary Veno-Occlusive Disease

Pulmonary veno-occlusive disease has been described in neonates. In slightly older infants, the lesion has simulated sudden unexplained infant death. The characteristic fibrous obliteration of intrapulmonary veins may be overlooked unless the lesion is suspected and elastic tissue stains are used in interlobular septa [321–324]. Focal perivascular hemorrhages and iron-laden macrophages may also be a prominent feature (Fig. 19.39).

Pulmonary Emboli

Pulmonary emboli are not uncommon in the lungs of infants dying in the neonatal period. Often, foreign material, presumably fragments of catheters or other material used in life support, can be seen in association with a thrombus [116, 124]. Non-bacterial thrombotic encarditis may be the source of multiple thromboemboli in the lung [320]. Stocker et al reported several infants with peripheral subpleural lung

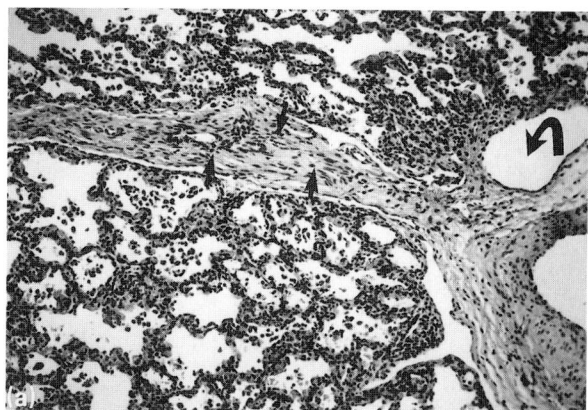

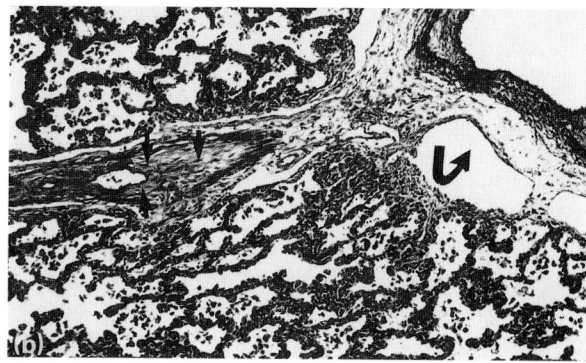

FIGURE 19.39.   *Pulmonary veno-occlusive disease (PVOD) is a rare cause of pulmonary hypertension in infants. Ordinary H&E stains (a) may show septal fibrosis (straight arrows), but the fact that the veins are occluded by fibrous tissue may be clear only with the use of elastic stains (b). Dilated septal and peribronchial lymphatics (curved arrows) and thick-walled pulmonary arteries (not shown) are also prominent features. (a and b, ×200.) (Case courtesy of Dr. Claire Langston, Houston, TX.)*

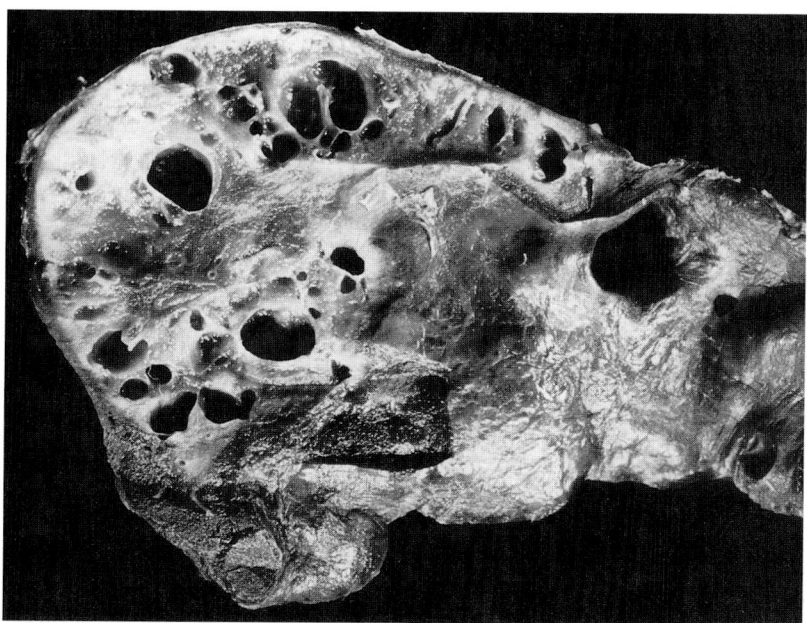

FIGURE 19.40.   *Peripheral subpleural lung cysts. These lesions are probably related to pulmonary artery occlusion and subsequent infarction. (Courtesy of Dr. JT Stocker, Washington, DC.)*

cysts (Fig. 19.40) that were thought to be related to pulmonary artery occlusion and lung infarction [325].

Cystic Fibrosis

Cystic fibrosis is a complex, inherited systemic disorder of exocrine glands with prominent involvement of the respiratory tract [326–328]. Hyperplasia of bronchial submucosal glands and inspissation of mucus may be seen in the newborn infant. Infection, pneumonia, or bronchitis can be seen in neonates but is often a complication of prior abdominal surgery, such as for treatment of meconium ileus.

DISORDERS OF THE DIAPHRAGM

Diaphragmatic Hernia

Congenital posterolateral diaphragmatic (Bochdalek's) hernia occurs in from 1:2000 to 1:5000 livebirths [329–338], but the incidence appears to be higher in stillborn infants and abortuses. At birth, left-sided hernia is much more common, but the incidence of right-sided hernia rises in older children. Overall, the incidence of associated anomalies may be as high as 20%, but infants surviving over 1 hour after birth rarely have other life-threatening malformations [329]. The etiology of the defect is unknown. A small number of familial cases have been reported [330]. There appears to be a notable association of pulmonary extralobar sequestration with diaphragmatic hernia, probably representing incidental early discovery of the lung lesion during diaphragmatic repair [7]. Attenuation rather than absence of the diaphragm is termed "eventration" [331].

Affected infants characteristically present with respiratory distress and bowel sounds in the chest. Most patients develop signs and symptoms at or shortly after birth, but delayed onset of clinical problems may occur [332]. Antenatal ultrasonic diagnosis has been reported. Silverman and Kopelman reported meconium pleuritis in a patient with diaphragmatic hernia and perinatal bowel perforation [333]. Interposition of the colon between the liver and diaphragm (Chilaiditi syndrome) may mimic a right-sided hernia [339]. One of the major complications of congenital diaphragmatic hernia is the development of persistent pulmonary hypertension in the newborn period—either directly at birth or after a "honeymoon" period of normal vascular resistance [334].

Morphological features of congenital diaphragmatic hernia include gross reduction in size of the ipsilateral lung (Fig. 19.41); the contralateral lung shows a varying degree of hypoplasia as well. Morphometric study has shown a reduction in the number of bronchial branches and of pulmonary arteries. The number of alveoli per acinus is normal but the total alveolar number is reduced because there are fewer acinar units [55, 59]. These changes are most marked in the ipsilateral lung but occur in the contralateral lung as

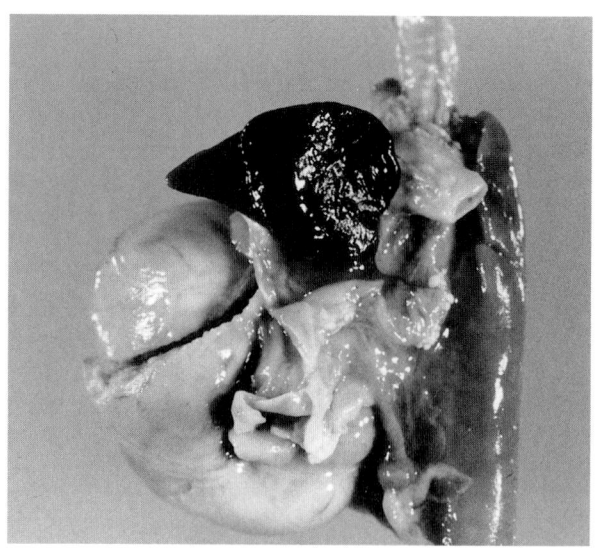

FIGURE 19.41.   *Pulmonary hypoplasia in a patient with left diaphragmatic hernia. The specimen is seen from the posterior aspect.*

well. Reduction in cross-sectional area of the vascular bed produces pulmonary hypertension. In addition, recent studies have shown that infants who have no honeymoon period have excessive muscularization of the distal (intra-acinar) pulmonary arteries and increased medial thickness of pre-acinar arteries as compared to those infants with diaphragmatic hernia who do have an early period of normotensive pulmonary vascular flow [334].

The reported mortality of infants with congenital diaphragmatic hernia varies from 25% to 75%, with the worst outcome in infants symptomatic at or soon after birth [332]. In survivors after surgical repair, pneumothorax and pulmonary hypertension are early causes of mortality. Morphological study in a few survivors has shown destructive emphysema and diminished alveolar and bronchiolar number in the ipsilateral lung. There is a suggestion that compensatory alveolar multiplication may occur on the contralateral side [335]. Extracorporeal membrane oxygenation (ECMO) has been used successfully in treating these patients.

Accessory Diaphragm

Accessory diaphragm is a rare congenital anomaly in which a fibrous membrane divides the hemithorax into two compartments [340]. Most cases involve the right side and the entrapped pulmonary lobe or lobes may be hypoplastic. In some examples, a lower lobe is divided into two parts by the membrane. Associated malformations, such as anomalous venous return or aberrant systemic arterial supply to the lung, are frequent, as are cardiac defects. The disorder is usually diagnosed in adults and is ordinarily not fatal.

Chest-wall anomalies may restrict lung growth but, other than as a feature of dwarfism or "short-rib" syndromes are more likely to be a problem in adolescents or young adults [7]. Apical pneumatoceles, however, do occur in children. In this entity, weakness in or absence of Sibson's fascia is associated with a cervical bulge representing herniation [341].

REFERENCES

1. Dehner LP. *Pediatric Surgical Pathology*. 2nd ed. Baltimore: Williams & Wilkins, 1987.
2. Dehner LP. Tumors and tumor-like lesions of the lung and chestwall in childhood: clinical and pathologic review. In: Stocker JT, ed. *Pediatric Pulmonary Disease*. New York: Hemisphere, 1989, pp. 207–67.
3. Pettinato G, Manivel JC, Saldana MJ, et al. Primary bronchopulmonary fibrosarcoma of childhood and adolescence: reassessment of a low-grade malignancy. Clinicopathologic study of five cases and review of the literature. *Hum Pathol* 1989; 20:463–71.
4. Bluestone CD, Stool SE, eds. *Pediatric Otolaryngology*. Philadelphia: W.B. Saunders, 1983.
5. Ferguson CF, Kendig EL, Jr. *Pediatric Otolaryngology, Vol. II. Disorders of the Respiratory Tract in Children*. Philadelphia: W.B. Saunders, 1972.
6. Kissane JM. *Pathology of Infancy and Childhood*. 2nd ed. St. Louis: C.V. Mosby, 1975.
7. Landing BH, Dixon LG. Congenital malformations and genetic disorders of the respiratory tract (larynx, trachea, bronchi and lungs). *Am Rev Respir Dis* 1979; 120:151–85.
8. Landing BH, Wells TR. Tracheobronchial anomalies in children. *Perspect Pediatr Pathol* 1973; 1:1–32.
9. Gilbert EF, Opitz JM. Malformations and genetic disorders of the respiratory tract. In: Stocker JT, ed. *Pediatric Pulmonary Disease*. New York: Hemisphere, 1989, pp. 29–100.
10. Zaw-Tun HIA. Development of congenital laryngeal atresias and clefts. *Ann Otol Rhinol Laryngol* 1988; 97:353–8.
11. Smith II, Bain AD. Congenital atresia of the larynx. A report of 9 cases. *Ann Otol Rhinol Laryngol* 1965; 74:338–49.
12. Cohen SR, Eavey RD, Desmond MS, May BC. Endoscopy and tracheotomy in the neonatal period. A 10-year review 1967–1976. *Ann Otol Rhinol Laryngol* 1977; 86:1–7.
13. Smith RJH, Catlin FI. Congenital anomalies of the larynx. *Am J Dis Child* 1984; 138:35–9.
14. Fox H, Cocker J. Laryngeal atresia. *Arch Dis Child* 1964; 39:641–5.
15. Silver MM, Thurston WA, Patrick JE. Perinatal pulmonary hyperplasia due to laryngeal atresia. *Hum Pathol* 1988; 19:110–13.
16. Wigglesworth JS, Desai R, Hislop AA. Fetal lung growth in congenital laryngeal atresia. *Pediatr Pathol* 1987; 7:515–25.
17. Benjamin B. Congenital laryngeal webs. *Ann Otol Rhinol Laryngol* 1983; 92:317–26.
18. Hannallah R, Rosales JK. Laryngeal web in an infant with tracheoesophageal fistula. *Anesthesiology* 1975; 42:96–7.
19. Holinger LD, Wong HW, Hemenway WG. Simultaneous glottic and supraglottic laryngeal webs. Report of a case. *Arch Otolaryngol* 1975; 101:496–7.
20. Jazbi B, Goodwin C, Tackett D, Faulkner S. Idiopathic subglottic stenosis. *Ann Otol Rhinol Laryngol* 1977; 86:644–8.
21. Peskine F, Latternand J, Guerrier B, Rodiene M, Brunel D. Membrane laryngie congenitale. A propos de deux observations. *Pediatrie* 1982; 37:391–599.
22. Constantinides CG, Cywes S. Complete median cleft of the mandible and aplasia of the epiglottis. A case report. *S Afr Med J*. 1983; 64:293–4.
23. Healy GB, Holt GP, Tucker JA. Bifid epiglottis: a rare laryngeal anomaly. *Laryngoscope* 1976; 86:1459–68.
24. Burroughs N, Leape LL. Laryngotracheoesophageal cleft: report of a case successfully treated and review of the literature. *Pediatrics* 1974; 53:516–22.
25. Phelan PD, Stocks JD, Williams HE, Danks DM. Familial occurrence of congenital laryngeal clefts. *Arch Dis Child* 1973; 48:275–8.
26. Pillsbury HC, Fischer ND. Laryngotracheoesophageal cleft. Diagnosis, management, and presentation of a new diagnostic device. *Arch Otolaryngol* 1977; 103:735–7.

27. Desanto LW, Devine KD, Weiland LH. Cysts of the larynx—classification. *Laryngoscope* 1970; 80:145–76.
28. Canty TG, Hendren WH. Upper airway obstruction from foregut cysts of the hypopharynx. *J Pediatr Surg* 1975; 10:807–12.
29. Solomons NB, Prescott CAJ. Laryngomalacia: a review and the surgical management of severe cases. *Int J Pediatr Otol Rhinol Laryngol* 1987; 13:31–9.
30. Gentile RD, Miller RH, Woodson GE. Vocal cord paralysis in children 1 year of age and younger. *Ann Otol Rhinol Laryngol* 1986; 95:622–5.
31. Dankle SK, Schuller DE, McLead RE. Risk factors for neonatal acquired subglottic stenosis. *Ann Otol Rhinol Laryngol* 1986; 95:626–30.
32. Dumas C, Patriguin HB, Pare C, Tetreault L. Iatrogenic lesions of the upper airway in the newborn. *J Can Assoc Radiol* 1983; 34:3–7.
33. Marcovich M, Pollauf F, Burian K. Subglottic stenosis in newborns after mechanical ventilation. *Prog Pediatr Surg* 1987; 21:8–19.
34. Lucaya J, Herrera M, Salcedo S. Traumatic pharyngeal pseudo-diverticulum in neonates and infants. Two case reports and review of the literature. *Pediatr Radiol* 1979; 8:65–9.
35. Jacobs RF, Yasida K, Smith AL, Benjamin DR. Laryngeal candidiasis presenting as respiratory stridor. *Pediatrics* 1982; 69:234–326.
36. Effmann EL, Spackman TJ, Berdon WE, Kuhn JP, Leonidas JC. Tracheal agenesis. *Am J Roentgenol Radium Ther Nucl Med* 1975; 125:767–81.
37. Haupt PA, Edwards WD. Two cases of tracheal agenesis. *Am J Dis Child* 1983; 137:498–501.
38. Warfel KA, Schultz DM. Agenesis of the trachea. Report of a case and review of the literature. *Arch Pathol Lab Med* 1976; 100:357–9.
39. Sankaran K, Bhagirath CP, Bingham WT, Hjertaas R, Haight K. Tracheal atresia, proximal esophageal atresia and distal tracheoesophageal fistula: report of two cases and review of the literature. *Pediatrics* 1983; 71:821–3.
40. Anderson CL, Ahmed G, Caldwell CC. Tracheal atresia associated with congenital absence of the radii. An addition to the VATER syndrome. *Clin Pediatr* 1981; 20:479–80.
41. Boutte P, Albertini M, Coussement A, Kreitmann P, Coubierc R, Mariani R. Stenose tracheale congenitale associée à une artere pulmonaire gauche aberrante. A propos d'une forme severe a revelation neonatale. *Pediatre* 1985; 40:539–644.
42. Voland JR, Benirschke K, Saunders B. Congenital tracheal stenosis with associated cardiopulmonary anomalies: report of two cases with a review of the literature. *Pediatr Pulmonol* 1986; 2:247–9.
43. Lacasse JE, Reilly BJ, Mancer K. Segmental esophageal trachea: a potentially fatal type of tracheal stenosis. *Am J Roentgenol* 1980; 134:829–31.
44. Greene DA. Congenital complete tracheal rings. *Arch Otolaryngol* 1976; 102:241–3.
45. Benjamin B, Pitkin J, Cohen D. Congenital tracheal stenosis. *Ann Otol Rhinol Laryngol* 1981; 90:364–71.
46. Maisel RH, Fried MP, Swain R, Spector G. Anomalous tracheal bronchus with tracheal hypoplasia. *Arch Otolaryngol* 1974; 100:69–70.
47. Sotomayor JL, Godinez RI, Borden S, Wilmott RW. Large-airway collapse due to acquired tracheo-bronchomalacia in infancy. *Am J Dis Child* 1986; 140:367–71.
48. Kushner DC, Clifton Harris GB. Obstructing lesions of the larynx and trachea in infants and children. *Radiol Clin N Am* 1978; 16:181–93.
49. Denson SE, Taussig LM, Pond GD. Intraluminal tracheal cyst producing airway obstruction in the newborn infant. *J Pediatr* 1976; 88:521–2.
50. Shikhani AH, Jones MH, Marsh BR, Holliday MJ. Infantile subglottic hemangiomas. An update. *Ann Otol Rhinol Laryngol* 1986; 95:336–47.
51. Close LG, Rosenberg HS, Vogler C, Warshaw HE. Neonatal laryngeal fibromatosis. *Otolaryngol Head Neck Surg* 1981; 89:992–7.
52. Zapf B, Lehmann WB, Snyder GG III. Hamartoma of the larynx: an unusual cause for stridor in an infant. *Otolaryngol Head Neck Surg* 1981; 89:797–9.
53. Cohen SR, Thompson JW. Lymphangiomas of the larynx in infants and children. A survey of pediatric lymphangioma. *Ann Otol Rhinol Laryngol* 1986; 95(Part 2, Suppl. 127):1–20.
54. Spooner BS, Wessells NK. Mammalian lung development: interactions in primordium formation and bronchial morphogenesis. *J Exp Zool* 1970; 875:445–54. 55. Reid LM. Lung growth in health and disease. *Br J Dis Chest* 1984; 78:113–34.
55. Reid LM. Lung growth in health and disease. *Br J Dis Chest* 1984; 78:133–34.
56. Reid LM, Rubino M. The connective tissue septa in the foetal human lung. *Thorax* 1959; 14:3–13.
57. Nelson GH (ed.). *Pulmonary Development. Transition from Intrauterine to Extrauterine Life*. New York: Marcel Dekker, 1985.
58. Langston C, Kida K, Reed M, Thurlbeck WM. Human lung growth in late gestation and in the neonate. *Am Rev Respir Dis* 1984; 129:607–13.

59. Langston C, Thurlbeck WM. Lung growth and development in late gestation and early postnatal life. *Perspect Pediatr Pathol* 1982; 7:203–35.

60. Cooney TP, Thurlbeck WM. The radial alveolar count method of Emery and Mithal: a reappraisal. 1. Postnatal lung growth. *Thorax* 1982; 37:572–9.

61. Cooney TP, Thurlbeck WM. The radial alveolar count method of Emery and Mithal: a reappraisal 2. Intrauterine and early postnatal lung growth. *Thorax* 1982; 37:580–3.

62. Farrell PM. Lung development: *Biological and Clinical Perspectives.* 2 vols. New York: Academic Press, 1982.

63. Thurlbeck WM. Postnatal human lung growth. *Thorax* 1982; 37:564–71.

64. Langston C. Prenatal lung growth and pulmonary hypoplasia. In: Stocker JT, ed. *Pediatric Pulmonary Disease.* New York: Hemisphere, 1989, pp. 1–92.186. Stocker JT. Sequestrations of the lung. *Semin Diagn Pathol* 1986; 3:106–21.

65. Campiche MA, Gautier A, Hernandez EI, Raymond A. An electron microscope study of the fetal development of human lung. *Pediatrics* 1963; 32:976–94.

66. Hage E. The morphological development of the pulmonary epithelium of human foetuses studied by light and electron microscopy. *Z Anat Entwicklungsgesch* 1973; 140:271–9.

67. Adamson IYR, Bowden DH. Derivation of type I epithelium from type 2 cells in the developing rat lung. *Lab Invest* 1975; 32:736–45.

68. Askin FB, Kuhn C. The cellular origin of pulmonary surfactant. *Lab Invest* 1971; 25:260–68.

69. Ballard PL. *Hormones and Lung Maturation.* Berlin: Springer-Verlag, 1986.

70. D'Ercole AJ, Underwood LE. Somatomedin in fetal growth. *Pediatr Pulmonol* 1985; 1:599–606.

71. Hallman M. Fetal development of surfactant: considerations of phosphatidylcholine, phosphatidylinositol and phosphatidylglycerol formation. *Prog Respir Res* 1981; 15:27–40.

72. Robertson B, Van Golde LMG, Batenburg JJ, eds. *Pulmonary Surfactant.* Amsterdam: Elsevier, 1984.

73. Solomon S (ed). Fetal lung development. Proceedings of a workshop held on June 1–3, 1982, ur Val David, Quebec, Canada. *Pediatr Pulmonol* 1985; 1:51–122.

74. Devi B, More JRS. Total tracheopulmonary agenesis associated with asplenia, agenesis of umbilical artery and other anomalies. *Acta Paediatr Scand* 1966; 55:107–16.

75. Booth JB, Berry CL. Unilateral pulmonary agenesis. *Arch Dis Child* 1967; 2:361–73.

76. Mygrind H, Paulsen SM. Agenesis of the right lung. *Arch Pathol Lab Med* 1980; 104:444.

77. Mardini MK, Nyhan WL. Agenesis of the lung. Report of four patients with unusual anomalies. *Chest* 1985; 87:522–7.

78. Ryland D, Reid L. Pulmonary aplasia—a quantitative analysis of the development of the single lung. *Thorax* 1971; 26:602–9.

79. Brereton RJ, Rickwood AMK. Esophageal atresia with pulmonary agenesis. *J Pediatr Surg* 1983; 18:618–20.

80. Josephsen L, Josephsen P, Bistsch KR. Agenesis of the lung. *Pediatr Radiol* 1986; 16:334.

81. Meehan PL, Lovell WW, Ahn JI. Congenital absence of the lung. *J Pediatr Orthop* 1985; 7:708–10.

82. Ostor AG, Stillwell R, Fortune DW. Bilateral pulmonary agenesis. *Pathology* 1978; 10:243–8.

83. Storey CF, Marrangoni AG. Lobar agenesis of the lung. *J Thorac Surg* 1954; 28:536–43.

84. Landing BH. Five (malformation complexes) of pulmonary symmetry, congenital heart disease, and multiple spleens. *Pediatr Pathol* 1984; 2:125–51.

85. Foster-Carter AF. Bronchopulmonary abnormalities. *Br J Tuberc Dis Chest* 1946; 40:111–24.

86. Maesen FPV, Santana B, Lamers J, Brekel B. A supernumerary bronchus of the right upper lobe. *Eur J Respir Dis* 1983; 64:473–6.

87. Lesbros D, Ferran J-L, Rieu D, Jean D. Stenose tracheale congenitale et bronche surnumeraire. *Arch Fr Pediatr* 1979; 36:703–8.

88. Cope R, Campbell JR, Wall M. Bilateral tracheal bronchi. *J Pediatr Surg* 1986; 21:443–4.

89. Remy J, Smith M, Marache P, Nuyts JP. La bronche "tracheale" gauche pathogene. Revue de la litterature à propos de 4 observations. *J Radiol* 1977; 58:621–30.

90. Siegel MJ, Shackleford DG, Francis RS, McAlister WH. Tracheal bronchus. *Radiology* 1979; 130:353–5.

91. Starshak RJ, Sty JR, Woods G, Keitzer FV. Bridging bronchus: a rare airway anomaly. *Radiology* 1981; 140:95–6.

92. Odell J. Anomalous origin of the anterior segmental bronchus of the right upper lobe. *Thorax* 1980; 35:213–4.

93. Chang N, Hertzler JH, Gregg RH, Olfti MW, Brough AJ. Congenital stenosis of the right mainstem bronchus. A case report. *Pediatrics* 1968; 41:739–42.

94. Chan YT, Ng WD, Tymak WP, Kwong ML, Chow CG. Congenital bronchobiliary fistula associated with biliary atresia. *Br J Surg* 1984; 73:240–1.

95. Kalayoglu M, Olcay I. Congenital broncho-biliary fistula association with esophageal atresia and tracheo-esophageal fistula. *J Pediatr Surg* 1976; 11:463–4.

96. Frank JL, Poole CA, Rasas G. Horseshoe lung: clinical, pathologic and radiologic features and a new plain film finding. *Am J Roentgenol* 1986; 146:217–26.

97. Freedom RM, Burrows PE, Moes CAG. "Horseshoe" lung: report of five new cases. *Am J Roentgenol* 1986; 146:211–5.

98. Smith KP, Cavett CM. Segmental bronchomalacia: successful surgical correction in an infant. *J Pediatr Surg* 1985; 20:240–1.

99. Agosti E, DeFilippi G, Fiom R, Chursi F. Generalized familial broncho-malacia. *Acta Paediatr Scand* 1974; 63:616–8.

100. Ramet J, Byloos J, Debree M, Sacro L, Clement P. Neonatal diagnosis of the immotile cilia syndrome. *Chest* 1986; 89:138–40.

101. Page DV, Stocker JT. Anomalies associated with pulmonary hypoplasia. *Am Rev Respir Dis* 1982; 125:216–21.

102. Askenazi SS, Perlman M. Pulmonary hypoplasia: lung weight and radial alveolar count as criteria of diagnosis. *Arch Dis Child* 1979; 54:614–8.

103. Wigglesworth JS, Desai R, Guerrini P. Fetal lung hypoplasia: biochemical and structural variations and their possible significance. *Arch Dis Child* 1981; 56:606–15.

104. Buolley AM, Imbert MC, Dehan M, et al. Hypoplasie pulmonaire bilaterale du nouveaune. Etude clinique et anatomo-pathologique. A propos de 17 cas. *Arch Fr Pediatr* 1982; 125:216–21.

105. Cooney TP, Dimmick JE, Thurlbeck WM. Increased acinar complexity with polyhydramnios. *Pediatr Pathol* 1986; 5:183–97.

106. Cooney TP, Thurlbeck WM. Pulmonary hypoplasia in Down's Syndrome. *N Engl J Med* 1982; 307:1170–3.

107. Davies G, Reid L. Effect of scoliosis on growth of alveoli and pulmonary arteries and on right ventricle. *Arch Dis Child* 1971; 46:623–32.

108. Detroyer A, Yernault J-C, Englert M. Lung hypoplasia in congenital pulmonary valve stenosis. *Circulation* 1977; 56:647–51.

109. Elias S, Boelen L, Simpson JL. Syndrome of camptodactyly, multiple ankylosis, facial anomalies and pulmonary hypoplasia. *Birth Defects, Orig Article Ser* 1978; 14(6B):243–51.

110. Fewell JE, Hislop AA, Ketterman JA, Johnson P. Effect of tracheostomy on lung development in fetal lambs. *J Appl Physiol* 1983; 55:1103–8.

111. Hislop A, Hey E, Reid L. The lungs in congenital bilateral renal agenesis and dysplasia. *Arch Dis Child* 1979; 54:32–8.

112. Langer R, Kaufman HJ. Primary (isolated) bilateral pulmonary hypoplasia: a comparative study of radiologic findings and autopsy results. *Pediatr Radiol* 1986; 16:175–9.

113. Nakayama DK, Glick PL, Harrison MR, Villa RL, Noall R. Experimental pulmonary hypoplasia due to oligohydramnios and its reversal by relieving thoracic compression. *J Pediatr Surg* 1983; 18:347–53.

114. Thibeault DW, Beatty EG Jr, Hall RT, Bowar SK, O'Neill DH. Neonatal pulmonary hypoplasia with premature rupture of fetal membranes and oligohydramnios. *J Pediatr* 1985; 107:273–7.

115. Wigglesworth JS, Desai R. Is fetal respiratory function a major determinant of perinatal survival? *Lancet* 1982; i:264–7.

116. Wigglesworth JS. *Perinatal Pathology.* Philadelphia: W.B. Saunders, 1984.

117. Blott M, Greenough A, Nicolaides KH, Moscoso G, Gibb D, Campbell S. Fetal movements as predictor of favourable pregnancy outcome after oligohydramnios due to membrane rupture in the second trimester. *Lancet* 1987; ii:129–31.

118. Moessinger AC, Fox HE, Higgins A, Rey HR, Al-Haideri M. Fetal breathing movements are not a reliable predictor of continued lung development in pregnancies complicated by oligohydramnios. *Lancet* 1987; ii:1297–300.

119. Currarino G. Williams hypoplasia: a study of 33 cases. *Pediatr Radiol* 1985; 15:15–24.

120. Bozic C. Ectopic fetal adrenal cortex in the lung of a newborn. *Virchows Arch A* 1974; 363:371–4.

121. Chi JG, Shong Y-K. Diffuse striated muscle heteroplasia of the lung. An autopsy case. *Arch Pathol Lab Med* 1982; 106:641–4.

122. Remberger K, Hubner G. Rhabdomyomatous dysplasia of the lung. *Virchows Arch A* 1974; 363:363–9.

123. Campo E, Bombi JA. Central nervous system heterotopia in the lung of a fetus with cranial malformations. *Virchows Arch A* 1981; 391:117–22.

124. Valdes-Dapena M. Iatrogenic disease in the perinatal period as seen by the pathologist. In: Naeye RL, Kissane JM, Kaufman N, eds. *Perinatal Disorders.* Baltimore: Williams & Wilkins, 1981, pp. 382–418.

125. Janny CG, Askin FB, Kuhn CK III. Congenital alveolar dysplasia—an unusual cause of respiratory distress in the newborn. *Am J Clin Pathol* 1981; 76:722–7.

126. Wagenvoort CA. Misalignment of lung vessels: a syndrome causing persistent neonatal pulmonary hypertension. *Hum Pathol* 1986; 17:727–30.

127. Sirkin W, O'Hare BP, Cox PN, et al. Alveolar capillary dysplasia: lung biopsy diagnosis, nitric oxide responsiveness, and bronchial generation count. *Pediatric Pathology & Laboratory Medicine* 1997; 17:125–32.

128. Rutledge JC, Jensen P. Acinar dysplasia: a new form of pulmonary maldevelopment. *Hum Pathol* 1986; 17:1290–3.

129. Stocker JT. Congenital and developmental disease. In: Dail DH, Hammar SP, eds. *Pulmonary Pathology.* 2nd ed. New York: Springer Verlag 1994:155–90.

130. Abe T, Kuribayashi R, Sato M, Nieda S. Direct communication of the right pulmonary artery with the left atrium. *J Thorac Cardiovasc Surg* 1972; 64: 38–44.

131. Berdon WE, Baker DH. Vascular anomalies and the infant lung: rings, slings and other things. *Semin Roentgenol* 1972: 7:39–64.

132. Brundage BH, Gomez AC, Cheitlin MD, Gmelich JT. Systemic artery to pulmonary vessel fistulas. Report of two cases and a review of the literature. *Chest* 1972: 62:19–23.

133. Burn J. Williams syndrome. *J Med Genet* 1986; 23:389–95.

134. Dines DE, Seward JB, Bernatz PE. Pulmonary arterio-venous fistulas. *Mayo Clin Proc* 1983; 58:176–81.

135. Freedman RM, Culhan JAG, Moes CAF. *Angiocardiography of Congenital Heart Disease.* New York: Macmillan, 1984.

136. Goldstein JD, Rabinovitch M, Van Praagh R, Reid L. Unusual vascular anomalies causing persistent pulmonary hypertension in a newborn. *Am J Cardiol* 1979; 43:962–8.

137. Grote WR, Tenholder MF. Pulmonary artery malformation syndrome. *South Med J* 1984; 77:1139–43.

138. Haworth SG, Reid L. Quantitative structural study of pulmonary circulation in the newborn with pulmonary atresia. *Thorax* 1977; 32:129–33.

139. Hislop A, Sanderson M, Reid L. Unilateral congenital dysplasia of lung associated with vascular anomalies. *Thorax* 1973; 28:435–41.

140. Kamio A, Fukushima K, Takebayashi S, Toshima H. Isolated stenosis of the pulmonary artery branches—an autopsy case with review of the literatures. *Jpn Circ J* 1978; 42:1289–96.

141. Keith JD, Rowe RD, Vlad P. *Heart Disease in Infancy and Childhood.* 3rd ed. New York: Macmillan, 1978.

142. Penkoske PA, Castaneda AR, Fyler DC, Van Praagh R. Origin of pulmonary artery branch from ascending aorta. Primary surgical repair in infancy. *J Thorac Cardiovasc Surg* 1983; 85:537–45.

143. Presbitero P, Bull C, Haworth SG, deLaval MR. Absent or occult pulmonary artery. *Br Heart J* 1984; 52:178–85.

144. Pryzbojewski JZ, Maritz F. Pulmonary arteriovenous fistulas. A case presentation and review of the literature. *S Afr Med J* 1980; 57:366–72.

145. Rabinovitch M, Grady S, David I, et al. Compression of intrapulmonary bronchi by abnormally branching pulmonary arteries associated with absent pulmonary valves. *Am J Cardiol* 1982; 50:804–13.

146. Taylor GA. Pulmonary arteriovenous malformation: an uncommon cause for cyanosis in the newborn. *Pediatr Radiol* 1983; 13:339–41.

147. Utzon F, Brandrup F. Pulmonary arteriovenous fistulas in children. A review with special reference to the disperse telangiectatic type illustrated by report of a case. *Acta Paediatr Scand* 1973; 62:422–32.

148. Tang JS, Kauffman SL, Lynfield J. Hypoplasia of the pulmonary arteries in infants with congenital rubella. *Am J Cardiol* 1971; 27:491–96.

149. Pernot C, Deschamps J-P, Didier F. Stenose de l'artere pulmonaire, taches cutaneus pigmentaires et anomalies du squelette. Quatre observations. *Arch Fr Pediatr* 1979; 28:593–603.

150. Haworth SG, Reid L. Structural study of pulmonary circulation and of heart in total anomalous pulmonary venous return in early infancy. *Br Heart J* 1977; 39:80–92.

151. Lucas RV Jr. Anomalous venous connections, pulmonary and systemic. In: Adams FH, Emmanouilides GC, eds. *Moss' Heart Disease in Infants, Children and Adolescents.* 3rd ed. Baltimore: Williams & Wilkins, 1983, pp. 458–500.

152. Godwin JD, Tarver RD. Scimitar syndrome: four new cases examined with CT. *Radiology* 1986; 159:15–20.

153. Mardini MK, Sakati NA, Lewall DB, Christie R, Nylan WL. Scimitar syndrome. *Clin Pediatr* 1982; 21:350–4.

154. Alivizatos P, Cheatle T, deLaval M, Stark J. Pulmonary sequestration complicated by anomalies of pulmonary venous return. *J Pediatr Surg* 1985; 20:76–9.

155. Hawker RE, Celermajer JM, Gengos DC, Cartmill TB, Bowdler JD. Common pulmonary vein atresia. Premortem diagnosis in two infants. *Circulation* 1972; 46:368–74.

156. Presibitero P, Bull C, MacCartney FJ. Stenosis of pulmonary veins with ventricular septal defect. A cause of premature pulmonary hypertension in infancy. *Br Heart J* 1983; 49:600–3.

157. Sade RM, Freed MD, Matthews EC, Castaneda AR. Stenosis of individual pulmonary veins. Review of the literature and report of a surgical case. *J Thorac Cardiovasc Surg* 1974; 67:953–62.

158. Swischuk LE, L'Heureux P. Unilateral pulmonary vein atresia. *Am J Roentgenol* 1980; 135:667–72.

159. Perelman R, Gauthier N, Nathanson M, et al. Varice pulmonaire chez l'enfant. A propos d'un cas. Revue de la litterature. *Ann Pediatr* 1975; 22:411–20.

160. Benson JE, Olsen MM, Fletcher BD. A spectrum of bronchopulmonary anomalies associated with tracheoesophageal malformations. *Pediatr Radiol* 1985; 15:377–80.

161. Corrin B, Danel C, Allaway A, Warner JO, Lenney W. Intralobar pulmonary sequestration of ectopic pancreatic tissue with gastropancreatic duplication. *Thorax* 1985; 40:637–8.

162. Flye MW, Izant RJ. Extralobar pulmonary sequestration with oesophageal communication and complete duplication of the colon. *Surgery* 1972; 71:744–52.

163. Gabrielle OF. Arterial supply to the lung via the celiac axis. *Am J Roentgenol Radium Ther Nucl Med* 1970; 169:522–7.

164. Goldblatt E, Vimpani G, Brown JH. Extralobar pulmonary sequestration. Presentation as an arteriovenous aneurysm with cardiac failure in infancy. *Am J Cardiol* 1972; 29:100–3.

165. Heithoff KB, Sane SM, Willims HJ, et al. Bronchopulmonary foregut malformations. A unifying etiological concept. *Am J Roentgenol* 1976; 126:46–55.

166. Hoeffel JC, Bernard C, Richer R, Bretagne MC, Gautry P, Olive D, Pernot C. Pulmonary sequestrations of the upper lobe in children: three presentations. *Forschr Rontgenstr* 1986; 144:542–5.

167. Karp W. Bilateral sequestration of the lung. *Am J Roentgenol* 1977; 128:513–15.

168. Leithiser RE Jr, Capitanio MA, Macpherson RI, Wood BP. "Communicating" bronchopulmonary foregut malformations. *Am J Roentgenol* 1986; 146:227–31.

169. Lewis JE, Murray RE. Pulmonary sequestration with bronchoesophageal fistula. *J Pediatr Surg* 1968; 3:575–9.

170. Lucaya J, Carcia-Conesa JA, Bernado L. Pulmonary sequestration associated with unilateral pulmonary hypoplasia and massive pleural effusion. A case report and review of the literature. *Pediatr Radiol* 1984; 14:228–9.

171. Masaoka A, Maeda M, Monden Y, Nakahara K, Tani Y. Total lung ectoplasia with systemic arterial supply. *Ann Thorac Surg* 1979; 27:76–9.

172. Case records of the Massachusetts General Hospital (Case 18–1981). *N Eng J Med* 1981; 304:1090–6.

173. Case records of the Massachusetts General Hospital (Case 48–1983). *N Eng J Med* 1983; 306:1374–81.

174. Maull KI, McElvein RB. Infarcted extralobar pulmonary sequestration. *Chest* 1975; 68:98–9.

175. Rodgers BM, Harman PK, Johnson AM. Bronchopulmonary foregut malformations. The spectrum of anomalies. *Ann Surg* 1986; 203:517–24.

176. Savic B, Birtel FJ, Knoche R, Tholen W, Schild H. Pulmonary sequestration. *Ergebn Kinderheilk* 1979; 43:58–92.

177. Stocker JT, Drake RM, Madewell JE. Cystic and congenital lung disease in the newborn. *Persp Pediatr Pathol* 1978; 4:93–154.

178. Stocker JT, Kagan-Hallet K. Extralobar pulmonary sequestration. Analysis of 15 cases. *Am J Clin Pathol* 1979; 72:917–25.

179. Stocker JT, Malczak HT. A study of pulmonary ligament arteries. Relationship to intralobar pulmonary sequestration. *Chest* 1984; 86:611–5.

180. Telander RL, Lennox C, Sieber W. Sequestration of the lung in children. *Mayo Clin Proc* 1976; 51:578–84.

181. Thilenius OG, Ruschaput DG, Replogle RL, Bharati S, Herman T, Arcilla RA. Spectrum of pulmonary sequestration: association with anomalous pulmonary venous drainage in infants. *Pediatr Cardiol* 1983; 4:97–103.

182. Thornhill BA, Cho KC, Morehouse HT. Gastric duplication associated with pulmonary sequestration: CT manifestations. *Am J Roentgenol* 1982; 138:1168–71.

183. Werthammer JW, Hatten HP Jr, Blake WB Jr. Upper thoracic extralobar pulmonary sequestration presenting with respiratory distress in a newborn. *Pediatr Radiol* 1980; 9:116–7.

184. Yabek SM, Burstein J, Berman W Jr, Dillon T. Aberrant systemic arterial supply to the left lung with congestive heart failure. *Chest* 1981; 80:636–7.

185. Clements BS, Warner JO. Pulmonary sequestration and related congenital bronchopulmonary–vascular malformations: nomenclature and classification based on anatomical and embryological considerations. *Thorax* 1987; 212:401–5.

186. Stocker JT. Sequestrations of the lung. *Semin Diagn Pathol* 1986; 3:106–21.

187. Loyer EM. Case of the season: congenital left broncho-esophageal fistula. *Semin Roentgenol* 1986; 21:169–71.

188. Allain O, Monatagne JP, Balquet P, Baudin P, Sardet A. Les manifestations radiologiques des kystes bronchogeniques de la carene chez l'enfant. A propos de 5 observations. *Arch Fr Pediatr* 1982; 39:803–6.

189. Amendola MA, Shirazi KK, Brooks J, Agha FP, Dutz W. Transdiaphragmatic bronchopulmonary foregut anomaly: "dumbbell" bronchogenic cyst. *Am J Roentgenol* 1982; 138:1165–7.

190. Case records of the Massachusetts General Hospital (Case 1–1984) *N Engl J Med* 1984; 310:36–41.

191. Dubois P, Belanger R, Wellington JL. Bronchogenic cyst presenting as a supra-clavicular mass. *Can J Surg* 1981; 24:530–1.

192. Reed JC, Sobonya RE. Morphologic analysis of foregut cysts in the thorax. *Am J Roentgenol* 1974; 120:851–60.

193. Salyer DC, Salyer WR, Eggleston JC. Benign developmental cysts of the mediastinum. *Arch Pathol Lab Med* 1977; 101:136–9.

194. DM. The lining of healed but persistent abscess cavities in the lung with epithelium of the ciliated columnar type. *J Pathol Bacteriol* 1948; 60:259–65.

195. Gerbeaux J, Couvreur J, Tournier G, eds. *Pediatric Respiratory Disease.* 2nd ed. New York: Wiley, 1982.

196. Kendig EL Jr, Chernick V, eds. *Disorders of the Respiratory Tract in Children.* 4th ed. Philadelphia: W.B. Saunders, 1983.

197. Weinberg AG, Zumwalt RE. Bilateral nephromegaly and multiple pulmonary cysts. *Am J Clin Pathol* 1977; 67:284–8.

198. Adzick NS, Harrison MR, Glick PL. Fetal cystic adenomatoid malformation: prenatal diagnosis and natural history. *J Pediatr Surg* 1985; 20:483–8.

199. Alt B, Shikes RH, Stanford RE, Silverberg S. Ultrastructure of congenital cystic adenomatoid malformation of lung. *Ultrastr Pathol* 1982; 3:217–28.

200. Avitabile AM, Greco MA, Hulnick DH, Feiner HD. Congenital cystic adenomatoid malformation of the lung in adults. *Am J Surg Pathol* 1984; 8:193–202.

201. Bale PM. Congenital cystic malformation of the lung. A form of congenital bronchiolar ("adenomatoid") malformation. *Am J Clin Pathol* 1979; 71:411–20.

202. Craig JM. Kirkpatrick J, Neuhauser EBD. Congenital cystic adenomatoid malformation of the lung in infants. *Am J Roentgenol Radium Ther Nucl Med* 1956; 76:516–26.

203. Daroca PJ Jr. Mucogenic cells of congenital adenomatoid malformation of lung. *Arch Pathol Lab Med* 1979; 103:258–60.

204. Fischer JE, Nelson SJ, Allen JE, Holzman RS. Congenital cystic adenomatoid malformation of the lung. A unique variant. *Am J Dis Child* 1982; 136:1071–74.

205. Gaisie G, Oh KS. Spontaneous pneumothorax in cystic adenomatoid malformation. *Pediatr Radiol* 1983; 13:281–3.

206. Glaves J, Baker JC. Spontaneous resolution of maternal hydramnios in congenital cystic adenomatoid malformation of the lung. Antenatal ultrasound features. Case report. *Br J Obstet Gynaecol* 1983; 90:1065–8.

207. Hutchin P, Friedman PJ, Saltzstein SL. Congenital cystic adenomatoid malformation with anomalous blood supply. *J Thorac Cardiovasc Surg* 1974; 62:220–5.

208. Miller RK, Sieber WK, Yunis EJ. Congenital adenomatoid malformation of the lung. A report of 17 cases and review of the literature. *Pathol Annu* 1980; 15(1):387–407.

209. Stocker JT, Madewell JE, Drake RM. Congenital adenomatoid malformation of the lung: classification and morphologic spectrum. *Hum Pathol* 1977; 8:155–71.

210. Tucker TT, Smith WL, Smith JA. Fluid-filled cystic adenomatoid malformation. *Am J Roentgenol* 1977; 129:323–5.

211. Cachia R, Sobonya RE. Congenital cystic adenomatoid malformation of the lung with bronchial atresia. *Hum Pathol* 1981; 12:947–50.

212. Holland-Moritz RM, Heyn RM. Pulmonary blastoma associated with cystic lesions in children. *Med Pediatr Oncol* 1984; 12:85–8.

213. Krous HF, Sexauer CL. Embryonal rhabdomyosarcoma arising within a congenital bronchogenic cyst in a child. *J Pediatr Surg* 1981; 16:506–8.

214. Baltaxe HA, Lee JG, Ehlers KH, Engle MA. Pulmonary lymphangiectasis demonstrated by lymphangiography in two patients with Noonan's syndrome. *Radiology* 1975; 115:149–53.

215. Bhatti MAK, Ferrante JW, Gielchinsky I, Norman JC. Pleuropulmonary and skeletal lymphangiomatosis with chylothorax and chylopericardium. *Ann Thorac Surg* 1985; 40:398–401.

216. Gardner TW, Domm AC, Brock CE, Pruitt AW. Congenital pulmonary lymphangiectasis. A case complicated by chylothorax. *Clin Pediatr* 1983; 22:75–8.

217. Hernandez RJ, Stern AM, Rosenthal A. Pulmonary lymphangiectasis in Noonan's syndrome. *Am J Roentgenol* 1980; 134:75–80.

218. Case records of the Massachusetts General Hospital (Case 30–1980). *N Engl J Med* 1980; 303:270–6.

219. Shannon MP, Grantmyre EB, Reid WD, Wotherspoon AS. Congenital pulmonary lymphangiectasis. Report of two cases. *Pediatr Radiol* 1974; 2:235–40.

220. Huret C, Montoya F, Sibille G, Bonnet H. Agenesie des valves pulmonaires et emphyseme lobaire geant. Une association non exceptionnelle. *Pediatrie* 1984; 39:267–72.

221. Katzenstein A-L A, Askin FB. *Surgical Pathology of Non-neoplastic Lung Disease.* Philadelphia: W.B. Saunders, 1982.

222. Knudson RJ, Lindgren I, Gaensler EA. Accessory lung (or extrapulmonary sequestration) as a cause of lobar emphysema. *Med Thorac* 1966; 23:52–62.

223. Case records of the Massachusetts General Hospital (Case 41–1979). *N Eng J Med* 1979; 301:829–35.

224. Munnell ER, Lambird PA, Austin RL. Polyalveolar lobe causing lobar emphysema of infancy. *Ann Thorac Surg* 1973; 16:624–8.

225. Powell HC, Eliott JL. Congenital lobar emphysema. *Virchows Arch A* 1977; 374:197–203.

226. Stanger P, Lucas RV Jr, Edwards JE. Anatomic factors causing respiratory distress in acyanotic congenital cardiac disease: special reference to bronchial obstruction. *Pediatrics* 1969; 43:760–9.

227. Sulayman R, Thilenius O, Replogle R, Arcilla RA. Unilateral emphysema in total anomalous pulmonary venous return. *J Pediatr* 1975; 87:433–5.

228. Wall, MA, Eisenberg JD, Campbell JR. Congenital lobar emphysema in a mother and daughter. *Pediatrics* 1982; 70:131–3.

229. Weichert RF, III, Lindsey ES, Pearce LW, Waring WW. Bronchogenic cyst with unilateral obstructive emphysema. *J Thorac Cardiovasc Surg* 1970; 59:287–91.

230. Swischuk LE. Respiratory system. In: *Radiology of the Newborn and Young Infant.* 2nd ed. Baltimore: Williams & Wilkins, 1980, pp. 1–190.

231. Morgan WJ, Lemen RJ, Rojas R. Acute worsening of congenital lobar emphysema and subsequent spontaneous improvement. *Pediatrics* 1983; 71:844–8.

232. Miller KE, Edwards DK, Hilton S, Collins D, Lynch F, Williams R. Acquired lobar emphysema in premature infants with bronchopulmonary dysplasia: an iatrogenic disease? *Radiology* 1981; 138:589–92.

233. Nagaraj HS, Shott R, Fellows R, Yacoub U. Recurrent lobar atelectasis due to acquired bronchial stenosis in neonates. *J Pediatr Surg* 1980; 15:411–15.

234. Jederlinic PJ, Sicilian LS, Baigelman W, Gaensler EA. Congenital bronchial atresia. A report of 4 cases and a review of the literature. *Medicine* 1987; 66:73–83.

235. Day DL, Burke BA. Pulmonary emphysema in a neonate with Marfan syndrome. *Pediatr Radiol* 1986; 16:518–21.

236. Comroe JH Jr. Premature science and immature lungs (Parts I–III). *Am Rev Respir Dis* 1977; 116:127–35, 311–23, 497–518.

237. Raivio KO, Hallman N, Kouvalainen K, Valimaki I, eds. *Respiratory Distress Syndrome.* London: Academic Press, 1984.

238. Rooney SA. The surfactant system and lung phospholipid biochemistry. *Am Rev Respir Dis* 1985; 131:439–60.

239. Creuwels LA, van Golde LM, Haagsman HP. The pulmonary surfactant system: biochemical and clinical aspects. *Lung* 1997; 175:1–39.

240. Chapman JF, Herbert WNP. Current methods for evaluating fetal lung maturity. *Lab Med* 1986; 17:597–602.

241. de la Fuente AA, Voorhout WF, deMello DE. Congenital alveolar proteinosis in the Netherlands: a report of five cases with immunohistochemical and genetic studies on surfactant apoproteins. *Pediatr Pathol Lab Med* 1997; 17:221–31.

242. deMello DE, Nogee LM, Heyman S, et al. Molecular and phenotypic variability in the congenital alveolar proteinosis syndrome associated with inherited surfactant protein B deficiency. *J Pediatr* 1994; 125:43–50.

243. Nogee LM. Surfactant protein-B deficiency. *Chest* 1997; 111:129–35.

244. Whitsett JA, Nogee LM, Weaver TE, Horowitz AD. Human surfactant protein B: structure, function, regulation, and generic disease. *Physiol Rev* 1995; 75:749–57.

245. James DK, Chiswick ML, Harkes A, Williams M, Hallworth J. Non-specificity of surfactant deficiency in neonatal respiratory disorders. *Br Med J* 1984; 288:1635–8.

246. Lauweryns JM. "Hyaline membrane disease" in newborn infants. Macroscopic radiographic and light and electron microscopic studies. *Hum Pathol* 1970; 1:175–204.

247. Perelman RH, Palta M, Kirby R, Faffell PM. Discordance between male and female deaths due to the respiratory distress syndrome. *Pediatrics* 1986; 78:238–44.

248. Rosan RC. Hyaline membrane disease and a related spectrum of neonatal pneumonopathies. *Perspect Pediatr Pathol* 1975; 2:15–60.

249. Singer DB. Morphology of hyaline membrane disease and its pulmonary sequelae. In: Stern L, ed. *Hyaline Membrane Disease. Pathogenesis and Pathophysiology.* Orlando, FL: Grune & Stratton, 1984, pp. 63–96.

250. Shanklin DR. Criteria for diagnosis of hyaline membrane disease. *Arch Pathol* 1975; 99:345–6.

251. Stark AR, Frantz ID III. Respiratory distress syndrome. *Pediatr Clin N Am* 1986; 38:533–44.

252. Gruenwald P. Exaggerated atelectasis of prematurity. A complication of recovery from the respiratory distress syndrome. *Arch Pathol* 1968; 86:81–5.

253. Doshi N, Klionsky B, Kanbour A. Yellow hyaline membrane disease in neonates: clinical diagnosis by tracheal aspiration cytology. *Pediatr Pathol* 1983; 1:193–8.

254. Boss JH, Craig JM. Reparative phenomena in lungs of neonates with hyaline membranes. *Pediatrics* 1962; 29:890–8.

255. Perkin RM, Anas NG. Pulmonary hypertension in pediatric patients. *J Pediatr* 1984; 105:511–22.

256. Benjamin DR, Wiegenstein L. Necrosis of the ductus arteriosus in premature infants. *Arch Pathol* 1972; 94:340–2.

257. Gersony WM. Patent ductus arteriosus in the neonate. *Pediatr Clin North Am* 1986; 33:545–60.

258. Gittenberger-de Groot AC, vanErtbruggen I, Moulaert AJMG, Harinck E. The ductus arteriosus in the preterm infant: histologic and clinical observations. *J Pediatr* 1980; 96:88–93.

259. Green TP, Thompson RT, Johnson DE, Lock JE. Furosemide promotes patent ductus arteriosus in premature infants with the respiratory-distress syndrome. *N Engl J Med* 1983; 208:743–8.

260. Jacob J, Gluck L, DiSessa T, Edwards D, Kulovich M, et al. The contribution of PDA in the neonate with severe RDS. *J Pediatr* 1980; 96:79–87.

261. King DT, Emmanouilides GC, Andrews JC, Hirose FM. Morphologic evidence of accelerated closure of the ductus arteriosus in preterm infants. *Pediatrics* 1980; 65:872–80.

262. Kirks DR, McCook TA, Serwer GA, Oldham HN Jr. Aneurysm of the ductus arteriosus in the neonate. *Am J Roentgenol* 1980; 134:573–6.

263. Nickerson BG. Bronchopulmonary dysplasia. Chronic pulmonary disease following neonatal respiratory failure. *Chest* 1984; 87:528–35.

264. O'Brodovich HM, Mellins RB. Bronchopulmonary dysplasia. Unresolved neonatal acute lung injury. *Am Rev Respir Dis* 1985; 132:694–709.

265. Anderson WR, Engel RR. Cardiopulmonary sequelae of reparative stages of bronchopulmonary dysplasia. *Arch Pathol Lab Med* 1983; 107:603–8.

266. Ahlstrom H, Mortenson W, Robertson B. Alveolar lesions in broncho-pulmonary dysplasia. *OPMEAR* 1984; 29:102–5.

267. Stocker JT. Pathologic features of long-standing "healed" bronchopulmonary dysplasia: a study of 28 3- to 40-month-old infants. *Hum Pathol* 1986; 17:943–61.

268. Sobonya RE, Logvinoff MM, Taussig LM, Theriault A. Morphometric analysis of the lung in prolonged bronchopulmonary dysplasia. *Pediatr Res* 1982; 16:969–72.

269. Tou SS, Farrell PM, Leavitt LA, Samuels DP, Edwards DK. Clinical and roentgenographic scoring systems for assessing bronchopulmonary dysplasia. *Am J Dis Child* 1984; 138:581–5.

270. Merritt TA, Puccia JM, Stuard ID. Cytologic evaluation of pulmonary effluent in neonates with respiratory distress syndrome and bronchopulmonary dysplasia. *Acta Cytol* 1981; 25:631–9.

271. Edwards DK, Jacob J, Gluck L. The immature lung: radiographic appearance, course and complications. *Am J Roentgenol* 1980; 135:659–66.

272. McKay CA Jr, Faulkner CS II, Edwards WH. Unusual pulmonary reaction to respiratory therapy in a premature newborn. *Hum Pathol* 1985; 16:629–31.

273. Hodgman JE, Mikity VG, Tatter D, Cleland RS. Chronic respiratory distress in the premature infant. Wilson-Mikity syndrome. *Pediatrics* 1969; 44:179–95.

274. Goetzman BW. Understanding broncho-pulmonary dysplasia. *Am J Dis Child* 1986; 140:332–4.

275. O'Bara H, Pappas CT, Northway WH Jr, Bensch KG. Comparison of the effect of two and six week exposure to 80% and 100% oxygen of the lung of the newborn mouse: a quantitative SEM and TEM correlative study. *Int J Radiat Oncol Biol Phys* 1985; 11:285–98.

276. Berman W Jr, Katz R, Yabek SM, Dillon T, Fripp RR, Papile L. Long term follow-up of bronchopulmonary dysplasia. *J Pediatr* 1986; 109:45–50.

277. Bertrand J-M, Riley SP, Popkin J, Coates AL. The long-term pulmonary sequelae of prematurity: the role of familial airway hyperreactivity and the respiratory distress syndrome. *N Engl J Med* 1985; 312:742–5.

278. Levine MI, Batisti O. Wigglesworth JS, et al. A prospective study of intrapulmonary fat accumulation in the newborn lung following intralipid infusion. *Acta Paediatr Scand* 1984; 73:454–60.

279. Werthammer J, Brown ER, Neff RK, Taeusch HW Jr. Sudden infant death syndrome in infants with bronchopulmonary dysplasia. *Pediatrics* 1982; 69:301–4.

280. Boros SJ, Mammel MC, Lewallen PK, Coleman JM, Gordon MJ, Ophoven J. Necrotizing tracheobronchitis: a complication of high-frequency ventilation. *J Pediatr* 1986; 109:95–100.

281. Escobedo MB, Gonzalez A. Bronchopulmonary dysplasia in the tiny infant. *Clin Perinatol* 1986; 13:315–26.

282. Farrell PA, Fiascone JM. Bronchopulmonary dysplasia in the 1990s: a review for the pediatrician. *Curr Probl Pediatr* 1997; 27:129–63.

283. Clarke TA, Edwards DK. Pulmonary pseudocysts in newborn infants with respiratory distress syndrome. *Am J Roentgenol* 1979; 133:417–21.

284. Levine DH, Trump DS, Waterkotte G. Unilateral pulmonary interstitial emphysema: a surgical approach to treatment. *Pediatrics* 1981; 68:510–4.

285. Madansky DL, Lawson EE, Chernick V, Taeusch HW Jr. Pneumothorax and other forms of pulmonary air leak in newborns. *Am Rev Respir Dis* 1979; 120:729–37.

286. Mayo P, Saha SP. Spontaneous pneumothorax in the newborn. *Am Surg* 1983; 49:192–5.

287. Oppermann HC, Wille L, Obladen M, Richter E. Systemic air embolism in the respiratory distress syndrome of the newborn. *Pediatr Radiol* 1979; 8:139–45.

288. Plenat F, Vert P, Didier F, Andre M. Pulmonary interstitial emphysema. *Clin Perinatol* 1978; 5:351–75.

289. Smith TH, Currarino G, Rutledge JC. Spontaneous occurrence of localized pulmonary interstitial and endolymphatic emphysema in infancy. *Pediatr Radiol* 1984; 14:142–5.

290. Wood BP, Anderson VM, Mauk JE, Merritt TA. Pulmonary lymphatic air: locating "pulmonary interstitial emphysema" of the premature infant. *Am J Roentgenol* 1982; 138:809–14.

291. Zimmermann H. Progressive interstitial pulmonary lobar emphysema. *Eur J Pediatr* 1982; 138:258–62.

292. Askin FB. Pulmonary interstitial air and pneumothorax in the neonate. In: Stocker JT, ed. *Pediatric Pulmonary Disease.* New York: Hemisphere, 1989, pp. 165–74.

293. Esterly JR, Oppenheimer EH. Massive pulmonary haemorrhage in the newborn. I. Pathologic considerations. *J Pediatr* 1966; 69:3–11.

294. Castile RG, Kleinberg F. The pathogenesis and management of massive pulmonary hemorrhage in the neonate. Case report of a normal survivor. *Mayo Clin Proc* 1976; 51:155–8.

295. Fedrick J, Butler NR. Certain causes of neonatal death. Massive pulmonary haemorrhage. *Biol Neonat* 1971; 18:243–62.

296. Kotas RV, Wells TJ, Mims LC, Trainor EJ, Wiles CL. A new model for neonatal pulmonary haemorrhage research. *Pediatr Res* 1975; 9:161–5.

297. Trompter R, Yu VYH, Aynsley-Green A, Roberton NRC. Massive pulmonary haemorrhage in the newborn infant. *Arch Dis Child* 1975; 50:123–7.

298. Bacsik RD. Meconium aspiration syndrome. *Pediatr Clin N Am* 1977; 24:463–79.

299. Hoffman RR Jr, Campbell RE, Decker JP. Fetal aspiration syndrome. Clinical, roentgenologic and pathologic features. *Am J Roentgenol* 1974; 122:90–6.

300. Jose JH, Schreiner RL, Lemons JA, et al. The effect of amniotic fluid aspiration on pulmonary function in the adult and newborn rabbit. *Pediatr Res* 1983; 17:976–81.

301. Manning FA, Schreiber J, Turkel SB. Fatal meconium aspiration "in utero": a case report. *Am J Obstet Gynecol* 1978; 132:111–13.

302. Murphy JD, Vawter GF, Reid LM. Pulmonary vascular disease in fatal meconium aspiration. *J Pediatr* 1984; 104:758–62.

303. Ohlsson A, Cumming WA, Najjar H. Neonatal aspiration syndrome due to vernix caseosa. *Pediatr Radiol* 1985; 15:193–5.

304. Baker C. Group B streptococcal infections. *Adv Int Med* 1980; 25:475.

305. Craig JM. Group B beta hemolytic streptococcal sepsis in the newborn. *Persp Pediatr Pathol* 1982; 6:139.

306. Naeye RL, Tafari N. *Risk Factors in Pregnancy and Diseases of the Fetus and Newborn.* Baltimore: Williams & Wilkins, 1983.

307. Remington JS, Klein JO (eds). *Infectious Diseases of the Fetus and Newborn Infant.* 2nd ed. Philadelphia: W.B. Saunders, 1983.

308. Rhine WD, Arvin AM, Stevenson DK. Neonatal aspergillosis. A case report and review of the literature. *Clin Pediatr* 1986; 25:400–3.

309. Sun C-C J, Duara S. Fatal adenovirus pneumonia in two newborn infants, one case caused by adenovirus type 30. *Pediatr Pathol* 1985; 4:247–55.

310. Wilfert CM, Gutman LT. Chlamydia trachomatis infections of infants and children. *Adv Pediatr* 1986; 33:49–76.

311. Baley JE, Kliegman RM, Fanaroff AA. Disseminated fungal infections in very low birthweight infants: clinical manifestations and epidemiology. *Pediatrics* 1984; 73:144–52.

312. Fox WW, Duara S. Persistent pulmonary hypertension in the neonate: diagnosis and management. *J Pediatr* 1983; 103:505–14.

313. Geggel RL, Reid LM. The structural basis of PPHN. *Clin Perinatol* 1984; 11:525–49.

314. Haworth SG. Primary and secondary pulmonary hypertension in childhood: a clinicopathological reappraisal. *Curr Top Pathol* 1983; 73:92–152.

315. Haworth SG. Pulmonary vascular disease in different types of congenital heart disease. Implications for interpretation of lung biopsy findings in early childhood. *Br Heart J* 1984; 52:551–71.

316. Rabinovitch M, Keane JF, Norwood WI, Castaneda AR, Reid L. Vascular structure in lung tissue obtained at biopsy correlated with pulmonary hemodynamic findings after repair of congenital heart defects. *Circulation* 1984; 69:655–67.

317. Rudolph AM. High pulmonary vascular resistance after birth. 1. Pathophysiologic considerations and etiologic classification. *Clin Pediatr* 1980; 19:585–90.

318. Stenmark KR, James SL, Voelkel NF, Toews WH, Reeves JT, Murphy RC. Leukotrienes C_4 and D_4 in neonates with hypoxia and pulmonary hypertension. *N Engl J Med* 1983; 309:77–80.

319. Yazbeck S, Clouthier R, Laberge JM. La hernie diaphragmatique congenitale: les resultats changent ils vraiment? *Chic Pediatr* 1986; 27:37–40.

320. Levin DL, Weinberg AG, Perkin RM. Pulmonary microthrombi syndrome in newborn infants with unresponsive pulmonary hypertension. *J Pediatr* 1983; 102:299–303.

321. Cagle P, Langston C. Pulmonary veno-occlusive disease as a cause of sudden infant death. *Arch Pathol Lab Med* 1984; 108:338–40.

322. Stoler MH, Anderson VM, Stuard ID. A case of pulmonary veno-occlusive disease in infancy. *Arch Pathol Lab Med* 1982; 106:645–7.

323. Voordes CG, Kuipers JRG, Elema JD. Familial pulmonary veno-occlusive disease: a case report. *Thorax* 1977; 32:763–6.

324. Wagenvoort CA, Wagenvoort N. The pathology of pulmonary veno-occlusive disease. *Virchows Arch Pathol Anat Histol* 1974; 364:69–79.

325. Stocker JT, McGill LC, Orsini EN. Post-infarction peripheral cysts of the lung in pediatric patients: a possible cause of idiopathic spontaneous pneumothorax. *Pediatr Pulmonol* 1985; 1:1–18.

326. Bedrossian CWM, Greenberg SD, Singer DB, Hansen JJ, Rosenberg HS. The lung in cystic fibrosis. A quantitative study including prevalence of pathologic findings among different age groups. *Hum Pathol* 1976; 7:195–204.

327. Oppenheimer EH, Esterly JR. Pathology of cystic fibrosis. Review of the literature and comparison with 146 autopsied cases. *Persp Pediatr Pathol* 1975; 2:241–78.

328. Sturgess J, Imrie J. Quantitative evaluation of the development of tracheal submucosal glands in infants with cystic fibrosis and control infants. *Am J Pathol* 1982; 106:303–11.

329. Puri P, Gorman F. Lethal nonpulmonary anomalies associated with congenital diaphragmatic hernia: implications for early intrauterine surgery. *J Pediatr Surg* 1984; 19:29–32.

330. Wolff G. Familial congenital diaphragmatic defect: review and conclusions. *Hum Genet* 1980; 54:1–5.

331. Paris F, Blasco E, Canto KA, Tarazona V, Casillas M. Diaphragmatic eventration in infants. *Thorax* 1973; 28:66–72.

332. Cullen ML, Clein MD, Philippart AI. Congenital diaphragmatic hernia. *Surg Clin N Am* 1985; 65:1115–38.

333. Silverman JF, Kopelman AE. Meconium pleuritis: cytologic diagnosis in a neonate with perforated sigmoid colon and diaphragmatic hernia. *Pediatr Pathol* 1986; 6:325–33.

334. Geggel RL, Murphy JD, Langleben D, Crone RK, Vacanti PJ, Redia LM. Congenital diaphragmatic hernia: arterial structural changes and persistent pulmonary hypertension after surgical repair. *J Pediatr* 1985; 107:457–64.

335. Thurlbeck WM, Kida K, Langston C, et al. Postnatal lung growth after repair of diaphragmatic hernia. *Thorax* 1979; 34:338–43.

336. Siegel MJ, Shackleford GD, McAlister WH. Left-sided congenital diaphragmatic hernia: delayed presentation. *Am J Roentgenol* 1981; 137:43–6.

337. Srousi M, Buck B, Downes JJ. Congenital diaphragmatic hernia: deleterious effects of pulmonary interstitial emphysema and tension extrapulmonary air. *J Pediatr Surg* 1981; 16:45–54.

338. Stahl GE, Warren WS, Rosenberg H, Spackman TJ, Schnaufer L. Congenital right diaphragmatic hernia. A case report and review of the literature. *Clin Pediatr* 1981; 20:422–5.

339. Gillot F, Quezede J, Sellah A. L'interposition hepatodiaphragmatique du colon chez l'enfant. Syndrome de Chilaiditi. *Arch Fr Pediatr* 1977; 34:248–57.

340. Hart JC, Cohen IT, Ballantine TVN, Varrano LF. Accessory diaphragm in an infant. *J Pediatr Surg* 1981; 16:947–9.

341. Devgan BK, Brodeur AE. Apical pneumatocele. *Arch Otolaryngol* 1975; 102:121–3.

The Cardiovascular System

Harvey S. Rosenberg   William H. Donnelly

INTRODUCTION

The cardiovascular system in the infant and child has been the subject of a number of scholarly works, particularly those of Edwards [1], Becker and Anderson [2], Arey [3], Freedom et al [4], Moller and Neal [5], and Clark and Takao [6], providing a base for a focus on the diseases affecting the neonate.

Malformations may appear as isolated, single defects or as part of complex alterations involving several components. Recognition of the complexities may be a prime requisite for appreciation of the malformations, but their interpretation has resulted in development of a variety of different terminologies depending largely on the observer's concepts of embryogenesis and development. Each new terminology may appear to clarify the older concepts, only to introduce new conceptual problems. Our comprehension of cardiovascular disease in infants and children remains in dynamic flux.

Altered cardiovascular morphology and function result from intranatal and postnatal events such as anoxia and infection. Cardiovascular involvement in generalized metabolic disease is not uncommon—e.g., the mucopolysaccharidoses—but only a few of the disorders affect the neonate—e.g., Pompe disease. Interpretation of the enigmatic cardiomyopathies remains essential but difficult due to the hereditary implications and the potentially hazy diagnostic criteria. Despite their rarity in the neonate, cardiovascular tumors require recognition because of their accessibility to surgical removal.

CARDIOVASCULAR DEVELOPMENT AND NORMAL ANATOMY

Morphogenesis

Salient features of cardiogenesis correlate with several embryonal markers: the age of the embryo after fertilization, the number of somites, the crown-rump length, and the stage (formerly known as the horizon) [7]. O'Rahilly related each change in the first 56 days of postovulatory life to a stage of development based on several criteria, including the length of the embryo [8]. Data on the development during fetal life, the period between 56 days and birth, have not been delineated so clearly. Because of the many overlapping terms used to describe embryonal structures, O'Rahilly introduced four terms to consolidate and clarify the description of embryonic cardiac structures: trabeculated left ventricle, trabeculated right ventricle, conus cordis, and truncus arteriosus (Fig. 20.1; Table 20.1) [8].

Morphogenesis, particularly cardiogenesis, relates to two processes: cellular growth and tissue deformation. Growth results from cellular hypertrophy and hyperplasia and the elaboration and accumulation of extracellular material. Since growth rarely proceeds at a uniform rate, both addition and deletion of tissues cause remodeling. Deformation from physical pressure on the developing organs combined with growth dictate heart shape; deformation causes rapid changes, and cell growth causes slower changes. The heart may loop to the right, loop to the left, or remain midline, principally due to deformation with an undetermined,

Table 20.1.   Glossary of embryonic cardiac structures

O'Rahilly	Other terms applied to the same structure
Trabeculated left ventricle	Primary heart tube
	Ventricle
	Ventricle, proampulla
	Primitive left ventricle
Trabeculated right ventricle	Primary heart tube
	Bulbus cordis
	Ventricle, metampulla
	Bulbus cordis, primitive right ventricle
Conus cordis	Primary heart tube
	Bulbus cordis
	Bulbus
	Conus arteriosus
	Bulbus cordis, conus cordis
	Infundibulum
Truncus arteriosus	Primary heart tube
	Aortic bulb
	Truncus
	Bulbus cordis, truncus arteriosus

From O'Rahilly [8].

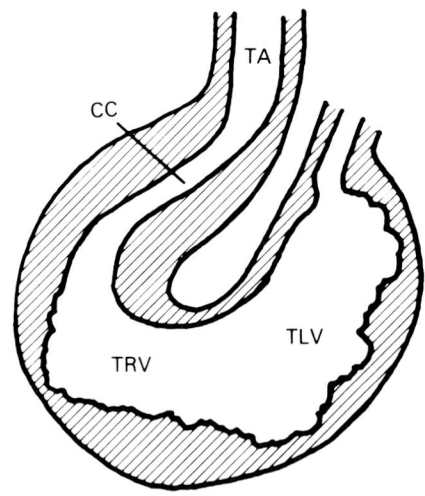

FIGURE 20.1.   *The embryonal cardiac tube has four principal segments: trabeculated left ventricle (TLV), trabeculated right ventricle (TRV), conus cordis (CC), and truncus arteriosus (TA). (After O'Rahilly [8].)*

perhaps passive role of cellular growth (Fig. 20.2). The regulation of looping has been attributed to a physical deformation and an interaction between cytodifferentiation and matrix production, rather than a result of differential growth [9].

The space between the myoepithelial mantle and the primitive heart tubes contains the cardiac jelly, a nonhomogeneous material made up of a radially oriented system of filaments, consisting largely of glycosaminoglycans which can expand and contract with changes in ionic strength (Fig. 20.3). Variations in the degree of hydration give the cardiac jelly a role in deformation of the heart [9].

Biochemical antecedents may integrate organogenesis in general and cardiogenesis and looping in particular. Using molecular approaches to determine tissue and stage-specific expression [10, 11], neural cell adhesion molecule [12], genes [13, 14, 14a], and growth factors [15, 15a, 15b] have been

identified in embryonal myocardium, indicating a determining or modulating role for these factors during cardiogenesis. Although cytodifferentiation may contribute to heart shape, the physical and chemical properties of the matrix generate the deforming force and regulate the direction of looping. The heart's form results from the independent action of cytodifferentiation, matrix maturation, and fibrillogenesis [9].

Neural Crest Contribution to Cardiogenesis
The mesoderm forms much of the heart, but the endoderm of the foregut influences cardiac shape through its proximity to the developing heart and the ectoderm contributes to the migration of neural crest elements. Using quail-chick chimera embryos to study neural crest migration because of structural differences of the interphase nuclei of chicks and quail [16], neural crest cells have been identified migrating

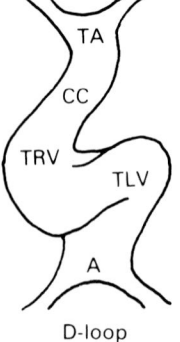

D-loop

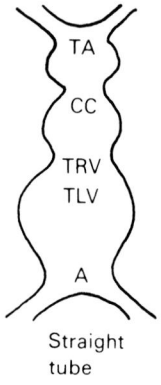

Straight tube

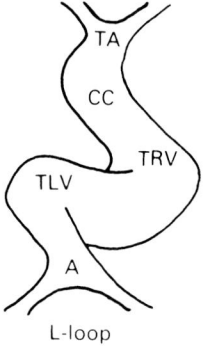

L-loop

FIGURE 20.2.   *Deformation of the primitive heart tube determines cardiac shape through looping of the tube to the right (d-loop), forming situs solitus, or to the left (l-loop), forming situs inversus. A—atria; TLV—trabeculated left ventricle; TRV—trabeculated right ventricle; CC—conus cordis; TA—truncus arteriosus.*

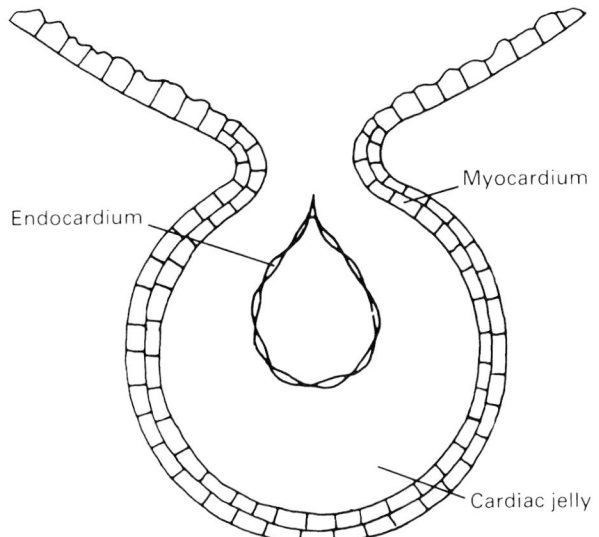

FIGURE 20.3. *The cardiac jelly, a filamentous layer between the myocardium and endocardium of the embryonic heart, contributes to cardiac shape by its capacity to respond to physical and chemical influences. (After Manasek [9].)*

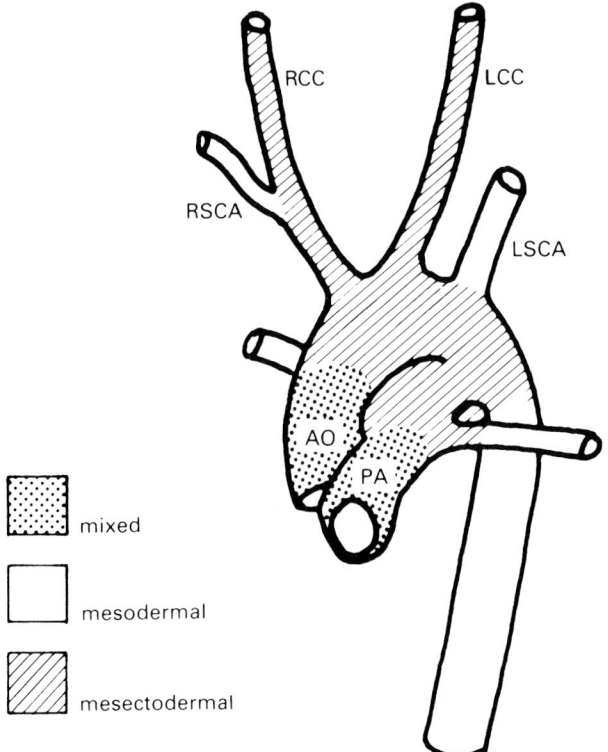

FIGURE 20.4. *Ectodermally derived mesenchyme contributes to formation of the pulmonary artery, ductus arteriosus, aortic arch, and the carotid arteries. Ao—aorta; PA—pulmonary artery; RSCA—right subclavian artery; RCC—right common carotid artery; LCC—left common carotid artery; LSCA—left subclavian artery.*

to the region of the aorticopulmonary septum [17]. Cells from the cardiac jelly, the endocardium, and the sixth aortic arch form the division of the truncus arteriosus [18]. Cardiac parasympathetic postganglionic neurons derive from the occipital neural crest while the heart is in the simple tube stage and may also seed the mesoderm cells, which are essential for proper septation since experimental removal of the region results in persistent truncus arteriosus, transposition of the great arteries, and interruption of the aortic arch [16, 19, 20]. The role of the neural crest elements in dysmorphogenesis may relate to altered hemodynamics in the embryo with dilatation of the ventricular portion of the cardiac tube and a decreased ejection fraction leading to malalignment and consequent malformations [21, 22].

The terms "mesectoderm" and "mesentoderm" have been proposed to distinguish the mesenchymes derived from ectoderm and mesoderm. Except for the endothelium, the walls of the large arteries derived from aortic arches III, IV, and VI originate entirely from mesectoderm: common carotids, pulmonary arteries, and the aortic arch (Fig. 20.4). The aortic and pulmonary arterial trunks derive from a mixture of mesectoderm and mesentoderm. The dorsal aorta, the coronary arteries, and the subclavian arteries derive entirely from mesoderm [16, 22a].

Cardiac morphogenesis usually completes by the 6th week of gestation, but varying from 38–44 days or more depending on the membranous portion of the ventricular septum, which may not close until after birth [22b].

Stages of Cardiogenesis

The lack of experimental precision in timing of morphogenesis by dates in humans led to the concept of stages, which was introduced by Streeter in his landmark studies [7]. This concept was augmented in the early embryo by O'Rahilly and others (Table 20.2) [8].

Valvulogenesis

Heart valves develop from modification of the endocardial cushion at the downstream end of the cardiac tube and grow by cellular proliferation at the margins [23]. Valvulogenesis begins at stage 15 with four mounds of endocardial tissue consisting of stellate and spindle-shaped cells in a loose matrix and covered by a single endothelial layer. By stage 17, the valves contain slender, unorganized elastic fibers with endothelium that is flattened proximally and cuboidal distally; slender, unorganized elastic fibers also appear in the media of the great arteries. By stage 21, the short, thick valve leaflets have a progressive cellularity with spindle cells perpendicular to the leaflet axis.

Conotruncal septation occurs in stage 15, well-formed semilunar valves appear in stage 17, and the septum closes in stage 18 [23]. After completion of cardiogenesis in stage 18, valvular organization continues. The leaflets gradually become thinner and more delicate, with a progressive increase, and then decrease in mucopolysaccharide deposits

Table 20.2.   Stages of cardiogenesis

Stage	Size (mm)	Age (days)	Development
1–8	—	1–20	During the precardiac time between fertilization and initiation of cardiogenesis, the blastocyst develops, followed by implantation at about 7 days, development of the extraembryonal structures trophoblast and yolk sac, and differentiation of the embryo into a trilaminar structure.
9	1.5–2.5	20	The two primordial cardiogenic cords fuse to form a single heart tube and promptly develop the sulci that determine the future components of the heart: atrioventricular, interventricular, bulboventricular, conotruncal, and infundibulotruncal. From thickened mesenchyme, a myoepithelial layer develops, separated from the lumen by the cardiac jelly, and forms the myocardium and epicardium, while the inner tube forms the endocardium. The pericardial cavity forms.
10	2.0–3.5	22	The pericardial cavity enlarges, and looping of the heart to the right begins in a d-loop pattern. Although the heart probably starts beating at this time, blood flows back and forth, because the cardinal veins are not yet attached to permit circulation. The cardiac asymmetry appears from the formation of an S-shaped heart through counterclockwise rotation of the tube as viewed from the front, the d-loop dictating the shape of the heart as it changes from the primitive tube to the complex four-chambered structure.
11	2.5–4.5	24	The tube elongates, looping to the right continues, the ventricular apex orients to the right, and both atria empty into a left ventricle through a common atrioventricular canal, resembling the circulation in the congenitally malformed heart with tricuspid valve atresia. The first aortic arch appears, and dilatations in the heart tube form the bulbus cordis, ventricles, atria, truncus, and sinus venosus.
12	3–5	26	The sinus venosus connects to the atrial end of the tube and circulation begins, although in series: right atrium–left atrium–left ventricle–right ventricle, rather than in parallel as in the fully developed heart. The ventricular apex rotates from the right to the midline. The truncus continues from the bulbus cordis to the aortic sac, and the sinus venosus receives blood from umbilical (chorion), vitelline (yolk sac), and common cardinal (embryo) veins.
13	4–6	28	Circulation changes from series to parallel with the formation of the septa, the endocardial cushions of the atrioventricular canal, the conal and septal cushions of the semilunar valves, the pulmonary veins, and aortic arches III (brachiocephalic and carotid), IV (aortic arch), and VI (pulmonary arteries and ductus arteriosus).
14	5–7	32	The ventricles form, and the trabeculae in the small right ventricle simulate the configuration of a univentricular malformed heart with a rudimentary right ventricular outflow chamber. The smaller right ventricle lies posterior to the left ventricle, and the atrioventricular canal lies between the left atrium and left ventricle. A common pulmonary vein joins the atria to the left of the septum primum.
15	7–9	33	The ventricular apex directs to the left, the ventricular septum appears, and the undivided atrioventricular canal opens into both the right and left ventricles. Fusion of the spiral truncal cushions with the semilunar valve cushions divide the aorta and pulmonary arteries. The septum primum in the atria now has an ostium secundum.
16	8–11	37	The tricuspid and mitral valvular orifices appear, and the ostium primum closes as the septum primum fuses with the endocardial cushions of the atrioventricular canal. The pulmonary artery arises from the right ventricle and the aorta arises from the left ventricle, separating the systemic and pulmonary circulations. The anterior pulmonary artery connects with the dorsal aortic arch VI and the posterior aorta joins the anterior aortic arch IV, resulting in a crossing of the circulations as the pulmonary goes from anterior to posterior and the aorta does the reverse, from posterior to anterior.
17	11–14	41	The semilunar valve leaflets appear as thick, cellular structures. Atrial septation is complete, but the cephalad portion of the ventricle remains incomplete.
18	13–17	44	The membranous septum fuses with the endocardial cushions and the conal cushions. Closure, which usually takes place at this point, may be delayed for some time, even after birth, accounting for examples of postnatal spontaneous closure of clinically recognized ventricular septal defects.
19–23	16–31	47–57	Morphogenesis is complete at this time. Subsequent changes in the heart involve growth, differentiation of the valves, and organization of the conduction system.

during weeks 6 to 16 of gestation. Collagen in distinct lamellae appears at the annulus and in the adventitia at 8 weeks and occupies the proximal third of the valve leaflets, the arterial media, and valve commissures by the 12th week. Subendocardial elastic fibers extend to the ventricular aspect of the valve leaflets by week 13, and the valves have a dense collagen core with loose connective tissue on the ventricular aspect by week 19. The subendocardial elastic tissue gradually extends around the valves at both the ventricular and arterial aspects.

A highly organized network of collagen fibers is present in the left ventricle. The network surrounds groups of myocytes, extends as struts between basal laminae of contiguous myocytes, and extends from the basal laminae of all capillaries to the basal laminae of all adjacent myocytes. Although the function of the network is not well defined, it apparently contributes to the elastic and viscous properties of the heart [24].

The valves have no blood vessels at any time. The pulmonary artery and aorta and their semilunar valves are structurally identical up to birth. The valvular endothelium is flat proximally and cuboidal distally, conforming to high and low shear forces. The aortic and pulmonic trunks develop when separate ventricular ejection streams appear, with the fibrous and elastic layers developing later in relation to fluctuating and static tensions [23].

The truncal septum seems to be mesenchyme filling the path between two bloodstreams rather than a distinct structure dividing the truncus into two vessels. Based on studies in the chick embryo, Thompson and Fitzharris conclude that truncal mesenchyme derives from two sources: a portion migrating caudally into the cardiac jelly of the distal truncus from the nearby aortic arch region, which coincides with the slowing of the anterior elongation of the heart tube; and a portion derived from endocardium, which fills the conus and proximal truncus radially, coinciding with the expansion of the bulbus cordis [25]. After it condenses, the truncal mesenchyme forms semilunar valves, the aorticopulmonary septum, and the media of the aorta and pulmonary artery.

Normal Morphology
(Including Segmental Analysis)

In the study of cardiovascular disease in the neonate, any deviation from the norm signals a major or minor malformation. The orientation of the heart may be situs solitus (normal), inversus, or ambiguous. With situs solitus, the heart occupies the midline with the apex (Fig. 20.5) directed toward the left, the right atrium on the right border, the right ventricle making up the major portion of the anterior surface, and the left ventricle forming the left one-third of the anterior surface and the apex. On the anterior surface, the anterior descending branch of the left coronary artery demarcates the position of the ventricular septum. Of the left atrium, only the atrial appendage appears on the anterior surface. The left atrium, which lies posteriorly, receives the pulmonary veins on its posterior surface. The pulmonary artery arises anterior and to the left of the aorta and branches into a left pulmonary artery, which gives off the

ductus arteriosus to join the aorta just distal to the origin of the left subclavian artery, and a right pulmonary artery, which passes posterior to the ascending aorta as it extends to the hilus of the right lung. The branches from the aortic arch are the brachiocephalic artery, which divides into the right subclavian and carotid arteries; the left carotid artery; and the left subclavian artery. Smaller branches may arise directly from the aortic arch between the carotid and subclavian arteries to supply the thyroid or vertebral arterial circulation. Identification of these branches in their normal positions precludes any of the several anomalies of the aortic arch.

The inferior vena cava (IVC) joins the right atrium promptly after penetrating the diaphragm with only a few millimeters of supradiaphragmatic IVC between the ostium of the hepatic vein and the entrance to the right atrium. The superior vena cava (SVC) drains the right and left innominate veins, which in turn drain the corresponding jugular and subclavian veins. The left innominate vein crosses the midline to join the right, forming the SVC. The thymus lies on the anterior surfaces of the pericardium and of the left innominate vein. If the left innominate vein does not cross the midline, it joins a left vertical vein, forming a persistent left SVC, which usually drains into the right atrium through the coronary sinus and may accompany other venous anomalies.

Within the right atrium (Fig. 20.6), the orientation of the atrial septum and the fossa ovalis direct flow from the SVC toward the tricuspid valve orifice and flow from the IVC toward the fossa. The foramen ovale remains patent for months and years. It is permanently patent in about 20% of adults. A valve covers the orifice of the foramen ovale, with the valve's free margin approximating the left side of the atrial septum.

The normal relative pressure gradient between the left and right atria closes the valve of the foramen ovale;

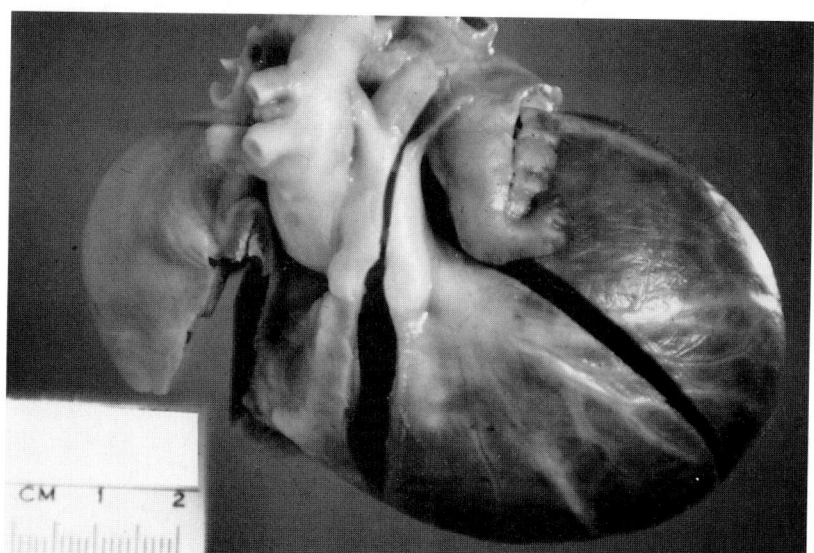

FIGURE 20.5. *The normal exterior markings of the anterior surface of the heart include the blunt right and hooked left atrial appendages, the anterior descending branch of the left coronary artery marking the position of the ventricular septum, and the ligamentum arteriosum joining the left pulmonary artery to the aortic arch distal to the origin of the left subclavian artery.*

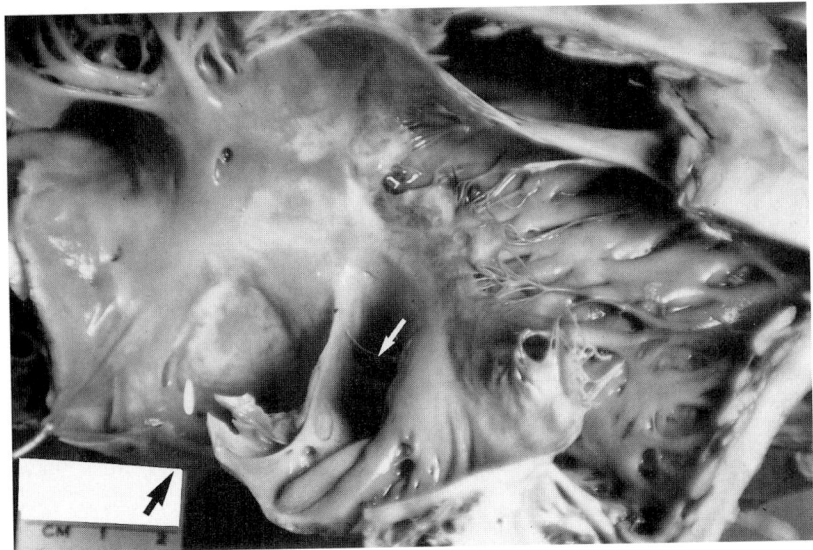

FIGURE 20.6.   *In the opened right atrium and ventricle, the orifice of the inferior vena cava (large arrow) lies beneath the fossa ovalis, and the veil-like eustachian valve (small arrow) guards the ostium of the coronary sinus. The tricuspid valve leaflets are inconspicuously separated from each other. Thick, fleshy trabeculae mark the right ventricle.*

increased right atrial pressure may reopen the orifice. Competence of the valve of the foramen ovale expresses the discordance between anatomic patency and function. A valve-competent foramen ovale has a normally formed valve and a higher left atrial pressure than right. A valve-incompetent foramen ovale has a fenestrated valve or one too small to cover its orifice, a form of foramen secundum atrial septal defect.

The coronary sinus, guarded by the frequently attenuated and inconspicuous eustachian valve, enters the right atrium inferior and posterior to the fossa ovalis. The usually small lumen becomes large if the coronary vein carries an excess flow as from drainage of a left SVC. The position of the ostium of the coronary sinus serves as a landmark for the atrioventricular (AV) node, which is not grossly visible. The AV node lies in the atrial myocardium, usually closer to the right side, anterior to the coronary sinus and inferior to the fossa ovalis. The bundle of His, also not grossly visible, extends anteriorly and inferiorly from the AV node to the central fibrous body, the junction of the tricuspid, mitral, and aortic valves, which it pierces to enter the ventricular septum.

The three leaflets of the tricuspid valve are not conspicuously separated from each other. Two right ventricular papillary muscles serve as landmarks: the anterior papillary muscle extends from the anterior leaflet to the apex of the ventricular septum, where it joins the moderator band, which, in turn, joins the septal limb of the crista supraventricularis; the small but constant papillary muscle of the conus (muscle of Lancisi), which serves as a landmark for the right branch of the conduction bundle and which arises from the septum inferior to the crista, attaches to the septal and anterior leaflets of the tricuspid valve (Fig. 20.7). After the conduction bundle penetrates the central fibrous body and splits into right and left bundles, the right branch curves around the papillary muscle of the conus.

The muscular wall of the right ventricle has thick trabeculae and small papillary muscles arising from both pari-

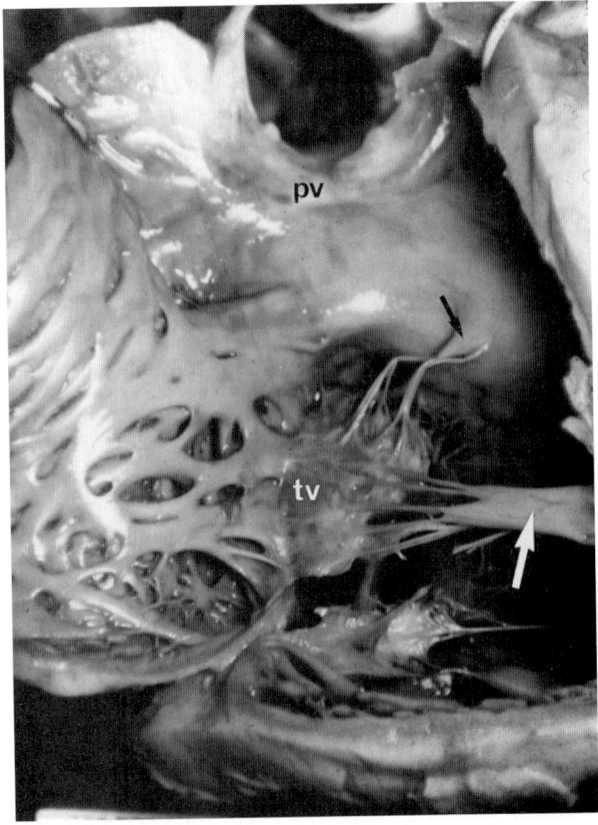

FIGURE 20.7.   *Landmarks of the outflow portion of the right ventricle include the anterior papillary muscle (large white arrow), the papillary muscle of the conus (small dark arrow), and the crista supraventricularis, which separates the tricuspid (tv) and pulmonary (pv) valves.*

etal and septal walls. The left ventricle has only parietal attachments for the papillary muscles and none from the septum. The distinctive outflow of the right ventricle differs from the outflow of the left ventricle by the crista supraventricularis, which crosses the basilar portion of the right ven-

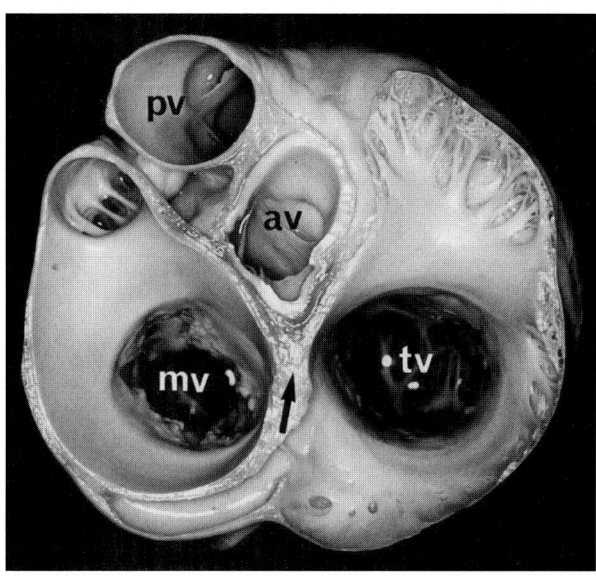

FIGURE 20.8. *A view of the base of the heart with much of the atria and great arteries removed reveals the junction of the mitral (mv), tricuspid (tv), and aortic (av) valves at the central fibrous body (arrow) but separated from the anteriorly placed pulmonary (pv) valve.*

Table 20.3. Definitions

Term	Anatomic regions to which the term has been applied
Conus	1. A clearly defined embryonic structure
	2. The subpulmonic area of the right ventricle
	3. The entire right ventricular outflow tract
	4. The portion of the right ventricle derived from the embryonic conus
Septal limb of the crista	Infundibular or conus septum
Conotruncus	Conus and truncus arteriosus

From Goor et al [27].

tricle, separating the tricuspid from the pulmonary valve and the pulmonary valve from the central fibrous body (Fig. 20.8).

Because the term "crista" has been applied loosely and inconsistently to different and similar structures partly due to controversies in concepts of cardiogenesis, Anderson et al [26] propose a restrictive terminology, replacing "conus" with "infundibulum" and "septal band of the crista" with "trabecula marginalis," stressing the necessity to identify each structure in malformed hearts:

1. *Crista supraventricularis:* the muscle mass that lies between the inflow and outflow of a normal right ventricle.
2. *Infundibular septum:* the muscle separating the pulmonary from the aortic valves.
3. *Ventriculoinfundibular fold:* the muscle separating the tricuspid from the pulmonary valve in a normal right ventricle.
4. *Trabecula septomarginalis:* the extensive septal trabeculation of the right ventricle.

Although the conus is clearly distinguished from the remainder of the right ventricle in the embryo, the name has been applied to three right ventricular structures: the subpulmonic area, the outflow tract, and that portion of the right ventricle considered to have been derived from the embryonic conus: the septal and parietal limbs of the crista. The septal limb of the crista has also been referred to as the "infundibular septum" or "conus septum"; "conotruncus" has been used as a collective term for the conus and the truncus arteriosus (Table 20.3) [27].

The pulmonary valve cusps have no continuity with the AV valve leaflets. The main pulmonary artery divides into two main branches and gives rise to the ductus on the left just distal to the bifurcation. The relation of the pulmonary arteries to the bronchi at the hilus of each lung is a key to determining visceral situs. On the right, a branch from the mainstem bronchus, the eparterial bronchus, lies superior to the pulmonary artery. The remaining bronchi on the right and left, the hyparterial bronchi, lie inferior to the corresponding artery. The eparterial bronchus identifies a morphologic right lung: with situs inversus, the morphologic right lung is on the left; with situs ambiguous, both lungs have an eparterial bronchus (right pulmonary isomerism) or both lungs lack an eparterial bronchus (left pulmonary isomerism).

While the descriptions of the cardiovascular system found here follow traditional anatomic dissections, anatomic tomographic study can enhance correlation with the clinical demonstration of disease by echocardiography, magnetic resonance imaging (MRI), and radiologic computed tomography (CT) [28]. Because the heart's position does not conform to the standard anatomic planes designated by the usual descriptive terminology, schematic diagrams illustrating the route of circulation are inherently anatomically inaccurate [29]. Although the four parts of the ventricular septum—inlet, trabecular, infundibular, and membranous—are usually diagrammed as a straight line, the septum actually occupies a triangular plane, which bows to the right, resulting in the conical left and crescentic right ventricles [29].

The pulmonary veins form one or more veins on either side and enter the dorsal aspect of the left atrium. The left atrium is more spherical and has a smoother endocardium than the right atrium. The large anterior and small posterior leaflets of the mitral valve attach to two corresponding papillary muscles by thin, delicate chordae. The left ventricular lining has fine trabeculae in contrast with the large, fleshy trabeculae of the right ventricle. In contrast to the relation between the tricuspid and pulmonary valve leaflets, the anterior leaflet of the mitral valve has fibrous continuity with the left and noncoronary cusps of the aortic valve.

Although the mitral and aortic valves appear continuous, a thin fibrous connective tissue band separates the anterior leaflet of the mitral valve from the adjacent sinuses of the aortic valve to form a normal spectrum of mitral and aortic valve discontinuity. The anterior mitral valve leaflet and the left and noncoronary cusps of the aortic valve have a variable relationship in normal hearts and a prominent separation in some malformations due to a muscular band interpreted as either persistence of the aortic conus or the bulboventricular flange [30].

Valve annular size in infants as measured in formalin-fixed hearts has not correlated well with the same measurement by two-dimensional echocardiography, differing by an average of 17%. Valve dimensions by two-dimensional echocardiography correlate well with body weight, forming a basis for determining valvular adequacy [30a].

The coronary arteries arise from the corresponding valve leaflet's sinus, but with considerable anatomic variation, without altering normal coronary arterial blood flow. The normal ascending aorta and aortic arch have a perceptibly larger cross-sectional diameter than the isthmus, which is that portion of the aorta between the left subclavian artery and the junction with the ductus arteriosus. At the isthmus, considerable activity during morphogenesis makes it a potential site for malformations secondary to diminished blood flow through the ascending aorta—e.g., coarctation, tubular hypoplasia, and interruption of the aortic arch. Although variable, the ductus arteriosus may be straight, mildly curved (C-shaped), or markedly curved (S-shaped), tending toward greater curvature as pregnancy proceeds [30b]. An abnormally S-shaped kinking of the ductus arteriosus has been related to fetal right atrial and ventricular dilatation, and transient tricuspid and pulmonary valve insufficiency [30c].

Segmental Analysis

In an attempt to group the combinations of congenital cardiovascular malformations rather than empirically tabulate them, Van Praagh [31] and others identify each cardiovascular segment, providing a uniform, less complex, descriptive classification. The eight developmental units of the heart representing anatomic units with an embryologic connotation (Table 20.4) are condensed to three for a descriptive classification: the visceroatrial situs, the ventricular loop, and the conotruncus. Each segment indicates the location of a major portion of the cardiovascular system: the visceroatrial situs locates the viscera and atria, the ventricular loop locates the ventricles, and the conotruncus locates the infundibulum and great arteries [21, 32].

Visceroatrial Situs The three potential types of situs are solitus, the usual or ordinary; inversus, the mirror image of the usual; and ambiguous, an ambiguous situs frequently accompanied by an anomalous visceral arrangement best characterized by the visceral arrangement in asplenia. With uncommon exceptions, atrial morphology determines visceral situs. The IVC connection to the right atrium is a

Table 20.4. Developmental units of the cardiovascular system

1. Sinus venosus	Venae cavae
	Coronary sinus
	Venous portion of the right atrium
2. Common pulmonary vein	Pulmonary veins
	Venous portion of the left atrium
3. Primitive atrium	Right and left atrial appendages
4. AV canal	Mitral and tricuspid valves
5. Ventricle	Left ventricle
6. Proximal bulbus cordis	Right ventricle
7. Distal bulbus cordis	Conus or infundibulum
8. Truncus	Aorta and pulmonary artery

From Van Praagh [31].

good marker for situs; the SVC connection is less reliable since it may join either atrium. In the absence of the IVC, usually restricted to absence of the segment receiving the renal and hepatic veins, the venous drainage goes to the azygous system [31].

Ventricular Loop Classification according to ventricular looping is based on variations of the normal fold to the right of the primitive cardiac tube, forming a d-loop; a fold to the left is designated an l-loop. As a result of looping, the proximal bulbus cordis (the primitive right ventricle) lies to the right of the future left ventricle with a d-loop; the converse with an l-loop. This interpretation of embryogenesis of the heart leads to Van Praagh's loop rule:

1. *d-loop:* The great arteries have their normal relationship, with the right ventricle on the right; with d-transposition of the great arteries, the aortic valve is to the right of the pulmonic valve.
2. *l-loop:* The great arteries have an inverse relationship, with the right ventricle on the left; with l-transposition of the great arteries indicated by an inverse relationship of the great arteries, the aortic valve is to the left of the pulmonic valve.

Although the loop rule has exceptions, particularly with single ventricle and dextrocardia, the distribution of the coronary arteries distinguishes the exceptions [31]. With a d-loop, the left anterior descending artery arises from the left coronary artery; with an l-loop, it originates from the right. Because of exceptions to the loop rule with transposition of the great arteries, complete transposition may be identified by the position of the right atrium and the aorta on the same side, and corrected transposition by the right atrium and aorta on opposite sides [31].

Conotruncus The conotruncus may take one of four configurations:

1. *Subpulmonary conus:* The normal pattern of a conus on the right between the tricuspid and pulmonic

valves; fibrous continuity of the mitral and aortic valves. The subpulmonic conus may be under-developed in tetralogy of Fallot and truncus arteriosus.
2. *Subaortic conus:* Absence of fibrous continuity between aortic and mitral valves characterizes the typical d- or l-transposition, whether complete or corrected.
3. *Bilateral conus:* Absence of fibrous continuity between either semilunar valve and either AV valve characterizes a number of malformations such as double-outlet right ventricle, transposition of the great arteries with pulmonary infundibular stenosis or atresia, and the ambiguous hearts of the asplenia syndromes.
4. *Absence of conal muscle beneath both great arteries:* Bilateral fibrous continuity between semilunar and AV valves in a case of double-outlet left ventricle [31].

While acknowledging the advantages of a segmental approach, Tynan et al avoid the dependence on changing concepts of embryology by describing the connections between the cardiac segments, their morphology, and their relations, and tabulating additional anomalies [33]. The discrete steps in the segmental approach require an assessment of each junction of the cardiac segments, the atria with the ventricles and the ventricles with the great arteries using four steps: the type of connection, the mode of connection, the morphology of the ventricles, and the relation of the ventricles to each other [33]. The segmental classification has utility with simple as well as complex malformations [34, 35].

Definition of normal valves and ventricles aids segmental classification. A normal ventricle has three components:

1. The inlet lies distal to the AV valve with or without a patent valve.
2. The trabecular component, distinctive for each ventricle, lies distal to the insertion of the papillary muscles independent of both the inlet and outlet.
3. The outlet or infundibular component, muscular on the right and attenuated on the left, supports the semilunar valve.

A ventricle need not have an outlet component but must have, at the very least, an inlet and a trabecular portion; a rudimentary chamber has no inlet and only a trabecular portion. An outlet chamber has trabecular and outlet components. A trabecular pouch has only the trabecular component.

Chambers and valves may be related in various defined ways:

1. Both inlet and outlet ventricular portions may be straddled by a valve.
2. A valve is arbitrarily assigned to a ventricle that has more than half its annulus.

3. A chamber has an inlet when it connects to more than half of an AV valve.
4. A rudimentary outlet chamber supports more than half of an arterial valve annulus.
5. A trabecular pouch connects to less than half of an AV and arterial valve.

With a common AV valve, the ventricles are considered separate, although a rudimentary chamber has less than a fourth of the valvular annulus.

The segmental analysis of Tynan et al [33] has four descriptive steps:

1. Atrial situs
2. AV junction
   a. AV connections
   b. Mode of connection
   c. Ventricular morphology
   d. Relation of ventricular chambers to each other
3. Ventriculoarterial junction
   a. Arterial connections
   b. Arterial relations
   c. Morphology of the outflow tracts.
4. Additional anomalies

Atrial situs—situs solitus, inversus, or ambiguous—describes the visceral situs established from the bronchial anatomy as its most reliable guide [33].

AV Junction
AV connections: A heart with two atria and two ventricles may have concordant, discordant, or ambiguous AV connections. An ambiguous connection implies an inability to identify the atria. With only one ventricle, the AV junction may be a double inlet or the absence of one connection, as with a valvular atresia.
Mode of connection: The connection may be with or without straddling by the tricuspid valve, mitral valve, or a common AV valve. A heart with a single ventricle may have two valves one of which may straddle, a common valve that may straddle, or one patent and one atretic valve.
Ventricular morphology: Features of the trabecular zone and the septal orientation designate a ventricle as right or left regardless of the connections. The coarse trabeculations, particularly of the septum, identify the right ventricle; the fine trabeculations and smooth septum identify the left ventricle. A rudimentary chamber may be indeterminate, but its trabecular arrangement is usually the converse of that of the main chamber.
Relation of ventricular chambers: A rudimentary chamber may be right of, left of, anterior to, posterior to, superior to, or inferior to the main ventricle.

Ventriculoarterial Junctions
Arterial connections: The four types of ventriculoarterial connections are concordant, discordant, double-outlet ventricle or chamber, and single-outlet heart. In a

concordant connection, the aorta arises from the left ventricle or left outlet chamber and the pulmonary artery arises from the right ventricle or right outlet chamber; in a discordant connection, the converse origins obtain. More than half of both aorta and pulmonary artery arising from a chamber constitutes a double outlet. A single-outlet heart may have a truncus arteriosus, pulmonary artery, or aortic valvular atresia.

Arterial relations: The relative positions of the aortic and pulmonary valves to each other in the anterior-posterior and lateral planes determine the relations of the great arteries.

Morphology of outflow tracts: Either or both semilunar valves may have a complete infundibulum or fibrous continuity with an AV valve. Outflow tract morphology is independent of both the connections and the relations of the great arteries and their valves.

Additional cardiovascular anomalies include abnormalities of venous connection, anomalous arterial origins, septal defects, and intracardiac obstructions [33].

Changes in the Circulation at Birth

Changes in circulation at birth accommodate the fetus emerging from a liquid, amniotic fluid environment to an air-breathing status (Fig. 20.9). In the fetus, the placenta pro-vides sustenance for growth, and maintains respiratory function by providing relatively well-oxygenated blood with a Po_2 (as measured in the fetal lamb) of about 30 mm Hg via the umbilical vein [36]. In the fetus, the umbilical vein becomes the ductus venosus, which extends about 1 to 2 cm along the inferior surface of the liver to join the hepatic vein after receiving a few anastomoses with the portal vein. About one half of the umbilical venous blood goes through the liver, while the remainder bypasses the liver through the ductus venosus to enter the inferior vena cava.

The eustachian valve guarding the entrance of the inferior vena cava into the right atrium directs the blood toward the atrial septum, where the crista dividens (the anterior limb) of the foramen ovale deflects most of it into the left atrium, leaving only a small proportion to enter the right atrium and join the venous return from the superior vena cava to enter the tricuspid valve. The crista interveniens, an indentation of the atrium between the orifices of the inferior and superior venae cavae, directs the blood from the superior vena cava entering the right atrium through the tricuspid valve to the right ventricle, with only about 2–3% entering the left atrium through the foramen ovale, resulting in a higher Po_2 in left atrial and ventricular blood since most of the relatively well-oxygenated blood from the umbilical vein ends up on the left [36].

Only about 10–15% of the stroke volume from the right ventricle enters the lung through the pulmonary artery; the

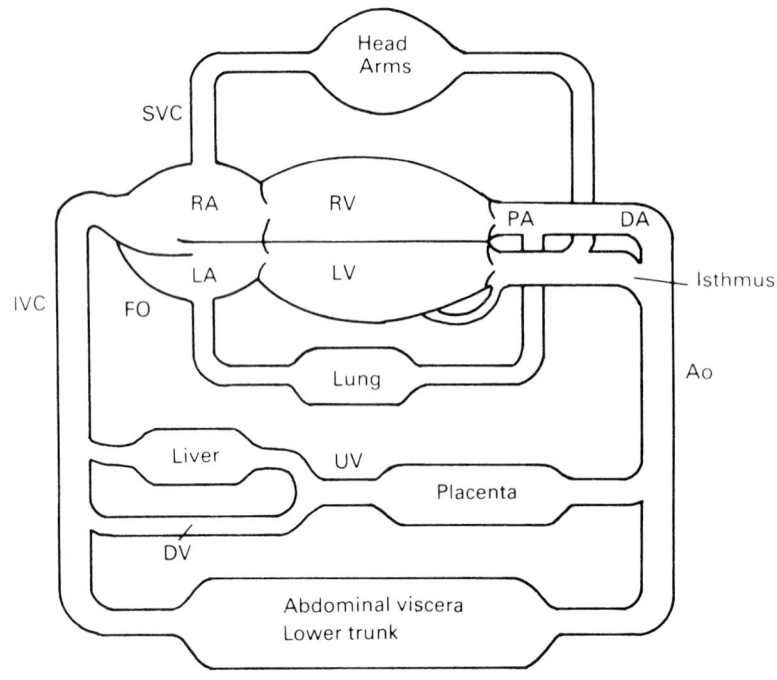

RV = Right ventricle
LV = Left ventricle
PA = Pulmonary artery
DA = Ductus arteriosus
Ao = Aorta
UV = Umbilical vein

DV = Ductus venosus
SVC = Superior vena cava
IVC = Inferior vena cava
FO = Foramen ovale
RA = Right atrium
LA = Left atrium

FIGURE 20.9. *Fetal circulation provides for the placental contribution to respiration and nutrition. Changes at birth must accommodate loss of the placenta, pulmonary expansion, and left ventricular support of the systemic circulation. (After Rudolph [36].)*

remainder goes through the ductus arteriosus to the descending aorta [36, 36a]. The preferential flow of the right ventricular blood through the ductus into the aorta relates to the unexpanded fetal lungs and the medial hypertrophy of the high-resistance pulmonary arteries. As a result of blood flow through the ductus, right ventricular blood perfuses the aorta and its branches distal to the left subclavian artery supplying the trunk, abdominal organs, lower extremities, and umbilical arteries. The high resistance may relate to the perfusion of the lung with the blood from the superior vena cava with its relatively low Po$_2$, high Pco$_2$, and low pH rather than the higher Po$_2$ of blood from the IVC.

The fetal pulmonary arteries develop a thickened medial layer in response to high pulmonary arterial pressures and to hypoxic induced constriction. The hypertrophy progressively increases during the latter half of gestation without precise correlation to functional changes, since resistance remains constant and pulmonary blood flow may increase. Circumstances that accentuate the low Po$_2$ of the pulmonary blood have no known effect on pulmonary vascular development, although postnatally the pulmonary vascular resistance drops more slowly at high altitudes or with a ventricular septal defect [36].

Postnatal Changes in the Pulmonary Circulation

The rise in Po$_2$ of the pulmonary arterial blood with the onset of respiration accompanies a reduction in the pulmonary arterial resistance. Endogenous nitric oxide (endothelium-derived relaxing factor) from normal vascular endothelium affects the normal decline in pulmonary vascular resistance at birth by modifying vascular tone in the fetal and postnatal lung [36b]. In the fetus at sea level, pulmonary vascular resistance drops in the first 2 to 3 days of life, accompanying constriction of the ductus, and reaches adult levels at about 2 weeks [36].

The paired umbilical arteries branch from the internal iliac arteries to ascend along the internal surface of the abdominal wall, separated by the urachus, to traverse the umbilicus and enter the umbilical cord, returning the oxygen-poor blood to the placenta and completing the fetoplacental circulation.

The well-oxygenated blood shunted through the foramen ovale joins the relatively small pulmonary venous return in the left atrium, traversing the mitral valve and left ventricle to supply the aorta and its branches proximal to the ductus—the coronary, brachiocephalic, left carotid, and left subclavian arteries. This route of circulation supplies the coronary arteries and brain with blood at a higher Po$_2$ value than that of the distal body organs and returns the unoxygenated blood to the placenta via the umbilical arteries. The left ventricle supplies the ascending aorta and aortic arch to the orifice of the left subclavian artery but proximal to the ductus arteriosus, and the right ventricle supplies the aorta distal to the ductus, leaving a stagnant segment of aorta—the aortic isthmus—between the left subclavian artery and

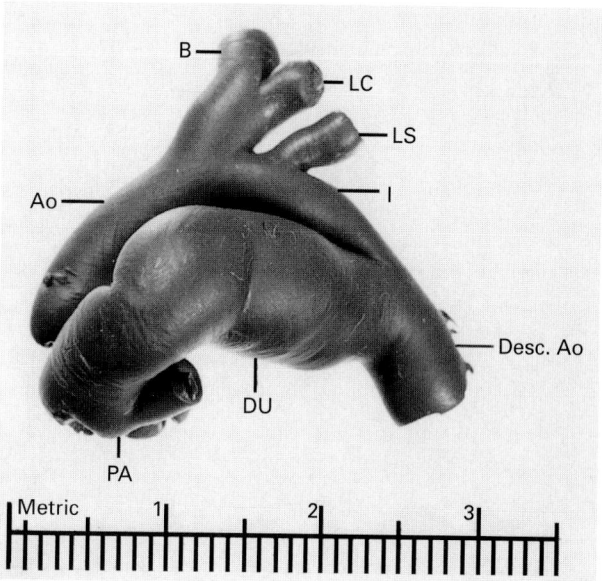

FIGURE 20.10. *A cast of the great arteries of a neonate illustrates the smaller diameter of the aortic isthmus as compared with the ascending or descending aorta or the ductus arteriosus. Ao—ascending aorta; PA—pulmonary artery; DU—ductus arteriosus; B—brachiocephalic artery; LC—left common carotid artery; LS—left subclavian artery; I—aortic isthmus; Desc. Ao—descending aorta. (Reproduced with permission from: Rosenberg HS. Coarctation of the aorta: morphology and pathogenetic considerations. In: Rosenberg HS, Bolande RP, eds.* Perspectives in Pediatric Pathology. *vol. 1. Chicago: Year Book Medical, 1973, p. 350.)*

the ductus, which remains smaller in diameter than the aorta proximal or distal to it (Fig. 20.10). Developmentally, the isthmus represents the junction of the fourth aortic arch, the distal portion of the sixth aortic arch (the ductus), and the descending aorta.

At birth, anatomic changes follow the functional changes, some taking place immediately and some delayed for days, weeks, months, or years.

1. The umbilical arteries and vein are severed, and their lumina obliterate. Separation of the placenta with its low vascular resistance increases systemic vascular resistance and consequently left ventricular pressure. Even before the umbilical cord is cut, the fetal lifeline [37] has been interrupted by separation of the placenta; any continued pulsations in the umbilical cord represent fetal circulation and not support from the placenta. Umbilical arterial and venous lumina remain patent for several days after birth (up to 4 days for the arteries, even longer for the veins), allowing access into the neonatal circulation during much of the first week of life. The ductus venosus closes functionally during the first 24 hours of life but remains patent since it has little muscle in its wall other than at its junction with the portal sinus.

2. The foramen ovale closes. The expanded lung and the reduced pressure on the right side of the heart functionally close the foramen ovale by allowing the increased left-sided pressure to close the flap forming the valve of the foramen ovale, although temporary incompetence at birth may allow a brief left-to-right shunt. Despite the functional closure of the foramen ovale, the valve does not seal promptly and the lumen remains patent (competent) in almost 50% of children at age 5 years and approximately 20% of otherwise normal adults.

3. The lungs expand. Expansion of the lungs begins with the first breath and is completed after several breaths. With expansion, the air spaces dilate, the lungs occupy a greater volume, and the pulmonary arteries traverse a greater distance, forcing them to uncoil and contribute to a decreased vascular resistance.

4. The small muscular arteries of the lungs lose their muscular mass (Fig. 20.11). The immediate expansion of the lungs accompanies a prompt drop in pulmonary vascular resistance, but the small pulmonary arteries retain their thick muscular walls of fetal life for several weeks [37a]. The medial thickness does not decrease uniformly through-out the lungs. Most arteries assume a mature configuration within 6 weeks after birth, but since others within the same lung may retain their thick media for an additional several weeks, medial hypertrophy cannot be considered pathologic until 12 weeks of age.

Because retention of medial hypertrophy in the small pulmonary arteries after birth may be prolonged with hypoxia or left-to-right shunts, left ventricular failure is rare prior to 4 to 12 weeks of life. The mechanism for controlling the medial

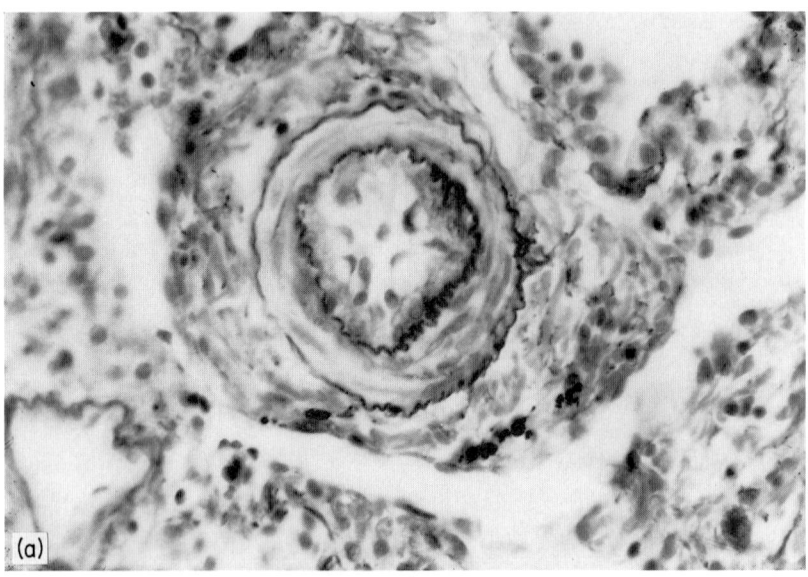

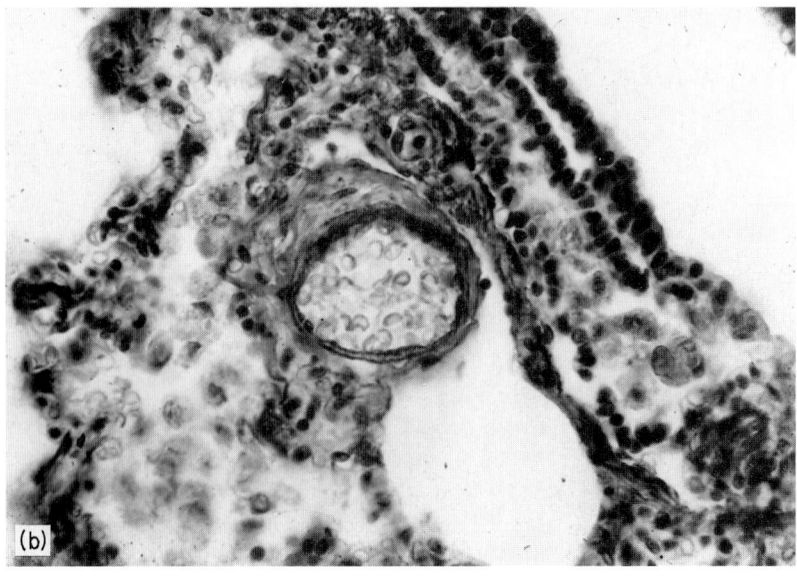

FIGURE 20.11.   *In small pulmonary muscular arteries of comparable size, the neonatal artery (a) has a greater amount of medial muscle than an artery at 3 months of age (b). (Verhoeff–van Gieson, ×100).*

thickness remains unknown, but hypoxia from any cause—e.g., alveolar hypoventilation or low environmental oxygen at high altitudes—delays maturation. Mechanisms of control have a species variation, and perhaps an intraspecies variation as well—e.g., calves hyperreact to hypoxia, whereas other species react little [38]. During the perinatal period of persistent medial smooth muscle thickness, the vessels have increased reactivity to hypoxia and acidemia. Since pulmonary arterial smooth muscle in the fetus increases with advancing gestational age, premature infants have less medial smooth muscle than full-term infants, may have a more rapid drop in vascular resistance, and are susceptible to an earlier onset of failure [36].

At birth, the prompt change in pulmonary arterial pressure with expansion of the lung contrasts with the gradual change in elastic tissue in the pulmonary artery. The pulmonary artery loses its high-pressure compact elastic laminar structure as the fibers break into smaller fragments separated by smooth muscle and collagen, forming a filigree pattern [39].

5. The left ventricle assumes its predominance and its muscle hypertrophies. The right and left ventricular myocardial fibers of the fetus are equal in size and in their respective muscular masses, representing the equal resistance to flow to each ventricle without the disparity of decreased resistance through an expanded lung (Fig. 20.12). During fetal life, the right ventricle gradually assumes predominance, being smaller than the left ventricle in the first trimester and of equal size in the second trimester. Although the left ventricle begins its work

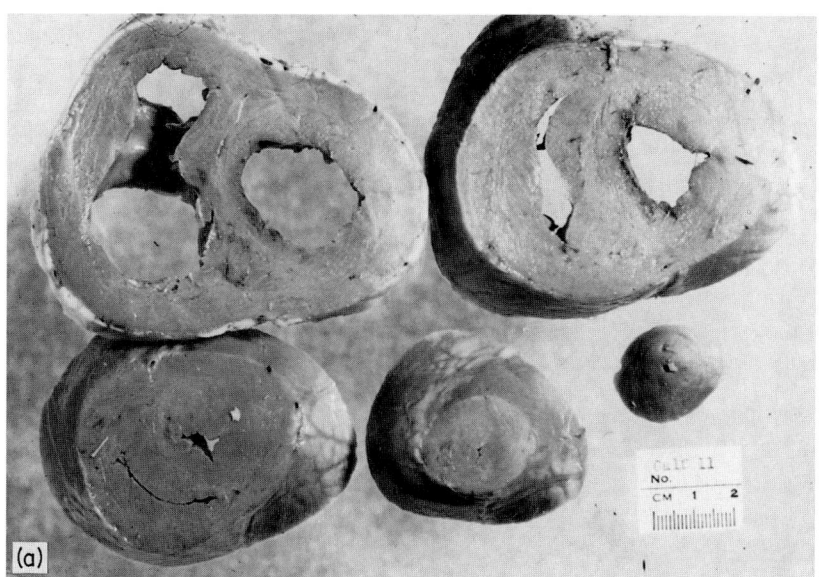

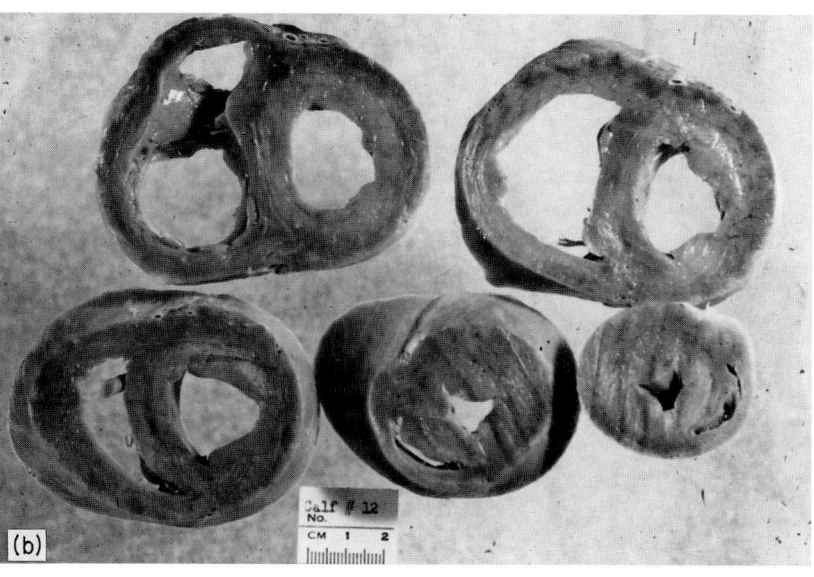

FIGURE 20.12. *At birth, the right and left ventricular muscle masses in the calf (as in the human) are equal (a). At 3 months of age, the left ventricle has assumed its predominance (b).*

overcoming systemic resistance with the first breath and closure of the ductus, the relative muscular hypertrophy is gradual. During fetal life, most hearts have a disproportionate ventricular septal thickening, defined as a septal–free wall ratio equal to or greater than 1.3. In more than a third of fetuses, this ratio may exceed 2.0. This proportion may be present at birth, but usually disappears by about 2 weeks of age. After birth, the free wall thickens at a faster rate than the septum [40].

At birth, the right and left ventricular muscular weights are equal. By about 12 weeks, the adult configuration is reached, with the weight of the right ventricle being one-half that of the left ventricle, and one-third of the total ventricular muscular mass [41].

6. The ductus arteriosus closes. Blood flow through the ductus arteriosus slows and stops with the development of a gradient between the high aortic pressure and the lower pulmonary arterial pressure. Before the ductus closes at 10 to 15 hours, the fetal right-to-left shunt has reversed to left-to-right; after closure of the ductus, the pulmonary arterial pressure drops and the systemic pressure rises. Since the structural orientation of the ductus favors flow from the pulmonary artery to the aorta and not the reverse, flow becomes stagnant and then stops in the first days of life, and anatomic closure follows at about 2 weeks of age.

7. The aortic isthmus begins its expansion with the closure of the ductus arteriosus and continues over several years of life [42].

The Ductus Arteriosus

The morphology of normal closure of the ductus arteriosus has been imprecisely understood, since most studies have been based on autopsy material, necessarily including infants who had been hypoxic for variable periods of time, which has a profound effect on the ductus [43]. Prostaglandin E_2, generated in the fetus and placenta, maintains patency of the fetal ductus [44]. Premature closure of the ductus may accompany tetralogy of Fallot or therapeutic administration of prostaglandin synthetase inhibitors for tocolysis. When the fetal ductus closes prematurely, as it rarely does, fetal distress [44a] or congestive heart failure and fetal hydrops [45, 45a] may result. Many factors influence normal closure of the ductus: prematurity, prenatal hypoxia, fetal infections such as rubella, heredity, birth at high altitude, prostaglandins, serum calcium concentration, and fluid intake. Postnatal oxygen is a potent stimulus to ductal contraction. Although unexplained, in premature infants the ductus may remain patent, may close immediately, or may close and then reopen in the first 2 weeks of life, allowing systemic-to-pulmonary shunting [35, 46]. Abnormal patency of the ductus with a lumen capable of passing a 1-mm probe has been defined as failure of closure during the first year of life [47].

Morphologically, the ductus has the three characteristic layers of a muscular artery. The intima rests directly on the internal elastic membrane or an intimal cushion made of a smooth muscle, elastic, and collagen bundle of variable size usually arranged longitudinally. Cushions, which appear as early as the 16th week of gestation and become progressively more extensive with advancing gestation, appear earliest and the most prominent in the pulmonary arterial aspect of the ductus. The internal elastic membrane is intact beneath the endothelium but may fragment beneath the cushions [48].

Histologically, the ductal intima consists of a single layer of endothelium separated from the underlying media by an internal elastic membrane. The loosely arranged smooth muscle fibers of the media lie in a connective tissue matrix with a few fine, wavy elastic fibers. The media has two indistinctly separated layers: an outer one-third with a spiral pattern penetrated by small groups of longitudinal fibers and an inner layer with fibers arranged in an oblique-to-longitudinal pattern with penetrating longitudinal fibers. No external elastic membrane lies between the media and the poorly defined adventitial fibrous tissue containing vasa vasorum and nerves. Elastic lamellae and collagen extend into the ductus from both the aorta and the pulmonary artery, seemingly supporting the ductal muscle [48].

Most ductuses have mounds of the inner media protruding into the lumen penetrating through gaps in the internal elastic membrane and covered by endothelium (Fig. 20.13). Muscle fibers in the inner media appear degenerated. In ducts with narrow lumina, the smooth muscle cells become inconspicuous. As the duct closes, the cellular elements are lost and the ligamentum becomes a hyalinized cord. A few ducts with patent lumina have thickened intima, a less dense media, increased ground substance, and increased elastic fibers. Ducts remaining patent beyond 1 year of life have a persistent internal elastic membrane without protrusion of the medial elements into the lumen [47] and a close relation of endothelial cells to subendothelial elastic lamina [48a].

Gradual closure with increased ground substance accompanying the mounds of proliferating intima or media has been interpreted as the mechanism of normal closure. Fragmentation of the internal elastic membrane accompanies the appearance of mucoid-filled spaces. Medial proliferation rather than intimal changes affects closure, with the changes beginning during fetal life [47].

Pathologic lesions in the ductus include intimal fibrinous deposits, focal hemorrhage, and dissecting aneurysms [48]. Subendothelial fibrin appears in patent ductus, in contrast with the intraluminal thrombi of contracting ductus. Most infants with ductal hemorrhage have been hypoxemic and acidotic. Dissecting aneurysms, frequently covered at the intimal aspect by fibrin, extend short and straight, circumferentially through the media, or track through the adventitia [48]. Ductal histology in growth-retarded premature infants has been marked by an increased incidence of frag-

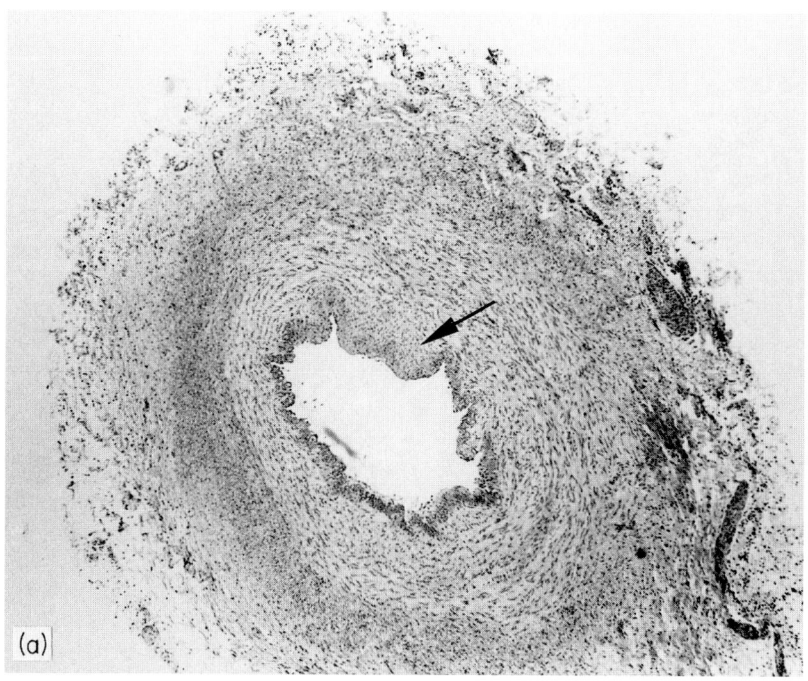

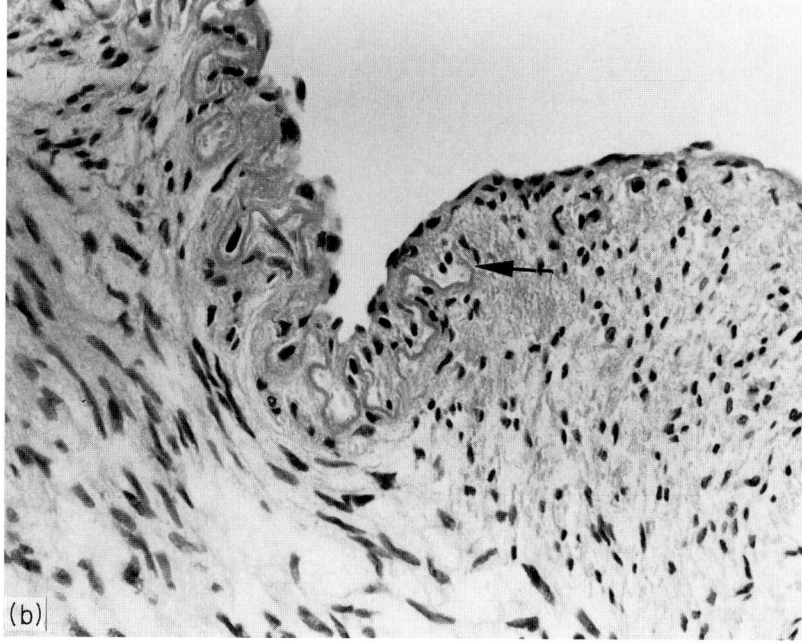

FIGURE 20.13. *(a) Mounds of media protruding into the lumen of the ductus arteriosus (arrow) result in an irregular inner boundary (H&E, ×40). (b) The mounds, which have an endothelial covering, focally penetrate toward the lumen through breaks (arrow) in the internal elastic membrane (H&E, ×100).*

mentation and coagulation necrosis of the intimal elastic lamina and of hemorrhage [48b].

The ductus remains functionally patent in most premature infants for the first 2 or 3 days of life, but persistent patency is a major cause of morbidity, causing prolonged respiratory compromise during the recovery phase of infantile respiratory distress syndrome (RDS). According to a national collaborative study, treatment with indomethacin effectively closes the ductus and decreases morbidity [49]. Pharmacologic closure of the ductus is not always successful, and even if closure is achieved, the ductus may reopen [50]. Ductal morphology in infants treated with prostaglandin has been marked by an increased incidence of pathologic lesions [48, 51, 51a, 51b]. The prognosis of premature infants with a patent ductus relates to the status of the respiratory distress; the prognosis is bad only if the respiratory distress is progressive [52].

MALFORMATION COMPLEXES

Atrial Septal Defects

The several malformations of the atrial septum—defects in the fossa ovalis, foramen primum defects, premature closure of the foramen ovale, and aneurysms of the fossa ovalis—account for an estimated 7% of congenital heart disease (CHD) in children, but they rarely affect the neonate. The most common malformation of the atrial septum, a defect in the fossa ovalis, may have a variety of configurations, but all have the same functional effect (Fig. 20.14). Recognizing the development of the atrial septum aids the distinction between an atrial septal defect (ASD) and a functionally patent but normal foramen ovale.

As the endocardial cushions fuse with the septum primum to close the foramen primum between the two primitive atria, perforations appear in the septum primum that coalesce to form the ostium secundum. The septum secundum extends anteriorly and inferiorly from the superior and posterior regions of the right atrium, covering the ostium secundum but leaving an interatrial communication, the foramen ovale. The septum secundum lies on the right side of the atrial septum, and the septum primum on the left. The opening in the septum primum does not coincide with the foramen ovale, resulting in the oblique passageway closed by the septum primum serving as a valve flap. The leading edge of the septum secundum forms the crista dividens, which diverts the fetal blood flow from the IVC through the foramen ovale into the left atrium.

With the changes in the cardiovascular pressure relationships at birth, the increasing left atrial pressure forces the septum primum against the septum secundum, functionally closing the oblique passage through the foramen ovale, although a potential passage remains. The foramen ovale closes after about a month, but remains patent in about half of 5-year-old children and about one-fourth of adults.

Defects in the fossa ovalis, known as secundum or fossa

Table 20.5.　Types of atrial septal defects in infants less than 1 year of age

Form of defect in the atrial septum	Incidence (%) among all atrial septal defects		
Fossa ovalis defects			93
Valve incompetent foramen ovale		88	
Associated malformations	85		
No associated malformations	3		
Fenestrated valve of the foramen ovale		5	
Other defects			6
Sinus venosus defect		5	
Single atrium		1	

From Tandon and Edwards [54].

ovalis defects, may result from an oversize ostium secundum, an undersize septum secundum, or fenestrations in the portion of the septum secundum covering the foramen ovale (Fig. 20.15; Table 20.5) [53, 54]. From among the multifactorial causes of congenital cardiovascular malformations, first-trimester maternal alcohol consumption and the fetal alcohol syndrome stand out as risk factors for ASDs as well as other malformations [55, 56].

Defects in the atrial septum other than in the fossa ovalis affect the atrial inlet (sinus venosus defect) and outlet (atrioventricular canal, or AVC, defect):

1. Septum primum defects virtually always accompany defects in the AV valves forming the spectrum of AVC defects.
2. Sinus venosus defect, which accounts for 2–3% of ASD, adjoins the ostium of the SVC and is usually

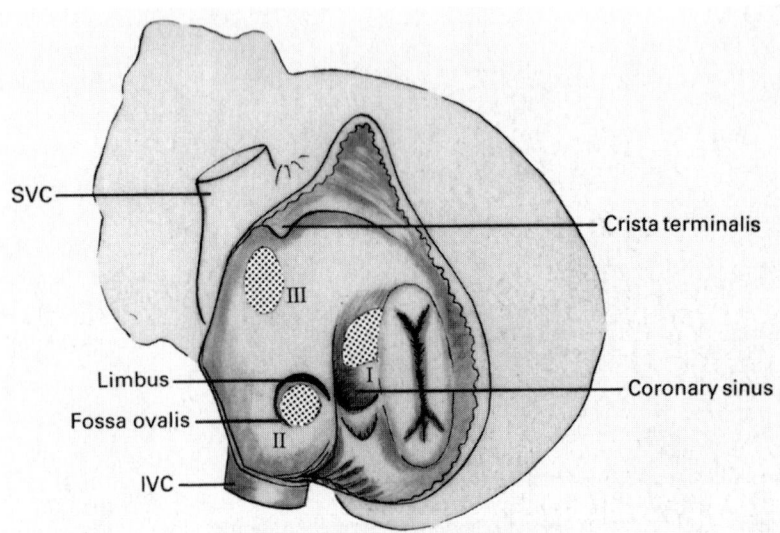

FIGURE 20.14.　*Atrial septal defects, as they relate to the anatomic landmarks of the right atrium, are primum defects (I) at the inferior margin of the septum adjoining the annulus of the tricuspid valve, secundum defects (II) in the fossa ovalis, and less common sites (III) adjacent to the ostium of the superior vena cava. IVC—inferior vena cava; SVC—superior vena cava.*

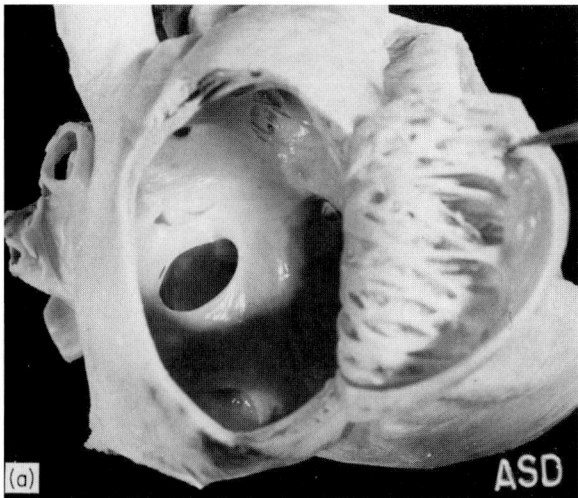

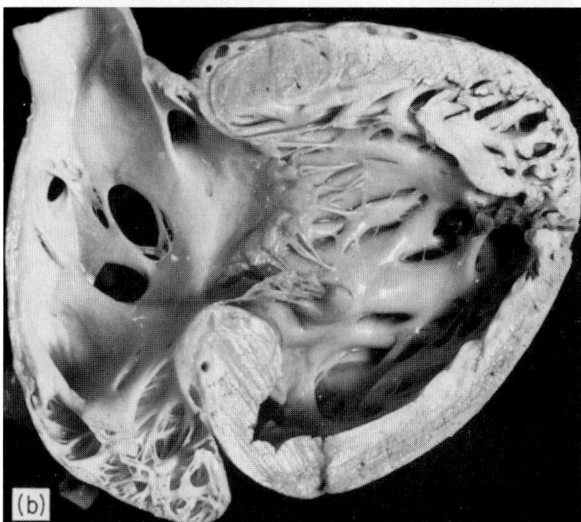

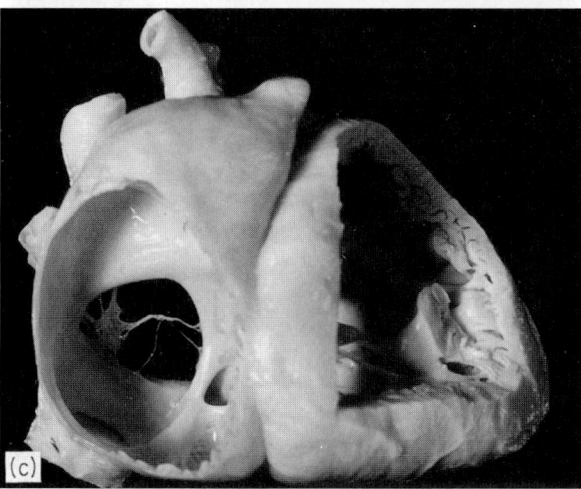

FIGURE 20.15. *Secundum ASDs may result from absence of the valve of the foramen ovale (a), or fenestrations of the valve of the foramen ovale, leaving the foramen partially (b) or completely (c) unguarded.*

associated with anomalous pulmonary venous drainage from the right upper lobe [53].

3. Coronary sinus defect has been attributed to persistence of the left SVC entering the right atrium and an absent coronary sinus.

4. An IVC defect lies low in the atrial septum adjacent to the ostium of the IVC.

Although isolated ASDs are among the most common cardiac malformations, they rarely cause symptoms in the neonate, and the malformation may escape detection during the first year of life. Much more commonly, an ASD identified in an infant, usually a secundum defect or a valve-incompetent foramen ovale, accompanies other malformations. Of infants 6 months of age or less with CHD identified at autopsy, about one-third have ASDs that do not appear to have contributed to the fatalities. Infants with secundum ASDs and failure to thrive often have noncardiac bases for their symptoms [56a].

Since a major factor relating to poor outcome from management of ASD is pulmonary hypertension, intervention is usually directed toward prevention of the long-term complications of chronic left-to-right shunting [57, 58]. The choice of the method of closure has resulted in closer scrutiny of the size of the ASD and its site in the fossa ovalis. Based on the relation of the size of the ASD to its natural history, Radzik et al concluded that defects less than 3mm in diameter had a virtual 100% spontaneous closure rate by 18 months of age [59]. Considering the high rate of spontaneous closure of the small defects and the failure to conform to the usual female preponderance for ASD, Radzik et al questioned whether defects measuring less than 3mm should be considered malformations. Only defects larger than 8mm were considered unlikely to close spontaneously. Those with diameters of 3 to 5mm and 5 to 8mm had closure rates of 87% and 80%, respectively [59]. Based on the usual site of the ASD within an undistorted fossa ovalis, an estimated 50–68% of children with ASDs should be candidates for transcatheter closure [60, 61].

Functional changes relate to the size of the defect in the septum. With a large defect, pressures in the atria equalize, while a small defect usually permits a left-to-right shunt, depending on the resistance to ventricular inflow. A transient left-to-right shunt at birth may result from a stretched flap of the foramen ovale, but a major shunt usually implies an associated malformation—mitral or aortic valve atresia, coarctation, transposition of the great arteries, or patent ductus arteriosus. Rarely, an ASD may be responsible for a right-to-left shunt, cardiomegaly, and failure in the neonate [62] with symptoms appearing at birth or during the first week of life [63–65]. More often, failure takes place well after the newborn period, frequently from associated malformations causing left ventricular obstruction, such as mitral valve or supravalvular stenosis or left ventricular cardiomyopathy. If the ASD was due to a dilated atrium and the dilatation is relieved, the ASD may close spontaneously.

Premature Closure of the Foramen Ovale

The foramen ovale may close prematurely, inhibiting venous return from the IVC to the left atrium in the normal fetal circulation, resulting in fetal hydrops, polyhydramnios, an underdeveloped left atrium, ventricle, and aorta, and stillbirth or rapidly fatal congestive heart failure at birth [66, 67, 68, 68a]. Several infants with premature closure of the foramen ovale have also had gonadal dysgenesis or the XO karyotype [69, 70].

Developmentally, premature closure may result from failed development of the ostium secundum in the septum primum, excessive growth of the septum secundum, or premature fusion of the septum primum and septum secundum, resulting in absence of the fossa ovalis, a normal but imperforate fossa ovalis, or a minute orifice. Premature closure of the foramen ovale may result in an aneurysm of the fossa ovalis (which may also accompany tricuspid valve atresia) and may accompany obstructive lesions on the left side of the heart—e.g., aortic or mitral valvular atresia or stenosis, bicuspid aortic valve, or coarctation [69].

Atrioventricular Canal Defects

Inclusion of atrioventricular canal (AVC) defects among disorders of the atrial septum is arbitrary, since canal defects comprise a spectrum of malformations that may include a defect in the inferior part of the atrial septum, abnormality of one or both AV valves, and a defect in the ventricular septum (Fig. 20.16). Because of the varied appearance of components of the spectrum, alternative terms and synonyms abound, further modified as complete, partial, intermediate, transitional, or primitive: Examples include canalis atrioventricularis communis, endocardial cushion defect, persistent atrioventricular ostium (or canal) malformation, ostium primum septal defect with cleft mitral valve, atrioventricular defect, atrioventricular septal defect, and atrioventricular canal [71–73].

While acknowledging good reasons from all sides for proper designation, we elect to use atrioventricular canal (AVC) defect for the entire spectrum. The complex origin of this malformation relates to failure of partition of the common channel between the embryonic atria and ventricles. Although the atrial septum is typically deficient in its lower portion, where it would have been contiguous with the AV valves, the site of the embryonic ostium primum and the source of its designation as an ostium primum defect, AVC defect involves more than persistence of the ostium primum [71]. The precise mechanism of this failure remains unknown, but Hutchins et al present the innovative concept of absence of the necessary compression of the atria in embryonic stages 13 to 18, rather than an inadequate growth of the endocardial cushions [73].

Titus and Rastelli divided the AVC complex into two groups: complete and incomplete based on the association of defects in the atrial and ventricular septa. Complete AVC has both an atrial and a ventricular septal defect; incomplete forms may have one or the other, or neither (Table 20.6) [71].

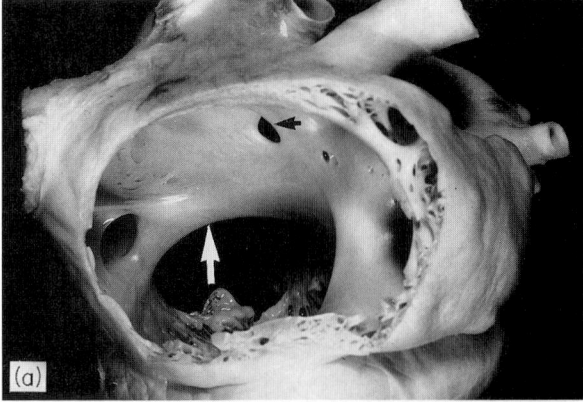

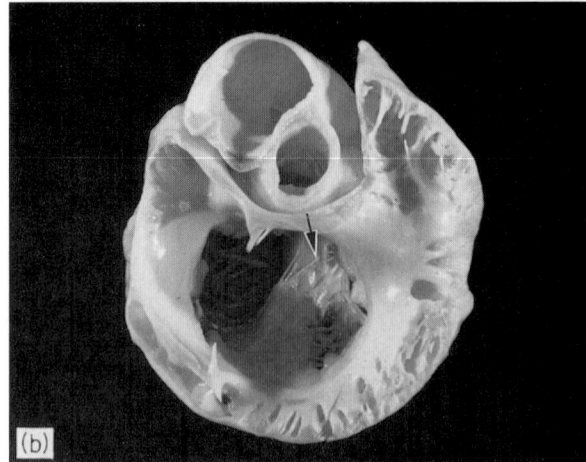

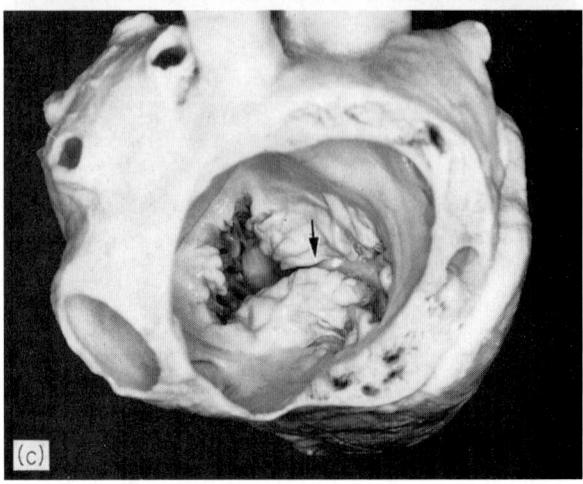

FIGURE 20.16.   *As viewed from the unroofed right atrium, (a) the foramen primum of an AVC defect has a crescentic superior edge (single arrow) forming the inferior margin of the atrial septum, which also has a secundum ASD (double arrow). The undivided common anterior leaflet may either attach (arrow) (b) or remain unattached (arrow) (c) to the superior margin of the ventricular septum.*

Complete defects, which make up about 20% of all AVC defects, have an atrial and ventricular communication and are subdivided into three groups on the basis of the anatomy of the AV valve leaflets. The grouping depends on whether

Table 20.6.   Classification of AVC defects (Titus and Rastelli [71])

I. Complete (type I)
  A. Anterior common leaflet divided, attached to the ventricular septum
  B. Anterior common leaflet divided, unattached to the ventricular septum
  C. Anterior common leaflet undivided, unattached to the ventricular septum
II. Incomplete (type II)
  A. Without a ventricular septal defect
    1. Partial: ostium primum ASD and cleft mitral valve
    2. Common atrium with AV valve deformity
    3. Isolated primum defect
    4. Isolated cleft of anterior leaflet of mitral valve
    5. Isolated cleft tricuspid valve
  B. With a ventricular septal defect
    1. AV canal type VSD and normal AV valves
    2. AV canal type VSD and abnormal AV valves including straddling

the common leaflet, the hallmark of the spectrum, has right and left components and whether they attach to the basal portion of the ventricular septum. The most common form is the incomplete (type II), partial AVC defect, which has an atrial but not a ventricular septal defect and a deformed anterior leaflet of the mitral valve. Type II defects more commonly accompany trisomy 21 while type I defects more commonly accompany other malformations, including the visceral symmetry-splenic malformation syndromes.

Infants with AVC defects may present during the neonatal period or develop heart failure and succumb to the disease during the first year depending on the extent of the malformation, accounting for 1.3% of all fatalities due to CHD in the first 3 months of life. Beyond the neonatal period, patients with complete AVC defects develop progressive, inexorable pulmonary vascular obstructive disease. The earlier development of pulmonary vascular disease in patients with Down syndrome than in those with normal karyotypes has been held responsible for the difference in survival rates between these groups [74, 75]. Since the vascular disease arises early, corrective surgery has been advocated during infancy to reduce the time of exposure of the pulmonary bed to high pressure and flow through the pulmonary artery [76].

AVC defect accompanies syndromes other than trisomy 21. AVC defect has been found to affect females more often than males, to affect blacks more often than whites [77], and to accompany increased fetal nuchal translucency [77a]. Genetic linkage analysis in patients with the Holt-Oram syndrome, who may have one of several types of malformations, including AVC, has indicated a gene locus at chromosome 12q2 [78]. The association between trisomy 21 and a high incidence of AVC defect has raised the likelihood of a locus on chromosome 21 for AVC defect. In a study of familial AVC defects not associated with trisomy 21, chromosome 21 was eliminated as the genetic locus in that family group, suggesting involvement of another gene, not on chromosome 21, in development of AVC defect [79].

The ASD has a superior atrial crescentic margin and a concave lower ventricular margin. The lower margin is lined by the endocardium of the summit of the ventricular septum. The remainder of the atrial septum may be normal, with a fossa ovalis or a secundum ASD [71].

The VSD, which is unique to both the complete and partial AVC types, presents on the right in the muscular aspect of the ventricular septum, posterior and inferior to the crista supraventricularis, with its superior boundary at the tricuspid valve ring. From the left, the basal part of the muscular portion of the ventricular septum has a scooped-out, concave appearance. The defect lies in the outflow of the left ventricle near the anterior leaflet of the mitral valve, with an upper border of muscular or membranous septum, in contrast with the usual VSD, which lies close to the anterior border of the left ventricle and borders on the basilar attachment of the right and noncoronary cusps of the aortic valve [71].

The mitral valve is always abnormal, with a cleft in the anterior leaflet dividing it into two portions. The cleft may vary from just a notch to complete separation of the leaflet. The designation of endocardial cushion defect relates partially to the defect in the mitral valve, but only a small portion of the atrioventricular valves derives from the endocardial cushions. Even so, proper fusion of the tubercles must occur to form the normal anterior leaflet of the mitral valve [71, 72].

Symptoms appear early when an AVC has an accompanying left ventricular outflow obstruction (Fig. 20.17) [80]. An AVC defect consisting of a primum ASD, a small VSD, an AV valve abnormality, and underdevelopment of the left ventricle results in severe intractable failure in the neonate with onset from 1 day to 1 month and survival from 1 day to 8 months [80A]. Most of the infants have an obstructive lesion in the aortic arch and a small left ventricle without endocardial sclerosis, representing one of the malformations

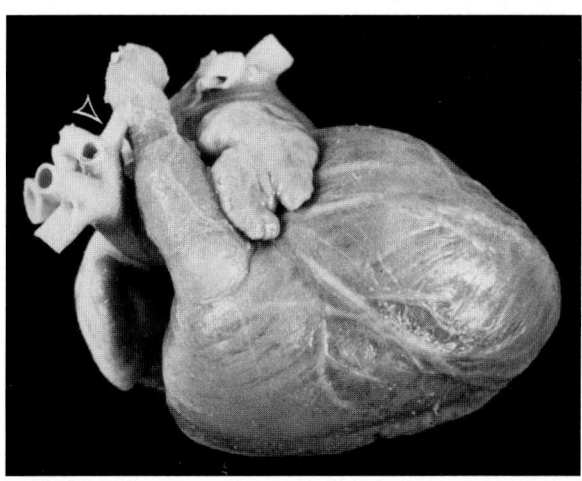

FIGURE 20.17.   *Tubular hypoplasia of the aortic arch (arrow), coarctation of the aorta, and an AVC defect cause an early onset of symptoms in the neonate.*

causing subaortic stenosis in infancy. Adherence of AV valve tissue to the left ventricular outflow tract narrows the subaortic area. Aortic arch obstruction is usual, consisting of isthmic hypoplasia, coarctation, and interruption [81].

Ventricular Septal Defects

VSDs account for about 25% of all CHD, cause considerable morbidity in infancy and childhood, but usually present after the perinatal period. The seed for problems from VSD later in life is nurtured during fetal and neonatal life, and the malformation forms an essential component of perinatal pathology. Functional abnormality from VSD in the neonate comes less from the isolated defect than when it forms part of a malformation complex (double-outlet right ventricle, single ventricle, truncus arteriosus, tetralogy of Fallot, and tricuspid atresia) or accompanies another type of CHD, not as part of a complex (ASD, AVC defect, ductus arteriosus, subaortic stenosis, coarctation, or d- and l-transposition) [82] (Table 20.7).

Many infants with VSDs have associated noncardiovascular malformations, with the functional effects of the VSD dominating the clinical syndrome [83, 84]. Syndromes in which an isolated VSD is prominent include trisomy 13, trisomy 18, trisomy 21, Turner syndrome, Marfan syndrome, and complex malformation syndromes.

Incidence

VSD has an incidence of about 2 in 1000 births, four to five times higher in prematurely born infants than in term infants, but drops to about 1 in 1000 by school age and even lower in adults due to spontaneous closure and to attrition from the mortality [83, 85]. Membranous and perimembranous defects are the most common large defects, accounting for two-thirds of the total; about 6% have multiple VSDs.

Anatomic Classification

Soto et al [86] identify four types of VSDs: a perimembranous defect involving the membranous septum and adjacent myocardium and three muscular defects affecting the inlet, trabecular, and infundibular components of the ventricular septum (Fig. 20.18). Most defects are membranous, followed in incidence by those in the trabecular septum, inlet, and infundibulum [86]. Because a supracristal defect has a roof made up of the joined aortic and pulmonic valves, providing access to both the pulmonary and aortic valve orifices, Anderson et al describe it as "doubly committed" [82].

Natural History of VSD in Infancy

VSD is not usually lethal during infancy. Doubly committed subarterial VSD may cause severe congestive heart failure in infancy, but most VSDs produce diagnostic symptoms during the first year of life and almost all VSDs do so by age 5 [83, 85, 87, 88]. Of those infants with VSDs who die in infancy, most are less than 5 months of age and have additional malformations, diseases, or malformation complexes.

Table 20.7. Incidence of cardiovascular malformations associated with VSD

Malformation	Percent
Isolated	82
ASD	6
Ductus arteriosus	4
Mitral insufficiency	1
Pulmonary valve insufficiency	1
Tricuspid valve insufficiency	<1
Right aortic arch	2
Partial anomalous pulmonary venous return	<1
SVC anomaly	2
Pulmonary artery branch stenosis	<1

From Corone et al [83].

Those VSDs that are fatal in infancy are relatively larger than those that are fatal at later ages, even when they accompany other malformations or chromosomal abnormalities [84]. The location of the defect influences the course of the disease much less than the size. Large septal defects, defined as at least 1.0 cm in diameter or half the size of the aortic valve orifice make up an estimated 10% of all defects [89]. Most VSDs in infants are in the muscular septum and have a high rate of spontaneous closure, usually in the first 6 months of life [90, 91], in contrast to the perimembranous defects, which rarely close spontaneously [92].

Spontaneous Closure

The greater incidence of VSD among infants than among older children has been attributed in part to spontaneous closure of the defect (Fig. 20.19). Although the ventricular

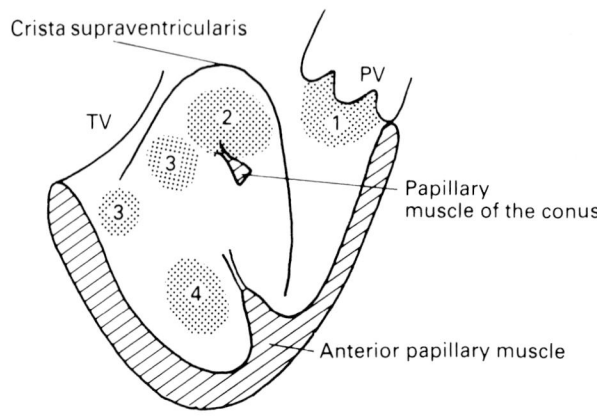

FIGURE 20.18. *The several defects in the ventricular septum may be designated by their relationships to the crista supraventricularis and the membranous septum as supracristal or infundibular (1), membranous (2), inlet (3), and muscular or trabecular (4).*

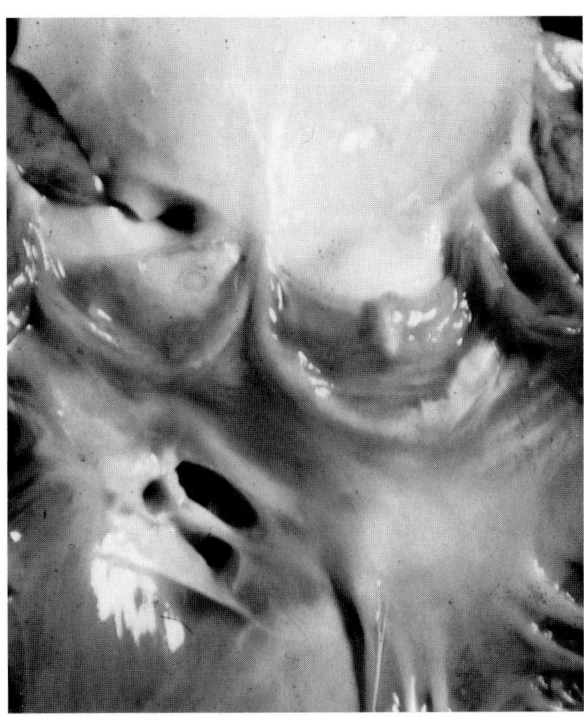

FIGURE 20.19.   *As viewed from the left ventricle of an older child, a spontaneously closed VSD persists as invaginations into the ventricular septum beneath the aortic valve and closed by connective tissue.*

septum usually forms completely by the 7th week of gestation, it may remain incomplete at birth and then close spontaneously, not in the first month of life, but during childhood—usually by age 5 or 6 years [83]. Small, but occasionally large, muscular or perimembranous defects intimately related to the tricuspid valve are most likely to close spontaneously [82, 93]. Defects may spontaneously close by adherence of the overlying septal leaflet of the tricuspid valve [93a], localized hypertrophy of muscle bundles, plugging of the defect by fibrous tissue, or prolapse of aortic valve tissue [82, 85]. Closure of a perimembranous septal defect may result in the septal configuration known as aneurysm of the ventricular septum with a potential for conduction defect [94, 95].

Symptomatic VSD, Congestive Heart Failure, and Pulmonary Hypertension in the Neonate

Of the fewer than half of premature and full-term infants developing symptoms from VSD in the first year of life, about 10% may do so in the first week and 40% in the first month of life [85]. Congestive heart failure with VSD is usually nonlethal and peculiar to infancy, affecting about 4% of symptomatic infants with VSDs and large shunts [83]. The development of congestive heart failure in premature and full-term infants with VSDs relates to the changes in somatic and cardiac growth, pulmonary vascular resistance, and the

nature and quantity of hemoglobin [85]. With postnatal body growth and decreased resistance of the pulmonary vascular bed, blood shunting from left to right through the defect results in low output failure and pulmonary edema [96]. The overall mortality from congestive heart failure in infants with VSD and pulmonary hypertension, sometimes potentiated by associated defects such as coarctation or by multiple VSDs, is less than 15% [93].

Infants with VSDs who die in failure in the first 2 months of life have normal medial muscle in the small pulmonary arteries, but those dying after 2 months have hypertrophic muscle [97]. Infants with small VSDs have little apparent change in the pulmonary vascularity from normal, although a large VSD may be associated with increased muscular mass. With pulmonary hypertension, the preacinar and acinar vessels have an increased muscular mass, but, for unknown reasons, intra-acinar vessels fail to increase in size or number [97]. As the earliest change in the blood vessels, muscle extends along the axes of the arteries beyond the normal degree for the age, presumably stimulated by the increase in pulmonary blood flow.

Double-Outlet Right Ventricle

While infants with double-outlet ventricles may present with symptoms in the neonatal period, the malformation has so many potential variations and associations that the designation has become more a description than an identification of a specific malformation. Double-outlet ventricle is not particularly common, accounting for 1–3% of CHD in the neonate in several series [98]. Double-outlet ventricle represents a heterogeneous group of malformations linked by the connection of the aorta and pulmonary artery to the same, usually right, ventricle. An essential feature of this group of malformations is the dependence on a VSD to maintain circulation [98a]. Based on four possible positions of the VSD and four possible relationships of the great arteries, Sridaromont et al [99] identified 16 potential variants of double-outlet ventricle.

A long-held marker for the double-outlet configuration has been absence of the normal continuity between the aortic and mitral valves, resulting in a bilateral infundibulum. In large measure, this marker has been replaced by consideration of the ventricular connections of the great arteries. Becker and Anderson designate a double-outlet ventricle if more than half of each arterial valve connects to the same ventricle, forming a spectrum of ventriculoarterial connections with many variations of visceral situs, AV valve concordance or discordance, site of the VSD, anomalies of the semilunar or AV valves, or relationships of the great arteries—e.g., tetralogy of Fallot would be a double-outlet ventricle if more than half of the overriding aortic valve arose from the right ventricle [100].

Lev and Bharati classify double-outlet ventricle as simple, making up 75% of cases, and complicated, making up the remaining 25% [98]. Simple forms have VSDs at a variety of sites—subaortic, subpulmonary, doubly committed, or noncommitted—but the remaining features in segmental analysis are normal. The complicated forms, which are more likely to affect the neonate, may include total anomalous pulmonary venous return, AVC defects, and mitral or aortic valve atresia or stenosis and obstruction to the aortic arch. Double-outlet ventricle with obstruction to flow from the left ventricle and causing symptoms in the neonate presents morphologically with a small left ventricle, an abnormal mitral valve, a subpulmonary VSD, and an obstructive lesion in the aortic arch.

Tricuspid Valve Atresia

The forms of CHD associated with atresia of the tricuspid valve produce symptoms in infancy but uncommonly in the neonate and make up about 5% of all cyanotic CHD, 1.5–3.0% of all CHD, and 1.5–2.0% of CHD identified and presenting in the neonatal period [101]. Although unusual, tricuspid valve atresia has been reported in multiple members of a family [101a, 101b].

The two clinical patterns of cyanotic CHD with tricuspid valve atresia relate to diminished or increased pulmonary blood flow, with reduced pulmonary blood flow affecting most cases and most likely to cause early symptoms and death in the neonatal period. Cyanosis, which reflects the degree of pulmonary blood flow, may appear on the first day of life and become intense with closure of the ductus. The severe symptoms reflect the obstruction to pulmonary blood flow whether or not the great arteries are transposed.

Tricuspid valve atresia with transposition of the great arteries has a high association with obstruction of the aortic arch due to coarctation, isthmic hypoplasia, or interruption. Congestive heart failure, which usually develops after the first month of life, may develop earlier in the neonate with an associated coarctation and has a particularly high mortality [102].

Constant features accompanying tricuspid valve atresia are an atrial communication, a patent left AV valve, hypoplastic or absent right ventricle, and a hypertrophic left ventricle with a large cavity (Fig. 20.20). Variable features with tricuspid valve atresia are the relation of the great arteries as normal, transposed, truncus, or double-outlet attachment; a normal, stenotic, or atretic pulmonary valve; and a VSD [102]. Rarely, an Ebstein-like membrane may form the atresia between the right atrium and the right ventricle [103].

A shallow depression or dimple in the floor of the dilated right atrium is the residual of the absent right AV valve. If the foramen ovale remains closed, leaving no exit for right atrial blood to the left atrium, the atrial septum may bulge as an aneurysm into the left atrium.

The right ventricle has an outflow area with no papillary muscles and with hypertrophied infundibular muscles. With an intact septum and pulmonary valve atresia, the right ventricle is minute and pulmonary blood flow depends on a patent ductus. Obstruction to the pulmonary blood flow

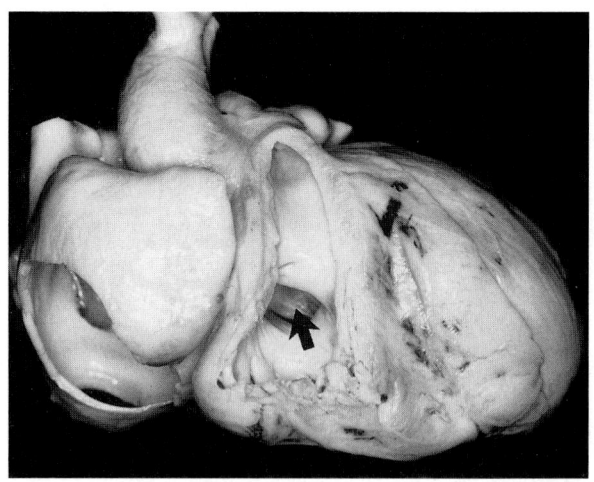

FIGURE 20.20.   *The small right ventricle accompanying tricuspid valve atresia has a patent pulmonary valve and a VSD through which a portion of the mitral valve (arrow) is visible.*

may be at the valve, at the subvalvular level, or, in older children, at a progressively narrowed VSD. With transposition, aortic obstruction may be a coarctation, tubular hypoplasia, or interruption of the aortic arch. Aside from right aortic arch, tricuspid valve atresia has few accompanying malformations.

Despite the clarity of the usual form of tricuspid valve atresia, controversy over terminology persists, based on the usual clashes over embryology, the anatomic connections, and perceptions of where the atretic valve really attaches [103a]. The original straightforward classification based on the association of pulmonary valve obstruction and a normal or transposed relationship of the great arteries has been expanded to include all the potential relationships and connections [102].

Since tricuspid atresia may accompany a variety of ventricular morphology and arterial connections, and since the arterial connections make up the cornerstone of the classifications, Becker and Anderson recommend segmental analysis for the malformation complex rather than an alphanumeric classification [103, 104].

Tetralogy of Fallot

Morphology

Tetralogy of Fallot (t/F) occurs in an incidence of about 1 in 4000 births but makes up fewer than 10% of neonates with cyanotic CHD. In the usual t/F, a subaortic VSD accompanies underdevelopment or malalignment of the subpulmonary conus. The infracristal defect occupies the membranous septum, separated from the pulmonary valve by the crista, and lies beneath the right cusp of the aortic valve and behind the septal leaflet of the tricuspid valve (Fig. 20.21). Despite the overriding aorta, mitral and aortic valves retain fibrous continuity, providing the sometimes contentious distinction between t/F and double-outlet right ventricle [105].

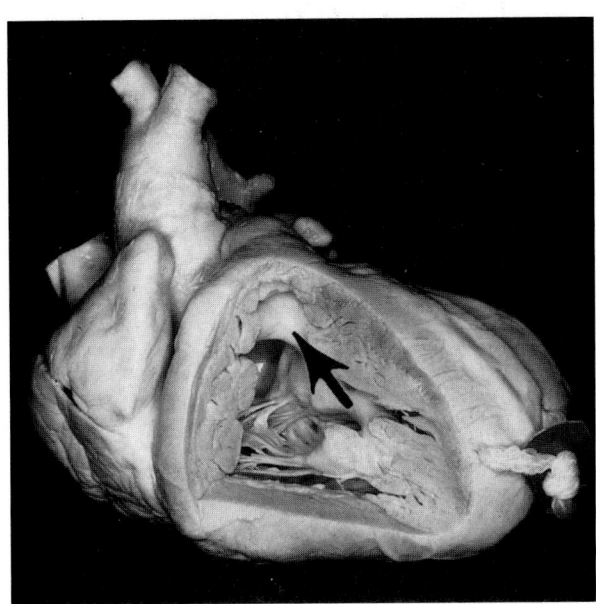

FIGURE 20.21.   *In a tetralogy of Fallot, the crista supraventricularis (arrow) extends into and obstructs the outflow from the right ventricle and provides the anterior border for the VSD.*

The morphologic and functional variations of t/F relate to the degree of the right ventricular outlet obstruction, which varies from mild obstruction to atresia. The pulmonary valve may be normal, bicuspid, atretic, or absent, and the pulmonary artery and its branches may be normal, stenotic, or atretic [106]. The infundibular septum lies in the outflow of the right ventricle due to an anterior, superior, and leftward deviation from its usual position, forming the VSD, the infundibular stenosis, and the overriding of the aorta; the right ventricular myocardium hypertrophies secondary to the obstruction to the right ventricle and systemic vascular resistance imposed by the overriding aorta. Infundibular obstruction may serve as the only source of obstruction or may be augmented by obstruction at other sites, but infundibular obstruction, which may develop postnatally, even late in life, is basic and other obstructive sites are superimposed or additional [107]. Accompanying an atretic pulmonary artery, the pulmonary blood supply comes from either the ductus or the bronchials via anastomoses with the intraparenchymal pulmonary arteries.

In contrast to the appearance of thin-walled pulmonary arteries in the older child with t/F, Hislop and Reid found the pulmonary arteries of infants with t/F to be more muscular, with muscular mass extending farther out into smaller vessels than normal. Although the vessel walls were thicker than normal, they had still decreased in size from the normal size at birth [108].

Presentation in the Neonate

The age at onset of symptoms in infants with t/F relates to the degree of the severity of obstruction to the right ventricular outflow. Symptoms in an infant with t/F may appear early in the first year of life, usually as a result of pulmonary

valve atresia or severe stenosis, with a variable period of good pulmonary flow relating to ductal flow. With outflow atresia, symptoms may appear within 1 to 2 days of life, presumably in relation to diminished flow through the ductus. Patients with t/F are not usually severely cyanotic at birth, but become so over the first few months of life [107]. Cyanosis with right-to-left shunting is uncommon in the first 1 to 2 months of life, but usually appears later in the first year. While the traditional management of t/F in infancy with palliative shunting followed at an older age by staged repair has its adherents [108a], primary repair of the lesion in the neonate has been associated with good early and midterm results [108b, 108c, 108d].

Pathogenesis

Tetralogy of Fallot has been considered to result from unequal division of the conus producing a small infundibulum with a membranous defect. Winn and Hutchins propose that t/F results from obstruction of the pulmonary blood flow in embryonic life, diverting right ventricular output through a VSD into the aorta, followed by postnatally acquired progressive infundibular stenosis. In most cases, a malformed stenotic pulmonary valve accounts for the diversion of the right ventricular stream and serves as the primary lesion. This causes the persisting patency of the VSD. The small infundibulum is the result of the decreased flow and not the cause. According to this concept, isolated pulmonary valve stenosis develops after closure of the ventricular septum [107].

Associated Malformations and Variants of t/F

When t/F is accompanied by an absent pulmonary valve, the infundibular stenosis is mild and, unlike classic t/F, the infant is prone to develop congestive heart failure (Fig. 20.22). The valve ring has no structural feature of a valve, consisting only of nodular tissue. The hypoplastic annulus may cause obstruction. The pulmonary artery may be dilated, and the right ventricle may dilate as a result of pulmonary arterial regurgitation. An initial right-to-left shunt is followed by a reversal to left to right as the neonatal pulmonary arterial resistance drops.

Variants and cardiovascular malformations with t/F include a right aortic arch, double-outlet right ventricle with pulmonary valve stenosis, t/F with an AVC defect, single ventricle with pulmonary valve stenosis with or without transposition, and transposition of the great arteries with pulmonary valve stenosis and a VSD [105]. Extracardiac anomalies that may be encountered are tracheoesophageal fistula, Down syndrome, components of the transplacental rubella syndrome, and occasional multiple malformation syndromes.

Single Ventricle

The terminology for single ventricle varies, but several terms have more or less widespread use, each with its own advocate: single ventricle, common ventricle, primitive ventricle,

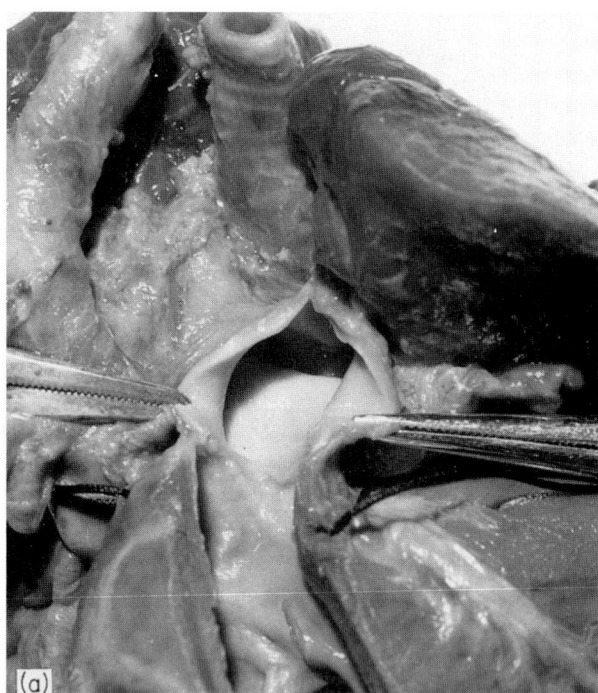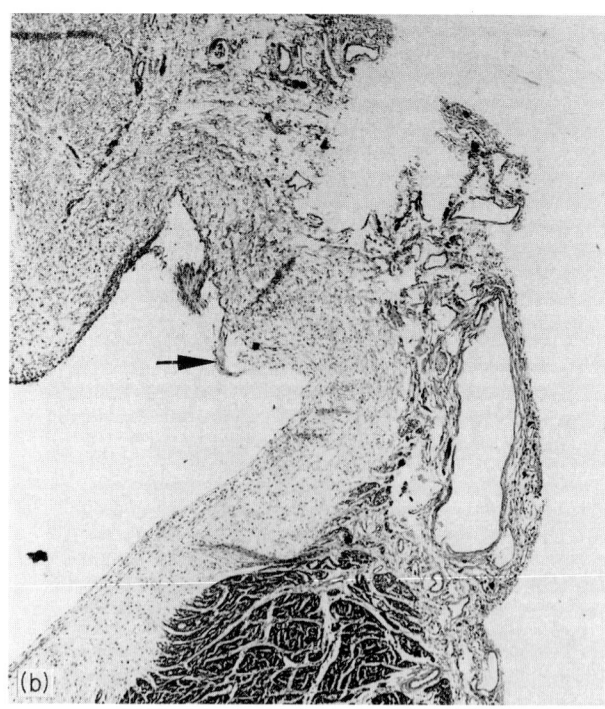

FIGURE 20.22.   *In a tetralogy of Fallot with absent pulmonary valve, (a) only a nubbin of connective tissue (arrow) instead of a valve protrudes into the lumen of the pulmonary artery at its origin from the right ventricle. (b) Histologically, a mound of connective tissue at the site of the absent valve is continuous with the right ventricular endocardium (Gomori's trichrome, ×40).*

double-inlet left ventricle, and univentricular heart [109–111]. "Single ventricle" is probably the most widely used term, advocated by those seeing no overriding reason to change. "Univentricular heart" has the same connotation as single ventricle, and each term carries the caveat that the name does not sufficiently characterize the malformation without specifying the associated connections and malformations. The designation "primitive ventricle" has been derided as neither necessary nor accurate, while "common ventricle" may refer to a particularly large VSD without the complexities usually accompanying single ventricle [110, 112].

The malformations making up single ventricle account for about 1% of all cardiac anomalies and about 4% of neonates with CHD, and have a wide range of survival. Some affected infants do not survive the first day of life, while others may live into the second decade [112, 113]. Those forms of single ventricle that affect the neonate have either severely reduced pulmonary blood flow, an increased blood flow with or without left ventricular outflow obstruction blood flow, severe AV valve regurgitation, or severe pulmonary venous congestion due to obstruction of the left AV valve and a restrictive foramen ovale. Single ventricle accounts for a high incidence of pulmonary congestion among forms of complex CHD with a bidirectional shunt in the first year of life [114].

In a heart with a single ventricle, the entire atrial flow enters a single ventricular chamber and may be a single left ventricle or a single right ventricle with or without a rudimentary chamber or a single ventricle of indeterminate type [115, 116]. Both single right and single left ventricles usually have a rudimentary outflow chamber with features of the opposite ventricle. The wide variety of combinations and intracardiac relationships with each variety of single ventricle requires a sequential nomenclature based on morphology, connections, and intracardiac relationships. Rudimentary chambers may vary according to their relations to the great arteries: either single right or single left ventricle may support either or both great arteries, or the rudimentary chamber may consist instead only of a trabecular pouch with no outlet to a great artery. With any variety, the rudimentary chamber may be right or left. It usually lies anterior to a single right ventricle, whereas it usually lies posterior to a single left ventricle [115, 117]. A heart with a single ventricle has as its hallmark the absence of the inlet septum that normally separates the inlet portions of the two ventricles and that normally carries the AV conduction bundle [118]. Virtually all single ventricles have a rudimentary chamber, although some may be inconspicuous and thus overlooked.

A single ventricle may have any of several AV connections: a double AV inlet may have two valves, a common valve, one imperforate valve, or a straddling valve; a single AV inlet may have only a right or left AV connection [115, 117]. Of the three parts of a ventricle—an inlet, a trabecular portion, and an outlet—a chamber achieves status as a ventricle when it has at least an inlet and a trabecular portion. A rudimentary chamber lacks an inlet portion. Either a single ventricle or a rudimentary chamber may have a right or left ventricular trabecular portion [117].

The great arteries may have any of several relationships: double outlet from the ventricle, concordant arterial connection with the aorta arising posteriorly from the outlet chamber, or atresia of one semilunar valve, usually the pulmonary [118].

Uhl Anomaly

In the Uhl anomaly (parchment right ventricle), the anterior wall of a greatly dilated right ventricle consists of endocardium, epicardium, and a small amount of intervening connective tissue but either no myocardium or only occasional small persistent muscle bundles. The dilated right atrium, the left atrium, and the left ventricle have normal or hypertrophic myocardium.

Neither the etiology, pathogenesis, nor establishment of the Uhl anomaly as a nosologic entity has been determined. The malformation has been described at all ages; about 15% of the reported cases have been in neonates with a uniformly fatal course regardless of the mode of treatment [119]. In the usual form of the anomaly, a neonate with absent right ventricular myocardium has normal cardiac situs and connections.

Infants and children with dysplastic right ventricular myocardium, unlike adults, have a high incidence of associated cardiovascular malformations, perhaps accounting for the relatively high incidence in the neonate [120]. The thin myocardium in infants with associated malformations may show signs of acute degeneration with inflammation and calcification, raising the question of a similar morphology but with different pathogenesis. The usual associated malformations affect the right side of the heart: tricuspid valve agenesis with hypoplasia of the cusps and papillary muscles and pulmonary valve atresia [121] or stenosis. Less commonly associated malformations include foramen secundum atrial septal defect, patent ductus arteriosus, and anomalous coronary arteries. In making a distinction, the absence of the right ventricular myocardium characterizes the Uhl anomaly.

Yet another clinical and morphologic presentation has raised the question of whether dysplastic right ventricular myocardium is a single disorder or several disorders with morphologic similarities [122, 123]. Although usually affecting young adults with conduction defects or sudden death, and variously called Uhl's anomaly or arrhythmogenic right ventricular dysplasia, a patchy distribution of fat replaces the myocardium, contrasting with the diffuse bland myocardial absence in the neonate [124, 124a]. Since arrhythmogenic dysplasia carries a genetic potential, a distinction is critical [125].

The distinction between Uhl anomaly and arrhythmogenic right ventricular dysplasia (or cardiomyopathy) (ARVD) currently rests on morphology and the age range at the time of clinical presentation. The Uhl anomaly presents in infancy, while ARVD rarely presents earlier than the latter half of the second decade of life. ARVD has at least two morphologic patterns: fatty and fibrofatty replacement of the right ventricular myocardium, which may represent separate disorders or variants of the same process [125a]. The recognized familial occurrence of ARVD and the identification of gene markers 14q23–q24 [125b] and 1q42–q43 [125c] in some but not all families with ARVD may provide a positive means of distinction.

Tricuspid Valve Dysplasia Including Ebstein's Anomaly

Ebstein's anomaly forms part of a spectrum of malformed tricuspid valve that includes both downward displacement of the valve and dysplastic leaflets. The leaflets in Ebstein's anomaly are dysplastic and displaced. Dysplastic leaflets that are not displaced make up other malformations in the spectrum. The dysplasia consists of focal or diffuse thickening of the valve leaflets, deficient chordae or papillary muscles, fusion of the valve leaflet with the ventricular wall, and focal agenesis of the leaflet [126]. Microscopically, the leaflets contain loose edematous connective tissue with collagen but no inflammation [127].

Ebstein's anomaly affects only the tricuspid valve, whether the valve is concordant or discordant (corrected transposition). As its common anatomic feature, the septal and posterior leaflets of the tricuspid valve displace downward into the right ventricular chamber, resulting in the proximal portion of the right ventricle remaining in continuity with the right atrium without an intervening valve (Fig. 20.23). The tricuspid valve orifice extends no farther than the junction of the inlet and the trabecular zones of the right ventricle [128]. The commissure between the posterior and septal leaflets extends to the maximum depth, leaving a normal origin of an enlarged anterior leaflet thickened with fibrous connective tissue and sometimes muscle [129]. The valve is usually incompetent, but it may be stenotic or even atretic, forming a variety of tricuspid valve atresias [128]. An ASD or patent foramen ovale frequently accompanies the greatly dilated right atrium and proximal right ventricle.

In the neonate, the normally elevated pulmonary vascular resistance accentuates the incompetence of the anomalous valve, often resulting in congestive heart failure, which may revert when pulmonary vascular resistance decreases. Because of the great variation in the anatomic and physiologic abnormality of the anomaly, Ebstein's anomaly may be lethal in the neonate or permit great longevity into adult life. The rarity of the anomaly in the neonate may be a paradox of the high rate of intrauterine mortality. Based on intrauterine diagnosis, tricuspid valve dysplasia may make up more than 8% of cardiovascular malformations, although fewer than 5% may survive the perinatal period [130, 131].

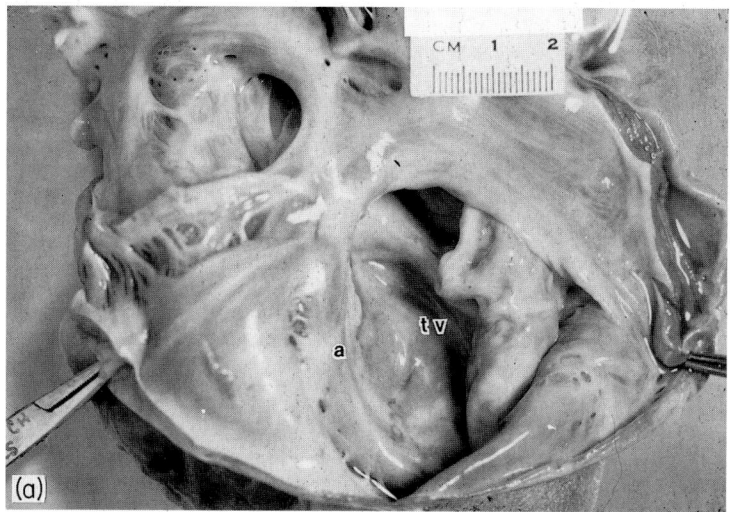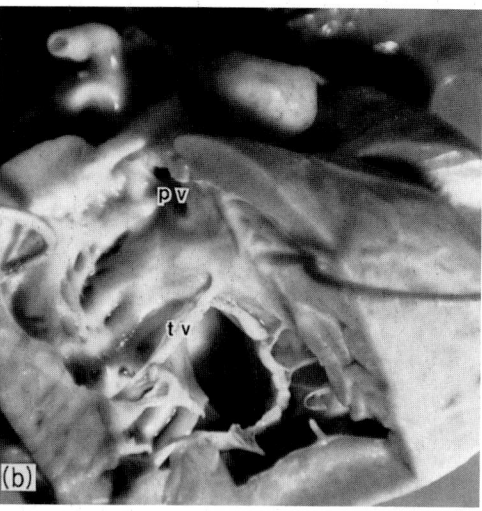

FIGURE 20.23.   *In Ebstein's anomaly, (a) the origin of the posterior and septal leaflets of the tricuspid valve are displaced inferiorly, leaving the proximal portion of the right ventricle in continuity with the right atrium without an intervening AV valve, and (b) reducing the size of the outflow portion of the right ventricle. a—annulus; tv—tricuspid valve; pv—pulmonary valve.*

Cardiovascular anomalies that may accompany Ebstein's anomaly include pulmonary valve stenosis or atresia, ductus arteriosus, VSD, tetralogy of Fallot, coarctation, transposition, and primum ASD, any of which increases the hazard to the neonate. Patients with Ebstein's anomaly are prone to the Wolff-Parkinson-White syndrome and supraventricular tachycardia [132]. The association with pulmonary valve stenosis and an intact ventricular septum or with sclerotic pulmonary valve leaflets presents early and affects the neonate [126, 127, 133].

Pulmonary Valve Stenosis and Atresia with an Intact Ventricular Septum

Morphology of the Pulmonary Valve

Pulmonary valve (PV) atresia more commonly affects the neonate than PV stenosis; other PV abnormalities produce disease in the neonate as they resemble PV atresia in their most severe aspects. Most PV abnormalities other than atresia, however, allow greater longevity, producing disease in the older infant, child, or adult. Sequentially, hearts with PV atresia usually have situs solitus, d-loop ventricular relationship, and a normal relationship of great arteries to each other.

In its usual form, the atretic PV has a hypoplastic annulus and an imperforate membrane forming a nipple-like dome projecting into the pulmonary artery, surrounded by three sinuses of Valsalva and with three raphae marking the sites of the commissures [134]. Of those with tiny right ventricles, most have atretic infundibula, but stenosis or atresia may accompany larger or even normal-sized right ventricles [135].

Stenosis and Atresia

Malformations at the valve, at the infundibulum, or in the peripheral arteries may obstruct the right ventricular outflow, but only valvular lesions aggravated by infundibular obstruction have consequence to the neonate. As isolated malformations, neither peripheral obstruction nor infundibular stenosis troubles the neonate. Symptomatic infants with PV stenosis presenting in the first month of life have critical PV stenosis defined as right ventricular pressure equal to or greater than systemic pressure and a right-to-left shunt [136]. Because of the difference in management of PV stenosis and somewhat better outcome, distinction from PV atresia is critical.

PV stenosis may have one of two anatomic forms: a dome with raphe similar to PV atresia but with a lumen of variable size, or sclerotic but well-formed leaflets (Fig. 20.24). Poststenotic dilatation of the pulmonary artery, progressive after birth, occurs with a dome-shaped valve but not with sclerotic leaflets. In severe PV stenosis, the tricuspid valve may be dysplastic. Right ventricular hypertrophy and increased myocardial oxygen demand may lead to myocardial dysfunction, infarction, and fibrosis, usually in the right ventricle [137].

Although the valve leaflets become progressively thicker and more sclerotic with age, they never calcify in the neonate and cause severe obstruction. Since the size of the orifice determines the course, a pinpoint orifice has an effect resembling PV atresia. Survivors have a larger valvular lumen. Although the ductus uncommonly remains patent, an interatrial communication is constant—usually a patent foramen ovale, and less often a secundum ASD.

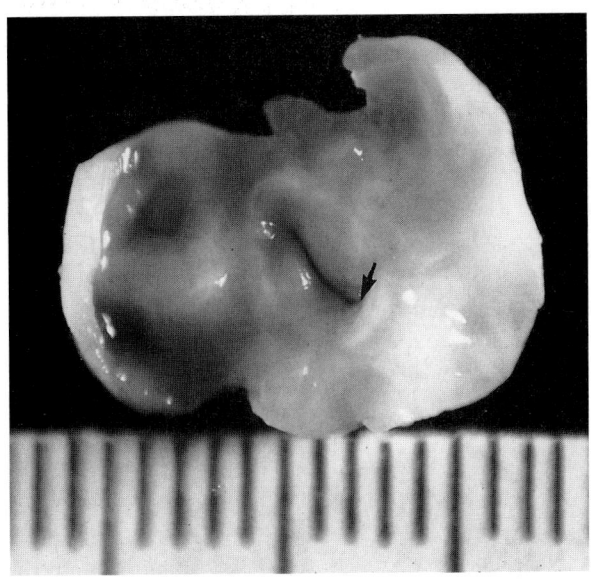

FIGURE 20.24. *A bicuspid, stenotic pulmonary valve has residual raphae between the cusps.*

Classification

Right ventricular size, which varies from tiny to enlarged, affects the prognosis, because the form most likely to affect the neonate has a small or diminutive right ventricle [138]. Although marked hypoplasia of the right ventricle is the most frequent form, it accounts for only slightly more than half the cases [139] (Table 20.8). The size of the right ventricle relates closely to the size and configuration of the tricuspid valve, with an enlarged right ventricle accompanying a dysplastic valve or Ebstein's anomaly (Fig. 20.25) [140]. An insufficient tricuspid valve with PV obstruction resembles the Ebstein's anomaly, with a small or a minute orifice and either normal or shortened leaflets with a slight downward shift [135, 141].

Coronary Arteries

The coronary arteries may have thick walls and small lumina presenting as tortuous vessels on the epicardial surface at the apex of the right ventricle. A fistulous connection between the sinusoids of the hypertrophic right ventricle and the coronary arteries may serve as the source of a shunt and egress of blood from the obstructed right ventricle.

Myocardial infarcts, ischemia, and dysfunction have been attributed to compromise of coronary circulation by the high pressure, by a fistula, and by abnormal capillary distribution in the right ventricular myocardium [142, 142a]. Although previously considered a complication of a shunt procedure, the pulmonary arteries in infants with congenital pulmonary atresia may spontaneously become distorted and discontinuous, possibly related to the effect of prostaglandin E_1 administration on ductal tissue [142b].

Table 20.8. Classification of pulmonary valve obstruction according to right ventricular size (Van Praagh [139], Freedom [140])

Right ventricular size	Incidence
1. Normal	8%
2. Enlarged (all had Ebstein's anomaly)	10%
3. Hypoplastic	
a. Moderate	28%
b. Marked	46%
c. Absent	7%

Pulmonary Vasculature

The pulmonary trunk usually extends in a funnel shape from the stenotic valve and gives off normal right and left pulmonary arteries, contrasting with the hypoplastic trunk accompanying PV atresia and a VSD. Occasional cases exhibit abnormalities of the main pulmonary artery or branches of the pulmonary arteries, such as a hypoplastic left pulmonary artery, diminutive main or right pulmonary artery, or absence of the main pulmonary artery. The small pulmonary arteries usually have a thin media and, in older patients, a diminished number of intra-acinar arteries [143].

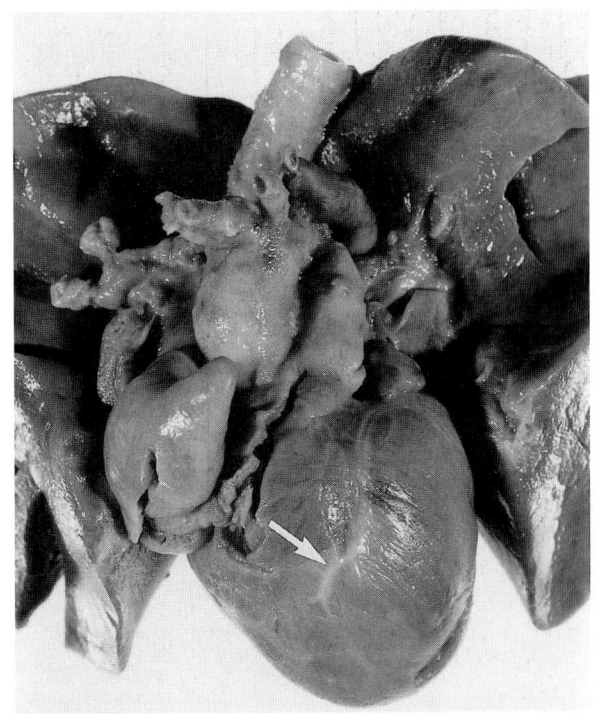

FIGURE 20.25. *On the anterior surface of a heart with pulmonary atresia, a tortuous, sclerotic anterior branch of the left coronary artery (arrow) marks the site of a coronary artery fistula to the right ventricle and demarcates the hypoplastic right ventricle from the enlarged left ventricle.*

Associated Defects

With the exception of the usual patent foramen ovale and occasional secundum atrial septal defect, few patients with isolated PV stenosis or atresia have an associated defect. When associated with the tetralogy of Fallot, pulmonary valve atresia has been identified with genetic syndromes, notably the CATCH syndrome (**C**ardiac defects, **A**bnormal facies, **T**hymic hypoplasia, **C**left palate, and **H**ypocalcemia) and deletion of chromosome 22q11 [143a, 143b].

Prognosis and Treatment

Of infants presenting with pulmonary atresia, usually symptomatic from cyanosis or in heart failure, about 60% survive at least 1 year, including the effects of surgery [143c]. Successful surgery may be precluded by a right ventricle too small to survive valvotomy or by a severe tricuspid valve regurgitation [135].

Mitral Valve Malformations

Excluding cases in which mitral valve abnormalities accompany aortic valve atresia and hypoplastic left ventricle, infants with symptoms referable to mitral valve disease have an almost equal division between those due to malformations (53%) and those due to infarcted papillary muscle (47%) [144]. Of the leaflet malformations, only Ebstein's anomaly of the left AV valve in corrected transposition affects the neonate with early left atrial hypertension [145], but other malformations such as commissural fusion, and abnormally long chordae with Marfan syndrome, may become symptomatic later in infancy [144].

The most frequent mitral valve abnormalities, those of the papillary muscles, may produce disease in the neonate by obstructing pulmonary venous return. Mitral valve regurgitation in infancy may accompany AVC defects, chordal and leaflet defects, Marfan syndrome, and the effects of bacterial endocarditis and anomalous left coronary artery [146, 147]. An anomalous arcade forms a fibrous connective tissue ridge at the free edge of the mitral valve leaflets and extending between the papillary muscles. A parachute mitral valve in which a single papillary muscle replaces the normal two with chordae extending to both leaflets usually accompanies other malformations obstructing left ventricular outflow. An abnormal position of the papillary muscle implies a high origin, as encountered in endocardial fibroelastosis with dilatation of the left ventricle. A bulky, but otherwise normal papillary muscle protruding into the orifice of the mitral valve serves as an "obstructing papillary muscle" [144].

Other mitral valve abnormalities obstructing pulmonary venous return include a hypoplastic valve with symmetric or asymmetric papillary muscles, and a double-orifice valve. Left atrial lesions that mimic mitral stenosis include a supravalvar mitral ring and cor triatriatum [147a].

With a normal aortic root, mitral valve atresia may accompany either normal or transposed great arteries and a left ventricle that may be absent, hypoplastic, normal, or even enlarged. The mitral valve usually consists of a dimple in the floor of the left atrium, although rarely with valve tissue and chordae tendineae [148]. Most cases have a small membranous VSD and an atrial communication—usually a patent foramen ovale, and less often a secundum or primum ASD. Maintenance of circulation requires an alternative pathway for pulmonary venous return: a collateral vein between the left atrium or pulmonary vein and the innominate vein, total anomalous pulmonary venous return, or a coronary sinus–left atrial fistula. Associated malformations include ductus arteriosus, coarctation, cor triatriatum, and a right aortic arch.

The pulmonary outflow may be normal or obstructed. With mitral atresia, the best prognosis accompanies a normal aortic root and moderate right ventricular obstruction; the worst prognosis accompanies pulmonary valve atresia or severe stenosis [149].

Aortic Valve Atresia

Terminology

Although the designation "hypoplastic left ventricle" has clinical value, each component of the several malformations that cause the small ventricle requires precise designation of its role in the complex [150]. Although both aortic valve atresia and stenosis may have an associated small left ventricle, the ventricular size has great variation, obviating synonymity between hypoplastic left ventricle and aortic valve abnormalities. The aortic valve abnormalities with hypoplastic left ventricle form a continuum including variation in the nature of the aortic and mitral valves, the size of the left ventricle, the integrity of the atrial septum, the pathway of pulmonary venous return to the right heart, and associated malformations.

Anatomy of Aortic Valve Atresia

The atretic valve usually projects slightly over the aortic ring as a dome into the ascending aorta whose caliber varies from diminutive to nearly normal, sometimes with dilated aortic sinuses about the atretic valve. The hypoplastic ascending aorta serves only as a conduit for the coronary arteries, since all the systemic arteries are supplied in a retrograde direction via the ductus.

The left ventricular cavity may be hypoplastic or so small that it is no more than a potential space requiring histologic examination for its identification (Fig. 20.26). The small left ventricle is delineated on the epicardium by the coronary arteries, which may include a tortuous left anterior descending artery. The thick left ventricular myocardium may contain sinusoidal spaces connecting to the coronary venous system, sometimes visible grossly. About half the cases have endocardial fibroelastosis, but only with a patent mitral valve. With mitral valve atresia, which affects about a fourth of the cases, the left ventricle has a flattened, small lumen [151]. The annulus of the mitral valve is small, and the mitral valve is hypoplastic. The disoriented fiber arrangement in

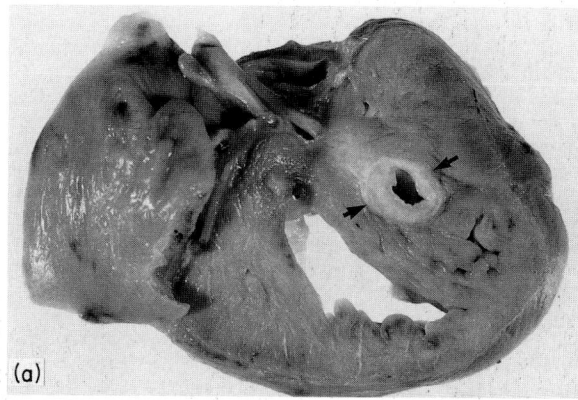

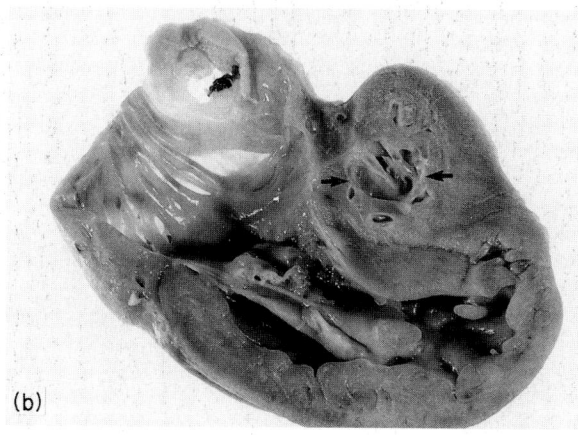

FIGURE 20.26. *As a result of aortic valve atresia and a diminutive mitral valve, the hypoplastic left ventricle (arrow) as seen in a frontal plane is maintained in dilatation and lined by a sclerotic layer of endocardium, more prominent in the outflow (a) than in the inflow (b).*

the ventricular myocardium resembles asymmetric septal hypertrophy, interpreted as secondary to the effect of large isometric contraction on the small chamber [152]. Subendocardial myocardial fibrosis and focal calcification affecting the inner third of the left ventricle conform to the effects of decreased subendocardial blood flow [153].

Associated Malformations

As the most frequent associated malformation, coarctation of the aorta adds no impediment to blood flow beyond that produced by the aortic atresia [154]. Other accompanying malformations of the aortic arch include aortopulmonary fenestrations and interrupted aortic arch. In the presence of a VSD, affecting about 10% of cases, the left ventricular size may approach normal [155, 156]. An ASD is almost universal—usually a patent foramen ovale—but other sites of communication include a defect in the valve of the fossa ovalis, a single atrium, a foramen primum, or a ventricular defect [151, 157]. Within the left atrium, the limbus of the foramen ovale is often hypoplastic, rotated, and deviated

toward the superior vena caval orifice while the eustachian valve of the inferior vena cava is usually absent or small but may be enlarged and redundant [157a]. Noncardiovascular malformations are not common, but aortic atresia may accompany the asplenia syndrome. Hypertrophy of the frenulum separating the alveolar portion of the maxillary palatine suture was identified in a fetus and in several children with hypoplastic left heart syndrome (HLHS) but not in children with other cardiovascular malformations [157b]. HLHS has been identified in siblings in a pattern suggesting autosomal recessive inheritance [157c]. Deletions on chromosomes 11q and 22q have been reported in several patients with HLHS [157d, 157e].

Pulmonary Venous Return

As one of the few malformations that alters the fetal circulation, aortic valve atresia must have a pathway for blood flow from the lung to the right side of the heart even in fetal life. Paths of egress from the left atrium include a patent mitral valve when there is a VSD, communication between the left atrium and the coronary sinus, anomalous pulmonary venous connection, fistula between the myocardial sinusoids and the coronary veins, and a levoatriocardinal vein from the left atrium or the pulmonary veins and a systemic vein [158, 159].

Classification

Of all cases of CHD, aortic atresia makes up only slightly more than 1%, but in the neonate it makes up almost 10% and is the most common fatal cardiovascular malformation in the first week of life. As with all types of aortic valve disease, both congenital and acquired, the gender incidence is overwhelmingly male [151, 154].

Classified according to the size of the left ventricular cavity, most cases have a hypoplastic left ventricle and an intact septum. Most of those with a hypoplastic left ventricle have a patent but diminutive mitral valve, and the remainder have mitral valve atresia. Few have a VSD and a well-developed left ventricle [151, 155, 156]. Many infants with aortic atresia do not survive the first week [159a]; most of those with a VSD do not survive the first month [151]. Attempts at surgical repair require recognition of the variation in size of the left ventricle, since an adequate ventricular size may improve the chances of survival [160, 161]. Despite inevitable congestive heart failure, a few affected infants survive beyond the neonatal period [162].

Pulmonary Vascularity

Pulmonary arteries may have the usual medial or increased medial muscular mass in the small muscular arteries. The status of the pulmonary arteries has been related to the integrity of the atrial septum, since the tortuosity of intrapulmonary arteries indicating pulmonary hypertension accompanies an intact atrial septum, in contrast to a diminished tortuosity with an atrial septal communication [163].

Aortic Valve Stenosis

Aortic Stenosis as a Component of Complexes

Symptomatic stenosis in the neonate usually forms part of a malformation complex that may include a hypoplastic aortic valve annulus, hypoplastic mitral valve, endocardial fibroelastosis, and obstructive lesions of the aortic arch, resulting in a range of disorders from underdeveloped left ventricles to almost normal hearts [163a]. Even severe aortic valvular stenosis identified in infancy may not produce symptoms for years [164]. Fewer than 10% of all cases of aortic valve stenosis produce symptoms in the neonate, although in cases of severe stenosis the symptoms, including congestive heart failure, appear early and carry a poor prognosis.

Morphology

The valve leaflets fuse at the commissures, forming a dome with two or three raphae and an eccentric orifice that frequently lies between the left coronary and noncoronary cusps. The thickened, deformed leaflets are of unequal size and may present as nodular valvular tissue projecting from a hypoplastic aortic ring. The valve may be bicuspid, unicommissural, or just a membrane with a narrow central hole.

The enlarged left ventricle usually has a hypertrophic myocardium lined by endocardial fibroelastosis, frequently with infarcts in the subendocardium and papillary muscles [165]. The left ventricular cavity may vary in size from small and hypoplastic through normal to enlarged. When accompanied by endocardial fibroelastosis, which is not restricted to only the small chambers, symptoms may appear in the first week of life.

Prognosis

Prognosis varies with the size of the aortic valve orifice. Mild to moderate stenosis of the aortic valve may have a good prognosis. Those in the first weeks of life with respiratory distress have large hearts and left ventricular hypertrophy.

Supravalvular Aortic Stenosis

Supravalvular aortic stenosis uncommonly produces symptoms in the neonate. The supravalvular obstruction contributes to a complex including supravalvular stenosis of the pulmonary artery and aorta, valvular dysplasia, and stenosis of the ostia of the coronary arteries and of the aortic arch branches, although not every case necessarily has all of these features [166]. Babies with Williams syndrome frequently have supravalvular aortic stenosis (see Chap. 13).

Transposition of the Great Arteries

Definition and Terminology

Transposition of the great arteries (TGA) describes an abnormal relationship between the great arteries, not a specific malformation. In the most common of at least three forms of TGA, the aorta arises from the right ventricle over a subaortic conus. Less common forms include a bilateral conus lacking fibrous continuity between either aortic or pulmonary semilunar valve and an AV valve, and a rare form with a foreshortened subpulmonary conus and a tenuous fibrous connection between the aortic and atrioventricular valves [167].

An alternative definition of TGA centers about the relationship of the aorta and pulmonary artery to each other and their relationship to the ventricles, requiring a segmental analysis in each case of the connection, the morphology of the outflow and of the ventricles, and the relation of the arterial valves [168].

Incidence

As the most frequent cardiovascular malformation causing cyanosis in the neonate, TGA accounts for up to 8% of CHD producing symptoms and morbidity in the first days and weeks of life, but not a high mortality during the first month of life. With the greater degree of recognition of the malformations in recent years, palliation followed by definitive surgical correction has resulted in prolonged survival of most affected infants. TGA is more common in males, in a ratio of 2:1.

Morbidity in the Perinatal Period

The hemodynamics and life expectancy of TGA depend on associated defects. With no associated defects, life expectancy would not exceed a few hours, but most affected infants have at least a patent foramen ovale and a patent ductus arteriosus. The parallel circulation of TGA resembles that of the early embryo, rather than the normal circulation in series. With an intact ventricular septum, only the foramen ovale and ductus provide mixing of blood. A VSD provides the greatest degree of mixing. With an intact septum, cyanosis appears on the first day of life; with a VSD, cyanosis may delay its appearance for about 2 weeks. In one study, infants with TGA with or without VSD had a mean survival time of $3\frac{1}{2}$ months [169]. With the introduction of palliative surgery in the mid-1960s, now utilized only for complex malformations, the mortality decreased from 100% to current rates of less than 20% [169a]. In many centers, the arterial switch procedure has been feasible in most forms of transposition in neonates for primary and definitive repair [169b]. Even the progressive pulmonary vascular disease in surgically unrepaired transposition has been inhibited by neonatal surgical repair, leaving only a small subgroup of infants with TGA and pulmonary vascular disease, possibly related to antenatal constriction of the ductus arteriosus [169c].

Morphology

The finite number of types of transposition relates to the limiting aspects of situs, ventricular loop, and relation of arteries to each other, resulting in five basic types of general relationships: normal, transposition, corrected transposition, double-outlet right ventricle, and double-outlet left ventricle, [167, 169d]. The most common form, complete or d-loop TGA, has either an intact ventricular septum, a VSD, or outflow stenosis of the left ventricle to the pulmonary artery. Slightly more than half of TGA cases have an intact ventricular septum, few with subpulmonic stenosis. Of those with a VSD, almost one-third have pulmonic stenosis.

Corrected transposition usually has an associated malformation, most often a VSD, pulmonary valve stenosis, insufficiency of the left AV valve, or cardiac malposition. Morphologically, the aorta lies anterior to and to the left of the pulmonary artery. The ventricles are inverted with the morphological left ventricle on the right and the right ventricle on the left. The atria retain their normal situs, connected to the inverted ventricles. The inverted ventricles have an l-loop pattern [170]. Although most symptoms develop in the first year of life, corrected TGA does not commonly cause problems in the perinatal period.

Truncus Arteriosus

Morphology
Narrowly defined, a truncus arteriosus, which accounts for less than 1% of all CHD, is a single vessel arising from the heart with a single truncal valve, supplying the pulmonary, systemic, and coronary circulations. This narrow definition excludes those malformations in which a patent vessel arises from the heart accompanied by an atretic vessel, as with aortic or pulmonary arterial atresia [171]. Although the truncus may arise predominantly from either the right or left ventricle with a restrictive VSD, most arise in continuity with a supracristal VSD (Fig. 20.27), reflecting the

concept of failed development of the aortopulmonary septum [172].

The positions of coronary orifices and the distribution of the coronary arteries are aberrant [173, 174]. The truncal valve may have two to five cusps with abnormalities causing morbidity by stenosis or insufficiency of the valve. The cusps may be sclerotic, have unequal size, prolapse into the ventricle, or have imperfectly formed commissures [175].

The origin of the pulmonary arteries from the truncus serves to classify the malformation into four varieties (Fig. 20.28) [176]:

I. A single artery to the lungs branching from the truncus and then dividing into two pulmonary arteries
II. Two pulmonary arteries arising independently from the truncus but in close proximity
III. Two pulmonary arteries arising from the truncus at some distance from each other
IV. Pulmonary arteries arising from the thoracic artery distal to the left subclavian artery

From this classification, types II and III are sufficiently similar to provide little clinical or morphologic distinction, and type IV represents an extreme form of pulmonary arterial atresia with the pulmonary blood supply coming from

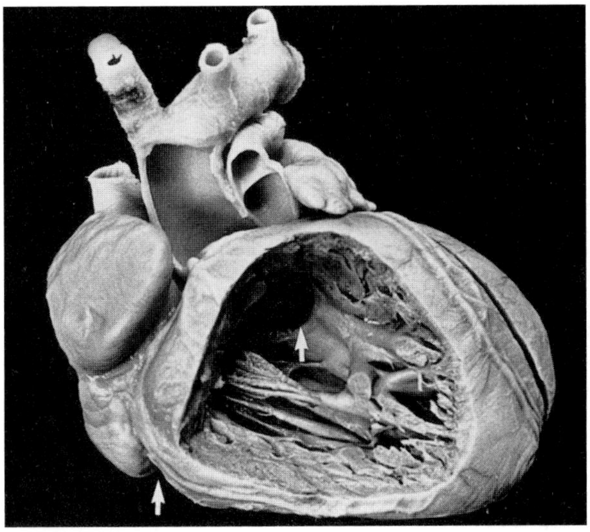

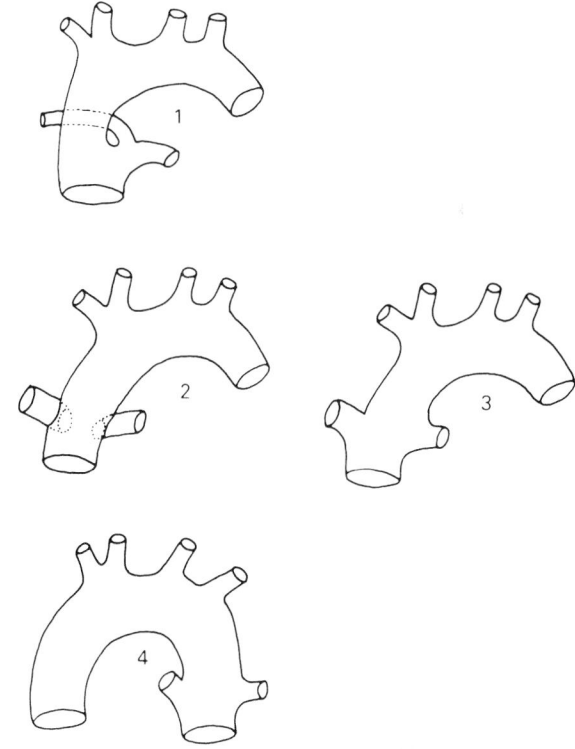

FIGURE 20.27. *Truncus arteriosus arises from both ventricles over a supracristal VSD (arrow), in this case with a single pulmonary artery with right and left branches.*

FIGURE 20.28. *In persistent truncus arteriosus, the pulmonary arteries may branch from a single main artery (1), as independent widely separated (2) or adjacent arteries (3), or as enlarged bronchial arteries from the descending aorta (4).*

enlarged bronchial arteries arising from the thoracic aorta. In some cases, the pulmonary artery may be absent on the side of the aortic arch.

Morbidity

Although patients with truncus arteriosus may survive to adult life, many infants survive only a few weeks to 6 months without surgical repair in early infancy. Risk factors for perioperative death include severe truncal valve regurgitation, interrupted aortic arch, coronary artery anomalies, and repair after 100 days of life [177].

Associated Malformations

Cardiovascular malformations commonly associated with truncus arteriosus include right aortic arch, coarctation, and interruption of the aortic arch, usually with a left aortic arch. The association with the DiGeorge anomalad emphasizes the abnormal neural crest origin of the malformation [177a]. Other extracardiac malformations include absent or hypoplastic kidney, absent gallbladder, unilateral pulmonary hypoplasia, cleft palate, and bony abnormalities [171].

Obstructive Lesions of the Aortic Arch: Coarctation, Tubular Hypoplasia, and Interruption

Coarctation, tubular hypoplasia, and interruption of the aortic arch share a number of features including their location in the aortic arch and the high incidence of associated malformations (Fig. 20.29). Of the three, only coarctation may occur with no associated malformations. The same types of obstructive malformations occur proximal to each of the three malformations [178]. The association of left ventricular outflow obstruction supports the concept that the aortic arch lesion results from the decreased flow through the aortic isthmus in fetal life, accentuating the isthmus and persisting as a functional obstruction. Particularly with interruption of the arch, the cardiac anatomy with left ventricular outflow obstruction favors preferential flow from the pulmonary artery through the ductus into the descending aorta [179].

Despite the anatomic similarities between tubular hypoplasia and coarctation, they must be distinguished from each other, since they may appear independently although they often coexist [180, 180a].

Coarctation

Incidence   Including all its varieties, coarctation is the fifth most common malformation among CHD [181]. Genetic transmission of coarctation is uncommon [181a], and monozygotic twins are not concordant if one twin has a coarctation [182]. Seasonal peaks in incidence of coarctation have been described between September and November and between January and March [183]. Symptoms appear early. Of 203 surgically resected coarctations, 13% were in the first month of life; of 70 coarctations identified at autopsy,

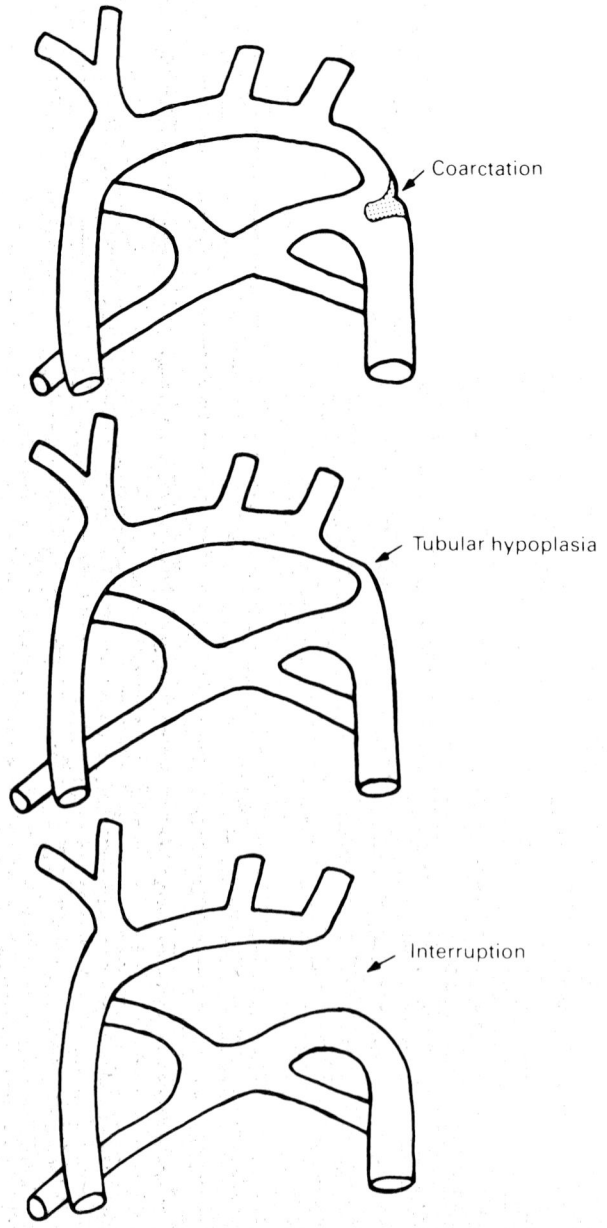

FIGURE 20.29.   *Coarctation, tubular hypoplasia, and interruption affect the aortic arch at the isthmus, usually slightly proximal to the ductus arteriosus.*

83% were in the first year and 43% were in the first month [184].

Classification   In the adult type of coarctation there is a sharply localized obstruction of the aortic arch in the region of the ductus, usually associated with either a ligamentum or a proximal patent ductus arteriosus. In the infantile type, there is an elongated narrowing of the distal aortic arch with a distal patent ductus arteriosus connecting to the descending aorta. A more precise anatomic classification designates the localized narrowing of the adult type as localized coarctation and the elongated infantile type as tubular hypoplasia. Tubular hypoplasia may appear with or without a coarctation; a localized coarctation, particularly in the neonate, frequently has an associated tubular hypoplasia. Since all localized coarctations approximate the ductus, they may carry the further designation of preductal, juxtaductal, or postductal depending on how they relate to the ductal orifice. The relative incidences of the individual types vary in different series [184, 185].

Further variations among coarctations relate to associated positional anomalies of the central vessels with stenosis or atresia of the left or right subclavian arteries, and origin of left subclavian or retroesophageal right subclavian artery distal to the coarctation [181, 186]. Coarctations that occur in atypical locations, such as the abdominal aorta, usually present in older infants and children but rarely in the neonate [187, 188].

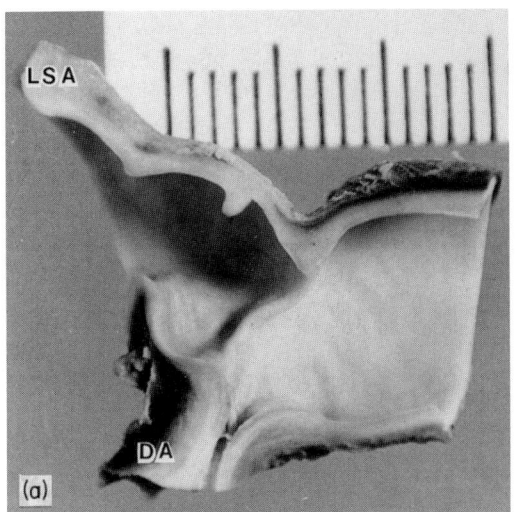

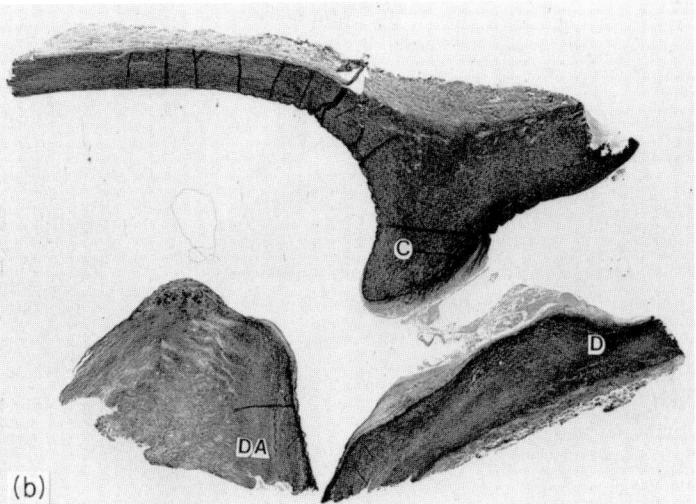

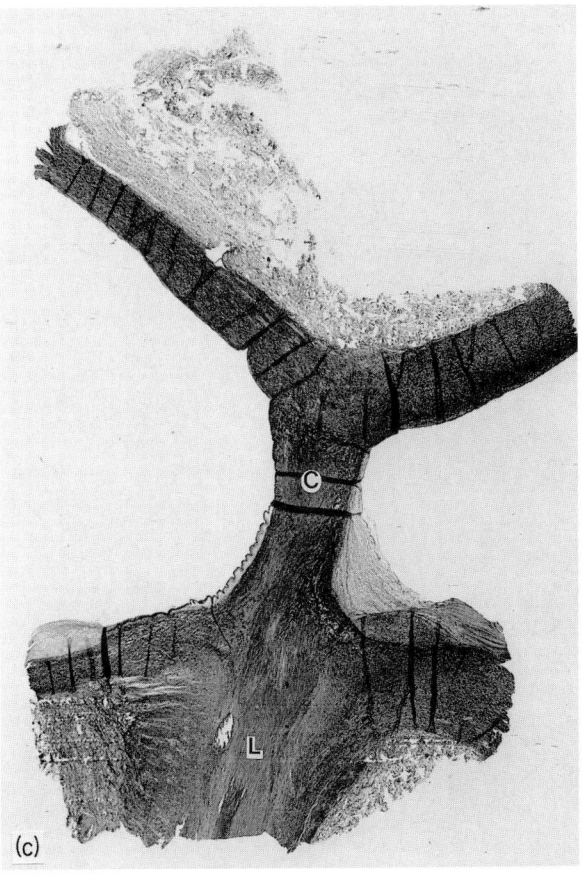

FIGURE 20.30. *(a) The curtain of the coarctation extends from the cephalad and posterior wall of the aorta to the ostium of the ductus arteriosus (DA). The origin of the left subclavian artery (LSA) lies at the proximal margin of the specimen at the left. (b) Histologically, the curtain (C) protrudes into the aortic lumen toward the ductus (DA), covered on its inferior and distal aspects by a sclerotic plaque that also affects the inferior wall of the aorta distal (D) to the coarctation. (c) A section of the coarctation tangential to the aortic wall reveals the continuity of the curtain with the wall of the ligamentum (L). (Reproduced with permission from: Rosenberg HS. Coarctation of the aorta: morphology and pathogenetic considerations. In: Rosenberg HS, Bolande RP, eds. Perspectives in Pediatric Pathology. vol. 1. Chicago: Year Book Medical, 1973, p. 354.)*

Morphology The external wall of an aorta with a localized coarctation has an obtuse indentation on its posterolateral surface. Within the lumen, an eccentric shelf protrudes from the superior wall opposite the orifice of the ductus arteriosus (Fig. 20.30). As the ductus closes, it constricts the aortic orifice, accentuating the aortic obstruction. Proximal to the coarctation, the aortic arch has either a normal caliber or a slight degree of tubular hypoplasia; distally, the aorta may have a poststenotic dilatation. The left subclavian artery may arise at or proximal to the coarctation. Coarctation may result in congestive heart failure, dilatation of the left atrium and ventricle, hypertrophy of the myocardium, left ventricular endocardial fibroelastosis, and abnormal papillary muscles resulting in mitral valvular insufficiency.

The curtain forming the coarctation consists of smooth muscle and fibrous and elastic tissue with a superimposed intimal sclerosis varying in degree but appearing as early as the first month of life. Eventually, the intima of the aorta distal to the coarctation becomes sclerotic. The distal aortic media is thicker, with more muscle and less compact elastic tissue, than proximal to the coarctation. This disparity in size between the aortic wall proximal and distal to the coarctation appears as early as 1 month of life, reflecting the damped systolic pressure and narrow pulse pressure distal to the curtain [184].

Associated Malformations Of infants less than 6 months of age with coarctation, most have additional cardiovascular malformations, usually tubular hypoplasia of the arch. Virtually all infants with combined coarctation and tubular hypoplasia have associated malformations [185]. Bicuspid aortic valve occurs in a particularly high incidence, up to 85% in some series. The association of coarctation and bicuspid aortic valve with syndromes involving pharyngeal structures has led to the hypothesis of disordered neural crest migration as a common factor in the genesis of the cardiovascular and noncardiovascular malformations [189].

The association of coarctation and aortic valve abnormality with Turner (45,XO) syndrome, more often in those with congenital neck webbing than in those with mosaic monosomy X [189a], led to the suggestion of lymphangiectasia as the common mechanism for most of the syndrome's phenotypic features [190]. The constancy of the relationship led Kalousek and Seller to consider the triad of cervical cystic hygroma, subcutaneous edema, and coarctation in a female as probably diagnostic of the lethal form of 45,XO syndrome [191].

Coarctations do not accompany malformations producing a left-to-right shunt through the ductus—e.g., tricuspid atresia, t/F, or pulmonary stenosis or atresia [184]. Collateral vessels about the coarctation usually develop postnatally, but have been identified in the neonate.

Pathogenesis The isthmus normally retains a smaller dimension than the remainder of the aortic arch well into postnatal life, particularly in prematurely born infants and in the presence of a ductus arteriosus [192]. A congenitally malformed heart with a reduced pulmonary arterial blood flow has a wider aortic isthmus than normal, since the isthmus must carry more blood in the fetus to compensate for the diminished flow through the ductus, thereby overcoming the usual isthmic stagnation. In contrast, obstruction of left ventricular outflow accentuates the narrowing of the isthmus, which remains underdeveloped postnatally [193].

The curtain of the coarctation enters the aortic wall at the entrance of the ductus, leading to the interpretation of ductal tissue forming the coarctation [194]. In 1855, Skoda recognized the aortic isthmus and, acknowledging Rokitansky's concept of coarctation as a retardation of normal development, suggested that ductal tissue spread into the aorta and transferred ductal shrinkage into the aorta [195]. Although extension of ductal tissue into the aorta may not produce the coarctation, the closure of the aortic orifice of the ductus reduces the aortic lumen size at the coarctation site, accounting for the abrupt postnatal onset of symptoms [196]. Considering its location at the junction of the aortic isthmus and the ductus arteriosus and the continuity of the ductal wall with the fibromuscular curtain, coarctation may be interpreted as the result of diminished flow through the fetal aorta, leading to the persistence of the normally narrow isthmus and subsequent development of the curtain [197].

Coarctation at the isthmus correlates with the functional aspect of the isthmus in the fetus. As determined in the fetal lamb, the ductus carries almost half the combined ventricular output to the descending aorta, with the isthmus carrying only one-fourth [196]. The low flow through the isthmus corresponds to the small size of the isthmus relative to the ascending and descending aorta.

The association of other cardiovascular malformations with coarctation is skewed toward those with small left ventricle and the development of tubular hypoplasia: large VSD, double-outlet right ventricle, and the Taussig-Bing malformation. Conversely, the isthmus has the same size as the descending aorta, with decreased pulmonary and ductal flow, as in pulmonary stenosis or atresia. With a right aortic arch, the ductus is usually small, and tubular hypoplasia and coarctation are virtually unknown [196].

Histologically, ductal tissue is readily distinguishable from aortic tissue at the site of a coarctation, blending into and forming a sling about the aortic wall. The curtain of the coarctation suspends from the superoposterior aortic wall with a less prominent protrusion laterally and medially [180].

Tubular hypoplasia represents exaggeration of the isthmus associated with a proximal obstruction, contrasting with the localized obstruction of a coarctation (Fig. 20.31) [180, 198]. Sometimes a coarctation at the distal end of a tubular hypoplasia requires histologic identification. Coarctation in the neonate has some degree of tubular hypoplasia, although mild, but the converse is not true—tubular hypoplasia may occur without a coarctation [199]. The curtain of the coarc-

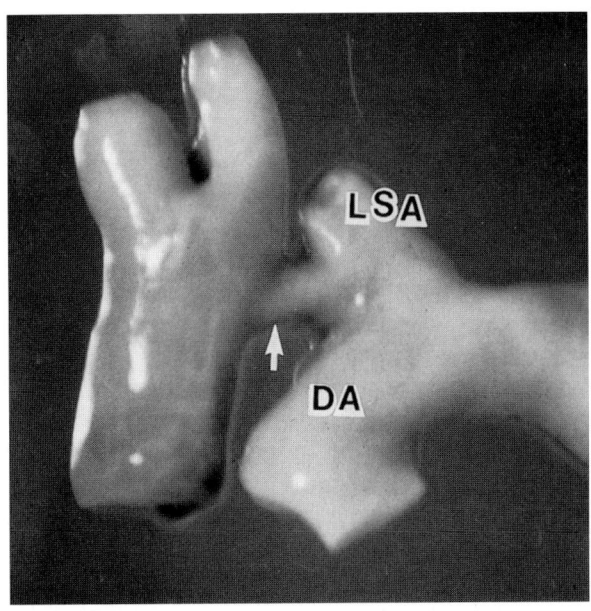

FIGURE 20.31.   *Tubular hypoplasia of the aortic arch (arrow) with a patent ductus arteriosus (DA) and origin of the left subclavian artery (LSA) distal to the hypoplastic segment.*

tation is not an ectopic fibromuscular bundle but represents the original wall of the distal left sixth aortic arch (the ductus) [184].

Hemodynamics Neither coarctation nor interruption of the aortic arch seems to interfere with fetal development, since both are compatible with normal fetal circulation. Symptoms appear within days or weeks of birth, relating to the closure of the ductus and the loss of the aortic orifice of the ductus and accentuating the small size of the lumen at the coarctation [196, 200].

Tubular Hypoplasia

Malformations frequently coexist with tubular hypoplasia, usually obstructing aortic outflow. Tubular hypoplasia without a coarctation always has associated malformations, usually a ductus arteriosus, ASD or VSD, aortic valve stenosis, TGA with tricuspid valve atresia, or single ventricle [199]. With or without associated malformations, the mortality rate and the operative mortality for patients with tubular hypoplasia are high [186].

Interruption of the Aortic Arch

Classification Interruption of the aortic arch, although uncommon, accounts for about 1% of all CHD and almost invariably presents in the neonatal period. Classified on the basis of the site relative to the arteries arising from the aortic arch, interruption consists of three major types [201]:

A. Distal to the left subclavian artery
B. Distal to the left common carotid artery
C. Distal to the brachiocephalic artery

Each type may be subclassified to indicate association with a truncus arteriosus, an aortopulmonary artery window, origin of a retroesophageal right subclavian artery distal to the left subclavian artery, or a right subclavian artery arising from the right pulmonary artery via a right ductus arteriosus [179]. In one group of 115 cases, 40% were type A, 56.5% were type B, and 3.5% were type C [202]. Recurrence of interruption of the aortic arch in siblings is more often of type B than of type A [202a].

Morphology An interrupted aortic arch lacks continuity between the aortic arch and the distal aorta, with the proximal aorta ending blindly proximal to the entrance of the ductus arteriosus (Fig. 20.32). The distal aorta is continuous with the pulmonary artery via the ductus arteriosus. The ductal morphology varies from the thick wall of a normally constricting ductus to the thin wall of an abnormally persistent patent ductus [179].

Associated Malformations A VSD, which is almost universal, usually lies within the conal septum, less often in the membranous or muscular septum, or in an AVC position [203]. A PDA, which is universal, may be constricted. Those few cases without a VSD have a window between the aorta and the pulmonary artery. Obstructive lesions in the left

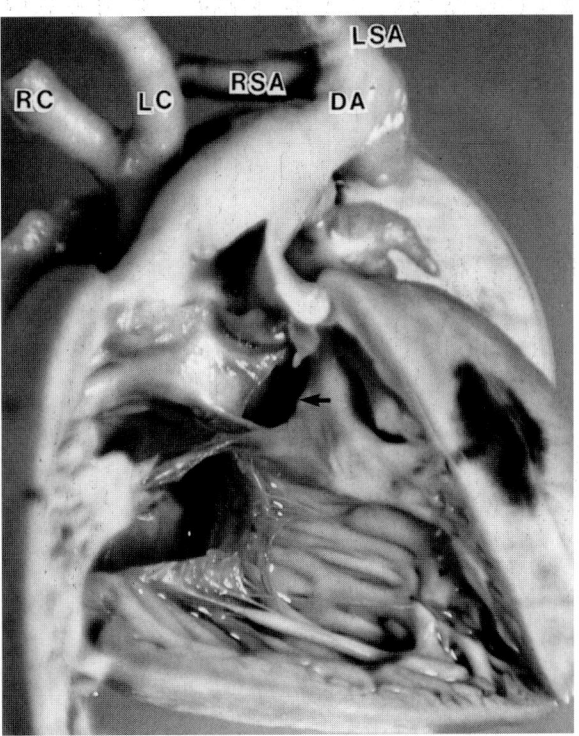

FIGURE 20.32.   *Proximal to the interruption in the aortic arch, the ascending aorta gives off the right carotid (RC) and left carotid (LC) arteries. The distal aorta continues with the ductus arteriosus (DA) and gives off the left subclavian artery (LSA) and a retroesophageal right subclavian artery (RSA). The ventricular septum has a supracristal defect (arrow).*

ventricular outlet, which are frequent, may consist only of a leftward-displaced septum and a conal septal defect, but other forms of left ventricular outlet obstruction accompany the other types of VSD, although the type of VSD has no relation to the type of interruption [203]. Other malformations accompanying interruption include transposition, truncus arteriosus, corrected transposition, straddling tricuspid valve, tricuspid atresia, and double-outlet right ventricle [179, 202]. About 50% have a bicuspid aortic valve.

About two-thirds have only a VSD and a PDA, making them potential candidates for surgery. Type B interruption has a greater tendency to have VSD as the only associated defect, in contrast to the more complex malformations associated with type A [179, 202]. The association of Type B interruption with the DiGeorge anomalad has led to the suggestion of a defect in neural crest migration in the pathogenesis of the heart lesion as well as the other components [204, 205].

Hemodynamics   With interruption of the aortic arch, increased pulmonary blood flow usually results from an accompanying VSD. The circulation resembles the fetal circulation with the descending aorta supplied from the right ventricle via the ductus arteriosus, differing from the fetal circulation by the absence rather than the diminution of isthmic blood flow. The affected infant may remain asymptomatic at birth but develops failure within 2 weeks of life with the postnatal decrease in pulmonary vascular resistance and closure of the ductus.

Survival to several months may occur with a combination of associated malformations, notably d-transposition, VSD, and ductus arteriosus [206]. With no intracardiac defect and only a PDA, the patient may survive for years with a functional syndrome resembling a coarctation [207]. A small number of cases have been successfully palliated or repaired surgically [202, 208].

Vascular Rings

To form a vascular ring, an aortic arch artery passes posterior to the esophagus, joining with other aortic arch branches to encircle the trachea and esophagus. The most common vascular ring is a double aortic arch with branches passing anterior and posterior to the trachea and esophagus and causing early symptoms [209, 209a, 209b]. Although the posterior arch encroaches on the dorsal esophageal wall, the earliest effects are on the trachea, initially resulting in respiratory distress due to expiratory airway resistance [210] and followed later by recurrent pulmonary infections [211] and effects of esophageal compression.

Retroesophageal vessels need not cause symptoms. As the most common aortic arterial abnormality, a retroesophageal right subclavian artery occurs at an incidence estimated at 1 in 200 individuals and is usually discovered incidentally, either clinically by its indentation of the posterior wall of the esophagus or at autopsy [212]. A retroesophageal right subclavian artery arises from the descending aorta distal to the left subclavian artery and proceeds retroesophageally to its normal distribution. Despite its anomalous position, the retroesophageal artery does not close the ring, leaving an open segment on the right of the trachea and esophagus.

The hypothetical model of Edwards, assuming the presence of a double aortic arch with a right- and left-sided ductus, enhances comprehension of the multiple forms of vascular ring (Fig. 20.33) [213]. Although the precise pattern of the model has not been identified in a human, it illustrates the distribution and connection of the arches, the origin of the great arteries from the aortic arch, and the potential components of a vascular ring. During cardiogenesis, the distal portion of the sixth aortic arches forms a ductus arteriosus on either side. Normally, one or the other ductus disappears and the descending aorta deviates to one

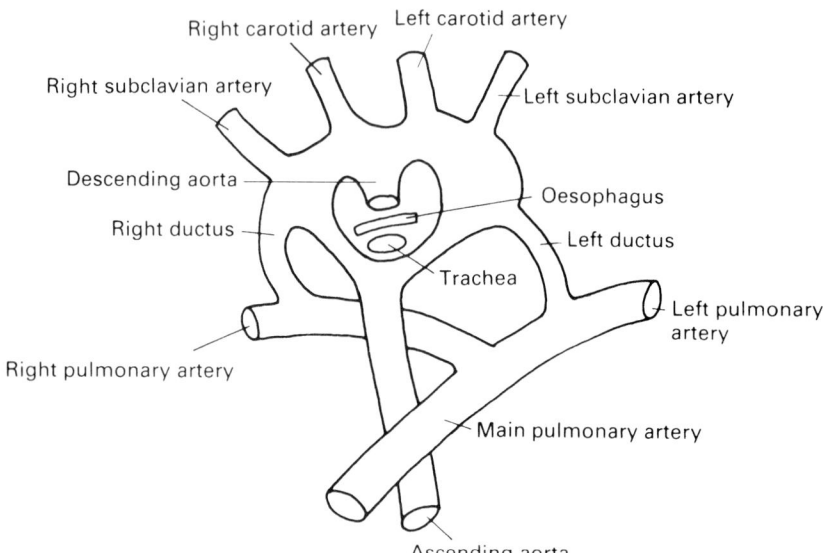

FIGURE 20.33.   *The hypothetical double arch of Edwards can be used to reconstruct most aortic arch configurations or vascular rings— e.g., the normal anatomy is revealed by deleting the right ductus arteriosus and the posterior arch between the right and left carotid arteries, retaining the connection between the left portion of the arch and the descending aorta (After Edwards [213]).*

side or the other. Persistence of a ductus or a branch that normally disappears results in one of four basic types of vascular ring: a left- or right-sided ductus, each with either a left- or right-sided descending aorta [213]. With any pattern, a double aortic arch with a retroesophageal branch may capture the trachea and esophagus in a ring.

A pulmonary artery sling does not usually form a ring but produces symptoms and a high mortality in the neonate. The malformed left pulmonary artery arises from the posterior aspect of the right main pulmonary artery, crosses the right mainstem bronchus, and passes between the trachea and the esophagus to reach the hilum of the left lung. The crossing left pulmonary artery may indent the esophagus, but it compresses the trachea and right main stem bronchus. A left ductus may connect from the right main pulmonary artery to the aorta but captures the trachea and bronchus in a sling rather than a complete ring.

Patients with pulmonary artery sling have associated cardiovascular malformations of no specific type and a particularly high incidence of tracheobronchial anomalies such as a hypoplastic trachea, hypoplastic bronchus, or complete cartilaginous rings [214]. Pulmonary artery sling usually produces symptoms at birth or by 1 month, with a mortality rate of about 50% relating to the tracheobronchial obstruction or to the associated malformations. The poor results of surgical repair result from the combination of the tracheobronchial malformation and the difficulty in reconstructing the pulmonary artery [215].

Anomalous Pulmonary Venous Connections and Return

Total Anomalous Pulmonary Venous Return

Incidence   A relatively uncommon malformation, total anomalous pulmonary venous return (TAPVR) makes up about 1–2% of CHD cases, occurring more often in males and frequently with a variety of associated congenital heart malformations [216]. Although usually occurring without a family history and with a low recurrence risk, a family has been reported in which TAPVR segregated as an autosomal dominant trait with decreased penetrance and a potential gene locus in the centromeric region of chromosome 4 [216a, 216b].

Classification   Since TAPVR has a variety of anatomic and physiologic combinations consequent to the developmental failure of incorporation of the common pulmonary vein into the left atrium, the circulation depends on a persistent fetal structure for pulmonary venous return to the heart [217]. Classified according to the anatomic site of the pulmonary venous return to the heart, TAPVR may be cardiac, supracardiac, or infracardiac (Fig. 20.34). The functional consequences of TAPVR are cyanosis with increased pulmonary blood flow or pulmonary hypertension due to obstructed pulmonary venous return. These functional abnormalities correlate imperfectly with the morphologic classification. Obstruction to venous return may accompany any of the

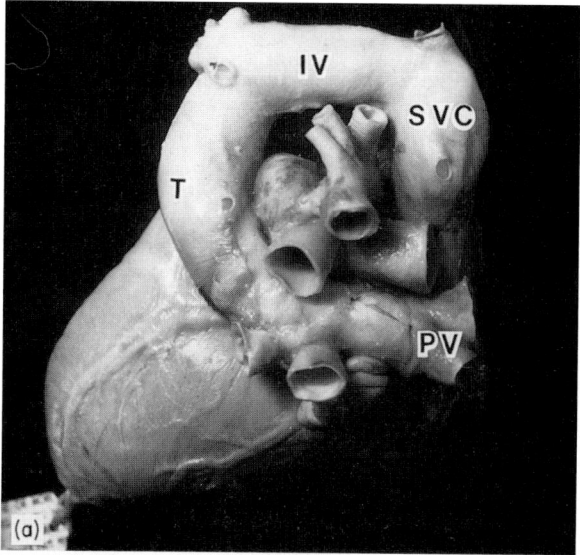

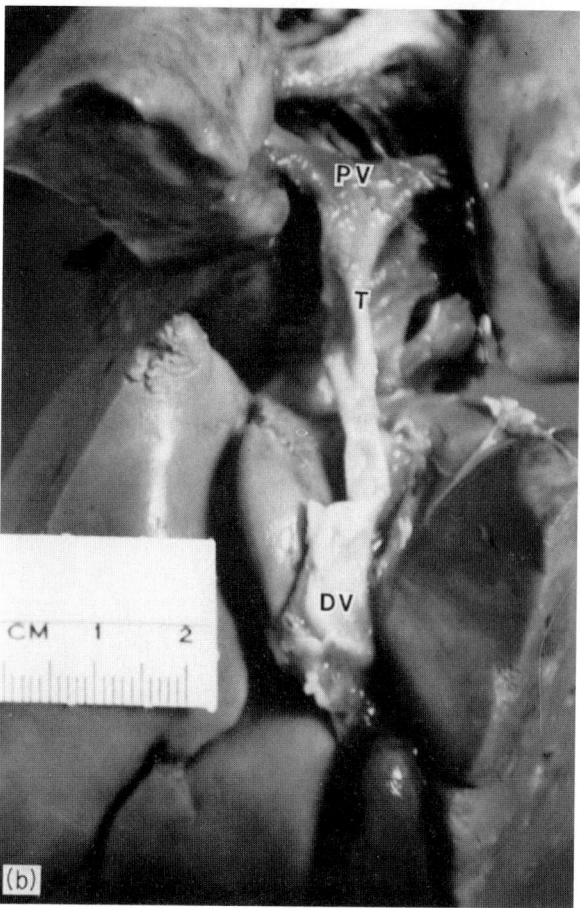

FIGURE 20.34.   *In malformations resulting in anomalous pulmonary venous return to the right atrium, the pulmonary veins (PV) may join to form a common trunk (T), which (a) ascends to join the innominate vein (IV) proximal to its junction with the superior vena cava (SVC) or (b) descends through the diaphragm to join the ductus venosus (DV), which traverses the liver and joins the inferior vena cava.*

morphologic types of TAPVR, but more likely in the infra-diaphragmatic types and less likely in the supradiaphragmatic and intracardiac types. Infradiaphragmatic TAPVR connects to the portal vein at its junction with the splenic and superior mesenteric veins, the ductus venosus, the hepatic vein, or the inferior vena cava.

Supracardiac TAPVR may connect on the right to a vena cava or azygous vein or on the left to a vena cava, coronary sinus, or left innominate vein, with a higher incidence of obstruction and mortality in those draining on the right to the vena cava or azygous vein [218, 219]. With infradiaphragmatic TAPVR, the potential sites of obstruction are the hepatic vascular bed, the junction of the anomalous channel with the portal vein or ductus venosus, and extrinsic compression at the diaphragm. Supradiaphragmatic obstruction may result from compression of the channel between the left pulmonary artery and the left mainstem bronchus, intrinsically within the vertical vein, or at the junction with the innominate vein or the right superior vena cava. The obstructing lesion may not be readily apparent on gross examination [220].

With obstruction, TAPVR causes symptoms in the neonate and, if not corrected, death within the first 2 months of life, sometimes occurring suddenly without prior significant symptoms [221]. The pulmonary arterial pressure remains high and does not fall postnatally. The pulmonary hypertension, pulmonary parenchymal status, and small left atrium are the source of morbidity [222], although they are not identified as risk factors for poor surgical outcome [223, 224]. The clinical effects of TAPVR depend on the degree of pulmonary venous obstruction, the pulmonary vascular resistance, and pulmonary blood flow [217]. Without surgical correction, patients with pulmonary venous obstruction, pulmonary hypertension, and decreased pulmonary blood flow—usually those with infradiaphragmatic TAPVR—rarely survive more than 2 to 3 weeks.

Structural changes appear very early in the pulmonary circulation with TAPVR and increase with age. Thick-walled blood vessels have an increased muscularity, and muscle extends farther into smaller arteries than normal. The obstructed veins have a well-defined external elastic lamina, giving them an arterialized appearance [220].

Cor Triatriatum

When the pulmonary veins join but are not completely incorporated into the left atrium, an accessory chamber forms from the common pulmonary vein, simulating three atrial chambers, cor triatriatum (Fig. 20.35). Unlike other malformations with obstruction to pulmonary venous return, symptoms of cor triatriatum frequently do not start until after the perinatal period [220]. The connection between the common pulmonary vein and the left atrium may have one or more orifices as small as 2 mm in diameter. The left atrium remains small and retains the appendage, which never arises from the proximal pulmonary venous chamber. The fossa ovalis also connects to the lower, left

atrial chamber, although the upper chamber may have a communication with the right atrium chamber (Fig. 20.36) [225–227].

Cor triatriatum may have one of three types of connection between the common pulmonary vein and the left atrium: diaphragm, hourglass, or tubular [228]. With the diaphragm type, a transverse septum consisting of a single layer of myocardium and perforated by one or more small openings separates the common pulmonary vein from the left atrium [229]. Associated CHD, more common with the hourglass and tubular types than with the diaphragm type, includes TAPVR [228].

Pulmonary Vein Stenosis and Atresia

Whereas cor triatriatum represents stenosis of the common pulmonary vein, all or only some individual pulmonary veins may be stenotic or atretic at their junctions with the left atrium (Fig. 20.37) [229, 230]. At the obstructive site, the venous wall has an intrinsic thickening, which may extend in a retrograde direction into the intraparenchymal veins. The venous obstruction induces right ventricular dilatation and hypertrophy. The infant with stenosis may survive a few months but has a poor prognosis with only transient alleviation from dilatation of the stenosis [229].

The common pulmonary vein may have an atretic orifice, connected to the left atrium by a residual fibrous band, but with no pulmonary venous return to the heart other than through small vascular channels to the esophageal and mediastinal veins and presumably the bronchial venous system [231, 232]. The pulmonary parenchyma has prominent lymphangiectasia. Symptoms begin promptly at birth, followed by congestive heart failure. Successful surgical repair involves both direct venous anastomoses and concurrent lung transplantation [223–235].

Pulmonary Veno-occlusive Disease

With pulmonary veno-occlusive disease, the small intraparenchymal veins are occluded by a combination of cellular proliferation and intimal fibrosis progressing from the small to the large veins. Pulmonary veno-occlusive disease usually affects older infants and children, and only rarely the neonate [236, 236a].

Ectopia Cordis

Classification

A heart unconfined to its usual position in the thorax may occupy ectopic sites—cervical, thoracic, or abdominal—most commonly a combined thoracic and abdominal location and rarely, if ever, one of the other sites [237, 238]. At a thoracoabdominal site, ectopia cordis has five malformations (Cantrell's pentad), although not all are necessarily present in each case [239]:

1. A midline supraumbilical abdominal defect extending caudally to the umbilicus as either a ventral

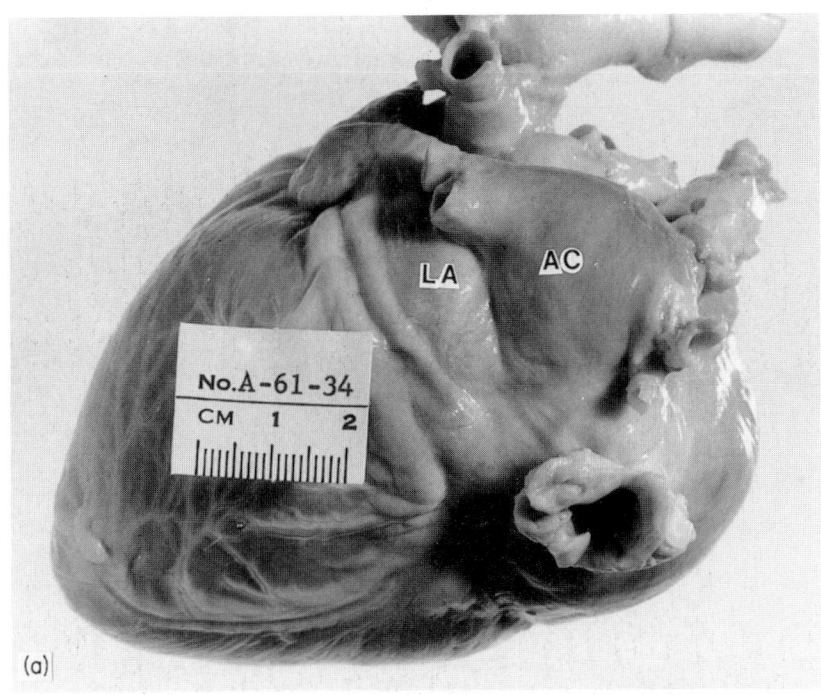

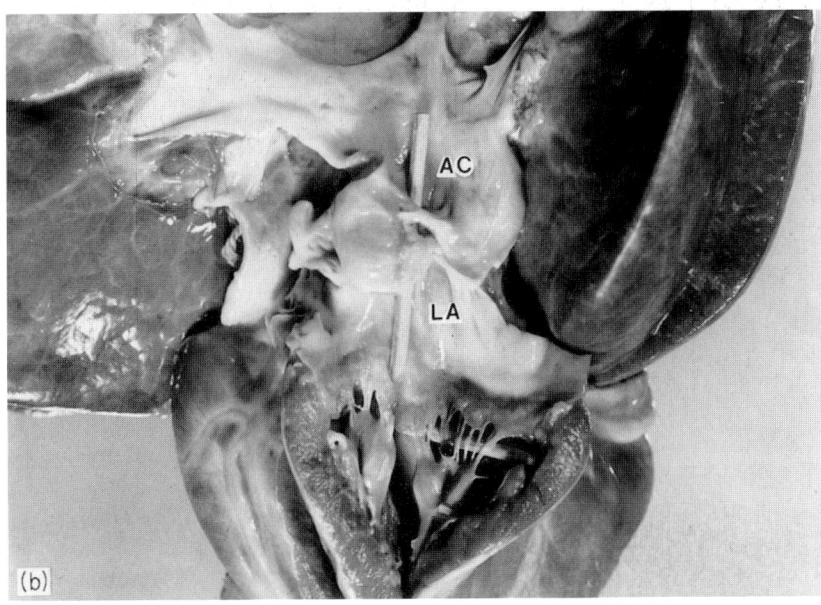

FIGURE 20.35.   *(a) The pulmonary veins join to form an accessory chamber (AC) on the posterior aspect of the left atrium (LA), forming a cor triatriatum, demarcated on the external surface by a shallow groove. (b) Several small communications (one holds a probe) extend through the septum between the accessory chamber and the left atrium.*

hernia with diastasis of the rectus abdominis muscles or an omphalocele

2. A lower sternum that may be normal, may be split, or may have absent segments
3. A V-shaped defect in the anterior diaphragm, not present in all patients
4. A defect in the diaphragmatic aspect of the pericardium affecting about 20% of cases
5. Various forms of congenital heart disease

The pentad has a varied expression from partial to complete, with partial expression including a normal heart or no

diaphragmatic defect [239]. The malformation complex usually appears as an isolated, sporadic event, but has been recorded in families [240] and associated with consanguinity [241], triploidy [241a], and trisomy 18 [242, 243].

Morphology

Defects in the overlying thoracic or abdominal wall include deficiency or absence of the sternum, pericardium, and skin. Thoracic or thoracoabdominal ectopia may have a partial or complete midline sternal cleft, an intact or partially or completely absent pericardium, and intact or absent overlying skin. In the extremely rare cervical form, an anterior

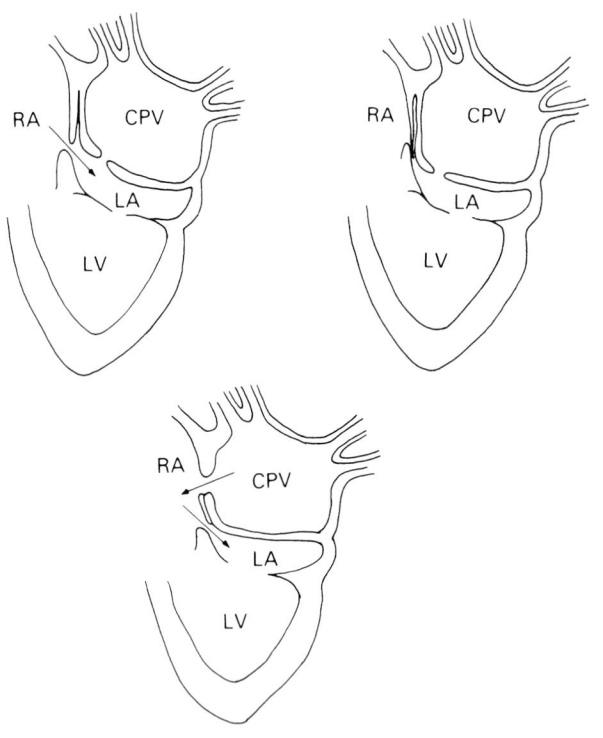

FIGURE 20.36.   *With cor triatriatum, the foramen ovale (upper left) or fossa ovalis (upper right) connects the common pulmonary venous trunk to the left atrial chamber. Connection of the common pulmonary venous trunk to the right atrium represents an associated anomalous pulmonary venous connection and return (lower left). RA—right atrium; LA—left atrium; LV—left ventricle; CPV—common pulmonary venous trunk. (Reproduced with permission from: Jordan JD, McNamara DG, Marcontell J, Rosenberg HS. Cor triatriatum. Cardiovasc Res Cent Bull 1963; 1:79–85.)*

cervical fissure, a sternal defect, and an inverted heart make for a difficult distinction between cervical and thoracic ectopia [244].

Associated Defects

About 90% of ectopia patients have associated cardiovascular malformations, which determine the prognosis [245, 246]. The associated malformations include VSD in three-fourths of the cases, ASD in half the cases, and sporadic examples of pulmonary valve atresia, patent or absent ductus arteriosus, truncus, single ventricle, cardiac diverticulum, AVC defect, anomalous venous return, aortic valve stenosis, right and left superior venae cavae, tricuspid valve atresia, t/F, and TGA [237, 239, 247, 248]. Associated noncardiovascular malformations include an absent or abnormal left lung and cranial or facial anomalies such as hydrocephalus, cleft palate, anencephaly, and meningocele.

Prognosis

The prognosis is generally poor, with fatality, before or immediately after birth, usually due to the associated malformations. In the thoracoabdominal type, those with umbilical hernia have a better prognosis than those with omphalocele [247]. Those cases with ectopia and no or mild associated CHD are potential survivors after successful surgical closure of the thoracic and abdominal defects [249].

Syndromes of Abnormal Symmetry, Abnormal Spleen, and Congenital Heart Disease

Following the initial report of the association of multiple, complex cardiovascular malformations associated with asplenia [250], similar malformation syndromes have been identified in which the spleen persists, most often as a cluster of

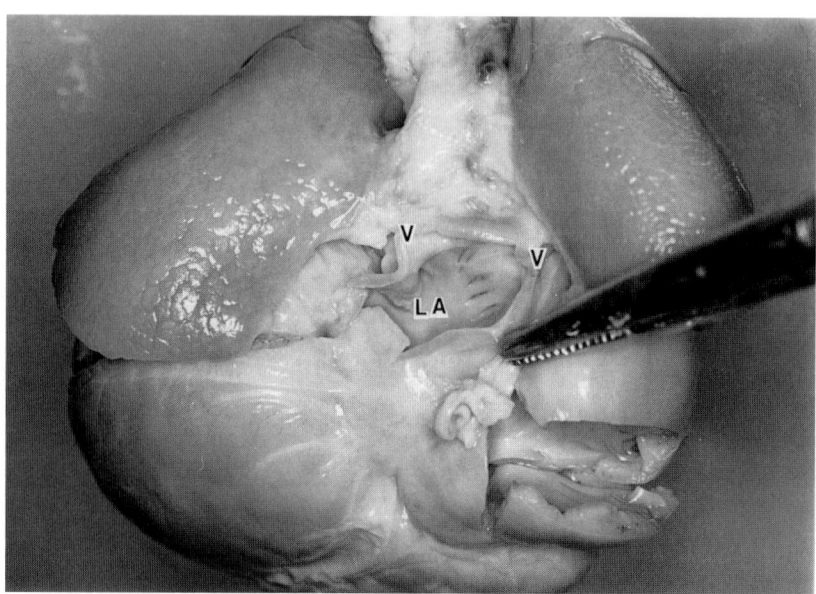

FIGURE 20.37.   *The pulmonary veins (V) are stenotic at their junction with the left atrium (LA), resulting in a small left atrium.*

small spleniculi. Asplenia and polysplenia syndromes have been estimated to occur in 1 in 1750 autopsies, 1 in 40,000 births, and 35% of cardiovascular malformations with malposition [251]. Other malformations in the syndromes include those of the gut and genitourinary system, but the cardiovascular malformations account for the mortality rates of greater than 95% for asplenia and 60% for polysplenia in the first year of life [252].

The spectrum of laterality disorders, or heterotaxy, has been identified in family groups with individual members expressing different anatomic arrangements including situs inversus, asplenia, and TAPVR with X-linked recessive [252a], autosomal dominant, and autosomal recessive patterns of inheritance [252a, 252b, 252c].

Several of the features of both right and left symmetry syndromes represent persistent undifferentiated symmetry of the embryo rather than abnormal sidedness—e.g., bilateral SVC, hepatic isomerism, and persistence of the proximal IVC and contralateral hepatic vein in asplenia and bilateral hepatic veins in polysplenia [253]. The absence of the spleen has been related to its status as the only major left-sided viscus; with bilateral right symmetry and no left side, a spleen cannot develop. Phoon and Neill hypothesized that most defects in the asplenia syndrome originate in the embryo at Streeter horizon XIII [253a].

The lack of the normal human asymmetry results in two basic syndromes with mirror-image symmetry: bilateral left symmetry and bilateral right symmetry (Fig. 20.38). Despite the cogent reasoning of Van Praagh and Van Praagh in rejecting the concept of atrial isomerism [254], the cardiac atria and the bronchial distribution reflect this symmetry, providing the diagnostic criteria for the two syndromes. In bilateral right symmetry, each atrial appendage has a right configuration and each lung has the bronchial distribution of a right lung; conversely, in bilateral left symmetry, each atrial appendage has a left configuration and each lung has the bronchial distribution of a left lung [255]. With notable exceptions, mirror-image right symmetry accompanies asplenia, and mirror-image left symmetry accompanies polysplenia.

The asplenia syndrome has several recurring features; the malformations are complex including anomalies of systemic and pulmonary venous return, a common atrium, endocardial cushion defects, TGA, stenosis or atresia of the pulmonary artery, often a single ventricle, and aorticocaval juxtaposition. Both atria resemble right atria, sometimes with bilateral sinoatrial nodes. The left and right lungs and the left and right lobes of the liver are mirror images of each other. With asplenia, abdominal heterotaxia includes hepatic isomerism as a rule. The stomach may be right, left, or midline. Some degree of malrotation of the small intestine is virtually universal, varying from partial malrotation to lack of any rotation with a midline mesentery attached to the entire small and large intestines [253].

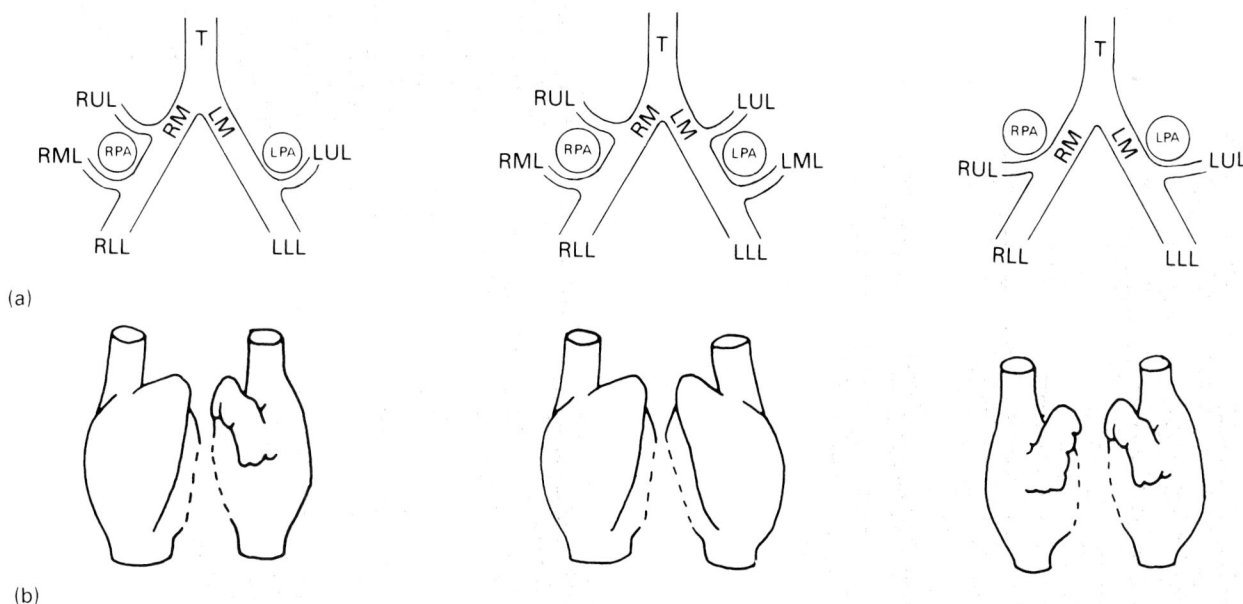

FIGURE 20.38. (a) The normal bronchial distribution (upper left) has an eparterial bronchus (RUL) on the right; bilateral eparterial bronchi characterize right pulmonary isomerism (upper center), and bilateral absence of an eparterial bronchus characterizes left pulmonary isomerism (upper right). (b) In the normal heart (bottom left), the atrial appendage is broad and blunt on the right and narrow and angulated on the left; bilateral broad appendages characterize right isomerism (bottom center), and bilateral angulated appendages characterize left isomerism (bottom right). T—trachea; RPA—right pulmonary artery; LPA—left pulmonary artery; RM—right mainstem bronchus; LM—left mainstem bronchus; RUL—right upper lobe; RML—right middle lobe; RLL—right lower lobe; LUL—left upper lobe; LLL—left lower lobe.

The varied cardiovascular malformations do not affect each case. About two-thirds of the cases have bilateral superior venae cavae, and the remaining third may have right or left superior venae cavae. The inferior vena cava may enter either the right or left atrium accompanied by a contralateral common hepatic vein entering independently in about one-third of cases. The common hepatic vein has been interpreted as the persistence, bilaterally, of the proximal segments of the embryonic vitelline venous system. In virtually all cases, the inferior vena cava and the aorta approximate each other on the same side of the vertebral bodies in a pattern designated aorticocaval juxtaposition [253]. The pulmonary veins drain anomalously in most cases, infradi-

aphragmatic to the portal vein or to one or more systemic veins, often with obstruction of the pulmonary veins [256a, 256b, 256c]. The great arteries are transposed in about two-thirds of cases. About three-fourths of the cases have stenosis or atresia of the pulmonary artery [256]. About two-thirds have the aortic arch on the left, one-third on the right.

About one-third have dextrocardia with the cardiac apex on the right. The usually absent coronary sinus represents failure of another left-sided structure, the left sinus horn. By definition of the right symmetry syndrome, right atrial isomerism is universal. The usual ASD varies in degree from a residual septum consisting of a strand of muscle to absence

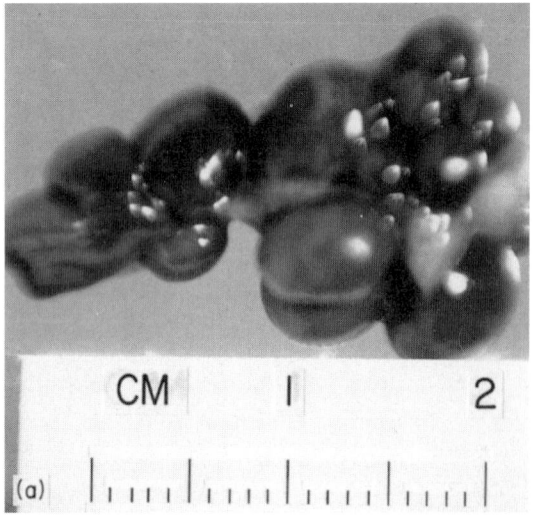

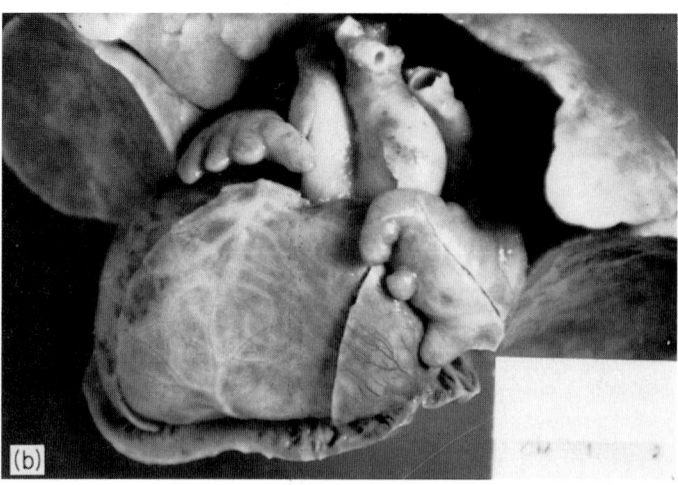

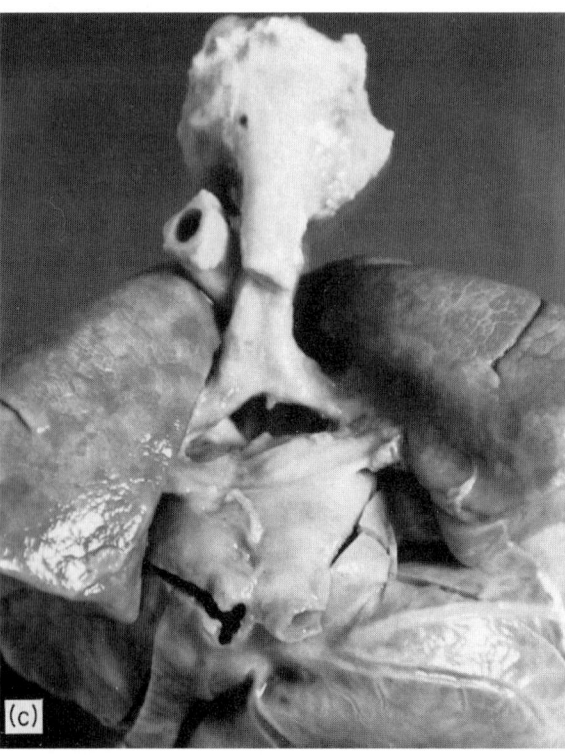

FIGURE 20.39. *An infant with left isomerism had (a) polysplenia with multiple spleniculi of equal size, (b) left atrial isomerism with bilateral, sharply angulated atrial appendages, and (c) left pulmonary isomerism with absence of an eparterial bronchus on either side.*

of the septum. The ASD accompanies an equal incidence of AVC defects. The cases are about equally divided between those with one and two ventricles. Notoriously, a rudimentary configuration of the ventricles may defy identification as right or left [253].

The AV junction usually has a common AV valve, a single valve orifice, or an ambiguous, rudimentary connection. The right ventricle may have a d- or l-loop. The rarely concordant ventriculo-arterial connections are most commonly arranged in a double-outlet right ventricle or with pulmonary valve atresia. The cardiac orientation may be right, left, or midline [257].

Polysplenia and other splenic abnormality syndromes with left symmetry may have less complex cardiovascular malformations than those with asplenia and right isomerism (Fig. 20.39). The heart may even be normal. Unlike right isomerism, left isomerism has an equal gender incidence. About 60% of affected infants die within the first year of life. Interruption of the inferior vena cava with drainage via the azygous system and aorticocaval juxtaposition are frequent [253]. The absent inferior vena cava, which is derived from a right-sided structure, results in venous return via the azygous system.

Landing et al define a syndrome of bilateral right sidedness and a bifurcated or lobed spleen with one or more main and accessory spleens—a syndrome that they call anisosplenia [258]. With an anisosplenic configuration similar to that in males, females with the syndrome had left symmetry, not notably different from the polysplenic syndromes, although the cardiovascular malformations did not include symmetric pulmonary venous return, double-outlet right ventricle, or an AVC defect [258].

In left isomerism, the narrow, hooked atrial appendages resemble a normal left appendage joining the atria along a narrow front with no crista between the trabecular and smooth portions of the atria. In contrast with right isomerism, left atrial isomerism is more likely to have a better-formed septum. The superior vena cava, frequently bilateral, has no crista guarding the junction with the atrium. Hepatic veins are frequently bilateral. The interrupted inferior vena cava results in drainage into a left or right azygous system. The pulmonary veins may drain normally or into each atrium. The variable AV connections are similar to those of right isomerism, including an occasional AVC defect. The right ventricle may have a d- or l-loop. Double-inlet left ventricle and single ventricle are less frequent than in right isomerism. Ventricular morphology may be ambiguous and indeterminate. The ventriculoarterial connections are frequently concordant [257].

Pericardium

Pericardial malformations, including partial or complete defects, cysts, and diverticula, except as they accompany other malformations, are usually asymptomatic, making them unlikely to play a role in perinatal disease. With the exception of the pericardial defect accompanying the acardiac malformation, pericardial malformations usually appear as incidental findings or as mediastinal tumors by diagnostic imaging [259, 260, 260a]. Partial defects present more often on the right than on the left, occasionally allowing herniation and potential strangulation of a portion of atrial appendage or ventricle [261]. Even less commonly, defects on the diaphragmatic aspect of the pericardium are associated with midline abdominal and sternal defects [262].

Pericardial cysts and diverticula are more often unilocular than multilocular, have thin walls lined by mesothelium, are usually on the right, and rarely produce symptoms [261, 262].

CARDIOMYOPATHIES

Histiocytoid Cardiomyopathy

A myocardial disorder of unknown etiology, pathogenesis, and incidence has been described under a variety of names reflecting the appearance of large, vacuolated cells within the myocardium. This disorder, evidently unique to the first 2 years of life and predominantly affecting females, usually presents clinically with a rapidly lethal arrhythmia, with no signs of other heart disease, and frequently preceded by signs attributed to a viral infection: vomiting, diarrhea, upper respiratory symptoms, and varicella. Until recently, most cases had been reported at autopsy and some still present as sudden death [263, 264, 264a, 264b]. Recognition of the association with tachyarrhythmias has led to electrophysiologic mapping and successful ablation of the lesion [265]. The vacuolated cells in the myocardium and their relationship to conduction tissue have led to an interpretation as myocardial hamartoma [266, 266a] or to names reflecting an unsubstantiated attribution to a lipidosis: cardiac lipidosis, xanthomatous cardiomyopathy, and lipid histiocytosis [267].

Grossly, the enlarged heart has a yellow-white myocardium, no malformations or coronary artery disease, and occasionally mural thrombi, small intramural nodules in or near the valves, and endocardial fibroelastosis.

Microscopically, the myocardium contains focal aggregates of large cells with finely granular, vacuolated cytoplasm containing few or no myofibrils and large numbers of mitochondria (Fig. 20.40) [268]. The foam cells appear at most sites—subendocardial, intramural, subepicardial, and all chambers and valves—but affect the left ventricle, right ventricle, and atria in decreasing incidence, and the conduction bundles in about half the cases [269]. The round or oval cells measure 20 to 40 μm in diameter (about three to eight times the size of the adjacent myocardial fibers), have smooth borders, one or two indented nuclei, and lightly staining eosinophilic cytoplasm. The cells, which resemble foamy or lipid-filled histiocytes, contain a variable amount of glycogen, lipid droplets, and lipofuscin. Similar cells have been identified in other tissues, notably exocrine and endocrine

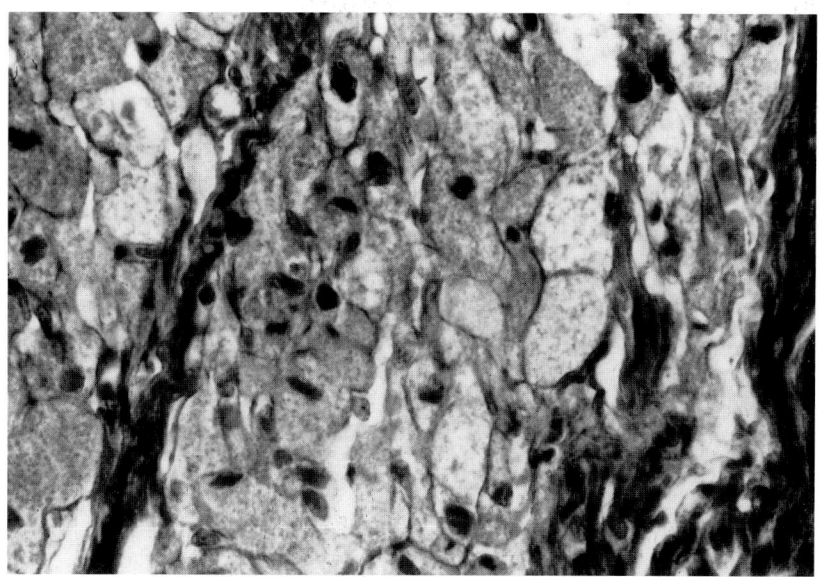

FIGURE 20.40. *The large cells of histiocytoid CMP, several times larger than the adjacent preserved, striated muscle fibers, have a foamy cytoplasm attributed to an increased concentration of mitochondria. (Gomori's trichrome, ×160.)*

cells [270, 271]. The myocardium may contain chronic inflammatory cells not associated with tissue necrosis [267].

Ultrastructurally, the cells have the configuration of abnormal muscle cells with a reduced number of myofibrils, an increased number of mitochondria, but little lipid [269]. The cells have smooth borders without microvilli or peripheral microprojections of macrophages. Although they have desmosomes, they lack the usual interdigitations of adjacent myocardial fibers. The numerous mitochondria that fill the cytoplasm contain a variety of inclusions: stacks of dense cristae, glycogen, and dense bodies resembling lipid. No viral particles have been identified [267, 270]. The name of the disorder has not been resolved, and its nature as a malformation or a metabolic or postinfectious defect remains speculative [269, 270, 272].

Hypertrophic and Other Cardiomyopathies

The 1995 WHO classification of the cardiomyopathies (CMPs) has shifted the definition from a focus on heart muscle diseases of unknown cause to diseases of myocardium associated with cardiac dysfunction with or without a known etiology. By introducing current concepts of etiology and pathogenesis, the new classification focuses on cardiac dysfunction rather than the older focus on unknown etiology. The revised classification preserves the original three types of CMP (Fig. 20.41)—dilated (congestive), hypertrophic, and restrictive (obliterative)—and adds a fourth, arrhythmogenic right ventricular CMP. The distinctions among the types are based on the dominant pathophysiology, the etiology, and the pathogenesis when known [272a].

The morphologic identification of CMPs poses a particular problem in the neonate due to the frequently unanticipated findings in association with clinical presentation of arrhythmia, sudden death, stillbirth, absence of recognized familial pattern, multiple etiologies, and the lack of specific anatomic features. Morphologic features attributed to the CMPs may overlap features of normal development. However, the clinical implications of several CMPs, notably autosomal dominant hypertrophic CMP, require recognition, distinction from normal maturation, and an alert to the genetic potential, since features of CMP have been identified in many genetic disorders—autosomal, recessive, and X-

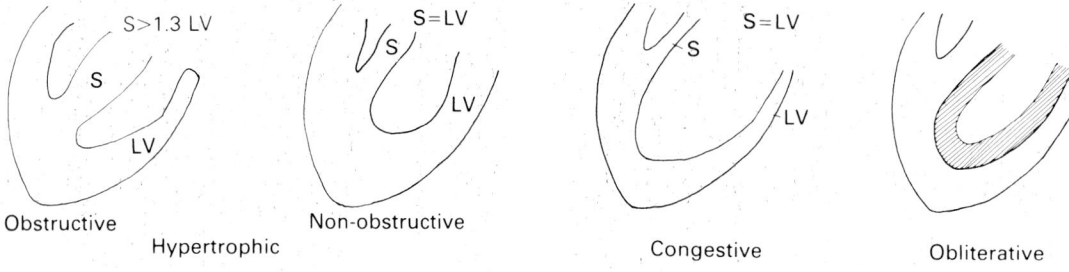

FIGURE 20.41. *Based on morphology, a CMP may be hypertrophic, congestive (dilated), or obliterative (restricted), with hypertrophic cardiomyopathy defined as obstructive on the basis of a septal–left ventricular wall ratio greater than 1.3 and nonobstructive with a ratio of 1.3 or less.*

linked [272b]—including glycogeneses and mitochondrial disorders [272c, 272d, 272e, 272f].

Dilated CMP, which includes toxic, infectious, and familial disorders, is characterized by diminished left ventricular systolic force and ventricular dilatation and hypertrophy without obstruction. Hypertrophic CMP is marked by diminished diastolic filling of the left ventricle, rigidity of the hypertrophic muscle, and thickening of the free wall and ventricular septum of the left ventricle. Hypertrophic CMP, known by many names, has ventricular hypertrophy concentrated in the ventricular septum, transmits genetically with substantial heterogeneity [273], occurs at all ages in both genders, has a propensity for sudden death in older patients [274], and presents clinically with or without obstruction of left ventricular outflow. In obliterative CMP, typified by endomyocardial fibrosis of the tropics [275] and Loeffler's eosinophilic CMP of temperate zones, fibrous tissue obliterates the ventricular cavities, frequently aggravated by intraluminal thrombi [276]. Arrhythmogenic right ventricular CMP has been distinguished from the Uhl anomaly presenting in infancy (see page 617) by the morphology and the age of presentation.

Although hypertrophic CMP had been recognized since the late 1950s under a variety of names, including idiopathic hypertrophic subaortic stenosis (IHSS), muscular subaortic stenosis, and hypertrophic obstructive cardiomyopathy (HOCM), its morphologic features were not characterized until the demonstration of its unique asymmetric septal hypertrophy [277]. The distinctive feature, whether or not it causes obstruction to left ventricular outflow, is a disproportionately thickened ventricular septum, yielding a ratio equal to or greater than 1.3 when comparing the maximum ventricular septal thickness with the thickness of the posterobasal left ventricular wall 3 mm below the mitral valve annulus [278]. Asymmetric septal hypertrophy (ASH) unifies the concept of hypertrophic CMP by identifying both its transmission as an autosomal dominant trait and its potential to remain preclinical and asymptomatic [277].

Obstruction results from narrowing of the left ventricular outflow tract when the anterior leaflet of the mitral valve apposes the hypertrophic ventricular septum. Hypertrophy confined to the septum does not lead to the obstruction associated with more extensive myocardial disease [277]. Most patients with ASH do not have left ventricular obstruction [279]. With obstruction, the hypertrophied free wall resembles the results of aortic valvular obstruction. Without obstruction, the free wall behind the posterior leaflet of the mitral valve remains normal or thin. The abnormality leading to obstruction has been attributed to disease localized in the septum, contrasting with the diffuse involvement without obstruction [279, 280].

Hypertrophic CMP in the first year of life is more likely to present with congestive heart failure than the sudden death of later life. The septal hypertrophy obstructs the left ventricle in infancy, but, unlike its effect in later life, it may also obstruct the right ventricle, clinically simulating pulmonary valve obstruction. Symptoms referable to hypertrophic CMP have been identified as early as 1 day of life. Morphologically, the same septal–free wall hypertrophy holds, with ratios greater than 1.3 [281].

Histologically, the myocardial cells exhibit several abnormalities that are more prevalent in the septum than in the left ventricular free wall: intracellular disarray of myofibrils and myofilaments, disorganized cellular arrangement with abnormal cell contacts, and enlarged, bizarrely shaped muscle cells [282]. Landing et al [272b] identified a distinctive bandlike pattern of myocardial fiber hypertrophy (differential myocardial fiber bundle hypertrophy) in an autopsy series of children, many of whom died suddenly, raising the question of an unsuspected hypertrophic CMP. Others have challenged the specificity, reliability, and pertinence of the difference in distribution of abnormal cells in distinguishing nonobstructive from obstructive CMP, since obstruction may develop in patients who were initially unobstructed [283, 284].

Since a developing heart may have a disproportionately thickened septum with a septal–free wall ratio approaching 1 in the first weeks of life, and perhaps persisting as long as 2 years, Maron and colleagues [281, 285] suggest several criteria for identifying ASH in infants:

1. A thickened septum in absolute terms, 8 to 30 mm thick with hypertrophic CMP
2. No associated heart lesion or other disease—e.g., insulin-dependent maternal diabetes, capable of producing septal thickening
3. Prominent histologic disorganization in the septum
4. Genetic transmission in first-degree relative

Infants with ASH and an affected first-degree relative died as a consequence of the disease in the first 5 months of life. The liveborns had heart failure, and each had septal thickening and the disorderly arrangement of hypertrophied muscle cells. In those with outflow obstruction, the septum had more prominent disarray than the free wall; those without obstruction had more diffuse disarray [278, 281].

Transient ASH has been demonstrated on ultrasound examination in neonates receiving steroids, with or without insulin therapy [285a], for respiratory disease, usually with resolution after cessation of therapy [285b, 285c]. Although hypertrophic CMP was considered to have contributed to the mortality in several cases [285d], postmortem examination often failed to confirm residual hypertrophy.

Endocardial Fibroelastosis

A thickened sclerotic endocardium due to deposition of collagen and elastic fibers usually accompanies other cardiac disease as a secondary change, but it may also affect the left ventricle in the absence of an obvious associated lesion [286]. The variable association with other diseases provides a pathogenetic classification of endocardial fibroelastosis (EFE)—primary and secondary—and the size of the left ventricular chamber affected by EFE provides a morphologic classification—dilated or constricted. The pathogenetic and morphologic classifications are usually in accord, since the constricted form of EFE accompanies a hypoplastic left ventricle or semilunar valvular stenosis and the dilated form of EFE accompanies myocardial disease of known (secondary) or unknown (primary) nature. Although thickening and sclerosis of the endocardium may occur at any age due to myocardial anoxia or hypoperfusion, the fibroelastic reaction of EFE seems to have a characteristic confinement to fetal and early infantile life, suggesting a relationship to growth and development [287].

A heart with constrictive EFE has a diminutive but normal mitral valve; short, thick chordae; a normal, sometimes bicuspid aortic valve; and a small ascending aorta (Fig. 20.42). The thickened endocardium extends as perivascular fibrosis about the intramyocardial vessels accompanied by myocardial infarcts with fibrosis and calcification. Whereas the dilated form of EFE has been considered a dilated form of CMP, the constricted form without valvular atresia may represent an intrauterine cardioendomyopathy with the EFE

resulting secondarily in the hypoplasia and underdevelopment of the ascending aorta [288]. Progression, verified by echocardiography, from a dilated left ventricle in a fetus at 20 weeks' gestation to a constricted left ventricle at 40 weeks suggests a close relationship between the two forms of EFE [289].

EFE accompanies ventricular outflow obstruction such as atresia or severe stenosis of the aortic or pulmonary valves, but only with a patent AV valve. EFE does not occur when AV valve atresia accompanies semilunar valvular atresia or stenosis. Other than semilunar valve abnormalities, including an estimated 18% incidence of bicuspid aortic valve, congenital malformations are uncommon in patients with EFE [287]. The most common associated malformation—coarctation, sometimes with a bicuspid aortic valve—affects fewer than 10% of cases, but the cause and effect of the coarctation and the EFE remain obscure and unsettled. Other disorders presumed responsible for the development of EFE are premature closure of the foramen ovale, anomalous origin of the left coronary artery from the pulmonary artery, medial calcification and intimal proliferation of the coronary arteries, and myocarditis.

Clinical

Primary EFE may occur sporadically or as part of syndromes with the genetic implications relating to the underlying disorder. In a population-based study, CMPs without cardiovascular structural abnormalities were identified in 1 in 10,000 live births, of which EFE made up less than 10% [290]. Although the primary form of EFE carries a mortality rate of up to 75% during the first year of life and usually produces symptoms prior to 6 months of age, symptoms are rare in the perinatal period. Uncommonly, older infants may have a prolonged course; more commonly, both the onset and course are acute and short.

Morphology

EFE predominantly affects the mural endocardium of the left ventricle, with infrequent involvement of the mitral valve. The globular heart has a rounded apex, increased size and weight, dilated left ventricle, uncommonly a dilated left atrium, and myocardial hypertrophy. The diffusely thickened, gray-to-white, opaque, sclerotic endocardium affects the ventricular septum somewhat more than the parietal wall (Fig. 20.43). The thickened endocardium accentuates the trabeculae, forming deep, narrow intertrabecular clefts. Occasionally, papillary muscles may exhibit necrosis, fibrosis, and calcification. Occasionally, a left ventricular mural thrombus may serve as the source of systemic emboli. The coronary arteries in the epicardium are characteristically normal. The right ventricle may have a patchy distribution of sclerotic endocardium, but it lacks the diffuse involvement of the left ventricle.

A deposition of collagen and elastic fibers thickens the endocardium, with the greatest concentration of elastic fibers adjacent to the myocardium. As the sclerotic endo-

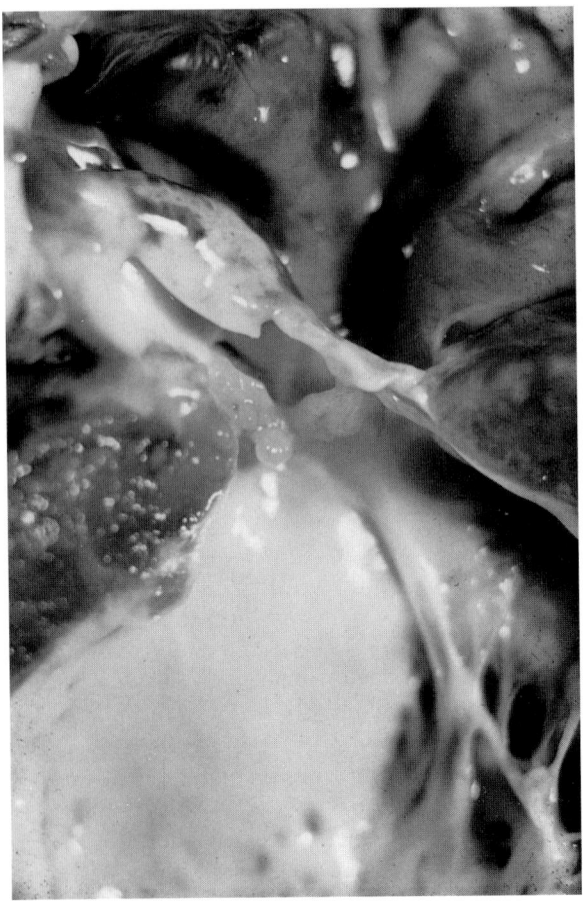

FIGURE 20.42. *Left ventricular EFE accompanies a bicuspid, sclerotic aortic valve.*

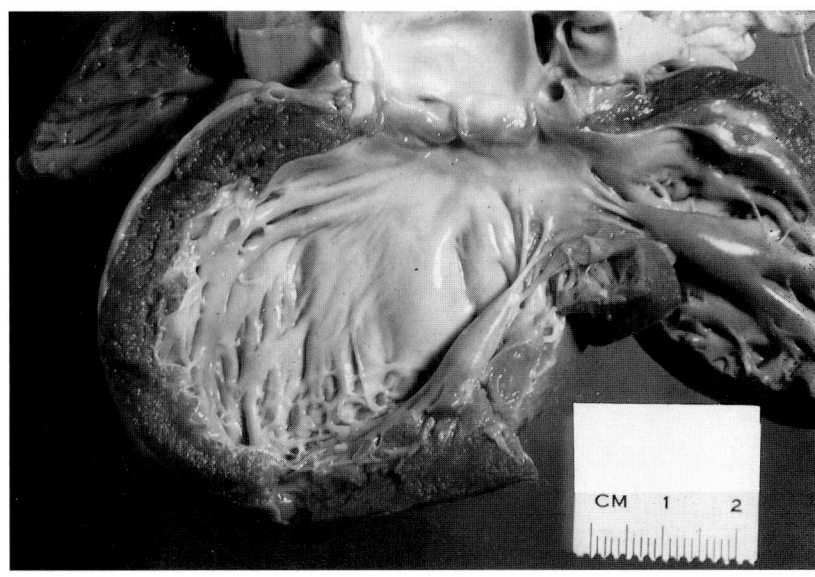

FIGURE 20.43. *The thickened, opaque, sclerotic endocardium of EFE affects the septum to a greater degree than the free wall of the left ventricle and forms deep clefts in the myocardium by surrounding the individual trabeculae.*

cardium extends into the underlying myocardium, it surrounds and isolates groups of myocardial fibers. The subendocardial myocardial cells have a swollen, vacuolated cytoplasm that contains a modest increase in glycogen. Ultrastructurally, the vacuoles are of two types: paranuclear vacuoles with membrane-bound granular material; and vacuoles that contain degenerated mitochondria, membranous whorls, and lysosomes [291].

Etiology and Pathogenesis

EFE has been attributed to anoxia, infection, metabolic disease, lymphatic obstruction, a nonspecific response to intramyocardial tension, and genetic mechanisms in the rare familial forms [288]. Black-Schaffer proposed that the tensions imposed on the endocardium of the dilated heart initiate both the dilated and constricted forms of EFE [292]. The concept of EFE as a nonspecific response to myocardial stress receives support from its identification in infants with both immune and nonimmune fetal hydrops [293], hereditary myopathies [294, 295], mucopolysaccharidosis [296], familial carnitine deficiency [297, 297a], and following myocarditis [298].

Of the suggested etiologies, a possible relationship to fetal infection remains unverified. Although infection has not been confirmed by culture, intranuclear viral particles have been related to coxsackievirus [291]. In myocarditis, virus has been localized by polymerase chain reaction and in situ hybridization [299, 299a].

Infants of Diabetic Mothers

An infant of a diabetic mother (IDM) has an increased susceptibility to congenital cardiovascular malformations and at least two forms of CMP, one dilated and congested and the other hypertrophic with or without left ventricular outflow obstruction [300].

Congenital malformations of the heart affect IDMs four to five times more frequently than the general population, with reported incidences of 1.7–4.0% clinically and, since the malformations are frequently lethal, as high as 20% when assessed in autopsy series [301–303]. The malformations in IDMs are notable for their variety, affecting the atrial and ventricular septa, the great arteries, the coronary arteries, and each valve with no particular malformation predominating, although VSD and TGA occur slightly more frequently than other defects [301, 303].

The increased heart weight among IDMs of two to three times the expected weight has been attributed to the generalized visceromegaly of IDMs, since it does not relate to malformations, hepatomegaly, edema as a sign of failure, or increased erythropoiesis [301, 303]. An increased mass of myocardial nuclei and sarcoplasm led Naeye to attribute the increased heart size to a combination of hypertrophy and hyperplasia [304].

About 50% of all IDMs have cardiomegaly clinically [300], but only a few have symptoms relating to defective left ventricular function, resembling the obstructive form of hypertrophic CMP [305]. The symptomatic infants develop a transient congestive heart failure and left ventricular outflow obstruction with resolution of the myocardial hypertrophy after a few months [306–308]. Although the ventricular walls are increased in thickness, the septum undergoes the most pronounced thickening, again resembling the asymmetric septal hypertrophy of hypertrophic CMP (Fig. 20.44) but with a lesser degree of myocardial fiber disarray [309]. Wolfe and Way [300] identify a second type of cardiomyopathy in IDMs consisting of ventricular dilatation attributed to a respiratory, metabolic, or hematologic basis with resolution within 72 hours of birth. In appropriately sized IDMs the cardiomegaly due to ventricular dilatation resolves promptly with control of hypoglycemia and acidosis [310].

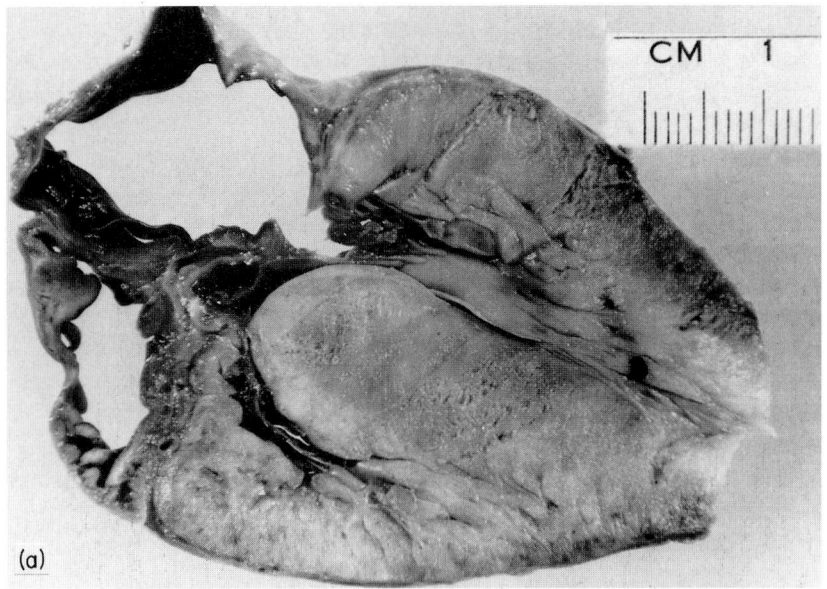

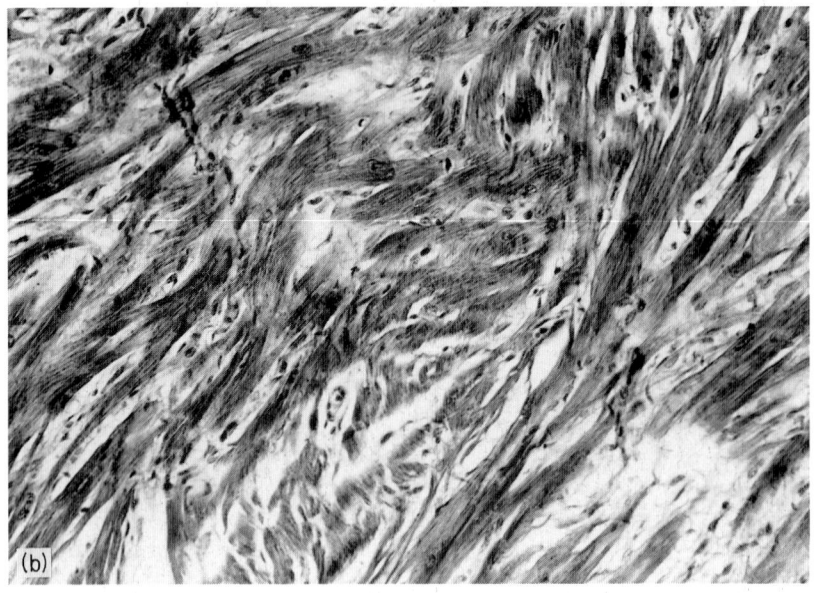

FIGURE 20.44. *(a) The heart of an infant of a diabetic mother who died of sepsis had asymmetric septal hypertrophy and (b) foci of irregular and disorderly muscle fibers in the septum. (H&E, ×100.) (Reproduced with permission from: Gutgesell HP, Speer ME, Rosenberg HS. Characterization of the cardiomyopathy in infants of diabetic mothers. Circulation 1980; 61:441–50.)*

Pompe Disease

Type II glycogenosis (Pompe disease) is unusual among metabolic diseases in affecting the neonatal heart. This disease results from a deficiency of lysosomal alpha-glucosidase (acid maltase), with a consequent accumulation of glycogen in lysosomes. Diagnosis is based on both the biochemical demonstration of the enzyme deficiency and the ultrastructural feature of lysosomal storage of glycogen [311–314]. The disorder is usually inherited as an autosomal recessive trait, and occasionally as a mutation [314a]. Clinically heterogeneous, Pompe disease has both early- and late-onset phenotypes, sometimes in the same family [314b, 314c]. The outcome relates to the age at onset and the tissue involvement, ranging from an infantile onset with rapid pro-

gression and early death to an adult onset with slow progression to myopathy and respiratory insufficiency [314d]. During infancy, the affected infant acquires the distinctive clinical syndrome of heart failure, intermittent cyanosis, neuromuscular weakness, and impaired respiratory function, usually leading to death before 2 years of age. Both bradycardia and supraventricular tachycardia, described in the neonate [315, 316], are attributed to glycogen storage in cells of the conduction system.

Grossly, the globular, enlarged heart has a firm, waxy, pale myocardium and is four to five times the expected weight (Fig. 20.45). Hypertrophy affects both ventricles, most prominently the left, and the atria to a lesser degree. The myocardial hypertrophy may lead to obstruction of the left ventricular outflow as with IDM or genetic hypertrophic

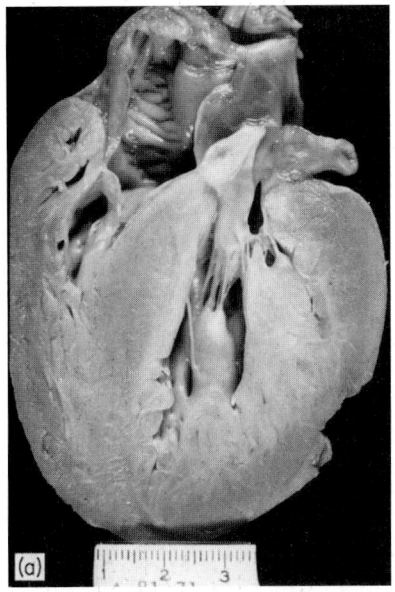

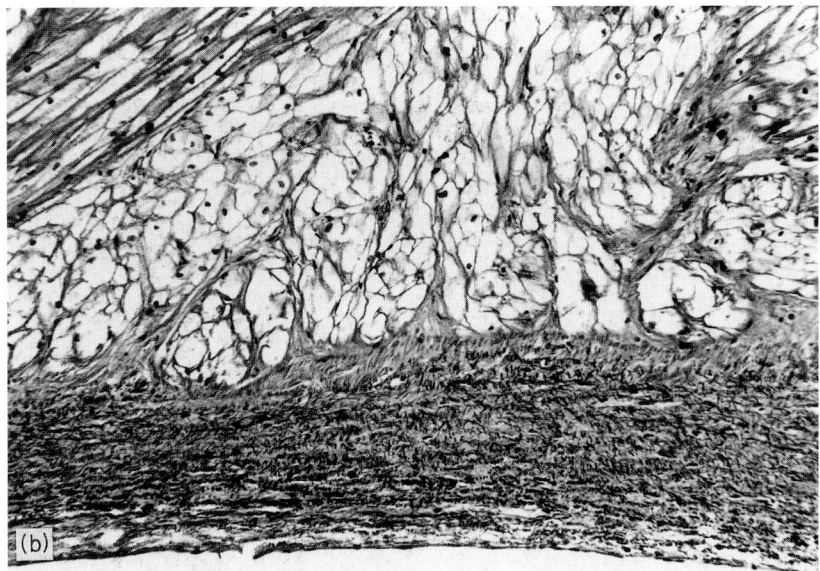

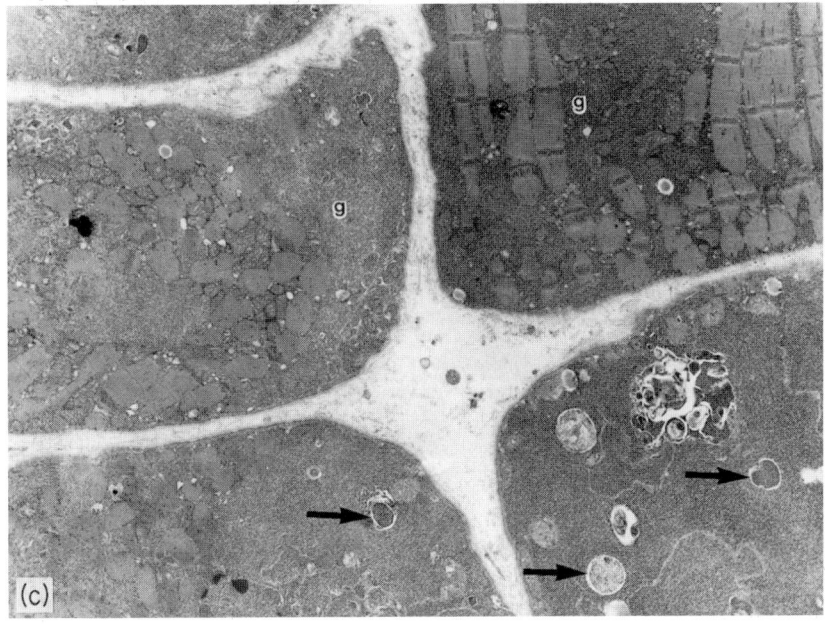

FIGURE 20.45. *(a) The myocardial hypertrophy of Pompe disease affects both ventricles but more prominently the left ventricle. (b) Clear, glycogen-filled cytoplasm surrounds the centrally placed nuclei of the myocardial fibers. The thickened, sclerotic endocardium results from the deposition of fibrous and elastic connective tissue (Verhoeff–van Gieson, ×40). (c) Ultrastructurally, the muscle fibers are separated by abundant, free, cytoplasmic glycogen (g) plus the characteristic intralysosomal glycogen (arrows) of Pompe disease. (The electron microscopic illustration of skeletal muscle graciously provided by Dr. George Hug, Department of Enzymology, Children's Hospital Medical Center, Cincinnati, Ohio.)*

CMP [317]. Although the infant may remain asymptomatic for several months of life, the cardiomegaly may appear during the first week of life. About 20% of affected infants have EFE in the left ventricle interpreted as secondary to the prolonged ventricular dilatation and myocardial weakness from the glycogen deposition and myofibrillar disruption. The enzyme deficiency is in all tissues. Despite the variation in clinical expression, the morphologic findings are fairly uniform.

Histologically, the enlarged, centrally vacuolated myocardial fibers form a distinctive lacework pattern. A sleeve of glycogen surrounds the centrally placed, glycogen-free nuclei, forming a hollow cylinder surrounded by a thin cap of peripherally placed cytoplasm containing the myofibrils.

Glycogen may be stored in the smooth muscle of the coronary arteries. Skeletal muscle, from which biopsy may be used diagnostically, shows vacuolation of most fibers. The muscle fibers contain numerous PAS-positive droplets, some of which resist digestion by pretreatment with malt diastase, perhaps representing the nonglycogen polysaccharides that have been identified in Pompe disease [318, 319]. Identification of intralysosomal glycogen by electron microscopy remains the morphologic hallmark of Pompe disease. In addition to the characteristic glycogen in membrane-bound vesicles, cells may have an increased amount of lipid and metachromatic stored material that does not stain with Alcian blue, variously interpreted as mucopolysaccharide, glycolipid, or glycoprotein [320].

INFLAMMATIONS

Myocarditis

Of the many infectious and toxic agents that may cause myocarditis, a few affect infants—notably coxsackie B virus, *Toxoplasma gondii*, rubella virus, and *Treponema pallidum*; less frequently other viruses such as herpes simplex virus, cytomegalovirus [320a], mumps, adenovirus [321], and parvovirus [322, 323]; and sometimes maternal lupus erythematosus [324] as well as bacteria and Candida accompanying generalized sepsis [325]. Since most myocarditis has no distinctive morphology, establishing the etiology requires identification of the agent. Failure to identify an organism is not uncommon in patients with myocarditis, nor does such failure exclude infection as the cause [326]. A virus is rarely cultured from an infected heart after the second week of infection [327], but a virus may be identified in myocardium by polymerase chain reaction (PCR) and in situ hybridization long after the acute phase has ended [328, 329, 329a, 329b].

Coxsackie B Virus

Serotypes of coxsackie B virus are the principal pathogens for myocarditis in infancy, with a peak incidence during the first month of life [330]. The prevalence of myocarditis in the first weeks of life, its epidemic nature, and its relation to systemic disease including hepatitis and meningoencephalitis had been recognized long before the association with coxsackievirus was established [331]. Clinical diagnosis has been established by classic viral isolation, by PCR, and by identification of coxsackie B-specific immunoglobulin M (IgM) antibodies [332, 332a, 332b]. Congestive heart failure, which usually occurs in the first 10 days of the illness, accompanies most fatal myocarditis.

Morphologically, the pericardial sac contains excess fluid, and petechiae cover the epicardium. The dilated and slightly enlarged heart has flabby, thickened muscle with pale brown and yellow mottling [333]. Mural thrombi may adhere to the endocardium over sites of necrotic myocardium [331]. Histologically, there is no distinction between the myocarditis due to coxsackievirus and that due to other viruses [334]. The myocardium exhibits patchy degeneration, focal necrosis, and a pleomorphic inflammatory cell infiltrate consisting of polymorphonuclears, lymphocytes, eosinophils, macrophages, and plasma cells. Dystrophic calcification in the myocardium has been identified as a poor prognostic sign [334a]. The muscle cells lose their striations, swell, and become eosinophilic. Interstitial edema and inflammation may extend to the endocardium.

Ultrastructural changes in myocardial cells vary from mild to severe. Necrosis and cytolysis appear within 24 hours of infection and tend to have a patchy distribution. The mitochondria swell and accumulate fluid between the cristae. Virus appears as crystalline particles. Sarcoplasmic reticulum dilates and large vesicles develop. The Z bands are the first to change, followed by alteration of the sarcomere [335].

Toxoplasmosis

Even when the CNS involvement dominates both the clinical and morphologic patterns, *Toxoplasma gondii* frequently involves the myocardium, potentially leading to congestive heart failure. In a widespread distribution, small vascular channels have thrombi, necrotic walls, and organisms in the lumina, endothelium, muscular wall, or perivascular tissues [336]. Grossly, the dilated, flabby heart exhibits interstitial hemorrhage in an appearance that differs from diffuse myocarditis only by small yellow necrotic foci.

Microscopically, all areas of the heart may have an interstitial inflammatory cell infiltrate of lymphocytes, plasma cells, eosinophils, and macrophages that may aggregate into granulomas. Necrotic, hyalinized, and fragmented myocardial fibers are separated by edema and the inflammatory cell infiltrate. With regeneration, myocardial cells have an increased number of nuclei and occasional mitoses.

Free or intracellular organisms appear at the edges of necrotic foci but not usually at inflammatory sites; encysted parasites occupy myocardial fibers, uncommonly lying free in the interstitium [336]. Parasitic cysts in the myocardial cells are accompanied by alterations in the cells. Parasites occur in large aggregates within muscle cells or in cysts, usually peripheral to the sites of inflammation. Single parasites occur in the centers of small areas of necrosis and at the peripheries of large areas. Inflammation probably comes from rupture of the muscle cells rather than as a response to the parasite.

Syphilis

In congenital syphilis, an inflammatory cell infiltrate extends from the epicardium into the underlying myocardium. The myocarditis has no characterizing pattern: interstitial inflammation or fibrosis extends in a perivascular distribution around coronary arteries or arterioles with atrophic muscle fibers from compression by the inflammatory cell infiltrate [337].

Rubella

Cardiovascular and systemic abnormalities in congenital rubella fall into three categories: transient, permanent, and delayed [338]. Each category has cardiovascular effects. Myocarditis is transient. Several forms of CHD, such as patent ductus arteriosus and pulmonary artery branch stenosis, are permanent. Various vascular diseases appear as delayed responses [339].

The incidence of CHD with transplacental rubella varies from 30 to 90%. The most common cardiovascular lesion due to rubella is ductus arteriosus, followed closely in frequency by pulmonary artery branch stenosis, systemic arterial sclerosis, and myocarditis [340–342]. The ductus has a thin media with abundant collagen, very little elastic tissue, and an attenuated internal elastic lamina [343]. Less common lesions include ASD, VSD, t/F, supravalvular aortic stenosis, retroesophageal right subclavian artery, multivalvular sclerosis, coarctation, truncus, TGA, anomalous venous return, and tricuspid valvular atresia [339]. Myocardial necrosis and degeneration with or without inflammation may affect stillborns and newborns, but without distinguishing morphologic features [344]. Arterial hypoplasia and fibromuscular intimal proliferation affect systemic and pulmonary arteries [345]. The aorta may have intimal sclerosis consisting of a proliferation of loose fibrous connective tissue in a mucopolysaccharide stroma as well as vacuolation, fragmentation, and diminution of elastic fibers in the media.

Pericarditis

Pericarditis, which infrequently affects the neonate, usually results from extension of infection from an extrapericardial focus, the myocardium or the mediastinum, or an infected catheter [346]. Pericarditis may complicate neonatal sepsis [347], but more often it accompanies pneumonia or follows direct extension or hematogenous spread [348]. Occasionally, purulent pericarditis may appear in a neonate or a stillborn, presumably the result of intrauterine infection [349]. Of the several bacteria that may cause pericarditis, *Staphylococcus aureus* is the most common [349a], but other organisms that have caused pericarditis include *Streptococcus pneumoniae* and other species, *Haemophilus influenzae*, *Neisseria meningitidis*, several gram-negative bacilli, and cytomegalovirus [349b]. The poor survival rate of prior years has been greatly improved by the combination of antibiotic therapy and surgical drainage [349c]. Even less frequent forms of epicarditis accompany maternal lupus [350], malformation complexes [351], and an enigmatic granulomatous epicarditis localized to the base of the heart near the origin of the great arteries [352].

Endocarditis

The rarity of infective endocarditis in the infant, and particularly in the neonate, has changed in the years associated with successful maintenance of the severely stressed neonate [353]. Although the precise mechanisms remain unclear, the incidence of severely hypoxic neonates with fibrinous, sometimes infected endocardial vegetations appears to be increasing. Endocarditis in the neonate takes several forms, which may have some common pathogenetic factors. The infant may have one of at least three types of valvular vegetations: the infective endocarditis usually associated with abnormal valves, the nonbacterial platelet–fibrin vegetation of nonbacterial endocarditis (NBE), and an infected fibrin vegetation that may represent a complication of NBE.

Infective Endocarditis

The main risk factors for infective endocarditis in the neonate are central venous catheters and congenital heart malformations, including PDA [354, 355, 356, 356a]. The endocardial infection is usually associated with skin or umbilical infections, necrotizing enterocolitis [356b],

osteomyelitis, meningitis, pneumonia, and peritonitis. A variety of organisms cause the few cases: most often *Staphylococcus aureus* and *Candida* sp. [356a, 357]; less often group B hemolytic streptococcus [358, 359], *Streptococcus pneumoniae*, *Neisseria gonorrhoeae*, and *Pseudomonas aeruginosa*. All valves, but more frequently the AV valves, may be affected. Several infants have been successfully managed by surgical replacement of the affected valve [360, 361, 361a].

Microscopically, the vegetations of infective endocarditis differ from NBE vegetations by the appearance of polymorphonuclear leukocytes and the organisms mixed with the fibrin and platelets, usually on the mural surface. Granulation tissue appears at the bases of the infected vegetations, again unlike the vegetations of NBE.

In contrast to the predisposition of the older infant or child with a preexisting rheumatic or congenitally malformed valve to endocarditis [362], most infants with infective or nonbacterial endocarditis have structurally normal hearts. Despite the rarity of infective endocarditis in the neonate, indwelling catheters and parenteral alimentation play a role in candidal endocarditis [363], and CHD in the presence of bacteremia seems to predispose to endocarditis, particularly in the older infant, but in the neonate as well [354, 363a].

Nonbacterial Endocarditis

Nonbacterial or aseptic vegetations affect the heart valves of newborns, usually those of greater than 34 weeks' gestation [364]. Although no infant is immune from the development of NBE, most have some disorder causing hypoxia [365, 366]. CHD provides no predisposition to the development of NBE. The maternal phospholipid antibody syndrome with recurrent pregnancy loss, thrombocytopenia, and venous or arterial thrombi may be associated with fetal vascular thrombi, although not with NBE [366a].

Affected infants may have a syndrome of NBE, thromboemboli, thrombocytopenia, and persistent pulmonary hypertension [364, 367]. The relation between the components of the syndrome represents either individual disorders common to the severely stressed, hypoxic infant or a link between the hypoxia and altered hemodynamics and the activation of vasoactive and platelet aggregation factors [368]. A common factor triggering the platelet aggregates and the pulmonary vasoconstriction has been proposed [364]. Potential pathogenetic mechanisms include fibrin deposition consequent to disseminated intravascular coagulation initiated by hypoxia, and direct trauma from umbilical vein catheters [355, 369]. Although 80% of neonates with endocarditis studied by Symchych et al had disseminated intravascular coagulation, so did 55% of infants who had intracardiac catheters but no vegetations—not a statistically significant difference [369]. With sepsis, bacteria may seed the thrombi, initiating microabscesses on the valve leaflets without antecedent NBE [355, 370]. Both infective and nonbacterial endocarditis relate to umbilical venous and central venous catheters [366].

The vegetations, which measure from 0.1 to more than 1.0 cm, attach to the atrial surfaces of the AV valves at the line of closure—usually the tricuspid valve, less often the mitral valve, but sometimes both—and to the right side of the atrial septum adjacent to the fossa ovalis [370]. The right ventricular and left atrial endocardium occasionally have NBE, but the left ventricle and pulmonary and aortic valve leaflets are spared (Fig. 20.46) [369, 370].

The vegetations, which are distinct from and unrelated to the common blood cysts, comprise thrombi adherent to the valve leaflet, usually at a site where the endothelium has been denuded. The vegetation contains a varying mixture of fibrin and platelets with only few trapped red and white blood cells. With the variation in composition, some vegetations may be almost exclusively either platelet aggregates or fibrin. With organization, older lesions may have an endothelial covering [370]. By definition, bacterial cultures and stains are uniformly negative. Pulmonary and systemic thromboemboli, sometimes with infarcts, are frequent with NBE. The emboli have the same histologic structure as the vegetations [364, 371].

CARDIAC TUMORS

Incidence

Several types of cardiac tumors are peculiar to children, and others may occur at any age, including childhood. Most are benign and intracavitary, have little tendency for growth, produce symptoms from obstruction or compression, and are often amenable to surgical excision [372, 372a]. Rhabdomyoma, teratoma, and fibromatosis made up almost 90% of cardiac tumors in infants during the first year of life, not necessarily confined to the perinatal period, at the Armed Forces Institute of Pathology (AFIP), with isolated cases of myocardial hemangioma, mesothelioma of the AV node, rhabdomyosarcoma, and fibrosarcoma [373].

Uncommon Types: Myxoma, Mesothelioma, and Hemangioma

Myxoma, the most common heart tumor of the adult, rarely affects children [374, 374a]. Hemangioma and hemangiopericytoma may occupy the epicardium, where they may

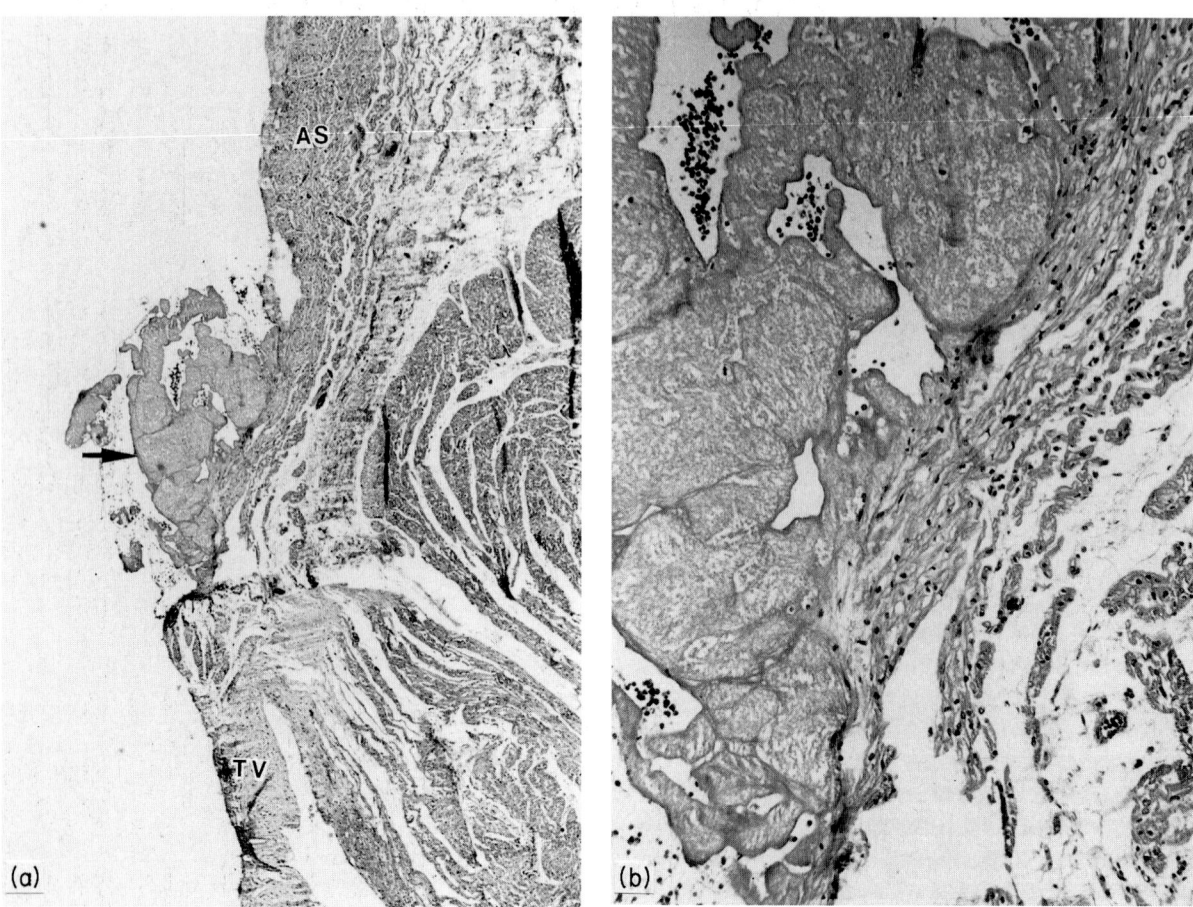

FIGURE 20.46.   (a) A fibrinous vegetation (arrow) adheres to the surface of the tricuspid valve (TV) and adjacent endocardium of the atrial septum (AS) (H&E, ×25). (b) The vegetation consists of fibrin with only a few trapped peripheral blood cells but no inflammatory cells (H&E, ×40).

bleed, resulting in hemorrhage and tamponade, or may occupy the atrial myocardium, where they may protrude into and obstruct the chamber and cause congestive heart failure [375, 375a, 375b].

Mesothelioma of the heart exclusively occupies the AV node, occurs only rarely in infancy, and expresses clinically as complete or partial heart block. The poorly circumscribed tumor produces a slight elevation in the atrial septum and consists of mesothelial cell nests forming small cystic spaces resembling those in the similar tumors of the testis and ovary. The polygonal, alcianophilic cells lining the cysts may be interrupted by squamous metaplasia [376].

Rhabdomyoma

Clinical Patterns

Rhabdomyoma presents predominantly in infants and children, with frequent identification by echocardiography in the fetus, neonate, and infant [377]. The functional effects of rhabdomyoma include cardiomegaly, conduction defects, congestive heart failure, fetal hydrops, and chamber obstruction. Each of several potential clinical effects of rhabdomyoma relating to the anatomic site of the tumor may affect the neonate. A clinical pattern that affects only the neonate results in either fetal hydrops and death or early fatality due to a conduction disturbance or an intracavitary tumor obstructing blood flow through the heart and resulting in congestive heart failure [378–380].

An estimated 50–85% of cardiac rhabdomyomas are associated with the tuberous sclerosis complex, although, since the tumor often precedes the cutaneous and neurologic findings, tuberous sclerosis may be difficult to establish in the neonate [381, 382, 382a]. Rhabdomyoma serves as a secondary feature in the diagnosis of the tuberous sclerosis complex, requiring other criteria to establish the diagnosis [382b]. Since most cardiac rhabdomyomas show some degree of regression over time, usually by age 6 years, surgical intervention has been reserved for those with refractory dysrhythmias or severe hemodynamic compromise [383, 384, 384a, 384b].

Morphology

Most cardiac rhabdomyomas are multiple, are white to yellow-tan, are circumscribed but unencapsulated, and vary from less than 1 mm to several centimeters in diameter. They may arise anywhere in the atrial or ventricular myocardium, usually the ventricle, but not from a valve, and many project into a cardiac chamber. Occasionally the tumor cells diffusely infiltrate the myocardium without forming a distinct tumor nodule [385].

Microscopically, the individual cells may be quite large, measuring up to 80 μm in diameter (Fig. 20.47). The characteristic spider cell has a peripheral cytoplasm filled with glycogen or eccentrically oriented strands traversing the cell. Extramedullary hematopoiesis may accompany the tumor.

Ultrastructurally, cellular junctions resemble intercalated discs, but arranged about the periphery of the cell—unlike normal myocardium, which has intercalated discs at the cellular poles [386]. The large, round, or polygonal tumor cells contain abundant monoparticulate glycogen. Few myofibrils, sometimes with Z-band masses, lie beneath the plasma membrane or radiate to the central area [387].

Morphogenesis

Rhabdomyoma has been considered a tumor of Purkinje's cells, a tumor of nonspecialized myocardium, and a localized form of glycogen storage disease, but with the resemblance of the tumor cells to ovoid cardiac myoblasts with peripheral intercalated discs, rhabdomyoma conforms to a hamartoma derived from embryonal myoblasts [388].

Teratoma

A teratoma of the heart usually occupies the pericardium, remains extracardiac, and produces ill effects by pericardial effusion or by compressing the heart or the airways [389]. Although uncommon, most cardiac teratomas affect infants or children, and sometimes the fetus or neonate [390, 390a]. Intrapericardiac teratomas typically arise at the base of the heart from the root of the pulmonary artery and aorta. They share the features of teratomas at other sites with cysts lined by a variety of epithelium, solid areas containing neural tissue, a variety of acinar and glandular elements, and a malignant potential, notably yolk sac tumor [390b].

Fibroma

Morphology

Fibromas are usually solitary; may become quite large, exceeding 10 cm in diameter; and occupy the anterior and lateral walls of the left ventricle, less often the septum, and rarely the right ventricular or the posterior wall of the left ventricle (Fig. 20.48) [391, 391a]. Because of their localization, myocardial fibromas may be successfully excised.

Histologically cardiac fibromas have the same localized but unencapsulated configuration as fibromatoses at other soft tissue and visceral sites. Peripherally, the fibrous tissue interdigitates with the myocardium; centrally, it may hyalinize and calcify. Component cells have the ultrastructure of myofibroblasts with pinocytotic vesicles, myofibrils, and portions of basement membrane [391, 392].

Functional Effects

Fibromatoses may affect the heart at any age, but they are the second most common tumor of the heart in children [393]. They may be associated with arrhythmias and heart block. Some occur in the first 3 months of life, but they are exceedingly rare in the perinatal period. Depending on the location, cardiac fibroma may cause failure, obstruct flow, or interrupt electrical conductivity and cause sudden death [394–396]. They are infrequently associated with congenital

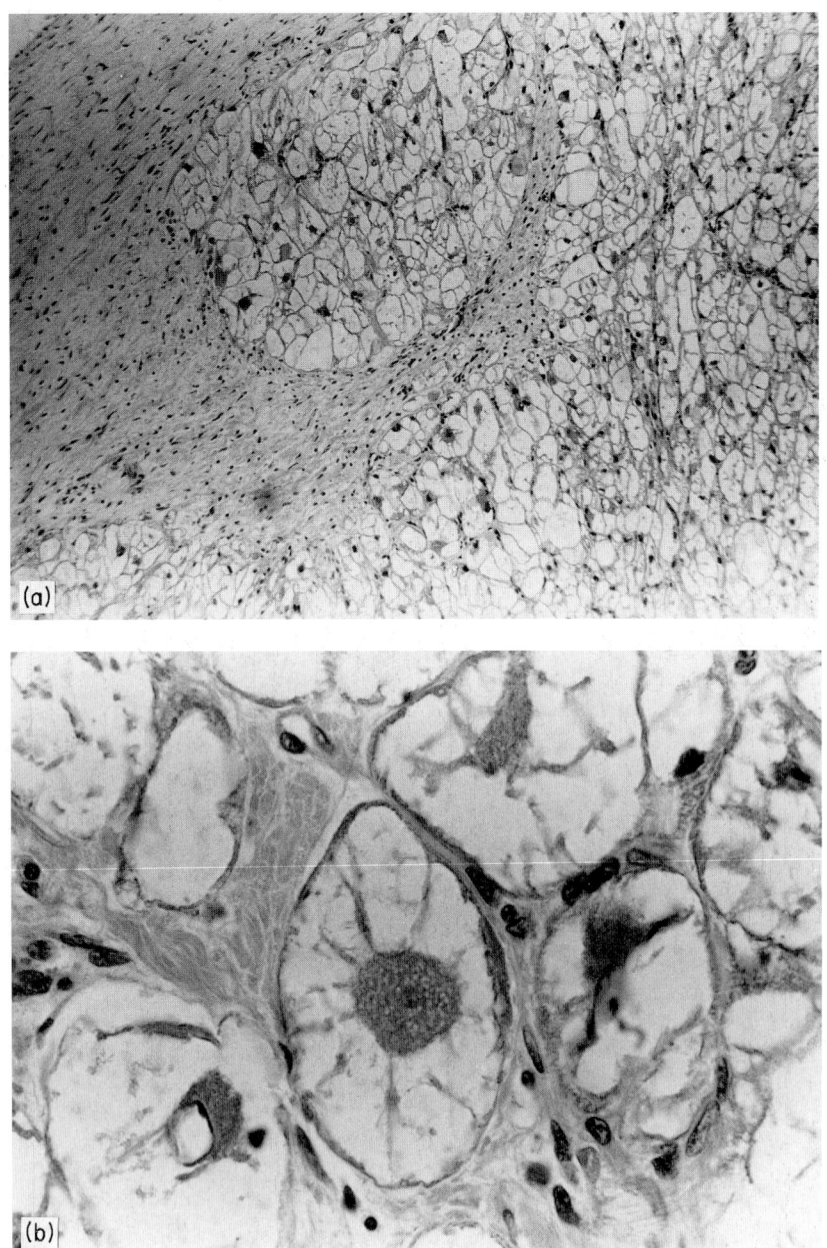

(a)

(b)

FIGURE 20.47. *(a) The rhabdomyoma lies in poorly demarcated clusters surrounded and separated by thin strands of connective tissue and cardiac muscle (H&E, ×40). (b) Thin strands of cytoplasm traversing the cell from the nucleus to the periphery form the characteristic spider cell of a cardiac rhabdomyoma (H&E, ×100).*

heart malformations. Multiple fibromas may occupy the myocardium in the form of congenital generalized fibromatosis with a visceral distribution pattern [391]. The cardiac fibromas with congenital generalized fibromatosis may be distinct by their appearance in the atrial myocardium, in contrast to localized fibromatosis, which predominates in the ventricle [397].

Blood Cysts

Blood cysts, arbitrarily included among cardiac tumors, occur on the valvular endocardium of newborn infants as small endothelium-lined cysts affecting more than one-half of stillborns, newborns, and infants from 6 months' gesta-

tion to 1 year as judged from autopsy data (Fig. 20.49) [398]. The cysts are usually multiple, may occur in clusters, and measure less than 1 mm in diameter. Most are on the atrial surfaces of the AV valve leaflets, and much less commonly on the ventricular surfaces, of the semilunar valve cusps. Histologically, the endothelium-lined cysts initially contain liquid blood without hemorrhage or inflammation, and eventually disappear with growth of the cusp and obliteration of the invagination. Pathogenetically, the cysts are variously interpreted as the result of dilatation of normal invaginations of the valve cusps [398], pressure gradient across the valve cusp causing a bulge and forming a cyst [399], and communication with the microcirculation of the valve cusp [400]. Despite their frequency and usual lack of

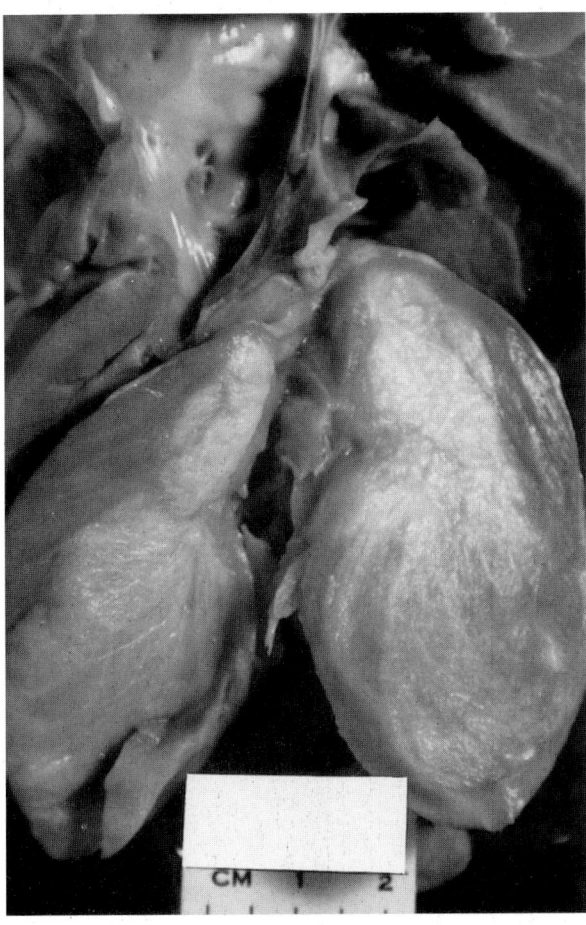

FIGURE 20.48. *A localized but poorly circumscribed fibromatosis occupies the free wall of the left ventricle. (Reproduced with permission from: Rosenberg HS, Stenback WA, Spjut HJ. The fibromatoses of infancy and childhood. In: Rosenberg HS, Bolande RP, eds.* Perspectives in Pediatric Pathology. *vol. 4. Chicago: Year Book Medical, 1973.)*

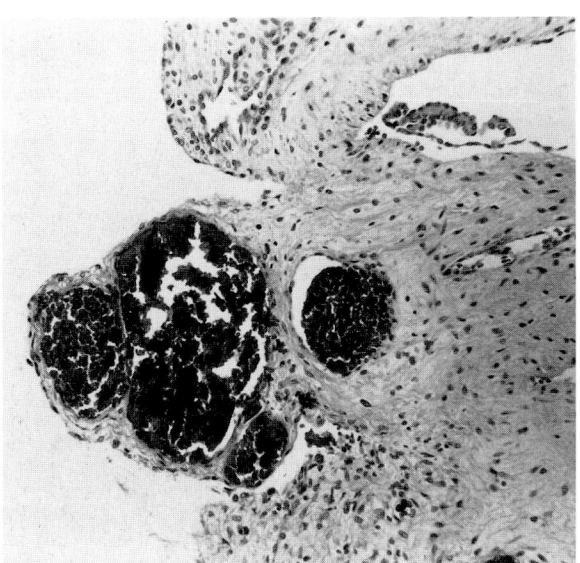

FIGURE 20.49. *A blood cyst in an AV valve leaflet consists of an endothelium-lined channel filled with noncoagulated blood (H&E, ×40).*

clinical relevance, blood cysts occasionally exhibit persistent growth and obstruct valve orifices [401–403].

ANATOMY AND EXAMINATION OF THE CONDUCTION SYSTEM

The conduction system is not the legendary enigma that most pathologists perceive it to be. When examined routinely in a practical manner, its anatomy and variations become familiar. The value of negative findings is not to be dismissed. Persistence will reward the examiner by unmasking an infarct, hemorrhage, or other pathology which explains a complex dysrhythmia or an unexpected cardiac death.

The Normal Heart

The specialized cells of the conduction system lie buried within the heart, itself a conducting system [404]. In a normally formed heart, the system's anatomy and vascular supply are rather constant; except for the sinoatrial (SA) node, most of the conduction cells lie within or near the atrial and ventricular septa [405], but the patterns vary widely [406]. In common cardiac malformations, the aberrant location of conduction tissues can be predicted with some accuracy unless there is discordance between the atria and ventricles, specific types of single ventricle, or abnormal atrioventricular valvular configuration.

Examination of the conduction system requires a careful technique. The approach to tissue sampling described by Davies et al [405] has proved optimal when examining the normal or malformed perinatal heart. In a normally formed perinatal heart, the chambers should be opened in the fresh state along the pathway of blood flow using one of the axial methods but preferably in a manner that protects the sinoatrial node, cardiac septa, and the structural relations [407]. Abnormally formed hearts can be opened in a similar manner or may be perfused prior to dissection. After fixation it is helpful to remove the free ventricular walls completely from the septa to allow orientation during the tissue sampling (see below). Transverse sections of the ventricles should not be made except in cases of cardiomyopathy or asymmetrical septal hypertrophy [407]. The right atrial incision should begin at the edge of the inferior vena cava and continue across the anterior wall of the right atrium to the tip of the right atrial appendage. This allows complete access to the chamber without compromising the SA node.

The spindle-shaped SA node, or pacemaker node, lies immediately beneath the epicardium of the sulcus terminalis at the lateral junction of the superior vena cava and the right atrium. In approximately 10% of cases, the SA node has a horseshoe shape that straddles that junction [408]. The node consists of small cells arranged in serpentine interwoven fascicles surrounded by dense fibrous tissue, and its tail extends out into the atrial myocardium. The nodal components lie around a central artery or contain ramifying small arteries. At the margins, the nodal cells merge abruptly with atrial myocardium. Their cytoplasm stains more lightly with eosin than the other atrial cells. Although striated after birth, no intercalated discs are visible by light microscopy.

The AV node is a relatively large plexiform arrangement of striated cells slightly smaller than those in the atrial walls. It has four parts: a transitional cell zone, compact atrioventricular node, penetrating atrioventricular (His) bundle, and branching atrioventricular bundle [409]. In the normal heart, the components of the AV node lie beneath the right atrial septal endocardium and within an area known as Koch's triangle above the insertion of the medial leaflet of the tricuspid valve. The triangle's base extends from the posterior edge of the coronary sinus to the tricuspid valve annulus. The superior leg of the triangle is the Tendon of Todaro, often visible as a curvilinear ridge extending anteriorly from the rostral side of the coronary sinus to nearly

join the tricuspid valve annulus in a region known as the central fibrous body. The inferior leg is the attachment of the tricuspid valve. The compact portion of the AV node, the largest, and most recognizable segment lies near the apex of Koch's triangle, next to the posterior border of the membranous ventricular septum. The left side of the compact node abuts the collagenous base of the mitral annulus (Fig. 20.50).

At the apex of Koch's triangle, the anterior aspect of the deep portion of the compact AV node forms the penetration (His) bundle—a dense aggregate of parallel fibers surrounded by fibrous tissue. The bundle penetrates the central fibrous body and continues forward on the right side of the membranous portion of the interventricular septum at its junction with the crest of the muscular portion of the septum, gradually crossing to the left side of the septum. The penetrating bundle branches along the crest of the muscular septum below the commissure of the posterior (noncoronary) and right coronary cusps of the aortic valve. Here, the bundle gives off fascicles of the left main bundle branch (LMBB). These exit beneath the membranous septum and continue down the left side of the ventricular septum

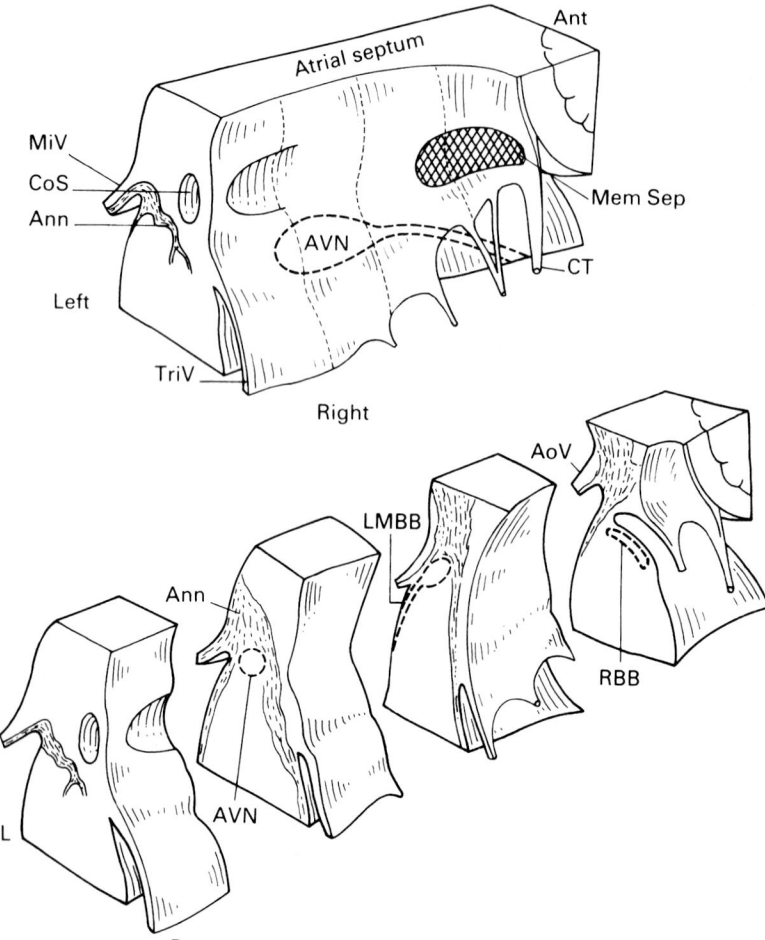

FIGURE 20.50.   *Schematic outline of the conduction system region with a sampling method, as viewed from the right side. Ann = annulus of atrioventricular valve; Ant = anterior; AoV = aortic valve; AVN = atrioventricular node; Cos = coronary sinus; CT = chorda tendinea; LMBB = left main bundle branch; Mem Sep = membranous septum; MiV = mitral valve; RBB = right bundle branch; TriV = tricuspid valve.*

beneath the endocardium, often dividing into wide branches or swaths that enter the bases of the anterior and posterior papillary muscles. The anterior radiation is smaller than the posterior. Both give off radiating branches that form a plexiform net of large, pale, clear Purkinje cells with round-to-oval nuclei in the apical region.

The remainder of the penetrating bundle passes toward the right to become the right bundle branch (RBB), which roughly follows a line drawn from the apex of Koch's triangle to the right medial papillary muscle. In contrast to the LMBB, the RBB continues downward and forward as a single bundle across the surface of the septum to the base of the right anterior papillary muscle, and on to the anterior wall of the right ventricle. The position of the branch is quite variable.

The SA node receives its blood supply via a rather large first atrial branch of the right coronary artery in approximately 55% of cases, via a comparable branch from the left coronary in about 35% of cases, and from a dual origin in approximately 10% [404]. The blood supply to the AV node arises from the epicardial coronary artery that provides the major supply to the posterior of the heart, i.e., the right coronary artery in 80–90% of cases [410]. The terminal ramifications of the AV nodal artery in infants are quite variable; they provide branches to the posterior interventricular septum in most hearts, to the interatrial septum in nearly half, reach the AV node in 90% of cases, and the penetrating bundle in little more than half [411, 412].

Removal and Preparation for Histology

Using Hudson's methods [413], the SA node can be sectioned perpendicularly or parallel to the long axis of the superior vena cava as either a single or multiple sequential blocks. The four parts of the AV node lie along the atrioventricular junction and require examination of those portions of the atrial and ventricular septa that begin at the coronary sinus and continue anteriorly along the entire length of the central fibrous body and beyond. In the procedure of Davies et al [405], using an upper and lower block, the upper block should extend anteriorly past the medial papillary muscle of the right ventricle and include at least one centimeter of atrium and ventricular septum above and below the tricuspid valve. The lower block includes the apical half of the ventricular septum. The upper block contains the atrioventricular node, the main bundle, and the origin of the bundle branches. For convenient automatic processing, this block is divided into sequential blocks [404] cut perpendicular to the tricuspid valve and serially sectioned from the posterior aspect (see Fig. 20.50). The lower block contains the peripheral portions of the left and right bundle branches and is sectioned horizontally, parallel to the plane of the tricuspid valve. Swabbing the left ventricular wall and aortic valve with india ink serves to orient the examiner at the microscope.

Slow processing to paraffin prevents distortion. Every tenth or twentieth section should be examined with hematoxylin and eosin. Special stains, such as elastic-van Gieson or Masson trichrome, occasionally provide an advantage, particularly for photography. Thorough study of the conduction system may require study of 200 to 300 sections. Specific conduction problems, such as the Wolff-Parkinson-White syndrome, or congenital heart disease, may require submission of both AV rings [404].

Development and Innervation of the Conduction System

The early fetal heart has a functioning conduction system before the cardiac autonomic nerve supply is complete. The embryologic origin of the conduction system components remains controversial [414–416]. The specialized myocardium of the early embryo's conduction system cannot be distinguished readily from the surrounding myocardium with the light microscope without specific monoclonal antibodies [416, 417] until relatively advanced stages of development, when the heart has developed a definitive form [418]. The innervation of the mature heart has been examined in a variety of mammals, but is less understood in humans [417].

PATHOLOGIC ANATOMY OF CONDUCTION ABNORMALITIES

Most fetal dysrhythmias are functional disorders with specific electrocardiographic criteria (Table 20.9). Except for those associated with congenital heart disease or fetal hydrops, few have structural counterparts [419, 420].

In both the fetus and neonate, supraventricular tachycardia, atrial flutter, and atrial fibrillation, or ventricular tachycardia, often are associated with severe congestive heart failure and may be caused by myocarditis or complex congenital heart disease. Ventricular fibrillation is extremely rare in the fetus and usually is associated with myocardial necrosis. Complete heart block is rare and may be due to viral myocarditis, congenital heart disease, or maternal connective tissue disease (see below).

Abnormal Conduction in the Normal Heart

Sinus dysrhythmias usually indicate extracardiac problems in the newborn infant due to the effect of placentally transferred maternal medication, fever, sepsis, severe hypoxemia, digitalis toxicity, hypoglycemia, metabolic or endocrine abnormality, or central nervous system deficit. Inherited conduction abnormalities are exceptionally rare [421].

Transient bradycardia is common in normal immature newborn infants and may be of little significance. Severe bradycardia is common in infants born of complicated pregnancies and deliveries that involve low Apgar scores,

Table 20.9.   Dysrhythmias in the fetus and newborn infant

Sinus node disorders
Sinus tachycardia
Sinus bradycardia
Sinus arrhythmia
Sino-atrial (SA) block

Supraventricular dysrhythmias
Premature supraventricular systoles
Escape beats
Supraventricular tachycardia
    with Wolff-Parkinson-White syndrome (WPW)
    with conduction system hypoplasia
    with congenital heart disease
Atrial flutter and fibrillation

Ventricular dysrhythmias
Premature ventricular systoles
Ventricular tachycardia
Ventricular fibrillation

Atrioventricular (AV) block (congenital heart block)
Normal heart–abnormal conduction system
    discontinuity between atrial myocardium and compact
    AV node
    discontinuity between AV node and penetrating bundle
Congenitally malformed heart

Miscellaneous
Abnormal pulse rhythm intervals
    glycogen storage disease, type 2 (Pompe)
Bundle branch block
    tumours

Modified from Shenker L. Fetal cardiac arrhythmias. *Surv Obstet Gynecol* 1979; 34:561–72; and Guntheroth and Motolsky [421].

repeated episodes of hypotension, persistent hypoxemia, acidosis, increased intracranial pressure, and intracranial hemorrhage. Singer reported six immature or premature perinates with bradycardia who had a variety of substantial hemorrhages in the SA or AV node and the bundle branches [422]. Survivors of such problems may have an increased risk of sudden death.

Supraventricular tachycardia, the most common and most serious tachydysrhythmia in the prenatal period, is usually associated with severe congestive failure [423]. In the normally formed heart, myocarditis, Wolff-Parkinson-White pre-excitation syndrome (WPW) or congenital hypoplasia of the conducting system may be the underlying cause. In WPW, a strand of cardiac muscle connects atrial muscle with ventricular muscle, bypassing the atrioventricular sulcus and AV nodal delay and providing faster conduction through an accessory pathway [405]. Congenital hypoplasia of the conducting system was reported in three perinates with fatal supraventricular tachycardia, including one identified in utero [424]. All had structurally normal hearts, but every SA and AV node was hypoplastic and contained little fibrous

tissue and fewer cells than normal. In two cases, the entire conduction system was smaller than normal.

Ventricular tachycardia is rare in the normal newborn heart. Cardiomegaly may be the only other abnormal sign recognized during life despite electrocardiography, echocardiography, or angiographic study. When these features are the only clues, and the heart appears otherwise normal on postmortem examination, the examiner should be alert to causes such as myocarditis, congestive or hypertrophic cardiomyopathy, cardiac tumor, or histiocytoid cardiomyopathy.

Spontaneous ventricular fibrillation should alert the examiner to possible severe acute myocardial ischemic injury or myocardial rupture.

Third-degree (complete) atrioventricular heart block is known as congenital heart block (CHB) when present at birth in normally formed and malformed hearts, and is defined as a complete lack of conduction of atrial depolarizations to the ventricles. Ventricular control is exercised by pulses arising "below" the AV node, usually in the bundle of His. Most cases of CHB are sporadic [421]. The condition may occur in 1:20,000 live births, according to Michaelsson and Engle, who reviewed 599 cases in an international study [425]. Of 418 patients with normal hearts, only 32 (7.9%) died, but of 181 with congenital heart disease, 53 (29%) died.

Few anatomic studies of CHB in otherwise normal perinatal hearts have been reported. In 1970, Sotelo-Avila et al reported an infant with an abnormal AV node and penetrating bundle of His distorted by dense bands of collagen and amorphous non-calcified tissues infiltrated by mononuclear cells, which they suggested was due most likely to a non-infective inflammatory process [426]. Calcification of the AV node may also cause CHB [420]. CHB in normally formed hearts may be associated with discontinuity between the atrial and ventricular conduction tissues, or with discontinuity between the AV node and His's bundle [427]. It also has a high association with maternal connective tissue disease, especially systemic lupus erythematosus (SLE) [428–432].

The recognition of a soluble tissue ribonucleoprotein antigen, Ro(SS-A), in the serum of mothers of infants with CHB, and the presence of IgG and IgA in the endocardium and interstitium suggest that an immunologically based inflammation may be an important causal mechanism of CHB [430, 432]. The postmortem examination of every infant with CHB may reasonably include a maternal serum study for ANA and Ro antibodies, and preparation of the SA and AV nodal areas for immunologic evaluation.

Short-pulse rhythm intervals have been described repeatedly in infants with glycogen storage disease, type 2 (Pompe disease): the few histologic studies of the conduction system reported have shown enlarged vacuolated cells filled with stainable glycogen throughout the conduction system [433].

Conduction defects occur in about 20% of cases of primary EFE and include WPW, left bundle branch blocks, complete heart block, and a variety of supraventricular and ventricular dysrhythmias [434].

Conduction Abnormalities in the Malformed Heart

Hearts with congenital malformations may have any of the conduction abnormalities described in Table 20.9. They also may have unusual conduction system pathways and patterns, which result from a variety of malpositions and misalignments during development. In many malformations, the conduction system anatomy may be predicted accurately.

Because most malformed hearts have normal atria, the SA node usually lies in the normal location and injury to its blood supply is possible whenever surgery involves the right atrium, e.g., atrial septectomy, or repair of transposition of the great arteries. In cases with right atrial isomerism and asplenia, each atrium usually has a superior vena cava, and the SA node usually occupies each sulcus terminalis at the junction of the superior vena cava and the atrial appendage [435]. With left atrial isomerism and polysplenia,the SA nodes may not be detectable or may lie near the AV junction [436].

Whenever the internal arrangement of the heart is abnormal, the AV node and penetrating bundle may have unusual locations or pathways. If septal components are normally aligned but have an isolated ventricular septal defect (VSD), the compact portion of the AV node is usually found in its normal position. However, the non-branching bundle may lie adjacent to a perimembranous or muscular inlet defect, but it might be present near any other types of isolated VSD [437]. The VSD of tetralogy of Fallot may be perimembranous or, occasionally, involve the muscle of the infundibulum. In each type, the right bundle branch may be subject to more injury than the left during surgical repair. With an atrioventricular septal defect, whether partial or total, the AV node and bundle locations are markedly displaced posteriorly and inferiorly, lying in the septal tissues or beneath bridging portions of the AV valve. Complete heart block may occur during surgical repair [438].

In hearts with only one functional chamber, with or without a rudimentary contralateral chamber, the inlet septum is the signpost to the position of the conducting tissues [439]. If that segment is absent, the AV node lies in the anterolateral position; if that part of the septum is present, it carries the AV bundle. The exact location depends on whether the right or left chamber predominates.

Arrhythmias Following Cardiac Surgery

Cardiac surgery involves a wide range of possible incisions and reconstructive changes and virtually any dysrhythmia can develop. The most common problems involve sinus node abnormalities after atrial surgery and complete atrioventricular (AV) block.

In the past, hearts with TGA repaired with Mustard's operation often had a substantial incidence of damage to the node or its vascular supply [440]. The incidence seems less with newer procedures. Evaluation may require postmortem coronary angiography.

Intra-operative conduction system mapping has led to fewer instances of postoperative complete AV block. Yet, knowledge of the conduction system anatomy often cannot prevent temporary or complete AV block during repair of complex congenital heart lesions. The confluence of the aortic, tricuspid, and mitral valves is the vulnerable point in the repair of perimembranous septal defects [438], whether isolated or in the tetralogy of Fallot.

Ventricular fibrillation may occur spontaneously during cardiac surgery, at times without apparent provocation. Ischemic myocardial injury, or direct injury such as a perforation during cardiac catheterization, may cause ventricular fibrillation. If the electrocardiogram suggests acute ischemic injury and death occurs within 2–6 hours, the use of tetrazolium compounds [441, 442] may help to identify myocardial infarction because, except for obvious hemorrhage or suture material, little histologic change is demonstrable until more than 6 hours after the ischemic event [443, 444].

Conduction System in Sudden Unexpected Infant Death

Of the many theories offered in the explanation of sudden infant death syndrome (SIDS), the conduction system findings have had a controversial history. James, on one hand, champions the position that the AV node and the bundle of His undergo a number of normal sporadic morphologic changes from the time of birth through the first year of life, in which irregular fronds or strands of conduction tissue are gradually destroyed and resorbed [445–447]. Others, examining similar cases, did not reach the same conclusion [405, 448–451]. Studies of individual regions [452–454] have occasionally demonstrated differences, but departures from the normal are common in this age group [455].

Myocardial Injury

Ischemic myocardial necrosis (IMN) is the most common perinatal myocardial injury, and occurs in normal and malformed hearts of stillborn and liveborn babies [456, 457]. In most instances the cause is underperfusion of the subendocardium and papillary muscles. In contrast to adults, coronary artery injury, thrombosis, and transmural infarcts are rare in this age group [458–461]. IMN may contribute to the deaths of one-quarter of the affected infants (Table 20.10). Identifying the presence and extent of IMN requires systematic examination of the myocardium, including all papillary muscles [407, 443, 444].

The asphyxiated perinate is particularly susceptible to ischemic myocardial injury [407, 443, 462], and the infant

Table 20.10.   Perinatal conditions associated with myocardial dysfunction and injury

Birth asphyxia (one minute Apgar <4)
Persistent fetal circulation (PFC)
Diaphragmatic hernia
Meconium aspiration syndrome
Congenital heart disease
    Aortic atresia/stenosis (hypoplastic left heart)
    Pulmonary atresia
    Anomalous pulmonary venous return
Sepsis
Fluid overload
Fetal hydrops
Maternal–fetal infectious disease (e.g., TORCH)
Disseminated intravascular coagulation
Protein C and S deficiencies
Multiple congenital anomalies
Fetomaternal transfusion syndrome

most vulnerable is the hemodynamically unstable newborn with hypotension, rales, tachypnea, hepatomegaly, a gallop rhythm, and other signs of cardiogenic shock [463, 464]. These infants with structurally normal hearts may suffer significant myocardial ischemia associated with Q-waves or ST-T wave electrocardiographic changes, and develop persistent tricuspid or mitral valve insufficiency murmurs [465, 466], along with elevated serum concentrations of creatine phosphokinase-M and -B fractions [467]. Premature infants surviving with severe lung disease, multiple episodes of bradycardia, hypotension, or cardiac arrests, and full-term infants with persistent pulmonary hypertension may have a range of acute or healed myocardial lesions, including infarcts, fibrotic scars, and dystrophic calcification [407, 443, 468–470].

Ischemic myocardial necrosis consistently affects hearts with congenital aortic and pulmonary outflow obstruction [471, 472], excessive venous return to the right heart due to anomalous pulmonary venous return [473], or congenital arteriovenous malformations of the vein of Galen [474]. Hearts with uncomplicated tetralogy of Fallot or transposition of the great vessels are affected less frequently.

Pathology

Ischemic myocardial necrosis occurs in both ventricles with near-equal frequency, most commonly in anterior papillary muscles, and less commonly in the posterior papillary muscles [407, 475]. Severely asphyxiated perinates often have multifocal ischemic injuries throughout the heart [407, 468]. Right ventricular injury is common when pulmonary hypertension is caused by severe pulmonic outflow obstruction in the presence of an intact ventricular septum, by anomalous pulmonary venous return to the right atrium [471, 472], by bronchopulmonary dysplasia, or persistent

fetal circulation [475]. Left ventricular injury is more likely in infants with aortic atresia or stenosis, or anomalous origin of the left coronary artery from the pulmonary trunk [471, 473]. Infants suffering severe bradycardia and shock after major cerebral intraventricular hemorrhage or abdominal catastrophes may have only left ventricular injury. Maternal cocaine use or certain medications may be associated with IMN [457, 476].

Myocardial damage is often subtle and its discovery requires systematic examination of the myocardium, including all papillary muscles and the coronary arteries [444, 457]. Because the myocardial fibers of the papillary muscles and ventricular subendocardium are oriented generally in the longitudinal axis of the ventricle [477], and since IMN in the perinatal heart is more easily recognized in longitudinally oriented fibers than those cut transversely, sections of the heart should be taken in the longitudinal axis [444]. Sections that include the atrial wall and the coronary artery, the AV ring and valve elements, and the ventricular wall with the papillary muscle, all in one block are the most economical and rewarding.

The injury may range from a distinctly ischemic focus in the apical position of a papillary muscle (Fig. 20.51) or the subendocardium, a massive hemorrhagic infarct of an entire papillary muscle, or multiple infarcts in several papillary muscles, along with septal and subendocardial necrosis of both ventricular free walls [407, 475]. Severely asphyxiated infants may have a "geographical" injury pattern of multiple infarcts in the middle and outer thirds of the ventricular wall [468]. Isolated transmural or massive septal injury is rare in the absence of a coronary thrombosis, infection, embolus, or trauma. The largest septal infarcts occur near the AV ring and may involve the AV node; longitudinal sections through the septum expose them.

With certain notable exceptions, the histologic appearance of acute perinatal IMN resembles that in the adult human and the experimental animal, although the chronology of the perinatal repair process has not been well defined. The stressed premature infant has a delayed inflammatory response, frequent dystrophic myocardial calcification, and rarely wavy fibers or contraction band necrosis. Aside from occasional thromboemboli within necrotic capillaries, occlusive thrombi are rare in coronary vessels.

Coagulation necrosis is the predominant ischemic injury found in perinates, although "contraction band" necrosis (coagulative myocytolysis) and myocytolysis (colliquative myocytolysis; vacuolar degeneration) do occur, as in adults [478]. Wavy fibers, said to be an early sign of ischemic injury in adults [479], rarely occur without other histologic signs of ischemic injury [457]; they are often difficult to identify with certainty in perinates because myocardial fiber separation is so common [443].

Coagulation necrosis develops in the myocardium of adults and infants within 12 hours of the onset of ischemia; in perinates, it may be the only finding after 24–30 hours. The earliest changes include swelling of myocardial cells and

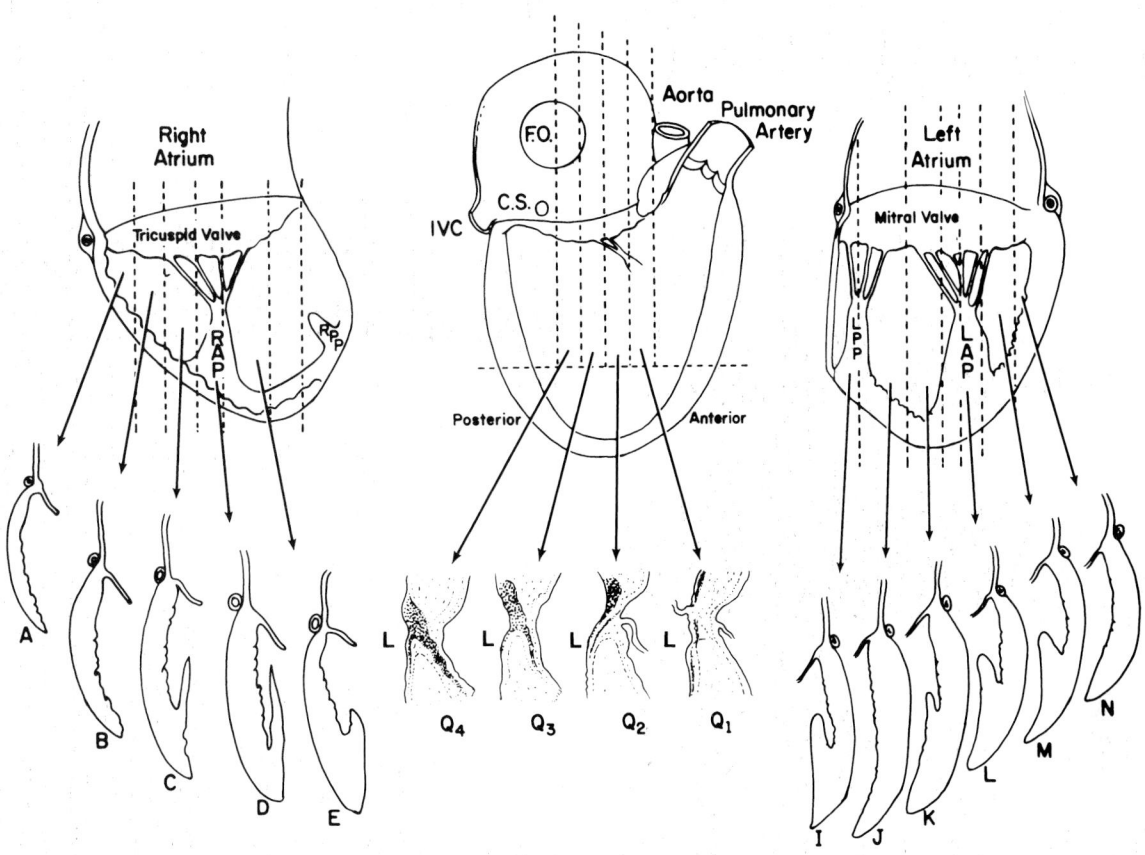

FIGURE 20.51. *Diagram for systematic histologic sampling of normally formed perinatal heart allows for consistent selection of identifiable locations in the heart [444]. Samples of right and left heart should include atrial wall, the AV ring with coronary artery, ventricular wall, and papillary muscle. The conduction system samples (Q1–Q4) are taken from the right side of septum in this approach. Routinely marking one side of septum with india ink helps orientation.*

crenation of their nuclear membranes. Thereafter, cell cytoplasm becomes increasingly granular, then glassy and increasingly eosinophilic. Eventually, nuclei become pyknotic or lysed. The myofibrils appear elongated and lose their cross-striations, but striations may persist for several days. Infants less than 30 weeks' gestational age have less obvious myofibrillar change than do older infants.

Contraction band necrosis, also called "coagulative myocytolysis" or "myofibrillar degeneration," is characterized by hypercontracted myocardial cells with large irregular transverse bands of shortened sarcomeres, appears at the edges of recently infarcted myocardium [457, 480], and is possibly mediated by altered cellular calcium metabolism and response to catecholamines [481]. The bands are aggregates of disorganized actinomycin filaments associated with myoplasm that lacks myofilaments. Myocardial contraction bands without other changes are uncommon in the perinate [443]. However, they may be the only finding in a stillborn infant or in a newborn infant dying after profound shock, asphyxia, or repeated resuscitative efforts involving exogenous catecholamines. While readily identifiable in

H&E stained materials, the Lendrum's Martius Scarlet Blue [468], any of the trichrome stains, or modified luxol fast blue [482] vividly demonstrate them. In early stages nuclei may remain, but time and progressive loss of the contractile apparatus leave an empty sarcolemmal tube containing pigmented yellow-brown macrophages.

Myocytolysis, also called "vacuolar degeneration" or "colliquative" myocytolysis, is the progressive loss of myofibrils resulting in a vacuolated muscle sarcoplasm having only a nucleus within the sarcolemmal tube [483]. Occurring in the presence of acute and chronic myocardial ischemia, cardiomyopathies, myocarditis, endocarditis, and in stillborns [457] myocytolysis has been considered the result of intracellular edema with the potential for healing without an inflammatory response or proliferation of granulation tissue [479]. In contrast to cells with necrosis, those with myocytolysis retain creatine phosphokinase-M and -B, LDH-1, aspartate aminotransferase, and myoglobin in the thin margins of the sarcoplasm surrounding the vacuole but not in the vacuoles, suggesting an intact sarcolemmal membrane and the potential for reversibility [483].

Compared to adults, defining the chronology of myocardial repair in the perinate is difficult because a precise starting point may not be evident from clinical observations. The character of the cellular exudate may serve to date an adult's infarct, but the perinate commonly has no interstitial acute inflammatory cell response during the first 24–36 hours after an ischemic insult. Later, the mononuclear, vascular, and fibroblastic responses may be slowed by associated systemic problems [475].

One rarely finds any histologic evidence of myocardial injury in infants dying within 9–12 hours of birth [407, 475] and wavy fibers are difficult to identify in the perinatal heart, especially after prolonged or repeated resuscitation. If death occurs in a premature baby within 24–48 hours after an acute obstetrical catastrophe, cytoplasmic eosinophilia, granularity, and nuclear pyknosis may be the only signs found. Cross-striations may persist in necrotic fibers or be absent. Despite necrosis and even hemorrhage, marginated polymorphonuclear cells in capillaries may be the only neutrophilic response in stressed neonates whose granulocytes do not respond to chemotactic stimuli at the same rate as those of older infants and children [484]. Thereafter, polymorphonuclear cells slowly infiltrate the margins of necrotic foci, become most intense by 72–96 hours, and apparently decline. Dissolution of transverse and longitudinal striations, karyolysis, and karyorrhexis follow. Basic fuchsin and the tetrazolium dyes do not uniformly accentuate myocardial necrosis in the perinate [462], nor does fluorescence microscopy identify changes not identifiable with H&E stains [475].

Dystrophic calcification is common in the usual sites of myocardial injury, and calcium granules may outline the sarcolemmal membrane or striations of myocardial cells when no other signs are present [469, 470, 475]. It is not unusual to find dystrophic calcification and acute necrosis or fibrosis in the same site with no attendant acute or chronic inflammatory response [469, 470].

Thrombosis of epicardial coronary arteries is rare except with severe disseminated intravascular coagulation or vegetative left heart endocarditis [485], but small fibrin-platelet thrombi may be found in small arterioles, capillaries, and venules within or around injury sites [456, 469].

Perinates dying more than 1 week after a stormy course involving asphyxia, cardiac arrest, repeated bradycardia, and hypotension may have acute myocardial injury in one site as well as scattered lymphocytes and plasma cells among proliferating fibroblasts and vessels elsewhere [475]. Fibrovascular granulation tissue in papillary muscles is a feature of long-term survivors, not the newborn infant.

Pathogenesis

The rarity of major coronary artery thrombosis and the common presence of damage in papillary muscles and subendocardium suggests that low perfusion underlies most

perinatal ischemic myocardial injury [407, 462–466, 475]. Although global myocardial ischemia is usual, the papillary muscles and subendocardium are more vulnerable than the outer subepicardial myocardium because: 1) they lie at the end of the coronary artery circulation; 2) they have a lower oxygen tension, lower oxygen tissue saturation, and lower levels of metabolic components; 3) by autoregulation, their vessels undergo maximum vasodilatation in response to progressive lowering of coronary artery pressure before the vessels of the other myocardial layers; 4) during systole the pressures in the subendocardium rises to equal intracavitary pressures, thereby reducing subendocardial flow, while those in the subepicardium approach zero [486, 487].

The fetal heart is more vulnerable because it functions at maximum efficiency to keep pace with the considerable demands for growth in a stable system [488]. Premature delivery disrupts that stability and magnifies the demands upon the immature heart, even without the added stress of asphyxia or hypoxia [489]. The asphyxiated perinate with a normal or malformed heart and congestive failure is at high risk without treatment because of the continuous high-energy demands and large oxygen extraction by the myocardium. Lactate metabolism sustains the myocardium to a point, but beyond that level of resistance to hypoxic injury the risk of myocardial necrosis escalates [489].

The frequency of right heart injury associated with sustained pulmonary hypertension from bronchopulmonary dysplasia or congenital heart disease may relate to the compressive effects of high intracavitary pressure on the blood vessels in the right ventricular subendocardium and anterior papillary muscle [475]. The direct effect of oxygen on the pulmonary arteries and even coronary arteries in these cases has not been explored. Intramural coronary vascular injury may be associated with abnormal prostaglandin effects on coronary vessels (e.g., vasospasm) and platelet aggregation; both effects seem to play roles in myocardial necrosis [475, 485].

ARTERIES AND VEINS

Spontaneous thrombosis of major arteries and veins is rare in the normal neonate. However, local or massive thrombosis from a variety of causes may result in the death of a critically ill neonate (Table 20.11). The basis for increased thrombosis during the neonatal period is not clear [490]. The newborn with homozygous protein C or protein S deficiency may develop catastrophic purpura and thrombosis [491–493]. Intrauterine thrombosis of major arteries and veins creates major diagnostic dilemmas [492–496].

In-dwelling plastic catheters for blood gas, electrolyte and chemical monitoring, administration of nutrients, and fluid management are key elements in the care of critically ill neonates [464, 497]. In experienced hands, complications of their use have diminished. Prolonged use of in-dwelling catheters is associated with recognized risks of cardiac and

Table 20.11. Causes and associations of neonatal arterial and venous thrombosis

Prolonged vascular catheterization
Sepsis
Maternal diabetes mellitus
Pregnancy hypertension and toxemia
Hypoxic tissue injury
Disseminated intravascular coagulation (DIC)
Necrotizing enterocolitis
Dehydration
Cold injury
Thrombocytopenia
Thrombotic thrombocytopenia
Hyperviscosity (polycythemia)
Congenital nephrotic syndrome

vascular thromboses and their complications, risks that increase with asphyxia, severe acidosis, shock, sepsis, or disseminated intravascular coagulation [464, 497, 498].

After death, all in-dwelling vascular catheters should be left in place for postmortem examination. The incidence of associated thrombosis ranges from 3.6% to 59% in different series [499]. Dissection of the umbilical and iliac arteries, aorta, and umbilical vein allows identification of most thrombi. Postmortem blood clots are commonly found extending from the end of a catheter left in place. In the case of tiny infants or if the catheter has been dislodged or removed, serial transverse sections of the vascular bundle after fixation may prove more fruitful than dissection.

The umbilical artery is the main access to the vascular system with the tip advanced in the aorta above the level of the renal arteries or farther up within the thoracic aorta. Perforation and perivascular dissection by the catheter during placement are common but usually of little consequence. However, undetected perforation of one of these arteries within the abdomen may cause massive hemorrhage.

With time, a thrombus forms around any catheter, leaving a sheath in place when the catheter is withdrawn. Catheter tips can be thrombogenic [500, 501] or directly damage the vascular endothelium and promote mural thrombosis. Retrograde or antegrade propagation of the thrombus or thromboembolization can cause ischemic injury, paraplegia, intestinal necrosis, renal hypertension [502], or death [503].

Damage to the umbilical vein, ductus venosus, or right atrium can occur during catheter placement for exchange transfusion. Thrombosis of the umbilical vein is much less common than in an umbilical artery because catheters are seldom left in the umbilical vein for prolonged periods. The risk of portal vein thrombosis and hepatic injury is high, especially with instillation of hypertonic fluids [504, 505].

Thromboses form in more than 15% of newborn infants of diabetic mothers, even when catheterization is not involved; their calcification suggests an intrauterine origin [506]. Plasma coagulation factors are not involved, but mild thrombocytopenia is a common premonitory sign.

Thrombosis of the renal and adrenal veins, the inferior vena cava, and even the sagittal sinus is sometimes associated with severe dehydration or sepsis.

Long-term central catheterization of the superior vena cava (SVC) for intravenous feeding [507] may be complicated by retrograde propagation of thrombus and partial or total occlusion of the innominate and jugular veins with development of clinical superior vena cava syndrome. A central venous catheter in the SVC or within the right atrium can cause local or massive thrombosis of the atrial wall and tricuspid valve [485, 508], and multifocal embolization to peripheral pulmonary arteries. Fatal cardiac tamponade may occur if the line accidentally perforates the right atrial or ventricular wall [509].

Bacterial or fungal contamination of in-dwelling catheters often results in septic embolization and arteritis. Venous occlusions may occur in pulmonary veins [510] or in hepatic veins [511].

Systemic Hypertension

While generally rare in the newborn infant at term, systemic hypertension has become a well-recognized problem in neonatal intensive-care units [512, 513]. The advent of ultrasound and intra-arterial blood pressure monitoring devices has allowed early identification of the hypertensive neonate and has led to earlier corrective therapy. Many cases are due to total or partial thrombotic occlusion of the main renal artery following the use of arterial catheters, while others result from congenital narrowing or hypoplasia of aorta or renal arteries, or have no identifiable cause. Congenital heart disease or patent ductus arteriosus is a common association. About two-thirds of the patients have nonspecific symptoms and signs, including cardiomegaly, hepatosplenomegaly, hematuria, and proteinuria. However, while their urea nitrogen, creatinine, catecholamine, and corticosteroid levels are normal, most have elevated renin levels.

Portal Hypertension

In the perinatal period, portal hypertension is due to propagation of an umbilical vein thrombus into the portal venous tract. Congenital Budd–Chiari syndrome usually presents with ascites at birth [511]. Acute omphalitis or thrombosis about an umbilical venous catheter is the most frequent underlying cause [514]; congenital portal vein abnormalities are extremely rare [511]. Diffuse hepatic necrosis or pulmonary thromboembolism may follow [515]. We, and others [505], have encountered fatal acute hypertension due to massive thrombosis following administration of hypertonic solutions through an umbilical venous catheter. Acute splenomegaly and hematemesis have been reported as late complications [504]. Hepatic veno-occlusive disease of the newborn is rare [516].

Idiopathic Infantile Arterial Calcification

This rare condition of both live and stillborn infants usually involves the aorta, its major branches, and coronary arteries in a focal or diffuse fashion [517–519]. The extent is best demonstrated with standard radiographic or xerographic techniques. The heart is enlarged and coronary involvement is usually pronounced and may be associated with myocardial necrosis. Cerebral vessels are seldom damaged. The brittle vessels crackle when compressed. The arteries usually have plaques and larger vessels have overlying intimal proliferation. Lymphocytic infiltrates are often present in plaques or in the adventitia. Ultrastructurally there is distinctive calcification of the elastic laminae as well as in collagen fibers, smooth muscle, and fibroblasts [517]. Ischemic injury in other organs is uncommon. Fetal hydrops may be present [518]. At least seven reports involve siblings [517, 520].

Dystrophic Calcification and Vascular Foreign Materials

Large and small vessels may become calcified after being occluded by thrombi, especially those that have contained in-dwelling catheters for extended periods of time (e.g., superior vena cava, aorta, and umbilical artery). The small vessels that filter embolic fragments and foreign materials (e.g., renal and peripheral pulmonary arteries) develop granulomatous foreign body reactions as well as calcifications [521, 522]. Experimental studies have raised the possibility of pulmonary microangiopathy subsequent to prostaglandin E$_1$ treatment [523].

Arteritis and Phlebitis

In the neonate, arteritis and phlebitis are usually due to direct invasion by organisms from a nearby site of infection or from an infection of an existing vascular damage site (e.g., thrombus). The major complications involve embolization and mycotic aneurysms. The appearance of the inflamed vessel depends on the infectious agent and ranges from acute necrotizing inflammation to caseous necrosis seen with pathogenic bacteria and fungi or obliterative chronic inflammation with repair encountered with active syphilis or rubella [524]. Syphilitic vascular damage is characterized by adventitial and perivascular infiltrates of lymphocytes and plasma cells and eventually a laminated thickening of the adventitia [525]. Rubella infection produces focal fibromuscular intimal proliferation but little damage to the internal elastic laminae and tunica media [526].

Congenital Dilatations

Congenital dilatations and aneurysms of arteries and veins are rare in the perinate. Poststenotic dilatations may resemble aneurysms. Dissecting aneurysms of the ductus arteriosus have been described in neonates [527–529]. Aneurysms in other sites often have an underlying infectious or traumatic cause [530–532]. Esophageal varices seldom become symptomatic before 6 months of age.

Lymphedema

Congenital or acquired lymphedema is due to deficiency, obstruction, or disruption of the lymphatic drainage from the distal portion of an extremity, the genital area, face, neck, or trunk. Defects may range from a small cutaneous change to a severe diffuse involvement of one or more entire limbs. If the obstruction involves the abdominal or thoracic drainage, chylous ascites or chylothorax may be present. Opitz considers congenital lymphedema to be a common finding and one that represents variable rates of lymphatic maturation [533]. Infants with congenital lymphedema tend to have cutis marmorata. Abnormal reversal of cutaneous hair patterns may overlie a nuchal cystic hygroma (see discussion in Chap. 14).

Pulmonary Hypertension

Pulmonary arterial hypertension (PAH) (Table 20.12) results from either a sustained increase in pulmonary blood flow or an increased pulmonary arterial resistance from functional or structural changes in the pulmonary vascular bed or parenchyma. In the newborn, it represents a failure of the fetal pulmonary circulation to adapt to extra-uterine life and

Table 20.12.   Pulmonary hypertension in the newborn

PRIMARY
    Persistent fetal circulation
    Primary pulmonary hypertension
SECONDARY
    Cardiovascular anomalies
        Hypoplastic left heart
        Severe coarctation
        Pulmonary venous obstructions
        Transposition of great vessels
        Total anomalous pulmonary venous return
        Cerebral arteriovenous malformation
    Meconium aspiration
    Pneumonia and sepsis
    Bronchopulmonary dysplasia
    Pulmonary hypoplasia
        Diaphragmatic hernia
        Oligohydramnios sequence
    Misalignment of pulmonary veins with alveolar capillary dysplasia
    Metabolic cardiomyopathy (e.g., glycogenosis type II)

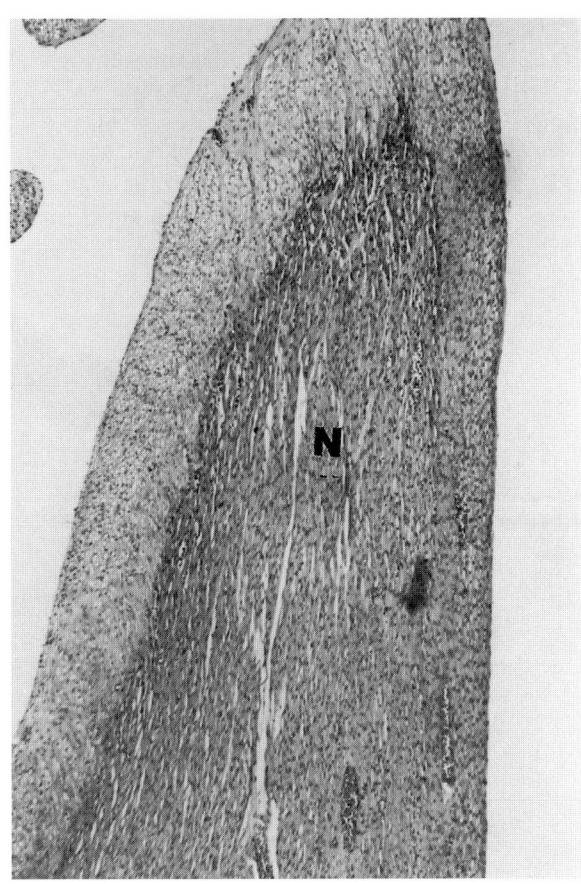

FIGURE 20.52. *Apical half of left posterior papillary muscle with ischemic necrosis of the center (N) and preservation of the subendocardial myocardium. Postmature infant with severe meconium aspiration, asphyxia, and persistent pulmonary hypertension survived 3 days. (H&E, original magnification ×30.)*

is associated with right-to-left shunting of deoxygenated blood through the foramen ovale, a patent ductus arteriosus, the lungs, or a combination of them all. Diverse conditions may affect pulmonary blood flow in utero or after birth and cause a reduction in the cross-sectional area of the pulmonary arteriolar bed with resultant increased pulmonary arterial resistance (Fig. 20.52).

The muscular arteries in the periphery of the lung regulate the flow of blood through the pulmonary microcirculation. In the perinate, structural changes in hypertensive pulmonary vessels are related to the stage of development of the lung and its vessels at birth, and the added effects of the cause of the hypertension. However, relationships between hemodynamic function and vessel structure in neonates are not as predictable as in older children or adults [534], and morphologic evaluation of pulmonary arteries in perinates can be difficult. Factors causing PAH can induce anatomic changes in the vessels which may augment the hypertension, and also sustain it when the original stimulus is removed [535].

The overall development of the pulmonary arteries and veins in utero is closely tied to that of the bronchial tree, which is completely formed by the 16th week of gestation [536–538]. The acinus, the functional unit of the mature lung, is supplied by a terminal bronchiole and consists of several generations of respiratory bronchioles, alveolar ducts, alveolar sacs, and alveoli. The preacinar arteries lie proximal to or accompany the terminal bronchioles and are the main resistance vessels that control pulmonary arterial pressure. The parallel branching pattern of preacinar pulmonary arteries and veins, termed *conventional vessels*, is recognizable by 14 weeks' gestation. Intra-acinar arteries accompany respiratory bronchioles and alveolar ducts and lie within alveolar walls. The development of terminal bronchioles, respiratory bronchioles, and saccules is accompanied by the appearance of the *supernumerary* arterial and venous branches that project at right angles from the conventional vessels to directly supply and drain the alveolar regions near the airways [536, 537]. In early fetal life, vessel branches increase in number, while in late fetal life, they increase in size and length. The diameters of proximal preacinar vessels increase faster than in the distal segments [536]. After birth, alveoli and associated supernumerary vessels normally continue to develop and increase in numbers [538]. The lung and its vascular bed undergo dramatic growth and remodeling during infancy and childhood [539].

Because of differences in the sizes and components at different ages, fetal and infant pulmonary arteries are not routinely classified as elastic or muscular merely by their size. The main intrapulmonary arteries of fetuses and adults are elastic arteries with internal and external elastic laminae and up to seven additional elastic laminae [536]. The arteries narrow toward the periphery and the number of elastic laminae decreases until only muscle separates the internal and external elastic laminae of truly muscular arteries in the fetus and infant. Thereafter, the circumferential muscular component thins until only an incomplete spiral of muscle separates the laminae. The most peripheral vessels have no muscle and only a single elastic lamina lies outside the endothelial sheath [537]. "Population studies" of the different types of perfused arteries in fetal lungs indicate that most of those larger than 175 μm in diameter are muscular. Of those between 175 and 87 μm, 63% are partly muscular, and most arteries smaller than 87 μm are non-muscular. At birth there is little muscle in normal arterial walls beyond the level of the terminal bronchioles [536]. The fetal pulmonary arterial wall is about twice the thickness of that in the adult, and the thickness is higher relative to external diameter. The total smooth muscle in pulmonary arteries had been thought to increase during gestation [540, 541]. However, studies of perfused vessels have shown that muscular pulmonary arteries are confined to the preacinar group in fetal life and that, within the respiratory unit, development of intra-acinar artery muscularity did not keep pace with that of the pulmonary saccules [537]. In the lung periphery, the normally circumferential muscular pattern changes to one in which the muscle cells are arrayed in a spiral. Between the muscle cells, and in distal continuations, the vessels have what amounts to a non-muscular capillary pattern [536, 537]. In the non-muscular segments of the vessels, two additional types of cells are identifiable within the interrupted elastic laminae: a pericyte and an intermediate cell with features of both smooth muscles and pericytes [542, 543].

Pathologic Changes and Causes of PAH

In the neonate PAH is more properly called *persistent pulmonary hypertension (PPHN)*, and the commonest pathophysiologic element is increased pulmonary vascular resistance, not increased pulmonary blood flow [544]. PPHN may be primary or secondary, and depending upon the cause and duration of hypertension, there may be pulmonary arterial muscular hyperplasia or hypertrophy [545–547]. Thickening of the tunica media in preacinar pulmonary arteries is the most common feature of pulmonary hypertension; it is difficult to evaluate in the newborn, especially the premature, without standardized preparations and data from normal infants [534].

Preacinar vascular pulmonary arteries are extremely sensitive to hypoxia, as well as to a variety of hormones, histamines, sympathetic and parasympathetic vasoactive amines [548, 549], prostaglandins [550–552], and vasoactive medications [553]. They may contract and give the tunica media a thickened appearance even in the absence of clinically evident PAH. Increased muscular artery tone may lead to increased pressure in the main pulmonary trunk and also in the muscular arteries themselves [554]. Increased left atrial or pulmonary venous pressure may cause pulmonary arteries to constrict and thereby restrict flow.

The relationship between the pulmonary and systemic vascular resistance affects blood flow through the ductus arteriosus and the foramen ovale, and the neonate with PPHN may have a right-to-left shunt at either site. Before birth, the airless fetal lungs filled with amniotic fluid are perfused through markedly constricted pulmonary arteries. The systemic circulation, including the placenta, has a lower resistance and shunts blood away from the lungs through the ductus arteriosus and the foramen ovale. After birth the ductus arteriosus and foramen ovale gradually close. Because the pulmonary resistance falls immediately after birth and the ductus closes within 1 or 2 days, there is no significant shunting in the newborn. The foramen ovale may remain patent for months or even indefinitely, but the normal pressure relationships prevent significant shunting. Right-to-left shunting across fetal channels may persist if resistance to pulmonary blood flow remains elevated after birth and cyanosis develops when pulmonary resistance exceeds systemic resistance. Ductal shunting may be intermittent or absent when resistances are relatively balanced. However, because right ventricular compliance continues to be lower than normal, a right-to-left shunt across the foramen ovale may persist if pulmonary arterial pressure is less than systemic levels [517].

Primary PPHN

The primary form of PPHN has no apparent pulmonary or cardiovascular cause and may be rapidly fatal. The typical infant is born at or near term and has central cyanosis associated with right-to-left shunting at the ductus arteriosus or foramen ovale, increased pulmonary vascular resistance, decreased pulmonary blood flow, and hypoxemia but no parenchymal lung disease or congenital heart defect. The hemodynamics mimic the fetal circulation, and these infants are said to have "persistence of fetal circulation" (PFC) [555]. The term "persistent hypertension of the newborn" [548] has been used interchangeably with PFC, but should be reserved for broader application because the PAH may have one or more specific causes [544]. Occasional cases may not show signs until after the first week of life [549].

Infants dying with primary PPHN usually have normal sized lungs, and a widely patent ductus arteriosus, with or without a significant patent foramen ovale. Their preacinar muscular arteries have quantifiable muscular thickening and there is muscle cell "extension" into the tunica media of nonmuscular intra-acinar arteries ($<30\,\mu m$ external diameter), which accompany respiratory bronchioles and supply the alveolar ducts and alveoli [556, 557]. Many of those arterial walls have double the normal thickness and associated narrow lumina. The arterial changes may begin in utero, possibly from increased sensitivity to hypoxia or stress, from alterations in the flow characteristics of the fetal pulmonary vascular bed, or from primary failure of mechanisms governing arterial muscularization and tone [546, 557]. Other possibilities include effects of maternal or fetal vasoactive substances on vascular development [556].

Secondary PPHN

The clinical [553, 558] and arterial changes found in the primary PPHN and PFC also occur in other newborn conditions associated with PAH. Term newborns who have massive meconium aspiration often develop PPHN and have comparable changes in the intra-acinar vessels [559–561]. The peripheral vascular muscular development suggests that the process begins in utero. Thrombocytopenia and pulmonary artery thromboemboli are occasional components. The possibility exists that vasoactive substances including prostaglandins may play roles in the development of the muscularization of intra-acinar vessels and abnormal platelet aggregation [557, 562, 563].

Patients with bronchopulmonary dysplasia with damage to intrapulmonary arteries and capillaries may develop PAH with right ventricular hypertrophy and ischemic injury [475]. Long-term survivors have a wide range of changes, including reduced numbers of arterial profiles due to destruction of the vascular bed, thickened muscular arterial walls, and abnormal muscularization of peripheral intra-acinar arteries [564–567]. Animal studies suggest that oxygen damage in the newborn period is associated with decreased DNA synthesis, delayed alveolar maturation, and dysplastic pulmonary vascular development [564, 568]. Comparable destruction to the vascular bed occurs in acute respiratory distress syndromes (ARDS) where the microvascular changes in the various stages include extension of muscle into small peripheral arterioles, reduced number and volumes of small arteries, medial hypertrophy, and widespread thromboembolic occlusions of arteries [569].

A variety of cardiac and vascular anomalies and metabolic cardiomyopathies can mimic PFC [570–576]. In terms of their pathophysiology, they include conditions with 1) pulmonary venous hypertension as with hypoplastic mitral valve; 2) increased pulmonary blood flow as in transposition of the great arteries and aneurysms of the vein of Galen [474]; and 3) isolated ventricular septal defects [555]. Many of these conditions are associated with changes in the muscularity of preacinar and intra-acinar arteries.

A decreased pulmonary vascular bed due to pulmonary hypoplasia in a newborn infant usually causes a clinical picture resembling PFC. Probably the most common cause is congenital diaphragmatic hernia. The pleuroperitoneal canals close between 6 and 7 weeks after ovulation and the fetal midgut recoils from the umbilical coelom into the fetal abdominal cavity sometime between the 7th and 9th weeks after ovulation. If the closure of the pleuroperitoneal canals is delayed, or if the gut returns to the pleuroperitoneal cavity too early, the peritoneal contents may herniate into the affected pleural cavity and compromise pulmonary development. At birth, the infant promptly develops cyanosis, respiratory distress, and acidosis. The involved lung has markedly decreased pulmonary airways and vascular bed, a decrease in number of vessels per unit of lung tissue, and increased arterial wall thickness [577, 578]. Infants with surgically correctable defects may survive without complication or for an extended "honeymoon" period before succumbing with PAH, hypoxemia, and acidosis (579). Those with extremely large defects may succumb rapidly with persistent hypoxemia, acidosis, and severe pulmonary hypertension ("no honeymoon period"). All these lungs are smaller than normal and have fewer bronchial generations and alveoli than normal lungs of comparable age. The "no-honeymoon" lungs have a smaller pulmonary vascular bed with smaller intra-acinar arteries with thicker walls due to abnormal muscularization of the tunica media and resultant reduced vascular lumina [579]. The lungs of infants with oligohydramnios sequence associated with renal agenesis or dysplasia have features comparable to those of other underdeveloped lungs [580].

An unusual anomalous development of the pulmonary microcirculation recognized only at autopsy but presenting clinically with "idiopathic" and uncorrectable PPHN is termed *misalignment of pulmonary veins with alveolar capillary dysplasia*. The condition is characterized histologically by failure of the formation and ingrowth of alveolar capillaries that do not make contact with alveolar epithelium, thickening of the medial muscular layer of the pulmonary arterial branches, muscularization of intra-acinar arteries, thickened alveolar walls, and anomalously located pulmonary veins that accompany the pulmonary arteries within the same adventitial sheaths [581–584]. About half of the reported cases also have cardiovascular, gastrointestinal, genitourinary, and other anomalies. Familial cases [584, 585] and examples with phocomelia have been described [583, 585, 586].

REFERENCES

1. Gould SE, ed. *Pathology of the Heart and Blood Vessels*. 3rd ed. Springfield, IL: Charles C Thomas, 1968.
2. Becker AE, Anderson RH. *Pathology of Congenital Heart Disease*. London: Butterworths, 1981.
3. Arey JB. *Cardiovascular Pathology in Infants and Children*. Philadelphia: WB Saunders, 1984.
4. Freedom RM, Benson LN, Smallhorn JF. *Neonatal Heart Disease*. London: Springer-Verlag, 1992.
5. Moller JH, Neal WA. *Fetal, Neonatal, and Infant Cardiac Disease*. Norwalk, CT: Appleton and Lange, 1990.
6. Clark EB, Takao A. *Developmental Cardiology. Morphogenesis and Function*. Mount Kisco, NY: Futura, 1990.
7. Streeter GL. Developmental horizons in human embryos. *Contrib Embryol Carnegie Inst Wash* 1942; 30:211–45.
8. O'Rahilly R. The timing and sequences of events in human cardiogenesis. *Acta Anat* 1971; 79:70–5.
9. Manasek FJ. Determinants of heart shape in early embryos. *Federation Proc* 1981; 40:2011–6.
10. Sweeney LJ. A molecular view of cardiogenesis. *Experientia* 1988; 44:930–6.
11. Parker TG. Molecular biology of cardiac growth and hypertrophy. *Herz* 1993; 18:245–55.
12. Watanabe M, Timm M, Fallah-Najmabadi H. Cardiac expression of polysialylated NCAM in the chicken embryo: correlation with the ventricular conduction system. *Dev Dynam* 1992; 194:128–41.
13. Ganim JR, Luo W, Ponniah S, et al. Mouse phospholamban gene expression during development in vivo and in vitro. *Circ Res* 1992; 71:1021–30.
14. O'Brien TX, Lee KJ, Chien KR. Positional specification of ventricular myosin light chain 2 expression in the primitive murine heart tube. *Proc Natl Acad Sci USA* 1993; 90:5157–60.
14a. Mably JD, Liew CC. Factors involved in cardiogenesis and the regulation of cardiac-specific gene expression. *Circ Res* 1996; 79:4–13.
15. Akhurst RJ, Fitzpatrick DR, Fowlis DJ, et al. The role of TGF-beta s in mammalian development and neoplasia. *Mol Reprod Dev* 1992; 32:127–35.
15a. Mima T, Ueno H, Fischman DA, Williams LT, Mikawa T. Fibroblast growth factor receptor is required for in vivo cardiac myocyte proliferation at early embryonic stages of heart development. *Proc Natl Acad Sci USA* 1995; 92:467–71.
15b. Pennica D, King KL, Shaw KJ, et al. Expression cloning of cardiotrophin 1, a cytokine that induces cardiac myocyte hypertrophy. *Proc Natl Acad Sci USA* 1995; 92:1142–6.
16. Le Lievre CS, Le Douarin NM. Mesenchymal derivatives of the neural crest: analysis of chimaeric quail and chick embryos. *J Embryol Exp Morph* 1975; 34:125–54.
17. Kirby ML, Gale TF, Stewart DE. Neural crest cells contribute to normal aorticopulmonary septation. *Science* 1983; 220:1059–61.
18. Rychter Z. Analysis of relations between aortic arches and aorticopulmonary septum. *Birth Defects; OAS* 1978; XIV:443–8.
19. Kirby ML. Role of extracardiac factors in heart development. *Experientia* 1988; 44:944–51.
20. Kirby ML. Neural crest and the morphogenesis of Down syndrome with special emphasis on cardiovascular development. *Prog Clin Biol Res* 1991; 373:215–25.
21. Tomita H, Connuck DM, Leatherbury L, Kirby ML. Relation of early hemodynamic changes to final cardiac phenotype and survival after neural crest ablation in chick embryos. *Circulation* 1991; 84:1289–95.
22. Leatherbury L, Connuck DM, Kirby ML. Neural crest ablation versus sham surgical effects in a chick embryo model of defective cardiovascular development. *Pediatr Res* 1993; 33:628–31.
22a. Waldo KL, Kumiski DH, Kirby ML. Association of the cardiac neural crest with development of the coronary arteries in the chick embryo. *Anatom Rec* 1994; 239:315–31.
22b. Leatherbury L, Waldo K. Visual understanding of cardiac development: the neural crest's contribution. *Cell Mol Biol Res* 1995; 41:279–91.

23. Maron BJ, Hutchins GM. The development of the semilunar valves in the human heart. *Am J Pathol* 1974; 74:331–44.

24. Borg TK, Caulfield JB. The collagen matrix of the heart. *Federation Proc* 1981; 40:2037–41.

25. Thompson RP, Fitzharris TP. Morphogenesis of the truncus arteriosus of the chick embryo heart: its formation and migration of mesenchymal tissue. *Am J Anat* 1979; 154:545–56.

26. Anderson RH, Becker AE, Van Mierop LHS. What should we call the "crista"? *Br Heart J* 1977; 39:856–9.

27. Goor DA, Dische R, Lillehei CW. The conotruncus. I. Its normal inversion and conus absorption. *Circulation* 1972; 46:375–84.

28. Ackermann DM, Edwards WD. Anatomic basis for tomographic analysis of the pediatric heart at autopsy. *Perspect Pediatr Pathol* 1988; 12:44–68.

29. Edwards WD, Tajik AJ, Seward JB. Standardized nomenclature and anatomic basis for regional tomographic analysis of the heart. *Mayo Clin Proc* 1981; 56:479–97.

30. Rosenquist GC, Clark EB, Sweeney LJ, McAllister HA. The normal spectrum of mitral and aortic valve discontinuity. *Circulation* 1976; 54:298–301.

30a. Tacy TA, Vermilion RP, Ludomirsky A. Range of normal valve annulus size in neonates. *Am J Cardiol* 1995; 75:541–3.

30b. Benson CB, Brown DL, Doubilet PM, et al. Increasing curvature of the normal fetal ductus arteriosus with advancing gestational age. *Ultrasound Obstet Gynecol* 1995; 5:95–7.

30c. Mielke G, Peukert U, Krapp M, Schneider-Pungs J, Gembruch U. Fetal and transient neonatal right heart dilatation with severe tricuspid valve insufficiency in association with abnormally S-shaped kinking of the ductus arteriosus. *Ultrasound Obstet Gynecol* 1995; 5:338–41.

31. Van Praagh R. The segmental approach to diagnosis in congenital heart disease. *Birth Defects: OAS* 1972; 8(5):4–23.

32. Becker AE, Anderson RH. Cardiac pathology. In: Berry CL, ed. *Paediatric Pathology*. Berlin: Springer-Verlag, 1981.

33. Tynan MJ, Becker AE, Macartney FJ, et al. Nomenclature and classification of congenital heart disease. *Br Heart J* 1979; 41:544–53.

34. Calcaterra G, Anderson RH, Lau KC, Shinebourne EA. Dextrocardia—value of segmental analysis in its categorization. *Br Heart J* 1979; 42:497–507.

35. Berry CL. The examination of embryonic and fetal material in diagnostic histopathology laboratories. *J Clin Pathol* 1980; 33:317–26.

36. Rudolph AM. The changes in the circulation after birth. *Circulation* 1970, 41:343–59.

36a. Friedman AH and Fahey JT. The transition from fetal to neonatal circulation: normal responses and implications for infants with heart disease. *Semin Perinatol* 1993; 17:106–21.

36b. Abman SH. Pathogenesis and treatment of neonatal and postnatal pulmonary hypertension. *Curr Opin Pediatr* 1994; 6:239–47.

37. Gruenwald P. Fetal deprivation and placental pathology: concepts and relationships. *Perspect Pediatr Pathol* 1975; 2:101–50.

37a. Basu S, Datta BN and Khandelwal N. Morphologic changes in pulmonary vasculature with arteriographic correlation. *Angiology* 1996; 47:375–80.

38. Vogel JNK, McNamara DG, Hallman G, et al. Effects of mild chronic hypoxia on the pulmonary circulation in calves with reactive pulmonary hypertension. *Circ Res* 1967; 661–9.

39. Heath D, Edwards JE. Configuration of elastic tissue of pulmonary trunk in idiopathic pulmonary hypertension. *Circulation* 1960; 21:59–62.

40. Maron BJ, Verter J, Kapur S. Disproportionate ventricular septal thickening in the developing normal heart. *Circulation* 1978; 57:520–6.

41. Groves BM, Greenberg SD, Rosenberg HS, McCrady JD. Variation in ventricular weights of calf hearts at sea level. *Exper Mol Pathol* 1964; 3:230–4.

42. Rosenberg HS, Klima T, Henderson S, McNamara DG. Maturation of the aortic isthmus. *Cardiovasc Res Cent Bull* 1971; 10:47–56.

43. Benjamin DR, Wiegenstein L. Necrosis of the ductus arteriosus in premature infants. *Arch Path* 1972; 94:340–2.

44. Tynan M. The ductus arteriosus and its closure. *N Engl J Med* 1993; 329:1570–2.

44a. Chao RC, Ho ES, Hsieh KS. Doppler echocardiographic diagnosis of intrauterine closure of the ductus arteriosus. *Prenat Diagn* 1993; 13:989–94.

45. Harlass FE, Duff P, Brady K, Read J. Hydrops fetalis and premature closure of the ductus arteriosus: a review. *Obstet Gynecol Surv* 1989; 44:541–3.

45a. Downing GJ, Thibeault DW. Pulmonary vasculature changes associated with idiopathic closure of the ductus arteriosus. *Pediatr Cardiol* 1994; 15:71–5.

46. Bell EF, Warburton D, Stonestreet BS, Oh W. Effect of fluid administration on the development of symptomatic patent ductus arteriosus and congestive heart failure in premature infants. *N Engl J Med* 1980; 302:598–604.

47. Ho SY, Anderson RH. Anatomical closure of the ductus arteriosus: a study in 35 specimens. *J Anat* 1979; 128:829–36.

48. Silver MM, Freedom RM, Silver MD, Olley PM. The morphology of the human newborn ductus arteriosus: a reappraisal of its structure and closure with special reference to prostaglandin E1 therapy. *Hum Pathol* 1981; 12:1123–36.

48a. Slomp J, van Munsteren JC, Poelmann RE, et al. Formation of intimal cushions in the ductus arteriosus as a model for vascular intimal thickening. An immunohistochemical study of changes in extracellular matrix components. *Atherosclerosis* 1992; 93:25–39.

48b. Ibara S, Tokunaga M, Ikenoue T, et al. Histologic observation of the ductus arteriosus in premature infants with intrauterine growth retardation. *Perinatol* 1994; 14:411–6.

49. Dudell GG, Gersony WM. Patent ductus arteriosus in neonates with severe respiratory disease. *J Pediatr* 1984; 104:915–20.

50. Ghosh PK, Lubliner J, Mogilner M, Yakirevich V, Vidne BA. Patent ductus arteriosus in premature infants. *Tex Heart Inst J* 1986; 13:163–8.

51. Gittenberger-de Groot AC, van Ertbruggen I, Moulaert AJMG, Harinck E. The ductus arteriosus in the preterm infant: histologic and clinical observations. *J Pediatr* 1980; 96:88–93.

51a. Korula A, Calder AL, Neutze JM. Effects of prostaglandin E1 given in low doses on the histopathology of the arterial duct. *Int J Cardiol* 1991; 33:215–24.

51b. Gittenberger-de Groot AC, Strengers JL. Histopathology of the arterial duct (ductus arteriosus) with and without treatment with prostaglandin E1. *Int J Cardiol* 1988; 19:153–66.

52. Kitterman JA, Edmunds LH, Gregory GA, et al. Patent ductus arteriosus in premature infants. Incidence, relation to pulmonary disease and management. *N Engl J Med* 1972; 287:473–7.

53. Becker AE, Anderson RH. Atrial septal defects. In: *Pathology of Congenital Heart Disease*. London: Butterworths, 1981, pp. 67–75.

54. Tandon R, Edwards JE. Atrial septal defect in infancy: common association with other anomalies. *Circulation* 1974; 49:1005–10.

55. Loser H, Pfefferkorn JR, Themann H. Alcohol in pregnancy and fetal heart damage. *Klin Paediatr* 1992; 204:335–9.

56. Tikkanen J, Heinonen OP. Risk factors for atrial septal defect. *Eur J Epidemiol* 1992; 8:509–15.

56a. Mainwaring RD, Mirali-Akbar H, Lamberti JJ, Moore JW. Secundum-type atrial septal defects with failure to thrive in the first year of life. *J Card Surg* 1996; 11:116–20.

57. Mandelik J, Moodie DS, Sterba R, et al. Long-term follow-up of children after repair of atrial septal defects. *Cleve Clin J Med* 1994; 61:29–33.

58. Meijboom F, Hess J, Szatmari A, et al. Long-term follow-up (9 to 20 years) after surgical closure of atrial septal defect at a young age. *Am J Cardiol* 1993; 72:1431–4.

59. Radzik D, Davignon A, van Doesburg N, et al. Predictive factors for spontaneous closure of atrial septal defects diagnosed in the first 3 months of life. *J Am Coll Cardiol* 1993; 22:851–3.

60. Ferreira SM, Ho SY, Anderson RH. Morphological study of defects of the atrial septum within the oval fossa: implications for transcatheter closure of left-to-right shunt. *Br Heart J* 1992; 67:316–20.

61. Chan KC, Godman MJ. Morphological variations of fossa ovalis atrial septal defects (secundum): feasibility for transcutaneous closure with the clam-shell device. *Br Heart J* 1993; 69:52–5.

62. Philips SJ, Okies JE, Henken D, Sunderland CO, Starr A. Complex of secundum atrial septal defect and congestive heart failure in infants. *J Thorac Cardiovasc Surg* 1975; 70:696–700.

63. Toews WH, Nora JJ, Wolfe RR. Presentation of atrial septal defect in infancy. *JAMA* 1975; 234:1250–1.

64. Spangler JG, Feldt RH, Danielson GK. Secundum atrial septal defect encountered in infancy. *J Thorac Cardiovasc Surg* 1976; 71:398–401.

65. Hunt CE, Lucas RV Jr. Symptomatic atrial septal defect in infancy. *Circulation* 1973; 47:1042–8.

66. Wigglesworth JS. Abnormalities of atrial chambers. In: *Perinatal Pathology*. Philadelphia: WB Saunders, 1984, pp. 217–19.

67. Porcelli PJ Jr, Saller DN Jr, Duwaji MS, Cowett RM. Nonimmune fetal hydrops with isolated premature restriction of the foramen ovale. *J Perinatol* 1992; 12:37–40.

68. Bharati S, Patel AG, Varga P, Husain AN, Lev M. In utero echocardiographic diagnosis of premature closure of the foramen ovale with mitral regurgitation and large left atrium. *Am Heart J* 1991; 122:597–600.

68a. Coulson CC, Kuller JA. Nonimmune hydrops fetalis secondary to premature closure of the foramen ovale. *Am J Perinatol* 1994; 11:439–40.

69. Arey JB. Malformations of the atrial septum. In: *Cardiovascular Pathology in Infants and Children*. Philadelphia: WB Saunders, 1984, pp. 55–76.

70. Suzuki K, Doi S, Oku K, et al. Hypoplastic left heart syndrome with premature closure of foramen ovale: report of an unusual type of totally anomalous pulmonary venous return. *Heart Vessels* 1990; 5:117–19.

71. Titus JL, Rastelli GC. Anatomic features of persistent common atrioventricular canal. In: Feldt RH, ed. *Atrioventricular Canal Defects*. Philadelphia: WB Saunders, 1976.

72. Becker AE, Anderson RH. Atrioventricular septal defects: what's in a name? *J Thorac Cardiovasc Surg* 1982; 83:461–9.

73. Hutchins GM, Liebman MA, Moore GW, Gharagozloo F. Atrioventricular canal malformations interpreted as secondary to reduced compression upon the developing heart. *Am J Pathol* 1979; 95:579–96.

74. Yamaki S, Yasui H, Kado H, et al. Pulmonary vascular disease and operative indications in complete atrioventricular canal defect in early infancy. *J Thorac Cardiovasc Surg* 1993; 106:398–405.

75. Rizzoli G, Mazzucco A, Maizza F, et al. Does Down syndrome affect prognosis of surgically managed atrioventricular canal defects? *J Thorac Cardiovasc Surg* 1992; 104:945–53.

76. Fyfe DA, Buckles DS, Gillette PC, Crawford FC. Preoperative prediction of postoperative pulmonary arteriolar resistance after surgical repair of complete atrioventricular canal defect. *J Thorac Cardiovasc Surg* 1991; 102:784–9.

77. Storch TG, Mannick EE. Epidemiology of congenital heart disease in Louisiana: an association between race and sex and the prevalence of specific cardiac malformations. *Teratology* 1992; 46:271–6.

77a. Hyett JA, Moscoso G, Nicolaides KH. First-trimester nuchal translucency and cardiac septal defects in fetuses with trisomy 21. *Am J Obstet Gynecol* 1995; 172:1411–13.

78. Basson CT, Cowley GS, Solomon SD, et al. The clinical and genetic spectrum of the Holt-Oram syndrome. *N Engl J Med* 1994; 330:885–91.

79. Cousineau AJ, Lauer RM, Pierpont ME, et al. Linkage analysis of autosomal dominant atrioventricular canal defects: exclusion of chromosome 21. *Hum Genet* 1994; 93:103–8.

80. Wright JS, Newman DC. Complete and intermediate atrioventricular canal in infants less than a year old: observations of anatomical and pathological variants in left ventricular outflow tract. *Ann Thorac Surg* 1982; 33:171–3.

80a. Giamberti A, Marino B, di Carlo D, et al. Partial atrioventricular canal with congestive heart failure in the first year of life: surgical options. *Ann Thorac Surg* 1996; 62:151–4.

81. Freedom RM, Bini M, Rowe AD. Endocardial cushion defect and significant hypoplasia of the left ventricle: a distinct clinical and pathological entity. *Eur J Cardiol* 1978; 7:263–81.

82. Anderson RH, Lenox CC, Zuberbuhler JR. The morphology of ventricular septal defects. *Perspect Pediatr Pathol* 1984; 8:235–68.

83. Corone P, Douon F, Gaudeau S, et al. Natural history of ventricular septal defect. *Circulation* 1977; 55:908–15.

84. Becu LM, Fontana RS, DuShane JW, et al. Anatomic and pathologic studies in ventricular septal defect. *Circulation* 1956; 14:349–64.

85. Hoffman JIE, Rudolph AM. The natural history of ventricular septal defects in infancy. *Am J Cardiol* 1965; 16:634–53.

86. Soto B, Becker AE, Moulaert AJ, Lie JT, Anderson RH. Classification of ventricular septal defects. *Br Heart J* 1980; 43:332–43.

87. Hislop A, Haworth SG, Shinebourne EA, Reid L. Quantitative structural analysis of pulmonary vessels in isolated ventricular septal defect in infancy. *Br Heart J* 1975; 37:1014–21.

88. de Leval MR, Pozzi M, Starnes V, et al. Surgical management of doubly committed subarterial ventricular septal defects. *Circulation* 1988; 78(suppl III):40–6.

89. Arey JB. Malformations of the ventricular septum. In: *Cardiovascular Pathology in Infants and Children*. Philadelphia: WB Saunders, 1984, pp. 77–111.

90. Hiraishi S, Agata Y, Nowatari M, et al. Incidence and natural course of trabecular ventricular septal defect: two-dimensional echocardiography and color Doppler flow imaging study. *J Pediatr* 1992; 120:409–15.

91. Suzuki H, Minami Y, Maeda J, et al. Spontaneous closure of muscular ventricular septal defect during early infancy: a report of three cases. *J Cardiol* 1989; 19:647–53.

92. Trowitzsch E, Braun W, Stute M, Pielemeier W. Diagnosis, therapy, and outcome of ventricular septal defects in the 1st year of life: a two-dimensional colour-Doppler echocardiography study. *Eur J Pediatr* 1990; 149:758–61.

93. Nadas AS. Ventricular septal defect. Report on the joint study on the natural history of congenital heart disease. Summary and conclusions. *Circulation* 1977; 56(suppl 1):70–1.

93a. Nir A, Driscoll DJ, Edwards WD. Intrauterine closure of membranous ventricular septal defects: mechanism of closure in two autopsy specimens. *Pediatr Cardiol* 1994; 15:33–7.

94. Graffigna A, Minzioni G, Ressia L, Vigano M. Surgical ablation of ventricular tachycardia secondary to congenital ventricular septal aneurysm. *Ann Thorac Surg* 1994; 57:921–4.

95. Tandon R, Edwards JE. Aneurysm-like formations in relation to membranous ventricular septum. *Circulation* 1973; 47:1089–97.

96. Unsigned editorial. Natural history of ventricular septal defect. *Br Med J* 1971; 4:571–2.

97. Hoffman JIE, Rudolph AM, Heymann MA. Pulmonary vascular disease with congenital heart lesions: pathologic features and causes. *Circulation* 1981; 64:873–7.

98. Lev M, Bharati S. Double outlet right ventricle. Association with other cardiovascular anomalies. *Arch Pathol* 1973; 95:117–22.

98a. Anderson RH, Ho SY, Wilcox BR. The surgical anatomy of ventricular septal defect part IV: double outlet ventricle. *J Card Surg* 1996; 11:2–11.

99. Sridaromont S, Ritter DG, Feldt RH, Davis GD, Edwards JE. Double-outlet right ventricle. *Mayo Clin Proc* 1978; 53:555–77.

100. Becker AE, Anderson RH. Double outlet ventricles. In: *Pathology of Congenital Heart Disease*. London: Butterworths, 1981, pp. 297–307.

101. Arey JB. Tricuspid atresia. In: *Cardiovascular Pathology in Infants and Children*. Philadelphia: WB Saunders, 1984, pp. 141–8.

101a. Kumar A, Victorica BE, Gessner IH, Alexander JA. Tricuspid atresia and annular hypoplasia: report of a familial occurrence. *Pediatr Cardiol* 1994; 15:201–3.

101b. Grant JW. Congenital malformations of the tricuspid valve in siblings. *Pediatr Cardiol* 1996; 17:327–9.

102. Tandon R, Edwards JE. Tricuspid atresia. A re-evaluation and classification. *J Thorac Cardiovasc Surg* 1974; 67:530–42.

103. Anderson RH, Wilkinson JL, Gerlis LM, Smith A, Becker AE. Atresia of the right atrioventricular orifice. *Br Heart J* 1977; 39:414–28.

103a. Orie JD, Anderson C, Ettedgui JA, Zuberbuhler JR, Anderson RH. Echocardiographic-morphologic correlations in tricuspid atresia. *J Am Coll Cardiol* 1995; 26:750–8.

104. Becker AE, Anderson RH. Absent right atrioventricular connection. In: *Pathology of Congenital Heart Disease*. London: Butterworths, 1981, pp. 261–8.

105. Becker AE, Anderson RH. Tetralogy of Fallot. In: *Pathology of Congenital Heart Disease*. London: Butterworths, 1981, pp. 191–8.

106. Burke EC, Kirklin JW, Edwards JE. Sites of obstruction to pulmonary blood flow in the tetralogy of Fallot. *Bull Staff Meet Mayo Clin* 1951; 26:498–504.

107. Winn KJ, Hutchins GM. The pathogenesis of tetralogy of Fallot. *Am J Pathol* 1973; 73:157–72.

108. Hislop A, Reid L. Structural changes in the pulmonary arteries and veins in tetralogy of Fallot. *Br Heart J* 1973; 35:1178–83.

108a. Vobecky SJ, Williams WG, Trusler GA, et al. Survival analysis of infants under age 18 months presenting with tetralogy of Fallot. *Ann Thorac Surg* 1993; 56:944–50.

108b. Sousa Uva M, Chardigny C, Galetti L, et al. Surgery for tetralogy of Fallot at less than six months of age. Is palliation "old-fashioned"? *Eur J Cardiol Thorac Surg* 1995; 9:453–60.

108c. Seliem MA, Wu YT, Glenwright K. Relation between age at surgery and regression of right ventricular hypertrophy in tetralogy of Fallot. *Pediatr Cardiol* 1995; 16:53–5.

108d. Reddy VM, Liddicoat JR, McElhinney DB, et al. Routine primary repair of tetralogy of Fallot in neonates and infants less than three months of age. *Ann Thorac Surg* 1995; 60(suppl 6):S592–6.

109. Anderson RH, Becker AE, Freedom RM, et al. Problems in the nomenclature of the univentricular heart. *Herz* 1979; 4:97–106.

110. Van Mierop LHS. Embryology of the univentricular heart. *Herz* 1979; 4:78–85.

111. de la Cruz MV. Different concepts of univentricular heart. *Herz* 1979; 4:67–72.

112. van Praagh R, Plett JA, van Praagh S. Single ventricle. Pathology, embryology and classification. *Herz* 1979; 4:113–50.

113. Van Praagh R, Van Praagh S, Vlad P, Keih JD. Diagnosis of the anatomic types of single or common ventricle. *Am J Cardiol* 1965; 15:345–66.

114. Quero-Jimenez M, Cameron AH, Acerete F, Quero-Jimenez C. Univentricular hearts: pathology of the atrioventricular valves. *Herz* 1979; 4:161–5.

115. Anderson RH, Tynan M, Freedom RM, et al. Ventricular morphology in the univentricular heart. *Herz* 1979; 4:184–97.

116. Wilkinson JL, Becker AE, Tynan M, et al. Nomenclature of the univentricular heart. *Herz* 1979; 4:107–12.

117. Wilkinson JL, Keeton B, Dickinson DF, et al. Morphology and conducting tissue in univentricular hearts of right ventricular type. *Herz* 1979; 4:151–60.

118. Becker AE, Wilkinson JL, Anderson RH. Atrioventricular conduction tissues in univentricular hearts of left ventricular type. *Herz* 1979; 4:166–75.

119. Corazza G, Soliani M, Bava GL. Uhl's anomaly in a newborn. *Eur J Pediatr* 1981; 137:347–52.

120. Vecht RJ, Carmichael DJS, Gopal R, Philip G. Uhl's anomaly. *Br Heart J* 1979; 41:676–82.

121. Descalzo A, Canadas M, Cintado C, et al. Uhl's anomaly associated with pulmonary atresia. *Hum Pathol* 1980; 11(suppl):575–6.

122. Gerlis LM, Schmidt-Ott SC, Ho SY, Anderson RH. Dysplastic conditions of the right ventricular myocardium: Uhl's anomaly vs arrhythmogenic right ventricular dysplasia. *Br Heart J* 1993; 69:142–50.

123. Gruter J, Jornod J, Enrico JF, Baumann RP. Arrhythmogenic ventricular dysplasia or Uhl's disease? *Schweiz Med Wochenschr* 1989; 119:582–7.

124. Tabib A, Loire R. Anatomoclinical study of 100 cases of hypoplasia of the right ventricular muscle (including 89 unexpected sudden deaths). Relation with Uhl's anomaly. *Arch Mal Coeur Vaiss* 1992; 85:1789–95.

124a. Daliento L, Turrini P, Nava A, et al. Arrhythmogenic right ventricular cardiomyopathy in young versus adult patients: similarities and differences. *J Am Coll Cardiol* 1995; 25:655–64.

125. Solenthaler M, Ritter M, Candinas R, et al. Right ventricular dysplasia (right ventricular cardiomyopathy). Clinical aspects, diagnosis and course in 15 patients from the Zurich area. *Schweiz Med Wochenschr* 1993; 123:1604–14.

125a. Basso C, Thiene G, Corrado D, et al. Arrhythmogenic right ventricular cardiomyopathy. Dysplasia, dystrophy, or myocarditis? *Circulation* 1996; 94:983–91.

125b. Rampazzo A, Nava A, Danieli GA, et al. The gene for arrhythmogenic right ventricular cardiomyopathy maps to chromosome 14q23–q24. *Hum Mol Genet* 1994; 3:959–62.

125c. Rampazzo A, Nava A, Erne P, et al. A new locus for arrhythmogenic right ventricular cardiomyopathy (ARVD2) maps to chromosome 1q42–q43. *Hum Mol Genet* 1995; 4:2151–4.

126. Becker AE, Becker MJ, Edwards JE. Pathologic spectrum of dysplasia of the tricuspid valve. Features in common with Ebstein's malformation. *Arch Pathol* 1971; 91:167–78.

127. Bogren HG, Ikeda R, Riemenscheider TA, Merten DF, Janos GG. Massive congenital tricuspid insufficiency in the newborn. *Acta Radiologica Diagn* 1979; 20:261–72.

128. Zuberbuhler JR, Allwork SP, Anderson RH. The spectrum of Ebstein's anomaly of the tricuspid valve. *J Thorac Cardiovasc Surg* 1979; 77:202–11.

129. Anderson KR, Zuberbuhler JR, Anderson RH, Becker AE, Lie JT. Morphologic spectrum of Ebstein's anomaly of the heart. *Mayo Clin Proc* 1979; 54:174–80.

130. Sharland GK, Chita SK, Allan LD. Tricuspid valve dysplasia or displacement in intrauterine life. *J Am Coll Cardiol* 1991; 17:944–9.

131. Hornberger LK, Sahn DJ, Kleinman CS, Copel JA, Reed KL. Tricuspid valve disease with significant tricuspid insufficiency in the fetus: diagnosis and outcome. *J Am Coll Cardiol* 1991; 17:167–73.

132. Perry JC, Garson A Jr. Supraventricular tachycardia due to Wolff-Parkinson-White syndrome in children: early disappearance and late recurrence. *J Am Coll Cardiol* 1990; 16:1215–20.

133. Stellin G, Santini F, Thiene G, et al. Pulmonary atresia, intact ventricular septum, and Ebstein anomaly of the tricuspid valve. Anatomic and surgical considerations. *J Thorac Cardiovasc Surg* 1993; 106:255–61.

134. Moore GW, Hutchins GM, Britq JC, Kang H. Congenital malformations of the semilunar valves. *Hum Pathol* 1980; 11:367–72.

135. Zuberbuhler JR, Anderson RH. Morphological variations in pulmonary atresia with intact ventricular septum. *Br Heart J* 1979; 41:281–8.

136. Freed MD, Rosenthal A, Bernhard WF, Litwin SB, Nadas AS. Critical pulmonary stenosis with a diminutive right ventricle in neonates. *Circulation* 1973; 48:875–81.

137. Harinck E, Becker AE, Gittenberger-De Groot AC, Oppenheimer-Dekker A, Versprille A. The left ventricle in congenital isolated pulmonary valve stenosis. *Br Heart J* 1977; 39:429–35.

138. Shams A, Fowler RS, Trusler GA, Keith JD, Mustard WT. Pulmonary atresia with intact ventricular septum: report of 50 cases. *Pediatrics* 1971; 47:370–7.

139. Van Praagh R, Ando M, Van Praagh S, et al. Pulmonary atresia: anatomic considerations. In: Kidd BSL, Rowe RD, eds. *The Child with Congenital Heart Disease After Surgery.* Mt. Kisco, NY: Futura, 1976, p. 103.

140. Freedom RM, Dische RM, Rowe RD. The tricuspid valve in pulmonary atresia and intact ventricular septum. *Arch Pathol Lab Med* 1978; 102:28–31.

141. Bharati S, McAllister HA, Chiemmongkoltip P, Lev M. Congenital pulmonary atresia with tricuspid insufficiency: morphologic study. *Am J Cardiol* 1977; 40:70–5.

142. Freedom RM, Harrington DP. Contributions of intramyocardial sinusoids in pulmonary atresia and intact ventricular septum to a right-sided circular shunt. *Br Heart J* 1974; 36:1061–5.

142a. Oosthoek PW, Moorman AF, Sauer U, Gittenberger-de Groot AC. Capillary distribution in the ventricles of hearts with pulmonary atresia and intact ventricular septum. *Circulation* 1995; 91:1790–8.

142b. Waldman JD, Karp RB, Gittenberger-de Groot AC, Agarwala B, Glagov S. Spontaneous acquisition of discontinuous pulmonary arteries. *Ann Thorac Surg* 1996; 62:161–8.

143. Shapira N, Heidelberger K, Behrendt D, Rosenthal A. The pulmonary vasculature in pulmonary valvar stenosis. *Am J Cardiol* 1980; 45:450.

143a. Seaver LH, Pierpont JW, Erickson RP, Donnerstein RL, Cassidy SB. Pulmonary atresia associated with maternal 22q11.2 deletion: possible parent of origin effect in the conotruncal anomaly face syndrome. *J Med Genet* 1994; 31:830–4.

143b. Digilio MC, Marino B, Grazioli S, et al. Comparison of occurrence of genetic syndromes in ventricular septal defect with pulmonic stenosis (classic tetralogy of Fallot) versus ventricular septal defect with pulmonic atresia. *Am J Cardiol* 1996; 77:1375–6.

143c. Bull K, Somerville J, Ty E, Spiegelhalter D. Presentation and attrition in complex pulmonary atresia. *J Am Coll Cardiol* 1995; 25:491–9.

144. Davachi F, Moller JH, Edwards JE. Diseases of the mitral valve in infancy. An anatomic analysis of 55 cases. *Circulation* 1971; 43:565–79.

145. Sreeram N, Walsh K, Nobre A, et al. Absent left-sided atrioventricular connexion, with right atrium connected to left ventricle: prospective diagnosis in infancy, and outcome. *Int J Cardiol* 1992; 34:7–19.

146. Kadoba K, Jonas RA, Mayer JE, Castaneda AR. Mitral valve replacement in the first year of life. *J Thorac Cardiovasc Surg* 1990; 100:762–8.

147. Hurwitz RA, Caldwell RL, Girod DA, Brown J, King H. Clinical and hemodynamic course of infants and children with anomalous left coronary artery. *Am Heart J* 1989; 118:1176–81.

147a. Moore P, Adatia I, Spevak PJ, et al. Severe congenital mitral stenosis in infants. *Circulation* 1994; 89:2099–106.

148. Moreno F, Quero M, Diaz LP. Mitral atresia with normal aortic valve. A study of eighteen cases and a review of the literature. *Circulation* 1976; 53:1004–10.

149. Mickell JJ, Mathews RA, Park SC, et al. Left atrioventricular valve atresia: clinical management. *Circulation* 1980; 61:123–7.

150. Noonan JA, Nadas AS. The hypoplastic left heart syndrome. *Pediatr Clin N Am* 1958; 5:1029–56.

151. Roberts WC, Perry LW, Chandra RS, et al. Aortic valve atresia: a new classification based on necropsy study of 73 cases. *Am J Cardiol* 1976; 37:753–6.

152. Bulkley BH, Weisfeldt ML, Hutchins GM. Isometric cardiac contraction. A possible cause of the disorganized myocardial pattern of idiopathic hypertrophic subaortic stenosis. *N Engl J Med* 1977; 296:135–9.

153. Cheitlin MD, Robinowitz M, McAllister H, et al. The distribution of fibrosis in the left ventricle in congenital aortic stenosis and coarctation of the aorta. *Circulation* 1980; 62:823–30.

154. Mahowald JM, Lucas RV Jr, Edwards JE. Aortic valvular atresia. Associated cardiovascular anomalies. *Pediatr Cardiol* 1982; 2:99–105.

155. Freedom RM, Williams WG, Dische MR, Rowe RD. Anatomical variants in aortic atresia. Potential candidates for ventriculoaortic reconstitution. *Br Heart J* 1976; 38:821–6.

156. Thiene G, Gallucci V, Macartney FJ, et al. Anatomy of aortic atresia. Cases presenting with a ventricular septal defect. *Circulation* 1979; 59:173–8.

157. van der Horst RL, Hastreiter AR, DuBrow IW, Eckner FAO. Pathologic measurements in aortic atresia. *Am Heart J* 1983; 106:1411–15.

157a. Remmell-Dow DR, Bharati S, Davis JT, Lev M, Allen HD. Hypoplasia of the eustachian valve and abnormal orientation of the limbus of the foramen ovale in hypoplastic left heart syndrome. *Am Heart J* 1995; 130:148–52.

157b. Lovell MA, McDaniel NL. Association of hypertrophic maxillary frenulum with hypoplastic left heart syndrome. *J Pediatr* 1995; 127:749–50.

157c. Grobman W, Pergament E. Isolated hypoplastic left heart syndrome in three siblings. *Obstet Gynecol* 1996; 88:673–5.

157d. Consevage MW, Seip JR, Belchis DA, et al. Association of a mosaic chromosomal 22q11 deletion with hypoplastic left heart syndrome. *Am J Cardiol* 1996; 77:1023–5.

157e. Guenthard J, Buehler E, Jaeggi E, Wyler F. Possible genes for left heart formation on 11q23.3. *Ann de Genetique* 1994; 37:143–6.

158. Beckman CB, Moller JH, Edwards JE. Alternate pathways to pulmonary venous flow in left-sided obstructive anomalies. *Circulation* 1975; 52:509–16.

159. O'Connor WN, Cash JB, Cottrill CM, Johnson GL, Noonan JA. Ventriculocoronary connections in hypoplastic left hearts: an autopsy microscopic study. *Circulation* 1982; 66:1078–86.

159a. Abu-Harb M, Wyllie J, Hey E, Richmond S, Wren C. Presentation of obstructive left heart malformations in infancy. *Arch Dis Child* 1994; 71:F179–83.

160. BuLock FA, Joffe HS, Jordan SC, Martin RP. Balloon dilatation (valvoplasty) as first line treatment for severe stenosis of the aortic valve in early infancy: medium term results and determinants of survival. *Br Heart J* 1993; 70:546–53.

161. Bogers AJ, Sreeram N, Hess J, Sutherland GR, Quaegebeur JM. Aortic atresia with normal left ventricle: one-stage repair in early infancy. *Ann Thorac Surg* 1991; 51:312–14.

162. Norwood WI, Lang P, Hansen DD. Physiologic repair of aortic atresia–hypoplastic left heart syndrome. *N Engl J Med* 1983; 308:23–6.

163. Grant CA, Robertson B. Microangiography of the pulmonary arterial system in hypoplastic left heart syndrome. *Circulation* 1972; 45:382–8.

163a. Gaynor JW, Elliott MJ. Congenital left ventricular outflow tract obstruction. *J Heart Valve Dis* 1993; 2:80–93.

164. Berman W Jr, Yabek SM, Fripp RR, et al. Medical management of three asymptomatic infants with severe valvar aortic stenosis. *Pediatr Cardiol* 1988; 9:237–42.

165. DuShane JW, Edwards JE. Congenital aortic stenosis in association with endocardial sclerosis of the left ventricle. *Proc Staff Meet Mayo Clin* 1954; 29:102–8.

166. Blieden LC, Lucas RV Jr, Carter JB, Miller K, Edwards JE. A developmental complex including supravalvular stenosis of the aorta and pulmonary trunk. *Circulation* 1974; 49:585–90.

167. Houyel L, Van Praagh R, Lacour-Gayet F, et al. Transposition of the great arteries [S,D,L]. Pathologic anatomy, diagnosis, and surgical management of a newly recognized complex. *J Thorac Cardiovasc Surg* 1995; 110:613–24.

168. Tynan MJ, Anderson RH. Terminology of transposition of the great arteries. In: Godman MJ, Marquiz RM, eds. *Paediatric Cardiology, Vol. 2: Heart Disease in the Newborn.* Edinburgh: Churchill Livingstone, 1979.

169. Rashkind WJ. The natural and unnatural history of transposition of the great arteries. *Birth Defects: OAS* 1972; 8:35–43.

169a. Gilljam T. Transposition of the great arteries in western Sweden 1964–83. Incidence, survival, complications and modes of death. *Acta Paediatrica* 1996; 85:825–31.

169b. Serraf A, Lacour-Gayet F, Bruniaux J, et al. Anatomic correction of transposition of the great arteries in neonates. *J Am Coll Cardiol* 1993; 22:193–200.

169c. Kumar A, Taylor GP, Sandor GG, Patterson MW. Pulmonary vascular disease in neonates with transposition of the great arteries and intact ventricular septum. *Br Heart J* 1993; 69:442–5.

169d. Pasquini L, Sanders SP, Parness IA, et al. Conal anatomy in 119 patients with d-loop transposition of the great arteries and ventricular septal defect: an echocardiographic and pathologic study. *J Am Coll Cardiol* 1993; 21:1712–21.

170. Van Praagh R, Durnin RE, Jockin H, et al. Anatomically corrected malposition of the great arteries (SDL). *Circulation* 1975; 51:20–31.

171. Victorica BE, Krovetz LJ, Elliott LP, et al. Persistent truncus arteriosus in infancy. *Am Heart J* 1969; 77:13–25.

172. Bartelings MM, Gittenberger-de-Groot AC. Morphogenetic considerations on congenital malformations of the outflow tract. Part 1: Common arterial trunk and tetralogy of Fallot. *Int J Cardiol* 1991; 32:213–30.

173. Suzuki A, Ho SY, Anderson RH, Deanfield JE. Coronary arterial and sinusal anatomy in hearts with a common arterial trunk. *Ann Thorac Surg* 1989; 48:792–7.

174. de la Cruz MV, Cayre R, Angelini P, Noriega-Ramos N, Sadowinski S. Coronary arteries in truncus arteriosus. *Am J Cardiol* 1990; 66:1482–6.

175. Fuglestad SJ, Puga FJ, Danielson GK, Edwards WD. Surgical pathology of the truncal valve: a study of 12 cases. *Am J Cardiovasc Pathol* 1988; 2:39–47.

176. Collett RW, Edwards JE. Persistent truncus arteriosus: a classification according to anatomic types. *Surg Clin N Amer* 1949; 29:1245–70.

177. Hanley FL, Heinemann MK, Jonas RA, et al. Repair of truncus arteriosus in the neonate. *J Thorac Cardiovasc Surg* 1993; 105:1047–56.

177a. Gamallo C, Garcia M, Palacios J, Rodriguez JI. Decrease in calcitonin-containing cells in truncus arteriosus. *Am J Med Genet* 1993; 46:149–53.

178. Moene RJ, Oppenheimer-Dekker A, Moulaert AJ, et al. The concurrence of dimensional aortic arch anomalies and abnormal left ventricular muscle bundles. *Pediatr Cardiol* 1982; 2:107–14.

179. Oppenheimer-Dekker A, Gittenberger-de Groot AC, Roozendaal H. The ductus arteriosus and associated cardiac anomalies in interruption of the aortic arch. *Pediatr Cardiol* 1982; 2:185–93.

180. Ho SY, Anderson RH. Coarctation, tubular hypoplasia, and the ductus arteriosus. *Br Heart J* 1979; 41:268–74.

180a. Zannini L, Gargiulo G, Albanese SB, et al. Aortic coarctation with hypoplastic arch in neonates: a spectrum of anatomic lesions requiring different surgical options. *Ann Thorac Surg* 1993; 56:288–94.

181. McNamara DG, Rosenberg HS. Coarctation of the aorta. In: Watson H, ed. *Paediatric Cardiology.* London: Lloyd-Luke, 1968, pp. 175–223.

181a. Gerboni S, Sabatino G, Mingarelli R, Dallapiccola B. Coarctation of the aorta, interrupted aortic arch, and hypoplastic left heart syndrome in three generations. *J Med Genet* 1993; 30:328–9.

182. Morgan J. Evidence of non-genetic origin of coarctation of the aorta. *Can Med Assoc J* 1969; 100:1134–8.

183. Miettinen OS, Reiner ML, Nadas AS. Seasonal incidence of coarctation of the aorta. *Br Heart J* 1970; 32:103–7.

184. Rosenberg HS. Coarctation of the aorta: morphology and pathogenetic considerations. *Perspect Pediatr Pathol* 1973; 1:339–68.

185. Becker AE, Becker MJ, Edwards JE. Anomalies associated with coarctation of aorta. Particular reference to infancy. *Circulation* 1970; 41:1067–75.

186. Edwards JE, Carey LS, Neufeld HH, Lester RG. Coarctation of the aorta. In: *Congenital Heart Disease.* Philadelphia: WB Saunders, 1965, pp. 677–703.

187. Riemenschneider TA, Emmanouilides GC, Hirose F, Linde LM. Coarctation of the abdominal aorta in children: report of three cases and review of the literature. *Pediatrics* 1969; 44:716–26.

188. Dean RH, Scott HW Jr. Subisthmic aortic coarctations. In: Dean RH, O'Neill JA Jr, eds. *Vascular Disorders of Childhood.* Philadelphia: Lea and Febiger, 1983, pp. 51–66.

189. Kappetein AP, Gittenberger-de Groot AC, Zwinderman AH, et al. The neural crest as a possible pathogenetic factor in coarctation of the aorta and bicuspid aortic valve. *J Thorac Cardiovasc Surg* 1991; 102:830–6.

189a. Gotzsche CO, Krag-Olsen B, Nielsen J, Sorensen KE, Kristensen BO. Prevalence of cardiovascular malformations and association with karyotypes in Turner's syndrome. *Arch Dis Child* 1994; 71:433–6.

190. Lacro RV, Jones KL, Benirschke K. Coarctation of the aorta in Turner syndrome: a pathologic study of fetuses with nuchal cystic hygromas, hydrops fetalis, and female genitalia. *Pediatrics* 1988; 81:445–51.

191. Kalousek DK, Seller MJ. Differential diagnosis of posterior cervical hygroma in previable fetuses. *Am J Med Genet* 1987; 3(suppl):83–92.

192. Rosenberg HS, Klima T, Henderson SR, McNamara DG. Maturation of the aortic isthmus. *Cardiovasc Res Cent Bull* 1971; 10:47–56.

193. Rudolph AM, Heymann MA, Spitznas U. Hemodynamic considerations in the development of narrowing of the aorta. *Am J Cardiol* 1972; 30:514–24.

194. Wielenga G, Dankmeijer J. Coarctation of the aorta. *J Pathol Bacteriol* 1968; 95:265–74.

195. Skoda J. Protokoll der Sections-Sitzung fur Physiologie and pathologie, am 19. October 1855. *Wbl Z KK Ges Aerzte Wien* 1855; 1:720–5.

196. Rudolph AM, Heymann MA. Coarctation of the aorta in the fetal and neonatal periods. *Birth Defects: OAS* 1972; 8:19–21.

197. Rosenberg HS. Coarctation as a deformation. *Pediatr Pathol* 1990; 10:103–15.

198. Ho SY, Anderson RH. Coarctation of the aorta. In: Godman MJ, Marquiz RM, eds. *Paediatric Cardiology,* vol. 2, *Heart Disease in the Newborn.* Edinburgh: Churchill Livingstone, 1979, pp. 173–86.

199. Sinha SN, Kardatzke ML, Cole RB, et al. Coarctation of the aorta in infancy. *Circulation* 1969; 40:385–98.

200. Petracek MR, Hammon JW Jr. Thoracic aortic (isthmic) coarctation. In: Dean RH, O'Neill JA Jr, eds. *Vascular Disorders of Childhood.* Philadelphia: Lea and Febiger, 1983, pp. 36–50.

201. Celoria GC, Patton RB. Congenital absence of the aortic arch. *Am Heart J* 1959; 58:407–13.

202. McNama.a DG, Rosenberg HS. Interruption of the aortic arch. In: Watson H, ed. *Paediatric Cardiology.* London: Lloyd-Luke, 1968, pp. 224–32.

202a. Nakada T, Yoneska S. Interruption of aortic arch type A in two siblings. *Acta Paediatrica Japonica* 1996; 38:63–5.

203. Freedom RM, Bain HH, Esplugas E, Dische R, Rowe RD. Ventricular septal defect in interruption of aortic arch. *Am J Cardiol* 1977; 39:572–82.

204. Van Mierop LHS, Kutsche LM. Cardiovascular anomalies in DiGeorge syndrome and importance of neural crest as a possible pathogenetic factor. *Am J Cardiol* 1986; 58:133–7.

205. Clark EB. Mechanisms in the pathogenesis of congenital cardiac malformations. In: Pierpont ME, Moller JH, eds. *The Genetics of Cardiovascular Disease.* Boston: Martinus Nijhof, 1986, pp. 3–11.

206. Esplugas E. Interruption of the aorta—anatomical, clincal [sic] and angiocardiographic observations. In: Dean RH, O'Neill JA Jr, eds. *Vascular Disorders of Childhood*. Philadelphia: Lea and Febiger, 1983, pp. 187–95.

207. Dische MR, Tsai M, Baltaxe HA. Solitary interruption of the arch of the aorta. *Am J Cardiol* 1975; 35:271–7.

208. Losman JG, Joffe HS, Beck W, Barnard C. Successful total repair of interrupted aortic arch associated with ventricular septal defect and large patent ductus arteriosus. *Am J Cardiol* 1974; 33:566–71.

209. Ledwith MV, Duff DF. A review of vascular rings 1980–1992. *Irish Med J* 1994; 87:178–9.

209a. Roberts CS, Othersen HB Jr, Sade RM, et al. Tracheoesophageal compression from aortic arch anomalies: analysis of 30 operatively treated children. *J Pediatr Surg* 1994; 29:334–7.

209b. Anand R, Dooley KJ, Williams WH, Vincent RN. Follow-up of surgical correction of vascular anomalies causing tracheobronchial compression. *Pediatr Cardiol* 1994; 15:58–61.

210. Thomson AH, Beardsmore CS, Firmin R, Leanage R, Simpson H. Airway function in infants with vascular rings: preoperative and postoperative assessment. *Arch Dis Child* 1990; 65:171–4.

211. van Aalderen WM, Hoekstra MO, Hess J, Gerritsen J, Knol K. Respiratory infections and vascular rings. *Acta Paediat Scand* 1990; 79:477–80.

212. Edwards JE. Anomalies of the aortic arch system. *Birth Defects: OAS* 1977; 13:47–63.

213. Edwards JE. Vascular rings. In: Gould SE, ed. *Pathology of the Heart and Blood Vessels*. 3rd ed. Springfield, IL: Charles C Thomas, 1968, pp. 433–44.

214. Landing BH, Wells TR. Tracheobronchial anomalies in children. *Perspect Pediatr Pathol* 1973; 1:1–32.

215. Sade RM, Rosenthal A, Fellow K, Castenada AR. Pulmonary artery sling. *J Thorac Cardiovasc Surg* 1975; 69:333–46.

216. Bove KE, Geiser EA, Meyer RA. The left ventricle in anomalous pulmonary venous return. *Arch Pathol* 1975; 99:522–8.

216a. Bleyl S, Ruttenberg HD, Carey JC, Ward K. Familial total anomalous pulmonary venous return: a large Utah-Idaho family. *Am J Med Genet* 1994; 52:462–6.

216b. Bleyl S, Nelson L, Odelberg SJ, et al. A gene for familial total anomalous pulmonary venous return maps to chromosome 4p13–q12. *Am J Hum Genet* 1995; 56:408–15.

217. Gersony WM. Presentation, diagnosis and natural history of total anomalous pulmonary venous drainage. In: Godman MJ, Marquis RM, eds. *Paediatric Cardiology*. vol. 2. *Heart Disease in the Newborn*. Edinburgh: Churchill Livingstone, 1979, pp. 463–73.

218. McNamara DG, Mullins CE, El-Said G. The unnatural history of total anomalous pulmonary venous return: medical management in the young infant. *Birth Defects: OAS* 1972; 8:32–4.

219. Neill CA. Development of pulmonary veins: with reference to the embryology of anomalies of pulmonary venous return. *Pediatrics* 1956; 18:880–7.

220. Haworth SG, Reid L. Structural study of pulmonary circulation and of heart in total anomalous pulmonary venous return in early infancy. *Br Heart J* 1977; 39:80–92.

221. James CL, Keeling JW, Smith NM, Byard RW. Total anomalous pulmonary venous drainage associated with fatal outcome in infancy and early childhood. *Pediatr Pathol* 1994; 14:665–78.

222. Engle ME. Total anomalous pulmonary venous drainage. *Circulation* 1972; 46:209–11.

223. Raisher BD, Grant JW, Martin TC, Strauss AW, Spray TL. Complete repair of total anomalous pulmonary venous connection in infancy. *J Thorac Cardiovasc Surg* 1992; 104:443–8.

224. Lupinetti FM, Kulik TJ, Beekman RH III, Crowley DC, Bove EL. Correction of total anomalous pulmonary venous connection in infancy. *J Thorac Cardiovasc Surg* 1993; 106:880–5.

225. Jordan JD, McNamara DG, Marcontell J, Rosenberg HS. Cor triatriatum: an anatomic and physiologic study. *Cardiovasc Res Cent Bull* 1963; 1:79–85.

226. van Son JA, Danielson GK, Schaff HV, et al. Cor triatriatum: diagnosis, operative approach, and late results. *Mayo Clin Proc* 1993; 68:854–9.

227. Nagatsu-M. Clinical classification and surgical treatment of cor triatriatum. *Nippon Kyobu Geka Gakkai Zasshi (Journal of the Japanese Association for Thoracic Surgery)* 1992; 40:473–84.

228. Marin-Garcia J, Tandon R, Lucas RV Jr, Edwards JE. Cor triatriatum: study of 20 cases. *Am J Cardiol* 1975; 35:59–66.

229. Driscoll DJ, Hesslein PS, Mullins CE. Congenital stenosis of individual pulmonary veins: clinical spectrum and unsuccessful treatment by transvenous balloon dilation. *Am J Cardiol* 1982; 49:1767–72.

230. Bini RM, Cleveland DC, Cebalos R, et al. Congenital pulmonary vein stenosis. *Am J Cardiol* 1984; 54:369–75.

231. Becker AE, Becker MJ, Edwards JE. Occlusion of pulmonary veins, "mitral" insufficiency, and ventricular septal defect. *Am J Dis Child* 1970; 120:557–9.

232. Rywlin AM, Fojaco RM. Congenital pulmonary lymphangiectasis associated with a blind common pulmonary vein. *Pediatrics* 1968; 41:931–4.

233. Hawker RE, Celermajer JM, Gengos DC, Cartmill TB, Bowdler JB. Common pulmonary vein atresia. Premortem diagnosis in two infants. *Circulation* 1972; 46:368–74.

234. Shimazaki Y, Nakano S, Kato H, et al. Mixed type of total anomalous pulmonary venous connection with hemi-pulmonary vein atresia. *Ann Thorac Surg* 1993; 56:1399–1401.

235. Spray TL, Mallory GB, Canter CB, Huddleston CB. Pediatric lung transplantation. Indications, techniques, and results. *J Thorac Cardiovasc Surg* 1994; 107:990–9.

236. Moragas A, Huguet P, Toran N, Rona V. Morphogenesis of pulmonary veno-occlusive disease in a newborn. *Path Res Pract* 1983; 176:176–84.

236a. Justo RN, Dare AJ, Whight CM, Radford DJ. Pulmonary veno-occlusive disease: diagnosis during life in four patients. *Arch Dis Child* 1993; 68:97–100.

237. Muller G, Schaller A. Ectopia cordis cervicalis. *Teratology* 1982; 25:277–81.

238. Geva T, Van Praagh S, Van Praagh R. Thoracoabdominal ectopia cordis with isolated infundibular atresia. *Am J Cardiol* 1990; 66:891–3.

239. Toyama WM. Combined congenital defects of the anterior abdominal wall, sternum, diaphragm, pericardium, and heart. *Pediatrics* 1972; 50:778–92.

240. Martin RA, Cunniff C, Erickson L, Jones KL. Pentalogy of Cantrell and ectopia cordis, a familial developmental field complex. *Am J Med Genet* 1992; 42:839–41.

241. Van Allen MI, Myhre S. New multiple, congenital anomalies syndrome in a stillborn infant of consanguinous parents and a prediabetic pregnancy. *Am J Med Genet* 1991; 38:523–8.

241a. Sepulveda W, Weiner E, Bower S, et al. Ectopia cordis in a triploid fetus: first-trimester diagnosis using transvaginal color Doppler ultrasonography and chorionic villus sampling. *J Clin Ultrasound* 1994; 22:573–5.

242. Fox JE, Gloster ES, Mirchandani R. Trisomy 18 with Cantrell pentalogy in a stillborn infant. *Am J Med Genet* 1988; 31:391–4.

243. Bick D, Markowitz RI, Horwich A. Trisomy 18 associated with ectopia cordis and occipital meningocele. *Am J Med Genet* 1988; 30:805–10.

244. Arey JB. Ectopia cordis. In: *Cardiovascular Pathology in Infants and Children*. Philadelphia: WB Saunders, 1984, pp. 37–39.

245. Medina-Escobedo G, Reyes-Mugica M, Arteaga-Martinez M. Ectopia cordis: autopsy findings in four cases. *Pediatr Pathol* 1991; 11:85–95.

246. Bogers AJ, Hazebroek FW, Hess J. Left and right ventricular diverticula, ventricular septal defect and ectopia cordis in a patient with Cantrell's syndrome. *Eur J Cardiothorac Surg* 1993; 7:334–5.

247. Jones AF, McGrath RL, Edwards SM, Lilly JR. Immediate operation for ectopia cordis. *Ann Thorac Surg* 1979; 28:484–6.

248. Van Der Horst RL, Mitha AS, Chesler E. Ectopia with single ventricle and a diverticulum. *S Afr Med J* 1975; 40:109–11.

249. Tachibana H, Gan K, Oshima Y, et al. Thoracoabdominal ectopia cordis with single ventricle and pulmonary stenosis. *Nippon Kyobu Geka Gakkai Zasshi (Journal of the Japanese Association for Thoracic Surgery)* 1989; 37:148–53.

250. Ivemark BI. Implications of agenesis of the spleen on the pathogenesis of conotruncus anomalies in childhood: an analysis of the heart malformations in the splenic agenesis syndrome with fourteen new cases. *Acta Paediatr* 1955; 44(suppl 104):1–56.

251. Monie IW. The asplenia syndrome: an explanation for the absence of the spleen. *Teratology* 1982; 25:215–19.

252. Freedom RM. The asplenia syndrome: a review of significant extracardiac structural abnormalities in 29 necropsied patients. *J Pediatr* 1972; 81:1130–3.

252a. Casey B, Devoto M, Jones KL, Ballabio A. Mapping a gene for familial situs abnormalities to human chromosome Xq24–q27.1. *Nat Genet* 1993; 5:403–7.

252b. Casey B, Cuneo BF, Vitali C, et al. Autosomal dominant transmission of familial laterality defects. *Am J Med Genet* 1996; 61:325–8.

252c. Devriendt K, Casaer A, Van Cauter A, et al. Asplenia syndrome and isolated total anomalous pulmonary venous connection in siblings. *Eur J Pediatr* 1994; 153:712–14.

253. Van Mierop LHS, Gessner IH, Schiebler GL. Asplenia and polysplenia syndrome. *Birth Defects: OAS* 1972; 8(1):74–82.

253a. Phoon CK, Neill CA. Asplenia syndrome: insight into embryology through an analysis of cardiac and extracardiac anomalies. *Am J Cardiol* 1994; 73:581–7.

254. Van Praagh R, Van Praagh S. Atrial isomerism in the heterotaxy syndromes with asplenia, or polysplenia, or normally formed spleen: an erroneous concept. *Am J Cardiol* 1990; 66:1504–6.

255. Ho SY, Cook A, Anderson RH, Allan LD, Fagg N. Isomerism of the atrial appendages in the fetus. *Pediatr Pathol* 1991; 11:589–608.

256. Vitiello R, Moller JH, Marino B, et al. Pulmonary circulation in pulmonary atresia associated with the asplenia cardiac syndrome. *J Am Coll Cardiol* 1992; 20:363–5.

256a. Heinemann MK, Hanley FL, Van Praagh S, et al. Total anomalous pulmonary venous drainage in newborns with visceral heterotaxy. *Ann Thorac Surg* 1994; 57:88–91.

256b. James CL, Keeling JW, Smith NM, Byard RW. Total anomalous pulmonary venous drainage associated with fatal outcome in infancy and early childhood: an autopsy study of 52 cases. *Pediatr Pathol* 1994; 14:665–78.

256c. Rubino M, Van Praagh S, Kadoba K, Pessotto R, Van Praagh R. Systemic and pulmonary venous connections in visceral heterotaxy with asplenia. Diagnostic and surgical considerations based on seventy-two autopsied cases. *J Thoracic Cardiovasc Surg* 1995; 110:641–50.

257. Becker AE, Anderson RH. Atrial isomerism ("situs ambiguus"). In: *Pathology of Congenital Heart Disease*. London: Butterworths, 1981.

258. Landing BH, Hatayama C, Wells TR, Diehl EJ, Lee T-YK. Five syndromes (malformation complexes) of pulmonary symmetry, congenital heart disease, and multiple spleens. *Pediatr Pathol* 1984; 2:125–51.

259. Gupta R, Carachi R. Pseudopericardial cyst in a neonate—a case report and review of the literature. *Z Kinderchir* 1989; 44:162–3.

260. Schiavone WA, Rice TW. Pericardial disease: current diagnosis and management methods. *Cleve Clin J Med* 1989; 56:639–45.

260a. Lu C, Ridker PM. Echocardiographic diagnosis of congenital absence of the pericardium in a patient with VATER association defects. *Clin Cardiol* 1994; 17:503–4.

261. Arey JB. Defects of the parietal pericardium. In: *Cardiovascular Pathology in Infants and Children*. Philadelphia: WB Saunders, 1984, pp. 200–1.

262. Becker AE, Anderson RH. The pericardium. In *Pathology of Congenital Heart Disease*. London: Butterworths, 1981, pp. 413–15.

263. Prahlow JA, Teot LA. Histiocytoid cardiomyopathy: case report and literature review. *J Foren Sci* 1993; 38:1427–35.

264. Jacob B, Haarhoff K, Neuen-Jacob E, et al. Unexpected infant death attributable to cardiac tumor or cardiomyopathy. Immunohistochemical and electron microscopical findings in three cases. *Zeitschrift fur Rechtsmedizin (Journal of Legal Medicine)* 1990; 103:335–43.

264a. Koponen MA, Siegel RJ. Histiocytoid cardiomyopathy and sudden death. *Hum Pathol* 1996; 27:420–3.

264b. Ruszkiewicz AR, Vernon-Roberts E. Sudden death in an infant due to histiocytoid cardiomyopathy. A light-microscopic, ultrastructural, and immunohistochemical study. *Am J Foren Med Pathol* 1995; 16:74–80.

265. Gharagozloo F, Porter CJ, Tazelaar HD, Danielson GK. Multiple myocardial hamartomas causing ventricular tachycardia in young children: combined surgical modification and medical treatment. *Mayo Clin Proc* 1994; 69:262–7.

266. Kearney DL, Titus JL, Hawkins EP, Ott DA, Garson A Jr. Pathologic features of myocardial hamartomas causing childhood tachyarrhythmias. *Circulation* 1987; 75:7905–10.

266a. Malhotra V, Ferrans VJ, Virmani R. Infantile histiocytoid cardiomyopathy: three cases and literature review. *Am Heart J* 1994; 128:1009–21.

267. Ferrans VJ, McAllister HA Jr, Haese WH. Infantile cardiomyopathy with histiocytoid change in cardiac muscle cells. *Circulation* 1976; 53:708–19.

268. Haese WH, Maron BJ, Mirowski M, Rowe RD, Hutchins GM. Peculiar focal myocardial degeneration and fatal ventricular arrhythmias in a child. *N Engl J Med* 1972; 287:180–1.

269. Witzleben CL, Pinto M. Foamy myocardial transformation in infancy: "lipid" or "histiocytoid" myocardiopathy. *Arch Pathol Lab Med* 1978; 102:306–11.

270. Silver MM, Burns JE, Sethi RK, Rowe RD. Oncocytic cardiomyopathy in an infant with oncocytosis in exocrine and endocrine glands. *Hum Pathol* 1980; 11:598–605.

271. Franciosi RA, Singh A. Oncocytic cardiomyopathy syndrome. *Hum Pathol* 1988; 19:1361–2.

272. Amini M, Bosman C, Marino B. Histiocytoid cardiomyopathy in infancy: a new hypothesis? *Chest* 1980; 77:556–8.

272a. Richardson P, McKenna W, Bristow M, et al. Report of the 1995 World Health Organization/International Society and Federation of Cardiology Task Force on the Definition and Classification of Cardiomyopathies. *Circulation* 1996; 93:841–2.

272b. Landing BH, Recalde AL, Lawrence TY, Shankle WR. Cardiomyopathy in childhood and adult life, with emphasis on hypertrophic cardiomyopathy. *Pathol Res Prac* 1994; 190:737–49.

272c. Tang TT, Segura AD, Chen YT, et al. Neonatal hypotonia and cardiomyopathy secondary to type IV glycogenosis. *Acta Neuropathologica* 1994; 87:531–6.

272d. Pitkanen S, Merante F, McLeod DR, et al. Familial cardiomyopathy with cataracts and lactic acidosis: a defect in complex I (NADH-dehydrogenase) of the mitochondria respiratory chain. *Pediatr Res* 1996; 39:513–21.

272e. Ozawa T. Mitochondrial DNA mutations in myocardial diseases. *Eur Heart J* 1995; 16(suppl O):10–14.

272f. Orstavik KH, Skjorten F, Hellebostad M, Haga P, Langslet A. Possible X linked congenital mitochondrial cardiomyopathy in three families. *J Med Genet* 1993; 30:269–72.

273. Thierfelder L, MacRae C, Watkins H, et al. A familial hypertrophic cardiomyopathy locus maps to chromosome 15q2. *Proc Natl Acad Sci USA* 1993; 90:6270–4.

274. Shah PM. IHSS-HOCM-MSS-ASH. *Circulation* 1975; 51:577–80.

275. Kawai C, Takatasu T. Clinical and experimental studies on cardiomyopathy. *N Engl J Med* 1975; 293:592–7.

276. Goodwin JF. Prospects and predictions for the cardiomyopathies. *Circulation* 1974; 50:210–19.

277. Henry WL, Clark CE, Epstein SE. Asymmetric septal hypertrophy (ASH): the unifying link in the IHSS disease spectrum. *Circulation* 1973; 47:827–32.

278. Maron BJ, Edwards JE, Henry WH, et al. Asymmetric septal hypertrophy (ASH) in infancy. *Circulation* 1974; 50:809–20.

279. Henry WL, Clark CE, Roberts WC, Morrow AG, Epstein SE. Differences in distribution of myocardial abnormalities in patients with obstructive and nonobstructive asymmetric septal hypertrophy. *Circulation* 1974; 50:447–55.

280. Maron BJ, Ferrans VJ, Henry WL, et al. Differences in distribution of myocardial abnormalities in patients with obstructive and nonobstructive asymmetric septal hypertrophy (ASH). *Circulation* 1974; 50:436–46.

281. Maron BJ, Tajik AJ, Ruttenberg HD, et al. Hypertrophic cardiomyopathy in infants: clinical features and natural history. *Circulation* 1982; 64:7–15.

282. Maron BJ, Roberts WC. Quantitative analysis of cardiac muscle cell disorganization in the ventricular septum of patients with hypertrophic cardiomyopathy. *Circulation* 1979; 59:680–706.

283. Edwards WD, Zakheim R, Mattioli L. Asymmetric septal hypertrophy in childhood. *Hum Pathol* 1977; 8:277–84.

284. Olsen EGJ. The pathology of idiopathic hypertrophic subaortic stenosis (hypertrophic cardiomyopathy). *Am Heart J* 1980; 100:553–62.

285. Maron BJ, Edwards JE, Moller JH, Epstein SE. Prevalence and characteristics of disproportionate ventricular septal thickening in infants with congenital heart disease. *Circulation* 1979; 59:126–33.

285a. Gill AW, Warner G, Bull L. Iatrogenic neonatal hypertrophic cardiomyopathy. *Pediatr Cardiol* 1996; 17:335–9.

285b. Weiner JC, Sicard RE, Hansen TW, et al. Hypertrophic cardiomyopathy associated with dexamethasone therapy for bronchopulmonary dysplasia. *J Pediatr* 1992; 120:286–91.

285c. Bensky AS, Kothadia JM, Covitz W. Cardiac effects of dexamethasone in very low birth weight infants. *Pediatrics* 1996; 97(6 Pt 1):818–21.

285d. Israel BA, Sherman FS, Guthrie RD. Hypertrophic cardiomyopathy associated with dexamethasone therapy for chronic lung disease in preterm infants. *Am J Perinatol* 1993; 10:307–10.

286. Craig JM. Congenital endocardial sclerosis. *Bull Int Assoc Med Museums* 1949; 30:15–67.

287. Neill CA, Ursell P. Endocardial fibroelastosis and left heart hypoplasia revisited. *Int J Cardiol* 1984; 5:547–50.

288. Ursell PC, Neill CA, Anderson RH, et al. Endocardial fibroelastosis and hypoplasia of the left ventricle in neonates without significant aortic stenosis. *Br Heart J* 1984; 51:492–7.

289. Carceller AM, Maroto E, Fouron JC. Dilated and contracted forms of primary endocardial fibroelastosis: a single fetal disease with two stages of development. *Br Heart J* 1990; 63:311–13.

290. Ferencz C, Neill CA. Cardiomyopathy in infancy: observations in an epidemiologic study. *Pediatr Cardiol* 1992; 13:65–71.

291. Factor SM. Endocardial fibroelastosis: myocardial and vascular alterations associated with viral-like nuclear particles. *Am Heart J* 1978; 96:791–801.

292. Black-Schaffer B. Infantile endocardial fibroelastosis. *Arch Pathol* 1957; 63:281–306.

293. Newbould MJ, Armstrong GR, Barson AJ. Endocardial fibroelastosis in infants with hydrops fetalis. *J Clin Pathol* 1991; 44:576–9.

294. Orstavik KH, Skjorten F, Hellebostad M, Haga P, Langslet A. Possible X linked congenital mitochondrial cardiomyopathy in three families. *J Med Genet* 1993; 30:269–72.

295. Ades LC, Gedeon AK, Wilson MJ, et al. Barth syndrome: clinical features and confirmation of gene localisation to distal Xq28. *Am J Med Genet* 1993; 45:327–34.

296. Stephan MJ, Stevens EL Jr, Wenstrup RJ, et al. Mucopolysaccharidosis I presenting with endocardial fibroelastosis of infancy. *Am J Dis Child* 1989; 143:782–4.

297. Tripp ME, Katchur ML, Peters HA. Systemic carnitine deficiency presenting as familial endocardial fibroelastosis. *N Engl J Med* 1981; 305:385–90.

297a. Bennett MJ, Hale DE, Pollitt RJ, Stanley CA, Variend S. Endocardial fibroelastosis and primary carnitine deficiency due to a defect in the plasma membrane carnitine transporter. *Clin Cardiol* 1996; 19:243–6.

298. Hutchins GM, Vie S. The progression of interstitial myocarditis to idiopathic endocardial fibroelastosis. *Am J Pathol* 1972; 66:483–96.

299. Hilton DA, Variend S, Pringle JH. Demonstration of coxsackievirus RNA in formalin-fixed tissue sections from childhood myocarditis cases by in situ hybridization and the polymerase chain reaction. *J Pathol* 1993; 170:45–51.

299a. Ni J, Bowles NE, Kim YH, et al. Viral infection of the myocardium in endocardial fibroelastosis. Molecular evidence for the role of mumps virus as an etiologic agent. *Circulation* 1997; 95:133–9.

300. Wolfe RR, Way GL. Cardiomyopathies in infants of diabetic mothers. *Johns Hopkins Med J* 1977; 140:177–80.

301. Driscoll SG, Benirschke K, Curtis GW. Neonatal deaths among infants of diabetic mothers. *Am J Dis Child* 1960; 100:818–35.

302. Neave C. Congenital malformation in offspring of diabetics. *Perspect Pediatr Pathol* 1984; 8:213–22.

303. Rowland TW, Hubbell JP Jr, Nadas AS. Congenital heart disease in infants of diabetic mothers. *J Pediatr* 1973; 83:815–20.

304. Naeye RL. Infants of diabetic mothers: a quantitative, morphologic study. *Pediatrics* 1965; 35:980–8.

305. Gutgesell HP, Speer ME, Rosenberg HS. Characterization of the cardiomyopathy in infants of diabetic mothers. *Circulation* 1980; 61:441–50.

306. Morriss FH Jr. Infants of diabetic mothers: fetal and neonatal pathophysiology. *Perspect Pediatr Pathol* 1984; 8:223–34.

307. Breitweiser JA, Meyer RA, Sperling MA, et al. Cardiac septal hypertrophy in hyperinsulinemic infants. *J Pediatr* 1980; 96:536–9.

308. Reller MD, Kaplan S. Hypertrophic cardiomyopathy in infants of diabetic mothers: an update. *Am J Perinatol* 1988; 5:353–8.

309. McMahon JN, Berry PJ, Joffe HS. Fatal hypertrophic cardiomyopathy in an infant of a diabetic mother. *Pediatr Cardiol* 1990; 11:211–12.

310. Halliday HL. Hypertrophic cardiomyopathy in infants of poorly-controlled diabetic mothers. *Arch Dis Child* 1981; 56:258–63.

311. Jones CJ, Lendon M, Chawner LE, Jauniaux E. Ultrastructure of the human placenta in metabolic storage disease. *Placenta* 1990; 11:395–411.

312. Zhong N, Martiniuk F, Tzall S, Hirschhorn R. Identification of a missense mutation in one allele of a patient with Pompe disease, and use of endonuclease digestion of PCR-amplified RNA to demonstrate lack of mRNA expression from the second allele. *Am J Hum Genet* 1991; 49:635–45.

313. Hermans MM, de Graaff E, Kroos MA, et al. Identification of a point mutation in the human lysosomal alpha-glucosidase gene causing infantile glycogenosis type II. *Biochem Biophys Res Commun* 1991; 179:919–26.

314. Park HK, Kay HH, McConkie Rosell A, Lanman J, Chen YT. Prenatal diagnosis of Pompe's disease (type II glycogenosis) in chorionic villus biopsy using maltose as a substrate. *Prenat Diagn* 1992; 12:169–73.

314a. Huie ML, Chen AS, Brooks SS, Grix A, Hirschhorn R. A de novo 13 nt deletion, a newly identified C647W missense mutation and a deletion of exon 18 in infantile onset glycogen storage disease type II (GSDII). *Hum Mol Genet* 1994; 3:1081–7.

314b. Kroos MA, Van der Kraan M, Van Diggelen OP, Kleijer WJ, Reuser AJ. Two extremes of the clinical spectrum of glycogen storage disease type II in one family: a matter of genotype. *Hum Mutation* 1997; 9:17–22.

314c. Reuser AJ, Kroos MA, Hermans MM, et al. Glycogenosis type II (acid maltase deficiency). *Muscle Nerve* 1995; 3:S61–9.

314d. Raben N, Nichols RC, Boerkoel C, Plotz P. Genetic defects in patients with glycogenosis type II (acid maltase deficiency). *Muscle Nerve* 1995; 3:S70–4.

315. Van Maldergem L, Haumont D, Saurty D, Jauniaux E, Loeb H. Bradycardia in a case of type II glycogenosis (Pompe's disease) revealing in early neonatal period. *Acta Clin Belg* 1990; 45:412–14.

316. Fung KP. Lo RN, Ho HC. Pompe's disease presenting as supraventricular tachycardia. *Aust Paediatr J* 1989; 25:101–2.

317. Seifert BL, Snyder MS, Klein AA, et al. Development of obstruction to ventricular outflow and impairment of inflow in glycogen storage disease of the heart: serial echocardiographic studies from birth to death at 6 months. *Am Heart J* 1992; 123:239–42.

318. Martin JJ, de Barsy T, van Hoff F, Palladini G. Pompe's disease. *Acta Neuropathol (Berl)* 1973; 23:229–44.

319. Eto K, Takeuchi T. An autopsy case of glycogen and nonglycogen polysaccharide storage disease with cardiomegaly. *Acta Pathol Jpn* 1973; 23:189–209.

320. Hudgson P, Fulthorpe JJ. The pathology of type II skeletal muscle glycogenosis. *J Pathol* 1975; 116:139–47.

320a. Schonian U, Crombach M, Maser S, Maisch B. Cytomegalovirus-associated heart muscle disease. *Eur Heart J* 1995; 16(suppl O):46–9.

321. Towbin JA, Griffin LD, Martin AB, et al. Intrauterine adenoviral myocarditis presenting as nonimmune hydrops fetalis: diagnosis by polymerase chain reaction. *Pediatr Infect Dis J* 1994; 13:144–50.

322. Saint Martin J, Bonnaud E, Morinet F, Choulot JJ, Mensire A. Acute parvovirus myocarditis with fatal outcome. *Pediatrie (Bucur)* 1991; 46:597–9.

323. Berry PJ, Gray ES, Porter HJ, Burton PA. Parvovirus infection of the human fetus and newborn. *Semin Diagn Pathol* 1992; 9:4–12.

324. Buyon JP. Neonatal lupus syndromes. *Am J Reprod Immunol* 1992; 28:259–63.

325. Rosenberg HS. Cardiovascular effects of congenital infections. *Am J Cardiovasc Pathol* 1987; 1:147–56.

326. Woodruff JF. Viral myocarditis. *Am J Pathol* 1980; 101:427–79.

327. Rose NR, Wolfgram LJ, Herskowitz A, Beisel KW. Postinfectious autoimmunity: two distinct phases of coxsackievirus B3-induced myocarditis. *Ann NY Acad Sci* 1986; 475:146–56.

328. Bowles NE, Richardson PJ, Olsen EG, Archard LC. Detection of coxsackie-B-virus-specific RNA sequences in myocardial biopsy samples from patients with myocarditis and dilated cardiomyopathy. *Lancet* 1986; 1:1120–3.

329. Foulis AK, Farquharson MA, Cameron SO, et al. A search for the presence of the enteroviral capsid protein VP1 in pancreases of patients with type 1 (coinsulin-dependent) diabetes and pancreases and hearts of infants who died of coxsackieviral myocarditis. *Diabetologia* 1990; 33:290–8.

329a. Martin AB, Webber S, Fricker FJ, et al. Acute myocarditis. Rapid diagnosis by PCR in children. *Circulation* 1994; 90:330–9.

329b. Nicholson F, Ajetunmobi JF, Li M, et al. Molecular detection and serotypic analysis of enterovirus RNA in archival specimens from patients with acute myocarditis. *Br Heart J* 1995; 74:522–7.

330. Rosenberg HS, McNamara DG. Acute myocarditis in infancy and childhood. *Prog Cardiovasc Dis* 1964; 7:179–97.

331. Saphir O, Cohen NA. Myocarditis in infancy. *Arch Pathol* 1957; 64:446–56.

332. Haddad J, Gut JP, Wendling MJ, et al. Enterovirus infections in neonates. A retrospective study of 21 cases. *Eur J Med* 1993; 2:209–14.

332a. Fujioka S, Koide H, Kitaura Y, et al. Molecular detection and differentiation of enteroviruses in endomyocardial biopsies and pericardial effusions from dilated cardiomyopathy and myocarditis. *Am Heart J* 1996; 131:760–5.

332b. Leparc I, Aymard M, Fuchs F. Acute, chronic and persistent enterovirus and poliovirus infections: detection of viral genome by seminested PCR amplification in culture-negative samples. *Mol Cell Probes* 1994; 8:487–95.

333. Gear JHS, Measroch V. Coxsackie virus infections of the newborn. *Prog Med Virol* 1973; 15:42–62.

334. Hosier DM, Newton WA Jr. Serious coxsackie infections in infants and children. *Am J Dis Child* 1958; 96:251–67.

334a. Stallion A, Rafferty JF, Warner BW, Ziegler MM, Ryckman FC. Myocardial calcification: a predictor of poor outcome for myocarditis treated with extracorporeal life support. *J Pediatr Surg* 1994; 29:492–4.

335. Burch GE. Ultrastructural myocardial changes produced by viruses. *Recent Adv Stud Card Struct Metab* 1975; 6:501–23.

336. Dische MR, Gooch WM III. Congenital toxoplasmosis. *Perspect Pediatr Pathol* 1981; 6:83–113.

337. Oppenheimer EH, Dahms BB. Congenital syphilis in the fetus and neonate. *Perspect Pediatr Pathol* 1981; 6:115–38.

338. Cooper LZ. Congenital rubella in the U.S. In: Krugman S, Gershon AA, eds. *Infections of the Fetus and Newborn Infant*. New York: Alan R Liss, 1975.

339. Rosenberg HS, Oppenheimer EH, Esterly JR. Congenital rubella syndrome: the later effects and their relation to early lesions. *Perspect Pediatr Pathol* 1981; 6:183–202.

340. Tang JS, Kaufman SL, Lynfield J. Hypoplasia of the pulmonary arteries in infants with congenital rubella. *Am J Cardiol* 1971; 27:491–6.

341. Singer DB, Rudolph AJ, Rosenberg HS, Rawls WE, Boniuk M. Pathology of the congenital rubella syndrome. *J Pediatr* 1967; 71:665–75.

342. Fortuin NJ, Morrow AG, Roberts WC. Late vascular manifestations of the rubella syndrome. *Am J Med* 1971; 51:134–40.

343. Cambell PE. Vascular abnormalities following maternal rubella. *Br Heart J* 1965; 27:134–8.

344. Rowe RD. Cardiovascular disease in the rubella syndrome. *Cardiovasc Clin* 1973; 5:61–80.

345. Esterly JR, Oppenheimer EH. Vascular lesions in infants with congenital rubella. *Circulation* 1967; 36:544–54.

346. Lawrenz Wolf B, Herrmann B. Pericardial tamponade caused by catheter infection in an extremely small premature infant. *Monatsschr Kinderheilkd* 1993; 141:932–5.

347. Kanarek KS, de Brigard T, Coleman J, Silbiger ML. Purulent pericarditis in a neonate. *Pediatr Infect Dis J* 1991; 10:549–50.

348. Gersony WM, McCracken GH Jr. Purulent pericarditis in infancy. *Pediatrics* 1967; 40:224–32.

349. Valdes-Dapena M, Miller WH. Pericarditis in the newborn. *Pediatrics* 1955; 16:673–6.

349a. Friedland IR, du Plessis J, Cilliers A. Cardiac complications in children with *Staphylococcus aureus* bacteremia. *J Pediatr* 1995; 127:746–8.

349b. Campbell PT, Li JS, Wall TC, et al. Cytomegalovirus pericarditis: a case series and review of the literature. *Am J Med Sci* 1995; 309:229–34.

349c. Dupuis C, Gronnier P, Kachaner J, et al. Bacterial pericarditis in infancy and childhood. *Am J Cardiol* 1994; 74:807–9.

350. Doshi N, Smith B, Klionsky B. Congenital pericarditis due to maternal lupus erythematosus. *J Pediatr* 1980; 96:699–701.

351. Pinar H, Rogers BB. Renal dysplasia, situs inversus totalis, and multisystem fibrosis: a new syndrome. *Pediatr Pathol* 1992; 12:215–21.

352. Moragas A, Vidal M-T. Granulomatous eosinophilic epicarditis in the newborn. *Arch Pathol* 1969; 88:459–62.

353. Millard DD, Shulman ST. The changing spectrum of neonatal endocarditis. *Clin Perinatol* 1988; 15:587–608.

354. Johnson DH, Rosenthal A, Nadas AS. Bacterial endocarditis in children under 2 years of age. *Am J Dis Child* 1975; 129:183–6.

355. Edwards K, Ingall D, Czapek E, Davis AT. Bacterial endocarditis in 4 young infants. *Clin Pediatr* 1977; 16:607–9.

356. Blieden LC, Morehead RR, Burke B, Kaplan EL. Bacterial endocarditis in the neonate. *Am J Dis Child* 1972; 124:747–9.

356a. Daher AH, Berkowitz FE. Infective endocarditis in neonates. *Clin Pediatr* 1995; 34:198–206.

356b. Rastogi A, Luken JA, Pildes RS, Chrystof D, LaBranche F. Endocarditis in neonatal intensive care unit. *Pediatr Cardiol* 1993; 14:183–6.

357. Perez-Benavides F, Park JM, Myers MK, Graham SC, Shehata BM. Sudden death in neonate with staphylococcal endocarditis. *J Perinatol* 1993; 13:285–7.

358. Weinberg AG, Laird WP. Group B streptococcal endocarditis detected by echocardiography. *J Pediatr* 1978; 92:335–6.

359. Franzek DA, Engle WA, Caldwell RL. Neonatal bacterial endocarditis of the pulmonary valve: report of two cases. *J Perinatol* 1987; 7:292–5.

360. Tulloh RM, Silove ED, Abrams LD. Replacement of an aortic valve cusp after neonatal endocarditis. *Br Heart J* 1990; 64:204–5.

361. Charaf L, Hallberg M, Henze A. Neonatal endocarditis requiring surgery. *Scand J Thorac Cardiovasc Surg* 1989; 23:79–80.

361a. Nomura F, Penny DJ, Menahem S, Pawade A, Karl TR. Surgical intervention for infective endocarditis in infancy and childhood. *Ann Thorac Surg* 1995; 60:90–5.

362. Johnson DH, Rosenthal A, Nadas AS. A forty-year review of bacterial endocarditis in infancy and childhood. *Circulation* 1975; 51:581–8.

363. Mendelsohn G, Hutchins GM. Infective endocarditis during the first decade of life. *Am J Dis Child* 1979; 133:619–22.

363a. Saiman L, Prince A, Gersony WM. Pediatric infective endocarditis in the modern era. *J Pediatr* 1993; 122:847–53.

364. Morrow WR, Haas JE, Benjamin DR. Nonbacterial endocardial thrombosis in neonates: relationship to persistent fetal circulation. *J Pediatr* 1982; 100:117–22.

365. Krous HF. Neonatal nonbacterial thrombotic endocarditis. *Arch Pathol Lab Med* 1979; 103:76–8.

366. McGuinness GA, Schieken RM, Maguire GF. Endocarditis in the newborn. *Am J Dis Child* 1980; 134:577–80.

366a. Tabbutt S, Griswold WR, Ogino MT, et al. Multiple thromboses in a premature infant associated with maternal phospholipid antibody syndrome. *J Perinatol* 1994; 14:66–70.

367. Oelberg DG, Fisher DJ, Gross DM, Denson SE, Adcock EW III. Endocarditis in high-risk neonates. *Pediatrics* 1983; 71:392–7.

368. Menahem S, Robbie MJ, Rajadurai VS. Valvar vegetations in the neonate due to fetal endocarditis. *Int J Cardiol* 1991; 32:103–5.

369. Symchych PS, Krauss AN, Winchester P. Endocarditis following intracardiac placement of umbilical venous catheters in neonates. *J Pediatr* 1977; 90:287–9.

370. Favara BE, Franciosi RA, Butterfield LJ. Disseminated intravascular and cardiac thrombosis of the neonate. *Am J Dis Child* 1974; 127:197–204.

371. Oppenheimer EH, Esterly JR. Nonbacterial thrombotic vegetations. Occurrence in neonate, infant, and child, and relation to valvular lesions in cardiac defects. *Am J Pathol* 1968; 53:63–73.

372. Bertolini P, Meisner H, Paek SU, Sebening F. Special considerations on primary cardiac tumors in infancy and childhood. *Thorac Cardiovasc Surg* 1990; 38(suppl 2):164–7.

372a. Takach TJ, Reul GJ, Ott DA, Cooley DA. Primary cardiac tumors in infants and children: immediate and long-term operative results. *Ann Thorac Surg* 1996; 62:559–64.

373. McAllister HA Jr, Fenoglio JJ Jr. Tumors of the cardiovascular system. In: *Atlas of Tumor Pathology*, Second series, Fascicle 15. Washington: Armed Forces Institute of Pathology, 1978.

374. Pasaoglu I, Demircin M, Ozkutlu S, Bozer AY. Right atrial myxoma in an infant. *Jpn Heart J* 1991; 32:263–6.

374a. Talmor D, Caspi J, Feuering S, et al. Surgical treatment of right ventricular myxoma in infancy. *Ann Thorac Surg* 1996; 61:1835–6.

375. Becker AE, Anderson RH. Cardiac tumours or tumour-like lesions. In: *Pathology of Congenital Heart Disease*. London: Butterworths, 1981, pp. 419–30.

375a. Cartagena AM, Levin TL, Issenberg H, Goldman HS. Pericardial effusion and cardiac hemangioma in the neonate. *Pediatr Radiol* 1993; 23:384–5.

375b. Kawakami K, Horigome H, Tsuchida M, et al. Right atrial hemangio-pericytoma with hemopericardium during infancy. *Pediatr Cardiol* 1995; 16:48–50.

376. Arey JB. Tumors of the heart and pericardium. In: *Cardiovascular Pathology in Infants and Children*. Philadelphia: WB Saunders, 1984, pp. 372–83.

377. Watson GH. Cardiac rhabdomyomas in tuberous sclerosis. *Ann NY Acad Sci* 1991; 615:50–7.

378. Ostor AG, Fortune DW. Tuberous sclerosis initially seen as hydrops fetalis. *Arch Pathol Lab Med* 1978; 102:34–9.

379. Massumi RA, Adkins PC, Reichelderfer TR, Fraga JR, Sampson R. Congenital rhabdomyoma of the heart. *J Thorac Cardiovasc Surg* 1968; 55:711–18.

380. Calhoun BC, Watson PT, Hegge F. Ultrasound diagnosis of an obstructive cardiac rhabdomyoma with severe hydrops and hypoplastic lungs. *J Reprod Med* 1991; 36:317–9.

381. Harding CO, Pagon RA. Incidence of tuberous sclerosis in patients with cardiac rhabdomyoma. *Am J Med Genet* 1990; 37:443–6.

382. Bosio M, Vitali GM, Pandolfi M, Pastori P. Cardiac rhabdomyoma in tuberous sclerosis. A report of five cases and review of the literature. *Minerva Pediatr* 1992; 44:305–11.

382a. Jozwiak S, Kawalec W, Dluzewska J, et al. Cardiac tumours in tuberous sclerosis: their incidence and course. *Eur J Pediatr* 1994; 153:155–7.

382b. Roach ES, Smith M, Huttenlocher P, et al. Diagnostic criteria: tuberous sclerosis complex. Report of the diagnostic criteria committee of the National Tuberous Sclerosis Association. *J Child Neurol* 1992; 7:221–4.

383. Smythe JF, Dyck JD, Smallhorn JF, Freedom RM. Natural history of cardiac rhabdomyoma in infancy and childhood. *Am J Cardiol* 1990; 66:1247–9.

384. De Conti F, Piovesana P, Viena P, Pantaleoni A. The complete regression of multiple cardiac rhabdomyomas in childhood. *G Ital Cardiol* 1993; 23:793–6.

384a. DiMario FJ Jr, Diana D, Leopold H, Chameides L. Evolution of cardiac rhabdomyoma in tuberous sclerosis complex. *Clin Pediatr* 1996; 35:615–19.

384b. Bosi G, Lintermans JP, Pellegrino P, Svaluto-Moreolo G, Vliers A. The natural history of cardiac rhabdomyoma with and without tuberous sclerosis. *Acta Paediatrica* 1996; 85:928–31.

385. Shrivastava S, Jacks JJ, White RS, Edwards JE. Diffuse rhabdomyomatosis of the heart. *Arch Pathol Lab Med* 1977; 101:78–80.

386. Fenoglio JJ Jr, Diana DJ, Bowen TE, McAllister HA, Ferrans VJ. Ultrastructure of a cardiac rhabdomyoma. *Hum Pathol* 1977; 8:700–6.

387. Silverman JF, Kay S, Chang CH. Ultrastructural comparison between skeletal muscle and cardiac rhabdomyomas. *Cancer* 1978; 42:189–93.

388. Fenoglio JJ Jr, McAllister HA Jr, Ferrans VJ. Cardiac rhabdomyoma: a clinicopathologic and electron microscopic study. *Am J Cardiol* 1976; 38:241–51.

389. Osmerova M, Nicovsky J, Necasova A, Balcarkova H, Jelinek Z. Pericardial teratoma in an infant. *Cesk Pediatr* 1990; 45:24–5.

390. Lakhoo K, Boyle M, Drake DP. Mediastinal teratomas: review of 15 pediatric cases. *J Pediatr Surg* 1993; 28:1161–4.

390a. Perez-Aytes A, Sanchis N, Barbal A, et al. Non-immunological hydrops fetalis and intrapericardial teratoma: case report and review. *Prenat Diagn* 1995; 15:859–63.

390b. Cowley CG, Tani LY, Judd VE, McGough EC, Minich LL. Intracardiac yolk sac tumor: echocardiographic evaluation. *Pediatr Cardiol* 1996; 17:196–7.

391. Rosenberg HS, Stenback WA, Spjut HJ. The fibromatoses of infancy and childhood. *Perspect Pediatr Pathol* 1978; 4:269–348.

391a. Beghetti M, Haney I, Williams WG, et al. Massive right ventricular fibroma treated with partial resection and a cavopulmonary shunt. *Ann Thorac Surg* 1996; 62:882–4.

392. Turi GK, Albala A, Fenoglio JJ Jr. Cardiac fibromatosis: an ultrastructural study. *Hum Pathol* 1980; 11(suppl):577–80.

393. Cooley DA. Surgical treatment of cardiac neoplasms. *Thorac Cardiovasc Surg* 1990; 38(suppl 2):176–82.

394. Yabek SM, Isabel-Jones J, Gyepes MT, Jarmakani JM. Cardiac fibroma in a neonate presenting with severe congestive heart failure. *J Pediatr* 1977; 91:310–12.

395. Rose AG. Fibrous histiocytoma of the heart. *Arch Pathol Lab Med* 1978; 102:389.

396. Filiatrault M, Beland MJ, Neilson KA, Paquet M. Cardiac fibroma presenting with clinically significant arrhythmias in infancy. *Pediatr Cardiol* 1991; 12:118–20.

397. Feldman PS, Meyer MW. Fibroelastic hamartoma (fibroma) of the heart. *Cancer* 1976; 38:314–23.

398. Begg JG. Blood-filled cysts in the cardiac valve cusps in foetal life and infancy. *J Pathol Bacteriol* 1964; 87:177–8.

399. Zimmerman KG, Paplanus SH, Dong S, Nagle RB. Congenital blood cysts of the heart valves. *Hum Pathol* 1983; 14:699–703.

400. Takeda T, Makita T, Nakamura N, Kimizuka G. Morphologic aspects and morphogenesis of blood cysts on canine cardiac valves. *Vet Pathol* 1991; 28:16–21.

401. Miles VN, Favara BE, Morriss JH, Prevedel AE, Hawes CR. Giant blood cyst and congenital pulmonic stenosis. *Am J Dis Child* 1975; 129:1079–81.

402. Xie SW, Lu OL, Picard MH. Blood cyst of the mitral valve: detection by transthoracic and transesophageal echocardiography. *J Am Soc Echocardiogr* 1992; 5:547–50.

403. Salas Valien JS, Ribas Arino MT, Palau Benavides MT, Gonzalez Moran MA. Varix of the heart causing outflow tract obstruction. *Histol Histopathol* 1991; 6:439–42.

404. Anderson RH, Ho SY, Smith A, Wilkinson JL. Study of the cardiac conduction tissues in the paediatric age group. *Diagn Histopathol* 1981; 4:3–15.

405. Davies MJ, Anderson RH, Becker AE. *The Conduction System of the Heart.* Boston: Butterworth, 1983.

406. Crick SC, Wharton J, Sheppard MN, et al. Innervation of the human cardiac conduction system. A quantitative immunohistochemical and histochemical study. *Circulation* 1994; 89:1697–1708.

407. Donnelly WH, Bucciarelli RL, Nelson RM. Ischemic papillary muscle necrosis in stressed newborn infants. *J Pediatr* 1980; 96:295–300.

408. Anderson KR, Ho SY, Anderson RH. The location and vascular supply of the sinus node in the human heart. *Br Heart J* 1979; 41:28–32.

409. Anderson RH, Becker AE. The morphology of the normal conducting system. In: Van Mierop LHS, Oppenheimer-Dekker A, Bruins CLD Ch, eds. *Embryology and Teratology of the Heart and Great Arteries.* Leiden: Leiden University Press, 1978, pp. 25–33.

410. Rombilt DW, Hackel DB, Estes EH Jr. Origin and blood supply of the sinoauricular and atrioventricular node. *Am Heart J* 1968; 75:279–80.

411. Anderson KR, Murphy JG. The atrioventricular node artery in the human heart. *Antgiology* 1983; 34:711–16.

412. Van der Hauwaert LG, Stroobrandt R, Verhaeghe L. Arterial blood supply of the atrioventricular node and main bundle. *Br Heart J* 1972; 34:1045–51.

413. Hudson REB. The human conduction system and its examination. *J Clin Pathol* 1963; 16:492–8.

414. Forsgren S, Carlsson E, Strehler E, Thornell L-E. Ultrastructural identification of human Purkinje fibers—a comparative immunocytochemical and electron microscopic study of composition and structure of myofibrillar M-regions. *J Mol Cell Cardiol* 1982; 14:437–49.

415. Forsgren S, Eriksson A, Kjorell U, Thornell L-E. The conduction system in the human heart at midgestation—immunohistochemical demonstration of the intermediate filament protein skeleton. *Histochemistry* 1982; 75:43–52.

416. Wessels A, Vermeulen JLM, Verbeek FJ, et al. Spatial distribution of "tissue-specific" antigens in the developing human heart and skeletal muscle. III. An immunohistochemical analysis of the distribution of the neural tissue antigen GIN2 in the embryonic heart; implications for the development of the atrioventricular conduction system. *Anat Rec* 1992; 232:97–111.

417. Ikeda T, Iwasaki K, Shimokawa I, et al. Leu-7 immunoreactivity in human and rat embryonic hearts, with special reference to the development of the conduction system. *Anat Embryol Berl* 1990; 182:553–62.

418. Wenink ACG. Development of the human cardiac conducting system. *J Anat* 1976; 121:617–31.

419. Hutchison ASA, Yu UY, Fortune DW. Non-immunological hydrops fetalis. A review of 61 cases. *Obstet Gynecol* 1982; 59:347–52.

420. Bridge JA, McManus BM, Remmenga J, Cuppage FP. Complete heart block in 18p syndrome. Congenital calcification of the atrioventricular node. *Arch Pathol Lab Med* 1989; 113:539–41.

421. Guntheroth WG, Motolsky AG. Inherited disorders of cardiac rhythm and conduction. *Prog Med Genet* 1983; 5:581.

422. Singer DB. Hemorrhage in cardiac conduction tissue of premature infants. *Arch Pathol Lab Med* 1985; 109:1093–6.

423. Newburger J, Keane JF. Intrauterine tachycardia. *Pediatrics* 1979; 95:780–6.

424. Ho SY, Mortimer G, Anderson RH, Pomerance A, Keeling JW. Conduction system defects in three perinatal patients with arrhythmia. *Br Heart J* 1985; 53:158–63.

425. Michaelsson M, Engle MA. Congenital complete heart block: an international study of the natural history. *Cardiovasc Clin* 1972; 4:85–102.

426. Sotelo-Avila C, Rosenberg HS, McNamara DG. Congenital heart block due to a lesion in the conduction system. *Pediatrics* 1970; 45:640–50.

427. Anderson RH, Wenink ACG, Losekoot TC, Becker AE. Congenitally complete heart block. Developmental aspects. *Circulation* 1977; 56:90–101.

428. Escher E, Scott JS. Congenital heart block and maternal systemic lupus erythematosus. *Br Med J* 1979; 1:1235–8.

429. Kasinath BS, Katz AI. Delayed maternal lupus after delivery of offspring with congenital heart block. *Arch Intern Med* 1982; 142:2317.

430. Litsey SE, Noonan JA, O'Connor WN, et al. Maternal connective tissue disease and congenital heart block. Demonstration of immunoglobulin in cardiac tissue. *N Engl J Med* 1985; 312:98–100.

431. McCue CM, Mantakas ME, Tingelstad JB, Ruddy S. Congenital heart block in newborns of mothers with connective tissue disease. *Circulation* 1977; 56:82–90.

432. Scott JS, Maddison PJ, Taylor PV, et al. Connective tissue disease, antibodies to ribonucleoprotein, and congenital heart block. *N Engl J Med* 1983; 309:209–312.

433. Bharati S, Serratto M, Dubrow I, et al. The conduction system in Pompe's disease. *Pediatr Cardiol* 1982; 2:25–32.

434. Vlad P, Rowe RD, Keith JD. The electrocardiogram in primary endocardial fibroelastosis. *Br Heart J* 1955; 17:189–97.

435. Van Mierop LHS, Wigglesworth FW. Isomerism of the cardiac atria in the asplenia syndrome. *Lab Invest* 1962; 11:1303–15.

436. Dickinson DF, Wilkinson JL, Anderson KR, et al. The cardiac conduction system in situs ambiguus. *Circulation* 1979; 59:879–85.

437. Milo S, Ho SY, Wilkinson JL, Anderson RH. The surgical anatomy and atrioventricular conduction tissues of hearts with isolated ventricular septal defects. *J Thorac Cardiovasc Surg* 1980; 79:244–55.

438. Thiene G, Wenink ACG, Frescura C, et al. The surgical anatomy of conduction tissues in atrioventricular septal defects. *J Thorac Cardiovasc Surg* 1981; 82:928–37.

439. Anderson RH, Wilkinson JL, Becker AE. Conducting tissues in the univentricular heart. In: Van Mierop LHS, Oppenheimer-Dekker A, Bruins CLD Ch, eds. *Embryology and Teratology of the Heart and Great Arteries.* Leiden: Leiden University Press, 1978, pp. 62–8.

440. El-Said G, Rosenberg HS, Mullens CS, et al. Dysrhythmias after Mustard's operation for transposition of great arteries. *Am J Cardiol* 1972; 30:526–32.

441. Fishbein MC, Meerbaum S, Rit J, et al. Early phase acute myocardial infarct size and quantification: validation of the triphenyltetrazolium chloride tissue enzyme staining technique. *Am Heart J* 1981; 101:593–600.

442. Vivaldi MT, Kloner RA, Schoen FJ. Triphenyl-tetrazolium staining of irreversible ischemic injury following coronary artery occlusion in rats. *Am J Pathol* 1985; 121:524–30.

443. DeSa DJ, Donnelly WH. Myocardial necrosis in the newborn. *Perspect Pediatr Pathol* 1984; 8:295–311.

444. Donnelly WH, Hawkins H. Optimum examination of the normally formed perinatal heart. *Hum Pathol* 1987; 18:55–60.

445. James TN. Cardiac conduction system: fetal and postnatal development. *Am J Cardiol* 1970; 25:213–26.

446. James TN. Crib death (Editorial). *J Am Coll Cardiol* 1985; 5:1185–7.

447. James TN. Sudden death in babies: new observation in the heart. *Am J Cardiol* 1968; 22:479–506.

448. Anderson RH, Bouton J, Burrow CT. Sudden death in infancy: a study of cardiac specialized tissue. *Br Med J* 1974; 2:135–9.

449. Lie JT, Rosenberg HS, Erickson EE. Histopathology of the conduction system in the sudden infant death syndrome. *Circulation* 1976; 53:3–8.

450. Valdes-Dapena MA. Are some crib deaths sudden cardiac deaths? *J Am Coll Cardiol* 1985; 5:113B–17B.

451. Valdes-Dapena MA, Greene M, Basavanand N, et al. The myocardial conduction system in sudden death in infancy. *N Engl J Med* 1973; 289:1179–80.

452. Anderson KR, Hill RW. Occlusive lesions of cardiac conducting tissue arteries in sudden infant death syndrome. *Pediatrics* 1982; 69:50–52.

453. Bharati S, Krongrad E, Lev M. Sudden infant death syndrome: conduction system study. *Circulation* 1983; 68(III):268 (Abstr).

454. Kozakewich HPW, McManus BM, Vawter GF. The sinus node in sudden infant death syndrome. *Circulation* 1982; 65:1242–6.

455. Marino TA, Kane BM. Cardiac atrioventricular junctional tissues in hearts from infants who died suddenly. *J Am Coll Cardiol* 1985; 5:1178–84.

456. DeSa DJ. Coronary arterial lesions and myocardial necrosis in stillbirths and infants. *Arch Dis Child* 1979; 54:918–30.

457. Young NA, Mondestin MAJ, Bowman RL. Ischemic changes in fetal myocardium. An autopsy series. *Arch Pathol Lab Med* 1994; 118:289–92.

458. Chiu T, Garrison RD, Miller RH, Saffos R. Neonatal coronary thrombosis. *South Med J* 1982; 75:749–51.

459. Gerlis LM, Gibbs JL, Williams GJ, Thomas GD. Coronary sinus orifice atresia and persistent left superior vena cava. A report of two cases, one associated with atypical coronary artery thrombosis. *Br Heart J* 1984; 52:648–53.

460. Bernstein D, Finkbeiner WE, Soifer S, Teitel D. Perinatal myocardial infarction: a case report and review of the literature. *Pediatr Cardiol* 1986; 6:313–7.

461. Lucas VW Jr, Burchfield DJ, Donnelly WH. Multiple coronary thromboemboli and myocardial infarction in a newborn infant. *J Perinatol* 1994; 14:145–9.

462. Setzer E, Ermocilla R, Tonkin I, et al. Papillary muscle necrosis in a neonatal autopsy population: incidence and associated manifestations. *J Pediatr* 1980; 96:289–94.

463. Cabal L, Devaskar U, Siassi B, et al. Cardiogenic shock associated with perinatal asphyxia in preterm infants. *J Pediatr* 1980; 96:705–10.

464. Lees MH. Perinatal asphyxia and the myocardium (Editorial). *J Pediatr* 1980; 96:675–8.

465. Bucciarelli RL, Nelson RM, Egan EA II, et al. Transient tricuspid insufficiency of the newborn: a form of myocardial dysfunction in stressed newborns. *Pediatrics* 1977; 59:330–7.

466. Rowe RD, Hoffman T. Transient myocardial ischemia of the newborn infant. A form of severe cardiorespiratory distress in full-term infants. *J Pediatr* 1972; 81:243–50.

467. Nelson RM, Bucciarelli R, Eitzman DV, et al. Serum creatine phosphokinase MB fraction in newborns with transient tricuspid insufficiency. *N Engl J Med* 1978; 28:146–9.

468. DeSa DJ. Myocardial changes in immature infants requiring prolonged ventilation. *Arch Dis Child* 1977; 52:138–47.

469. Donnelly WH. Ischemic myocardial injury. The histopathologic spectrum in 167 cases. *Lab Invest* 1982; 46:5P (Abstr.).

470. Topaz O. Myocardial calcification in neonates and infants. A unique tissue reaction. *South Med J* 1991; 84:891–5.

471. Esterly JR, Oppenheimer EH. Some aspects of cardiac pathology in infancy and childhood. IV. Myocardial and coronary lesions in cardiac malformations. *Pediatrics* 1967; 39:896–903.

472. Franciosi RA, Blanc WA. Myocardial infarction in infants and children. I. A necropsy study in congenital heart disease. *J Pediatr* 1968; 73:309–19.

473. Esterly JR, Oppenheimer EH. Some aspects of cardiac pathology in infancy and childhood. I. Neonatal myocardial necrosis. *Bull Johns Hopkins Hosp* 1966; 119:19–24.

474. Jedeikin R, Rowe RD, Freedom RM, et al. Cerebral arterial venous malformation in neonates. The role of myocardial ischemia. *Pediatr Cardiol* 1983; 4:29–35.

475. Donnelly WH. Papillary muscle dysfunction. *Am J Cardiovasc Pathol* 1987; 1:173–88.

476. Fletcher SE, Fyfe DA, Case CL, et al. Myocardial necrosis in a newborn after long-term maternal subcutaneous terbutaline infusion for suppression of pre-term labor. *Am J Obstet Gynecol* 1991; 165:1401–4.

477. Streeter DD. Gross morphology and fiber geometry of the heart. In: Berne RM, Seperlakin N, eds. *Handbook of Physiology. The Cardiovascular System*, Vol. I, Chapter 4. Bethesda: American Physiology Society, 1979, pp. 61–122.

478. Baroldi G. Different types of myocardial necrosis in coronary artery disease: a pathophysiologic review of their functional significance. *Am Heart J* 1975; 89:742–52.

479. Bouchardy B, Majno G. A new approach to the histologic diagnosis of early myocardial infarcts. *Cardiology* 1971; 56:327–32.

480. Ganote CE. Contraction band necrosis and irreversible myocardial injury (Editorial). *J Mol Cell Cardiol* 1983; 15:67–73.

481. Karch SB, Billingham ME. Myocardial contraction bands revisited. *Hum Pathol* 1986; 17:9–13.

482. Arnold G, Kaiser C, Fischer R. Myofibrillar degeneration—a common type of myocardial lesion and its selective identification by a modified Luxol Fast Blue stain. *Pathol Res Pract* 1985; 180:405–15.

483. Ewalds GM, Said JW, Block MI, et al. Myocytolysis (vacuolar degeneration) or myocardium: immunohistochemical evidence of viability. *Hum Pathol* 1984; 15:753–6.

484. Miller ME. Pathology of chemotaxis and random mobility. *Semin Hematol* 1975; 12:59–82.

485. Favara BE, Franciosi RA, Butterfield LJ. Disseminated intravascular and cardiac thrombosis of the neonate. *Am J Dis Child* 1974; 127:197–204.

486. Hoffman JIE. Determinants and prediction of transmural myocardial perfusion. *Circulation* 1978; 58:381–91.

487. Hoffman JIE, Buckberg GD. Transmural variations in myocardial perfusion. In: Yu D, Goodwin JF, eds. *Progress in Cardiology*. Philadelphia: Lea & Febiger, 1976, pp. 37–89.

488. Friedman WF. The intrinsic physiological properties of the developing heart. *Prog Cardiovasc Dis* 1972; 15:87–111.

489. Friedman WF, Kirkpatrick SE. Fetal cardiovascular adaptation to asphyxia. In: Gluck L, ed. *Intrauterine Asphyxia and the Developing Fetal Brain*. Chicago: Year Book, 1978, pp. 149–65.

490. Schmidt B, Zipursky A. Thrombotic disease in newborn infants. *Clin Perinatol* 1984; 11:461–88.

491. Tarras S, Gadia C, Meister L, Roldan E, Gregorios JB. Homozygous protein C deficiency in a newborn. Clinicopathologic correlation. *Arch Neurol* 1988; 45:214–6.

492. Marlar RA, Neumann A. Neonatal purpura fulminans due to homozygous protein C or protein S deficiencies. *Semin Thromb Hemost* 1990; 16:299–309.

493. Haffner D, Wuhl E, Zieger B, et al. Bilateral renal venous thrombosis in a neonate associated with resistance to activated protein C. *Pediatr Nephrol* 1996; 10:737–9.

494. Ahmadi A, Furste HO, Pringsheim W, et al. Congenital aortic thrombosis with complete obliteration of the aortic arch and the great vessels. *Thorac Cardiovasc Surg* 1983; 31:256–9.

495. Pierce RN, Dunn L, Knisely AS. Consumptive coagulopathy in utero associated with multiple vascular malformations. *Pediatr Pathol* 1992; 12:67–71.

496. Pilossoff W, Schober JG, Muller KD, et al. Complete thrombotic obliteration of the ascending aorta and the aortic arch as a cause of acute heart failure in a newborn. *Eur J Pediatr* 1988; 148:11–4.

497. Wigger HJ, Bransilver BR, Blanc WA. Thrombosis due to catheterization in infants and children. *J Pediatr* 1970; 76:1–11.

498. Vailas GA, Brouillette RT, Scott JP, et al. Neonatal aortic thrombosis: recent experience. *J Pediatr* 1986; 109:101–8.

499. Tyson JE, Desa DJ, Moore S. Thromboatheromatous complications of umbilical artery catheterization in the newborn period: clinical pathological study. *Arch Dis Child* 1976; 51:744–54.

500. Clawson CC, Baros SJ. Surface morphology of polyvinyl chloride and silicone elastomere umbilical artery catheters by scanning microscopy. *Pediatrics* 1978; 62:702–5.

501. Hecker JF. Thrombogenicity of tips of umbilical catheters. *Pediatrics* 1960; 67:467–71.

502. O'Neil JA, Neblett WW, Born ML. Management of major thromboembolic complications of umbilical artery catheters. *J Pediatr Surg* 1981; 16:972–8.

503. Gonzalez R, Schwartz S, Sheldon CA, Fraley EE. Bilateral renal vein thrombosis in infancy and childhood. *Urol Clin North Am* 1982; 9:279–83.

504. Junker P, Egeblad M, Nielson O, Kamper J. Case report. Umbilical vein catheterization and portal hypertension. *Acta Paediatr Scand* 1976; 65:499–504.

505. Kitterman JA, Phibbs RH, Tooley WH. Catheterisation of umbilical vessels in newborn infants. *Pediatr Clin North Am* 1970; 17:897–912.

506. Oppenheimer EM, Esterly JR. Thrombosis in the newborn: comparison between infants of diabetic mothers and non-diabetic mothers. *J Pediatr* 1965; 67:549–56.

507. Mulvihill SJ. Complications of superior versus inferior vena cava occlusion in infants receiving central total parenteral nutrition. *J Pediatr Surg* 1984; 19:452–7.

508. Marsh D, Wilkerson SA, Cook LN, Pietsch JB. Right atrial thrombus formation screening using two-dimensional echocardiograms in neonates with central venous catheters. *Pediatrics* 1988; 81:284–6.

509. Bayard R, Bourne AJ, Moore L, Little KET. Sudden death in early infancy due to delayed cardiac tamponade complicating central venous catheterization. *Arch Pathol Lab Med* 1992; 116:654–6.

510. Moragas A, Huguet P, Toran N, Rona V. Morphogenesis of pulmonary veno-occlusive disease in a newborn. Image analysis study. *Pathol Res Pract* 1983; 176:176–84.

511. Jaffe R, Yunis EJ. Congenital Budd-Chiari syndrome. *Pediatr Pathol* 1983; 1:187–92.

512. Abman SH, Warady BA, Lum GM, Koops BL. Systemic hypertension in infants with bronchopulmonary dysplasia. *J Pediatr* 1984; 104:928–31.

513. Bauer SB, Feldman SM, Gelis SS, Retick AB. Neonatal hypertension: a complication of umbilical artery catheterization. *N Engl J Med* 1975; 293:1032–3.

514. McClead RE. Budd-Chiari syndrome in a premature infant receiving total parenteral nutrition. *J Pediatr Gastroenterol Nutr* 1986; 5:655–8.

515. Larroche JC. Umbilical catheterisation: its complications. *Biol Neonat* 1970; 16:101–16.

516. Siebold-Weiger K, Vochem M, Mackensen-Haen S, Speer C. Fatal hepatic veno-occlusive disease in a newborn infant. *Am J Perinatol* 1997; 14:107–11.

517. Anderson KA, Burbach JA, Fenton LJ, et al. Idiopathic arterial calcification of infancy in newborn siblings with unusual light and electron microscopic manifestations. *Arch Pathol Lab Med* 1985; 109:838–42.

518. Jones DED, Pritchard KI, Gioannini CA, et al. Hydrops fetalis associated with idiopathic arterial calcification. *Obstet Gynecol* 1972; 39:435–40.

519. Milner LS, Heitner R, Thomson PD, et al. Hypertension as the major problem of idiopathic arterial calcification of infancy. *J Pediatr* 1984; 105:934–7.

520. Bellah RD, Zawodniak L, Librizz RJ, Harris MC. Idiopathic arterial calcification of infancy: prenatal and postnatal effects of therapy in an infant. *J Pediatr* 1992; 121:930–3.

521. Walley VM, Stinson WA, Upton C, et al. Foreign materials found in the cardiovascular system after instrumentation or surgery (including a guide to their light microscopic identification). *Cardiovasc Pathol* 1993; 2:157–85.

522. Puntis JW, Wilkins KM, Ball PA, et al. Hazards of parenteral treatment: do particles count? *Arch Dis Child* 1992; 67:1475–7.

523. Goddard-Finegold J, Langston C, Hawkins EP, et al. Prostaglandin E1-associated pathology of pulmonary microvasculature in newborn pups: similarity to findings in prostaglandin E1-treated human newborns. *Pediatr Pathol* 1989; 9:251–60.

524. Davies B. Aortitis and large vessel arteritis in a newborn [letter]. *Hum Pathol* 1985; 16:1284.

525. Oppenheimer EH, Hardy JB. Congenital syphilis in the newborn infant: clinical and pathological features in recent cases. *J Hopkins Med J* 1971; 129:63–82.

526. Esterly JR, Oppenheimer EH. Intrauterine rubella infection. *Perspect Pediatr Pathol* 1973; 1:313–38.

527. Fripp RR, Whitman V, Waldhausen JA, Boal DK. Ductus arteriosus aneurysm presenting as pulmonary artery obstruction: diagnosis and management. *J Am Coll Cardiol* 1985; 6:234–6.

528. Gillan JE, Costigan DC, Keeley FW, Rose T, Cutz E, Rose V. Spontaneous dissecting aneurysm of the ductus arteriosus in an infant with Marfan syndrome. *J Pediatr* 1984; 105:952–5.

529. Malone PS, Cooper SG, Elliott M, Kiely EM, Spitz L. Aneurysm of the ductus arteriosus. *Arch Dis Child* 1989; 64:1386–8.

530. Guzzetta PC. Congenital and acquired aneurysmal disease. *Semin Pediatr Surg* 1994; 3:97–102.

531. Esper E, Krabill KA, St-Cyr JA, et al. Repair of multiple mycotic aortic aneurysms in a newborn. *J Pediatr Surg* 1993; 28:1553–6.

532. Roques X, Choussat A, Bourdeaud'hui A, et al. Aneurysms of the abdominal aorta in the neonate and infant. *Ann Vasc Surg* 1989; 3:335–40.

533. Opitz JM. On congenital lymphedema. *Am J Med Gene* 1986; 24:127–9.

534. Haworth SG. Primary and secondary pulmonary hypertension in childhood: a clinicopathological reappraisal. *Curr Top Pathol* 1983; 73:91–152.

535. Perkin RM, Anas NG. Pulmonary hypertension in pediatric patients. *J Pediatr* 1984; 105:511–22.

536. Hislop A, Reid LM. Formation of the pulmonary vasculature. In: Hodson WA, ed. *Development of the Lung.* New York: Marcel Dekker, 1977, pp. 37–86.

537. Hislop A, Reid LM. Intrapulmonary arterial development during fetal life—branching pattern and structure. *J Anat* 1972; 113:35–48.

538. Reid LM. The pulmonary circulation: remodeling in growth and disease. The 19th J. Burns Amberson Lecture. *Am Rev Resp Dis* 1979; 119:531–46.

539. Reid L. Bronchopulmonary dysplasia: pathology. *J Pediatr* 1979; 195:836.

540. Naeye RL. Arterial changes during the perinatal period. *Arch Path Lab Med* 1961; 71:121–8.

541. Levin DL, Rudolph AM, Heymann MA, Phibbs RH. Morphologic development of the pulmonary vascular bed in fetal lambs. *Circulation* 1976; 53:144–51.

542. Meyrick B, Reid LM. The effect of continued hyperoxia on rat pulmonary arterial circulation. *Lab Invest* 1978; 38:188–200.

543. Meyrick B, Reid LM. Hypoxia induced structural changes in the media and adventitia of the rat hilar pulmonary artery and their regression. *Am J Pathol* 1980; 100:151–69.

544. Gersony WM. Neonatal pulmonary hypertension: pathophysiology, classification, and etiology. *Clin Perinatol* 1984; 11:517–24.

545. Geggel RL, Reid LM. The structural basis of persistent pulmonary hypertension of the newborn. *Clin Perinatol* 1984; 11:525–49.

546. Levin DL, Fixler DE, Morriss FC, Tyson J. Morphologic analysis of the pulmonary vascular bed in infants exposed in utero to prostaglandin synthetase inhibitors. *J Pediatr* 1978; 92:478–83.

547. Spitzer AR, Davis J, Clarke WT, et al. Pulmonary hypertension and persistent fetal circulation in the newborn. *Clin Perinatol* 1988; 15:389–410.

548. Levin DL, Heymann MA, Kitterman JA, et al. Persistent pulmonary hypertension of the newborn. *J Pediatr* 1976; 89:626–30.

549. Raine J, Hislop AA, Redington AN, et al. Fatal persistent pulmonary hypertension presenting late in the neonatal period. *Arch Dis Childhood* 1991; 66:398–402.

550. Rudolph AM, Heymann MA. Effects of prostaglandins and inhibitors of prostaglandin synthesis in the fetus and newborn infant. *J Perinatal Med* 1981; 9(suppl 1):91–2.

551. Levin DL, Mills LJ, Weinberg AG. Hemodynamic pulmonary vascular and myocardial abnormalities secondary to pharmacologic constriction of the fetal ductus arteriosus. *Circulation* 1979; 60:360–4.

552. Leffler CW, Hessler JR, Green RS. The onset of breathing at birth stimulates pulmonary vascular prostacyclin synthesis. *Pediatr Res* 1984; 18:938–42.

553. Fox WW, Duara S. Persistent pulmonary hypertension in the neonate: diagnosis and management. *J Pediatr* 1983; 103:505–14.

554. Baylen BG, Emmanouilides GC, Juratsch CE, et al. Main pulmonary artery distention: a potential mechanism for acute pulmonary hypertension in the human newborn infant. *J Pediatr* 1980; 96:540–4.

555. Gersony WM, Duc CV, Sinclair JD. "PFC" syndrome (persistence of the fetal circulation). *Circulation* 1969; 40(Suppl III):87.

556. Levin DL, Hyman AI, Heymann MA, Rudolph AM. Fetal hypertension and the development of increased pulmonary vascular smooth muscle. A possible mechanism for persistent pulmonary hypertension of the newborn infant. *J Pediatr* 1978; 92:265–9.

557. Murphy JD, Rabinovitch M, Goldstein JD, Reid L. Structural basis of persistent pulmonary hypertension of the newborn infant. *J Pediatr* 1981; 98:962–7.

558. Drummond WH, Peckham GJ, Fox WW. The clinical profile of the newborn with persistent pulmonary hypertension. *Clin Pediatr* 1977; 16:335–41.

559. Fox WW, Gewitz MH, Dinwiddie R, et al. Pulmonary hypertension in the perinatal aspiration syndromes. *Pediatrics* 1977; 59:205–11.

560. Murphy JD, Vawter GF, Reid L. Pulmonary vascular disease in fatal meconium aspiration. *J Pediatr* 1984; 104:758–62.

561. Perlman EJ, Moore GW, Hutchins GM. The pulmonary vasculature in meconium aspiration. *Hum Pathol* 1989; 20:701–6.

562. Levin DL, Weinberg AG, Perkin RM. Pulmonary microthrombi syndrome in newborn infants with unresponsive persistent pulmonary hypertension. *J Pediatr* 1983; 102:299–303.

563. Segall ML, Goetzman BW, Schick JB. Thrombocytopenia and pulmonary hypertension in perinatal aspiration syndrome. *J Pediatr* 1980; 96:724–30.

564. Reid LM. The Third Grover Conference on the pulmonary circulation. The control of cellular proliferation in the pulmonary circulation. *Am Rev Respir Dis* 1989; 140:1490–3.

565. Hislop AA, Haworth SG. Pulmonary vascular damage and the development of cor pulmonale following hyaline membrane disease. *Pediatr Pulmonol* 1990; 9:152–61.

566. Bush A, Busst CM, Knight WB, et al. Changes in pulmonary circulation in severe bronchopulmonary dysplasia. *Arch Dis Childhood* 1990; 65:739–45.

567. Gorenflo M, Vogel M, Obladen M. Pulmonary vascular changes in bronchopulmonary dysplasia. A clinicopathologic correlation in short and long term survivors. *Pediatr Pathol* 1991; 11:851–66.

568. Shaffer SG, O'Neill D, Bodt SK, Thibeault DW. Chronic vascular pulmonary dysplasia associated with neonatal hyperoxia exposure in the rat. *Pediatr Res* 1987; 21:14–20.

569. Snow RL, Davies P, Pontoppidan H, et al. Pulmonary vascular remodeling in adult respiratory distress syndrome. *Am Rev Respir Dis* 1982; 126:887.

570. Naeye RL. Perinatal vascular changes associated with underdevelopment of the left heart. *Am J Pathol* 1962; 41:287–93.

571. Haworth SG, Sauer U, Buehlmeyer C, Reid L. Development of the pulmonary circulation in ventricular septal defect: a quantitative structural study. *Am J Cardiol* 1977; 40:781–8.

572. Haworth SG, Reid L. Quantitative structural study of pulmonary circulation in the newborn with aortic atresia, stenosis, or coarctation. *Thorax* 1977; 32:121–8.

573. Rabinovitch M, Reid LM. Quantitative structural analysis of the pulmonary vascular bed in congenital heart defects. *Cardiovasc Clin* 1981; 11:149–69.

574. Hoffman JIE, Rudolph AM, Heyman MA. Pulmonary vascular disease with congenital heart disease: pathologic features and causes. *Circulation* 1981; 64:873–7.

575. Haworth SG. Pulmonary vascular disease in different types of congenital heart disease. Implications for interpretation of lung biopsy findings in early childhood. *Br Heart J* 1984; 52:557–71.

576. Galt B, Shikes RH. Pulmonary hypertension in congenital heart disease: irreversible vascular changes in young infants. *Pediatr Pathol* 1983; 1:423–4.

577. Naeye RL, Shochat SJ, Whitman V, Maisels MJ. Unsuspected pulmonary vascular abnormalities associated with diaphragmatic hernia. *Pediatrics* 1976; 58:902–6.

578. Levin DL. Morphologic analysis of the pulmonary vascular bed in congenital left-sided diaphragmatic hernia. *J Pediatr* 1978; 92:805–9.

579. Geggel RL, Murphy JD, Langleben D, et al. Congenital diaphragmatic hernia: arterial structural changes and persistent pulmonary hypertension after surgical repair. *J Pediatr* 1985; 107:457–64.

580. Hislop A, Hey E, Reid L. The lungs in congenital bilateral renal agenesis and dysplasia. *Arch Dis Child* 1979; 54:32–8.

581. Janney CG, Askin FB, Kuhn C III. Congenital alveolar capillary dysplasia— an unusual cause of respiratory distress in the newborn. *Am J Clin Pathol* 1981; 76:722–7.

582. Wagenvoort CA. Misalignment of lung vessels: a syndrome causing persistent neonatal pulmonary hypertension. *Hum Pathol* 1985; 17:727–30.

583. Cullinane C, Cox PN, Silver MM. Persistent pulmonary hypertension of the newborn due to alveolar capillary dysplasia. *Pediatr Pathol* 1992; 12:499–514.

584. Boggs S, Harris MC, Hoffman DJ, et al. Misalignment of pulmonary veins with alveolar capillary dysplasia: affected siblings and variable phenotypic expression. *J Pediatr* 1994; 124: 125–8.

585. Haraida S, Lochbühler H, Heger A, et al. Congenital alveolar capillary dysplasia: rare cause of persistent pulmonary hypertension. *Pediatr Pathol* 1997; 17:959–75.

586. Simonton S, Chrenka B. Familial persistent pulmonary hypertension in two siblings with phocomelia and alveolar capillary dysplasia (ACD*): a new syndrome? *Mod Pathol* 1993; 6:9P. [Abstract]

The Central Nervous System

Jeanne-Claudie Larroche   Ferechte Encha-Razavi

Jonathan S. Wigglesworth

PART I
DEVELOPMENT

JEANNE-CLAUDIE LARROCHE

A description of some landmarks of the developing brain is important to aid assessment of the age of a given embryo or fetus and to allow better understanding of morphogenetic disorders and specific pathologic conditions. Several monographs may be recommended for more detailed descriptions [1–6].

FORMATION OF THE MAIN STRUCTURES

For descriptive convenience, the development of the central nervous system (CNS) can be divided into four successive periods, bearing in mind that these periods overlap slightly.

First Period (Neurulation)

In the first 4 weeks of embryonic life, the neural plate, formed by repeated mitotic divisions of neuroepithelial cells (programmed to be neurons, glial cells, and ependymal cells), tends to form a groove that closes progressively and gives origin to the neural tube. The closure of the groove starts at 22 days in the dorsal region and proceeds bidirectionally: the anterior pore is closed at 24 days and the posterior neuropore at 26 days. Recent experiments in mice have shown concomitant multiple sites of closure [7], and, in humans, this hypothesis is consistent with neuropathologic observations of multiple neural tube defects in the same patient. All neural tube defects or dysraphic states take place during this brief early period.

Second Period (Formation of the Cerebral Vesicles)

At 4 to 7 weeks, while the neuroepithelium thickens due to repetitive mitoses, the neural tube enlarges in its rostral part to form three vesicles. The anterior vesicle (forebrain), or prosencephalon, evaginates to form two "hemispheres" with their respective ventricles and the diencephalon; the intermediate (midbrain), or mesencephalon, gives origin to the cerebral peduncles and to the lamina quadrigemina; the caudal vesicle (hindbrain), or rhombencephalon, gives origin to the pons, cerebellum, and medulla oblongata. The olfactory bulbs and optic vesicles evaginate; basal ganglia and hypothalamus are formed. Anomalies of the holoprosencephaly group and arrhinencephalia develop during this period.

Third Period (Corticogenesis)

At 8 to 16 weeks, divisions of neuroepithelial cells (stem cells) in the ventricular zone and their migration to form the cortical plate are the two salient events. Cell differentiation in ependymal cells, glial cells, and neurons that acquire their separate morphologic attributes also takes place during this period. Any adverse condition interfering at that time may lead to cortical abnormalities. The corpus callosum is the last gross structure to develop, and total or partial agenesis occurs during this period.

Fourth Period

The fourth period spans the second half of fetal life. This period is characterized by a progressive increase in the volume of neurons and of their processes, with the development of afferent fibers and proliferation of glial cells. These events lead to a spectacular increase in the cortical surface within a minimal intracranial volume. Formation of sulci and convolutions provides the solution to this geometric problem. Two-thirds of the cortical surface is thus buried within the sulci, the folding phenomenon implying a harmonious cell ratio between the superficial and deep layers of the cortex [8].

Intense proliferation of capillaries is an additional factor in the increasing volume of the cortical plate.

Finally, myelination, which commences in the spinal cord and brainstem, reaches the basal part of the brain by the end of fetal life.

Environmental factors and pathologic processes, either vascular or infectious, occurring during this period are more likely to produce clastic lesions. In some instances, cortical scars may mimic malformations. Maternal renal diseases, hypertension, and placental diseases leading to intrauterine growth retardation (IUGR) also lead to subtle and nonspecific effects on the brain with unknown implications on the future neurobehavioral status of the child.

After Birth

Myelogenesis and glial cell proliferation are the most prominent events.

CELL DEATH

Cell death in the CNS has been observed in various settings such as hypoxia-ischemia, genetic disorders, and toxic or degenerative processes. Recently, researches have been focused on cell death that occurs during normal development—i.e., apoptosis. Molecular biology, allowing studies on the various phases of cell death in nematodes, may provide new insights on causes, mechanisms, and eventually means of preventing neuronal degeneration.

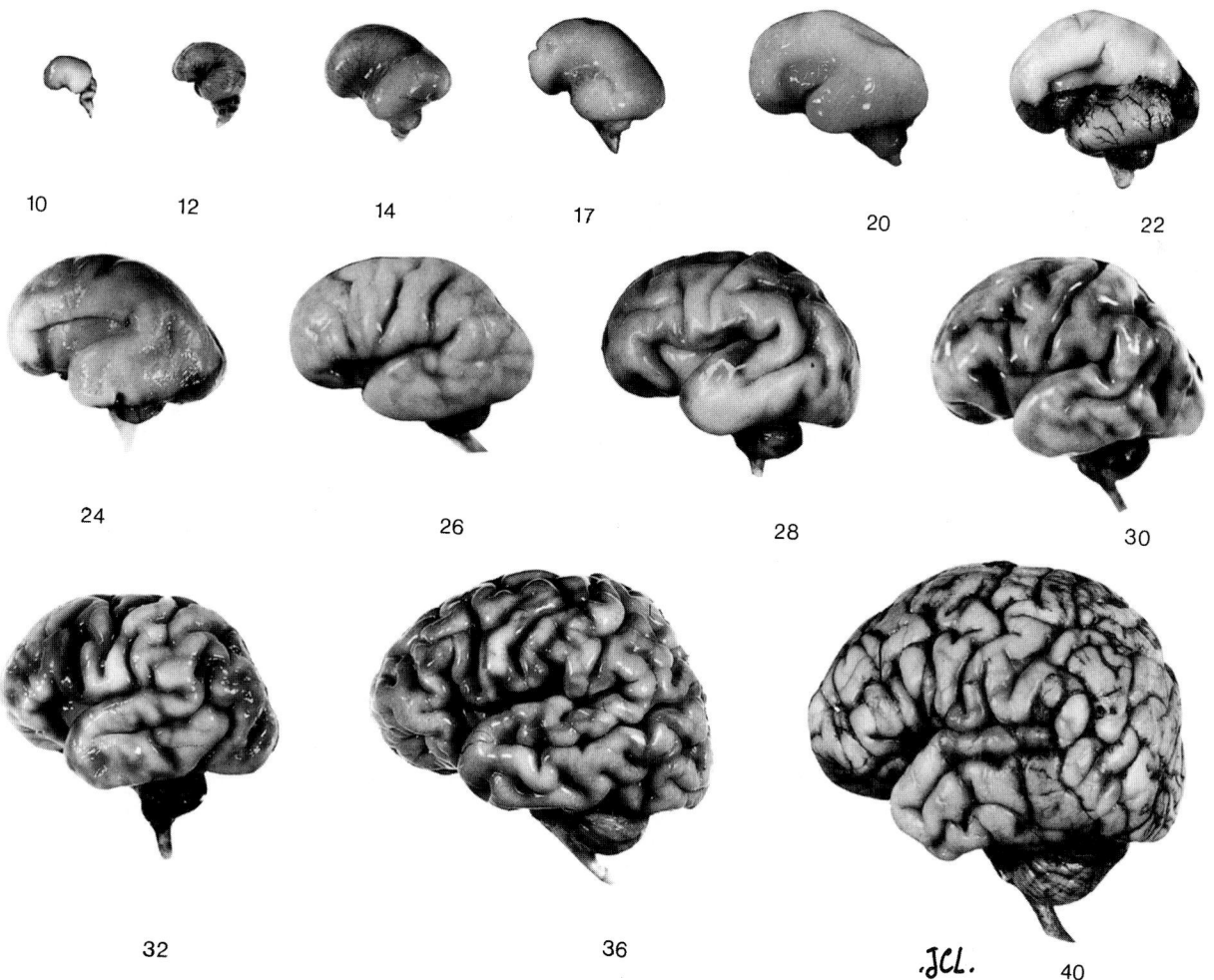

FIGURE 21.1. *External view of the developing brain from 10 to 40 weeks.*

GROSS MORPHOLOGY

During fetal life, the brain weight represents 10–14% of total body weight, while in the adult it represents only 2% of total body weight.

External Configuration

In spite of the increasing weight, the surface configuration of the brain does not change significantly until 20 to 22 weeks (Figs. 21.1 and 21.2). The hemispheres are smooth, and a diagnosis of agyria cannot be made on the basis of ultrasound study or, at autopsy, on gross appearance only. Other criteria, such as early enlargement of the ventricles and cortical dysplasia, must be used. The primary fissures and, after 28 weeks, the secondary sulci are good landmarks for gestational age estimation, although there may be a slight difference in pattern between the two hemispheres. The left hemisphere is usually longer than the right, which tends to be shifted forward. Sulci on the left hemisphere show a slight advance in development. On the lateral surfaces of the hemispheres, the sylvian fissure, widely open and shallow at 14 weeks, leaving the insula exposed, progressively deepens.

Due to the increasing bulk of the temporal and parietal lobes, the posterior part of the insula is covered first, while the anterior part remains visible until 36 weeks. The rolandic fissure, a short and shallow groove by 22 weeks, extends downward and posteriorly to reach the interhemispheric fissure by 30 weeks. The temporal lobe is smooth until 26 weeks, when a dimple indicates the first temporal sulcus, which is constantly visible on both sides at 28 weeks. On the medial surfaces of the hemispheres, the parieto-occipital sulcus first appears, forming with the calcarine fissure the characteristic Y-shaped complex by 18 to 19 weeks. From 14 weeks on, the sulcus of the corpus callosum and the sulcus cinguli extend backward as the corpus callosum develops. At the base of the brain, the olfactory sulci are visible by 18 to 20 weeks. From 28 weeks onward, the secondary sulci appear according to a rather strict schedule.

Corpus Callosum

The corpus callosum develops first anteriorly, by 12 weeks, within the massa commissuralis (lamina reuniens) [9]. Then, from the isocortical plate of the telencephalic vesicles, com-

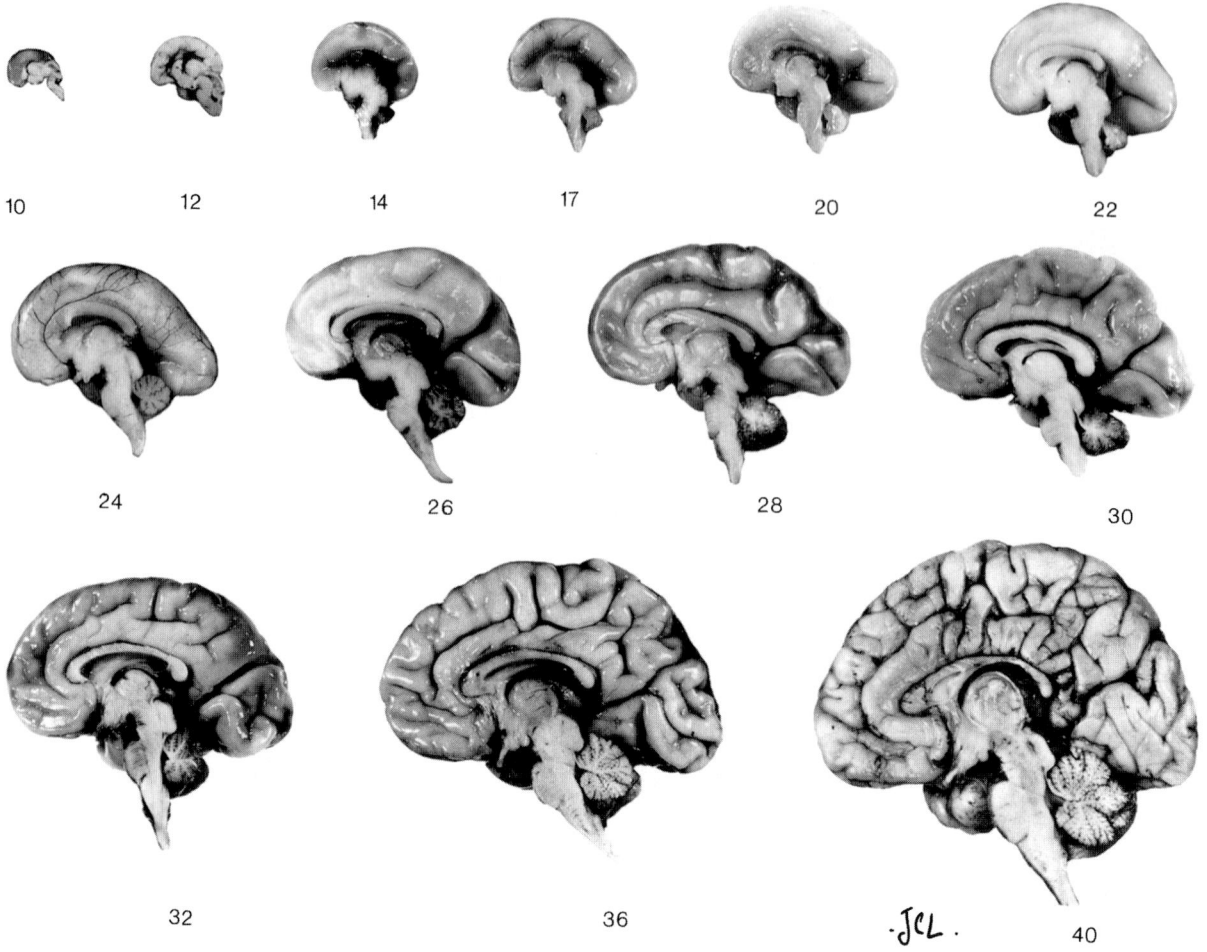

FIGURE 21.2. *Midsagittal view of the developing brain from 10 to 40 weeks.*

missural fibers cross the midline, forming successively the genu and rostrum, the body and splenium of the corpus callosum. By 18 weeks, the anterior part with the cavum septi pellucidi is visible on ultrasound. By 22 weeks, its form and position are those of the adult brain.

Septum Pellucidum

The development of the septum and of the midline cavities is linked to the development of the corpus callosum, although a septum lucidum-like structure has been noted in agenesis of the corpus callosum [3]. The cavum septi pellucidi is always present in fetuses and progressively decreases until term [10]. It may extend posteriorly, below the splenium to form the cavum Vergae. There is no ependymal lining in the cavum. Both cavities are visible on ultrasound, at 18 and 22 weeks, respectively.

Cerebellum

Initially forming as an exposed structure, the cerebellum is covered by the enlarging cerebral hemispheres by 14 to 15 weeks. Subsequently, its development lags behind that of the cerebrum and its posterior margin is far from the occipital pole. In young fetuses, its weight represents less than 4% of the total brain weight and progressively increases from 4.5%

at 28 weeks to 6.5% at term, 9% in the first months of life, and 12% after 1 year. Since cerebellar malformations and hypoplasia are rather common in fetal pathology, standard growth curves of the cerebellum and differential growth curves of the cerebrum and cerebellum should be used [11, 12].

HISTOLOGIC FEATURES

The Neocortex of the Cerebrum

In the 4-week-old embryo, the neural tube, formed by neuroepithelial cell proliferation, is a rather homogeneous pseudostratified structure (Fig. 21.3a). At these early stages of neural tube formation, undifferentiated stem cells extend from the ventricle to the pial surface. These cells have been termed radial-glial cells. During the mitotic cycle, the synthesis of DNA takes place in the apical, external part of the cell, then the nucleus of the cell migrates to the inner, subependymal zone and divides. The nuclei of the daughter cells return to the periphery to undergo a further duplication of DNA and so on until their genetically programmed division activity is exhausted. The apical processes of the "ependymoglial cells" form the external subpial boundary of the nervous tissue and, at the ventricular wall, some of them acquire the attributes of ependymal cells,

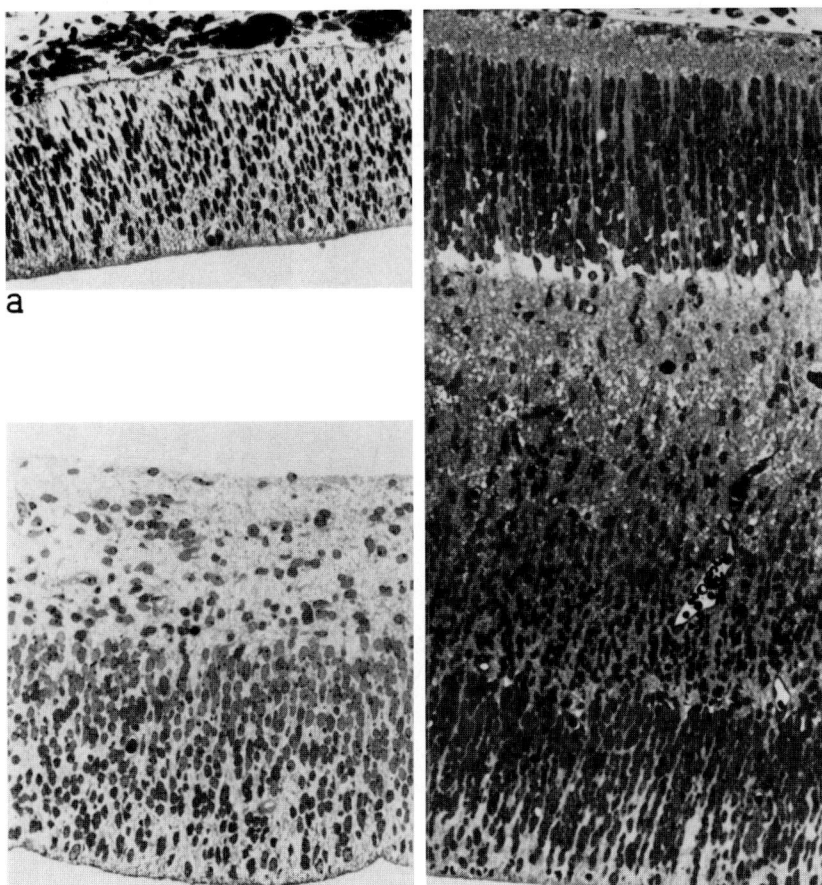

a

b   c

FIGURE 21.3. *Neocorticogenesis. External wall of the anterior vesicle (semithin sections). (a) At 5 weeks: pseudostratified epithelium. (b) At 7 weeks, the wall is a two-layered structure: the matrix or ventricular zone and the external marginal layer. (c) At 9 to 10 weeks, there are five layers: matrix or ventricular zone, subventricular and intermediate zones, and cortical plate and external marginal zone or molecular layer.*

following a caudocephalic gradient around the neural tube [13].

At 4 to 7 weeks, the wall of the anterior vesicle thickens and becomes progressively a two-layered structure: an inner matrix or ventricular zone with many mitoses in a columnar arrangement of the nuclei, and a less cellular external marginal layer (Fig. 21.3b). This layer consists of afferent processes from diencephalic structures, distributed tangentially and perpendicular to the apical processes of the glio-ependymal-radial glial cells, thus forming a plexiform layer. Large and mature neurons, the so-called Cajal-Retzius cells, and axodendritic synapses can be seen already in this layer [14]. In the ventricular zone, some of the daughter cells have been programmed to differentiate into neurons and others into glial cells.

At 7 to 8 weeks, the cortical plate appears within the marginal layer. The cortical plate forms by an inside-out process, as first shown by the autographic study of Angevine and Sidman [15] in mice. The first young neurons that migrate form the deep cortical layers and are then bypassed by later-formed neurons that pile up on those that migrated earlier. This process of migration probably provides early contacts and recognition between cells. Before birth, the programmed quota of neurons is attained and the neurons have reached their assigned position. The external part of the marginal layer is called molecular layer or layer I. The inner part or deep layer VI [16] is now known as the subplate. This layer is the site of termination of catecholaminergic afferent fibers that do not enter the cortical plate until their target neurons have reached their final position in the cortex. The subplate is thus considered a transient or "waiting" layer, but its role is not yet well established.

The radial-glial fibers and their role as a guide for migrating neurons have been demonstrated in newborn monkeys [17] and, more recently, in human fetuses [18–21] by electron microscopy, with Golgi impregnations and on immunohistologic preparations. Young neurons migrate along the apical process of the glial fibers, which stretch to the pial surface, thus forming parallel columns easily visible in the matrix as well as in the cortical plate (Fig. 21.3c). On arrival in the cortical plate, the neuron loses its glial attachment. Until 16 weeks, the radial-glial fibers are grouped in fascicles of five to eight [22] and, with their respective neurons, form neuroradial units with specific and programmed distribution. Anomalies of glial cells, or disturbances in their guiding role, may cause cytoarchitectonic disorders such as cortical dysplasia, heterotopias, and anarchic orientation of the neurons (see Part II, on CNS malformations). The migration of neurons follows such a rigid tempo that it may be possible, in certain types of cortical anomalies, to date the occurrence of the morphopathologic event.

In addition to this radiating pattern, in early fetal life, migrating neurons can be found around blood vessels and should not be mistaken for inflammatory cells. They may also take the form of strata in the frontal and occipital white matter and may account for hyperechoic zones visible on ultrasound. Other granular neurons, generated in the basal insular areas, migrate tangentially over the hemispheres, forming a transitory subpial layer whose fate is unknown [23].

In this period, the primitive glial cells differentiate into astrocytes, following a ventriculofugal gradient, with detachment of the ventricular pole and resorption of the apical

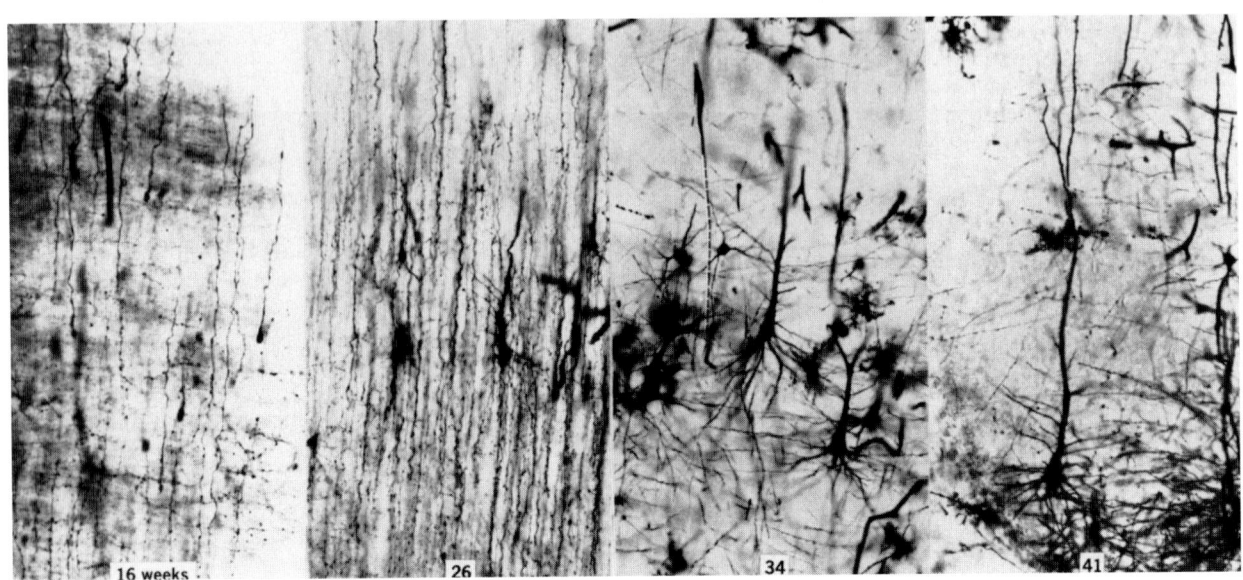

FIGURE 21.4. *Maturation of neurons in the cortical plate (motor area); development of the soma, dendrites, and axons. Golgi-Cox preparations at 16 weeks, 26 weeks, 34 weeks, 41 weeks.*

process [24]. Oligodendrocytes are also derived from radial-glial cells [25].

The ventricular matrix zone is the site of origin of nearly all neurons destined for the cortical plate until 16 weeks; thereafter, when mitotic activity is exhausted, the relative volume of the matrix decreases. Masses of cells still persist until 32 to 33 weeks, over the head of the caudate nucleus, in the thalamostriate groove about the foramen of Monro, in the roof of the temporal horn and in the external wall of the occipital horn. These zones contain small neurons and glial cells and are often the sites of hemorrhages in preterm neonates (see Part III, on fetal and perinatal brain damage).

Young neurons, initially bipolar during their migration, acquire progressively their triangular adult shape; the cytoplasm enlarges and shows characteristic organelles; axons and dendrites develop (Fig. 21.4). The process of "maturation" starts within the deep and early-formed layers, before the completion of the cortical plate.

Horizontal cortical lamination is visible when neurons forming layer II have reached their final position, a process that varies according to cortical areas, thus allowing a cytoarchitectonic map of the hemispheres to be drawn. At a histologic level, the motor cortex (area 4) and visual cortex (area 17), for example, are the most suitable sites for estimating the age of a fetus during the second half of gestation (Fig. 21.5).

Synapses

We know very little about human synaptogenesis. The first axodendritic synapses have been identified in the external marginal layers of embryos as early as 7 weeks, before the formation of the cortical plate [14], and then, just below the cortical plate, in the inner part of the primitive marginal layer or subplate, by 10 weeks. We first saw synapses at 15 to 16 weeks in the deep layers, along with the growing axons, while others [26] noticed them only at 23 weeks. Most quantitative data derive from investigations in primate brains, and results have been extrapolated to humans. Following a phase of overproduction around birth, there is a plateau phase during infancy and adolescence, then a decline in synaptic density.

The Cerebellum

The cytoarchitectonic development of the cerebellar cortex is spread over a longer period of time than that of the cerebral cortex and seems more complicated [27, 28]. In fact, the rigid and orderly displacement of the cells can be used readily as an index of maturation (Fig. 21.6).

The rhombencephalon is initially composed of a ventricular germinal layer and a marginal sparsely cellular external layer, as in any other part of the neural tube.

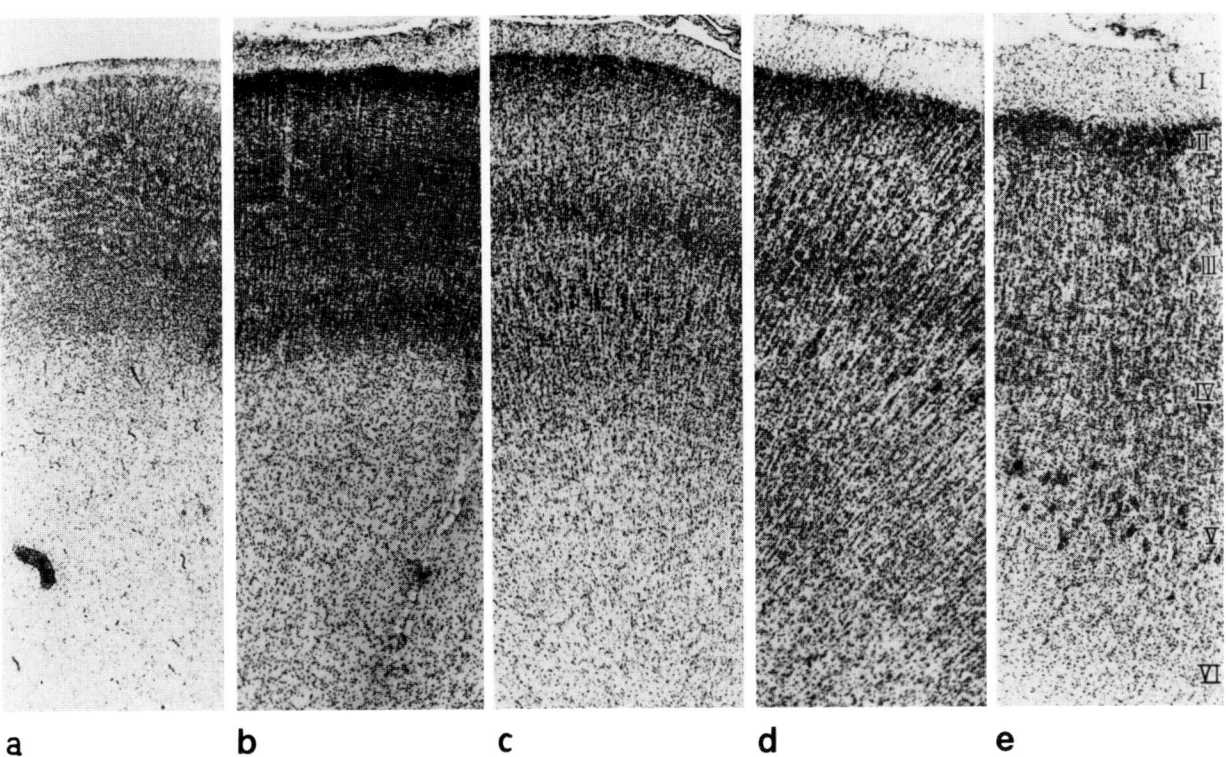

a   b   c   d   e

FIGURE 21.5.   *Development of the cortical plate (area 4); horizontal lamination and neuronal maturation at (a) 24 weeks, (b) 28 weeks, (c) 32 weeks, (d) 36 weeks, (e) 40 weeks.*

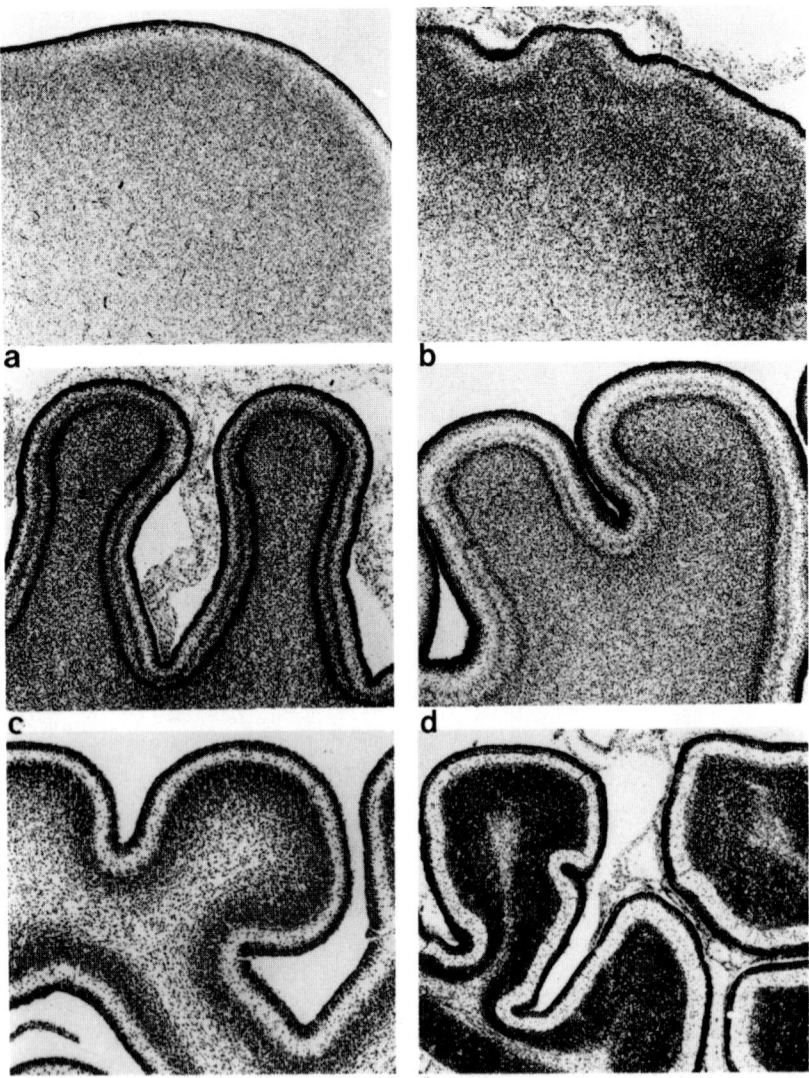

FIGURE 21.6. *Development of the cerebellar cortex: (a) 13 weeks, (b) 16 weeks, (c) 24 weeks, (d) 32 weeks, (e) 36 weeks, (f) 40 weeks.*

Neuroepithelial cells proliferate in the ventricular zone and then migrate outward. Five periods can be recognized according to the successive stages of development.

1. *3 to 8 weeks, two-layer stage.* An intermediate and highly cellular layer differentiates from the ventricular layer, while the marginal layer is still barely cellular.

2. *9 to 10 weeks, three-layer stage.* From the matrix, cells migrate tangentially to the surface, outside the marginal layer, to form a transient external granular layer, which progressively thickens by repeated mitoses. Thus, the marginal or molecular layer lies between the external granular layer and the deep cellular layer or intermediate zone. At 13 to 14 weeks, this intermediate zone becomes less cellular and receives a new population of large neurons, which form the dentate and roof nuclei.

3. *20 weeks, five-layer stage.* A remarkable clearing, known as "lamina dissecans" appears in the external part of the intermediate zone; the inner part forms the internal granular layer, which is lined by the Purkinje's cells. From 28 to 32 weeks, the thickness of the lamina dissecans decreases.

4. *32 weeks to term, four-layer stage.* The lamina dissecans becomes attenuated and disappears completely. The Purkinje's cells stand clearly above the internal granular layer. After birth, the external granular layer slowly decreases, and by 7 months only a few vestigial cells remain under the pia.

5. *End of first year, three-layer stage.* The cerebellar cortex has reached its adult pattern.

These sequences of differentiation are valid for all the folia, with slight advances in the paleocerebellum, vermis, and flocculus.

MYELINATION

Myelination is a late process that begins during the second half of pregnancy and continues during the first years of life [1, 4, 5]. It is said to be achieved by 7 years, but association fibers are fully myelinated only during the fourth decade.

Myelination can be appreciated by light microscopic examination of thick preparations stained with Luxol fast blue or by the Loyez method. These classic histologic techniques allow recognition of a useful and reliable schedule for myelination. However, thin tissue sections, studied with immunohistochemistry and electron microscopic techniques, indicate a schedule that starts earlier in fetal life.

Study of myelination is difficult, because each system of fibers follows its own pattern of myelination in terms of starting point and direction, in terms of time (i.e., beginning of the process), and finally, in terms of speed, all of which Yakovlev and Lecours [1] have called "cycles of myelination." However, assessment of the degree of myelination in a given fiber system is a reliable method for gestational age evaluation.

1. In the peripheral nervous system, the ventral roots myelinate earlier (22 weeks) than the dorsal roots.
2. In the spinal cord, myelination of spinothalamic fibers (deep sensation) progresses slowly in a caudocephalic direction: fasciculus cuneatus at 24 weeks; gracilis at 26 weeks; medial lemniscus at 26 weeks, up to the thalamus at 34 weeks. Fiber systems conducting pain, temperature, and light touch are myelinated later.
3. In contrast, the statoacoustic system, medial longitudinal fasciculus, and lateral lemniscus myelinate early and rapidly by 24 weeks.
4. Myelination of the pyramidal tract begins in the pons at 36 weeks and then proceeds caudally and rostrally. At term, the ventral corticospinal tract is myelinated to as far as the cervical region.
5. In the hemispheres, myelination of the thalamo-cortical fibers begins by the end of fetal life in the pre- and postcentral cortices and seems to be synchronized with the myelination of the corticospinal fibers. It is completed by the age of 1 year.
6. The extrapyramidal system (fibers of the pallidum, ansa lenticularis, and subthalamic nucleus) is myelinated early and rapidly, at 30 weeks.
7. In the brainstem, the early (24 weeks) and rapid myelination of the statoacoustic system contrasts with the late myelination of the optic system, which begins in the chiasma at 30 weeks. In the cortex of the temporal lobe, the myelination of the acoustic analyzers starts several weeks after birth and continues until after the first postnatal year, while myelination of the geniculocalcarine tract (optic radiations) starts just before birth and is completed rapidly. Acoustic and gravitational stimuli during fetal life may elicit early myelination at a subcortical level. However, a premature infant cannot orient its head toward a noise, although it is able to fix and choose between two different objects. It is difficult, therefore, to establish a parallel between the degree of myelination of a fiber system and its function. The development of muscle tone seems to be in better conformity with the chronology and direction of the myelination processes. In premature infants, the tone is controlled mainly by spinal and brainstem pathways that myelinate in a caudorostral direction, and flexion of the legs precedes flexion of the arms. However, it has now been demonstrated by ultrasound examinations that fetuses of 14 to 19 weeks can exhibit "spontaneous" movements, such as rotation and ante- or retroflexion of the head as well as movements of the arms and trunk.
8. The corpus callosum begins to myelinate at about 4 months postnatally.
9. Finally, some association fibers are not completely myelinated until the fourth decade.

Thus, even at term, the hemispheres are almost totally devoid of myelin, and the white matter, which contains a large amount of water, is barely distinguishable from the adjacent cortex. These features probably account for the extreme fragility of the immature brain and for its specific pathology.

REFERENCES: DEVELOPMENT OF THE CNS

1. Yakovlev PI, Lecours AR. The myelogenetic cycles of regional maturation of the brain. In: Minkowski A, ed. *Regional Development of the Brain in Early Life*. Oxford: Blackwell Scientific, 1967, pp. 3–70.
2. Rorke LB, Riggs H, eds. *Myelination of the Brain in the Newborn*. Philadelphia: JB Lippincott, 1969, p. 108.
3. Lemire RJ, Loeser DJ, Leech RW, Alvord EC, eds. *Normal and Abnormal Development of the Human Nervous System*. New York: Harper and Row, 1975, p. 421.
4. Larroche JC, ed. *Developmental Pathology of the Neonate*. Amsterdam: Excerpta Medica, 1977, p. 525.
5. Gilles FH, Leviton A, Dooling EC, eds. *The Development of the Human Brain. Growth and Epidemiologic Neuropathology*. Boston: John Wright, 1983, p. 349.
6. Feess-Higgins A, Larroche JC, eds. *Development of the Human Foetal Brain. An Anatomical Atlas*. Paris: INSERM-CNRS, 1987.
7. Van Allen MI, Kalousek DK, Chernoff GF, et al. Evidence for multi-site closure of the neural tube in humans. *Am J Med Genet* 1993; 47:723–43.
8. Richman DP, Stewart RM, Hutchinson JW. Mechanical model of brain convolutional development. *Science* 1975; 189:18–21.
9. Rakic P, Yakovlev PI. Development of the corpus callosum and cavum septi in man. *J Comp Neurol* 1968; 132:45–72.
10. Larroche JC, Baudey J. Cavum septi lucidi, cavum Vergae, cavum veli interpositi. Cavités de la ligne médiane. Etude anatomique et pneumoencéphalographique dans la période néonatale. *Biol Neonate* 1961, 3:196–236.
11. Roessmann U. Weight ratio between the infratentorial and supratentorial portions of the central nervous system. *J Neuropathol Exp Neurol* 1974; 33:164–70.
12. Guihard-Costa AM, Larroche JC. Differential growth between the fetal brain and its infratentorial part. *Early Hum Dev* 1990; 23:27–40.
13. Sarnat HB. Regional differentiation of the human fetal ependyma. *J Neuropathol Exper Neurol* 1992; 51:58–75.
14. Larroche JC. The marginal layer in the neocortex of a 7 week old human embryo. A light and electron microscopic study. *Anat Embryol* 1981; 162:301–12.

15. Angevine JB, Sidman RL. Autoradiographic study of cell migration during histogenesis of cerebral cortex in the mouse. *Nature* 1961; 192:766–8.

16. Marin-Padilla M. Dual origin of the mammalian neocortex and evolution of the cortical plate. *Anat Embryol* 1976; 152:109–26.

17. Rakic P. Mode of cell migration to the superficial layers of the fetal monkey neocortex. *J Comp Neurol* 1972; 145:61–84.

18. Choi BH, Lapham LW. Radial glia in the human fetal cerebrum: a combined Golgi, immunofluorescent and electron microscopic study. *Brain Res* 1978; 148:295–311.

19. Larroche JC, Privat A, Jardin L. Some fine structures of the human fetal brain. In: Minkowski A, ed. *Physiological and Biochemical Basis for Perinatal Medicine.* Basel: Karger, 1981, pp. 350–8.

20. Larroche JC, Houcine O. Le neocortex chez l'embryon et le foetus humain. Apport du microscope électronique et du Golgi. *Reprod Nutrition Dévelop* 1982; 22:163–70.

21. Gadisseux JF, Evrard PH. Glial-neuronal relationship in the developing CNS. A histochemical electron microscopic study of radial glial cell particulate glycogen in normal reeler mice and in the human fetus. *Dev Neurosci* 1985; 7:12–37.

22. Gressens P, Evrard PH. The glial fascicle: an ontogenetic and phylogenetic unit guiding, supplying and distributing mammalian cortical neurones. *Dev Brain Res* 1993; 76:272–7.

23. Brun A. The subpial granular layer of the fetal cerebral cortex in man. *Acta Pathol Microbiol Scand* 1965; 179(suppl):3–98.

24. Wilkinson M, Hume R, Strange P, Bell JE. Glial and neuronal differentiation in the human fetal brain 9–23 weeks gestation. *Neuropathol Appl Neurobiol* 1990; 16:196–204.

25. Choi BH, Lapham LW. Do radial glia give rise to both astroglial and oligodendroglial cells? *Dev Brain Res* 1983; 8:119–30.

26. Molliver ME, Kostovic I, Van Der Loos H. The development of the synapses in cerebral cortex of human fetus. *Brain Res* 1973; 50:403–7.

27. Larroche JC. Quelques aspects anatomiques du développement cérébral. *Biol Neonate* 1962; 4:126–53.

28. Rakic P, Sidman RL. Histogenesis of cortical layers in human cerebellum particularly the lamina dissecans. *J Comp Neurol* 1970; 13:473–500.

PART II
MALFORMATIONS

JEANNE-CLAUDIE LARROCHE   FERECHTE ENCHA-RAZAVI

Malformations of the CNS are considered to be "deviations in form and structure from the genetically determined pattern, exceeding the range of normal variability" [1], but the borderline between CNS malformations and other brain disorders is still a matter of discussion [2–5]. Brain malformations, exhaustively described in the past, should be considered as disorders of the developing brain and studied with special attention to the causes and their prevention.

CAUSES OF CNS MALFORMATIONS

CNS malformations are classified into primary and secondary malformations. Primary malformations are considered to result from genetic or chromosomal disorders and represent together 8.1% of all malformations. Secondary malformations result from interference with normal developmental processes and depend on exogenous causes such as infection, teratogen, or trauma. They represent 12% of all malformations [6]. By definition, secondary malformations cannot be inherited. However, genetic factors can predispose to, and influence the occurrence of, such malformations. These so-called multifactorial causes acount for 20% of all malformations. In 60% of all malformations, the cause remains undetermined. Similar structural abnormalities may be produced by genetic, chromosomal, or exogenous causes. Therefore, it may be very difficult to prove that a given agent is teratogenic, and genetic counseling becomes a great challenge.

Monogenic Causes

Cerebral malformations due exclusively to mutant genes are rare. Autosomal recessive microcephaly vera, autosomal dominant paralysis of the 7th cranial nerve, and X-linked hydrocephalus are the most common forms. Mutation of neurogenic genes has been demonstrated in lower species and raises the question of the existence of analogous genes controlling CNS development in humans [7]. In practice, except for a few cases, the hereditary occurrence of CNS malformations is difficult to establish because of the variable penetrance and polygenic nature of the gene disorder, the development of new mutations, and the smallness of the pedigrees.

Chromosomal Causes

Chromosome disorders are usually responsible for mental retardation, but their association with CNS malformations is inconstant and semispecific. Chromosome aberrations have been found in 40% of spontaneous abortuses with CNS malformations [8], but in another series, more than two-thirds of fetuses and infants with chromosomal anomalies had no brain malformations [9]. CNS malformations usually are not associated with specific chromosomal syndromes. Their appearance follows patterns of semispecificity. If a strong association exists between some chromosome aberrations such as trisomy 13 and holoprosencephaly, not all the brains in individuals with trisomy 13 will present holoprosencephaly, and this anomaly is also observed in partial monosomy of chromosome 13, in trisomy 18, and in triploidy [10].

Other chromosome aberrations (autosomal or gonosomal) can be associated, occasionally, with CNS malformations [11].

The semispecificity of chromosome aberrations and the related CNS malformations has yet to be explained.

Recently, with the introduction of high-resolution techniques, minute chromosome defects that previously were unidentifiable have been detected. The Miller-Dieker syndrome, for example, consisting of microcephaly, lissencephaly, and multiple dysmorphic features, which was previously considered to be an autosomal recessive disorder, may be related, at least in some cases, to a partial monosomy of chromosome 17 [12, 13].

Inborn Errors of Metabolism

Among inborn errors of metabolism, only the association of gyral abnormalities and subcortical neuronal heterotopias with peroxisome defect and impaired oxidation of very-long-chain fatty acids (VLCFAs) in Zellweger cerebrohepatorenal syndrome has been established [14].

Exogenous Causes

Classically, the critical period in teratogenesis of the CNS is from the 3rd to the 6th week of the embryonic period. However, teratogenic agents acting during late embryonic and fetal life or in the early postnatal period may interfere with brain development and cell differentiation.

The teratogenic effects of some infectious agents such as rubella, herpes simplex, and cytomegalovirus or *Toxoplasma gondii* are now well established. However, two questions still remain unanswered: how often during pregnancy does infection with teratogenic organisms occur, and how often do such organisms cause malformations? In addition, in several animal species, antenatal viral infection can selectively destroy a cell population without leaving any trace. For example, a form of cerebellar ataxia in cats, previously considered to be a genetically transmitted disease, is in fact due to the feline panleukopenic virus [15], and, in hamsters, mumps virus can attack the ependyma without inflammation, leaving a narrowed aqueduct [16]. In maternofetal transmission of human immunodeficiency virus (HIV) infection, intrauterine growth retardation, microcephaly, and developmental delay have been reported [17]. A few neuropathologic studies have shown decreases in cell population, edema, and microglial-like cell proliferation [18]. However, the relationship between these lesions and HIV infection has not yet been demonstrated. It is well known that, during pregnancy, associated factors such as alcohol and drug abuse, other viral or parasitic infections, and poor health conditions can damage the developing brain. In HIV-infected mothers, neuropathologic studies of the "noninfected fetuses" have failed to show specific changes [19]. Nests of migrating cells and cerebellar heterotopias found in most cases were considered as common findings in the fetal brain.

Among the noninfectious maternal illnesses, diabetes [20] and phenylketonuria may be associated with CNS malformations, mainly with neural tube defects and cerebellar heterotopias.

Among environmental substances suspected of causing brain malformations, only mercury is a proven human teratogen causing neuronal migration abormalities. Various syndromes, including microcephaly, facial dysmorphia, and mental retardation, have been described in relation to a number of drugs such as phenytoin (hydantoin) and warfarin (coumarin) and to alcohol abuse [21]. The use of large doses of vitamin A and certain vitamin deficiencies can also interfere with CNS development [22].

Ionizing radiation is a potent teratogen, acting on neuron proliferation and migration, with subsequent microcephaly and mental retardation.

MECHANISMS OF BRAIN MALFORMATIONS

The mechanism by which brain malformations occur is still unknown. Mutation of genes and chromosome aberrations probably operate through excessive cell death, failure of cell interaction, reduced biosynthesis, and impaired morphogenetic movement.

In chromosomal monosomies, only half of the expected normal amount of gene is present, whereas in trisomy, one and a half times the normal amount of gene is present, reflecting the fact that a triple dose of gene results in a tripling of the amount of gene product over monosomy.

Exogenous causes and early direct injury to the brain may impair cell division, radial glial cell function, and neuronal migration as well as all connections.

CLASSIFICATION

The final morphology of some malformations obviously depends on the time of occurrence of the "insult" and the stage of development of the CNS.

For instance:

neurulation failure occurs during the 4 embryonic weeks
neural tube growth failure occurs up to 10 weeks
cytoarchitectonic abnormalities up to 16 to 18 weeks

In addition, early destructive lesions may mimic malformations.

Malformations Related to Neurulation Failure

Faulty Neural Induction
This anomaly is extremely rare and results in the absence of formation of the CNS, especially the cranial part. The head is then rudimentary or absent such as in holocardius twins.

Neural Tube Defects (NTD) or Dysraphia
The term "NTD" or "dysraphic state" [23] is applied to a variety of malformations resulting from incomplete to total absence of closure of the neural tube. It includes exencephaly, anencephaly, encephalocele, meningocele, and meningomyelocele—anomalies that can occur singly or in association. Their etiology is multifactorial [24] including

both genetic and environmental factors. In addition, there exist ethnic and geographic variations in the frequency of occurrence of the malformations [25].

The precise mechanism of NTD formation is not yet well understood. The concept of secondary rupture of the neural tube [23] has been ruled out, and primary nonclosure of the opposing neural folds is demonstrated in experimental models [2, 22, 26]. In recent years, multisite initiation of neural tube closure has been suggested to occur also in humans [27]. This is consistent with the recognition by fetopathologists of multisite neural tube defects. Primary mesodermal insufficiency [28] or abnormal arterial patterns in the territories corresponding to the NTD [29] may be implicated in the initiation of the disorder.

Prenatal detection of NTD is possible by ultrasonography as early as 12 weeks for anencephaly and by estimation of maternal serum values of alpha-fetoprotein (AFP) between 16 and 18 weeks. A raised level of acetyl-cholinesterase in amniotic fluid is also associated with open spina bifida.

Prevention of NTD seems to be possible with improvement of the maternal diet and preconceptional therapy with folic acid and multivitamin preparations.

Exencephaly and Anencephaly *Exencephaly* has rarely been described in human pathology. The scalp and calvarium are missing, and the "hemispheres" are covered by a dura-mater-like membrane. Exencephaly is said to be found only in young fetuses because of the rapid necrosis of brain tissue when exposed to amniotic fluid, subsequently leading to anencephaly. However, in our cases [30], including both immature fetuses and full-term infants, the hemispheres consisted of a large mass of anarchic nervous tissue with a superficial polymicrogyric cortex and large nodules of heterotopic cells. The hippocampal structures were in an ectopic position.

In *anencephaly*, by definition, the calvarium is absent. In some cases, however, the "cerebral" tissue may be partially covered by a rudiment of bony vault and scalp. The base of the skull is coarse and flattened, and there is a constant anomaly of the sphenoid bone. The orbits are shallow, causing protrusion of the eyes (Fig. 21.7). The forebrain is replaced by an angiomatous mass with multiple cavities containing cerebrospinal fluid (CSF). In the rudimentary posterior fossa, a disorganized structure resembling brainstem and cerebellum can be found. Absent calvarium may be associated with a spinal defect, producing a craniorachischisis.

Histologic examination of the "cerebral" mass reveals a dense meshwork of connective tissue containing thin-walled veins and capillaries. Communication with the systemic circulation is minimal. Nodules of glial tissue, ependyma-like epithelium, choroid plexuses, and trigeminal ganglia are usually found. The anterior pituitary gland, although hypoplastic, is present, while the intermediate and posterior lobes are always missing. The absence of these structures and of the hypothalamus is responsible for the hypoplastic

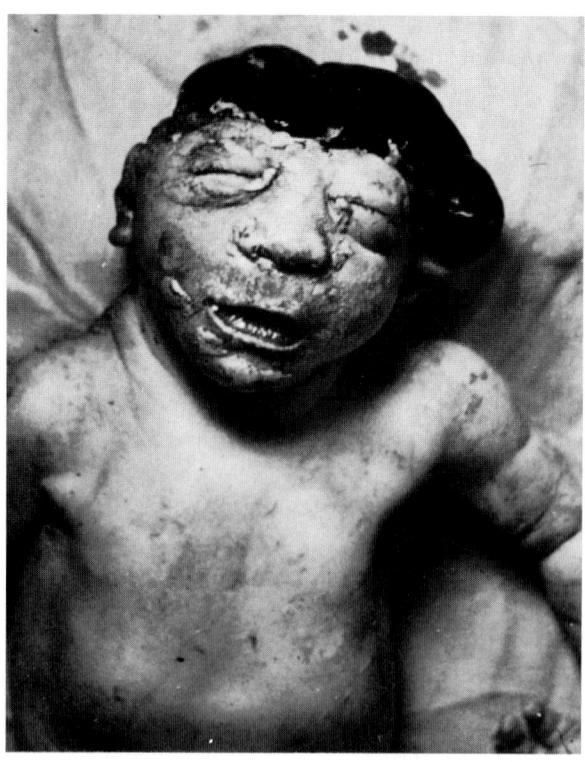

FIGURE 21.7.   *Anencephalic full-term stillborn with a large mass of angiomatous tissue.*

adrenal cortex. Anencephaly may be associated with spina bifida and with visceral anomalies such as large thymus and hypoplastic lungs.

Cranial Meningocele and Encephalocele These malformations occur most frequently, in 75–80% of cases, in the occipital region. The cranial defect is usually at or below the inion. Anterior (Fig. 21.8) and parietal encephaloceles are much less common. The herniated mass is totally or partially covered with normal skin and hair and is attached to one hemisphere by a narrow pedicle. The lesion may consist only of meninges and CSF or of disorganized fibrous and vascular tissue. It may contain brain tissue as well. The size of the herniated mass varies from case to case; when a significant portion of the brain, or all of it, is included in the cephalocele, the cranial vault is extremely reduced in size and the gross appearance of the infant's face mimics that of anencephaly. The herniated neural tissue may show small convolutions with normally laminated or polymicrogyric cortex and white matter, which may or may not surround a cavity, which in turn may or may not communicate with the main ventricular system. The cephaloceles are also found in the nasal, pharyngeal, and sphenoidal areas.

Certain occipital encephaloceles are a component of Meckel syndrome, which also includes polydactyly and polycystic kidney. The malformation my also be a part of the amniotic band syndrome.

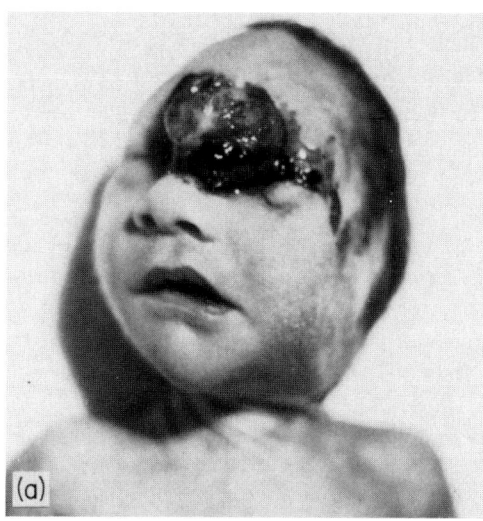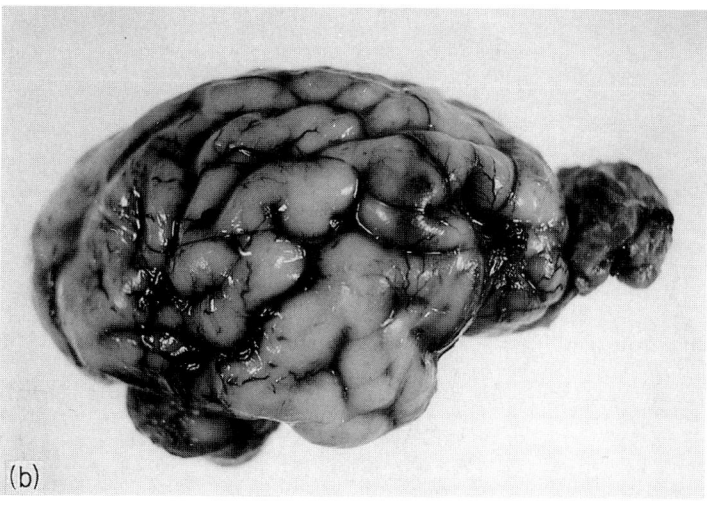

FIGURE 21.8.   *Anterior encephalocele: (a) general view; (b) brain after dissection with the anterior herniated mass.*

Spinal Meningocele and Myelomeningocele   Meningocele and myelomeningocele represent the most common NTD, with a female-to-male ratio of 4:1. They are associated with a defect in the vertebrae that consists of a lack of fusion or absence of the vertebral arches (spina bifida) with varying degrees of severity. The defect is most commonly lumbar or sacral (Fig. 21.9). In *meningocele*, the herniated meninges are covered with normal skin or with a thin membrane. The lesion may be ulcerated and flat, or may form a bulging sac filled with CSF. Usually, above the lesion, the spinal cord shows abnormalities such as syringomyelia, hydromyelia, diastematomyelia, or diplomyelia [31].

In *meningomyelocele*, the spinal cord is flattened and dysplastic, with an open central canal or disorganized ependymal structures, glial tissue, and angiomatous formation as in anencephaly; it blends progressively into the surrounding normal skin. In the malformed area, the spinal roots either traverse the cystic cavity or run along the wall. Above the defect, the spinal cord also shows a great variety of abnormalities [31].

Hydrocephalus is often associated with one of these defects, but the relationships between the two anomalies are not clearly understood.

Arnold-Chiari Malformation   The Arnold-Chiari malformation is almost constantly present in patients with meningomyelocele. In this complex anomaly, deformities of brainstem and cerebellum can be found in various combinations and degrees of severity. Four types have been described under this double eponym.

Type I consists of herniation of the cerebellar tonsils. This lesion afflicts adults and may be a cause of late-onset hydrocephaly; there is no spina bifida.

Type II is by far the most common type, encountered in neonates and fetuses (Fig. 21.10a); it is almost always associated with lumbosacral myelomeningocele and is now recognized as the Arnold-Chiari malformation. It consists of cranial bone and brainstem-cerebellum abnormalities. The bones of the vault show variations in thickness known as craniolacunia, and the posterior fossa is small and shallow with a low position of venous sinuses and torcula. The

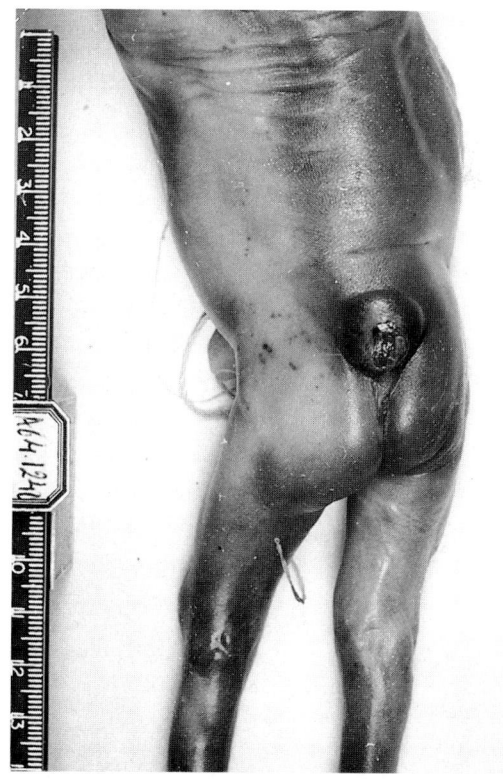

FIGURE 21.9.   *Lumbosacral meningomyelocele in a 25-week-old fetus.*

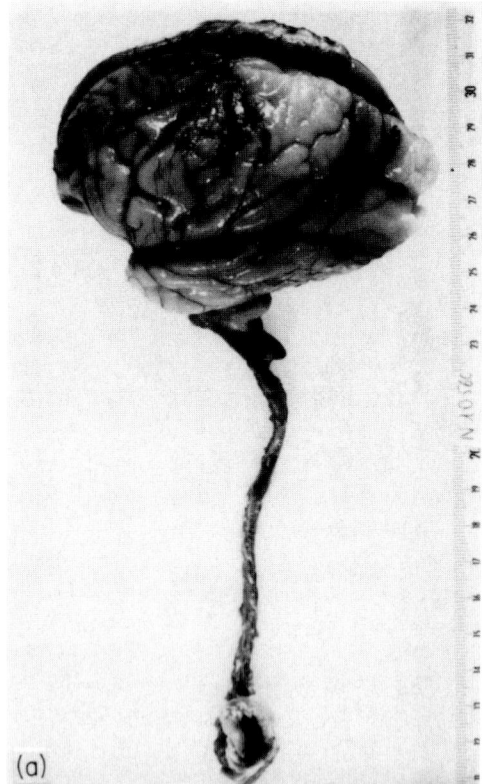

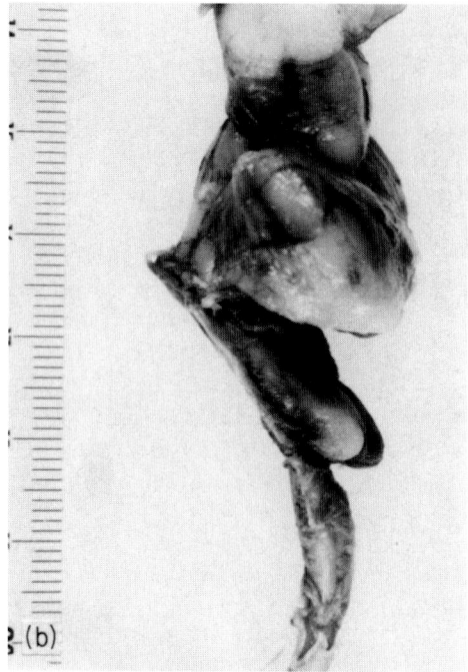

FIGURE 21.10.   *Arnold-Chiari malformation: (a) general view; (b) note flattened cerebellum and Z-shaped upper spinal cord.*

insertion of the tentorium, which may be rudimentary, is low, and the foramen magnum is enlarged.

Brainstem, pons, and medulla oblongata are elongated; the caudal portion of the vermis and the amygdalae are dis-

placed downward and herniated through the foramen magnum; the medulla oblongata, which seems too long, overrides the posterior cervical segments of the spinal cord, giving, on sagittal view, a characteristic Z-shaped appearance (Fig. 21.10b). The vermis is buried between the hemispheres, which are often asymmetric and flattened. Tufts of choroid plexus and hypervascularized meninges surround the herniated cerebellum, which is usually necrosed. Large heterotopic cell nodules are common findings in the cerebellum.

At the level of the cerebral peduncles, the quadrigeminal plate shows a beak-shaped deformity, and the aqueduct of Sylvius is often atretic.

Hydrocephalus is the most common associated abnormality, caused either by herniation of tissue through the foramen magnum or by a dysmorphic aqueduct. The surfaces of the hemispheres exhibit small gyria (microgyria), but on microscopic examination there is no true polymicrogyria [32].

In the spinal cord, hydromyelia, diastematomyelia, syringomyelia, diplomyelia, and asymmetry or absence of the ventral pyramidal tracts may be found.

Type III consists of cervical spina bifida with herniation of the cerebellum through the bony defect.

Type IV is cerebellar hypoplasia.

The cause and the pathogenesis of the malformation are still under discussion. Several theories have been proposed, such as downward traction of the cord due to its fixation in the myelomeningocele, deformity secondary to hydrocephalus, primary developmental disorder of the brainstem and cerebellum, failure of formation of the pontine flexure, and overgrowth of the cerebellum. The only common denominator among the first three types is a disproportion between the sizes of the cerebellum and the posterior fossa, which is always small.

Other Abnormalities of the Spinal Cord   Myelodysplasias are often associated with myelomeningocele and Arnold-Chiari malformation but may also be an incidental finding on systematic histologic examination of the spinal cord.

Hydromyelia is an overdistension of the central canal as a result of persistent embryonal state. In the neonate, isolated hydromyelia is asymptomatic and may be associated with a cyst of the ventriculus terminalis [33].

Syringomyelia, which may develop in adults, is hardly differentiated from hydromyelia in its congenital form. The abnormal syrinx may or may not be lined by ependyma; it may form a diverticulum of hydromyelia or be totally separated from the central canal.

Duplication of the central canal, usually associated with myelomeningocele, may be a fortuitous discovery on systematic examination of fetal spinal cords.

Diastematomyelia consists of two hemicords either contained in a single dural sac or separated by vascular and connective tissue, or contained in two distinct dural sacs between which may be a bony septum. Both hemicords are often rotated, facing each other, each with its own spinal artery. The malformation is often associated with bone anomalies in Klippel-Feil syndrome. Symptoms do not develop until childhood.

Diplomyelia represents a duplicate spinal cord instead of two facing hemicords.

Malformations Related to Failure of Neural Tube Growth

Prosencephalon Growth Failure

Prosencephalon growth failure covers a large group of heterogeneous anomalies whose classification is difficult. After Jellinger and Gross [34], Leech and Shuman [35] proposed to group together all those malformations sharing defects of median and paramedian structures of the prosencephalon and adjacent rostral structures. The group includes aprosencephaly, holoprosencephaly, septo-optic dysplasia and commissural agenesis (corpus callosum and anterior commissure), and isolated arhinencephaly. In spite of its historical connotation, the term "arhinencephaly" should not be used as a synonym for "holoprosencephaly." From cytoarchitectonic and-mapping studies of Yakovlev [36], it became clear that the only missing architectonic fields are those characteristic of the frontal lobes, anterior to the motor area.

In this large spectrum, any malformation can develop by itself or in association with others.

Holoprosencephaly *Holoprosencephaly* is a complex malformation that was subdivided by DeMyer et al [37] into three main forms, according to their severity.

The alobar form (Fig. 21.11a, b, and c), with no distinct interhemispheric fissure, absence of corpus callosum and septum, single ventricle with roofed membrane, unseparate thalami, and hippocampi in dorsal position is the most severe form.

The semilobar form shows rudimentary hemispheric lobes, incomplete interhemispheric fissure, and absence of olfactory bulbs.

Lobar holoprosencephaly shows well-formed hemispheric lobes, complete or incomplete separation of the neocortex across the midline, and a single ventricular system. In fact, there is a continuum among these three groups, with a great variety of intermediate forms [1]. Fetal and postnatal ultrasound scans show the characteristic features (Fig. 21.11d).

Brain anomalies are often associated with midline facial defects, including cyclopia, ethmocephaly, cebocephaly, premaxillary agenesis, and other minor facial features [38].

Histologically, in the most severe form with cyclopia, cortical lamination is abnormal [33]. It consists of a normal molecular layer, a superficial layer with a nodular distribution of large neurons, a sparsely cellular layer, a thick homogeneous cellular layer, and a deep layer devoid of cells that blends into the subcortical white matter. The meninges around the brainstem are thickened and contain a large amount of extracerebral glial tissue. The cerebellum may be hypoplastic, and there are always large heterotopic nodules of cells dispersed preferentially in the white matter and in the nuclei.

Holoprosencephaly is not uncommon. The risk is estimated at more than 1 in 16,000 births. It occurs sporadically or in a variety of chromosomal anomalies [39, 40], such as trisomy 13 most frequently, but also trisomy 18, trisomy 21, triploidy, the 18p- syndrome, and the 13q- syndrome. Some familial cases have been reported, suggesting an autosomal recessive inheritance. Diabetic mothers have a risk at least 200 times higher than that of the general population.

Aprosencephaly *Aprosencephaly* refers to an extreme reduction of the prosencephalon with fusion of the thalami.

Agenesis of the Corpus Callosum Total or partial agenesis of the corpus callosum may be an incidental finding in the otherwise normal brain or be associated with a large number of complex cerebral malformations [41], such as holoprosencephaly with absence of the anterior commissure and/or septum pellucidum, Dandy-Walker syndrome, cerebellar hypoplasia, arthrogryposis multiplex congenita, and Aicardi syndrome [42], as well as with skeletal and/or visceral malformations. Agenesis of the corpus callosum is generally sporadic, but familial cases have been reported. Although the malformation in humans often appears to be autosomal recessive as in mice, afflicting either boys or girls [43, 44], an X-linked mode of inheritance has also been suggested [45]. Partial agenesis of the corpus callosum most often affects the posterior part of the structure, but not exclusively (Fig. 21.12). In total absence of the corpus callosum, the medial surfaces of the hemispheres have an abnormal gyral pattern. The cingulum is poorly outlined, and most gyri extend perpendicularly to the roof of the third ventricle. On coronal sections of the brain, no midline structure separates the lateral ventricles, which present a characteristic horn shape. Callosal fibers that did not cross the midline form an anteroposterior structure known as Probst's bundle. The fornix is displaced laterally, and the septum is classically absent. However, septum pellucidum-like tissue may be found between Probst's bundle and the fornix [46]. When hydrocephalus is associated with the malformation, the roof of the third ventricle, formed by a pial-arachnoid and ependymal tissue, bulges between the hemispheres and may be mistaken for an arachnoid cyst.

Agenesis of the corpus callosum can be detected by ultrasound in fetuses of 18 weeks only indirectly when the cavum septi pellucidi is not visible. In neonates, ultrasound is the method of first choice for detecting the malformation [47] (Fig. 21.13).

Anomalies of the Septum Pellucidum One or both leaves of the septum may be absent with a normal corpus callosum, indicating a relative independence of the two structures [48]. Agenesis of the septum pellucidum (Fig. 21.14) may be an isolated finding or may be associated with optic nerve anomalies and hypopituitarism known as septo-optic dysplasia [49] or with porencephalies [50].

Anomalies of the Wall of the Lateral Ventricles Anomalies of ventricular shape with supernumerary cavities have been

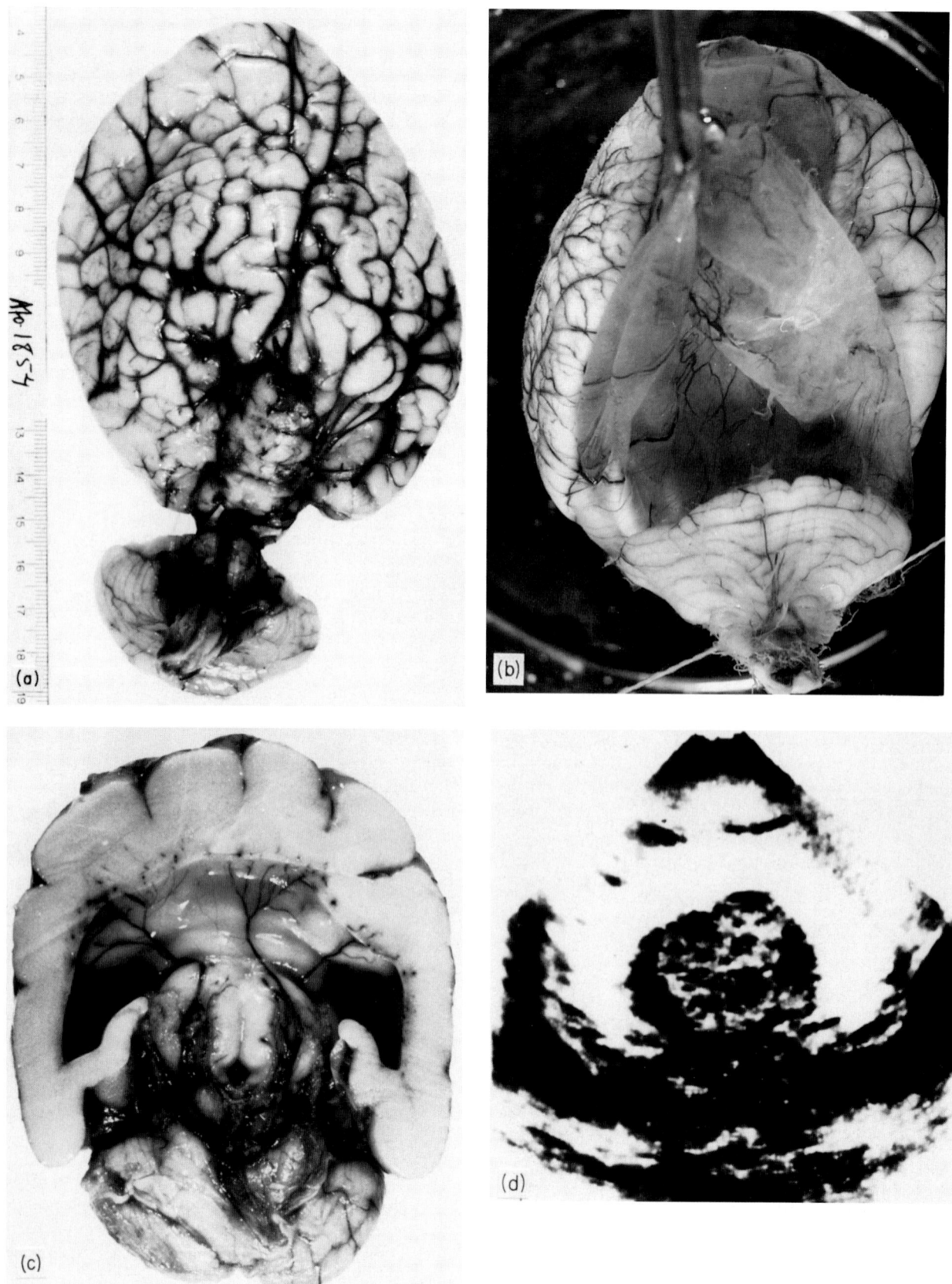

FIGURE 21.11.   *Holoprosencephaly: (a) basal view; (b) superior view showing distended thin membrane-roofed single ventricle; (c) coronal section of the brain showing horseshoe-shaped ventricle and temporal lobes; (d) ultrasound image of the malformation.*

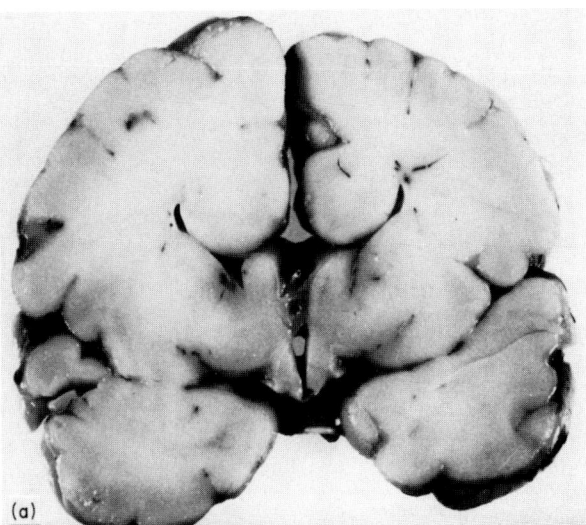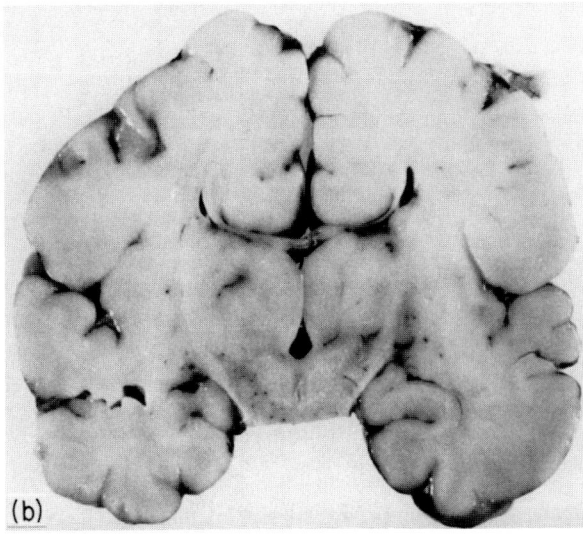

FIGURE 21.12.   *Partial agenesis of the corpus callosum: (a) anterior section—agenesis; (b) median section—the corpus callosum is hypoplastic but present.*

described under a variety of names, such as coarctation [51] and coaptation [52]. The affected ventricle may be reduced in size, and the contralateral one may be enlarged. The supplementary cavities may be closed or in communication with the main ventricular system. On microscopic examination, the surfaces of the cavities are lined with ependymal cells or a dense glial network with tufts of remaining germinal cells [33]. Possible causative factors include an early inflammatory process with secondary adhesion between two

facing ventricular walls, and early hypoxic-ischemic destruction of subependymal cells with subsequent cavitation.

Brainstem and Cerebellum Growth Failure

Brainstem Abnormalities   Brainstem anomalies are often associated with other brain abnormalities. In Arnold-Chiari malformation, the quadrigeminal plate often shows a beaklike deformity above the cerebellum. In posterior encephalocele, the defect may originate from the quadrigeminal plate and include part or all of the cerebellum.

Abnormalities of the aqueduct of Sylvius, such as slitlike shape, forking, atresia, and absence with multiple rosette formations, are often associated with gross anomalies of the

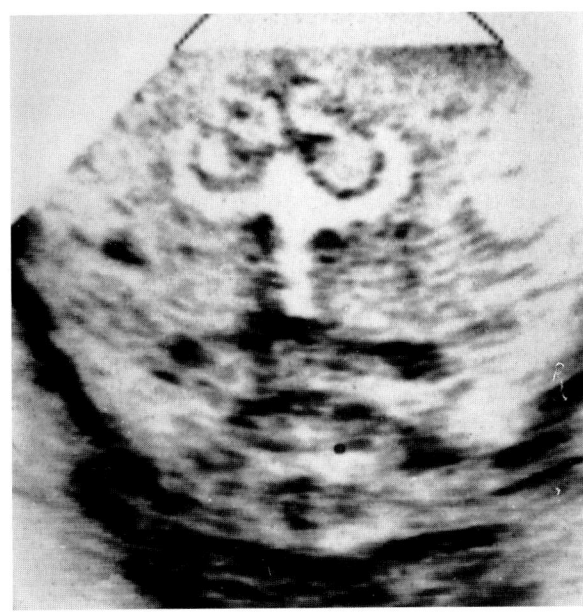

FIGURE 21.13.   *Ultrasound view of total agenesis of the corpus callosum.*

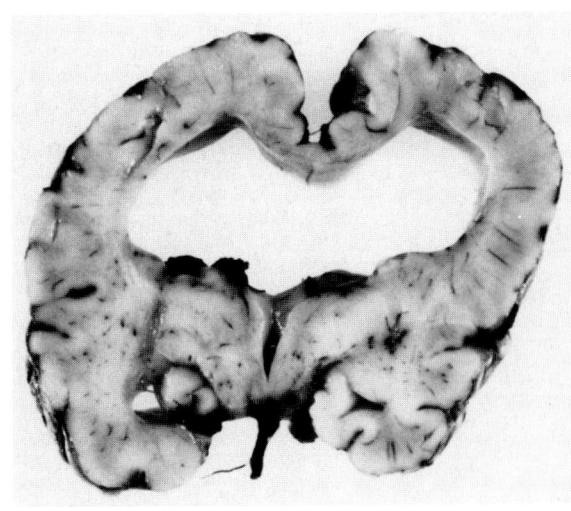

FIGURE 21.14.   *Agenesis of the septum pellucidum.*

brainstem. Stenosis of the aqueduct, following Russel's definition, is rare, and has been reported in an X-linked syndrome including deformed thumbs and anomalies of the pyramidal tracts.

Malformations of the Cerebellum *Agenesis* of the entire cerebellum [53] (Fig. 21.15) or of one hemisphere is very uncommon and has been described in a heterogeneous group of patients; it may be associated with other malformations such as agenesis of the corpus callosum. The inferior olives and pons are hypoplastic.

Hypoplasia of the cerebellum is observed in a great variety of situations. One hemisphere or the entire cerebellum may be hypoplastic.

Granular cell hypoplasia has been found in some cases of amaurotic idiocy. A similar anomaly, described in Weaver mutant mice, can be induced experimentally by injecting cycasin into newborn mice [54]. It is considered as an arrest of development of the external granular cells during early life [55]. Histologically, the molecular layer is usually wide and gliotic, and myelination is poor. Purkinje's cells are mildly affected, with anarchic growth of dendrites and an excess of dendritic spines. Disordered formation of Bergmann's glia is probably the cause of the failure of migration and death of granular cells.

In pontocerebellar hypoplasia, only the lateral lobes of the cerebellum are hypoplastic. The vermis and flocculi are usually well developed. The dentate nuclei are fragmented into isolated nuclear clumps, and pontine nuclei are markedly reduced in number. In the brainstem, nuclei with cerebellar connections are either absent or poorly developed. The ventral pons shows a marked reduction in the number of transverse fibers and cells. Severe neuronal loss of the inferior olives has also been reported. A retardation in development or a degenerative process is considered to be the cause of the anomaly.

In fetuses and neonates, hypoplasia and atrophy of the cerebellum are often associated with encephaloceles, holoprosencephalies, and trisomy 18 and 21. Later in life, hypoplasia may follow severe neonatal anoxic-ischemic episodes. It is also observed in Werdnig-Hoffmann disease.

Total or partial absence of the vermis occurs as an isolated feature; as part of a syndrome, as in Walker-Warburg syndrome or Dandy-Walker malformation; or in association with other disorders such as encephalocele, holoprosencephaly, fusion of the thalami, polymicrogyria, and hypoplastic corpus callosum. The posterior part of the vermis is usually missing. In some cases, the cerebellar hemispheres are fused in the midline as well as the dentate nuclei. Aplasia of the vermis is also described in familial Joubert syndrome, which includes episodic hyperpnea, abnormal eye movements, ataxia, and mental retardation.

Cysts of the cerebellum are very unusual. In the neonatal period, they may occur as a feature of Von Hippel-Lindau disease with multiple angiomas. In older patients, cystic lesions are secondary to infarction or hemorrhage.

Dandy-Walker malformation is an entity that associates posterior fossa "cyst" corresponding to the distended roof of the fourth ventricle (Fig. 21.16a) and hypoplasia of the vermis [56, 57] (Fig. 21.16b). The posterior fossa is enlarged, with high insertion of the sinuses and tentorium. The cerebellar hemispheres are usually normal in size but, because of the frequently associated hydrocephalus, are flattened. The wall of the cyst is made of an ependymal-meninges-like membrane with connective tissue and ectopic cerebellar cells. It progressively blends with the meninges of the hemispheres. Associated malformations, such as total or partial callosal defect, and abnormal cerebral gyral pattern with polymicrogyria and heterotopias, are common. The inferior olives are often malformed and in an ectopic position. At birth, infants with this malformation have a large head with noticeable bulging of the occipital region and raised intracranial pressure.

Pathogenesis of the Dandy-Walker syndrome is unknown. Prenatal diagnosis is possible by ultrasonography (Fig. 21.16c).

Cerebral Cysts

Arachnoid Cysts Arachnoid cysts [58] are formed by splitting of the arachnoid membrane, which is reinforced by a thick layer of collagen. The wall of the cyst is totally independent of the inner layer of the dura, and the fine structure of the cells forming the membrane is similar to that of normal trabecular arachnoid cells. Arachnoid cysts are found most commonly in the sylvian fissure or in the hippocampal fissure; they are rare in neonates. Lourie and Berne [59]

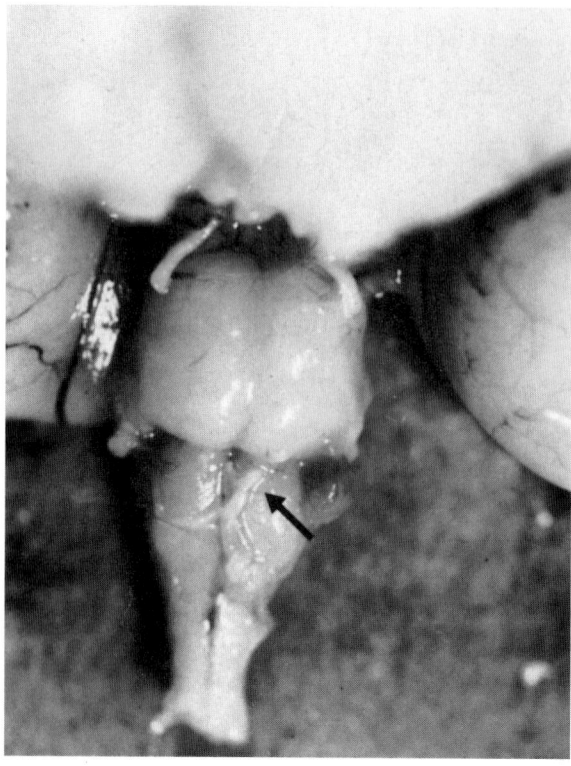

FIGURE 21.15. *Agenesis of the cerebellum. Basal view with basilar artery (arrow).*

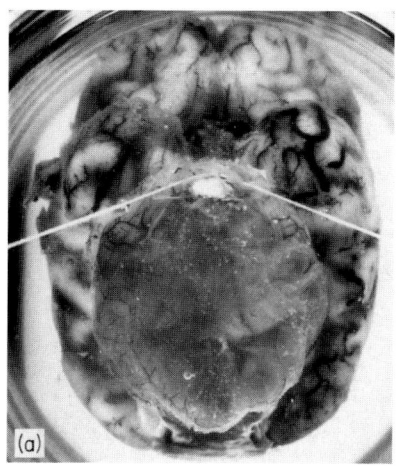
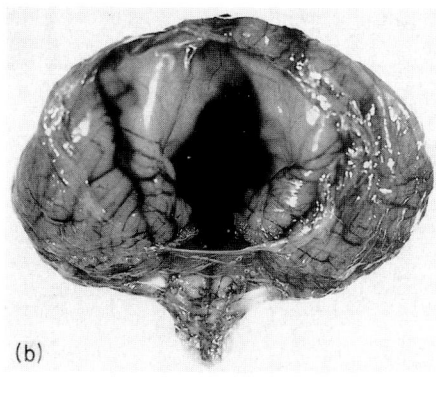
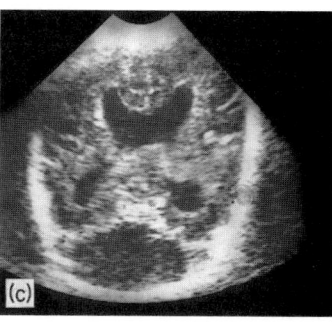

FIGURE 21.16. *Dandy-Walker malformation: (a) basal view under water shows the large cyst with floating membranes; (b) the cyst is open, showing agenesis of the vermis; (c) ultrasound shows the empty posterior fossa and enlarged ventricles.*

reported a case of congenital hydrocephalus due to a hemorrhagic arachnoid cyst located over the cerebral peduncles. Multiple arachnoid cysts, attached to the inferior and posterior margins of the falx cerebri (Fig. 21.17), may be associated with other brain malformations [46]. The cysts can be diagnosed by ultrasonography and computed tomography (CT).

Choroid Plexus Cysts Choroid plexus cysts, rare in neonates, are seen more frequently in fetal brains by ultrasonography; they tend to disappear on advancing age (Fig. 21.18).

Subependymal Pseudocysts Subependymal pseudocysts are described in Part III.

Arteriovenous Malformations

Aneurysmal malformation of the vein of Galen is a true embryopathy that consists of the persistence of the embryonic vascular pattern [60]. It is the most frequent arteriovenous malformation observed in neonates [61]. Aneurysms of the vein of Galen are generally supplied by blood from one or both posterior cerebral arteries or from one of their

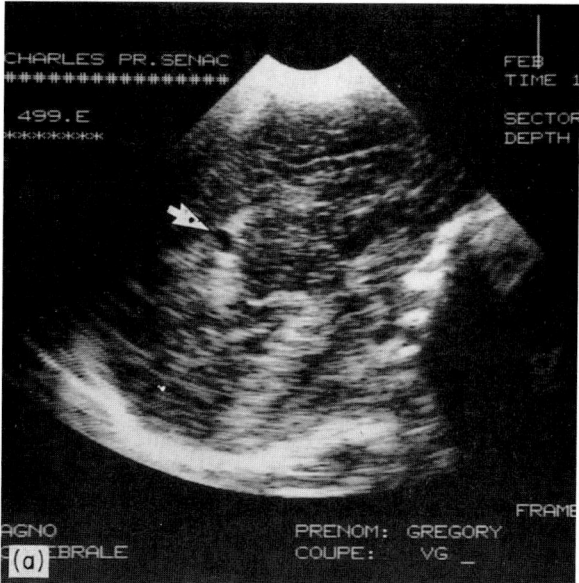

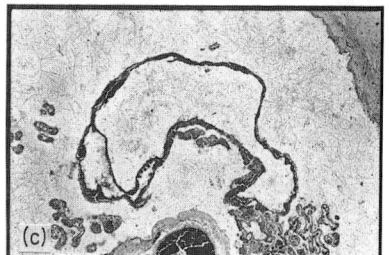
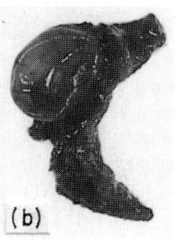

FIGURE 21.17. *Multiple arachnoid cysts attached to the inferior margin of the falx cerebri.*

FIGURE 21.18. *Choroid plexus cyst: (a) fetal ultrasound, showing cyst formation within the echoic plexus; (b) and (c) gross and microscopic appearance of a cyst.*

branches and less frequently from small posterior branches of the middle cerebral arteries. These aneurysms may also be fed by anomalous branches of the carotid and/or basilar circulation. The vessels may have a normal architecture, but more often a lacelike network of tortuous vessels empties into the saccular vein of Galen; the caliber of the distended vein may be up to several centimeters in diameter. The entire venous system, including the transverse and straight sinuses, is dilated. The upper vertebral and basilar arteries and the circle of Willis are often also tortuous, with thick walls.

Large shunts lead to cardiomegaly and congestive cardiac failure soon after birth. Various cerebral lesions, either in the territories of the corresponding arteries or elsewhere, occur in association with this vascular malformation. Periventricular infarction and intraventricular hemorrhage due to compression by the tumor-like vascular mass and periventricular calcification have been described. The aneurysm itself may become thrombosed or calcified.

Other arteriovenous malformations may occur elsewhere, probably resulting from failure of the primary vessels to differentiate into mature arterial and venous channels.

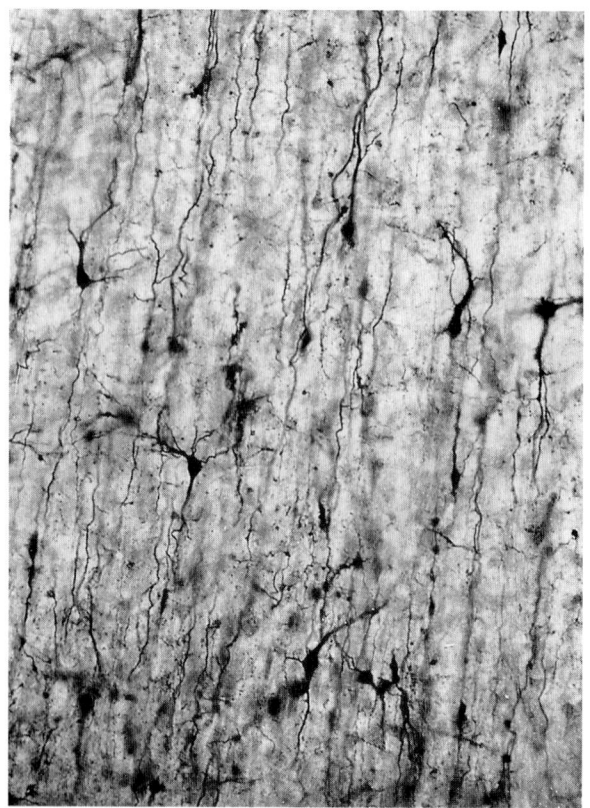

FIGURE 21.19. *Reverse orientation of neurons (Golgi-Cox preparation).*

Cytoarchitectonic Abnormalities

The cytoarchitectonic development of the brain depends on temporal and spatial sequences of cell multiplication and migration, which imply complex mechanisms and perfect neuron-glial interactions [62]. Failures or errors during this program result in a large spectrum of anomalies ranging from minute heterotopias in the otherwise normal brain to complex syndromes with agyria or polymicrogyria and microcephaly.

Heterotopias

Heterotopias refer to cells or groups of cells that have failed to migrate toward their assigned locations. They may be found anywhere in the cerebrum and cerebellum.

In the *subependymal zone*, heterotopic nodules of cells bulge into the ventricular cavity and can be seen by CT and ultrasound. Histologic study differentiates them from Bourneville's tuberous sclerosis. Even in young fetuses, in addition to characteristic morphologic features of the cells, the glial fibrillary acidic protein (GFAP) reaction is positive in tuberous sclerosis, and negative in heterotopias.

In the *white matter*, isolated heterotopic neurons are fairly common findings in otherwise normal brains. Large nodules of heterotopic cells are usually associated with other brain anomalies.

In the *cortex*, protrusion of groups of neurons of layer II (?) or isolated neurons in the molecular layer may have no significance, but large heterotopias are usually associated with complex anomalies. Neurons, obliquely oriented or in reverse position (Fig. 21.19), may be found in normal brains [63] or in association with other cortical dysplasias.

In the *meninges*, isolated neurons or small heterotopic nodules may be found on routine examination of immature brains (Fig. 21.20). However, large extracerebral glial or neuronal heterotopias are common in malformations such as microcephaly and holoprosencephaly and in viral fetal encephalopathies [64]. They are characteristic of the so-called dysplastic cortex of lissencephaly type II (Walker-Warburg syndrome) (see below).

In the *cerebellum*, heterotopias occur occasionally in normal fetuses and neonates and are found constantly in association with chromosomal aberrations such as trisomy 13 and trisomy 18 or with other complex cerebral malformations. Three types of cells—granular, spindle, and ganglionic cells—have been described [65, 66], usually grouped in clusters of homogeneous or heterogeneous components (Fig. 21.21). Each type tends to be located in specific sites: in folia or dentate and other nuclei, or in white matter.

Abnormalities of the Cortical Plate and Agyria-Pachygyria

A large spectrum of cortical anomalies are to be found in association with lissencephalies (agyria/pachygyria) [67–69]. However, three main types may be recognized based on the

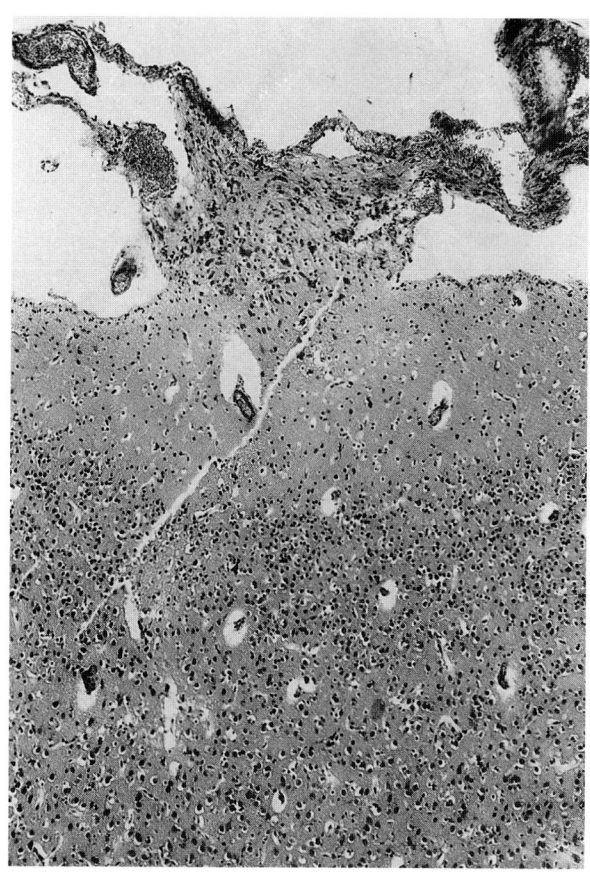

FIGURE 21.20. *Nodule of ectopic neurons in the meninges.*

external appearance of the brain, the pattern of the associated cortical anomalies, and other phenotypic characters. The third type is dominated by micrencephaly [70].

Lissencephaly Type I–Four-Layered Cortex–Miller-Dieker Syndrome The classical four-layered cortex of Bielschowsky [71], particularly well described by Crome in 1956 [72], is characteristic of lissencephaly type I found in the Miller-Dieker syndrome. The surface of the brain is smooth (Fig. 21.22a), and the cytoarchitectural anomaly consists of a reversed ratio between gray and white matter (Fig. 21.22b). The gray matter forms the main bulk of the wall of the hemispheres around a narrow rim of white matter.

Histologically, the "cortex" is characterized by: a marginal, molecular layer; a second, highly cellular layer made of medium-sized and large pyramidal cells and polymorphic neurons found in layers III, V, and VI of normal cortex; a third, sparsely cellular layer with a large number of tangential fibers and, in children, some poorly myelinated radial fibers; and a fourth, thick and deep cellular layer with neurons of varying size arranged in columns or in concentric rows. The narrow rim of periventricular white matter may contain dense islands of heterotopic neurons (Fig. 21.22c).

Other anomalies, such as ectopic inferior olives, are always found. In addition, large foci of calcification, either in the midline [33] (Fig. 21.22b) or close to the ventricles, have been reported. Apart from the smooth surface, the brain is always small with large ventricles.

The morphopathogenesis of this disorder is unclear. Arrest of neuronal migration is considered to be the basic mechanism leading to the cytoarchitectonic abnormalities specific to the Miller-Dieker syndrome [73, 74]. This syndrome includes characteristic phenotypic features such as small head, dysmorphic face, low-set ears, and small mandibles. Familial occurrence suggests a genetic transmission of the anomaly. In some cases of Miller-Dieker syndrome, deletion of the L1S1 gene located on 17p13 has been demonstrated [75]. Other clinicopathologic variants of type I lissencephaly, such as the Norman-Roberts syndrome [76] and the isolated lissencephaly syndrome (ILS) [77], have been identified. In the last group, chromosomal anomalies are not constant.

Lissencephaly Type II–Cortical Dysplasia–Walker-Warburg Syndrome The term "cortical dysplasia" refers to a peculiar disorder characteristic of lissencephaly type II. In addition to the smooth appearance of the brain and cerebellum (Fig. 21.23a), the leptomeninges appear thickened and whitish, and tightly adherent to the brain, particularly so at the base and around the brainstem (Fig. 21.23d). The frontal poles may be fused. On section of the brain, the ventricles are enlarged, and a number of heterotopic nodules bulge into the cavities (Fig. 21.23b).

Histologically, the cortical dysplasia consists of obliteration of the arachnoid space by neurons and glial cells and an absence of cortical lamination [64, 78, 79] (Fig. 21.23c). In the thick, extracortical neuroglial tissue, GFAP-positive glial cells are seen, with intense vascularization, enhanced by reticulin staining [79]. This outer band of tissue is separated from the inner part of the "cortex" by a layer of vascular connective tissue or primitive meninges. Groups of neurons appear to have been arrested by these meninges, while others have burst into the extracerebral space through defects in the meningovascular barrier (Fig. 21.23c). The inner part of the mantle consists of scattered nodules of heterotopic neurons and of a thin rim of white matter around the ventricles.

This form of cortical dysplasia, seen in lissencephaly type II, is characteristic of the *Walker-Warburg syndrome*. The malformation was first identified by Walker in 1942 [78], then considered by Chemke et al [80] as a possible autosomal recessive disorder. Later, Warburg [81] drew attention to the retinal dysplasia. The syndrome includes hydrocephaly, agyria, and retinal dysplasia (or abnormal anterior chamber, cataract microphthalmia, etc.), with or without encephalocele, hence the acronym HARD + E [82]. In 1984, Williams et al [83] proposed the dual eponym of Walker-Warburg syndrome (WWS) or cerebro-ocular dysgenesis. Other associated anomalies include dysplastic aqueduct of Sylvius and quadrigeminate plate, small cerebellum with micropolygyric

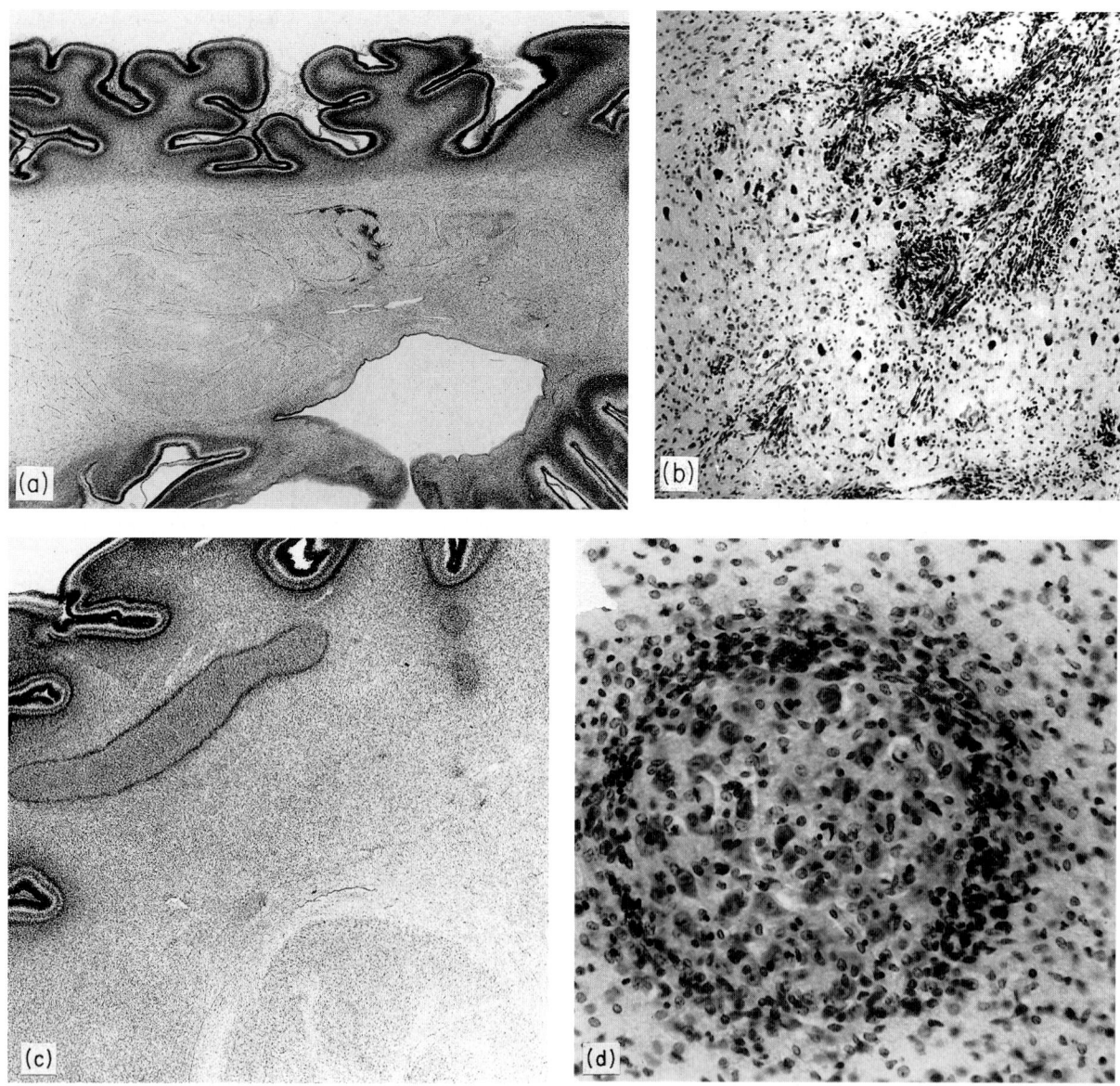

FIGURE 21.21.   *Cerebellar heterotopias: spindle cells in the dentate nucleus at low (a) and high (b) magnification; heterotopic nodule in the white matter at low (c) and high (d) magnification.*

folia, and hypoplastic vermis. All these features have been described in fetuses as young as 20 weeks [84].

In classic WWS, the cortical dysplasia is diffuse, involving the entire surface of the brain. However, the abnormal cell migration may be nodular and segmental, involving stripes of mantle, from the ependyma to the surface [85]. This type of cortical dysplasia suggests several possible types of pathomorphogenesis: a defect of the pial/glial membrane, which normally forms the external barrier to the migrating neurons, or an early ependymoglial defect impeding neuronal migration.

Related syndromes, described as cerebro-oculo-muscular syndrome (COMS) [86], a possible variant of Fukuyama

congenital muscular dystrophy (FCMD) [87], Tanaka syndrome [88], and muscle-eye-brain (MEB) disease [89], have been identified.

Lissencephaly Type III–Micrencephaly–Cytoarchitectonic Anomalies   In fetuses presenting the akinesia sequence (FAS) (Neu-Laxova, Pena-Shokier type II syndrome), heterogeneous cortical changes have been reported [90, 91], in association with severe micrencephaly-lissencephaly and external-internal hydrocephaly, features that may be grouped as lissencephaly type III. In addition, in most of our cases, there were multiple subependymal pseudocysts. The main histologic features are an immature cortical plate with focal polymicrogyria, hypoplastic basal ganglia, and brain-

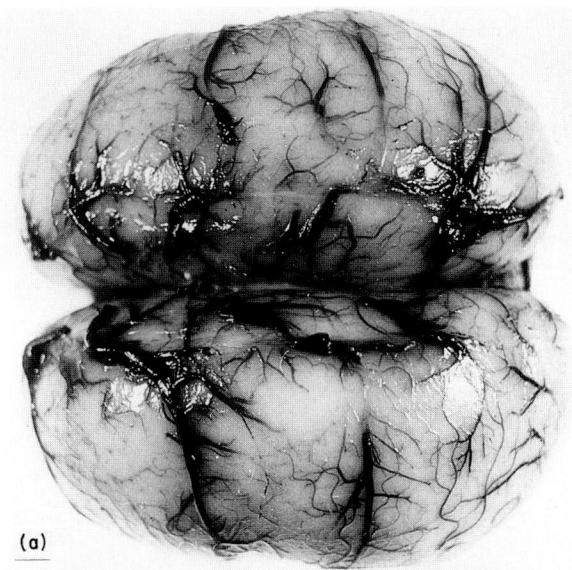

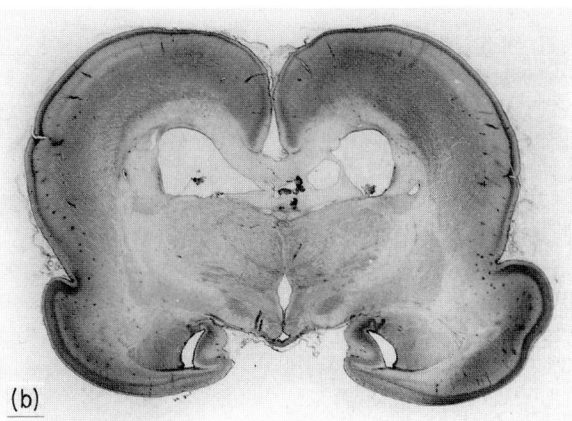

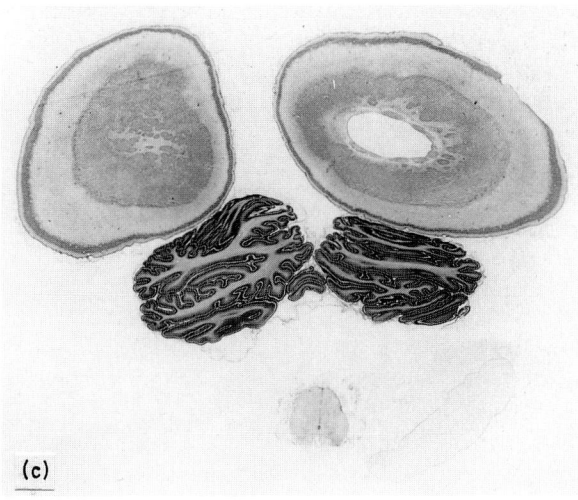

FIGURE 21.22. *Lissencephaly type I, Miller-Dieker syndrome in a 38-week-old fetus: (a) upper view of the agyric hemispheres; (b) coronal celloidin section (CV stain) shows the thick abnormal cortex and calcifications in the midline structure; (c) occipital lobes with massive periventricular heterotopias.*

stem and medulla with severe cell loss and proliferation of GFAP stellar astrocytes, associated with a possible secondary reduction of fiber tracts. All these features suggest a process of abnormal apoptosis or abnormal neurotrophic growth factors.

Microgyria

Microgyria describes an abnormality of the surface configuration of the brain consisting of a reduction in size and an increase in the number of gyri. The distribution of this pattern varies from case to case and may be associated with other brain abnormalities. In Arnold-Chiari malformation, the surface of the brain is often microgyric, but the underlying cortex is usually normal [32]. Microgyria must be differentiated from ulegyria or atrophic gyri secondary to anoxic-ischemic necrosis.

Pseudomicrogyria is described in fetal brains; when the meninges are peeled off during fixation, the surface of the brain often appears wrinkled. Histologically, the cortex is normal (Fig. 21.24).

Polymicrogyria

Polymicrogyria refers to microscopic anomalies of the cerebral and cerebellar cortex that at times may underlie a normal or even agyric surface.

Histologically, the classic polymicrogyric cortex [71] has four layers: 1) a sparsely cellular marginal or molecular layer; 2) an irregular, festoon-like superficial cellular layer with small round cells in the external part and multipolar or pyramidal cells in the inner part; 3) an acellular layer composed mainly of horizontal fibers that are myelinated in older infants; and 4) a deep cellular layer containing pyramidal and round cells. The polymicrogyric cortex may form deep indentations underneath a smooth surface of the brain and is often juxtaposed to normal cortex without transition (Fig. 21.25). This form is thought to be secondary to postmigratory laminar necrosis.

However, polymicrogyria, found adjacent to infarcts that developed early in fetal life (see Part III), may not show the four-layered type and may be associated with heterotopias. This feature is also seen in intrauterine infections due to cytomegalovirus, toxoplasmosis, and syphilis. In those cases, it seems that the hypoxic-ischemic insult has occurred before or during cell migration.

Another form of polymicrogyria without a clear layer or acellular layer (Figs. 21.25 and 21.26) is found in cases with complex malformations and large heterotopias, in thanatophoric dwarfism [30, 92, 93], or in metabolic disorders such as Zellweger syndrome [14]. This form may be considered as primary polymicrogyria.

In *cerebellar* polymicrogyria or cortical dysplasia (Fig. 21.27), the usual laminar cell pattern is disturbed: the external granular layer is disrupted with protrusion of neural cells in the arachnoid spaces. Purkinje cells and internal granular cells show a patchy or anarchic distribution, often associated with multiple foci of heterotopic cells in the white matter

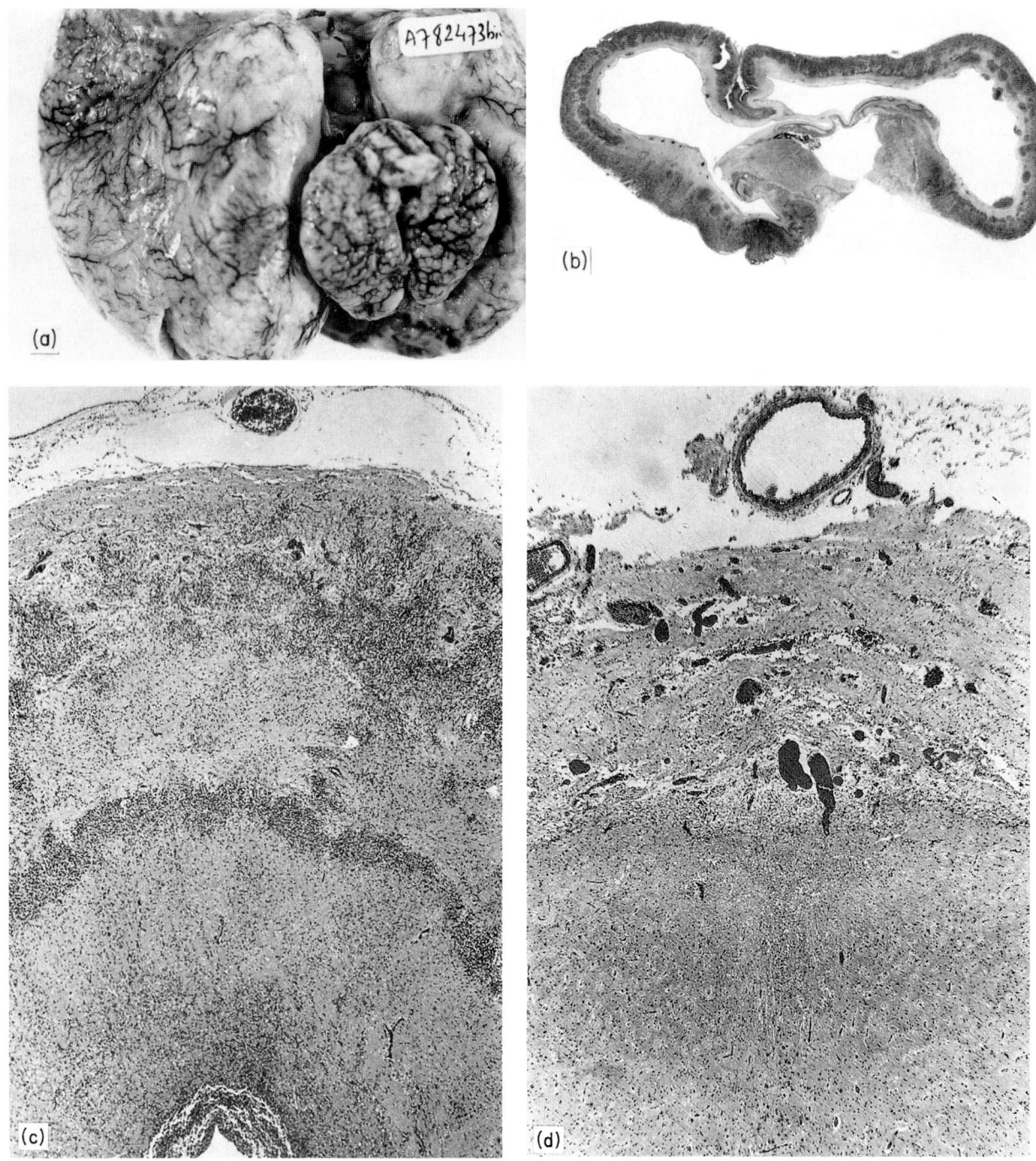

FIGURE 21.23.   *Lissencephaly type II, Walker–Warburg syndrome: (a) full-term brain with thickened whitish meninges; (b) coronal section (CV stain) showing the anarchic distribution of the neurons and large nodules of heterotopias; (c) microscopic view of the dysplastic cortex of a 20-week-old fetus, showing the external half of the mantle made of extracerebral neural tissue; (d) brainstem of the same fetus with thickened meninges, invaded by gliovascular tissue.*

or dentate and other nuclei. This is a common feature in lissencephaly type II, Walker–Warburg syndrome.

Status Verrucosus Simplex

Status verrucosus simplex, status pseudo verrucosus, or papillae of Retzius is an irregular pattern of layer II with

protrusion of cells into the molecular layer (Fig. 21.28). This puzzling appearance is often depicted in fetuses of about 20 weeks, and its significance has been diversely interpreted as a normal stage of cortical plate development or as a form of cortical dysplasia. Observation of a large number of serial sections of fetal brains from 10 to 40 weeks led us to

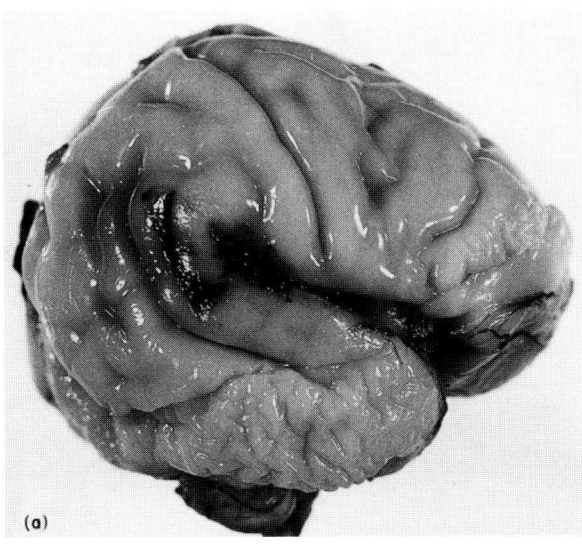

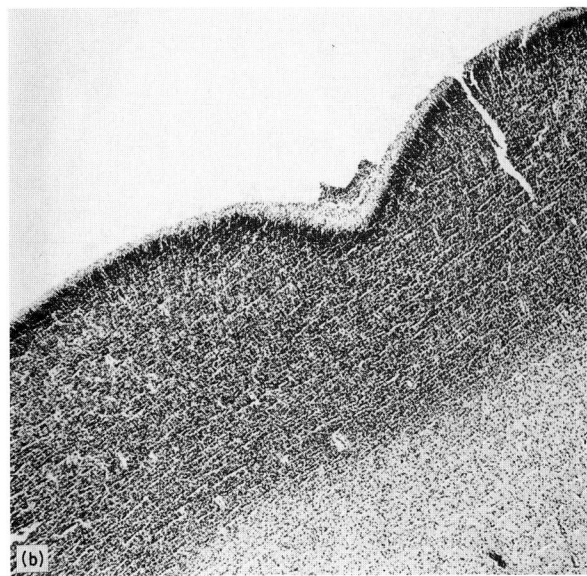

FIGURE 21.24. *Pseudomicrogyria in a 27-week-old fetus: (a) fine wrinkles over the temporal lobe; (b) underlying normal cortex.*

the conclusion that status verrucosus simplex is an artifact: the feature is not constant, as one would expect if it were a normal stage of cortical development; it is observed in fetuses of 10 to 28 weeks' gestation; it is not associated with other cortical anomalies; and its severity increases with the delay between death of the fetus and fixation of the brain.

Microcephaly and Micrencephaly

"Microcephaly" means "small head," and "micrencephaly" has been used to describe a small brain less than 2 SD below

the mean [94] but today usually describes a brain less than 3 SD below the mean. Both names are descriptive terms and do not refer to a particular etiology. For the genetic counsellor, it is important to distinguish between genetic or primary microcephaly and secondary or environmental microcephaly due to prenatal infections, drugs and chemical agents, and intrauterine growth retardation.

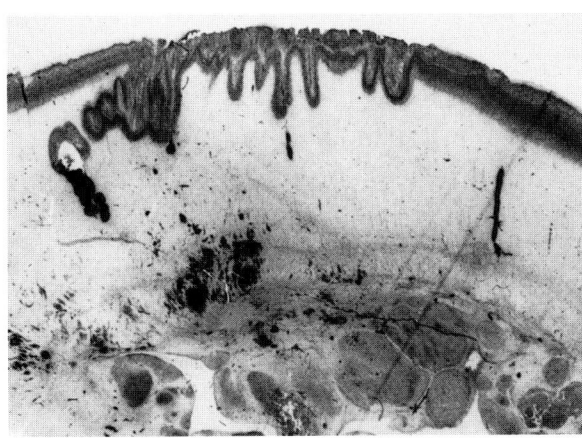

FIGURE 21.25. *Polymicrogyria, neuronal heterotopias, and calcifications in a severely malformed brain.*

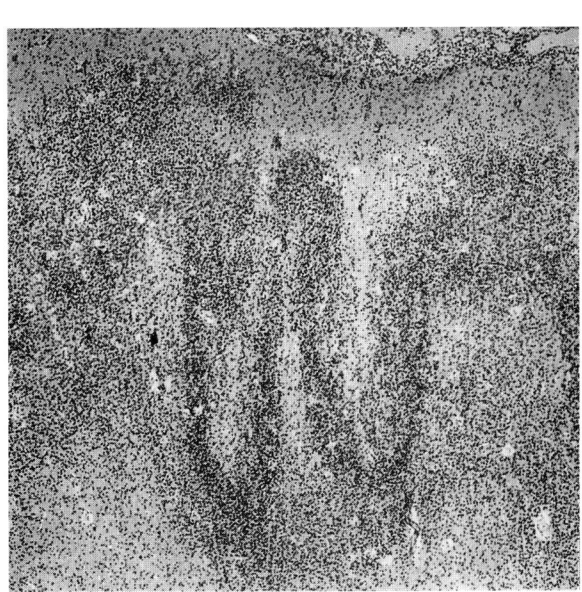

FIGURE 21.26. *Polymicrogyria in a fetus with cytomegalovirus infection.*

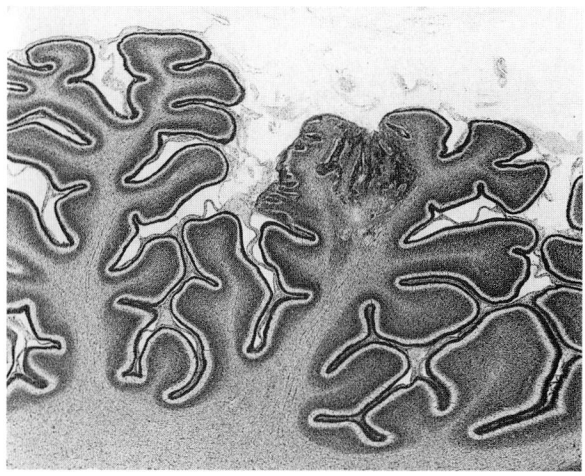

FIGURE 21.27.   *Cerebellar polymicrogyria (cortical dysplasia).*

Among genetically determined micrencephaly, "microcephaly vera" is an autosomal recessive disorder that includes dysmorphic features, mental retardation, and abnormal neurologic signs. The gross appearance of the "miniature brain" varies slightly from case to case. The frontal lobes are particularly reduced, and the gyri are often broad (Fig. 21.29). The gray/white matter ratio is either normal or in favor of the gray matter. There are voluminous heterotopic nodules of neurons (Fig. 21.30), and the cortex may be focally polymicrogyric.

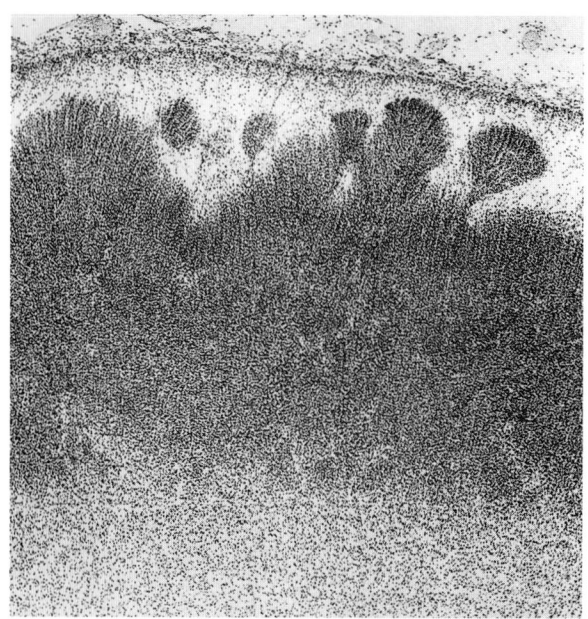

FIGURE 21.28.   *Status verrucosus simplex in a 24-week-old fetus.*

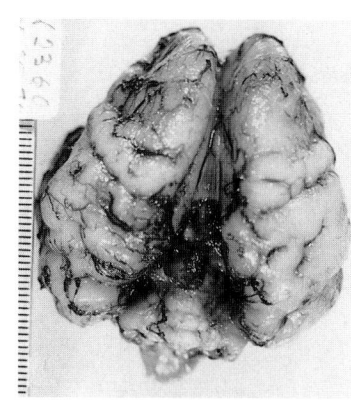

FIGURE 21.29.   *Micrencephaly: upper view of the brain of a 37-week-old fetus. Brain weight, 37 grams.*

Rare cases of autosomal dominant and X-linked microcephaly have been reported.

Micrencephaly is also a feature of many malformation syndromes, such as Cockayne syndrome, de Lange syndrome, Meckel syndrome, fetal akinesia sequence with lissencephaly type III, and some chromosome aberrations. In addition, most malformed brains are small.

Megalencephaly

"Megalencephaly" means "large brain," 2.5 SD above the mean for age and sex. Three main categories have been described by Dekaban and Sakuragawa [95].

Primary megalencephaly refers to a heterogeneous group of disorders such as achondroplasia, campomelic dwarfism, and endocrine disorders, in which the brain is symmetrically enlarged. Other anomalies such as corpus callosum defect or abnormal gyration, external hydrocephalus, heterotopias, and polymicrogyria may be associated findings. The hypothetical mechanism is an abnormal neuronal proliferation. Clinically, mental retardation and neurologic disorders are present in the majority of patients.

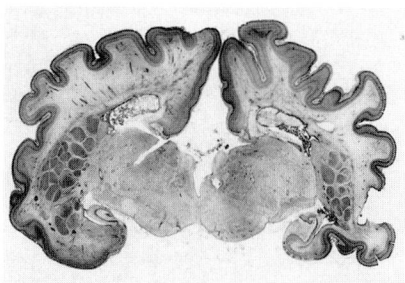

FIGURE 21.30.   *Coronal celloidin section (CV stain) of another case of micrencephaly, showing a normal cortical pattern and massive neuronal heterotopias.*

Secondary megalencephaly is found in metabolic disorders such as sphingolipidoses, mucopolysaccharidoses, amaurotic idiocy, various forms of leukodystrophy, and neurocutaneous syndromes.

Cerebral gigantism or Sotos syndrome is a heterogeneous condition suggested by a large baby at birth, advanced bone age, and dysmorphic features. Environmental and genetic factors are probably implicated.

Unilateral megalencephaly, found in unilateral hypertrophy of the body, in Sturge-Weber syndrome, may be associated with gross and microscopic abnormalities.

Congenital Hydrocephalus

Hydrocephalus consists of expansion of the cerebrospinal fluid (CSF), usually at the expense of brain tissue and with an increased CSF pressure. Many classifications of this condition have been proposed, according to:

1. *Localization*—i.e., in the ventricles (internal hydrocephalus) or in the subarachnoid spaces (external hydrocephalus), or in both compartments.
2. *Causes and mechanisms*, such as overproduction of CSF (tumors of the choroid plexus), decreased absorption about the pacchionian granulations, destruction of a significant amount of brain tissue (termed *ex vacuo*), impaired circulation of the CSF, or obstructive hydrocephalus. The latter is one of the most frequent mechanisms.

Obstructive Hydrocephalus

Obstruction in the flow of CSF may be in the posterior fossa, in the aqueduct of Sylvius, or at the foramen of Monro. Hydrocephalus commonly accompanies meningomyelocele and Arnold-Chiari malformation. Years ago, when infants survived with open meningomyelocele, subsequent meningitis was thought to be the cause of hydrocephalus; we know now that, even in young aborted fetuses, hydrocephalus is a frequent associated feature, partly due to herniation of tissue into the malformed posterior fossa and partly to a dysplastic aqueduct and quadrigeminal plate.

A few cases of tumors or neoplasms in the posterior fossa or in the cerebral peduncles, such as gliomas and ependymomas, aneurysm of the vein of Galen, angiomas or in cysts in Von Hippel-Lindau disease, and teratomas, have been reported in fetuses.

Hydrocephalus may result from gliosis formed around the aqueduct of Sylvius, gradually occluding the lumen. This feature is common in toxoplasmosis and cytomegalovirus infection, but in many other cases it is difficult to ascertain whether the obstruction is a true malformation or is due to secondary gliosis.

In fetuses and neonates, obstructive hydrocephalus may be posthemorrhagic or postinflammatory with arachnoiditis and ependymitis (see Part III).

Hydrocephalus Associated with Brain Malformations

Hydrocephalus is often associated with the Dandy-Walker malformation and with agenesis of the corpus callosum. In the latter condition, the roof of the dilated ventricle often bulges between the two hemispheres and should not be mistaken for an arachnoid cyst of the midline. In other complex malformations, the aqueduct may show various forms of dysplasia, such as atresia, forking, or ependymal rosette-like structures (Fig. 21.31).

Hydrocephalus with Genetically Transmitted Disorders

Hydrocephalus is associated with a variety of syndromes:

1. *Autosomal recessive syndromes* associated with hydrocephalus include Walker-Warburg syndrome, Meckel-Gruber syndrome, VATER syndrome, Seckel bird-headed dwarfism, Dandy-Walker syndrome, and neurocutaneous syndromes. In the majority of forms of recessive autosomal hydrocephaly, the aqueduct of Sylvius is dysplastic.
2. *Autosomal dominant syndromes*, such as thanatophoric dwarfism, may be associated with ventriculomegaly.
3. *X-linked hydrocephalus* was described by Bickers and Adams in 1949 [96] and by Holmes et al in 1973 [97]. This genetically determined hydrocephalus is due to stenosis of the aqueduct of Sylvius and is associated with corticospinal tract hypoplasia. According to the classic definition of Russell [98], stenosis means decreased size but normal appearance. For the pathologist, the diagnosis of stenosis is the most difficult task because the size of the lumen varies according to the age of the fetus and to the site of measurement. Histologically, the aqueduct

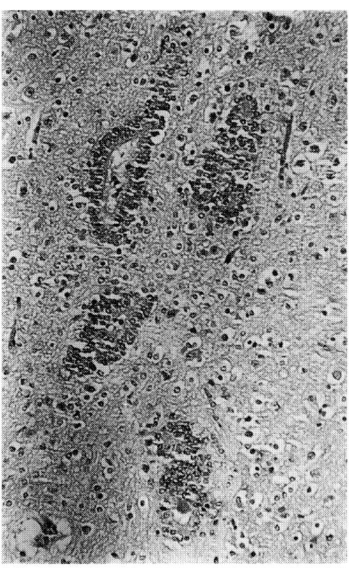

FIGURE 21.31. *Dysplastic aqueduct made of several rosette-like formations.*

may be a narrow slit rather than the normal shield shape. In some affected infants, flexed adducted thumbs are noted [99] and other members of the family may be mentally retarded. Although, classically, only boys are affected, familial cases of affected girls have been reported, suggesting possible autosomal recessive transmission. More recently, the stenosis has been considered as a consequence of the hydrocephalus [100].

4. *Chromosome aberrations*, such as trisomy 13 and 18, 13q− and 14q+ syndrome, and deletion and 17p in Miller-Dieker lissencephaly, may also be associated with hydrocephalus.

REFERENCES: MALFORMATIONS

1. Probst FP. *The Prosencephalies*. Berlin: Springer-Verlag, 1979.
2. Warkany J. *Congenital Malformations*. Chicago: Year Book Medical, 1971, p. 1309.
3. Myrianthopoulos NC. Concepts, definitions and classifications of congenital and developmental malformations of the central nervous system and related structures. In: Vinken PJ, Bruyns GW, eds. *Handbook of Clinical Neurology*. vol. 30. Amsterdam: North-Holland, 1977, pp. 1–14.
4. Smith DW. *Recognizable Patterns of Human Malformations*. 5th ed. Philadelphia: WB Saunders, 1997, p. 857.
5. Norman MG, Ludwin SK. Brain malformations. The problems. In: Arima M, Suzuki Y, Yabuuchi H, eds. *The Developing Brain and Its Disorders*. Tokyo: University of Tokyo, 1984, pp. 15–27.
6. Katler H, Warkany J. Congenital malformations. Etiologic factors and their role in prevention. *New Engl J Med* 1983; 308:424–31.
7. Rorke L. A perspective: the role of disordered genetic control of neurogenesis in the pathogenesis of migration disorders. *J Neuropathol Exp Neurol* 1994; 53:105–17.
8. Creasy MR, Alderman ED. Congenital malformations of the central nervous system in spontaneous abortions. *J Med Genet* 1976; 13:9–16.
9. Gulotta F, Rehdoer H, Gropp A. Descriptive neuropathology of chromosomal disorders in man. *Hum Genet* 1981; 5:337–44.
10. Raravi-Encha F, Gonzales M, Larroche JC, Migne G, Mulliez N. Cerebral malformations in chromosome disorders. *J Neuropathol Exp Neurol* 1988; 47:368.
11. de Grouchy J, Turleau C. *Atlas des Maladies Chromosomiques*. 2 ème éd. Paris: Expansion Scientifique, 1982, p. 489.
12. Dobyns WB, Stratton RF, Parke JT, et al. Miller-Dieker syndrome: lissencephaly and monosomy 17p. *J Pediatr* 1983; 102:552–8.
13. Dhellemmes C, Girard S, Dulac O, et al. Agyria-pachygyria and Miller-Dieker syndrome: clinical, genetic and chromosome studies. *Hum Genet* 1988; 79:163–7.
14. Volpe JJ, Adams RD. Cerebro-hepato-renal syndrome of Zellweger: an inherited disorder of neuronal migration. *Acta Neuropathol* 1972; 20:175–98.
15. Kilham L, Margolis G. Viral etiology of spontaneous ataxia of cats. *Am J Pathol* 1966; 48:991–1011.
16. Johnson RT. *Infections of the Nervous System*. New York: Raven, 1982.
17. Iosub S, Bamji M, Stone RK. More on human immunodeficiency virus embryopathy. *Pediatrics* 1987; 80:512–16.
18. Lyman WD, Soeiro R, Rashbaum K. HIV-1 infection of human fetal central nervous system tissue. In: Kozlowski PB, Snider DA, Vietze PM, Wisniewski HM, eds. *Brain in Pediatric AIDS*. Basel: Karger, 1990, pp. 183–96.
19. Encha-Razavi F, Larroche JC, Vazeaux R, Roume J, Mulliez N. Correlation between HIV infection and central nervous system changes in fetal life. *J AIDS* 1991; 4:540.
20. Barr M Jr, Hanson JW, Currey K, et al. Holoprosencephaly in infants of diabetic mothers. *J Pediatr* 1983; 102:565–8.
21. Hill LM, Kleinberg F. Effects of drugs and chemicals on the fetus and the newborn. *Mayo Clin Proc* 1984; 59:755–65.
22. Giroud A. Anencephaly. In: Vinken PJ, Bruyn GW, eds. *Handbook of Clinical Neurology*. vol. 30. Amsterdam: North-Holland, 1977, pp. 173–208.
23. Gardner W. *The Dysraphic States from Syringomyelia to Anencephaly*. Amsterdam: Excerpta Medica, 1975.
24. Carter CO. Clues to the aetiology of neural tube malformation. *Dev Med Child Neurol* 1974; 32(suppl 16):3–15.
25. Laurence KM. Antenatal detection of neural tube defects. In: Barson AJ, ed. *Fetal and Neonatal Pathology*. New York: Praeger, 1982, pp. 75–102.
26. Wood LR, Smith MT. Generation of anencephaly: aberrant neurulation and conversion of exencephaly to anencephaly. *J Neuropathol Exp Neurol* 1984; 4:620–33.
27. Van Allen MI, Kalousek DK, Chernoff GF, et al. Evidence for multi-site closure of the neural tube in human. *Am J Med Genet* 1993; 47:723–43.
28. Marin-Padilla M. Notochordal basichondrium relationships: abnormalities in experimental axial skeletal (dysraphic) disorders. *J Embryol Exp Morphol* 1979; 53:15–38.
29. Stevenson RE, Kelly JC, Aylsworth AS. Vascular basis for neural tube defects: a hypothesis. *Pediatrics* 1987; 80:102–6.
30. Larroche JC, Encha-Razavi F, de Vries L. Central nervous system. In: Gilbert-Barnes E, ed. *Potter Pathology of the Fetus and Infant*. Philadelphia: Mosby Year Book, 1997, pp. 1028–150.
31. Emery JL, Lendon RG. The local cord lesions in neurospinal dysraphisms (meningomyelocele). *J Pathol* 1973; 11:83–96.
32. Friede RL. *Developmental Neuropathology*. Vienna: Springer Verlag, 1975, p. 524.
33. Larroche JC. *Developmental Pathology of the Neonate*. Amsterdam: Excerpta Medica, 1977.
34. Jellinger K, Gross H. Congenital telencephalic midline defects. *Neuropediatrics* 1973; 4:446–52.
35. Leech RW, Shuman RM. Holoprosencephaly and related midline cerebral anomalies: a review. *J Child Neurol* 1986; 1:3–18.
36. Yakovlev PI. Pathoarchitectonic studies of the cerebral malformations. III Arhinencephalies (holoprosencephalies). *J Neuropathol Exp Neurol* 1959; 18:22–55.
37. DeMyer W, Zeman W, Palmer CG. The face predicts the brain: diagnostic significance of median facial anomalies for holoprosencephaly (arhinencephaly). *Pediatrics* 1964; 35:256–63.
38. Delezoide AL, Narcy F, Larroche JC. Cerebral midline developmental anomalies: spectrum and associated features. *Genet Counsel* 1991; 1:190–210.
39. Cohen M. Perspectives on holoprosencephaly. Part I: Epidemiology, genetics and syndromology. *Teratology* 1989; 40:211–35.
40. Cohen M. Perspectives on holoprosencephaly. Part III: Spectra, distinctions, continuities and discontinuities. *Am J Med Genet* 1989; 34:271–88.
41. Jeret JS, Serur D, Wisniewski KE, Lubin RA. Clinico-pathological findings associated with agenesis of the corpus callosum. *Brain Dev* 1987; 9:255–64.
42. Aicardi J, Chevrie JJ. Le syndrome agénésie calleuse, spasmes en flexion, lacunes choriorétiniennes. *Arch Franç Pédiatr* 1969; 26:7–12.
43. Shapiro Y, Cohen T. Agenesis of the corpus callosum in two sisters. *J Med Genet* 1973; 10:266–9.
44. Cao A, Cianchetti C, Signorini E. Agenesis of the corpus callosum, infantile spasms, spastic quadriplegia, microcephaly and severe mental retardation in three siblings. *Clin Genet* 1977; 1:290–6.
45. Menkes JH, Philipart M, Clark DB. Hereditary partial agenesis of corpus callosum. *Arch Neurol* 1964; 11:198–208.
46. Lemire RJ, Loeser JD, Leech RW, Alvord EC Jr. *Normal and Abnormal Development of the Human Nervous System*. Hagerstown, NY: Harper and Row, 1975, p. 421.
47. Fawer CL, Calame A, Anderegg A. Agenesis of the corpus callosum: real-time ultrasonographic diagnosis and autopsy findings. *Helv Paediatr Acta* 1985; 40:371–80.
48. Bruyn GW. Agenesis septi pellucidi, cavum septi pellucidi and cavum vergae, and cavum veli interpositi. In: Vinken PJ, Bruyn GW, eds. *Handbook of Clinical Neurology*. vol. 30. Amsterdam: North-Holland, 1977, pp. 299–336.
49. De Morcier G. Agénésie du septum pellucidum avec malformation du tractus optique (la dysplasie septo-optique). *Schweiz Arch Neurol Neurochir Psychiatr* 1956; 77:267–92.
50. Aicardi J, Goutières F. Syndrome of absence of the septum pellucidum with porencephalies and other developmental defects. *Neuropediatrics* 1981; 12:319–29.
51. Davidoff LM. Coarctation of the walls of the lateral angles of the lateral ventricles. *J Neurosurg* 1946; 3:250–6.
52. Bates JI, Netsky MG. Developmental anomalies of the horns of the lateral ventricles. *J Neuropathol Exp Neurol* 1955; 14:316–25.
53. Larroche JC. Malformations of the nervous system. In: Hume-Adams J, Corsellis JAN, Duchen LW, eds. *Greenfield's Neuropathology*. London: Edward Arnold, 1984, pp. 385–450.
54. Hirano A, Dembitzer M, Jones M. An electron microscopic study of cycasin induced cerebellar alterations. *J Neuropathol Exp Neurol* 1972; 31:113–25.

55. Rakic P, Sidman RL. Sequence of developmental abnormalities leading to granule cell deficit in cerebellum cortex of weaver mutant mice. *J Comp Neurol* 1973; 152:103–32.

56. Tal Y, Freigung B, Dunn HG. Dandy-Walker syndrome: analysis of 21 cases. *Dev Med Child Neurol* 1980; 22:189–201.

57. Hirsch JF, Pierre-Kahn A, Renier D. The Dandy-Walker malformation. *J Neurosurg* 1984; 61:515–22.

58. Shaw CM, Alvord EC. Congenital arachnoid cysts and their differential diagnosis. In: Vinken PJ, Bruyn GW, eds. *Handbook of Clinical Neurology.* vol. 31. Amsterdam: North-Holland, 1977, pp. 75–135, 137–209.

59. Lourie H, Berne A. A contribution on the etiology and pathogenesis of congenital communicating hydrocephalus. *Biol Neonat* 1961; 15:815–22.

60. Lasjaunias P. Contribution à l'étude et au traitement des malformations artérioveineuses cérébrales de l'enfant. *Rivista Neuroradiol (Ital)* 1993; 4:399–492.

61. Lagos JC. Congenital aneurysms and arteriovenous malformations. In: Vinken PJ, Bruyn GW, eds. *Handbook of Clinical Neurology.* vol. 30. Amsterdam: North-Holland, 1977, pp. 137–209.

62. Rakic P. Cell migration and neuronal ectopias in the brain. *Birth Defects Orig Artic Ser* 1975; 11:95–129.

63. Larroche JC. Early human neocorticogenesis. In: Arima M, Suzuki Y, Yabuuchi H, eds. *The Developing Brain and Its Disorders.* Tokyo: University of Tokyo, 1984, pp. 3–13.

64. Choi BH, Matthias SC. Cortical dysplasia associated with massive ectopias of neurons and glial cells within the subarachnoid space. *Acta Neuropathol* 1987; 73:105–9.

65. Rorke LB, Fogelson MH, Riggs H. Cerebellar heterotopias in infancy. *Dev Med Child Neurol* 1958; 10:644–50.

66. Larroche JC. Cytoarchitectonic abnormalities. In: Vinken PJ, Bruyn GW, eds. *Handbook of Clinical Neurology.* vol. 30. Amsterdam: North-Holland, 1977, pp. 479–506.

67. Dambska M, Wisniewski K, Sker JH. Lissencephaly: two distinct clinicopathological types. *Brain Dev* 1983; 5:302–10.

68. Dobyns WB, Gilbert EF, Opitz JM. Letter to the editor: further comments on the lissencephaly syndrome. *Am J Med Genet* 1985; 22:197–211.

69. Aicardi J. The agyria-pachygyria complex; a spectrum of cortical malformations. *Brain Dev* 1991; 13:1–8.

70. Larroche JC. The lissencephalies: a large spectrum of morphological abnormalities. *Neuropathology* 1991; 4(suppl): 434–7.

71. Bielschowsky M. Uber die Oberflächen-gestaltung des Grosshirnmantels bei Pachygyrie, Mikrogyrie und bei normaler Entwicklung. *J Psychol Neurol Leipzig* 1923; 30:29–76.

72. Crome L. Pachygyria. *J Pathol Bacteriol* 1956; 71:335–52.

73. Miller J. Lissencephaly in two siblings. *Neurology* 1963; 13:841–50.

74. Dieker H, Edwards RH, Zu Rhein G, et al. The lissencephaly syndrome. *Birth Defects Orig Artic Ser* 1969; 5:53–64.

75. Dobyns WB, Reiner O, Carrozzo R, Ledbetter DH. Lissencephaly. A human brain malformation associated with deletion of the LIS1 gene located on the chromosome 17p 13. *JAMA* 1993; 270:2838–42.

76. Norman MG, Roberts J, Siroid J. Lissencephaly. *J Can Sci Neurol* 1976; 3:39–46.

77. Dobyns WB, Stratton RF, Greenberg F. Syndrome with lissencephaly I: Miller-Dieker and Norman-Roberts syndromes and isolated lissencephaly. *Am J Med Genet* 1984; 18:509–26.

78. Walker AE. Lissencephaly. *Arch Neurol Psychiatr* 1942; 48:13–29.

79. Squier MV. Development of the cortical dysplasia type II lissencephaly. *Neuropathol Appl Neurobiol* 1993; 19:209–13.

80. Chemke J, Czernobilsky B, Mundel G, Barishak YR. A familial syndrome of central nervous system and ocular malformations. *Clin Genet* 1975; 7:1–7.

81. Warburg M. Hydrocephalus, congenital retinal non attachment and congenital falciform fold. *Am J Ophthalmol* 1978; 85:88–94.

82. Pagon RA, Chandler JW, Collie WR, et al. Hydrocephaly, agyria, retinal dysplasia, encephalocele (HARD+E) syndrome; an autosomal recessive condition. *Birth Defects Orig Artic Ser* 1978; 14:233–41.

83. Williams RS, Swisher CN, Jennings M, Ambler M, Caviness VS Jr. Cerebro-ocular dysgenesis (Walker-Warburg syndrome): neuropathologic and etiologic analysis. *Neurology* 1984; 34:1531–41.

84. Larroche JC, Razavi-Encha F. *Walker-Warburg Malformation in Young Fetuses.* Southampton: British Neuropath Society, 1987.

85. Larroche JC, Nessmann C. Focal cerebral anomalies and retinal dysplasia in a 23–24 week-old fetus. *Brain Dev* 1993; 15:51–6.

86. Damska M, Wisniewski KE, Sher JH, Solish G. Cerebro-oculo muscular syndrome: a variant of Fukuyama congenital cerebromuscular dystrophy. *Clin Neuropathol* 1982; 1:93–8.

87. Fukuyama Y, Osawa M, Suzuki H. Congenital progressive muscular dystrophy of the Fukuyama type: clinical, genetic and pathological considerations. *Brain Dev* 1981; 3:1–29.

88. Takada K, Nakamura H, Tanaka J. Cortical dysplasia in congenital muscular dystrophy with central nervous system involvement (Fukuyama type). *J Neuropathol Exp Neurol* 1984; 43:395–407.

89. Santavuori P, Somer H, Sainio K, et al. Muscle-Eye-Brain disease (MEB). *Brain Dev* 1989; 11:147–53.

90. Larroche JC, Razavi-Encha F, Squier W. The lissencephalies: a large spectrum of morphological abnormalities. In: Proc XIth International Congress of Neuropathology. Neuropathology (suppl 4) 1991:434–7.

91. Spearritt DJ, Tannenberg AEG, Payton DJ. Lethal multiple pterygium syndrome: report of a case with neurological anomalies. *Am J Med Genet* 1993; 47:45–9.

92. Goutières F, Aicardi J, Farkas-Bargeton E. Une malformation particulière associée au nanisme thanatophore. *Rev Neurol* 1971; 125:435–40.

93. Wongmongkolrit T, Bush M, Roessman U. Neuropathological findings in thanatophoric dysplasia. *Arch Pathol Lab Med* 1983; 107:132–5.

94. Ross JJ, Frias JL. Microcephaly. In: Vinken PJ, Bruyn GW, eds. *Handbook of Clinical Neurology.* vol. 30. Amsterdam: North-Holland, 1977, pp. 507–24.

95. Dekaban AS, Sakuragawa N. Megalencephaly. In: Vinken PJ, Bruyn GW, eds. *Handbook of Clinical Neurology.* vol. 30. Amsterdam: North-Holland, 1977, pp. 647–60.

96. Bickers DS, Adams RA. Hereditary stenosis of the aqueduct of Sylvius as a cause of congenital hydrocephalus. *Brain* 1949; 72:246–62.

97. Holmes LB, Nash A, ZuRhein GM, Levin M, Opitz JM. X-linked aqueductal stenosis: clinical and neuropathological findings in two families. *Pediatrics* 1973; 51:697–704.

98. Russell D. *Observations on the Pathology of Hydrocephalus.* Medical Research Council Special Report Series, No. 265. London: His Majesty's Stationery Office, 1949, p. 138.

99. Edwards JH, Norman RM, Roberts JM. Sex-linked hydrocephalus. Report of a family with 15 affected members. *Arch Dis Childhood* 1961; 36:481–5, 486–93.

100. Van Egmond-Linden A, Wladimiroff JW, Jahoda MGJ, et al. Prenatal diagnosis of X-linked hydrocephalus. *Prenat Diag* 1983; 3:245–8.

PART III
FETAL AND PERINATAL BRAIN DAMAGE

JEANNE-CLAUDIE LARROCHE

INTRACRANIAL HEMORRHAGE (ICH)

This term covers a wide spectrum of different forms of hemorrhage, regardless of pathogenesis. In this chapter, ICH is described according to the site; at-risk situations and possible causes are discussed, bearing in mind that the same cause can produce different effects at different gestational ages as the brain matures, and that various causes can produce similar lesions.

Extradural and Subdural Hemorrhage

Both of these localizations are usually secondary to mechanical difficulties during delivery and will be discussed in a different chapter. Subdural hemorrhage, however, has been described in hemophilic newborn infants [1–3] and in cases of thrombocytopenia (Fig. 21.32). CT scanning and ultrasound cannot differentiate subdural hematoma from subarachnoid hematoma (see below).

Thrombosis of Sinuses and Cerebral Veins

In the past, thrombosis of sinuses and cerebral veins was often described in association with sepsis, dehydration, and congenital heart disease, conditions that are better controlled today [1, 4, 5]. Bacterial meningitis and meningoencephalitis may, however, still be complicated by microthrombi, leading to hemorrhagic encephalopathy. This is particularly true in sepsis due to gram-negative organisms. Classically, in the case of thrombosis of the sagittal sinus, hemorrhagic infarcts occur symmetrically in both hemispheres and involve cortex and white matter.

Subarachnoid Hemorrhage

Extravasations of blood into the subarachnoid space are common in both premature and full-term infants. They may be of traumatic origin in cases of forceps or vacuum extraction or may result from asphyxia. The hemorrhage may be focal or diffuse. Blood often collects in the wide sylvian fissure or in the basal cisterns. When blood diffuses into the posterior fossa, around the cerebellum and brainstem, it must be differentiated from an extension of an intraventricular hemorrhage. Occasionally, hydrocephalus may develop secondary to arachnoid thickening and occlusion of the foramina of Luschka and Magendie [6].

Subarachnoid Hematoma

Subarachnoid hematoma is a well-circumscribed collection of blood lying over one or several lobes. The thickness may vary from several millimeters to 1 cm. The underlying brain is either normal or the site of hemorrhagic necrosis. In the author's series (60 cases out of 2000 postmortem examinations), subarachnoid hematoma was found more often over the left hemisphere, particularly over the temporal lobe (Fig. 21.33). The pathogenesis is not known. However, since the majority of infants in this group, before 1980, received exchange transfusions either for blood group incompatibility or septicemia, hemostatic failure and/or thromboembolism have been suggested as underlying factors [1]. CT scanning and ultrasound barely distinguish this collection of blood from subdural hematoma (Fig. 21.33a).

Subpial Hemorrhage

Subpial hemorrhage can be diagnosed only on histologic examination. According to Friede [7], subpial hemorrhage occurs in 15% of cases of perinatal intracranial hemorrhage. In the author's experience, subpial hemorrhage is usually associated with subarachnoid hemorrhage and has little or no specific significance.

Intracerebral Hemorrhage

The site of the hemorrhage within the cerebral hemispheres, and the variety of causes, makes it difficult to describe hemorrhages under a single entity. In fact, intracerebral hemorrhage often complicates a number of other lesions. These include secondary hemorrhage in an ischemic infarct (arterial occlusion) or leukomalacia, extension of an intraventricular hemorrhage with mechanical pressure, occlusion of the sagittal sinus, meningoencephalitis, and blood dyscrasia. These aspects will be described in their respective sections.

A primary and isolated hemorrhagic infarct of the white matter is rare. However, the fanlike venous network, directed toward the ventricle, presents no anastomosis between its branches; therefore, during severe episodes of asphyxia with venous stasis, the thin-walled veins may be distended and disrupted before their confluence around the subependymal matrix, and the hemorrhage often presents a triangular shape with an external base. In addition, a large intraventricular hemorrhage may compress the deep veins, impeding normal return of blood flow [8] (see section below on IVH).

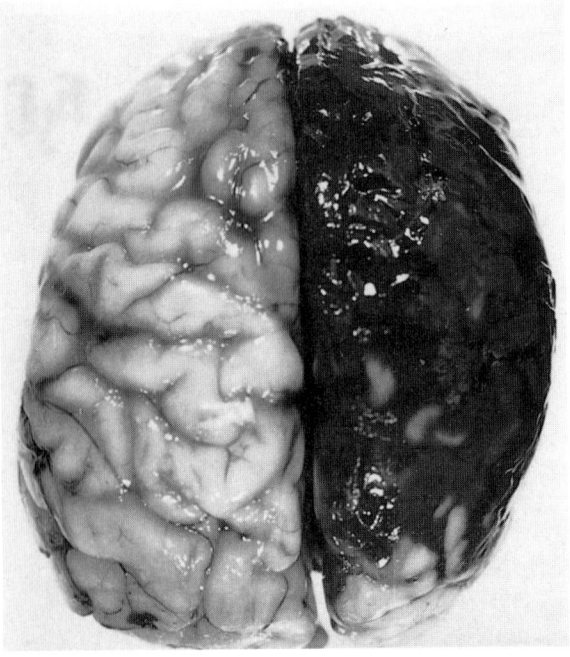

FIGURE 21.32. *Subdural hemorrhage in a newborn infant with severe thrombocytopenia.*

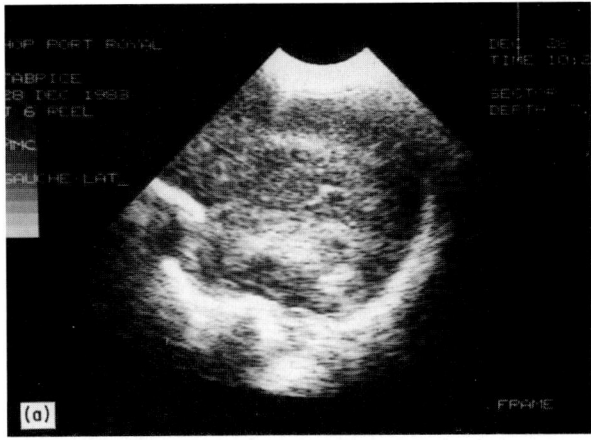

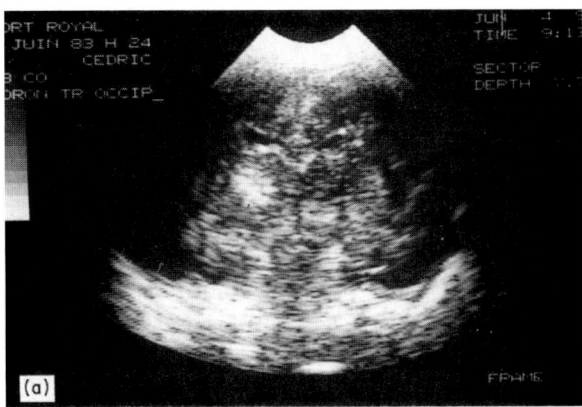

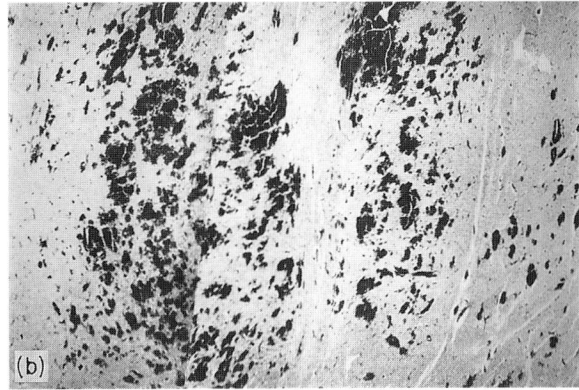

FIGURE 21.34. *Thalamic infarct: (a) ultrasound—echo-dense area in the left basal ganglia; (b) histologic preparation shows the confluent petechial hemorrhages in the striatum.*

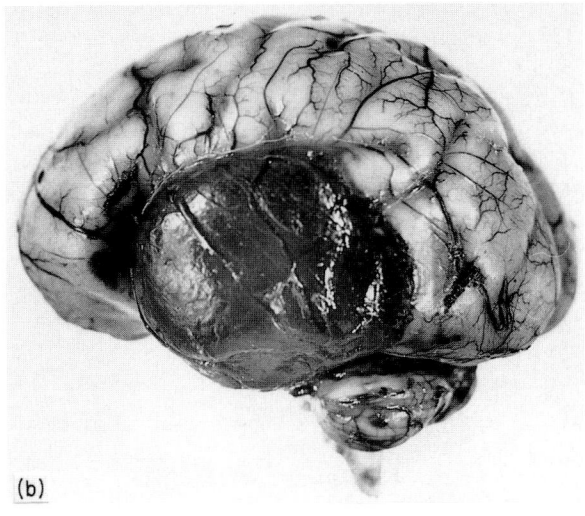

FIGURE 21.33. *Subarachnoid hematoma: (a) ultrasound—echo-dense area over the left temporal lobe; (b) lateral view of the brain after fixation.*

Hemorrhagic infarcts of the basal ganglia and thalamus have been described in a number of various pathologic conditions, such as blood group incompatibility, meningo-encephalitis with vascular occlusions, arteriovenous malformations, and tumors. Nowadays, thalamic hemorrhages can be diagnosed in vivo by real-time ultrasound and CT scanning. They have been described in asphyxiated newborn infants [9–11] (Fig. 21.34) and may be secondary events in an area of ischemic necrosis.

Germinal Matrix Hemorrhage (GMH) and Intraventricular Hemorrhage (IVH)

Although several articles and monographs [12–14] have drawn attention to these forms of cerebral bleeding in premature infants, it was the introduction of CT [15] and ultrasonography [16, 17] that led to renewed interest in and general recognition of these lesions. Despite the wealth of data on the localization, size, frequency, and evolution of the

hemorrhages, their pathogenesis is still uncertain and their treatment is unsatisfactory.

Germinal Matrix and Vascularization of the Area

The subependymal germinal matrix is a transient structure whose characteristics may explain its vulnerability. As soon as the cortical plate is formed (16–18 weeks), the relative size of the periventricular matrix progressively decreases. A conspicuous mass of cells still persists in three major sites until 33 to 34 weeks, over the head of the caudate nucleus, in the groove between the caudate nucleus and the thalamus, in the roof of the temporal horn, and in the external wall of the occipital horn. At this stage, the matrix consists of compactly arranged cells—mainly glial cells and small neurons with scanty cytoplasm and short processes.

During the period of mitotic activity, the microvascularization of the matrix increases but the capillaries cannot be differentiated from small veins. After 18 weeks, the number of "capillaries" per surface area decreases, while a spectacular proliferation of capillaries takes place in the cortex. Endothelial cells and pericytes, basal lamina, and glial perivascular end-feet are mature by 20 weeks (Fig. 21.35). In the endothelial cells, peculiar features, such as large numbers of organelles, intraluminal microvilli, and rod-

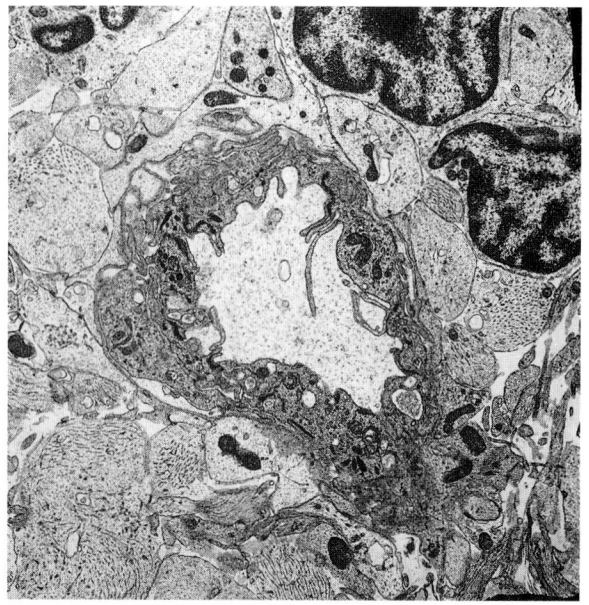

FIGURE 21.35.   *Capillary in the subependymal matrix of a 20-week-old fetus. Electron microscopy, ×4500.*

shaped bodies, can be seen [18, 19]. The latter structures may be linked to thromboplastic and clotting activity. In addition, in premature infants, the relative paucity of the arterial capillary bed of the matrix has been demonstrated in microangiographs, while in venographs there exists a rich subependymal venous network [20]. Furthermore, experimental studies have shown that the arterial blood flow was low in the matrix of the beagle pup [21]. After 26 weeks, the deep venous system of Galen becomes more apparent, draining blood from the expanding hemispheres. The veins, at first converging toward the foramen of Monro, form the two internal veins of Galen that flow backward to the sinus rectus. This sharp angle is a weak point in cases of venous stasis.

The Hemorrhages

The main source of intraventricular hemorrhage is a primary bleeding in the germinal matrix. Other sources of hemorrhage (in about 15% of cases, the choroid plexus or the tela choroidea) are rarely isolated.

Hemorrhage can occur at one or several sites of the matrix, usually anteriorly, at the level of the foramen of Monro, much less often in the roof of the temporal horn or in the external wall of the occipital horn; it may be unilateral or bilateral. The hemorrhage often destroys the whole structure while the surrounding tissue is spared. The thin veins, not only in the matrix but also in the septum pellucidum, the tela choroidea, and the plexuses, are usually congested and small thrombi are observed in about 15% of cases. Ruptured vessels are more difficult to identify; although, in normal conditions, capillaries are very resistant

[22], they are often damaged in asphyxiated neonates. Electron micrographs show swollen glial end-feet, thickened and cloudy basal lamina, and dislocation of endothelial cells with extravasation of blood. In addition, ischemic infarcts [5, 23], with proliferations of GFAP-positive glial cells, are often observed, predating or accompanying the hemorrhage.

The germinal matrix hemorrhage may be held temporarily by the surrounding structures and the ependymal lining. When the latter ruptures, the blood fills the entire ventricular system (Fig. 21.36) and collects in the subarachnoid spaces of the posterior fossa, before extending anteriorly to the basal cisterns and posteriorly to the spinal canal.

When the ventricles are overdistended, the blood may dissect into the parenchyma. This event is not always simply mechanical; in fact, the ependyma is usually altered and the underlying white matter is often the site of an ischemic infarct, resulting in decreased resistance of the brain tissue; alternatively, a hemorrhagic infarct of the white matter may rupture into the ventricle.

Time of Occurrence

Intraventricular hemorrhage usually develops a few hours after birth [24, 25]. However, delayed IVH in premature infants has been observed; since the germinal matrix regresses postnatally at the same speed as in utero, hemodynamic defects can lead to IVH as long as the matrix persists. Hemorrhage of the matrix and IVH can also occur during fetal life (see section below).

Antecedents and Pathogenesis

The only obstetric condition considered to be a risk factor is vaginal breech delivery, a rather common occurrence in preterm birth. It is now well established that IVH is related

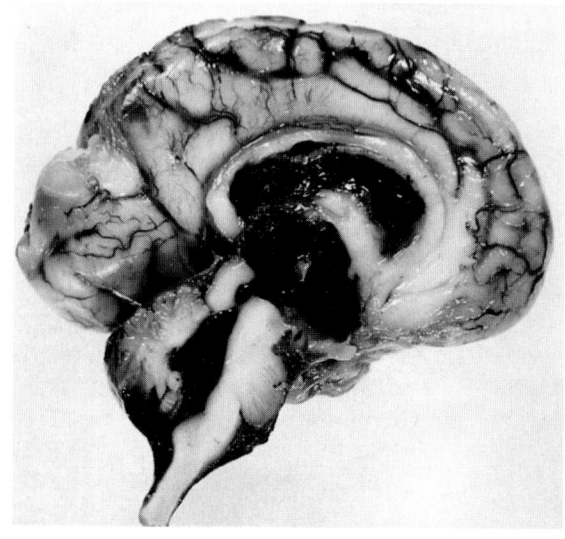

FIGURE 21.36.   *IVH. Midsagittal view of the brain: blood fills the entire ventricular system.*

to immaturity, and the morphologic characteristics of the subependymal matrix explain, in part, why bleeding occurs so often in this particular site. However, the etiology of the hemorrhage is probably multifactorial.

A variety of conditions that disturb cerebral blood flow, such as hyaline membrane disease with hypoxia [17, 26, 27], hypothermia, hypercapnia and acidosis, blood pressure instability [28, 29], and occurrence of a pneumothorax, are common findings before or during the development of an IVH. Raised intracranial venous pressure [30] and increased pressure in the right atrium [8] have been reported in the course of mechanical ventilation, and, in fetal sheep [31], IVH occurred after production of asphyxia and increased venous pressure. As a result of postmortem injection studies, Hambleton and Wigglesworth [32] suggested that the hemorrhage was due to rupture of capillaries and capillary-venous junctions, secondary to increased pressure in the territory of Heubner's artery, a branch of the anterior cerebral artery, of the lateral striate branches of the middle cerebral artery, and of the anterior choroidal artery.

In addition, Lou et al [33] demonstrated that in the asphyxiated neonate, autoregulation of cerebral blood flow is impaired, and blood pressure instability has indeed been reported in infants with IVH [28, 29]. When there is no mechanism to compensate for fluctuations in the systemic blood pressure, the vulnerability of the CNS is increased. Furthermore, when vascular walls have been damaged by hypoxia, they can be disrupted easily as a result of hypertensive episodes. Increased fibrinolytic activity in the matrix [34] could account for the rapid extension of the hemorrhage.

All these factors, acting on the brain and its vasculature, have been integrated by Wigglesworth and Pape [35] and by Pape and Wigglesworth [36] in a schematic model to explain hemorrhagic and ischemic lesions (Fig. 21.37).

Experimental Studies

The development of an appropriate animal model for IVH has been difficult because of major differences between humans and animals in the degree of immaturity of the brain, the presence of a large matrix in human infants, and the vascular pattern of the vulnerable area. However, in sheep fetuses [31] and in beagle pups [37], it was demonstrated that intermittent modifications of arterial and venous pressure, when associated with asphyxia, led to hemorrhages in the germinal layer, tela choroidea, and plexuses, similar to those described in the brains of newborn infants.

Diagnosis

During the first hours of life, respiratory distress is usually predominant while silent bleeding develops within the matrix. The signs of deterioration, including seizures or coma, cardiorespiratory failure, and metabolic and hematologic disorders, reflect the rupture of the ependyma and ventricular flooding. When severe parenchymal lesions are

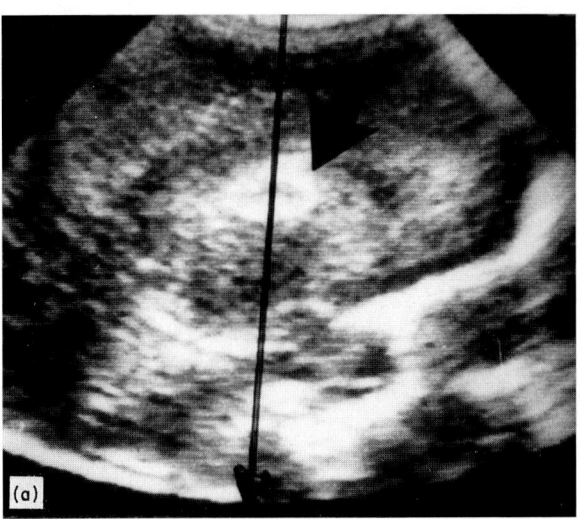

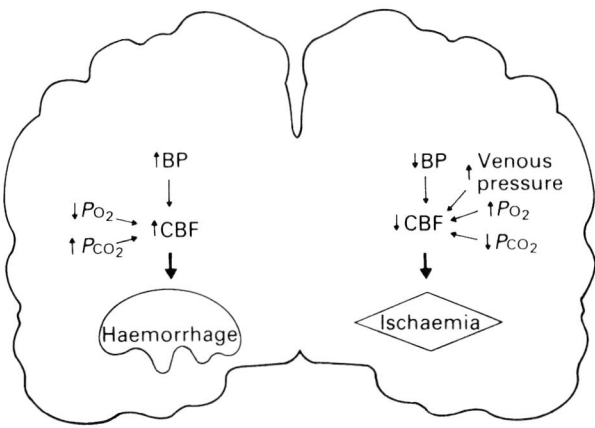

FIGURE 21.37.   *Basic two-part model for hemorrhage and ischemia in the newborn infant brain (from Pape and Wigglesworth [36]).*

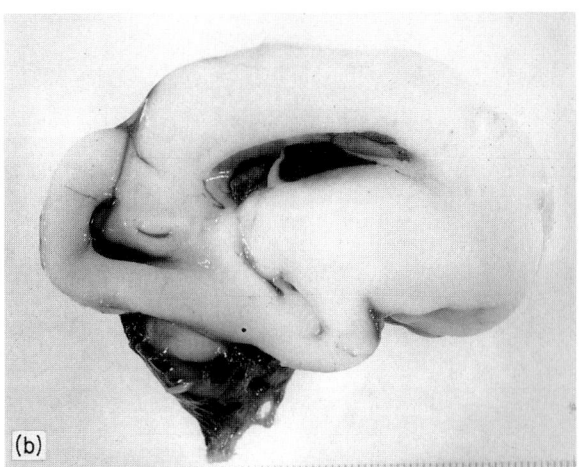

FIGURE 21.38.   *Subependymal hemorrhage: (a) ultrasound; (b) sagittal view of the brain after fixation.*

associated with IVH, the EEG often shows rolandic spikes or more diffuse electrical anomalies. In cases of severe IVH, the anterior fontanelle may be tense. However, there may be no abnormal increase in the head circumference [6, 38]. In premature infants, the arachnoid spaces over the convexity and the basal cisterns are wide and easily accommodate the enlarging brain. In addition, the unmyelinated brain tissue in the hemispheres can be compressed and thinned as the ventricles expand.

With transfontanellar real-time ultrasonography, performed in the incubator, the diagnosis of IVH can be made rapidly and easily, with evaluation of the site and size of the bleeding (Figs. 21.38–21.41). The classification based on CT findings proposed by Papile et al [39] is also valid for ultrasound:

Stage I: hemorrhage in the matrix
Stage II: IVH without ventricular dilatation

Stage III: IVH with enlarged ventricles
Stage IV: IVH with parenchymal hemorrhage

Epidemiology

Prior to the use of mechanical ventilation, most infants suffering from hyaline membrane disease (HMD) and IVH died, and the diagnosis of IVH was based on clinical and laboratory data and was confirmed at postmortem examination. In the University Clinic of Baudelocque in Paris, IVH occurred in 20% of infants of less than 36 weeks' gestation and in 2% over 36 weeks, with a maximum of 35% between 28 and 32 weeks. Fedrick and Butler [26], using data from the British Perinatal Mortality Survey, estimated the incidence to be 45 per 1000 livebirths at less than 32 weeks and 0.4 per 1000 livebirths at over 35 weeks. Improved resuscitation and supportive measures for respiratory distress syndrome (RDS), while decreasing the mortal-

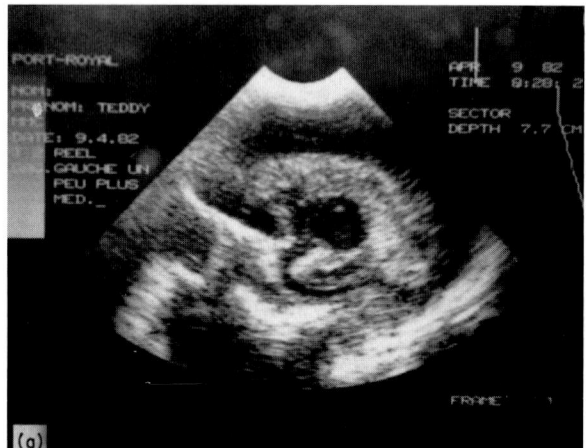

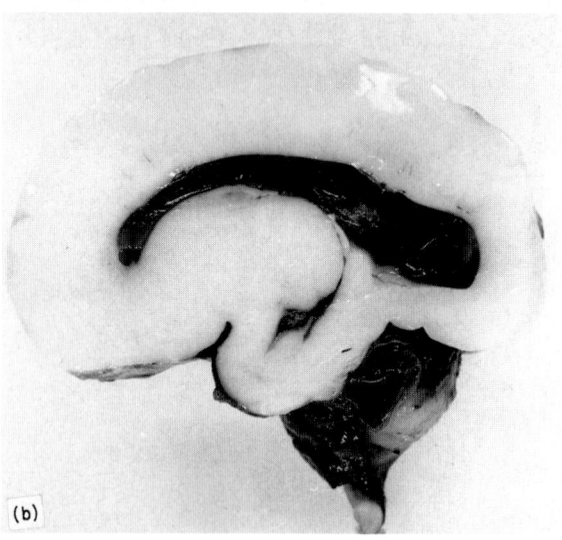

FIGURE 21.39.   *Intraventricular hemorrhage, sagittal view: (a) ultrasound; (b) the brain after fixation.*

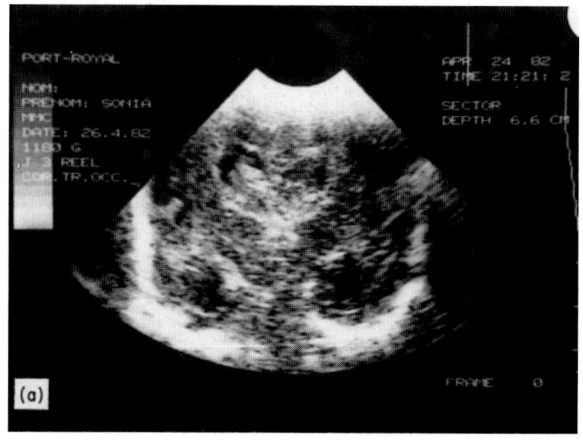

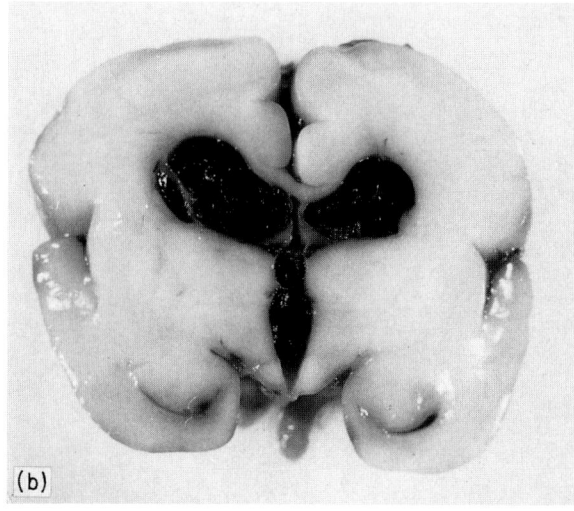

FIGURE 21.40.   *Intraventricular hemorrhage, coronal view: (a) ultrasound; (b) the brain after fixation.*

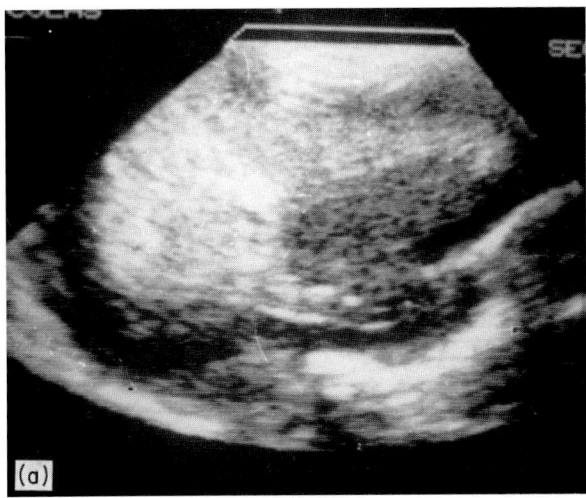

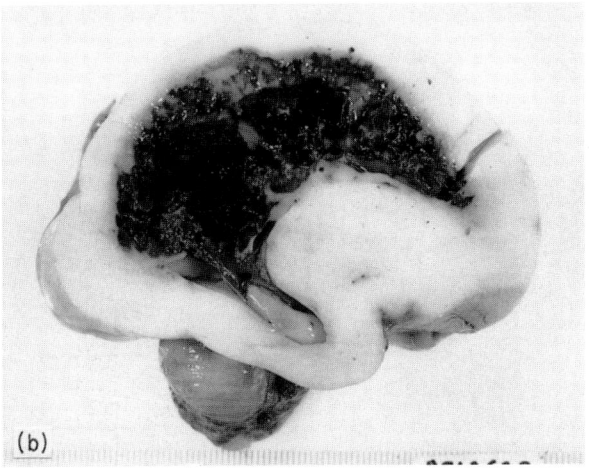

FIGURE 21.41. *Intraventricular hemorrhage and periventricular necroticohemorrhagic lesions, sagittal view: (a) ultrasound; (b) the brain after fixation.*

ity rate, have modified the pattern of perinatal pathology. A large number of infants treated with mechanical ventilation have overcome their lung problems, which may have been associated with IVH, and survived. It has, therefore, been difficult to evaluate the incidence of IVH. Nowadays, with ultrasound, the rate of IVH is estimated to be 40–50% in infants with a birth weight of less than 1500 grams, with a preponderance of stages I and II [40]. In recent years however, better treatment of RDS has not only decreased the incidence and severity of respiratory disease in premature infants, but has also significantly reduced the incidence and severity of IVH, a clear demonstration of the close link between the two disorders.

Evolution

Subependymal Pseudocyst Small hemorrhages in the matrix are clinically silent, but the implications of neuronal and glial destruction for the later development of the infant

are unknown. If death occurs, due to intercurrent disease, the presence of macrophages loaded with iron pigment and of subependymal pseudocyst formation (Fig. 21.42) indicate the site of previous bleeding [41, 42]. Hemorrhages and cysts may also be detected by ultrasound.

Posthemorrhagic Hydrocephaly With improved general care, the number of cases, seen by the author at postmortem examination after surviving for more than 10 days, has increased from 8% during the years 1956 to 1966 in a nursery department, to 12% in an intensive care unit before utilization of constant positive pressure (1967 to 1973), and to 25% from 1974 to 1985. The pattern of pathology in this condition has, therefore, changed. In the old statistics, before mechanical ventilation, posthemorrhagic hydrocephalus, for example (Fig. 21.43), occurred in 2% of cases in which IVH was found at postmortem examination. With prolonged survival, this complication is found in 30% of cases. Of course, these figures may vary from one department to another, depending on the population studied and on ethical considerations.

Blood clot in the posterior fossa is hemolyzed and resorbed within about a week, but a cellular reaction and hemosiderin-laden macrophages thicken the meninges, impeding the normal circulation of CSF and leading to the development of obstructive hydrocephalus. At postmortem examination, a rusty discoloration of the meninges over the brainstem and basal part of the cerebellum indicates previous hemorrhage. On section of the brain, the entire ventricular system usually is dilated, the occipital horns are affected more severely than the frontal and temporal horns, and the lateral ventricles become distended before the third and fourth ventricles. The ependyma is covered with a fine

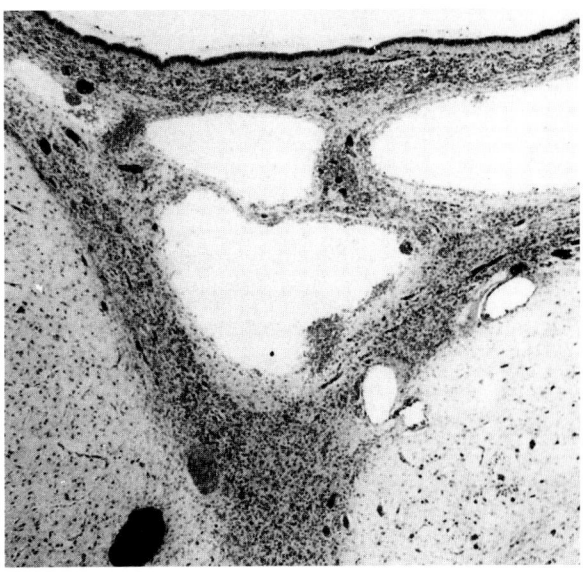

FIGURE 21.42. *Pseudocystic lesions in the matrix with iron pigment.*

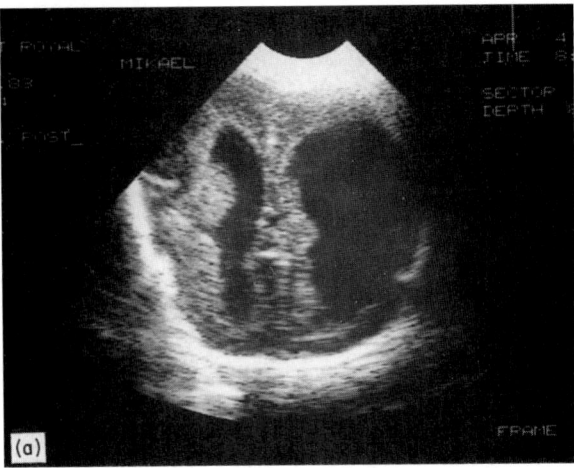

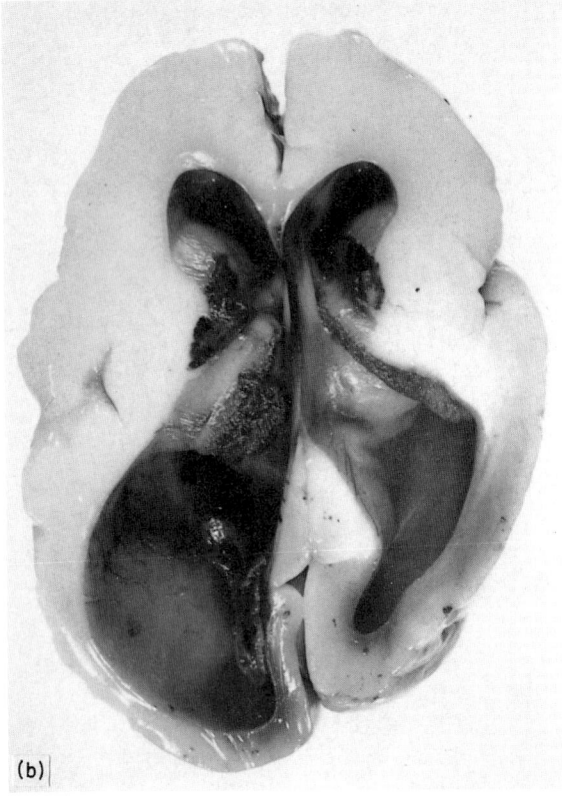

FIGURE 21.43.   *Posthemorrhagic hydrocephalus: (a) ultrasound, coronal view; (b) horizontal section of the brain after fixation.*

granular and rusty deposit containing macrophages laden with hemosiderin. The choroid plexuses are brown, with a firm consistency in the case of hemorrhage. Occasionally, when necrotic debris occludes the aqueduct, the fourth ventricle may be of normal size.

In cases of severe bleeding, the ventricles may be distended quite rapidly, leading to "hemocephaly," with the clotted blood forming a large cast of the cavities. The persistence of large blood clots within the ventricles during the

development of hydrocephalus may be described as "hemohydrocephalus" (Fig. 21.44).

On histologic examination, the primary site of bleeding can be identified, in the surviving matrix, by the findings of hemolyzed blood, iron pigment, or cavities [5, 41, 42]. The ependyma is usually destroyed, not only at the site of the hemorrhage but also elsewhere, or it may become buried beneath proliferating glial cells, forming rosette-like structures (Fig. 21.45).

IVH is often associated with damage of the white matter. Whether due to ischemia and/or hemorrhage, cavitation (often misnamed "porencephaly") and ventricular diverticulum may develop [43, 44] (Fig. 21.46).

In survivors, correlations of neuropathologic findings and neurologic follow-up studies are quite accurate when they are based on consecutive ultrasounds over the first month of life [45, 46]. The neurologic sequelae depend on the

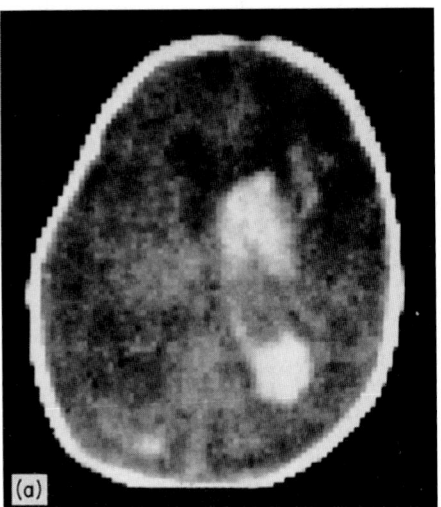

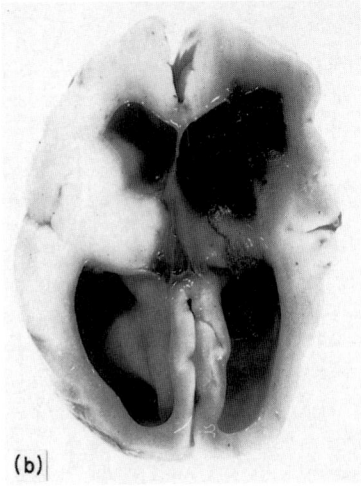

FIGURE 21.44.   *Hemohydrocephalus: (a) CT scan showing large ventricles with blood and necrosis of the parenchyma; (b) horizontal section of the brain.*

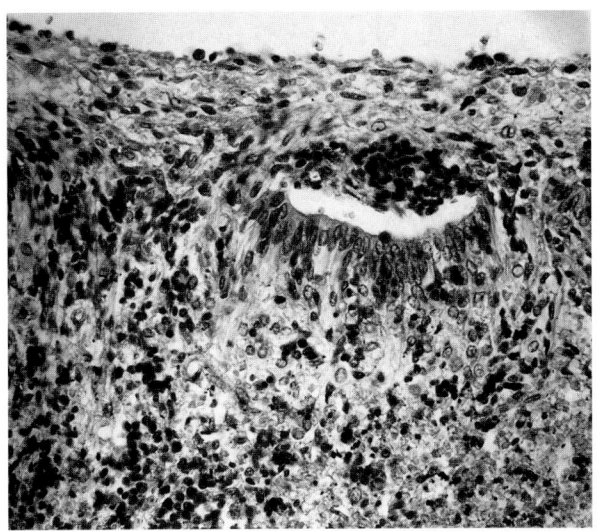

FIGURE 21.45.   *Posthemorrhagic hydrocephalus: destruction of the ependyma with glial reaction and rosette-like formation.*

severity of the hemorrhage and associated parenchymal lesions. Two major groups emerge:

1. Noncomplicated IVH, grades I and II of Papile [39]: matrix or ventricular hemorrhage without dilatation or parenchymal lesions carry a good prognosis.
2. Complicated IVH, grades III and IV of Papile: posthemorrhagic hydrocephalus, general atrophy of the brain, multicystic encephalopathy, and hydrocephalus ex vacuo. In this group, neurologic sequelae occur in 30–60% of cases, depending on the extent of the lesions.

In the full-term newborn infant, IVH can occur, but there are very few data concerning its frequency [2, 47, 48]. The source of the bleeding is usually the choroid plexus, a vascular malformation, extension of a parenchymal hemorrhage into the ventricle, or blood dyscrasia.

Cerebellar Hemorrhage

Subarachnoid hemorrhage over the cerebellum is fairly common in premature infants; it occurs alone or in association with supratentorial subarachnoid hemorrhage. Blood may collect over one hemisphere and destroy the underlying foliae (Fig. 21.47a). Small hemorrhages and hematomas occur frequently within the foliae but less often in the white matter and deep nuclei, where they are seen only on section of the cerebellum. Extension of hematomas into the vermis, with disruption of the wall of the dilated fourth ventricle, is seen in cases of severe IVH.

In the author's experience, the incidence increased from 7% (1961 to 1966) to 15% (1968 to 1984) in relation to

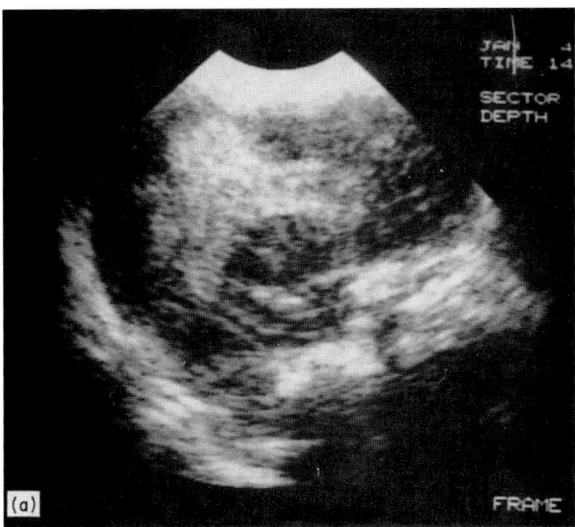

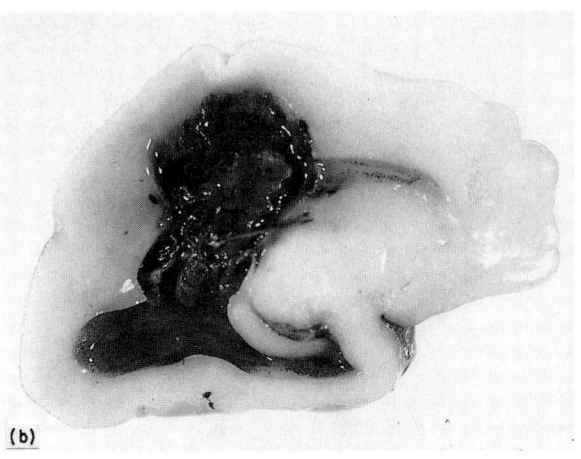

FIGURE 21.46.   *Intraventricular hemorrhage and intraparenchymal diverticulum, sagittal view: (a) ultrasound; (b) the brain after fixation.*

the changing population admitted to an intensive care unit. Since then, the number of cases is decreasing as well as that of IVH.

The pathogenesis of the bleeding is poorly understood [49, 50]. It has been suggested that hemorrhages in the immature cerebellar foliae could be related to the poorly formed capillary bed in this region [36]. In infants who survive for a few weeks, collected hemorrhages appear as golden or olive green staining of the meninges, which may resemble pus; cystic degeneration and atrophy of the involved hemisphere are seen in severe forms. Intracerebellar hematomas can be detected by CT scanning [51] and by ultrasound [52, 53].

Petechial hemorrhages are often associated with bacterial sepsis, in a context of hemorrhagic encephalopathy (Fig. 21.47b). Hemosiderin-laden macrophages, gliosis, and neuronal necrosis of varying extent are found on microscopic examination (Fig. 21.47c).

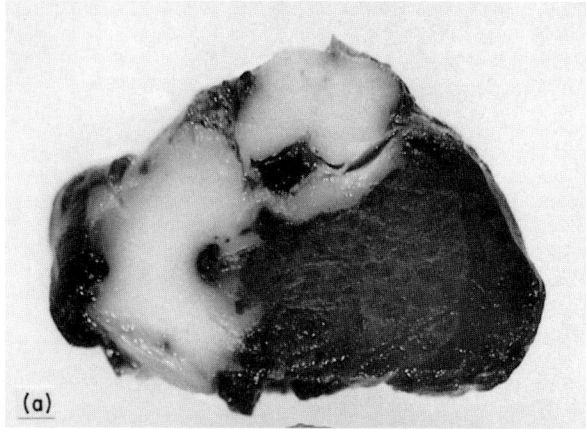

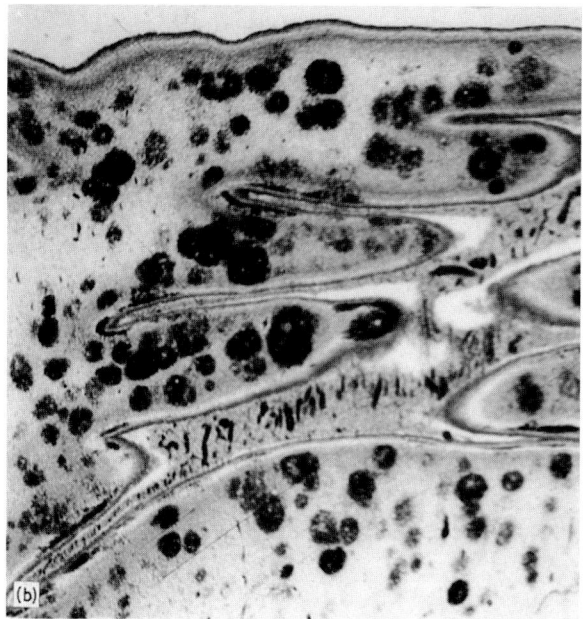

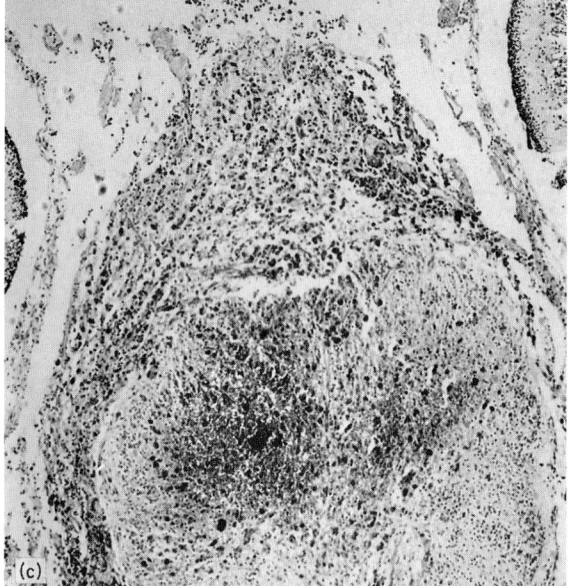

FIGURE 21.47.   *Hemorrhage of the cerebellum: (a) large hematoma; (b) multiple microscopic hemorrhages (staphylococcal septicemia); (c) old hematoma with gliosis and iron pigments.*

HYPOXIC-ISCHEMIC ENCEPHALOPATHY (HIE)–NEURONAL NECROSIS IN FULL-TERM NEONATES

The term "hypoxic-ischemic encephalopathy" (HIE), as it is used in the literature, is rather confusing, since clinical signs as well as pathologic anatomy are described under the same label that covers almost the entire spectrum of perinatal cerebral pathology, including hemorrhages. Therefore, we shall describe separately, first, the HIE that is observed in full-term neonates, within a rather well-defined framework of asphyxia, and, second, periventricular leukomalacia (PVL), which occurs mainly in preterm infants in a different setting.

In full-term infants, several clinical classifications, based on the severity of the encephalopathy, have been proposed [8, 54–57].

- In stage I or mild HIE, muscle tone abnormality and excessive responsiveness to stimulation are

maximal during the first day after birth and then progressively diminish; there is no evidence of neuronal necrosis or raised intracranial pressure. The prognosis is good.

- In stage II, or moderate HIE, the infant is lethargic or hypotonic; isolated convulsions and EEG abnormalities are present over the first 48 to 72 hours. The encephalopathy then either regresses or progresses to stage III.

- Stage III is the most severe situation for which we have reliable neuropathologic documentation. We shall limit our description to this form.

Severe hypoxic-ischemic encephalopathy usually occurs in the course of difficult labor and/or delivery [58, 59], such as occipitoposterior and occipitotransverse position, breech presentation in primipara, antepartum hemorrhage due to placenta previa or abruptio placentae, prolapsed umbilical cord or tight cord around the neck, labor of less than 3 hours in primipara or more than 15 hours in multipara or primipara, a prolonged second stage of labor (more than 1.5 hours), or difficult forceps delivery. In large maternity hospitals, the risk of grade III HIE in full-term infants has been reduced by virtue of better antenatal and perinatal care. Figures given by Amiel-Tison and Stewart (60) are as follows: 1.6 per 1000 livebirths in the years 1962 to 1964, 1.3 per 1000 in the 1970s, and less than 1 per 1000 today.

Clinical and Brain Imaging Data

A newborn infant with severe hypoxic-ischemic encephalopathy is stuporous or comatose after birth. The Apgar score is less than 3, and the infant requires resuscitation and mechanical ventilation. Convulsions occur within a few hours in about 50% of cases, progressing to status epilepticus. Seizures may not be apparent clinically, but the EEG shows bursts of paroxysmal activity or is inactive [61]. Abnormal eye movements, dilated pupils, inappropriate sucking, or subtle movements of the chin are seizure equivalents. The fontanelles are tense and the sutures are separated. It is often impossible to obtain CSF at lumbar puncture because of cerebral edema.

CT scanning and ultrasound show narrow ventricles and sometimes hypodense areas, which may represent edematous unmyelinated white matter or severe malacia. In such circumstances the prognosis is very poor. Radionuclide brain scanning [62] and positron emission tomography (PET) scan

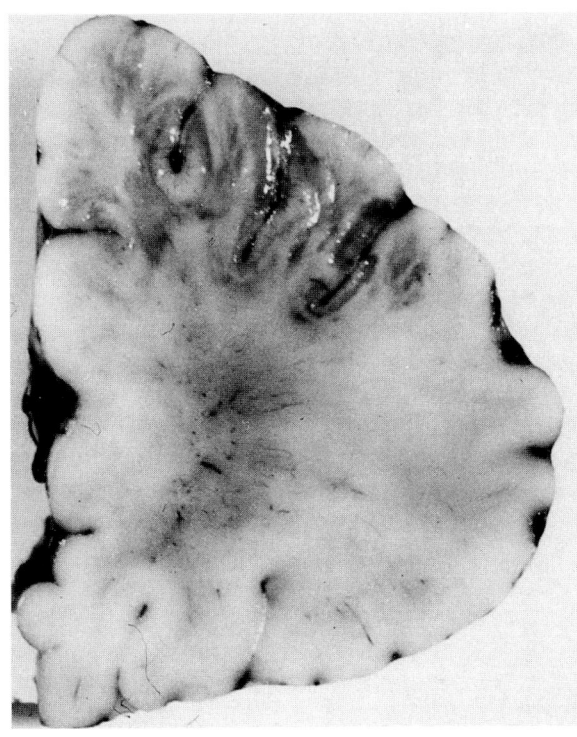

FIGURE 21.48.   *Cortical necrosis in a full-term infant with tissue disintegration (frontal lobe).*

[63] have demonstrated hypoxic-ischemic lesions in the parasagittal regions of both hemispheres. These areas correspond to the border zone at the terminal territories of the anterior, middle, and posterior cerebral arteries. In animal experiments, these regions are most vulnerable to conditions of reduced cerebral blood flow and oxygen supply. In infants who die in similar conditions, the lesions are often symmetric but usually extend well beyond the parasagittal zones and involve the basal ganglia, thalamus, and brainstem as well.

Pathologic Anatomy

At postmortem examination, there is no CSF in the arachnoid space, the brain is edematous and abnormally heavy, the gyri are flattened and the sulci are narrowed, and there is herniation of the uncus toward the midline and of the cerebellar tonsils through the foramen magnum. On section, the brain may be pale and dry or watery, with a tendency to disintegrate (Fig. 21.48). The ventricles are compressed, and the infundibulum often protrudes into the interpeduncular cistern. At first the cortex is pale, contrasting with the more congested white matter and giving a "ribbon effect" [1]. At times, the cortex, the deep gray matter, and the brainstem nuclei, essentially the inferior colliculi, may be grayish brown (Figs. 21.49a, 21.50a, and 21.51a) due to necrosis and capillary proliferation. The basal parts of the temporal lobes are usually spared.

On histologic examination, cortical necrosis may be focal or diffuse, patchy or columnar in distribution. It is often more pronounced in the depth of the sulci than on the crest of the gyri (Fig. 21.49b). Necrosis may be laminar [58, 64], preferentially involving layers III and V (Fig. 21.52) where oxidative enzyme activity first develops in the full-term infant [65]. Neuronal necrosis is characterized by a pyknotic nucleus, an acidophilic or vacuolated cytoplasm, margination of Nissl substance, and tigrolysis. Karyorrhexis or fragmentation of nuclei is a prominent feature in the neonate, observed mainly in the subiculum, griseum pontis, and internal granular layer of the cerebellum.

In the thalamus, basophilic neurons and, at times, neuronophagia can be seen (Fig. 21.50b). In the brainstem, the most striking feature is necrosis of the inferior colliculi, characterized by loss of neurons, glial reaction, and prominent capillaries (Fig. 21.51b); these lesions are very similar to those described in asphyxiated newborn monkeys [66] and may be related to the rich vascularization, an advanced state of myelination, and requirement of high levels of glucose. Selective necrosis of cranial nerve nuclei (VI and VII) is responsible for the so-called Möbius syndrome. Incrusted neurons and cavitations involve the reticular formation as well.

In the cerebellar cortex, apart from karyorrhexis of the internal granular layer cells, the Purkinje's cells are pyknotic or swollen and then disintegrate, being replaced by a regular row of optically empty spaces (Fig. 21.53). The phylogenet-

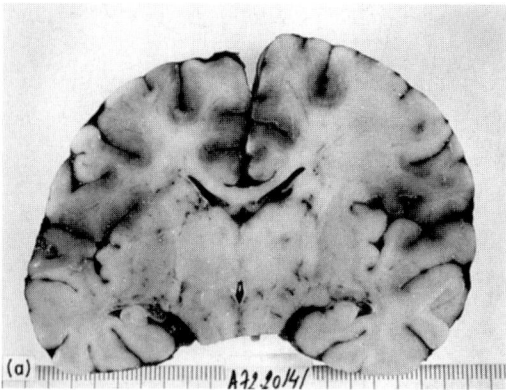
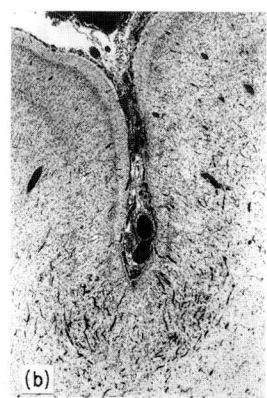

FIGURE 21.49. *Cortical necrosis: (a) coronal section—the necrosis is most severe in the depth of the sulci; (b) histologic view.*

ically older the structures, the greater their vulnerability. The dentate nucleus is usually affected with gliosis and/or liquefaction of the hilus.

The white matter of the hemispheres may be involved as well; with specific stains, the early myelinated tracts are poorly stained and, on microscopic examination, the fibers appear swollen and fragmented.

In this form of severe HIE, all neuronal structures may be involved, with varying severity. In a series of 40 affected full-term infants, three dominant topographic patterns were observed: in 23 cases the lesions were diffuse; in 12 cases the lesions were predominantly situated in the basal ganglia, thalamus, and brainstem, as already described by others [67,

68]; and in four cases the cortex alone was damaged. In the last case, severe lesions were restricted to the brainstem but were associated with a large subdural hematoma and cerebral edema; the lesions may have been at least partially due to compression.

Apart from this well-defined entity based on clinical-electrical and anatomic findings, another form of anoxic encephalopathy with lesions restricted to the pontosubicular regions has been described [69] in premature and full-term infants who have presented with RDS. A similar distribution was found by Ahdab-Barmada et al [70] in severely asphyxiated neonates who were subjected to episodes of hyperoxemia.

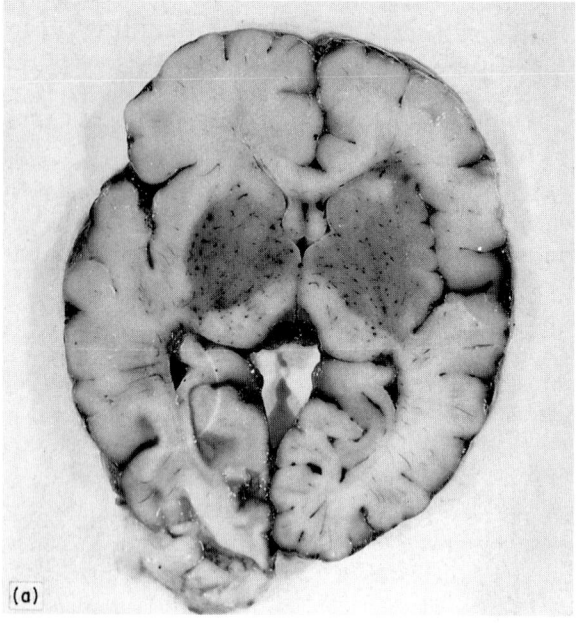
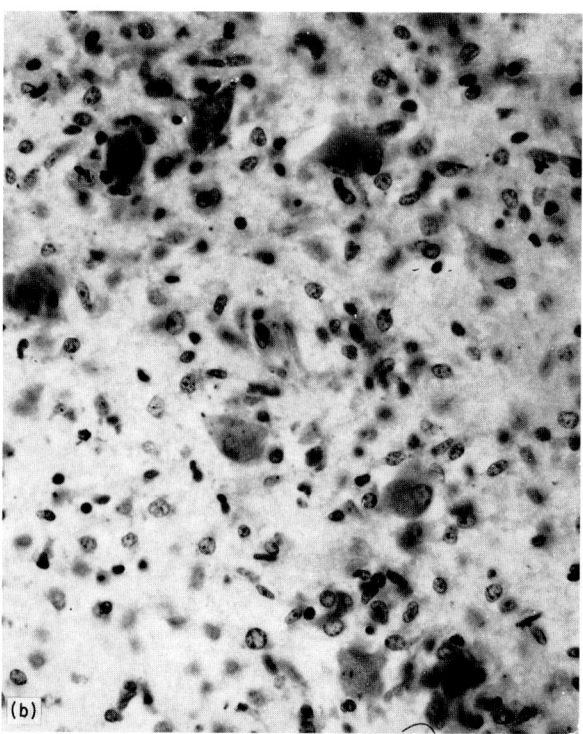

FIGURE 21.50. *Necrosis of the deep gray nuclei: (a) horizontal section of the brain; (b) histologic neuronal necrosis and neuronophagia.*

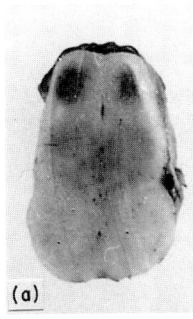

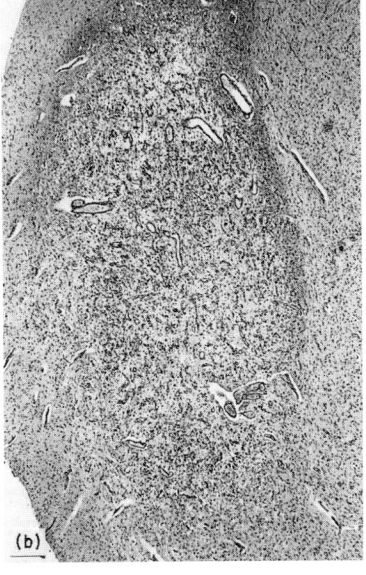

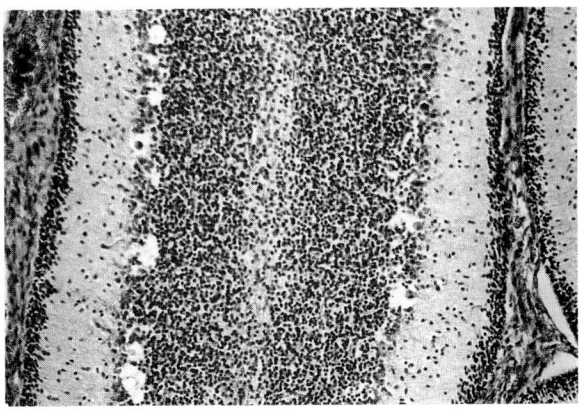

FIGURE 21.53. *Necrosis of cerebellar lamellae; note the absence of Purkinje's cells.*

FIGURE 21.51. *Necrosis of the inferior colliculi: (a) grayish brown discoloration of the structure after fixation; (b) microscopically, the necrosis is strictly limited to the inferior colliculi.*

surviving animals and described structural abnormalities that closely mimic the pathologic findings in human neonates. Several patterns of lesions were produced in the newborn monkey:

1. Total asphyxia caused by clamping of the umbilical cord and prevention of the onset of respiration, leading to brainstem damage with a particularly high frequency of involvement of the inferior colliculi
2. Partial asphyxia caused by reduction of placental perfusion, leading to cerebral edema and cortical necrosis
3. Partial asphyxia without acidosis, leading to lesions involving mainly the white matter

Experimental Data and Pathogenesis

Many experiments have been developed in order to understand the mechanisms by which hypoxic-ischemic states act on the brain [71, 72]. In a large series of experiments conducted over many years, Myers et al [73] accumulated laboratory data and clinical reports on the development of

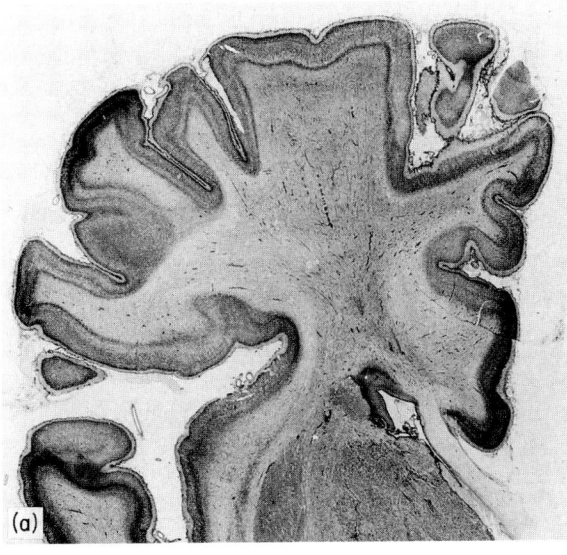

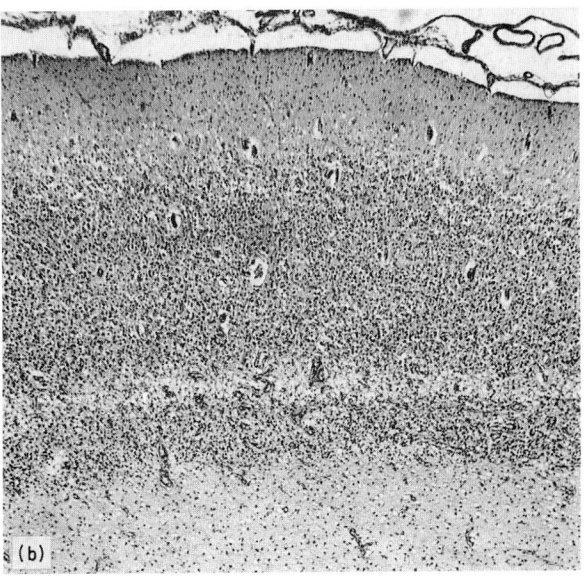

FIGURE 21.52. *Cortical laminar necrosis: (a) large celloidin section (CV stain); (b) histologic preparation of another case with necrosis of layer V.*

4. Partial asphyxia followed by total asphyxia, leading to necrosis of the basal ganglia and sometimes the cortex

In addition, Myers emphasized the deleterious role of lactate accumulation in the brain, the production of which is related not only to the level of oxygen delivery but also to the quantity of blood glucose and glycogen storage in the different areas of the brain.

Recently, in animal experiments, cellular mechanisms and other biochemical changes have been demonstrated during hypoxic-ischemic states. Accumulation of excitatory amino acid (EAA) receptors [74, 75] and increased free radical production with cell membrane damage may lead to cell death. Furthermore, different types of agonists of EAAs or potential neuroprotective agents, given before or sometimes shortly after hypoxic-ischemic insult, could improve cerebral outcome. Unfortunately, none of these treatments can be applied to neonates at the present time.

Sequelae of Hypoxic-Ischemic Encephalopathy

After an apparent clinical improvement and restoration of vital functions, surviving infants may develop signs of persistent neurologic disorder, such as spastic paraplegia or quadriplegia with or without choreoathetosis, seizures, and severe mental retardation and microcephaly. CT scanning shows cerebral atrophy with enlarged ventricles. However, the ex vacuo hydrocephalus observed in full-term infants who sustain this form of HIE is usually less pronounced than that observed in preterm infants who survive with severe leukomalacia [76] (see below).

The structural sequelae vary from case to case. The brain may undergo extensive disintegration and liquefaction (Figs. 21.48 and 21.54a). The progression to cavitation (multicystic encephalomalacia) may be explained by the presence of an associated edema in the early phase of the disease. When necrosis is predominant in the cortex with neuronal loss and poor myelination, the convolutions become shrunken or atrophic and the sulci widen [77, 78]; this sequel is known as ulegyria, which should not be confused with microgyria (Fig. 21.54b). Laminar necrosis and nodular atrophy are best seen on sections stained for myelin or by Holzer's method for fibrillary astrocytes. Similar glial scars or "plaques fibromyeliniques" in the basal ganglia are described as status marmoratus or "état marbré" [79, 80]. The apparent increase of myelin staining is now thought to be due to a disturbance of myelin formation by glial cells [81] and disoriented myelinated fibers crossing the scarred tissue [82]. In addition to neuronal devastation, incrusted or ferruginated neurons or cavitation may also be observed and seen in vivo with imaging techniques.

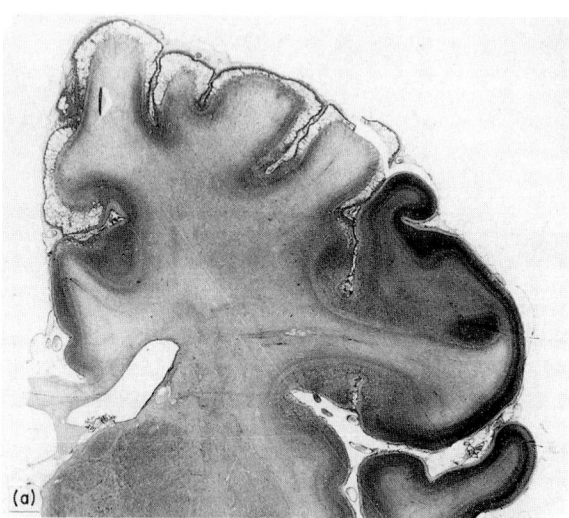
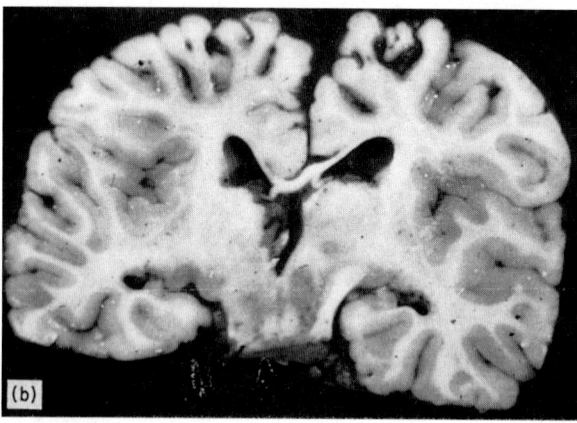

FIGURE 21.54. *Sequela of severe asphyxia neonatorum: (a) lacelike appearance of the cortex and disintegration of the white matter in a 15-day-old infant; (b) ulegyria in a 5-month-old child. (Courtesy of Dr. E. Farkas.)*

PERIVENTRICULAR LEUKOMALACIA (PVL)

Periventricular leukomalacia, or necrosis of the white matter, was first described by Virchow in 1867 [83] in infants born of mothers suffering from smallpox or syphilis. At the same time, Parrot [84, 85] found similar lesions in small debilitated infants. Later, the lesions were related to venous circulatory impairment during the birth process or in the neonatal period [12]. In 1962, Banker and Larroche [86] described the lesions in detail, mainly in preterm infants, and considered them to be the morphopathologic basis for the spastic mono- and diplegia reported by Little in 1861 [87]. They emphasized the anoxic-ischemic character of the lesions and their stereotyped topography (Fig. 21.55) in the border zones among the three main arterial territories. A number of articles and monographs have been published since, and should be consulted [88–90].

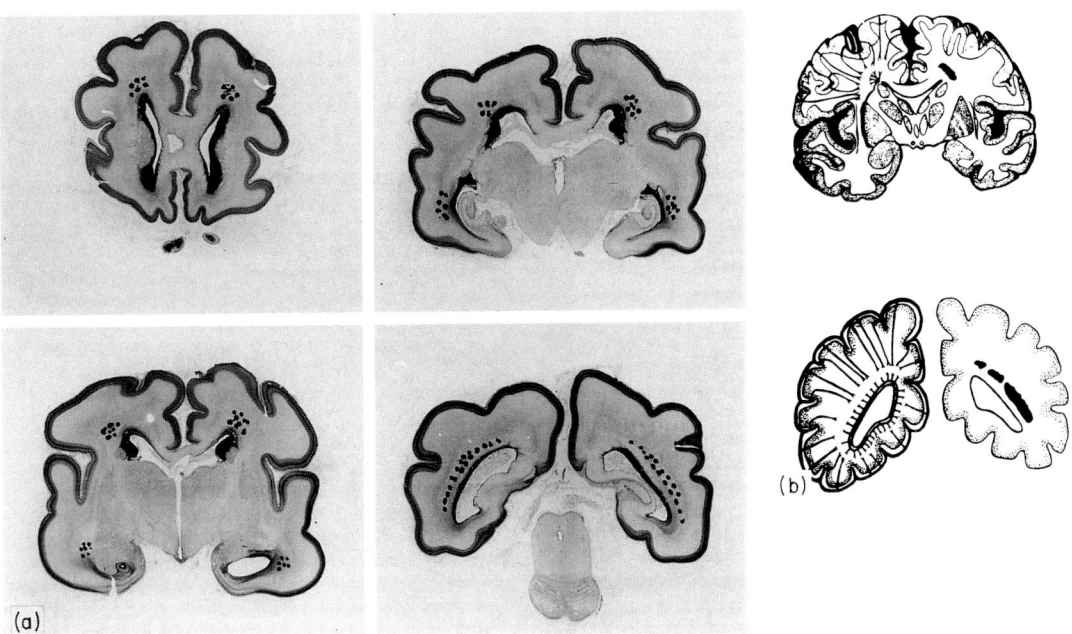

FIGURE 21.55.   *Leukomalacia: (a) schematic representation of the preferential localization of the lesions; (b) relationship between leukomalacia and vascularization. (From Ref. 92.)*

Pathologic Anatomy

On sections of the fixed brain, ill-defined "white spots" measuring one to several millimeters in diameter are seen in a pale, watery, unmyelinated white matter; these areas of necrosis may be single or multiple, and are often symmetric in the corona radiata, near the external angle of the lateral ventricle, in the temporal acoustic radiations, and posteriorly in the tapetum and optic radiations (Fig. 21.56a). Initially homogeneous, they subsequently become outlined by a chalky white ring (Fig. 21.56b) and often become centrally cavitated. In infants who present with severe biliru-

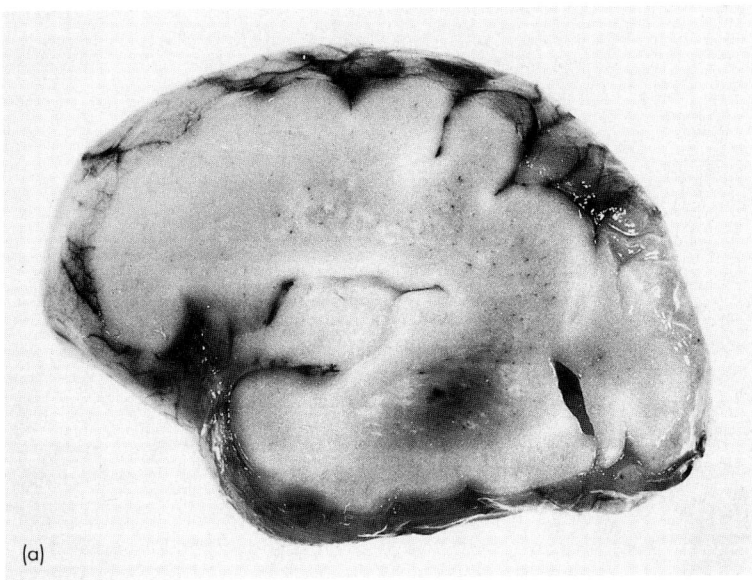
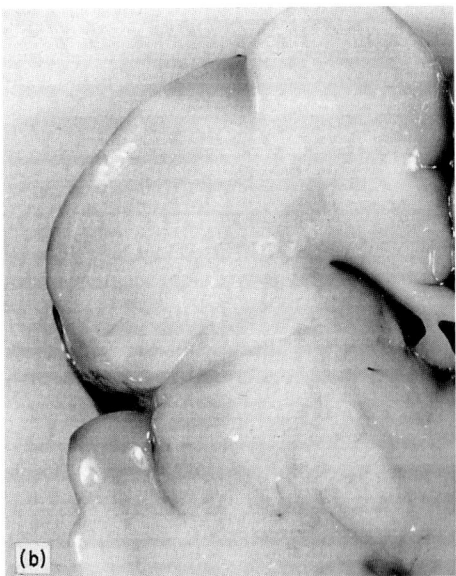

FIGURE 21.56.   *Leukomalacia: (a) parasagittal section showing the lesions in the periventricular white matter; (b) coronal section showing "white spots" in the corona radiata with a chalky white ring.*

binemia, and when the pigment is fixed by macrophages, the "white spots" may be stained yellow.

Microscopic examination of the earliest stage of the lesion reveals areas of coagulation necrosis (Fig. 21.57a) well stained by PAS and Luxol fast blue. Within 24 to 48 hours, round bodies and parallel fibrillary structures appear at the periphery of the necrosis. Microglia, large astrocytes, and macrophages soon proliferate. Silver impregnation shows the characteristic features of axonal disintegration—i.e., swollen,

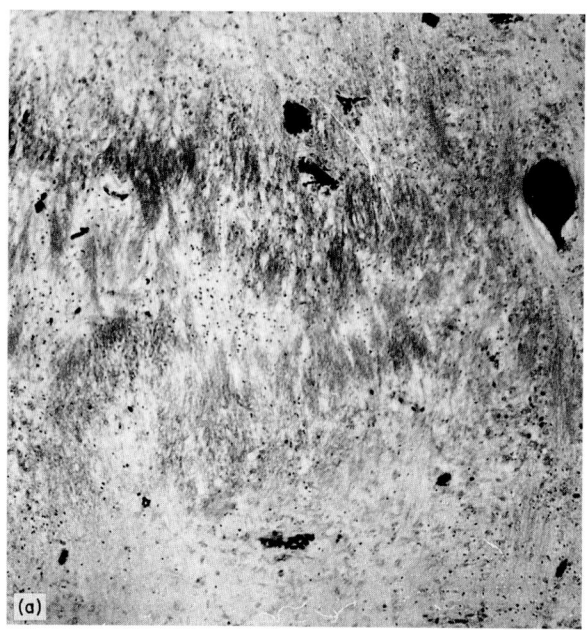

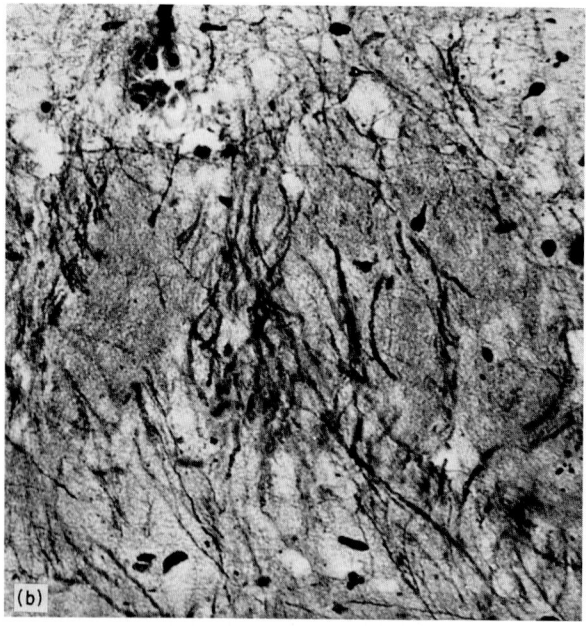

FIGURE 21.57.   *Leukomalacia: (a) coagulation necrosis brightly stained with PAS; (b) swollen and fragmented axons (silver impregnation).*

fragmented, clublike structures and retraction balls (Fig. 21.57b). The ependyma near the necrotic areas is usually destroyed. In addition, neuronal necrosis may be found in various sites of the brain, such as globus pallidus, subiculum, dentate nucleus, and brainstem nuclei.

Pathophysiology

In spite of the considerable importance of this pathologic entity in neonatal medicine, one must admit that its pathophysiogenesis is poorly understood. Various hypotheses on the causes and mechanisms have been proposed over more than a century. The hypothesis of hypoxic encephalopathy and of vulnerable territories in the border zones among the three main cerebral arteries was first proposed by Banker and Larroche [86]. Later, border zones between ventriculopetal and ventriculofugal arteries were demonstrated [90–92], but recently this arterial network has been denied [93–95]. However, combining histologic techniques and radioangiographs, Takashima and Tanaka [96] demonstrated leukomalacia in these poorly vascularized zones. In addition, when brain arterial perfusion is reduced in experimental animals, similar white matter necrosis develops [97–99]. Similarly, in distressed premature infants, with episodes of hypotension and recurrent apnea, impaired cerebral blood flow auto-regulation would affect preferentially these terminal arterial territories. Furthermore, the white matter of these areas is in the process of early myelination and might be particularly vulnerable.

In older series that included more infants beyond 36 weeks' gestation than are seen today, other pathologic conditions, such as congenital heart malformations and intrauterine growth retardation with hypoglycemia, were often associated with leukomalacia and might have taken part in its genesis [86].

In both age groups of infants, leukomalacia is often associated with sepsis and meningoencephalitis. In these conditions, cardiovascular collapse, damage to the capillary walls, and various metabolic disorders may also enhance the injury of the white matter. A related form of leukomalacia named "telencephalic leukoencephalopathy" was indeed reproduced in kittens by intraperitoneal administration of *E coli* endotoxin [100].

Recently, a new hypothesis has been proposed [101]. It was suggested that a number of cytokines, proteins produced and released by macrophages during infections in pregnancy, might have deleterious effects on the immature brain. One of these cytokines, tumor necrosis factor (TNF), would be particularly involved [102]. TNF, stimulated by endotoxin, induces hypotension and promotes disseminated intravascular coagulation, vasoconstriction, and cellular changes such as destruction of oligodendrocytes and proliferation of astrocytes. In human infants, however, the pathogenesis of PVL remains unclear and is probably multifactorial.

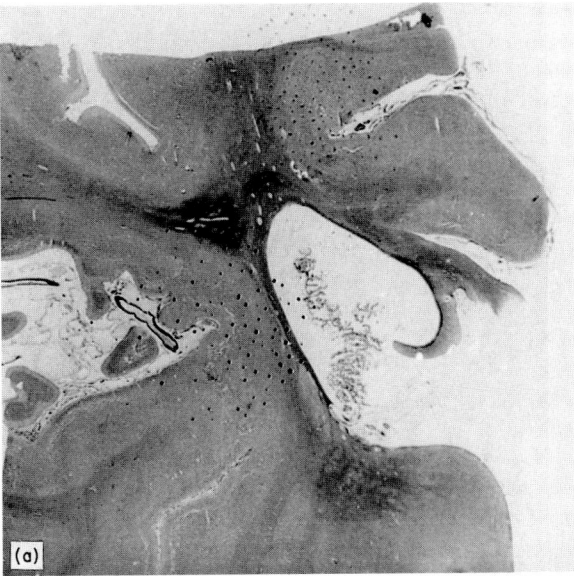
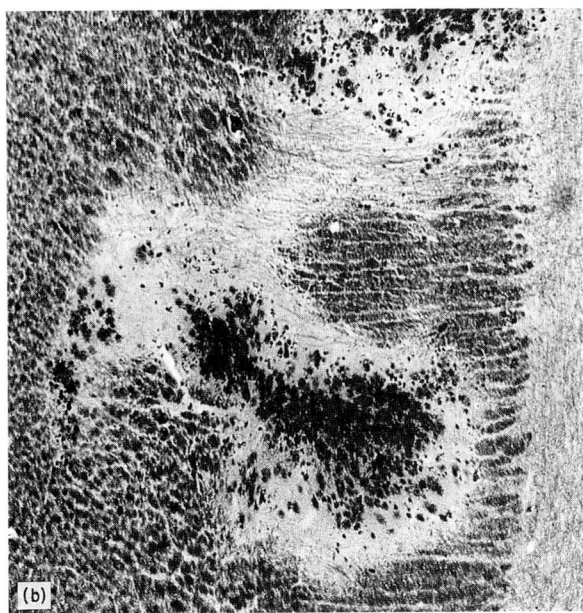

FIGURE 21.58.   *Sequelae of leukomalacia: (a) sclerosis of the centrum semiovale with fibrillary gliosis (courtesy of Dr. E. Farkas); (b) focal absence of myelin and fat-laden macrophages in the stratum sagittale of an 8-month-old infant (frozen section and Sudan black stain).*

Evolution of the Lesions

When the infant survives the acute phase, two different and unpredictable forms of sequelae occur. One form is sclerosis of the centrum semiovale [103–105], which includes fibrillary gliosis (Fig. 21.58a) and calcium deposits or mummified cells, accumulation of macrophages, and lack of myelination (Fig. 21.58b). White matter sclerotic atrophy is compensated by ex vacuo hydrocephalus.

The other form of sequelae is multicystic encephalopathy or polyporencephaly [106], resulting from disintegration of the brain tissue (Fig. 21.59). Astrocytic gliosis,

macrophages, and calcium deposits surround the cavities (Fig. 21.60). Evolution to this form with cavitation may be related to the severity of edema accompanying the primary necrosis. This loss of brain tissue is associated with ex vacuo hydrocephalus as well, which may be uni- or bilateral, symmetric or asymmetric, and usually more pronounced on the side showing severe cavitation.

Clinical and Brain Imaging Data

During the first week of life, there are no specific neurologic abnormalities associated with the pure form of leuko-

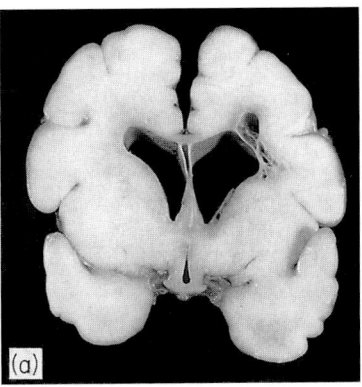
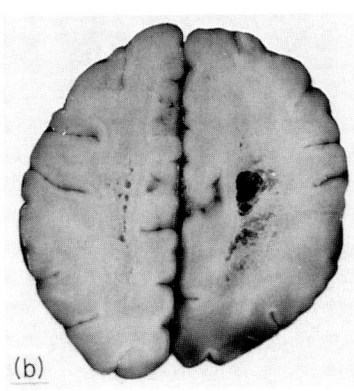
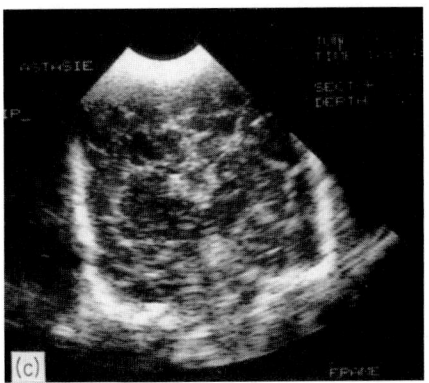

FIGURE 21.59.   *Multicystic leukomalacia: (a) coronal section showing multiple cavitations in the right periventricular white matter with ipsilateral ventricular dilatation in a 20-day-old premature infant; (b) horizontal section in a 5-week-old premature infant; (c) ultrasound in a surviving premature infant shows bilateral periventricular cavitations.*

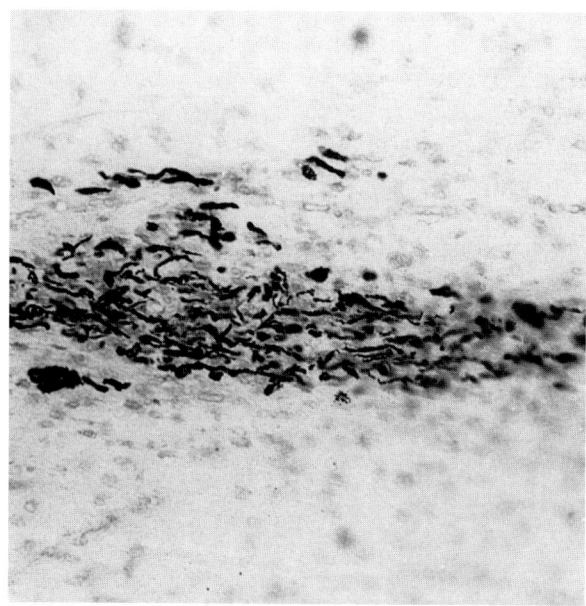

FIGURE 21.60.   *Pleiomorphic gliosis and calcium deposits in the walls of the cavities.*

malacia (the infant tends to be hypotonic and lethargic), and the diagnosis is based on presumption in infants who present repeated apneas and bradycardia, low blood pressure, and no evidence of IVH. With the new generation of high-resolution transducers, it is possible to make the diagnosis of the early stage of PVL on the basis of increased periventricular echogenicity (PVE) at the external angle of the lateral ventricle [107–113]. Small cysts develop 2 to 3 weeks after the onset of PVE, and within 2 to 3 months they may no longer be visible. In severe forms, they may become confluent, and, due to tissue loss, ex vacuo hydrocephalus develops. Nuclear magnetic resonance permits differentiation between gliosis and hemorrhage [114], and poor myelination can be assessed [115, 116] later in life.

Epidemiology

Thirty years ago, PVL was found in the brains of about 20% of preterm infants, usually as an isolated feature; necrosis in the basal ganglia, brainstem, and dentate nucleus were, however, sometimes described in association. In full-term infants, PVL occurred in 15%, but in this group the lesions were usually associated with neuronal necrosis in the setting of hypoglycemia and growth retardation, in congenital heart disease and in meningoencephalitis. Since then, with intensive-care support, 30% of infants who die have survived for more than 10 days, and the frequency of leukomalacia at postmortem examination has increased to 30–40%. In other series of high-risk infants, it is more than 80% [89]. In addition, the leukomalacia-meningoencephalitis associa-

tion has increased from 8% to 20% in the author's experience. Meanwhile, because of the long survival of many infants, the natural history of leukomalacia—i.e., sclerosis of the centrum ovale and multicystic encephalomalacia—is being described in an increasing number of cases: 2.2% from 1956 to 1966; 7.2% from 1967 to 1973; 14.4% from 1974 to 1980; and recently about 25% in our population. These data reflect the evolution of perinatal pathology, which parallels the modifications of our technology and the management of the smallest and most seriously ill patients.

Other Types of Leukomalacia

Leukomalacia and Meningoencephalitis

In *meningoencephalitis*, the white matter is usually severely involved. On section of the brain, the yellowish white matter, with or without localized foci of "white spots," contrasts with the light gray color of the cortex and basal ganglia and may disintegrate rapidly (Fig. 21.61). Histologic study shows intense proliferation of hypertrophic, GFAP-positive astrocytes. Similar leukoencephalopathy was reproduced experimentally in newborn kittens by intraperitoneal injections of *E coli* endotoxin into pregnant

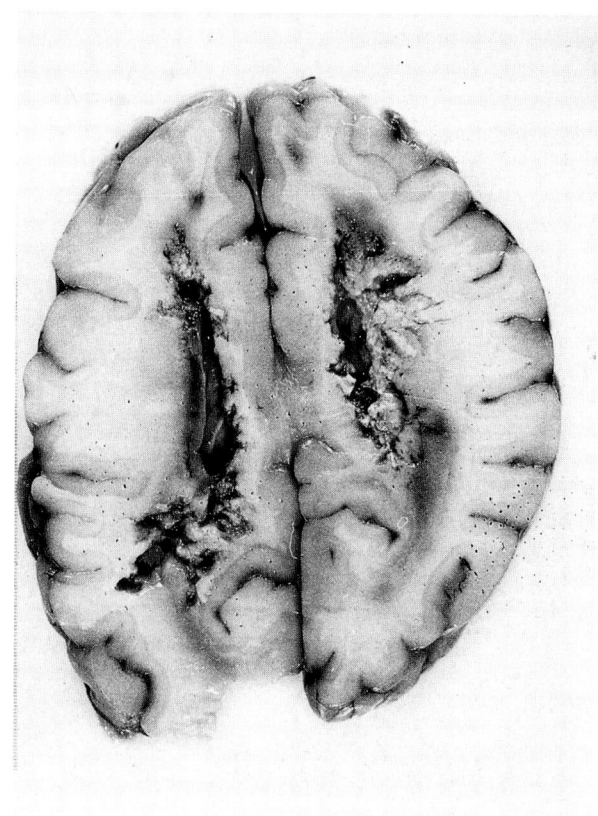

FIGURE 21.61.   *Leukomalacia and meningoencephalitis with disintegration of the white matter.*

animals [100] or following neonatal injection of similar endotoxine [117]. Necrosis of the capillary walls and diffuse petechial hemorrhages are often associated with this form of leukomalacia.

Subcortical Leukomalacia

Subcortical leukomalacia is seen more frequently in mature newborn infants than in preterm infants and is often associated with edema. The subcortical white matter (the site of the U fibers) is disintegrated. Microscopic study reveals the edematous tissue with a honeycomb appearance and glial reaction (Fig. 21.62). This lesion develops in the subcortical, poorly vascularized, triangular arterial territory [118]. After survival for several weeks or months, subcortical cystic lesions may be seen at autopsy [119] and detected by ultrasonography [120].

Hemorrhagic Leukomalacia

In preterm infants, leukomalacia was first described as a hypoxic-ischemic event. However, more recently, with ultrasonography, echo-dense areas have been described in the same sites as PVL and correspond to *hemorrhagic periventricular leukomalacia* (Fig. 21.63). In fact, the primary lesion is usually ischemic [88]. According to various authors [107, 110], such hemorrhages occur in 7–25% of cases, when vascular walls and surrounding tissues are severely damaged. The evolution of the lesion can be followed by ultrasound.

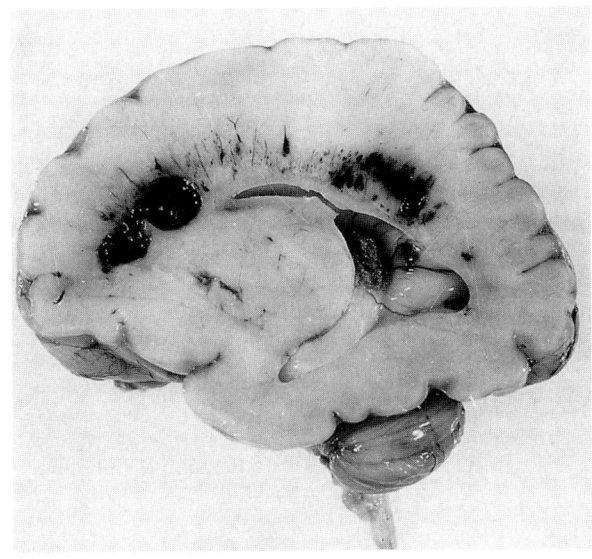

FIGURE 21.63. *Hemorrhagic leukomalacia.*

ARTERIAL OCCLUSION

Until recently, due to the paucity of clinical symptoms, the diagnosis of arterial occlusion in the neonate was made only at postmortem examination [121]. Availability of new imaging techniques now allows rapid diagnosis of arterial infarct [122] (Fig. 21.64). Prenatal diagnosis can be made as well [123], and the large number of reports confirms that the accident occurs during fetal life more frequently than was once thought.

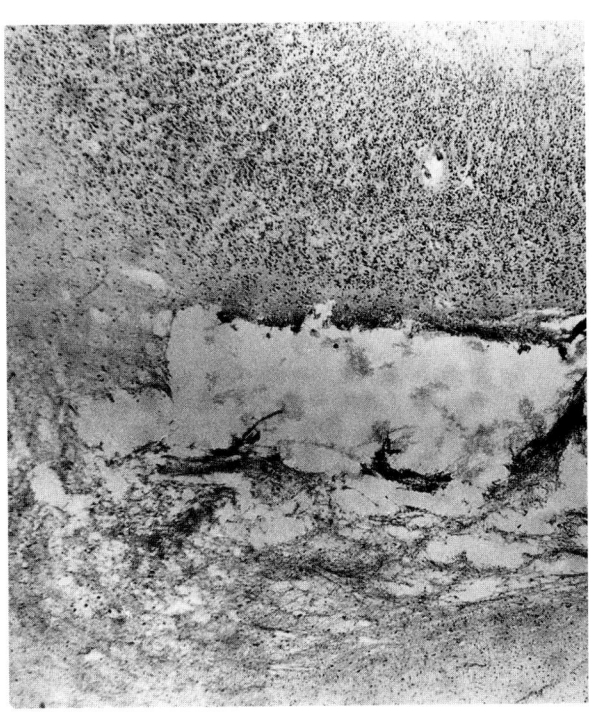

FIGURE 21.62. *Subcortical leukomalacia in a full-term infant with honeycomb appearance of the tissue.*

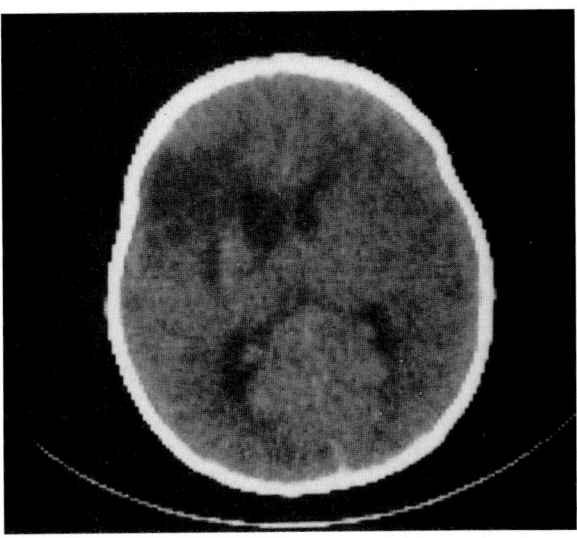

FIGURE 21.64. *CT scan of a 2-day-old infant: infarct in the territory of the left middle cerebral artery.*

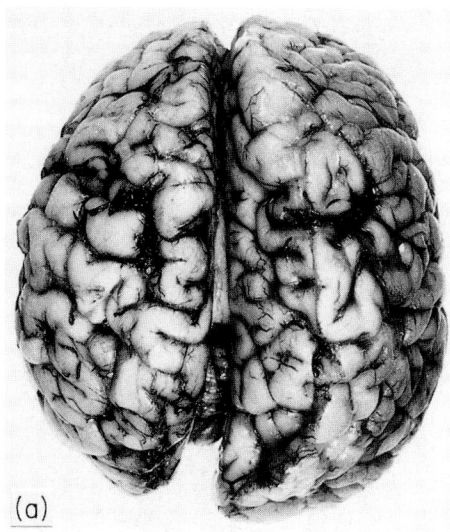

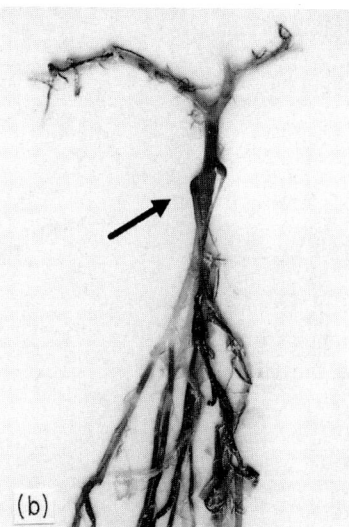

FIGURE 21.65.   *Arterial occlusion: (a) the right hemisphere is enlarged and edematous due to an ischemic and hemorrhagic infarct: (b) large embolus in the proximal part of the right middle cerebral artery after exchange transfusion (arrow).*

Pathologic Anatomy

At autopsy, when death occurs soon after the accident, the infarcted hemisphere is enlarged and edematous (Fig. 21.65a). Dissection of large vessels may reveal a thrombus or an embolus, but the procedure is time-consuming and uncertain (Fig. 21.65b). In the neonate, it is noteworthy that the infarcted area is often hemorrhagic and the diagnosis may be missed. However, the sharp apposition of normal and infarcted cortices suggests a primary arterial infarct (Fig. 21.66). On histologic examination, the neurons are poorly stained or pyknotic; within a few days, glial proliferation takes place, and lipid phagocytes and prominent endothelial cells are observed.

When the vascular accident has occurred in utero, long before birth, the affected hemisphere is atrophic, with narrow convolutions—i.e., the features of ulegyria. On sections of the brain, the infarcted area consists of multiple cavities of varying size, crossed by trabeculae (Fig. 21.67a); the ventricle of the damaged hemisphere is enlarged. The cerebral peduncles, pons, and medulla oblongata may be asymmetric, with marked atrophy of the pyramidal tract (Fig. 21.67b).

On histologic examination, the characteristic attributes of old infarct are to be found: necrosis of the cortex with a relatively preserved molecular layer, multiple cavities limited by glial tissue and macrophages loaded with iron pigment and lipids, and encrusted neurons. At the border of the infarct, heavily myelinated glial plaques (Fig. 21.68), similar to those described by Borit and Hemdon [81], and polymicrogyric cortex [1] can be found. The classic four-layered cortex of polymicrogyria, supposed to be secondary to postmigratory laminar necrosis, may not be found. The presence of an unlayered cortex, associated with a cell migration disorder, suggests that the injury occurred before or during neuronal migration (see fetal vascular encephalopathies, page 721).

Pathogenesis of Arterial Occlusion

The pathogenesis of arterial occlusion in the neonate is not well understood. In one of the first descriptions, Clark and Linell [124] incriminated emboli arising from the fetal veins or placenta. In survivors, when intracardiac shunts are still present, occlusion of a major vessel, most often the middle cerebral artery, can occur in the course of transfusion, exchange transfusion [1, 121], or indwelling catheters [125], and in cardiac right-to-left shunt [126]. In a large series of neonatal brains, Barmada and Moosy [127] found infarcts in 5.4% of cases. Severe infection with possible disseminated

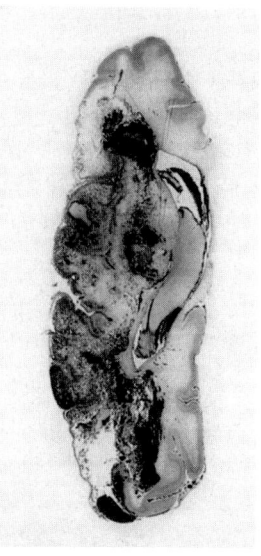

FIGURE 21.66.   *Horizontal serial celloidin section shows a sharp apposition of normal and infarcted cortices and hemorrhagic white matter.*

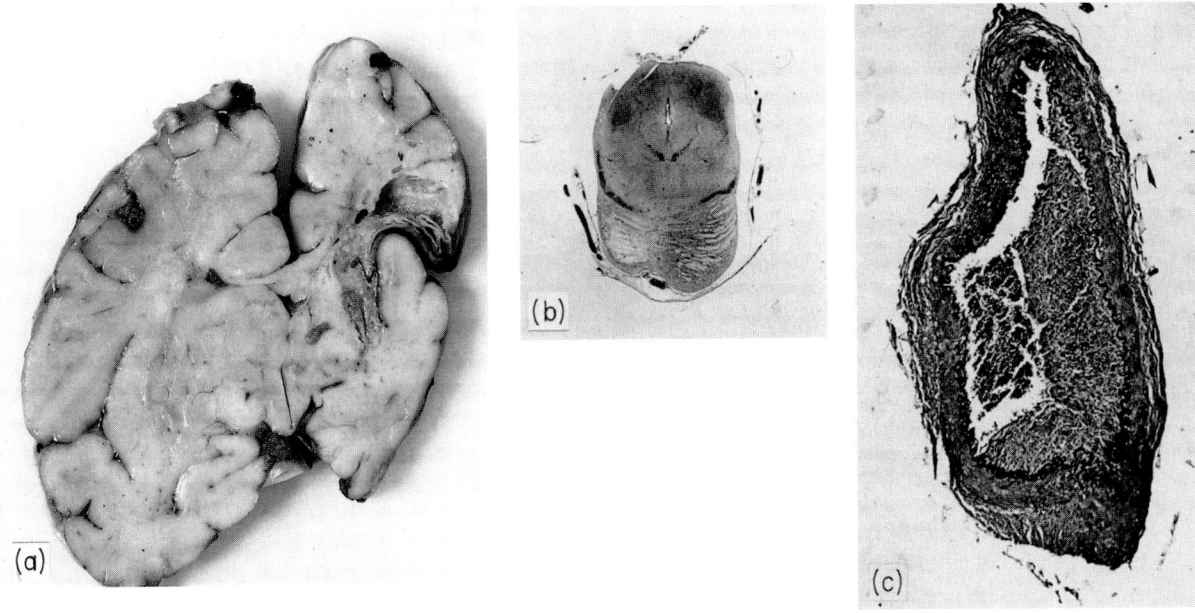

FIGURE 21.67.   *Occlusion in utero of the middle cerebral artery: (a) old and multicystic infarct; (b) atrophy of the pyramidal tract; (c) artery partly occluded by an organized thrombus.*

intravascular coagulation may account for this high frequency.

The pathogenesis of isolated occlusion occurring in utero is even more difficult to establish. In one of the author's cases,

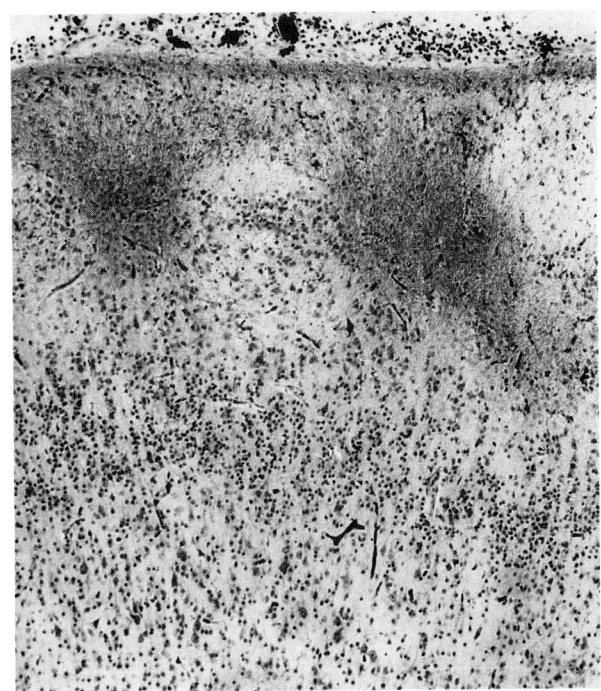

FIGURE 21.68.   *Heavily myelinated plaques close to the infarct.*

a full-term stillborn fetus [121], the middle cerebral artery was dissected and cut in serial sections and had an old and well-organized thrombus (Fig. 21.67c) of unknown cause.

Cerebral infarcts occurring in twin fetuses will be discussed later in this chapter.

FETAL VASCULAR ENCEPHALOPATHIES

This is a heterogeneous group of lesions that occur in utero and are, in their majority, similar to those previously described in the neonate. Hypoxic-ischemic lesions, including PVL and multicystic encephalopathy, neuronal necrosis, and infarct due to arterial occlusion, are most frequent, while hemorrhagic lesions are rare.

An additional group of abnormalities, such as cavities and clefts (porencephaly-schizencephaly, hydranencephaly) and polymicrogyria, occurring exclusively in fetal life, will be described in this chapter.

The lesions can be due to different factors related to maternal conditions (systemic disorders, trauma, gas poisoning, and drug intoxication or abuse), maternofetal conditions (isoimmune hemolytic disease and isoimmune thrombocytopenia), fetal conditions (twinning, nonimmune hydrops, coagulopathy, and cardiomyopathy), and placental pathology. It is important to recognize that these conditions are potentially harmful to the fetus, and to perform or repeat fetal ultrasound and/or imaging studies of the fetus and of the neonate. Once identified, the lesions and subsequent neurologic disorders will be attributed no longer to difficult labor and birth. Unfortunately, in a number of cases, the lesion is a fortuitous discovery at autopsy or on ultrasonogram.

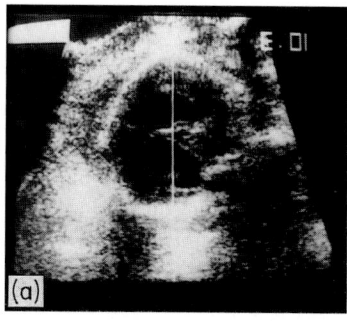

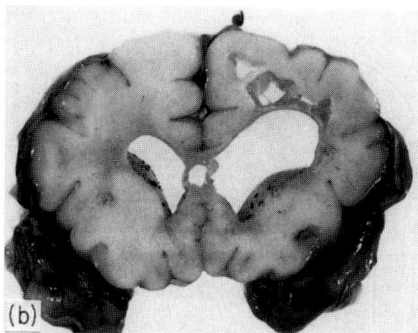

FIGURE 21.69. *Hydrocephalus and multicystic leukomalacia after an automobile accident without direct trauma to the mother: (a) ultrasound of the fetus 3 weeks after the accident; (b) section of the brain of the stillborn infant a week later.*

Maternal Pathologic Conditions

Systemic Disorders

Toxemia with hypertension [128], recurrent urinary tract infections [129], and severe anemia or maternal cardiorespiratory arrest [130] have been incriminated by pathologists in the pathogenesis of fetal cerebral damage. More recently, fetal ultrasonograms have shown a close relationship between maternal circulatory disturbances in a case of anaphylactic shock [131], or severe cardiorespiratory failure [132], and the development of multicystic lesions in the fetus, the lesions being confirmed at autopsy. Maternal blood dyscrasias, such as idiopathic thrombocytopenia [133] or anticoagulant therapy [134], may cause intracranial hemorrhage in the fetus.

Maternal Trauma

A number of maternal physical injuries may lead to various types of fetal brain damage. Direct trauma to the mother may lead to cephalohematoma of the fetus. In one such case, the bleeding, diagnosed in utero by ultrasound and confirmed at birth, resolved completely within 3 weeks [135]. Similarly, a subdural hematoma occurred following a fall by the mother. More frequently, ischemic lesions with multicystic encephalopathy and hydranencephaly have been reported after automobile and aircraft accidents [136–138]. Severe maternal injuries with cardiovascular shock might have led to fetal brain perfusion failure. An automobile accident without direct trauma to the mother, but only stress, was also thought to be the cause of fetal brain damage (Fig. 21.69) and posed a difficult medicolegal problem [138]. In fact, it has been demonstrated, in the pregnant rhesus monkey [139], that maternal psychological stress produces catecholamine discharges, leading to uterine vasoconstriction and impaired intervillous perfusion with subsequent fetal ischemic brain damage similar to that observed in human pathology.

Gas Intoxication

In the old literature, cases of fetal cerebral damage in both white and gray matter and neurologic disorders in survivors [140] have been reported following inhalation of carbon monoxide during pregnancy. In addition, polymicrogyria

was described after such accidents early in pregnancy [141]. Attempted suicide of a pregnant woman by inhalation of butane gas illustrates the effects on the fetus of pure anoxia followed by prolonged cardiovascular collapse [142]. The infant was born alive 4 weeks after the accident and survived for a few hours. On postmortem examination, there were anoxic-ischemic lesions of the kidneys and severe multicystic encephalomalacia, compatible with a process of several weeks' duration (Fig. 21.70). When such lesions can be identified in utero by ultrasound, the question of therapeutic abortion may be raised.

Drug Intoxication and Abuse

Direct implication of drugs in brain injuries is not yet well documented. A few cases of cocaine exposure during pregnancy have been reported as the cause of cerebral infarction [143, 144].

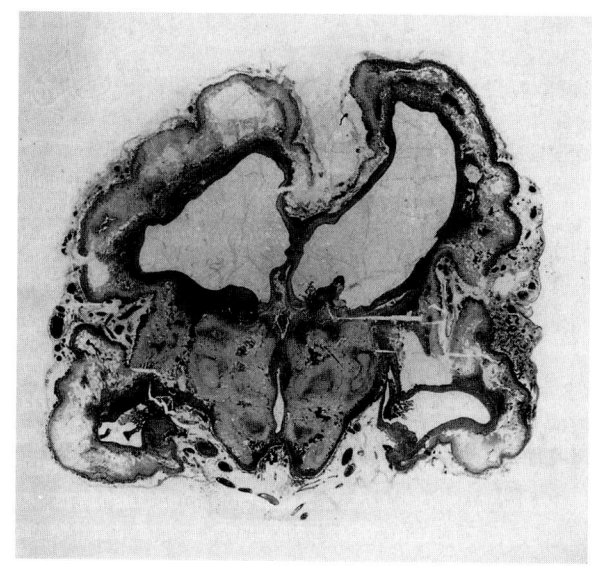

FIGURE 21.70. *Butane gas intoxication 4 weeks before delivery; severe cerebral malacia.*

Maternofetal Conditions

Isoimmune hemolytic disease, once a very common pathologic situation, is associated with a bleeding tendency, mostly in cases that present with hydrops [145].

Isoimmune thrombocytopenia was recently reported as a cause of intracranial hemorrhagic complications with consequent porencephaly [146]. The diagnosis can be made with imaging techniques performed within the first few hours of life [147, 148] or in utero [149, 150].

Fetal Conditions

Twinning

In monochorial twin placentae, vascular anastomoses between the two circulations may be vein to vein, artery to artery, or artery to vein. In the last situation, differences in

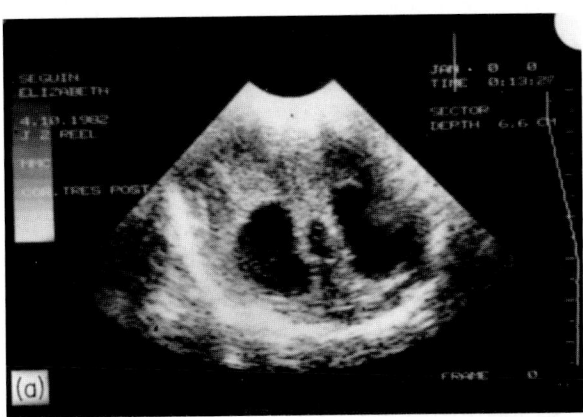

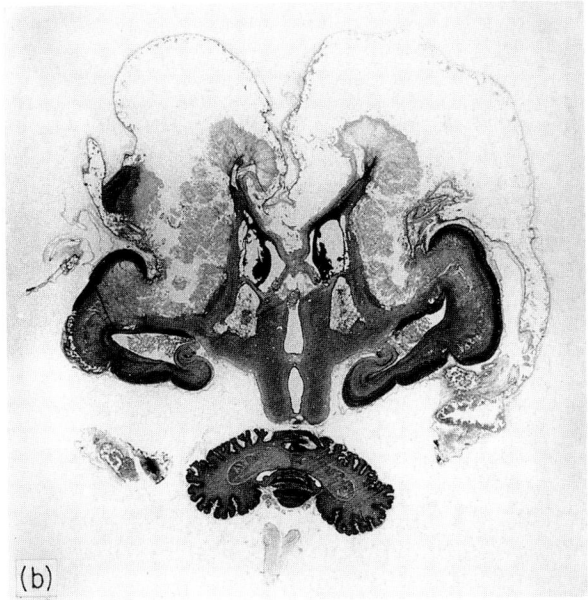

FIGURE 21.71. *Fetal vascular accident in a twin born alive; the co-twin was stillborn and macerated: (a) ultrasound shows enlarged ventricles and inhomogeneous white matter; (b) coronal celloidin section shows the brain lesions (hydranencephaly).*

blood pressure between the two vascular compartments can lead to disparate growth of the fetuses, a condition known as twin-twin transfusion syndrome. In addition, hemodynamic disorders can lead to brain and/or visceral damage. Several situations are observed depending on whether one or both fetuses die in utero or are born alive, and whether both fetuses or only one is affected.

In the classic situation, the donor is hypovolemic, hypotensive, and anemic, dies in utero, and subsequently becomes macerated. In such a case, autopsy is often not performed, and lesions, if any, are missed. The recipient twin survives and is most often affected; a large spectrum of lesions may develop, including ischemic infarcts, leukomalacia, and multicystic encephalopathy [151–153], and less commonly hemorrhage. Cavitation can be detected in utero and postnatally with ultrasonography [152–154]. The extreme form of brain damage with tissue loss is described as hydranencephaly [155].

When delivery occurs in the course of polyhydramnios, for example, with both fetuses alive, it is possible to find lesions in both of them, and even calcified leukomalacia, as early as 22 weeks [153].

Current debate focuses on the pathogenesis of the lesions that often develop in a surviving twin after death of the co-twin in utero. It was classically thought that necrotic or thrombotic material passed from the macerated fetus to the surviving one, causing disseminated intravascular coagulation [156, 157] or occlusion of large arteries [155]. More likely, other mechanisms are involved [153]. The donor twin being in a state of chronic distress, the fluctuations of its blood pressure may be transmitted to the recipient co-twin, leading to episodic brain perfusion failure and hypoxic-ischemic damage. In addition, when the donor twin dies in utero, the co-twin is suddenly deprived of a large amount of blood and may develop hypoxic-ischemic lesions. Moreover, the recipient twin may be exsanguinated into the co-twin, a low-pressure compartment.

Depending on the time of the vascular accident and its severity, the lesions range from localized brain infarcts to hydranencephaly (see Figs. 21.71a and b and 21.72). In addition, abnormal cell migration resulting in cortical disorganization with polymicrogyria may be related to such accidents when they occur early in fetal life before the cortical plate is completed [158–160].

In infants who survive, a wide range of psychomotor handicaps develop, depending on the extent of the lesions and on their localization [161, 162].

Nonimmune Hydrops Fetalis

In cases of nonimmune hydrops fetalis, due to a variety of causes, anemia, hypoproteinemia, heart failure, and subsequent hypotension are often associated conditions that may impair brain perfusion and cause hypoxic-ischemic damage. The lesions occur mostly in the white matter, which is particularly vulnerable in young fetuses. Leukomalacia with cavitation, diffuse gliosis and microcalcification of the white

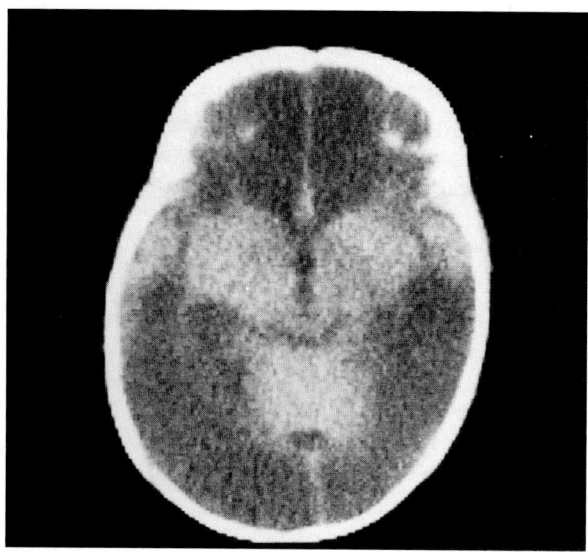

FIGURE 21.72. *CT scan of a surviving twin (macerated co-twin); thalami and brainstem are relatively spared.*

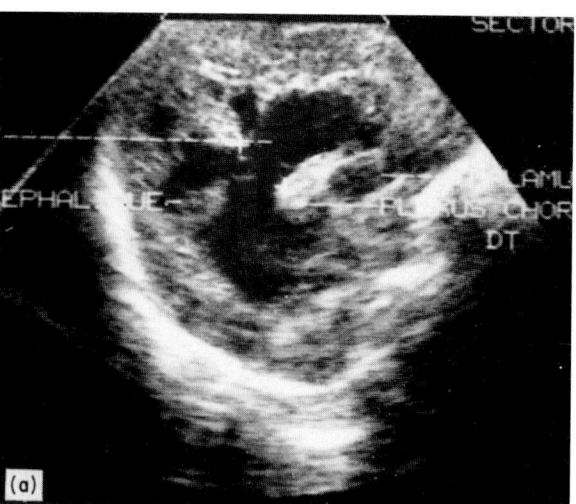

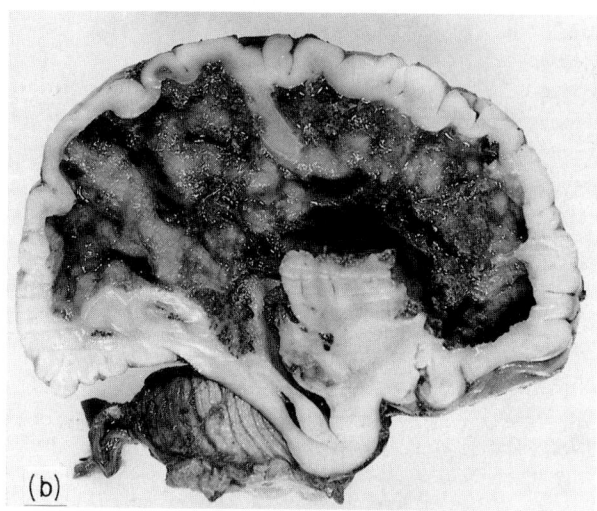

FIGURE 21.73. *Fetal thrombopathy: (a) ultrasound in a 2-day-old infant shows enlarged ventricles and severe destruction of the surrounding parenchyma; (b) parasagittal section of the brain on the third day.*

matter, and disseminated microinfarcts have been recently described [163]. Large injuries may be detected in utero with ultrasound [163].

Coagulopathy

This situation is poorly documented, although systematic autopsies of stillborns or neonates reveal a number of cases with vascular thromboses that have occurred in utero. Fetal thrombopathy with cerebral and multivisceral hemorrhages was observed by the author in a neonate without history of infection or blood incompatibility. At birth, CT scan revealed enlarged ventricles with irregular contours and severe parenchymal damage (Fig. 21.73a); at autopsy, there was a diffuse parenchymal hemorrhagic necrosis with disseminated venous thromboses (Fig. 21.73b).

Factor V [164] and factor X [165] deficiencies have been reported as causes of fetal cerebral hemorrhage.

Placental Anomalies

One must stress the importance of examining the placenta and cord, at least when the infant presents difficulties at birth. In one case seen by the author [138], severe placental calcification was associated with hypoxic-ischemic brain damage. CT scanning revealed diffuse hypodensities compatible with the diagnosis of hydranencephaly (Fig. 21.74a). The infant died on the second day of life. On postmortem examination, the brain was edematous but grossly normal (Fig. 21.74b). However, histologic study revealed a near-total loss of neurons (Fig. 21.74c). In the event of longer survival, such an infant may develop hydranencephaly.

Unknown Causes

Finally, an increasing number of cases of fetal intracranial injuries, without apparent cause, have been diagnosed recently by ultrasonography and/or described on post-mortem examination [166–173].

SPECIFIC FORMS OF FETAL BRAIN DAMAGE: PORENCEPHALY-SCHIZENCEPHALY, HYDRANENCEPHALY, AND POLYMICROGYRIA

Porencephaly

There has been much confusion about the definition of the term "porencephaly," which refers to a congenital cerebral defect with communication between the ventricle and the

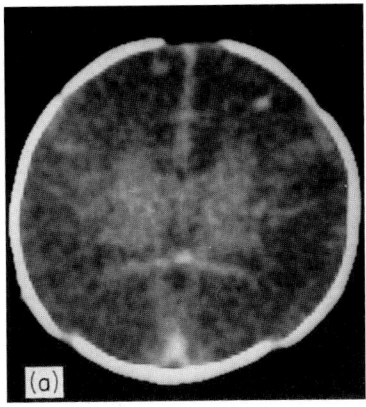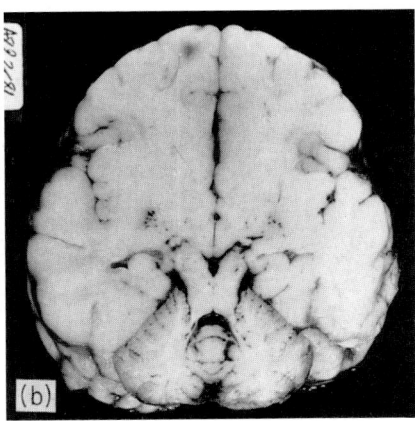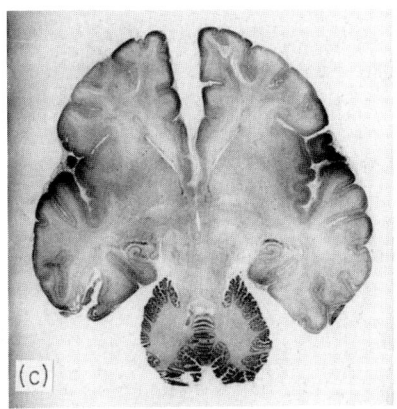

FIGURE 21.74.   *Chronic hypoxia associated with calcification of the placenta: (a) CT scan at 2 days shows hydranencephaly (?); (b) edematous but grossly normal brain; (c) near-total loss of neurons.*

surface of the brain. The defect usually involves the pre- and postcentral gyri and the insula. The surface of the porus is covered by the pia-arachnoid membrane, which is often torn during manipulations. Porencephaly can be unilateral or bilateral, symmetric or asymmetric. Bilateral and symmetric cavitations are rare and are known as "basket brain" (Fig. 21.75). The septum pellucidum is always absent, and its association with porencephaly has been described as a distinct syndrome [174]. Microscopic examination shows polymicrogyric cortex at the margin of the cavities [175–179] and in the contralateral hemisphere.

Schizencephaly

The term "schizencephaly" or "cleft brain" was introduced by Yakovlev and Wadsworth [180] to described morphologic anomalies, usually bilateral, without cavitation (fused lips) or with cavitation (lips separated), and characterized by cortical dysplasia. The form with fused lips is extremely rare. The form with lips separated is synonymous with porencephaly. Both types are said to be as a consequence of early vascular injury in utero, although a few familial cases have been reported.

Hydranencephaly

Hydranencephaly is the most severe form of brain destruction that can occur in utero as a result of hypoxic-ischemic infarction [155], although a few familial cases have been reported due to proliferative vasculopathy [181]. The skull is filled with CSF maintained by the pia-arachnoid membrane. The remaining brain consists of basal ganglia and thalami, brainstem, and cerebellum (Fig. 21.76). In less dramatic forms, which occur later in fetal life, the basal parts of the frontal, temporal, and occipital lobes are relatively preserved (see section on twins).

Polymicrogyria

Polymicrogyria as a primary anomaly occurs in association with complex brain malformations, in exencephaly, micrencephaly, thanatophoric dwarfism, and Zellweger syndrome (see Part II). A second form of polymicrogyria develops later in fetal life, resulting from hypoxic-ischemic postmigratory laminar necrosis. However, the time of occurrence of this abnormal cortical pattern is still debated [158, 159, 160].

KERNICTERUS (BILIRUBIN ENCEPHALOPATHY)

Bile pigment in the basal ganglia was known in the nineteenth century, but the term "kernicterus" was coined in

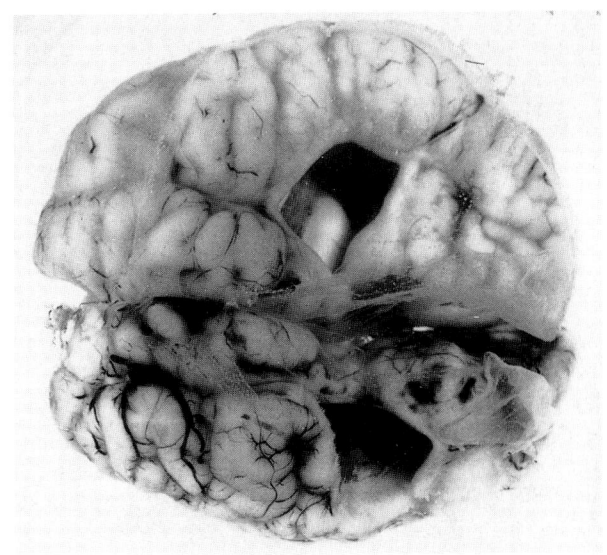

FIGURE 21.75.   *Basket brain with two symmetric frontoparietal cavities.*

1903 by Schmorl [182]. Since then, kernicterus (KI), as a clinicopathologic entity, has been described extensively in a number of articles and monographs [183, 184], but today it is a rather historical disease.

Bilirubin Metabolism

In the newborn infant, 75% of bilirubin is derived from the normal destruction of circulating erythrocytes in the liver and spleen. Bilirubin, bound to albumin, is conjugated in the liver with glucuronic acid by the enzyme uridine diphosphoglucuronyl transferase, passes in the bile to the intestine, and is eliminated. In the neonate, the bilirubin-glucuroconjugation enzyme in the liver is low, and jaundice results mainly from incapacity of the liver to conjugate an overload of bilirubin. This may be the case after abnormal hemolysis due to various pathologic conditions, such as blood incompatibilities, resorption of hematomas, and sepsis, or from impaired function of the liver after administration of certain drugs, necrosis of the parenchyma, and deficiency of glucose-6-phosphate dehydrogenase, or to a lesser degree from an increased intestinal reabsorption of bilirubin.

In full-term infants, a free bilirubin level in the blood of less than 20 mg/100 mL is considered to be a safe threshold; however, in asphyxiated and acidotic preterm infants and in cases of bacterial meningoencephalitis, KI is observed with levels as low as 10 to 12 mg/100 mL. Free bilirubin, a lipid-soluble compound with free access to the brain tissue, is thought to be the toxic fraction to neurons, but it is not yet known why certain neurons within particular structures fix the pigment and are damaged.

Since the introduction of anti-D prophylactic measures, the incidence of KI due to blood incompatibility has decreased significantly. In low-birth-weight infants, the incidence of KI varied from 6.4% [185] to absence [186] at postmortem examinations in some series.

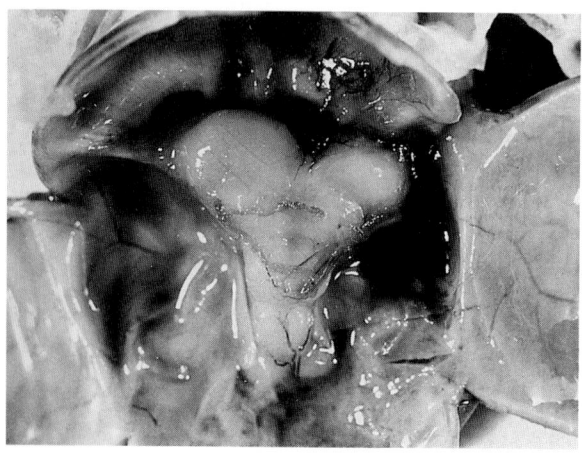

FIGURE 21.76.   *Hydranencephaly; thalami and brainstem are the only remnant structures at the base of the skull.*

Pathologic Features

In KI, the brightest coloration was first described in infants with hemolytic disease. At autopsy, the CSF and meninges, vermis, flocculus, and parahippocampal gyrus might have a yellow tinge. On sections of the brain, most of the deep gray nuclei were stained yellow, symmetrically, including the corpus luysi, globus pallidus, and lateral nuclei of the thalamus. The lateral geniculate bodies and the putamina were affected less frequently. In the brainstem, all the cranial nerve nuclei, nucleus gracilis, and cuneatus could be affected together with the anterior horn cells of the spinal cord. Rarely, the pigment diffused to other structures, such as the hippocampus, fornix, mamillary bodies, and habenula. The ependyma and choroid plexuses could also be pigmented. In a few cases, sensorimotor, insular, and visual cortices were also yellow, but no lesions were detected on microscopic study [187].

In preterm infants, the color is much less intense and is restricted to a smaller number of structures, such as third nerve nuclei, lateral nuclei of the thalamus, and, less frequently, nucleus subthalamicus and other cranial nerve nuclei. Therefore, KI can easily be missed.

On histologic preparations, when KI is severe, only part of the pigment is dissolved during the course of paraffin wax or celloidin processing; a whole area or some neurons may remain yellow; with light microscopy, most neurons are pyknotic and fusiform, with loss of Nissl bodies, while others look normal. Biochemical studies and electron microscopy observations have shown alterations of mitochondria, impaired oxidative phosphorylation processes, and, finally, cell loss [188, 189].

Kernicterus corresponds to the acute phase of bilirubin encephalopathy, and the yellow tinge of the nuclei disappears by the end of the first postnatal week. The neurologic signs consist of hypertonia, particularly of the neck and extensor muscles of the back, attacks of opisthotonos with extension and adduction of lower limbs, flexion of the elbows, or slow athetoid movements of the upper extremities. An abnormality of gaze, with the eyes looking downward, is known as the setting sun sign. This form of the disease has practically disappeared, but the problem remains unsolved in the susceptible low-birth-weight infant, and the diagnosis of bilirubin encephalopathy is rarely certain in the neonatal period.

ACKNOWLEDGMENTS

The author thanks Professors J.P. Relier and J. Vignaud for permission to use the ultrasound and CT scan documents.

REFERENCES: FETAL AND PERINATAL BRAIN DAMAGE

1. Larroche JC. *Developmental Pathology of the Neonate.* Amsterdam: Elsevier, 1977, p. 525.

2. Larroche JC. Perinatal brain damage. In: Hume Adams J, Corsellis JAN, Buchen LW, eds. *Greenfield's Neuropathology*. 4th ed. London: Edward Arnold, 1984, pp. 451–89.

3. Volpe JJ, Manica JP, Land VJ, Coxe WS. Neonatal subdural hematoma associated with severe hemophilia. *Am J Pediatr* 1976; 88:1023–5.

4. Friede RL. *Developmental Neuropathology*. Vienna: Springer-Verlag, 1975.

5. Rorke LB. *Pathology of Perinatal Brain Injury*. New York: Raven, 1982.

6. Larroche JC. Post-haemorrhagic hydrocephalus in infancy. Anatomical study. *Biol Neonat* 1972; 20:287–99.

7. Friede RL. Subpial hemorrhage in the newborn. *J Neuropathol Exp Neurol* 1972; 31:548–56.

8. Volpe JJ. *Neurology of the Newborn*. 2nd ed. Philadelphia: WB Saunders, 1987, p. 716.

9. Kotagal S, Toce S, Kotagal P, Archer C. Symmetrical bithalamic and striatal hemorrhage following perinatal hypoxia in a term infant. *J Comp Assist Tom* 1983; 7:353–5.

10. Trounce JQ, Fawer LL, Punt J, et al. Primary thalamic haemorrhage in the newborn: a new clinical entity. *Lancet* 1985; i:190–2.

11. de Vries L, Smet G, Goesmans N, et al. Unilateral thalamic haemorrhage in the pre-term and full-term newborn. *Neuropediatrics* 1992; 23:153–6.

12. Schwartz P. *Birth Injury of the Newborn: Morphology, Pathogenesis, Clinical Pathology and Prevention*. New York: Hafner, 1961.

13. Larroche JC. Les hémorragies cérébrales intraventriculaires chez le prématuré. I Anatomie et physiopathologie. *Biol Neonat* 1964; 7:26–56.

14. Dekaban A. Cerebral birth injury. Pathology of hemorrhagic lesions. *Ment Retard* 1962; 39:196–227.

15. Flodmark O, Becker LE, Harwood-Nash DC, et al. Correlation between computed tomography and autopsy in premature and full-term neonates that have suffered perinatal asphyxia, *Radiology* 1980; 137:93–103.

16. Couture A, Cadier L. *Echographie cérébrale par voie transfontanellaire*. Paris: Vigot, 1983.

17. Levene MI, Williams JL, Fawer IL. Ultrasound of the infant brain. In: *Clinics in Developmental Medicine*. No. 92. Oxford: Blackwell Scientific, 1985, p. 148.

18. Larroche JC. The fine structure of the matrix capillaries in human embryos and young fetuses. In: *The Second Ross Conference on Intraventricular Hemorrhage, Washington, DC*. Columbus, OH: Ross Laboratories, 1982, pp. 1–5.

19. Povlishock JT, Martinez AJ, Moosy J. The fine structure of blood vessels of the telencephalic germinal matrix in the human fetus. *Am J Anat* 1977; 149:439–52.

20. Takashima S, Tanaka K. Microangiography and vascular permeability of the subependymal matrix in the premature infant. *Can J Neurol Sci* 1978; 5:45–50.

21. Pasternak JF, Groothius DR, Fischer JM, Fischer DP. Regional cerebral blood flow in the newborn beagle pup: the germinal matrix is a "low-flow" structure. *Pediatr Res* 1982; 16:499–503.

22. Goldstein GW. Pathogenesis of brain edema and hemorrhage: role of the brain capillary. *Pediatrics* 1979; 64:357–60.

23. Towbin A. Cerebral intraventricular hemorrhage: subependymal matrix infarction in the fetus and premature newborn. *Am J Pathol* 1968; 52:121–40.

24. Tsiantos A, Victorin L, Relier JP, et al. Intracranial hemorrhage in the prematurely born infant: timing of clots and evaluation of clinical signs and symptoms. *J Pediatr* 1974; 85:854–9.

25. Funato M, Tamai H, Kodaka FW, *et al.* The moment of intraventricular hemorrhage. *Brain Dev* 1988; 10:325–7.

26. Fedrick J, Butler NR. Certain causes of neonatal death: II. Intraventricular haemorrhage. *Biol Neonat* 1970; 15:257–90.

27. Leech RW, Kohnen P. Subependymal and intraventricular hemorrhage in the newborn. *Am J Pathol* 1974; 77:465–76.

28. Moriette G, Relier JP, Larroche JC. Les hémorragies intraventriculaires au cours de la maladie des membranes hyalines. *Arch Fr Pédiatr* 1977; 34:492–504.

29. Thorburn JR, Lipscomb AP, Stewart AL, Reynolds EOR, Hope PL. Timing and antecedents of periventricular haemorrhage and cerebral atrophy in very preterm infants. *Early Hum Dev* 1982; 7:221–38.

30. Vert P, Monin P, Sibout M. Intracranial venous pressure in newborns: variations in physiologic state and in neurologic and respiratory disorders. In: Stern L, ed. *Intensive Care in the Newborn*. New York: Masson, 1975, pp. 185–96.

31. Reynolds ML, Evans CAN, Reynolds ED, et al. Intracranial hemorrhage in the preterm sheep foetus. *Early Hum Dev* 1979; 3:163–86.

32. Hambleton G, Wigglesworth JS. Origin of intraventricular haemorrhage in the preterm infant. *Arch Dis Child* 1976; 51:651–9.

33. Lou HC, Lassen NA, Friis-Hansen B. Impaired autoregulation of cerebral blood flow in the distressed newborn infant. *J Pediatr* 1979; 94:118–21.

34. Gilles F, Price R, Kevy S, Berenberg W. Fibrinolytic activity in the ganglionic eminence of the premature human brain. *Biol Neonat* 1971; 18:426–32.

35. Wigglesworth JS, Pape KE. An integrated model for haemorrhage and ischaemic lesions in the newborn brain. *Early Hum Dev* 1978; 2:179–99.

36. Pape KE, Wigglesworth JS. *Haemorrhage, Ischaemia and the Perinatal Brain*. London: Heinemann, 1979.

37. Goddard J, Lewis RM, Alcala H, Zeller RS. Intraventricular hemorrhage. An animal model. *Biol Neonat* 1980; 37:39–52.

38. Volpe JJ, Pasternak JF, Allan WC, Ventricular dilatation preceding rapid head growth following neonatal intracranial hemorrhage. *Am J Dis Child* 1977; 131:1212–15.

39. Papile LA, Burstein J, Burstein R, Koffler H. Incidence and evolution of subependymal and intraventricular hemorrhage: a study of infants with birth weight less than 1000 g. *J Pediatr* 1978; 92:529–34.

40. Levene M. Incidence of intraventricular hemorrhage. In: Levene MI, Lilford RJ, eds. *Fetal and Neonatal Neurology and Neurosurgery*. 2nd ed. London: Churchill Livingstone, 1997, p. 730.

41. Larroche JC. Subependymal pseudocysts in the newborn. *Biol Neonat* 1972; 21:170–83.

42. Takashima S, Armstrong D, Becker LE. Old subependymal necrosis and hemorrhage in the prematurely born infant. *Brain Dev* 1979; 1:299–304.

43. Donn SM, Bowerrnan RA. Neonatal posthemorrhagic porencephaly. Ultrasonographic features. *Am J Dis Child* 1982; 136:707–9.

44. Grant EG, Kerner M, Schellinger D, et al. Evolution of porencephalic cysts from intraparenchymal hemorrhage in neonates: sonographic evidence. *Am J Radiol* 1982; 3:47–50.

45. McMenamin JB, Shakelford GD, Volpe JJ. Outcome of neonatal intraventricular hemorrhage with periventricular echodense lesions. *Ann Neurol* 1984; 15:285–90.

46. Stewart AL. Early prediction of neurological outcome when the very preterm infant is discharged from the intensive care unit. *Ann Pediatr* 1985; 32:27–38.

47. Lacey DJ, Terplan K. Intraventricular hemorrhage in full term neonates. *Dev Med Child Neurol* 1982; 24:332–7.

48. Bergman J, Balier RE, Barmada MA, et al. Intracerebral hemorrhage in the fulfilterm neonatal infant. *Pediatrics* 1985; 75:488–96.

49. Grunnet ML, Shields WD. Cerebellar hemorrhage in the premature infant. *J Pediatr* 1976; 88:605–8.

50. Martin R, Roessmann U, Fanaroff A. Massive intracerebellar hemorrhage in low-birth-weight infants. *J Pediatr* 1976; 89:290–3.

51. Rom S, Serfontein GL, Humphreys RP. Intracerebellar hematoma in the neonate. *J Pediatr* 1978; 93:486–8.

52. Perlman JM, Nelson JS, McAlister WH, Volpe JJ. Intracerebellar hemorrhage in a premature newborn: diagnosis by real-time ultrasound and correlation with autopsy findings. *Pediatrics* 1983; 71:159–62.

53. Reeder JD, Setzer ES, Kande JV. Ultrasonic detection of perinatal intracerebellar hemorrhage. *Pediatrics* 1982; 70:385–6.

54. Amiel-Tison C. Cerebral damage in fullterm newborn; aetiological factors, neonatal status and long term follow-up. *Biol Neonat* 1969; 14:234–50.

55. Brown JK, Purvis RJ, Forfar JO, Cockburn F. Neurological aspects of perinatal asphyxia. *Dev Med Child Neurol* 1974; 16:567–80.

56. Fenichel GM. Hypoxic-ischemic encephalopathy in the newborn. *Arch Neurol* 1983; 40:261–6.

57. Sarnat HB, Sarnat MS. Neonatal encephalopathy following fetal distress. A clinical and electroencephalographic study. *Arch Neurol* 1975; 33:696–705.

58. Larroche JC. Nécrose cérébrale massive chez le nouveau-né. Ses rapports avec la maturation; son expression clinique et bioélectrique. *Biol Neonat* 1968; 13:340–60.

59. Terplan KL. Histopathologic brain changes in 1152 cases of the perinatal and early infancy period. *Biol Neonat* 1967; 11:348–66.

60. Amiel-Tison C, Stewart A. *The newborn infant. One brain for life*. Paris: INSERM, Doin, 1994.

61. Dreyfus-Brisac C, Monod N. Electroclinical studies of status epilepticus and convulsions in the newborn. In: Kellaway P, Petersen I, eds. *Neurologic and Electroencephalographic Correlative Studies in Infancy*. New York: Grune & Stratton, 1964.

62. O'Brien MJ, Ash JM, Gilday DL. Radionuclide brain scanning in perinatal hypoxia/ischemia. *Dev Med Child Neurol* 1979; 21:161–73.

63. Volpe JJ, Herscovitch P, Perlman JM, Kreusser KL, Raichle M. Positron emission tomography in the asphyxiated term newborn: parasagittal impairment of cerebral blood flow. *Ann Neurol* 1985; 17:187–96.

64. Courville CB. Etiology and pathogenesis of laminar cortical necrosis. *Arch Neurol Psychol* 1958; 79:17–30.

65. Hopkins I, Farkas-Bargeton E, Larroche JC. Neonatal neuronal necrosis: its relationship to the distribution and maturation of oxidative enzymes of newborn cerebral and cerebellar cortex. *Early Hum Dev* 1980; 4:51–60.

66. Ranck JB, Windle WF. Brain damage in the monkey *Macaca mulatta* by asphyxia neonatorum. *Exp Neurol* 1959; 1:130–54.

67. Leech RW, Alvord EC. Anoxic-ischemic encephalopathy in the human neonatal period. *Arch Neurol* 1977; 34:109–13.

68. Schneider H, Ballowitz L, Schachinger H, Hanefeld F, Drözus JU. Anoxic encephalopathy with predominant involvement of basal ganglia, brainstem and spinal cord in the perinatal period. *Acta Neuropathol* 1975; 33:287–98.

69. Friede RL. Ponto-subicular lesions in perinatal anoxia. *Arch Pathol (Chicago)* 1972; 94:343–54.

70. Ahdab-Barmada M, Moosy J, Painter M. Pontosubicular necrosis and hyperoxemia. *Pediatrics* 1980; 66:840–7.

71. Brierly JB, Meldrum BS. *Brain Hypoxia*. London: Heinemann, 1971.

72. Duffy ThE, Vannuci RC. Metabolic aspects of cerebral anoxia in the fetus and the newborn. In: Berenberg SR, ed. *Brain: Fetal and Infant*. The Hague: Martinus Nijhoff, 1977, pp. 316–23.

73. Myers RE, de Courten Myers GM, Wagner KR. Effect of hypoxia on fetal brain. In: Beard RW, Nathanielsz PW, eds. *Fetal Physiology and Medicine*. 2nd ed. New York: M. Dekker, 1984, pp. 419–58.

74. McDonald JW, Johnston MV. Physiological and pathological roles of excitatory amino acids during central nervous system development. *Brain Res Rev* 1990; 15:41–70.

75. Delivoria-Papadopoulos M, Cortey A. Mécanismes neuroprotecteurs dans les lésions cérébrales hypoxiques du nouveau-né. In: Relier JP, ed. *Progrés en Néonatologie Karger* 1994; 14:39–45.

76. Kulakowski S, Larroche JCl. Cranial computerized tomography in cerebral palsy. An attempt at anatomoclinical and radiological correlations. *Neuropediatrics* 1980; 11:339–53.

77. Courville CB. Pathogenesis of nodular atrophy of the cerebral cortex. A common cortical change found in cases of cerebral palsy. *Arch Pediatr* 1960; 77:101–29.

78. Norman RM. Atrophic sclerosis of the cerebral cortex associated with birth injury. *Arch Dis Child* 1944; 19:111–21.

79. Malamud N. Status marmoratus: a form of cerebral palsy following either birth injury or inflammation of the central nervous system. *J Pediatr* 1950; 37:610–19.

80. Norman RM. Etat marbré of the corpus striatum following birth injury. *J Neurol Neurosurg Psychiatr* 1947; 10:12–25.

81. Borit A, Hemdon RM. The fine structure of plaques fibromyéliniques in ulegyria and in status marmoratus. *Acta Neuropathol* 1970; 14:304–31.

82. Friede RL, Schachenmayr W. Early stages of status marmoratus. *Acta Neuropathol* 1977; 38:123–7.

83. Virchow R. Zur pathologischen anatomie des gehirns. I Congenitale encephalitis und myelitis. *Virch Arch Pathol Anat* 1867; 38:129–42.

84. Parrot J. Etude sur le ramollissement de l'encéphale chez le nouveau-né. *Arch Physiol Norm Pathol (Paris)* 1873; 5:59–73; 176–95; 283–303.

85. Parrot J. *Clinique du nouveau-né. L'athrepsie.* Paris: Masson, 1877.

86. Banker BQ, Larroche JCl. Periventricular leukomalacia of infancy: a form of neonatal anoxic encephalopathy. *Arch Neurol* 1962; 7:386–410.

87. Little W. The influence of abnormal parturition, difficult labours, premature birth and asphyxia neonatorum on the mental and physical condition of the child, especially in relation to deformities. *Trans Obstet Soc London* 1861; 3:293–344.

88. Armstrong D, Norman HG. Periventricular leucomalacia in neonates. Complication and sequelae. *Arch Dis Child* 1974; 49:367–75.

89. Shuman RM, Selednik LJ. Periventricular leukomalacia. A one year autopsy study. *Arch Neurol* 1980; 37:231–5.

90. de Reuck J, Chattha AS, Richardson EP. Pathogenesis and evolution of periventricular leukomalacia in infancy. *Arch Neurol* 1972; 27:229–36.

91. van den Bergh R, van der Eecken H. Anatomy and embryology of cerebral circulation. In: Luyendijk W, ed. *Cerebral Circulation. Progress in Brain Research.* vol. 30. Amsterdam: Elsevier, 1968, pp. 1–25.

92. van den Bergh R. The periventricular intracerebral blood supply. In: Meyer JS, Lechner H, Eichhom O, eds. *Research on the Cerebral Circulation.* Springfield IL: Charles Thomas, 1969, pp. 52–65.

93. Kuban KCK, Gilles FH. Human telencephalic angiogenesis. *Ann Neurol* 1985; 17:539–48.

94. Moody DM, Bell MA, Challa VR. Anatomic features of the cerebral vascular pattern that predict vulnerability to perfusion or oxygenation deficiency. *Am J Neuroradiol* 1990; 11:431–9.

95. Nelson MD, Gonzalez-Gomez I, Gilles FH. The search for human telencephalic ventriculofugal arteries. *Am J Neuroradiol* 1991; 12:215–22.

96. Takashima S, Tanaka K. Development of cerebrovascular architecture and its relationship to periventricular leukomalacia. *Arch Neurol* 1978; 35:11–16.

97. Abramowitz A. The pathogenesis of experimental periventricular necrosis and its possible relationship to the periventricular leucomalacia of birth trauma. *J Neurol Neurosurg Psychiatr* 1964; 27:85–95.

98. Young RSK, Hernandez MJ, Yagel SK. Selective reduction of blood flow to white matter during hypotension in newborn dogs: a possible mechanism of periventricular leukomalacia. *Ann Neurol* 1981; 12:445–8.

99. Ment LR, Stewart WB, Duncan CC, et al. Beagle puppy model of perinatal cerebral infarction: acute changes in cerebral blood flow and metabolism during hemorrhagic hypotension. *J Neurosurg* 1985; 63:441–7.

100. Gilles FH, Averill DR, Kerr CS. Neonatal endotoxin encephalopathy. *Ann Neurol* 1977; 2:49–56.

101. Adinolfi M. Infectious diseases in pregnancy. Cytokines and neurological impairment: an hypothesis. *Dev Med Child Neurol* 1993; 35:549–58.

102. Leviton A. Preterm birth and cerebral palsy: is tumor necrosis factor the missing link? *Dev Med Child Neurol* 1993; 35:549–58.

103. Foix CH, Bariety M, Baruch H, Marie J. A propos d'un nouveau cas de sclérose intracérébrale centro-lobaire et symétrique. *Rev Neurol* 1926; 33:930–42.

104. Marie J, Lyon G, Bargeton E. La sclérose cérébrale centro-lobaire. A propos de l'étude anatomo-clinique d'un cas de diplégie spasmodique congénitale. (Syndrome de Little). *Presse Méd* 1959; 60:2286–9.

105. Larroche JC, Amiel C, Relier JP, Korn G. Leucomalacie et avenir cérébral en relation avec les soins intensifs néonataux. *J Anesth* 1975; 16:171–5.

106. Crome L. Multilocular cystic encephalopathy of infants. *J Neurosurg Psychiatr (London)* 1958; 21:146–52.

107. Levene MI, Wigglesworth JS, Dubowitz V. Haemorrhagic periventricular leukomalacia in the neonate: a real time ultrasound study. *Pediatrics* 1983; 71:794–7.

108. Delaporte B, Cherinat C, Sidibe M. Aspect échographique des lésions ischémiques et/ou anoxiques non hémorragiques du nouveau-né prematuré. *Arch Fr Pédiatr* 1984; 41:222–3.

109. Nwaesei CG, Pape KE, Martin DJ, Becker LE, Fitz CR. Periventricular infarction diagnosed by ultrasound. A post mortem correlation. *J Pediatr* 1984; 105:106–10.

110. Rushton DI, Preston PR, Durbin GM. Structure and evolution of echo dense lesions in the neonatal brain. *Arch Dis Child* 1985; 60:798–808.

111. Fawer CL, Calame A, Parentes E, Anderegg A. Periventricular leukomalacia: a correlation study between real-time ultrasound and autopsy findings. *Neuroradiology* 1985; 27:292–300.

112. de Vries LS, Wigglesworth JS, Regeg R, Dubowitz LMS. Evolution of periventricular leukomalacia during the neonatal period and infancy: correlation of imaging and postmortem findings. *Early Hum Dev* 1988; 17:205–19.

113. de Vries LS, Eken P, Dubowitz LMS. The spectrum of leukomalacia using cranial ultrasound. *Behav Brain Res* 1992; 49:1–6.

114. Schouman-Claeys E, Henry-Feugeas MC, Roset F, et al. Periventricular leukomalacia: correlation between MR imaging and autopsy findings during the first 2 months of life. *Radiology* 1993; 189:59–64.

115. Dubowitz LMS, Bydder GM, Mushin J. Developmental sequence of periventricular leukomalacia. *Arch Dis Child* 1985; 60:319–55.

116. de Vries LS, Eken P, Groenendaal F, Haastert IC, van Meiners LC. Correlation between the degree of periventricular leukomalacia diagnosed using cranial ultrasound and MRI later in life in children with cerebral palsy. *Neuropediatrics* 1993; 24:263–8.

117. Gilles FH, Averill DR, Kerr CS. Neonatal endotoxine encephalopathy. *Ann Neurol* 1977; 2:49–56.

118. Takashima S, Armstrong DL, Becker LE. Subcortical leukomalacia; relationship to development of the cerebral sulcus and its vascular supply *Arch Neurol* 1978; 35:470–2.

119. Smith JF. *Pediatric Neuropathology*. New York: McGraw-Hill, 1974.

120. Trounce JQ, Levene MI. Diagnosis and outcome of subcortical cystic leucomalacia. *Arch Dis Child* 1985; 60:1041–4.

121. Larroche JC, Amiel C. Thrombose de l'artère Sylvienne à la période néonatale. Etude anatomique et discussion pathogénique des hémiplégies dites congénitales. *Arch Fr Pédiatr* 1966; 23:257–74.

122. Wiklund LM, Uvebrant P, Flodmark O. Computed tomography as an adjunct in etiological analysis of hemiplegic cerebral palsy. I. Children born preterm. *Neuropediatrics* 1990; 22:121–8.

123. Amato M, Hüppi P, Herschkowitz N, Huber P. Prenatal stroke suggested by intrauterine ultrasound and confirmed by magnetic resonance imaging. *Neuropediatrics* 1991; 22:100–2.

124. Clark RM, Linell EA. Case report: prenatal occlusion of the internal carotid artery. *J Neurol Neurosurg Psychiatr* 1954; 17:295–7.

125. Ruff RL, Shaw CM, Beckwith JB, Iozzo RV. Cerebral infarction complicating umbilical catheterization. *Ann Neurol* 1979; 6:85–8.

126. Pellicer A, Cabanas F, Garcia-Alix A, Perz-Higueras A, Quero J. Stroke in neonates with cardiac right to left shunt. *Brain Dev* 1992; 14:381–5.

127. Barmada MA, Moosy J. Cerebral infarcts with arterial occlusion in neonates. *Ann Neurol* 1979; 6:495–502.

128. Courville CB. Antenatal and perinatal circulatory disorders as a cause of cerebral damage in early life. *J Neuropath Exp Neurol* 1959; 18:115–39.

129. Rizzuto N, Martin L. Le problème de l'encéphalopathie foetale kystique survenant au cours du deuxième tiers de la grossesse. *Biol Neonat* 1967; 11:115–27.

130. Gallaway PG, Roessmann U. Neuronal karyorrhexis in Sommer's sector in a 22-week stillborn. *Acta Neuropathol* 1986; 70:343–4.

131. Erasmus C, Blackwood W, Wilson J. Infantile multicystic encephalomalacia after maternal bee sting anaphylaxis during pregnancy. *Arch Dis Child* 1982; 57:785–7.

132. Goodlin RC, Heidrick WP, Papenfuss HL, Kubitz RL. Fetal malformations associated with maternal hypoxia. *Am Obstet Gynecol* 1984; 149:228–9.

133. Levene MI. *Neonatal Neurology*. Edinburgh: Churchill Livingstone, 1987.

134. Robinson MJ, Cameron MD, Smoth MF, Ayers AB. Fetal subdural haemorrhage presenting as hydrocephalus. *Br Med J* 1980; 281:35.

135. Grylack L. Prenatal sonographic diagnosis of cephalohematoma due to prelabor trauma. *Pediatr Radiol* 1982; 12:145–7.

136. Coignet J, Palix C, Tommasi C, Raybaud C. Apport de la scanographie dans la souffrance cérébrale du nouveau-né. *Pediatrie* 1979; 34:787–97.

137. Fowler M, Brown C, Cabrera KF. Hydranencephaly in a baby after an aircraft accident to the mother: case report and autopsy. *Pathology* 1971; 3:21–30.

138. Larroche JC. Fetal encephalopathies of circulatory origin. *Biol Neonat* 1986; 50:61–74.

139. Myers RE. Maternal psychological stress and fetal asphyxia: a study in the monkey. *Am J Obstet Gynecol* 1975; 122:47–59.

140. Beau A, Neimann N, Pierson M. Du rôle de l'intoxication oxycarbonée gravidique dans la genèse des encéphalopathies néo-natales. A propos de trois observations. *Arch Fr Pédiatr* 1956; 13:130–43.

141. Bankl H, Jellinger K. Zentralnervose Schäden nach fetaler Kohlenoyd-vergiftung. *Beitr Pathol Anat* 1967; 135:350–76.

142. Gosseye S, Golaire MC, Larroche JCI. Cerebral, renal and splenic lesions due to fetal anoxia and their relationship to malformations. *Dev Med Child Neurol* 1982; 4:510–18.

143. Chasnoff IJ, Bussey ME, Savich R, Stack CM. Perinatal cerebral infarction and maternal cocaine abuse. *J Pediatr* 1986; 108:456–9.

144. Dixon SD, Bejar R. Echoencephalographic findings in neonates associated with maternal cocaine and methamphetamine use: incidence and clinical correlates. *J Pediatr* 1989; 115:770–8.

145. Bose C. Hydrops fetalis and in utero intracranial hemorrhage. *J Pediatr* 1978; 93:1023–4.

146. Jesurum CA, Levin GS, Sullivan WR, Stevens O. Intracranial hemorrhage in utero and thrombocytopenia. *J Pediatr* 1980; 97:695–6.

147. Zalneraitis EL, Young RSK, Krishnamoorthy KS. Intracranial hemorrhage in utero as a complication of isoimmune thrombocytopenia. *J Pediatr* 1979; 95:611–14.

148. Magny JF, Vial M, Bessis R, et al. Hémorragie cérébrale anténatale et incompatibilité plaquettaire foetomaternelle. *Arch Fr Pédiatr* 1984; 41:711–12.

149. de Vries LS, Connel J, Bydder GM, Dubowitz LMS. Recurrent intracranial haemorrhage in utero in an infant with alloimmune thrombocytopenia. Case report. *Br J Obstet Gynaecol* 1988; 95:299–302.

150. Khun MJ, Couch SM, Binstadt DH, et al. Prenatal recognition of central nervous system complication of alloimmune thrombocytopenia. *Comp Med Imag Graph* 1992; 16:137–42.

151. Choulot JJ, Leclerc MA, Saint-Martin J. Malformation cérébrale et jumeau survivant. *Arch Fr Pédiatr* 1982; 39:105–7.

152. Scymonowitz W, Preston H, Yu VYH. The surviving monozygotic twin. *Arch Dis Child* 1986; 61:454–8.

153. Larroche JC, Droullé P, Delezoide AL, Narcy F, Nessmann C. Brain damage in monozygous twins. *Biol Neonat* 1990; 57:261–78.

154. Hugues HE, Miskin M. Congenital microcephaly due to vascular disruption: in utero documentation. *Pediatrics* 1986; 78:85–7.

155. Yoshioka H, Kadomoto Y, Mino M, et al. Multicystic encephalomalacia in liveborn twin with a stillborn macerated co-twin. *J Pediatr* 1979; 95:798–800.

156. Moore CM, McAdams AJ, Sutherland J. Intrauterine disseminated intravascular coagulation: a syndrome of multiple pregnancy with a dead twin fetus. *J Pediatr* 1969; 74:523–8.

157. Choulot JJ, Fescharek R, Saint-Martin J. Mort d'un jumeau in utero et complications cérébrales chez le survivant. *Presse Méd* 1985; 14:1077–80.

158. Norman MG. Bilateral encephaloclastic lesions in a 26 week gestation fetus: effect on neuroblast migration. *J Can Sci Neurol* 1980; 7:191–4.

159. Barth PG, Van der Harten J. Parabiotic twin syndrome with topical isocortical disruption and gastroschisis. *Acta Neuropathol* 1985; 67:345–9.

160. Larroche JC, Girard N, Narcy F, Fallet C. Abnormal cortical plate (polymicrogyria), heterotopias and brain damage in monozygous twins. *Biol Neonat* 1994; 65:343–52.

161. Aicardi J, Goutières F. Multicystic encephalomalacia of infants and its relation to abnormal gestation and hydranencephaly. *J Neurol Sci* 1972; 15:357–73.

162. Enbom JA. Twin pregnancy with intrauterine death of one twin. *Am J Obstet Gynecol* 1985; 152:424–9.

163. Larroche JC, Aubry MC, Narcy F. Intrauterine brain damage in nonimmune hydrops fetalis. Biol Neonat 1992; 61:273–80.

164. Whitelaw A, Haines ME, Bolsover W, Harris E. Factor V deficiency and antenatal intraventricular haemorrhage. *Arch Dis Child* 1984; 59:997–9.

165. De Souza C, Clark T, Bradshaw A. Antenatal diagnosed subdural haemorrhage in congenital factor X deficiency. *Arch Dis Child* 1988; 63:1168–74.

166. Bondurant S, Boehm FH, Fleischer AC, Machin JE. Antepartum diagnosis of fetal intracranial hemorrhage by ultrasound. *Obstet Gynecol* 1984; 63:25–7.

167. Donn SM, Barr M, McLeary RD. Massive intracranial hemorrhage in utero: sonographic appearance and pathologic correlation. *Obstet Gynecol* 1984; 63:285–305.

168. Hill A, Rozdilsky B. Congenital hydrocephalus secondary to intra-uterine germinal matrix intraventricular haemorrhage. *Dev Med Child Neurol* 1984; 26:524–7.

169. Sims ME, Beckwitt-Turkel S, Halterman G, Paul RH. Brain injury and intrauterine death. *Am J Obstet Gynecol* 1985; 151:721–3.

170. Jackson JC, Blumhagen JD. Congenital hydrocephalus due to prenatal intracranial hemorrhage. *Pediatrics* 1983; 72: 344–6.

171. Ellis WG, Goetzman BW, Lindenberg JA. Neuropathologic documentation of prenatal brain damage. *Am J Dis Child* 1988; 142:858–66.

172. Bejar R, Wosniak P, Allard M, et al. Antenatal origin of neurologic damage in newborn infants. *Am J Obstet Gynecol* 1988; 159:357–63.

173. Squier M, Keeling JW. The incidence of prenatal brain injury. *Neuropathol Appl Neurobiol* 1991; 17:29–38.

174. Aicardi J, Goutières F. The syndrome of absence of the septum pellucidum with porencephalies and other developmental defects. *Neuropediatrics* 1981; 12:319–24.

175. Dekaban A. Large defects in cerebral hemispheres associated with cortical dysgenesis. *J Neuropath Exp Neurol* 1965; 24:512–30.

176. Lyon G, Robain O. Etude comparative des encéphalopathies circulatoires prénatales et para-natales (hydranencéphalies, porencéphalies et encéphalomalacies kystiques de la substance blanche). *Acta Neuropathol* 1967; 9:79–98.

177. Barth PG. Prenatal clastic encephalopathies. *Clin Neurol Neurosurg* 1984; 86:65–75.

178. Larroche JC. Fetal cerebral pathology of circulatory origin. In: Levene ML, Lilford J, eds. *Fetal and Neonatal Neurology and Neurosurgery*. 2nd ed. London: Churchill Livingstone, 1997, pp. 1028–150.

179. Larroche JC, Encha-Razavi F, de Vries LS. The central nervous system. In: Gilbert E, ed. *Potter Pathology of the Fetus and the Newborn*. Philadelphia: Mosby, 1997, pp. 321–33.

180. Yakovlev PI, Wadsworth RC. Schizencephalies. A study on the congenital clefts in the cerebral mantle. I. Clefts with fused lips. II. Clefts with hydrocephalus and lips separated. *J Neuropathol Exp Neurol* 1946; 5:116–30; 169–206.

181. Harper C, Hockey A. Proliferative vasculopathy and an hydranencephalic-hydrocephalic syndrome: a neuropathological study of two siblings. *Dev Med Child Neurol* 1983; 25:232–44.

182. Schmorl G. Zur Kenntnis des ikterus neonatorum. *Verh Dtsch Pathol Gesamte* 1903; 6:109–15.

183. Boreau T, Martin L, Larroche JC, Sautriot G. Etude clinique et anatomique de quelques cas d'ictère nucléaire du nouveau-né par maladie hémolytique à évolution rapidement mortelle. *Gynécol Obstét* 1964; 63:289–336.

184. Haymaker W, Margoles C, Pentschew A, et al. Patholoy of kernicterus and posticteric encephalopathy. Presentation of 87 cases with a consideration of pathogenesis and etiology. In: *Kernicterus and Its Importance in Cerebral Palsy*. Springfield, IL: Charles Thomas, 1961, pp. 21–228.

185. Gartner LM, Snyder RN, Chabon RS, Bernstein J. Kernicterus: high incidence in premature infants with low serum bilirubin concentration. *Pediatrics* 1970; 45:906–17.

186. Pearlman MA, Gartner LM, Lee KS, Morecki R, Horoupian DS. Absence of kernicterus in low birth weight infants; from 1971 through 1976: comparison with findings in 1966 and 67. *Pediatrics* 1978; 62:460–4.

187. Martin L, Larroche JC. Incidence et interprétation des lésions corticales dans l'ictère nucléaire. *Rev Neurol* 1964; 6:545–55.

188. Mustapha MG, Cowger ML, King TE. Effects of bilirubin on mitochondrial reactions. *J Biol Chem* 1969; 244:6403–14.

189. Schutta HS, Johnson L, Neville HE. Mitochondrial abnormalities in bilirubin encephalopathy. *J Neuropathol Exp Neurol* 1970; 29:296–305.

PART IV
MISCELLANEOUS CONDITIONS AFFECTING THE FETUS AND NEONATE

JONATHAN S. WIGGLESWORTH

This section will consider conditions that affect the CNS in the fetal and newborn periods and that are not fully covered elsewhere.

INFECTIVE LESIONS:
MENINGITIS AND MENINGOENCEPHALITIS

The effects of individual infectious agents on various organs, including the brain, are described in Chapter 17, and discussion here is limited to description of the major pathologic processes.

Viral Infections

The CNS is one of the major sites of damage by viruses in the perinatal period. Rubella virus, cytomegalovirus, herpesviruses I and II, coxsackievirus B, and echoviruses all cause significant perinatal brain lesions. Most perinatal brain damage from these viral agents results from intrauterine transplacental infection. More detailed descriptions of the pathologies of these lesions are given in Chapter 17, but some general points may be made here.

The main brain lesion caused by fetal viral infection is a meningoencephalitis. In rubella infection there tends to be a relatively low-grade inflammatory reaction with perivascular lymphocytic cuffing and glial proliferation affecting the cortex, but more specifically involving basal ganglia, midbrain, and brainstem. Disruption of capillaries is seen with mineralization in and around the capillary walls. Late stages may be associated with microcephaly [1]. As the cerebral lesions of rubella are due to vasculitis, it may be difficult sometimes on a histopathological basis to differentiate them from those of a pure anoxic-ischemic or hemorrhagic origin.

The meningoencephalitis of cytomegalovirus and herpesvirus infections is often of a far more acute and destructive nature, with extensive neuronal necrosis and ventriculitis. Microcephaly, hydrocephaly, or porencephaly may ensue.

Typical inclusions are sometimes present during the acute phase in cases of cytomegalovirus, and periventricular calcification may be observed at a late stage, although this is far less marked than in cases of toxoplasmosis.

Similar lesions are described in cases of infection with coxsackievirus and echovirus.

Protozoal Infection

Toxoplasmosis is a major cause of perinatal brain damage in some populations, particularly in the southern USA and Europe. The most severe lesions are associated with infection of a previously uninfected mother in early pregnancy (see Chap. 17).

Infants who die in the perinatal period often show extensive cerebral destruction involving the cortex, periventricular region, and basal ganglia. The pattern of discrete patches of yellow-white necrosis affecting these separate regions may be quite distinctive, as is the powdery calcification seen on microscopy (Fig. 21.77). A granulomatous meningoencephalitis is characteristic and trophozoites are seen either singly or in groups, with intracellular cysts usually recognizable at the peripheries of lesions or in uninvolved white matter (Fig. 21.78). Microcephaly, hydrocephaly, or porencephaly with dystrophic calcification is seen at a late stage.

Bacterial Infections

The most common form of cerebral pathology due to perinatal bacterial infection is meningitis, although a meningoencephalitis is characteristic of some organisms.

Bacterial Infection at Birth

Listeria monocytogenes most frequently infects the fetus in utero, and at stillbirth or early neonatal death there may be a fully developed meningitis or meningoencephalitis. The most characteristic feature of infection with this organism in the brain, as elsewhere, is the presence of multiple pinhead-sized white or gray granulomatous lesions with little surrounding flare. On microscopy, these lesions show necrosis and infiltration with mononuclear cells. A purulent meningitis may be seen in acute perinatal infections. In an untreated case, the gram-positive diphtheroid organisms are usually readily identified.

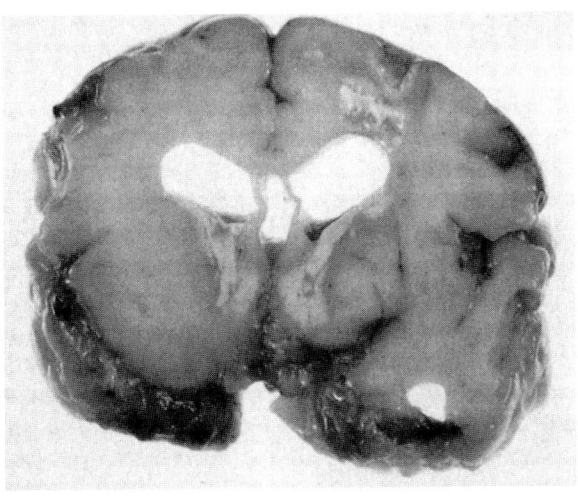

FIGURE 21.77. *Coronal section of the brain of a 34-week-gestation infant with congenital toxoplasmosis who died on the second day of life. Chalky white areas of necrosis involve the cortex and periventricular regions.*

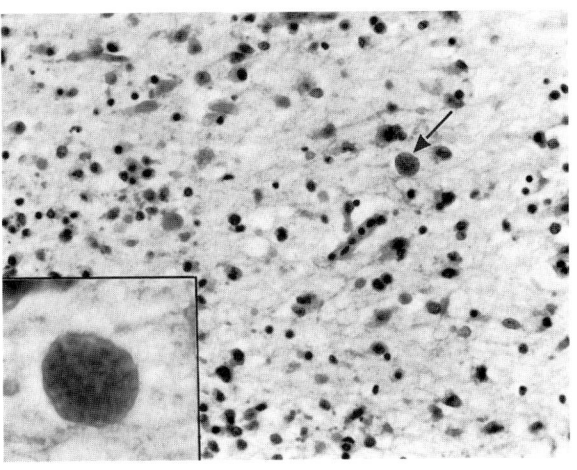

FIGURE 21.78. *Histological appearance at the margin of the necrotic cortex in the brain shown in Fig. 21.77. H&E, ×350. There is a non-specific inflammatory infiltrate and one* Toxoplasma *cyst (arrow). Inset shows the cyst. ×1300.*

Bacterial Infection of Neonatal Origin

Bacterial meningitis is characteristically a form of late-onset sepsis, developing some days or weeks after birth as a result of intrapartum or nosocomial infection. Meningitis is reported in about 0.4 per 1000 births in most series and may be due to any one of a wide variety of gram-positive and gram-negative organisms. Despite modern antibiotic regimens, there is still a mortality rate of 15–40% and a frequency of neurologic abnormality of up to 50% in survivors [2, 3].

The most comprehensive description of the pathology of neonatal meningitis is that given by Berman and Banker [4] based on a study of 25 cases at postmortem examination. The early stages of meningitis present as slight thickening and opacification of the meninges over the base of the brain, with a varying quantity of dull yellow to gray-green exudate in the developed stage. Exudate is particularly abundant in cases of meningitis due to *E coli* (Fig. 21.79). Exudate may fill the sulci and basal cisterns and is often most prominent over the inferior surface of the cerebellum, although

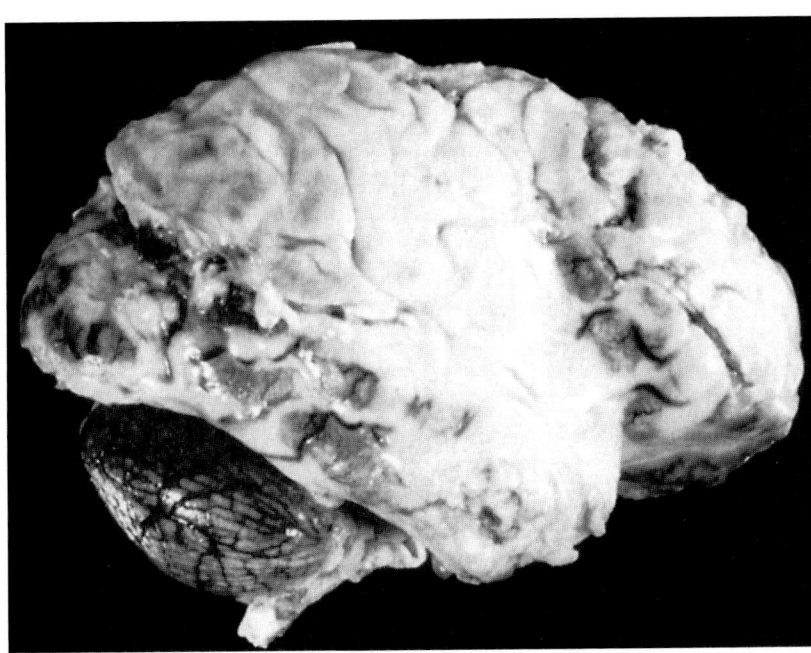

FIGURE 21.79. *Brain of a 37-week-gestation infant who suffered perinatal brain damage and died with* E. coli *meningitis at 13 weeks of age. Florid exudate covers the atrophic cerebral hemispheres.*

sometimes it may be seen predominantly over the convexity. Over the convexity, the exudate is closely related to the pial and subarachnoid vessels in the depths of the fissures.

In the acute stage of the disease, the underlying brain was found to be swollen and hyperemic and the lateral ventricles were often small, although herniation of cerebral or cerebellar tissue was not observed [4]. There is commonly an accompanying ventriculitis, particularly in gram-negative infections [5], with envelopment of the choroid plexus in purulent exudate in some instances. The acute stage of the infection (up to the end of the first week) is characterized by a polymorphonuclear exudate within a fibrin network. This gradually changes, as in other sites of acute bacterial infection, to a mononuclear cellular infiltrate in those infants who survive for 2 to 3 weeks. At several weeks after onset of infection, the pia-arachnoid may be thickened by fine fibrous trabeculations with thick collagenous strands radiating from the thickened adventitia of blood vessels. Glial bridges may narrow and partition the aqueduct of Sylvius and obliterate the rhomboid fossa in the fourth ventricle. Cerebral blood vessels characteristically show phlebitis and arteritis.

Acute obstructive hydrocephalus may ensue if cellular debris or organizing granulation tissue occludes the aqueduct or the foramina of the fourth ventricle.

Communicating hydrocephalus may also be seen as a sequel to impaired resorption of CSF by a chronic inflammatory reaction.

Parenchymal changes include a glial reaction in areas directly subjacent to the inflammatory exudate, a diffuse encephalopathy, and cerebral infarction resulting from the vascular changes.

The encephalopathy described in all cases studied by Berman and Banker [4] is of the pattern seen in anoxic-ischemic injury with karyorrhexis and loss of nerve cells involving the deeper layers of the cortex, Sommer's sector of the hippocampus, and, less often, the basal ganglia, thalamus, and dentate nuclei. In preterm infants, PVL frequently is present in addition.

The thrombophlebitis may lead to widespread thrombosis of cerebral veins with resultant venous infarction. The cerebral vein thrombosis can sometimes spread to intracranial sinuses. Other complications include brain abscess [6] and otis interna. Given the mixture of sclerotic and infarctive lesions, it is not surprising that survivors may show cystic changes within the cerebral parenchyma [7].

Hemorrhagic Meningoencephalitis

Hemorrhagic and necrotic features predominate in some cases of gram-negative bacterial infection, usually in association with venous thrombosis [8, 9]. Organisms involved have included *Pseudomonas aeruginosa*, *Proteus*, and *Serratia marcescens*. There may be no surface exudate, but the brain is swollen and edematous, with purplish discoloration

or areas of obvious hemorrhagic necrosis. Microscopy confirms the presence of extensive necrosis with masses of organisms around the vessels diffusely infiltrating the cerebral substance.

LYSOSOMAL ENZYME DEFICIENCIES

Most of these conditions present after the neonatal period, although a few, such as Gaucher disease, sialidosis, and mucopolysaccharidosis VII, are sometimes manifested as nonimmunologic hydrops at birth (see Chap. 14) or may present at birth with dysmorphic facial features, hepatosplenomegaly, and failure to thrive (e.g., GM$_1$ gangliosidosis).

An increasing number of such cases may now present as fetuses to the pathologist following prenatal diagnosis and termination.

Macroscopic brain abnormalities are not features of such cases, but histologic and ultrastructural evidence of abnormal brain storage has been described in a variety of lysosomal disorders.

Thus, in Niemann-Pick disease type A, there may be ballooning of neurons and glia with gliosis and storage cells in the white matter by term [10]. Electron microscopy at 19 weeks' gestation has shown lamellated lipid cytosomes in neurons of the basal ganglia and storage bodies in endothelial cells and pericytes of the vessels [11].

In GM$_1$ gangliosidosis, electron microscopy at 17 weeks showed the beginning of neuronal storage, with typical zebra bodies in the dorsal root ganglia and less-well-developed membrane-bound inclusions in neurons of the cerebral cortex and cerebellum [12].

Similar inclusions were seen in Tay-Sachs disease at 18 to 21 weeks' gestation [13].

In a case of mucopolysaccharidosis II, zebra bodies were present in the brainstem and spinal cord as early as 15 weeks' gestation [14].

Fetuses affected with Krabbe's leukodystrophy show globoid cells in the pontine tegmentum, medulla, and spinal cord. The peripheral nerves may also be involved by 23 weeks' gestation [15].

It is evident that the influence of lysosomal disorders on the developing brain commences well before birth, although in most instances the newborn infant would not show signs of the disorder.

AMINOACIDURIAS

Inborn errors of amino acid metabolism have severe effects on the brain, but the lesions, including spongy change, delayed myelination, or gliosis, are relatively nonspecific and may be difficult to recognize in the perinatal period. There are occasional reports of well-developed lesions of prenatal origin observed in the early neonatal period [16].

NEONATAL HYPOGLYCEMIA

Neonatal hypoglycemia may develop in growth-retarded infants with low carbohydrate stores if feeding is delayed. It is also a feature of infants of diabetic mothers and some inborn errors of carbohydrate metabolism. The study by Anderson et al [17] reported widespread damage involving the cortex, basal ganglia, internal granular layer of the cerebellum, and spinal cord. Neuronal damage was characterized by pyknosis and karyorrhexis. This study was carried out at a time when low blood sugar levels (20 mg/100 mL or less) were being recognized but not yet adequately treated. Shortly thereafter, the prevention and correct management of neonatal hypoglycemia became standard practice in perinatal units throughout the developed world. Severely hypoglycemic infants are unlikely now to die untreated; most will have received ventilatory and cardiovascular support. Consequently, any such infants who do eventually die will have been exposed to episodes of severe cerebral anoxia and ischemia in addition to the initial hypoglycemia.

As the lesions caused by hypoxia-ischemia and those caused by hypoglycemia are similar, the possibility of recognizing pure hypoglycemic lesions in the human infant now seems remote. It may well be true, as suggested by Banker [18], that the end result of hypoglycemia would be the production of a small brain with large ventricles, but without any focal lesions. It seems unlikely that this will now be possible to prove.

TUMORS OF THE CNS IN THE FETUS AND NEWBORN INFANT

These tumors are discussed in Chapter 15, to which the reader is referred.

REFERENCES: MISCELLANEOUS

1. Weil ML, Itabashi HH, Cremer NE, et al. Chronic progressive panencephalitis due to rubella virus simulating subacute sclerosing panencephalitis. *N Engl J Med* 1975; 292:994–8.
2. McCracken GH, Threlkeld N, Mize SG, et al. Moxalactam therapy for neonatal meningitis due to gram negative enteric bacilli: a prospective controlled evaluation. *J Am Med Assoc* 1984; 252:1427–32.
3. Siegel JD. Neonatal sepsis. *Semin Perinatol* 1985; 9:20–8.
4. Berman PH, Banker BQ. Neonatal meningitis: a clinical and pathological study of 29 cases. *Pediatrics* 1966; 38:6–24.
5. Lee EL, Robinson MJ, Thong ML, et al. Intraventricular chemotherapy in neonatal meningitis. *J Pediatr* 1977; 91:991–5.
6. Graham DR, Bard JD. *Citrobacter diversus* brain abscess and meningitis in neonates. *J Am Med Assoc* 1981; 245:1923–5.
7. Brown LW, Zimmerman RA, Bilanuik LT. Polycystic brain disease complicating neonatal meningitis: documentation of evolution by computed tomography. *J Pediatr* 1979; 94:757–9.
8. Cussen LJ, Ryan GB. Haemorrhagic cerebral necrosis in neonatal infants with enterobacterial meningitis. *J Pediatr* 1967; 71:771–6.
9. Ragazzini F, La Cauza C, Ferrucci I. Infection by *Serratia marcescens* in premature children. *Ann Pediat* 1965; 205:289–300.
10. Burne JC. Niemann-Pick disease in a foetus. *J Pathol Bacteriol* 1953; 66:473.
11. Schneider EL, Ellis WG, Brady RO, McCulloch JR, Epstein CJ. Prenatal Niemann-Pick disease: biochemical and histologic examination of a 19 gestational week fetus. *Pediatr Res* 1972; 6:720–9.
12. Lowden JA, Cutz E, Conen PE, Rudd N, Doran TA. Prenatal diagnosis of GM₁ gangliosidosis. *N Engl J Med* 1973; 288:225–8.
13. O'Brien JS, Okada S, Fillerup DL, et al. Tay-Sachs disease: prenatal diagnosis. *Science* 1972; 172:61–4.
14. Lake BD. Lysosomal enzyme deficiencies. In: Adams JH, Corsellis JAN, Duchen LW, eds. *Greenfield's Neuropathology*. 4th ed. London: Edward Arnold, 1984, pp. 491–572.
15. Ellis WG, Schneider EL, McCulloch JR, Suziki K, Epstein CJ. Fetal globoid cell leukodystrophy (Krabbe disease). *Arch Neurol* 1973; 29:253–7.
16. Filloux F, Townsend JJ, Leonard C. Ornithine transcarbamoyl deficiency: neuropathologic changes acquired in utero. *J Pediatr* 1986; 108:942–5.
17. Anderson JM, Milner RDG, Strich SJ. Effects of neonatal hypoglycaemia on the nervous system: a pathological study. *J Neurol Neurosurg Psychiatr* 1967; 30:295–310.
18. Banker BQ. The neuropathological effects of anoxia and hypoglycaemia in the newborn. *Dev Med Child Neurol* 1967; 9:544–50.

The Orofacial Region

Robert J. Gorlin   M. Michael Cohen, Jr.

Craniofacial birth anomalies are frequent. Akimoto et al [1], in a review of over 10,000 Japanese fetal and newborn post-mortem examinations, noted that about 5% had craniofacial and oral malformations.

CRANIOFACIAL EMBRYOLOGY

Neural Crest

Emigration of neural crest cells cranial to the otocyst begins before neural tube closure. As the neural folds elevate, crest cells at the junction between the surface ectoderm and the neural plate leave the ectoderm. In the head region, most skeletal and connective tissue is derived from neural crest. Derivatives include cartilage, bone, dentin, connective tissue surrounding blood vessels, glands, connective tissue of the dermis, smooth muscle, and adipose tissue. In addition, the meninges of the forebrain, corneal endothelium and stroma, and most of the sclera and ciliary muscle are of neural crest origin [2].

Calvaria and Sutures

The neurocranium is divided into a calvarial component of flat bones, which have intramembranous bone formation, and a cranial base component, which arises from endo-chondral bone formation. The sides and roof of the skull arise as membranous ossification centers characterized by needle-like bone spicules that radiate peripherally. At the margins of the frontal, parietal, and occipital bones, presumptive sutures and fontanelles appear.

Sutures develop initially by a wedge-shaped proliferation of cells at the periphery of the extending bone fields, the osteogenic front [3]. Osteogenic fronts appear to govern morphogenetic determination of sutural architecture [4, 5].

They approximate each other in one of two ways. They may overlap each other, forming a beveled suture, or they may approximate each other in the same plane, with an intervening zone of immature fibrous connective tissue, which leads to an end-to-end type of suture [5, 6].

End-to-end sutures are formed in the midline. All other sutures [7, 8]—e.g., the coronal and frontozygomatic—are of the beveled type. Initiation in the midline may be end-to-end, because the biomechanical forces on either side of the initiating suture are likely to be equal in magnitude. In contrast, sutures away from the midline have biomechanical forces of unequal magnitude acting on them and hence are of the overlapping, beveled type [9].

Face and Upper Lip (Primary Palate)

By the end of the 4th week, the maxillary swellings appear lateral to, and the mandibular swellings caudal to, the stomodeum. Above, the frontal prominence forms by proliferation of mesenchyme ventral to the brain vesicles. Nasal placodes arise as ectodermal thickenings on either side of the frontal prominence. During the 5th week, a horseshoe-shaped ridge, consisting of medial and lateral nasal swellings, surrounds each nasal placode. As mesenchyme elevates the ridges, the nasal pits form (Fig. 22.1). By the 6th week, with continued growth of the maxillary swellings, the nasal and maxillary swellings become separated by deep furrows. During the 6th and 7th weeks, the maxillary swellings fuse with the medial nasal swellings and both medial nasal swellings merge with each other. The deep furrow separating the lateral nasal swelling and the maxillary swelling, the nasolacrimal groove, develops a solid epithelial cord that detaches from the overlying ectoderm in the furrow (Fig. 22.2). Following canalization of the cord, the nasolacrimal duct forms and widens at its upper end to create the

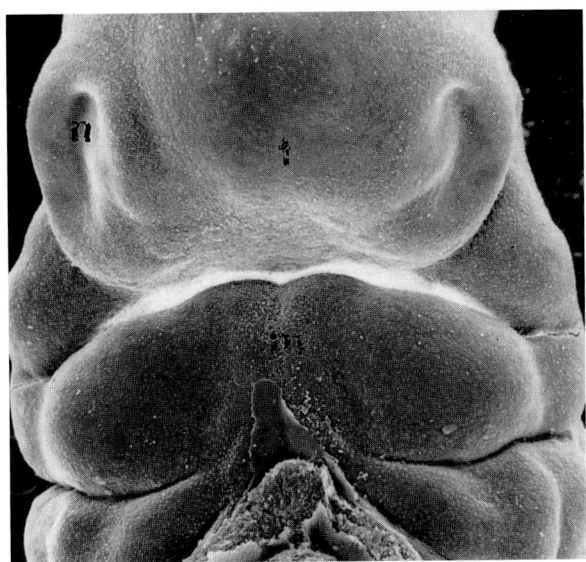

FIGURE 22.1. *Scanning electron microscopy (SEM) image of face of 5-week-old embryo. Note olfactory pits developing on lateral portions of frontonasal prominence. f = frontonasal prominence, n = nasal pit, m = mandibular prominence. (Courtesy of K Sulik, Chapel Hill, North Carolina.)*

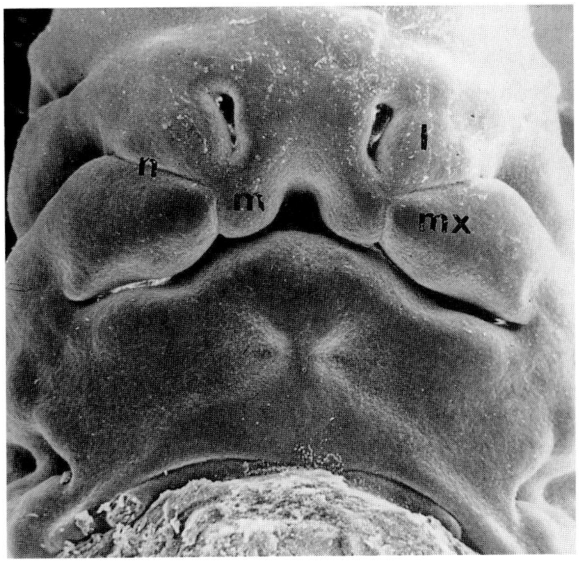

FIGURE 22.2. *SEM image of 6-week-old embryo. Note that notched median nasal prominences have not yet fused with maxillary processes. Midline notch is evanescent. m = median nasal prominence, mx = maxillary prominence, l = lateral nasal prominence, n = nasolacrimal groove. (Courtesy of K Sulik, Chapel Hill, North Carolina.)*

lacrimal sac. Following detachment of the cord, the lateral nasal and maxillary swellings fuse to form the alae of the nose [10, 11].

The fusion of the medial nasal swellings with the maxillary swellings and the merging of the medial nasal swellings with each other produce the primary palate or intermaxillary segment, which is composed of three parts: 1) a labial component later forming the philtrum; 2) a medial section—the future dental arch containing the four maxillary incisor teeth; and 3) a triangular palatal component, extending posteriorly to the incisive foramen [10, 11].

Secondary (Definitive) Palate

The definitive palate is formed from two shelflike outgrowths of the maxillary swellings (Fig. 22.3). These are the vertical palatine shelves, which appear during the 6th week and elevate to a horizontal position during the 7th week. The shelves fuse with the triangular portion of the intermaxillary segment and fuse with each other by programmed cell death of the medial edges, allowing mesenchyme to join in the midline. Complete fusion occurs by the 10th week. The soft palate and uvula form by merging [10, 12].

Nasal Cavities

During the 6th week, the nasal pits deepen, in part because of penetration into the underlying mesenchyme. An oronasal

membrane separates the pits from the primitive oral cavity. Following rupture, the primitive nasal chambers open into the oral cavity through the newly formed primitive choanae [11].

Salivary Glands

The salivary glands develop from oral epithelial buds invaginating into the underlying mesenchyme. The buds branch and extend as solid cords making up a duct system with acini. The cords canalize by degeneration of central cells to form ducts and the secretory portion of the acini.

The parotid gland anlagen develop from groovelike invagination of ectoderm at the junction of the maxillary or mandibular swellings (see Fig. 22.3). As the embryo grows, the duct opening is transferred to the inner surface of the cheek. Similar invaginations into the oral floor and paralingual sulci give rise to the submandibular and sublingual salivary glands, respectively.

The parotid gland ducts develop in the 6th fetal week, the submandibular gland ducts soon thereafter, and the sublingual glands during the 8th week. However, the acini do not develop until the 5th month in utero. Although the parotid glands develop earliest, their capsular development is delayed, which allows lymphoid tissue and oral epithelial entrapment within lymph nodes to be incorporated into the gland [13].

The parotid gland is composed of serous acini, and the submandibular gland consists mostly of mucous acini with

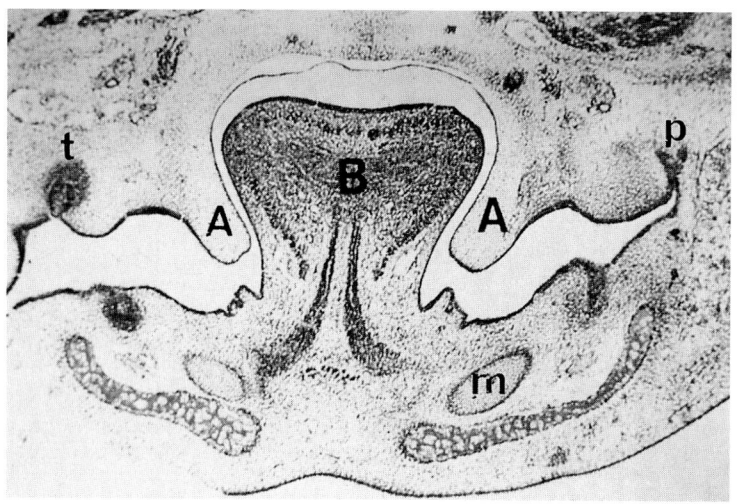

FIGURE 22.3.   *Frontal section through head of 8-week-old embryo. Palatal shelves (A) are on sides of tongue (B). Note also developing tooth buds (t), Meckel's cartilage (m), and anlage of parotid gland (p). As face widens and grows forward, tongue will drop and the two palatal shelves will fuse in the midline above the tongue.*

serous demilunes but also with some serous acini. The sublingual gland is made up mostly of mucous acini.

Teeth

Teeth arise from the dental lamina, a C-shaped epithelial structure in the upper and lower jaws that forms around the 6th week. Tooth buds begin to develop at 8 weeks (see Fig. 22.3). The lamina invaginates to form a cap stage followed by a bell stage at around 10 weeks. In the bell stage, an enamel organ is composed of an inner and outer enamel epithelium with a stellate reticulum between and a stratum intermedium adjacent to the inner enamel epithelium. A mesenchymal proliferation forms the dental papilla in the concave opening of the enamel organ. The inner enamel epithelium differentiates into ameloblasts while the subjacent cells of the dental papilla become odontoblasts. Through a process of induction and interaction, the odontoblasts form dentin and the ameloblasts form enamel. At the lowermost portion of the enamel organ, the inner and outer enamel epithelia are in direct contact with each other without intervening stellate reticulum. This becomes the epithelial diaphragm, which forms the tooth root. Mesenchyme surrounding the developing tooth becomes cementum, periodontal ligament, and alveolar bone.

Branchial Arches

The branchial arches appear during the 4th and 5th weeks of development. Deep branchial clefts separate the bars of mesenchyme. Accompanying the arches and the externally located clefts, internal outpocketings known as pharyngeal pouches appear along the lateral walls of the pharyngeal portion of the gut. At the end of the 4th week, the central portion of the face is formed by the stomodeum surrounded by the first pair of branchial arches. The maxillary and mandibular swellings develop from the first (mandibular)

arch [2, 11]. The various branchial arches and their derivative nerves, muscles, cartilages, bones, ligaments, and branchial pouches are summarized in Table 22.1.

The ears develop from six mesenchymal proliferations, the auricular hillocks, three on each side of the first branchial cleft. The definitive auricle results from fusion of the hillocks. With development of the mandible, the ears, which initially form in the lower neck region, ascend to the sides of the head at the level of the eyes [14].

The second branchial arch grows down over the third and fourth arches, leaving a space that becomes the cervical sinus. The inferior parathyroid gland and thymus arise from the third pharyngeal pouch, the superior parathyroid gland and ultimobranchial body arising from the fourth to sixth pharyngeal pouches. The thymus migrates caudally and medially, pulling the parathyroid along with it. The thymus then fuses with its counterpart from the opposite side [11].

The tongue begins to form ventrally at approximately 4 weeks. The two lateral lingual tubercles and the medial tuberculum impar arise from the first arch. A second medial swelling, the copula, is formed from the second, third, and fourth arches. A third medial swelling, formed by the posterior part of the fourth arch, develops into the epiglottis [11].

The thyroid gland arises as an epithelial proliferation of the pharyngeal floor between the tuberculum impar and the copula (later marking the foramen cecum). Subsequently, the thyroid migrates downward as a bilobed diverticulum to reach its final position in front of the trachea during the 7th week [11].

CRANIOFACIAL TERATOGENS

Fetal Alcohol Syndrome

The fetal alcohol syndrome is the most important human teratogenic condition known today. It occurs with a birth

Table 22.1. Branchial arch derivatives

Branchial arches	Nerves	Muscles	Skeletal, cartilaginous, and ligamentous structures	Branchial pouches
First (mandibular)	Trigeminal (V)	Mastication (temporalis, masseter, medial and lateral pterygoids), mylohyoid, anterior belly of digastric, tensor palatini, tensor tympani	Meckel's cartilage, sphenomandibular ligament, malleus, incus	Eustachian tubes
Second (hyoid)	Facial (VII)	Facial expression (buccinator, auricularis, frontalis orbicularis oculi, orbicularis oris), posterior belly of digastric, stylohyoid, stapedius	Styloid process, stapes, stylohyoid ligament, lesser cornua of hyoid, upper portion of body of hyoid	Palatine tonsils
Third	Glossopharyngeal (IX)	Stylopharyngeus	Greater cornua of hyoid, lower portion of body of hyoid	Thymus, inferior parathyroid glands
Fourth, fifth, and sixth	Superior laryngeal branch and recurrent laryngeal branch of vagus (X)	Levator veli palatini, pharyngeal constrictors	Laryngeal cartilages	Superior parathyroid glands (fourth), ultimobranchial body (fifth)

prevalence of 1 in 500 in the United States. One in 30 pregnancies is characterized by excess alcohol intake, and of the resultant births, about 6% have clinically recognizable fetal alcohol syndrome [15].

Major features include growth deficiency of prenatal onset persisting into postnatal life, developmental delay, microcephaly, short palpebral fissures, epicanthal folds, midface hypoplasia, short nose, long flat philtral area, convex upper lip with thin vermilion border, micrognathia in some cases, joint abnormalities, alterations of the palmar creases, and cardiac defects—especially atrial and ventricular septal defects (Fig. 22.4). Hypoplastic labia may occur. Hypospadias and renal malformations are less common. In early life, poor coordination, hypotonia, neonatal irritability, and hyperactivity are characteristic. Ptosis and strabismus may also be observed, and approximately 15% of patients have cleft palate. Embryonal tumors have been noted on occasion [15, 16].

Fetal Hydantoin Syndrome

The fetal hydantoin syndrome consists of growth deficiency of prenatal onset persisting into postnatal life, microcephaly, developmental delay with dull mentality or frank mental retardation, and dysmorphic features including short nose, low nasal bridge, mild hypertelorism, ptosis of eyelids, strabismus, wide mouth, sutural ridging, and short neck with mild webbing. Less commonly observed are limb anomalies such as hypoplastic nails and distal phalanges, finger-like thumbs, and low-arch dermal ridge patterns on the fingers. Congenital heart defects (especially ventricular septal defect), renal malformations, and hypospadias have been observed in some patients.

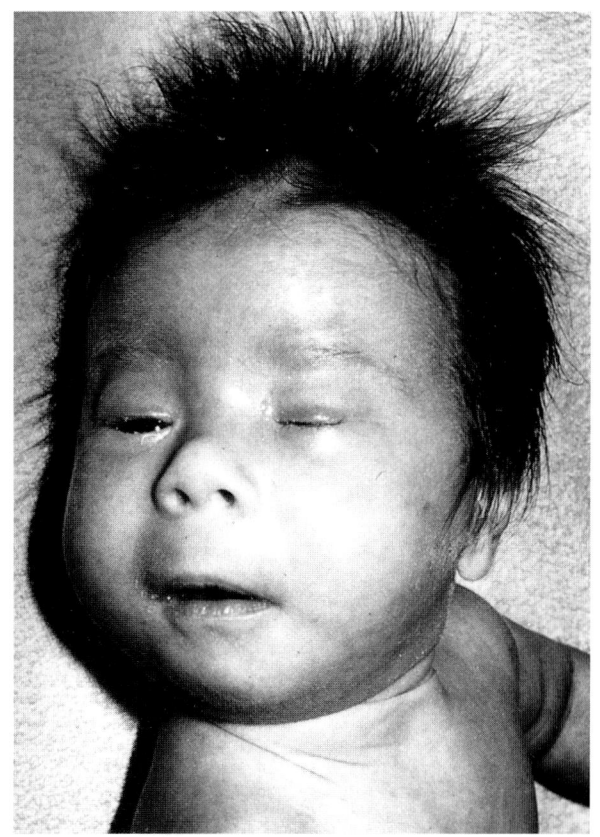

FIGURE 22.4. *Alcohol embryopathy. Facies is characterized by narrow palpebral fissures, indistinct philtrum, narrow vermilion, and small nose with anteverted nares. (Courtesy of F Majewski, Tübingen, Germany.)*

Cleft lip with or without cleft palate occurs rarely. A number of embryonal neoplasms have been reported [16, 17].

Fetal Trimethadione Syndrome

Major features of the fetal trimethadione syndrome include mental deficiency, speech disorders, prominent forehead, V-shaped eyebrows, epicanthic folds, low-set ears with anteriorly folded helices, highly arched palate, and micrognathia. In some instances, features may include intrauterine growth retardation, short stature, microcephaly, cardiac defects, ambiguous genitalia, hypospadias, strabismus, ptosis of eyelids, and single palmar creases [18, 19].

Fetal Valproate Syndrome

The fetal valproate syndrome phenotype consists of developmental delay or neurologic abnormality, midface hypoplasia, short nose with broad or flat nasal bridge, epicanthal folds, minor anomalies of the ear, long or flat philtrum, thin vermilion border, and micrognathia. Prominent metopic ridge, outer orbital ridge deficiency or bifrontal narrowing,

and various major anomalies such as tracheomalacia, talipes equinovarus, and lumbosacral meningomyelocele seem peculiar to infants with valproic acid exposure in utero [20].

Warfarin Embryopathy

Characteristic features of warfarin embryopathy include chondrodysplasia punctata with stippling of uncalcified epiphyses radiographically, nasal hypoplasia, low nasal bridge, and deep groove between the alae nasi and the nasal tip (Fig. 22.5). Pathogenesis is based on maternal intake of the oral anticoagulant warfarin, which results in bleeding into the embryonic and fetal tissues [21, 22].

Retinoic Acid Embryopathy

Characteristic features of retinoic acid embryopathy include central nervous system (CNS) abnormalities such as hydrocephalus, lissencephaly, cerebral dysgenesis, and heterotopias. Other findings include small malformed ears, micrognathia, ocular abnormalities, cleft palate in some instances, conotruncal heart defects, aortic arch abnormalities, and DiGeorge sequence [23] (Fig. 22.6).

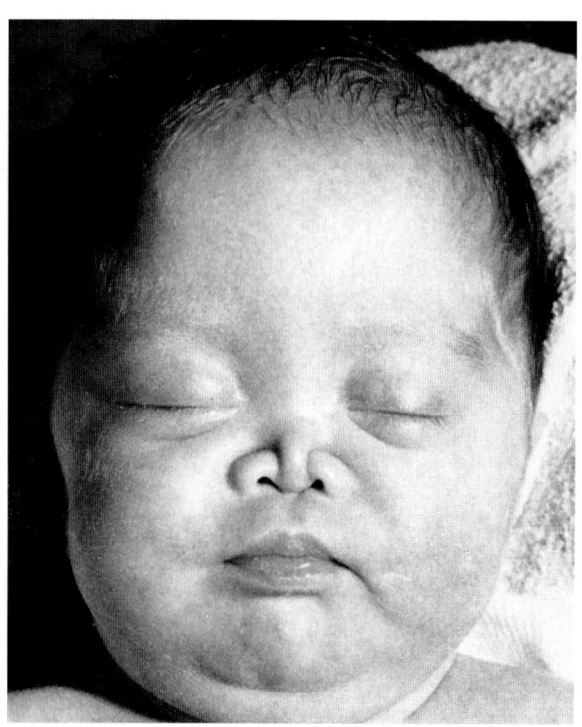

FIGURE 22.5. *Warfarin embryopathy. Nose is small with grooves between nasal alae and nasal tip.*

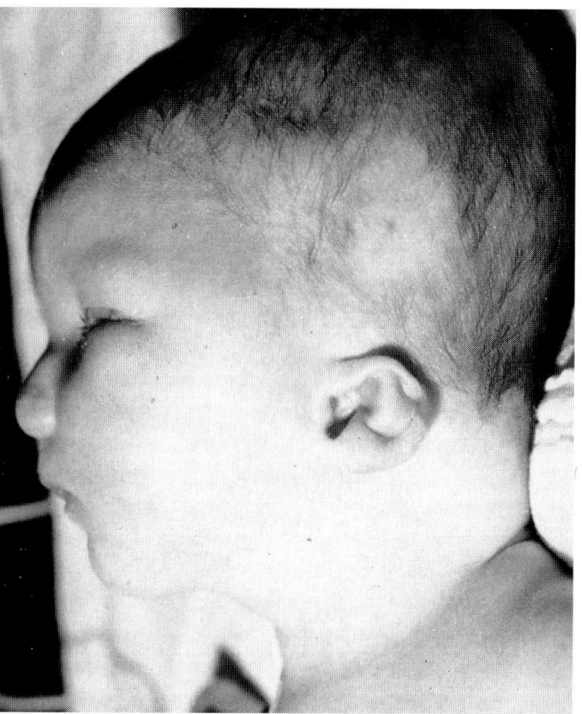

FIGURE 22.6. *Retinoic acid embryopathy. Small and low-set dysmorphic ear. (Courtesy of P Fernhoff, Atlanta, Georgia.)*

Table 22.2. Holoprosencephalic facies

Facial type*	Main facial features	Brain
Cyclopia	Median monophthalmia, synophthalmia, or anophthalmia; proboscis may be single or absent; hypognathism in some cases	Alobar holoprosencephaly
Ethmocephaly	Ocular hypotelorism with proboscis	Alobar holoprosencephaly
Cebocephaly	Ocular hypotelorism and blind-ended, single-nostril nose	Usually alobar holoprosencephaly
Median cleft lip	Ocular hypotelorism, flat nose, and median cleft lip	Usually alobar holoprosencephaly
Less severe facial dysmorphism	Variable features including ocular hypotelorism or hypertelorism, flat nose, unilateral or bilateral cleft lip, iris coloboma, or other anomalies; minimal facial dysmorphism in some cases	Semilobar or lobar holoprosencephaly

* Transitional facial forms are known to occur.
Modified after DeMyer et al [37], Cohen [32], and Cohen et al [327].

Rubella Embryopathy

Clinical manifestations of congenital rubella syndrome are widespread and have been noted in the cardiovascular system, CNS, eyes, ears, blood, liver, and bones. Features include intrauterine growth retardation, microcephaly, mental deficiency, cataracts, microphthalmia, deafness, patent ductus arteriosus, septal defects, thrombocytopenia, and osteolytic metaphyseal lesions [24].

Radiation Embryopathy

Characteristic radiation effects include malformations, particularly microcephaly and eye defects; intrauterine growth retardation; and embryonic death [25]. Studies in Hiroshima and Nagasaki established a definite relationship between irradiation and microcephaly. The highest frequency of microcephaly was found in those individuals who had been exposed before the 18th week of intrauterine life, especially between the 3rd and 15th weeks. Associated mental deficiency was common [26]. The dose-response relationship was dramatically shown by Blot [27].

Diabetic Embryopathy

In diabetic embryopathy, craniofacial malformations have included microcephaly, anencephaly, holoprosencephaly, ear anomalies, and cleft lip/palate.

Folate Antagonist Embryopathy

Aminopterin and methotrexate exposure during the 8th to 10th weeks may result in growth deficiency of prenatal onset, hydrocephalus, patent cranial sutures, craniolacunae, abnormal skull shape, neural tube defects, hypertelorism, auricular anomalies, and reduction defects of distal extremities [12].

HOLOPROSENCEPHALY

Holoprosencephaly is a malformation sequence in which impaired midline cleavage of the embryonic forebrain is the basic feature. The prosencephalon fails to cleave sagittally into cerebral hemispheres, transversely into telencephalon and diencephalon, and horizontally into olfactory and optic bulbs. The condition can be graded according to the degree of severity as alobar, semilobar, or lobar holoprosencephaly. Various gradations of facial dysmorphism are commonly associated with holoprosencephaly, including cyclopia, ethmocephaly, cebocephaly, median cleft lip, and less severe facial dysmorphism (Fig. 22.7; Table 22.2).

Birth Prevalence

The estimate of one holoprosencephalic infant per 16,000 livebirths by Roach et al [28] is based on nonchromosomal cases only and would be considerably higher if chromosomal holoprosencephaly were taken into account. The frequency is much higher in embryos than in liveborn infants, indicating that most holoprosencephalic embryos are eliminated prenatally. In the large study of Matsunaga and Shiota [29], in which 36,380 conceptuses were obtained by induced abortion, the prevalence of holoprosencephalic embryos was 1 in 250.

Etiology

Mutations in the human *Sonic Hedgehog* gene at chromosome 7q36 have been demonstrated [30, 31]. Well over 60 syndromes with holoprosencephaly or arhinencephaly

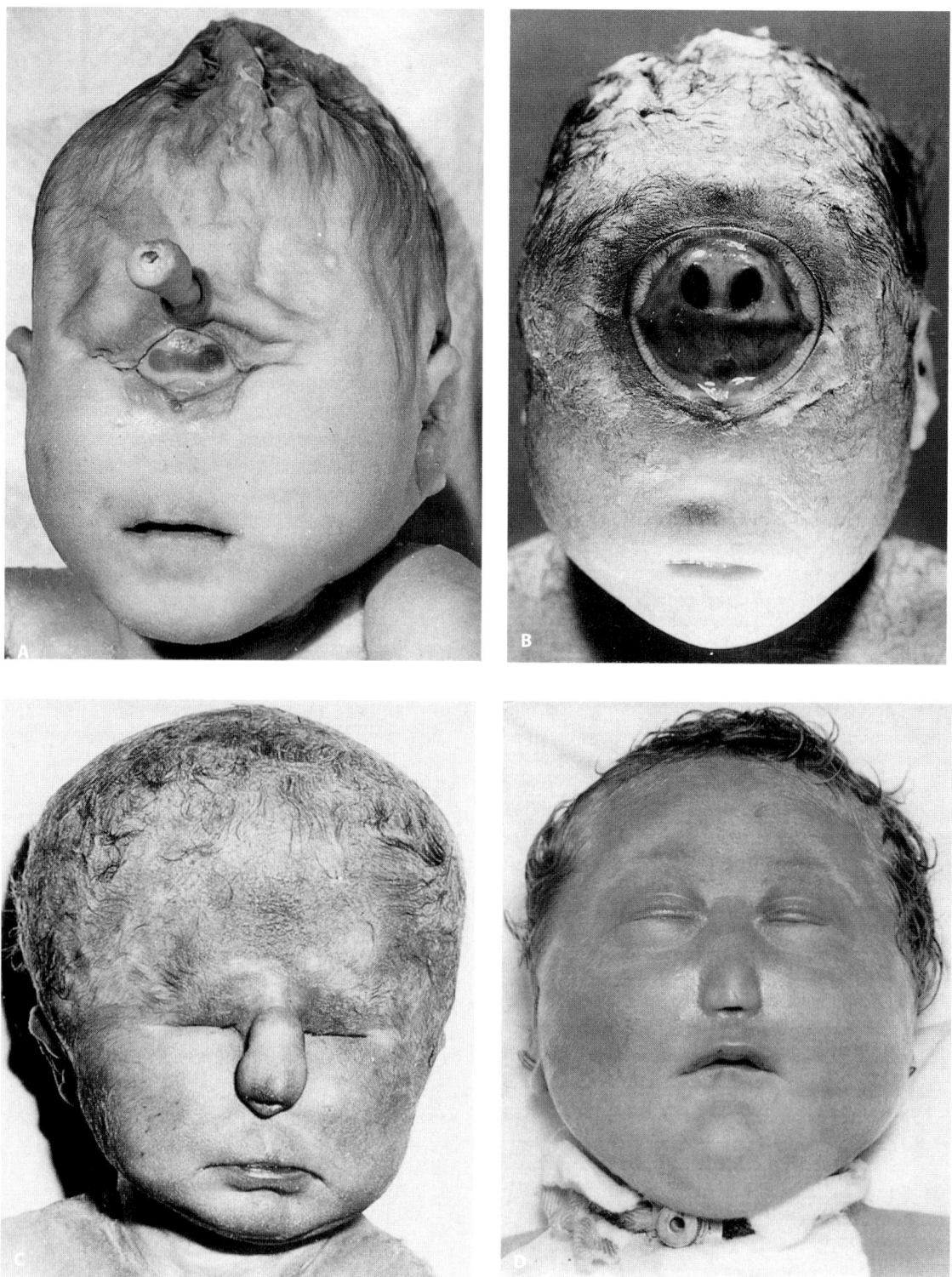

FIGURE 22.7. *Holoprosencephaly. Spectrum of dysmorphic facies associated with holoprosencephaly. (A) Cyclopia with proboscis. (B) Cyclopia without proboscis. (C) Ethmocephaly; note separate eye sockets. (D) Cebocephaly; note hypotelorism and centrally situated blind-ended nostril. (E) Premaxillary agenesis form. (F) Facies associated with some degree of formation of corpus callosum and septum pellucidum.*

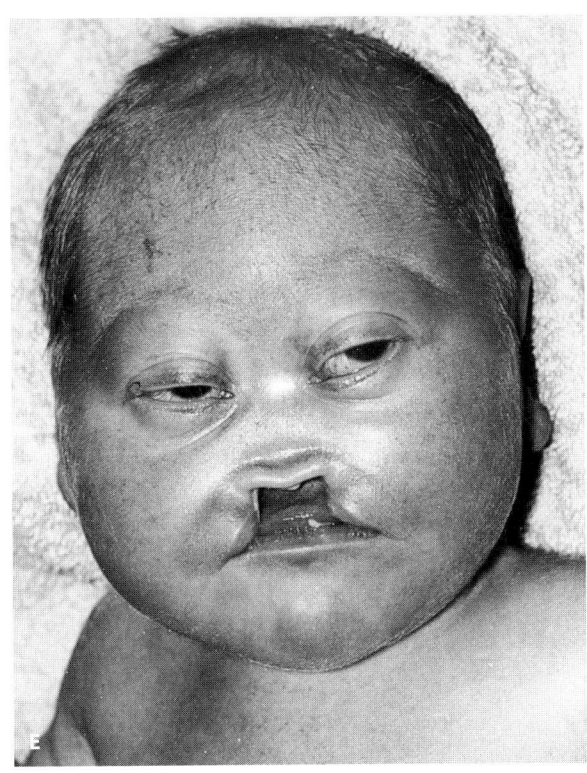
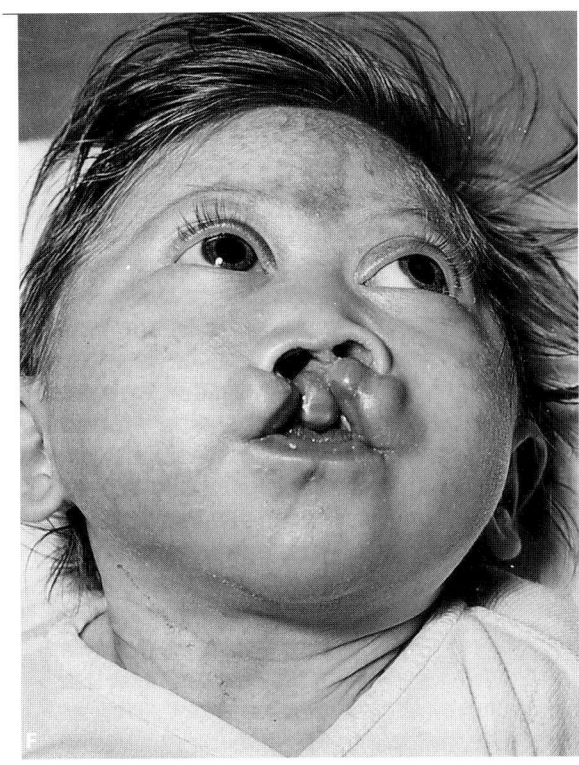

FIGURE 22.7. *Continued*

(absence of olfactory tracts and bulbs) have been delineated [32–34]. Several of the most important [35, 36] are summarized in Table 22.3.

Facial Anomalies

The face usually, but not always, predicts the brain [37]. In the severe forms of holoprosencephaly, and specifically excluding microforms, the face predicts the brain about 80% of the time. In the other instances of severe holoprosencephaly, the face is nondiagnostic. Less severe facial dysmorphism has variable features, including mild hypotelorism or hypertelorism, iris colobomas, flat nose, midface hypoplasia, unilateral or bilateral cleft lip, and/or single maxillary central incisor. Some patients are so mildly affected that they may go undetected without careful scrutiny [32]. Many cases of median cleft lip *without* holoprosencephaly have been recorded. Patients may have normal mentation or retardation, and a clinical clue during infancy is often a *normal head circumference* [38].

Cyclopia

In cyclopia, a single median eye with no evidence of duplication is rare. Although the optic nerve is always single,

Table 22.3.   Some causes of holoprosencephaly

Chromosomal
Trisomy 13
Trisomy 18
Triploidy
Monogenic
del(2)(p21)[HPE2][a]
dup(3pter)
del(7)(q36)[HPE3;AD][a,b]
del(13q)
del(18p)[HPE4][a]
del(21)(q22.3)[HPE1][a]
Autosomal recessive
Meckel's syndrome [AR][c]
Pseudotrisomy 13 syndrome [AR][c,d]
Teratogenic
Diabetic embryopathy

[a]   HPE1, HPE2, HPE3 and HPE4 = four designated genes for holoprosencephaly (Muenke [35] and Belloni et al [30]).
[b]   AD = autosomal dominant. Many, but not all, families with autosomal dominant inheritance have del(7)(q36).
[c]   AR = autosomal recessive inheritance.
[d]   Many cases represent autosomal recessive inheritance, but the possibility of etiologic heterogeneity in pseudotrisomy 13 syndrome cannot be entirely ruled out at present.

duplication of the intrinsic ocular structures is the rule. Two gradients of organization are evident. First, the anterior part of the eye is usually paired and tends to be well differentiated. In contrast, a single, more disorganized, posterior compartment is usually observed. Second, lateral components show more advanced differentiation than medial parts of the eye [39]. The eye socket is usually diamond-shaped with two upper and two lower eyelids. In some instances, the two upper or two lower eyelids may be fused into one, resulting in a triangular-shaped eye socket. The upper palpebrae do not always meet in the midline, but the two lower ones do, with a lacrimal punctum or double puncta appearing at their junction. The eyelids are normally short or even absent. There may be a single eyebrow over the cyclopic eye, two eyebrows, or no eyebrows at all.

A single, blind-ended, medially placed proboscis located above the eye is characteristic in most cases of cyclopia,

although the proboscis is absent in some instances, particularly in hypognathic cyclopia (see Fig. 22.7A,B). Sometimes the canal of the proboscis may be partially partitioned by septa. Histologic examination has shown keratinized squamous epithelium covering the cutaneous surface and continuing for a short distance into the canal, where it may merge with ciliated pseudostratified epithelium. Sections of proboscis wall may contain numerous subsurface skin appendages, including hair follicles and sweat glands. Within the proboscis wall may be observed collagen, striated muscle, cartilage, adipose tissue, blood vessels, nerves, pigmented cells on occasion, and minor salivary glands [39].

Skull bones of the frontonasal prominence, including the ethmoid, presphenoid, vomer, inferior turbinates, nasal bones, lacrimal bones, and premaxilla, are absent. With absent ethmoids, the frontal bones unite across the midline. Similarly, with absent median facial bones, the maxillae unite across the midline. The nasal cavity is completely absent, so the fused maxillae form the floor of the median orbit and the palatal roof of the oral cavity. The roof of the central orbit is formed by fusion of the orbital processes of the frontal bones, the floor by fusion of the two maxillae, and the lateral parts by the zygomatic bones and great wings of the sphenoid. A single, central optic foramen is present. The anterior cranial base is extremely small, and the middle cranial fossa is narrow [40, 41]. The cerebrum corpora striata and thalami are uncleft in midline. No septum pellucidum and corpus callosum are formed (Fig. 22.8).

The mandible is usually of normal size but may be hypoplastic or absent in cyclopia. The mouth may also be small, and in some instances astomia may occur. The ears are malformed, ventrally placed, and approach each other or fuse in the midline. Agnathia or hypognathia may also occur with cebocephaly on occasion or with a normal brain, as in otocephaly [32].

BRANCHIAL ARCH/POUCH ANOMALIES

Abnormal Pinnae

Malformations of the pinnae may vary from bilaterally asymmetric ears, microtia, minor degrees of dysmorphism such as prominent or hypoplastic anthelix or duplication of the lobule, to complete absence. Some instances are associated with abnormalities of the ossicles and/or absence of the external auditory meatus. Ear tags may be associated but may also occur together with an otherwise normal ear. Tags may be single, multiple, unilateral, or bilateral. They occur anywhere along a line from the tragus to the corner of the mouth (Fig. 22.9). Ear tags may occur with hemifacial microsomia and with branchio-oto-renal syndrome.

Aural Sinuses

Congenital aural sinuses are located at the root of the helix and are blind-ended. They may be unilateral or bilateral, may

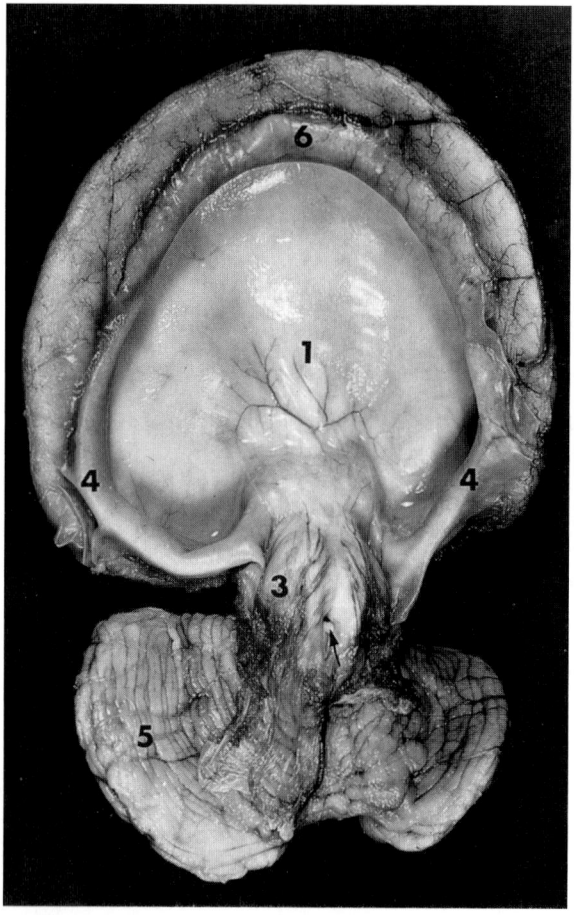

FIGURE 22.8. *Holoprosencephaly, dorsal view of brain. Cerebrum is uncleft. Note cavity of single ventricle (1); corpora striata, uncleft in midline (2); uncleft thalami (3); hippocampi, dorsal rather than rotated backward, downward, and forward into temporal lobes (4); normal-appearing cerebellum (5); mesopallium bordering entopallium and ectopallium (6). (From DeMyer et al [37].)*

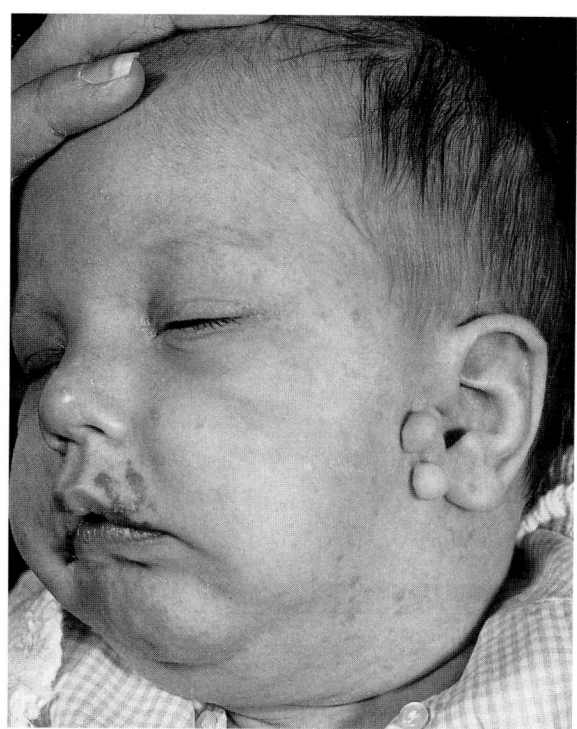

FIGURE 22.9. *Ear tags. Note superficial hemangioma of upper lip.*

be associated with presternocleidomastoid sinuses, and may have autosomal dominant inheritance.

Oculoauriculovertebral Spectrum

Oculoauriculovertebral spectrum is also known as hemifacial microsomia, Goldenhar syndrome, and the first and second branchial arch syndrome. Hemifacial microsomia affects aural, oral, and mandibular development. The disorder varies from mild to severe, and facial involvement is limited to one side in many cases, although bilateral involvement may also occur with more severe expression on one side. Goldenhar syndrome is characterized additionally by vertebral anomalies and epibulbar dermoids and is a variant of hemifacial microsomia (Fig. 22.10A). Since no valid distinction can be made between them, they are grouped under the term oculoauriculovertebral spectrum [42].

Some degree of facial and bony asymmetry is evident in 65% of the cases (Fig. 22.10B). The asymmetry may not be apparent in the infant or young child, but becomes evident with growth, usually by 4 years of age. Adequate overlying soft tissue may mask the skeletal asymmetry. Conversely, deficient soft tissue overlying adequate bony structures may result in facial asymmetry [43].

Malformations of the external ears may vary from anotia to a hypoplastic mass of tissue that is displaced anteriorly

and inferiorly, to a mildly dysmorphic ear (Fig. 22.10C,D). Occasionally, both ears may be malformed. Preauricular tags and sinuses may be observed. Narrow external auditory canals are found in mild cases with atretic canals in more severe cases. Conductive or, less frequently, sensorineural hearing deficit may be a feature. Causes include lesions of the middle and external ears, hypoplasia or agenesis of the ear ossicles, aberrant facial nerves, patulous eustachian tubes, and/or deformed skull base [32, 43].

A variety of other anomalies may be found, including, among others, cleft lip/palate, microphthalmia, vertebral anomalies, congenital heart defects, and CNS malformations [32].

Oculoauriculovertebral spectrum is etiologically heterogeneous. Many cases are sporadic, but a few families have autosomal dominant inheritance. Different chromosomal anomalies have been reported in some cases. Several human teratogenic agents are known; the condition can be found in infants of diabetic mothers, and some features of hemifacial microsomia have been reported with thalidomide and retinoic acid embryopathies.

Poswillo [44] reported a phenocopy of hemifacial microsomia in mice, following maternal administration of triazene, and in monkeys, following maternal ingestion of thalidomide. He proposed that pathogenesis was based on embryonic hematoma formation arising from the anastomosis that precedes formation of the stapedial artery stem. The severity of hemifacial microsomia varied with the size and extent of the hematoma, with large hematomas interfering more severely with branchial arch growth by taking longer to resolve than small hematomas.

Hematoma formation itself has heterogeneous causes including hypoxia, hypertension, pressor agents, salicylates, and anticoagulants [44]. While embryonic hematoma formation may explain some cases of hemifacial microsomia, it does not explain all cases. Affected relatives may have only preauricular tags. In minimally affected individuals, the ear and mandible are well formed, and the preauricular tag seems to represent an accessory auricular hillock. To postulate separate pathogenetic mechanisms to explain instances of hemifacial microsomia and accessory ear tags in the same family seems unnecessarily complicated.

Another example that shows the limitation of the hematoma hypothesis is a true malformation syndrome in which hemifacial microsomia is only one component, such as a patient with hemifacial microsomia, occipital encephalocele, hypoplastic lung, vertebral anomalies, and renal agenesis. These anomalies most likely have a common cause (although unknown) rather than being caused by different factors acting independently. Whatever mechanism is responsible for one malformation should be responsible for the others. To date, there is no experimental evidence that hematoma formation can cause encephalocele or renal agenesis. Therefore, it seems likely that hematoma formation has nothing to do with the pathogenesis of this recurrent pattern syndrome [32].

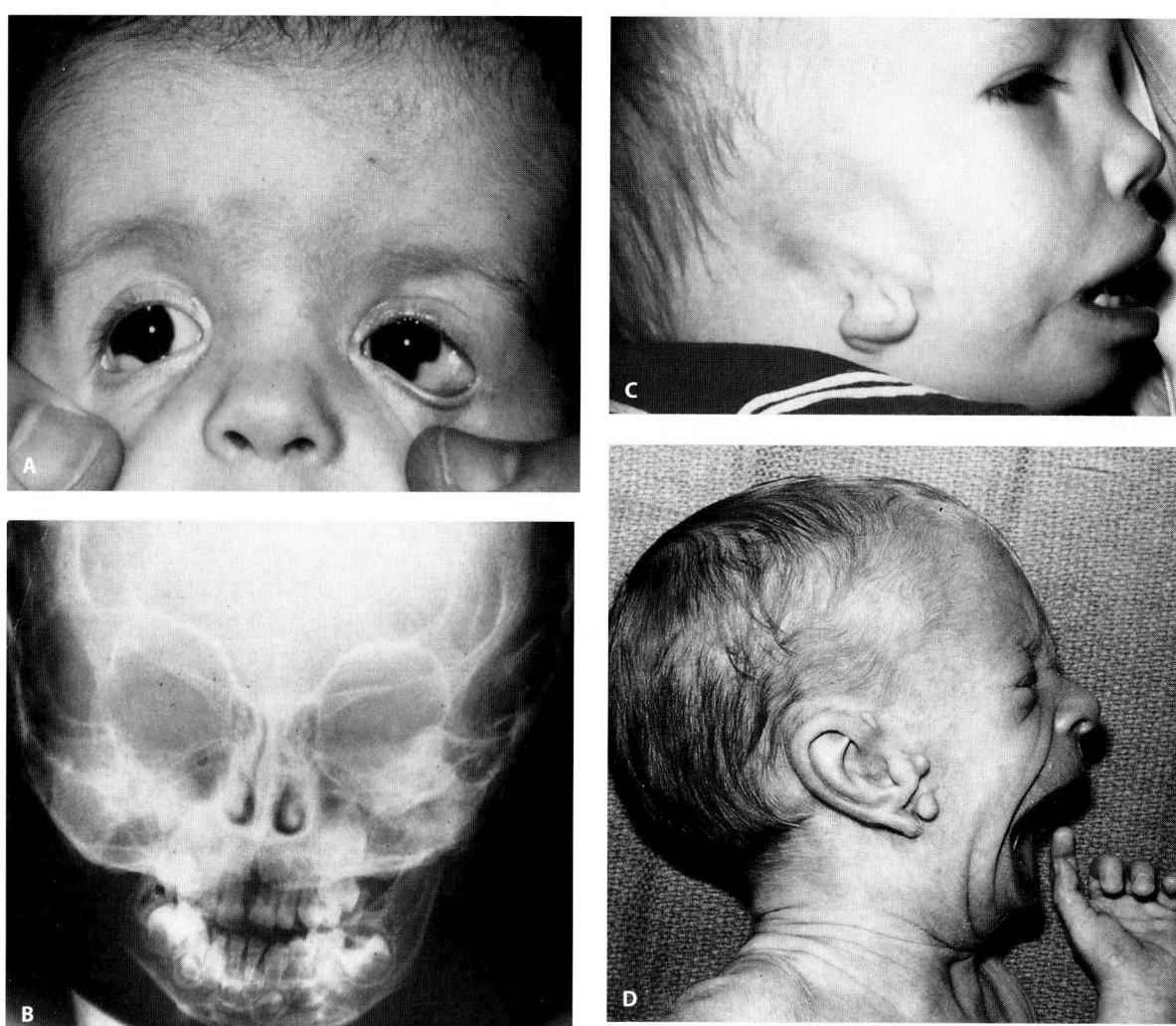

FIGURE 22.10.   *Oculoauriculovertebral syndrome. (A) Epibulbar dermoids. (B) Absence of ramus of mandible on right side. (C) Absent external auditory canal and mastoid, and markedly reduced pinna. Macrostomia has been repaired. (D) Abnormally formed and angulated pinna; ear tags.*

Mandibulofacial Dysostosis

Mandibulofacial dysostosis (Treacher Collins syndrome), involving the first and second branchial arches, is characterized by bilateral zygomatic hypoplasia, downslanting palpebral fissures, hypoplastic ears, and micrognathia (Fig. 22.11). The mastoids may be hypoplastic or absent. There is narrowing or absence of the external auditory canals, and malformed malleus, incus, and stapes. The palate is cleft in about 35% of cases [12].

Inheritance is autosomal dominant, the gene being localized to 5q31.3–q33.3 [45]. There may also be an autosomal recessive type [46].

Poswillo [47], Sulik et al [48], and Wiley et al [49], using mouse, rat, and hamster models, gave teratogenic doses of vitamin A or isotretinoin and produced a mandibulofacial dysostosis-like phenotype. Histologic studies showed deficiency of neural crest in the zygomatic area. The principal defect is unknown. It may involve migration, it may involve differentiation of ectomesenchymal cells or their death in the condensing trigeminal ganglia, or it may produce an effect on first and second arch placodal cells.

Branchial Cleft Duplication

There are two types of duplication anomalies. Type I, which is ectodermal, involves duplication of the first branchial cleft. Type II, which exhibits both ectodermal and mesodermal components, has contributions from the first and second branchial clefts (Fig. 22.12). Type I lesions course medially, inferiorly, and posteriorly to the pinna. Extension may occur anterior to the ear lobe. Drainage from a sinus tract may occur at any site. Type II lesions are more common and

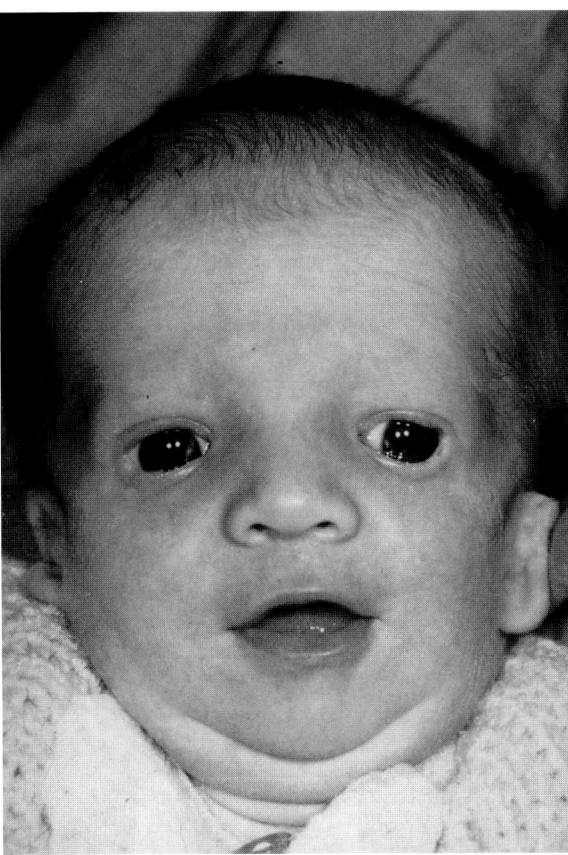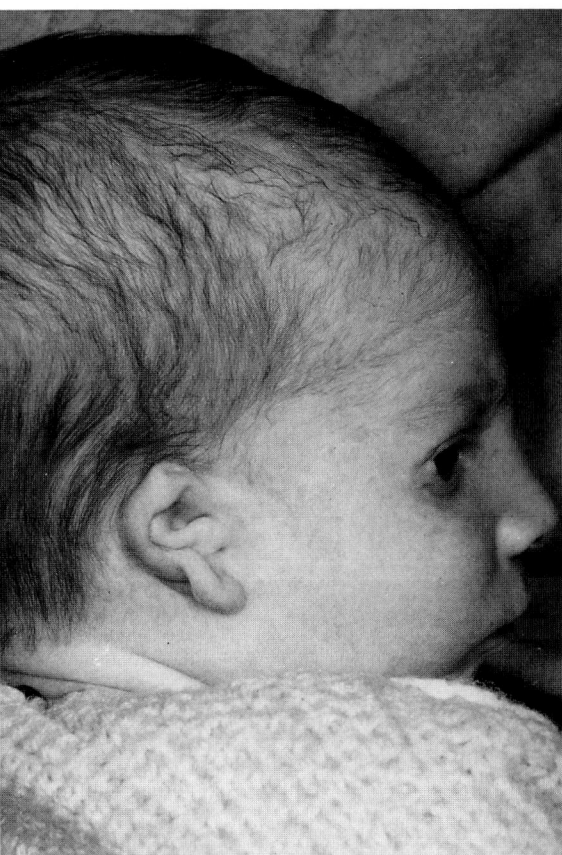

FIGURE 22.11.   *Mandibulofacial dysostosis. Observe downslanting palpebral fissures, micrognathia, and bilateral microtia.*

contain adnexal structures and cartilage. The lesion may extend from soft tissue superficial to the angle of the mandible upward through the parotid gland and may connect as a sinus tract opening into the external auditory canal [50].

Branchial Sinus Tracts and Fistulas

If the second branchial arch fails to overgrow completely the third and fourth arches, branchial sinuses or fistulas may result. Externally, they may appear anywhere along a line just anterior to the sternocleidomastoid muscle. The openings, which may be unilateral or bilateral, connect to a narrow canal that may be blind-ended or may, by disruption, break through a branchial pouch, establishing an internal-to-external draining fistula. Internal communication with drainage is most common around the palatine tonsil area [50].

Branchial sinus tracts and fistulas should be distinguished from so-called "branchial cleft cysts," which are usually said to arise from the cervical sinus. However, there is good evidence to suggest that these cysts are lymphoepithelial cysts arising from enclavement of salivary duct elements in lymph nodes of the neck [51]. Most examples superficially situated

near the angle of the mandible are found lying on the carotid sheath covered only by the sternocleidomastoid muscle. Probably there are a few examples of true branchial cleft cysts derived from the cervical sinus. For this to occur, the cyst must be deep to the derivatives of the hyoid arch—that is, beneath the stylohyoid ligament, external carotid artery, stylohyoid muscle, and hypoglossal nerve [52].

Cervical Prolongation of the Thymus

As the thymus descends from the third branchial pouch to the mediastinum, it may leave a thymic nodule or larger portion of thymic tissue along its path of descent. There are several types of cervical prolongation of the thymus. In Figure 22.13, types 3 and 4 are the most common [53]. Such thymic nodules may be solid or cystic. When they are cystic, the epithelial lining may be squamous or cuboidal and the cyst wall may contain cholesterol clefts and foreign body reaction [50].

Parathyroid Cysts

Microscopic parathyroid cysts are frequent findings. They present as solitary masses in the inferior lobe of either side

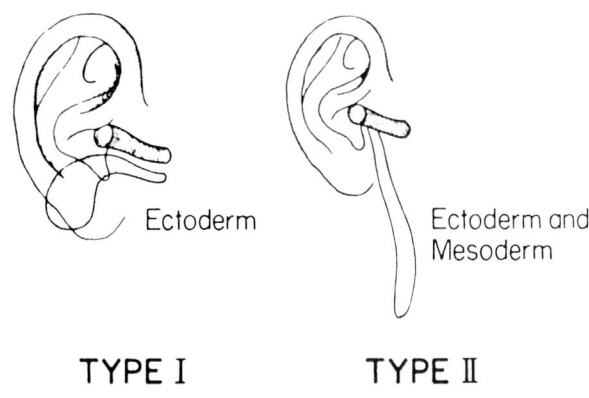

TYPE I   TYPE II

FIGURE 22.12.   *Branchial cleft duplication. Type I, which is ectodermal, courses medially, inferiorly, and posteriorly to the pinna. The more common type II is both ectodermal and mesodermal and often contains adnexal structures and cartilage. (From Batsakis [281].)*

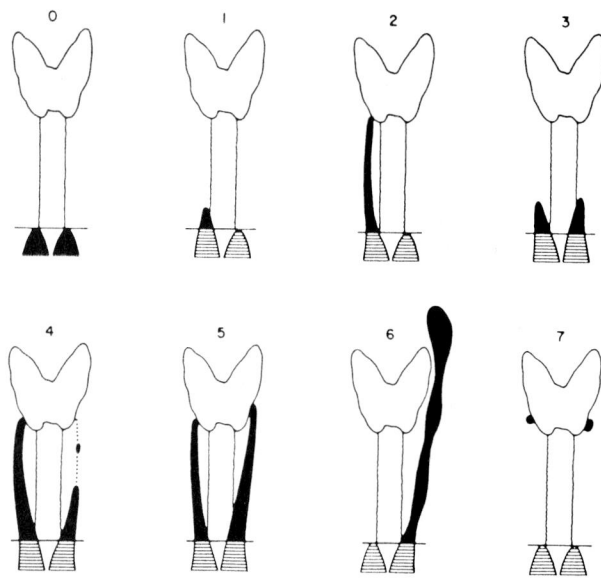

FIGURE 22.13.   *Cervical prolongation of thymus. Types 3 and 4 are the most common types. (From Maisel et al [53].)*

of the thyroid gland. The origin of such cysts is obscure [50].

DiGeorge Sequence

The DiGeorge sequence is expressed as a III–IV branchial pouch complex of absent or hypoplastic thymus and/or parathyroid glands. Cardiovascular defects—particularly interrupted aortic arch and truncus arteriosus—may be associated. Various craniofacial anomalies occur in about 60% of cases. The DiGeorge sequence is etiologically heterogeneous [54, 55]. Some cases have been mapped to 22q11.2. The velocardiofacial syndrome, an autosomal dominant condition also mapped to 22q11.2, is associated with the DiGeorge sequence in approximately 10% of cases.

CRANIOSYNOSTOSIS

The term "craniosynostosis" indicates premature fusion of one or more cranial sutures. Craniosynostosis may be of prenatal or postnatal onset and may involve one, several, or all cranial sutures. The earlier that synostosis takes place, the greater the effect on skull shape, and, conversely, the later that synostosis occurs, the less the effect on skull shape. Reddy et al [56] reported a series of patients with delayed and progressive multiple sutural synostosis. The mean age at presentation for the progressive synostosis group was 64 months.

Skull shape depends on the order and rate of progression of sutural synostosis. When the coronal suture is involved, a brachycephalic skull shape results. Premature closure of the sagittal suture results in a dolichocephalic head shape. Unilateral involvement of the coronal or lambdoid suture produces plagiocephaly. Metopic fusion produces trigonocephaly. Multiple sutural synostosis may also occur.

Birth Prevalence

Prevalence of all types of craniosynostosis, both isolated and syndromic, is 343 per one million births. About 15 per million have Apert syndrome [57], and about the same birth prevalence holds for Crouzon disease [58].

Etiologic Pathogenesis

The craniosynostoses are both etiologically and pathogenetically heterogeneous [9, 59, 60] (Fig. 22.14). By 1991, 90 syndromes with craniosynostoses had been delineated [9], and a number of others have emerged since then. Several syndromes have been mapped and the genes identified (Table 22.4). A variety of chromosomal anomalies have also been reported in association with craniosynostosis (Table 22.5). Secondary synostosis may be observed with several teratogenetically induced conditions, metabolic disorders, hematologic disorders, and malformations [61] (Table 22.6).

Heterogeneity is illustrated diagrammatically in Figure 22.14. For example, craniosynostosis may be caused in some cases by an autosomal dominant gene, in other cases by hyperthyroidism, and in still other cases by microcephaly. The pathogenesis in these cases is also heterogeneous. For example, it may be a defect in the mesenchymal blastema, accelerated osseous maturation, or lack of growth stretch across the sutures. In some cases, there may be a common pathogenesis. Both microcephaly and low-pressure shunting for hydrocephalus may occur with craniosynostosis secondary to lack of growth stretch across the sutures. In other cases, the pathogenesis may be similar. For example, craniosynostosis may accompany α-L-iduronidase deficiency and

Table 22.4. Craniosynostosis syndromes

Condition	Chromosome localization[a]	Gene[a]
Craniosynostosis, Boston type	5qter	MSX2
Greig cephalopolysyndactyly	7p13[b]	GL13
Saethre-Chotzen syndrome	7p21[c]	?
Crouzon syndrome	10q23–q26	FGFR2
Jackson-Weiss syndrome	10q23–q26	FGFR2
Pfeiffer syndrome	8p11.2–P12[d]	FGFR1
	10q23–q26[d]	FGFR2
Apert syndrome	10q23–q26[e]	FGFR2

[a] Data from Jabs et al [328, 329], Vortkamp et al [330], Lewanda et al [331], Preston et al [332], Li et al [333], Robin et al [334], Muenke et al [36], Rutland et al [335], Wilkie et al [336], and Schell et al [337].
[b] Only about 5% of cases have craniosynostosis [330].
[c] Reid et al [253] suggested that there may be more than one locus for Saethre-Chotzen syndrome on 7p.
[d] Pfeiffer's syndrome is etiologically heterogeneous.
[e] Data from Wilkie et al [336].
From Cohen and Kreiborg [338] and Cohen [339].

Table 22.5. Chromosomal anomalies associated with craniosynostosis

del(1q)	dup(8q)	45,X
del(2q)	del(9p)	45,X/46,X + frag
del(3q)	del(9q)	46,fraX(q27.3)Y
dup(3p)	del(11q)	47,XX + cen frag/46/XX
dup(3q)	del(12p)	Triploidy
dup(5p)	del(13q)	Tetrasomy 14q
del(6q)	dup(13q)	
dup(6p)	del(15q)	
dup(6q)	dup(15q)	
del(7p)	del(17p)	
dup(7p)		

From Cohen [60].

also ß-glucuronidase deficiency [9]. Although little is known about pathogenesis, fibroblast growth factors and their receptors, insulin-like growth factor 2, and transforming growth factors β play roles in suture closure [62].

Sutural Pathology

With respect to midline, end-to-end sutures and nonmidline, beveled sutures of the calvaria, two different architectural forms of craniosynostosis seem to occur. Midline calvarial (sagittal, metopic) synostosis is much more likely to produce significant ridging than nonmidline (coronal, lambdoid) synostosis. Because craniosynostosis begins at one point and then spreads along the suture, a series of distinct zones of alteration can be identified. At the center of the fused portion is a zone of complete osseous obliteration characterized by nonlamellar bone across the sutural space. Farther away from the central portion is a zone of partial osseous union in which initial fusion of nonlamellar bone is found together with some connective tissue portions of the suture. The initial point of fusion can take place at either the ectocranial or endocranial margin of a suture and then

spread gradually toward the other margin. Still farther away is a zone of impending osseous union characterized by marked changes in the ossifying margins and narrowing of the connective tissue portion of the suture. Abnormal changes are least apparent in the zone of minimal alteration characterized by a prominent band of connective tissue across the sutural space [63].

Simple Craniosynostosis

Sagittal synostosis is the most common type, accounting for about 57% of all cases. Males are affected much more often than females. Coronal synostosis occurs less frequently, with estimates ranging from 18–29%. Females are affected slightly more commonly than males. Metopic synostosis, lambdoid synostosis, oxycephaly, and other sutural combinations occur with lower frequency. Isolated craniosynostosis occurs more commonly than syndromic synostosis [59].

Most cases of simple craniosynostosis are sporadic. Of patients with sagittal synostosis, about 2% are familial. Most of these cases are due to mutations in fibroblast growth factor receptors 2 and 3 [64]. Of patients with coronal synostosis, approximately 8% are familial. Mixtures of bilateral and unilateral coronal synostosis are common within families. Unilateral involvement is not observed in all affected members. In familial instances, the ratio of bilateral to unilateral coronal involvement is approximately 3:1, in contrast to the nonfamilial group ratio of 1:1 [65, 66].

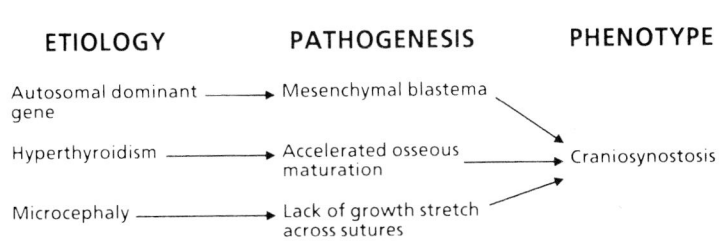

FIGURE 22.14. *Etiologic and pathogenetic heterogeneity of craniosynostosis. Various causes effect essentially the same end result. (From Cohen [9].)*

Table 22.6. Known causes of craniosynostosis

Monogenic conditions*
Chromosomal syndromes
Metabolic disorders
   Hyperthyroidism
   Rickets
Mucopolysaccharidoses
   Hurler syndrome
   Morquio syndrome
   β-glucuronidase deficiency
Mucolipidoses
   Mucolipidosis III
Hematologic disorders
   Thalassemias
   Sickle cell anemia
   Congenital hemolytic icterus
   Polycythemia vera
Teratogens
   Aminopterin
   Diphenylhydantoin
   Retinoic acid
   Valproic acid
Malformations
   Microcephaly
   Encephalocele
   Shunted hydrocephalus
   Holoprosencephaly

* There are many distinct monogenic conditions. Some involve isolated craniosynostosis and others are syndromic. The gene for craniosynostosis, Boston type, has been assigned to 5qter. The gene locus for Greig cephalopolysyndactyly has been pinpointed to 7p13. Localization of the gene for Saethre-Chotzen syndrome is in the 7p21–p22 region [340]. Reproduced from Cohen [9] with permission of the publisher.

One form, the Boston type, has been mapped to the terminal portion of the long arm of chromosome 5 (see Table 22.4).

Cloverleaf Skull

The cloverleaf skull is etiologically and pathogenetically heterogeneous. Variability in the degree of severity occurs, and different sutures may be involved in different patients. The cloverleaf skull may occur as an isolated anomaly or as part of a syndromic pattern—most commonly thanatophoric dysplasia and Pfeiffer syndrome, occasionally with amniotic bands (Fig. 22.15). The large number of conditions that accompany cloverleaf skull have been reviewed elsewhere [67].

Apert Syndrome

Apert syndrome is characterized by craniosynostosis, ocular proptosis, hypertelorism, midface deficiency, and symmetric syndactyly of the upper pand lower limbs minimally involving digits 2, 3, and 4 (Fig. 22.16). A widely patent midline

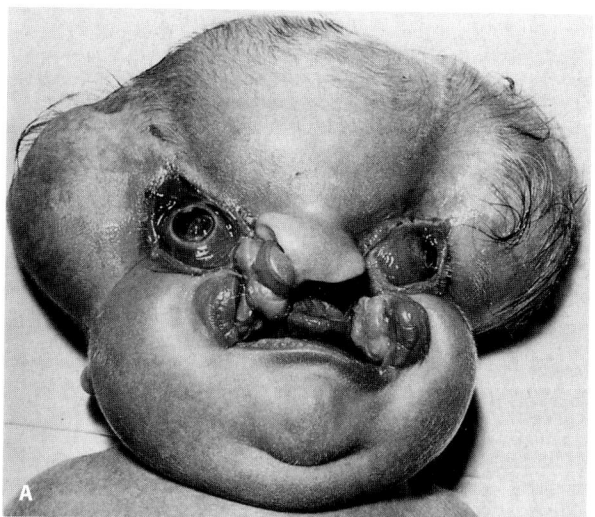

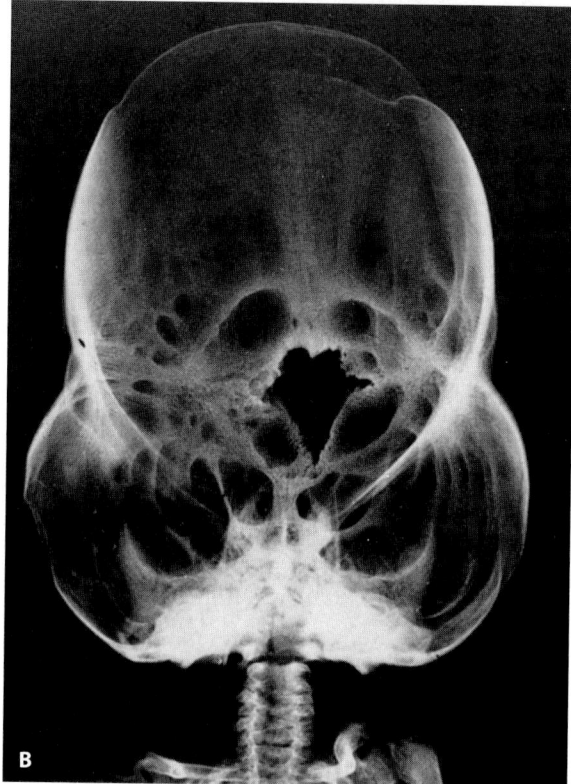

FIGURE 22.15. *Cloverleaf skull. (A) Infant with bilateral oblique facial clefts and cloverleaf skull. Child also had amniotic bands of extremities. (From Schuch A, Pesch HJ.* Z Kinderheilkd *1971; 109:187.) (B) Radiograph showing classic trilobar skull. (From Partington MW et al.* Arch Dis Child *1971; 46:656.)*

calvarial defect extending from the glabella to the posterior fontanelle is observed during infancy, but is obliterated during the first few years of life by coalescence of bony islands that form in the defect. No proper suture formation occurs in the metopic and sagittal zones that later go on to fuse prematurely. Thus, the term "craniosynostosis" is a misnomer for the midline calvarial defect and its closure in

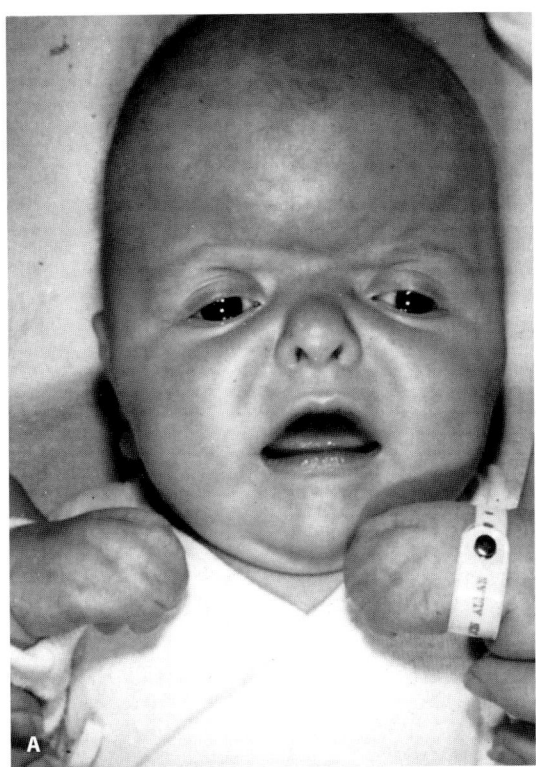

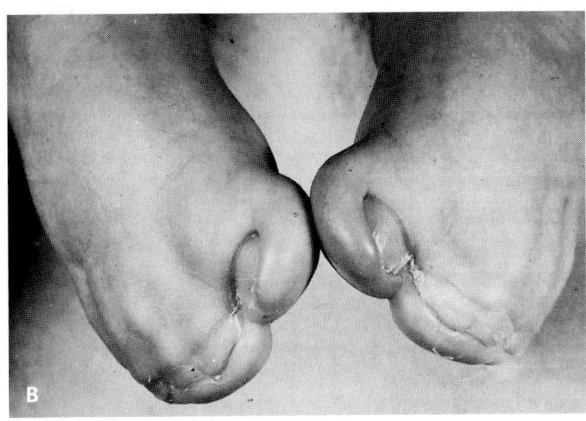

FIGURE 22.16.   *Apert syndrome. (A) Craniosynostosis, ocular hypertelorism, downslanting palpebral fissures, and syndactyly of hands. (B) Syndacytyly of feet.*

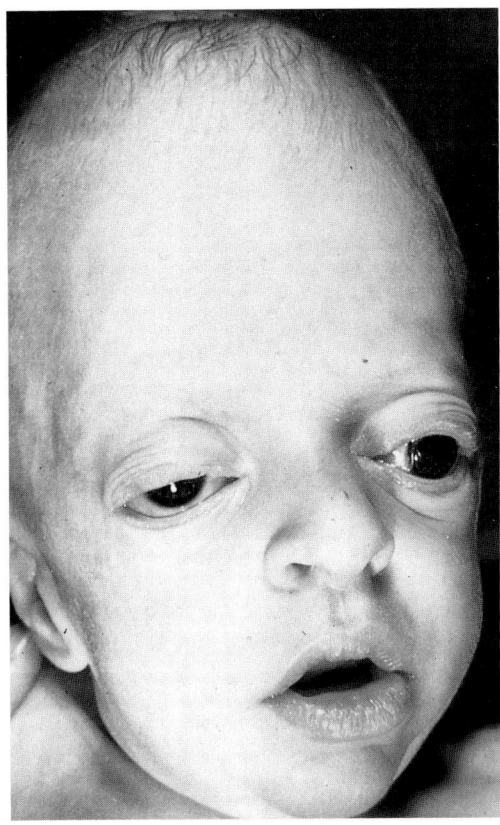

FIGURE 22.17.   *Crouzon syndrome. Note ocular hypertelorism, exorbitism, and exotropia.*

Apert syndrome [68, 69]. Although the syndrome has autosomal dominant inheritance, it is rarely transmitted because of the frequently associated mental retardation and dysmorphic state. The gene has been mapped to the long arm of chromosome 10 at 10q25 (see Table 22.4). New mutations are exclusively of paternal origin [70].

Crouzon Syndrome

Crouzon syndrome consists of craniosynostosis, midface deficiency, and pronounced ocular proptosis (Fig. 22.17). Inheritance is autosomal dominant [71]. It is one of the more common craniosynostosis syndromes and, like Apert

syndrome, is due to a mutation in fibroblast growth factor receptor 2 gene at 10q25 (see Table 22.4) [58].

Pfeiffer Syndrome

Pfeiffer syndrome comprises craniosynostosis, hypertelorism, midface deficiency, broad thumbs, broad great toes, and frequently partial soft tissue syndactyly of the hands and symphalangism of the hands and feet. Cloverleaf skull deformity and radiohumeral or radioulnar synostosis are variable features. Inheritance is autosomal dominant. There is genetic heterogeneity, the defect being due to defects in fibroblast growth receptor genes 1 and 2 at 8p11.2 and 10q25, respectively (see Table 22.4) [72].

NOSE

Choanal Atresia

Choanal atresia refers to congenital obstruction of one or both posterior choanae with connective tissue (10%) or bone (90%). It occurs in about 1 in 5000 live births and is thought to result from failure of breakdown of the oronasal membrane. However, Hengerer and Strome [73] suggested that it results from misdirection of ectomesenchymal elements that originate in the neural crest. There is a 2M:1F gender predilection [9, 74].

Obstruction, depending on the degree of narrowing and whether one or both sides fail to be patent, can result in severe respiratory distress. Choanal atresia is usually demonstrated by failure to pass a rubber or metal catheter more than 32 mm into each nostril. About 50% of infants with choanal atresia have associated findings, among them CHARGE association, warfarin embryopathy, Antley-Bixler syndrome, Crouzon syndrome, mandibulofacial dysostosis, Lenz-Majewski syndrome, and Schinzel-Giedion syndrome [12].

A lateral radiograph using radiopaque dye will demonstrate dye in the nasal cavities and in the nonoccluded nasopharynx but none behind the obstruction. Computed tomography (CT) and magnetic resonance imaging (MRI) scans are helpful.

Frontonasal Malformation

Frontonasal malformation is a nonspecific developmental field defect characterized by ocular hypertelorism, broad nasal root, lack of nasal tip, widow's peak, and anterior cranium bifidum occultum (Fig. 22.18). It represents a clinical spectrum.

Etiology rests in failure of the nasal capsule to develop properly. As a result, the primitive brain vesicle then fills the space and results in hypertelorism and cranium bifidum. The widow's peak is secondary to hypertelorism, the two fields of hair-growth suppression failing to overlap sufficiently high on the forehead.

Almost all cases are sporadic, but the condition has been seen in two generations [75]. There is a distinct subgroup at the severe end of the spectrum. Associated anomalies include epibulbar dermoids, agenesis of the corpus callosum, tibial hypoplasia, and bilateral polydactyly of the halluces [12, 76].

Aplasia of the Entire Nose (Arhinia) or Half of the Nose (Hemirhinia)

Arhinia and hemirhinia are usually isolated findings but may be found in association with other anomalies of the facial region, especially hypoplasia of the midface [77–79]. A lateral nasal proboscis or tissue tag rarely may be present (vide infra). In some, there is no nose; in others, a blind-ended nasal pit is present [80]. Ipsilaterally displaced eye, ocular colobomata, microphthalmia, anophthalmia, congenital cataract, and absence of olfactory bulbs and tracts and of the nasolacrimal duct have been noted [81, 82] (Fig. 22.19). A few patients have associated cleft palate [78]. Intelligence has been normal. Arhinia has been reported in sisters [83].

Radiographic changes include missing nasal septum, conchae, maxillary incisors, paranasal sinuses, hypoplastic nasal and maxillary bones, absence of lacrimal, ethmoid, and vomer bones, and choanal atresia [84].

As indicated earlier in this chapter, by the end of the 6th embryologic week, neural crest cells have migrated into the medial and lateral nasal processes, forming bilateral horseshoe-shaped nasal ridges. The cartilaginous septum is formed by neural crest cells that persist between the two nasal sacs—i.e., posterior extensions of the nasal pits. At the deepest portions of the sacs, there is the oronasal membrane, which normally ruptures during the second month [85]. Rupture is necessary for patency of the nostrils; otherwise, choanal atresia results. Cells from the frontonasal prominence form the external nose. The primitive nostrils then fill with epithelial plugs. Failure of one or both sacs to form or failure of the plugs to resorb results in arhinia or hemirhinia [86].

Lateral Nasal Proboscis

Lateral nasal proboscis is characterized by a tubular proboscis-like structure (similar to that seen in the midline above the eye in cyclopia), usually 2 to 4 cm in length and 0.5 to 1.0 cm in width extending from an area just lateral to the nasal root [87] (Fig. 22.20A). Ocular hypertelorism may be present. Lateral nasal proboscis is accompanied by agenesis of one-half of the nose. Rarely, the proboscis is located in the midline. In a few cases, there has been normal nose formation [88]. Bilateral proboscides have also been described [89] (Fig. 22.20B).

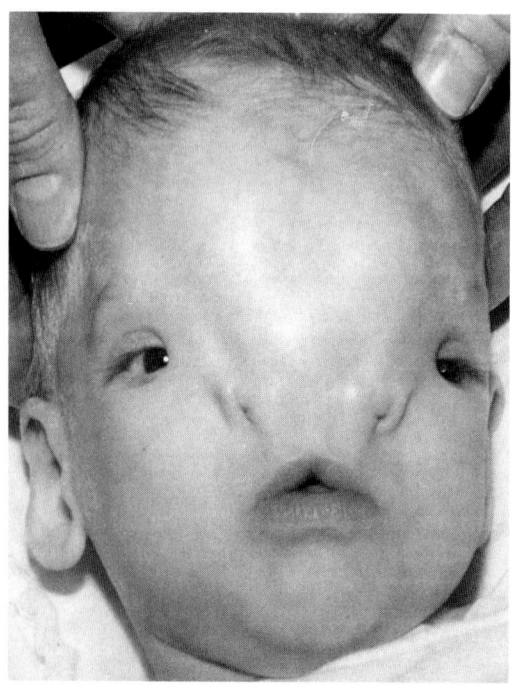

FIGURE 22.18. *Frontonasal malformation. Ocular hypertelorism, very broad nasal root, widow's peak, and anterior cranium bifidum occultum.*

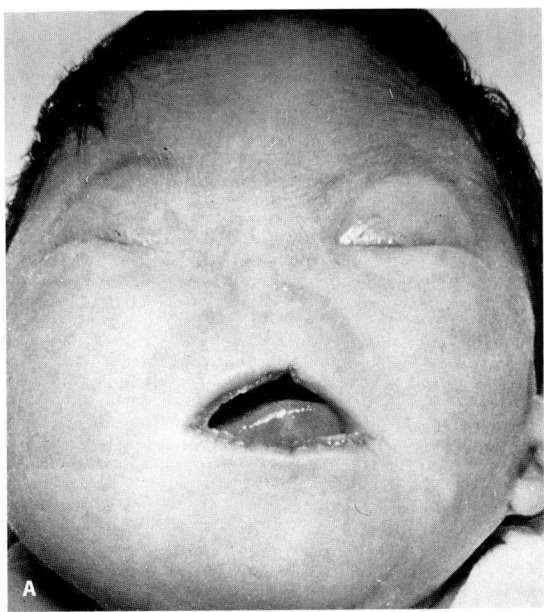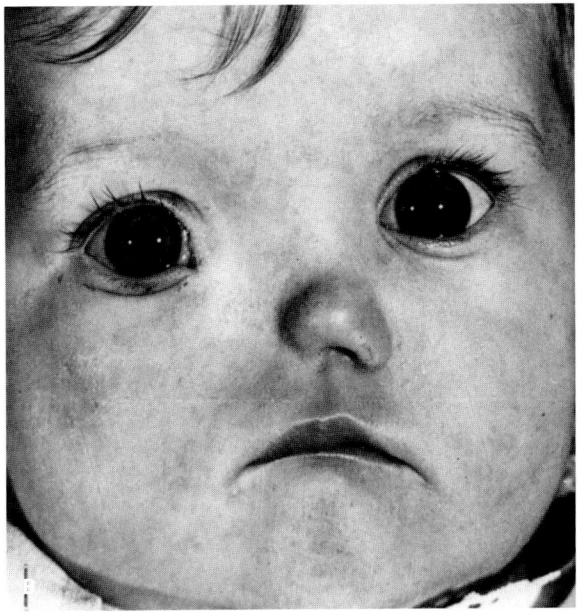

FIGURE 22.19.   *Arhinia and hemirhinia. (A) Absence of nose. Note notch in upper lip. (B) Half the nose is missing. Ipsilateral eye is laterally displaced. (Courtesy of J O'Connor, Helena, Montana.)*

The proboscis is usually blind-ended, and rarely solid. It represents the missing nostril and lateral half of the nose [90]. The lacrimal duct, nasal bone, vomer, maxillary sinus, cribriform plate, and ethmoid cells are often missing on the involved side, and there may be unilateral choanal atresia. Colobomas of the iris and upper and lower eyelids have been noted [91]. The olfactory bulb is usually rudimentary on the involved side [88].

The frequency has been estimated to be less than 1 in 100,000 liveborn infants. There is no gender or racial predilection.

Embryologically, as indicated earlier, the external nose is derived from the medial and lateral nasal prominences. Each median nasal prominence gives rise to half of the septum and the medial crus of the lower lateral cartilage. Each lateral nasal prominence forms the nasal bone, the lateral crus of the lower lateral cartilage, the upper lateral cartilage, and the anterior end of the lower turbinal complex. The lateral nasal proboscis arises from defective formation of the lateral nasal prominence sometime during the 4th or 5th week of embryonal life.

Bifid Nose and Duplication of the Nose

The nose may be bifurcated (or even trifurcated) by a groove resulting from infolding of the median nasal prominence [92]. Some clefts are extremely mild [93]; others extend to the upper lip [94]. Folded nose may be seen in association with frontonasal dysplasia [95].

Rarely there may be true duplication (rhinodymia) with two separate noses, each with two nostrils. An associated condition is marked ocular hypertelorism [96, 97].

Three nostrils have been reported in a child with anophthalmia [98]. Other patients have had supernumerary nostrils, one above the other [99].

Doubling of one side of the nose was described by Winkler [100]. A nose within a nose was reported by Ungerecht [101]. Wilke [102] and Morgan and Evans [103] noted transitional forms between doubling of one side of the nose and lateral nasal proboscis.

Weaver and Bellinger [94] and Erich [96] described embryologic errors that may explain these defects.

Although all these anomalies are usually isolated in occurrence, Anyane-Yeboa et al [93] reported bifid-tipped nose as an autosomal dominant trait.

Lateral Nasal Cleft

The lateral nasal cleft is a rare triangular defect involving the ala of the nose. The apex of the cleft is directed upward, beginning in the midportion of the ala nasi. It may be unilateral or bilateral [104] (Fig. 22.21).

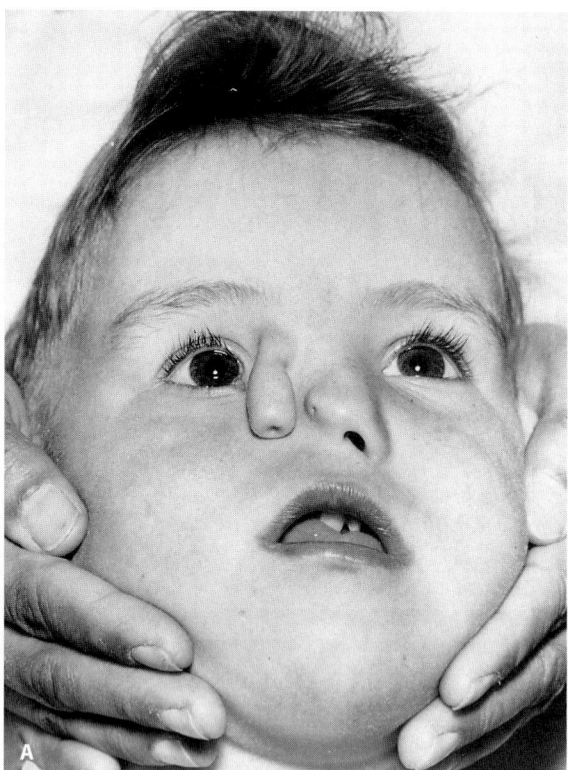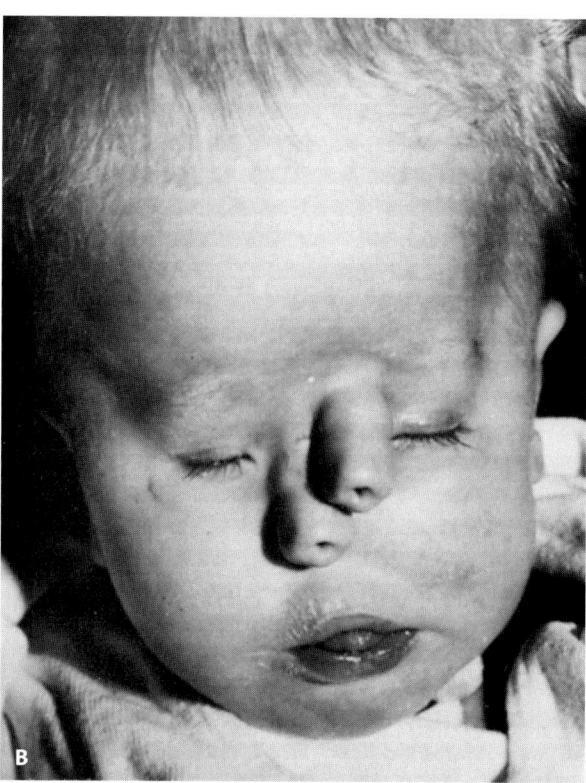

FIGURE 22.20.   *Lateral nasal proboscis. (A) Tubular proboscis attached medial to inner canthus of eye. Also note nasal pit on ipsilateral side. (B) Bilateral proboscides.*

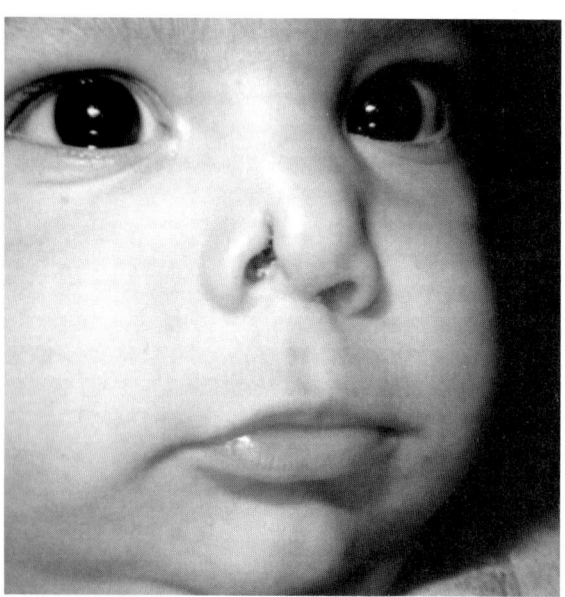

FIGURE 22.21.   *Lateral nasal cleft. This cleft is often isolated but may be associated with ipsilateral microphthalmia or anophthalmia.*

The cleft may be isolated or may be associated with anophthalmia or microphthalmia, or with lower lid coloboma. We view this anomaly as an incomplete (naso-ocular) oblique facial cleft [105].

Nasal Dermoid Cyst

Nasal dermoid cysts (nasal dermoids) constitute about 1–3% of all congenital dermoid cysts, and 3–12% of those located in the head and neck.

The nasal dermoid is often (40–50%) manifested as a single, rarely multiple, dimple, indentation, comedo, or pimple located midsagittally on the nose anywhere between the glabella and the nasal tip [106, 107]. It is most often located at the mid-dorsum or glabella. When superficial, the nasal dermoid is a painless firm mass. The indentation is blind-ended or may extend to a cystic space beneath the nasal bone, but does not communicate with the nasal cavity proper [108]. Extension to the basisphenoid or crista galli occurs in at least 10% of cases [109] and can be demonstrated by CT scan [110]. Hairs may protrude from the midline fistula, and sebaceous debris may exude. Associated broadening of the nasal bridge may be found [111, 112]. The nasal dermoid does not transilluminate and does not enlarge when the baby cries.

A 2M:1F gender predilection has been noted. Although usually an isolated defect, nasal dermoid cyst has been seen in identical twin males [113], and there have been a few reports in more than one generation of a family [111, 112].

The origin of the nasal dermoid rests in defective embryogenesis [107]. During the first stage of development, the nose consists of ectoderm, mesoderm, and underlying cartilaginous capsule. After 60 days' gestation, the frontal and nasal bones have differentiated from the mesoderm by intramembranous ossification but remain separated by a space (fonticulus nasofrontalis) that spans from the skull base to the nasal tip (Fig. 22.22A). Into this space extends a small piece of dura that initially contacts the skin but becomes separated from it with growth of the nasal process. The dural projection becomes encircled by an opening in the frontal bone called the foramen cecum (Fig. 22.22B). This opening eventually fuses with the fonticulus nasofrontalis near the site of the future cribriform plate, obliterating any nasoectodermal connections. If this process is incomplete, dermal contact may occur from the nasal tip to the intracranial space through the foramen cecum.

About 10% of nasal dermoids become superficially infected. Frontal lobe abscess may occur in those with intracranial extension. Patients with deep pits have a higher rate of extension to the cranium.

Microscopically, the cyst is similar to that of any other dermoid cyst. It is lined by stratified squamous epithelium and is surrounded by a capsule of fibrous connective tissue. Within the cyst wall are hair follicles and sebaceous and sweat glands. The lumen is filled with caseous material and hairs.

Nasal Hemangioma

The nasal hemangioma is about one-half as frequent as the nasal dermoid cyst. Among examples, it is present at birth in 10–30%; the rest usually appear within the first few weeks of life. It may be firm to the touch and is only partially blanchable. Distinction from nasal glioma is difficult because both may have surface telangiectasia. The nasal hemangioma

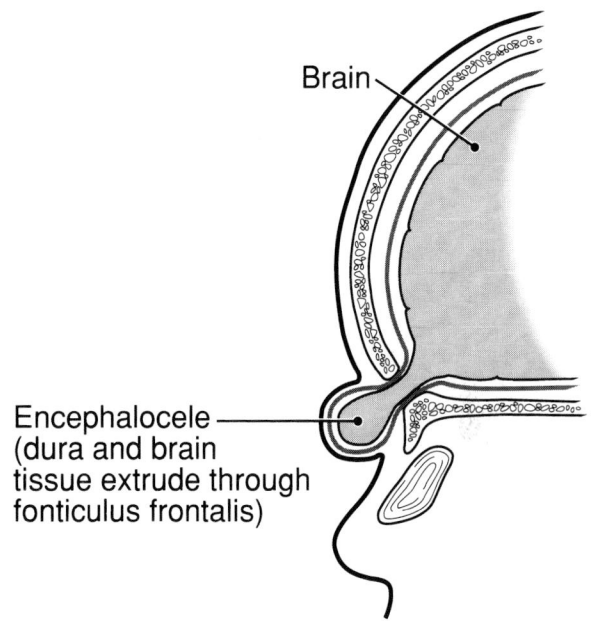

FIGURE 22.23. *Nasal encephalocele. Note extension of dura and brain through fonticulus frontalis. (From Kennard and Rasmussen [114].)*

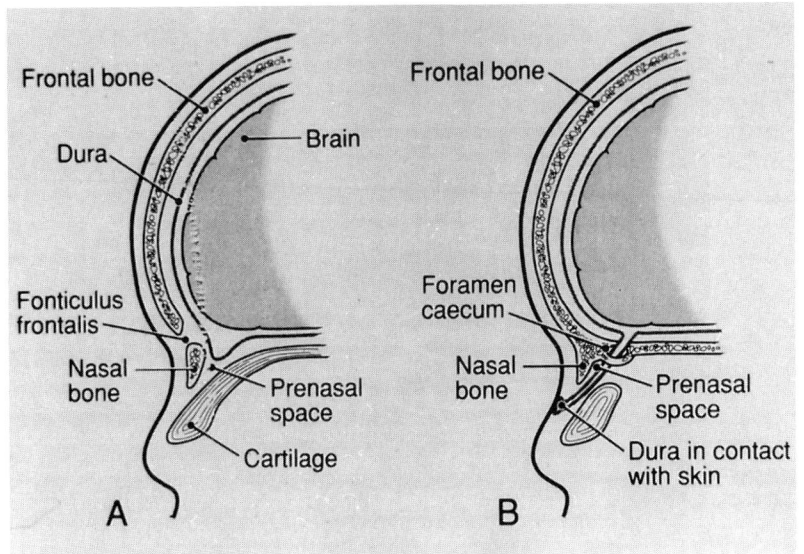

FIGURE 22.22. *Embryologic development of nose and frontobasal skull. (A) Note potential spaces: fonticulus nasofrontalis and prenasal space. (B) Foramen cecum develops by partial fusion of nasal bone with frontobasal skull. Note extension of dural process to nasal skin. (From Kennard and Rasmussen [114].)*

is characterized by rapid growth. Some cases exhibit break-down of the overlying skin [114].

Nasal Encephalocele

Nasal encephalocele is noted in 1 in 3500 to 1 in 4000 births. Intracranial connection is present in all infants with nasal encephalocele [115] (Fig. 22.23). Broadening of the nasal bridge is observed in about 65% of the cases. The encephalocele is often blue, pulsatile, and reducible, and often (50%) transilluminates (in contrast with the nasal dermoid). Nasal encephaloceles are not as firm as nasal gliomas or nasal dermoids and tend to enlarge when the

infant cries or when the jugular veins are compressed (Furstenberg test) [114]. The nasal encephalocele is easily demonstrated in CT or MRI studies [116]. The foramen cecum is enlarged, the crista galli distorted, and the nasal septum widened. Ocular hypertelorism is often found. Frequently there is erosion of contiguous bones. Midline examples may present as either frontoethmoid or nasofrontal masses. The former herniate through the ethmoid plate behind the crista galli, the latter in front of the crista galli.

Association with other midline defects, especially facial clefts, is not rare (15%).

Both nasal gliomas and nasal encephaloceles exhibit similar histopathologic changes—i.e., interweaving strands of

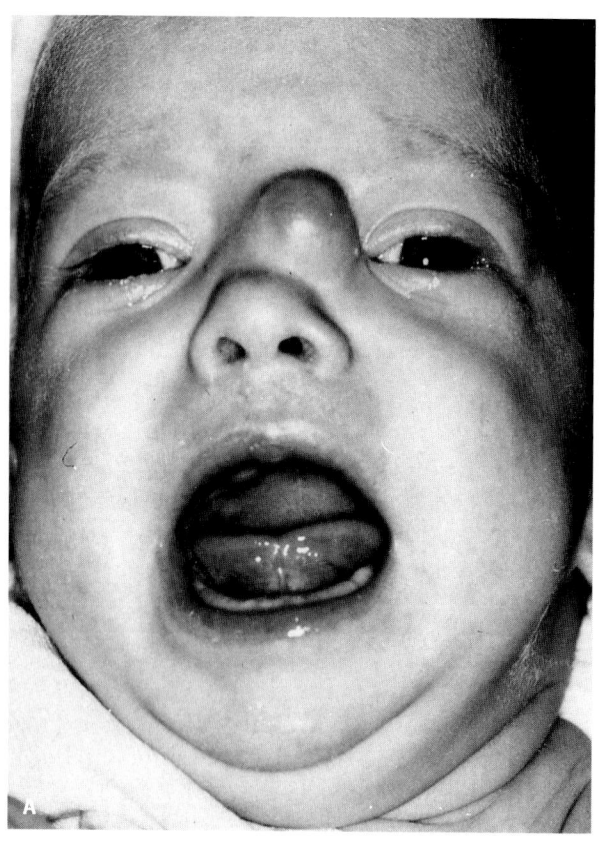

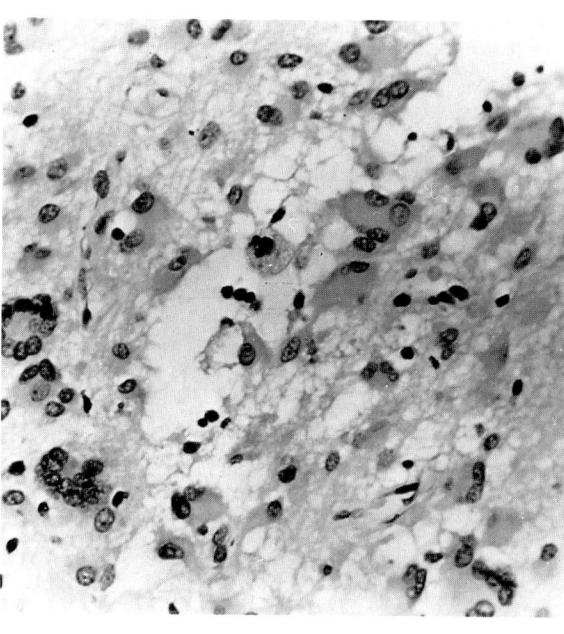

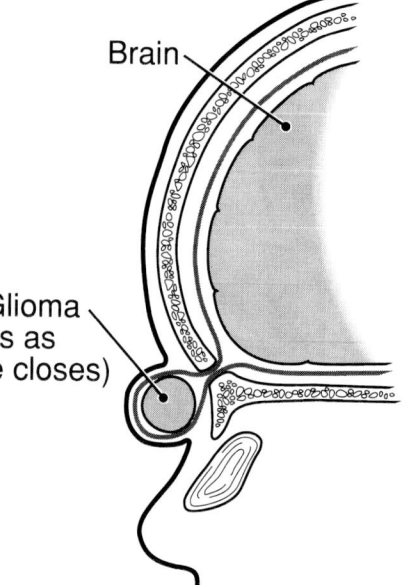

FIGURE 22.24.   *Nasal glioma. (A) Usual site is just lateral to nasal root. (B) Gemistocytic astrocytes and multinucleated cells. (C) Embryologic derivation of nasal glioma. (From Kennard and Rasmussen [114].)*

neural and fibrous tissue glial cells (astrocytes), loose textured glial substance, and occasionally nerves.

For theory of origin, see the discussion under Nasal Dermoid Cyst.

Nasal Glioma

Nasal gliomas represent ectopic neural tissue. They are located at or just lateral to the nasal root [117] (Fig. 22.24A,B). Extensive lacrimation may be present on the involved side. Nasal gliomas produce slow asymmetric expansion of the nasal bridge. A slight (3:2) male gender predilection has been noted. About 60% are external (lying outside the nasal bone), 30% are internal, and 10% have both internal and external elements (dumbbell form). External examples are often reddish with overlying telangiectasia and may be mistaken for hemangiomas. The nasal glioma is firm and noncompressible, does not increase in size with crying or with compression of the jugular veins (Furstenberg test), and does not transilluminate [118].

The nasal glioma is usually present at birth or appears during the neonatal period. It is firm, rounded, and attached to the nasal skeleton. Ocular hypertelorism is not produced unless it is located within the nasal cavity proper.

For theory of origin, see the discussion under Nasal Dermoid Cyst (Fig. 22.24C).

Unusually Shaped Noses

Some noses are so characteristic, even at birth, that they can strongly suggest a disorder or syndrome. Other than the conditions noted above, we suggest that the reader consult a comprehensive text for the following, inter alia:

alpha-thalassemia/X-linked mental retardation syndrome (hypoplastic septum and columella), de Lange syndrome (small nose with anteverted nostrils), Johanson-Blizzard syndrome (very hypoplastic alae), Hallermann-Streiff syndrome (thin and pointed), trichorhinophalangeal syndrome (hypoplastic alae, broad root), Waardenburg syndrome (hypoplastic alae), Rubinstein-Taybi syndrome (hyperplastic septum), Williams syndrome (small nose with anteverted nostrils), and oculodento-osseous syndrome (narrow nose with alar hypoplasia) [12, 119].

A separate dominant disorder is characterized by short nose, retracted columella, broad bridge, flat tip, and widened, outwardly directed nostrils [120]. Still another autosomal dominant disorder is identified by broad columella, septum, nasal tip, and bridge. The outer wall of the nose balloons out. There are no nasal bones, the lateral wall being composed of an ill-defined cartilaginous mass [121].

Small nose, while seen in several disorders noted above (e.g., Williams syndrome and de Lange syndrome), may be an isolated finding. The similarity of the diminutive nasal form in three disorders—warfarin embryopathy, chondrodysplasia punctata, and Binder syndrome—cause us to believe that they share the same pathogenetic mechanisms [12, 119].

MOUTH

Commissural Lip Pits

Commissural lip pits, resulting from minor failure of penetration of mesenchyme at the junction of the maxillary and mandibular prominences, are seen as unilateral or bilateral (25%) indentations at the commissures of the mouth. They

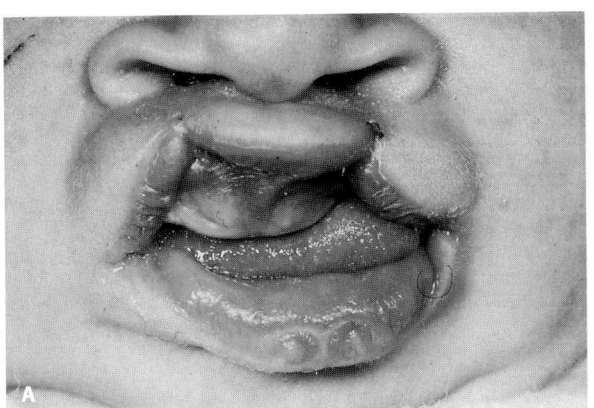
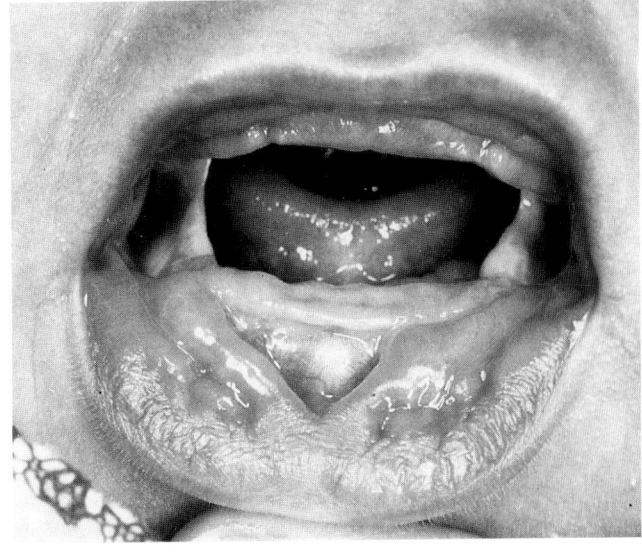

FIGURE 22.25. *Paramedian pits of lower lip. (A) Infant with bilateral symmetric paramedian pits of lower lip. Patient also had bilateral cleft lip (Van der Woude syndrome). (B) Lateral grooves of lower lip and syngnathia in popliteal pterygium syndrome.*

are present in about 12% of whites, in 20% of blacks, and in 6% of Japanese [122]. The pits range in depth from 0.5 to 2.5 cm. Rarely, they may be fistulous and/or infected [123] and have been reported with accessory bone and teeth [124] as a minor expression of lateral facial cleft.

Everett and Wescott [125] suggested single gene dominant inheritance, but we do not believe that there is single gene inheritance. Commissural pits may be associated with pretragal pits with higher than chance frequency.

Microscopically, the pits are lined by stratified squamous epithelium. In the underlying connective tissue, there is often a chronic inflammatory infiltrate.

Paramedian Pits of the Lower Lip (Van der Woude Syndrome)

Paramedian pits of the lower lip vary in size from small bilateral dimples on the vermilion border to large snoutlike structures in the midline to lateral grooves in the lower lip. Resulting fistulas are lined by stratified squamous epithelium and are connected at the base with the mucous glands of the lip by means of communicating ducts. Mucus may exude from the openings [12].

The pits may occur alone or in combination with cleft palate or cleft lip and agenesis of the second premolars as part of Van der Woude syndrome (Fig. 22.25A). Inheritance is autosomal dominant with variable expressivity [126]. The gene has been mapped to 1q23. Pits may also be seen in autosomal dominant popliteal pterygium syndrome [12] (Fig. 22.25B).

Lateral Sinus of the Upper Lip

The lateral sinus of the upper lip is located along the line of fusion of the median nasal and maxillary prominences—i.e., along the line of closure of the lip, probably represent-

ing a microform of cleft lip [127] (Fig. 22.26). It may be located in the vermilion and associated with minor salivary glands or may even extend into a palatal cyst. Bilateral sinuses have been reported [128].

Midline (Philtral) Sinus

The midline sinus is misnamed, being actually situated in the philtral area, ranging from the base of the nose to the vermilion of the upper lip [129] (Fig. 22.27). Only rarely is it situated within the vermilion [130].

The unbranched blind sinus extends to the anterior nasal spine. The sinus tract is lined by stratified squamous epithelium and, in some cases, is associated with skin appendages or even hyaline cartilage. Associated anomalies have included cleft palate, double frenulum, short frenulum, nasal dermoid, and sinus of the frenulum [131].

Although one cannot be certain, the midline sinus is probably formed by a relative paucity of ectomesenchyme in the midline at the point at which the two median nasal prominences merge [132]. This seems to be borne out by the combination of midline cleft of the upper lip and a philtral pit below the columella [133].

Sebaceous Glands of the Labial and Oral Mucosa (Fordyce's Granules)

Sebaceous glands on the lips or buccal mucosa (Fordyce's granules) are so common as to be usual rather than exceptional [134]. They occasionally present in the fetus or newborn [135].

Median Nodule of the Upper Lip

Autosomal dominant inheritance of median nodule of the upper lip has been reported [136, 137].

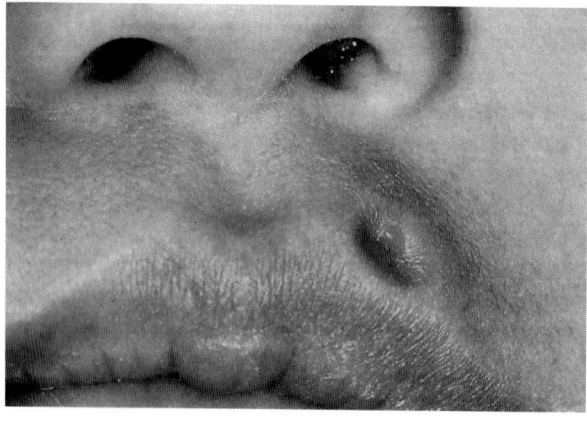

FIGURE 22.26.   *Lateral sinus of upper lip. Sinus is located at junction of median nasal and maxillary prominences.*

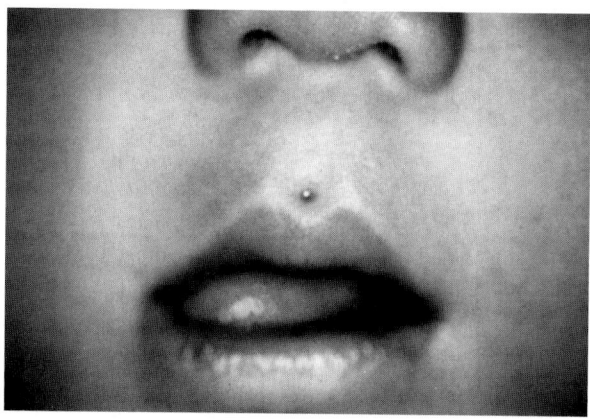

FIGURE 22.27.   *Midline (philtral) sinus. The pit may be located from the base of the nose to the vermilion of the upper lip.*

Upper Labial Frenum Anomalies

The upper labial frenum is a single structure in only about 60% of patients. About 20% have a small mucosal appendix, and another 10% have a nodule. In about 3%, the frenum is bifid. The frenum is absent in holoprosencephalic disorders. Less common anomalies include a hole or recess in the frenum (2.5%), persistent tectolabial frenum (2.5%), and duplicated frenum (0.5%). The most thorough study has been published by Sewerin [138].

Median Cleft of the Upper Lip, Double Frenum, and Hamartoma of the Columella and/or Anterior Alveolar Ridge

A median cleft of the upper lip may extend through the vermilion [139]. The cleft is associated with duplication of the maxillary median frenum [140]. There is a pedunculated club-shaped mass attached to the nasal septum and a similar mass attached to the midanterior alveolar process [141] (Fig. 22.28). Microscopically, it consists of fibrous connective tissue, adipose tissue, and striated muscle [103]. This represents a malformation of the primary palate [142]. A lipoma may be found in the corpus callosum or in the spinal canal [143].

The suggestion that this condition has autosomal dominant inheritance, we believe, is weak [139, 144].

Double Upper Lip

Double upper lip is not a true duplication of the lip. Although present at birth, it usually does not become apparent until the teeth have erupted [12, 145].

So-called double lip is characterized by a horizontally running groove located between the inner (pars villosa) and

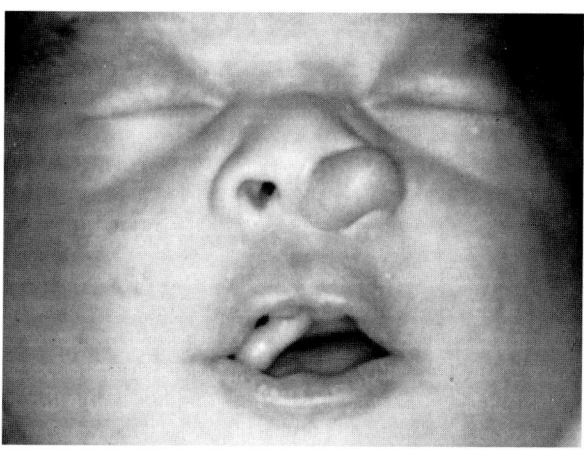

FIGURE 22.28. *Median cleft of upper lip, double frenum, and hamartoma of columella and/or anterior alveolar ridge. Masses extend from columella and from anterior alveolar process. Note subtle midline cleft of upper lip. (Courtesy of J Nakamura, Tokyo, Japan.)*

outer (pars glabrosa) parts. The inner fold cannot be seen when the lips are closed [146].

Gingival Cyst of Infancy (Bohn's Nodules, Dental Lamina Cysts)

Gingival cysts, 2 to 3 mm in diameter on or near the gingival surface, probably arise from cyst formation within the remnants of the dental lamina (Serres' glands) [147]. They may occur in both the free and attached gingiva or in the gingival papilla [148]. More commonly they are found on the maxillary gingiva and are multiple [149].

The cysts are lined by a thin layer of stratified squamous epithelium, and often are filled with concentric layers of parakeratin.

I-Cell Disease (Mucolipidosis II)

In I-cell disease, in addition to mental and somatic retardation and hypotonia, there are typical orofacial changes (flat supraorbital ridges, puffy eyelids, copious nasal discharge, full pink cheeks with overlying fine telangiectasia, and marked enlargement of the gingiva and alveolar processes), especially from the fourth month on. There is anterior open bite and macroglossia. The teeth are often buried. Storage material surrounds the crowns of unerupted molars.

Congenital Granular Cell Epulis

Congenital epulis (granular cell tumor) is a rare benign congenital growth of the anterior gingiva occurring almost exclusively in female infants (10F : 1M) (Fig. 22.29A). The maxilla is the site of the growth about twice as often as the mandible, but an infant may have lesions in both jaws [150]. Epulis has been detected in utero due to associated polyhydramnios [151]. The lesion does not grow after birth and does not recur even if incompletely resected. Spontaneous regression has been recorded [152].

The epulis arises at the gingival crest and is polypoid with a broad base, pink-red in color, nonulcerated, and 0.5 to 9.0 cm in size. It has no connection with the underlying bone or developing teeth.

Microscopically, the epulis consists of sheets of large, closely packed polyhedral cells with acidophilic granular cytoplasm and a delicate plexiform network of capillaries (Fig. 22.29B). A few strands of odontogenic epithelium may be seen. The nucleus is small, somewhat pyknotic, and eccentrically placed, and usually contains a single small nucleolus. The cytoplasmic granules are PAS-positive and diastase-resistant. Phosphatase activity is strong within the cytoplasm of the granular cells. In contrast to granular cell schwannoma, there is no overlying pseudoepitheliomatous hyperplasia and no demonstrable neural component. However, staining characteristics of the granular cells are similar in the two lesions when trichrome and PAS stains are used.

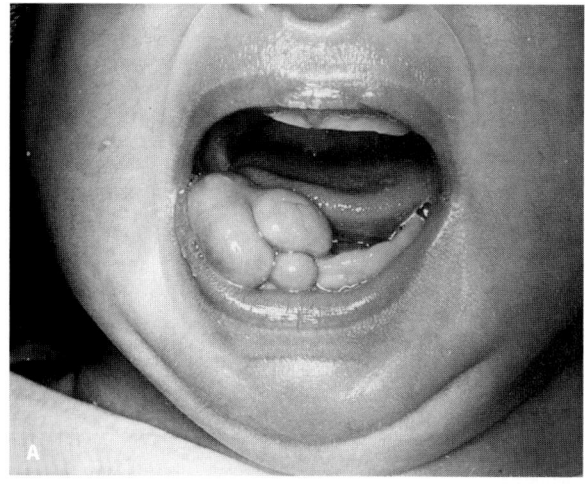

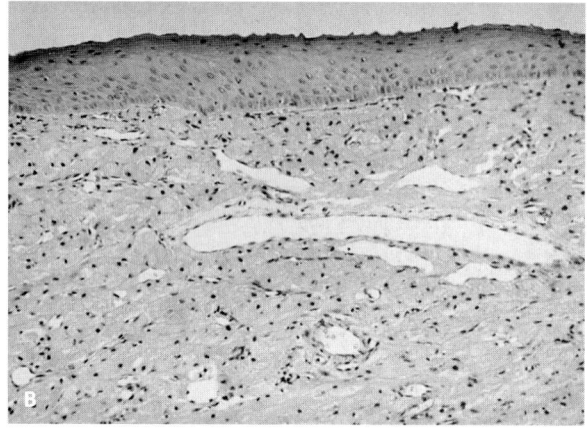

FIGURE 22.29.   *Congenital granular cell epulis.*
(A) Three-day-old female with multiple polypoid growths of anterior
mandibular gingiva. (B) The epulis consists of sheets of large, closely
packed polyhedral cells with acidophilic granular cytoplasm. (From
Silver HK, Simon JL. Am J Dis Child 1953; 93:687.)

There is a lack of positivity for S-100 protein (in contrast to granular cell schwannoma) and a positive reaction for carcinoembryonic antigen [150, 153].

Ultrastructural findings suggest an origin from mesenchymal cells—i.e., gingival stromal cells [154].

Melanotic Neuroectodermal Tumor of Infancy

The melanotic neuroectodermal tumor of infancy is a rare, usually benign, rapidly growing lesion of neural crest origin, largely seen in the anterior maxilla (75%) of infants [155] (Fig. 22.30A). Although usually a single lesion, multiple examples have been reported [156]. A few examples of aggressive spread have been recorded [157]. At the time of discovery of the tumor, the infant is frequently a few months of age. The tumor may rapidly enlarge and interfere with nursing. There is no gender predilection. Local recurrence rate is about 15%. In a survey of 195 cases, Mosby et al

[158] reported similar tumors in the calvaria (anterior fontanel) (10%), mandible (6%), epididymis (5%), brain (5%), mediastinum, and other sites. Borello and Gorlin [159] demonstrated that the tumor occasionally (2.5%) may elaborate vanilmandelic acid. They suggested neural crest origin and proposed the name "melanotic neuroectodermal tumor of infancy." Ultrastructural and histochemical evidence supports this view. CT and MRI aid in diagnosis [160].

Intrabony lesions are radiolucent with or without irregular margins ("sunray pattern").

Grossly, the tumor is often irregularly pigmented and well circumscribed, although no well-defined capsule is present. Microscopically, the tumor consists of fibrous connective tissue stroma in which tubules or spaces are present in large numbers. The spaces are lined by a single layer of large cuboid cells with abundant cytoplasm in which are found numerous melanin granules. The spaces frequently are filled with many deeply staining neuroblast-like cells that are smaller than the mural cells and contain much less cytoplasm (Fig. 22.30B). At the periphery, new bone is often formed [161]. The small dark cells are positive for neuron-specific enolase, synaptophysin, and dopamine β-hydroxylase [162]. The large cuboidal mural cells are cytokeratin-, vimentin-, and enolase-positive and exhibit melanosomes and tonofilaments [163]. Rare examples have been S-100 protein-positive, but most have been negative [158, 164]. Alphafetoprotein has been elevated in a few cases [164]. The few malignant examples have shown the same histologic picture as that of benign examples.

Orofacial Clefting

Orofacial clefting is extremely complex. Cleft lip is a cleft of the primary palate, while cleft palate is a cleft of the secondary palate. Microforms include bifid uvula, linear lip indentation, submucous cleft palate, and subepithelial cleft (intrauterine healed cleft) [165]. Combined clefts of the primary and secondary palates (cleft lip/palate) constitute 50%, while isolated cleft lip and isolated cleft palate each represent 25%. Cleft lip is usually unilateral and is twice as common on the left as on the right side [12, 166]. Soft tissue bridges (Simonart's bands) occur in 20–30% of those with otherwise complete clefts of the lip and palate [167].

There is also gender predilection. Cleft lip with or without cleft palate is etiologically distinct from isolated cleft palate and is twice as common in males as in females. Conversely, complete cleft palate is twice as common in females as in males.

The distinction between cleft lip with or without cleft palate [CL(P)] and isolated cleft palate has been confirmed [168]. Although an individual with CL(P) has a greater chance of having a child with the same anomaly, there is no more than a normal chance of having an offspring with isolated cleft palate. The same rule applies to a patient with isolated cleft palate. However, this rule breaks down when one deals with single gene cleft disorders such as Van der

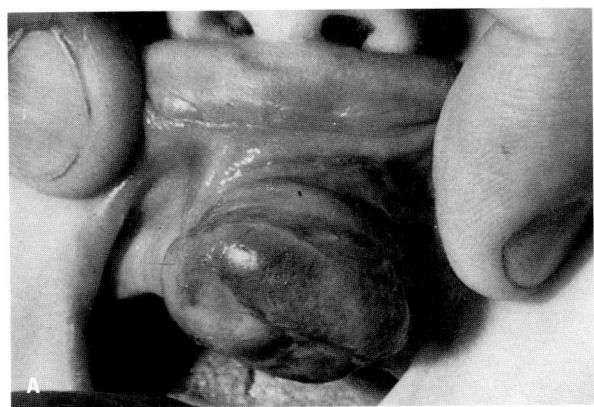

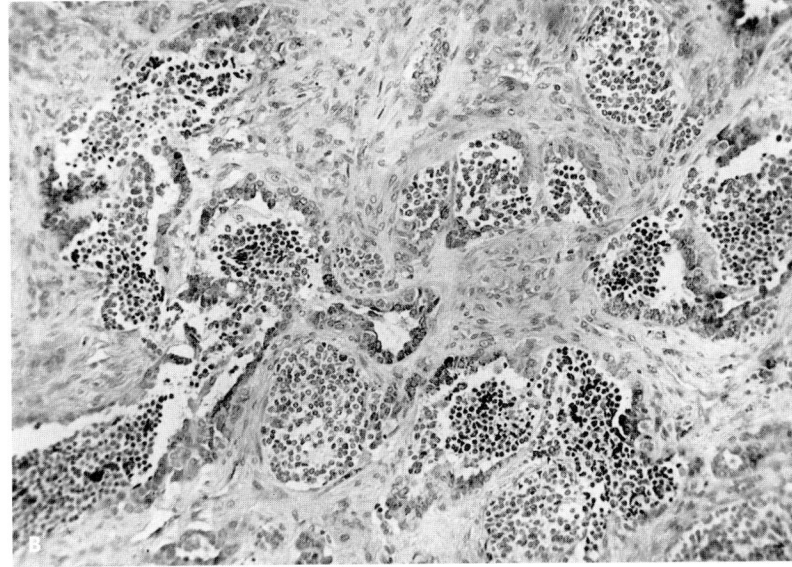

FIGURE 22.30. *Melanotic neuroectodermal tumor of infancy. (A) Pigmented solid mass of maxillary anterior gingiva. (B) Note spaces lined by large cuboidal cells with melanotic neuroblast-like cells within spaces. (From Borello and Gorlin [159].)*

Woude syndrome. Patients with this autosomal dominant syndrome of paramedian pits of the lower lip may have children with pits only or with cleft lip/palate or with isolated cleft palate with or without lip pits.

Embryology

Cleft of the primary palate involves failure of fusion of the median nasal prominence with the maxillary prominence, unilaterally or, less often, bilaterally. Fusion occurs during the 7th week embryologically. The primary palate consists of a philtral part and an alveolar part. The alveolar portion contains the maxillary central and lateral incisor teeth. The most posterior point of the primary palate is marked by the incisive papilla. In the case of bilateral cleft, the primary palate is suspended from the nasal septum and is often anteriorly displaced.

The secondary palate is formed from the palatine processes of the maxilla that are vertically directed to the side of the tongue. Closure of the secondary palate involves movement of the palatal shelves from this vertical orientation to the horizontal above the tongue, where they extend to the midline to meet and fuse. This complex process involves two factors: an intrinsic force in the shelves caused by increased turgidity following build-up of glycosaminoglycans which imbibe water; and tongue growth forward and downward, moving out of the space between the shelves, thereby reducing the tongue's resistance to the shelf force. Prior to the meeting of the shelves, the covering epithelia have undergone programmed cell death. Fusion thus entails the flow of ectomesenchyme from one side to the other following the death of the covering epithelium [10].

If the shelves do not meet each other at a fixed time, they will not fuse, either because they are too far apart to fuse or because the stage of epithelial breakdown has passed. Factors that delayed horizontal movement of the palatal shelves (diminished shelf force, increased tongue resistance) promote cleft palate.

In mice, major teratogens, mutant genes, or a combination of genetic or environmental factors result in cleft palate [169]. Humans, being composed of several subpopulations, have variable genetic liabilities. Based on animal models, we find attractive the notion that cleft lip and palate also fit a multifactorial threshold model.

Epidemiology

Clefts of the primary and secondary palates are among the more common congenital anomalies, representing causally heterogeneous developmental field defects. There is pronounced racial predilection. CL(P) is found in 1 in 1000 white births (range 0.0006–0.0013), in 1 in 600 births in Orientals, in 1 in 2500 births in blacks, and in 1 in 280 births in Native Americans [12, 166, 170] (Fig. 22.31A,B).

Isolated cleft palate has been reported to occur at rates from 1 in 2000 to 2 in 2500 births in both whites and blacks [12] (Fig. 22.31C). Submucous cleft palate is found in 1 in 1200 adults and in 3–7% of patients presenting at cleft palate clinics. Cleft uvula is seen in 2% of whites [12].

Heredity

Much has been written about oral clefts representing the interactions of genes and environment that determine susceptibility [171]. This has been borne out in studies of experimentally produced cleft palate in mice and in various combined human twin studies. In twins with CL(P), there is 60% concordance in monozygotic (MZ) twins and 10% in dizygotic (DZ) twins. In those with isolated cleft palate, concordance is about 25% in MZ twins compared with 5% in DZ twins [172]. In conjoined twins, clefting has nearly always been discordant [173].

There have been advocates for 1) polygenic inheritance (a large number of genes, each with small and equal effect), 2) oligogenic inheritance (major autosomal recessive gene, with or without additional polygenic variation), and 3) a mixed model [174–177].

An association between cleft lip and certain alleles of transforming growth factor-alpha (TGF-α) has been confirmed [178], but linkage has not been found [179]. TGF-α, which maps to 2p13, has been shown to be a potent epithelial mitogen, and plays a role in palatal development [180].

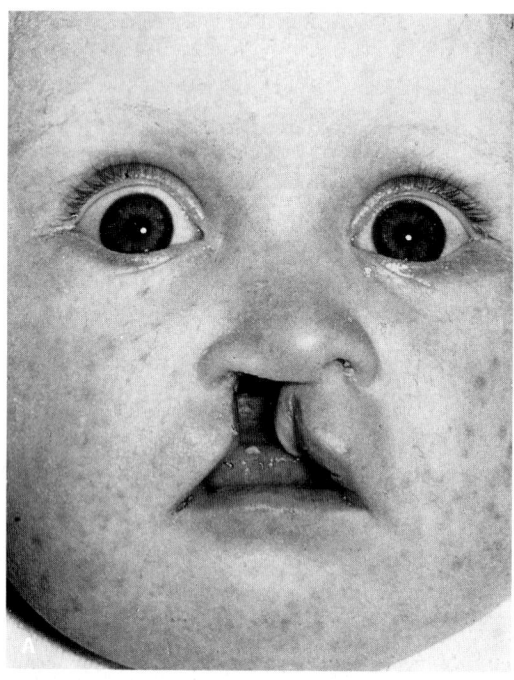
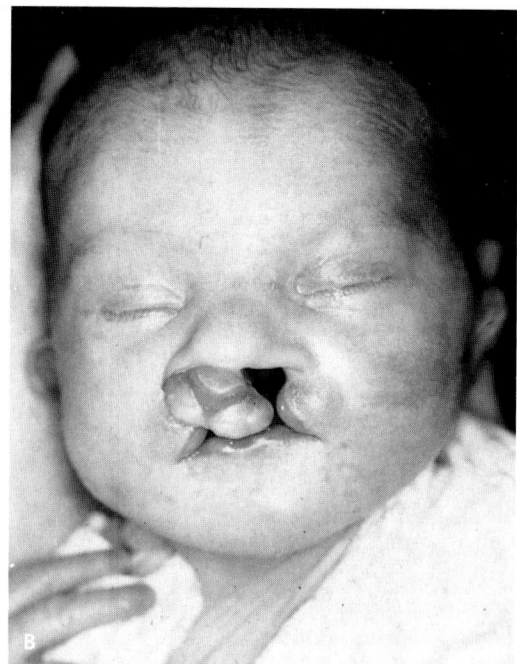
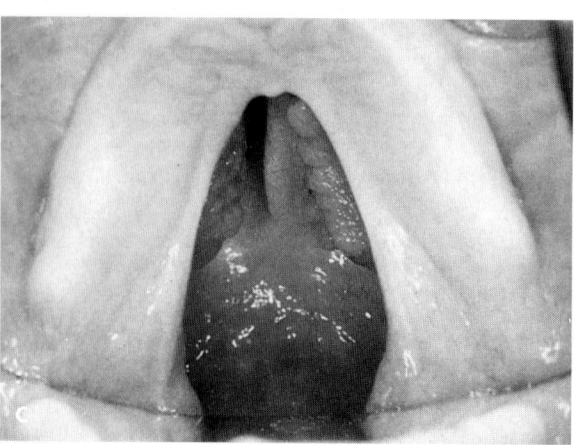

FIGURE 22.31.   *Common facial clefts. (A) Unilateral cleft lip/palate. (B) Bilateral cleft lip/palate. Note primary palate attached to nasal septum. Both alveolar and philtral portions are evident. (C) Cleft palate. Horseshoe-shaped complete cleft extends to incisive papilla.*

Risk of Recurrence

Based on the general concept of liability, one would expect that probands from different subpopulations will have different genetic liability. For example, an affected proband with an affected sib or an affected parent will have a greater liability than one who has normal parents and normal sibs. Further, those with more severe clefts would have a greater liability, and the recurrence risk would be greater than for those with clefts of mild degree [181].

Many investigations have provided us with enough data to provide families with empirical estimates of recurrence risks. These are, however, averages, not adjusted for individual family patterns. In general, the average risk for a male offspring of a parent affected with cleft lip is about 4%, but this increases to about 10% if the unaffected spouse has an affected sib [182]. The more severe the cleft, the greater the recurrence risk in a sib [181]. Cleft palate has lower heritability and lower recurrence risks.

In addition to the mixed model of inheritance discussed above, there have been several large families with X-linked cleft palate with or without ankyloblepharon [183, 184]. Female heterozygotes have variable expression. However, there is clearly genetic heterogeneity: the German and Icelandic families map to Xq21.3–q22 [185], while a native British Columbian kindred map to Xq13–q21.31 [183]. There are even families with autosomal dominant inheritance of clefting [186].

Several cleft syndromes have been mapped: Van der Woude syndrome to 1q32 [187]; Stickler syndrome and spondyloepiphyseal dysplasia congenita to 12q13.11 [188, 189], and cleft palate with or without ankyloglossia, as noted above, to Xq13 [184] and Xq21.3 [185].

Associated Anomalies

The frequency and types of anomalies that accompany orofacial clefting have been well documented [12]. Isolated cleft palate is associated much more commonly (13–50%) with other congenital anomalies than is isolated cleft lip (7–13%) or cleft lip/palate (2–11%) [12]. Although no definite data exist, cleft palate appears to be more highly syndromal.

Clefting syndromes probably number in excess of 350 but, in aggregate, constitute only about 5% of cases of orofacial clefting.

It appears that Robin sequence is heterogeneous, both etiologically and pathogenetically. Robin sequence (cleft palate, micrognathia, and glossoptosis) may occur by itself or in association with numerous other anomalies such as Stickler syndrome and velocardiofacial syndrome (Fig. 22.32).

Because the number of cleft syndromes is legion and the nature of this chapter is synoptic, the reader is referred to books and chapters that are more comprehensive [12, 169].

Unusual Forms of Orofacial Clefting

Unusual forms of orofacial clefting include median cleft of the upper lip, median cleft of the lower lip (discussed else-

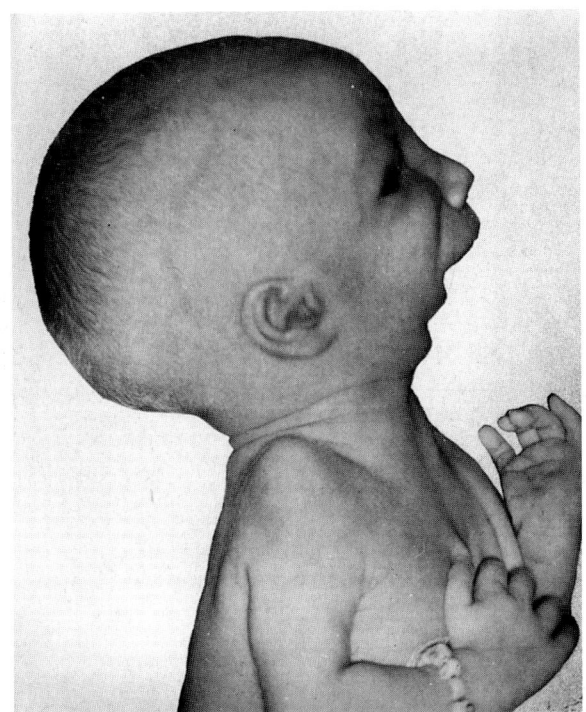

FIGURE 22.32. *Robin sequence. Extreme smallness of mandible is usually associated with cleft palate and glossoptosis. Many syndromes are associated with Robin sequence, principally Stickler syndrome and velocardiofacial syndrome.*

where in this chapter), and oblique and lateral facial clefts (Fig. 22.33).

Median cleft of the upper lip is a heterogeneity [190]. One form, often associated with holoprosencephaly, is characterized by failure of formation of the primary palate. The second type, resulting from persistence of the intranasal furrow, is observed in association with frontonasal dysplasia. A third type, caused by insertion of the maxillary labial frenum into the middle part of the upper lip, is encountered in such conditions as Ellis-van Creveld syndrome; the various orofaciodigital syndromes; Majewski short-rib polydactyly syndrome; and median cleft of the upper lip, double frenum and hamartoma of the columella and/or the anterior alveolar ridge [12].

Lateral facial cleft extends from the angle of the mouth toward the ear. It is somewhat variable in extent and direction, producing macrostomia. To a minor degree it may be seen in the oculoauriculovertebral spectrum, as an isolated phenomenon or with an accessory maxilla [191]. It represents clefting between the maxillary and mandibular prominences.

Oblique facial cleft is also extremely variable in degree and extent. It extends toward the eye from the lateral upper lip along the nasolacrimal canal—i.e., at the junction between the lateral nasal and maxillary prominences. It may accompany amniotic rupture sequence.

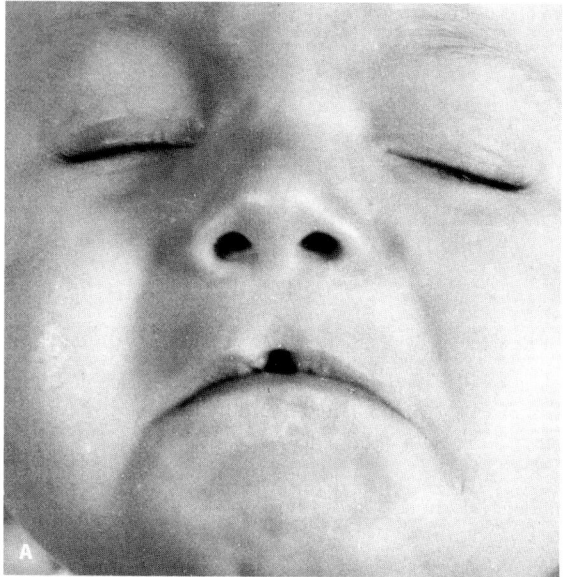

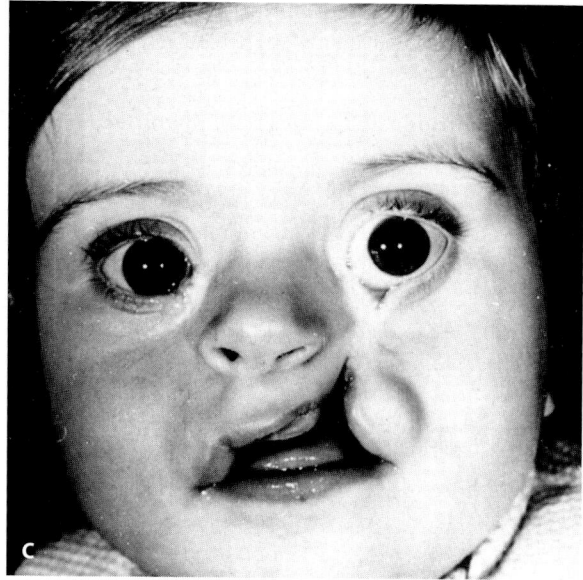

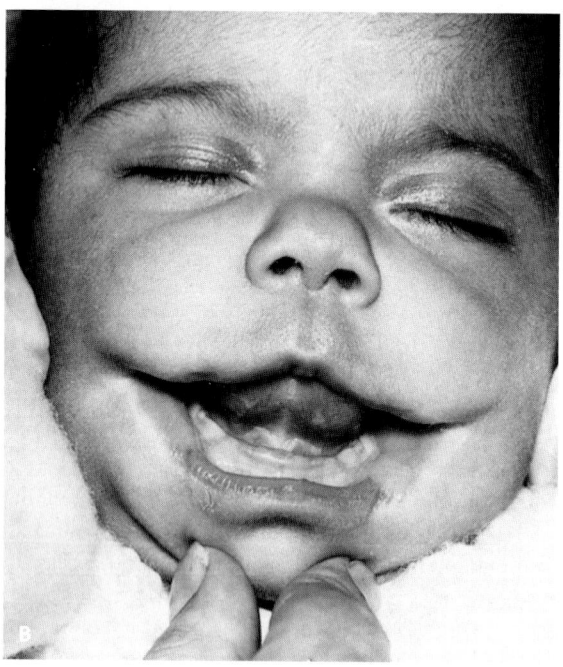

FIGURE 22.33. *Unusual orofacial clefts. (A) Median cleft of upper lip. (B) Lateral facial clefts. May be unilateral or bilateral, producing marked macrostomia. (C) Oblique facial cleft. Note that the cleft skirts the nose as it extends to the eye. There is a mild notch in contralateral portion of upper lip.*

Neither the lateral nor the oblique facial cleft appears to have single gene inheritance, nor are we aware of any evidence of oligofactorial inheritance for either cleft, resulting in increased recurrence risks.

Median Mandibular Cleft

Some examples of median mandibular cleft are very mild, involving only the lower lip and sparing the bone (Fig. 22.34). Most are more extensive, about 35% cleaving the tongue and producing ankyloglossia, the tongue tip being attached to the cleft by a broad frenum. On the other hand, the cleft may be very extensive, bifurcating the mandible, the tongue, and structures of the midneck down to the

hyoid bone. The hyoid bone and, rarely, the manubrium of the sternum are absent. About 100 examples have been published [192, 193].

Absence of the Vestibular Sulcus

Attachment of the labial mucosa to the free margin of the gingiva in the anterior region is essentially limited to the Ellis–van Creveld syndrome (chondroectodermal dysplasia) [12]. This disorder consists of bilateral manual postaxial polydactyly, chondrodysplasia of long bones resulting in acromelic dwarfism, hypoplastic nails, dysplastic teeth, and, less often, congenital heart malformations. The syndrome exhibits autosomal recessive inheritance.

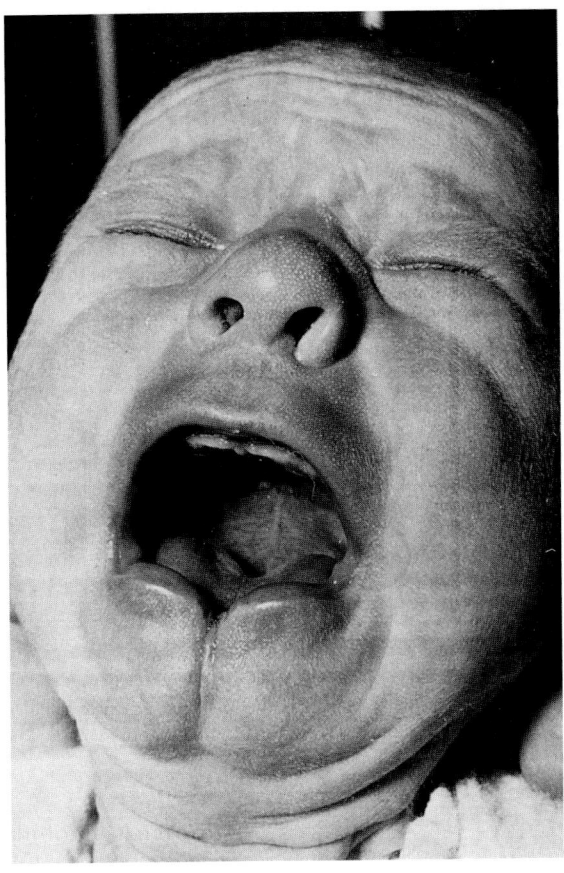

FIGURE 22.34. *Cleft mandible. Extremely variable in expression, cleft mandible ranges from a notch in the midline of the lower lip to a cleft that extends to the manubrium of the sternum.*

Associated oral anomalies include midline defect of the upper lip, natal teeth, teeth with conical crown form, and serration of the lower alveolar process.

Midpalatal Raphe Cyst of Infancy (Epstein's Pearls)

Nearly all humans after the 4th month of fetal life, and at least 80% of newborn infants, have small nodules or cysts (Epstein's pearls) at the junction of the hard and soft palates near the median raphe [194]. These nodules, usually several in number and white to yellowish white, are small epithelial inclusion cysts resulting from incorporation of epithelium during the embryonic process of palatal fusion [195]. Thus, they are fissural cysts. These cysts become superficial and rupture, usually within the first few weeks of life [196]. They are usually about 1 mm or less in diameter, are lined by a thin layer of stratified squamous epithelium, and often are filled with concentric layers of parakeratin.

Agnathia (Otocephaly)

The combination of agnathia, microstomia, hypoglossia, and synotia is known as otocephaly [197] (Fig. 22.35). Agnathia

(failure of formation of the mandibular arch), or, more often, hypognathia associated with synotia (fusion of external ears) in the midline region normally occupied by the mandible, is quite striking. A remnant of the tongue base is frequently present low in the pharynx. Microphthalmia may be noted [198]. The parotid and submandibular salivary glands are absent [199]. Although the oral opening may be missing (astomia), more often it is minute—i.e., 2 to 3 mm in diameter with the long axis usually rotated 90°. In some cases, there is no communication with the pharynx, possibly as a result of persistence of the buccopharyngeal membrane. The soft palate may be deficient as well. This condition is incompatible with life. Nearly all cases have been associated with hydramnios [199]. Agnathia has been diagnosed in utero [200], and more than 80 cases have been reported.

There have been several reports of agnathia in combination with cyclopia (hypognathic cyclopia) [201]. These cases differ from classic cyclopia in that the proboscis-like structure usually located above the centrally located eye is absent (Fig. 22.36). Otocephaly may be associated with various anomalies of the viscera [202]. Familial occurrence has been reported [201].

Lateral Palatal Synechiae

Unilateral or bilateral bands of mucosa, extending from the edges of a palatal cleft to the lateral margins of the tongue or oral floor, are called lateral palatal synechiae. This syndrome has variable expressivity [203].

It has been assumed that this condition has autosomal dominant inheritance [203], but Nakata et al [204] described it in sibs, suggesting autosomal recessive inheritance; however, gonadal mosaicism cannot be excluded.

Oromandibular-Limb Hypogenesis Syndrome

Included within this spectrum are glossopalatine ankylosis, hypoglossia-hypodactylia, Hanhart syndrome, Möbius syndrome, and other variants [12].

Attachment of the tip of the tongue to the hard palate (glossopalatine ankylosis) may be associated with other congenital anomalies (ankyloglossum superior syndrome). The tongue tip is attached to the hard palate or upper alveolar ridge, or, in the case of cleft palate, to the lower edge of the nasal septum [205]. The mandible is underdeveloped. Hypodontia principally affecting the incisors is frequent. Ankylosis of the temporomandibular joint has been mentioned in a few cases.

Frequently associated are digital anomalies, often asymmetric: syndactyly, hypoplasia of the thumb, clinodactyly, peromelia, absence of nails, ectrodactyly, and absence of tarsal bones. The combination of peromelia and micrognathia is termed Hanhart syndrome.

When cranial nerve involvement is present (VI and VII; less often III, V, IX, and XII), the condition is called Möbius syndrome [206].

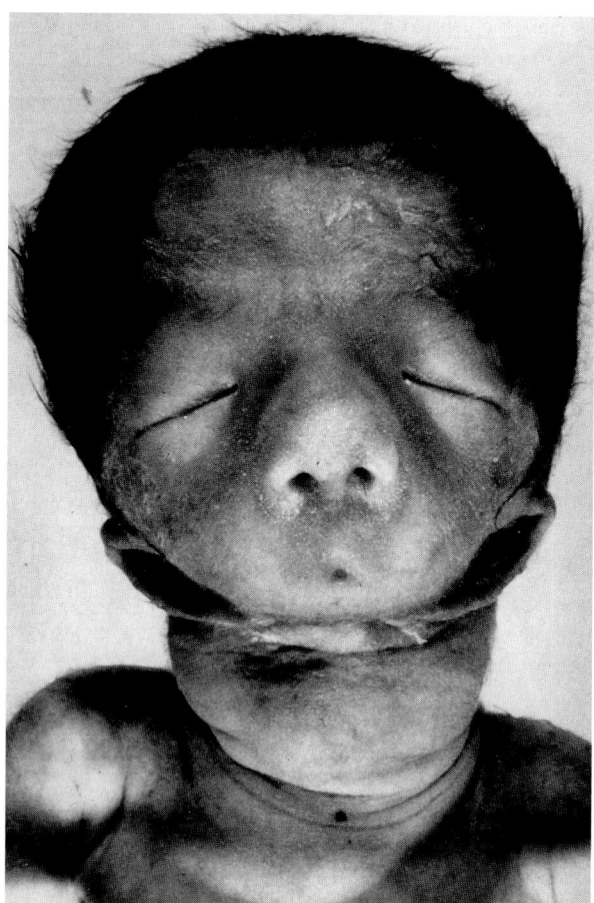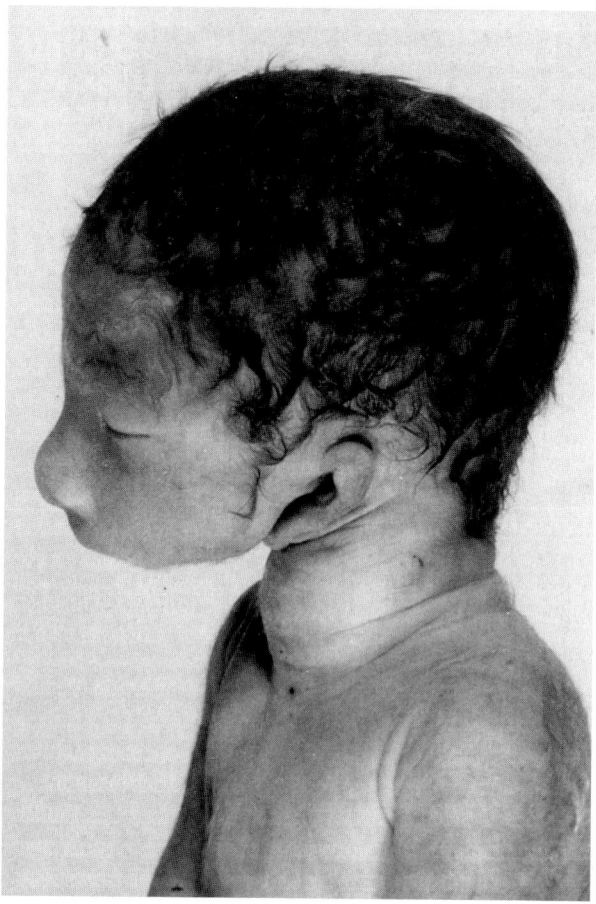

FIGURE 22.35. *Agnathia. Absence of mandible. Note microstomia and synotia.*

Familial transmission has been reported in a few cases in which no limb abnormalities have been found. Otherwise, the recurrence risk has been about 2% [207].

There has been a recent suggestion that limb hypogenesis occurs more often than chance in association with chorionic villus sampling at 55 to 65 days [208], but disagreement is abundant.

Patent Nasopalatine Ducts

Rarely reported, patent nasopalatine ducts, either unilateral or bilateral, are epithelial-lined canals that connect the oral cavity with the vomeronasal olfactory organs of Jacobson. These vestigial bodies normally disappear before birth in humans. The canals, usually two, are located at the site of fusion of the primary and secondary palates. Rarely the ducts are not totally patent.

The nasopalatine ducts are lined with respiratory epithelium, epithelial remnants (pearls), and mucous glands. Cysts that develop later in this area are known as cysts of the nasopalatine canal or cysts of the incisive papilla depending on the oral/nasal location [209].

There appears to be a significant (10:3) male predilection [210].

Fistulas of the Lateral Soft Palate

Unilateral or, more often, bilateral symmetric defects of the soft palate may occur as isolated anomalies or with absence of one or both palatine tonsils [211].

Supernumerary Mouth and/or Jaw

Supernumerary mouth and/or jaw is rare indeed (Fig. 22.37). While examples are sufficiently different from one another to make each unique, for purposes of discussion we will consider four forms: 1) single mouth with replication of mandibular segments containing teeth, 2) supernumerary mouth laterally placed with rudimentary mandible, 3) single mouth with duplication of maxillary arch, and 4) true facial duplication (diprosopus) with or without anencephaly. Barr [212] proposed a different classification.

Duplication probably arises from various causes: forking of notochord, doubling of prosencephalon, doubling of

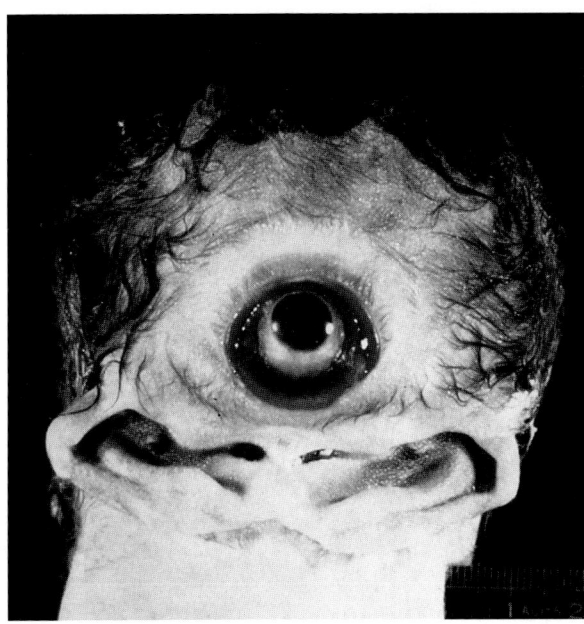

FIGURE 22.36. *Hypognathic cyclopia. This condition is a combination of cyclopia and agnathia. Proboscis is absent in this disorder.*

olfactory placodes, and duplication of maxillary and/or mandibular growth centers around the stomadeal plate [12]. A case of replication of the jawbone segments containing teeth (polygnathism) in which there was a single oral cavity has been reported [213]. There appears to be a 2:1 female predilection.

An accessory blind-ended mouth that contained bits of mandible and teeth has been described. Often there has been an accessory tongue [161, 214]. The mouth, surrounded by functional lips, has been laterally positioned, often below the angle of the normal mouth. Even an example in the temporal region has been found [215]. Two pituitary glands were noted by Bacsich et al [161].

There have been several examples of children with two palates, a double set of maxillary teeth, and a grooved or trifurcated tongue (due to failure of fusion of the three tubercules) [196, 216]. Even more complex cases of midfacial duplication have been reported by other authors [212, 217].

Diprosopus, the most extreme form of doubling, is usually characterized by two lateral eyes, a median eye, and doubling of the hypophysis, mouth, and nose [218]. A somewhat intermediate example has been described by Obwegeser et al [219]. Some examples have also been anencephalic [220]. One case with epignathus has been reported [221].

Supernumerary Tongue

Supernumerary tongue represents partial or complete duplication. It is often part of supernumerary mouth [222].

Although there are many examples, each case is unique. In some cases there is a single mouth with replication of mandibular segments. Others present a supernumerary mouth laterally placed, often with a rudimentary mandible. Finally, there is true facial duplication (diprosopus) with or without anencephaly. An extra tonguelike process may extend from the tonsillar area in the oculoauriculovertebral spectrum [223].

Tongue duplication has been discordant in identical twins [217]. It has been reported in association with cleft palate [224].

Syngnathia

Syngnathia refers to fusion of the upper and lower jaws by either fibrous or bony adhesions (see Fig. 22.25B). Bony attachment is much rarer than fibrous union [225]. Association with cleft palate has been well demonstrated [12]. Presumably, the primary defect is fusion between gingivae or alveolar processes, which in turn prevents the tongue from dropping and thereby preventing closure of the palatal shelves.

The mandible is usually small (micrognathia). In cases of firm bony fusion, the temporomandibular joint is usually ankylosed because movement is necessary during the developmental period [226].

Intraoral adhesions may also be associated with paramedian pits of the lower lip (Van der Woude syndrome), popliteal pterygium syndrome, lateral palatal synechiae and cleft palate, and posterior palatal synechiae and cleft palate [12].

Infantile Cortical Hyperostosis (Caffey-Silverman Disease)

Although infantile cortical hyperostosis principally affects infants under 6 months of age, there are several examples of this disorder being identified at birth or even prenatally. The most constant features are bilateral swelling over the mandible or other bones, radiograph evidence of new bone formation in the area, hyperirritability, and mild fever. Autosomal dominant inheritance has been repeatedly demonstrated [227]. Saul et al [228] indicated that familial infantile cortical hyperostosis seems to differ in several respects from sporadic instances, the former having an earlier onset of disease (25% at birth), less frequent mandibular, ulnar, and clavicular involvement, no involvement of ribs and scapulae, and more frequent lower extremity involvement. There is reason to believe that the sporadic form is disappearing [12]. Onset is about 10 weeks in the sporadic form and about 7 weeks in the familial form, but there has been radiographic evidence of disease as early as 5 weeks prenatally to 20 months after birth [227]. Cayler and Peterson [229] estimated that the disorder is found in three of every 1000 registered patients under 6 months of age. It has been suggested the pathogenesis is based on congenital abnormality

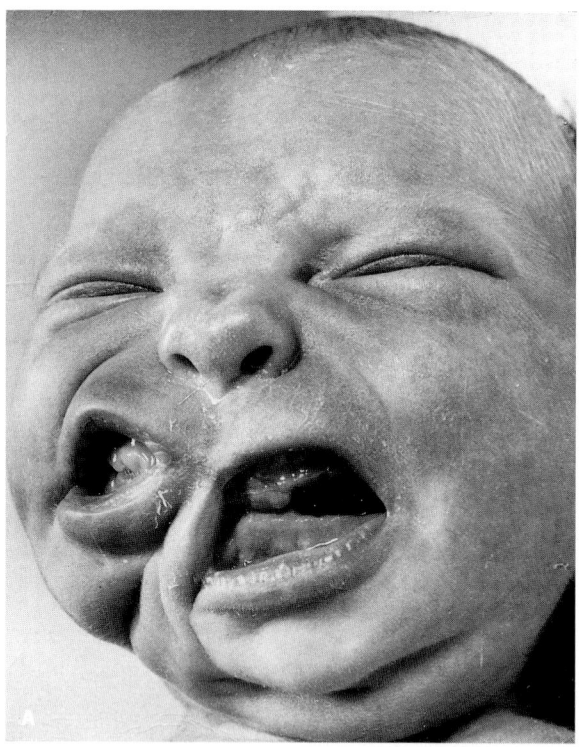

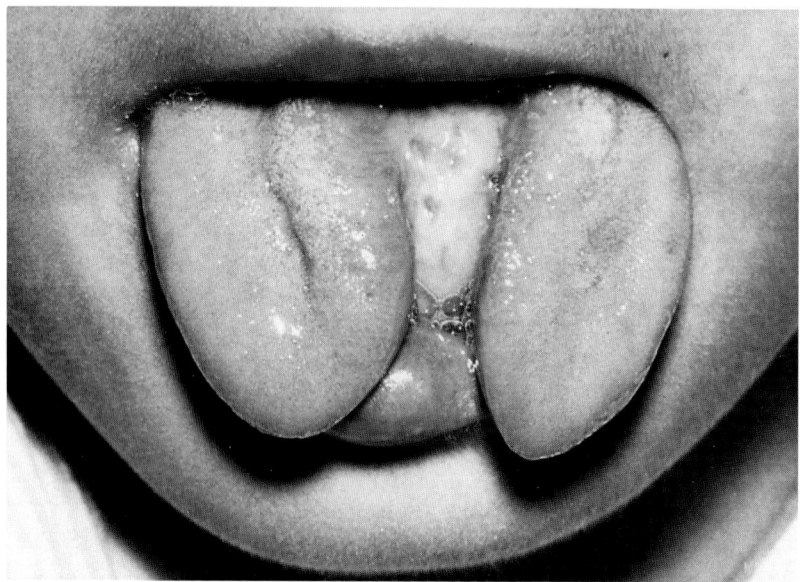

FIGURE 22.37. *Duplication. (A) Partial doubling of lower face with two mouths. (B) Doubling of tongue. (From Bacisch et al [161].)*

of vessels supplying the periosteum of the involved bones, with the hypoxia effecting focal necrosis of the overlying soft tissues and resulting in new subperiosteal bone formation [230].

Anemia, leukocytopenia, and elevation of the sedimentation rate occur in more than half the patients [12].

Congenital Oral Teratoma

"Epignathus," "episphenoid," "epipalatus," "palatopagus," and "sphenopagus parasiticus" are terms that have been employed to describe a teratoma arising in the region of Rathke's pouch and projecting into and filling the pharynx

or oral cavity between the palatal halves and at times protruding from the mouth and causing airway obstruction [231] (Fig. 22.38). About 50% of affected infants live beyond the neonatal period [232].

At times, the base of the skull is intact, but usually the base is separated, the teratoma having an hourglass shape, with intracranial and extracranial portions. Some teratomas, arising at the sphenoid, bulge into the cheek. Still others have no connection with the sphenoid bone [233, 234].

Because about 50% of these teratomas are attached to the sphenoid, 25% to the lateral wall of the epipharynx near the opening of the eustachian tube, and the rest to the soft palate or hard palate, the term "epignathus" is ill-chosen and

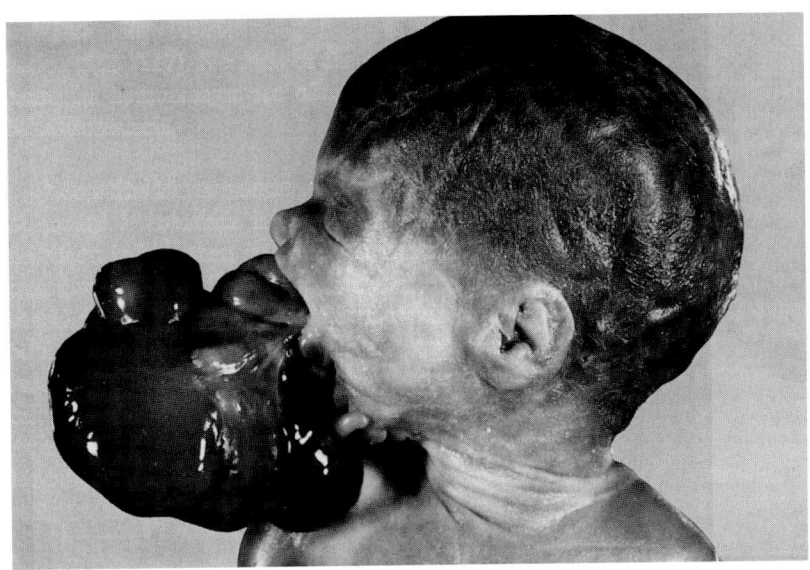

FIGURE 22.38. *Oropharyngeal teratoma. Protrusion of teratoma through mouth. (From Conran RM et al. Am J Perinatol 1993; 10:71.)*

should be abandoned. Congenital oral teratomas appear to have some female predilection [235].

Oral teratomas have varied considerably in structure. In one case, a well-formed finger was found on the upper surface of a small, grapefruit-sized teratoma [236]. Most have been somewhat cystic, lined by skin and cutaneous appendages, and composed of connective tissue. Cysts lined by columnar epithelium with smooth muscle in the walls, bones (with and without joints), embryonal neural epithelium, cartilage, liver, intestinal epithelium, etc., have been found in these teratomas. Rarely, oral and paraoral teratomas have contained teeth [237]. Theories of their origin have been legion [238]. We prefer to believe that they arise from fetal totipotential cells that have become isolated and undergo unrestricted growth.

Fetal ultrasound may provide adequate warning. CT or MRI scans should rule out encephalocele [239, 240].

Natal Teeth

Rarely (1 in 2000 white infants), teeth are present at birth (natal teeth) or within the first month (neonatal teeth) (Fig. 22.39). In 90%, the teeth are part of the normal deciduous dentition. Natal teeth may be an isolated finding or, occasionally, may be found in association with other anomalies (chondroectodermal dysplasia, pachyonychia congenita, Wiedemann-Rautenstrauch syndrome, and oculomandibulodyscephaly) [12].

Hypoglossia and Microglossia (Aglossia)

Hypoglossia and microglossia are rare congenital anomalies. Severe hypoglossia is often associated with other defects, especially diminution of the extremities (oromandibular-limb hypogenesis syndromes; hypoglossia-hypodactyly syndrome) [223]. The term "aglossia" is not accurate, because a small nubbin of tongue is always present. It is located pos-

teriorly at the level of the genioglossal processes and consists essentially of that part normally developed from the copula. Cleft palate and bony fusion of the jaws have been associated with microglossia [12].

Macroglossia

The term "macroglossia" is nonspecific, referring only to the presence of an enlarged tongue. This term is used erroneously when it refers to a normal-sized tongue in a small

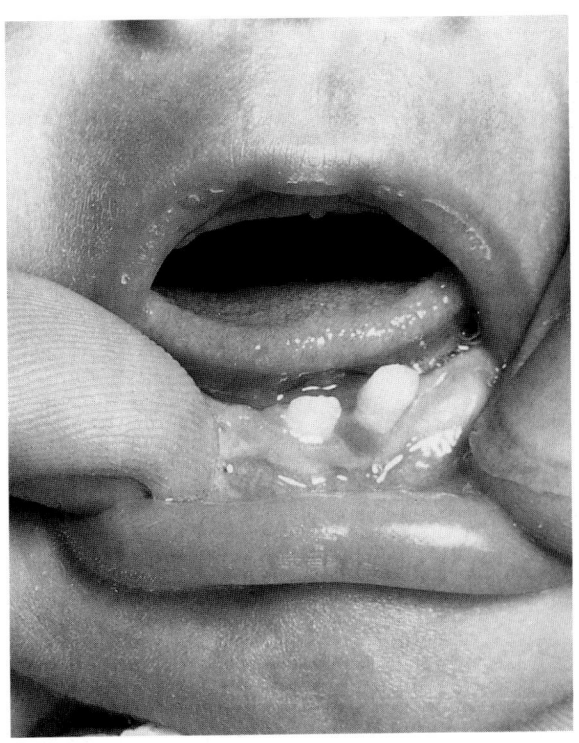

FIGURE 22.39. *Natal teeth. Natal teeth are usually part of the normal deciduous dentition.*

mouth (relative macroglossia) [241]. In cases observed at birth or in the neonatal period, the usual cause is lymphangioma or hemangiolymphangioma [242]. Rarely there may be true muscular hypertrophy or an increase in size due to neurofibromatosis. Enlargement of half the tongue occurs in congenital hemifacial hyperplasia (Fig. 22.40). The tongue may protrude from the mouth in trisomy 21, congenital hypothyroidism, Hurler syndrome, Beckwith-Wiedemann syndrome, Pompe disease (glycogen storage disease, type 2), GM_1 gangliosidosis, mannosidosis, hereditary angioedema, I-cell disease, and many other conditions [12, 223].

Respiratory Epithelium or Nonciliated Columnar Epithelial Lined Cyst of the Tongue

A cyst of the tongue that contains respiratory epithelium would be classified as a choristoma. As with the more numerous enterogenous cyst of the tongue, a cyst lined by either ciliated or nonciliated epithelium is entirely enclosed within the body of the tongue [243]. Like enterogenous cysts, these cysts represent foregut epithelial remnants having the potential to differentiate into this form of epithelium. The same explanation may be given for lingual cysts lined by nonkeratinized stratified squamous epithelium. It should be borne in mind that the primitive foregut gives rise to parts of both the digestive system and the respiratory tract. A similar example has been reported in the skin of the chin [244].

Epidermoid and Dermoid Cysts of the Tongue

Both epidermoid and dermoid cysts of the anterior half of the tongue in the newborn are rare. They may be large

and may interfere with feeding [245]. Congenital cysts located at the base of the tongue are usually thyroglossal duct cysts [246]. However, in the case of Howell and Prince [247], there was no evidence to suggest that this was the case.

As in other areas, the epidermoid cyst is lined by stratified squamous epithelium [248], while dermoid cysts are lined by stratified squamous epithelium plus skin derivatives [249]. Some are lined by a combination of stratified squamous and ciliated columnar epithelium [250].

Oral Cysts with Gastric, Intestinal, and/or Respiratory Epithelium

Heterotopic islands of gastric, intestinal, and/or respiratory epithelium (enterocytomas) have been found throughout the gastrointestinal tract, and a large number have been reported in the tongue or oral area [251]. A similar entity has been described in the lip [252].

The choristomatic cyst may be entirely enclosed within the body of the tongue (most often), oral floor, lip, hypopharynx, submandibular gland, or (rarely) anterior neck [253, 254]. The cystic wall may be composed of highly differentiated and organized tissues, partly of stratified squa-

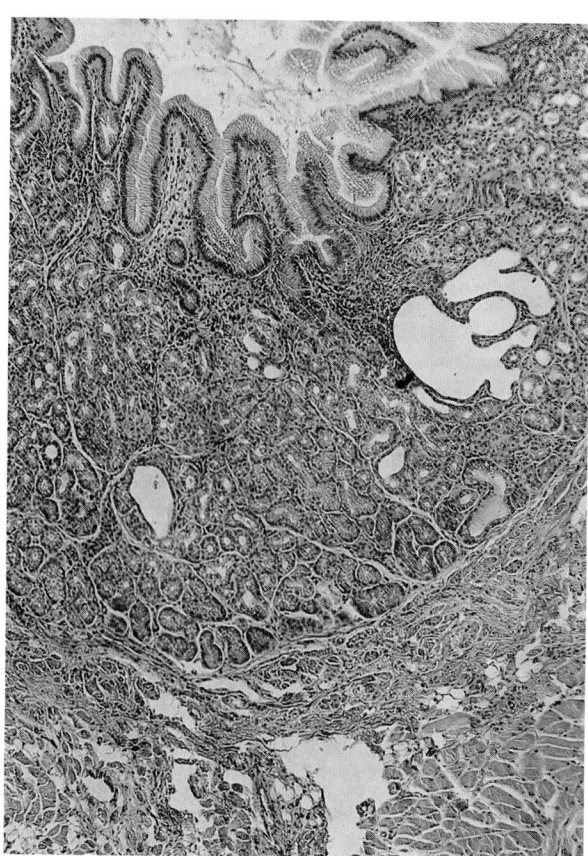

FIGURE 22.41.   *Oral cyst with gastric mucosa. Mucosa of both fundic and body type are present.*

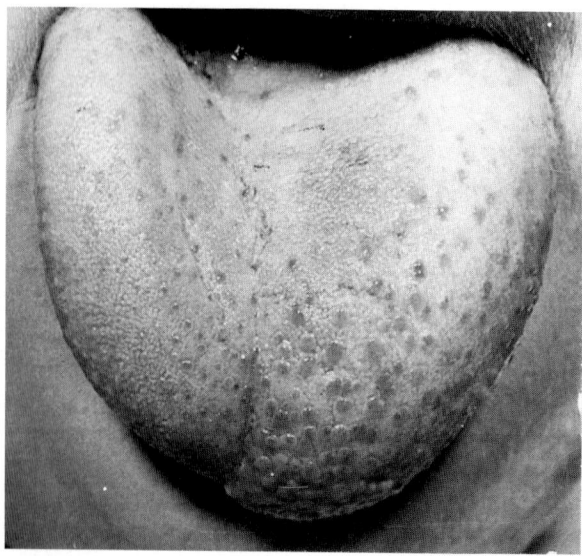

FIGURE 22.40.   *Hemihyperplasia of tongue. Note enlarged fungiform papillae of left half of tongue as well as absolute enlargement.*

mous and partly (or, in rare cases, totally) of gastric mucosa of the type seen in the body and fundus of the stomach or of the intestinal mucosa [255] (Fig. 22.41). Occasionally, Brunner's glands are noted. Oral dermoid cyst and choristomatous cyst can occur together [256]. In cases where there is a tube extending from the cyst to the oral mucosa, sebaceous glands have emptied into the tube. Some are partly lined by pseudostratified ciliated columnar epithelium, which we suspect is derived from displacement of embryonal rests and represents their pluripotentiality.

Hamartoma of the Tongue: Mixed Type

Mixed-type hamartoma of the tongue is a benign lesion consisting of oddly arranged, focally overgrown, mixed tissue elements indigenous to the tongue [257]. The hamartoma usually presents as a spherical mass covered by normal oral mucosa. It has limited growth capacity and does not invade surrounding tissues. Microscopically, it consists of mucous salivary glands, adipose tissue, nerves, smooth muscle, connective tissue, and blood vessels [258]. It is difficult to separate this lesion from the so-called benign mesenchymoma of the tongue. Most examples have been found incidentally, often due to interference with feeding, and have been located at the base of the tongue in the foramen cecum area. Exceptions to this rule are lingual hamartomas associated with orofaciodigital syndromes, such as that noted by Ishii et al [259].

Lingual Thyroid

Lingual thyroid should be suspected when a mass or nodule is located at the level of the foramen cecum in front of the terminal sulcus of the tongue. Radioactive iodine 123 or technetium 99m scanning and CT scan are used to demonstrate the presence of thyroid tissue at the lingual location.

Lingual thyroid generally presents as a round, purplish, firm nodule, 2 to 3cm in diameter. Ninety percent of cases occur at the level of the foramen cecum, but some patients may present thyroid tissue embedded in the body of the tongue, sublingually, or, rarely, in the anterior portion of the tongue [260] (Fig. 22.42). Some patients may have obstructive problems such as dysphagia (50%), dysphonia (44%), or dyspnea (28%). More than 70% of patients with lingual thyroid have total absence of the normally located thyroid gland. Infants with lingual thyroid may present symptoms of hypothyroidism [261].

The thyroid gland is formed during weeks 3 to 4 of embryonal development by invagination of proliferating endoderm in the floor of the pharynx at the level of the future foramen cecum on the dorsal surface of the tongue, between the tuberculum impar and the copula. This tissue descends in front of the pharyngeal gut but remains attached to the tongue by a thin evanescent canal known as the *thyroglossal duct*. Ectopic thyroid tissue can be found at different levels of the duct, from the tongue base to the neck. Failure of descent of this epithelial proliferation results in ectopic thyroid.

More than 400 cases of this anomaly have been reported in the literature, with a 4–5F:1M gender predilection [261]. Residual thyroid tissue has been found in the vicinity of the foramen cecum in 10% of 200 routine autopsies, with equal distribution between the genders [262]. Williams et al [263] reported the frequency of lingual thyroid at 1.3 per 10,000 births.

Nearly all examples of lingual thyroid have been isolated. However, there are a few examples in siblings [264–266]. Sensorineural hearing loss has been an associated finding in a few cases [267].

Lymphangioma of the Tongue

Congenital lymphangioma of the anterior two-thirds of the tongue may occur alone or, more often, in combination with involvement of the oral floor (Fig. 22.43). About 5% are associated with cystic hygroma of the neck. The tongue

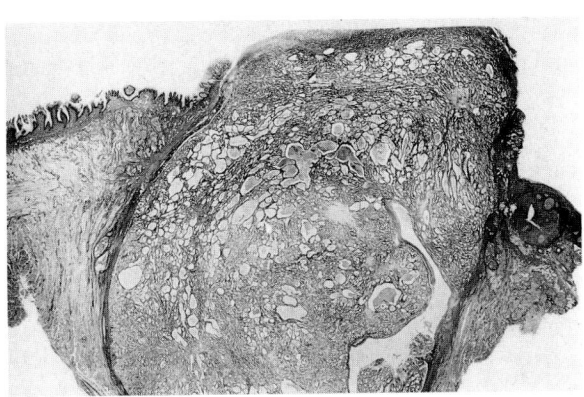

FIGURE 22.42. *Lingual thyroid. Nodule of thyroid rises above surface of tongue at site of foramen cecum.*

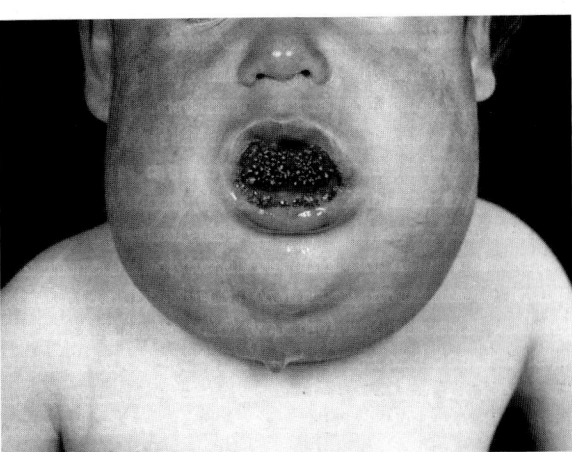

FIGURE 22.43. *Lymphangioma of tongue. The lymphangioma also involves the oral floor.*

surface is covered with nodular masses, 1 to 3 mm in diameter, composed of lymph-filled vesicles of various sizes. Some rupture, and others become papillomatous, almost grapelike in size. Most are pink, although some are purplish, indicating a hemangiolymphangiomatous component. Superficial ulceration and infection with subsequent macroglossia are common following trauma [223].

Presenting at birth, the lesions grow slowly and remain essentially quiescent. Some are relatively localized, but about 40% are diffuse, involving more than one-half the dorsal surface. There is no gender predilection [268].

Microscopically, the oral lymphangioma is composed of large, thin-walled, lymph-containing, endothelial-lined spaces located within a stroma of thin, fibrous connective tissue. Some spaces are quite superficial, being covered by only a thin layer of stratified squamous epithelium. Others are deeply situated between muscle bundles.

Teratoma of the Tongue

Although teratomas of the head and neck constitute 3–9% of all teratomas, very few examples in the tongue have been reported. Some have been enclosed within the body of the tongue; others have been attached to the tongue base or side by a pedicle [269, 270].

In contrast to epidermal cysts and dermoid cysts, teratoid cysts exhibit all three germ layer derivatives. Most contain immature neuroectodermal tissue, but bone, cartilage, skin, muscle, and cystlike structures lined by various types of epithelia, including ependyma, have been seen. There has been neither gender nor racial predilection [271].

Size has ranged from a few centimeters to 10 cm in diameter. Associated anomalies have included umbilical and/or inguinal hernia and cleft palate. All examples have been benign.

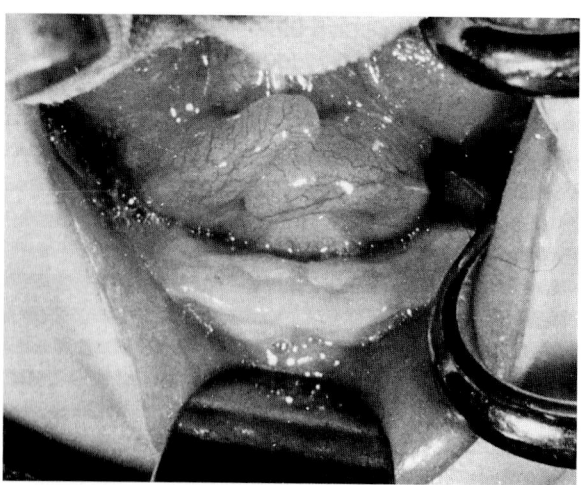

FIGURE 22.44.   *Imperforate submandibular ducts.*

SALIVARY GLANDS

Agenesis of the Salivary Glands and Ducts

The major salivary glands or one or more lobes may be symmetrically aplastic or severely hypoplastic. Duct orifices may be missing, but the ducts may be present [272]. Not infrequently, the lacrimal glands also fail to develop [273]. Lack of secretions causes severe dryness of the oral and conjunctival mucosae. The teeth have extensive caries and often fracture at the neck.

Several reports indicate autosomal dominant inheritance [274, 275]. Nuclear medicine scanning and MRI are ideal to detect function and to define anatomy of the glands [276]. Aplasia of salivary glands may also be found in lacrimoauriculodentodigital (LADD) syndrome [12]. Unilateral parotid aplasia may occur as an isolated finding or may be seen in oculoauriculovertebral spectrum (hemifacial microsomia) [12] and agnathia [199].

Agenesis of duct openings may be reported as "congenital ranula" [277] (Fig. 22.44).

Accessory Salivary Ducts

Supernumerary salivary ducts of the submandibular gland are rare congenital anomalies [278]. The ducts usually share a common orifice. They are usually discovered incidentally later in life [279]. Occasionally the supernumerary duct is associated with a supernumerary gland [272].

Salivary Gland and Duct Heterotopia

Submandibular salivary gland tissue may be included in the mandible, usually near the angle, where it may be seen as "Stafne's cyst." Sublingual gland tissue may be found in the symphysis and premolar region [280].

Rare heterotopias of salivary gland tissue include the hypophysis, external and middle ears, thyroglossal duct, capsules of the thyroid and parathyroid glands, tonsils, lymph nodes, and upper and lower neck regions [281]. Salivary ducts incorporated in lymph nodes give rise to Warthin's tumor (papillary cystadenoma lymphomatosum) later in life. Accessory parotid tissue may be found along the parotid duct in 20% of patients [282].

Congenital salivary fistulas have been associated with the parotid gland, the submandibular gland, and especially the ectopic salivary gland [283]. The sites of opening have been retroauricular, cheek, oral mucosa, and cervical skin [284]. We suspect that a number of these cases represent oculoauriculovertebral spectrum.

Epidermal Cysts of the Salivary Glands

Epidermal cysts of the salivary glands are extremely rare. A few examples have been reported in the parotid gland [285].

Neonatal Parotitis

Acute parotitis is characterized by sudden onset of swelling associated with purulent drainage from Stensen's duct. Diffuse, firm, smooth, tender swelling typically involves the entire gland. Low-grade fever and variable leukocytosis are noted. About 200 cases have been reported in neonatal infants [286, 287]. Çoban et al [288] suggested that it is a vanishing disease.

In newborns, *Staphylococcus aureus* is the principal pathogen. Other organisms include *Escherichia coli*, *Pseudomonas aeruginosa*, *Neisseria catarrhalis*, and *Klebsiella pneumoniae*. Dehydration is a common predisposing condition, the infection taking place by bacteria ascending the duct. Septicemia is another possible route.

Although initially believed to be limited to the salivary and lacrimal glands, cytomegalic inclusion disease is now recognized as a generalized condition [122]. (See Chap. 17.)

Congenital Angiomas of the Salivary Glands

During infancy, vascular lesions are the most common tumors of salivary glands. At least 80% are hemangiomas, and the remaining 20% are lymphangiomas. Most hemangiomas regress before age 5 years, making aggressive growth and cosmesis the only indications for surgical removal [289].

Hemangiomas of the parotid gland are more common in female infants (3F:1M) [290]. Grossly, they are usually diffuse and have a glistening pink appearance on sectioning [291]. Microscopically, the vascular tumor replaces the acini, leaving only a few isolated ducts lined by columnar or cuboidal epithelium. The lobular architecture of the gland is preserved. Hemangiomas of the parotid gland may be associated with facial angiomatosis, supraumbilical raphe, and nonunion of the sternum as a syndrome.

As indicated under Cystic Hygroma, most lymphangiomas of the parotid gland are extensions of lesions of the neck. Rarely, the submandibular gland is involved. Clinically, lymphangiomas are usually softer than hemangiomas and more often transilluminate. While hemangioma infiltrates the salivary glands, lymphangioma compresses the glandular parenchyma. Spontaneous regression does not occur [292]. Grossly, the lymphangioma is cystic and grayish.

Sialoblastoma

Sialoblastoma has been called by a large number of names, such as "embryoma," "monomorphic adenoma," "basaloid congenital basal cell adenoma," "congenital adenoid cystic carcinoma," and "congenital carcinoma" [293]. About 30 examples have been reported [294]. We prefer the term "sialoblastoma" because it reflects the resemblance of the tumor to the developing salivary gland [295].

Sialoblastoma presents at birth in both the parotid and submandibular glands, far more often in the former. Among the 25 reports, sialoblastoma has ranged from 1 to 15 cm in diameter, with an occasional example being so large as to cause dystocia [143]. On gross examination, it is tan-gray to yellow, lobulated, and occasionally cystic due to focal necrosis, but it is generally well circumscribed.

Microscopically, the tumor is formed from solid nests of epithelial cells that contain small ductlike structures, which in turn are surrounded by narrow bands of fibrous connective tissue. The tumor cells have round to oval nuclei with one or more large nucleoli. The cytoplasm is pale-staining. Mitoses are not rare [296] (Fig. 22.45).

Immunohistochemical studies indicate that the luminal ductal cells are positive for cytokeratins 3, 5, 6, 7, 13, and 19 [294]. However, both ductal cells and epithelial cells express vimentin. The myoepithelial cells stain positively

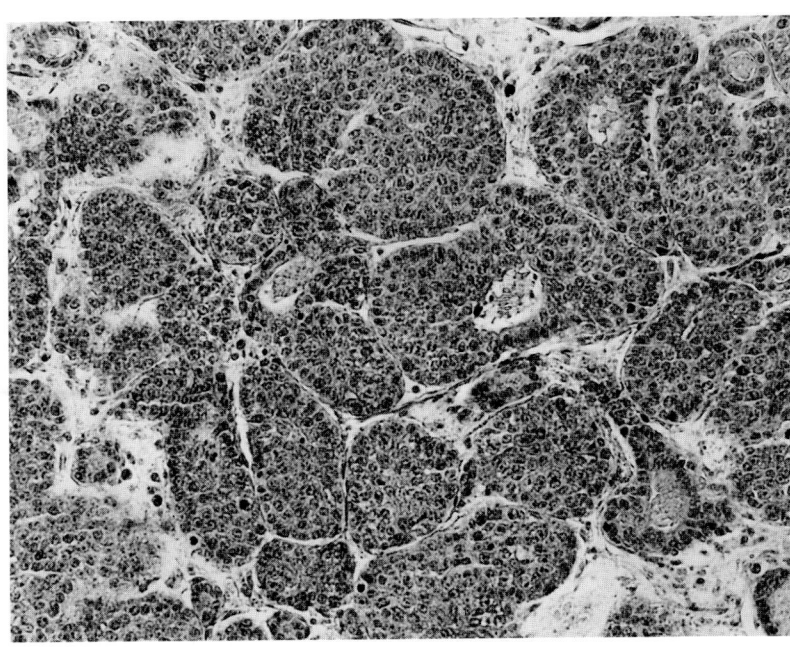

FIGURE 22.45. *Sialoblastoma. Predominant tumor pattern shows ductal structures budding from solid nests of cells. (From Taylor [143].)*

with smooth muscle actin, S-100, myosin, cytokeratin 14, and vimentin [294].

On electron microscopic study, the epithelial cells exhibit small oval nuclei, numerous ribosomes, abundant endoplasmic reticulum, and few primitive cell junctions. The ductal epithelial cells have irregular nuclei, less prominent cytoplasm with numerous lysosomes, and free ribosomes, tight junctions, and microvilli.

Occasionally, there is local recurrence, but no distant metastasis or death has been reported.

Congenital Pleomorphic Adenoma

Congenital pleomorphic adenoma is a polypoid hamartoma of minor salivary glands of the nasopharynx. It obstructs the airway in the first few days or weeks of life. Examples have also been called "salivary gland anlage tumor" and "undifferentiated carcinoma of the parotid gland" [297, 298].

Only nine examples of this tumor have been reported, and it is difficult to generalize, but the tumors have usually been polypoid lesions measuring 1 to 3 cm in diameter attached to the posterior pharyngeal wall by a pedicle. Dehner et al [297] describe a 7M:2F gender predilection. Excision has resulted in cure.

Microscopically, the tumor is composed of epithelial tubular and myoepithelial elements. The histologic pattern is biphasic with squamous nests and ductlike structures at the periphery blended into solid, predominantly mesenchymal-appearing nodules centrally (Fig. 22.46).

The peripheral epithelial structures are positive for cytokeratin and epithelial membrane antigen. The central stroma-like cells are variably positive for cytokeratin, vimentin, and muscle-specific actin. Both areas stain for salivary gland amylase.

Ultrastructurally, some of the strandlike cells resemble myoepithelial cells.

Other Congenital Salivary Gland Tumors

A few other salivary gland tumors meeting none of the criteria for any of the above-mentioned neoplasms or hamartomas have been reported. They have been described as undifferentiated carcinoma, characterized by rapid localized invasion and local and distant metastases [299, 300]. Survival is extremely rare.

Other rare congenital salivary gland tumors include pleomorphic adenoma [299], hemangiopericytoma [301], and juvenile xanthoma [292].

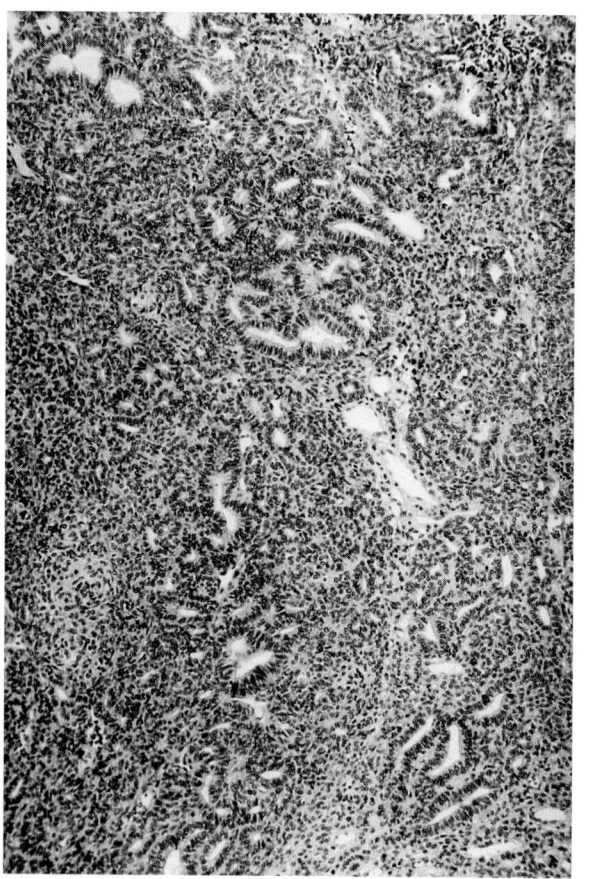
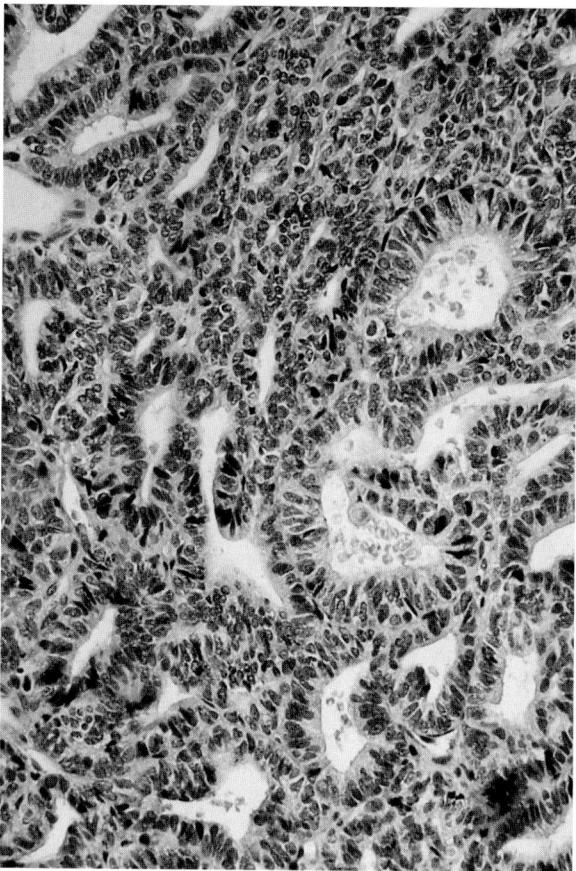

FIGURE 22.46.   *Congenital pleomorphic adenoma. Tumor consists of epithelial tubular and myoepithelial elements. (Courtesy of A Perez-Atayde, Boston, Massachusetts.)*

NECK

Lateral Cervical and Pharyngeal (Branchial Cleft) Fistulas and Sinuses

Normally, the second branchial arch grows caudally, covering the third and fourth arches and fusing with the neck. In so doing, it buries the cervical sinus. If the second arch fails to overgrow the other arches entirely, then a branchial fistula will extend from the lateral surface of the neck, between the internal and external carotid arteries, to the region of the cervical sinus.

Preauricular fistulas accompany cervical fistulas in perhaps 30% of the cases. The pinnae may be malformed. They also may be in binary combination with conductive and/or sensorineural hearing loss and renal anomalies, in which case the condition is known as branchio-oto-renal syndrome. This combination has autosomal dominant inheritance [302].

Rarely, a fistula can be observed arising from failure of closure of the first branchial cleft. This fistula opens behind, above, or in front of the ear, runs parallel to or enters the external auditory canal, and extends to the nasopharynx or lateral aspect of the neck [303].

Fistulas are lined by either stratified squamous or ciliated columnar epithelium. Those on the lower neck commonly secrete a mucoid material.

An internal branchial fistula may result from rupture of a membrane between the second branchial arch and the pharyngeal pouch, forming a tract that opens into the tonsillar fossa [304]. Rarely, a branchiogenic sinus extends from the lateral aspect of the neck to the pharynx [305].

Many investigators contend that failure or disappearance of the cervical sinus results in branchial cleft cyst, a view not shared by us. We believe that these cysts are really lymphoepithelial cysts that have resulted from entrapment of salivary duct epithelium within lymph nodes.

Branchial fistulas are occasionally bilateral [306]. There does not appear to be a gender predilection.

Congenital Midline Cervical Cleft, Web, or Cord

At least 30 patients have been described in whom there was a midline blind-ended cervical cleft extending, at times, from the lower border of the mandible to the suprasternal notch [307, 308]. In others, there have been midline subcutaneous webs or cords cephalad to the defect that may tether the mandible, producing a torticollis-like anomaly. A skin tag or cartilaginous nodule may be located at the upper end of the cleft or cord (Fig. 22.47). A submental bone spur appears at the attachment of the cervical cord [309]. A superb review is that of Kriens and Schuchardt [310]. In one patient there was an associated midline cyst of the mandible [311]. In our survey, there was a 10F:1M gender predilection.

The anomaly appears to result from failure of the branchial arches to close in the midline. Normally the arches merge in a cephalad-to-caudal direction. Prior to fusion, mesoderm migrates between the arches, pushing ectoderm outward to flatten the ventral groove [312]. Microscopic changes include absence of epithelial adnexa in the dermis. Fibrous connective tissue replaces superficial musculature [313].

Congenital Teratoma of the Neck

Congenital cervical teratoma is relatively rare, constituting about 3% of teratomas presenting in infancy [314]. Some assume massive dimensions. In more than 40%, the tumor is larger than 10 cm (Fig. 22.48). A history of polyhydramnios is obtained in about half of this latter group. About 30% of the babies are either stillborn or premature [315]. Another third die of respiratory obstruction soon after birth [314]. There is no gender predilection, but about half of the patients are black, suggesting increased racial predilection.

Grossly, the mass is usually semicystic but may be solid or multiloculated and is nearly always encapsulated. Wiatrak et al [240] described MRI as useful in differential diagnosis.

Microscopically, all three embryonal layers are represented [316]. Fetal brain tissue is especially common (about 70%).

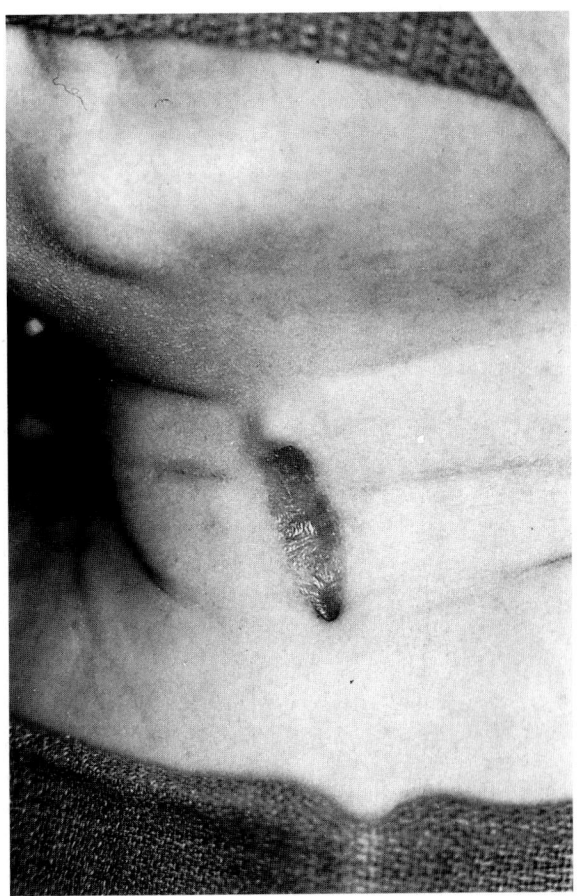

FIGURE 22.47. *Congenital midline cervical cleft. Note deficiency of skin in midline, and nodule at cephalic end of defect.*

Thyroid tissue has been noted in 30%. Nearly all congenital cervical teratomas have been benign [317], in contrast to those of the neck in adults, which are probably always malignant [318].

Alphafetoprotein levels may occasionally be elevated [314].

Cystic Hygroma

The cystic hygroma or diffuse lymphangioma is a rather poorly defined, soft, fluctuant cervical tissue mass, usually located behind the sternocleidomastoid muscle (Fig. 22.49). It may be noted before birth, be evident at birth, or manifest within the first 2 years of life. Cystic hygroma presenting in the fetus has a different natural history and prognosis from one appearing postnatally. Most fetal examples are diagnosed before 30 weeks' gestation and present with hydrops or diffuse lymphangiomatosis. Prognosis is poor. Cervical cystic hygroma, which becomes evident late

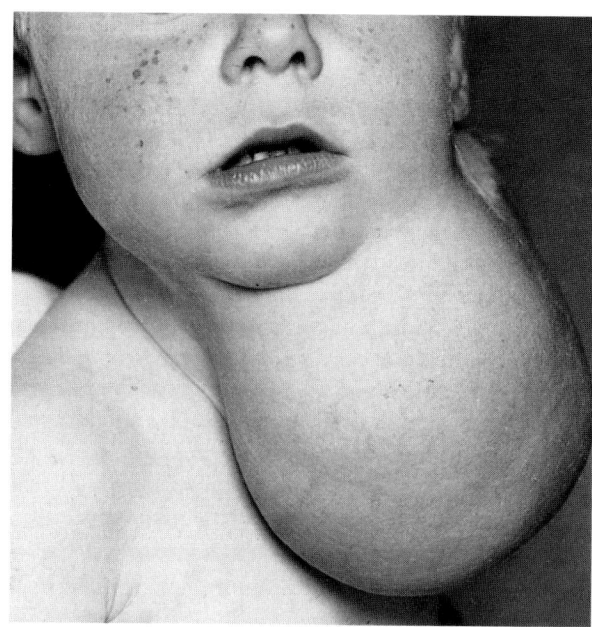

FIGURE 22.49. *Cystic hygroma. Child died from massive hemorrhage into hygroma. (Courtesy of IW Broomhead, Edinburgh, Scotland.)*

in pregnancy, is rather rare [319]. It probably represents a developmental anomaly, and prognosis is more favorable [320]. Ultrasonography is of considerable value [321].

About 20% of cystic hygromas extend to involve the axilla, mediastinum, cheek, tongue, oral floor, or parotid gland [125]. Approximately 15% resolve spontaneously, and about 30% become infected, causing dysphagia and toxemia [322].

Among those seen before birth, about 50% have 45,X Turner syndrome. An occasional fetus will have Down syndrome. Fetuses with abnormal karyotypes rarely have polyhydramnios. Those with normal karyotypes often (about 65%) have additional abnormalities (cardiac anomaly, hydronephrosis, neural tube defect, cleft lip/palate, multiple pterygium syndrome, etc.) [323, 324].

Microscopically, the cystic hygroma consists of numerous endothelium-lined lymphatic spaces with size ranging from microscopic (cavernous lymphangioma) to large (cystic lymphangioma) in a loose connective tissue stroma.

Recurrence is high after surgical removal [325].

Aspiration can distinguish the cystic hygroma from the ranula by the finding of low total protein and low amylase in the cystic hygroma [326].

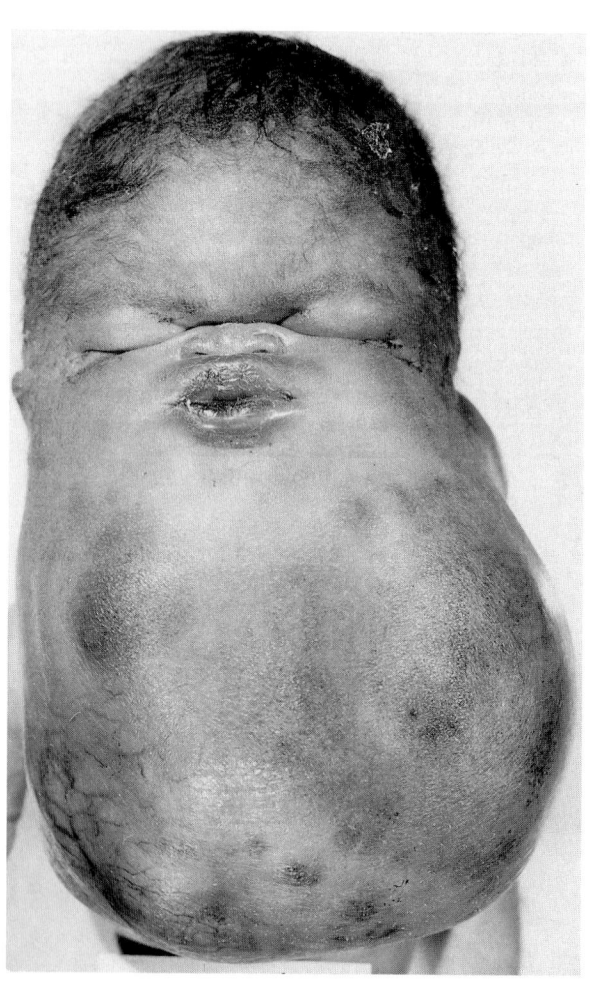

FIGURE 22.48. *Congenital teratoma of neck. Large, rounded cystic tumor projects from anterior neck. (From Hajdu S. Am J Dis Child 1966; 111:412.)*

REFERENCES

1. Akimoto N, Ikeda T, Satow Y, Lee JY, Okamoto N. Craniofacial and oral malformations in an autopsy population of Japanese human fetuses and newborns. *J Craniofac Genet Dev Biol* 1986; 2(suppl):213–33.

2. Sulik KK. Craniofacial embryogenesis and dysmorphogenesis. In: Siebert JR, Cohen MM Jr, Sulik KK, Shaw C-M, Lemire RJ, eds. *Holoprosencephaly: An Overview and Atlas of Cases.* New York: Wiley-Liss, 1990, pp. 59–98.

3. Decker JD, Hall SH. Light and electron microscopy of the newborn sagittal suture. *Anat Rec* 1985; 212:81–9.

4. Hall SH, Decker JD. Calvarial suture morphogenesis: cellular and molecular aspects. In: Persing JA, Edgerton MT, Jane JA, eds. *Scientific Foundations and Surgical Treatment of Craniosynostosis.* Baltimore: Williams & Wilkins, 1989, pp. 29–37.

5. Johansen V, Hall SH. Morphogenesis of the mouse coronal suture. *Acta Anat* 1982; 114:58–67.

6. Furtwangler JA, Hall SH, Koskinen-Moffett LK. Sutural morphogenesis in the mouse calvaria: the role of apoptosis. *Acta Anat* 1985; 124:74–80.

7. Kokich VG. Age changes in the human frontozygomatic suture. *Am J Orthod* 1976; 69:411–30.

8. Koskinen L. Adaptive sutures: changes after unilateral masticatory muscle resection in rats. A microscopic study. *Proc Finn Dent Soc* 1977; 73(suppl X):1–79.

9. Cohen MM Jr. Sutural biology and the correlates of craniosynostosis. *Am J Med Genet* 1993; 47:581–616.

10. Gorlin RJ, Slavkin HC. Embryology of the face. In: Tewfik TL, Der Kaloustian VM, eds. *Congenital Anomalies of the Ear, Nose and Throat.* New York: Oxford University, 1997.

11. Larsen WJ. *Human Embryology.* New York: Churchill Livingstone, 1993.

12. Gorlin RJ, Cohen MM Jr, Levin LS. *Syndromes of the Head and Neck.* 3rd ed. New York: Oxford University, 1990.

13. Ten Cate AR. *Oral Histology.* 4th ed. St. Louis: CV Mosby, 1994.

14. Sulik KK, Cotanche DA. Embryology of the ear. In: Gorlin RJ, Toriello HV, Cohen MM Jr, eds. *Hereditary Hearing Loss and Its Syndromes.* New York: Oxford University, 1995, pp. 22–42.

15. Hanson JW, Streissguth AP, Smith DW. The effects of moderate alcohol consumption during pregnancy on fetal growth and morphogenesis. *J Pediatr* 1978; 92:457–60.

16. Cohen MM Jr. Neoplasia and the fetal alcohol and hydantoin syndromes. *Neurobehav Toxicol Teratol* 1981; 3:161–2.

17. Hanson JW, Smith DW. The fetal hydantoin syndrome. *J Pediatr* 1975; 87:285–90.

18. Feldman GL, Weaver DD, Lourien EW. The fetal trimethadione syndrome. *Am J Dis Child* 1977; 131:1389–92.

19. Zackai EH, Mellman WJ, Neiderer B, Hanson JW. The fetal trimethadione syndrome. *J Pediatr* 1975; 87:280–4.

20. Ardinger HH, Atkin JF, Blackston RD, et al. Verification of the fetal valproate syndrome phenotype. *Am J Med Genet* 1988; 29:171–85.

21. Hall JG, Pauli RM, Wilson KM. Maternal and fetal sequelae of anticoagulation during pregnancy. *Am J Med* 1980; 68:122–40.

22. Pauli RM, Madden JD, Kranzler KJ, Culpepper W, Port R. Warfarin therapy initiated during pregnancy and phenotypic chondrodysplasia punctata. *J Pediatr* 1976; 88:506–8.

23. Lammer EJ, Chen DT, Hoar RM, et al. Retinoic acid embryopathy. *N Engl J Med* 1985; 313:837–41.

24. Warkany J. *Congenital Malformations: Notes and Comments.* Chicago: Year Book Medical, 1971.

25. Brent RL. Radiation teratogenesis. In: Sever JL, Brent RL, eds. *Teratogen Update: Environmentally Induced Birth Defect Risks.* New York: Alan R. Liss, 1986, pp. 145–63.

26. Cohen MM Jr. *Craniosynostosis: Diagnosis, Evaluation, and Management.* 2nd ed. New York: Oxford University, 1998.

27. Blot WJ. Growth and development following prenatal and childhood exposure to atomic radiation. *J Radiat Res* 1975; 16(suppl):82–8.

28. Roach E, DeMyer W, Palmer K, Connelly M, Merritt A. Holoprosencephaly: birth data, genetic and demographic analysis of 30 families. *Birth Defects* 1975; 11(2):294–313.

29. Matsunaga E, Shiota K. Holoprosencephaly in human embryos: epidemiologic studies of 150 cases. *Teratology* 1977; 16:261–72.

30. Belloni E, Muenke M, Roessler E, et al. Identification of *Sonic hedgehog* as a candidate gene responsible for holoprosencephaly. *Nature Genet* 1996; 14:353–6.

31. Roessler E, Belloni E, Gaudenz K, et al. Mutations in the human *Sonic Hedgehog* gene cause holoprosencephaly. *Nature Genet* 1996; 14:357–60.

32. Cohen MM Jr. Perspectives on holoprosencephaly. Part III. Spectra, distinctions, continuities, and discontinuities. *Am J Med Genet* 1989; 34:271–88.

33. Cohen MM Jr, Sulik KK. Perspectives on holoprosencephaly. Part II. Central nervous system, craniofacial anatomy, syndrome commentary, diagnostic approach, and experimental studies. *J Craniofac Genet Dev Biol* 1992; 12:196–244.

34. Siebert JR, Cohen MM Jr, Sulik KK, Shaw C-M, Lemire RJ, eds. *Holoprosencephaly: An Overview and Atlas of Cases.* New York: Wiley-Liss, 1990.

35. Muenke M. Holoprosencephaly as a genetic model for normal craniofacial development. *Dev Biol* 1994; 5:293–301.

36. Muenke M, Schell U, Hehr A, et al. A common mutation in the fibroblast growth factor receptor 1 gene in Pfeiffer syndrome. *Nature Genet* 1994; 8:269–74.

37. DeMyer WE, Zeman W, Palmer CG. The face predicts the brain: diagnostic significance of median facial anomalies for holoprosencephaly (arhinencephaly). *Pediatrics* 1964; 34:256–63.

38. Gorlin RJ, Cohen MM Jr. Median facial dysplasia in unilateral and bilateral cleft lip and palate: a subgroup of median cerebrofacial malformations. Discussion. *Plast Reconstr Surg* 1993; 91:1006–7.

39. Torczynski E, Jacobiec FA, Johnston MC, Font RL, Madewell JA. Synophthalmia and cyclopia: a histopathologic, radiographic and organogenetic analysis. *Doc Ophthalmol* 1977; 44:311–78.

40. Kokich VG, Ngim C-H, Siebert JR, Clarren SK, Cohen MM Jr. Cyclopia: an anatomic and histologic study of two specimens. *Teratology* 1982; 26:105–13.

41. Smith S, Boulgakow B. A case of cyclopia. *J Anat* 1927; 61:105–11.

42. Cohen MM Jr, Rollnick BR, Kaye CI. Oculoauriculovertebral spectrum: an updated critique. *Cleft Palate J* 1989; 26:276–86.

43. Figueroa AA, Pruzansky S. The external ear, mandible and other components of hemifacial microsomia. *J Max Fac Surg* 1982; 10:200–11.

44. Poswillo D. The pathogenesis of the first and second branchial arch syndrome. *Oral Surg* 1973; 35:302–29.

45. Jabs EW, Li X, Coss CA, et al. Mapping of the Treacher-Collins syndrome locus to 5q31.3 → 5q33.3. *Genomics* 1991; 11:193–8.

46. Richieri-Costa A, Bortolozo MA, Lauris JRP, et al. Mandibulofacial dysostosis: report on two Brazilian families suggesting autosomal recessive inheritance. *Am J Med Genet* 1993; 46:659–64.

47. Poswillo D. The pathogenesis of the Treacher Collins syndrome (mandibulofacial dysostosis). *Br J Oral Surg* 1975; 13:1–26.

48. Sulik KK, Johnston MC, Smiley SJ, Speight HS, Jarvis BE. Mandibulofacial dysostosis (Treacher Collins syndrome): a new proposal for its pathogenesis. *Am J Med Genet* 1987; 27:359–72.

49. Wiley MJ, Cauwenbergs P, Taylor IM. Effects of retinoic acid on the development of the facial skeleton in hamsters: early changes involving cranial neural crest cells. *Acta Anat* 1983; 116:180–92.

50. Batsakis JG. *Tumors of the Head and Neck.* 2nd ed. Baltimore: Williams & Wilkins, 1979.

51. Bhaskar SN, Bernier JL. Histogenesis of branchial cysts: a report of 468 cases. *Am J Path* 1959; 35:407–24.

52. Gorlin RJ. Cysts of the jaws, oral floor, and neck. In: Gorlin RJ, Goldman HM, eds. *Thoma's Oral Pathology.* 6th ed. St. Louis: CV Mosby, 1970.

53. Maisel H, Yoshihara H, Waggoner D. The cervical thymus. *Mich Med* 1975; 74:259–61.

54. Cohen MM Jr, Cole DEC. Origins of recognizable syndromes: etiologic and pathogenetic mechanisms and the process of syndrome delineation. *J Pediatr* 1989; 115:161–4.

55. Lammer EJ, Opitz JM. The DiGeorge anomaly as a developmental field defect. *Am J Med Genet Suppl* 1986; 2:113–27.

56. Reddy K, Hoffman HJ, Armstrong D. Delayed and progressive multiple suture craniosynostosis. *Neurosurgery* 1990; 26:442–8.

57. Cohen MM Jr, Kreiborg S, Lammer EJ, et al. Birth prevalence study of the Apert syndrome. *Am J Med Genet* 1992; 42:665–9.

58. Cohen MM Jr, Kreiborg S. Birth prevalence studies of the Crouzon syndrome: comparison of direct and indirect methods. *Clin Genet* 1992; 41:12–15.

59. Cohen MM Jr. Craniosynostosis and syndromes with craniosynostosis: incidence, genetics, penetrance, variability, and new syndrome updating. *Birth Defects* 1979; 15(5B):13–63.

60. Cohen MM Jr. Craniosynostosis update: 1986–1987. *Am J Med Genet Suppl* 1988; 4:99–148.

61. Cohen MM Jr. Etiopathogenesis of craniosynostosis. *Neurosurg Clin N Am* 1991; 2:507–13.

62. Cohen MM Jr. Transforming growth factor βs and fibroblast growth factors and their receptors: role in sutural biology and craniosynostosis. *J Bone Mineral Res* 1997; 12:322–31.

63. Kokich VG, Moffett BC, Cohen MM Jr. The cloverleaf skull anomaly: an

anatomic and histologic study of two specimens. *Cleft Palate J* 1982; 19:89–99.

64. Gorlin RJ. Fibroblast growth factors, their receptors and receptor disorders. *J Craniomaxillofac Surg* 1997; 25:69–79.

65. Hunter AGW, Rudd NL. Craniosynostosis I. Sagittal synostosis: its genetics and associated clinical findings in 214 patients who lacked involvement of the coronal suture(s). *Teratology* 1976; 14:185–93.

66. Hunter AGW, Rudd NL. Craniosynostosis II. Coronal synostosis: its familial characteristics and associated clinical findings in 109 patients lacking bilateral polysyndactyly or syndactyly. *Teratology* 1977; 15:301–10.

67. Cohen MM Jr. The cloverleaf skull anomaly: managing extreme cranio-orbito-facio-stenosis: discussion. *Plast Reconstruct Surg* 1993; 91:10–14.

68. Kreiborg S, Cohen MM Jr. Characteristics of the infant Apert skull and its subsequent development. *J Craniofac Genet Dev Biol* 1990; 10:399–410.

69. Kreiborg S, Marsh JL, Cohen MM Jr, et al. Comparative three-dimensional analysis of CT-scans of the calvaria and cranial base in Apert and Crouzon syndromes. *J Craniomaxillofac Surg* 1993; 21:181–8.

70. Moloney DM, Staney SF, Oldridge M, et al. Exclusive paternal origin of new mutations in Apert syndrome. *Nature Genet* 1996; 13:48–51.

71. Kreiborg S. Crouzon syndrome. *Scand J Plast Reconstr Surg Suppl* 1981; 18:1–98.

72. Cohen MM Jr. Pfeiffer syndrome update, clinical subtypes, and guidelines for differential diagnosis. *Am J Med Genet* 1993; 45:300–7.

73. Hengerer AS, Strome M. Choanal atresia: a new embryologic theory and its influence on surgical management. *Laryngoscope* 1982; 92:913–21.

74. Maniglia AJ, Goodwin WJ. Congenital choanal atresia. *Otolaryngol Clin N Am* 1981; 14:167–73.

75. Fryburg JS, Persing JA, Link Y. Frontonasal dysplasia in two successive generations. *Am J Med Genet* 1993; 46:712–4.

76. Sedano HO, Cohen MM Jr, Jirasek J, Gorlin RJ. Fronto-nasal dysplasia. *J Pediatr* 1970; 76:906–13.

77. Cohen D, Goitein K. Arhinia revisited. *Rhinology* 1987; 25:237–44.

78. Lütolf U. Bilateral aplasia of the nose. *J Maxillofac Surg* 1976; 4:245–9.

79. Van Kempen AAMW, Nabben FAE, Hamel BCJ. Heminasal aplasia: a case report and review of the literature of the last 25 years. *Clin Dysmorphol* 1997; 6:147–52.

80. Gifford GH, Swanson L, MacCollum DW. Congenital absence of the nose and anterior nasopharynx. *Plast Reconstr Surg* 1972; 50:5–12.

81. Navarro-Vila C, Cuestas Matras G, Carlos Martinez G. Congenital absence of the nose and nasal fossae. *J Craniomaxillofac Surg* 1991; 19:56–60.

82. Weinberg A, Neuman A, Benmeir P, Lusthaus S, Wexler MR. A rare case of arhinia with severe airway obstruction: case report and review of the literature. *Plast Reconstr Surg* 1993; 91:146–9.

83. Ruprecht KW, Majewski F. Familiäre Arhinie mit Peterscher Anomalie und Kiefermissbildungen, ein neues Fehlbildungssyndrom. *Klin Mbl Augenheilkd* 1978; 172:708–15.

84. Cole RR, Myer CM, Bratcher GO. Congenital absence of the nose. *Int J Pediatr Otolaryngol* 1989; 17:171–7.

85. Mühlbauer W, Schmidt A, Fairley J. Simultaneous construction of an internal and external nose in an infant with arhinia. *Plast Reconstr Surg* 1993; 91:720–5.

86. Nishimura Y. Embryological study of nasal cavity development in human embryos with reference to congenital nostril atresia. *Acta Anat* 1993; 147:140–4.

87. Mahindra S, Daljit R, Jamwal N, Mathew M. Lateral nasal proboscis. *J Laryngol Otol* 1973; 87:177–81.

88. Skevas A, Tsoulias T, Papadopoulos N, Assimakopoulos D. Proboscis lateralis, a rare malformation. *Rhinology* 1990; 28:285–9.

89. Rosen Z, Gitlin G. Bilateral nasal proboscis. *Arch Otolaryngol* 1959; 70:545–50.

90. Dasgupta G. Proboscis. *J Laryngol Otol* 1971; 85:401–6.

91. Maguers A, Guillen G, Migueis C. Surgical treatment of proboscis lateralis. *Rev Laryngol* 1993; 114:193–5.

92. Bumba J, Lucksch F. Ein Fall von Doggennase. *Virchows Arch Path Anat* 1927; 264:554–62.

93. Anyane-Yeboa K, Raifman MA, Berant M, Frogel MP, Travers J. Dominant inheritance of bifid nose. *Am J Med Genet* 1984; 17:561–3.

94. Weaver DF, Bellinger DH. Bifid nose associated with midline cleft of the upper lip. *Arch Otolaryngol* 1946; 44:480–2.

95. Krikun LA. Clinical features of median cleft of nose. *Acta Chir Plast* 1972; 14:137–48.

96. Erich JB. Nasal duplication. Report of a patient with two noses. *Plast Reconstr Surg* 1962; 29:159–66.

97. Yadava VNS. Duplication of the nose with unilateral complete cleft lip, alveolus, and palate in a male child. *Plast Reconstr Surg* 1990; 85:953–4.

98. Holmes EM. Congenital triple nares. *Arch Otolaryngol* 1950; 52:70–3.

99. Coessens B, De Mey A, Lejour M. Correction of supernumerary nostrils. *Int J Pediatr Otorhinolaryngol* 1992; 23:275–80.

100. Winkler E. Zur Frage der Entstehung und chirurgischer Behandlung von Missbildungen der Nase. *Bruns Beitr Klin Chir* 1959; 198:358–73.

101. Ungerecht K. Teilweise Verdoppelung der äusseren Nase Infolge Missbildung. *Arch Ohren Nasen Kehlkopfheilkd* 1951; 157:674–8.

102. Wilke J. Beitrag zum Problem der Nasendoppelbildungen. *Z Laryngol Rhinol Otol* 1958; 37:770–4.

103. Morgan DW, Evans JNG. Developmental nasal anomalies. *J Laryngol Otol* 1990; 104:393–403.

104. Mullin WR, Millard DR Jr. Management of congenital bilateral cleft nose. *Plast Reconstr Surg* 1985; 75:255–7.

105. Thompson HG, Sleightholm R. Isolated naso-ocular cleft: a one-stage repair. *Plast Reconstr Surg* 1985; 76:534–8.

106. Ghestem M, Dhellemes P, Pellerin P. Kystes et fistules dermöides congénitaux du dos du nez. *Ann Chir Plast Esthét* 1991; 36:183–91.

107. Paller AS, Pensler JM, Tomita T. Nasal midline masses in infants and children. Dermoids, encephalocoeles and gliomas. *Arch Dermatol* 1991; 127:363–6.

108. Vibe P, Løntoft E. Congenital nasal dermoid cysts and fistulas. *Scand J Plast Reconstr Surg* 1985; 19:105–7.

109. Wardinsky TD, Pagon RA, Kropp RJ, Hayden PW, Clarren SK. Nasal dermoid sinus cysts: association with intracranial extension and multiple malformations. *Cleft Palate Craniofac J* 1991; 28:87–95.

110. Posnick JC, Bortoluzzi P, Armstrong DC, Drake JM. Intracranial nasal dermoid sinus cysts: computed tomographic scan findings and surgical results. *Plast Reconstr Surg* 1994; 93:745–54.

111. Khan MA, Gibb AG. Median dermoid cysts of the nose. Familial occurrences. *J Laryngol Otol* 1970; 84:709–18.

112. Mühlbauer W, Dittmar W. Hereditary median dermoid cysts of the nose. *Br J Plast Surg* 1976; 29:334–40.

113. Furness FW. Mesial dermoid cyst of the nose occurring in twin boys. *J Laryngol Otol* 1938; 53:314–15.

114. Kennard CD, Rasmussen JE. Congenital midline nasal masses. *J Derm Surg Oncol* 1990; 16:1025–36.

115. Bagger-Sjöbäck D, Bergastrand G, Edner G, Anggård A. Nasal meningoencephalocele: a clinical problem. *Clin Otolaryngol* 1983; 8:329–35.

116. Lusk RP, Lee PC. Magnetic resonance imaging of congenital midline nasal masses. *Otolaryngol Head Neck Surg* 1986; 95:303–5.

117. Gorenstein A, Kern EB, Facer GW, Laws ER. Nasal gliomas. *Arch Otolaryngol* 1980; 106:536–40.

118. Bradley PJ, Singh SD. Nasal glioma. *J Laryngol Otol* 1985; 99:247–52.

119. Cohen MM Jr. The nose. In: Stevenson RE, Hall JG, Goodman RM, eds. *Human Malformations and Related Anomalies.* New York: Oxford University, 1993, pp. 323–39.

120. Toriello HV, Higgins HV, Walen A, Waterman DF. Familial occurrences of a developmental defect of the medial nasal processes. *Am J Med Genet* 1985; 21:131–5.

121. Nieuwenhuijse AC. Continuation of the pedigree of hereditary potato nose (Benjamins-Stibbe). *Acta Otolaryngol* 1950; 38:112–19.

122. Gorlin RJ. Developmental anomalies of the face and oral structures. In: Gorlin RJ, Goldman HM, eds. *Thoma's Oral Pathology.* 6th ed. St. Louis: CV Mosby, 1970.

123. Ohishi M, Yamamoto K, Higuchi Y. Congenital dermoid fistula of the lower lip. *Oral Surg Oral Med Oral Pathol* 1991; 71:203–5.

124. Stoneman DW. Congenital facial fistula with formation of accessory bone and teeth. *Oral Surg* 1978; 45:150–4.

125. Everett FG, Wescott WB. Commissural lip pits. *Oral Surg* 1961; 14:202–9.

126. Shprintzen RJ, Goldberg RB, Sidoti EJ. The penetrance and variable expression of the Van der Woude syndrome: implications for genetic counseling. *Cleft Palate J* 1980; 17:52–7.

127. Calderon S, Garlick JA. Surgical excision of a congenital lateral fistula of the upper lip. *J Craniomaxillofac Surg* 1988; 16:46–8.

128. Radcliffe R. Rare congenital malformation of the upper lip. *Br J Surg* 1940; 28:329–30.

129. Sakamoto H, Imar Y, Asakura A. Congenital midline sinus of the upper lip. *Int J Oral Maxillofac Surg* 1992; 21:10–11.

130. Mizuki H, Shimizu M, Danjo T. Congenital fistula with an island of vermilion epithelium in the paramidline of the upper lip. *J Craniomaxillofac Surg* 1993; 21:22–4.

131. Grenman R, Salo H, Rintala A. Midline sinuses of the upper lip. *Scand J Plast Surg* 1985; 19:215–19.

132. Miller CJ, Smith JM. Midline sinus of the upper lip and a theory concerning etiology. *Plast Reconstr Surg* 1980; 65:674–5.

133. Eppley BL, Sadove AM, Goldenberg J. Philtral fistula in median cleft lip: cause and effect or coincidence? *Ann Plast Surg* 1992; 29:263–5.

134. Sewerin I. The sebaceous glands in the vermilion border of the lips and in the oral mucosa of man. *Acta Odont Scand Suppl* 1975; 68:1–226.

135. Guiducci AA, Hyman AB. Ectopic sebaceous glands, a review of the literature regarding their occurrence, histology and embryonic relationships. *Dermatologica (Basel)* 1962; 125:44–63.

136. Prystowsky SD, Rogers JG. A median nodule of the upper lip as a familial trait. *Oral Surg* 1976; 42:653–5.

137. Tsukahara M, Fernandez I, Sugio Y, Shiota K. Median nodule of the upper lip: an autosomal dominant trait. *Am J Med Genet* 1994; 51:13–15.

138. Sewerin I. Prevalence of variations and anomalies of the upper labial frenum. *Acta Odont Scand* 1971; 29:487–96.

139. Pai GS, Levkoff AH, Leithiser RE. Median cleft of the upper lip associated with lipomas of the central nervous system and cutaneous polyps. *Am J Med Genet* 1987; 26:921–4.

140. Lewin ML. Median cleft lip with pedunculated skin masses. *Plast Reconstr Surg* 1987; 79:843–4.

141. Reardon W, Jones B, Baraitser M. Median clefting of the upper lip associated with cutaneous polyps. *J Med Genet* 1990; 27:337–8.

142. Nakamura J, Tomonari H, Goto S. True median cleft of the upper lip associated with three pedunculated club-shaped skin masses. *Plast Reconstr Surg* 1985; 75:727–31.

143. Taylor GP. Case 6. Congenital epithelial tumor of the parotid-sialoblastoma. *Pediatr Pathol* 1988; 8:447–52.

144. Rudnik-Schöenborn S, Zerres K. A further patient with Pai syndrome with autosomal dominant inheritance? *J Med Genet* 1994; 31:497–8.

145. Benmeir P, Weinberg A, Neuman A, Eldad A. Congenital double lip: report of five cases and a review of the literature. *Ann Plast Surg* 1992; 28:180–2.

146. Reddy KA, Rao AK. Congenital double lip: a review of seven cases. *Plast Reconstr Surg* 1989; 84:420–3.

147. Peters RA, Schock RK. Oral cysts in newborn infants. *Oral Surg* 1971; 32:10–14.

148. Cataldo E, Berkman M. Cysts of the oral mucosa in newborns. *Am J Dis Child* 1968; 116:44–8.

149. Jorgenson RJ, Shapiro SD, Salinas CF, Levin LS. Intraoral findings and anomalies in neonates. *Pediatrics* 1982; 69:577–82.

150. Zuker RM, Buenechea R. Congenital epulis: review of the literature and case report. *J Oral Maxillofac Surg* 1993; 51:1040–3.151. McMahon MG, Mintz S. In utero diagnosis of a congenital gingival granular cell tumor and immediate postnatal surgical management. *J Oral Maxillofac Surg* 1994; 52:496–8.

151. McMahon MG, Mintz S. In utero diagnosis of a congenital gingival granular cell tumor and immediate postnatal surgical management. *J Oral Maxillofac Surg* 1994; 52:496–8.

152. Lack E, Crawford BE, Worsham GF, Vawter GF, Callihan MD. Gingival granular cell tumors of the newborn (congenital "epulis"). *Am J Surg Pathol* 1981; 5:37–46.

153. Stewart CM, Watson RE, Eversole LR, Fischlschweiger W, Leider AS. Oral granular cell tumor: a clinicopathologic and immunohistochemical study. *Oral Surg Oral Med Oral Pathol* 1988; 65:427–35.

154. Lack EE, Perez-Atayde AR, McGill TJ, Vawter GF. Gingival granular cell tumor of the newborn (congenital "epulis"): ultrastructural observations relating to histogenesis. *Hum Pathol* 1981; 13:686–9.

155. Carpenter BF, Jiminez C, Robb IA. Melanotic neuroectodermal tumor of infancy. *Pediatr Pathol* 1985; 3:227–44.

156. Steinberg B, Shuler C, Wilson S. Melanotic neuroectodermal tumor of infancy: evidence for multicentricity. *Oral Surg Oral Med Oral Pathol* 1988; 66:666–9.

157. Dehner LP, Sibley RK, Sauk JJ, et al. Malignant melanotic neuroectodermal tumor of infancy. A clinical, pathologic, ultrastructural and tissue culture study. *Cancer* 1979; 43:1389–1410.

158. Mosby EL, Lowe MW, Cobb CM, Ennis RL. Melanotic neuroectodermal tumor of infancy. *J Oral Maxillofac Surg* 1992; 50:886–94.

159. Borello E, Gorlin RJ. Melanotic neuroectodermal tumor of infancy—a neoplasm of neural crest origin: report of a case with associated high urinary excretion of vanilmandelic acid. *Cancer* 1966; 19:196–206.

160. Atkinson GO Jr, Davis PC, Patrick LE, et al. Melanotic neuroectodermal tumor of infancy. MR findings and review of the literature. *Pediatr Radiol* 1989; 20:20–2.

161. Bacsich P, Dennison WM, McDonald AM. A rare case of duplicitas anterior: a female infant with two mouths and two pituitaries. *J Anat* 1964; 98:292–3.

162. Stirling RW, Powell G, Fletcher CDM. Pigmented neuroectodermal tumor of infancy: an immunohistochemical study. *Histopathology* 1988; 12:425–35.

163. Melissari M, Tragni G, Gaetti L, et al. Melanotic neuroectodermal tumour of infancy. Immunohistochemical and ultrastructural study of a case. *J Craniomaxillofac Surg* 1988; 16:330–6.

164. Pettinato G, Manivel C, d'Amore ESG, Jaszcz W, Gorlin RJ. Melanotic neuroectodermal tumor of infancy. A reexamination of a histogenetic problem based on immunohistochemical, flow cytometric, and ultrastructural study of 10 cases. *Am J Surg Pathol* 1991; 15:233–45.

165. Martin RA, Jones KL, Benirschke K. Extension of the cleft lip phenotype: the subepithelial cleft. *Am J Med Genet* 1993; 47:744–7.

166. Wyszynski DF, Beaty TH, Maestri NE. Genetics of nonsyndromic oral clefts revisited. *Cleft Palate Craniofac J* 1996; 33:406–17.

167. Silva Filho O, Christovão RM, Semb G. Prevalence of a soft tissue bridge in a sample of 2014 patients with complete unilateral clefts of the lip and palate. *Cleft Palate Craniofac J* 1994; 31:122–4.

168. Fogh-Andersen P. *Inheritance of Harelip and Cleft Palate.* Copenhagen: Nyt Fordisk Forlag, 1942.

169. Cohen MM Jr, Gorlin RJ, Fraser FC. Craniofacial disorders. In: Rimoin DL, Connor JM, Pyeritz RE, eds. *Emery and Rimoin's Principles and Practice of Medical Genetics.* 3rd ed. New York: Churchill Livingstone, 1997.

170. Vanderas AP. Incidence of cleft lip, cleft palate, and cleft lip and palate among races: a review. *Cleft Palate J* 1987; 24:216–25.

171. Townsley JD, Johnston MC, eds. Research advances in prenatal craniofacial development. *J Craniofac Genet Dev Biol* 1991; 11:181–378.

172. Christiansen K, Fogh-Andersen P. Cleft lip (± cleft palate) in Danish twins, 1979–1990. *Am J Med Genet* 1993; 47:910–16.

173. Seller MJ. Conjoined twins discordant for cleft lip and palate. *Am J Med Genet* 1990; 37:530–1.

174. Farrall M, Holder S. Familial recurrence-pattern analysis of cleft lip with or without cleft palate. *Am J Hum Genet* 1992; 50:270–7.

175. Fraser FC. The genetics of cleft lip and cleft palate. *Am J Hum Genet* 1970; 33:336–52.

176. Marazita ML, Hu DN, Spence A, Liu YE, Melnick M. Cleft lip with or without cleft palate in Shanghai, China: evidence for an autosomal major locus. *Am J Hum Genet* 1992; 51:648–53.

177. Melnick M. Cleft lip (± cleft palate) etiology: a search for solutions. *Am J Med Genet* 1992; 42:10–14.

178. Sassani R, Bartlett SP, Feng H, et al. Association between alleles of the transforming growth factor-alpha locus and the occurrence of cleft lip. *Am J Med Genet* 1993; 45:565–9.

179. Vintiner GM, Holder SE, Winter RM, Malcolm S. No evidence of linkage between the growth factor—alpha gene in families with apparently autosomal dominant inheritance of cleft lip and palate. *J Med Genet* 1992; 29:393–7.

180. Dixon MJ, Garner J, Ferguson MWJ. Immunolocalization of epidermal growth factor (EGF), EGF receptor and transforming growth factor alpha (TGFα) during murine palatogenesis in vivo and in vitro. *Anat Embryol* 1991; 194:83–91.

181. Mitchell LE, Risch N. Correlates of genetic risk for non-syndromic cleft lip with or without cleft palate. *Clin Genet* 1993; 43:255–60.

182. Tolarová M, Morton NE. Cleft lip and palate—recurrence risk and genetic counseling. *Acta Chir Plast (Prague)* 1975; 17:97–111.

183. Gorski SM, Adams KJ, Birch PH, Friedman JM, Goodfellow PJ. The gene responsible for X-linked cleft palate (CPX) in a British Columbia native kindred is localized between PGK1 and DXYS1. *Am J Hum Genet* 1992; 50:1129–36.

184. Moore GE, Ivens A, Chambers J, et al. Linkage of an X-chromosome cleft palate gene. *Nature* 1987; 326:91–2.

185. Mandel JL, Willard HE, Nussbaum RL, et al. Report of the committee on the genetic constitution of the X chromosome. *Cytogenet Cell Genet* 1989; 51:384–437.

186. Temple K, Calvert M, Plent B, Thompson E, Pembrey M. Dominantly inherited cleft lip and palate in two families. *J Med Genet* 1989; 26:386–9.

187. Murray JC, Nishimura DY, Buetow KH, et al. Linkage of an autosomal dominant clefting syndrome (van der Woude) to loci on chromosome 1q. *Am J Hum Genet* 1990; 46:486–91.

188. Ahmad NN, Ala-Kokko L, Knowlton RG, et al. Stop codon in the procollagen II gene (COL2A1) in a family with the Stickler syndrome. *Proc Nat Acad Sci USA* 1991; 88:6624–7.

189. Tiller GE, Rimoin DI, Murray LW, Cohn DH. Tandem duplication within a type II collagen gene (COL2A1) exon in an individual with spondyloepiphyseal dysplasia. *Proc Natl Acad Sci USA* 1990; 87:3889–93.

190. Wiemer DR, Hardy SB, Spira M. Anatomic findings in median cleft of upper lip. *Plast Reconstr Surg* 1978; 62:866–9.

191. Cheung LK, Samman N, Tideman H. Bilateral transverse facial clefts and

accessory maxillae—variant or separate entity? *J Craniomaxillofac Surg* 1993; 21:163–7.

192. Chidzonga MM, Shija JK. Congenital median cleft of the lower lip, bifid tongue with ankyloglossia, cleft palate, and submental epidermal cyst. *J Oral Maxillofac Surg* 1988; 46:809–12.

193. Park S, Takushima A. Median cleft of the lower lip, mandible and manubrium. *J Craniomaxillofac Surg* 1993; 21:189–91.

194. Monteleone L, McLellan MS. Epstein's pearls (Bohn's nodules) of the palate. *J Oral Surg* 1964; 22:301–4.

195. Burdi AR. Distribution of midpalatine cysts: a reevaluation of human palatal closure mechanisms. *J Oral Surg* 1968; 26:41–5.

196. Chandra R. Congenital duplication of lip, maxilla, and palate. *Br J Plast Surg* 1978; 31:46–7.

197. Black FO, Myers EN, Rorke LB. Aplasia of the first and second branchial arches. *Arch Otolaryngol* 1973; 98:124–8.

198. Pfeiffer RL, Bouldin RW, Huffines WD, Sulik KA. Ocular malformations associated with agnathia. *J Craniofac Genet Dev Biol* 1992; 12:55–60.

199. Ursell W. Hydramnios associated with congenital microstomia, agnathia, and synotia. *J Obstet Gynaecol Br Commonw* 1972; 79:185–6.

200. Scholl HW Jr. In utero diagnosis of agnathia, microstomia and synotia. *Obstet Gynecol* 1977; 49(suppl 1):81–3.

201. Pauli RM, Patterson JK, Arya S, Gilbert EF. Familial agnathia-holoprosencephaly. *Am J Med Genet* 1983; 14:677–98.

202. Pauli RM, Graham JM Jr, Barr M Jr. Agnathia, situs inversus, and associated malformations. *Teratology* 1981; 23:85–93.

203. Fuhrmann W, Koch F, Schweckendiek W. Autosomal dominante Vererbung von Gaumenspalte und Synechien zwischen Gaumen und Mundboden oder Zunge. *Humangenetik* 1972; 14:196–203.

204. Nakata NMK, Guion-Almeida ML, Richieri-Costa A. Cleft palate-lateral synechiae syndrome: report on three new patients with additional findings and evidence for variability and heterogeneity. *Am J Med Genet* 1993; 47:330–2.

205. Gima H, Yamashiro M, Toshitatsu Y. Ankyloglossum superius syndrome. *J Oral Maxillofac Surg* 1987; 45:158–61.

206. Sudarshan A, Goldie WD. The spectrum of congenital facial diplegia (Moebius syndrome). *Pediatr Neurol* 1985; 1:180–9.

207. MacDermot KD, Winter RM, Taylor D, Baraitser M. Oculofacialbulbar palsy in mother and son: review of 26 reports of familial transmission within the Möbius spectrum of defects. *J Med Genet* 1990; 28:18–26.

208. Firth HV, Boyd PA, Chamberlain P, Huson SM. Oromandibular hypogenesis syndromes, limb reduction defects, and chorionic villus sampling. *J Med Genet* 1992; 29:274–5.

209. Farman AG, Gould AR, Schuler ST. Patent nasopalatine ducts: a developmental anomaly. *JADA* 1982; 105:473–5.

210. Götzfried HF. Bilateral patent nasopalatine ducts. *J Maxillofac Surg* 1986; 14:113–15.

211. Miller AS. Lateral soft palate fistula. *Arch Otolaryngol* 1970; 91:200.

212. Barr M. Facial duplications. Case review and embryogenesis. *Teratology* 1982; 25:153–8.

213. Akpuaka FC, Nwozo JC. Reduplication of the mouth and mandible. *Plast Reconstr Surg* 1990; 86:971–2.

214. Wittkampf ARM, van Limborgh J. Duplication of structures around the stomatodeum. *J Maxillofac Surg* 1984; 12:17–20.

215. Borçbakan C. An accessory mouth. *Plast Reconstr Surg* 1978; 61:778–80.

216. Robertson NRE. Apparent duplication of the upper alveolar process and dentition. *Br Dent J* 1970; 129:333–4.

217. Verdi GD, Hersh JH, Russell LJ. Partial duplication of the face: case report and review. *Plast Reconstr Surg* 1991; 87:759–82.

218. Turpin IM, Furnas DW, Amlie RN. Craniofacial duplication (diprosopus). *Plast Reconstr Surg* 1981; 67:139–42.

219. Obwegeser HL, Weber G, Freihofer HP, Sailer HF. Facial duplication—the unique case of Antonio. *J Maxillofac Surg* 1978; 6:179–98.

220. Changaris DG, McGavran MH. Craniofacial duplication (diprosopus) in a twin. *Arch Pathol Lab Med* 1976; 100:392–4.

221. Steinhilber W. Partielle Doppelanlage des Unterkiefers mit Epignathus. Zwischenkieferbürzel und Zungenspalte. *Z Kinderheilkd* 1972; 112:171–6.

222. McLaughlin CR. Reduplication of mouth, tongue and mandible. *Br J Plast Surg* 1948; 1:89–92.

223. Gorlin RJ, Sedano HO. The tongue: In: Stevenson RE, Hall JG, Goodman RM, eds. *Human Malformations and Related Anomalies.* New York: Oxford University, 1993.

224. Bartholdson L, Hellström SOM, Soderberg O. A case of double tongue. *Scand J Plast Reconstr Hand Surg* 1991; 25:93–6.

225. Agrawal K, Chandra SS, Sreekumar NS. Congenital bilateral intermaxillary bony fusion. *Ann Plast Surg* 1993; 30:163–6.

226. Valnicek SM, Clarke HM. Syngnathia: a report of two cases. *Cleft Palate Craniofac J* 1993; 30:582–5.

227. Fried K, Manor A, Pajewski M, Starinski R, Vure E. Autosomal dominant inheritance with incomplete penetrance of Caffey disease (infantile cortical hyperostosis). *Clin Genet* 1981; 19:271–4.

228. Saul RA, Lee WH, Stevenson RE. Caffey's disease revisited. *Am J Dis Child* 1982; 136:56–60.

229. Cayler GC, Peterson CA. Infantile cortical hyperostosis: report of 17 cases. *Am J Dis Child* 1956; 91:119–25.

230. MacLachlan AK, Gerrard JW, Houston CS, Ives EG, et al. Familial infantile cortical hyperostosis in a large Canadian family. *Can Med Assoc J* 1984; 130:1172–4.

231. Sciubba JJ, Younai F. Epipalatus: a rare intraoral teratoma. *Oral Surg Oral Med Oral Pathol* 1991; 71:476–81.

232. Katona G, Hirschberg J, Hosszu Z, Kiraly L. Epipharyngeal teratoma in infancy. *Int J Pediatr Otorhinolaryngol* 1992; 24:171–5.

233. Conran RM, Kent SG, Wargatz ES. Oropharyngeal teratomas. A clinico-pathological study of four cases. *Am J Perinatol* 1993; 10:71–5.

234. Rybak LP, Rapp MF, McGrady MD, et al. Obstructing nasopharyngeal teratoma in the neonate. *Arch Otolaryngol Head Neck Surg* 1991; 117:1411–15.

235. Ward RF, April M. Teratomas of the head and neck. *Otolaryngol Clin N Am* 1989; 22:621–9.

236. Wynn SK, Waxman S, Ritchie G, Askotzky M. Epignathus. *Am J Dis Child* 1956; 91:495–7.

237. Wen IC. A note on an epignathous teratoma. *Chin Med J* 1933; 47:674–9.

238. Mills R. Teratomas of the head and neck in infancy and childhood. *Int J Pediatr Otorhinolaryngol* 1984; 8:177–80.

239. Calderon S, Kaplan I, Gornish M. Epignathus. *Int J Oral Maxillofac Surg* 1991; 20:322–6.

240. Wiatrak B, Myer C, Bratcher G. Report of a nasopharyngeal teratoma evaluated with MRI. *Otolaryngol Head Surg* 1990; 102:186–90.

241. Rizer FM, Schechter GL, Richardson MA. Macroglossia. Etiologic considerations and management techniques. *Int J Pediatr Otolaryngol* 1985; 8:225–36.

242. Vogel JE, Mulliken JB, Kaban LB. Macroglossia. A review of the condition and a new classification. *Plast Reconstr Surg* 1986; 78:715–23.

243. Baile BMW. A detached bronchogenic cyst occurring in the tongue of a neonate. *Br J Oral Surg* 1982; 20:288–93.

244. Ambiavagar PC, Rosen Y. Cutaneous ciliated cyst of the chin. *Arch Dermatol* 1979; 115:895–6.

245. Quinn JH. Congenital epidermoid cyst of anterior half of tongue. *Oral Surg* 1960; 13:1283–7.

246. La Bagnara J. Cysts of the base of the tongue in infants: an unusual cause of neonatal airway obstruction. *Otolaryngol Head Neck Surg* 1989; 101:108–11.

247. Howell JA, Prince TC. Congenital cyst of the base of the tongue. *Ann Otol Rhinol Laryngol* 1953; 62:896–9.

248. Calderon S, Kaplan I. Concomitant sublingual and submental epidermoid cysts. *J Oral Maxillofac Surg* 1993; 51:790–2.

249. Flom GS, Donovan TJ, Landgraf JR. Congenital dermoid cyst of the anterior tongue. *Otolaryngol Head Neck Surg* 1989; 101:388–91.

250. Dahlman B, Livaditis A. Congenital cyst of the anterior half of the tongue. *Z Kinderchir* 1980; 29:244–7.

251. Gorlin RJ, Jirasek JE. Oral cysts containing gastric or intestinal mucosa. Unusual embryologic accident or heterotopia? *J Oral Surg* 1970; 28:9–11.

252. Bite U, Cramer HM. Mixed heterotopic gastrointestinal and respiratory cyst of the lip: case report and review of the literature. *Plast Reconstr Surg* 1992; 90:1068–72.

253. Katz A, Aimi K, Skolnick EM. Enterocystomas of the head and neck. *Laryngoscope* 1980; 90:1441–4.

254. Oygür T, Dursun A, Uluoglu O, Dursun G. Oral congenital dermoid cyst in the floor of the mouth of a newborn. *Oral Surg Oral Med Oral Pathol* 1992; 74:627–30.

255. Lipsett J. Sparnon AL, Byard RW. Embryogenesis of enterocystomas—enteric duplication cysts of the tongue. *Oral Surg Oral Med Oral Pathol* 1993; 75:626–30.

256. Eppley BL, Bell MJ, Sclaroff A. Simultaneous occurrences of dermoid and heterotopic intestinal cysts in the floor of the mouth of a newborn. *J Oral Maxillofac Surg* 1985; 43:880–3.

257. Freedman PD, Chou MD, Diner H, Lumerman H. Benign mesenchymoma of the oral soft tissues. *Oral Surg* 1982; 53:606–10.

258. Demuth RJ, Johns DF. Recurrent aspiration pneumonitis in a cleft palate child with hamartoma of the tongue. *Cleft Palate J* 1979; 18:299–303.

259. Ishii T, Takemori S, Suzuki J. Hamartoma of the tongue. *Arch Otolaryngol* 1968; 88:171–3.

260. Chanin LR, Greenberg LM. Pediatric upper airway obstruction due to ectopic thyroid: classification and case reports. *Laryngoscope* 1988; 98:422–7.

261. van der Wal N, Wiener JD, van der Waal I. Lingual thyroid. A clinical and postmortem study. *Int J Oral Maxillofac Surg* 1986; 15:431–6.

262. Sauk JJ. Ectopic lingual thyroid. *Pathology* 1970; 102:239–43.

263. Williams ED, Toyn CE, Harach HR. The ultimobranchial gland and congenital thyroid abnormalities in man. *J Pathol* 1989; 159:135–42.

264. Kaplan M, Kauli R, Raviv U, Lubin E, Laron Z. Hypothyroidism due to ectopy in siblings. *Am J Dis Child* 1977; 131:1264–5.

265. Orti E, Castells S, Qazzi GH, et al. Familial thyroid disease. Lingual thyroid in two siblings and hypoplasia of a thyroid lobe in a third. *J Pediatr* 1971; 78:675–7.

266. Rosenberg T, Gilboa Y. Familial thyroid ectopy and hemiagenesis. *Arch Dis Childh* 1980; 55:639–41.

267. Elidan J, Chisin R, Gay I. Lingual thyroid, sensorineural hearing loss and mental retardation: a coincidental association? *J Laryngol Otol* 1983; 97:539–42.

268. Brandrup F. Lymphangioma circumscriptum of the tongue. *Dermatologica* 1976; 153:191–5.

269. Antoine GA, White JD, Heffner PK. Teratoma of the tongue. *Laryngoscope* 1985; 95:1262–3.

270. Ashley JV, Shafer AD. Teratoma of the tongue in a newborn. *Clev Clin Q* 1983; 50:34–6.

271. Lalwani AK, Engel TL. Teratoma of the tongue: a case report and review of the literature. *Int J Pediatr Otolaryngol* 1992; 24:261–8.

272. Pownell PH, Brown OE, Pransky SM, Manning SC. Congenital abnormalities of the submandibular duct. *Int J Pediatr Otorhinolaryngol* 1992; 24:164–9.

273. Higashino H, Tsuguo H, Yoshiaki O. Congenital absence of lacrimal puncta and of all major salivary glands. *Clin Pediatr* 1987; 26:366–8.

274. Caccamise WC, Townes PL. Congenital absence of lacrimal puncta associated with alacrima and aptyalism. *Am J Ophthalmol* 1980; 89:62–5.

275. Wiesenfeld D, Iverson ES, Ferguson MM, et al. Familial parotid gland aplasia. *J Oral Med* 1985; 40:84–5.

276. Milunsky JM, Lee VW, Siegel BS, Milunsky A. Agenesis or hypoplasia of major salivary and lacrimal glands. *Am J Med Genet* 1990; 37:371–4.

277. Rees RT. Congenital ranula. *Br Dent J* 1979; 146:345–6.

278. Towers JF. Duplication of the submandibular salivary duct. *Oral Surg* 1977; 44:326.

279. Myerson M, Crelin ES, Smith HW. Bilateral duplication of the submandibular ducts. *Arch Otolaryngol* 1966; 83:488–90.

280. Miller AS, Winnick M. Salivary gland inclusions in the anterior mandible. *Oral Surg* 1971; 31:790–7.

281. Batsakis JG. Heterotopic and accessory salivary tissues. *Ann Otol Rhinol Laryngol* 1986; 95:434–5.

282. Frommer J. The human accessory parotid gland: its incidence, nature, and significance. *Oral Surg* 1977; 43:671–6.

283. Arriaga MA, Dindzans LJ, Bluestone CD. Parotid duct communicating with a labial pit and ectopic salivary cyst. *Arch Otolaryngol Head Neck Surg* 1990; 116:1445–7.

284. Yamasaki H, Tashiro H, Watanabe T. Congenital parotid gland fistula. *Int J Oral Maxillofac Surg* 1986; 15:492–4.

285. Brennan MF, Gwynne JF, Macbeth WA. Simple parotid cysts. *Aust NZ J Surg* 1970; 40:15–19.

286. Kugelmass IN. Suppuration of the salivary glands in the newborn. *New York J Med* 1951; 51:613–17.

287. Leake D, Leake R. Neonatal suppurative parotitis. *Pediatrics* 1970; 46:203–7.

288. Çoban A, Ince Z, Ücsel R, Özgeneci A, Can G. Neonatal suppurative parotitis: a vanishing disease? *Eur J Pediatr* 1993; 152:1004–5.

289. Nussbaum M, Tan S, Som ML. Hemangiomas of the salivary glands. *Laryngoscope* 1976; 86:1015–59.

290. Mantravadi J, Roth LM, Kafwawy AH. Vascular neoplasms of the parotid glands. *Oral Surg Oral Med Oral Pathol* 1993; 75:70–5.

291. Weber TR, Connors RH, Tracy TF Jr, Bailey PV. Complex hemangiomas of infants and children. *Arch Surg* 1990; 125:1017–20.

292. Bhaskar SN, Lilly GE. Salivary gland tumors of infancy; report of twenty-seven cases. *J Oral Surg* 1963; 21:305–12.

293. Casas LA, Gonzalez-Crussi F, Pensler JM. Monomorphic adenoma of the parotid in a premature neonate. *Ann Plast Surg* 1989; 22:47–9.

294. Seifert G, Donath K. The congenital basal cell adenoma of salivary glands. Contribution to the differential diagnosis of congenital salivary gland tumours. *Virchows Arch* 1997; 430:311–19.

295. Batsakis JG, Frankenthaler R. Embryoma (sialoblastoma) of salivary glands. *Ann Otol Rhinol Laryngol* 1992; 101:958–60.

296. Adkins GF. Low-grade basaloid adenocarcinoma of salivary gland in childhood: the so-called hybrid basal cell adenoma-adenoid cystic carcinoma. *Pathology* 1990; 22:187–90.

297. Dehner LP, Valbuena L, Perez-Atayde A, et al. Salivary gland anlage tumor ("congenital pleomorphic adenoma"): a clinicopathologic immuno-histochemical and ultrastructural study of nine cases. *Am J Surg Pathol* 1994; 18:25–36.

298. Stillwater LB, Fee WE. Squamous cell proliferative lesion of the nasopharynx in a newborn. *Otolaryngol Head Neck Surg* 1980; 88:240–7.

299. Luna MA, Batsakis JG, El Naggar AK. Salivary gland tumors in children. *Ann Otol Rhinol Laryngol* 1991; 100:869–71.

300. McKnight HA. Malignant parotid tumor in newborn. *Am J Surg* 1939; 45:128–30.

301. Bailey PV, Weber TR, Tracy TF, O'Connor DM, Sotelo-Avila C. Congenital hemangiopericytoma: an unusual vascular neoplasm of infancy. *Surgery* 1993; 114:936–41.

302. Gorlin RJ, Toriello HV, Cohen MM Jr. *Hereditary Hearing Loss and Its Syndromes*. New York: Oxford University, 1995.

303. Lincoln JCR. Cervico-auriculo fistulas. *Arch Dis Child* 1965; 40:218–23.

304. Boysen ME, deBesche A, Djupesland G, Thorud E. Internal cysts and fistulae of branchial origin. *J Laryngol Otol* 1979; 93:533–9.

305. Kinder CH. Branchial cyst and lateral cervical fistula. *Br J Surg* 1954; 42:53–6.

306. Jacobs PH, Shafer JC, Higdon RS. Congenital branchiogenous anomalies. *JAMA* 1959; 169:442–6.

307. Nicklaus PJ, Forte V, Friedberg J. Congenital midline cervical cleft. *J Otolaryngol* 1992; 21:241–3.

308. van der Staak FHJ, Prusczynski M, Severijnen RS, van de Kaa CA, Festen C. The midline cervical cord. *J Pediatr Surg* 1991; 26:1391–3.

309. Gargan TJ, McKinnon M, Mulliken JB. Midline cervical cleft. *Plast Reconstr Surg* 1985; 76:225–9.

310. Kriens O, Schuchardt K. Die oberflächliche mediane Halsspalte. *Chir Plast Reconstr* 1969; 6:235–54.

311. Wynn-Williams D. Congenital midline cervical cleft. *Br J Plast Surg* 1952; 5:87–93.

312. Fincher SG, Fincher GG. Congenital midline cervical cleft with subcutaneous fibrous cord. *Otolaryngol Head Neck Surg* 1989; 101:339–401.

313. Maddalozzo J, Frankel A, Holinger LD. Midline cervical cord. *Pediatrics* 1993; 92:286–7.

314. Jordan RB, Gauderer MWL. Cervical teratomas: an analysis. Literature review and proposed classification. *J Pediatr Surg* 1988; 23:583–91.

315. Byard RW, Jiminez CL, Carpenter BF, Smith CR. Congenital teratomas of the neck and nasopharynx: a clinical and pathological study of 18 cases. *J Paediatr Child Health* 1990; 26:12–16.

316. Jaarsma AS, Tamminga RYJ, de Langen Z, et al. Neonatal teratoma presenting as hyroma colli. *Eur J Pediatr* 1994; 153:276–8.

317. Bale GF. Teratoma of the neck in the region of the thyroid gland. *Am J Pathol* 1950; 26:565–79.

318. Roediger WE, Spitz L, Schmaman A. Histogenesis of benign cervical teratomas. *Teratology* 1974; 10:111–18.

319. Emery PJ, Bailey CM, Evans JNG. Cystic hygroma of the head and neck: a review of 37 cases. *J Laryngol Otol* 1984; 98:613–19.

320. Langer JC, Fitzgerald PG, Desa D, et al. Cervical cystic hygroma in the fetus: clinical spectrum and outcome. *J Pediatr Surg* 1990; 25:58–62.

321. Goshen S, Ophir D. Cystic hygroma of the parotid gland. *J Laryngol Otol* 1993; 107:855–7.

322. Ninh TN, Ninh TX. Cystic hygroma in children: a report of 126 cases. *J Pediatr Surg* 1974; 9:191–5.

323. Elejalde BR, de Elejalde M, Leno J. Nuchal cysts syndrome: etiology, pathogenesis, and prenatal diagnosis. *Am J Med Genet* 1985; 21:417–32.

324. Lyngbye T, Haugaard L, Klebe JG. Antenatal sonographic diagnoses of giant cystic hygroma of the neck. *Acta obstet Gynecol Scand* 1986; 65:873–5.

325. Ricciardelli EJ, Richardson MA. Cervicofacial cystic hygroma: patterns of recurrence and management of the difficult case. *Arch Otolaryngol Head Neck Surg* 1991; 117:546–53.

326. Osborne TE, Haller TA, Levin LS, Lattle BJ, King KE. Submandibular cystic hygroma resembling a plunging ranula in a neonate. *Oral Surg Oral Med Oral Pathol* 1991; 71:16–20.

327. Cohen MM Jr, Jirásek JE, Guzman RT, Gorlin RJ, Peterson MQ. Holoprosencephaly and facial dysmorphia: nosology, etiology and pathogenesis. *Birth Defects* 1971; 7(7):125–35.

328. Jabs EW, Li X, Scott AF, et al. Jackson-Weiss and Crouzon syndromes are allelic with mutations in fibroblast growth factor receptor 2. *Nature Genet* 1994; 8:275–9.

329. Jabs EW, Müller U, Li X, et al. A mutation in the homeodomain of the human MSX2 gene in a family affected with autosomal dominant craniosynostosis. *Cell* 1993; 75:443–50.

330. Vortkamp A, Gessler M, Grzeschik KH. GL13 zinc finger gene interrupted by translocations in Greig syndrome families. *Nature* 1991; 352:539–40.

331. Lewanda AF, Cohen MM Jr, Jackson CE, et al. Genetic heterogeneity among craniosynostosis syndromes: mapping the Saethre-Chotzen syndrome locus between D7S513 and D7S516 and exclusion of Jackson-Weiss and Crouzon syndrome loci from 7p. *Genomics* 1994; 19:115–19.

332. Preston RA, Post JC, Keats BJB, et al. A gene for Crouzon craniofacial dysostosis maps to the long arm of chromosome 10. *Nature Genet* 1994; 7:149–53.

333. Li X, Lewanda AF, Eluma F, et al. Two craniosynostotic syndrome loci, Crouzon and Jackson-Weiss, map to chromosome 10q13–q26. *Genomics* 1994; 22:418–24.

334. Robin NH, Feldman GJ, Mitchell HF, et al. Linkage of Pfeiffer syndrome to chromosome 8 centromere and evidence for genetic heterogeneity. *Hum Mol Genet* 1994; 3:2153–8.

335. Rutland P, Pulleyn LJ, Reardon W, et al. Identical mutations in the FGFR2 gene cause both Pfeiffer and Crouzon syndrome phenotypes. *Nature Genet* 1995; 9:173–6.

336. Wilkie AOM, Staney SF, Oldridge M, et al. Apert syndrome results from localized mutations of FGFR2 and is allelic with Crouzon syndrome. *Nature Genet* 1995; 9:165–72.

337. Schell U, Hehr A, Feldman GJ, et al. Mutations in FGFR1 and FGFR2 cause familial and sporadic Pfeiffer syndrome. *Hum Molec Genet* 1995; 4:323–8.

338. Cohen MM Jr, Kreiborg S. Hands and feet in the Apert syndrome. *Am J Med Genet* 1995; 57:82–96.

339. Cohen MM Jr. *The Child with Multiple Birth Defects.* 2nd ed. New York: Oxford University, 1997.

340. Reid CS, McMorrow LE, McDonald-McGinn DM, et al. Saethre-Chotzen syndrome with familial translocation at chromosome 7p22. *Am J Med Genet* 1993; 47:637–9.

The Eye

ALEC GARNER

DEVELOPMENT

First Month

Ocular development [1–4] begins with outpouching of the anterior neural folds on either side of the midline to form pits by the 3-mm stage (day 21). Within the next day or so, each pit expands into a vesicle, which, subsequent to thickening of the overlying surface ectoderm to form the future lens plate, commences to invaginate to create a double-layered optic cup. In addition to the indentation at the distal end of the vesicle, there is a simultaneous invagination from below to form a groove by the 7-mm stage (day 28) (Fig. 23.1). Very soon, however, the margins of the groove or optic fissure come together and begin to fuse, the process normally being complete by the 18-mm stage (week 6). The outer layer of the optic cup acquires melanin pigment to constitute the future retinal pigment epithelium, which, in turn, induces formation of the choroidal vascular coat on its external aspect. Vascularization of the loose mesenchymal tissue filling the cavity of the optic cup develops toward the end of the first month by virtue of a branch of the ophthalmic artery known as the hyaloid artery, entering through the as yet unclosed posterior part of the optic fissure.

Second Month

The lens plate, having induced invagination of the optic vesicle, continues to grow and itself invaginates into the opening of the optic cup (Fig. 23.2). Early in the second month of gestation (10-mm stage), the lens vesicle separates from the surface ectoderm to form a rudimentary lens (Fig. 23.3) and almost immediately it becomes invested by blood vessels derived from the hyaloid artery (Fig. 23.4). The inner layer of the optic cup begins to separate into its definitive neuroblastic layers, while the optic stalk connecting the original optic vesicle to the forebrain gives rise to the optic nerve as axons from the ganglion cells of the retina extend centripetally to the optic disk.

Directly after the lens vesicle has separated, the cornea begins to form, the surface ectoderm providing an epithelial covering for a substantia propria formed by ingrowth of mesoderm from the proximity of the rim of the optic cup (Fig. 23.5). This occurs at the 21- to 26-mm stage (6th to 7th week). A second, more posterior, wave of mesodermal invasion provides a pupillary membrane, which is the anlage for the future iris stroma. The anterior chamber emerges toward the end of the month as a cleft between the cornea and the pupillary membrane. Adnexal structures, such as the lacrimal gland, nasolacrimal drainage system, extraocular muscles, and bony orbits, begin to develop at about this time. The first vestiges of the eyelids also emerge during the second month as a circular fold of mesenchyme covered by ectoderm.

Third Month

Axial extension of the epithelial margins of the optic cup along the back of the pupillary membrane not only contributes to the further development of the iris but also serves to separate the latter from the lens and create the posterior chamber of the eye. The ciliary body also begins to appear at this time, the cilary processes deriving from the margins of the optic cup and the smooth muscle component differentiating from the paraxial mesoderm.

Condensation of the mesoderm surrounding the developing eye commences next with the production of collagen fibers and proceeds to form a fibrous shell subsequently

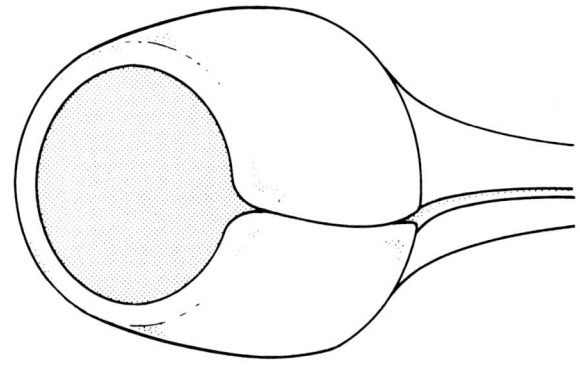

FIGURE 23.1.   *Diagrammatic representation of invaginated optic vesicle (7-mm embryo) with inferior groove.*

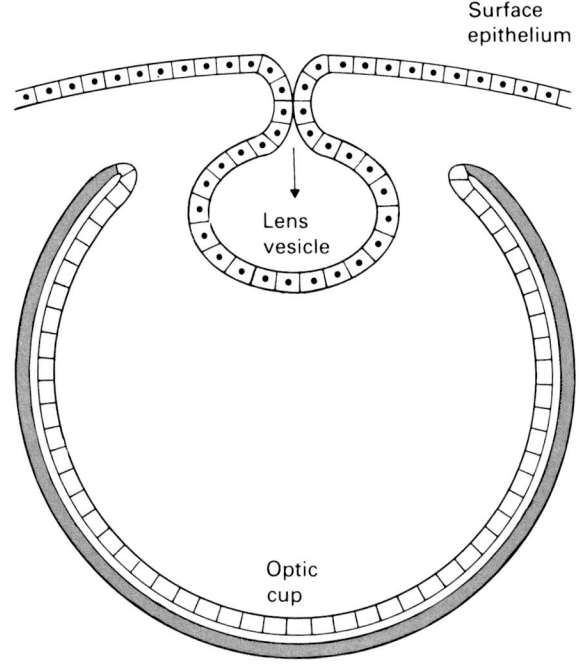

FIGURE 23.2.   *A 9-mm embryo. Invagination of the surface ectoderm overlying the optic cup produces a vesicle that separates to constitute the primitive lens.*

identified as the sclera. Further neuroretinal differentiation occurs, and vascularization of the anterior segment also proceeds.

The eyelids, which began as an ever diminishing circular hole in front of the eye, grow rather unequally, with the effect that the hole is converted into a transverse slit: toward the end of the third month the margins of the ectoderm above and below the slit fuse.

Fourth Month

By the fourth month blood vessels originating from the base of the involuting hyaloid artery start to invade the inner layers of the retina. The suspensory ligaments of the lens become established by the outgrowth of filamentous material (the so-called tertiary vitreous) from the tips of the ciliary body processes, which fuse with the lens capsule.

Fifth Month

The cornea increases in curvature and development of the choroid and sclera nears completion.

Sixth Month

Muscular elements of the ciliary body and iris undergo further development and the eyelids reopen. Pigmentation of the uveal stroma begins in the choroid and gradually spreads anteriorly to involve the ciliary body and iris.

From the time of fusion toward the end of the third month, the ectodermal covering of the rudimentary eyelids undergoes progressive differentiation. That on the outer surface is converted to epidermis, the keratinization and subsequent exfoliation of which lead to separation of the fused lid margins. Specialized hairs (eyelashes or cilia) form close to the lid margins. The ectoderm lining the inner surface of the lids acquires some features of squamous epithelium and goblet cells appear; but, being continuously moist, it does

not keratinize and comes to constitute the palpebral conjunctiva.

Seventh Month

The formation and organization of the anterior chamber and other anterior segment structures approach completion.

Eighth Month

Maturation of the retina reaches completion in all areas apart from the fovea, which is only just beginning to differentiate at this time. The hyaloid artery is totally atrophied.

Ninth Month

The pupillary membrane disappears to leave a clear pupil, and myelinization of the optic nerve reaches the lamina cribrosa.

Situation at Birth

The eye at term has an anteroposterior diameter of 17.5 mm, compared with an average 24.1 mm in adult life; its volume is 2.4 mL relative to 6.9 mL when fully developed [5]. Thus, while the eye continues to grow until adolescence, the changes are fairly small and the definitive structure of

Chapter 23 The Eye

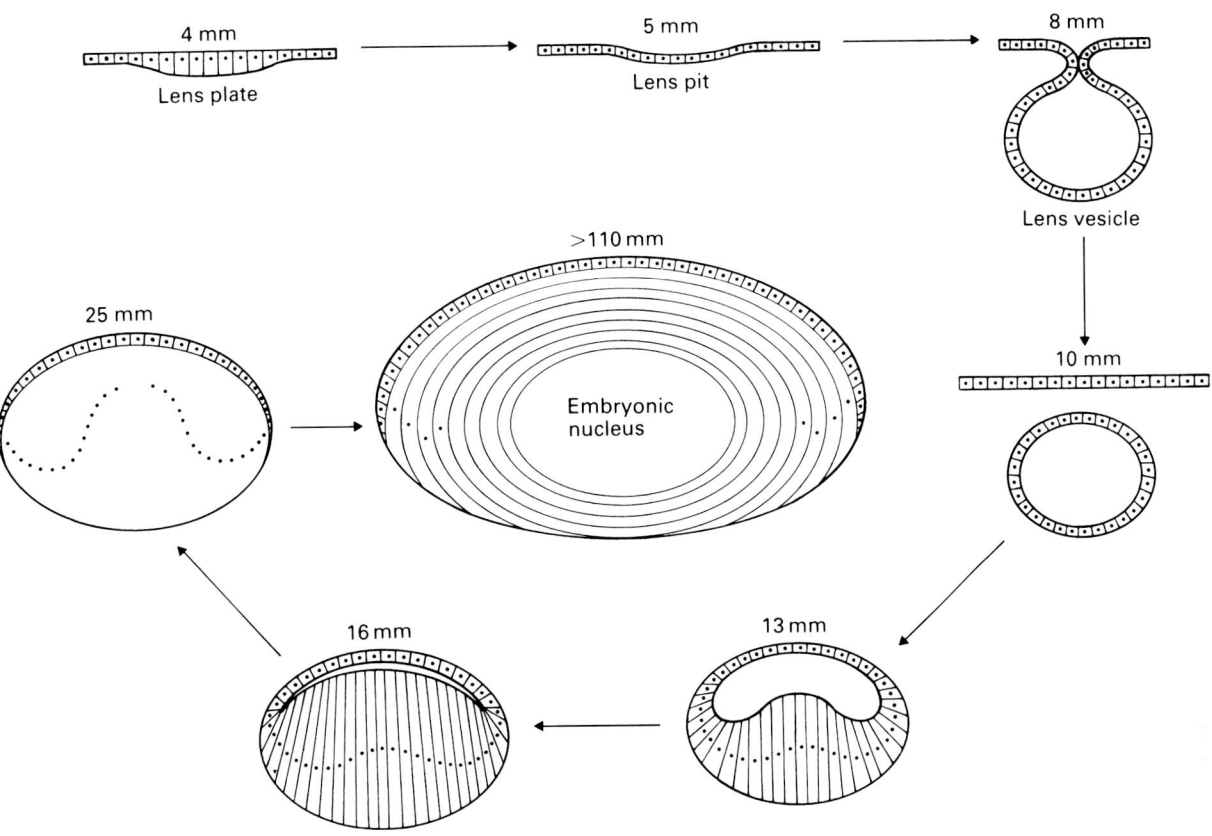

FIGURE 23.3. *Diagrammatic representation of lens development. Beginning at the 4-mm stage of embryogenesis, the surface epithelium adjacent to the optic vesicle thickens to form the primordial lens plate, which soon invaginates to form a vesicle. The vesicle separates from the surface at about the 10-mm stage. Thereafter, continued proliferation of the lens epithelium results in obliteration of the cavity of the vesicle by the 20-mm stage. The embryonic nucleus formed in this way then becomes encapsulated by successive layers of secondary lens fibers derived from the migration and differentiation of epithelium at the equator, a process that continues slowly throughout life.*

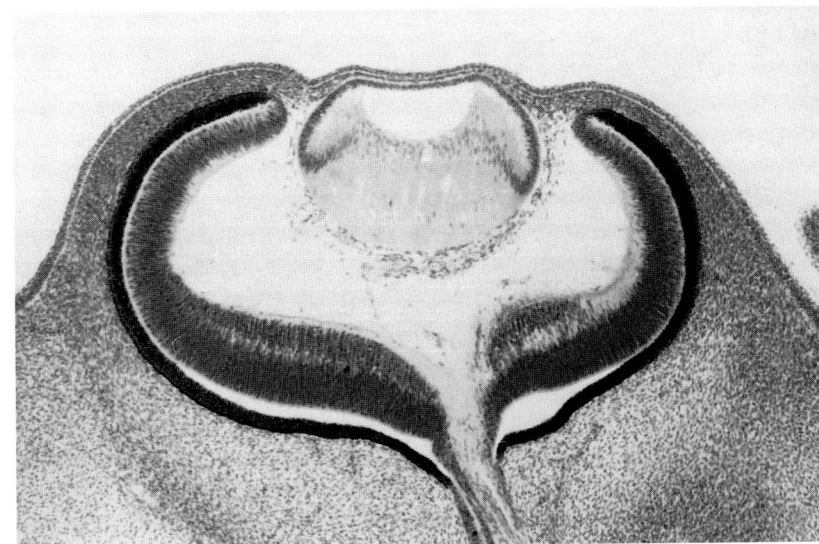

FIGURE 23.4. *Histological section of 20-mm (6 weeks') embryo showing optic cup with clearly defined pigment epithelium in the outer layer and developing retina on the inner aspect. The cavity of the developing lens is near obliteration. (H&E, ×80.)*

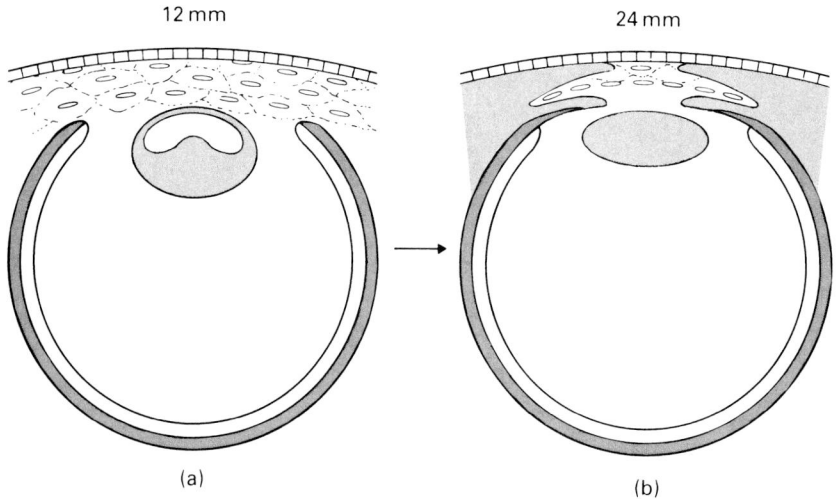

12 mm   24 mm

(a)   (b)

FIGURE 23.5. *Development of cornea and iris. (a) Diagram of eye at 12-mm stage, showing a loose matrix beneath the surface epithelium with mesothelial precursors of the endothelium responsible for laying down Descemet's membrane to delineate the deep surface of the cornea. There is no iris development at this stage. (b) By the 24-mm stage, a second wave of stromal tissue invades the space between the surface epithelium and the lips of the optic cup in a two-pronged manner to form the substantia propria of the cornea and the stroma of the iris, which lines the anterior surface of the centripetal extension of the pigmented layer of the optic cup.*

the eye is virtually established at birth. Even so, some post-natal development does take place:

1. *Cornea:* Descemet's membrane measures 2 to 3 μm at birth and only gradually reaches its final thickness of 8 to 16 μm in adult life [6].
2. *Iris:* Pigmentation of the stroma begins at about the time of birth and may continue for several months. Remnants of the pupillary membrane may persist.
3. *Ciliary body:* Fibers of the oblique part of the ciliary muscle remain to be formed.
4. *Lens:* Slow growth continues throughout life.
5. *Retina:* Macular development, essential for visual acuity, having commenced in the eighth month, continues for another 4 or 5 months.

The histological structure of a mature eye is shown in Figure 23.6.

CONGENITAL ANOMALIES

Whole Eye

Anophthalmos

Complete absence of the eye is extremely rare. More often there is an inapparent microphthalmic globe, in which case the term "clinical anophthalmos" is nearer the mark. True anophthalmos does occur, however, generally because of failure of the optic vesicle either to form or to invaginate. It is usually associated with other maldevelopments of the brain and may be linked with a variety of chromosomal disorders [7].

Microphthalmos

An abnormally small eye results when the area of contact between the optic vesicle and the surface ectoderm (7-mm stage) is less than usual. Alternatively, microphthalmos can

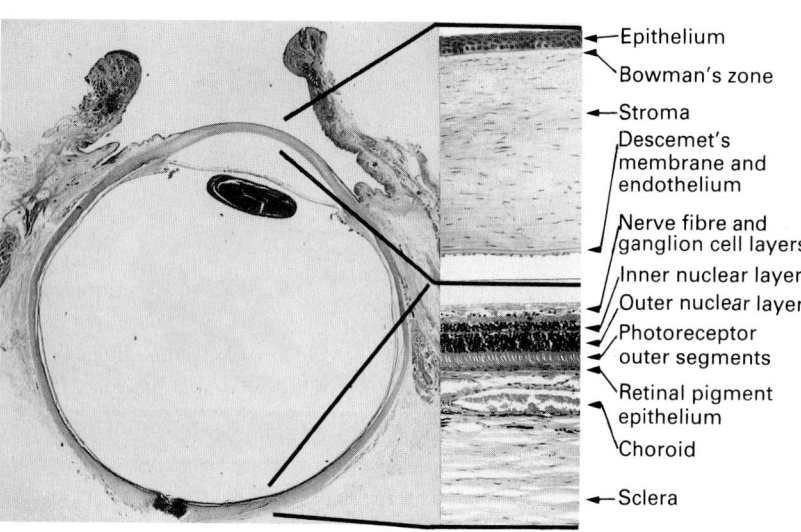

←Epithelium
Bowman's zone
←Stroma
Descemet's membrane and endothelium
Nerve fibre and ganglion cell layers
Inner nuclear layer
Outer nuclear layer
Photoreceptor outer segments
Retinal pigment epithelium
Choroid
←Sclera

FIGURE 23.6. *Developed eye. Vertical and slightly oblique section passing through the optic disk but to the side of the pupil, with upper and lower eyelids in position. Inset shows the cornea and posterior coats of the eye in greater detail. (H&E, ×2.1. Insets: ×67.)*

occur at a later stage should the vitreous fail to accumulate to the required degree, since it is this that is largely responsible for expanding the outer scleral coat of the globe. The eyeball may be small but functional and structurally almost normal (nanophthalmos); or there may be associated ocular abnormalities, especially coloboma, in which case the eye is blind. Microphthalmos can occur as a solitary finding, or, rather more commonly, as part of a systemic maldevelopment syndrome and may be attributable to infection, maternal radiation, and a range of chromosomal and genetic disturbances [7]. Angle-closure glaucoma is a well-recognized complication of nanophthalmos and in some cases is probably due to compression by a disproportionately large lens [8].

Cryptophthalmos

In this usually bilateral condition the anterior surface of the eye is fused with the adjacent skin to produce the semblance of a thin scar where the palpebral fissure would be expected. There are no eyelashes or eyebrows. Anomalous development of the eye and subsequent xerosis of the cornea are frequent, although reduced size is uncommon. The condition can occur as an isolated event or as part of a multisystem disorder.

Synophthalmos and Cyclopia

Fusion of the eyeballs is linked with malformation of the forebrain, allowing the optic vesicles to merge during the first month of gestation [9]. The fusion can vary in extent from a structure in which there is duplication of most of the intraocular tissues (synophthalmos) (Fig. 23.7) to a truly single eye (cyclopia) in the midline. In both situations there is always a single optic nerve and no chiasm. Cyclopia is usually associated with death in the first trimester, whereas synophthalmic fetuses may be born alive only to die moments later because of the accompanying severe maldevelopment of the nasopharynx.

Coloboma

Invagination of the optic vesicle at about the 7-mm stage is accompanied by simultaneous indentation from below to create a cup with an inferior fissure. This optic or retinal fissure subsequently closes as the opposed edges come together. Failure of the fissure to close constitutes a coloboma and this may extend along the entire length of the fissure from the site of the future iris to the optic nerve, or it may involve just a part (Fig. 23.8). Colobomas formed in this way are situated inferiorly and slightly nasally.

Colobomas of the choroid and retina are seen histologically as areas devoid of pigment epithelium and choroidal stroma, straddled by an attenuated layer of atrophic neuroretina. Disproportionate development of the inner layer of the optic cup can herniate through the unclosed fissure and produce an extraocular (orbital) cyst.

Iris colobomas are the most common and a proportion are atypical in that they occur other than in an inferonasal

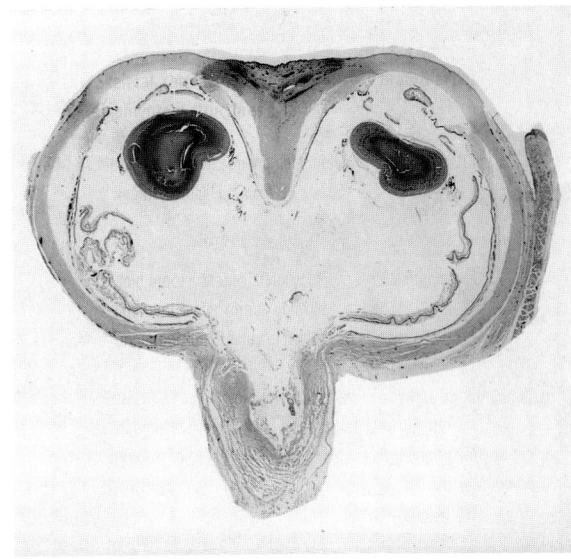

FIGURE 23.7. *Synophthalmos. There is separate development of the anterior segments of the conjoined eyes but the posterior segments ate totally fused. (H&E, ×3.)*

position. This type of defect reflects abnormal development after the optic fissure has closed [6]. It seems that persistence of the vascular anastomosis between the hyaloid system as it arborizes around the lens and the vessels at the rim of the optic cup can prevent the rim from growing forward to form the iris epithelium and musculature.

Coloboma formation is usually bilateral, although not necessarily symmetrical, and may be linked with other ocular abnormalities. Genetic defects are common, especially those of an autosomal dominant character, but a wide range of exogenous causative agents has also been implicated.

Amniotic Bands

Through direct contact and interference with development, amniotic bands may give rise to congenital corneal leukomas and eyelid colobomas as extensions of facial clefts. Hypertelorism is common in these situations. Postnatal corneal opacities may occur as a result of exposure secondary to eyelid maldevelopment [10].

Fetal Alcohol Syndrome

More than three-quarters of babies subject to the effects of maternal alcohol consumption have short palpebral fissures. Eyelid ptosis and epicanthal folds are also well recognized. Less commonly reported complications include microphthalmia, blepharophimosis, and hypoplasia of the optic nerve [11].

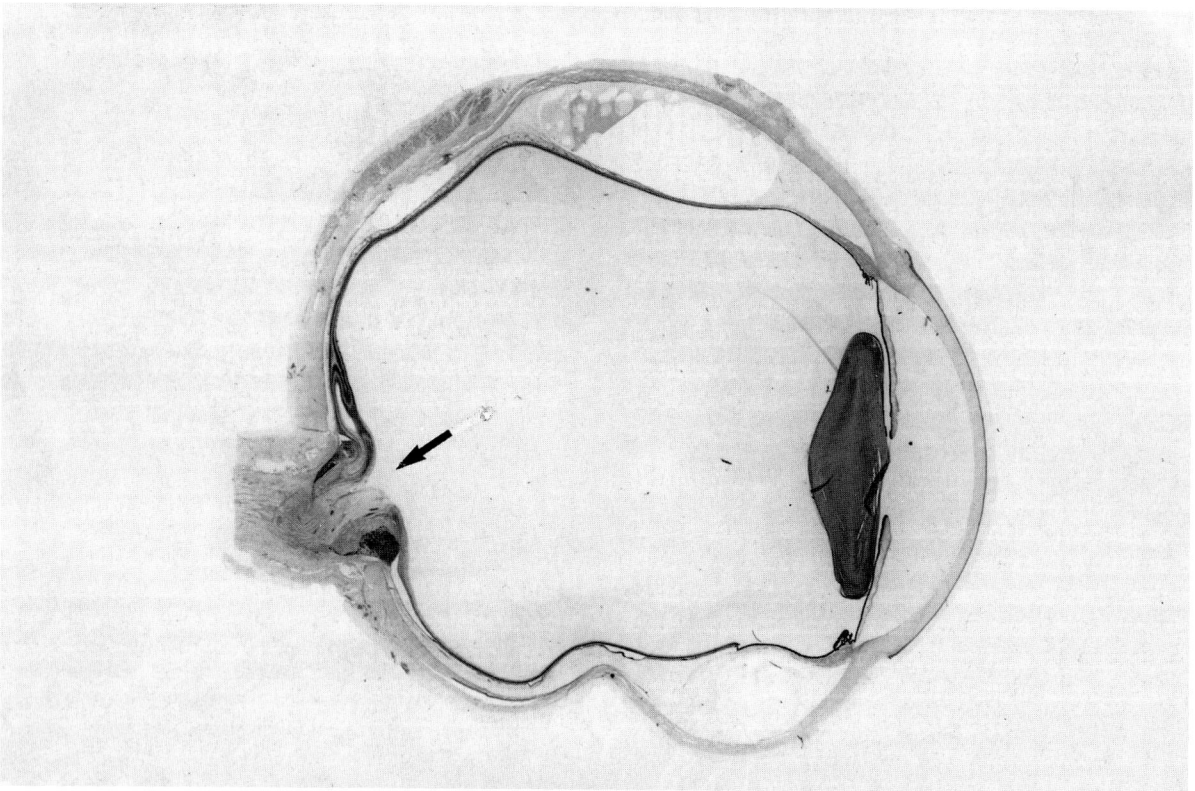

FIGURE 23.8.   *Optic nerve coloboma. The head of the optic nerve shows a deep congenital pit (arrow), which is associated with incomplete formation of the adjacent sclera. (H&E, ×4.5.)*

Cornea

Sclerocornea

The wave of mesoderm that is the progenitor of the definitive corneal stroma differentiates in a quite exceptional manner, such that parallel lamellae of identical collagen fibers are deposited in a pattern that simulates a diffraction grating. Rarely, this special differentiation fails to occur and the resultant fibrils vary in caliber and have a more random alignment (Fig. 23.9). In consequence, the affected cornea resembles the contiguous opaque sclera, the extent of the scleralization ranging from a rim at the periphery to involvement of the entire cornea. Vascularization of the stroma may be a further feature. Histological examination also reveals absence of Bowman's zone beneath the epithelium; defects in Descemet's membrane are also not uncommon [12]. Known as *sclerocornea*, the condition may be unilateral or bilateral, sporadic or inherited.

Megalocornea and Microcornea

In megalocornea the diameter of the cornea exceeds 13 mm, and in microcornea the diameter is less than 11 mm by the end of the first year of life. Sex-linked recessive inheritance (Xq21.3–q22) is common in megalocornea, whereas microcornea is usually linked with an autosomal dominant gene defect. Neither situation involves any histological abnormality or loss of transparency [7], although both are frequently associated with other ocular abnormalities, particularly of the anterior segment.

Dermoids

The favored site for epibulbar dermoid formations is at the corneo-conjunctival limbus. They represent developmental sequestrations of primitive tissue and appear clinically as white or tan-colored firm nodules. Histologically they are composed of hair follicles with sebaceous and, less commonly, sweat gland acini in a fibroadipose stroma (Fig. 23.10). The surface epithelium is often keratinized. Occasionally, non-dermal tissue, such as cartilage or smooth muscle, is seen and for these circumstances the term "complex choristoma" is appropriate [13].

Most epibulbar dermoids are solitary lesions, but they may also present as part of Goldenhar's oculoauriculovertebral dysplasia and in association with microphthalmos [14].

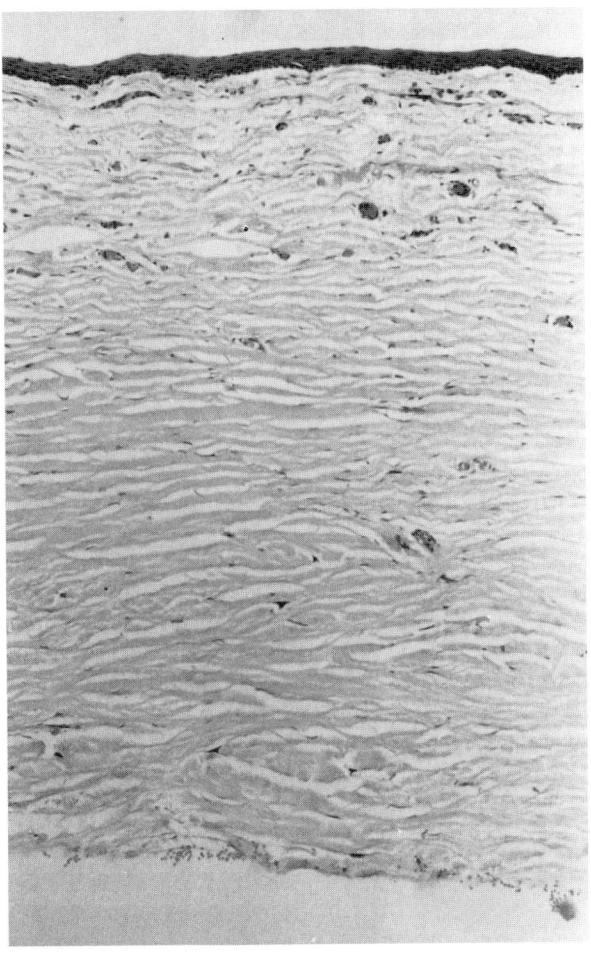

FIGURE 23.9. *Sclerocornea. Section through the cornea showing absence of Bowman's layer and Descemet's membrane, and vascularization of the substantia propria, the collagen bundles of which lack the normal laminar alignment. (H&E, ×90.)*

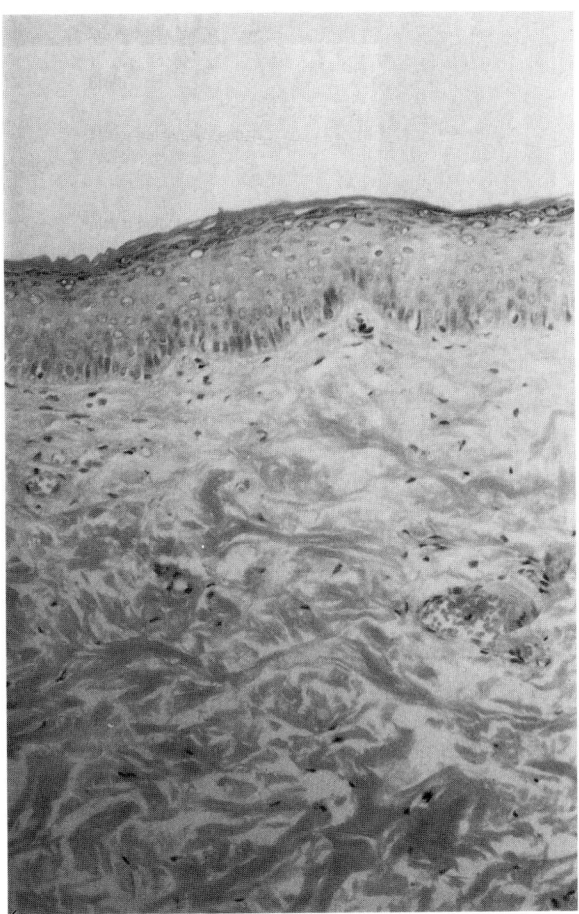

FIGURE 23.10. *Limbal dermoid. The epithelium resembles normal epidermis in having a well-defined stratum granulosum and surface keratinization. The normally loose underlying stroma is replaced by dense, randomly aligned collagen bundles. (Adnexal skin structures are not seen in this case.) (H&E, ×180.)*

Anterior Chamber

The cleft that is to develop into the aqueous-filled anterior chamber of the eye starts to form around the 26-mm stage through a process of presumed rarefaction of the mesenchyme between the Descemet's membrane of the cornea and the secondary wave of mesoderm responsible for the iridial stroma. Anomalous development can occur toward the periphery [15] or more centrally [16].

Schwalbe's Line

Alternatively known as posterior embryotoxon, Schwalbe's line is a concentric ring of corneal opacification near to the periphery, produced by mesenchymal tissue at the margin of Descemet's membrane. Histologically, it is seen as a ridge projecting from the back of the cornea into the anterior chamber.

Axenfeld's Anomaly

In Axenfeld's anomaly Schwalbe's line is connected intermittently along its circumference to the iris by delicate strands of connective tissue (Fig. 23.11).

Rieger's Anomaly

Rieger's anomaly is comparable to Axenfeld's anomaly, with the addition of marked hypoplasia of the iridial stroma. Deletion of either the short or long arm of chromosome 4 (4p- or 4q-) may be featured [17, 18], in which case the corneal abnormality tends to be part of a generalized systemic disturbance. Duplication of the short arm of chromosome 3 (3p+) is also described.

Peters Anomaly

Peters anomaly is a central dysgenesis, bilateral in 80% of cases, in which the lens and/or the iris are attached to the

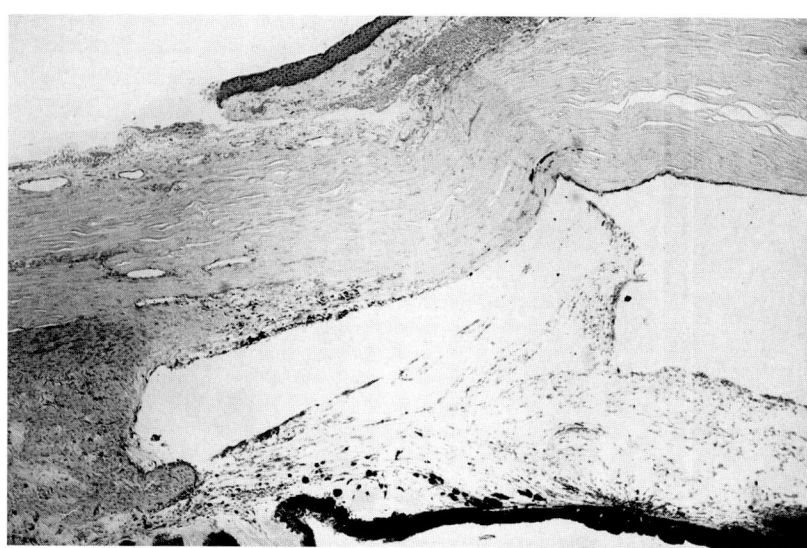

FIGURE 23.11.   *Axenfeld's anomaly. Strands of loose connective tissue run from the iris to the posterior surface of the cornea. (H&E, ×51.)*

cornea. Descemet's membrane is deficient in the axial region due either to failure of the primitive mesenchyme, from which it arises, to reach the center or to incomplete separation of the lens vesicle from the surface ectoderm. Chromosomal abnormalities are a well-recognized accompaniment, with associated systemic abnormalities in the form of a ring chromosome 18, partial trisomy 16q, or deletions (13 and 18q-) [7, 19].

Congenital Glaucoma

Anomalous development of the angle of the anterior chamber can interfere with the outflow of aqueous to a level that elevates the intraocular pressure sufficiently to damage the retina [20]. The nature of the maldevelopment is uncertain and may vary, but several reports describe insertion of the longitudinal fibers of the ciliary muscle so far forward that they obstruct the scleral trabecular meshwork through which aqueous drainage mainly occurs. Autosomal recessive inheritance is a feature of some cases.

The structural damage to the eye as a consequence of unrelieved ocular hypertension includes corneal haziness due to waterlogging, enlargement of the entire globe (buphthalmos) through stretching of the immature corneoscleral envelope (Fig. 23.12), pressure atrophy of the choroid and retina, and indentation (cupping) of the optic disc.

Although the seeds of the condition are present at birth, clinical manifestation may be delayed until infancy.

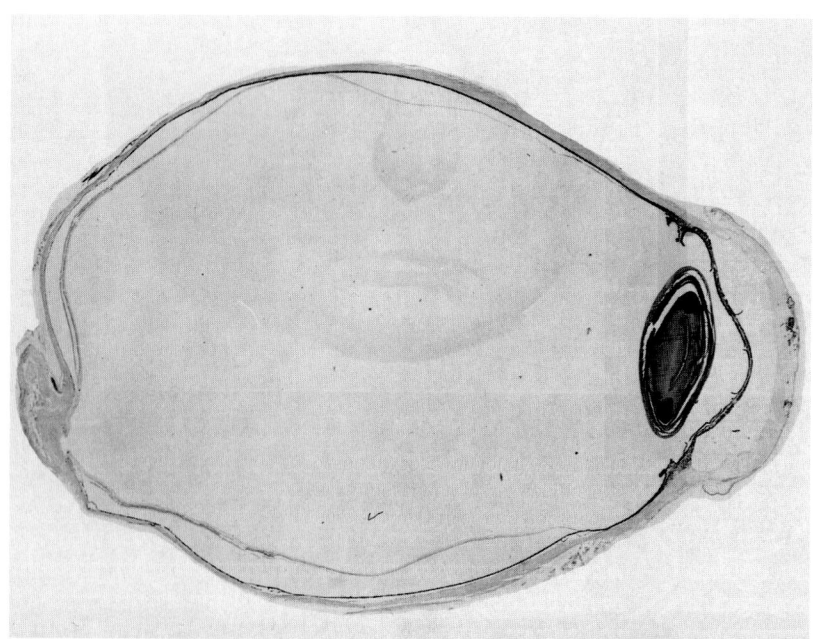

FIGURE 23.12.   *Buphthalmos. The increased intraocular pressure associated with congenital glaucoma has produced distension of the corneoscleral envelope. Enlargement is greatest in the anteroposterior diameter. Some cupping of the optic nerve head is also present. (H&E, ×3.)*

Iris

Aniridia

Despite its designation aniridia usually has some rudimentary iris formation; rarely is the iris totally absent [21]. It is almost always bilateral and generally accompanied by a variety of other developmental ocular abnormalities. Both sporadic and familial forms are recognized, the former being linked to chromosomal defects, especially deletion of the short arm of chromosome 11, and the latter showing autosomal dominant inheritance. Aniridia linked to genetic disturbance at the 11p13 locus commonly occurs in association with Wilms' tumor as part of the Wilms' tumor-aniridia-gonadoblastoma-retardation syndrome [22]. Some observers have regarded aniridia as a subtotal form of atypical coloboma [23].

Persistent Pupillary Membrane

The mesoderm responsible for forming the stroma of the iris extends across the midline during embryogenesis and the definitive pupil does not develop until late in pregnancy. Remnants of the vascularized fibrous tissue are not uncommon at birth but occasionally can be more extensive and cause partial, rarely complete, occlusion of the pupil. Sometimes the remnants are simultaneously attached to the lens or cornea.

Heterochromia

Differing degrees of pigmentation between the iris of one eye and its fellow may be inherited as an autosomal dominant disorder. In later life, inflammation, melanosis, and hemorrhage may produce the same result. Heterochromia iridis may occasionally be a feature of certain more widespread developmental defects, such as syringomyelia, Waardenberg syndrome, and congenital Horner syndrome. The difference in pigmentation relates to the stroma melanocytes as opposed to the pigment epithelium of the iris.

Lens

Lens abnormalities identifiable at birth include complete absence (aphakia), duplication, variations in shape, microphakia, ectopia, and cataract.

Congenital Cataract

Lens opacification is one of the more common congenital ocular defects and can have a variety of causes [24]. The defect may be unilateral or bilateral, inherited (approximately 25%) or secondary, and can represent either anomalous development or intrauterine degeneration of otherwise normally formed lens tissue.

Cataract morphology depends as much, if not more, on the timing of the insult as on its nature. Commonly recognized morphological types of congenital cataract are summarized below.

Lamellar (Zonular) Cataracts Lamellar cataracts are characterized by a zone of opaque fibers produced during a transient episode of defective development in an otherwise normal evolution. This results in clear tissue on either side of the opacity, which, although starting superficially beneath the capsule, comes to lie deeper within the lens as growth proceeds. Histologically, the affected fibers are replaced by degenerate lens material and amorphous debris.

Nuclear Cataracts Nuclear cataracts may develop in the first 2 months of gestation, when the embryonal nucleus is still forming: this produces a small (less than 1 mm) opacity in the center of the lens (embryonal nuclear cataract). An insult in the third month leads to opacification at the level of the anterior and posterior Y-shaped sutures (fetal nuclear cataract).

Polar Cataracts Polar cataracts are frequently associated with defects of the vascular network surrounding the lens.

Anterior polar cataracts represent either disturbed formation and persistence of the pupillary membrane or defective separation of the lens vesicle from the surface ectoderm. The opacity is immediately subcapsular and caused by proliferation and fibrous metaplasia of the subcapsular epithelium.

Posterior polar cataracts occur where the hyaloid artery arborizes into the tunica vasculosa lentis and results in a minute white spot (Mittendorf's dot) over the center of the capsule covering the back of the lens. Occasionally, the affected capsule may rupture (it is particularly prone to do so if associated with a persistent hyperplastic primary vitreous) and lead to more extensive lens opacification. Autosomal dominant inheritance is usual.

Ring Cataracts Ring cataracts develop when the primary lens cells fail to develop or if later resorption occurs due to rubella virus infection or some other cause. The absence of a nucleus around which the secondary lens cells can grow produces a doughnut-shape, with the central part consisting of apposed anterior and posterior capsular tissue (Fig. 23.13). Ring cataracts are seen also in the Hallermann-Streiff syndrome, when they are associated with other ocular and craniofacial abnormalities [25].

Coronary Cataracts Coronary cataracts are small punctate opacities, often greenish blue (cerulean cataract), arranged in a ring when the lens is viewed from front. The opacities lie under the capsule near the equator of the lens and, histologically, are seen as PAS-positive excrescences on the deep surface of the capsule. With time, the excrescences disintegrate and move into the cortex as fine granules. Coronary cataracts are often seen in Down syndrome children [26].

Vitreous

Persistent Hyperplastic Primary Vitreous

The primary vitreous develops soon after the formation of the optic cup as a loose mesenchymal matrix that is

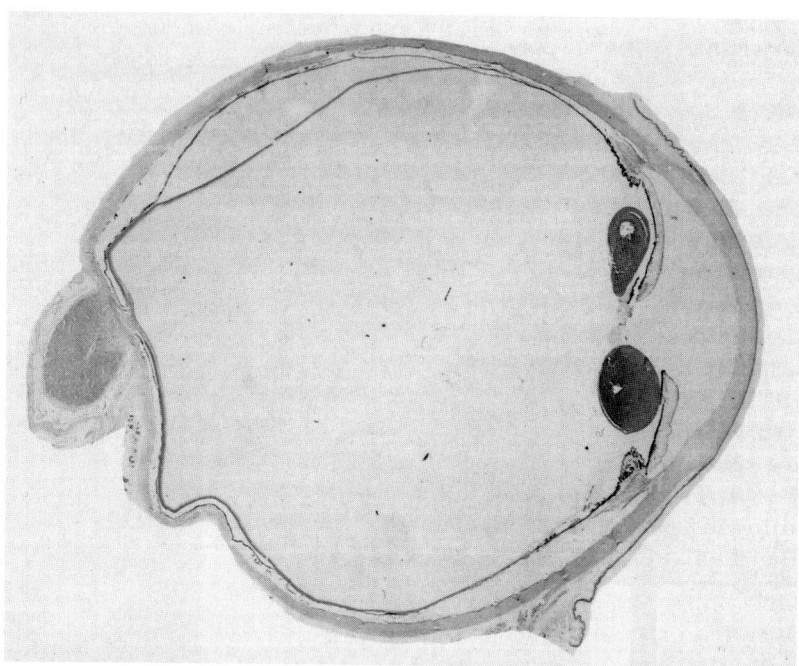

FIGURE 23.13. *Congenital ring cataract. The central part of the lens has failed to form and there has been irregular development of the secondary lens fibers in a circumferential manner toward the equator. (H&E, ×3.5.)*

vascularized by branches of the hyaloid artery (Fig. 23.14). Subsequently, in the 50 to 60 mm stage, cells presumed to derive from the retina begin to secrete glycosaminoglycan, which eventually constitutes the definitive secondary vitreous. Contemporaneous with this process is gradual involution of the hyaloid vascular system until the sole remaining branches of the hyaloid artery are those at its terminus, where it ramifies over the back of the lens. Eventually, these too atrophy so that by the eighth month all that remains is a filmy condensation of collagen at the interface between the primary and secondary vitreous, which invests the erstwhile hyaloid artery to constitute the canal of Cloquet.

Very occasionally, the involutional process is arrested [27] and the vessels adjacent to the lens persist and may be a cause of intraocular hemorrhage in early infancy (Fig. 23.15). The vessels are accompanied by fibrous tissue, and it is this that probably causes the frequently observed rupture of the posterior part of the lens capsule, which, in turn, predisposes to degenerative cataractogenesis. Cicatrization of the fibroblastic tissue is also the likely explanation for the elongated ciliary processes seen extending over the back of the lens. Rarely, the fibrovascular tissue behind the lens contains fat or cartilage [28]. In addition to cataract, glaucoma is a recognized complication of persistent hyperplastic primary vitreous by virtue of undue enlargement of the lens and its impinging on the iris to narrow the filtration angle of the anterior chamber. The condition is almost always unilateral.

2nd–3rd month   8th month

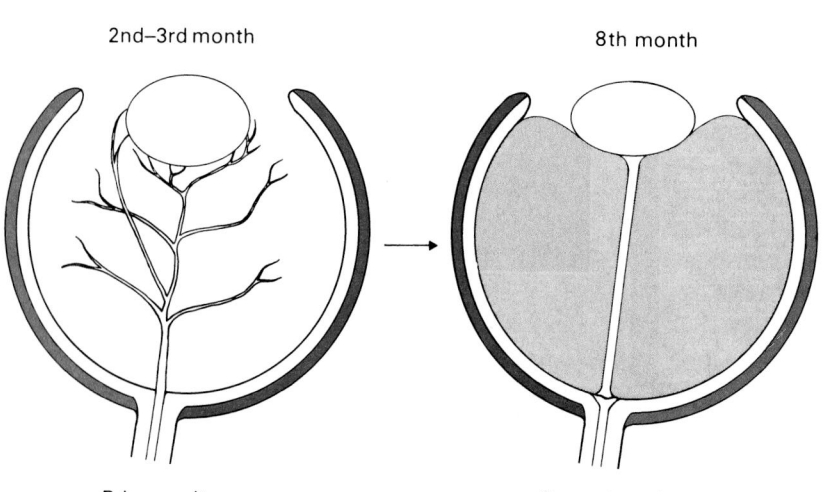

Primary vitreous   Secondary vitreous

FIGURE 23.14. *Vitreous development. At about the 30-mm stage, the cavity of the optic cup is filled by loose primitive connective tissue vascularized by branches of the hyaloid artery. Subsequently, the vascularized primary vitreous is replaced by an accumulation of hyaluronic-acid–rich proteoglycan gel. The course of the hyaloid artery is represented by the canal of Cloquet running from the optic nerve head toward the lens.*

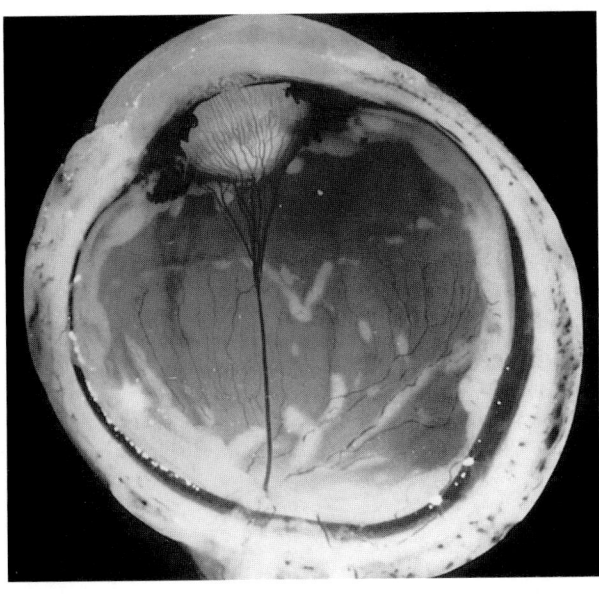

FIGURE 23.15. *Persistent hyperplastic primary vitreous. The hyaloid artery has persisted into postnatal life and is seen ramifying over the posterior surface of the lens, where it is attached to elongated processes of the ciliary body. (H&E, ×4.4.)*

Retina

Retinal Dysplasia

Retinal dysplasia represents disturbed organization of the neuroretina (Fig. 23.16). It may be an isolated finding but is also a feature of other ocular maldevelopments, especially microphthalmos. Bilaterality is common, and an association with trisomy 13 is well documented [29]. The outstanding histological finding is the presence of rosettes (Fig. 23.17) wherein the differentiating cell layers are arranged in a circle around an inner rim representing the outer limiting membrane of the retina [30]. Coordination of retinal growth depends, in large part, on an intimate relationship between the inner (primitive neuroretina) and outer (primitive pigment epithelium) layers of the optic cup; dysplasia can result from deficiencies in either, particularly the latter.

Congenital Retinal Detachment

Retinal detachment represents separation of the neuroretina from the retinal pigment epithelium but it is possible that most instances of congenital detachment are strictly examples of nonattachment, in that incomplete invagination of the optic cup has meant that the two layers were never

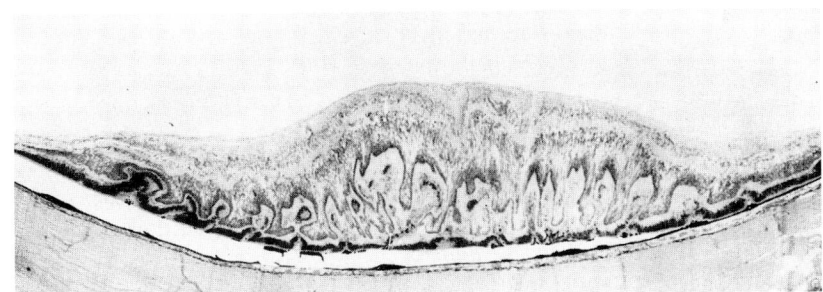

FIGURE 23.16. *Retinal dysplasia. The affected retina is incompletely organized and is thickened and folded. (H&E, ×7.5.)*

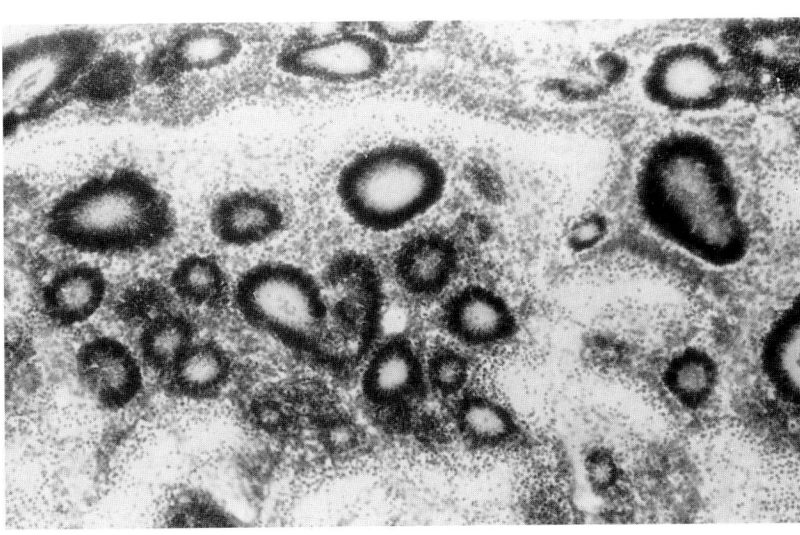

FIGURE 23.17. *Retinal dysplasia. There is absence of the normal stratification of the neuroretina. Instead, abortive and incomplete attempts at maturation have produced multiple rosettes composed of primitive photoreceptor cells. (H&E, ×128.)*

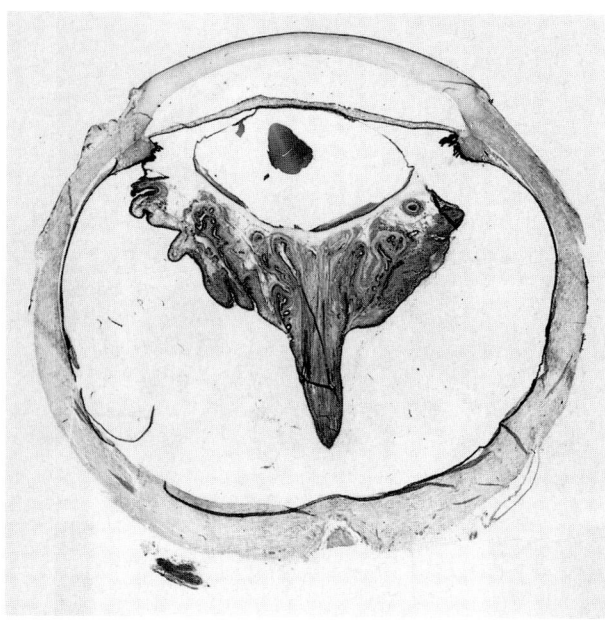

FIGURE 23.18.   *Retinopathy of prematurity. In the terminal phase, the totally detached retina is bound to the back of the lens by vascularized fibrous tissue (the lens substance has been largely lost in sectioning). (H&E, ×5.)*

together in the first place. Not unexpectedly, dysplasia is a common accompaniment in such cases. The retina may fail to attach to the pigment epithelium as an isolated event or in combination with other ocular maldevelopments [6]. The nonattachment may be complete or limited to a fold that usually originates at the optic disc. Multiple mechanisms may be involved, with theories including disproportionate growth rates between the two layers of the optic cup, and deficiency of the glycosaminoglycan considered to help

retinal adhesion. Tears due to persistent foci of vascularized primary vitreous may produce true detachment.

Retinopathy of Prematurity

Retinopathy of prematurity is a bilateral blinding condition affecting premature babies [31] in which postnatal formation of blood vessels on the retinal surface leads to the latter's detachment. In its fully fledged form, the retina is completely detached and bound to the back of the lens by fibrous tissue accompanying the neovascularization: the term "retrolental fibroplasia" is applicable to such cases (Fig. 23.18). The condition first achieved prominence over 50 years ago: the subsequent realization, born from clinical experience [32] and confirmed by animal experimentation [33], that overenthusiastic oxygen supplementation in the management of respiratory distress was a key factor soon led to a dramatic drop in its incidence.

The observed preretinal neovascularization is related to inadequate perfusion of the underlying retina and consequent tissue hypoxia (Fig. 23.19). The finding that reducing the amount of oxygen reduced the incidence of retinal disturbance fostered the concept that newly formed blood vessels—and those of the retina in particular—were in some way damaged by oxygen. Oxygen in excess injures the endothelial lining of the immature vessels, such as are to be found in the still-developing preterm baby's retinal circulation, with the result that the vessels are irretrievably damaged. Consequently, when the oxygen supplementation is discontinued, the retina is under-vascularized. Blood vessels in the fully developed circulation pertaining at term are much less vulnerable. Evidence is accumulating that angiogenic factors are released in hypoxic situations of the sort described [34, 35]; a fraction diffuses into the largely stagnant vitreous where it accumulates and exercises a chemotactic effect on residual vessels close to the inner surface of the retina (Fig. 23.20). Later cicatrization of the

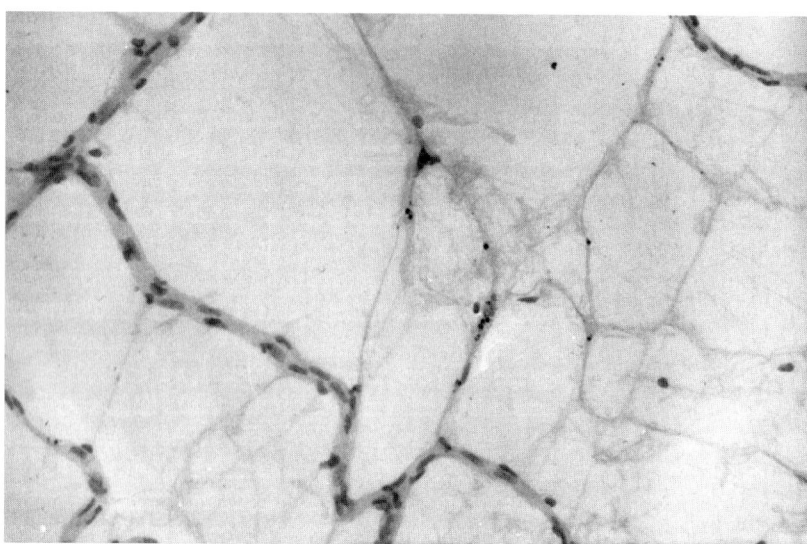

FIGURE 23.19.   *Retinopathy of prematurity. Flat preparation of the retina showing the vascular bed, the neural components having been removed by proteolytic enzyme digestion. Many of the capillaries are reduced to acellular basement membrane residues as a consequence of oxygen-induced vaso-obliteration. (H&E, ×126.)*

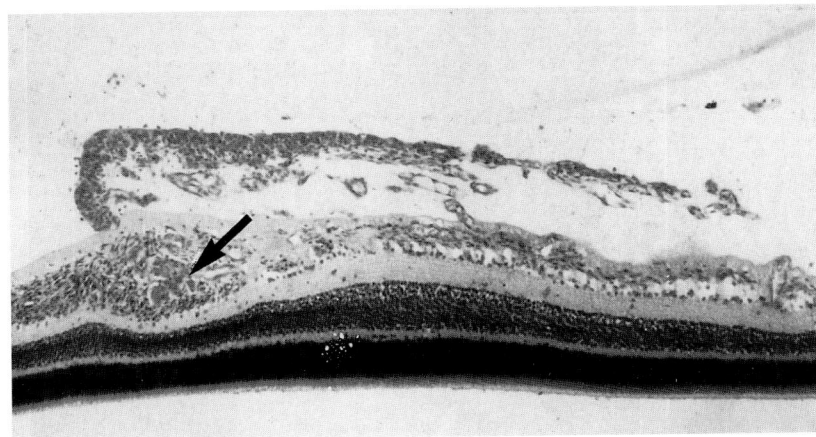

FIGURE 23.20.   *Retinopathy of prematurity. In the postobliterative phase, the ischemic retina provokes a vasoproliferative response that invades the vitreous space, here seen as newly formed capillaries on the surface of the retina. The boundary between the avascular and vascularized retina is seen as a thickening of the inner retina (arrow). (H&E, ×84.)*

fibrous tissue that forms around the intravitreal vessels promotes tractional detachment of the underlying retina.

Despite the awareness that retinopathy of prematurity is in part an iatrogenic disorder, occasional cases continue to present even in the absence of supplemental oxygen. In some such cases it is conceivable that retinal hypoxia directly related to respiratory dysfunction and hypoxemia could be involved [36], given that the immediate stimulus to neovascularization is hypoxia and only indirectly hyperoxia. However, in that case some evidence of cerebral hypoxia might also be anticipated. Another suggestion is that the relative hyperoxia experienced in the transition from intra- to extrauterine conditions may be sufficient to damage the retinal vasculature [37].

In recent years there has been a mild resurgence of the disorder, particularly in the United States, despite rigorous attention to oxygen levels [38]. The reason for the increase is not entirely clear, but it is probably significant that the vast majority of affected babies have very low birth weights (<1000 g), babies for whom adequate support systems did not exist until recent times. It is possible that the retinal vessels of these babies are vulnerable to levels of oxygen previously considered safe, because it is clear that the susceptibility to oxygen-induced damage is a function of vessel and/or retinal maturity.

The relevance of the frequently observed acidosis and hypercapnia to the risk of provoking retinopathy of prematurity is unresolved. There is no evidence of direct toxicity on the part of carbon dioxide, but animal experiments involving newborn lambs suggest that hypercapnia induces dilatation of the retinal vessels, which, in the presence of concomitant hyperoxemia, could serve to increase blood flow and the delivery of oxygen to the retina [39].

Clearly, there are residual problems surrounding the pathogenesis of retinopathy of prematurity, and factors relating to the effect of strong light, blood transfusion, and infection cannot be excluded. The action of free oxygen

radicals may prove to be the final common pathway (see Chap. 3).

INFECTIONS

Rubella

Infection by the rubella virus is transplacental. Infections that occur in the first trimester have the most serious consequences for most organs, including the eye.

Infection early in the first trimester may cause microphthalmia or lens cataract [40]. Cataracts are usually bilateral, and, although they may be evident at birth, they can take up to 2 years to become manifest. They are typically nuclear and involve entry by the virus between the 4th and 7th weeks of gestation—that is, after the lens vesicle has separated from the surface ectoderm but before the lens capsule has formed. Histology shows karyorrhetic or pyknotic nuclei in the central part of the lens (Fig. 23.21).

Later infection can cause an iridocyclitis leading to necrosis of the iridial stroma and pigment epithelium and, eventually, glaucoma. Pigmentary retinopathy is observed in over 70% of cases and may be the only manifestation of infection. It can develop as late as the 5th month of gestation. The clinical picture of stippling is represented at the tissue level by alternating foci of atrophy and hypertrophy of the retinal pigment epithelium, with evidence of underlying choroiditis.

The virus can persist in the ocular tissues for up to 3 years after birth [41].

Syphilis

Interstitial keratitis complicates 10% to 15% of children with congenital syphilis but is rarely evident before the age of 2 years. Microscopy reveals stromal scarring, vascularization, and focal lymphocytic and plasma cell infiltration in the

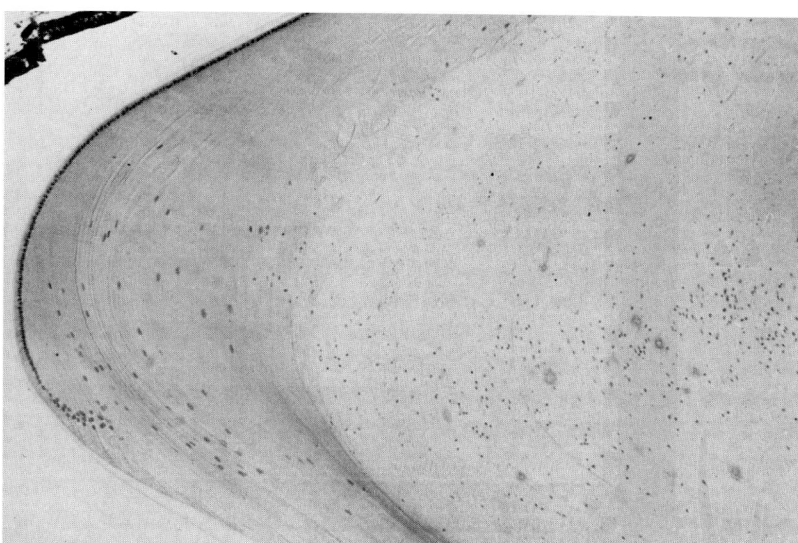

FIGURE 23.21. *Rubella cataract. Histological section showing the characteristic persistence of pyknotic nuclei in the central part of the lens. Normally nucleated lens fibers are seen in the lens cortex. (H&E, ×80.)*

absence of epithelial damage [42]. Acute iritis may be present at birth but is more usual after the first 6 months, while patchy chronic choroidoretinitis may also occur. Optic neuritis is a further complication.

Toxoplasmosis

Ocular toxoplasmosis is a complication of transplacental infection occurring late in pregnancy. Early infection usually results in developmental defects that are incompatible with life.

Focal necrotizing retinitis is the characteristic ocular lesion (Fig. 23.22). The macular area is at particular risk, and involvement may be unilateral or bilateral. Healed lesions present as choroidoretinal scars in which a loss of retinal tissue and pigment produces a clinically whitish area sur-

rounded by an irregular zone of increased pigmentation. The latter is the result of melanin dispersion and reactive hyperplasia of the pigment epithelium. Occasionally, the retinal involvement is more extensive and generalized rather than focal. Other complications include microphthalmia, secondary cataract, and congenital retinal detachment.

The tissue damage is attributed to direct effects of the toxoplasmal protozoa, but recurrent lesions developing after the neonatal period are considered to be largely a result of hypersensitivity to residual organisms [43, 44].

Ophthalmia Neonatorum

The term *ophthalmia neonatorum* covers any hyperacute purulent conjunctivitis occurring in the first 10 days of life. As such it may be infective or non-infective.

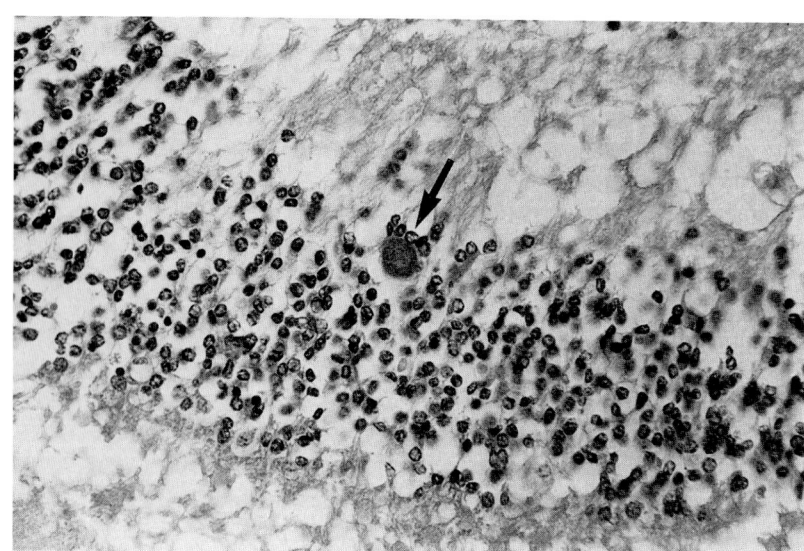

FIGURE 23.22. *Congenital toxoplasmic retinitis. A solitary toxoplasma cyst is seen in a moderately degenerate retina (arrow), although there is no sign of active inflammation. (H&E, ×350.)*

Chemical Toxicity

Where it is the practice to use topical applications of silver nitrate in the prophylaxis of gonococcal conjunctivitis, a sterile inflammatory response is not infrequent; until recently some 6% of all neonates in the United States were said to have been affected to some degree [45].

Gonococcal Infection

When the outer eye is infected by *Neisseria gonorrhoeae* during passage through an affected birth canal, it is usually manifest 24 to 28 hours later [45]. The conjunctiva lining the eyelids is acutely inflamed and gives rise to serosanguineous exudation. In neglected cases, exudations are followed by corneal involvement, which can culminate in perforation. The intense fibrinous exudation may present as a pseudomembrane on the surface of the conjunctiva and cornea. The tissue damage is a direct result of gonococcal exotoxin release and proteolytic enzyme activation.

Other Bacterial Infections

Staphylococcus pyogenes, streptococci, pneumococci, and coliform bacilli have each been implicated in ophthalmia neonatorum, although they have less tendency to involve the cornea than do gonococci infections.

Trachoma-Related Inclusion Conjunctivitis (TRIC)

Trachoma-related inclusion conjunctivitis (TRIC) ophthalmia neonatorum is caused by specific serotypes of *Chlamydia trachomatis* that inhabit the genitourinary tract. Infection is contracted during birth and presents as an acute purulent conjunctivitis some 5 to 12 days later [46] with papillary hypertrophy of the mucosal surface. After about 3 weeks the inflammation gradually subsides to leave a chronic follicular conjunctivitis that can persist for several months. Smears from the conjunctiva stained by the Giemsa method can be expected to show basophilic inclusion bodies in the cytoplasm of the infected epithelium [47].

Congenital Cytomegalic Inclusion Disease

Infection with cytomegalovirus is transplacental. In the eye, it manifests as a retinochoroiditis in the form of multiple, small, nonpigmented lesions, which may ultimately coalesce. Histology shows extensive necrosis of the retina, including the underlying pigment epithelium, with a chronic inflammatory cell response in the adjacent choroid [48] (Fig. 23.23). In the acute phase, enlarged cells with both intranuclear and cytoplasmic inclusions may be seen, but in the later stages the necrotic tissue is replaced by glial scar tissue.

TUMORS

Ocular and orbital neoplasia presenting at birth or shortly afterwards is rare. The intact gene has an integral role in cell cycle regulation, triggering apoptotic removal of cells with impaired replication control [49]. Its absence or inactivation has a permissive effect on tumor growth.

Retinoblastoma

The incidence of retinoblastomas varies from 1 in 15,000 to 1 in 34,000 live births, and the average age of the patient at diagnosis is 18 months. Hereditary tumors present a little earlier [50] and sporadic tumors a little later than the median, but recognition at birth, exceptionally in association with prematurity, is not unknown. Neonatal retinoblastomas are usually inherited.

There is now unequivocal evidence of an association between retinoblastoma development and gene disturbance at the 14q locus on chromosome 13 [51]. Although this appears to be due to gene mutation in most cases, it can be due to chromosomal abnormality when, as in the 13q deletion syndrome, retinoblastoma development is linked to other developmental anomalies. The defective gene behaves in a recessive manner such that both alleles need to be

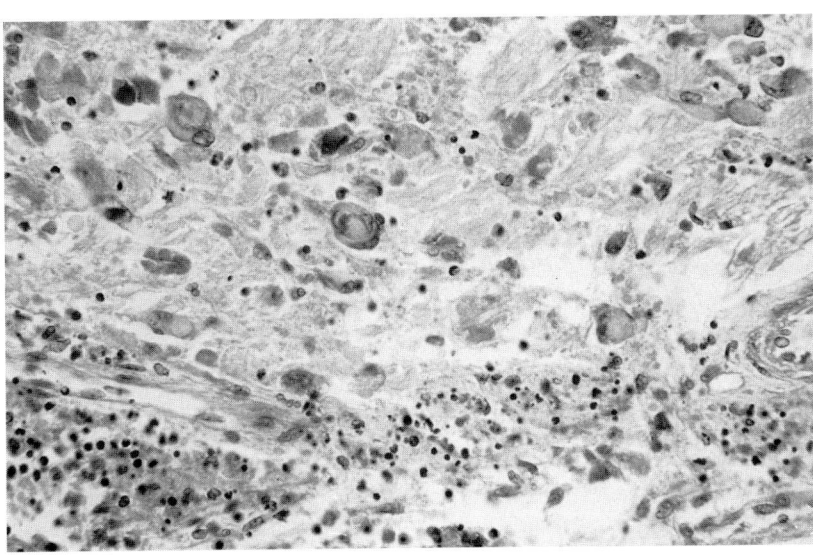

FIGURE 23.23. *Cytomegalic virus retinitis. The retina, which is artefactually detached from the underlying choroid, is totally necrotic with loss of structural organization and is infiltrated by cells containing intranuclear and intracytoplasmic inclusions. (H&E, ×131.)*

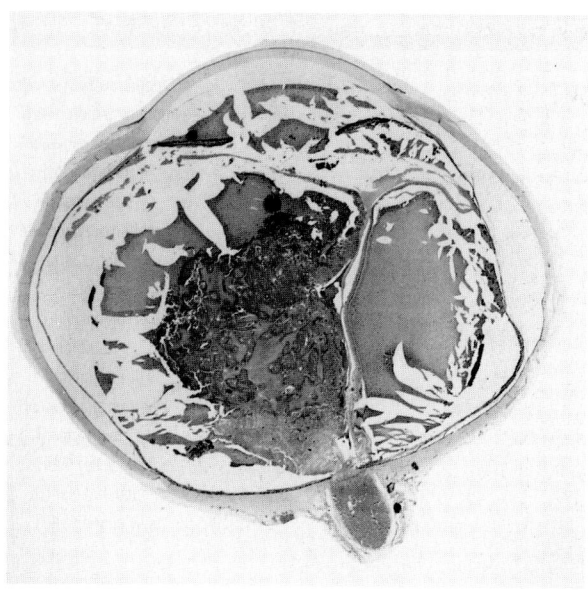

FIGURE 23.24. *Retinoblastoma. Much of the posterior segment of the eye is occupied by tumor and there is detachment of the residual retina, the result of an exophytic growth pattern. (H&E, ×3.)*

Retinoblastomas are considered to be essentially of neuronal derivation; however, since evidence of glial differentiation may also be evident, a more primitive precursor cell origin is likely [54]. The tumors are commonly multicentric. Occasionally, they grow diffusely through the retina but more often they proliferate into the vitreal cavity (endophytic growth) or on the outer surface of the retina into the potential retinal space (exophytic growth) (Fig. 23.24). The latter pattern is associated with retinal detachment, which can obscure the causative tumor and hinder ophthalmoscopic diagnosis.

Histologically, the tumor cells are small with round or ovoid hyperchromatic nuclei and scanty cytoplasm. The better differentiated tumors show orientation of the cells into rosettes around a central space in a semblance of retinal organization (Fig. 23.25). The individual cells represent a degree of photoreceptor specialization: the presence of rosettes confers a relatively favorable prognosis following treatment. More complete photoreceptor differentiation to form "fleurettes" is associated with even better prognosis [55], and tumors composed entirely of such elements have been termed *retinomas* or *retinocytomas* [56, 57]. Extensive necrosis is usual (Fig. 23.26) in retinoblastomas and focal calcification is common.

Spread can occur into the vitreal cavity and seedling deposits may eventually enter the anterior chamber (this allows for cytological diagnosis following an aqueous tap). Such a development carries a poor prognosis, as does massive infiltration of the choroid, the latter predisposing to hematogenous metastasis to bone and other sites. Particularly serious is optic nerve invasion since this is a forerunner of intracranial spread, whether directly via the neural tissue or through the cerebrospinal fluid. The overall mortality in treated cases is less than 10%, provided the optic nerve is not involved. Mortality increases to 65% if tumor cells are present at the surgical resection margin of the nerve in enucleated specimens [58].

defective or deleted before neoplasia can ensue. Babies with hereditary tumors have inherited one retinoblastoma gene from one or other parent and then succumbed to a subsequent somatic mutation of the second gene. It is implicit that all the body cells in these children will have the inherited retinoblastoma gene; correspondingly, infants who may have been successfully treated for their retinal tumors are at a much greater risk of developing non-ocular cancers at a later date. This is particularly true of those treated by irradiation, with a cited incidence of 35% after 30 years' follow-up [52, 53].

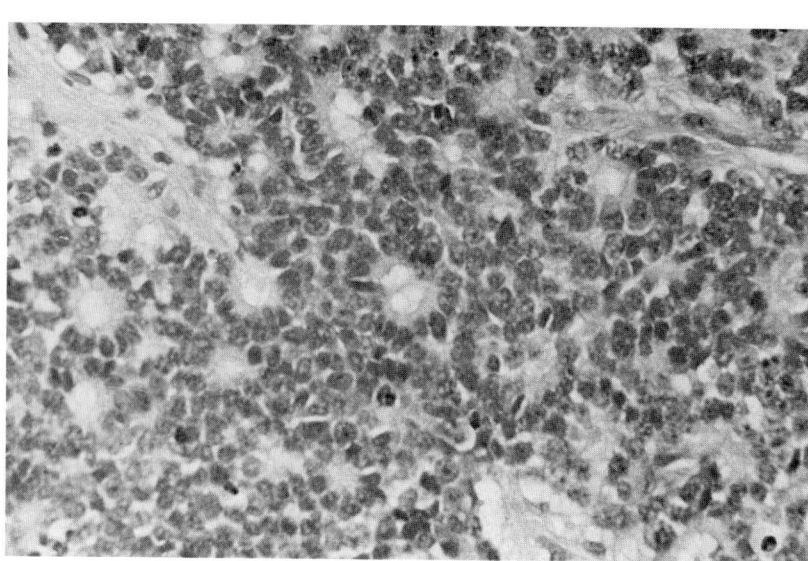

FIGURE 23.25. *Retinoblastoma. Well-differentiated tumor showing rosette formation. (H&E, ×95.).*

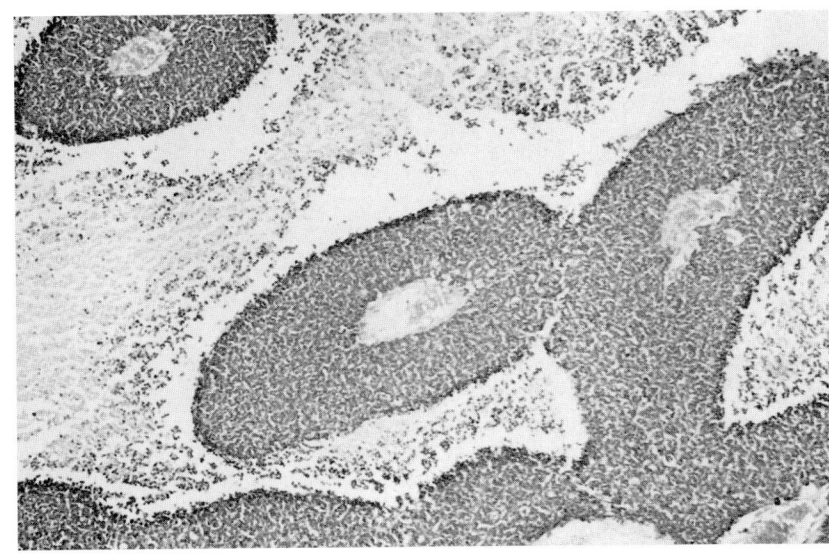

FIGURE 23.26. *Retinoblastoma. There is considerable necrosis, and the viable cells, here showing little differentiation as evidenced by rosette formation, are grouped around the vascular supply to the tumor. (H&E, ×80.)*

In recent years it has been established that a tumor equivalent to a retinoblastoma can involve the pineal gland in hereditary cases, thus constituting a so-called "trilateral" retinoblastoma [59]. Such a development is rare, but may account for some cases reported as having an extensive intracranial tumor in the absence of detectable optic nerve involvement on the part of the ocular tumors.

Medulloepithelioma

A medulloepithelioma (alternatively, but less appropriately, termed "diktyoma") closely resembles the medullary epithelioma of the brain and embryonal optic cup [60]. It is a tumor of childhood: presentation before the age of 6 months is rare and chiefly involves the ciliary body as opposed to the more posteriorly located primitive optic cup.

The constituent cells are cuboidal and are arranged in convoluted sheets which, in histological section, produce tubular and papillary structures (Fig. 23.27). A degree of polarization is usual, with alcianophilic glycosaminoglycan mimicking the vitreous on one aspect of the epithelial sheets, and intercellular junctional complexes reminiscent of the so-called outer limiting membrane of the retina on the other. Occasional tumors include foci of cartilaginous, neural, or skeletal muscle differentiation, in which case they are termed teratoid medulloepitheliomas [61].

Most medulloepitheliomas are benign, but local invasion can sometimes occur. Such tumors show cytological evidence suggestive of malignancy. Distant metastasis is exceptional.

Glioneuroma

Glioneuroma is a rare, benign, and probably choristomatous lesion. Histologically, it presents as a circumscribed proliferation of well-differentiated glial cells and neurons, including

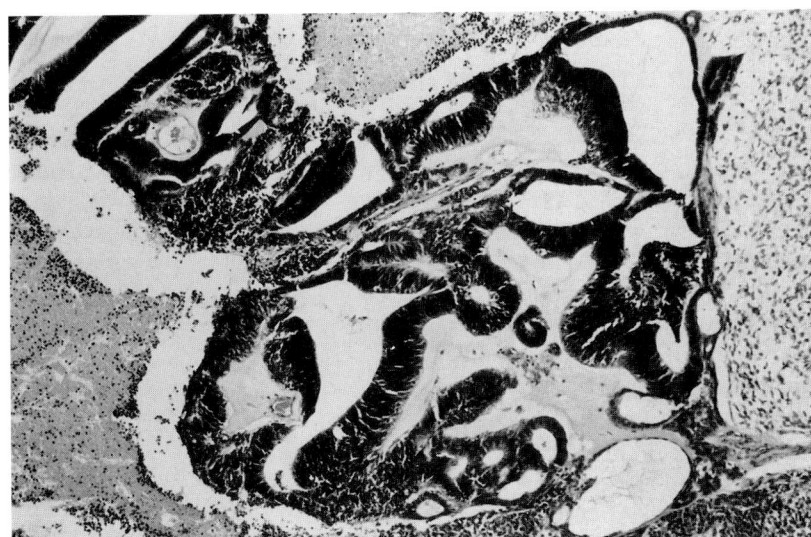

FIGURE 23.27. *Medulloepithelioma of the ciliary body. The cells are arranged in cords that are frequently folded. Many form tubules. The surrounding, loose, mucinous stroma includes cells with glial characteristics. (H&E, ×95.)*

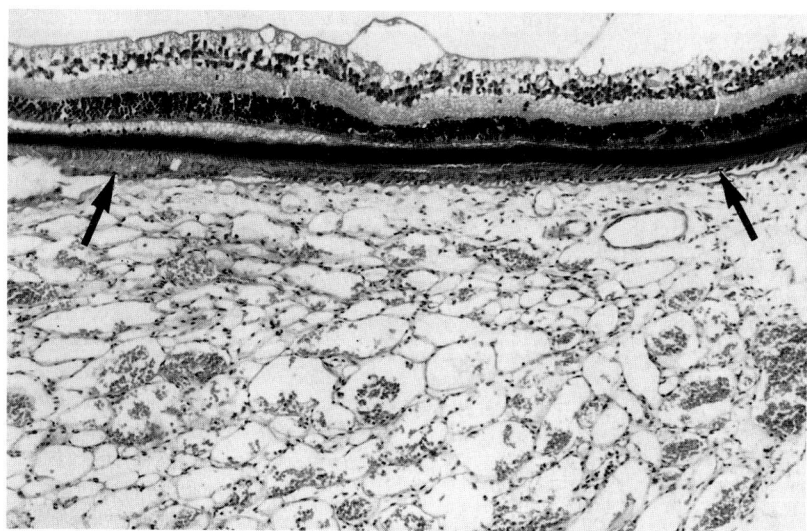

FIGURE 23.28.   *Choroidal hemangioma. The tumor is composed of large, thin-walled, vascular channels and is associated with atrophy of the overlying retinal pigment epithelium (arrow). The neuroretina is essentially intact. (H&E, ×80.)*

ganglion cells, within the retina. Glioneuromas have been observed at birth, when they may be associated with malformation of a sector of the embryonic cup, especially a coloboma [62].

Astrocytic Hamartoma of the Retina

An astrocytic hamartoma is a localized proliferation of fibrous astrocytes within the retina or overlying the optic disk as a congenital lesion, commonly in combination with either tuberous sclerosis or, less often, generalized neurofibromatosis. Such hamartomas grow slowly in childhood, and have no malignant potential.

Choroidal Hemangioma

Cavernous hemangiomas in the choroid (Fig. 23.28) may be isolated lesions but commonly present in conjunction with

ipsilateral facial and intracranial hemangiomas as part of the Sturge-Weber syndrome. About one-third of the children subsequently develop glaucoma, but the causative mechanism is obscure [63].

Embryonal Rhabdomyosarcoma of the Orbit

Embryonal rhabdomyosarcoma is a highly malignant tumor arising from presumed mesenchymal tissue, with a tendency toward skeletal muscle differentiation. The cells have round or pleomorphic hyperchromatic nuclei and the cytoplasm, while often sparse, may be elongated to form characteristic strap-shaped cells (Fig. 23.29) that, exceptionally, exhibit cross-striations. Mitotic activity is conspicuous.

Many tumors show little or no muscle differentiation and have been referred to simply as embryonal sarcomas. The cells in these cases are usually round with scanty cytoplasm (Fig. 23.30) and, superficially, many resemble a lymphoma.

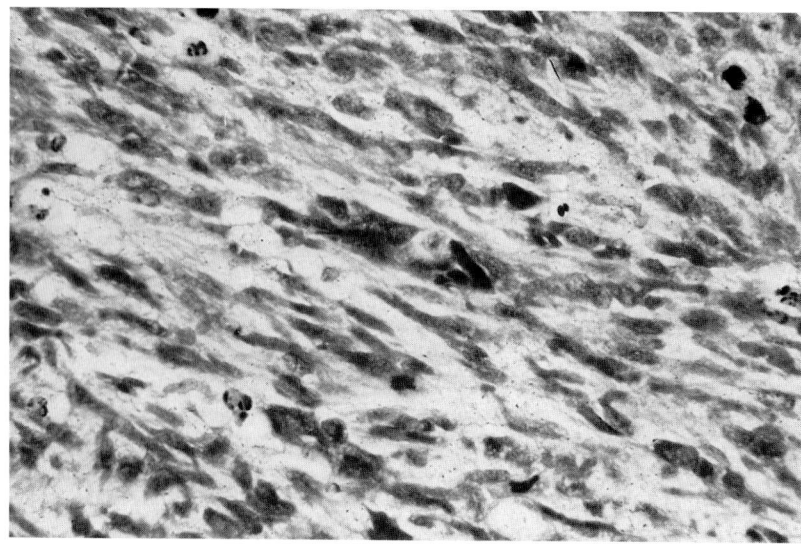

FIGURE 23.29.   *Embryonal rhabdomyosarcoma of the orbit. Many of the cells are strap-shaped, but others are pleomorphic with nuclear irregularity. Mitotic figures are also present. (H&E, ×328.)*

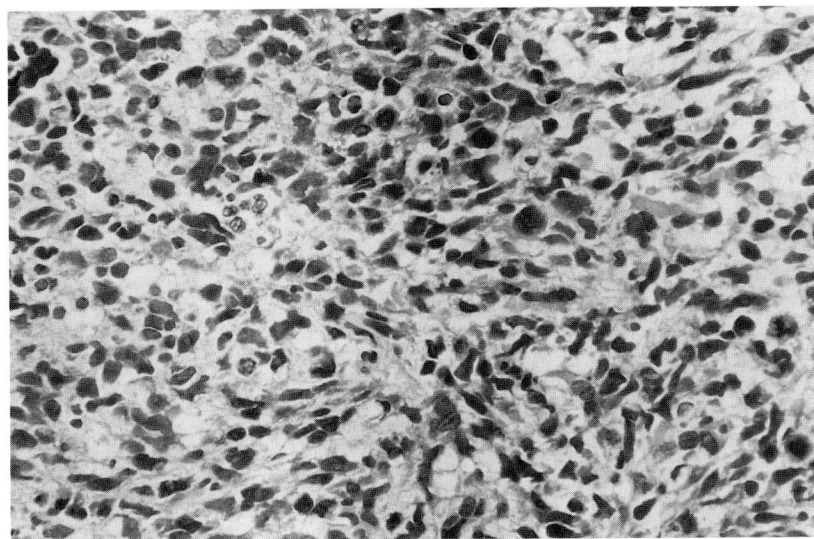

FIGURE 23.30. *Embryonal rhabdomyosarcoma of the orbit. There is considerable cellular pleomorphism and nuclear irregularity, with little or no attempt at differentiation. Such tumors have been referred to as undifferentiated rhabdomyosarcoma or more simply as embryonal sarcoma. (H&E, ×328.)*

Immunohistochemical demonstration of alpha-sarcomeric actin or desmin can be helpful in difficult cases.

Embryonal rhabdomyosarcoma is essentially a tumor of childhood: 75% of cases occur within the first decade, and it is occasionally present at birth [64]. Any part of the orbit may be involved and, in the absence of treatment, local spread into the brain or hematogenous metastasis to the lungs rapidly leads to a fatal outcome. In recent years, however, due to the introduction of combined chemotherapeutic and radiotherapeutic regimes, the situation has improved dramatically.

REFERENCES

1. Jakobiec FA. *Ocular Anatomy, Embryology and Teratology.* Philadelphia: Harper & Row, 1982.
2. Mann I. *The Development of the Human Eye.* 3rd ed. London: British Medical Association, 1964.
3. McCartney ACE. Embryological development of the eye. In: Garner A, Klintworth GK, eds. *Pathobiology of Ocular Disease: A Dynamic Approach.* 2nd ed. New York: Marcel Dekker, 1994, pp. 1255–84.
4. O'Rahilly R. The prenatal development of the human eye. *Exp Eye Res* 1975; 21:91–112.
5. Duke-Elder S, Cook C. *System of Ophthalmology. Vol. 3. Normal and Abnormal Development. Part 1. Embryology.* London: Kimpton, 1963.
6. Mullaney J. Curious colobomata. *Trans Ophthalmol Soc UK* 1977; 97:517–22.
7. Torczynski E. Developmental anomalies of the eye. In: Garner A, Klintworth GK, eds. *Pathobiology of Ocular Disease: A Dynamic Approach.* 2nd ed. New York: Marcel Dekker, 1994, pp. 1285–344.
8. Calhoun FP Jr. The management of glaucoma in nanophthalmos. *Trans Am Ophthalmol Soc* 1975; 73:97–122.
9. Torczynski E, Jakobiec FA, Johnston MC, Font RL, Madewell JA. Synophthalmia and cyclopia: a histopathologic, radiographic and organogenetic analysis. *Doc Ophthalmol* 1977; 44:61–73.
10. Miller MT, Deutsh TA, Cronin C, Keys CL. Amniotic bands as a cause of ocular anomalies. *Am J Ophthalmol* 1987; 104:270–9.
11. Stromland K. Ocular involvement in the fetal alcohol syndrome. *Surv Ophthalmol* 1987; 31:277–83.
12. Rodrigues MM, Waring GO, Laibson PR, Weinreb S. Endothelial alterations in congenital corneal dystrophies. *Am J Ophthalmol* 1975; 80:678–89.
13. Mansour AM, Barber JC, Reinecke RD, Wang FM. Ocular choristomas. *Surv Ophthalmol* 1989; 33:339–58.
14. Casey RJ, Garner A. Epibulbar choristoma and microphthalmia. *Br J Ophthalmol* 1992; 75:247–50.
15. Townsend WM, Font RL, Zimmerman LE. Congenital corneal leukomas. 3. Histopathologic findings in 13 eyes with no central defect in Descemet's membrane. *Am J Ophthalmol* 1974; 77:400–12.
16. Townsend WM, Font RL, Zimmerman LE. Congenital corneal leukomas. 2. Histopathologic findings in 19 eyes with central defect in Descemet's membrane. *Am J Ophthalmol* 1974; 77:192–206.
17. McKusick VA. *Mendelian Inheritance in Man. Catalogs of Autosomal Dominant, Autosomal Recessive and X-linked Phenotypes.* 10th ed. Baltimore: Johns Hopkins University Press, 1992.
18. Musarella MA. Gene mapping of ocular diseases. *Surv Ophthalmol* 1992; 36:285–312.
19. Wilcox LM Jr, Bercovitch D, Howard RO. Ophthalmic features of chromosome deletion 4p (Wolf-Hirschorn syndrome). *Am J Ophthalmol* 1978; 86:834–9.
20. Kwitko ML. *Glaucoma in Infants and Children.* Norwalk, CT: Appleton-Century Crofts, 1973.
21. Nelson LB, Spaeth GL, Nowinski TS, Margo CE, Jackson L. Aniridia: a review. *Surv Ophthalmol* 1984; 28:621–42.
22. Harley RD. *Paediatric Ophthalmology.* London: W.B. Saunders, 1975.
23. Grant WM, Walton DS. Progressive changes in the angle in congenital aniridia, with development of glaucoma. *Am J Ophthalmol* 1974; 78:842–7.
24. Klintworth GK, Garner A. The causes, types, and morphology of cataracts. In: Garner A, Klintworth GK, eds. *Pathobiology of Ocular Disease: A Dynamic Approach.* 2nd ed. New York: Marcel Dekker, 1994, pp. 481–532.
25. Steele RW, Bass JW. Hallermann-Streiff syndrome. *Am J Dis Child* 1970; 120:462–5.
26. Cogan DG, Kuwabara T. Pathology of cataracts in mongoloid idiocy: a new concept of pathogenesis of cataracts of the coronary-cerulean type. *Doc Ophthalmol* 1962; 16:73–80.
27. Manschot WA. Persistent hyperplastic primary vitreous. *Arch Ophthalmol* 1958; 59:188–203.
28. Font RL, Yanoff M, Zimmerman LE. Intraocular adipose tissue and persistent hyperplastic primary vitreous. *Arch Ophthalmol* 1969; 82:43–50.
29. Hoepner J, Yanoff M. Ocular anomalies in trisomy 13–15: an analysis of 13 eyes with two new findings. *Am J Ophthalmol* 1972; 74:729–37.
30. Lahav M, Albert DM, Wyand S. Clinical and histopathological classification of retinal dysplasia. *Am J Ophthalmol* 1973; 75:648–67.
31. Garner A. The pathology of prematurity of retinopathy. In: Silverman W, Flynn JT. eds. *Retinopathy of Prematurity.* Boston: Blackwell Scientific, 1985, pp. 21–54.
32. Patz A, Hoeck LE, de la Cruze E. Studies of the effect of high oxygen administration in retrolental fibroplasia. 1. Nursery observations. *Am J Ophthalmol* 1952; 37:513–20.
33. Ashton N, Ward B, Serpell G. Role of oxygen in the genesis of retrolental fibroplasia: preliminary report. *Br J Ophthalmol* 1953; 37:513–20.
34. Kissun RD, Hill CR, Garner A, et al. A low molecular weight angiogenic factor in cat retina. *Br J Ophthalmol* 1982; 66:165–9.
35. Taylor CM, Weiss JB, Kissun RD, Garner A. Effect of oxygen tension on the quantities of procollagenase activating angiogenic factor present in the developing kitten retina. *Br J Ophthalmol* 1986; 70:162–5.
36. Lucey JF, Horber JD, Osishi MJ. Cerebral and retinal hypoperfusion as a

possible cause of retrolental hyperplasia: hypothesis to explain non-oxygen related RLF. *Pediatr Res* 1981; 15:670. Abstract.

37. Patz A. The role of oxygen in retrolental fibroplasia. *Trans Am Ophthalmol Soc* 1968; 66:940–85.

38. Phelps DL. Retinopathy of prematurity; an estimate of vision loss in the United States—1979. *Pediatrics* 1981; 67:924–6.

39. Milley JR, Rosenberg AA, Jones MD. Retinal and choroidal blood flow in hypoxic and hypercarbic newborn lambs. *Pediatr Res* 1984; 18:410–4.

40. Zimmerman LE. Histopathologic basis for ocular manifestation of congenital rubella syndrome. *Am J Ophthalmol* 1968; 65:837–62.

41. Rawls WE, Phillips CA, Melwick JL, Desmond MM. Persistent virus infection in congenital rubella. *Arch Ophthalmol* 1967; 77:430–3.

42. Westcamp C. Histopathology of interstitial keratitis due to congenital syphilis. *Am J Ophthalmol* 1949; 32:793–806.

43. Dutton GN, Garner A. Protozoal infections. In: Garner A, Klintworth GK, eds. *Pathobiology of Ocular Disease: A Dynamic Approach.* 2nd ed. New York: Marcel Dekker, 1994, pp. 335–50.

44. Frenkel JK. Pathogenesis of toxoplasmosis with a consideration of cyst rupture in Besnoitia infection. *Surv Ophthalmol* 1961; 6:799–825.

45. Scheie HG, Albert DM. *Textbook of Ophthalmology.* 9th ed. Philadelphia: W.B. Saunders, 1977.

46. Rees E, Tait AI, Hobson D, Johnson FWA. Perinatal chlamydial infection. In: Hobson D, Holmes KK, eds. *Nongonococcal Urethritis and Related Infections.* Washington, DC: American Society for Microbiology, 1977, pp. 323–7.

47. Darougar S, Dwyer RSHC, Treharne JD, et al. A comparison of laboratory methods of diagnosis of chlamydial infection. In: Nichols RL, ed. *Trachoma and Related Disorders.* Amsterdam: Excerpta Medica, 1971, pp. 445–60.

48. Smith ME, Zimmerman LE, Harley RD. Ocular involvement in congenital cytomegalic disease. *Arch Ophthalmol* 1966; 76:696–9.

49. Riley DJ, Lee EY-HP, Lee WH. The retinoblastoma protein: more than a tumor suppressor. *Annu Rev Cell Biol* 1994; 10:1–29.

50. Warburg M. Retinoblastoma. In: Goldberg M, ed. *Genetic and Metabolic Disease.* Boston: Little, Brown, 1974, pp. 447–61.

51. Sahel JA, Albert DM. Tumors of the retina. In: Garner A Klintworth GK, eds. *Pathobiology of Ocular Disease: A Dynamic Approach.* 2nd ed. New York: Marcel Dekker, 1994, pp. 1479–522.

52. Abramson DH, Ellsworth RM, Zimmerman LE. Non-ocular cancer in retinoblastoma survivors. *Trans Am Acad Ophthalmol Otolarlyngol* 1976; 81:454–6.

53. Roarty JD, McLean IW, Zimmerman LE. Incidence of second neoplasms in patients with bilateral retinoblastoma. *Ophthalmology* 1988; 95:1583–7.

54. Terenghi G, Polak JM, Ballesta J, et al. Immunocytochemistry of neuronal and glial markers in retinoblastoma. *Virchows Arch A* 1984; 404:61–73.

55. Tso MOM, Zimmerman LE, Fine BS, Ellsworth RM. A cause of radio-resistance in retinoblastoma: photoreceptor differentiation. *Trans Am Acad Ophthalmol Otolaryngol* 1970; 74:959–69.

56. Margo C, Hidayat A, Kopelman J, Zimmerman LE. Retinocytoma: a benign variant of retinoblastoma. *Arch Ophthalmol* 1983; 101:1519–31.

57. Zimmerman LE. Retinoblastoma and retinocytoma. In: Spencer WH, ed. *Ophthalmic Pathology: An Atlas and Textbook.* Philadelphia: W.B. Saunders, 1985, pp. 1292–351.

58. Sang DN, Albert DM. Retinoblastoma: clinical and histopathologic factors. *Hum Pathol* 1982; 13:133–47.

59. Bader JL, Miller RW, Meadows AT, et al. Trilateral retinoblastoma. *Lancet* 1980; 2:582–3.

60. Broughton WL, Zimmerman LE. A clinicopathologic study of 56 cases of intraocular medulloepithelioma. *Am J Ophthalmol* 1978; 85:407–18.

61. Zimmerman LE. Verhoeff's "terato-neuroma," a critical reappraisal in light of new observations and current concepts of embryonic tumors. *Am J Ophthalmol* 1971; 72:1039–57.

62. Spencer WH, Jesberg DO. Glioneuroma (choristomatous malformation of the optic cup margin): a report of two cases. *Arch Ophthalmol* 1973; 89:387–92.

63. Font RL Ferry AP. The phakomatoses. *Int Ophthalmol Clin* 1972; 12:1–50.

64. Ellenbogen E, Lasky MA. Rhabdomyosarcoma of the orbit in the newborn. *Am J Ophthalmol* 1975; 80:1024–7.

Pathology of the Alimentary Tract

Derek J. deSa

GENERAL DEVELOPMENT OF THE GASTROINTESTINAL TRACT

The first stage at which a "primitive gut" can be recognized is during the 4th week of development [1]. The head, tail, and lateral folds of the embryo incorporate the dorsal segment of the yolk sac into an elongated tube extending the length of the embryo. The tube is lined by endoderm, and its walls are derived from the splanchnopleuric mesoderm. The endoderm provides most of the epithelial and glandular elements of the gastrointestinal tract while the splanchnopleuric mesoderm provides the muscular, fibrous, and visceral peritoneal coats.

It is useful to divide the primitive gut into three segments: 1) the *foregut*, incorporating that segment of the gut delineated by the head fold; 2) the *midgut*, delineated by the segment caudal to the head fold, but cephalad to the tail fold; and 3) the *hindgut*, demarcated by that portion of the primitive gut that lies within the tail fold. Different components of the gastrointestinal tract and its related organs are derived from each segment, and each has its distinctive blood supply.

The foregut derivatives include 1) the buccal cavity and pharynx, 2) the esophagus, larynx, trachea, and lungs, 3) the stomach and duodenum up to the opening of the common bile duct, 4) the liver, gall bladder, and biliary tract, and 5) the pancreas. The pharynx, lower respiratory tract, and esophagus are supplied by the arteries of the branchial arches; the coeliac artery supplies the other foregut derivatives.

The midgut derivatives include the duodenum distal to the bile duct orifice, the jejunum, ileum, appendix, cecum, ascending colon, and the proximal one-half to two-thirds of the transverse colon. These structures are supplied by the superior mesenteric artery.

The hindgut derivatives include the distal transverse colon, descending colon, sigmoid colon, rectum, cephalad segment of the anal canal, urinary bladder, and most of the urethra. With the exception of the urinary bladder and urethra, these structures are supplied by the inferior mesenteric artery. The exact site of transition between midgut and hindgut is variable and poorly defined, but it lies between the fields of distribution of the superior and inferior mesenteric arteries.

The main developmental thrust varies in each segment. The foregut derivatives require a complex series of steps in differentiation (e.g., branchial arch derivatives, liver, pancreas, larynx, and lung), while the elongation of the midgut derivatives leads to the rotation and fixation of the small and large bowels. The development of the caudad hindgut derivatives requires sequential and complex septation with division of the cloaca, which may be affected in turn by changes in adjacent organs, such as the spinal canal and sacrum.

The development of each organ (esophagus, stomach, small and large bowel) is considered under their individual sections. This section contains general comments regarding the development of autonomic innervation and the enterochromaffin system.

Innervation of the Bowel Wall

Early observations based on extirpation of the neural crest in chick embryos directed attention to the crucial importance of this structure in the development of the autonomic innervation of the bowel. The extensive studies of Okamoto and Ueda [2] on human embryos have shown that vagal fibers extending to the esophagus can be seen at 5 weeks' gestation. Neuroblasts appear within the esophagus by about 6 weeks; by 8 weeks' gestation, all but the distal colon is colonized by neuroblasts. By 12 weeks, innervation is complete. The neuroblasts lie outside the circular layer and differentiate there into the ganglion cells of the myenteric plexus. Neuroblasts are not seen in the mesentery. At any stage of development, immature ganglia appear more numerous in proximal segments of the alimentary tract, and craniocaudal development is suggested. The submucosal plexus develops from centripetal migration of the neuroblasts from the region of the myenteric plexus. However, Okamoto and Uda [2] do not provide details regarding the development of innervation between the 8th and 12th weeks. During this period, the sites of predilection for Hirschsprung disease—the distal colon and rectum—are innervated.

Andrew [3] had shown that in early chick embryos, the caudal neural crest can innervate the bowel, independently of the cephalic neural crest. The possibility exists that, in the chicken embryo at least, the distal bowel's autonomic ganglia may be derived directly from the distal neural crest, without craniocaudal migration.

In a series of elegant experiments, Kapur [4] demonstrated that vagal-derived enteric neurons can colonize the entire length of the gut in a craniocaudal manner. All vagal-derived enteric neuroblasts express catecholamines transiently and this includes dopamine beta-hydroxylase (DBH). A colony of transgenic mice was created that carried recombinant DNA for promoter sequences that control expression of DBH linked to a bacterial "reporter" gene that encoded for the enzyme beta-galactosidase. This DBH-nlacZ gene was expressed in transiently catecholaminergic cells and could be demonstrated by staining of the whole gut, or histological sections, with X-gal, a specific substrate for beta-galactosidase. Using "lethal spotted" (ls/ls) mice with the DBH-nlacZ transgene, Kapur [4] was able to show that colonization of the gut seemed to halt at the ileocecal junction, whereas in heterozygote (ls/+) or wild embryos bearing the transgene the colonization proceeded in a manner that allowed the hindgut to become colonized. Sacral enteric neurons never displayed this transient catecholaminergic phase, and the presence of reactive cells in the hindgut of wild-type embryos was interpreted to mean that colonization had been by vagal enteric neurons. Thus, the two separate populations of enteric neural cells (vagal and sacral) that appear to be of great importance in avian embryology may not be relevant to mammalian development. Obviously this work is of great relevance to an understanding of Hirschsprung disease.

The Enterochromaffin System

The enterochromaffin system is made up of groups of cells with endocrine characteristics and can be identified in the embryonic gut at 16 weeks' gestation. The cells are known to secrete a large number of polypeptide hormones [5, 6] and probably act as paracrine glands with specific local actions—regulating blood flow and secretory activity. Earlier

studies suggested that these cells were derived from the neural crest [6, 7], but, as shown in Lewin's review [8], it is much more likely that enterochromaffin cells develop by differentiation in situ. Some of these cells are argentaffin in nature, capable of reducing silver salts after formalin fixation without extraneous reduction [9]; these cells contain 5-hydroxytryptamine (5HT). Other cells of this diffuse endocrine system secrete numerous peptide hormones; the ever-growing list includes enteroglucagon, motilin, vasoactive intestinal peptide, and many others. These cells can be stained with silver salts following extraneous reduction—the argyrophil reaction. In current practice, the cell types can be identified by the ultrastructural characteristics of the granules and immunochemical methods [10–13]. An interesting and detailed review of the evolutionary and phylogenetic aspects of this system is provided by Falkmer and Wilander [14].

THE ESOPHAGUS

Development and Structure

The esophagus and trachea develop from a common anlage at the cranial end of the foregut, in continuity with the pharyngeal floor and the caudal branchial arches. A pair of lateral constricting grooves form a septum that divides the foregut into a ventral groove destined to become the trachea, and a dorsal segment that will form the esophagus. The lateral grooves fuse to complete the separation of the trachea from the esophagus [1]. The cephalic end of the ventral groove differentiates further to form the lower segment of the larynx. As these changes occur, there is concomitant elongation of the tube, due to the development of the lung and midgut. The development of the trachea, larynx, and esophagus from a common anlage explains why congenital anomalies affecting all three structures coexist, and why so many variants of tracheoesophageal fistula are found [15].

The structure of the esophagus is defined at a relatively early stage of gestation. The mucosa, muscularis mucosa, submucosa, and muscularis propria can be identified in the embryo by the latter half of the 3rd month [16]. However, alterations in the structure of the mucosa occur. In the 3rd month of gestation, the mucosa of the foregut is made up of a thin layer of columnar epithelium with scattered ciliated cells. By the 11th week, the mucosal layer is greatly thickened and is thrown into shallow, multilayered folds (Fig. 24.1). Squamous epithelial islands appear in the midzone of the esophagus at about 20 weeks, and the squamous transformation is complete by about 25 weeks [17]. A layer of muscularis mucosa is identified readily in the neonatal esophagus, and simple mucus-secreting glands with long ducts that penetrate the mucosa may be seen scattered through the submucosa as early as at 21 weeks' gestation (Fig. 24.2). The upper cervical segment of the esophagus is innervated by the recurrent laryngeal nerves and cervical

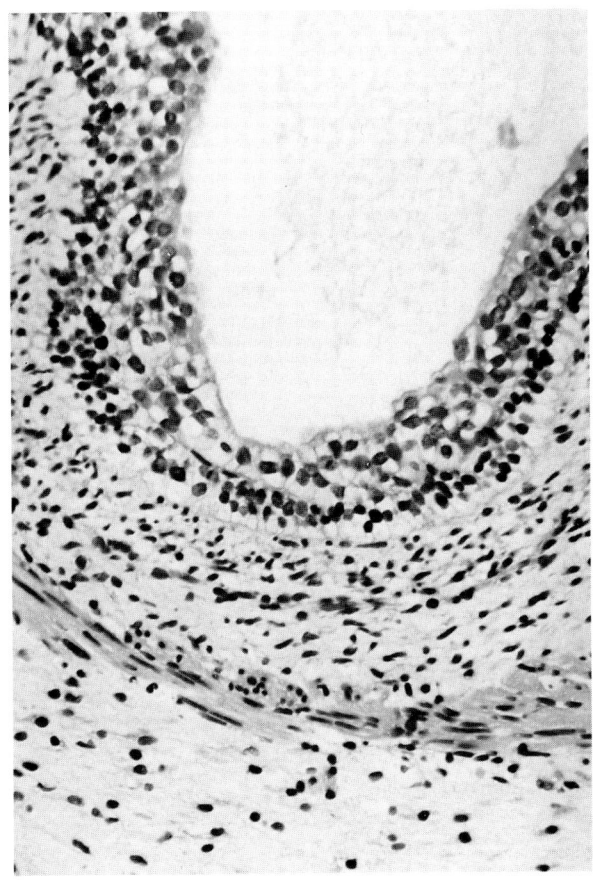

FIGURE 24.1. *Developing esophagus of a 9-mm embryo showing the multilayered epithelium, developed muscularis propria, and developing muscularis mucosa.*

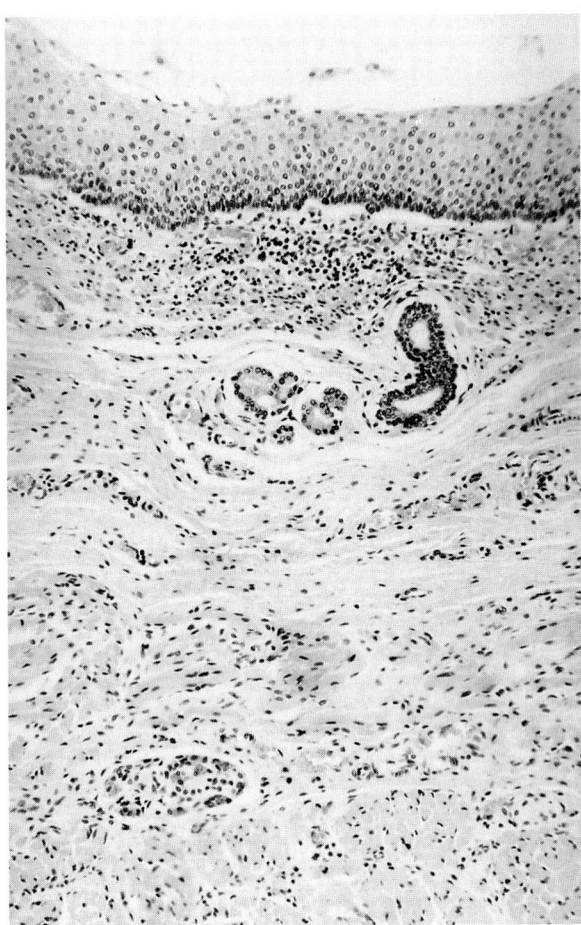

FIGURE 24.2. *Cervical esophagus from an infant of 24 weeks showing a well-developed stratified squamous epithelium, muscularis mucosa, muscularis propria, autonomic nervous system ganglion, and submucosal gland.*

sympathetic chain, while the thoracic segment receives branches from the vagus and esophageal plexus, as well as from recurrent branches of the splanchnic nerves. These nerves form a plexus with ganglion cells and nerve fibers between the two layers of the muscular coat, as well as a submucous plexus [18]. The upper third of the muscularis propria of the esophagus is skeletal (striated) in type, while in the lower third only smooth muscle is seen. There is a gradual transition in the middle third between these types of muscle, with a progressive increase of smooth-muscle cells toward the caudal end of this zone.

Congenital Anomalies

Heterotopic Gastric Mucosa
Islands of gastric surface epithelium may be an incidental finding in many neonates, infants, and even adults [19, 20]. They are usually seen in the upper third of the esophagus, and do not have any relationship to Barrett's esophagus. (Barrett's esophagus will be discussed in a later section.) In addition to surface columnar epithelium of gastric type, cil-

iated epithelium may also be found, and actual gastric glands with parietal cells may be present (Fig. 24.3).

Tracheoesophageal Fistula, Esophageal Atresia, and Related Variants
Tracheoesophageal fistula, esophageal atresia, and variants of these conditions form a malformation spectrum that accounts for the vast majority of congenital anomalies of the trachea and esophagus, found in approximately 1:1000 to 1:2000 births. Several different malformation patterns are seen and different classifications are current. The earlier classifications of Vogt [21] and Ladd [22] were melded into the widely accepted classification devised by Gross [23]. Type III of Ladd [22], type IIIb of Vogt [21], or type C of Gross [23] (Fig. 24.4) account for the vast majority of cases. Vogt's classification includes the exceptionally rare anomaly of the absence of the esophagus (Vogt type I). Ladd's classification distinguishes between those infants where a fistula between trachea and esophagus opens above the carina, and those

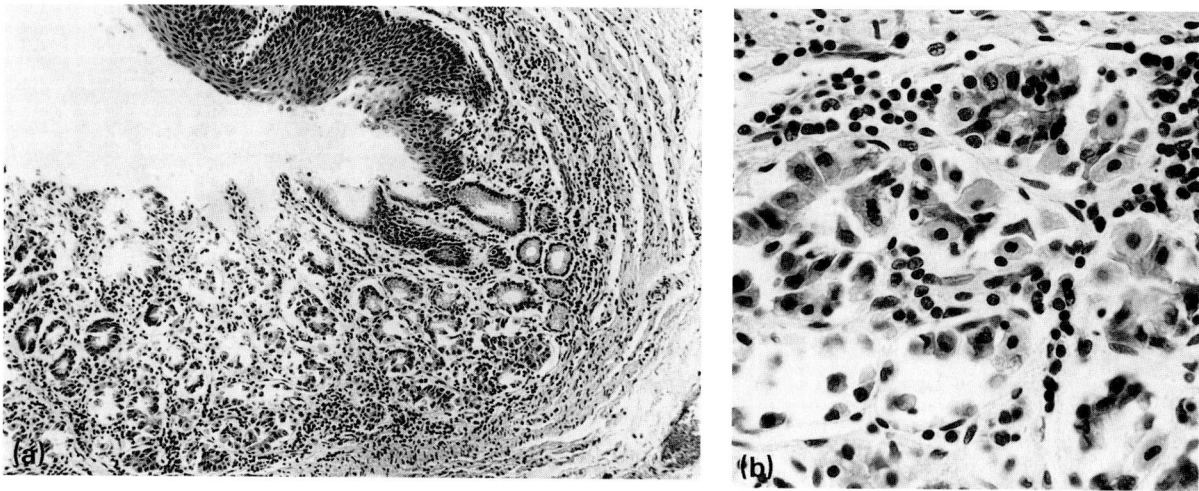

FIGURE 24.3. *Heterotopic gastric mucosa in a term infant (a) found incidentally in the upper cervical esophagus. Parietal cells were present in the gland units (b).*

where the orifice is at the carina (Ladd type IV). Gross' simplified classification [23] does not include absence of the esophagus, nor does it distinguish between fistulae that open above or at the carina. These descriptions give some idea of the complex patterns of malformation that may be present.

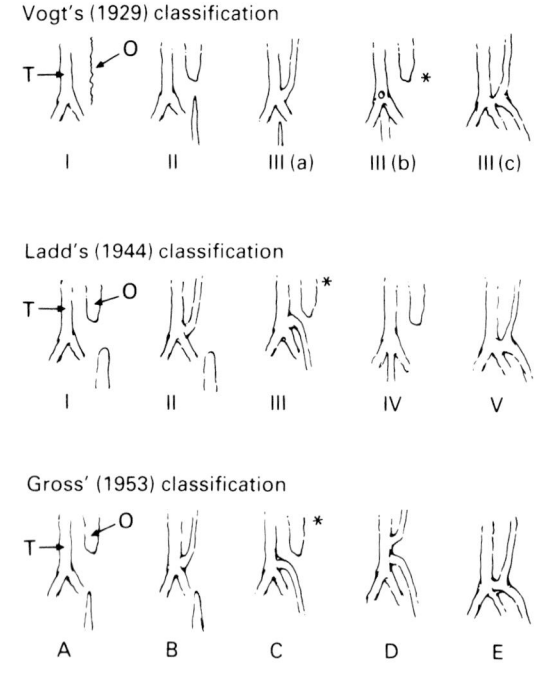

FIGURE 24.4. *A comparison of the different classifications of tracheoesophageal fistulae. Lesions marked with an asterisk are found most frequently [21–23].*

For practical purposes, I prefer using an anatomical description of these lesions rather than a specific numerical identifier.

The tracheal and esophageal anomalies may coexist with laryngeal malformations, producing some extremely bizarre results [15]. A tracheoesophageal fistula may be combined with laryngeal atresia, stenosis, or clefting, and a common passage for the larynx, trachea, and upper esophagus may be present (Fig. 24.5). The trachea and esophagus may fail to separate throughout their length [24], or multiple tracheoesophageal obstructions may be present [25, 26]. The malformation complex arises very early in development, probably before the 6th week of life, and a 9-mm embryo with an established tracheoesophageal fistula and esophageal atresia (corresponding to Ladd type III or Gross type C) has been described [27]. As Rosenthal [28] has shown, the defect occurs before the vascular tree is fully developed.

In very rare instances, congenital tracheoesophageal (and bronchoesophageal) fistulae have been described in an older child or adult [29, 30]. These cases, of course, are not associated with esophageal obstruction. Robb's case [30] was associated with an esophageal diverticulum. The fistulae, though small, can be associated with hemoptysis and aspiration pneumonia.

The development of the entire spectrum of malformations can be explained by disorders in the formation of the lateral grooves that separate the trachea and esophagus, which is accentuated by the downward growth of the developing lung. In those cases complicated by additional malformations of the larynx, the added failure of union between the foregut tube and the caudal branchial arches (and their mesodermal components) must be implicated.

The fistula is lined by a mucosal layer between trachea and esophagus, and the muscle layers of the trachea, fistula,

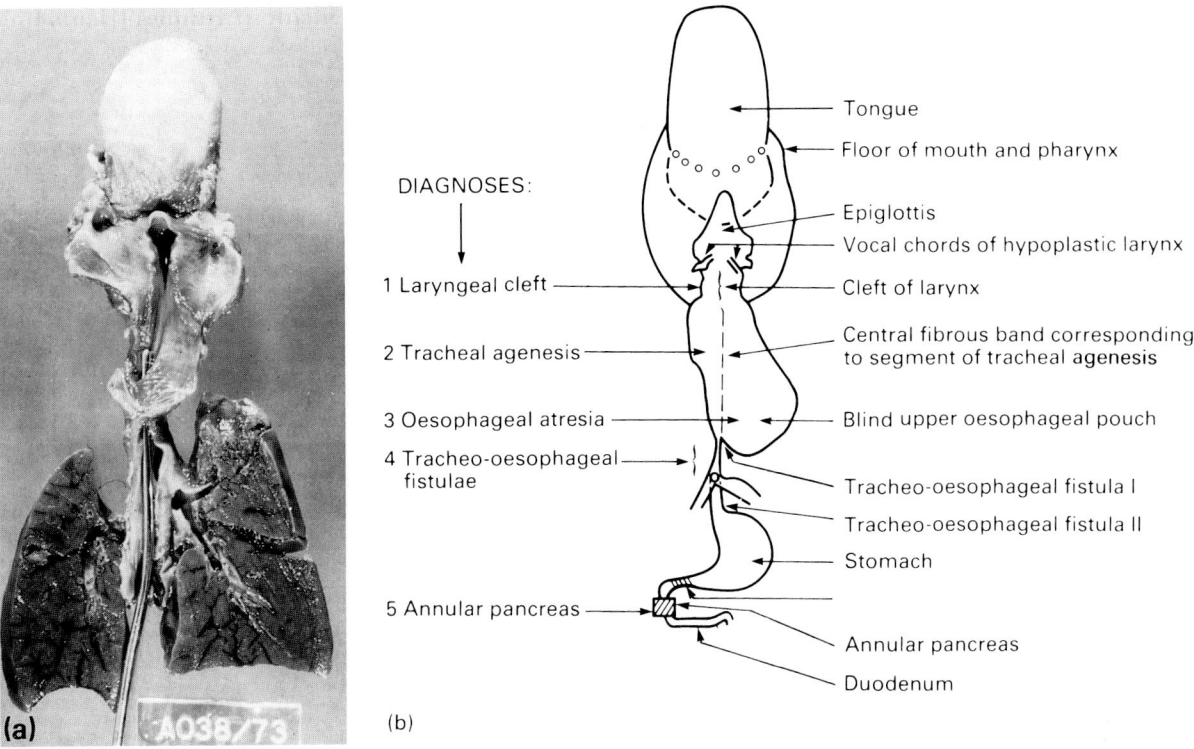

FIGURE 24.5. *(a) A complex malformation that includes laryngotracheal clefting, tracheal agenesis, esophageal atresia, and tracheoe-sophageal fistula. (b) The diagrammatic representation includes duodenal obstruction due to annular pancreas, which is not depicted in (a). (Courtesy of Paes et al [15].)*

and esophagus are often in direct continuity. Stratified squamous epithelium may extend into the trachea, and islands of respiratory epithelium can be seen in the esophagus.

The clinical consequences in the neonate are easy to predict. Difficulty in feeding, excessive drooling of saliva, respiratory distress, and coughing in the newborn period are explained readily on the basis of the malformations. If the malformations are not treated, dehydration, aspiration of gastric juice, and pneumonitis are to be expected. Early radiological diagnosis searching for gaseous overdistension of the stomach in plain films of the abdomen is now the rule. It is clear from the pathologic anatomy that not all cases will show this sign. A knowledge of the many variants that may be encountered can help in making an early diagnosis. When a diagnosis has been made at an early stage of postnatal life, interruption of the fistula and the creation of feeding gastrotomies has led to improved survival.

The malformation complex of esophageal atresia and a tracheoesophageal fistula is often associated with maternal polyhydramnios [31]. The failure to swallow amniotic fluid [32] cannot be the entire explanation for the association, since hydramnios can be associated with laryngotracheoesophageal anomalies in the absence of any obstruction to the ingestion of amniotic fluid [15].

The exact incidence of congenital anomalies associated with the tracheoesophageal spectrum is not known. Series of cases based on autopsy findings are likely to be biased by the exclusion of uncomplicated cases that survive surgical correction, but the presence of a tracheoesophageal fistula should lead one to investigate the infant for the presence of other abnormalities. While occasionally seen in infants with trisomy 18 and Down syndrome, there is a high frequency of anomalies of the trachea and esophagus in singleton infants with a single umbilical artery [33, 34]. In some of these latter infants there may be associated abnormalities of the genitourinary tract, especially renal dysplasia. Other frequently associated anomalies include imperforate anus and cloacal anomalies, and many abnormalities of the heart and great vessels [35]. The eponym "VATER" (or "VACTERL") anomalad has been used to describe an association of *v*ertebral, *a*nal, *c*ardiac, *t*racheoesophageal, *r*enal and genital anomlies, and *l*imb anomalies [32].

While it is difficult to be certain about their exact significance, anomalies in the blood supply to the esophagus have been described in infants with a single umbilical artery and the tracheoesophageal malformation complex [36]. In the report by Lister [36], these vascular deficiencies are interpreted as having etiological significance. While the vascular basis of the malformation complex offers an attractive pathogenetic mechanism, the evidence is not conclusive. The lesion develops very early in embryonic life, and the abnormal blood supply could represent an effect of the lesion [28]. However, a vascular contribution to the development of the syndrome cannot be excluded with certainty [37].

While there has not been any convincing evidence of a familial trait, families with more than one affected sibling are known, and probable identical twins with esophageal atresia have been described [38, 39], though more often than not monozygotic twins are discordant for the anomalad [40]. Occasional clustering of cases has been described, which, along with the uncommon association of thalidomide embryopathy and esophageal atresia without fistulae [31], has suggested that the majority of cases are acquired in some currently unknown fashion. A tracheoesophageal fistula has been produced in the offspring of vitamin A–deficient maternal rats, and esophageal atresia has been produced in the embryos of riboflavin-deficient mice [41, 42].

Other Congenital Abnormalities of the Esophagus

Many of these lesions may present for the first time after the neonatal period, even in adults. Examples of either local of total esophageal duplication are reported [43, 44]. The etiology of duplications is not known, but they are probably derived from the epithelial islands that may be seen near the developing foregut and midgut in early embryos [45]. These lesions may be difficult to distinguish clinically from enterogenous cysts of the posterior mediastinum, with which they may share a common pathogenesis [46, 47]. The duplications and cysts may be lined with esophageal or gastric epithelium (of cardiac type) and foci of ciliated epithelium are not infrequent. In exceptional instances pancreatic tissue has been identified in the wall. Silverman and Roy [48] provide a good review of gastrointestinal duplications; about 20% are located in the thorax. These lesions may be noted either as incidental findings in perinatal postmortem examinations, or they may become distended with mucus and cause respiratory embarrassment, leading to surgical excision. Peptic ulceration may also occur.

Enterogenous cysts of the posterior mediastinum in close proximity to the carina, esophagus, and pericardium are not uncommonly associated with severe respiratory embarrassment. The cysts are fluid-filled and may be lined by an admixture of esophageal, gastric, or respiratory epithelium. Their walls may contain cartilage and striated and smooth muscle. Their origin in the posterior mediastinum may become obscured by their progressive enlargement and subsequent displacement of the adjacent structures. Hemorrhage and peptic ulceration into the esophagus or trachea may occur; erosion of major vessels is fortunately rare [49]. Many of these lesions may be associated with a vertebral anomaly, especially hemivertebra. Veeneklaas and others have suggested that adhesions between the notochord and developing gut draw out and sequester islands of developing foregut—the split notochord concept [50–52].

Rarely, a sequestered (Rokitansky) pulmonary lobe can arise from the esophagus. The bronchus supplying the lobe has no connection with the bronchial tree [53]. Rarely a

main branch may arise from the esophagus, a situation that is often associated with cardiac abnormalities [54].

Intramural Esophageal Cysts

These lesions lie within the wall of the esophagus and may distort the lumen or bulge toward the external aspect of the esophagus. The lining of these cysts may be very varied with squamous, cuboidal, transitional or ciliated epithelium, or a mixture of all three. Vertebral anomalies are rare with these cysts. Rarely gastric epithelium may be present in the cyst wall, particularly near the gastroesophageal junction. Occasionally true bronchogenic cysts, with cartilage, bronchial glands, and ciliated epithelium, may be seen in the esophagus.

As mentioned earlier, these lesions may be symptomatic by virtue of their size or because of ulceration, and many of them present in later life (including among adults). They may therefore be part of the differential diagnosis of posterior mediastinal masses. The author's collection includes an example of a 35-year-old female with a posterior mediastinal cyst lying near the esophagus that had dysplastic glandular epithelium in its lining. Other areas showed a mixture of squamous and glandular epithelium of gastric type. Two years following cyst resection she died of a disseminated adenocarcinoma involving the lower third of the esophagus.

Congenitally Short Esophagus

In some older infants, symptoms of projectile vomiting dating back to the newborn period may be encountered. A minority of these infants may be shown at surgery to have a short lining of esophageal epithelium, with much of the lower one-third to one-half of the dilated "esophagus" being lined by an orderly gastric epithelium. This syndrome has been given the name of "congenitally short esophagus" or "partial thoracic stomach." Neither the nomenclature nor the explanation for its development is satisfactory. Some authorities attribute the partial thoracic stomach to reflux complicating the relatively common occurrence of a sliding hiatal hernia. Botha [55], however, has argued that the occurrence of a partial thoracic stomach represents a major derangement in the development of the cardioesophageal region and diaphragm. Others have emphasized the importance of associated malformations, especially those of the aortic arch (such as the right-sided aortic arch) [56]. However, not all infants with this syndrome have associated major malformations, and the exact etiology is uncertain. The overlap with Barrett's esophagus is obvious [57] but in the short esophagus the epithelium is orderly and the glands contain parietal cells.

Displacement of the Esophagus

The esophagus may be displaced and kinked by a variety of intrathoracic space-occupying lesions. In infants with the relatively common left-sided diaphragmatic hernia, the esophagus is often drawn to the left but rarely is there any kinking. Other causes of displacement include enterogenous cysts and very rare congenital mediastinal tumours, such as neuroblastoma and teratoma. These lesions may be associated with obstruction due to compression. The esophagus may be crossed by abnormal great vessels, such as an aberrant aortic arch or an aberrant right subclavian artery (dysphagia lusoria). These latter lesions rarely cause symptoms in the newborn.

Esophageal Erosions and Ulcers

Mucosal erosions are common lesions that may be found in many perinatal infants dying from acute asphyxial causes (especially antepartum hemorrhage and cord prolapse) or in overwhelming neonatal sepsis. They have been seen in up to 30% of all neonatal postmortem examinations [58] and in stillbirths (Fig. 24.6). The upper third of the organ is affected most commonly, and the erosions may coexist with multiple petechial hemorrhages on the visceral pleura, epicardium, thymic cortex, and the mucosa of the gastrointestinal tract. Microscopically, they are characterized by mucosal epithelial loss, capillary dilatation, and rupture, with only a minimal cellular inflammatory response. They are usually limited to the mucosal folds, but on rare occasions ulceration may extend into the submucosa. Rarely, necrosis of the muscular elements of the wall may be associated with the epithelial changes. The esophageal lesions resemble the mucosal petechiae seen in the small and large bowel in early ischemia. Erosions have been identified in stillbirths and other infants who have never been intubated. Trauma, therefore, cannot be the sole factor in their development, but the passage of a nasogastric tube can exacerbate the lesion and may account for some of the larger lesions. In most instances they are asymptomatic, but they may be colonized by pathogenic organisms in the newborn (Fig. 24.7).

Isolated examples of spontaneous bleeding from deeper esophageal ulcers have been described. These symptomatic lesions are usually seen in the lower third of the esophagus above the cardia. They are not necessarily associated with intubation, but are probably related to peptic ulceration secondary to gastroesophageal reflux [59].

Spontaneous Rupture of the Esophagus (Boerhaave Syndrome)

Linear rupture sites in the lower third of the esophagus may be encountered in some early neonatal deaths. Fortunately, this is a rare event and few adequate pathological descriptions are available [60, 61]. The syndrome is associated with vomiting and the rapid development of a hydropneumothorax and mediastinitis. In a review by Hohf et al [62], only one case was associated with esophageal obstruction. The etiology is uncertain and a relationship with mucosal erosions is not established. There is no known association with ectopic gastric mucosa or partial thoracic stomach, but the lack of detailed pathological reports hinders our understanding of this problem. Clearly, surgery offers the only hope of survival, but survivors may develop strictures.

Traumatic Lesions of the Esophagus

The esophagus may be damaged by attempts at endotracheal intubation or by the passage of nasogastric tubes. Fortunately, the incidence of serious complications (laceration or perforation) is low. Minor degrees of mucosal abrasion confined usually to the upper esophagus and the pyriform fossa of the pharynx are common. Since access to the larynx and trachea may be restricted, problems of this nature are more likely to occur in the very tiny immature baby, but not exclusively. Difficulty in intubation of the airway may be

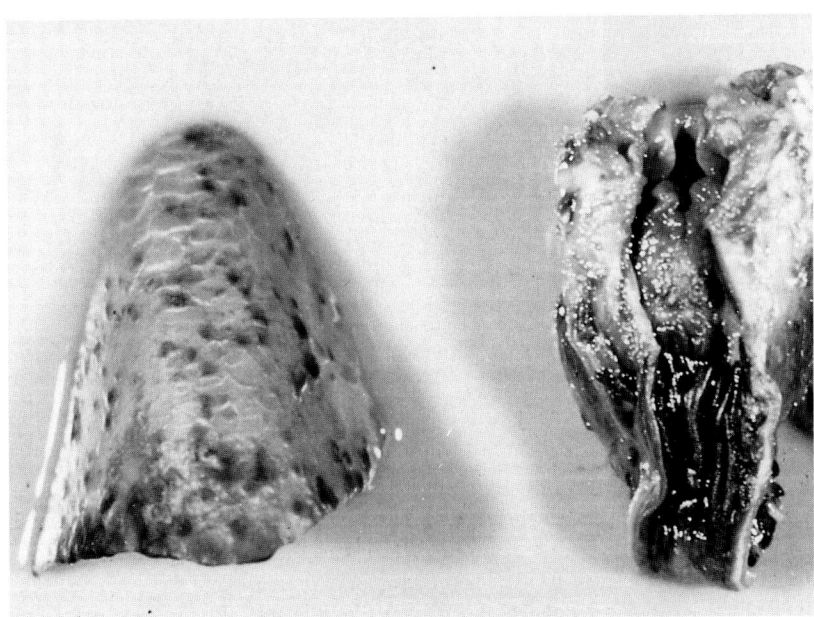

FIGURE 24.6.   *Hemorrhagic esophageal erosions* (right) *coexisting with visceral pleural petechiae* (left) *from an infant of 37 weeks' gestation who was stillborn following an antepartum hemorrhage. (Approx. 1.1.)*

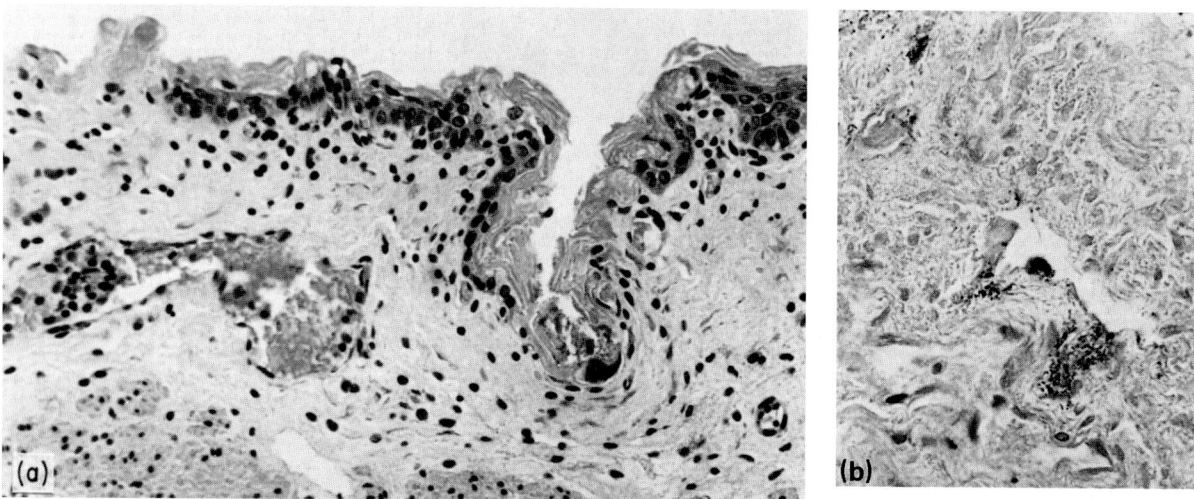

FIGURE 24.7. *(a) Histological appearance of an esophageal erosion with dilated capillaries below a focus of coagulative necrosis of the epithelium, devoid of any significant inflammatory response. (b) Among the debris of the epithelium, scattered clusters of organisms (in this instance* Escherichia coli*) are present.*

encountered in larger infants, especially those with any form of laryngotracheal obstruction or deformity. With more extensive damage, a false passage extending downward into the mediastinum parallel to the esophagus may be produced [63].

Traumatic lesions due to the passage of a nasogastric tube are infrequent, but may be extensive. Any zone of the esophagus may be damaged, including the usually "physiologically" narrowed sites (opposite the aortic arch and carina and at the diaphragmatic opening). Extensive linear lacerations of varying depth (including complete perforation) may occur [63]. More commonly, large mucosal and submucosal hematomata may be seen. Prolonged intubation of the esophagus may lead to stenosis [63].

Inflammatory Lesions of the Esophagus

The esophagus may show focal ulceration in many perinatal infections. Conversely, acute erosions of the esophagus may become colonized with organisms (Fig. 24.7).

Two specific infections of the esophagus in the perinatal period merit attention. Candidial (monilial) infections of the esophagus may be part of the syndrome of congenital candidiasis [64], or part of a widespread systemic disease which may arise from ulcers related to prolonged intubation [67]. The lesions vary from small superficial foci to larger confluent granular plaques. In congenital candidiasis, the yeasts do not usually penetrate deeply into the esophagus (Fig. 24.8). Penetration into the deeper layers of the esophagus, with extensive necrosis of the epithelium, is more common in cases with widespread systemic disease, suggesting an infection that overwhelms host defenses [65, 66].

Vesicles may be seen in the esophageal epithelium in congenital herpetic infections [67]. Esophageal involvement

is merely part of a widespread dissemination, with lesions in the lungs, liver, central nervous system, and occasionally other sites in the gastrointestinal tract.

Rubella esophagitis [68] has been described, and the esophageal surface epithelium and glands may show the presence of the pathognomonic "owl's-eye" intranuclear inclusions of cytomegalovirus [69]. Rarely, fatal neonatal varicella infection may be associated with esophageal lesions (Fig. 24.9).

Congenital syphilis may involve the entire gastrointestinal tract, but specific esophageal lesions have not been reported [70].

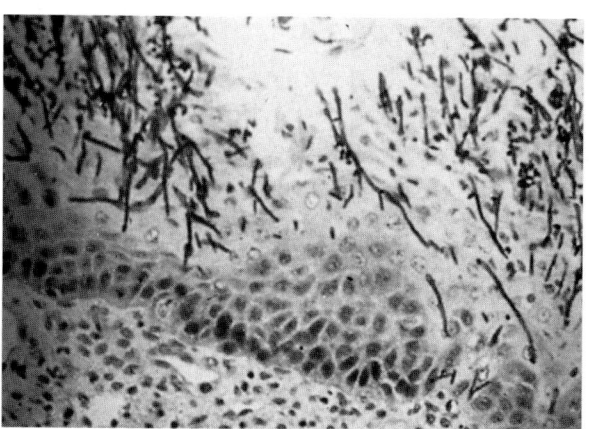

FIGURE 24.8. *The esophageal epithelium in a case of congenital candidiasis shows pseudohyphae in and among the epithelial cells. No inflammatory response is seen. (Periodic acid-Schiff after diastase [D-PAS].)*

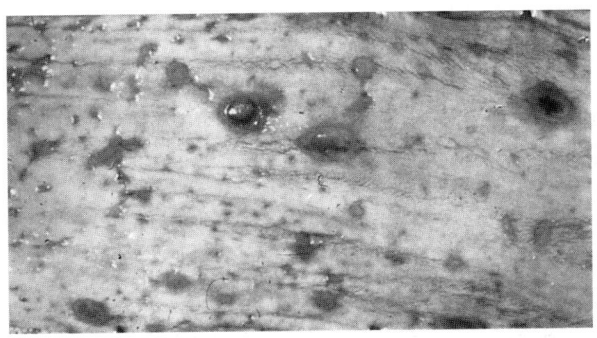

FIGURE 24.9. *Vesicles in the esophageal epithelium are seen in an infant born at term who died aged 10 days. The mother had a severe varicella infection at the time of delivery, which she had contracted from her older child. (Case provided by Dr. Hans Lucke, Hamilton, Ontario.)*

Functional Disorders of the Esophagus

In the newborn period and in later life, a variety of disorders characterized by incoordinate esophageal contraction may be encountered. The frequency of these disorders is not known and their etiology and pathogenesis are uncertain. Irregularity of esophageal contraction and gastroesophageal reflux may persist for a varying length of time following surgical correction of esophageal atresia and a tracheoesophageal fistula [59]. No appropriate explanation is available; the irregular contractions are usually a short-lived phenomenon and scarring at the site of anastomosis in the reconstructed esophagus is not likely to be the entire explanation. The esophagus has a pattern of autonomic innervation that is similar to that seen in the lower gastrointestinal tract [18]. Sphincter dysfunction of the lower esophagus has been described in some affected infants [71], but the anatomical basis is not defined.

Reflux Esophagitis

In recent years a great deal of attention has been directed toward problems of spontaneously occurring gastroesophageal reflux in the newborn, and mucosal biopsies of the esophagus in very young children including infants are more frequent [59, 72–74]. On the basis of these reports it is clear that esophagitis complicating reflux, which may begin in the newborn period, is not uncommon. There is even a report of the development of Barrett's esophagus in the newborn [75]. Regurgitation and apnea have been linked in some reports [76, 77], though evidence of gastroesophageal reflux was present in only 21% of infants presenting with the sudden infant death syndrome (SIDS) [78].

The role of mucosal biopsy in the study of esophageal problems in infants and children is reviewed by Dahms and Rothstein [79]. It is clear that this is an expanding field of interest [80], but as yet this author has not been able to study examples of esophageal mucosal biopsies from the newborn.

In the condition of megaesophagus, the esophagus is dilated and shows muscular hyperplasia. Despite the clinical evidence of poor esophageal contraction, with its associated regurgitation of feeds or gastric contents, routine microscopic preparations have shown normal autonomic innervation [81].

Other Lesions of the Esophagus

Isolated instances of stenosing esophageal mucosal webs, with neither tracheoesophageal fistulas nor any other associated anomalies, may be encountered in the newborn period [82]. No adequate explanation of their pathogenesis is available, but their frequent occurrence in the middle third of the esophagus recapitulates the commonest site of involvement of the tracheoesophageal fistula complex. Symptoms may be delayed until adult life is reached [83].

In some infants, esophageal stenosis has been associated with the same cluster of anomalies in other viscera as seen

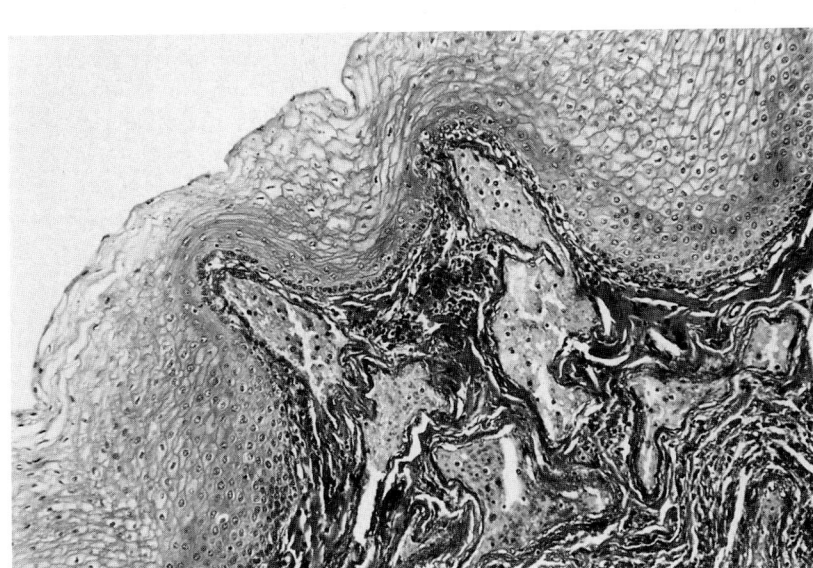

FIGURE 24.10. *Large dilated vessels in the mucosa of an infant with diffuse neonatal angiomatosis. Similar lesions were found in the small bowel and colon, and some of the latter had bled profusely. (Masson's trichrome.)*

in esophageal atresia [31]. The author's collection includes an instance of a $3\frac{1}{2}$-week-old child with an esophageal stricture involving the middle third of the organ, and no other anomalies detected clinically. The surgically resected specimen had an intact epithelium, but the muscular layer was focally deranged by irregularly placed bundles of scar tissue. The child had never been intubated and the etiology was never discovered.

Tracheobronchial remnants are choristomatous lesions of the distal esophagus and are a rare cause of esophageal stenosis and dysphagia. They are made up of a circumferential arrangement of tracheal seromucous glands, cartilaginous bars or rings with prominent lymphoid tissue [82, 84, 85].

The esophagus may be involved in epidermolysis bullosa, of either the "letalis" or "dystrophica" type, where the characteristic features of the bullous skin lesions may be duplicated in the stratified squamous epithelium of the esophagus [86].

Mucosal and submucosal angiomata may be found in cases of diffuse neonatal hemangiomatosis [87]. The angiomata vary from tight clusters of capillaries to dilated channels that produce mucosal blebs (Fig. 24.10).

Esophageal varices may be a delayed complication of prolonged umbilical venous catheterization [88, 89], or as a complication of severe liver disease [90].

The esophagus may be involved in congenital fibromatosis, and a good pictorial example is provided by Stout and Lattes [91].

The submucosal esophageal glands may be distended in cases of cystic fibrosis of the pancreas (Fig. 24.11), but these incidental and asymptomatic lesions are overshadowed by the extensive pathology in other organs.

THE STOMACH

Development

The stomach can be identified as a fusiform dilatation of the foregut appearing caudad to the developing lung buds. With the progressive elongation of the midgut and the development of the lung buds, the primordial stomach is displaced even more caudally [1]. The final disposition of the stomach is determined by disproportionate growth of the posterior segment, as well as the progressive elongation of the midgut. These changes result in the pyloric region of the stomach being displaced to the right of the midline and the stomach undergoing its own separate rotation so that the dorsal border is displaced laterally and to the left of the midline. The ventral border is destined to become the lesser curvature, and the disproportionately elongated dorsal border forms the greater curvature. The pyloric sphincter is recognizable as a denser condensation of mesenchyme near the caudal end. The arterial blood supply of the stomach is derived from the coeliac axis through large anterior (right) and posterior (left) gastric arteries. The development and enlargement of the spleen in the posterior mesogastrium and the liver in the septum transversum lead to the coeliac axis branches becoming remodeled to achieve the "adult" conformation.

At first the stomach is lined by a simple columnar epithelium (Fig. 24.12), but by the end of the 14th week the rudiments of gastric pits and branching glands appear [92]. Differentiation of parietal (oxyntic) cells appear by the 16th week. Elementary rugal folds can be defined in fetuses at 20 weeks, but the complexity of these folds varies considerably even in much older children and adults.

Congenital Anomalies

Absence of the stomach has been reported in acardius acephalus and this may be associated with other multiple malformations of the alimentary tract, including multiple atretic segments in the small and large bowel [93].

The stomach is the least frequent site of obstructive lesions in the neonatal period. Hypertrophic pyloric stenosis, though obviously of congenital origin, rarely if ever pre-

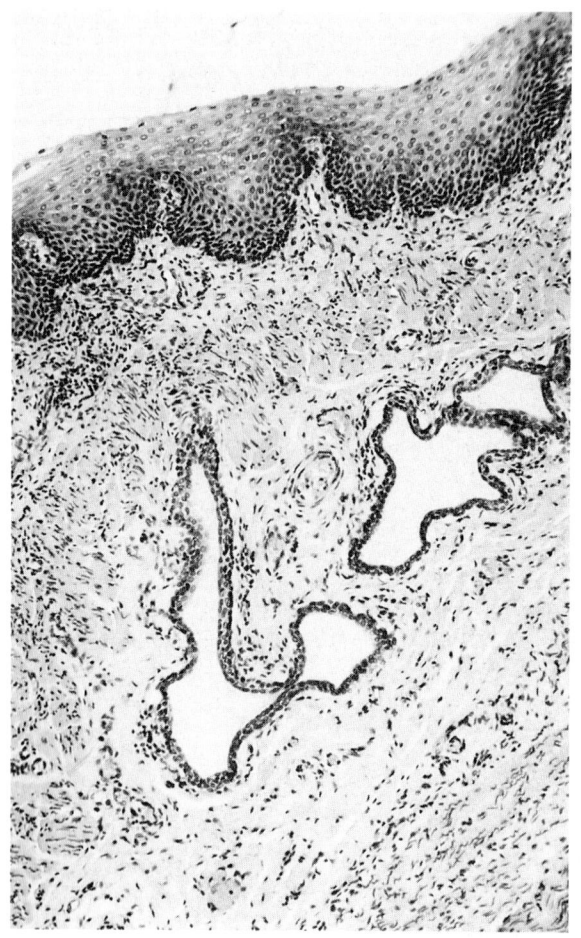

FIGURE 24.11. *Dilated ducts and glands in the esophagus of an infant who presented with meconium ileus, perforated small bowel, and meconium peritonitis.*

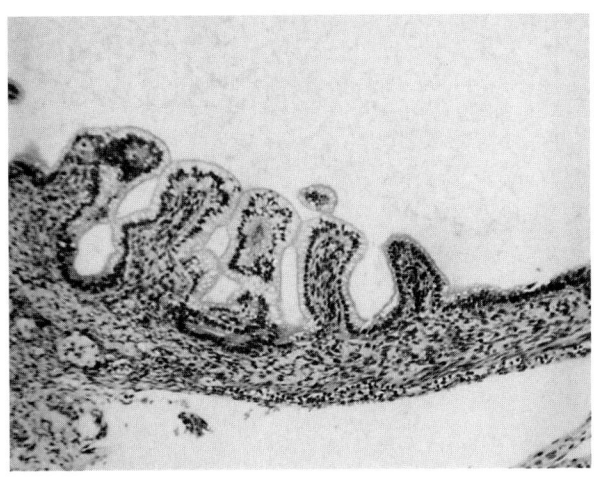

FIGURE 24.12. *Simple columnar epithelium lines the stomach of a 9-mm fetus. Note also the recognizable muscle layer and autonomic innervation.*

sents in the neonatal infant. Even cases of congenital "hourglass stomach" are, most often, examples of duodenal obstruction (either due to atresia or an annular pancreas) with the lower chamber of the hourglass being identified, incorrectly, as the pyloric end of the stomach.

Apart from abnormalities of position, associated with diaphragmatic hernia or situs inversus, and the problems of the "short esophagus–thoracic stomach" variety, congenital abnormalities of the stomach are uncommon. In the peri-

natal period, duplications and enterogenous cysts of the stomach are often asymptomatic [94, 95] but may present as pyloric stenosis (Fig. 24.13). These duplications are usually localized and consist of an outpouching of gastric mucosa of pyloric type with an incomplete replica of the layers of the stomach, including muscularis propria [96]. They tend to be commoner near the pyloric sphincter [97], but there may be total duplication of the stomach and the sausage-shaped lesions may extend into the chest [47, 94, 98]. The larger lesions may be associated with angulation of the esophagus, diaphragmatic elevation, and even displacement of mediastinal structures. Enterogenous cysts may present in a similar fashion to duplications. They consist of cysts that distort the pyloric region, which are lined by epithelium and have irregular muscle bundles in their walls. The lining of cysts may include pancreatic and intestinal epithelium (Fig. 24.14).

Both types of lesions are uncommon, and a detailed analysis of any associated malformations is not possible. However, the presence of associated hemivertebrae has been recorded, and in an infant with Turner syndrome, renal dysplasia was associated with gastric duplication [98]. Gastric duplications may remain asymptomatic until adult life, when they may be associated with epigastric pain and vomiting; in one such lesion, the wall of the duplicated segment was calcified (Fig. 24.15).

Closely related to duplications and cysts are the far less frequent congenital gastric diverticula. These lesions are found near the pyloric sphincter but are not symptomatic in the newborn. They may be lined by attenuated gastric epithelium of pyloric type [99].

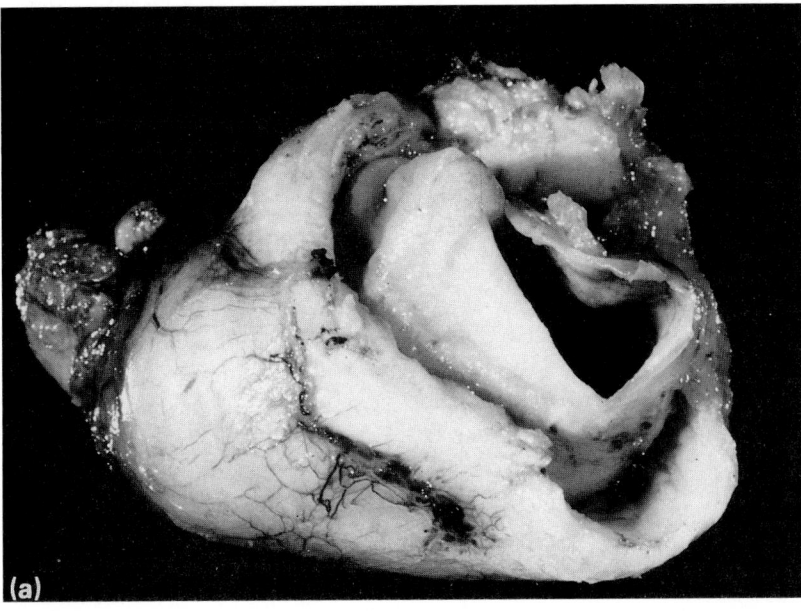

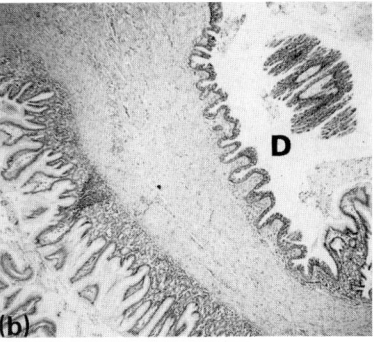

FIGURE 24.13. *A resected, partly opened, sausage-shaped duplication of the pyloric end of the stomach, which was removed from a 6-week-old infant who presented with a clinical picture of pyloric stenosis. (a) The pylorus was removed with the duplication. (b) The septum between the pylorus and the duplication (D). Note the simplified appearance of the epithelium in this duplication.*

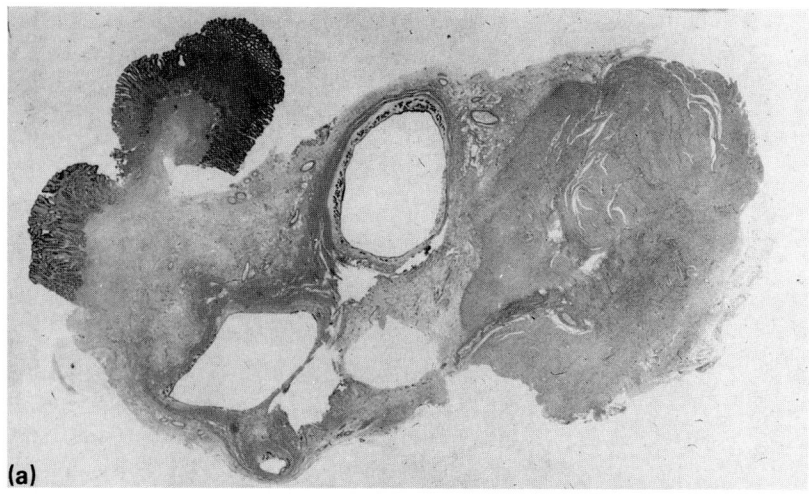

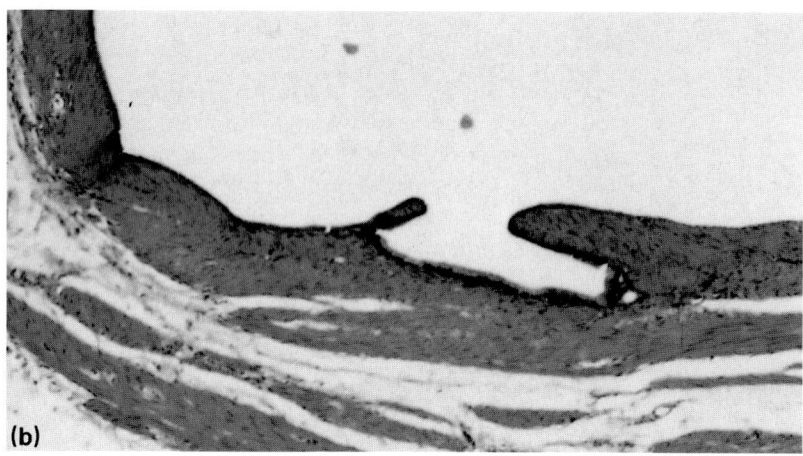

FIGURE 24.14.   *A whole-mount preparation of a resected cystic mass of the pylorus of a 3-week-old infant. (a) Several scattered intramural cysts are seen. (b) Histologically they were lined by a flattened cuboidal epithelium, with occasional bands of poorly defined muscle supporting the lining epithelium, diagnostic of an "enterogenous" gastric cyst. (D-PAS.)*

A good review of the problems posed by gastric duplications and cysts and diverticula is provided by Wieczorek et al [100]. These authors showed that 39/109 genuine duplications were seen in infants under 3 months of age. They also defined differences between cysts and duplication.

However, it may be difficult to be certain of the exact type of lesion in every instance.

A small hypoplastic stomach may be a concomitant finding in association with a tracheoesophageal fistula, but rare examples of microgastria without esophageal obstruc-

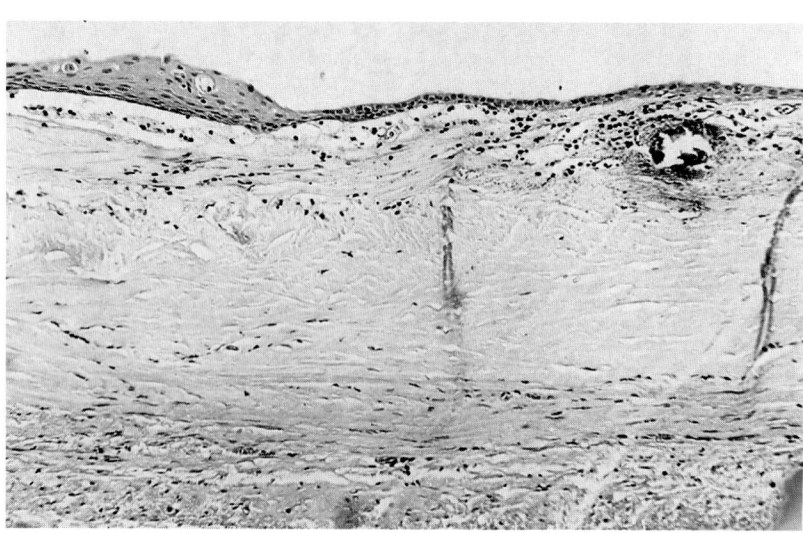

FIGURE 24.15.   *The wall of a gastric duplication resected from a 24-year-old male shows a squamous epithelial lining, and marked scarring of the wall in which foci of darkly staining dystrophic calcification can be seen.*

tion or a fistula may be encountered [112]. The lesion may form part of Ivemark asplenia-polysplenia syndrome [101–103]. The stomach is small, lies in the midline, and is a simple tubular structure without a fundus or antrum [104], and the esophagus may be dilated.

Small, heterotopic islands of small-intestine-type mucosa, Brunner's glands, or exocrine pancreatic tissue are occasional, incidental, histological findings in the stomach [93, 105, 106]. They are rarely, if ever, symptomatic until later life, when they may present with pyloric obstruction or as polypoidal lesions.

Dextroposition of the stomach may occur in association with situs inversus [107] and in other syndromes with abnormal situs. Rarely, isolated dextroposition of the stomach may occur [108].

Pyloric Atresia and Antral Webs

Pyloric atresia is an exceptionally rare event probably occurring in less than one birth in a million [109–111]. The pylorus may be blocked by an imperforate mucosal diaphragm just before the pylorus, or there may be two diaphragms that produce the false impression of a duplication, or there may be complete fibrous interruption of the pyloric area (sometimes called pyloric aplasia) [112]. While the membranous variety probably represents an untoward fusion of the mucosal folds, the more drastic variety of pyloric aplasia may represent the sequel of a vascular injury [112]. Familial cases and an autosomal recessive pattern of inheritance have been reported [112, 113]. Hydramnios may be an accompanying feature [114, 115]. Antral webs represent an incomplete variant of membranous pyloric atresia [116–118] which usually present in later childhood and young adults. Clearly, some of these may represent a reaction to prior repeated episodes of peptic ulceration leading to obstruction.

Congenital Hypertrophic Pyloric Stenosis

This lesion may have a congenital origin but it is uncommon for it to present in the neonatal period. The condition is the commonest major gastric lesion seen in infancy, and affects boys more than girls in a ratio of 4:1. The incidence of the lesion varies from about 1.25 to 4 per 1000 in different white populations, but is found in only 0.48 per 1000 among blacks. There is therefore considerable variation in the incidence of this lesion; there may even be some variation over time [119].

The thickened pylorus may be present at birth, but symptoms are rarely encountered before 2 or 3 weeks after birth [120]. The pylorus is increased in length, has a firm consistency, is white in color, and is gristly in appearance and texture. The circular muscle layer is enlarged and thickened, and the longitudinal layer is only slightly affected. The lesion is usually sharply demarcated at its duodenal end, but may taper gradually into the adjacent tissue at its proximal gastric margin. Histologically, the muscle cells appear normal, but the mucosa is usually edematous and swollen with a mild inflammatory infiltrate. The pyloric obstruction leads to profuse vomiting that progressively becomes projectile, and often the thickened pylorus can be palpated through the abdominal wall between bouts of vomiting. At least one example of congenital hypertrophic pyloric stenosis has been preceded by massive bleeding from a peptic ulcer [121].

The etiology of the condition is not known. Only on rare occasions are there other associated malformations [120]. The role of the autonomic nervous system in the pyloric region is not clearly defined [122–126]. The role of a deficiency of vasoactive peptides in the circular muscle (but not in the myenteric plexus) remains to be assessed fully [123, 125].

The importance of genetic factors in the development of the syndrome is accepted, but the exact mechanisms are not clear. It is known that siblings born after a first affected child have a 19-fold greater risk of being affected, and the offspring of previously affected children have a 12-fold greater risk of being affected. However, there is no increased incidence of parental consanguinity, and the incidence of pyloric stenosis in siblings of the propositi is only 1:20 as opposed to an expected 1:4 for a recessive condition [127]. Clearly, the simple explanation of recessive inheritance is inapplicable. McKeown et al [128] showed that birth rank played no role in infants who were symptomatic immediately after birth, whereas those who had symptoms later in the newborn period or infancy were more likely to be the first born. Carter's studies of the sex ratios of children of patients with pyloric stenosis [129] are of interest: males who survived had 7% affected boys and 1.5% affected girls. The female patients also had four times as many affected children. These findings have been developed to suggest that the disease is due to a dominant gene but with a considerable degree of background modification of its effects. The sex of the infant was one of these modifying factors, but most are unknown [129]. The development of symptoms about 2 to 3 weeks after birth in the majority of instances suggests that mucosal edema is the first step leading to obstruction. However, the trigger stimulus is not known, and though gastrin oversecretion has been suggested [130], it is not thought to be a major factor now. San Filippo reported five cases that appeared to develop following treatment with erythromycin [131].

Hypertrophic pyloric stenosis has been associated with Down syndrome and thalidomide embryopathy [127]. An unusual case of pyloric stenosis, Hirschsprung disease, and an additional chromosome (probably 16) was reported by Butler et al [132]. Ahmed [133] and Dodge [134] have described several isolated congenital anomalies associated with pyloric stenosis, including esophageal atresia, Meckel's diverticulum, malrotation of the small bowel, and diaphragmatic hernia. Turner syndrome and the Smith-Lemli-Opitz syndrome may be complicated by pyloric stenosis [134].

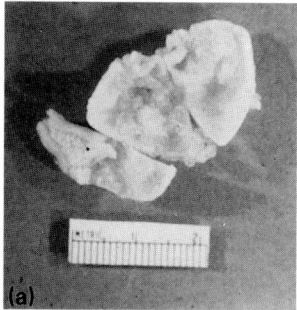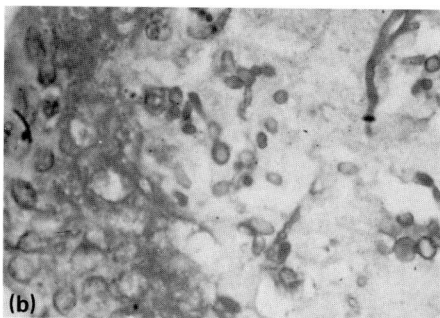

FIGURE 24.16. *The stomach from a case of congenital candidiasis in a 20-week-fetus is filled with a felted mucoid mass (a) in which yeasts and pseudohyphae can be demonstrated histologically (b). (B, PAS.)*

Gastric Perforation in the Newborn

Braunstein [135] described a spontaneous perforation of the stomach in an infant that was ascribed to a defect in the muscularis propria. Subsequently, other reports have appeared that indicate that most of the affected infants have been of low birth weight [136, 137]. These spontaneous perforations are associated with increasing neonatal respiratory embarrassment, abdominal distension, and radiographic demonstration of free air in the abdomen [138–140]. Unless urgent surgical correction is undertaken, the condition will prove fatal. The exact nature of this condition remains controversial. There are no convincing reports that describe congenital deficiencies of the smooth muscle of the gastric wall in the absence of perforation. It has been assumed that the perforation is due to the muscular defect, but Shaw et al [137] have shown that potential weaknesses exist in the muscle layers due to their complex arrangement. Most tears due to overdistension have a linear pattern [138]. Overdistension with fluid or air from any cause could possibly lead to mucosal prolapse and rupture. The muscular anomalies described with gastric perforation are thought to be produced by the perforation, with subsequent distortion of the adjacent muscle bundles due to irregular contraction. The possibility of ischemia producing perforation is suggested by some workers [139–142].

Functional abnormalities of the stomach with overdistension and regurgitation of feeds are encountered on occasion [137]. The exact incidence of these abnormalities is not known, nor is there any information regarding their pathological basis. It is worth noting, however, that a review of the clinical features of those infants who have gastric perforations suggests that several, if not all, had some functional anomaly with delayed emptying prior to the development of a perforation.

Traumatic Gastric Perforation

With the advent of neonatal intensive care and concomitant therapeutic interventions, traumatic gastric perforation with the passage of a nasogastric tube may be encountered. Fortunately, this is a very rare event, even with very firm nasogastric tubes. Overdistension of the stomach by air, as may occur during vigorous resuscitation procedures, may be an additional contributory factor.

Infections and Inflammatory Lesions of the Stomach

In congenital candidiasis, felted masses of yeast, hyphae, and mucin are seen in the stomach (Fig. 24.16) and may even be found as far distally as the colon and appendix [143]. No inflammatory reaction is present and there is no evidence of tissue penetration by the organisms.

Intranuclear inclusions have been seen in the epithelial cells in cases of cytomegalovirus infections of the neonate (Fig. 24.17) and in congenital neonatal herpes simplex infections [67].

Ulcers of the stomach have been seen in disseminated candidiasis and group B streptococcal sepsis [63].

Mucosal Erosions and Ulcers in the Newborn

Hemorrhagic mucosal erosions and petechiae are common findings at the summit of rugal folds in the stomach of the

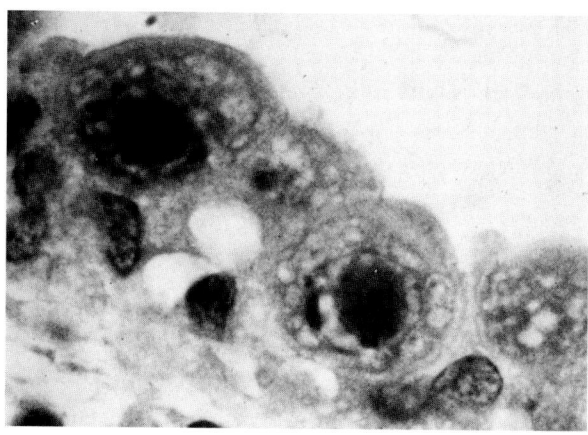

FIGURE 24.17. *Cytomegalovirus inclusion bodies are seen in the superficial gastric epithelium from an infant of 31 weeks' gestation. Similar cells were seen in the kidney, pancreas, lung, adrenal, liver, parotid, and thyroid, and a dense plasmacytic villitis with inclusion bodies was seen in the placenta.*

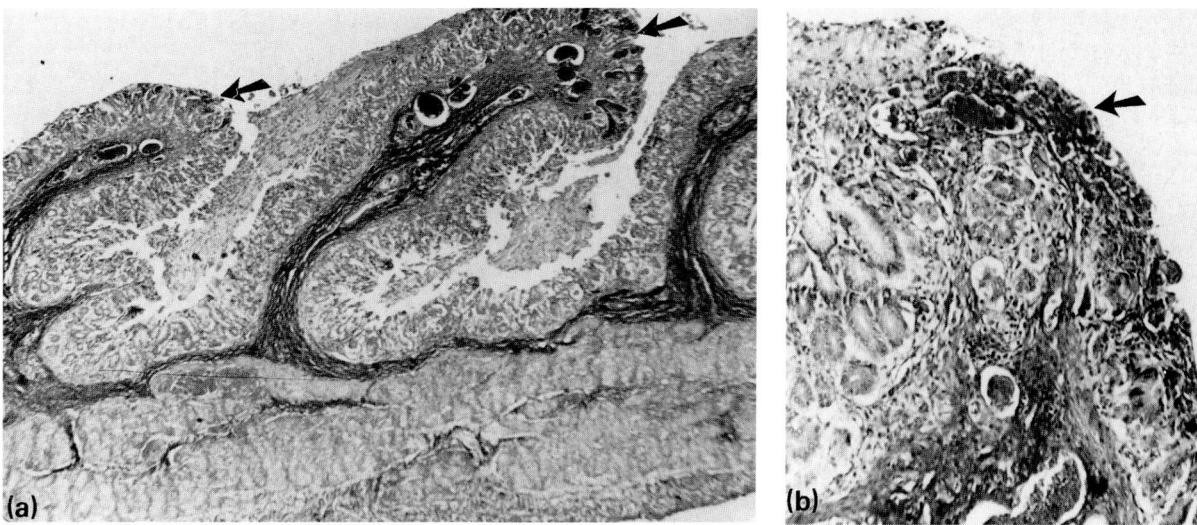

FIGURE 24.18.   *(a) Low-power and (b) high-power views of a hemorrhagic gastric mucosal erosion. Note the localization of the lesion (arrow) near the summit of the rugal fold. (Masson's trichrome.)*

newborn. They may coexist with similar lesions of the esophagus and with ischemic lesions of the small and large bowel, with which they probably share a similar pathogenesis (Fig. 24.18). They are found commonly in severely asphyxiated babies, and in infants with overwhelming sepsis, when organisms may be seen in the bed of the lesions (Fig. 24.19). Larger peptic ulcers of the stomach are described only occasionally in the newborn period [144], but are commoner in older children. Their etiology is not known. The ulcers may cause severe hemorrhage, even to the point of exsanguination, and perforation may occur without prior hematemesis [145]. Kelsey et al [121] have described an infant with massive hemorrhage from an ulcer that presented in the newborn period. The infant was readmitted at 3 weeks with classic pyloric stenosis. They offer a reasonable explanation that both the ulceration and the later pyloric stenosis may be effects of hyperacidity.

The use of the alpha-adrenergic blocking agent tolazoline in infants with pulmonary hypertension has been linked to the development of severe gastric ulceration [146]. Since the drug has a chemical structure that resembles histamine, this complication may have been predicted but unavoidable, since the structural mimicry may be the basis for the vasodilatory effect of the drug.

Miscellaneous Lesions

Gastric volvulus may occur as an uncommon complication of a diaphragmatic hernia in the neonate. Secondary ischemia may lead to perforation, requiring emergency surgery [147].

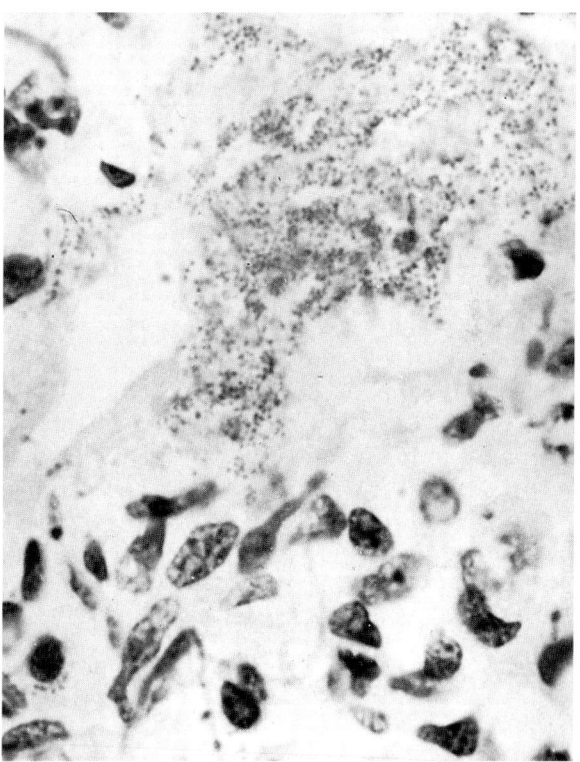

FIGURE 24.19.   *Clusters of organisms (in this instance Streptococci) are seen in the sludged vessels below an erosion in a case of severe group B streptococcal sepsis in a preterm 27-week neonate.*

Gastric infarction has been seen as a complication of umbilical arterial and aortic catheterization for monitoring arterial blood gases in the newborn period [148] (Fig. 24.20). The arterial catheter tip, invariably, has been placed high in the aorta, well above the 12th thoracic vertebral body.

Pyloric atresia has been described as a complication of epidermolysis bullosa [86, 149]. Microscopic distension of pyloric mucous glands has been seen in mucoviscidosis (cystic fibrosis) [150]. Gastric angiomata have been noted in neonatal angiomatosis and in infantile angiodysplasia [87, 151]. Serosal deposits of neuroblastoma have been seen in some infants with congenital neuroblastomas [152]. In familial hemophagocytic reticulosis, submucosal infiltrates may be present.

Rarely, examples of hypertrophic gastropathy may present in the newborn [153]. The syndrome mimics Ménétrier disease, and the obstruction to the gastric outlet that may complicate prostaglandin E_1 therapy [154].

Very rare gastric teratomas are reported [155, 156].

Small heterotopic islands may be noted as incidental findings in children and adults. Large heterotopic pancreatic nodules may be asymptomatic or associated with outlet obstruction or even ulceration [112, 157]. Islets of Langerhans may accompany the exocrine tissue. Adenomyomata of the pyloric end of the stomach are hamartomatous collections of simple mucinous glands, and occur in the mucosa and submucosa. They rarely, if ever, present in the newborn.

THE SMALL INTESTINE

Development of the Small Bowel

The small intestine extends from the pylorus to the ileocecal valve. With the exception of the proximal segment of the duodenum, the small bowel is a midgut derivative, and since the superior mesenteric artery is the artery of the midgut, most of the small bowel is supplied by that vessel [1]. The proximal segment of duodenum is supplied by branches from the right gastric vessels that arise ultimately from the coeliac artery.

In early fetal life the yolk sac communicates freely with the midgut loops, but the patent, originally tubular, connection is reduced to a narrow stalk, the vitello-intestinal duct, which has usually disappeared completely by the time the midgut loops return to the abdominal cavity. The midgut is suspended from the dorsal abdominal wall by a mesentery, which carries the superior mesenteric artery and its branches (including the vitelline vessels to the yolk sac). The midgut loop has a cranial (pre-arterial) limb and a caudal (post-arterial) limb at this stage and the vitello-intestinal duct arises from the apex of the loop where the two limbs join. The disproportionate growth of the pre-arterial limb of the midgut gives rise to the many loops of the small bowel, while the post-arterial limb is recognizable by the presence of a small outpouching just distal to the attachment of the vitello-intestinal duct. This is the cecal diverticulum, the primordium of the cecum, and appendix, and it serves to identify the post-arterial limb.

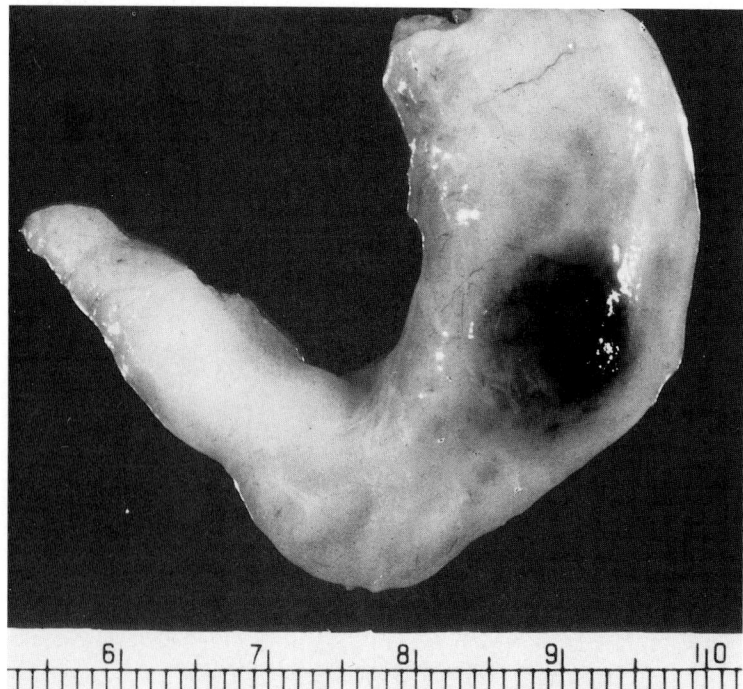

FIGURE 24.20. *A sharply demarcated zone of infarction is seen on the anterior wall of the stomach from an infant of 27 weeks' gestation with a high placement of an umbilical arterial catheter tip, opposite the ductus arteriosus. Contact thrombi were present along the aortic wall and umbilical artery as well as around the catheter.*

The central issue in the development of the small bowel concerns the rotation of the midgut, since this defines its anatomical situs. The relatively rapid elongation of the midgut, as well as the development of the large hepatic and renal primordia, outstrips the capacity of the developing abdomen; consequently, the loops of the developing midgut prolapse into the umbilical opening along with the vitello-intestinal duct (and its related vessels) [1]. At about the 6th week of development, due to the rapid elongation of the pre-arterial limb, the midgut undergoes a counterclockwise rotation through 90 degrees (when viewed from the ventral aspect) (Fig. 24.21). The two limbs lie beside each other within the umbilical opening and extra-embryonic coelom. Further elongation of both limbs occurs, with the growth in the pre-arterial limb exceeding that of the post-arterial limb. Contemporaneously, the abdominal cavity is enlarging, the pace of growth of the liver and kidneys is slowing, and eventually by 10 weeks' gestation the abdomen can accommodate the midgut loops. The loops of the pre-arterial limb return first, its proximal segments pushing to the left and dorsal to the axis of the superior mesenteric artery. The loops of the post-arterial limb are forced through a further 90 degree counterclockwise rotation to the right and ventral to the arterial axis, which eventually carries the cecal diverticulum into a subhepatic position. Later, further elongation of the colon carries the cecum downward into its normal anatomical site. This final phase of colonic descent occurs relatively late in pregnancy and many immature infants (of less than 28 weeks' gestation) have an incompletely descended colon.

Midgut development is characterized, therefore, by rapid asymmetrical growth of the pre-arterial and post-arterial

limbs, leading to physiological herniation and counterclockwise rotation through approximately 270 degrees. This results in the most proximal segment of the pre-arterial limb, the future third part of the duodenum, being placed across the midline behind the superior mesenteric artery, and leads to the "peripheral" distribution of the large bowel around the abdomen in a plane ventral to the superior mesenteric artery. While it is convenient to think of these events as specific steps, it is important to realize that the process is continuous, with many of the changes arising as a consequence of the rapid intrinsic growth of the pre-arterial limb of the midgut. This sequence can, of course, be interrupted at any point. By the end of the 10th week, rotation of the midgut is complete, except for the final repositioning of the cecum.

Duodenal development warrants separate consideration not only because the organ is derived from both the caudad foregut and the cephalad midgut, but also because it is the site from which the hepatic and pancreatic primordia arise (Fig. 24.22) and its anatomical site is affected by the rotation of the stomach and the midgut. The site of the junction between the foregut and the midgut is just distal to Vater's ampulla and the opening of the common bile duct. The rotation of the stomach carries the cephalad duodenal segment to the right of the midline, and the return of the midgut loops carries the caudad segment of the duodenum to the left of the midline. The dorsal mesentery of the duodenum becomes incorporated into the posterior abdominal wall, causing the duodenum to become a retroperitoneal organ. Apart from the small segment that forms the anterior border of the aditus to the lesser sac of the peritoneum (epiploic, or Winslow's, foramen), the ventral mesentery of the duodenum (drawn out by the developing hepatic primordium) disappears. Persistence of the ventral mesentery of the duodenum may result in aberrant peritoneal bands that lie across the ventral aspect of the duodenum (Ladd's bands), and these may be a cause of obstruction [158].

Details of hepatic and pancreatic development are found in the relevant chapters on those organs.

Differentiation of the Small Bowel

At 6 weeks the small bowel is a simple tube lined by a single-layered epithelium and surrounded by a mesenchymal collar. By 8 weeks the epithelium has proliferated to become a lining that is several cells thick. With the exception of the duodenum, this epithelial proliferation never occludes the lumen completely; in the duodenum there is a temporary period of occlusion during the 9th week caused by rapid epithelial growth. This epithelial plug breaks down normally by about the middle of the 10th week [159, 160]. In the more distal segments of the small bowel, the lumen is continuous and there is no convincing evidence that it is ever occluded. Villi begin to appear in the duodenum and upper jejunum by the latter part of the 9th week and a circular layer of muscularis propria appears at about the same time.

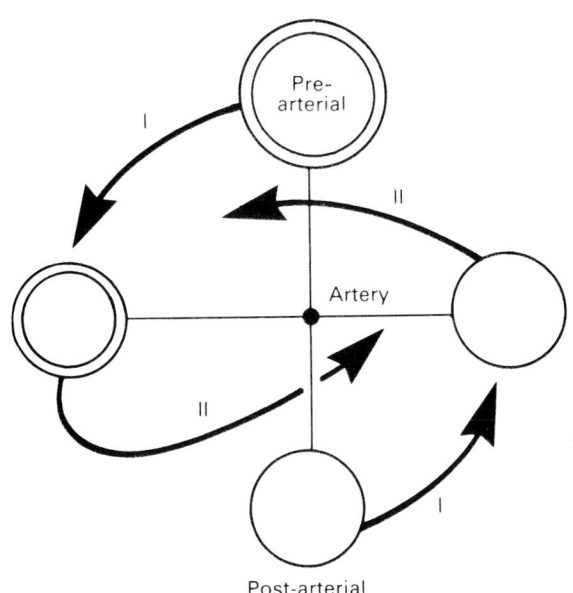

FIGURE 24.21. *A simplified scheme indicating the rotation of the gut.*

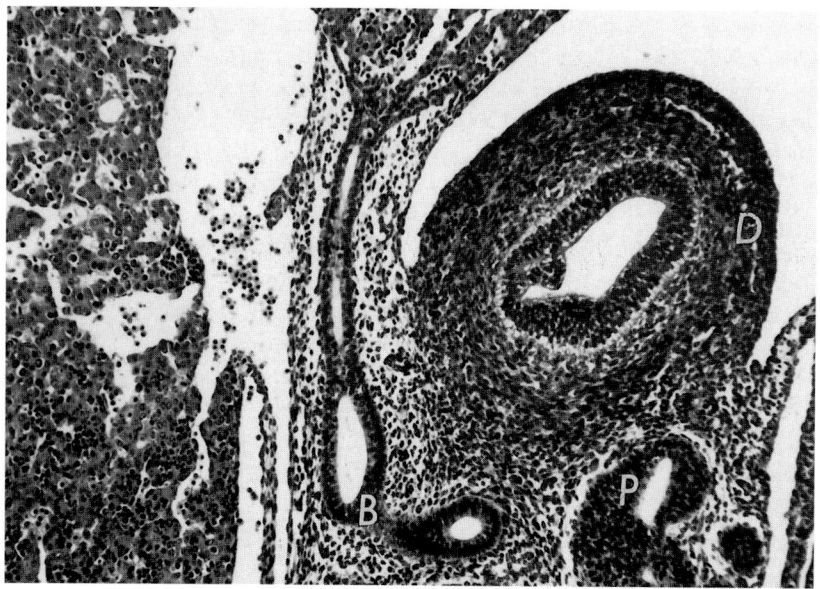

FIGURE 24.22. *Transverse section of duodenum from 55-mm embryo showing duodenum (D) with developing liver, bile ducts (B), and pancreatic duct (P).*

The crypts of Lieberkuhn appear in the proximal small bowel during the latter half of the 3rd month, but gastrin-producing cells can be seen in the duodenum at a slightly earlier stage [10, 161, 162]. Goblet cells and a longitudinal layer of muscularis propria appear during the 3rd month, as the epithelium thins into a single layer [162]. During the latter part of the 3rd month and early part of the 4th month, episodic rhythmic contractions may be noted and a myenteric plexus becomes recognizable. By the 78-mm stage (latter half of the 4th month), villi are present in the entire small intestine, and circular folds are present in the mucosa (Fig. 24.23). Brunner's glands appear in the duodenum at this stage. Peristaltic activity can be identified and Meissner's plexus is detectable at the 65-mm stage. Meconium accumulates in the gut lumen, made up of desquamated cells and amorphous debris. Paneth cells are present by the middle of the 5th month. In the 6th month, mast cells and lymphoid aggregates can be found and a muscularis mucosa is evident for the first time [15].

Congenital Anomalies of the Small Bowel

Malrotation

From what has been said earlier, it is apparent that growth and rotation of the small bowel involves a complex series of steps that may be interfered with at any point. In a classic paper, Snyder and Chaffin [163] showed that abnormalities of rotation could produce many varied anatomical arrangements of the bowel. Their review of 40 cases of malrotation indicated that the main clinical problems stemmed from the presence of a redundant unfixed mesentery and anomalous peritoneal bands. Both these elements can cause obstruction, either by encouraging volvulus and compromising the vascular pedicle in the case of infants with a redundant mesen-

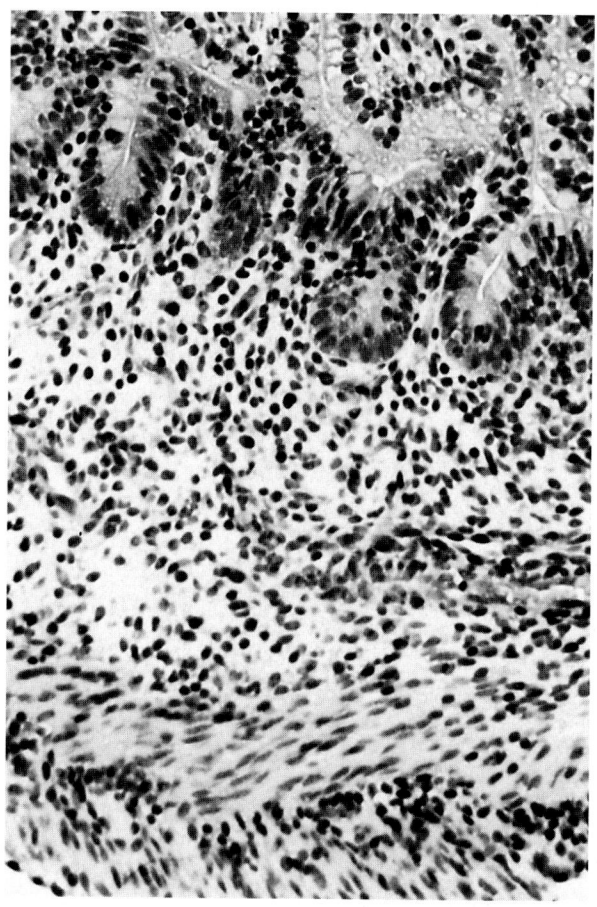

FIGURE 24.23. *Developing small bowel from 85-mm embryo showing muscularis propria and ganglia of myenteric plexus, villi, but no muscularis mucosa.*

tery, or by the presence of peritoneal bands across the duodenum and jejunum (i.e., Ladd's bands) [158]. Frequently, volvulus of the midgut is the presenting sign of malrotation [164], and bowel necrosis due to obstruction of the vessels in the vascular pedicle may be a dreaded complication (Fig. 24.24). Duodenal obstruction due to Ladd's bands may be an additional complicating feature in some cases. Omphalocele and gastroschisis are associated frequently with malrotation, as are many cases of the short bowel syndrome.

Malrotation occurs in approximately 1% of all newborn babies [163], but in only half of these infants are there any symptoms during the newborn period. In many patients, malrotation may be completely asymptomatic. There is a male predominance [163, 165, 166]. Malrotation is a common finding in infants with trisomy 18 [167], but can be seen in association with trisomy 13, Down syndrome, triploidy, de Lange syndrome, partial trisomy 10q, and early urethral obstruction sequences [167–170]. Less frequently, malrotation of the small bowel may be an associated finding in Marfan syndrome [171] and as part of the asplenia/polysplenia syndromes [172, 173].

In addition to volvulus, malrotations may be associated with duodenal atresia in infants with Down syndrome [174] and occasionally with anal atresia [175].

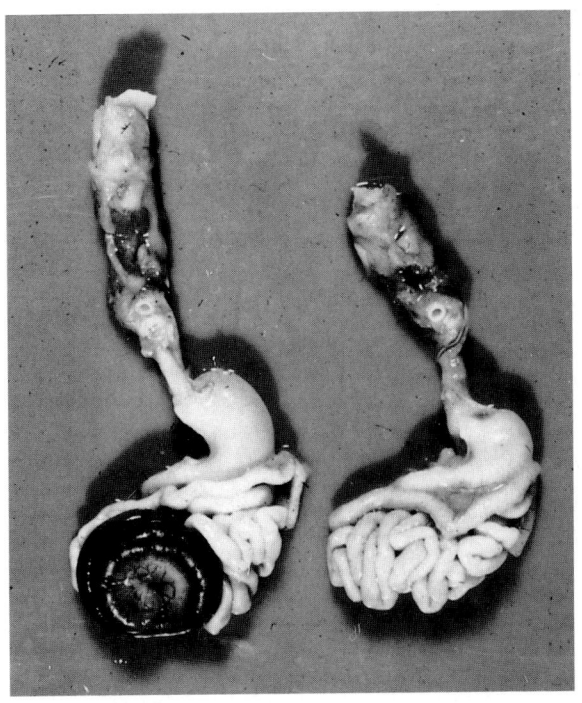

FIGURE 24.24. *Volvulus and bowel infarction complicating malrotation in one of monozygous twins. (Courtesy of the publishers of deSa [211].)*

Congenital Short Bowel

Congenital short bowel is a relatively rare syndrome that is associated with malrotation in many instances. Instead of having a normal bowel length of approximately 250 cm at term [176], the small bowel may be as short as 24 cm [177–180]. An excellent study of the normal growth of the fetal gastrointestinal tract is provided by Fitzsimmons et al [181]. Growth is linear with respect to gestational age (determined by foot length). Fetuses with omphaloceles tended to have shorter guts. Infants with congenital heart defects had guts shorter than the mean, but rarely were they as short as infants with omphalocele. Aneuploid fetuses had lengths of gut within normal limits until 20 weeks of gestation, after which the rate of linear growth decreased. Some workers have claimed that fetuses with congenital heart defects have an abnormally elongated intestine [182].

It is important to draw a distinction between a small bowel that is intrinsically shorter than normal, and those cases where multiple or extensive surgical resection results in a reduction of the length of the small bowel. In the first group, symptoms date from birth and include failure to gain weight, profuse diarrhea, and poor feeding with vomiting. Parenteral alimentation is needed, either as a supplementary measure or as the sole source of nutrition, and it may be life saving. In infants where surgical resection of the bowel has been undertaken, the age at presentation will vary. Excellent clinicopathological reviews of this latter form of shortened bowel are provided by Klish and Putnam [183], Schwartz and Maeda [184], and Grosfeld et al [185].

Malrotation and incomplete fixation of the bowel is an associated finding in many infants with intrinsically short bowel, and there may be an associated omphalocele. Siebert [176] shows that there is considerable variation in small bowel length, and not all cases of malrotation have a short small intestine. However, Reiquam et al [182] found that of the 16 children they studied who had a small bowel length that was shorter than expected for the crown–rump length, seven had malrotation and/or omphalocele. In view of the importance of small bowel growth in initiating and sustaining the process of rotation, the association of a congenitally short bowel with malrotation or an omphalocele should not be too surprising. Nevertheless, the causes of an intrinsically short bowel are not known. Apart from villous atrophy, the intrinsically short small bowel appears histologically normal and appropriately differentiated [180].

Among the causes of extensive bowel resection that may lead to a short bowel syndrome, neonatal volvulus due to malrotation and bowel ischemia ("necrotizing enterocolitis") loom large. Other causes, including inflammatory lesions and vascular insults, may be seen in older infants and children. In those who survive resection of large amounts of small bowel, varying degrees of adaptation may be seen in the remaining bowel, including longitudinal growth, increased diameter of the bowel, and an increase in the total villous surface area. A reduction in the length of the jejunum can be tolerated better than the loss of an equivalent length of ileum [183–185].

The Undifferentiated Bowel

Bennington and Haber [186] described an example of a newborn child in whom the gut failed to differentiate into large and small bowel. The infant died after protracted vomiting and diarrhea. Postmortem examination revealed a malrotated gut with an overall length of 75 cm from pylorus to anus. The normally expected length from Siebert's data [176] would be approximately 200 cm for the small bowel alone. The muscular pattern resembled the small intestine without tenia coli, and the mucosa showed poorly formed villi with relatively few Paneth cells and a deficiency of distal myenteric ganglia. There was neither a cecum nor an appendix, and no ileocecal valve. The case was complicated further by the presence of a cartilaginous choristoma just distal to the pylorus. This unique case probably represents the result of an even earlier insult than those causing a congenitally short bowel.

Reverse Rotation

Reverse rotation is a rare phenomenon that has the duodenum and superior mesenteric artery lying anterior to the transverse colon. This may cause extrinsic obstruction of the colon [187].

Duodenal Atresia and Intrinsic Obstruction

Relative to its length, the duodenum is a very frequent site of obstruction of the small bowel, especially atresias. It is useful to separate duodenal obstruction from other obstructive lesions of the small bowel, as the duodenum is the only segment of the small bowel that is obliterated at some stage of its normal development [159, 160]. It is appropriate, therefore, to invoke failure of recanalization of the lumen as one of the mechanisms for duodenal atresia. The failure of recanalization may be related to the relatively massive degree of mesenchymal and epithelial activity in this area, brought about by the development of the liver and pancreas. Relatively few cases of atresia, however, occur at the level of Vater's ampulla. The obstructing lesion is a membranous partition of varying thickness, usually distal to the point of entry of the bile duct. The proximal duodenum and the stomach are dilated and ballooned, leading to the characteristic "double-bubble" sign on a plain x-ray of the abdomen [188].

In duodenal atresia, symptoms usually occur shortly after birth (even within a few hours in some instances), with abdominal distension and vomiting. Many infants may present antenatally due to maternal polyhydramnios. There is an approximately equal sex distribution. Bodian et al [174] drew attention to the high incidence of Down syndrome in infants with duodenal atresia; 10 of their 32 cases of duodenal obstruction were infants with the stigmata of trisomy 21. Boggs and Bishop [189] found that just under half of

their cases of duodenal atresia had Down syndrome. However, less than 1% of infants with Down syndrome have duodenal atresia [169].

About 40% to 50% of all cases of duodenal atresia have an associated congenital anomaly. These include malrotation, tracheoesophageal atresia and fistula complex, biliary atresia, and congenital heart disease of different types [190–196]. Duodenal atresia has been seen in thalidomide embryopathy [197]. Many infants with duodenal atresia are premature [198].

While most cases of duodenal atresia are associated with a membrane separating the dilated proximal from the collapsed distal segments, some cases have segments linked by a fibrous cord. Willis [199] illustrated a case of an anencephalic infant with posterior protrusion of the stomach and spleen through a cervicothoracic spinal cleft, accompanied by duodenal atresia. The atretic segment was represented by a fibrous cord, which apparently spanned the region of Vater's ampulla.

Atresia is not the only intrinsic cause of duodenal obstruction. Other lesions include stenosis of the duodenum (with symptoms and pathology similar to atresia), and duplication cysts of the duodenum. Wilkinson [195] includes annular pancreas as an "intrinsic" cause of duodenal obstruction, since the symptoms are identical to those of atresia. In most cases the lumen of the duodenum has been reduced to the dimension of a pinhole, with pancreatic tissue below the duodenal surface mucosa (Fig. 24.25). Patton [200] described two infants with muscular hypertrophy of the duodenum that resembled pyloric stenosis, both clinically and pathologically. A muscle-splitting procedure was curative in these cases.

Extrinsic causes of duodenal obstruction include volvulus and malrotation, compression by Ladd's bands, and compression of the duodenum by related structures like a hydronephrotic kidney or choledochal cyst [195]. Rarely, the bowel may be compressed by a superior mesenteric artery [201], a lesion usually found in older infants and children.

Obstruction of the Jejunum and Ileum

A very large number of conditions may be associated with obstruction of the small bowel. In the perinatal period the most important lesions include atresia and stenosis of the jejunum and ileum, duplications of the small bowel, volvulus, and meconium ileus. Rare causes include internal and external hernias, intussusceptions (more common in older infants and children), defects of the muscularis propria, and rare tumors, usually hamartomatas. Hirschsprung disease (aganglionosis) may affect the small bowel in very extensive examples of that condition.

Atresia and Stenosis of Jejunum and Ileum

The presence of an atretic or stenosed segment of the jejunum or ileum constitutes the most frequently encountered cause of small bowel obstruction in the neonatal

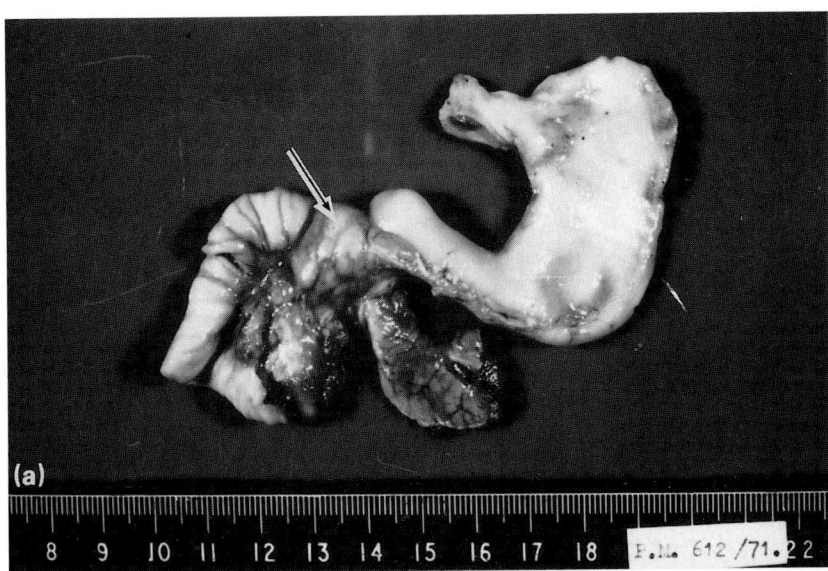

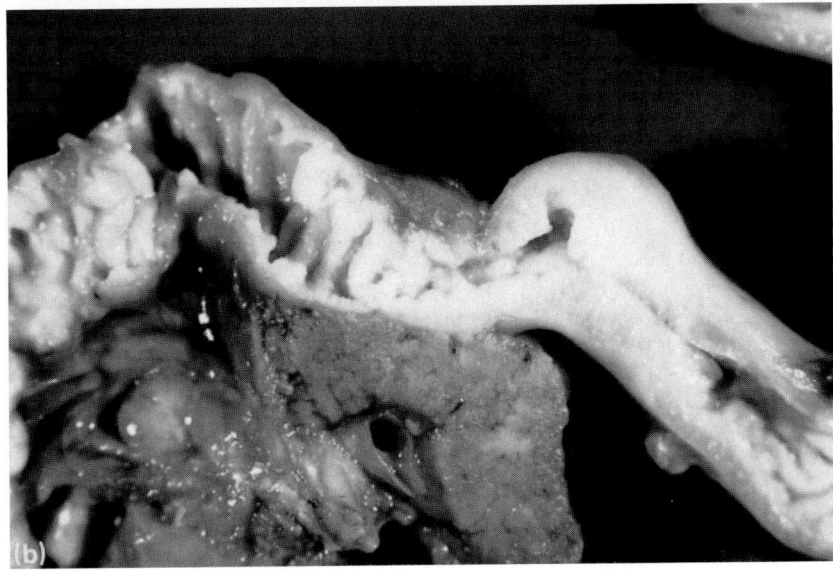

FIGURE 24.25. *(a) Annular pancreas (arrow) in a case of de Lange syndrome (scale in cm). (b) A closer view of the dissected specimen shows the marked narrowing of the duodenum.*

period. Symptoms related to obstruction may be present within hours of birth and are usually well developed in the first 24 hours. Symptoms present earlier in patients with proximal lesions, and they include vomiting of bile-stained fluid and abdominal distension with no demonstrable colonic gas pattern on a plain x-ray of the abdomen. Some infants may present in utero with polyhydramnios.

Most workers have found that the ileum is affected more often than the jejunum, but Grosfeld [202] found no particular predilection for the ileum. Most patients (about 90%) have a single lesion, but there are several reports and reviews of multiple lesions [203–205] (Fig. 24.26).

Two major classifications of intestinal atresia and stenosis are used, those of Louw [198] and of Martin and Zerella [206]. As seen in the diagrams in Figures 24.27 and 24.28, Louw's simpler classification [198] includes stenoses, while Martin and Zerella [206] provide a more detailed and

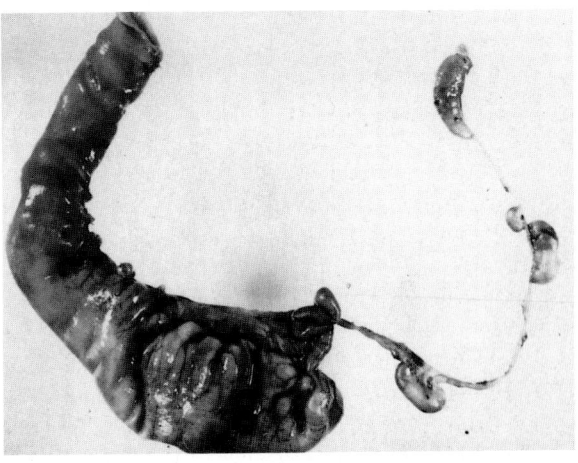

FIGURE 24.26. *Resected specimen of multiple congenital intestinal atresia. (Approx. ×4.)*

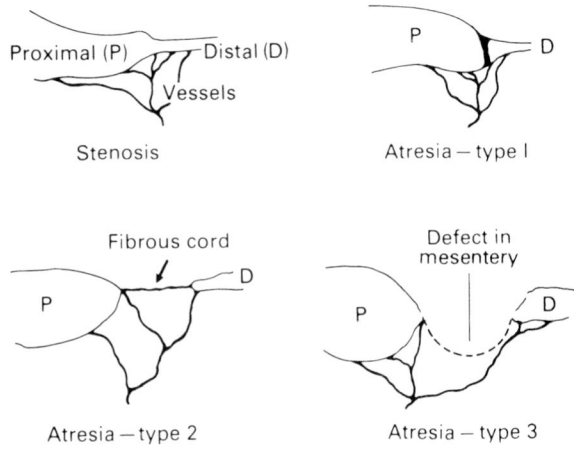

FIGURE 24.27. *A schematic representation of Louw's classification of stenosis and atresia [198].*

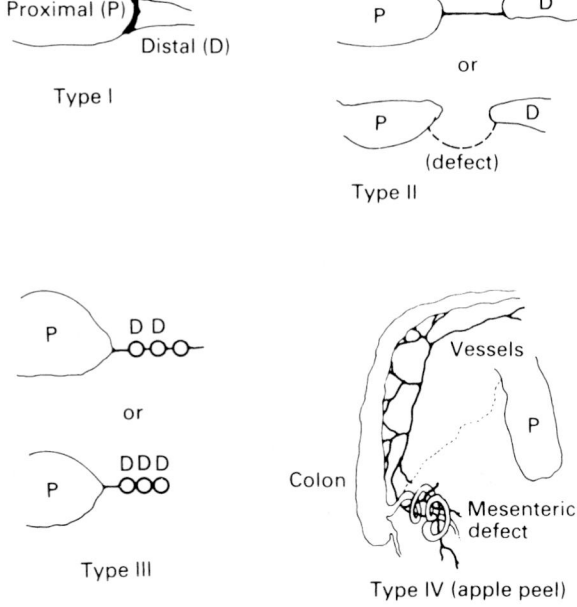

FIGURE 24.28. *Martin and Zerella's classification of atresia [206] depicted in diagrammatic fashion.*

complex classification of atresia but do not include stenosis. They do include "apple peel" atresia, originally described by Santulli and Blanc [207]. A brief review of Figures 24.27 and 24.28 should suffice to outline the many macroscopic patterns that may be encountered at laparotomy or postmortem examination. Variations on these basic patterns include an association with meconium peritonitis, omphalocele, and the changes of cystic fibrosis [149, 198, 206]. Daneman and Martin [208] described extensive intraluminal calcification in the intervening patent segments of bowel in their series of multiple atresias.

The proximal segment of bowel appears dilated and bulbous, but there may be considerable variation in what is encountered distal to the most proximal site of obstruction (see Figs. 24.27 and 24.28). The site of obstruction may be scarred and calcified due to old meconium peritonitis [198] and in many cases the mesentery may appear redundant.

"Apple peel" atresia [207] represents a special, and fortunately uncommon, variant of atresia of the bowel. The continuity of the bowel is completely interrupted (usually in the distal duodenum or proximal jejunum), with absence of the dorsal mesentery and obliteration of most of the superior mesenteric artery, while the distal small bowel is shortened and coiled around a narrow nutrient vessel arising as a branch from the ileocolic vessels.

The comments regarding etiology and pathogenesis that follow apply equally to intestinal and colonic atresia/steno-

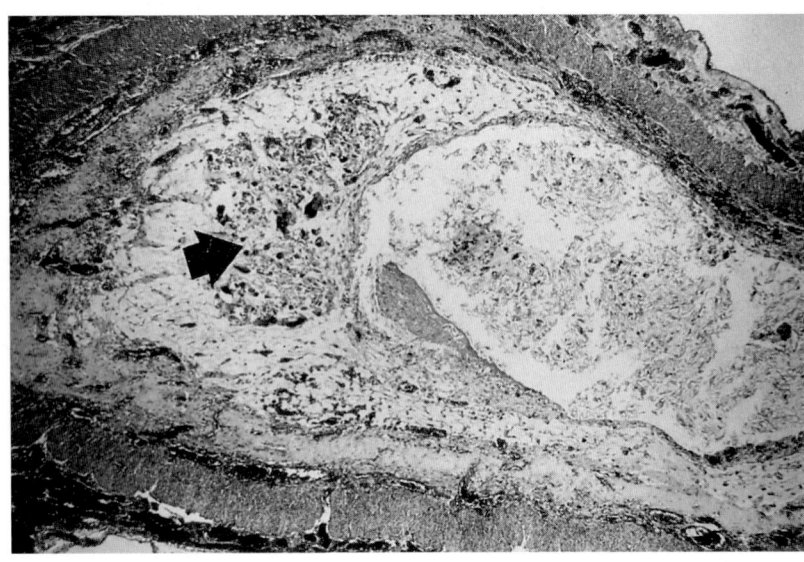

FIGURE 24.29. *The contents of one of the distal loops in Figure 24.26. Note the normal musculature, fibrosed submucosa with a granulomatous response to lanugo hairs (arrow). Lanugo hairs fill the lumen.*

sis, with the exception of duodenal atresia and anorectal lesions in which special considerations apply.

Microscopic findings in cases of small bowel atresia or stenosis are not always reported in detail. In several instances, all that can be seen is a thick fibrous cord linking the two segments of atretic bowel. However, hemosiderin-laden macrophages in the partitioning membrane or fibrous cord, scarring of the mucosa, muscularis mucosa and muscularis propria, and irregular villous configurations and fibrosis of the lamina propria have all been found consistently [209,

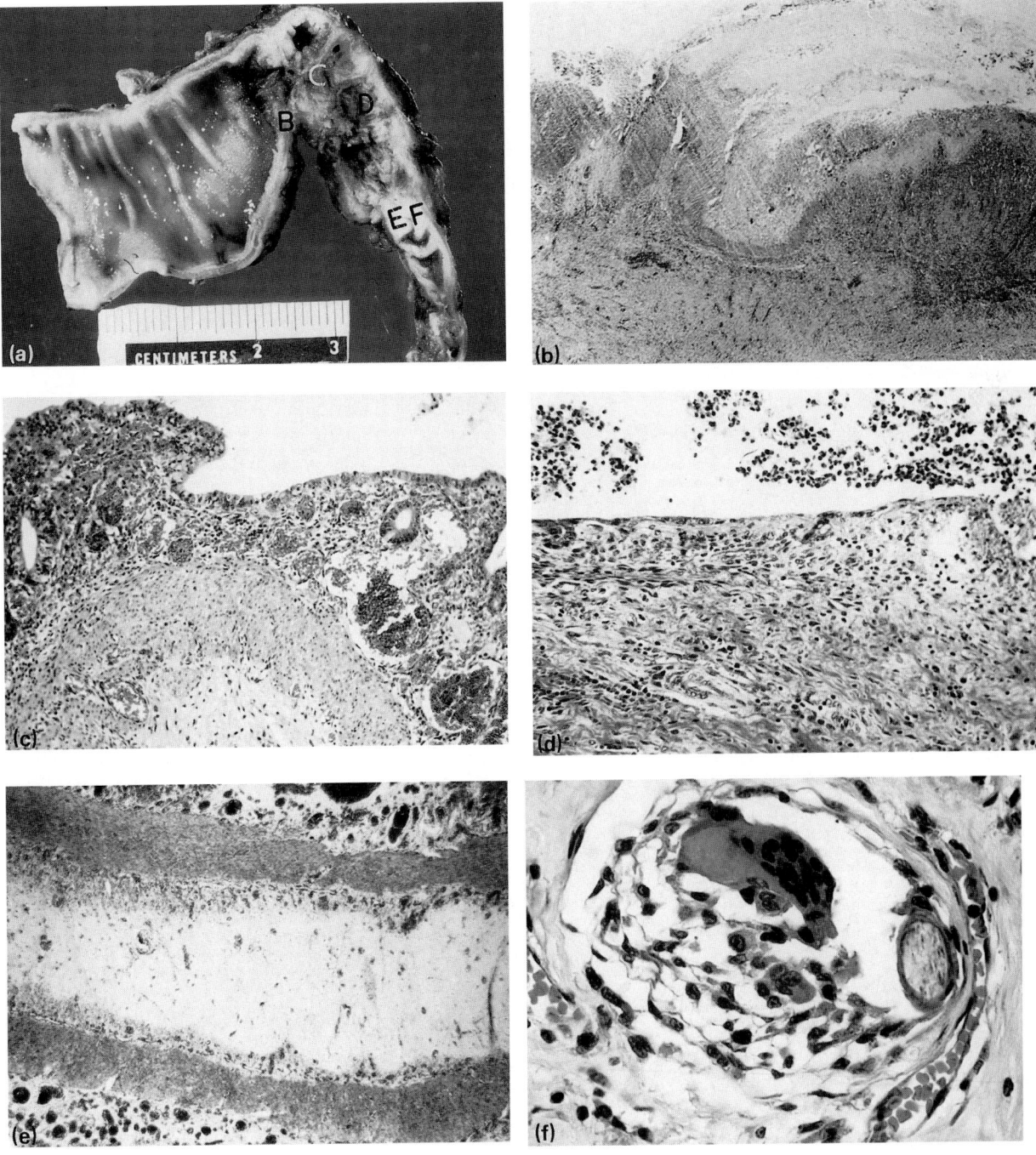

FIGURE 24.30. *(a) A resected loop of terminal ileum showing dilatation proximal to an area of irregular obstruction leading down to a zone of complete occlusion. (b) Ischemic necrosis of mucosa and muscularis is seen in zone B of the specimen. (Attwood's stain.) (c) Focal irregularity of the mucosal architecture with loss of villi, and thickened muscularis mucosa in zone C. (Attwood's stain.) (d) Granulation and scar tissue with regenerating epithelium in zone D. (Masson's trichrome.) (e) The atretic segment (zone E) shows replacement of the lumen by dense collagenous tissue. (Attwood's stain.) (f) In the atretic zone (F) a small granuloma in relation to a lanugo hair is seen. (Attwood's stain.)*

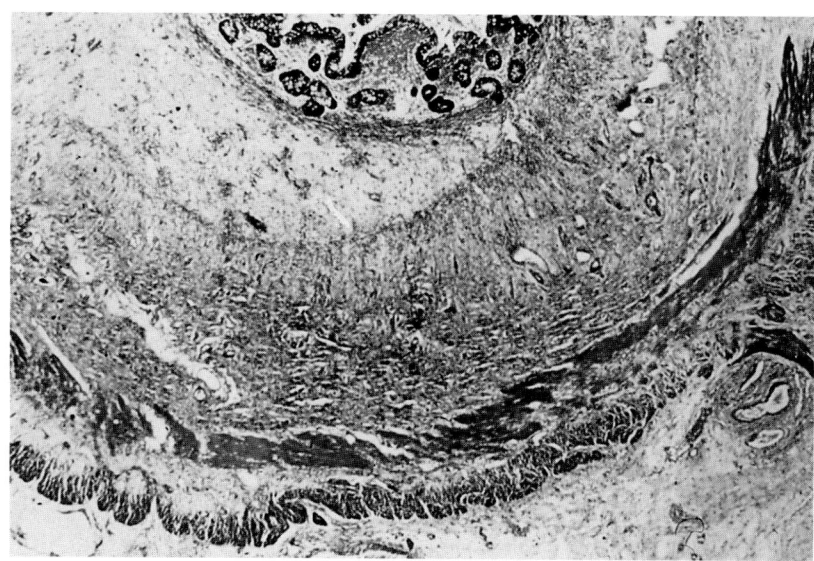

FIGURE 24.31.   *Extensive scarring of the muscularis mucosa is seen in this transverse section of a stenotic lesion of jejunum. The muscularis mucosa is split into two component layers. Note the simplified mucosal pattern. (Masson's trichrome.) (Courtesy of the publishers of deSa [209].)*

210]. Subepithelial calcification, presumably following previous mucosal ulceration, may be present either focally [211] or extensively [208]. Santulli and Blanc [207] described lanugo hairs distal to the site of the atresia. Some of these features of atresia/stenosis are illustrated in Figures 24.29 through 24.31.

The microscopic findings in the bowel suggest most strongly that intestinal stenosis and atresia are related to an intrauterine vascular accident, as suggested by Louw [212, 213]. Several reports have described individual cases of stenosis complicating previous bowel ischemia [214–217], and bowel stenosis due to previous ischemic bowel disease is a recognized complication in adults [218]. A series of infants who were followed closely after neonatal ischemic bowel injury—so-called "necrotizing enterocolitis" demonstrated a high incidence of stenotic and atretic lesions as late complications. The spectrum of abnormalities found in the survivors mimicked that seen in classic congenital stenosis or atresia of the bowel [219–225].

It appears that ischemia from any cause may produce stenosis or even atresia if there is sufficient damage to the mucosa and deeper layers, and provided the bowel is able to recover from the insult. Viewed from this perspective, the finding of stenosis/atresia of the bowel in association with intussusception [226] (Fig. 24.32), umbilical hernia with strangulation, gastroschisis [227], strangulated mechanical obstruction in utero [215, 228], or intrauterine volvulus is understandable. The association of cystic fibrosis with bowel stenosis/atresia may be due to an interplay of several factors, including the likelihood of volvulus or perforation with scarring [149, 229].

Single small bowel atresias have been described in two brothers in the same family [230]. Guttman [231] described a syndrome of multiple hereditary atresias of small bowel; a second family with a similar syndrome was reported by Arnal-Monreal et al [232]. Kao et al [204] provide a detailed description of a case they studied with multiple complex membranous partitions producing multiple atresias of the jejunum, ileum, and colon. A sibling had died previously with similar pathology. The membranous septa contained epithelial inclusion cysts and the muscularis mucosa appeared to form part of the walls of the cysts and partitions. Though there were patent areas of bowel between the septa, no keratinized squamae or lanugo hairs were seen distal to the most proximal atretic segments. They suggested that these hereditary septal atresias were the result of failure of recanalization, but it appears to this author that the evidence for such a conclusion is not overwhelming. The pres-

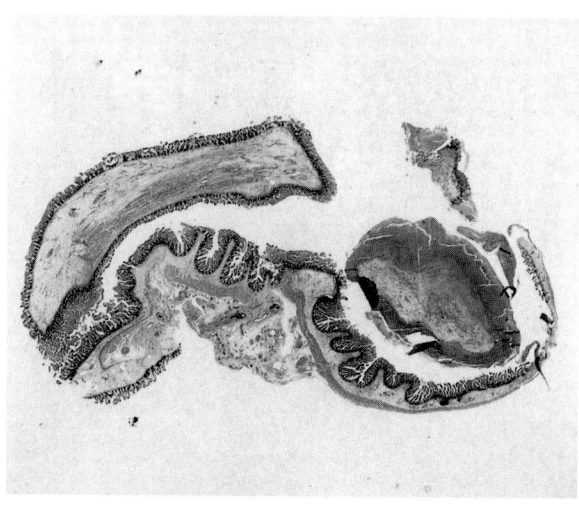

FIGURE 24.32.   *Longitudinal section through "atretic" segment of jejunum, showing a prolapsed fibrotic and hemorrhagic segment of bowel filling the lumen. This was interpreted as probably representing an example of intrauterine intussusception with secondary necrosis. (Attwood's stain.)*

ence of muscularis mucosa around the septal cysts and in the bowel between the cysts argues for the lesion occurring relatively late in development; the absence of lanugo hair in distal segments may indicate only that the jejunal lesions occurred before the colonic ones.

Collins et al [233] have described an association of multiple intestinal atresias with amyoplasia congenita in four unrelated infants. Ileocecal atresia has been observed in identical twins in one family [234]. In another family one monozygotic twin had multiple intestinal atresias while the other had an umbilical hernia and colonic atresia [235]. It is possible that a genetic component may be present in a few cases of atresia/stenosis of the small bowel, but in most instances no genetic influences are discernible.

The exact nature of any intrauterine vascular accident that may produce stenosis is likely to be uncertain in any given case. Louw [198] mentioned the coexistence of a redundant mesentery in many cases and suggested that torsion of a vascular pedicle may have been an important factor. Earlam suggested that torsion may occur in the stage of "physiological umbilical hernia" [236]. Portal emboli from thrombi in fetal placental veins have been described in some infants [237, 238], and though these cases did not have stenosis/atresia of the bowel, several had mild ischemic bowel damage [238]. Placental findings in cases of bowel stenosis are not usually documented, but the possibility remains that emboli from the placental circulation may cause vascular damage in the mesenteric circulation. Placental thrombi with embolism to the superior mesenteric artery could explain the findings in some rare examples of neonatal bowel infarction presenting at birth.

A history of bleeding during pregnancy, or prematurity, or possible intrauterine growth retardation has been reported in several infants with stenosis or atresia [198, 206, 209].

Unlike duodenal atresia, jejunal and ileal atresia/stenosis is not usually associated with anomalies in organ systems other than those directly concerned with the bowel (i.e., omphalocele, gastroschisis, malrotation, cystic fibrosis). Isolated examples of intestinal atresia associated with cardiovascular anomalies are known, but unless associated with duodenal atresia or hindgut abnormalities, jejunal or ileal atresias usually occur as independent single abnormalities.

Duplication of the Small Bowel

The small bowel is the most common site for duplications of the gastrointestinal tract and nearly 60% of all duplications of the gastrointestinal tract occur in the small bowel [47]. The duodenum is the least common site affected, while the ileum is the site affected most often [42, 239]. Males are affected more often than females [240]. The lesions present as single (or, rarely, multiple) tubular or sausage-shaped cystic structures that do not communicate, usually, with the bowel lumen (Fig. 24.33). While jejunal lesions may be lined by a small-bowel-type mucosa, the distal lesions are usually lined

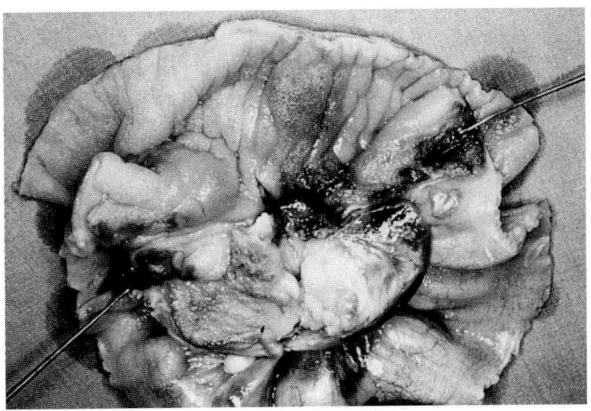

FIGURE 24.33.   *View of a duplication of small bowel in a 4-month-old child viewed from the mesenteric aspect. The small bowel has been opened and placed mucosal surface down. The irregular sausage-shaped lesion on the mesenteric aspect can be seen.*

by a nondescript columnar epithelium, with neither villi nor the specialized cells of the ileum. Occasionally, duplications may be lined by heterotopic gastric or colonic mucosa. The muscular coat is present but very often it is an incomplete layer. The lesions are almost invariably on the mesenteric aspect, and either are intimately apposed to the bowel or form part of its wall. Some may lie in the mesentery a few centimeters away from the bowel. Since the vessels supplying the bowel cross the duplication, resection of the duplication usually involves sacrificing the adjacent small bowel as well.

Total tubular duplication of the small intestine was described by Jewett [241]. This lesion communicated with the distal ileum near the ileocecal valve, and mucosal ulceration led to melena.

Not all bowel duplications produce symptoms in the perinatal period; surprisingly, many duodenal duplications do, even though they occur less frequently. Many of these duodenal duplications lie within the submucous layer of the bowel [242]. The duodenal lesions produce obstruction, with abdominal distention and vomiting, which can be mistaken for pyloric stenosis or duodenal atresia. As noted earlier in the section discussing the stomach (and later in the section on the large bowel), duplications of the intestine may be associated with spinal cord and vertebral body defects. It is important, therefore, to exclude spinal anomalies in infants or children with duplications [49, 243].

A discussion of the origins of duplications of the intestinal tract is to be found in the section on the large bowel; in the large bowel, these lesions may be part of an extremely complex malformation sequence.

Diverticula

Diverticula lesions rarely present in the perinatal infant but may be seen in older infants, children, and adults. Classically, they are situated on the antimesenteric border of the bowel,

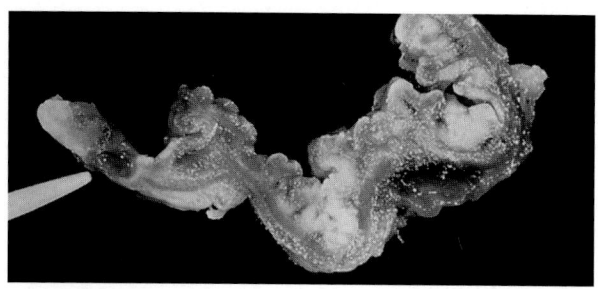

FIGURE 24.34. *Opened segment of small bowel showing a small intramural diverticulum (at tip of pointer). This lesion was an incidental finding in a 16-year-old boy whose bowel was resected after a motor vehicle accident.*

and are associated with a poorly formed muscle coat. They can be found anywhere in the small bowel [244]. In some cases, the diverticula remain predominantly intramural, producing a largely submucous cyst with an attenuated muscle coat (Fig. 24.34). These cases may be difficult to separate from duplications. The origin of diverticula of the small intestine is not known; whether or not they represent a type of duplication is uncertain.

Abnormal Regression of the Vitellointestinal Duct

The vitellointestinal (omphalomesenteric) duct is the narrowed remnant of the tubular communication between the

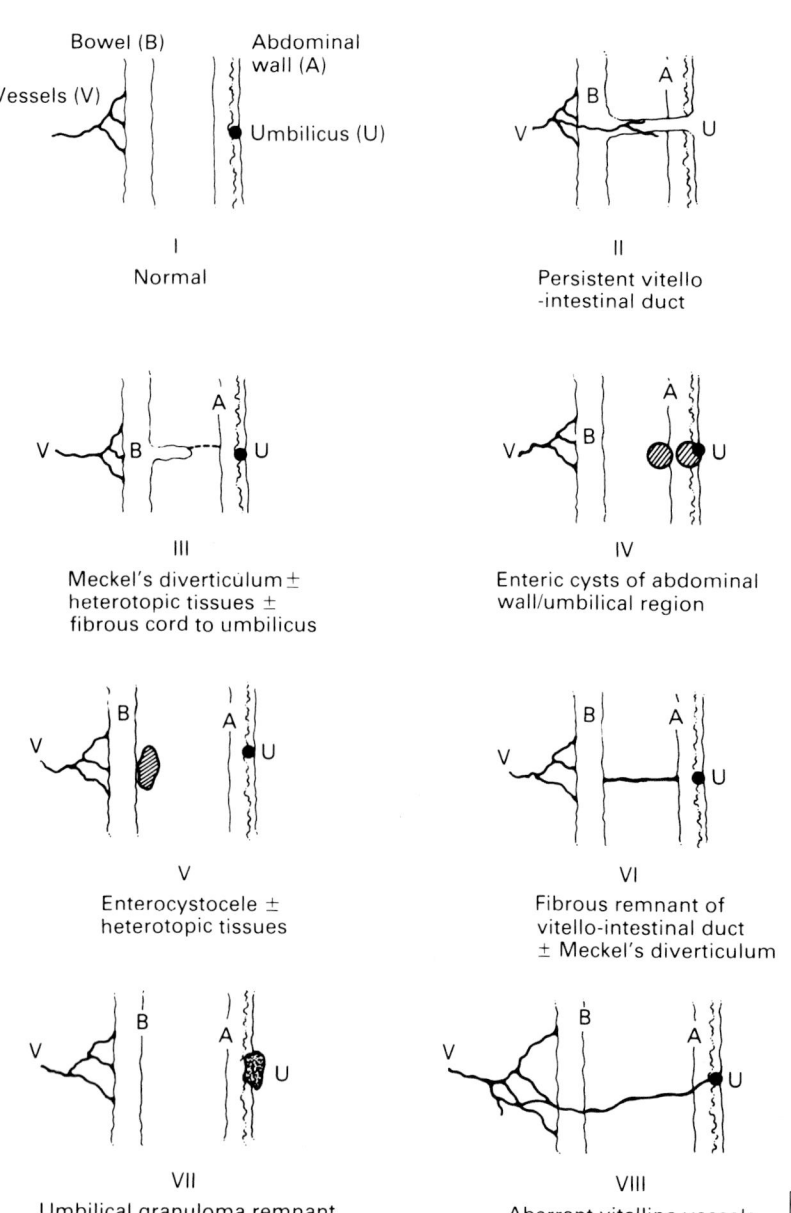

FIGURE 24.35. *Schematic representation of the changes associated with abnormal persistence of the vitello-intestinal duct.*

yolk sac and the midgut. Originally, it has the same diameter as the midgut, but it decreases rapidly in size to a thin cord-like structure. By the 10th week it has disappeared in most infants, though scattered cystic remnants may be encountered in the umbilical cord [245] or at the umbilicus. Some of these umbilical and cord lesions may be large and may even contain gastric mucosa and pancreatic tissue; there is a case report of fatal exsanguination due to peptic ulceration of the umbilical vessels [246].

A Meckel's diverticulum is by far the commonest remnant of the vitellointestinal duct. There are, however, several uncommon anomalies that may be encountered due to persistence of vitellointestinal duct remnants (Fig. 24.35).

Meckel's diverticulum may be found in up to 2% of the population [247], and in the majority of affected patients it does not produce symptoms [248]. The blunt, blind diverticulum arising from the antimesenteric border of the terminal ileum may be lined by ileal-type mucosa, but heterotopic gastric and pancreatic tissues are found frequently in symptomatic patients. While it is rare for a Meckel's diverticulum to be symptomatic in the perinatal period, in Japan most symptomatic cases have been diagnosed by 2 years of age [249]. The clinical presentation can be varied: as a leading point of an intussusception, in association with volvulus, as a cause of painless rectal bleeding, or with evidence of peptic ulceration and even perforation (Fig. 24.36). Meckel's diverticula probably occur with equal frequency in males and females [247], but among symptomatic patients there is a marked male predominance (around 3:1) [250].

Most diverticula are less than 5 cm in diameter, with a narrow opening into the ileum of approximately 2 cm in diameter. So-called "giant Meckel's diverticula," whose dimensions exceed those given above and which have a wide opening into the ileum, may be encountered on rare occasions in infants [251, 252].

A rarity that does not figure prominently in reported series is the presence of mucosal diverticula occurring in a Meckel's diverticulum (Fig. 24.37). Several examples have been seen in one institution over the last 10 years [253].

Many of the less-frequent variants of vitellointestinal duct remnants may present in later infancy or childhood, although a persistently patent duct (see Fig. 24.35, II) and the umbilical granuloma (see Fig. 24.33, II) are present at birth. Other variants may present as abdominal wall masses (see Fig. 24.35, IV), or masses resembling duplications but on the antimesenteric border (see Fig. 24.35, V). In those rare examples where all that remains of the vitellointestinal duct is a fibrous cord, strangulation and volvulus of the bowel may occur [244, 248, 254, 255]. Tumors, both benign (adenomata) and malignant (carcinomata), may arise in adults with a Meckel's diverticulum [248].

Adenomyomata (foregut choristomata) [256] may occur, and we have seen an example associated with a Meckel's diverticulum in an infant.

Absence of the Muscle Layer of the Small Bowel
Emanuel et al [257] described a neonatal infant with intestinal obstruction that was felt clinically to be due to atresia or stenosis of the bowel. At laparotomy, multiple dilated

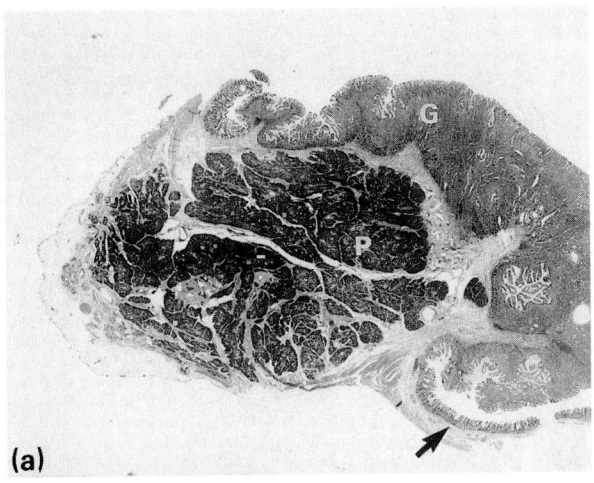

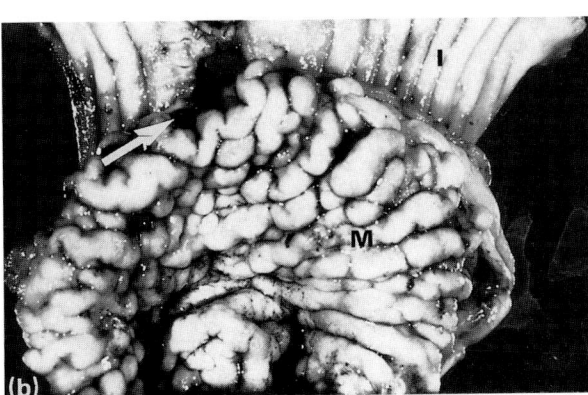

FIGURE 24.36. *(a) Histological section through the wall of a Meckel's diverticulum found incidentally at postmortem examination. Pancreatic (P) and gastric tissue (G) are seen, and differ from the ileal mucosa (arrow). (b) At the junction of a Meckel's diverticulum (M) with the ileum (I) a perforation (arrow) is seen. The diverticulum was lined in its entirety by gastric mucosa (14-month-old female infant).*

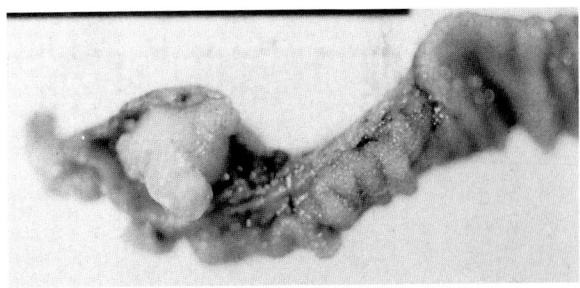

FIGURE 24.37. *An opened Meckel's diverticulum from which protrudes a firm tubular nodule lined by a mucosa continuous with the main diverticulum (diverticulosis of Meckel's diverticulum).*

loops of bowel with interspersed normal bowel were seen *without* evidence of perforation. Multiple segments of the ballooned areas of bowel were resected, and the intervening loops of normal bowel were anastomosed. Histological examination of the resected loops showed that the dilated bowel had no muscularis propria, but did have a muscularis mucosa. At the margins of the resected segments the muscularis propria layer tapered until it disappeared, and this was associated with marked dilatation of the abnormal bowel. Following this report, several other examples have been reported [258–262]. These highly unusual cases share several features in common, namely ballooned segments of bowel with intervening normal bowel, clinical signs of intestinal obstruction, no evidence of perforation, a relatively sharply demarcated junction between normally muscularized bowel and abnormal bowel, absence of the myenteric plexus in the abnormal bowel, and an atrophic (but not ischemic) mucosa. My personal experience is confined to a single case (Fig. 24.38) which shared all these features. The normal segments

do not appear to be scarred or fibrosed. Unlike the situation in the stomach, defects of the small bowel musculature (as in the cases cited above) cannot be attributed to either a histological artefact or to the secondary effects of perforation. In my view the condition of "segmental absence of muscularis propria of the small bowel" appears to be a true, albeit extremely rare, entity.

The etiology and pathogenesis of this bizarre anomalad is not known. Since the muscularis mucosa appears to be present in the abnormal segment in all cases, deficient myogenesis of the muscularis propria appears to be unlikely. The muscularis mucosa develops after the muscularis propria [15], so a primary segmental deficiency of myogenesis appears to be an unlikely explanation. Classically, ischemia of the bowel tends to affect the mucosa preferentially, and can in all probability be excluded as a major cause. A solitary case in my collection of a muscularis propria defect associated with a sealed perforation mimicking this condition is published elsewhere [63]. Experimentally, isolated

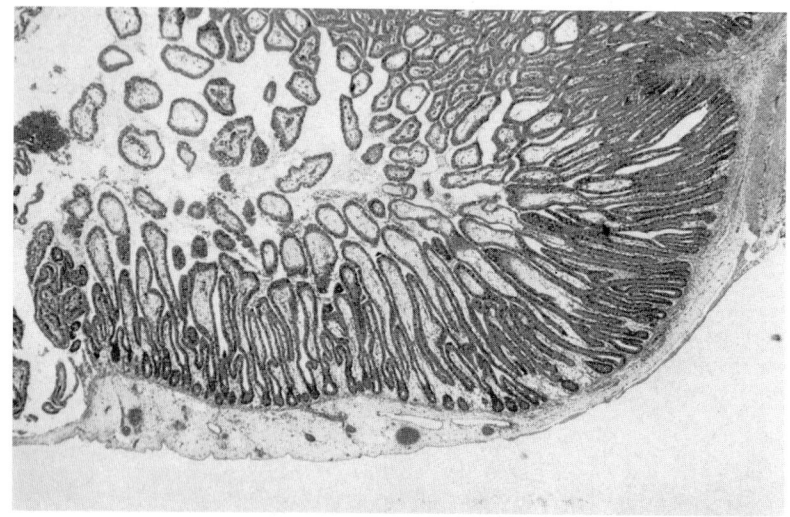

(a)

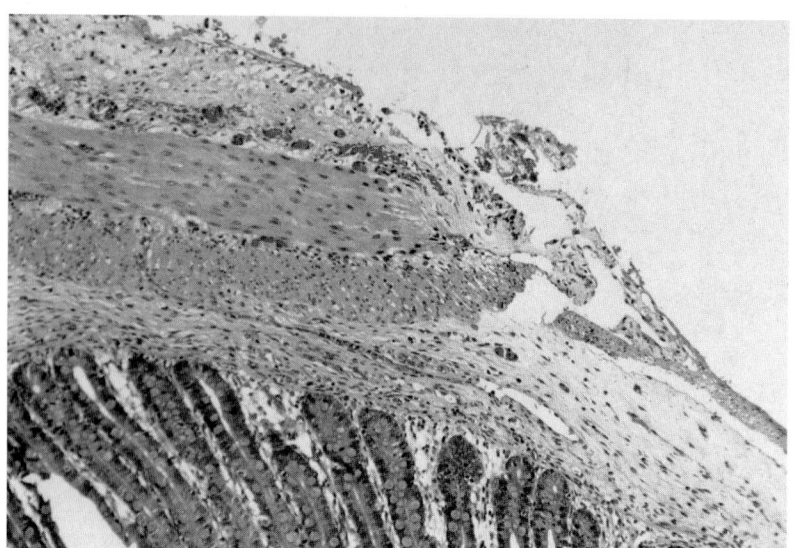

(b)

FIGURE 24.38.   *(a) Section of small bowel wall from term newborn infant delivered after a normal pregnancy. Progressive abdominal distension at day 3 led to laparotomy investigation which showed dilated loops of small bowel but no perforation. Note the intact mucosa and deficient muscularis propria. (b) View of the muscularis propria deficiency showing the muscle defect and the disappearance of the myenteric plexus.*

perfusion of toxins into peripheral branches of the mesenteric vessels can damage both muscle and nerve cells [263], but these procedures do not produce the severe degree of ablation of nerve or muscle seen in the cited cases and they may in fact produce muscular hypertrophy as the bowel heals. At least one case [258] was associated with volvulus.

Litwin et al [264] found three infants with perforations of the ileum who also showed deficiencies of the muscular layer with preserved mucosa in the bowel away from the site of perforation. These cases are more difficult to evaluate, since the thin layer of muscle found in their case 3 could be due to dilatation of the bowel. Two of their infants appear to be similar to the cases cited in the earlier reports; however, they do not describe any alteration in nerve cells in the affected segments of their cases. Future cases will need a detailed study of the innervation of the bowel. To date, the cases reported do not appear to be associated with any consistent pattern of complications of pregnancy or maternal exposure to teratogenic agents.

Alvarez et al [265] described segmental absence of muscle coats associated with atresia, but in my view their cases resemble extreme examples of stenosis following ischemia. Humphrey et al [266] have reported a case with a defect of the circular muscle in a 1-year-old child—a finding that is even more difficult to explain.

Meconium Ileus and Gastrointestinal Changes in Cystic Fibrosis of the Pancreas

For all practical purposes, meconium ileus is a syndrome associated with cystic fibrosis (mucoviscidosis) of the pancreas [149]. Characteristically, the absence of pancreatic enzymes and the high proteinaceous content contribute to a greatly increased viscosity, leading to the obstruction of the lower ileum by thick, tarry meconium. Affected infants are usually symptomatic within the first 24 to 48 hours of life, with abdominal distension, poor feeding, and bile-stained vomit. Rectal passage of meconium is either absent or delayed and sparse. Visible peristalsis may be seen, and palpable masses due to dilated loops of bowel filled with thick, inspissated (and often calcified) meconium may be noted. Radiographically, dilated loops of bowel, usually without air–fluid interfaces, are seen but a granular opacification of the lower abdomen and the right lower quadrant is characteristic. At laparotomy or postmortem examination, the proximal jejunum and ileum are dilated, with thickened hypertrophied walls that taper down to the narrower terminal ileum and collapsed "microcolon." Perforation with meconium peritonitis—and, in boys, meconium-related calcified scrotal hydroceles—may be seen. The meconium has an almost solid consistency, and often calcific gritty material is admixed with it. Emptying the bowel of meconium may be a difficult task and a variety of surgical irrigating solutions, usually incorporating acetylcysteine, have been used to relieve the obstruction.

The bowel wall shows considerable inspissation of mucin within the lumen and in the crypts—especially in the ileum,

appendix, and colon (Fig. 24.39). Muscle hypertrophy is a prominent feature, especially in the terminal ileum. The staining properties of the mucin are not abnormal for the area of affected bowel. The discovery and sequencing of the mutant gene makes it likely that a greater understanding of the pancreatic pathology and, possibly, treatment for the condition is within reach [267].

Meconium ileus may be complicated by atresia/stenosis, perforation, or volvulus [149, 229]. Neonatal volvulus in the absence of malrotation should raise a strong suspicion of meconium ileus. In a personal series of five such infants, evidence of cystic fibrosis was available in three. Since the vast majority of cases have been associated with cystic fibrosis, the overall prognosis of meconium ileus is affected not only by the surgical feasibility of relieving the obstruction but also by the overall prognosis of cystic fibrosis.

Rickam and Boeckmann [268] reported on seven cases with a clinical syndrome resembling meconium ileus, none of whom had evidence of cystic fibrosis on follow-up. Six

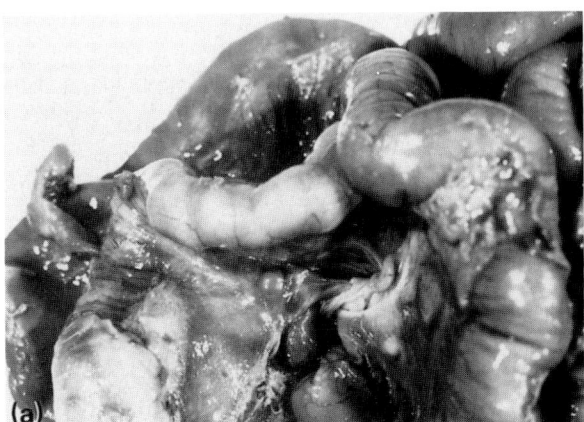

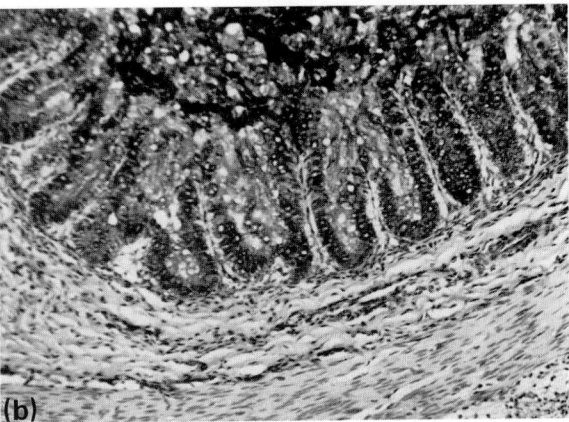

FIGURE 24.39. *(a) Postmortem specimen from an example of meconium peritonitis complicating the perforation of the ileum in a case of meconium ileus, showing the matted loops of bowel with dark discoloration of the peritoneum. (b) A section of the terminal ileum shown in (a) demonstrates distension of the crypts, obliteration of the villous pattern, and filling of the lumen with inspissated mucin. (Maxwell's stain.)*

of the seven infants had calcified, white tarry meconium in their proximal jejunum and ileum, with inspissated meconium in the colon. In the seventh case, only the proximal jejunum was involved. Calcification of the contents, sufficient to produce radiopaque bowel casts, was noted in one infant. Five of the seven infants survived; two of the deaths were attributable to delayed complications. The surviving children are alive and well.

Dolan and Touloukian [269] described two brothers who presented with classic meconium ileus, responded well to surgical evacuation of the terminal ileum, and made uneventful recoveries with sustained postoperative growth. The reports of these exceptional cases point out the need for a thorough investigation of all children with the syndrome of meconium ileus, since a small proportion do not have evidence of cystic fibrosis of the pancreas. While the clinical features may be similar, these unusual cases of meconium ileus should be distinguished from meconium plug syndrome, which affects the colon.

Ischemic Bowel Disease ("Necrotizing Enterocolitis")

Ischemic lesions may affect both the small and large bowel in the newborn and are an important cause of mortality and morbidity. Considerable controversy remains over the etiology of the condition. It is the author's view that much of the controversy arises from an incomplete appreciation of the range of the pathological findings and from a bemused inertia induced by the use of the term "necrotizing enterocolitis."

Mizrahi et al [270] used the term *necrotizing enterocolitis* to describe a condition seen in sick, shocked infants with bowel distension, vomiting, and gastrointestinal bleeding. Their criteria relied heavily on the much earlier description of the clinical signs and symptoms of neonatal peritonitis and bowel perforation described by Thelander [271]. Despite the evidence that necrotizing enterocolitis is in fact the condition previously identified by Thelander, the catchy neologism reinforced the conviction among neonatologists that it is a new disease.

Spontaneous neonatal bowel perforation is a disease of considerable antiquity, with examples in the medical museums of Europe dating at least as far back as 1823 [211, 271]. Ischemic bowel disease ("necrotizing enterocolitis") cannot be considered a disease of recent times, nor can any hypothesis based solely on conditions in the modern nursery be considered as complete.

A logical approach to the problem can be mapped out: 1) neonatal ischemic bowel disease and spontaneous bowel perforations are part of the same pathological process, 2) ischemic bowel disease may complicate a variety of therapeutic maneuvers, 3) ischemic bowel disease may complicate obstruction of the bowel from any cause, and 4) ischemic bowel disease can appear de novo in the newborn. The overlap between neonatal perforation of the bowel and

primary ischemic bowel disease has now finally been accepted [139, 214, 222, 272–274].

Ischemic bowel disease with perforation has been reported as a complication of exchange transfusion [275]. The affected infants have usually been subjected to late transfusions, usually after 24 hours' postnatal age, and often require multiple transfusions. Portal vein thrombosis has been seen [214], reflecting the fact that in late exchange transfusions the catheter tip may reach down into the portal vein [276, 277]. With the inevitable postnatal closure of the ductus venosus, the portal venous sinus in the liver undergoes retraction, producing a narrower structure [278]. Late transfusions are likely to be traumatic and may lead to vascular damage in the portal system.

Bowel ischemia and perforation have been seen as a complication of umbilical arterial and aortic catheterization in the newborn, a procedure used to monitor arterial oxygen tensions [147]. The affected infants usually can be identified by the presence of arterial thrombi in many different divisions of the superior and inferior mesenteric arteries [211], a histological finding that is shared by this group of infants with those neonates who have systemic arterial emboli associated with non-bacterial endocarditis [279, 280]. It is notable that not all infants with arterial thrombi develop infarcts [147], reflecting the importance of a background of mesenteric hypoperfusion in affected infants.

On purely epidemiological grounds, the likelihood of noxious substances leaked out of the catheters being responsible for damaging the bowel in a substantial number of cases is unlikely [281, 282].

Gastrointestinal perforation has been reported in premature infants following enteral indomethacin therapy to close a persistently patent ductus arteriosus [283–285]. This change has usually been considered to represent a toxic effect of the drug. Indomethacin has been shown to cause a sharp drop in mesenteric perfusion in dogs [286], and parenteral indomethacin in hypoxic lambs can be associated with myocardial necrosis (personal unpublished observations). Bauer's meta-analysis has shown that the case for a specific association of indomethacin and bowel perforation is unproven [287].

Ischemic bowel disease can complicate a variety of obstructive lesions, including volvulus, strangulated intussusception, strangulated omphalocele or gastroschisis, strangulated internal hernia [211], and Hirschsprung disease [288, 289]. In Hirschsprung disease, extensive colonic necrosis can be present (Fig. 24.40), but the complication is seen only rarely in those infants where relief of obstruction is achieved in early neonatal life. In the other varieties of obstruction cited, direct mechanical compression and occlusion of the vascular pedicle can be demonstrated, even though the vessels may not show histological evidence of occlusion.

Finally, ischemic bowel disease can occur de novo and most controversy centers around this group of infants. Before discussing these cases any further it is perhaps appro-

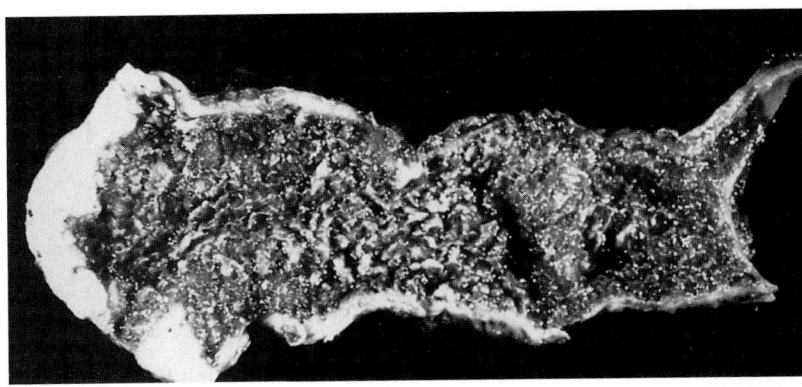

FIGURE 24.40. *A resected length of colon in a 30-day-old male infant with Hirschsprung disease, showing extensive hemorrhagic necrosis with some residual, paler, normal mucosa.*

priate to consider the pathological aspects of ischemic bowel disease in the newborn.

In the newborn infant, as in the adult, the effects of ischemia will depend on the differing sensitivities to hypoxia of the many tissues within the organ. In turn, the changes depend on the severity of the changes and the rapidity with which ischemia supervenes, and acute fulminant lesions will differ from those with a slower evolution or one of lesser severity. The bowel environment in the newborn infant is unique, since in the normal newborn infant the contents can be expected to be sterile in utero; therefore, the pattern of bacterial colonization of the bowel following delivery can be expected to play a part in the overall clinical and histological picture. In turn, ischemia may affect the pattern of colonization, and it has been known for several years that the changes of ischemia are diminished considerably in a bowel washed free of bacteria, bile, and enzymes [290]. Finally, in the hypoxic newborn infant a splanchnic shunt mechanism can be demonstrated in which the less vital organs, such as the gut, undergo a reduction of blood flow to protect the brain and heart. The early hypothesis [139] has been shown to be true by later experimental studies

[291, 292]. The role of the collateral circulation and local interruption has also been emphasized in experimental models [293, 294].

Gross Pathology

Macroscopically, in ischemia bowel involvement may be focal or diffuse and may involve multiple segments, with single or multiple perforations. In its least severe form, ballooned congested segments of bowel may be found (Fig. 24.41) or there may be closely aligned bands of vascular congestion [211]. Perforations (single or multiple) with an associated peritonitis may be a complication (Fig. 24.42). The most common site of involvement is the terminal ileum followed by the adjacent colon, but any site of the small and large bowel may be involved, either as a single focus or as part of multifocal disease. In cases with multifocal involvement, there is often some degree of variation in the severity of the lesion from one area to the next.

Histological Findings

The mucosa is the site affected first in cases of ischemia, and the earliest stage consists of capillary dilatation and

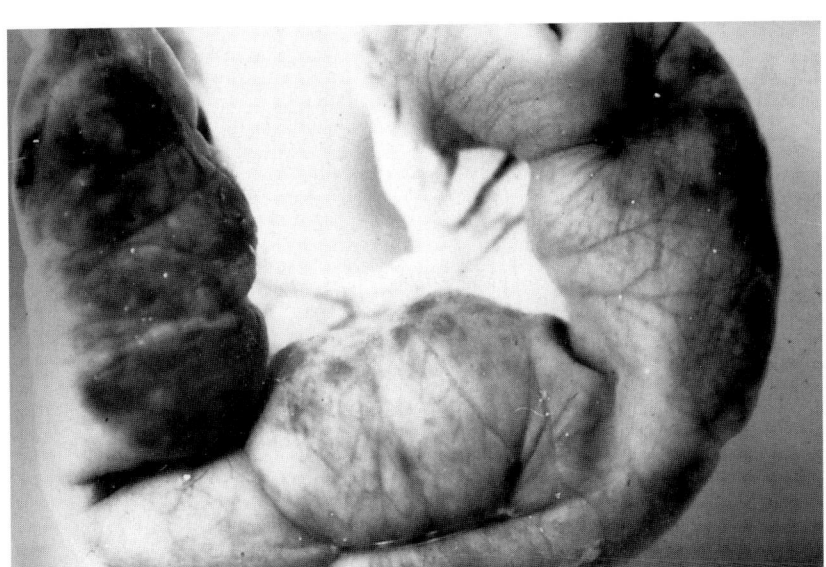

FIGURE 24.41. *Ballooned and congested bowel loops in a 29-week-gestation male infant with respiratory distress syndrome, who developed abdominal distension and passage of rectal blood.*

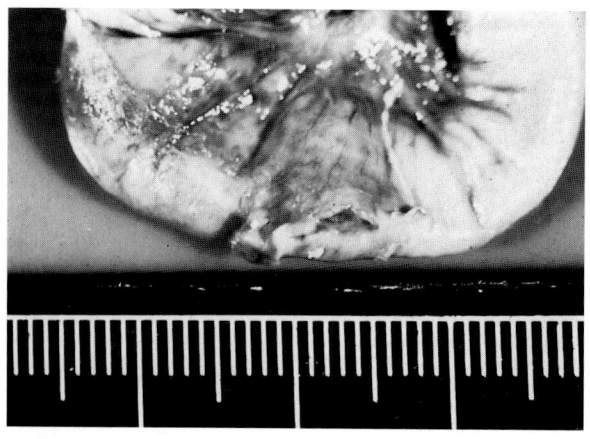

FIGURE 24.42. *Perforation of the bowel surrounded by vascular dilatation and fibrinous exudate (scale in cm).*

rupture near the tips of the villi or the surface of the mucosa (Fig. 24.43). Later, there is progressive necrosis with desquamation of the epithelial cells progressing from the lumen through to the deeper layers. The change is seen best in surgically resected samples, since considerable distortion may be encountered in postmortem material due to congestion and autolysis. Early in the course of ischemia, erythrocytes may be seen in the capsular sinus of the lymph nodes draining the affected segment; when present, the change can be useful in differentiating between simple congestion and early ischemia.

With the progression of the lesion, coagulative necrosis of the mucosa occurs, which in its earlier stages manifests as lysis of red cells and blurring of epithelial cell outlines, usually with some preservation of the ghosted outlines of the mucosal structure. A variable degree of inflammatory response may be present, and a pseudomembranous exudate

of necrotic debris may replace the damaged mucosa. With more extensive ischemia there is hemorrhagic necrosis of the submucosa and later the circular muscle. With the most severe degree of ischemia there is full-thickness necrosis. Curiously, autonomic nervous system ganglion cells seem to be capable of resisting ischemic damage, and their anatomical integrity is matched by their capacity to remain functional despite several hours of ischemic deprivation, an observation of considerable antiquity [290, 295] but confirmed easily by an examination of ischemic bowel (Fig. 24.44).

In full-thickness necrosis the changes in the bowel wall can vary due, presumably, to the rapidity with which ischemia supervenes. In some infants the appearances suggest a fulminant course with extensive hemorrhagic full-thickness necrosis, with little or no inflammatory response of any type, even though there may be scattered areas of less severely involved bowel near zones of imminent perforation (Fig. 24.45). Pneumatosis, characterized by the presence of intramural gas-filled cysts, is often seen in ischemic bowel in the neonatal period (Fig. 24.46); however, in most series, cases without pneumatosis are recorded, and in some reviews up to 14% of cases do not show the change [272]. In our experience, with cases followed by sequential x-rays, pneumatosis is not an invariable feature of early ischemic change and appears later in the course of the disease [296]. Twenty percent of our cases did not show any evidence of pneumatosis. Gas-filled cysts may dissect along the course of the bowel until there is almost total pneumatosis. However, much of the bowel so affected may be intrinsically normal apart from the presence of intramural gas (Fig. 24.47). In our experience, microorganisms of mixed type are demonstrated, usually with ease, in virtually all cases with pneumatosis (Fig. 24.48). It follows, therefore, that the extent of pneumatosis does not correlate with the extent of disease, nor is it a necessary diagnostic feature of ischemic bowel

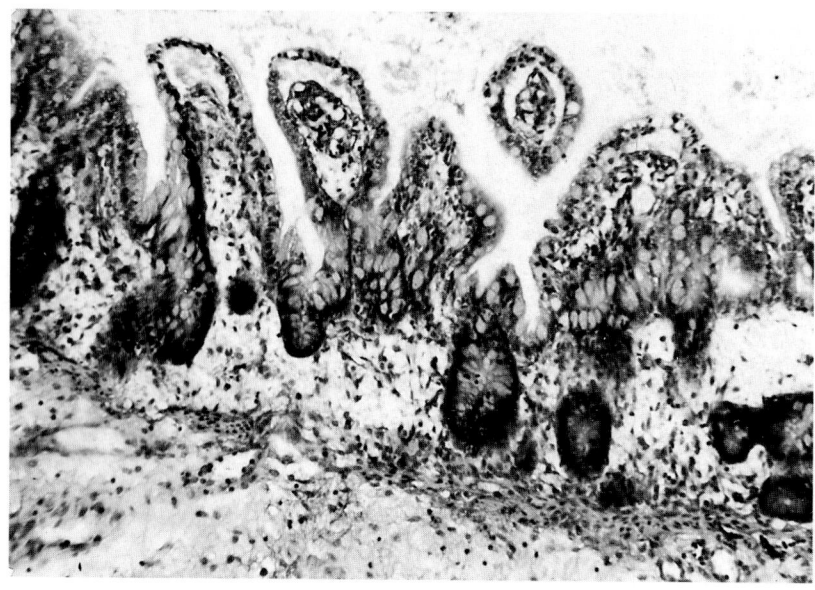

FIGURE 24.43. *Early ischemic change is characterized by mucosal capillary dilatation and interstitial hemorrhage into the lamina propria. (Picro Mallory. Courtesy of the publishers of deSa [211].)*

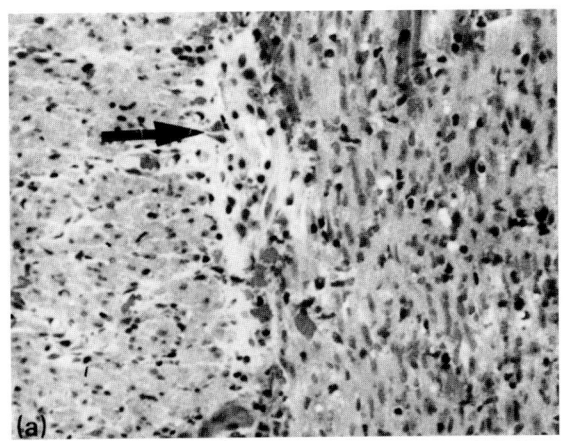

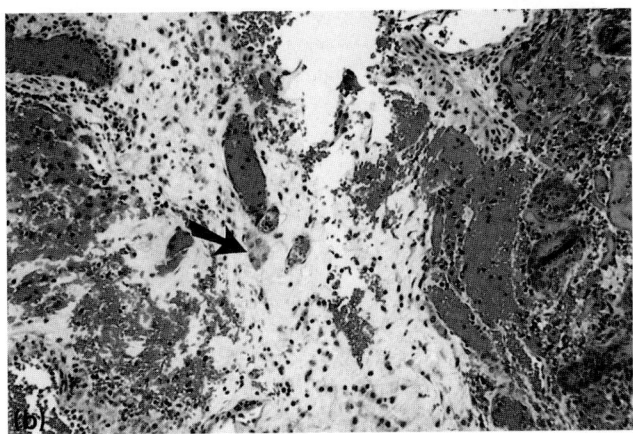

FIGURE 24.44. *Surviving autonomic ganglia of the myenteric plexus (a) and submucosal plexus (b) in a segment of ischemic bowel.*

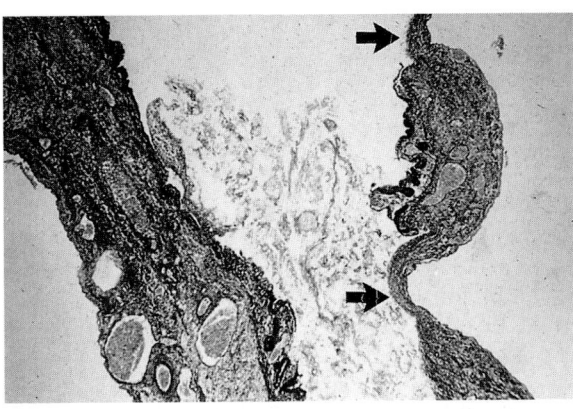

FIGURE 24.45. *A longitudinal section through a zone of ischemic bowel showing acute fulminant changes, without pneumatosis or inflammatory reaction, but with areas of imminent perforation (arrow). The bowel wall shows ischemic change of varying severity. (Picro Mallory. Courtesy of publishers of deSa [211].)*

furthermore, that pneumatosis supervenes in those cases of bowel ischemia where the course is relatively slower (compare Fig. 24.45 with Fig. 24.46).

Repair of Ischemic Necrosis

Reparative phenomena following ischemic bowel damage have been described by several workers following the earlier descriptions [214, 216, 297] and can progress to stricture formation, or even atresia [219]. Tongues of mucosa appear on the edges of ulcerated zones of bowel and spread over the inflammatory granulation tissue that contemporaneously replaces necrotic debris. The regenerating epithelium is low cuboidal in type, and lacks mucin or zymogen granules. As the gap is bridged, small glandular structures develop, and they appear even before the mucosal defect is covered [209]. The redevelopment of brush borders and villi takes longer; incomplete regeneration of villi may be responsible for the

damage. In my view, pneumatosis does imply that there is an abnormal proliferation of organisms within the lumen and wall of the bowel and that there is ulceration, albeit of a size that may not be demonstrated readily. It would appear,

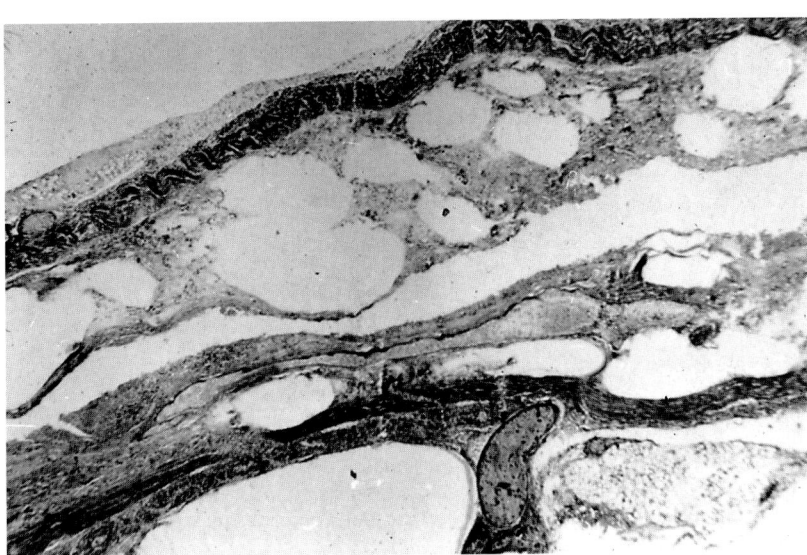

FIGURE 24.46. *A longitudinal section through terminal ileum in a resected specimen of ileum, cecum, ascending colon, and appendix showing numerous intramural gas-filled cysts (pneumatosis intestinalis). In this segment the mucosa and submucosa appear necrotic. (Picro Mallory. Courtesy of publishers of deSa [58].)*

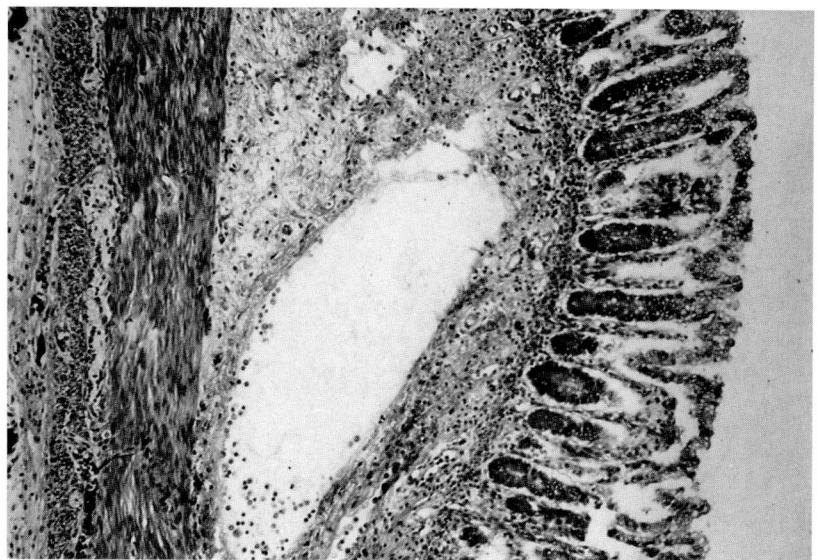

FIGURE 24.47.   *Same case as Figure 24.46. In the distal margin of the resected bowel, blebs of submucosal gas are seen beneath normal mucosa of the colon. (Picro Mallory.)*

various disaccharide intolerances and malabsorption that may persist for weeks after ischemic damage [219, 298, 299].

The process of repair extends through the lamina and muscularis mucosa, with variable scarring of these structures, and may produce extensive widening and splitting of the muscularis mucosa into its longitudinal and circular muscular components (Fig. 24.49). Repair of damage to the circular layer of the muscularis propria usually produces a peculiar moth-eaten appearance in that structure, and often there is fusion of the muscularis propria with the scarred muscularis mucosa producing a stricture (Fig. 24.50). Expectant medical management in the author's institution has yielded some unusual examples of repair of ischemic bowel damage, including a sealed perforation (Fig. 24.51) and a walled abscess (Fig. 24.52), indicating the great regenerative capacity of the bowel. There is also an example of a muscle defect [28]. These changes occur under favorable conditions, such as when oral feeding is restricted and bacterial overgrowth is dampened by antibiotic cover. Occasionally, the

reparative process is associated with the production of a picture indistinguishable from "congenital" atresia (Fig. 24.53).

Clinical Features of Acute Ischemic Bowel Damage in the Newborn

A large number of studies and reviews indicate clearly that the majority of infants who are likely to develop ischemic bowel disease in the absence of mechanical lesions or therapeutic maneuvers are immature infants who are subjected to a perinatal hypoxic stress [139, 214, 270, 272, 300–305]. In these infants, hypoperfusion of the mesenteric circulation via a splanchnic shunt may be expected. Severe hypoxia may also be associated with myocardial damage, and in this setting intestinal ischemia may form part of a syndrome of cardiovascular collapse [306, 307]. Many of the most severely affected infants nowadays are extremely immature [308, 309].

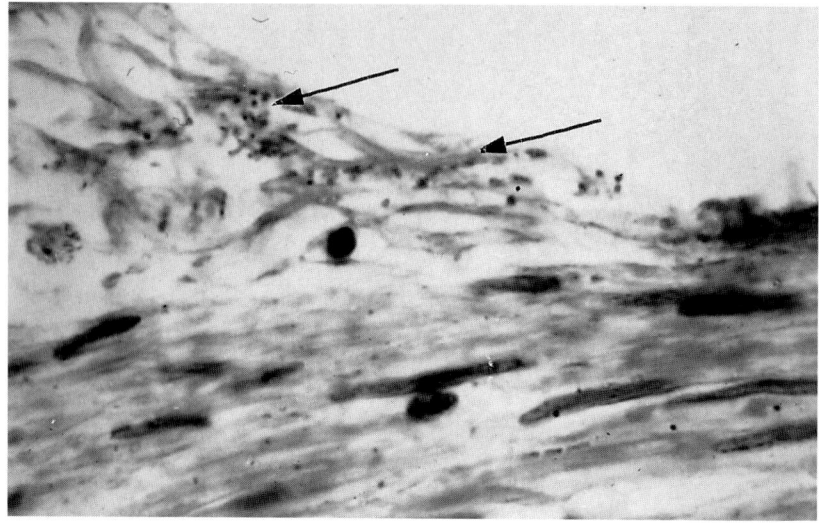

FIGURE 24.48.   *Rod-like organisms (arrow) are seen in the walls of many cysts in pneumatosis intestinalis. Gram's stain showed the organisms to be Gram-positive: they can be seen on routine preparations. (Picro Mallory.)*

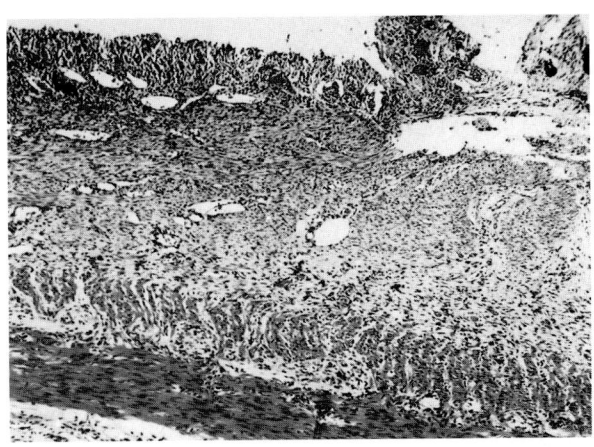

FIGURE 24.49. *Repair following ischemic damage is seen in this segment of bowel removed from a 34-day-old infant who developed a stricture following neonatal necrotizing enterocolitis. The thickened muscularis mucosa is splayed out and merges with the granulation tissue of the submucosa and scarred circular muscle layer. (Attwood's stain.)*

The incidence of affected infants in neonatal intensive-care units has varied from 2% to 8% of admissions, and the mortality from the disease in most centers is now less than 15% compared to initial figures of as high as 60%. Ischemic damage is not confined to immature infants, however, and larger infants may be affected, as may infants of high gestation who are growth-retarded [216]. This is reflected in some experimental work on term piglets, where low birth weight at term predisposed to bowel necrosis [310]. Yu et al [311] describe a curious relationship between birth weight and onset of symptoms from ischemic bowel disease: larger infants present at an earlier age than immature infants.

Perforation and peritonitis with supervening sepsis remain dreaded complications, but the overall management of infants with ischemic bowel damage has benefited greatly from the application of staging criteria [312, 313]. Portal vein gas due to extension of the pneumatosis was once considered an invariably fatal sign, but this is not borne out in recent studies [303, 314–316]. In our series [296], three of eight infants with this sign died; all had extensive bowel involvement, with perforation progressing to peritonitis.

Most of the infants, as may be expected, have abdominal distension progressing to absent bowel sounds and blood in stools (either overt or occult). Many of these infants also have a wide range of nonspecific signs, including lethargy and poor feeding. Many appear in a shocked state with apneic and bradycardic episodes.

Rare cases of neonatal appendicitis [317] have been described, and the only case personally studied had a perforated appendix as part of a multifocal ischemic insult.

Epidemic Case-Clusters of "Necrotizing Enterocolitis"

Several reports describe clusters of cases with bloody stools and pneumatosis occurring in nurseries [318–325]. These infants have usually been more mature and show less evidence of hypoxia than the usual infants with ischemic bowel damage. In most instances, their course has been relatively mild with fewer serious complications and a lower mortality than expected.

In such a clinical setting, the likelihood of a specific infectious agent causing an epidemic is an obvious cause for concern. The search for such an infectious agent has been, almost invariably, unsuccessful. Most of the cases do not show evidence of case-to-case transmission or a common source of origin. It is not clear from the published reports whether all the infants suffered from the same disease. The pathological diagnosis of "necrotizing enterocolitis," as outlined earlier, consists of a full and varied spectrum of ischemic bowel damage, but it cannot be said that either bloody stools, or pneumatosis, or both in combination are always ischemic in origin. A detailed review of the infectious aspects of necrotizing enterocolitis shows that the bacteriological studies have been contradictory. Even prominent candidates for the role of a primary agent, such as the *Clostridium* species [326–328], have been shown to be normal colonizers of the neonatal gut [329–332]. There is doubt whether the detection of the presence of cytopathic toxins is an abnormal phenomenon [330–333]. Lawrence et al [334], however, were able to show bacterial synergism between *Staphylococcus aureus* and *Bacillus cereus* species on the one hand, and *Klebsiella* species on the other in experimental animals. Prior inoculation with *S. aureus* or *B. cereus* followed 24 hours later by *Klebsiella* produced a picture of mucosal hemorrhagic ulceration compatible with necrotizing enterocolitis. Similarly, Gonzalez-Crussi and Hsueh [335] produced ischemic bowel necrosis using platelet-activating factor and bacterial lipopolysaccharide in rats. It appears likely, therefore, that abnormal bacterial colonization with cytopathic toxin-producing strains may produce a syndrome resembling classic ischemic bowel damage [324]. However, epidemic cases of necrotizing enterocolitis fortunately do not seem to progress to the picture of generalized infection with meningitis and other widely disseminated infections, which would be expected if there were devitalized bowel with an increased population of toxin-producing organisms in the lumen. Liver damage in these infants appears only infrequently.

In some unusual settings, a primary insult by a bacterial toxin can damage the bowel. Such a condition is *pigbel*, which does not affect newborns, but is brought on by massive ritual consumption of improperly cooked pork. Here, a clostridial toxin is of fundamental importance [336].

Obviously, there are conditions that can mimic the clinical picture of ischemic bowel disease, and some of the "epidemics" may represent a mixture of true cases of ischemic bowel disease and contemporaneous infections. Viruses have not been studied systematically as a potential cause of bowel necrosis or any of the syndromes that may mimic it in the newborn. Reports of rotavirus or coronavirus infection in the newborn are available [337, 338]. These infections could

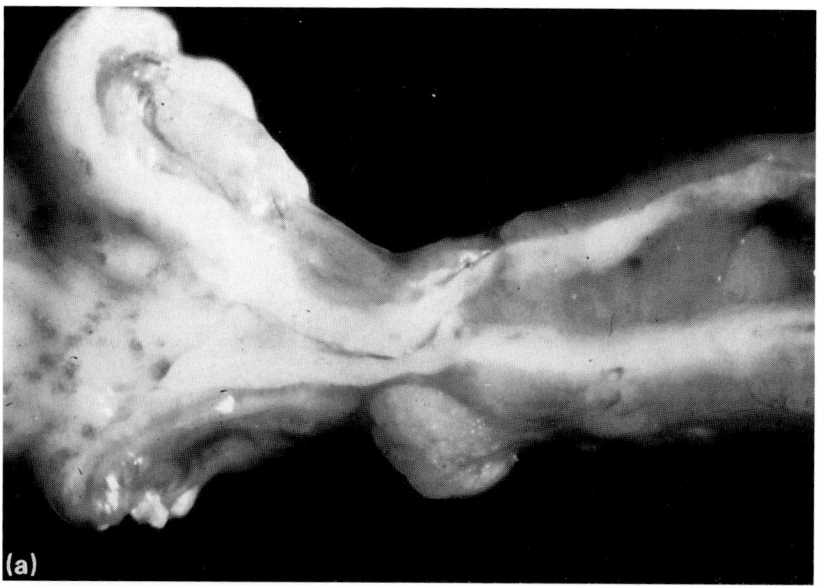

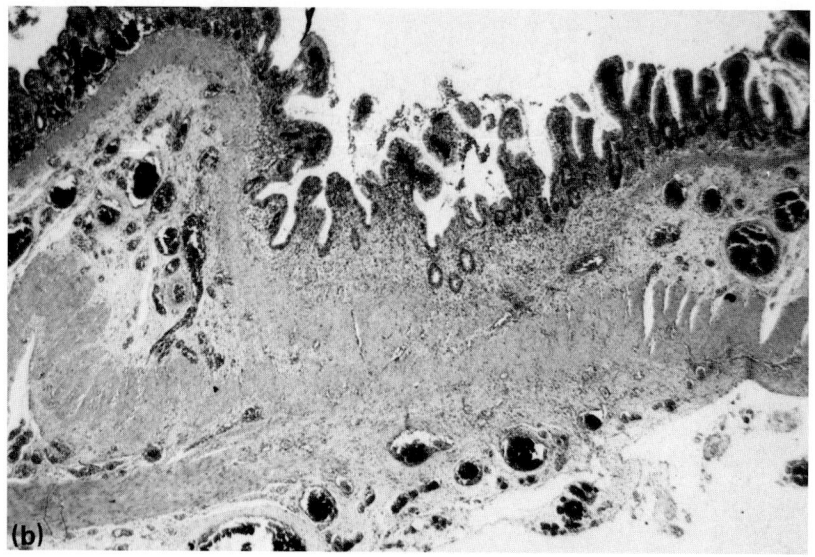

FIGURE 24.50. *(a) A strictured segment of bowel removed from a 48-day-old infant with prior ischemic bowel damage. The opened bowel shows obvious narrowing of the lumen and scarring. (b) A section through the area stricturing shows disorganization of the wall with fusion of the muscularis mucosa and the circular muscular layer with the scarred submucosa. Note the distorted villus architecture. (Attwood's stain.)*

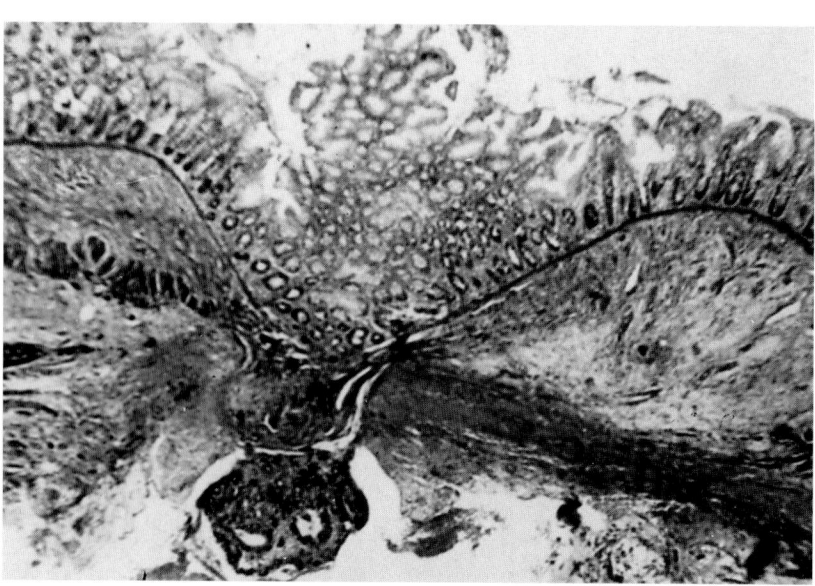

FIGURE 24.51. *A sealed perforation plugged by a nodule made up of mucosal epithelium and granulation tissue from a 51-day-old infant with previous ischemic bowel damage. (Clinical signs of bowel perforation were transient.)*

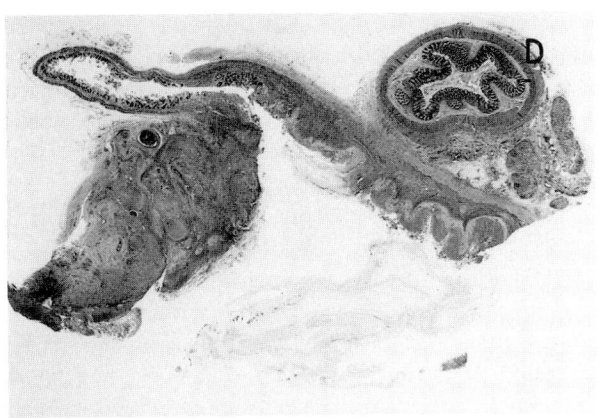

FIGURE 24.52. *Part of the wall of a loculated abscess (partly sealed perforation) found at postmortem examination of a 78-day-old infant with previous ischemic bowel damage. The abscess was peeled off the lateral abdominal wall (not in picture), and the walls were made up of sigmoid colon with evidence of ischemic damage and repair. The lesion overlay the descending colon (D), which led into the abscess.*

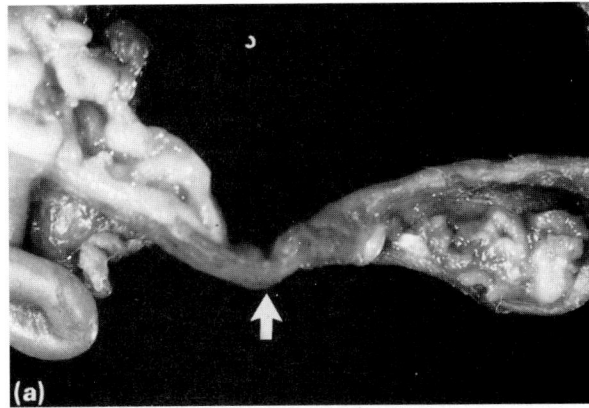

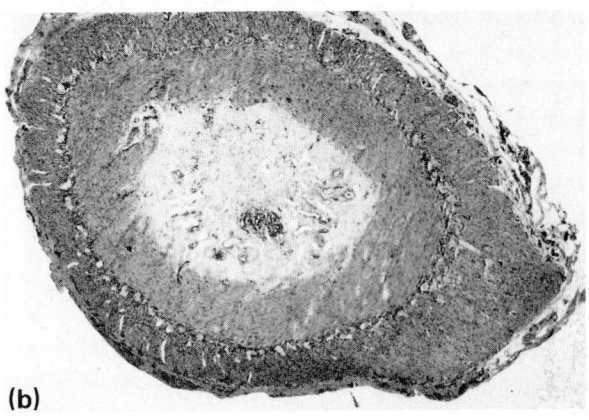

FIGURE 24.53. *(a) A thread-like atretic segment of ileum in an 82-day-old infant is shown (arrow). (Approx. ×4.) The proximal segment is filled with inspissated fecal debris while the distal segment was filled with glairy mucin (removed). (b) The infant had severe ischemic bowel damage in the newborn period. A transverse section of the thread-like segment shows complete obliteration of the lumen (acquired atresia). (Attwood's stain.)*

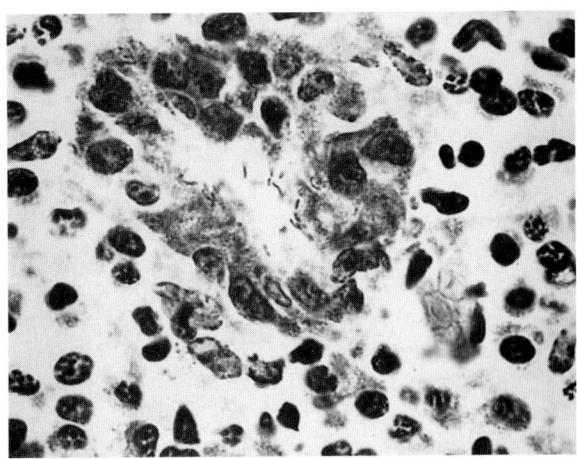

FIGURE 24.54. Campylobacter *organisms seen among the crypts of a colonic biopsy in a case of bloody neonatal diarrhea and colonic pneumatosis. The infant's mother had an episode of diarrhea previously. (Warthin-Starry stain.)*

represent a potential cause of microscopic ulceration that would allow secondary bacterial invaders to produce a syndrome with an associated pneumatosis.

The increasing recognition of *Campylobacter* enteritis in neonates (Fig. 24.54) should be emphasized [339–344]. Infections with this group of organisms may result in bloody stools, but the severity of the symptomatology can vary. Coello-Ramirez et al [345] reported a series of Mexican infants with diarrhea from varied causes, pneumatosis, and a 30% to 40% mortality. Increasingly, enterotoxigenic strains of bacteria, including *Aeromonas* and *Yersinia*, have been described in children, and it is reasonable to suggest that they also may be of importance in neonates, especially in those instances where cases occur in clusters [346].

Several problems related to the study of the etiology of ischemic bowel disease remain unanswered. It is useful to consider the result of any disease as reflecting a balance between "soil and seed" interaction. An ischemic background may be considered to represent the "soil" while abnormal bacterial overgrowth may be thought of as the "seed." Additional modifiers of both the soil and seed may include the effects of feeding (either breast milk or hyperosmolar fluids), but their overall contribution is uncertain [347]. It may be that, as argued by Kosloske [304], a combination of ischemia, pathogenic flora, and an excess of "substrate" is required for the development of the full spectrum. Modifying any two of the three components may change the outcome. It remains unclear, however, why some infants at risk develop ischemic bowel damage while others do not. Recent experimental models developed by the group in Chicago [348–352] have emphasized the interaction of hypoxia, bacterial lipopolysaccharide, endogenous nitric oxide production, tumor necrosis factor alpha, and platelet-activating factors in triggering a cascade of necrosis and inflammation. Their models appear very promising and reproducible.

Rarer Causes of Ischemic Bowel Disease in the Newborn

Periarteritis (polyarteritis) nodosa has been reported in neonates [353–355] and may involve the intestine. Bjarke et al described two infants with aortic thrombosis, possibly related to antithrombin III deficiency, one of whom had bowel infarction at postmortem examination [356]. Homocystinuria [357] can cause ischemia due to platelet aggregates occluding small vessels, and a case of bowel infarction in a 3-week-old male infant has been described [211].

Intestinal Involvement in Neonatal Systemic Disease

Ulceration and even perforation of the small bowel may be seen in several generalized neonatal infections, including listeriosis, congenital syphilis, herpes simplex infections, cytomegalovirus, toxoplasmosis, and *Candida* infections [63, 66, 68, 69, 358]. In these instances, however, the intestinal lesions are overshadowed by the changes in other organs. Intestinal lesions may be part of Langerhans cell histiocytosis [359].

Primary Abnormalities of the Enterocyte

Several workers [360–362] have drawn attention to a wide spectrum of ultrastructural abnormalities of the intestinal epithelial cells. Affected infants are symptomatic from birth, with severe diarrhea. Histologically, they have a flat mucosa with hypoplastic villous atrophy and abnormal mucin. This has been called congenital microvillus atrophy or familial enteropathy. A wide range of abnormalities in microvillus architecture may be found, ultrastructurally, and the cases are heterogeneous [362]. The author has little personal experience in this group of conditions, but with the improving outlook for all sick infants, and the progressive reduction in neonatal mortality from other causes, these enterocyte abnormalities will assume increasing importance. The cited studies indicate the importance of ultrastructural studies in patients who present in infancy with intractable diarrhea and failure to thrive. In the past, it is likely that many cases with this clinical presentation have not been diagnosed with accuracy due to the lack of detailed study [363, 364].

Tumors of the Small Intestine

Rare examples of congenital, probably hamartomatous tumors of the small bowel presenting in the newborn include a congenital hemangiopericytoma of the duodenum [365], solitary fibromatosis [366, 367], neonatal angiomatosis [87], and angiodysplasia [151]. An intestinal ganglioneuroblastoma has been found in a 22-week fetus [368].

Neonatal mucormycosis and non-syphilitic spirochetosis have been described in neonates and fetuses [369, 370].

Peritoneal Lesions

Reference was made earlier to meconium peritonitis, and the peritonitis complicating intestinal ischemic damage. Peritonitis in the newborn is a secondary phenomenon in the vast majority of cases, one that invariably complicates perforation of the stomach and small or large intestine from any cause. Bile peritonitis may complicate surgery on the biliary tract. Recently, starch particles have assumed importance in many centers as a cause of postoperative peritonitis. Peritonitis can, of course, occur as a complication of any systemic hematogenous infection. In males, extension of the exudate into the scrotum may occur.

Mesenteric cysts that may mimic an ascitic effusion [371] may be encountered in neonates, albeit rarely. These cysts are now considered to be derived from lymphatic vessels. Gonzalez-Crussi et al [372] described omental and mesenteric myxoid hamartomatas that were misdiagnosed clinically as neuroblastomas or other malignant tumors.

GENERAL FEATURES, DEVELOPMENT, AND ANATOMY OF THE LARGE BOWEL

The large intestine includes the cecum, vermiform appendix, colon, rectum, and anal canal. As reflected by their blood supply, these structures are derived from three distinct components. The cecum, vermiform appendix, ascending colon, and the proximal two-thirds of the transverse colon arise from the midgut and are supplied by branches of the superior mesenteric artery. The remainder of the transverse colon distally to the lower third of the anal canal develops from the hindgut and is supplied by the inferior mesenteric artery. The lower third of the anal canal is derived from the proctodeum and receives its blood supply from the inferior rectal arteries, as well as branches of the (somatic) internal pudendal arteries. The exact point of transition between the midgut and hindgut derivatives may vary between patients, but the site is indicated by the zone of overlap between the territories of distribution of the superior and inferior mesenteric artery.

Development of the Large Bowel

The components of the large intestine that are derived from the midgut are affected by the "physiological hernia" that occurs when excessive growth of loops of midgut outstrip the capacity of the developing abdomen [373]. Like the small intestinal derivatives of the midgut, the future cecum, vermiform appendix, and ascending colon prolapse into the sac of the omphalocele. The growth of the abdominal cavity is associated with the rotation of the bowel and the return of the midgut loops. The rotation of the midgut fixes the cephalad segment of the midgut to the right of the midline and, as a consequence, the caudad loops are displaced to the left. The cecum and the future ascending and transverse colon initially lie on the left of the midline following the return of the midgut. There now ensues a further period of rapid growth of both the developing "midgut-derived" colon, as well as the hindgut-derived segments of colon, which leads to the repositioning of the cecum, first across the midline to the right and then caudally to its normal anatomical site in the right iliac fossa.

Initially the large bowel retains a mesocolon, but eventually as the pace of growth slows (and with it the consequent repositioning of the bowel), the mesocolon is fixed to the parietal peritoneum of the posterior abdominal wall. With the cecum in its normal anatomical position, the sites of fixation are the ascending colon and the descending colon since these are the areas in direct contact with the parietal peritoneum. There is, however, considerable variation in the degree of fixation of the large bowel, and a definite ascending and/or descending mesocolon is a common variant in neonatal and adult autopsy material. The sigmoid mesocolon undergoes some reduction in its overall length during the fixation of the other segments. The length and redundancy of the sigmoid mesocolon varies considerably between different patients, however, and this may have an important bearing on the problem of volvulus of the sigmoid colon.

The early stages of the development of the large bowel are a relatively straightforward process of growth and repositioning of a tubular structure. However, the later development of the distal hindgut involves a complex series of steps with coordinated changes in many adjacent structures. These include the development of the bladder, the uterus and adnexal structures, the sacrococcygeal region of the spine, as well as the cloacal membrane and external genitalia [373, 374]. As a consequence, congenital anomalies of the anorectal region are relatively frequent, and they may form part of extremely complex malformation sequences.

Development of the Rectum and Anal Canal

The terminal portion of the hind-gut is the *cloaca*. This cavity is lined by endoderm and comes in contact with the ectoderm in an area known as the *cloacal membrane*. The cloacal membrane forms the base of a shallow depression known as the *anal pit* or *proctodeum*. Ventrally the cloaca is in continuity with the allantois, while the mesonephric ducts open into the lateral aspect of the cloaca. A short, blind prolongation of the hindgut into the tail fold is known as the *tailgut*, and initially this communicates with the cloaca.

A sheet of mesenchyme develops in the coronal plane between the allantois and the hindgut. This *urorectal septum* grows caudally toward the cloacal membrane separating the dorsal (alimentary) structures from the ventral (genitourinary) derivatives. The alimentary derivatives are the rudimentary rectum and the upper two-thirds of the anal canal. Simultaneously with the development of the urorectal septum, the mesenchyme around the cloacal membrane proliferates leading to the development of the genital tubercles and the deepening of the anal pit, on the floor of which is the cloacal membrane. The deep anal pit so produced is now known as the proctodeal canal, and its development is accompanied by the shrinkage, and ultimate disappearance, of the tail fold and the tailgut. In the female the paramesonephric ducts that are the progenitors of the fallopian tubes, uterus, cervix, and upper vagina develop within the urorectal septum. By the end of the 7th week the urorectal septum has reached and fused with the cloacal membrane.

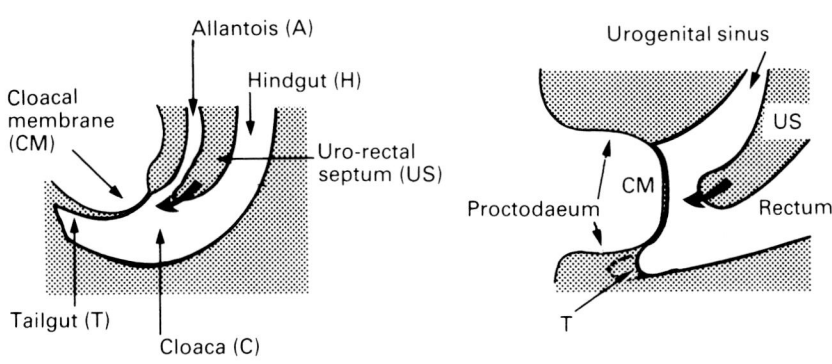

(I) 4 weeks approx.   (II) 6 weeks approx.

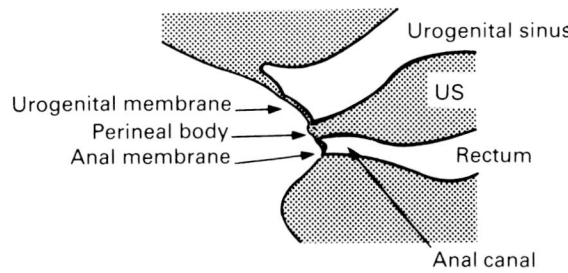

(III) 7 weeks approx.

FIGURE 24.55.   *A diagrammatic representation of the division of the cloaca by the urorectal septum and the disappearance of the tailgut. For the sake of clarity only the status in the male is shown.*

The point of fusion is marked by the perineal body or central perineal tendon. The cloacal membrane is now divided into an anal membrane posteriorly and a larger urogenital membrane anteriorly. In the male the urogenital membrane, when it disintegrates, is incorporated into the urethral floor, while in the female it contributes to the hymen (Fig. 24.55).

In the fetus, therefore, the hindgut communicates with the dorsal segment of the cloaca and is separated from the exterior only by the anal membrane. When the anal membrane breaks down, the hindgut opens to the exterior; this step is complete by 51 days [375].

The anal canal of the fetus has two components. The upper two-thirds arise from the cloacal component, while the proctodeal component forms the lower third. In the adult organ, their junction, the site of the anal membrane, is defined by the pectinate line and anal valves. The pectinate line should not be confused with the anocutaneous junction or "white line" where the anal canal epithelium changes from stratified squamous to a keratinized type. The change from the mucus-producing columnar epithelium of the hindgut to the anal skin is not accomplished in a series of distinct clear-cut anatomical lines. In many infants the anal canal above the anal valves is lined by a narrow zone of mucosa with reduced numbers of goblet cells and islands of stratified squamous epithelium or by "transitional" epithelium (Fig. 24.56). Transitional epithelium can be seen, almost invariably, lining the anal crypts. This transitional epithelium shows an increase in the numbers of basally situated polygonal cells and no squamous stratification. Several authors use the term "cloacogenic epithelium" to describe the transitional epithelium. The term appears tautologous since the upper two-thirds of the anal canal is entirely cloacal in origin, irrespective of the nature of its epithelial lining. Below the pectinate line the mucosa shows increasing keratinization, and at the anal margin, primitive dermal appendages may be present.

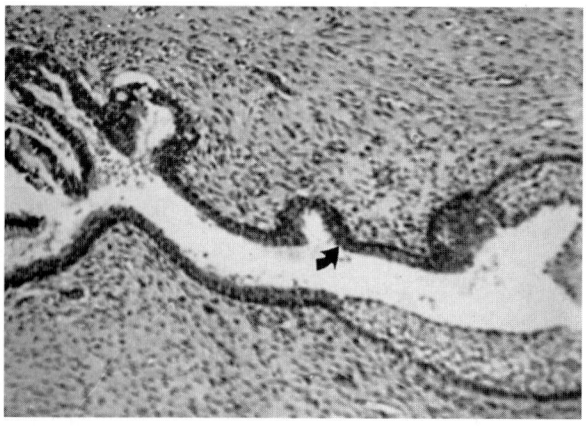

FIGURE 24.56.   *The anal canal in a 15-week fetus with transitional epithelium (arrow) extending into the lower rectum (on left).*

The urorectal septum is the sole partition that separates the lower gastrointestinal tract from the genitourinary tract, and the development of a normal anal canal depends on the coordinated development of the proctodeum with the urorectal septum. All the developmental anomalies that are associated with fistulae between the two systems, in either sex, are related to defects in the formation of the urorectal septum. The site of the fusion between the urorectal septum and the cloacal membrane is marked by the perineal body in both sexes, and the absence of the perineal body indicates failure in the coordinated development of the urorectal septum with the cloacal membrane [376].

The normal development of the anal canal and lower rectum depends on at least two more factors: the regression of the tail and the tailgut, and the normal development of the sacrococcygeal vertebrae and lower spinal cord. Aberrant development of the lower spine or persistence of the tailgut and vestigial tail-like appendages may be associated with malformations of the anal canal and rectum. The tailgut is a blind extension of the hindgut into the tail-fold just distal to the cloacal membrane. With the growth of the fetus and the development of the proctodeum, the tailgut is progressively resorbed and taken up into the lower cloaca. This process is complete by 56 days [375]. Remnants of this structure may persist, however, and form one variety of duplication or cyst of the presacral or retrorectal region. In their early developmental stages the anlages of the neural tube and the hindgut are anatomically adjacent to each other, becoming separated only later by the development of the notochord and somitic mesoderm. In association with abnormal development of the lower spinal cord and sacrococcygeal vertebrae, small columns of tissue linking the developing neural tube and hindgut may remain, giving rise to neurenteric fistula and posterior enteric cysts.

Finally, anomalies of the anal canal and rectum may be part of malformation syndromes where abnormal development of many organ systems may exist in a bewildering number of combinations. Many of these syndromes are associated with lethal malformations but formes frustes do exist. Since they may be associated with a very wide range of malformations, finding any anorectal anomaly is an indication for a detailed investigation of the affected patient [377].

Innervation of the Bowel

Though reference has been made to it in earlier sections, perhaps nowhere else does the autonomic innervation of the bowel assume as much importance as it does in the large bowel. Our knowledge of this facet of the anatomy of the large bowel stems from the pioneering work of Yntema and Hammond [378], who studied avian embryos. By removing the cephalic neural crest, ganglionic development in the gastrointestinal tract was halted. These researchers suggested that the autonomic innervation of the bowel depended on migration of neural crest cells to the developing gastrointestinal tract along the vagal trunks. Okamoto and Ueda [2] examined human embryos with silver impregnation studies of celloidin-embedded sections and confirmed the earlier results of Yntema and Hammond [378]. At 5 weeks' gestation, paired vagal fibers extended to the cervical esophagus, but intramural ganglia were absent. Immature ganglion cells were seen along the vagal trunks. The esophagus was colonized with neuroblasts by 6 weeks, and by the eighth week a wave of immature ganglion cells could be seen up to the distal half of the colon. The cells were not seen in the mesentery and this suggested craniocaudal migration and development along the gastrointestinal tract. By 12 weeks the entire bowel was innervated. Okamoto and Ueda [2] did not specify whether they studied embryos between 8 and 12 weeks of gestation—the period during which the colon is innervated. Andrew [379], however, was able to show that in chick embryos, at least, the distal neural crest—if it remains in anatomical continuity with the distal somites—can be a source of neuroblasts (and ganglia) to the distal gut. These experiments left open the question of craniocaudal migration of neural crest–derived neuroblasts in humans, and in particular the innervation of the distal large bowel. This apparent divergence between vagal-derived enteric neuroblasts and sacral-derived neuroblasts is of fundamental importance when considering Hirschsprung disease and its variants and mimics [380–382].

Reference was made earlier to the elegant fundamental work of Kapur [4]. Working with a transgenic mouse model he showed that craniocaudal migration does occur, and the process can be visualized with ease. In the mammalian gut the sacral-derived enteric neuroblast contribution does not appear to have the same importance as it may have in avian embryos.

The submucosal (Meissner's) plexus develops from neuroblasts that migrate across the muscularis from the intermuscular, myenteric (Auerbach's) plexus. This phase also occurs in a craniocaudal fashion during the third and fourth months [2]. In addition to these intrinsic nerve plexuses, extrinsic nerves may enter the bowel wall from the sympathetic and parasympathetic nerve plexuses in relation to blood vessels.

Traditional anatomical descriptions of the orientation of the myenteric and submucosal plexuses in the bowel are based on either tangentially cut or transversely cut sections [380]. Wells et al [383] have developed microdissection techniques that provide a dramatic flat-mount preparation, thereby permitting detailed quantitative analysis of the myenteric plexus in different selected areas of the bowel. The normal myenteric plexus appears as a network of nerve fibers and ganglia with ganglion cells concentrated along the margins of the strands of nerve fibers [380, 383]. The space between the units of the network varies in different segments of the gut, indicating a varying density of autonomic nervous system components. The variation in the pattern of the myenteric plexus in different sectors of the bowel has been interpreted as an indicator of differences in the biochemical induction or maturation of control signals in different gut segments [383]. The network pattern allows nerve

transmission to be unaffected by stretching or distension; it may also permit the transmission of impulses over alternate network pathways.

Smith [384] has provided useful data regarding intestinal neuronal density in childhood. The study, based on neuronal counts of transverse and longitudinal sections, covers the small and large intestine, and, when taken with Wells' work [383], provides a much needed baseline for any future studies of the innervation of the bowel.

Anatomy of the Large Bowel and Anus

The anatomy of the colon and rectum reflects their primary physiologic functions—the absorption of water and the expulsion of feces. The general tubular structure of the bowel is maintained with a mucosal layer, a muscularis mucosa, a submucosal layer, a muscularis propria, and serosa. A timetable of differentiation of the bowel in the fetus is provided by Semba et al [15].

The lumen is lined by a simple columnar absorptive epithelium that dips down into the lamina propria to produce simple tubular glands, with a progressive increase in the proportion of goblet cells in the epithelium from the cecum to the rectum. The columnar epithelial cells do not have zymogen granules, but in neonatal infants occasional Paneth cells may be seen in the crypts. Enterochromaffin cells are also present [7]. The lamina propria carries the mucosal plexus of vessels and a variable and mixed population of inflammatory cells. In the normal neonatal infant most of these cells are lymphocytes with scattered mast cells. The muscularis mucosa is a well-defined structure even in the developing fetal bowel and similar in structure to that seen in small bowel. In the junctional plane between the muscularis mucosa and the submucosa, primary lymphoid follicles are commonly present and the mucosa overlying them is attenuated. The dimpling of the mucosa over the lymphoid follicles produces the "innominate grooves" seen on double-contrast radiographic studies of the colon [385]. Though less marked than in older children, lymphoid follicles can be prominent in neonates [386]. Even in the neonatal infant, occasional lymphoid follicles may be seen in the vermiform appendix but usually only in infants near term. As in the small bowel the submucosa contains the larger vessels. The circular muscle is a complete layer, but the longitudinal muscle is aggregated into three bundles—the tenia coli—over most of the large bowel. They fuse together to form a complete layer in the appendix and rectum.

Since the anal canal is derived from both the cloaca and the proctodeum, the pectinate line, which defines the site of the anal membrane, is an important landmark. The line represents the approximate site of anastomosis between the branches of the superior, middle, and inferior hemorrhoidal arteries. Similarly, the region of the pectinate line represents a watershed between the cephalad areas that drain to the portal system of veins and pararectal lymph nodes, and the caudal areas that drain to the systemic veins and inguinal lymph nodes. The line also represents the approximate lower end of the internal sphincter muscles (supplied by the autonomic nervous system's nervi erigentes derived from S2–3 or 3–4) and the junction between the subcutaneous and superficial muscles of the external sphincter muscle (supplied by inferior hemorrhoidal nerves derived from S3–4). Above the pectinate line the mucosa is relatively insensitive, whereas below the line the mucosa is extremely sensitive. These observations were made over 60 years ago but their validity remains [387].

The sphincter mechanism consists of the puborectalis sling of the levator ani muscle (supplied by S3–4) and the internal and external sphincters. The internal sphincter is a condensation and concentration of the circular smooth muscle, arranged in a spiral fashion around the anal canal's upper two-thirds. Above, it is continuous with the circular muscle of the rectum. The external sphincter muscle has three components: the subcutaneous fibers, the superficial layer, and the deep bands. The subcutaneous muscle lies around the anal verge and does not contribute greatly to sphincteric integrity. The superficial layer surrounds the internal sphincter, acting as a spiral constrictor of the anal canal. The deepest muscle bundles merge above with the puborectalis sling. The external sphincter receives its nerve supply from S3–4 segments.

The anal glands are small aggregates of ducts, lined by transitional epithelium which open behind the cusps of the anal valves and pass into the submucosa, sometimes beyond the internal sphincter. The secretory component of the anal glands is a mucus-secreting epithelium arranged in a simple acinar fashion, surrounded by variable amounts of lymphoid tissue.

Congenital Anomalies of the Colon

While the most frequent malformations of the large bowel are found in the anorectal region, the colon may be affected by many of the abnormalities seen in the small bowel and a brief discussion of these lesions seems appropriate.

Malrotation

If rotation of the bowel has been incomplete, the position of the large bowel is abnormal. The cecum and vermiform appendix may, therefore, be found in several different areas of the abdomen, depending on the extent to which bowel rotation and growth have occurred. The most frequent aberration is the subhepatic cecum, but the cecum may be found in the left upper quadrant, and very rarely the entire colon may be found on the left side of the abdomen. A complete reversal of visceral situs can be seen in cases of complete *situs inversus*, and in syndromes such as Kartagener's triad where situs inversus is a feature [168]. Malrotation of the colon may be encountered frequently in association with urethral obstruction in utero [388], and in some infants with trisomy 13, trisomy 18, triploidy, Zellweger syndrome, de Lange syndrome, Down syndrome, and partial trisomy 10q syndrome [166–169].

Lack of Fixation of Large Bowel

It is not uncommon to find some mesocolon attached to the ascending and descending colon in addition to the normal sigmoid mesocolon, but a large redundant mesocolon is not normal. In many instances the condition is asymptomatic, but it may predispose the large bowel to volvulus, especially of the sigmoid colon. The preferential involvement of the sigmoid colon in volvulus of the large bowel may be related to the increasingly solid nature of its contents; the combined effects of a redundant mesocolon, active peristalsis, and inspissated contents could lead to torsion of the bowel around its vascular pedicle.

Stenosis and Atresia of Large Bowel

Although they are less frequent than similar lesions of the small bowel, stenosis and atresia do occur in the large bowel, and probably have the same ischemic origin [215]. Certainly the long-term follow-up of survivors of necrotizing enterocolitis in infancy yielded a high proportion (around 25%) of stenotic and atretic lesions, which included the large bowel, as well as sealed perforations [219].

Large Bowel Hamartomata

Most hamartomatous lesions of the large bowel rarely present in the neonatal period, but are mentioned here since they may occasionally be seen in autopsy material.

Hamartomatous ganglioneuromatous polyposis has now been described on many occasions, not only in association with von Recklinghausen neurofibromatosis but with juvenile polyposis [389, 390] or adenomatous polyps [391]. In neurofibromatosis, serosal lesions are common and diffuse plexiform involvement may be seen [392–394]. In multiple endocrine neoplasia 2B, ganglioneuromatous polyposis is well recognized [395, 396]. These lesions virtually never present in neonatal infants, but Berry et al [397] described a family with familial megacolon that mimicked Hirschsprung disease, while the bowel showed neuromatosis.

Hemangiomas may be seen as incidental findings, but may also cause bleeding, even when small [392]. Several types of vascular hamartomata may be a cause of rectal bleeding in the newborn period. Colonic mucosal lesions of diffuse neonatal angiomatosis [87], blue rubber-bleb nevus syndrome [398], and hereditary hemorrhagic telangiectasia [399] have been reported, but in these rare conditions, colonic involvement is only seen with extensive disease. When present, these lesions can bleed profusely, and repeated episodes of bleeding may be life-threatening. The commonest cavernous angiomas of the colon are usually localized, but the entire colon may be involved [400]. The abnormal vessels in larger lesions involve the pericolic and perirectal tissues, and resection of the lesion involves sacrificing the segment of gut.

Hamartomatous polyps of the epithelium (e.g., juvenile and Peutz-Jeghers syndrome) are not seen in neonates.

Congenital fibromatosis may involve the large bowel, causing obstruction in the neonatal period and potentially even leading to perforation [366, 401].

Metabolic Diseases and the Large Bowel

In meconium ileus with cystic fibrosis the colon may be small (microcolon, hypoplastic colon). Intussusception may be a complication in older infants, as may rectal prolapse and colonic perforation [402, 403]. Giant diverticula have been seen in some older patients with mucoviscidosis (Mancer, personal communication). In all patients, goblet cell hyperplasia and dilatation is a striking finding (Fig. 24.57), and inspissation of mucus in the appendix of a newborn or infant can be a useful diagnostic finding [404]. An extensive literature exists on the role of rectal biopsy in the diagnosis of lipid storage disorders, mucopolysaccharidoses, gangliosidoses, neuronal ceroid lipofuscinosis, and cystinosis [405–409], and a recent comprehensive review is provided by Lake [410]. The diagnosis in these disorders depends on identifying the characteristic storage cells or crystals (Fig. 24.58).

Duplications of the Large Bowel

Duplications of the large bowel fall into two separate categories [411]. By far, the more common variety consists of large, spherical, or sausage-shaped mucus-filled cystic structures, with a muscular wall of varying thickness and completeness, lying within the mesocolon parallel to the normal loop of bowel. Only rarely do these structures communicate with the lumen of the bowel. The vascular supply to the normal bowel usually runs on the walls of the anomalous gut, so surgical removal of the anomaly requires sacrificing normal bowel as well. Usually the duplication is localized, but rarely the entire colon may be affected. Even when extensive, these duplications are *not* associated with

abnormalities of the bladder and urethra and the anatomy of the lower rectum, anal canal, and sphincters is normal. This is in sharp contrast to the next category.

In the second, rarer variety of duplication of the colon the anorectal region is *always* involved and there are abnormalities of the bladder, müllerian structures, and external genitalia [377, 411, 412]. This complex of malformations affecting the urinary and anal passages is the subject of an excellent review by Stephens and Smith [377] who analyzed 32 cases in the literature. Females are affected more often than males (22:10), and while most cases presented in the newborn period or early childhood, 6 of the 32 presented in adult life (one at 62 years of age!). Depending on the number of duplicated ani, three types of lesions were identified: double perineal ani opening externally (12 cases), double ani with fistulae of one or both duplicated segments to the genitourinary tract (11 cases), and one external anus and one imperforate within the pelvis (9 cases). The female preponderance in the series is explained entirely by an increased number of cases in the first two categories; the

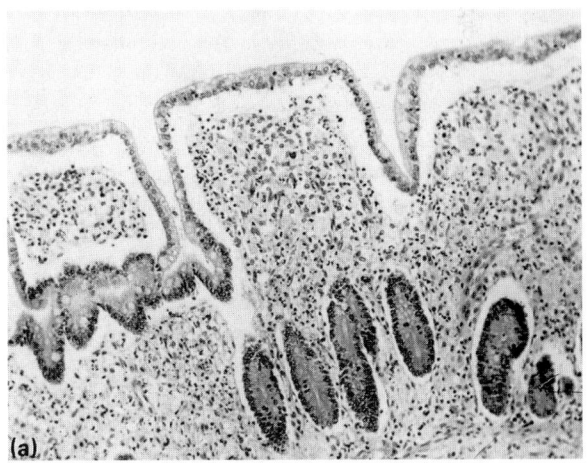

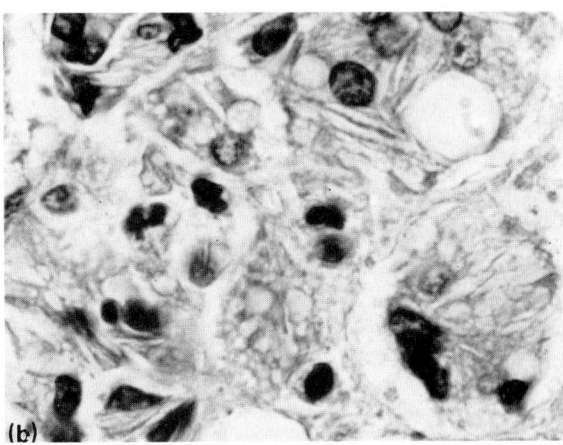

FIGURE 24.58.   (a) Colonic mucosa in a case of Wolman's disease shows wide separation of glands by foamy histiocytic cells. (b) At a higher magnification the characteristic cholesterol clefts are seen in the cytoplasma. (H&E, slide from a case of Dr. J. Hoogstraten, Childen's Hospital, Winnipeg, Manitoba.)

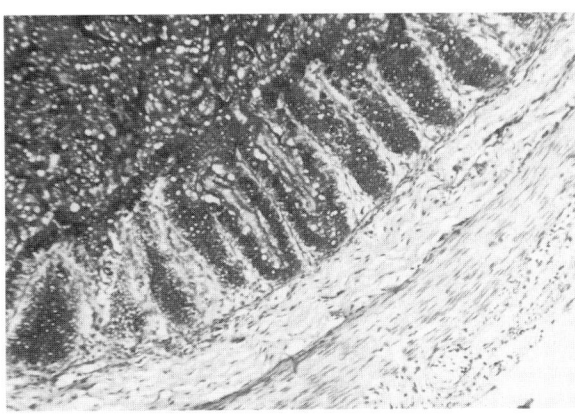

FIGURE 24.57.   The rectum in meconium ileus is plugged with darkly stained alcianophilic mucin that distends the gland units as well. Alcian Blue—Periodic acid-Schiff.

third category appears to be common in males. However, the patterns are not exclusive to any one sex. The bladder may be duplicated or septate with double urethral openings. There may be two uteri and duplication of the vagina. There may be two penes, or two clitorides, or combinations of the above. Anomalies outside the pelvis and pelvic area are frequent and were found in 14 of the cases; in five reports no structures outside the pelvis were mentioned, and 13 infants were otherwise normal. The associated abnormalities ranged from a single instance of Meckel's diverticulum [377], two examples of double-headed infants [413, 414], an example of double hemi-liver with duplication of the lumbar spine but absent sacrum and anterior myelomeningocele [415], and an infant with four lower limbs [416]. Somewhat surprisingly, associated renal anomalies were not frequent: there were two examples of horseshoe kidneys—one draining with a single ureter to the left half of a double bladder [417], the other with three ureters [418]; two cases with unilateral absence of a kidney [419, 420]; a single dysplastic kidney [421]; and a single example of unilateral bifid ureters draining a duplex kidney [415].

The anal component of the duplication may be separated from the normal bowel only by a thin septum, and in Van Zwalenburg's case [411] this septum had been resected in childhood. The anal openings may be on either side of the midline, but may also occur in the midline [422].

Micturition is normal in those infants without neurological problems or fistulae, and menstrual flow did not appear to be impeded in those patients who presented in adult life.

The extent of duplicated bowel varies from duplication of the entire alimentary system [413, 414], or duplication of the entire colon from the cecum onward (in 12 patients) or of the terminal ileum onward [419–421], with the remainder showing lesser degrees of duplication. Fourteen of the infants are specifically mentioned as having double vermiform appendices. There is even a single case of triplication of the entire large intestine where two patent colonic structures emptied into the rectum and a normal anus, while a large dilated cul-de-sac, paralleling the double-barreled colon, ended blindly at the rectosigmoid junction. All three "colons" received fecal material at the ileocecal valve. Ovaries were present but no uterus was seen and there was exstrophy of the bladder [423].

The simple (and fortunately commoner) variety of duplication, even though it may be extensive, is amenable (potentially) to simple surgical removal. Infants with multiple severe malformations affecting bladder, urethra, and anal canal pose more complex problems of management. Many of the malformation sequences are likely to be lethal; in the review by Stephens and Smith [377], there were two stillbirths and 11 deaths related to the malformations, despite attempted surgical correction. Recent reviews of this problem [48] have added more cases but the general pattern remains unchanged.

Duplications of the large bowel are therefore a heterogeneous collection of abnormalities that share the common feature of their proximity to the large bowel and an epithelial lining similar to that seen in the normal large bowel. The very different associated malformations of the two groups make it likely that duplications of the large bowel develop as a response to a variety of insults that may vary from case to case. In those cases with double-headed malformations an abnormal postzygotic event affecting the entire embryonic disk appears to be the most likely event. Infants with complicated malformation sequences in other organs as well as the hindgut have clearly been subjected to mutant stimuli affecting several developmental areas either simultaneously or in sequence.

The mode of development of the duplicated bowel is not known with certainty [424]. Lewis and Thyng [45] had described small diverticula and epithelial islands within the mesentery of the developing small gut in the embryo of pigs, rabbits, and humans, and their observations have been used to explain the development of isolated duplications of the bowel that are *not* associated with bladder anomalies [411]. However, these embryonic structures have not been seen in relation to the developing hindgut, and while they offer an attractive explanation for the development of duplications within the mesentery, they cannot be accepted unequivocally as the origin of the colonic lesions.

The development of an anomalous septum or sequestration of a tubular segment of bowel has been offered as an explanation for the extensive duplications of the colon [421], but it is difficult to see how this would explain an isolated segmental duplication. The usually extensive duplications of the bowel seen in the second group of cases (with multiple associated anomalies including the bladder) are, conceivably, due to a teratogenic insult that exerts its influence over an extensive segment of developing bowel, including the caudal section of midgut (i.e., terminal ileum and colonic segments), as well as the entire hindgut including the cloaca.

Anorectal Anomalies (Other Than Duplications)

As the development of the anal canal and rectum shows, a complex series of steps have to be coordinated before the cloaca can be divided into the ventral genitourinary structures and the dorsal anorectal structures. This involves the urorectal septum, the proctodeum, and in the female the development of the müllerian structures that are destined to form the female genital tract. If these steps become deranged in their sequence or are executed incompletely, many malformations may result.

To provide a rational approach to malformations in this area several attempts have been made at classifying the lesions. Historically, the earliest attempt was made by Ladd and Gross [425] who recognized four different types. This classification was adopted by most North American studies, but other classifications were developed in Europe and elsewhere [426–430]. The literature on the confusing subject of anorectal anomalies was confounded with several different systems of incompletely described nomenclature, making a true assessment of prognosis and the effects of surgical procedures almost impossible. In the 1960s, Stephens [431] summarized the extensive experience in the Royal Children's Hospital, Melbourne (Australia), and indicated the incomplete nature of all the classifications then current. This led to the development of an International Classification of Anorectal Anomalies that has received a wide measure of acceptance among pediatric surgeons [432]. The descriptive classification recognizes several discriminants which include the level of the abnormality in the anus or rectum, the site of the anal opening, the presence of fistulae, and the recording of the organs involved; it also distinguishes between the patterns seen in the two sexes. The descriptive terminology of the International Classification offers an accurate method for comparing the data from different areas (Table 24.1; Figs. 24.59 and 24.60). The classification does *not* include duplications with fistulae, nor does it include lesions derived from tailgut remnants or those associated with cloacal agenesis [375].

The level of the anomaly is defined by the situation of the lesion relative to the levator ani muscle. The importance of this anatomical landmark lies in the bearing that it has on reconstructive surgery and sphincteric function [377]. The classification of the site of the lesion does not have any embryological significance, other than the fact that all lesions above the line of the anal valves occur in structures derived from the cloaca.

Low Deformities

Low deformities are lesions occurring below the level of the levator ani musculature. They are subdivided into whether or not the anus is normally located. Lesions associated with a *normal sited* anus include the "completely covered anus" and "anal stenosis." The designation of lesions as being "covered" indicates that no opening can be seen. Some of these lesions may occur in both sexes. The anus may be *ectopically* situated at the site of the perineal body, and in both sexes two conditions are delineated: the anterior perineal anus and the covered anus with an anterior anocutaneous fistula. A more anteriorly sited anus in the female is known as the vestibular anus.

In females, additional "low" malformations are seen: 1) the anovulvar fistula where no anus is present and the anal canal opening may be hidden by a fold of the fourchette, and 2) the anovestibular fistula where the anus opens above the vestibule. The latter lesion is said to be the commonest variety of anal anomaly in the female [377].

From an embryological point of view these lesions are predominantly related to the incomplete or inappropriate development of the anal canal and anal membrane, coupled

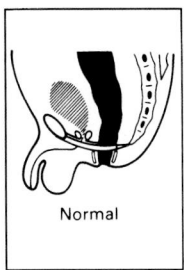 Normal	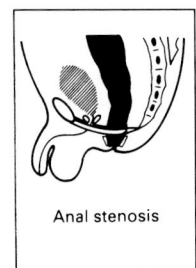 Anal stenosis	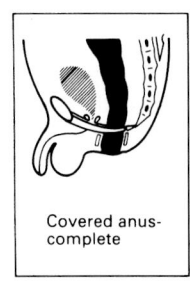 Covered anus-complete
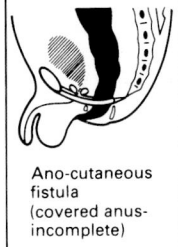 Ano-cutaneous fistula (covered anus-incomplete)	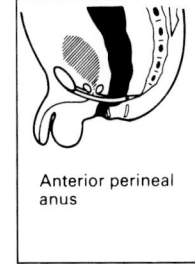 Anterior perineal anus	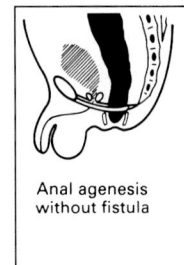 Anal agenesis without fistula
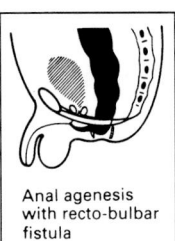 Anal agenesis with recto-bulbar fistula	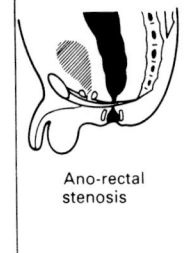 Ano-rectal stenosis	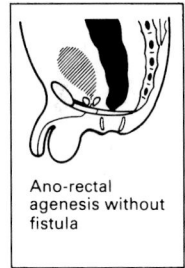 Ano-rectal agenesis without fistula
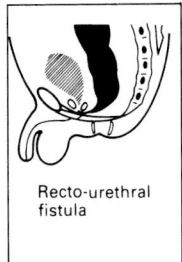 Recto-urethral fistula	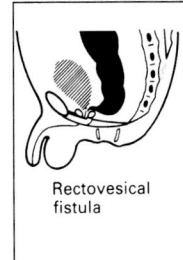 Rectovesical fistula	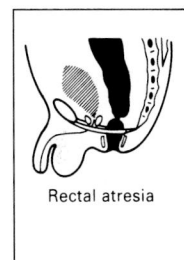 Rectal atresia

FIGURE 24.59. *Line drawings of the spectrum of anorectal anomalies as seen in male infants [377, 432].*

with prominent genital folds that contribute to the covered appearance. The persistence of the anal membrane in both covered anus and anal stenosis is stressed by Magnus and Stephens [433] (whose detailed study of serial sections of a case of complete covered anus includes the interesting observation that part of the blind rectum, above the anal canal, was covered by an epithelium that many would regard as being of transitional type). Anocutaneous, anovulvar, and anovestibular fistulae are associated with an upper anal canal of normal dimensions that tapers abruptly into a narrow tubular channel that runs forward to the ostia.

In these low abnormalities the sphincteric mechanisms are intact in both sexes, and these patients are continent.

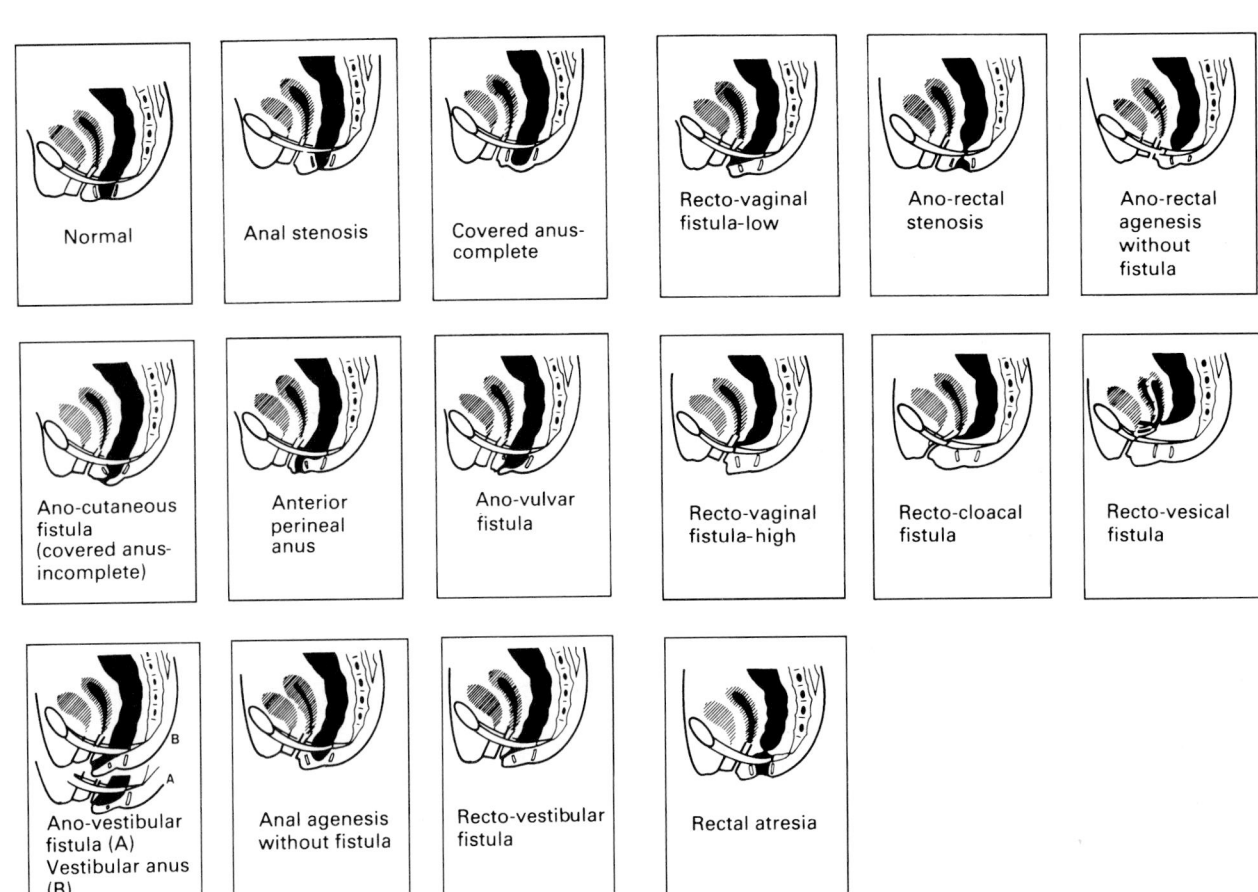

Intermediate Anomalies

Intermediate anomalies occur where the blind segment ends at the level of the levator ani muscle and at the level of a line joining the ischial tuberosities, as seen on a plain x-ray of the pelvis (ischial line) [377]. In males, three types of lesions are seen: anal agenesis without fistula formation, anal agenesis with rectobulbar fistula, and anorectal stenosis. In the female, the general pattern of malformation is along similar lines, but instead of a rectobulbar fistula a low rectovaginal or rectovestibular fistula may be seen. Anorectal stenosis is found in both sexes.

Anal agenesis—or, more correctly, anal canal agenesis—occurs almost exclusively in male infants [377]. The blind and dilated rectal pouch often has a small anterior protrusion at its lower end. In addition, the anal dimple may be flattened or absent. With rectobulbar fistula (a much less frequent anomaly than agenesis without fistula) the dilated rectal pouch leads through a fistulous track to the cavernous tissue of the urethral bulb. Some fistulae may be relatively wide; others may be threadlike. In both of the anomalies described above, the internal sphincter is absent, and the poorly formed external sphincter is not an effective control mechanism. In addition, the urethral floor is often very thin and friable and intimately attached to the anterior wall of the rectum. Penile hypospadias may occur in association with a rectobulbar fistula.

Anorectal stenosis occurring at a level 4 cm above the anus is an extremely rare lesion and must be distinguished from the incomplete covered low lesions mentioned earlier which are far more superficial. The bowel wall in this condition may show a tubular stenotic segment with variably increased amounts of connective tissue. Stephens and Smith [377] suggest that this lesion has an ischemic basis. The sphincters are intact in this anomalad.

In females, the low rectovaginal and rectovestibular fistula are usually associated with a normal appearing vulva and hymen. Usually the fistulae open in the lower third of the vagina and vestibule and in the midline. With low rectovaginal fistulae the rectal opening into the vagina is usually wide, but the opening of a rectovestibular fistula may be a narrow, threadlike tube running downward and anteriorly from the dilated rectal pouch. The internal sphincter is not present and the external sphincter is as poorly defined as it is in males with rectobulbar fistulae.

Table 24.1.   International classification of anorectal abnormalities

	Male	Female
Low (Translevator)	1. Normal and site 　a) Anal stenosis 　b) Covered anus complete 2. Perineal site 　a) Anocutaneous fistula 　　(covered anus incomplete) 　b) Anterior perineal anus	1. Same 　a) Same 　b) Same 2. Same 　a) Same 　b) Same 3. At vulvar site 　a) Anovulvar fistula 　b) Anovestibular fistula 　c) Vestibular anus
Intermediate	1. Anal agenesis 　a) Without fistula 　b) With rectobulbar fistula 　c) Rectovaginal fistula (low) 2. Anorectal stenosis	1. Same 　a) Same 　b) Rectovestibular fistula 2. Same
High (Supralevator)	1. Anorectal agenesis 　a) Without fistula 　b) With rectourethral fistula 　c) With rectovesical fistula 　d) Rectovesical fistula 2. Rectal atresia	1. Same 　a) Same 　b) With rectovaginal fistula (high) 　c) Rectocloacal fistula 2. Same
	Both Sexes	
Miscellaneous	Imperforate anal membrane Cloacal exstrophy Others	

Source: Santulli TV, Kieswetter WB, Bill AH Jr [432].

High Malformations

High malformations are a group of anomalies characterized by the presence of a blind rectal pouch with or without a fistulous track, above the level of the levator ani muscle's puborectalis sling. In addition to the blind rectal pouch, the upper anal canal is absent as well. In the male, several patterns are seen. In the main group, that of *anorectal agenesis*, the large bowel ends blindly at the level of a line joining the lower end of the pubis with the coccyx, as seen on a plain x-ray of the pelvis (the pubococcygeal line), and there is no anal dimple. Anorectal agenesis may exist without a fistula but there is usually either a rectovesical or rectourethral fistula. Less frequently in rectal atresia, an anal canal is connected by a membranous or string-like cord of tissue with a blind rectal pouch that may even lie above the pubococcygeal line. Several workers believe this malformation to be a postischemic lesion [428, 434, 435].

In anorectal agenesis the internal and external sphincter muscles are not formed. In rectal atresia the sphincteric mechanisms are intact.

In females, anorectal agenesis without fistula or with a rectovesical fistula may be present. These anomalies are identical to those seen in the male. However, in females several other anomalies may be present in association with anorectal agenesis. A rectocloacal fistula may be found where the rectal pouch, vagina, and urethra all empty into a common cloacal channel with a single perineal opening. In addition, high rectovaginal fistulae with openings near the posterior fornix may be present. Variations on rectocloacal and rectovaginal fistulae of high type are encountered and may be the source of considerable confusion [436]. Much of the confusion centers around rectocloacal fistula formation. In some cases of this anomaly the cloaca may appear to be a direct continuation of the vagina, whereas in others it may appear to be a direct continuation of the urethra. However, if a single perineal opening drains all these viscera, it satisfies the criteria for a cloacal opening, and any lesion with such a pattern is best regarded as a rectocloacal fistula.

Rectal atresia has been found in females as well as males. As in the male, rectal atresia is the only category of high malformation that is associated with an intact sphincteric mechanism.

This review of the commoner malformations indicates the importance of the level of the lesion and the complex nature of fistulae associated with anal anomalies. The International Classification scheme [432] is valuable and consistent, but not complete. The "Miscellaneous" and "Other" categories (see Table 24.1) [432] include imperforate anal membrane and anal membrane stenosis in both sexes, where the distinction from complete covered anus and incomplete covered anus is based solely on the relatively thinner membranes in the former pair of conditions. Stephens and Smith [377] also include perineal grooves and canals in their classification, lesions not described by others.

Other rare abnormalities, which may be found in a bewildering number of combinations, are well outlined and summarized by Stephens and Smith [377]. These vary from double fistulae (rectourethral and rectovesical, rectovesical and rectoperineal), fistulae into ectopia vesicae, and lesions as complicated as the vesicointestinal fissure or exstrophy of the cloaca [437].

In vesicointestinal fissure the bladder, vagina (if present), and intestine all open onto the anterior abdominal wall [401]. The bladder is usually bifid and in the central opening there is a double-barrel opening of bowel, the rostral opening of which discharges intestinal contents while the lower end is usually blind. No hindgut or anus is present, but variable lengths of colon may be present. An omphalocele may be present above the exstrophy. There are often multiple renal anomalies such as hydronephrosis or dysplasia. The lesion is seen in both sexes; in males there is a high incidence of cryptorchidism, and the phallus is duplicated. Magnus [438] has suggested that the lesion is due to a strangulation of the physiological hernia of the midgut combined with another separate insult to the hindgut. Clearly, the defect must involve the development of the anterior abdominal wall at an early stage of development, and many of the features are similar to those seen in the "OEIS" syndrome [439] (Table 24.2).

The embryologic explanation for the main anomalies outlined here centers on the urorectal septum. All the anomalies in the male can be explained by aberrations in the fusion of the urorectal septum with the cloacal membrane, or in the disordered formation of the urorectal septum. The anomalies in the female are somewhat more complex since the müllerian ducts develop not just as offshoots of the anterior urinary chamber but within the urorectal septum initially [373].

The relative incidence of the various types of abnormalities is difficult to ascertain. Reported series, particularly in recent years, might lead one to believe that the very rare anomalies are commoner than may be the case. Large series collected in different centers are sometimes difficult to compare due to the several classifications used. The Melbourne series of Stephens and Smith [377] suggests that anal anomalies are commoner than rectal anomalies in male

infants (95 to 64) and that covered anus with anocutaneous fistula (37) and covered anal stenosis (23) are the commonest anal lesions. Rectourethral fistula with rectal agenesis was the commonest single rectal high anomaly in males (44 cases). An analysis of 92 female patients showed that anal anomalies were commoner than rectal anomalies (59 to 28) with anovestibular fistula by far the commonest lesion (22 cases). Of rectal anomalies, rectocloacal fistula and rectovaginal fistulae (both high and intermediate) were equally frequent (8 cases each). Stephens and Smith's [377] analysis of the data from eight other authors, reclassified according to the International Classification, suggests that the Melbourne series offers a good approximation of the general pattern seen throughout the world.

Agenesis of the Cloacal Membrane

Agenesis of the cloacal membrane is an unusual malformation sequence in which neither an anal opening nor a urethral opening is present, and in females the vagina ends blindly. The rectum, urethra, and vagina end blindly or empty into a chamber of varying depth that does *not* communicate with the surface. The infants do not have a perineal body or median perineal raphe, indicating that the most probable primary abnormality is agenesis of the cloacal membrane. Robinson and Tross [375] provide a detailed description of five infants with this pattern of anomaly, and cite reports of seven other affected infants between the years 1926 and 1980. Choisy [440] reviewed several cases from the early European literature. Others have seen isolated cases or small series in different North American centers [401, 441, 442]. Many other cases probably go unreported. This lesion has only been seen in autopsy material, and detailed dissections of these infants have yielded a remarkably precise and consistent pattern of anomalies that Robinson and Tross [375] have classified into 1) primary malformations of the cloacal membrane, and 2) deformations of the other organs due to the effects of external compression of the fetus and internal distension.

The primary malformations associated with the absence of a cloacal membrane include incomplete division of the cloaca (2 of 5 patients), blind termination of the rectum and bladder, and lack of a perineal body or median perineal raphe (all patients). The agenesis of the cloacal membrane is accompanied by failure to form a vaginal vestibule and labia minora (in female infants) or anus. Distal urethral development was rudimentary in all and there was no connection with the exterior. All infants (male and female) had a rudimentary phallic structure. The deformation sequences included massive bladder and ureteric distension with hydronephrosis and renal dysplasia in all except one infant with renal agenesis and bladder hypoplasia. Other deformities included cephalad displacement of the massively dilated rectum, distension of the abdominal wall in all cases (leading to rupture in one infant), and compression deformities of the limbs. In the three females the uterus and vagina were also affected, with vaginal duplication in one case or vaginal

T a b l e 2 4 . 2 .   Anal anomalies in multiple malformation syndromes

Syndrome	Other Core Anomalies	References
1. Rear (Townes) syndrome	Radial and thumb anomalies	537
	Ear anomalies, renal anomalies	538
2. Schinzel syndrome	Ulnar deletion of hand, laryngeal stenosis, microphallus	539
3. Kaufman Syndrome	Postaxial polydactyly, vaginal atresia, congenital heart disease	540
4. "C" syndrome	Postaxial polydactyly/syndactyly, fusion of metopic suture, multiple frenula; genu recurvatum; hypoplastic kidneys	541
5. "FG" syndrome	Broad thumbs, syndactyly, agenesis of corpus callosum, congenital heart disease, megacolon	544
6. Meckel-Gruber syndrome	Postaxial polydactyly, renal dysplasia, hepatic fibrosis, occipital encephalocele, congenital heart disease, microphthalmus	543, 544
7. Noonan-Saldino syndrome	Postaxial polydactyly, renal dysplasia, vaginal atresia, microphallus, congenital heart disease, hemivertebrae, chest abnormalities	545
8. Cryptophthalmos (Fraser syndrome)	Cryptophthalmos, laryngeal atresia/stenosis, renal agenesis/dysplasia, cleft lip/palate, deafness, syndactyly	546, 547
9. Laurence-Moon-Bardet-Biedl syndrome	Obesity, retinitis pigmentosa, postaxial polydactyly, syndactyly, nephritis and renal anomalies, hypogonadism, mental retardation	548
10. "G" syndrome (Opitz-Frias syndrome)	Short limbs, congenital heart disease, hypospadias, hypertelorism, laryngeal cleft	549, 550
11. Opitz syndrome [BBB syndrome]	Hypospadias, hypertelorism, cryptorchidism	551
12. Johanson-Blizzard syndrome	Hypothyroidism, deafness, hypoplastic alae nasi, absent permanent teeth, microcephaly, pancreatic insufficiency, scalp defects	552, 553
13. "4H-RALPH-MISHAP"	Hypothalamic hamartoblastoma, syndactyly, polydactyly, hypopituitarism, microphallus, abnormal lung lobulation	467
14. OEIS complex	Omphalocele, extrophy of bladder, spinal abnormalities	439
15. VATER complex + single umbilical artery	Vertebral, cardiac, tracheoesophageal, renal, and radial abnormalities	33, 554
16. Apert syndrome	Irregular craniostenosis, cleft palate, syndactyly, fused fingers, congenital heart disease	555
17. Thanatophoric dwarfism	Thanatophoric dwarfism, cloverleaf skull, pulmonary hypoplasia	168
18. Caudal dysplasia syndrome (caudal regression)	Variable absence of limb structures, absent external genitalia, absent internal genitalia, limb fusion, sacral vetebral abnormalities	456, 457
19. Familial hemisacrum I and II	Hemisacrum, anterior meningocele, presacral teratoma	464, 465
20. 13q⁻ syndrome	Absent thumbs, eye anomalies, retinoblastoma, holoprosencephaly, hypertelorism	169
21. Trisomy 18 syndrome	Polydactyly, syndactyly, meningomyelocele, renal dysplasia, cardiac defects, cryptorchidism	169
22. Cat's-eye syndrome (trisomy 22)	Colobomata of eye, hypertelorism, cardiac defects, renal agenesis	168, 169
23. Fetal hydantoin effect	Rib anomalies, hypertelorism, umbilical and inguinal hernias, hip dislocation, cryptorchidism, duodenal atresia	556
24. Monozygous/Conjoined malformation sequences	Gastroschisis, porencephaly, aplasia cutis	168, 557
25. Sling pulmonary artery	Abnormal trachea and bronchi, abnormal aortic arch, pulmonary artery abnormalities	558

hypoplasia and partial incorporation of the vaginal wall into the bladder in the other cases; bicornuate atrophic uteri with slit-like lumina were found in all three females.

Not surprisingly, anomalies in other sites were present. Three infants had sacrococcygeal dimples; one had multiple spina bifida of lumbar, thoracic, and sacral vertebrae. All infants had abnormal numbers of umbilical vessels. In four infants, a single umbilical artery was present while in the fifth infant one artery was hypoplastic. Single examples of rectal duplication, esophageal atresia, and tracheoesophageal fistula, ventricular septal defect, and septum primum defect were present.

The initial cluster of cases occurred over a 7½ month period in a relatively localized area of northeastern Ohio, and Robinson and Tross [375] advanced a plausible case for their suggestion that exposure to a single drug available in numerous proprietary, non-prescription cold and cough remedies may have been implicated in their particular group of cases. Whatever the etiology, this important series of cases illustrates the crucial importance of the cloacal membrane,

and the bizarre pattern of malformations that may result when the development of the urorectal septum and the cloacal membrane is not coordinated. Our own studies of a series of 11 cases [401, 442] have included infants with the OEIS syndrome [439] and hemisacrum anomalies, and were notable for the almost inevitable association of spinal and vertebral anomalies.

Spinal Defects and Anorectal Anomalies

Many of the anomalies discussed in the preceding sections may be associated with abnormalities of the lower half of the skeleton, especially spina bifida or hemivertebrae. Two important subgroups of anorectal anomalies warrant special discussion: the lesions associated with defects of the sacrum and those associated with caudal dysplasia (or caudal regression) and homologous anomalies [443].

Abnormalities of the sacral vertebrae, either in the form of large defects in bifid vertebrae or smaller defects in hemivertebrae, may coexist with a variety of hindgut enteric fistulae. Bale [374] has provided an outstanding review of these lesions based on material in the Royal Alexandra Hospital for Children in Sydney, Australia. Loops of hindgut may herniate through sacral vertebral defects to open directly onto the skin surface with the distal limb of the loop opening at the anus, or the hindgut may end at the skin surface with the anus being imperforate. Rectal duplications associated with an otherwise normal rectum and anus are also described. Portions of a rectal duplication may persist as either presacral, intraspinal, or postsacral enteric cysts, or a fistula between the rectum and the postsacral skin may be present. These uncommon malformations all pose the hazard of superadded meningitis in addition to the neurological and anorectal deficits that may be present.

The structure of these hindgut malformations varies. They usually have a muscular wall of variable thickness and an epithelial lining that may contain epithelium identifiable as either colonic, small intestinal [51], gastric [444], or mixed with some structures resembling esophageal and bronchial epithelium [445, 446]. Bale [374] describes tissue resembling pancreas in one instance. The presence of aberrant cartilaginous and adipose tissue nodules [447, 448] has been noted. These enteric sinuses may be associated with a presacral teratoma [449], but obviously many of these hindgut-derived presacral cysts may be mistaken for a teratoma at first [450].

The pathogenesis of these lesions is believed to be related to adhesions between ectoderm and entoderm developing in the caudal end of the early embryonic disk. This interferes with notochordal development and leads to splitting of the notochord to bypass the adhesion. In turn, the notochordal split is associated with a defect of mesenchyme that allows the endodermal and ectodermal adhesions to persist. This view [56, 444, 445] has gained considerable acceptance and is often described as "the split notochord syndrome" [446, 450]. An alternative view that the lesions are teratomatous in nature [445] should not be dismissed out of hand, however. Bale [374] cites an unusual case of a teenager with a presacral enteric cyst, presumably present since birth, who developed teratoma at the same site a year later. In addition to the already cited example of a presacral teratoma with an enteric sinus [447], Bentley and Smith [52] include a case of a hindgut malformation associated with a postsacral dermoid with a rudimentary tooth! There is a relationship between teratogenesis and oncogenesis in all sites [451], but nowhere is the overlap greater than in the sacrococcygeal area.

Caudal Dysplasia (Regression) and Anorectal Anomalies

The syndrome of caudal dysplasia is associated with sacral vertebral anomalies, abnormalities in the pelvis and lower limbs, and other anomalies such as meningomyelocele, anal and genital defects, absent fibula, and short femora [452, 453]. The upper limbs are rarely involved. Congenital anomalies of the heart and great vessels and tracheoesophageal fistula may be noted [454, 455]. Its most extreme form is sirenomelia [456, 457]. The mothers of affected infants may

show minor sacral anomalies [458]. In this unusual constellation of anomalies, anal malformations figure prominently and several variants exist. The commonest lesions recorded are complete covered anus with or without fistula, and rectal atresia, but any of the many varieties of anorectal anomalies described earlier may be seen [456].

The justification for the separate discussion of this group of anorectal anomalies is provided by the fact that many cases of caudal dysplasia may be associated with maternal diabetes or prediabetes [452, 453]. Wilson and Vallance-Owen [459] have suggested that the syndrome is related to the presence of insulin antagonists in diabetics. Landauer and Clark [460] described the development of a syndrome superficially similar to caudal dysplasia called "rumplessness" in chick embryos who received insulin. This argument was used to incriminate insulin therapy of gestational diabetics in the development of caudal dysplasia, but the occurrence of caudal dysplasia in prediabetic women argues against such a relationship. Studies in fetal rats suggest that fetal insulin production may have a role in the production of sacral defects [461]. It is unlikely that these experimental results can be applied to humans, since the dysmorphic lesions that are present indicate an intrauterine insult that predates the onset of fetal insulin production (which normally only begins at week 10). The exact mechanisms that predispose infants of diabetic and prediabetic mothers to develop caudal dysplasia is unknown at present, but the association is important [458]. The occurrence of very rare familial cases of caudal dysplasia syndrome [462, 463] suggests that genetic factors may also play a "conditioning" role in the development of caudal dysplasia. The overall low incidence of caudal dysplasia among infants of diabetic mothers (even though greater than in the nondiabetic population) and the rare occurrence of familial caudal dysplasia have led Welch and Aterman [458] to suggest that a combination of both a "diabetogenic trend" and unrelated genes coding for skeletal differentiation is required for the fully developed caudal dysplasia syndrome. These two factors may both be related to genes of the HLA-DR system.

A group of syndromes that are superficially very similar to the caudal dysplasia syndrome are grouped together under the heading of "familial sacral dysgenesis." These disorders include the Cohn-Bay-Nielsen syndrome of familial hemisacrum (type 1) and the Ashcraft syndrome of familial hemisacrum (type 2) [458, 464, 465]. In familial hemisacrum I there is unilateral hemisacrum affecting all members of the family. Anal stenosis and rarely complete covered anus was seen in some of the affected siblings in some subsequent sibships. These affected members also had an anterior meningocele, and the inheritance pattern suggests an autosomal dominant gene. In Ashcraft syndrome [465] the unilateral hemisacrum is associated with presacral teratomata (sometimes malignant) rather than anterior meningocele, but the distinction between the two hemisacral syndromes may not be an absolute one. Anal stenosis and complete covered anus were seen in the signal family.

Anorectal Abnormalities and Multiple Malformation

Anorectal abnormalities are an important component of numerous multiple malformation syndromes (see Table 24.2). It would be pointless to attempt to discuss them all or the multiplicity of fine points that differentiate between them. Detailed references are cited in most standard works on malformation syndromes [169], and many are available in the excellent reviews by Pinsky [466] and Hall et al [467]. Although this discussion is not complete, and could not attempt to be, certain general comments should be made.

There appears to be an increasing number of syndromes, while simultaneously several previously separate syndromes have been collapsed into new entities. Since the pattern of inheritance of these disorders is unknown in most cases and can vary from autosomal dominant to autosomal recessive, to X-linked, to sporadic, it is mandatory that individual cases are not placed arbitrarily in any one category. Only if the "fit" is good with a detailed study of all the organ systems and a karyotype has been obtained should cases be assigned to any single category. Some syndromes appear to merge with each other (e.g., Opitz-Frias and Opitz syndrome—see Table 24.2, nos. 10 and 11); many overlap with each other (e.g., the single umbilical artery–associated malformation sequences overlap with VATER association—see Table 24.2). Finally, some of these malformation syndromes may result from a preventable teratogenic influence (e.g., fetal hydantoin effect). The development of banks of dysmorphic syndromes, accessible by computer and electronic media, has probably rendered many of these lists obsolete. We use the GDB-DMIM database of Johns Hopkins University, and "POSSUM" of the Royal Children's Hospital of Melbourne. Both resources are invaluable.

In sirenomelia the absence of the hindgut derivatives, accompanied by renal agenesis, has been explained in part by the fact that the single umbilical artery that is present arises high on the dorsal aorta. This abnormal vessel represents the continuation of the dorsal aorta (and may be a persistent vitelline artery). The distal vessels are rudimentary at best, and it has been said that this may lead to agenesis of the organs they should supply in more normal circumstances. Though it is attractive, this explanation is unduly simplistic [401].

Hirschsprung Disease and Related Disorders

Since it was first described in 1887 by Harald Hirschsprung [468], the problem of aganglionic megacolon has attracted a considerable degree of attention. However, it was only when Whitehouse and Kernohan [469] and Zuelzer and Wilson [470] reported the absence of ganglion cells in the spastic bowel that a proper understanding of the pathogenesis of this disease entity began to emerge. This concept of aganglionosis as the basis for Hirschsprung disease was established, even more firmly, when Bodian et al [471] were able to demonstrate that other causes of megacolon did not have abnormalities of autonomic innervation. This enabled Hirschsprung disease to be separated from other causes of megacolon.

The disease presents in a neonate with either a prolonged delay in the passage of meconium or overt obstruction. Older infants may present with abdominal distension and severe chronic constipation. Ehrenpreis' monograph [472], based on a very extensive experience and literature review, indicates an incidence of approximately 1:5000 live births, but there is considerable variation in the incidence of the disease based on a review of different reports [473]. An overwhelming male preponderance (in excess of 80% of cases) is known to exist in affected infants. Cases with extensive aganglionosis of the colon (long segment disease) and familial cases are also described; in these rarer variants the males and females are more equally affected [474]. Sibling involvement occurs in about 4% of cases, but as Passarge [475] has shown, only 2.7% of the sibs of male index cases are affected, while 7.2% of sibs of female index patients are affected. The inheritance pattern of Hirschsprung disease cannot, therefore, be explained solely on the basis of one form or another of simple Mendelian inheritance, and must be multifactorial.

The proximal colon in Hirschsprung disease is distended, often massively, while the distal colon is usually spastic and has a smaller luminal diameter (microcolon). A transitional zone of varying length is usually present, and here there is progressive bowel dilatation from below upwards. This characteristic appearance can be demonstrated by barium enema and is virtually pathognomonic of the disease. The appearances at surgery and radiology may be modified considerably if an enterocolitis supervenes [288], which often is associated with bowel dilatation.

The length of the "microcolon" is related to the degree of aganglionosis present and helps to classify the disease. Most frequently, the aganglionic segments of bowel are limited to the anal canal, rectum, and sigmoid and this "limited segment" disease produces the classic clinical picture; approximately 80% of cases fall into this category [380]. "Ultrashort" segment disease is a term used to describe involvement confined to the distal rectal segment and the anus. This category is the most difficult to diagnose clinically and pathologically, and consequently estimates of its frequency vary. "Subtotal" involvement is a term used to designate extension of aganglionosis above the sigmoid colon; "total" or "long segment" disease refers to involvement of the entire colon. Finally, there are cases with extension into the small intestine, even reaching the duodenum [476].

Pathology of Hirschsprung Disease

The essential abnormality of Hirschsprung disease is the absence of ganglion cells in the myenteric and submucosal plexuses and the presence of thicker *preganglionic* fibers replacing the thinner nerve strands of these plexuses. The abnormal fibers have a thicker perineural sheath, with demonstrable collagen and parallel orientation of Schwann cells (Fig. 24.61). These preganglionic fibers are cholinergic and can be demonstrated to contain acetylcholinesterase (AChE), thereby forming the basis of a method of diagnosis. These thick nerve trunks can be demonstrated in the submucosa in mucosal suction biopsies [380], and AChE staining shows in addition a thick coarse network of fibers around the muscularis mucosa and mucosa [477, 478] (Fig. 24.62). Nerve fibers and ganglion cells can be demonstrated using immunoperoxidase techniques with antibodies directed against S-100 protein and neuron-specific enolase. These techniques may be useful in very immature infants with poorly defined ganglion cells, but are no substitute for AChE staining, since they do not detect the *qualitative* difference that is the hallmark of Hirschsprung disease.

Full-thickness biopsies are still used by many surgeons, and while submucosal suction biopsies are usually adequate in experienced hands (both surgical and pathological), there are many surgeons who vary their choice of biopsy with full thickness biopsies at laparatomy and mucosal biopsies at the bedside.

Problems encountered in the diagnosis of Hirschsprung disease in newborns are legion. Apart from the technical problems encountered in cutting frozen sections of very small (and often inadequate) mucosal biopsies, it may be difficult to identify ganglion cells in the immature infant. Problems are invariably encountered when the mucosal biopsy is taken from a site in close proximity to the anal canal. In this region there is a normal submucosal "hypoganglionosis," but the ganglion cells in Auerbach's plexus extend farther down (in the muscle layer) than the ganglion cells in Meissner's plexus [479]. This zone of physiological hypoganglionosis extends to about 1 cm above the pectinate line. Yet it is precisely this area that must be biopsied if cases of ultrashort segment disease are to be diagnosed. Matters are not helped by the fact that this is an area where a precisely directed mucosal biopsy is difficult to achieve [480].

Hypoganglionosis

Weinberg [380] defines hypoganglionosis as a marked reduction in the number of ganglion cells within the enteric

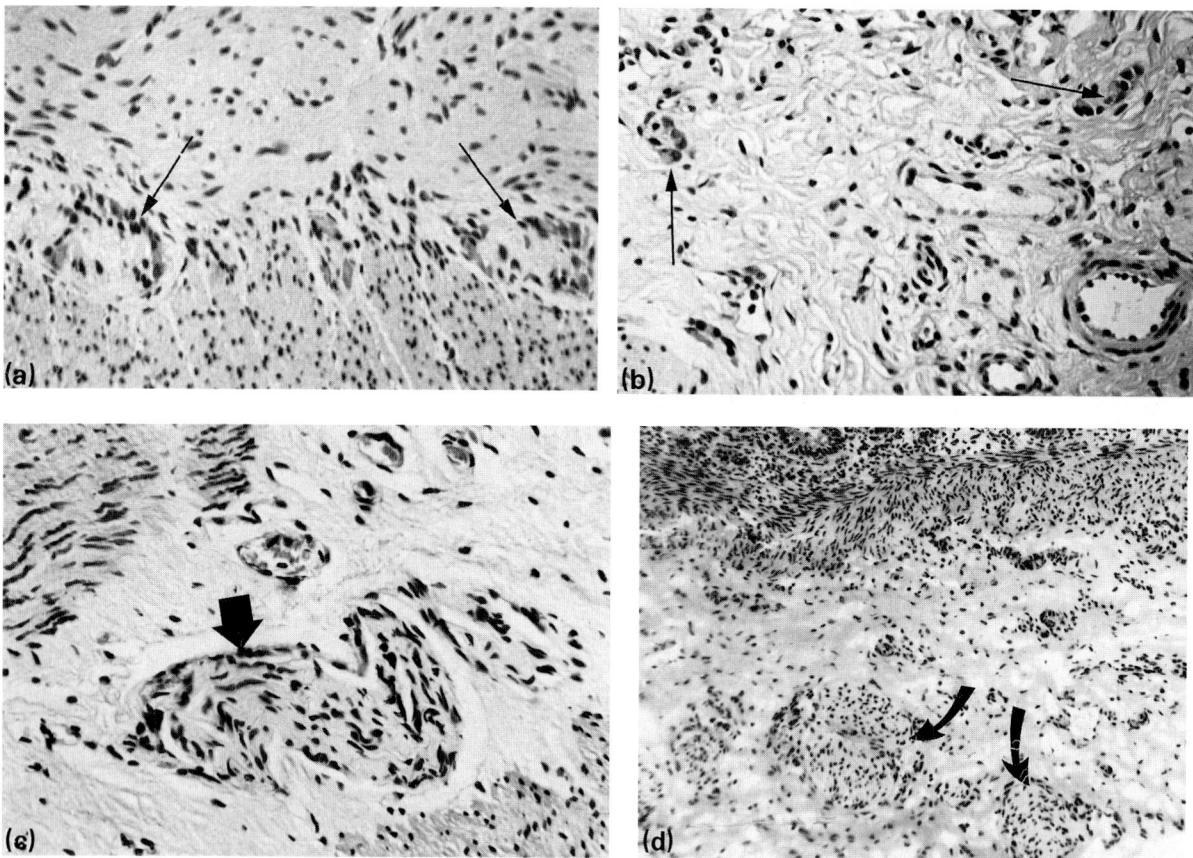

FIGURE 24.61.   *Hirschsprung disease. (a) Normal myenteric plexus and ganglia (arrows). (b) Normal submucosal ganglia (arrows). (c) Abnormal thick nerve trunks (arrow) in aganglionic bowel in intermuscular plane (compare with a). (d) Abnormal thick nerve bundles in submucosa (arrows).*

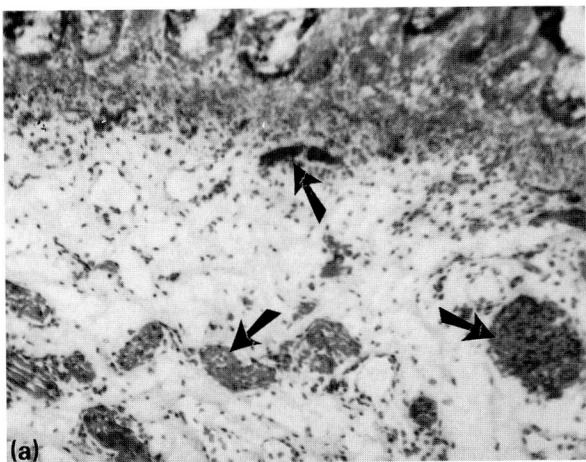

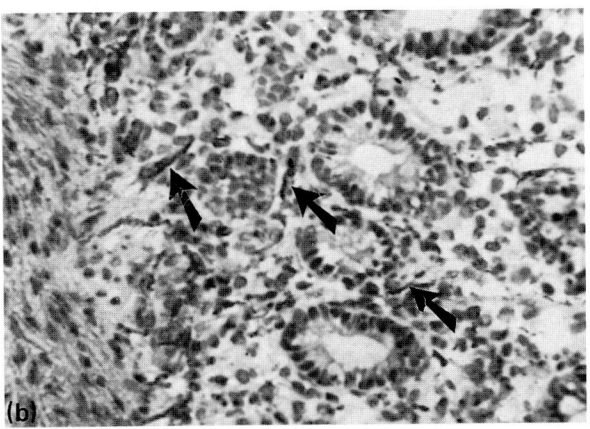

FIGURE 24.62. *(a) Frozen section stained for cholinesterase activity shows thick, positively stained nerve trunks in submucosa of aganglionic segment (arrows). (b) Frozen section showing nerve fibers (arrows) stained positively for cholinesterase in mucosa of aganglionic segment.*

plexuses; the original definition is not precise. The data of Smith [384] offer the potential for a more accurate definition in the future. The "circuit diagram" approach of Wells et al [383] demonstrates elegantly that the plexuses are designed to remain functional despite considerable distension (a situation when ganglion cell density per mm of colon might be expected to decrease).

Despite these caveats, relative hypoganglionosis exists in the transitional zone of the bowel between the aganglionic and normally innervated colonic segments. In this area there may be small, widely separated ganglion cells that do not appear to form ganglia. Within the transitional zone there is a gradual increase (from distal to proximal ends) in the numbers of cells in the myenteric plexus and (higher up and later) in the submucosal plexus. Occasionally, long transitional zones are found in association with relatively short zones of distal aganglionosis. Rarely, hypoganglionosis has been the sole abnormality in infants presenting with otherwise classical Hirschsprung disease but without any area of

aganglionosis. However, as Weinberg [380] points out, cases of hypoganglionosis have to be accepted with considerable caution. Many cases of hypoganglionosis are accompanied by illustrations of remarkably normal-appearing ganglia, suggesting that the lesion may have been misdiagnosed.

The absence of ganglion cells and the presence of abundant cholinergic fibers helps to explain the distal colonic spasm in Hirschsprung disease, since denervated smooth muscle is prone to spasm in response to minimal stimulation. Gannon et al [481] have drawn attention to the importance of adrenergic innervation of the bowel in Hirschsprung disease. The presence of adrenergic fibers may be expected to contribute to the spasm, since even though the adrenergic fibers normally exert an inhibitory effect on smooth muscle contraction, this is achieved by acting on ganglion cells first. Burnstock [482] has proposed a separate subgroup of "purinergic" inhibitory neurons which are, of course, not present in aganglionosis. Finally, the role of the numerous peptide hormones, especially vasoactive intestinal peptide, which can be produced by the abnormal nerve fibers in Hirschsprung disease, has never been adequately assessed. The role of the noncholinergic, nonadrenergic mediators probably relates to internal communication between the various groups of ganglia and plexuses [410].

The pathophysiology of the colonic spasm in Hirschsprung disease has been studied using rectal manometry, and the abnormal muscle activity has been used as an aid to diagnosis of aganglionosis. Adherents of this investigative tool appear completely convinced of its value in diagnosis. Others have experienced an unacceptably large number of false-positive and false-negative results [483].

Zonal Aganglionosis

The term *zonal aganglionosis* is somewhat of a misnomer: most of the affected cases had a small segment of normally innervated bowel, usually in the ascending colon and vicinity of the hepatic flexure, in otherwise classical long segment aganglionosis. This runs against the usual pattern of craniocaudal migration, and consequently, the existence of this condition has been questioned by many authors. Yunis et al [381] reviewed the world literature and accepted two cases in the earlier literature with well-documented zonal aganglionosis to which they added four cases of their own. Kapur et al have now updated this experience [484].

These infants present with classic symptoms of Hirschsprung disease. The distal colon is found to be aganglionic, and a site of normally innervated bowel is found for the colostomy. The subsequent course is fairly characteristic. The colostomy does not function postoperatively, leading to a second laparotomy to "release adhesions." Despite a relative lack of adhesions the bowel appears obstructed, and in a personally studied case, an incidental appendectomy (which revealed aganglionosis in the appendix) provided the major diagnostic clue. In that case a terminal ileostomy was required to relieve the obstruction [484].

Kapur et al [484] have suggested that this phenomenon occurs due to an unusually persistent block in neuroblast migration in the area of the ileocecal junction. Based on Kapur's work [3] with transgenic mice destined to develop short-segment aganglionosis (Ls/Ls, homozygous lethal spotted mice), there is a transient period when the vicinity of the cecum and ascending colon is not colonized by neuroblasts, but the distal colon is. A persistence of this stage, followed by a lack of any distal migration, could be the basis for the presence of an innervated zone in the middle of an otherwise classic area of aganglionic bowel.

MacIver and Whitehead [485] reported four infants in whom zones of aganglionosis were seen in apparently normal bowel, and reviewed the earlier literature for rare cases with similar pathology. This report has engendered considerable controversy and even skepticism, but reports of acquired aganglionosis with progressive ganglion cell loss [486–489] would suggest that the final chapters on aganglionosis and variants remain to be written. These "skip" lesions, whether of ganglion cells being found in a zone of aganglionosis or aganglionic stretches of bowel in otherwise normally innervated bowel, lead one to suggest that ganglion cells can be destroyed once formed. Dimmick and Bove [382] reported a particularly intriguing case of cytomegalovirus infection associated with aganglionosis, and reviewed other possible causes of "acquired" aganglionosis. Cytomegalovirus infection, in particular, is an intriguing candidate as a cause for an acquired aganglionosis [489].

Hirschsprung disease may be a feature of Down syndrome. The disease may also be associated with a variety of congenital cardiac defects, ventilatory dysautonomia, Werner mesomelic dysplasia, and Waardenburg syndrome [169, 490–492]. Chatten and Witzleben [493] described the coexistence of neuroblastoma and Hirschsprung disease. Shocket and Teloh [494] describe an unusual combination of Hirschsprung disease, megaloureter, pheochromocytoma, and neurofibroma; and Swenson and Fisher [495] drew attention to the coexistence of megacolon and megaloureter. In this latter report the ureter and bladder problems persisted after surgical correction of the intestinal anomaly. Skinner and Irvine [496] reported a series of unrelated patients with congenital nerve deafness and Hirschsprung disease. Fibromuscular dysplasia of arteries in association with Hirschsprung disease has been reported [497]. In many of these reports it is difficult to be certain what links (if any) exist between the different components of the malformation complex. It is easier to see a relationship with intestinal abnormalities [288] and Hirschsprung disease, and a persuasive case can be made for the association of Hirschsprung disease and other anomalies related to neural crest–derived cells and tissues. In many other instances, however, the relationship is far from clear; since many reports are of single cases, any association could be coincidental.

Pseudo-Hirschsprung Disease

When cases of aganglionosis and its variants are excluded, there are a large number of conditions that mimic Hirschsprung disease both clinically and radiographically. These cases have been designated as examples of "pseudo-Hirschsprung disease" and are obviously not a homogeneous group. Some cases may well represent unrecognized examples of zonal aganglionosis or, less convincingly, hypoganglionosis. Others are examples of qualitative defects in innervation such as those now classed as colonic neuronal dysplasia [498–501]. Other cases may represent examples of an entity now known as familial hollow visceral myopathy [502–504].

Colonic neuronal dysplasia is described as a developmental disorder with excessive numbers of nerve fibers that are abnormally distributed, affecting the myenteric and submucosal plexus. It may coexist with aganglionosis in the distal colon. Several morphologic variants are known and they include hyperplasia of the submucosae and myenteric plexuses with ganglioneuromatosis, or ganglion cells in the lamina propria and muscularis mucosa, or abnormal innervation of the myenteric plexus. Scharli and Meier-Rouge [500] classified the hyperplasias of the myenteric plexus into a sympathetic form (intestinal neurofibromatosis), and a parasympathetic form (neuronal colonic dysplasia). Aganglionosis of the distal colon may coexist with the parasympathetic form. Some cases of disseminated neuronal dysplasia have been described as megacystis-microcolon-hypoperistalsis syndrome and this syndrome is reviewed by Gillis and Grantmyre [505]. In colonic neuronal dysplasia, extensive arborization of nerve fibers can be seen in the muscularis propria and abnormal fibers may extend into the lamina propria (Fig. 24.63). When significant numbers of ganglion cells are admixed with the abnormal nerve fibers, the resemblance to neurofibromatosis and/or multiple endocrine neoplasia 2B may be striking. Some examples of intestinal hypoperistalsis have been shown to be examples of axonal dystrophy [506], and there are other examples of so-called neuronal intranuclear inclusion disease that have been grouped with neuronal dysplasia of the colon (even though there is no history of chronic constipation) [507].

It is clear that there are very many variants of abnormal enteric nerve fibers and classifications must be regarded as somewhat tentative. However, the existence of the variants serves to emphasize the complex nature of neuronal development in the enteric plexus, and conversely makes it difficult to assess where deficiencies in argyrophil neurons [508] belong in the spectrum. Scarred bowel, especially in the newborn, may show a pattern of hypertrophy of nerves that can mimic neuronal dysplasia, and be a further source of confusion; as discussed by Yunis and Schofield [509], neuronal dysplasia is not a clearly defined entity.

Hollow visceral myopathy may well be one of the commonest causes of chronic intestinal pseudo-obstruction. While ganglion cells are present and apparently normal,

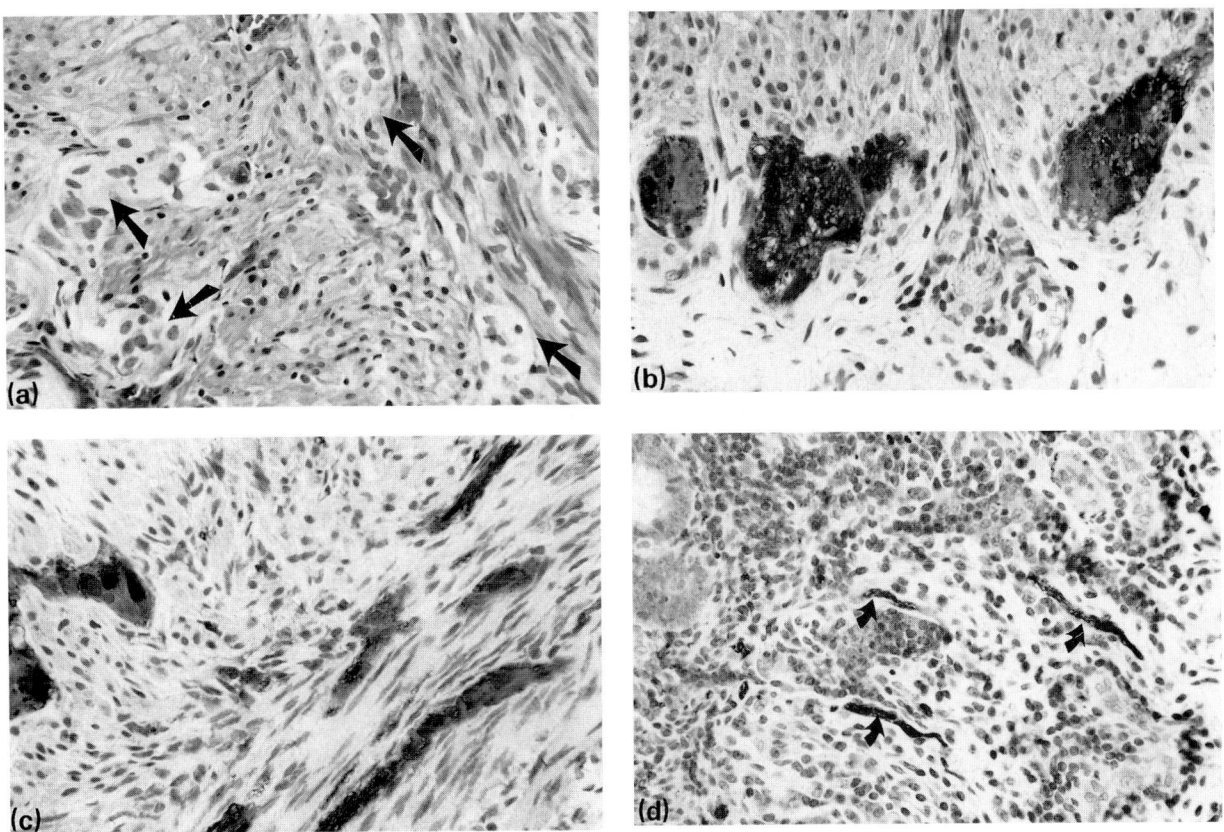

FIGURE 24.63. *(a) A case of colonic neuronal dysplasia shows abnormally large and abundant ganglia (arrows). (b) These ganglia stain positively with neuron-specific enolase. (c) Abundant dark-stained nerve fibers are present in the muscularis propria (C), and submucosa (not shown). (d) Thick, dark-stained nerve fibers (arrows) are seen in the lamina propria (cut tangentially in this section). (a, H&E; b, c, d, Immunoperoxidase staining for neuron-specific enolase—NSE.)*

there is progressive degeneration and fibrosis of muscularis propria [510], associated with marked loss of myofilaments (Fig. 24.64). The change may affect the external layer exclusively, so that mucosal suction biopsies may not be able to provide a diagnosis. The disease is related to a deficiency of smooth muscle alpha-actin [511], a feature readily demonstrated by the use of immunohistochemistry (see Fig. 24.64). The early stages of the disease are difficult to diagnose and, understandably, may be missed on a small biopsy of muscularis propria. Murray et al [512] showed that changes in rectal muscularis propria that mimicked hollow visceral myopathy could occur in chronically constipated children, irrespective of its origin. It is important to stress, however, that in true hollow visceral myopathy the change is diffuse and there is usually small bowel dysfunction as well (see Fig. 24.65 for a *small* intestine example).

A disuse atrophy with an excess of interstitial fibrous tissue has been seen in some infants on prolonged parenteral hyperalimentation [63]. However, the muscle cells have normal amounts of actin, and the muscle fiber degeneration

seen in Figure 24.64 is not present. Schuffler's review of neuromuscular abnormalities of the gut is recommended as a broad general reference, but many of the conditions described are not applicable to the newborn [513].

Idiopathic small left colon syndrome [514] is a rare cause of functional obstruction of unknown etiology, though an association with maternal diabetes mellitus was found in 40% of cases in the original series. Barium enema may be curative, and there is no abnormality detectable in either the ganglion cells or muscle. There is a similarity to the meconium plug syndrome [515], which is a transient obstructive phenomenon. Radiologically, both the idiopathic microcolon and the meconium plug syndrome may resemble Hirschsprung disease.

Despite the increasing number of cases (and causes) of pseudo-Hirschsprung, it remains true that the majority of infants who present with a clinical picture of Hirschsprung disease have aganglionosis. Mucosal and full thickness biopsies, therefore, remain as useful as ever, despite the many difficulties that may be encountered.

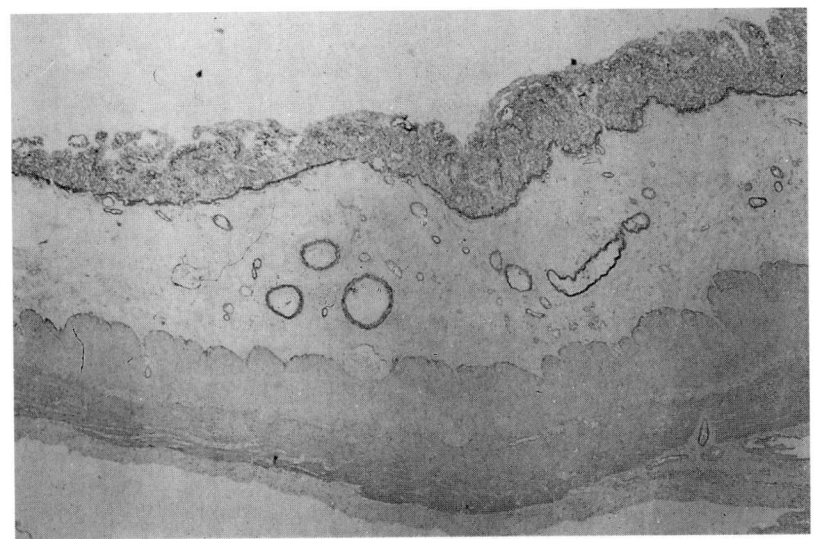

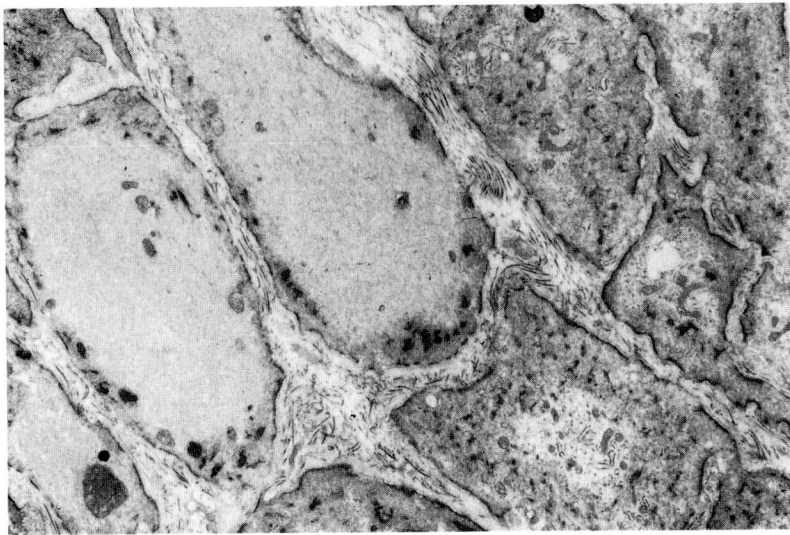

FIGURE 24.64. *(a) Hollow visceral myopathy specimen of small bowel stained with antibody against muscle-specific actin. (HHF 35, Dako.) Note the pale staining of much of the circular muscle layer, while the muscularis mucosa and vascular muscle stains well. (b) Ultrastructurally, there is marked loss of myofilaments in the affected cells (on right of field), accompanied by increased intercellular collagen. Two normal cells are seen on the left of the field.*

Enteric Cysts and Tailgut Cysts of the Anorectal Region

A variety of cystic lesions may occur in the presacral and coccygeal region. They are derived from sequestered duplications of the bowel, tailgut remnants, or as part of the complex of neurenteric fistulae and sinuses associated with sacral anomalies. The presacral cysts may impinge on the anus and rectum or be intimately attached to the wall of these organs, and they may be associated with intraspinal and postsacral cysts as outlined earlier. The cysts may be large multilocular and single, or multiple and small. The cysts contain mucin, but their lining may include ciliated and squamous epithelium. Cysts of the hindgut are said to be larger, while cysts derived from tailgut remnants are usually smaller with satellite cysts [374]. Hindgut cysts are surrounded by a muscle layer of varying thickness and completeness that resembles a sequestered duplication. Tailgut cysts may contain isolated bundles of muscle but a clearly defined wall of smooth muscle is not seen. Squamous epithelium when present has been attributed to metaplasia in the presence of inflammation, but Bale [374] has shown that it may be present in the lining of cysts found in infants without evidence of inflammation. She suggests that it indicates differentiation toward an anal epithelium. A hindgut cyst with pancreatic epithelium in the wall has been reported [401].

Unless they are associated with sacral defects, intraspinal lesions or posterior rectocutaneous fistula (all features seen more frequently in sequestered duplications of hindgut origin), cysts of the presacral area rarely present in infants or children. Tailgut cysts usually present in adult life as "abscesses" in association with constipation, or as an incidental rectal mass during childbirth or a gynecologic examination [516–524]. These lesions have sometimes been designated as retrorectal cyst hamartomata [525] and are usually benign; rarely an adenocarcinoma has developed in a precoccygeal tailgut cyst [525–528].

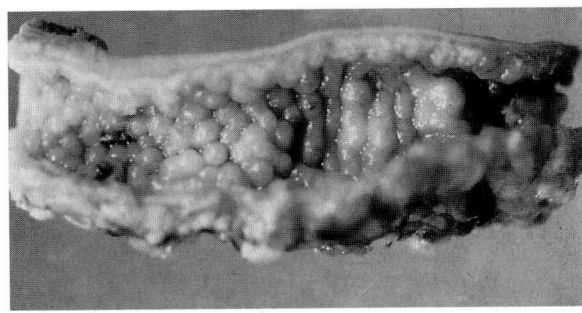

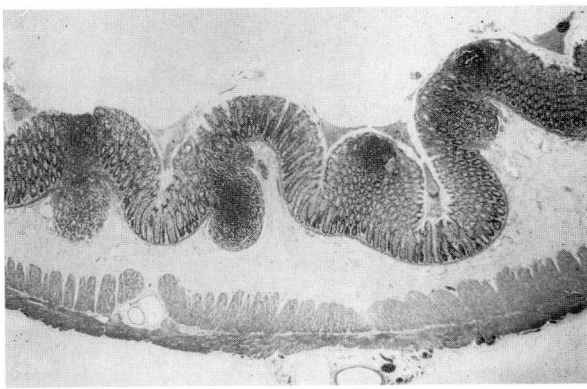

FIGURE 24.65. *(a) Very extensive granularity of the mucosa in a diverted aganglionic segment of Hirschsprung disease. (b) Histologically, the intramucosal lymphoid tissue is particularly prominent, and appears to represent an extension and enlargement of the lymphoid aggregates normally present.*

Sacrococcygeal Tumors and Anorectal Lesions

An example of a "dermoid cyst" of the presacral region associated with rectal stenosis and rectovaginal fistula is recorded by Bale [374], and the author has autopsied a stillbirth with anorectal agenesis and rectovesical fistula with a large sacrococcygeal teratoma [401].

Heterotopia

Heterotopic epithelium in the anorectal regions is rare, and usually presents in adults [401]. Gastric epithelium is the commonest variety [529–531], and it may present as a polyp or as a cause of bleeding [529]. Gastric mucosa may line a duplication, and salivary acinar tissue may be seen as well [532–534]. Sun et al [535] described renal tissue in the rectum in a case of caudal regression.

Miscellaneous

Prominent lymphoglandular complexes may occur in the aganglionic segment of Hirschsprung disease [536]. This is more than a marked accentuation of the normal lymphoid follicular pattern [386], with intramucosal lymphoid aggregates (Fig. 24.65). A similar change can occur in any diverted loop of colon, and the lesion represents an example of diversion colitis.

REFERENCES

1. Moore KL. *The Developing Human: Clinically Oriented Embryology*. 3rd ed. Philadelphia: WB Saunders, 1982, pp. 227–54.
2. Okamoto E, Ueda T. Embryogenesis of intramural ganglia of the gut and its relation to Hirschsprung's disease. *J Pediatr Surg* 1967; 2:437–43.
3. Andrew A. The origin of intramural ganglia. IV. The origin of enteric ganglia: a critical review and discussion of the present state of the problem. *J Anat* 1971; 108:169–84.
4. Kapur RP. Contemporary approaches towards understanding the pathogenesis of Hirschsprung's disease. *Pediatr Pathol* 1993; 13:83–100.
5. Dawson I. The endocrine cells of the gastrointestinal tract and the tumours that arise from them. *Curr Top Pathol* 1976; 63:221–58.
6. Pearse AGE. The endocrine cells of the GI tract: origins, morphology and functional relationships in health and disease. *Clin Gastroenterol* 1974; 3:491–510.
7. Pearse AGE. The cytochemistry and ultrastructure of polypeptide hormone producing cells (the APUD series) and the embryologic, physiologic and pathologic implications of the concept. *J Histochem Cytochem* 1969; 17:303–13.
8. Lewin KJ. The endocrine cells of the gastrointestinal tract: the normal endocrine cells and their hyperplasias. Part I. *Pathol Ann* 1986; 21:1–27.
9. Barter R, Pearse AGE. Mammalian enterochromaffin cells as the source of serotonin (5-hydroxytryptamine). *J Pathol Bacteriol* 1955; 69:25–31.
10. Forsmann WG, Orci L, Pictet R, Renold AE, Roviller C. The endocrine cells in the epithelium of the gastrointestinal mucosa of the rat. *J Cell Biol* 1969; 40:692–715.
11. Moxey PC, Trier JS. Endocrine cells in the human fetal small intestine. *Cell Tissue Res* 1977; 183:33–50.
12. Polak JM, Bloom SR, Kuzio M, Pearse AGE. Cellular localisation of gastric inhibitory polypeptide in the duodenum and jejunum. *Gut* 1973; 14:284–8.
13. Robinson G, Dawson I. Immunochemical studies of the endocrine cells of the gastrointestinal tract. II. An immunoperoxide technique for the localisation of secretin-containing cells in the human duodenum. *J Clin Pathol* 1975; 28:631–5.
14. Falkmer S, Wilander E. The endocrine cell population. In: Whitehead R, ed. *Gastrointestinal and Oesophageal Pathology*. 2nd ed. Edinburgh: Churchill-Livingstone, 1995, p. 63.
15. Paes BA, deSa DJ, Hitch DA. Fatal malformations of the larynx and upper trachea. *Laryngoscope* 1984; 94:1477–81.
16. Semba R, Tanaka O, Tanimura T. Digestive system. In: Nishimura H, ed. *Atlas of Human Prenatal Histology*. Tokyo: Igaku-Shoin, 1983, pp. 171–234.
17. John BAE. Developmental changes in the esophageal epithelium in man. *J Anat* 1952; 86:431–2.
18. Smith RB, Taylor IM. Observations on the intrinsic innervation of the foetal oesophagus between the 10 mm and 140 mm crown-rump length stages. *Acta Anat* 1972; 81:127–38.
19. Rector LF, Connerley ML. Aberrant mucosa in the esophagus of infants and in children. *Arch Pathol* 1941; 31:285–94.
20. Willis RA. Developmentally heterotopic tissues. In: *The Borderland of Embryology and Pathology*. London: Butterworth, 1958, pp. 306–40.
21. Vogt EC. Congenital esophageal atresia. *Am J Roentgenol Radium Ther* 1929; 22:463–5.
22. Ladd WE. The surgical treatment of esophageal atresia and tracheo-esophageal fistulas. *N Engl J Med* 1944; 230:625–37.
23. Gross RE. *Surgery of Infancy and Childhood*. Philadelphia: WB Saunders, 1953, pp. 75–102.
24. Griscom NT. Persistent esophagotrachea: the severest form of laryngotracheoesophageal cleft. *Am J Roentgenol Radium Ther Nucl Med* 1966; 97:211–15.
25. Eckstein HB, Somasundaram K. Multiple tracheoesophageal fistulas without atresia. *J Pediatr Surg* 1966; 1:381–3.
26. Rehbein F. Oesophageal atresia with double tracheo-oesophageal fistula. *Arch Dis Child* 1964; 39:138–42.
27. Gruenwald P. Case of atresia of esophagus combined with tracheoesophageal fistula in a 9 mm human embryo and its embryological explantation. *Anat Rec* 1940; 78:293–302.
28. Rosenthal AH. Congenital atresia of the esophagus with tracheoesophageal fistula. Report of eight cases. *Arch Pathol* 1931; 12:756–72.
29. Berman JK, Test PS, McArt BA. Congenital esophago-bronchial fistula in an adult. *J Thorac Surg* 1952; 24:493–501.
30. Robb D. Congenital tracheo-oesophageal fistula without atresia with a large oesophageal diverticulum. *Aust NZ J Surg* 1952; 22:120–2.

31. Warkany J. *Congenital Malformations*. Chicago: Year Book Medical, 1971, pp. 678–86.

32. Smith DW. *Recognizable Patterns of Human Malformation: Genetic, Embryologic, and Clinical Aspects*. 3rd ed. Philadelphia: WB Saunders, 1982, pp. 517–19.

33. Ainsworth P, Davies PA. The single umbilical artery: a five year survey. *Dev Med Child Neurol* 1969; 11:297–302.

34. Heifetz SA. Single umbilical artery: a statistical analysis of 237 autopsy cases and review of the literature. *Perspect Pediatr Pathol* 1984; 8:345–78.

35. Mellins RB, Blumenthal S. Cardiovascular anomalies and esophageal atresia. *Am J Dis Child* 1964; 107:160–4.

36. Lister J. The blood supply of the oesophagus in relation to oesophageal atresia. *Arch Dis Child* 1964; 39:131–7.

37. Fluss Z, Poppen KJ. Embryogenesis of tracheo-esophageal fistula and esophageal atresia: a hypothesis based on associated vascular anomalies. *Arch Pathol* 1951; 52:168–81.

38. Grieve JG, McDermott JG. Congenital atresia of the esophagus in two brothers. *Can Med Assoc J* 1939; 41:185–6.

39. Hausmann PF, Close AS, Williams LP. Occurrence of tracheoesophageal fistula in three consecutive siblings. *Surgery* 1957; 41:542–8.

40. Haight C. Some observations on esophageal atresias and tracheoesophageal fistulas of congenital origin. *J Thorac Surg* 1957; 34:141–72.

41. Kilter H, Warkany J. Congenital malformation in inbred strains of mice induced by riboflavin-deficient, galactoflavin-containing diets. *J Exp Zool* 1957; 136:531–53.

42. Warkany J, Roth CB, Wilson JG. Multiple congenital malformations: a consideration of etiologic factors. *Pediatrics* 1948; 1:462–71.

43. Favara BE, Franciosi RA, Akers DR. Enteric duplications, thirty-seven cases: a vascular theory of pathogenesis. *Am J Dis Child* 1971; 122:501–6.

44. Grosfeld JL, O'Neill JA Jr, Clatworthy HW Jr. Enteric duplication of infancy and childhood: an 18 year review. *Ann Surg* 1970; 172:83–90.

45. Lewis JH, Thyng FW. The regular occurrence of intestinal diverticula in embryos of the pig, rabbit and man. *Am J Anat* 1908; 7:505–19.

46. Kirwan WO, Walbaum PR, McCormack RJM. Cystic intrathoracic derivatives of the foregut and their complications. *Thorax* 1973; 28:424–8.

47. Reed JC, Sobonya RE. Morphologic analysis of foregut cysts in the thorax. *Am J Roentgenol Radium Ther Nucl Med* 1974; 120:851–60.

48. Silverman A, Roy CC. *Pediatric Clinical Gastroenterology*. 3rd ed. St Louis: CV Mosby, 1983, pp. 75–80.

49. Bourne AJ. The oesophagus. In: Whitehead R, ed. *Gastrointestinal and Oesophageal Pathology*. 2nd ed. Edinburgh: Churchill-Livingstone, 1995, p. 277.

50. Veeneklaas GMH. Pathogenesis of intrathoracic gastrogenic cysts. *Am J Dis Child* 1952; 83:500–7.

51. Bremer JL. Dorsal intestinal fistula: accessory neurenteric canal; diastematomyelia. *Arch Pathol* 1952; 54:132–8.

52. Bentley JFR, Smith JR. Developmental posterior enteric remnants and spinal malformations: the split notochord syndrome. *Arch Dis Child* 1960; 35:76–86.

53. Louw JH, Cywes S. Extralobar pulmonary sequestration communicating with the oesophagus and associated with a strangulated congenital diaphragmatic hernia. *Br J Surg* 1962; 50:102–5.

54. Lacina S, Townley R, Radecki L, Stockinger F, et al. Esophageal lung with cardiac abnormalities. *Chest* 1981; 79:468–70.

55. Botha GSM. The gastro-oesophageal region in infants. *Arch Dis Child* 1958; 33:78–94.

56. Williams ER. A case of right-sided aortic arch associated with congenital short oesophagus and partial thoracic stomach. *Br J Radiol* 1945; 18:323–6.

57. Spechler SJ, Goyal RK. Barrett's oesophagus. *N Engl J Med* 1986; 315:362–71.

58. Merriam JC Jr, Benirschke K. Esophageal erosions in the newborn. *Lab Invest* 1959; 8:39–47.

59. Groben PA, Siegal GP, Shub MD, Ulshen MH, Askin FB. Gastroesophageal reflux and esophagitis in infants and children. *Perspect Pediatr Pathol* 1987; 11:124–51.

60. Harell GS, Friedland GW, Daily WJ, Cohn RB. Neonatal Boerhaave's syndrome. *Radiology* 1970; 95:665–8.

61. Myers NA, Hiller HG. Neonatal rupture of the esophagus: the radiological diagnosis of a cause of acute respiratory distress in neonates. *Aust Pediatr J* 1973; 9:106–8.

62. Hohf RP, Kimball ER, Ballenger JJ. Rupture of the esophagus in the neonate. *J Am Med Assoc* 1962; 181:939–43.

63. deSa DJ. *The Pathology of Neonatal Intensive Care*. London: Chapman & Hall Medical, 1995, pp. 113, 115, 118.

64. Whyte RK, Hussain Z, deSa DJ. Antenatal infections with Candida species. *Arch Dis Child* 1982; 57:528–35.

65. Hood IC, deSa DJ, Whyte RK. The inflammatory response in candidal chorioamnionitis. *Hum Pathol* 1983; 14:984–90.

66. Hood IC, Browning D, deSa DJ, Whyte RK. Fetal inflammatory response in second trimester candidal chorioamnionitis. *Early Hum Dev* 1985; 11:1–10.

67. Singer DB. Pathology of neonatal herpes simplex virus infection. *Perspect Pediatr Pathol* 1981; 6:243–78.

68. Chatty EM, Tomeh MO, Mercer RD, Osborne DG. Congenital rubella with viral esophagitis. *Cleveland Clin Q* 1971; 38:73–8.

69. Becroft DMO. Prenatal cytomegalovirus infection: epidemiology, pathology and pathogenesis. *Perspect Pediatr Pathol* 1981; 6:203–41.

70. Oppenheimer EH, Dahms BB. Congenital syphilis in the fetus and neonate. *Perspect Pediatr Pathol* 1981; 6:115–38.

71. Shermeta DW, Whitington PF, Seto DS, Haller JA. Lower esophageal sphincter dysfunction in esophageal atresia. Nocturnal regurgitation and aspiration pneumonia. *J Pediatr Surg* 1977; 12:871–6.

72. Dahms BB, Rothstein FC. Barrett's esophagus in children: a consequence of chronic gastroesophageal reflux. *Gastroenterology* 1984; 86:318–23.

73. Hassall E, Weinstein WM, Ament ME. Barrett's esophagus in childhood. *Gastroenterology* 1985; 89:1331–7.

74. Biller JA, Winter HS, Grand RJ, Alfred EN. Are endoscopic changes predictive of histologic esophagitis in children? *J Pediatr* 1983; 103:215–8.

75. Robins DB, Zaino RJ, Ballantine TVN. Barrett's esophagus in a newborn. *Pediatr Pathol* 1911; 11:663–7.

76. Menon AP, Schefft GL, Thach BT. Apnea associated with regurgitation in infants. *J Pediatr* 1985; 106:625–9.

77. Gaultier CL. Interference between gastroesophageal reflux and sleep in near miss SIDS. *Clin Rev Allergy Immunol* 1990; 8:395–401.

78. Byard RW, Moore L. Gastroesophageal reflux and sudden infant death syndrome. *Pediatr Pathol* 1993; 13:55–7.

79. Dahms BB, Rothstein FC. Mucosal biopsy in the esophagus of children. *Perspect Pediatr Pathol* 1987; 11:97–123.

80. DiGiorgio CJ, Orenstein SR, Shalaby TM, Mahoney TM, et al. Quantitative computer-assisted image analysis of suction biopsy in pediatric gastroesophageal reflux. *Pediatr Pathol* 1994; 14:653–64.

81. Blank E, Michael TD. Muscular hypertrophy of the esophagus. *Pediatrics* 1963; 32:595–8.

82. Greenough WG. Congenital esophageal strictures. *Am J Roentgenol Radium Ther Nucl Med* 1964; 92:994–9.

83. Adler RH. Congenital esophageal webs. *J Thorac Cardiovasc Surg* 1963; 45:175–85.

84. Ishida M, Tsuchida Y, Saito S, Tsunoda A. Congenital oesophageal stenosis due to tracheobronchial remnants. *J Pediatr Surg* 1969; 4:339–45.

85. Rose JS, Kassner EG, Jurgens KH, Farman J. Congenital oesophageal strictures due to cartilaginous rings. *Br J Radiol* 1975; 48:16–18.

86. Chang C-H, Perrin EV, Bove KE. Pyloric atresia associated with epidermolysis bullosa: special reference to pathogenesis. *Pediatr Pathol* 1983; 1:449–57.

87. Holden KR, Alexander F. Diffuse neonatal hemangiomatosis. *Pediatrics* 1970; 46:411–21.

88. Lauridsen UB, Enk B, Gammeltoft A. Oesophageal varices as a late complication to neonatal umbilical vein catheterization. *Acta Paediatr Scand* 1978; 67:633–6.

89. Stahlman M, Hedwall G, Dolanski E, et al. A six year follow up of clinical hyaline membrane disease. *Pediatr Clin North Am* 1973; 20:443–6.

90. Hoogstraten J, deSa DJ, Knisely AS. Fetal liver disease may precede extrahepatic siderosis in neonatal hemochromatosis. *Gastroenterology* 1990; 98:1699–701.

91. Stout AP, Lattes R. Tumors of the esophagus. In: *Atlas of Tumor Pathology*. Series I, Fascicle 20. Washington, DC: Armed Forces Institute of Pathology, 1957, p. 36.

92. Nishimura N, ed. *Atlas of Human Prenatal Histology*. Tokyo: Igaku-Shoin, 1983, pp. 171–234.

93. Willis RA. *The Borderland of Embryology and Pathology*. 2nd ed. London: Butterworths, 1962, pp. 139, 306.

94. Goon CD. Duplication of the stomach with extension into the chest. *Am Surgeon* 1953; 19:721–7.

95. Kiesewetter WB. Duplication of the stomach. *Ann Surg* 1957; 146:990–3.

96. Grosfeld JL, Boles ET Jr, Reiner C. Duplication of the pylorus in the newborn: a rare cause of pyloric obstruction. *J Pediatr Surg* 1970; 5:365–9.

97. Berg HF, Marx K. Duplication of the stomach. *J Pediatr* 1952; 40:334–8.

98. Gould RJ, Toffler AH. Duplication of the stomach: a case report. *Radiology* 1961; 76:79–94.

99. Eras P, Beranbaum SL. Gastric diverticula: congenital and acquired. *Am J Gastroenterol* 1972; 57:120–32.

100. Wieczorek RL, Seidman I, Ranson JHC, Ruoff M. Congenital duplication of the stomach: case report and review of the English literature. *Am J Gastroenterol* 1984; 79:597–602.
101. Blank E, Chisolm AJ. Congenital microgastria: a case report with a 26-year follow up. *Pediatrics* 1973; 51:1037–41.
102. Putschar WG, Manion WC. Congenital absence of the spleen and related anomalies. *Am J Clin Pathol* 1956; 26:429–70.
103. Rose V, Izukawa T, Moes CAF. Syndromes of asplenia and polysplenia: a review of cardiac and non-cardiac malformation in 60 cases with special reference to diagnosis and prognosis. *Br Heart J* 1975; 37:840–52.
104. Shackelford GD, McAlister WH, Brodeur AE, Ragsdale EF. Congenital microgastria. *Am J Roentgenol Radium Ther Nucl Med* 1973; 118:72–6.
105. Berant M, Aviad I, Jacobs J. Heterotopic duodenal mucosa in the stomach. *Am J Dis Child* 1965; 110:566–9.
106. Martinez NS, Morlock CG, Dockerty MB, Waugh JM, Weber HM. Heterotopic pancreatic tissue involving the stomach. *Ann Surg* 1958; 147: 1–12.
107. Landing BH, Wells TR. Tracheobronchial anomalies in children. *Perspect Pediatr Pathol* 1973; 1:1–32.
108. Teplick JG, Wallmer RJ, Levine AH, Haskin ME. Isolated dextrogastria: report of two cases. *Am J Radiol* 1979; 132:124–6.
109. Parrish RA, Kanavage CB, Wells JA, Moretz WH. Congenital antral membrane. *Surg Gynecol Obstet* 1978; 127:999–1004.
110. Bronsther B, Nadeau MR, Abrams MW. Congenital pyloric atresia: a report of three cases and a review of the literature. *Surgery* 1971; 69:130–6.
111. Saw EC, Arbegast NR, Comer TP. Pyloric atresia: a case report. *Pediatrics* 1973; 51:574–7.
112. Kissane JM. *Pathology of Infancy and Childhood.* 2nd ed. St. Louis: Mosby, 1975, p. 175.
113. Olsen L, Grotte G. Congenital pyloric atresia: report of a familial occurrence. *J Pediatr Surg* 1976; 11:181–4.
114. Benson CD, Coury JJ. Congenital intrinsic obstruction of the stomach and duodenum in the newborn. *Arch Surg* 1951; 62:856–66.
115. Touroff ASW, Sussman RM. Congenital prepyloric membranous obstruction in a premature infant. *Surgery* 1940; 8:739–55.
116. Haddad V, Macon WL, Islami MH. Mucosal diaphragm of the gastric antrum in adults. *Surg Gynecol Obstet* 1981; 152:227–33.
117. Tunell WP, Smith EI. Antral web in infancy. *J Pediatr Surg* 1980; 15:152–5.
118. Sheinfeld A, Olsha O, Rivkin L, Dolberg OM. Prepyloric diaphragm, an unusual cause of gastric outlet syndrome. *Isr J Med Sci* 1982; 18:1044–7.
119. Incidence of infantile hypertrophic pyloric stenosis. *Lancet* 1984; 1:888–9.
120. Spicer RP. Infantile hypertrophic pyloric stenosis: a review. *Br J Surg* 1982; 69:128–35.
121. Kelsey D, Stayman W Jr, McLaughlin ED, Mebane W. Massive bleeding in a newborn infant from a gastric ulcer associated with hypertrophic pyloric stenosis. *Surgery* 1968; 64:979–82.
122. Belding HH, Kernohan JW. A morphologic study of the myenteric plexus and musculature of the pylorus with special reference to the changes in hypertrophic pyloric stenosis. *Surg Gynecol Obstet* 1953; 97:322–34.
123. Wattchow DA, Cass DT, Furness JB, et al. Abnormalities of peptide-containing nerve fibres in infantile hypertrophic pyloric stenosis. *Gastroenterology* 1987; 92:443–8.
124. Challa VR, Jona JZ, Markesberg WR. Ultrastructural observations of the myenteric plexus of the pylorus in infantile hypertrophic pyloric stenosis. *Am J Pathol* 1977; 88:309–15.
125. Malmfor G, Sundler PF. Peptidergic innervation in infantile hypertrophic pyloric stenosis. *J Pediatr Surg* 1986; 21:303–6.
126. Tam PKG. An immunohistochemical study with neuron specific enolase and substance P of human enteric innervation—the normal developmental pattern and abnormal deviations in Hirschsprung's disease and pyloric stenosis. *J Pediatr Surg* 1986; 21:227–32.
127. Warkany J. *Congenital Malformations.* Chicago: Year Book Medical, 1971, pp. 686–90.
128. McKeown T, MacMahon B, Record RG. Evidence of post-natal environmental influence in the aetiology of infantile pyloric stenosis. *Arch Dis Child* 1952; 27:386–90.
129. Carter CO. The inheritance of congenital pyloric stenosis. *Br Med Bull* 17:251–4.
130. Rogers IM, Macgillion F, Drainer JK. Congenital hypertrophic pyloric stenosis: a gastrin hypothesis pursued. *J Pediatr Surg* 1976; 11:173–6.
131. San Filippo JA. Infantile hypertrophic pyloric stenosis related to ingestion of erythromycine estolate: a report of five cases. *J Pediatr Surg* 1976; 11:177–80.
132. Butler LJ, France NE, Russell A, Sinclair L. A chromosomal aberration associated with multiple congenital anomalies. *Lancet* 1962; 1:1242.
133. Ahmed S. Infantile pyloric stenosis associated with major anomalies of the alimentary tract. *J Pediatr Surg* 1970; 6:660–6.
134. Dodge JA. Infantile hypertrophic pyloric stenosis. In: Rotter JI, Samloff IM, Rimoin DL, eds. *Genetics and Heterogeneity of Common Gastrointestinal Disorders.* New York: Academic Press, 1980, pp. 419–39.
135. Braunstein H. Congenital defect of the gastric musculature with spontaneous perforation. *J Pediatr* 1954; 44:55–63.
136. Reams G, Unaway JB, Walls WL. Neonatal gastric perforation with survival. *Pediatrics* 1963; 31:97–102.
137. Shaw A, Blanc WA, Santulli TV, Kaiser G. Spontaneous rupture of the stomach in the newborn: a clinical and experimental study. *Surgery* 1965; 58:561–71.
138. Pochaczevsky R, Bryk D. New roentgenographic signs of neonatal gastric perforation. *Radiology* 1972; 102:145–7.
139. Helardot PG, Elkoubi P, Grapin C, Bargy F, Bienayme J. Les perforations gastriques neonatales. *Chir Pediatr* 1984; 25:169–75.
140. Lloyd JR. The etiology of gastrointestinal perforations in the newborn. *J Pediatr Surg* 1969; 4:77–84.
141. Rees JR, Redo SF. Neonatal gastric necrosis and perforation treated by gastrectomy and esophagogastric anastomosis. *Surgery* 1968; 64:472–4.
142. Sanz S, Corral T, Laplana R, Tejedor FR. Perforacion gastrica neonatal. *Bol So Vasonav Pediatr* 1967; 2:41–7.
143. Whyte RK, Hussain Z, deSa DJ. Antenatal infections with Candida species. *Arch Dis Child* 1982; 57:528–35.
144. Watt J. The pathology of multiple gastric ulceration in the newborn infant. *J Pathol Bacteriol* 1966; 91:105–16.
145. Bird CE, Limper MA, Mayer JM. Surgery of peptic ulceration of stomach and duodenum in infants and children. *Ann Surg* 1941; 114:526–42.
146. Goetzman BW, Sunshine P, Johnson JD, et al. Neonatal hypoxia and pulmonary vasospasm: response to tolazoline. *J Pediatr* 1978; 89:617–21.
147. Idowu J, Aitken DR, Georgeson KE. Gastric volvulus in the newborn. *Arch Surg* 1980; 116:1046–9.
148. Tyson JE, deSA DJ, Moore S. Thromboatheromatous complications of umbilical arterial catheterization in the newborn period. *Arch Dis Child* 1976; 51:744–54.
149. Bull MJ, Norins AL, Weaver DD, Weber T, Mitchell M. Epidermolysis bullosa pyloric atresia. *Am J Dis Child* 1983; 137:449–51.
150. Oppenheimer EH, Esterly JR. Pathology of cystic fibrosis: review of the literature and comparison with 146 autopsied cases. *Perspect Pediatr Pathol* 1975; 2:241–78.
151. Odell JM, Haas JE, Tapper D, Nugent D. Infantile hemorrhagic angiodysplasia. *Pediatr Pathol* 1987; 7:629–36.
152. Smith CR, Chan HSL, deSa DJ. Placental involvement in congenital neuroblastoma. *J Clin Pathol* 1981; 34:785–9.
153. Beneck D. Hypertrophic gastropathy in a newborn: a case report and review of the literature. *Pediatr Pathol* 1994; 14:213–21.
154. Peled N, Dagan O, Babyn P, Silver MM, et al. Gastric-outlet obstruction produced by prostaglandin therapy in neonates. *N Engl J Med* 1992; 327:505–10.
155. Matias K, Huang YC. Gastric teratoma in infancy: report of a case and review of the world literature. *Ann Surg* 1973; 178:631–6.
156. Selman AN. Complex tridermal teratoma of stomach (benign): case report. *Am J Surg* 1943; 59:567–70.
157. Barrocas A, Fontenelle LJ, Williams MJ. Gastric heterotopic pancreas: a case report and review of the literature. *Am J Surg* 1973; 39:361–5.
158. Ladd WE. Congenital obstructions of the duodenum in children. *N Engl J Med* 1932; 206:277–80.
159. Boyden EA, Cope JG, Bill AH Jr. Anatomy and embryology of congenital intrinsic obstruction of the duodenum. *Am J Surg* 1967; 114:190–202.
160. Johnson FP. The development of the mucous membrane of the esophagus, stomach and small intestine in the human embryo. *Am J Anat* 1910; 20:521–61.
161. Dubois PM, Paulin C, Chayvialle JA. Identification of gastrin-secreting cells and cholecystokinin-secreting cells in the gastrointestinal tract of the human fetus and adult man. *Cell Tissue Res* 1976; 175:31–56.
162. Moxey PC, Trier JS. Specialized cell types in the human fetal small intestine. *Anat Rec* 1978; 191:269–85.
163. Snyder WJ Jr, Chaffin L. Embryology and pathology of the intestinal tract: presentation of 40 cases of malrotation. *Ann Surg* 1954; 140:368–79.
164. Andrassy RJ, Mahour GH. Malrotation of the midgut in infants and children. A 25 year review. *Arch Surg* 1981; 116:158–60.
165. Bill AH Jr. Malrotation of the intestine. In: Ravitch MM, Welch KJ, Benson CD, Aberdeen E, Randolph JG, eds. *Pediatric Surgery.* 3rd ed. Vol. 2. Chicago: Year Book Medical, 1979, pp. 912–23.

166. Estrada R. *Anomalies of Intestinal Rotation and Fixation.* Springfield, IL: CC Thomas, 1968.

167. Warkany J, Passarge EB, Smith LB. Congenital malformations in autosomal trisomy syndromes. *Am J Dis Child* 1966; 112:502–17.

168. Klep de Pater JM, Bijlsma JB, de France HF, et al. Partial trisomy 10q. A recognisable syndrome. *Hum Genet* 1979; 45:29–40.

169. Smith DW. Recognizable patterns of human malformation: *Genetic, Embryologic, and Clinical Aspects.* 3rd ed. Philadelphia: WB Saunders, 1982, pp. 13–20.

170. Yunis J. *New Chromosomal Syndromes.* New York: Academic Press, 1977, pp. 69–71, 221–34.

171. Ross LJ. Arachnodactyly. Review of recent literature and report of a case with cleft palate. *Am J Dis Child* 1949; 78:417–36.

172. Freedom R. The asplenia syndrome. *J Pediatr* 1972; 81:1130–33.

173. van Mierop LHS, Gessner IH, Schiebler GL. Asplenia and polysplenia syndromes. *Birth Defects: Original Article Series* 1972; 8:74–80.

174. Bodian M, White LL, Carter CO, Louw JH. Congenital duodenal obstruction and mongolism. *BMJ* 1952; 1:77–8.

175. Gustavson K-H, Finley SC, Finley WH, Jalling B. A 4–5/2–22 chromosomal translocation associated with multiple congenital anomalies. *Acta Paediatr* 1964; 53:172–81.

176. Siebert JR. Small intestine length in infants and children. *Am J Dis Child* 1980; 134:593–95.

177. Hamilton JR, Reilly BJ, Morecki R. Short small intestine associated with malrotation: a newly described congenital cause of intestinal malabsorption. *Gastroenterology* 1969; 56:124–36.

178. Konvolinka CW. Congenital short small intestine: a rare occurrence. *J Pediatr Surg* 1970; 5:574.

179. Tiu CM, Chou YH, Pan HB, Chang T. Congenital short bowel. *Pediatr Radiol* 1984; 14:343–5.

180. Yutani C, Sakurai M, Miyaj T, Okuno M. Congenital short intestine: a case report and review of the literature. *Arch Pathol* 1973; 96:81–2.

181. Fitzsimmons J, Chinn A, Shepard TH. Normal length of the human fetal gastrointestinal tract. *Pediatr Pathol* 1988; 8:633–41.

182. Reiquam CW, Allen RP, Akers DR. Normal and abnormal small bowel. *Am J Dis Child* 1965; 109:447–51.

183. Klish WJ, Putnam TC. The short gut. *Am J Dis Child* 1981; 135:1056–61.

184. Schwartz MZ, Maeda K. Short bowel syndrome in infants and children. *Pediatr Clin North Am* 1985; 32:1265–79.

185. Grosfield JL, Rescoria FJ, West KW. Short bowel syndrome in infancy and children: analysis of 60 patients. *Am J Surg* 1986; 151:41–6.

186. Bennington J, Haber SL. The embryologic significance of an undifferentiated intestinal tract. *J Pediatr* 1964; 735–9.

187. Kieswetter WB, Smith JW. Malrotation of the midgut in infancy and childhood. *Arch Surg* 1958; 77:483–91.

188. Taybi H. *Radiology of Syndromes.* Chicago: Year Book Medical, 1975, p. 53.

189. Boggs TR Jr, Bishop H. Neonatal hyperbilirubinemia associated with high obstruction of the small bowel. *J Pediatr* 1965; 66:349–56.

190. Fonkalsrud EW, de Lorimier AA, Hays DM. Congenital atresia and stenosis of the duodenum. *Pediatrics* 1969; 43:79–83.

191. Girvan DP, Stephens CA. Congenital intrinsic duodenal obstruction: a twenty year review of its surgical management and consequences. *J Pediatr Surg* 1974; 9:833–9.

192. Jona JZ, Belin RP. Duodenal anomalies and the ampulla of VATER. *Surg Gynecol Obstet* 1976; 143:565–9.

193. Longo MF, Lynn HB. Congenital duodenal obstruction: review of 29 cases encountered in a 30 year period. *Mayo Clin Proc* 1967; 42:423–30.

194. Spitz L, Ali M, Brereton RJ. Combined esophageal and duodenal atresia: experience of 18 patients. *J Pediatr Surg* 1981; 16:4–7.

195. Wilkinson AW. Congenital causes of duodenal obstruction. *J R Coll Surg Edinb* 1973; 18:197–208.

196. Young DG, Wilkinson AW. Abnormalities associated with neonatal duodenal obstruction. *Surgery* 1968; 63:832–6.

197. Warkany J. *Congenital Malformations: Notes and Comments.* Chicago: Year Book Medical, 1971, pp. 694–96.

198. Louw JH. Jejunoileal atresia and stenosis. *J Pediatr Surg* 1966; 1:8–23.

199. Willis RA. *The Borderland of Embryology and Pathology.* 2nd ed. London: Butterworth, 1962, p. 161.

200. Patton EF. Congenital hypertrophic stenosis of the duodenum. *J Pediatr* 1948; 32:301–3.

201. Appell RG, Bolkenius M. Arteriomesenteric occlusion of the duodenum in infants and adolescents: a rare form of intestinal obstruction. *Z Kinderchir* 1984; 39:310–4.

202. Grosfeld JL. Atresia and stenosis of the jejunum and ileum. In: Ravitch MM, Welch KJ, Benson CD, Aberdeen E, Randolph JG, eds. *Pediatric Surgery.* 3rd ed. Vol 2. Chicago: Year Book Medical, 1979, pp. 933–43.

203. de Lorimier AA, Fonkalsrud EW, Hays DM. Congenital atresia and stenosis of the jejunum and ileum. *Surgery* 1969; 65:819–27.

204. Kao KJ, Fleischer R, Bradford WD. Multiple congenital septal atresias of the intestine: histomorphologic and pathogenetic considerations. *Pediatr Pathol* 1983; 1:443–8.

205. Teja D, Schnatterly P, Shaw A. Multiple intestinal atresias: pathology and pathogenesis. *J Pediatr Surg* 1981; 16:194–9.

206. Martin LW, Zerella JT. Jejunoileal atresia: a proposed classification. *J Pediatr Surg* 1976; 11:399–403.

207. Santulli RV, Blanc WA. Congenital atresia of the intestine: pathogenesis and treatment. *Ann Surg* 1961; 154:939–48.

208. Daneman A, Martin DJ. A syndrome of multiple gastrointestinal atresias with intraluminal calcification. *Pediatr Radiol* 1979; 8:222–9.

209. deSa DJ. Congenital stenosis and atresia of the jejunum and ileum. *J Clin Pathol* 1972; 25:1063–70.

210. Lafferty K, Brereton RJ, Wright VM. Necrotising enterocolitis in small bowel atresia. *Z Kinderchir* 1983; 38:224–8.

211. deSa DJ. The spectrum of ischemic bowel disease in the newborn. *Perspect Pediatr Pathol* 1976; 3:273–309.

212. Louw JH. Congenital intestinal atresia and severe stenosis in the newborn. *S Afr J Clin Sci* 1952; 3:109–29.

213. Louw JH, Barnard CN. Congenital intestinal atresia. *Lancet* 1955; 2:1065–7.

214. deSa DJ, Mucklow ES, Gough MH. Neonatal gut infarction. *J Pediatr Surg* 1970; 5:454–9.

215. Erskine JM. Colonic stenosis in the newborn: the possible thromboembolic etiology of intestinal stenosis and atresia. *J Pediatr Surg* 1970; 5:321–33.

216. Joshi VV, Winston YE, Kay S. Neonatal necrotizing enterocolitis: histologic evidence of healing. *Am J Dis Child* 1973; 126:113–16.

217. Rabinowitz JG, Wolf BS, Feller MR, Krasna I. Colonic changes following necrotizing enterocolitis in the newborn. *Am J Roengenol Radium Ther Nucl Med* 1968; 103:359–65.

218. Marston A, Pheils MT, Thomas ML, Morson BC. Ischaemic colitis. *Gut* 1966; 7:1–15.

219. Virjee JP, Gill GJ, deSa D, Somers S, Stevenson GW. Strictures and other late complications of neonatal necrotizing enterocolitis. *Clin Radiol* 1979; 30;25–31.

220. Shackelford G. Intestinal stricture in necrotizing enterocolitis. *J Pediatr Surg* 1976; 11:319–27.

221. Cikrit D, West KW, Schreiner R, Grosfeld JR. Longterm follow up after surgical management of necrotizing enterocolitis: sixty-three cases. *J Pediatr Surg* 1986; 21:533–5.

222. Dudgeon DL, Schneider PA, Colombani P, et al. Neonatal necrotizing enterocolitis: an update. *South Med J* 1984; 77:1389–92.

223. Pokorny WJ, Harr VL, McGill CW, Harberg FJ. Intestinal stenosis resulting from necrotizing enterocolitis. *Am J Surg* 1981; 142:721–24.

224. Stevenson DK, Kerner JA, Malachowski N, Sunshine P. Late morbidity among survivors of necrotizing enterocolitis. *Pediatrics* 1980; 66:925–7.

225. Gough MH. The perinatal aspects of intestinal ischemia. *Clin Gastroenterol* 1973; 1:675–87.

226. Parkkulainen KV. Intrauterine intussusception as a cause of intestinal atresia: a contribution to the etiology of intestinal atresias. *Surgery* 1958; 44:1106–11.

227. Tibboel D, Kluck P, Molenaar JC, Gaillard JLJ. A comparative investigation of the bowel wall in gastroschisis and omphalocele. *Pediatr Pathol* 1987; 7:277–85.

228. Nixon HH. Intestinal obstruction in the newborn. *Arch Dis Child* 1955; 30:13–22.

229. Bernstein J, Vawter G, Harris GB, Young V, Hillman LS. The occurrence of intestinal atresia in newborns with meconium ileus: the pathogenesis of an acquired anomaly. *Am J Dis Child* 1960; 99:804–18.

230. Winter ST, Zeltzer M. Congenital atresia of the ileum in two brothers. *J Pediatr* 1956; 49:194–6.

231. Guttman FM. Multiple atresias and a new syndrome of hereditary multiple atresias involving the gastrointestinal tract from stomach to rectum. *J Pediatr Surg* 1973; 8:633–40.

232. Arnal-Monreal F, Pombo F, Capderila-Puerta A. Multiple hereditary gastrointestinal atresias: study of a family. *Acta Paediatr Scand* 1983; 72:773–7.

233. Collins DL, Kimura K, Morgan A, et al. Multiple intestinal atresia and amyoplasia congenita in four unrelated infants: a new association. *J Pediatr Surg* 1986; 21:331–3.

234. Lewis FJ. Intestinal atresia in identical twins. *Surgery* 1953; 33:121–5.

235. Denney ES, Sloan LH. Congenital intestinal malformations in identical twins (monozygotic twins) with closely related developmental defects; one of extreme rarity. *Surg Clin North Am* 1932; 12:227–40.

236. Earlam RJ. A study of the aetiology of congenital stenosis of the gut. *Ann R Coll Surg Engl* 1972; 5:126–30.

237. Blanc WA. The future of antepartum morphologic studies. In: Adamsons K, ed. *Diagnosis and Treatment of Fetal Disorders*. New York: Springer-Verlag, 1968, pp. 15–49.

238. deSa DJ. Intimal cushions in foetal placental veins. *J Pathol* 1973; 110:347–52.

239. Leffal LS Jr, Jackson M, Press H, Syphax B. Duplication cyst of the duodenum. *Arch Surg* 1967; 94:30–4.

240. Mellish RWP, Koop CE. Clinical manifestations of duplication of the bowel. *Pediatrics* 1961; 27:397–407.

241. Jewett TC. Duplication of the entire small intestine with massive melena. *Ann Surg* 1958; 147:239–44.

242. Schuler HW, Schuler B. Beitrag zur Klinik der duodenalen duplicaturen. *Z Kinderheilkd* 1967; 100:291–6.

243. Nathan MT. Cysts and duplications of neurenteric origin. *Pediatrics* 1959; 23:476–84.

244. Bremer JL. *Congenital Anomalies of the Viscera—Their Embryological Basis*. Cambridge, MA: Harvard University Press, 1957.

245. Heifetz S, Rueda-Pedraza ME. Omphalomesenteric duct cysts of the umbilical cord. *Pediatr Pathol* 1983; 1:325–35.

246. Blanc WA, Allan GW. Intrafunicular ulceration of persistent omphalomesenteric duct with intra-amniotic hemorrhage and fetal death. *Am J Obstet Gynecol* 1961; 82:1392–6.

247. Jackson RH, Bird AR. Meckel's diverticulum in childhood. *BMJ* 1961; 2:1399–1402.

248. Brown R.G. Meckel's curious anomaly. *Med Clin North Am* 1953; 37:227–35.

249. Yamaguchi M, Takeuchi S, Awazu S. Meckel's diverticulum: investigation of 600 patients in Japanese literature. *Am J Surg* 1978; 136:247–9.

250. de Bartolo HM Jr, van Heerden JA. Meckel's diverticulum. *Ann Surg* 1976; 183:30–3.

251. Cross VF, Wendth AJ, Phelan JJ, Goussous H, Moriarity DJ. Giant Meckel's diverticulum in a premature infant. *Am J Roentgenol Radium Ther Nucl Med* 1970; 108:591–7.

252. Miller DH, Becker MH, Eng K. Giant Meckel's diverticulum: a cause of intestinal obstruction. *Radiology* 1981; 140:93–4.

253. Kamel M, Heggtveit HA. Diverticulosis of Meckel's Diverticulum. Banff, Alberta: Congress of Laboratory Medicine, 1993. Abstract.

254. Christie A. Meckel's diverticulum: pathologic study of sixty-three cases. *Am J Dis Child* 1931; 42:544–53.

255. Kleinhaus S, Cohen MI, Boley SJ. Vitelline artery and vein remnants as a cause of intestinal obstruction. *J Pediatr Surg* 1974; 9:295–9.

256. Kim CJ, Choe GY, Chi JG. Foregut choristoma of the ileum (adenomyoma): a case report. *Pediatr Pathol* 1990; 10:799–805.

257. Emanuel B, Gault J, Sanson J. Neonatal intestinal obstruction due to absence of intestinal musculature: a new entity. *J Pediatr Surg* 1967; 2:332–35.

258. Carroll RL Jr. Absence of musculature of the distal ileum: a cause of neonatal intestinal obstruction. *J Pediatr Surg* 1973; 8:29–31.

259. Dhall JC, Khatri HL, Jaiswal TS, Sekkhon GS. Congenital segmental absence of intestinal musculature: a rare cause of intestinal obstruction in a neonate. *Am J Gastroenterol* 1978; 70:401–3.

260. Solowiejczyk M, Koren E, Deligdish L, Loewenthal M. Congenital absence of the muscle coats in the intestinal wall. *Int Surg* 1974; 59:367–8.

261. Steiner DH, Maxwell JG, Rasmussen BL, Jones R. Segmental absence of intestinal musculature. *Am J Surg* 1969; 118:964–7.

262. Husáin AN, Hong HY, Gooneratne S, Muraskas J, et al. Segmental absence of small intestinal musculature. *Pediatr Pathol* 1992; 12:407–15.

263. Okamoto E, Iwasaki T, Kakatani T, Ueda T. Selective destruction of the myenteric plexus: its relation to Hirschsprung's disease, achalasia of the esophagus and pyloric stenosis. *J Pediatr Surg* 1967; 2:444–54.

264. Litwin A, Avidor I, Schujman E, et al. Neonatal intestinal perforation caused by congenital defects of the intestinal musculature. *Am J Clin Pathol* 1984; 81:77–80.

265. Alvarez SP, Greco MA, Genieser NB. Small intestinal atresia and sequential absence of muscle coats. *Hum Pathol* 1992; 13:948–51.

266. Humphrey A, Mancer K, Stephens CA. Obstructive circular muscle defect in a one-year old child. *J Pediatr Surg* 1980; 15:197–9.

267. Welsh MJ, Tsui L-C, Boat AF, Beaudet AL. Cystic fibrosis. In: Scriver C, Beaudet AL, Sly WS, Valle D, eds. *Molecular and Metabolic Basis of Inherited Disease*. Philadelphia: McGraw-Hill, 1995, pp. 3799–877.

268. Rickham P, Boeckmann CR. Neonatal meconium obstruction in the absence of mucoviscidosis. *Am J Surg* 1965; 109:173–7.

269. Dolan TF Jr, Touloukian RJ. Familial meconium ileus not associated with cystic fibrosis. *J Pediatr Surg* 1974; 9:821–4.

270. Mizrahi A, Barlow O, Berdon W, Blanc WA, Silverman WA. Necrotizing enterocolitis in premature infants. *J Pediatr* 1965; 66:697–706.

271. Thelander HE. Perforation of the gastrointestinal tract of the newborn infant. *Am J Dis Child* 1939; 58:371–93.

272. Kliegman RM, Fanaroff AA. Necrotizing enterocolitis. *N Engl J Med* 1984; 310:1093–103.

273. Ricketts RR. Surgical therapy for necrotizing enterocolitis. *Ann Surg* 1984; 190:653–7.

274. Waldhausen JA, Herendeen T, King H. Necrotizing colitis of the newborn: common cause of perforation of the colon. *Surgery* 1963; 54:365–372.

275. Touloukian RJ, Kadar A, Spencer RP. The gastrointestinal complications of neonatal umbilical venous exchange transfusion: a clinical and experimental study. *Pediatrics* 1973; 51:36–43.

276. Diamond LK, Allen FH Jr, Thomas WO Jr. Erythroblastosis foetalis: treatment with exchange transfusion. *N Engl J Med* 1951; 244:39–49.

277. Peck DR, Lowman RM. Roentgen aspects of umbilical vascular catheterization in the newborn: the problem of catheter placement. *Radiology* 1967; 89:874–7.

278. Meyer WW, Lind J. Postnatal changes in the portal circulation. *Arch Dis Child* 1966; 41:606–12.

279. Ling E, deSa DJ. Nonbacterial thrombotic endocarditis of the tricuspid valve. *Lab Invest* 1970; 40:307–8. Abstract.

280. Morrow WR, Haas JE, Benjamin DR. Nonbacterial endocardial thrombosis in neonates: relationship to persistent fetal circulation. *J Pediatr* 1982; 100:117–22.

281. Rogers AF, Dunn PM. Intestinal perforation, exchange transfusion and P.V.C. *Lancet* 1969; 2:1246.

282. Hey EN, Ellis MI, Walker W. Ileocolitis following exchange transfusion. *Lancet* 1972; 1:266.

283. Alpan G, Eyal F, Vinograd I, et al. Localized intestinal perforations after enteral administration of indomethacin in premature infants. *J Pediatr* 1983; 106:277–81.

284. Kuhl G, Wille L, Bolkenius M, Seyberth HW. Intestinal perforation associated with indomethacin treatment in premature infants. *Eur J Pediatr* 1985; 143:213–16.

285. Nagaraj HS, Sandhu AS, Cook LN, Buchino JJ, Gross DB. Gastrointestinal perforation following indomethacin therapy in very low birth weight infants. *J Pediatr Surg* 1981; 16:1003–7.

286. Cronen PW, Nagaraj HS, Janik JS, et al. Effect of indomethacin on mesenteric circulation in mongrel dogs. *J Pediatr Surg* 1982; 17:474–78.

287. Bauer CR. Necrotizing enterocolitis. In: Sinclair JC, Bracken MB, eds. *Effective Care of the Newborn Infant*. Oxford: Oxford University Press, 1992, pp. 602–16.

288. Bill AH Jr, Chapman ND. The enterocolitis of Hirschsprung's disease. *Am J Surg* 1962; 103:70–4.

289. Fraser GC, Berry CL. Mortality in neonatal Hirschsprung's disease: with particular reference to enterocolitis. *J Pediatr Surg* 1967; 2:205–11.

290. Khanna SD. An experimental study of mesenteric occlusion. *J Pathol Bacteriol* 1959; 77:575–90.

291. Alward CR, Hook JB, Helmrath TA, Mattison JC, Baillie MD. Effects of asphyxia on cardiac output and organ blood flow in the newborn piglet. *Pediatr Res* 1978; 12:824–27.

292. Touloukian RJ, Posch JN, Spencer R. The pathogenesis of selective ischemic gastro-enterocolitis of the neonate: selective mucosal gut ischemia in asphyxiated neonatal piglets. *J Pediatr Surg* 1972; 7:194–205.

293. Sibbons PD, Spitz L, van Velzen D. Collateral blood flow in the distal ileum of neonatal piglets: a clue to the pathogenesis of necrotizing enterocolitis. *Pediatr Pathol* 1992; 12:15–27.

294. Sibbons PD, Spitz L, van Velzen D. Necrotizing enterocolitis induced by local circulatory interruption in the ileum of neonatal piglets. *Pediatr Pathol* 1992; 12:1–4.

295. Cannon WP, Burket IR. The endurance of anemia by nerve cells in the myenteric plexus. *Am J Physiol* 1913; 32:247–52.

296. Virjee J, Somers S, deSa D, Stevenson G. Changing patterns of neonatal necrotizing enterocolitis. *Gastrointest Radiol* 1979; 4:169–75.

297. Berry CL. Persistent changes in the large bowel following the enterocolitis associated with Hirschsprung's disease. *J Pathol* 1969; 97:731–32.

298. O'Neill JA Jr. Neonatal necrotising enterocolitis. *Surg Clin North Am* 1981; 61:1013–22.

299. Rickham P. Massive small intestinal resection in newborn infants. *Ann R Coll Surg Engl* 1967; 41:480–92.

300. Bell MJ, Shackelford P, Feigin RD, Ternberg JL, Brotherton T. Epidemiologic and bacteriologic evaluation of neonatal necrotizing enterocolitis. *J Pediatr Surg* 1979; 14:1–4.

301. Berdon WE, Grossman H, Baker DH, et al. Necrotizing enterocolitis in the premature infant. *Radiology* 1964; 83:879–87.

302. de Louvois J. Necrotising enterocolitis. *J Hosp Infect* 1986; 7:4–12.

303. Frantz ID, L'Heureux P, Engel RR, Hunt CE. Necrotizing enterocolitis. *J Pediatr* 1975; 86:259–63.

304. Kosloske AM. Pathogenesis and prevention of necrotizing enterocolitis. *Pediatrics* 1984; 74:1086–92.

305. Yu VY, Tudehope D. Neonatal necrotizing enterocolitis. II. Perinatal risk factors. *Med J Aust* 1977; 1:688–93.

306. deSa DJ, Donnelly WH. Myocardial necrosis in the newborn. *Perspect Pediatr Pathol* 1984; 8:295–311.

307. deSa DJ, Zipursky A. Myocardial necrosis and hypofibrinogenemia: a syndrome of cardiovascular collapse? *Lab Invest* 1980; 42:171. Abstract.

308. Uauy R, Fanaroff AA, Korones S, Philips EA, et al. Necrotizing enterocolitis in very low birthweight infants: biodemographic and clinical correlates. *J Pediatr* 1991; 119:630–38.

309. Rowe MI, Reblock KK, Kurkchubasche AG, Healey PJ. Necrotizing enterocolitis in the extremely low birth weight infant. *J Pediatr Surg* 1994; 29:987–91.

310. Sibbons P, Spitz L, van Velzen D, Bullock GR. Relationship of birth weight to the pathogenesis of necrotizing enterocolitis in the neonatal piglet. *Pediat Pathol* 1988; 8:151–62.

311. Yu VY, Tudehope D, Gill G. Neonatal necrotizing enterocolitis. I. Clinical aspects. *Med J Aust* 1977; 1:685–88.

312. Bell MJ, Ternberg JL, Feigin RD. Neonatal necrotizing enterocolitis. Therapeutic decisions based upon clinical staging. *Ann Surg* 1978; 187:1–7.

313. Walsh MC, Kliegman RM. Necrotizing enterocolitis treatment based on staging criteria. *Pediatr Clin North Am* 1986; 33:179–201.

314. Toma MJ, Delmos RA, Rogers JR, Diserens HM. Necrotizing enterocolitis in infants: analysis of 45 consecutive cases. *Am J Surg* 1973; 126:758–64.

315. Touloukian RJ, Berdon WE, Amoury RA, Santulli TU. Surgical experience with necrotizing enterocolitis in infants. *J Pediatr Surg* 1967; 2:389–401.

316. Wolfe JN, Evans WA. Gas in the portal veins of the liver in infants. *Am J Roentgenol Radium Ther* 1955; 74:486–90.

317. Firor HV, Myers HAP. Perforating appendicitis in premature infants. *Surgery* 1964; 56:581–83.

318. Bhargava SK. An outbreak of necrotizing enterocolitis in a special care newborn nursery. *Indian Pediatr* 1973; 10:551–53.

319. Brown EG, Sweet AY. Neonatal necrotizing enterocolitis. *Pediatr Clin North Am* 1982; 29:1149–70.

320. Guinan M, Schaberg D, Bruhn FW, Richardson CJ, Fox WW. Epidemic occurrence of neonatal necrotizing enterocolitis. *Am J Dis Child* 1979; 133:594–97.

321. Kliegman RM, Fanaroff AA. Neonatal necrotising enterocolitis: a nine year experience. I. epidemiology and uncommon observations. *Am J Dis Child* 1981; 135:603–7.

322. Polin RA, Pollack PF, Barlow B, et al. Necrotizing enterocolitis in term infants. *J Pediatr* 1976; 89:460–62.

323. Stein H. Gastroenteritis with necrotizing enterocolitis in premature babies. *BMJ* 1972; 2:616–19.

324. Takayanagi K, Kapila L. Necrotizing enterocolitis in older infants. *Arch Dis Child* 1981; 56:468–71.

325. Virnig NL, Reynolds JW. Epidemiological aspects of neonatal necrotizing enterocolitis. *Am J Dis Child* 1974; 128:186–90.

326. Cashore WJ, Peter G, Lavermann M, Stonestreet BS, Oh M. Clostridial colonization and clostridial toxin in neonatal necrotizing enterocolitis. *J Pediatr* 1981; 98:308–11.

327. Howard FM, Bradley JM, Flynn DM, Noone P, Szawatkowski M. Outbreak of necrotising enterocolitis caused by *Clostridium butyricum*. *Lancet* 1977; 2:1099–102.

328. Kliegman RM. Neonatal necrotising enterocolitis: implications for an infectious disease. *Pediatr Clin North Am* 1979; 36:327–44.

329. Bolton RP, Tait SK, Dear PRF, Losowsky MS. Asymptomatic neonatal colonisation by *Clostridium difficile*. *Arch Dis Child* 1984; 59:466–72.

330. Richardson SA, Alcock PA, Gray J. Clostrdium difficile and its toxin in healthy neonates. *BMJ* 1983; 2:878–9.

331. Smith MF, Borriello SP, Clayden GS, Casewell MW. Clinical and bacteriological findings in necrotising enterocolitis: a controlled study. *J Infect* 1980; 2:23–31.

332. Michel MF, Mettau J. Quantitative study of the aerobic and anaerobic faecal flora in neonatal necrotizing enterocolitis. *Arch Dis Child* 1983; 58:523–38.

333. Rietra PJGM, Slaterus KW, Zanen HC, Meuwissen SGM. Clostridial toxin in feces of healthy infants. *Lancet* 1978; 2:1319.

334. Lawrence G, Bates J, Gaul A. Pathogenesis of neonatal necrotising enterocolitis. *Lancet* 1982; 1:137–9.

335. Gonzalez-Crussi F, Hsueh W. Experimental model of ischemic bowel necrosis. *Am J Pathol* 1983; 112:127–35.

336. Cooke RA. Pig-bel. *Perspect Pediatr Pathol* 1979; 5:137–52.

337. Mogilner BM, Bar-Yochai A, Miskin A, Shie I, Aboudi Y. Necrotising enterocolitis associated with rotavirus infection. *Isr J Med Sci* 1983; 19:894–6.

338. Roussett S, Moscovici O, Lebon P et al. Intestinal lesions containing coronavirus-like particles in neonatal necrotizing enterocolitis: an ultrastructural analysis. *Pediatrics* 1984; 73:218–24.

339. Anders BJ, Lauer BA, Paisley JW. Campylobacter gastroenteritis in neonates. *Am J Dis Child* 1981; 135:900–2.

340. Buck GE, Kelly MT, Pichanick AM, Pollard TG. *Campylobacter jejuni* in newborns: a cause of asymptomatic bloody diarrhoea. *Am J Dis Child* 1982; 136:774.

341. Karmali MA, Tan YC. Neonatal campylobacter enteritis. *Can Med Assoc J* 1980; 122:192–3.

342. Mawer SL, Smith BAM. Campylobacter infection of premature baby. *Lancet* 1979; 1:1041.

343. Vesikari K, Chan KN, Ribeiro CD. *Campylobacter jejuni/coli* meningitis in a neonate. *BMJ* 1980; 280:1301–2.

344. Youngs ER, Roberts C, Davidson DC. Campylobacter enteritis and bloody stools in the neonate. *Arch Dis Child* 1985; 60:480–1.

345. Coello-Ramirez P, Gutierres-Topete G, Lifshitz F. Pneumatosis intestinalis. *Am J Dis Child* 1970; 120:3–9.

346. Gracey M. Bacterial diarrhoea. *Clin Gastroenterol* 1986; 15:21–37.

347. Lake AM, Walker WA. Neonatal necrotizing enterocolitis: a disease of altered host defences. *Clin Gastroenterol* 1977; 6:463–80.

348. Hsueh W, Gonzalez-Crussi F, Arroyave JL. Platelet-activating factor is an endogenous mediator in endotoxin induced bowel necrosis. *FASEB J* 1987; 1:403–5.

349. Hsueh W, Gonzalez-Crussi F, Arroyave JL. Sequential release of leukotrienes and norepinephrine in rat bowel after platelet activating factor: a mechanistic study of platelet-activating factor-induced bowel necrosis. *Gastroenterology* 1988; 94:1412–18.

350. Caplan M, Kelly A, Hsueh W. Endotoxin and hypoxia-induced intestinal necrosis in rats: the role of platelet activating factor. *Pediatr Res* 1992; 31:428–34.

351. Caplan M, Hedland E, Hill N, Mackendrick, W. The role of the endogenous nitric oxide and platelet activating factor in hypoxia-induced intestinal injury in rats. *Gastroenterology* 1994; 106:346–52.

352. Sun X, Caplan MS, Liu Y, Hsueh W. Endotoxin resistant mice are protected from PAF-induced shock, tissue injury and death. Roles of TNF_1 complement activation and endogenous PAF production. *Digest Dis Sci* 1995; 40:495–502.

353. Johansmann RJ, Zeek P. Periarteritis nodosa in a week-old infant. *Arch Pathol* 1954; 58:207–13.

354. Roberts FB, Fetterman GH. Polyarteritis nodosa in infancy. *J Pediatr* 1963; 63:519–29.

355. Willmer HA. Two cases of periarteritis nodosa occurring in the first month of life. *Bull Johns Hopkins Hosp* 1945; 77:275–86.

356. Bjarke B, Herin P, Blomback M. Neonatal aortic thrombosis: a possible manifestation of congenial anti-thrombin III deficiency. *Acta Pediatr Scand* 1974; 63:297–301.

357. Cusworth DC, Dent CE. Homocystinuria. *Br Med Bull* 1969; 25:42–7.

358. Dische MR, Gooch WM III. Congenital toxoplasmosis. *Perspect Pediatr Pathol* 1981; 6:83–114.

359. Boccon-Gibod L, Krichen HA, Cartier-Mercier LMB, Salaun JF, et al. Digestive tract involvement with exudative enteropathy in Langerhans cell histiocytosis. *Pediatr Pathol* 1992; 12:515–24.

360. Carruthers L, Dourmashkin R, Phillips A. Disorders of the cytoskeleton of the enterocyte. *Clin Gasteroenterol* 1986; 15:105–20.

361. Davidson GP, Cutz E, Hamilton JR, Gall DG. Familial enteropathy: a symptom of protracted diarrhoea from birth, failure to thrive and hypoplastic villous atrophy. *Gastroenterology* 1978; 75:783–90.

362. Phillips AD, Jenkins P, Rafaat F, Walker-Smith JA. Congenital microvillus atrophy: specific diagnostic features. *Arch Dis Child* 1985; 60:135–9.

363. Avery GB, Villavicencio O, Lilly JR, Randolph JG. Intractable diarrhoea in early infancy. *Pediatrics* 1968; 41:712–22.

364. Lloyd-Still JD, Schwachman H, Filler RM. Protracted diarrhoea in infancy treated with intravenous alimentation. I. Clinical studies of 16 infants. *Am J Dis Child* 1973; 125:358–64.

365. Hammoudia SM, Corkey JJ. Congenital hemangiopericytoma of the duodenum. *J Pediatr Surg* 1985; 20:559–60.

366. Srigley JR, Mancer K. Solitary intestinal fibromatosis with perinatal bowel obstruction. *Pediatr Pathol* 1984; 2:249–58.

367. Canioni D, Fekete C, Nezelof C. Solitary intestinal fibromatosis: a rare cause of neonatal obstruction. *Pediatr Pathol* 1989; 9:719–24.

368. Kapur RP, Shepard TH. Intestinal ganglioneuroblastoma in a 22-week fetus. *Pediatr Pathol* 1992; 12:583–92.

369. Reimund E, Ramos A. Disseminated neonatal gastrointestinal mucomycosis: a case report and review of the literature. *Pediatr Pathol* 1994; 14:385–9.

370. Abramowsky C, Beyer-Patterson P, Cortinas E. Nonsyphilitic spirochaetosis in second-trimester fetuses. *Pediatr Pathol* 1991; 11:827–38.

371. Molander M-L, Mortensson W, Uden R. Omental and mesenteric cysts in children. *Acta Paediatr Scand* 1982; 71:227–9.

372. Gonzalez-Crussi F, de Mello DE, Sotelo-Avila C. Omental-mesenteric myxoid hamartomas: infantile lesions simulating malignant tumours. *Am J Surg Pathol* 1983; 7:567–78.

373. Moore KL. *The Developing Human: Clinically Oriented Embryology.* 3rd ed. Philadelphia: WB Saunders, 1982, pp. 204, 227–54.

374. Bale PM. Sacrococcygeal developmental abnormalities and tumours in children. *Perspect Pediatr Pathol* 1984; 8:9–56.

375. Bruyere HJ Jr, Arya S, Kozel JS, Gilbert EF, et al. The value of examining spontaneously aborted human embryos and placentas. *Birth Defects— Original Article Series* (National Foundation: March of Dimes) 1987; 23(1):169–78.

376. Robinson HB Jr, Tross K. Agenesis of the cloacal membrane: a probable teratogenic anomaly. *Perspect Pediatr Pathol* 1984; 8:79–96.

377. Stephens FD, Smith ED. *Anorectal Malformations in Children.* Chicago: Year Book Medical, 1971.

378. Yntema CL, Hammond WS. The origin of intrinsic ganglia of trunk viscera from vagal neural crest in the chick embryo. *J Comp Neurol* 1954; 101: 515–41.

379. Andrew A. The origin of intramural ganglia. IV. The origin of enteric ganglia: a critical review and discussion of the present state of the problem. *J Anat* 1971; 108:169–84.

380. Weinberg AG. Hirschsprung's disease: a pathologist's view. *Perspect Pediatr Pathol* 1975; 2:207–39.

381. Yunis EJ, Sieber WJ, Akers DR. Does zonal aganglionosis really exist? Report of a rare variety of Hirschsprung's disease and review of the literature. *Pediatr Pathol* 1983; 1:33–49.

382. Dimmick JE, Bove KE. Cytomegalovirus infection of the bowel in infancy: pathogenetic and diagnostic significance. *Pediatr Pathol* 1984; 2:95–102.

383. Wells TR, Landing BH, Ariel I, Nadorra R, Garcia C. Normal anatomy of the myenteric plexus of infants and children: demonstration by flat-mount (circuit diagram) preparations. *Perspect Pediatr Pathol* 1987; 11:152–74.

384. Smith VV. Intestinal neuronal density in childhood: a baseline for the objective assessment of hypo- and hyperganglionosis. *Pediatr Pathol* 1993; 13:225–37.

385. Cole FM. Innominate grooves of the colon: morphological characteristics and etiologic mechanisms. *Radiology* 1978; 128:41–3.

386. Laufer I, deSa DJ. Lymphoid follicular pattern: a normal feature of the pediatric colon. *Am J Roentgenol Radium Ther Nucl Med* 1978; 130:51–5.

387. McGregor AL. A synopsis of surgical anatomy. 8th ed. Bristol: John Wright, 1957, p. 99.

388. Pagon RA, Smith DW, Shepard TH. Urethral obstruction malformation complex: a cause of abdominal muscle deficiency and the prune belly. *J Pediatr* 1979; 94:900–6.

389. Donnelly WH, Sieber WK, Yunis EJ. Polypoid ganglioneurofibromatosis of the large bowel. *Arch Pathol* 1969; 87:537–41.

390. Mendelsohn G, Diamond MP. Familial ganglioneuromatous polyposis of the large bowel: report of a family with associated juvenile polyposis. *Am J Surg Pathol* 1974; 8:515–20.

391. Weidner N, Flanders DJ, Mitros FA. Mucosal ganglioneuromatosis associated with multiple colonic polyps. *Am J Surg Pathol* 1984; 8:779–86.

392. Morson BC, Dawson IMP. *Gastrointestinal Pathology.* 2nd ed. Oxford: Blackwells, 1979, pp. 500, 687.

393. Hochberg FH, Dasilva AB, Galdabini J, Richardson EP. Gastrointestinal involvement in von Recklinghausen's neurofibromatosis. *Neurology* 1974; 24:1144–51.

394. Raszkowski HJ, Hufner RF. Neurofibromatosis of the colon: a unique manifestation of von Recklinghausen's disease. *Cancer* 1971; 27:134–42.

395. Carney JA, Go VLW, Sizemore GW, Hayles AB. Alimentary tract ganglioneuromatosis. A major component of the syndrome of multiple endocrine neoplasia, type 2B. *N Engl J Med* 1976; 295:1287–91.

396. Carney JA, Hayles AB. Alimentary tract malformations of multiple endocrine neoplasia, type 2B. *Mayo Clin Proc* 1977; 52:543–8.

397. Berry PJ, Favara BE, Burrington JD, Waddell WR. Familial megacolon with neuromatosis of the myenteric plexus. *Pediatr Pathol* 1984; 2:491. Abstract.

398. Fretzin DF, Potter B. Blue rubber bleb nevus syndrome. *Arch Intern Med* 1965; 116:924–9.

399. Halpern M, Turner AF, Citron BP. Hereditary hemorrhagic telangiectasia: an angiographic study of abdominal visceral angiodysplasias associated with gastrointestinal hemorrhage. *Radiology* 1968; 90:1143–9.

400. Westerholm P. A case of diffuse haemangiomatosis of the colon and rectum. *Acta Chir Scand* 1966; 133:173–6.

401. deSa DJ. The large bowel, rectum and anus. In: Whitehead R, ed. *Gastrointestinal and Oesophageal Pathology.* 2nd ed. Edinburgh: Churchill-Livingstone, 1995, p. 303.

402. Mullins F, Talamo R, di Sant' Agnese PA. Late intestinal complications of cystic fibrosis. *JAMA* 1965; 192:741–6.

403. Lloyd-Still J, Klaw KT, Shwachman H. Problems of rectal prolapse. *BMJ* 1971; 1:110.

404. Esterly JR, Oppenheimer EH. Pathology of cystic fibrosis: review of the literature and comparison with 146 autopsied cases. *Perspect Pediatr Pathol* 1975; 2:241–78.

405. Brett EM, Berry CL. Value of rectal biopsy in pediatric neurology. *BMJ* 1967; 3:400–3.

406. Kamoshita S, Landing BH. Distribution of lesions in myenteric plexus and gastrointestinal mucosa in lipidosis and other neurologic diseases of children. *Am J Clin Pathol* 1968; 49:312–18.

407. Holtzapple PG, Genel M, Yakovac WC, Hummeler K, Segal S. Diagnosis of cystinosis by rectal biopsy. *N Engl J Med* 1969; 281:143–5.

408. Flynn DM, Lake BD, Boothby CB, Young EP. Gut lesions in Fabry's disease without a rash. *Arch Dis Child* 1972; 47:26–33.

409. Myers GJ, Hedley-Whyte ET, Fagan ME. Reevaluation of role of rectal biopsy in diagnosis of pediatric neurologic disorders. *Neurology* 1973; 23:27–34.

410. Lake BD. Storage disorders involving the alimentary tract. In: Whitehead R, ed. *Gastrointestinal and Oesophageal Pathology.* 2nd ed. Edinburgh: Churchill-Livingstone, 1995, p. 343.

411. Van Zwalenburg BR. Double colon: differentiation of cases into two groups. *Am J Roentgenol Radium Ther* 1952; 68:22–7.

412. Smith ED. Duplications of the anus and genitourinary tracts. *Surgery* 1969; 66:909–21.

413. Smith S, Boulgakov B. A case of dicephalus dibrachius dipygus showing certain features of embryologic interest. *J Anat* 1926; 61:94–107.

414. Beischer NA, Fortune DW. Double monsters. *Obstet Gynecol* 1968; 32:158–70.

415. Mysorekar VR, Kolte DT, Shirole DB. A case of intestinal and urogenital duplication. *J Obstet Gynaecol Brit Commonwlth* 1967; 74:596–602.

416. Rowe MI, Ravitch MM, Ranniger K. Operative correction of caudal duplication (dipygus). *Surgery* 1968; 63:840–8.

417. Volpe M. Dell'asta Doppia. *Il Policlin Roma* 1903; 10:46–52.

418. Smith ED. Urinary anomalies and complications in imperforate anus and rectum. *J Pediat Surg* 1968; 3:337–49.

419. Weber HM, Dixon CF. Duplication of entire large intestine (colon duplex): report of a case. *Am J Roentgenol Radium Ther* 1946; 53:319–24.

420. Van Velzer DA, Barrick CW, Jenkinson EL. Duplication of the colon: a case presentation. *Am J Roentgenol Radium Ther* 1956; 75:349–53.

421. Ravitch MM, Scott WW. Duplication of the entire colon, bladder and urethra. *Surgery* 1953; 34:843–58.

422. Abrami G, Dennison WM. Duplication of the stomach. *Surgery* 1961; 49:794–801.

423. Gray AW. Triplication of the large intestine. *Arch Pathol* 1940; 30:1215–22.

424. Smith JR. Accessory enteric remnants: a classification and nomenclature. *Arch Dis Child* 1960; 35:87–9.

425. Ladd WE, Gross RE. Congenital malformations of the anus and rectum: report of 162 cases. *Am J Surg* 1934; 23:167–83.

426. Browne D. Some congenital deformities of the rectum, anus, vagina and urethra. *Ann R Coll Surg Engl* 1951; 8:173–92.

427. Gough MH. Congenital anomalies of the anus and rectum. *Arch Dis Child* 1961; 36:146–51.

428. Nixon HH. Imperforate anus. In: *British Surgical Practice.* (Surgical Progress). London: Butterworths, 1961.

429. Louw JH. *Congenital Abnormalities of the Rectum and Anus.* Chicago: Year Book Medical, 1965.

430. Romualdi P. Classification of the ano-rectal abnormalities. *Riv Chir Pediat* 1965; 7:1–7.

431. Stephens FD. *Congenital Malformations of the Rectum, Anus and Genitourinary Tract*. Edinburgh: E&S Livingstone, 1963.

432. Santulli TV, Kiesewetter WB, Bill AH Jr. Anorectal anomalies: a suggested international classification. *J Pediatr Surg* 1970; 5:281–7.

433. Magnus RV, Stephens FD. Imperforate anal membrane: the anatomy and function of the sphincters of the anal canal. *Aust Paediatr J* 1966; 2:165–72.

434. Partridge JP, Gough MH. Congenital abnormalities of the anus and rectum. *Br J Surg* 1961; 49:37–50.

435. Magnus RV. Rectal atresia as distinguished from rectal agenesis. *J Pediat Surg* 1968; 3:593–8.

436. Snyder WH Jr. Some unusual forms of imperforate anus in female patients. *Am J Surg* 1966; 111:319–25.

437. Johnston JH, Penn IA. Exstrophy of the cloaca. *Brit J Urol* 1966; 30:302–6.

438. Magnus RV. Ectopia cloacae—a misnomer. *J Pediat Surg* 1969; 4:511–19.

439. Carey JC, Greenbaum B, Hall BD. The OEIS complex (Omphalocele, exstrophy, imperforate anus, spinal defects). *Birth Defects—Original Article Series* 1978; 14(6B):253–63.

440. Choisy R. Sur l'absence des organes genitaux externes et la peritonite externe. *Gynecol Obstet* 1926; 13:177–82.

441. Gale DH, Stocker JT. Cloacal dysgenesis with urethral, vaginal outlet and anal agenesis and functioning internal genitourinary excretion. *Pediatr Pathol* 1987; 7:457.

442. Miarczynski D, deSa DJ. Agenesis of the cloacal membrane: analysis of the malformation complex. Banff: Canadian Congress of Laboratory Medicine, June 1993. Abstract.

443. Currarino G, Weinberg A. From small pelvic outlet syndrome to sirenomelia. *Pediatr Pathol* 1991; 11:195–210.

444. Prop N, Frensdorf EL, van der Stadt FR. A post-vertebral entodermal cyst associated with axial deformities: a case showing the entodermal-ectodermal adhesion syndrome. *Pediatrics* 1967; 39:555–62.

445. Cameron AH. Malformations of the neuro-spinal axis, urogenital tract and foregut in spina bifida attributable to disturbances in the blastophore. *J Pathol Bacteriol* 1957; 73:213–21.

446. Burrows FGO, Sutcliffe J. The split notochord syndrome. *Br J Radiol* 1968; 41:844–7.

447. Keen WW, Coplin ML. Sacrococcygeal tumour (teratoma) with an opening entirely through the sacrum, and a sinus passing through this opening and communicating with the rectum, the sinus resembling a bronchus. *Surg Gynecol Obstet* 1906; 3:661–76.

448. Rosselet PJ. A rare case of rhachisis with multiple malformations. *Am J Roentgenol Radium Ther* 1955; 73:235–40.

449. Esterly JR, Baghdassarian OM. Presacral neurenteric cyst. An unusual malformation resulting from persistence of the neurenteric canal. *Bull Johns Hopkins Hosp* 1963; 113:202–10.

450. Faris JC, Crowe JE. The split notochord syndrome. *J Pediatr Surg* 1975; 10:467–72.

451. Bolande RP. Neoplasia of early life and its relationship to teratogenesis. *Perspect Pediatr Pathol* 1976; 3:145–83.

452. Blumel J, Evans EB, Eggers GWN. Partial and complete agenesis or malformation of the sacrum with associated anomalies. *J Bone Joint Surg Am* 1959; 41A:497–518.

453. Passarge E, Lenz W. Syndrome of caudal regression in infants of diabetic mothers: observations of further cases. *Pediatrics* 1966; 37:672–4.

454. Smith ED. Congenital anomalies of the sacrum. *Aust NZ J Surg* 1959; 29:165–76.

455. Rusnak SL, Driscoll SG. Congenital spinal anomalies in infants of diabetic mothers. *Pediatrics* 1965; 35:989–95.

456. Duhamel B. From the mermaid to anal imperforation: the syndrome of caudal regression. *Arch Dis Child* 1961; 36:152–5.

457. Stocker JT, Heifetz SA. Sirenomelia. A morphological study of 33 cases and review of the literature. *Perspect Pediatr Pathol* 1987; 10:7–50.

458. Welch JP, Aterman K. The syndrome of caudal dysplasia: a review including etiologic considerations and evidence of heterogeneity. *Pediatr Pathol* 1984; 2:313–27.

459. Wilson JSP, Vallance-Owen J. Congenital deformities and insulin antagonism. *Lancet* 1966; 2:940–2.

460. Landauer W, Clarke EM. Teratogenic interaction of insulin and 2-deoxy-D-glucose in chick development. *J Exp Zool* 1962; 151:245–62.

461. Deuchar EM. Experimental evidence relating fetal anomalies to diabetes. In: Sutherland HW, Stowers JM, eds. *Carbohydrate Metabolism in Pregnancy and the Newborn 1978*. New York: Springer-Verlag, 1979, pp. 247–63.

462. Finer NN, Bowen P, Dunbar LG. Caudal regression anomalad (sacral agenesis) in siblings. *Clin Genet* 1978; 13:353–8.

463. Stewart JM, Stoll S. Familial caudal regression anomalad and maternal diabetes. *J Med Genet* 1979; 16:17–20.

464. Cohn J, Bay-Nielsen E. Hereditary defect of the sacrum and coccyx with anterior sacral meningocele. *Acta Pediatr Scand* 1969; 58:268–74.

465. Ashcraft KW, Holder TM, Harris DJ. Familial presacral teratomas. *Birth Defects: Original Article Series XV* (National Foundation: March of Dimes) 1975; 11(5):143–6.

466. Pinsky L. The community of human malformation syndromes that shares ectodermal dysplasia and deformities of the hands and feet. *Teratology* 1975; 11:227–42.

467. Hall JG, Pallister PD, Clarren SK, et al. Congenital hypothalamic hamartoblastoma, hypopituitarism, imperforate anus, and post axial polydactyly—a new syndrome? *Am J Med Genet* 1980; 7:47–74.

468. Hirschsprung H. Stuhltrageit neugeborener in folge von dilatation und hypertrophie des colons. *Jahrb Kinderheilk* 1887; 27:1–42.

469. Whitehouse FR, Kernohan JW. Myenteric plexus in congenital megacolon. *Arch Intern Med* 1948; 82:75–111.

470. Zuelzer WW, Wilson JL. Functional intestinal obstruction on neurogenic basis in infancy. *Am J Dis Child* 1948; 75:40–64.

471. Bodian M, Stephens FD, Ward BCH. Hirschsprung's disease and idiopathic megacolon. *Lancet* 1949; 1:6–11.

472. Ehrenpreis T. *Hirschsprung's Disease*. Chicago: Year Book Medical, 1970.

473. Warkany J. *Congenital Malformations*. Chicago: Year Book Medical, 1971, pp. 704–9.

474. Bodian M, Carter CO. A family study of Hirschsprung's disease. *Ann Hum Genet* 1963; 26:261–77.

475. Passarge E. The genetics of Hirschsprung's disease. Evidence of hetero-geneous etiology and a study of sixty families. *N Engl J Med* 1967; 276:138–43.

476. Madsen CM. *Hirschsprung's Disease: Congenital Intestinal Aganglionosis*. Springfield, IL: Thomas, CC. 1964.

477. Lake BD, Puri P, Nixon HH, Claireaux AE. Hirschsprung's disease: an appraisal of histochemically demonstrated acetylcholinesterase activity in suction rectal biopsy specimens as an aid to diagnosis. *Arch Pathol Lab Med* 1978; 102:244–7.

478. Wakely PE Jr, McAdams AJ. Acetylcholinesterase histochemistry and the diagnosis of Hirschsprung's disease: a $3\frac{1}{2}$ year experience. *Pediatr Pathol* 1984; 2:35–46.

479. Venugopal S, Mancer K, Shandling B. The validity of rectal biopsy in relation to morphology and distribution of ganglion cells. *J Pediatr Surg* 1981; 16:433–7.

480. Chow CW, Campbell PE. Short segment Hirschsprung's disease as a cause of discrepancy between histologic, histochemical and clinical features. *J Pediatr Surg* 1977; 12:675–80.

481. Gannon BJ, Noblet HR, Burnstock G. Adrenergic innervation of the bowel in Hirschsprung's disease. *BMJ* 1968; 1:487–9.

482. Burnstock G. Purinergic nerves. *Pharmacol Rev* 1972; 24:509–81.

483. Aaronson I, Nixon HH. A clinical evaluation of anorectal pressure studies in the diagnosis of Hirschsprung's disease. *Gut* 1972; 13:138–46.

484. Kapur RP, deSa DJ, Luquette M, Jaffe R. Hypothesis: pathogenesis of skip areas in long-segment Hirschsprung's disease. *Pediatr Pathol Lab Med* 1995; 15:23–37.

485. MacIver AG, Whitehead R. Zonal colonic aganglionosis, a variant of Hirschsprung's disease. *Arch Dis Child* 1972; 47:233–7.

486. Touloukian RJ, Duncan R. Acquired aganglionic megacolon in a premature infant: report of a case. *Pediatrics* 1975; 56:459–62.

487. Dimler M. "Acquired" Hirschsprung's disease. *J Pediatr Surg* 1981; 16:844–5.

488. Weinberg RJ, Klish WJ, Smalley JR, Brown MR, Putnam TC. Acquired distal aganglionosis of the colon. *Pediatrics* 1982; 101:406–9.

489. Tam PKH, Quint WGV, Van Velzen D. Hirschsprung's disease: a viral etiology? *Pediatr Pathol* 1992; 12:807–10.

490. Stern M, Hellwege HH, Gravinghoff L, Lambrecht W. Total aganglionosis of the colon (Hirschsprung's disease) and congenital failure of automatic ventilation (Ondine's curse). *Acta Paediatr Scand* 1981; 70:121–4.

491. Hall CM. Werner's mesomelic dysplasia with ventricular septal defect and Hirschsprung's disease. *Pediatr Radiol* 1981; 10:247–9.

492. Mallory SB, Weiner E, Nordlund JJ. Waardenburg's syndrome with Hirschsprung's disease: a neural crest defect. *Pediatr Dermatol* 1986; 3:119–24.

493. Chatten J, Witzleben CL. Neuroblastoma and Hirschsprung's disease. *Am J Pathol* 1975; 78:2a. Abstract.

494. Shocket E, Teloh HA. Aganglionic megacolon, pheochromocytoma, megaloureter and neurofibroma. *Am J Dis Child* 1957; 94:185–91.

495. Swenson O, Fisher JH. The relation of megacolon and megaloureter. *N Engl J Med* 1955; 253:1147–50.

496. Skinner R, Irvine D. Hirschsprung's disease and congenital deafness. *J Med Genet* 1973; 10:337–9.

497. Taguchi T, Tanaka K, Ikeda K. Fibromuscular dysplasia of arteries in Hirschsprung's disease. *Gastroenterology* 1985; 88:1099–103.

498. Saul RA, Sturner RA, Burger PC. Hyperplasia of the myenteric plexus: its association with early infantile megacolon and neurofibromatosis. *Am J Dis Child* 1982; 136:852–4.

499. Puri P, Lake BD, Nixon HH. Adynamic bowel syndrome: report of a case with disturbance of the cholinergic innervation. *Gut* 1977; 18:754–9.

500. Scharli AF, Meier-Ruge W. Localized and disseminated forms of neuronal intestinal dysplasia mimicking Hirschsprung's disease. *J Pediatr Surg* 1981; 16:164–70.

501. Schuffler MD, Bird TD, Sumi SM, Cook A. A familial neuronal disease presenting as intestinal pseudo-obstruction. *Gastroenterology* 1978; 75:889–98.

502. Byrne WJ, Cipel L, Euler AR, Halpin TC, Ament ME. Chronic idiopathic intestinal pseudo-obstruction syndrome in children—clinical characteristics and prognosis. *J Pediatr* 1977; 90:585–9.

503. Kaschula ROC, Cywes S, Katz A. Louw JH. Degeneration leiomyopathy with massive myacolon. *Perspect Pediatr Pathol* 1987; 11:193–213.

504. Nonaka M, Goulet O, Arahan P, Fekete C, et al. Primary intestinal myopathy: a cause of chronic idiopathic intestinal pseudo-obstruction syndrome (CIPS). *Pediatr Pathol* 1989; 9:409–24.

505. Gillis DA, Grantmyre EB. Megacystis-microcolon-intestinal hypoperistalsis syndrome: survival of a male infant. *J Pediatr Surg* 1985; 20:279–81.

506. Al-Rayess M, Ambler MW. Axonal dystrophy presenting as the megacystis-microcolon-intestinal hypoperistalsis syndrome. *Pediatr Pathol* 1992; 12:743–50.

507. Goutieres F, Mikol J, Aicardi J. Neuronal intranuclear inclusion disease in a child: diagnosis by rectal biopsy. *Ann Neurol* 1990; 27:103–6.

508. Tanner MS, Smith B, Lloyd JK. Functional intestinal obstruction due to deficiency of argyrophil neurons in the myenteric plexus. *Arch Dis Child* 1976; 51:837–41.

509. Yunis EJ, Schofield DE. Intestinal neuronal dysplasia in a case of sigmoid stenosis. *Pediatr Pathol* 1992; 12:275–80.

510. Mitros FA, Schuffler MD, Teja K, Anuras S. Pathologic features of familial visceral myopathy. *Hum Pathol* 1982; 13:825–33.

511. Smith VV, Lake BD, Kamm MA, Nicholls RJ. Intestinal pseudo-obstruction with deficient smooth muscle action. *Histopathology* 1992; 21:535–42.

512. Murray RD, Qualman SJ, Powers P, Caniano DA, et al. Rectal myopathy in chronically constipated children. *Pediatr Pathol* 1992; 12:787–98.

513. Schuffler MD. Neuromuscular abnormalities of small and large intestine. In: Whitehead R, eds. *Gastrointestinal and Oesophageal Pathology*. 2nd ed. Edinburgh: Churchill-Livingstone, 1995, p. 407.

514. Davis WS, Allen RP, Favara BE, Slovis TL. Neonatal small left colon syndrome. *Am J Roentgenol Radium Ther Nucl Med* 1974; 120:322–9.

515. Berdon WE, Slovis TL, Campbell JB, Baker DH, Haller JO. Neonatal small left colon syndrome: its relationship to aganglionosis and meconium plug syndrome. *Radiology* 1977; 125:457–62.

516. Hjernstad BM, Helwig EB. Tailgut cysts: report of 53 cases. *Am J Clin Pathol* 1988; 89:139–47.

517. Gius JA, Stout AP. Perianal cysts of vestigial origin. *Arch Surg* 1938; 37:268–87.

518. Hawkins WJ, Jackman RJ. Developmental cysts as a source of perianal abscesses and fistulas. *Am J Surg* 1953; 86:678–83.

519. Laird DR. Presacral cystic tumours. *Am J Surg* 1954; 88:793–7.

520. Edwards M. Multilocular retrorectal cystic disease—cyst hamartoma: report of twelve cases. *Dis Colon Rectum* 1961; 4:103–10.

521. Guillermo C, Grossman IW. Presacral cyst. *Am Surg* 1972; 38:448–50.

522. Campbell WL, Wolff M. Retrorectal cysts of developmental origin. *Am J Roentgenol Radium Ther Nucl Med* 1973; 117:307–13.

523. Caropreso PR, Wengert PA Jr, Milford EH. Tailgut cyst—a rare retrorectal tumour. *Dis Colon Rectum* 1975; 18:597–600.

524. Uhlig BE, Johnson RL. Presacral tumors and cysts in adults. *Dis Colon Rectum* 1975; 18:581–96.

525. Marco V, Autonell J, Farre J, Fernandez-Layos M, Doncel M. Retrorectal cyst-hamartomas: report of two cases with adenocarcinoma developing in one. *Am J Surg Pathol* 1982; 6:707–14.

526. Crowley LV, Page HG. Adenocarcinoma arising in presacral enterogenous cyst. *Arch Pathol* 1960; 69:64–6.

527. Spencer RJ, Jackman RJ. Surgical management of pre-coccygeal cysts. *Surg Gynecol Obstet* 1962; 115:449–52.

528. Colin JF, Branfoot AC, Robinson KP. Malignant change in rectal duplication. *J R Soc Med* 1979; 72:935–7.

529. Picard EJ, Picard JJ, Jorissen J, Jardon M. Heterotopic gastric mucosa in the epiglottis and rectum. *Am J Diag Dis* 1978; 23:217–21.

530. Edouard A, Jouanelle A, Amar A, Doutone P, et al. Ulcerated heterotopic gastric mucosa located in the rectum. *Gastroenterol Clin Biol* 1983; 7:39–42.

531. Castellanos D, Menchen P, Lopez de la Riva M, et al. Heterotopic gastric mucosa in the rectum. *Endoscopy* 1984; 16:197–9.

532. Schwarzenburg SJ, Whitington PF. Rectal gastric mucosa heterotopia as a cause of hematochezia in an infant. *Dig Dis Sci* 1983; 28:470–2.

533. Shindo K, Bacon HE, Holmes EJ. Ectopic gastric mucosa and glandular tissue of a salivary type in the anal canal concomitant with a diverticulum in hemorrhoidal tissue: report of a case. *Dis Colon Rectum* 1972; 15:57–62.

534. Weitzner S. Ectopic salivary gland tissue in submucosa of rectum. *Dis Colon Rectum* 1983; 26:814–17.

535. Sun CC, Raffel LJ, Wright LL, Mergner WL. Immature renal tissue in colonic wall of patient with caudal regression syndrome. *Arch Pathol Lab Med* 1986; 110:653–5.

536. Drut R, Drut RM. Hyperplasia of lymphoglandular complexes in colon segments in Hirschsprung's disease. *Pediatr Pathol* 1992; 12:575–81.

537. Townes PL, Brocks ER. Hereditary syndrome of imperforate anus with hand, foot and ear anomalies. *J Pediatr* 1972; 81:321–6.

538. Kurnit DM, Steele MW, Pinsky L, Dibbins A. Autosomal dominant transmission of a syndrome of anal, ear, renal and radial congenital malformations. *J Pediatr* 1978; 93:270–3.

539. Temtamy S. Schinzel syndrome of ulnar ray defects, hypogenitalism and anal atresia. *Birth Defects: Original Article Series* 1978; 14:156–7.

540. Dungy C, Aptekar RG, Cann HM. Hereditary hydrometrocolpos with polydactyly in infancy. *Pediatrics* 1971; 47:138–41.

541. Pinsky L. The syndromology of anorectal malformation (atresia, stenosis, ectopia). *Am J Med Genet* 1978; 1:461–74.

542. Riccardi V, Hassler E, Lubinsky M. The FG syndrome: further characterization, report of a third family, and of a sporadic case. *Am J Med Genet* 1977; 1:47–58.

543. Mecke S, Passarge E. Encephalocele, polycystic kidneys, and polydactyly as an autosomal recessive trait simulating certain other disorders. The Meckel syndrome. *Ann Genet* 1971; 14:97–103.

544. Hsia YE, Bratu M, Herbordt A. Genetics of the Meckel syndrome (dysencephalia splanchnocystica). *Pediatrics* 1971; 48:237.

545. Saldino RM, Noonan C. Severe thoracic dystrophy with striking micromelia, abnormal osseous development, including the spine, and multiple visceral anomalies. *Am J Roentgenol Radium Ther Nucl Med* 1972; 114:257–63.

546. Fraser CR. Our genetical "load." A review of some aspects of genetical variation. *Ann Hum Genet* 1962; 25:387–415.

547. Azvedo ES, Biondi J, Ramaldo LM. Cryptophthalmos in two families. *J Med Genet* 1973; 10:389–92.

548. Toledo SA, Medeiros-Neto GA, Knobel M, Matler E. Evaluation of the hypothalamic-pituitary-gonadal function in Bardet-Biedl syndrome. *Metabolism* 1977; 26:1277–91.

549. Little JR, Opitz JM. Case reports: the G syndrome. *Am J Dis Child* 1971; 121:505–7.

550. Frias JL, Rosenbloom AL. Two new familial cases of the "G" syndrome. *Birth Defects: Original Article Series* 1975; 11(2):54–7.

551. Opitz JM, Summitt RL, Smith DW. The BBB syndrome, familial telecanthus with associated anomalies. *Clinical Delineation of Birth Defects* (National Foundation—March of Dimes) 1969; 5:86–94.

552. Johanson A, Blizzard R. A syndrome of congenital aplasia of the alae nasi, deafness, hypothyroidism, dwarfism, absent permanent teeth, and malabsorption. *J Pediatr* 1971; 79:982–7.

553. Daentl DL, Frias JL, Gilbert EF, Opitz JM. The Johanson-Blizzard syndrome: case report and autopsy findings. *Am J Med Genet* 1979; 3:129–35.

554. Quan L, Smith DW. The VATER association: vertebral defects, anal atresia, T-E fistula with esophageal atresia, radial and renal dysplasia: a spectrum of associated defects. *J Pediatr* 1973; 82:104–7.

555. Blank CE. Apert's syndrome (a type of acrocephalo-syndactyly) obser-

vations on British series of thirty-nine cases. *Ann Hum Genet* 1960; 24: 151–64.

556. Hanson JW, Myrianthopoulos NC, Harvey MAS, Smith DW. Risks to the offspring of women treated with hydantoin anticonvulsant, with emphasis on the fetal hydantoin effect. *J Pediatr* 1976; 89:662–8.

557. Tan KL, Tan R, Tan SH, Tan AM. The twin transfusion syndrome. *Clin Pediatr* 1979; 18:111–14.

558. Wells TR, Gwinn JL, Landing BH. Sling left pulmonary artery: two diseases, one with bridging bronchus, absence of pars membranacea and high incidence of imperforate anus. *Lab Invest* 1987; 56:7P. Abstract.

Liver Disease in the Perinatal Infant

JAMES E. DIMMICK   GARETH P. JEVON

INTRODUCTION

In assessing fetal and neonatal liver disease, the pathologist must understand developmental changes and how they relate to injury in early life.

EMBRYOLOGY

The liver originates from a diverticulum of the foregut in the middle of the third week of embryonic development. This hepatic primordium of endodermal cells lies between the pericardial cavity and the yolk sac, and has cephalic and caudal portions, the former producing the common bile duct and liver, and the latter forming the cystic duct and gallbladder. Endodermal epithelial clusters proliferate on the cap of the cephalic part of the diverticulum and invade the septum transversum, preexisting vascular spaces, and hematopoietic cells. These features are shared with mesoderm of the adjacent yolk sac. Branches of paired lateral vitelline veins immerse in the proliferating parenchyma, forming primitive sinusoids. The relatively large blood supply may contribute to rapid liver growth and incorporation of the laterally placed paired umbilical veins. Through anastomoses and atrophy involving the caudal portions of the left and right vitelline veins, the S-shaped portal vein forms. This vein is composed of the right cranial component of the distal vitelline vein and an anastomotic channel dorsal to the foregut. Anomalous development during this phase may result in an anteriorly positioned preduodenal portal vein associated with such anomalies as polysplenia, intestinal malrotation, and biliary atresia. The distal portion of the portal vein joins the superior mesenteric and splenic veins. The proximal or cephalic residue of the vitelline veins drains the hepatic sinusoids to the sinus venosus. Ultimately,

the left vitelline vein atrophies and the right contributes to the formation of the hepatic veins. With the disappearance of the right umbilical vein and acquisition of substantial blood flow through the left umbilical vein, the ductus venosus develops by enlargement of sinusoidal passages. The left umbilical vein gives off branches predominantly to the left lobe, which is perfused with richly oxygenated blood. The right lobe receives lesser amounts of the umbilical flow but more of the less oxygenated portal venous supply. This vascular asymmetry accounts for differences in pathology occurring in left and right lobes in stillbirths and newborn infants, and reminds us that in a postmortem examination one should sample both the left and right lobes of the liver [1].

The ductus venosus shunts the majority of umbilical blood to the inferior vena cava until birth, when it closes functionally. The ductus may reopen with hypoxia, and shunting then may be responsible for transient hyperammonemia of the neonate.

Hepatic arteries are less conspicuous than veins in early gestation. Similarly, portal vein branches, as one might expect from the relative lack of intestinal function, are small and peripherally approach the small size of arterioles. Hepatic vein growth exceeds that of the portal vein, and the lobular microscopic spatial arrangement of the adult liver is lacking.

The common bile duct forms from the cephalic hepatic diverticulum. The lumen is obliterated by proliferating epithelial cells, then is recanalized; this observation is contradicted by some who refute a "solid phase" [2]. Smaller inter- and intralobular ducts develop through induction of embryonic hepatocytes [3–9]. The portal vein develops from the hilum to the hepatic periphery, with an enveloping cuff of mesenchyme. Embryonic hepatocytes encountering the mesenchyme transform into a ductal plate, which is initially a single cell layer (Fig. 25.1) [10]. The induced cells increasingly produce cytokeratins that are distinct from adjacent hepatocytes, lose carcinoembryonic antigen, and exhibit epithelial membrane antigen. The plate becomes bilayered focally, then forms a lumen. Mesenchymal cells increase in the adjoining portal tract, and laminin appears at the interface with the newly formed duct. Ultrastructurally, the duct cells are enclosed by a basement membrane. Through focal dissolution and mesenchymal interposition, the ductal plate network is progressively reduced and transformed into the intrahepatic duct system, which is ultimately invested in an arterial plexus. Interlobular ducts are rare at 13 weeks, becoming more numerous as gestation progresses [7]. Genesis of the intralobular ducts and ductules is critical to an understanding of the mechanisms by which abnormalities, such as autosomal recessive polycystic kidney disease and paucity of intrahepatic ducts, evolve.

The canaliculus, the finest extracellular component of the biliary system, is present very early in hepatogenesis. Based on studies of fetal and neonatal rat liver, canaliculi at first are primitive invaginations of adjacent cell membranes and later develop microvilli [11, 12]. By showing that rat fetal hepatocytes lack canalicular contractions seen in adult cells, Phillips suggests that this functional immaturity may be significant in neonatal cholestasis [13].

Hematopoiesis becomes pronounced by the third month in hepatic cords, gaining access to the sinusoids through large gaps between Kupffer's cells, which also become increasingly prominent. Hematopoiesis is more pronounced in the right lobe than in the left. Following birth, hematopoiesis progressively disappears, regardless of the length of gestation at the time of delivery. A few pockets of erythroid cells persist in the lobule, and some myeloid cells linger in the portal tracts into early infancy, but usually little remains after the seventh postpartum day [14].

Hemosiderin occurs normally, but in widely varying quantities, in fetal hepatocytes, especially the periportal cells [15]. Hemosiderin tends to be more abundant in the left lobe than in the right. Those not familiar with normal fetal and neonatal liver histology may misinterpret hemosiderin as pathologic, especially when it is abundant.

Developing human hepatocytes have a microvillus intercellular and sinusoidal border. Sinusoid walls are at first incomplete, but a continuous lining of endothelial and Kupffer's cells is established by 6 to 8 weeks of gestation. Rough endoplasmic reticulum is prominent by the seventh week, peroxisomes by the eighth week, and the Golgi apparatus, which is perinuclear at 4 weeks, moves to the pericanalicular zone in the third month at about the time bile formation commences [16]. Phagocytic activity of the Kupffer's cells is evident in the third month. Smooth endoplasmic reticulum becomes prominent at the 12th week, coincident with glycogen deposits and bile formation. Significant amounts of glycogen accumulate prior to birth. Following delivery, glycogen is utilized and the hepatocyte volume increases with an abundance of rough endoplasmic reticulum, mitochondria, lysosomes, peroxisomes, and Golgi apparatus.

Ultrastructural heterogeneity of hepatocytes with corresponding functional zonation is seen through the lobule in the adult liver but is not present in the fetus or neonate. This lack of morphologic zonation implies that functional homogeneity exists in the immature fetal liver lobule, and

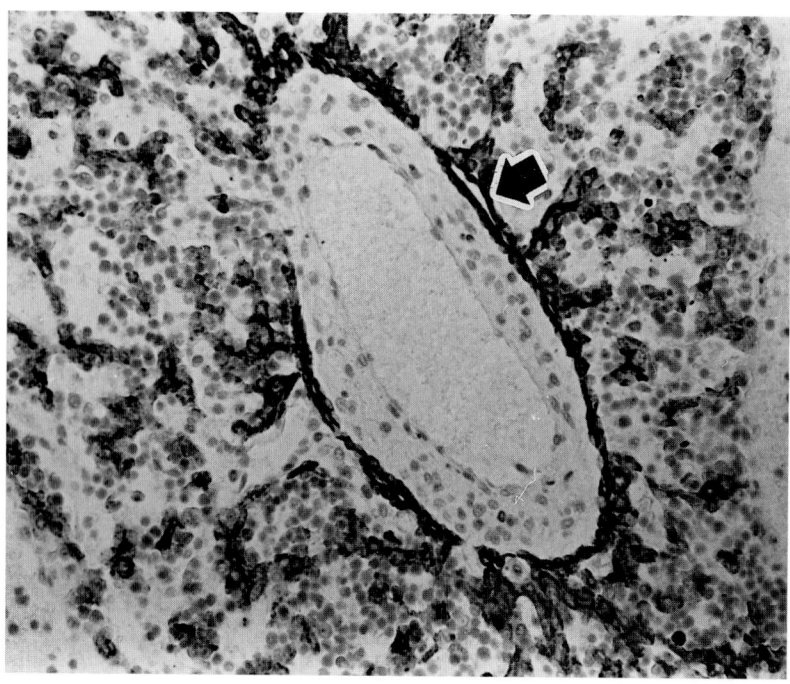

FIGURE 25.1.   *Liver of a 17-week-gestation fetus. The ductal plate is labeled with anticytokeratin antibody in an immunoperoxidase reaction. Note that the plate is partly a single and partly a double layer. A lumen is present at one point (arrow). ×100.*

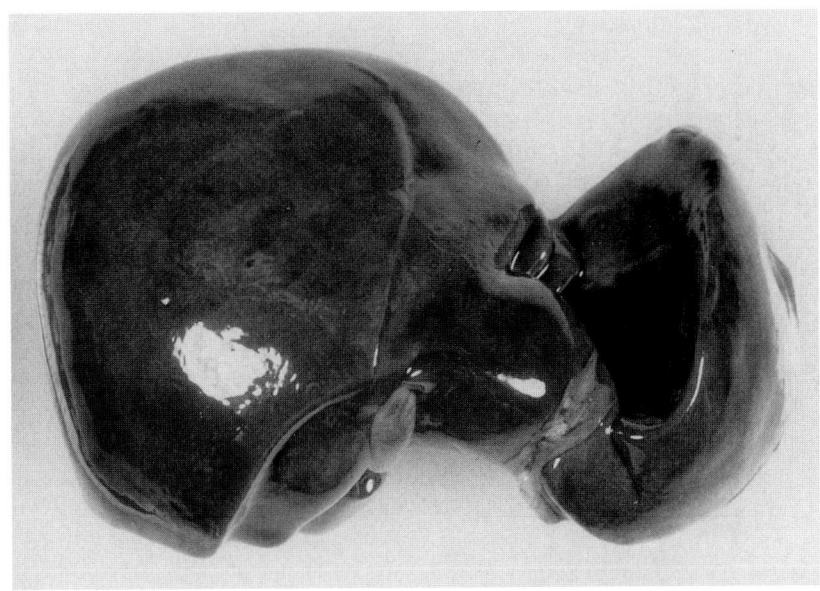

FIGURE 25.2. *Left diaphragmatic hernia. The left hepatic lobe is folded into the pleural space.*

in fact has been demonstrated for urea cycle enzymes [17]. Functional immaturity affects bilirubin and bile acid metabolism after birth. The fetal liver is capable of catabolizing xenobiotics. In the first phase, the P-450 system is present, particularly in the left lobe, and the fetal liver has oxidation reduction drug metabolizing reactions. The second phase of conjugation reactions is immature, suggesting that the fetus could be susceptible to xenobiotic injury from toxic metabolites generated from first-phase reactions [18, 19].

Anatomic anomalies of the liver include abnormalities of position and lobation. In syndromes of abnormal situs (situs inversus, polysplenia, and asplenia), the liver may be left-sided or symmetrically disposed. The left lobe folds around the residuum of diaphragm into the left pleural space in the most common form of diaphragmatic hernia (Fig. 25.2). In the rare occurrence of bilateral diaphragmatic hernias, both lobes extend cephalad, simulating inversion of the liver (Fig. 25.3). The liver also protrudes into the pleural cavity in diaphragmatic eventration, although a thin membrane, sometimes bearing islands of hepatocytes, intervenes. The liver may also extrude into an omphalocele or gastroschisis, and then is globular. In the acardiac chorangiopagus twin, the liver may be absent. Liver parenchyma rarely occurs ectopically in gallbladder, pancreas, splenic capsule, adrenal gland, umbilicus, gastroesophageal junction, pylorus, lung, and retroperitoneum [20]. Hepatic parenchyma without portal tracts occasionally occurs in teratomas. A hepatic adenoma (monodermal teratoma) in placenta has been reported [21].

PERINATAL HEPATITIDES

Many infectious agents cause hepatitis, but the majority of cases with histologically defined hepatitis as yet have no known etiology. Hepatic pathology need not be due to an infectious agent (Table 25.1). Metabolic disturbances (see later) are important causes, as exemplified by alpha$_1$-antitrypsin deficiency, Niemann-Pick type C, and hepatitis associated with some chromosomal errors. The diversity of associations is further illustrated by infants with neonatal lupus erythematosus who may have cholestatic liver disease with pathologic changes of neonatal hepatitis. The pathogenesis is unknown, although, hypothetically, transplacental maternal antibody may cause the injury [22, 23].

Hepatitis of infectious etiology is acquired in utero via the placenta, from an ascending genital tract infection, and during or after birth. Generally, the risk of transplacental fetal infection increases with gestation. Thus, the risk of infection of the fetus is low in the first trimester of

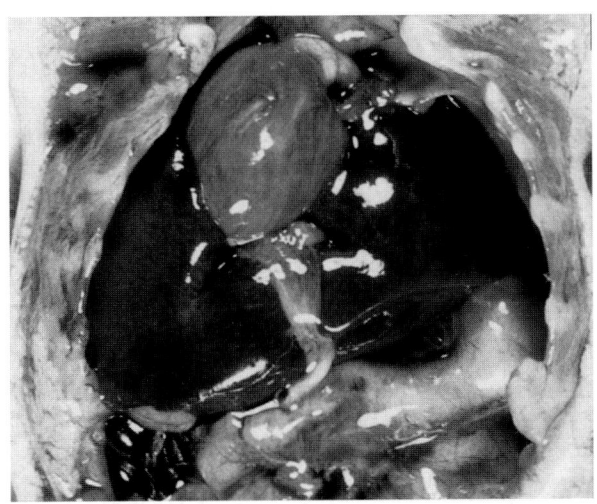

FIGURE 25.3. *Bilateral diaphragmatic hernias: both hepatic lobes extend into the pleural spaces.*

Table 25.1.   Perinatal hepatitides (histologic hepatitis)

Idiopathic group
Idiopathic neonatal hepatitis
Infectious group
Viral hepatitides: cytomegalovirus; rubella virus; reovirus 3; hepatitis viruses (A, B, C): Echovirus; coxsackievirus ; herpesvirus; varicella virus; adenovirus; parvovirus B19; HIV
Bacterial hepatitides: Listeria monocytogenes; Mycobacterium tuberculosis; Treponema pallidum; bacterial sepsis-associated hepatitis
Protozoan hepatitis: Toxoplasma gondii
Metabolic group
Alpha$_1$-antitrypsin deficiency; Niemann-Pick disease type C; cystic fibrosis; bile acid synthesis disorders (some); mitochondriopathies (some); peroxisomopathies (some); tyrosinemia
Miscellaneous group
Idiopathic neonatal iron storage syndrome; familial cholestasis and bile duct paucity syndromes (some); neonatal lupus erythematosis; trisomy 21, 18, and 4 del

pregnancy for such agents as toxoplasmosis and hepatitis B [24]. Infectious agents of the genital tract, such as herpesvirus, take an ascending route to the fetus, even through intact placental membranes, and easily contaminate the infant during birth. Infection of the infant by hepatitis B virus from maternal blood also occurs during delivery [24]. Routes of postnatally acquired infections are breast feeding, umbilical sepsis, instrumentation, and the common pathways recognized for infections of older infants.

Idiopathic Neonatal Hepatitis Syndrome

Idiopathic neonatal hepatitis (INH) is a clinical pathologic syndrome separate from cholestatic liver disease due to biliary atresia [25, 26]. Hepatitis virus, once considered the probable etiology, is only an exceptional cause. Landing suggested that neonatal hepatitis, biliary atresia, and choledochal cysts are pathophysiologically related and probably due to

viral infection, modified in some patients by coexistent metabolic disease [27].

In large studies of cholestasis in infants with patent extrahepatic ducts, approximately 70% have INH (Table 25.2) [28, 29]. Of 1086 infants with all forms of liver disease, INH comprised 30% [30].

Clinically, INH is characterized by cholestasis, hepatic dysfunction, hepatomegaly, splenomegaly, and failure to thrive. Acholic stools may occur, and there may be evidence of hemolysis. Infants are likely to be preterm, of small birth weight, and male. There is a familial occurrence, and the recurrence risk in siblings is one in seven [28]. The incidence of INH in southeast England is 21 per 100,000 livebirths [31].

In INH, the lobular architecture is retained, but there is hepatocellular unrest and usually giant-cell transformation, which distorts the hepatic cord pattern. Cytoplasmic and canalicular cholestasis is prominent. There is hepatocellular necrosis, with acidophilic bodies. Kupffer's cells are stimulated. Granules of hemosiderin and foci of erythropoiesis are present in the lobule. There is a modest portal lymphocytic infiltrate. Portal and lobular fibrosis may occur, but this is variable. Ductular proliferation is usually absent or minimal, and bile thrombi and bile duct proliferation are rare (Fig. 25.4).

Diagnosis of INH is necessarily one of exclusion. It is important to distinguish idiopathic hepatitis from biliary atresia. Infectious and metabolic causes and other diseases with similar histology should be excluded (see Table 25.1). The distinction between biliary obstructive disease and hepatocellular disorders can be made accurately by liver biopsy; in 93.3% of cases in the study by Brough and Bernstein, and 96.8% of cases noted by Lai et al [32, 33].

The nature and pathogenesis of giant-cell transformation, which occurs commonly in idiopathic neonatal hepatitis, are controversial. These hepatocytes are characterized by three or four (or more) nuclei and by fine granular cytoplasm often stained with bile, hemosiderin, or lipofuscin, and they are not mitotically active. It has been proposed that they are

Table 25.2.   Neonatal cholestasis with patent extrahepatic ducts

	Alagille [36]	Danks et al [28]	Mowat et al [29]
Idiopathic neonatal hepatitis	169	69	71
Infections	18	22	6
Cytomegalovirus	5	13	1
Rubella	4	3	2
Toxoplasmosis	3	2	1
Syphilis	4	1	—
Hepatitis B	—	1	2
Coxsackie	—	2	—
Metabolic	16	14	26
Other	21	—	—

formed by cell fusion (possibly virus induced) or by amitotic division [34]. Ruebner and Thaler suggested that giant cells form through fusion of hepatocytes that have undergone pseudoductular formation [35]. Hepatocellular giant cells are seen in many diseases of the infant liver (Table 25.3) and are nonspecific [34]. They are, however, particularly common in INH and are less obvious in other disorders causing conjugated hyperbilirubinemia. Hepatocellular giant cells disappear with resolution of cholestasis.

Infants with INH recover completely (50%), die acutely or within the first year (25%), or develop chronic liver disease (25%), including cirrhosis and paucity of intrahepatic ducts [36–40]. Hepatitis may recur in some patients following orthotopic liver transplantation [41]. Death in the first year, or later in some cases, may be due to associated diseases [37]. The prognosis for infants with a history positive for familial hepatitis is worse, as is the prognosis for those with very severe cholestasis and those with biopsy

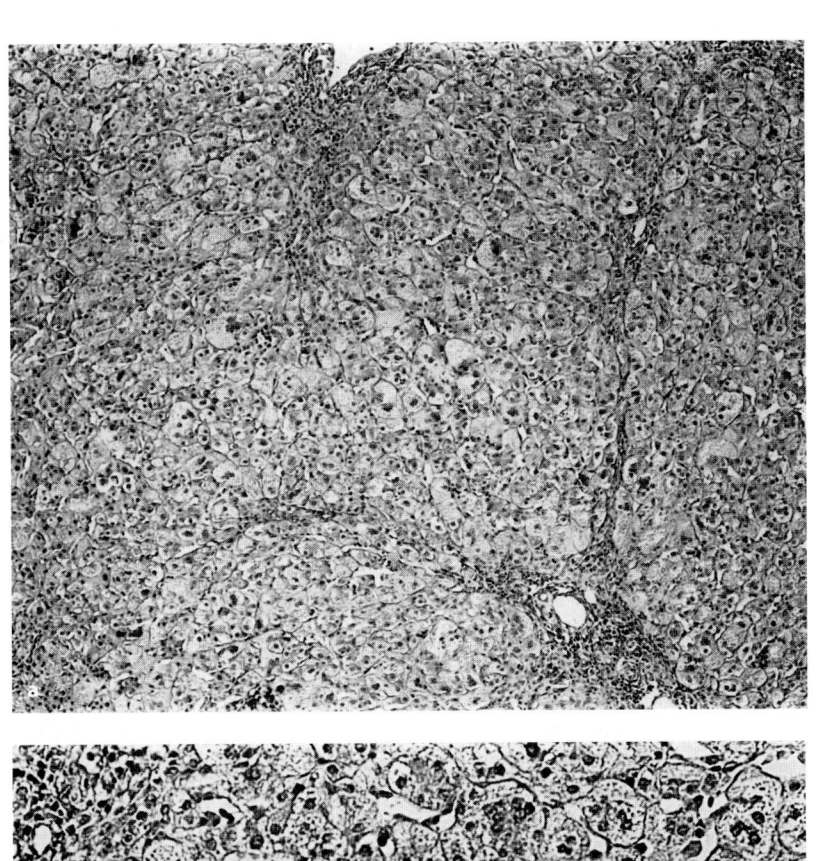

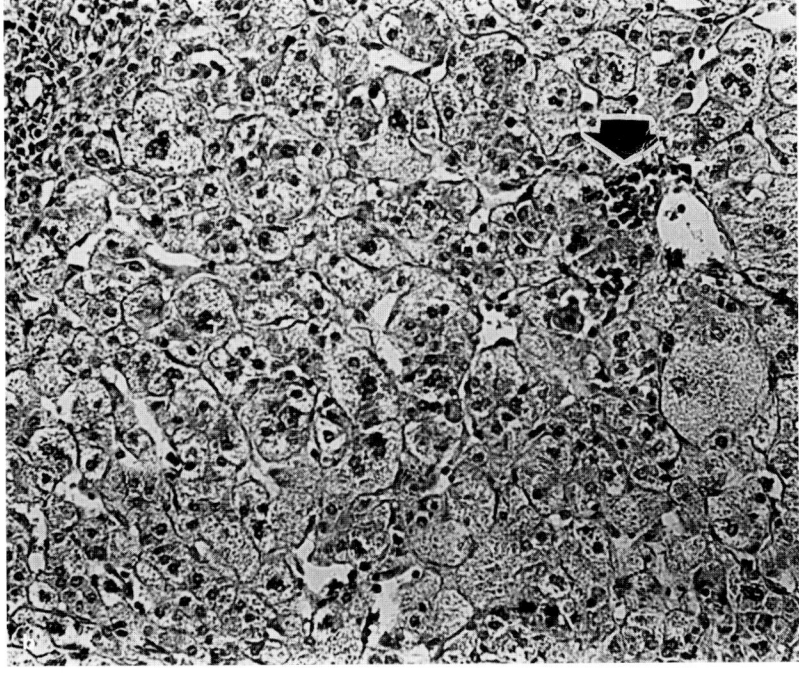

FIGURE 25.4. *Idiopathic neonatal hepatitis. (a) Giant-cell transformation prominently developed in the lobule, mild septal fibrosis, and portal inflammation. H&E, ×40. (b) At higher magnification, one can readily identify the multinucleate giant cells. Granular quality of the cytoplasm is largely due to cholestasis. A portal tract lies at the upper left; a hepatic vein with an adjacent cluster of erythroid cells lies at mid-right (arrow). H&E, ×200.*

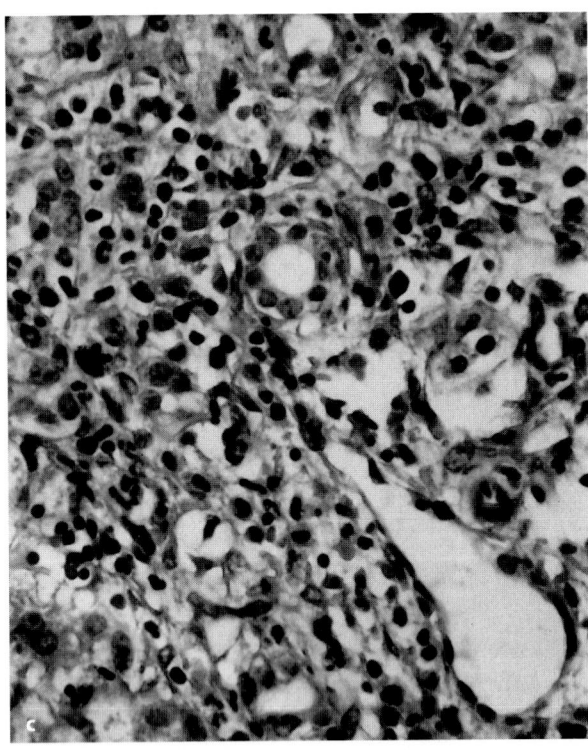

FIGURE 25.4. *Continued.* *(c) Portal tract inflamed with lymphocytes. There is no ductular or ductal proliferation. H&E, ×160.*

Table 25.3. Giant cell transformation and associations (modified from Montgomery and Ruebner [34])

Infantile obstructive cholangiopathy complex
Idiopathic neonatal hepatitis; biliary atresia; choledochal cyst; intrahepatic bile
 duct paucity
Infections (see Table 25.1)
Metabolic
Alpha₁-antitrypsin deficiency; Niemann-Pick disease type C; cystic fibrosis; Gaucher
 disease; galactosemia; mucolipidosis; bile acid synthesis disorders (some);
 mitochondriopathies (some); peroxisomopathies (some); tyrosinemia
Chromosomal errors
Trisomy 21, trisomy 18, monosomy X
Associations with anomalies
Endocardial cushion defect; anomalous pulmonary venous return; Arnold-Chiari
 malformation
Miscellaneous
Idiopathic neonatal iron storage syndrome; familial cholestasis syndromes; Alagille
 syndrome; neonatal lupus erythematosus, immunohemolytic disorders

evidence of diminished intralobular bile ducts [38]. Worse outcome for infants who have undergone surgical exploration for diagnosis than for those who have not is attributed to the known poor outcome of familial hepatitis rather than to the surgery [40, 42]. Regardless, it is preferable to do a needle rather than a surgical biopsy for diagnosis if possible.

Perinatal Hepatitides of Infectious Etiology

Cytomegalovirus (CMV) infection of the liver is usually part of a generalized infection arising in utero or postnatally. Symptomatic infants are jaundiced with conjugated hyperbilirubinemia and hepatosplenomegaly. Hepatic pathology varies considerably [43, 44]. Few viral inclusions may be found in bile duct epithelial cells in an otherwise normal liver from an asymptomatic infant. On the other hand, cholangitis, hepatitis with giant-cell transformation, periportal and lobular fibrosis, and cirrhosis may occur, although CMV-induced cirrhosis is not accepted by all (Figs. 25.5 and 25.6) [43]. There may be ductular proliferation and steatosis [43, 44]. Viral inclusions are found in hepatocytes, in Kupffer's cells, and especially in the biliary epithelium.

In addition to hepatitis, extrahepatic biliary atresia and paucity of intrahepatic bile ducts have been attributed to or associated with CMV infection [45–48].

CMV hepatitis may persist for several months, but despite this there is no significant residual liver disease in most infants [44]. Periportal and subcapsular calcification may be the sole residuum of intrauterine infection. Diagnosis of CMV hepatitis requires demonstration of the virus by culture or histology. Viral inclusions, however, may be sparse. Immunoperoxidase antibody or DNA techniques are helpful.

Intrauterine rubella infection causes hepatosplenomegaly and conjugated hyperbilirubinemia. Clinical signs of liver dysfunction may persist for months. Early manifestations of rubella liver disease include focal hepatocellular necrosis, cholestasis, excessive hematopoiesis, portal mononuclear inflammation, periportal fibrosis, ductular proliferation, and giant-cell transformation of hepatocytes [49, 50]. The pathology may be indistinguishable from idiopathic neonatal hepatitis, requiring serologic investigations to establish the diagnosis. There appear to be few late effects, although cirrhosis and biliary atresia have occurred [50].

In infants, hepatitis B causes hepatitis (sometimes severe), causes cirrhosis, induces a carrier state, and predisposes the patient to hepatocellular carcinoma [51–53]. Hepatitis B surface and core antigens have been identified with unexpected frequency in the livers of Japanese patients with neonatal hepatitis, biliary atresia, and choledochal cyst [54].

In a review of icteric hepatitis B in 40 infants, 14 died and seven developed cirrhosis [24]. The risk of hepatitis in the infant is related to the timing of the maternal infection and the antigen and antibody status of the mother [24]. Acute hepatitis B of the mother in the third trimester yields a 70% risk of fetal transmission; within 8 weeks of delivery, an 80% risk; and first-trimester hepatitis, a 5% risk [24].

Mothers who are carriers of HBsAg and HBeAg transmit the virus with a frequency of 85–100%, and hepatitis

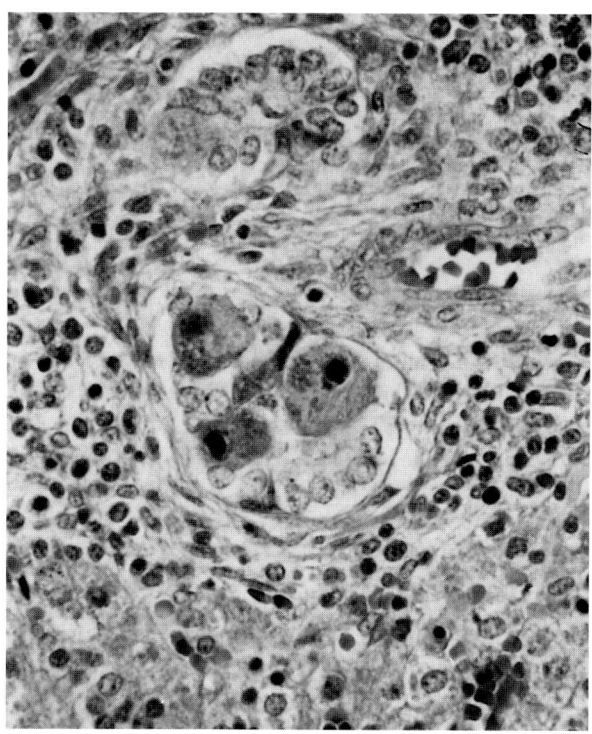

FIGURE 25.5.   *Cytomegalovirus hepatitis. Note viral inclusions in duct epithelium. ×160.*

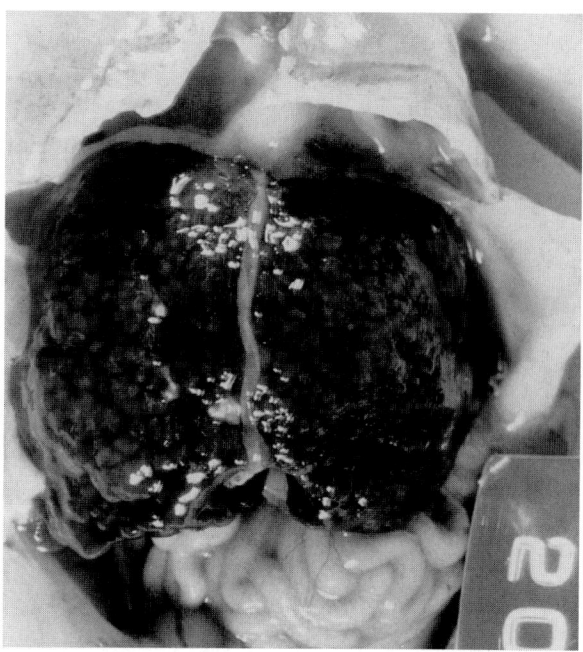

FIGURE 25.6.   *Eighteen-week-gestation fetus with severe cytomegalovirus hepatitis.*

and a carrier state may develop in the infants. Should the mother also have anti-HBe antibody, the transmission rate falls to less than 10%, with no carriers created and only mild hepatitis occurring in the offspring [24]. Maternal carriers lacking both the Hbe antigen and antibody offer a 20% risk of the carrier state for their infants. The overall risk for clinical hepatitis in infants infected perinatally is 3–5% [24]. The liver in those infected varies from normal histology to massive necrosis. Dupuy et al described massive liver necrosis, absent inflammation, and pale hepatocytes in the acute phase, with periportal fibrosis and multinucleated cells appearing later [51]. Delta agent associated with severe hepatitis B in the adult is transmitted with hepatitis B from mother to infant [24].

Hepatitis A and E are usually not transmitted to the fetus [53]. Hepatitis A infection in the neonate generally follows a benign course with asymptomatic seroconversion, although in one nursery outbreak of clinical hepatitis an infant with hepatic necrosis died [55]. Vertical hepatitis C transmission from mother to infant is more likely when the mother is HIV positive. Infection in the infant is usually silent clinically, although a carrier state or, rarely, symptomatic hepatitis may arise [56, 57].

Infants with congenital toxoplasmosis with either generalized or neurologic disease usually have hepatomegaly and jaundice. Hepatic pathology is not specific. Excessive hematopoiesis is the most constant abnormality [58]. There

is minimal focal or diffuse hepatitis, focal necrosis and cholestasis, ductal proliferation, and periportal fibrosis. Giant-cell transformation and cirrhosis may develop [58]. Calcification occurs in the liver parenchyma and in vessel walls. Parasites are seen rarely in endothelium, Kupffer's cells, and foci of necrosis.

Herpesvirus, echovirus, varicella, coxsackievirus, and adenovirus hepatic infections share pathologic similarities. All, and particularly the first two, are frequently associated with fulminant disease with massive hepatic necrosis. Herpesvirus hepatitis is the most common of this group. Acquired from a genital tract infection, herpes hepatitis is part of a generalized infection. The liver shows massive coagulative necrosis and hemorrhage but little inflammatory reaction (Fig. 25.7) [59]. There is no zonal predilection. Multinucleate hepatocytes occur [59]. Intranuclear viral inclusions, present in remaining viable hepatocytes at the margins of necrosis or around portal tracts, are homogeneous and faintly basophilic, and push the chromatin to the nuclear membrane. Only a few inclusions have halos about them. Pathology of echovirus and herpesvirus hepatitis is the same, but inclusions are not seen by light microscopy in the former [60, 61]. Similar necrotizing hepatitis occurs in congenital varicella infection. Viral nuclear inclusions are found in hepatocytes and particularly in the bile duct epithelium. Coxsackieviral hepatic necrosis without viral inclusions and inflammation has been reported [44]. Adenovirus also produces massive necrosis of the infant liver. Both hepatocytes and ducts are involved; surviving liver cells contain intranuclear inclusions bounded by a halo, and the cytoplasm may contain lipid droplets. Infants reported with adenovirus hepatic necrosis have been immunodeficient. Foci of dystrophic calcification may be the only marker of an intrauterine viral hepatitis [62].

Parvovirus B19 infection of the fetus usually manifests as hydrops fetalis. The liver rarely may be the site of hepatitis with giant-cell transformation, cholestasis, duct proliferation, and periportal fibrosis [63].

Reovirus 3 is associated with neonatal hepatitis, biliary atresia, and choledochal cyst, but an etiologic relationship has not been confirmed [64]. Beyond the neonatal period, giant-cell transformation and hepatitis occur in some infants with HIV infection [65, 66].

Bacterial hepatitis is rare. *Listeria monocytogenes*, *Treponema pallidum*, and *Mycobacterium tuberculosis* directly infect the liver, but the so-called toxic hepatitis associated with gram-negative bacterial sepsis is encountered more commonly. Infants with this form of toxic hepatitis frequently have conjugated hyperbilirubinemia and hepatomegaly. The pathology is similar to that of idiopathic neonatal hepatitis. Cholestasis is cytoplasmic and canalicular, rarely ductular. Bile duct proliferation is minimal, as is portal fibrosis, and mild portal inflammation, hepatocellular unrest, and giant-cell transformation occur. Congenital listeriosis and tuberculosis both cause multiple foci of necrosis (miliary abscesses), which are obvious both grossly and microscopically. Organisms may be demonstrated in the lesions with Gram's and Ziehl-Neelsen stains. Mononuclear inflammatory cells without histiocytic giant cells surround the necrotic foci [67]. In congenital syphilis, there are focal or diffuse mononuclear inflammation and hepatocellular necrosis. Focal or diffuse fibrosis and giant-cell transformation

may occur throughout the lobule where, before treatment, spirochetes abound in the space of Disse [68].

PERINATAL CHOLANGIOPATHIES

Some instances of extrahepatic biliary atresia, choledochal cyst, and paucity of intrahepatic bile ducts originate in the fetus, and then the pathologic expression is dependent on the timing of the insult to the biliary system or programming error in development [69, 70]. Disorders of the intrahepatic and extrahepatic bile ducts are listed in Table 25.4.

Extrahepatic Biliary Atresia

Biliary atresia occurs less frequently than idiopathic neonatal hepatitis. An incidence of 1 in 8000 for hepatitis is compared with 1 in 14,000 for atresia [28]. In southeast England, the incidences are 21 and 8 per 100,000 livebirths for hepatitis and atresia, respectively [31]. The occurrence of biliary atresia in Japan is also approximately 1 per 10,000 livebirths [71].

Unlike INH, there is a preponderance of female infants in most series of biliary atresia. The infants are of normal weight and full-term gestation, and familial occurrence is rare, with only 11 instances reported since 1855 [28, 72]. The infant with biliary atresia has acholic stools at birth or soon thereafter and becomes progressively jaundiced. Although the infant thrives initially, growth and well-being soon cease and biliary cirrhosis and complications evolve if the condition is not treated. The major differential diagnosis is INH. Uncommonly, a patent small-caliber extrahepatic duct may progressively obliterate in an infant with clinical

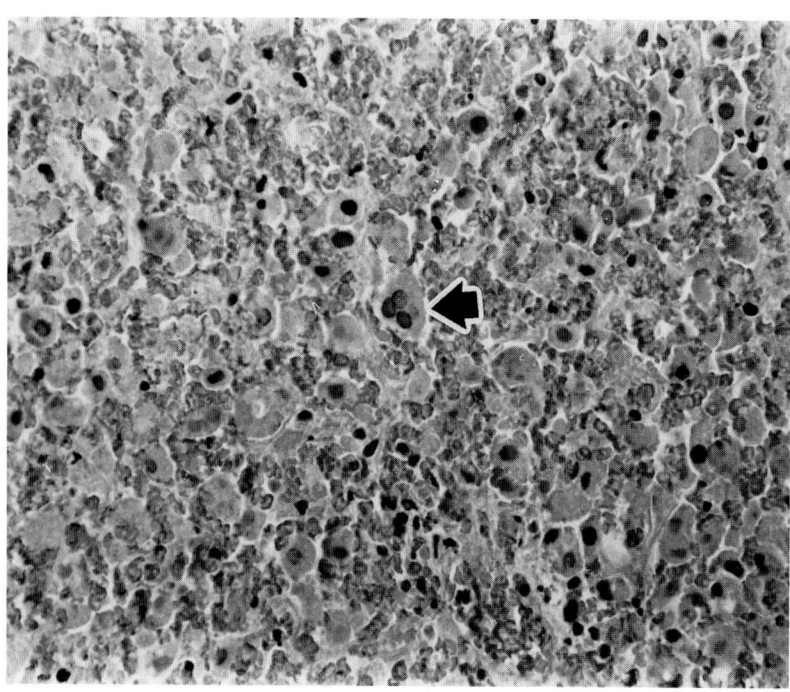

FIGURE 25.7. *Herpesvirus hepatitis in a newborn infant. There is extensive hepatocellular necrosis. In the center, a trinuclear hepatocyte (arrow) contains intranuclear inclusions displacing the chromatin to form a ring at the nuclear margin. H&E, ×200.*

Table 25.4. Perinatal cholangiopathies

Extrahepatic biliary atresia
Isolated
With syndromes (polysplenia, Alagille syndrome)
With chromosomal errors (trisomy 18, triploidy)
With metabolic disorders (alpha$_1$-antitrypsin deficiency, cystic fibrosis, Niemann-
 Pick disease)
With infections (rubella, cytomegalovirus, reovirus 3, L. monocytogenes)
With multiple anomaly complexes
Choledochal cyst
Isolated
With biliary atresia
With choledochopancreatic junction anomalies
With intrahepatic duct dilatation
With duodenal atresia
Paucity of intrahepatic bile ducts
Syndromic (Alagille syndrome)
Nonsyndromic
With extrahepatic biliary atresia
With metabolic disorders (alpha$_1$-antitrypsin deficiency, THCA excess, Zellweger
 syndrome)
With chromosomal errors (trisomy 18, trisomy 21, partial trisomy 11, monosomy X,
 partial deletion chromosome 20)
With infections (cytomegalovirus, rubella)
With graft-versus-host disease
Portal-biliary dysgenesis (ductal plate malformation)
Autosomal recessive polycystic kidney disease
Meckel syndrome
Ivemark syndrome (renal-hepatic-pancreatic dysplasia)
Beckwith-Wiedemann syndrome
With skeletal disorders
 Chondrodysplasias (Saldino-Noonan syndrome, Elejalde syndrome, Ellis–van
 Creveld syndrome, Jeune syndrome, Majewski syndrome)
Roberts syndrome
With chromosomal errors (trisomy 9, trisomy 13)
With metabolic disorders (glutaric aciduria type II, Zellweger syndrome)
Other
Duplications of duct system
Spontaneous perforation of bile duct
External compression of common duct
Luminal obstruction of common duct

neonatal hepatitis, or an early neonatal onset may occur for those in whom ductal atresia has occurred in utero. Among infants and children with sclerosing cholangitis, onset occurs in the neonatal period in 27% [73].

The etiology of extrahepatic biliary atresia is unknown. Circumstantial evidence suggests that there is an insult to previously normally formed ducts [74]. Biliary atresia is usually not associated with malformations and is rare in stillborn infants. Inflammation, ductal epithelial destruction, and ongoing fibrosis are found in the excised duct remnant. Acholic stools may follow an initial short period in which bile has been seen, indicating that the duct was previously patent [74].

A viral etiology is considered to be the most likely. Hepatitis A and Epstein-Barr virus have not been implicated. Rubella virus, hepatitis B, and CMV are uncommon causes [48, 54, 74]. We failed to identify CMV DNA in a polymerase chain reaction–based study of 12 cases [75]. Reovirus 3 has a serologic association but remains unproved as an etiology. One case of congenital *Listeria monocytogenes* infection possibly caused biliary atresia [76].

Evidence for an inflammatory pathogenesis includes immunoglobulin on the basement membrane of periductal gland remnants and a higher-than-expected frequency of HLA B12 in infants with biliary atresia [77, 78]. Toxin-mediated duct injury has been proposed but has little support as a cause.

Errors of duct development occur in a minority of cases in which failed recanalization (if an epithelial solid phase does indeed occur) or discordant epithelial–mesenchymal longitudinal growth could result in a solid cord, discontinuous duct, or membranous diaphragmatic obstruction [79, 80]. Biliary atresia occasionally concurs with membranous duodenal atresia, a recanalization defect [81].

A vascular accident–ischemia hypothesis is supported by experimental evidence [82]. There are, however, few reported concurrences of intrauterine ischemic injury of the bowel or other sites with atresia of the extrahepatic duct.

Anomalies associated with biliary atresia are listed in Table 25.4. In three series of infants with biliary atresia, the percentages with polysplenia syndrome were 7.5% of 308, 17% of 35, and 20% of 29 infants [83–85]. Among 51 infants with atresia of the biliary tract and developmental anomalies, the laterality sequence (polysplenia syndrome) was present in 15, another six probably had limited expression of the same syndrome, and the remaining 30 had various nonsyndromic anomalies with probable etiologic heterogeneity [86].

Based on knowledge of aberrant vascular patterns in the polysplenia syndrome, Witzleben speculated that an intrauterine vascular accident may be responsible for biliary atresia [87]. Others suggest that abnormal cilia found in some infants with polysplenia may in some way be implicated during embryogenesis [88].

A small number of affected infants have trisomy 18, triploidy, and duplications of chromosomes 10 and 22 [69].

Therefore, there are multiple etiologies of biliary atresia, and different expressions, depending on the time of insult to the liver and duct system.

The liver becomes enlarged, green, and increasingly firm and fibrous as biliary cirrhosis evolves. Early microscopic pathology consists of hepatocellular cytoplasmic and canalicular cholestasis. Ductular proliferation is usually not prominent until approximately 4 weeks of postnatal age (Figs. 25.8–25.10). The exception is found in early onset cases when ductular proliferation and, sometimes, a ductal-plate-type anomaly may be present. The lobular architecture is maintained at first. Giant-cell transformation occurs in about 15% of cases, and there is variable portal inflammation and

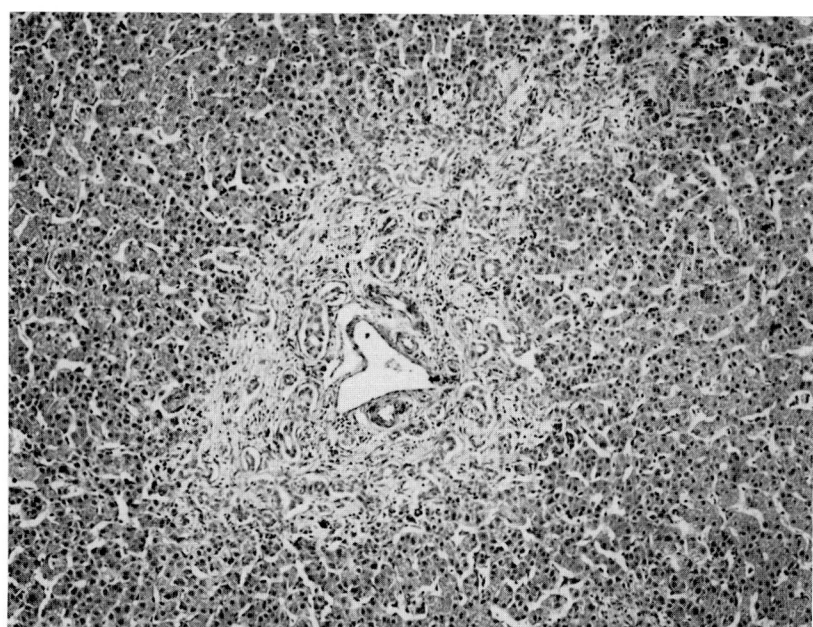

FIGURE 25.8. *Extrahepatic biliary atresia in 1-month-old infant. There are ductal and ductular proliferation and moderate portal fibrosis. ×27.*

fibrosis, which progresses to a concentric pattern different from the radiating septal pattern of hepatitis. Bile stasis is present in ductules and ducts. Hepatocellular necrosis occurs focally; extramedullary erythropoiesis is less prominent than in INH. As the disease unfolds, ductal proliferation peaks at about 7 months, and then the ducts and ductules progressively disappear. The features in biopsies that are most valuable in distinguishing biliary obstruction from hepatitis are ductular proliferation and ductular and ductal bile stasis. These features may not be fully evident before 4 to 6 weeks of age.

Pathology of the extrahepatic duct varies. In correctable forms, the proximal duct is patent, and when this is anastomosed to the bowel, bile flow is reestablished. These forms constituted a minority of cases (8.1%) in a compilation of 596 patients [89]. The majority, which were noncorrectable

cases, had totally obliterated ducts (61.9%), and 18.3% were patent distally. The typical remnant consists of a thin, fibrous strand culminating in a broad, fibrous mass in the porta hepatis. The gallbladder is often small. Histologic studies of the surgically excised extrahepatic duct have shown obliteration of the lumen at some level, and most have been inflamed [90, 91]. The porta hepatis may show inflammation with fibrous tissue replacing the duct. In some cases, the porta hepatis contains scattered periductal glands and their ductules, and in others a true biliary duct is seen. Early attempts to correlate the histology of the proximal tissues with bile flow following hepatic portoenterostomy [90–92] showed a negative correlation with obliterative fibrous pathology, but more recent evaluations have related positive bile flow to the presence of true biliary duct structures [92]. There is controversy as to whether or not the size of the

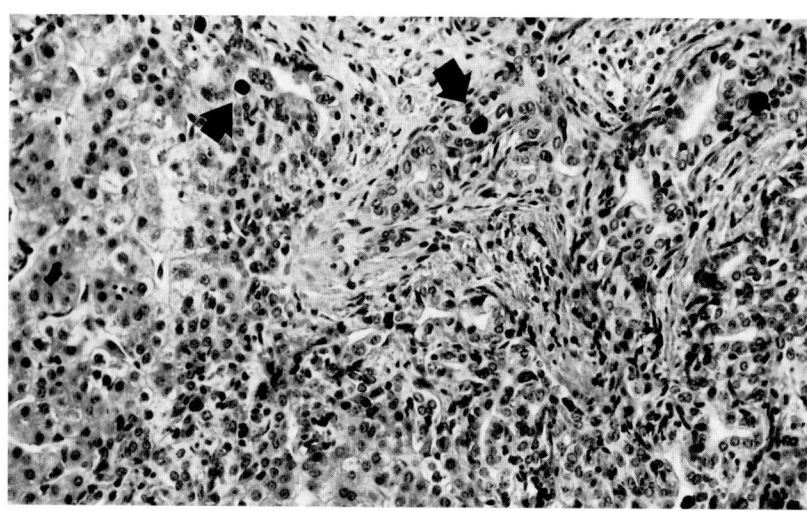

FIGURE 25.9. *Extrahepatic biliary atresia. Ductal and ductular proliferation; note the bile plugs (arrows) ×140.*

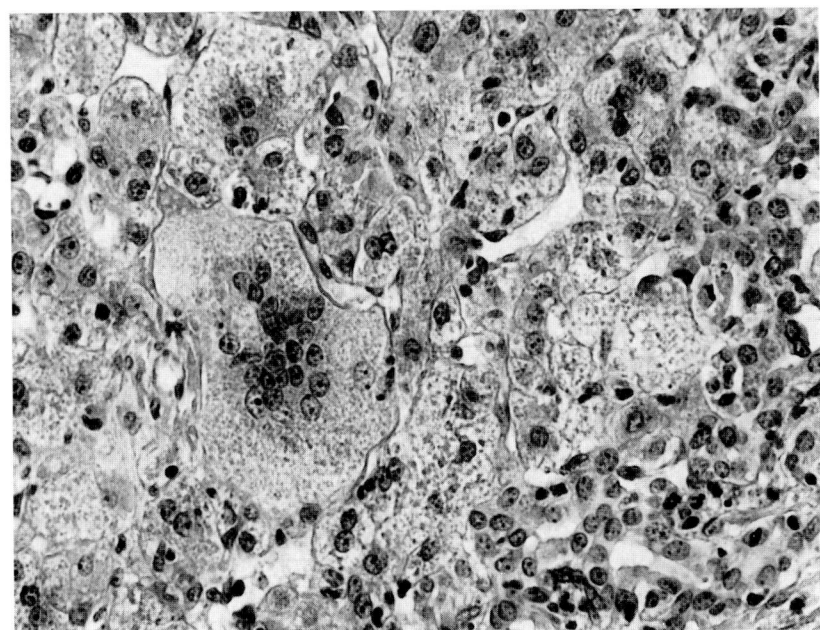

FIGURE 25.10. *Extrahepatic biliary atresia. Giant-cell transformation. ×140.*

residual duct has any correlation with outcome. Timing of portoenterostomy is important to outcome; those undergoing surgery before 2 months of age have a 90% chance of having bile flow reestablished. There is no success when surgery is delayed beyond 5 months [93].

The untreated infant with extrahepatic biliary atresia dies from complications of biliary cirrhosis. Hepatic portoenterostomy has improved longevity, but there are significant complications, including progressive destruction of intrahepatic bile ducts and cirrhosis [94]. Liver transplantation is now used to treat selected patients with biliary atresia, both before and after portoenterostomy.

Choledochal Cyst

Choledochal cysts are less common than INH or biliary atresia but occur over a broader age span. Seventy-one percent are found in the first year of life [95]. Although described in the fetus, most choledochal cysts present after the neonatal period [96]. The high female predominance in biliary atresia is repeated with choledochal cysts. Obstructive jaundice with hepatomegaly and, less often, symptoms of cholangitis and an abdominal mass constitute the major manifestations, which may be indistinguishable clinically from neonatal hepatitis and biliary atresia [95].

The most common type of lesion is cystic dilatation of the common bile duct. Dilatated intrahepatic ducts are frequently associated and usually resolve after successful operative correction. Less often, ectasia of the hepatic duct and stenosis or atresia of the gallbladder, cystic duct, or common bile duct may coexist. Diverticular cysts and choledochocele are rare. An undetermined number of infants with choledochal cysts have developmental anomalies of the hepatopancreatic duct junction, a finding of pathogenetic importance [97].

Once considered to be a developmental anomaly, most choledochal cysts are now regarded as secondary to destruction of the bile duct wall. Coexistence of choledochal cyst with giant cell hepatitis and biliary atresia supports Landing's concept of infantile obstructive cholangiopathy in which an infectious agent is proposed [27]. On the other hand, an abnormal extraduodenal union of the common bile duct and pancreatic duct would allow pancreatic reflux into the bile duct, causing chemical injury to the bile duct wall [97]. The association of choledochal cyst with duodenal atresia and agenesis of the gallbladder suggests that some cases are due to maldevelopment [98]. Finally, a similarity to Hirschsprung disease is raised with the description of hypoganglionosis in the narrow distal part of the duct in some cases [99].

Excised choledochal cysts are composed of a dense collagenous wall with focal or no residual biliary epithelium (Fig. 25.11). In infancy, the liver pathology is more prominent and severe than in older patients. There is a high incidence of cirrhosis, but fibrosis and hepatitis with giant-cell transformation also occur, creating a histologic overlap with biliary atresia and neonatal hepatitis.

Paucity of Intrahepatic Bile Ducts

Intrahepatic biliary atresia (see Table 25.4) or hypoplasia has been recognized for many years but is uncommon [100]. Alagille and colleagues first defined a group of children with chronic cholestasis and intrahepatic bile duct paucity, some with associated anomalies [101]. These latter patients were categorized as syndromic, and those who did not have the

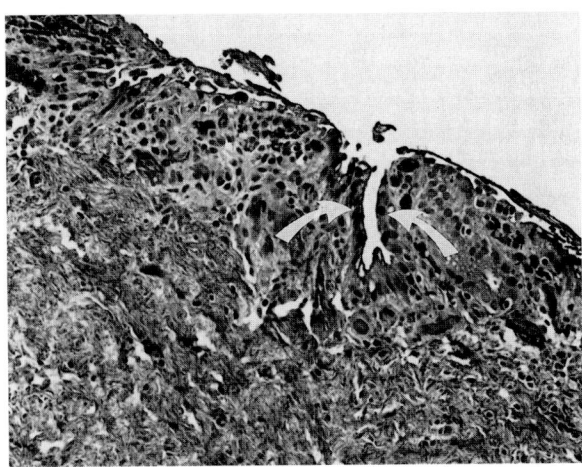

FIGURE 25.11. *The scarred wall of a choledochal cyst. Note minimal residual epithelium (arrows). ×80.*

associated features, who were a more diverse group, were classified as nonsyndromic [102]. Similar cases were subsequently reported as arteriohepatic dysplasia [103–105]. The associated anomalies in Alagille syndrome are pulmonary arterial stenosis, vertebral arch defects, hypogonadism, mental and physical retardation, and abnormalities of the retina and anterior chamber of the eye. These features occur to varying extents in affected patients [106].

Alagille syndrome has an autosomal dominant genetic pattern with variable penetrance and expression. Deletion of the short arm of chromosome 20 and balanced translocation of 2;20 have been documented [107, 108]. Importantly, the liver pathology is often nonprogressive, whereas aggres-

sive disease is associated more often with the nonsyndromic group. And yet, Alagille syndrome is not entirely benign, having a mortality of approximately 25% (cardiac, 35%; hepatic, 12%; other causes, 53%) [106].

Pathology is characterized by paucity of interlobular bile ducts, and there may be diminished portal tracts [109]. Biopsies taken early in infancy may show hepatitis with giant-cell transformation and normal interlobular bile ducts. Duct inflammation and degeneration have also been found [103]. The diminished population of interlobular ducts in the absence of inflammation is noted later in infancy and childhood (Fig. 25.12). Variable portal fibrosis and even cirrhosis occur. The extrahepatic bile duct may be of small caliber or, rarely, atretic, and extrahepatic biliary atresia has occurred in siblings of patients with Alagille syndrome [102].

Originally regarded as a possible failure of development of the interlobular bile ducts, Alagille syndrome now appears to be due to an insult, infectious or otherwise, to the duct, which may begin in utero [103]. Ultrastructural absence of biliary material in the Golgi apparatus suggests that obstruction in the intracellular bile secretory process with reduced bile flow may lead to duct atrophy [110].

Diagnosis of Alagille syndrome may not be possible in biopsies from young infants if hepatitic features exist and bile ducts are present in normal numbers. In this situation, identification of the associated clinical anomalies will assist, and sequential liver biopsies should be considered. After this transitional phase, a morphologic diagnosis is more readily reached.

Confirmation of bile duct paucity depends on quantitation of the interlobular bile duct in relation to portal tracts. The ratio of interlobular bile ducts to portal tracts is normally 0.9 to 1.8, and there are 8.2 ± 4.3 portal tracts in 10

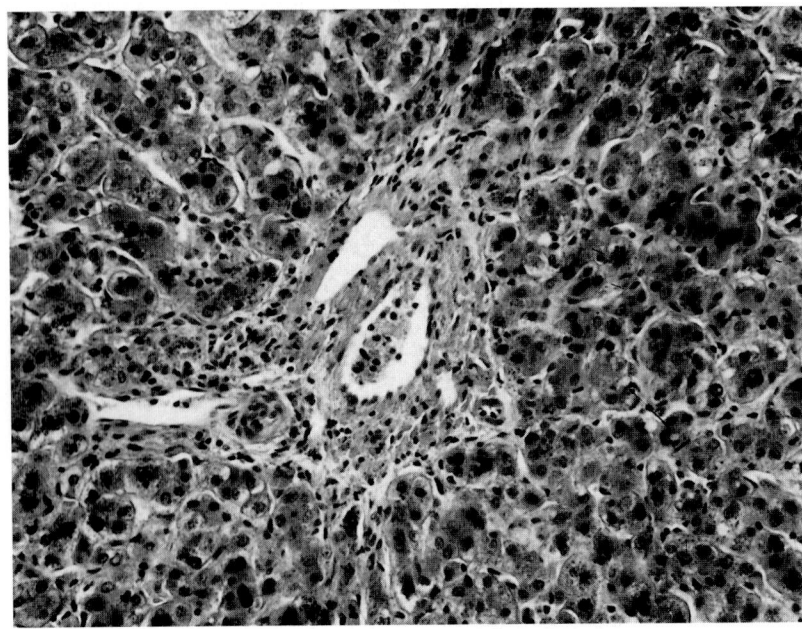

FIGURE 25.12. *Alagille syndrome in a 6-week-old infant. The portal tract lacks bile ducts; no inflammation is present; cholestasis is evident in the hepatocytes and canaliculi. ×140.*

mm² [101, 109]. In Alagille syndrome, the ratio of interlobular ducts to portal tracts is 0 to 0.4; portal tracts may be reduced to 4.5 ± 2.9 per 10 mm². To accomplish an accurate quantitation, an open surgical biopsy may be needed to obtain a sufficient number of portal tracts. Alagille recommended biopsy of both left and right lobes of the liver [102]. A satisfactory number of portal tracts for examination ranges from 5 to 20; Witzleben prefers the latter number [111]. One must recall that the intrahepatic biliary system continues its development through and beyond full gestation, and thus reference to established normal values or use of age-matched normal controls is imperative when evaluating the livers of premature and neonatal infants [104].

Recognition of paucity of intrahepatic bile ducts does not in itself define Alagille syndrome (see Table 25.4). The nonsyndromic group with bile duct paucity is diverse [101]. Among this group are patients with alpha₁-antitrypsin deficiency and, rarely, cystic fibrosis [112]. In disorders of bile acid metabolism, one might anticipate bile duct epithelial toxic injury. Such a mechanism may occur in coprostanic acidemia in which there is bile duct paucity with portal fibrosis, progressing to cirrhosis [113]. Similarly, paucity of ducts occurs in the cerebrohepatorenal syndrome of Zellweger, a peroxisomal disorder with abnormal bile acid metabolism, and in syndromes of progressive familial intrahepatic cholestasis of unknown cause. The initial presentation and liver pathology may masquerade as neonatal hepatitis, as may occur in Alagille syndrome [114, 115].

Intrahepatic bile duct destruction by CMV infection in utero may result in paucity [45, 47]. Congenital rubella, trisomy 18, trisomy 21, monosomy X, and graft-versus-host disease are other documented associations or causes of ductopenia [111, 116]. Diminished interlobular bile ducts are described but not quantitated in partial trisomy 11 and in a syndrome of multiple anomalies with renal tubular dysfunction, cholestasis, and dysmorphism [117, 118].

Portal-Biliary Dysgenesis (Ductal Plate Malformation, Fibrocystic Cholangiopathy)

Autosomal recessive polycystic kidney disease (ARPKD) and congenital hepatic fibrosis (CHF), also autosomal recessive, share a similar hepatic lesion termed congenital hepatic fibrosis or ductal plate malformation [10, 119]. Several other, less common syndromes have similar liver lesions (see Table 25.4). In perinatal pathology, only autosomal recessive polycystic kidney disease, Meckel syndrome, and other uncommon lethal syndromes of multiple anomalies are of concern. Although the pathology of CHF is present in the neonatal period and earlier, the manifestations of hepatomegaly and portal hypertension, with or without renal dysfunction, usually do not occur until after the first year of life. On the other hand, newborn infants with ARPKD have hepatomegaly and nephromegaly and die of renal and respiratory failure.

The hepatic anomaly consists of excessive, bland, fibrous tissues expanding the portal tract and an increase in microscopically dilated bile ducts and ductules, which may be isolated within the lobule (Fig. 25.13). Ducts are often tortuous and oddly shaped, and do not appear proliferative. In some tracts, there are too few ducts. The portal lobular boundary is sharp; there is usually no inflammation in the neonatal liver, and the connective tissue is not suggestive of reactive fibrosis. Hepatocytes and hepatic veins are normal, but portal veins may be reduced or compressed, probably responsible in part for portal hypertension, which may be a clinical problem beyond infancy.

The hepatic lesion, portal-biliary dysgenesis, suggests an error in mesenchymal-epithelial interaction with retention of the primitive ductal plate and, in some, inadequate development of interlobular ducts [10, 120]. Desmet notes that the ductal plate anomaly is often associated with abnormal development of the portal vein, which should have a tree-like branching pattern. Instead, he likens the portal vein development to a "pollard willow" with branches of small caliber arising close together and resulting in a large, abnormal portal tract [120, 121].

Both Meckel and Jeune syndromes have liver lesions with excessive connective tissue and ducts. In Meckel syndrome the tracts are more fibrous than in ARPKD, and in Jeune syndrome the portal areas are smaller (Fig. 25.14). Similar dysgenetic biliary lesions occur in the chondrodysplasia syndromes of Majewski and Saldino-Noonan and of Ellis-van Creveld and Elejalde, and in trisomy 9, trisomy 13, glutaric aciduria type II, Beckwith-Wiedemann syndrome, and Ivemark renal-hepatic-pancreatic dysplasia [122] (Table 25.4).

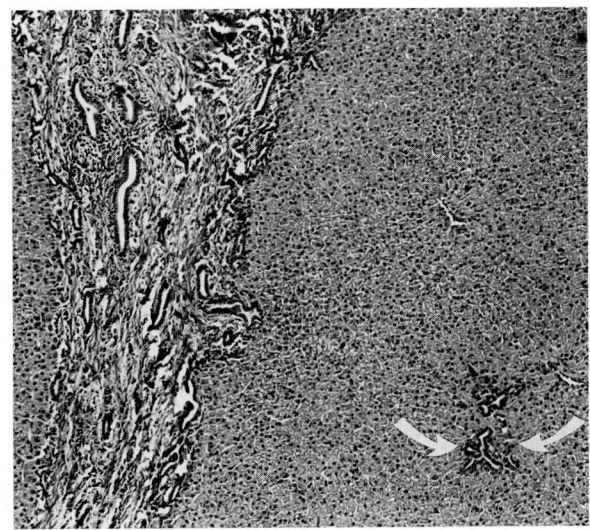

FIGURE 25.13. *Infantile polycystic disease. Note excess portal collagen, ducts, and ductular structures. Intralobular ductules are present. ×29.*

Other Cholangiopathies

Caroli disease (dilatation of intrahepatic ducts) is not a clinical problem in the perinatal period. However, prominent intrahepatic cystic dilatation of ducts occurs in newborn infants with Ivemark syndrome, Meckel syndrome, and rarely autosomal recessive polycystic kidney disease [123, 124]. Mucin inspissation may produce major duct obstruction in cystic fibrosis. In hemolytic disease, bile plugs and choledocholithiasis rarely occur. Spontaneous perforation of the extrahepatic bile duct, producing cholestasis, is an unusual event in early infancy.

INBORN ERRORS OF METABOLISM

Inherited metabolic disorders that involve the liver of the perinatal infant are listed in Table 25.5. The liver may or may not be the sole focus of pathology in these diseases. The reader should refer to Chapter 18 for a broader dissertation on metabolic diseases.

From the perspective of hepatic histopathology, inborn metabolic diseases fall into three categories, albeit with some overlap: those with nonspecific pathology, those with nondiagnostic but suggestive features, and a small group of diseases with diagnostic lesions. As examples, in alpha$_1$-antitrypsin deficiency, storage material may interfere with cellular metabolism; ATP depletion from phosphate sequestration in hereditary fructose intolerance explains steatosis and cholestasis; cellular toxicity is attributed to accumulated metabolites of tyrosine degradation in hereditary tyrosinemia; and steatosis arises in the fatty acid oxidative disorders when the pathways to oxidation are defective. The mecha-

nisms fall into three broad groups: those involving intracellular storage, generally with insidious courses; those acutely manifesting with interferences in energy metabolism; and those expressed acutely or chronically by toxic metabolites. These mechanisms, and others, operating during embryofetal development, may produce metabolic dysplasias of the hepatobiliary or other systems.

Metabolic Diseases with Nonspecific Pathology

Organic acidemias are associated with nonspecific liver pathology. Hepatomegaly and steatosis occur in isovaleric, propionic, and methylmalonic acidemia. Glutaric aciduria type II has been reported with nonspecific steatosis and with portal-biliary dysgenesis [122]. Most of the aminoacidopathies, with the exception of hereditary tyrosinemia, also have nonspecific or no identifiable hepatic lesions. In maple syrup urine disease and nonketotic hyperglycinemia, steatosis with or without hepatomegaly is the sole feature. Similarly, in lysinuric protein intolerance, nonspecific fat deposition is present in the livers of neonatal cases, but clusters of pale hydropic hepatocytes occur in older patients [125].

Urea cycle disorders have nonspecific liver pathology in the neonatal age group. No pathology, steatosis, focal hepatocellular necrosis, or focal hemorrhage is identified. In the urea cycle disorders, reports of ultrastructural appearances of mitochondria are numerous, and the results are variable. Normal mitochondria are reported in carbamylphosphate synthetase deficiency and ornithine transcarbamylase deficiency [126, 127]. However, abnormal mitochondria,

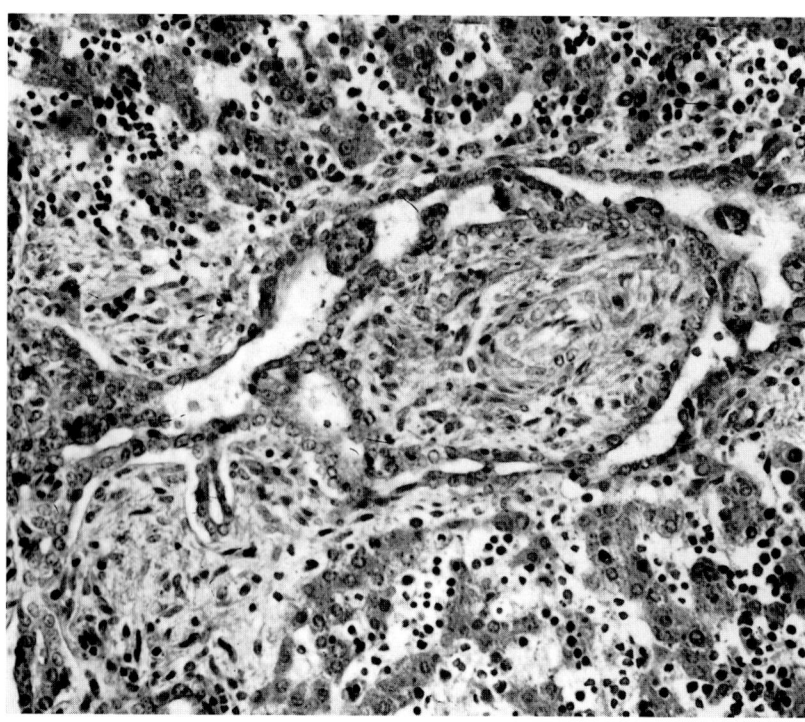

FIGURE 25.14.   *The liver of an 18-week-old fetus with Meckel syndrome, showing ductal plate malformation. ×75.*

Table 25.5. Perinatal inherited metabolic disorders

	Histologic diagnostic specificity	Disorder
Organic acidemia	Nonspecific	Proprionic acidemia
		Methylmalonic acidemia
		Isovaleric acidemia
		Multiple carboxylase deficiency
		Pyruvate dehydrogenase deficiency
	Nondiagnostic suggestive	Glutaric aciduria II
		Pyruvate carboxylase deficiency
		Fatty acid oxidative disorders
Aminoacidopathy	Nonspecific	Maple syrup urine disease
		Nonketotic hyperglycinemia
		Hypervalinemia
		Hyper-beta-alaninemia
		Lysinuric protein intolerance
	Nondiagnostic suggestive	Tyrosinemia type I
Carbohydrate disorders	Nonspecific	Fructose-1,6-diphosphatase deficiency
	Nondiagnostic suggestive	Hereditary fructose intolerance
		Galactosemia
	Diagnostic	Glycogen storage disease I
		Glycogen storage disease III
		Glycogen storage disease IV
Lysosomopathy	Nondiagnostic suggestive	GM$_1$ gangliosidosis type I
		Mucopolysaccharidoses, I, II, VII
		Sialidosis
		Sialic acid storage disease, severe infantile form
		Mucolipidosis II
	Diagnostic	Niemann-Pick disease
		Gaucher disease
		Wolman disease
		Cholesteryl ester storage disease
		Glycogen storage disease II
Other	Nonspecific	Urea cycle disorders
	Nondiagnostic suggestive	Mitochondrial respiratory chain disorders
		Dubin-Johnson syndrome
		Chronic familial cholestatic syndromes
		THCA excess (trihydroxycoprostanic acid)
		Bile acid synthesis disorders
	Diagnostic	Alpha$_1$-antitrypsin deficiency
		Cystic fibrosis
		Neonatal iron storage syndrome
		Peroxisomal deficiency disorders

swollen and increased in number or pleomorphic, may occur in all the neonatal urea cycle disorders [126–128], but do not resemble those seen in Reye syndrome. Both qualitative and quantitative abnormalities of peroxisomes are noted in ornithine transcarbamylase deficiency and citrullinemia [126, 128, 129].

Among the inherited disorders of carbohydrate metabolism, fructose-1,6-diphosphatase deficiency has the most nonspecific morphology. Steatosis alone occurs.

Many metabolic disorders of bilirubin metabolism have nonspecific liver pathology or no histologic changes. Crigler-Najjar syndrome type I causes serious unconjugated hyperbilirubinemia in the newborn infant but has no significant liver pathology. Patients with Gilbert syndrome are usually identified well beyond the perinatal period, but some infants with prolonged hyperbilirubinemia after the 10th day of life have been described [130]. The very rare Rotor syndrome, producing predominantly conjugated hyperbilirubinemia, has no hepatic pathology by light microscopy [131].

Metabolic Disorders with Nondiagnostic Suggestive Pathology

Fatty acid oxidative defects and mitochondrial respiratory chain abnormalities are recently appreciated metabolic diseases of the fetus and neonate. Hepatic steatosis varies from minimal to marked and from micro- to macrovesicular or mixed. Therefore, the histopathology may be nonspecific or, with prominent steatosis, suggestive of this diagnosis. Mixed micro- and macrovesicular steatosis, with ultrastructurally normal mitochondria, occurs in carnitine palmitoyl transferase II deficiency, which may present in the neonate and be lethal [132]. Short-chain acyl-CoA dehydrogenase deficiency occurs rarely in this age group, but a few infants with hepatic steatosis have been described [133]. Medium-chain acyl-CoA dehydrogenase deficiency usually manifests in later infancy or early childhood; neonatal death rarely occurs. There is macrovesicular, microvesicular, or mixed hepatic steatosis; mitochondria do not resemble those of Reye syndrome, but may be enlarged, with crystalloids, increased matrix density, and dilated cristae [134, 135]. Deficiency of long-chain acyl-CoA dehydrogenase may affect the pregnant mother and infant. Heterozygous mothers carrying homozygous fetuses have an unexpectedly high occurrence of fatty liver and HELLP (hemolysis, elevated liver enzymes, low platelet count) syndrome. Affected neonates have hepatomegaly with macro- or mixed micro- and macrovesicular steatosis, and may later develop portal fibrosis [136, 137].

Among mitochondrial respiratory chain disorders, defects of complex IV predominate in the fetal-neonatal age group. Fetal ascites, neonatal liver failure, and death occur. Microvesicular steatosis is common, but cytoplasmic and canalicular cholestasis, giant-cell transformation, ductular proliferation, fibrosis, and even cirrhosis are reported [138–142]. Important to the identification of these disorders are the observations that mitochondrial number in hepatocytes is increased and that these mitochondria show qualitative abnormalities [138].

Since it is rare in early infancy, Reye syndrome should be diagnosed with caution. Thorough investigation should exclude inherited metabolic errors. Mitochondrial changes of Reye syndrome are helpful if present, since they are not known to be mimicked by inborn metabolic disorders. The same concern applies to the diagnosis of sudden infant death syndrome (SIDS) in very young infants. A clinical history of failure to thrive and hepatic steatosis should call attention

to diagnoses other than SIDS. One should consider acquired conditions causing steatosis in this age group, such as hypoxemia, drug intoxication, and the effects of intravenous alimentation. There are published protocols for postmortem biochemical evaluation of suspected disorders of fatty acid metabolism [143, 144].

The onset of Dubin-Johnson syndrome is variable, occurring rarely in newborn infants when there is a predominantly conjugated hyperbilirubinemia [145]. In the adult, the liver is black due to the deposition of dark pigment in centrilobular hepatocytes. In the neonate, the liver is yellow-brown but otherwise normal. The pigment is unknown but stains like melanin and is intralysosomal. Similar black pigmentation of the liver in association with arthrogryposis, renal dysfunction, and hepatic cholestasis has been described in four infants by Nezelof et al [146]. Coprostanic acidemia, an autosomal recessive abnormality in bile acid synthesis, is characterized by cholestasis and increased amounts of trihydroxycoprostanic acid (THCA) [147]. Affected infants have paucity of interlobular bile ducts. Cirrhosis and liver failure occur terminally. Disorders of bile acid metabolism, detected with fast atom bombardment–mass spectrometry, may manifest pathologically with neonatal hepatitis [148–150]. Ultrastructurally, complex membrane contours and diverticula of the hepatocyte canaliculus are seen in Δ-4-3 oxysteroid 5β reductase deficiency [148].

There are other cholestatic syndromes with presumed metabolic bases. Aagenaes et al and others have described siblings with initial giant-cell transformation of the liver, chronic cholestasis, and lymphedema of the legs later in childhood [151, 152]. Liver pathology is nonspecific but with suggestive features, showing giant-cell transformation, subsequent hepatocellular and canalicular cholestasis, and slight progressive portal fibrosis. Benign recurrent familial cholestasis, manifesting later in infancy or in childhood, has a nonspecific pathology [153]. "Progressive familial cholestasis" and "familial cholestatic cirrhosis" are synonyms for a syndrome complex of progressive cholestasis, which may commence in the neonatal period although more commonly after 3 months of age. Among this group of cholestatic syndromes is the Byler kindred. The liver changes in this group of disorders generally proceed from cytoplasmic to canalicular and cytoplasmic cholestasis with progressive portal fibrosis, culminating in cirrhosis sometimes complicated by hepatocellular carcinoma. Giant-cell hepatitis is the presenting pathology in early biopsies of some patients [154]. Ultrastructurally, canalicular distension with particulate matter, diminished microvilli, and canalicular membrane interruption have been noted [154]. Broadening of the pericanalicular microfilamentous zone has been observed. Similar pericanalicular accentuation was reported in North American Indian children with a progressive disease beginning as giant-cell hepatitis and terminating in cirrhosis [155].

In the lysosomal disorders, mucopolysaccharidoses I, II, and VII, sialidosis, mucolipidosis II, and generalized GM1 gangliosidosis, the liver pathology is sufficiently distinct to indicate a storage disease but is inadequate for definitive diagnosis. These lysosomopathies may present in the neonatal period, but mucopolysaccharidosis type VII (β-glucuronidase deficiency) is the most likely to do so and can cause hydrops fetalis [156]. Kupffer's cells and hepatocytes are vacuolated, and the storage product may be demonstrated with colloidal iron stains. Ultrastructurally, one may see scant, nonspecific intralysosomal fibrillogranular material. Portal fibrosis is variable but may be marked in older patients, and cirrhosis may evolve [157]. We have examined two neonates with hydrops fetalis who had mucopolysaccharidosis type VII. The liver was moderately increased in size and was finely pebbled and firm. Cellular vacuolation was most pronounced in Kupffer's cells and was only modestly present in hepatocytes (Fig. 25.15).

The sialidoses, formerly classified as mucolipidosis I, constitute a group of diseases involving the storage of sialic acid, free and bound. The infantile dysmorphic type may present in the neonatal period with hydrops fetalis or congenital ascites [158]. These infants have biochemical evidence of liver dysfunction, hepatomegaly, and prominent vacuoles in Kupffer's cells and hepatocytes with PAS-positive diastase-resistant staining. Ultrastructurally, lysosomes contain sparse nonspecific granular and fibrillar material. Portal fibrosis may be marked, approaching the appearance of cirrhosis, although in one case that we examined the extensive fibrosis was not diffusely present in the liver. A similar clinical and pathologic picture has been reported in one infant with free sialic acid storage [159]. In mucolipidosis II (I-cell disease), there is vacuolation of fibroblasts in the portal tracts and foamy histiocytes. There may be vacuolation of hepa-

tocytes, which stain positively for neutral lipid, and involvement of Kupffer's cells. Ultrastructurally, the vacuoles are single membrane bound, are often electron lucent, or contain reticulogranular or membranous material [160]. Involvement of mesenchymal structures, particularly fibroblasts and endothelial cells, predominates.

Generalized GM_1 gangliosidosis in the neonatal period may present with hydrops fetalis or ascites [158]. The liver is enlarged with vacuolation of Kupffer's cells and hepatocytes. Ultrastructurally, nonspecific fibrillogranular material is present in the vacuoles.

In pyruvate carboxylase deficiency, the liver is enlarged and lipid laden and has similarities to hereditary fructose intolerance [161]. Macrovesicular steatosis occurs in all but the periportal hepatocytes, with cholestasis, ductular proliferation, minimal portal septal fibrosis, and acinar transformation of hepatocytes. Liver cells are swollen but not necrotic and have prominent nucleoli.

Liver pathology is variable in hereditary fructose intolerance [157, 162]. In young infants in whom the clinical presentation is likely to be most severe, there is panlobular macrovesicular steatosis, portal fibrosis, ductular proliferation, cholestasis, fine lobular fibrosis, and acinar transformation of hepatocytes (Fig. 25.16). A few necrotic hepatocytes may be seen. Nuclear anisocytosis and prominent nucleoli are present. In older infants the pathology is generally less pronounced, being one of variable steatosis and portal fibrosis. Cirrhosis occurs rarely in hereditary fructose intolerance [163]. Steatosis may persist even following fructose exclusion, and, interestingly, infants treated with a fructose-free diet from birth may have fatty vacuolation of liver cells [162]. Ultrastructural pathology of the liver occurs acutely after fructose ingestion, with membranous arrays and cytoplasmic rarefaction, attributed to altered hydration and degranulation of the rough endoplasmic reticulum secondary to ATP depletion, which may explain the cholestasis and steatosis [164].

Two metabolites of galactose, galactitol, and galactose 1-phosphate appear to account for the tissue toxicity in classic galactosemia. The initial hepatic lesion is panlobular steatosis (Fig. 25.17). This is followed by cholestasis, ductular proliferation, and acinar transformation of hepatocytes; later, atrophy and focal hepatocellular necrosis precede stromal collapse, with the ultimate development of cirrhosis. Regenerative nodules are common. Inflammatory cells sparsely infiltrate the fibrous portal septa, and giant-cell transformation has been noted. Initially, the liver in classic galactosemia is enlarged and yellow; later it has a typical cirrhotic appearance [157, 165].

Hepatic pathology of hereditary tyrosinemia type I is sufficiently distinctive to suggest the disease but is still not pathognomonic [157, 166, 167]. The liver is often of normal size, particularly in patients dying early in infancy, and it may be brown and bile stained. It is usually not yellow, although regenerative nodules, which are especially prominent in this disease (Fig. 25.18), may be lipid laden and have varying

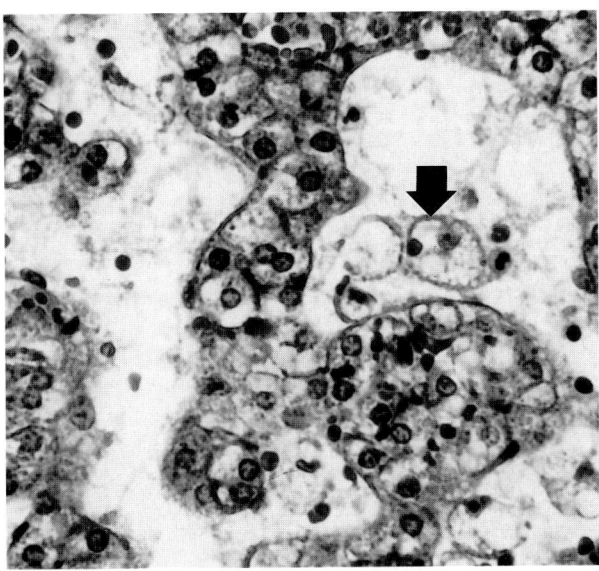

FIGURE 25.15. *Liver in mucopolysaccharidosis type VII. Sinusoids are dilated and contain vacuolated Kupffer's cells (arrow). Hepatocytes also are vacuolated.* ×160.

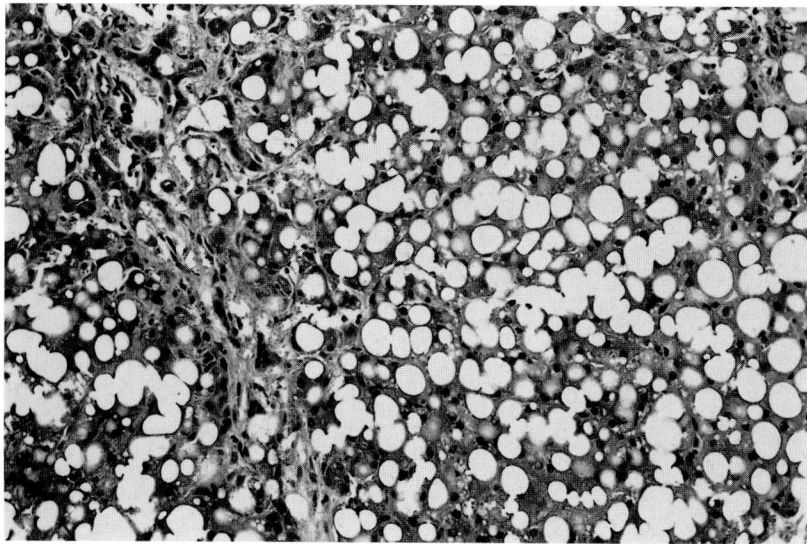

FIGURE 25.16. *Hereditary fructose intolerance. Note macrovesicular steatosis, fine portal fibrosis, and ductular proliferation. ×75.*

colors. The normal hepatic architecture is distorted by progressive acinar transformation of hepatocytes, accompanied by intralobular and portal fibrosis (Fig. 25.19). Hepatocellular necrosis is not a prominent feature, nor is inflammation. Hepatocellular and Kupffer's cell iron may be prominent. Nuclear atypicality in regenerative nodules may be striking, and, not surprisingly, aneuploidy is present in some, probably a harbinger of hepatocellular carcinoma known to occur in 37% of infants who survive the acute disease (Fig. 25.20) [166, 168]. The degradation products of tyrosine, maleyl- and fumarylacetoacetate accumulate when the final enzyme in the pathway is deficient and they alkylate DNA. Eliminating these degradation products by blocking the more proximal pathway reduces liver injury [169, 170].

Metabolic Disorders with Diagnostic Pathology

Inherited glycogen storage disease, types I to IV, may present in the neonatal period. The pathology of the glycogen storage diseases has been documented thoroughly by McAdams et al, who propose that the hepatic pathologic features are sufficiently distinctive to permit a presumptive diagnosis [171]. Our experience is similar, but others disagree [172]. Regardless, morphologic diagnoses must be confirmed by appropriate biochemical tests.

Glycogen storage disease type I can present in the neonatal period. In one case, fetal growth retardation and bradycardia were attributed to marked hypoglycemia, a common

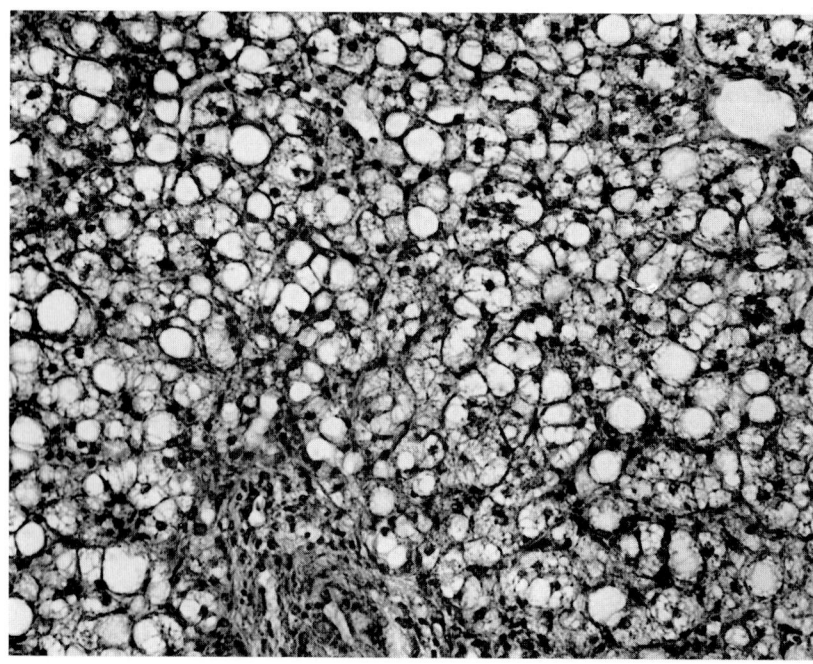

FIGURE 25.17. *Galactosemia. The early lesion of steatosis is seen in the liver of a neonate. Portal tract, lower left; hepatic vein, upper right. ×70.*

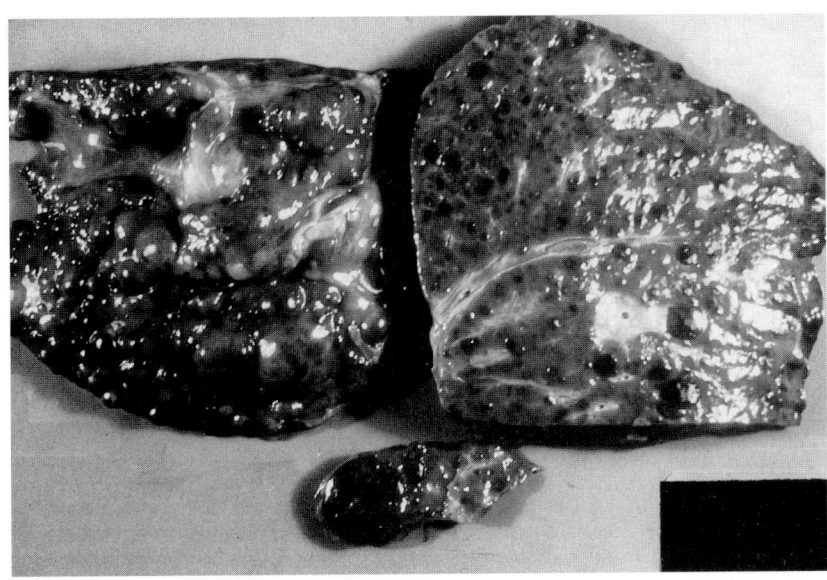

FIGURE 25.18. *Tyrosinemia in an 11-week-old infant. Multiple regenerative nodules are present. ×27.*

manifestation of the disorder [173, 174]. The liver is large, and hepatocytes are swollen and assume a mosaic pattern; large vacuolar steatosis is prominent. Nuclear hyperglycogenation is significant. There is no portal or lobular fibrosis. Ultrastructurally, normal glycogen is abundant, displaces cytoplasmic organelles, and is within hepatic nuclei. Lipid droplets are also present. The liver in glycogen storage type IB has a nonuniform mosaic hepatocellular pattern without nuclear hyperglycogenation but with the same degree of steatosis as type I [175].

On first examination, the liver in Pompe disease (glycogen storage disease type II) may appear normal. The lobular architecture is retained, usually with no septal fibrosis or steatosis and with no exaggerated nuclear glycogenation. On close inspection, the hepatocytes are finely vacuolated due to intralysosomal glycogen accumulation, which is demonstrated even better ultrastructurally (Fig. 25.21).

Glycogen storage disease type III is unlikely to be identified in the perinatal period, but diagnosis was made in one neonate who had persistent hepatomegaly detected initially

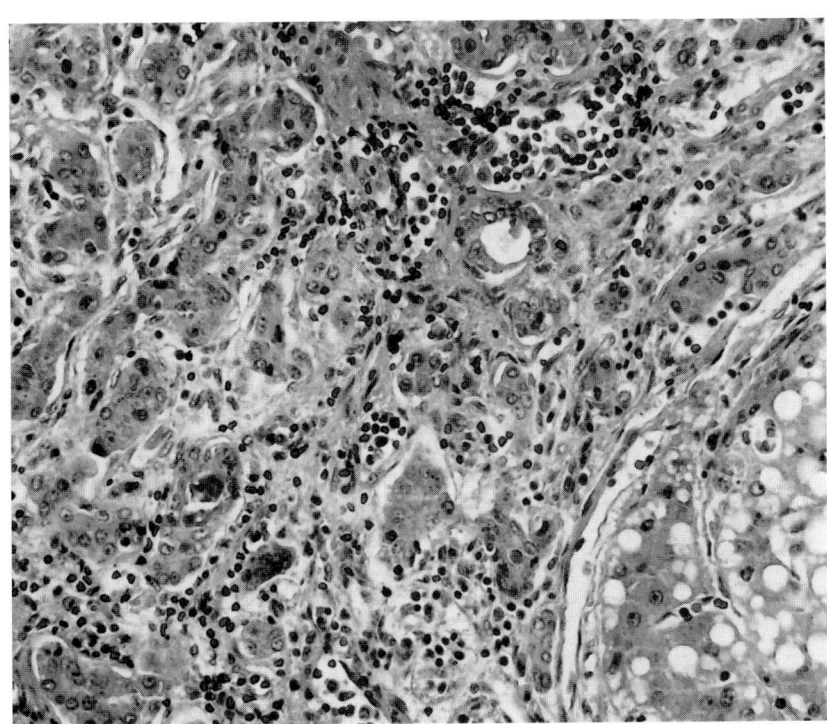

FIGURE 25.19. *Tyrosinemia. Note the lobular fibrosis and acinar transformation of hepatocytes. ×100.*

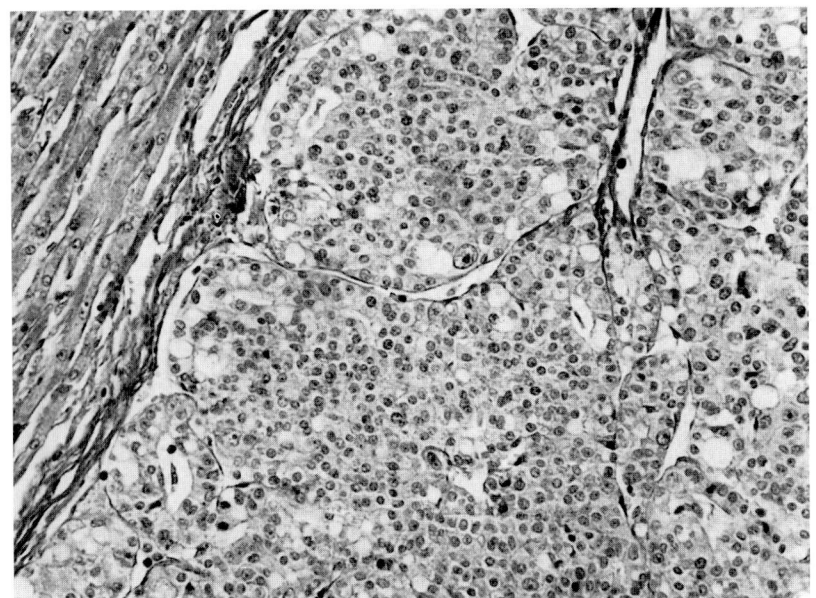

FIGURE 25.20. *Tyrosinemia. An incipient hepatoma. ×80.*

at 28 weeks' gestation [176]. Pathology is similar to glycogen storage disease type I, but fibrous portal septa are present [171].

In type IV glycogenosis, abnormal glycogen is formed and cirrhosis evolves [171] aggressively from portal fibrosis. Hepatocytes bear PAS-positive diastase-resistant amphophilic inclusions that are most prominent in the periportal hepatocytes (Fig. 25.22). The deposits do not stain for alpha₁-antitrypsin and in frozen section are lavender when

stained with Lugol's iodine. Ultrastructurally, the abnormal glycogen has a fibrillar structure. Presentation is usually in infancy or early childhood, but a congenital form is also described [177].

Of the lysosomopathies, Niemann-Pick disease, Wolman disease, Gaucher disease, and Pompe disease may be diagnosed morphologically. In the perinatal period, the pathologist may encounter Niemann-Pick disease type A (type I) or type C (type II). Hepatomegaly is a common feature of type A in which, with age, Niemann-Pick cells progressively increase within hepatic sinusoids. These cells may be infrequent in very young infants. Hepatocellular vacuolation is variable. As the storage process advances, hepatic lobules become progressively distorted. Portal septal fibrosis, cholestasis, and giant-cell transformation have also been noted [178]. Prolonged cholestasis and severe clinical liver disease may occur in infants with Niemann-Pick disease type C [179, 180]. Ultrastructural appearances of the cytosomes in Niemann-Pick disease are diagnostically useful (Fig. 25.23). Biliary material in cholestasis may be confused with the Niemann-Pick storage product.

The acute neuronopathic form of Gaucher disease occurs in early infancy; hepatomegaly is prominent, and there may be hydrops fetalis [158]. In the liver, one finds Gaucher's cells. In young infants, however, the wrinkled cytoplasmic appearance may not be evident. The cells are PAS-positive, and there may be portal and intralobular fibrosis. The ultrastructural appearance of the Gaucher's cell is typical and diagnostic. Clumps of Gaucher's cells lodged in and obstructing hepatic veins and sinusoids likely contribute to ascites. Progressive accumulation of Gaucher's cells, with encroachment on hepatocytes, leads to compression atrophy, progressive fibrosis, and, later, cirrhosis [157].

In Wolman disease, the liver is large and yellow due to extensive lipid deposits. One finds portal and periportal

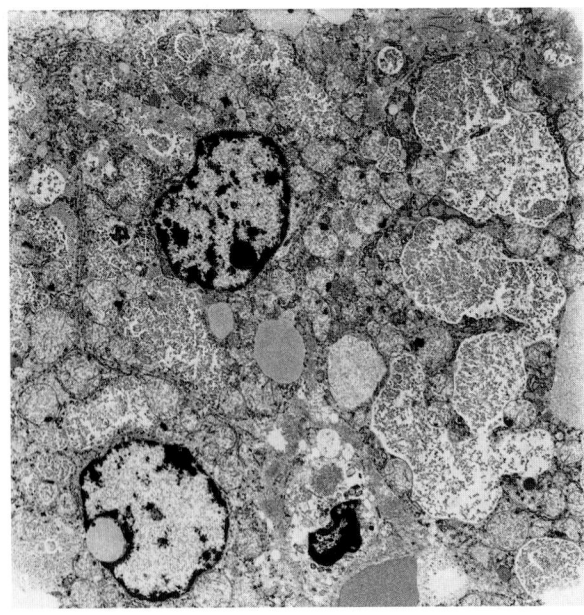

FIGURE 25.21. *Glycogen storage disease type II. Note lysosomal-bound glycogen in liver cells. ×6400.*

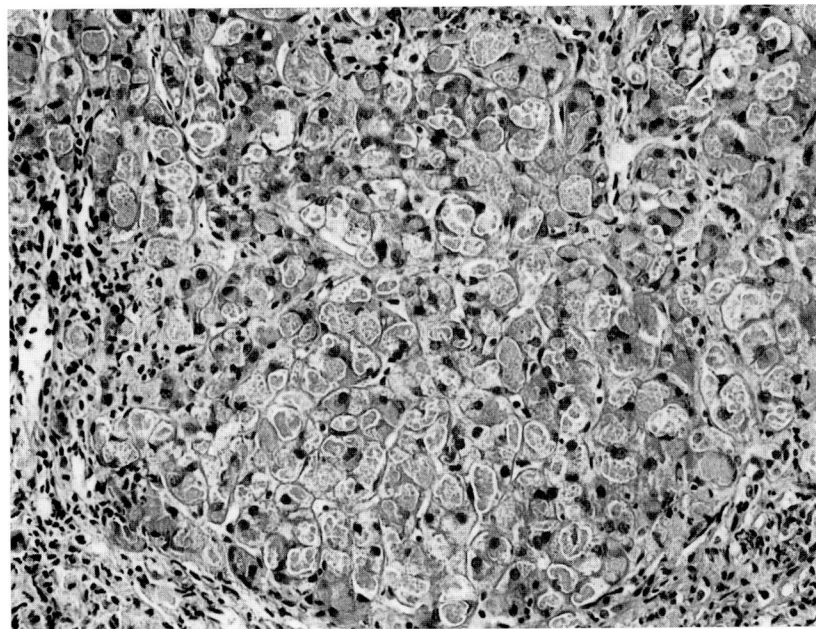

FIGURE 25.22. *Glycogen storage disease type IV in a 2-month-old infant. The liver is cirrhotic; hepatocytes contain amylopectin aggregates. ×70.*

fibrosis. Foamy histiocytes contain triglycerides and cholesteryl ester. Hepatocytes and Kupffer's cells are vacuolated and ultrastructurally contain lipid droplets. Cholesteryl ester crystal clefts appear in histiocytic lysosomes. Also, there is cholestasis and ductular proliferation [181].

Focal biliary fibrosis or "cirrhosis" is the diagnostic lesion of cystic fibrosis in the neonatal age group, but this lesion occurs infrequently in newborn infants. The incidence of focal biliary fibrosis is 10.8% among infants up to age 3 months and 26.8% in infants over 1 year of age [182]. The lesion may be present in utero. Focal biliary fibrosis is made up of ducts with inspissated eosinophilic mucin, ductular proliferation, chronic inflammation, and portal fibrosis. Marked hepatic steatosis and multilobular biliary cirrhosis,

which evolve from expansion of focal biliary fibrosis, occur in older patients with cystic fibrosis. Extrahepatic biliary tract obstruction, clinically suggesting biliary atresia, is rare in infancy and is due to severe mucous inspissation, duct inflammation with ampullary obstruction, or extraluminal compression by pancreatic fibrosis [183]. Biliary atresia may also coexist very rarely with cystic fibrosis. More commonly, in young infants, nonspecific portal inflammation, edema, cholestasis, and mild portal fibrosis are noted. Rarely, giant-cell hepatitis may be the sole pathology [184].

Idiopathic neonatal iron storage syndrome (neonatal hemochromatosis) is an uncommon clinicopathologic entity distinct from genetic hemochromatosis. It is very likely a manifestation of serious fetal liver injury of differing causes

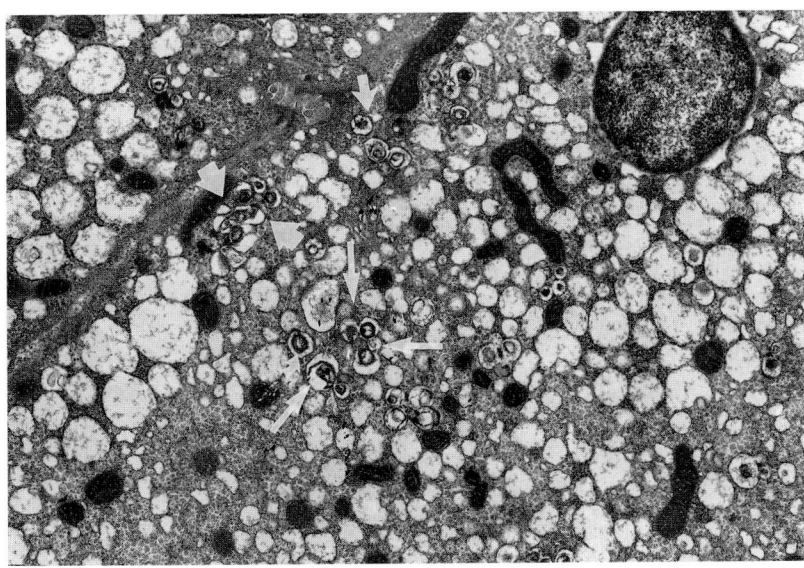

FIGURE 25.23. *Inclusions characteristic of Niemann-Pick disease type C (arrows). Original magnification, ×10,800. (Photograph courtesy of Katrine Hansen, MD, Providence, RI.)*

with secondary disturbance of iron metabolism [185–188]. A metabolic disorder of iron remains possible for some patients. A similar histopathology occurs in some infants with Down syndrome who have megakaryocytic dyshemopoiesis [189, 190]. The clinical course is rapidly progressive, with liver failure and death sometimes occurring immediately after birth. The liver is firm, is of normal or increased size, and may be red-brown or green, and ascites may be present. These are extensive intralobular fibrosis, hepatocellular atrophy, focal necrosis, acinar transformation of hepatocytes, cholestasis, and hemosiderin storage predominating in hepatocytes (Fig. 25.24). Extramedullary hematopoiesis persists in variable amounts, and there is no inflammation. Hepatic vein sclerosis is common. Giant-cell transformation may occur. Regenerative nodules, some with atypicality, occur variably. Completing the picture are extensive hemosiderin deposits in parenchymal cells, particularly in the pancreas, heart, stomach, and endocrine and exocrine glands. The reticuloendothelial system contains little or no hemosiderin.

Hepatic hemosiderin deposition is common in neonatal liver disease occurring, for example, in erythroblastosis fetalis, hereditary tyrosinemia, cerebrohepatorenal syndrome of Zellweger, and neonatal hepatitis. The liver in trisomy 22 may also contain abundant hepatocellular iron, but there is no other pathology [191].

Of peroxisomal disorders with neonatal liver involvement, the most common are the cerebrohepatorenal syndrome of Zellweger and neonatal adrenoleukodystrophy [192, 193]. Infants with Zellweger syndrome develop hepatomegaly and jaundice in the first few weeks of life. Pathology is varied and progressive, with giant-cell transformation, cholestasis, diminished bile ducts in some, variable

steatosis, portal and lobular fibrosis, and cirrhosis [192]. In neonatal adrenoleukodystrophy, cirrhosis and extensive portal fibrosis, sometimes with PAS-positive macrophages, have been described [192]. Of two infants we studied, one rapidly developed micronodular cirrhosis. The other had only transient hepatocellular swelling, and the liver appeared normal with the exception of a few PAS-positive macrophages. These macrophages contained trilaminate lysosomal inclusions, thought to be derived from very-long-chain fatty acids. Peroxisomal immunohistochemistry (for catalase and other peroxisomal enzymes) and electron microscopy are useful in demonstrating deficiency of the peroxisomes [193].

Alpha$_1$-antitrypsin deficiency is an important cause of neonatal liver disease, particularly for infants with the Pi ZZ phenotype. In a large Swedish study, 125 Pi ZZ infants were detected among 200,000 newborns [194]. Eleven percent developed neonatal cholestasis, and approximately 50% of the remaining asymptomatic infants had abnormal liver function tests. At 4 years of age, a full 45% of infants with Pi ZZ phenotype had abnormal hepatic enzyme activity [195]. However, the 8-year follow-up suggested that, based on clinical studies, liver disease may not be as significant as originally thought. Eighty-three percent of children had no clinical evidence of hepatic disease [196]. The earliest morphologic evidence of alpha$_1$-antitrypsin deficiency was in a 20-week-old fetus with immunoperoxidase and electron microscopic evidence of alpha$_1$-antitrypsin retention [197]. No other liver abnormality was evident. In contrast, two siblings with the Pi SZ phenotype died, in the neonatal period, of cirrhosis, which must have evolved in utero [198]. However, the majority of newborn infants with alpha$_1$-antitrypsin deficiency are asymptomatic. Those symptomatic

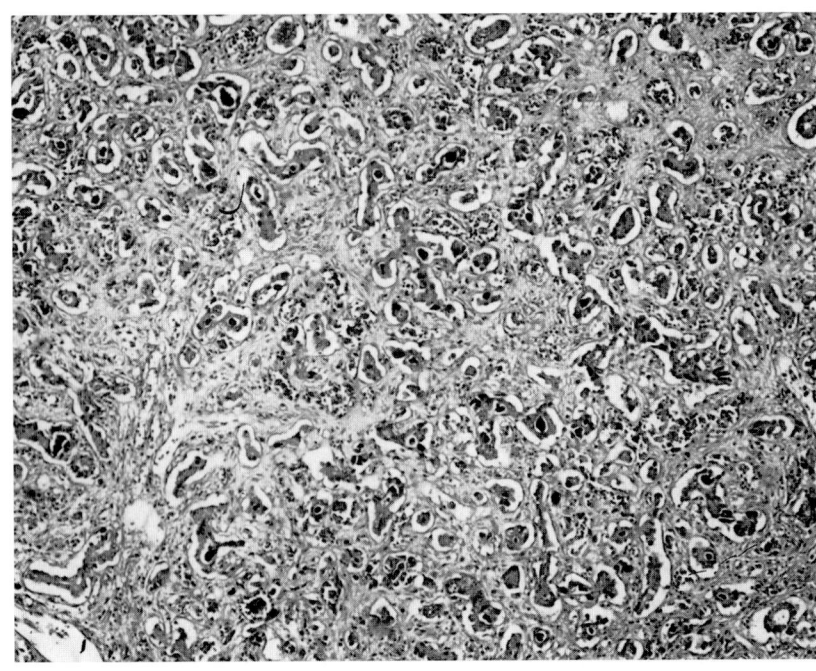

FIGURE 25.24.   *Neonatal iron storage syndrome. The liver is extensively fibrotic, and hepatocytes are sparse and atrophic. ×28.*

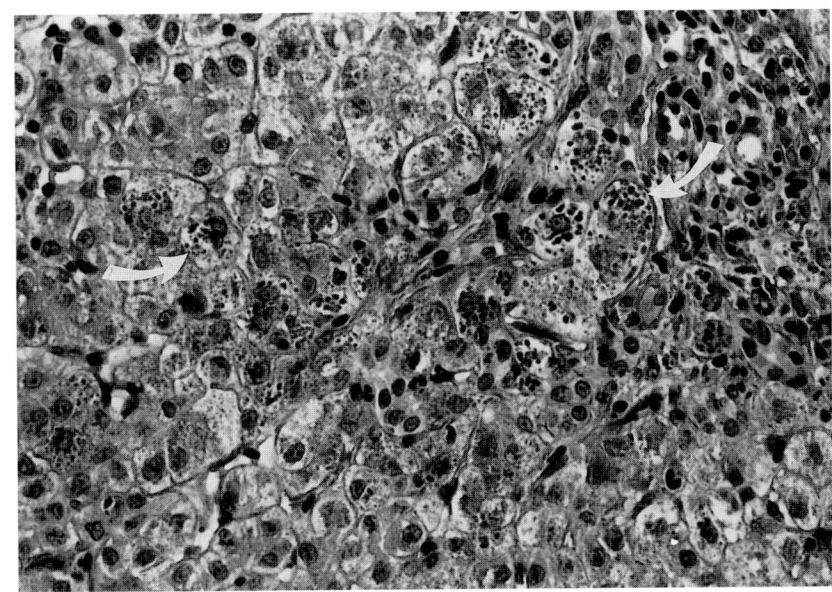

FIGURE 25.25.   *Alpha₁-antitrypsin deficiency in a 3-month-old infant. Note the cytoplasmic granules (arrows). PAS-diastase, ×180.*

with neonatal cholestasis may have INH. In one study, 29% of patients with the neonatal hepatitis syndrome had alpha₁-antitrypsin deficiency [199]. Liver pathology in a few infants will suggest major duct obstruction, and extrahepatic biliary atresia may rarely coexist [199]. A small number of infants have paucity of intrahepatic bile ducts. Histologic diagnosis of alpha₁-antitrypsin deficiency may be particularly difficult in the newborn. Typical PAS-positive diastase-resistant globules are less frequent in young infants and may be masked by similarly staining material occurring in cholestasis (Fig. 25.25). Immunofluorescent antibody and immunoperoxidase methods (Fig. 25.26) may be excessively sensitive, resulting in positive staining in livers with a normal alpha₁-antitrypsin phenotype. Such normal staining tends to be finer and to

be dispersed rather than globular. In the neonate, ultrastructural granular deposits are found in cisternae of the endoplasmic reticulum (Fig. 25.27). Morphologic studies should be supported by alpha₁-antitrypsin quantitation and Pi typing.

The mutant alpha₁-antitrypsin protein is not easily transported in the endoplasmic reticulum, which becomes obstructed. Consequently, significant accumulation of the protein may interfere with cellular metabolism. This pathogenetic theory is supported by a transgenic mouse model bearing the mutant Pi Z allele; such mice develop a neonatal hepatitis syndrome [200].

Prognostically, 25% of infants with alpha₁-antitrypsin deficiency and neonatal cholestasis will recover, with no

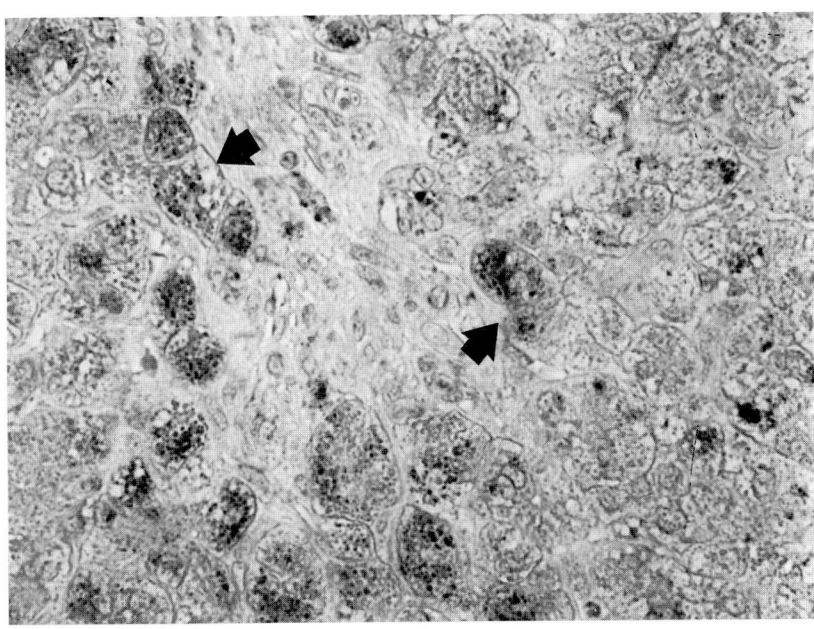

FIGURE 25.26.   *Immunoperoxidase stain for alpha₁-antitrypsin in a 4-week-old infant (Pi ZZ). Positive granules are present in only moderate numbers in several periportal hepatocytes (arrows). ×300.*

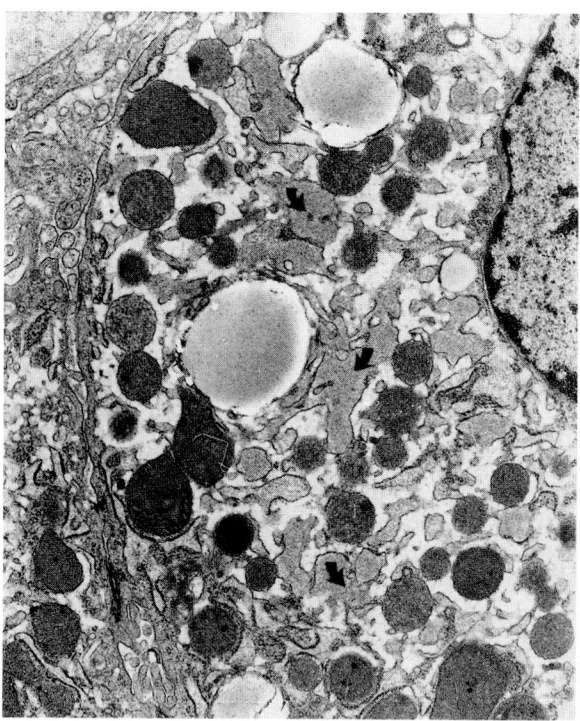

FIGURE 25.27. *Alpha₁-antitrypsin deficiency. Granular material is seen expanding the endoplasmic reticulum. ×10,680.*

evidence of chronic liver disease; 50% will progress at a variable pace to become cirrhotic and 25% will have minimal liver dysfunction [201]. These figures seem more foreboding than those of Sveger [196] but illustrate that one cannot predict outcome from the biopsy for infants with neonatal cholestasis. There may be a correlation with the degree of duct proliferation, portal fibrosis, and paucity of intrahepatic bile ducts [202].

HEPATIC CIRRHOSIS

Cirrhosis is usually a problem of the older pediatric patient and not the perinatal infant, but it may evolve in utero and manifest dramatically at birth (Fig. 25.28). In our experience, one affected infant died at 42 hours of age from massive gastrointestinal hemorrhage due to ruptured esophageal varices [157].

Cirrhosis in pediatric patients has been reviewed previously [157] (Table 25.6). In all series, secondary biliary cirrhosis is the predominant type, followed by posthepatitic and metabolic cirrhosis. Cardiac and idiopathic forms constitute the bulk of the remainder. In the perinatal period, the etiologic spectrum differs from that of older infants, largely because of the later occurrence of biliary cirrhosis. Cirrhosis of unknown cause is more common in the perinatal period. Thaler documented 24 cases in a 23-year period, and similar examples have been reported subsequently [157, 203]. In the perinatal age group, cirrhosis with known etiology includes alpha₁-antitrypsin deficiency, erythroblastosis fetalis, cardiac disease, and idiopathic neonatal iron storage syndrome. Undoubtedly, some cases follow infections such as CMV.

VASCULAR AND RELATED DISORDERS

Perinatal hypoxic hepatocellular degeneration is recognized by cellular glycogen depletion, vacuolation, steatosis, or foci of necrosis. Sinusoidal congestion may be prominent. In utero, the left lobe, being protected by oxygen-rich umbilical blood, may be affected less by asphyxia. This asymmetry is observed microscopically and by gross examination, the right lobe being pale and the left darker. Postnatally, the left lobe appears to be more susceptible to injury than the right [1].

Hepatocellular necrosis and sinusoidal fibrin thrombi may occur in infants dying of hyaline membrane disease. We have

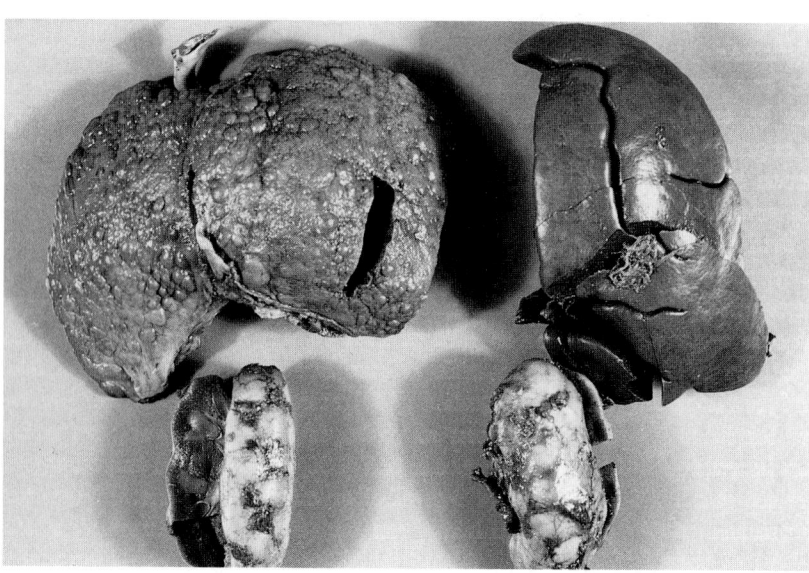

FIGURE 25.28. *Congenital cirrhosis and splenomegaly; kidneys in lower field. (Courtesy of Year Book Medical Publishers, Chicago.)*

Table 25.6. Cirrhoses of infancy

Obstructive biliary
Biliary atresia/obstruction; choledochal cyst; bile duct paucity
Posthepatitic
Idiopathic neonatal hepatitis; infectious
Metabolic
Hereditary tyrosinemia; alpha₁-antitrypsin; galactosemia; peroxisomal deficiency
    diseases (some); Wolman disease; sialidosis (incomplete cirrhosis);
    mitochondrial respiratory complex disorder (some); bile acid synthesis disorder
    (some); hereditary fructose intolerance
Cardiac
Hematologic
Erythroblastosis fetalis; congenital leukemia (including megakaryocytic)
Iatrogenic
Intravenous alimentation
Miscellaneous
Idiopathic; idiopathic neonatal iron storage syndrome; familial chronic cholestasis
    syndromes

encountered hepatic infarcts in an infant with chorionic vascular thromboses, implying multifocal thromboses or embolism. More widespread midzonal and centrilobular hepatic necrosis, steatosis, and sinusoidal thrombi occur in infants with congenital heart disorders in which visceral perfusion is dependent on the ductus arteriosus [204, 205]. Hepatic pathology in this setting is due to hypoperfusion rather than congestive heart failure. Similar lesions are seen in cases of shock. Thickening of the walls of terminal hepatic veins in infants with hypoplastic left heart syndrome is probably due to increased hepatic venous pressure in utero. Hepatic necrosis and infarcts may also follow umbilical venous catheterization [206]. Massive hepatic necrosis is infrequent in the neonate. Cases with unknown etiology have been reported, and extensive destruction may occur with a variety of viral infections (see Perinatal Hepatitides of Infectious Etiology) [207].

Subcapsular hematoma of the liver is not as common a clinical or pathologic finding as it once was, but still may be a cause of hypovolemic shock. In our experience, the incidence was 1.2% in fetal and neonatal deaths over a span of 15 years [69]. Hepatic congestion, hypoxia, and manipulation are pertinent pathogenetic factors [208]. Typically, the hematoma lies along the anterior edge of the right lobe and is enclosed by the thin hepatic capsule (Fig. 25.29), but it may be found at other sites, including the inferior surface. When ruptured, the source of the hemoperitoneum may not be obvious.

Portal hypertension in children often has an extrahepatic cause—particularly portal vein thrombosis, which may result from omphalitis, abdominal sepsis, dehydration, or umbilical venous catheterization [209]. Causes of portal hypertension in the neonatal period include cirrhosis and metabolic diseases in which storage cells block sinusoids or obstruct hepatic veins. A similar pathogenesis may occur with excess

intralobular extramedullary erythropoiesis. Veno-occlusive disease and Budd-Chiari syndrome rarely occur in infancy. Portal hypertension from noncirrhotic sinusoidal fibrosis due to CMV hepatitis has been reported in the neonate [210, 211].

Peliosis hepatis is very rare in early infancy [212].

TUMORS

Hepatic tumors are uncommon in the perinatal period [213–215]. Of 240 congenital tumors, Wells in 1940 tallied 19 (7.9%) in the liver [216]. Fifteen were hemangioendotheliomas. Hepatic tumors may be asymptomatic, but most produce abdominal masses, and some cause cardiac failure, jaundice, or metabolic or hormonal abnormalities [217–219]. Acute polyhydramnios has been reported in a fetus with a large hepatoblastoma [220]. Some infants with liver tumors have associations such as hemihypertrophy or the Beckwith-Wiedemann syndrome.

The most common liver tumors in the perinatal age group are mesenchymal hamartomas, hemangioendotheliomas, hepatoblastomas, and cavernous hemangiomas (Table 25.7) [218]. Metastatic neuroblastomas and congenital leukemia are the most common secondary malignancies.

Mesenchymal Hamartoma

This lesion is presumably an abnormality of development, perhaps due to defective vascularization. Seventy-five to eighty-five percent occur in infants less than 1 year of age [217]. Most present as asymptomatic abdominal masses, and they rarely present with heart failure or neonatal ascites due

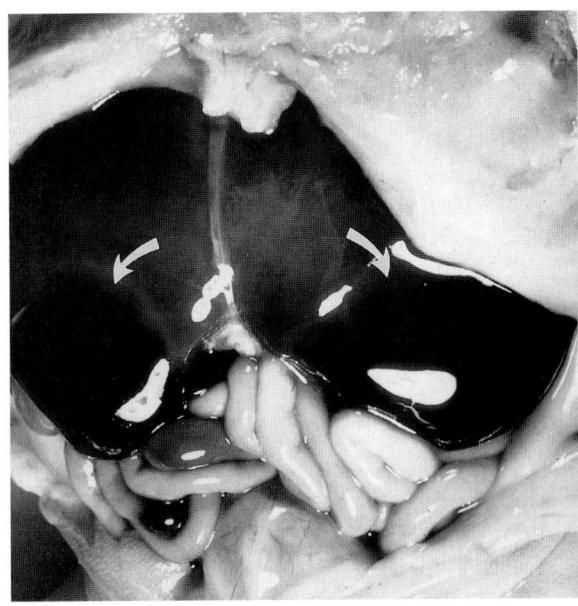

FIGURE 25.29. *Bilateral subcapsular hematoma of liver.*

Table 25.7. Liver tumors in the perinatal period

Malignant tumors	Benign tumors
Hepatoblastoma	Mesenchymal hamartoma
Metastatic neuroblastoma	Hemangioendothelioma
Congenital leukemia	Hemangioma
Undifferentiated embryonal	Focal nodular hyperplasia
sarcoma	Hepatic adenoma
Hepatocellular carcinoma	Teratoma
Lymphoma	Primary cysts
	Langerhans cell histiocytosis

to rupture. The tumor is well demarcated, intrahepatic or sometimes pedunculated, and usually solitary in the right lobe. A mixed cystic and solid pattern is typical. The hamartoma has been compared in appearance to a fibroadenoma of the breast. Microscopically, the predominant feature is loose, often myxomatous, connective tissue containing irregular bile ducts, blood vessels, and lymphatic spaces (Fig. 25.30). Hematopoietic foci may be present. Hepatocytes reside in the intervening zones. Cyst formation occurs in the stroma and lymphatics and through dilatation of the ducts. Whereas the blood vessels do not have an angiomatous appearance, some mesenchymal hamartomas are impressively vascular. The hypothetical "premalignant" relationship of mesenchymal hamartoma to undifferentiated (embryonal) sarcoma of the liver is unproved but worthy of continued consideration in view of the recent finding of the two tumors in one child [221]. Further, two hamartomas

have displayed 11–19 chromosomal translocations, and aneuploidy has been demonstrated [222, 223]. Seven to seventeen percent of infants with mesenchymal hamartomas in one series died from intraoperative and postoperative complications [224].

Hemangioendothelioma

Hemangioendotheliomas of the liver occur almost exclusively in early infancy (87% in the first 6 months) [225, 226]. Asymptomatic hepatomegaly, cardiac failure, thrombocytopenia, and intraperitoneal hemorrhage are the manners of presentation. Partial biliary obstruction with cholestasis may occur. Antenatally, these lesions may produce hydrops and polyhydramnios, probably from high-output cardiac failure. Often, the gross appearance belies the vascular nature of the tumor. Thirty to forty percent are multicentric, and the nodules are solid, yellow to tan or gray, and unencapsulated [225]. The surgeon may misinterpret the lesions as metastatic neuroblastomas. The microscopic appearance also may not be recognized as vascular by the casual observer. Compact endothelial cells are separated by fine reticulin, and bile ducts are intermixed. Larger, more obvious angiomatous structures often are present. Central hemorrhage, calcification, and scarring develop as involution proceeds. Mitoses are rare. Distinction of two histologic types, one more worrisome with anastomosing vascular channels and atypical endothelial cells, seems to offer no value in predicting behavior [225, 226]. The relatively common concurrence (11% of cases) of hemangiomas elsewhere in patients with hemangioendotheliomas should not be misconstrued as evidence of metastases.

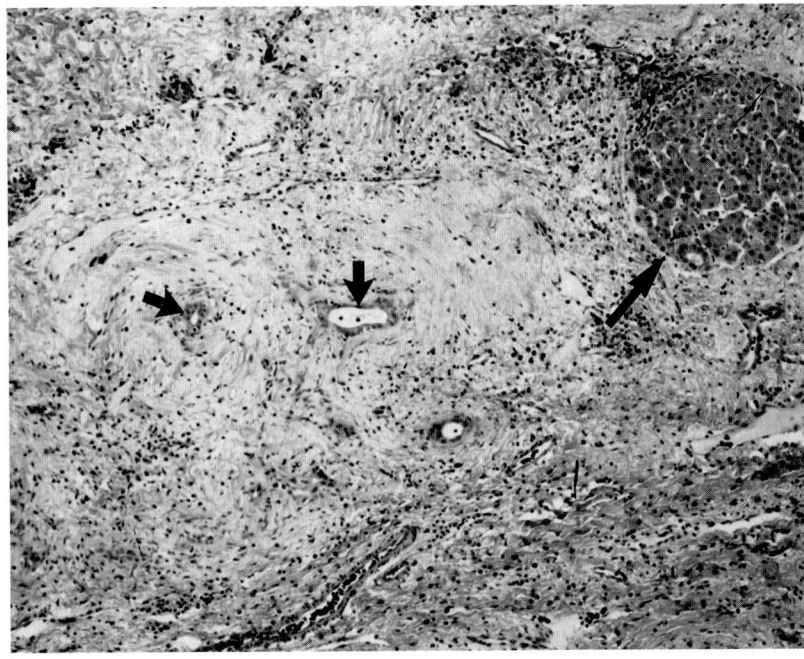

FIGURE 25.30. *Mesenchymal hamartoma of liver. Note the ducts (small arrows); a nodule of hepatocytes is incorporated (large arrow). ×28.*

Cavernous Hemangioma

This lesion does not differ from those in other locations. It is usually asymptomatic and most often is found incidentally at postmortem examination (Fig. 25.31).

Hepatoblastoma

The hepatoblastoma is usually a solitary, large, lobulated gray tumor of the right hepatic lobe. Males predominate, and the tumor is uncommon beyond the age of 3 years [218, 219]. It may present in utero, causing hydrops fetalis, or it may be found at birth in an infant with an abdominal mass or, rarely, with placental metastases [227, 228]. A small number of patients have hemihypertrophy or the Beckwith-Wiedemann syndrome. Of the latter, a few have 11p15 deletions in the hepatoblastoma. An important association exists with familial adenomatous polyposis, when children are at risk for hepatoblastoma [229]. Other associations identified in case reports are with Aicardi syndrome, fetal alcohol syndrome, trisomy 18, maternal use of oral contraceptives, and, in a broad survey, recognition of parental exposure to petroleum products and metals [212–232]. Alphafetoprotein is produced by 84–91% of tumors, particularly the better-differentiated types, and is therefore of value for both diagnosis and follow-up. Grossly, the tumor resembles a Wilms' tumor, having a pseudocapsule, lobularity, soft gray consistency, and areas of hemorrhage and necrosis (Fig. 25.32). The pattern is multinodular or diffuse in 15–30% of cases [218]. The adjacent liver is not cirrhotic. Hepatoblastomas are either pure epithelial or mixed, containing both epithelial and mesenchymal elements. The latter account for 30% of cases, although this determination is clearly dependent on the thoroughness of sampling [219]. Epithelial subtypes include fetal, embryonic, and small-cell undifferentiated patterns. In any one case, tumor epithelium may be comprised of one or a mixture of types. The fetal type, mimicking fetal liver, is composed of cells identifiable as hepatocytes but distinctly smaller and arranged in cords, sometimes with recognizable canaliculi. Neither normal hepatic lobular architecture nor portal tracts are present. The cells are deceptively regular, with little variation in nuclear size, and the incidence of mitoses is less than two per 10 high-power fields. Cells may have a granular or clear cytoplasm. Hematopoiesis is consistently present. The less differentiated embryonic hepatoblastoma is composed of more primitive cells with less cytoplasm, common mitoses, and nuclear variability. The tumor occurs in sheets, tubules, or pseudorosette patterns, thus mimicking the primitive embryonic liver, but hematopoiesis is absent. The small-cell undifferentiated variant occurs in young infants, disseminates widely, and may be confused with neuroblastoma. Another undifferentiated tumor with a rhabdoid phenotype arises in the liver and may be associated with primitive neuroectodermal tumor of the brain [233]. In addition, there is a macrotrabecular type of hepatoblastoma that is reminiscent of a hepatocellular carcinoma and that has a poor prognosis compared with the standard fetal epithelial subtype [234]. The mesenchymal component in the hepatoblastoma is usually primitive; when differentiated, osteoid predominates. Rhabdomyoblastic differentiation occurs infrequently.

Histologic typing of hepatoblastomas for prognostic purposes is considered valid, but not by everyone [235–239]. Early reviews indicating that fetal epithelial tumors have the best outlook are supported by the acknowledgment that the tumor should be exclusively fetal in type. A dissenting conclusion in a recent review of 105 cases indicates that the prognosis relates significantly to stage at presentation, and not with histologic type [238].

Other Tumors

Hepatocellular carcinoma is very rare under the age of 5 years. In our registry, the youngest child is a 4-year-old girl with hepatitis B, likely acquired by blood transfusion when she was a premature infant. Hepatocellular carcinoma of childhood has many associations, which are reviewed elsewhere [215, 240]. Of these, the relationship to hepatitis B virus is the most significant. Early exposure through vertical transmission to the infant results in greater viral genome incorporation into the host DNA and greater risk for hepatocarcinoma than would occur at an older age. Successful vaccination of infants or carrier mothers has resulted in reduction of the carrier state and tumor frequency in infants [241].

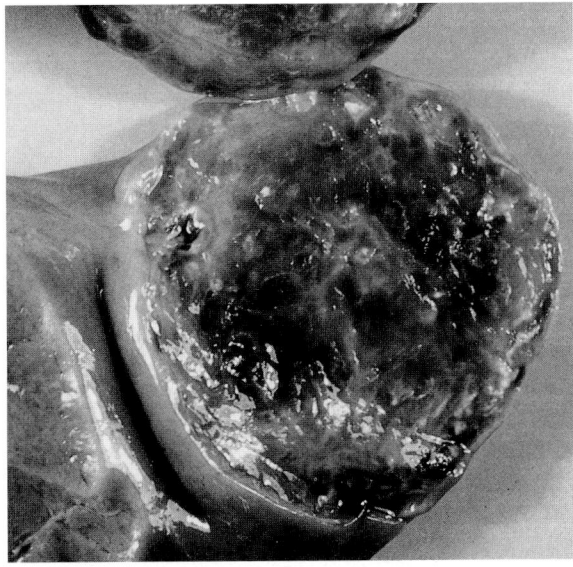

FIGURE 25.31. *Cavernous hemangioma of liver discovered incidentally in newborn infant.*

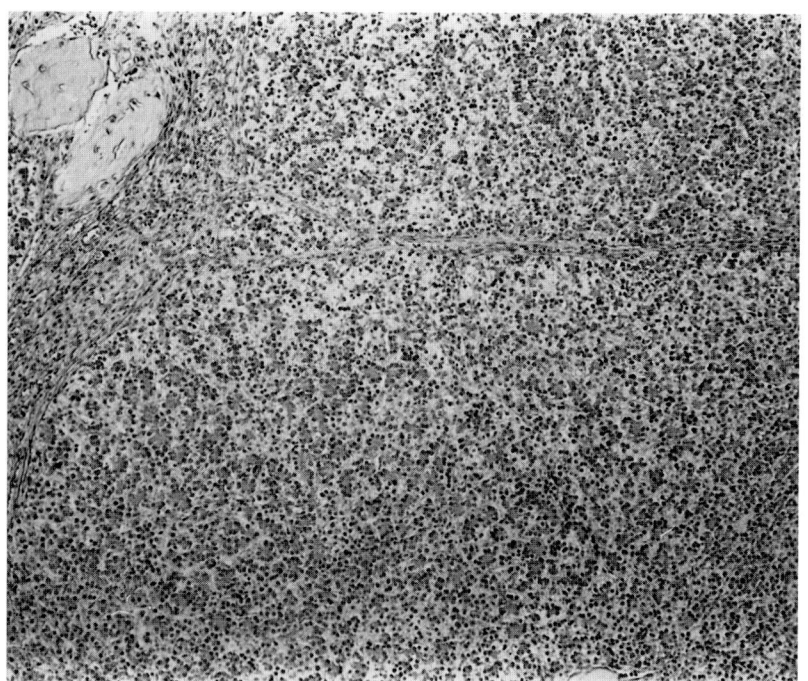

FIGURE 25.32.   *Hepatoblastoma. The pattern is mixed epithelial-mesenchymal. In this field, the epithelial type is fetal, and in the upper left there are two islands of osteoid. H&E, ×40.*

Focal nodular hyperplasia is generally appreciated as a nonneoplastic entity and does not differ grossly or microscopically from the adult counterpart. Stocker and Ishak, reporting a large pediatric experience, note the same female predominance as is seen in adults, but with a lack of associated hepatic angiomas [242]. Their cases include one neonate with multiple malformations.

The rare hepatic adenoma of the type found in patients with glycogen storage disease type I has been reported in an infant with galactosemia, and may be found in patients treated with anabolic steroids [219].

Hepatic teratomas occur in neonates and stillborn infants [243]. These tumors should not be confused with so-called teratoid hepatoblastomas, which contain neural elements. We have experienced a primary choriocarcinoma in the liver of a 2-month-old infant without evidence of hepatoblastoma or placental primary trophoblastic tumor [215].

The undifferentiated (embryonal) sarcoma of liver occurs predominantly in the pediatric age group but is rare in the neonate [244]. This tumor is a pleomorphic sarcoma, solid and cystic, with an aggressive behavior. The tumor is highly mitotic and contains anaplastic, giant, and stellate tumor cells and benign ductal structures entrapped at the tumor periphery. It has been compared to malignant fibrous histiocytoma, but ultrastructural and immunohistochemical studies do not clarify the origin beyond its being mesenchymal [244].

Histiocytosis X involving the liver may cause cholestasis, but not usually in the neonatal period.

Rhabdomyosarcomas of the biliary tract occur in older infants and young children.

MISCELLANEOUS CONDITIONS

Erythroblastosis fetalis due to immunohemolysis is now uncommon. Stillborn or neonatal infants have accentuated hematopoietic activity in the fetal liver, and there is a shift to early erythroid precursors (Fig. 25.33). Parenchymal and Kupffer's cell iron stores are increased, and hepatic fibrosis, giant-cell transformation, neonatal hepatitis, and cirrhosis have been recorded in some infants [245]. Cholestasis occurring in infants with severe erythroblastosis fetalis was known as the inspissated bile syndrome. In some infants with hemolytic disease, bile plugging of major ducts may mimic extrahepatic biliary atresia both clinically and pathologically. Exaggerated hepatic iron deposits, uncommon in biliary atresia, may assist in the differential diagnosis. Increase in hepatic erythropoietic activity is not confined to erythroblastosis fetalis but occurs with other causes of erythrocyte destruction (parvovirus B19 infection) or loss (fetomaternal hemorrhage), in hemoglobinopathies (alpha thalassemia), and in maternal diabetes mellitus, where hypoxemia or hyperinsulinemia may be causative.

Abnormalities of the liver and biliary system occasionally occur with chromosomal errors [69]. As examples, extrahepatic biliary atresia, paucity of intrahepatic bile ducts, giant-cell transformation, and neonatal hepatitis may occur in trisomy 18 [111, 246]. Both intrahepatic bile duct paucity and giant-cell transformation are recorded in trisomy 21 and in monosomy X (Turner syndrome) [111]. In trisomy 9, intrahepatic bile ducts appear excessive and proliferative [247]. We have observed portal fibrosis and ductal proliferation in a newborn infant with 3-14 translocation, and in

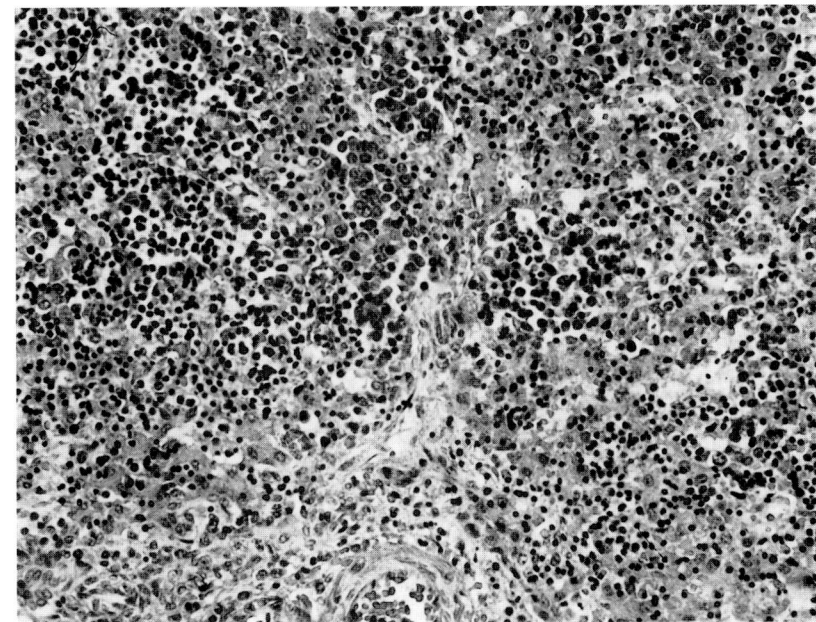

FIGURE 25.33.   *The liver in erythroblastosis fetalis. There is exaggerated erythropoiesis with a "left shift." Portal tract, lower center. ×70.*

one premature infant with triploidy there was atresia of the gallbladder and extrahepatic bile ducts. We also have seen prominent hepatic hemosiderosis in three newborn infants with trisomy 22.

Drug-induced hepatic injury is a matter of concern in the perinatal infant because of the immaturity of drug-metabolizing processes. This and other iatrogenic insults are presented fully elsewhere [248]. However, it is pertinent to discuss the liver pathology of parenteral alimentation [249]. Variable liver morphology occurs, ranging from steatosis to canalicular and cytoplasmic cholestasis to cirrhosis. Portal fibrosis may be minimal or marked, with bridging from

portal tract to portal tract and with bile duct proliferation and periductal inflammation. Both giant-cell and acinar transformation of hepatocytes may be present. The liver pathology in fact can simulate major duct obstruction, leading to an erroneous diagnosis of extrahepatic biliary atresia (Fig. 25.34). Eosinophils infiltrate the portal tracts in some cases. Cholelithiasis may develop in chronically intravenously fed infants, and infants have developed hepatocellular carcinomas following prolonged therapy [250]. Pathogenetic mechanisms involved in liver toxicity in infants receiving parenteral nutrition are probably multiple. Toxicity of the administered substances and superimposed

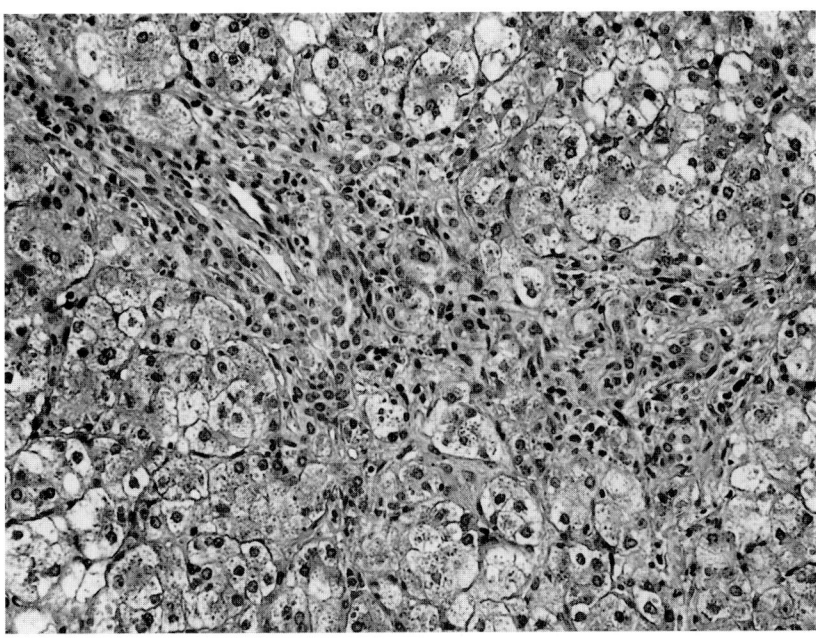

FIGURE 25.34.   *The liver in chronic intravenous alimentation in a 4-week-old infant. Note portal fibrosis, ductular proliferation, cholestasis, and steatosis. ×70.*

Table 25.8.   Neonatal cholestasis

Hepatitides (see Table 25.1)
Idiopathic
Known etiology
Cholangiopathies (see Table 25.4)
Extrahepatic biliary atresia
Choleductal cyst
Paucity of intrahepatic ducts
Other: duct perforation, external and internal obstruction
Metabolic diseases (see Table 25.5)
Chromosomal errors
Turner syndrome
Trisomy 18, trisomy 21
Drug toxicity
Parenteral alimentation
Erythromycin
Endocrine disorders
Hypothyroidism
Hypopituitarism
Other
Erythroblastosis fetalis
Intestinal obstruction
Hepatic tumors
Maternal Dubin-Johnson syndrome
Shock

sepsis are implicated, and lack of oral feeding may result in failed stimulation of bile flow.

GALLBLADDER DISORDERS

The gallbladder is rarely abnormal in newborn infants. In our experience, the most common abnormality is absence of the structure, most often seen in infants with lethal malformation syndromes. An incidence of 0.38% is reported in pediatric postmortem examinations; in our experience, the rate is 1.25% [69, 251]. The gallbladder may be duplicated, sometimes with biliary obstruction, embedded in hepatic parenchyma, pendulous, or inflamed and hydropic. In extrahepatic biliary atresia, the gallbladder is often small, even absent. In cystic fibrosis, the gallbladder may be mucin-filled, and in metachromatic leukodystrophy, lysosomal storage is apparent in the mucosa. Cholelithiasis and choledocholithiasis, and attendant complications, sometimes are recognized in the fetus and newborn infant [252, 253]. Calculi are of pigment type. Intravenous alimentation is occasionally associated with marked distention of the gallbladder and cholelithiasis.

CONCLUDING REMARKS

Jaundice, which is an exceedingly common finding in newborn infants, is categorized as unconjugated or conjugated hyperbilirubinemia. In most instances, unconjugated hyperbilirubinemia does not indicate liver disease, whereas conjugated bilirubin in excess should always be regarded as pathologic and most often signifies neonatal cholestasis [254].

Differential diagnosis of neonatal cholestasis is particularly important for the pathologist. The multiple etiologies dictate different therapies (Table 25.8). Thus, precise diagnosis is required. The collaborative use of clinical, biochemical, and radiologic information assists in the interpretation of morphologic findings in the liver. The pathologist can distinguish extra- and intrahepatic cholestatic disease and can detect metabolic disorders, specific infectious diseases, and abnormalities of portal, vascular, and intrahepatic ductal structures. Interpretation of pathologic findings is important for immediate care of the infant, prognostication, and genetic counseling.

REFERENCES

1. Emery JL. Asymmetrical liver disease in infancy. *J Pathol Bacteriol* 1995; 69:219–20.
2. Tan CE, Driver M, Howard ER, Moscosa GJ. Extrahepatic biliary atresia; a first trimester event? *J Pediatr Surg* 1994; 29:808–14.
3. Blankenberg T, Lund JK, Ruebner BH. Normal and abnormal development of human intrahepatic bile ducts. An immunohistochemical perspective. *Perspect Pediatr Pathol* 1991; 14:143–67.
4. Shah KD, Gerber MA. Development of intrahepatic bile ducts in humans. *Arch Pathol Lab Med* 1989; 114:597–600.
5. Shah KD, Gerber MA. Development of intrahepatic bile ducts in man: possible role of laminin. *Hepatology* 1989; 10:605.
6. Ruebner B, Blankenberg TA, Burrows D, Soo Hoo W, Lund J. Development and transformation of the ductal plate in the developing human liver. *Pediatr Pathol* 1990; 10:55–68.
7. Kahn E, Markowitz J, Aiges H, Daum F. Human ontogeny of the bile duct to portal space ratio. *Hepatology* 1989; 10:21–3.
8. Reif S, Lebenthal E. Extracellular matrix modulation of liver ontogeny. *J Pediatr Gastroenterol Nutr* 1991; 12:1–4.
9. Van Eyken P, Desmet VJ. Cytokeratins and the liver. *Liver* 1993; 13:113–22.
10. Jorgensen MJ. The ductal plate malformation. *Acta Pathol Microbiol Scand Suppl* 1977; 257:1–88.
11. De Wolf-Peeters C, De Vos R, Desmet V. Electron microscopy and histochemistry of canalicular differentiation in fetal and neonatal rat liver. *Tissue Cell* 1972; 4:379–88.
12. De Wolf-Peeters C, De Vos R, Desmet V. Electron microscopy and morphometry of canalicular differentiation in fetal and newborn rat liver. *Exp Mol Pathol* 1974; 21:339–50.
13. Phillips MJ. Microanatomy of bile secretion. In: Adcock EW, Lester R, eds. *Neonatal Cholestasis: Causes, Syndromes, Therapies*. Report of the 87th Ross Conference on Pediatric Research. Columbus, OH: Ross Laboratory Publications, 1984, pp. 24–31.
14. Singer DB. Hepatic erythropoiesis in infants of diabetic mothers: a morphometric study. *Pediatr Pathol* 1986; 5:471–9.
15. Faa G, Sciot R, Farci A, et al. Iron concentration and distribution in the newborn liver. *Liver* 1994; 14:193–9.
16. Tanikawa K. *Ultrastructural Aspects of the Liver and Its Disorders*. Tokyo: Igaku-Shoin, 1979, pp. 82–6.
17. Moorman AFM, Vermeulen JLM, Charles R, Lamers WH. Localization of ammonia-metabolizing enzymes in human liver: ontogenesis of heterogeneity. *Hepatology* 1989; 9(3):367–72.
18. Sano K, Fujioka Y, Nagashima K, et al. Distributional variation of P-450 immunoreactive hepatocytes in human liver disorders. *Hum Pathol* 1989; 20:1015–20.
19. Riggs BS, Bronstein AC, Kulig K, Archer PG, Rumack BH. Acute acetaminophen overdose during pregnancy. *Obstet Gynecol* 1989; 74:247–52.
20. Buck FS, Koss MN. Heterotopic liver in an adrenal gland. *Pediatr Pathol* 1988; 8:535–40.
21. Chen KTK, Ma CK, Kassel SH. Hepatocellular adenoma of the placenta. *Am J Surg Pathol* 1986; 10:436–40.

22. Laxer RM, Roberts EA, Gross KR, et al. Liver diseases in neonatal erythematosus. *J Pediatr* 1990; 116:238–42.

23. Evans N, Gaskin K. Liver disease in association with neonatal lupus erythematosus. *J Pediatr Child Health* 1993; 29:478–80.

24. Flower AJE, Tanner MS. Perinatal transmission of hepatitis B. In: Tanner MS, Stocks RJ, eds. *Neonatal Gastroenterology, Contemporary Issues.* Newcastle-upon-Tyne, UK: Intercept, 1984, pp. 155–77.

25. Stokes J, Wolman IH, Blanchard MC, Farquhar JD. Viral hepatitis in the newborn: clinical features, epidemiology and pathology. *Am J Dis Child* 1951; 82:213–16.

26. Craig J, Landing BL. Form of hepatitis in neonatal period simulating biliary atresia. *Arch Pathol* 1954; 54:321–33.

27. Landing BH. Considerations of the pathogenesis of neonatal hepatitis, biliary atresia and choledochal cyst—the concept of infantile obstructive cholangiopathy. *Prog Pediatr Surg* 1974; 6:113–39.

28. Danks DM, Campbell PE, Jack I, Rogers J, Smith AL. Studies of the etiology of neonatal hepatitis and biliary atresia. *Arch Dis Child* 1977; 52:360–7.

29. Mowat AP, Psacharopoulos HT, Williams R. Extrahepatic biliary atresia versus neonatal hepatitis: review of 137 prospectively investigated patients. *Arch Dis Child* 1976; 51:736–70.

30. Mieli-Vergani G, Howard ER, Mowat AP. Liver disease in infancy: a 20 year perspective. *Gut* 1991; 32(suppl):S123–28.

31. Psacharopoulos HT, Mowat AP. Incidence and early history of obstructive jaundice in infancy in southeast England. In: Javitt N, ed. *Neonatal Hepatitis and Biliary Atresia.* Washington: NIH DHEW, 1979, pp. 167–71.

32. Brough AJ, Bernstein J. Conjugated hyperbilirubinemia in early infancy, a reassessment of liver biopsy. *Hum Pathol* 1974; 5:507–16.

33. Lai MN, Chang MH, Hsu SC, et al. Differential diagnosis of extrahepatic biliary atresia from neonatal hepatitis: a prospective study. *J Pediatr Gastroenterol Nutr* 1994; 18:121–7.

34. Montgomery CK, Ruebner BH. Neonatal hepatocellular giant cell transformation: a review. In: Rosenberg HS, Bolande RP, eds. *Perspectives in Pediatric Pathology.* vol. 3. Chicago: Year Book Medical, 1976, pp. 85–101.

35. Ruebner BH, Thaler MM. Giant-cell transformation in infantile liver disease. In: Javitt N, ed. *Neonatal Hepatitis and Biliary Atresia.* Washington: NIH DHEW, 1979, pp. 299–311.

36. Alagille D. Clinical aspects of neonatal hepatitis. *Am J Dis Child* 1972; 123:287–91.

37. Deutsch J, Smith AL, Danks DM, Campbell PE. Longterm prognosis for babies with neonatal liver disease. *Arch Dis Child* 1985; 60:447–51.

38. Odievre M, Hadchouel M, Landrieu P, Alagille D, Eliot N. Long-term prognosis for infants with hepatic cholestasis and patient extrahepatic biliary tract. *Arch Dis Child* 1981; 56:373–6.

39. Thaler MM, Gellis SS. Studies in neonatal hepatitis and biliary atresia. I. Long-term prognosis of neonatal hepatitis. *Am J Dis Child* 1968; 116:257–61.

40. Thaler MM, Gellis SS. Studies in neonatal hepatitis and biliary atresia. II. The effect of diagnostic laparotomy on long-term prognosis of neonatal hepatitis. *Am J Dis Child* 1968; 116:262–70.

41. Pappo O, Yunis E, Jordan J, et al. Recurrent and de novo giant cell hepatitis after orthotopic liver transplantation. *Am J Surg Pathol* 1994; 18:804–13.

42. Lawson EE, Boggs JD. Long-term follow up of neonatal hepatitis: safety and value of surgical exploration. *Pediatrics* 1974; 53:650–5.

43. Becroft DMO. Prenatal cytomegalovirus infection: epidemiology, pathology and pathogenesis. In: Rosenberg HS, Bolande RP, eds. *Perspectives in Pediatric Pathology.* vol. 6. New York: Masson, 1981, pp. 203–41.

44. Rosenberg HS, Kohl S, Vogler C. Viral infections of the fetus and neonate. In: Naeye RL, Kissane JM, Kaufmann N, eds. *Perinatal Diseases.* Baltimore: Williams & Wilkins, 1981, pp. 133–200.

45. Finegold MJ, Carpenter RJ. Obliterative cholangitis due to cytomegalovirus: a possible precursor of paucity of intrahepatic bile ducts. *Hum Pathol* 1986; 13:662–5.

46. Oppenheimer EH, Esterly JR. Cytomegalovirus: a possible cause of biliary atresia. *Am J Pathol* 1973; 71:22.

47. Dimmick JE. Intrahepatic bile duct paucity and cytomegalovirus infection. *Pediatr Pathol* 1993; 13:847–52.

48. Hart M, Kaufman S, Vanderhoof J, et al. Neonatal hepatitis and extrahepatic biliary atresia with CMV infection in twins. *Am J Dis Child* 1991; 145:302–5.

49. Esterly JR, Oppenheimer EH. Intrauterine rubella infection. In: Rosenberg HS, Bolande RP, eds. *Perspectives in Pediatric Pathology.* vol. 1. Chicago: Year Book Medical, 1973, pp. 313–18.

50. Rosenberg HS, Oppenheimer EH, Esterly JR. Congenital rubella syndrome: the late effects and their relation to early lesions. In: Rosenberg HS, Bolande RP, eds. *Perspectives in Pediatric Pathology.* vol. 6. New York: Masson, 1981, pp. 183–202.

51. Dupuy JM, Frommel D, Alagille D. Severe viral hepatitis in infancy. *Lancet* 1975; i;191–4.

52. Mulligan MJ, Stiehm ER. Neonatal hepatitis B infection: clinical and immunologic considerations. *J Perinatol* 1994; 14:2–9.

53. Simms J, Duff P. Viral hepatitis in pregnancy. *Semin Perinatol* 1993; 17:384–93.

54. Tanaka M, Ishikawa T, Sakaguchi M. The pathogenesis of biliary atresia in Japan: immunohistochemical study of HBV-associated antigen. *Acta Pathol Japon* 1993; 43:360–6.

55. Balaraman V, Wilson C, Nakamura K, et al. Severe neonatal hepatitis (HAV) infection in the newborn. *Pediatr Res* 1991; 29:279A.

56. Novati R, Theirs V, Monforte A, et al. Mother-to-child transmission of hepatitis C detected by nested polymerase chain reaction. *J Infect Dis* 1992; 165:720–2.

57. Nagat Y, Tanaka Y, Okada T. Mother-to-infant transmission of hepatitis C virus. *J Pediatr* 1992; 120:432–4.

58. Dische MR, Gooch WM. Congenital toxoplasmosis. *Perspect Pediatr Pathol* 1981; 6:83–113.

59. Singer DB. Pathology of neonatal herpes simplex virus infection. In: Rosenberg HS, Bolande RP, eds. *Perspectives in Pediatric Pathology.* vol. 6. New York: Masson, 1981, pp. 242–78.

60. Hughes JR, Wilfert CM, Moore M, Benirschke K, de Hayos-Guevara E. Echovirus 14 infection associated with fatal neonatal hepatic necrosis. *Am J Dis Child* 1981; 123:61–7.

61. Mostoufizadeh M, Lack E, Gang DL, Perez-Atayde R, Driscoll SG. Postmortem manifestations of echovirus 11 sepsis in five newborn infants. *Hum Pathol* 1983; 14:818–23.

62. Robertson NJ, McKeever PA. Fetal and placental pathology in two cases of maternal varicella infection. *Pediatr Pathol* 1992; 12:545–50.

63. Metzman R, Anand A, DeGialo P, Knisely A. Hepatic disease associated with intrauterine parvovirus B19 infection in a newborn premature infant. *J Pediatr Gastroenterol Nutr* 1989; 9:112–14.

64. Richardson SC, Bishop RF, Smith AL. Reovirus serotype 3 infection in infants with extrahepatic biliary atresia or neonatal hepatitis. *J Gastroenterol Hepatol* 1994; 9:264–8.

65. Witzleben C, Marshall GS, Wenner W, Piccoli DA, Barbour SD. HIV as a cause of giant cell hepatitis. *Hum Pathol* 1988; 19:603–5.

66. Kahn E, Greco M, Daum F, et al. Hepatic pathology in pediatric AIDS. *Hum Pathol* 1991; 22:1111–9.

67. Vawter GF. Perinatal listeriosis. In: Rosenberg HS, Bolande RP, eds. *Perspectives in Pediatric Pathology.* vol. 6. New York: Masson, 1981, pp. 153–66.

68. Oppenheimer EH, Barrett Dahms B. Congenital syphilis. In: Rosenberg HS, Bolande RP, eds. *Perspectives in Pediatric Pathology.* vol. 6. New York: Masson, 1981, pp. 115–38.

69. Dimmick JE. Hepatobiliary system. In: Dimmick JE, Kalousek DK, eds. *Developmental Pathology of the Embryo and Fetus.* Philadelphia: JB Lippincott, 1992, pp. 545–78.

70. Desmet VJ. The cholangiopathies. In: Suchy FJ, ed. *Liver Disease in Children.* St. Louis: Mosby, 1994, pp. 145–65.

71. Shiraki K, Okaniwa M, Landing BH. Cholestatic syndromes of infancy and childhood. In: Zakim D, Boyer TD, eds. *Hepatology.* Philadelphia: WB Saunders, 1982, pp. 1176–92.

72. Cunningham M, Sybert V. Idiopathic extrahepatic biliary atresia: recurrence in sibs in two families. *Am J Med Genet* 1988; 31:421–6.

73. Debray D, Pariente D, Urvaas E, Hadchouel M, Bernard O. Sclerosing cholangitis in children. *J Pediatr* 1994; 124:49–56.

74. Stern H, Tucker SM. Cytomegalovirus infection in the newborn and in early childhood. Three atypical cases. *Lancet* 1965; 2:1268–71.

75. Jevon GP, Dimmick JE. Biliary atresia and cytomegalovirus infection: a PCR based study. *Mod Pathol* 1995; 8:4p.

76. Becroft DMO. Biliary atresia associated with prenatal infection by *Listeria monocytogenes. Arch Dis Child* 1972; 47:656–60.

77. Hadchouel M, Hugon RN, Odievre M. Immunoglobulin deposits in the biliary remnants of extrahepatic biliary atresia: a study by immunoperoxidase staining in 128 infants. *Histopathology* 1981; 5:217–21.

78. Silveira TR, Salzano FM, Donaldson PT, et al. Association between HLA and extrahepatic biliary atresia. *J Pediatr Gastroenterol Nutr* 1993; 16:114–17.

79. Stowens D. Congenital biliary atresia. *Am J Gastroenterol* 1959; 32:57.

80. Fisher MM, Chen S-H, Dekker A. Congenital diaphragm of the common hepatic duct. *Gastroenterology* 1968; 54:605–10.

81. LeCoultre C, Fete R, Cuendet A, Berclaz J-P. An unusual association of small bowel atresia and biliary atresia: a case report. *J Pediatr Surg* 1983; 18:136–7.

82. Pickett L, Briggs H. Biliary obstruction secondary to hepatic vascular ligation in fetal sheep. *J Pediatr Surg* 1969; 4:95–100.

83. Dimmick JE, Bove KE, McAdams AJ. Extrahepatic biliary atresia and the polysplenia syndrome. *J Pediatr* 1975; 86:644–5.

84. Maksem JA. Polysplenia syndrome and splenic hypoplasia associated with extrahepatic biliary atresia. *Arch Pathol Lab Med* 1980; 104:212–14.

85. Davenport M, Savage M, Mowat AP, Howard ER. Biliary atresia splenic malformation syndrome: an etiologic and prognostic subgroup. *Surgery* 1993; 113:662–8.

86. Carmi R, Magee CA, Neill CA, Karre FM. Extrahepatic biliary atresia and associated anomalies: etiologic heterogeneity suggested by distinctive patterns of associations. *Am J Med Genet* 1993; 45:683–93.

87. Witzleben CL. Extrahepatic biliary atresia: concept of cause diagnosis and management. In: Rosenberg HS, Bolande RP, eds. *Perspectives in Pediatric Pathology*. vol. 5. New York: Masson, 1979, pp. 41–62.

88. Teichberg S, Markowitz J, Silverberg M, et al. Abnormal cilia in a child with the polysplenia syndrome and extrahepatic biliary atresia. *J Pediatr* 1982; 100:399–401.

89. Lilly JR, Stellin G, Pau CML, Ohi R. Historical background of the biliary atresia registry. In: Dahm F, ed. *Extrahepatic Biliary Atresia*. New York: Dekker, 1983, pp. 73–7.

90. Chandra RS, Altman RP. Ductal remnants in extrahepatic biliary atresia: a histopathologic study with clinical correlation. *J Pediatr* 1978; 93:196–200.

91. Gautier M, Jehan P, Odievre M. Histologic study of biliary fibrous remnants in 48 cases of extrahepatic biliary atresia. *J Pediatr* 1976; 89:704–9.

92. Chandra RS. Bile duct and hepatic morphology in biliary atresia: correlations with bile flow following portoenterostomy. In: Dahm F, ed. *Extrahepatic Biliary Atresia*. New York: Dekker, 1983, pp. 43–63.

93. Nelson R. Managing biliary atresia. *Br Med J* 1989; 298:1471–2.

94. Kobayashi A, Itabashi F, Ohbe Y. Long-term prognosis in biliary atresia after hepatic portoenterostomy: analysis of 35 patients who survived beyond 5 years of age. *J Pediatr* 1984; 105:243–6.

95. Kim SH. Choledochal cysts: survey by the surgical section of the American Academy of Pediatrics. *J Pediatr Surg* 1981; 16:402–7.

96. Bancroft JD, Bucuvalas JC, Ryckman FC, Schwartz KB. Antenatal diagnosis of choledochal cyst. *J Pediatr Gastroenterol Nutr* 1994; 18:142–5.

97. Miyano T, Suruga K, Shimomura H, Nittono H, Matsumoto M. Chole-dochopancreatic elongated common channel disorders. *J Pediatr Surg* 1984; 19:165–70.

98. Reid IS. Biliary tract anomalies associated with duodenal atresia. *Arch Dis Child* 1973; 48:592–7.

99. Kusunoki M, Saitoh N, Yamamura T, et al. Choledochal cysts: oligoganglionosis in the narrow zone of the choledochus. *Arch Surg* 1988; 123: 984–6.

100. Woolf GM, Vierling JM. Disappearing intrahepatic bile ducts: the syndromes and their mechanisms. *Semin Liver Dis* 1993; 13:261–75.

101. Alagille D, Odievre M, Gautier M, Dommergues JP. Hepatic ductular hypoplasia associated with characteristic facies, vertebral malformations, retarded physical, mental and sexual development and cardiac murmur. *J Pediatr* 1975; 86:63–71.

102. Alagille D, Odievre M. *Liver and Biliary Tract Disease in Children*. New York: Wiley-Flammarion, 1978, pp. 180–92.

103. Dahms BB, Petrelli M, Wyllie R, et al. Arteriohepatic dysplasia in infancy and childhood: a longitudinal study of six patients. *Hepatology* 1982; 2:350–8.

104. Markowitz J, Daum F, Kahn EI, et al. Arteriohepatic dysplasia. I. Pitfalls in diagnosis and management. *Hepatology* 1983; 1:74–6.

105. Watson GH, Miller V. Arteriohepatic dysplasia. *Arch Dis Child* 1973; 48:459–66.

106. Mueller RF, Pagon RA, Tepin MG, et al. Arteriohepatic dysplasia: phenotypic features and family studies. *Clin Genet* 1984; 25:323–31.

107. Byrne J, Harrod M, Friedman J, Howard-Peebles P. del(20p) with mani-festations of arteriohepatic dysplasia. *Am J Med Genet* 1986; 24:673–8.

108. Spinner NB, Fortina P, Genin A, Taub R. Cytogenetically balanced t(2:20) in a two-generation family with Alagille syndrome: cytogenetic and molecular studies. *Am J Hum Genet* 1994; 55:238–43.

109. Alagille D, Hadchouel M, Hugon RN, Gautier M. Reduced ratio of portal tracts to paucity of intrahepatic bile ducts. *Arch Pathol Lab Med* 1978; 102:402.

110. Valenci-Mayoral P, Weber J, Cutz E, Edwards VD, Phillips MJ. Possible defect in the bile secretory apparatus in arteriohepatic dysplasia (Alagille syndrome): a review with observations on the ultrastructure of liver. *Hepatology* 1984; 4:691–8.

111. Witzleben CL. Bile duct paucity ("intrahepatic atresia"). In: Rosenberg HS, Bolande RP, eds. *Perspectives in Pediatric Pathology*. vol. 7. New York: Masson, 1982, pp. 185–202.

112. Furuya K, Roberts E, Canny G, Philips MJ. Neonatal hepatitis syndrome in paucity of interlobular bile ducts in cystic fibrosis. *J Pediatr Gastroenterol Nutr* 1991; 12:127–30.

113. Hanson RF, Isenberg JN, Williams GC, et al. The metabolism of 3-alpha 7-alpha 12-alpha-trihydroxy 5-beta cholestan-26-oic acid in two siblings with cholestasis due to intrahepatic bile duct anomalies. *J Clin Invest* 1975; 56:577–87.

114. Kimura A, Yuge K, Yukizane S, et al. Abnormal low ratio of cholic acid to chenodeoxycholic acid in a cholestatic infant with severe hypoglycemia. *J Pediatr Gastroenterol Nutr* 1991; 12:383–7.

115. Alanso E, Snover D, Montag R, Freese D, Whitington P. Histologic pathology of the liver in progressive familial intrahepatic cholestasis. *J Pediatr Gastroenterol Nutr* 1994; 18:128–33.

116. Kahn E. Paucity of interlobular bile ducts: arteriohepatic dysplasia and nonsyndromatic duct paucity. *Perspect Pediatr Pathol* 1991; 14:168–215.

117. Mikati MA, Barakat AY, Sulh HB, Der Kaloustian VM. Renal tubular insufficiency, cholestatic jaundice and multiple congenital anomalies—a new multisystem syndrome. *Helv Paediatr Acta* 1984; 39:463–71.

118. Wales JK, Walker V, Moore IE, Clayton PT. Bronze baby syndrome, biliary hypoplasia, incomplete Beckwith-Weidemann syndrome and partial trisomy 11. *Eur J Pediatr* 1986; 145:141–3.

119. Witzleben CL. Cystic disease of the liver. In: Zakim D, Boyer TD, eds. *Hepatology*. Philadelphia: WB Saunders, 1982, pp. 1193–212.

120. Desmet VJ. Congenital diseases of intrahepatic ducts: variations on the theme "ductal plate malformation." *Hepatology* 1992; 16:1069–83.

121. Desmet VJ. What is congenital hepatic fibrosis? *Histopathology* 1992; 20:465–77.

122. Bernstein J. Hepatic and renal involvement in malformation syndromes. *Mt Sinai J Med* 1986; 53:421–8.

123. Strayer DS, Kissane JM. Dysplasia of the kidneys, liver and pancreas: report of a variant of Ivemark syndrome. *Hum Pathol* 1979; 10:228–34.

124. Blankenberg TA, Ruebner BH, Ellis WG, Bernstein J, Dimmick JE. Pathology of renal hepatic anomalies in Meckel syndrome. *Am J Med Genet* 1987; 3(suppl):395–410.

125. Perheentupa J, Rapola J, Visakorpi JK, Eskelin L-E. Lysinuric protein intolerance. *Am J Med* 1975; 59:229–40.

126. Hug G, Kline J, Schubert W. Liver ultrastructure: dissimilarity between Reye's syndrome and hereditable defects of carbamylphosphate synthetase or ornithine transcarbamylase. *Pediatr Res* 1978; 12:437.

127. Zimmerman A, Bachman C, Colombo JP. Ultrastructural pathology in congenital defects of the urea cycle: ornithine transcarbamylase and carbamyl phosphate synthetase deficiency. *Virchows Arch A* 1981; 393:321–31.

128. Leibowitz J, Wick H, Mihatsch MJ, et al. Liver morphology in a case of citrullinemia (a light and electron microscopic study). *Beitr Pathol* 1974; 151:200–7.

129. Landrieu P, Francois B, Leon G, Van Hoof F. Liver peroxisome damage during acute hepatic failure in partial ornithine transcarbamylase deficiency. *Pediatr Res* 1982; 16:977–81.

130. Alagille D, Odievre M. *Liver and Biliary Tract Disease in Children*. New York: Wiley-Flammarion, 1978, p. 35.

131. Scharschmidt BF, Gollan JL, Wolkoff AW. Inheritable disorders manifested by conjugated hyperbilirubinemia. *Semin Liver Dis* 1983; 3:65–72.

132. Hug G, Bove K, Soukop S. Lethal neonatal multiorgan deficiency of carnitine palmitoyl transferase II. *N Engl J Med* 1991; 325:1862–4.

133. Amendt BA, Greene C, Sweetman L, et al. Short-chain acyl-CoA dehydrogenase deficiency: clinical and biochemical studies in two patients. *J Clin Invest* 1988; 81:171–5.

134. Treem WR, Witzleben C, Piccoli DA, et al. Medium-chain and long-chain acyl CoA-dehydrogenase deficiency: clinical, pathology, and ultrastructural differentiation from Reye syndrome. *Hepatology* 1986; 6:1270–8.

135. Leung K-C, Hammond JW, Chabra S, et al. A fatal neonatal case of medium chain acyl-coenzyme A dehydrogenase deficiency in homozygous A-G985 transition. *J Pediatr* 1992; 121:965–8.

136. Wilken B, Leung K-C, Hammond J, Kamath R, Leonard J. Pregnancy and fetal long chain 3-hydroxyacyl coenzyme A dehydrogenase deficiency. *Lancet* 1993; 341:407–8.

137. Treem W, Rinaldo P, Hale D, et al. Acute fatty liver of pregnancy and long chain 3-hydroxyacyl coenzyme A dehydrogenate deficiency. *Hepatology* 1994; 19:339–45.

138. Bioulac-Sage P, Parrot-Roulard F, Mazat P, et al. Fatal neonatal liver failure and mitochondrial cytopathy (oxidative phosphorylation deficiency): light and electron microscopy study of the liver. *Hepatology* 1993; 18:839–46.

139. Van Ekeren GS, Tadhouders A, Smeitink J, Sengers R. A retrospective study of patients with the hereditary syndrome of congenital cataracts, mitochondrial myopathy of heart and skeletal muscle and lactic acidosis. *Eur J Pediatr* 1993; 152:255–8.

140. Fayon M, Lamireau T, Biolac-Sage P, et al. Fatal neonatal liver failure and mitochondrial cytopathy: an observation with antenatal ascites. *Gastroenterology* 1992; 103:1332–5.

141. Mazziotta M, Ricci E, Bertini E, et al. Fatal infantile liver failure associated with mitochondrial DNA depletion. *J Pediatr* 1992; 121:896–901.

142. Cormier V, Rustin P, Bonnefont J-P, et al. Hepatic failure in disorders of oxidative phosphorylation with neonatal onset. *J Pediatr* 1991; 119:951–4.

143. Bennett MJ, Powell S. Metabolic disease and sudden death. *Hum Pathol* 1994; 25:742–6.

144. Boles RG, Martin SK, Blitzer MG, Rinaldo P. Biochemical diagnosis of fatty acid oxidation disorders by metabolite analysis of postmortem liver. *Hum Pathol* 1994; 25:735–41.

145. Nakata F, Oyanagi K, Fujiwara M. Dubin-Johnson syndrome in a neonate. *Eur J Pediatr* 1979; 132:299–301.

146. Nezelof C, Dupart MC, Jaubert F, Eliachar E. A lethal familial syndrome associating arthrogryposis multiplex congenita, renal dysfunction and cholestatic and pigmentary liver disease. *J Pediatr* 1979; 94:258–60.

147. Freeze DK, Hanson RF. Neonatal cholestatic syndromes associated with alterations and bile acid synthesis. *J Pediatr Gastroenterol Nutr* 1983; 2:374–80.

148. Daugherty C, Setchell K, Heubi J, Balistreri W. Resolution of liver biopsy alterations in three siblings with bile acid treatment of an inborn error of bile acid metabolism (delta-4-3-oxosteroid 5 beta-reductase deficiency). *Hepatology* 1993; 18:1096–1101.

149. Horslem S, Lawson A, Malone M, Clayton P. 3 beta-hydroxy-delta 5-C27-steroid dehydrogenase deficiency: effects of chenodeoxycholic acid therapy on liver histology. *J Inherit Metab Dis* 1992; 15:38–46.

150. Suchy F. Bile acids for babies? Diagnosis and treatment of metabolic liver disease. *Hepatology* 1993; 18:1274–7.

151. Aagenaes O, Van der Hagen CB, Refsum S. Hereditary recurrent intrahepatic cholestasis from birth. *Arch Dis Child* 1968; 43:646.

152. Sharp H, Krivit W. Hereditary lymphedema and obstructive jaundice. *J Pediatr* 1971; 78:491–6.

153. Finegold MJ. Cholestatic syndromes in infancy. In: Rosenberg HS, Bolande RP, eds. *Perspectives in Pediatric Pathology*. vol. 3. Chicago: Year Book Medical, 1976, pp. 41–84.

154. Linarelli LG, Williams CN, Phillips MJ. Byler's disease: fatal intrahepatic cholestasis. *J Pediatr* 1972; 81:484–92.

155. Weber AM, Tuchweber B, Yousef I, et al. Severe familial cholestasis in North American Indian children: a clinical model of microfilament dysfunction? *Gastroenterology* 1981; 81:653–62.

156. Irani D, Kim H-S, El-Hibri H, et al. Postmortem observations on beta glucuronidase deficiency presenting as hydrops fetalis. *Ann Neurol* 1983; 14:486–90.

157. Hardwick DF, Dimmick JE. Metabolic cirrhoses of infancy and early childhood. In: Rosenberg HS, Bolande RP, eds. *Perspectives in Pediatric Pathology*. vol. 3. Chicago: Year Book Medical, 1976, pp. 103–44.

158. Gillan JE, Lowden JA, Gaskin K, Cutz E. Congenital ascites as a presenting sign of lysosomal storage disease. *J Pediatr* 1984; 104:225–31.

159. Hancock LW, Thaler MM, Horwitz AL, Dawson G. Generalized N-acetylneuraminic acid storage disease: quantitation and identification of a monosaccharide accumulating in brain and other tissues. *J Neurochem* 1982; 38:803–9.

160. Gilbert EF, Dawson G, Zu Rhein GM, Opitz JM, Spranger JW. I-cell disease, mucolipidosis II. *Z Kinderheilkd* 1973; 114:259–92.

161. Wong LT, Davidson AGF, Applegarth DA, et al. Biochemical and histologic pathology in an infant with CRM(−) pyruvate carboxylase deficiency. *Pediatr Res* 1986; 20:274–9.

162. Odievre M, Gentil C, Gautier M, Alagille D. Hereditary fructose intolerance in childhood. *Am J Dis Child* 1978; 132:605–8.

163. Dubois R, Loeb H, Malaisse-Lagae F, Toppet M. Etude clinique et anatomopathologicque de deux cas d'intolerance congenitale au fructose. *Pediatrie* 1965; 20:5–14.

164. Yu DT, Burch HB, Phillips MJ. Pathogenesis of fructose hepatotoxicity. *Lab Invest* 1974; 30:85–91.

165. Dennehi PH, O'Shea PA, Abuelo DN. A newborn infant with bilious vomiting and jitteriness. *J Pediatr* 1985; 106:161–6.

166. Weinberg AG, Mize CE, Worthen HG. The occurrence of hepatoma in a chronic form of hereditary tyrosinemia. *J Pediatr* 1976; 88:434–8.

167. Russo P, O'Regan S. Visceral pathology of hereditary tyrosinemia, type 1. *Am J Hum Genet* 1990; 47:317–24.

168. Zerbini C, Weinberg DS, Hollister KA, Perez-Atayde AR. DNA ploidy abnormalities in the liver of children with hereditary tyrosinemia type 1. Correlation with histopathologic features. *Am J Pathol* 1992; 140:1111–9.

169. Laberg C, Lescault A, Tanguay RM. Hereditary tyrosinemia (type 1): a new vista on tyrosine toxicity and cancer. *Adv Exp Biol Med* 1986; 206:209–21.

170. Lindstedt S, Holme E, Lock EA, Hjalmarson O, Strandvik B. Treatment of hereditary tyrosinemia type 1 by inhibition of 4-hydroxyphenol pyruvate dioxygenase. *Lancet* 1992; 340:872–3.

171. McAdams AJ, Hug G, Bove KE. Glycogen storage disease types I to X. *Hum Pathol* 1974; 5:463–87.

172. Jevon GP, Finegold MJ. Reliability of histological criteria in glycogen storage disease of the liver. *Pediatr Pathol* 1994; 14:709–21.

173. Hufton BR, Wharton BA. Glycogen storage disease (type I) presenting in the neonatal period. *Arch Dis Child* 1982; 57:309–19.

174. Burchell A, Waddell ID, Stewart L, Hume R. Perinatal diagnosis of type 1c glycogen storage disease. *J Inherit Metab Dis* 1989; 12(suppl 2):315–7.

175. Buchino JJ, Brown BI, Volk DM. Glycogen storage disease type Ib. *Arch Pathol Lab Med* 1983; 107:283–5.

176. Reifen RM, Nadjari M, Hurvitz H, Barash V, Gutman A. Hepatomegaly *in utero* in type III glycogenosis. *Acta Paediatr Scand* 1989; 78:954–5.

177. van Noort G, Straks W, Van Diggelen OP, Hennekam RCM. A congenital variant of glycogenosis type IV. *Pediatr Pathol* 1993; 13:685–98.

178. Ivemark BI, Svennerholm L, Thoren C, Tunell R. Niemann Pick disease in infancy. *Acta Paediatr* 1963; 52:291–404.

179. Buchino JJ. Niemann-Pick type C. *Pediatr Pathol* 1993; 13:841–5.

180. Kelly DA, Portmann B, Mowat AP, Sherlock S, Lake BD. Niemann-Pick disease type C: diagnosis and outcome in children with particular reference to liver disease. *J Pediatr* 1993; 123:242–7.

181. Miller R, Bialer MG, Rogers JF, et al. Wolman disease. *Arch Pathol Lab Med* 1982; 106:41–5.

182. Oppenheimer EH, Esterly JR. Pathology of cystic fibrosis. In: Rosenberg HS, Bolande RP, eds. *Perspectives in Pediatric Pathology*. vol. 2. Chicago: Year Book Medical, 1975, pp. 241–78.

183. Vitullo BB, Seemayer TA, Beardmore H, deBelle RC. Intrapancreatic compression of the common bile duct in cystic fibrosis. *J Pediatr* 1978; 93:1060–1.

184. Rosenstein BJ, Oppenheimer EH. Prolonged obstructive jaundice and giant cell hepatitis in an infant with cystic fibrosis. *J Pediatr* 1977; 91:1022–3.

185. Knisely AS. Neonatal hemochromatosis. *Adv Pediatr* 1992; 39:383–403.

186. Witzleben CL, Uri A. Perinatal hemochromatosis: entity or end result? *Hum Pathol* 1989; 20:335–40.

187. Hoogstraten J, deSa D, Knisely AS. Fetal liver disease may precede extrahepatic siderosis in neonatal hemochromatosis. *Gastroenterology* 1990; 98:1699–701.

188. Silver MM, Valberg L, Cutz E, Lines L, Phillips MJ. Hepatic morphology and iron quantitation in perinatal hemochromatosis. *Am J Pathol* 1993; 143:1312–25.

189. Ruchelli ED, Uri A, Dimmick JE, et al. Severe perinatal liver disease and Down syndrome: an apparent relationship. *Hum Pathol* 1991; 22:1274–80.

190. Becroft DMO. Fetal megakaryocytic dyshemopoiesis in Down syndrome: association with hepatic and pancreatic fibrosis. *Pediatr Pathol* 1993; 13:811–20.

191. Dimmick JE, Pantzar T, Taylor GP, Norman M. Complete trisomy 22: pathologic analysis of three neonates. *Lab Invest* 1985; 52:4p.

192. Dimmick JE, Applegarth DA. Pathology of peroxisomal disorders. *Perspect Pediatr Pathol* 1993; 17:45–98.

193. Roels F, Espeel M, Poggi F, et al. Human liver pathology in peroxisomal diseases: a review including novel data. *Biochemie* 1993; 75:281–92.

194. Sveger T. Alpha 1 antitrypsin deficiency in early childhood. *Pediatrics* 1978; 62:22–5.

195. Sveger T, Thelin T. Four year old children with alpha 1 antitrypsin deficiency. Clinical followup and parental attitudes towards neonatal screening. *Acta Paediatr Scand* 1981; 70:1–7.

196. Sveger T. Prospective study of children with alpha 1 antitrypsin deficiency: eighty-year old followup. *J Pediatr* 1984; 104:91–3.

197. Roberts PF. Pi ZZ alpha 1 antitrypsin deficiency in a 20 week fetus. *Hum Pathol* 1985; 16:188–90.

198. Wilkinson EJ, Raab K, Browning CA, Hosty TA. Familial hepatic cirrhosis in infants associated with alpha 1 antitrypsin SZ phenotype. *J Pediatr* 1974; 85:159–64.

199. Cutz E, Cox DW. Alpha 1 antitrypsin deficiency: the spectrum of pathology and pathophysiology. In: Rosenberg HS, Bolande RP, eds. *Perspectives in Pediatric Pathology*. vol. 5. New York: Masson, 1979, pp. 1–39.

200. Dycaico JM, Grant SGN, Felts K, et al. Neonatal hepatitis induced by alpha-1-antitrypsin: a transgenic mouse model. *Science* 1988; 242:1409–12.

201. Sharp HL. Alpha 1 antitrypsin: an ignored protein in understanding liver disease. *Semin Liver Dis* 1982; 2:314–28.

202. Nebbia G, Hadchouel M, Odievre M, Allagille D. Early assessment of evolution of liver disease associated with alpha-1-antitrypsin deficiency in childhood. *J Pediatr* 1983; 102:661–5.

203. Thaler MM. Fatal neonatal cirrhosis: entity or end result. *Pediatrics* 1964; 33:721–34.

204. Coen R, McAdams AJ. Visceral manifestation of shock in congenital heart disease. *Am J Dis Child* 1970; 119:383–9.

205. Weinberg AG, Bolande RP. The liver and congenital heart disease. *Am J Dis Child* 1970; 119:390–4.

206. Larroche J-C. Umbilical catheterization: its complications, anatomical study. *Biol Neonat* 1970; 16:101.

207. Ruebner BH, Bhagavan BS, Greenfield AJ, Campbell P, Danks DM. Neonatal hepatic necrosis. *Pediatrics* 1969; 43:963–70.

208. French CE, Waldstein G. Subcapsular hemorrhage of the liver in the newborn. *Pediatrics* 1982; 69:204–8.

209. Bernard O, Alveras F, Brunelle F, Hadchouel P, Alagille D. Portal hypertension in children. *Clin Gastroenterol* 1985; 14:333–55.

210. Ghishan FK, Greene HL, Halter S, Barnard JA, Moran JR. Non-cirrhotic portal hypertension in congenital cytomegalovirus infection. *Hepatology* 1984; 4:684–6.

211. Jaffe R, Yunis EJ. Congenital Budd-Chiari syndrome. *Pediatr Pathol* 1983; 1:187–92.

212. Nuernberger SP, Ramos CV. Peliosis hepatis in an infant. *J Pediatr* 1975; 87:424–6.

213. Finegold MJ. Tumors of the liver. *Semin Liver Dis* 1994; 14:270–81.

214. Magee JF, McFadden DE, Pantzar JT. Congenital tumors. In: Dimmick JE, Kalousek DK, eds. *Developmental Pathology of the Embryo and Fetus.* Philadelphia: Lippincott, 1992, pp. 235–70.

215. Dimmick JE, Rogers PCJ, Blair G. Hepatic tumors. In: Pochedly C, ed. *Neoplastic Diseases of Childhood.* Chur, Switzerland: Harwood Academic, 1994, pp. 973–1010.

216. Wells HG. Occurrence and significance of congenital malignant neoplasms. *Arch Pathol* 1940; 30:535–601.

217. Dehner LP. Hepatic tumors in the pediatric age group. In: Rosenberg HS, Bolande RP, eds. *Perspectives in Pediatric Pathology.* vol. 4. Chicago: Year Book Medical, 1978, pp. 217–68.

218. Dehner LP. Neoplasms of the fetus and neonate. In: Naeye RL, Kissane JM, Kaufman N, eds. *Perinatal Diseases.* Baltimore: Williams & Wilkins, 1981, pp. 286–345.

219. Weinberg AG, Feingold MJ. Primary hepatic tumors of childhood. *Hum Pathol* 1983; 14:512–37.

220. Van de Bor M, Verwey RA, van Pel R. Acute polyhydramnios associated with fetal hepatoblastoma. *Eur J Obstet Gynecol Reprod Biol* 1985; 20:65–9.

221. de Chadarevian J-P, Faerber EN, Weintraub H. Undifferentiated (embryonal) sarcoma arising in conjunction with mesenchymal hamartoma of the liver. *Mod Pathol* 1994; 7:490–3.

222. Mascarello JT, Krous HF. Second report of a translocation involving 19q 13.4 in a mesenchymal hamartoma of the liver. *Cancer Genet Cytogen* 1992; 58:141–2.

223. Otal TM, Hendricks JB, Pharis P, Donnelly WH. Mesenchymal hamartoma of the liver. DNA flow cytometric analysis of eight cases. *Cancer* 1994; 74:1237–42.

224. Stocker JT, Ishak KG. Mesenchymal hamartoma of the liver: report of 30 cases and review of the literature. *Pediatr Pathol* 1983; 1:245–67.

225. Dehner LP, Ishak KG. Vascular tumors of the liver in infants and children. *Arch Pathol* 1971; 92:101–11.

226. Selby D, Stocker JT, Waclawiw M, Hitchcock C, Ishak K. Infantile hemangioendothelioma of the liver. *Hepatology* 1994; 20:39–45.

227. Kazzi NJ, Chang C-H, Roberts EC, Shankaran S. Fetal hepatoblastoma presenting as non-immune hydrops. *Am J Perinatol* 1989; 6:278–80.

228. Robinson HB, Bolande RP. Case 3: fetal hepatoblastoma with placental metastases. *Pediatr Pathol* 1985; 4:163–7.

229. Hughes LJ, Michels VV. Risk of hepatoblastoma in familial adenomatous polyposis. *Am J Med Genet* 1992; 43:1023–5.

230. Mamlock V, Nichols M, Lockart L, Mamlock R. Trisomy 18 and hepatoblastoma. *Am J Med Genet* 1989; 33:125–6.

231. Tanaka T, Takakura S, Kodama T, Hasegawa H. A rare case of Aicardi syndrome with severe brain malformation and hepatoblastoma. *Brain Dev* 1985; 7:507–12.

232. Buckley JD, Sather H, Raccione K, et al. A case control study of risk factors for hepatoblastoma. *Cancer* 1989; 64:1169–73.

233. Chang C-H, Ramirez N, Sakr WA. Primitive neuroectodermal tumor of the brain associated with malignant rhabdoid tumor of the liver. *Pediatr Pathol* 1989; 9:307–19.

234. Gonzales-Crussi F, Upton MP, Maurer HS. Hepatoblastoma: attempt at characterization of histologic subtypes. *Am J Surg Pathol* 1982; 6:599–612.

235. Kasai M, Watanabe I. Histologic classification of liver cell carcinoma in infancy and childhood and its clinical evaluation. A study of 70 cases collected in Japan. *Cancer* 1970; 25:551–63.

236. Haas JE, Muczynski KA, Krailo M, et al. Histopathology and prognosis in childhood hepatoblastoma and hepatocarcinoma. *Cancer* 1989; 64:1082–95.

237. Lack EE, Neave C, Vawter GF. Hepatoblastoma: a clinical and pathological study of 54 cases. *Am J Surg Pathol* 1982; 6:693–705.

238. Conran RM, Hitchcock CL, Stocker JT, Ishak KG. Hepatoblastoma: the prognostic significance of histologic type. *Pediatr Pathol* 1992; 12:167–83.

239. Douglass EC, Reynolds M, Finegold M, Cantor A, Glicksman A. Cisplatin, vincristine and fluorouracil therapy for hepatoblastoma: a pediatric oncology group study. *J Clin Oncol* 1993; 11:96–9.

240. Finegold MJ. Liver tumors. In: Walker-Smith JA, Watkins JB, eds. *Pediatric Gastrointestinal Disease.* Philadelphia: BC Decker, 1991, pp. 914–26.

241. Chen D-S. From hepatitis to hepatoma: lessons from type B viral hepatitis. *Science* 1993; 262:369–70.

242. Stocker JT, Ishak KG. Focal nodular hyperplasia of the liver: a study of 21 pediatric cases. *Cancer* 1981; 48:336–45.

243. Witte DP, Kissane JM, Askin FB. Hepatic teratomas in children. *Pediatr Pathol* 1983; 1:81–92.

244. Lack EE, Schloo BL, Azumi N, et al. Undifferentiated (embryonal) sarcoma of the liver: clinical and pathologic study of 16 cases with emphasis on immunohistochemical features. *Am J Surg Pathol* 1991; 15:1–16.

245. Craig JM. Sequences in the development of cirrhosis of the liver in cases of erythroblastosis fetalis. *Arch Pathol* 1950; 49:665.

246. Alpert LI, Strauss L, Hirschhorn K. Neonatal hepatitis and biliary atresia associated with trisomy 17–18 syndrome. *N Engl J Med* 1969; 280:14–19.

247. Kurnick J, Atkins L, Finegold M, Hills J, Devorak A. Trisomy 9: predominance of cardiovascular, liver, brain and skeletal anomalies in the first diagnosed case. *Hum Pathol* 1974; 5:223–32.

248. Kassner EG. *Iatrogenic Disorders of the Fetus, Infant and Child.* New York: Springer-Verlag, 1985, pp. 277–9.

249. Mullick FG, Moran CA, Ishak KG. Total parenteral nutrition: a histopathologic analysis of the liver changes in 20 children. *Mod Pathol* 1994; 7:190–4.

250. Patterson K, Kapur SP, Chandra RS. Hepatocellular carcinoma in a noncirrhotic infant after prolonged parenteral nutrition. *J Pediatr* 1985; 106:797–9.

251. Stolkind E. Congenital abnormalities of the gallbladder and extrahepatic ducts. Review of 245 reported cases with reports of 31 unpublished cases. *Br J Child Dis* 1939; 36:150, 182, 295.

252. Descos B, Bernard O, Brunelle F, et al. Pigment gallstones of the common bile duct in infancy. *Hepatology* 1984; 4:678–83.

253. Klingensmith WC, Cioffi-Ragan DT. Fetal gallstones. *Radiology* 1988; 167:143–4.

254. Watkins JB. Neonatal cholestasis: developmental aspects and current concepts. *Semin Liver Dis* 1993; 13:276–88.

FURTHER READING

Bakker HD, Scholte HR, Dingemans KP, et al. Depletion of mitochondrial deoxyribonucleic acid in a family with fatal neonatal liver disease. *J Pediatr* 1996; 128:683–7.

Bioulac-Sage P, Parrot-Roulaud F, Mazat JP, et al. Fatal neonatal liver failure and mitochondrial cytopathy (oxidative phosphorylation deficiency): a light and electron microscopic study of the liver. *Hepatology* 1993; 18:839–46.

Bull LN, Carlton VE, Stricker NL, et al. Genetic and morphological findings in progressive familial intrahepatic cholestasis (Byler disease [PFIC-1] and Byler syndrome); evidence for heterogeneity. *Hepatology* 1997; 26:155–64.

Capistrano-Estrada S, Marsden DL, Nyhan WL, et al. Histopathological findings in a male with late-onset ornithine transcarbamylase deficiency. *Pediatr Pathol* 1994; 14:235–43.

Favara BE. Histopathology of the liver in histiocytosis syndromes. *Pediatr Pathol Lab Med* 1996; 16:413–33.

Hale LP, van de Ven CJ, Wenger DA, et al. Infantile sialic acid storage disease: a rare cause of cytoplasmic vacuolation in pediatric patients. *Pediatr Pathol Lab Med* 1995; 15:443–53.

Klenn PJ, Rubin R. Hepatic fibrosis associated with hereditary cystinosis: a novel form of noncirrhotic portal hypertension. *Mod Pathol* 1994; 7:879–82.

Lamps LW, Gray GF, Scott MA. The histologic spectrum of hepatic cat scratch disease. A series of six cases with confirmed *Bartonella henselae* infection. *Am J Surg Pathol* 1996; 20:1253–9.

Lykavieris P, Bernard O, Hadchouel M. Neonatal cholestasis as the presenting feature in cystic fibrosis. *Arch Dis Child* 1996; 75:67–70.

Ludwig J, Moyer TP, Rakela J. The liver biopsy diagnosis of Wilson's disease. Methods in pathology. *Am J Clin Pathol* 1994; 102:443–6.

Maaswinkel-Mooij PD, Van den Bogert C, Scholte HR, et al. Depletion of mitochondrial DNA in the liver of a patient with lactic acidemia and hypoketotic hypoglycemia [see comments]. *J Pediatr* 1996; 128:679–83.

Pandit A, Bhave S. Present interpretation of the role of copper in Indian childhood cirrhosis. *Am J Clin Nutr* 1996; 63:830S–5S.

Pradhan AM, Bhave SA, Joshi VV, et al. Reversal of Indian childhood cirrhosis by D-penicillamine therapy. *J Pediatr Gastroenterol Nutr* 1995; 20:28–35.

Takahashi T, Akiyama K, Tomihara M, et al. Heterogeneity of liver disorder in type B Niemann-Pick disease. *Hum Pathol* 1997; 28:385–8.

Tanner MS, Taylor CJ. Liver disease in cystic fibrosis. *Arch Dis Child* 1995; 72:281–4.

Teckman JH, Qu D, Perlmutter DH. Molecular pathogenesis of liver disease in alpha₁-antitrypsin deficiency. *Hepatology* 1996; 24:1504–16.

Chapter

The Pancreas

RONALD JAFFE

ORGANOGENESIS AND EXOCRINE HISTOGENESIS

The ventral foregut, early in the 5th week of gestation, gives rise to two pancreatic buds, which arise laterally to the junction of the hepatic duct and the gut (see McLean [1] for a review). The ventral lobe in the human is said to be bilobed, its left lobe regressing early. Only the right portion of the ventral bud persists, and its duct system joins that of the hepatic duct (Fig. 26.1). A larger dorsal pancreatic bud arises more rostrally and grows rapidly into the dorsal mesentery. The hepatic duct and the ventral bud take part in the clockwise rotation of the gut tube as the stomach forms, and they migrate dorsally to occupy the space immediately caudal to the larger dorsal pancreas. The duodenum at this time, having rotated to the right, comes into contact with the retroperitoneum and loses its mesentery, thus becoming, in part, retroperitoneal. Both dorsal and ventral pancreatic primordia now occupy the concavity of the duodenum.

The duct of the dorsal pancreas opens more proximally in the duodenum. The duct of the small ventral pancreas, together with the common bile duct, opens more distally in the duodenum. At about 7 weeks of gestation, the two primordia fuse, their duct systems anastomose, and, in general, the duct of the ventral pancreas becomes the main pancreatic duct of Wirsung. The duct of the dorsal portion often remains patent, as the minor duct of Santorini. In 5–10% of cases, ductal fusion may be incomplete or absent, with resulting separate drainage of dorsal and ventral derivatives—the so-called pancreas divisum [2].

In this manner, then, the lower part of the pancreatic head and the uncinate process derive from the primordial ventral pancreas, whereas the rest of the head, the body, and the tail derive from the original dorsal bud.

The pancreatic elements, both exocrine and endocrine, develop from a ramifying tubular epithelial system that grows into the mesenchymal pancreatic stroma. Buds of cuboidal cells at the ends of the branching epithelial tube form the first recognizable acinar units by the 10th week of gestation, and by this time endocrine elements are also present. Lobular configuration is evident by 12 to 14 weeks. It must be remembered that pancreatic acinar development, like pulmonary alveolar development, is largely a postnatal event. The appearance of the pancreas from 10 weeks to term, as illustrated in Figure 26.2, represents progressive branching of the duct system, with only minimal acinar development, but there is extensive endocrine development. The amount of mesenchyme, always prominent in the fetus, becomes less so with progressive ductular budding. The ratio of acinar to connective tissue volume (a measure of acinar growth) increases in a linear manner from 0.5 at 32 weeks of intrauterine life to 2.0 at 52 weeks postconception [3]. Calculating from the controls of Imrie et al [3], the acinar to connective tissue ratio is 0.78 at 2 days, 0.99 at 6.8 days, and 1.57 at 55 days after birth, reflecting the rapid postnatal acquisition of acinar tissue. In assessment of the maturation of the pancreas, it is important that the length of postnatal survival be taken into account. In other words, the exocrine pancreas of an infant born at 30 weeks' gestation who survives for 5 weeks will be far better developed than that of a stillborn of 35 weeks' gestation.

Zymogen granules are evident by 12 weeks of age. These early granules are not round but are elongated, spindle shaped, or elliptical [4]. The complexity of lateral cell membrane interdigitations and the Golgi apparatus increases from 12 to 20 weeks, at which time the endoplasmic reticulum is prominent and zymogen granules appear to be larger, rounder, and more mature. By 20 weeks, the acinar cells

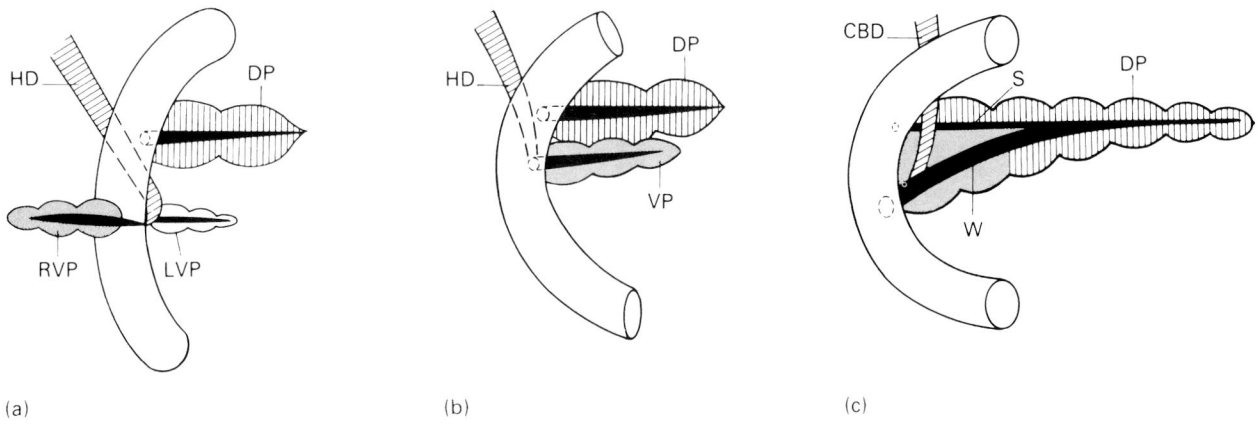

(a)   (b)   (c)

FIGURE 26.1. *(a) right and left ventral pancreatic buds (RVP, LVP) form in close association with the hepatic duct (HD). (b) As the LVP regresses, the duodenum rotates, carrying the RVP posteriorly to abut the dorsal pancreas (DP). (c) Dorsal and ventral primordia fuse; the duct of the RVP becomes dominant as the duct of Wirsung (W), entering the duodenum with the common bile duct (CBD). The remnant of the DP duct enters the duodenum more proximally (when present) as the duct of Santorini (S). VP = ventral pancreas. (Redrawn from Refs. 1, 45, 47, and 225.)*

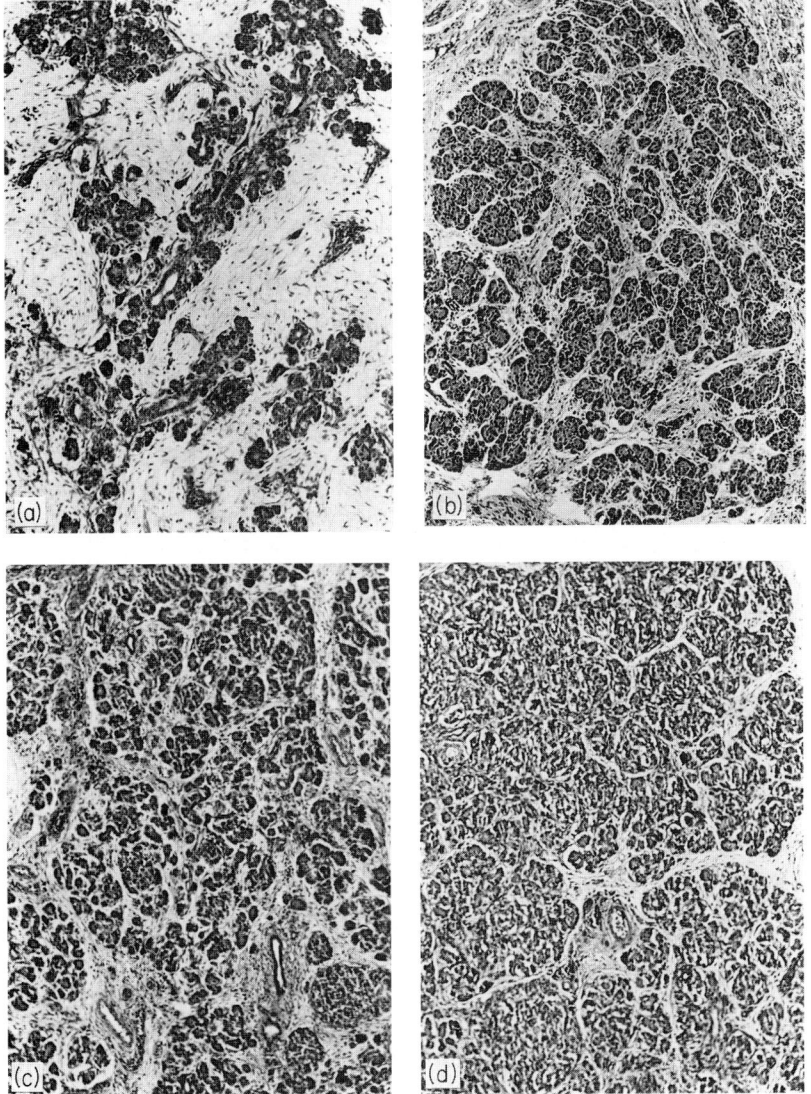

FIGURE 26.2. *Pancreatic development. (a) 10 weeks: a simple branching duct system has rudimentary buds in a bed of mesenchyme. (b) 20 weeks: progressive acinar and endocrine development forms clear lobules with diminution of the mesenchymal element. (c) 34 weeks, survived 14 hours: apart from some further loss of mesenchyme, the pancreas is not much changed. (d) 34 weeks, survived 21 days: the early postnatal burst of acinar development is reflected in the more mature appearance. H&E, ×115.*

have assumed their polarization with apically situated zymogen granules [5]. The developing ductal and exocrine cells are rich in glycogen, a feature distinguishing them in the first trimester from endocrine cells. Ductal, centroacinar, and acinar cells are clearly recognizable at 20 weeks, and glycogen disappears first from the larger ducts and then from progressively smaller ones.

Congenital Malformations

Agenesis and Hypoplasia

The term "primary agenesis of the pancreas" is applied only to those instances in which both exocrine and endocrine elements are totally lacking. This serves to distinguish agenesis from exocrine aplasia, in which the ducts and islets of Langerhans are preserved, or pure endocrine agenesis, both of which are discussed later. The void left by the absence of a pancreas in primary agenesis is occupied by fat that contains vessels and nerves, and the appearance by computed tomography (CT) can simulate a pancreatic lipomatosis [6]. It must be cautioned that the premature and newborn pancreas are normally hyperechoic relative to liver, and that this does not signify absence of the organ [7]. A patient is described who was homozygous for a point deletion of the human insulin promoter factor 1 (IPF1) gene, at 13q12.1 [7a]. The gene is known to be critical for pancreatic development in the mouse, and this autosomal recessive mutation has now been shown to be of importance in humans too. The clinical presentation of agenesis in the newborn is that of diabetes mellitus and malabsorption [8–11]. Absence of the gallbladder and paucity of intrahepatic bile ducts were observed in some of these cases, and total agenesis has been reported also in association with diaphragmatic hernia [12].

More commonly, the pancreas is misshapen without being truly hypoplastic and is described as short, stubby, or globular (Fig. 26.3a). Some are isolated instances and have been described as partial agenesis of the pancreas in which one of the primordia, dorsal or ventral, failed to develop [13–16]. Short pancreas is more commonly part of a wider malformation complex that encompasses defects of lateralization, congenital heart disease, multiple or lobulated

spleens, and intestinal malrotation [17, 18] (Fig. 26.3b). Extrahepatic biliary atresia is seen in association with this same spectrum of malformations, and we have observed an instance of extrahepatic biliary atresia, short pancreas, and polysplenia. Short pancreas has been noted in complete trisomy 22 syndrome [19].

Familial instances of congenital combined exocrine and endocrine hypoplasia with an autosomal recessive pattern present clinically with pancreatic hypofunction rather than with organ failure. The amylase and trypsin levels are reduced, and C peptide and glucagon levels are low but not absent. For this reason, hypoplasia may be diagnosed only later in life [20, 21]. A syndrome of hereditary pancreatic hypoplasia and congenital heart disease is described [21a].

Pancreatic Enlargement

The pancreas is occasionally described as being larger than usual. Pancreatic weights are given in Fig. 26.4 [22]. A large pancreas in the newborn may be encountered in the Beckwith-Wiedemann syndrome, in which case endocrine hyperplasia is often accompanied by acinar hypoplasia [23]. Congenital syphilis is characteristically associated with pancreatomegaly due to inflammation and an increase in interstitial fibrous tissue [24]. Congenital leukemia may have massive pancreatic infiltration, and erythroblastosis fetalis and nonimmune hydrops lead to pancreatic enlargement by extensive extramedullary hematopoiesis. Down syndrome with congenital megakaryoblastic leukemia and pancreatic fibrosis has been reported [25]. Massive fatty replacement of the exocrine portion of the pancreas has been termed "lipomatous pseudohypertrophy" [26], and is seen in the Shwachman and Johanson-Blizzard syndromes.

Some of the cystic disorders to be discussed are characterized by an enlarged pancreas, as are pancreatic tumors.

Abnormalities of Position

The pancreas is normally fixed in the retroperitoneal position. Abnormalities of fixation and position are often associated with left-sided diaphragmatic hernias, but a "floating" pancreas on a mesentery has been described in the absence of a diaphragmatic hernia [27]. Partial situs inversus, in

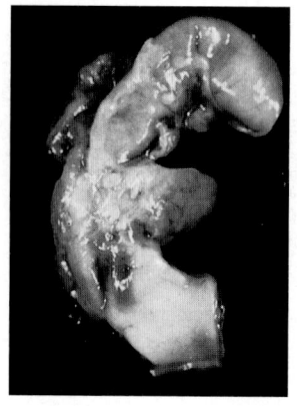
(a)

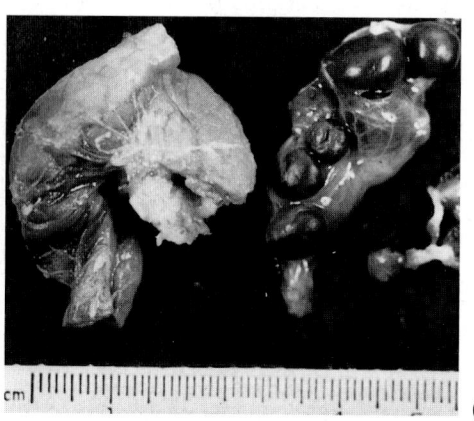
cm
(b)

FIGURE 26.3. *(a) A malformed, short pancreas that was associated with a bilobed spleen in a term newborn. (b) A short pancreas in an infant who had situs inversus and 16 small spleens. (From Drut RM, Drut R, Gilbert-Barness E, Reynolds JF Jr. Abnormal spleen lobulation and short pancreas. In: Blastogenesis: Normal and Abnormal. March of Dimes Birth Defects Foundation, 1993, pp. 345–52. Reprinted by permission.)*

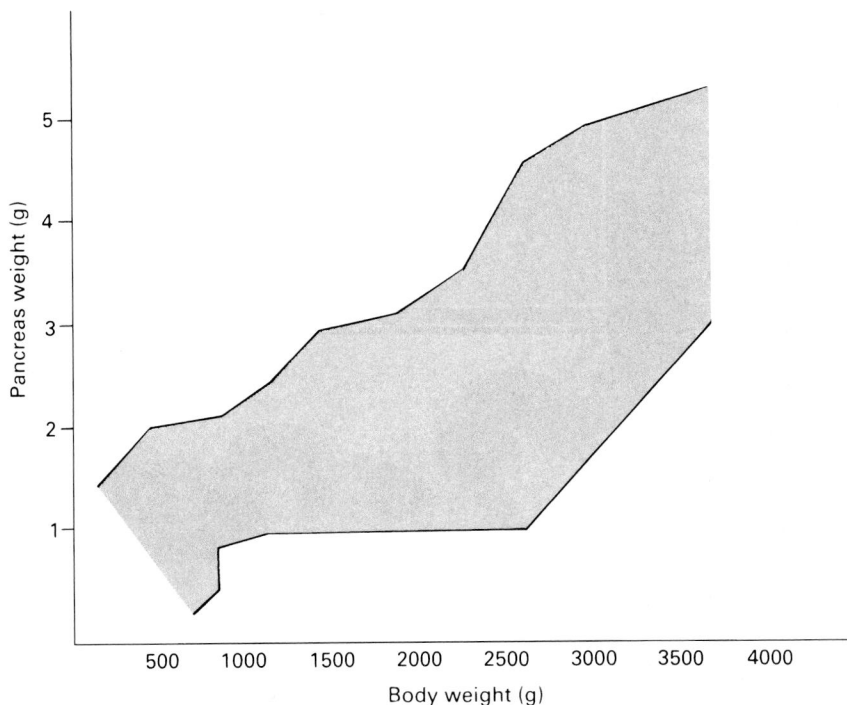

which the cardiac position is normal but the abdominal organs including the pancreas are inverted, has been associated with annular pancreas [28].

Annular Pancreas

In annular pancreas, a ring of pancreas encircles the duodenum, usually in its second part (Fig. 26.5). Presentation in the fetus with polyhydramnios, and in the neonate with bile-stained vomiting, depends on the degree of obstruction. In those rare instances in which the constriction is above the ampulla, the vomitus may not be bile stained and the clinical situation then mimics pyloric stenosis. The duodenal obstruction is an associated malformation, and the clinical picture is not due simply to mechanical constriction produced by the annular pancreas [29]. The annulus is sometimes extramural, in which case it can be peeled off the surface, and the ducts run around to join the main pancreatic duct. Alternatively, the annulus can be intramural, intimately bound within elements of the duodenal wall, and small ducts drain directly to the duodenum [30]. Twenty to thirty percent of infants with annular pancreas have trisomy 21 [31]. Conversely, about 8% of children with trisomy 21 may have annular pancreas or duodenal stenosis. Annular pancreas may also be associated with other intestinal malformations, such as tracheoesophageal fistula, duodenal atresia, intestinal malrotation, and Meckel's diverticulum [28, 32]. Twenty-one percent of the cases described by Merril and Raffensperger [31] had congenital heart disease. Annular pancreas has been observed in a single instance of Rothmund-Thomson syndrome [33], and has been identified in the fetus [34, 35].

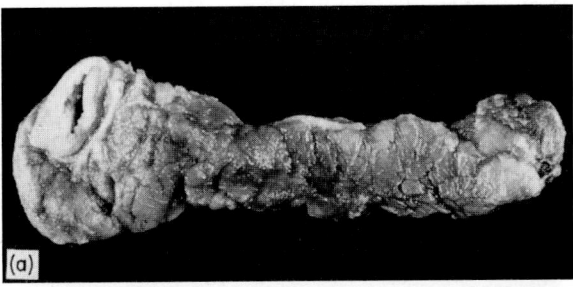

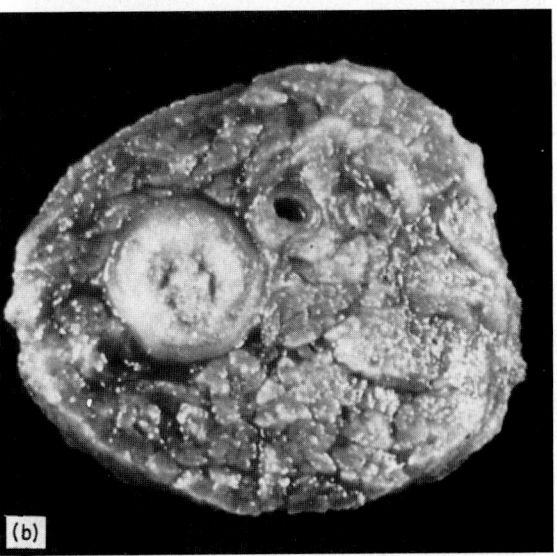

FIGURE 26.5. *Annular pancreas. (a) The pancreatic head envelops the duodenum. (b) Cross-section of the pancreas surrounding the duodenum.*

The occurrence of annular pancreas is ascribed to a failure of the ventral pancreatic bud to migrate posteriorly and to take up its position as the posterior part of the head of the pancreas. Alternatively, fixation of the tip of the ventral anlage to the duodenal wall prior to rotation would result in the anlage being stretched circumferentially [35]. A portion of the head of the pancreas, the PP lobe, is characterized by a large number of pancreatic polypeptide-containing islets of Langerhans [36]. The endocrine cell content of the annular pancreas resembles that of the normal pancreatic polypeptide-rich portion of the ventral head of the pancreas [37]. Although the malformation is usually sporadic, familial instances have been reported [38–41].

Variations in the Pancreatic Ducts

After fusion of the dorsal and central anlage, the dorsal duct becomes the accessory duct of Santorini and the ventral duct becomes the main draining duct of the pancreas, the duct of Wirsung. The accessory duct may be obliterated in 20% of the cases but occasionally functions as the main duct. Two separate and similarly sized ducts are seen in 10% of patients, the so-called pancreas divisum, and a number of other ductal variations occur in up to 30% of cases [42, 43].

Pancreas divisum is silent in the neonate, and there is considerable debate about its clinical relevance in producing pancreatitis later in life.

Stenosis of the ampulla may present with pancreatitis, but in the newborn it more commonly manifests as bile duct perforation without pancreatitis, possibly due to pancreatic juice reflux [44]. Wong and Lister demonstrated in fetuses that the normal choledochopancreatic junction migrates inward toward the duodenal lumen [45]. Arrested migration leads to an elongated common choledochopancreatic duct, with the junction lying outside the circular muscle. This may produce an abnormally long common channel so that the sphincter of Oddi cannot prevent reflux up the ducts. The elongated common channel syndrome has been implicated in instances of recurrent pancreatitis in older children and adults, and in cystic, inflammatory disorders of the extra-hepatic biliary tree in infants [46].

Ectopic Pancreas

Ectopic pancreatic tissue that has no connection to the pancreas is a common finding generally restricted to the gastrointestinal tract. It is estimated that heterotopic pancreas may be present in 2% of all postmortem examinations [47],

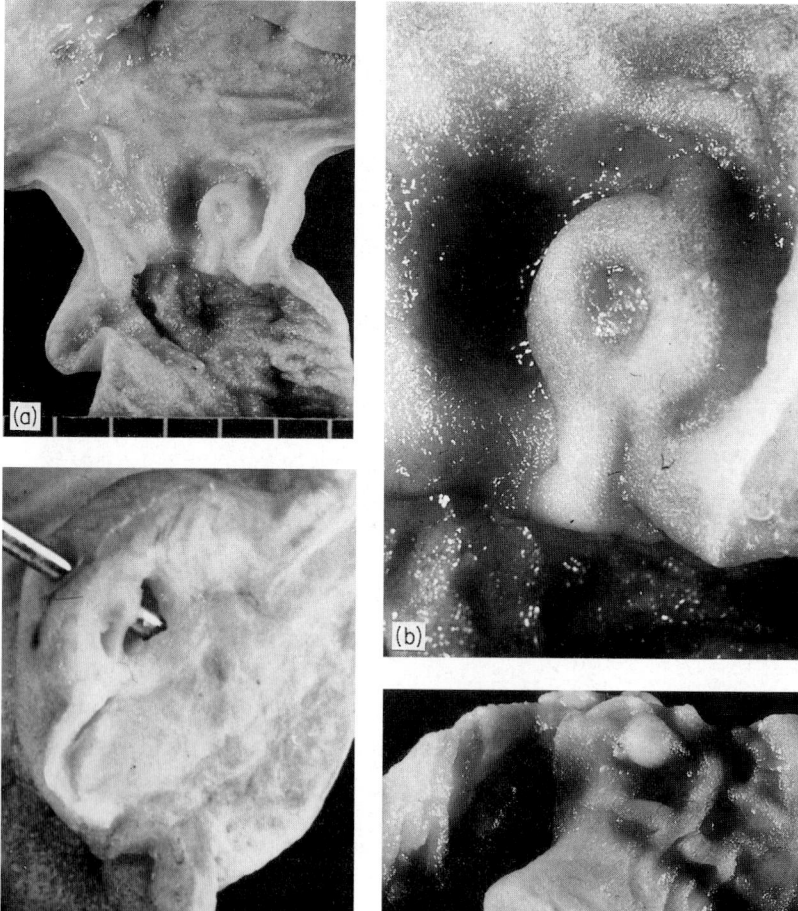

FIGURE 26.6.   *Ectopic pancreas. (a and b) Ectopic pancreas at the pylorus has a characteristic button-like shape with a central depression. (c) Pylorus. A probe is present in a duct remnant. The thick muscularis contains lobules of pancreatic tissue (see Fig. 26.7b). (d) Jejunum containing a submucosal nodule of ectopic pancreas.*

but the true incidence in neonates is probably higher if the condition is specifically sought [48]. Pancreatic tissue is most frequently found in the wall of the stomach, duodenum, and jejunum. In the stomach it is not unusual to find a nodule that has a central pit or ulceration projecting into the lumen, with an underlying localized thickening of the gastric wall (Fig. 26.6). The greater curvature of the antrum (65%), followed by the pyloric region (20%), are the most usual sites for ectopic pancreas according to Seifert [47], who describes three types of ectopic pancreatic tissue:

1. Ectopic tissue with acini, ducts, and islets of Langerhans (Fig. 26.7).
2. Ectopic tissue with incomplete lobular arrangement that contains only a few acini and multiple ducts. Endocrine elements are absent.
3. Ectopic tissue consisting of proliferating ducts only. Both exocrine acini and endocrine elements are lacking. These aggregates of ducts within the muscle are usually called adenomyomas, the ducts being nondescript.

To these three types of ectopic pancreas must be added another common appearance, residual ductal and islet tissue after scarring and involution of the acinar portion, recapit-ulating the process seen in the pancreas following duct obstruction. Immunostaining for pancreatic endocrine hormones in heterotopic lesions has demonstrated relatively normal distribution of all endocrine cell types [49].

Pancreatic tissue can be found in the hilus of the liver or within the liver substance [50] (Fig. 26.8). An unusual hepatopancreatic duplication obstructed the pylorus in the first week of life [51]. Ectopic pancreas has been found in the mesentery and in association with duplication cysts of the gut [52–54], Meckel's diverticulum and vitelline duct [55], fallopian tube [56], and even the umbilical cord [57]. Intrasplenic islands of pancreas are common in trisomies 13 and 15 but are also found rarely in the absence of a trisomy. Gastrointestinal aberrant pancreas is usually silent in neonates but may serve as a lead for an intussusception or become symptomatic later in life.

Pancreatic tissue, both acinar and endocrine, is found quite often in teratomas (Fig. 26.9). Mediastinal teratomas may have large amounts of pancreatic tissue [58], as opposed to gonadal teratomas in which pancreas is said to be infrequent or even absent [59, 60]. One partially removed mediastinal cyst had only pancreatic elements [55], and an insulin-secreting pancreas-rich mediastinal teratoma has been described [61]. Mediastinal pancreatic pseudocysts have

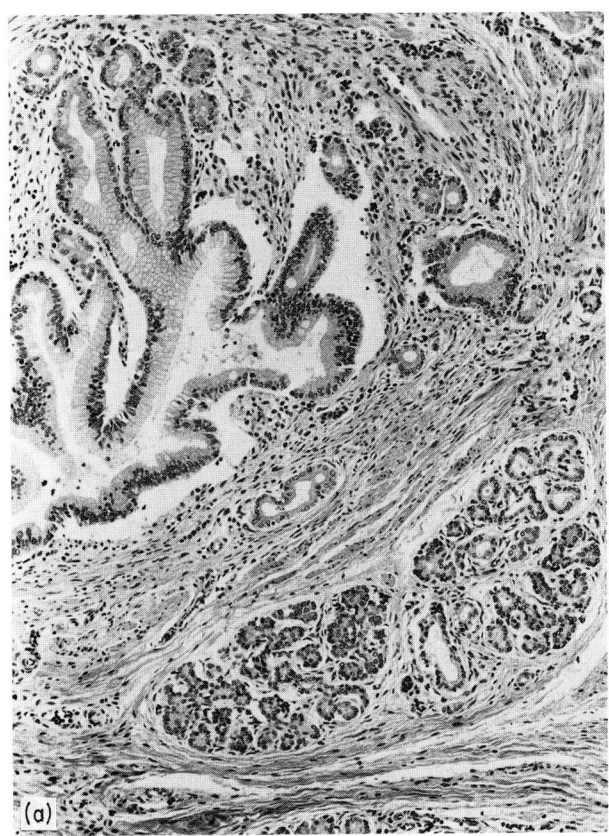

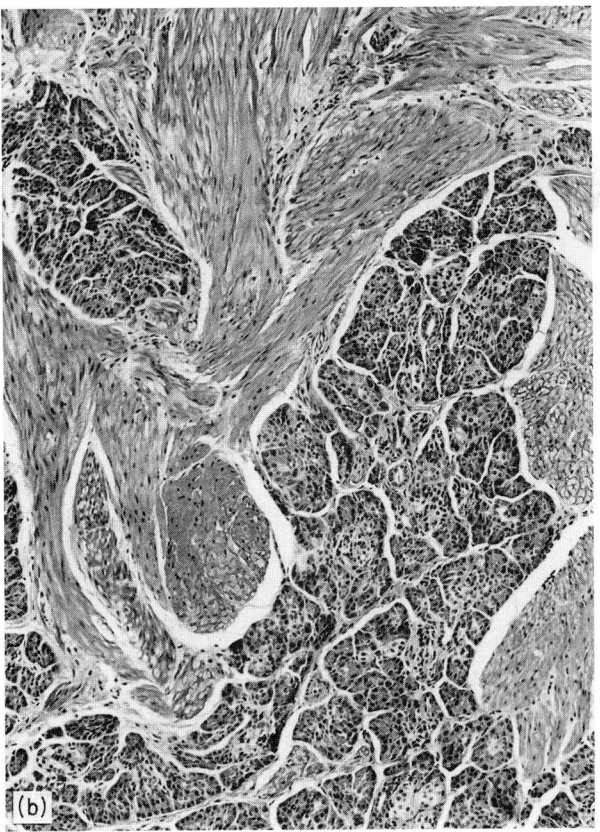

FIGURE 26.7. *(a) Ectopic pancreatic tissue is associated with a duct in this lesion from the pylorus. (b) Pancreatic lobules lie in the disorganized bundles of muscularis from the pylorus (see Fig. 26.6c). H&E, ×124.*

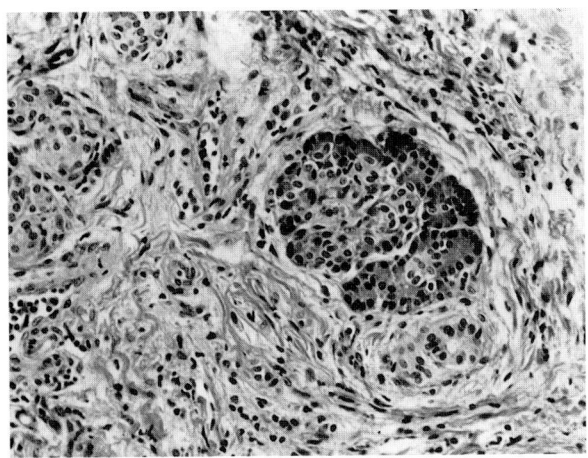

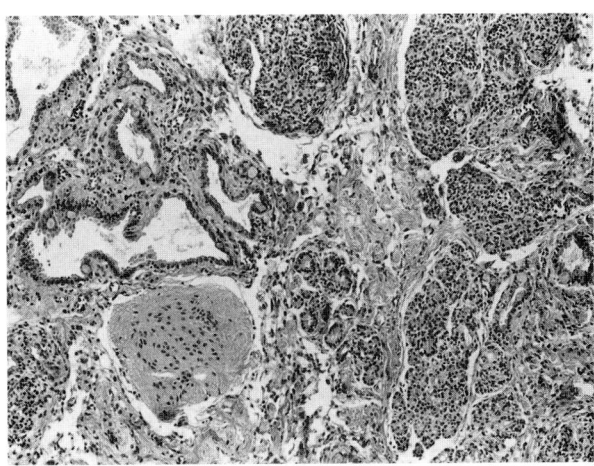

FIGURE 26.8.   *Ectopic pancreas, hilus of liver. It is not uncommon to find tiny islands of pancreas, including endocrine cells, in the hepatic hilus if it is sectioned extensively. In later life this is said to be a metaplastic change. H&E, ×155.*

FIGURE 26.9.   *Pancreatic tissue in a teratoma. Lobules of pancreatic tissue, acini with ducts, and endocrine elements lie near a glial island in a mediastinal teratoma. H&E, ×66.*

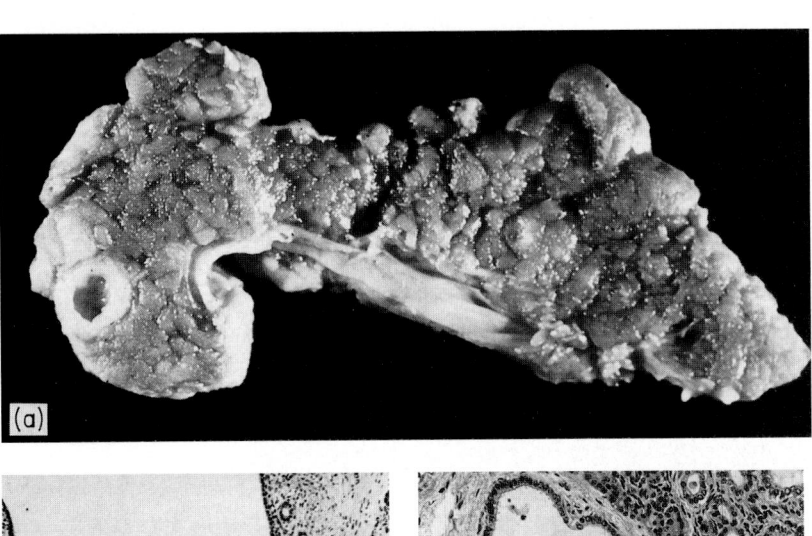

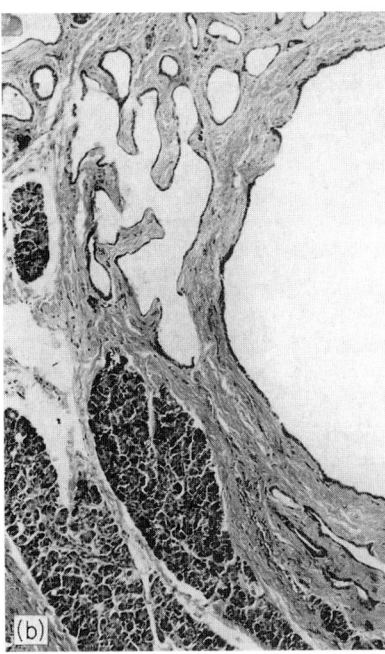

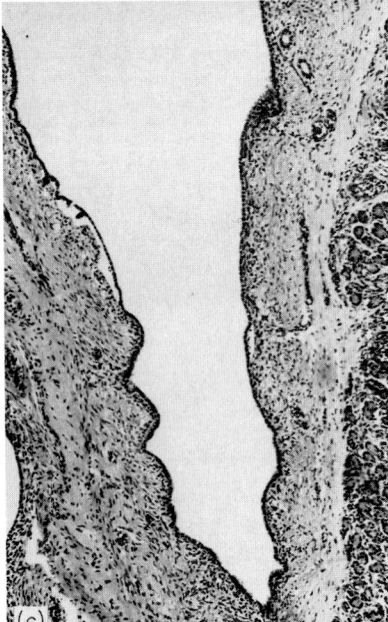

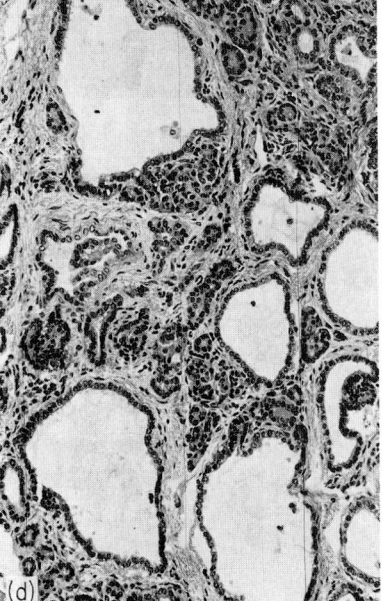

FIGURE 26.10.   *Pancreatic cysts. (a) A circumscribed cystic lesion in the head of the pancreas from a child with trisomy 13. (b) Ramifying interconnected cystic spaces in the pancreas of a child with infantile-type cystic disease of the kidney and liver. H&E, ×70. (c) Large cystic spaces lined by a simple cuboidal epithelium in the pancreatic cyst of a child with Meckel-Gruber syndrome. H&E, ×70. (d) Cystic lesion of the head of the pancreas of a child with trisomy 13 (cystadenoma). H&E, ×97.*

been reported [62], most of which arose below the diaphragm, but isolated thoracic forms do exist, and intrapulmonary (enteric) cysts have been shown to contain pancreatic tissue [63, 64]. Most of the lesions described above did not present clinically in the newborn period but are included here as probable congenital lesions.

Quantitative immunohistochemical studies on mediastinal and sacrococcygeal teratomas [60, 65, 66] have been interpreted as showing functional immaturity of the endocrine tissue, with a prominence of somatostatin-containing cells. Endocrine islets in teratomas may show an intrinsic organization and cell type distribution identical to that seen in the developing normal pancreas [60].

Peripancreatic intestinal and gastric duplications may have communications with the pancreatic duct. The duplications are usually lined by acid-producing gastric mucosa and have muscular walls. They do not usually become symptomatic until later in life, when they can be mistaken for pancreatic pseudocysts [54, 67, 68].

Congenital Pancreatic Cysts and Cystic Pancreatic Dysplasia

Simple epithelial-lined or multilocular cysts of the fetal and neonatal pancreas are not commonly reported [69–74], but the advent of sonography will undoubtedly reveal more unsuspected congenital cysts including antenatal detection [73, 74a]. Pancreatic pseudocysts are only rarely described in the newborn. Two cases that were detected prenatally had pseudocysts with scar and inflammation, but no epithelial lining. No cause was suggested for either [74b]. Pancreatic involvement in both adult and infantile-type polycystic

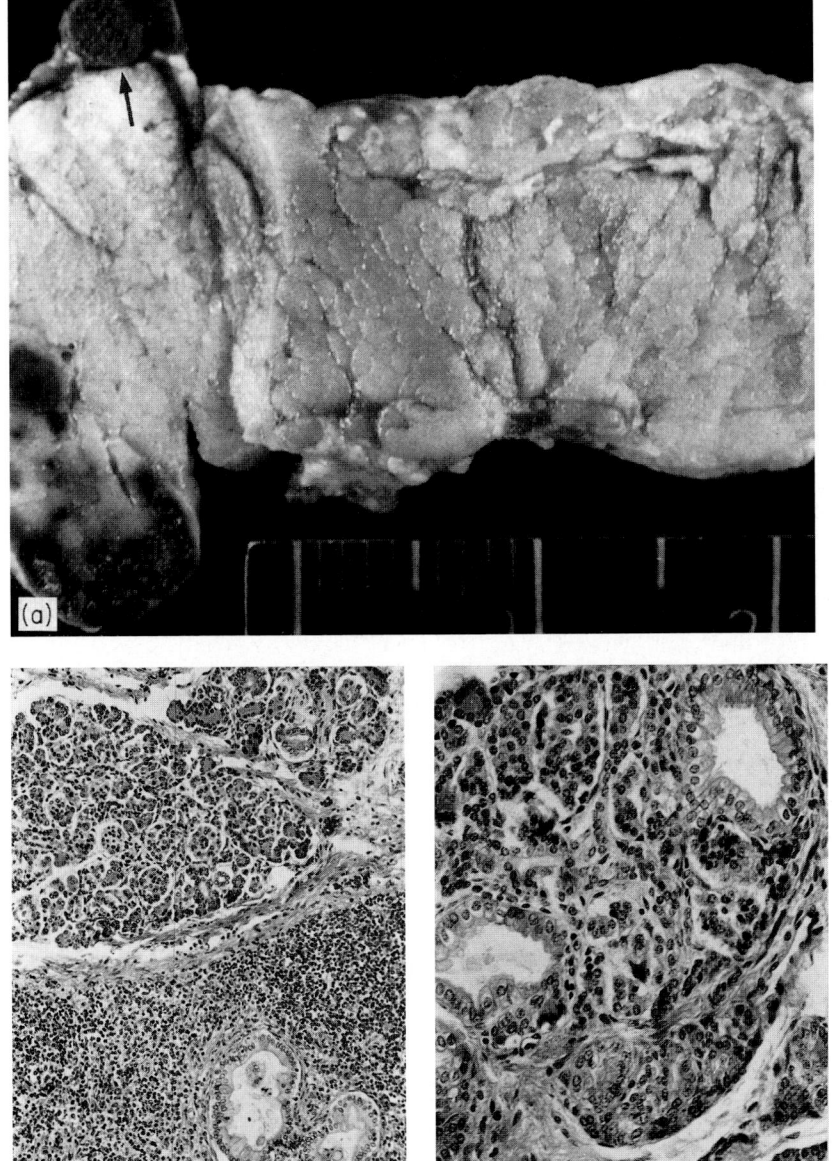

FIGURE 26.11. *Trisomy 13. (a) Accessory spleen (arrow) as well as diffuse splenosis of the pancreatic tail. (b) Poorly circumscribed splenic stroma extends into the pancreas, and epithelium-lined spaces with goblet cells are found in the splenic tissue. H&E, ×98. (c) Tall columnar cells line ducts within the pancreatic lobules. H&E, ×160.*

disease of the kidney is encountered [69], but is rare, occurring in only 2 of 370 cases encountered by Potter and Craig [75] (Fig. 26.10). In a study of 18 cases of Meckel-Gruber syndrome, the pancreases of 11 were normal, and the other seven had only duct dilatation and periductal fibrosis. The pancreas was grossly normal in all 18 [76]. Cysts are occasionally encountered in the Meckel-Gruber syndrome [69] (see Fig. 26.10).

Ivemark et al, in 1959, described a familial form of renal, hepatic, and pancreatic cystic dysplasia (the other Ivemark syndrome) [77], and other such cases (single or familial) have been reported but generally without cytogenetic information [78–80]. The pancreas has fibrosis, dilated ducts, and cysts, and an inflammatory component may be present. Rare cases with situs inversus, a feature of the other Ivemark syndrome, have been reported [81]. Earlier publications reporting pancreatic cysts in association with widespread malformations are more suggestive of trisomies 13 or 15 [82, 83]. Cystic lesions, particularly microcysts and cystadenomas, are distinctive features of trisomy 13 [84] (see Fig. 26.10). Cystadenomas of the pancreas have been reported [85], some in association with cytomegalovirus (CMV) infection [86, 87], and we have also seen one such instance in a newborn. It is probable that the viral infection is the cause of an acquired "cystadenomatous" change. Seifert [47] describes two instances of polycystic involvement of the pancreas in association with renal cysts, generalized chondrodysplasia, and thoracic dystrophy. Although these are called Jeune's syndrome, they are difficult to distinguish from cases of the short-rib polydactyly syndrome type I, in which pancreatic cysts have also been described [88, 89]. Bernstein et al [90] emphasize that renal-hepatic-pancreatic dysplasia is not a single entity, but may represent any one of the conditions already mentioned, as well as Elejalde syndrome and glutaric aciduria.

Pancreatic Pathology in Trisomies

Lesions of the pancreas in trisomy 13 appear to be quite distinctive [84] and were well illustrated long before the chromosomal defect was identified [69]. Multiple, poorly demarcated aggregates of splenic tissue are present and contain pancreatic acini, islets, and knots of ducts lined by tall columnar epithelium rich in goblet cells (Fig. 26.11). Focal microcystic change is also a feature, often unassociated with inspissation [91] (see Fig. 26.10). Ectopic splenic tissue in the gastric fundus, and in the upper pole of the kidney, contained pancreatic elements in two cases of trisomy 13 [92].

The pancreas in trisomy 18 reveals lobular fibrosis and focal fibrous nodules in which clusters of ducts and atrophic acini are found [93]. Microcystadenomas and inflammatory aggregates suggest obstructive changes [84]. Annular pancreas may be present in up to 8% of infants with trisomy 21 [31]. A short pancreas has been observed in trisomy 22 [20], and pancreatic anomalies including atresia have

been reported in some fetuses or infants with triploidy [94].

THE EXOCRINE PANCREAS

Functional Development of the Exocrine Pancreas

The exact time and sequence in which the enzymes of pancreatic exocrine secretion appear in the human fetal pancreas are not known [95]. By approximately 16 weeks, lipase is detectable in pancreatic homogenate and amylase is demonstrable by immunohistochemistry in the pancreas [96]. Amylase becomes detectable in the amniotic fluid at about the same time. Trypsin, chymotrypsin, lipase, and phospholipase have been shown to increase slowly from 20 to 32 weeks in pancreatic homogenates, with a more rapid rise thereafter until birth [97]. Lee and Lebenthal [95] describe minimal or absent amylase at birth despite its presence in the amniotic fluid, a low lipase, and a moderate trypsinogen content of the pancreas. Duodenal levels of amylase and lipase remain low for the first year, while trypsin and chymotrypsin reach adult levels [98]. This relative neonatal deficiency in pancreatic amylase may be compensated for by the high levels of mammary amylase in milk [99].

Pancreatic secretion is influenced largely by neural (cholinergic) stimulus, cholecystokinin-pancreozymin, and secretin. In adults, pancreozymin is responsible for pancreatic enzyme release, while secretin promotes fluid and electrolyte release. Gastrin and cholecystokinin have been demonstrated in human small bowel by 10 weeks of age [100]. The neonatal pancreas is unresponsive to pancreozymin and fully responsive only by the age of 2 years [98]. Neonatal response to secretin is also incomplete. Premature and full-term newborn infants may respond to pancreozymin and secretin but fail to differentiate between the stimuli, producing the same response to each until 1 week of age [101].

Controversy has existed over the mechanism of secretion of enzymes from pancreatic exocrine cells. The "parallel process" propounded by Palade [102] described the synthesis, intracellular segregation, apical storage, and eventual exocytic release of a number of pancreatic enzymes. Rothman [103, 104] pointed out that enzyme-specific secretion did occur and suggested an "equilibrium hypothesis" in which individual enzymes are released from the acinar cell in a regulated fashion. Scheele [105] has described specific hormone-receptor interactions that lead to selective regulation of pancreatic gene expression through different second messenger pathways in the pancreatic acinar cell. The centroacinar cells are also said to have some control over exocrine secretion, proliferation, and differentiation [106].

There is accumulating evidence (in rabbits) for both processes, the pancreas being a heterogeneous organ secreting digestive enzymes from different sources within the gland [107]. There may also be functional (and possibly morphologic) differences between peri-insular and teleinsular cells, and an islet-acinar portal vascular system is said to allow insulin to act as a regulator of exocrine function [108]. Basal secretion refers to the ongoing amount of pancreatic secretion, possibly under neural control. Basal unstimulated pancreatic enzyme secretion is present at birth, rising within the first month [101, 109]. The content of individual enzymes varies in the basal secretion [98], amylase being absent even at age 1 month and lipase being low.

Abnormalities of the Exocrine Pancreas

Isolated Enzyme Deficiencies

Isolated enzyme deficiencies are comprehensively detailed by Lerner and Lebenthal [110]. Isolated trypsinogen deficiency, leading to malabsorption, growth failure, anemia, and hypoproteinemia, has been described [111]. The association with imperforate anus [112] is reminiscent of the same association in cases of Shwachman syndrome (see below). Congenital enterokinase deficiency mimics cystic fibrosis, with diarrhea, vomiting, hypoproteinemia, and failure to thrive [113]. Isolated lipase deficiency presents with severe steatorrhea soon after birth without failure to thrive, presumably due to the presence of effective nonpancreatic lipases [114]. Isolated amylase deficiency is not diagnosed in newborn infants because of the normal physiologic absence of this enzyme [115]. No pancreatic pathology has been reported in patients with isolated enzyme deficiency, although the pancreases of the siblings of children with trypsinogen deficiency have been described as having immature acini without zymogen granules [111].

Exocrine Atrophy without Fibrosis

Exocrine atrophy, which is synonymous with lipomatous atrophy [47] or lipomatous pancreatic pseudohypertrophy [26], refers to a pathologic finding that may be common to a number of disease processes.

Shwachman-Diamond Syndrome

Shwachman-Diamond syndrome is the second most common cause of pancreatic insufficiency in early life after cystic fibrosis. Although this syndrome was defined by Shwachman et al [116], prior cases had been described [26, 117–119], and these earlier cases were reviewed in detail by Bodian et al [120]. Shwachman-Diamond syndrome is inherited as an autosomal recessive disorder. Pancreatic exocrine insufficiency is accompanied by growth retardation, bone marrow dysfunction with neutropenia, and skeletal changes, predominantly metaphyseal dysostosis. The sweat test is normal. Cases have been associated with anal atresia [117, 121], Hirschsprung disease [122], and asphyxiating thoracic dystrophy [123]. The marrow dysfunction progresses in some instances to aplastic anemia or leukemia,

usually nonlymphatic [119, 124–127]. Cases have been reported in which the clinical onset of pancreatic insufficiency occurred soon after birth [120]. Abnormally low levels of trypsin in some infants suggest that the pancreatic acinar insufficiency begins early [128]. Mack et al [128a] have followed a cohort of patients and have documented that the exocrine deficiency is invariable but that the other clinical manifestations vary widely in occurrence and severity.

Bodian et al [120] reviewed those cases in which histologic evidence of pancreatic disease was obtained and biopsies were performed. Older children have been studied at postmortem examination. In general, there is agreement that the bulk of the pancreas is replaced by fatty tissue, which may give the appearance of lipomatous pseudohypertrophy [26]. Acinar tissue is absent, and there is preservation of pancreatic ducts as well as endocrine elements [26] (Fig. 26.12). The exception is a biopsy description of one of the cases described by Shwachman et al [116], in which acinar cells were not only preserved but described as being large and devoid of secretory granules. The nuclei were also large and irregular, with prominent nuclear membranes, pale nucleoplasm, and striking intranuclear "structures." A biopsy performed early in life by Burke et al [122] showed only inspissation but an otherwise intact pancreas. The question as to whether the pancreatic morphology in Shwachman syndrome represents primary hypoplasia or secondary degeneration is discussed by Nezelof and Watchi [119] and by Aggett et al [127], who suggest that a primary microtubular or microfilament dysfunction was responsible.

Johanson-Blizzard Syndrome

The autosomal recessive syndrome of congenital aplasia of the alae nasi, deafness, hypothyroidism, dwarfism, absent permanent teeth, and malabsorption described by Johanson and Blizzard [129] is associated with pancreatic insufficiency presenting within the first few weeks of life [110, 130–132]. One case had XXY Kleinfelter syndrome [133]. A postmortem report on a 15-month-old child revealed complete replacement of the pancreas with adipose tissue and a few remaining islets with connective tissue around the ducts [134]. Overlap between the Shwachman and Johanson-Blizzard syndromes has been noted as the spectrum of abnormalities found in affected families has increased [127].

A patient described by Szilagyi et al [135] had features in common with the Shwachman-Diamond syndrome, the Johanson-Blizzard syndrome, and leprechaunism; both hypopituitarism and growth hormone deficiency have been observed in the Johanson-Blizzard syndrome [136].

Exocrine Atrophy with Fibrosis

Exocrine atrophy with fibrosis is a common consequence of ductal obstruction and chronic pancreatitis. Pancreatic ductal ligation is the prototype for this process.

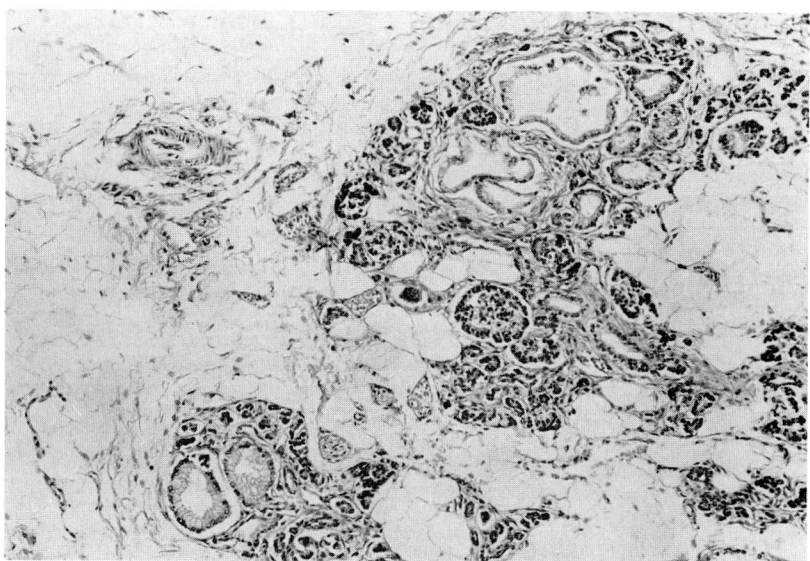

FIGURE 26.12. *Shwachman-Diamond syndrome, age 10 months. Dilated ducts are surrounded by wispy fibrosis and endocrine elements, almost all acinar tissue having been replaced by fat. H&E, ×120.*

Cystic Fibrosis

Fanconi et al [137] and Andersen [138], in investigating causes of malabsorption, delineated a group of patients with what they called "cystic fibrosis" of the pancreas; recognition of the pancreatic lesion thus preceded full clinical definition of the disease. Farber [139] invoked plugging of mucus-secreting glands (mucoviscidosis) as the common pathogenetic mechanism. The more general term "cystic fibrosis" now refers to an autosomal recessively inherited disease affecting serous as well as mucous glands. The historical background has been well covered by Taussig [140].

Cystic fibrosis has been shown to be a defect in the cystic fibrosis transmembrane conductance regulator (CFTR) gene responsible for chloride transport, and the gene has been localized to the long arm of chromosome 7q31, cloned and sequenced [141–143]. The ΔF508 single mutation has been found in 70–75% of instances, but more than 100 different mutations account for the rest, making genetic diagnosis difficult. Kerem et al [144] claimed that pancreatic involvement occurred earlier in ΔF508 homozygotes, and with a 99% incidence as opposed to 72% pancreatic involvement in heterozygotes and 36% in other genotypes. This segregation has not held up well, and pancreas sparing is seen with various alleles, including ΔF508.

Not all patients with clinically diagnosed cystic fibrosis develop pancreatic insufficiency, although 85% are said eventually to do so [145], and 93% of children with cystic fibrosis at postmortem examination have morphologic evidence of disease demonstrable by histology [146] or by morphometric methods [147]. In general, there is wide variation in the severity of the disease at any age, although the disease is progressive and causes increasingly severe changes with time [146].

About half the infants with cystic fibrosis diagnosed by neonatal screening for immunoreactive trypsin have adequate pancreatic function, and 28% of these have reduced function within the next 2 years [148].

It has also been said that 25–30% of infants below the age of 6 weeks with other evidence of cystic fibrosis have little or no pancreatic disease at postmortem examination. This has been challenged on morphometric grounds, where it can be shown that, even before 40 weeks of gestation, the pancreas that is affected in cystic fibrosis can be distinguished from those of normal controls [5, 147, 149]. The ratio of acinar to connective tissue volume is 0.5 at 32 weeks postconception, increasing in a linear fashion to 2.0 at 52 weeks in normal controls [3]. In the cystic fibrosis pancreas, the ratio of acinar to connective tissue, low to begin with, *decreases* from 0.5 at 35 weeks to 0.3 at 52 weeks postconception. Thus, the lack of exocrine tissue is demonstrable before birth, and further degeneration supervenes postnatally. In one study, the volume of the lobular ducts in the least affected pancreases increased 250% by 5 months of age in cystic fibrosis, and that of the main duct increased 1700% over normal controls, emphasizing the early and primary role of duct obstruction in the pathogenesis of the disease [149].

CFTR mRNA has been mapped in the human fetus, and the highest levels have been found in the pancreas, liver, gallbladder, and intestine, with lower levels in the lung and trachea. The expression correlates well with the tissue targets of the disease [150, 151].

The earliest visible lesions are similar in second-trimester fetuses and in newborns, and there are focal eosinophilic concretions in acini and ductules, which may lead to acinar or ductular dilatation and flattening of the lining epithelium [150, 152] (Fig. 26.13). The concretions are generally PAS-positive and contain calcium. The change may be very focal in preterm infants and in the mildest cases. The pathogenetic train of inspissation, obstruction, dilatation, epithelial

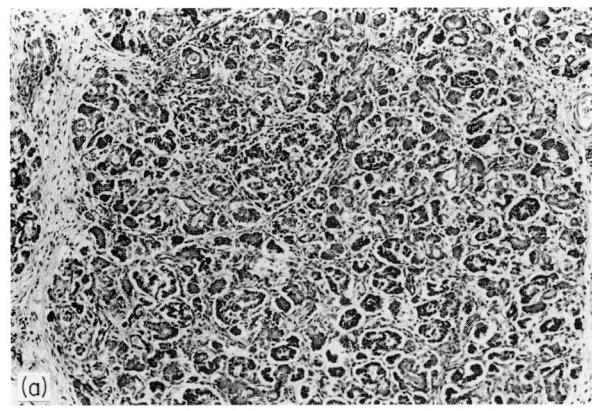

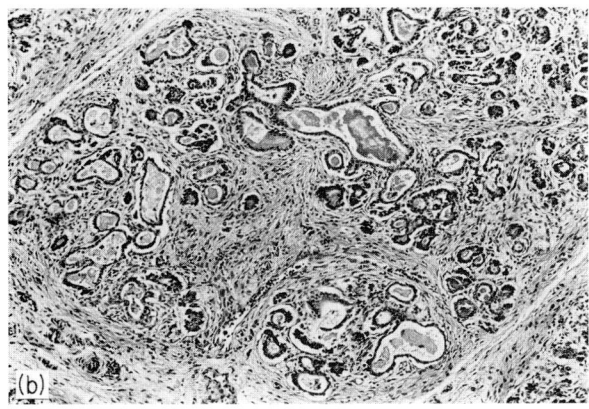

FIGURE 26.13. *Cystic fibrosis. A wide range of pathologic severity is displayed; the pancreas may be normal at birth. (a) A child aged 3 months shows mild interstitial fibrosis with inconspicuous duct dilatation and inspissation. H&E, ×80. (b) At 2.5 months, the pancreas has extensive fibrosis, cystic ductal and ductular change, and acinar atrophy. H&E, ×80.*

damage, atrophy, cell destruction, and fibrosis with minimal inflammation is accelerated postnatally, and this leads to progressive acinar loss with fibrosis. The range of pathology present within 6 weeks of birth varies widely. The lipomatous replacement so characteristic of late lesions of the pancreas in older children with cystic fibrosis is not seen in early life [69]. Generalized luminal dilatation, duct ectasia, inspissation and acinar disorganization, and interlobular and intralobular fibrosis, together with other ultrastructural changes, have been observed in fetuses with cystic fibrosis [147, 153], and it has been suggested that the secretions precipitate because of the presence of pancreatic stone-thread proteins [154], a major constituent of the exocrine secretion possibly encoded by the reg (regenerating) gene [155].

Perinatal Hemochromatosis

There appears to be a clinically homogeneous group of infants who have perinatal onset of severe liver disease for which no etiologic agent or metabolic cause has been found [156]. Vast amounts of iron have been documented in the exocrine glands of the pancreas, in the heart, in the liver, and in endocrine cells. Islet cells are involved, but only very mildly relative to the acinar cells [157–160]. Exocrine accumulation of iron is not, however, diagnostic of hemochromatosis but is common to all forms of liver injury in the perinatal period, and no etiologic role for the iron has been found. Functional pancreatic impairment has not been noted [156, 159, 161].

Pearson Syndrome

Pearson et al [162] described a syndrome of refractory sideroblastic anemia with variable neutropenia, thrombocytopenia, and pancreatic insufficiency. Presentation in the neonatal period has been reported. A high lactate pyruvate molar ratio in plasma led Rötig et al [163] to postulate a mitochondrial disorder as the cause, and indeed, a number of different mitochondrial DNA deletions have subsequently been reported [163–165]. Morikawa et al [165] described a neonate with Pearson syndrome and diabetes mellitus, and pointed out that diabetes mellitus is sometimes seen in the Kearns-Sayre syndrome, a mitochondrial myopathy. Patients who survive Pearson syndrome may later develop a clinical picture of the Kearns-Sayre syndrome [164, 166].

The pancreas in Pearson syndrome, unlike that in the Shwachman syndrome, has acinar atrophy *with* fibrosis [162], and in Morikawa's diabetic infant [165] who died at 26 months, fibrosis and acinar atrophy were associated with depletion of B cells in the islets.

We have noted striking oncocytic changes of the ducts and centroacinar cells in a child with mitochondrial myopathy, lactic acidosis, and ragged red muscle fibers.

Other Associations with Exocrine Hypoplasia

A child with neonatal onset of pancreatic insufficiency had clinical features of cutis laxa. The pancreatic pathology is unknown and the association may be fortuitous [167]. A tyrosinemia-like syndrome with hepato-pancreato-renal features and neuropathy was said to have islet cell hyperplasia and exocrine hypoplasia [168].

Inspissation of Pancreatic Secretions

Baggenstoss [169] reported inspissation of secretions in centroacinar-lined ductules, and this observation is not restricted to uremia but may be seen in children with acidosis, dehydration, cardiac failure, and sepsis [47]. Inspissation may be observed in infants undergoing hyperalimentation, but they generally have many of the above-mentioned conditions as well, particularly endotoxemia.

Pancreatitis

Hereditary Pancreatitis

Hereditary pancreatitis may be a diverse group of disorders. Familial pancreatitis with autoimmune phenomena, including intractable enteritis and nephritis, was described in two newborn cousins [170] (Fig. 26.14). A review of large

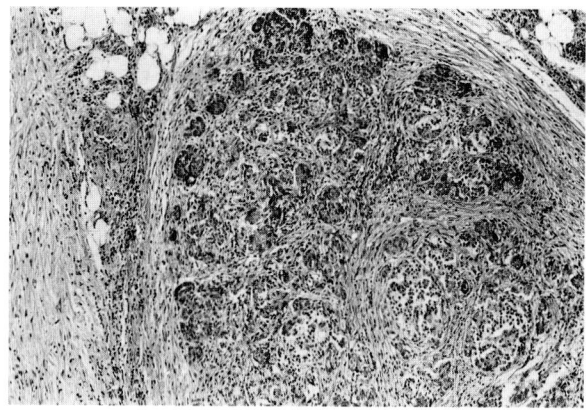

FIGURE 26.14.   *Familial pancreatitis. A whorling fibrosing reaction envelops entire lobules. Squamous metaplasia (not shown) was a prominent feature of the duct. H&E, ×58.*

numbers of patients from a number of kindreds has shown that infants of families with hereditary pancreatitis may occasionally be affected [171]. The pancreases from these children show extensive fibrosis, acinar atrophy, and prominent ductular dilatation with calcification. The molecular basis of hereditary pancreatitis has been delineated, the locus being on chromosome 7q35, which also contains other pancreatic-specific products including trypsinogen and carboxypeptidase genes [172]. The mutation lies in the cationic trypsinogen and is thought to alter the normal feedback of trypsin activation leading to pancreatic autodigestion [172a]. Some of the patients who presented in the past with a clinical picture of hereditary pancreatitis may have had an undiagnosed metabolic disease. Reference has already been made to the pancreatic disorder of Pearson marrow/pancreas syndrome. Kahler et al [173] demonstrated that acute or chronic pancreatitis may be symptomatic in children who have branched-chain organic acidemias, methylmalonic acidemia, isovaleric acidemia, and maple syrup urine disease. Onset varied from prenatal to 6 years of age.

Congenital and Neonatal Infections

The pancreas may be the incidental site of involvement in most disseminated viral (herpes, CMV) or bacterial diseases, but only rarely is bona fide pancreatitis encountered [174]. The association between neonatal CMV and cystadenoma has been mentioned [86, 87].

Rubella

Interstitial pancreatitis has been noted in cases of congenital rubella syndrome [175], and exocrine pancreatic insufficiency with some recovery has been reported soon after birth [176]. The onset of diabetes has been documented before 2 years of age [177].

Mumps

A potent cause of pancreatitis later in life, mumps can rarely cause pancreatitis in neonates [178].

Coxsackievirus

Pancreatic involvement is usually noted at postmortem examination but not clinically. There may be exocrine [179, 180] and selective endocrine involvement in neonates [174, 181, 182]. A 2-day-old infant with chronic interstitial pancreatitis but without meningo-encephalo-myocarditis has been reported [183].

Parainfluenza 3

Parainfluenza 3 pancreas involvement with multinucleated giant cells has been described in a child with severe combined immunodeficiency [184], and later confirmed by immunostaining [185].

Syphilis

Congenital syphilis usually involves the pancreas. Gummas are rare [186], but pancreatitis with ductular obliteration, acinar loss, and exuberant interstitial fibrosis with concentric perivascular accentuation are the usual findings [24] (Fig. 26.15).

E. coli

Pancreatitis, whether clinically evident or noted only at postmortem examination, may accompany *E. coli* septicemia [187, 188] (Fig. 26.16).

Drug-Related and Toxic Pancreatitis

A large number of drugs can cause pancreatic damage, although none has been implicated in neonatal disease or in causing congenital malformations involving the pancreas in humans.

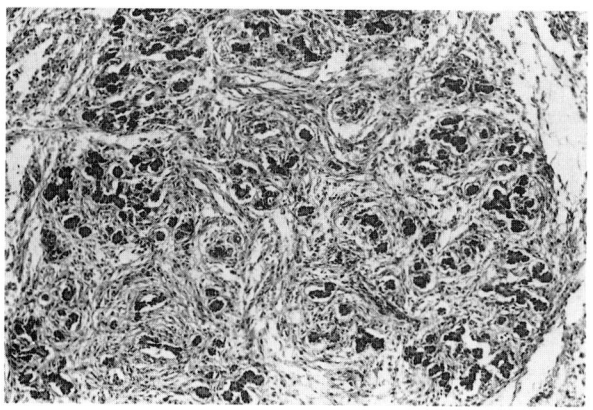

FIGURE 26.15.   *Congenital syphilis. An extensive interstitial fibrosis surrounds atrophic acini. H&E, ×80.*

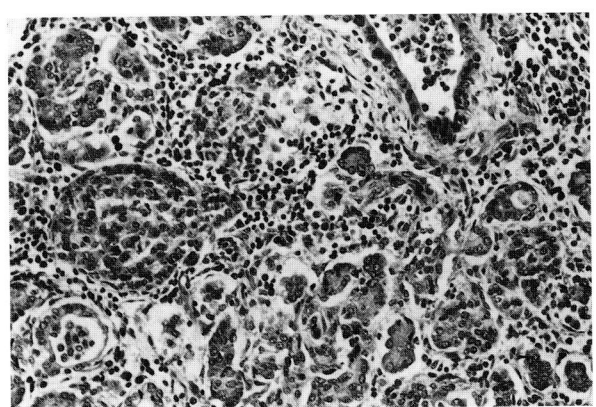

FIGURE 26.16. *Acute pancreatitis. A neutrophilic infiltrate fills the ducts while neutrophils, mononuclear cells, and hematopoiesis were noted in the interstitium. E. coli sepsis. H&E, ×140.*

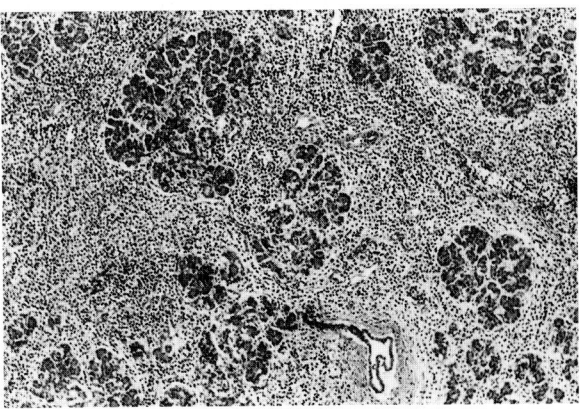

FIGURE 26.17. *Congenital leukemia. Lobules of pancreatic tissue are widely separated by a massive infiltrate. Most other organs were similarly affected in this instance of acute granulocytic leukemia. H&E, ×58.*

Boric Acid Toxicity

Boric acid, used for the treatment of eczema and diaper rash, is absorbed through the skin and may cause symptomatic disease in newborns within a week of use. The pancreas shows intracytoplasmic, rounded, homogeneous, eosinophilic inclusions in acinar cells [189].

Interstitial Infiltrates

Lymphoid

Focal lymphoid infiltrates, often quite large and on occasion surrounding interlobular ducts, are common in the developing pancreas [69, 75, 190]. Characterization of these lymphoid accumulations reveals T cells with high endothelial venules and interdigitating dendritic cells [191]. Their significance is not known, although Liu and Potter [192] suggested that they were involved in the degeneration of primary islets. These lymphoid aggregates are not seen outside the neonatal period. Follicular aggregates are described in congenital diabetes with autoimmune manifestations [193, 194]. Acute graft-versus-host disease can occur in the neonatal period following transfusions in immune-deficient children [185].

Hematopoietic Infiltrates

Erythropoiesis may be noted in the interstitium of the pancreas in hemolytic disease of the newborn [69, 195]. Hematopoiesis is also a component of inflammatory infiltrates in the fetus and newborn and accompanies most intrauterine inflammatory processes involving the pancreas.

Leukemia

The pancreas appears to be a site of predilection for congenital leukemia, mostly nonlymphoid leukemia that may cause considerable enlargement of the organ [195] (Fig. 26.17).

Accessory Spleen

Accessory spleen is not uncommonly found within the tail of the pancreas, and is generally well encapsulated [196]. Intrapancreatic accessory spleens should be distinguished from the poorly encapsulated intrapancreatic aggregates of splenic tissue (splenosis) that, together with pancreatic exocrine dysplasia, characterize trisomy 13 [84].

Congenital Tumors

Cysts and duplications have already been mentioned. Burt et al [197] reported a hamartoma of the head of the pancreas, with ductal and connective tissue elements. A hamartomatous 9-cm mass contained exocrine elements, fibrous tissue, fat, and cysts. Endocrine cells were scattered, but islets were not demonstrable [198]. A pancreatic mass weighing 120 grams was a presenting feature in a premature newborn with the Beckwith-Wiedemann syndrome; the histology was described as a "cystic dysplasia" in which ductular and endocrine elements predominated and acini were scanty [199]. A hemangioendothelioma of the pancreas, which obstructed the bile duct and duodenum, presented at 3 months of age and underwent some regression [200], and a newborn with a pancreatic hemangioendothelioma who had the Kasabach-Merritt syndrome has been documented [201]. The kaposiform hemangioendothelioma of infancy is often retroperitoneal and may involve the pancreas [202]. Benign teratomas—specifically, dermoid cysts—have been reported [203], but the youngest presented at 2 years of age with a cyst bearing skin, hair, and teeth [204]. There have been reports of "lymphosarcomas" of the pancreas in newborn infants [205, 206], but these are old reports and it is not clear that the lesions were truly lymphoid in nature. The pancreatoblastomas are similar to other embryomas in having both epithelial and mesenchymal elements, and may

---

include heterologous tissue—particularly squamous elements [207]. Most have occurred in males. The occurrence of pancreatoblastomas in neonates with the Beckwith-Wiedemann syndrome has been reported, and the diagnosis has been made intrauterine at 32 weeks' gestation in association with the Beckwith-Wiedemann syndrome [208–211], although the morphology of the lesion designated as a pancreatoblastoma in this context must be differentiated clearly from the florid diffuse adenomatosis or cystic dysplasia seen in some Beckwith-Wiedemann infants. Most reports of carcinomas or adenocarcinomas in newborns are determined to be pancreatoblastomas when the descriptions or illustrations are reviewed [212].

THE ENDOCRINE PANCREAS

Histogenesis and Development

The islets of Langerhans and pancreatic endocrine cells are part of the diffuse neuroendocrine cell system. Morphologic descriptions of islet development in the human have been described in detail [4, 192, 213–216]. The major cell types recognized in the endocrine pancreas are the B cell producing insulin, the A cell producing glucagon, the D cell producing somatostation, and the PP cell producing pancreatic peptide [217, 218] (Fig. 26.18).

Islet cells in humans are derived from the pancreatic ducts [219, 220]. No immunoreactive endocrine cells are found at 7 weeks of gestation [221]. Using electron microscopy, Like and Orci [216] identified A cells first at 9 weeks' gestation. At 10 weeks, endocrine cells form about 2% of the pancreatic volume density, and immunoreactive B cells are sparse, solitary, and confined to the epithelial ducts. By 12 weeks, the endocrine volume density is 6%, and small groups of B cells surround ducts. By 14 weeks, the volume density is 20%, and there are now large B cell clusters near the ducts and solitary cells in acini [222]. Robb [214] described budding of islet cells from the pancreatic duct into the adjacent mesenchyme, visible by light microscopy at 10.5 weeks' gestation. The knot of endocrine cells loses its

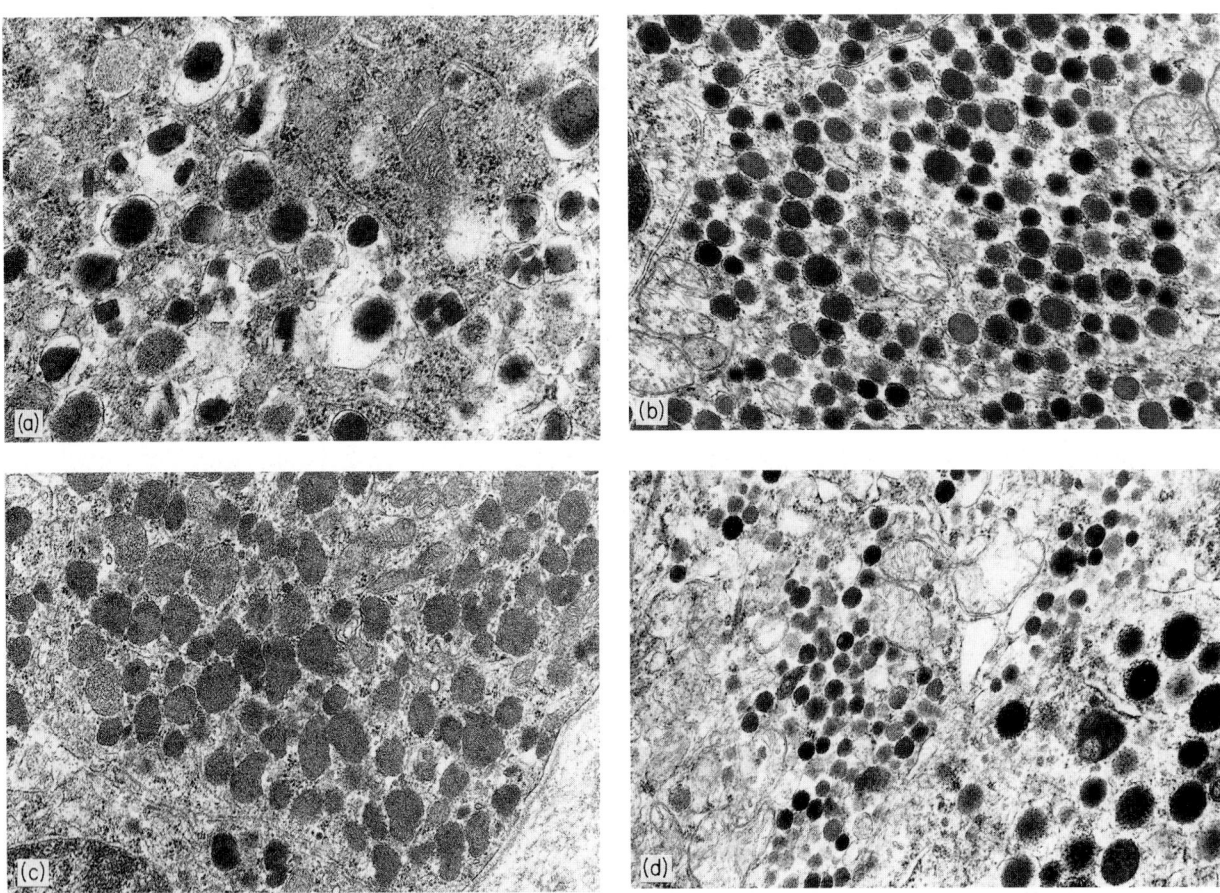

FIGURE 26.18. *Islet cell granules. (a) B cell, showing large, finely granular insulin granules and dense angular crystalloids, with an empty space separating the core from the limiting membrane. The largest granules here measure 385 nm. ×29,250. (b) The A cell has a granule with a dense core and a less dense periphery. The largest granules here measure 335 nm. ×16,350. (c) D cell. Somatostatin granules are larger and less dense than glucagon granules, are irregular in shape, and fill the limiting membrane. The largest D granules here measure 410 nm, compared with the 250-nm A granules in the adjacent cell. ×20,480. (d) PP cell. Pancreatic peptide granules are small with uniformly dense, round granules having a tight-fitting membrane. The largest granules here measure 200 nm, while the A granules on the right measure 470 nm. ×16,350.*

connection with the duct and becomes vascularized by a central capillary. The enlarging islets seen in the mesenchyme may show segregation of cell types. The mantle islet has centrally placed B cells surrounded by a mantle of A cells, while the bipolar islet has polar aggregates of A and B or A and D cells. By 30 weeks' gestation, the mature trabecular arrangement is noted around a well-formed capillary network, with the A cells and D cells arranged marginally while the B cells are central in the cord (Fig. 26.19).

Liu and Potter [192] claim that the interstitial islets are primary islets, some of which degenerate by birth, and that persistent primary islets, often attended by lymphoid aggregates, are present in the premature infant. This process of degeneration of primary islets and development of a second, definitive intra-acinar generation has not been confirmed by others [216, 223–225]. Emery and Bury [223] did observe

some hemorrhagic islets in premature neonates but related the finding to changing endocrine demands rather than to systematic insular involution.

The endocrine tissue in the developing pancreas can be seen to lie centrally within the developing lobules, close to the ductal system. The larger and better-formed islets of Langerhans form the stalk of the lobule (Fig. 26.20). Smaller aggregates and even single endocrine cells (the secondary islets of Liu and Potter) bud off within the more peripheral centroacinar tissues so that the distribution of endocrine tissue within the late fetal pancreas is characteristic [218, 226]. At term, these small peripheral clusters of endocrine cells may be numerous, and the nonislet (or preislet) endocrine cells may constitute much of the endocrine component of the newborn pancreas (Fig. 26.21). The centroacinar cells are said to have a role in endocrine cell proliferation, differentiation, and function [106].

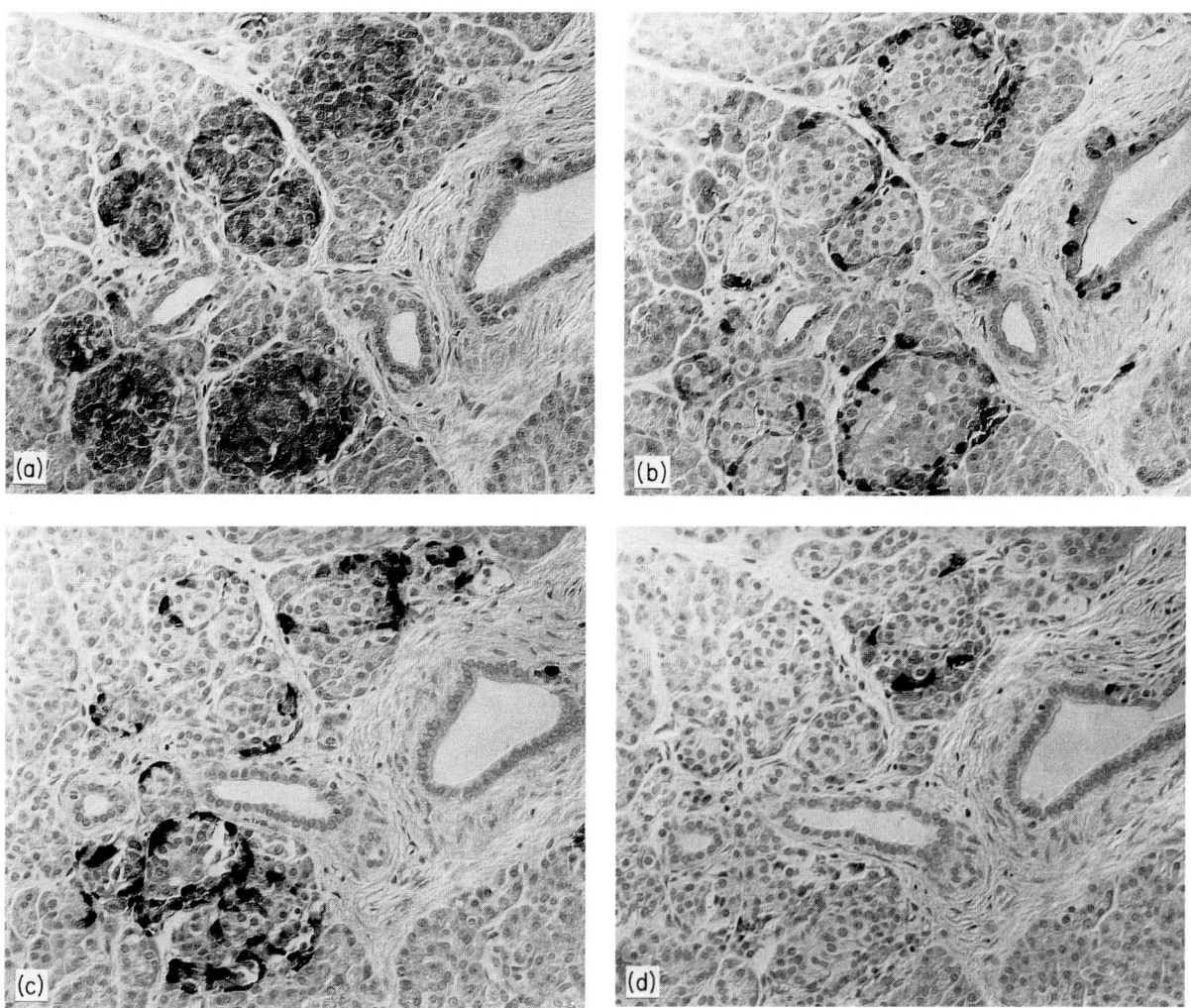

FIGURE 26.19. *Arrangement of cells within the islet. Adjacent sections are immunostained to reveal: (a) insulin—the central B cells in the islets contain insulin; (b) glucagon—peripheral and marginal A cells contain glucagon; (c) somatostatin—the distribution of D cells, like that of glucagon, is marginal in the islet; (d) pancreatic peptide—in the PP-poor region of the body, only isolated PP cells are noted in the islets. Note the duct-related endocrine cells of all kinds. Immunostain, ×160.*

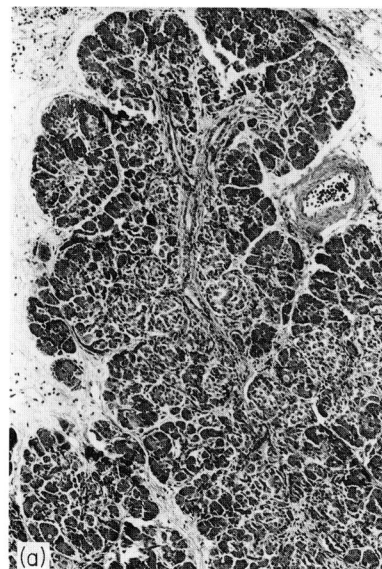
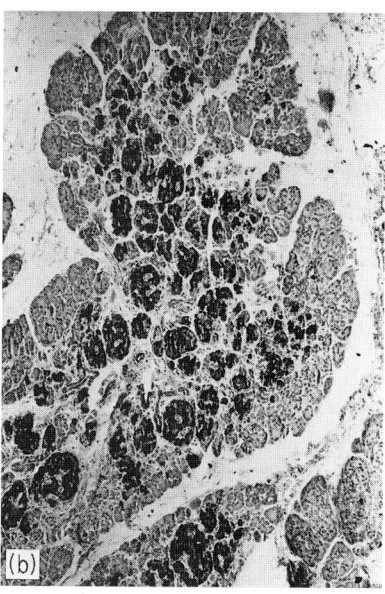

FIGURE 26.20.   *Endocrine tissue in the newborn pancreas, showing the lobular arrangement of developing endocrine tissue. (a) Normal full-term pancreas, when cut longitudinally, demonstrates a central branching duct system with most of the endocrine tissue clustered around the duct system, the acinar tissue being more peripheral. H&E, ×84. (b) A similar field, immunostained to demonstrate all endocrine cells simultaneously. Larger islets are central; smaller islets and endocrine cell clusters are peripheral. Immunostain for insulin + glucagon + somatostatin + pancreatic peptide, ×84.*

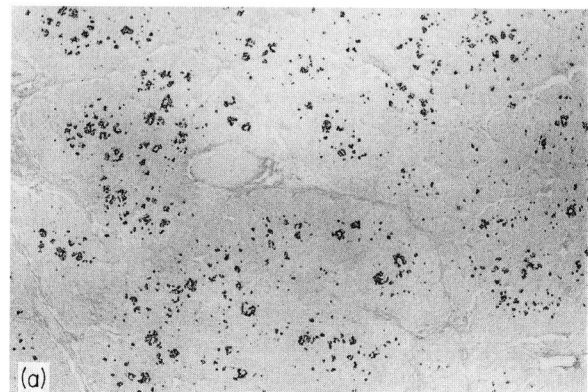
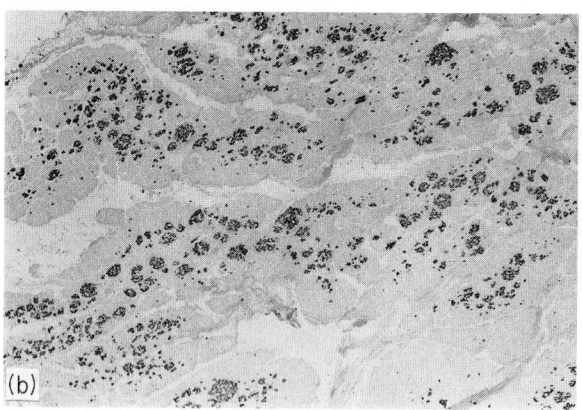

FIGURE 26.21.   *Extrainsular endocrine cells. (a) At birth, the normal pancreas has a generous sprinkling of single endocrine cells and cell clusters in addition to the islets. (b) By 6 weeks, the islets are larger and more consolidated. Note the distribution in the center of the lobular stalk. Immunostain for insulin, ×58.*

The literature regarding islet cell production in postnatal life, mostly from rodent experiments, has been summarized by Bouwens and Klöppel [226a]. Multipotential stem cells are found throughout life in, or associated with, the pancreatic ductules and resemble the oval stem cells of the liver. The mechanisms that regulate islet neogenesis from progenitor cells are still unknown.

Unfamiliarity with this morphologic pattern of dispersion of endocrine cells in the neonatal pancreas has led to the pathologic diagnosis of "nesidioblastosis." Nesidioblastosis, or the process of budding of new islets from ducts, is the normal developmental process at this stage of life. Pathologic—that is, persistent and excessive—nesidioblastosis will be discussed under hyperinsulinemic hypoglycemia.

Like other cells of the diffuse neuroendocrine system, islet cells can be shown to have epithelial cytokeratins as well as a number of neural attributes [227]. The cells have neuron-like electrical excitability, express adrenergic enzymes during development, and contain neuron-specific enolase and protein gene product (PgP) 9.5. There remains some controversy around the embryologic derivation of the islet cells. Some possibilities are as follows:

1. The cells are of endodermal origin, and both exocrine and endocrine cells share a common precursor. Islet cells are induced by local factors to express neuroendocrine differentiation [225].
2. The cells are endodermally derived but are not regular endodermal cells. Instead, the endocrine cells are programmed from the epiblast and committed to neuroendocrine differentiation. Exocrine and endocrine cells, therefore, have no common

precursor but are embryologically predetermined to go their own ways [228].

3. Ductal and acinar cells retain their capacity and the plasticity to interchange as conditions demand. The centroacinar cells may function as a reservoir, and the presence of hybrid intermediate acinar-islet cells is adduced as evidence of this possibility [106, 229]. Changing genetic expression throughout life can determine the fate of new cellular differentiation. Plasticity of the rat pancreatic ductal cells has been demonstrated by co-culture of adult pancreatic duct epithelium with fetal mesenchyme; insulin- and glucagon-secreting islets formed and became vascularized [230].

Functional Maturation, Morphology, and Morphometry

A cells appear before other cell types at 9 weeks' gestation [216], followed in short order by D and B cells at 10.5 weeks and lastly by PP cells [218]. Transcriptional levels of insulin are detectable by 12 weeks, but are lower in the fetus than in the adult, whereas the transcriptional levels of glucagon and somatostatin mRNA are higher after 14 weeks' gestation than they are postnatally [155]. The distribution of the various islet cells is not homogeneous throughout the pancreas [231]. A portion of the head of the pancreas that is apparently derived from a ventral anlage, the so-called PP lobe, is rich in PP-containing islets [232] (Fig. 26.22). In the fetus and neonate, the number of somatostatin-containing D cells is greater than later in life [233], and the distribution of B cells shows large numbers of peripherally placed aggregates in the normal neonate [234].

There is a large body of literature on the quantitation of endocrine tissue in the developing pancreas [222, 234–240];

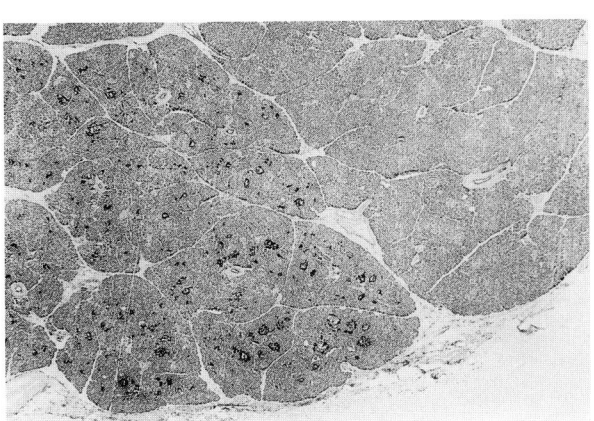

FIGURE 26.22. *The PP lobe. Large, irregular islets in the PP lobe are rich in pancreatic peptide cells while the rest of the pancreas is PP-poor. Immunostain for PP, ×29.*

Table 26.1 summarizes some of the attempts at quantitation. Most of the older literature gives figures that are unacceptably low for the newborn pancreas, a time of life when the pancreas is rich in endocrine and mesenchymal tissue and before the acinar tissue develops. It is important to note that, in general, the quantitation compares endocrine to total exocrine epithelial tissue, a feature that varies considerably with postnatal survival, as does the amount of mesenchyme. Some point-counting methods may exclude the mesenchyme from consideration, so that the various methods are not strictly comparable, and this is reflected in the widely divergent results.

The general pattern of development can be clearly seen in Table 26.1: much of the endocrine tissue is present in the third trimester. Acinar growth and development with concomitant loss of mesenchyme constitute a postnatal phenomenon. The relative amount of endocrine tissue is thus greatest in the pancreas of a third-trimester infant, diminishing rapidly after birth as the acinar tissue expands.

Relative proportions of various islet types in the PP-rich and PP-poor portions of the pancreas are given in Table 26.2, derived from a composite of figures [218, 221].

Abnormalities of the Endocrine Pancreas

Islet Hypertrophy

Islet size varies with age. Jaffe et al [234] found that in normal controls, below the age of 2 months, only 3.5% of all islets measured greater than 200 μm in diameter. Single islets, often large septal islets, can measure up to 700 μm in diameter (Fig. 26.23). There is no evidence that these large islets are the cause of hyperinsulinism [238]. Islet hypertrophy should thus refer to the percentage of all islets greater than 200 μm. Borchard and Müntefering [241] have given values for the sizes of islets at different stages of gestation. Islet hypertrophy is seen in infants of diabetic mothers and, less commonly, in infants with erythroblastosis fetalis. For a review, see Wellmann and Volk [242] and Hultquist and Olding [243].

Endocrine Hyperplasia

Hyperplasia refers to an increase in endocrine bulk due to an increase in the number of cells. Hyperplasia and hypertrophy usually occur together in the endocrine pancreas, but not necessarily, and it is worth considering them separately since much of the endocrine mass in the developing human occurs outside the islets. The determination of endocrine hyperplasia is made by comparing a given mass with the established values for a child of the same gestational age and the same length of postnatal development and presumably by making some adjustment for body weight. Since no such tables exist, crude approximations must be made, bearing in mind the relatively large contribution that the endocrine mass makes to the normal infant pancreas. A potential source of error is the presence of chronic

Table 26.1.   Quantitation of the endocrine component of the developing pancreas

Reference	Gestational Age	Method	No. of Specimens Examined	Site	Results (%)
Grotting et al [235]	8 months' gestation to 1 month postnatal	Linear scan, islet volume	12		8.21 ± 2.63
Jaffe et al [234]	Birth to 2 months	Direct area	6		6.1–12.9
	2–8 months	Direct area	7		5.1–7.7
Rahier et al [236]	Neonates	Point counting Volume density	6	Head (posterior)	6.5–20.8
				Head (anterior)	11.4–19.6
				Isthmus	8.0–20.7
				Body	9.2–22.1
				Tail	8.2–25.4
Milner et al [237]	26–44 weeks	Quantimet	9	PP-rich	5.4 ± 0.53
		Fractional surface area and point counting	12	PP-poor	5.48 ± 0.25
Witte et al [238]	24 weeks to 1 month postnatal	Point counting Volume density	31		24 weeks,* 1month*
				Head	38.6, 18.2
				Body	26.5, 12.4
				Tail	32.8, 13.8
Goudswaard et al [239]	15–17 weeks	Point counting	5		4.3 ± 0.4
	Neonates	Total endocrine area	9		7.7 ± 0.9
Hahn von Dorsche et al [222]	10 weeks	Volume density	4		2
	12 weeks		7		6
	14 weeks		7		20
Van Assche et al [240]	32–37 weeks	Point counting, volume to density	10		5.1 ± 1.4

*   Representative values at these ages, not averages.

pancreatitis (see Table 26.1) [244]. Since surface area or volumetric determinations of endocrine mass are expressed relative to the acinar mass, any diminution in exocrine tissue will reveal an apparent proportionate increase in the endocrine bulk. Table 26.3 lists those conditions in which endocrine hyperplasia has been claimed to exist, some after formal quantitation, most without [157, 234, 237, 243, 245–255].

Table 26.2.   Relative proportions of the various cell types in the developing pancreas [218, 221]

Region of Pancreas	Cell Type	20 weeks (Head of Pancreas)	Neonate	Infant
PP-rich	A	2.8	1–10	1–10
	B	21.8	10–30	25–35
	D	33.8	10–30	15–25
	PP	41.5	35–70	40–60
PP-poor	A	41.2	15.30	10.25
	B	28.8	40.50	50.70
	D	27.0	25.35	20.30
	PP	3.0	0.1–1.0	0.1–1.0

Endocrine Aplasia and Hypoplasia

There have been several reports of children with congenital diabetes who had no pancreatic islets [193, 194, 256, 257] (Fig. 26.24). Whether this represents true agenesis or is secondary to destruction has been controversial.

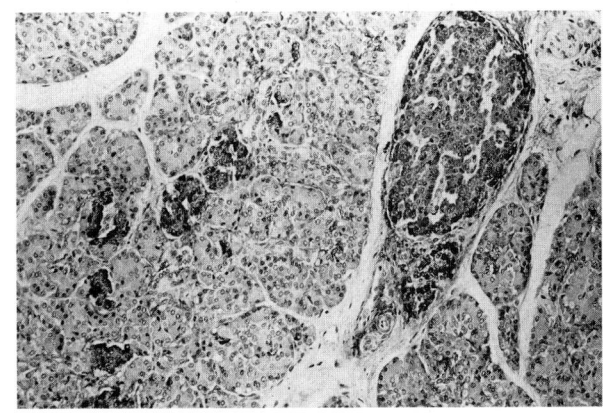

FIGURE 26.23.   *Large septal islets. Gigantic septal islets are seen during the first few years. Immunostain for insulin + glucagon + somatostatin + pancreatic peptide, ×137.*

Table 26.3.   Endocrine hyperplasia of the neonatal pancreas

Condition	Reference
Demonstrated	
Infant of diabetic mother	Hultquist and Olding [243], Milner et al [237]
Adenomatosis (focal nesidioblastosis)	Klöppel et al [245], Jaffe et al [234]
Erythroblastosis fetalis	Van Assche et al [240], Hultquist and Olding [243], Van Assche and Gepts [246]
Nonimmune hydrops fetalis	Van Assche et al [240], Mostoufi-Zadeh et al [247]
Claimed, but without quantitation, or not universally present	
Hereditary tyrosinemia	Hardwick and Dimmick [248], Perry et al [249]
Donohue syndrome	Rosenberg et al [250]
Zellweger syndrome	Zellweger [251]
Multiple endocrine neoplasia (MEN 2)	Vance et al [252]
Familial pheochromocytoma syndrome	Carney et al [253]
Endocrine cell dysplasia (diffuse nesidioblastosis)	Jaffe et al [234], Heitz et al [254]
Neonatal hemochromatosis	Blisard and Bartow [158]
Perlman syndrome	Greenberg et al [255]

In three of these families, male siblings were affected [193, 194, 257], and in two, secretory diarrhea was a feature [193, 194]. The intestines in some of these boys were lined by a simplified secretory-type epithelium devoid of crypts of Lieberkühn and villi.

Wong et al [258] described a newborn who survived for 3 days before dying of diabetes. Although all other islet hormones were demonstrable, no B cells were found, prompting the claim that they were congenitally absent. The authors conceded that the picture was likely to represent a late gestational onset of diabetes mellitus with B cell destruction. A 16-day-old female who had methylmalonic acidemia had no B cells demonstrable by electron microscopy, immunohistochemistry, or in situ hybridization. The child was diabetic and was also shown to have paternal isodisomy of chromosome 6 [259]. Congenital absence of A cells has been reported [260], and few A cells were found in an infant with normoinsulinemic hypoglycemia [261]. Paucity of somatostatin-containing D cells has been implicated in cases of neonatal hypoglycemia [262, 263]. An overall reduction in endocrine pancreatic tissue has been claimed for growth-retarded fetuses [264].

Infant of the Diabetic Mother

Detailed reviews have considered the older literature, much of it contradictory [265]. The changes listed in Table 26.4 occur in the pancreases of about 85% of the children of diabetic mothers, some features being more constant than others [243]. The variety of findings can be explained, in part, by the fact that maternal diabetes may be type I or type II, and that some are treated while others are not. The time of onset of the diabetes during pregnancy and the fetal response to the hyperglycemia are also variables, since glucose freely crosses the placenta but insulin does not, unless complexed to anti-insulin antibody [266, 267]. The glucose transporter genes and glucokinase mRNA are detectable by 13 weeks of gestation, so that the relative insensitivity of the fetal B cell to glucose is not due to a lack of glucose sensors [155]. Identical features may be seen in the pancreases of the offspring of prediabetic mothers, which may account for at least some of the reports of diabetic-type pathology occurring in the pancreases of infants of ostensibly normal mothers.

The most detailed statistical observations have been those of Hultquist and Olding [243]. Pancreatic weight was greater in normal newborn infants than in newborn infants of mothers with diabetes, especially those mothers with severe complications, after differences in body weight were taken

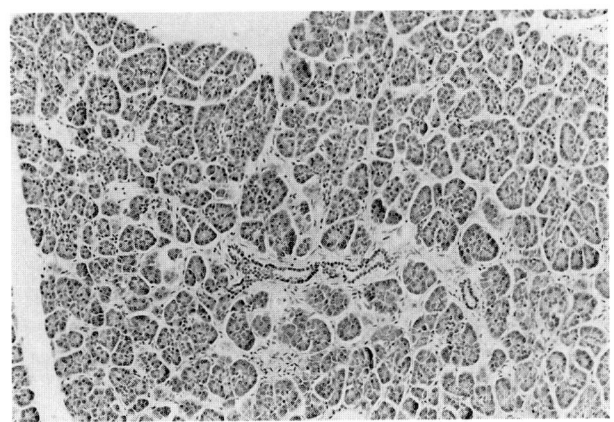

FIGURE 26.24.   *Congenital diabetes mellitus, died at 10 months. A lobule immunostained with PgP 9.5 that highlights most endocrine cells in the normal pancreas. Note the complete absence of endocrine cell staining and no visible islets. PgP ×113. (Section courtesy of Dr. J Searle, Brisbane, Australia.)*

Table 26.4.   Features of the pancreas of the infant of a diabetic mother

Islet hypertrophy (>10% over 200 μm)
Increased islet cell volume
Pleomorphism of B cell nuclei
Eosinophilic insulitis of large islets
Peri- and intrainsular fibrosis

into account. The first suggestion that maternal hyperglycemia led to islet hypertrophy in the fetus was made by Dubreuil and Anderodias [268]. Total islet volume was found to be greater in the infants of diabetic mothers when birth weight was greater than 2.25 kg, and was greater in infants of diabetic mothers after 34 weeks of gestation. The increase in islet volume held true only for infants of mothers with mild and uncomplicated diabetes, since only this group had large babies. No difference in islet volume was detected between infants of normal mothers and those with severe and complicated diabetes. An increase in mean islet diameter was more characteristic of the infant of the diabetic

mother than an increase in the number of islets [241] (Fig. 26.25).

The increase in endocrine volume is due to an increase in the B cell mass, from about 40% of all endocrine cells to 60% [264]. Milner et al [237], using immunocytochemical stains and automated quantitation in part, concluded that relative B cell area was higher in infants of diabetic mothers in both the PP-rich and PP-poor regions of the pancreas. They, however, concluded that the hyperplasia was not limited to the B cell mass alone, but that A cell bulk was increased in the PP-rich areas. The increase of B cell mass is said to be a more sensitive accompaniment of maternal diabetes than islet hypertrophy, since it occurs more frequently and is not a feature of erythroblastosis fetalis [264].

A strong correlation between increased islet volume and pleomorphism of B cell nuclei has been demonstrated [243], and is associated with increased B cell response to glucose stimulation. In contrast to total islet volume, B cell pleomorphism was a feature of the pancreas of infants of mothers who had severe diabetes with complications.

Infiltration of the pancreatic mesenchyme by inflammatory cells, particularly eosinophils and lymphocytes, is seen in the infants of diabetic mothers (see Wellmann and Volk [242] for a review). The eosinophilic infiltrate has been shown to be associated with the largest islets [243] (Fig. 26.26). Eosinophilic myelocytes, as well as Charcot-Leyden crystals, can be found, and the infiltrate is said to disappear within a few days of birth [242]. Careful examination of the pancreas of the fetus, even when macerated, may reveal eosinophils, and the presence of Charcot-Leyden crystals can persist even after all other clues are gone (Fig. 26.27). Klöppel [269] suggested that the infiltrate is a local reaction to insulin-containing immune complexes formed when maternal anti-insulin antibodies bind to fetal insulin. The eosinophilic peri-insulitis occurs in about half of the infants with maternal diabetes, and is seen in the children of

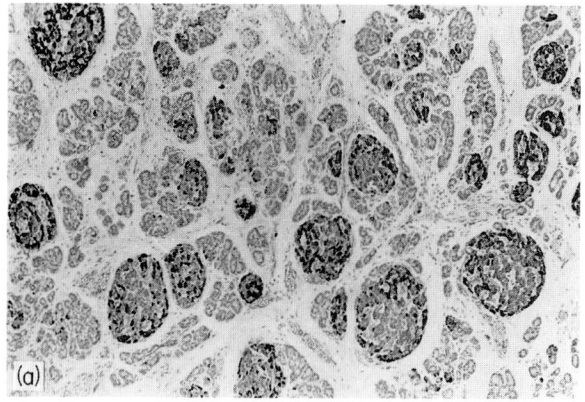

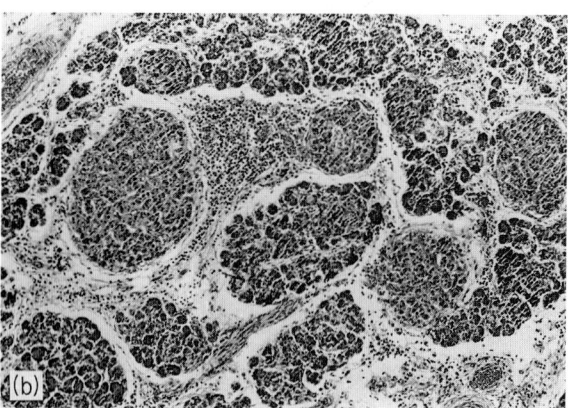

FIGURE 26.25.   *Infant of diabetic mother. (a) Large numbers of oversized islets are noted in this newborn infant. Immunostain for glucagon, ×58. (b) Many of the gigantic islets are stromal and associated with a cellular (eosinophilic) infiltrate. H&E, ×80.*

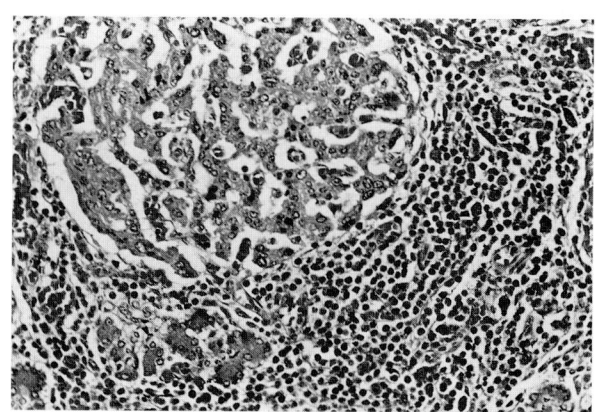

FIGURE 26.26.   *Infant of diabetic mother. Eosinophilic peri-insulitis. The largest islets are, on occasion, surrounded by an infiltrate of eosinophils. H&E, ×137.*

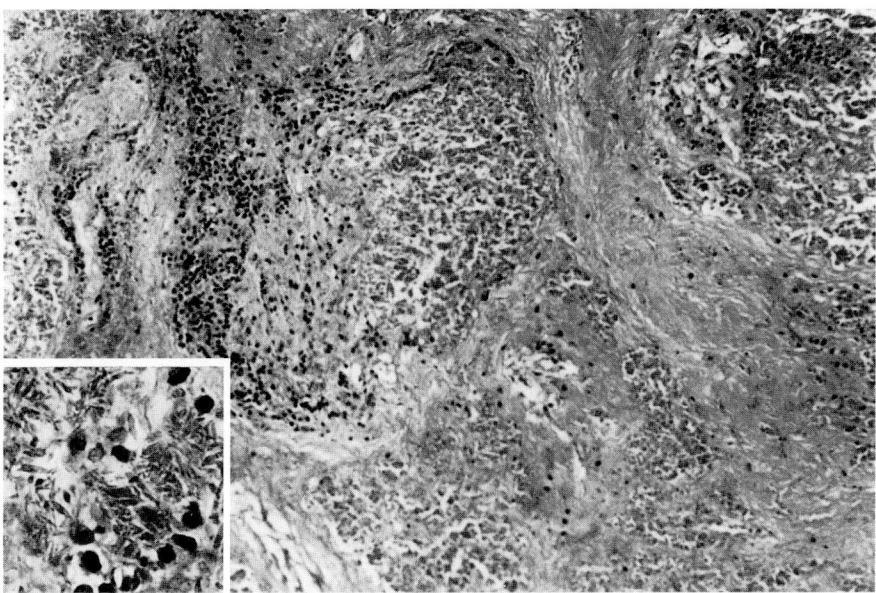

FIGURE 26.27. *Infant of diabetic mother. Macerated fetal pancreas. Some eosinophils survive and are still recognizable* (arrows). *H&E, ×97. Inset: Charcot-Leyden controls are stacked in arrays, giving a morphologic clue to the cause of death even in a macerated pancreas. H&E, ×480. (Sections courtesy of Dr. E. Popek, Houston, TX.)*

mothers who were receiving insulin as well as those not on insulin.

A close relationship exists among eosinophilic infiltration, large islets, and peri-insular as well as intrainsular fibrosis [243]. Nelson et al [270] confirmed the presence of fibrosis but found it to be early and, in their material, independent of eosinophilia. They suggested that the fibrosis was largely an in utero phenomenon rather than a perinatal acquisition. Other findings in the pancreases of infants of diabetic mothers [242] include an increase in the mitotic index, degranulation of B cells (not a constant finding), lymphocyte infiltration (not confirmed by Hultquist and Olding [243]), islet edema, hydropic swelling of islet cells, ribbon-like transformation of islet cells, necrosis, thickened intrainsular capillaries, and thickened interstitial fibrous septa.

It has been suggested that an intact hypothalamo-hypophyseal axis is required for the development of pancreatic changes, since the anencephalic offspring of diabetic mothers failed to show pancreatic changes [246]. Correlation between the degree of islet hyperplasia and the chemical control of maternal diabetes is low. Islet volume has been found to correlate with high maternal blood glucose in the 24 hours preceding delivery only, and not with the mean gestational level. The mechanism of changes in the pancreases of offspring of prediabetic mothers remains to be elucidated.

Diabetes Mellitus

Diabetes that occurs within the first few weeks of life and lasts for more than 2 weeks, requiring insulin treatment, has a clinically variable course [271, 272]. It manifests with

hyperglycemia, glycosuria, and dehydration, but ketosis and ketonuria are generally mild, and remission or recovery occurs in about half of the cases [272]. Some of these are instances of the Wolcott-Rallison syndrome of multiple epiphyseal dysplasias with early-onset diabetes mellitus [273].

Pancreatic pathology has been reported from a small number of children who succumbed, but these may not all represent the transitory neonatal form of diabetes mellitus, since pancreatic hypoplasia [21, 274] and aplasia are reported and these conditions are more likely to result in permanent diabetes [8–10, 275]. Pancreatic histology has been described as normal [276], having reduced numbers of islet cells [277, 278], or even an excess of islets [279]. Permanent diabetes mellitus has developed years after a previous transient neonatal diabetes [272, 280].

The absence of B cells described by Wong et al [258] is more in keeping with the appearance of an intrauterine-onset type I diabetes mellitus than a primary congenital agenesis of B cells alone. A number of familial cases have been reported [193, 194, 257, 281, 282], mostly X-linked with autoimmune phenomena, and the pancreases lacked, or were relatively deficient in, islet cells (see Fig. 26.24). The presence of insulitis is not commonly mentioned, but large follicular lymphoid aggregates are. An association of methylmalonic acidemia and diabetes mellitus with absent B cells is reported, with paternal disomy of chromosome 6 [259].

Neonatal Hyperinsulinemic Hypoglycemia

Most causes of hypoglycemia in the newborn are transient; only relatively few conditions are associated with a more

Table 26.5.   Pancreatic findings in infants who present under the age of 2 months with hyperinsulinemic hypoglycemia, compiled from 13 personal cases

Finding*	Association	Relative Incidence (n = 13)
No or minor pathologic change	Sporadic	2
Endocrine cell dysplasia (diffuse nesidioblastosis)	Most familial	3
Unifocal adenomatosis (focal nesidioblastosis)	Sporadic or familial	4
Multifocal adenomatosis (focal nesidioblastosis)	Familial, multiple endocrine neoplasia (MEN2)	1
Diffuse adenomatosis (confluent nesidioblastosis)	Beckwith-Wiedemann syndrome	3
Adenoma	—	0

* Synonyms are given in parentheses (Goossens et al [292]).

persistent hypoglycemia, and among these, hyperinsulinism is of most interest here because of the associated pancreatic changes. Hyperinsulinemic hypoglycemia in the newborn includes familial cases with an autosomal recessive inheritance pattern and persistent familial hyperinsulinemic hypoglycemia of infancy (FHHI) [283–287], and in some families the diagnosis has been made in utero in a subsequent child [288]. In some families the disorder has been linked to chromosome 11p14–15.1 [289], and mutations have been detected in the sulfonylurea receptor gene [290, 290a]. Apparently, sporadic cases also fit the autosomal recessive pattern, and the claim is made that persistent FHHI is a fairly homogeneous inherited condition [291]. Identification of a responsible gene is a major advance in unscrambling the relationship between form and dysfunction in this intriguing condition.

The earlier literature was confounded by a plethora of descriptive terms and synonyms, and the term "nesidioblastosis," the neoformation of endocrine elements from the pancreatic ducts, was applied too loosely for a condition that is essentially normal for this stage of human development. Over the past decade, however, there has been a clearer understanding of what constitutes the ongoing development of the fetal and neonatal pancreas when contrasted with the findings in children who have undergone pancreatic resection for hyperinsulinism. The papers of Goossens and colleagues [292, 293] serve as a good basic summary of the field, and their terminology is adopted here, with explanation.

It should be borne in mind that despite the following anatomic discussion, the relationship to insulin secretion is unclear [234, 294]. Thornton et al [291] found that the histologic changes were not consistent among different patients in the same family, and an abnormality of a regulatory protein is strongly suspected; in this instance, mutations in the sulfonylurea receptor described by Thomas et al [289] are thought to act in a manner similar to the CFTR muta-

tions in cystic fibrosis. The mutations lead to chronic depolarization and hypersecretion of the B cells.

Table 26.5 presents the frequency of the various findings in pancreases from infants with hyperinsulinism, derived from our own material and from a review of descriptions in the literature. There are essentially five main morphologic patterns:

1. No change, very minor nondiagnostic changes ("normal"), or centroacinar cell hyperplasia
2. Endocrine cell dysplasia, nesidiodysplasia, or islet cell dysmaturation (diffuse nesidioblastosis)
3. Unifocal adenomatosis (focal nesidioblastosis)
4. Multifocal adenomatosis (focal nesidioblastosis)
5. Diffuse adenomatosis (confluent nesidioblastosis)

In a comprehensive review of 234 published cases, Goossens et al [293] found that 22% of reported cases had features of the focal or multifocal kind and that 78% could be classified as diffuse nesidioblastosis, although in their own material they claim the incidence of focal and diffuse disease to be about equal [293].

In some infants, particularly older ones, the resected pancreas has shown no detectable endocrine change [226]. One infant with pancreatomegaly on CT scan had a diffuse increase in centroacinar cells (best seen by cytokeratin immunostaining) with a subtle increase in small clusters of endocrine, especially insulin-containing, cells. It is important to use endocrine immunostained age-matched controls in this circumstance because of the large number and peculiar distribution of extrainsular endocrine cells in the normal newborn pancreas. B cell nucleomegaly may be an isolated finding [238]. It is most likely that in this group the defect is a purely regulatory one and that medical therapy is likely to be of value although the hypothesis is not easily tested.

The largest group has the changes of endocrine cell dysplasia [234]—that is, nesidioblastosis that is *persistent* and *excessive*, also described as diffuse nesidioblastosis [292], nesidiodysplasia [295], or the islet cell dysmaturation syndrome [296]. The findings are visible on routine pancreas sections, but are best appreciated when immunostained sections of pancreas highlight the endocrine cells (PgP 9.5, neuron-specific enolase, or just insulin) and are contrasted with similarly stained age-matched controls (Fig. 26.28). Islets are of varying size, often poorly defined and tailing off into the acinar parenchyma. There is an excessive budding of small endocrine clusters within acini and around intralobular ducts, noted diffusely throughout the pancreas. All cell types are involved, not only B cells [234, 255, 293, 295]. B cell volume may be increased, and nuclear hypertrophy is a prominent finding and in some instances the only finding. Nuclear surface area and volume of the B cells is increased [297], and the hypertrophied B cell nuclei are probably tetraploid [298]. Reports of a relative deficiency of extractable somatostatin [262] or a paucity of somatostatin-containing cells remain controversial: most deny the finding [234, 238, 254, 292, 295, 299], but Marks claims that it is indeed the paracrine relationship of the B and D cells that is disturbed [263], and perfusion of islet-like cell clusters in

vitro reveals that insulin release by cells derived from persistently hyperinsulinemic infants is poorly stimulated by glucose and effectively blocked by somatostatin, suggesting that there may indeed be a functional somatostatin deficiency in vivo [300].

Ductuloinsular complexes are tangles of ducts, ductules, and intervening endocrine cells within and around the ductules (see Fig. 26.28). Goossens et al [292] point out that the ductuloinsular complex is not found in the normal developing infant and is characteristic of the pancreas with hyperinsulinism. There appears to be wide case-to-case variation in the extent of the endocrine proliferation in diffuse nesidioblastosis. An overall excess of endocrine tissue may occur [238], but this excess is not invariable and is not required for the diagnosis. Rather, the qualitative change in endocrine cell distribution is the more characteristic feature [234, 293]. Centroacinar hyperplasia is commonly noted in the rest of the pancreas [226].

Electron microscopy has revealed no characteristic findings but has suggested the occurrence of intermediate hybrid acinar-endocrine cells, with the inference that reserve

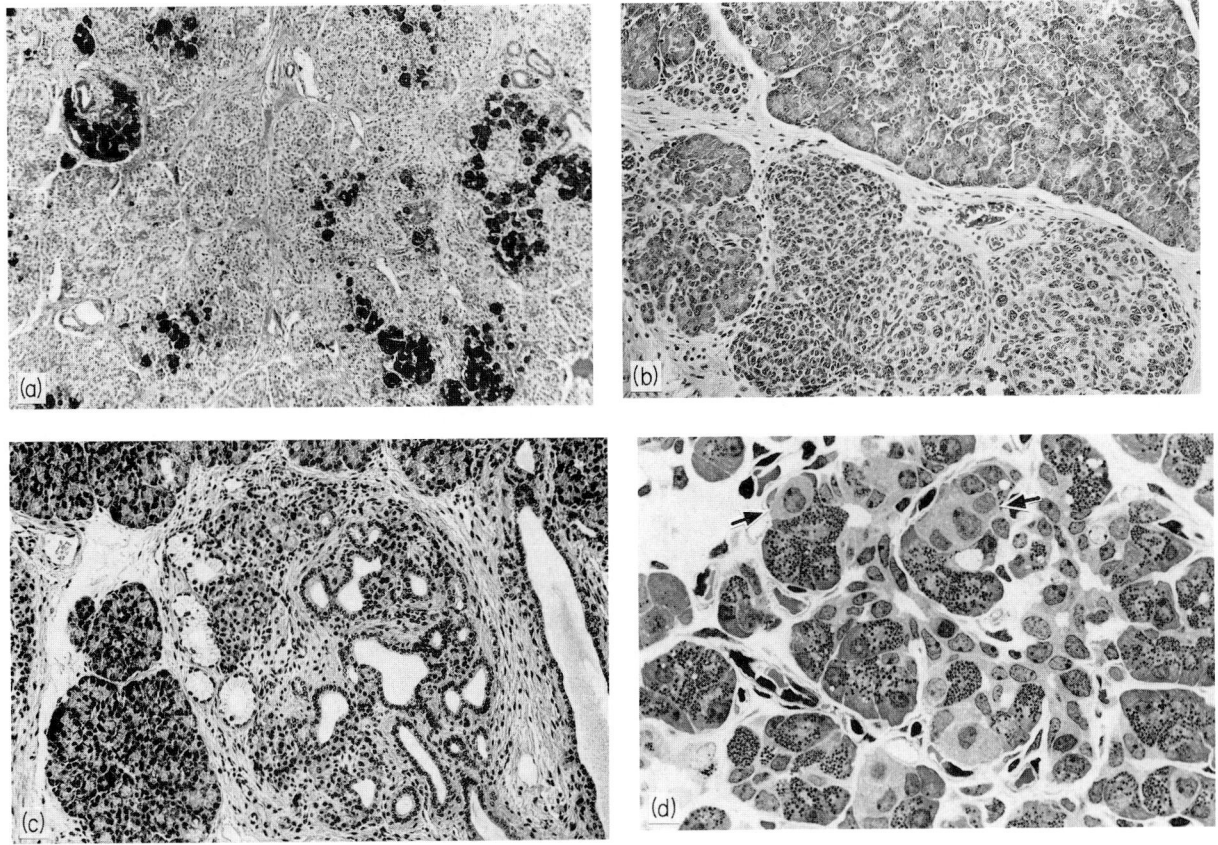

FIGURE 26.28. *Endocrine cell dysplasia (diffuse nesidioblastosis). (a) Immunostain demonstrates a qualitative abnormality. Islets are misshapen and irregular in contour, and there are some lobules with large islets while others contain only endocrine cell clusters. Immunostain for insulin + somatostatin + pancreatic peptide, ×58. (b) Large, complex septal islets have prominent nuclear hypertrophy. H&E, ×95. (c) The ductuloinsular complex consists of knots of ductules, some with mucus-secreting cells, together with intervening endocrine cells. H&E, ×97. (d) Endocrine cells (arrows) insinuate themselves widely between the granular acinar cells. 1 μm, polychrome, plastic-embedded.*

cells can mature in two directions or that acinar-endocrine transformation is possible [229, 234, 238, 295, 301, 302].

Adenomatosis (focal nesidioblastosis) [245] is an excessive proliferation of islet cells (usually more than 40% of all cells in a given area), pushing the exocrine elements aside or haphazardly incorporating them. Neoproliferation from ducts, ductuloinsular complexes, are always an integral component, and all cell types are represented. The proliferation most characteristically recapitulates islet formation, with the pattern of A and D cells being peripheral to more centrally aggregated B cells (Fig. 26.29).

The focal lesion is restricted to one discrete area of the pancreas, and the rest of the pancreas is generally normal. Importantly for diagnosis and therapy, such a lesion may occasionally bulge from the surface of the pancreas, lie adjacent to the pancreas, or even be ectopic [293, 303–305]. Venous sampling [306] may be successful in detecting the focal intrapancreatic lesions not noted on ultrasound examination, and intraoperative ultrasonography has been used successfully to detect and remove focal lesions [307].

Multifocal adenomatosis (multifocal nesidioblastosis) represents the preceding lesion occurring in multiple discrete sites throughout the pancreas. The practical implication of the distinction of multifocal adenomatosis from the focal variety is that variants of the multiple endocrine adenoma syndrome are likely to be represented in the pancreas by multifocal adenomatosis (although the tumors are also described as "adenomas with multiple cell types") [252].

Diffuse adenomatosis (confluent nesidioblastosis) is the occurrence of a florid endocrine overgrowth that has ductuloinsular complexes and in which islet morphology is recapitulated. Acinar tissue may be deficient. This is characteristic of some cases of the Beckwith–Wiedemann syndrome [199, 226].

Adenomas are extraordinarily rare in infants. Adenomas are well demarcated and differ from adenomatosis in being devoid of admixed acinar tissue. The adenoma does not contain all islet cell types in normal proportions, even though more than one cell type is usually represented. Most importantly, the adenoma lacks the characteristic recapitula-

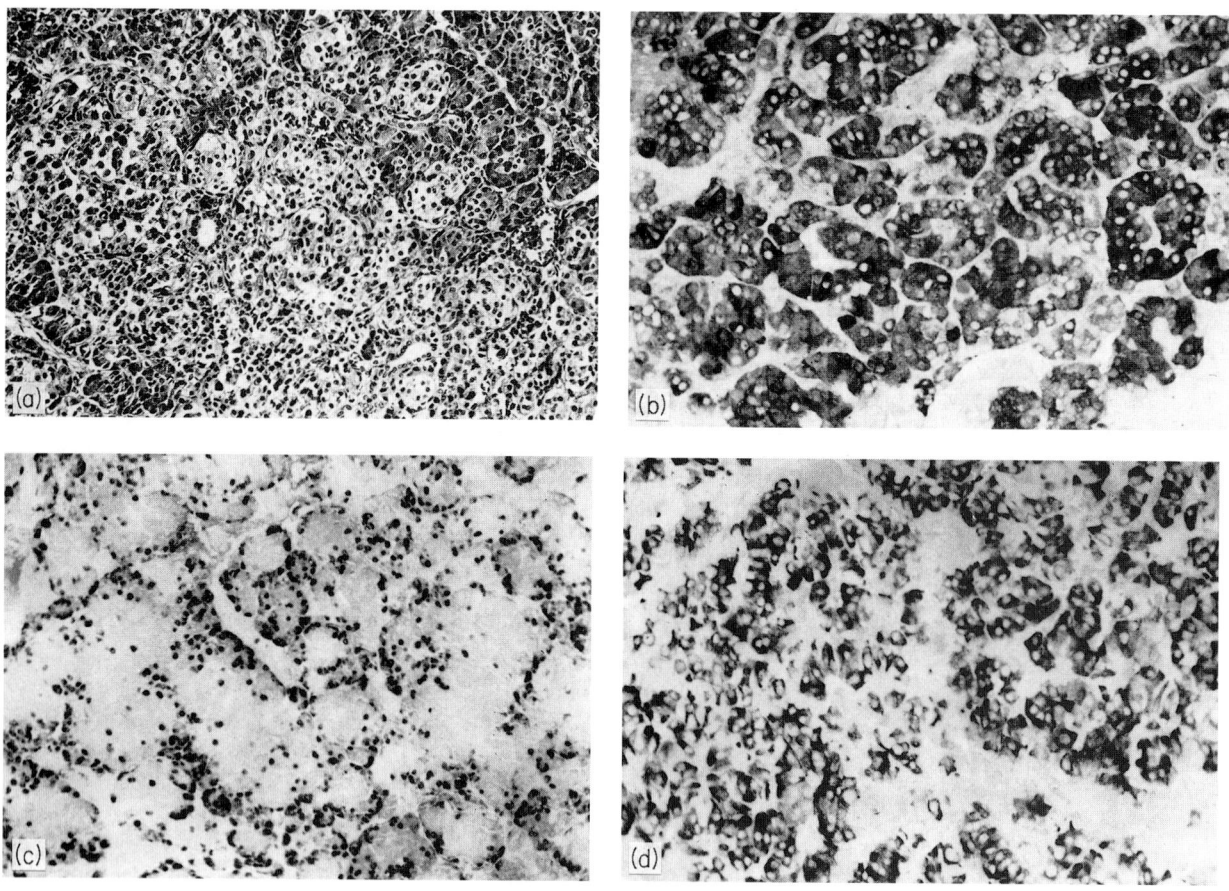

FIGURE 26.29.   *Focal adenomatosis (focal nesidioblastosis). (a) Most of the field is occupied by endocrine tissue. The endocrine cells are arranged as compact and adjacent mini-islets. H&E, ×98. (b) Large fields of endocrine cells are highlighted by their staining for the presence of neuron-specific enolase (NSE). Immunostain for NSE, ×184. (c) Immunostain for pancreatic peptide shows the distribution of the cells at the outer margins of the islet-like aggregates. Immunostain for pancreatic peptide ×184. (d) Insulin immunostain on sections adjacent to (b) and (c). Immunostain for insulin ×184.*

tion of the islet arrangement. Most previous lesions described as adenomas in infants appear to be instances of adenomatosis when the illustrations are reviewed [308].

The cause of the hyperinsulinism is not yet known, and the relationship to the morphologic abnormalities is not clear [294]. Some children with hyperinsulinism have no detectable lesions. Others who presumably do can be managed medically, even for years [309], and the hyperinsulinism can disappear. What happens to the endocrine pancreas in these children over time is not known. The most flagrant example of the dissociation between the function and the anatomy is the Beckwith-Wiedemann syndrome, in which the pancreas may be profoundly "adenomatous" but the hyperinsulinism only transient.

Despite this pathogenetic uncertainty, the current classification lends itself to a more rational approach to the diagnosis and treatment of hyperinsulinism. If the diagnosis of hyperinsulinism is made by finding insulin levels too high for a given level of hypoglycemia [310], treatment is immediately instituted with frequent feeds; intravenous glucose, often by central line; and medical manipulation using adrenaline, glucocorticoids, glucagon, and diazoxide [311]. More recently, short- and long-term treatment with the somatostatin analogue octreotide has been instituted [309, 312]. An abdominal ultrasound examination can be done to find the rare instance of focal nesidioblastosis that bulges from the pancreatic surface or abuts the organ. If such a lesion is present, its resection may be curative. If such a lesion is not found, selective venous sampling is indicated to document the presence of a focal lesion that is amenable to surgery. Even if a focal lesion is present, surgery is indicated only if the hypoglycemia cannot be managed medically. Should surgery be indicated, visual inspection and intraoperative ultrasound can be used to detect and remove a focal lesion. The pathologist should be prepared to confirm a diagnosis of focal adenomatosis (focal nesidioblastosis) at frozen section. If no focal lesion is detected, it can be assumed that the disorder is a diffuse nesidioblastosis. Current surgical opinion holds that if medical management is unsuccessful, a full 95% pancreatectomy is the treatment of choice [313]. Although the 95% pancreatectomy leaves only a rim of pancreas around the bile duct, sonography has shown that regeneration is rapid [314] and that the functional outcome for exocrine and endocrine pancreatic function is excellent [313, 314].

Recent reviews that include longer follow-up, however, have questioned this approach, documenting a high incidence of B cell dysfunction and frank diabetes in the survivors [315, 315a].

Viral Infection and the Endocrine Pancreas

Viral infection of B cells has been considered to be one of the triggers of diabetes mellitus in human leukocyte antigen (HLA) susceptible hosts, although substantive evidence in humans is sparse. In the neonate, selective damage to islet cells has been noted in coxsackievirus B infections [174, 181, 182]. The islets may be involved nonselectively, together

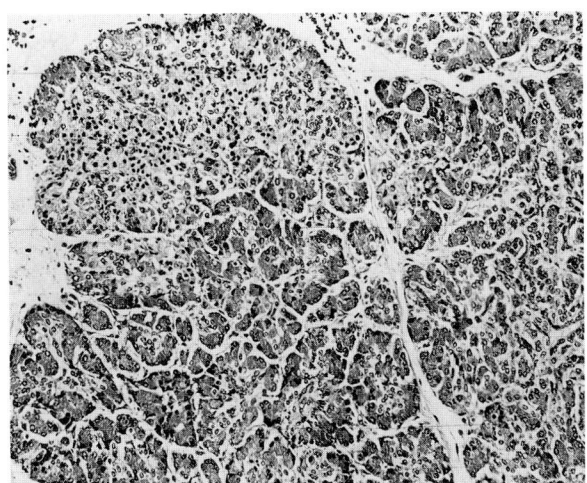

FIGURE 26.30. *Ischemic necrosis. Lobular or sublobular zonal necrosis is not uncommon in infants with shock or severe congenital heart disease. H&E, ×90.*

with acinar tissue, in disseminated herpes virus, CMV, varicella zoster, and rubella infections [175], and necrosis may also be found at postmortem examination of infants who died in shock or from severe congenital heart disease [316, 317] (Fig. 26.30). Caution should be exercised, therefore, in ascribing the necrosis to a virus. It is probable that in genetically susceptible persons, viruses may cause alterations in B cells, leading to immune damage.

Familial Disorders and Congenital Malformation Syndromes Involving the Endocrine Pancreas

Beckwith-Wiedemann Syndrome

The Beckwith-Wiedemann syndrome of macrosomia, macroglossia, omphalocele, and visceromegaly is accompanied in about 50% of cases by transient hypoglycemia attributed to hyperinsulinism [318, 319]. Macrosomia is not necessarily accompanied by hypoglycemia or by increased insulin levels [320]. The features of the pancreas are those of diffuse adenomatosis, some nodules of which may form large or even palpable masses [321]. Immunohistochemistry has shown, in one case, markedly increased numbers of B and A cells with fewer D or PP-containing cells; a lack of segregation of A and PP cells to appropriate parts of the gland was noted [322]. In some cases, the endocrine overgrowth is accompanied by a concomitant hypoplasia of exocrine components (Fig. 26.31). Focal areas of necrosis may be round within larger endocrine nodules, and microcysts are a feature of the dysplastic organ [199]. The unusual appearance and size of the Beckwith-Wiedemann pancreas should not be confused with pancreatoblastoma, an embryoma that may arise in association with the syndrome [208–211]. Even though hypoglycemia is transient, Sotelo-Avila and Gooch [323] found islet cell hyperplasia on postmortem examination of five children with the

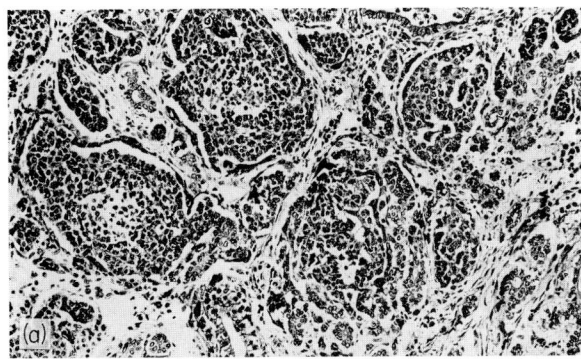

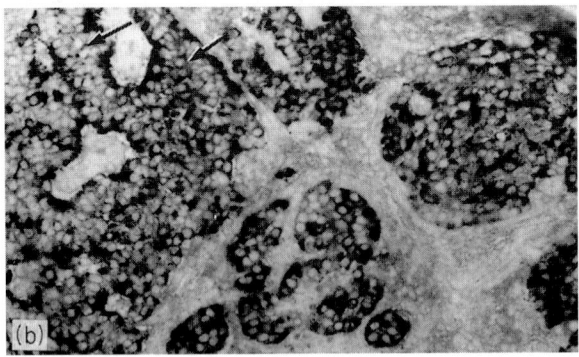

FIGURE 26.31.   *Beckwith-Wiedemann syndrome. (a) The pancreatic features may be those of diffuse adenomatosis, most of the parenchyma being formed by large irregular islet-like endocrine aggregates. Acinar hypoplasia is also present. Trichrome, ×98. (b) Insulin-glucagon double stain reveals the vast amount of endocrine tissue organized along the lines of normal islets, with the A cells lying peripheral to the lighter-staining B cells (arrows). Immunostain for insulin + glucagon, ×137.*

Beckwith-Wiedemann syndrome who died later in life with neoplasms.

Perlman Syndrome

Perlman syndrome is an autosomal recessively inherited disorder with macrosomia, visceromegaly, and unusual facies, with nephroblastomatosis, renal hamartomas, Wilms' tumor, cryptorchidism in males, polyhydramnios, and fetal ascites. About half the described cases are said to have islet cell hyperplasia, and one was clinically hypoglycemic [255].

Leprechaunism

Donohue [324] described infants with a characteristic facies, hirsutism, enlarged genitalia, decreased muscle, and subcutaneous tissue and "dysendocrinism." Intermittent hypoglycemia with hyperinsulinism may be present, and 67% of cases in a selected review of the literature had islet cell hyperplasia described at postmortem examination [250]. A defect in the insulin receptor gene has been reported (see Chap. 2).

Neurocristopathies

Endocrine overgrowth has been described in association with congenital neuroblastomas [235, 325]. Multiple endocrine neoplasia (MEN type 1) is characterized by tumors of the pituitary, parathyroids, and endocrine pancreas. Islet cell hyperplasia, adenomas with hyperplasia, multiple micro- and macroadenomas, and islet cell carcinomas have all been reported [252, 326]. Nesidioblastosis is not a feature in the adults studied. MEN type 2 is characterized by pheochromocytomas, medullary thyroid carcinomas, and pancreatic adenomas. Families with features of both MEN 1 and 2 have been described with familial pheochromocytomas and islet cell tumors [252], and all symptomatic patients have been more than 14 years of age.

Congenital Heart Disease

A nonquantitative study without documentation of hyperinsulinism describes the association of nesidioblastosis and congenital heart malformation [327].

Hereditary Tyrosinemia

This condition may be associated with glycosuria and refractory hypoglycemia. The pancreas has been shown to contain many large islets, occasionally with mitotic activity and hyalinization [248, 249]. A hepato-pancreato-renal disorder with neuropathy and abnormal polyunsaturated acids shares the hypoglycemia and islet cell hyperplasia of tyrosinemia, but the metabolic defect is different [168].

The Endocrine Pancreas in Sudden Infant Death Syndrome (SIDS)

The role of the endocrine pancreas in SIDS appears still to be a controversial area. In order to establish that a morphologic pancreatic finding was responsible for the death, it is essential that hypoglycemia and hyperinsulinism be documented. The presumption of cause based on pancreatic findings alone is insufficient, because it has been clearly documented that there is a dichotomy between the structure and the function; hyperinsulinism can occur with a normal-looking pancreas, and hyperinsulinism can be transient and disappear while the pancreatic endocrine hyperplasia persists. Worse yet, the normal newborn pancreas, rich in endocrine tissue and with its own peculiar distribution of cells, can be mistaken for pathologic nesidioblastosis. No pancreatic pathology was reported in reviews of the postmortem findings of SIDS victims [328], and detailed examination of the endocrine pancreas did not reveal suggestive features [329]. Hisaoka et al [330] claim to have found the morphologic changes of endocrine cell dysplasia (i.e., pathologic nesidioblastosis) in two of 15 SIDS cases, but again, no hypoglycemia or hyperinsulinism was documented. There are other cases in the literature in which undocumented hyperinsulinism was attributed to the finding of islet cell changes [331, 332]. On the other hand, hyperinsulinemic hypoglycemia *can* present as sudden unexplained death [333].

Endocrine Tumors

Most prior reports of adenomas in the fetus and neonate appear to be examples of focal adenomatosis. True adenomas may occur, but metastasizing endocrine carcinomas appear to be undocumented in this age group.

REFERENCES

1. McLean JM. Embryology of the pancreas. In: Howat HT, Sarles H, eds. *The Exocrine Pancreas*. Philadelphia: WB Saunders, 1979, pp. 3–13.
2. Opie EL. *Disease of the Pancreas, Its Cause and Nature*. Philadelphia: JB Lippincott, 1910.
3. Imrie JR, Fagan DG, Sturgess JM. Quantitative evaluation of the development of the exocrine pancreas in cystic fibrosis and control infants. *Am J Pathol* 1979; 95:697–707.
4. Laitio M, Lev R, Orlic D. The developing human fetal pancreas: an ultrastructural and histochemical study with special reference to exocrine cells. *J Anat* 1974; 117:619–34.
5. Lebenthal E, Lev R, Lee PC. Perinatal development of the exocrine pancreas. In: Lebenthal E, ed. *Textbook of Gastroenterology and Nutrition in Infancy*. New York: Raven, 1981, pp. 149–65.
6. Dupont C, Sellier N, Chochillon C, et al. Pancreatic lipomatosis and duodenal stenosis or atresia in children. *J Pediatr* 1989; 115:603–5.
7. Walsh E, Cramer B, Pushpanathan C. Pancreatic echogenicity in premature and newborn infants. *Pediatr Radiol* 1990; 20:323–35.
7a. Stoffers DA, Zinkin NT, Stanojevic V, et al. Pancreatic agenesis attributable to a single nucleotide deletion in the human IPF1 gene coding sequence. *Nat Genet* 1997; 15:106–10.
8. Dourov N, Buyl-Strouvens ML. Agenesie du pancreas. Observation anatomo-clinique d'un cas de diabete sucre, avec steatorhee et hypotrophie, chez un nouveau-ne. *Arch Fr Pediatr* 1969; 26:641–50.
9. Mehes K, Vamos K, Goda M. Agenesis of pancreas and gallbladder in an infant of incest. *Acta Paediatr Acad Sci Hung* 1976; 17:175–6.
10. Topke B, Menzel K. Die Pancreasagenesie des Neugenborenen, ein seltenes, klinisch aber charakteristisches Krankheitsbild. *Acta Paediatr Acad Sci Hung* 1976; 17:147–51.
11. Wright NM, Metzger DL, Borowitz SM, Clarke WL. Permanent neonatal diabetes mellitus and pancreatic exocrine insufficiency resulting from congenital pancreatic agenesis. *Am J Dis Child* 1993; 147:606–9. Letter.
12. Lemons JA, Ridenour R, Orsini EN. Congenital absence of the pancreas and intrauterine growth retardation. *Pediatrics* 1979; 64:255–7.
13. Hammar A. Ein Fall von Aplasie der Gallenblase und des Pankreas ventrale, sowie von Uberentwicklung der primären Gallengansplatte bei einen 7.2 mm langen Menschenembryo. *Z Mikrosk Anat Forsch* 1926; 5:90–4.
14. Kriss B. Zur kenntnis der Hypoplasie des Pankreas. *Virch Arch A* 1927; 263:591–8.
15. Welch KJ. The pancreas. In: Ravich M, ed. *Pediatric Surgery*. Chicago: Year Book Medical, 1979, pp. 857–61.
16. Wang JT, Lin JT, Chuang CN, et al. Complete agenesis of the dorsal pancreas—a case report and review of the literature. *Pancreas* 1990; 5:493–7.
17. Hatayama C, Wells TR. Syndrome of externally bilobed lungs with normal bronchial branch pattern, congenital heart disease, multiple spleens, intestinal malrotation and short pancreas: an apparently hitherto undefined malformation complex. *Pediatr Pathol* 1984; 2:127–33.
18. Drut RM, Drut R, Gilbert-Barness E, Reynolds JF Jr. Abnormal spleen lobulation and short pancreas. *Birth Defects* 1993; 29:345–52.
19. Dimmick JE, Pantzar T, Taylor GP, Norman M. Complete trisomy 22: pathologic analysis of three neonates. *Lab Invest* 1985; 52:4P–5P. Abstract.
20. Sherwood WC, Chance WG, Hill DC. A new syndrome of familial pancreatic agenesis: the role of insulin and glucagon in somatic and cell growth. *Pediatr Res* 1974; 8:360. Abstract.
21. Winter WE, McClaren NK, Riley WJ, et al. Congenital pancreatic hypoplasia: a syndrome of exocrine and endocrine pancreatic insufficiency. *J Pediatr* 1986; 109:465–8.
21a. Yorifuji T, Matsumura M, Okuno T, et al. Hereditary pancreatic hypoplasia, diabetes mellitus, and congenital heart disease: a new syndrome? *J Med Genet* 1994; 31:331–3.
22. Baldwin VJ, Kalousek DK, Dimmick JE, Applegarth DA, Hardwick DF. Diagnostic pathologic investigation of the malformed conceptus. *Perspect Pediatr Pathol* 1982; 7:65–108.
23. Sotelo-Avila C, Singer DB. Syndrome of hyperplastic fetal visceromegaly and neonatal hypoglycemia (Beckwith's syndrome). A report of 7 cases. *Pediatrics* 1970; 46:240–51.
24. Oppenheimer EH, Hardy JB. Congenital syphilis in the newborn infant: clinical and pathological observations in recent cases. *Johns Hopkins Med J* 1971; 129:63–82.
25. Becroft DM, Zwi LJ. Perinatal visceral fibrosis accompanying megakaryoblastic leukemoid reaction of Down syndrome. *Pediatr Pathol* 1990; 10:397–406.
26. Høyer A. Lipomatous pseudohypertrophy of the pancreas with complete absence of exocrine tissue. *J Pathol Bacteriol* 1949; 61:93–100.
27. Kissane JM. *Pathology of Infancy and Childhood*. 2nd ed. St. Louis: CV Mosby, 1975, p. 329.
28. Adeyemi SD. Combination of annular pancreas and partial situs inversus: a multiple organ malrotation syndrome associated with duodenal obstruction. *J Pediatr Surg* 1988; 23:188–91.
29. Elliot GB, Kliman MR, Elliot KA. Pancreatic annulus: a sign or a cause of duodenal obstruction? *Can J Surg* 1968; 11:357–64.
30. Johnston DW. Annular pancreas: a new classification and clinical observation. *Can J Surg* 1978; 21:241–4.
31. Merril JR, Raffensperger JG. Pediatric annular pancreas: twenty years' experience. *J Pediatr Surg* 1976; 11:921–5.
32. Kiernan PD, ReMine SG, Kiernan PC, ReMine WH. Annular pancreas: Mayo Clinic experience from 1957 to 1976 with review of the literature. *Arch Surg* 1980; 115:46–50.
33. Blaustein HS, Stevens AW, Stevens PD, Grossman ME. Rothmund-Thomson syndrome associated with annular pancreas and duodenal stenosis: a case report. *Pediatr Dermatol* 1993; 10:159–63.
34. Weissberg H. Ein Pancreas annulare bei einem menschlichen Embryo von 16 mm Länge. *Anat Anz* 1935; 79:296–301.
35. Ikeda Y, Irving IM. Annular pancreas in a fetus and its three-dimensional reconstruction. *J Pediatr Surg* 1984; 19:160–4.
36. Baetens D, Malaisse-Lagae F, Perrelet A, Orci L. Endocrine pancreas: three-dimensional reconstruction shows two types of islets of Langerhans. *Science* 1979; 206:1323–5.
37. Sessa F, Fiocca R, Tenti P, et al. Pancreatic polypeptide rich tissue in the annular pancreas. A distinctive feature of ventral primordium derivates. *Virch Arch A Pathol Anat Histopathol* 1983; 399:227–32.
38. Montgomery RC, Poindexter MH, Hall GH, Leigh JE. Report of a case of annular pancreas of the newborn in two consecutive siblings. *Pediatrics* 1971; 48:148–50.
39. Jackson LG, Apostolides P. Autosomal dominant inheritance of annular pancreas. *Am J Med Genet* 1978; 1:319–21.
40. MacFayden UM, Young ID. Annular pancreas in mother and son. *Am J Med Genet* 1987; 27:987–8. Letter.
41. Hendricks SK, Sybert VP. Association of annular pancreas and duodenal obstruction—evidence for mendelian inheritance? *Clin Genet* 1991; 39:383–5.
42. Millbourn E. On the excretory ducts of the pancreas in man, with special reference to their relations to each other, to common bile duct and to duodenum. Radiological and anatomical study. *Acta Anat* 1950; 9:1–34.
43. Berman LG, Prior JT, Abramow SM, Ziegler DD. A study of the pancreatic duct system in man by the use of vinyl acetate casts of postmortem preparations. *Surg Gynecol Obstet* 1960; 110:391–403.
44. Donahoe PK, Hendren WH. Bile duct perforation in a newborn with stenosis of the ampulla of Vater. *J Pediatr Surg* 1976; 11:823–5.
45. Wong KC, Lister J. Human fetal development of the hepato-pancreatic duct junction—a possible explanation of congenital dilatation of the biliary tract. *J Pediatr Surg* 1981; 16:139–45.
46. Cangiarella J, Thomas PA, Genieser NB, Greco MA. Pancreatitis due to anomalous junction of the pancreaticobiliary ductal system. *Pediatr Pathol* 1993; 3:853–61.
47. Seifert G. Congenital anomalies. In: Klöppel G, Heitz PU, eds. *Pancreatic Pathology*. New York: Churchill Livingstone, 1984, pp. 22–6.
48. Lai EC, Tompkins PK. Heterotopic pancreas: review of a 26 year experience. *Am J Surg* 1986; 151:697–700.
49. Hara M, Tsutsumi Y. Immunohistochemical studies of endocrine cells in heterotopic pancreas. *Virch Arch A Pathol Anat Histol* 1986; 408:385–94.

50. Mobini J, Krouse TB, Cooper DR. Intrahepatic pancreatic heterotopia: review and report of a case presenting as an abdominal mass. *Am J Dig Dis* 1974; 19:64–70.

51. Gonzalez OR, Hardin WD Jr, Isaacs H Jr, Lally KP, Brennan LP. Duplication of the hepatopancreatic bud presenting as pyloric stenosis. *J Pediatr Surg* 1988; 23:1053–4.

52. Gruenwald P, Levine W, Zeichner S. Enterogenous cyst and cystadenoma of the omentum. *Am J Surg* 1954; 87:775–9.

53. Spence RK, Schnaufer L, Mahboubi S. Co-existent gastric duplication and accessory pancreas: clinical manifestations, embryogenesis and treatment. *J Pediatr Surg* 1986; 21:68–70.

54. Black PR, Welch KJ, Eraklis AJ. Juxtapancreatic intestinal duplications with pancreatic ductal communication: a cause of pancreatitis and recurrent abdominal pain in childhood. *J Pediatr Surg* 1986; 21:257–61.

55. Willis RA. *The Borderland of Embryology and Pathology*. London: Butterworth, 1958, p. 285.

56. Mason TE, Quagliarello JR. Ectopic pancreas in the fallopian tube: report of a first case. *Obstet Gynecol* 1976; 48:70S–75S.

57. Harris LE, Wenzl JE. Heterotopic pancreatic tissue and intestinal mucosa in the umbilical cord. Report of a case. *N Engl J Med* 1963; 268:721–2.

58. Schumberger HG. Teratoma of the anterior mediastinum in the group of military age, study of 16 cases and review of theories of genesis. *Arch Pathol* 1946; 41:398–444.

59. Abell MR, Johnson VJ, Holtz F. Ovarian neoplasms in childhood and adolescence. 1. Tumors of germ cell origin. *Am J Obstet Gynecol* 1965; 92:1059–81.

60. Resnick JM, Manivel JC. Immunohistochemical characterization of teratomatous and fetal neuroendocrine pancreas. *Arch Pathol Lab Med* 1994; 118:155–9.

61. Honicky RE, dePapp EW. Mediastinal teratoma with endocrine function. *Am J Dis Child* 1973; 126:650–3.

62. Jaffe BM, Ferguson TB, Holtz S, Shields JB. Mediastinal pancreatic pseudo-cysts. *Am J Surg* 1972; 124:600–6.

63. Beskin CA. Intralobar enteric sequestration of the lung containing aberrant pancreas. *J Thorac Cardiovasc Surg* 1961; 41:314–17.

64. Corrin B, Danel C, Allawoy A, Warner J, Lenney W. Intralobar pulmonary sequestration of ectopic pancreatic tissue with gastropancreatic duplication. *Thorax* 1985; 40:637–8.

65. Hodes JE, Hull MT, Mirkin LD, Hodes ME. Immunohistochemical demonstration of altered functional differentiation of pancreatic tissue in sacrococcygeal teratomas. *Hum Pathol* 1983; 14:724–6.

66. Dunn PJ. Pancreatic endocrine tissue in benign mediastinal teratoma. *J Clin Pathol* 1984; 37:1105–9.

67. Akers DR, Favara BE, Franciosi RA, Nelson JM. Duplications of the alimentary tract: report of three unusual cases associated with bile and pancreatic ducts. *Surgery* 1972; 71:817–23.

68. Wold M, Callery M, White JJ. Ectopic gastric-like duplication of the pancreas. *J Pediatr Surg* 1988; 23:1051–2.

69. Seifert G. *Die Pathologie des Kindlichen Pankreas*. Leipzig: Geory Thieme, 1956.

70. Miles RM. Pancreatic cyst in a newborn. *Ann Surg* 1959; 149:576–81.

71. Carcassone M, Delarue A, Ille O, et al. Lesions kystiques du pancreas de l'enfant. *Chirurgie* 1971; 110:143–58.

72. Mares AJ, Hirsch M. Congenital cysts of the head of the pancreas. *J Pediatr Surg* 1977; 12:547–52.

73. Baker LL, Hartman GE, Northway WH. Sonographic detection of congenital pancreatic cysts in the newborn: report of a case and review of the literature. *Pediatr Radiol* 1990; 20:488–90.

74. Auringer ST, Ulmer JL, Sumner TE, Turner CS. Congenital cyst of the pancreas. *J Pediatr Surg* 1993; 28:1570–1.

74a. Crowley JJ, McAlister WH. Congenital pancreatic pseudocyst: a rare cause of abdominal mass in a neonate. *Pediatr Radiol* 1996; 26:210–11.

74b. Daher P, Diab N, Melki I, et al. Congenital cyst of the pancreas. Antenatal diagnosis. *Eur J Ped Surg* 1996; 6:180–2.

75. Potter EL, Craig JM. *Pathology of the Fetus and Infant*. 3rd ed. Chicago: Year Book Medical, 1975, p. 349.

76. Rapola J, Salonen R. Visceral anomalies in the Meckel syndrome. *Teratology* 1985; 31:193–201.

77. Ivemark BI, Oldfelt V, Zetterstrom R. Familial dysplasia of kidneys, liver and pancreas: a probably genetically determined syndrome. *Acta Pediatr* 1959; 48:1–11.

78. Crawfurd MD. Renal dysplasia and asplenia in two sibs. *Clin Genet* 1978; 14:338–44.

79. Strayer DS, Kissane JM. Dysplasia of the kidneys, liver and pancreas: report of a variant of Ivemark's syndrome. *Hum Pathol* 1979; 10:228–34.

80. Yeoh GP, Bannatyne PM, Russel P, Storey B. Combined renal and pancreatic dysplasia in the newborn. *Pathology* 1985; 17:658–67.

81. Hiraoka K, Haratake J, Horie A, Miyagawa T. Bilateral renal dysplasia, pancreatic fibrosis, intrahepatic biliary dysgenesis and situs inversus totalis in a boy. *Hum Pathol* 1988; 19:871–3.

82. De Lange C, Janssen TA. Large solitary cyst and other developmental errors in a premature infant. *Am J Dis Child* 1948; 75:587–94.

83. Gibb B. Das angeborne Zystenpankreas. *Zentralbl Allg Pathol Anat* 1962; 103:524–8.

84. Hashida Y, Jaffe R, Yunis EJ. Pancreatic pathology in trisomy 13: specificity of the morphologic lesion. *Pediatr Pathol* 1983; 1:169–78.

85. Jenkins JM, Othersen HB Jr. Cystadenoma of the pancreas in a newborn. *J Pediatr Surg* 1992; 27:1569.

86. Amir G, Hurvitz H, Neeman Z, Rosenmann E. Neonatal cytomegalovirus infection with pancreatic cystadenoma and nephrotic syndrome. *Pediatr Pathol* 1986; 6:393–401.

87. Chang CH, Perrin EV, Hertzler J, Brough AJ. Cystadenoma of the pancreas with cytomegalovirus infection in a female infant. *Arch Pathol Lab Med* 1980; 104:7–8.

88. Hopper MS, Boultbee JE, Watson AR. Polyhydramnios associated with congenital pancreatic cysts and asphyxiating thoracic dysplasia. A case report. *S Afr Med J* 1979; 56:32–3.

89. Bernstein R. Short rib polydactyly syndrome, type I. In: Buyse ML, ed. *Birth Defects Encyclopedia*. vol 2. Cambridge: Blackwell, 1990, pp. 1528–9.

90. Bernstein J, Chandra M, Creswell J, et al. Renal-hepatic-pancreatic dysplasia: a syndrome reconsidered. *Am J Med Genet* 1987; 26:391–403.

91. Marin-Padilla M, Hoefnagel D, Benirschke K. Anatomic and histopathologic study of two cases of D₁ (13–15) trisomy. *Cytogenetics* 1964; 3:258–84.

92. Mottet NK, Jensen H. The anomalous embryonic development associated with trisomy 13–15. *Am J Clin Pathol* 1965; 43:334–47.

93. Rohde RA, Hodgman JE, Cleland RS. Multiple congenital anomalies in the E₁-trisomy (group 16–18) syndrome. *Pediatrics* 1964; 33:258–70.

94. Doshi N, Surti U, Szulman AE. Morphologic anomalies in triploid liveborn fetuses. *Hum Pathol* 1983; 14:716–23.

95. Lee PC, Lebenthal E. Prenatal and postnatal development of the human exocrine pancreas. In: Go VLW, DeMagno EP, Gardner JD, et al, eds. *The Pancreas: Biology, Pathobiology and Disease*. 2nd ed. New York: Raven, 1993, pp. 57–73.

96. Davis MM, Hodes ME, Munsick RA, Ulbright TM, Goldstein DJ. Pancreatic amylase expression in human pancreatic development. *Hybridoma* 1986; 5:137–45.

97. Track NS, Creutzfeldt C, Bokermann M. Enzymatic, functional and ultrastructural development of the exocrine pancreas. II. The human pancreas. *Comp Biochem Physiol A* 1975; 51(1A):95–100.

98. Lebenthal E, Lee PC. Development of functional responses in human exocrine pancreas. *Pediatrics* 1980; 66:556–60.

99. Heitlinger LA, Lee PC, Dillon WP, Lebenthal E. Mammary amylase: a possible alternate pathway of carbohydrate digestion in infancy. *Pediatr Res* 1983; 17:15–18.

100. Dubois PM, Paulin C, Chayvialle JA. Identification of gastrin secreting cells and cholecystokinin secreting cells in the gastrointestinal tract of the human fetus and adult man. *Cell Tissue Res* 1976; 175:351–6.

101. Zoppi G, Andreotti G, Pajno-Ferrara F, Bellini P, Gaburro D. The development of specific responses of the exocrine pancreas to pancreozymin and secretin stimulation in newborn infants. *Pediatr Res* 1973; 7:198–203.

102. Palade GE. Intracellular aspects of the process of protein synthesis. *Science* 1975; 189:347–58.

103. Rothman SS. Protein transport by the pancreas. *Science* 1975; 190:747–53.

104. Rothman SS. Independent secretion of different digestive enzymes by the pancreas. *Am J Physiol* 1976; 231:1847–51.

105. Scheele GA. Regulation of pancreatic gene expression in response to hormone and nutritional substrates. In: Go VLW, DeMagno EP, Gardner JD, et al, eds. *The Pancreas: Biology, Pathobiology and Disease*. 2nd ed. New York: Raven, 1993, pp. 103–34.

106. Pour P. Pancreatic centroacinar cells. The regulator of both exocrine and endocrine function. *Int J Pancreatol* 1994; 15:51–64.

107. Adelson JW, Miller PE. Pancreatic secretion by nonparallel exocytosis: potential resolution of a long controversy. *Science* 1985; 228:993–6.

108. Williams JA, Goldfine ID. The insulin-acinar relationship. In: Go VLW, DeMagno EP, Gardner JD, et al, eds. *The Pancreas: Biology, Pathobiology and Disease*. 2nd ed. New York: Raven, 1993, pp. 789–802.

109. Lieberman J. Proteolytic enzyme activity in fetal pancreas and meconium. Demonstration of plasminogen and trypsinogen activators in pancreatic tissue. *Gastroenterology* 1966; 50:183–90.

110. Lerner A, Lebenthal E. Hereditary diseases of the pancreas. In: Go VLW, DeMagno EP, Gardner JD, et al, eds. *The Pancreas: Biology, Pathobiology and Disease.* 2nd ed. New York: Raven, 1993, pp. 1083–94.

111. Townes PL. Trypsinogen deficiency disease. *J Pediatr* 1965; 66:275–85.

112. Morris MD, Fisher DA. Trypsinogen deficiency disease. *Am J Dis Child* 1967; 114:203–8.

113. Lebenthal E, Antonowicz I, Shwachman H. Enterokinase and trypsin activities in pancreatic insufficiency and diseases of the small intestine. *Gastroenterology* 1976; 70:508–12.

114. Figarella C, De Caro A, Leupold D, Poley JR. Congenital pancreatic lipase deficiency. *J Pediatr* 1980; 96:412–16.

115. Lilibridge CB, Townes PL. Physiologic deficiency of pancreatic amylase in infancy: a factor in iatrogenic diarrhea. *J Pediatr* 1973; 82:279–82.

116. Shwachman H, Diamond LK, Oski FA, Khaw KT. The syndrome of pancreatic insufficiency and bone marrow dysfunction. *J Pediatr* 1964; 65:645–63.

117. Lumb G, Beautyman W. Hypoplasia of the exocrine tissue of the pancreas. *J Pathol Bacteriol* 1952; 64:679–86.

118. Seifert G. Lipomatöse cystiche Pankreasfibrose und lipomatöse Pankreatrophie des Kindesalters. *Beitr Pathol Anat* 1959; 121:64–80.

119. Nezelof C, Watchi M. L'hypoplasie congénitale lipomateuse du pancreas exocrine chez l'enfant. Deux observations et revue de la litteratuer. *Arch Fr Pediatr* 1961; 18:1135–72.

120. Bodian M, Sheldon W, Lightwood R. Congenital hypoplasia of the exocrine pancreas. *Acta Paediatr (Stockholm)* 1964; 53:282–93.

121. Townes PL. Proteolytic and lipolytic deficiency of the exocrine pancreas. *J Pediatr* 1969; 75:221–8.

122. Burke V, Colebatch JH, Anderson CM, Simons MJ. Association of pancreatic insufficiency and chronic neutropenia in childhood. *Arch Dis Child* 1967; 42:147–57.

123. Karjoo M, Koop CE, Cornfeld D, Holtzapple PG. Pancreatic exocrine enzyme deficiency associated with asphyxiating thoracic dystrophy. *Arch Dis Child* 1973; 48:143–6.

124. Huijgens PC, van der Veen EA, Meijer S, Muntinghe OG. Syndrome of Shwachman and leukemia. *Scand J Haematol* 1977; 18:20–4.

125. Strevens MJ, Lilleyman JS, Williams RB. Shwachman's syndrome and acute lymphoblastic leukaemia. *Br Med J* 1978; 2:18.

126. Caselitz J, Klöppel G, Delling G, et al. Shwachman's syndrome and leukaemia. *Virch Arch A Pathol Anat Histopathol* 1979; 385:109–16.

127. Aggett PJ, Cavanagh NP, Matthew DJ, et al. Shwachman's syndrome. A review of 21 cases. *Arch Dis Child* 1980; 55:331–47.

128. Dossetors JF, Spratt HC, Rolles CJ, Seem CP, Heely AF. Immunoreactive trypsin in Shwachman's syndrome. *Arch Dis Child* 1989; 64:395–6.

128a. Mack DR, Forstner GG, Wilschanski M, et al. Schwachman syndrome: exocrine pancreatic dysfunction and variable phenotypic expression. *Gastroenterology* 1996; 111:1593–602.

129. Johanson A, Blizzard R. A syndrome of congenital aplasia of the alae nasi, deafness, hypothyroidism, dwarfism, absent permanent teeth and malabsorption. *J Pediatr* 1971; 79:982–7.

130. Schussheim A, Choi SJ, Silverberg M. Exocrine pancreatic insufficiency with congenital abnormalities. *J Pediatr* 1976; 89:782–4.

131. Daentl DL, Frias JL, Gilbert EF, Optiz JM. The Johanson-Blizzard syndrome: case report and autopsy findings. *Am J Med Genet* 1979; 3:129–35.

132. Gershoni-Baruch R, Lerner A, Braun J, et al. Johanson-Blizzard syndrome: clinical spectrum and further delineation of the syndrome. *Am J Med Genet* 1990; 35:546–51.

133. Grand RJ, Rosen SW, Di Sant'Agnese PA, Kirkham WR. Unusual case of XXY Kleinfelter's syndrome with pancreatic insufficiency, hypothyroidism, deafness, chronic lung disease, dwarfism and microcephaly. *Am J Med* 1966; 41:478–85.

134. Moeschler JB, Polak MJ, Jenkins JJ III, Amato RS. The Johanson-Blizzard syndrome: a second report of full autopsy findings. *Am J Med Genet* 1987; 26:133–8.

135. Szilagyi PG, Corsetti J, Callahan CM, McCormick K, Metlay LA. Pancreatic exocrine aplasia, clinical features of leprechaunism and abnormal gonadotropin regulation. *Pediatr Pathol* 1987; 7:51–61.

136. Sandhu BK, Brueton MJ. Concurrent pancreatic and growth hormone insufficiency in Johanson-Blizzard syndrome. *J Pediatr Gastroenterol Nutr* 1989; 9:535–8.

137. Fanconi G, Uehlinger E, Knauer C. Das Coeliakiesyndrom dei angeborener zystischer Pankreasfibromatose und Bronchiektasien. *Wien Med Wchnschr* 1936; 86:753–6.

138. Andersen DH. Cystic fibrosis of the pancreas and its relation to celiac disease: clinical and pathologic study. *Am J Dis Child* 1933; 56:344–99.

139. Farber S. Pancreatic function and disease in early life; pathologic changes associated with pancreatic insufficiency in early life. *Arch Pathol* 1944; 37:238–50.

140. Taussig LM. *Cystic Fibrosis.* New York: Thieme-Stratton, 1984.

141. Kerem B, Rommens JM, Buchanan JA, et al. Identification of the cystic fibrosis gene: genetic analysis. *Science* 1989; 245:1073–80.

142. Riordan JR, Rommens JM, Kerem B, et al. Identification of the cystic fibrosis gene: cloning and characterization of complementary DNA. *Science* 1989; 245:1066–73.

143. Rommens JM, Iannuzzi MC, Kerem B, et al. Identification of the cystic fibrosis gene: chromosome walking and jumping. *Science* 1989; 245:1059–65.

144. Kerem E, Corey M, Kerem BS, et al. The relationships between genotype and phenotype in cystic fibrosis; analysis of the most common mutation (▲F508). *N Engl J Med* 1990; 323:1517–22.

145. Shwachman H, Dooley RR, Guilmette F, et al. Cystic fibrosis of the pancreas with varying degrees of pancreatic insufficiency. *Am J Dis Child* 1956; 92:347–68.

146. Oppenheimer EH, Esterly JR. Pathology of cystic fibrosis. Review of the literature and comparison with 146 autopsied cases. *Perspect Pediatr Pathol* 1975; 2:241–78.

147. Sturgess JM. Structural and developmental abnormalities of the exocrine pancreas in cystic fibrosis. *J Pediatr Gastroenterol Nutr* 1984; 3(suppl 1):S55–S66.

148. Gaskin K, Waters D, Dorney S, et al. Assessment of pancreatic function in screened infants with cystic fibrosis. *Pediatr Pulmonol* 1991; 7(suppl): 69–71.

149. Kopito LE, Shwachman H, Vawter GF, Edlow J. The pancreas in cystic fibrosis. Chemical composition and comparative morphology. *Pediatr Res* 1976; 10:742–9.

150. Tizzano EF, Chitayat D, Buchwald M. Cell-specific localization of CFTR mRNA shows developmentally regulated expression in human fetal tissues. *Hum Mol Genet* 1993; 2:219–24.

151. Foulkes AG, Harris A. Localization of expression of the cystic fibrous gene in human pancreatic development. *Pancreas* 1993; 8:3–6.

152. Ornoy A, Arnon J, Katznelson D, et al. Pathological confirmation of cystic fibrosis in the fetus following prenatal diagnosis. *Am J Med Genet* 1987; 28:935–47.

153. Gosden CM, Gosden JR. Fetal abnormalities in cystic fibrosis suggest a deficiency in proteolysis of cholecystokinin. *Lancet* 1984; 2:541–6.

154. Forstner GG, Vesely SM, Durie PR. Selective precipitation of 14 kDa stone thread proteins by concentration of pancreaticobiliary secretions: relevance to pancreatic ductal obstruction, pancreatic failure and CF. *J Pediatr Gastroenterol Nutr* 1989; 8:313–20.

155. Mally M, Otonkoski T, Lopez AD, Hayek A. Developmental gene expression in the human fetal pancreas. *Pediatr Res* 1994; 36:537–44.

156. Silver MM, Valberg LS, Cutz E, Lines LD, Phillips MJ. Hepatic morphology and iron quantitation in perinatal hemochromatosis. Comparison with a large perinatal control population, including cases with chronic liver disease. *Am J Pathol* 1993; 143:1312–25.

157. Goldfischer S, Grotsky HW, Chang CH, et al. Idiopathic neonatal iron storage involving the liver, pancreas, heart and endocrine and exocrine glands. *Hepatology* 1981; 1:58–64.

158. Blisard KS, Bartow SA. Neonatal hemochromatosis. *Hum Pathol* 1986; 17:376–83.

159. Knisely AS, Magid MS, Dische MR, Cutz E. Neonatal hemochromatosis. *Birth Defects* 1987; 22:75–102.

160. Silver MM, Beverley DW, Valberg LS, et al. Perinatal hemochromatosis. Clinical morphologic and quantitative iron studies. *Am J Pathol* 1987; 128:538–54.

161. Singla PN, Gupta VK, Agarwal KN. Storage iron in human foetal organs. *Acta Paediatr Scand* 1985; 74:701–6.

162. Pearson HA, Lobel JS, Kocoshis SA, et al. A new syndrome of refractory sideroblastic anemia with vacuolization of marrow precursors and exocrine pancreatic dysfunction. *J Pediatr* 1979; 95:976–84.

163. Rötig A, Cormier V, Blanche S, et al. Pearson's marrow-pancreas syndrome. A multisystem mitochondrial disorder in infancy. *J Clin Invest* 1990; 86:1601–8.

164. McShane MA, Hammans SR, Sweeney M, et al. Pearson syndrome and mitochondrial encephalomyopathy in a patient with a deletion of mtDNA. *Am J Hum Genet* 1991; 48:39–42.

165. Morikawa Y, Matsuura N, Kakudo K, et al. Pearson's marrow/pancreas syndrome: a histological and genetic study. *Virch Arch A Pathol Anat Histopathol* 1993; 423:227–31.

166. Larsson NG, Holme E, Kristiansson B, Oldfors A, Wilinius M. Progressive increase of the mutated mitochondrial DNA fraction in Kearns-Sayre syndrome. *Pediatr Res* 1990; 28:131–6.

167. Kocoshis SA, McGuire JS, Arulananthan K, Flynn FJ Jr, Gryboski JD. Congenital cutis laxa associated with exocrine pancreatic insufficiency. *J Clin Gastroenterol* 1981; 3(suppl 1):69–71.

168. Sharp HL, Lindahl A, Freese DK, et al. A new hepato-pancreato-renal disorder resembling tyrosinemia involving neuropathy and abnormal metabolism of polyunsaturated acids. *J Pediatr Gastroenterol Nutr* 1988; 7:167–76.

169. Baggenstoss AH. The pancreas in uremia. *Am J Pathol* 1947; 23:908–9.

170. Ellis D, Fisher SE, Smith WI Jr, Jaffe R. Familial occurrence of renal and intestinal disease associated with tissue autoantibodies. *Am J Dis Child* 1982; 136:323–6.

171. Kattwinkel J, Lapey A, Di Sant'Agnese PA, Edwards WA. Hereditary pancreatitis: three new kindreds and a critical review of the literature. *Pediatrics* 1973; 51:55–69.

172. Whitcomb DC. A gene for hereditary pancreatitis maps to chromosome 7q35. *Gastroenterology* 1996; 110:1975–80.

172a. Whitcomb DC. Hereditary pancreatitis is caused by a mutation in the cationic trypsinogen gene. *Nat Genet* 1996; 14:141–5.

173. Kahler SG, Sherwood WG, Woolf D, et al. Pancreatitis in patients with organic acidemias. *J Pediatr* 1994; 124:239–43.

174. Jenson AB, Rosenberg HS, Notkins AL. Pancreatic islet-cell damage in children with fatal viral infections. *Lancet* 1980; 2:354–8.

175. Bunnell CE, Monif GR. Interstitial pancreatitis in the congenital rubella syndrome. *J Pediatr* 1972; 80:465–6.

176. Donowitz M, Gryboski JD. Pancreatic insufficiency and congenital rubella syndrome. *J Pediatr* 1975; 87:241–3.

177. Johnson GM, Tudor RB. Diabetes mellitus and congenital rubella infection. *Am J Dis Child* 1970; 120:453–5.

178. Sibert JR. Pancreatitis in children. A study in the North of England. *Arch Dis Child* 1975; 50:443–8.

179. Kibrick S, Benirschke K. Severe generalized disease (encephalohep-atomyocarditis) occurring in the newborn period and due to infection with Coxsackie virus, group B; evidence of intrauterine infection with this agent. *Pediatrics* 1958; 22:857–75.

180. Koch F, Enders-Ruckle G, Wokittel E. Coxsackie B5-Infektionen mit signifikanter Antikörperentwicklung bei Neugeborenen. *Arch Kinderheilk* 1962; 165:245–58.

181. Gladisch R, Hofmann W, Waldherr R. Myokarditis und Insulitis nach Coxsackie Virus-Infekt. *Z Kardiol* 1976; 65:837–49.

182. Ujevich MM, Jaffe R. Pancreatic islet cell damage. Its occurrence in neonatal coxsackievirus encephalomyocarditis. *Arch Pathol Lab Med* 1980; 104:438–41.

183. Winsser J, Altieri RH. A three-year study of coxsackie virus, group B, infection in Nassau County. *Am J Med Sci* 1964; 274:269–73.

184. Frank JA Jr, Warren RW, Tucker JA, Zeller J, Wilfert CM. Disseminated parainfluenza infection in a child with severe combined immunodeficiency. *Am J Dis Child* 1983; 135:1172–4.

185. Washington K, Gossage DL, Gottfried MR. Pathology of the pancreas in severe combined immunodeficiency and DiGeorge syndrome: acute graft-versus-host disease and unusual viral infections. *Hum Pathol* 1994; 25:908–14.

186. Raeburn C. Gumma of the pancreas in a premature infant. *J Pathol Bacteriol* 1951; 63:158–9.

187. Blumenthal HT, Probstein JG. Acute pancreatitis in the newborn, in infancy and in childhood. *Am Surg* 1961; 27:533–9.

188. Frey C, Redo SF. Inflammatory lesions of the pancreas in infancy and childhood. *Pediatrics* 1963; 32:93–102.

189. Valdes-Dapena MA, Arey JB. Boric acid poisoning. Three fatal cases with pancreatic inclusions and a review of the literature. *J Pediatr* 1962; 61:531–46.

190. Nakamura N. Untersuchungen über Pankreas bei Föten, Neugeborenen, Kindern und in Pubertätsalter (Mit einem Anhang: Fälle mit Diabetes und Glykosurie). *Virch Arch A* 1924; 253:286–349.

191. Jansen A, Voorbij HA, Jeucken PH, et al. An immunohistochemical study on organized lymphoid cell infiltrates in fetal and neonatal pancreas. A comparison with similar infiltrates found in the pancreas of a diabetic infant. *Autoimmunity* 1993; 15:31–8.

192. Liu HM, Potter EL. Development of the human pancreas. *Arch Pathol* 1962; 74:439–52.

193. Jonas MM, Bell MD, Eidson MS, Koutouby R, Hensley GT. Congenital diabetes mellitus and fatal secretory diarrhea in two infants. *J Pediatr Gastroenterol Nutr* 1991; 13:415–25.

194. Roberts J, Searle J. Neonatal diabetes mellitus associated with severe diarrhea, hyperimmunoglobulin E syndrome, and absence of islets of Langerhans. *Pediatr Pathol* 1995; 15:477–83.

195. Schulz DM, Giordano DA, Schulz DH. Weights of organs of fetuses and infants. *Arch Pathol* 1962; 74:244–50.

196. Eraklis AJ, Filler RM. Splenectomy in childhood: a review of 1413 cases. *J Pediatr Surg* 1977; 7:382–8.

197. Burt TB, Condon VR, Matlak ME. Fetal pancreatic hamartoma. *Pediatr Radiol* 1983; 13:287–9.

198. Flaherty MJ, Benjamin DR. Multicystic pancreatic hamartoma: a distinctive lesion with immunohistochemical and ultrastructural study. *Hum Pathol* 1992; 23:1309–12.

199. Stiegman CK, Uri AK, Chatten J, Peckham GJ. Beckwith-Wiedemann syndrome with unusual hepatic and pancreatic features: a case expanding the phenotype. *Pediatr Pathol* 1990; 10:593–600.

200. Tunell WP. Hemangioendothelioma of the pancreas obstructing the common bile duct and duodenum. *J Pediatr Surg* 1976; 11:827–30.

201. Villegas-Alvarez F, de Léon-Bojorge BY. Hemangioendotelioma del páncreas y colédoco, como couse de sindromes colestásico neonatal y de Kasabach-Merritt. *Bol Med Hosp Infant Mex* 1989; 46:672–5.

202. Zukerberg LR, Nickoloff BJ, Weiss SW. Kaposiform hemangioendothelioma of infancy and childhood. An aggressive neoplasm associated with Kasabach-Merritt syndrome and lymphangiomatosis. *Am J Surg Pathol* 1993; 17:321–8.

203. Assawamatiyanont S, King AD Jr. Dermoid cysts of the pancreas. *Am Surg* 1977; 43:503–4.

204. DeCourcy JL. Dermoid cyst of the pancreas: case report. *Ann Surg* 1943; 118:394–5.

205. Eichler P. Ein Fall von Kongenitalem Lymphosarkom des Pancreas. *Frankf Z Pathol* 1928; 36:326–33.

206. L'Huillier A. Uber Einen Fall von Kongenitalem lymphosarkom des pankreas. *Virch Arch* 1904; 178:507–9.

207. Horie A. Pancreatoblastoma. Histopathologic criteria based upon a review of 6 cases. In: Humphrey GB, Grindey GB, Dehner LP, Acton RT, Pyscher TJ, eds. *Pancreatic Tumors in Children.* vol. 8. *Cancer Treatment and Research.* The Hague: Martinus Nijhoff, 1982, pp. 159–66.

208. O'Hara D. Pancreatoblastoma—does it exist? *Pediatr Pathol* 1985; 3:118–19. Abstract.

209. Koh TH, Cooper JE, Newman CL, et al. Pancreatoblastoma in a neonate with Wiedemann-Beckwith syndrome. *Eur J Pediatr* 1986; 145:435–8.

210. Potts SR, Brown S, O'Hara MD. Pancreatoblastoma in a neonate associated with Beckwith-Wiedemann syndrome. *Z Kinderchir* 1986; 41:56–7.

211. Drut R, Jones MC. Congenital pancreatoblastoma in Beckwith-Wiedemann syndrome. An emerging association. *Pediatr Pathol* 1988; 8:331–9.

212. Kissane JM. Pancreatoblastoma and solid and cystic papillary tumor: two tumors related to pancreatic ontogeny. *Sem Diagn Pathol* 1994; 11:152–63.

213. Ferner H, Stoeckinius W Jr. Die Cytogenese des Inselsystems beim Menschen. *Z Zellforsch Mikrosk Anat* 1950; 35:147–75.

214. Robb P. The development of the islets of Langerhans in the human foetus. *Q J Exp Physiol* 1961; 46:335–43.

215. Conklin JL. Cytogenesis of the human fetal pancreas. *Am J Anat* 1962; 111:181–93.

216. Like AA, Orci L. Embryogenesis of the human pancreatic islets. A light and electron microscopic study. *Diabetes* 1972; 2:511–34.

217. Erlandsen SL. Types of pancreatic islet cells and their immunocytochemical identification. In: Fitzgerald PJ, Morrison AB, eds. *The Pancreas.* Baltimore: Williams & Wilkins, 1980, pp. 140–55.

218. Klöppel G, Lenzen S. Anatomy and physiology of the endocrine pancreas. In: Klöppel G, Heitz PU, eds. *Pancreatic Pathology.* New York: Churchill Livingstone, 1984, pp. 133–53.

219. Le Douarin NM. On the origin of pancreatic endocrine cells. *Cell* 1988; 53:169–71.

220. Dubois PM. Ontogeny of the endocrine pancreas. *Horm Res* 1989; 32:53–60.

221. Clark A, Grant AM. Quantitative morphology of endocrine cells in human fetal pancreas. *Diabetologia* 1983; 25:31–5.

222. Hahn von Dorsche H, Fält K, Titebach M, et al. Immunohistochemical, morphometric and ultrastructural observations of the early development of insulin, somatostatin, glucagon and PP cells in the foetal human pancreas. *Diabetes Res* 1989; 12:51–6.

223. Emery JL, Bury HPR. Involutionary changes in the islets of Langerhans in the foetus and newborn. *Biol Neonat* 1964; 6:16–25.

224. Falin LI. The development and cytodifferentiation of the islets of Langerhans in human embryos and foetuses. *Acta Anat* 1967; 68:147–68.

225. Pictet R, Rutter WJ. Development of the embryonic pancreas. In: Greep RO, Astwood EB, eds. *Handbook of Physiology.* sec. 7. *Endocrinology.* vol. 1. Washington: American Physiological Society, 1972, pp. 25–66.

226. Jaffe R, Hashida Y, Yunis EJ. The endocrine pancreas of the neonate and infant. *Perspect Pediatr Pathol* 1982; 7:137–65.

226a. Bouwens L, Klöppel G. Islet cell neogenesis in the pancreas. *Virch Arch* 1996; 427:553–60.

227. Meittinen M, Lehto V-P, Dahl D, Virtanen I. Varying expression of cytokeratin and neurofilaments in neuroendocrine tumors of the human gastrointestinal tract. *Lab Invest* 1985; 52:429–36.

228. Pearse AG, Takor T. Embryology of the diffuse neuroendocrine system and its relationship to the common peptides. *Fed Proc* 1979; 38:2288–94.

229. Cossel L. Intermediate cells in the adult human pancreas. Contribution to the transformation of differentiated cells in vertebrates. *Virch Arch B* 1984; 47:313–88.

230. Dudek RW, Lawrence IE Jr, Hill RS, Johnson RC. Introduction of islet cytodifferentiation by fetal mesenchyme in adult pancreatic ductal epithelium. *Diabetes* 1991; 40:1041–8.

231. Stefan Y, Grasso S, Perrelet A, Orci L. A quantitative immunofluorescent study of the endocrine cell populations in the developing human pancreas. *Diabetes* 1983; 32:293–301.

232. Rahier J, Wallon J, Gepts W, Haot J. Localization of pancreatic polypeptide cells in a limited lobe of the human neonate pancreas: remnant of the ventral primordium? *Cell Tissue Res* 1979; 200:359–66.

233. Rahier J, Wallon J, Henquin JC. Abundance of somatostatin cells in the human neonatal pancreas. *Diabetologia* 1980; 18:251–4.

234. Jaffe R, Hashida Y, Yunis EJ. Pancreatic pathology in hyperinsulinemic hypoglycemia of infancy. *Lab Invest* 1980; 42:356–65.

235. Grotting JC, Kassel S, Dehner LP. Nesidioblastosis and congenital neuroblastoma. A histologic and immunocytochemical study of a new complex neurocristopathy. *Arch Pathol Lab Med* 1979; 103:642–6.

236. Rahier J, Wallon J, Henquin JC. Cell populations in the endocrine pancreas of human neonates and infants. *Diabetologia* 1981; 20:540–6.

237. Milner RD, Wirdnam PK, Tsanakas J. Quantitative morphology of B, A, D, and PP cells in infants of diabetic mothers. *Diabetes* 1981; 30:271–4.

238. Witte DP, Greider MH, DeSchryver-Kecskemeti K, Kissane JM, White MH. The juvenile human endocrine pancreas: normal v. idiopathic hyperinsulinemic hypoglycemia. *Semin Diagn Pathol* 1984; 1:30–42.

239. Goudswaard WB, Houthoff HJ, Koudstaal J, Zwierstra RP. Nesidioblastosis and endocrine hyperplasia of the pancreas: a secondary phenomenon. *Hum Pathol* 1986; 17:46–54.

240. Van Assche FA, Aerts L, Holemans K, Vercruysse L. The endocrine pancreas in nonimmune hydrops fetalis. *Am J Obstet Gynecol* 1994; 171:236–8.

241. Borchard F, Müntefering H. Beitrag zur quantitativen morphologie der Langerhanschen inseln bei früh und neugeborenen. *Virch Arch A* 1969; 346:178–98.

242. Wellmann KF, Volk BW. The islets of infants of diabetic mothers. In: Volk BW, Wellmann KF, eds. *The Diabetic Pancreas.* New York: Plenum, 1977, pp. 365–80.

243. Hultquist GT, Olding LB. Endocrine pathology of infants of diabetic mothers. A quantitative morphological analysis including comparison with infants of iso-immunized and of non-diabetic mothers. *Acta Endocrinol Suppl* 1981; 241:1–202.

244. Bartow SA, Mukai K, Rosai J. Pseudoneoplastic proliferation of endocrine cells in pancreatic fibrosis. *Cancer* 1981; 47:2627–33.

245. Klöppel G, Altenähr E, Menke B. The ultrastructure of focal islet cell adenomatosis in the newborn with hypoglycemia and hyperinsulinism. *Virch Arch A Pathol Anat Histol* 1975; 366:223–36.

246. Van Assche FA, Gepts W. The cytological composition of the foetal endocrine pancreas in normal and pathological conditions. *Diabetologia* 1971; 7:434–44.

247. Mostoufi-Zadeh M, Weiss LM, Driscoll SG. Nonimmune hydrops fetalis: a challenge in perinatal pathology. *Hum Pathol* 1985; 16:785–9.

248. Hardwick DF, Dimmick JE. Metabolic cirrhoses of infancy and early childhood. *Perspect Pediatr Pathol* 1976; 3:103–44.

249. Perry TL, Hardwick DF, Dixon GH, Dolman CL, Hansen S. Hypermethioninemia: a metabolic disorder associated with cirrhosis, islet cell hyperplasia and renal tubular degeneration. *Pediatrics* 1965; 36:236–50.

250. Rosenberg AM, Haworth JC, Degroot GW, Trevenen CL, Rechler MM. A case of leprechaunism with severe hyperinsulinemia. *Am J Dis Child* 1980; 134:170–5.

251. Zellweger H. Cerebro-hepato-renal syndrome. In: Buyse ML, ed. *Birth Defects Encyclopedia.* vol. 1. Cambridge: Blackwell, 1990, pp. 302–4.

252. Vance JE, Stoll RW, Kitabchi AE, et al. Familial nesidioblastosis as the predominant manifestation of multiple endocrine adenomatosis. *Am J Med* 1972; 52:211–17.

253. Carney JA, Go VL, Gordon H, et al. Familial pheochromocytoma and islet cell tumor of the pancreas. *Am J Med* 1980; 68:515–21.

254. Heitz PU, Klöppel G, Häcki WH, Polak JM, Pearse AG. Nesidioblastosis: the pathologic basis of persistent hyperinsulinemic hypoglycemia in infants.

Morphologic and quantitative analysis of seven cases based on specific immunostaining and electron microscopy. *Diabetes* 1977; 26:632–42.

255. Greenberg F, Copeland K, Gresik MV. Expanding the spectrum of the Perlman syndrome. *Am J Med Genet* 1988; 29:773–6.

256. Moore RA. Congenital aplasia of islands of Langerhans with diabetes mellitus. *Am J Dis Child* 1936; 52:627–32.

257. Dodge JA, Laurence KM. Congenital absence of islets of Langerhans. *Arch Dis Child* 1977; 52:411–13.

258. Wong KC, Tse K, Chan JKC. Congenital absence of insulin-secreting cells. *Histopathology* 1988; 12:541–5.

259. Abramowicz MJ, Andrien M, Dupont E, et al. Isodisomy of chromosome 6 in a newborn with methylmalonic acidemia and agenesis of pancreatic beta cells causing diabetes mellitus. *J Clin Invest* 1994; 94:418–21.

260. Gotlin RW, Silver HK. Neonatal hypoglycaemia, hyperinsulinism and absence of pancreatic alpha-cells. *Lancet* 1970; 1:1346.

261. Barresi G, Inferrera C, de Luca F, Gemelli M, Bussolati G. Persistent neonatal normoinsulinaemic hypoglycaemia. *Histopathology* 1981; 5:45–52.

262. Bishop AE, Polak JM, Chesa PG, et al. Decrease of pancreatic somatostatin in neonatal nesidioblastosis. *Diabetes* 1981; 30:122–6.

263. Marks V. Hypoglycemia in childhood. In: Marks V, Rose FC, eds. *Hypoglycemia.* Oxford: Blackwell, 1991, p. 219.

264. Van Assche FA. The fetal endocrine pancreas. In: Sutherland HW, Stowers JM, eds. *Carbohydrate Metabolism in Pregnancy and the Newborn: Incorporating the Proceedings of the International Colloquium at Aberdeen, Scotland, July, 1973.* Edinburgh: Churchill Livingstone, 1975, pp. 68–82.

265. Haust MD. Maternal diabetes mellitus—effects on the fetus and placenta. *Monogr Pathol* 1981; 22:201–85.

266. Steel RB, Mosley JD, Smith CH. Insulin and placenta: degradation and stabilization, binding to microvillous membrane receptors, and amino acid uptake. *Am J Obstet Gynecol* 1979; 135:522–9.

267. Bauman WA, Yalow RS. Transplacental passage of insulin complexed to antibody. *Proc Natl Acad Sci USA* 1981; 78:4588–90.

268. Dubreuil G, Anderodias J. Illots de Langerhans geants chez un nouveau ne issue de mere glucosurique. *C R Soc Biol (Paris)* 1920; 83:1490–3.

269. Klöppel G. Experimental insulitis. In: Podolsky S, Viswanathan M, eds. *Secondary Diabetes: The Spectrum of the Diabetic Syndromes.* New York: Raven, 1980, pp. 493–501.

270. Nelson L, Turkel S, Shulman I, Gabbe S. Pancreatic islet fibrosis in young infants of diabetic mothers. *Lancet* 1977; 2:362–3.

271. Gepts JC, Cornblath M. Transient diabetes of the newborn. In: Schulman I, ed. *Advances in Pediatrics.* vol. 16. Chicago: Year Book Medical, 1969, pp. 345–63.

272. von Mühlendahl KE, Herkenhoff H. Long-term course of neonatal diabetes. *N Engl J Med* 1995; 333:704–8.

273. Wolcott CD, Rallison ML. Infancy-onset diabetes mellitus and multiple epiphyseal dysplasia. *J Pediatr* 1972; 80:292–7.

274. Devine J. A case of diabetes mellitus in a young infant. *Arch Dis Child* 1938; 13:189–92.

275. Howard CP, Go VL, Infante AJ, et al. Long-term survival in a case of functional pancreatic agenesis. *J Pediatr* 1980; 97:786–9.

276. Hickish G. Neonatal diabetes. *Br Med J* 1956; 1:95–6.

277. Lewis E, Eisenberg H. Diabetes mellitus neonatorum. Report of probable case. *Am J Dis Child* 1935; 49:408–10.

278. Tidd JT, Stanage WF. Congenital diabetes mellitus: a case report. *S D J Med* 1965; 18:15–19.

279. Osborne GR. Congenital diabetes. *Arch Dis Child* 1965; 40:332. Abstract.

280. Weimerskirch D, Klein DJ. Recurrence of insulin-dependent diabetes mellitus after transient neonatal diabetes: a report of two cases. *J Pediatr* 1993; 122:598–600.

281. Powell BR, Buist NR, Stenzel P. An x-linked syndrome of diarrhea, polyendocrinopathy, and fatal infection in infancy. *J Pediatr* 1982; 100:731–7.

282. Meyer B, Nezelof C, Lemoine M, et al. A propos de du cas de diabète néonatale. *Ann Pediatr* 1970; 17:569–73.

283. Woo D, Scopes JW, Polak JM. Idiopathic hypoglycaemia in sibs with morphological evidence of nesidioblastosis of the pancreas. *Arch Dis Child* 1976; 51:528–31.

284. Schwartz SS, Rich BH, Lucky AW, et al. Familial nesidioblastosis; severe neonatal hypoglycaemia in two families. *J Pediatr* 1979; 95:44–53.

285. Wüthrich CH, Schubiger G, Zuppinger K. Persistent neonatal hyperinsulinemic hypoglycemia in two siblings successfully treated with diazoxide. *Helv Paediatr Acta* 1986; 41:455–9.

286. Moreno LA, Turck D, Gottrand F, et al. Familial hyperinsulinism with nesidioblastosis of the pancreas. Further evidence for autosomal recessive inheritance. *Am J Med Genet* 1989; 34:584–6.

287. Woolf DA, Leonard JV, Trembath RC, Pembrey ME, Grant DB. Nesidioblastosis: evidence for autosomal recessive inheritance. *Arch Dis Child* 1991; 66:529–30.

288. Bianchi C, Corbella E, Beccaria L, Bolla P, Chiumello G. A case of familial nesidioblastosis: prenatal diagnosis of foetal hyperinsulinism. *Acta Pediatr* 1992; 81:853–5.

289. Thomas PM, Cote GJ, Hallman DM, Mathew PM. Homozygosity mapping, to chromosome 11p, of the gene for familial persistent hyperinsulinemic hypoglycemia of infancy. *Am J Hum Genet* 1995; 56:416–21.

290. Thomas PM, Cote GJ, Wohllk N, et al. Mutations in the sulfonylurea receptor gene in familial persistent hyperinsulinemic hypoglycemia of infancy. *Science* 1995; 268:426–9.

290a. Dunne MJ, Kane C, Sheperd RM, et al. Familial persistent hyperinsulinemic hypoglycemia of infancy and mutations in the sulphonylurea receptor. *N Engl J Med* 1997; 336:703–5.

291. Thornton PS, Sumner AE, Ruchelli ED, et al. Familial and sporadic hyperinsulinism: histopathologic findings and segregation analysis support a single autosomal recessive disorder. *J Pediatr* 1991; 119:721–4.

292. Goossens A, Gepts W, Saudubray JM, et al. Diffuse and focal nesidioblastosis. A clinicopathological study of 24 patients with persistent neonatal hyperinsulinemic hypoglycemia. *Am J Surg Pathol* 1989; 13:766–75.

293. Goossens A, Heitz P, Klöppel G. Pancreatic endocrine cells and their non-neoplastic proliferation. In: Y Dayal, ed. *Endocrine Pathology of the Gut and Pancreas*. Boca Raton, FL: CRC, 1991, pp. 69–104.

294. Rahier J. Relevance of endocrine pancreas nesidioblastosis to hyperinsulinemic hypoglycemia. *Diab Care* 1989; 12:164–5.

295. Gould VE, Memoli VA, Dardi LE, Gould NS. Nesidiodysplasia and nesidioblastosis of infancy: structural and functional correlations with the syndrome of hyperinsulinemic hypoglycemia. *Pediatr Pathol* 1983; 1:7–31.

296. Gabbay HK. Case records of the Massachusetts General Hospital. Weekly clinicopathological exercises. Case 30-1978. *N Engl J Med* 1978; 299:241–8.

297. Rahier J, Fält K, Müntefering H, et al. The basic structural lesion of persistent neonatal hypoglycaemia with hyperinsulinism: deficiency of pancreatic D cells or hyperactivity of B cells? *Diabetologia* 1984; 26:282–9.

298. Falkmer S, Askensten U. Disturbed growth of the endocrine pancreas. In: Lefebvre PJ, Pepeleers DG, eds. *The Pathology of the Endocrine Pancreas in Diabetes*. Berlin: Springer-Verlag, 1988, p. 125.

299. Klöppel G, Heitz PU. Persistent hyperinsulinaemic hypoglycemia in infancy. In: Klöpple G, Heitz PU, eds. *Pancreatic Pathology*. Edinburgh: Churchill Livingstone, 1984, pp. 193–203.

300. Otonkoski T, Andersson S, Simell O. Somatostatin regulation of beta-cell function in the normal human fetuses and in neonates with persistent hyperinsulinemic hypoglycemia. *J Clin Endocrinol Metab* 1993; 76:184–8.

301. Bani D, Bani Sacchi T, Biliotti G. Nesidioblastosis and intermediate cells in the pancreas of patients with hyperinsulinemic hypoglycemia. *Virch Arch B Cell Pathol* 1985; 48:19–32.

302. Melmed RN. Intermediate cells of the pancreas. An appraisal. *Gastroenterology* 1979; 76:196–201.

303. Kirkland J, Ben-Menachem Y, Akhtar M, Marshall R, Dudrick S. Islet cell tumor in a neonate. Diagnosis by selective angiography and histological findings. *Pediatrics* 1978; 61:790–1.

304. Seki S, Ikenoue T, Murakami N, et al. Ectopic nesidioblastosis. *Acta Paediatr Jpn* 1990; 32:308–10.

305. Taguchi T, Suita S, Hirose R. Histological classification of nesidioblastosis: efficacy of immunohistochemical study of neuron-specific enolase. *J Pediatr Surg* 1991; 26:770–4.

306. Brunelle F, Negre V, Barth MO, et al. Pancreatic venous samplings in infants and children with primary hyperinsulinism. *Pediatr Radiol* 1989; 19:100–3.

307. Telander R, Charbonneau JW, Haymond MW. Intraoperative ultrasonography of the pancreas in children. *J Pediatr Surg* 1986; 21:262–6.

308. Bordi C, Ravazzola M, Pollak A, Lubec G, Orci L. Neonatal islet cell adenoma: a distinct type of islet cell tumor. *Diab Care* 1982; 5:122–5.

309. Thornton PS, Alter CA, Katz LE, Baker L, Stanley CA. Short- and long-term use of octreotide in the treatment of congenital hyperinsulinism. *J Pediatr* 1993; 123:637–43.

310. Cornblath M, Schwartz R. *Disorders of Carbohydrate Metabolism in Infancy*. 3rd ed. Boston: Blackwell Scientific, 1991, p. 79.

311. Thomas CG Jr, Underwood LE, Carney CN, Dolcourt JL, Whitt JJ. Neonatal and infantile hypoglycemia due to insulin excess. New aspects of diagnosis and surgical management. *Ann Surg* 1976; 185:505–17.

312. Delemarre-van de Waal HA, Veldekamp EJM, Schrander-Stumpel CTRM. Long term treatment of an infant with nesidioblastosis using a somatostatin analogue. *N Engl J Med* 1987; 316:222–3. Letter.

313. Spitz L, Bhargava RK, Grant DB, Leonard JV. Surgical treatment of hyperinsulinaemic hypoglycaemia in infancy and childhood. *Arch Dis Child* 1992; 67:201–5.

314. Schonau E, Deeg KH, Huemmer HP, Akcetin YZ, Bohles HJ. Pancreatic growth and function following surgical treatment of nesidioblastosis in infancy. *Eur J Pediatr* 1991; 150:550–3.

315. Shilyansky J, Fisher S, Cutz E, Perlman K, Filler RM. Is 95% pancreatectomy the procedure of choice for treatment of persistent hyperinsulinemic hypoglycemia of the neonate? *J Pediatr Surg* 1997; 32:342–6.

315a. Liebowitz G, Glaser B, Higazi AA, et al. Hyperinsulinemic hypoglycemia of infancy (nesidioblastosis) in clinical remission: high incidence of diabetes mellitus and persistent β-cell dysfunction at long term follow up. *J Clin Endocrinol Metab* 1995; 80:386–92.

316. Bernstein J. Renal tubular and pancreatic islet necrosis in newly born infants. *Am J Dis Child* 1958; 96:705–10.

317. Seemayer TA, Osborne C, DeChadarevian J-P. Shock-related injury of pancreatic islets of Langerhans in newborn and young infants. *Hum Pathol* 1985; 16:1231–4.

318. Filippi G, Mckusick VA. The Beckwith-Wiedemann syndrome. *Medicine* 1970; 49:279–98.

319. Butler MG. Beckwith-Wiedemann syndrome. In: Buyse ML, ed. *Birth Defects Encyclopedia*. vol. 1. Cambridge: Blackwell, 1990, pp. 218–19.

320. Van Assche FA, Spitz B, Sieprath P, Eggermont E, DeVlieger H. More on the Beckwith-Wiedemann syndrome. *Diabetologia* 1986; 29:468. Letter.

321. Roe TF, Kershnar AK, Weitzman JJ, Madrigal LS. Beckwith's syndrome with extreme organ hyperplasia. *Pediatrics* 1973; 52:372–81.

322. Stefan Y, Bordi C, Grasso S, Orci L. Beckwith-Wiedemann syndrome: a quantitative, immunohistological study of pancreatic islet cell populations. *Diabetologia* 1985; 23:914–19.

323. Sotelo-Avila C, Gooch WM III. Neoplasms associated with the Beckwith-Wiedemann syndrome. *Perspect Pediatr Pathol* 1976; 3:255–72.

324. Donohue WL. Clinicopathological conference at the Hospital for Sick Children, Toronto, Ontario. Dysendocrinism. *J Pediatr* 1948; 32:739–48.

325. Shuangshoti S, Ekaraphanich S. Congenital neuroblastoma and hyperplasia of islets of Langerhans in an infant. *Clin Pediatr* 1972; 11:241–3.

326. Simmons PS, Telander RL, Carney JA, Wold LE, Haymond MW. Surgical management of hyperinsulinemic hypoglycemia in children. *Arch Surg* 1984; 119:520–5.

327. de Morais CF, Lopes EA, Bisl H, Alves VA, de Macedo Santos RT. Nesidioblastosis associated with congenital malformations of the heart—morphological and immunohistochemical study of necropsy cases. *Pathol Res Pract* 1986; 181:175–80.

328. Naeye RL. The sudden infant death syndrome. A review of recent advances. *Arch Pathol Lab Med* 1977; 104:165–7.

329. Loo SWH, Kozakewich HPW, Wald RA, Vawter GF. Sudden infant death syndrome and nesidioblastosis: no evidence for pathologic relationship. *Lab Invest* 1982; 46:10P. Abstract.

330. Hisaoka M, Haratake J, Nakamura Y, Itoh Y. Pancreatic islet abnormalities in sudden infant death syndrome. *Acta Pathol Jpn* 1992; 42:870–5.

331. Polak JM, Wigglesworth JS. Islet-cell hyperplasia and sudden infant death. *Lancet* 1976; 2:570–1.

332. Cox JN, Guelpa G, Terrapon M. Islet cell hyperplasia and sudden infant death. *Lancet* 1976; 2:739–40. Letter.

333. Aynsley-Green A, Polak JM, Keeling J, Gough MH, Baum JD. Averted sudden neonatal death due to pancreatic nesidioblastosis. *Lancet* 1978; 1:550–1. Letter.

Pathology of the Adrenal Glands

Derek J. deSa

DEVELOPMENT AND GROWTH OF THE FETAL ADRENAL GLANDS

The adrenal gland is made up of two separate components: a cortex derived from embryonic mesoderm that secretes steroid hormones, and a medulla that arises from the neural crest and secretes catecholamines. The adrenal gland develops in the intermediate mesoderm, lateral to the dorsal mesentery and medial to the mesonephros. A zone of celomic mesothelial proliferation can be identified at approximately 4 weeks of gestation, and shortly thereafter the surface polygonal cells migrate downward into the mesoderm. The cells become arranged in cords and trabeculae, which are the precursors of the developing fetal cortex of the adrenal gland [1]. At this stage of development, three main sources of blood supply to the developing primordium can be identified. Branches from an artery derived from a segmental aortic branch to the septum transversum are destined to become the superior adrenal artery, and its parent vessel becomes the inferior phrenic artery. A segmental branch arising directly from the aorta supplies the gland directly and forms the middle adrenal artery. The inferior adrenal arteries are derived from blood vessels that supply both the developing kidneys and the adrenal. Initially, due to its relatively larger size in comparison with the developing kidney, the branches to the adrenal gland are larger. In later embryonic life, the branches to the rapidly enlarging metanephros become remodeled into the renal artery, and in the term fetus the parent vessel can be identified as the adrenal branch of the renal artery.

The medulla is derived from neural crest cells that migrate anteriorly into the medial aspect of the developing adrenal cortical primordium (Fig. 27.1) which engulfs the invaginating cells. In their migration, the adrenal medullary cells draw with them their preganglionic nerve fibers. The cells of the adrenal medulla therefore have many of the characteristics of postganglionic cells of the autonomic nervous system. The development of the adrenal medulla is associated with contemporaneous forward migration of other neural crest derivatives that will form the para-aortic paraganglionic tissues, including the organs of Zuckerkandl. Clusters of chromaffin cells lying medial to the adrenal gland are seen frequently in autopsy material.

Relative to body size, the adrenal gland in the fetus is 10 to 20 times larger than in the adult [2], due to a large fetal zone of cortex that is the most prominent histologic feature of the gland. A detailed study of the development of the adrenal cortex during the second trimester of gestation provides useful indices of the length, height, and thickness of the gland between 15 and 27 weeks [3]—data that are of use to both ultrasonographers and pathologists. In the initial phases of development, mitotic activity can be seen throughout the primordium, and this hyperplasia is associated with the rapid development of a proportionately massive fetal cortex. By the 12th week of gestation, mitotic activity is markedly reduced [1] and is confined almost entirely to the peripheral outer rim of the gland.

The cortex has therefore two distinct components: a large, deeper fetal zone and a smaller peripheral rim of definitive cortex. The definitive cortex forms less than one-fifth of the overall thickness of the gland [3]. These zones are readily recognizable after the 12th week of gestation. The fetal cortical cells are larger, with abundant eosinophilic cytoplasm, and contain more lipid in the resting state. The peripherally located, definitive cortical cells are smaller and contain much less lipid. The increase in cortical mass is associated with a change in the shape of the gland, and the adrenal assumes an extended, flattened appearance. This

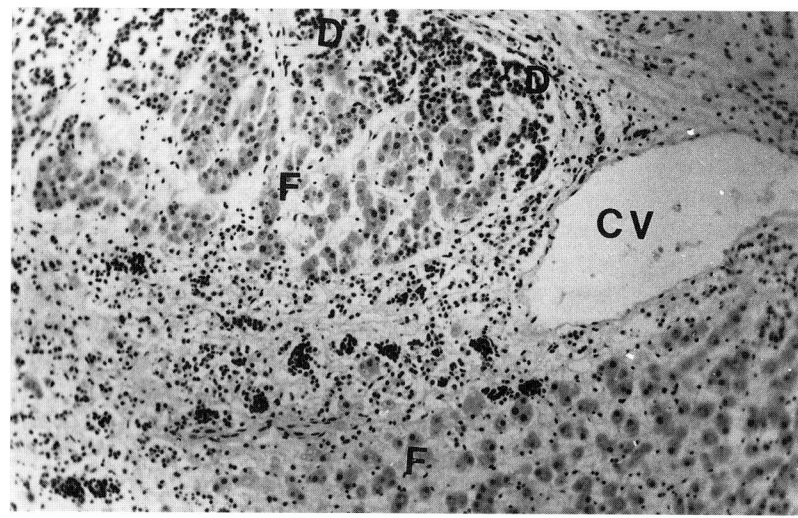

FIGURE 27.1. *Darkly staining clusters of neuroblasts can be seen invaginating the developing adrenal cortex of a fetus of 14 weeks. CV = central vein, D = definitive cortex, F = fetal cortex. H&E, ×40.*

permits growth without any increase in cortical thickness, and therefore equalization of cortical perfusion. In the infant at term, the medulla is made up predominantly of pheochromocytes that are polygonal cells with granular cytoplasm that can secrete adrenaline and noradrenaline. They are arranged in packets surrounded by a rich capillary network. Adrenal medullary cells are concentrated in the head of the gland and are *not* uniformly distributed throughout the gland, and, unless the head of the adrenal gland is sampled, the adrenal medulla may not be identified. This problem of identification of the adrenal medulla is encountered most often in smaller preterm infants.

Faye-Petersen and Parker [4, 5] have provided newer insights into adrenal development. Using a range of antibodies to neuronal/neuroendocrine markers, they have been able to show a distinction between the development of the neuroblastic cells and of pheochromocyte precursors that are present in the developing medullae of fetuses between 11

and 41 weeks' gestation. Between 15 and 23 weeks' gestation, the neuroblasts traverse the cortex, as well as showing medullary clusters, which progressively decrease in size and number after 24 weeks' gestation. Pheochromocytic precursors, originally widely scattered in the cortex between 11 and 14 weeks, coalesce around the central veins after 24 weeks' gestation. At first, in close association with the neuroblasts, the pheochromocyte precursors outnumber the neuroblasts in later gestation [4]. The same authors also showed that cells containing synaptophysin (or a synaptophysin-like protein) were not restricted to the medulla, but could be present in a Golgi-related distribution, as well as on cytoplasmic membranes, in cells of the definitive cortex after 24 weeks' gestation [5]. The functional significance of these changes is not known at present, but they are of relevance in understanding the presence of "ectopic" chromaffin tissue and apparently "heterotopic" islands of pheochromocytes in the adrenal cortex (Fig. 27.2).

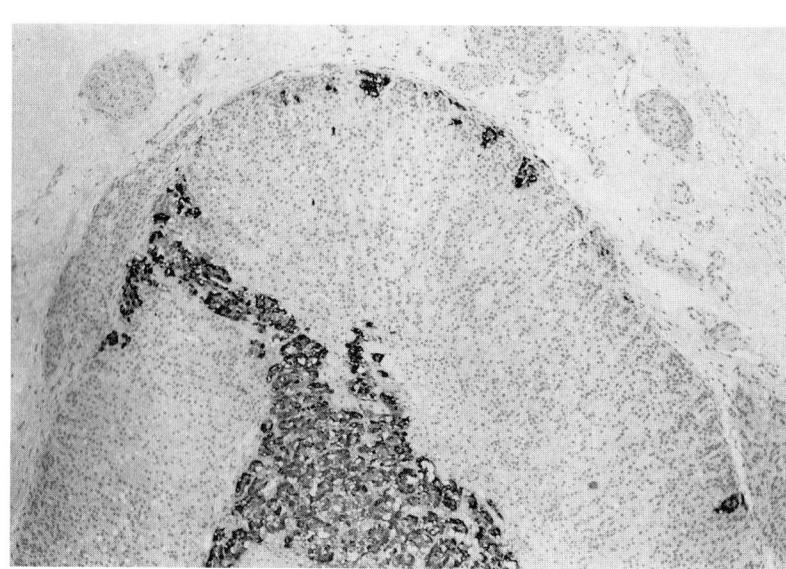

FIGURE 27.2. *Aberrant neuroblastic migration in one alar segment of an adrenal gland. The darkly stained islands can be seen in the subcapsular cortex and deeper cortex. Streptavidin-biotin technique with primary antibody to neuron-specific enolase. ×15.*

Distribution of Blood Vessels in the Adrenal Gland

The adrenal gland is supplied through a vascular plexus situated in the capsule to which all three arteries contribute. This plexus provides a means of equalizing and redistributing blood flow through the gland. Penetrating branches from the capsular plexus enter the gland, and, after coursing through the capillaries, blood is drained through a complex system of veins. While the majority of the blood flow is drained through the tributaries of the central vein, numerous small veins can be seen in the capsule of the gland. This implies some venous return, almost as a countercurrent, to capsular veins. The central vein of the medulla appears almost completely ensheathed by the medullary cells, apart from occasional small clusters of cortical cells destined to form the "cortical collars" of the vein in the adult adrenal gland [6] (Fig. 27.3).

Function of the Fetal Cortex in the Fetus and Newborn

The large size of the fetal adrenal gland is due to the presence of a thick layer of fetal cortex, but following birth there is rapid involution of this layer. Most of this involution is complete by 2 to 3 weeks' postnatal age, but the process can be irregular and haphazard [7], and it is not uncommon to find isolated islands of surviving fetal cortex in infants more than 4 weeks of age. Until recently there has been no satisfactory explanation for the prominence of the fetal zone or its postnatal involution. In recent years, however, a greater understanding of fetal adrenal physiology has provided a rational explanation for the changes seen in the adrenal cortex [8–10].

Close metabolic interrelationships exist between the placenta and the adrenal gland, for it is known that dehydroepiandrosterone (DHEA) and other Δ^5-3β-hydroxysteroids are produced in large quantities by the adrenal and are metabolized by the fetal liver and placenta. This led to the earlier concept of a fetoplacental unit [11] where the fetal adrenal cortex was seen as a producer of DHEA, which in turn was regarded as an essential substrate for placental estrogen synthesis.

By term, the fetal adrenals produce between 100 and 200 mg of steroid daily—a much higher rate than that of a normal adult [8]. The adrenal gland can synthesize cholesterol or extract it from low-density lipoprotein (LDL)–bound cholesterol that is derived from the fetal liver. However, the fetal adrenal gland has a relatively low level of activity of 3β-hydroxysteroid dehydrogenase (3β-HSD) activity. Thus, while small amounts of cortisol are produced, quantitatively the major end product of adrenal steroidogenesis is DHEA, which is rapidly sulfurylated (particularly by the cells of the inner fetal cortex). Cortisol is formed in an "inefficient" manner (and is rapidly cleared by the placenta), and probably less than 75% of plasma cortisol in the fetus comes from its adrenal cortex [12].

The major tropic drive that regulates steroidogenesis in the fetal adrenal gland is fetal pituitary adrenocorticotropic hormone (ACTH) stimulation, and the feedback mechanisms that exist in normal adults also operate in the fetus. The relatively low unit output of cortisol induces an ACTH-triggered hypertrophy of the gland, especially the cells of the fetal zone [9].

The inhibition of 3β-HSD activity is brought about in large measure by rising levels of estrogen and other steroids in utero [10]. Following delivery, and removal from the uteroplacental environment, these inhibitory factors are not

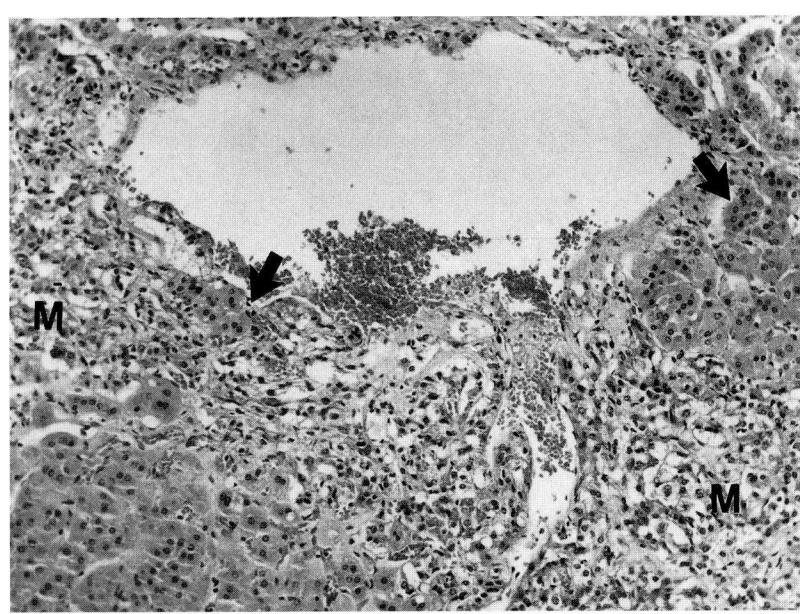

FIGURE 27.3. *Islands of cortical tissue (arrows) abutting on the central vein in the adrenal gland of a term infant. M = medullary cells. H&E, ×40.*

effective. The output of cortisol rises as a consequence, leading to a "physiologic involution" of the fetal zone. The fetal zone cells were at first thought to disappear completely, but it is likely that, with postnatal "involution," a progressive remodeling of the "fetal" zone into the zonae fasciculata and reticularis occurs [13], and that postnatal involution is really a phase of functional regression due to the appropriate reduction of the ACTH drive.

The phenomenon of apoptosis is thought to be the morphologic indicator of a physiologic reduction in the numbers of cells in an organ, and a means whereby cells that have reached the end of their life cycle may be removed and replaced without tissue breakdown. This phenomenon has been described in detail in the adrenal cortex of the neonatal rat, where it occurs in the deeper layers of the involuting fetal cortex [14]. Similar histologic changes can be seen in the adrenal glands of human neonates, even in those born in the second trimester [3], but the process has not been studied in depth.

The adrenal medulla is functionally a part of the sympathetic nervous system and the related ganglia. The ability of this group of organs to respond to stress, such as hypoxia, is established early in development [15].

CONGENITAL ANOMALIES

Absence of the Adrenal Glands

Absence of one or both adrenal glands is extremely rare and usually occurs only in association with multiple major congenital malformations [16]. The only case personally studied by the author was in an infant with a single umbilical artery, hydrocephalus due to aqueduct stenosis, truncus arteriosus, and renal dysplasia. Dunn, however, reported an infant

without any cranial abnormalities but lacking both an adenohypophysis and both adrenal glands [17]. Without appropriate replacement therapy, this condition is *not* compatible with life.

Ectopic and Heterotopic Adrenal Tissue

Due to the close developmental relationship with the gonad and its duct, it is not surprising that ectopic islands of adrenal cortical tissue have been found in very many sites, from the para-aortic region to the gonad. Adrenal cortical rests may be seen in the epididymal region of the testes, in the hilar region of the ovary (Fig. 27.4), above the diaphragmatic opening for the aorta within the thorax on both the right and left side, and anywhere in between. Small nests of adrenal cortical tissue may be seen under the renal capsule. Surgeons often encounter small nests of ectopic adrenal cortical tissue during inguinal herniorrhaphy. Wright and Gillis offer a useful review of this topic, and report a mediastinal foregut cyst with an adrenal cortical rest [18]. In almost all instances, ectopic cortical tissue is not accompanied by medullary tissue, but an example of a formed adrenal gland within the skull was described by Wiener and Dallgaard [19]. Ectopic adrenal cortical tissue was found in the liver of a neonatal infant [20], and adrenal tissue may be seen rarely in the wall of the gallbladder [21]. Qureshi and Jacques reported two cases in which the placenta contained islands of cells resembling adrenocortical tissue, and speculated on the histogenesis [22]. Intrapulmonary adrenal cortical nests [23, 24] have been noted, but no adequate explanation of their histogenesis exists. Unlike the others, Armin and Castelli's report [24] emphasizes the presence of adrenal cytomegaly, indicating a responsiveness to ACTH stimulation.

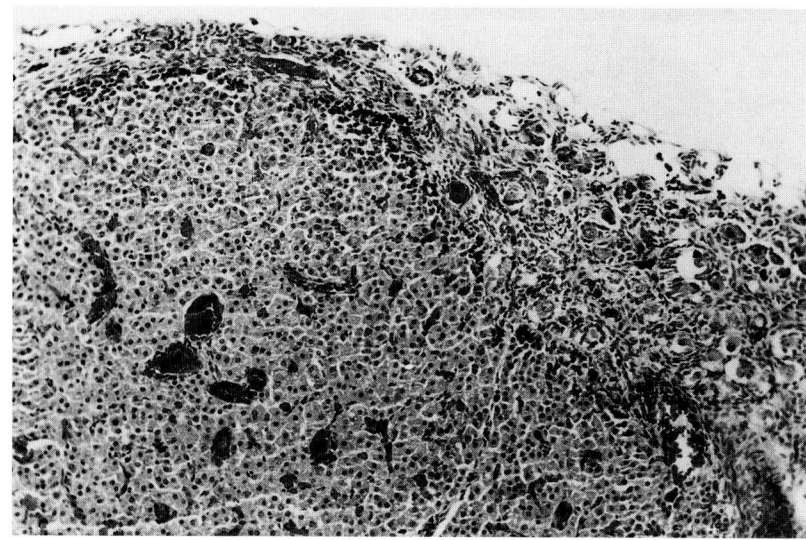

FIGURE 27.4.   *Part of a large hilar nodule of adrenal cortical tissue in the ovary of a term female stillborn infant. H&E, ×40.*

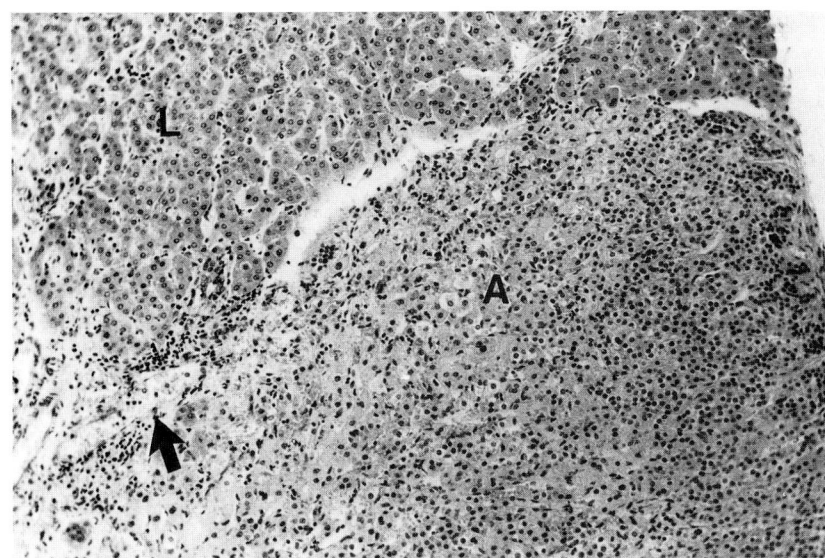

FIGURE 27.5. *Fusion of the adrenal cortex (A) and liver tissue (L). Note shared vessels (arrow). H&E, ×40.*

FUSION WITH OTHER ORGANS

In rare cases, fusion of the adrenal gland with other organs may occur, especially with the upper pole of the kidneys, and examples in which the right adrenal gland may have included segments of liver tissue (Fig. 27.5) have been described [25]. This may help explain the ectopic adrenal tissue seen in the liver by Vestfrid [20]. There are usually other associated anomalies in these infants, and in the illustrated example the infant's karyotype was 47XY, 18+ (trisomy 18). Combined adrenorenal and adrenohepatic fusion was described by Honore and O'Hara [26]. Lockitch et al [27] have described examples of pulmonary and adrenal fusion associated with body wall defects and diaphragmatic hernia. Islands of chromaffin tissue embedded in the outer cortex of the adrenal gland may also occur, and the author has seen three such examples, all occurring in infants without any malformations in other organs.

Fusion of the Adrenal Glands

Fusion of the two adrenal glands (Fig. 27.6) has been described in de Lange syndrome (Amsterdam dwarfism), in the caudal regression syndrome [28–30], and in other malformation syndromes including spinal dysraphism [31]. The reader's attention is drawn to the excellent review by Kelly et al [32], which provides an interesting analysis of fusion in paired organs and outlines the several conditions that may be associated with fused adrenal glands.

Abnormalities of Shape of the Adrenal Gland

While abnormalities in adrenal cortical function such as those observed in congenital adrenal hyperplasia (see below) are associated with abnormal adrenal morphology, there is

one situation in which the shape of the adrenal is always abnormal. The definitive configuration of the disciform adrenal gland depends on its molding in relation to the immediately caudad, developing normal kidney. In instances of renal agenesis or ectopia of the kidney, the adrenal gland assumes a nondescript, flattened, discoid appearance on the affected side (Fig. 27.7). In the presence of markedly distorted kidney masses, as may be seen in renal dysplasia, the adrenal gland may be intimately enfolded into the irregular outline produced by the cysts in that organ, resulting in an adrenal cast of the outline of the upper pole of the kidney. In some of these infants, there may be foci of fusion of the adrenal cortex and renal tissue.

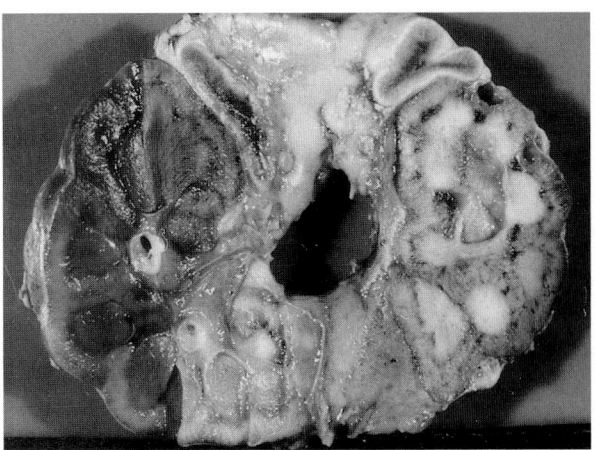

FIGURE 27.6. *Fused adrenal glands above a horseshoe kidney in an infant with de Lange syndrome.*

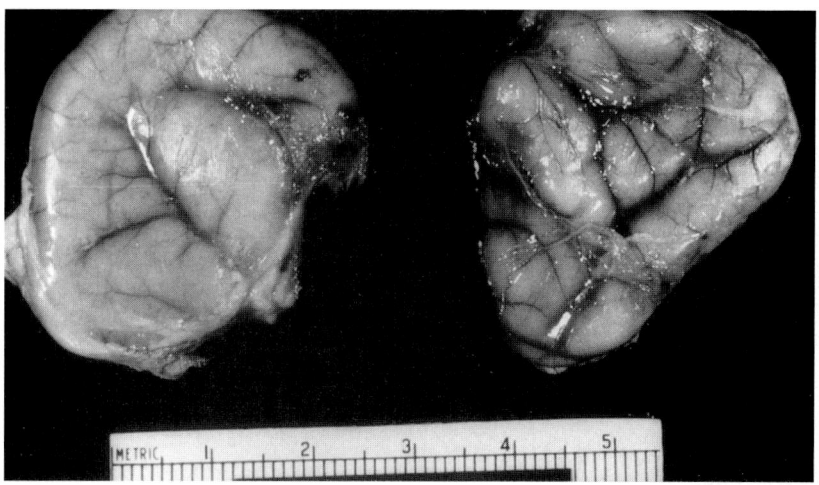

FIGURE 27.7.   *Flattened adrenal glands from a case of bilateral renal agenesis.*

HEMORRHAGE AND NECROSIS OF THE ADRENAL GLAND

Hemorrhagic necrosis of the adrenal gland has been described under many synonyms by different authors [6]. There is, however, a spectrum of changes from massive, predominantly hemorrhagic lesions of the adrenal gland to focal segmental necrosis of one wing of the gland, and, since it emphasizes the ischemic nature of the process, this author prefers the term "hemorrhagic necrosis." Bilateral hemorrhagic necrosis of the entire gland (with or without a central hematoma), and hemorrhagic necrosis of one gland with an intact gland contralaterally, are the least common manifestations, accounting for a total of 25% of all cases in a large series. Segmental involvement was by far the most common lesion [33].

Traditionally, many of these lesions have been ascribed to birth trauma, and in earlier descriptions [25] there has been a noticeable association of the more massive (and presumably more noteworthy) examples of hemorrhagic necrosis with breech deliveries and other varieties of severe birth trauma. However, a critical analysis of the entire spectrum of hemorrhagic necrosis of the adrenal gland in stillborns and neonatal infants shows that the most important factors in its development (even in the presence of massive birth trauma) are severe intrauterine and intrapartum asphyxia, leading to hypotension, and thus diminished perfusion of the adrenal cortex. Consequently, the fact that cortical necrosis is seen most frequently in severely asphyxiated infants with severe cardiovascular collapse [34] should not be surprising.

True traumatic lesions of the adrenal gland (without convincing evidence of underlying necrosis) do occur, but in these cases the damage is not confined to the adrenal gland alone and usually involves the adjacent abdominal wall musculature and perinephric and retroperitoneal tissues. In the past, these lesions were more common in term infants when labor was obstructed, but fortunately, due to improved obstetric management, instances of traumatic damage to the adrenal gland are very infrequent today.

The earliest histologic lesion consists of irregular zones of hemorrhage in one or more alae of the adrenal cortex, accompanied by varying amounts of coagulative necrosis within the hemorrhagic foci. The lesions progress through focal segmental areas of necrosis to massive involvement of a wing or the entire gland (Figs. 27.8–27.10). Rupture of the gland with retroperitoneal hemorrhage may occur. Occlusive lesions of arteries are uncommon in this author's experience, except in association with high placement within the aorta of an umbilical arterial catheter [35] (see below). In the venules draining necrotic areas, early thrombi may be seen (Fig. 27.11); these thrombi are similar to those observed in other necrotic tissues and probably represent thrombi developing as a result of hypoperfusion. Focal calcification of the thrombus and necrotic cells may occur. Capillary thrombi within the adrenal sinusoids have been reported in some hydropic infants with rhesus isoimmunization and in infants with overwhelming sepsis [33].

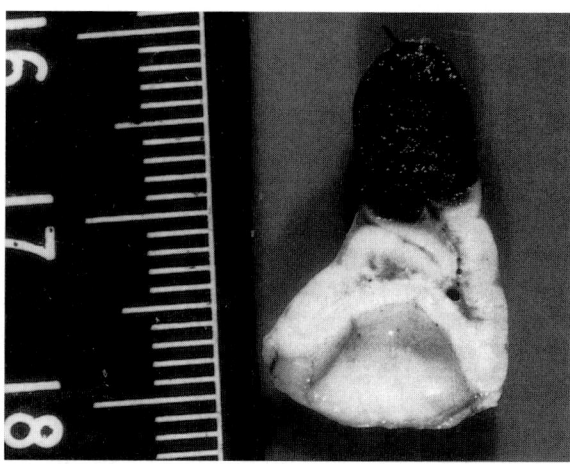

FIGURE 27.8.   *Segmental necrosis involving the superior segment of the right adrenal gland. This was the only area involved.*

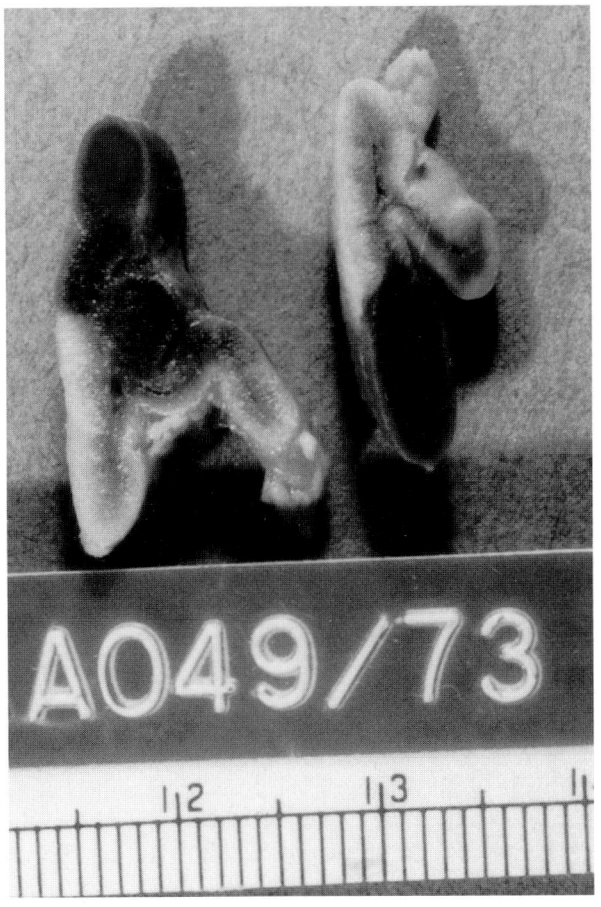

FIGURE 27.9. *Bilateral segmental necrosis involving different areas of both glands.*

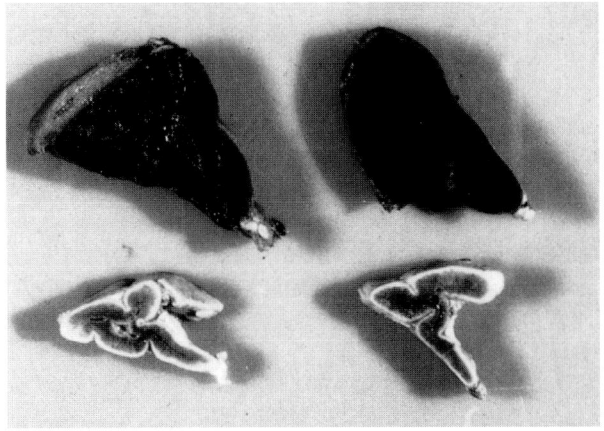

FIGURE 27.10. *Bilateral hemorrhagic necrosis involving both adrenal glands (upper) contrasted with normal glands (lower). Approximately ×3. (From deSa and Nicholls [33], with permission.)*

Hemorrhagic necrosis of the adrenal glands may be part of the spectrum of lesions seen in gram-negative septicemias and group B streptococcal sepsis in the newborn infant. However, there are no specific histologic features that distinguish necrosis in association with sepsis from that observed in severe intrapartum asphyxia. In fact, in many cases of severe neonatal sepsis with acute peripheral circulatory collapse, necrosis of the adrenal gland may be absent, and massive necrosis of the adrenal gland is even less common.

Adrenal infarcts have been described as a complication of umbilical arterial and aortic catheterization, with high placement of the catheter tip within the aorta [35]. Thrombi can be seen in capsular arteries and their intracortical branches in these infants [36]. The thrombi may show varying degrees of organization and incorporation into the wall of the vessel, suggesting asynchrony of the embolic lesions. Paradoxically, capsular thrombi can be present without infarction of the adrenal cortex, suggesting that a considerable reduction in overall perfusion must be present before infarction occurs [35]. This discrepancy between embolism and infarction emphasizes the great importance of the capsular cortical plexus in stabilizing cortical blood flow;

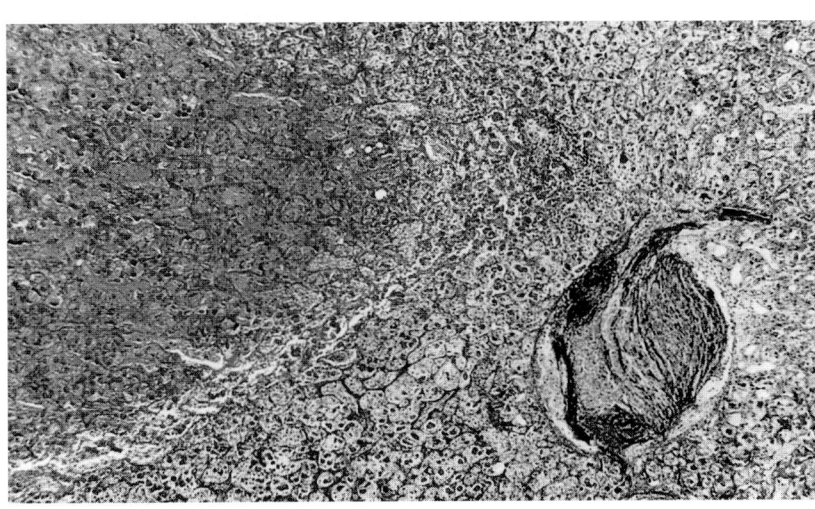

FIGURE 27.11. *Early thrombosis of venule draining area of established coagulative necrosis. Picro-Mallory, ×120. (From deSa and Nicholls [33], with permission.)*

conversely, finding necrosis without vascular obstruction indicates the overall decrease in perfusion.

Some infants with adrenal necrosis have presented with clinical signs mimicking those seen in infants with intraventricular hemorrhages and cyanotic heart disease. In most infants, however, adrenal necrosis is not associated with specific signs, and this may be due to the fact that the other signs and symptoms of severe asphyxia (or, less commonly, sepsis) assume overwhelming importance. Fever of unknown origin, tachypnea, pallor, and cyanosis, associated with abdominal distension and abdominal pseudotumors, have all been described in infants with adrenal hemorrhage [37, 38]. In some nonlethal examples of adrenal hemorrhagic necrosis, jaundice and hyperbilirubinemia, even necessitating exchange transfusion, may be presenting signs and may constitute the most common clinical presentations [39, 40].

Adrenal hemorrhage is not necessarily fatal and, in infants who have recovered a variety of different pathologic sequelae, may be seen in the adrenal. These sequelae include focal areas of calcification [41, 42] and nodular adrenocortical hyperplasia [33], and small scars [36]. Cysts are much rarer in neonatal material than in adults [36]. Surprisingly, there is little evidence to show that glands that have been the sites of previous necrosis are functionally deficient. In one infant, rupture of the adrenal gland was associated with hemorrhagic necrosis, and surgical evacuation of the hematoma led to a good recovery, without any subsequent evidence of adrenal hypocorticalism [38].

Some examples of adrenal hemorrhage have been detected antenatally [43, 44], lending weight to the importance of the decreased vascular perfusion of the gland in the pathogenesis of the lesion.

Renal vein thrombosis and coexistent adrenal hemorrhage have been described recently [45–47], and an association with intestinal lesions has been documented [48, 49], supporting some earlier observations [33]. The advent of newer imaging techniques has provided a broader view of the clinical spectrum of the lesion as well as an opportunity for closer monitoring, as shown by the case report of neonatal adrenal hemorrhage presenting with a scrotal mass [50].

Stress Changes in the Developing Adrenal Gland

The histologic changes of a stress reaction have been described by several workers [51–55], although their association with stress has not always been recognized. Macroscopically, the glands appear congested and depleted of cortical lipid, and have a red-brown color. Histologically, there is depletion of lipid, and the cells have a compact, densely eosinophilic cytoplasm (Figs. 27.12 and 27.13). There is an increased amount of pyroninophilic material in the cytoplasm and a depletion in the amount of refractile cholesterol identifiable in the adrenal gland. Ultrastructurally, there is a marked depletion of lipid vacuoles and an increase

in granular endoplasmic reticulum (Fig. 27.14). These changes are more marked in the fetal cortex than in the definitive cortex. In extremely immature infants, cytolysis of the definitive cortex, producing the classic "pseudofollicular" pattern [56, 57], may occur. These pseudofollicular changes have been interpreted, fancifully, as representing the differentiation of a "zona glomerulosa," but ultrastructural studies show that the "follicles" are formed by the cytolysis of severely stressed cells (Fig. 27.15) and filled with a variety of debris and extravasated red cells [57]. Rarely, the changes can be present in ectopic cortical rests as well [58].

In some infants, a pattern identical to "clear-cell reversal" in adults [6] is seen. Instead of diffuse depletion of adrenal cortical lipid, there is retention of lipid in the central zones of the fetal cortex, with depletion of the outer layers (Fig. 27.16). There are small foci of transition in these glands, where diffuse depletion of lipid may be adjacent to areas showing lipid retention in the deeper layers. In all probability, the apparent lipid retention in the deeper layers represents the reaccumulation of lipid in cells that were once depleted. The lipid vacuoles in these deeper cells are smaller than expected, and the cells display the pyroninophilia of a "stressed" cell.

The diffuse pattern of depletion of adrenal cortical lipid is seen in stillbirths dying from acute antepartum hemorrhage, acute cord prolapse, acute infections in utero, or other "acute" causes of death. It coexists with other "acute" signs,

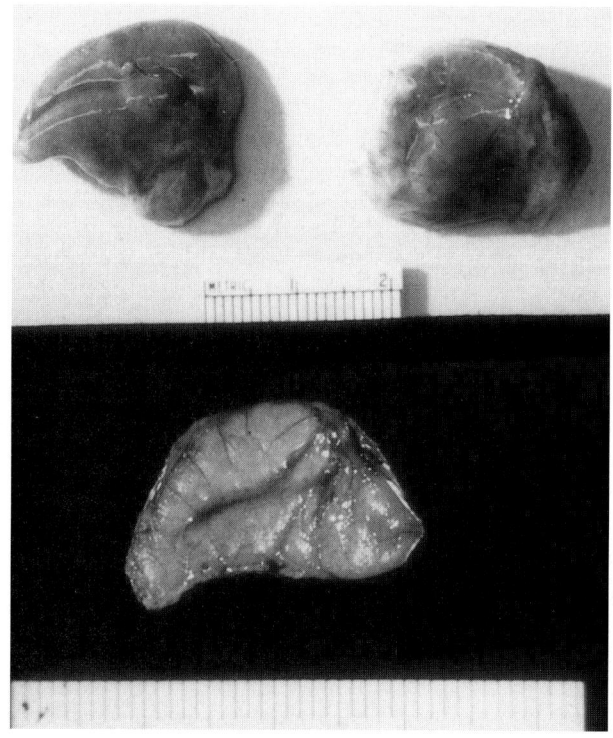

FIGURE 27.12. *Dark red stressed glands (above) contrast with lipid-rich normal gland (below).*

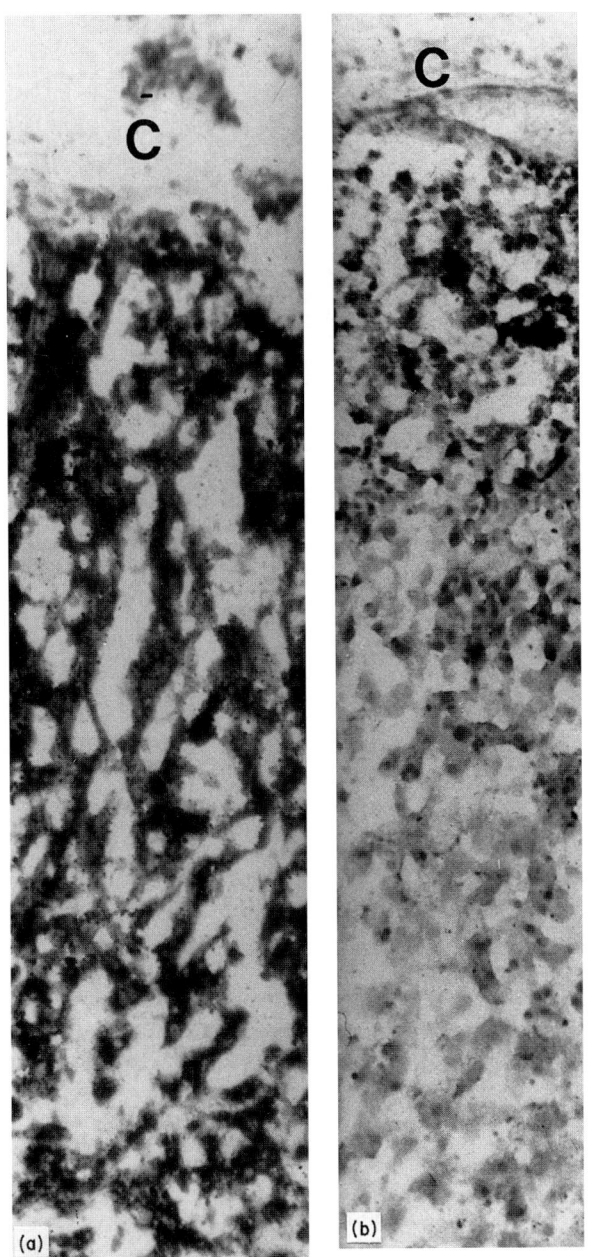

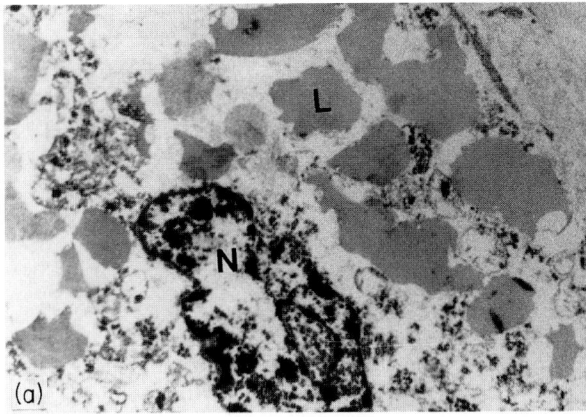

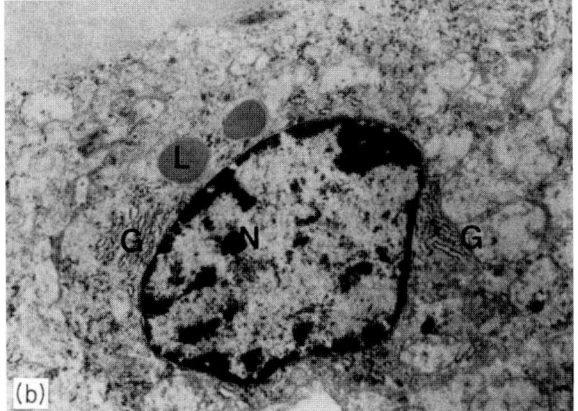

FIGURE 27.14.   *Ultrastructural appearances of a lipid-rich cell (a) and a stressed lipid-depleted cell (b), showing the decrease in lipid content and increase in granular endoplasmic reticulum in the stressed cell. N = nucleus, L = lipid, G = granular endoplasmic reticulum. Lead citrate, uranyl acetate; ×18,000. (Courtesy of deSa [57].)*

FIGURE 27.13.   *Frozen section of lipid-rich unstressed gland (a) contrasted with lipid depletion in an acutely stressed gland (b). C = capsule. Oil red O, ×450.*

such as serosal petechiae, thymic petechiae, and "starry-sky" change in the thymic cortex. The "clear-cell" reversal pattern is seen most frequently in association with intrauterine growth retardation and hydrops fetalis. In hydrops fetalis, this change may be very extensive indeed and may even be associated with microcalcification (Fig. 27.17).

Becker and Becker [59] have shown that the patterns of lipid depletion help in identifying "acute" and "chronic" modes of death in stillbirths. While this is a helpful concept in the study of fresh stillbirths, this author has found the Beckers' scheme to be less reliable in severely macerated stillbirths. However, the pattern of adrenal lipid distribution may be useful in assessing which one of multiple obstetric complications may have been of particular importance in causing a stillbirth. In a stillbirth born to a mother with hypertension and an antepartum hemorrhage, an "acute" stress reaction could suggest that the antepartum hemorrhage was of greater immediate importance, while a "chronic" pattern could indicate that "chronic" placental hypoperfusion may have been of greater significance than the hemorrhage. The Beckers' scheme [59] has been said to be unreliable when studying fetuses in the second trimester [3], but material from these fetuses seems to show a range of lipid patterns that are comparable to those seen in older fetuses. There does not seem to be any definite reason why the general principle should not apply to them as well.

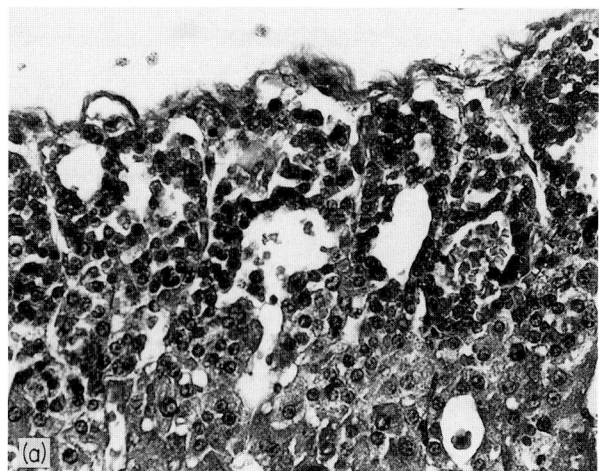
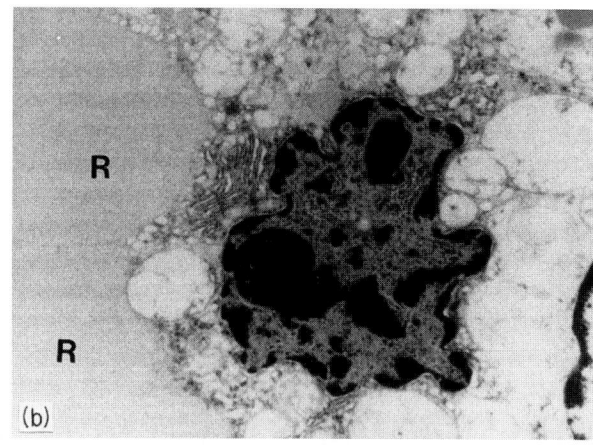

FIGURE 27.15.   (a) Pseudofollicular pattern in stressed adrenal cortex. H&E, ×100. (b) Ultrastructurally, the "follicles" are produced by cytolysis of stressed cells, and the follicles contain red cells and debris (R). ×14,000. (Courtesy of deSa [57].)

THE ADRENALS IN ANENCEPHALY AND OTHER MAJOR MALFORMATIONS OF THE CENTRAL NERVOUS SYSTEM

In anencephalic infants, outside the central nervous system (CNS), the most consistent anomaly is the presence of extremely small "hypoplastic" adrenal glands. The adrenal glands are markedly reduced in size and may be so minute that they are difficult to identify. In addition to the obvious reduction in size, there is an extremely important qualitative difference between the adrenal glands of anencephalics and those of normal infants. At term, the fetal adrenal gland in the anencephalic has a severely reduced or absent fetal cortex (Fig. 27.18). It can be shown that in anencephalics

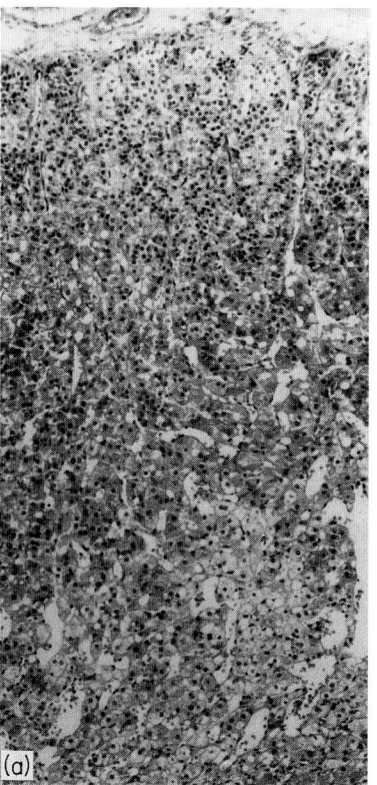
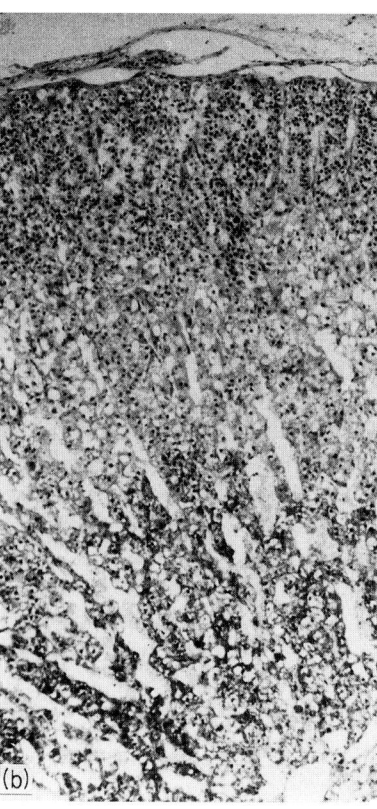

FIGURE 27.16.   The "clear-cell reversal" pattern is characterized by (a) vacuolated lipid-rich cells deep in the fetal cortex and more superficial stressed cells. H&E, ×40. (b) Frozen sections stained with oil red O reveal the darkly staining lipid. Oil red O, ×40.

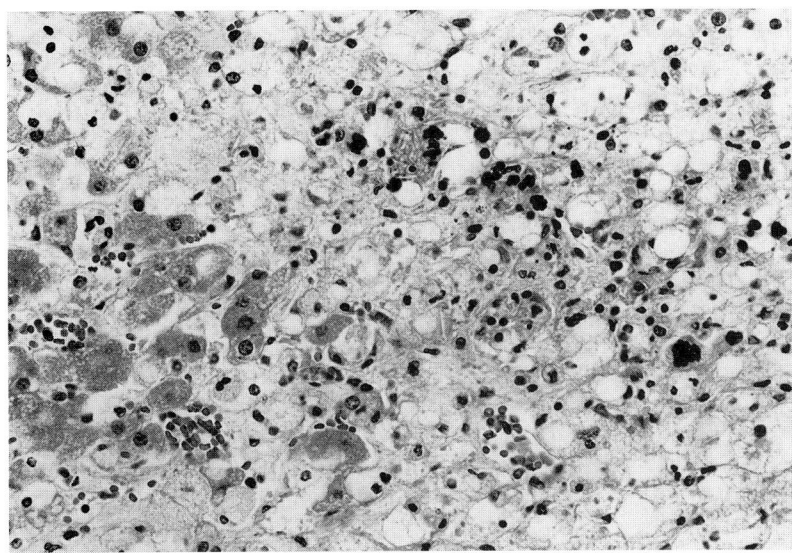

FIGURE 27.17. *A view of the deeper layers of the fetal cortex in an infant with Rhesus isoimmunization and hydrops fetalis. Swollen lipid-rich cells are visible, and there is spotty microcalcification (seen as darkly stained masses). H&E, ×150.*

the adrenal gland develops normally until the 20th week of gestation and then atrophies progressively to term [3, 60]. Experimentally, the fetal cortex can be made to atrophy by transection of the pituitary stalk or hypothalamic damage in animals, and the marked reduction in the fetal cortex seen in anencephalics is directly related to the intrinsic abnormality of the hypothalamic-pituitary axis, with lack of ACTH stimulation. The fetal cortex can be "restored" to normal size by the administration of ACTH [61]. Despite the reduced overall mass and hypoplastic fetal cortex of their adrenals, anencephalic infants do not suffer from deficiency of cortisol, since sufficient maternal cortisol can cross the placenta to meet the needs of the fetus. However, pregnancies with anencephalic fetuses that are *not* complicated by hydramnios are often prolonged [62], and, by analogy with results in sheep, this is linked to a failure of adrenal steroid production [63]. It is more likely, however, that prolongation of pregnancy in anencephalics is due to many factors

other than failure of adrenal steroid production. These factors include deficient estriol production [64], which appears to make the myometrium less sensitive to the action of prostaglandins, especially $PGF_{2\alpha}$.

Changes identical to those seen in anencephalic infants may be seen in the adrenal cortices of infants with other major malformations of the CNS, such as severe hydrocephalus [16]. The adrenal changes in such infants are invariably associated with pituitary lesions and disruption of the hypothalamus-hypophyseal portal system of vessels (see Pituitary), and have sometimes been described as forming one variant of adrenal hypoplasia (see below).

ADRENAL CYTOMEGALY

In the Beckwith-Wiedemann syndrome, there is a triad of lesions characterized by exomphalos, visceromegaly (when organ weights of affected infants are compared with

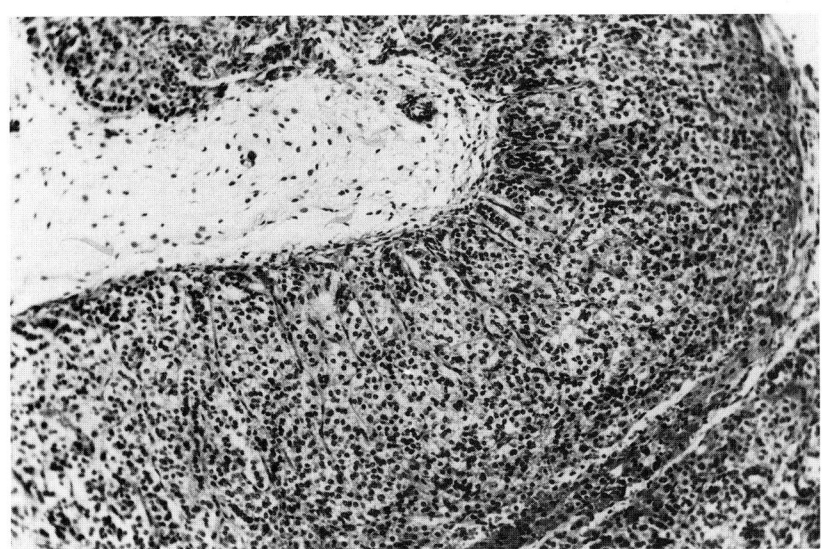

FIGURE 27.18. *Adrenal gland of an anencephalic fetus delivered at 42 weeks' gestation. Note the poorly developed fetal cortex. H&E, ×32.*

unaffected infants of comparable gestation and age), and macroglossia [65, 66]. The adrenal glands are not only enlarged, but are the sites of one of the most striking and consistent histologic hallmarks of the syndrome [67]. There is massive enlargement of the fetal zone, with numerous and diffusely scattered cortical cells with enlarged nuclei (two to three times the normal size). The nuclei are hyperchromatic, and they may be irregular in shape, with pseudoinclusions and intranuclear vacuoles (Fig. 27.19). Cytomegalovirus is *not* found in these cells. When ectopic adrenal tissue is present, it may show similar changes.

Recently, the gene for Beckwith-Wiedemann syndrome (BWS) has been linked to the short arm of chromosome 11 (11p). Trisomy of 11p has been described in some cases of Beckwith-Wiedemann syndrome [68, 69]. In a case personally studied by the author, the diagnosis of Beckwith-Wiedemann syndrome was made in an infant of 22 weeks' gestation who presented with exomphalos, massive cytomegaly of adrenal cortical cells, pancreatic islet cell hyperplasia, renal dysplasia, interstitial cell hyperplasia of the testis with cytomegaly, and a reciprocal translocation of 11p and 16q.

Only a very small minority of infants with Beckwith-Wiedemann syndrome die in the neonatal period (due to a concomitant islet cell hyperplasia of the pancreas, leading to hyperinsulinemia and hypoglycemia). In survivors, there is an appreciably increased risk of developing Wilms' tumor of the kidney (also linked to chromosome 11), adrenal cortical carcinoma, and an expanding range of tumors including pancreatoblastoma and hepatic tumors [70–75]. It has been suggested that this proclivity to develop a wide range of tumors in the Beckwith-Wiedemann syndrome is related to the proximity of the BWS gene on chromosome 11p to insulin-like growth factor II and the HRAS-1 oncogene [71].

The reason(s) for the development of the very striking adrenal nuclear enlargement in the Beckwith-Wiedemann syndrome is not known, but it may be that it represents an

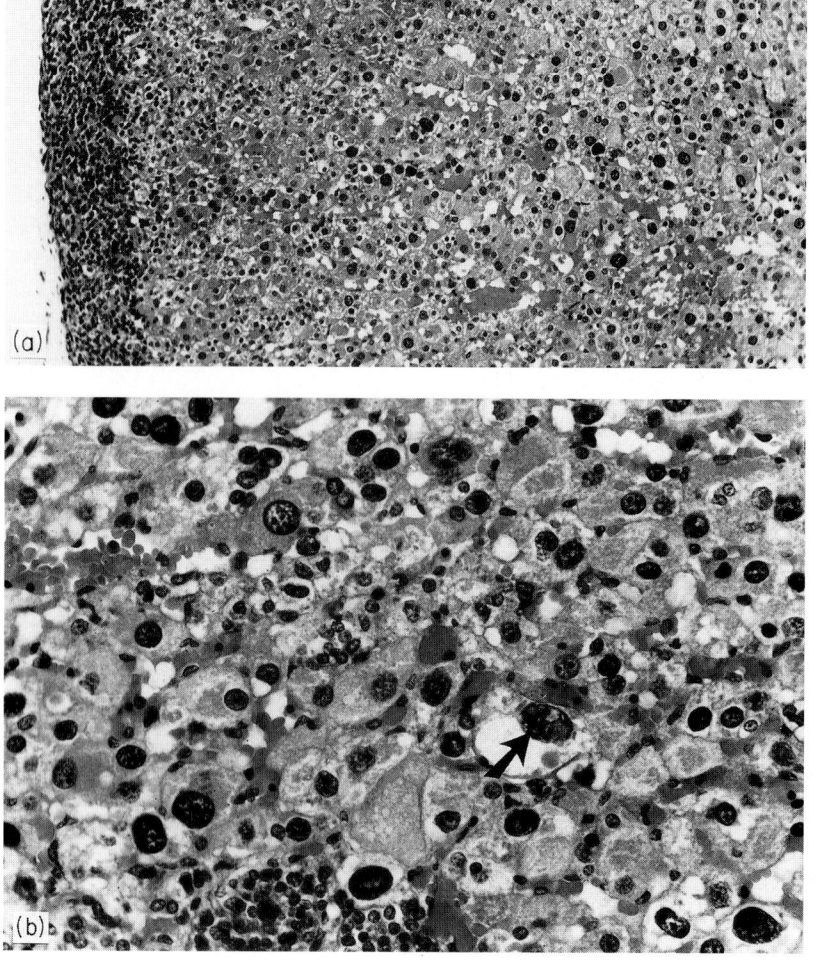

FIGURE 27.19.   *The adrenals in Beckwith-Wiedemann syndrome. (a) Large hyperchromatic nuclei are visible in the fetal cortex. H&E, ×40. (b) At a higher magnification, the bizarre nature of the nuclei is obvious. Note pseudoinclusion (arrow). H&E, ×150.*

exaggerated response to ACTH stimulation with an underlying intrinsic defect linked to damage to the short arm of chromosome 11. Pituitary amphophil hyperplasia has been described in some infants with Beckwith-Wiedemann syndrome [67], suggesting that a pituitary component may be involved in the development of the adrenal nuclear changes.

Other Causes of Adrenal Cytomegaly

Scattered foci of adrenal cortical cells displaying the characteristic features of adrenal cytomegaly may be seen in a number of other clinical settings. In these infants, they usually occur as small focal aggregates, distinct from the diffuse involvement observed in Beckwith-Wiedemann syndrome, and the adrenal glands are not enlarged. The changes may be unilateral or bilateral. Focal adrenal cytomegaly has been reported as occurring in several different intrauterine viral infections, including rubella [76], and in association

with extensive hemolysis (as seen in conditions as disparate as rhesus isoimmunization, congenital lupus erythematosus, and erythropoietic porphyria). The polyploidy represents protracted stimulation in cells unable to divide [77–80]. Cytomegaly may also be seen in association with trisomy 13 and trisomy 18 (sometimes in very small glands) [58]. Ectopic adrenal tissue, on very rare occasions, may show a similar change. This list of additional causes is incomplete, since increasing attention to the adrenal gland will undoubtedly reveal more associations.

ADRENAL INVOLVEMENT IN SPECIFIC SYSTEMIC INFECTIONS

Reference has been made to the occurrence of hemorrhagic necrosis of the adrenal glands in infants with bacterial sepsis and to the "stress pattern" that may be present in those infants and fetuses that have experienced a gestation

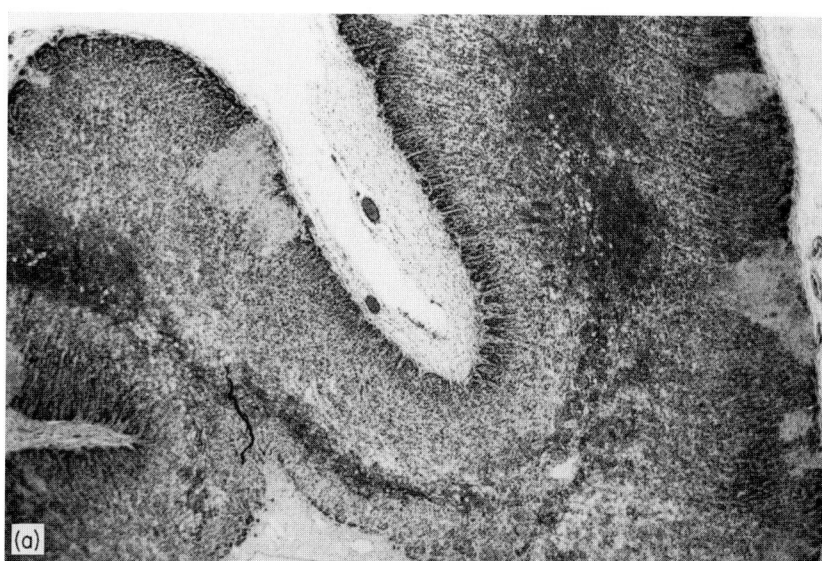

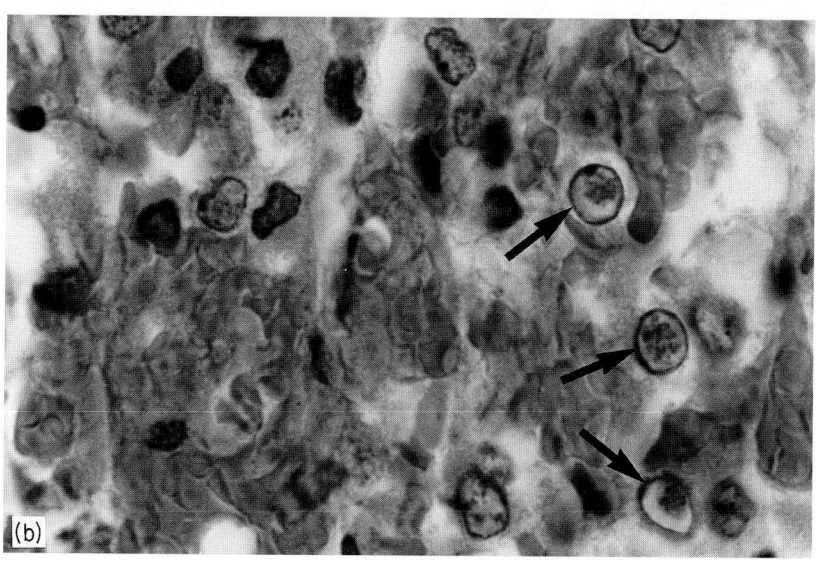

FIGURE 27.20. *(a) Pale, sharply demarcated necrotic foci are seen in a case of neonatal herpes simplex II infection. H&E, ×15. (b) In viable cells adjacent to the necrosis, intranuclear inclusions are visible (arrowheads) as well as smudged "ground-glass" nuclei. H&E, ×800.*

complicated by chorioamnionitis in utero. Septic necrosis of the adrenal gland may be seen in cases of systemic infections with gram-negative organisms, especially *Pseudomonas* species, or in generalized listeriosis. The lesions are sharply demarcated, and histologically, organisms may be seen in the affected tissues. In infections with gram-negative organisms, there is often invasion of the walls of blood vessels in the capsule. Very similar lesions may be found in disseminated candidiasis (36). A bland capsular and cortical fibrosis may occur in congenital syphilis. There is, however, considerable variation among cases, and in many examples of disseminated infections, apart from a stress reaction, the adrenal is uninvolved.

Many *viral* infections damage the adrenal gland, and necrotic lesions may accompany congenital infections due to herpes simplex (Fig. 27.20), coxsackie B infections, and echovirus infections [81, 82]. The lesions vary in severity from sharply punched-out necrotic foci to diffuse destruction. Occasionally, intranuclear inclusions may be present without evidence of tissue necrosis as in many infants with congenital cytomegalovirus infections.

Adrenal Abscesses

Adrenal abscesses are rare but may develop on a background of hemorrhagic necrosis (with secondary bacterial colonization) or as a complication of any of the infections previously noted [36].

CONGENITAL ADRENAL HYPERPLASIA

Several enzyme deficiencies block the ability of the fetal adrenal gland to produce any cortisol, and this leads to the production of a variety of other steroids, including androgens [83]. In these conditions, there is no "negative feed-back," and fetal pituitary ACTH continues to be secreted. The adrenal glands, acting under the unopposed influence of the abundant ACTH output, undergo an extreme degree of hyperplasia. The gland is enlarged and heavier than expected, but in addition the cortical cells are thrown into a complex undulating ribbon that produces a characteristically "cerebriform" appearance in the intact gland. The cerebriform convolutions of the cortex are especially obvious when the cut surface of the gland is examined (Figs. 27.21

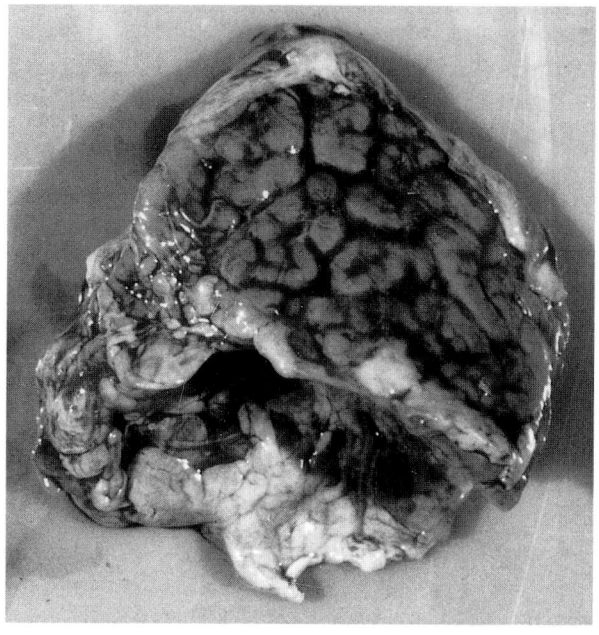

FIGURE 27.21. *An adrenal from a case of salt-losing adrenal hyperplasia due to 21-hydroxylase deficiency. ×3.*

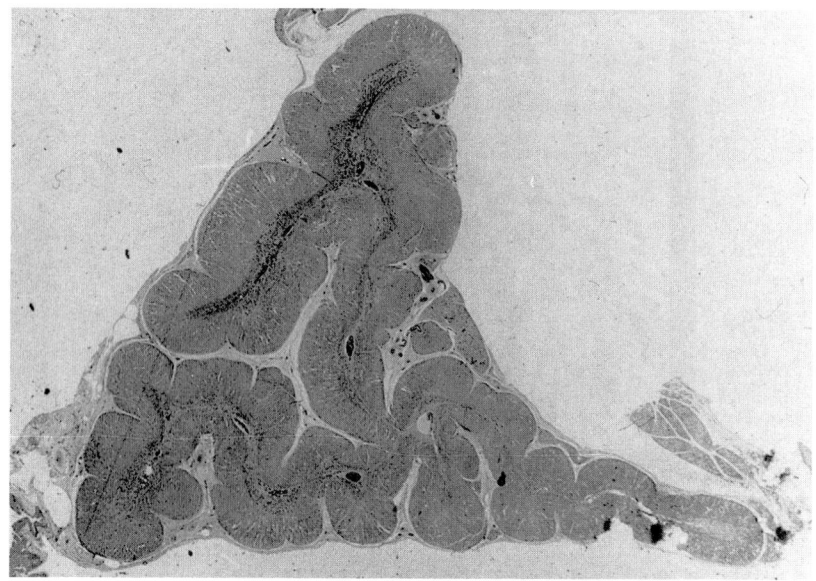

FIGURE 27.22. *A low-power view of the adrenal gland shown in Fig. 27.21, showing the cerebriform convolutions of adrenal cortex. ×9.*

Table 27.1.   Salient clinical features of disorders of steroidogenesis. (After New et al [83])

Enzyme Defect*	Newborn Sexual Ambiguity (occurs in)	Salt Wasting	Hypertension	Postnatal Virilization
1. 21α-Hydroxylase				
a) Simple virilizing	Females	++	0	+
b) Salt-losing	Females	++	0	+
2. 11β-Hydroxylase ("Hypertensive")	Females	0	++	+
3. 3β-Hydroxysteroid dehydrogenase	Both males and females	+	0	0
4. 17α-Hydroxylase	Females	0	+	0
5. Cholesterol desmolase (congenital lipid hyperplasia)	Males	0	+	0
6. 18-Hydroxylase (aldosterone defect)	—	++	0	0
7. Methyl oxidase type II (18-dehydrogenase of 18-hydroxycorticosterone)	—	++	0	0
8. 17β-Hydroxysteroid dehydrogenase	Males, possibly females	0	0	+ (Pubertal males)

*   Enzyme defects 1–4 are associated with classic congenital adrenal hyperplasia; defect 5 is associated with lipid hyperplasia. Disorders associated with enzyme defects 6–8 are not known to cause adrenal hyperplasia, but they can be confused with those that do.

and 27.22). The complex infolding ensures that an extremely large increase in cortical mass is *not* associated with any increase in the distance between the capsular surface and the deep tributaries of the central vein.

The several enzymic deficiencies are associated in most cases with identical macroscopic appearances in congenital adrenal hyperplasia (Table 27.1). With the exception of "congenital lipid hyperplasia," there are no macroscopic features that are pathognomonic of any specific deficiency, and distinction among the different states depends on detailed biochemical studies of corticosteroid metabolism. There are clinical features such as virilization and sodium loss that may suggest what the deficiency in any particular case may be, but a definitive diagnosis always requires detailed biochemical study. Detailed descriptions of the various clinical states are available [27, 83], but it is worth emphasizing that, during the first few days of life, many of the infants are not distressed, due to protective levels of circulating maternal cortisol.

The clinical and biochemical changes generally conform to expectations based on accumulation of precursors and deficiency of products distal to the site of action of the absent enzyme. The three most common defects (21α-hydroxylase, 11β-hydroxylase, and 3β-hydroxysteroid dehydrogenase deficiencies) are associated with virilization of the female fetus as a result of overproduction of testosterone and its precursors, one of which, dehydroepiandrosterone, is also a major fetal precursor to maternal estriol production. With the rarer enzyme defects (17α-hydroxylase and desmolase deficiencies), both glucocorticoid and sex steroid production are reduced. Hardy et al [84] describe a case of desmolase deficiency in a female fetus associated with low maternal estriol levels.

New et al [83] have postulated a functional separation between the zona fasciculata and glomerulosa in the devel-

oping adrenal. This "two-gland" hypothesis draws support from the infants with 21α-hydroxylase deficiency, some of whom may have salt wasting while others do not. In infants *without* salt wasting, the enzyme defect is found only in cells of the fasciculata. The development of salt wasting is attributed to the enzyme defect being expressed in cells of both the glomerulosa and fasciculata.

Microscopically, the hyperplastic adrenal cortical cells in congenital adrenal hyperplasia show an irregular pattern of lipid retention and depletion, but the cells do not appear unusual in any other way. Ultrastructural studies have shown variable results, with some cases showing mitochondrial ballooning and prominence of rough endoplasmic reticulum, while other cases have shown only modest deviations from normal.

Cortisol therapy has turned a life-threatening situation into an eminently salvageable condition. The importance of early diagnosis is, of course, self-evident, and delay in reaching a diagnosis can still lead to death by electrolyte depletion. It is notable, however, that few affected fetuses die in utero, reemphasizing the protective role of maternal cortisol production.

Congenital Lipid Hyperplasia

In this variety of congenital adrenal hyperplasia, the changes in the adrenal gland appear to be sufficiently distinctive to suggest the diagnosis. The glands are enlarged, the cortex is pale and nodular, and appropriate stratification is not seen. The cortical cells are large and lipid-filled and cholesterol may be present. The deficiency may affect any of three enzymes [83], and there is an inability to synthesize many steroids, including androgens. The failure to produce androgens is associated with the development of a female genital tract in affected male fetuses [85].

Enlargement of the Adrenal Glands

The adrenal glands may appear enlarged and fat laden in hydropic infants [58]. Gaillard et al [3] described an increase in adrenal gland weight in some second-trimester fetuses suffering from "hypoxia" of variable origin. The adrenal gland undergoes some enlargement in adults exposed to prolonged stress [6], and Gaillard's observations [3] are intriguing since they would suggest that a similar phenomenon is present very early in development. (In view of the development of adrenal cytomegaly, another probable response to chronic stress, this should not occasion too much surprise.) Nodular hyperplasia as a response to previous scarring has been referred to [33]. Swollen adrenal glands may also be seen in some storage diseases (see below).

HYPOPLASIA OF ADRENAL GLANDS

Adrenal hypoplasia is a field of considerable complexity and some controversy, which has received some welcome clarification. Lockitch et al [27] offer a classification of primary and secondary hypoplasia and link these anomalies to their patterns of inheritance where appropriate. Three histologic patterns are observed: "anencephalic," "cytomegalic," and "miniature" types. The lesions may be inherited as an X-linked, autosomal recessive, or variable trait, or may occur sporadically.

Anencephalic-Type Hypoplasia

Very occasionally, infants without any anatomic malformation of the hypothalamo-hypophyseal region are found to have extremely small adrenal glands (usually less than 2 gm total weight) at autopsy. Structurally, the glands have a poorly developed fetal cortex, resembling that seen in anencephalic infants, and the bulk of the gland is made up of definitive cortex. These otherwise anatomically normal infants may be considered to have the "anencephalic" variant of adrenal hypoplasia. (This variety may of course also be present in infants with pituitary/hypothalamic anomalies.) It is worth emphasizing that the size of the fetal adrenal gland reflects the combination of effects due to an inhibitor of cortisol production and a sustained ACTH output. In the absence of pituitary or hypothalamic lesions, the "hypoplastic" adrenal could indicate an inability to respond to ACTH. The otherwise normal development of these infants in utero reflects protection by maternal cortisol production. Symptoms present shortly after birth, with early death if untreated; survivors may have hypogonadism at puberty [86].

Cytomegalic-Type Hypoplasia

A second variety of adrenal hypoplasia is associated with an abnormal histologic pattern similar to that seen in adults with primary Addison disease or neonatal leukodystrophy

(Fig. 27.23). The cortex is shrunken and of irregular width; the cells are arranged in nodules, with clusters of enlarged cells with abundant eosinophilic cytoplasm and occasional lymphoid aggregates. The nuclei may be enlarged with pseudoinclusions similar to but less marked than those found in "cytomegaly." The only example personally studied by the author was from an infant born to a mother with gestational diabetes mellitus, and the possibility of an autoimmune destructive phenomenon was considered but never proved. Weiss and Mellinger [87] described an X-linked recessive trait in their patients with the cytomegalic form of adrenal hypoplasia, but many cases appear to be sporadic in nature [88]. Some of these individuals have an associated myopathy and glycerol kinase deficiency [89], but detailed biochemical analyses do not appear to be available for most cases.

Miniature-Type Hypoplasia

One of the more disturbing and distressing findings at autopsy in some neonates is the presence of quantitatively small adrenal glands (less than 2 gm total mass) that, nevertheless, show relatively normal proportions of fetal and definitive cortex on histologic examination. This quantitative reduction in the presence of apparently normal differentiation is difficult to explain. While some cases have been described in triploidy [90], very many cases do not have any obvious association with malformation syndromes or karyotypic abnormalities. Favara et al [91] reported finding small adrenal glands in five neonatal infants who died suddenly. Two were born to hypertensive mothers and were small for gestational age. None of the five neonates (nor any of the five older infants in this report) showed any evidence of chronic adrenocortical insufficiency, so that it is unlikely that hypofunction of the adrenal cortex played a significant role. However, as the authors indicate, the rapid deterioration in these infants suggests an inability to cope with an acute stress. Brown and Singer [92] described similar findings in the infants of mothers with pregnancy-induced hypertension.

No adequate explanation for the changes exists, since the presence of a well-defined fetal zone (albeit quantitatively reduced) implies an effective ACTH drive; the presence of such a drive would lead one to expect an adrenal gland of normal size. The observations of Gaillard et al [3] should be recalled, since in early gestation some (but not all) infants suffering from hypoxia showed adrenal *enlargement*. The possibility exists that the "hypoplasia" may represent atrophy following previous hypertrophy, but there is no conclusive evidence on this point.

Hereditary unresponsiveness to ACTH may mimic the clinical picture of adrenal hypoplasia [93–95]. However, the pathology of the adrenal glands in neonatal infants with this condition is not described fully, and the patterns of inheritance are uncertain. Older infants have an atrophic zona fasciculata in a small gland, but the zona glomerulosa is intact.

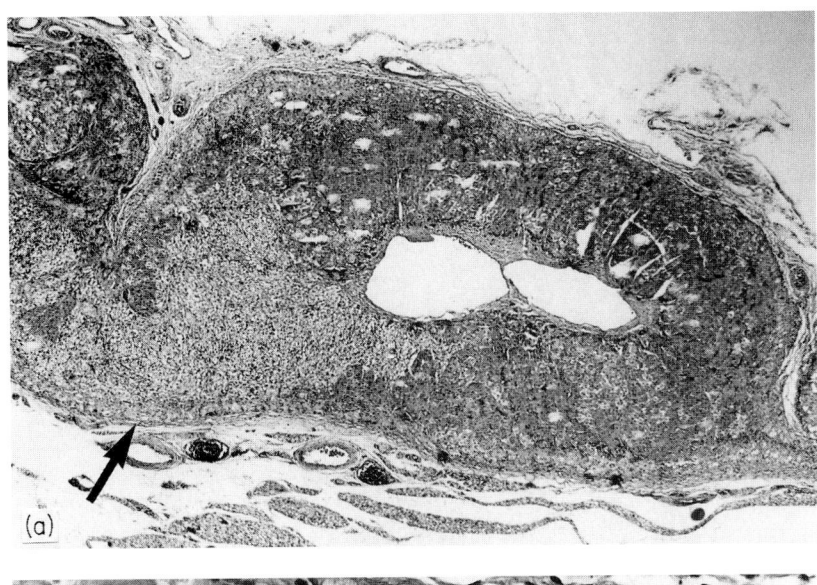

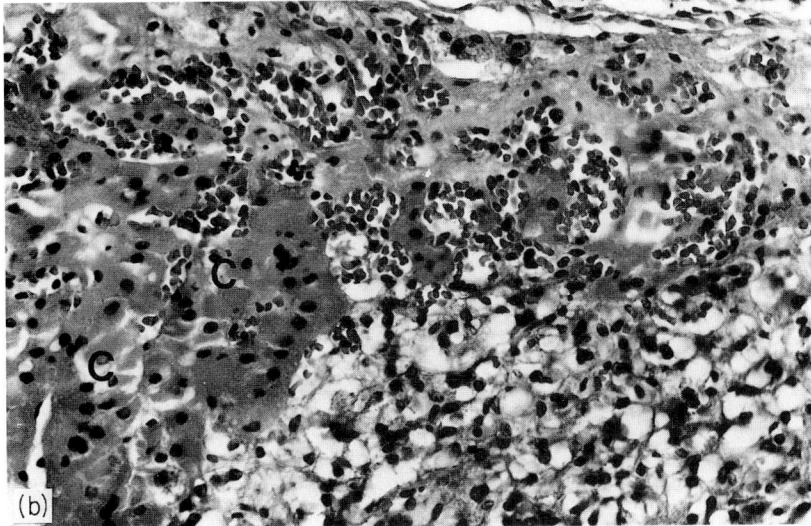

FIGURE 27.23. *A small adrenal gland (<2 gm) from a case of adrenal hypoplasia of the "cytomegalic" type. (a) The darker-staining cortex is of irregular thickness, with baring of the medulla (arrow). H&E, ×40. (b) At a higher magnification, the cortical cells (C) are plump and show darkly staining nuclei. C = cortical cells, M = medulla. H&E, ×150.*

Whether or not this represents the effect of steroid therapy is uncertain. Finally, some familial cases of adrenal hypoplasia defy classification due to incomplete histologic details, but probably fall into the "miniature" type [96]. Some examples of "anencephalic"-type hypoplasia may have occasional cytomegalic cells. Therefore, no classification covers all the details or is completely satisfactory [97].

ADRENAL INVOLVEMENT IN METABOLIC STORAGE DISEASE

While most patients with Wolman disease (cholesterol-ester storage due to acid lipase deficiency) do not die in the newborn period, they may present in the newborn period with hepatosplenomegaly and calcification in the adrenal gland [98]. The glands are enlarged, and the cut surface has a chalky-yellow color with a gritty consistency. Calcifica-

tion may be scattered throughout the gland, but is more obvious in the deeper layers. As well as the adrenal cortical cells, the sinusoidal lining cells are swollen, and the characteristic profiles of cholesterol crystals can be identified within their cytoplasm (Fig. 27.24). Cholesterol can be demonstrated in frozen sections studied with polarized light, and by staining the same sections with Sudan dyes or oil red O. Detailed biochemical studies of the distribution of cholesterol and lipid storage were reported by Lough et al [99] and by Beaudet et al [100].

Adrenal involvement has been seen rarely in other storage diseases in older children [31], but lesions in the neonatal period do not appear to have been reported.

Adrenal cortical cells and endothelial cells may show an increase in stainable iron in the uncommon neonatal disorder of iron storage known as "idiopathic neonatal iron storage disease" [101–105].

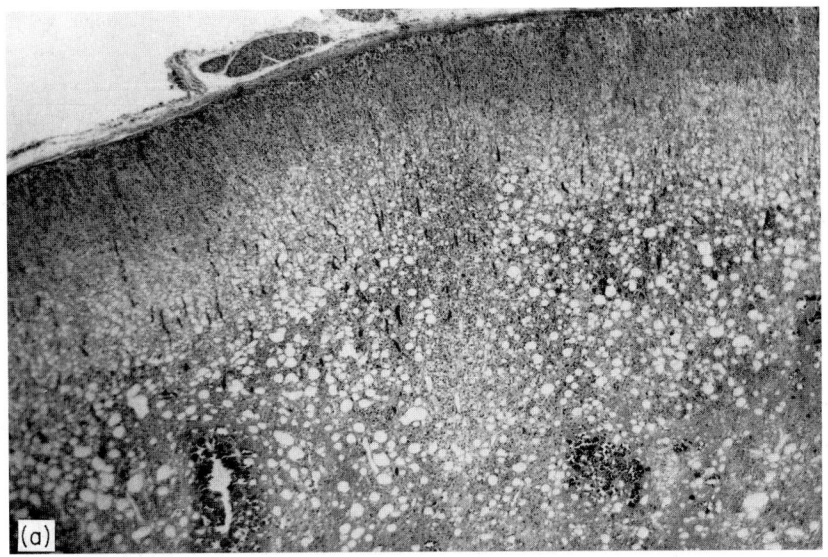

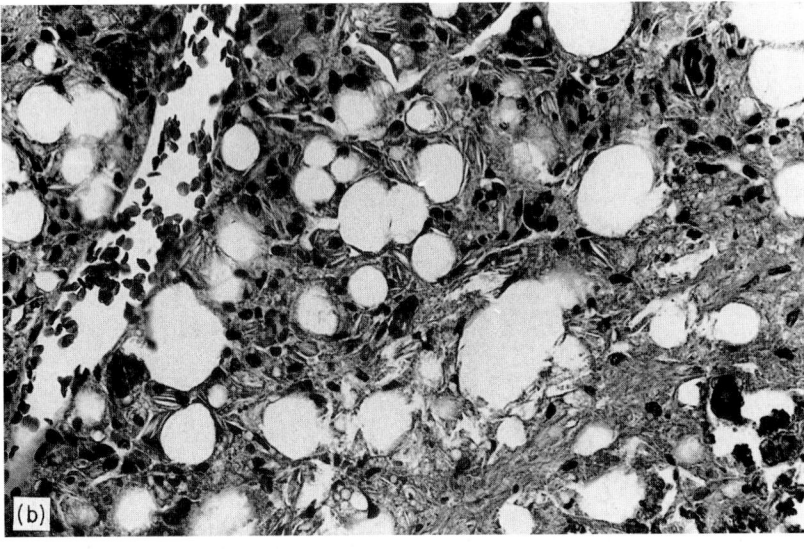

FIGURE 27.24.   *(a) Swollen adrenal glands with focal calcification characterize Wolman disease. H&E, ×10. (b) At a higher magnification, the calcification is associated with foamy macrophages and giant cells related to needle-like cholesterol crystals. H&E, ×150.*

Accelerated Maturation of the Adrenal Medulla

In a study that needs to be confirmed, accelerated maturation of the adrenal medulla was reported in anencephalics [106]. This provocative observation raises questions about the potential interrelationship between adrenocortical cells and medullary development. It would be of interest also to know the status of the other chromaffin tissues in anencephalics.

TUMORS OF THE ADRENAL GLAND

Isolated clusters and rosettes of neuroblastic cells, *rarely more than 100 μm in overall diameter*, are a frequent histologic finding in the adrenal glands of very immature fetuses. They may be associated with areas of marked sinusoidal dilatation (mimicking hemorrhagic foci), and, at a microscopic level, the resemblance to neuroblastomata is striking [107]. They

are not true tumors, but they represent islands of aberrant migration of sympathogonia as distinct from pheochromocyte precursors [4]. Beckwith and Perrin [108] described discrete nodular lesions of immature neuroblasts, *usually in excess of 2 mm in diameter*, in the adrenal glands of several infants. They called these much larger lesions "in situ neuroblastomata" and discussed their possible relationship to true invasive neuroblastomata. The lesions were found incidentally at autopsy, and metastatic spread had not occurred. Many of the infants had anomalies of the CNS. The "in situ neuroblastomata" are large, vascular, clearly delineated, discrete nodules, and are recognizable on gross inspection (Fig. 27.25). While it is possible that these neuroblastomata are derived from the aberrant foci of sympathogonia, it is difficult to assess their overall potential with regard to growth, differentiation, and metastatic spread. Some have, however, shown ganglion-cell-like differentiation. It may be that these collections of small cells and neuroblastomata in situ mature

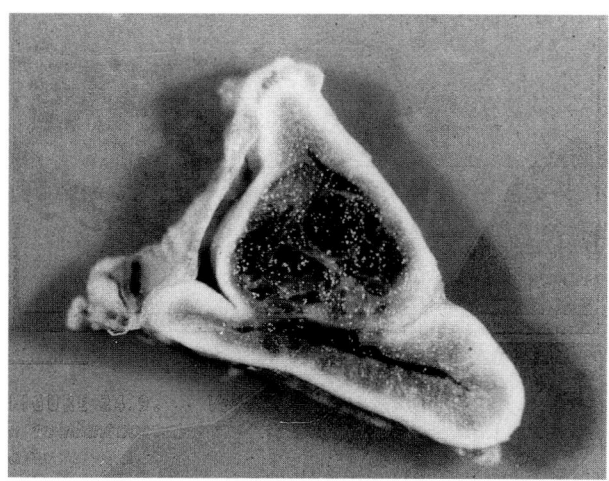

FIGURE 27.25. *A hemorrhagic tumor nodule in the adrenal of an infant who died of myocarditis at 3 days of age. Histologically, the lesion was a neuroblastoma with numerous dilated vessels. No metastases were seen. ×3.*

into the irregularly distributed foci of medullary and chromaffin tissue that may be encountered in sections of the adrenal gland in both infants and adults. Some neuroblastomata in situ may undergo regression and calcify, accounting for the presence of some calcific foci in areas of necrosis with ghost cells.

Congenital Disseminated Neuroblastoma (IV-S Neuroblastoma)

This relatively uncommon form of disseminated neuroblastoma may present in the newborn period. Adrenal involvement is always present, and multiple "hemorrhagic" nodules may be seen in the skin, viscera, and bone marrow (but there is no bony destruction). The placenta may be enlarged and bulky and may show neuroblastic cells in (fetal) villous capillaries, but without invasion of the (maternal) intervillous space or (fetal) stroma [109]. When biopsied, the lesions in the skin and viscera may mimic an undifferentiated metastatic neoplasm, but mitotic rates are usually low. Despite the extensive involvement, many of the infants recover spontaneously and show no residual ill effects. This decidedly unusual behavior suggests that the lesion is not a true neoplasm, but rather a generalized hamartomatosis [110]. It has been suggested that there is an analogy between the aberrant migration of neural crest cells, as seen in the adrenal gland in many fetuses, and the more diffuse aberrant migration as seen in IV-S congenital neuroblastoma. There may be a link with von Recklinghausen's neurofibromatosis [111]. While there is no satisfactory explanation at present for the behavior of congenital disseminated neuroblastomata, Bolande has produced some elegant experimental evidence to show that the cytolytic form of regression of

these congenital tumors may be mediated by an IgM-complement-mediated reaction [112].

Not all cases of congenital neuroblastoma survive. Some may have massive liver and/or cardiac involvement and present as examples of nonimmune hydrops fetalis, which may be refractory to treatment [109].

Chromosomal anomalies have been described in truly malignant neuroblastomata with metastases, but as yet the karyotype of congenital neuroblastomata has been firmly established. In one example personally studied by the author, a normal 46XX karyotype was found in 25 of 26 cells. In the remaining cell, a balanced translocation between 7p and 17p was found. Neuroblastomata have occurred in more than one member of a family, sometimes with anomalies of other organs [113–116]. A pedigree with segregation of Hirschsprung disease and neuroblastomata has been described by Chatten and Witzleben [117]. Overall, the vast majority of neuroblastomata are sporadic. Ten of the 55 cases of familial neuroblastomata (from 23 familiar aggregations) have presented as IV-S congenital cases [118].

Other Tumors of the Adrenal Gland

Rarely, retroperitoneal teratomata may involve and replace the adrenal gland. These tumors of aberrant totipotent germ cells are invariably large and not confined to the adrenal gland alone. Adenomata and carcinomata of the adrenal cortex are rare in neonates [119, 120]. Potter and Craig [55] describe a pheochromocytoma near the adrenal gland of a newborn infant.

REFERENCES

1. Crowder RE. The development of the adrenal gland in man, with special reference to origin and ultimate location of cell types and evidence in favour of the cell migration theory. *Carnegie Contr Embryol* 1957; 36:193–217.
2. Neville AM, O'Hare MJ. *The Human Adrenal Cortex.* Berlin: Springer-Verlag, 1982, p. 12.
3. Gaillard DA, Lallemand AV, Moirot HH, et al. Fetal adrenal development during the second trimester of gestation. *Pediatr Pathol* 1990; 10:335–50.
4. Faye-Petersen O, Parker CR Jr. Histomorphologic and immunohistochemical studies of human adrenal medullary ontogeny. *Pediatr Pathol* 1995; 15:349–50. Abstract.
5. Faye-Petersen O, Parker CR Jr. Adrenal cortical expression of cytokeratin, vimentin, and synaptophysin during human fetal development. *Pediatr Pathol* 1995; 15:350. Abstract.
6. Symington T. *Functional Pathology of the Human Adrenal Gland.* Edinburgh: Livingstone, 1970, pp. 70, 174.
7. Hayes MMM, Kaschula ROC. Studies on the rate of regression of the fetal adrenal cortex. *Pediatr Pathol* 1987; 7:128. Abstract.
8. Winter JSD. The adrenal cortex in the fetus and neonate. In: Anderson DC, Winter JSD, eds. *Adrenal Cortex.* London: Butterworths, 1985, pp. 32–56.
9. Fujieda K, Faiman C, Reyes FI, Winter JSD. The control of steroidogenesis in human fetal adrenal cells in tissue culture. I. Responses to adrenocorticotropin. *J Clin Endocrinol Metab* 1981; 53:34–8.
10. Fujieda K, Faiman C, Reyes FI, Winter JSD. The control of steroidogenesis in human fetal adrenal cells in tissue culture. IV. The effect of exposure to placental steroids. *J Clin Endocrinol Metab* 1982; 54:89–94.
11. Diczfalusy E. Steroid metabolism in the foeto-placental unit. *Excerpta Med Int Congr Series* 1969; 183:65–109.
12. Davies J. The fetal adrenal. In: Tulchinsky D, Ryan KJ, eds. *Maternal-Fetal Endocrinology.* Philadelphia: WB Saunders, 1980, p. 242.

13. McNulty WP. Postnatum evolution of the adrenal glands of rhesus macaques. In: Novy MJ, Resko JA, eds. *Fetal Endocrinology*. New York: Academic Press, 1981, pp. 53–64.

14. Wyllie AR, Kerr JFR, Currie AR. Cell death in the normal neonatal rat adrenal cortex. *J Pathol* 1973; 111:255–61.

15. Dawes GS. *Foetal and Neonatal Physiology*. Chicago: Year Book Medical, 1968, pp. 74, 184.

16. Benirschke K, Bloch E, Hertig AT. Concerning the function of the fetal zone of the human adrenal gland. *Endocrinology* 1956; 58:598–625.

17. Dunn JM. Anterior pituitary and adrenal absence in a live-born normocephalic infant. *Am J Obstet Gynecol* 1966; 96:893–4.

18. Wright JR Jr, Gillis DA. Mediastinal foregut cyst containing an intramural adrenal cortical rest: a case report and review of supradiaphragmatic adrenal rests. *Pediatr Pathol* 1993; 13:401–7.

19. Wiener MF, Dallgaard SA. Intracranial adrenal gland. A case report. *Arch Pathol* 1959; 67:228–33.

20. Vestfrid MA. Ectopic adrenal cortex in neonatal liver. *Histopathology* 1980; 4:669–72.

21. Busuttil A. Ectopic adrenal within the gall-bladder wall. *J Pathol* 1974; 113:231–3.

22. Qureshi F, Jacques SM. Adrenocortical heterotopia in the placenta. *Pediatr Pathol* 1995; 15:51–6.

23. Bozic C. Ectopic fetal adrenal cortex in the lung of a newborn. *Virch Arch [Pathol Anat]* 1974; 363:371–4.

24. Armin A, Castelli M. Congenital adrenal tissue in the lung with adrenal cytomegaly. *Am J Clin Pathol* 1984; 82:225–8.

25. Stowens D. *Pediatric Pathology*. 2nd ed. Baltimore: Williams & Wilkins, 1966, pp. 33, 43, 71.

26. Honore LH, O'Hara KE. Combined adrenorenal fusion and adrenohepatic adhesion: a case report with review of the literature and discussion of pathogenesis. *J Urol* 1976; 115:323–5.

27. Lockitch G, Halstead AC, Dimmick JE. Endocrine system. In: Dimmick JE, Kalousek DK, eds. *Developmental Pathology of the Embryo and Fetus*. Philadelphia: JB Lippincott, 1992, p. 707.

28. Gans B, Thurston JGB. De Lange's Amsterdam dwarf syndrome. *Dev Med Child Neurol* 1965; 7:42–5.

29. D'Cruz C, Huff D, deSa D, Zaeri N. Fused adrenals in the Cornelia de Lange syndrome. *Lab Invest* 1987; 56:1p. Abstract.

30. D'Cruz CA, Patel RB. Caudal regression syndrome: the spectrum of anomalies. *Lab Invest* 1985; 52:3p. Abstract.

31. Lack E, Kozakewich HPW. Embryology, developmental anatomy, and aspects of non-neoplastic pathology. In: Lack E, ed. *Pathology of the Adrenal Glands*. New York: Churchill-Livingstone, 1990, p. 24.

32. Kelly DR, Mroczek EC, Galliani CA, et al. Horseshoe lung and crossover lung segments: a unifying concept of fusion events in the lungs and other paired organs. *Perspect Pediatr Pathol* 1995; 18:183–213.

33. deSa DJ, Nicholls S. Haemorrhagic necrosis of the adrenal gland in perinatal infants: a clinico-pathological study. *J Pathol* 1972; 106:133–49.

34. deSa DJ, Zipursky A. Myocardial necrosis and hypofibrinogenemia: a syndrome of cardiovascular collapse? *Lab Invest* 1980; 42:171p.

35. Tyson JE, deSa DJ, Moore S. Thromboatheromatous complications of umbilical arterial catheterization in the newborn period. *Arch Dis Child* 1976; 51:744–54.

36. deSa DJ. *The Pathology of Neonatal Intensive Care*. London: Chapman & Hall Medical, 1995, p. 101.

37. Marin HM, Graham JH, Kirknam CJE. Adrenal hematoma simulating tumour in a newborn. *Arch Surg* 1955; 71:941–5.

38. Ausserer O, Ortore PG, Sarra A, von Fioreschy G. Adrenal hemorrhage in the newborn. *Progr Pediatr Surg* 1983; 16:107–11.

39. Rose J, Berdon WE, Sullivan T, Baker DH. Prolonged jaundice as presenting sign of massive adrenal hemorrhage in newborn. *Radiology* 1971; 98:263–72.

40. Stejskal J, Fucik P. Je krvaceni do nadledvin u novorozencu vzache (Is adrenal hemorrhage rare in neonates?). *Cesk Pediatr* 1989; 44:120–2.

41. Stevens RC, Tomsykoski AJ. Bilateral adrenal hemorrhage and calcification. *Am J Dis Child* 1954; 87:475–7.

42. Donn SM, Pollack LD, Roloff DW. Calcified neonatal adrenal hemorrhage: diagnostic and therapeutic considerations. *Am J Perinatol* 1983; 1:36–9.

43. Suda H, Matsuda I, Chida S, Maeta H. Neonatal adrenal hemorrhage detected antenatally. *Acta Paediatr Jpn* 1992; 34:606–10.

44. Marino J, Martinez-Urrutia MJ, Hawkins F, Gonzalez A. Encysted adrenal hemorrhage: prenatal diagnosis. *Acta Paediatr Scand* 1990; 79:230–1.

45. Demirci A, Selcuk MB, Yazicioglu I. Bilateral adrenal hemorrhage associated with bilateral renal vein and vena cava thrombosis. *Pediatr Radiol* 1991; 21:130.

46. Veiga PA, Springate JE, Brody AS, et al. Coexistence of renal vein thrombosis and adrenal hemorrhage in two newborns. *Clin Pediatr* 1992; 31: 174–6.

47. Brill PW, Jagannath A, Winchester P, Markisz J, et al. Adrenal hemorrhage and renal vein thrombosis in the newborn: MR imaging. *Radiology* 1989; 170:95–8.

48. Cheves H, Bledsoe F, Rhea WG, Bomar W. Adrenal hemorrhage with incomplete rotation of the colon leading to early duodenal obstruction: case report and review of the literature. *J Pediatr Surg* 1989; 24:300–2.

49. Levine C. Intestinal obstruction in a neonate with adrenal hemorrhage and renal vein thrombosis. *Pediatr Radiol* 1989; 19:477–8.

50. Putnam MH. Neonatal adrenal hemorrhage presenting as a right scrotal mass. *JAMA* 1989; 261:2958.

51. Elliot TR, Armour RC. The development of the cortex in the human suprarenal glands and its condition in hemicephaly. *J Pathol Bacteriol* 1911; 15:481–8.

52. Da Costa AC. Les formations vesiculeuses dans les glandes endocrines. *Comptes Rend del'Assoc Anatom* 1928; 23:69–75.

53. Gruenwald P. Embryonic and postnatal development of the adrenal cortex, particularly the zona glomerulosa and accessory nodules. *Anat Rec* 1946; 95:391–421.

54. Oppenheimer EH. Cyst formation in the outer adrenal cortex: studies in the human fetus and newborn. *Arch Pathol* 1969; 87:653–9.

55. Potter EL, Craig JM. *Pathology of the Fetus and the Infant*. 3rd ed. Year Book Medical, 1975, pp. 334, 342.

56. deSa DJ. Adrenal changes in chorioamnionitis. *Arch Dis Child* 1974; 49:149–51.

57. deSa DJ. Stress response and its relationship to cystic (pseudofollicular) change in the definitive cortex of the adrenal gland in stillborn infants. *Arch Dis Child* 1978; 53:769–76.

58. deSa DJ. The endocrine organs. In: Gilbert-Barness E, Opitz JM, eds. *Potters Pathology of the Fetus and Newborn Infant*. Philadelphia: Mosby-Year Book, 1995; pp. 1178–94.

59. Becker MJ, Becker AE. Fat distribution in the adrenal cortex as an indication of the mode of intrauterine death. *Hum Pathol* 1976; 7:495–504.

60. Nichols J. Observations on the adrenal of the premature anencephalic fetus. *Arch Pathol* 1956; 62:312–17.

61. Johannisson E. The foetal adrenal cortex in the human. Its ultrastructure at different stages of development and in different functional states. *Acta Endocrinol* 1968; 58(suppl):130.

62. Milic AB, Adamsons K. The relationship between anencephaly and prolonged pregnancy. *J Obstet Gynaecol Br Commonw* 1969; 76:102–11.

63. Liggins GC. Premature delivery of foetal lambs infused with glucocorticoids. *J Endocrinol* 1969; 45:515–23.

64. Ryan KJ. Placental synthesis of steroid hormones. In: Tulchinsky D, Ryan KJ, eds. *Maternal-Fetal Endocrinology*. Philadelphia: WB Saunders, 1980, pp. 8–9.

65. Beckwith JB. Macroglossia, omphalocele, adrenal cytomegaly, gigantism, and hyperplastic visceromegaly. *Birth Defects Orig Artic Ser* 1969; 5:188–96.

66. Wiedemann HR. Complex familial avec hernie ombilicale et macroglossie— un "syndrome nouveau." *J Genet Hum* 1964; 13:223–32.

67. Smith DW. *Recognizable Patterns of Human Malformations*. 2nd ed. Philadelphia: WB Saunders, 1976, pp. 130–1.

68. Waziri M, Patil SR, Hanson JW, Bartley JA. Abnormality of chromosome 11 in patients with features of Beckwith-Wiedemann syndrome. *J Pediatr* 1983; 102:873–6.

69. Turleau C, de Grouchy J, Chavin-Colin F, et al. Trisomy 11p15 and Beckwith-Wiedemann syndrome. A report of 2 cases. *Hum Genet* 1984; 67:219–21.

70. Sotelo-Avila C, Gooch WM III. Neoplasms associated with Beckwith-Wiedemann syndrome. *Perspect Pediatr Pathol* 1976; 3:255–72.

71. Koh TH, Cooper JE, Newman CL, et al. Pancreatoblastoma in a neonate with Wiedemann-Beckwith syndrome. *Eur J Pediatr* 1986; 145:435–8.

72. Drut R, Jones MC. Congenital pancreatoblastoma in Beckwith-Wiedemann syndrome: an emerging association. *Pediatr Pathol* 1988; 8:331–9.

73. Orozco-Florian R, McBride TA, Favara BE, et al. Congenital hepatoblastoma and Beckwith-Wiedemann syndrome: a case study including DNA ploidy profiles of tumour and adrenal cytomegaly. *Pediatr Pathol* 1991; 11:131–42.

74. Drut R, Drut RM, Toulouse JC. Hepatic hemangioendotheliomas, placental chorangiomas, and dysmorphic kidneys in Beckwith-Wiedemann syndrome. *Pediatr Pathol* 1992; 12:197–204.

75. Coffin CM, Dehner LP. Congenital tumours. In: Stocker JT, Dehner LP, eds. *Pediatric Pathology*. Philadelphia: JB Lippincott, 1992, p. 326.

76. Esterly JR, Oppenheimer EH. Intrauterine rubella infection. *Perspect Pediatr Pathol* 1973; 1:313–38.

77. Aterman K, Kerenyi N, Lee M. Adrenal cytomegaly. *Virch Arch A* 1972; 355:105–22.

78. Camuto PM, Wolman SR, Perle MA, Greco MA. Flow cytometry of fetal adrenal glands with adrenocortical cytomegaly. *Pediatr Pathol* 1989; 9:551–8.

79. Favara BE, Steele A, Grant JH, Steele P. Adrenal cytomegaly: quantitative assessment by image analysis. *Pediatr Pathol* 1991; 11:521–36.

80. Nakamura Y, Komatsu Y, Yano Y, et al. Non-immunologic hydrops fetalis: a clinicopathologic study of 50 autopsy cases. *Pediatr Pathol* 1987; 7:19–30.

81. Singer DB. Neonatal herpes simplex virus infection. *Perspect Pediatr Pathol* 1981; 6:243–78.

82. Berry PJ, Nagington J. Fatal infection with echovirus II. *Arch Dis Child* 1982; 57:22–9.

83. New MI, Dupont B, Grumbach K, Levine LS. Congenital adrenal hyperplasia and related conditions. In: Stanbury JB, Wyngaarden JB, Fredrickson DS, Goldstein JL, Brown MS, eds. *The Metabolic Basis of Inherited Disease*. 5th ed. New York: McGraw-Hill, 1983, pp. 973–1000.

84. Hardy MJ, Ragbeer MS, Goodwin JW. Low maternal blood estriol levels resulting from congenital adrenal hyperplasia in a female baby. *J Obstet Gynecol* 1984; 5:84–6.

85. Siebenmann RE. Die Kongenitale Lipoidhyperplasie der Nebennierenrinde mit Nebennierenrindeninsuffizienz. *Schweiz Z Allg Pathol Bakteriol* 1957; 20:77–86.

86. Laverty CRA, Fortune DW, Beischer NA. Congenital idiopathic adrenal hypoplasia. *Obstet Gynecol* 1973; 41:655–64.

87. Weiss L, Mellinger RC. Congenital adrenal hypoplasia: an X-linked disease. *J Med Genet* 1970; 7:27–32.

88. Oppenheimer EH. Adrenal cytomegaly: studies by light and electron microscopy. *Arch Pathol* 1970; 90:57–64.

89. Francke U, Harper JF, Darras BT, et al. Congenital adrenal hypoplasia, myopathy and glycerol kinase deficiency: molecular genetic evidence for deletions. *Am J Hum Genet* 1987; 40:212–17.

90. Kalousek DK. Adrenal hypoplasia in triploidy. *Pediatr Pathol* 1984; 2:359–62.

91. Favara BE, Franciosi RA, Miles V. Idiopathic adrenal hypoplasia in children. *Am J Clin Pathol* 1972; 57:287–96.

92. Brown W, Singer DB. Pregnancy-induced hypertension and congenital adrenal hypoplasia. *Obstet Gynecol* 1988; 72:190–4.

93. Davidai G, Kahana L, Hochberg Z. Glomerulosa failure in congenital adrenocortical unresponsiveness to ACTH. *Clin Endocrinol* 1984; 20:515–20.

94. Migeon CJ, Kenny FM, Kowarski A, et al. The syndrome of congenital unresponsiveness to ACTH: report of six cases. *Pediatr Res* 1968; 2:501–13.

95. Kelch RP, Kaplan S, Biglieri EG, et al. Hereditary adrenocortical unresponsiveness to adrenocorticotrophic hormone. *J Pediatr* 1972; 81:726–36.

96. Roselli A, Barbosa LT. Congenital hypoplasia of the adrenal gland: report of two cases in sisters with necropsy. *Pediatrics* 1965; 35:70–5.

97. Kerenyi N. Congenital adrenal hypoplasia. Report of a case with extreme adrenal hypoplasia and neurohypophyseal aplasia, drawing attention to certain aspects of etiology and classification. *Arch Pathol* 1961; 71:336–43.

98. Wolman M, Sterk VV, Gatt SL, Frenkel M. Primary familial xanthomatosis with involvement and calcification of the adrenals: report of 2 more cases in siblings of a previously described infant. *Pediatrics* 1961; 28:742–57.

99. Lough J, Fawcett J, Wiegensberg B. Wolman's disease: an electron microscopic, histochemical and biochemical study. *Arch Pathol* 1970; 89:103–10.

100. Beaudet AL, Ferry GD, Nicholas BL Jr, Rosenberg HS. Cholesterol ester storage disease: clinical, biochemical and pathological studies. *J Pediatr* 1977; 90:910–14.

101. Goldfischer S, Grotsky HD, Chang CH, et al. Idiopathic neonatal iron storage involving the liver, pancreas, heart, and endocrine and exocrine glands. *Hepatology* 1981; 1:58–64.

102. Jacknowe G, Johnson D, Freese D, et al. Idiopathic neonatal iron storage disease. *Lab Invest* 1983; 48:7p.

103. Silver MM, Valberg LS. Tissue iron quantitation in five cases of perinatal hemochromatosis. *Lab Invest* 1986; 54:9p.

104. Witzleben CL, Uri AK. "Infantile hemochromatosis"—pathogenetic entity or non-specific response. *Lab Invest* 1986; 54:70A.

105. Hoogstraten J, deSa DJ, Knisely AS. Fetal liver disease may precede extra-hepatic siderosis in neonatal hemochromatosis. *Gastroenterol* 1990; 98:1699–1701.

106. Namnoum A, Hutchins GM. Accelerated maturation of the adrenal medulla in anencephaly. *Pediatr Pathol* 1990; 10:895–900.

107. Turkel SB, Itabashi HH. The natural history of neuroblastic cells in the fetal adrenal gland. *Am J Pathol* 1974; 76:225–44.

108. Beckwith JB, Perrin EV. In situ neuroblastomas: a contribution to the natural history of neural crest tumors. *Am J Pathol* 1963; 43:1089–1104.

109. Smith CR, Chan HSL, deSa DJ. Placental involvement in congenital neuroblastoma. *J Clin Pathol* 1981; 34:785–9.

110. Bolande RP. The neurocristopathies: a unifying concept of disease arising in neural crest maldevelopment. *Hum Pathol* 1974; 5:409–29.

111. Bolande RP, Towler WF. A possible relationship of neuroblastoma to von Recklinghausen's disease. *Cancer* 1970; 26:162–75.

112. Bolande RP. Spontaneous regression of neuroblastoma: an experimental approach. *Pediatr Pathol* 1990; 10:195–206.

113. Wagget J, Aherne G, Aherne WA. Familial neuroblastoma: report of 2 sib pairs. *Arch Dis Child* 1973; 48:63–6.

114. Chatten J, Voorhess ML. Familial neuroblastoma: report of a kindred with multiple disorders. *N Engl J Med* 1967; 227:1230–6.

115. Griffin ME, Bolande RP. Familial neuroblastoma with regression and maturation to ganglioneurofibroma. *Pediatrics* 1969; 43:377–82.

116. Knudson AG, Strong L, Anderson DE. Heredity and cancer in man. *Progr Med Genet* 1973; 9:113–58.

117. Chatten J, Witzleben CL. Neuroblastoma and Hirschsprung's disease. *Am J Pathol* 1975; 78:2a.

118. Bolande RP. The prenatal origins of cancer. In: Reed GB, Claireaux AE, Cockburn F, eds. *Diseases of the Fetus and Newborn*. London: Chapman & Hall Medical, 1995, p. 72.

119. Hayles AB, Hahn HB Jr, Sprague RG, Bahn RC, Priestley JT. Hormone-secreting tumours of the adrenal cortex in children. *Pediatrics* 1966; 37:19–25.

120. Artigas JLR, Niclewicz EDA, Silva AdePG, Ribas DB, Athayde SL. Congenital adrenal cortical carcinoma. *J Pediatr Surg* 1976; 11:247–52.

Pathology of the Pituitary, Thyroid, and Parathyroid Glands

Derek J. deSa

PART I
THE PITUITARY GLAND

In light of the crucial role of the pituitary gland of the newborn infant in the regulation of endocrine activity, it is surprising how little attention is paid to the changes that may occur in this gland. While this attitude may have been justified in the past, the improved survival of sick newborns makes it increasingly important to study the pathologic lesions of the pituitary, since survivors may have suffered pituitary damage. In turn, this could influence their growth and development during infancy.

DEVELOPMENT OF THE PITUITARY

The pituitary sits in the sella turcica capped by the diaphragma sellae, a fold of dura mater that effectively separates the pituitary from the subarachnoid space [1]. The gland has two anatomic components that develop from two separate ectodermal tissues [2]. The adenohypophysis arises from an outpouching of ectoderm (Rathke's pouch) anterior and cephalad to the stomatodeal membrane [3]. This outpouching, which is apparent by 28 days [4], grows toward the developing diencephalon. It eventually becomes pinched off from the ectoderm by the development of the membranous bones of the base of the skull. Rathke's pouch grows toward a ventral projection of the floor of the diencephalon, which it enfolds. This projection of the floor of the diencephalon is visible by 37 days [5], and it gives rise to the median eminence of the hypothalamus, the infundibulum, the pituitary stalk, and the pars nervosa (neurohypophysis) [1, 6]. This traditional explanation of the origin of the adenohypophysis has been challenged. In birds,

there is evidence to suggest that the cells that form Rathke's pouch are of neuroectodermal origin, arising from the ventral neural ridge [7]. Pearse and colleagues [7–9] have advanced the view that the adenohypophysis is of neuroectodermal origin. This would link the adenohypophysis with the neural crest structures and the amine precursor uptake and decarboxylation (APUD) system and imply that the entire pituitary gland is derived from neuroectoderm. Whether or not the mammalian pituitary gland has the same embryologic derivation as the avian gland is uncertain. However, the hypothesis developed by Pearse and colleagues raises the interesting possibility of a link between the endocrine system and the "paracrine system" [10], and could explain some of the complex endocrine changes that may be associated with parenteral alimentation in infancy [11, 12].

With the growth of the adenohypophysis on its ventral aspect, the cystic pouch of Rathke "collapses," and the original lumen is represented as the interglandular cleft of the definitive gland. The posterior wall of the cyst can be identified as the pars intermedia of the adult gland. The neurohypophysis receives the axons of the supraoptic-hypophyseal tract and their supporting glial fibers. There is an increase in the cellular content of the neurohypophysis between 60 and 100 days.

Blood Supply to the Pituitary Gland

The blood supply to the pituitary gland is a reflection of the functional integration of the pituitary and the nuclei of the hypothalamus [1, 13, 14]. The vessels supplying the diencephalic outpouching are destined to become the superior hypophyseal arteries, and they supply the hypothalamic nuclei of the median eminence, as well as the supraoptic and paraventricular nuclei through a system of complex convoluted capillaries, the gomitoli [1]. The vessels draining these sites run down the developing pituitary stalk and, when they merge with the capillaries in the pars distalis (adenohypophysis), form the "long portal vessels" of a hypothalamic-hypophyseal portal system. The pars distalis receives an additional blood supply from branches of the inferior hypophyseal arteries, which, after they ramify in the neurohypophysis, drain through a second set of "short portal vessels" to the parenchyma of the adenohypophysis. There they branch and divide into a network of capillaries that completes the hypothalamic-hypophyseal portal system. There are virtually no direct arterial channels to the pars distalis; even the trabecular artery, a branch of the superior hypophyseal artery, described by McConnell [15] and by Stanfield [16], usually passes through the pars distalis to anastomose with the long portal vessels in the lower infundibulum [4]. However, capsular branches of the hypophyseal arteries in the dura mater may send small branches into the adenohypophysis.

The pituitary as a whole drains by way of small dural veins to the venous sinuses of the base of the skull. The anatomic relationships of the adenohypophysis and neurohypophysis are integrated functionally by the hypothalamic-hypophyseal portal system of vessels, linking the nuclei in the floor of the diencephalon with the hypophysis. This portal system of vessels allows the hypothalamic peptidergic hormones to act on the adenohypophysis [17]; the dual nature of the arterial blood supply to the long portal vessels and the separate arterial supply of the short portal vessels ensures adequate oxygen tensions in the blood coursing through the sinusoids. There is, however, an apparent discrepancy between the size of the arterial vessels and the size of the veins draining the pituitary. This has led to the view that, through a reversal of flow in the portal system, the pituitary may be able to secrete directly to the hypothalamus, with the neurohypophysis playing a key role in the direction of blood flow [18, 19].

The vascular architecture is complete by midgestation [2, 20]. The long descending vessels form a pair of "vascular hila" on each side of the midline of the adenohypophysis, from which the vessels are distributed in a radial fashion.

FUNCTIONAL DIFFERENTIATION OF THE CELLS OF THE ADENOHYPOPHYSIS

At term, by conventional histology, most (60%) of the cells of the adenohypophysis appear to be undifferentiated. Eosinophils (30%) are sparsely distributed, and basophils are even more difficult to identify [21]. Pearse [22], using the PAS and trichrome staining methods, demonstrated muco-

protein cells (the probable precursors of basophils) as early as the 8th week, and eosinophils by the 11th week. The development of immunofluorescent techniques allowed Ellis et al [23] to demonstrate true human growth hormone (hGH) in the fetal pituitary. Cells containing hGH were consistently present in fetuses of 17 weeks' gestation or more. The overwhelming majority of these cells could be identified as acidophils (eosinophils) by conventional staining of the same slides used for the immunofluorescent studies. Ultrastructurally, somatotropes are identifiable by 12 weeks, and lactotropes can be identified by immunocytochemistry by 19 weeks [24, 25]. Reliable details of the development of luteinizing hormone (LH) and follicle-stimulating hormone (FSH) cells are not available due to differences in assay specificity and problems of nonspecific cross-reactions [26].

When the tissues are studied by electron microscopy, it is possible to identify the different varieties of cells in the pars distalis by the sizes of the granules in their cytoplasm. Precise identification of cells using ultrastructural methods combined with immunostaining is now possible. Detailed studies of the development of the human pituitary gland using these techniques have not been published to date, since the technical problems are formidable [27, 28].

A discussion of the considerable volume of data on the functional development of the adenohypophysis, and its interrelationship with the developing hypothalamic nuclei, is beyond the scope of this chapter. Excellent reviews are available [29, 30]. Several hypothalamic hormones act as "releasing hormones" that facilitate the secretion of pituitary hormones. These hormones include thyrotropin-releasing hormone (TRH), gonadotropin-releasing hormone (Gn-RH), corticotrophin-releasing hormone (CRH), and growth hormone–releasing hormone (GH-RH). The anterior lobe hormones include growth hormone, prolactin, and the pituitary gonadotropins (LH and FSH), as well as the common precursor molecule that gives rise to β-lipotropin (β-LPH) and adrenocorticotropic hormone (ACTH). ACTH in turn contains within its primary structure the amino acid sequence for α-melanocyte-stimulating hormone (α-MSH) and corticotropin-like intermediate lobe peptide (CLIP). β-LPH contains the amino acid sequence for β-endorphin, met-enkephalin, and β-MSH.

Several hypothalamic and pituitary hormones have their counterparts in placental hormones. Homology exists between the hypothalamic and placental forms of TRH and Gn-RH. Chorionic somatomammotropin (CS) shares a 96% homology with growth hormone, and peptide hormones resembling ACTH, FSH, and β-endorphin have been detected in amniotic fluid; prolactin exists in very high concentration in amniotic fluid. The exact significance of this overlap is not known, but it is obvious that there is interaction between the placenta and the fetal hypothalamic-pituitary axis. The postulated common endocrine system of Pearse and Takor Takor [9] provides an intriguing, although unproven, embryologic link.

ABNORMALITIES OF THE PITUITARY

Agenesis and Duplication

Complete absence of the pituitary gland has been described in a cyclopic infant [31]. In rare instances, pituitary agenesis may be familial [32]. Rarely, the pituitary gland has been minute or even absent in infants with normal skulls [33, 34], when it can be associated with one variety of congenital hypopituitarism. In contrast to pure adrenal hypoplasia, in hypopituitarism there is an additional associated hypogonadism, and the thyroid is hypoplastic [35, 36]. Pituitary hypofunction may be associated with major craniofacial anomalies (e.g., facial clefts and alobar holoprosencephaly), and the gland may be minute [37]. Infants with isolated pituitary aplasia [38] may have normal intrauterine growth but present with symptoms of hypoglycemia in the newborn period.

Incomplete duplication of the pituitary and sella turcica has been reported, and has been interpreted as an unsuccessful attempt at twinning [39]. Duplication of the gland has been described in association with some extremely complex neural tube defects [40, 41]. In a detailed study of a janiceps twin, however, no adenohypophyseal tissue was observed [42].

The Pharyngeal Pituitary

Small nodules of adenohypophyseal tissue are reported to occur in the posterior nasopharynx in many normal patients at all ages. These structures lie high in the nasopharynx below the mucoperiosteum and between the sphenoid and vomer bones, a site not usually sampled in many routine studies [43]. Removal of a pharyngeal pituitary leading to hypopituitarism was reported by Weber et al [44]. The pharyngeal pituitary has been reported to be comparable in size to the developing adenohypophysis in very early gestation, but diminishes in size as the full vascular and cytologic architecture of the normally sited pituitary develops. In anencephalics, the pharyngeal pituitary may be enlarged.

A poorly defined pituitary stalk in association with hydrocephalus has been described as "dystopia" of the pituitary [45]. This lesion was not associated with functional insufficiency, due to the presence of a functioning hypothalamic-hypophyseal system of vessels.

The Pituitary in Anencephaly

In anencephaly, a characteristic anomaly of the pituitary is found (Fig. 28.1). The sella turcica may be shallow or obliterated by vascular tissue that covers the base of the skull. Embedded in the vascular tissue, the adenohypophysis can usually be identified as a small, congested disc of tissue. With conventional staining techniques, the well-developed cell cords show some differentiation into acidophils and basophils, and ultrastructural studies demonstrate normal differentiation of somatotropes, lactotropes, and gonadotropes.

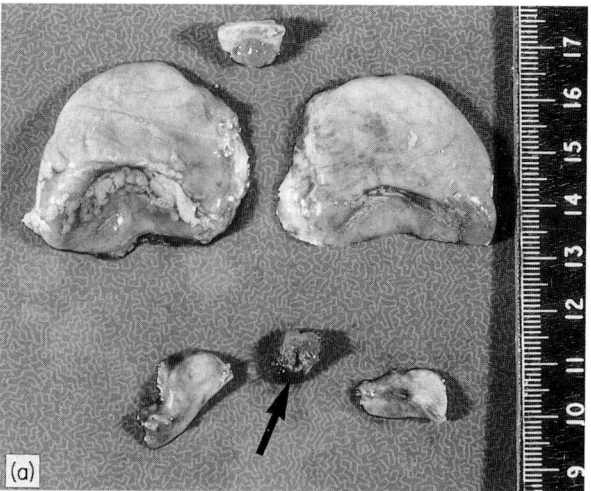

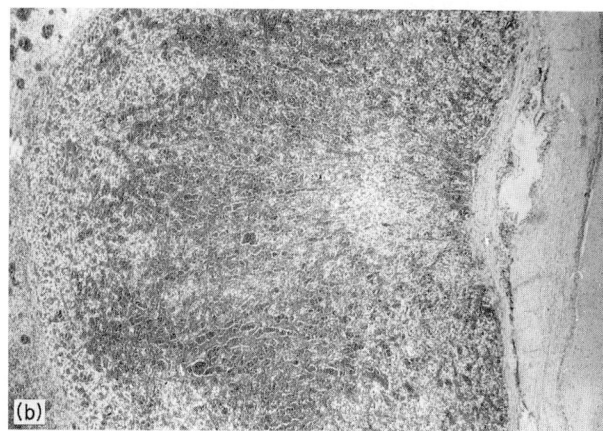

FIGURE 28.1. *(a) The pituitary and adrenal glands from a normal term infant (top), contrasted with hypoplastic adrenals and congested small pituitary (arrow) of an anencephalic infant born at 42 weeks' gestation. (b) Histologically, the pituitary gland of the anencephalic infant shown in (a) has a congested adenohypophysis, but no neurohypophysis can be seen here. H&E, ×60.*

There are markedly reduced numbers of corticotropes [46–48]. No true neurohypophysis is seen; nodules of glial tissue may be found in the vicinity of the adenohypophysis in approximately 25% of anencephalics and have been described as representing hypoplastic and/or deformed neurohypophyseal remnants [49]. The crucial abnormality, however, is the absence of any direct functional link between the adenohypophysis and the neural elements, since, despite the presence of numerous irregularly arranged telangiectatic vessels, there is no hypothalamic-hypophyseal portal system of vessels. When present, the "neurohypophyseal" elements lack detectable neurosecretory material [50].

The absence of a neurohypophysis is related to the lack of development of the forebrain and hypothalamus, and of itself is not surprising. However, the finding of an adenohypophysis in an appropriate anatomic site in anencephalics is of interest, since it implies that whatever factors were involved in the eventual production of the anencephalic state must have occurred relatively late in development and had essentially local effects, which spared Rathke's pouch and allowed its migration.

The abnormal hypothalamic-neurohypophyseal unit and the absence of hypothalamic-hypophyseal portal vessels are reflected in the "cortical hypoplasia" seen in the adrenal gland. The lack of an ACTH drive results in marked reduction in the fetal zone of cortex. This reduction is most apparent after 20 weeks' gestation, and in experimental animals the reduction in the fetal adrenal cortex can be reversed by the administration of ACTH [51, 52]. Other endocrine organs appear to be affected less or not at all. In some anencephalic infants, the colloid of the thyroid gland has been described as being more "prominent" than expected [53], but the weight of the gland usually lies within normal limits. Claims that there are changes in the gonads of male and female anencephalic infants are difficult to evaluate since they do not appear to take gestational differences into account [54, 55]. Undescended testes are a common finding. It is obvious that, with the striking exception of the corticotropes [46–48], a functioning hypothalamus is not necessary for the functional differentiation of the adenohypophysis.

Even more surprising is the fact that fetal growth in anencephalics is not significantly reduced—after due allowance is made for the mass of lost cerebral and cranial tissue. In anencephalics with associated maternal hydramnios, birth weights were surprisingly close to normal [56]. Obviously, fetal growth can occur in the absence of an anatomically normal pituitary. Some anencephalic fetuses appear to have an excess of subcutaneous fat; this has been attributed to increased insulin levels. In experimental animals (decapitated fetuses), the development of increased subcutaneous fat can be blocked by ACTH [57, 58]. Other detailed studies of the fetal pituitary-endocrine axis in anencephalics [59–63] indicate that, despite the importance of the pituitary gland in fetal life, growth hormone has little effect on fetal growth.

Pituitary Anomalies in Other Malformation Complexes

In some infants with holoprosencephaly, there may be an anatomic and functional dissociation of the pituitary gland from the hypothalamus, due to an abnormal stalk and poorly developed portal vessels [64, 65]. The pituitary gland is small, with a rudimentary neurohypophysis, and the fetal zone of the adrenal cortex is reduced in size. Similar lesions of the pituitary stalk have been described in association with septo-optic dysplasia [66–69]. In some of these malformation complexes, in addition to pituitary and cerebral anomalies, there may be associated defects of bones in the base of the skull. The true incidence of anomalies of the pituitary in association with malformation complexes of the central nervous system is not known; in particular, studies of the cytologic differentiation of the adenohypophysis do not appear to have been performed in these infants.

Isolated growth hormone deficiency has been reported in some infants with cleft palate, but the adenohypophyseal abnormality is not described in any detail [70, 71].

Other Irregularities of Pituitary Development

A number of minor irregularities of development may be seen on histologic examination of the pituitary. By far the most common anomaly is an extension of acinar tissue derived from the posterior regions of the interglandular cleft into the neurohypophysis (Fig. 28.2). The process may lead to the envelopment of the entire neurohypophysis by acini, or isolated clusters of glandular epithelium may be seen within the neurohypophysis (Fig. 28.3). In sections taken in

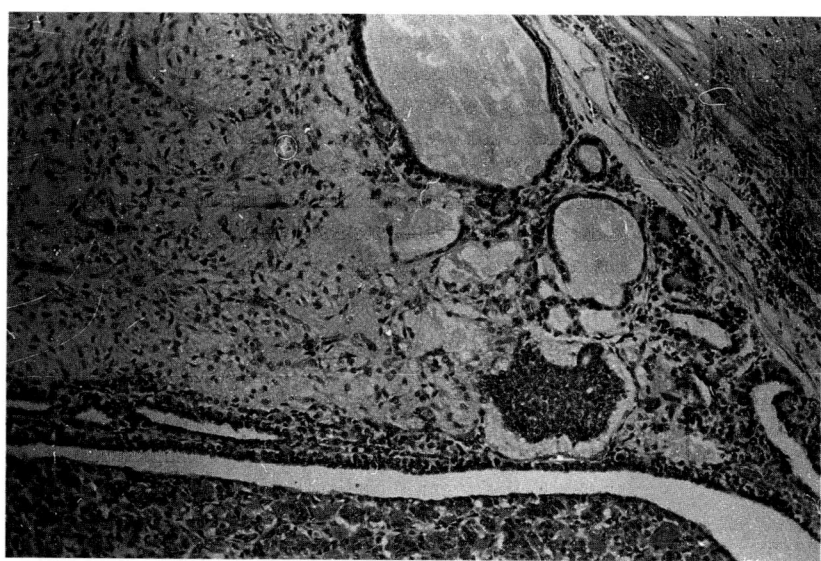

FIGURE 28.2.   *Extension of the glandular elements of the pars intermedia around and into the neurohypophysis. H&E, ×250.*

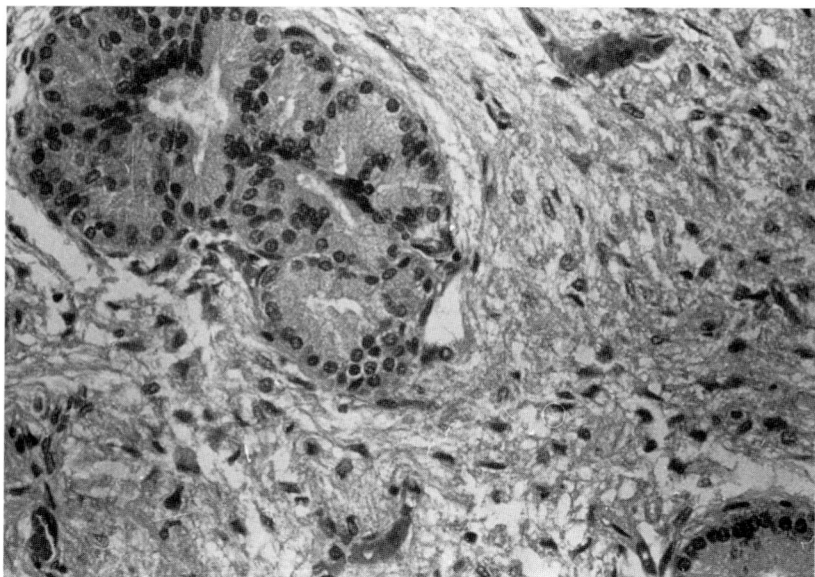

FIGURE 28.3. *Isolated clusters of glandular cells in the neurohypophysis of a term infant. H&E, ×800.*

the horizontal plane, the glandular elements may appear to form a collar around the neurohypophysis, but there is no interruption of the continuity of the neurohypophysis with the hypothalamus or any interruption of the hypothalamic-hypophyseal vascular connections. The lesions are, therefore, of no functional significance.

Occasionally, small psammoma-like calcific concretions may be seen in the adenohypophysis (Fig. 28.4). Their significance is uncertain. Barson and Symonds [72] demonstrated that the lesions rarely occurred in infants over 6 months of age, and suggested that the phenomenon was analogous to the development of Crooke's hyaline change. In the author's material, the lesions contain as much iron as calcium (Fig. 28.5), as well as laminin, and they resemble mineralized redundant basement membrane material [73].

A less frequent anomaly is the misplacement of glial tissue in the adenohypophysis (Fig. 28.6). The lesion probably represents the effects of irregular fusion of the two components of the gland, and no functional significance can be attributed to the lesion. Small aggregates of granular cells with sharply defined cytoplasmic borders have been seen in the neurohypophyses of some infants and adults. These choristomas are of no functional significance [74].

The density of glial fibers and nuclei in the neurohypophysis appears to vary from case to case (Fig. 28.7). In adults, this has been interpreted as one feature of atrophy of the neurohypophysis—especially when the lesion has been found in cases of postpartum panhypopituitarism [1, 75]. In the newborn infant, the significance of the variation in fiber density is less clear.

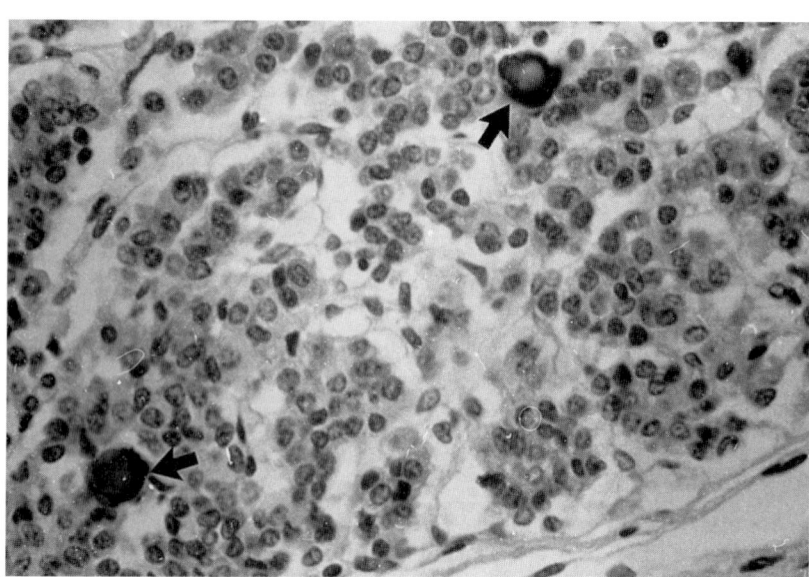

FIGURE 28.4. *"Psammoma" bodies (arrows) in the adenohypophysis of an infant of 30 weeks' gestation with Rhesus isoimmunization. H&E, ×1000.*

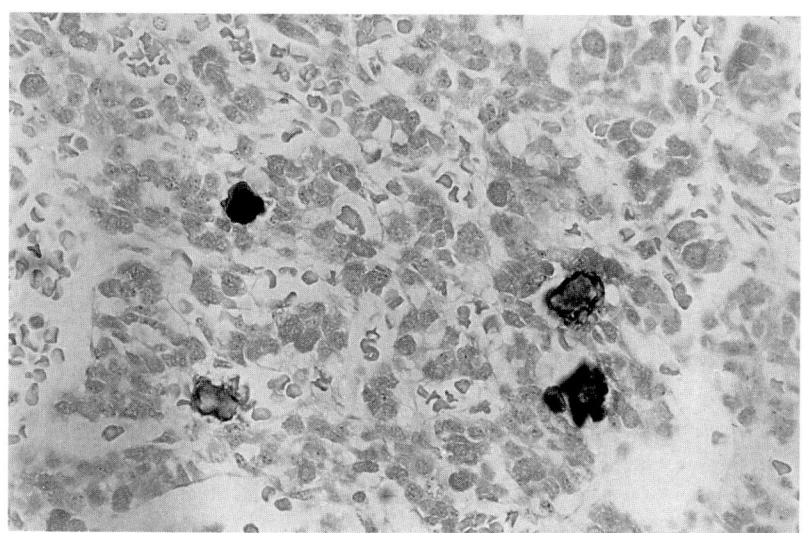

FIGURE 28.5.   *Concretions in the adenohypophysis, stained strongly with Perls' Prussian blue, indicating the presence of iron. Perls' Prussian blue, ×1000.*

PITUITARY DAMAGE IN THE PERINATAL PERIOD

The Effects of Severe Intrapartum Anoxia and Raised Intracranial Tension on the Pituitary

In most instances of perinatal deaths related to severe intrapartum anoxia, the pituitary gland shows an intense, although focal, dilatation of vessels within the adenohypophysis. The congestion may be so marked that the epithelial elements appear to be compressed between the dilated vessels, and there may be areas of rupture of the capillaries (Fig. 28.8). In its most severe form, the lesion resembles the development of early ischemic damage in other sites such as the mucosa of the bowel [76], where capillary dilatation and rupture are the earliest indicators of ischemic injury. There appears to be a spectrum of findings ranging from focal congestion of capillaries (the mildest form of the lesion) to a hemorrhagic gland with ruptured capillaries.

A similar range of vascular changes may be present in the pituitary glands of many neonatal infants who were found to have elevated intracranial pressure during life, characterized by a tense anterior fontanelle, retinal venous engorgement, or a measured rise in cerebrospinal fluid pressure. Obviously, many of the infants in this category also suffered from intrapartum or antepartum hypoxia. The more immature infants may have developed large intraventricular or intracerebral hematomas, or both, while the larger infants may exhibit thalamic and brainstem lesions with generalized brain swelling [77–79]. These infants may have some of the most severe examples of pituitary damage, although the overall incidence may not be easy to assess. In a review of 54 cases with severe intrapartum anoxia *and* elevated

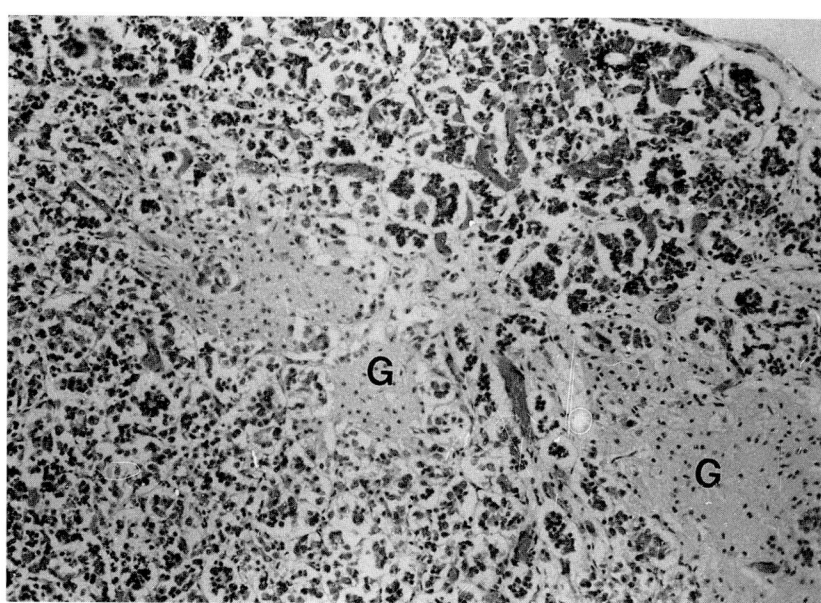

FIGURE 28.6.   *Glial islands (G) in the adenohypophysis of a neonatal death (36 weeks' gestation; group B streptococcal sepsis). H&E, ×250.*

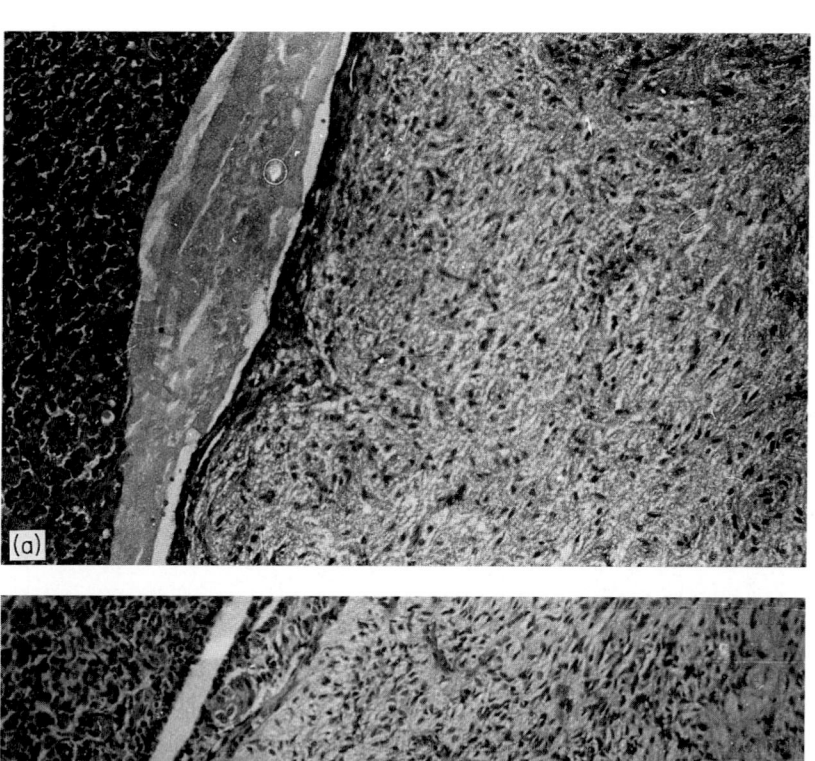

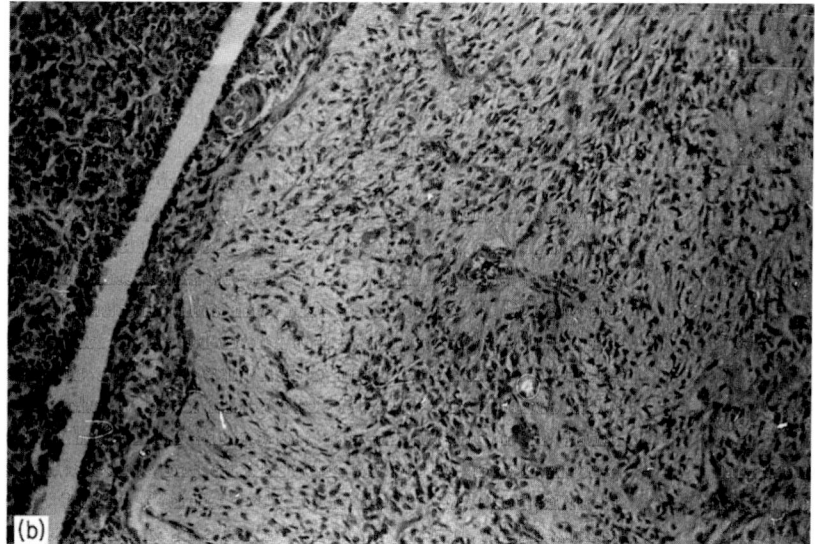

FIGURE 28.7.   *Two examples of neurohypophyseal areas in infants of 41 (a) and 42 (b) weeks' gestation. Note the variation in density of the cells. H&E, ×250.*

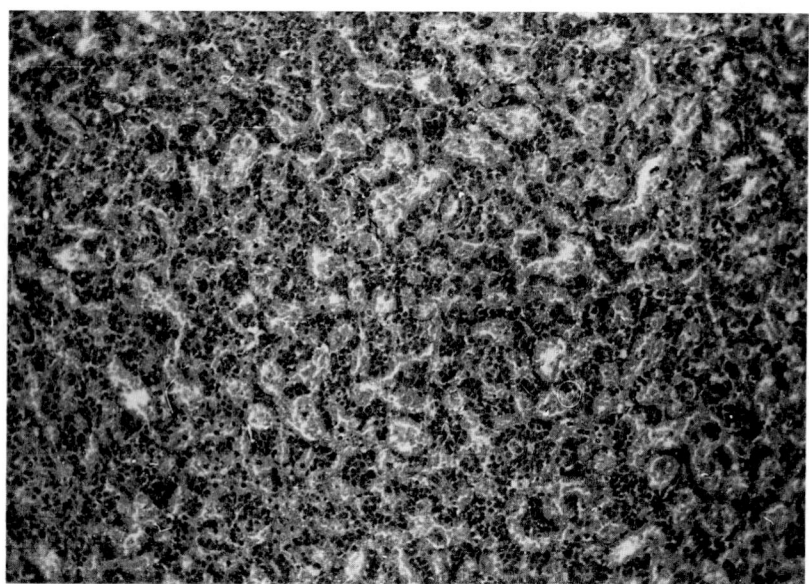

FIGURE 28.8.   *Extreme congestion of the adenohypophysis in an infant with severe intrapartum asphyxia due to bleeding from placenta previa. H&E, ×250.*

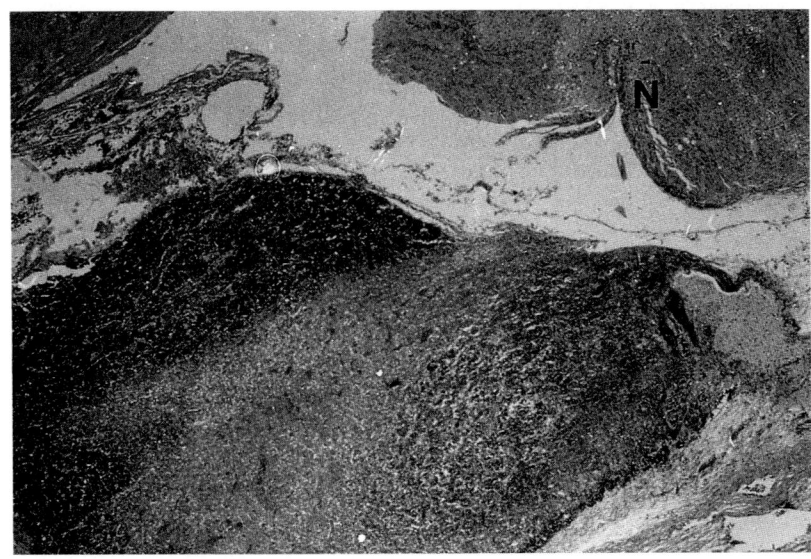

FIGURE 28.9. *Massive necrosis of the pituitary gland (seen as pale-staining area involving most of the adenohypophysis). The neurohypophysis (N) is relatively intact but separated from the adenohypophysis by artifact. Severely asphyxiated 29-week gestation with myocardial necrosis. H&E, ×60.*

intracranial pressure, there were 12 cases of pituitary necrosis [80]. Usually, the lesions were small foci situated in the central areas of the adenohypophysis, adjacent to the central vascular hilum. These lesions could be overlooked. There were, however, four cases of extensive pituitary necrosis (Fig. 28.9) in which the bulk of the adenohypophysis was necrotic. Similar necrotic lesions of the pituitary have been described in adults and children with elevated intracranial pressure and cardiac anomalies, maintained on ventilators [14]. It appears reasonable to suggest that in infants, as in adults, elevated intracranial pressure, if unchecked, leads to a decrease in intracranial perfusion. Their unusual anatomy probably makes the vessels of the stalk (long portal vessels) particularly susceptible to rises in intracranial pressure. A further contributory factor to the development of pituitary necrosis in these infants is the fact that many infants suffering from intrapartum hypoxia and intracranial pathology had

ischemic myocardial damage [81] that could be expected to lead to hypoperfusion. Some surviving islands of pituitary tissue may be found; these areas usually correspond to the zones of the gland supplied by the short portal vessels, which are relatively better protected from rises in intracranial pressure since they lie below the diaphragma sellae. The survival of a thin peripheral rim of adenohypophysis may indicate some oxygenation due to reflux of venous blood [14] or anastomoses with capsular arterial vessels [1].

Very extensive pituitary damage can be seen in infants who develop hydrocephalus following a large intraventricular/intracerebral hemorrhage. Obstruction of the circulation of cerebrospinal fluid occurs due to organization of the hematoma in the vicinity of the cerebellomedullary and basal cisterns. In those infants in whom there is extensive accumulation of clotted blood in the basal cistern, the pituitary stalk and its vessels may be compromised, and

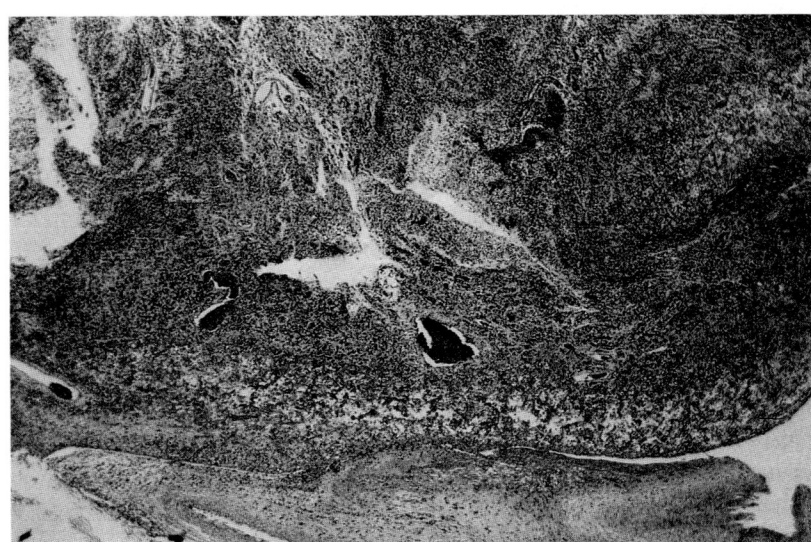

FIGURE 28.10. *An organized hematoma in the sella turcica in an infant with massive intracerebral and subarachnoid hemorrhage, associated with complete destruction of the gland. H&E, ×60.*

necrosis of the gland may occur. The organization of the hematoma can therefore be associated with massive destruction of the entire gland (Fig. 28.10).

THE NEUROHYPOPHYSIS IN THE PERINATAL PERIOD

In contrast to the many excellent studies on the physiology of the gland [29, 30, 58, 82, 83], the neurohypophysis receives relatively little attention in the pathologic literature.

Neurohypophyseal Hormones

Three neurohypophyseal hormones have been identified, either in tissue or in plasma, in the perinatal period in mammals. These peptides are arginine vasotocin (AVT), arginine vasopressin (AVP), and oxytocin (OT). Each has a similar amino acid sequence consisting of a six-membered amino acid ring with a disulfide bridge from position 1 to position 6, and a three-membered carboxyl-terminal side chain. The peptides differ in the identities of the amino acids at positions 3 and 8. In AVT and OT, the amino acid in position 3 is isoleucine, while in AVP it is phenylalanine. In OT, leucine is substituted for arginine in position 8. AVT has been found in the human fetal hypothalamus from 11 to 19 weeks' gestation, but whether or not it is secreted in the newborn is not known. AVP is detectable at 10 to 12 weeks' gestation in the human fetal neurohypophysis, and OT is found from 11 to 15 weeks' gestation onward [84].

The functional significance of these fetal hormones in the perinatal period is not known. There are numerous factors that stimulate AVP release in adults, including changes in extracellular fluid volume or blood pressure, activation of the renin-angiotensin system, hypoglycemia, prostaglandins, and surgery [82, 83]. Many of these factors can be shown to be effective in fetal sheep, but their effects on plasma levels of AVP in the human fetus remain unknown. AVP levels are elevated in umbilical arterial blood during labor (indicating fetal production), but the relatively low levels of AVP in cord plasma make it unlikely that the hormone has any role to play in the initiation of labor. Prolonged labor is associated with elevated levels possibly related to compression of the fetal head [85]. OT levels are also increased in cord blood following labor, but the exact significance of this change is not known [86]. In fetal sheep, hemorrhage can cause an increase in AVP and OT secretion, and in this animal at least, the mechanism of control of neurohypophyseal activity is fully developed at term [87].

Some newborn infants with intracranial hemorrhage develop a syndrome of inappropriate secretion of antidiuretic hormone associated with fluid retention and hyponatremia [88]. The pathologic basis for these changes has not been documented clearly in humans. In monkeys, acute elevation of intracranial pressure by inflation of balloons placed in the subdural space causes a sharp rise in AVP secretion [89]. Presumably, a similar rise in intracranial pressure leads

to inappropriate secretion of AVP in the newborn infant, but the mechanisms of inappropriate AVP secretion in infants with intracranial hemorrhage are not understood.

With the exception of massive necrotic lesions, the neurohypophysis usually appears to be uninvolved in many infants with adenohypophyseal damage. It is possible, however, that the variation of density of fibrillary material and glial cells in the neurohypophysis referred to earlier (see Fig. 28.7) may reflect a pattern of response to ischemic/hypoxic injury in some infants.

DIFFUSE PITUITARY DAMAGE

Pituitary Damage in Meningitis

The location of the pituitary fossa renders it susceptible to damage due to accumulations of meningitic inflammatory exudates. In patients with abundant purulent exudates in the basal cisterns of the brain, there may be secondary involvement of the pituitary stalk and fossa [73]. In a few instances we have found microscopic abscesses of the pituitary gland in infants with basal meningitis. Pituitary lesions affecting both anterior and posterior lobes of the gland have been found in infants with severe meningitis (associated with ulcerated meningomyeloceles and with ventriculitis complicating the Arnold-Chiari malformation complex). Very rare examples of pituitary abscesses in neonates with group B streptococcal meningitis and sepsis have been reported. The exact frequency of pituitary involvement in neonatal meningitis can only be estimated, since detailed surveys have never been published. The diaphragma sellae help to separate the pituitary capsule from the subarachnoid space, thereby offering some protection from direct spread of infection. When present, lesions in the pituitary in meningitis are almost inevitably due to damage to the long portal vessels. These destructive lesions of the pituitary gland have been identified at autopsy, and while there has been no indication that they have been of clinical significance, evidence of pituitary damage in these patients has not been sought. The possibility of pituitary damage in those who survive neonatal meningitis is considered only on rare occasions [90].

While it may appear that finding pituitary damage in anoxic infants or infants with intracranial pathology may be of interest solely to pathologists, it is obvious that the existence of a wide range of destructive lesions, including several focal lesions, raises the possibility that some survivors may have a similar range of lesions. In most survivors, evidence for or against hypopituitarism as a cause of growth disorders has not always been sought during life. Multiple hormone deficiency has been linked to "traumatic" or breech delivery [10], and Piccolo et al [91] showed that one-fifth of their patients with hypopituitarism and growth hormone deficiency had been delivered by the breech.

Isolated growth hormone deficiency has been reported in an 8-year-old girl with perinatally acquired human immunodeficiency virus (HIV) infection [92], but the

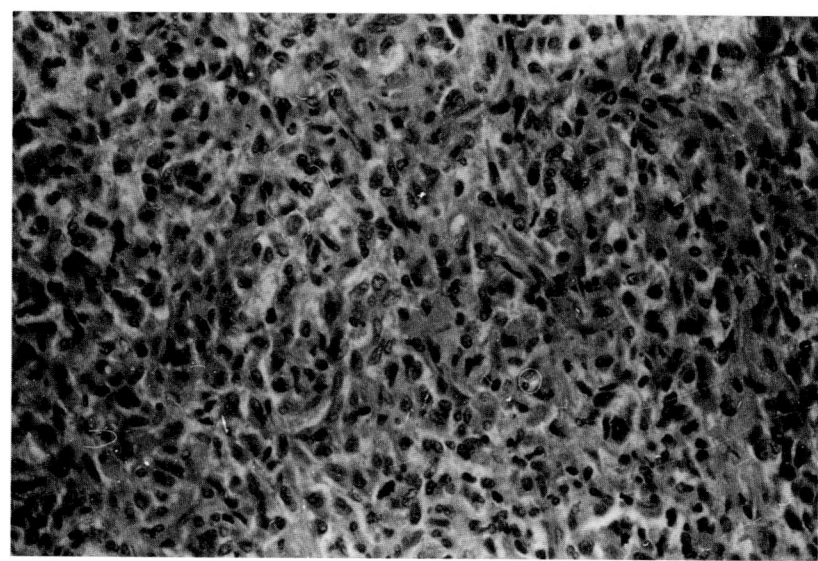

FIGURE 28.11.   *Extensive infiltration of the neurohypophysis in histiocytosis X. The 3-week-old infant also had extensive infiltration of the floor of the middle fossae, cavernous sinus, and petrous temporal bones. H&E, ×800.*

pathology of the gland does not receive much attention. Cytomegalovirus and rubella are other viral infections that may damage the pituitary [10], and Preece et al [93] reported isolated growth hormone deficiency in association with the congenital rubella syndrome.

Pituitary Involvement in Disseminated Disease

With the recognition of Langerhans-Birbeck granules as the best cytologic marker for the characteristic cells that make up the bulk of the infiltrating cells in histiocytosis X, classification and identification of the numerous "histiocytosis" syndromes are undergoing a welcome rationalization [94–97]. Several cases of disseminated histiocytosis X have presented in the early neonatal period, with characteristic

skin lesions and, eventually, widespread visceral lesions that have led to death. The pituitary fossa is involved in many fatal cases, with an extensive infiltration of the dura mater and petrous temporal bone in the base of the skull (Fig. 28.11). In the newborn, symptoms of panhypopituitarism or diabetes insipidus are usually overshadowed by the extensive multisystem involvement. Initially, the infiltrate is confined to the capsule of the gland and the cavernous sinus wall, with spread into the parenchyma of the gland occurring much later and only in unusual circumstances. The neurohypophysis is affected more severely than the adenohypophysis.

In older infants with the Hunter-Hurler syndromes of mucopolysaccharidosis, the parenchymal cells of the adenohypophysis are swollen and enlarged (Fig. 28.12), but there is rarely any evidence of functional derangement.

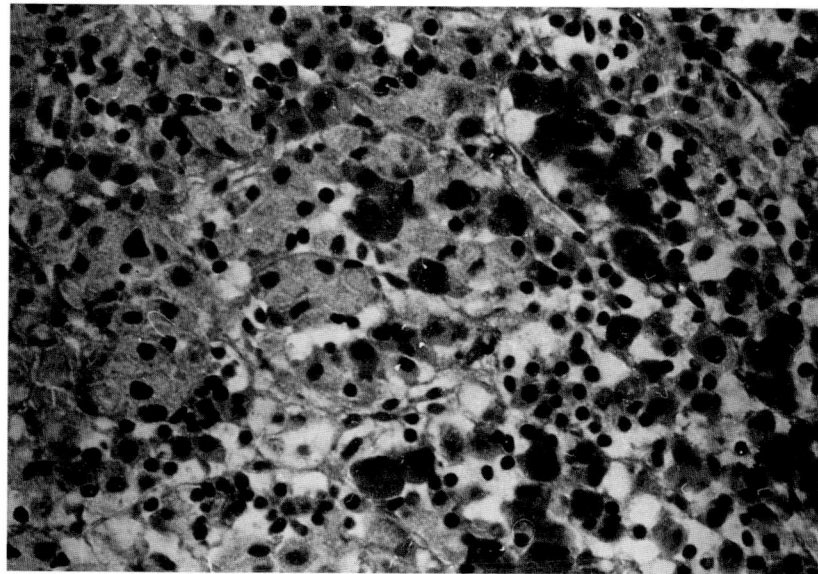

FIGURE 28.12.   *Swollen pale cells in the adenohypophysis of a 4-week-old infant with Hunter syndrome (mucopolysaccharidosis I). ×1000.*

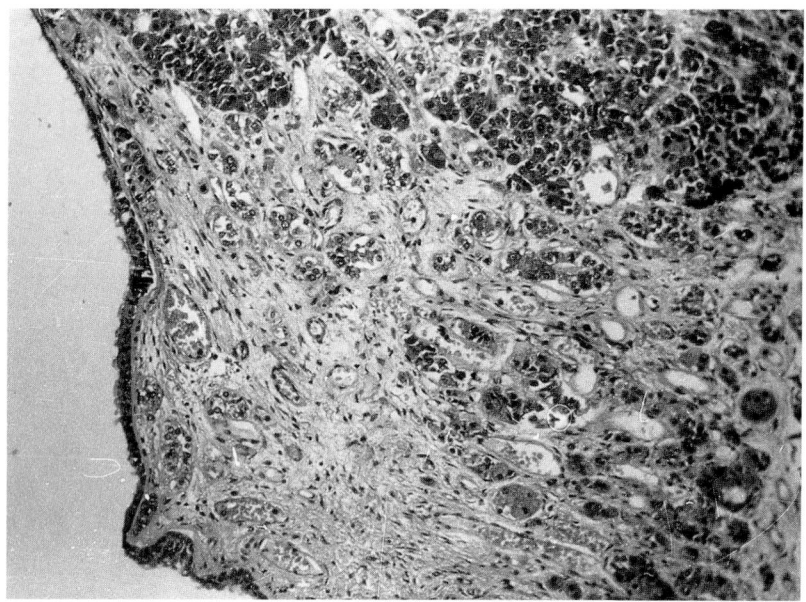

FIGURE 28.13. *A cyst of the anterior border of the adenohypophysis lined by respiratory epithelium and derived from Rathke's pouch, found incidentally in a neonatal death at $2^1/_2$ weeks. H&E, ×250.*

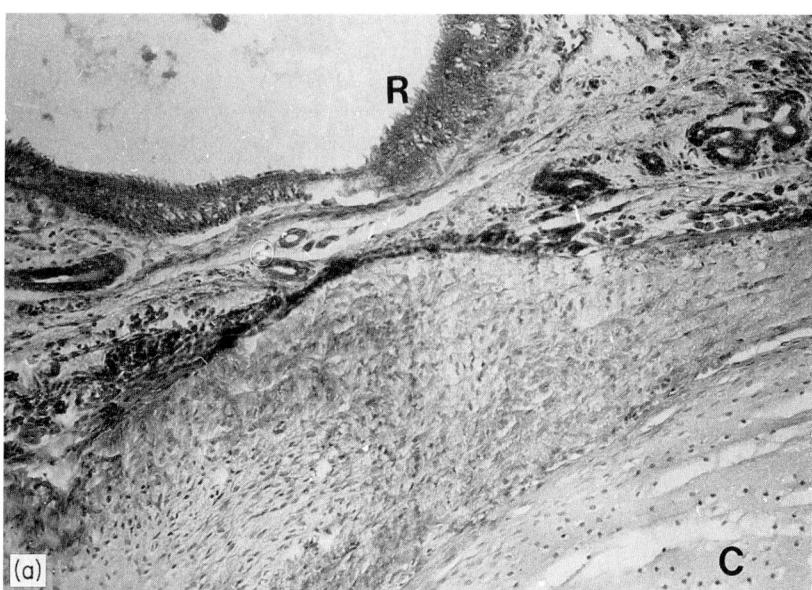

(a)

R

C

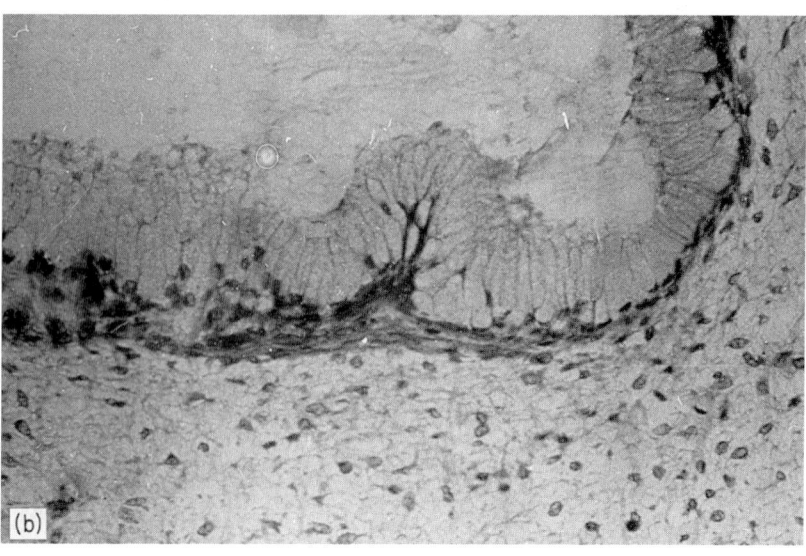

(b)

FIGURE 28.14. *(a) A semisolid teratoma of the pituitary region in a stillborn infant containing respiratory epithelium (R), cartilage (C), glandular epithelium, and collagenous and glial tissue. (b) Mucous epithelium and myxoid tissue in other area. H&E, (a) ×250; (b) ×800.*

CYSTS AND TUMORS OF THE PITUITARY AND PARAPITUITARY REGION

Cysts of the remnants of Rathke's pouch are a frequent finding in general autopsy material in adults, and microscopic cysts have been seen in up to 20 of 100 randomly selected glands [98]. A similar review of neonatal material is not available, although microscopic cysts derived from Rathke's pouch are occasionally identified in the neonatal pituitary (Fig. 28.13). The characteristic ciliated epithelial lining of the cyst may be admixed with foci of squamous epithelium, and the cyst has a collagenous wall.

Parapituitary craniopharyngiomas have been described in children, and rarely in neonatal material [74]. These cysts and tumors originate in embryonic structures but manifest themselves only in later life. A better estimate of the frequency of their occurrence is needed, and this can be obtained only by a study of neonatal material. Teratomas replacing the pituitary gland have occasionally been found in neonates (Fig. 28.14) as an incidental finding. Examples of secondary destruction of the pituitary by hypothalamic hamartoblastomas [99, 100], and a large intracerebral teratoma [101], have been reported.

Rare gangliogliomas of the hypothalamus may compromise pituitary function, but in the neonatal infant these lesions are incidental findings that are not usually symptomatic. Occasionally they may present as one cause of precocious puberty in infants [74].

MISCELLANEOUS

Iron deposition in the acinar cells of the adenohypophysis has been described in the enigmatic condition of "neonatal hemochromatosis" [73, 102]. In the presence of severe liver disease, pituitary siderosis may be a more frequent finding than is realized.

Diabetes insipidus of central origin has been reported as a complication of massive intraventricular hemorrhage [103], but the pituitary was not described.

REFERENCES

1. Daniel PM, Prichard MML. *Studies of the Hypothalamus and the Pituitary Gland.* Oxford: Alden, 1975, pp. 27–40, 89–107.
2. Moore KL. The developing human. In: *Clinically Oriented Embryology.* 3rd ed. Philadelphia: WB Saunders, 1982, pp. 396–8.
3. Conklin JL. The development of the human fetal adenohypophysis. *Anat Rec* 1968; 160:79–92.
4. Falin LI. The development of human hypophysis and differentiation of cells of its anterior lobe during embryonic life. *Acta Anat* 1961; 44:188–205.
5. Yokoh Y. The early development of the nervous system in man. *Acta Anat (Basel)* 1968; 71:492–518.
6. Daughaday WH. The adenohypophysis. In: Williams RH, ed. *Textbook of Endocrinology.* 6th ed. Philadelphia: WB Saunders, 1981, pp. 73–116.
7. Takor Takor T, Pearse AGE. Neuroectodermal origin of avian hypothalamo-hypophyseal complex: the role of the ventral neural ridge. *J Embryol Exp Morphol* 1975; 34:311–25.
8. Pearse AGE. The diffuse neuroendocrine system and the APUD concept. *Med Biol* 1977; 55:115–25.
9. Pearse AGE, Takor Takor T. Embryology of the diffuse neuroendocrine system and its relationship to the common peptides. *Fed Proc* 1979; 38:2288.
10. Gray ES. The endocrine system. In: Keeling J, ed. *Fetal and Neonatal Pathology.* 2nd ed. London: Springer-Verlag, 1993, pp. 499–528.
11. Adrian TE, Lucas A, Bloom SR, Aynesly-Green A. Growth hormone response to feeding in term and preterm neonates. *Acta Paediatr Scand* 1983; 72:251–4.
12. Lucas A, Bloom SR, Aynesly-Green A. Metabolic and endocrine consequences of depriving preterm infants of enteral nutrition. *Acta Paediatr Scand* 1983; 72:245–9.
13. Niemineva K. Observations on the development of the hypophysial-portal system. *Acta Paediatr Scand* 1950; 39:366–77.
14. Daniel PM, Spicer EJF, Treip CS. Pituitary necrosis in patients maintained on mechanical respirators. *J Pathol* 1973; 111:135–8.
15. McConnell EM. The arterial blood supply of the human hypophysis cerebri. *Anat Rec* 1953; 115:1175–1204.
16. Stanfield JP. The blood supply of the human pituitary gland. *J Anat (London)* 1960; 94:257–73.
17. Gay VL. The hypothalamus: physiology and clinical use of releasing factors. *Fertil Steril* 1972; 23:50–63.
18. Bergland RM, Page RB. Can the pituitary secrete directly to the brain? (affirmative anatomical evidence). *Endocrinology* 1978; 102:1325–38.
19. Bergland RM, Page RB. Pituitary-brain vascular relations: a new paradigm. *Science* 1979; 204:18–24.
20. Espinasse PG. The development of the hypophysio-portal system in man. *J Anat* 1933; 68:11–18.
21. Rasmussen AT. Changes in the proportion of cell types in the anterior lobe of the human hypophysis during the first nineteen years of life. *Am J Anat* 1950; 86:75–89.
22. Pearse AGE. Cytological and cytochemical investigations on the foetal and adult hypophysis in various physiological and pathological states. *J Pathol Bacteriol* 1953; 65:355–70.
23. Ellis ST, Beck JS, Currie AR. The cellular localization of growth hormone in the human foetal adenohypophysis. *J Pathol Bacteriol* 1966; 92:179–83.
24. Li JY, Dubois MP, Dubois PM. Somatotrophs in the human fetal anterior pituitary. *Cell Tissue Res* 1977; 181:545–52.
25. Baker RL, Jaffe RB. The genesis of cell types in the adenohypophysis of the human fetus as observed with immunocytochemistry. *Am J Anat* 1975; 143:137–48.
26. Gluckman PD, Grumbach MM, Kaplan SN. The human fetal hypothalamus and pituitary gland. In: Tulchinsky D, Ryan KJ, eds. *Maternal-Fetal Endocrinology.* Philadelphia: WB Saunders, 1980, pp. 196–232.
27. Horvath E, Kovacs K. Pathology of the pituitary gland. In: Ezrin C, Horvath E, Kaufmann B, Kovacs K, Weiss MH, eds. *Pituitary Diseases.* Boca Raton, FL: CRC, 1980, pp. 1–83.
28. Kovacs K, Horvath E. *Tumors of the Pituitary Gland.* fasc. 21, ser. 2. Washington: Armed Forces Institute of Pathology, 1986, p. 6.
29. Gluckman PD. The fetal neuroendocrine axis. *Curr Top Exp Endocrinol* 1983; 5:1–42.
30. Goodyer CG. Ontogeny of pituitary hormone secretion. In: Collu R, Ducharme JR, Ghyda HA, eds. *Pediatric Endocrinology.* 2nd ed. New York: Raven, 1989:125–34.
31. Edmonds HW. Pituitary, adrenal and thyroid in cyclopia. *Arch Pathol* 1950; 50:727–35.
32. Jost A. Anterior pituitary function in foetal life. In: Harris GW, Bonovan BT, eds. *The Pituitary Gland.* London: Butterworths, 1966, pp. 299–323.
33. Brewer DB. Congenital absence of the pituitary gland and its consequences. *J Pathol Bacteriol* 1957; 73:59–67.
34. Reid JD. Congenital absence of the pituitary gland. *J Pediatr* 1960; 56:658–64.
35. Blizzard RM, Alberts M. Hypopituitarism, hypoadrenalism and hypogonadism in the newborn infant. *J Pediatr* 1956; 48:782–92.
36. Mosier HD. Hypoplasia of the pituitary and adrenal cortex. *J Pediatr* 1956; 48:633–9.
37. Lockitch G, Halstead A, Dimmick JE. Endocrine system. In: Dimmick JE, Kalousek DK, eds. *Developmental Pathology of the Embryo and Fetus.* Philadelphia: JB Lippincott, 1992, pp. 707–48.
38. Moncrieff MW, Hill DS, Archer J, Arthur LJH. Congenital absence of the pituitary gland and adrenal hypoplasia. *Arch Dis Child* 1972; 47:136–7.
39. Morton WRM. Duplication of the pituitary and stomatodeal structures in 38 week male infant. *Arch Dis Child* 1987; 32:135–41.
40. Roessman U. Duplication of the pituitary gland and spinal cord. *Arch Pathol Lab Med* 1985; 109:518–20.
41. Tagliarini F, Pilleri G. Mammilo-hypophyseal duplication. *Acta Neuropathol* 1986; 69:38–44.
42. Sperberg GH, Machin GA. Microscopic study of midline determinants in janiceps twins. *Birth Defects Orig Artic Ser* 1987; 23:243–75.

43. McPhie, Beck JS. The histological features and human growth hormone content of the pharyngeal pituitary gland in normal and endocrinologically-disturbed patients. *Clin Endocrinol (Oxford)* 1973; 2:157–73.

44. Weber FT, Donnelly WH, Bejar RL. Hypopituitarism following extirpation of a pharyngeal pituitary. *Am J Dis Child* 1977; 131:525–8.

45. Lennox B, Russell DS. Dystopia of the neurohypophysis. Two cases. *J Pathol Bacteriol* 1951; 63:485–90.

46. Satow Y, Okamoto N, Ikeda T, Ueno T, Miyabra S. Electron microscopic studies of the anterior pituitaries and adrenal cortices of normal and anencephalic human fetuses. *J Electron Microsc* 1972; 21:29–37.

47. Osamura RY. Functional prenatal development of anencephalic and normal anterior pituitary glands. *Acta Pathol Jpn* 1977; 27:495–509.

48. Hatakeyama S. Electron microscopic study of the anencephalic adenohypophysis with reference to the adrenocorticotrophs and their correlation with the functional differentiation of the hypothalamus during the foetal life. *Endocrinol Jpn* 1969; 187–203.

49. Lemire RJ, Beckwith JB, Warkany J. *Anencephaly.* New York: Raven, 1978.

50. Pinner-Poole B. Absence of neurosecretory material in the pituitary glands in anencephaly. *J Neuropathol Exp Neurol* 1967; 26:117(a).

51. Nichols J. Observations on the adrenal of the premature anencephalic fetus. *Arch Pathol* 1956; 62:312–17.

52. Johannisson E. The foetal adrenal cortex in the human. Its ultrastructure at different stages of development and in different functional states. *Acta Endocrinol* 1968; 58(suppl):130.

53. Morison JE. *Foetal and Neonatal Pathology.* 3rd ed. London: Butterworths, 1970, pp. 420–2.

54. Ch'in KY. The endocrine glands of anencephalic foetuses. *Chinese Med J* 1938; 2(suppl):63–8.

55. Bearn JG. Anencephaly and the development of the male genital tract. *Acta Paediatr (Acad Sci Hung)* 1968; 9:159–80.

56. Sagar HJ, deSa DJ. The relationship between hydramnios and some characteristics of the infant in pregnancies complicated by fetal anencephaly. *J Obstet Gynaecol Br Commonw* 1973; 80:429–32.

57. Naeye RL, Blanc WA. Organ and body growth in anencephaly: a quantitative morphological study. *Arch Pathol* 1971; 91:140–7.

58. Jack PMG, Milner RDG. Effect of decapitation and ACTH on somatic development of the rabbit fetus. *Biol Neonate* 1975; 26:195–204.

59. Gray ES, Abramovich DR. Morphologic features of the anencephalic adrenal gland in early pregnancy. *Am J Obstet Gynecol* 1980; 137:491–5.

60. Kaplan SL, Grumbach MM, Aubert ML. The ontogenesis of pituitary hormones and hypothalamic factors in the human fetus: maturation of central nervous system regulation of anterior pituitary function. *Recent Prog Horm Res* 1976; 32:161–84.

61. Allen JP, Greer MA, McGilvra R, Castro A, Fisher D. Endocrine function in an anencephalic infant. *J Clin Endocrinol Metab* 1974; 38:94–8.

62. Grasso S, Filetti S, Mazzone D, et al. Thyroid-pituitary function in eight anencephalic infants. *Acta Endocrinol* 1980; 93:396–401.

63. Begeot M, Dubois MP, Dubois PM. Growth hormone and ACTH in the pituitary of normal and anencephalic human fetuses: immunocytochemical evidence of hypothalamic influences during development. *Neuroendocrinology* 1977; 24:208–20.

64. Haworth JC, Medovy H, Lewis AJ. Cebocephaly with endocrine dysgenesis. *J Pediatr* 1961; 59:726–33.

65. Hintz RL, Menking M, Sotos JF. Familial holoprosencephaly with endocrine dysgenesis. *J Pediatr* 1968; 72:81–7.

66. de Morsier G. Agenesie due septum pellucidum avec malformation du tractus optique. La dysplasie septo-optique. *Schweiz Arch Neurol Psychiatr* 1956; 77:267–73.

67. Stanhope R, Preece MA, Brock CGD. Hypoplastic optic nerves and pituitary dysfunction. *Arch Dis Child* 1984; 59:111–14.

68. Margalith D, Tze WJ, Jan JE. Congenital optic nerve hypoplasia with hypothalamic-pituitary dysplasia. *Am J Dis Child* 1985; 139:361–6.

69. Costin G, Murphree AL. Hypothalamic-pituitary function in children with optic nerve hypoplasia. *Am J Dis Child* 1985; 139:249–54.

70. Rudman D, Davis T, Priest JH, et al. Prevalence of growth hormone deficiency in children with cleft lip of palate. *J Pediatr* 1978; 93:378–82.

71. Duncan PA, Shapiro LR, Soley RL, Turet SE. Linear growth patterns in patients with cleft lip or palate or both. *Am J Dis Child* 1983; 137:159–63.

72. Barson AJ, Symonds J. Calcified pituitary concretions in the newborn. *Arch Dis Child* 1977; 52:642–5.

73. deSa DJ. *Pathology of Neonatal Intensive Care: An Illustrated Reference.* London: Chapman and Hall Medical Publications, 1995, pp. 98–9.

74. Sheehan HL, Kovacs K. Neurohypophysis and hypothalamus. In: Bloodworth JMB Jr, ed. *Endocrine Pathology.* 2nd ed. Baltimore: Williams & Wilkins, 1982, p. 45.

75. Sheehan HL, Whitehead R. The neurohypophysis in postpartum hypopituitarism. *J Pathol Bacteriol* 1963; 85:145–69.

76. deSa DJ. The spectrum of ischemic bowel disease in the newborn. *Perspect Pediatr Pathol* 1976; 3:273–309.

77. Harding B. The brain. In: Reed GB, Claireaux AE, Cockburn F, eds. *Diseases of the Fetus and Newborn.* 2nd ed. London: Chapman and Hall Medical Publications, 1995, pp. 413–64.

78. Norman MG. Perinatal brain damage. *Perspect Pediatr Pathol* 1978; 4:41–92.

79. Laroche JC. The central nervous system: fetal and perinatal brain damage. In: Wigglesworth JS, Singer DB, eds. *Textbook of Fetal and Perinatal Pathology.* Oxford: Blackwell Scientific Publications, 1991, pp. 807–38.

80. deSa DJ. Necrosis of the pituitary gland in neonatal infants. *Mod Pathol* 1990; 3:3p. Abstract.

81. deSa DJ, Donnelly WH. Myocardial necrosis in the newborn. *Perspect Pediatr Pathol* 1984; 8:295–311.

82. Leake RD, Weitzman RE. The fetal-maternal neurohypophyseal system. In: Tulchinsky D, Ryan KJ, eds. *Maternal-Fetal Endocrinology.* Philadelphia: WB Saunders, 1980, pp. 233–41.

83. Milner RDG, Hill DJ. Interaction between endocrine and paracrine peptides in prenatal growth control. *Eur J Pediatr* 1987; 146:113–22.

84. Skowsky WR, Fisher DA. Fetal neurohypophyseal arginine vasotocin in man and sheep. *Pediatr Res* 1977; 11:627–30.

85. Hadeed AJ, Leake RD, Weitzman RE, Fisher DA. Possible mechanisms of high blood levels of vasopressin during the neonatal period. *J Pediatr* 1979; 94:805–8.

86. Kumaresan P, Anandarangam PB, Dianzon W, Vasicka A. Plasma oxytocin levels during human pregnancy and labor as determined by radioimmunoassay. *Am J Obstet Gynecol* 1974; 119:215–23.

87. Alexander DP, Bashore RA, Britton HG, Forsling ML. Antidiuretic hormone and oxytocin release and antidiuretic hormone turnover in the fetus, lamb and ewe. *Biol Neonate* 1976; 30:80–7.

88. Anast CS. Disorders of the adrenal glands and sodium metabolism. In: Avery ME, Taeusch WH Jr, eds. *Schaffer's Diseases of the Newborn.* 5th ed. Philadelphia: WB Saunders, 1984, pp. 488–9.

89. Gaufin L, Skowsky WR, Goodman SJ. Release of antidiuretic hormone during mass-induced elevation of intracranial pressure. *J Neurosurg* 1977; 46:627–37.

90. Pai KG, Rubin HM, Wedemeyer PP, Linarelli LG. Hypothalamic-pituitary dysfunction following group B beta-hemolytic streptococcal meningitis in a neonate. *J Pediatr* 1976; 88:289–91.

91. Piccolo F, Pasquino AM, Boscherini B, et al. Hypopituitary dwarfism and breech delivery. *Arch Dis Child* 1979; 54:485–6.

92. Jospe N, Powell KR. Growth hormone deficiency in an 8 year old girl with human immunodeficiency virus infection. *Pediatrics* 1990; 86:309–12.

93. Preece MA, Kearney PJ, Marshall WC. Growth hormone deficiency in congenital rubella. *Lancet* 1977; ii:842–4.

94. Favara B. Definition of the histiocyte in Sydney Farber Workshop, Part I: definitions, patterns, prognosis. *Pediatr Pathol* 1984; 2:387–95.

95. Jaffe RB. Pathology of histiocytosis X. *Perspect Pediatr Pathol* 1987; 9:4–47.

96. Landing B. Lymphohistiocytosis in childhood: pathologic comparison with fatal Letterer-Siwe disease. *Perspect Pediatr Pathol* 1987; 9:48–74.

97. Jaffe RB. Review of human dendritic cells: isolation and culture from precursors. *Pediatr Pathol* 1993; 13:821–37.

98. Shanklin WH. Incidence and distribution of cilia in the human pituitary with a description of micro-follicular cysts derived from Rathke's cleft. *Acta Anat* 1951; 11:361–82.

99. Hall JG, Pallister PD, Clarren SK, et al. Congenital hypothalamic hamartoblastoma, hypopituitarism, imperforate anus and postaxial polydactyly—a new syndrome? Part I: clinical, causal and pathogenetic considerations. *Am J Med Genet* 1980; 7:47–74.

100. Clarren SK, Alvord EC Jr, Hall JG. Congenital hypothalamic hamartoblastoma, hypopituitarism, imperforate anus and postaxial polydactyly—a new syndrome? Part II. Neuropathological considerations. *Am J Med Genet* 1980; 7:75–83.

101. Paes BA, deSa DJ, Hunter DJS, Pirani M. Benign intracranial teratoma: prenatal diagnosis influencing delivery. *Am J Obstet Gynecol* 1982; 143:600–1.

102. Hoogstraten J, deSa DJ, Knisely AJ. Fetal liver disease may precede extrahepatic siderosis in neonatal hemochromatosis. *Gastroenterology* 1990; 98:1699–1701.

103. Adams JM, Kenny JD, Rudolph AJ. Central diabetes insipidus following intraventricular hemorrhage. *J Pediatr* 1976; 88:292–4.

PART II
THE THYROID GLAND

The thyroid gland is functional in utero and plays an important role in neonatal thermogenesis, but there is a relative dearth of information on the pathologic changes that take place in the newborn period [1].

DEVELOPMENTAL ANATOMY OF THE THYROID GLAND

The thyroid gland develops about the 24th day from a median thickened area of foregut endoderm in the floor of the primitive pharynx [2]. This area of thickening lies caudad to the first pharyngeal pouch and the developing tuberculum impar of the tongue. The thickening soon produces a cellular downgrowth known as the thyroid diverticulum, which descends into the neck as the embryo elongates and assumes a flasklike vesicular structure. This vesicle retains its connection with the floor of the pharynx by a narrow canal, the thyroglossal duct, which becomes resorbed in later stages of development. The site of origin of the thyroid diverticulum is recognizable as the foramen cecum of the adult tongue, and the residuum of the caudal end of the duct is represented by the occasional finding of a pyramidal lobe arising from the isthmus of the thyroid gland.

Due to the growth and elongation of the body and floor of the pharynx, the primordium of the thyroid gland lies near the levels of the laryngeal primordium by the end of the 7th week [3]. The gland is bilobed at this stage with a narrow isthmus, and what was originally a midline structure assumes the configuration of a paired gland. While the thyroid is descending caudally, the paired derivatives of the median thyroid incorporate the ultimobranchial bodies, the so-called "lateral components," into the lateral lobes of the definitive gland. The ultimobranchial bodies develop from the ventral elongated part of the fourth pharyngeal pouch and may incorporate the rudimentary fifth pharyngeal pouch as well [2, 3].

The descent of the thyroglossal duct is modified by the development of the hyoid bone, which develops later than the thyroid primordium at a site near the midpoint of the course of the thyroglossal duct. The duct envelops the anterior, inferior, and posterior aspects of the hyoid bone (Fig. 28.15) and may even appear to traverse the bone itself.

An excellent timetable of the differentiation and development of the thyroid gland is provided by Tanimura and Shiota [4]. The empty vesicle becomes filled with proliferating endodermal cells, and by 9 weeks the thyroid is a relatively compact mass of cells arranged in sheets and cords with loose intervening stroma. At about 10 weeks, a pattern of cords and tubular structures is seen with well-defined mesodermal septa, but there is no colloid (the precolloid stage). By 12 weeks the peripheral areas of the cords are arranged in follicles with early colloid secretion of a non-iodinated protein with low molecular weight (the colloid stage). Colloid development proceeds apace, and by 16 weeks noniodinate thyroglobulin is present in many of the widely dispersed follicular spaces. Development continues with the appearance of increasing numbers of colloid-filled spaces and the establishment of a capillary plexus; biochemically, there is increasing evidence of concentration of iodide. Ultrastructurally, rough-surfaced endoplasmic reticulum can be seen in follicular cells around 18 weeks' gestation, and thyroxine is present by the end of the 5th month.

Much of our knowledge of the fate of the cells developed from the ultimobranchial body is based on the study of medullary carcinomas of the thyroid by Williams [5, 6] and on the cytochemical work of Pearse and Polak [7]. It is now known that the parafollicular cells of the thyroid, which secrete calcitonin (and hence are occasionally designated as C cells), form a separate endocrine entity, and they are considered by some workers to form part of the APUD (amine precursor uptake and decarboxylation) system of neural-crest-derived cells [7]. Cells migrate from the neural crest into the developing ultimobranchial body and become incorporated into the lateral lobes of the thyroid gland.

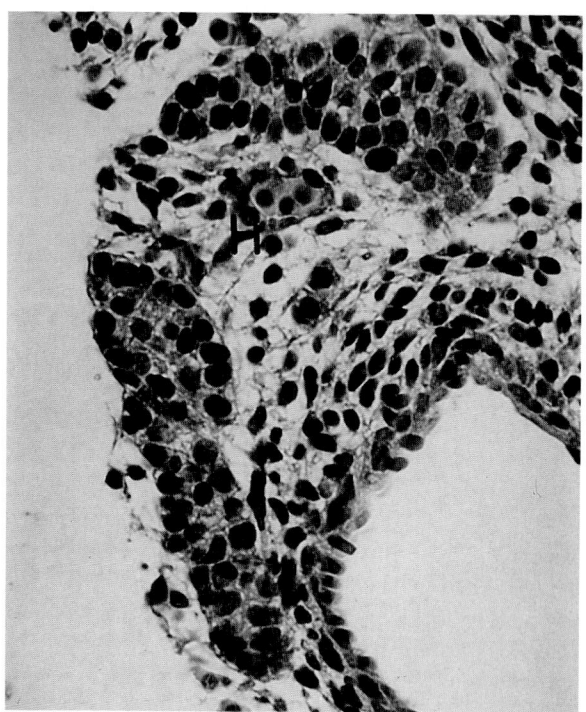

FIGURE 28.15.   *The curved course of the thyroglossal duct in a 9-mm embryo. The ventral and cephalic margins of the mesenchymal primordium of the hyoid bone (H) are bounded by the cord of cells that make up the duct. H&E, ×800.*

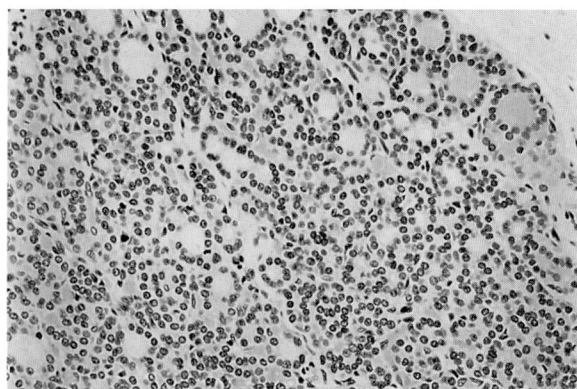

FIGURE 28.16.   *The thyroid gland of an infant of 23 weeks' gestation, showing poorly developed follicles and relatively little colloid. H&E, ×500.*

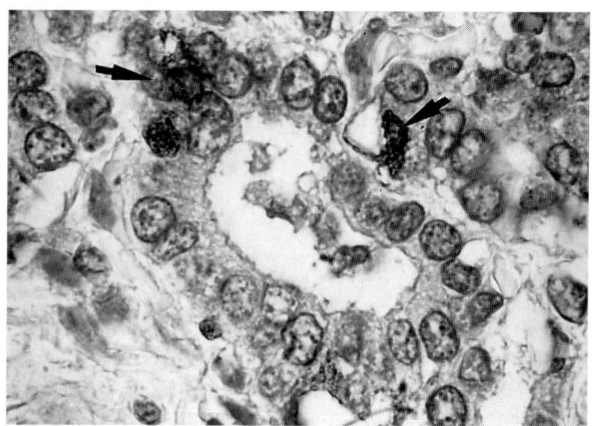

FIGURE 28.18.   *Thyroid gland in an infant of 29 weeks' gestation, stained by the peroxidase-antiperoxidase method using an initial antibody against calcitonin. A small group of darkly staining C cells is visible (arrow). ×2000.*

Parafollicular cells may be identified tentatively by light microscopy around the 12th week, but the characteristic neurosecretory granules are found at the earliest around the 16th week. The cells can be identified confidently as "C" cells by about 20 weeks. Pueblitz et al [8] have shown that there is good evidence to suggest that some C cells are derived from thyroid endoderm.

In its fully developed state, the thyroid gland is represented by two symmetric lobes on either side of the larynx connected by an isthmus. Each lobe is divided into lobules by vascular septa that carry numerous capillaries, making the thyroid gland one of the most vascular organs of the body. The follicles are lined by a cuboidal to low columnar epithelium and contain variable amounts of iodine-rich eosinophilic thyroglobulin depending on the gestational age (Figs. 28.16 and 28.17). Within the walls of the follicles lie

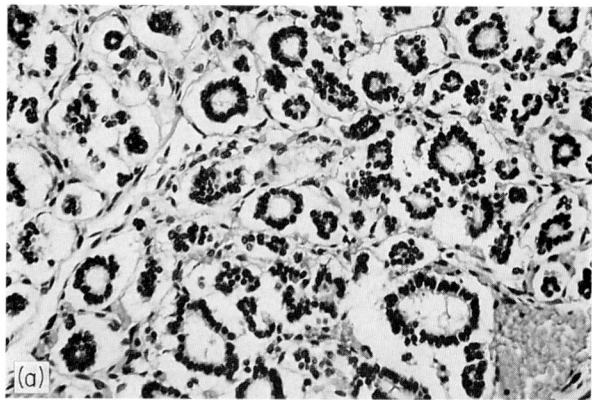

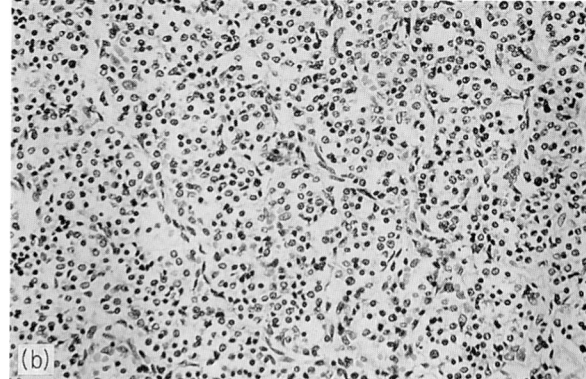

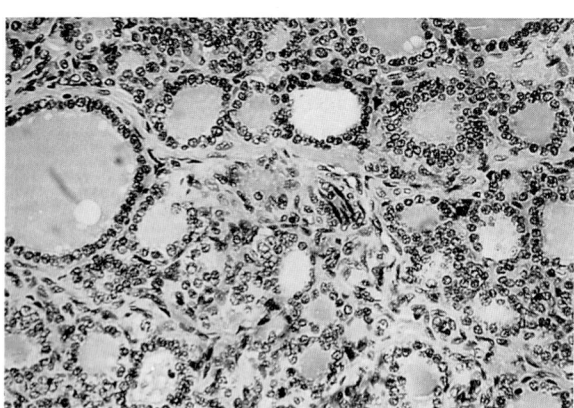

FIGURE 28.17.   *The thyroid gland of a term infant. Note the variability in the size of the follicles, height of the epithelium, and amount of colloid present. H&E, ×500.*

FIGURE 28.19.   *Examples of autolysis disproportionately affecting the thyroid gland in infants without evidence of significant autolysis elsewhere. There is a separation of cells from the basement membrane (a) and disruption and desquamation of cells into the lumen of the follicles with total disorganization (b). H&E, ×500.*

the relatively polygonal, paler-staining "C" cells, which may be identified by their position between the basement membrane and the follicular epithelium. They can be demonstrated with silver stains, but are best revealed with immunocytochemical techniques designed to identify calcitonin (Fig. 28.18).

Follicular size and colloid content vary from lobe to lobe and within each lobule, even in the absence of abnormal thyroid function, and may well reflect fluctuations in the activity of each follicle. An irregular depletion of colloid, with desquamation of epithelium and masses of pyknotic debris between follicles, that Sagreiya and Emery [9] have described as "perinatal discharge," occurs in autopsy material. This colloid depletion has been ascribed to the stress of delivery and release of thyroxine [10]. Alternatively, the changes seen in postmortem material with variable degrees of autolysis can lead to a range of unusual histologic appearances (Fig. 28.19). Desquamation of epithelial cells and the retraction from the basement membrane may occur in infants without significant autolysis in other organs. These autopsy-related findings may explain most of the changes described by earlier workers.

FUNCTIONAL DEVELOPMENT OF THYROID SECRETION

It is not the purpose of this section to provide a detailed review of thyroid hormone synthesis, but Lockitch et al [11] provide a good introduction to the functional development of triiodothyronine during gestation. It is necessary, however, to discuss briefly the control of thyroid hormone production.

For all practical purposes, once normal organogenesis of the hypothalamus, pituitary, and thyroid is complete, the thyroid gland is under autonomous fetal control. In the normal state, maternal thyroid-stimulating factors do not have an effect on fetal thyroid function [12]. Hypothalamic thyrotropin-releasing hormone (TRH) is present by about 8 to 10 weeks' gestation, and pituitary thyroid-stimulating hormone (TSH) is present at the same time. TSH levels rise to a plateau at about 28 weeks, preceded by a sharp rise around 16 to 18 weeks [13]. This is associated with a surge of iodine uptake by the fetal thyroid at 20 weeks' gestation, which in turn corresponds approximately to the development of the hypothalamic-hypophyseal system of portal vessels. Thyroid stimulation by TRH and TSH is associated with increasing fetal serum thyroxine (T4 or tetraiodothyronine) levels, especially between 20 and 30 weeks of gestation. The increase in the level of T4 is associated with an increase of thyroid-binding globulin (TBG) levels during the same period. After 30 weeks, TBG levels tend to remain constant while T4 levels rise, leading to an elevation of free T4 levels in the serum. As the free T4 level rises, there is a negative feedback, and TSH levels drop [1], indicating that a hypothalamic-pituitary-thyroid axis exists in utero. Despite this, however, absence of the hypothalamus (as in an anencephalic infant) does not appear to impede thyroid growth in the same fashion (unlike the effect on the adrenal cortex; see Chap. 27, and Part I of the present chapter), presumably implying that TSH can be produced in the absence of a hypothalamus if the pituitary is intact [12, 14–17].

The thyroid gland releases thyroxine after delivery, and there is a surge of fetal TSH at birth [18]. Some of the release of thyroid hormones may occur in response to norepinephrine, and there is synergism in the actions of the catecholamines and T4 in the elevation of basal metabolic rate and nonshivering thermogenesis. This allows the human newborn to increase heat production after delivery [1, 19].

CONGENITAL ANOMALIES OF THE THYROID

Absence of the Thyroid Gland (Thyroid "Aplasia," "Athyreosis," "Cryptothyroidism")

Various terms have been used to describe the state of the thyroid gland in sporadic nongoitrous cretinism. In most of these infants, thyroid tissue cannot be palpated in its usual site in the neck. These cases of "aplasia," "absent thyroid gland," or "athyreosis" were always assumed to be due to a failure to form the median component of the thyroid gland. However, with the use of scintiscan techniques, Little et al [20] demonstrated that, in almost all the cases they studied, small remnants of thyroid tissue were found in the lingual region. These nodules could trap radioactive iodine and produce thyroxine, but their overall size was too small to prevent cretinism. Most cases would satisfy the *clinical* criteria of athyreosis suggested by Carr et al [21] despite the fact that the ectopic foci were under maximal stimulation of TSH [20, 22]. Little and colleagues [20] believe that the real failure in this group of cases is a failure of descent (and, therefore, differentiation) of the thyroid gland, and they draw a parallel with the cryptorchid state to support their use of the term "cryptothyroidism." However, it must be remembered that the major impetus for the "descent" of the thyroid gland is the progressive elongation of the body and floor of the pharynx. It would appear, therefore, that despite the apparent lack of "descent," some intrinsic abnormality of the thyroid primordium must be postulated.

Some true examples of thyroid aplasia are cited by Warkany [23] in the literature of an earlier period—a time when the tissues of the neck were sectioned in a semiserial fashion. Gabr [22] found no thyroid tissue, even after scanning, in 18 of 35 patients with sporadic nongoitrous cretinism, while Hutchinson [24] could not demonstrate thyroid tissue in 16 of 39 patients. More recently, Bamforth et al [24a] could not find evidence of thyroid tissue in 10 of 19 infants with nongoitrous cretinism. Most instances of true athyreosis have occurred in females, and there was reduced life expectancy.

Therefore, absence of thyroid tissue does occur, but it is obvious that small residua of thyroid tissue may be present in infants who do not have any palpable thyroid gland in the neck. Most of these ectopic islands are in the lingual region (Fig. 28.20), but in many others the ectopic thyroid tissue may be scattered over a wide area, along the course of the descent of the thyroglossal duct and even the anterior mediastinum [25].

Partial agenesis of one lobe of a thyroid gland has been reported [26], and this hemiaplasia of the gland may be associated with normal function or hypothyroidism. The missing thyroid lobe may be replaced by mucinous glands and crypts set in a fibrous stroma. This is not a problem usually encountered in the perinatal period, since it is found most often in autopsy material or at surgery in older children and young adults. Absence of the thyroid isthmus and a portion of a lobe may be part of the constellation of anomalies that make up the DiGeorge III–IV pharyngeal pouch syndrome [27]. The C cell population may be depleted in this syndrome [28], but, as noted earlier, the presence of some C cells indicates that some of these cells may arise from thyroid endoderm.

ANOMALIES OF THE THYROGLOSSAL DUCT

It is not uncommon to find small islands of ductlike structures as an incidental histologic finding near the base of the tongue, near the hyoid bone, and above the thyroid isthmus. They represent remnants of the thyroglossal duct, and the ducts are lined by a respiratory or low cuboidal epithelium with occasional acinar groups around central ducts. Variable amounts of lymphoid tissue may surround the remnants. These remnants rarely pose problems during the perinatal

period, but they may enlarge in later life and present as cysts of the thyroglossal duct. Secondary changes of squamous metaplasia, or even destruction of the epithelium, may be present, usually accompanied by obvious signs of infection of the cyst contents. Unless the skin overlying them has broken down, thyroglossal duct cysts do *not* open onto the skin. Due to the complex pathway of migration of the duct in relation to the hyoid bone, excision of remnants of the thyroglossal duct necessitates sacrificing the median zone of the hyoid bone and the adjacent soft tissue, since persistent ductal elements have been seen above, below, behind, and even within the hyoid bone.

Absence of the isthmus of the thyroid gland is very occasionally encountered at autopsy or in patients undergoing surgery and represents an exaggerated degree of obliteration of the thyroglossal duct. It is commonly observed in cases of DiGeorge syndrome [27].

ECTOPIC THYROID TISSUE

Reference has been made to the presence of small, functional (although ineffectual) islands of thyroid tissue in cases of sporadic nongoitrous cretinism. Islands of ectopic functional thyroid tissue may be found in both hypothyroid and euthyroid patients in the same sites as the islands of thyroglossal duct remnants, from which they may be distinguished by the presence of thyroid follicles (Fig. 28.21). In most patients there is no symptomatology, and only rarely are there any problems in the perinatal period. Larger ectopic foci at the base of the tongue may cause problems in swallowing. Instead of being centered around the larynx, thyroid tissue may extend into the superior mediastinum, where enlargement at puberty may cause respiratory embarrassment. Occasionally, isolated ectopic nodules of thyroid tissue with a separate blood supply may be seen in the mediastinum.

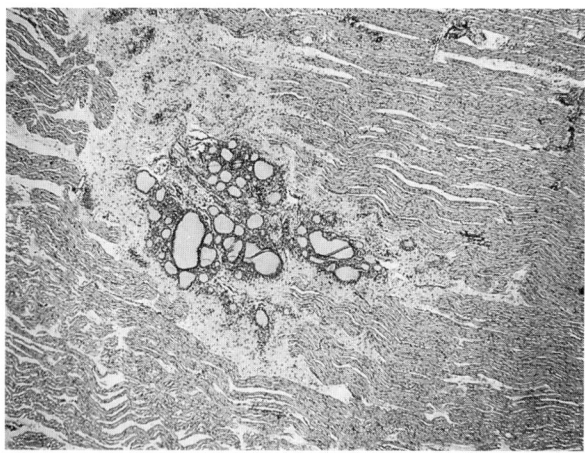

FIGURE 28.20. *Remnants of thyroid tissue in the base of the tongue of an infant of 6 months who presented with congenital athyreotic hypothyroidism. (Slide kindly provided by Dr. Hans Lucke, Hamilton, Ontario.) H&E, ×50.*

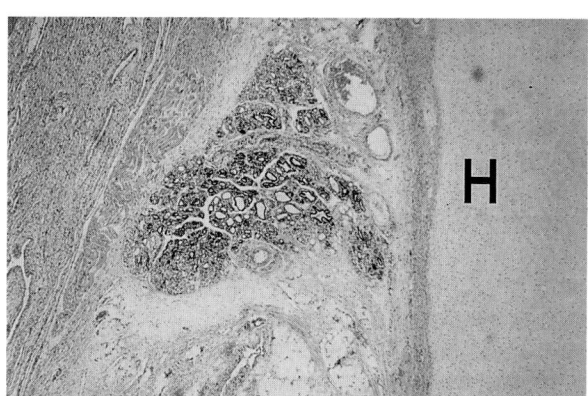

FIGURE 28.21. *A nodule of thyroid acinar tissue anterior to the hyoid bone (H) in an infant of 38 weeks' gestation. A normal gland was present in the neck. H&E, ×50.*

Ectopic thyroid tissue may be observed in cervical lymph nodes in as many as 3% of normal people [27], and these foci may be readily confused with metastases from small, well-differentiated follicular carcinomas in the main gland.

In perinatal autopsy material, thyroid tissue may be seen infiltrating the strap muscles (Fig. 28.22). The fate of these foci in adults is not known. Similarly, thyroid glandular tissue may extend into the trachea without causing any symptoms.

CONGENITAL HYPOTHYROIDISM

Approximately 1 in every 4000 to 5000 livebirths suffers from congenital hypothyroidism, making this the most common single cause of preventable mental retardation [29].

The signs and symptoms detectable in the newborn period include prolonged gestation, large size at birth, large posterior fontanelle, respiratory distress, hypothermia, peripheral cyanosis, poor motor activity, poor feeding, delay in passage of meconium (in excess of 20 hours postnatal), umbilical hernia, abdominal distension with vomiting, prolonged icterus (in excess of 3 days' duration), and edema of eyelids, labia, and face [30]. In most affected infants, many of these features are present, and many infants may exhibit evidence of a delay in skeletal maturation [31]. Respiratory distress and circulatory problems have also been noted, including respiratory distress associated with a patent ductus arteriosus in infants weighing more than 2.5 kg at birth [32]. There is therefore a very wide range of symptoms, and early diagnosis in the neonate may be difficult.

The need for early diagnosis of congenital hypothyroidism emphasizes the role of screening programs. Many screening procedures have been developed, including filter paper spot sampling of heel-prick specimens for T_4 levels, filter paper spot tests for TSH levels, cord blood serum TSH levels, and cord blood serum T_4 levels, with some variation from center to center. The experience of the oldest North American programs, outlining the results of screening more than a million infants [29], yields an incidence and pattern

of results that are similar to those reported in Wales [23], Belgium [33], Hong Kong [34], and Australia [35]. Hypothyroidism is a worldwide problem.

The causes of hypothyroidism vary [29]. The vast majority of the cases are due to primary thyroid disorders, while only 10 of 284 infants had either pituitary or hypothalamic causes, so-called "secondary" or "tertiary" hypothyroidism, respectively. Of the primary thyroid disorders, approximately 60% were found to have the spectrum of changes of athyreosis (as previously discussed). Fourteen percent were found to have normal or enlarged thyroid glands associated with dyshormonogenesis, while ectopic thyroid glands (usually lingual) were associated with hypothyroidism in approximately 25% of cases. Isolated cases of maternal goitrogen exposure were also noted, usually due to maternal iodide or propylthiouracil intake. Occasionally, infants have transient elevations of cord TSH and low cord sera T_4 levels, whereas others exhibit normal T_4 levels but elevated TSH levels. There may even be a discrepancy between monozygotic twins with regard to the effects of maternal drug exposure on the thyroid [21].

Severe fetal iodine deficiency from any cause, including a deficiency of the levels in maternal drinking water in early pregnancy, can cause severe, irreparable brain damage that does not respond to postnatal therapy [36]. These infants present with euthyroid goitrous enlargement with neurologic damage. Since a deficiency of iodine in maternal drinking water can be a common problem worldwide, its contribution to the overall problem of neonatal mental damage may be enormous—and easily underdiagnosed.

GOITROUS HYPOTHYROIDISM IN THE NEWBORN

While it is likely that cases of goitrous hypothyroidism represent thyroid dyshormonogenesis, most cases have not been studied in detail.

Dyshormonogenesis usually reflects an abnormality in the synthesis and metabolism of T_4 and T_3 [37]. The majority of cases present at puberty. Defects may occur in iodide transport, in the conversion of iodide to organically bound iodine in the thyroid (peroxidase defect), in deiodination of monoiodotyrosine and diiodotyrosine (halogenase defect), or in the synthesis of thyroglobulin and iodothyronine. Most of these defects are inherited as autosomal recessive conditions [38], but abnormalities of thyroglobulin synthesis represent a heterogeneous group that in some families appear to be inherited in an autosomal dominant fashion [39]. The impact of any defect in iodide transport or any halogenase defect may be masked by a high dietary iodine intake, but Couch et al [40] have described a neonate with hypothyroidism due to defective iodide transport. Peroxidase defects [41] often present with severe cretinism in the newborn period, and Pendred's syndrome (deaf-mutism, hypothyroidism, and probable peroxidase defect) represents a special variant. An isolated sibship with unresponsiveness

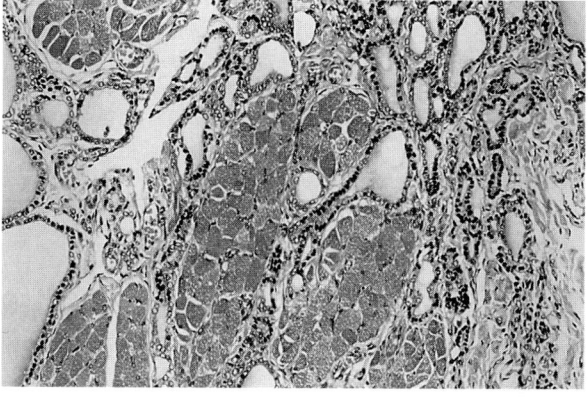

FIGURE 28.22. *Thyroid tissue in strap muscles of an immature neonate. H&E, ×200.*

to circulating thyroid hormone, severe deaf-mutism, delayed bone maturation, stippled epiphyses, normal metabolic rate, and elevated thyroxine levels has been recorded [38]. Perelman et al [42] described examples of polyhydramnios and goiter associated with peroxidase deficiency. Some cases were treated successfully with intra-amniotic T₄.

Only in very rare instances is the neonatal thyroid gland available for histologic study in cases of goitrous cretinism [37], and such cases have shown varying degrees of hyperplasia (Fig. 28.23). Since the effect of TSH stimulation on the histology of the gland appears to be cumulative, the histologic changes in the newborn are not likely to be as severe as those seen in older patients with these disorders [43].

Congenital, transient, neonatal hypothyroidism due to maternal ingestion of goitrogenic drugs (such as propyl-

thiouracil) has been recognized as a hazard of this form of therapy for many years. Maternal ingestion of iodides has also been known to produce congenital hypothyroidism, as has maternal exposure to contrast media during pregnancy, or even topical applications of iodine. The ease with which iodine crosses the placenta makes it a very strong potential candidate for otherwise unexplained transient congenital hypothyroidism [29, 44–47].

Congenital hypothyroidism of a transient nature may be present in infants born to mothers with IgG-class immunoglobulins that block TSH-stimulated iodine binding. These antibodies may be present even in the absence of maternal autoimmune thyroiditis [48], although they are much more common in patients with this condition [49–51]. However, the contribution of this group of

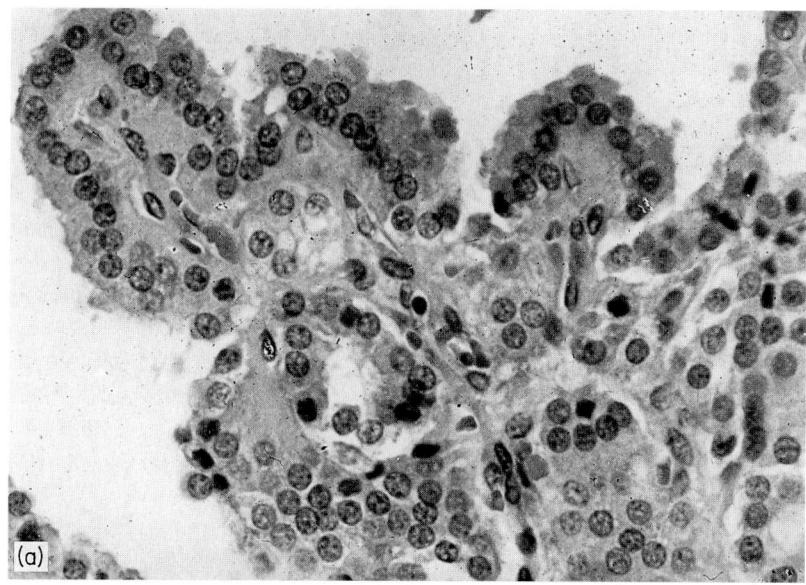

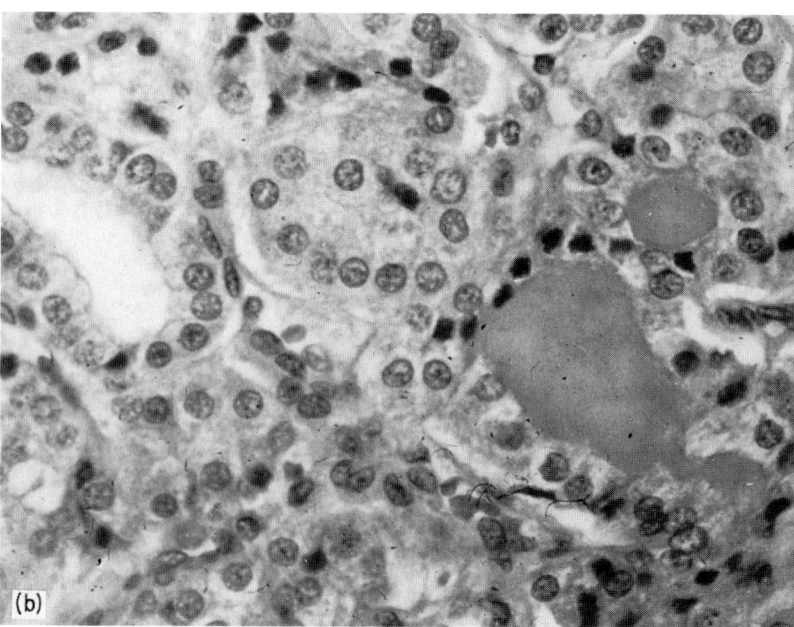

FIGURE 28.23. *Papillary (a) and hyperplastic (b) cellular foci in a biopsy of the thyroid gland in a 3-year-old child who presented with congenital goitrous hypothyroidism of unknown type. (Slide kindly provided by Dr. Hans Lucke, Hamilton, Ontario.) H&E, ×800.*

cases to the overall incidence of hypothyroidism is small [48].

In all cases, goitrous enlargement may compromise the airway, especially if there is a complicating hemorrhage.

Since there are many different varieties of neonatal hypothyroidism with greatly differing clinical courses and genetic patterns, an accurate diagnosis of the cause in each individual case is necessary. The variety of etiologies helps to explain the great variation in the pathology of these glands. Most glands appear atrophic and fibrotic, but with residual adenomatous areas. These changes are usually described in adult autopsy material, and the appearances in the newborn period are likely to be quite different [21].

Eayrs [52] has shown that hypothyroidism in utero interferes with protein synthesis in the developing brains of rat fetuses, associated with hypoplasia of the perikarya and neuropil in the developing cortex. In humans, the exact cause of the mental retardation is not known, but the damage to the developing brain is no less definite; in some cases, even postnatal therapy may be ineffective [36]. Early diagnosis and treatment can alter the otherwise gloomy prognosis in the majority of cases [53]. Some have even suggested intrauterine therapy with intramuscular T_4 to the fetus in those pregnancies at high risk for congenital hypothyroidism [54].

Hypothyroidism may be part of other malformation syndromes, being a frequent finding in the Johanson-Blizzard syndrome of hypoplastic alae nasi, deafness, prenatal growth retardation, and variable urogenital and anorectal abnormalities [55, 56]. Hypothyroidism may be present also as part of Down syndrome, Turner syndrome, and Albright's hereditary osteodystrophy [57–59]. In these syndromes, the presence of hypothyroidism may be masked by the other abnormalities. Winter et al [60] have described a case of congenital hypothyroidism associated with a ring chromosome 18, and have reviewed other abnormalities of this chromosome associated with hypothyroidism.

Finally, not all hypothyroid neonates have neuronal damage and the full clinical picture of cretinism, which has been ascribed to the protective effect of maternal thyroxine [61]. This view could explain why the severity and incidence of cretinism are higher when the mother herself is hypothyroid.

CONGENITAL HYPERTHYROIDISM

Congenital hyperthyroidism is encountered much less commonly than is hypothyroidism. Affected infants are usually born to mothers with clinically active Graves disease, but examples of affected infants being delivered to mothers whose hyperthyroidism has been controlled by drugs or surgery are also known [62, 63]. The incidence of thyrotoxicosis in pregnancy is low (0.047% of all pregnant mothers), and only 1 in 70 newborns of thyrotoxic mothers develop signs and symptoms [64]. However, the immediate morbidity and even mortality in the newborn period overshadows the rarity of the condition.

Infants are often delivered prematurely. The affected infants usually show evidence of tachycardia, increased irritability, failure to thrive, diarrhea, and vomiting. Thyroid enlargement, although frequent, may have to be sought for specifically, and while exophthalmos may be present, the finding is not invariable. In most infants (about 60%), the disease is transient, with symptoms subsiding spontaneously and complete recovery occurring by 3 months [12]. In about 20%, death may result with a clinical syndrome resembling high-output cardiac failure. In the remaining 20%, symptoms may persist well beyond 6 months and require prolonged treatment.

The study of neonatal hyperthyroidism has lent support to the concept of the role of long-acting thyroid stimulators (LATS) in the development of thyrotoxicosis. These thyroid-stimulating immunoglobulins of the IgG class can cross the placenta and can stimulate thyroid tissue in vitro as well as secretion of thyroid hormone in normal volunteers [65]. At least two main groups of thyroid-stimulating immunoglobulins are known. There is a LATS that acts in experimental assays on the thyroid glands of guinea pigs and mice, but whose titer does not always correlate well with the degree of thyroid hyperactivity. There is a second group of immunoglobulins, present in the sera of thyrotoxic patients, that can stimulate the human thyroid but that blocks the uptake of classic LATS and is known by some as "LATS-protector" or "LATS-P" [66]. A new terminology has been espoused to avoid the confusion inherent in the earlier system of nomenclature. All thyroid-stimulating immunoglobulins or antibodies are referred to as "TsAb" or better as "TSI" (thyroid-stimulating immunoglobulin); "LATS" becomes mouse thyroid stimulator (MTS), and "LATS-P" becomes human thyroid stimulator (HTS). Both MTS and HTS may be present in the same sera [12, 67]. The half-life of transplacental TSI is approximately 2 weeks. The natural decay of these maternally derived immunoglobulins in the fetus explains the transient course of most cases of neonatal thyrotoxicosis.

There remains a group of cases that present with thyrotoxic symptoms in the newborn period and in which symptoms persist well after 6 months of age. A convincing case can be made for the belief that these infants have inherited Graves disease [68, 69]. Infants with neonatal thyrotoxicosis should therefore be assessed with care, bearing in mind the possibility of HTS-triggered, inherited disease becoming unmasked at an early age [70].

In fatal cases, the affected gland is larger than expected, intensely congested, and very firm. Often the enlargement of the gland may be surprising (Fig. 28.24). Histologically, the acinar colloid is depleted and the follicles are lined by tall columnar cells that may fill the lumina of the gland (Fig. 28.25). The appearances mimic the exaggerated hyperplastic change seen in glands exposed to thiouracil derivatives.

The changes in other organs are variable but usually include an excessive degree of extramedullary erythropoiesis

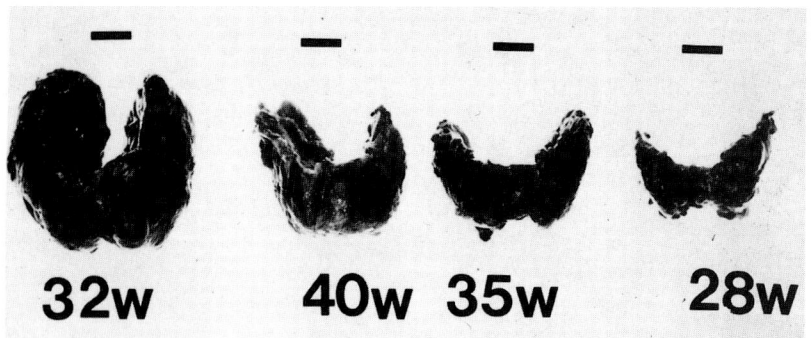

FIGURE 28.24. *Neonatal thyrotoxicosis in an infant of 32 weeks' gestation associated with a very obvious degree of thyroid enlargement (when compared to infants of 40, 35, and 28 weeks' gestation). The bar represents 1 cm.*

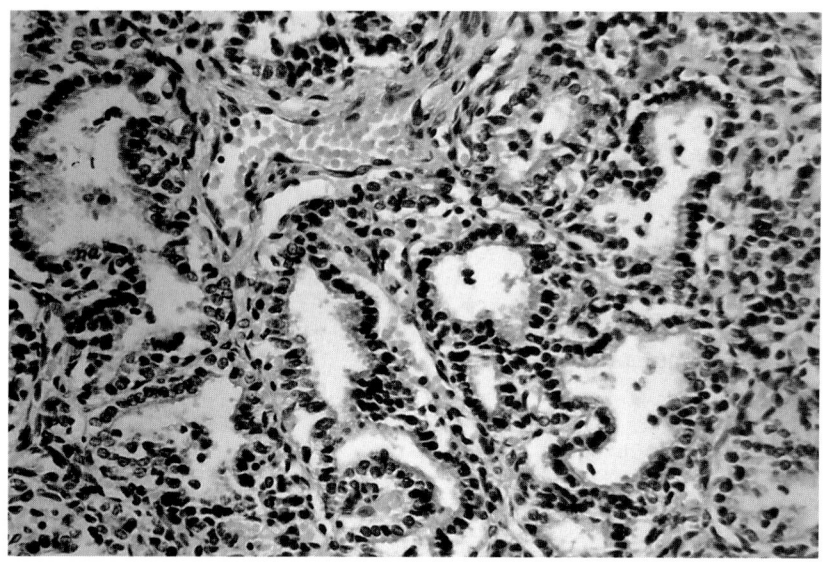

FIGURE 28.25. *In neonatal thyrotoxicosis, the thyroid acini are depleted of colloid and lined by tall columnar epithelium (same case as Fig. 28.24); compare with Fig. 28.17). H&E, ×500.*

for the stage of gestation. In fatal cases, variable amounts of subendocardial and interstitial scarring and necrosis of the myocardium have been observed [71]. In infants with prolonged neonatal thyrotoxicosis, premature cranial synostosis may occur [69].

TUMORS OF THE THYROID GLAND

In addition to dyshormonogenetic goiters associated with cretinism, on rare occasions tumors of the thyroid may be found in the neonatal period. By far the most frequent tumors are teratomas that may virtually replace the entire gland (Fig. 28.26). The tumors present as large neck masses that may interfere with the progress of labor since they may cause the head to present in the deflexed position. Tracheal deviation and esophageal compression may result. Many of the larger tumors are associated with hydramnios. Histologically, the majority of the tumors are well differentiated [72], usually with abundant glial components, cartilage, and clefts lined by respiratory epithelium. All three germ layers

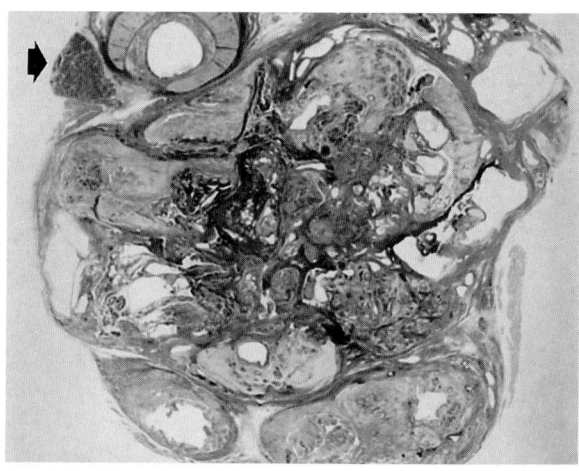

FIGURE 28.26. *A whole mount preparation of a large cervical teratoma involving the thyroid in a stillborn term infant associated with persistent occipitoposterior position and obstructed labor. A small nodule of residual thyroid is visible (arrow), but the tumor replaced the rest of the gland. Goldner's trichrome, ×5.*

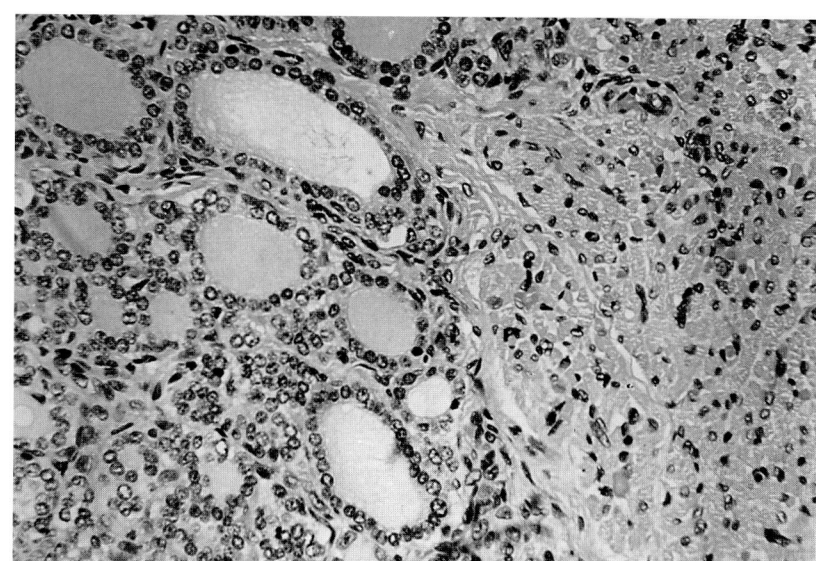

FIGURE 28.27.   *A nodule of smooth and striped muscle in the lateral lobe of the thyroid. H&E, ×500.*

are represented, and there may be entrapped thyroid acini, or thyroid epithelium may be part of the tumor [73]. An example of a metastasizing cervical/thyroid teratoma has been reported [74]. While the exact frequency of this complication is uncertain [75], it is obviously very rare.

Hamartomas of the thyroid gland have been reported in newborn infants [76]. These relatively large nodular masses differ histologically from teratomas by the absence of tissues derived from all three germ layers, and are made up of lobules of fibrous tissue with nodules of metaplastic cartilage. Entrapped thyroid acini appear compressed and contain variable amounts of colloid. The small mucinous acini seen on rare occasions in the thyroid probably represent choristomatous lesions.

Winship and Chase [77] reviewed 285 cases of thyroid carcinoma in childhood, and their series included a tumor in an infant of 4 weeks. A later review [78] of 562 collected cases revealed 12 cases where there had been a thyroid nodule at birth that later proved to be a carcinoma. This incidence, although relatively low, would make the thyroid gland the most common site for a carcinoma in infancy. There is a case report of a congenital occult papillary carcinoma in a newborn [79]. It is not always clear whether these are examples of dyshormonogenesis or true tumors, particularly since intrauterine exposure to iodine can occasionally produce hyperplastic changes in the glands of some infants [80].

Studies on survivors of the Chernobyl nuclear disaster suggest that both dyshormonogenetic changes and true tumors of the thyroid gland may occur [81, 82]. While neonatal infants are not mentioned specifically in these reports, it seems possible that hyperplastic changes were present in infancy, since many of the children with true tumors were very young.

HETEROTOPIC TISSUES IN THE THYROID

Intrathyroidal thymic rests near the lower pole of the thyroid are common incidental findings that are rarely symptomatic [83]. Nodules of striated and striped muscle within the lateral lobes of the gland are occasional incidental findings (Fig. 28.27). Intrathyroidal parathyroid glands may be encountered in some neonatal infants [84].

MISCELLANEOUS

The thyroid gland may be affected in congenital cytomegalovirus infections [85], when the pathognomonic inclusion-bearing cells are usually obvious.

The prolonged use of skin-cleansing solutions containing iodine may lead to the development of hypothyroidism in the postnatal period [86, 87]. This is fortunately a rare event in modern practice.

The thyroid vessels may be the lodging sites for emboli from the mitral valve or even various intravenous lines [88].

A lateral neck cyst with features combining a branchial cyst, a bronchogenic cyst, and a thyroglossal cyst was reported by Tyson and Graff [89]. The possibility of such lateral cysts being derived from the laterally situated ultimobranchial bodies should be remembered. In a provocative review, Williams et al [90] have provided evidence that the ultimobranchial body's contributions to the thyroid gland (including its follicular components) may be more complex and critical than formerly believed.

REFERENCES

1. Fisher DA, Klein AH. The ontogenesis of thyroid function and its relationship to neonatal thermogenesis. In: Tulchinsky D, Ryan KJ, eds. *Maternal-Fetal Endocrinology*. Philadelphia: WB Saunders, 1980, pp. 281–93.

2. Moore KL. *The Developing Human: Clinically Oriented Embryology*. 3rd ed. Philadelphia: WB Saunders, 1982, pp. ••–••.

3. Corliss CE. *Patten's Human Embryology. Elements of Clinical Development*. New York: McGraw-Hill, 1976, pp. 330–2.

4. Tanimura T, Shiota K. Endocrine system. In: Nishimura H, ed. *Atlas of Human Prenatal Histology*. Tokyo: Igaku-Shoin, 1983, pp. 267–76.

5. Williams ED. Histogenesis of medullary carcinoma of the thyroid. *J Clin Pathol* 1966; 19:114–18.

6. Williams ED. Medullary carcinoma of the thyroid. In: Harrison CV, Weinbren K, eds. *Recent Advances in Pathology*. no 9. Edinburgh: Churchill-Livingstone, 1975, pp. 156–82.

7. Pearse AGE, Polak J. Cytochemical evidence for the neural crest origin of mammalian ultimobranchial C cells. *Histochemie* 1971; 27:96–102.

8. Pueblitz S, Weinberg AG, Albores-Saavedra J. Thyroid C-cells in the DiGeorge anomaly: a quantitative study. *Pediatr Pathol* 1993; 13:463–73.

9. Sagreiya K, Emery JL. Perinatal thyroid discharge: a histological study of 1225 infant thyroids. *Arch Dis Child* 1970; 4:746–54.

10. Larroche JC. *Developmental Pathology of the Neonates*. Amsterdam: Excerpta Medica, 1977, pp. 225–31.

11. Lockitch G, Halstead AC, Dimmick JE. Endocrine system. In: Dimmick JE, Kalousek DK, eds. *Developmental Pathology of the Embryo and Fetus*. Philadelphia: JB Lippincott, 1992, pp. 707–48.

12. Jost A. Full or partial maturation of foetal endocrine systems under pituitary control. *Perspect Biol Med* 1968; 11:371–5.

13. Fisher DA. Hyperthyroidism: pediatric aspects. In: Werner SC, Ingbar SH, eds. *The Thyroid*. 4th ed. New York: Harper & Row, 1978, pp. 805–13.

14. Jost A. Hormones in development: past and prospects. In: Hamburgh M, Barrington EJ, eds. *Hormones in Development*. New York: Appleton-Century-Crofts, 1971, pp. 1–18.

15. Bamforth JS, Hughes I, Lazarus J, John R. Congenital anomalies associated with hypothyroidism. *Arch Dis Child* 1986; 61:608–9.

16. Gluckman PD. The fetal neuroendocrine axis. *Curr Top Exp Endocrinol* 1993; 5:1.

17. Kaplan SL, Grumbach MM, Aubert ML. The ontogenesis of pituitary hormones and hypothalamic factors in the human fetus: maturation of central nervous system regulation of anterior pituitary function. *Recent Prog Horm Res* 1976; 32:161–243.

18. Fisher DA, Odell WD. Acute release of thyrotropin in the newborn. *J Clin Invest* 1969; 48:1670–7.

19. Bruck K. Temperature regulations in the newborn infant. *Biol Neonate* 1961; 3:65–119.

20. Little G, Meador CK, Cunningham R, Pittman JA. "Cryptothyroidism" the major cause of "athyreotic" cretinism. *J Clin Endocrinol Metab* 1965; 25:1529–36.

21. Carr EA Jr, Beierwaltes WH, et al. The various types of thyroid malfunction in cretinism and their relative frequency. *Pediatrics* 1961; 28:1–16.

22. Gabr M. The role of thyroid dysgenesis and maldescent in the etiology of sporadic cretinism. *J Pediatr* 1962; 60:830–5.

23. Warkany J. *Congenital Malformations: Notes and Comments*. Chicago: Year Book, 1971, pp. 102, 437.

24. Hutchinson JH. The aetiology and diagnosis of nongoitrous hypothyroidism in childhood. In: Mason AS, ed. *The Thyroid and Its Diseases*. London: JB Lippincott, 1963, pp. 39–60.

24a. Bamforth JS, Hughes I, Lazarus J, John R. Congenital anomalies associated with hypothyroidism. *Arch Dis Child* 1986; 61:608–9.

25. Willis RA. *The Borderland of Embryology and Pathology*. London: Butterworths, 1962, p. 320.

26. Huckel R. Die entwicklungstorungen der schilddruse. In: Schwalbe S, ed. *Die Morphologie der Missbildungen des Menschen und der Tiere*. vol. 3, pts. 12–15. Jena: Gustav Fischer, 1932, pp. 600–1.

27. Robinson HB Jr. DiGeorge's or the III–IV pharyngeal pouch syndrome: pathology and a theory of pathogenesis. *Perspect Pediatr Pathol* 1975; 3:173–206.

28. Daentl DL, Frias JL, Gilbert EF, Opitz JM. The Johanson-Blizzard syndrome: case report and autopsy findings. *Am J Med Genet* 1979; 3:129–35.

29. Fisher DA, Dussault JH, Foley TP Jr, et al. Screening for congenital hypothyroidism. Results of screening 1 million North American infants. *J Pediatr* 1979; 94:700–5.

30. Smith DW, Klein AM, Henderson JR, Myrianthopoulos NC. Congenital hypothyroidism—signs and symptoms in the newborn period. *J Pediatr* 1975; 87:958–62.

31. Smith DW, Popich G. Large fontanels in congenital hypothyroidism: a clue to earlier recognition. *J Pediatr* 1972; 80:753–6.

32. Fisch RO, Bilek MM, Miller LD, Engel RR. Physical and mental status at four years of age of survivors of respiratory distress syndrome. *J Pediatr* 1975; 86:497–503.

33. Chanoine JP, Bourdoux P, Delange F. Congenital anomalies associated with hypothyroidism. *Arch Dis Child* 1986; 61:1147. Letter.

34. Low LCK, Lin HJ, Cheung PT, et al. Screening for congenital hypothyroidism in Hong Kong. *Aust Paediatr J* 1986; 22:53–6.

35. Connelly J. Congenital hypothyroidism. *Aust Paediatr J* 1986; 22:165–6.

36. Pharoah POD, DeLange F, Fierro-Benitez R, Stanbury JB. Endemic cretinism. In: Stanbury JB, Hetzel BS, eds. *Endemic Goiter and Endemic Cretinism*. New York: Wiley, 1980, p. 395.

37. Stanbury JB. Inborn errors of the thyroid. In: Steinberg AG, Bearn AG, eds. *Progress in Medical Genetics*. vol. C. New York: Grune & Stratton, 1974, p. 55.

38. Zonana J, Rimoin DL. Genetic disorders of the thyroid. *Med Clin N Amer* 1975; 59:1263–74.

39. Couch RM, Hughes IA, deSa DJ, et al. An autosomal dominant form of adolescent multinodular goiter. *Am J Hum Genet* 1986; 39:811–16.

40. Couch RM, Dean HJ, Winter JSD. Congenital hypothyroidism caused by defective iodide transport. *J Pediatr* 1985; 106:950–3.

41. Maenpaa J. Congenital hypothyroidism. Aetiological and clinical aspects. *Arch Dis Child* 1972; 47:914–23.

42. Perelman AH, Johnson RL, Clemons RD, et al. Intrauterine diagnosis and treatment of fetal goitrous hypothyroidism. *J Clin Endocrinol Metab* 1990; 71:618–21.

43. Kennedy JS. The pathology of dyshormonogenetic goitre. *J Pathol* 1969; 99:251–64.

44. Danziger Y, Pertzelan A, Mimouri M. Transient congenital hypothyroidism after topical iodine in pregnancy and lactation. *Arch Dis Child* 1987; 62:295–6.

45. DeWolf D, DeSchepper J, Verhaaren H, et al. Congenital hypothyroid goitre and amiodarone. *Acta Paediatr Scand* 1988; 77:616–18.

46. Uhrmann S, Marks KH, Maisels MJ, et al. Frequency of transient hypothyroxinemia in low birth weight infants. *Arch Dis Child* 1981; 56:214–17.

47. Green HG, Gareis FJ, Shepard TH, Kelley VC. Cretinism associated with maternal I[31] therapy during pregnancy. *Am J Dis Child* 1971; 122:247–9.

48. Ginsberg J, Walfish PG, Rafters DJ, von Westarp C, Ehrlich RM. Thyrotrophin blocking antibodies in the sera of mothers with congenitally hypothyroid infants. *Clin Endocrinol* 1986; 25:189–94.

49. Matsuura N, Yamada Y, Nohara Y, et al. Familial neonatal transient hypothyroidism due to maternal TSH-binding inhibitor immunoglobulin. *N Engl J Med* 1980; 303:738–41.

50. Takasu N, Naka M, Mori T, Yamada T. Two types of thyroid function blocking antibodies in autoimmune atrophic thyroiditis and transient neonatal hypothyroidism due to maternal IgG. *Clin Endocrinol* 1984; 21:345–55.

51. Van der Gaag RD, Drexhage HA, Dussault JH. Role of maternal immunoglobulins blocking TSH-induced thyroid growth in sporadic forms of congenital hypothyroidism. *Lancet* 1985; 1:246–50.

52. Eayrs JT. Thyroid and developing brain: anatomical and behavioural effects. In: Hamburgh M, Barrington EJW, eds. *Hormones in Development*. New York: Appleton-Century-Crofts, 1971, pp. 345–55.

53. Klein AH, Meltzer S, Kenny FM. Improved prognosis in congenital hypothyroidism treated before age three months. *J Pediatr* 1972; 81:912–15.

54. Van Herle AJ, Young RT, Fisher DA, et al. Intrauterine treatment of a hypothyroid fetus. *J Clin Endocrinol Metab* 1975; 40:474–7.

55. Johanson A, Blizzard R. A syndrome of congenital aplasia of the alae nasi, deafness, hypothyroidism, dwarfism, absent permanent teeth and malabsorption. *J Pediatr* 1971; 79:982–7.

56. Smith DW. *Recognizable Patterns of Human Malformation*. 3rd ed. Philadelphia: WB Saunders, 1982, p. 10.

57. Brook CGD, Murset G, Zachmann M, Prader A. Growth in children with 45XO Turner syndrome. *Arch Dis Child* 1974; 49:789–95.

58. Marx SJ, Hershman JM, Aurbach GD. Thyroid dysfunction in pseudohypoparathyroidism. *J Clin Endocrinol Metab* 1971; 33:822–8.

59. Winter JSD, Ahluwalia K, Ray W. Congenital hypothyroidism in association with a ring chromosome 18. *J Med Genet* 1972; 9:122–6.

60. Hetzel BS, Mano MT. A review of experimental studies of iodine deficiency during fetal development. *J Nutr Sci* 1989; 119:145–51.

61. Lewis IC, MacGregor AG. Congenital hyperthyroidism. *Lancet* 1957; 1:14–16.

62. Javett SN, Senior B, Braudo JL, Heymann S. Neonatal thyrotoxicosis. *Pediatrics* 1959; 24:65–73.

63. Hawe P, Francis HH. Pregnancy and thyrotoxicosis. *Br Med J* 1962; 2:817–22.

64. Adams DD, Fastier FN, Howie JB, et al. Stimulation of the human thyroid by infusions of plasma containing LATS protector. *J Clin Endocrinol Metab* 1974; 39:826–32.

65. Adams DD, Kennedy TH. Occurrence in thyrotoxicosis of a gamma globulin which protects LATS from neutralization by an extract of thyroid gland. *J Clin Endocrinol Metab* 1967; 27:173–7.

66. Green WL. Humoral and genetic factors in thyrotoxic Graves disease and neonatal thyrotoxicosis. *JAMA* 1976; 235:1449–50.

67. Hollingsworth DR, Mabry CC. Congenital Graves disease. Four familial cases with long-term follow up and perspective. *Am J Dis Child* 1976; 130:148–55.

68. Hollingsworth DR, Mabry CC, Eckerd JM. Hereditary aspects of Graves disease in infancy and childhood. *J Pediatr* 1972; 81:446–59.

69. Solomon DH, Chopra IJ. Graves disease. *Mayo Clin Proc* 1972; 47:803–13.

70. Farber S, Craig JM. Clinical pathological conference (neonatal hyperthyroidism). *J Pediatr* 1959; 54:829–38.

71. Gonzalez-Crussi F. Extragonadal teratomas. In: *Atlas of Tumor Pathology.* fasc. 18, 2nd ser. Washington: Armed Forces Institute of Pathology, 1982, p. 118.

72. Vujanic GM, Harach HR, Minic P, Vuckovic N. Thyroid/cervical teratomas in children: immunohistochemical markers for specific thyroid epithelial cell markers. *Pediatr Pathol* 1994; 14:369–75.

73. Baumann FR, Nerlich A. Metastasizing cervical teratoma of the fetus. *Pediatr Pathol* 1993; 13:21–7.

74. Vujanic GM. Cervical teratomas. *Pediatr Pathol* 1955; 15:221–2. Letter.

75. Willis RA. *The Pathology of the Tumours of Children.* Edinburgh: Oliver & Boyd, 1962, p. 107.

76. Winship T, Chase WW. Thyroid carcinoma in children. *Surg Gynecol Obstet* 1955; 101:217–24.

77. Winship T, Rosvoll RV. Childhood thyroid carcinoma. *Cancer* 1961; 14:734–43.

78. Mills SE, Allen MS. Congenital occult papillary carcinoma of thyroid gland. *Hum Pathol* 1986; 17:1179–81.

79. Becroft DMO, Smeeton WMI, Stewart JH. Fetal thyroid hyperplasia, rhesus isoimmunisation, and amniography. *Arch Dis Child* 1980; 55:213–17.

80. Nikiforov Y, Gnepp DR. Pediatric thyroid cancer after the Chernobyl disaster: pathomorphological study of 84 cases from the Republic of Belarus. *Mod Pathol* 1994; 11:55A. Abstract.

81. Nikiforov Y, Gnepp DR. Characteristics of nonmalignant changes in thyroid glands of children and adolescents exposed to radiation after the Chernobyl disaster. *Mod Pathol* 1994; 11:55A. Abstract.

82. Harach HR, Vujanic GM. Intrathyroidal thymic tissue: an autopsy study in fetuses with some emphasis on pathological implications. *Pediatr Pathol* 1993; 13:431–4.

83. Harach HR, Vujanic GM. Intrathyroidal parathyroid. *Pediatr Pathol* 1993; 13:71–4.

84. Becroft DMO. Prenatal cytomegalovirus infection. *Perspect Pediatr Pathol* 1981; 6:203–41.

85. Castaing H, Fournet JP, Leger FA, et al. Thyroid of the newborn and postnatal iodine overload. *Arch Fr Pediatr* 1979; 36:356–68.

86. Chabrolle JP, Rossier A. Goitre and hypothyroidism in the newborn after cutaneous absorption of iodine. *Arch Dis Child* 1978; 53:495–8.

87. Pyati SP, Ramamurthy RS, Kraw MT, Pildes RS. Absorption of iodine in the neonate following topical use of providone-iodine. *J Pediatr* 1977; 91:825–8.

88. deSa DJ. *Pathology of Neonatal Intensive Care.* London: Chapman & Hall, 1995, p. 101.

89. Tyson RW, Groff DB. An unusual lateral neck cyst with the combined features of a bronchogenic, thyroglossal, and branchial cleft origin. *Pediatr Pathol* 1993; 13:567–72.

90. Williams ED, Toyn CE, Harach HR. The ultimobranchial gland and congenital thyroid anomalies in man. *J Pathol* 1989; 159:135–41.

PART III
THE PARATHYROID GLAND

DEVELOPMENT AND STRUCTURE

The human parathyroid glands were studied extensively by Norris [1], who provided much of the basis for our current knowledge. The glands are first identifiable at the 8-to-9-mm stage, as bilateral clusters of cells arising from the third and fourth branchial pouches. The dorsal parathyroid primordium associated with the third pouch (parathyroid III) is attached to the ventrally located primordium of the thymus. The "descent" of the heart into the thoracic region draws down the thymus and parathyroid III. Parathyroid IV (the primordium derived from the fourth pouch) remains in close proximity to the developing lateral lobe of the thyroid gland and ultimobranchial body. At about the 18-mm stage, the parathyroid III rudiment separates from the thymus and settles near the lower pole of the thyroid as the inferior parathyroid gland. Parathyroid IV remains closely related to the upper pole of the thyroid as the superior parathyroid gland. This orderly pattern of migration can be interrupted in many ways, with premature separation of parathyroid III, subdivision of either parathyroid III or IV, or failure of parathyroid III to separate from the thymic anlage. These derangements help to explain the anomalous anatomic locations of the parathyroid glands, the presence of supernumerary glands, and even intrathymic parathyroids (Fig. 28.28). The various anatomic locations of the parathyroid glands are the subject of an outstanding review by Wang [2].

Sequential differentiation of the various cellular components of the gland is well delineated by Tanimura and Shiota [3]. From the earliest stage, the parathyroid glands are recognizable as clusters of polygonal cells (Fig. 28.29), which become progressively vascularized (by the 15-mm stage) prior to separation from either the thymic or the ultimobranchial body. Parathyroid hormonal activity is detectable by the end of the third month, and clusters of polygonal cells with glycogen-rich cytoplasm are recognizable by the middle of the fourth month of gestation; true vesicle-bearing cells, the forerunners of the chief cells of the fully formed gland, are seen in the sixth month, and at term, the gland is made up of chief cells set in an areolar vascular stroma with only a very few fat cells (Fig. 28.30). True oxyphil cells appear only after a few years of postnatal life and are well developed at puberty [4]. Colloid retention in the gland is seen only after late adolescence. Significant accumulations of fat within the gland appear near puberty, becoming more prominent in later life.

The staining characteristic of the main cells of the gland can vary—even in infancy—and although it has never been studied in neonatal material, the variation is probably related to the cyclic activity of individual cells, as described by Shannon and Roth [5]. This is reflected in the varying proportion of chief cells (Fig. 28.31). The parathyroid gland of the fetus can respond to changes in ionic calcium concentrations, with an increase in gland size when calcium levels fall in the mother, and secondary hyperparathyroidism can

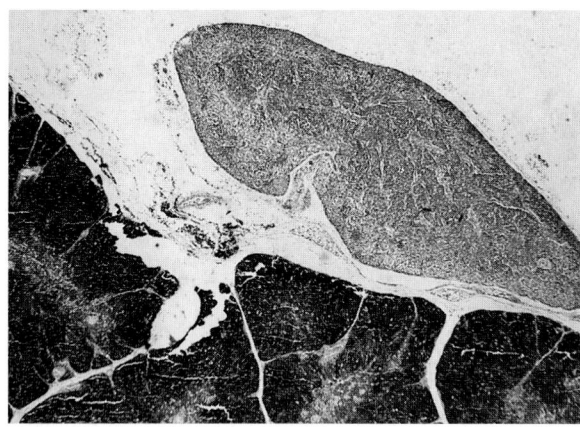

FIGURE 28.28. *A parathyroid gland found in a random section of the thymus in an infant of 31 weeks' gestation. H&E, ×50.*

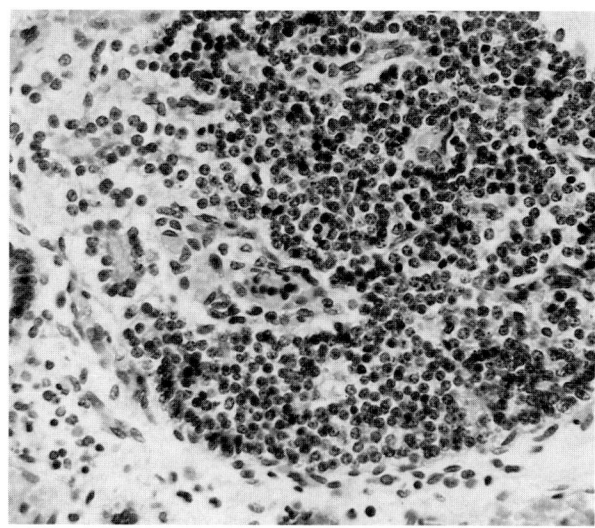

FIGURE 28.29. *Developing parathyroid gland of a 20-week fetus, showing the arrangement of cells and early vascularization. H&E, ×50.*

develop in infants of hypoparathyroid mothers [6]. This may account for the variation in the size of the gland in the neonate [7]; however, a good study of the normal size of the neonatal gland has not been conducted, due in large measure to the difficulty of identifying all four glands in every autopsy.

ABSENCE OF THE PARATHYROID GLANDS

Abnormalities of the parathyroid gland are common in DiGeorge syndrome (the III–IV pharyngeal pouch syndrome). The abnormalities vary from functional deficits to a complete absence of parathyroid tissue. In a review of 25 cases, the glands were absent in 13 infants, and only minute hypoplastic remnants were found in another case [8]. In all 25 infants, functional hypoparathyroidism was present and all infants had neonatal tetany. In Robinson's excellent review [8], the possible relationship of this syndrome to pre-

mature involution of the thyroidea ima artery (the principal artery supplying the region of the third and fourth pouches in the embryo) is presented with great clarity and force. Abnormalities of this artery are often associated with abnormalities of the aortic arch (which may actually lead to the involution of the thyroidea ima artery). Early involution of the thyroidea ima artery and the fourth left aortic arch is postulated to lead to damage and destruction of the primordia of the thymus and parathyroid glands.

In addition to the parathyroid abnormalities, thymic abnormalities (absence or extreme hypoplasia), aortic arch abnormalities, and abnormal facies may be present. Other commonly associated anomalies include tracheoesophageal abnormalities, partial thyroid aplasia, and absence of the thyroid isthmus, with depletion of the lymphocyte popula-

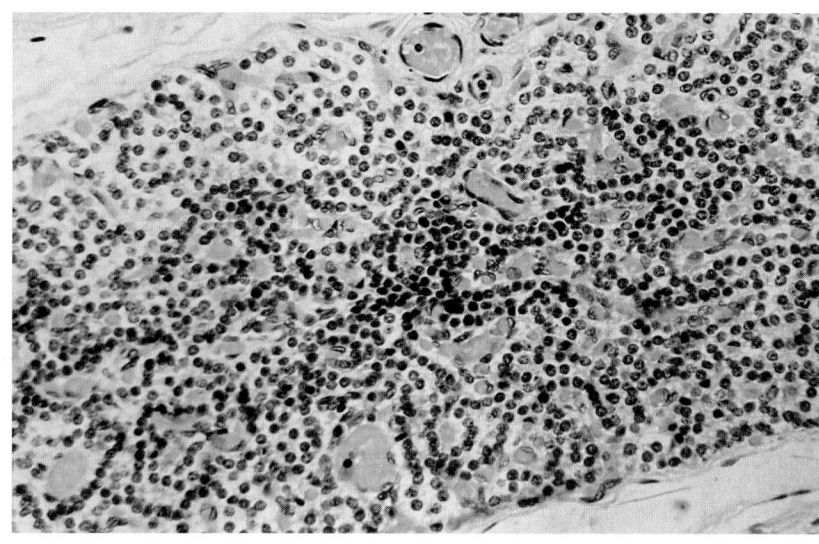

FIGURE 28.30. *Parathyroid gland of a 29-week infant, showing the increased vascularity of the gland. H&E, ×500.*

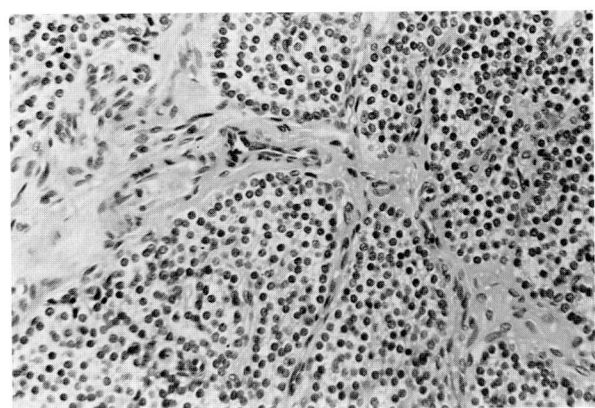

FIGURE 28.31.   *Parathyroid gland of a term infant, showing segments of several lobules made up of pale-staining chief cells. H&E, ×500.*

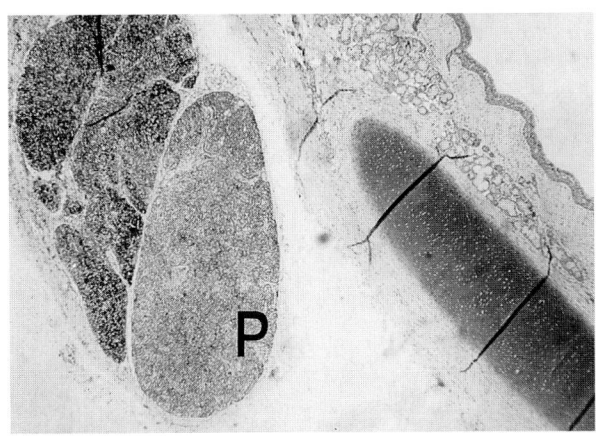

FIGURE 28.32.   *Parathyroid (P) and thymic tissue near the tracheal bifurcation; an incidental finding in an infant of 11 months. H&E, ×50.*

tion in thymic-dependent areas of lymph nodes and spleen. Robinson [8] suggested that there may be a functional deficit in thyroid "C" cells due to damage to the ultimobranchial body. C cells are not always absent, although they may be reduced in number [9, 10].

ABERRANT MIGRATION AND ECTOPIA

In general, detailed anatomic studies of the parathyroid glands do not feature prominently in either neonatal autopsy reports or reviews of malformation complexes. DiGeorge syndrome is a notable exception, but considering the frequency of aortic arch abnormalities in neonatal malformation complexes, one would expect that more examples of parathyroid abnormalities would be reported. Like many other colleagues, this author has great difficulty in identifying the parathyroid glands at the time of gross dissection and has come to rely on embedding a block of tissue that includes the larynx, thyroid, and trachea and then examining, in a semiserial fashion, multiple slices taken through the block. Even with this practice, one is often unsure of the true state of the parathyroids if one is unable to identify all four glands. This uncertainty is fed by the studies of Wang [2] and Akerstrom et al [11], who have clearly demonstrated that the parathyroid glands may be found in multiple sites.

The complex embryology of the parathyroid glands (with particular reference to their "migration") means that parathyroid tissue may be found in the mediastinum or thymus, attached to the pericardium, or in a paratracheal position (Fig. 28.32), in retropharyngeal or retroesophageal tissue, or even in the wall of a thymic duct cyst (duct of Kursteiner cyst) [2, 11, 12]. Some of these abnormalities may represent abnormal or aberrant migration, but many are probably due to premature (or repeated) subdivision of the primordium [2].

Functional parathyroid cysts [13, 14], and this includes examples in the mediastinum encountered in young adults, are a reflection of the problems that may arise from ectopic parathyroid tissue. The diagnostic problems that they pose are matched only by the complexity of their management.

Intrathyroidal parathyroid tissue was observed in 13 of 58 fetal thyroid glands by Harach and Vujanic [15]. The parathyroid tissue varied in size, and was found either just below the capsule of the gland or within the gland itself.

SUPERNUMERARY GLANDS

While most humans have four parathyroid glands, some have five and, exceptionally, some have 11 or 12 glands strung out like a "string of pearls" [16]. These cases are probably examples of a combination of repeated premature subdivision and aberrant migration. Some supernumerary glands lie very close to normally sited glands.

Bizarre Heterotopias

Rare examples of parathyroid heterotopia have included functioning parathyroid tissue in the vagina of a 3-year-old [17], and Lack et al [18] found minute foci of parathyroid tissue in the vagus nerve or below the epineurium in 4 of 64 infants under 1 year of age. The finding of parathyroid tissue in either site is not explained by our current knowledge of the glands' development and migration.

FUNCTIONAL ABNORMALITIES

Most instances of altered calcium and phosphorus metabolism in infancy are not due to primary parathyroid disorders, which are very uncommon overall.

HYPOPARATHYROIDISM

Hypoparathyroidism may occur in the newborn as a reactive condition in response to maternal hypercalcemia or latent hyperparathyroidism. Some such infants may present with tetany and seizures toward the end of the first week of postnatal life, but others may present later with convulsions precipitated by feeds of milk formula. Prolonged therapy with vitamin D and calcium may be needed before recovery occurs [19, 20]. Parathyroid function may be suppressed for as long as 3 months [21]. A syndrome of transient idiopathic hypoparathyroidism is also known to occur [22, 23]. This entity has a short, self-limited course and occurs in infants born to mothers who do not have hypercalcemia. Primary familial hypoparathyroidism has been reported [24], as has a rare congenital, X-linked recessive hypoparathyroidism [25]. The pathologic changes in these rare conditions are not known, since detailed histologic studies are not available.

Burke [26] has provided an excellent tabulated summary of causes of hypoparathyroidism in infancy and childhood. This includes the very rare examples of failure of parathyroid hormone action, deficiency of secretions of parathormone, and hereditary variants. Most of these conditions do not cause problems in neonates, but the association of hypoparathyroidism with a ring chromosome 16 or 18, Kenny syndrome [27], and mitochondrial myopathy [28] is of importance to neonatologists.

Primary hyperparathyroidism in infancy is extremely rare and has been the subject of only isolated reports [29–32], and at least one report provides ultrastructural evidence of hyperplasia [33]. Hillman et al reported two siblings of a consanguineous marriage with symptomatic hyperparathyroidism in the newborn period [34]. One sibling died of massive parathyroid hyperplasia; the other recovered after subtotal parathyroid removal. In this setting, the infants are usually asymptomatic at birth, and hypercalcemia becomes evident after about a week [35]. Skeletal x-rays may show presymptomatic demineralization and osteopenia: fractures and renal calcinosis may be present. Histologically, the glands have diffuse hyperplasia, and there is a high degree of recurrence if only three glands are removed. Treatment requires resection of at least three glands plus up to 75% of the fourth gland [36].

Primary hyperparathyroidism may have an autosomal dominant or recessive pattern of inheritance [26, 36], and this field is one of considerable complexity that, in this author's view, has not been fully elucidated. There are many more examples of secondary hyperparathyroidism, and the list includes cases associated with vitamin D deficiency rickets, vitamin-D-dependent rickets due to 1α-hydroxylase deficiency, hepatic diseases, renal diseases, maternal hypoparathyroidism, furosemide therapy, and feeding of infants with humanized cow's milk formula (with a high phosphorus load) [36–38]. The bone lesions and renal calcinosis may be as evident as in any example of primary hyperparathyroidism. The full clinical manifestations of these conditions are not evident in the newborn period, or may be masked by other serious illness. This phenomenon may acquire greater significance in the future as more sick newborns receive intensive care (including parenteral hyperalimentation and diuretic therapy).

HEMORRHAGE AND SIDEROSIS OF PARATHYROID GLANDS

Knisely and his colleagues have drawn attention to hemorrhage and siderosis in the parathyroid glands [39]. They found lysis and hemorrhage in the glands of four infants with perinatally lethal osteogenesis imperfecta who died after surviving 9 days or more, and suggested that the parathyroid damage was related to problems in maintenance of calcium homeostasis. This may probably be accentuated by the lack of calcium reserves in bone, since hypocalcemia was observed in two of the infants studied. The changes were not seen in infants who died within 2 hours of birth, and only minor foci of hemorrhage were reported in 3 of 170 parathyroid glands from "control" infants. In addition to recent hemorrhage, evidence of siderosis (indicating older episodes of hemorrhage) was seen in the parathyroid but not in the adjacent thyroid epithelium. Knisely et al [39] present a good case for believing that destructive lesions of the parathyroid gland could produce hypercalcemia and be a precipitating cause of death.

Knisely et al [39] refer, in passing, to occasional examples of siderosis of the parathyroid gland in neonatal hemochromatosis and erythroblastosis.

HYPOCALCEMIA IN THE NEWBORN

Hypocalcemia is not always associated with parathyroid disease, but may be associated, in rare instances, with delayed development of a renal parathyroid receptor in preterm babies [40] or with elevated calcitonin levels [41]. The vast majority of cases, however, occur in infants fed formulas that do not meet their calcium and phosphorus requirements [35–37]. Some of these infants may even develop tetany. Stimmler et al [42] described defects in the enamel of the primary dentition of infants who had suffered from neonatal hypocalcemia, and the changes were said to resemble those seen in congenital hypoparathyroidism. The anomalies of the enamel were thought to predispose to premature development of dental caries in the primary dentition. This fascinating observation has not been followed systematically, even though it has been demonstrated that the primordia of the teeth are susceptible to any generalized insult suffered by the fetus and newborn [43].

REFERENCES

1. Norris EH. The parathyroid glands and the lateral thyroid in man: their morphogenesis, histogenesis, topographic anatomy and prenatal growth. *Contrib Embryol* 1937; 159:247–94.

2. Wang C-A. The anatomic basis of parathyroid surgery. *Ann Surg* 1983; 183:271–5.

3. Tanimura T, Shiota K. Endocrine system. In: Nishimura H, ed. *Atlas of Human Prenatal Histology.* Tokyo: Igaku-Shoin, 1983, p. 267.

4. Valdes-Dapena MA. *Histology of the Fetus and Newborn.* Philadelphia: WB Saunders, 1979, p. 126.

5 Shannon WA, Roth SI. An ultrastructural study of acid phosphatase activity in normal, adenomatous and hyperplastic (chief-cell type) human parathyroid glands. *Am J Pathol* 1974; 77:493–506.

6. Sann L, David L, Frederich A, Chapuy M, Francois R. Congenital hyper-parathyroidism and vitamin D deficiency secondary to maternal hypoparathy-roidism. *Acta Paediatr Scand* 1976; 65:381–5.

7. Castleman B, Roth SI. Tumors of the parathyroid glands. In: *Atlas of Tumor Pathology.* fasc. 14, 2nd ser. Washington: Armed Forces Institute of Pathology, 1978, pp. 3–20.

8. Robinson HB Jr. DiGeorge's or the III–IV pharyngeal pouch syndrome: pathology and a theory of pathogenesis. *Perspect Pediatr Pathol* 1975; 3:173–206.

9. Pueblitz S, Weinberg A, Albores-Saavedra J. Thyroid C cells in the DiGeorge anomaly: a quantitative study. *Pediatr Pathol* 1993; 13:463–73.

10. Burke BA, Johnson D, Gilbert E, et al. Thyrocalcitonin containing cells in the DiGeorge anomaly. *Hum Pathol* 1987; 18:355–60.

11. Akerstrom G, Malmaens J, Bergstrom R. Surgical anatomy of human parathy-roid glands. *Surgery* 1984; 95:14–21.

12. Silver WE. Cervical mediastinal thymic parathyroid cyst. *Otolaryngol Head Neck Surg* 1980; 88:403–8.

13. Ramos-Gabatin A, Mallette LE, Bringhurst FR, Draper MW. Functional mediastinal parathyroid cyst. *Am J Med* 1985; 79:633–9.

14. Calandra DB, Shah KH, Prinz RA, et al. Parathyroid cysts: a report of eleven cases including two associated with hyperparathyroid crisis. *Surgery* 1983; 94:887–92.

15. Harach HR, Vujanic GM. Intrathyroidal parathyroid. *Pediatr Pathol* 1993; 13:71–4.

16. Grimelius L, Akerstrom G, Johansson H, Bergstrom A. Anatomy and histopathology of human parathyroid glands. *Pathol Ann* 1981; 2:1–24.

17. Kurman RJ, Prabha AC. Thyroid and parathyroid glands in the vaginal wall: report of a case. *Am J Clin Pathol* 1973; 59:503–7.

18. Lack EE, Delay S, Linnoila RI. Ectopic parathyroid tissue within the vagus nerve: incidence and possible clinical significance. *Arch Pathol Lab Med* 1988; 112:304–6.

19. Wagner G, Transbol I, Melchior JC. Hyperparathyroidism and pregnancy. *Acta Endocrinol* 1964; 47:549–64.

20. Jacobsen BB, Terslev E, Lund B, Sorensen OH. Neonatal hypocalcemia associated with maternal hyperparathyroidism. *Arch Dis Child* 1978; 53:308–11.

21. Better OS, Levi J, Greif E, et al. Prolonged neonatal parathyroid suppression. *Arch Surg* 1973; 106:722–4.

22. Fanconi A, Prader A. Transient congenital idiopathic hypoparathyroidism. *Helv Paediatr Acta* 1967; 22:342–59.

23. Rosenbloom AL. Transient congenital idiopathic hypoparathyroidism. *South Med J* 1973; 66:666–70.

24. Gorodischer R, Aceto T, Terplan K. Congenital familial hypoparathyroidism. *Am J Dis Child* 1970; 119:74–8.

25. Peden VH. True idiopathic hypoparathyroidism as a sexlinked recessive trait. *Am J Hum Genet* 1960; 12:323–37.

26. Burke B. The pituitary, pineal, adrenal, thyroid and parathyroid glands. In: Stocker J, Dehner LP, eds. *Pediatric Pathology.* Philadelphia: JB Lippincott, 1992, p. 980.

27. Fanconi S, Fischer JA, Wieland P, et al. Kenny syndrome: evidence for idiopathic hypoparathyroidism in two patients and for abnormal parathyroid hormone in one. *J Pediatr* 1986; 109:469–75.

28. Toppet M, Telerman-Toppet N, Szilwowski B, et al. Oculocranio-somatic neuromuscular disease with hypoparathyroidism. *Am J Dis Child* 1977; 131:437–42.

29. Pratt EL, Geren BB, Neuhauser EBD. Hypercalcemia and idiopathic hyperplasia of parathyroid glands in infant. *J Pediatr* 1947; 30:388–99.

30. Philips RN. Primary diffuse parathyroid hyperplasia in infant of 4 months. *Pediatrics* 1948; 2:428–34.

31. Randall C, Lauchlan SC. Parathyroid hyperplasia in infant. *Am J Dis Child* 1963; 105:364–7.

32. Goldbloom RB, Gillis DA, Prasad M. Hereditary parathyroid hyperplasia: a surgical emergency of early infancy. *Pediatrics* 1972; 49:514–23.

33. Garcia-Bunuel R, Kutchemeshgi A, Brandes D. Hereditary hyper-parathyroidism: the fine structure of the parathyroid gland. *Arch Pathol* 1974; 97:399–403.

34. Hillman DA, Scriver CR, Pedius S, Shragovitch I. Neonatal familial primary hyperparathyroidism. *N Engl J Med* 1954; 270:483–90.

35. Anast CS. Disorders of mineral and bone metabolism. In: Avery ME, Taeusch TW, eds. *Schaeffer's Diseases of the Newborn.* Philadelphia: WB Saunders, 1984, p. 464.

36. Tsang RC, Venkataraman P. Pediatric parathyroid and vitamin D related disorders. In: Kaplan SD, ed. *Clinical Pediatric and Adolescent Endocrinology.* Philadelphia: WB Saunders, 1982, p. 246.

37. Venkataraman PS, Tsang RC, Greer FR, et al. Late infantile tetany and secondary hyperparathyroidism in infants fed humanized cow milk formula. *Am J Dis Child* 1985; 139:664–8.

38. Venkataraman PS, Han BK, Tsang RC, Daugherty CC. Secondary hyper-parathyroidism and bone disease in infants receiving long term furosemide therapy. *Am J Dis Child* 1983; 137:1157–61.

39. Knisley AS, Magid MS, Felix JC, Singer DB. Parathyroid gland hemorrhage in perinatally lethal osteogenesis imperfecta. *J Pediatr* 1988; 112:720–5.

40. Mallet E, Basuyau JP, Brunelle P, et al. Neonatal parathyroid secretion and renal receptor maturation in premature infants. *Biol Neonate* 1978; 33:304–8.

41. Venkataraman PS, Tsang RC, Chen IW, Sperling MA. Pathogenesis of early neonatal hypocalcemia: studies of serum calcitonin, gastrin, and plasma glucagon. *J Pediatr* 1987; 110:599–603.

42. Stimmler L, Snodgrass GJ, Jaffe E. Dental defects associated with neonatal symptomatic hypocalcemia. *Arch Dis Child* 1973; 48:217–20.

43. Newton RW, Levine RS, Turner EP, Barson AJ. The sensitivity of the tooth germ to systemic disturbances. *Early Hum Dev* 1984; 9:269–73.

Chapter

29

The Kidneys and Urinary Tract

Juhani Rapola

DEVELOPMENT OF THE KIDNEY

The development of the human excretory system is described in traditional embryological texts as the formation of three temporally and spatially different successive "organs": the pronephros, mesonephros, and metanephros. This sequence of development might also be viewed as a continuum in which the earliest primitive stages of differentiation give rise to the formation of the next more complex structure until the final structurally and functionally effective metanephros or permanent kidney begins to develop.

This continuous development includes the disappearance or modification of structures that do not participate in the formation of the permanent kidney.

The first signs of differentiation of the kidney appear on both sides in the mesoderm between the ventrolateral aspect of the somites and the coelom during the latter part of the third postconceptional week in embryos of 8 to 9 somites. About seven pairs of the pronephric tubules appear at the level of 4 to 14 somites before the end of the 4th week. The ends of the lateral tubular parts turn caudally, fuse together, and form the pronephric duct. The pronephric ducts give rise to the important mesonephric duct, while the rest of the pronephric structures degenerate rapidly in the order of their appearance. The paired mesonephric ducts grow rapidly on the dorsolateral part of the nephrogenic cord and reach the cloaca before the end of the 4th week.

The mesonephric (wolffian) duct is the central part of the developing excretory system. It acts as an inducer of the mesonephric nephrons [1], drains the excretions of the mesonephros, gives rise to the ureteric bud, and ultimately, forms the major part of the vas deferens.

The mesonephros is present between the 9th and 13th somite in the 20-somite embryo. Altogether, 40 pairs of

mesonephric nephrons are formed, but because the most cranial degenerate as the most caudal ones develop, a full set of mesonephric nephrons is never present at the same time. Topographic anatomy of the pronephros and mesonephros indicates that the former is a cervical "organ" and the latter is formed in the thoracic region (Fig. 29.1). The mesonephros, however, shifts caudally due to the process of regression at the cephalic end, with continued growth at the caudal end. Most mesonephric nephrons have disappeared by the 12th week.

Permanent Kidney (Metanephros)

The permanent kidney develops from two components, the metanephrogenic mesenchyme (blastema) and the ureteric bud which is derived from the mesonephric duct.

In the 5th week a small bud emerges near the lower ends of both mesonephric ducts. The buds grow and elongate dorsally, and come into contact with the caudal end of the nephrogenic mesenchyme. When contact is established, the expanded end of the ureteric bud is surrounded by a condensed mass of mesenchymal cells.

The present knowledge of organogenesis of the kidney has its origin in the extensive microdissection studies of Osathanondh and Potter [2] and that of Oliver [3], whose reviews deal with the subject thoroughly. The ureteric bud within the mantle of the mesenchymal cells divides dichotomously and the branches grow toward the periphery.

The first division of the ureteric bud results in two branches that grow in opposite directions. The early divisions are more rapid at the poles of the developing organ, causing the elongated shape of the kidney. The first few generations of the branches expand to form the renal pelvis and the subsequent three generations develop into calices and

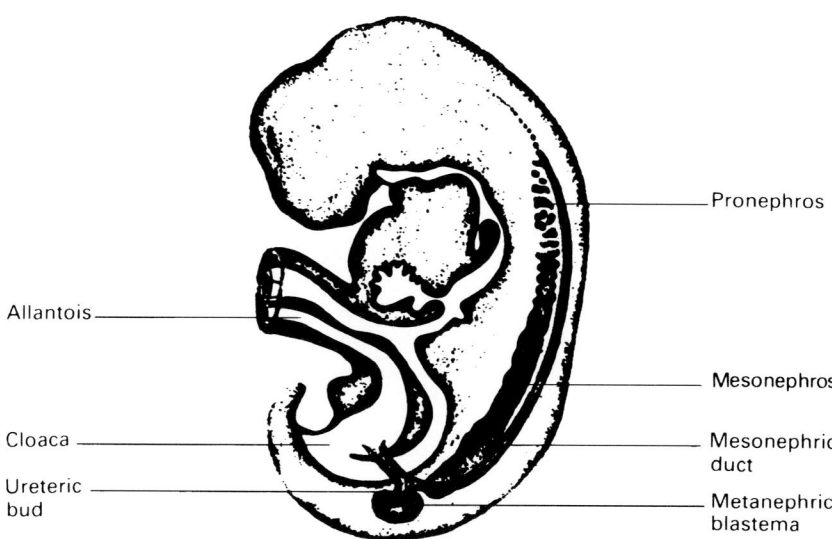

Allantois

Cloaca

Ureteric
bud

Pronephros

Mesonephros

Mesonephric
duct

Metanephric
blastema

FIGURE 29.1. *Diagram illustrating the developing urinary system in the human embryo about 5–6 weeks old.*

papillae. The following 7 to 8 branches form the collecting ducts.

Further ramification of the collecting system and nephron formation takes place in three successive stages that are important for the spatial arrangement of the renal structure. The first stage is characterized by successive branching at the widened tips of "ampullae." The ampullae both divide and induce the adjacent mesenchyme to form the first anlagen of nephrons. The prospective nephron becomes connected to the ampullary part of the collecting duct. At this stage, one nephron is attached to one branch of the collecting ducts and this continues until 6 to 8 generations of nephrons are produced. The newly formed nephron remains attached to the ampullary part of the growing and dividing collecting duct, and is carried with it into the cortex of the developing kidney. The ampullary branching of the collecting ducts decreases and virtually ends after the 20th week of fetal life. The development of the nephrons now enters the second stage. At this stage, the non–dividing ampullae continue to induce nephrons. One ampulla is capable of inducing more than one nephron. The first nephron attaches initially to the ampulla, but after the induction and ampullary connection of the second nephron the older one

shifts its point of attachment to the connecting piece of the newly formed nephron. As the process goes on, 4 to 6 nephrons are attached to one another by their connecting pieces (Fig. 29.2). These formations are known as *arcades*. During the final stage of nephron formation, the collecting duct grows in length toward the periphery and a series of 4 to 6 nephrons become connected individually to the ampulla and remain connected at regular intervals directly to the terminal part of the collecting duct. Nephron formation comes to an end at 32–36 weeks of fetal life.

Nephrogenesis

The ureteric bud exerts profound cellular and biochemical changes on the surrounding mesenchyme when the two components meet. The induction of the nephrons is, however, the final morphogenetic inductive action of the ureteric bud branches. The prospective nephron appears first as a dense cell cluster at the side of the ampullary tip of the collecting duct. It soon develops into the familiar S-shaped tubule. The upper part of the S-shaped body connects with the collecting duct, and the middle part elongates and forms the loop of Henle and the proximal tubule. The lower limb

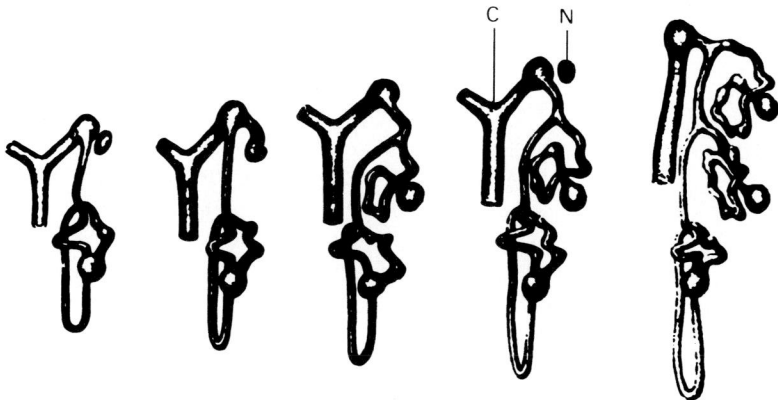

C   N

FIGURE 29.2. *Diagram of the formation of the nephronic arcades. C = branching point of the collecting duct; N = cell cluster of a future nephron. Modified from Ref. 13.*

of the "S" begins to form a Bowman's capsule and renal glomerulus.

Descriptive organogenesis and classic embryological mechanisms such as the induction and morphogenetic movements of early renal development have been well explained in the past [1]. More recently, the molecular biology of renal differentiation has been studied intensely. Several growth factors and their receptors seem to be instrumental in the early differentiation of the nephrons [4–6]. Transgenic animals are useful in elucidating gene function in normal and abnormal renal differentiation [7, 8]. While many of the growth factors and their receptors functioning in the differentiating kidney are universal message mediators, and thus unspecific, the Wilms' tumor–associated tumor suppressor gene *WT-1* is closely related to urinary tract organogenesis and its absence or mutation renders the individual susceptible to Wilms' tumor (see Chapter 15). The *WT-1* gene is expressed in the metanephric mesenchymal cells at the time of their first signs of nephron differentiation (cell clusters) and in the early stages of developing nephric tubules and glomeruli [9, 10]. Germ line mutations of *WT-1* are associated with urogenital malformations, specifically with Denys-Drash syndrome [11]. Constitutional chromosomal deletion 11p13 affects the structural integrity of the *WT-1* gene and leads to the WAGR syndrome (Wilms' tumor, aniridia, genitourinary malformations, mental retardation) (see Chap. 15). Introducing a mutation into the mouse *WT-1* gene results in excessive apoptosis of the metanephric blastema and failure of the ureteric bud to grow [8]. The molecular building blocks of the kidney are thus gradually being understood [12].

The early development of the human kidney takes place in the pelvic region. Between the 5th and 8th weeks of intrauterine life the kidneys rise to their final position at the level of the upper lumbar vertebrae. In the course of this ascent, the kidneys undergo an axial rotation of 90 degrees. The renal hilus faces originally toward the ventral aspect of the body and turns toward the midline during the rotation.

Renal Maturation and the Kidney of the Newborn

Potter [13] estimated that 8 to 12 generations of nephrons are formed in each human kidney, totalling 1 million nephrons. Since new nephrons are formed up to the 36th week of gestation, renal histology provides an index of fetal maturity in the preterm infant. In premature neonates, nephron formation continues after birth until the full number is achieved. Nephrogenic mesenchyme, immature tubules, and glomeruli are evident in the subcapsular cortex of such infants who die in the neonatal period (Fig. 29.3).

The exact time of onset of fetal urine production is not known, but it is generally assumed to take place after the first nephrons attain morphological maturity at about the 10th week of fetal life [14]. Renal function in the fetus has little, if any, homeostatic function, which is performed by the placenta. Fetal urine is voided into the amniotic sac. During the latter half of pregnancy, a large proportion of the amniotic fluid is derived from the fetal urine. Any pathological condition that prevents fetal urination decreases the amniotic fluid, with serious consequences to fetal development.

The kidney of the full-term newborn infant is still immature compared to the kidneys of older children. Macroscopically, it shows lobation of the surface, which disappears in the first year of life (Fig. 29.4). Microscopically,

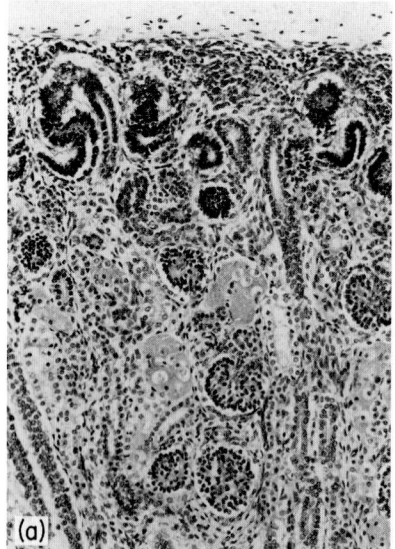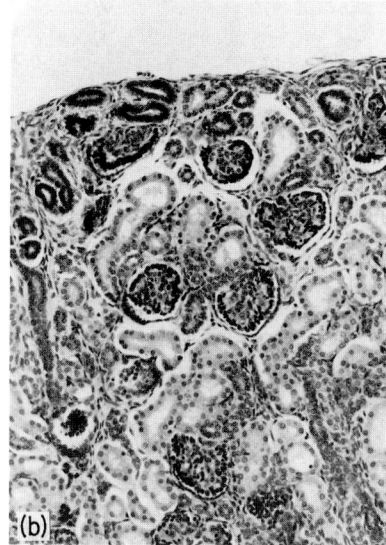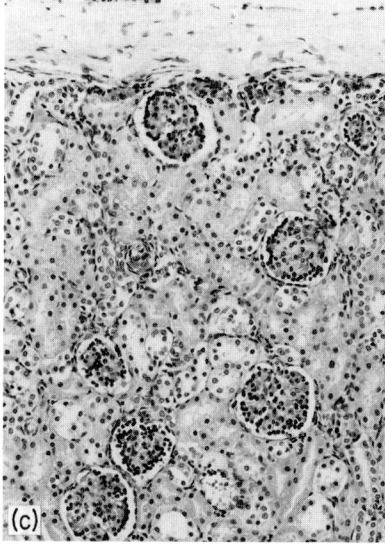

FIGURE 29.3.   *Kidney at different stages of maturation: (a) 25 weeks; (b) 32 weeks; (c) 40 weeks of gestation. Nephrons showing S-shaped tubules are forming in (a). A few immature tubules are present in (b), and all immature elements have disappeared in (c). H&E, ×55.*

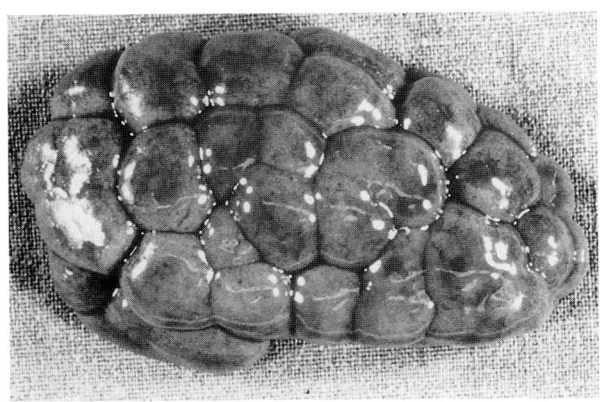

FIGURE 29.4. *Fetal lobation of the kidney in a preterm infant.*

Table 29.1. Malformations of the kidney

Abnormalities in amount of renal tissue
  Bilateral renal agenesis
  Unilateral renal agenesis
  Renal hypoplasia
  Supernumerary kidneys
  Nephromegaly
Renal ectopia, malrotation, and fusion

the glomeruli are of various sizes but generally are well developed at birth. The tubules of the nephrons are underdeveloped compared to the glomeruli. The mean diameter of the glomeruli increases twofold from the newborn to the adult, while the length of the proximal tubules increases tenfold [15].

The newborn kidney shows some peculiar features that are not seen in the kidneys of older children. A small number of sclerotic and hyalinized glomeruli are often found in infant kidneys that are otherwise normal. Emery and MacDonald [16] demonstrated two populations of sclerotic glomeruli. A few, large, hyalinized glomeruli were found at the juxtamedullary portion of the kidney. Smaller sclerotic glomeruli were present in the subcapsular layer of the renal cortex. The pathogenesis of the infantile sclerotic glomeruli remains speculative. The juxtamedullary glomeruli may represent the early-formed nephrons that failed to be carried by the collecting duct ampullae into the outer part of the kidney. The subcapsular sclerotic glomeruli belong, supposedly, to the last generation of the nephrons and either have not established proper continuity with the collecting ducts or remained without vascularization. Glomerular sclerosis is rare in fetuses and newborn infants. The number of scarred glomeruli increases to about 2% of all the glomeruli between the ages of 6 months and 2 years.

MALFORMATIONS OF THE KIDNEY

Malformations of the urinary system occur in approximately 10% of all newborn infants [17, 18]. These vary in severity from minor abnormalities to malformations incompatible with prolonged extrauterine life. Many renal and urinary tract malformations render the kidneys susceptible to secondary pyelonephritis, hypertension, and lithiasis. Several hereditary and non-hereditary malformation syndromes include abnormalities in the kidneys, and a very large proportion of the patients with renal malformations have concomitant anomalies in the urinary tract or elsewhere in the

body. In Table 29.1 the malformations of the kidneys are grouped together according to the anatomical similarities. Some malformations are not dealt with further because even if they are developmental in origin, they will become manifest later in childhood or in adult life.

Abnormalities in Amount of Renal Tissue

Bilateral Renal Agenesis

The term defines a total absence of any renal structures. The diagnosis is valid only after microscopic investigation of all suspected rudiments in the place of the kidneys. The ureters and renal arteries are also absent. The bladder is hypoplastic or absent and the urethra is often defective in development. In a study of 625,000 consecutive births in British Columbia, the incidence of bilateral renal agenesis (BRA) was $147.2/10^5$ and that of unilateral renal agenesis (URA) $187.2/10^5$ [19]. The ratio of males to females is about 2.5 : 1. In perinatal postmortem series, slightly less than half of the bilateral agenesis cases are observed in stillborns. Liveborn infants are small for gestational age and usually die within 1 or 2 days after birth. Death is attributed to the respiratory difficulties caused by pulmonary hypoplasia.

Infants with no kidneys show a pattern of abnormalities and dysmorphic features, known as *Potter sequence*. The full-blown features include absence of the kidneys, hypoplasia of the lungs, characteristic features of the head, bowing of the legs with talipes, broad spade-like hands, abundant loose skin, and growth retardation (Fig. 29.5). The non-renal features of Potter sequence are also present with any condition preventing fetal urination, such as severe renal dysplasia (RD) and urinary tract obstruction. The features of Potter sequence are secondary to oligohydramnios, which in turn is caused by lack of fetal urination.

There are descriptions of rare occasions in which bilateral agenesis was associated for various reasons with a normal amount of amniotic fluid and no features of Potter sequence were present [20]. On the other hand, chronic leakage of amniotic fluid will cause more or less developed features of the syndrome in a fetus with normal kidneys and urinary tract [20, 21].

The pathogenesis of BRA has been explained as a developmental field defect [22]. The most restricted defect is limited to the ureteric buds and small portions of the distal mesonephric and paramesonephric ducts, resulting in BRA

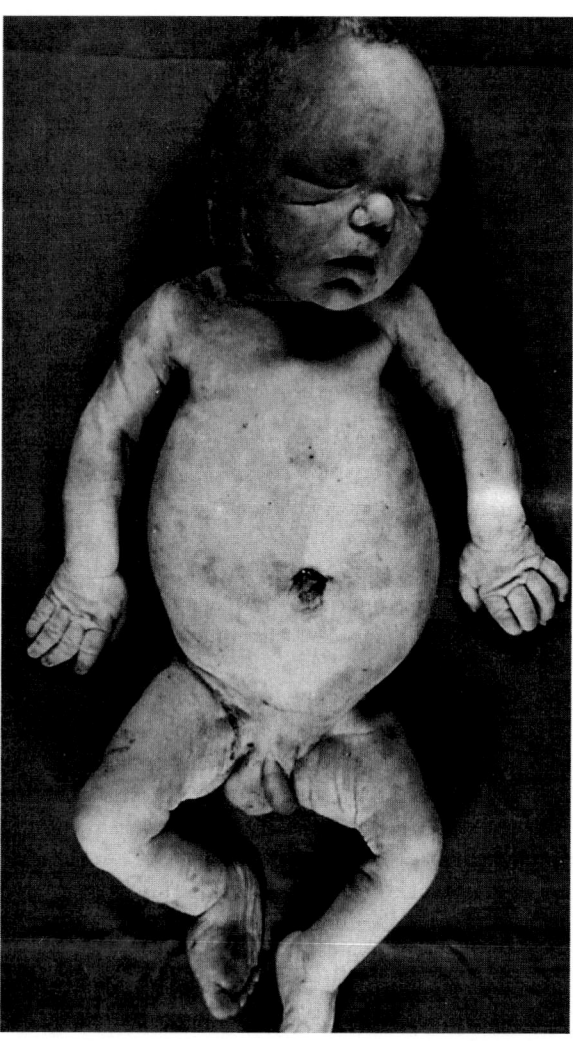

FIGURE 29.5.   *Potter sequence. Note the V-shaped epicanthic fold, low nasal bridge, receding chin, loose skin, and inward rotation of the right foot.*

and anomalies of the internal genitalia, including anomalies of the uterus and vagina in females and abnormalities of the epididymis and vas deferens in males. A wider field defect would cause anomalies of the hindgut and lower urinary tract and the most extensive defect is postulated to affect the entire caudal part of the embryo and lead to sirenomelia. Extensive hindgut and bladder malformations are uncommon and sirenomelic monsters are rare.

Most cases of BRA are sporadic, but several familial cases are known and are discussed in the section on hereditary renal adysplasia.

Unilateral Renal Agenesis

URA is more common than the bilateral form, but because this condition is compatible with normal life it is relatively rare in perinatal postmortem series. In a sonographic study

of almost 700 asymptomatic persons of all ages, the absence of one kidney was found in 0.3% [23]. The condition appears to be about equally common in both genders.

Ipsilateral ureter and hemitrigone of the bladder are usually absent, although a short distal ureter may be present in some patients. The single kidney is usually in its normal position and shows compensatory hypertrophy.

At perinatal postmortem examinations, URA is often a secondary finding, and the infant died because of major malformations in organs other than the kidney. A solitary kidney indicates the possibility of various hereditary and non-hereditary malformation syndromes [22]. About half of the females with URA have associated anomalies in the reproductive organs [17, 24]. They include ipsilateral absence of the fallopian tube, and unicornuate and bicornuate uterus. In about 10% of affected males, homolateral vas deferens and testis are absent or hypoplastic [24]. Malformations in organs other than the genitourinary tract are also common. Frequently encountered anomalies include esophageal atresia, congenital heart disease, meningomyelocele, and aplasia of the homolateral adrenal gland [19].

Hereditary Renal Dysplasia

URA and BRA as well as RD are usually sporadic conditions, but several reports showed them to run in families. Buchta et al [25] coined the term *hereditary renal adysplasia* (HRA) in two families showing absence, dysplasia, and hypoplasia of the kidneys. The presence of BRA, URA, and RD was found in several pedigrees and is also referred to as *familial renal adysplasia* [23, 26, 27]. Autosomal dominant inheritance with variable penetrance [25, 28], autosomal recessive inheritance [29], and X-linked [30] inheritance have all been suggested as modes of transmission.

Roodhooft et al [23] showed that 9% of parents and siblings of patients with bilateral severe renal malformation including BRA, URA with renal adysplasia, or bilateral severe RD had asymptomatic renal malformations. An empiric risk for recurrence of BRA or lethal aplasia in siblings is about 3.5% [31, 32]. The risk of severe bilateral adysplasia is up to 20% in offsprings of affected HRA patients [28].

It seems that BRA, URA, and HRA have a common ontogenetic origin [33], most likely related to the failure of the inductive interaction of the ureteric bud and metanephrogenic mesenchyme. Recent experimental results with transgenic mice lend support to this concept. Mice with targeted homozygous mutation of the c-*ret* proto-oncogene (*ret-k*⁻) show the whole spectrum of renal malformations typical for HRA. They include BRA, URA with severe RD of the contralateral kidney, and bilateral severe RD. The *ret-k*⁻ mice are also devoid of enteric autonomic ganglions [7]. The c-*ret* gene is normally expressed in the ureteric bud and the results suggest that the *ret-k* mutation prevents the reciprocal inductive action of the ureteric bud and the mesenchyme.

Renal Hypoplasia

Renal hypoplasia is defined as a congenitally abnormally small kidney. The arbitrary limit is at or below 2 standard deviations of the expected weight. The number of lobes (reniculi) is usually reduced to 5 or less instead of the normal complement of 10 [17]. The most extreme form of hypoplasia is a kidney with only one lobe and a single papilla, called *unirenicular* or *unipapillary kidney* [34]. The definition of *hypoplasia* excludes kidneys showing dysplasia or any acquired lesion such as scarring or atrophy.

Renal hypoplasia is occasionally found in several malformation syndromes [22]. It seems to be common in Down syndrome, with a frequency of approximately 15% of the patients [35].

In the older literature, any small kidneys were called *hypoplastic*. Closer examination, however, may disclose RD, or atrophy due to hydronephrosis or some acquired lesion, to be the cause of the small kidney. The term *hypodysplasia* is suggested for kidneys that are small and show dysplastic changes [36]. In this chapter, such kidneys are included in the RD group of malformations. Using strict criteria, true hypoplastic kidneys are considered to be rare. However, since the definition relies on a statistical concept of renal size, "small kidneys" are found relatively frequently in some postmortem series. Rubenstein et al [18] reported 55 bilateral and 3 unilateral hypoplastic kidneys in a postmortem series of more than 2000 infants and children. In their series, the weight of the kidneys fell within the range for the lowest fifth percentile of the population. In this series, the small kidneys were rarely associated with urinary tract abnormalities, but malformations of other organs were common.

Unilateral renal hypoplasia is a cause of hypertension and predisposes the kidneys to chronic pyelonephritis [34]. The clinical consequences of the bilateral hypoplasia depend on the amount of functional renal parenchyma present. In severe cases, the individuals have renal insufficiency and die in infancy. In less severe cases, growth retardation, signs of chronic renal insufficiency, and mental retardation are found [34].

Oligomeganephronic Renal Hypoplasia This uncommon congenital disorder was first described by Royer et al in 1962 [37] and several cases have been reported more recently [38, 39]. The disorder is characterized by the presence of a small number of hypertrophic nephrons, in contrast with the simple hypoplasia showing a reduced number of normal-sized nephrons.

The kidneys are extremely small; a renal weight of 1.5 grams was recorded in one neonate [38]. The number of lobes is reduced and may be only 1 or 2. The glomeruli are increased in size and the tubules are dilated with hypertrophic epithelium. The juxtaglomerular apparatuses are prominent and the interstitium shows focal fibrosis. Microdissected nephrons have a 12-fold increase in the glomerular volume and the volume of the proximal tubules is 17 times larger than expected [39]. Moerman et al [38]

observed in two infants only 3 layers of glomeruli instead of the usual 7 to 10, suggesting premature cessation of glomerulogenesis during fetal development. The children have chronic renal insufficiency and reach the terminal stage at the end of the first decade. Patients with the most severely impaired kidneys may die in infancy or in the neonatal period. Most cases are sporadic, but the condition is occasionally found in siblings [38].

Oligomeganephronic hypoplasia is rarely associated with extrarenal malformations, but a few affected patients have chromosomal 4p monosomy [40].

Nephromegaly

A single kidney usually shows compensatory hypertrophy and may approach the weight of two normal kidneys. Bilateral nephromegaly due to the increased number or size of normally developed nephrons hardly exists except in connection with malformation syndromes or general disorders. Renal tubular dysgenesis with nephromegaly is discussed later in this chapter.

Hyperplastic kidneys with an increased number of lobes and normal histological differentiation have been described in association with the Beckwith-Wiedemann (B-W) syndrome [41–43] and with hemihypertrophy, which in turn is sometimes a part of the B-W syndrome.

Kidneys are large when affected by nephroblastomatosis or hamartomatous tumors in association with B-W syndrome and Perlman syndrome [44]. These conditions are described in Chapter 15.

Statistically significant enlargement of kidneys has also been observed with congenital nephrosis of the Finnish type [45]. The number of nephrons is increased in this disorder, approximately by a factor of 1.5 [46, 47].

Supernumerary Kidney

Supernumerary kidney is a rare anomaly consisting of one or several separate ectopic kidneys in addition to the 2 normal ones. It is essential that no parenchymal connection exists between the 2 nearest situated kidneys [17]. Duplication of the renal pelvis and ureter is a relatively common anomaly and it is sometimes difficult to differentiate it from a supernumerary kidney on the basis of radiographic investigations.

A supernumerary kidney usually lies caudal to the normal kidney and is hypoplastic with a reduced number of lobes. The supernumerary kidney has its own pelvis and a ureter that usually drains to the ipsilateral ureter of the normal kidney.

Renal Ectopia, Malrotation, and Fusion

As mentioned in the section dealing with renal development, the kidneys rise during development from their pelvic position to the lumbar level and rotate 90 degrees during the ascent. This process is normally completed by the 8th intrauterine week. During the ascent the kidneys receive their vascular supply from different neighboring arteries until, at the final position, normal renal arteries are established. This complex development is susceptible to various disturbances, as evidenced by the relative frequency of abnormalities in the position and form of the kidneys.

Congenital malposition of the kidneys is called *renal ectopia*. *Simple ectopia* is the malposition of a normally lateralized kidney, while *crossed ectopia* denotes a situation in which both kidneys are located on the same side and the ureter of the ectopic kidney crosses the midline before entering the bladder.

A normal kidney, but more often an ectopic kidney, may show malrotation. Theoretically, the rotation could be incomplete, reverse, or excessive. Persistent ventral position (i.e., insufficient or incomplete rotation) of the renal hilus is the usual form of malrotation. Reverse and excessive rotations are very rare.

The most common type of simple ectopia is the pelvic kidney (Fig. 29.6). Its frequency in a large pediatric postmortem series was 1 in 730 [48]. The pelvic kidney is also usually malrotated and shows abnormal configuration. Its pelvicaliceal system is often distorted, and RD is not an uncommon feature. Associated malformations are common in patients with pelvic kidney. Hypospadias in males and vaginal abnormalities in females are the most common genitourinary malformations. Skeletal anomalies are found in more than 50% of the patients with pelvic kidney, and congenital heart disease is likewise common [49]. The high frequency of widespread malformations in patients with pelvic kidney indicates that the teratogenic influence on the developing organism has been more general than that of simply preventing the ascent and rotation of the kidney.

High ectopia of the kidney is very rare. Intrathoracic kidney is usually on the left side, but bilateral cases have also been reported [49].

In crossed renal ectopia, the ectopic kidney usually lies caudal to the normal kidney. Both kidneys are usually fused together, forming bizarre configurations. S-shaped and L-shaped kidneys are some common forms of crossed fusion (Fig. 29.7). The incidence of crossed renal ectopia in postmortem examinations has been reported to be 1 in 7500 [17]. Crossed ectopia with fusion is approximately 10 times more common than without fusion [49]. As in simple renal ectopia, pelvicaliceal abnormalities and malformations elsewhere in the body are common.

Renal fusion of the normally lateralized kidneys is a relatively common malformation, the horseshoe kidney being the most familiar type (Fig. 29.8). It was found once in 312 pediatric postmortem examinations [48] but appears to be even more common in perinatal postmortem examinations.

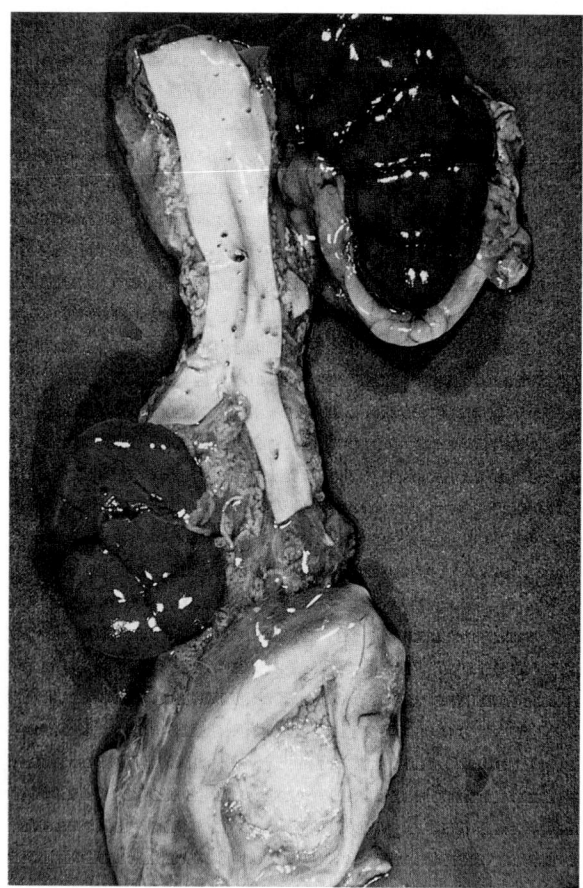

FIGURE 29.6.   *Normally located left kidney and pelvic right kidney. (Courtesy of Dr. R Herva.)*

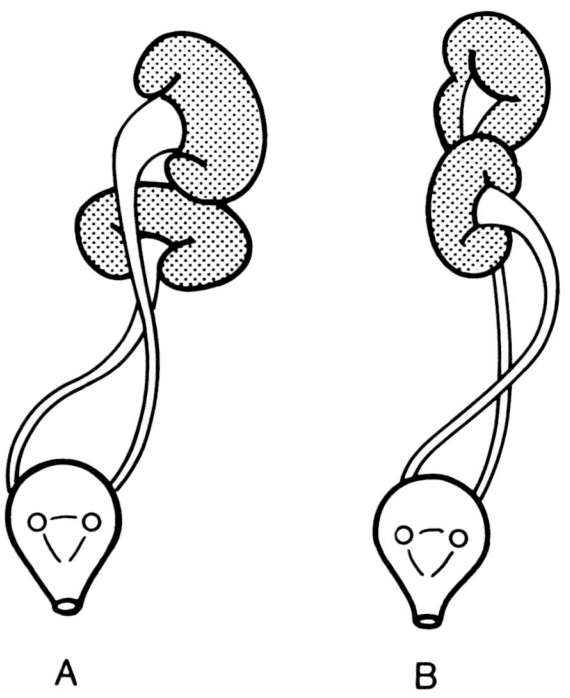

A   B

FIGURE 29.7.   *Diagram of L-shaped (A) and S-shaped (B) crossed kidneys with fusion.*

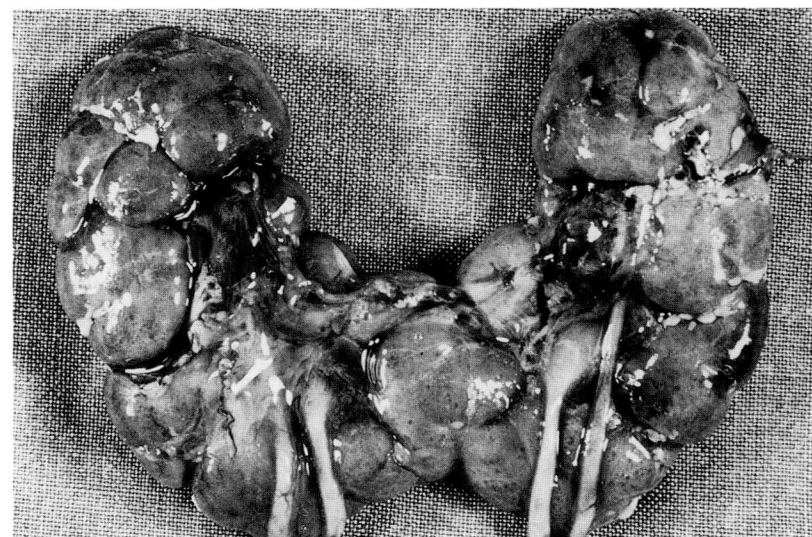

FIGURE 29.8. *Horseshoe kidney with bilateral duplex ureters. The renal hilus faces anteriorly.*

In the vast majority of horseshoe kidneys there is fusion at the lower poles of the kidneys. The kidney is situated at a lower level than normal. The isthmus is usually just below the inferior mesenteric artery and it has been thought that this artery prevents the ascent of the fused kidneys. The rotation of the two halves of the horseshoe kidney is incomplete, and both pelves lie more or less on the anterior aspect of the kidney. Rare variations of horseshoe kidney include fusion of the upper poles or both upper and lower poles, the so-called doughnut kidney.

The relative frequency of horseshoe kidneys in perinatal postmortem examinations is due to associated anomalies. The kidney itself is an innocuous, albeit easily recognizable, marker of a malformation syndrome. Urogenital anomalies are often present and include duplications, cryptorchidism, and urethral abnormalities [49]. The horseshoe kidney is also frequently a feature of chromosomal anomalies, most notably Turner syndrome and trisomy 18 [50]. Anomalies associated with horseshoe kidney are less common in older children and adults.

Another uncommon condition is fused pelvic kidneys. Both kidneys are fused into a mass of irregular configuration. It is referred to as a cake or disk kidney depending on its shape. The fused pelvic kidney is usually located low in the pelvic and the renal pelves and ureters lie on the anterior surface.

CYSTIC RENAL DISEASE

Renal cysts in the fetus and newborn comprise a heterogeneous group of parenchymal lesions. This is due to the fact that cyst formation is one of the main consequences of deviant renal differentiation and maturation.

Cystic kidneys may be classified purely on the basis of their microanatomy. This approach, with the aid of microdissection, has led to a widely applied classification elaborated

Table 29.2. Cystic renal disease

Renal dysplasia
Polycystic kidney disease
Autosomal recessive polycystic kidney disease (ARPKD)
Autosomal dominant polycystic kidney disease (ADPKD)
Glomerulocystic kidney disease
Medullary cystic disorders
Cortical microcysts and simple cysts
Multilocular cyst
Cystic disease and renal cysts in malformation syndromes and hereditary disorders

by Osathanondh and Potter and often referred to as *Potter's classification* [13]. The essential component of this classification is the description of the anatomical lesion. Clinical and genetic implications are not included, with occasional exceptions. The contemporary classifications are more clinically oriented, but the basic anatomical lesions of Potter's classification characterize many of the clinical and genetic entities [51].

Classification of cystic kidneys is sometimes confused by loose use of descriptive terminology. As an example, the term *polycystic kidney (disease)* is, in current terminology, confined to 2 genetically different diseases—autosomal recessive polycystic kidney disease (ARPKD) and dominant polycystic kidney disease (ADPKD)—and should not be used with kidneys displaying merely numerous cysts. Similarly the term *multicystic kidney* is confined to a type of RD.

A classification of the cystic diseases of the kidney is presented in Table 29.2.

Renal Dysplasia

Renal dysplasia is defined as abnormal differentiation of the metanephric parenchyma. It consists of microscopic

Table 29.3.   Morphological classification of renal dysplasia

Total
   Multicystic kidney
      Unilateral
      Bilateral
   Hypoplastic-aplastic dysplasia
   Diffuse dysplasia
Partial
   Focal and segmental dysplasia
      Cortical
      Medullary
      Combined

Table 29.4.   Clinical and genetic classification of renal dysplasia

Sporadic renal dysplasia
Hereditary renal adysplasia
Renal dysplasia associated with obstructive lesions of the urinary tract
Renal dysplasia in malformation syndromes and inherited metabolic syndromes

structures not found in normal nephrogenesis [34, 52]. According to the microdissection studies of Osathanondh and Potter [2], their type 2 cystic kidneys result from reduced branching of ampullae of the collecting ducts and failure to induce the formation of nephrons. The sparse collecting ducts are increased in diameter and often terminate in cysts. In histological sections, the essential feature of RD is the presence of so-called primitive ducts, ducts lined by cuboidal/columnar epithelium, which may even be ciliated (Fig. 29.9). The ducts are encircled by concentric layers of mesenchyme containing collagen fibers and smooth muscle. Further features include poorly developed "fetal" tubules, loose and fibrotic mesenchyme, sinusoidal blood spaces, hematopoietic tissue, and often spicules of cartilage. Fetal glomeruli and more or less developed nephric tubules are mixed with the above-mentioned dysontogenic components. The cysts vary in size and are lined by flat or columnar epithelium.

The definition of RD does not imply the presence of cysts. Solid non-cystic dysplasia does exist, and such a kidney is known as *aplastic* or *adysplastic*. On the other hand, dys-

plastic kidneys are usually grossly cystic and, conversely, most perinatal cystic kidneys are dysplastic [53].

The anatomical manifestation of RD is extremely variable. The kidney may be a huge non-reniform mass of cysts or a small nub of immature ducts. The dysplasia may be total, cortical, medullary, segmental, or focal, depending on how large a portion of the parenchyma is replaced by the dysplastic elements. It may also be bilateral or unilateral. A morphological classification of RD is presented in Table 29.3.

Non-syndromatic RD is usually sporadic; hereditary renal adysplasia has already been mentioned. The most common associations with RD are obstructive or non-obstructive malformations of the urinary tract [54–56]. RD may also be a part of a number of general malformation syndromes or inherited metabolic disorders [22]. Clinical associations with RD are presented in Table 29.4.

Multicystic Kidney

This represents the extreme form of RD. The cysts are large and tend to be distributed peripherally (Fig. 29.10). Corticomedullary and lobar organization is totally or severely distorted in a multicystic kidney. The kidney often gives an appearance of a "bunch of grapes" (Fig. 29.11). A multicystic kidney may be huge, manifesting as an abdominal mass, or it may be smaller than a normal kidney. It is a common experience that nephrectomized multicystic kidneys are

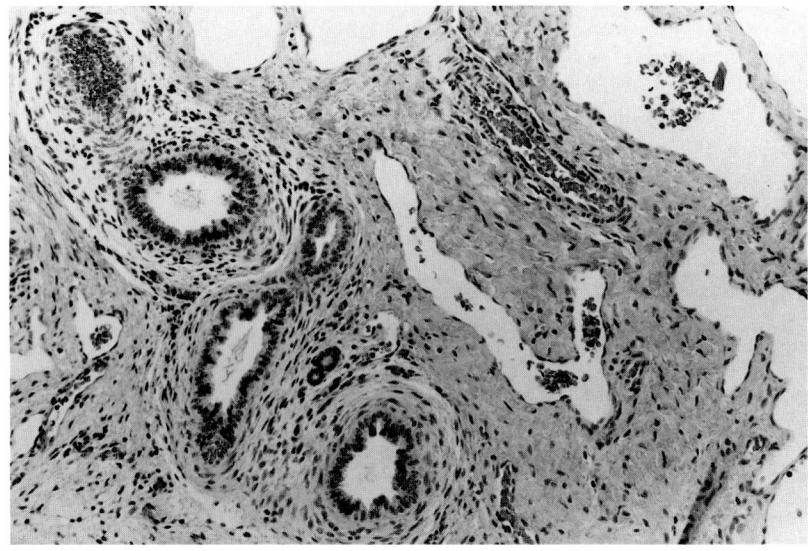

FIGURE 29.9.   *Primitive ducts in renal dysplasia. Note also sinusoidal blood spaces. H&E, ×70.*

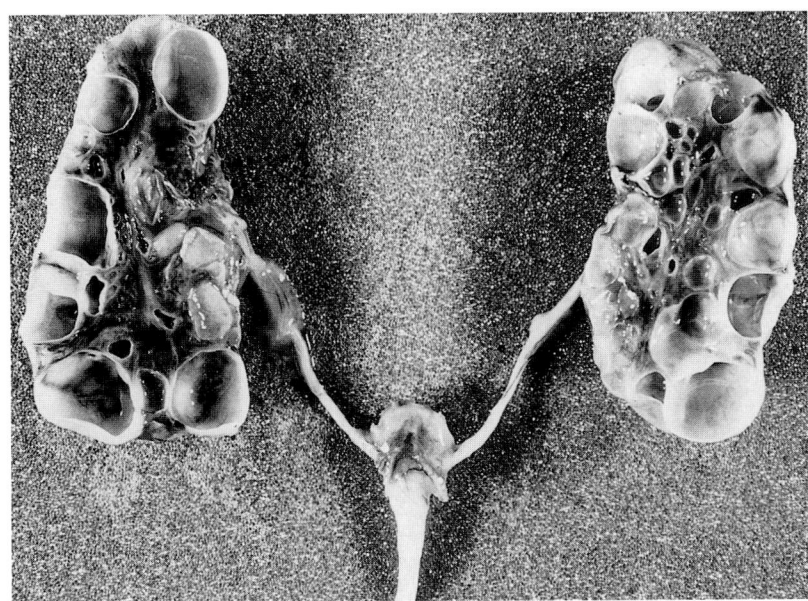

FIGURE 29.10. *Congenital bilateral multicystic kidney showing large peripheral cysts, stenotic but patent ureters, and hypoplastic bladder.*

often larger than those found at postmortem examination [56]. The ureter of the multicystic kidney is atretic or absent (Fig. 29.12). Histologically, the cysts are lined by flat epithelium. The stroma between the cysts varies in amount, and the dysplastic elements are usually found in the middle of the kidney.

Multicystic kidney is most often unilateral. The contralateral kidney frequently shows abnormalities, such as hydronephrosis due to obstruction at different levels of the urinary tract [56]. Bilateral multicystic kidney is incompatible with extrauterine life and the infants show external and internal features of Potter sequence. Perinatal bilateral multicystic kidneys quite often have patent ureters in the normal position.

Aplastic Kidney

There is a continuum of large multicystic kidneys to hypoplastic and aplastic forms. Aplastic kidney is a small nub of tissue containing immature ducts and microscopic cysts within fibrous stroma. The ureter is atretic or very severely stenotic. Aplastic kidney represents the most severe form of RD without gross cysts. At postmortem examination, careful histological study is required to distinguish it from renal agenesis.

Renal Dysplasia Associated with Urinary Tract Abnormalities

Congenital anomalies of the upper and the lower urinary tract are both numerous and relatively common. Many of them cause obstruction of the urinary flow [57]. Total obstruction of the urinary tract due to urethral agenesis, atresia, or stricture is almost invariably associated with RD of a severe degree. The less severe obstruction is also often associated with dysplasia but of variable degree.

Total duplication of the renal pelvis and ureter with ectopia of the vesical orifice of one of the ureters presents a classic example of segmental dysplasia. The pole of the kidney draining to the ectopic ureter is dysplastic. The upper

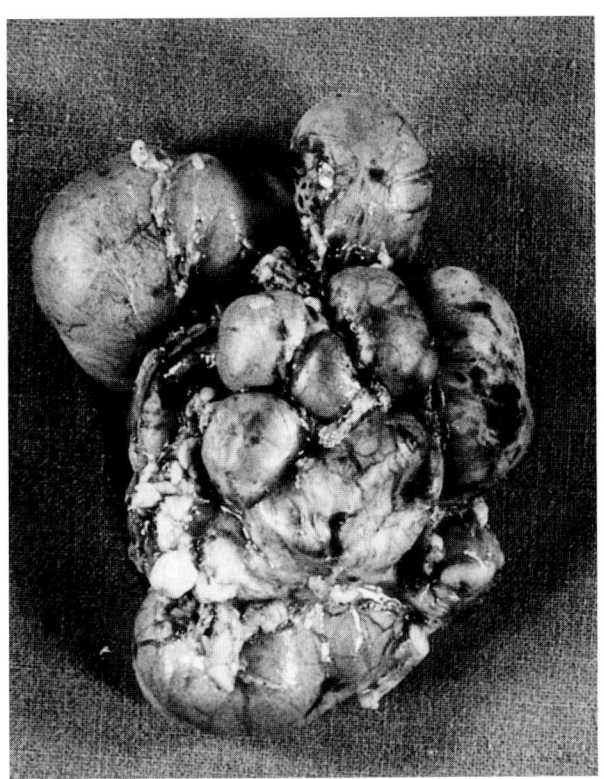

FIGURE 29.11. *Unilateral multicystic kidney. The reniform shape is lost.*

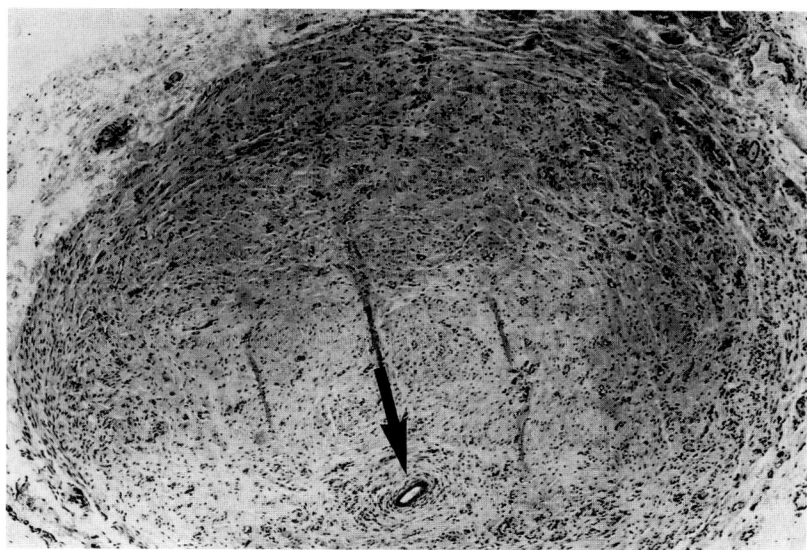

FIGURE 29.12. *Atretic ureter of a multicystic kidney. Note the small remnant of the ureteric lumen (arrow), which disappears in the more distal sections. H&E, ×22.*

pole is usually affected, but when the ectopic ureter drains the lower pole the dysplasia is more severe. It has been postulated that the site of the ectopic ureteric orifice in the bladder determines the extent of the RD and hypoplasia [58–60]. The extent of deviation of the ureteral orifice from normal is directly related to the severity of dysplasia (Fig. 29.13). The uncommon ureteral ectopia without duplication is also associated with focal or segmental RD.

Obstruction of the lower urinary tract of variable degree is usually associated with cortical dysplasia characterized by subcortical cysts with variable degrees of dysplastic elements (Fig. 29.14). It appears that the last generations of the nephrons have not differentiated normally. This type of dysplasia in Potter's classification is designated as type 4 [13]. The common lesions associated with subcortical dysplasia or cysts are posterior urethral valves, megacystis-megaureter syndrome, and prune-belly syndrome. In all these cases hydronephrosis is usually present and often clinically more important than the dysplasia. This applies also to the common stenosis or atresia of the ureteropelvic junction that causes hydronephrosis but seldom shows dysplastic lesions of the renal parenchyma.

Renal Dysplasia Associated with Malformation Syndromes (Diffuse Cystic Dysplasia)

Cystic kidneys, some of them dysplastic, are seen in association with several malformation syndromes and in some inherited metabolic disorders. The most common syndromes are discussed separately (see page 997). The renal abnormality is often described as diffuse cystic dysplasia [54, 61]. The

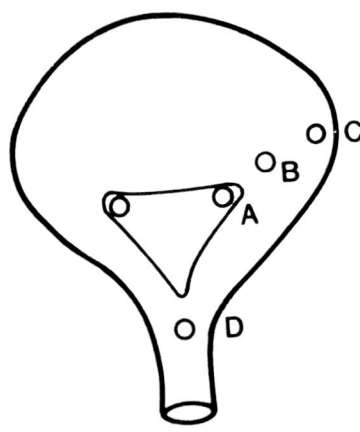

FIGURE 29.13. *Diagram illustrating the ectopic positions of the ureteric orifice in the bladder: (A) normal position; (B) mild lateral position; (C) lateral ectopia associated with renal dysplasia; (D) medial ectopia of double ureters. (Modified from Ref. 60.)*

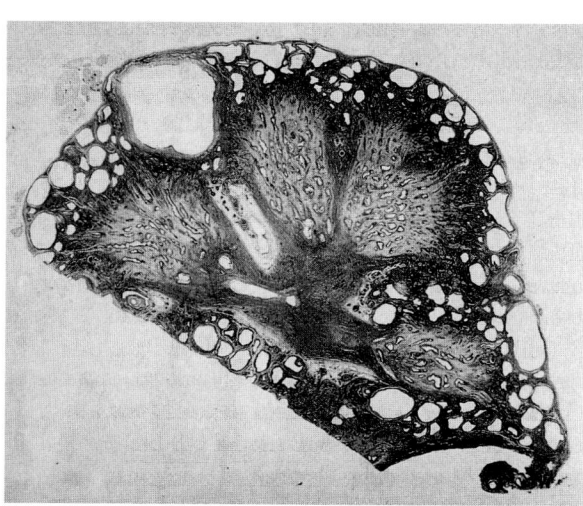

FIGURE 29.14. *Section of Potter type 4 kidney associated with partial urinary tract obstruction. The largest cysts are located beneath the capsule. H&E, ×3.5.*

term denotes kidneys that show loss of lobar and corticomedullary demarcation with a poorly developed caliceal system and renal pelvis. Ureters are patent, but hypoplastic, as is the urinary bladder. The renal parenchyma is studded by spherical cysts showing microscopically nondescript epithelium and separated by ample connective tissues. A small number of poorly developed nephrons are sometimes present. Diffuse cystic dysplasia is occasionally encountered without any signs of a syndrome or metabolic disease.

An important practical aspect of diffuse cystic dysplasia is its separation from perinatal forms of autosomal recessive and dominant polycystic kidneys. All these cystic kidneys have retained their reniform shape, and are enlarged and diffusely cystic. Separation of ARPKD and dysplasia is relatively easy based on both macroscopic and microscopic features, as shown in Figs. 29.17 and 29.18 (ARPKD) and Figs. 29.25 and 29.26 (Meckel syndrome). The neonatal form of ADPKD may be more confusing, because the medulla in this condition is deceptively "dysplasia like" (see Fig. 20.21). The microanatomy of the cortex is, however, quite different in these disorders (see Fig. 29.20).

Pathogenesis of Renal Dysplasia

Osathanondh and Potter [2, 13] believed that dysplasia is caused primarily by failure of the ampullae of the fetal collecting ducts to induce formation of the nephrons in the apposed mesenchyme. The frequent association of obstructive urinary tract lesions with dysplastic kidneys led Bernstein [34, 55] to hypothesize that the obstruction might be the primary event or at least an integral part in the pathogenesis of dysplasia. Another theory, based on the observation that the location of the misplaced ureteric orifice of a single or duplex ectopic ureter determines the extent of the dysplasia, brings the primary pathogenetic event back to early embryonic development of the ureteric bud [58, 59, 62, 63]. The embryonic ureteric bud arises from the caudal part of the mesonephric duct (Fig. 29.15). During the subsequent development, both ducts separate and will be absorbed by the bladder wall. According to the "bud theory" an ectopic ureteric orifice reflects a misplaced origin of the ureteric bud from the mesonephric duct, with the consequence that the union of the bud and the metanephric mesenchyme will not occur at the right time and place. The bud theory and that of Osathanondh and Potter [2] are not mutually exclusive.

The failure of nephron formation may be due to either deficient inductive action or unresponsiveness of the mesenchyme. In vitro cultivation of chicken embryonic explants before grafting them on the chorioallantoic membrane causes disappearance of the nephrogenic mesenchyme around the branches of the ureteric bud and results in an organ rudiment closely resembling human RD [64]. These experimental results are compatible with the bud theory, suggesting that lack of synchronization in the contact of the ureteric bud and the mesenchyme may result in impaired responsiveness of the mesenchyme and maldifferentiation of the kidney.

The occurrence of HRA with cases of renal agenesis and dysplasia in the same family argues strongly in favor of a defect in the reciprocal inductive action of the ureteric bud and the metanephrogenic mesenchyme. Support of this theory is gained from the experiments with c-ret-k⁻ mice [7]. The frequent presence of extrarenal malformations in association with RD implies a teratogenic action of wider influence than the impairment of the ureteral bud–mesenchyme interaction.

The "bud failure" theory does not explain diffuse cystic dysplasia with or without syndromatic association. Its pathogenesis remains unknown.

Polycystic Renal Disease

The term *polycystic renal disease* is reserved for two different hereditary conditions, both of which show considerable variation in the age of manifestation, gross and microscopic pathology, and severity of the clinical course.

Autosomal Recessive Polycystic Kidney Disease

This disease is transmitted as an autosomal recessive trait [65, 66]. The gene defect associated with ARPKD has been

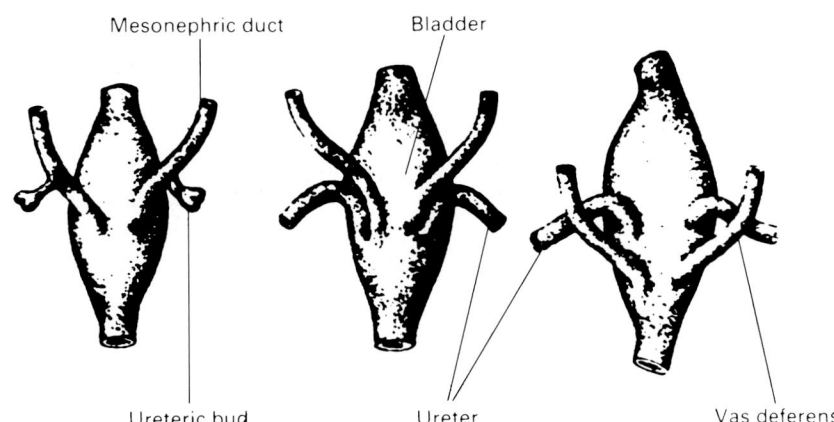

FIGURE 29.15. *Diagram illustrating the separation of the ureter from the mesonephric duct in the formation of the ureteric orifices in the bladder.*

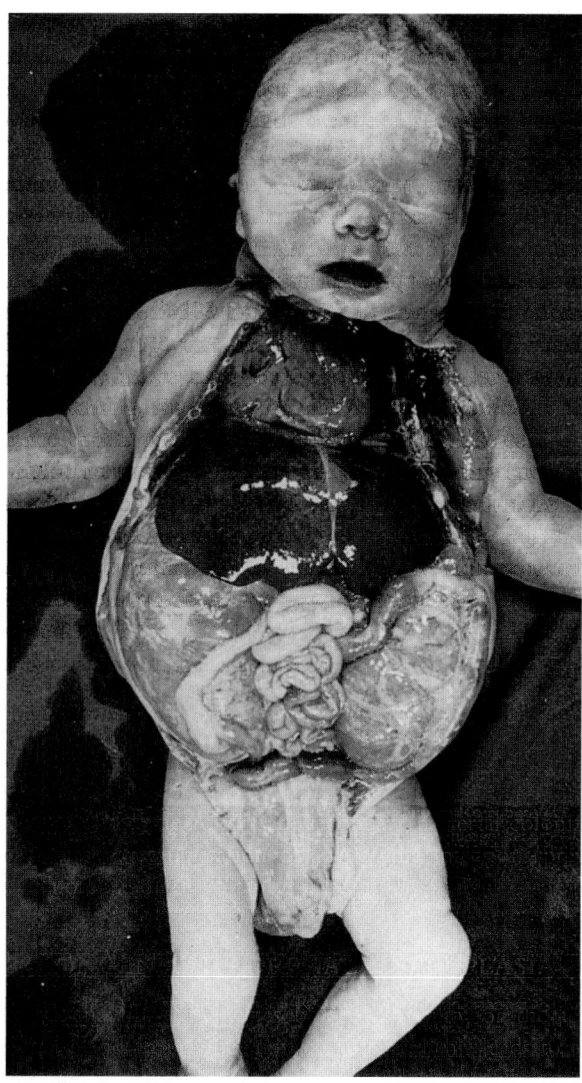

FIGURE 29.16.   *Large cystic kidneys in the perinatal form of ARPKD.*

localized in a number of families to chromosomal region 6p21-cen [67]. The identification of the gene and the pathogenesis of the disease wait further clarification.

ARPKD usually manifests at birth or infancy, and it is therefore also known as *infantile polycystic disease*. Since this form of polycystic kidney disease may escape detection until adolescence or early adulthood, terminology indicating the mode of inheritance is to be preferred. The disease is one of the most common forms of inherited nephropathy in infancy, but as such is relatively rare. In the series of Potter and Craig [68], 22 cases were found among 6000 postmortem examinations of newborn babies and infants. In the postmortem series of over 6000 children of all ages in our hospital, 15 cases were found [53].

The pathology of ARPKD in the newborn child is very characteristic. Huge bilateral symmetric reniform masses distend the abdomen (Fig. 29.16). Viewed through the

capsule, the surface is filled by innumerable miniature cysts about 1 mm in diameter. On section, the corticomedullary demarcation is obscured or absent. A diagnostic feature is the radiation of closely apposed fusiform or cylindrical dilated ducts from the medullary part to the subcapsular area (Fig. 29.17). Larger and more spherical cysts may be seen in the medullary portion of the kidney. In histological sections, the elongated cysts are lined by a single layer of cuboidal epithelium. The cysts constitute more than 90% of the renal parenchyma (Fig. 29.18). Normal glomeruli and nephric tubules are disposed between the cysts. Especially in the medullary portion of the kidney, the loose interstitial connective tissue is abundant. In Potter's classification the lesion constitutes type 1.

The evidence that the cysts in ARPKD are derived from the collecting ducts comes from three sources. The main evidence is presented by the microdissection studies of Osathanondh and Potter [2]. It is augmented by the histological demonstration of branches in the cysts [34]. Branching of the ducts is a feature confined exclusively to the collecting ducts in the normal kidney. The histochemical approach using lectins with selective binding to various parts of the renal structures also confirmed the collecting duct origin of the cysts in ARPKD [69, 70].

The liver in ARPKD shows characteristic and constant changes. The cut surface may show macroscopic cysts a few millimeters in diameter, but more often the changes are apparent only in histological sections. The lobular architecture of the liver is preserved, but all portal areas are expanded and contain tortuous, slightly dilated intrahepatic bile ducts, particularly at the borders of the lobules and portal areas. Dilated ducts are occasionally found within the lobules, as well. The ducts are accompanied by an increased amount of collagenous mesenchyme containing numerous small blood vessels (Fig. 29.19). Stereological studies have indicated that the "ducts" are in fact cisterns communicating with each other. Jörgensen [71] called this arrangement of the cisterns *ductal plate malformation*. Very similar hepatic changes are found also in a number of syndromes affecting both the kidneys and the liver including Meckel syndrome, Zellweger syndrome, Jeune syndrome, and occasionally juvenile nephronophthisis [72, 73]. Malformations in organs other than the kidney, liver, and occasionally the pancreas are very rare. ARPKD in newborn infants is incompatible with life and they die within hours or days in respiratory difficulties. Features of Potter sequence are often present, but rarely fully developed.

ARPKD is not confined to the newborn child. When the renal lesions are less extensive, the children live longer. Many clinical, pathological, and genetic problems are associated with patients manifesting ARPKD later in childhood or adolescence [65, 66, 74–76].

Autosomal Dominant Polycystic Kidney Disease

ADPKD is a common hereditary disease and an important cause of renal failure in adults. In white populations, the

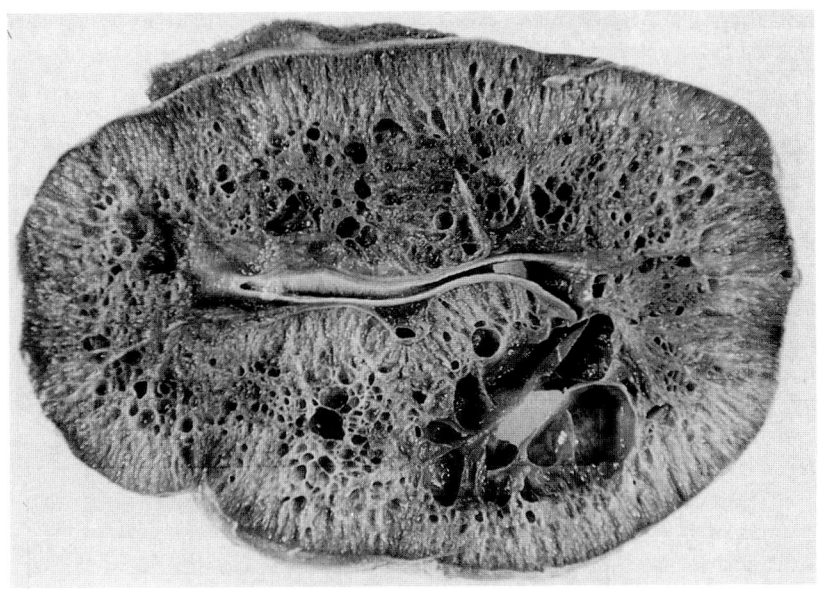

FIGURE 29.17.   *Cut surface of the kidney in perinatal ARPKD.*

published incidences range from 1 in 400 to 1 in 1000 people. The incidence varies in different populations [77, 78]. Older patients with ADPKD frequently show a variable clinical course with hypertension, renal failure, renal cancer, and several extrarenal manifestations including cardiovascular abnormalities [77, 79].

Although ADPKD is also known as an adult polycystic disease, it occurs occasionally in newborn infants and fetuses. It is important to separate the neonatal form of ADPKD from ARPKD and some types of cystic RD

because the clinical and genetic implications are different in these disorders. In 1964, Mehrizi et al [80] first reported on a newborn child with polycystic kidneys of adult type and the affected father. An increasing number of affected fetuses and newborn infants are found because offsprings in families known to carry the disease are subjected to sensitive imaging and gene linkage studies [81].

The pathological manifestations of fetal and neonatal ADPKD include small cysts in normal-sized kidneys [82–84] or greatly enlarged cystic kidneys incompatible with

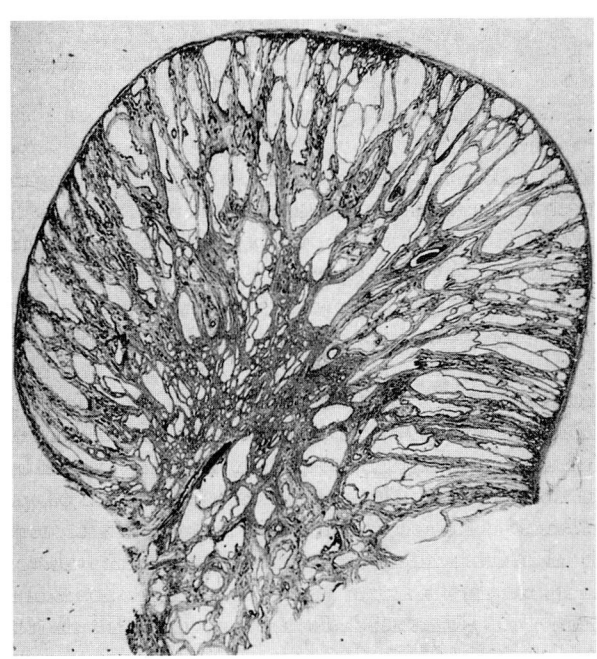

FIGURE 29.18.   *Typical arrangement of cylindrical cysts in perinatal ARPKD. H&E, ×5.*

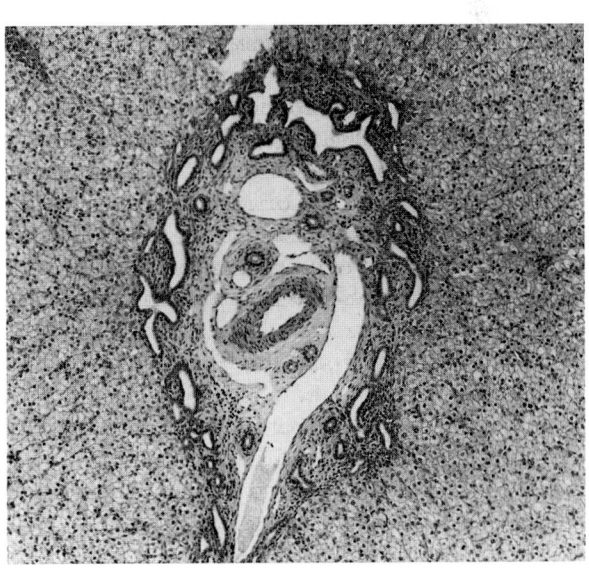

FIGURE 29.19.   *Ductal plate malformation of a hepatic portal tract in ARPKD. Note the dilated biliary cisterns at the border of the liver lobes. The blood vessels are located in the middle of the portal tract. H&E, ×22.*

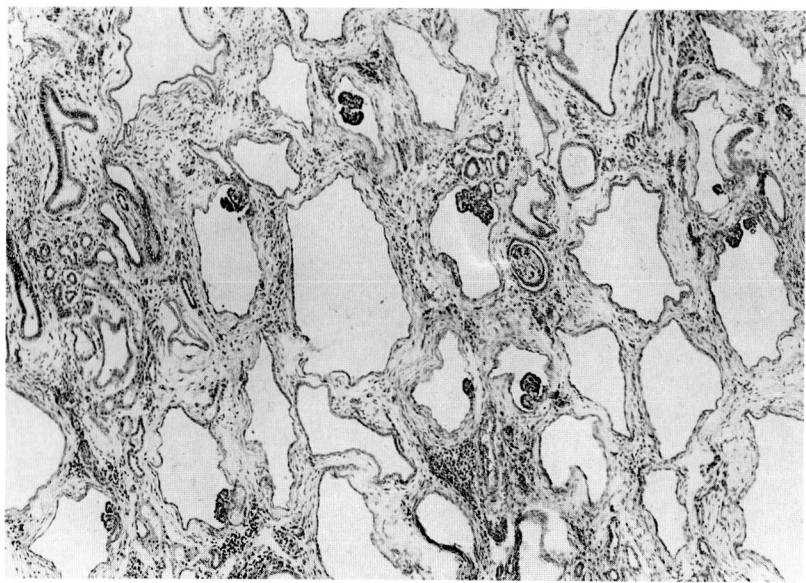

FIGURE 29.20.   *Histological section of a kidney with neonatal ADPKD. The cysts are more roundish than in ARPKD and several glomerular cysts are present. H&E, ×75.*

prolonged life [83, 85–88]. The kidneys of the latter type have retained their reniform shape, but their weight is up to 10 times more than normal. They may be grossly and unevenly cystic or contain diffusely distributed minute cysts. In such cases the macroscopic picture is deceptively similar to that of ARPKD [85, 88]. Histological investigation discloses ovoid to roundish cysts of variable size in the cortex and medulla. The corticomedullary demarcation is often obscured. Diagnostically important are numerous glomerular cysts in the cortex [88] (Fig. 29.20). Glomerular cysts are sometimes the most prevalent types of cysts in fetal and neonatal ADPKD kidneys [81, 82]. Tubular cysts are also common, and it seems that cysts arise in all parts of the nephrons and collecting ducts. The cystic lesion of ADPKD is the archetype of Potter type 3 kidneys. The medulla of diffusely cystic large fetal kidneys has roundish cysts with flat epithelium separated by ample connective tissue (Fig. 29.21). This picture may be confused with non-syndromatic diffuse dysplasia. Although ADPKD in older children and adults is often associated with extrarenal abnormalities including hepatic cysts, the neonatal liver is usually normal [82, 83, 87, 88]. Histological investigation of the liver is a useful adjunct in separating ADPKD and ARPKD, the latter showing consistently the ductal plate malformation. However, in a few families with neonatal ADPKD, congenital hepatic fibrosis has been reported [89].

A gene linked with ADPKD was mapped to chromosome 16p [90]. This gene is known as *PKD1*. Some families with less severe disease do not show the 16p linkage. Another gene locus for ADPKD has been localized to chromosome 4p [91, 92] (*PKD2*). Neither of these genes has been cloned. Families with *PKD1* appear to be most frequent in white populations.

The pathogenesis of ADPKD has been subject to several studies and speculations. They include tubular cell hyperplasia, fluid accumulation in the cysts, abnormalities of the cell polarity, non-differentiation of tubular cells, and abnormalities of the extracellular matrix [93, 94]. The understanding of the pathogenesis awaits identification of the structure and the function of the mutant genes of ADPKD.

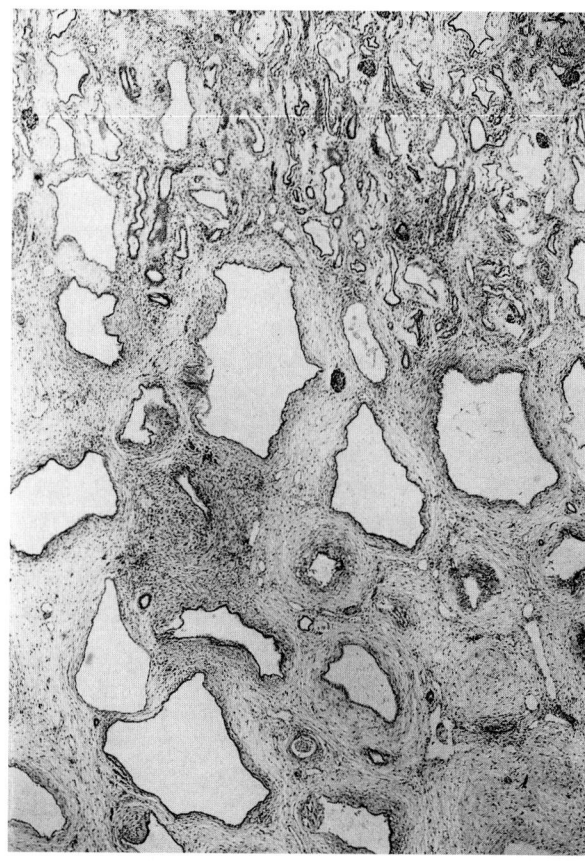

FIGURE 29.21.   *Histological section of the medullary part of a neonatal ADPKD kidney resembling renal dysplasia. H&E, ×50.*

Glomerulocystic Kidney

Distended Bowman capsules with shrunken capillary tufts are frequently found in many cystic disorders of the kidney including inherited malformation syndromes and RD. They are frequent or even predominant lesions in tuberous sclerosis, orofaciodigital syndrome, and Zellweger syndrome [95]. Taxy and Filmer [96] coined the term *glomerulocystic kidney* to designate cystic small kidneys with predominantly glomerular cysts. Most cases of so-called glomerulocystic kidney disease with a positive family history appear to be ADPKD. Sporadic cases are morphologically indistinguishable from familial ones [95]. Another type of glomerulocystic disease shows small kidneys and abnormal calices besides the glomerular cysts. The disease leads to chronic renal failure [97, 98].

Medullary Cystic Disorders

Medullary cystic disorders are rarely a concern in perinatal pathology. Juvenile nephronophthisis manifests in later childhood [99]. Rare cases of juvenile nephronophthisis-like disorder with onset in infancy and a severe clinical course have been reported [100]. This disorder is sometimes associated with congenital hepatic fibrosis [73, 100]. Medullary cysts are seen as a part of several cystic diseases including RD, ADPKD, and several inherited malformation syndromes [101].

Cortical Microcysts and Simple Cysts

Besides the cortical cystic lesion seen in association with relative urinary obstruction (Potter type 4), microscopic cysts scattered in the subcapsular cortex are seen relatively often in neonatal kidneys. The cysts are usually of unknown origin with low epithelium and surrounding connective tissue. Glomerular cysts are seen occasionally. The cortical microcysts appear to be associated with hereditary malformation syndromes, chromosomal aberrations (e.g., trisomies 13, 18, and 21) and in many undefined malformation conditions [36, 53]. The cortical microcysts appear not to have clinical importance.

Simple cysts are very rare in neonatal kidneys, contrasting with their frequency in adults [17]. They may be located either in the cortex or in the medulla. Large simple cysts may rupture and bleed, in which case they cause clinical symptoms such as abdominal mass, hematuria, urinary tract infection, and hypertension [56].

Multilocular Cyst

This uncommon lesion may manifest at any age, from newborn infant to adult. It is a relatively easily defined pathological entity, but its origin and nature remain controversial. It has been thought to be an unusual manifestation of RD [13, 102], hamartomatous malformation [103], or true neoplasia [104–106]. Confused terminology of the condition reflects the opinions of the authors. Cystic mesoblastic nephroma [105], cystic partially differentiated nephroblastoma [106], and benign multilocular cystic nephroma [107] are some examples of the various designations. Whether the multilocular cyst is a true neoplasia or malformation has not been finally settled.

A multilocular cyst is usually unilateral, solitary, and massive (Fig. 29.22). Pathological criteria include multilocular cysts without communication with each other or the renal pelvis, loculi lined by regular epithelium, no differentiated elements within the cysts or septa, and normal structure of the remaining kidney [107]. The capsule and the septa are composed of spindle-cell mesenchyme, and occasional foci of cartilage have been reported [17, 105].

The multilocular cyst in infancy presents usually as an abdominal mass. The clinical alternatives include massive hydronephrosis, multicystic kidney, nephroblastoma, and mesoblastic nephroma. Sonographic and computed tomography investigations differentiate readily the first two alternatives mentioned [56], but the pathologist has to distinguish between a multilocular cyst and a nephroblastoma. Sampling of a large number of blocks for histological investigation is highly advisable to exclude a nephroblastoma with cystic degeneration. The prognosis is excellent after the nephrectomy, regardless of the presence or absence of true neoplastic foci. Congenital renal tumors, other than multilocular cyst, are discussed in Chapter 15.

Cystic Disease and Renal Cysts in Malformation Syndromes and Hereditary Disorders

A number of hereditary syndromes transmitted as autosomal recessive or X-linked traits carry renal cysts as a part of the syndrome. Chromosomal anomalies are associated very often with cystic and other renal malformations (see Chap. 12).

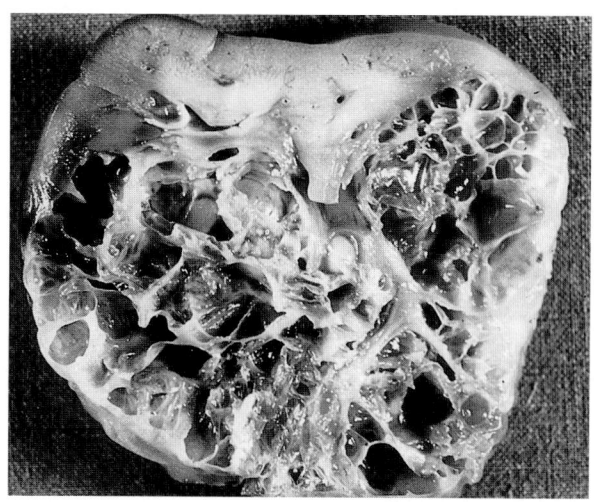

FIGURE 29.22.   *Cut surface of a multilocular cyst. Normal kidney structures are seen in the upper part of the picture.*

Finally, many syndromes or malformation associations of unknown etiology are accompanied by cystic lesions in the kidneys. RD appears to be the most common type of lesion in many syndromes. In several syndromes, however, morphological classification of the renal cysts is difficult or impossible. The cystic manifestation within a syndrome may be variable or the cysts simply do not fit into any of the main categories of the prevailing classifications. In the unravelling of a complex malformation syndrome, the other features of the syndrome provide more diagnostic information than do the renal cysts [108].

In this section only a small number of syndromes presenting in the neonate will be dealt with. For the rest, the reader is referred to the appropriate reviews [22, 33, 51].

Tuberous Sclerosis

This is a neurocutaneous disorder transmitted as an autosomal dominant trait. It is characterized by various cutaneous lesions, epilepsy, mental retardation, and visceral hamartomas. Renal lesions occur in 50–100% of the patients [109, 110]. The common lesions are angiomyolipomas and cysts or a combination of both. The kidneys in tuberous sclerosis may be grossly cystic early in infancy [111]. Cystic kidneys are typical in children, while angiomyolipomas are found more often in adults [112]. The cysts in tuberous sclerosis have distinctive microscopic characteristics. They appear to arise from proximal tubules, but glomerular cysts may also be numerous. The epithelium is locally hyperplastic and stratified and piles up to form polypoid or small papillary projections that protrude into the lumens of the cyst. The cells are fairly large, pale, and eosinophilic [112]. Hyperplastic tubular epithelium is sometimes conspicuous without actual cyst formation (Fig. 29.23). In an infantile case with grossly enlarged kidneys, the papillary projections obliterated the cystic spaces to create an adenoma-like appearance [111]. The hyperplastic epithelium of the cysts in tuberous sclerosis readily distinguishes it from all other types of cystic renal disease in infancy.

Meckel Syndrome

This syndrome consists of posterior encephalocele, cystic kidneys, and postaxial polydactyly (Fig. 29.24). The latter is tetramelic in over 90% of patients [113]. A further constant abnormality is the hepatic involvement, which is histologi-

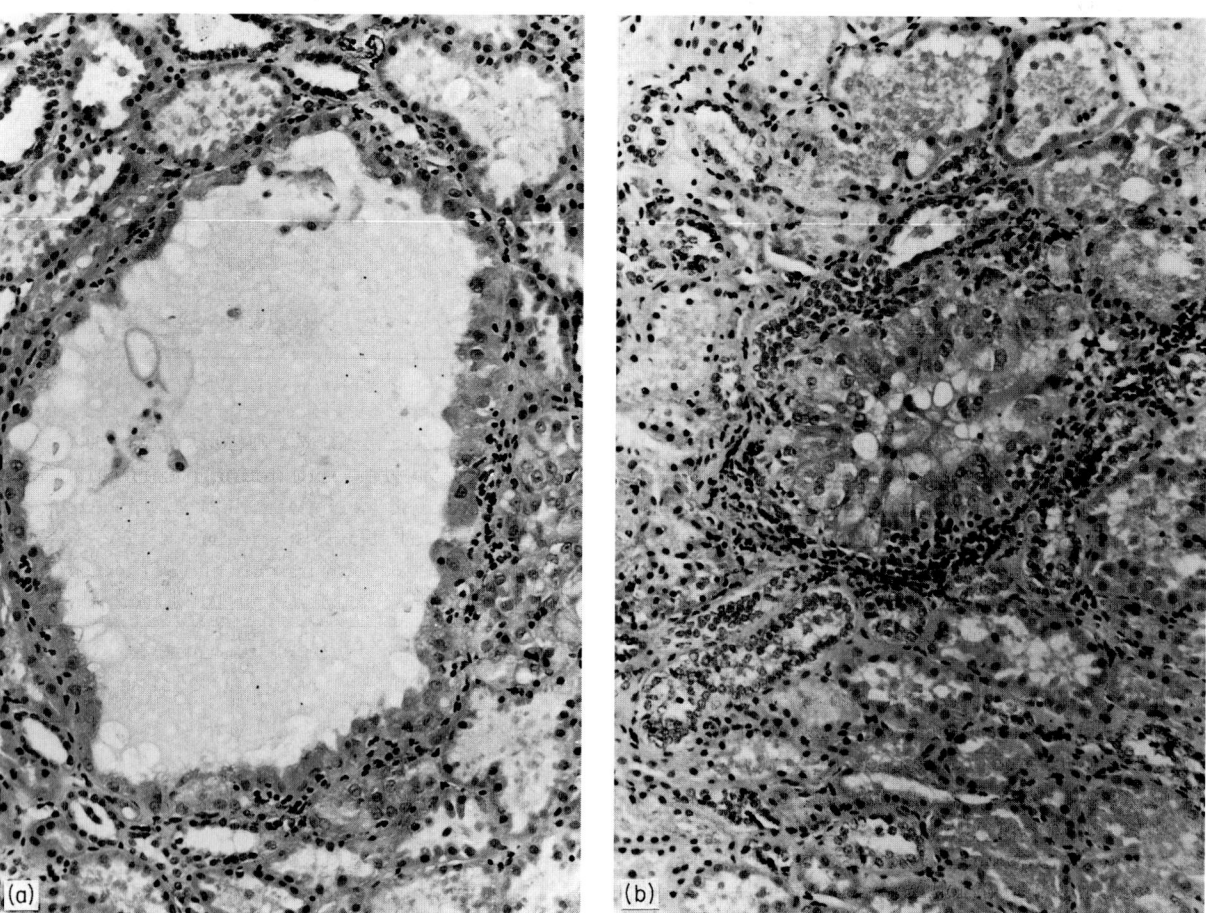

FIGURE 29.23. *Renal cysts in tuberous sclerosis: (a) a cyst with hypertrophic epithelium; (b) hyperplastic epithelium of a dilated non-cystic tubule. H&E, ×80.*

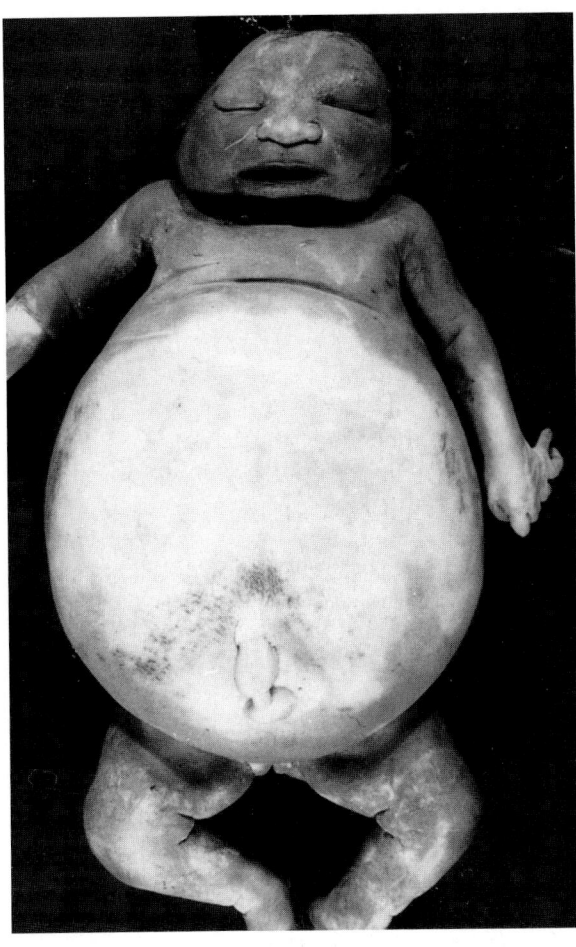

FIGURE 29.24. *Meckel syndrome. The abdomen is distended by huge cystic kidneys. The facial expression is characteristic and different from the Potter sequence (see Fig. 29.5) and that of ARPKD (see Fig. 29.16). Postaxial polydactyly is seen in the left hand.*

cally similar to that in ARPKD [114]. Almost all males show severe underdevelopment of the external genitalia, causing difficulties in gender determination at birth. In a few cases, uterus and fallopian tubes have been recorded in the presence of testes, constituting male pseudohermaphroditism [113, 114]. Full-blown Meckel syndrome is incompatible with prolonged life and the patients either are stillborn or die soon after birth.

The syndrome is transmitted as an autosomal recessive trait. The gene defect associated with Meckel syndrome has been localized to chromosomal region 17q21–q24 [115]. It occurs in about 1 in 10,000 births but this varies in different populations [113]. This incidence may even exceed that of the better-known ARPKD [51].

Because many of the abnormalities of Meckel syndrome share features with other malformation syndromes, a considerable number of articles deal with differential diagnostic problems, "atypical syndromes," "variants," or "minimal diagnostic criteria" of Meckel syndrome [116, 117].

In most cases the kidneys are bilaterally enlarged, causing abdominal distention resembling that of the perinatal form of ARPKD. Occasional asymmetry has been found, but the histological lesions are always bilateral. On a cut surface the kidneys show roundish cysts ranging in size from a few millimeters to several centimeters (Fig. 29.25). The microcysts appear to be under the capsule and the large cysts are situated in the inner and medullary parts of the kidney. Corticomedullary demarcation is usually abolished. Pelvicaliceal structures are distorted or absent, but thin patent ureters and hypoplastic bladders are present. Histologically, the renal parenchyma is studded by cysts of various shapes, forms, and sizes (Fig. 29.26). The single-layered epithelium of the cysts varies from cuboidal to columnar, and occasional glomerular cysts are observed. Cysts layered by transitional urothelium have been described [118, 119]. The stroma between the cysts is abundant, loose, fetal-like mesenchyme.

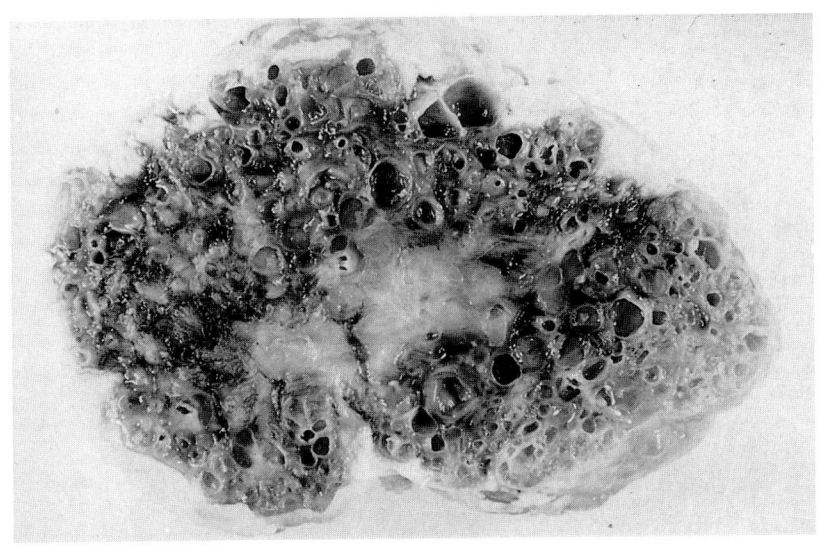

FIGURE 29.25. *Cut surface of a cystic kidney in Meckel syndrome. Note the difference from ARPKD (see Fig. 29.17).*

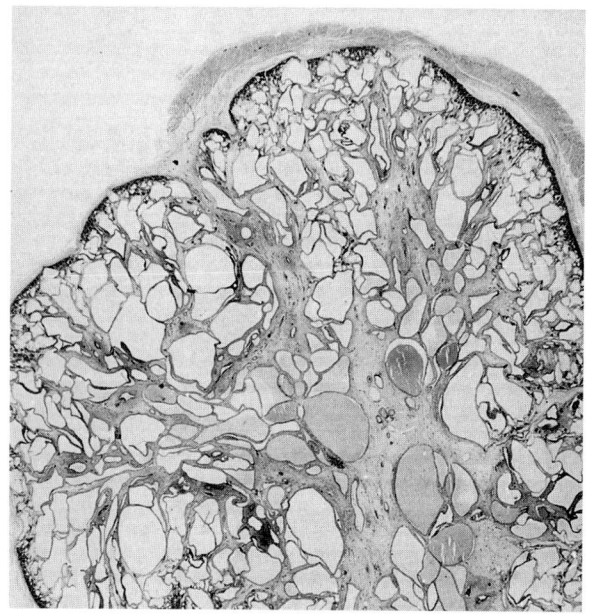

FIGURE 29.26.   *Histological section of a kidney in a patient with Meckel syndrome. The cysts are spherical and increase in size from the subcapsular area toward the middle of the kidney. H&E, ×4.5.*

The kidneys of Meckel syndrome have been considered a prototype of diffuse RD [54, 61]. Microscopic investigation of fetal kidneys affected by Meckel syndrome has thrown light on the cystogenesis of this disorder. While the kidneys in newborn infants show nothing but cysts separated by the loose mesenchyme, the picture in second-trimester fetuses is different. The medullary parts are diffusely cystic, but nephrogenesis in the periphery of the renal lobes takes place in normal fashion (Fig. 29.27). As

soon as the nephrons are formed, they display cystic dilatation, which is also seen in the branching collecting ducts. Cystogenesis is seen in Meckel syndrome kidneys as early as the 10th week of gestation [120]. The nascent cysts attain and retain, at least for some time, their differentiation of proximal and distal tubules as well as collecting ducts as evidenced by histology and histochemical differentiation markers [70, 121]. The pathogenesis of the RD of Meckel syndrome, if it is dysplasia, is obviously quite different from that of more common dysplasias. This is probably the case also in many of the hereditary syndromes other than Meckel syndrome.

Cerebrohepatorenal Syndrome of Zellweger

This syndrome consists of craniofacial and limb malformations, anomalies in the central nervous system, joint calcifications, hepatic fibrosis, and cysts in the kidneys. The affected children are hypotonic and mentally retarded and usually die within 6 months. The disorder is transmitted as an autosomal recessive trait [122, 123]. The molecular defect appears to be a mutation of the gene responsible for peroxisomal assembly located on chromosome 8q21.1 [124, 125].

In the vast majority of patients, scattered cortical cysts of tubular and glomerular origin are present. The size of the cysts ranges from microscopic to 1 cm in diameter. The cysts are often associated with increased stroma containing remnants of immature tubuli. Extensive dysplastic changes have been found in a few patients [126] while some authors consider the cystic changes more like those of polycystic kidney disease (Potter, type 3) [127]. Hepatic fibrosis and accumulation of hemosiderin in liver are found to a varying extent [122].

The liver and kidney cells are devoid of peroxisomes on electron microscopy [128]. Cerebrohepatorenal (CHR) syn-

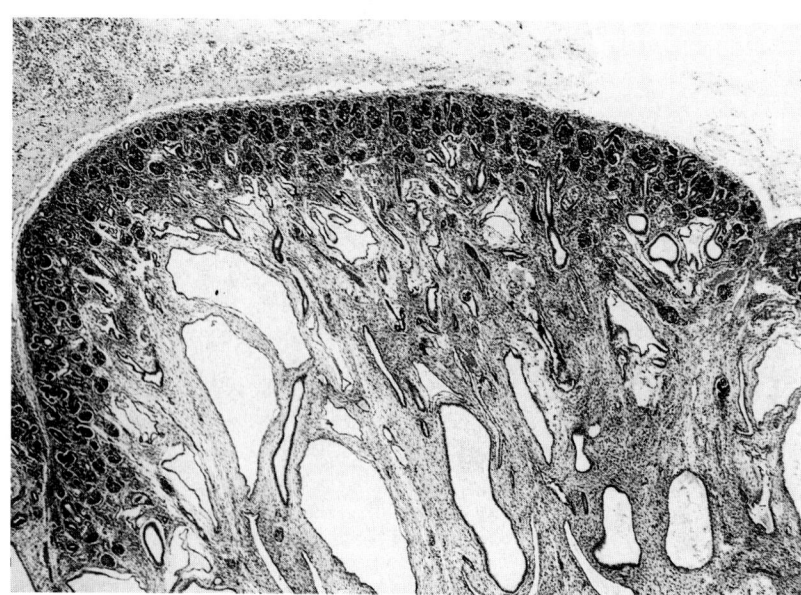

FIGURE 29.27.   *Histological section of a kidney from an 18-week fetus with Meckel syndrome. Note the normal nephrogenesis at the periphery of the renal lobe. Cysts appear in the center of the lobe. H&E, ×38.*

drome is one of several disorders with impaired peroxisomal function. The cells accumulate very-long-chain fatty acids and are deficient in plasmalogens [129].

Prenatal diagnosis of CHR syndrome is possible by demonstration of fatty acid abnormalities from cultured amniotic cells or chorionic villus biopsy specimens [127]. In such a study, the affected fetuses of 13–21 weeks' gestational age showed macroscopic and microscopic lesions typical for CHR syndrome. The findings included numerous cystic dilatations of the renal cortical tubules [127].

Asphyxiating Thoracic Dystrophy of Jeune

This disorder is included in the group of skeletal chondrodysplasias [130]. Short-limbed dwarfism is accompanied by short horizontal ribs, making the thoracic cage narrow. The infants have severe respiratory difficulties and many die in early infancy. The disease is transmitted as an autosomal recessive trait.

The renal lesions in infancy vary from almost constant cortical cysts to diffuse cystic disease and frank cystic dysplasia [126]. The cysts appear to arise from nephronic elements and collecting ducts. Extrarenal visceral lesions include pancreatic microcysts and hepatic fibrosis with bile duct increase, similar to those in ARPKD.

The renal disease in the survivors is characterized by progressive tubular dysfunction, glomerular hyalinization, fibrosis, and interstitial nephritis [131, 132]. The pathogenesis of asphyxiating thoracic dystrophy of Jeune is unknown. It seems probable that the renal changes in this inherited disorder reflect the underlying metabolic defect, resulting in different morphological manifestations at different stages of development.

Glutaric Aciduria Type II

Glutaric aciduria type II is a rare metabolic disorder causing respiratory distress, hypotonia, metabolic acidosis, nonketotic hypoglycemia, and hyperammonemia. Its neonatal syndromatic form includes several dysmorphic features, cerebral and visceral abnormalities including large cystic kidneys [133, 134]. The disorder is caused by a defect in electron-transferring flavoprotein (ETF) or ETF-ubiquinone oxidoreductase, leading to multiple acyl coenzyme A dehydrogenation deficiencies [135].

Glutaric aciduria type II is one of the uncommon causes of cystic renal disease with known biochemical background. The kidneys are variably enlarged and overall cystic and contain glomerular and tubular cysts with dysplastic elements [134, 136]. Most of them belong to the group of diffuse RDs.

CONGENITAL RENAL TUBULAR DYSGENESIS

In 1983 Allanson et al [137] described 2 stillborn siblings showing oligohydramnios, Potter sequence, and normal-sized kidneys, with absence of proximal tubules on histol-

ogy. The authors suggested a new autosomal recessive disorder. Recent reports suggested that the anatomical lesion of absent or nearly absent renal proximal tubules in newborn infants is not a very rare condition [138, 139].

In most cases, the kidneys are of normal shape and size or moderately enlarged [140, 141]. The main lesion is the absence or paucity of proximal tubules, leading to a crowding of normal-appearing glomeruli (Fig. 29.28). The tubular lesion is easy to observe in ordinary sections and may be confirmed by appropriate tubule-specific immunohistochemical markers [141, 142].

Atrophy of the medullary pyramids and collecting ducts [140] and squamous metaplasia of the pelvic transitional epithelium are noted in some patients [142]. Large cranial fontanels, hypoplasia of calvarial bone [141, 144, 145], and severe neonatal liver disease with hemochromatosis [142] can be found as extrarenal manifestations of congenital tubular dysgenesis.

The presence of male and female affected siblings in the family has suggested autosomal recessive inheritance [137, 140, 146, 147].

The absence of proximal tubules of the neonatal kidney may also be secondary to some general malformation or disease. Genest and Lage [139] reported 6 neonatal autopsy cases, 4 of which were from monochorionic twin pregnancies, 1 an acardiac fetus, and 1 a stillborn with trisomy 21. Renal hypoperfusion was suggested as the common denominator of all these cases. Renal vein thrombosis [141, 145] and abnormal glomerular vasculature as shown by microdissection [140] may support the hypoperfusion hypothesis.

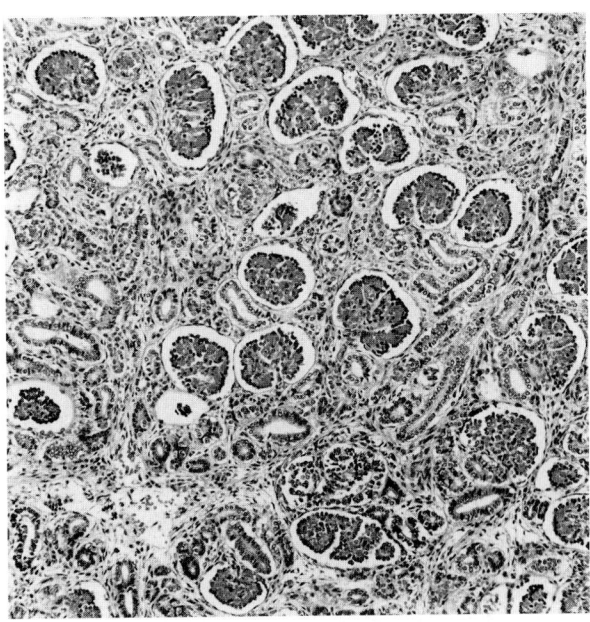

FIGURE 29.28. *Histological section of a kidney from a patient with congenital renal dysgenesis. Crowding of the glomeruli and absence of proximal tubules are demonstrated. H&E, ×250.*

RENAL LESIONS OF
ASPHYXIA AND ISCHEMIA

In the past, renal lesions caused by diminished blood flow were relatively common in the perinatal period. Perinatal asphyxia and hypoxia were responsible for acute renal failure and necrosis [148–151]. In a more recent autopsy study, about half of the renal necroses were associated with congenital heart disease. Asphyxia, septic infection, major malformations, and anemic shock were principal causes for the rest [152]. Renal venous thrombosis [153] and thrombosis associated with indwelling umbilical artery catheters [154] are also well-known causes of renal necrosis. Prematurity and respiratory distress syndrome are commonly associated features. Hypoxemia, acidosis, increased renal vascular resistance, and disseminated intravascular coagulation are considered to be the main pathogenetic pathways to renal ischemia.

The pathological lesions caused by ischemia vary in severity and location. Peculiar to neonatal kidneys is the frequency of medullary necrosis. In older children and adults acute ischemia causes tubular and cortical necrosis, whereas in the neonate, medullary necrosis is about as common as cortical necrosis [148, 155, 156]. This may be related to the different distribution of intrarenal blood flow in the neonate as compared with the adult. The medulla receives its perfusion from the efferent arterioles of the juxtamedullary glomeruli, which are more mature in the newborn infant than the peripheral ones. Consequently, the blood flow in the kidney of a newborn infant is more effective in the deep cortex and medulla than in the outer cortex [157]. Medullary congestion and microscopic hemorrhages are common findings during postmortem examinations of asphyxiated infants. Possibly related to these considerations is the observation that the cortical necrosis of neonates tends to be located in the deep cortex with a spared peripheral zone [155].

Renal necrosis in the newborn infant may be ischemic or hemorrhagic (Fig. 29.29). Fresh medullary lesions are usually hemorrhagic [156], as are the necroses associated with venous thrombosis. Renal necrosis is commonly associated with necrotic foci in other organs, for example, the liver, adrenal, myocardium, and gut (necrotizing enterocolitis) [151, 155]. Some infants who survive severe perinatal asphyxia but die later show regenerative changes in the medulla. The ducts are lined by tall hyperchromatic and sometimes pseudostratified epithelium and the interstitial connective tissue is increased. Infants recovering from acute neonatal renal failure show pelvicaliceal abnormalities, cortical atrophy, and calcifications in subsequent radiographic investigations [148].

RENAL INFECTIONS

Pathological lesions caused by bacteria are rare in perinatal kidneys, although significant bacteriuria has been found in about 1% of all newborn infants [158]. Congenital pyelonephritis is uncommon [159]. Necrotic lesions of listeriosis are less common in the kidneys than in the liver and adrenal glands, and the kidney may also be involved in generalized candidiasis (see Chap. 17).

Interstitial nephritis in the newborn infant is usually caused by infectious agents known by the acronym TORCH (see Chap. 17). The kidney, however, is only one of the organs affected and in most patients the lesions are more obvious in organs other than the kidney.

Perinatal toxoplasmosis affects the kidneys of neonates relatively often, although the lesions are overshadowed by those found in the central nervous system and eyes [160]. Interstitial nephritis with infiltrates of lymphocytes, plasma cells, and eosinophils is present. Encysted *Toxoplasma* organisms can seldom be demonstrated in the kidney. Rare lesions include necrotizing glomerulonephritis with trophozoites in

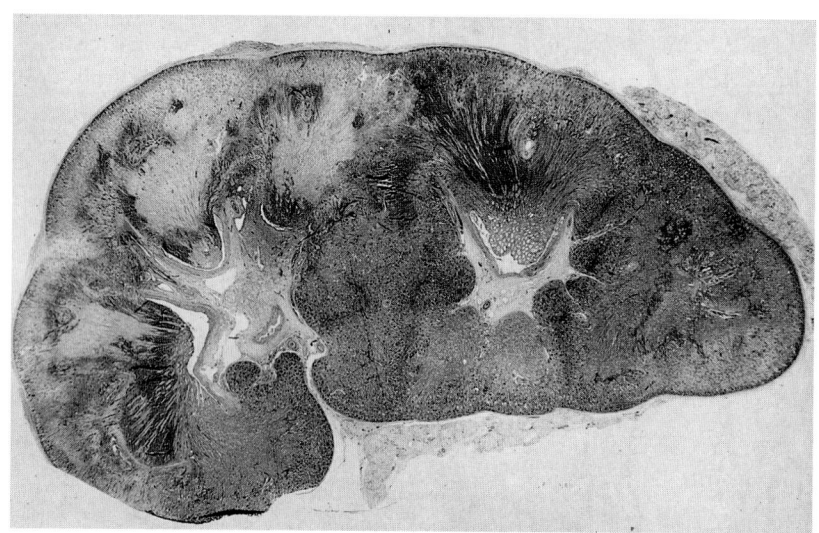

FIGURE 29.29.   *Histological section of the kidney from a premature infant showing cortical and medullary necrosis. Note that the pale necrotic area spares the tips of the pyramids and the outer rim of the cortical tissue. H&E, ×4.*

the necrotic glomeruli. Nephrotic syndrome associated with renal *Toxoplasma* infection has been reported [161].

Congenital rubella infection is characterized by general growth retardation and immaturity of various organs [162]. This is reflected in the kidney by the persistence of extramedullary hematopoiesis [163]. Focal cortical glomerulonephritis with mononuclear cell infiltration has occurred in some infants with congenital rubella infection. Nephrotic syndrome with membranous glomerulonephritis is a rare complication [163].

In 60–90% of newborn infants with clinically significant cytomegalovirus infection, the kidneys show characteristic lesions [164, 165]. Classic inclusion-bearing cells are seen most frequently in the epithelial cells of the distal convoluted tubules and collecting ducts. Focal interstitial nephritis is frequently associated with renal cytomegalovirus infection (Fig. 29.30). An association of neonatal cytomegalovirus infection and congenital nephrosis has been reported [166].

Kidneys are occasionally affected by congenital herpes simplex virus infection. Intranuclear inclusions and multinucleated cells have been found in cortical tubules and parietal epithelium of the glomeruli. Focal medullary hemorrhages without necrosis have also been described [167].

Congenital syphilis causes generalized infection affecting all visceral organs in the fetus and the newborn infant. The organs are more immature than expected from the gestational age. Persistent glomerulogenesis and extramedullary hematopoiesis are present in kidneys. Heavy infiltrates of mononuclear cells and macrophages compress the tubules, which may become atrophic [168]. Immunocomplex disease causing infantile glomerulonephritis and nephrotic syndrome appears in infants older than 1 month [169].

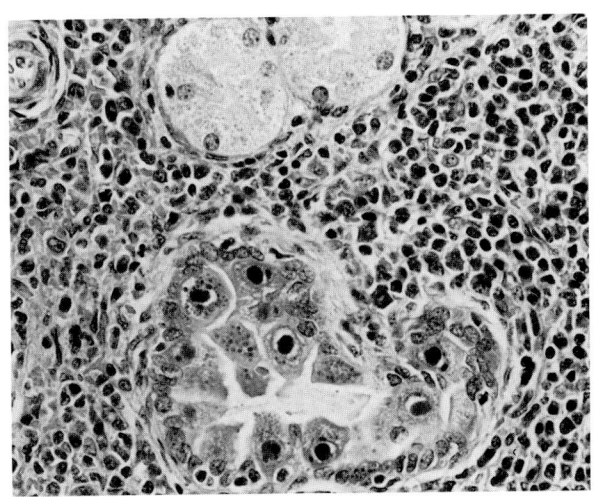

FIGURE 29.30. *Perinatal renal cytomegalovirus infection. The cells of the distal tubule show both intranuclear and cytoplasmic inclusions. Two spared proximal tubules are in the upper part of the picture. Extensive interstitial inflammation is present. H&E, ×155.*

The acquired immunodeficiency syndrome (AIDS) caused by the human immunodeficiency virus (HIV) is associated with distinct nephropathy (HIVN) including proteinuria, nephrotic syndrome, progressive azotemia, and rapid progression to end-stage renal disease [170]. Renal pathology is characterized by focal and segmental glomerular sclerosis (FSGS), global glomerular sclerosis, diffuse mesangial sclerosis, vacuolization of the podocytes, dilated nephric tubules with degenerative epithelial changes, and interstitial inflammation. Tubuloreticular inclusions are found in the glomerular endothelial cells [171]. HIVN has been encountered less commonly in children and affected children are usually older than 1 year, but some infants with HIVN have been reported [172–174]. The disease in children is usually less fulminant than in adults and the cause of death is often other than nephropathy [175]. Histological lesions are similar, but often less severe than in adults.

CONGENITAL NEPHROTIC SYNDROME

Best known of the glomerular diseases of the neonatal period is congenital nephrotic syndrome. In order to separate the idiopathic form that is manifested already in utero from the disorders with onset in infancy, and from the acquired forms, the term *congenital nephrosis of Finnish type* (CNF) has been used [176]. CNF is inherited as an autosomal recessive trait and its incidence in Finland is several times higher than elsewhere in the world. The gene locus of CNF has been assigned to the long arm of chromosome 19 (19q12–g13.1) [177]. Identification of the gene locus is of great importance for the differential diagnosis of congenital nephrotic syndrome other than CNF. It can also be used for prenatal diagnosis.

CNF has a very characteristic clinical picture. The infants are usually born a few weeks before term. They are slightly small for gestational age and often show mild birth asphyxia. The most striking finding at birth is the large placenta. The placental weight is always more than 25%, and may be up to 60%, of the birth weight of the infant [178]. Postural deformities, including talipes calcaneovalgus and contractures of the large limb joints, are common and probably due to the voluminous placenta. The main nephrotic signs, proteinuria and edema, are present at birth or develop in the first week of life in at least half of CNF patients. Urinary protein loss is heavy throughout the life of the patients, but they do not develop renal insufficiency or hypertension. Without contemporary treatment the disorder is fatal within the first 2 years of life and half of the patients die in the first 6 months [178]. Active treatment to alleviate the consequences of the urinary protein loss, avoidance of infections, and renal transplantation have radically changed the prognosis of CNF [179].

The kidneys in CNF are large and pale, partly due to the edema and dilated tubules, but an increased number of nephrons have been documented [46, 47].

Light microscopic changes are limited to the renal cortex. The most characteristic lesion is tubular dilatation, which primarily affects the proximal tubules. Because this feature is very striking in many patients, CNF has also been called *microcystic disease*, and even listed in the classifications of cystic renal disease [36]. The cystic dilatations, however, are often sparse in very young CNF infants and limited to the deep cortex [45] (Fig. 29.31). Dilated tubules are present in infantile nephropathies other than CNF. They are probably secondary to the heavy protein load leaking from the glomeruli. Therefore, the term *microcystic disorder* should not be used, to avoid confusion with genuine congenital renal cystic malformations. From a few weeks of age the dilated tubules spread radially from the deep cortex toward the periphery. Later the whole cortex appears cystic and is accompanied by interstitial fibrosis and inflammation [45]. Glomerular changes in the neonate are subtle. Mesangial hypercellularity with wide and even ectatic capillaries is the principal finding (Fig. 29.32). Progressive glomerular sclerosis and fibrosis are found in older patients. On electron

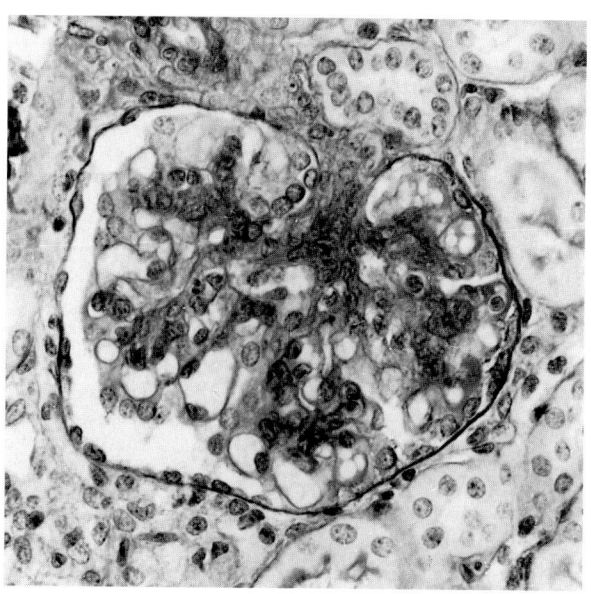

FIGURE 29.32.   *A glomerulus of a 2-week-old infant with congenital nephrotic syndrome. Mesangial hypercellularity is present, but the capillaries are wide open. PAS & H, ×330.*

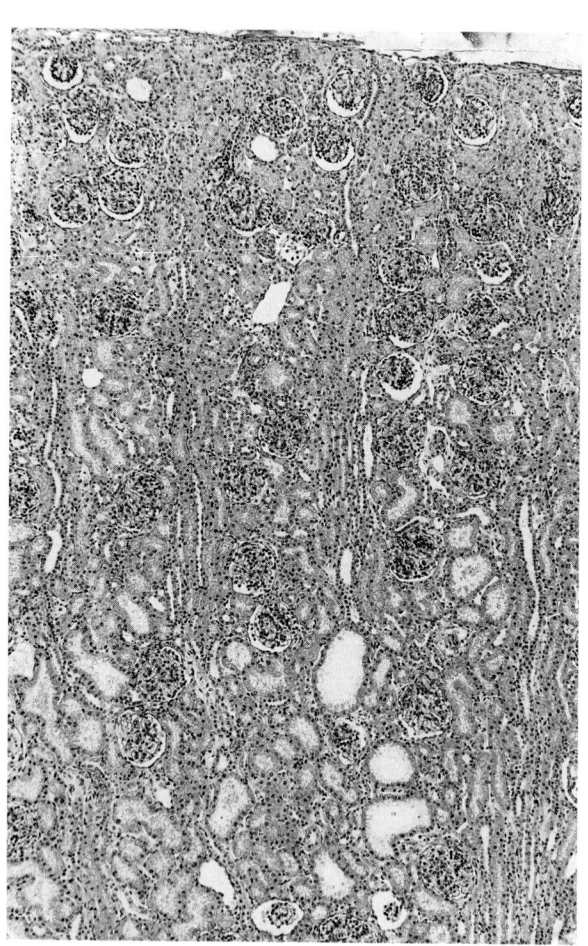

FIGURE 29.31.   *Renal cortex in a 2-week-old infant with congenital nephrotic syndrome. The cystic changes are mild and located in the deep cortex. H&E, ×90.*

microscopy, the glomerular basement membrane is thin without any deposits suggesting immunological injury. Visceral epithelial cells (podocytes) are edematous, show numerous microvilli, and have lost their foot processes.

The onset of proteinuria takes place in CNF fetuses before midterm. Fetal proteinuria can be demonstrated by showing an increase in alpha-fetoprotein (AFP) in the amniotic fluid [180]. Since AFP is the major fetal serum protein, it is separated easily from the maternal proteins of the amniotic fluid and can be used for the demonstration of fetal proteinuria, with the provision that open neural tube defect, exomphalos, and other rare conditions associated with an increase in AFP are excluded. The kidneys in midterm fetuses with CNF show scattered dilated tubules with flat epithelium and filled by eosinophilic colloid-like material in the deep cortex [181] (Fig. 29.33). On electron microscopy the most mature glomeruli situated near the corticomedullary junction show loss of the foot processes as the morphological counterpart of fetal proteinuria [182].

The pathogenesis of CNF is unknown. One hypothesis postulates a metabolic error in the heparan sulfate–rich sites of the glomerular basement membrane. This would alter the electrically charged barrier to anionic proteins in the basement membrane, allowing increased passage of proteins through the membrane [183]. Recent studies did not confirm this hypothesis [184, 185].

Nephrotic syndrome from causes other than CNF is rare in the neonate. After the age of 1 month a number of uncommon disorders can cause nephrotic syndrome. Diffuse mesangial sclerosis [186], various idiopathic glomerular disorders [187], and nephrotic syndrome secondary to perina-

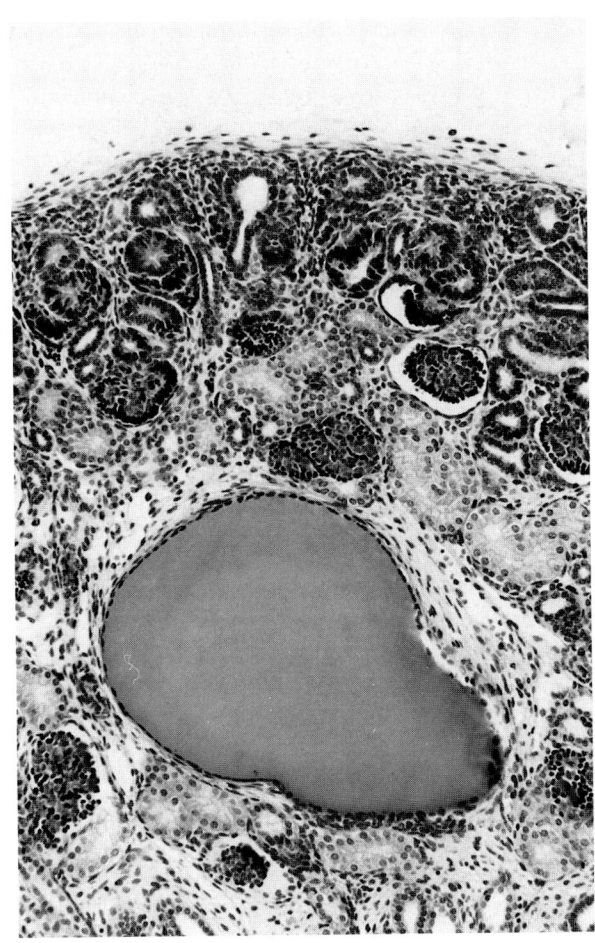

FIGURE 29.33.   *Renal cortex of a 17-week-old fetus with CNF. A cyst filled with brightly eosinophilic colloid-like material is found in the deep cortex. Note normally proceeding nephrogenesis in the outer cortex. H&E, ×105.*

tal infections, most often syphilis, are the best-known examples [176]. Clinical presentation of these disorders may overlap with CNF and cause diagnostic difficulties in later infancy.

Denys-Drash syndrome [188, 189] including male pseudohermaphroditism (XY), glomerulopathy, and Wilms' tumor sometimes presents as congenital nephrotic syndrome [176]. The glomerular pathology is that of diffuse mesangial sclerosis [187]. Diffuse mesangial sclerosis has also been the underlying glomerular abnormality in the rare type of syndromatic congenital nephrosis with microcephaly [190].

RENAL PELVIS AND URETER

Development of Ureters and the Lower Urinary Tract

As already mentioned, the renal pelvis develops from the space formed after the first divisions of the tip of the ureteric bud, and the ureter is the derivative of the unbranched portion of the ureteric bud. The embryonic development of the lower part of the ureter, bladder, and urethra is closely related to the development of a vestigial cloaca. At the end of the 4th postconceptional week in embryos 4 mm long, the cloaca is continuous with three tube-like spaces: hindgut, allantois, and mesonephric duct. It is separated from the outer surface of the embryo by a cloacal membrane, which occupies a large part of the abdominal wall below the umbilicus (Fig. 29.34). During the 7th week the urorectal septum separates the cloaca into the hindgut and the urogenital sinus continuous with the allantois. The upper part of the urogenital sinus will become the bladder. The membranous urethra and the prostatic part of the male urethra develop from the pelvic part of the urogenital sinus and the penile urethra arises from the phallic

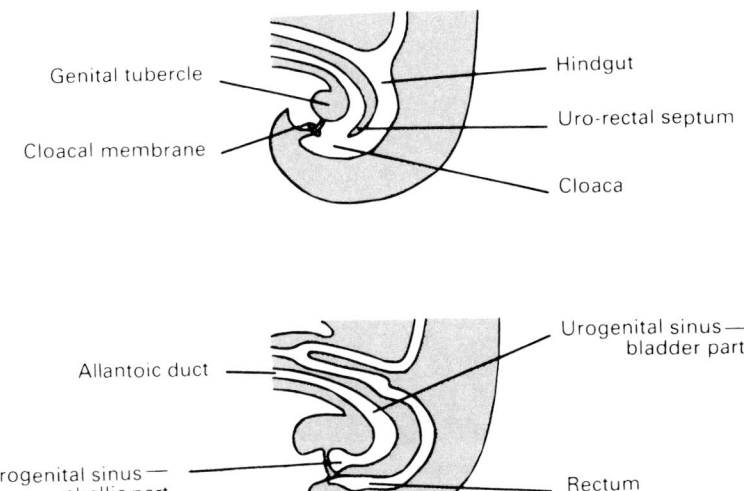

FIGURE 29.34.   *Diagram illustrating the development of the lower urinary tract.*

part of the definitive urogenital sinus. The lumen of the allantois will be obliterated and forms a fibrous chord, the urachus, connecting the apex of the bladder and umbilicus. Ureteric buds originate from the cloacal part of the mesonephric ducts. The part distal to the origin of the ureteric bud is incorporated into the wall of the urogenital sinus, resulting in separate openings for ureters and mesonephric ducts. The part of the urogenital sinus wall between these openings becomes the trigone of the bladder (see Fig. 29.15). This part of the mesonephric ducts eventually forms ejaculatory ducts in males and disappears in females. Disturbances in the development of the distal mesonephric duct and the ureteric bud result in ureteric ectopia.

Anomalies in the Renal Pelvis and Ureters

Hydronephrosis is the most common abnormality of the renal pelvis. It is defined as a dilatation of the renal pelvis and calices to form a fluid-filled sac that may exceed the size of the kidney. Hydronephrosis causes atrophy and flattening of the renal pyramids, and in extensive cases the whole parenchyma of the kidney is severely atrophic. Hydronephrosis is always secondary to urinary tract obstruction [57]. Pelviureteral stenosis or stricture is the most common cause of congenital hydronephrosis, but obstruction at any level of the urinary tract results in hydronephrosis and will be referred to with individual disorders.

Duplication of the renal pelvis and ureter is one of the most common anomalies of the urinary tract. It is more common in females than males [191]. Two ureteric buds arising from one mesonephric duct result in complete duplication of the ureters. The upper ureter remains attached longer to the mesonephric duct and will be carried with it to a more caudal and medial location in relation to the bladder, compared to its mate arising more caudally from the mesonephric duct. As a result, the ureter draining the upper segment of the kidney has a more medial and inferior bladder orifice than does the ureter draining the lower segment. The upper segment may be ectopic outside the bladder and open to the vaginal vestibulum, vagina, or urethra in females and prostate, urethra, or ejaculatory ducts in males. The ureter of the upper segment is also prone to obstruction.

Partial duplication of the ureters is embryologically explained by precocious branching of the ureteric bud. The bifurcation may be located at any place between the bladder wall and the renal pelvis, most commonly, however, in the lower part of the ureter. The duplicated ureter is associated with various anomalies in the renal pelvis.

One kidney with two separate pelvicaliceal systems is called a *duplex kidney* (Fig. 29.35). The most common duplex kidney consists of a smaller upper pelvis with only 1 or 2 minor calices. Severe obstruction in utero may cause fetal hydronephrosis. The clinical consequences of the

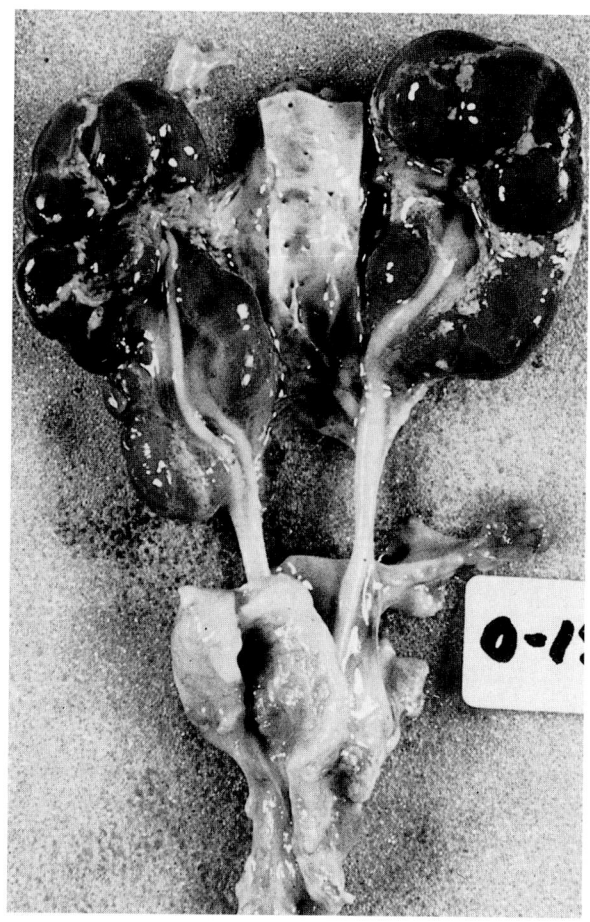

FIGURE 29.35.   *Right duplex kidney with partial duplication of the ureter. The lower pole also shows malrotation.*

duplex kidney and ureter are vesicoureteral reflux and chronic infection in childhood.

Ureterocele is a congenital cystic dilation of the terminal ureter. Simple ureterocele is the dilation of the ureter at the normally positioned ureteric orifice. In ectopic ureterocele the cystic part of the ureter bulges either inside or outside the bladder wall and terminates in an ectopic ureteric orifice at the neck of the bladder or urethra. In most patients, ectopic ureterocele is associated with the upper segment of the duplex kidney.

Anomalies of the Bladder and Urethra

Agenesis of the bladder is an extremely rare anomaly and is usually associated with various urogenital malformations [192].

Exstrophy of the bladder, epispadias, and cloacal exstrophy are related malformations and are due to the failure of the cloaca and cloacal membrane to develop normally. In the early embryo, the cloacal membrane occupies most of the lower abdominal wall below the umbilicus. Ingrowth of the mesoderm separates the ectodermal and endodermal layers of the membrane and simultaneously limits its relative size. The membrane will become circumscribed by mesodermal masses forming genital tubercles, genital swellings, and urethral folds closely related to the development of the outer genitalia (see Chap. 30). When the cloacal membrane ruptures during the 6th week, the abdominal wall is well developed and the opening is into the subphallic urogenital sinus. The basic embryological failure in the exstrophy complex is considered to result from an excessively large cloacal membrane that fails to regress in the normal fashion. Consequently, the lower abdominal wall, outer bladder wall, urethral folds, and the ventral skeleton of the pelvis are prevented from developing normally. When the abnormally large cloacal membrane ruptures, the exposed bladder will evert to form the exstrophy [193]. The pathogenesis of cloacal exstrophy is similar, with the addition of defective formation of the urorectal septum. Bladder exstrophy is an uncommon anomaly, with a 3:1 male predominance [192].

A protruding polypoid red mass with an open or bifid urethra is the classic picture of bladder exstrophy. The pubic symphysis remains open. The degree of exstrophy may range from a small exposed trigone to a huge eversion occupying most of the lower abdominal wall. Epispadias accompanies the bladder exstrophy, but it may also occur as an independent malformation. Embryologically, it is explained by less severe persistence of the cloacal membrane. Epispadias includes the complete (penopubic), glandular, or merely balanitic form, depending on the extent of the open urethral groove. Cloacal exstrophy, known also as a vesicointestinal fissure, consists of an enormous eversion of two halves of the bladder separated by a central exstrophied bowel area (Fig. 29.36). Cloacal exstrophy is associated with severe genital anomalies. Urachal anomalies are among the common malformations of the urinary tract. They result from incomplete obliteration of the allantoic duct. Depending on the location and degree of the defect in the closure, four basic forms of urachal anomaly are known: patent urachus, vesicourachal diverticulum, urachal cyst, and urachal sinus. The rare malformations of the bladder include duplication, various forms of septation, and multilocular bladder [57, 192]. Complete duplication of the bladder consists of two bladders, each having its own ureter and urethra. Double external genitalia and duplication of the hindgut are associated anomalies. Incomplete duplication and various forms of septation often cause obstruction of urinary flow, with consequent hydronephrosis and dysplastic changes in the kidneys.

Bladder Outlet Obstruction

The most common obstruction of bladder drainage is caused by posterior urethral valves in males. Their embryology is poorly known and a controversial issue [194]. Young et al [195] classified posterior urethral valves into three types. Type 1 valves pass from the verumontanum to the anterolateral part of the urethral wall. The normal male urethra has a pair of mucosal folds corresponding to the location of type 1 valves. It is considered that the type 1 valves are formed by exaggeration of the growth of these folds. Type 2 valves run from the verumontanum toward the neck of the bladder. Type 3 valves consist of a diaphragm with a small opening either above or below the level of the verumontanum. The type 1 valves are considered to be the most common type, whereas controversy exists over the significance and existence of type 2 and 3 valves. Part of this confusion is due to the dissection technique commonly used in neonatal postmortem examinations. Robertson and Hayes

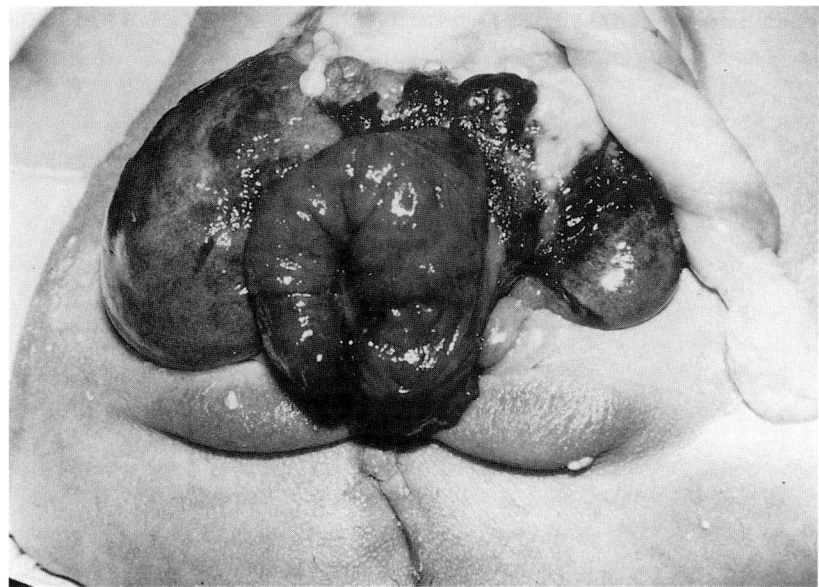

FIGURE 29.36. *Cloacal exstrophy of a newborn infant. Protruding gut is in the middle, and everted halves of the bladder on both sides. Note the scrotal swellings below the everted organs. The infant had testicles but no development of the external genitalia.*

[196] demonstrated that if the wall of the proximal urethra is opened carefully by removing the anterior wall instead of performing the usual incision with scissors, the obstruction is composed of a diaphragm with a slitlike opening across the lower prostatic urethra. With this approach the structure of the valve is close to type 3 of Young's classification, whereas the ordinary anterior incision produced a picture of type 1 valves.

The consequences of valvular obstruction depend on the severity of the lesion. With severe lesions, the proximal urethra is dilated. The bladder neck becomes hypertrophic and the bladder is distended, trabeculated, and thick walled. A bilateral hydroureter and hydronephrosis are present. The kidneys often show cortical dysplasia of Potter type 4.

Prune-Belly Syndrome

Prune-belly syndrome consists of a congenital defect or hypoplasia of the abdominal musculature, large hypotonic bladder, dilated and tortuous ureters, hydronephrosis, and bilateral cryptorchidism in males [197]. The incidence of prune-belly syndrome is 1 in 35,000 to 50,000 livebirths [198]. The pregnancies are often complicated by oligohydramnios with consequent pulmonary hypoplasia of the newborn infant. The abdominal wall is thin and lax and tends to wrinkle, resembling a wizened prune. The kidneys show hydronephrotic atrophy and dysplastic changes of varying severity. Tortuous thin-walled megaureters may attain the size of intestines. Ureteric orifices are unobstructed, but often lie at the edges of the greatly distended trigone. The bladder neck is hypertrophic and dilated. Histology of the abdominal wall discloses absence or atrophy of the muscle fibers in various degrees. The absence of muscle may actually represent a large diastasis recti, pushing the rectus abdominis muscles far laterally where they may be found with attenuated fibers.

The cause of prune-belly syndrome is considered to be bladder outlet obstruction, and several patients with urethral valves, stenosis, or atresia have been described. However, in most patients there is no clear evidence of anatomical obstruction [197]. This finding has challenged the pathogenetic explanation of prune-belly syndrome in terms of outflow obstruction.

The anatomy of the bladder neck including the internal sphincter, prostatic urethra, and the prostate gland is abnormal in prune-belly syndrome. The prostatic urethra is dilated and funnel shaped to the extent that the border of the bladder and the urethra is obscured [199]. Hypoplasia of the prostate is found in many patients [199–201]. It has been postulated that the development of the urogenital sinus with contributing lateral mesoderm is defective, resulting in abnormalities of the prostate and urethra [201]. Moerman et al [200] emphasized the lack of prostatic smooth muscle, causing a flap valve mechanism that closed the narrow membranous urethra. The outflow obstruction would thus be relative and functional rather than anatomical. Approxi-

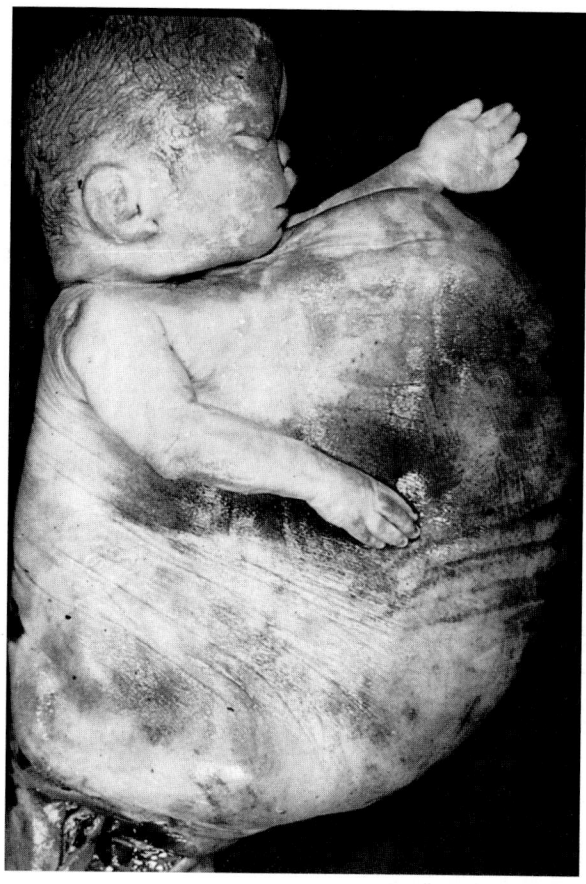

FIGURE 29.37.   *A stillborn infant with prune-belly syndrome showing extensive ascites, which distends the abdomen.*

mately 3% of prune-belly syndrome patients are female. They show urethral atresia, duplication of the uterus, and various anorectal anomalies [202], suggesting maldevelopment of the urogenital sinus and cloaca.

Severe cases of prune-belly syndrome cause perinatal death, but the less affected boys live longer and surgical correction is frequently difficult. The cases seen at perinatal postmortem examinations are in either stillborn or liveborn infants showing lesions of extreme severity. Fetal ascites is an impressive finding in some patients [200, 203] (Fig. 29.37).

PRENATAL DIAGNOSIS OF RENAL AND URINARY TRACT ABNORMALITIES

Suspected urinary tract abnormalities are common indications for prenatal diagnosis. Various diagnostic techniques may be applied to the urinary tract.

Sonography is the usual method of detecting gross malformations of the kidneys and the urinary tract during the second and third trimesters of pregnancy. The kidneys, dilated ureters, bladder, and amniotic fluid are readily visualized [204]. Grossly cystic kidneys, severe hydronephrosis, renal agenesis, megacystis, megaureter, and tumors can be diagnosed by sonography [204, 205]. An agreement of fetal sonographic findings and postnatal findings is found in more than two-thirds of cases [206, 207]. ARPKD is difficult to detect early in pregnancy. It appears that the kidneys enlarge and the echogenicity increases after 22–24 gestational weeks [208, 209]. In one series some suspected cases of ARPKD were detected by 22 weeks, but in 1 infant, it was not seen before 30 weeks [210].

Another less commonly used method is fetoscopy with thin fiberoptics. Meckel syndrome with polydactyly and occipital encephalocele has been visualized at 10 to 11 gestational weeks [120, 211].

If the chromosomal site of the gene locus is known, prenatal diagnosis is possible from chorionic villus specimens usually at 8 to 10 weeks. This method has been applied to ADPKD [81] and should be available soon for diagnosing an increasing number of diseases inherited as mendelian traits.

Disorders with known metabolic derangement are detectable by examination of chorionic villus or amniotic fluid samples. Zellweger syndrome [127] and glutaric aciduria type II [134] are examples of disorders detectable by biochemical assays.

Congenital nephrotic syndrome of Finnish type has been diagnosed by demonstration of elevated AFP levels in the maternal serum and the amniotic fluid [180], but much more elegant DNA haplotype analysis is becoming available [177].

Whatever methods of prenatal diagnosis have been used, clinicians and pathologists must be aware of them and be able to confirm or reject the results by appropriate investigations after birth.

REFERENCES

1. Saxen L. *Organogenesis of the Kidney.* Cambridge: Cambridge University Press, 1988.
2. Osathanondh V, Potter EL. Pathogenesis of polycystic kidneys. *Arch Pathol* 1964; 77:459–512.
3. Oliver J. *Nephrons and Kidneys: A Quantitative Study of Development and Evolutionary Mammalian Renal Architectonics.* New York: Harper & Row, 1968.
4. Goodyer PR, Cybulski A, Goodyer C. Expression of the epidermal growth factor receptor in fetal kidney. *Pediatr Nephrol* 1993; 7:612–15.
5. Hammerman MR, Rogers SA, Ryan G. Growth factors and kidney development. *Pediatr Nephrol* 1993; 7:616–20.
6. Sariola H, Saarma M, Sainio K, et al. Dependence of kidney morphogenesis on the expression of nerve growth factor receptor. *Science* 1991; 254:571–3.
7. Schuchardt A, D'Agati V, Larsson BL, et al. Defects in the kidney and enteric nervous system of mice lacking the tyrosine kinase receptor Ret. *Nature* 1994; 367:380–3.
8. Kreidberg JA, Sariola H, Loring JM, et al. WT-1 is required for early kidney development. *Cell* 1993; 74:679–91.
9. Armstrong JF, Pritchard-Jones K, Bickmore WA, et al. The expression of the Wilms' tumor gene WT1 in the developing mammalian embryo. *Mech Dev* 1992; 40:85–97.
10. Pelletier J, Schalling M, Buckler AJ, et al. Expression of the Wilms' tumor gene WT1 in the murine urogenital system. *Genes Dev* 1991; 5:1345–56.
11. Pelletier J, Bruening W, Kashtan CE, et al. Germline mutations in the Wilms' tumor suppressor gene are associated with abnormal urogenital development in Denys-Drash syndrome. *Cell* 1991; 67:437–47.
12. Davies J. How to build a kidney. *Semin Cell Biol* 1993; 4:213–19.
13. Potter EL. *Normal and Abnormal Development of the Kidney.* Chicago: Year Book Medical, 1972.
14. Gersh I. The correlation of structure and function in the developing mesonephros and metanephros. *Contrib Embryol Carnegie Inst Wash* 1937; 26:33–58.
15. Fetterman GH, Shuplock NA, Phillip FJ, Gregg HS. The growth and maturation of human glomeruli and proximal convolutions from term to adulthood: studies by microdissection. *Pediatrics* 1965; 35:601–19.
16. Emery JL, MacDonald MS. Involuting and scarred glomeruli in the kidneys of infants. *Am J Pathol* 1960; 36:713–23.
17. Kissane JM. Congenital malformations. In: Heptinstall RH, ed. *Pathology of the Kidney.* Boston: Little, Brown, 1983, pp. 83–140.
18. Rubenstein M, Meyer R, Bernstein J. Congenital abnormalities of the urinary tract. I. A postmortem survey of developmental anomalies and acquired congenital lesions in a children's hospital. *J Pediatr* 1961; 58:356–66.
19. Wilson RD, Baird PA. Renal agenesis in British Columbia. *Am J Med Genet* 1985; 21:153–65.
20. Thomas IT, Smith DW. Oligohydramnios, cause of the nonrenal features of Potter's syndrome, including pulmonary hypoplasia. *Pediatrics* 1974; 84:811–14.
21. Bendon RW, Ray MB. The pathologic findings of the fetal membranes in very prolonged amniotic fluid leakage. *Arch Pathol Lab Med* 1986; 110:47–50.
22. Gilbert-Barness E, Opitz JM. Renal abnormalities in malformation syndromes. In: Edelmann CM, ed. *Pediatric Kidney Disease*, vol. 2. 2nd ed. Boston: Little, Brown, 1992, pp. 1067–119.
23. Roodhooft AM, Bimholz JS, Holmes LB. Familial nature of congenital absence and severe dysgenesis of both kidneys. *N Engl J Med* 1984; 310:1341–5.
24. Thompson DP, Lynn HB. Genital anomalies associated with solitary kidney. *Mayo Clin Proc* 1966; 41:538–48.
25. Buchta RM, Visekul C, Gilbert EF, et al. Familial bilateral renal agenesis and hereditary renal adysplasia. *Z Kinderheilk* 1973; 115:111–29.
26. Biedel CW, Pagon RA, Zapata JO. Mullerian anomalies and renal agenesis: autosomal dominant urogenital adysplasia. *J Pediatr* 1984; 104:861–4.
27. Murugasu B, Cole BR, Hawkins EP, et al. Familial renal adysplasia. *Am J Kidney Dis* 1991; 18:490–4.
28. McPherson E, Carey J, Kramer A, et al. Dominantly inherited renal adysplasia. *Am J Med Genet* 1987; 26:863–72.
29. Cain DR, Griggs D, Kagan BM. Familial renal agenesis and total dysplasia. *Am J Dis Child* 1974; 128:377–80.
30. Pashayan HM, Dowd T, Nigro AV. Bilateral absence of the kidneys and ureters: three cases reported in one family. *J Med Genet* 1977; 14:205–9.
31. Carter CO, Evans K, Pescia G. A family study of renal agenesis. *J Med Genet* 1979; 16:176–88.
32. Bankier A, DeCampo M, Newell R, et al. A pedigree study of perinatally lethal renal disease. *J Med Genet* 1985; 22:104–11.
33. Gilbert E, Opitz JM. Renal involvement in genetic hereditary malformation syndromes. In: Hamburger J, Crosnier J, Grünfield JP, eds. *Nephrology.* New York: Wiley-Flammarion, 1979, pp. 909–44.
34. Bernstein J. Developmental abnormalities of the renal parenchyma—renal hypoplasia and dysplasia. *Pathol Annu* 1968; 3:213–47.
35. Ariel I, Wells TR, Landing BH, Singer DB. The urinary system in Down syndrome: a study of 124 autopsy cases. *Pediatr Pathol* 1991; 11:879–88.
36. Glassberg KI, Stephens FD, Lebowitz RL, et al. Renal dysgenesis and cystic disease of the kidney. A report of the Committee on Terminology, Nomenclature and Classification, Section on Urology, American Academy of Pediatrics. *J Urol* 1987; 138:1085–92.
37. Royer P, Habib R, Mathieu H, Courtecruisse V. L'hypoplasie rénale bilatérale congénitale avec réduction du nombre et hypertrophie des néphrons chez l'enfant. *Ann Pediatr (Paris)* 1962; 38:753–66.
38. Moerman P, van Damme B, Proesmans W, et al. Oligomeganephronic renal hypoplasia in two siblings. *J Pediatr* 1984; 105:75–7.
39. Fetterman GH, Habib R. Congenital bilateral oligonephronic renal hypoplasia with hypertrophy of nephrons (oligomeganephronie). Studies by microdissection. *Am J Clin Pathol* 1969; 52:199–207.
40. Park SH, Chi JG. Oligomeganephronia associated with 4p deletion type chromosomal anomaly. *Pediatr Pathol* 1993; 13:731–40.
41. Beckwith JB. Macroglossia, omphalocele, adrenal cytomegaly, gigantism and hyperplastic visceromegaly. *Birth Defects* 1969; 2:188–96.
42. Roe TF, Kershnar AK, Weitzmann JJ, Salinas-Madrigal L. Beckwith's syndrome with extreme organ hyperplasia. *Pediatrics* 1973; 52:372–81.
43. Sotelo-Avila C, Singer DB. Syndrome of hyperplastic fetal visceromegaly and neonatal hypoglycemia (Beckwith's syndrome): a report of seven cases. *Pediatrics* 1970; 46:240–51.

44. Perlman M, Goldberg GM, Bar-Ziv J, Danowitch G. Renal hamartomas and nephroblastomatosis with fetal gigantism. A familial syndrome. *Pediatrics* 1973; 83:414–18.

45. Huttunen N-P, Rapola J, Vilska J, Hallman N. Renal pathology in congenital nephrotic syndrome of Finnish type: a quantitative light microscopic study of 50 patients. *Int J Pediatr Nephrol* 1980; 1:10–16.

46. Tryggvason K. Morphometric studies on glomeruli in the congenital nephrotic syndrome of the Finnish type. *Nephron* 1978; 22:544–50.

47. Tryggvason K, Kouvalainen K. Number of nephrons in normal human kidneys and kidneys of patients with the congenital nephrotic syndrome. *Nephron* 1975; 15:62–8.

48. Campbell MF. Embryology and anomalies of the urogenital tract. In: *Clinical Pediatric Urology*. Philadelphia: WB Saunders, 1951, pp. 159–353.

49. Kelalis PP. Anomalies of the urinary tract. The kidney. In: Kelalis PP, King LR, Belman AB, eds. *Clinical Pediatric Urology*. Philadelphia: WB Saunders, 1985, pp. 643–72.

50. Egli F, Stalder G. Malformations of kidney and urinary tract in common chromosomal aberrations. I. Clinical studies. *Humangenetik* 1973; 18:1–15.

51. Zerres K, Völpel M-C, Weiss H. Cystic kidneys. Genetics, pathologic anatomy, clinical picture, and prenatal diagnosis. *Hum Genet* 1984; 68:104–35.

52. Kissane JM. The morphology of renal cystic disease. In: Gardner KDJ, ed. *Cystic Diseases of the Kidney*. New York: Wiley, 1976, pp. 31–63.

53. Mir S, Rapola J, Koskimies O. Renal cysts in pediatric autopsy material. *Nephron* 1983; 33:189–95.

54. Bernstein J, Gilbert-Barness E. Congenital malformations of the kidney. In: Tisher CG, Brenner BM, eds. *Renal Pathology with Clinical and Functional Correlations*, vol. 2. 1st ed. Philadelphia: JB Lippincott, 1989, pp. 1278–308.

55. Bernstein J. Renal hypoplasia and dysplasia. In: Edelman CM, ed. *Pediatric Kidney Disease*, vol. 2. 2nd ed. Boston: Little, Brown, 1992, pp. 1121–37.

56. Glassberg KI, Filmer RB. Renal dysplasia, renal hypoplasia, and cystic disease of the kidney. In: Kelalis PP, King LR, Belman AB, eds. *Clinical Pediatric Urology*. Philadelphia: WB Saunders, 1985, pp. 922–71.

57. Bernstein J, Churg J, eds. *Urinary Tract Pathology; An Illustrated Practical Guide to Diagnosis*. New York: Raven, 1992.

58. Schwarz RD, Stephens FD, Cussen LJ. The pathogenesis of renal dysplasia. I. Quantification of hypoplasia and dysplasia. *Invest Urol* 1981; 19:94–6.

59. Schwarz RD, Stephens F, Cussen LJ. The pathogenesis of renal dysplasia. II. The significance of lateral and medial ectopy of the ureteric orifice. *Invest Urol* 1981; 19:97–100.

60. Schwarz RD, Stephens F, Cussen LJ. The pathogenesis of renal dysplasia. III. Complete and incomplete urinary obstruction. *Invest Urol* 1981; 19:101–3.

61. Kissane JM. Renal cysts in pediatric patients. A classification and overview. *Pediatr Nephrol* 1990; 4:69–77.

62. Hennebery MO, Stephens FD. Renal hypoplasia and dysplasia in infants with posterior urethral valves. *J Urol* 1980; 123:912–15.

63. Mackie GG, Stephens FD. Duplex kidneys: a correlation of renal dysplasia with position of the ureteral orifice. *J Urol* 1975; 114:274–80.

64. Maizels M, Simpson SB. Primitive ducts of renal dysplasia induced by culturing ureteral buds denuded of condensed renal mesenchyme. *Science* 1983; 219:509–10.

65. Kaplan BS, Fay J, Shah V, et al. Autosomal recessive polycystic kidney disease. *Pediatr Nephrol* 1989; 3:43–9.

66. Zerres K. Autosomal recessive polycystic kidney disease. *Clin Invest* 1992; 70:794–801.

67. Zerres K, Mücher G, Bachner L, et al. Mapping of the gene for autosomal recessive polycystic kidney disease (ARPKD) to chromosome 6p21-cen. *Nat Genet* 1994; 7:429–32.

68. Potter EL, Craig JM. *Pathology of the Fetus and the Infant*. 3rd ed. Chicago: Year Book Medical, 1975.

69. Faraggiana T, Bernstein J, Strauss L, Churg J. Use of lectins in the study of histogenesis of renal cysts. *Lab Invest* 1985; 53:575–9.

70. Holthöfer H, Kumpulainen T, Rapola J. Polycystic disease of the kidney. Evaluation and classification based on nephron segment and cell-type specific markers. *Lab Invest* 1990; 62:363–9.

71. Jörgensen MJ. The ductal plate malformation. *Acta Pathol Microbiol Scand Sect A* 1977; 257:1–88.

72. Bernstein J. Hepatic involvement in hereditary renal syndromes. *Birth Defects Orig Article Ser* 1987; 23:115–30.

73. Witzleben CL, Sharp AR. "Nephronophthisis–congenital hepatic fibrosis". An additional hepatorenal disorder. *Hum Pathol* 1982; 13:728–33.

74. Blyth H, Ockenden BG. Polycystic disease of kidneys and liver presenting in childhood. *J Med Genet* 1971; 8:257–84.

75. Gang DL, Herrin JT. Infantile polycystic disease of the liver and kidneys. *Clin Nephrol* 1986; 25:28–36.

76. Lieberman E, Salinas-Madrigal L, Gwinn JL, et al. Infantile polycystic disease of kidneys and liver: clinical, pathological and radiological correlations and comparisons with congenital hepatic fibrosis. *Medicine (Baltimore)* 1971; 50:277–318.

77. Gabow PA. Autosomal dominant polycystic kidney disease. *N Engl J Med* 1993; 329:332–42.

78. Dalgaard OZ. Bilateral polycystic disease of kidneys: a follow-up of two hundred eighty-four patients and their families. *Acta Med Scand* 1957; 328:1–255.

79. Fick GM, Gabow PA. Natural history of autosomal dominant polycystic kidney disease. *Annu Rev Med* 1994; 45:23–9.

80. Mehrizi A, Rosenstien BJ, Pusch A, et al. Myocardial infarction and endocardial fibroelastosis in children with polycystic kidneys. *Bull Johns Hopkins Hosp* 1964; 115:92–8.

81. Michaud J, Russo P, Grignon A, et al. Autosomal dominant polycystic kidney disease in the fetus. *Am J Med Genet* 1994; 51:240–6.

82. Bengtsson U, Hedman L, Svalander C. Adult type of polycystic kidney disease in newborn child. *Acta Med Scand* 1975; 197:447–50.

83. Ross DG, Travers H. Infantile presentation of adult-type polycystic kidney disease in a large kindred. *J Pediatr* 1975; 87:760–3.

84. Eulderink F, Hogewind BL. Renal cysts in premature children. *Arch Pathol Lab Med* 1978; 102:592–5.

85. Proesmans W, Van Damme B, Casaer P, Marchal G. Autosomal dominant polycystic kidney disease in the neonatal period: association with a cerebral arteriovenous malformation. *Pediatrics* 1982; 70:971–5.

86. Shokeir MHK. Expression of "adult" polycystic renal disease in the fetus and newborn. *Clin Genet* 1978; 14:61–72.

87. Chevalier RL, Garland TA, Buschi AJ. The neonate with adult-type autosomal dominant polycystic kidney disease. *Int J Pediatr Nephrol* 1981; 2:73–7.

88. Rapola J, Kääriäinen H. Polycystic kidney disease. Morphological diagnosis of recessive and dominant polycystic kidney disease in infancy and childhood. *APMIS* 1988; 96:68–76.

89. Cobben JM, Breuning MH, Schoots C, et al. Congenital hepatic fibrosis in autosomal-dominant polycystic kidney disease. *Kidney Int* 1990; 38:880–5.

90. European Polycystic Kidney Consortium. The polycystic kidney disease 1 gene encodes a 14 kb transcript and lies within a duplicated region on chromosome 16. *Cell* 1994; 77:881–94.

91. Kimberling WJ, Kumar S, Gabow PA, et al. Autosomal dominant polycystic kidney disease: localization of the second gene to chromosome 4q13–q23. *Genomics* 1993; 18:467–72.

92. Mochizuki T, Wu G, Hayashi T, et al. PKD2, a gene for polycystic kidney disease that encodes an integral membrane protein. *Science* 1996; 272:1339–42.

93. Wilson PD, Burrow CR. Autosomal dominant polycystic kidney disease: cellular and molecular mechanisms of cyst formation. *Adv Nephrol Necker Hosp* 1992; 21:125–42.

94. Carone FA, Bacallao R, Kanwar YS. Biology of polycystic kidney disease. *Lab Invest* 1994; 70:437–48.

95. Bernstein J. Glomerulocystic kidney disease nosological considerations. *Pediatr Nephrol* 1993; 7:464–70.

96. Taxy JB, Filmer RB. Glomerulocystic kidney. *Arch Pathol Lab Med* 1976; 100:186–8.

97. Rizzoni G, Loirat C, Levy M, et al. Familial hypoplastic glomerulocystic kidney. A new entity? *Clin Nephrol* 1982; 18:263–8.

98. Kaplan BS, Gordon I, Pincott J, Barrat TM. Familial hypoplastic glomerulo-cystic disease: a definite entity with dominant inheritance. *Am J Med Genet* 1989; 34:569–73.

99. Waldherr R, Lennert T, Weber H-P, et al. The nephronophthisis complex: a clinicopathologic study in children. *Virchows Arch A Pathol Anat Histopathol* 1982; 394:235–54.

100. Gagnadoux MF, Bacri JL, Broyer M, Habib R. Infantile chronic tubulo-interstitial nephritis with cortical microcysts: variant of nephronophthisis or new disease entity? *Pediatr Nephrol* 1989; 3:50–5.

101. Bernstein J. A classification of renal cysts. In: Gardner KD, Bernstein J, eds. *The Cystic Kidney*. London: Kluwer Academic, 1990, pp. 147–70.

102. Johnson DE, Ayalal AG, Medellin H, Wilbur J. Multilocular renal cystic disease in children. *J Urol* 1973; 109:101–3.

103. Arey JB. Cystic lesions of the kidney in infants and children. *J Pediatr* 1959; 54:429–45.

104. Fowler M. Differentiated nephroblastoma: solid, cystic or mixed. *J Pathol* 1971; 105:215–8.

105. Ganick DJ, Gilbert EF, Beckwith JB, Kiviat N. Congenital cystic mesoblastic nephroma. *Hum Pathol* 1981; 12:1039–43.

106. Joshi W. Cystic partially differentiated nephroblastoma. An entity in the spectrum of infantile renal neoplasia. *Perspect Pediatr Pathol* 1979; 5:217–35.

107. Boggs LK, Kimmelstiel P. Benign multilocular cystic nephroma: report of two cases of so-called multilocular cyst of the kidney. *J Urol* 1956; 76:530–41.

108. Schimke RN. Genetics in cystic kidney disease. In: Gardner KDJ, ed. *Cystic Diseases of the Kidney*. New York: Wiley, 1976, pp. 83–90.

109. Chonko AM, Weiss SM, Stein JH, Ferris TF. Renal involvement in tuberous sclerosis. *Am J Med* 1974; 56:124–32.

110. Zimmerhackl LB, Rehm M, Kaufnehl K, et al. Renal involvement in tuberous sclerosis complex: a retrospective survey. *Pediatr Nephrol* 1994; 8:451–7.

111. Stapleton FB, Johnson D, Kaplan GW, Griswold W. The cystic renal lesion in tuberous sclerosis. *J Pediatr* 1980; 97:574–9.

112. Bernstein J. Renal cystic disease in the tuberous sclerosis complex. *Pediatr Nephrol* 1993; 7:490–5.

113. Salonen R. The Meckel syndrome: clinicopathological findings in 67 patients. *Am J Med Genet* 1984; 18:671–89.

114. Rapola J, Salonen R. Visceral anomalies in the Meckel syndrome. *Teratology* 1985; 31:193–201.

115. Paavola P, Salonen R, Weissenbach J, Peltonen L. The locus for Meckel syndrome with multiple congenital anomalies maps to chromosome 17q21–q24. *Nat Genet* 1995; 11:213–15.

116. Lowry RB, Hill RH, Tischler B. Survival and spectrum of anomalies in the Meckel syndrome. *Am J Med Genet* 1983; 14:417–21.

117. Wright C, Healicon R, English C, Burn J. Meckel syndrome: what are the minimum diagnostic criteria? *J Med Genet* 1994; 31:482–5.

118. Anderson VM. Meckel syndrome: morphologic considerations. *Birth Defects* 1982; 18:45–60.

119. Rehder H, Labbe F. Prenatal morphology in Meckel's syndrome. *Prenat Diagn* 1981; 1:161–72.

120. Dumez Y, Dommergues M, Gubler MC, et al. Meckel-Gruber syndrome: prenatal diagnosis at 10 menstrual weeks using embryoscopy. *Prenat Diagn* 1994; 14:141–4.

121. Rapola J. Kidneys in Meckel's syndrome as a model of abnormal renal differentiation. *Int J Dev Biol* 1989; 33:177–82.

122. Danks DM, Tippet P. Adams C, Campbell P. Cerebro-hepato-renal syndrome of Zellweger. A report of eight cases with comments upon the incidence, the liver lesion, and fault in picrocolic acid metabolism. *J Pediatr* 1975; 86:382–7.

123. Passarge E, McAdams AJ. Cerebro-hepato-renal syndrome. *J Pediatr* 1967; 71:691–702.

124. Shimozawa N, Tsukamoto T, Suzuki Y, et al. A human gene responsible for Zellweger syndrome that affects peroxisome assembly. *Science* 1992; 255;1132–4.

125. Masuno M, Shimozawa N, Suzuki Y, et al. Assignment of the human peroxisome assembly factor-1 gene (PXMP3) responsible for Zellweger syndrome to chromosome 8q21.1 by fluorescence in situ hybridization. *Genomics* 1994; 20:141–2.

126. Bernstein J, Brough AJ, McAdams AJ. The renal lesions in syndromes of multiple congenital malformations. Cerebrohepatorenal syndrome; Jeune asphyxiating thoracic dystrophy; tuberous sclerosis; Meckel syndrome. *Birth Defects* 1974; 10:34–53.

127. Powers JM, Moser HW, Moser AB, et al. Fetal cerebrohepatorenal (Zellweger) syndrome: dysmorphic, radiologic, biochemical, and pathologic findings in four affected fetuses. *Hum Pathol* 1985; 16:610–20.

128. Goldfischer S, Powers JM, Johnson AB, et al. Peroxisomal and mitochondrial defects in the cerebrohepatorenal syndrome. *Science* 1973; 182:62–4.

129. Schutgens RBH, Heymans HSA, Wanders RJA, et al. Peroxisomal disorders: a newly recognized group of genetic diseases. *Eur J Pediatr* 1986; 144:430–40.

130. Yang S-H, Heidelberger KP, Brough AJ, et al. Lethal short-limbed chondrodysplasia in early infancy. *Perspect Pediatr Pathol* 1976; 3:1–40.

131. Edelson PJ, Spachman TJ, Belliveau RE, Mahoney MJ. A renal lesion in asphyxiating thoracic dysplasia. *Birth Defects* 1974; 10:51–6.

132. Herdman RC, Langer LO. The thoracic asphyxiant dystrophy and renal disease. *Am J Dis Child* 1968; 116:192–201.

133. Wilson GN, de Chadarevian J, Kaplan P, et al. Glutaric aciduria type II: review of the phenotype and report of an unusual glomerulopathy. *Am J Med Genet* 1989; 32:395–401.

134. Hockey A, Knowles S, Davies D, et al. Glutaric aciduria type II, an unusual cause of prenatal polycystic kidneys: report of prenatal diagnosis and confirmation of autosomal recessive inheritance. *Birth Defects* 1993; 29:373–82.

135. Loehr JP, Goodman SI, Frerman FE. Glutaric acidemia type II: heterogeneity of clinical and biochemical phenotypes. *Pediatr Res* 1990; 27:311–15.

136. Kamiya M, Eimoto T, Kishimoto H, et al. Glutaric aciduria type II: autopsy study of a case with electron-transferring flavoprotein dehydrogenase deficiency. *Pediatr Pathol* 1990; 10:1007–19.

137. Allanson JE, Pantzar JT, MacLeod PM. Possible new autosomal recessive syndrome with unusual renal histopathological changes. *Am J Med Genet* 1983; 16:57–60.

138. Allanson JE, Hunter AG, Mettler GS, Jimenez C. Renal tubular dysgenesis: a not uncommon autosomal recessive syndrome: a review. *Am J Med Genet* 1992; 43:811–14.

139. Genest DR, Lage JM. Absence of normal-appearing proximal tubules in the fetal and neonatal kidney: prevalence and significance. *Hum Pathol* 1991; 22:147–53.

140. Voland RV, Hawkins EP, Wells TR, et al. Congenital hypernephronic nephromegaly with tubular dysgenesis: a distinctive inherited renal anomaly. *Pediatr Pathol* 1985; 4:231–45.

141. Metzman RA, Husson MA, Dellers EA. Renal tubular dysgenesis: a description of early renal maldevelopment in siblings. *Pediatr Pathol* 1993; 13:239–48.

142. Bale PM, Kan AE, Dorney SF. Renal proximal tubular dysgenesis associated with severe neonatal hemosiderotic liver disease. *Pediatr Pathol* 1994; 14:479–89.

143. Moldavsky M, Shahin A, Turani H. Renal tubular dysgenesis present in a newborn with meconium ileus. *Pediatr Pathol* 1994; 14:245–51.

144. Russo R, D'Armiento M, Vecchione R. Renal tubular dysgenesis and very large cranial fontanels in a family with acrocephalosyndactyly. S.C. type. *Am J Med Genet* 1991; 39:482–5.

145. Barr MJ, Cohen MMJ. ACE inhibitor fetopathy and hypocalvaria: the kidney-skull connection. *Teratology* 1991; 44:485–95.

146. Schwartz BR, Lage JM, Pober BR, Driscoll SG. Isolated congenital renal tubular immaturity in siblings. *Hum Pathol* 1986; 17:1259–63.

147. Swinford AE, Bernstein J, Toriello HV, Higgins JV. Renal tubular dysgenesis: delayed onset of oligohydramnios. *Am J Med Genet* 1989; 32:127–32.

148. Anand SK, Northway JD, Gussi FG. Acute renal failure in newborn infants. *J Pediatr* 1978; 92:985–8.

149. Chevalier RL, Campbell F, Brenbridge AN. Prognostic factors in neonatal acute renal failure. *Pediatrics* 1984; 74:265–72.

150. Dauber IM, Krauss AN, Symchych PS, Auld PA. Renal failure following perinatal anoxia. *J Pediatr* 1976; 88:851–5.

151. Kozlowski K, Brown RW. Renal medullary necrosis in infants and children. *Pediatr Radiol* 1978; 7:85–9.

152. Lerner G, Kurnetz R, Bernstein J, et al. Renal cortical and renal medullary necrosis in the first 3 months of life. *Pediatr Nephrol* 1992; 6:516–18.

153. Arneil GC, MacDonald AM, Murphy AV, Sweet EM. Renal venous thrombosis. *Clin Nephrol* 1973; 1:119–31.

154. Wigger HJ, Bransilver BR, Blanc WA. Thromboses due to catheterization in infants and children. *J Pediatr* 1970; 76:1–11.

155. Bernstein J, Meyer R. Congenital abnormalities of the urinary system. II. Renal cortical and medullary necrosis. *J Pediatr* 1961; 59:657–68.

156. Davies DJ, Kennedy A, Roberts C. Renal medullary necrosis in infancy and childhood. *J Pathol* 1969; 99:125–30.

157. Spitzer A. Renal physiology and functional development. In: Edelmann CHJ, ed. *Pediatric Kidney Disease*. Boston: Little, Brown, 1978, pp. 25–128.

158. Edelman CMJ, Ogwo JE, Fine BP, Martinez AB. The prevalence of bacteriuria in full-term and premature infants. *J Pediatr* 1973; 82:125–32.

159. Porter KA, Giles HMC. A pathological study of pyelonephritis in the newborn. *Arch Dis Child* 1956; 31:303–9.

160. Dische MR, Manford Gooch WI. Congenital toxoplasmosis. *Perspect Pediatr Pathol* 1981; 6:83–113.

161. Shahin B, Papadopoulou ZL, Jenis EH. Congenital nephrotic syndrome associated with congenital toxoplasmosis. *J Pediatr* 1974; 85:366–70.

162. Singer DB, Rudolph AJ, Rosenberg HS, et al. Pathology of the congenital rubella. *J Pediatr* 1967; 71:665–79.

163. Esterly JR, Oppenheimer EH. Pathological lesions due to congenital rubella. *Arch Pathol* 1969; 87:380–8.

164. Becroft DMO. Prenatal cytomegalovirus infection: epidemiology, pathology and pathogenesis. *Perspect Pediatr Pathol* 1981; 6:203–41.

165. Medearis DNJ. Cytomegalic inclusion disease. *Pediatrics* 1957; 19:467–80.

166. Batisky DL, Roy S, Gaber LW. Congenital nephrosis and neonatal cytomegalovirus infection: a clinical association. *Pediatr Nephrol* 1993; 7:741–3.

167. Singer DB. Pathology of neonatal herpes simplex virus infection. *Perspect Pediatr Pathol* 1981; 6:243–78.

168. Oppenheimer EH, Dahms BB. Congenital syphilis in the fetus and neonate. *Perspect Pediatr Pathol* 1981; 66:115–38.

169. Wiggelinkhuizen J, Kaschula ROC, Uys CJ, et al. Congenital syphilis and glomerulonephritis with evidence for immune pathogenesis. *Arch Dis Child* 1973; 48:375–81.

170. Rao TKS. Clinical features of human immunodeficiency virus associated nephropathy. *Kidney Int Suppl* 1991; 35:S13–18.
171. Bourgoignie JJ, Pardo V. The nephropathology in human immunodeficiency virus (HIV-1) infection. *Kidney Int Suppl* 1991; 35:S19–23.
172. Strauss J, Abitbol C, Zilleruelo G, et al. Renal disease in children with the acquired immunodeficiency syndrome. *N Engl J Med* 1989; 321:625–30.
173. Connor E, Gupta S, Joshi V, et al. Acquired immunodeficiency syndrome-associated renal disease in children. *J Pediatr* 1988; 113:39–44.
174. Foster S, Hawkins E, Hanson CG, Shearer W. Pathology of the kidney in childhood immunodeficiency: AIDS-related nephropathy is not unique. *Pediatr Pathol* 1991; 11:63–74.
175. Strauss J, Zilluruelo G, Abitbol C, et al. Human immunodeficiency virus nephropathy. *Pediatr Nephrol* 1993; 7:220–5.
176. Rapola J. Congenital nephrotic syndrome. *Pediatr Nephrol* 1987; 1:441–6.
177. Kestilä M, Männikkö M, Holmberg C, et al. Congenital nephrotic syndrome of the Finnish type maps to the long arm of chromosome 19. *Am J Hum Genet* 1994; 54:757–64.
178. Huttunen N-P. Congenital nephrotic syndrome of Finnish type. Study of 75 cases. *Arch Dis Child* 1976; 51:344–8.
179. Holmberg C, Jalanko H, Koskimies O, et al. Renal transplantation in small children with congenital nephrotic syndrome of the Finnish type. *Transplant Proc* 1991; 23:1378–9.
180. Ryynänen M, Seppälä M, Kuusela P, et al. Antenatal screening for congenital nephrosis in Finland by maternal serum alpha-fetoprotein. *Br J Obstet Gynaecol* 1983; 90:437–42.
181. Rapola J. Renal pathology of fetal congenital nephrosis. *Acta Pathol Microbiol Immunol Scand Sect A* 1981; 89:63–4.
182. Rapola J, Sariola H, Ekblom P. Pathology of fetal congenital nephrosis: immunohistochemical and ultrastructural studies. *Kidney Int* 1984; 25:701–7.
183. Vernier RL, Klein DJ, Sisson S, et al. Heparan sulfate-rich anionic sites in the human glomerular basement membrane. *N Engl J Med* 1983; 309:1001–9.
184. Ljungberg P. Glycosaminoglycans in urine and amniotic fluid in congenital nephrotic syndrome of the Finnish type. *Pediatr Nephrol* 1994; 8:531–6.
185. Heuvel LPWJ van den, Born J van den, Jalanko H, et al. The glycosaminoglycan content of renal basement membranes in the congenital nephrotic syndrome of the Finnish type. *Pediatr Nephrol* 1992; 6:10–5.
186. Habib R, Bois E. Heterogeneite des syndromes nephrotiques a debut precoce du nourrison (syndrome nephrotique "infantile"). *Helv Pediatr Acta* 1973; 28:91–107.
187. Habib R. Nephrotic syndrome in the 1st year of life. *Pediatr Nephrol* 1993; 7:347–53.
188. Denys P, Malvaux P, Van den Berghe H, et al. Association d'un syndrome anatomopathologique de pseudohermaphrodisme masculin, d'une tumeur de Wilms, d'une néphropathie parenchymateuse et d'un mosaicisme. *Arch Fr Pediatr* 1967; 24:729–39.
189. Drash A, Sherman F, Hartmann W, Blizzard RM. A syndrome of pseudohermaphroditism, Wilms' tumor, hypertension and degenerative renal disease. *J Pediatr* 1970; 76:585–93.
190. Koskimies O, Sariola H, Holmberg C, Rapola J. Clinical quiz. *Pediatr Nephrol* 1991; 5:433–5.
191. Kelalis PP. Renal pelvis and ureter. In: Kelalis PP, King LR, Belman AB, eds. *Clinical Pediatric Urology*. Philadelphia: WB Saunders, 1985, pp. 672–725.
192. Duckett JW, Caldamore AA. Bladder and urachus. In: Kelalis PP, King LR, Belman AB, eds. *Clinical Pediatric Urology*. Philadelphia: WB Saunders, 1985, pp. 726–51.
193. Muecke EC. The role of the cloacal membrane in exstrophy: the first successful experimental study. *J Urol* 1984; 92:659–67.
194. Brock WA, Kaplan GW. Anomalies of the upper urinary tract. In: Edelmann CM, ed. *Pediatric Kidney Disease*, vol. 2. 2nd ed. Boston: Little, Brown, 1992, pp. 2023–36.
195. Young HH, Frontz WA, Baldwin JC. Congenital obstruction of the posterior urethra. *J Urol* 1919; 3:289–365.
196. Robertson WB, Hayes JA. Congenital diaphragmatic obstruction of the male posterior urethra. *Br J Urol* 1969; 41:592–8.
197. Wigger HJ, Blanc WA. The prune-belly syndrome. *Pathol Annu* 1977; 12:17–39.
198. Woodard JR. Prune-belly syndrome. In: Kelalis PP, King LR, Belman AB, eds. *Clinical Pediatric Urology*. Philadelphia: WB Saunders, 1985, pp. 805–24.
199. Popek EJ, Tyson RW, Miller GJ, Caldwell SA. Prostate development in prune belly syndrome (PBS) and posterior urethral valves (PUV): etiology of PBS-lower urinary tract obstruction or primary mesenchymal defect? *Pediatr Pathol* 1991; 11:1–29.
200. Moerman P, Fryns J-P, Goddeeris P, Lauweryns M. Pathogenesis of the prune-belly syndrome: a functional urethral obstruction caused by prostatic hypoplasia. *Pediatrics* 1984; 73:470–5.
201. Manivel JC, Pettinato G, Reinberg Y, et al. Prune belly syndrome: clinicopathologic study of 29 cases. *Pediatr Pathol* 1989; 9:691–711.
202. Reinberg Y, Shapiro E, Manivel JC, et al. Prune belly syndrome in females: a triad of abdominal musculature deficiency and anomalies of the urinary and genital systems. *J Pediatr* 1991; 118:395–8.
203. Monie IW, Monie BJ. Prune-belly syndrome and fetal ascites. *Teratology* 1979; 9:111–8.
204. Hadlock FP, Deter RL, Carpenter RJ. Sonography of the fetal genitourinary tract. *Semin Ultrasound CT MR* 1984; 5:213–28.
205. Fourcroy JL, Blei CL, Glassman LM, White R. Prenatal diagnosis by ultrasonography of genitourinary abnormalities. *Urology* 1983; 22:223–9.
206. Barakat AJ, Butler MG, Cobb CG, et al. Reliability of ultrasound in the prenatal diagnosis of urinary tract abnormalities. *Pediatr Nephrol* 1991; 5:12–4.
207. Korantzis A, Cardamakis E, Apostolidis C. Prenatal diagnosis of fetal urinary pathology with ultrasound. *Eur J Obstet Gynecol Reprod Biol* 1993; 52:169–74.
208. Zerres K, Hansmann M, Mallmann R, Gembruch U. Autosomal recessive polycystic kidney disease. Problems of prenatal diagnosis. *Prenat Diagn* 1988; 8:215–29.
209. Mahony BS, Gallen PW, Filly RA, Golbus MS. Progression of infantile polycystic kidney disease in early pregnancy. *J Ultrasound Med* 1984; 3:277–9.
210. Reuss A, Wladimiroff JW, Stewart PA, Niermeijer MF. Prenatal diagnosis by ultrasound in pregnancies at risk for autosomal recessive polycystic kidney disease. *Ultrasound Med Biol* 1990; 16:355–9.
211. Quintero RA, Abuhamad A, Hobbins JC, Mahoney MJ. Transabdominal thin-gauge embryofetoscopy: a technique for early prenatal diagnosis and its use in the diagnosis of a case of Meckel-Gruber syndrome. *Am J Obstet Gynecol* 1993; 168:1552–7.

Chapter

30

The Reproductive System

STUART C. LAUCHLAN   HALIT PINAR

GENDER DIFFERENTIATION

In order for an infant to develop as a phenotypically complete male or female, a cascade of complex molecular and morphological events must occur at the appropriate time and in the correct sequence during ontogeny. The guidelines that govern gender differentiation are essentially those deduced and demonstrated by Jost [1]. Initially both genders share a common genital development and a common undifferentiated gonad. This undifferentiated gonad develops at about 32 days of ovulation age when gonadal ridges appear on the medial aspect of the mesonephros. Germ cells migrate to this region from the yolk sac [2]. The arrival of the primordial germ cells in the area of the future gonads, at about the 10th thoracic level, induces cells in the mesonephros and adjacent coelomic epithelium to proliferate and form a pair of genital ridges just medial to the developing mesonephroi (Fig. 30.1). After the proliferation of the surface coelomic mesothelium that follows, toothlike projections of this mesothelium (the sex cords) extend into the developing gonadal ridges [3] (Fig. 30.2). The indifferent stage of the gonad lasts about 12 days [4]. At the end of this stage (i.e., at about 44 days following ovulation), the gonad destined to become an ovary continues to develop without major changes, but the appearance of testicular differentiation heralds significant histological and endocrine deviation from the preceding common developmental pathway.

The male embryo's genetic gender is determined by its chromosomal contents, the most important of which is the gender-determining gene, or what used to be called the testis-determining factor (TDF), on the Y chromosome. This gene, called SRY for sex-determining region of the Y, is specific to the Y chromosome of all mammals studied and is highly conserved [5–8]. It thus remains the best plausible candidate for the TDF gene [7]. Male gonadal gender, or testis formation, is subsequently thought to be determined by this gene and by other secondary pathways. The male gonad, in turn, normally produces hormones such as testosterone and müllerian-inhibiting substance (MIS) that regulate differentiation of the internal and external genitalia, thus determining phenotypic gender. The MIS gene, which was cloned in 1986 [9] and subsequently mapped to the short arm of chromosome 19 in 1987 [10], belongs to a superfamily of growth factors important in cell growth, differentiation, and regulation. This family includes transforming growth factor (TGF)-β, inhibin, and activin.

The traditional view of passive female gender differentiation in the absence of the SRY gene, the associated hormones, and the growth factors such as MIS is being challenged by recent advances in molecular genetics. Bardoni et al investigated cases of male to female gender reversal in individuals with duplications of the short arm of the X chromosome [8, 11]. They demonstrated that gender reversal results from the presence of 2 active copies of an Xp locus rather than from its rearrangement, and alterations at this locus constituted one of the causes of gender reversal in individuals with a normal 46,XY karyotype. They named this locus DSS (dosage-sensitive sex reversal) and localized it to a 160-kilobase region of chromosome Xp21. The identification of male individuals in whom DSS is deleted suggested that this locus is not required for testis differentiation. This evidence suggests strongly that female gender differentiation is an active process rather than a passive one as previously suggested (Fig. 30.3).

The absence of the SRY gene and the presence of the DSS gene allow the slow completion of ovarian differentiation and the organization of the müllerian ducts into an effective internal genital system in the female. When the

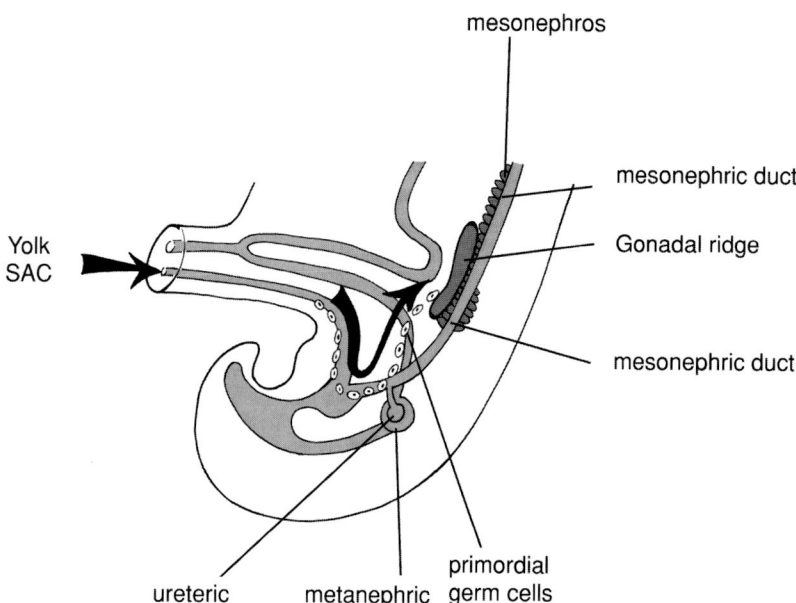

FIGURE 30.1.   *The migration of primordial germ cells from the yolk sac to the gonadal ridge in a 5-week postconceptional embryo. (Modified from Moore KL, Persaud TVN. The Developing Human: Clinically Oriented Embryology. Philadelphia: W.B. Saunders, 1993. Fig. 13.20.)*

ovary develops on its own, memory of its origin from the genital ridge is perpetuated throughout fetal life by its slender, elongated shape (Fig. 30.4). By the 3rd month, contrasting with the smooth surface of the testis's tunica albuginea, the ovarian surface has a few deep sulci and a number of shallow depressions, which contribute to an irregular surface [12] (Fig. 30.5).

FEMALE GENITAL DEVELOPMENT

In the developing ovary the germ cells, the ova-to-be, are enclosed by granulosa cells, usually, though not universally [13, 14], considered to be derived from the sex cords. The theca cells, peripheral to the granulosa, originate in the mes-

enchyme of the genital ridge. The rete ovarii, non-functional and sparse, is regularly present in the female. A few sex cords, with Leydig cells, normally persist in the ovarian medulla throughout life. Certain virilizing tumors of adult females are thought to arise from persistent Leydig cells.

The müllerian (paramesonephric) ducts appear at 6 weeks when the testis is becoming distinguishable from the indifferent gonad (see Fig. 30.2) [15]. The initial invagination of coelomic mesothelium occurs in both genders [16]. The growth of the müllerian duct depends on and is guided by the mesonephric duct [17]. Congenital absence or experimental section of the mesonephric duct will lead to absence of müllerian-derived structures (oviduct, uterus, etc.) from that side. This explains the common conjunction

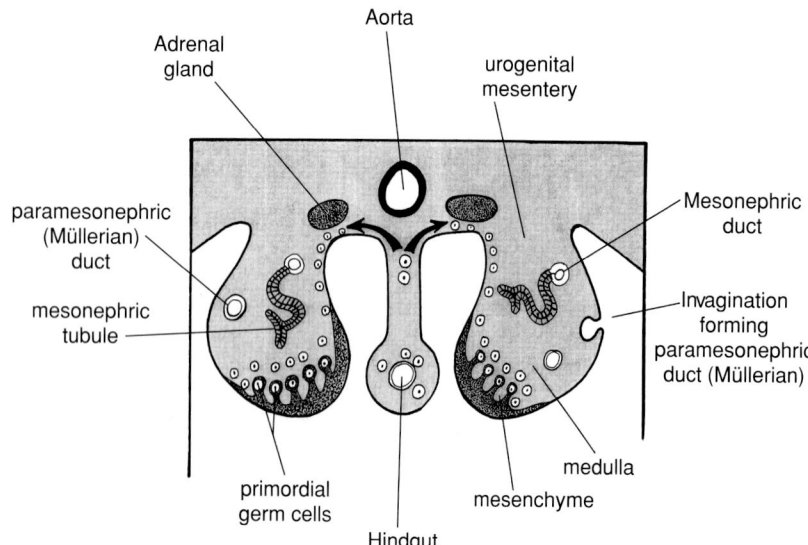

FIGURE 30.2.   *Principal constituents and relations of the developing gonad in the embryonic gonadal ridge at 6 weeks after conception. (Modified from Moore KL, Persaud TVN. The Developing Human: Clinically Oriented Embryology. Philadelphia: W.B. Saunders, 1993. Fig. 13.20.)*

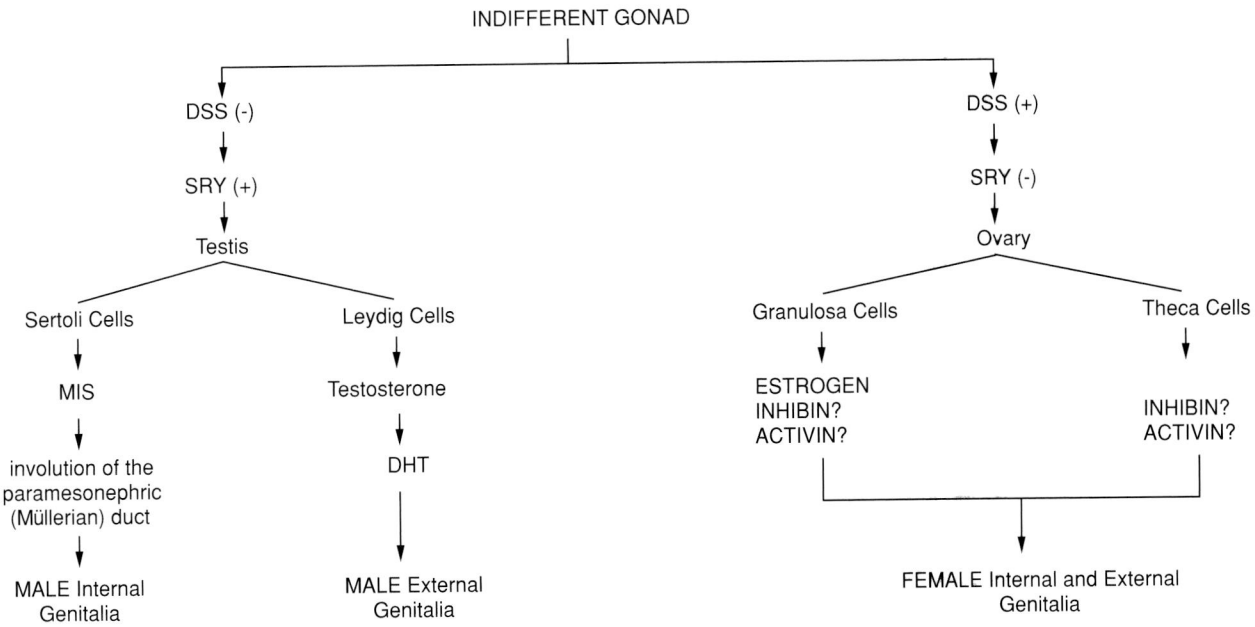

FIGURE 30.3. *Diagram of gender differentiation beginning with an indifferent gonad at about 44 days after conception. DSS = dosage sensitive sex reversal; SRY = sex-determining region of the Y chromosome; MIS = müllerian-inhibiting substance; DHT = dihydrotestosterone.*

of unilateral renal and ureteral aplasia with ipsilateral unicornuate uterus.

The müllerian ducts approach each other, passing anterior to the mesonephric ducts, and fuse in the midline to form an unpaired canal, which will develop into the uterus, cervix, and vagina.

The form of the oviduct, uterus, cervix, and vagina found at term develops gradually during fetal life by the differentiation of epithelia and the acquisition and growth of smooth muscle. The oviduct has an increasingly complex, folded, pseudostratified, and ciliated epithelium. The endometrium has a simple low columnar epithelium and a sparse, simple stroma while the cervix has prominent branching glands (Fig. 30.6). In the later weeks of gestation, the tall columnar epithelial cells accumulate abundant mucus. The locations and features of tubal, endometrial, and endocervical epithelia are fairly straightforward though they may be mixed unexpectedly. The glandular epithelium on the surface of the cervix extends onto the portio for varying distances (Fig. 30.7a). In later development, squamous epithelial metaplasia replaces the columnar epithelium on the portio and the junctional zone gradually migrates to the endocervical area a few millimeters above the external cervical os, forming the junctional zone (Fig. 30.7b).

Caudally, the fused ducts reach the urogenital sinus at 8 weeks at the site of the so-called Müller's tubercle. The tubercle has been termed a "site at which three types of epithelium meet and very likely mingle" [18]. Tracing the derivatives of these three epithelia—sinusal, mesonephric, and müllerian—has provided abundant fuel for scholarly dispute. This major epithelial puzzle is concerned with the origin and development of the epithelium of the vagina.

It is generally agreed that the vaginal portion of the fused müllerian ducts is initially lined by a pseudostratified columnar epithelium of müllerian origin. On contact with the epithelium of Müller's tubercle, this epithelium is replaced by a stratified squamous epithelium, a process starting caudally and extending in a cranial direction [19]. At about the

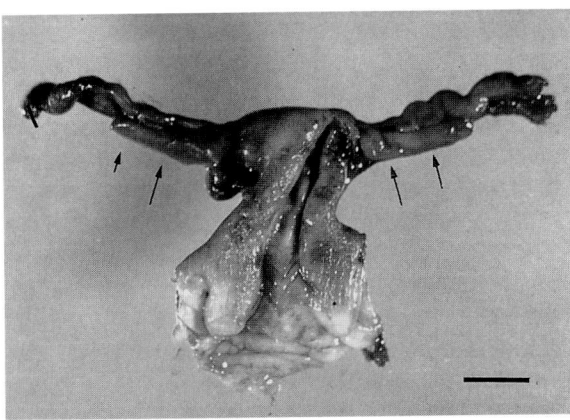

FIGURE 30.4. *Neonatal female internal genitalia. The ovaries (arrows) are elongated narrow structures suspended beneath the tortuous oviducts. The uterine corpus is small compared to the cervix. The exocervix and vagina are lined by squamous epithelium, which is thickened under the influence of maternal estrogens. Bar = 1 cm.*

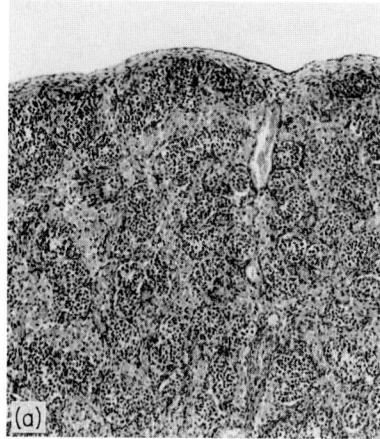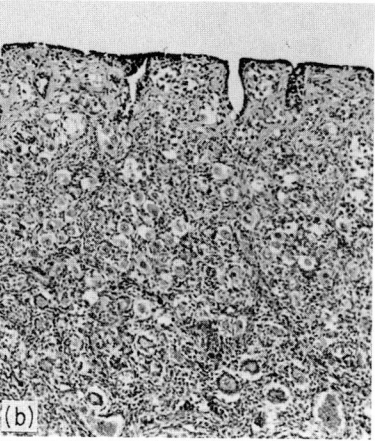

FIGURE 30.5. *(a) Testis from fetus at 14 weeks' gestation. The tunica albuginea has a smooth surface. (b) Ovary from a fetus at 16 weeks' gestation. The surface is punctuated by narrow grooves. H&E, ×148.*

same time a solid epithelial proliferation, the vaginal plate, appears between the urogenital sinus and the uterovaginal canal (Fig. 30.8). This cellular plate advances cranially, obliterating the existing vaginal lumen [15]. At its caudal extremity the plate begins to cavitate, forming a new lumen, the lining of which is formed by epithelium derived from the vaginal plate. Arrest of, or another distortion of, this process may produce obstructive lesions ranging from imperforate hymen and hydrocolpos to more serious forms of vaginal stenosis or atresia.

The origin of the plate itself is disputed. On morphological and histochemical grounds, Forsberg [19] considered it to be of mesonephric origin, whereas Vilas thought it to be derived from the epithelium of the sinus [20], reaching cranially well into the endocervical canal. Clearly, however, the vaginal epithelium is not normally of müllerian origin. As the fetus approaches term gestation, the vaginal epithelium accumulates glycogen and is thrown into prominent white folds (see Figs. 30.4 and 30.7). After birth, the squamous epithelium gradually thins as the effects of the mater-

nal estrogen wear off. (The urothelium in the bladder undergoes similar but milder changes in both male and female fetuses and neonates.) The hymen forms from a thickened, rolled fold of tissue along the dorsal aspect of the vaginal opening.

Having guided and perhaps contributed to the müllerian ducts, the mesonephric ducts in the female are of no further practical concern, and are largely discarded. Vestiges of the duct and the mesonephric tubules may persist and give rise to cystic swellings in the lateral walls of the vagina (Gartner's duct cysts), and persistence in the cervix, the lateral uterine wall, or the broad ligament is not uncommon [21].

By the end of the 10th week of gestation, the ovarian cortex contains numerous mitotically dividing germ cells called *oogonia*. The number of oogonia increases exponentially by mitotic division until approximately the 20th week, when the maximal number of germ cells, oogonia and oocytes, is about 7 million [22]. Extensive degeneration will, however, reduce the number of germ cells drastically during the rest of fetal life.

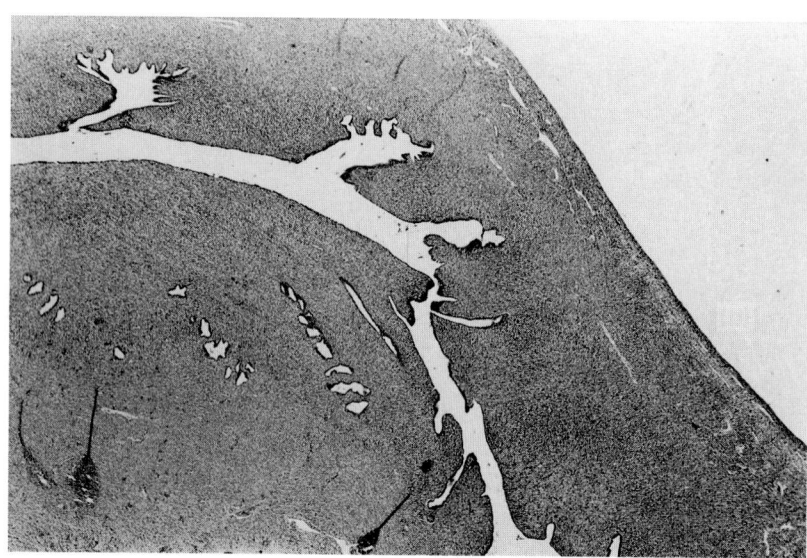

FIGURE 30.6. *Branching glands of the cervix in a fetus at 20 weeks' gestation. H&E, ×15.*

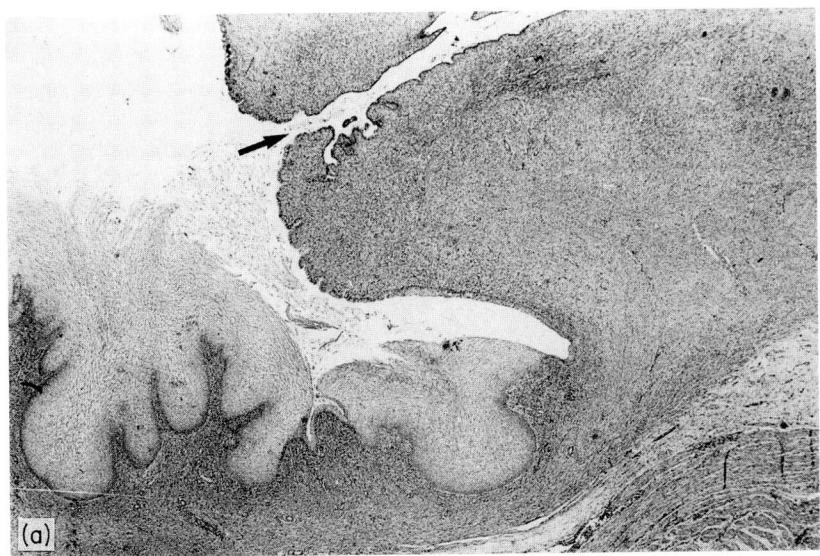

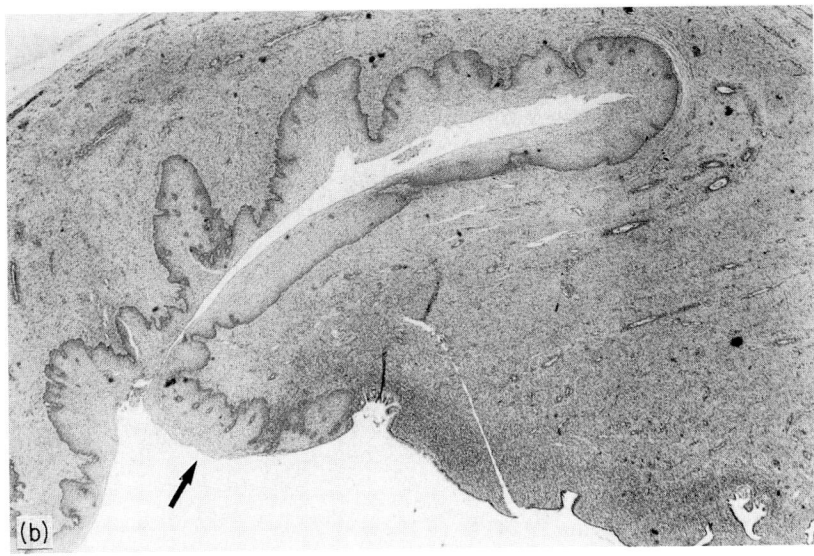

FIGURE 30.7.   *(a) In the later weeks of gestation the fornix and vagina have squamous epithelium, while columnar epithelium covers most of the portio of the cervix. The external os of the cervix is indicated by an arrow. H&E, ×15. (b) the distal endocervix, portio, fornix, and vagina are covered by squamous epithelium. The external os of the cervix is indicated by an arrow. H&E, ×15.*

When oogonia stop dividing and enter meiosis, they are termed *oocytes*. The first oocytes in the human ovary are seen during the 11th week of fetal life. Transformation of an oogonium into an oocyte and then into an ovum with a haploid number of chromosomes denotes oogenesis.

Meiosis begins with premeiotic DNA synthesis, followed by the transitory stages of the meiotic prophase. The first meiotic division is arrested when the diplotene stage is reached. The oocyte resumes meiosis just before ovulation or degenerates and may thus last for the whole fertile life span. Oocyte degeneration may occur at any time during development. With ovulation, first meiotic division resumes and proceeds with the second meiotic division, resulting in 23 chromosomes at the time of fertilization.

The maturation of individual follicles after puberty depends on multiple endocrine factors including recently described regulatory peptides such as activin and inhibin

[23–25]. Mature inhibin is a 32-kd glycoprotein that has been isolated from ovarian follicular fluid and is composed of a common α-subunit and two β-subunits, β_A and β_B [26–29]. Treatment of pituitary cell cultures with inhibin suppresses follicle-stimulating hormone (FSH) secretion, whereas treatment with the homodimeric β_A, β_A form of inhibin, termed *activin*, stimulates FSH release [30]. It is still uncertain whether the effects of inhibin and activin on pituitary FSH release in vitro reflect physiologically important functions of these proteins in the human endocrine system. However, intragonadal functions for inhibin and activin seem very likely, as suggested by the high degree of homology with the growth factors of the same family such as TGF-β and MIS [31, 32]. There is evidence that inhibin and activin may play a role in the selection of the dominant follicle in the menstrual cycle and also in controlling the follicular estrogen synthesis [23, 33, 34].

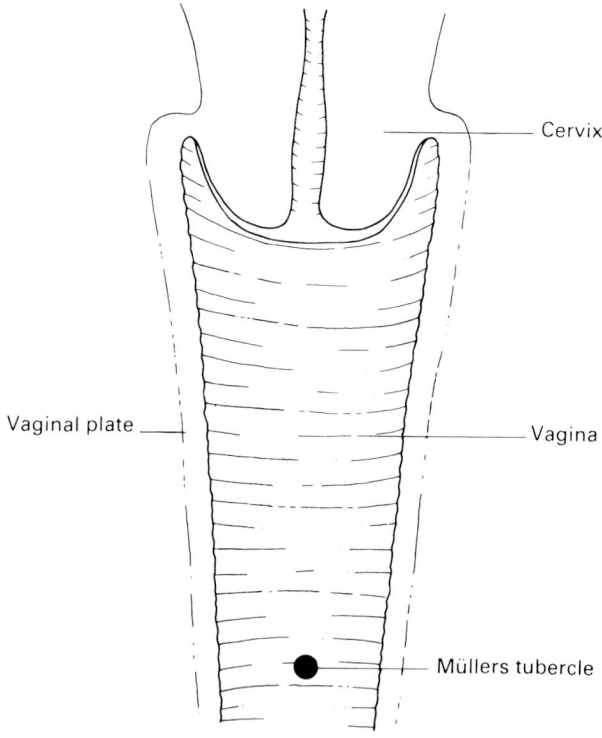

Cervix

Vaginal plate

Vagina

Müllers tubercle

FIGURE 30.8.   *Diagrammatic representation of the extent of müllerian contribution to vaginal development. The cells in the vaginal plate may originate from the urogenital sinus, or mesonephros.*

MALE GENITAL DEVELOPMENT

Normal testicular development depends on the presence of a Y chromosome, where the *SRY* gene is located. This factor is responsible for testicular differentiation [7, 8]. The tissue specificity and complementary ontogeny of *SRY* and *MIS* expression suggest that *SRY* may induce *MIS* transcription and that MIS may then act to support continued testicular and gender differentiation [7, 8]. Development of the associated male internal and external genitalia in turn depends on hormone production by the fetal testis. Thus, induction of testicular differentiation by the *SRY* gene is the initial regulatory event leading to the development of the entire male genital tract.

Even before morphological differentiation of the testis, the fate of the gonad has already been determined. The gonad that is to develop into a testis grows more rapidly than that destined to be an ovary [35]. Although this growth spurt is presumably under the control of the *SRY* gene, the gene clearly does not work alone and in some circumstances is not even essential for testicular formation [36].

Jost [37] summarized the morphological development of the testis and the male reproductive system as occurring in three phases: the beginning differentiation of the seminiferous tubules (15–17-mm stage or 47–49 days), the appearance of interstitial cells (28–30 mm or 55–56 days), and masculine organization of the genital tract.

The seminiferous tubules are composed of prespermatogonia and Sertoli (sustentacular) cells. Spermatogonia are the sparsely distributed large germ cells preceding meiosis. Secondary spermatogonia are not present in fetuses and neonates; they are the result of reduction division (meiosis) with a haploid set of chromosomes [38].

The secretory activity of the testis becomes quickly evident. In the rabbit embryo the onset of virilization of the male genital tract occurs approximately 1 day after the histological differentiation of the testis [39]. This virilization is effected in part by testosterone synthesis in the interstitial (Leydig) cells, the male analogue of theca cells, which differentiate from the stromal cells. In the human the peak of testosterone secretion occurs between 12 and 16 weeks [40].

Testosterone, incorporated into a target cell, may be converted to dihydrotestosterone by 5α-reductase. In general terms, testosterone is responsible for the utilization and virilization of the mesonephric ducts, and dihydrotestosterone for the virilization of the external genitalia [41]. Thus, absence of testosterone leads to a failure of the formation of both internal and external male genitalia whereas absence of the dihydrotestosterone leads to normal seminal vesicles, vasa deferentia, and prostatic tissues but feminized external genitalia.

Just as the developing ovary is faced with two sets of ducts, mesonephric and müllerian, so the testis is confronted by the same two sets. Its reaction is opposite to that of the ovary: The mesonephric duct is exploited and the müllerian ducts are largely discarded. The development of the mesonephric ducts is mediated by testosterone; the destruction of the müllerian ducts is the responsibility of MIS, a glycoprotein product of the Sertoli cells of the developing testis [7]. MIS remains at high levels in normal male serum for several years postnatally and by puberty it falls to a low baseline level, which is maintained throughout adult life [42]. In contrast, MIS is undetectable in newborn females but is measurable at low serum concentrations between puberty and the onset of menopause.

Regression of the müllerian ducts occurs prior to full development of the mesonephric ducts, beginning at the 30-mm stage [43]. The inhibiting substance, acting ipsilaterally, causes disappearance of all but the extreme cranial and caudal ends of the müllerian ducts. These persist as, respectively, the appendix testis and part of the prostatic utricle (uterus masculinus) [17].

The rete testis, formed in homologous fashion in both genders, establishes contact with the mesonephros, extending into the mesonephric stroma to link up with the mesonephric tubules. The tubules thus connected to the rete testis lose their glomeruli, but persist to form the efferent ductules that establish communication with the mesonephric duct. The efferent ductules, therefore, include the whole mesonephric unit—the glomerulus, tubule proper, and collecting tubule [3]. The mesonephric duct's fate is conversion to the exit passage for the male gametes— the epididymis, vas deferens, and seminal vesicles.

Table 30.1. Summary of embryonic urogenital structures and the adult derivatives

Male	Embryonic Structure	Female
Testis	Indifferent gonad	Ovary
Seminiferous tubules	Cortex	Ovarian follicles
Rete testis	Medulla	Rete ovarii
Gubernaculum testis	Gubernaculum	Ovarian ligament
		Round ligament of uterus
Ductuli efferentes	Mesonephric tubules	Epoöphoron
Paradidymis		Paroöphoron
Appendix of epididymis	Mesonephric duct	Appendix vesiculosa
Duct of epididymis		Duct of epoöphoron
Ductus deferens		Duct of Gartner
Ureter, pelvis, calyces, and collecting tubules		Ureter, pelvis, calyces, and collecting tubules
Ejaculatory duct and seminal vesicle		
Appendix of testis	Paramesonephric duct	Hydatid (of Morgagni)
		Uterine tube
		Uterus
Urinary bladder	Urogenital sinus	Urinary bladder
Urethra (except navicular fossa)		Urethra
Prostatic utricle		Vagina
Prostate gland		Urethral and paraurethral glands
Bulbourethral glands		Greater vestibular glands
Seminal colliculus	Sinus tubercle	Hymen
Penis	Phallus	Clitoris
Glans penis		Glans clitoridis
Corpus cavernosum penis		Corpora cavernosa clitoridis
Corpus spongiosum penis		Bulb of the vestibule
Ventral aspect of penis	Urogenital folds	Labia minora
Scrotum	Labioscrotal swellings	Labia majora

Modified from Moore KL, Persaud TVN. *The Developing Human: Clinically Oriented Embryology*. Philadelphia: W.B. Saunders, 1993. Table 13.1.

The differentiation of the testis is largely completed in the first third of gestation. In the final two thirds, the testis descends slowly toward an intrascrotal position—a descent that may possibly be initiated by MIS [39], and that may not be complete by birth.

DEVELOPMENT OF THE EXTERNAL GENITALIA

The development of the external genitalia is summarized in Figure 30.9. The external genitalia pass through a sexually undifferentiated stage. At 24 days following conception, a small protuberance, the genital tubercle, develops cranial to the cloacal membrane. Two sets of folds extend caudally from the genital tubercle; the external folds are the labioscrotal folds and the internal ones are the urogenital folds. The genital tubercle enlarges to form the phallus. At about 40–42 days following conception, the cloaca is divided into the urogenital sinus and the anorectal canal by the urorectal membrane, which fuses with and divides the cloacal membrane into the dorsal anal membrane and the ventral urogenital membrane. These membranes rupture at about 48–50 days. The urethral groove forms under the phallus and is continuous with the urogenital ostium.

Between 58 and 63 days following conception, the external genitalia begin to differentiate into male or female genitalia. In the male, testicular androgens cause the phallus to elongate, pulling the paired urogenital folds forward to form the lateral walls of the urethral groove on the undersurface of the penis. The folds fuse from the base toward the end (glans) of the phallus, thus forming the urethra. The end of the urethra is lined by an ectodermal epithelial derivative while along its length, the urethral epithelium is derived from the lining of the urogenital sinus (endoderm). A fold of skin grows over the glans to form the prepuce during the 12th week of gestation. It is loosely fused with the glans throughout gestation and for several weeks after birth. Corpora cavernosa and corpus spongiosum arise from the mesenchyme in the phallus. The lateral labioscrotal folds fuse in the sagittal plane to form the scrotum, a prominent raphe marking the course of fusion [44].

In the female, with the lack of testicular androgens, the phallus is small and becomes the clitoris. The urogenital folds become the labia minora and remain separated

Indifferent stage

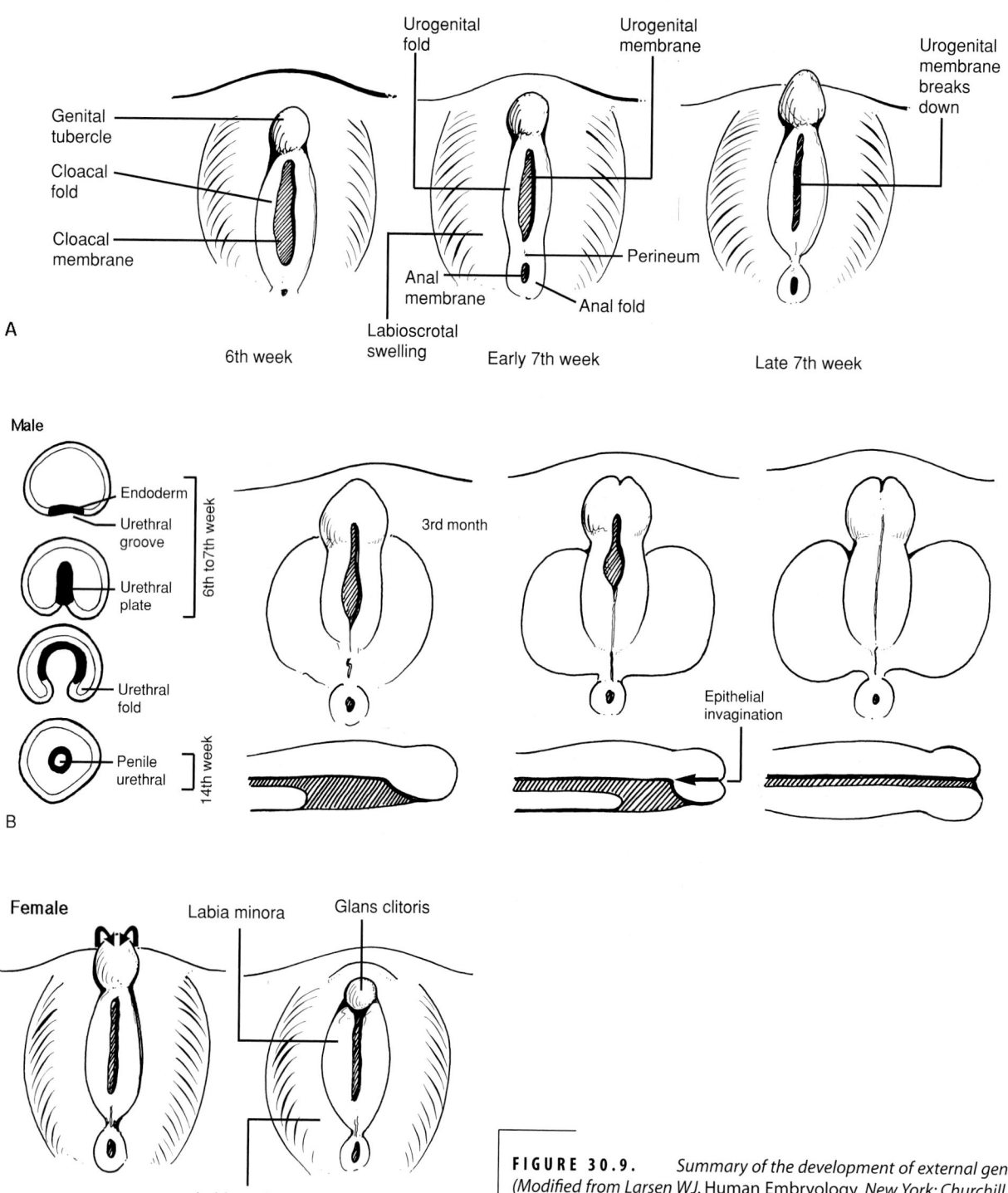

FIGURE 30.9.   *Summary of the development of external genitalia. (Modified from Larsen WJ. Human Embryology. New York: Churchill Livingstone, 1993. Fig. 10.18.)*

except just ventral to the anus. The urogenital sinus becomes the vaginal vestibule with the openings of the urethra, the vagina, and the vestibular glands. The major portions of the labioscrotal folds remain unfused except at the dorsal end

and at the ventral end, the latter contributing to the mons pubis.

Figure 30.10 illustrates the microscopic development of the ovary and testis through the later stages of fetal life.

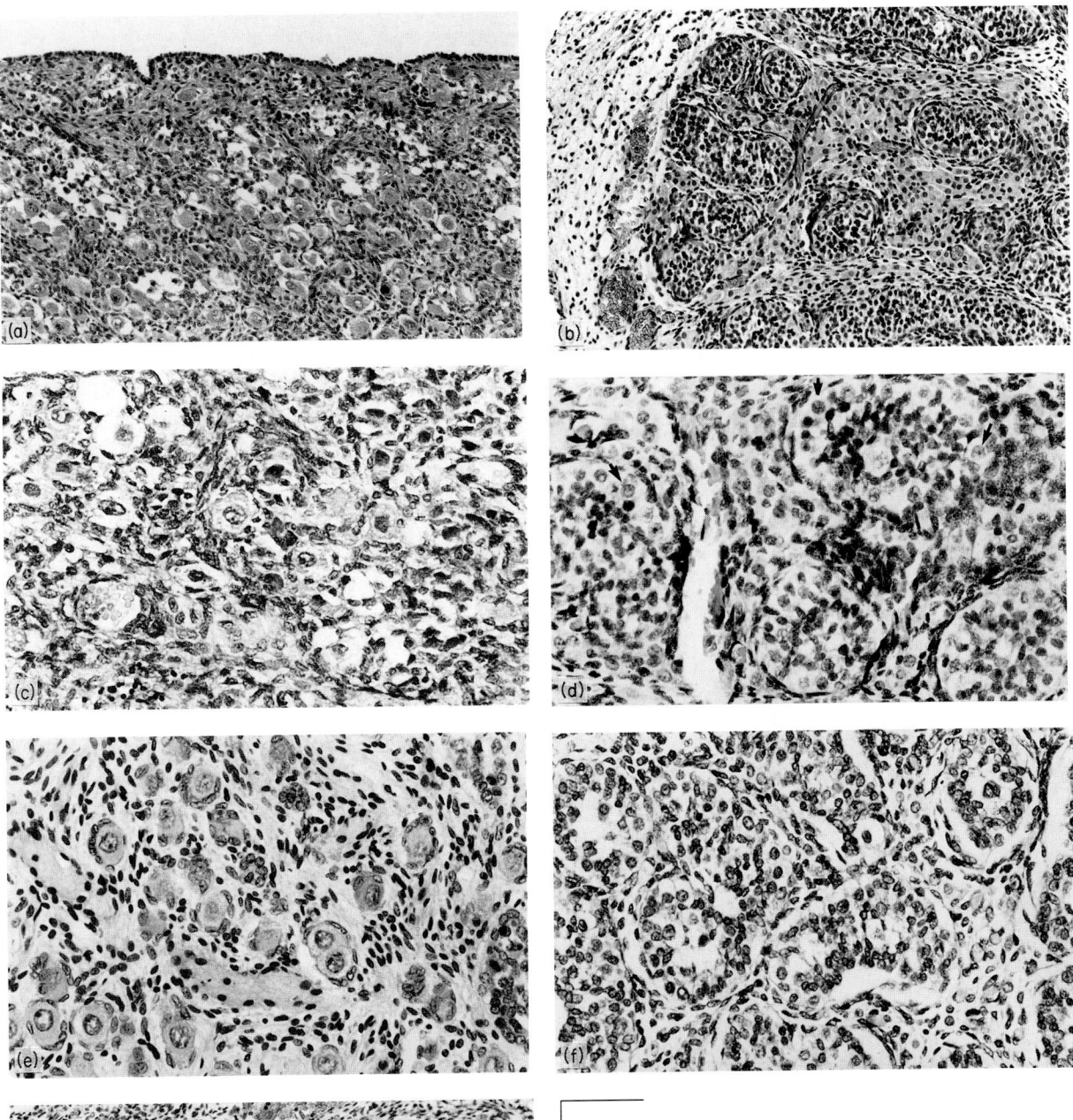

FIGURE 30.10.   *(a) Ovary from a fetus at 16 weeks' gestation. Primordial follicles are numerous but the oocytes are relatively small and granulosa cells are ill-defined. The stroma and indented surface epithelium (mesothelium) are prominent. H&E, ×108. (b) Testis from a fetus of 16 weeks' gestation. Seminiferous tubules are composed largely of Sertoli cells. Leydig cells, derived from the sex cords, are abundant. H&E, ×108. (c) Ovary from a fetus at 20 weeks' gestation. Primordial follicles are more clearly defined and granulosa cells are beginning to organize around the oocytes. H&E, ×204. (d) Testis from a fetus at 20 weeks' gestation. Seminiferous tubules are more cellular and a few spermatogonia are recognized (arrows). H&E, ×204. (e) Ovary from a newborn infant at 35 weeks' gestation. The primary follicles are well formed. Oocytes are still dividing— a follicle with 2 oocytes is found near the center of the photograph. H&E, ×204. (f) Testis from a newborn infant at 35 weeks' gestation. Spermatogonia are found in greater numbers. Tubular growth crowds the interstitium and Leydig cells are less conspicuous. H&E, ×204. (g) Ovary from an infant born at 40 weeks' gestation. In the deep cortex, some primary follicles have developed further. Some of these may enlarge to form macrosopic cysts. H&E, ×108.*

Table 30.1 summarizes the embryonic urogenital structures and the adult derivatives.

DISORDERS OF GENDER DEVELOPMENT

Gender determinants are multifaceted with several independent and interdependent sets to consider, namely, the external genitalia, the internal genitalia and duct differentiation, the gonads, the endocrine gender, genetic gender, nuclear gender, chromosomal gender, psychological gender, and social gender. Table 30.2 lists the conditions in which gender differentiation has the potential for disorder. It is clear, for example, that both 5α-reductase deficiency and androgen insensitivity are genetically controlled disease processes, and it seems probable that a similar genetic basis will ultimately be demonstrable for many disorders that, with present knowledge and understanding, are usually discussed on an anatomical or physiological level. Likewise, it seems equally reasonable to discuss Leydig cell agenesis as either an endocrine disorder (its most conspicuous manifestation) or a morphological gonadal disorder. The grouping of disorders in this section is based on the intersection of detectable disease processes, at whatever level, with the normal processes of differentiation. A number of chromosomal and genetic disorders may have gonadal or genital maldevelopment but are otherwise quite disparate, for example, micropenis in Prader-Willi syndrome and in some cases of Down syndrome; double uterus in both trisomy 13 and cryptophthalmia syndrome [45].

Disorders of Sex Chromatin

Monosomy Y

At least one X chromosome is essential for life. A pure YO constitution is lethal. It is not found even in teratomas. It is a biological non-entity.

Monosomy X (Turner Syndrome)

Monosomy X, commonly designated Turner syndrome, is a common sequela of conception and most affected embryos are spontaneously aborted [46]. Deficiency of cells with Barr bodies is almost always associated with a 45,X karyotype or with XX-XO mosaics [47]. In older children and adults, the classic gonad is the fibrous streak 2–3 cm long and about 0.5 cm thick, located at the usually expected site of the ovary. These streaks consist microscopically of recognizable ovarian stromal cells, a medulla, and a hilum. In the latter, both hilar (interstitial, Leydig) cells and a developed rete are present (Fig. 30.11).

The oocytes from the majority of XO gonads gradually disappear. In early embryonic and fetal development the gonad in the patient with Turner syndrome appears to be a normally developing ovary with a normal complement of oocytes. By the third trimester, however, a diminution of oocyte numbers is found [48]. This is attributed to ovarian dependence on the genetic activity of two X chromosomes,

Table 30.2. Disorder of gender differentiation

Disorders of sex chromatin
 Monosomy Y
 Monosomy X
 Polysomy X
  The XXX karyotype
  The XXY karyotype
 Polysomy Y
  The XYY karyotype
Disorders of the gonads
 Disorders of germ cell migration
 Dysgenetic ovaries and testes
  Mixed gonadal dysgenesis
  Pure gonadal dysgenesis
 Hermaphroditism
 Testicular regression syndromes
 Leydig cell agenesis
Endocrine disorders
 Persistent müllerian duct syndrome
 Central nervous system disorders
 Disorders of sex steroid function
  Disorders of steroid synthesis
Androgen resistance syndromes
 5α-Reductase deficiency
 Testicular feminization
Maternal endocrine disturbances
 Virilization during pregnancy
 Exogenous hormones
 Diethylstilbestrol
Ontogenic genitourinary anomalies
 Müllerian duct anomalies
 Urogenital sinus anomalies
 Sinus tubercle anomalies
 Phallic anomalies
 Cloacal anomalies
Miscellaneous genital disorders
 Tumors
 Trauma

both of which are in the active, non-condensed state in female germ cells [49].

Gonadal tumors in the neonate with Turner syndrome are never a problem, but in later life, gonadoblastoma [50], a mucinous cystadenoma with a Brenner tumor [51], and occasional tumors of the germ cell series [52] can occur. In older XO patients, endometrial carcinoma can develop after estrogen administration [53].

A large number and wide variety of phenotypic abnormalities occur in patients with Turner syndrome (see also Chap. 12). Among the more conspicuous in fetuses is lymph stasis of the hand or foot presenting as edema. Fluid accumulation around the neck is often a marked feature during fetal life, and at birth it is often represented by neck webbing, an involutionary residue. Coarctation of the aorta, ventricular septal defects, horseshoe kidney, double ureters,

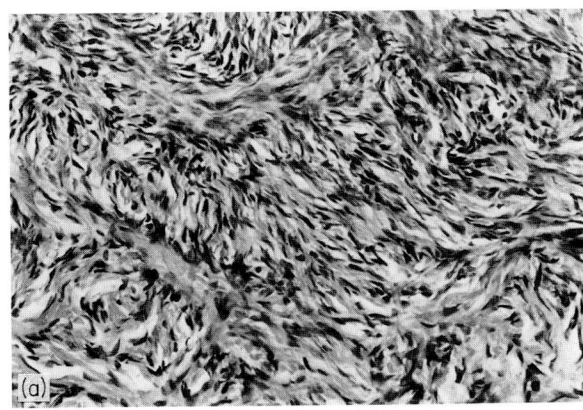

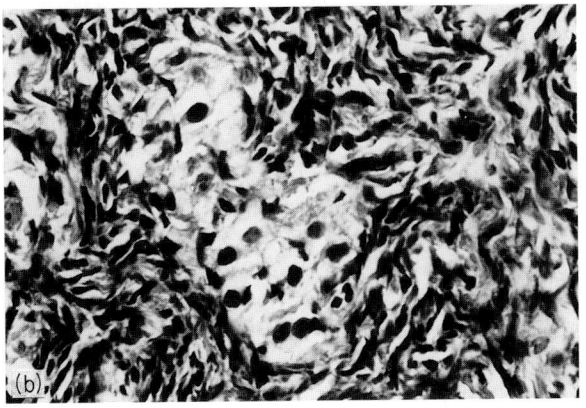

FIGURE 30.11. *(a) Ovarian stroma from a streak gonad in a child with Turner syndrome (45,XO). At birth, oocytes and follicles were most likely histologically normal but numerically deficient. H&E, ×180. (b) Leydig cells persist in the streak gonad. H&E, ×340.*

and minor renal rotational malformations are fairly common [54].

The most frequent karyotype in Turner syndrome is 45,X, that is, complete monosomy X (57%). Mosaic individuals may be 45,X/46,XX, in which case the effects of the monosomic cell line may be mitigated by the normal cell line. In addition, structural abnormalities of the X chromosome may produce partial monosomy of either the p or q arm or both. When one of the short arms is deleted, the Turner phenotype is always present, while normal gonadal development and function are generally preserved. However, this function is lost if the deletion extends to the proximal region of Xp11 [55]. Occasional patients with Turner syndrome menstruate and a few have become pregnant [56]. The 45,X/46,XY mosaicism is seen in 4% of Turner syndrome patients. The phenotype ranges from almost normal males with cryptorchidism or hypospadias to females indistinguishable from those with the 45,X Turner syndrome. On occasion this mosaicism may produce a phenotypically normal male, but if the gonads are intra-abdominal, they pose the hazard of germ cell tumor formation, and prophylactic gonadectomy must be considered [47].

Polysomy X

The XXX Karyotype Females with three X chromosomes may present with phenotypes ranging from mostly normal through mildly dysmorphic to severely retarded individuals. They may have hypertelorism, widely spaced nipples, skeletal anomalies, brachycephaly, and microcephaly that is associated with moderate to severe mental retardation. Infertility is a usual problem [57, 58].

This karyotype occurs in about 1 of every 1600 newborn females [47]. Diagnosis, when established at birth, is usually made purely by cytogenetic analysis. In later life the incidence of spontaneous abortion and pregnancy wastage is increased [59].

With increasing numbers of X chromosomes (XXXX or XXXXX), there is a consistently demonstrated mental retardation, and in some instances other phenotypic, often skeletal, abnormalities are present [60].

The XXY Karyotype (Klinefelter Syndrome) Barr bodies are found in approximately 1 out of 600 newborn males. Almost all of these children have the XXY karyotype (Klinefelter syndrome) and most are clinically normal at birth [47]. Occasional minor genital abnormalities (hypospadias) or extragenital manifestations are seen. The characteristic clinical features that become evident in adolescence are small atrophic testes, small penis, gynecomastia, incomplete virilization, variable eunuchoidism, and tendency to dull mentality. The main anatomical lesion of Klinefelter syndrome that occurs in adolescence or later is a testicular tubular degeneration with persisting Leydig cells [61].

Disorders of the Gonads

The important gonadal abnormalities are listed in Table 30.3.

Disorders of Germ Cell Migration

The failure of germ cells to migrate to the genital ridge will inevitably lead to agonadism [62]. Supernumerary or accessory gonads may be formed as a result of misguided migration of germ cells, or by a mechanism of detachment and reimplantation of gonadal ridge tissue after germ cell migration has been completed [63].

In an XX individual, bilateral agonadism seems likely to be the result of failed germ cell migration. In XY individuals a similar mechanism may be responsible, but in this case early testicular regression must also be considered. Sometimes germ cells migrate to extragonadal sites and this phenomenon may explain such lesions as sacrococcygeal teratoma [64].

Dysgenetic Ovaries and Testes

Mixed Gonadal Dysgenesis Mixed gonadal dysgenesis, the presence of a testis on one side and a fibrous streak on the other or bilateral dysgenetic testes and müllerian derivatives, is usually associated with 45,X/46,XY mosaicism but other combinations may be found. In the absence of appropriate

Table 30.3.   Gonadal anomalies

Gonadal agenesis
Small ovaries or testes
Supernumerary gonads
Dysgenetic ovaries or testes
Germinal and epithelial cysts of ovaries or testes
Ovotestes

gonadal induction as a testis, seminiferous tubular differentiation does not take place, and MIS is produced in only small amounts or not at all, resulting in retention of müllerian ducts. Leydig cell differentiation may also be deficient or delayed, which leads to subnormal or late production of testosterone and incomplete masculinization. There are three clinical categories. Ninety percent of the cases present with ambiguous genitalia and 10% present with unambiguous male or female external genitalia. Somatic features of Turner syndrome may be present. Gonadoblastomas may develop in the dysgenetic gonads. The *SRY* coding region is normal in the small number of patients studied thus far [7].

Pure Gonadal Dysgenesis (Swyer Syndrome)   The presence of bilateral streak gonads in a 46,XY individual with female external genitalia and normal müllerian derivatives is called pure gonadal dysgenesis. There are no somatic anomalies present. In older patients the external genitalia are female but have an infantile character. Breast development is minimal and axillary and pubic hair are sparse. Testosterone and estrogen levels may be decreased but FSH usually is more than 40 mIU/mL. Histologically the streak gonads have a similar appearance as those seen with Turner syndrome. Twenty percent to 30% of patients develop gonadal neoplasia in the dysgenetic gonads. Most of the neoplasias are gonadoblastomas. Dysgerminomas, juvenile granulosa tumors, seminomas, and mature and immature teratomas have been described. So far 11 mutations in the *SRY* region have been described. Not all patients with pure gonadal dysgenesis show these mutations [65, 66].

Other dysgenetic ovaries may be associated with chromosomal and non-chromosomal conditions. Potter [67] described one infant born at term with small cordlike ovaries that were normal in length but were only a fraction of normal in diameter. Rare germ cells were detected and no primordial or more advanced follicles were found. Ovarian hypoplasia with varying degrees of dysgenesis is described with both trisomy 13 and trisomy 18 [45]. We examined a term female infant with 4p-syndrome in whom the ovaries were narrow and had poorly developed oogonia and primordial follicles (Fig. 30.12).

Coerdt et al [64], using morphometric techniques, showed that the number and volume of testicular premeiotic germ cells from fetuses and neonates with trisomy 13, trisomy 18, or XYY are reduced by 50–75%. Impaired migration of germ cells to the gonadal ridge or decreased mitotic activity may account for these reductions. Anencephaly is said to cause reduced numbers of germ cells, probably on the basis of reduced Leydig cell numbers and activity [64].

Hermaphroditism

"True" gonadal hermaphroditism, the presence of both ovarian follicles and testicular tubules, may develop with bilateral ovotestes, an ovary on one side, usually the left, and a testis on the other, usually the right, or an ovotestis on one side may coexist with a streak gonad. Most often an

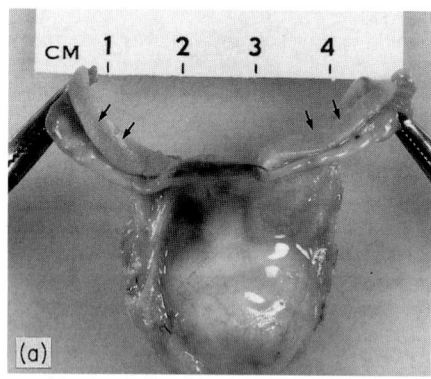

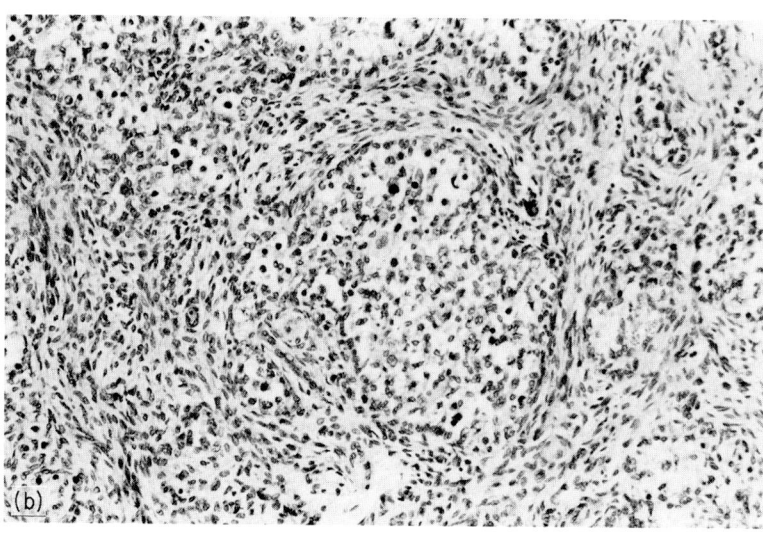

FIGURE 30.12.   *(a) Flattened ovaries (arrows) from a baby with 4p-syndrome. (b) The ovarian cortex is disorganized with ill-defined primordial follicles and small oogonia. H&E, ×180. DHEA = dehydroepiandrosterone.*

ovotestis is identified [68–70]. Ovotestes with more testicular than ovarian tissue are usually in an inguinal or scrotal position, whereas gonads with predominantly ovarian tissue are most often located intra-abdominally [69]. The incidence of gonadal hermaphroditism in postnatal subjects is about 0.2% but it is 5 to 6 times higher among embryos in the first 40–56 days of gestation [68].

The karyotype of true hermaphroditism is XX in 60% or more of patients but a few are 46,XY, 46,XX/46,XY, or 46,XX/47,XXY. Their external genitalia are usually ambiguous or predominantly male with hypospadias and bifid scrotum. A vagina and a well-differentiated uterus are usually present. A familial distribution is noted in some and others result from an autosomal recessive mutation [71].

Among patients with ostensibly an XX constitution the most common presentation of hermaphroditism is an ovary on one side and an ovotestis on the other [72]. Among 79 true hermaphrodites with a Y chromosome in van Niekerk and Retief's series [69], a testis was found in 48 (61%), a finding consistent with the concept that the presence of a Y chromosome increases the probability that a testis is one of the gonads present [69]. The presence of testicular tissue in individuals lacking a Y chromosome (i.e., 46,XX true hermaphrodites) could be explained in at least four ways: 1) undetected mosaicism or chimerism, presence of undetected 46,XY cells; 2) translocation of *SRY* gene locus to an X chromosome; 3) translocation of *SRY* gene locus to an autosome; 4) mutant gene(s). Each of these may explain certain cases but the most common etiology is still undetermined. The macroscopic appearance of an ovotestis is usually diagnostic, the ovarian and testicular tissue being arranged in an end-to-end fashion. The ovarian portion of an ovotestis has a convoluted surface, whereas the testicular component is smooth (see Fig. 30.5).

Phenotypic expression in true hermaphroditism ranges from almost normal female to almost normal male (Table 30.4). Approximately half of these patients are raised as males and half as females [69, 70, 72].

MIS produced by the testicular tissue will cause müllerian hypoplasia, persistence of the corpus alone, complete absence of the uterus, or unicornuate uterus in up to 90% of individuals. On the other hand, it should be noted that ovulation occurs in ovarian tissue and phenotypic females with hermaphroditism may be fertile [70, 73].

With a male phenotype, testosterone appears capable of differentiating the mesonephric (wolffian) duct, but dihydrotestosterone may be deficient, leading to poorly developed male external genitalia. In most cases only a partial virilization of the external genitalia is present. Production of spermatozoa has not been observed [70] and only 12% of patients have a penile urethra [69].

Testicular Regression Syndrome

Testicular regression syndrome can be defined as a total absence of testes in a 46,XY individual. The external genitalia may have varying degrees of male differentiation. The

Table 30.4. Classification of intersex

Ambiguous internal genitalia
  Gonadal hermaphroditism
  Testicular regression syndrome
  Persistent müllerian duct syndrome
  Testicular feminization
Ambiguous external genitalia
  45,X/46,XY mosaics (mixed gonadal dysgenesis)
  XXY (Klinefelter) syndrome
  Gonadal hermaphroditism
  Late testicular regression
  Leydig cell agenesis
  20,22-Desmolase deficiency
  3β-Hydroxysteroid dehydrogenase deficiency
  17α-Hydroxylase deficiency
  21α-Hydroxylase deficiency
  11β-Hydroxylase deficiency
  5α-Reductase deficiency
  Incomplete testicular feminization
  Maternal virilizing ovarian tumors
  Maternal ingestion of androgenic hormones
Phenotypic external male genitalia in gonadal and chromosomal female
  Maternal virilizing ovarian tumors
  Maternal ingestion of androgenic hormones
  21α-Hydroxylase deficiency
Phenotypic external female genitalia in gonadal and chromosomal male
  Gonadal hermaphroditism (rare)
  Testicular regression syndrome
  Leydig cell agenesis
  20,22-Desmolase deficiency
  17α-Hydroxylase deficiency
  17,20-Desmolase deficiency
  17-Ketosteroid reductase deficiency
  5α-Reductase deficiency
  Testicular feminization syndromes

presence of the *SRY* gene, which is located in the Y chromosome, is required for the undifferentiated gonad to become a testis. In the presence of this gene, a testis will form after 7 weeks' gestation and start secreting MIS and testosterone for the male differentiation of the external and internal genitalia. If, however, the testis degenerates and its function fails, depending precisely on the timing of testicular failure, both internal and external genitalia will reflect only that degree of masculinization appropriate to the stage of development at which testicular failure occurred.

Testicular failure prior to the secretion of MIS or testosterone will allow a continued feminine development. If a testis is formed and secretes MIS, the derivatives of the müllerian ducts, the oviducts, uterus, cervix, and vagina, will be compromised. If testosterone continues to be secreted, the external genitalia will be masculinized and the mesonephric duct will be fully developed. The same pathological lesion—testicular failure in XY agonadal individuals—may result in a phenotypic female at one extreme, a phenotypic male at the other, and a variety of intermediate forms, dependent solely on the precise timing of the failure of testicular secretions [74]. The name *testicular regression syndrome* encompasses a number of other designations such as pure gonadal dysgenesis, Swyer syndrome, vanishing testis, true agonadism, and familial anorchia.

Failure of testicular development may result from failure of germ cell migration to the genital ridge. If testicular formation is successfully initiated and is then followed by regression, the etiology is usually not known, but a notable familial incidence indicates a genetic basis for many of these cases.

Dating the onset of testicular failure is possible in the majority of affected individuals. If the phenotype is female and the internal genitalia are absent, then the damaging agent must have affected the genital ridge prior to the onset of müllerian differentiation (day 43 of development). Patients with rudimentary testes and a micropenis have normal mesonephric (wolffian) derivatives. In their case the damage occurred after 90 days when the mesonephric duct is completely developed and before 140 days when masculinization of the external genitalia is completed [75]. Onset may also be localized to the time frame between the initiation and the completion of the action of MIS or testosterone.

In some cases of late testicular regression, vessels extend to the termination of the vas, although the testis and epididymis are absent [76]. This suggests that the testis was originally present and was damaged at some point during descent.

Leydig Cell Agenesis
A rare disorder is the absence of Leydig (interstitial) cells and consequently a deficiency of testosterone [77]. In this condition the external genitalia are female as a result of the lack of testosterone, but with unimpaired production of MIS the derivatives of the müllerian ducts are absent. In older patients, markedly hyalinized seminiferous tubules are lined by normal Sertoli cells and occasional immature germ cells. No Leydig cells are identifiable by light or electron microscopy. The testosterone level is low despite elevated FSH and luteinizing hormone levels. A normal epididymis and vas deferens are present so that small amounts of testosterone, secreted by the adrenals and possibly by the Sertoli cells, are postulated for the development of these structures. Leydig cell agenesis is diagnosed at or before birth only if investigation is prompted by the detection of an XY chromosomal pattern in a phenotypic female.

Endocrine Disorders

Persistent Müllerian Duct Syndrome
Isolated persistence of müllerian duct derivatives in otherwise normal males results from failure of MIS. The action of MIS requires secretion of a biologically active compound, proper timing of the action, and acceptance by appropriate müllerian tissue receptors. Failure at any one of these steps

may be the basis of müllerian duct persistence. Evaluation of MIS in the sera of affected boys has been helpful in delineating the etiology of this disorder. Because these boys may have either normal or undetectable serum MIS levels, this disorder is believed to be heterogeneous, characterized by a defect in MIS secretion in some patients and by end-organ responsiveness in others [78]. In one study, testicular biopsy specimens from 5 patients with persistent müllerian duct syndrome were positive for MIS messenger RNA by Northern blot analysis, but only 2 of the 5 specimens were positive for bioactive MIS [79]. The remaining 3 patients were siblings who were later identified as having an *MIS* nonsense mutation. This point mutation produced a premature stop signal that interrupted the translation of the *MIS*, resulting in an inactive protein. The other MIS-positive patients probably have MIS receptor defects. Diagnosis may be made in male fetuses or neonates investigated for cryptorchidism or hernia, particularly if the syndrome has been discovered in the patient's male siblings. The müllerian ducts form a uterus with bilateral oviducts arising from the prostate and frequently dislocated into inguinal hernias [61]. The external genitalia are male, but most patients are cryptorchid either unilaterally or bilaterally, raising the question of a role for MIS in the normal descent of the testis [39, 80]. A familial incidence is most common [80, 81], but sporadic cases occur [82]. Testicular pathology is comparable to those of any cryptorchid testis and germ cell neoplasms are also a hazard in later life. The condition should be distinguished from mixed gonadal dysgenesis in which 45,XO/46,XY mosaicism may result in a testis on one side and a streak gonad on the other [83]. On the side of the streak gonad, müllerian structures may persist—a strictly unilateral phenomenon.

Central Nervous System Disorders
Disorders of reproductive organs can result from failures of gonadotropin production or release. Both defective gonadotropin and no gonadotropin at all have been reported [84]. A genetic basis, as for other causes of male pseudohermaphroditism, is postulated. These are rare disorders with the noteworthy exception of anencephaly, but in that condition the lack of cerebral tissue is likely to overshadow that of gonadal dysfunction [64].

Disorders of Sex Steroid Function
In spite of the ubiquity of estrogens during intrauterine life, or perhaps because of that very pervasiveness, estrogens play a limited role in the development of the reproductive system in either gender. Circulating estrogens are bound by fetoneonatal estrogen-binding protein, a compound closely related to or indistinguishable from α-fetoprotein. This protein, which circulates in high concentration during the latter part of gestation and then gradually disappears over the first few weeks of postnatal life, binds and deactivates the estrogens in the fetal and neonatal circulations, but it does not bind testosterone.

Paradoxically, the major developmental action of estradiol is in the "masculinization" of the central nervous system. In males testosterone is free to enter the brain where it is converted by local aromatization to estradiol. Circulating estradiol is prevented by protein binding from exercising this role [85]. Sex hormone disorders in utero and in the neonate, therefore, depend fundamentally on an excessive or on a deficient action of androgens, primarily testosterone. As usual, one must consider not only quantitative variations in the production of biologically active androgens, but also the timing of their appearance and the tissue response mediated by receptors.

Disorders of Steroid Synthesis

20,22-Desmolase Deficiency. The initial step in the construction of the endocrinologically active steroid molecule is the conversion of cholesterol to 5-pregnenolone under the influence of 20,22-desmolase (Fig. 30.13). Deficiency of this enzyme causes an accumulation of cholesterol and hence massive hyperplasia of the adrenals. The adrenal cells are markedly distended and filled with cholesterol. Synthesis of all gonadal and adrenal hormones is blocked, male

fetuses have female external genitalia, but since MIS production is not depressed, normal regression of the müllerian ducts occurs in these fetuses. In both genders there is severe adrenocortical insufficiency, and most individuals die in early infancy. Changes in the testis and ovary are, at best, minor and questionable.

3β-Hydroxysteroid Dehydrogenase Deficiency. Both adrenal and gonadal hormones are disturbed by deficiency of 3β-*OH* dehydrogenase, an enzyme that normally intersects at several points with steroid synthesis. Severe adrenocortical deficiency is the result with neonatal addisonian crises. Testosterone synthesis is disrupted and male external genitalia are not virilized. In this case, however, dihydroepiandrosterone, which is weakly androgenic, accumulates. It leads to genital ambiguity with hypospadias in males and to clitoromegaly without labial fusion in females. The genital anomaly may be compounded because the liver isoenzyme is not affected and some testosterone may be formed from accumulated precursors [86]. At autopsy the adrenals are enlarged and the cells are filled with lipid.

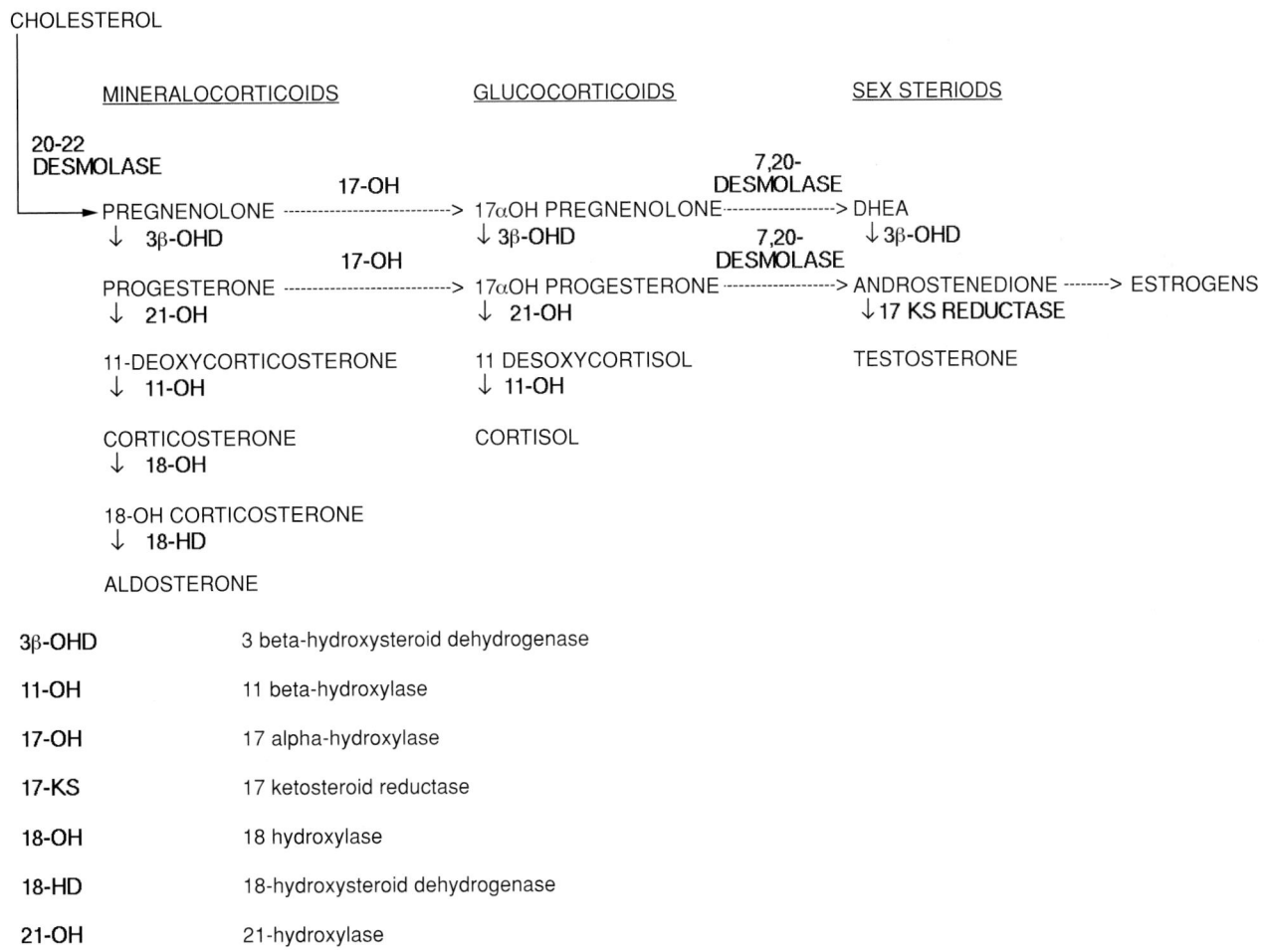

FIGURE 30.13. *Schema for the biosynthesis of steroids as the basis for the development of ambiguous genitalia.*

17α-Hydroxylase Deficiency. In deficiency of 17α-hydroxylase, the pathways leading to mineralocorticoid synthesis are unaffected, but those involved in the synthesis of cortisol, testosterone, and estrogens are blocked. Male infants usually show female external genitalia, with occasional ambiguous genitalia.

21α-Hydroxylase Deficiency. By far the most important enzyme deficiency in this group of disorders is deficiency of 21α-hydroxylase, accounting for 70% of female pseudohermaphroditism in the United States [87]. The deficiency is an autosomal recessive disorder. The responsible gene is located on chromosome 6. Homozygosity and heterozygosity can be determined by haplotyping [88]. Both the pathway leading to aldosterone synthesis and that leading to the production of cortisol are interrupted. Adrenocorticotropin hormone (ACTH) secretion is increased and the adrenals are enlarged 6 to 8 times. Hyperplastic accessory adrenocortical nodules are often found in the retroperitoneum, broad ligament, and mesovarium and adjacent to the testis and epididymis [61]. Normal steroidogenesis proceeds to the progesterone or 17-hydroxyprogesterone level before 21α-hydroxylase deficiency becomes apparent. Testosterone is derived from 17-hydroxyprogesterone by way of androstenedione, some of this conversion occurring in such locations as the liver [86]. Virilization of the female infant varies considerably depending both on the severity of the enzymatic defect and on the timing of the endocrine effects. The clitoris may be enlarged. The urethra and vagina may open together at the base of this enlarged clitoris, superficially suggesting hypospadias. In males the penis may be enlarged and the scrotum rugose. Rarely the gonads contain tumors or tumor-like nodules composed of testicular interstitial cells [89]. Salt loss may be life-threatening but there may be sufficient mineralocorticoid production to prevent salt loss (simple virilizing congenital adrenal hyperplasia).

11β-Hydroxylase Deficiency. In 11β-hydroxylase deficiency both deoxycorticosterone and deoxycortisol (compound S) accumulate behind the enzyme block. ACTH is secreted in excess in response to the deoxycorticosterone and a mineralocorticoid excess syndrome results. The excess deoxycortisol is transformed to androgens. The result is the presence of hypertension in both genders and ambiguous external genitalia in females [71]. In some cases virilization does not appear until after puberty, and in others hypertension is not a feature.

17,20-Desmolase and 17-Ketosteroid Reductase Deficiencies. Deficiencies of 17,20-desmolase and 17-ketosteroid reductase do not involve the adrenocortical hormones, but are confined to the pathways of gonadal hormone synthesis. In both deficiencies the effects are female external genitalia in an XY male, and in both the critical enzymatic deficiency can be determined by measurement of the accumulated precursors. 17-Ketosteroid reductase deficiency has been identified in some women with polycystic ovary disease.

Androgen Resistance Syndromes

The term *androgen resistance syndrome* denotes a group of disorders, of which the most important members are 5α-reductase deficiency and testicular feminization.

5α-Reductase Deficiency
The disorder now known as 5α-reductase deficiency was described in 1961 as a specific variety of hereditary male pseudohermaphroditism [90]. The name *pseudovaginal perineoscrotal hypospadias* was descriptive of the main clinical features. The disease is now almost invariably known as 5α-reductase deficiency [91–93] and is believed to represent the homozygous state of an autosomal recessive gene. Abnormal sexual development occurs only in males. Normal development and normal fertility are found in homozygous 46,XX individuals.

Testosterone converts to dihydrotestosterone as a result of 5α-reductase action [94]. In the presence of low levels or complete absence of this enzyme, the seminal vesicles, ejaculatory ducts, epididymes, and vasa deferentia are present but because of the reduced dihydrotestosterone, the external genitalia are generally female or ambiguous. The ejaculatory ducts open into a short vagina, implying that the failure of male gender differentiation is largely confined to derivatives of the urogenital sinus and the urogenital tubercle, fold, and swelling, areas in which dihydrotestosterone is considered to be the major intracellular hormonal agent [92]. The testes in these patients are relatively normal, and since there is ample MIS, the müllerian-derived structures are absent, other than the usual vestiges of normal males.

At puberty there may be variable degrees of virilization with lengthening of the penis, growth and pigmentation of the scrotum, and enlargement and descent of the testes. In a few cases, prepubertal enlargement of the penis may prompt reconsideration of the gender of the patient. Despite a female gender-of-rearing, subjects have a remarkable tendency to adopt a male sexual identity and orientation at puberty [95].

Complete Testicular Feminization
Testicular feminization has been recognized in genetic males since the pedigree analyses of Petterson and Bonner in 1937 [96]. The term *testicular feminization* was introduced in 1953 [97]. The main clinical features are regular and predictable [98]; the external genitalia are clearly female and the clitoris is not enlarged. Although the vagina is short and ends blindly and the karyotype is 46,XY, these patients are usually identified at birth as girls, and are so raised. The gonads, which may be found in the abdomen, in the inguinal canals, or in the labia majora, are testes. Testicular production of MIS is unimpaired so there are no female internal genitalia, save for occasional vestiges. Little is known of testicular histology at birth but later the findings are those of long-standing cryptorchidism of whatever cause. At puberty the

breasts, the distribution of body fat, and the general habitus are unmistakably feminine. Axillary and pubic hair, however, is scanty or absent. Amenorrhea is the single most common symptom for which these patients seek medical advice and on which the diagnosis is first suspected. Testicular feminization is a genetic X-linked disorder. The androgen receptor locus is X-linked in humans and mice, and a homologous disorder occurs in the Tfm mouse [99, 100]. A defect in the receptor protein that binds testosterone and dihydrotestosterone to target cells and transports these androgens to the nuclei has been demonstrated [101–104]. In patients who meet the clinical and endocrine criteria for complete androgen resistance, yet who do not appear to have abnormal receptor activity by current tests, androgen resistance may be due to still-unidentified faulty postreceptor or parareceptor factors.

Incomplete Testicular Feminization

An incomplete form of the disorder involves about 10% of patients, often in the same kindred as those with complete testicular feminization. In many respects this resembles the classic form of the disorder, save for some ambiguity of the external genitalia [105–107]. Pedigrees are compatible with an X-linkage and it is now generally accepted that the condition represents varying degrees of defects involving the androgen receptor protein. The most common presentation in a newborn male is perineoscrotal hypospadias, and sometimes a pseudovagina. Cryptorchidism with small testes is common. Some patients have wolffian duct abnormalities such as absence or severe hypoplasia of the vas deferens. In later life, defective spermatogenesis and the anatomical defects may contribute significantly to infertility. At puberty there is some virilization as well as the more usual feminization [108].

A variety of genetic defects in the androgen receptor gene have been characterized in individuals with testicular feminization syndromes. A point mutation [101] and a large deletion [102] in the androgen-binding domain of the receptor gene as well as aberrant splicing [103] and a premature termination codon in the messenger RNA [104] have been described. Most recently, X-linked spinal and bulbar muscular atrophy was found to be associated with an androgen receptor gene mutation [109].

Testicular germ cell neoplasia is not a concern in the neonate but is the most serious potential hazard of testicular feminization [110]. Castration after puberty is recommended for patients except for those with the incomplete form, in whom some androgenic effects may be best avoided by prepubertal castration [111].

Maternal Endocrine Disturbances

Unique among endocrine organs, the ovary is capable of endocrine activity in response to almost any intraovarian mass. This startling property is probably because the ovary responds to an expanding lesion just as it does normally to an expanding follicle, that is, by activation of theca cells or by conversion of stromal cells to functioning theca. The hormones produced may be estrogens or androgens. Estrogens are not important influences in gestation. Androgens may virilize the mother. They have no significant effect on a male fetus, the "infant Hercules" being a purely postnatal phenomenon, but on a female fetus the effects can be striking, and depend critically on the timing of the androgen exposure. When a virilizing ovarian lesion such as a polycystic ovary or a Sertoli-Leydig cell tumor antedates gestation, there may be significant alteration of the normal fetal female genitalia: When the virilization develops late in pregnancy, the effects may be limited to relatively mild enlargement of the clitoris or to mild rugation and occasionally fusion of the labia [112]. So far, no case of extraovarian disease causing virilization during pregnancy has been reported. All cases have been ovarian in origin with a wide variety of ovarian masses, but most commonly the so-called luteoma of pregnancy [112, 113]. With luteomas, raised levels of testosterone and dihydrotestosterone tend to occur only late in pregnancy with only mild degrees of fetal virilization. It is of interest, from the maternal point of view, that the changes induced in the mother by a lesion that has become actively virilizing as a result of the pregnancy tend to regress quickly when the pregnancy is over.

Exogenous Hormones

Oral contraceptives, usually taken inadvertently at the beginning of an unsuspected pregnancy, have been associated with reproductive system manifestations at birth. Those containing 19-nortestosterone derivatives may produce such mild virilizing changes as clitoral enlargement. Depending on the time of gestation at which the progestins were administered, there may be some labioscrotal fusion. Though the changes are usually mild, they may cause sexual ambiguity and rarely to male gender assignment. Other progestins such as medroxyprogesterone acetate have been similarly incriminated, but conclusive evidence is lacking. In the male fetus progestins may occasionally give rise to hypospadias [114]. In any case, the genital changes produced by exposure to exogenous progestins are limited to the period of exposure. When the agent is withdrawn, there is no progression of the disorder, and the gonads and internal genitalia are unaffected [58].

Diethylstilbestrol

In the 1940s diethylstilbestrol (DES) was administered to patients considered to be in danger of abortion. It was finally realized that, as a savior of precarious pregnancies, DES was ineffective. However, it appeared to do little harm and its use continued in the hope that it might possibly be doing some good. In 1970 there was a report of an unusual cluster of 7 cases of adenocarcinoma of the vagina in adolescents of which were clear-cell carcinomas [115]. One year later the intrauterine exposure of these patients to DES was confirmed [116]. Clear-cell carcinoma was a rare complication (about 1 case/1200 exposures), but vaginal adenosis was a common, almost constant, complication of intrauterine DES exposure and the lesion could be detected in fetuses from 29–36 weeks' gestational age [117–120]. Adenosis is the abnormal presence of glandular epithelium in the vagina (Fig. 30.14). The glandular cells may resemble those of the endocervix, or either tubal or endometrial cells, or an indeterminate "tuboendometrial" type. The epithelium might line superficially located glands or it might cover or replace the surface-stratified squamous epithelium. Adenosis is more common in the upper part of the vagina, and less so in the lower third. There is a difference in the distribution of glandular epithelium, all cases in the lower vagina being of the tuboendometrial type, while only 21% of this type of epithelium is found in adenosis of the upper vagina. Vaginal adenosis occurs in three-fourths of individuals whose mothers began taking DES in the first 2 months of pregnancy but in only 7% of those initially exposed in the 17th week or later. None of 19 subjects whose mothers began therapy in the 18th week or later were found to have adenosis [121]. The basis of DES action is believed to be related to the estrogen-binding protein (demonstrable in mice and rats), which effectively sequesters natural estrogens in the fetal and neonatal circulations [85]. Synthetic estrogens such as DES are much less effectively bound, and their estrogen effects are unfettered. The result, according to this widely held hypothesis, is the partial retention of müllerian epithelium in the fetal vagina. Stromal anomalies such as vaginal ridges and septa have been linked to the influence of mesenchyme on epithelial differentiation. This led to an alternative hypothesis that the primary DES-induced effect is the failure of segregation of the mesenchymal layers, which determine the ratio of mucinous to tuboendometrial epithelium in various parts of the genital tract [122].

Table 30.5. Developmental genital anomalies

Müllerian duct (uterine) anomalies
    Class I—segmental müllerian agenesis or hypoplasia. The location of the defect
      may be vaginal, cervical, fundal, or a combination of these.
    Class II—unicornuate uterus
    Class III—uterus didelphys
    Class IV—bicornuate uterus
    Class V—septate uterus
    Class VI—uterus with internal luminal changes (e.g., diethylstilbestrol)
Urogenital sinus anomalies
    Atresia of the urethra and vagina
    Exstrophy of the bladder
    Hypospadias
    Epispadias
Sinus tubercle anomalies
    Imperforate hymen
Phallic anomalies
    Absence of phallus
    Micropenis
Cloacal anomalies
    Cloacal dysgenesis

Ontogenic Genitourinary Anomalies

Table 30.5 lists the developmental genitourinary anomalies.

Müllerian Duct Anomalies

Anomalies of the müllerian ducts most commonly present as clinical problems during the reproductive years, when they may be responsible for amenorrhea, infertility, or obstetric problems. They may present in the newborn when secretions accumulate proximal to an atretic vagina, at autopsy when lesser anomalies are discovered, or in the course of investigating another, usually renal, problem.

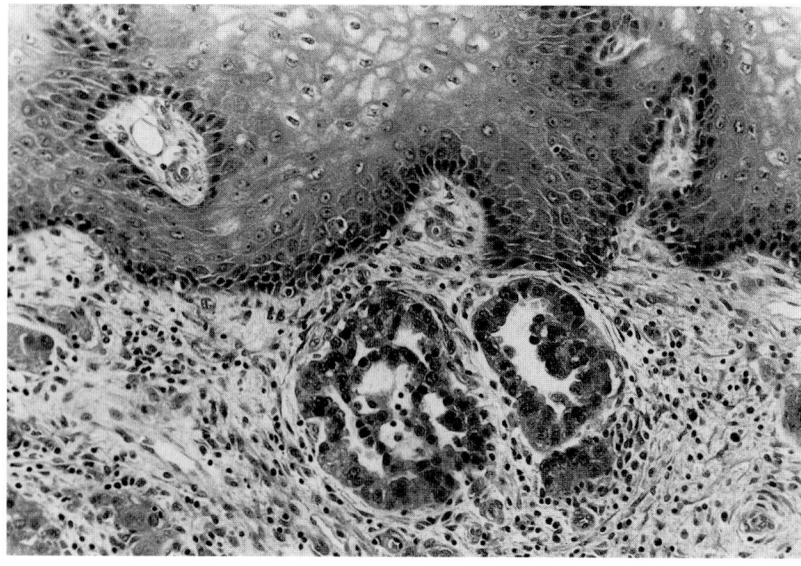

FIGURE 30.14. *Vaginal adenosis. H&E, ×94.*

There are a number of classifications of müllerian duct abnormalities, each charting an uneasy course between the Scylla of a too-simplistic approach and the Charybdis of unnecessary complexity. A recent and acceptable classification is that of Buttram and Gibbons [123] who list 6 major classes of anomaly, with numerous subdivisions (see Table 30.5).

Class I malformations are most often represented by some sort of vaginal malformation, such as imperforate hymen or the more severe vaginal agenesis, combined with a cervical or fundal abnormality or both. Vaginal atresia occurs about once in every 4000 or 5000 births. In the newborn period secretions proximal to an atretic vagina can cause massive abdominal swelling, which may be confused with or accompanied by acute urinary retention [124]. Approximately one-third of patients have an abnormal appearing intravenous pyelogram, and 12% have skeletal abnormalities. Other congenital abnormalities include congenital heart lesions and, occasionally, deafness [125].

A sagittal vaginal septum, which may be present alone or may coexist with other müllerian anomalies, is most often found concurrently with class III, IV, or V anomalies. Duplication of müllerian derivatives progresses in a cephalad-caudal direction with septa in the sagittal plane. When the uterus is duplicated, the cervix and vagina may be single; when both uterus and cervix are duplicated, the vagina may

be single, and so on (Fig. 30.15). Even when the uterus is duplicated, the more caudal double structures are often fused. Exceptions occur in exstrophy of the bladder, which is associated with widely separated duplicated vaginas and cervixes.

Absence of müllerian derivatives occurs with sirenomelia [67]. The urogenital sinus may remain undivided when the vesicovaginal and rectovesicle or rectovaginal septa fail to completely form (Fig. 30.16). This leaves a single cavity, the so-called persistent cloaca, into which the urinary, intestinal, and genital tracts empty. Any of these tracts may be obstructed due to stenosis or atresia of their openings into the common cavity.

Cloacal Dysgenesis Sequence

When the embryo is formed of 3 germ layers, the caudal and craniad ends of the endoderm fuse with the ectoderm to form membranes without intervening mesoderm. Interposition of mesoderm results in failure of ectodermal-endodermal fusion, varying degrees of cloacal dysgenesis, and agenesis of the caudal (cloacal) and the craniad (oropharyngeal) membrane (see Fig. 30.16) [126]. In the fetus and newborn, dysgenesis of the cloaca is reflected by absence of anal, genital, and urinary orifices in the perineum. Smooth intact skin is found in the region ordinarily occupied by the labia, vaginal vestibule, and anus in females and by the

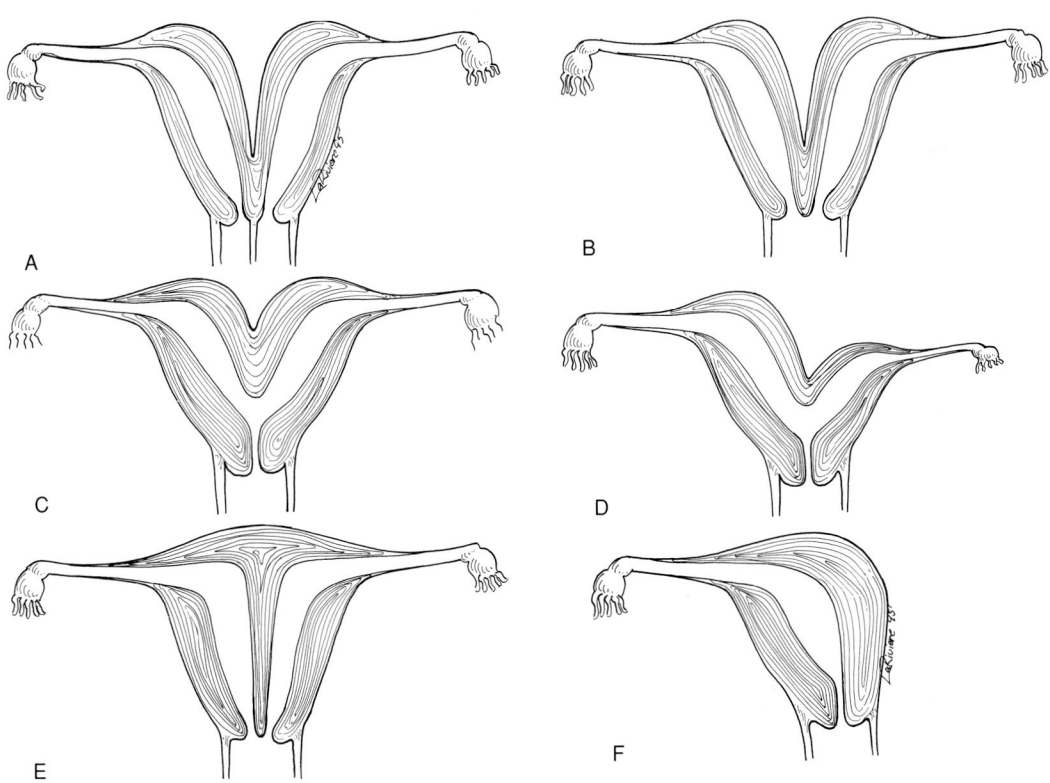

FIGURE 30.15. *Various types of congenital uterine anomalies: (A) double uterus (uterus didelphys) and double vagina; (B) double uterus with single vagina; (C) bicornuate uterus; (D) bicornuate uterus with a rudimentary left horn; (E) septate uterus; (F) unicornuate uterus.*

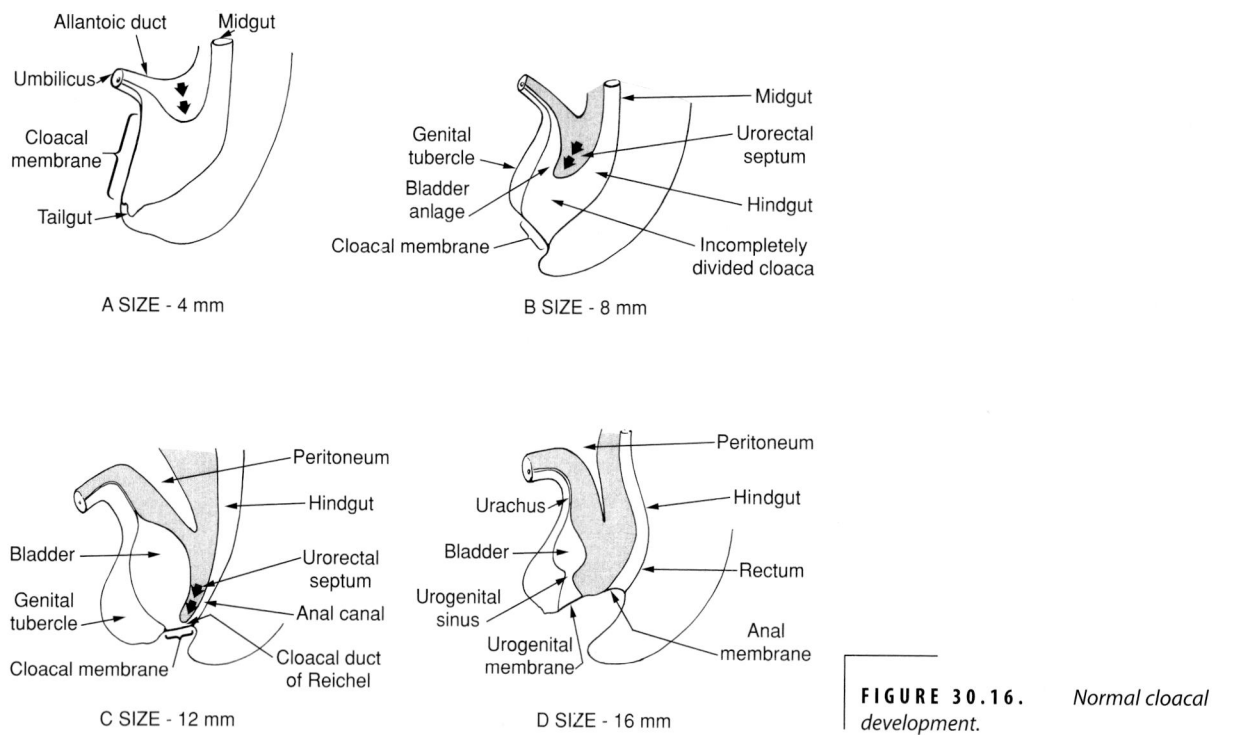

FIGURE 30.16.   *Normal cloacal development.*

scrotum, perineum, and anus in males. No median perineal raphe is present but a rudimentary phallus usually projects from the inferior border of the symphysis pubis (Fig. 30.17). Associated hindgut and genitourinary malformations are those associated with atresias of all the usual openings including those of the vestibular glands. In severe cases, the primitive cloaca where the rectum and the ureters drain may persist. In milder forms there may only be agenesis of the cloacal membrane with near-normal internal structures. Distention of the hollow viscera produces deformations such as patent urachus, megacystis, megaureters, renal dysplasia, hydrocolpos, and megacolon. Some viscera may perforate, leading to inflammatory lesions in the peritoneum or pelvis. Prune belly is an associated feature in either males or females (Fig. 30.18). Müllerian structures are sometimes duplicated. Testes are flattened and located in the abdomen and the vasa deferentia are attenuated or atretic. An anal dimple may be located in the skin high over the sacrum [127].

Hypospadias and Epispadias

If the embryonic urogenital folds do not entirely enclose the end of the urogenital sinus, varying degrees of hypospadias develop. These abnormally located urethral openings are among the most common of male genital malformations. In mild form the urethral meatus is located on the inferior aspect of the end of the penis, beneath the glans. In more severe forms, it develops closer to the base of the penile shaft and then the penis is usually shortened so that it may be mistaken for a clitoris. The scrotum may be prominently

cleft, resembling labia; testes may be undescended, making the assignment of gender a difficult task.

Epispadias is the opening of the urethra on the dorsal aspect of the penis. It may on occasion be associated with exstrophy of the bladder, and in this case the urethra is laid open to the exterior throughout its length. Occasionally a secondary meatus, communicating with an otherwise normal urethra, may be present on the dorsum of the penis.

Penile Agenesis and Micropenis

Complete absence of the penis is rare but not incompatible with life, except when associated with acardiac or sireniform anomalies. It results from failure in the development of the genital tubercle. Genitourinary abnormalities may include cryptorchidism; hypoplasia or agenesis of the prostate, kidneys, bladder, and ureters; polycystic kidneys; and abnormalities of renal location [128]. Anomalies of the anus, rectum, and lower colon may also be found. When the bladder is absent, the ureters usually open individually into the intestine, or may end blindly: When the bladder is normal, the urethra usually opens into the rectum. Micropenis is associated with many chromosomal, genetic, structural, and endocrine developmental defects [45] (Fig. 30.19).

Trauma

One of the major disadvantages of the ovary is its exposure, via the vagina and müllerian duct derivatives, to environmental agents, some of which may be carcinogenic. It is protected, on the other hand, from the day-to-day traumas that

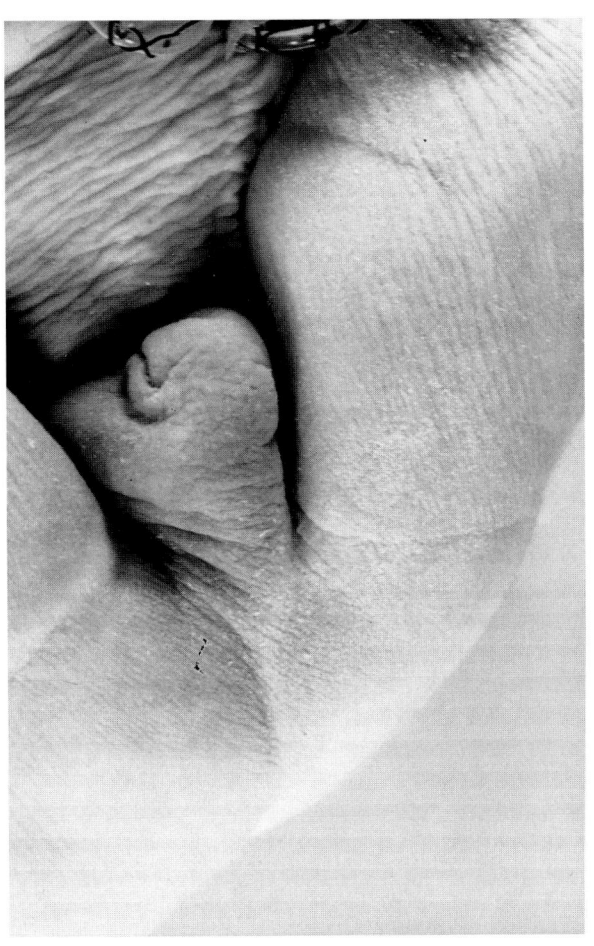

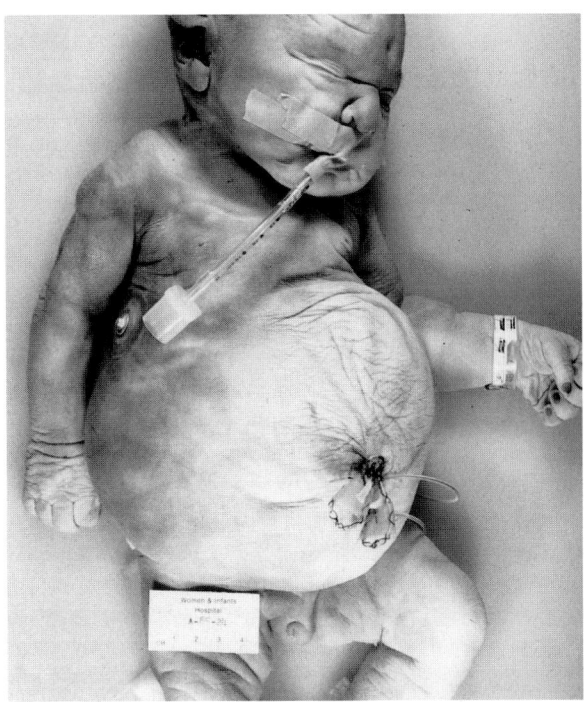

FIGURE 30.18.   *Prune-belly syndrome in a male with cloacal dysgenesis syndrome.*

FIGURE 30.17.   *The smooth perineum in a baby with cloacal membrane dysgenesis. A rudimentary phallus is present; wrinkled skin in the lower abdomen is reflective of the prune-belly syndrome.*

threaten the testis. Delivery, particularly when associated with a breech presentation, is a time of considerable testicular hazard. Congestion and edema of the scrotum may be associated with interstitial hemorrhage of the testis [129]. Frank infarction of the testis in the newborn is usually associated with torsion of the testis on the spermatic cord [130]. When the processus vaginalis communicates with the peritoneal cavity, then the testis is exposed to bleeding from whatever intra-abdominal source that may derive.

With perforation of the bowel wall in utero, meconium may gain access to the tunica vaginalis, with a resultant periorchitis, a differential in the diagnosis of neonatal scrotal lesions [131].

Neoplasms of the Reproductive System

Although ovarian enlargement due to non-neoplastic follicle retention cysts is relatively frequent, true neoplasms of the gonads are rare in the fetal or neonatal period. Each gonad, testis or ovary, is composed of three primary tissues—the surface epithelium (mesothelium), the sex cord–stroma complex, and the germ cells. Each of these tissues gives rise to its own characteristic tumor group, the differences between the tumors of the two genders being largely differences of incidence and prognosis, with only minor variations in histological appearances.

Ovarian follicle cysts are almost universally found in prepubertal girls. While less frequent in neonates and fetuses, they are found often enough to preclude alarm at their presence (Fig. 30.20). The follicle cysts may be single but are usually present in small numbers. In a baby with Donohue syndrome (leprechaunism), both ovaries were massive due to multiple follicular cysts (Fig. 30.21).

In the fetus or neonate the most characteristic neoplasm (or neoplasm-like lesion) is the gonadoblastoma [132] (Fig. 30.22). This is a proliferation of a mixture of cell types reminiscent of the cells involved in the formation of the early gonad. The cells include germ cells and smaller epithelial cells resembling immature Sertoli and granulosa cells. There may be luteinized stromal cells or cells indistinguishable from Leydig cells. In most cases, focal calcifications, often forming mulberry-like masses, are a conspicuous feature. The size of the tumors ranges from microscopic to 8 cm in diameter. The majority of patients with gonadoblastomas have a 46,XY karyotype or an 45,X/46,XY mosaic karyotype. They are, however, phenotypically female, with or without virilization. Only 13 of 74 patients in Scully's series were phenotypic males [132]. Gonadoblastoma usually

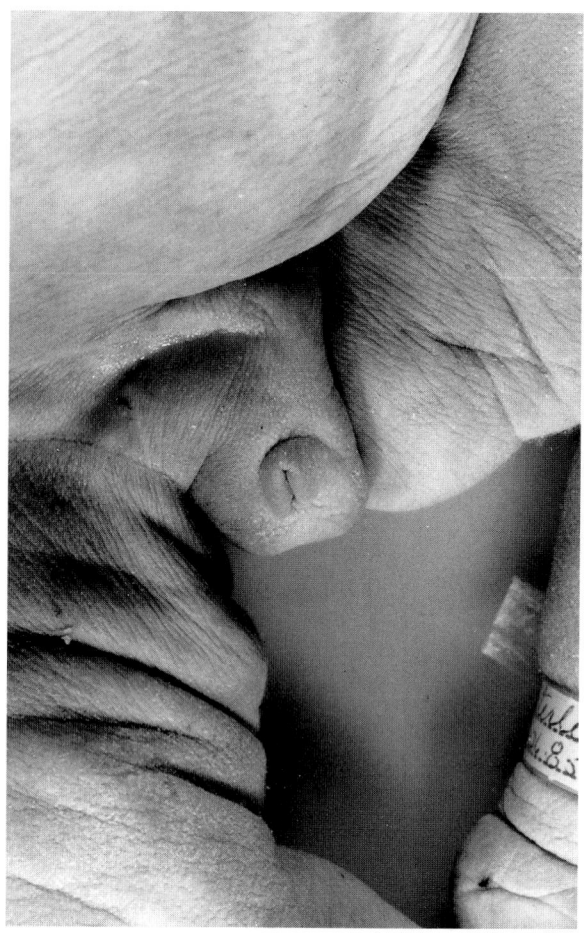

FIGURE 30.19. *Micropenis.*

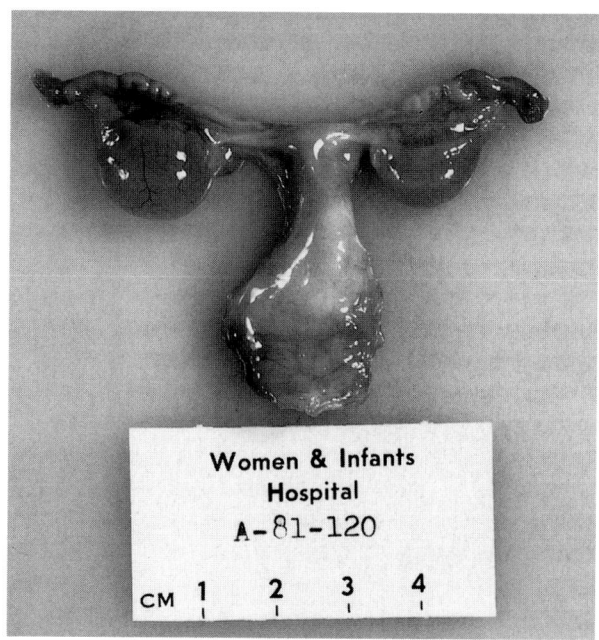

FIGURE 30.20. *A single large cystic follicle is found in each ovary from this newborn infant.*

develops in a dysgenetic gonad. The lesion, however, may be found in women who are capable of ovulation and occasionally of pregnancy [133]. The gonadoblastoma may be bilateral, but a pure gonadoblastoma never invades and never metastasizes. Its implicit menace lies in the germ cells that it contains. Alone of the constituent cells of a gonadoblastoma, these germ cells may show mitotic activity and may give rise to tumor of the germ cell series, usually a germi-

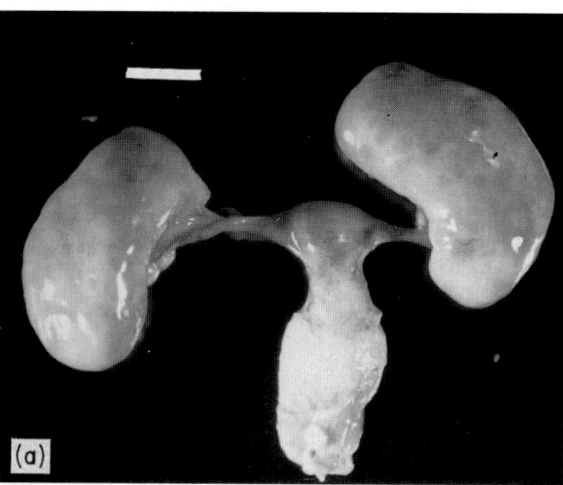

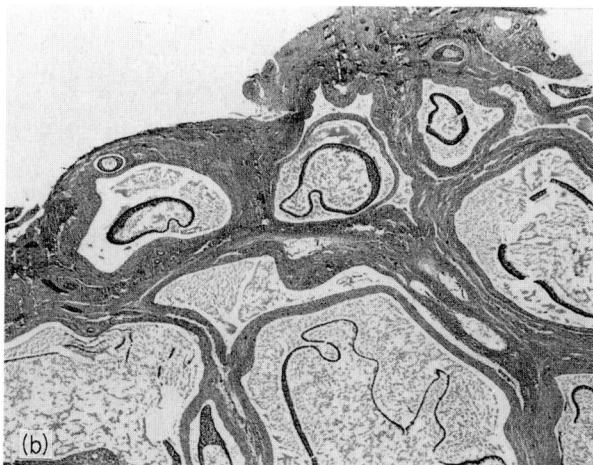

FIGURE 30.21. *(a) Massive enlargement of ovaries due to multiple cysts in a baby with Donohue syndrome (leprechaunism). (Case contributed by Dr. Milton Finegold, Houston, TX.) Bar = 1 cm. (b) The multiple follicle cysts are lined by granulosa cells that have separated from the theca and float in the follicular fluid. Primordial and primary follicles are sparsely distributed in the cortex. H&E, ×13.*

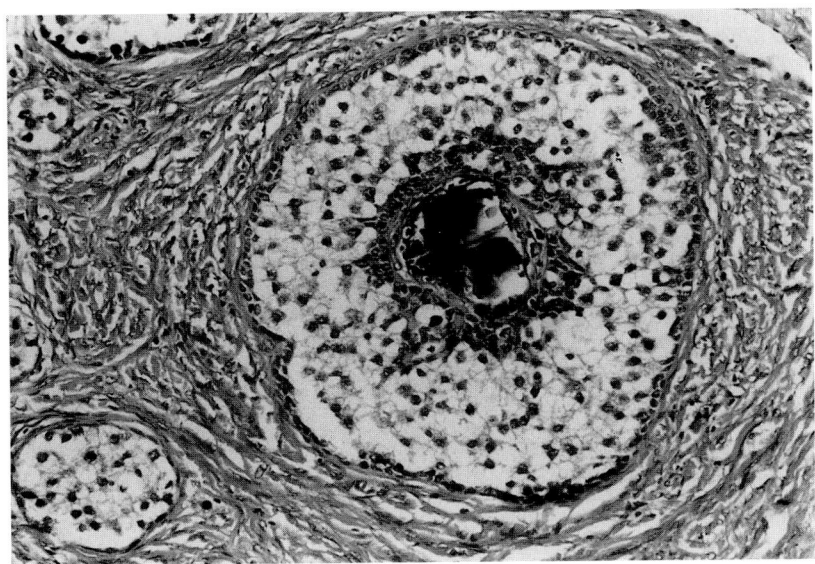

FIGURE 30.22.   *Characteristic microscopic appearance of gonadoblastoma. H&E, ×94.*

noma (dysgerminoma, seminoma), though such tumors as endodermal sinus tumors or choriocarcinoma may be found.

Epithelial Tumors

In the neonatal period and prepubertal child, testicular epithelial tumors are nonexistent. Ovarian epithelial tumors are rare before menarche and none have been reported in neonates [134, 135].

Sex Cord–Stroma Tumors

Sex cord–stroma tumors are rare, but not unknown, in the newborn. In one series 18 testicular sex cord–stroma tumors were found in children under 6 months old. Seven were found in liveborn neonates, and 1 in a stillborn with a gestational age of 30 weeks [136]. Of these 18 tumors, 14 had the pattern of juvenile granulosa cell tumor, a tumor type more commonly associated with the ovary. As in the adult type of granulosa cell tumor, granulosa cells and theca cells form a variety of solid and follicular patterns, and can be distinguished by reticulin staining. In the testis, no endocrine disturbances have been noted, and the prognosis has generally been good. In the neonatal ovary a similar tumor may be found [137]. The microscopic appearances of the tumors are similar, but in later years isosexual precocity and clinical malignancy may be found.

Pure neoplastic proliferations of Leydig cells or of theca cells may occasionally be encountered in the newborn period.

Germ Cell Tumors

Tumors of the germ cell series are the most commonly encountered gonadal neoplasms of infancy. Their frequency is relative rather than absolute, but of the tumors found, the endodermal sinus tumor is the most usual pattern [138]. This tumor is characterized microscopically by clear cells and a prominent perivascular arrangement of tumor cells with the appearance of "glomeruloid" Schiller-Duval bodies. It is also characterized by such tumor products as α-fetoprotein, as α_1-antitrypsin, albumin, and transferrin [139]. Although the endodermal sinus tumor is a feared malignancy in other situations, in the testis the prognosis during the first year of life is usually better than the histological features would suggest. About two-thirds of the patients survive.

Histologically malignant germ cell tumors of the gonads are more common in the testis than the ovary. This sexual bias is not reflected in the case of extragonadal germ cell tumors. The endodermal sinus tumor in the female may present as a polypoid vaginal mass [140]. Again, the prognosis in infancy may be better than initially expected.

Teratomas

Teratomas are considerably more common in extragonadal locations, such as the sacrococcygeal region, than in the gonads themselves. They are more common in females (ratio approximately 4 females to 1 male). Most sacrococcygeal teratomas in full-term infants are evident at birth [141] and if they are completely excised, the prognosis is excellent [142]. Delay in treatment may allow the emergence of malignant elements, especially the endodermal sinus tumor. As in adults, extragonadal teratomas may be found in a variety of other locations, usually in the midline.

Sarcoma Botryoides

Of the non-gonadal, non–germ cell tumors that may occasionally affect the reproductive system in both genders in the neonatal period, the most important is sarcoma botryoides. Grossly this tumor presents as an aggregation of fleshy polypoid masses arising in the neighborhood of the cervix or prostate. Microscopically, the tumor is an embryonal alveolar rhabdomyosarcoma, characterized by a so-called cambium layer underlying normal epithelium, and having a core of tumor cells, some of which may show cross-striations and in which myoglobin may be demonstrated by immunoperoxidase techniques.

The Mammary Glands

The mammary glands are first detectable in the 6th week of gestation as narrow, ribbon-like thickenings of the ectoderm extending ventrally from near the origin of the anterior limb buds to near the origin of the posterior. This so-called milk line is common to all mammals, and though normally in humans only a small area near the upper part of each line develops, supernumerary breast or nipple tissue may be found, usually, though not invariably, along the milk line.

Breast disease is extremely uncommon in the newborn, though expressible secretion may be present, and on occasion this may become infected. Hemorrhages and foci of extramedullary hemopoiesis may be found in the neonatal breast.

REFERENCES

1. Jost A. Problems of fetal endocrinology: the gonadal and hypophyseal hormones. *Recent Prog Horm Res* 1955; 8:379–418.
2. Witschli E. Migrations of the germ cells of human embryos from the yolk sac to the primitive gonadal folds. *Contrib Embryol Carnegie Inst* 1948; 32:67–80.
3. Gillman J. The development of the gonads in man with a consideration of the role of fetal endocrines and the histogenesis of ovarian tumors. *Contrib Embryol Carnegie Inst* 1948; 32:81–131.
4. O'Rahilly R. The timing and sequence of events in the development of the human reproductive system during the embryonic period proper. *Anat Embryol* 1983; 166:247–61.
5. Sinclair A, Berta P, Palmer M, et al. A gene from the human sex-determining region encodes a protein with homology to a conserved DNA-binding motif. *Nature* 1990; 346:240–4.
6. Whitfield L, Lovell-Badge T, Goodfellow P. Rapid sequence evolution of the mammalian sex-determining gene SRY. *Nature* 1993; 364:713–5.
7. Gustafson M, Donahoe P. Male sex determination: current concepts of male sexual differentiation. *Annu Rev Med* 1994; 45:505–24.
8. Haqq C, King C-Y, Ukiyama E, et al. Molecular basis of mammalian sexual determination: activation of müllerian inhibiting substance gene expression by SRY. *Science* 1994; 266:1494–500.
9. Cate R, Mattaliano R, Hession C, et al. Isolation of the bovine and human genes for müllerian inhibiting substance and expression of the human gene in animal cells. *Cell* 1986; 45:685–98.
10. Cohen-Hagenauer O, Picard J, Graciano A, et al. Mapping the gene for anti-müllerian hormone to the short arm of the human chromosome 19. *Cytogenet Cell Genet* 1987; 44:2–6.
11. Bardoni B, Zanaria E, Guioli S, et al. A dosage sensitive locus at chromosome Xp21 is involved in male to female sex reversal. *Nat Genet* 1994; 7:497–501.
12. van Wagenen G, Simpson M. *Embryology of the Ovary and Testis*. New Haven: Yale University Press, 1965.
13. Satoh M. Histogenesis and organogenesis of the gonad in human embryos. *J Anat* 1991; 177:85–107.
14. Byskov A. Differentiation of mammalian embryonic gonad. *Physiol Rev* 1986; 66:71–117.
15. O'Rahilly R. *The Embryology and Anatomy of the Uterus*. Baltimore: Williams & Wilkins, 1973.
16. Boyd E. *An Introduction to Human Biology an Anatomy for First Year Medical Students*. Denver: Child Research Council, 1952.
17. Gruenwald P. The relation of the growing müllerian duct to the Wolffian duct and its importance for the genesis of malformations. *Anat Rec* 1941; 81:1–19.
18. Glenister T. The development of the utricle and of the so-called "middle" or "median" lobe of the human prostate. *J Anat* 1962; 96:443–55.
19. Forsberg J. The origin of vaginal epithelium. *Obstet Gynecol* 1965; 25:787–91.
20. Vilas E. Uber die entwicklung der menschlichen scheide. *Z Anat Entwicklungsgesch* 1932; 98:263–92.
21. Huffman J. Mesonephric remnants in the cervix. *Am J Obstet Gynecol* 1948; 56:23–40.
22. Baker T. Oogenesis and ovarian development. In: Balin H, Glasser S, eds. *Reproductive Biology*. Amsterdam: Excerpta Medica, 1973, pp. 398–437.
23. Hillier S. Regulatory functions for inhibin and activin in human ovaries. *J Endocrinol* 1991; 131:171–5.
24. Dye R, Rabinovici J, Jaffe R. Inhibin and activin in reproductive biology. *Obstet Gynecol Surv* 1992; 47:173–85.
25. Hillier S, Miro F. Inhibin, activin and follistatin: potential roles in ovarian physiology. *Ann NY Acad Sci* 1993; 687:28–38.
26. Ling N, Ying S, Ueno N, et al. Isolation and partial characterization of a Mr 32,000 protein with inhibin activity from porcine follicular fluid. *Proc Natl Acad Sci USA* 1985; 82:7217–21.
27. Miyamato K, Hasegawa Y, Fukuda M, et al. Isolation of porcine follicular fluid inhibin of 32K daltons. *Biochem Biophys Res Commun* 1985; 129:396–403.
28. Rivier J, Spiess J, McClintock R, et al. Purification and partial characterization of inhibin from porcine follicular fluid. *Biochem Biophys Res Commun* 1985; 133:120–7.
29. Robertson D, Foulds L, Leversha L, et al. Isolation of inhibin from bovine follicular fluid. *Biochem Biophys Res Commun* 1985; 126:220–6.
30. Vale W, Rivier J, McClintock R, et al. Purification and characterization of an FSH releasing protein from porcine ovarian follicular fluid. *Nature* 1986; 321:776–9.
31. Roberts A, Flanders K, Kondaiah P, et al. Transforming growth factor β: biochemistry and roles in embryogenesis, tissue repair and remodeling, and carcinogenesis. *Recent Prog Horm Res* 1988; 44:157–97.
32. Robets A, Sporn M. Transforming growth factor βs. In: Sporn M, Roberts A, eds. *Handbook of Experimental Pharmacology*, vol. New York: Springer, 1990, pp. 419–72.
33. Brown J. Pituitary control of ovarian function: concepts derived from gonadotrophin therapy. *Aust NZ J Obstet Gynaecol* 1978; 18:46–54.
34. Schwall R, Mason A, Wilcox J, et al. Localization of inhibitor/activin subunit mRNAs within the primate ovary. *Mol Endocrinol* 1990; 4:75–9.
35. Mittwoch U, Delhanty J, Beck F. Growth of differentiating testes and ovaries. *Nature* 1969; 224:1323.
36. Mittwoch U. How do you get sex? *J Endocrinol* 1991; 128:329–31.
37. Jost A. A new look at the mechanisms controlling sex differentiation in mammals. *Johns Hopkins Med J* 1972; 130:38–53.
38. Moore K. *The Developing Human*. 2nd ed. Philadelphia: WB Saunders, 1973, pp. 13–15.
39. Wilson J, George F, Griffin J. The hormonal control of sexual development. *Science* 1981; 211:1278–84.
40. Voutilainen R. Differentiation of the fetal gonad. *Horm Res* 1992; 38(suppl):66–71.
41. Siiteri P, Wilson J. Testosterone formation and metabolism during male sexual differentiation. *J Clin Endocrinol Metab* 1974; 38:113–25.
42. Hudson P, Douglas I, Donahoe P, et al. An immunoassay to detect müllerian inhibiting substance in males and females during normal development. *J Clin Endocrinol Metab* 1990; 70:16–22.
43. Jirasek J. *Development of the Genital System and Male Pseudohermaphroditism*. Baltimore: Johns Hopkins Press, 1971.
44. Moore K. *The Developing Human*. 2nd ed. Philadelphia: WB Saunders, 1973, p. 411.
45. Smith D. *Recognizable Patterns of Human Malformation*. 3rd ed. Philadelphia: WB Saunders, 1982, pp. 639–41.
46. Hecht F, Macfarlane J. Mosaicism in Turner's syndrome reflects the lethality of XO. *Lancet* 1969; 2:1197–8.
47. Gerald P. Sex chromosome disorders. *N Engl J Med* 1976; 294:706–8.
48. Rivelis C, Coco R, Bergada C. Ovarian differentiation in Turner's syndrome. *J Genet Hum* 1978; 26:69–82.
49. Lyon M. Mechanisms and evolutionary origins of variable X-chromosome activity in mammals. *Proc R Soc Lond* 1974; 187:243–68.
50. Bonakdar M, Peisner D. Gonadoblastoma with XO karyotype. *Obstet Gynecol* 1980; 56:748–50.
51. Murphy G, Welch W, Urcuyo R. Brenner tumor and mucinous cystadenoma of borderline malignancy in a patient with Turner's syndrome. *Obstet Gynecol* 1979; 54:660–3.

52. Dominguez C, Greenblatt R. Dysgerminoma of the ovary in a patient with Turner's syndrome. *Am J Obstet Gynecol* 1962; 83:674–7.

53. Dowsett J. Corpus carcinoma developing in a patient with Turner's syndrome treated with estrogen. *Am J Obstet Gynecol* 1963; 86:622–5.

54. Polani P. Turner's syndrome and allied conditions. *Br Med Bull* 1961; 17:200–5.

55. Passarge P, Schmidt A. Functional consequences of X-chromosome loss in the human female. In: Sandberg A, ed. *Cytogenetics of the Mammalian X-Chromosome. Part B: X-Chromosome Anomalies and Their Clinical Manifestations.* New York: Alan R. Liss, 1983, pp. 301–20.

56. King C, Magenis E, Barnett S. Pregnancy and the Turner syndrome. *Obstet Gynecol* 1978; 52:617–24.

57. Barr M. The triple-X female: an appraisal based on a study of 12 cases and a review of the literature. *Can Med Assoc J* 1969; 101:247–58.

58. Tennes K, Puck M, Bryant K, et al. A developmental study of girls with trisomy X. *Am J Hum Genet* 1975; 27:71–80.

59. King C, Pernoli M. Sexual differentiation. *Obstet Gynecol Annu* 1984; 13:1–33.

60. Dryer R, Patil S, Zellweger H, et al. Pentasomy X with multiple dislocations. *Am J Med Genet* 1979; 4:313–21.

61. Siebenmann R. The pathology of gonads and adrenal cortex in intersex. *Prog Pediatr Surg* 1983; 36:149–93.

62. Kennedy J, Freeman M, Benirschke K. Ovarian dysgenesis and chromosome abnormalities. *Obstet Gynecol* 1977; 50:13–20.

63. Printz J, Choate J, Townes P, Harper RC. The embryology of supernumerary ovaries. *Obstet Gynecol* 1973; 61:246–52.

64. Coerdt W, Rehder H, Gausmann I, Johannison R, Gropp A. Quantitative histology of human fetal testes in chromosomal disease. *Pediatr Pathol* 1985; 3:245–59.

65. Hawkins J. Mutational analysis of SRY in XY females. *Hum Mutat* 1993; 2:347–50.

66. Guidozzi F, Ball J, Spurdle A. 46,XY Pure gonadal dysgenesis (Swyer-James syndrome)—Y or Y not?: a review. *Obstet Gynecol Surv* 1994; 49:138–46.

67. Potter E. *Pathology of the Fetus and Infant.* 2nd ed. Chicago: Year Book Medical, 1961, pp. 446ff.

68. Lee S. High incidence of true hermaphroditism in the early human embryo. *Biol Neonat* 1971; 18:418–25.

69. van Niekerk W, Retief A. The gonads of human true hermaphrodites. *Hum Genet* 1981; 58:117–22.

70. McKelvie P, Jaubert F, Nezelof C. Is true hermaphroditism a primary germ cell disorder? *Pediatr Pathol* 1987; 7:31–41.

71. Rosenfield R, Lucky A, Allen T. The diagnosis and management of intersex. *Curr Probl Pediatr* 1980; 10:3–66.

72. Hadjiathanasiou C, Brauner R, Lortat-Jacob S, et al. True hermaphroditism: genetic variants and clinical management. *J Pediatr* 1994; 125:738–44.

73. Williamson H, Phansey S, Mathur R. True hermaphroditism with term delivery and a review. *Am J Obstet Gynecol* 1981; 141:262–5.

74. Edman C, Winters A, Porter J, Wilson J, MacDonald P. Embryonic testicular regression. *Obstet Gynecol* 1977; 49:208–17.

75. Coulam C. Testicular regression syndrome. *Obstet Gynecol* 1979; 53:44–9.

76. Abeyaratne M, Aherne W, Scott J. The vanishing testis. *Lancet* 1969; 2:822–4.

77. Berthezène F, Forest M, Grimaud J, Claustrat B, Mornex R. Leydig cell agenesis. A cause of male pseudohermaphroditism. *N Engl J Med* 1976; 295:969–72.

78. Gustafson M. Lee M, Asmundson L, et al. Müllerian inhibiting substance in the diagnosis and management of intersex and gonadal abnormalities. *J Pediatr Surg* 1993; 28:439–44.

79. Guerrier D, Tran D, VanderWinden J, et al. The persistent müllerian duct syndrome: a molecular approach. *J Clin Endocrinol Metab* 1989; 68:46–52.

80. Brook C, Wagner H, Zachmann M, et al. Familial occurrence of persistent müllerian structures in otherwise normal males. *BMJ* 1973; 1:771–3.

81. Sloan W, Walsh P. Familial persistent müllerian duct syndrome. *J Urol* 1976; 115:459–61.

82. Shenoy S, Supe A, Voras I. Non-familial male hermaphrodite uterine hernia syndrome. *J Postgrad Med* 1984; 30:181–2.

83. Davidoff F, Federman D. Mixed gonadal dysgenesis. *Pediatrics* 1973; 52:725–42.

84. Park I, Aimakhu V, Jones HW Jr. An etiologic and pathogenetic classification of male pseudohermaphroditism. *Am J Obstet Gynecol* 1975; 123:505–18.

85. MacLusky N, Naftolin F. Sexual differentiation of the central nervous system. *Science* 1981; 211:1294–303.

86. Bongiovanni A, Eberlein W, Moshang TJ. Urinary excretion of pregnanetriol and Δ5-pregnanetriol in two forms of congenital adrenal hyperplasia. *J Clin Invest* 1971; 50:2751–4.

87. Federman D. *Abnormal Sexual Development.* Philadelphia: WB Saunders, 1967.

88. Dupont B, Zachmann M, Levine L, et al. Mapping of the 21-hydroxylase deficiency gene within the HLA complex. *Pediatr Res* 1978; 12:1088. Abstract.

89. Kirkland R, Kirkland J, Keenan B, et al. Bilateral testicular tumors in congenital adrenal hyperplasia. *J Clin Endocrinol* 1977; 44:369–78.

90. Nowakowski H, Lenz W. Genetic aspects in male hypogonadism. *Recent Prog Horm Res* 1961; 17:53–95.

91. Imperato-McGinley J, Guerero L, Gautier T, Peterson R. Steroid 5 alpha-reductase deficiency in man: an inherited form of male pseudohermaphroditism. *Science* 1974; 186:1213–15.

92. Walsh P, Madden J, Harrod M, et al. Familial incomplete male pseudohermaphroditism, type 2. Decreased dihydrotestosterone formation in pseudovaginal perineoscrotal hypospadias. *N Engl J Med* 1974; 291:944–9.

93. Peterson R, Imperato-McGinley J, Gautier T, Sturla E. Male pseudohermaphroditism due to steroid 5 alpha-reductase deficiency. *Am J Med* 1977; 62:170–91.

94. Griffin J, Wilson J. The syndromes of androgen resistance. *N Engl J Med* 1980; 302:198–209.

95. Imperato-McGinley J, Peterson R, Gautier T, Sturla E. Androgens and the evolution of male gender identity among male pseudohermaphrodites with 5 alpha-reductase deficiency. *N Engl J Med* 1979; 300:1233–7.

96. Peterson G, Bonner G. Inherited sex-mosaic in man. *Hereditas* 1937; 23:49–69.

97. Morriss J. The syndrome of testicular feminization in male pseudohermaphrodites. *Am J Obstet Gynecol* 1953; 65:1192–211.

98. Morriss J, Mahesh V. Further observations on the syndrome 'testicular feminization'. *Am J Obstet Gynecol* 1963; 87:731–48.

99. Lyon M, Hawkes S. X-linked gene for testicular feminization in the mouse. *Nature* 1979; 227:1217–9.

100. Bullock L, Bardin C, Ohno S. The androgen insensitive mouse: absence of intranuclear androgen retention in the kidney. *Biochem Biophys Res Commun* 1971; 44:1537–43.

101. Lubahn D, Brown T, Simental J, et al. Sequence of the intron/exon junctions of the coding region of the human androgen receptor gene and identification of a point mutation in a family with complete androgen insensitivity. *Proc Natl Acad Sci USA* 1989; 86:9534–8.

102. Brown T, Lubahn D, Wilson E, et al. Deletion of the steroid-binding domain of the human androgen receptor gene in one family with complete androgen insensitivity syndrome: evidence for further genetic heterogeneity in this syndrome. *Proc Natl Acad Sci USA* 1988; 85:8151–5.

103. Ris-Stalpers C, Kuiper G, Fabner P, et al. Aberrant splicing of androgen receptor mRNA results in synthesis of a nonfunctional receptor protein in a patient with androgen insensitivity. *Proc Natl Acad Sci USA* 1990; 87:7866–70.

104. Marcelli M, Tilley W, Wilson C, et al. Definition of the human androgen receptor gene structure permits the identification of mutations that cause androgen resistance: premature termination of the receptor protein at amino acid 588 causes complete androgen resistance. *Mol Endocrinol* 1990; 4:1105–16.

105. Griffin J, Punyashthiti K, Wilson J. Dihydrotestosterone binding by cultured human fibroblasts: comparison of cells from control subjects and from patients with hereditary male pseudohermaphroditism due to androgen resistance. *J Clin Invest* 1976; 57:1342–51.

106. Walker A, Stack E, Horsfall W. Familial male pseudohermaphroditism. *Med J Aust* 1970; 1:156–60.

107. Gardó S, Papp Z. Clinical variations of testicular intersexuality in a family. *J Med Genet* 1974; 11:267–70.

108. Winterborn M, France N, Raith S. Incomplete testicular feminization. *Arch Dis Child* 1970; 45:811–2.

109. LaSpada A, Wilson E, Lubahn D, et al. Androgen receptor gene mutations in X-linked spinal and bulbar muscular atrophy. *Nature* 1991; 352:77–9.

110. O'Connell M, Ramsey H, Whang-Peng J, Wiernik P. Testicular feminization syndrome in three sibs: emphasis on gonadal neoplasia. *Am J Med Sci* 1973; 265:321–33.

111. Manuel M, Katayama K, Jones HJ. The age of occurrence of gonadal tumors in intersex patients with a Y-chromosome. *Am J Obstet Gynecol* 1976; 124:293–300.

112. Novak D, Lauchlan S, McCawley J, Faiman C. Virilization during pregnancy. *Am J Med* 1970; 49:281–90.

113. Sternberg W, Barclay D. Luteoma of pregnancy. *Am J Obstet Gynecol* 1966; 59:165–84.

114. Aarskog D. Maternal progestins as a possible cause of hypospadias. *N Engl J Med* 1974; 300:75–6.

115. Herbst A, Scully R. Adenocarcinoma of the vagina in adolescence. *Cancer* 1970; 25:745–57.

116. Herbst A, Ulfelder H, Poskanzer D. Adenocarcinoma of the vagina: association of maternal stilbestrol therapy with tumor appearance in young women. *N Engl J Med* 1971; 284:878–81.

117. Kurman R, Scully R. The incidence and histogenesis of vaginal adenosis. *Hum Pathol* 1974; 5:265–76.

118. Kaufman R, Noller K, Adam E, et al. Upper genital tract abnormalities and pregnancy outcome on diethylstilbestrol-exposed progeny. *Am J Obstet Gynecol* 1984; 148:973–84.

119. McFarlane M, Feinstein A, Horwitz R. Diethylstilbestrol and clear cell vaginal carcinoma. *Am J Med* 1986; 81:855–63.

120. Stillman R. In utero exposure to diethylstilbestrol: adverse effects on the reproductive tract and reproductive performance in male and female offspring. *Am J Obstet Gynecol* 1982; 142:905–21.

121. Herbst A, Poskanzer D, Robboy S, Friedlander L, Scully R. Prenatal exposure to stilbestrol: a prospective comparison of exposed female offspring with unexposed controls. *N Engl J Med* 1975; 292:334–9.

122. Robboy S. A hypothetic mechanism of diethylstilbestrol (DES)-induced anomalies in exposed progeny. *Hum Pathol* 1983; 14:832–3.

123. Buttram VJ, Gibbons WE. Müllerian anomalies. A proposed classification. *Fertil Steril* 1979; 32:40–6.

124. Spence H. Congenital hydrocolpos. *JAMA* 1962; 180:1100–5.

125. Neinstein L, Castle G. Congenital absence of the vagina. *Am J Dis Child* 1983; 137:669–72.

126. Okonkwo J, Crocker K. Cloacal dysgenesis. *Obstet Gynecol* 1977; 50:97–101.

127. Robinson HJ, Tross K. Agenesis of the cloacal membrane. *Perspect Pediatr Pathol* 1984; 8:79–96.

128. Richart R, Benirschke K. Penile agenesis. *Arch Pathol* 1960; 70:252–60.

129. Dunn P. Testicular birth trauma. *Arch Dis Child* 1975; 50:744–5.

130. Longino L, Martin L. Torsion of the spermatic cord in the newborn infant. *N Engl J Med* 1955; 253:695–7.

131. Dehner L, Scott D, Stocker J. Meconium periorchitis: a clinicopathologic study of four cases with a review of the literature. *Hum Pathol* 1986; 17:807–12.

132. Scully R. Gonadoblastoma. *Cancer* 1970; 25:1340–56.

133. Bergher de Bacalao E, Dominguez I. Unilateral gonadoblastoma in a pregnant woman. *Am J Obstet Gynecol* 1969; 105:1279–81.

134. Abell M, Holtz F. Ovarian neoplasms in childhood and adolescence. *Am J Obstet Gynecol* 1965; 93:850–86.

135. Jensen R, Norris H. Epithelial tumors of the ovary. Occurrence in children and adults less than 20 years of age. *Arch Pathol* 1972; 94:29–34.

136. Lawrence W, Young R, Scully R. Juvenile granulosa cell tumor of the infantile testis. *Am J Surg Pathol* 1985; 9:87–94.

137. Young R, Dickersin G, Scully R. Juvenile granulosa cell tumor of the ovary. *Am J Surg Pathol* 1984; 8:575–96.

138. Brown N. Teratomas and yolk sac tumours. *J Clin Pathol* 1976; 29:1021–5.

139. Beilby J, Horne C, Milne G, et al. Alpha-fetoprotein, alpha-1-antitrypsin and transferrin in gonadal yolk sac tumours. *J Clin Pathol* 1977; 32:455–61.

140. Norris H, Bagley G, Taylor H. Carcinoma of the infant vagina. A distinctive tumor. *Arch Pathol* 1970; 90:473–9.

141. Berry C, Keeling J, Hilton C. Teratomata in infancy and childhood. A review of 91 cases. *J Pathol* 1969; 98:241–52.

142. Gonzalez-Crussi F, Winkler R, Mirkin D. Sacrococcygeal teratomas in infants and children. Relationship of histology and prognosis in 40 cases. *Arch Pathol Lab Med* 1976; 102:420–5.

The Skeletal System

S. Samuel Yang

In the past 3 decades the knowledge of constitutional bone diseases has greatly increased [1–4] and the significant contribution of chondro-osseous histopathology in defining these entities has been amply demonstrated [5–9]. This has coincided with an explosion of knowledge in human genetics and a greatly increased public interest in genetic and heritable conditions. Since virtually all constitutional diseases of bone require genetic counseling, pathological examination is now frequently requested to ascertain the diagnosis. Furthermore, because of recent advances in maternal-fetal medicine the fetuses with these disorders are frequently aborted and subjected to postmortem examination [10]. Consequently, pathologists must no longer ignore these conditions.

More than 40 constitutional diseases of bone are identifiable at birth [11] and the list is still rapidly expanding. Most of these disorders are not very common, though they are not rare as a whole, and therefore it may seem formidable to study them. In most instances, a reasonably accurate diagnosis can be rendered by the pathologist when the histopathological findings are combined with certain clinical and radiological features. Recent discoveries of collagenopathies in various skeletal dysplasias have been helpful in understanding the pathogenesis, but the diagnosis and prognosis still depend on the traditional clinical, radiological, and pathological findings.

Bone diseases caused by metabolic disorders are included in the osteochondrodysplasias in the latest classification. Systemic infections that may involve the skeletal system are also included in this chapter. Congenital malformations without significant systemic skeletal pathology are given brief mention only.

Proper sectioning of bone is important. An understanding of the normal development and the histology of chondro-osseous tissue is helpful in evaluating the pathology of skeletal growth. They are briefly described below.

PATHOLOGICAL EXAMINATION OF CHONDRO-OSSEOUS TISSUE—RECOMMENDED TECHNIQUE

Histopathological examination of the chondro-osseous tissue has been greatly facilitated by many commercially available rapid decalcifying solutions. Most bone tissue blocks now can be processed after overnight decalcification. Certain laboratories find glycol methacrylate sections without decalcification superior to the paraffin sections, despite some disadvantages.

Adequate histopathological examination of the systemic skeletal disorders requires, at a minimum, sections of ribs, vertebral bodies, and the proximal or distal end of the femur or humerus, with preservation of the cartilage–bone junction [12]. A single bone section is usually inadequate for postmortem pathological evaluation. The ribs are sectioned longitudinally across the cartilage–bone junction; the 5th and 6th ribs are preferred. For the vertebral bodies, 2 to 3 consecutive lumbar vertebrae (L2–L4) including the disks are sectioned sagittally at the midline. The humerus or femur is cut parallel to the plane of the shaft axis across the cartilage–bone junction. The specimens are sectioned while they are fresh. They are then fixed adequately with formalin, decalcified overnight with rapid decalcifying solution, and processed for paraffin sectioning. The costochondral junction, iliac crest, and proximal end of the tibia across the cartilage–bone junction are the preferred sites for biopsies.

Histopathological examination of the chondroosseous tissue with hematoxylin and eosin (H&E), periodic acid–Schiff (PAS) after diastase digestion, alcian blue stain (pH 1.8), and safranin O–fast green stains is usually sufficient for diagnostic purposes. However, electron microscopy, immunopathology, and biochemical analysis may produce additional information in some instances.

DEVELOPMENT OF BONES

There are two types of bone formation in the human skeletal system: endochondral ossification and membranous ossification [13, 14]. The bones that grow by endochondral ossification are always accompanied by some periosteal membranous ossification. One the other hand, no endochondral ossification is present in the bones that develop by membranous ossification. Both types are derived from the pluripotential primitive mesenchyme.

Endochondral Ossification

Most of the bones, except the cranial vault and most of the facial bones, grow by endochondral ossification. The vertebrae also develop in this fashion by way of several ossification centers. Early in evolution, these bones are preceded by a cartilage stage, which can be seen as early as the 6th week after ovulation. Endochondral ossification can be demonstrated in the clavicle, humerus, and femur by the end of the embryonic period. By 12 weeks, primary centers of ossification are present in nearly all bones of the limbs, although they are not present in some bones until several years after birth. At first, the chondrocytes in the middle of the cartilaginous shaft become hypertrophic and then undergo

degeneration. Meanwhile, calcium deposits in the intervening matrix, the corresponding perichondrium is transformed into periosteum, and its inner cambium layer develops a thin layer of cortical bone (Fig. 31.1a). Blood vessels of the periosteum then invade into the degenerated cartilage of the midshaft through the thin shell of membranous cortical bone (Fig. 31.1b). Osteoblasts accompany the blood vessels and lay osseous seams on the trabeculae of degenerated cartilaginous matrix. Multinucleated osteoclasts, originated from blood-borne monocytic cells, remodel the osseous seams. Chondroclasts identical to the osteoclasts are invariably seen on the cartilage trabeculae before ossification. The cartilage on both ends of the osseous shaft is now the epiphyseal cartilage. Physeal growth zones with proliferation and hypertrophy of chondrocytes are discernible at both ends of the osseous midshaft. The resting cartilage remains at the extreme ends of the bone. The endochondral ossification spreads from the center toward the ends of the shaft. The periosteal ossification likewise advances toward the ends and is always slightly in advance of the endochondral ossification. This produces a curved growth plate with the convexity toward the midshaft (diaphysis).

Membranous Ossification

The cranial vault and most of the facial bones develop by this type of ossification. These are not preceded by a cartilage stage; instead, the mesenchymal cells are directly transformed into osteoblasts, which lay down trabeculae of osteoid tissue. These osteoid trabeculae are rapidly mineral-

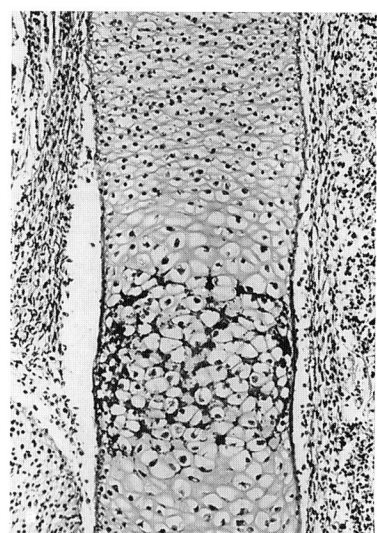
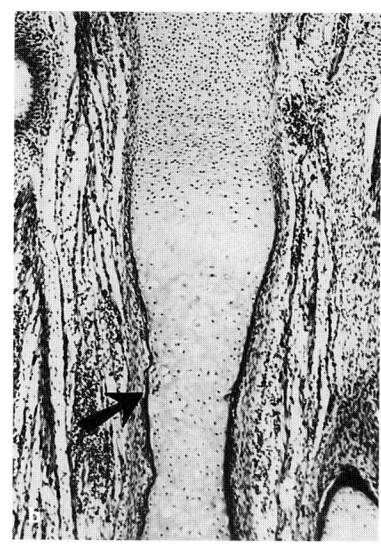

FIGURE 31.1.   *(a) The cartilaginous femur of an embryo. The midshaft shows calcification of the matrix and ballooning of the chondrocytes. The adjacent cartilage displays features of the physeal growth zone. A very thin layer of membranous bone is present beneath the perichondrium (periosteum). Undecalcified section, H&E, ×78. (b) A developing fetal metatarsal bone illustrating initiation of endochondral ossification. A small focus of periosteal vascular tissue is invading through the subperiosteal membranous bone into the degenerating cartilage of the midshaft (arrow). This invading vascular tissue will eventually create marrow spaces. The same tissue also carries osteoblastic and osteoclastic precursors for endochondral ossification. The subperiosteal membrane bone is evident, and a well-developed physeal growth zone is present above the degenerating cartilage of the midshaft in this photograph. H&E, ×50.*

ized and increase in size. The entrapped osteoblasts become osteocytes. The enlarging osseous trabeculae anastomose to form a lattice-like meshwork, and marrow tissue appears in the intervening spaces. Concomitantly, periosteal ossification participates in shaping the bone.

HISTOLOGY OF ENDOCHONDRAL OSSIFICATION

Endochondral ossification takes place principally in the physeal growth plates (zones) (epiphyseal growth plates), which are situated between the resting cartilage and the metaphysis. The chondrocytes in these plates proliferate in three poorly demarcated zones [13, 14] (Fig. 31.2). The first is the zone of proliferation, in which multiplying chondrocytes aggregate in small longitudinal columns. The second is the zone of hypertrophy, where chondrocytes become ballooned with clear glycogen-rich cytoplasm as they approach the metaphysis. Alkaline phosphatase activity is demonstrated in this zone. The third zone abuts the metaphysis and has degenerated chondrocytes, often without nuclei. This is designated the zone of degeneration. The studies by Cowell et al [15] suggest that the cells in this zone do not degenerate; they appear to synthesize and secrete macromolecules responsible for the mineralization of the matrix, capillary invasion, and formation of bone on the calcified cartilage. This zone and the adjacent portion of the zone of hypertrophy correspond to the zone of provisional calcification, which shows calcium deposition in the matrix. After decalcification, the color of this area frequently differs from that of the remaining cartilage. Spicules of calcified cartilage matrix remain between metaphyseal capillaries,

which invade the degenerating chondrocytic lacunae (primary spongiosa). These spicules become bony when osteoblasts form osteoid seams and osteoclasts remodel the structure. Cores of calcified cartilage matrix persist in this zone (secondary spongiosa). The primary and secondary spongiosa constitute the zone of provisional ossification (metaphysis, or zone of cartilage removal and bone deposition).

ELECTRON MICROSCOPY OF CARTILAGE

The resting (reserve) chondrocytes are plump, spindle-shaped, oval, or round [16]. They contain a few tubules of rough endoplasmic reticulum, which are focally distended with electron-dense material. Mitochondria are few and small. Occasional lipid droplets and inconspicuous Golgi zones are noted in resting cartilage. These ultrastructural features closely resemble those of fibroblasts. Chondrocytes also contain clear cytoplasmic vacuoles filled with small electron-dense granules and beaded filaments. Among these chondrocytes (chief cells) are less common dark cells with more dilated endoplasmic reticulum, prominent Golgi zones, electron-dense cytoplasm, and numerous slender cytoplasmic processes. Both types of cells participate in the formation of the physeal growth plate. The dark cells are probably the source of matrix vesicles and related to calcification of the cartilage. Most of the cells in the zone of proliferation are chief cells, and are characterized by the presence of clear non-membrane-bound cytoplasmic vacuoles, which contain beaded filaments and oval granules. The cytoplasmic ground substance becomes more compact with increased prominence of rough endoplasmic reticulum and Golgi zones. Mitochondria remain inconspicuous. In the zone of hypertrophy, the lacunar spaces rapidly increase in size. Half of the chief cells become markedly swollen with confluent non-membrane-bound vacuoles and widely dispersed organelles. The remaining chief cells fail to enlarge. The dark cells show an increasing number of large vacuoles filled with fibrillary or floccular material. Concomitantly, large numbers of cytoplasmic processes and dense vesicles sprout from the cell surface. The lacunar spaces of these cells are filled with abundant small stellate granules, which form a reticulated network. Occasional water-clear cells are also seen in this zone. The cartilage matrix is composed of randomly arranged collagen fibrils, matrix granules (glycosaminoglycan), and dense membrane-bound matrix vesicles that are more numerous in the physeal growth zone. The matrix vesicles may play a role in initiating calcification of the cartilage.

CONGENITAL ANOMALIES INVOLVING THE SKELETON WITHOUT SIGNIFICANT SYSTEMIC SKELETAL PATHOLOGY

Some localized skeletal malformations are characteristic of specific syndromes, for example, sacral hypoplasia and agenesis in the infant of a diabetic mother, while others, such

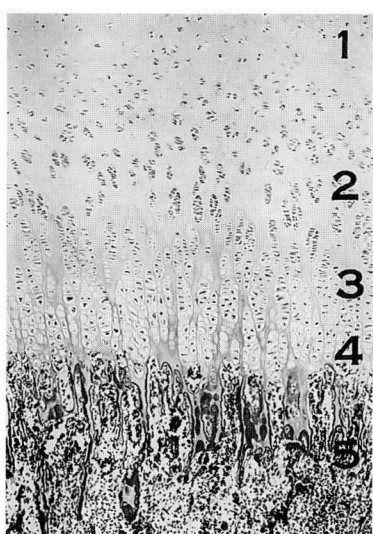

FIGURE 31.2. *Physeal growth zone with normal endochondral ossification. The physeal chondrocytes are arranged in columns: 1, resting cartilage; 2–4, physis; 2, zone of proliferation; 3, zone of hypertrophy; 4, zone of degeneration; 5, metaphysis. H&E, ×42.*

Table 31.1.   Selected anomalies involving the skeleton

Site	Syndrome	Features
Cranium	Synostosis syndromes: e.g., Carpenter syndrome and Apert syndrome	Variable cranial synostosis; both associated with characteristic forms of syndactyly and sometimes with fatal internal anomalies
Jaw anomalies	Pierre Robin syndrome	Micrognathia, cleft soft palate
Vertebral column	Neck: Klippel-Feil syndrome	Fusion of cervical vertebrae
	Thorax: Jarcho-Levin syndrome	Short thorax with decreased ribs and multiple vertebral defects
	Lumbosacral: caudal regression syndrome	Ranges from sacral hypoplasia or agenesis to sirenomelia
Limb anomalies	Holt-Oram syndrome	Upper limb deficiency with cardiac anomalies
	Roberts syndrome	Midfacial anomalies and hypomelia
	Facial limb disruption spectrum	Micrognathia, hypoglossia, and distal limb deficiencies
	Amniotic band syndrome	Limb amputations; sometimes cranial anomalies
	Radial aplasia in:	
	Radial aplasia–thrombocytopenia syndrome	TAR syndrome—thrombocytopenia, anemia, and radial hypoplasia or aplasia
	Fanconi pancytopenia syndrome	Radial hypoplasia or aplasia with pancytopenia and small stature; sometimes other internal anomalies
Syndromes with bony anomalies as one feature include:		
	VACTERL association	Vertebral, anal, cardiac, tracheoesophageal, rib, and limb anomalies
	MURCS association	Müllerian duct aplasia, renal aplasia, and cervicothoracic somite dysplasia

as hemivertebrae and a reduced complement of ribs, may be non-specific or seen as part of a number of malformation syndromes.

A small selection of those that may be of importance to the pathologist in the perinatal period are presented in Table 31.1. In most of them, the bone anomaly forms a small part of the syndrome, resulting from a primary deficit or vascular lesion affecting the field of origin within the mesenchyme or limb bud. Many of them are classified as dysostoses (malformation of individual bones, singly or in combination) in the 1983 International Nomenclature of Constitutional Diseases of Bone [17]. Some of the conditions are described elsewhere in texts on malformation syndromes [18–20].

CONSTITUTIONAL DISEASES OF BONE

In the 1983 international classification [17] constitutional diseases of bone were classified into the following 5 groups:

1. Osteochondrodysplasia
2. Dysostosis
3. Idiopathic osteolysis
4. Primary metabolic abnormalities
5. Miscellaneous disorders with osseous involvement

This classification was revised again in 1992, and in the latest version the groups of idiopathic osteolysis and primary metabolic abnormalities are included under osteochondrodysplasia [11]. The dysostoses are excluded because of insufficient information at the present time. Many of the osteochondrodysplasias including the primary metabolic diseases show significant chondro-osseous histopathological abnormalities, which are useful in diagnosis and for a better understanding of the disorders (Table 31.2). For the sake of completeness, certain secondary metabolic disorders and infectious diseases that may involve the skeletal system are included.

OSTEOCHONDRODYSPLASIAS

These entities include the disorders previously considered as chondrodystrophies, osteogenesis imperfecta (OI), osteopetrosis, and so on. Significant knowledge of these disorders has been gained in the last three decades, and numerous new entities have been separated from the original two conditions, achondroplasia and Morquio disease. The recent discoveries of collagenopathies in some of these entities do not alter the importance of pathological findings in diagnosis and prognostication [21, 22].

The conditions identifiable at birth are mostly chondrodysplasias, which are osteochondrodysplasias with defects of growth of tubular bones or axial skeleton or both [2]. These are further divided into 5 groups to facilitate differential diagnosis. This classification is based on morphological similarities and does not imply pathogenetic relationships within each group. A table of differential diagnosis is included with the descriptions of each group.

Osteochondrodysplasia with Defects of the Tubular Bones or Axial Skeleton (Chondrodysplasia)

Short-Trunk Chondrodysplasias

The disorders in this group result in a significantly short trunk. Radiologically, the vertebral bodies display variable abnormalities, ranging from their complete absence to vertebrae that are small and oval or variable in size and shape. The cartilage of these disorders mostly reveals either a significantly abnormal matrix or many PAS-positive, diastase-resistant cytoplasmic inclusions.

Achondrogenesis Types I and II   Achondrogenesis types I and II are well-established entities [3, 11, 23]. Borochowitz et al [24] further divided type I patients into IA (Houston-Harris) and IB (Fraccaro). Others attempted to subclassify achondrogenesis into 4 types and might have included hypochondrogenesis and spondyloepiphyseal dysplasia congenita [25, 26]. Grebe-Quelce-Salgado dysplasia has been designated as non-lethal achondrogenesis [27]; this is clinically not related to lethal types of achondrogenesis [23].

Achondrogenesis Type I (A and B). In 1952, Fraccaro [28] reported a case of achondrogenesis that he believed to be similar to the case reported by Parenti in 1936 [29]. The entity is the severest form of chondrodysplasia, and is uniformly fatal in the perinatal period [3, 23]. Genetically, the disorder is an autosomal recessive condition. The trunk is extremely short, as are the extremities (Fig. 31.3a). Congenital cardiac anomalies (patent ductus arteriosus, atrial septal defect, ventricular septal defect) have been reported. Radiological examination (Fig. 31.3b) reveals a characteristic absence of ossification in the ischia, pubis, and vertebral bodies. The lumbosacral region consistently lacks ossification. The ossification of cranial bones is deficient in type IA but adequate in IB. The ribs are thin with numerous fractures in type IA but there are no fractures in IB [24, 30]. The limb bones are extremely short with spike-like metaphyseal spurs.

Prenatal diagnosis of achondrogenesis can be achieved as early as 19 weeks of gestation with amniography, radiography, and real-time ultrasonography [31].

Histopathologically, the physeal growth zone of the cartilage is extremely retarded and disorganized in both subtypes (Fig. 31.3c). The resting chondrocytes in type IA frequently contain characteristic large PAS-positive, diastase-resistant cytoplasmic inclusions. They are spherical or oval, lying within membrane-bound vacuoles [32] (Fig. 31.3d). Ultrastructurally, the vacuoles correspond to markedly

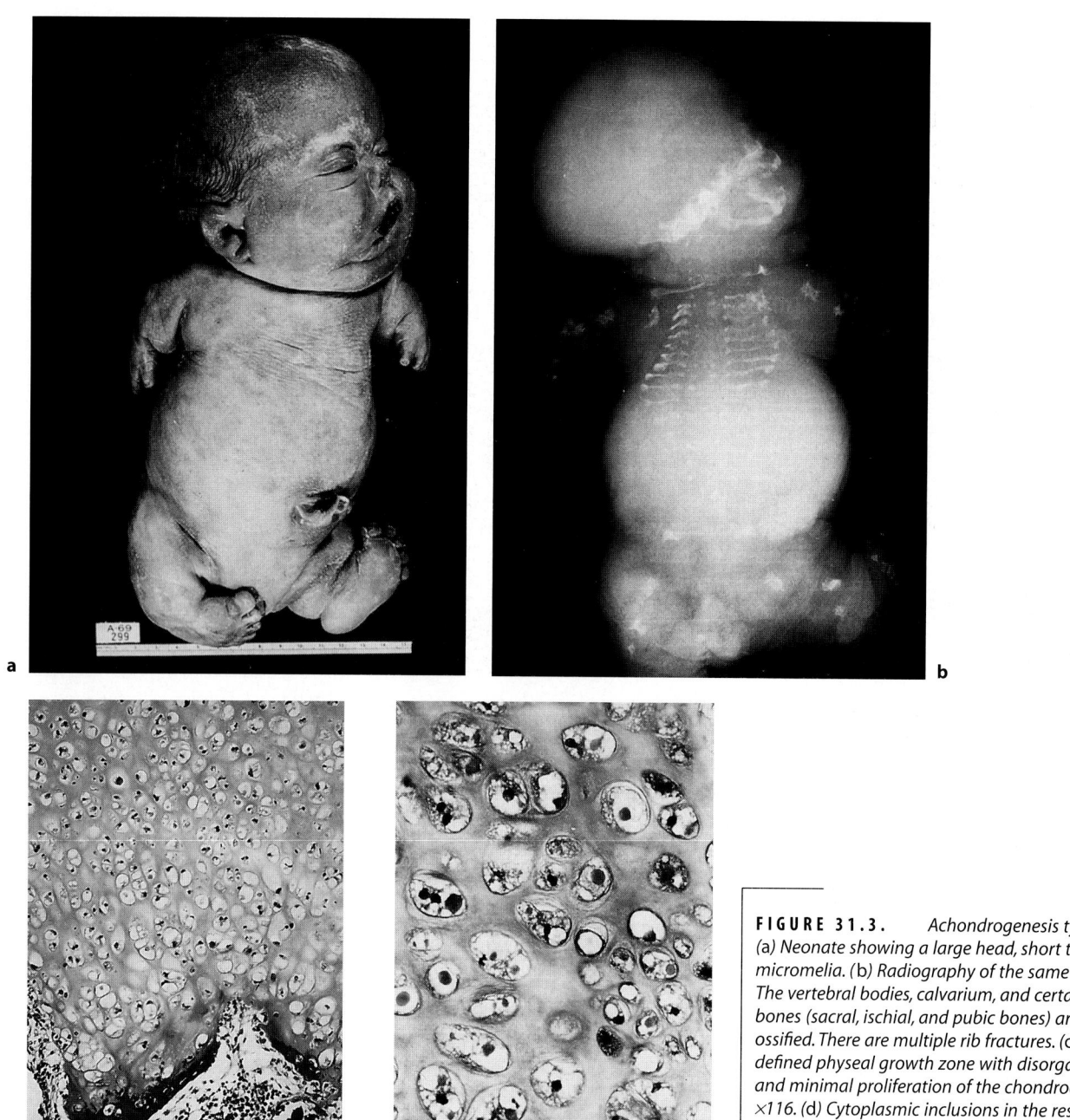

FIGURE 31.3.   *Achondrogenesis type IA. (a) Neonate showing a large head, short trunk, and micromelia. (b) Radiography of the same neonate. The vertebral bodies, calvarium, and certain pelvic bones (sacral, ischial, and pubic bones) are not ossified. There are multiple rib fractures. (c) Poorly defined physeal growth zone with disorganization and minimal proliferation of the chondrocytes. H&E, ×116. (d) Cytoplasmic inclusions in the resting chondrocytes. H&E, ×330. (From Yang et al [9, 23].)*

distended cisterns of rough endoplasmic reticulum, and the inclusions are globular masses of electron-dense material [33]. The inclusions of this condition are different from those seen in spondyloepiphyseal dysplasia congenita, Kniest dysplasia, pseudoachondroplasia, and an isolated case of short-rib dysplasia type III. Ornoy et al [34] noted enlarged cartilage matrix vesicles.

The resting cartilage in type IB is characterized by matrix deficiency and perichondrocytic collagen rings, which stain with trichrome, silver methenamine, and toluidine blue [24, 30]. Chondrocytic inclusions are absent in this subtype.

Achondrogenesis Type II. Clinically, this entity rivals achondrogenesis type I in severity (Fig. 31.4a). Originally, the two were considered a single entity. As with achondrogenesis type I (A and B), this type is also uniformly fatal in the perinatal period. Although type II had been reported in the past to transmit as an autosomal recessive trait [3, 6, 23], most recent reports now describe it as a type II collagenopathy and the result of an autosomal dominant mutation [4, 11, 22]. Fetal hydrops is frequently noted. Salient radiological findings [3, 23, 30] (Fig. 31.4b) include markedly deficient ossification in the vertebral bodies (frequently absent in the lumbosacral region), pubis, and

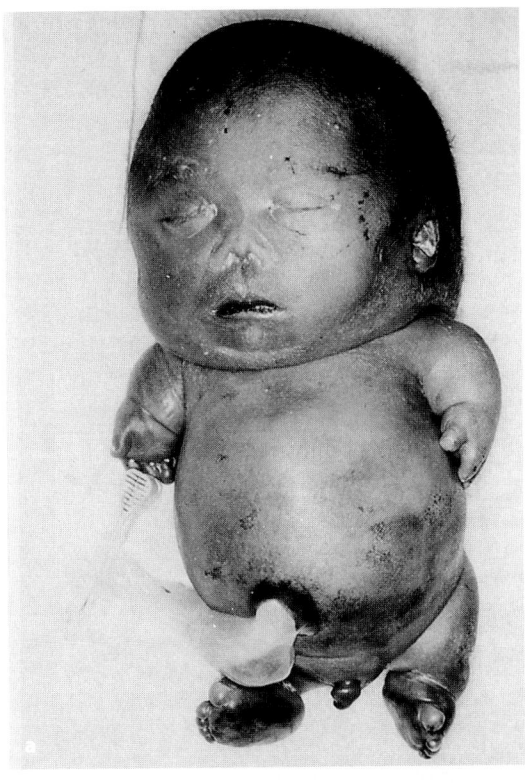
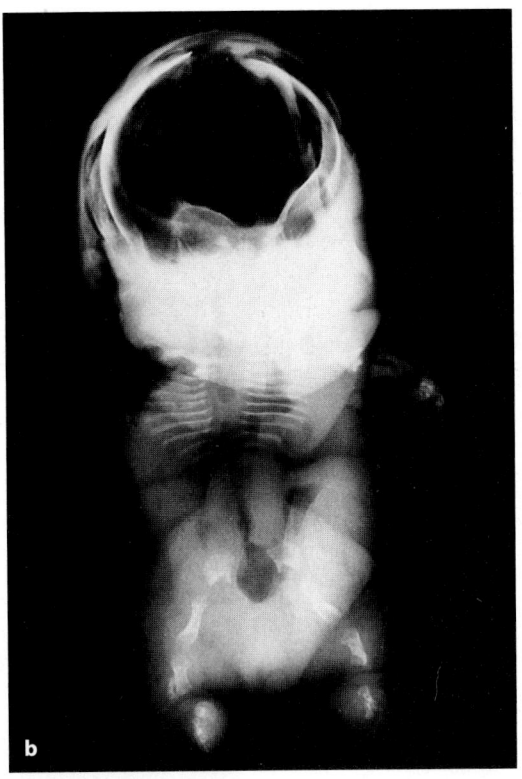
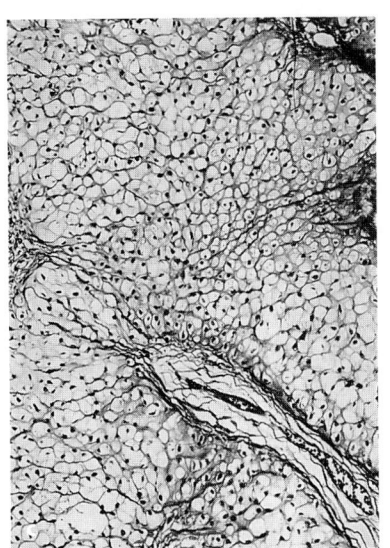
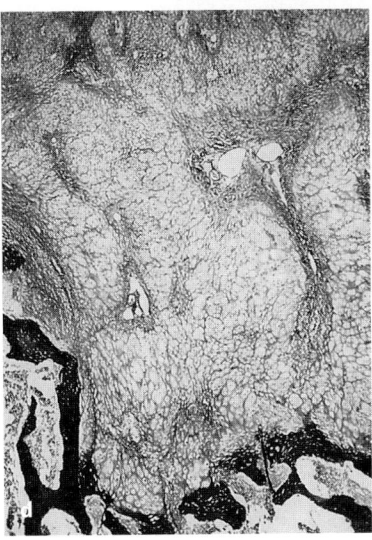

FIGURE 31.4. *Achondrogenesis type II. (a) Neonate showing a large head, short trunk, and severe micromelia. (b) Radiograph of another neonate with no ossification in the vertebral, ischial, and pubic bones. (c) Severe deficiency of cartilage matrix. D-PAS, ×78. (d) Poorly defined physeal growth zone and large stellate-shaped cartilage canals in the resting cartilage. D-PAS, ×21. ((b) and (d) from Yang et al [9, 23].)*

ischia, as in achondrogenesis type I. However, this type has better ossified ilia and limb bones, with flared and cupped metaphyseal ends. The cranial bones are well ossified, and there are no rib fractures.

This condition has been diagnosed as early as 12 weeks of gestation by vaginal ultrasonography [35].

Histopathological examination of the cartilage shows a characteristic generalized deficiency of the matrix with an increased number of markedly enlarged lacunae and chondrocytes that may contain abundant clear cytoplasm (Fig. 31.4c). The cartilage canals are markedly enlarged, stellate in shape, and fibrotic [23, 30]. The physeal growth zone is markedly retarded and disorganized, with closely arranged large chondrocytic lacunae and prominently deficient intervening matrix (Fig. 31.4d). Immunohistochemical and microchemical studies indicate that the predominant collagen of cartilage in this disorder is type I rather than type II as is normally found. The findings suggest a disorder of type II collagen biosynthesis or of chondrocytic differentiation [36].

Hypochondrogenesis On further examination of several patients with a mild form of achondrogenesis type II, Maroteaux et al [37] labeled the condition *hypochondrogenesis*. The survival period varied but did not exceed several months. They body configuration and the radiological findings of the skeletal system vary from those resembling achondrogenesis type II (Fig. 31.5a) to milder forms resembling spondyloepiphyseal dysplasia congenita. Additional reports suggest that the three conditions actually form a continuous spectrum [30, 38] and they all belong to type II collagenopathy with autosomal dominant trait [11, 22].

In general, the radiological findings of the skeletal system, especially the shape of the vertebral bodies, are similar to those of spondyloepiphyseal dysplasia congenita (Fig. 31.5b). The shape of the ilia may vary from that of achondrogenesis type II to that of spondyloepiphyseal dysplasia congenita.

Consequently, in the past some of these patients were considered to have fatal spondyloepiphyseal dysplasia congenita [37]. Careful examination of the bones across the cartilage–bone junction, including the vertebrae, is helpful in separating this entity from achondrogenesis type II and especially from spondyloepiphyseal dysplasia congenita; the latter condition is compatible with life.

Histopathological findings of the cartilage are similar to those of achondrogenesis type II, with matrix deficiency and large ballooned chondrocytic lacunae, though milder and focal in distribution [5, 39]. The abnormal changes are more consistently seen in the vertebral bodies (Fig. 31.5c).

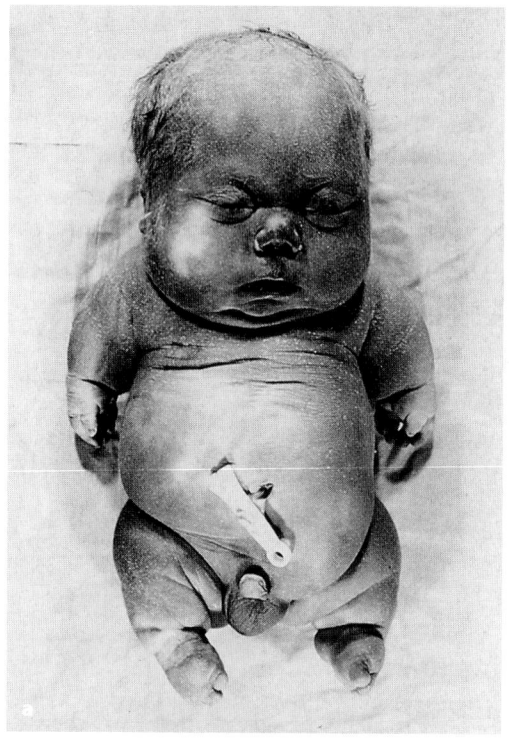

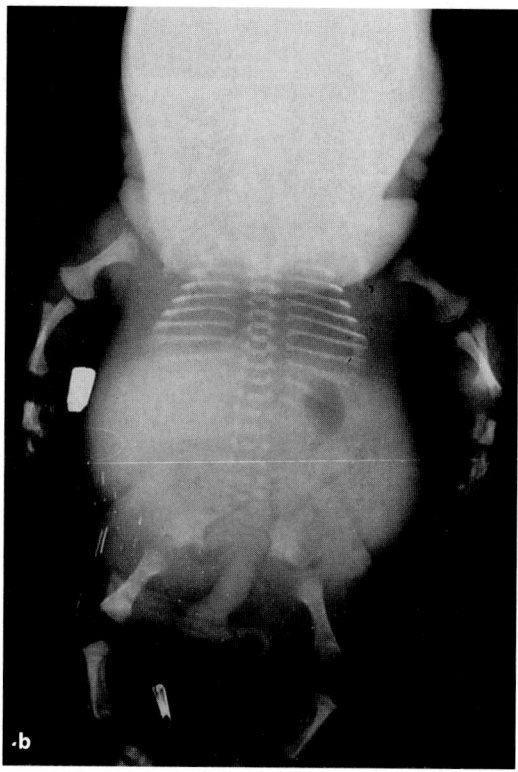

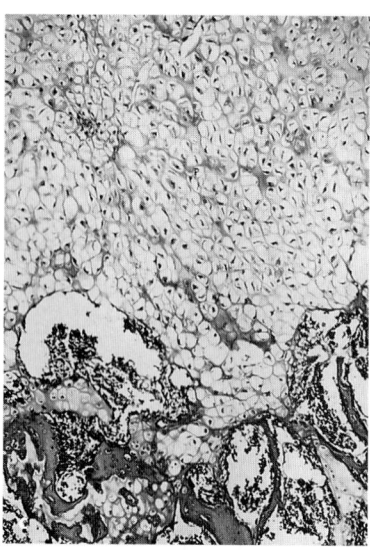

FIGURE 31.5. *Hypochondrogenesis. (a) Neonate with an appearance similar to achondrogenesis type II. (b) Skeletal radiograph of the same neonate showing better ossification than that seen in achondrogenesis type II and resembling spondyloepiphyseal dysplasia congenita. (c) Histopathology of the cartilage resembles that of achondrogenesis type II. This abnormality is focal in distribution. H&E, ×45. ((b) from Chen et al [39]. (a) and (c) from Gilbert et al [5].)*

Chondrocytic inclusions, which are seen in spondyloepiphyseal dysplasia congenita, are occasionally observed in this condition.

Spondyloepiphyseal Dysplasia Congenita The disorder was originally established by Spranger and Wiedemann in 1966 [40]. Genetically, this is an autosomal dominant condition; however, in many patients it is the product of dominant mutation [40]. Type II collagenopathy with genetic linkage to CoL2A1 was noted recently [22, 41]. Most of these patients survive, but a few die from respiratory insufficiency or idiopathic respiratory distress syndrome in the neonatal period. The fatal cases show rather uniform clinical manifestations [42], with a large head, flat face, short neck, short trunk, protuberant abdomen, and moderately shortened extremities (Fig. 31.6a). The radiological changes of the skeletal system are characteristic, with small oval vertebral bodies, vertically shortened reniform ilia, and mildly dysplastic limb bones (Fig. 31.6b). Ossification centers of the pubic bones and knee epiphyses are absent in infancy. On

gross pathological examination, the proximal femoral head is slightly flattened. Clinically it is difficult to separate the fatal cases and medically aborted fetuses of spondyloepiphyseal dysplasia congenita from those of hypochondrogenesis; the two conditions actually form a continuous spectrum.

Histopathological examination of the cartilage in the neonate shows a slightly to moderately disorganized physeal growth zone (Fig. 31.6c). The chondrocytes in the zone of proliferation and the adjacent resting cartilage contain many diastase-resistant, PAS-positive cytoplasmic inclusions [42] (Fig. 31.6d). Ultrastructurally, the inclusions correspond to the electron-dense granular material accumulated in the dilated cisterns of rough endoplasmic reticulum.

In most instances, histopathological examination of the cartilage is helpful in distinguishing spondyloepiphyseal dysplasia congenita from hypochondrogenesis. Later in life, mucopolysaccharidosis type IV (Morquio disease) may mimic this condition, but the histology of the cartilage is entirely different. During infancy, spondyloepiphyseal

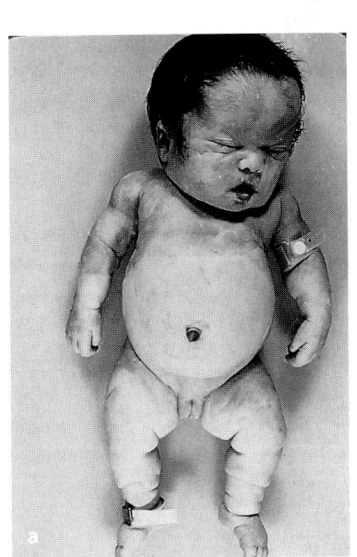
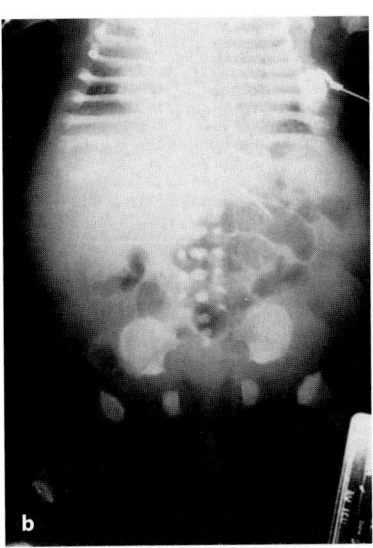
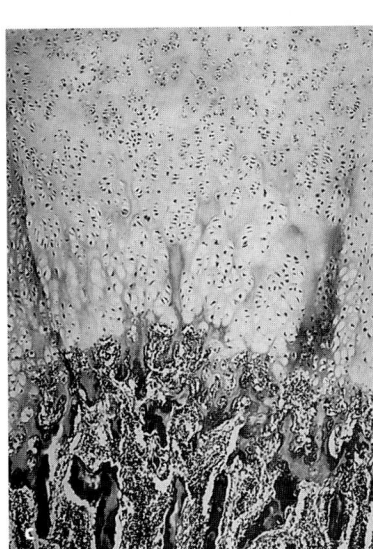
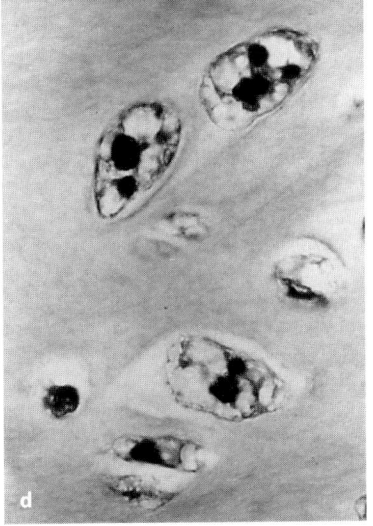

FIGURE 31.6. *Spondyloepiphyseal dysplasia congenita. (a) Neonate with a large head, flat face, short neck, short trunk, and moderately shortened extremities. (b) Radiograph of the skeletal system showing small oval vertebral bodies and vertically shortened reniform ilia. (c) Slightly disorganized physeal growth zone. H&E, ×42. (d) Cytoplasmic inclusions in the chondrocytes of resting cartilage and the zone of proliferation. D-PAS, ×1060. ((a) and (c) from Yang et al [42]. (a) and (b) from Gilbert et al [5].)*

dysplasia congenita is indistinguishable radiologically and histopathologically from the autosomal recessive spondylometepiphyseal dysplasia (Strudwick type) [41, 43].

Kniest Dysplasia Kniest [44] described this disorder (Kniest syndrome, pseudometatropic dwarfism, metatropic dwarfism type II) in 1952. This short-trunk chondrodysplasia is rarely fatal in the neonatal period. Most cases occur sporadically due to autosomal dominant mutation, and the familial cases are transmitted in autosomal dominant fashion [45, 46]. Type II collagen is abnormal [22, 47]. The body configuration (Fig. 31.7a) and the radiological changes of the skeletal system (Fig. 31.7b) are similar to those of spondyloepiphyseal dysplasia congenita, except for the dumbell-shaped limb bones, which are due to markedly enlarged metaphyses and resemble those of metatropic dysplasia. Coronal clefting of the lumbar vertebrae, cleft palate, and stiff joints may be present in infancy. Recurrent respiratory distress with tracheomalacia may occur in infancy.

Kyphoscoliosis, myopia, and hearing loss are observed later in life. Some patients excrete excess keratan sulfate although the results of urinary mucopolysaccharide screening tests are mostly negative [45].

Histopathologically, the cartilage in the neonate is hypercellular. The physeal growth zone is disorganized (Fig. 31.7c). The resting cartilage shows small foci of Swiss cheese–type myxoid and cystic degeneration. In addition, many chondrocytes contain cytoplasmic inclusions (Fig. 31.7d) similar to those of spondyloepiphyseal dysplasia congenita, as demonstrated in both light and electron microscopic preparations [48, 49]. In occasional cases the inclusions are absent.

Sconyers et al [50] reported 2 siblings with a severe lethal skeletal dysplasia, resembling Kniest dysplasia radiologically and pathologically. Genetic transmission may have been via an autosomal recessive trait. Limb bones in these patients were markedly shortened, with metaphyseal irregu-

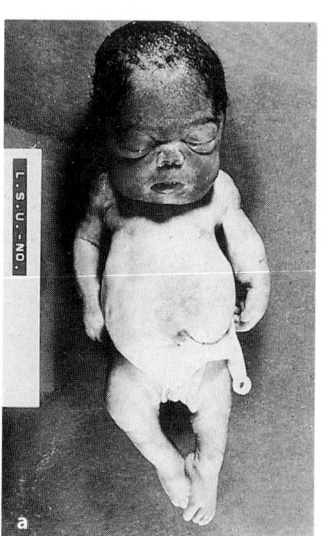
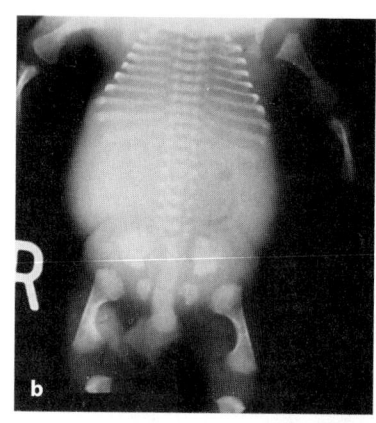
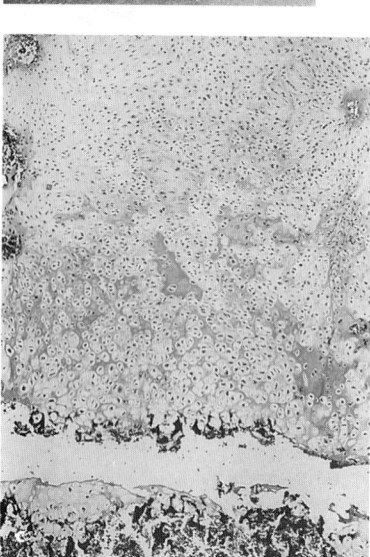
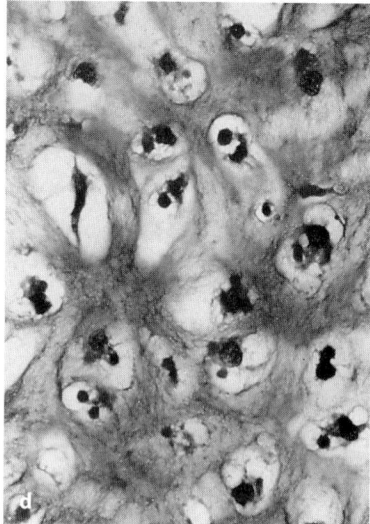

FIGURE 31.7. *Kniest dysplasia. (a) Infant appears similar to one with spondyloepiphyseal dysplasia congenita. In addition, the joints are prominent. (b) Skeletal radiograph of the same neonate is similar to that of spondyloepiphyseal dysplasia congenita except for the broad flared metaphysis. (c) The physeal growth zone of a neonate is hypercellular and disorganized. The transverse cleavage is an artifact. H&E, ×40. (d) Spherical cytoplasmic inclusions in the chondrocytes. D-PAS, ×620. (From Chen et al [48].)*

larity. There was platyspondyly with posterior exaggeration. In addition, there was brachydactyly, rib shortening, and anterior rib splaying. The cartilage of these 2 patients had "Swiss-cheese" degeneration and also clusters of large chondrocytes surrounded by fibrous-appearing matrix bands (seen in vertebrae) and a frayed or dense appearance of the matrix.

Dyssegmental Dysplasia This is an autosomal recessive lethal chondrodysplasia with some clinical features of Kniest dysplasia [51, 52]. A short trunk, short neck, and camptomelia characterize this condition (Fig. 31.8a). Radiologically the appendicular bones show large metaphyses, as in Kniest dysplasia, but there is a more pronounced bending of diaphyses (Fig. 31.8b). The vertebral bodies are irregular in size, frequently with separate ossifying masses. The ilia are small. Aleck et al [53] demonstrated at least two forms of this entity. The milder form, type Rolland-Desbuquois, is characterized by frequent survival beyond the newborn period and by radiological resemblance to Kniest dysplasia. The severe form, type Silverman-Handmaker, is characterized by perinatal death and by more severe radiographic changes.

Histopathological examination of the cartilage in the Silverman-Handmaker type demonstrates characteristic puddle-like spaces filled with mucoid material in the resting cartilage [51–53] (Fig. 31.8c). The physeal growth zone is significantly retarded and disorganized. There are large unfused calcospherites in the growth plate and calcifying zones. In the Rolland-Desbuquois type, the resting cartilage has prominent patches of broad collagen fibers but the growth plate is relatively normal [53].

Atelosteogenesis (Spondylohumerofemoral Hypoplasia) The condition was originally reported as giant-cell chondrodys-

plasia [54]. The term *atelosteogenesis* was coined by Maroteaux et al [55] to indicate incomplete ossification. This is a lethal chondrodysplasia without familial incidence, according to the few reported cases. Clinically, the affected infant shows an unusual facies, with a flat nose, depressed nasal bridge, micrognathia, and occasional cleft palate. The extremities display rhizomelic shortening, dislocation of elbows, and frog-like posture of lower extremities with talipes equinovarus (Fig. 31.9a). Radiologically (Fig. 31.9b), the vertebral bodies are markedly hypoplastic; some of them are entirely absent. The humeri and femora are very short and club-shaped, with a tapered distal segment. Occasionally, the entire humeri are unossified. The fibulae are usually absent [54–56]. The recently reported atelosteogenesis type II has many features of severe diastrophic dysplasia [57]. Omodysplasia types I and II may display limb bones similar to this condition [58–60].

Histopathologically, the physeal growth zone is slightly to moderately disorganized without significant retardation. It may be disrupted by acellular zones (Fig. 31.9c). Multinucleated giant chondrocytes are seen in some patients [54, 56] (Fig. 31.9d). Scattered small foci of myxoid degeneration are also observed in the resting cartilage.

Boomerang Dysplasia This achondrogenesis-like sporadic lethal disorder was described by Tenconi et al [61] in 1983. A similar case was reported earlier by Kozlowski et al [62]. This condition may overlap with atelosteogenesis [63, 64]. The affected patient has a short trunk, large head, and distinctly short limbs. Short ribs and polydactyly may be present [4]. Radiological examination shows achondrogenesis-like poor ossification and absence of vertebral bodies. However, the ribs, ilia, and ischia are well ossified

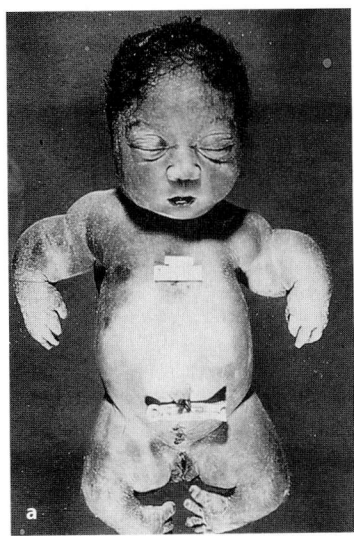
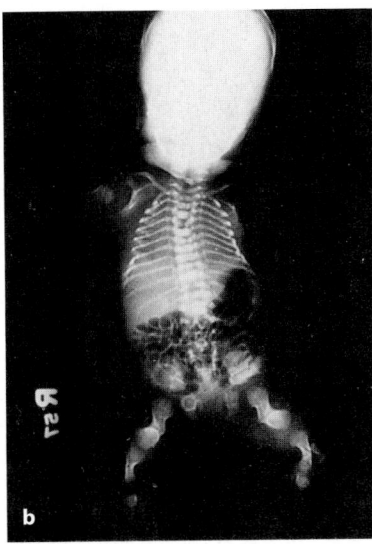
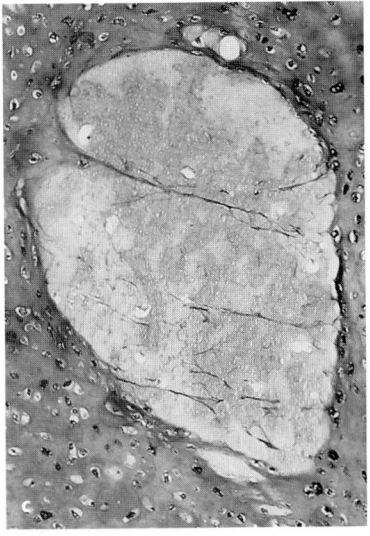

FIGURE 31.8. *Dyssegmental dysplasia. (a) An infant showing a short neck, trunk, and extremities with camptomelia. (b) Radiography of the same infant showing segmented irregular vertebral bodies and camptomelic limb bones with large metaphyses. (c) Resting cartilage with puddle-like spaces containing mucoid material. H&E, ×78. (From Greco et al [51].)*

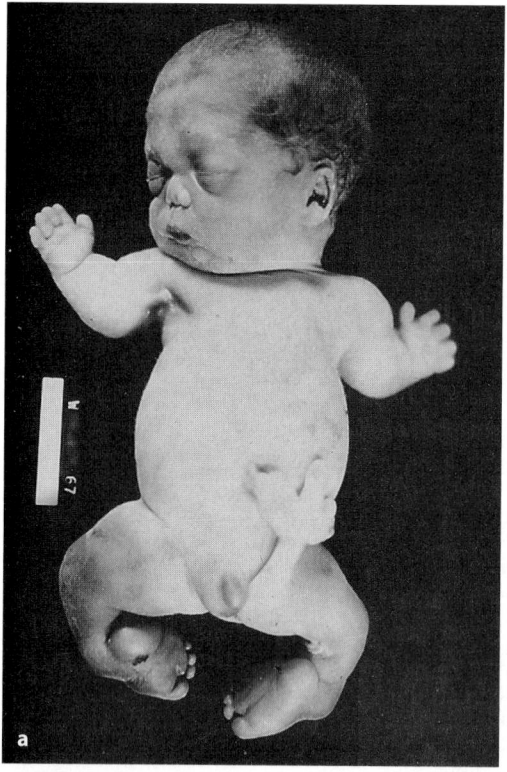
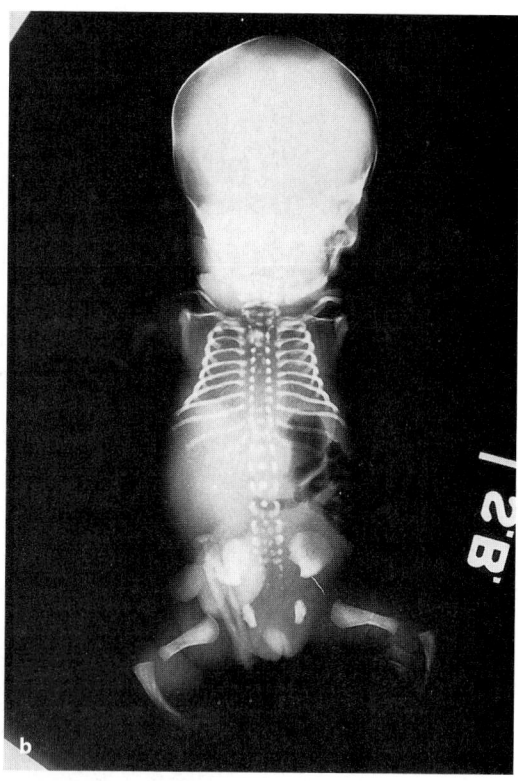
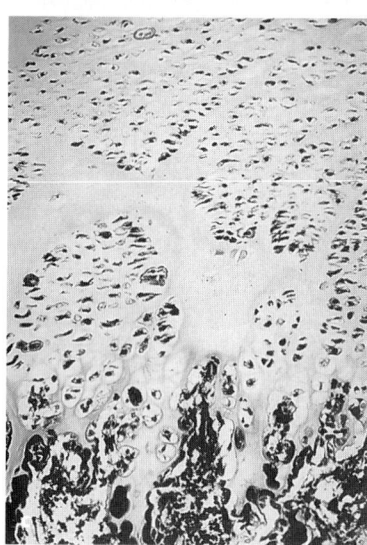
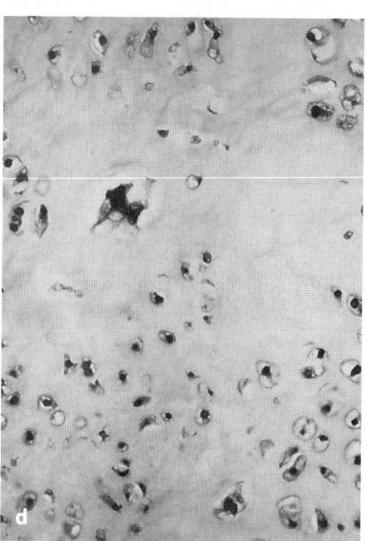

FIGURE 31.9. *Atelosteogenesis. (a) Neonate showing a flat face, depressed nasal bridge, micrognathia, and rhizomelic shortening of the extremities with talipes equinovarus. (b) Radiograph of the same neonate with poorly ossified vertebral bodies, club-shaped short humeri (barely visible in this picture), and femora with tapered distal segments. (c) Moderately disorganized physeal growth zone with acellular areas. H&E, ×90. (d) Giant cells in the resting cartilage. Small foci of myxoid degeneration are seen elsewhere. H&E, ×214. (From Yang et al [56].)*

and prominent. The lower portions of the ilia are narrow. The major limb bones are either unossified or very poorly ossified with a shape suggesting a boomerang.

Histopathologically, the resting chondrocytes are irregularly distributed, with focal acellularity. Multinucleated giant cells have been noted. The physeal growth zones are markedly retarded and disorganized. The unossified limb bones are entirely composed of cartilage.

Fibrochondrogenesis   Stanescu, Stanescu, and Maroteaux [7] should be credited for identifying this rare entity in 1977. This is a unique autosomal recessive rhizomelic short-trunk chondrodysplasia that is uniformly fatal in the peri-

natal period [65, 66]. The condition superficially resembles thanatophoric dysplasia (TD) and metatropic dysplasia. The liveborn babies always have respiratory difficulties. The disorder may affect identical twins [67]. Clinically, the patient's face is round, with protuberant eyes, wide flat nasal root, anteverted nares, microstomia, and cleft soft palate. Pinnae may be small and malformed. The neck and trunk are short. The extremities are markedly rhizomelic with large joints. There may be camptodactyly and clinodactyly. No anomalies are seen in the other viscera, except 1 patient showed unilateral cerebral atrophy and microgyria, and another had omphalocele. Radiological examination of the skeletal

Table 31.3. Differential diagnosis of short-trunk chondrodysplasias

	Radiography		Cartilage Histopathology
	Vertebra	**Metaphysis of Femora**	
Achondrogenesis I	Absent	Spikes	Chondrocytic inclusions (IA), perichondrocytic rings
Achondrogenesis II	Absent or small	Cupping	Matrix deficiency, large clear lacunae
Hypochondrogenesis	Small, oval	Large	Same as above, focal
Spondyloepiphyseal dysplasia congenita	Small, oval	Slightly abnormal	Chondrocytic inclusions
Kniest dysplasia	Small, oval	Large	Chondrocytic inclusions and Swiss cheese degeneration
Dyssegmental dysplasia			
SH	Irregular	Large, camptomelic	Puddle-like spaces
RD	Irregular (lat)	Large	Patches of broad collagen fibers in resting cartilage
Atelosteogenesis	Small to absent	Tapered distally	Giant cells and/or focal myxoid degeneration
Boomerang dysplasia	Small to absent	Absent or misshapen	Giant cells, irregularly distributed resting chondrocytes
Fibrochondrogenesis	Small, pear shaped	Large with flare	Fibrous
Schneckenbecken dysplasia	Small, flat (AP) Small, round (Lat)	Large with flare	Hypercellular resting cartilage with absence of lacunar space

AP = anteroposterior radiograph; Lat = lateral view radiograph; SH = Silverman-Handmaker type; RD = Rolland–Desbuquois type.

system shows shallow orbits, flat nasal bones, short ribs with widened and cupped anterior ends, small pear-shaped vertebral bodies with some sagittal midline clefts, small ilia with a relatively broad basilar portion, very small sacrosciatic notches, and metatropic dysplasia–like limb bones that are short, broad, and dumbbell-shaped. There are metaphyseal flares and peripheral spurs. The overall radiological features resemble those of metatropic dysplasia, Kniest dysplasia, or TD, especially the first disorder.

Histopathological changes of the cartilage are unique [7, 65, 66, 68]. They are characterized by interwoven fibrous septa and fibroblastic dysplasia of chondrocytes, which are often clustered in groups of 2–4 cells per lacuna (Fig. 31.10a). The physeal growth zone is markedly retarded and disorganized (Fig. 31.10b).

Schneckenbecken Dysplasia This entity was identified by Borochowitz et al in 1986 [59]. This is an autosomal recessive condition, and is included in the metatropic dysplasia

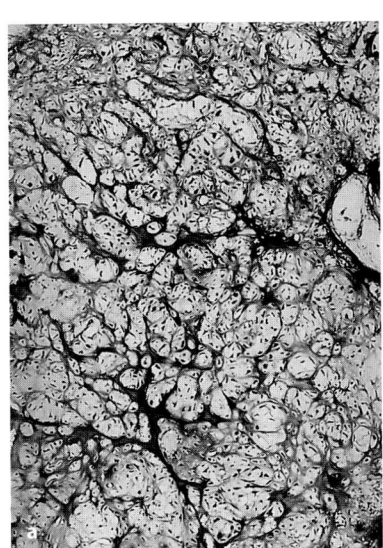
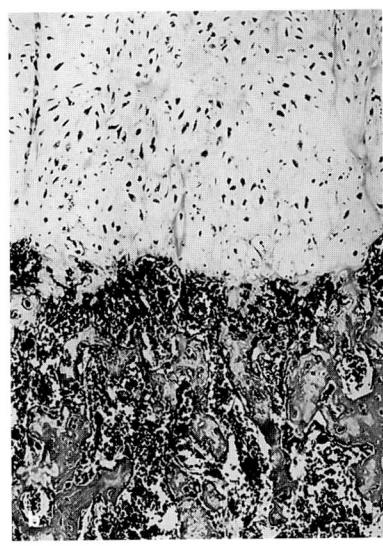

FIGURE 31.10. *Fibrochondrogenesis. (a) Resting cartilage showing interwoven fibrous septa and fibroblastic dysplasia of chondrocytes. D-PAS, ×31. (b) Poorly demarcated and disorganized physeal growth zone. Trichrome, ×57. (From Gilbert et al [5].)*

group in the 1992 classification [11]. Radiological findings of the skeletal system may suggest fibrochondrogenesis or spondylodysplasia of the Torrance or San Diego type, but there is a distinctive snail head–like projection at the medial margin of the ilium bilaterally. There is also precocious ossification of the talus.

Histopathological examination of the cartilage shows hypercellular resting chondrocytes that are spherical and the cells completely occupy the lacunae. The centrally located nuclei are relatively large. The physeal growth zone is thin and slightly irregular.

Differential Diagnosis   A simplified differential diagnosis of short-trunk chondrodysplasias is outlined in Table 31.3.

Non-Short-Trunk Chondrodysplasia with Platyspondyly

The entities in this group show a disproportionate short stature without significant shortening of the trunk. Radiologically, the vertebral bodies are markedly flattened. Histopathologically, the physeal growth zone is usually abnormal but the resting cartilage is free of significant abnormalities.

Achondroplasia (Heterozygous and Homozygous)   In the past, the term *achondroplasia* was applied indiscriminately to many short-limbed chondrodysplasias. The entity is now clearly defined [1, 3, 5, 6]. This is an autosomal dominant condition, with an 80% incidence of sporadic dominant mutation. The gene is probably within chromosome 4p [69, 70]. Unexpected recurrence of achondroplasia in infants of normal parents has been documented in several families [71, 72]. The heterozygous condition is compatible with survival into adulthood. Occasional patients may die as a

result of compression of the upper cervical spinal cord due to a small foramen magnum [73, 74]. The homozygous condition is mostly incompatible with life. Respiratory insufficiency due to a small thorax or upper cervical cord compression or both are the probable causes of death. A single patient survived beyond infancy following correction of the small foramen magnum by upper cervical laminectomy at age 4 months [75]. The clinical and radiological features of heterozygous (Fig. 31.11a,b) and homozygous (Fig. 31.12a,b) achondroplasia are, in general, identical except that the thorax is much smaller and there is more prominent platyspondyly in the homozygous form. The affected patient has a relatively normal trunk length, with narrow chest, rhizomelic shortening of the limbs, and a large head with frontal bossing and a depressed nasal bridge.

Salient radiological changes include a large head, platyspondyly, vertically shortened small square ilia, and short limb bones with metaphyseal flaring. Successful prenatal diagnosis with ultrasonography has been reported [76, 77].

Pathologically, the cartilage of heterozygous achondroplasia (Fig. 31.11c) shows a retarded but reasonably organized physeal growth zone [5, 78]. On the other hand, the physeal growth zone of homozygous achondroplasia (Fig. 31.12c,d) is markedly retarded and disorganized [9, 79].

Thanatophoric Dysplasia   Maroteaux et al [80] separated this most common lethal short-limbed chondrodysplasia from achondroplasia in 1967. The majority of cases have occurred sporadically and the most likely explanation is a new dominant mutation [6, 80]. Only one set of affected siblings

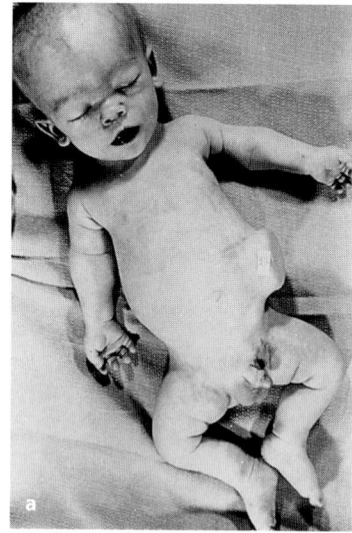
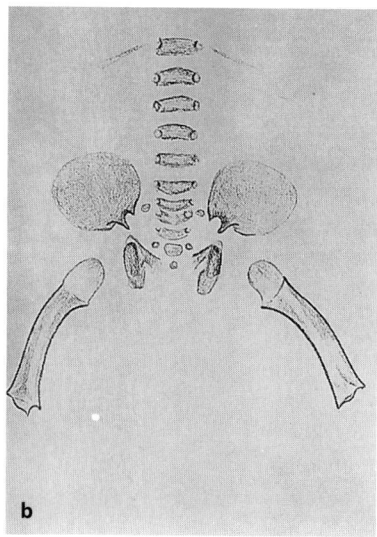
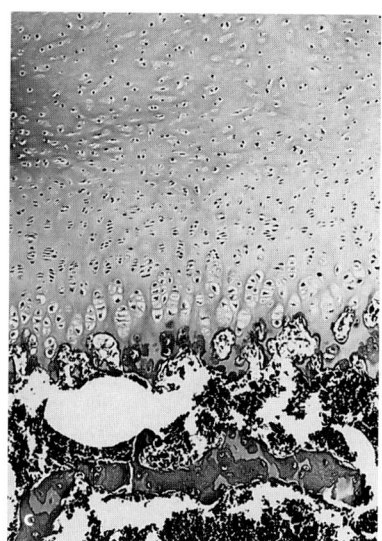

FIGURE 31.11.   *Achondroplasia, heterozygous. (a) An infant with a large head and rhizomelic dwarfism. A pacemaker was implanted in the left flank to combat arrhythmia caused by a small foramen magnum and cervical cord damage. (b) A tracing of the patient's radiograph showing platyspondyly, vertically shortened ilia, and short abnormal femora. (c) The physeal growth zone of femur is retarded but the chondrocytes are arranged in columns. H&E, ×57. ((a) and (c) from Gilbert et al [5].)*

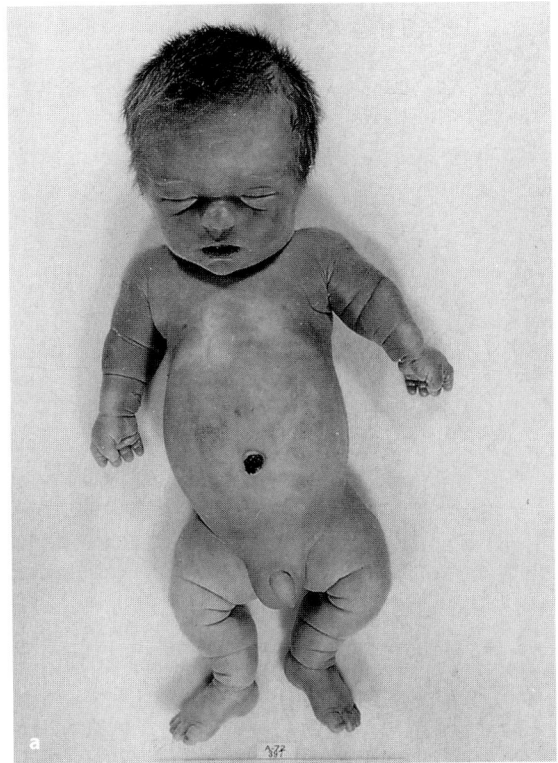
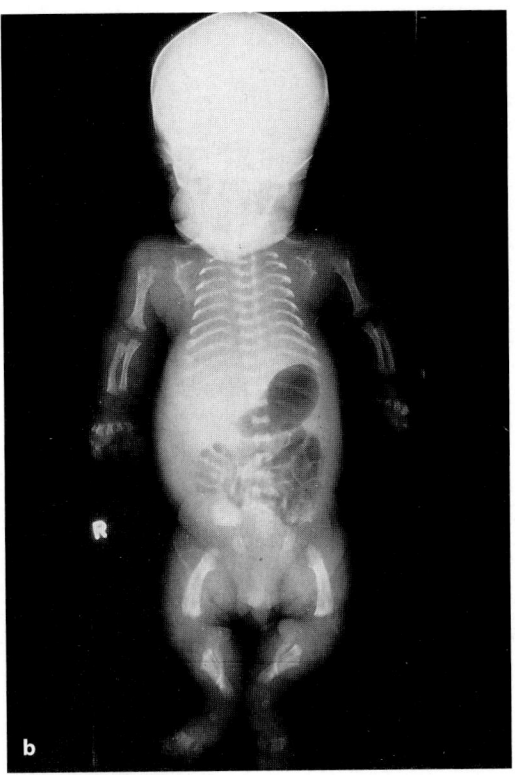
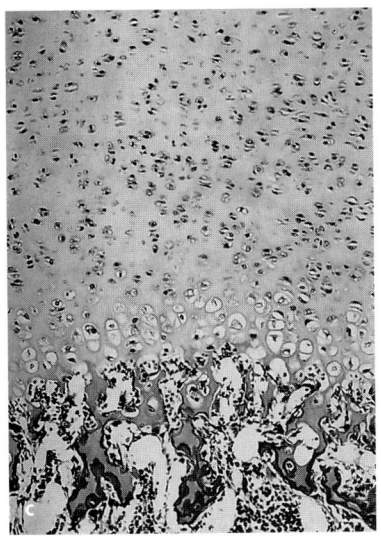
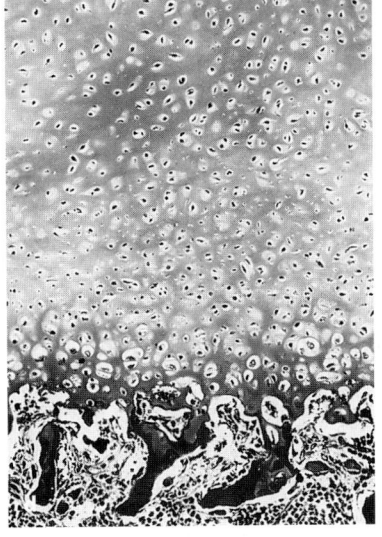

FIGURE 31.12. *Achondroplasia, homozygous. (a) A neonate of achondroplastic parents. The appearance is similar to both heterozygous achondroplasia and thanatophoric dysplasia, with a large head, small chest, and severe rhizomelic dwarfism. (b) Radiograph showing severe platyspondyly, hypoplastic ilia, and short limb bones. (c,d) Physeal growth zones of 2 siblings showing severe disorganization and retardation. H&E, ×104. (From Yang et al [9].)*

has been reported. The disorder may occasionally affect identical twins and triplets [81, 82]. Maroteaux et al [80] coined the term *thanatophore*, meaning "death-bearing" (Greek), to indicate its invariably fatal outcome in the perinatal period. The appearance of an affected baby is quite similar to that of one with homozygous achondroplasia (Fig. 31.13a). The trunk is approximately normal in length, with a narrow thorax, severe micromelia, and a large head with frontal bossing and a depressed nasal bridge.

The radiological findings (Fig. 31.13b) are diagnostic and include severe platyspondyly with H-shaped or inverted U-shaped vertebrae, markedly widened disk spaces, small ilia with narrow sacrosciatic notches, and markedly shortened limb bones with telephone receiver–like femora. The bending of femora in small fetuses less than 20 weeks' gestational age is not prominent and there is no telephone receiver–like configuration [83].

The following extraskeletal malformations have been observed in occasional patients: congenital heart disease (patent ductus arteriosus, atrial septal defect, and coarctation of aorta), and central nervous system (CNS) anomalies (megalencephaly, hydrocephalus, absence of corpus callosum, microgyria, dysmorphogenesis of temporal lobe and hippocampus, and herniation of the cerebellum) [84, 85]. Lung

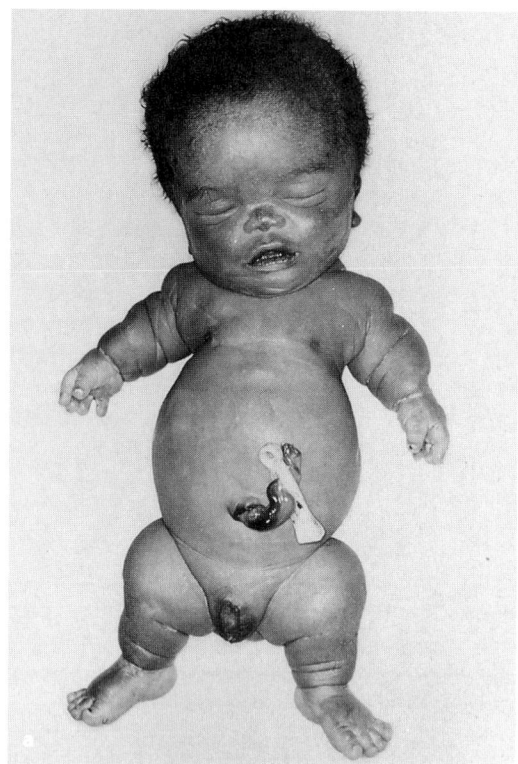
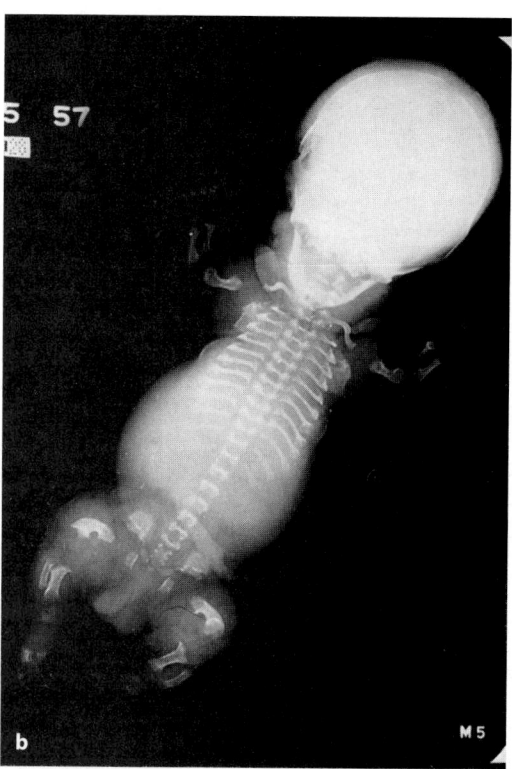

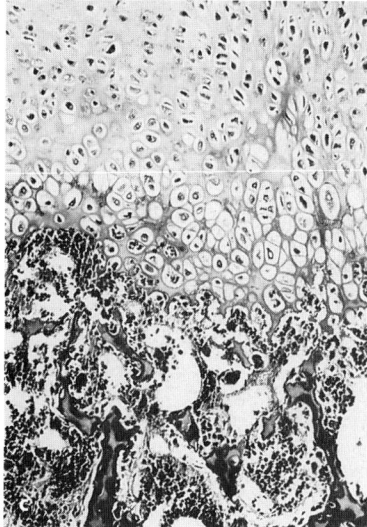
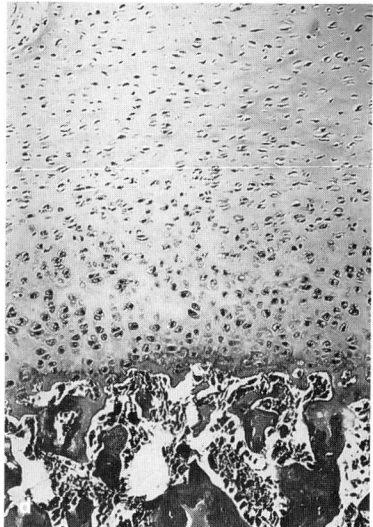

FIGURE 31.13.   *Thanatophoric dysplasia. (a) Neonate with severe micromelia, a large head, and narrow thorax. The trunk is relatively normal in length. (b) Radiograph showing severe platyspondyly, small ilia, and short limb bones with telephone receiver–like femora. (c,d) Physeal growth zones with a spectrum of disorganization and retardation. H&E, ×104. (From Yang et al [9].)*

hypoplasia occurs regularly as a result of a severe reduction in thoracic volume (see Chap. 19) and prevents survival after birth. Moreover, a small foramen magnum and spinal canal might compress the upper cervical cord and further aggravate the respiratory difficulties [86].

Prenatal diagnosis of TD by ultrasonography is now quite common [10], and the pregnancy is often terminated medically following multidisciplinary genetic counseling.

Histopathology of the cartilage (Fig. 31.13c,d) shows a severely retarded and disorganized physeal growth zone [6, 9]. The resting cartilage does not show significant abnormalities. The cartilage columns in the juxtaphyseal

primary spongiosa of the metaphysis are reduced in number and distorted; in severe cases, the metaphyseal surfaces of the physes are entirely covered by transverse plates of lamellar bone, indicating a virtual cessation of endochondral ossification. A study by Ornoy et al [87] showed abnormal mesenchyme-like tissue in the growth plate and periosteum, and this was the postulated mechanism for this abnormal bone formation.

Thanatophoric Dysplasia with Cloverleaf Skull (Kleeblattschaedell)   Cloverleaf skull may occur without chondrodysplasia. On the other hand, one should not confuse TD with hydrocephalus and TD with cloverleaf skull (TDCS)

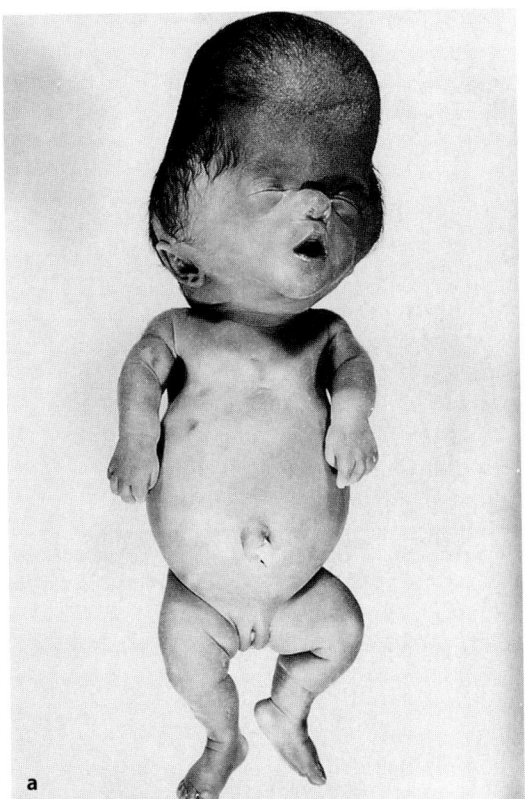

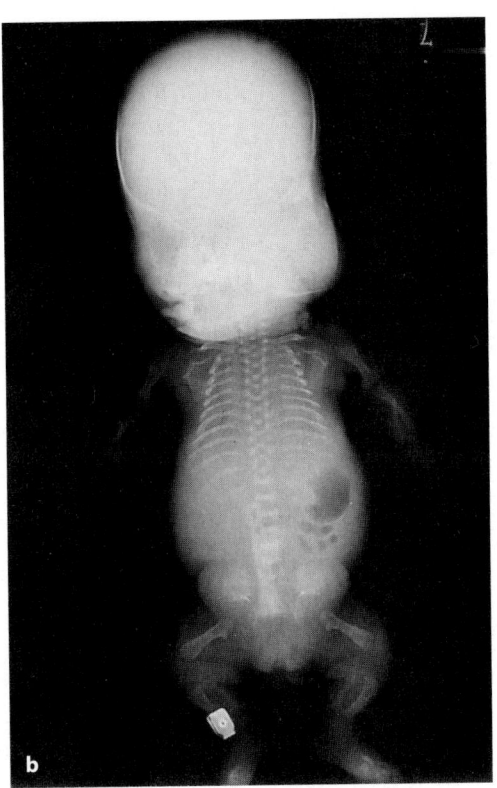

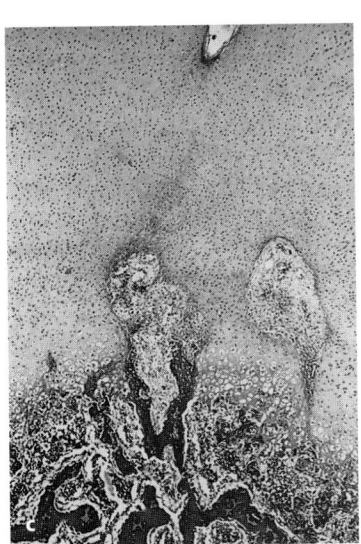

FIGURE 31.14. *Thanatophoric dysplasia with cloverleaf skull. (a) A thanatophoric dysplasia–like baby with a large, trilobed head. (b) Radiograph is similar to that of thanatophoric dysplasia. However, the femora do not show the telephone receiver–like configuration of classic thanatophoric dysplasia. (c) Ossified cartilage canals of the physis are more prominent. H&E, ×42. ((a) and (c) from Yang et al [9]. (b) from Gilbert et al [5].)*

[88] (Fig. 31.14a). Whether the TDCS and the classic TD without cloverleaf skull belong to a single entity or to two separate entities is controversial. Langer et al [89] suggested that there are probably 2 types of chondrodysplasias associated with cloverleaf skull. The first type shows a strikingly trilobed head with a towering forehead and straight or minimally curved femora (Fig. 31.14b). The platyspondyly is not as prominent as in the second type, which displays classic radiographic features of TD and less prominent cranial trilobe deformation. The second type is designated as an

atypical (mild) type (TDACS). The identical thanatophoric twins with cloverleaf skull reported by Corsello et al [83] and Horton et al [90] belong to the second type (TDACS). Careful evaluation of a typical case of TDCS did not show a small foramen magnum, a feature that is present in classic TD.

Histopathology of the cartilage in TDCS is quite similar to that of the classic TD and TDACS. Physeal growth zones are markedly retarded and disorganized; this similarity is, for some authorities, sufficient evidence to consider the two disorders as a single entity. Furthermore, the electrophoretic pattern of soluble type II collagen in the cartilage [91] and the pathological findings in the CNS [84] are identical in both conditions. However, there are subtle differences in the histopathology of the cartilage between these two conditions [89, 92]. The appendicular bones of TDCS show more prominently ossified cartilage canals vertically intersecting the physis (Fig. 31.14c). To demonstrate this particular feature, multiple sections must be evaluated. In addition, the physeal chondrocytes are larger and more vacuolated than those of TD; this difference is better shown in the vertebral bodies. On the other hand, TD frequently shows narrow bands of degeneration and fibrosis in the peripheral physis parallel to the cartilage–bone junction. Such changes are rarely seen in TDCS. The osseous portion of the vertebral bodies are thinner in TD and TDACS than in TDCS. Contrary to the gross findings, the bony spicules in the verte-

brae of TD and TDACS are thicker, longer, and more horizontally oriented than those of TDCS.

Metatropic Dysplasia   Maroteaux et al [93] described this disorder in 1966. Beck et al [94] revealed at least 3 genetic entities: 1) autosomal recessive non-lethal type, 2) dominant non-lethal type, and 3) lethal type with possibly autosomal recessive inheritance. Regardless of the different types, the body length of these patients is normal at birth, but later in life it becomes short with kyphoscoliosis. Characteristically, the baby's extremities are short, with bulbous enlargement of the joints accompanied by limitation of motion. A coccygeal tail or skin fold may be present.

Radiologically (Fig. 31.15a,b), the short limb bones demonstrate a striking barbell-like metaphyseal enlargement. The lethal form has more severely shortened tubular bones and more prominently enlarged metaphyses [94]. The vertebral bodies of this condition are thinner than

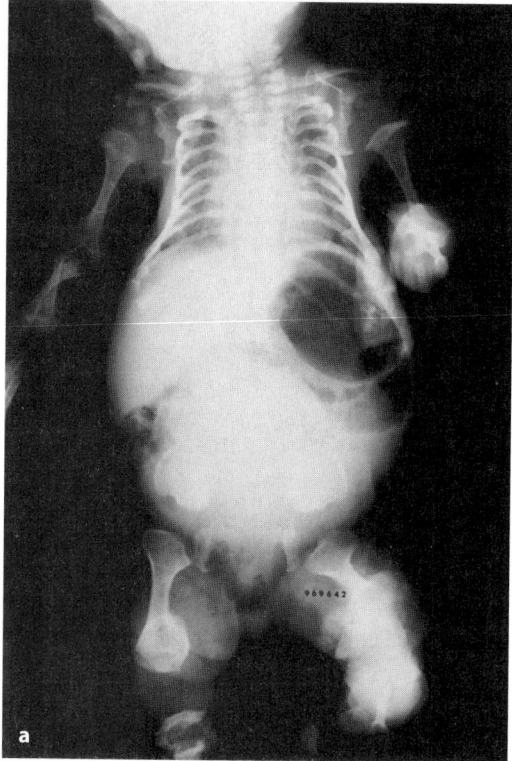
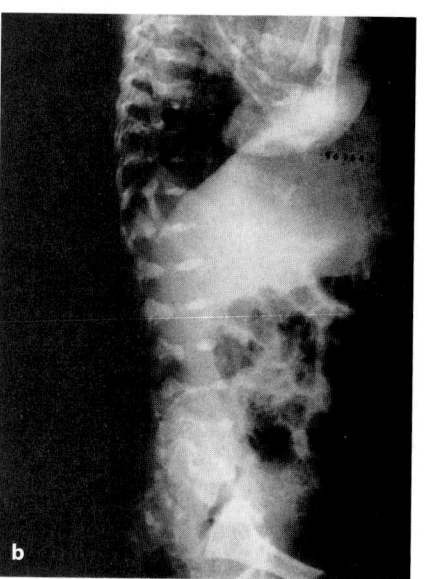
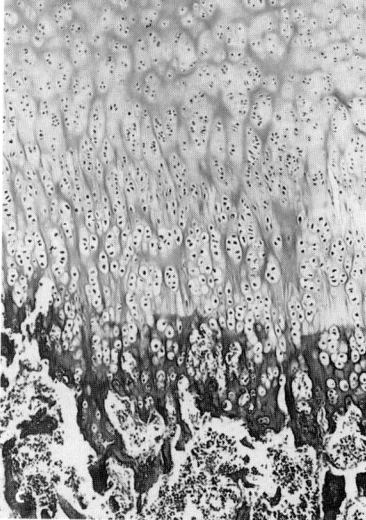

FIGURE 31.15.   *Metatropic dysplasia. (a) Radiograph of a 4-month-old infant who died of bronchopneumonia. Battle-axe–like ilia and barbell-like limb bones with large metaphyses are evident. (b) Lateral view radiograph. Platyspondyly is very prominent. (c) Physeal growth zone showing some columnization of chondrocytes and irregular vascular penetration. Cells in the zones of hypertrophy and degeneration are small. There is no band-like bone at the chondro-osseous junction in this case, but the zone of provisional calcification is prominent. H&E, ×49. ((a) and (c) from Gilbert et al [5].)*

Table 31.4.   Differential diagnosis of platyspondylic chondrodysplasias

	Radiography of Limb Bones	Histopathology of Physis
Achondroplasia, heterozygous	Slightly curved femora	Retarded with normal columnization
Achondroplasia, homozygous	Slightly curved femora	Severely retarded and disorganized
Thanatophoric dysplasia	Telephone receiver–like short femora	Severely retarded and disorganized
Cloverleaf skull with thanatophoric dysplasia	Straight short femora	Same as above but with more ossified cartilage canals
Spondylodysplasia		
San Diego type	Very short straight femora	Abnormal
Torrance type	Same as San Diego type	Normal*
Luton type	Short straight femora	Focally abnormal
Metatropic dysplasia	Dumbbell shape	Small hypertrophic chondrocytes with irregular vascular penetration
Opsismodysplasia	Very short and square bones of hands and feet	Wide hypertrophic zone with disorganization and irregular vascular penetration

*   May be abnormal [92].

those of TD. The ilia are battle-ax–like (halberd-like) in configuration.

The histopathology of the cartilage is characterized by uncoupling of endochondral (longitudinal) and perichondrial (circumferential) growth [95]. Since the endochondral ossification is abnormal, the relatively normal perichondrial ring structure with normal circumferential growth results in an unusually large metaphysis. Resting cartilage is unremarkable except that the chondrocytes are more vacuolated than normal, with metachromatic inclusions [7]. The physeal chondrocytes are either disorganized [96] or organized in columns [6] according to the previous reports. The cells in the zones of hypertrophy and degeneration are poorly developed and small. Vascular penetration of the physis is irregular [6] (Fig. 31.15c). The patients who survive beyond 2 months may show a discontinuous band of bone at the chondro-osseous junction. Primary spongiosa was absent in the metaphysis of a patient who died at age 7 months [95].

Opsismodysplasia   Three patients were described by Maroteaux et al in 1984 [97]. Two of the 3 died in infancy at ages 2 months and 6 months. The condition is believed to transmit in an autosomal recessive fashion [97, 98]. The Greek term *opsismodysplasia* is adopted to indicate a delay in bone maturation. The affected baby shows short stature, short hands, a short nose, and a depressed nasal bridge. The radiological changes of the skeletal system are characterized by severe retardation of bone maturation, with markedly shortened bones of the hands and feet, and thin lamellar vertebral bodies [97, 98].

Histopathological examination of the cartilage in 1 patient revealed a wide hypertrophic zone of physis with large groups of chondrocytes separated by septa of matrix. Irregular provisional calcification and vascular invasion are present. Type I collagen was detected in the hypertrophic zone with immunohistochemical and microchemical tests.

Spondylodysplasias of Torrance, San Diego, and Luton Types
The Torrance type and San Diego type were described by Horton et al in 1979 [91] as platyspondylic chondrodysplasias. They were not included in the international classification until 1992. The appearance of these patients is similar to that of those with TD.

Radiological changes of the skeletal system in both types are identical and differ from those of TD by having diminished ossification of the cranial base, extremely hypoplastic vertebral bodies (wafer-like to ovoid disks on lateral view), wider sacrosciatic notches, and wider but short straight long bones with more tubular contour.

The histopathology of the cartilage in both types shows large resting chondrocytes. The cellularity is normal in the San Diego type, but hypercellular in the Torrance type [91, 92]. The former is associated with poor columnization of the physeal chondrocytes, while normal column formation may [91] or may not [92] be present in the latter condition.

The Luton type was described by Winter and Thompson [99]. The radiological changes of the skeletal system are similar to the aforementioned 2 platyspondylic chondrodysplasias, with milder long-bone abnormalities and different pelvic configuration. The resting cartilage is hypercellular, and ballooned chondrocytes are arranged in clusters. The matrix shows patchy lobulation. The physeal chondrocytes are arranged in normal columns with focal disorganization.

Differential Diagnosis   A simplified differential diagnosis of the non-short-trunk platyspondylic chondrodysplasias is outlined in Table 31.4.

Short-Rib Dysplasias (With or Without Polydactyly)

The chondrodysplasias in this group are all autosomal recessive, and characterized by the presence of a narrow chest and short ribs with or without polydactyly. Except for asphyxiating thoracic dysplasia (ATD) of Jeune and short-rib dysplasia (polydactyly) [SR(P)] type IV (Beemer-Langer), polydactyly is almost a constant finding. The histopathology of the chondro-osseous tissue in this group is similar to that of the platyspondylic group. The physeal growth zone is abnormal but the resting cartilage is mostly unremarkable.

Asphyxiating Thoracic Dysplasia (Jeune)   Jeune et al [100] reported this disorder in 1955. Genetically, this is an autosomal recessive condition [101]. Approximately 60% of patients died of asphyxia in infancy because of a small chest [9, 102]. The typical patient has a severely narrowed chest

with mild acromelic shortening of the limbs. Polydactyly, congenital heart malformations, and abnormal nails and teeth are occasionally seen. Mild cystic renal dysplasia and hypoplasia are often present, and some patients may die from renal failure in later childhood [101]. Periportal fibrosis with bile duct proliferation (early cirrhosis) was reported recently [103]. This disorder is frequently confused with chondroectodermal dysplasia of Ellis–van Creveld (EVCD) [101, 102, 104].

Radiologically, the ribs are very short and the ilia are vertically shortened, but the vertebral bodies are normal. Prenatal diagnosis of ATD has been achieved with ultrasonography at 18 weeks' and 23 weeks' gestation [105, 106]. In our experience, ATD can be further divided into two types [107].

ATD (Jeune) Type I (Fig. 31.16a).   Radiologically, the vertical shortening of the ilia is more prominent in this type (Fig. 31.16b,c) than in type II. The metaphyseal ends of the limb bones are irregular. Histopathological examination of the physeal growth zone shows patchy distribution of endo-

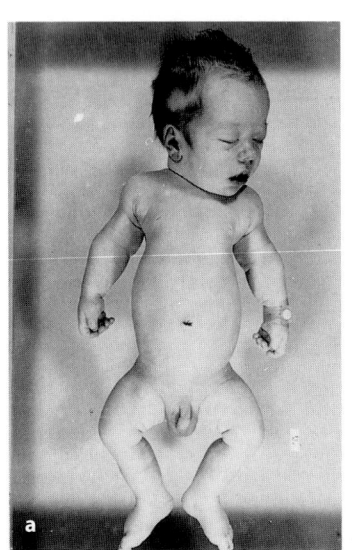
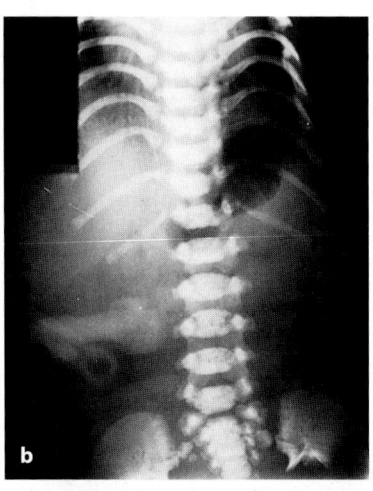
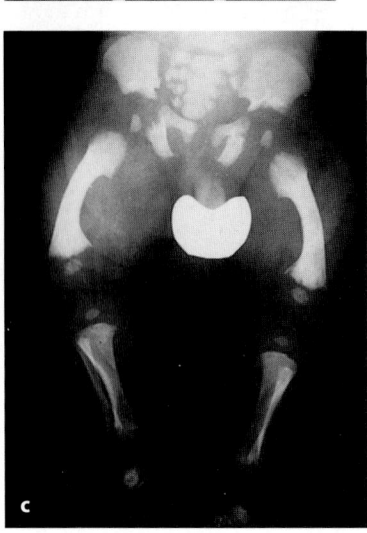
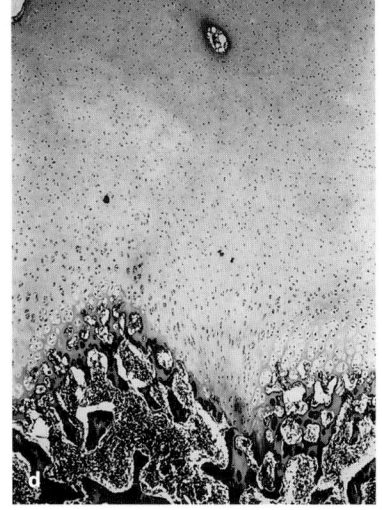

FIGURE 31.16.   *Asphyxiating thoracic dysplasia type I (Jeune). (a) Infant with a narrow chest and mild dwarfism. (b) Skeletal radiograph showing short ribs and normal vertebral bodies. (c) Vertically shortened ilia and abnormal femoral metaphyses. (d) Physeal growth zone with patchy cellular proliferation and irregular cartilage–bone junction. H&E, ×22. ((a) and (d) from Yang et al [9].)*

chondral ossification, with an irregular cartilage–bone junction (Fig. 31.16d). ATD type I is often confused with Verma–Naumoff type SR(P) dysplasia. The latter condition is perinatally fatal; the ribs and the limb bones are appreciably shorter, polydactyly is decidedly more common, and histopathology of the physis shows a mixed pattern of ATD type I and type II.

ATD (Jeune) Type II (Fig. 31.17a). Radiologically, the vertical shortening of the ilia is not as prominent as in type I. The metaphyseal ends of the limb bones are smooth and not irregular (Fig. 31.17b). Histopathological examination of the physeal growth zone invariably shows a diffuse disorganization and retardation (Fig. 31.17c). The cartilage–bone junction is not irregular. The primary spongiosa of the proximal end of the femur frequently demonstrates poorly ossified cartilage columns forming a lattice pattern. This last finding may not be seen in other bones. ATD type II may be confused with EVCD. In the latter condition, polydactyly is always present in at least one limb, and there is a higher incidence of congenital heart disease. Columnization of chondrocytes is seen in the central physis, despite growth retardation.

Ellis–van Creveld (Chondroectodermal) Dysplasia This autosomal recessive syndrome was established in 1940 by Ellis and van Creveld [108]. The patient's general appearance is similar to that of ATD (Jeune), with a small chest and acromelic shortening of the limbs [9, 101, 104, 109] (Fig. 31.18a). The radiograph of the skeletal system also appears quite similar to that of ATD (Jeune) (Fig. 31.18b). The patient with chondroectodermal dysplasia is always associated with postaxial polydactyly of the hands and ectodermal dysplasia, such as hypoplastic nails, thin hair, and

abnormal teeth. Neonatal teeth are common. The upper lip is usually short and bound down. Various congenital heart diseases occur in 50–60% of the patients, and these are the main determinants of longevity [110]. Using ultrasonography and fetoscopy, prenatal diagnosis of EVCD is possible at 17 weeks' gestation, with demonstration of polydactyly [111].

The physeal growth zones in the tubular bones and vertebrae show retardation without disorganization [6, 9] (Fig. 31.18c). Abnormal changes of endochondral ossification have been described by others [109, 112]. When the physeal growth zone is abnormal, the possibility of ATD must be considered. However, in the small fetus, disorganization of the physeal growth zone is frequently seen in the limb bones. Normal columnization of physeal chondrocytes is present only in the vertebral bodies [113].

Short-Rib Dysplasia (Polydactyly) Type I (Saldino-Noonan) Saldino and Noonan described this entity in 1972 [114]. Genetically, this is an autosomal recessive condition that is incompatible with life [115]. The affected babies are usually hydropic. Postaxial polydactyly is always present. Visceral anomalies are very common, involving especially the gastrointestinal, genitourinary, and cardiovascular systems [114–117].

Radiologically (Fig. 31.19a), the ribs are extremely short and the vertebral bodies and ilia are small and very dysplastic. The limb bones are markedly shortened, with pointed and jagged metaphyseal ends [114–117]. Oral and dental abnormalities are reported [116]. Ultrasound examination failed to demonstrate long bones or spine of 1 fetus in utero at 19, 20, and 23 weeks. A fetal radiograph at 29 weeks' gestation demonstrated unequivocal evidence of the

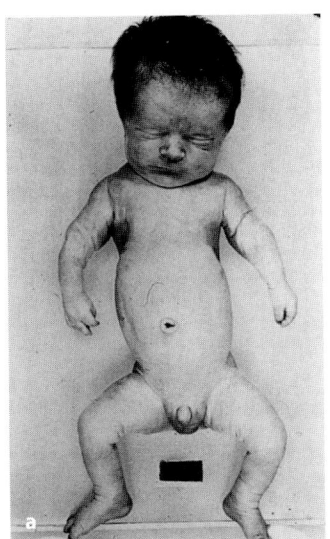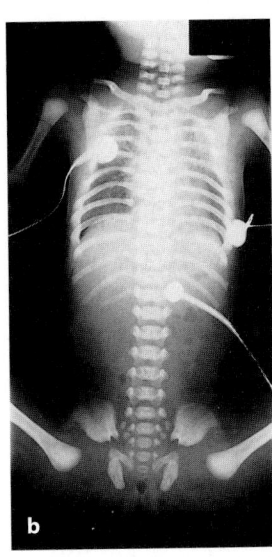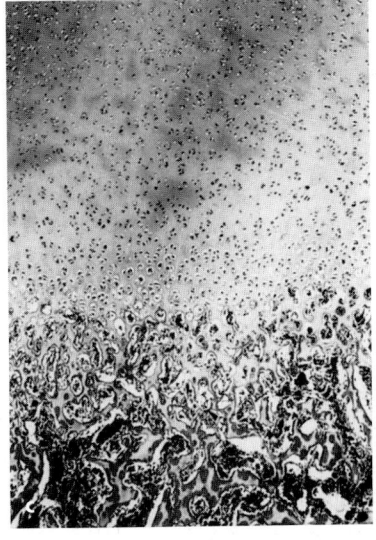

FIGURE 31.17. *Asphyxiating thoracic dysplasia type II (Jeune). (a) The neonate appears similar to a type I patient. The head appears large with a depressed nasal bridge. (b) Radiograph showing short ribs, normal vertebral bodies, and vertically shortened ilia. The metaphyses of limb bones are not irregular as seen in type I. (c) Diffusely retarded and disorganized physeal growth zone with lattice-like primary spongiosa. H&E, ×20. ((a) and (b) from Gilbert et al [5]. (c) from Yang et al [9].)*

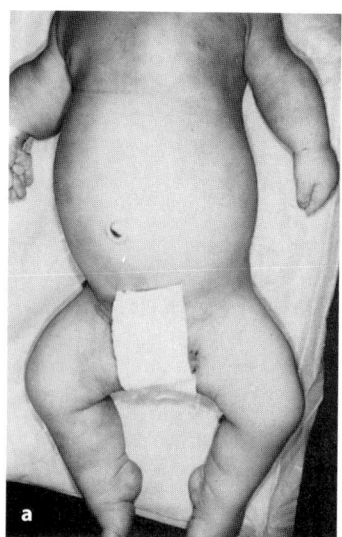
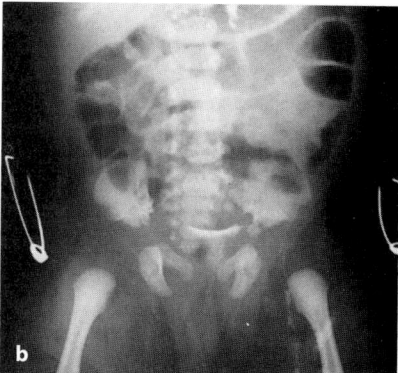
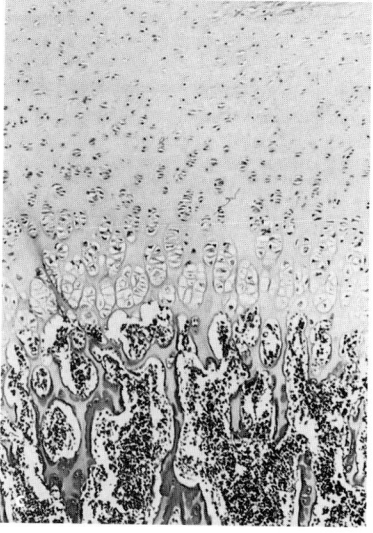

FIGURE 31.18. *Ellis–van Creveld dysplasia. (a) Infant with a small chest and mild dwarfism. (b) Skeletal radiograph showing normal vertebral bodies and vertically shortened ilia. Short ribs are not shown here. (c) Retarded but organized physeal growth zone. H&E, ×51. ((a) from Yang et al [9]. (b) and (c) from Gilbert et al [5].)*

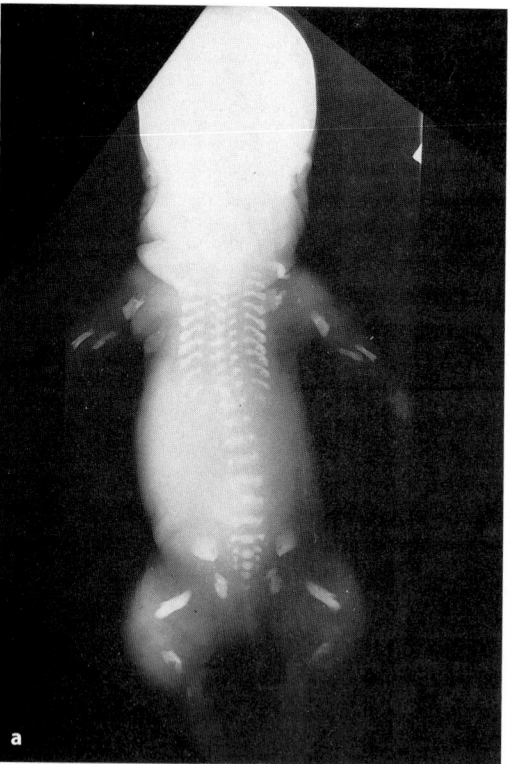
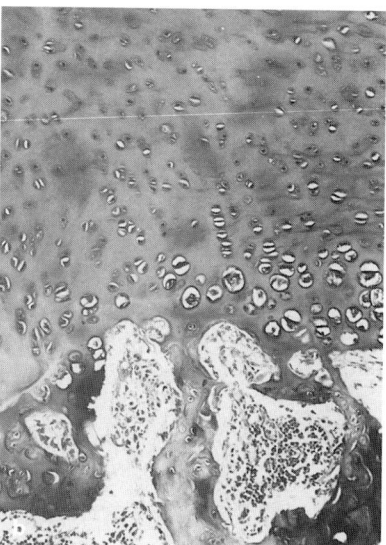
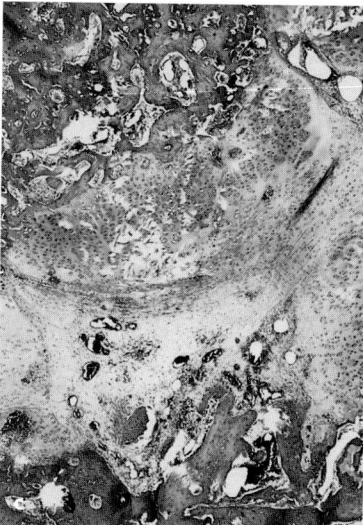

FIGURE 31.19. *Short rib (polydactyly) syndrome type 1 (Saldino-Noonan). (a) Skeletal radiograph showing extremely short ribs and small abnormal vertebral bodies and ilia. The limb bones are extremely dysplastic with irregular metaphyses. (b) Physeal growth zone of the distal end of the femur is markedly retarded and disorganized. H&E, ×91. (c) A large focus of fibrosis is present in the center of the proximal humeral physeal growth zone, and the remaining growth zone is markedly deranged. Similar changes are also seen in the proximal femora. H&E. A portion of premature ossification center is present in the upper part of this photomicrograph. H&E, ×23. (From Yang et al [9].)*

disease [117]. Fetoscopy offers an instant diagnosis; it demonstrated polydactyly as early as 15–16 weeks' gestation in a family with a previously afflicted infant [118].

Histopathologically, the physeal growth zone is markedly retarded and disorganized (Fig. 31.19b). The physeal growth zones of the proximal ends of the humeri and femora, in addition, show a large central fibrosis with converging disordered physeal chondrocytes [9] (Fig. 31.19c). Premature ossification centers are present in the proximal ends of the humeri and femora.

The differential diagnosis must include SR(P) type II (Majewski), EVCD, ATD, Meckel syndrome, and trisomy 13. Whether SR(P) type III (Verma-Naumoff) and SR(P) type I are single or separate entities is still controversial, and the problem is discussed in the section on SR(P) type III (Verma-Naumoff).

Short-Rib Dysplasia (Polydactyly) Type II (Majewski)   This entity was delineated by Majewski et al in 1971 [119]. This is probably an autosomal recessive condition and is uniformly fatal in the perinatal period [115, 119–122]. The patient shows an extremely narrow chest, protuberant abdomen, severe micromelia (Fig. 31.20a), and preaxial or postaxial polydactyly or both. The patient is often hydropic at birth. There is also a median cleft lip or palate, hypoplasia of the epiglottis and larynx, ambiguous genitalia, and renal tubular and glomerular cysts. The extraskeletal anomalies may resemble hydrolethalus syndrome [123]. A probable case of SR(P) type II with milder features was reported by Bidot-Lopez et al [124].

Radiologically, the ribs are extremely short, as in SR(P) type I. However, this type is distinguished from the latter condition by the presence of normal-appearing vertebrae

(anteroposterior view) and ilia (Fig. 31.20b). Characteristically, the tibiae are disproportionately shortened and oval. Fetoscopic demonstration of polydactyly may provide an instant prenatal diagnosis of this disease as early as 15–16 weeks' gestation in a family with a previously affected infant [118].

Histopathologically, the physeal growth zone is markedly retarded and disorganized [120–122] (Fig. 31.20c). The abnormal changes are especially prominent in the ribs, where enchondral ossification is almost absent. A normal physeal growth zone with only focal areas of disorganization was noted in the knee and ankle regions of 1 patient [5].

Short-Rib Dysplasia (Polydactyly) Type III (Verma-Naumoff)   This is a controversial entity [125, 126] that was included in SR(P) type I before the 1983 international nomenclature. Moreover, the short-rib syndrome type III (lethal thoracic dysplasia) of the 1983 international nomenclature was once considered identical to SR(P) type IV and created additional confusion [107]. The clinical features (Fig. 31.21a) and the prognosis are similar to those of SR(P) type I. However, this entity demonstrates better ossification of the ilia and limb bones (Fig. 31.21b) when compared with the classic SR(P) type I [127–129]. In addition, the incidence of gastrointestinal and genitourinary anomalies is much lower than that of SR(P) type I. The incidence of congenital heart disease is also lower and the nature of the anomalies is different from that of type I [129]. The difference between them is probably not due to relative prematurity in type I, as suggested by others. SR(P) type III also shares many clinicopathological features with ATD type I [107].

Histopathologically, the physeal growth zone is severely retarded and disorganized (Fig. 31.21c). The abnormalities

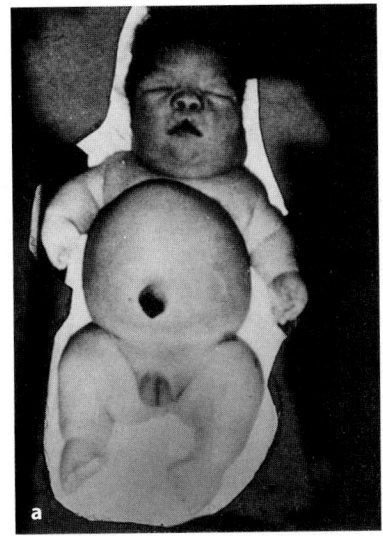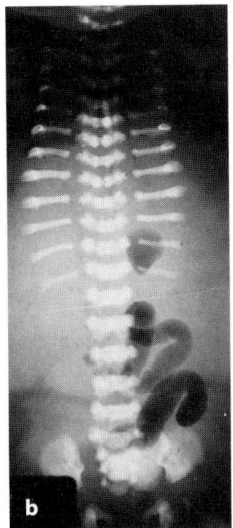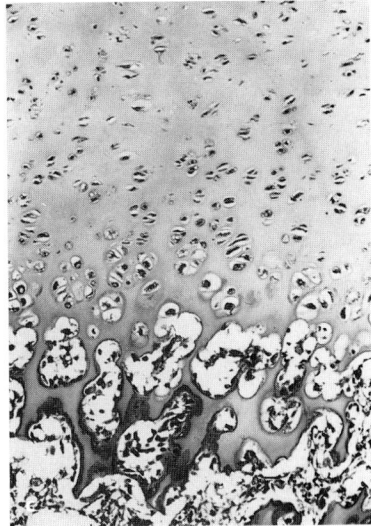

FIGURE 31.20.   *Short rib (polydactyly) syndrome type II (Majewski). (a) A hydropic neonate with severe dwarfism. Polydactyly is difficult to demonstrate in this photograph. (b) Radiograph showing extremely shortened horizontal ribs and normal-appearing vertebrae and ilia. Characteristic short oval tibiae are not shown in this picture. (c) A markedly retarded and disorganized physeal growth zone. H&E, ×78. (From Chen et al [120].)*

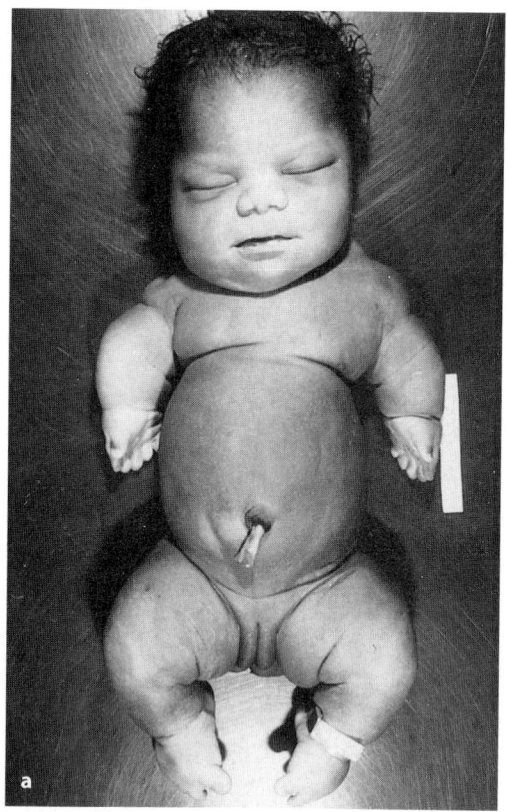
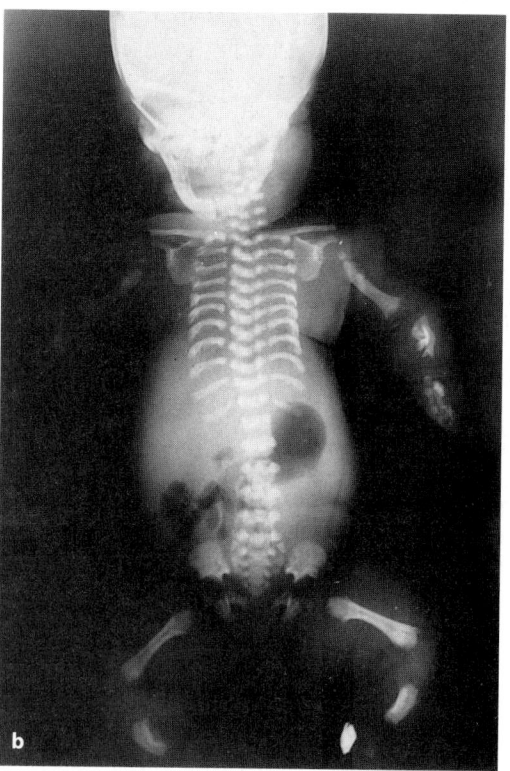
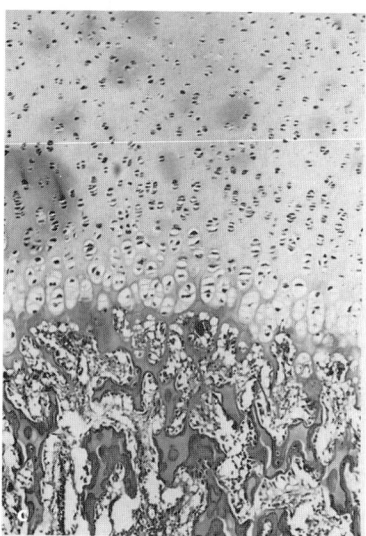

FIGURE 31.21.   *Short rib (polydactyly) syndrome type III. (a) A hydropic neonate with severely shortened extremities. Postaxial polydactyly of the hands is demonstrable. (b) Skeletal radiograph showing extremely shortened ribs, abnormal vertebral bodies, and vertically shortened ilia. The limb bones are not as dysplastic as those of short rib (polydactyly) syndrome type I. (c) The physeal growth zone is markedly retarded and disorganized, but not as severe as short rib (polydactyly) syndrome type I. H&E, ×50. (From Yang et al [129]. (c) from Gilbert et al [5].)*

are a mixture of those seen in types I and II ATD. A single patient showed chondrocytic inclusions [129] and might represent a separate entity [4, 130]. No fibrosis is present in the center of the proximal ends of the humeri or femora as in type I.

Short-Rib Dysplasia Type IV (Beemer-Langer) This entity was reported by Beemer et al in 1983 [131]. This is an autosomal recessive disorder. One recently described patient showed de novo paracentric inversion of chromosome 17q [132]. The clinical and radiological features resemble those

of ATD type II and SR(P) type II (Majewski), especially the latter condition. Lurie [133] used concordance rate analysis and separated this entity from SR(P) type II. Polydactyly is uncommon, although it may occur [134]. Cleft lip, ambiguous genitalia, and omphalocele are usually present. The extraskeletal anomalies resemble orofaciodigital syndrome [135], and overlap with midline malformation complexes [136]. Physes of tubular bones demonstrate a prominent but disorganized zone of hypertrophy and irregular vascular penetration [134].

Table 31.5.   Differential diagnosis of short-rib dysplasias (with or without polydactyly)

	Radiography		Histopathology of Physis
	Short Ribs	**Vertebrae**	
Asphyxiating thoracic dysplasia (Jeune), I	Severe	Normal	Patchy proliferation
Asphyxiating thoracic dysplasia (Jeune), II	Severe	Normal	Diffusely abnormal with lattice-like primary spongiosa
Ellis–van Creveld dysplasia	Mild to severe	Normal	Normal columnization, abnormal in periphery
SR(P) type I (Saldino-Noonan)	Extreme	Abnormal	Diffusely abnormal, focal fibrosis in proximal physis
SR(P) type II (Majewski)	Extreme	Normal	Diffusely abnormal
SR(P) type III (Verma-Naumoff)	Extreme	Abnormal	Mixed Jeune I and II histology
SR(P) type IV (Beemer-Langer)	Extreme	Abnormal	Prominent zone of hypertrophy wtih disorganization

SR(P) = short rib (polydactyly) syndrome.

Unclassified Short-Rib Dysplasias The SR(P) dysplasias may not be limited to the 4 types listed in the 1992 classification [4], and the classification of a given case may become controversial. Therefore, some authors suggested a single entity to encompass all types [132]. Single case reports that cannot be classified within the 1992 nomenclature are not enumerated in this chapter, except for the following case which was described in the previous edition.

In 1977, Piepkorn et al [137] described a patient with lethal SR(P) syndrome with severe deficiency of ossification in all bones except for the clavicles. The humeri, radii, ulnae, femora, tibiae, and fibulae were composed entirely of cartilage [137]. Cherstvoy et al [138] classified this case as type IV SR(P) syndrome. However, Spranger and Maroteaux [4] recently reclassified the case as a severe form of boomerang dysplasia.

Differential Diagnosis A simplified differential diagnosis of short-rib dysplasias is outlined in Table 31.5.

Miscellaneous Disorders

There are no common clinical features among the entities in this group. Except for diastrophic dysplasia, the physeal growth zones of these disorders reveal no significant abnormalities.

Chondrodysplasia Punctata (Stippled Epiphysis, Chondrodystrophia Calcificans Congenita) This group of disorders is characterized by stippled epiphyseal calcification in infancy. The entity was originally considered to be a variant of achondroplasia by Conradi in 1914 [139] and by Hünermann in 1931 [140]. According to the 1992 international nomenclature [11], there are 4 types: rhizomelic, X-linked dominant (Conradi-Hünermann), X-linked recessive, and tibia–metacarpal (MT) type. These different types share the following features in varying degrees and incidence: stippled epiphyses with dwarfism, flat facies with a depressed nasal

bridge, cataract, short neck, flexion contracture, foot deformity, and ichthyosiform dermatitis. Epiphyseal stippling also occurs in diastrophic dysplasia in infancy, and rarely with maternal use of warfarin, hypothyroidism, Zellweger syndrome, generalized GM_1 gangliosidosis, mucolipidosis II, anencephaly, Smith-Lemli-Opitz syndrome, fetal alcohol syndrome, and trisomies 18 and 21 [11, 141, 142]. Pauli and Haun [143] recently reviewed the probable pathogenesis of epiphyseal stippling in these various conditions.

Rhizomelic Type. This is an autosomal recessive disorder [141, 142]. The prognosis is poor; more than 60% of the patients die in the first year of life. The patient has microcephaly with chipmunk-like face, severe psychomotor retardation, and a high incidence of cataract. The stippled calcification may be absent after the age of 3.5 months [141]. Deficiency of multiple peroxisomal enzymes [144] and isolated deficiency of dihydroxyacetonephosphate acyltransferase [145] have been demonstrated, raising the possibility of prenatal detection of the disease by biochemical procedures. Greenberg dysplasia and dappled dysplasia must be excluded from this condition (see Unclassified or Unclassifiable Osteochondrodysplasia).

The salient radiological findings [141, 142] include severe symmetrical rhizomelic (proximal) shortening of the limb bones, with flared irregular metaphyses. Coronal clefting of the vertebral bodies is present in the lateral view, but there is no stippled calcification along the spine. There is trapezoid dysplasia of the upper part of the ilia.

Histopathological changes of the epiphyseal cartilage are characterized by subarticular myxoid and cystic degeneration of the epiphyseal cartilage with dystrophic calcification (Fig. 31.22a). Increased vascularization of resting cartilage has been reported [6]. The physeal growth zones of the long bones show normal columnization of the proliferating and hypertrophic chondrocytes (Fig. 31.22b). Focal disruption of

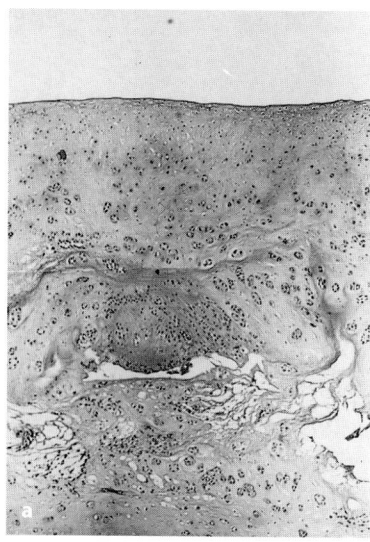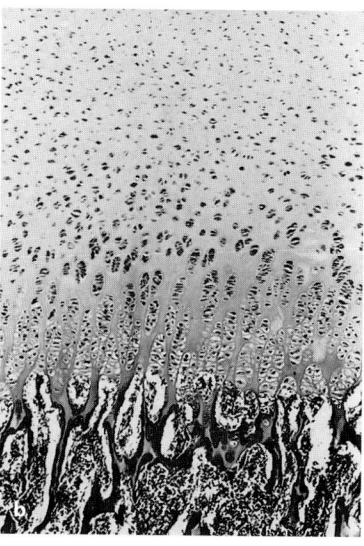

FIGURE 31.22. *Chondrodysplasia punctata, rhizomelic type. (a) Subarticular cystic degeneration and calcification. H&E, ×31. (b) Physeal growth zone shows no abnormalities. H&E, ×41. (From Gilbert et al [5].)*

normal physis by zones of proliferating connective tissue and ossification has been reported [141]. Both normal and abnormal growth zones may exist in the same patient in different areas [6].

X-Linked Dominant Type (Conradi-Hunermann). This entity was originally considered as an autosomal dominant instead of X-linked dominant disorder. It is seen exclusively in female patients (Fig. 31.23a), and is associated with normal intellect, normocephaly, and good prognosis. However, it is lethal in the affected hemizygous male fetuses [146–148]. Manzke et al [147] estimated that about one-fourth of all chondrodysplasia punctata patients have this type. Clinically, this type is characterized by punctate epiphyseal calcification (Fig.

31.23b), asymmetrical shortening of the limbs, asymmetrical cataracts, linear or whorled patches of ichthyosiform erythroderma or atrophoderma or both, and circumscribed cicatricial alopecia. The mosaic pattern of manifestations and the limitation of reported cases to females are considered to reflect lyonization. The family reported by Silengo et al [149] probably represents this type. Extensive punctate calcifications were shown in the aborted fetus at 16 weeks' gestation. A 2-year-old sister had milder calcifications, and the affected 27-year-old mother showed virtually no calcifications [149]. There have been a few reports of prenatally diagnosed chondrodysplasia punctata made by serendipity near term [149], or by a family history [10].

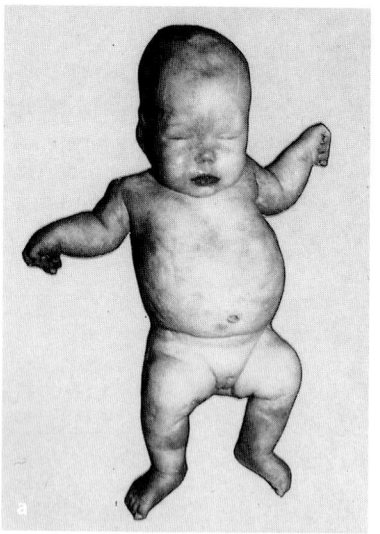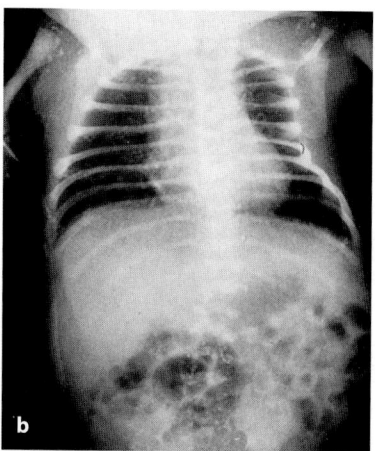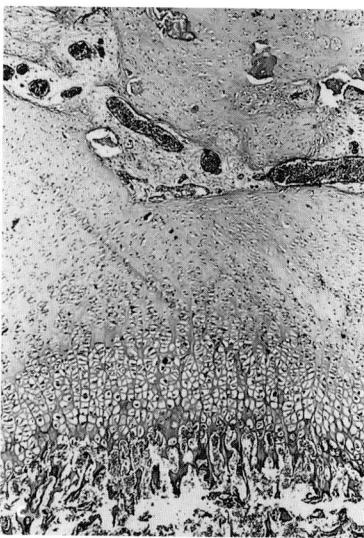

FIGURE 31.23. *Chondrodysplasia punctata, X-linked dominant. (a) Female infant showing severe dwarfism without microcephaly. Asymmetrical involvement is not prominent in this particular case. (b) The same infant's radiograph showing punctate calcification along the spine and epiphyseal regions of the humeri. (c) Physeal growth zone is normally organized. Multiple foci of calcification are seen in and about large cartilage canals. H&E, ×31. ((a) and (b) from Yang et al [9]. (c) from Gilbert et al [5].)*

Histopathological examination of the skeletal system shows normal proliferation of the physeal chondrocytes with columnization. A mild myxoid degeneration of the cartilage is common, especially in the zone of proliferation and the adjacent resting cartilage. Focal calcification is present in the cartilage adjacent to the physis, usually within and around cartilage canals (Fig. 31.23c) [9]. Calcification also occurs in the perichondrial and subsynovial soft tissue.

X-Linked Recessive Type. This type affects male offspring [150]. Cytogenetic examination demonstrated a deletion of the terminal short arm of the X chromosome in occasional patients [150, 151]. The clinical findings are similar to those of the X-linked dominant (Conradi-Hünermann) type, but mental retardation is consistently seen in this type. The infant shows a moderate degree of proportionately short stature with mild microcephaly, sparse and unruly hair, and mild generalized ichthyosis of skin. Severe nasal hypoplasia is common, which may improve later in childhood. Distal phalangeal hypoplasia has been noted in the fetus.

Radiological examination reveals symmetrical punctate stippling of multiple epiphyses, including the paravertebral epiphyses, and the laryngotracheal cartilage. Poorly developed small distal phalanges and metaphyseal cupping of the femora and tibiae have been noted in the fetus. The stippled calcification is not demonstrated in aborted fetuses at 14 and 22 weeks' gestation, and it is also absent after the age of 18 months [150, 151].

The osteochondral histopathology is yet to be delineated.

Tibia–Metacarpal Type. This sporadic disorder is compatible with life [152]. Clinically, the patient shows midfacial hypoplasia with a depressed nasal bridge, small mouth, and micrognathia. Radiological examination of the skeletal system shows punctate calcifications in the sacral, tarsal, and carpal regions. There is disproportionate shortening of the 4th metacarpals and tibiae. Short 3rd metacarpals, short broad proximal phalanges of the 2nd digits, deficient ossification of the cervical spine, coronal clefting of the vertebral bodies, distal hypoplasia of ulnae with bowing, and proximal dislocation of radii may be present.

Histopathological changes of the skeletal system are yet to be documented.

Camptomelic Dysplasia (Camptomelic Syndrome, Camptomelic Dwarfism, Camptomelic Syndrome) This autosomal recessive disorder was originally defined by Maroteaux et al [153] and Bianchine et al [154] in 1971. *Camptomelia* means "curved limb" in Greek. An abnormal chromosome 17 with de novo paracentric inversion or rearrangement of the long arm has been reported [132]. Recently the gene was mapped to 17q24.3–q25.1 [155]. Early death often occurs due to severe hypotonia, respiratory difficulties caused by tracheobronchial malacia and narrow chest, or aspiration pneumonia [156], usually within 1 month [157].

Clinically, the affected infant is usually born near term with a weight in the low-normal range. Polyhydramnios is seen in one-third of patients. The patient has a large dolichocephalic head, a small flat face with micrognathia and a cleft or high-arched palate, and short limbs with anterior bowing of the legs or thighs or both, frequently with pretibial cutaneous dimples [158] (Fig. 31.24a). Kyphoscoliosis and severe talipes equinovarus are common. Polyhydramnios may prompt fetal ultrasonography and radiography, which may demonstrate cervical hyperextension and an unusual presentation [157].

Radiological examination of the skeletal system [156–160] (Fig. 31.24b) shows anterior bowing of the shortened tibiae, fibulae, or femora; hypoplastic fibulae;

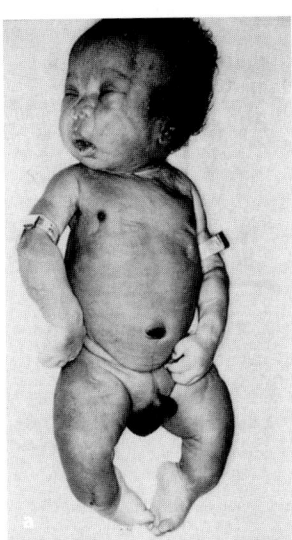 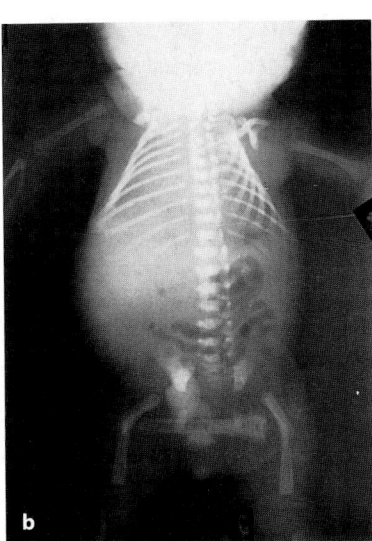 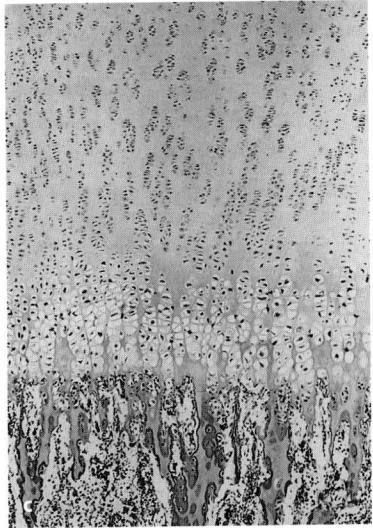

FIGURE 31.24. *Camptomelic dysplasia. (a) Infant with a large head, flat face, low-set ears, micrognathia, and bowed legs. (b) Skeletal radiograph of another patient showing bowed femora. (c) Physeal growth zone shows no appreciable abnormalities. H&E, ×41. (From Gilbert et al [5].)*

severely hypoplastic scapulae; hypoplastic pedicles of the thoracic vertebrae; retarded ossification of the sternum, cervical spine, tarsal, and knee epiphyses; and 11 paired thin ribs. The pelvis is narrow because of agenesis of the sacral wings, narrow small iliac wings, and poorly developed ischiopubic rami. Subluxation of the hips is common. Mild bowing is occasionally present in the humeri, ulnae, and radii. The neurocranium is large but the chondrocranium is small.

Extraskeletal findings include XY gonadal dysgenesis in some phenotypically female patients with lack of testis-organizing factor "H-Y" antigen [156, 157, 159], CNS anomalies (absence of olfactory nerves, macrocephaly, hydrocephalus, polygyria), congenital heart defects (patent ductus arteriosus, ventricular septal defect, coarctation of aorta), urinary system abnormalities (hydronephrosis, hydroureter, renal hypoplasia, medullary and glomerular cysts), other rarer anomalies, and secondary changes such as pulmonary hypoplasia and systemic changes of hypoxia.

Histopathological examination of the skeletal system shows no defect in bone collagen, ground substance, or mineralization, in spite of limb bowing [158]. Since a similar bowing is present in osteogenesis imperfecta (OI) and other entities, the camptomelia per se is considered a secondary phenomenon [160]. The resting cartilage is unremarkable. However, ultrastructurally there are more numerous dark cells, which are surrounded by granular and flocular materials [161]. The physeal growth zone is almost normal in most patients [6] (Fig. 31.24c). Occasional patients show mild retardation and even disorganization of the physes and osteoporosis [9, 156].

The differential diagnosis must include infantile hypophosphatasia, OI type II, and especially kyphomelic dysplasia. Many other conditions may show mild bowing of long bones [162].

Kyphomelic Dysplasia (Short-Limbed Camptomelic Dysplasia)
The entity [163], originally considered short-limbed camptomelic dysplasia [160, 164], is an autosomal recessive condition with good prognosis. This disorder is characterized by severely angulated short femora and a mild to moderate degree of platyspondyly. The patient shows other changes suggestive of camptomelic dysplasia, for example, congenital bowing of other long bones with skin dimples, narrow thorax, and micrognathia. However, kyphomelic dysplasia does not have the other changes of camptomelic dysplasia, such as hypoplasia of thoracic vertebral pedicles, hypoplasia of the scapulae, severe talipes equinovarus, mental retardation, fatal respiratory difficulties, and sex reversal with XY gonadal dysgenesis [163]. Prenatal diagnosis of this disorder has been achieved at 17 weeks' gestation [165].

Diastrophic Dysplasia Lamy and Maroteaux [166] delineated this autosomal recessive disorder in 1960. Type IX collagen of the cartilage is abnormal [167], and the gene of this disorder is mapped to the long arm of chromosome 5 [168]. Less than 10% of patients die in the neonatal period. Respiratory insufficiency and pneumonia are the causes of such

neonatal death. As the word *diastrophic* denotes "tortuous" in Greek, the disease is characterized by progressive kyphoscoliosis, bilateral clubfeet (pes equinovarus), and extreme short stature with micromelia. In the past, this was called *achondroplasia with clubbed feet*, or *cherub dwarf*. The disease is apparent at birth. The affected baby shows clubbed feet, and characteristic hand deformities including short fingers and proximally inserted "hitchhiker" thumbs. The toes are also similar in configuration. The simultaneous presence of contracture and dislocation of joints, and proximal symphalangism are commonly seen. Cleft palate is present in one-third to one-half of patients and is occasionally associated with hypoplasia of the mandible [1]. In more than 80% of patients, the ears develop intense inflammatory swelling within the first few days or weeks of life. After 3–4 weeks, it results in cauliflower-like deformity, calcification, and even ossification of the ears. Despite the severe debilitating skeletal deformities and the possibility of spinal cord compression, intellectual development and head size are normal.

Radiological examination of the skeletal system [1, 3] shows that the tubular bones are short and thick with broad metaphyses. The epiphyseal development is delayed, especially in the femora. This produces flat and irregular epiphyses. Stippled epiphyses are noted in early infancy. The 1st metacarpals are small and oval or triangular. Carpal ossification centers are present at birth. The lower lumbar spine shows moderate narrowing of the interpediculate distance. The iliac bones are normal at birth; later the acetabular roofs develop secondary changes.

Prenatal diagnosis of diastrophic dysplasia has been successful at 16 and 17 weeks' gestation [169, 170].

Histopathological examination of the cartilage in the fetal period shows significant deficiency of the matrix with irregular areas of myxoid and cystic degeneration. The perilacunar matrix is spared by the abnormal changes and appears more darkly stained [171] (Fig. 31.25). No appreciably abnormal changes are present in the physeal growth zones. After the neonatal period [8, 172, 173], the cartilage reveals a reduction in the number of chondrocytes in both resting cartilage and physeal growth zone. The latter is about one-half of the normal thickness, with short columns and fibrous stroma. The resting chondrocytes are irregular in distribution and aggregate in islands. The lacunae often contain 3 to 4 enlarged chondrocytes and are surrounded by pink matrix. Many of these cells appear degenerated with pyknotic nuclei. The cytoplasm, the lacunar area, and the immediate surrounding matrix are intensely stained with metachromatic stains, such as alcian blue, toluidine blue, azure A (pH 1.75), and PAS. Concentric metachromatic laminations of the lacunae are seen in plastic sections cut 1 μm thick. The abnormal changes may extend to the physeal growth zone in patchy areas. As in the fetal period the cartilage matrix is mostly deficient with areas of cystic degeneration. Silver methenamine stain clearly shows an abnormal collagen distribution. This is confirmed, ultrastructurally, by

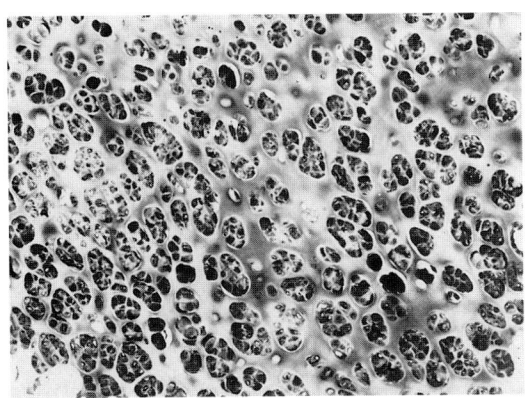

FIGURE 31.25. *Diastrophic dysplasia. The resting cartilage of a fetus showing matrix deficiency and cystic degeneration. The matrix surrounding the chondrocytes is prominently stained with PAS after diastase digestion. ×89. (Courtesy of F. Qureshi, MD, Hutzel Hospital, Detroit.)*

the presence of abnormally arranged thick bundles of collagen fibrils [8, 172, 174]. The abnormal collagen fibrils are also present in the lacunar spaces. Fibrovascular proliferation and ossification may occur. Since most of the above pathological changes are also observed in the tracheal [173] and earlobe cartilage, diastrophic dysplasia is considered a generalized disorder of cartilage [172].

The differential diagnosis must include achondroplasia, arthrogryposis multiplex, and spondyloepiphyseal dysplasia congenita. The lethal atelosteogenesis type II shows many of the same phenotypical and histopathological features as severe diastrophic dysplasia. The genetics of both entities are similar.

Larsen Syndrome In 1950 Larsen et al [175] described 6 unrelated patients with multiple congenital dislocations. Joint dislocations involved elbows, hips, and knees. There are both autosomal dominant and autosomal recessive forms. Clinically, the facial appearance is considered to be characteristically flat with a depressed nasal bridge, hypertelorism, and a prominent forehead [175, 176]. The fingers are cylindrical and nontapering, and the thumbs are spatulate. There is equinovarus or valgus deformity of the feet. Cleft palate or lip, genital anomalies, and syndactyly may be demonstrated.

Radiological examination of the skeletal system reveals multiple joint dislocations, epiphyseal dysplasia, short metacarpals with multiple ossification centers, delayed coalescence of calcaneal ossification centers, and abnormal segmentation of vertebrae, especially in the upper thoracic and cervical regions. The recessive form shows a more prominent short stature, epiphyseal dysplasia, and metacarpal shortness. Vertebral segmentation, syndactyly, cleft palate, and genital anomalies are also more common in this form. The dominant form shows a more striking flat face.

Histopathological examination of the tubular bones and vertebral bodies shows no significant abnormalities [177] (Fig. 31.26). However, electron microscopy of the resting chondrocytes demonstrates fairly abundant dilated rough endoplasmic reticulum containing moderately electron-dense proteinaceous material [177]. Tracheal cartilage rings are small, thin, and soft. The central portions of the cartilage rings are hypocellular, with a deficiency in hyaline matrix. The same areas stain intensely with PAS and are distinctly argyrophilic with reticulum stain. Ultrastructurally, mature collagen fibers are reduced in number, with a relative increase in small short fibers. Abnormal histochemical properties are also noted in the dermal connective tissue and joint capsules. The dermal collagen bundles are relatively broad and smudgy. Abundant elastic fibers are also seen.

Desbuquois Syndrome Desbuquois et al [178] reported this autosomal recessive condition in 1966. Some of the patients are detected prenatally. There is significant phenotypic variability. Clinically, the patient has a round flat face with severe micrognathia, severe rhizomelic shortening of the limbs, and severe joint laxity. Multiple joint dislocations are seen later in life [178, 179].

Radiological examination of the skeletal system shows a monkey wrench–like femoral neck because of an enlarged lesser trochanter and metaphyseal beaking. A supernumerary ossification center is present between the proximal phalanx of the index finger and the 2nd metacarpal, causing radial deviation of the same finger. This supernumerary bone fuses with the 2nd metacarpal later in life.

Histopathological examination of the cartilage shows abnormally narrow physeal growth zones with their chondrocytes arranged in ovoid groups. Hypertrophic

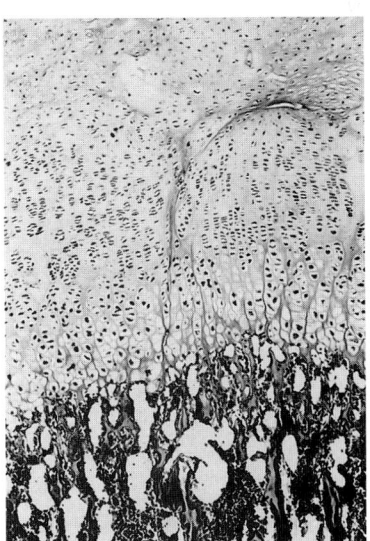

FIGURE 31.26. *Larsen syndrome. The physeal growth zone is mostly normal in appearance. Slight disorganization is present in focal areas. H&E, ×50. (Courtesy of C.-H. Chang, MD, Children's Hospital of Michigan, Detroit.)*

Table 31.6.   Differential diagnosis of miscellaneous chondrodysplasias

	Clinical	Histopathology of Cartilage
Chondrodysplasia punctata (4 types)	Stippled epiphyses	Focal calcification myxoid degeneration*
Camptomelic dysplasia	Bowing of limb bones	Mostly unremarkable
Kyphomelic dysplasia	Severely angulated short femora	
Diastrophic dysplasia	Short fingers and toes, hitchhiker thumbs (and toes), club feet	Perilacunar corona of collagen and matrix deficiency with cystic degeneration
Larsen syndrome	Multiple congenital joint dislocations	Unremarkable
Desbuquois syndrome	Severe joint laxity, very short limbs, and abnormal facies	Narrow physis with cells in ovoid groups, hypercellular large resting chondrocytes

* Rhizomelic type and Conradi–Hümermanm type.

chondrocytes are relatively small. The chondrocytes in the resting cartilage are large and numerous. Ultrastructural examination shows homogeneously dense inclusions in the rough endoplasmic reticulum of resting chondrocytes. There is reduction of collagen fibrils and proteoglycan in the cartilaginous matrix.

Differential Diagnosis   A simplified differential diagnosis of this miscellaneous group is outlined in Table 31.6.

Others

Mesomelic dysplasias (types Nievergelt, Langer, Robinow, Rheinhardt, and others), acromesomelic dysplasia, and otopalatodigital syndrome (types I and II) are also identifiable at birth [17]. The pathological changes of the skeletal system in these conditions are either unrecorded or insignificant.

Osteochondrodysplasias with Abnormal Bone Density

Osteogenesis Imperfecta

OI comprises a heterogeneous group of systemic collagen disorders characterized by osteopenia, multiple fractures, and blue sclerae. It is traditionally divided into two main clinical groups: OI congenita, which is a severe neonatal form, and OI tarda, a mild form in which the patient is apparently normal at birth. However, there is a wide spectrum of severity even in the same family. Studies by Sillence [180] suggested that there are at least 4 types, designated types I to IV. In this classification, OI type II and probably type III are equivalent to OI congenita. OI types I and IV are equivalent to OI tarda but may occasionally manifest in the perinatal period; they are usually not subjected to pathological examination.

OI Type II (OI Congenita, OI Fetalis, Perinatal Lethal OI, Vrolik Disease)   This type of OI is most commonly encountered at postmortem examination because of its uni-

formly lethal outcome during the perinatal period. The disease was first described by Vrolik in 1849 [1], and has been considered an autosomal recessive condition [180]. However, many sporadic severe cases are probably examples of autosomal dominant mutation [1, 181, 182]. In the past disturbances of collagen formation, organization, and chemical composition were suspected based on histopathological examination of the dermal connective tissue [183]. The observation was confirmed by recent biochemical studies that demonstrated abnormalities in the secretion of type I procollagen. One of the two pro-α_1 (I) chains of type I procollagen synthesized by fibroblasts is abnormally shortened. Such molecules are unstable and degrade intracellularly or after excretion [21]. Type I collagen of bone is markedly reduced. There is evidence of heterogeneity at the molecular level [184, 185]. Intracranial hemorrhage or respiratory insufficiency is the usual cause of death. Upper cervical cord compression might also be the cause of death [186]. The differential diagnosis includes lethal hypophosphatasia and achondrogenesis type IA.

Prenatal diagnosis of OI type II is possible before 17.5 weeks' gestation with ultrasonography [187, 188], and at 20–22 weeks' gestation with fetal radiography and biochemical analysis of cultured amniotic fluid cells for abnormal collagen chemistry [188].

Clinically the affected infant is small for gestational age. The cranial bones are small, soft, and mostly of the wormian type. The cranial sutures and fontanelles are widely open. The extremities are short and distorted because of multiple fractures (Fig. 31.27a). Extraskeletal manifestations include deep blue sclerae, hyperlaxity of joints, and hernia.

Radiologically, OI type II is further classified into 3 subgroups [189]. Type IIA patients (the most common group) show marked fragility of the skin and connective tissue, radiological changes of broad crumpled femora, and continuously beaded ribs (Fig. 31.27b). This subgroup is now considered an autosomal dominant disorder [182, 184, 185,

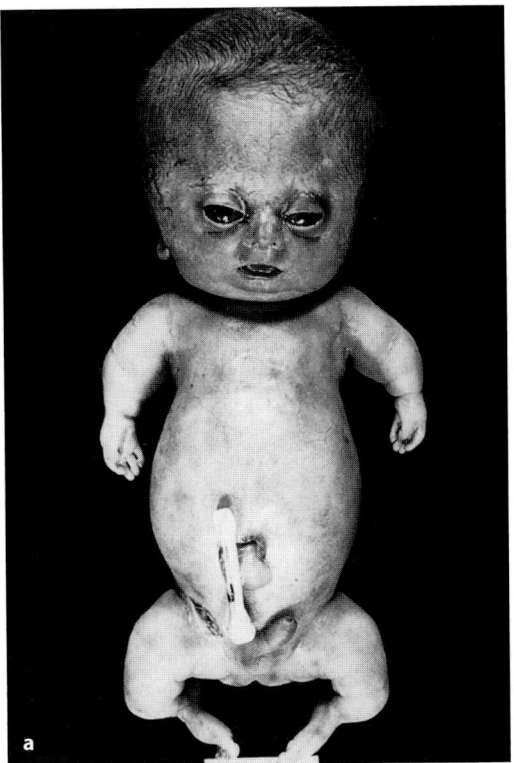

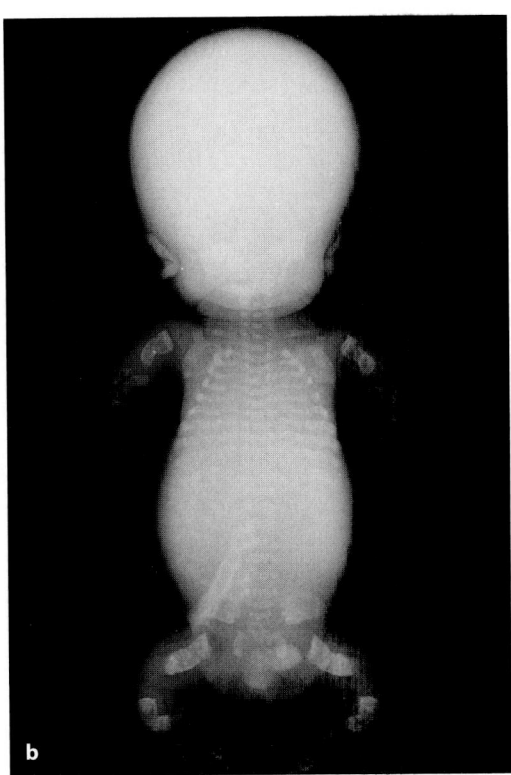

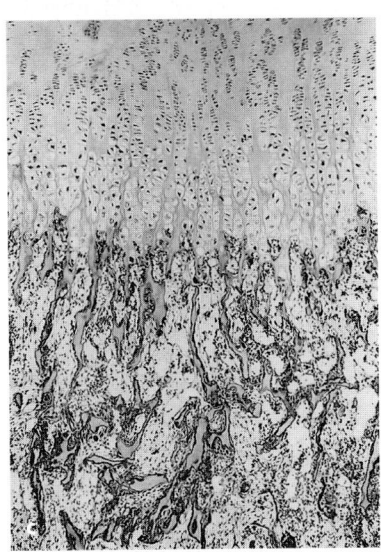

FIGURE 31.27. *Osteogenesis imperfecta type IIA. (a) Neonate showing a large soft head, deep blue sclerae, and short and deformed limbs. (b) The bones are osteopenic. Beaded ribs and thick crumpled limb bones due to fractures are evident. (c) The physeal growth zone is mostly normal. Bony spicules in the metaphysis are thin and severely deficient in ossification. They are mostly composed of cartilage. H&E, ×31. (From Gilbert et al [5].)*

190]. The recurrence rate among sibs is about 6% [185]. Type IIB patients also display broad crumpled femora, but the ribs show minimal or no fractures. Type IIC is characterized by thin beaded ribs and narrow femora with fractures. Types IIB and IIC are autosomal recessive in inheritance. There is a possibility of autosomal dominant mutation in type IIB, and this type is not necessarily lethal in the neonatal period [190].

Histopathological changes of the skeletal system are similar in types IIA and IIB [191]. The cartilage, including the physeal growth zone, is unremarkable. The principal change is severe deficiency of ossification in the metaphysis, diaphysis, and cortex. In the metaphysis, the columns of calcified cartilage matrix are narrow and covered by meager basophilic primitive woven (fiber) bone [13, 191] (Fig. 31.27c). The cartilage columns in type IIC are more broad with many interconnections [191]. The osteoblasts are spindle-shaped and not as plump as normally seen. The diaphyseal bony spicules are markedly reduced in number and size. These small medullary bony spicules and the abnormally thin cortex are composed of primitive woven (fiber) bone. The osteocytes are large and closely arranged because of matrix deficiency. In the fractured areas the bony spicules are disorganized and associated with fibrosis and callus formation.

Ultrastructurally, the collagen is scanty in the reticular dermis, and the diameters of the collagen fibrils are substantially reduced in size. There are no well-defined fibers of higher-order aggregates [188].

The unerupted teeth may show abnormal dentin formation, which is derived from mesoderm. The formation of enamel is affected only indirectly because it is derived from ectoderm [13].

OI Type III (Progressively Deforming OI with Normal Sclerae, OI Tarda Gravis) [180, 192]   Recent studies suggested that this is caused by autosomal dominant mutation of the *COL1A1* and *COL1A2* genes. The risk of recurrence is low [184], although there are exceptions [193]. There is a high mortality rate in childhood. Clinically, the patient may show numerous fractures at birth and mimic OI type IIB. However, the birthweight and length are normal. The osseous deficiency of cranial bones is not as severe, and the limbs are not as short and deformed as with OI type IIB. Postnatal growth failure and progressive skeletal deformation are striking. The sclerae are blue at birth, but become progressively less blue later in life.

Radiologically, the rib fractures do not show the continuous beading of type II. The long bones may show crumpling with metaphyseal flaring. Multiple small wormian bones are present along the wide cranial sutures.

Histopathological examination of the skeletal system shows an increased amount of woven bone and increased osteocytic cellularity. The metaphyseal histology is similar to that of OI types IIA and IIB [191].

Osteopetrosis (Albers-Schonberg Disease, Marble Bone Disease, Osteosclerosis Fragilis Generalisata)

This rare inborn skeletal disorder is associated with markedly decreased resorption of bone and cartilage due to osteoclastic dysfunction. The bones are dense and compact, but because of poor remodeling, they are brittle and susceptible to recurrent fractures [13, 194]. Albers-Schonberg [195] established the disorder as a clinical entity in 1904. Recent studies indicated that osteoclasts are derived from monocytes, and transplantation of HLA-identical bone marrow tissue corrects the skeletal aberrations, including the secondary hematopoietic disturbances [194, 196–198].

There are 4 types of osteopetrosis [17]: autosomal recessive lethal, intermediate recessive, autosomal dominant (osteopetrosis tarda), and recessive with tubular acidosis. Separation of these 4 types may not be distinct. The autosomal recessive lethal type is usually seen in the perinatal period.

Autosomal Recessive Lethal Osteopetrosis (Osteopetrosis with Precocious Manifestation, Osteopetrosis Fetalis, Osteopetrosis Congenita, Infantile Malignant Osteopetrosis)   The skeletal abnormality has been identified in utero, and the disease is well developed at birth. The affected fetus may die in the perinatal period [3, 13, 199]. Most patients die in infancy or early childhood of infection, bleeding, or both, due to marrow failure [194, 196]. If radiological examination is not done in such patients, the disease may not be detected at postmortem examination unless adequate bone examination is carried out [13]. Clinically there is growth retardation. Frontal and parietal bossing, hydrocephalus, hypertelorism, and flattening of the nose are common. The chest wall may show prominent costochondral junctions or a costal rosary. The patient who survives the neonatal period will show signs of encroachment on the marrow cavity by excess bone deposition. Progressive anemia, thrombocytopenia with ecchymoses, extramedullary hematopoiesis with hepatosplenomegaly, and lymphadenopathy are manifestations of this process. The excess bone also encroaches on cranial nerve foramina and causes blindness (associated with optic atrophy, exophthalmos, nystagmus, and strabismus), deafness, anosmia, and facial palsies. The encroachment of excess bone, however, does not entirely explain the myelophthisis, hydrocephalus, and cranial nerve deficiencies [194, 196]. Recurrent fracture and osteomyelitis of jaw bones secondary to dental infection are common. Serum calcium, phosphorus, and alkaline phosphatase levels are usually normal. The treatment of choice now is bone marrow transplantation. However, the foraminal constrictions causing cranial nerve deficits are often not reversed in time, and surgical decompression of the optic nerves continues to be the sight-saving measure [196].

Radiological changes of the skeletal system are characterized by a diffuse osteosclerosis, with loss of trabecular pattern and corticomedullary demarcation [3]. The metaphyses are frequently spared by the sclerosis. The sclerosis of the cranial base is usually more prominent than the vault, with a classic "sign of the mask." Metacarpals show 2 osteosclerotic cones facing one another by their tips. Metaphyseal remodeling defects are mild at first but later become prominent and club-shaped. The metaphyseal changes may suggest rickets [1]. Some patients actually develop rickets, which requires clinical and pathological verification [200]. In the later stage, transverse metaphyseal bands of tubular bones, arcuate bands of ilia, and bone-in-bone appearance (dense bone surrounded by bone of lesser density) may be seen. The vertebral bodies are sandwich-like, with excess sclerosis of the upper and lower plateaus [3].

Prenatal sonography of an affected fetus showed diagnostic skeletal hyperdensity at 18 weeks' gestation [199].

Gross pathology of the bones confirms the radiological changes. The medullary spongy bone is compact and at times cannot be distinguished from the thickened cortex [13, 194]. The histopathological changes of the bone formed by endochondral ossification are characterized by persistence of calcified cartilage matrix surrounded by excessive unresorbed and unremodeled primitive woven (non-lamellar) bone [13] (Fig. 31.28). Lamellar bone is rare [194]. Osteoclasts are increased in number [194], although occasionally the number is decreased [13]. In either case, osteoclastic resorption of bone is absent. Ultrastructurally,

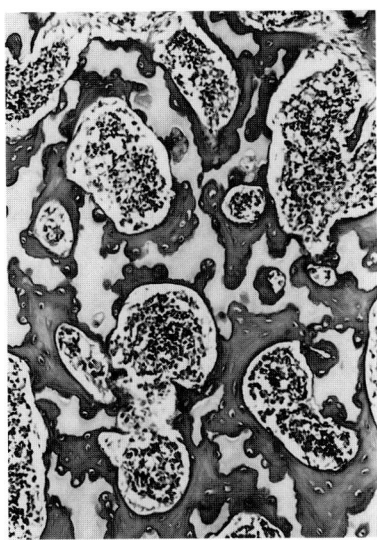

FIGURE 31.28. *Osteopetrosis. A photomicrograph of medullary spongy bone showing broad trabeculae of unresorbed cartilage surrounded by excessive primitive woven (non-lamellar) bone. H&E, ×78.*

the osteoclasts in most patients show an absence of normal clear zones and ruffled borders [194, 198]. Osteoblasts are normal. The thick abnormal bony trabeculae form a lattice meshwork, and the intervening marrow spaces are markedly obliterated. The cartilage, including the physeal growth zone, is generally normal. Distortion of the physeal growth zone is seen in occasional small areas and is probably a sequela of fracture [194]. The bones formed by intramembranous ossification are also composed of abnormal woven bone but are less atypical in appearance because of the absence of cartilage matrix [13].

The differential diagnosis of osteopetrosis includes pycnodysostosis, dominant osteosclerosis (type Stanescu), osteomyelosclerosis, and melorheostosis. The latter two conditions are not seen in infancy [1].

Pycnodysostosis

This condition was previously confused with osteopetrosis [1]. The disease is an autosomal recessive condition, is recognized at various ages, and is compatible with life. As in osteopetrosis, the bones are generally sclerotic and prone to fracture. Clinically, the infant shows growth retardation, a large head with frontal and occipital bossing, a large anterior fontanelle, blue sclerae, and a hypoplastic mandible. Anemia is rare. Hepatosplenomegaly and cranial nerve deficits are not seen.

Histopathological examination of the skeletal system [8] shows narrow physeal growth zones with small islets of cells instead of columns. The chondrocytes contain lipid inclusions, probably phospholipid. Ultrastructurally, these inclusions are single-membrane-bound and contain granu-

lar material and irregularly interwoven lamellar structures [8]. The matrix in the physeal growth zone is strongly metachromatic. The zone of provisional calcification is narrow with short, thick irregular primary trabeculae.

Dominant Osteosclerosis, Type Stanescu

Stanescu et al described an autosomal dominant disorder similar to pycnodysostosis but without fractures [1, 201]. Histopathological findings of the skeletal system are not available at the present time.

Infantile Cortical Hyperostosis (Caffey Disease)

This disease was clearly delineated in 1945 by Caffey and Silverman [202]. It is characterized by periosteal new bone formation and is associated with mild fever, irritability, loss of appetite, and vomiting. The etiology is unknown. Most of the familial cases have shown an autosomal dominant trait with variable expressivity [203]. The sporadic cases may be influenced by environmental factors. Allergy may play a role in precipitating the disease [204]. This condition is self-limited. A fatal outcome is rare [205]. Recently Kozlowski and Tsuruta [206] described a case of lethal dysplastic cortical hyperostosis with non-immune hydrops (see Unclassified or Unclassifiable Osteochondrodysplasia).

Clinically, the onset of disease is usually before the age of 5 months, and the latest onset is at the age of 46 weeks [203]. The disease is observed occasionally in newborn infants and rarely in fetuses [1, 203–205]. During the early stage of the disease, tender firm swellings of soft tissue develop over the cheek and mandibular bones, limb bones, ribs, clavicles, scapulae, and cranial bones [204]. The disease may involve single or multiple bones, and may be bilateral. Laboratory examination shows mild anemia, moderate leukocytosis, elevated red blood cell sedimentation rate, and serum alkaline phosphatase levels. The patient usually recovers before the age of 1 year. Occasionally the recovery may not occur until early childhood, or even until adulthood [1]. Steroid therapy may be indicated for relieving symptoms. Diaphyseal bowing, synostosis, persistent facial asymmetry, and exophthalmos are occasional complications [204].

The most notable radiological finding is striking periosteal new bone formation of the mandible and the diaphyses of limb bones (Fig. 31.29).

Histopathological changes are characterized by thickening of the periosteum, absence of cortical bone, intense proliferation of subperiosteal cells, and fibrosis of bone marrow [205]. The physeal growth zones are normal. However, persistent hypertrophic chondrocytes are seen in the metaphysis. The diaphyseal bony spicules are partially calcified and their large and round lacunae are irregularly distributed. The findings mimic OI, but there are no associated fractures [205]. In the early stage of the disease, the affected periosteum shows cellular fibrous tissue with scattered osteoid trabeculae, acute inflammatory infiltration, and microabscesses. The disease process extends into the adjacent muscle and erodes the underlying bone. Biopsy findings during this

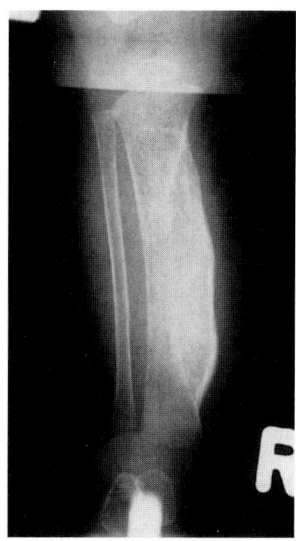

FIGURE 31.29.   *Infantile cortical hyperostosis. Skeletal radiograph of a 3-month-old girl's leg. The tibia shows striking periosteal new bone formation. The same patient's mandible showed a similar abnormality. (Courtesy of Alexander Cacciarelli, MD, William Beaumont Hospital, Royal Oak, Michigan.)*

acute stage may be confused with osteogenic sarcoma [207]. Later in the subacute stage, the acute inflammation subsides and the osteoid trabeculae of the periosteum are mineralized. These periosteal bony trabeculae are resorbed in the subsequent remodeling stage.

Osteochondrodysplasia with Defective Mineralization and Metabolic Abnormalities

Hypophosphatasia

This rare heritable metabolic disorder is characterized by rachitic change of the skeletal system, low serum and tissue alkaline phosphatase (bone/liver/kidney isoenzymes) levels, and increased blood and urine levels of phosphoethanolamine and inorganic pyrophosphate [208, 209]. The term *hypophosphatasia* was coined by Rathbun in 1948 when he reported a case study [210]. There are at least infantile, childhood, and adult forms, according to the age at onset and the severity of the disease. However, there is considerable overlap of these 3 forms [211], occasionally even in the same family [210].

Hypophosphatasia, Infantile (Congenital Lethal)   This is a lethal autosomal recessive condition with a point mutation or small deletion in the alkaline phosphatase gene and messenger RNA. The gene resides in the distal end of the short arm of chromosome 1 [209]. Most of the pregnancies reach term. Clinically the affected newborn infant (Fig. 31.30a) shows external features of both chondrodysplasia and rickets, with disproportionately shortened limbs, a costal rosary, and metaphyseal bulging. The head is globular but small and soft

(caput membranaceum). There is hypotonia. Irritability, anorexia, persistent vomiting, and mild pyrexia are common. Convulsions, attacks of cyanosis, and pneumonia are seen in severely affected infants. The patient may die from respiratory insufficiency because of poorly developed ribs, or intracranial hemorrhage within hours or days after birth. Few survive beyond the first year of life. Failure to thrive becomes evident before the age of 6 months. Hypercalcemia is common and may result in nephrocalcinosis. Serum phosphorus values are usually normal [210]. A recent attempt at enzyme replacement therapy with intravenous infusions of pooled plasma in a boy with infantile hypophosphatasia resulted in normalization of circulating bone alkaline phosphatase activity, followed by skeletal remineralization [212].

The radiological changes of the skeletal system are identical to those of severe rickets with a generalized deficiency of ossification (Fig. 31.30b). The tubular bones are thin, with severe metaphyseal cupping and irregularity. Fractures are common. The cranial bones are small and poorly mineralized [210, 211]. Severe cases may simulate achondrogenesis type I (Fig. 31.30c).

Ultrasonography as early as 16 weeks of gestation will disclose a poorly defined or apparently absent fetal skull. A normal value for alpha-fetoprotein in the amniotic fluid excludes anencephaly. Demonstration of low levels of alkaline phosphatase in cultured amniotic fluid cells is helpful in the prenatal diagnosis, but assay of alkaline phosphatase in the amniotic fluid itself is not informative [213].

Histopathological findings of severe skeletal rachitic changes in a newborn infant are characteristic of this disorder [13, 208, 210]. The resting cartilage is normal. The physeal growth zone in a 5-month-old fetus shows minimal changes [214]. However, in the neonatal period it is widened, thickened, and hypercellular with chondrocytic disarray. Alkaline phosphatase is greatly diminished in the physeal growth zone [214]. The primary spongiosa has broad columns of unmineralized cartilage with hypertrophic chondrocytes persisting deep into the metaphysis (Fig. 31.30d,e). In both the fetus and newborn infant, these metaphyseal columns of cartilage are covered with wide osteoid seams, which are also deficient in mineralization. Osteoblasts and osteoclasts are normal in number and morphology. Mineralized bone in the metaphysis frequently contains large proportions of woven bone. Mineralization of diaphyseal bone is reported to be normal [214]. Membranous bone is also affected and it too shows osteoid seams. The above changes are analogous to the changes of vitamin D–deficient rickets. The latter, however, is not associated with alkaline phosphatase deficiency.

The differential diagnosis must include achondrogenesis type I and OI type IIC because these conditions are characterized by multiple fractures or deficiency of ossification or both. However, the rachitic bone changes at birth, low serum and tissue alkaline phosphatase levels, and increased levels of phosphoethanolamine and inorganic pyrophosphate in blood and urine will separate hypophosphatasia from the

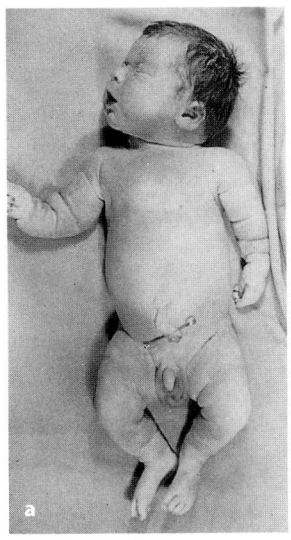
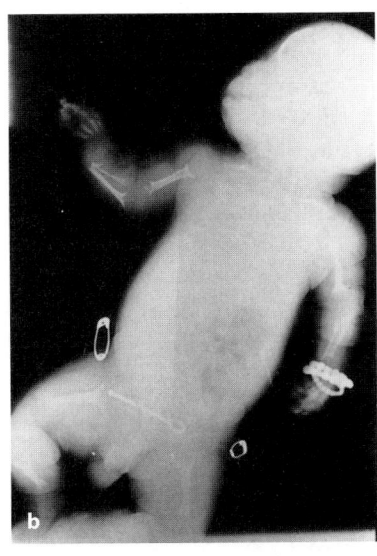
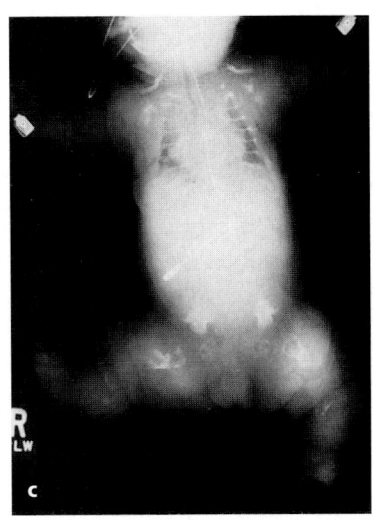

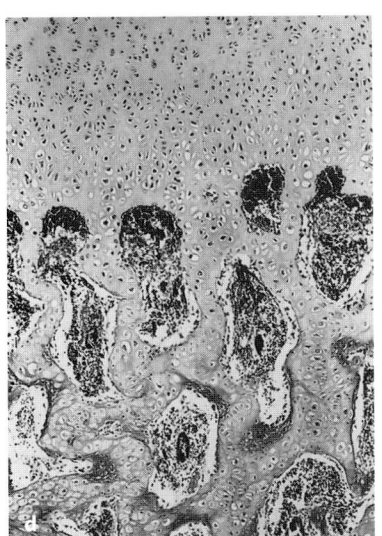
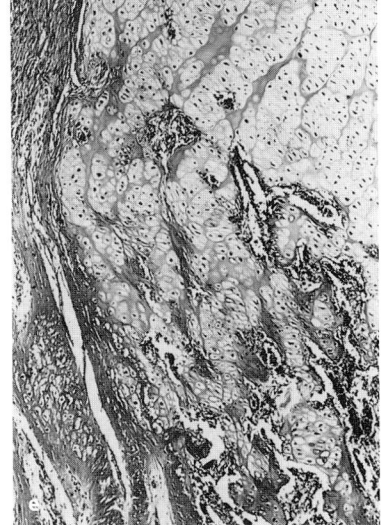

FIGURE 31.30. *Hypophosphatasia, congenital lethal type. (a) Neonate indistinguishable from one with chondrodysplasia. (b) Skeletal radiograph showing rickets-like distinct cupping of metaphyses. (c) Skeletal radiograph of severely affected patient showing changes suggestive of achondrogenesis type I. (d,e) Femur and rib showing disorganized physeal growth zone. Broad columns of hypertrophic chondrocytes persist into the metaphysis. The matrix of these cartilage columns and the surrounding osteoid seams are poorly mineralized. H&E, ×36 (d), ×31 (e). (From Gilbert et al [5].)*

other 2 entities. The presence of low serum levels of alkaline phosphatase in both parents is also helpful in the differential diagnosis.

Mucolipidosis II (I-Cell Disease)

This lysosomopathic disease has some features of mucopolysaccharidosis I (Hurler syndrome) and was discovered by Leroy and DeMars in 1967 [215]. This autosomal recessive condition is characterized by coarse cytoplasmic inclusions in the tissues, cultured skin fibroblasts, and amniotic fluid cells. Markedly increased amounts of many lysosomal enzymes are present in the serum, and the same enzymes are deficient in the lysosomes.

Clinically the disease may be evident at birth, with low birthweight, coarse facies, gingival hypertrophy, thick skin, mild hepatosplenomegaly, arachnodactyly of the fingers, and joint contractures [216].

Skeletal radiographs in the neonatal period demonstrate generalized demineralization, a coarse trabecular pattern, and

"cloaking" of the long tubular bones due to periosteal new bone formation. Similar findings are also seen in congenital syphilis, neonatal hyperparathyroidism, and GM_1 gangliosidosis. Epiphyseal stippling and pathological fractures may occur [217, 218].

Histopathological examination of the epiphyseal cartilage in a child (Fig. 31.31) showed markedly ballooned chondrocytes with abundant clear cytoplasm. The physeal growth zone was virtually absent. Other investigators noticed the same findings [219]. The large clear chondrocytes are probably present in the perinatal period because similar abnormal cells have seen observed in the placenta [220]. Furthermore, abnormal skeletal system has been detected at birth radiographically [218].

Others

Mucopolysaccharidosis VII (beta-glucuronidase deficiency), a rare storage disease, has been diagnosed postmortem [221]. The patient presented as a case of non-immunological

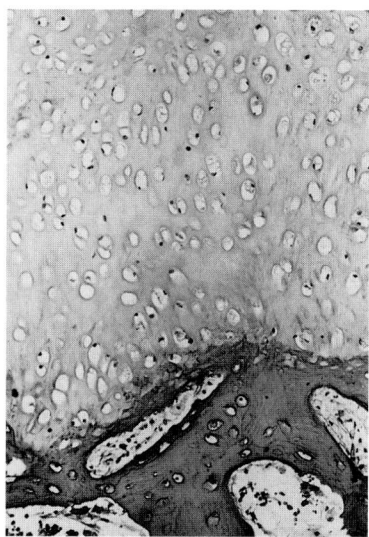

FIGURE 31.31. *Mucolipidosis II. A photomicrograph of epiphyseal cartilage from an 8-year-old girl showing ballooned chondrocytes with abundant clear cytoplasm. H&E, ×103. Similar changes should be evident in the perinatal period. The physeal growth zone is virtually absent in this patient.*

hydrops. A skeletal radiograph revealed thick ribs and poorly developed vertebral bodies. Histopathological examination of the bones showed foamy cells in the marrow. A similar presentation has been reported for Gaucher disease, generalized GM_1 gangliosidosis, and sialidosis. Other forms of mucopolysaccharidosis, mucolipidosis, and lipidosis may not be recognized at birth, and usually do not present to the pathologist in the perinatal period. However, advances in antenatal diagnosis may bring such cases to the attention of the perinatal pathologist [221].

Unclassified or Unclassifiable Osteochondrodysplasias

Atelosteogenesis type II (de la Chapelle) [57] is a controversial autosomal recessive disorder [11]. This is also labeled as *McAlister dysplasia* [4]. All reported patients died in the neonatal period. The entity shares many features with severe diastrophic dysplasia. Since de la Chapelle dysplasia [222] is also included in the atelosteogenesis type II by Sillence et al [11, 57], the condition may represent a heterogeneous group. The salient clinical findings include "hitchhiker" thumbs (and great toes), cleft palate, small thorax, moderately severe micromelia, small hands, and equinovarus. Radiologically, the ulnae and fibulae are reduced to triangular remnants. Metacarpals may [4, 57] or may not [223] be anarchic in appearance. Other long bones are short and bowed. Histopathologically, the physeal growth zone is more retarded than that seen in diastrophic dysplasia. As in diastrophic dysplasia, the cartilage matrix is deficient with focal

cystic degeneration, and the resting chondrocytes are surrounded by halos of denser matrix that is reactive to PAS and methenamine silver nitrate–alcian blue stain.

Koide et al [224] in 1983 described a lethal achondrogenesis-like short-limbed dwarfism that was identical to the Case 2 of new lethal neonatal dwarfism reported by Kozlowski et al earlier [62]. The limb bones of their patient were broad with smooth rounded ends. The distal humeri were pointed.

Glasgow round femoral inferior epiphysis chondrodysplasia is similar to TD, but there is only a mild degree of platyspondyly [225]. Well-developed round inferior epiphyses are present in the femora [226]. This is a sublethal recessive disorder. Histopathologically the physeal growth zones are retarded and disorganized. There are demasked fine fibers in the matrix. Irregular trabeculae are noted in the primary and secondary spongiosa.

Dappled diaphyseal dysplasia [227, 228] and *Greenberg dysplasia* [229] are characterized by features suggestive of severe chondrodysplasia punctata. Greenberg dysplasia may appear as a mild form of dappled diaphyseal dysplasia, but it is associated with severe non-immune hydrops. Radiographically the tubular bones are fragmented and mottled, especially at the ends. The dappled diaphyseal dysplasia shows radiographically unique multiple irregular ossification centers throughout the tubular bones. Both conditions are lethal and dappled diaphyseal dysplasia is autosomal recessive.

Lethal brittle bone syndrome with thin bones and multiple fractures is a new OI-like disorder. An increased amount of type V collagen was demonstrated by Bonaventure et al [230]. The possibility of OI was excluded by them.

Raine syndrome is a rare sclerotic bone dysplasia [231]. The condition is lethal in the neonatal period. There is a possibility of autosomal recessive inheritance. The neonate shows microcephaly, midface hypoplasia, exophthalmos, a small flattened nose, triangular mouth micrognathia, and shell-like low-set ears. Radiological examination of the skeletal system demonstrates a generalized increase in bone density with poor corticomedullary demarcation. Uneven ragged periosteal thickening may be present in the long tubular bones, especially in the ribs. Multiple pseudofractures of ribs have been noted. Histopathologically, the cartilage is unremarkable. However, bizarre large globules of mucoid substance and calcospherites with reactive giant cells are present in the periosteum and the adjacent soft tissue.

Dysplastic cortical hyperostosis reported by Kozlowski and Tsuruta [206] may suggest infantile cortical hyperostosis (Caffey disease). However, soft tissue induration is absent in this condition, and there is no periosteal thickening. Involvement of the skeletal system is symmetrical. This disorder is lethal and there is severe hydrops. Radiologically, the abnormal changes of the skeletal system are also similar to those of Raine syndrome [231], but the facial bones are normal in this condition.

Beemer et al [232] reported a lethal neonatal spondylometaphyseal dysplasia with narrow chest and advanced bone age. Radiologically it was similar to the rhizomelic form of chondrodysplasia punctata, but there was no epiphyseal stippling. The femora showed a retarded physeal growth zone and cellular resting cartilage.

Langer et al [233] reported a case of brachymesomelia-renal syndrome without skeletal histopathology. Juberg and Van Ness [234] described a new form of hereditary short-limbed dwarfism with microcephalus. There are many more reports of malformation syndromes that may include chondrodysplasia, for example, cerebro-oculo-facial-skeletal syndrome with chondrocytic necrosis [235].

Many additional unclassified disorders were summarized recently by Spranger and Maroteaux [4].

SECONDARY DISORDERS OF METABOLISM

Congenital and neonatal rickets, both of which have prominent chondro-osseous lesions, are described in this section.

Congenital and Neonatal Rickets

Congenital rickets may occasionally occur in babies born to mothers with undiagnosed malabsorption syndrome [236], deficiency of vitamin D intake [237], renal failure [238], and preeclampsia [239]. These infants show evidence of rickets on the first day of life.

Neonatal rickets develops after birth because of insufficient intake of vitamin D, calcium, and phosphorus, especially among premature infants of very low birthweight. The advances in the treatment of premature infants, with prolonged survival, have been associated with increased reports of rickets among these patients. Human milk and many commercially available formulas, including soy isolate formulas, do not provide sufficient calcium and phosphorus for these very small premature infants [240]. Premature infants on parenteral nutrition also have a high incidence of rickets, mostly due to hypophosphatemia. Superimposed diseases (congenital heart disease, respiratory disease, necrotizing enterocolitis) appear to increase the susceptibility to rachitic change [240, 241]. Delay in maturation of 1-hydroxylase enzymes has been suspected as one of the mechanisms in the development of rickets [242].

The affected infants may show rachitic rosaries; enlargement of wrists, knees, and ankles; and frontal bossing. Fractures may be the presenting symptoms [243]. The soft rib cage, fractures, and respiratory muscular weakness may result in late respiratory distress [244].

The most important radiological finding of the skeletal system is cupping of the ends of the tubular bones. It is best shown at the lower end of the ulna. Similar cupping occurs much later in the radius and other bones [13].

Histopathological examination of the chondro-osseous tissue shows widened and thickened physeal growth zones with irregular vascular invasions, and poor removal of cartilage with persistent hypertrophic chondrocytes in the zone

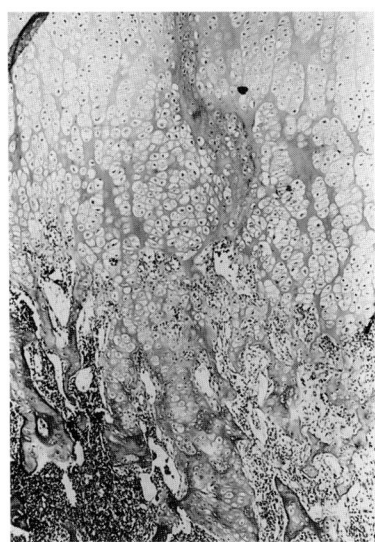

FIGURE 31.32.   *Neonatal rickets in one of a pair of premature twins delivered at 28 weeks' gestation who died at age 84 days. The physeal growth zone is thickened and there is irregular vascular penetration. Variously sized broad cartilage columns with persistent hypertrophic chondrocytes are present deep in the metaphysis. These cartilage columns demonstrate poorly defined broad osteoid seams. H&E, ×31.*

of provisional ossification (metaphysis). The abnormally large cellular metaphyseal cartilage columns are surrounded by broad osteoid seams (Fig. 31.32). This abnormal zone of provisional ossification is conspicuously widened and is called the *rachitic metaphysis* or *rachitic intermediate zone*. The cortex and the cancellous bone of diaphysis also demonstrate abnormal remodeling. Subperiosteal bone formation is less affected and overtakes endochondral ossification, consequently producing the cupping deformity. Oppenheimer and Snodgrass [245] noticed pathological differences between the form of neonatal rickets with phosphorus deficiency and the vitamin D–deficient type. The former showed reduced osteoblastic activity, while such activity was normal or increased in the latter. The phosphorus-deficient type also has better calcium deposition and thinner osteoid seams than did the vitamin D–deficient type in the zone of provisional ossification.

CONGENITAL INFECTIONS

Congenital Syphilis

The skeletal changes of congenital syphilis are part of a systemic disease (see Chap. 17). However, if the disease is mild, the only lesion that can be demonstrated is syphilitic osteochondritis [13]. In the patient with more advanced disease, syphilitic osteomyelitis can be demonstrated. Syphilitic osteoperiostitis usually appears after resolution of the osteochondritis, although it may be seen in the fetal period.

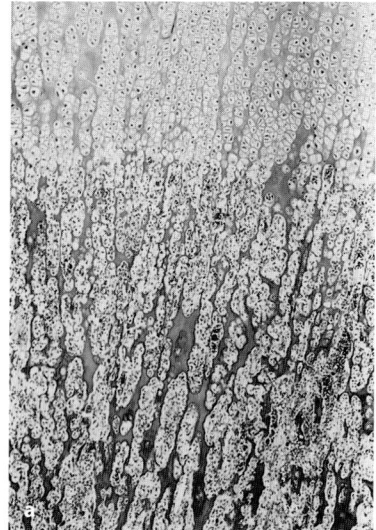
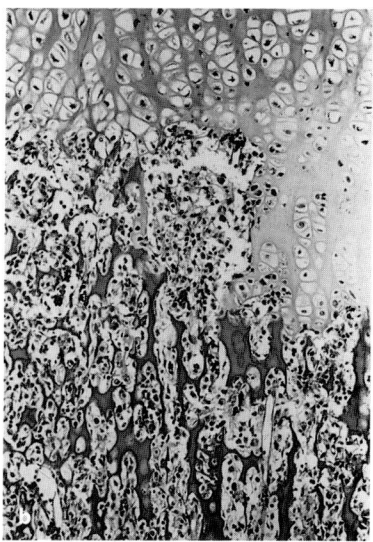

FIGURE 31.33.   *Syphilitic osteochondritis in 26-week gestational infant. (a) The metaphysis of the femur is composed of jagged cartilage columns that are devoid of ossification. The intervening marrow tissue is replaced by inflammatory granulation tissue. H&E, ×31. (b) A higher magnification from another area shows the inflammatory process extending into the physeal zone of degeneration. Osteoblasts and osteoclasts are difficult to demonstrate. H&E, ×78. (Courtesy of Jonathan S. Wigglesworth, MD, Royal Postgraduate Medical School, University of London.)*

Syphilitic osteochondritis occurs in the area of endochondral ossification. It affects virtually every bone, and is more prominent in the bones with more active growth. Radiologically, early syphilitic osteochondritis manifests as a transverse radiopaque band at the epiphyseal-metaphyseal junction, which is due to the widened provisional ossification zone. Later, it becomes radiolucent and grossly yellow-white. On microscopic examination, this abnormal zone (Fig. 31.33) is composed of jagged calcified cartilage columns with diminished osteoblastic and osteoclastic activities. New bone deposition is diminished or absent. Granulation tissue is present in the intervening spaces and is composed of vascular fibrous tissue and mixed leukocytes [13, 246]. The lesion is not dystrophic in nature, as Cremin and Fisher believed [247], because spirochetes might be demonstrated in the granulation tissue [13]. However, plasma cells are found with difficulty. Epiphyseal separation may occur in this area. Syphilitic osteochondritis must be distinguished from the metaphyseal lesions of rickets, congenital rubella, and cytomegalovirus infection.

Diaphyseal osteomyelitis is characterized by large foci of fibrohistiocytic granulation tissue, which are usually wedge-shaped with the base resting on the periosteum [13]. Such lesions may require a biopsy to exclude neuroblastoma, leukemia, and pyogenic osteomyelitis. These lesions heal very slowly after treatment [13].

Radiologically and pathologically, syphilitic periostitis presents as subperiosteal granulation tissue and new bone formation of the long bones [13, 246]. This lesion must be distinguished from infantile cortical hyperostosis and trauma [248], and also from mucolipidosis II.

Congenital Rubella Syndrome

Congenital rubella syndrome, reported by Gregg in 1941 [249], was reconfirmed and expanded in the worldwide epidemic of 1964–1965. The syndrome still occurs, despite widespread vaccination [250]. In addition, reinfection of the mother in the later stages of pregnancy with late-onset congenital rubella syndrome has been reported [251].

Radiological changes of the skeletal system were seen in 45–84% of patients with expanded congenital rubella syndrome [252, 253]. Abnormal bone changes were documented in a 19-week-old fetus [254]. Typically, the tubular bones of the newborn patient demonstrate celery stalk–like longitudinal radiolucencies in the metaphyses, especially in the distal end of the femur and proximal end of the tibia (Fig. 31.34a). These abnormal changes heal after 2–3 months, except in the patients who fail to thrive [253]. Less specific changes include a metaphyseal radiolucent band paralleling the growth plate, and alteration of the trabecular pattern. These latter changes are also seen in congenital syphilis, cytomegalovirus infection, erythroblastosis fetalis, and severe growth retardation [253].

Histopathological examination of the skeletal system (distal part of femur, proximal part of tibia, rib, and vertebrae) demonstrates malaligned metaphyseal cartilage spicules, with increased osteoblastic and osteoclastic activities and decreased osteoid deposition [252, 253, 255] (Fig. 31.34b). A brief survey of 9 cases from the Texas Children's Hospital (courtesy of Dr. Milton J. Finegold) and William Beaumont Hospital, Michigan, confirmed the previous observations that the lesions occur in infants who died before the age of 1 month and that they are inconspicuous in those who died after 3 months. Focal myxofibromatous changes may occur in the metaphysis [255]. The corresponding physeal growth zones show irregular areas of diminished activities and disorderly arrangement of the chondrocytes. In those patients older than 2 months, the metaphysis shows irregular foci of osteoporosis, with small cartilage spicules and reduced numbers of osteoblasts and osteoclasts (Fig. 31.34c). The skeletal lesions are considered

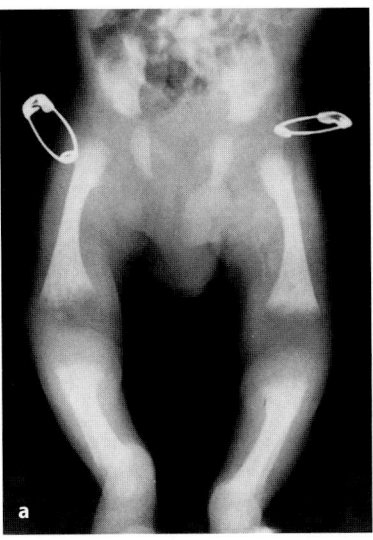 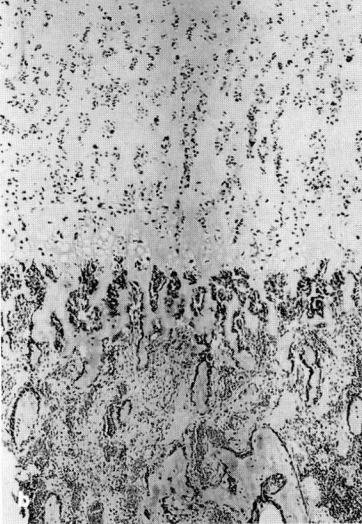 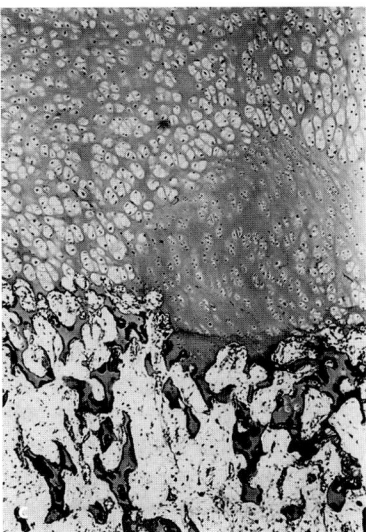

FIGURE 31.34. *Congenital rubella syndrome. (a) Skeletal radiograph of a male infant's lower extremities, showing celery stalk–like longitudinal radiolucencies in the distal femoral and proximal tibial metaphyses. (Courtesy of Alexander Cacciarelli, MD, William Beaumont Hospital, Royal Oak, Michigan.) (b) Photomicrograph of 1-month-old female neonate's bone showing malaligned metaphyseal cartilage columns with increased numbers of osteoblasts and osteoclasts. Paradoxically the osteoid deposition is diminished. The physis is retarded and disorganized. H&E, ×31. (Courtesy of Milton J. Finegold, MD, Texas Children's Hospital, Houston, Texas.) (c) Photomicrograph of bone from the patient whose radiograph is shown in (a). The patient died from pneumocystis pneumonia at age 4 months. The chondrocytic proliferation of the physeal growth zone is diminished and disorganized. A rare focus of growth arrest is present. The metaphyseal cartilage and bony spicules are disorganized with focal osteoporosis. H&E, ×31.*

to be the results of focal failure in bone formation secondary to retarded cell division caused by rubella infection [255].

Others

Rubella-like radiological bone changes have been associated with congenital cytomegalovirus infection [256]. However, no corresponding pathological findings are available. A review of the bone sections taken from fatal cases of congenital cytomegalovirus infection did not show significant pathological changes. Milgram [257] reported a case of congenital toxoplasmosis showing radiological metaphyseal lucency and irregularity of the line of provisional calcification at the epiphyseal plates. Metaphyseal cartilage columns were elongated, new bone formation was deficient, and mononuclear inflammatory cells infiltrated the marrow spaces. Occasional *Toxoplasma* pseudocysts were demonstrated in the marrow.

Suppurative osteomyelitis and purulent arthritis may occur in newborn infants with generalized sepsis, but are rare nowadays. The septic inflammation commences in the metaphysis. It may spread to the subperiosteal space rather than to the marrow cavity because of the vascularity and spongy structure of the cortical bone in the newborn infant. The most common causative agents are staphylococci and streptococci. Other agents include *Escherichia coli*, *Proteus* species, *Klebsiella pneumoniae*, *Pseudomonas* species, and *Salmonella* species [221].

ACKNOWLEDGMENTS

David Sillence, MD, of the School of Public Health and Tropical Medicine, Commonwealth Institute of Health, University of Sydney, lent his personal experience in osteogenesis imperfecta, hypophosphatasia, osteopetrosis, camptomelic dysplasia, and diastrophic dysplasia for the preparation of this chapter in the first edition. His assistance is gratefully acknowledged.

Permission to use copyrighted illustrations has been granted by Appleton-Century-Crofts (Pathology Annual, 1987; 22(2):281–345) for Figs. 31.5a,c; 31.6a,b; 31.8c; 31.10a,b; 31.11a,c; 31.14b; 31.15a,c; 31.17a,b; 31.18b,c; 31.21c; 31.22a,b; 31.23c; 31.24a,b,c; 31.25; 31.26; 31.27a,b,c; and 31.30a,b,c,d,e.

REFERENCES

1. Maroteaux P. *Bone Diseases of Children*. Philadelphia: JB Lippincott, 1979.
2. Rimoin DL, Lachman RS. The chondrodysplasias. In: Emery AEH, Rimoin DL, eds. *Principles and Practice of Medical Genetics*. 2nd ed. Edinburgh: Churchill Livingstone, 1990, pp. 895–932.
3. Spranger J, Langer LO Jr, Wiedemann H-R. *Bone Dysplasias: An Atlas of Constitutional Disorders of Skeletal Development*. Philadelphia: WB Saunders, 1974.
4. Spranger J, Maroteaux P. The lethal osteochondrodysplasias. *Adv Hum Genet* 1990; 19:1–103.
5. Gilbert EF, Yang SS, Langer L, et al. Pathologic changes of osteochondrodysplasia in infancy. A review. *Pathol Ann* 1987; 22:281–345.
6. Sillence DO, Horton WA, Rimoin DL. Morphologic studies in the skeletal dysplasia. *Am J Pathol* 1979; 96:813–60.
7. Stanescu V, Stanescu R, Maroteaux P. Morphological and biochemical studies of epiphyseal cartilage in dyschondroplasias. *Arch Fr Pediatr* 1977; 34:1–80.

8. Stanescu V, Stanescu R, Maroteaux P. Pathogenic mechanisms in osteochondrodysplasias. *J Bone Joint Surg Am* 1984; 66:817–36.

9. Yang SS, Heidelberger KP, Brough A, et al. Lethal short-limbed chondrodysplasia in early infancy. *Perspect Pediatr Pathol* 1976; 3:1–40.

10. Sharony R, Browne C, Lachman RS, Rimoin DL. Prenatal diagnosis of the skeletal dysplasias. *Am J Obstet Gynecol* 1993; 169:668–75.

11. Beighton P, Giedion A, Gorlin R, et al. International classification of osteochondrodysplasias. *Am J Med Genet* 1992; 44:223–9.

12. Yang SS, Kitchen E, Gilbert EF, Rimoin DL. Histopathologic examination in osteochondrodysplasia: time for standardization. *Arch Pathol Lab Invest* 1986; 110:10–2.

13. Jaffe HL. *Metabolic, Degenerative and Inflammatory Diseases of Bones and Joints.* Philadelphia: Lea & Febiger, 1972.

14. Kelly DE, Wood RL, Enders AL. *Bailey's Textbook of Microscopic Anatomy.* 8th ed. Baltimore: Williams & Wilkins, 1984, pp. 217–26.

15. Cowell HR, Hunziker EB, Rosenberg L. The role of hypertrophic chondrocytes in endochondral ossification and in the development of secondary centers of ossification. *J Bone Joint Surg Am* 1987; 69:159–61.

16. Hwang WS. Ultrastructure of human foetal and neonatal hyaline cartilage. *J Pathol* 1978; 126:209–14.

17. International Nomenclature of Constitutional Diseases of Bone. *Ann Radiol (Paris)* 1983; 26:457–62.

18. Buyse ML, ed. *Birth Defects Encyclopedia.* Cambridge, MA: Blackwell Science, 1990.

19. Gorlin RJ, Cohen MM, Levin LS. *Syndromes of the Head and Neck.* 3rd ed. New York: Oxford University Press, 1990.

20. Jones KL. *Smith's Recognizable Patterns of Human Malformation.* 4th ed. Philadelphia: WB Saunders, 1988.

21. Prockop DJ, Baldwin CT, Constantinou CD. Mutations in type I procollagen genes that cause osteogenesis imperfecta. *Adv Hum Genet* 1990; 19:105–32.

22. Spranger J, Winterpacht A, Zabel B. The type II collagenopathies: a spectrum of chondrodysplasias. *Eur J Pediatr* 1994; 153:56–65.

23. Yang SS, Brough AJ, Garewal GS, Bernstein J. Two types of heritable lethal achondrogenesis. *J Pediatr* 1974; 85:796–801.

24. Borochowitz Z, Lachman R, Adomian GE, et al. Achondrogenesis type 1: delineation of further heterogeneity and identification of two distinct subgroups. *J Pediatr* 1988; 112:23–32.

25. Kozlowski K, Masel J, Morris L, et al. Neonatal death dwarfism (report of 17 cases). *Australas Radiol* 1977; 21:164–83.

26. Whitley CB, Gorlin RJ, Achondrogenesis: new nosology with evidence of genetic heterogeneity. *Radiology* 1983; 148:693–8.

27. Garcia-Castro JM, Perez-Comas A. Nonlethal achondrogenesis (Grebe-Quelce-Salgado type) in two Puerto Rican sibships. *J Pediatr* 1975; 87:948–52.

28. Fraccaro M. Contributo allo studio della malattie del mesenchima osteopoietico l'acondrogenesi. *Folia Hered Pathol (Milano)* 1952; 1:190–207.

29. Parenti GC. La anosteogenesi (una varieta della osteogenesi imperfetta). *Pathologica* 1936; 28:447–62.

30. Van der Harten HJ, Brons JTJ, Dijkstra PF, et al. Achondrogenesis-hypochondrogenesis: the spectrum of chondrogenesis imperfecta. A radiological, ultrasonographic, and histopathologic study of 23 cases. *Pediatr Pathol* 1988; 8:232–52.

31. Benacerraf B, Osathanondh F, Bieber FR. Achondrogenesis type I: ultrasound diagnosis in utero. *J Clin Ultrasound* 1984; 12:357–9.

32. Yang SS, Heidellberger KP, Bernstein J. Intracytoplasmic inclusion bodies in the chondrocytes of type I lethal achondrogenesis. *Hum Pathol* 1976; 7:667–73.

33. Molz G, Spycher MA. Achondrogenesis type I: light and electron microscopic studies. *Eur J Pediatr* 1980; 134:69–74.

34. Ornoy A, Sekeles E, Smith P, et al. Achondrogenesis type I in three sibling fetuses, scanning and transmission electron microscopic studies. *Am J Pathol* 1976; 82:71–84.

35. Soothill PW, Vuthiwong C, Rees H. Achondrogenesis type 2 diagnosed by transvaginal ultrasound at 12 weeks' gestation. *Prenat Diagn* 1993; 13:523–8.

36. Horton WA, Machado MA, Cho JW, Campbell D. Achondrogenesis type II, abnormalities of extracellular matrix. *Pediatr Res* 1987; 22:324–9.

37. Maroteaux P, Stanescu V, Stanescu R. Hypochondrogenesis. *Eur J Pediatr* 1983; 141:14–22.

38. Borochowitz Z, Ornoy A, Lachman R, Rimoin DL. Achondrogenesis II–hypochondrogenesis: variability versus heterogeneity. *Am J Med Genet* 1986; 24:273–88.

39. Chen H, Liu CT, Yang SS. Achondrogenesis: a review with special consideration of achondrogenesis type II (Langer-Saldino). *Am J Hum Genet* 1981; 10:379–94.

40. Spranger J, Wiedemann HR. Dysplasia spondyloepiphysaria congenita. *Helv Paediatr Acta* 1966; 21:598–611.

41. Anderson IJ, Goldberg RB, Marion RW, et al. Spondyloepiphyseal dysplasia congenita: genetic linkage to type II collagen (COL2A1). *Am J Med Genet* 1990; 46:896–901.

42. Yang SS, Chen H, Williams P, et al. Spondyloepiphyseal dysplasia congenita. Comparative study of chondrocytic inclusions. *Arch Pathol Lab Med* 1980; 104:208–11.

43. Anderson CE, Sillence DO, Lachman RS, et al. Spondylometepiphyseal dysplasia, Strudwick type. *Am J Med Genet* 1982; 13:243–56.

44. Kniest W. Zur abgrenzung der dysostosis enchondrallis von der Chondrodystrophie. *Z Kinderheilkd* 1952; 70:633–40.

45. Kim HG, Beratis NG, Brill P, et al. Kniest syndrome with dominant inheritance and mucopolysacchariduria. *Am J Hum Genet* 1975; 27:755–64.

46. Maroteaux P, Spranger J. La maladie de Kniest. *Arch Fr Pediatr* 1973; 30:735–50.

47. Poole AR, Pidoux I, Reiner A, et al. Kniest dysplasia is characterized by an apparent abnormal processing of the C-propeptide of type II collagen resulting in imperfect fibril assembly. *J Clin Invest* 1988; 81:579–89.

48. Chen H, Yang SS, Gonzalez E. Kniest dysplasia: neonatal death with necropsy. *Am J Med Genet* 1980; 6:171–8.

49. Horton WA, Rimoin DL. Kniest dysplasia. A histochemical study of the growth plate. *Pediatr Res* 1979; 13:1266–70.

50. Sconyers SM, Rimoin DL, Lachman RS, et al. A distinct chondrodysplasia resembling Kniest dysplasia: clinical roentgenographic, histologic, and ultrastructural findings. *J Pediatr* 1983; 103:898–904.

51. Greco MA, Alvarez SP, Genieser NB, Becker MH. Dyssegmental dwarfism: a histologic study of osseous and nonosseous cartilage. *Hum Pathol* 1984; 15:490–3.

52. Gruhn JG, Gorlin RJ, Langer LO. Dyssegmental dwarfism. A lethal anisospondylic camptomicromelic dwarfism. *Am J Dis Child* 1978; 132:382–6.

53. Aleck KA, Grix A, Clericuzio C, et al. Dyssegmental dysplasia: clinical, radiographic, and morphologic evidence of heterogeneity. *Am J Med Genet* 1987; 295–312.

54. Sillence DO, Lachman RS, Jenkins T, et al. Spondylohumerofemoral hypoplasia (giant cell chondrodysplasia): a neonatally lethal short-rib skeletal dysplasia. *Am J Med Genet* 1982; 13:7–14.

55. Maroteaux P, Spranger J, Stanescu V, et al. Atelosteogenesis. *Am J Med Genet* 1982; 13:15–25.

56. Yang SS, Roskamp J, Liu CT, et al. Two lethal chondrodysplasias with giant chondrocytes. *Am J Med Genet* 1983; 15:615–25.

57. Sillence DO, Kozlowski K, Rogers JG, et al. Atelosteogenesis: evidence for heterogeneity. *Pediatr Radiol* 1987; 17:112–8.

58. Baxova A, Maroteaux P, Barosova J, Netriova I. Parental consanguinity in two sibs with omodysplasia. *Am J Med Genet* 1994; 49:263–5.

59. Borochowitz Z, Jones KL, Silbey R, et al. A distinct lethal neonatal chondrodysplasia with snail-like pelvis: Schneckenbecken dysplasia. *Am J Med Genet* 1986; 25:47–59.

60. Maroteaux P, Sauvegrain J, Chrispin A, Farriaux JP. Omodysplasia. *Am J Med Genet* 1989; 32:371–5.

61. Tenconi R, Kozlowski K, Largaiolli G. Boomerang dysplasia. A new form of neonatal death dwarfism. *ROEFO* 1983; 138:378–80.

62. Kozlowski K, Tsuruta T, Kameda Y, et al. New forms of neonatal death dwarfism; report of 3 cases. *Pediatr Radiol* 1981; 10:155–60.

63. Greally MT, Jewett T, Smith WL Jr, et al. Lethal bone dysplasia in a fetus with manifestation of atelosteogenesis I and boomerang dysplasia. *Am J Med Genet* 1993; 47:1086–91.

64. Hunter AGW, Carpenter BF. Atelosteogenesis I and boomerang dysplasia: a question of nosology. *Clin Genet* 1991; 39:471–80.

65. Eteson DJ, Adomian GE, Ornoy A, et al. Fibrochondrogenesis: radiologic and histologic studies. *Am J Med Genet* 1984; 19:277–90.

66. Whitley CB, Langer LO Jr, Ophoven J, et al. Fibrochondrogenesis: lethal, autosomal recessive chondrodysplasia with distinctive cartilage histopathology. *Am J Med Genet* 1984; 19:265–75.

67. Bankier A, Fortune D, Duke J, Sillence DO. Fibrochondrogenesis in male twins at 24 weeks gestation. *Am J Med Genet* 1991; 38:95–8.

68. Lazzaroni-Fossati F, Stanescu V, Stanescu R, et al. La fibrochondrogenese. *Arch Fr Pediatr* 1978; 35:1096–104.

69. Le Merrer M, Rousseau F, Legeai-Mallet L, et al. A gene for achondroplasia-hypochondroplasia maps to chromosome 4p. *Nat Genet* 1994; 6:318–21.

70. Velinov M, Slaugenhaupt SA, Stoilov I, et al. The gene for achondroplasia maps to the telomeric region of chromosome 4p. *Nat Genet* 1994; 6:314–7.

71. Opitz JM. "Unstable premutation" in achondroplasia: penetrance vs phenotrance. *Am J Med Genet* 1984; 19:251–4.

72. Reiser CA, Pauli RM, Hall JG. Achondroplasia: unexpected familial recurrence. *Am J Med Genet* 1984; 19:245–50.

73. Pauli RM, Scott CI, Wassman ER, et al. Apnea and sudden unexpected death in infants with achondroplasia. *J Pediatr* 1984; 104:342–8.

74. Yang SS, Corbett DP, Brough AJ, et al. Upper cervical myelopathy in achondroplasia. *Am J Clin Pathol* 1977; 68:68–72.

75. Hecht JT, Horton WA, Bulter IJ, et al. Foramen magnum stenosis in homozygous achondroplasia. *Eur J Pediatr* 1986; 145:545–7.

76. Filly RA, Golbus MS, Carey JC, Hall JG. Short limbed dwarfism: ultrasonic diagnosis by mensuration of fetal femoral length. *Radiology* 1981; 138: 653–6.

77. Leonard CO, Sanders RC, Lorrin Lau H. Prenatal diagnosis of the Turner syndrome, a familial chromosomal rearrangement and achondroplasia by amniocentesis and ultrasonography. *Johns Hopkins Med J* 1979; 145:25–30.

78. Rimoin DL, Hughes GN, Kaufman RL, et al. Endochondral ossification in achondroplasia dwarfism. *N Engl J Med* 1970; 283:728–35.

79. Aterman K, Welch JP, Taylor PG. Presumed homozygous achondroplasia. *Pathol Res Pract* 1983; 178:27–39.

80. Maroteaux P, Lamy M, Robert JM. Le nanisme thanatophore. *Presse Med* 1967; 75:2519–24.

81. Sabry A. Thanatophoric dwarfism in triplets. *Lancet* 1974; 2:533.

82. Serville F, Carles D, Maroteaux P. Thanatophoric dysplasia of identical twins. *Am J Med Genet* 1984; 17:703–6.

83. Corsello G, Maresi E, Rossi C, et al. Thanatophoric dysplasia in monozygotic twins discordant for cloverleaf skull: prenatal diagnosis, clinical and pathological findings. *Am J Med Genet* 1992; 42:122–6.

84. Ho KL, Chang CH, Yang SS, Chason JL. Neuropathologic findings in thanatophoric dysplasia. *Acta Neuropathol (Berl)* 1984; 63:218–28.

85. Knisely AS, Amber MW. Temporal-lobe abnormalities in thanatophoric dysplasia. *Pediatr Neurosci* 1988; 14:169–76.

86. Faye-Petersen OM, Knisely AS. Neural arch stenosis and spinal cord injury in thanatophoric dysplasia. *Am J Dis Child* 1991; 145:87–9.

87. Ornoy A, Adomian GE, Eteson DJ, et al. The role of mesenchyme-like tissue in the pathogenesis of thanatophoric dysplasia. *Am J Med Genet* 1985; 21:613–30.

88. Partington MW, Gonzalez-Crussi F, Khakee SG, Wollin DG. Cloverleaf skull and thanatophoric dwarfism: report of four cases, two in the same sibship. *Arch Dis Child* 1971; 46:656–64.

89. Langer LO, Yang SS, Gilbert EF, et al. Thanatophoric dysplasia (TD) and cloverleaf skull deformity (CSD). *Am J Med Genet* 1987; 3:167–79.

90. Horton WA, Harris DJ, Collins DL. Discordance for the kleeblattschadel anomaly in monozygotic twins with thanatophoric dysplasia. *Am J Med Genet* 1983; 15:97–101.

91. Horton WA, Rimoin DL, Hollister DW, Lachman RS. Further heterogeneity within lethal neonatal short-limbed dwarfism; the platyspondylic types. *J Pediatr* 1979; 94:736–42.

92. Van der Harten HJ, Brons JTJ, Dijkstra PF, et al. Some variants of lethal neonatal short-limbed platyspondylic dysplasia: a radiological, ultrasonographic, neuropathological and histopathological study of 22 cases. *Clin Dysmorphol* 1993; 2:1–19.

93. Maroteaux P, Spranger J, Wiedemann H-R. Der metatropische Zwergwuchs. *Arch Kinderheilkd* 1966; 173:211–26.

94. Beck M, Roubicek M, Rogers JG, et al. Heterogeneity of metatropic dysplasia. *Eur J Pediatr* 1983; 140:231–7.

95. Boden SD, Kaplan FS, Fallon MD, et al. Metatropic dwarfism. Uncoupling of endochondral and perichondral growth. *J Bone Joint Surg Am* 1987; 69:174–84.

96. Jenkins P, Smith MB, McKinnell JS. Metatropic dwarfism. *Br J Radiol* 1970; 43:561–5.

97. Maroteaux P, Stanescu V, Stanescu R, et al. Opsismodysplasia: a new type of chondrodysplasia with predominant involvement of the bones of the hand and the vertebrae. *Am J Med Genet* 1984; 19:171–82.

98. Beemer FA, Kozlowski KS. Additional case of opsismodysplasia supporting autosomal recessive inheritance. *Am J Med Genet* 1994; 49:344–7.

99. Winter RM, Thompson EM. Lethal, neonatal, short-limbed platyspondylic dwarfism: a further variant? *Hum Genet* 1982; 61:269–72.

100. Jeune M, Beraud C, Carron R. Dystrophie thoracique asphyxiante de caractere familial. *Arch Fr Pediatr* 1955; 12:886–91.

101. Langer LO Jr. Thoracic-pelvic-phalangeal dystrophy: asphyxiating thoracic dystrophy of the newborn, infantile thoracic dystrophy. *Radiology* 1968; 91:447–56.

102. Oberklaid F, Danks DM, Mayne V, Campbell P. Asphyxiating thoracic dysplasia: clinical, radiological, and pathological information on 10 patients. *Arch Dis Child* 1977; 52:758–65.

103. Hudgins L, Rosengren S, Treem W, Hyams J. Early cirrhosis in survivors with Jeune thoracic dystrophy. *J Pediatr* 1992; 120:754–6.

104. Kozlowski D, Szmigiel CA, Barylak A, Stopyrowa M. Difficulties in differentiation between chondroectodermal dysplasia (Ellis-van Creveld syndrome) and asphyxiating thoracic dystrophy. *Australas Radiol* 1972; 16:401–10.

105. Elejalde BR, Elejalde MM, Pansch D. Prenatal diagnosis of Jeune syndrome. *Am J Med Genet* 1985; 21:433–8.

106. Lipson M, Waskey J, Rice J, et al. Prenatal diagnosis of asphyxiating thoracic dysplasia. *Am J Med Genet* 1984; 18:273–7.

107. Yang SS, Langer LO, Cacciarelli A, et al. Three conditions in neonatal asphyxiating thoracic dysplasia (Jeune) and short rib-polydactyly syndrome spectrum: a clinicopathologic study. *Am J Med Genet* 1987; 3:191–207.

108. Ellis RWB, van Creveld S. A syndrome characterized by ectodermal dysplasia, polydactyly, chondrodysplasia and congenital morbus cordis. *Arch Dis Child* 1940; 15:65–84.

109. Bohm N, Fukuda M, Staudt R, Helwig H. Chondroectodermal dysplasia (Ellis-van Creveld syndrome) with dysplasia of renal medulla and bile ducts. *Histopathology* 1978; 2:267–81.

110. Da Silva EO, Janovitz D, De Albuquerque SC. Ellis-van Creveld syndrome: report of 15 cases in an inbred kindred. *J Med Genet* 1980; 17:349–56.

111. Mahoney MJ, Hobbins JC. Prenatal diagnosis of chondroectodermal dysplasia (Ellis-van Creveld syndrome) with fetoscopy and ultrasound. *N Engl J Med* 1977; 297:258–60.

112. Jequier S, Dunbar JS. The Ellis-van Creveld syndrome. *Prog Pediatr Radiol* 1973; 4:167–83.

113. Qureshi F, Jacques SM, Evans MI, et al. Skeletal histopathology in fetuses with chondroectodermal dysplasia (Ellis-van Creveld syndrome). *Am J Med Genet* 1993; 45:471–6.

114. Saldino RM, Noonan CD. Severe thoracic dystrophy with striking micromelia, abnormal osseous development, including the spine and multiple visceral anomalies. *AJR Am J Roentgenol* 1972; 114:257–63.

115. Spranger J, Grimm B, Weller M, et al. Short rib-polydactyly (SRP) syndromes, types Majewski and Saldino-Noonan. *Z Kinderheilkd* 1974; 116:73–94.

116. Koppang HS, Boman H, Hoel PS. Oral abnormalities in the Saldino-Noonan syndrome. *Virchows Arch A Pathol Anat Histopathol* 1983; 398:247–62.

117. Richardson MM, Beaudet AL, Wagner ML, et al. Prenatal diagnosis of recurrence of Saldino-Noonan dwarfism. *J Pediatr* 1977; 91:467–71.

118. Toftager-Larsen K, Benzie RJ. Fetoscopy in prenatal diagnosis of the Majewski and the Saldino-Noonan types of the short rib-polydactyly syndromes. *Clin Genet* 1984; 26:56–60.

119. Majewski F, Pfeiffer RA, Lenz W. Polysyndaktylie, verkurzte Gleidmassen und Genitalfehlbidungen: Kennzeiehen eines Selbstandigen syndroms. *Z Kinderheilkd* 1971; 11:118–38.

120. Chen H, Yang SS, Gonzalez E, et al. Short rib-polydactyly syndrome, Majewski type. *Am J Med Genet* 1980; 7:215–22.

121. McCormae RM, Flannery DB, Nakoneczna I, Kodroff MB. Short rib-polydactyly syndrome type II (Majewski syndrome): a case report. *Pediatr Pathol* 1984; 2:457–67.

122. Motegi T, Kusunoki M, Nishi T, et al. Short rib-polydactyly syndrome, Majewski type, in two male siblings. *Hum Genet* 1979; 49:269–75.

123. Sharma AK, Phadke S, Chandra K, et al. Overlap between Majewski and hydrolethalus syndrome. *Am J Med Genet* 1992; 43:949–53.

124. Bidot-Lopez P, Ablow RC, Ogden JA, Mahoney MJ. A case of short rib polydactyly. *Pediatrics* 1978; 61:427–32.

125. Bernstein R, Isdale J, Pinto M, et al. Short rib-polydactyly syndrome: a single or heterogeneous entity? A re-evaluation prompted by four new cases. *J Med Genet* 1985; 22:46–53.

126. Sillence D, Kozlowski K, Bar-Ziv J, et al. Perinatally lethal short rib-polydactyly syndromes. I. Variability in known syndromes. *Pediatr Radiol* 1987; 17:474–80.

127. Belloni C, Beluffi G. Short rib-polydactyly syndrome, type Verma-Naumoff. *Fortschraeb Roentgenstr* 1981; 134:431–5.

128. Habeck J-O, Kunzel W, Muller D, et al. Kurzrippen-polydaktylie-syndrom type III (Verma-Naumoff) mit zeichen einer ektodermalen dysplasie. *Zentralbl Gynaekol* 1982; 104:568–75.

129. Yang SS, Lin SC, Al Saadi A, et al. Short rib-polydactyly syndrome, type 3 with chondrocytic inclusions: report of a case and review of the literature. *Am J Med Genet* 1980; 7:205–13.

130. Erzen M, Stanescu R, Stanescu V, Maroteaux P. Comparative histopathology of

the growth cartilage in short-rib polydactyly syndromes type I and type III and in chondroectodermal dysplasia. *Ann Genet* 1988; 31:144–50.

131. Beemer FA, Langer LO Jr, Klep-de Pater JM, et al. A new short rib syndrome: report of two cases. *Am J Med Genet* 1983; 14:115–23.

132. Chen H, Mirkin D, Yang S. A de novo 17q paracentric inversion mosaicism in a patient with Beemer-Langer type short rib-polydactyly syndrome with a special consideration to the classification of short rib polydactyly syndrome. *Am J Med Genet* 1994; 53:165–71.

133. Lurie IW. Further delineation of the Beemer-Langer syndrome using concordance rates in affected sibs. *Am J Med Genet* 1994; 50:313–7.

134. Yang SS, Roth JA, Langer LO. Short rib syndrome Beemer-Langer type with polydactyly: a multiple congenital anomalies syndrome. *Am J Med Genet* 1991; 39:243–6.

135. Lin AE, Doshi N, Flom L, et al. Beemer-Langer syndrome with manifestations of an orofaciodigital syndrome. *Am J Med Genet* 1991; 39:247–51.

136. Hingorani SR, Pagon RA, Shepard TH, Kapur RP. Twin fetuses with abnormalities that overlap with three midline malformation complexes. *Am J Med Genet* 1991; 41:230–5.

137. Piepkorn M, Karp LE, Hickok D, et al. A lethal neonatal dwarfing condition with short ribs, polysyndactyly, cranial synostosis, cleft palate cardiovascular and urogenital anomalies and severe ossification defect. *Teratology* 1977; 16:345–50.

138. Cherstvoy ED, Lurie IW, Shved IA, et al. Difficulties in classification of the short rib-polydactyly syndromes. *Eur J Pediatr* 1980; 133:57–61.

139. Conradi E. Vorzeitiges Auftreten von Knochen und eigenartigen Verkalkungskernen bei Chondrodystrophia foetalis hypoplastica: Histologische und Rontgenuntersuchungen. *Z Kinderheilkd* 1914; 80:86–97.

140. Hünermann C. Chondrodystrophia calcificans congenita als abortive. From der Chondrodystrophie. *Z Kinderheilkd* 1931; 51:1–19.

141. Gillbert EF, Opitz JM, Spranger JW, et al. Chondrodysplasia punctata rhizomelic form: pathologic and radiologic studies of three infants. *Eur J Pediatr* 1976; 123:89–109.

142. Spranger JW, Opitz JM, Bidder U. Heterogeneity of chondrodysplasia punctata. *Humangenetik* 1971; 11:190–212.

143. Pauli RM, Haun JM. Intrauterine effects of coumarin derivatives. *Dev Brain Dysfunct* 1993; 6:229–47.

144. Heymans HSA, Oorthuys JWE, Nelck G, et al. Rhizomelic chondrodysplasia punctata: another peroxisomal disorder. *N Engl J Med* 1985; 313:187–8.

145. Wanders RJA, Schumacher H, Heikoop J, et al. Human dihydroxyacetonephosphate acyltransferase deficiency: a new peroxisomal disorder. *J Inherit Metab Dis* 1992; 15:389–9.

146. Happle R, Phillips RJS, Roessner A, Junemann G. Homologous genes for X-linked chondrodysplasia punctata in man and mouse. *Hum Genet* 1983; 63:24–7.

147. Manzke H, Christophers E, Wiedemann H-R. Dominant sex-linked inherited chondrodysplasia punctata: a distinct type of chondrodysplasia punctata. *Clin Genet* 1980; 17:97–107.

148. Mueller RF, Crowle PM, Jones RAK, Davison BCC. X-Linked dominant chondrodysplasia punctata: a case report and family studies. *Am J Med Genet* 1985; 20:137–44.

149. Silengo MC, Luzzatti L, Silverman FN. Clinical and genetic aspects of Conradi-Hünermann disease: a report of three family cases and review of the literature. *J Pediatr* 1980; 97:911–7.

150. Curry CJR, Magenis RE, Brown M, et al. Inherited chondrodysplasia punctata due to a deletion of the terminal short arm of an X chromosome. *N Engl J Med* 1984; 311:1010–5.

151. Maroteaux P. Brachytelephalangic chondrodysplasia punctata: a possible X-linked recessive form. *Hum Genet* 1989; 82:167–70.

152. Rittler M, Menger H, Spranger J. Chondrodysplasia punctata, tibia-metacarpal (MT) type. *Am J Med Genet* 1990; 37:200–8.

153. Maroteaux P, Spranger JW, Opitz JM, et al. Le syndrome campomelique. *Presse Med* 1971; 79:1157–62.

154. Bianchine JW, Risemberg HM, Kanderian SS, Harrison HE. Camptomelic dwarfism. *Lancet* 1971; 1:1017–8.

155. Tommerup N, Schempp W, Meinecke P, et al. Assignment of an autosomal sex reversal locus (SRA1) and campomelic dysplasia (CMPD1) to 17q24.3-q25.1. *Nat Genet* 1993; 4:170–4.

156. Becker MH, Finegold M, Genieser NB, et al. Campomelic dwarfism. *Birth Defects* 1975; 11:113–8.

157. Houston CS, Opitz JM, Spranger JW, et al. The campomelic syndrome: review, report of 17 cases, and follow-up on the currently 17-year-old first reported by Maroteaux et al. in 1971. *Am J Med Genet* 1983; 15:3–28.

158. Austin GE, Gold RH, Mirra JM, et al. Long-limbed campomelic dwarfism: a radiologic and pathologic study. *Am J Dis Child* 1980; 134:1035–42.

159. Hovmoller ML, Osuna A, Eklof O, et al. Campomelic dwarfism. A genetically determined mesenchymal disorder combined with sex reversal. *Hereditas* 1977; 86:51–62.

160. Khajavi A, Lachman R, Rimoin D, et al. Heterogeneity in the campomelic syndromes: long- and short-bone varieties. *Radiology* 1976; 120:641–7.

161. Hwang WS. Pathology of cartilage in camptomelic dwarfism. *Lab Invest* 1979; 40:305–6.

162. Hall BD, Spranger JW. Congenital bowing of the long bones: a review and phenotype analysis of 13 undiagnosed cases. *Eur J Pediatr* 1980; 133:131–8.

163. Maclean RN, Prater WK, Lozzio CB. Skeletal dysplasia with short, angulated femora (kyphomelic dysplasia). *Am J Med Genet* 1983; 14:373–80.

164. Hall BD, Spranger JW. Familial congenital bowing with short bones. *Radiology* 1979; 132:611–14.

165. Fryns JP, van den Berghe K, van Assche A, van den Berghe H. Prenatal diagnosis of campomelic dwarfism. *Clin Genet* 1981; 19:199–201.

166. Lamy M, Maroteaux P. Le nanisme diastrophique. *Presse Med* 1960; 68:1977–80.

167. Diab M, Wu J-J, Shapiro F, Eyre D. Abnormality of type IX collagen in a patient with diastrophic dysplasia. *Am J Med Genet* 1994; 49:402–9.

168. Hasbacka J, Kaitila I, Sistonen P, de la Chapelle A. Diastrophic dysplasia gene maps to the distal long arm of chromosome 5. *Proc Natl Acad Sci USA* 1990; 87:8056–9.

169. Gollop TR, Eigier A. Prenatal ultrasound diagnosis of diastrophic dysplasia at 16 weeks. *Am J Med Genet* 1987; 27:321–4.

170. Wladimiroff JW, Niermeijer MF, Laar J, et al. Prenatal diagnosis of skeletal dysplasia by real-time ultrasound. *Obstet Gynecol* 1984; 63:360–4.

171. Qureshi F, Jacques SM, Johnson SF, et al. Histopathology of fetal diastrophic dysplasia. *Am J Med Genet* 1993; 45:471–76.

172. Horton WA, Rimoin DL, Hollister DW, Silberg R. Diastrophic dwarfism: a histochemical and ultrastructural study of the endochondral growth plate. *Pediatr Res* 1979; 13:904–9.

173. Taber P, Freedman S, Lackey DA. Diastrophic dwarfism. *Prog Pediatr Radiol* 1973; 4:152–66.

174. Stoss H, Pesch H-J. Structural changes of collagen fibrils in skeletal dysplasia. *Virchows Arch A Pathol Anat Histopathol* 1985; 405:341–64.

175. Larsen LJ, Schottstaedt ER, Bost RC. Multiple congenital dislocations associated with characteristic facial abnormality. *J Pediatr* 1950; 37:574–81.

176. Latta RJ, Graham B, Aase J, et al. Larsen's syndrome: a skeletal dysplasia with multiple joint dislocations and unusual facies. *J Pediatr* 1971; 78: 291–8.

177. Chen H, Chang C-H, Perrin E, Perrin J. A lethal, Larsen-like multiple joint dislocation syndrome. *Am J Med Genet* 1982; 13:149–61.

178. Desbuquois G, Grener B, Michel J, et al. Chondrodystrophique avec ossification anarchique et poly-malformations chez deux soeurs. *Arch Fr Pediatr* 1966; 23:573–87.

179. Shohat M, Lachman R, Gruber HE, et al. Desbuquois syndrome: clinical, radiographic and morphologic characterization. *Am J Med Genet* 1994; 52:9–18.

180. Sillence DO. Osteogenesis imperfecta. An expanding panorama of variants. *Clin Orthop* 1981; 159:11–25.

181. Spranger J, Cremin B, Beighton P. Osteogenesis imperfecta congenita: features and prognosis of a heterogeneous condition. *Pediatr Radiol* 1982; 12:21–7.

182. Young ID, Thompson EM, Hall CM, Pembrey ME. Osteogenesis imperfecta type IIA: evidence for dominant inheritance. *J Med Genet* 1987; 24:386–9.

183. Follis RH Jr. Maldevelopment of the corium in the osteogenesis imperfecta syndrome. *Bull Johns Hopkins Hosp* 1953; 93:225–33.

184. Byers P. Osteogenesis imperfecta. In: Royce P, Steinmann B, eds. *Connective Tissue and Its Heritable Disorders.* New York: Wiley-Liss, 1993, pp. 317–50.

185. Byers PH, Tsipouras P, Bonadio JF, et al. Perinatal lethal osteogenesis imperfecta (OI): a biochemically heterogeneous disorder usually due to new mutations in the genes of type I collagen. *Am J Hum Genet* 1988; 42:237–48.

186. Pauli RM, Gilbert EF. Upper cervical cord compression as cause of death osteogenesis imperfecta type II. *J Pediatr* 1986; 108:579–81.

187. Elejalde R, Elejalde MM. Prenatal diagnosis of perinatally lethal osteogenesis imperfecta. *Am J Med Genet* 1983; 14:353–9.

188. Shapiro JE, Phillips JA III, Byers PH, et al. Prenatal diagnosis of lethal perinatal osteogenesis imperfecta (OI type II). *J Pediatr* 1982; 100:127–33.

189. Sillence DO, Barlow KK, Garber AP, et al. Osteogenesis imperfecta type II. Delineation of the phenotype with reference to genetic heterogeneity. *Am J Med Genet* 1984; 17:407–23.

190. Maroteaux P, Frezal J, Cohen-Solal L. The differential symptomatology of

errors of collagen metabolism: a tentative classification. *Am J Med Genet* 1986; 24:219–30.

191. Van der Harten HJ, Brons JTJ, Dijkstra PF, et al. Perinatal lethal osteogenesis imperfecta: radiologic and pathologic evaluation of seven prenatally diagnosed cases. *Pediatr Pathol* 1988; 8:232–52.

192. Sillence DO, Barlow KK, Cole WG, et al. Osteogenesis imperfecta type III. Delineation of the phenotype with reference to genetic heterogeneity. *Am J Med Genet* 1986; 23:821–32.

193. Wallis GA, Sykes B, Byers PH, et al. Osteogenesis imperfecta type III: mutations in the type I collagen structural genes, COL1A1 and COL1A2, are not necessarily responsible. *J Med Genet* 1993; 30:492–6.

194. Shapiro F, Glimcher MJ, Holtrop ME, et al. Human osteopetrosis. A histological, ultrastructural and biochemical study. *J Bone Joint Surg Am* 1980; 62:384–99.

195. Albers-Schonberg H. Rontgenbilder einer seltenen Knochenerkrankung. *Muench Med Wochenschr* 1904; 51:365–8.

196. Case records of the Massachusetts General Hospital (case 37-1982). *N Engl J Med* 1982; 307:735–43.

197. Coccia PF, Krivit W, Cervenka J, et al. Successful bone marrow transplantation for infantile malignant osteopetrosis. *N Engl J Med* 1980; 302:701–8.

198. Marks SC Jr. Congenital osteopetrotic mutations as probes of the origin, structure, and function of osteoclasts. *Clin Orthop* 1984; 189:239–63.

199. El Khazen N, Faverly D, Vamos E, et al. Lethal osteopetrosis with multiple fractures in utero. *Am J Med Genet* 1986; 23:811–9.

200. Reeves J, Arnaud S, Gordon S, et al. The pathogenesis of infantile malignant osteopetrosis: bone mineral metabolism and complications in five patients. *Metab Bone Dis Rel Res* 1981; 3:135–42.

201. Dipierri JE, Guzman JD. A second family with autosomal dominant osteosclerosis-type Stanescu. *Am J Med Genet* 1984; 18:13–8.

202. Caffey J, Silverman WA. Infantile cortical hyperostosis: preliminary report on new syndrome. *AJR Am J Roentgenol* 1945; 54:1–16.

203. Saul RA, Lee WH, Stevenson RE. Caffey's disease revisited. Further evidence for autosomal dominant inheritance with incomplete penetrance. *Am J Dis Child* 1982; 136:56–60.

204. Finsterbush A, Rang M. Infantile cortical hyperostosis. Follow-up of 29 cases. *Acta Orthop Scand* 1975; 46:727–36.

205. Pazzaglia UE, Byers PD, Beluffi G, et al. Pathology of infantile cortical hyperostosis (Caffey's disease). Report of a case. *J Bone Joint Surg Am* 1985; 67:1417–26.

206. Kozlowski K, Tsuruta T. Dysplastic cortical hyperostosis: a new form of lethal neonatal dwarfism. *Br J Radiol* 1989; 62:376–8.

207. Eversole SL Jr, Holman GH, Robinson RA. Hitherto undescribed characteristics of the pathology of infantile cortical hyperostosis (Caffey's disease). *Bull Johns Hopkins Hosp* 1957; 101:80–99.

208. Fallon MD, Teitelbaum SL, Weinstein RS, et al. Hypophosphatasia: clinicopathologic comparison of the infantile, childhood, and adult forms. *Medicine* 1984; 63:12–24.

209. Weiss MJ, Ray K, Fallon MD, et al. Analysis of liver/bone/kidney alkaline phosphatase mRNA and enzymatic activity in cultured skin fibroblasts in 14 unrelated patients with severe hypophosphatasia. *Am J Med Genet* 1989; 44:686–94.

210. Fraser D. Hypophosphatasia. *Am J Med* 1957; 22:730–46.

211. Macpherson RI, Kroeker M, Houston CS. Hypophosphatasia. *J Can Assoc Radiol* 1972; 23:16–26.

212. Whyte MP, Magill HL, Fallon MD, Herrod HG. Infantile hypophosphatasia: normalization of circulating bone alkaline phosphatase activity followed by skeletal remineralization. *J Pediatr* 1986; 108:82–8.

213. Mulivor RA, Mennuti M, Zackai EH, Harris H. Prenatal diagnosis of hypophosphatasia: genetic, biochemical, and clinical studies. *Am J Hum Genet* 1978; 30:271–82.

214. Ornoy A, Adomian GE, Rimoin DL. Histologic and ultrastructural studies on the mineralization process in hypophosphatasia. *Am J Med Genet* 1985; 22:743–58.

215. Leroy JG, DeMars RI. Mutant enzymatic and cytological phenotypes in cultured human fibroblasts. *Science* 1967; 157:804–6.

216. Spritz RA, Doughty RA, Spackman TJ, et al. Neonatal presentation of I-cell disease. *J Pediatr* 1978; 93:954–8.

217. Lemaitre L, Remy J, Farriaux JP, et al. Radiological signs of mucolipidosis II or I-cell disease. *Pediatr Radiol* 1978; 7:97–105.

218. Michels VV, Dutton RV, Caskey CT. Mucolipidosis II: unusual presentation with a congenital angulated fracture. *Clin Genet* 1982; 21:225–7.

219. Blank E, Linder D. I-cell disease (mucolipidosis II): a lysosomopathy. *Pediatrics* 1974; 54:797–805.

220. Powell HC, Benirschke K, Favara BE, et al. Foamy changes of placental cells in fetal storage disorders. *Virchows Arch A Pathol Anat Histopathol* 1976; 369:191–6.

221. Wigglesworth JS. *Perinatal Pathology*. Philadelphia: WB Saunders, 1984, p. 384.

222. Whitley CB, Burke BA, Granroth G, Gorlin RJ. de la Chapelle dysplasia. *Am J Med Genet* 1986; 25:29–39.

223. Nores JA, Rotmensch S, Romero R, et al. Atelosteogenesis II: sonographic and radiological correlation. *Prenat Diagn* 1992; 12:741–53.

224. Koide T, Katayama H, Sumi Y, Ishi K. A case of new chondrodystrophy. *Pediatr Radiol* 1983; 13:102–5.

225. Connor JM, Connor RAC, Sweet EM, et al. Lethal neonatal chondrodysplasias in the West of Scotland 1970–1983 with a description of a thanatophoric dysplasia like, autosomal recessive disorder, Glasgow variant. *Am J Med Genet* 1985; 22:243–53.

226. Maroteaux P, Stanescu R, Stanescu V, Cousin J. Recessive lethal chondrodysplasia, "round femoral inferior epiphysis type." *Eur J Pediatr* 1988; 147:408–11.

227. Carty H, Kozlowski K, Sillence D. Dappled diaphyseal dysplasias. *Fortschr Rontgenstr* 1989; 150:228–9.

228. Nairn ER, Chapman S. A new type of lethal short-limbed dwarfism. *Pediatr Radiol* 1989; 19:253–7.

229. Greenberg CR, Gruber HE, DeSa DJB, et al. A new autosomal recessive lethal chondrodystrophy with non-immune hydrops. *Am J Med Genet* 1988; 29:623–32.

230. Bonaventure J, Zylberberg L, Cohen-Solal L, et al. A new lethal brittle bone syndrome with increased amount of type V collagen in a patient. *Am J Med Genet* 1989; 33:299–310.

231. Kan AE, Kozlowski K. New distinct lethal osteosclerotic bone dysplasia (Raine syndrome). *Am J Med Genet* 1992; 43:860–4.

232. Beemer FA, Kramer PPG, van der Harten HJ, Gerards LJ. A new syndrome of dwarfism, neonatal death, narrow chest, spondylometaphyseal abnormalities, and advanced bone age. *Am J Med Genet* 1985; 20:555–8.

233. Langer LO Jr, Nishino R, Yamaguchi A, et al. Brachymesomelia-renal syndrome. *Am J Med Genet* 1983; 15:57–65.

234. Juberg RC, Van Ness MB. A new form of hereditary short limbed dwarfism with microcephalus. *Clin Genet* 1975; 7:111–9.

235. Hwang WS, Trevenen CL, Greenberg C, Reed MH. Chondro-osseous changes in cerebro-oculo-facial-skeletal (COFS) syndrome. *J Pathol* 1982; 138:33–40.

236. Begum R, Coutinho ML, Dormandy T, Yudkin S. Maternal malabsorption presenting as congenital rickets. *Lancet* 1968; 1:1048–52.

237. Moncrieff M, Fadahunsi TO. Congenital rickets due to maternal vitamin D deficiency. *Arch Dis Child* 1974; 49:810–1.

238. Kirk J. Congenital rickets—a case report. *Aust Paediatr J* 1982; 18:291–3.

239. Zeidan S, Bamford M. Congenital rickets with maternal pre-eclampsia. *J R Soc Med* 1984; 77:426–7.

240. Kulkarni PB, Dorand RD, Bridger WM, et al. Rickets in premature infants fed different formulas. *South Med J* 1984; 77:13–6, 20.

241. Masel JP, Tudehope D, Cartwright D, Cleghorn G. Osteopenia and rickets in the extremely low birth weight infant—a survey of the incidence and a radiological classification. *Australas Radiol* 1982; 26:83–96.

242. Kovar IZ, Mayne PD, Robbe I. Hypophosphataemic rickets in the preterm infant; hypocalcaemia after calcium and phosphorus supplementation. *Arch Dis Child* 1983; 58:629–31.

243. Gefter WB, Epstein DM, Anday EK, Dalinka MK. Rickets presenting as multiple fractures in premature infants on hyperalimentation. *Radiology* 1982; 142:371–4.

244. Glasgow JFT, Thomas PS. Rachitic respiratory distress in small preterm infants. *Arch Dis Child* 1977; 52:268–73.

245. Oppenheimer SJ, Snodgrass GJAI. Neonatal rickets: histopathology and quantitative bone changes. *Arch Dis Child* 1980; 55:945–9.

246. Oppenheimer EH, Dahms BB. Congenital syphilis in the fetus and neonate. *Perspect Pediatr Pathol* 1981; 6:115–38.

247. Cremin BJ, Fisher RM. The lesions of congenital syphilis. *Br J Radiol* 1970; 43:333–41.

248. Rosenfeld SR, Weinert CR, Kahn B. Congenital syphilis, a case report. *J Bone Joint Surg Am* 1983; 65:115–9.

249. Gregg NM. Congenital cataracts following German measles in the mother. *Trans Ophthalmol Soc Aust* 1941; 3:35–46.

250. Centers for Disease Control. Rubella and congenital rubella—United States, 1983. *JAMA* 1984; 251:2774–5, 2779.

251. Levine JB, Berkowitz CD, St. Geme JW Jr. Rubella virus reinfection during pregnancy leading to late-onset congenital rubella syndrome. *J Pediatr* 1982; 100:589–91.

252. Rosenberg HS, Kohl S, Vogler C. Viral infections of the fetus and neonate. In: Naeye RL, Kissane JM, Kaufman N, eds. *Perinatal Diseases*. Baltimore: Williams & Wilkins, 1981, pp. 133–200.

253. Rudolph AJ, Singleton EB, Rosenberg HS, et al. Osseous manifestations of the congenital rubella syndrome. *Am J Dis Child* 1965; 110:428–33.

254. Strauss L. Rubella symposium. *J Pediatr* 1965; 67:989–90.

255. Reed GB Jr. Rubella bone lesions. *J Pediatr* 1969; 74:208–13.

256. Graham CB, Thal A, Wassum CS. Rubella-like bone changes in congenital cytomegalic inclusion disease. *Radiology* 1970; 94:39–43.

257. Milgram JW. Osseous changes in congenital toxoplasmosis. *Arch Pathol* 1974; 94:150–1.

Chapter 32

Skeletal Musculature

BRIAN D. LAKE   J. PATRICK BARBET

The biomolecular structure and organization of the sarcolemmal membrane provides for classification of the genetically determined muscular dystrophies founded on the various defects in the sarcolemmal membrane subunits. The basis of many of the congenital myopathies and denervations is understood in molecular biological terms and the standard examination of muscle tissue has been modified to take these advances into account. Material must be preserved in an appropriate state for future investigations of the biochemistry and of the mutations that, if not already known, will no doubt be found in the future. Biochemical study of the components of the respiratory chain is also important in patients presenting with a metabolic acidosis, and this can now be done using as little as 50 mg of tissue.

STUDY OF SKELETAL MUSCLE

A neuromuscular disorder is best evaluated by a histochemical and electron microscopic approach [1], and samples of tissue should be reserved for biochemical and molecular biological studies. Although a certain amount of helpful information can be obtained from routine sections of formalin-fixed tissue, most of the congenital myopathies will be missed and fiber typing and immunohistochemistry, which are most important, will not be possible. In small neonates it is preferable not to use any muscle tissue for formalin fixation, but to rely on the frozen sections, which in the right hands are at least as good as paraffin sections. Routine paraffin sections of postmortem muscle will be helpful to supplement the information gained from cryostat sections, and have the advantage that larger areas can be sampled.

Tissue should be snap-frozen in such a manner as to prevent ice-crystal formation, and cryostat sections with thicknesses of 5–8 μm can then be cut from transversely oriented specimens. Staining techniques include, at a minimum, the modified Gomori trichrome method; a method (or methods) for typing muscle fibers as type 1, 2A, 2B, or 2C; and an NADH dehydrogenase method. Additional stains are hematoxylin and eosin, a fat stain, periodic acid–Schiff (PAS) to demonstrate glycogen, an acid phosphatase reaction, and, when necessary, reactions to demonstrate the activities of cytochrome oxidase, succinate dehydrogenase, phosphorylase, and phosphofructokinase. Immunohistochemical techniques may also be necessary to analyze the expression of different muscular proteins such as the myogenic factors, the slow and fast isoforms of the myosin heavy chains, and the sarcolemmal membrane proteins and glycoproteins dystrophin, merosin, spectrin, the sarcoglycans, and β-dystroglycan.

Fiber diameters are measured as the smallest diameter of a fiber and can be assessed adequately by using an eyepiece graticule or from a photograph. Fiber areas or diameters derived from computer-linked equipment are more accurate, but this approach is probably unnecessary for most purposes, since there is a wide range of normality. Fiber diameters measured in routine paraffin sections may only be 70–80% of those observed in cryostat sections, due to shrinkage during processing.

Tissue for electron microscopy can be fixed and processed by conventional means. Transverse sections generally give more information than longitudinally oriented blocks.

It must be said that the microscopic evaluation of skeletal muscle in the fetus and neonate is difficult and frustrating and poses many challenges to the pathologist.

DEVELOPMENT OF SKELETAL MUSCLE

An appreciation of the development of skeletal muscle during embryonic and fetal life [2–6] can help in the

1083

understanding of some of the congenital abnormalities and myopathies occurring in the neonatal period.

At the 2–3-week stage, somites form along each side of the axial line and differentiate into smooth muscle and mesenchymal structures. In the dorsomedial portion, mesodermal elements differentiate into skeletal muscles of the limb and trunks, while the branchial arches give rise to the cervical and craniobulbar muscles.

At 4–5 weeks the developing myoblasts unite with the laterally placed dermatomes to form the dermatomyotomes, each of which is innervated with a spinal nerve. The dermatomyotomes are arranged metamerically along each side of the spinal column and the segments grow dorsally and vertically to meet in the midline. The skeletal muscle is formed from the myotomes by fusion, splitting, and reorientation. The somites give rise to 2 distinct muscle populations. The first population differentiates within the somite itself, probably following induction from the neural tube or from the notochord. The process is locally mediated by diffusible factors (7) and this population forms the "myotomal" muscles (paravertebral and trunk muscles). Mononucleated cells from the second population do not differentiate within the somite but are able to migrate and to colonize different regions of the embryo such as the limb buds; they form the limb muscles. It is likely that the position of this second population of myogenic cells within the somite allows them to escape the effects of local induction factors and to migrate; it has been shown that the potential for these cells to migrate is accompanied by the transient expression of different factors such as pax3. In both precursor cell populations, the onset of the myogenic program involves the activation of several regulatory genes. Different regulatory proteins such as the myogenic factors (myf's) and the myogenic enhancer factor 2 (MEF2) seem to participate in a complex regulatory circuit involving direct and indirect positive feedback loops [8, 9]. Four main myogenic factors

(myf3, myf4, myf5, and myf6) in human muscle development have been described, corresponding to similar factors previously described in different species (respectively, myoD, myogenin, myf5, muscle regulatory factor 4 [MRF4]). These basic helix-loop-helix (bHLH) nuclear proteins are sequentially and transiently expressed during muscle cell formation: The factors myf5 and myf3, relatively redundant, are expressed early in mononucleated myoblasts; myf4 is expressed later and seems essential for the terminal differentiation of previously committed myoblasts (i.e., myogenic fusion); myf6 is expressed even later [9, 10]. When they are expressed, these factors probably activate the transcription of different muscle-specific proteins such as desmin and the sarcomeric proteins.

From the morphological point of view, myoblasts among other differentiating mesodermal cells have no particular microscopic appearance to allow their specific identification until about 6–7 weeks, when they synthesize myofilaments. Creatine kinase (CK) activity and acetylcholine receptors can also be detected. At 7–9 weeks the myoblasts proliferate, elongate, and fuse to form myotubes. The myotubes are multinucleate, the nuclei showing a prominent nucleolus, while the cytoplasm contains glycogen, mitochondria, and myofibrils which begin to organize into the sarcomeres of mature skeletal muscle. The primary myotubes occur in small clusters, and the spaces between the clusters contain less-differentiated mesodermal cells that later develop into fibroblasts and blood vessels.

Myotubes are present up to about 15 weeks of development (Fig. 32.1), when the nucleus becomes peripherally located and the muscle fibers have their own basal lamina rather than sharing with a group of myotubes. Undifferentiated mononuclear cells are found under the basal lamina and represent the satellite cells found in mature muscle fibers. At 15 weeks the muscle fibers all have characteristics of type 2C fibers. By about 20 weeks, scattered larger fibers,

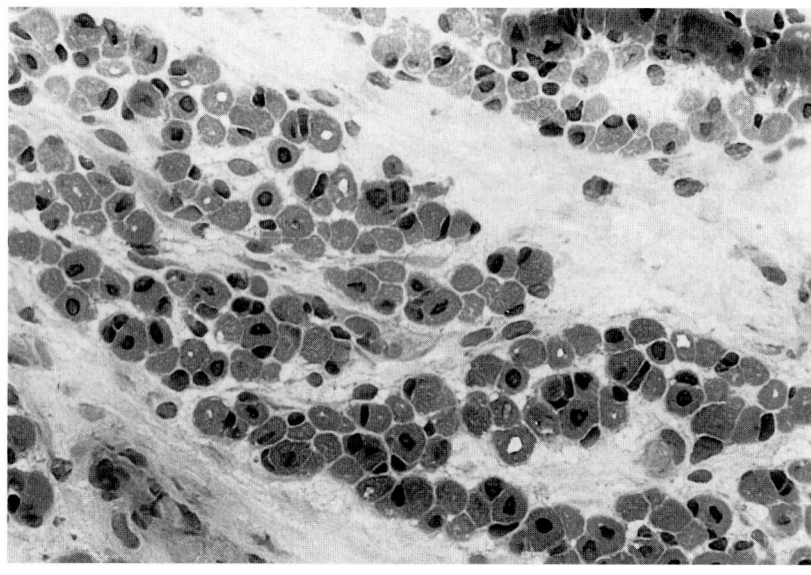

FIGURE 32.1.   *Fetal muscle, 15 weeks. Myotubes and central nuclei are evident. There is abundant loose connective tissue between small groups of fibers. Cryostat section, H&E, ×365.*

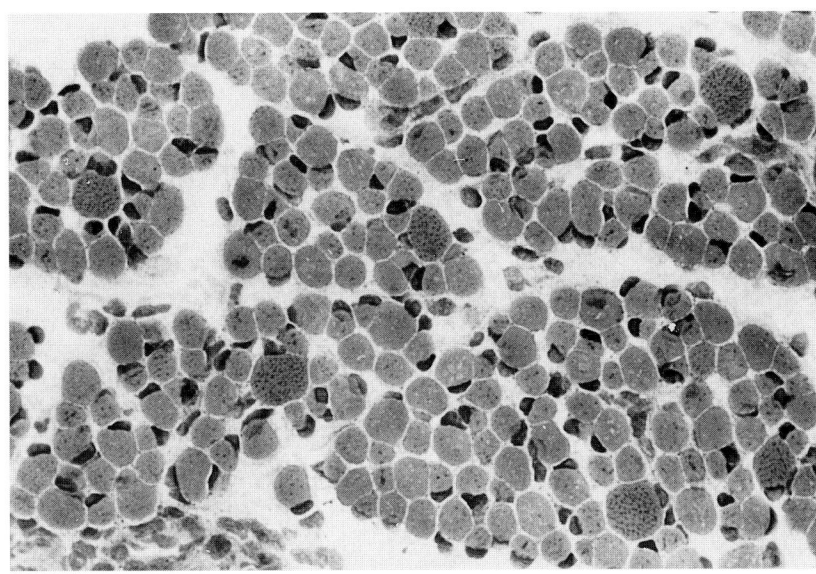

FIGURE 32.2. *Fetal muscle, 22 weeks. Most fibers are of a relatively uniform size, and the groups of fibers are larger than at earlier stages. The large fibers with discrete punctate staining are type 1 fibers and correspond to Wohlfart type B fibers. Cryostat section, trichrome, ×365.*

accounting for some 2% of the total, have type 1 fiber characteristics (Figs. 32.2 and 32.3). They correspond to Wohlfart type B fibers.

From the enzyme histochemical point of view, fiber type differentiation becomes apparent from 30 weeks, when small type 1 fibers appear (Fig. 32.4). Fibers with type 2B characteristics are seen soon after this and by about 35 weeks type 2A fibers are also present. At birth, fiber type differentiation is complete but there may be a variable proportion of type 2C fibers remaining, and this proportion may comprise up to 10% of the total [11]. Type 2C fibers are normally absent from muscle in infants older than 1 or 2 weeks.

Immunohistochemical study of the expression of diverse protein isoforms reveals differentiation of the muscle fibers even earlier than is possible with classic enzyme histochemistry [12–14]. The myosin heavy chains are of special interest as the expression of their different isoforms is clearly

developmentally regulated. In almost all muscle fibers, the developmental (embryonic and fetal) isoforms of the myosin heavy chains are progressively replaced either by the adult slow or by the adult fast isoform. Studies clearly suggest the existence of 2 distinct generations of muscle fibers in humans [12]. First-generation fibers form before 10 weeks, express the slow myosin heavy chain almost as soon as they form (which is prior to the establishment of motor innervation), and seem to give rise exclusively to slow fibers in the adult muscle. Second-generation fibers form asynchronously around the primary fibers and never express initially the slow myosin heavy chain but express a mixture of embryonic, fetal, and fast myosin heavy chains; their maturation after 20 weeks gives rise to both slow and fast fibers in the adult muscle. Epigenetic factors regulate both the maturation and the differentiation of the muscle fibers. In particular, the establishment of the motor innervation

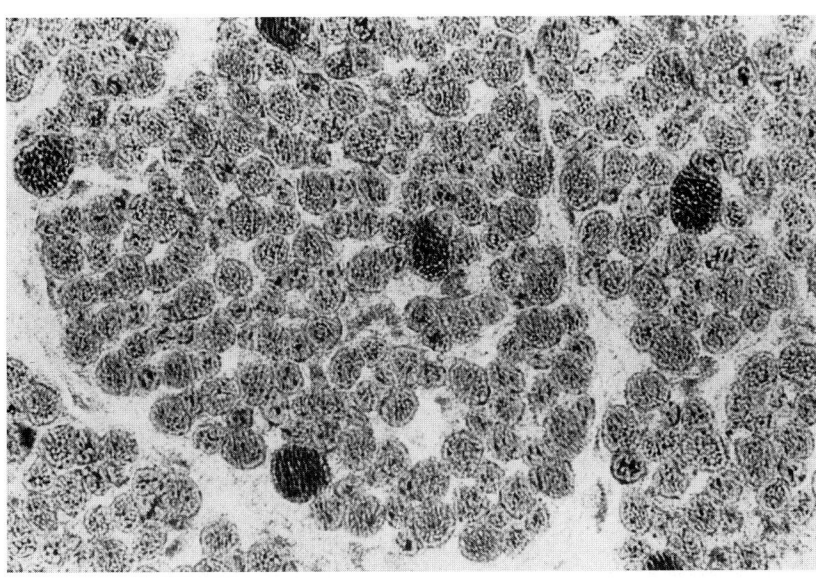

FIGURE 32.3. *Fetal muscle, 22 weeks. Same muscle as in Fig. 32.2. The larger fibers have strong NADH dehydrogenase activity and are scattered throughout the muscle. Cryostat section, NADH dehydrogenase, ×365.*

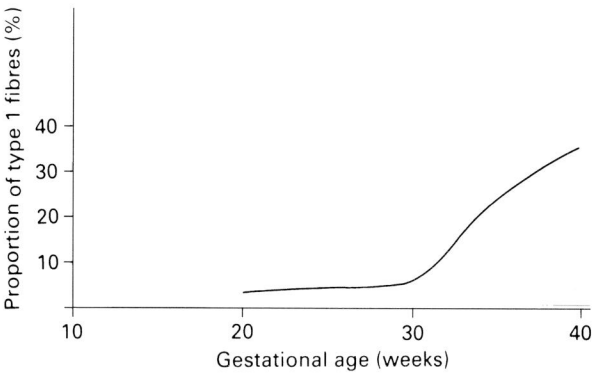

FIGURE 32.4.   *Graph showing proportion of type 1 fibers against gestational age. Between 20 and 30 weeks only about 2% of fibers have type 1 characteristics, and these are Wohlfart type B fibers. See Figs. 32.2 and 32.3.*

determines the establishment of the slow phenotype in the second-generation fibers whereas different factors such as thyroid hormone influence the level of expression of the fast myosin heavy chain and the establishment of the fast phenotype. The adenosine triphosphatase (ATPase) characteristics of the muscle fibers correspond to their myosin heavy chains. Immature type 2c fibers have a mixture of developmental and adult (either fast or slow) myosin heavy chains; mature type 1 fibers contain exclusively the adult slow myosin heavy chain; mature type 2 fibers contain exclusively an adult fast type of myosin heavy chain [15]. During fetal development, the first-generation fibers mature before 20 weeks (Fig. 32.5), corresponding to the first histochemically mature type 1 fibers (Wohlfart type B). The maturation of the second-generation fibers occurs later during development (Fig. 32.6) and is only totally achieved after birth [2, 12].

Fiber size, based on area or on the smallest diameter, varies with gestational age (Fig. 32.7). There is a wide range of diameters at the myotube stage, from as small as 5 μm up to 15 μm. This variability decreases to about 25–30 weeks, when fiber diameter becomes relatively uniform at around 9–10 μm. Toward term, the fiber diameters gradually increase, and at birth they are uniform in size and in the range of 12–15 μm. At around 12–15 weeks there is much connective tissue in areas corresponding to the perimysium and endomysium. The rounded fibers have become rounded polygonal fibers by term and there is no light microscopic evidence of endomysial connective tissue. Primitive neuromuscular contacts have been observed at about the 9th or 10th week. Certainly, myoblasts can fuse and produce myotubes without neural influences, since this can be observed in culture. The transition from myotubes to muscle fibers and their subsequent differentiation into fiber types depends on neural input, but how is not yet understood.

NORMAL MUSCLE

In the infant at term the muscle has acquired mature characteristics, unlike in the rat and mouse in which further differentiation takes place over several days after birth [3]. The muscle fascicles are separated by perimysial connective tissue, which varies quite considerably in density and width, and unless there is other pathology present, the amount of perimysial connective tissue is of no significance. Within the fascicles the muscle fibers are of uniform size and within the range of 12–15 μm. The fibers have a rounded polygonal shape and are all closely apposed without evidence of endomysial connective tissue, when studied by light microscopy (Fig. 32.8), although by electron microscopy a small amount of collagen usually can be seen. The rounded polygonal shape of the neonatal muscle fiber is in contrast with the more angular polygonal profiles found in older

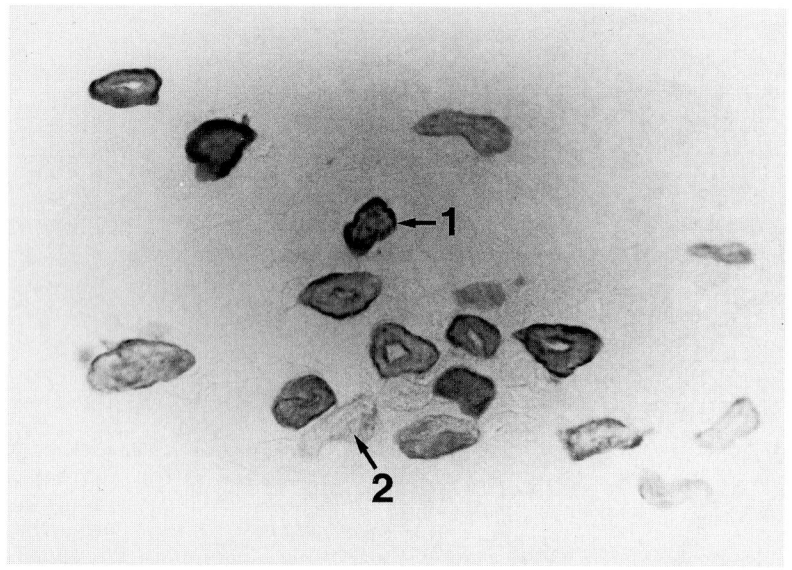

FIGURE 32.5.   *Fetal muscle, 12 weeks. The muscle is mainly composed of first-generation fibers (1) expressing the slow myosin heavy chain, whereas there are only a few second-generation fibers (2), which do not express the slow myosin heavy chain at this stage. Cryostat section, immunohistochemistry with an antibody specific for the slow myosin heavy chain revealed using a peroxidase antiperoxidase (PAP) technique, ×390.*

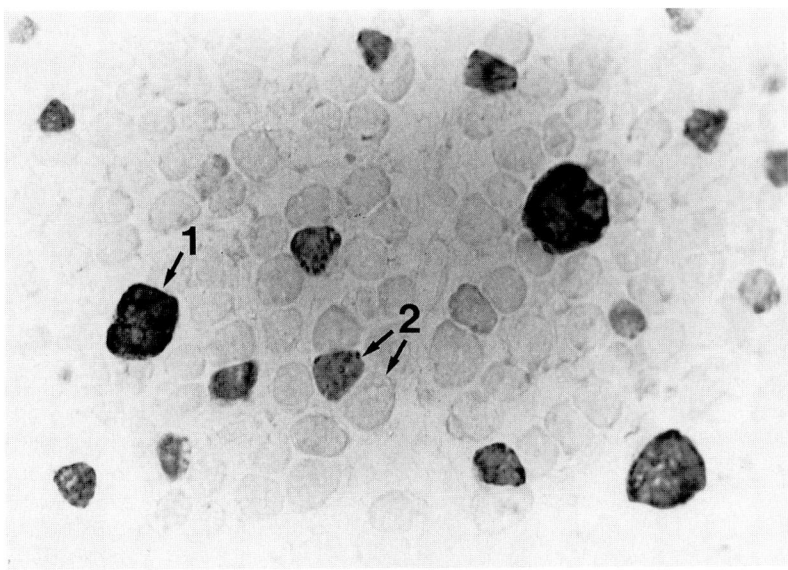

FIGURE 32.6. *Fetal muscle, 30 weeks. The first-generation fibers (1), corresponding to the Wohlfart type B fibers, express the slow myosin heavy chain. Some but not all of the second-generation fibers (2), corresponding to Wohlfart type A fibers, have started to express the slow myosin heavy chain. Cryostat section, immunohistochemistry with an antibody specific for the slow myosin heavy chain revealed using a PAP technique, ×390.*

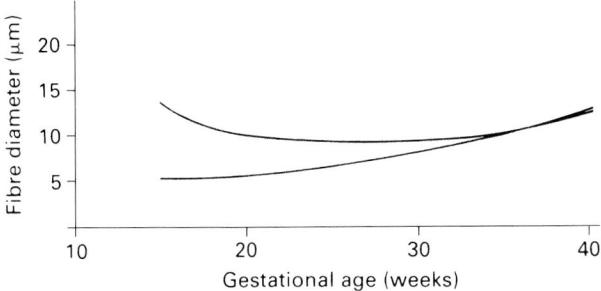

FIGURE 32.7. *Graph showing mean fiber diameters in relation to gestational age. There is a wide range of diameters at the earlier ages, but more uniformity is seen at term.*

children and adults (Fig. 32.9). Muscle fiber nuclei are at the periphery of the fiber and at this age usually only 1 nucleus per fiber is visible. In a given area of a section many fibers will contain no nuclei. Small capillaries scattered through the fascicles, and occasional nerve fibers also may be seen. Larger vessels and nerves may be present in the perimysium. Each myofiber is packed with myofibrils and the fibers are uniformly stained in hematoxylin and eosin and in trichrome preparations. In the trichrome stain, fibers with mainly type 1 characteristics show a scattering of fine red droplets, corresponding to mitochondria, but fiber type cannot be assessed reliably on this basis. Small accentuations of red staining may also be found in the paranuclear regions and close to capillaries. Glycogen is evenly distributed

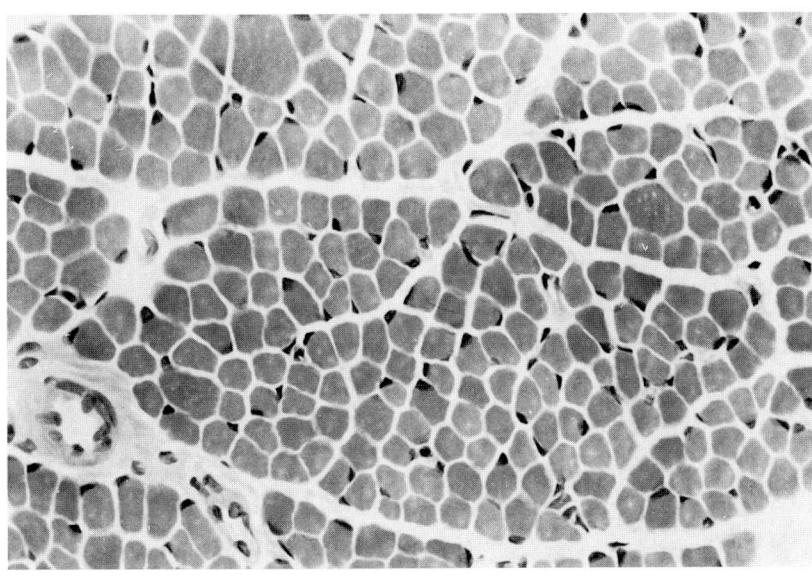

FIGURE 32.8. *Normal neonatal muscle, at age of 4 days. The fibers are mostly uniform and the nuclei are peripherally located. Occasional larger fibers may be present. Cryostat section, H&E, ×365.*

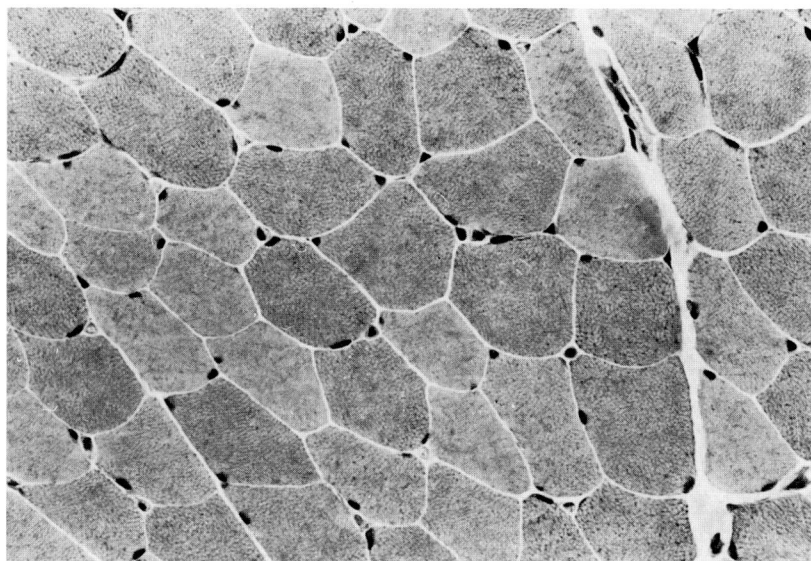

FIGURE 32.9. *Normal muscle from a 10-year-old boy. Uniform polygonal fibers are present with no evidence of endomysial connective tissue. Compare the size and shape of the fibers with those in Fig. 32.6. Cryostat section, trichrome, ×365.*

through the fibers, and is slightly more evident in type 2 fibers. In the neonate, neutral fat normally is not found in the fibers or in the perimysium.

Evaluation of mitochondrial enzyme activity with reactions for either succinate dehydrogenase, cytochrome oxidase, or NADH dehydrogenase (although this enzyme activity is present also in the sarcoplasmic reticulum) often reveals the centers of fibers to be more densely stained and a halo of weak staining under the sarcolemma. This appearance changes with age and the halo disappears after several weeks. The checkerboard appearance seen in children and adults using the NADH dehydrogenase reaction is usually less well defined in neonates.

Active regeneration as evidenced by basophilic fibers with plump nuclei and prominent nucleoli is not seen, and histiocytes, shown by a reaction for acid phosphatase activ-

ity, are generally absent although occasional single histiocytes may be found in the perimysium.

Fiber typing (Fig. 32.10) shows a distribution and proportion of types that will depend on the muscle sampled. Although there are guidelines published for individual muscles [16], there is quite a wide spectrum of normality, and interfascicular variability may be evident [11].

With the fiber typing methods that demonstrate ATPase activity, 2 patterns are found. Firstly, with the unreversed ATPase method the type 1 fibers are paler than type 2 fibers, and with the technically better preparations type 2B fibers are darker than type 2A fibers. Secondly, with the reversed ATPase method with acid preincubation (often erroneously referred to as ATPase at pH 4.3) the type 1 fibers are darkly stained, type 2A fibers are very pale, and type 2B fibers are intermediate in color. Type 2C fibers are

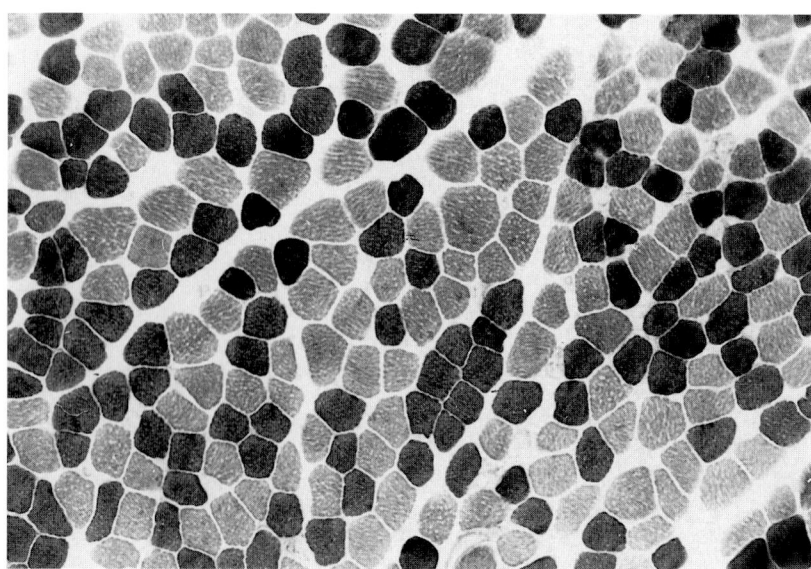

FIGURE 32.10. *Normal neonatal quadriceps muscle, at age of 4 days. Fiber types are randomly scattered without evidence of grouping. Type 1 fibers are pale, while type 2 fibers are dark. Cryostat section, unreversed ATPase, ×365.*

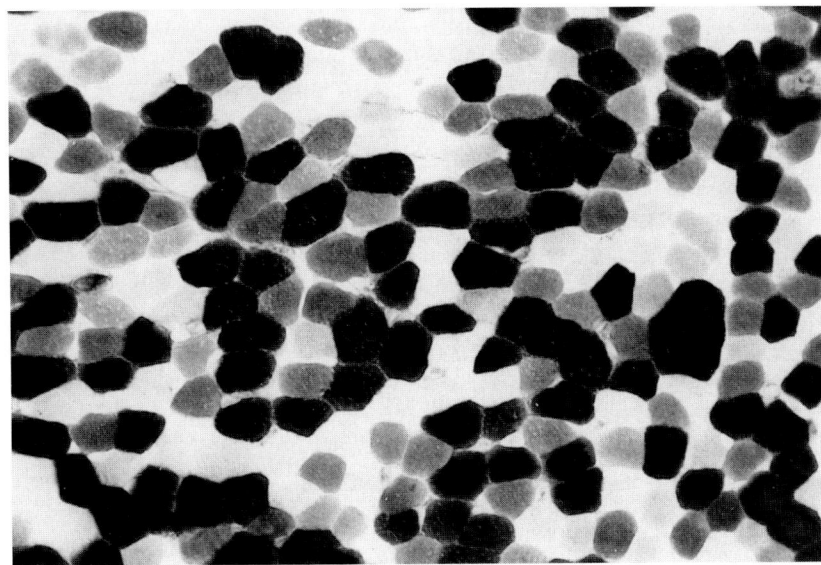

FIGURE 32.11. *Normal neonatal quadriceps muscle, at age of 4 days. The type 1 fibers, including the scattered larger fibers, are darkly stained while type 2B fibers are pale and type 2A fibers are unstained in this preparation. Cryostat section, ATPase after preincubation at pH 4.3, ×365.*

intermediate in color between type 1 and type 2B fibers and, unlike type 2B fibers, resist acid preincubation at pH 4.1. The pH at which the best reversal is seen is probably laboratory-related. The actual pH is immaterial and, as long as 3 fiber types can be shown clearly, it does not matter whether the pH is 4.3, 4.4, or 4.6 (Fig. 32.11). Reversal with a citrate buffer (0.1M) at pH 4.6 for 2 minutes 30 seconds gives consistent results, and is not temperature-dependent [17].

Immunocytochemical study of the myosin heavy chains demonstrates that the type 1 fibers contain exclusively the slow isoform whereas the type 2A/2B fibers contain exclusively an adult fast isoform. Only the rare type 2C fibers still contain a mixture of developmental and adult fast isoforms [2].

ABNORMALITIES OF MUSCLE DEVELOPMENT

Abnormalities of muscle development can be due to genetic, teratogenic, or neural influences. It may be possible to infer the etiology from the morphology as genetic and teratogenic causes generally lead to absence of muscle and substitution of fat and connective tissue, whereas a neural cause is suggested by the presence of abnormally small fibers.

Defects of muscle often are associated with abnormalities in other systems, which may be either the cause or the effect of the muscle disorder, or both may occur together as part of a complex malformation. For example, aplasia or hypoplasia of muscles of the lower limbs is found in association with agenesis of the lumbar or sacral vertebral segments, due to failure of development of the embryonic myotome at the same level as the absent vertebra. In place of muscle there is fat and connective tissue, in which may be found a few muscle fibers.

In the prune-belly syndrome, some patients have a pronounced diastasis recti with attenuated and stretched muscle fibers. Other have no rectus abdominis muscle. Both types are associated with hydronephrosis and renal tract abnormalities. Various theories have been proposed to explain the association. It has been suggested that pressure from the hydronephrotic kidney causes failure of normal development of the abdominal wall; or that the rectus abdominis deficiency is primary, with the renal tract abnormalities resulting from reduced intra-abdominal pressure; or that there is a primary muscle problem common to both bladder and abdominal wall. The absent muscle is replaced by connective tissue containing a few hypertrophic muscle fibers with central nuclei [18]. Fiber necrosis is seen, but no evidence of regeneration can be demonstrated. Muscles in other sites are normal.

An example of a neural cause of muscle abnormality is the rare amyoplasia or hypoplasia of muscle in the diaphragm, where agenesis of the phrenic nerve results in the lack of neural input necessary for the normal development of muscle. However, in most patients with amyoplasia or hypoplasia of the diaphragm, the phrenic nerve is normal. The deficiency of muscle in the diaphragm leads to eventration and secondary pulmonary hypoplasia. Lack of nervous input leading to failure of muscle development in other sites may also be caused by entrapment of ventral nerve roots by absent or poorly formed vertebral bodies.

In the Poland syndrome [19, 20] the unilateral absence of pectoralis minor and the sternal absence of pectoralis major are associated with ipsilateral symbrachydactyly, and it has been suggested that both result from abnormal development of the proximal subclavian artery, leading to an early reduction in blood flow to the affected side.

Congenital absence of one or more muscle groups may occur as an isolated anomaly. The pectoral muscles are the most commonly affected, and the condition may be unilateral or bilateral. Other muscles that may be absent congenitally are the trapezium, sternomastoid, serratus anterior, and quadriceps femoris.

Normal muscle development depends on normal skeletal growth, and agenesis of the long bones due to a genetic epiphyseal dysplasia or to a teratogen will lead to a reduction in muscle bulk without replacement by fat or connective tissue. Since modeling of bone is influenced by muscle tone, absence or weakness of muscle may lead to arthrogryposis or dysmorphic features. This secondary effect is noticed particularly in neurogenic disorders, where deformities of the fingers and hands are frequent. In some congenital myopathies, such as nemaline myopathy, a high-arched palate results from abnormal modeling and molding of the palatal bones. Similarly, other abnormalities of skull shape may also be due to muscle weakness or absence of particular muscle groups. Generalized myopathies produce delicate and gracile ribs and long bones.

ARTHROGRYPOSIS

Arthrogryposis occasionally is regarded as a disease entity but it should be considered the result of joint immobility during fetal development. Proper joints depend on their movement from about 8 weeks' gestation and failure to move leads to joint fixation. Limitation of movement can be due to many factors, the most common of which is a neurological deficit, including some gross brain defects (anencephaly, hydranencephaly, and holoprosencephaly), meningomyelocele, and anterior horn cell disease. Some muscle disorders related to failure of proper development or in some instances in connection with a congenital myopathy can also lead to arthrogryposis. Skeletal defects and disorders of connective tissue may produce limited joint movement, as can fetal crowding in multiple births or oligohydramnios.

With a wide spectrum of causes it is not surprising that the muscles examined show changes ranging from neurogenic atrophy to congenital myopathies or congenital muscular dystrophy (CMD). Muscles may show only minor non-specific changes or may even appear normal [21–23]. Porter [24] reviewed the pathology and pathogenesis of lethal arthrogryposis multiplex congenita (also known as the fetal akinesia deformation sequence, FADS), and emphasized the need to define the etiology as many of the cases are genetically determined. The lethal congenital contracture syndrome, as part of FADS, is an autosomal recessive disorder seen in Finland and elsewhere. A clinicopathological study of 83 cases of FADS in Finland [25] revealed that 67 patients had a neurogenic lesion, and of these, 41 were regarded as having the lethal contracture syndrome. The muscles of these showed extreme atrophy. Patients with the lethal pterygium syndrome had normal muscle histology. Nemaline myopathy was found in 1 patient. Neurogenic atrophy was seen in patients with anterior horn cell disease with arthrogryposis, which has now been mapped to the X

chromosome at p11.3–q11.2 [26]. In arthrogryposis associated with a congenital myasthenic syndrome, the muscle biopsy specimen appeared normal by light microscopy, but by electron microscopy there were abnormalities of the motor end plates with a paucity of synaptic folds [27].

DENERVATION

Denervating disorders presenting in the neonatal period are few and are mostly confined to disorders of the lower motor neuron, but the pathology may extend beyond the lower motor neuron territory [28]. An abnormality at any point tends to produce similar lesions and it is only from clinical evaluation and electromyography (EMG) studies that more precise diagnoses can be made. In general, spinal muscular atrophies (SMAs) are transmitted in an autosomal recessive manner; those cases where symptoms are detected first in the fetus or the newborn correspond, by definition, to Werdnig-Hoffmann disease (type 1 SMA). Infantile-onset (type 1 SMA), intermediate-childhood (type 2 SMA), Kugelberg-Welander (type 3 SMA), and adult spinal muscular atrophy result, in over 98% of patients, from a truncated or absent survival motor neuron gene (SMN) located on chromosome 5 at q12–q14 [29, 30]. Refined mapping shows that type 1 SMA also has a further deletion in the neuronal apoptosis inhibitory protein gene (NAIP), and this extra mutation is not seen in types 2 and 3 SMA [31].

Postmortem studies can show grossly thinned anterior nerve roots of the spinal cord, while posterior nerve roots are of normal thickness. Anterior horn cells are depleted in number, are smaller than those of a 16-week fetus, and show signs of immaturity [32]. There is also neuronophagia, supporting the evidence of a genetic defect affecting motor neurons. In other cases with loss of anterior horn cells there may also be pontocerebellar hypoplasia [33] or an absence of myelin in the central and peripheral nervous systems [34].

In neonates the classic large and small group atrophy may not be present, and biopsy changes are difficult to interpret. Changes similar to the originally described congenital fiber type disproportion with small type 1 fibers, and others with small type 2 fibers are seen in the neonatal period in some patients (Figs. 32.12 and 32.13). The classic changes may not appear until the age of 6 weeks (Figs. 32.14 and 32.15).

Denervation in the adult or in the experimental animal shows shrunken thin angular muscle fibers, while in the disorders of the lower motor neuron the changes are characterized by groups of small rounded fibers (5–9 μm in diameter) and groups of markedly hypertrophic fibers (up to 40 μm in diameter). These changes may serve to differentiate between acute and chronic denervation. The small fibers are mostly type 2 with scattered type 1 fibers, while the large fibers are almost invariably type 1 (see Fig. 32.15). No abnormality of the fibers (apart from smallness or hypertrophy) is seen and no target fibers are found in the acute Werdnig-Hoffmann form.

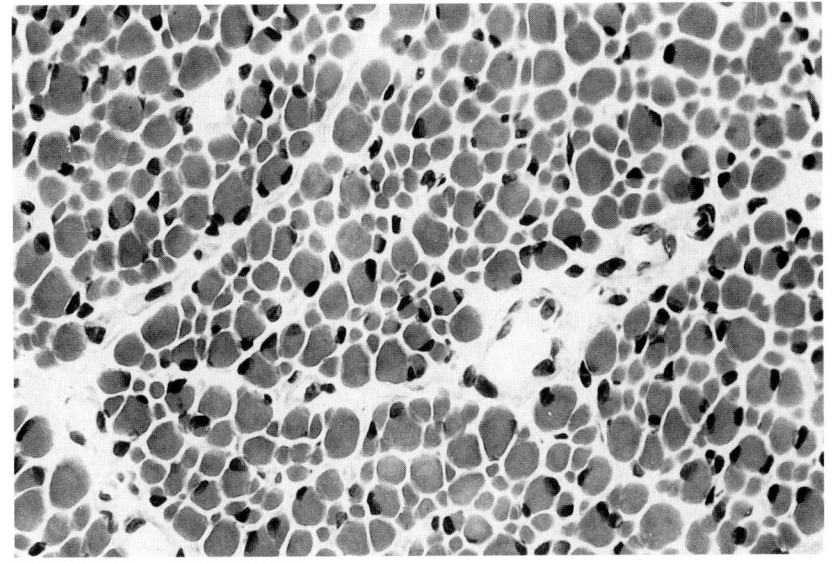

FIGURE 32.12. *Infantile spinal muscular atrophy (Werdnig-Hoffman). Quadriceps, postmortem sample. Small fibers are scattered throughout the fascicles with no evidence of grouping. This patient died at age 4 weeks and the clinical diagnosis was confirmed by neuropathological examination of the spinal cord. Cryostat section, H&E, ×365.*

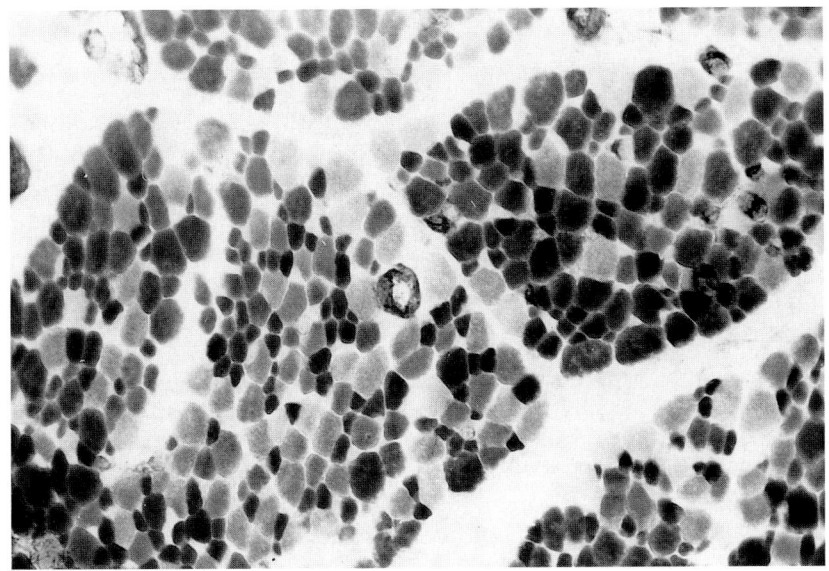

FIGURE 32.13. *Infantile spinal muscular atrophy. Same case as in Fig. 32.12. The scattered small fibers are mostly type 1, but some normal-sized type 1 fibers are also present. Compare with Fig. 32.15. Cryostat section, ATPase after preincubation at pH 4.3, ×365.*

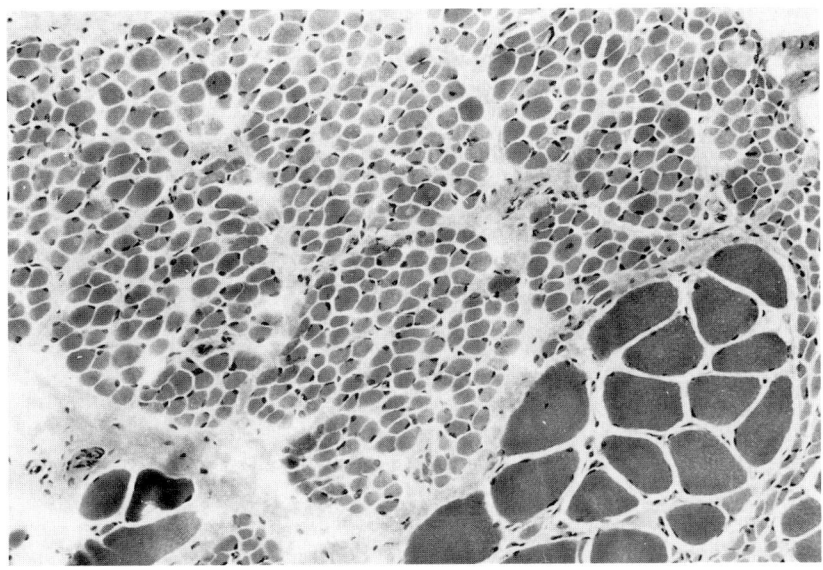

FIGURE 32.14. *Infantile spinal muscular atrophy. Muscle biopsy specimen. Groups of large fibers are present among the large groups of small fibers. This appearance is typical of established cases but may not be so clear in neonates (see Fig. 32.12). Cryostat section, H&E, ×145.*

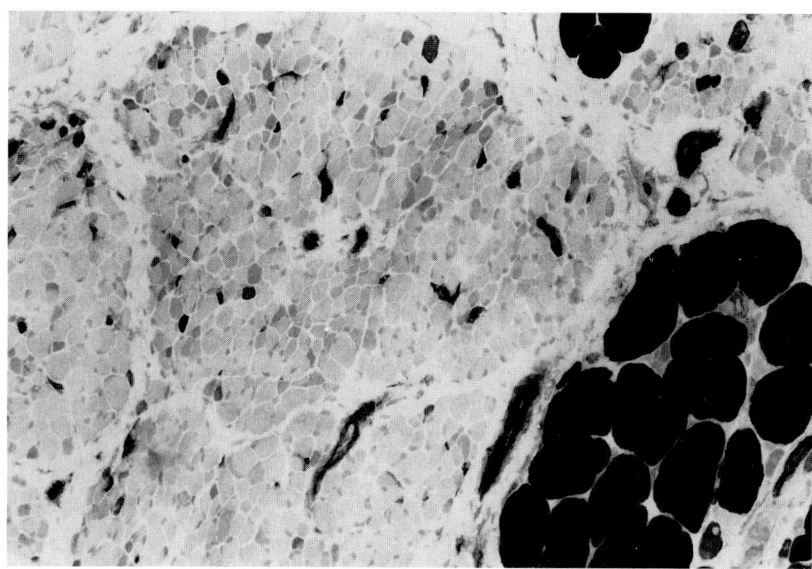

FIGURE 32.15.   *Infantile spinal muscular atrophy. Muscle biopsy specimen, same case as in Fig. 32.14. The large fibers are type 1 while the groups of small fibers contain mostly type 2 fibers with a scattering of type 1 fibers. Cryostat section, ATPase after preincubation at pH 4.3, ×145.*

Generally, endomysial connective tissue is normal although it may be increased in some patients with a chronic disorder, giving an appearance of CMD (see Fig. 32.17). In this condition the small fibers are mostly type 1, which should help to differentiate the 2 conditions. An increase in fat in perimysium is unusual but may occur with an increase in connective tissue in the chronic forms.

Arguments as to the significance of the small rounded fibers and whether they represent denervated fibers or whether they are fetal fibers that have never received a proper neural input have not been resolved. However, Hausmanowa-Petrusewicz et al [35] suggested that the biochemical and ultrastructural features are suggestive of a fetal defect not only for Werdnig-Hoffmann disease but also for the milder chronic Kugelberg-Welander form. The muscle fibers must have received some neural input, since fiber typing has post-36-week characteristics. Moreover, immunohistochemical studies of the metabolic differentiation of the fibers in Werdnig-Hoffmann disease did not confirm a simple blockage of their maturation at an early stage of development [36–38]. The changes are probably the result of a dynamic situation in the anterior horn cells and their survival varies according to the absence or reduced expression of the *SMN* gene.

MUSCULAR DYSTROPHIES

The muscular dystrophies are a heterogeneous group of disorders characterized by dystrophic changes in the skeletal muscles, theoretically with no involvement of the central nervous system (CNS). Recent advances in molecular genetics have made it possible to detect anomalies in proteins that are related to the cell membrane and that interact between the cytoskeleton of the muscle fibers and the extracellular matrix. The most important of these proteins

are dystrophin (coded by a gene located at p21 of the X chromosome), the protein and glycoproteins associated with dystrophin (dystroglycans, sarcoglycans, and syntrophins), and laminin [39–41].

Congenital Muscular Dystrophy

As the name implies, CMD is present from birth, and reduced fetal movements during pregnancy are noted frequently. Hypotonia and weakness of the limb, trunk, and facial muscles with absent reflexes are the presenting features. Sucking, swallowing, and respiratory difficulties are also common. Contractures of various muscles may be present at birth or may develop later [42–44]. No ptosis, ophthalmoplegia, or muscular hypertrophy is seen. The disorder (or disorders) is ill-defined and may be slowly progressive, or static, or may even improve. A proportion of patients have significant CNS involvement [45–47]. The muscle pathology is mixed. In the neonatal period the picture is usually of a marked increase in endomysial connective tissue (Fig. 32.16), with a marked reduction in the number and size of muscle fibers [48], although the biopsy specimen from 1 patient at Great Ormond Street Hospital showed no significant morphological changes at this age. Generally, there is no evidence of an active process, no regenerating fibers are seen, and there is no sign of fiber necrosis. The spectrum of change is so wide in the older patients that the changes in muscle may be so slight as to appear normal. In these older patients with milder disease, the designation CMD is perhaps misleading because, although the disorder might be labeled correctly as congenital, there is little evidence of a muscular dystrophic process.

In the neonate a strong similarity exists with some cases of chronic denervation if only routinely stained muscle sec-

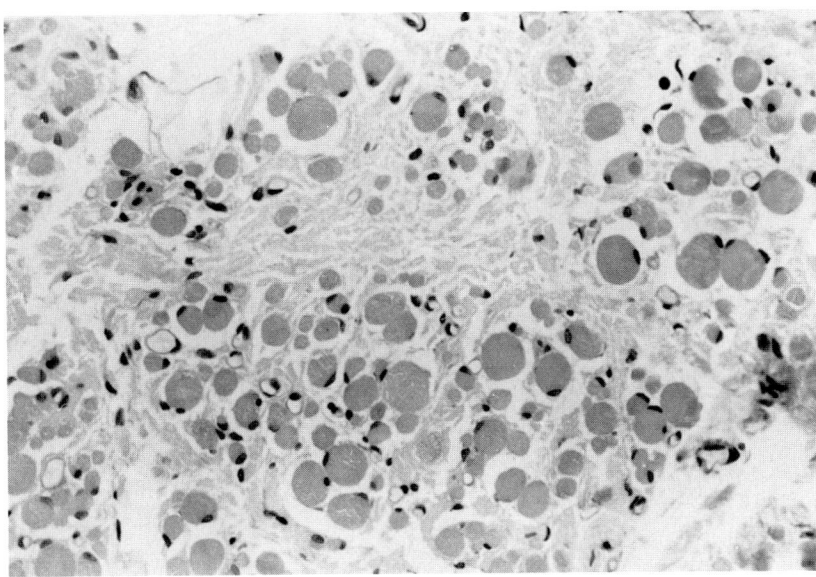

FIGURE 32.16. *Congenital muscular dystrophy. A gross excess of connective tissue is present not only between remaining fascicles but also between the fibers, which are rounded. Routine paraffin section, H&E, ×365.*

tions are examined (Fig. 32.17). In the dystrophic disorder the fibers generally have type 1 characteristics. However, in contrast, in the few instances where the balance of evidence was in favor of denervation, the fibers are mostly type 2. It should also be noted that an inflammatory process can give rise to a marked increase in perimysial and endomysial connective tissue, with reduced numbers of rounded muscle fibers. Thus, the pathology, which is generally regarded as that of CMD, may be truly that, the result of chronic denervation, or the result of an intrauterine infection. The latter itself may indeed be the initiating factor for a denervating condition.

The most classic, pure or type I forms of CMD share an autosomal recessive transmission but have variable patterns of evolution. In almost half of patients, the dystrophy is associated with an absence of expression of the extracellular matrix protein merosin (laminin 2), which is coded by a gene located in the region q22–q23 on chromosome 6 [49, 50]. Mutations in the α2 chain of merosin have been described [51]. The forms of CMD with absent merosin expression detected with antibodies to the C-terminus of merosin (CMD 1a) (Fig. 32.18) are associated with a more severe prognosis than are the forms in which there is an internal mutation in the merosin alpha 2 chain (CMD 1b) [51a]. A few patients with "pure" CMD (merosin-positive) have been shown to be deficient in a skeletal muscle isoform of α-actinin (α-actinin-3) by immunohistochemistry and Western blotting [52]. CMD type Ia can also be diagnosed using antibodies to merosin on cryostat sections of skin, where the dermoepidermal junction expresses merosin in the normal patient, and shows no expression in affected patients. Prenatal diagnosis is also possible on chorionic

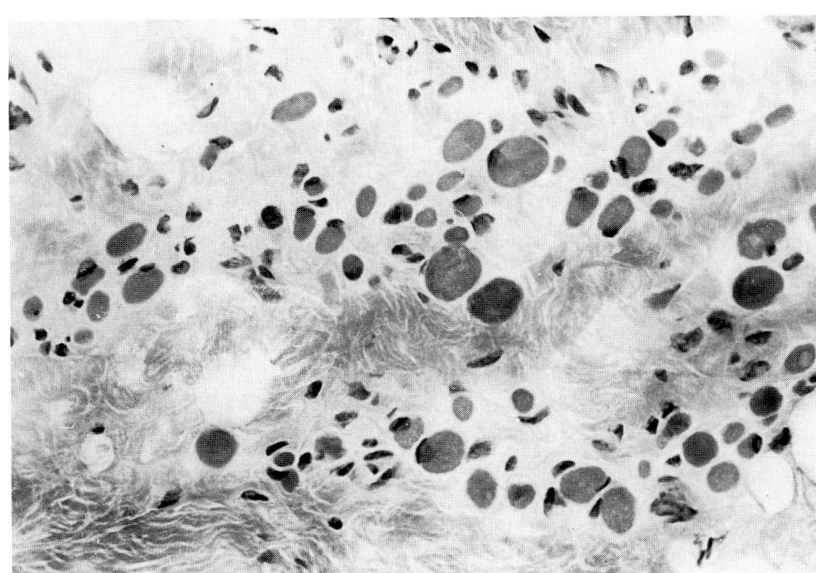

FIGURE 32.17. *Denervation. Some patients with a form of spinal muscular atrophy have a gross increase in endomysial connective tissue and the appearance is very similar to congenital muscular dystrophy. In this biopsy specimen the fibers were mostly type 2, in contrast to congenital muscular dystrophy where the fibers are mostly type 1. Compare with Figs. 32.12, 32.14, and 32.16.*

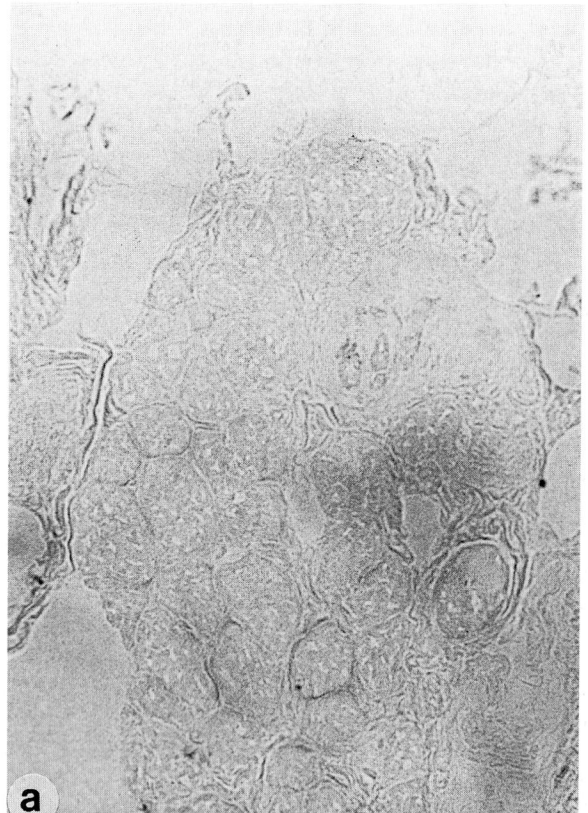
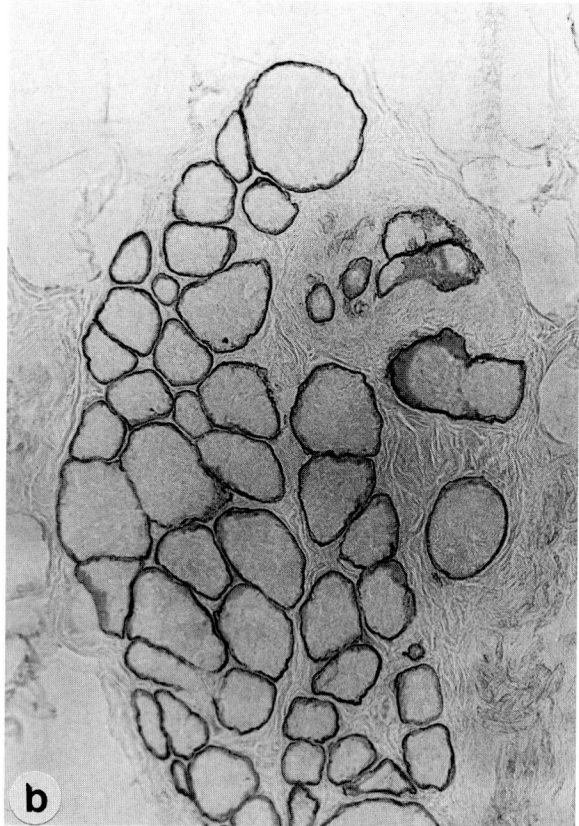

FIGURE 32.18.   *Congenital muscle dystrophy with absence of merosin. There is a total absence of immunoreactivity for merosin (a), whereas the expression of immunoreactive dystrophin is normal (b). Cryostat section, immunohistochemistry with an antibody specific for dystrophin revealed using a PAP technique, ×195.*

villus samples, as the normal trophoblast basement membrane expresses merosin [53, 54].

A separate distinct form of CMD is comparatively common in Japan. Fukuyama et al [55] reported on 15 patients and by 1985 some 266 patients had been studied. There is generalized weakness and floppiness, with wasting, particularly of the neck muscles. Contractures are present, beginning in the extremities and progressing to other joints. Generalized focal tonic fits occur in 50% of patients. There is no or only minor ocular involvement. The disorder is progressive and independent standing or walking is not achieved. Severe mental retardation is found in most but not all patients and is related to changes in the brain, such as polymicrogyria, pachygyria, and lack of myelin [56–58]. In contrast with type 1 CMD, the Fukuyama type always shows a high CK level, even in the patients surviving to their teens. The muscle biopsy specimen shows a marked increase in endomysial connective tissue surrounding small rounded muscle fibers. Muscle fiber hypertrophy is rare and no inflammatory cells or fiber grouping are found. As might be expected from the high persistent CK level, scattered necrotic fibers and regenerating fibers are present. Although prevalent in Japan, the Fukuyama type or CMD type II has

been reported from other countries [59]. It has an autosomal recessive mode of transmission and is linked to the defect of a gene located on chromosome 9 at q31–33 [60].

Several related disorders may or may not be allelic with Fukuyama CMD [61, 62] and involve other systems. These include Warburg syndrome (or CMD type III), the HARD syndrome, and the form of muscular dystrophy with distinct eye changes described by Santavuori et al [63, 64]. These can be classified as cerebro-ocular-muscular syndromes. An autosomal recessive pattern of inheritance is clear in some patients, while an intrauterine infection may be a factor in others. Cattle and hamsters infected with Akabane virus during pregnancy produce offspring that may have arthrogryposis and muscle changes that superficially resemble those in CMD [65].

Several male patients presenting in the neonatal period with congenital adrenal hypoplasia had high CK levels and glycerol kinase deficiency [66, 67]. Their muscle biopsy specimens showed a muscular dystrophy indistinguishable from the Duchenne type, including absent dystrophin staining, even at this early age. Congenital adrenal hypoplasia, glycerol kinase deficiency, and Duchenne dystrophy are all X-linked disorders and their association in several patients indicates that the gene loci are close. The gene for ornithine carbamoyltransferase is also in close proximity to this region [68].

The other forms of muscular dystrophy do not present in the neonatal period but the changes are present from a relatively early age, even though there are no clinical features.

Duchenne Muscular Dystrophy

This disease, due to a defect in the gene coding for the protein dystrophin located at p21 of the X chromosome, practically never shows any clinical manifestation during the fetal or neonatal period. A positive diagnosis should only be considered in exceptional cases. With classic histological techniques, there is no definite evidence of this disease in fetal muscle up to 21 weeks' gestation. The dystrophic lesions begin after birth. Prior to the age of 2 months, muscle biopsy specimens may appear essentially normal or show only focal lesions [69]. In some affected infants aged 2 months [70], the muscle fibers already show a variation in size, are rounded, and have increased endomysial connective tissue. Focal necrosis and regeneration are evident

[1]. In 1 patient whose CK level was high, a biopsy specimen obtained at age 2.5 weeks showed only occasional hyaline fibers, and the remainder of the specimens were normal. Further biopsy tissue obtained at age 3 years showed changes typical of Duchenne muscular dystrophy yet there were no clinical signs [69].

Conversely, the absence of immunoreactivity for dystrophin now makes it possible to establish a positive diagnosis in newborn infants [71] as well as prenatally on a fetal muscle biopsy specimen [72] in cases where no mutation in the dystrophin gene has been detected in the proband, despite absent dystrophin staining in the initial biopsy specimen. This is possible because of the changes in dystrophin immunoreactivity seen in fetal tissue obtained from therapeutic abortions after positive diagnosis of Duchenne muscular dystrophy by molecular techniques on chorionic villus samples (Fig. 32.19). However, it should be noted that during muscle development, dystrophin is only expressed in myotubes about 15 days after they have formed (myogenic fusion) and that it may therefore be difficult to assess very early biopsy samples. Reliable detection of dystrophin immunoreactivity is possible at 12 weeks' gestation, and possibly earlier.

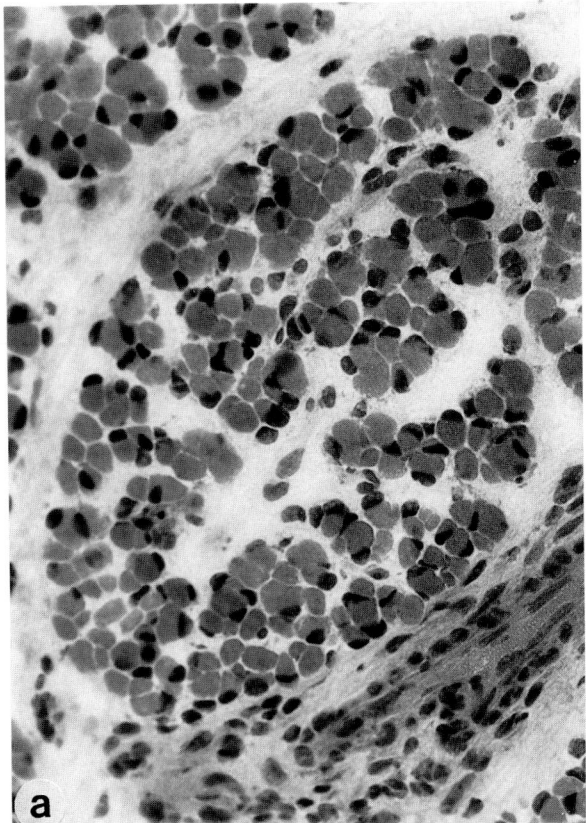 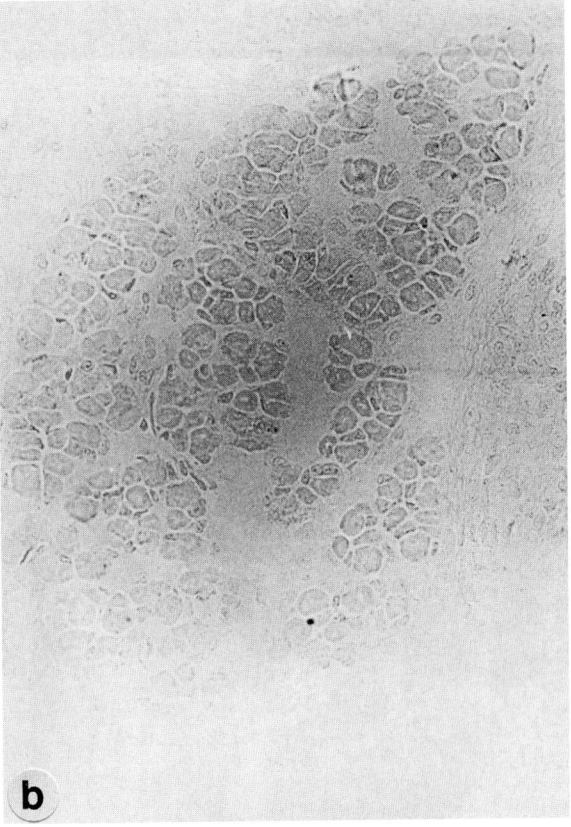

FIGURE 32.19.   *Fetal muscle at 20 weeks from the first of two twins genetically affected with Duchenne muscular dystrophy. The degree of muscle development is almost normal on the H&E preparation (a) whereas there is no immunoreactivity for dystrophin (b). Cryostat section, (a) H&E, (b) immunohistochemistry with an antibody specific for dystrophin revealed using a PAP technique, ×195.*

CONGENITAL MYOPATHIES

Centronuclear Myotubular Myopathy

Profound neonatal hypotonia is found in patients with centronuclear myotubular myopathy [73, 74] of early onset, and one separate subgroup of patients also has severe and usually fatal respiratory problems [75–77]. This latter group shows an X-linked pattern of inheritance while in the former there is no clear pattern and both autosomal recessive and autosomal dominant modes have been proposed. A genetic defect in the q27–q28 region on the X chromosome is responsible for the severe X-linked forms of the disease [78], and mutations in the myotubularin gene are reported [78a].

The term *myotubular myopathy* is used because the muscle fibers in this disorder have many characteristics of fetal myotubes (Fig. 32.20), not only the presence of central nuclei with the perinuclear halo of glycogen and mitochondria but also the ultrastructural characteristics with clusters of myoblasts and myotubes enclosed by a single basement membrane. The term *centronuclear myopathy* has been used to describe some of the forms with later onset and milder symptoms, and in other forms where the fibers with centrally located nuclei do not have all of the features of myotubes. The evidence in neonates of ultrastructural characteristics showing marked similarities to fetal muscle at 12–15 weeks' gestational age, and the EMG findings suggesting a neurogenic origin, led to the speculation that there is maturational delay due to impaired neural input [79]. The term *myotubular* may well be correct (and first) but since there is a well-established usage of *centronuclear*, it could be argued that the term *centronuclear myotubular myopathy* should be used, at least until a definitive etiology is found.

In neonates the muscle fibers are smaller than normal for age, with some fibers having diameters as small as 3 μm [76].

Central nuclei are present in 3–75% of fibers and there is always a myofibril-free halo around the nucleus. This zone extends down the fiber, and in the fibers without central nuclei the myofibril-free zone is visible and best demonstrated by its high glycogen content and relative abundance of mitochondria. Fiber typing usually shows a normal distribution of fiber types, often with a type 1 predominance. The hypotrophic fibers are type 1, and type 2 fibers also are often small. Motor end plates seem to be normal in number and intrafusal fibers are normal.

It may be difficult to differentiate between centronuclear myotubular myopathy of neonatal onset and infantile myotonic dystrophy based on biopsy findings. An increase in intrafusal fibers, especially at the polar regions [1], increased acid phosphatase activity in muscle fibers, and a wider range of stages of muscle fiber development are more usually associated with infantile myotonic dystrophy; these features may help in the differential diagnosis. Studying the expression of the slow myosin heavy chain by immunohistochemistry is very useful, as the expression of this marker of muscle maturation is almost normal in myotubular myopathy (Fig. 32.21) whereas it is markedly delayed in myotonic dystrophy [2].

The changes in centronuclear myotubular myopathy are widespread and found in all skeletal muscles, but the degree of change can vary from muscle to muscle.

Central nuclei, myotubes, general fiber hypotrophy, and type 2 fiber predominance are also found in neonates with fetal alcohol myopathy who present with hypotonia and respiratory embarrassment [80]. One patient studied at 10 days showed no fiber type differentiation. Of the 3 patients reported with the facial stigmas of the fetal alcohol syndrome, born to mothers who drank heavily during pregnancy, 2 had died by the age of 8 months and the other patient was severely retarded at 16 months.

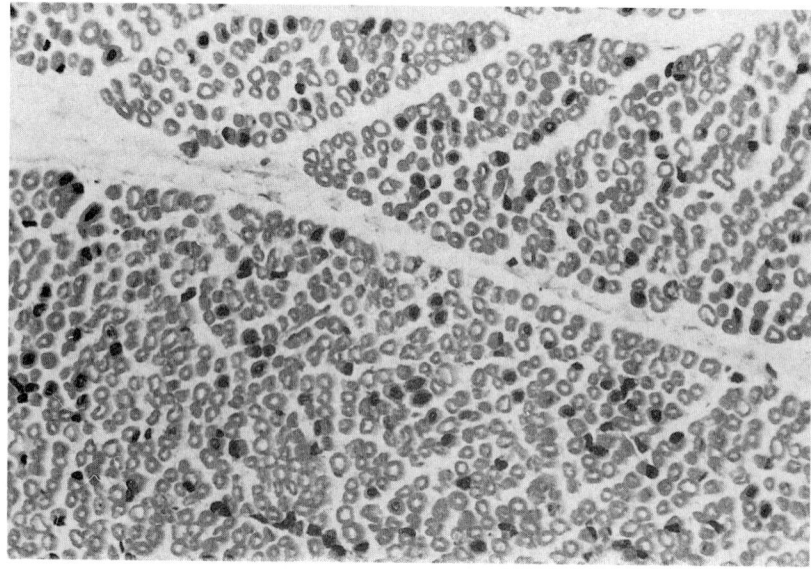

FIGURE 32.20.   *Centronuclear myotubular myopathy. The fibers are very small and nearly all of them appear as myotubes. The central nucleation is evident in many of them. The appearance is not always as clear as this and varies from one site to another. Routine paraffin section, H&E, ×365.*

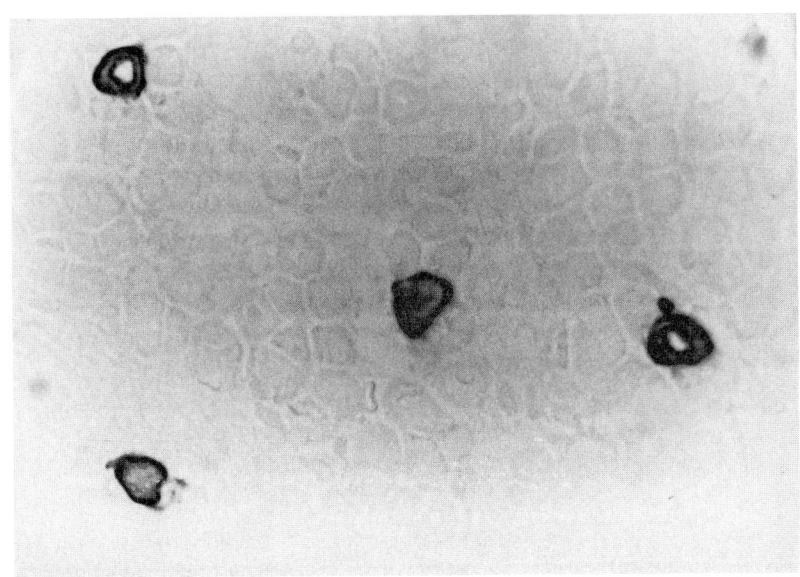

FIGURE 32.21. *Congenital myotonic dystrophy in a newborn premature child. There is a marked delay of maturation and only the first-generation fibers express the slow myosin heavy chain. Cryostat section, immunohistochemistry with an antibody specific for the slow myosin heavy chain revealed using a PAP technique, ×485.*

Congenital Myotonic Dystrophy

Myotonic dystrophy is caused by the anomaly of a gene located on q13 of chromosome 19. A dynamic mutation in this region results in the amplification of a trinucleotide sequence CTG in the 3′ noncoding region of a gene probably corresponding to a protein kinase known as myotonin [81, 82]. Neighboring genes may also be implicated in this disease, and anomalies of the corresponding messenger RNAs have even been suggested [83]. The degree of amplification of the trinucleotide repeat is perfectly correlated ("anticipation") with the symptomatology, especially in the usual adolescent or adult forms, sharing the classic autosomal dominant mode of transmission.

The severe congenital form of myotonic dystrophy corresponds to a very particular entity [84], being always maternally transmitted. The mother is always affected, although only mildly. It should be noted that not all affected mothers will necessarily have severely affected children [85]. This exclusive maternal transmission had suggested a role of environmental factors [86, 87] but instead seems now to be linked to limits of transmission of the genetic defect during meiosis. Indeed, the severe form is only found when there has been an extensive amplification resulting in the presence of more than 2000 copies of the trinucleotide repeat. It seems that such an important defect cannot be transmitted through male meiosis.

Clinically, the congenital form of myotonic dystrophy presents at birth with extreme hypotonia and weakness of pharyngeal and respiratory muscles, which lead to respiratory distress and difficulties with sucking and swallowing [88]. Facial diplegia with a tented upper lip is usually present and edema and arthrogryposis are often found. Pulmonary hypoplasia with a ratio of lung weight to body weight of less than 0.019 was observed in 2 infants and the hypopla-

sia was attributed to weakness and poor functioning of the diaphragm in utero [89]. Intestinal smooth muscle may be affected [90] and this can accentuate the feeding difficulties, which were alleviated by metoclopramide treatment in 1 patient with gastroparesis [91].

The mortality rate is about 50% and those who survive have marked mental and motor retardation. In the adult form, myotonia is rarely evident until about the age of 2 years.

The muscles show arrested or delayed maturation, with abnormalities ranging from myotubes to incomplete fiber type differentiation, and a general smallness of fibers [92]. The marked increase in numbers of central nuclei, nuclear chains, ring fibers, and inflammatory changes associated with the adult form are not found. The most immature fibers are in the muscles close to joint contractures and in the pharynx and diaphragm. Here, by electron microscopy, an increase in satellite cells, primitive myoblasts, and disordered myofilaments can be found. In the less severely affected muscles (e.g., the biceps), maturation arrest is less evident, but some degree of type 1 fiber hypotrophy may be seen. Fiber type is not clear in NADH dehydrogenase preparations and a subsarcolemmal halo of low activity is often prominent. The changes may be difficult to differentiate from X-linked severe myotubular myopathy. Carpenter and Karpati [1] and Karpati et al [93] found that many of the muscle fibers in patients with congenital myotonic dystrophy show acid phosphatase activity in subsarcolemmal areas up to $10\,\mu m$ in diameter. Immunocytochemical studies demonstrate a delay in the differentiation and maturation of the fast and slow fibers (Fig. 32.22), resulting in a pattern very different from that of myotubular myopathy at the same age. These anomalies suggest a transitory defect in the nerve–muscle contact in the pathogenesis of this congenital form of myotonic dystrophy [2, 94]. Intrafusal fibers of the polar regions of the

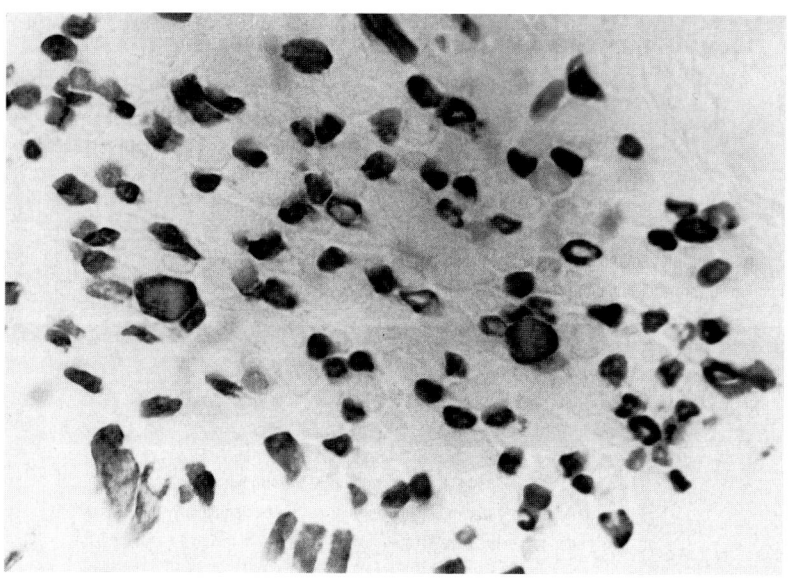

FIGURE 32.22.   *Severe X-linked form of myotubular myopathy in a newborn premature child. The slow myosin heavy chain is expressed both in the first- and in the second-generation fibers. This immunocytochemical pattern of expression of the slow myosin heavy chain is very different from that observed in myotonic dystrophy at the same age. Cryostat section, immunohistochemistry with an antibody specific for the slow myosin heavy chain revealed using a PAP technique, ×485.*

muscle spindle sometimes are increased in number in the adult form, and this increase may also be evident in the neonatal disorder.

Nemaline Myopathy

This used to be regarded as an essentially benign condition, but it is now clear that a neonatal onset may be fatal within the first year of life. Those most at risk of dying have extreme hypotonia as the presenting feature [95] and appear to have an autosomal recessive form mapped to chromosome 2 [96]. Other patients with milder symptoms have an autosomal dominant disease mapped to chromosome 1 at q22–q23, where a mutation in the α-tropomyosin gene *TPM3* has been found [96]. In addition to weakness, hypotonia, respiratory distress, feeding difficulties, and swallowing difficulties, other features include a high-arched palate, a weak cry, areflexia, and joint contractures [97, 98]. Nemaline myopathy has also been recorded in association with FADS [24, 25]. Progression after the neonatal period may be slow. These features are very similar to those of other congenital myopathies and a muscle biopsy is necessary for diagnosis. In many cases the CK level and EMG findings are normal.

The muscle biopsy specimen (Figs. 32.23 and 32.24) shows a wide variation in fiber diameters, with the type 1 fibers being atrophic or hypotrophic and the type 2 fibers of normal or increased size. Rods, shown in the modified trichrome stain, are present in small or large clusters mainly at the periphery of type 1 fibers, although type 2 fibers may be also involved. The rods, which generally are invisible in hematoxylin and eosin preparations, may be identified with

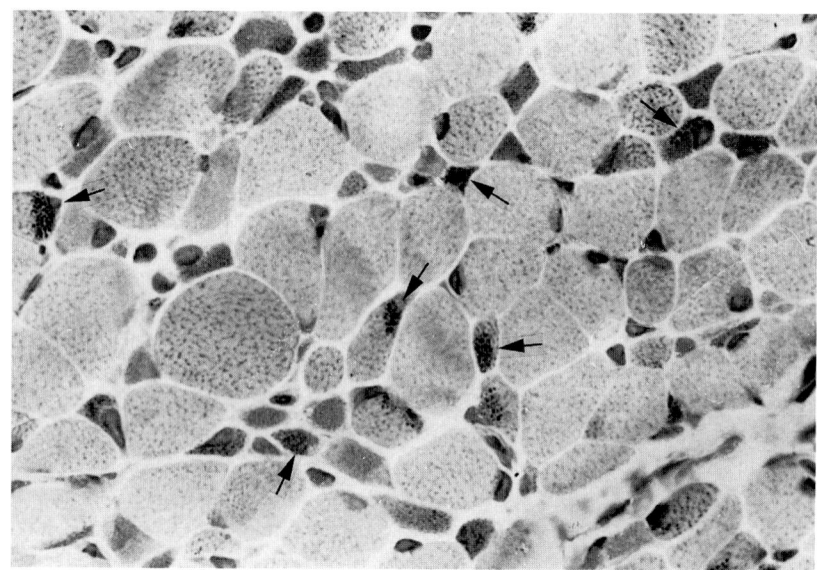

FIGURE 32.23.   *Neonatal nemaline myopathy. Collections of the nemaline (rod-like) bodies (arrows) are present mainly in the small fibers, although a few rods may be seen in the larger fibers in other areas. In a routine H&E-stained section the general impression may be of a congenital fiber type disproportion, and rods will not be seen unless the trichrome stain is used. Cryostat section, trichrome, ×585.*

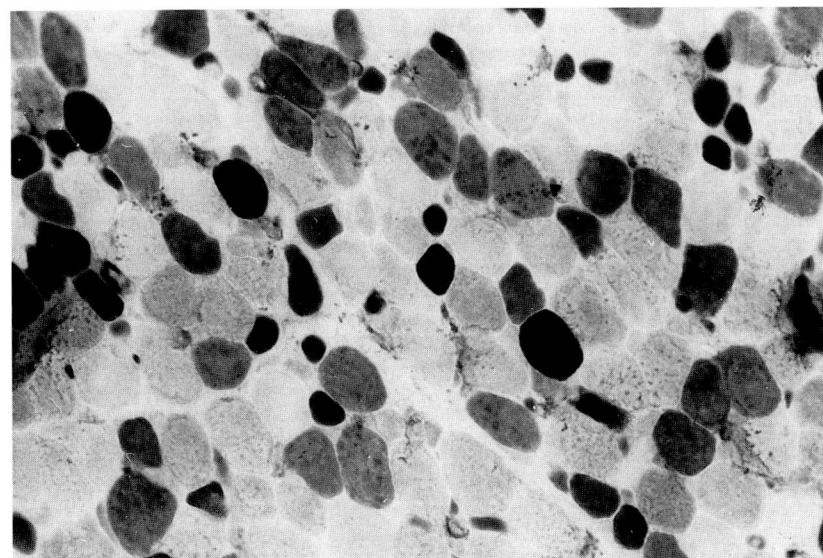

difficulty in phosphotungstic acid hematoxylin (PTAH)–, Masson trichrome–, or Martius, scarlet blue (MSB)–stained routine paraffin sections. A type 1 fiber predominance is usually found, but occasional cases have a predominance of type 2 fibers, of which more than 90% were type 2C fibers in 1 patient [99]. Some authors described many muscle fibers with fetal characteristics and with an increase in satellite cells and clusters of myocytes within a single basement membrane [100].

By electron microscopy, the rods measure 2–5 µm in length and have ultrastructural characteristics of Z-bands with parallel filaments and regular cross-striations. Continuity of Z-bands and rods may be found. Immunohistochemical studies show that the rods and Z-bands react with antibodies to α-actinin [101]. Nuclear rod material was observed in some severely affected neonates [102, 103].

In postmortem studies, all skeletal muscles are affected, although the degree varies from one muscle to another and there can be variation in the number of rods within a single muscle. Pharyngeal, diaphragm, and intercostal muscles are most severely affected [104], with degenerative changes in addition to the presence of rods [105]. Heart muscle and smooth muscle are not involved, although rods have been observed in the heart muscle of adults presenting initially with cardiomyopathy [106].

The question "How many rods are necessary for a diagnosis of nemaline myopathy?" is often posed. It has been reported that rods occur in a variety of conditions, including muscular dystrophy, denervation, and dermatomyositis, but the numbers of rods are small and in our experience the appearances are more rod-like than true rods. These may well represent Z-band streaming. Consequently, well-defined rods in a muscle fiber in the clinical context of a congenital myopathy are an important diagnostic feature, whether there are 1 or 2 or hundreds. In 1 patient,

a muscle biopsy sample from the quadriceps showed only 1 or 2 fibers containing a few rods, yet after this patient died of respiratory infection every other muscle examined contained abundant rods. This observation emphasizes the importance of only a few rods and reinforces the view that the number of rods bears no relation to the severity of the disease.

Occasionally both rods and cores have coexisted, and these observations, together with fetal characteristics, led to the hypothesis that many of the congenital myopathies are the result of impaired or altered maturation of fetal muscle [107, 108].

Central Core Disease

This well-known autosomal dominant congenital myopathy is very rarely seen in the neonate. Although it is congenital, it is generally mild and the symptoms are gradual in onset so that only the most severely affected patients are seen in the neonatal period. Biopsy samples obtained at an early age may or may not show a few scattered central (or peripheral) cores. The cores are invisible to routine hematoxylin and eosin preparations and are best demonstrated by methods that show mitochondrial enzyme activity. The core consists of disorganization of myofibrils with loss of mitochondria and hence shows as a region of pale or negative staining in an otherwise normally staining fiber. It has been noticed that with increasing age type 1 fibers tend to predominate and the proportion of cores increases. The severity of the disorder is unrelated to the number of cores. Associations with malignant hyperthermia and mutations in the ryanodine receptor gene have been found [109, 110]. Not all central core disease patients are susceptible to malignant hyperthermia, and not all malignant hyperthermia patients have central cores.

Congenital Fiber Type Disproportion

This term was used to describe the disproportion in sizes between fiber types and not, as is sometimes thought, a disproportion in composition of fiber types within a muscle. The essential features were a relative smallness of type 1 fibers whose size is uniform, and a normal or slightly increased size of uniform type 2 fibers (Fig. 32.25), with no other features present. In the original description by Brooke [110a], the difference in size between type 1 and type 2 fibers was greater than 12%. Although such a difference is readily appreciated in muscle from older children, in the neonate where fibers are only 12–15 µm normally, a 12% difference may not be recognized. The description *congenital fiber type disproportion* is only a histological description [111], as the same features occur in a wide variety of disorders, including infantile myotonic dystrophy, Krabbe's leukodystrophy, multiple sulfatase deficiency [112], and neurogenic disorders. The presence of fiber type disproportion gives no clue as to the nature of the underlying disease or to its prognosis [111, 113]. Although some patients with this label have improved, others have deteriorated or died. The appearance of fiber type disproportion may be as a result of altered neural influences during fetal development [114]. The term using the narrow definition of a 12% difference should be abandoned, and as Brooke said at the VIIth International Congress of Neuromuscular Diseases in Munich in 1990, reserved for those cases that show a difference in fiber type size of around 40%. These cases never occur in the neonatal period.

INFLAMMATORY MUSCLE DISEASE

Inflammatory myopathies range from the polymyositis/dermatomyositis group to the collagen vascular disorders, to parasitic and viral myositis. Inflammatory myositis is rarely encountered in the neonate. An infantile myositis presenting in the first year with neck and proximal muscle atrophy and weakness, and a grossly raised CK level, has been described [115]. The pathology is quite variable from one area to another and the findings may be entirely normal in distal muscles. Affected areas show large portions of fascicles replaced by connective tissue and the remaining fibers are smaller than normal and are rounded. Scattered lymphocytes are found in these areas. Elsewhere, large or small collections of mononuclear inflammatory cells can be found. Fibers undergo necrosis. With electron microscopy, intranuclear filaments and microtubules were found in 2 patients. Corticosteroid treatment may be effective.

METABOLIC MYOPATHIES

Pompe Disease

Pompe disease (glycogenosis II), with autosomal recessive inheritance and defective acid maltase activity caused by mutations at the locus on chromosome 17 [116], is characterized by hypotonia, weakness, hepatic enlargement, and a cardiomyopathy. The hypertrophic cardiomyopathy brings the patients to the attention of cardiologists soon after birth. Pompe disease is fatal but there are also less severe juvenile and adult forms with the same enzyme defect.

Skeletal muscle shows a gross vacuolar myopathy with massive amounts of glycogen, which is readily soluble so that unless great care is taken, the muscle will appear as a series of holes held together with sarcolemma and a little myofibrillar material (Fig. 32.26). No fat is found. In addition to the glycogen, many observers have commented on the presence of a metachromatic substance [117–119]. Many explanations, including multiple enzyme defects, have been proposed but it is probable that the metachromasia is induced by the binding of phosphate by aggregates of glyco-

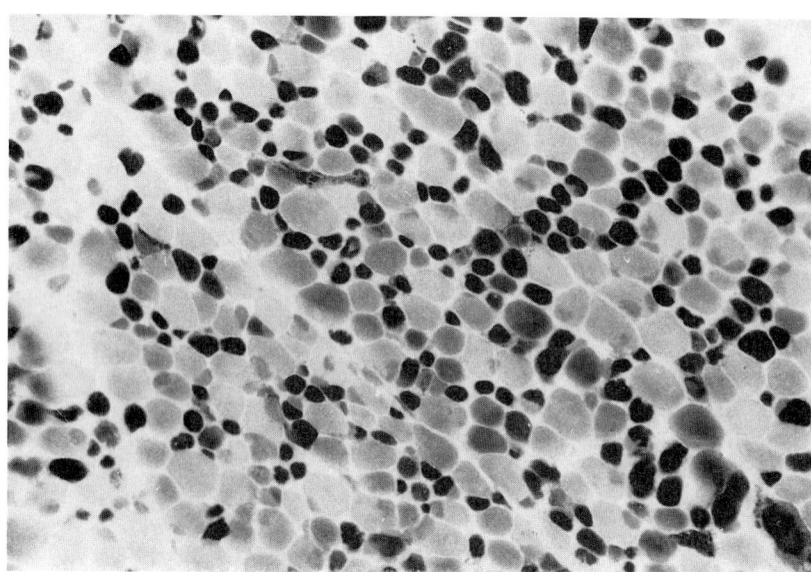

FIGURE 32.25. *Congenital fiber type disproportion. Although the appearance of the biopsy specimen fulfills the original criteria for congenital fiber type disproportion, the resemblance to denervation is strong (see Figs. 32.12 and 32.13). Cryostat section, ATPase after preincubation at pH 4.3, ×365.*

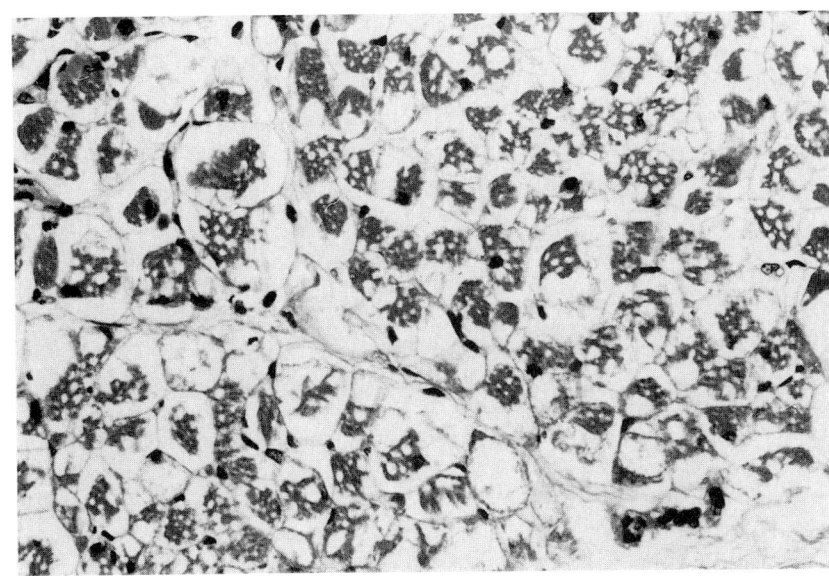

FIGURE 32.26. *Pompe disease, glycogen storage disease type 2. The muscle fibers are grossly vacuolated, making it difficult to appreciate that the tissue is muscle. The vacuoles are filled with glycogen. Routine paraffin section, H&E, ×365.*

gen. The muscle fibers show strong acid phosphatase activity within the vacuoles. Glycogen can also be found in the endothelial cells of capillaries and in the smooth muscle cells of vessel walls. Macrophages in the perimysium often accumulate glycogen.

Muscle biopsy is rarely necessary, the diagnosis being made by examination of peripheral blood films and detection of discrete glycogen deposits in lymphocytes [120]. The assay of acid α-1,4-glucosidase necessary for the confirmation of the diagnosis is performed on cultured skin fibroblasts.

Anterior horn cells are ballooned and filled with glycogen, and although their functions might be impaired, there is no evidence of denervation in the neonatal muscles. However, 1 patient with the adult form had chronic neurogenic muscular atrophy [121]. This is the exception rather than the rule.

Glycogen is found within the myofibers of the heart, the whole of which is affected. However, several other conditions have a near-identical microscopic appearance in the heart and the diagnosis of Pompe disease should not be made without biochemical evidence of deficient acid α-1,4-glucosidase activity. Ethanolaminosis [122] and low-molecular-weight glycogen storage [123] can be distinguished from Pompe disease by the diastase-resistant nature of the storage material in the former conditions. Debranching enzyme deficiency, while affecting skeletal muscle and sometimes giving rise to a cardiomyopathy, to date has not presented in the neonatal period, although infants may first present with hepatomegaly and hypoglycemia.

Phosphofructokinase Deficiency

Another glycogen storage disease that rarely presents with neonatal hypotonia is phosphofructokinase deficiency [124, 125]. There is a mixed population of small and larger rounded muscle fibers with no vacuolar change and no excess glycogen detected by light microscopy (in spite of a 1.5 to 3.0 times increase found on glycogen assay), but subsarcolemmal blebs containing glycogen were present in electron micrographs. The phosphofructokinase activity was about 1.5% of normal.

Myophosphorylase Deficiency

Myophosphorylase deficiency was reported as a fatal infantile disorder in 2 siblings who presented with floppiness and progressive respiratory distress [126, 127]. The muscle fiber diameters ranged from small to normal and numerous subsarcolemmal spaces containing glycogen were evident in each fiber type. The phosphorylase reaction was negative in muscle fibers but present in the smooth muscle of vascular walls, where a genetically different phosphorylase enzyme exists. Quantitatively, no phosphorylase activity could be detected and no enzyme protein was found on radial diffusion plates [127]. No fat was present and the acid phosphatase reaction was normal.

Branching Enzyme Deficiency

Intrauterine growth retardation and premature delivery and death, either in utero or very soon after birth, were features of 3 patients in whom a defect of branching enzyme activity was presumed. This was based on heterozygote values in the parents and normal values on antenatal testing in a later pregnancy that resulted in a normal child [128]. The 3 patients had pulmonary hypoplasia (lung/body ratio <0.010), and one of the fetuses had flexion contractures at the hips, knees, and feet. Paraffin sections of the muscles revealed severe fibrosis, and basophilic deposits in muscle fibers and macrophages that were PAS-positive (after digestion) and showed Maltese cross-birefringence. These deposits were identical in appearance to starch grains and are stained intensely blue-black with Lugol's iodine. Similar deposits were also found in the heart, liver, and brain.

Other Causes of Glycogen Deposition

In any patient presenting with hypotonia and hypoglycemia it is usual to give intravenous dextrose, which often leads to high glycogen concentrations not only in liver but also in muscle, giving the appearance of a glycogen storage problem.

Disorders of the Respiratory Chain and Lipid Metabolism

The finding of lipid droplets in muscle fibers presents great difficulties in interpretation. In muscle from the neonate and young infant, no lipid is usually found. However, in the presence of defects of the respiratory chain enzymes and of lipid metabolism an increase of lipid droplets is often seen. It should be noted that in any severely ill neonate an increase in lipid droplets may be the result of respiratory embarrassment. A dietary origin may also be possible.

The possibility of a mitochondrial problem should be considered in any patient with increased plasma lactate levels, and if the levels are increased, the cerebrospinal fluid lactate level should also be assessed. An increase in lactate is a sign of abnormal mitochondrial function and can be due to a wide range of defects, including disorders of lipid metabolism [129]. It should be noted that the classic ragged red fibers associated with mitochondrial cytopathies (Kearns-Sayre, MERRF, MELAS) are not found in any mitochondrial disorder in neonates. The ragged red fibers do not become apparent until after the ages of 5–7 years.

Lactic acidosis presenting in the first month with failure to thrive and renal dysfunction and characteristics of the De Toni-Fanconi-Debré syndrome has been observed in several patients [130–132]. Respiratory difficulties, ptosis, and diminished reflexes are combined with a deficiency of cytochrome-c oxidase activity in muscle but there is normal activity in the heart, brain, and liver. The enzyme protein may also be absent or decreased [133]. Most patients with cytochrome oxidase deficiency die early, but may survive up to 8 months with prolonged assisted ventilation.

Muscle biopsy specimens show normal-sized type 1 fibers containing lipid droplets and small type 2 fibers. Clumps of finely granular red-staining material in trichrome preparations (Fig. 32.27) and increased succinate dehydrogenase and NADH dehydrogenase activities are scattered throughout the fibers. This contrasts with the peripheral subsarcolemmal accumulations of mitochondrial cytopathy. These clumps correspond to an increased number of small and large mitochondria with disorganized cristae. Cytoplasmic bodies are also found frequently. Cytochrome oxidase activity is deficient in muscle fibers, as demonstrated by both histochemical (Fig. 32.28) and biochemical means. A similar deficiency of cytochrome oxidase was also found in muscles of older patients, one aged 8 years with the neuropathological diagnosis of Leigh disease at postmortem examination [134] and one who died of cardiac failure at 8 months [135]. Both had hypotonia and weakness but renal dysfunction was not found.

Congenital lactic acidosis, hypotonia, failure to thrive, and progressive liver disease are found in the mitochondrial DNA depletion syndrome [136–139]. In muscle there may be an increase in the red granularity seen with the trichrome stain, together with increased lipid droplets in some or many fibers. Cytochrome oxidase activity appears to be absent from some fibers and strong in others in some patients. Ultrastructural studies show proliferation of mitochondria

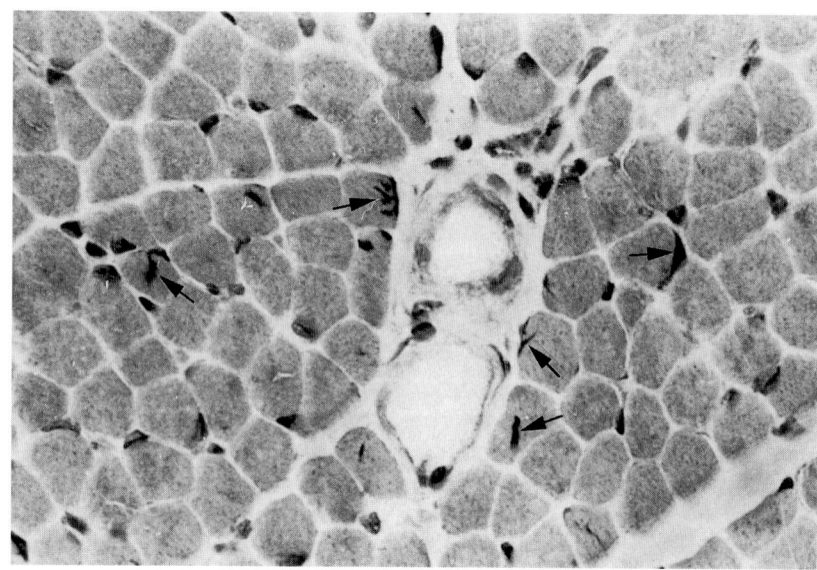

FIGURE 32.27.   *Cytochrome oxidase deficiency. Clumps of darkly staining material (arrows) are present mostly at the periphery of some fibers, but are also seen in more central locations. Cryostat section, trichrome, ×585.*

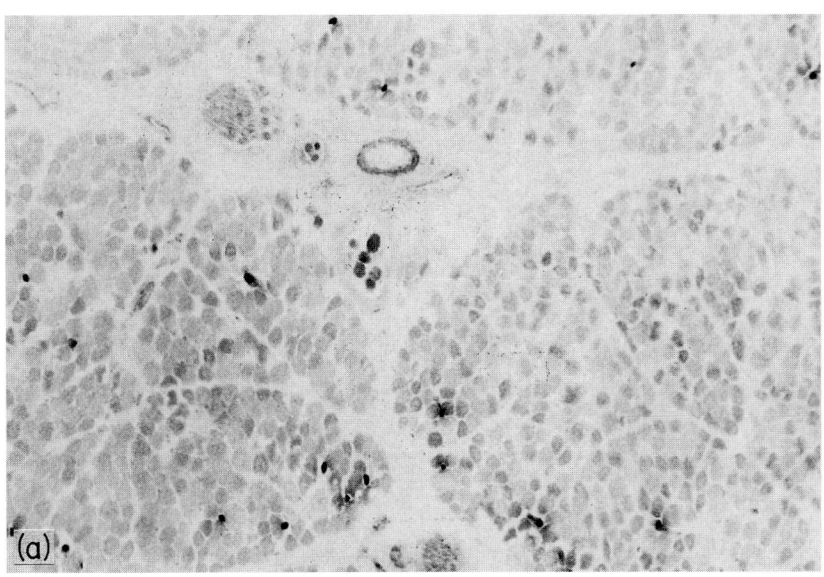

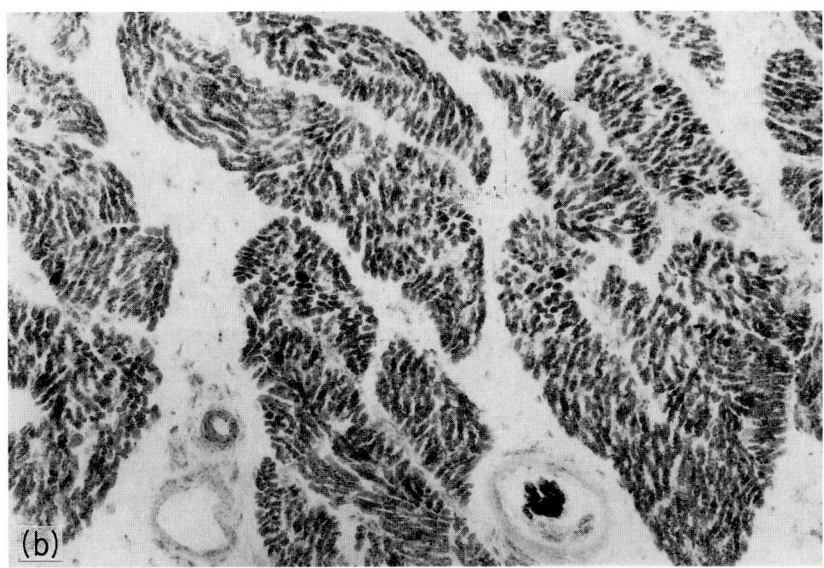

FIGURE 32.28. *Cytochrome oxidase deficiency. Activity of cytochrome oxidase is normally present in the mitochondria of muscle fibers and smooth muscle cells of blood vessels. Intrafusal fibers are strongly positive. (a) Postmortem muscle from a 4-day-old infant with deficient activity in muscle fibers. Capillaries and intrafusal fibers show activity. (b) Postmortem control muscle, matched for chronological age and time from death. Cryostat sections, cytochrome oxidase, ×145.*

and some bizarre large mitochondria containing membranous material. The depletion of mitochondrial DNA is severe in liver, but may be milder in the muscle where, in some patients, no morphological abnormality can be seen [138]. Encephalopathy and rapidly progressive hypotonia were features in an infant who died at 4 months. All muscle fibers were deficient in cytochrome oxidase activity and there was a 99% depletion of mitochondrial DNA in muscle as shown by Southern blotting [140]. The disorder is hereditary and is rapidly fatal.

A benign form of cytochrome oxidase deficiency in which the activity increases to normal over a period of years has been described [141–143]. The infants present with hypotonia and severe weakness of all but the extraocular muscles. There is marked lactic acidemia, which gradually normalizes, with slow clinical improvement to normality. Muscle biopsy specimens obtained at the early stage may

appear morphologically normal with no increase in fat and only occasional red spots in the trichrome preparation. Cytochrome oxidase activity is reduced, and can affect a small or large proportion of muscle fibers. In repeat biopsy samples, a few ragged red fibers are found, glycogen and fat are increased in some fibers, and a greater cytochrome oxidase activity is found. Later the biopsy specimen appears normal and all fibers show cytochrome oxidase activity. These cases bear some clinical similarities to mitochondrial-lipid-glycogen (MLG) disease [144], but differ in that muscle biopsy specimens from patients with MLG disease show severe changes, marked lipid and glycogen accumulation (Fig. 32.29), and grossly disorganized mitochondria. The lactic acidemia decreases and the patients improve from having severe hypotonia and feeding difficulties to near normality at 3 years. The biopsy also reveals normal findings. In 2 personally observed patients the cytochrome oxidase

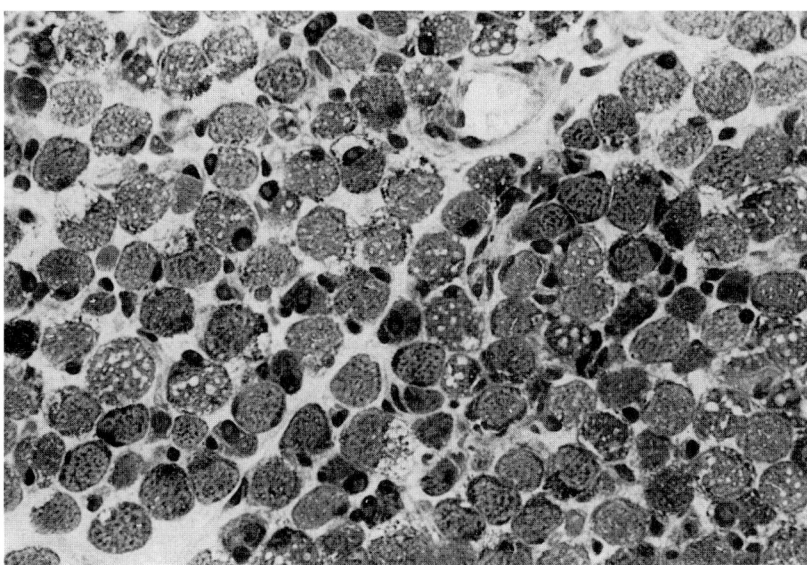

FIGURE 32.29. *Mitochondrial-lipid-glycogen disease. The fibers show vacuoles in which fat is present, and peripheral blebs are found to contain excess glycogen. Excessive red staining in fibers and around their periphery indicates an excess of mitochondria. Cryostat section, trichrome, ×365.*

activity was normal at the time of biopsy in the neonatal period, although published cases are reported retrospectively as showing deficient activity.

Lactic acidosis in association with hypotonia in the neonatal period is also reported in cytochrome-*c* deficiency (complex III deficiency) [96] and in complex I deficiency [144]. Severe respiratory distress and hypoglycemia are features in the first 24 hours of life. Glycogen and lipid accumulation in skeletal muscle with increased numbers of mitochondria, which were enlarged and had concentric cristae, was found in complex I deficiency. The heart in 1 patient showed normally structured mitochondria in myofibers that were distended with fat and glycogen.

Apart from the defect of cytochrome-*c* oxidase and MLG disease, lipid deposition in muscle fibers in the neonatal period has been associated with carnitine palmitoyltransferase deficiency presenting with hypotonia, retardation, and fits [145, 146]. In the group of disorders associated with defects of β-oxidation of fatty acids, deficiencies of short-, long-, and particularly medium-chain fatty acid acyl coenzyme A dehydrogenases have been found and lipid deposition in skeletal muscle fibres is prominent (Fig. 32.31). Marked lipid accumulation is also present in the liver, heart myofibers, and renal tubular epithelium. The patients may present with sudden infant death syndrome [147], while others present with severe hypoglycemia that does not

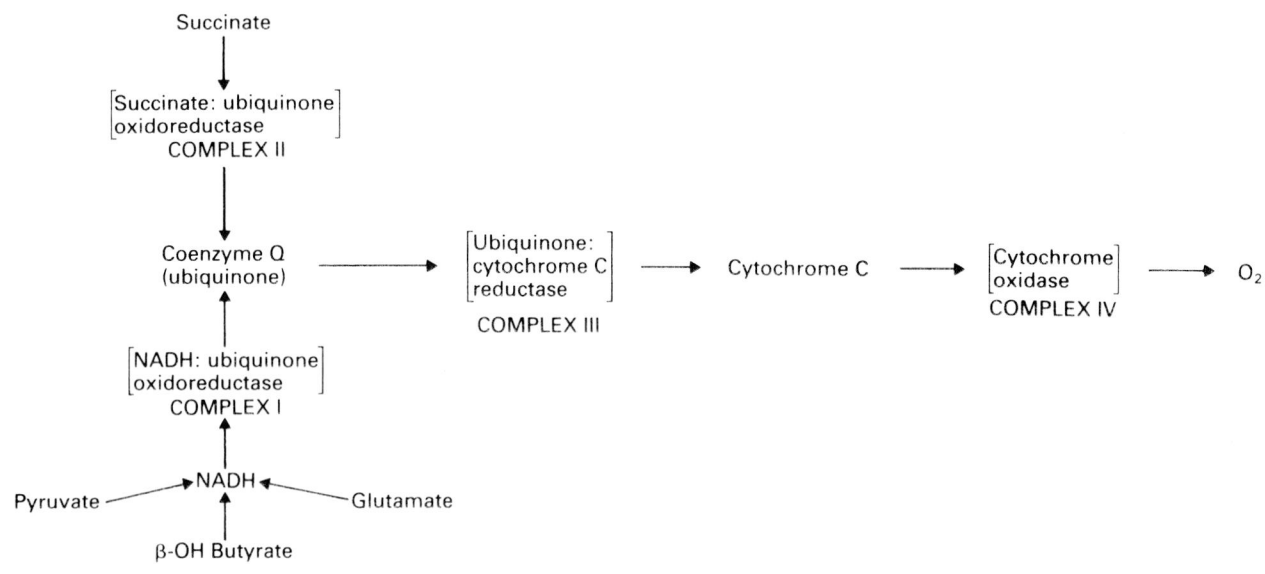

FIGURE 32.30. *Simplified diagram of electron transport in the respiratory chain. The arrows indicate the flow of electrons.*

respond to intravenous dextrose, and at postmortem examination no glycogen can be found in the liver or muscle. Patients with the milder forms of this group of disorders may have several episodes of hypoglycemia and hyperammonemia [148] and are often regarded as examples of "recurrent Reye syndrome." Treatment with oral carnitine and riboflavin may be of help, although the symptoms may spontaneously resolve and only reappear with stress.

A patient with absent 5,10-methylenetetrahydrofolate reductase activity who had a lipid storage myopathy associated with CNS deterioration responded with full recovery to treatment with folate, methionine, and carnitine [149]. A patient with severe X-linked cardiomyopathy described by Barth et al [150] had respiratory chain defects, a lipid storage myopathy, and deficient myoadenylate deaminase activity, the latter being relatively benign in older children.

A variety of other disorders presenting with a congenital lactic acidosis include glycogen storage disease type 1, the organic acidemias, phospho*enol*pyruvate carboxykinase deficiency, fructose-1,6-diphosphatase deficiency, and disorders of the pyruvate dehydrogenase complex. Muscle may or may not be involved. The various causes giving rise to Leigh syndrome have been examined and defects in respiratory chain enzymes and of the pyruvate dehydrogenase complex reported, together with mutations [151]. This group includes the NARP syndrome (neurogenic muscle weakness, ataxia, and retinitis pigmentosa) with the T8993G mutation, which can present at birth with lactic acidosis, respiratory difficulties, bulbar problems, and failure to thrive [151, 152]. The "milder" NARP mutation (T8993C) appears to present later.

Metabolic disorders that do not primarily affect muscle may show their influence on muscle. For example, in maple syrup urine disease a variation in fiber diameters and focal destruction of myofibrillar material were observed in 3 patients [153]. The changes are not usually of diagnostic significance.

MYASTHENIA

Transient Neonatal Myasthenia

A significant proportion (up to 15%) of infants born to myasthenic mothers (even those who are asymptomatic) may develop generalized weakness and hypotonia within the first few days of life, and the severity of the symptoms may be life-threatening. Tube feeding and respiratory assistance may be necessary but most infants recover completely within a few weeks. Antibodies to acetylcholine receptors in the maternal circulation cross the placenta and can be detected in the infant, and their disappearance correlates with clinical improvement. Antiacetylcholinesterase therapy or exchange transfusion [154] may be helpful in patients with severe disease.

Congenital Myasthenia

In contrast with the transient neonatal and adult types of myasthenia in which antibodies to acetylcholine receptors are present, no circulating or bound antibodies can be detected in the congenital myasthenic syndromes. The congenital myasthenic syndromes comprise a group of hereditary conditions affecting the neuromuscular junction, several distinct subgroups have been identified [27, 155, 156], and their means of investigation outlined [157, 158]. Any investigation will require, in addition to the confirmation that acetylcholine receptor antibodies are absent, specialized EMG studies [159]. A motor point muscle biopsy may be

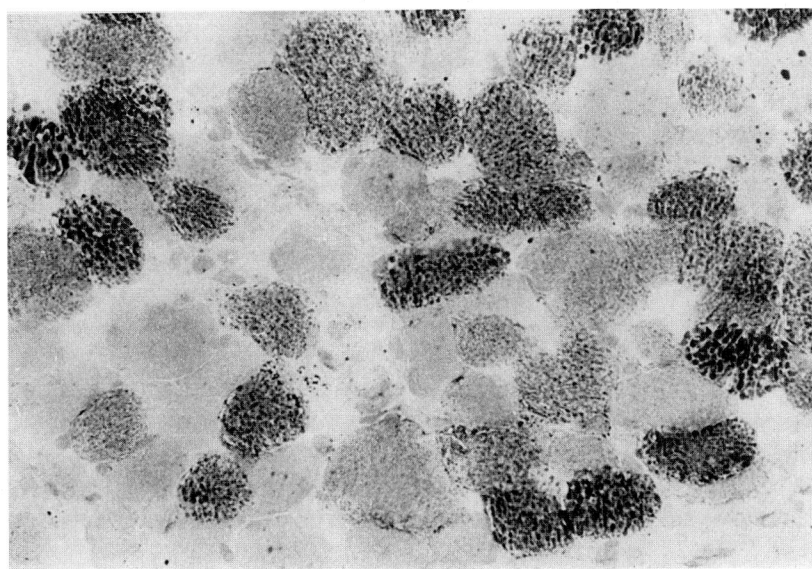

FIGURE 32.31.   *A lipid storage myopathy. Many fibers contain a marked excess of lipid droplets. This is the typical appearance of "carnitine deficiency," which results from a variety of disorders of lipid utilization. Lesser amounts of lipid are more difficult to interpret. Cryostat section, oil red O, ×365.*

necessary for the examination of the structure of the end plate, its enzyme activity, and the presence of acetylcholine receptors.

Defects have been identified as follows:

1. *Presynaptic defects*, with abnormal synaptic vesicles [160], or paucity of synaptic vesicles [161].
2. *End plate acetylcholinesterase deficiency*, in which no acetylcholinesterase activity can be found at the motor end plates [162, 163]. The acetylcholinesterase gene shows no abnormality in such patients [164].
3. *Postsynaptic defects*, with deficient or absent acetylcholine receptors. Mutations in the α and ε subunits of the receptor have been described [165, 166]. This group may also be referred to as slow channel syndromes. The motor end plates may appear abnormally elongated with acetylcholinesterase staining, and show atrophic changes on electron microscopy, or they may be normal [167].

Blocking of neuromuscular transmission, leading to a myasthenic syndrome, generally occurs in older patients and is uncommon in the neonatal period. Several cases of infantile botulism have been recorded, most in infants 1–8 months old. In vitro production of botulinus toxin in the gut is considered the cause. No toxin is found in the circulation. In older children a myasthenic syndrome may be induced by several of the antibiotics and by penicillamine.

REFERENCES

1. Carpenter S, Karpati G. *Pathology of Skeletal Muscle.* New York: Churchill Livingstone, 1984.
2. Barbet JP. Skeletal muscle and nerve. In: Keeling JW, ed. *Fetal and Neonatal Pathology.* 2nd ed. London: Springer, 1993, pp. 595–618.
3. Dubowitz V. Enzyme histochemistry of skeletal muscle. Part I. Developing animal muscle. Part II. Developing human muscle. *J Neurol Neurosurg Psychiatry* 1965; 28:516–24.
4. Farkas Bargeton E, Diebler MF, Arsenio Nunes ML, Wehrle R, Rosenberg B. Etude de la maturation histochimique quantitative et ultrastructurale du muscle foetal humain. *J Neurol Sci* 1977; 31:245–59.
5. Kumagai T, Hakamada S, Hara K. Development of human fetal muscles: a comparative histochemical analysis of the psoas and the quadriceps muscles. *Neuropediatrics* 1984; 15:198–202.
6. Schloon H, Schlottmann J, Lenard HG, Goebel HH. The development of skeletal muscles in premature infants. I. Fibre size and histochemical differentiation. *Eur J Pediatr* 1979; 131:49–60.
7. Buffinger N, Stockdale FE. Myogenic specification of somites is mediated by diffusible factors. *Dev Biol* 1995; 169:96–108.
8. Molkentin JD, Black BL, Martin JF, Olson EN. Co-operative activation of muscle gene expression by MEF2 and myogenic bHLH proteins. *Cell* 1995; 83:1125–36.
9. Olson EN, Klein WH. bHLH factors in muscle development. Deadlines and commitments, what to leave in and what to leave out. *Genes Dev* 1994; 8:1–8.
10. Buckingham M. Which myogenic factors make muscle? *Curr Biol* 1994; 4:61–3.
11. Vogler C, Bove KE. Morphology of skeletal muscle in children. An assessment of normal growth and differentiation. *Arch Pathol Lab Med* 1985; 109:238–42.
12. Barbet JP, Thornell L, Butler-Browne GS. Immunocytochemical characterisation of two generations of fibres during the development of the quadriceps muscle. *Mech Dev* 1991; 35:3–11.
13. Draeger A, Weeds AG, Fitzsimons RB. Primary, secondary and tertiary myotubes in developing skeletal muscle: a new approach to the analysis of human myogenesis. *J Neurol Sci* 1987; 31:245–59.
14. Thornell L, Billeter R, Butler-Browne GS, et al. Development of fibre types in human fetal muscle. An immunocytochemical study. *J Neurol Sci* 1984; 66:107–15.
15. Ennion S, Sant'Ana Periera J, Sargeant AJ, Young A, Goldspink G. Characterization of human skeletal muscle fibres according to the myosin heavy chains they express. *J Muscle Res Cell Motil* 1995; 16:35–43.
16. Johnson MA, Polgar J, Weightman D, Appleton D. Data on the distribution of fibre types in thirty-six human muscles. An autopsy study. *J Neurol Sci* 1973; 18:111–29.
17. Matoba H, Gollnick PD. Influence of ionic composition, buffering agent, and pH on the histochemical demonstration of myofibrillar actomyosin ATPase. *Histochemistry* 1984; 80:609–14.
18. Afifi AK, Rebeiz J, Mire J, Andonian J, Kaloustian VM. The myopathology of the prune belly syndrome. *J Neurol Sci* 1972; 15:153–65.
19. Bouvet JP, Maroteaux P, Briard Guillemot ML. [Poland's syndrome. Clinical and genetic studies; physiopathologic considerations]. *Nouv Presse Med* 1976; 5:185–90.
20. Mace JW, Kaplan JM, Schanberger JE, Gotlin RW. Poland's syndrome. Report of seven cases and review of the literature. *Clin Pediatr (Phila)* 1972; 11:98–102.
21. Banker BQ. Arthrogryposis multiplex congenita: spectrum of pathologic changes. *Hum Pathol* 1986; 17:656–72.
22. Strehl E, Vanasse M, Brochu P. EMG and needle muscle biopsy studies in arthrogryposis multiplex congenita. *Neuropediatrics* 1985; 16:225–7.
23. Uchida T, Nonaka I, Yokochi K, Kodama K. Arthrogryposis multiplex congenita: histochemical study of biopsied muscles. *Pediatr Neurol* 1985; 1:169–73.
24. Porter HJ. Lethal arthrogryposis multiplex congenita (fetal akinesia deformation sequence, FADS). *Pediatr Pathol* 1995; 15:617–37.
25. Vuopala K, Leisti J, Herva R. Lethal arthrogryposis in Finland. A clinico-pathological study of 83 cases during thirteen years. *Neuropediatrics* 1994; 25:308–15.
26. Kobayashi H, Baumbach L, Matise TC, et al. A gene for a severe lethal form of X-linked arthrogryposis (X-linked infantile spinal muscular atrophy) maps to human chromosome Xp11.3–q11.2. *Hum Mol Genet* 1995; 4:1213–6.
27. Vajsar J, Sloane A, MacGregor DL, et al. Arthrogryposis multiplex congenita due to congenital myasthenic syndrome. *Pediatr Neurol* 1995; 12:237–41.
28. Towfighi J, Young RS, Ward RM. Is Werdnig-Hoffmann disease a pure lower motor neuron disorder? *Acta Neuropathol (Berl)* 1985; 65:270–80.
29. Melki J, Shelti P, Abdfhak S. Mapping of acute (type 1) spinal muscular atrophy to chromosome 5q12–q14. *Lancet* 1990; 336:271.
30. Brahe C, Servidei S, Zappata S, et al. Genetic homogeneity between childhood-onset and adult-onset autosomal recessive spinal muscular atrophy. *Lancet* 1995; 346:741–2.
31. Burlet P, Burglen L, Clermont O, et al. Large scale deletions of the 5q13 region are specific to Werdnig-Hoffmann disease. *J Med Genet* 1996; 33:281–3.
32. Fidzianska A, Rafalowska J, Glinka Z. Ultrastructural study of motoneurons in Werdnig-Hoffmann disease. *Clin Neuropathol* 1984; 3:260–5.
33. Steiman GS, Rorke LB, Brown MJ. Infantile neuronal degeneration masquerading as Werdnig-Hoffmann disease. *Ann Neurol* 1980; 8:317–24.
34. Palix C, Coignet J. Un cas de polyneuropathie peripherique neo-natale par amyelinisation. *Pediatrie* 1978; 33:201–7.
35. Hausmanowa-Petrusewicz I, Fidzianska A, Niebroj Dobosz I, Strugalska MH. Is Kugelberg-Welander spinal muscular atrophy a fetal defect? *Muscle Nerve* 1980; 3:389–402.
36. Muruyama S, Boudin TW, Suzuki K. Immunocytochemical and ultrastructural studies of Werdnig-Hoffmann disease. *Acta Neuropathol (Berl)* 1991; 81:408–17.
37. Sawchak JA, Benoff B, Sher JH, Shafiq SA. Werdnig-Hoffmann disease. Myosin isoform expression not arrested at prenatal stage of development. *J Neurol Sci* 1990; 95:183–92.
38. Sewry CA. Contribution of immunocytochemistry to the pathogenesis of spinal muscular atrophy. In: Merlini L, Granata C, Dubowitz V, eds. *Current Concepts in Childhood Spinal Muscular Atrophy.* Bologna: Gaggi, 1989, pp. 57–68.
39. Worton R. Muscular dystrophies: diseases of the dystrophin-glycoprotein complex. *Science* 1995; 270:755–6.
40. Brown RH. Dystrophin-associated proteins and the muscular dystrophies: a glossary. *Brain Pathol* 1996; 6:19–24.
41. Hoffman EP. Clinical and histopathological features of abnormalities of the dystrophin-based membrane cytoskeleton. *Brain Pathol* 1996; 6:49–61.

42. Donner M, Rapola J, Somer H. Congenital muscular dystrophy: a clinico-pathological and follow-up study of 15 patients. *Neuropadiatrie* 1975; 6:239–58.

43. McMenamin JB, Becker LE, Murphy EG. Congenital muscular dystrophy: a clinicopathologic report of 24 cases. *J Pediatr* 1982; 100:692–7.

44. Topaloglu H, Yalaz K, Renda Y, et al. Occidental type cerebromuscular dystrophy; a report of eleven cases. *J Neurol Neurosurg Psychiatry* 1991; 54:226–9.

45. Leyten QH, Gabreels FJ, Renier WO, et al. White matter abnormalities in congenital muscular dystrophy. *J Neurol Sci* 1995; 129:162–9.

46. Barth PG, Fleury P, Oorthuys JW. Congenitale spierdystrofieen spectrum. *Tijdschr Kindergeneeskd* 1984; 52:209–12.

47. Egger J, Kendall BE, Erdohazi M, et al. Involvement of the central nervous system in congenital muscular dystrophies. *Dev Med Child Neurol* 1983; 25:32–42.

48. Zellweger H, Afifi A, McCormick WF, Mergner W. Severe congenital muscular dystrophy. *Am J Dis Child* 1967; 114:591–602.

49. Tome FMS, Evangelista T, Leclerc A, et al. Congenital muscular dystrophy with merosin deficiency. *C R Acad Sci Paris* 1994; 317:351–7.

50. Hillaire D, Leclerc A, Faure S, et al. Localization of merosin-negative congenital muscular dystrophy to chromosome 6q2 by homozygosity mapping. *Hum Mol Genet* 1995; 3:1657–61.

51. Helbling Leclerc A, Zhang X, Topaloglu H, et al. Mutations in the laminin alpha 2-chain gene (LAMA2) cause merosin-deficient congenital muscular dystrophy. *Nat Genet* 1995; 11:216–8.

51a. Allamand V, Sunada Y, Salih MA, et al. Mild congenital muscular dystrophy in two patients with an internally deleted laminin alpha 2 chain. *Hum Mol Genet* 1997; 6:747–52.

52. North KN, Beggs AH. Deficiency of a skeletal muscle isoform of α-actinin (α-actinin-3) in merosin-positive congenital muscular dystrophy. *Neuromuscul Disord* 1996; 6:229–35.

53. Leivo I, Engvall E. Merosin, a protein specific for basement membranes of Schwann cells, striated muscle, and trophoblast, is expressed late in nerve and muscle development. *Proc Natl Acad Sci USA* 1988; 85:1544–8.

54. Muntoni F, Sewry C, Wilson L, et al. Prenatal diagnosis in congenital muscular dystrophy. *Lancet* 1995; 345:591.

55. Fukuyama Y, Osawa M, Suzuki H. Congenital progressive muscular dystrophy of the Fukuyama type—clinical, genetic and pathological considerations. *Brain Dev* 1981; 3:1–29.

56. Aida N, Yagishita A, Takada K, Katsumata Y. Cerebellar MR in Fukuyama congenital muscular dystrophy: polymicrogyria with cystic lesions. *AJNR Am J Neuroradiol* 1994; 15:1755–9.

57. Takada K, Rin YS, Kasagi S, et al. Long survival in Fukuyama congenital muscular dystrophy: occurrence of neurofibrillary tangles in the nucleus basalis of Meynert and locus ceruleus. *Acta Neuropathol (Berl)* 1986; 71:228–32.

58. Takada K, Nakamura H, Tanaka J. Cortical dysplasia in congenital muscular dystrophy with central nervous system involvement (Fukuyama type). *J Neuropathol Exp Neurol* 1984; 43:395–407.

59. McMenamin JB, Becker LE, Murphy EG. Fukuyama-type congenital muscular dystrophy. *J Pediatr* 1982; 101:580–2.

60. Toda T, Ikegawa S, Okui K, et al. Refined mapping of a gene responsible for Fukuyama-type congenital muscular dystrophy: evidence for strong linkage disequilibrium. *Am J Hum Genet* 1994; 55:946–50.

61. Yoshioka M, Kuroki S. Clinical spectrum and genetic studies of Fukuyama congenital muscular dystrophy. *Am J Med Genet* 1994; 53:245–50.

62. Toda T, Yoshioka M, Nakahori Y, et al. Genetic identify of Fukuyama-type congenital muscular dystrophy and Walker–Warburg syndrome. *Ann Neurol* 1995; 37:99–101.

63. Ranta S, Pihko H, Santavuori P, Tahvanainen E, de la Chapelle A. Muscle-eye-brain disease and Fukuyama type congenital muscular dystrophy are not allelic. *Neuromuscul Disord* 1995; 5:221–5.

64. Santavuori P, Somer H, Sainio K, et al. Muscle-eye-brain disease (MEB). *Brain Dev* 1989; 11:147–53.

65. Saito K, Fukuyama Y, Ogata T, Oya A. Experimental intrauterine infection of akabane virus. Pathological studies of skeletal muscles and central nervous system of newborn hamsters with relevances to the Fukuyama type congenital muscular dystrophy. *Brain Dev* 1981; 3:65–80.

66. Dunger DB, Davies KE, Pembrey M, et al. Deletion on the X chromosome detected by direct DNA analysis in one of two unrelated boys with glycerol kinase deficiency, adrenal hypoplasia, and Duchenne muscular dystrophy. *Lancet* 1986; 1:585–7.

67. Renier WO, Nabben FA, Hustinx TW, et al. Congenital adrenal hypoplasia, progressive muscular dystrophy, and severe mental retardation, in

68. Hammond J, Howard NJ, Brookwell R, et al. Proposed assignment of loci for X-linked adrenal hypoplasia and glycerol kinase genes. *Lancet* 1985; 1:54. Letter.

69. Bradley WG, Hudgson P, Larson PF, Papapetropoulos TA, Jenkison M. Structural changes in the early stages of Duchenne muscular dystrophy. *J Neurol Neurosurg Psychiatry* 1972; 35:451–5.

70. Hudgson P, Pearce GW, Walton JN. Pre-clinical muscular dystrophy: histopathological changes observed on muscle biopsy. *Brain* 1967; 90:565–76.

71. Bieber FR, Hoffman EP, Amos JA. Dystrophin analysis in Duchenne muscular dystrophy. Use in fetal diagnosis and in genetic counselling. *Am J Hum Genet* 1989; 45:362–7.

72. Evans MI, Hoffman EP, Cadrin C, et al. Fetal muscle biopsy: collaborative experience with varied indications. *Obstet Gynecol* 1994; 84:913–7.

73. Heckmatt JZ, Sewry CA, Hodes D, Dubowitz V. Congenital centronuclear (myotubular) myopathy. A clinical, pathological and genetic study in eight children. *Brain* 1985; 108:941–64.

74. Pages M, Cesari JB, Pages AM. Centronuclear myopathy. Complete review of the literature apropos of a case. *Ann Pathol* 1982; 2:301–10.

75. Barth PG, Van Wijngaarden GK, Bethlem J. X-Linked myotubular myopathy with fatal neonatal asphyxia. *Neurology* 1975; 25:531–6.

76. Ambler MW, Neave C, Singer DB. X-Linked recessive myotubular myopathy: II. Muscle morphology and human myogenesis. *Hum Pathol* 1984; 15:1107–20.

77. Ambler MW, Neave C, Tutschka BG, et al. X-Linked recessive myotubular myopathy: I. Clinical and pathologic findings in a family. *Hum Pathol* 1984; 15:566–74.

78. Wallgren-Pettersson C, Clarke A, Samson F. The myotubular myopathies: differential diagnosis of the X-linked recessive, autosomal dominant and autosomal recessive forms and present state of DNA studies. *J Med Genet* 1995; 32:673–9.

78a. de Gouyon BM, Zhao W, Laporte J, et al. Characterization of mutations in the myotubularin gene in twenty-six patients with X-linked myotubular myopathy. *Hum Mol Genet* 1997; 6:1499–504.

79. Elder GB, Dean D, McComas AJ, Paes B, DeSa D. Infantile centronuclear myopathy. Evidence suggesting incomplete innervation. *J Neurol Sci* 1983; 60:79–88.

80. Adickes ED, Shuman RM. Fetal alcohol myopathy. *Pediatr Pathol* 1983; 1:369–84.

81. Brook JD, McCurrach ME, Harley HG. Molecular basis of myotonic dystrophy. Expansion of a trinucleotide CTG repeat at the 3′ end of the transcript encoding a protein kinase family member. *Cell* 1992; 68:799–808.

82. Buxton J, Shelbourne P, Davis J. Detection of an unstable fragment of DNA specific to individuals with myotonic dystrophy. *Nature* 1992; 355:547–8.

83. Wang J, Pegoraro E, Menegazzo E. Myotonic dystrophy: evidence for a possible dominant-negative RNA mutation. *Hum Mol Genet* 1995; 4:599–606.

84. Vanier TM. Dystrophia myotonica in childhood. *BMJ* 1960; 2:1284–8.

85. Glanz A, Fraser FC. Risk estimates for neonatal myotonic dystrophy. *J Med Genet* 1984; 21:186–8.

86. Farkas Bargeton E, Barbet JP, Dancea S, et al. Immaturity of muscle fibres in the congenital form of myotonic dystrophy. Its consequences and its origin. *J Neurol Sci* 1988; 83:145–59.

87. Harper PS, Dyken PR. Early-onset dystrophia myotonica. Evidence supporting a maternal environmental factor. *Lancet* 1979; 2:53–7.

88. Pearse RG, Howeler CJ. Neonatal form of dystrophia myotonica. Five cases in preterm babies and a review of earlier reports. *Arch Dis Child* 1979; 54:331–8.

89. Vilos GA, McLeod WJ, Carmichael L, Probert C, Harding PG. Absence or impaired response of fetal breathing to intravenous glucose is associated with pulmonary hypoplasia in congenital myotonic dystrophy. *Am J Obstet Gynecol* 1984; 148:558–62.

90. Lenard HG, Goebel HH, Weigel W. Smooth muscle involvement in congenital myotonic dystrophy. *Neuropadiatrie* 1977; 8:42–52.

91. Bodensteiner JB, Grunow JE. Gastroparesis in neonatal myotonic dystrophy. *Muscle Nerve* 1984; 7:486–7.

92. Silver MM, Vilos GA, Silver MD, Shaheed WS, Turner KL. Morphologic and morphometric analyses of muscle in the neonatal myotonic dystrophy syndrome. *Hum Pathol* 1984; 15:1171–82.

93. Karpati G, Carpenter S, Watters GV, Eisen AA, Andermann F. Infantile myotonic dystrophy. Histochemical and electron microscopic features in skeletal muscle. *Neurology* 1973; 23:1066–77.

association with glycerol kinase deficiency, in male sibs. *Clin Genet* 1983; 24:243–51.

94. Sarnat HB, Silbert SW. Maturational arrest of fetal muscle in neonatal myotonic dystrophy. *Arch Neurol* 1976; 33:466–74.

95. Martinez BA, Lake BD. Childhood nemaline myopathy. An analysis of clinical features in relation to outcome. *Dev Med Child Neurol* 1987; 29:815–20.

96. Wallgren-Pettersson C, Avela K, Marchand S, et al. A gene for autosomal recessive nemaline myopathy assigned to chromosome 2q by linkage analysis. *Neuromuscul Disord* 1995; 5:441–3.

97. Wallgren-Pettersson C. Congenital nemaline myopathy: a clinical follow-up study of twelve patients. *J Neurol Sci* 1989; 89:1–14.

98. Norton P, Ellison P, Sulaiman AR, Harb J. Nemaline myopathy in the neonate. *Neurology* 1983; 33:351–6.

99. Morimoto T, Nagao H, Sano N, et al. Impaired muscle fiber type differentiation in a child with nemaline myopathy. *J Pediatr* 1983; 103:268–70.

100. Nonaka I, Tojo M, Sugita H. Fetal muscle characteristics in nemaline myopathy. *Neuropediatrics* 1983; 14:47–52.

101. Wallgren-Pettersson C, Jasani B, Newman GR, et al. Alpha-actinin in nemaline bodies in congenital nemaline myopathy: immunological confirmation by light and electron microscopy. *Neuromuscul Disord* 1995; 5:93–104.

102. Rifai Z, Kazee AM, Kamp C, Griggs RC. Intranuclear rods in severe congenital nemaline myopathy. *Neurology* 1993; 43:2372–7.

103. Barohn RJ, Jackson CE, Kagan-Hallet KS. Neonatal nemaline myopathy with abundant intranuclear rods. *Neuromuscul Disord* 1994; 4:513–20.

104. Tachi N, Wakai S, Watanabe Y, et al. Severe neonatal nemaline myopathy—histological and histochemical studies of respiratory muscles. *Acta Paediatr Jpn* 1992; 34:139–43.

105. McMenamin JB, Curry B, Taylor GP, Becker LE, Murphy EG. Fatal nemaline myopathy in infancy. *Can J Neurol Sci* 1984; 11:305–9.

106. Meier C, Voellmy W, Gertsch M, Zimmermann A, Geissbuhler J. Nemaline myopathy appearing in adults as cardiomyopathy. A clinicopathologic study. *Arch Neurol* 1984; 41:443–5.

107. Fardeau M. Congenital myopathies. In: Mastaglia FL, Walton J, eds. *Skeletal Muscle Pathology.* Edinburgh: Churchill Livingstone, 1992, pp. 237–81.

108. van der Ven PF, Jap PH, ter Laak HJ, et al. Immunophenotyping of congenital myopathies: disorganization of sarcomeric, cytoskeletal and extracellular matrix proteins. *J Neurol Sci* 1995; 129:199–213.

109. Quane KA, Keating KE, Healy JM, et al. Mutation screening of the RYR1 gene in malignant hyperthermia detection of a novel Tyr to Ser mutation in a pedigree with associated central cores. *Genomics* 1994; 23:236–9.

110. Zhang Y, Chen HS, Khanna VK, et al. A mutation in the human ryanodine receptor gene associated with central core disease. *Nat Genet* 1993; 5:46–50.

110a. Brooke MH. Congenital fiber type disproportion. In: Kakulas BA, ed. *Clinical Studies in Mycology.* Amsterdam: Excerpta Medica, 1973, pp. 147–59.

111. Cavanagh NP, Lake BD, McMeniman P. Congenital fibre type disproportion myopathy. A histological diagnosis with an uncertain clinical outlook. *Arch Dis Child* 1979; 54:735–43.

112. Tachi N, Fujibayashi S, Wagatsuma K, Minami R, Imamura S. A case of multiple sulfatase deficiency with fiber type disproportion. *No To Hattatsu* 1984; 16:205–9.

113. Iannaccone ST, Bove KE, Vogler CA, Buchino JJ. Type 1 fiber size disproportion: morphometric data from 37 children with myopathic, neuropathic, or idiopathic hypotonia. *Pediatr Pathol* 1987; 7:395–419.

114. Argov Z, Gardner Medwin D, Johnson MA, Mastaglia FL. Patterns of muscle fiber-type disproportion in hypotonic infants. *Arch Neurol* 1984; 41:53–7.

115. Carpenter S, Karpati G. The major inflammatory myopathies of unknown cause. *Pathol Annu* 1981; 16:205–37.

116. Zhong N, Martiniuk F, Tzall S, Hirschhorn R. Identification of a missense mutation in one allele of a patient with Pompe disease, and use of endonuclease digestion of PCR-amplified RNA to demonstrate lack of mRNA expression from the second allele. *Am J Hum Genet* 1991; 49:635–45.

117. Griffin JL. Infantile acid maltase deficiency. III. Ultrastructure of metachromatic material and glycogen in muscle fibers. *Virchows Arch B Cell Pathol Incl Mol Pathol* 1984; 45:51–61.

118. Griffin JL. Infantile acid maltase deficiency. II. Muscle fiber hypertrophy and the ultrastructure of end-stage fibers. *Virchows Arch B Cell Pathol Incl Mol Pathol* 1984; 45:37–50.

119. Griffin JL. Infantile acid maltase deficiency. I. Muscle fiber destruction after lysosomal rupture. *Virchows Arch B Cell Pathol Incl Mol Pathol* 1984; 45:23–36.

120. Lake BD. Lysosomal and peroxisomal disorders. In: Graham D, Lantos P, eds. *Greenfield's Neuropathology,* vol. 1. 6th ed. London: Edward Arnold, 1996, pp. 658–753.

121. Pongratz D, Kotzner H, Hubner G, Deufel T, Wieland OH. Adult form of acid maltase deficiency presenting as progressive spinal muscular atrophy. *Dtsch Med Wochenschr* 1984; 109:537–41.

122. Vietor KW, Havsteen B, Harms D, Busse H, Heyne K. Ethanolaminosis. A newly recognized, generalized storage disease with cardiomegaly, cerebral dysfunction and early death. *Eur J Pediatr* 1977; 126:61–75.

123. Krivit W, Sharp HL, Lee JC, Larner J, Edstrom R. Low molecular weight glycogen as a cause of generalized glycogen storage disease. *Am J Med* 1973; 54:88–97.

124. Danon MJ, Carpenter S, Manaligod JR, Schliselfeld LH. Fatal infantile glycogen storage disease: deficiency of phosphofructokinase and phosphorylase b kinase. *Neurology* 1981; 31:1303–7.

125. Guibaud P, Carrier H, Mathieu M, et al. Observation familiale de dystrophie musculaire congenitale par deficit en phosphofructokinase. *Arch Fr Pediatr* 1978; 35:1105–15.

126. DiMauro S, Hartlage PL. Fatal infantile form of muscle phosphorylase deficiency. *Neurology* 1978; 28:1124–9.

127. Miranda AF, Nette EG, Hartlage PL, DiMauro S. Phosphorylase isoenzymes in normal and myophosphorylase-deficient human heart. *Neurology* 1979; 29:1538–41.

128. van Noort G, Straks W, Van Diggelen OP, Hennekam RCM. A congenital variant of glycogenosis type IV. *Pediatr Pathol* 1993; 13:685–98.

129. DiMauro S, Trevisan C, Hays A. Disorders of lipid metabolism in muscle. *Muscle Nerve* 1980; 3:369–88.

130. DiMauro S, Mendell JR, Sahenk Z, et al. Fatal infantile mitochondrial myopathy and renal dysfunction due to cytochrome-c-oxidase deficiency. *Neurology* 1980; 30:795–804.

131. Zeviani M, Nonaka I, Bonilla E, et al. Fatal infantile mitochondrial myopathy and renal dysfunction caused by cytochrome c oxidase deficiency: immunological studies in a new patient. *Ann Neurol* 1985; 17:414–7.

132. Minchom PE, Dormer RL, Hughes IA, et al. Fatal infantile mitochondrial myopathy due to cytochrome c oxidase deficiency. *J Neurol Sci* 1983; 60:453–63.

133. Bresolin N, Zeviani M, Bonilla E, et al. Fatal infantile cytochrome c oxidase deficiency: decrease of immunologically detectable enzyme in muscle. *Neurology* 1985; 35:802–12.

134. Willems JL, Monnens LA, Trijbels JM, et al. Leigh's encephalomyelopathy in a patient with cytochrome c oxidase deficiency in muscle tissue. *Pediatrics* 1977; 60:850–7.

135. Rimoldi M, Bottacchi E, Rossi L, et al. Cytochrome-c-oxidase deficiency in muscles of a floppy infant without mitochondrial myopathy. *J Neurol* 1982; 227:201–7.

136. Ricci E, Moraes CT, Servidei S, et al. Disorders associated with depletion of mitochondrial DNA. *Brain Pathol* 1992; 2:141–7.

137. Moraes CT, Shanske S, Tritschler HJ, et al. mtDNA depletion with variable tissue expression: a novel genetic abnormality in mitochondrial diseases. *Am J Hum Genet* 1991; 48:492–501.

138. Mazziotta MRM, Ricci E, Bertini E, et al. Fatal infantile liver failure associated with mitochondrial DNA depletion. *J Pediatr* 1992; 121:896–901.

139. Telerman Toppet N, Biarent D, Bouton JM, et al. Fatal cytochrome c oxidase-deficient myopathy of infancy associated with mtDNA depletion. Differential involvement of skeletal muscle and cultured fibroblasts. *J Inherit Metab Dis* 1992; 15:323–6.

140. Paquis Flucklinger V, Pellissier JF, Camboulives J, et al. Early-onset fatal encephalomyopathy associated with severe mtDNA depletion. *Eur J Pediatr* 1995; 154:557–62.

141. Zeviani M, Peterson P, Servidei S, Bonilla E, DiMauro S. Benign reversible muscle cytochrome c oxidase deficiency: a second case. *Neurology* 1987; 37:64–7.

142. DiMauro S, Nicholson JF, Hays AP, et al. Benign infantile mitochondrial myopathy due to reversible cytochrome c oxidase deficiency. *Ann Neurol* 1983; 14:226–34.

143. Salo MK, Rapola J, Somer H, et al. Reversible mitochondrial myopathy with cytochrome c oxidase deficiency. *Arch Dis Child* 1992; 67:1033–5.

144. Jerusalem F, Angelini C, Engel AG, Groover RV. Mitochondria-lipid-glycogen (MLG) disease of muscle. A morphologically regressive congenital myopathy. *Arch Neurol* 1973; 29:162–9.

145. Hermier M, Carrier H, Berthillier G, Feit JP, Jeune M. Hypotonie et encephalopathie convulsivante avec myopathie lipidique et deficit en palmityl carnitine transferase (PCT). Entite nouvelle? *Pediatrie* 1979; 34:503–18.

146. Land JM, Mistry S, Squier M, et al. Neonatal carnitine palmitoyltransferase-2 deficiency: a case presenting with myopathy. *Neuromuscul Disord* 1995; 5:129–37.

147. Howat AJ, Bennett MJ, Variend S, Shaw L. Deficiency of medium chain fatty acylcoenzyme A dehydrogenase presenting as the sudden infant death syndrome. *BMJ* 1984; 288:976.

148. Bougneres PF, Rocchiccioli F, Kolvraa S, et al. Medium-chain acyl-CoA dehydrogenase deficiency in two siblings with a Reye-like syndrome. *J Pediatr* 1985; 106:918–21.

149. Allen RJ, Wong P, Rothenberg S, DiMauro S, Headington J. Neonatal carnitine deficiency with muscle and CNS deterioration secondary to absent 5,10-methylene tetrahydrofolate reductase, responsive to substrate replacement. *Pediatr Res* 1981; 15:1556. Abstract.

150. Barth PG, Scholte HR, Berden JA, et al. An X-linked mitochondrial disease affecting cardiac muscle, skeletal muscle and neutrophil leucocytes. *J Neurol Sci* 1983; 62:327–55.

151. Rahman S, Blok RB, Dahl H, et al. Leigh syndrome: clinical features and biochemical and DNA abnormalities. *Ann Neurol* 1996; 39:343–51.

152. Makela Bengs P, Soumalainen A, Majander A, et al. Correlation between the clinical symptoms and the proportion of mitochondrial DNA carrying the 8993 point mutation in the NARP syndrome. *Pediatr Res* 1995; 37:634–9.

153. Ferriere G, de Castro M, Rodriguez J. Abnormalities of muscle fibers in maple syrup urine disease. *Acta Neuropathol (Berl)* 1984; 63:249–54.

154. Pasternak JF, Hageman J, Adams MA, Philip AG, Gardner TH. Exchange transfusion in neonatal myasthenia. *J Pediatr* 1981; 99:644–6.

155. Engel AG. Congenital myasthenic syndromes. *Neurol Clin* 1994; 12:401–37.

156. Middleton LT. Congenital myasthenic syndromes; workshop report. *Neuromuscul Disord* 1996; 6:133–6.

157. Vincent A, Newsom Davis J, Wray D, et al. Clinical and experimental observations in patients with congenital myasthenic syndromes. *Ann NY Acad Sci* 1993; 681:451–60.

158. Engel AG. The investigation of congenital myasthenic syndromes. *Ann NY Acad Sci* 1993; 681:425–34.

159. Harper CM. Neuromuscular transmission disorders in childhood. In: Jones HR, Bolton CF, Harper CM, eds. *Pediatric Clinical Electromyography.* Philadelphia: Lippincott-Raven, 1996, pp. 353–86.

160. Mora M, Lambert EH, Engel AG. Synaptic vesicle abnormality in familial infantile myasthenia. *Neurology* 1987; 37:206–14.

161. Walls TJ, Engel AG, Nagel AS, Harper CM, Trastek VF. Congenital myasthenic syndrome associated with paucity of synaptic vesicles and reduced quantal release. *Ann NY Acad Sci* 1993; 681:461–8.

162. Hutchinson DO, Engel AG, Walls TJ, et al. The spectrum of congenital endplate acetylcholinesterase deficiency. *Ann NY Acad Sci* 1993; 681:469–86.

163. Hutchinson DO, Walls TJ, Nakano S, et al. Congenital endplate acetylcholinesterase deficiency. *Brain* 1993; 116:633–53.

164. Camp S, Bon S, Li Y, et al. Patients with congenital myasthenia associated with end-plate acetylcholinesterase deficiency show normal sequence, mRNA splicing, and assembly of catalytic subunits. *J Clin Invest* 1995; 95:333–40.

165. Ohno K, Hutchinson DO, Milone M, et al. Congenital myasthenic syndrome caused by prolonged acetylcholine receptor channel openings due to a mutation in the M2 domain of the epsilon subunit. *Proc Natl Acad Sci USA* 1995; 92:758–62.

166. Sine SM, Ohno K, Bouzat C, et al. Mutation of the acetylcholine receptor alpha subunit causes a slow-channel myasthenic syndrome by enhancing agonist binding affinity. *Neuron* 1995; 15:229–39.

167. Engel AG, Uchitel OD, Walls TJ, et al. Newly recognized congenital myasthenic syndrome associated with high conductance and fast closure of the acetylcholine receptor channel. *Ann Neurol* 1993; 34:38–47.

Chapter

33

The Skin

Geoffrey A. Machin

HISTOGENESIS OF THE SKIN

A composite of ectodermal, ectomesenchymal, mesodermal, and bone marrow elements results in the formation of the skin and of the linings of associated structures (mouth, nose, paranasal sinuses, mammary gland, cornea, conjunctiva, lacrimal glands, salivary glands, tooth enamel, and adenohypophysis). Epidermis and amnion are continuous at the edges of the embryonal bilaminar disk (Fig. 33.1). The normal differentiation and determination of skin derivatives in an integrated fashion produce the wide variety of types of skin on the body, in terms of degrees of pigmentation, thickness of keratinization, and expression of secondary sexual characteristics. Inductive influences of dermis with epidermis are important in normal development, and are also germane to considerations of the genodermatoses and phakomatoses.

Dermal mesenchyme appears to have instructive inductive effects on embryonal epidermis that are time-dependent [1]. Chick embryo ectoderm is committed to keratinization by day 12; prior to that time, ectoderm can be programmed to produce other types of epithelia, for example, respiratory and gastric, if laid on the appropriate mesenchyme [1]. However, adult human ectoderm retains some plasticity, as corneal and conjunctival cells can be induced in vitro to differentiate into keratinocytes [2]. Transplantation experiments have shown that regional differences in epidermal characteristics such as hairiness and thickness of stratum corneum are determined by the dermis [3]. But it has also been shown that epidermal transplants of human lamellar ichthyosis skin to nude mice retain their ichthyotic characteristics; that is, determination of lamellar ichthyosis is strictly at an ectodermal level [4]. Similar work with other genodermatoses is revealing the extent to which dermal or epidermal determination applies.

NORMAL SKIN EMBRYOLOGY

With one major exception, the normal development of the epidermis proceeds temporally from the early appearance of the basal layer to the final emergence of the stratum corneum. The presence of the periderm complicates this otherwise simple picture (Fig. 33.2). In early human fetuses, at 5–6 weeks of gestation, the epidermis has 2 cell layers, the basal layer and the periderm (see Fig. 33.2). The latter persists until 22–23 weeks of gestation, when it is shed. The periderm closely resembles amniotic epithelium, with numerous microvilli and cytoplasmic vesicles, suggesting an exchange function with amniotic fluid [5].

By 10 weeks, the first layer of stratum intermedium is present, and has increased to 2 to 3 layers by 19 weeks (Fig. 33.3). Keratinization begins by about 22 weeks, with small keratohyaline granules apparent, and the beginnings of a stratum corneum proper. Melanocytes reach the epidermis by about 8–10 weeks in the head and neck region, but somewhat later more caudally. Langerhans' cells can be identified at 14 weeks.

NORMAL SKIN DYNAMICS AND STRUCTURE—SOME SELECTED TOPICS

The papillary infolding of the dermis and epidermis provides an enhanced surface area for bonding at the dermoepidermal junction [6]. Basal cells are attached to the basement membrane by hemidesmosomes with anchoring fibrils, while basal cells and spinous cells are attached to each other by numerous fully formed desmosomes. Structural epidermal protein synthesis occurs in the spinous layer. Tonofilaments about 0.8 nm in diameter are distributed within all suprabasal epidermal cells. They are composed of keratin, which remains within the cytoplasm. Tonofilaments

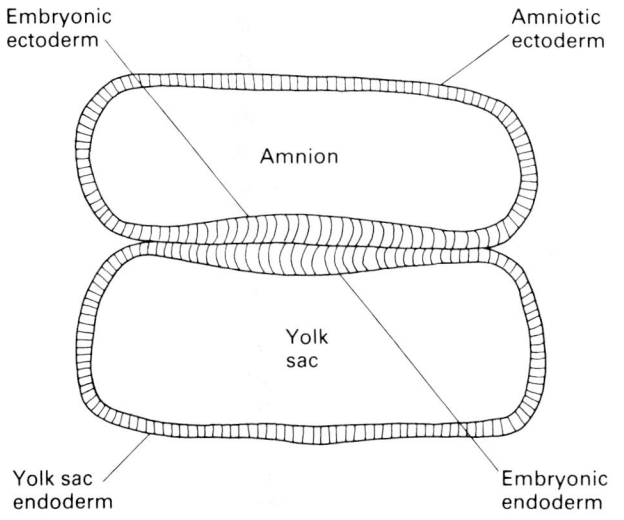

FIGURE 33.1. *Diagrammatic representation of the bilaminar disk, showing relationships of the ectoderm and endoderm.*

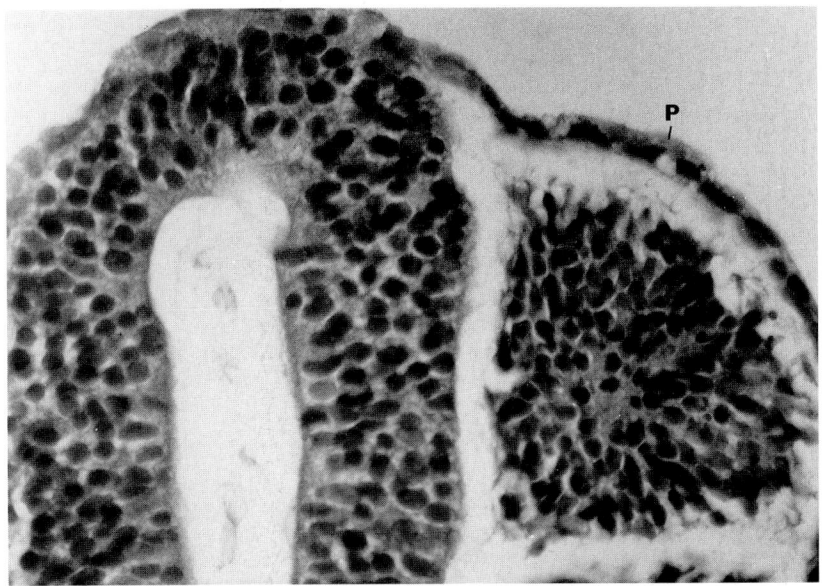

FIGURE 33.2. *An 8-mm fetus of an ectopic pregnancy. Peridermal cells (P) are still present. H&E, ×400.*

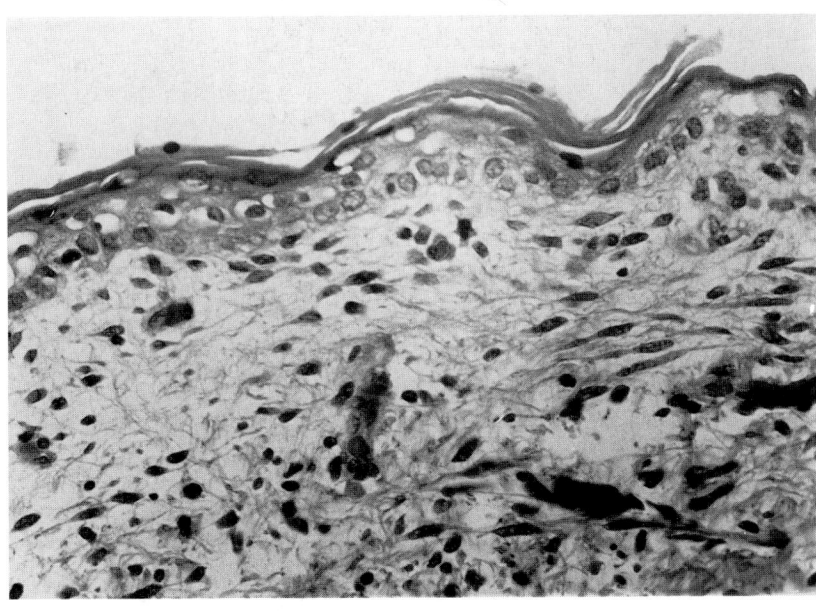

FIGURE 33.3. *Fetal skin at 19 weeks' gestation. Stratum intermedium is present, but keratinization has not yet commenced. Surface cells are flattened but not keratinized. H&E, ×100.*

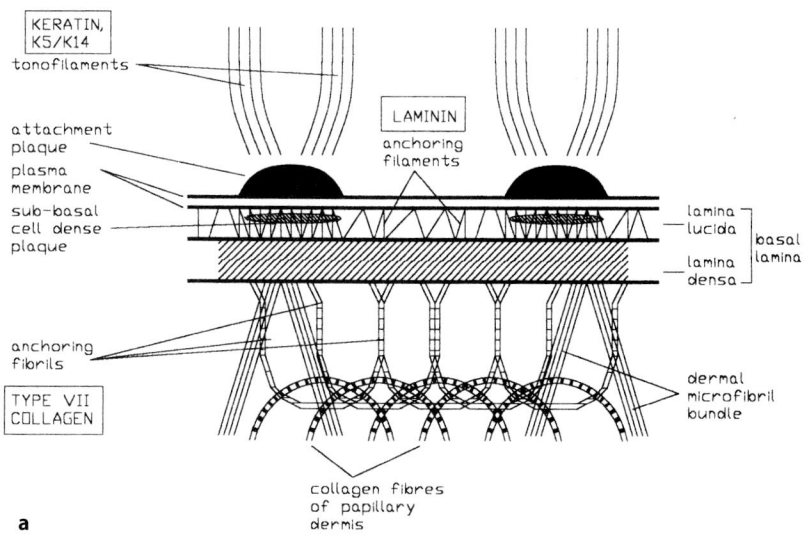

a

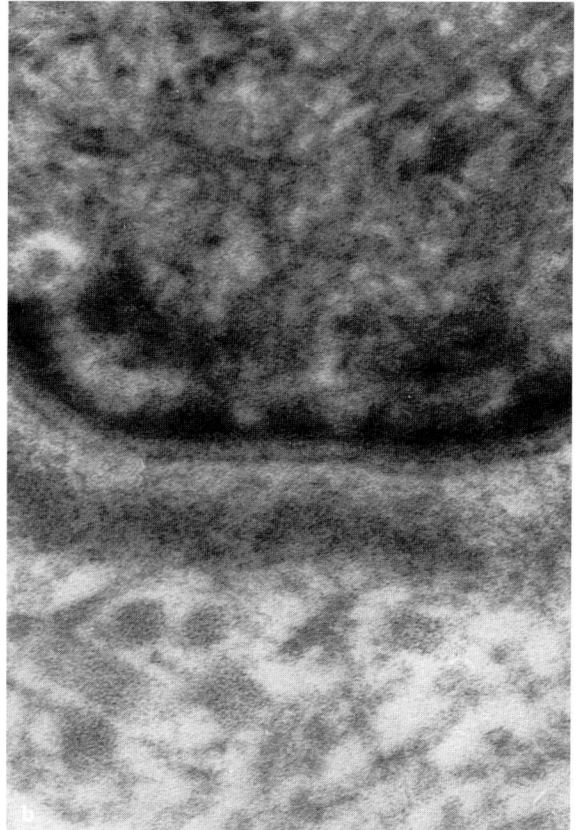

FIGURE 33.4. *(a) Diagrammatic representation of a hemidesmosome. The complexities of the relationship between the plasma membrane of the basal cell and the basal lamina are important in delineating the subtypes of epidermolysis bullosa (EB), further discussed in Fig. 33.9. The lamina lucida is a space between the plasma membrane and the basal lamina; junctional EB occurs at the level of the lamina lucida, with abnormal structure of the anchoring filaments. Dermal anchoring fibrils and microfibrils attach the dermis to the deep surface of the basal lamina. In the basal cell, tonofibrils (keratin filaments) are attached to desmosomes and hemidesmosomes at the attachment plaques. The dense plaques of the lamina lucida correspond with the attachment plaques, and mechanical forces are transmitted through the anchoring filaments to the dermal anchoring fibrils. (b) Electron micrograph of newborn epidermis. Compare with (a). ×300,000.*

are attached by plaques to the cytoplasmic aspects of the hemidesmosomes and desmosomes, hence forming a sort of intercytial skeleton (Fig. 33.4).

Keratohyalin granules are distinct organelles that develop as the cells come to constitute the stratum granulosum. Although keratin confers the tough texture of the desquamating stratum corneum, it seems that waterproofing principally results from the synthesis of lipids in membrane-coating granules that are extruded into the intercellular space at the base of the stratum corneum. The content of these Odland bodies also provides cohesion between cells in the lower stratum corneum. Steroid sulfatase and related enzymes remove the intercellular lipid in the upper stratum corneum, thus permitting desquamation. Thus, the structure of the epidermis depends on "bricks" (i.e., keratin) and "mortar" (i.e., intercellular lipids).

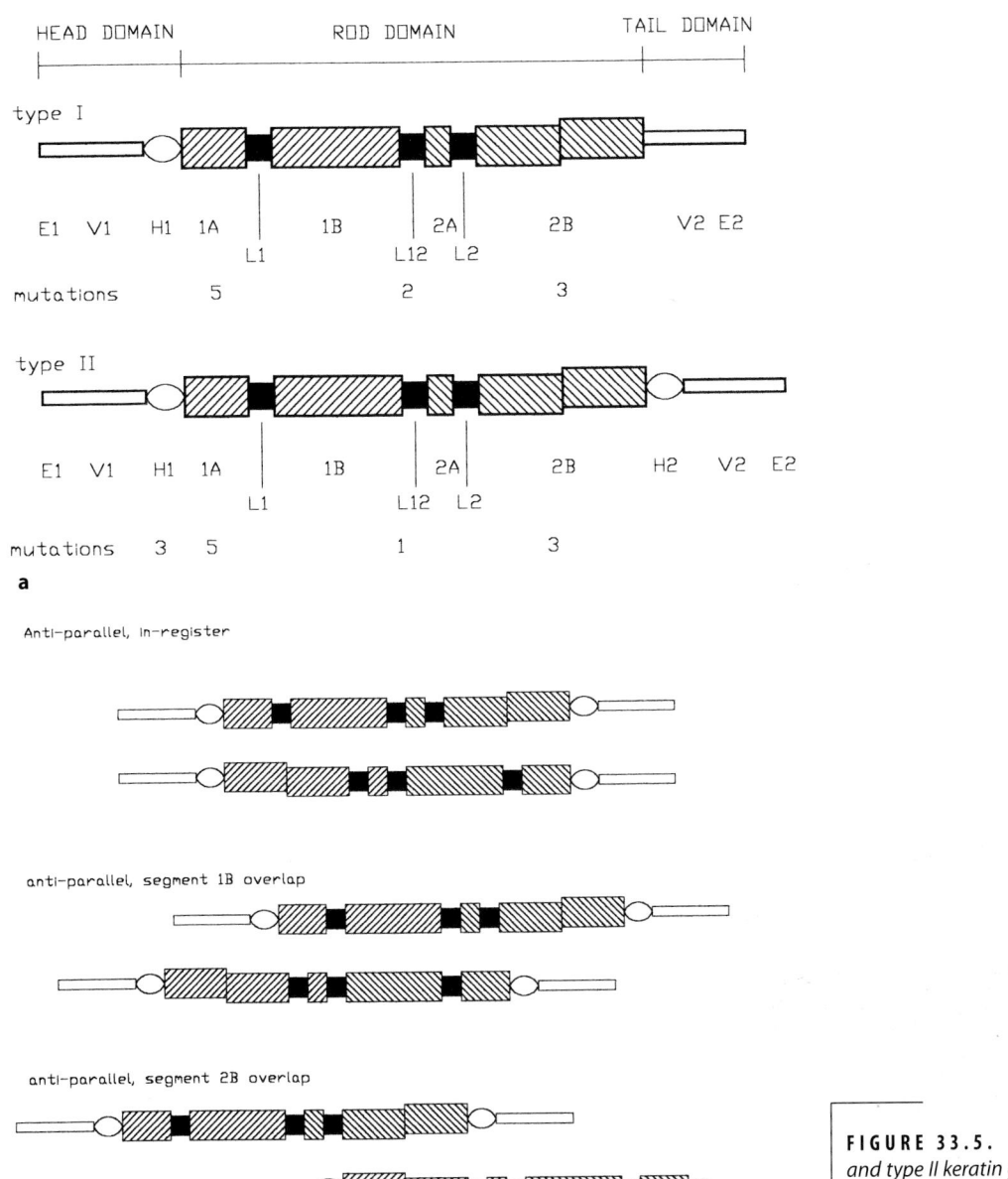

FIGURE 33.5. *(a) The domains of type I and type II keratin genes. (b) Possible antiparallel arrangements of keratin dimers.*

Transition from prekeratin to keratohyalin involves dephosphorylation and the action of a basic protein that is rich in histidine. The protein of the stratum corneum is highly insoluble, and techniques for solubilizing and analyzing it appear to have introduced artifactual biochemical changes. In terminal differentiation, protein is deposited on the intracellular aspect of the plasma membrane, and is termed the *cornified (or cross-linked) envelope*. This occurs by a process involving keratin transglutaminase.

Recently, the molecular biology of the keratins and the components of hemidesmosomes were clarified. Mutations have been found in genes coding for 6 different major structural proteins, distributed in the corresponding 3 major clinical types of epidermolysis bullosa (EB). Also, keratin gene mutations have been discovered for epidermolytic pal-

moplantar keratoderma (EPPK), a localized ichthyosis-like genodermatosis, as well as for generalized epidermolytic hyperkeratosis (EH). The molecular basis of X-linked ichthyosis has been attributed to mutations in the steroid sulfatase gene, and lamellar ichthyosis involves abnormal transglutamination during terminal differentiation.

Keratins are members of the intermediate filament (IF) family of cytoskeletal proteins [7]. All IF proteins have 3 major domains whereby a central α-helical rod domain is flanked by head and tail domains (Fig. 33.5a). Acidic (type I) and basic (type II) keratins differ; there are 2 H domains in type II keratins and only 1 H domain in type I keratins. Heterodimers are formed between type I and type II keratin molecules in antiparallel arrays with varying degrees of overlap of A and B regions (Fig. 33.5b) [8].

There are about 20 epithelial (soft) keratins and 10 hair and nail (hard) keratins. A wide array of keratins is expressed in fetal epidermal cells in the early and late periods of the second trimester. The expression is simpler in the skin of the neonate and adult, such that the keratin dimer K5/K14 is present in the basal layer, and K1/K10 in suprabasal cells.

Within the central rod domains of keratins, there are highly conserved sequences of about 310 amino acid residues arranged in 4 segments, 1A, 1B, 2A, and 2B. Within these segments, the amino acid residues are arranged as repeating heptads (-a-b-c-d-e-f-g-)^n, in which residues a and d are almost always hydrophobic and e and g residues are polar and oppositely charged. The central rod domains in their subsegments specify how keratin polypeptides interact during keratin IF formation; the other domains probably allow some flexibility in the macromolecules.

Keratin IFs characterize differentiation from stem cells in the basal layer to the cornified cells in the stratum corneum. Because keratin IFs are joined to desmosomes and hemidesmosomes, they form not only intracellular cytoskeletons but also intercellular and transcellular bridging network skeletons that resist deforming mechanical and tractional forces on the epidermis and other epithelial surfaces.

Since the keratin genes were isolated and sequenced, mutations in these genes have been identified in epidermolysis bullosa simplex (EBS) (including several clinical subtypes), EH, EPPK, and ichthyosis bullosa of Siemens.

In EBS, light microscopic and ultrastructural studies have shown blister formation within the subnuclear cytoplasm of the basal cells, accompanied by abnormal keratin IF clumping. Not surprisingly, mutations have been found in K5 and K14 genes, since these are the keratins expressed in basal cells [9].

In EH, vacuolation is seen in the first suprabasal spinous cell layer, and then increases in severity with progression through to the granular layer. Mutations have been found in the genes coding for K1 and K10, the keratins expressed in keratinocytes above the basal layer.

In EPPK, mutations are found in the gene coding for K9, a keratin expressed in the restricted zones of palms and soles.

Taken together with the mutations in laminin, bullous pemphigoid antigen 1, plectin, integrin and collagen types VII found in various subtypes of EB, respectively (see below), it seems likely that the molecular biology of 2 major groups of genodermatoses, EB and the ichthyoses, may soon be fully worked out.

Lipids account for 10–15% of the volume of the stratum corneum, and consist of neutral lipids, sphingolipids, and ceramides. Also present are small quantities of n-alkanes, which are of importance in the scaling disorders (see below).

Details of the structure of the basal lamina are important in understanding the differential diagnosis within the disease group of EB. The structure of desmosomes and hemidesmo-

somes is shown diagrammatically and ultrastructurally in Fig. 33.4.

The connective tissue of the mature dermis consists largely of collagen and glycosaminoglycan ground substance. In the papillary dermis, type I and type VII collagen are found, whereas the reticular dermis is composed largely of type I collagen.

Epidermal turnover time is about 30 days; basal cells function as stem cells, with a cell cycle time of several hundred hours.

SCALING CONDITIONS

The ichthyoses [10] (Table 33.1) are a group of disorders with chronic hyperkeratosis and the production of scales, fancifully likened to fish scales. Ichthyosis is a purely epidermal disorder, and therefore other ectodermal structures are largely spared. Ichthyoses exist as pure skin disorders and also as components of syndromes affecting other organ systems. The pure ichthyoses are genodermatoses and have been classified into 5 groups, based on clinical presentation, histopathology, and pattern of inheritance. The ichthyosis-related syndromes are discussed later. Of the genetic ichthyoses, all but ichthyosis vulgaris present regularly at birth.

The molecular basis of X-linked recessive ichthyosis has largely been determined. Deficiency of 3-β-hydroxy sulfatase is responsible for low maternal serum and urinary estriol levels, with difficulty in initiating labor; the same enzyme deficiency also causes the ichthyosis [11]. The steroid sulfatase deficiency was demonstrable widely in different tissues, including placenta, skin fibroblasts, cultured epidermal cells, callus and scale, and peripheral blood leukocytes. Prenatal diagnosis is available (see below), and the gene for X-linked ichthyosis has been cloned and sequenced [12]. Many patients show a very small deletion of the short arm of the X chromosome as part of a contiguous gene syndrome [13]. Others have point mutations [14, 15].

Features of classic lamellar ichthyosis, non-bullous ichthyosiform erythroderma, and EH are summarized in Table 33.1.

The non-bullous, autosomal recessive ichthyoses are beginning to be characterized (see Table 33.1). Classic lamellar ichthyosis has been strongly linked to the transglutaminase 1 gene, and mutations have been described [16, 16a].

Mutations in the genes coding for keratins K1 and K10 have been found in patients with EH [9, 17–20] (Fig. 33.6). These mutations mostly occur at sites of initiation of the helix in domain 1A or termination of the helix in 2B, without change in ionic status.

It is thought that the mutations in EH serve to destabilize the head-to-tail overlap of antiparallel keratin dimers, affecting epidermal cells in the acanthocytic layer and stratum granulosum, where K1/K10 keratins are expressed.

Table 33.1.   The ichthyoses

Name	Inheritance and Prevalence	Age at Onset	Clinical	Histology/Histogenesis
Ichthyosis vulgaris	AD 1/300	6 mo–3 yr	Fine, dry, brown scales; keratosis pilaris, sparing palms and soles	Decreased granular layer; normal turnover; delayed desmosomal dissolution in corneum
X-Linked ichthyosis	X-Linked recessive 1/6000 males	Birth–6 mo	Extensive dark scaling of distal extremities, not palms and soles; corneal opacities	Orthokeratotic hyperkeratosis; normal granular layer; normal turnover; retention hyperkeratosis (steroid sulfatase gene mutations)
Classic lamellar ichthyosis	AR	Birth	Severe generalized plate-like scales, including scalp, palms and soles; ectropion; mild erythroderma	Twofold thickening of corneum; psoriasiform rete ridges; no parakeratosis; normal granular layer, normal *n*-alkane content; raised sphingolipid and free sterols; normal turnover; linked to transglutaminase gene
Non-bullous ichthyosiform erythroderma	AR	Birth	Erythroderma; severe generalized scaling, fine on face, arms and trunk, plate-like on legs; some cases of ectropion	Acanthosis; variable parakeratosis; thickened corneum; focal parakeratosis; normal *n*-alkane content; raised sphingolipid and free sterols; high turnover
Epidermolytic hyperkeratosis (see Fig. 33.6)	AD 1/300,000	Birth	Erythroderma; accentuated creases; bullae; erosions; secondary staphylococcal infections	Swollen acanthocytes and granular cells; increased keratohyalin granules; compact hyperkeratosis; excessive tonofilaments; dissociation of desmosomes and tonofilaments; K1/K10 keratin gene mutations

AD = autosomal dominant; AR = autosomal recessive.

Ichthyosis bullosa of Siemens is a mild, blistering form of ichthyosis that develops in the first few months of life. Mutations in the 1A and 2B domains of keratin 2e have been reported [21, 22].

Ichthyosis hystrix is a subtype of EH in which the degree of hyperkeratosis is unevenly distributed. At its most severe, it takes the form of hypertrophic papillary excrescences that may be linear and that do not transgress the midline [23]. In this respect, ichthyosis hystrix appears to be an intermediate form between generalized EH and linear epidermal nevus (see below).

Two classic congenital presentations of ichthyosis are the collodion baby and the harlequin fetus. These disorders are quite distinct; collodion baby may be a manifestation of several different ichthyoses (or none), whereas the harlequin fetus is probably an entity separate from the other ichthyoses. Collodion babies are entirely covered by tight, shiny, parchment-like membranes; ectropion and eclabium are seen, and chest movement may be restricted (Fig. 33.7). Within a few days the membrane peels away, and the ultimate state of the skin is revealed. The majority of collodion babies develop classic lamellar ichthyosis, while some may evolve to X-linked or linear circumflex types; a few apparently have normal skin after separation of the membrane. Many collodion babies die in infancy [24]. The neuropathic (type 2) form of Gaucher disease may also present as a collodion fetus [25].

Harlequin ichthyosis is a far more serious type of congenital ichthyosis that is fatal in infancy [26, 27]. Extremely thick scales are separated by deep fissures that extend down into the dermis. There is massive hyperkeratosis with acan-

Table 33.2.   Syndromes with ichthyosis

Name	Features
Basex [30]	Follicular ichthyosiform disorder; follicular atrophoderma; multiple basal cell carcinomas
Rud [31]	Sexual infantilism; neurological abnormalities; autosomal recessive
KID (keratitis, ichthyosis, deafness) [32]	Vascularizing keratitis; neurosensory deafness; cutaneous bacterial and fungal infections; basket weave hyperkeratosis
Sjögren-Larsson [33]	Mental retardation; spastic degeneration; lamellar ichthyosis; autosomal recessive
Netherton's [34]	Trichorrhexis invaginata (bamboo deformity of hair shafts); ichthyosis linearis circumflexa; sparse hair and eyebrows; skin atrophy; autosomal recessive
Refsum [35]	Ichthyosis; retinitis pigmentosa; chronic polyneuritis; deafness; ataxia; flaccid paralysis; defect in α-hydroxylation of phytanic acid, autosomal recessive
Conradi-Hünermann [36]	Ichthyosis (collodion baby); dwarfism; flexion contractures of limbs; cataracts; stippled epiphyses; mental retardation

thosis. Harlequin ichthyosis probably represents a heterogeneous autosomal recessive group of diseases, universally fatal and distinct from the other ichthyoses. Because of its rarity, little is known about the histopathology or histogenesis; the few reported cases show a variety of histopathological fea-

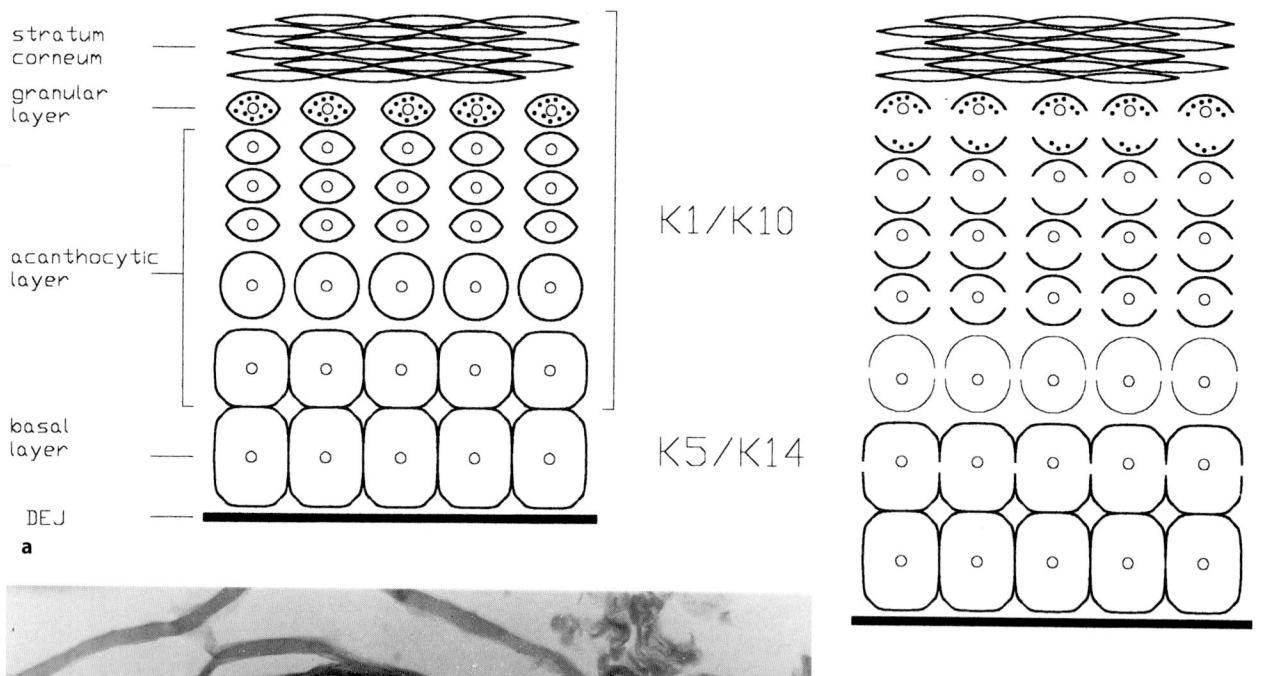

FIGURE 33.6. *(a) Keratin gene expression in the layers of the skin. DEJ = dermal-epidermal junction. (b) Epidermal cell lysis in epidermolytic hyperkeratosis. (c) Epidermolytic hyperkeratosis. Acanthocytes are swollen, keratohyaline granules are compact, and there is keratosis pilaris. H&E, ×100.*

tures, varying from grossly thickened stratum corneum, the presence of lipid vacuoles in cells of the stratum corneum, marked parakeratosis, numerous lysosomes, and varying results on keratin polyacrylamide gel electrophoresis (PAGE).

Another evolution of harlequin fetus is toward non-bullous congenital ichthyosiform erythroderma, with absence of demonstrable filaggrin [28, 29].

EPPK is a scaling condition of the palms and soles for which mutations have been found in the keratin 9 gene.

Ichthyosis occurs in a large number of syndromes, of which the more important are listed in Table 33.2 [30–36].

BULLOUS, VESICULAR, AND PUSTULAR DISEASES

Fluid-filled lesions are termed *pustules* when they contain pus, whereas those containing clear fluid are called *vesicles* if they measure less than 1 cm in diameter and *bullae* if they are larger. There are several interesting diseases of this type in the fetus and neonate, and it is important to distinguish between those that are transient and less clinically threatening (Table 33.3) [37–39], the serious acute infectious disorders, and those that herald chronic bullous disorders that are serious or lethal, often with a genetic background.

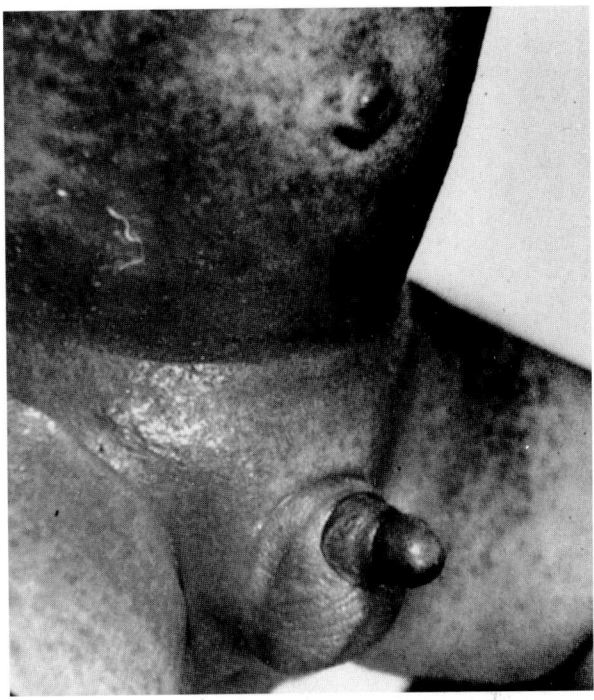

FIGURE 33.8. *Neonatal moniliasis of the diaper area.*

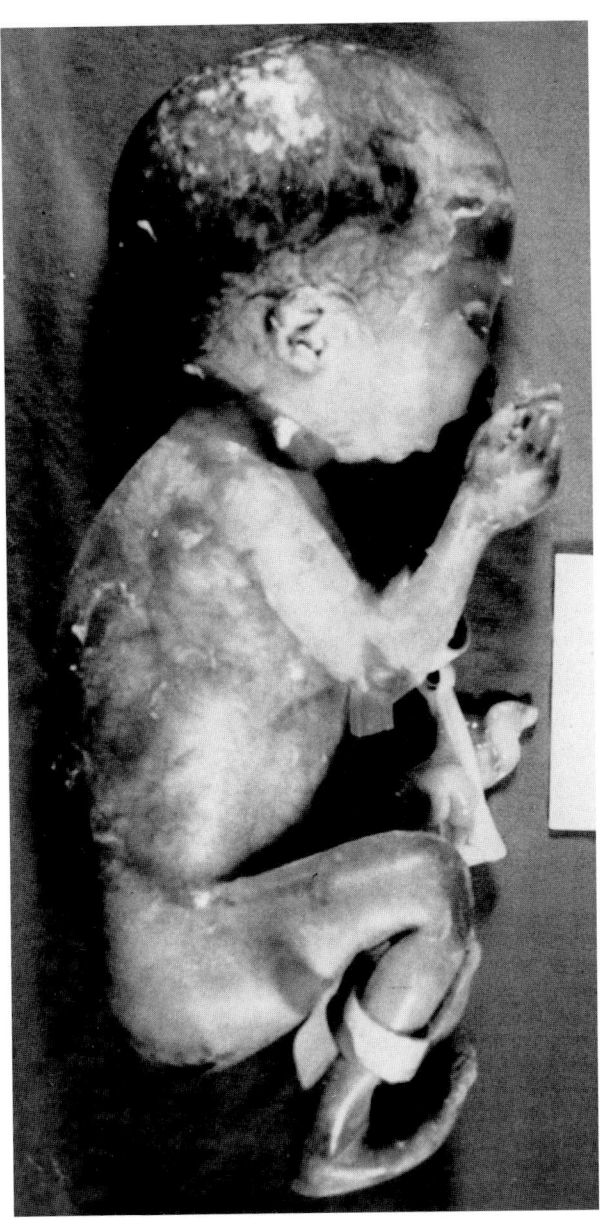

FIGURE 33.7. *Collodion baby with epidermolytic hyperkeratosis. This infant died at the age of 4 days, at which time the collodion membrane was beginning to peel around the neck and over the knees. This neonate shows evidence of a restrictive dermopathy with resulting flexion deformities.*

Milder Infectious Disorders

Candidiasis may be congenital or neonatal in onset. The congenital form is assumed to represent an ascending infection, already established prior to birth, while the neonatal form is acquired during passage through an infected birth canal, with clinical onset during the 2nd week postpartum. Congenital candidiasis is clinically detected at birth or within the first 12 hours as macules, papules, and vesicles on the face, chest, back, and extremities, unaccompanied by pyrexia [40]. Stool cultures are negative, and oral lesions are absent. Often there is a candidal chorioamnionitis [41]. A small proportion develop systemic candidiasis.

Neonatal candidiasis presents with typical oral thrush and extensive lesions in the diaper area, beginning as perianal vesicles and pustules (Fig. 33.8). The histopathology of both types of candidiasis is of subcorneal pustules containing pseudohyphae and spores.

Bullous impetigo neonatorum is a mild manifestation of skin infection with *Staphylococcus aureus*, occurring in the first 2 weeks of life, distributed in the diaper area, umbilicus, axillae, and neck. There are no systemic signs. Vesicles, pustules, and bullae develop on an erythematous base. Staphylococci of phage group II are usually isolated from these lesions, but all phage types may be found. Subcorneal pustules contain neutrophils and gram-positive cocci. Systemic spread may occur occasionally. These lesions denote the presence of staphylococci in the nursery, with the potential for epidemic but not serious infection in the newborn.

Serious Infectious Disorders

Staphylococcal Scalded Skin Syndrome

This disease has to be distinguished from toxic epidermal necrolysis (TEN), which occurs more often in adults, and is usually associated with antibiotic therapy or immunodeficiency. Staphylococcal scalded skin syndrome (SSS) primar-

Table 33.3.   Transient non-infectious disorders with good prognosis

Name	Age at Onset	Duration	Distribution	Lesions	Pathology
Acropustulosis of infancy [37]	Birth–10 mo	3 yr	Extremities	Red papules, evolving to pustular and vesicular over 24 hr	Subcorneal pustules, neutrophilic, occasionally eosinophilic
Erythema toxicum [38]	2–3 days	1 wk	Face, trunk, extremities	Red macules and papules; pink pustules and vesicles	Subcorneal eosinophilic pustules involving pilosebaceous apparatus; intradermal; inflammation
Miliaria crystallina	Within 7 days	Hours–days	Generalized	Clear superficial vesicles	Subcorneal vesicles associated with sweat ducts
Miliaria rubra	Within 7 days	Hours–days	Generalized	Grouped erythematous papules	Intraepidermal spongiosis; vesicles associated with sweat ducts
Transient neonatal pustular melanosis [39]	Birth–24 hr	3 mo	Head, neck, palms, and soles	Vesicles and papules desquamate to leave brown macules	Macules have basilar hyperpigmentation, intracorneal pustules, mixed infiltrate, mostly neutrophilic

ily affects children, including neonates, and is usually caused by staphylococcal colonizations or infections in non-cutaneous sites [42]. The skin disease is caused by liberation of an epidermolytic toxin which splits the epidermis at the level of the granular layer. Mucous membranes are not involved in SSS, but they are usually affected in TEN and erythema multiforme. It is thought that SSS occurs in young children because of inadequate renal clearance of the toxin. Clinical features are a generalized erythema, often leading to wrinkling and peeling of the superficial epidermis, large flaccid bullae, and eventual exfoliation. A septic focus may be found (conjunctiva, nasopharynx, stool, etc.), but the skin lesions themselves are sterile. The causative organism is *S. aureus*, group III most commonly, but group I occasionally. The cleavage plane is in the mid to upper epidermis, and this can be confirmed by frozen section of the roofs of the bullae [42], or by exfoliative cytology, which shows acantholytic cells. No inflammatory cells are present in the bulla walls or fluid, in contrast with TEN. Biopsy or cytological diagnosis is necessary because SSS should be treated with penicillinase-resistant penicillin analogues, whereas antibiotic therapy is contraindicated in TEN.

Other Infections

Several other bacterial and viral pathogens cause vesiculobullous lesions in the neonate. Of these, herpes simplex type 2 virus is numerically the most important in the present era of herpes genitalis [43]. Half of patients with neonatal herpes have skin manifestations; if not treated, half of these develop the severe sequelae of systemic herpes infection [44]. In vertex deliveries, the scalp is most commonly affected, and, conversely, the buttocks and perianal area are involved in breech-delivered neonates. Groups of tense vesicles develop on an erythematous base, but may progress to pustules and denudation. The Tzanck preparation is a poor method of diagnosis and newer fluorescent techniques are preferred. Herpes virus can also be diagnosed by cytopathic changes in tissue culture. Biopsy material is seldom seen.

Chronic Bullous Disorders (Epidermolysis Bullosa and Cutaneous Mastocytosis)

Epidermolysis Bullosa

EB is a heterogeneous group of genetically determined mechanobullous diseases in which trivial trauma causes blistering. Classification is complex, but is based on genetic, histological, and clinical parameters [45] (Table 33.4). There are 3 main histological types: non-scarring, epidermolytic (simplex) type with superficial planes of cleavage; junctional EB; and the scarring, dermolytic (dystrophic) type with dermal cleavage. The extent of distribution of bullae varies between the different disease entities, and some also involve the mucous membranes, thereby contributing significantly to morbidity and mortality. A simplified working classification of the principal subtypes of EB is given in Table 33.4 and the biochemical abnormalities underlying the subtypes of EB are now being determined. The spectrum of subtypes of EB will probably continue to increase.

Standard histological, ultrastructural, and antigenic studies can now be supplemented by the demonstration of mutations in 6 structural proteins in the 3 clinical subtypes of EB. In EBS, mutations have been discovered in the genes coding for keratins K14 and K5, which are expressed in basal epidermal cells (see Fig. 33.4).

The loss of normal keratin structure causes loss of stability of the basal cells, which vacuolate and lyse (Fig. 33.9). Clinical variants in the EBS groups have mutations in different domains of K14 and K5 [9, 46, 47]. Recessive EB simplex with late onset muscular dystrophy is associated with mutations in the plectin gene [47a].

In junctional EB, the structural abnormality is found in the anchoring filaments of the lamina lucida. These filaments contain laminin, a trimeric adhesion molecule that is ubiquitous to basement membranes. Many mutations have been found in the gene coding for the laminin component kallinin B2 [48, 49, 49a]. Laminin mutations in Herlitz type JEB involve premature chain termination, whereas those in

Table 33.4. Classification of epidermolysis bullosa (EB)

Disease	Inheritance	Onset	Clinical	Pathology/Histogenesis
EB simplex, localized (see Fig. 33.10b)	AD	Late childhood	Bullae of palms and soles, temperature-related?; not a serious disorder	Cytolysis of basal layer; suprabasal bullae
EB simplex, generalized (see Fig. 33.20)	AD	Neonatal	Widespread, most marked on extremities; mild mucosal and nail involvement, temperature-related?	As for EB simplex, localized; keratin 5/14 gene mutations
Recessive EB simplex with late onset muscular dystrophy	AR	Early	—	Plectrin gene mutations
Junctional EB, Herlitz variant	AR	Neonatal	Large erosions and granulation tissue, perioral and trunk; mouth and teeth involved; anemia and malnutrition; death usual at <2 yr	Subepidermal bullae above PAS-positive basement membrane; lamina lucida bullae; reduced hemidesmosomes by EM; laminin gene mutations
Junctional EB, generalized atrophic benign (GABEB)	AR	Neonatal	Serosanguineous blisters, temperature-related?; extremities most severe; nail dystrophy and mild mucosal involvement	As for junctional EB, Herlitz variant, laminin, COl7A1; laminin gene mutations
Junctional EB with pyloric atresia	AR	—	—	Mutations in β4 integrin gene
Dominant dermolytic EB, Cockayne-Touraine variant	AD	Early infancy	Generalized, most severe over bony prominences; dystrophic nails; healing by scarring; normal teeth; not life-threatening	Cleavage below basal lamina; decreased anchoring fibrils limited to bullous areas
Dominant dermolytic EB, Pasini variant	AD	Neonatal	Generalized, most marked on extremities; atrophic scarring; normal life span	Generalized abnormality of anchoring fibrils
Recessive dermolytic EB (see Fig. 33.10)	AR	Neonatal	Localized and generalized forms; bullae result in scarring, nail dystrophy and loss, fusion of digits (mitten deformity), flexural contractures, and esophageal, conjunctival, corneal, and urethral lesions; raised serum CEA; poor nutrition, anemia; reduced life expectancy	Cleavage below basal lamina; dermal collagen degeneration; generalized reduction in anchoring fibrils; type VII collagen gene mutations

AD = autosomal dominant; AR = autosomal recessive; CEA = carcinoembryonic antigen; PAS = periodic acid–Schiff; EM = electron microscopy.

GABEB are usually mis-sense mutations. The majority of cases of GABEB, however, are found to have mutations in the gene coding for bullous pemphigoid antigen 2 (BPAG2), also known as collagen type XVII [49b]. A further clinical subtype of JEB is associated with pyloric atresia and is attributable to mutations in the integrin β4 gene [50].

In dermolytic (dystrophic) EB (Fig. 33.10), mutations have been found in the genes coding for type VII collagen, a major constituent of the anchoring fibrils of the superficial dermis [51–54].

Mastocytosis

Cutaneous mastocytosis can present in 3 main clinical forms in the neonate: solitary mastocytosis, generalized urticaria pigmentosa, and diffuse cutaneous mastocytosis. It is a feature of these diseases that all 3 often display vesicular or bullous variants, presumably because of histamine-induced transudates. The basis of clinical diagnosis is Darier's urtication sign.

In solitary mastocytosis, patients have 1 lesion or a few isolated lesions that usually regress within a few years. They occur most frequently on the wrists, neck, and trunk, and are elevated light brown or tan plaques that may blister. Biopsy or excision is usually considered unnecessary [55].

Urticaria pigmentosa is the most common form of mastocytosis in childhood, and may have a dramatic presentation at birth, with generalized hyperpigmented macules, bullae, and erosions [56]. The prognosis is good.

Diffuse cutaneous mastocytosis is uncommon. The dermis is infiltrated by mast cells to such an extent that it becomes thickened and boggy, as well as pigmented. There is usually extensive bulla formation in the neonate, and there may also be signs of systemic histamine effects. In addition, there may be systemic mastocytosis, and the mortality from diffuse cutaneous mastocytosis is high [57].

The histological appearances are well known and are not discussed in detail here (Fig. 33.11). There are abnormal accumulations of dermal mast cells, and these infiltrations are particularly dense in neonates. Metachromatic stains are used to demonstrate the histamine granules. Ultrastructural studies are not usually necessary, but a familial type of

(a)

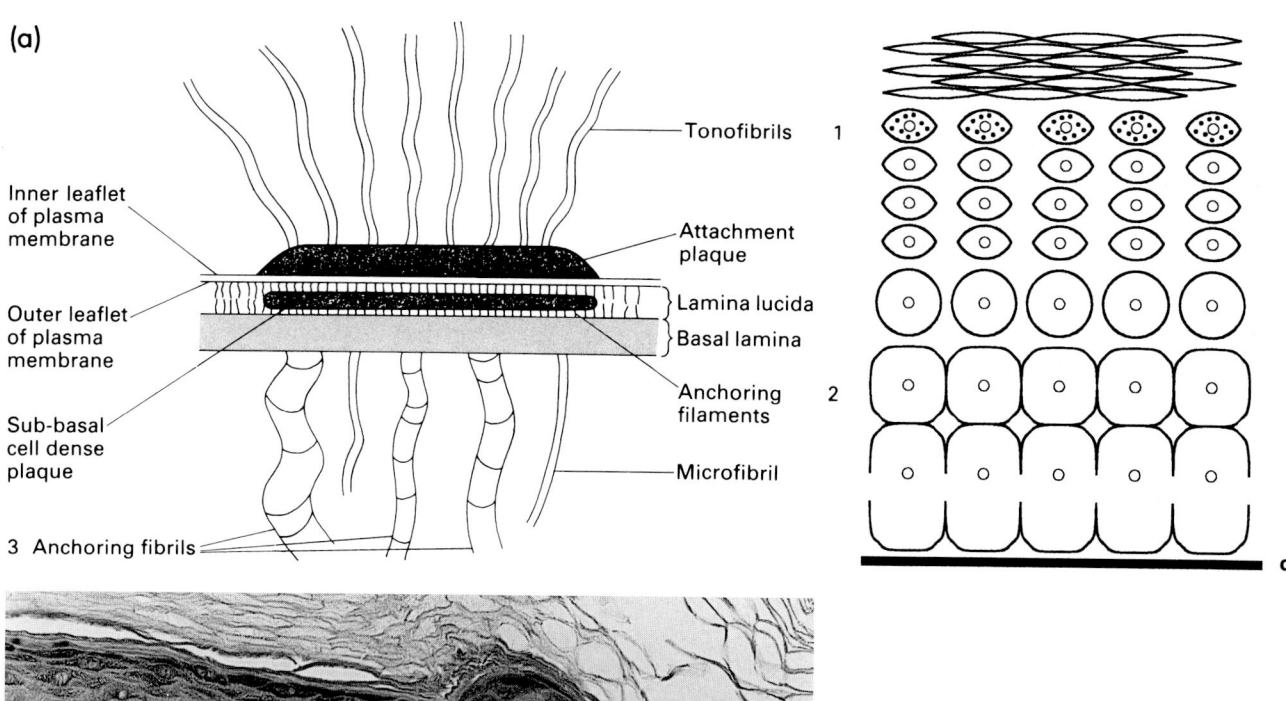

Tonofibrils

Inner leaflet of plasma membrane

Attachment plaque

Outer leaflet of plasma membrane

Lamina lucida

Basal lamina

Sub-basal cell dense plaque

Anchoring filaments

Microfibril

3 Anchoring fibrils

1

2

d

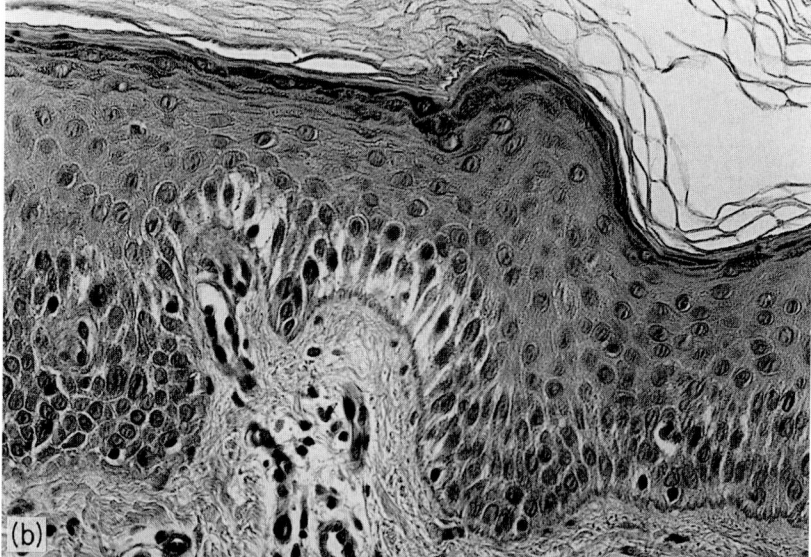

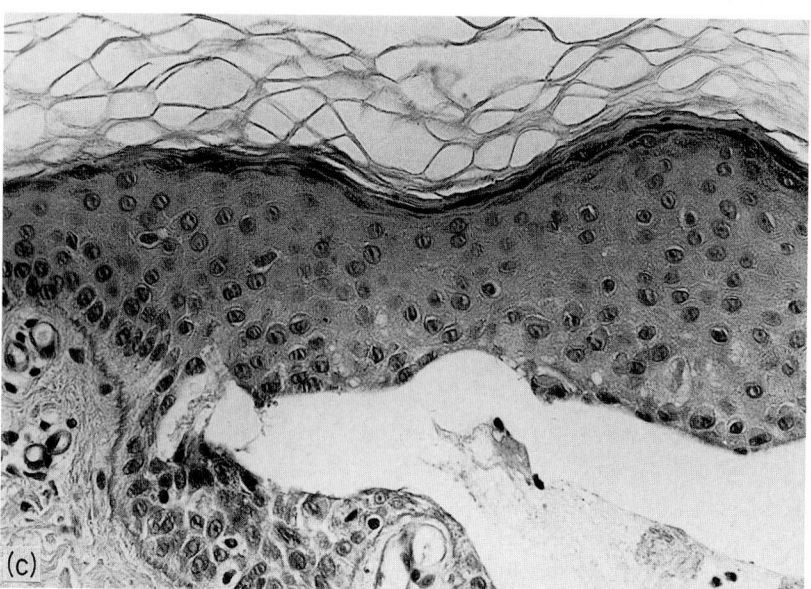

FIGURE 33.9. (a) Diagrammatic representation of the cleavage planes in the various subtypes of epidermolysis bullosa (EB). 1, intraepidermal splitting in EB simplex, localized and generalized; 2, reduced or absent anchoring fibrils in junctional EB; 3, abnormal collagen and/or collagenase activity in the dermolytic types of EB. (b) Early intraepidermal separation in generalized EB simplex. H&E, ×400. (c) Intraepidermal bulla formation in the same patient. H&E, ×400. (d) Mutations involve keratins K5 and K14, expressed in the basal layer.

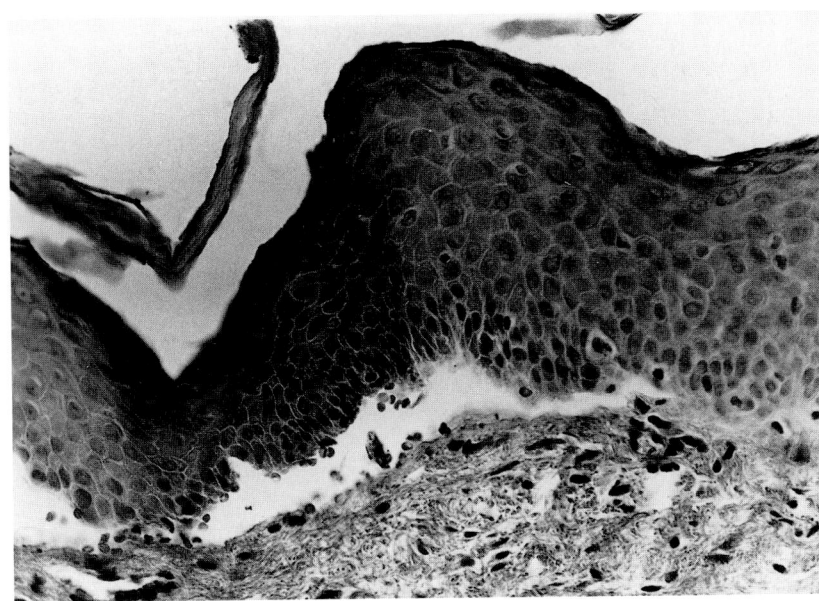

FIGURE 33.10. *Dermolytic bulla in recessive dermolytic epidermolysis bullosa. H&E, ×400.*

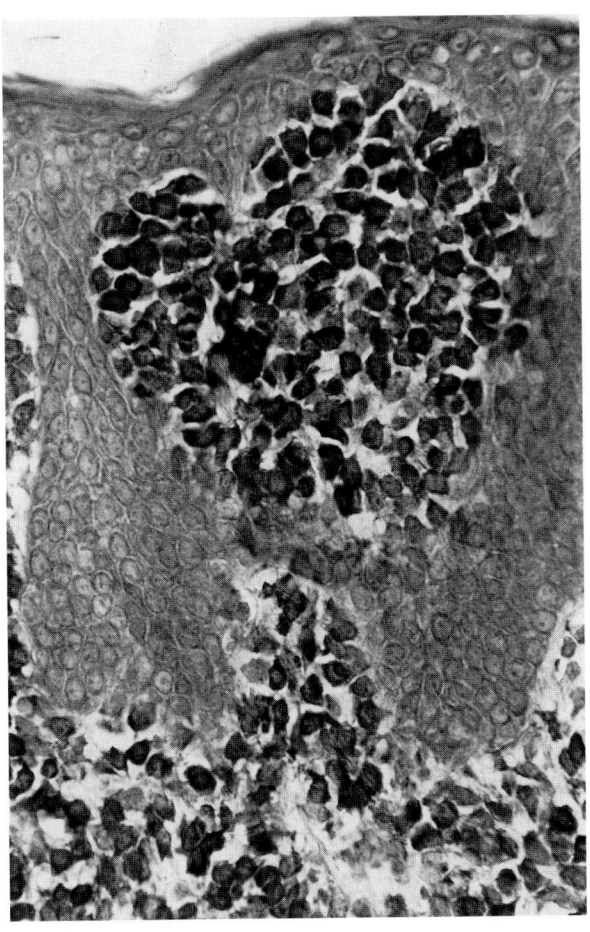

FIGURE 33.11. *Urticaria pigmentosa. The arrows indicate groups of mast cells around skin appendages and venules. H&E, ×100.*

urticaria pigmentosa has been described in which there are giant mast cell granules [58].

The etiology and pathogenesis of most cases of cutaneous mastocytosis are not known.

HAMARTOMATOUS DISORDERS

General Considerations

Hamartomas are errors of development resulting in the presence of abnormal mixtures of tissues appropriate to the part, often with excess of more than 1 component. While generally distinct from neoplasms, hamartomas may ultimately give rise to neoplasms; alternatively, both neoplasms and hamartomas may be expressions of abnormal maturation of tissues. One of the major concerns of the histopathologist is to predict the likelihood of the supervention of neoplasia in patients with certain histological patterns of hamartomas or hamartomatoses, particularly the congenital nevocytic nevi.

Skin hamartomas are of many types, including nevocytic nevi, keratinocytic (epidermal) and organoid ectodermal nevi, the various angiomas, and connective tissue nevi. Nevocellular nevi occur in 1.0–1.4% of neonates [59].

Pigmented Nevi

Congenital nevocellular nevi (CNN) are a focus of current interest and debate for 4 main reasons:

1. Classification by size may give indications of malignant potential; this is now a matter of great dispute. Obviously, size is also important in terms of feasibility of surgical resection.

2. The anatomical distribution of nevus cells in CNN is generally reported to be quite different from that seen in acquired nevi. This may be an expression of an abnormal centrifugal migration of neural crest rather than of the more commonly seen centripetal "dropping down" of nevocytes into the dermis as the result of junctional activity in the basal epidermal layer. This abnormal migration could also explain the frequent occurrence of deep dermal, subcutaneous, or other origins of neoplasia in association with the larger CNNs.

3. There is an association between giant CNN and leptomeningeal melanosis and malignant melanoma, a condition best considered as a phakomatosis. This association may be related to the abnormal migration just discussed.

4. Giant CNN appear to show evidence of "metastasis," with spontaneous regression. They therefore fall within the "oncogenic period of grace" [60].

CNN are fully formed early in gestation, as shown by the "divided" nevus of the eyelids [61] and of the fingers [62]. Studies of the prevalence of CNN are often flawed by a lack of adequate biopsy studies, since it is clear that the majority of pigmented hamartomas are not actually CNN. The survey by Alper and Holmes [59] involved over 4500 consecutive newborns, and gave a 1.1% prevalence of clinical CNN. The large survey by Castilla et al [63] involved 530,000 neonates, but the clinical ascertainment rate was variable between the different hospitals. In the best-monitored institution, the prevalence was 1.0%. This survey was of most value in ascertaining the 0.005% prevalence of CNN exceeding 10 cm in diameter.

Appropriate classification of pigmented nevi by size is accomplished using several different systems, making it difficult to compare reports. Most authors agree that small CNN (SCNN) are less than 2–3 cm in diameter, while giant CNN (GCNN) are recognized by their covering a very large anatomical area in the pattern of a garment, bathing trunk, vest, cape, coat sleeve, or stocking distribution. GCNN are sometimes unilateral, stopping at the midline, but often appear to have their origin in the midline. Lesions intermediate between SCNN and GCNN are vaguely termed *large*, and the SCNN and "large" CNN are the subject of lively dispute with regard to management from the point of view of malignant potential. In general terms, SCNN are removable by excision under local anesthesia, while the larger CNN require serial excision, often with the use of flap or graft techniques.

Although the potential for malignancy in GCNN is well recognized, the relatively much higher prevalence of SCNN could imply that they make a larger contribution to the development of malignant melanoma in children and adults. However, the premalignant status of SCNN is certainly not accepted by all authors. The risk of malignancy in GCNN is calculated as a minimum of 6% over a lifetime [64]. What gives urgency to the treatment of GCNN is the fact that malignancy supervenes at a surprisingly early age. The cumulative age risk for malignancy, based on 3 reports of literature surveys involving 58 cases [64–66] in which malignant change was documented in GCNN, is shown in Figure 33.12.

Estimates of the risk of malignancy in SCNN are based

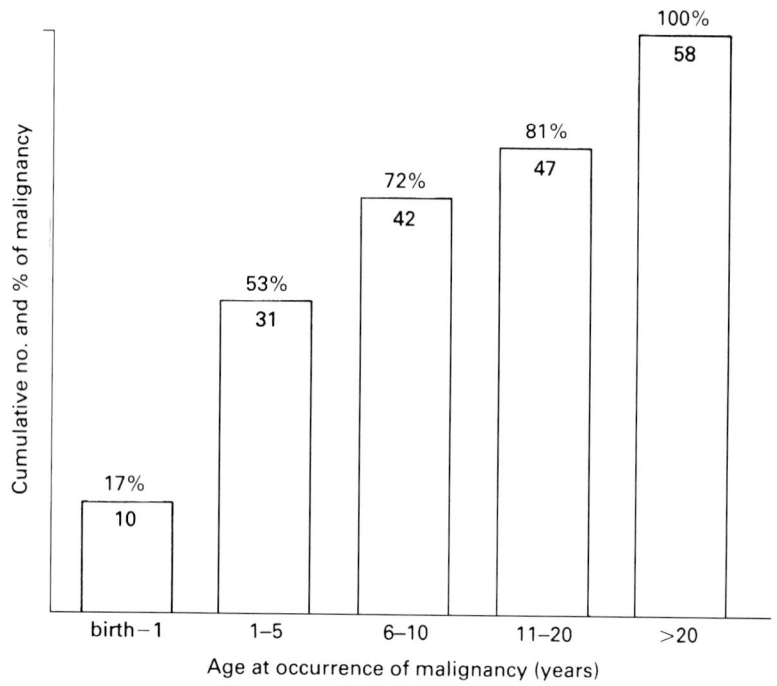

FIGURE 33.12. *Cumulative risk of development of malignancy in giant congenital nevocellular nevi (GCNN), analyzed by age (years) at onset of malignancy. About 6% of all patients with GCNN develop malignancy in a lifetime. This bar graph shows that more than 50% of these malignancies occur by the age of 5 years, indicating the need for early surgery.*

on indirect evidence in the absence of a prolonged prospective study. Criteria depending on a history of SCNN prior to the development of malignant melanoma, and of the presence of histological evidence of preexisting SCNN in or around overt malignant melanoma suggest that the risk of melanoma arising in SCNN is 10 to 20 times that in the general population [67].

It seems that at present the majority view favors the excision of small and large CNN in addition to GCNN, on the grounds that prevention should be highly effective [68, 69]. The relative risk of melanoma in different sizes of CNN may simply relate to the number of nevocytes (or stem cells) present in the lesions; as has been stated [69], there is no reason to suppose that CNN of different sizes are of different biological origin or behavior, and preventative treatment would seem appropriate and probably cost-effective when there are few reliable prospective data on CNN other than GCNN.

CNN are reported to have special histological features that distinguish them from acquired nevi. Classic histological appearances of CNN were described by Mark et al [70]:

1. The presence of nevus cells in the lower reticular dermis in the great majority of patients, and in the subcutis in more than 50% of patients. The papillary dermis is relatively less involved (Fig. 33.13a).
2. Distribution of nevus cells in an Indian file distribution between collagen bundles.
3. Distribution of nevus cells in the adventitia around skin appendages of the deep dermis and subcutis

(Fig. 33.13b). There may be marked neuroid differentiation.

These features were present in CNN of all sizes. The epidermal components of CNN do not differ from those of acquired nevocytic nevi. Blue nevi and areas of cartilage occur in a minority of GCNN [65].

Two features are important in the histopathology of malignancies arising on the basis of CNN. Such lesions are often deep (i.e., not epidermal), so that they can arise in subcutaneous tissues subsequent to the deep resection of CNN [64]. For this reason it is important to pay attention to the deep resection margins when reporting CNN; it has been recommended that resection of CNN should proceed as far as the fascia. A number of key questions concerning the histological appearance of CNN and its evolution to malignancy were reviewed authoritatively [71].

Neoplasms arising from GCNN are frequently not classic melanomas; in a series of 7 GCNN, Hendrickson and Ross [72] reported only 1 typical melanoma; other neoplasms included malignant cellular blue nevus and undifferentiated spindle cell, lipoblastic, rhabdomyoblastic, and atypical epithelioid lesions. The authors emphasized that the origin of melanoblasts from neural crest could explain the development of a number of neuroectodermal-ectomesenchymal neoplasms in the context of GCNN. GCNN of the cape or cloak distribution may be accompanied by leptomeningeal melanosis, which can be demonstrated by computed tomography (CT). This melanosis can affect intracranial and spinal meninges. Malignant melanoma may supervene in the meninges [73].

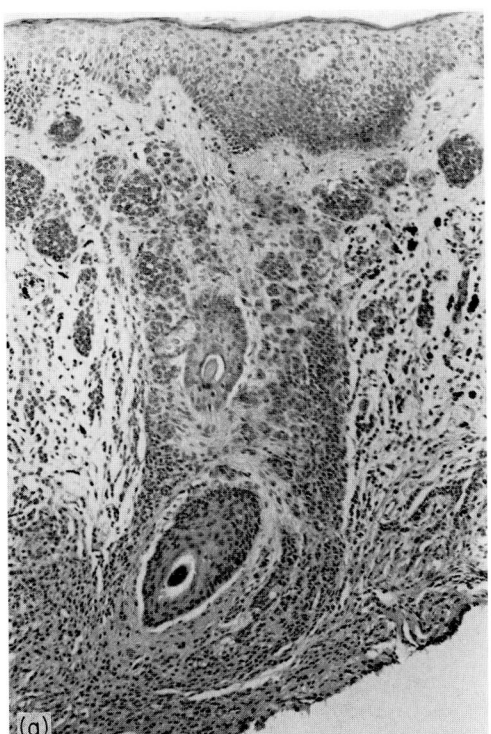

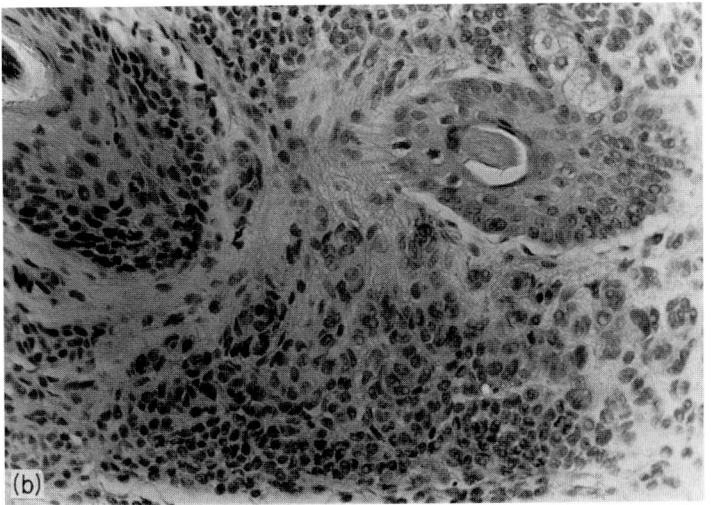

FIGURE 33.13.   *Congenital nevocellular nevus. (a) Low-power view shows sparing of epidermis and papillary dermis. H&E, ×25. (b) Typical distribution around skin appendages. H&E, ×400.*

Metastases from GCNN have been found in the chorionic villi of the placenta, furnishing evidence of prenatal metastatic behavior where clinical and histological findings did not show evidence of malignancy in the GCNN itself [74]. This phenomenon may simply represent maturation of the primary lesion, as is well known in neuroblastoma. Placental metastases may be regarded as melanoma "stage IVP," with good prognosis.

Congenital pigmented nevi occur in a number of syndromes, including Carney syndrome (with cardiac and cutaneous myxomas and endocrine abnormalities), premature aging syndromes, occult spinal dysraphism with tethering of the cord, and probably, neurofibromatosis type I [75].

Metastatic melanoma to the fetus can occur from maternal primary malignant melanoma. Trozak et al [66] validated 3 cases from the literature, of which the case of Brodsky et al [76] is the best documented. Multiple cutaneous metastases developed in the neonatal period, with death from melanomatosis occurring at the age of 48 days. Metastases were present in the maternal vascular spaces of the placenta.

Dysplastic nevus syndrome is not present in the neonate, and is not discussed here. Blue nevi are seldom present at birth, but in 1 case a very large occipital blue nevus caused dystocia and intrapartum death [77].

Lentigines may be present at birth or soon after (Fig. 33.14), whether or not they are a component of the multiple lentigines syndrome [78]. As with other phakomatoses, lentiginosis often respects the midline and is associated with other congenital dysplasias [79].

Dermal melanocytes are found in a number of congenital pigmented lesions apart from CNN and blue nevi. Other entities include the nevi of Ota [80] and of Ito [81], and mongolian blue spots.

Several chromosome abnormalities in hypomelanosis of Ito have recently been documented, in geographic patterns of somatic mosaicism. These include trisomy 18 [82], ring chromosome 22 [83], and X ring [84]. Various balanced autosomal translocations, triploidy mosaicism, ring 5 and ring 14, and upper X (autosomal) translocations have been found in pigmentary dysplasias.

Café au lait spots may be present at birth, and are well recognized as components of neurocutaneous syndromes, notably neurofibromatosis [85] and tuberous sclerosis [86].

Angiomatous Hamartomas

These lesions are less frequently sampled by biopsy than are nevocytic nevi, do not have malignant potential, and do not necessarily show good clinicopathological correlations. However, cutaneous hemangiomas are sometimes components of extensive or generalized neonatal hemangiomatosis; they may also be complicated by the development of Kasabach-Merritt syndrome.

Hemangiomas are classifed clinically as follows:

Flat Vascular Nevi, Involuting

1. Salmon patch occurs in over 40% of neonates, in the nape of the neck, midforehead, glabella, and upper eyelids. It is of no clinical significance.
2. Cutis marmorata telangiectatica congenita. This reticulate skin lesion may be localized or generalized. It generally fades with time. Fifty percent of patients have other anomalies, including hemihypertrophy, port-wine stains, other angiomas, and aplasia cutis congenita [87]. The skin appears bluish and mottled, and there may be ulceration. Examination of biopsy specimens shows dilated capillaries and veins in dermis and subcutis.

Flat Vascular Nevi, Non-involuting (Port-Wine Stain)

This lesion is often unilateral, respecting the midline, or else

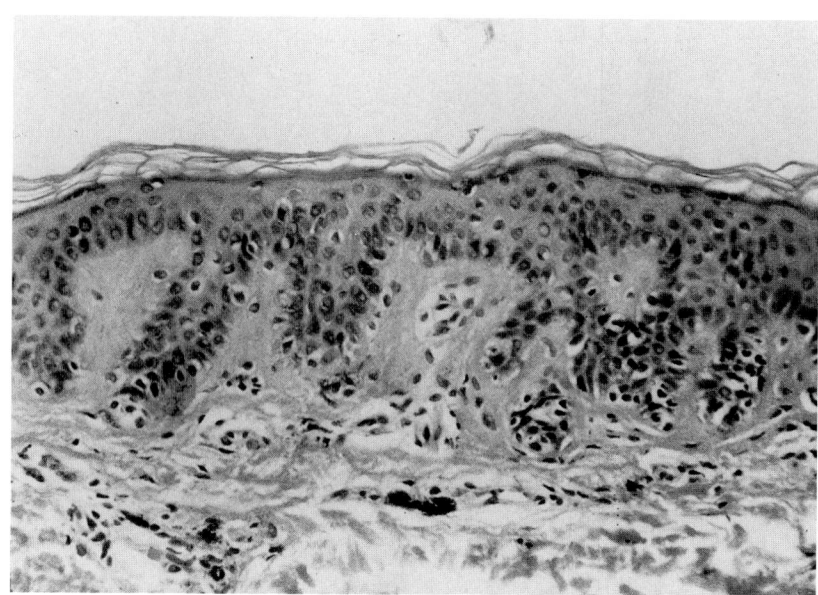

FIGURE 33.14.   *Multiple lentigines in a neonate with LEOPARD syndrome. There is an increase of pigmented cells in the epidermal basal layer, with considerable pigmentary incontinence. H&E, ×100.*

segmental, most commonly on the face and neck. At the time of birth, the lesion is light pink, but assumes its typical blue or purple hue later. It occurs in 0.3% of neonates. The histopathological basis for port-wine stains is the presence of dilated capillaries in the dermis. Connective tissue proliferation also occurs when the lesion is accompanied by overgrowth of a limb. Port-wine stains in the distribution of the ophthalmic division of the trigeminal nerve are associated with involvement of the leptomeninges and choroid vessels, leading to contralateral seizures and hemiplegia, together with ipsilateral congenital glaucoma (Sturge-Weber syndrome). The embryological rationale for this syndrome is the common origin of the vascular supply of the meninges, choroid, and skin of the scalp and upper face from a primordial superficial vascular plexus [88].

Raised Vascular Nevi, Involuting

The natural history of the "strawberry" type of nevus is well known. The lesion is present in 10% of neonates, and is first seen as a pink macule. There is no marked proliferation until the early months of infancy. Biopsy specimens show marked endothelial hyperplasia, a disturbingly high mitotic rate, and characteristic basement membrane thickening.

Raised Vascular Nevi, Non-involuting

The verrucous hemangioma has a characteristic combination of papillomatous epidermal hyperplasia and superficial dermal hemangioma [89]. All other angiomas in this class are lymphangiomas or hemangiolymphangiomas. Four clinical types are described: 1) Simple lymphangiomas are uncommon; they are solitary dermal or subdermal swellings. 2) Lymphangioma circumscriptum is the most common type, and is seen in the neck, tongue, buccal mucosa, and proximal areas of the limbs. 3) Cavernous lymphangiomas are diffuse, ill-defined cystic dilatations in dermis, subcutaneous tissue, and intermuscular septa. In all cases, the spaces are lined by endothelium, and the contents appear histologically as coagulated protein. Interstitial collections of lymphocytes may be present. The significance of nuchal cystic hygromas in prenatal diagnosis has been discussed [90].

Complications and Associations of Vascular Nevi

Klippel-Trenaunay syndrome consists of port-wine stains and limb hypertrophy, present at birth [91]. Maffucci syndrome includes hemangiomas, lymphangiomas, and dyschondroplasia, but is not generally apparent at birth [92].

In blue rubber bleb syndrome, compressible blue subcutaneous nodules appear. They may be multiple, often bleed easily, and can cause serious anemia [93].

Kasabach-Merritt syndrome can occur in any clinical subtype of hemangioma of considerable extent, including hemangiomatosis (see below). There is consumptive coagulopathy, with entrapment thrombocytopenia. Ecchymoses may be localized around the hemangioma or become more

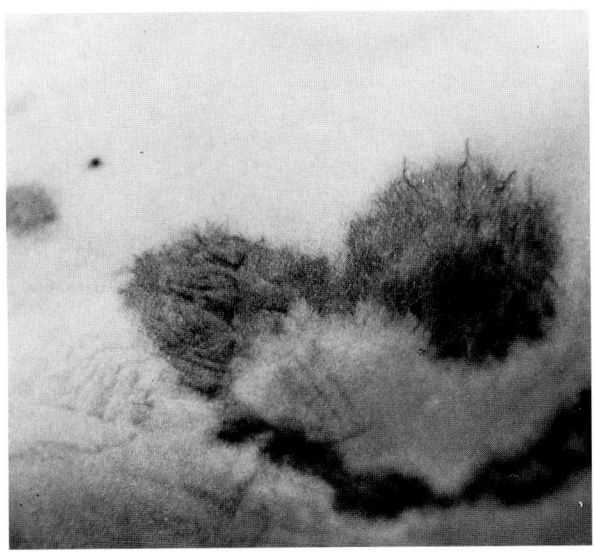

FIGURE 33.15.   *Anterior abdominal wall skin hemangiomatosis in a newborn who had ascites diagnosed prenatally by ultrasound. He developed Kasabach-Merritt syndrome. Extensive gastrointestinal hemangiomatosis was found at laparotomy, but the liver was not involved.*

generalized. Acute hemorrhage and space occupation can occur in the hemangioma or at any other site [94].

Riley-Day syndrome consists of macrocephaly, unusual cutaneous angiomatosis, and pseudopapilledema [95].

In Cobb syndrome there is a variety of cutaneous vascular nevi with associated spinal cord angioma [96]. The disease is a spinal equivalent of Sturge-Weber syndrome.

Diffuse or disseminated and eruptive hemangiomatosis is a dangerous disease in the newborn infant. It affects the skin, liver, gastrointestinal canal, lungs, and central nervous system [97] (Fig. 33.15). Cutaneous manifestations are disseminated, raised, small bright red lesions, usually numbering in the hundreds, but even the presence of a single eruptive hemangioma should cause concern about the possibility of hemangiomatosis. However, it should be recognized that there are cases in which skin only is affected (benign eruptive hemangiomatosis) [98], and also instances in which cutaneous involvement is absent but visceral hemangiomatosis is extensive (usually involving the liver). Hepatomegaly combined with cutaneous hemangiomas makes the diagnosis of disseminated eruptive hemangiomatosis highly likely. The mortality rate for untreated patients has been reported as 95%. Complications include high-output cardiac failure, cerebral hemorrhage, and Kasabach-Merritt syndrome. Hepatic artery ligation has been used successfully to control cardiac failure.

Epidermal and Organoid Nevi

This group of disorders has a confusing terminology, probably resulting from attempts to split these hamartomas artificially into small groups of distinct entities [99]. They are important because they may be components of phako-matoses and because early removal of the skin lesions may preempt the later development of adenomas and low-grade malignant lesions.

Epidermoid Neoplasms

Purely epidermal nevi may be thought of as hamartomas of the keratin, with little or no contribution from the skin appendages. In effect, they are localized hyperplasias of the epidermis, but there are undoubtedly considerable dermal contributions, since the nevi are fibroepithelial in character. They may be single (nevus verrucosus, Fig. 33.16), multiple, or widespread; sometimes may be linear; sometimes apparently may follow dermatoses or respect the midline (nevus unius lateris); or have a component of EH, thereby qualifying for the term *ichthyosis hystrix* (see ichthyosis section). In the neonate, epidermal nevi are flesh-colored or brown, with a velvety or granular surface. Whatever their distribution, they consist histologically of epidermal hyperplasia with papillary proliferation of the dermis but without an adnexal component. The inflammatory linear verrucous epidermal nevus appears as a linear, dermatitic, scaling, and erythematous lesion with histological components of focal hypergranulosis and hyperkeratosis alternating with focal loss of granular layer and parakeratosis [100].

Verrucous nevi may show chromosomal mosaicism [101].

The epidermal nevus syndrome [102] consists of a rather wide variety of anomalies, including kyphoscoliosis, vertebral defects, hemihypertrophy, phocomelia, skin angiomas, coarctation of the aorta, central nervous system involvement by angiomas and neoplasms, mental retardation, hydrocephalus, and seizures.

Supervention of carcinoma is reportedly rare in epidermal nevi, but basal cell carcinomas do occur.

Organoid nevi involve the epidermis and also adnexal structures such as pilosebaceous apparatus, and eccrine and apocrine sweat glands. Nevus sebaceus of Jadassohn is a hairless, yellowish circumscribed plaque with a flat velvety appearance. Prominent sebaceous gland proliferation does

not occur until puberty. In the neonate, the histological features resemble those of the pure epidermal nevus; that is, there is papillary epidermal proliferation. However, the hair follicles show poorly developed hair bulbs, and there may be an excess of sebaceous glands. The natural history of nevus sebaceus includes the development in adulthood of overt skin adnexal adenomas and carcinomas in about 10% of lesions [103] (Fig. 33.17). Excision prior to puberty is therefore the appropriate treatment.

The linear sebaceous nevus syndrome has been extensively reported [104]. Midline (often nasal tip) sebaceous nevi are strongly associated with widespread visceral malformations (leptomeningeal hemangioma, congenital heart disease, urinary tract malformations and nephroblastomatosis, hydrocephalus, vitamin D–resistant rickets, coloboma and ocular dermoids, seizures, and mental retardation), as well as with non-cutaneous neoplasms (acute lymphoblastic leukemia, rhabdomyosarcoma, ameloblastoma). The spectrum of these anomalies overlaps with that of linear epidermal nevus syndrome, but also has some unique features.

Nevus comedonicus is a rare organoid hamartoma in which grouped hair follicles are filled with horny plugs; half of the cases are congenital. Linear bands of comedones are found on the face, neck, upper arms, or trunk. Sweat gland adenomas may develop. The nevus comedonicus syndrome involves neurological, skeletal, and ocular defects [105].

Becker's nevus is a rather complex organoid hamartoma composed of mild hyperkeratosis, heavily pigmented basal cells, hyperplasia of hair follicles with large sebaceous glands, and proliferation of smooth muscle bundles; lesions may be present at birth [106]. The congenital pilar and smooth muscle nevus is a closely related entity [107].

A number of nevi of connective tissue (other than angiomas) are known as components of phakomatoses (e.g., tuberous sclerosis) [108]. Large lipomatous hamartomas are observed in the newborn [109].

ECTODERMAL DYSPLASIAS

This large group of over 150 dysplastic disorders includes 2 or more of the following components:

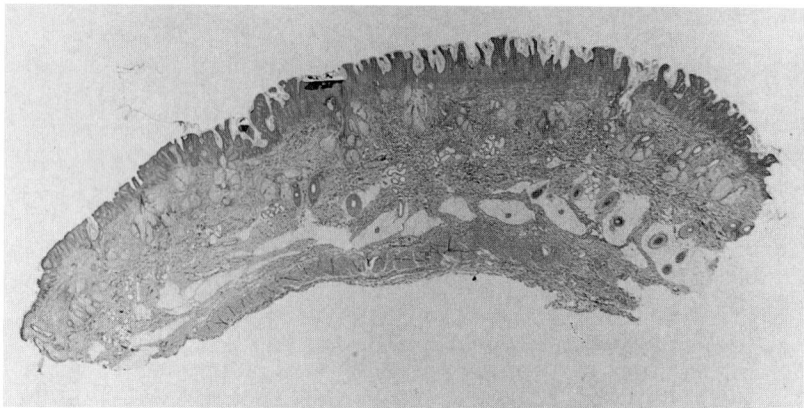

FIGURE 33.16.   *Nevus verrucosus type of epidermal nevus. ×6 life size, approximately.*

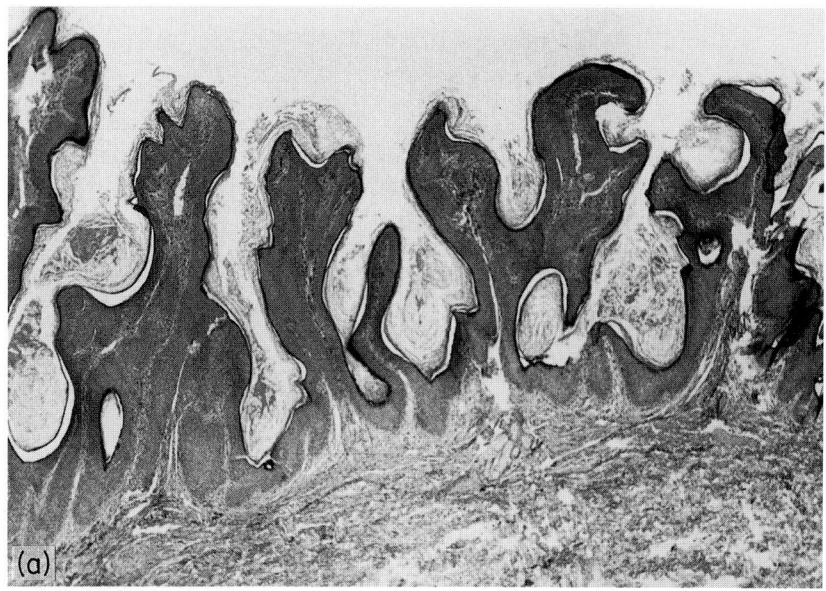

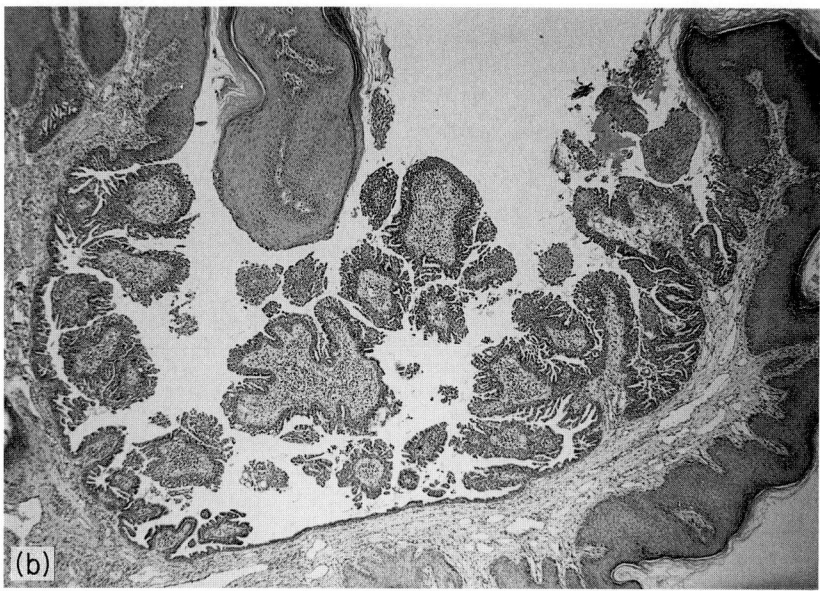

FIGURE 33.17. *Nevus sebaceus of the scalp in a newborn with linear sebaceous nevus syndrome. (a) At this stage, there is squamous papillomatosis only. H&E, ×100. (b) At the age of 6, this mentally retarded child developed a syringocystadenoma papilliferum in an extensive linear sebaceous scalp nevus. H&E, ×100.*

1. Trichodysplasia
2. Dental defects
3. Onychodysplasia
4. Dyshidrosis

These disorders are congenital and non-progressive and involve the whole skin surface [110, 111, 111a].

The consequences of trichodysplasia are sparse or absent eyebrows and eyelashes, with congenital baldness; the dental defects include absent or reduced deciduous and permanent teeth, abnormally shaped teeth, and accelerated dental caries. Onychodysplasia causes split nails. Dyshidrosis results in dry skin and neonatal hyperthermia. In some forms of anhidrotic ectodermal dysplasia, mucous glands of the pharynx and respiratory tract may be absent, and, as might

be expected, mammary glands and nipples are also absent. The histopathology varies according to how many of the 4 components are present. In most patients, there is hypoplasia of the pilosebaceous apparatus. In addition, patients with anhidrotic ectodermal dysplasia have severe hypoplasia or complete absence of eccrine sweat glands [112]. The first gene mutation in anhidrotic ectodermal dysplasia was recently reported [112a]. From the clinical standpoint, the ectodermal dysplasia diseases often include mental deficiency, hyperpigmentation, polydactyly, syndactyly, and deafness. It has been suggested that these diseases be classified according to how many of the 4 components are present [110]:

Components 1, 2, 3, and 4: 23 diseases, including focal

dermal hypoplasia (Goltz-Gorlin), dyskeratosis congenita, ectrodactyly–ectodermal dysplasia–clefting syndrome, Kid syndrome (see ichthyosis section), and hypomelanosis of Ito
Components 1, 2, and 3: 20 diseases, including Rothmund-Thomsom syndrome, incontinentia pigmenti, and Ellis–van Creveld syndrome

If this principle of classification is accepted, there are at present over 150 disease entities in the ectodermal dysplasia group. The following entities are of some importance: Goltz-Gorlin disease (focal dermal hypoplasia, X-linked dominant) is characterized by soft, fluctuant areas of herniation of subcutaneous fat covered by very thin cutis. There are also reticular areas of pigmentary change, and papillomas may be present. Additional features include syndactyly, polydactyly, oligodactyly, facial asymmetry, and anophthalmia [113]. The histopathological appearances are of a dermal defect, with accumulation of adult adipocytes that are only separated from the epidermis by a thin band of dermis.

The histopathological appearance of the skin in dyskeratosis congenita (X-linked recessive) is non-specific, with hydropic degeneration of basal epidermal cells, telangiectasia of superficial dermal capillaries, and homogenization of collagen. Clinical features include leukokeratosis of the oral mucosa, ectropion, urogenital anomalies, complete heart block, and Fanconi-type anemia. There is a high risk of blood dyscrasia and squamous carcinoma [114].

Hypomelanosis of Ito (neurocutaneous form) presents with pigmentary loss in early infancy, seizures, and skeletal abnormalities. The distribution of hypopigmentation is similar to the pattern of hyperpigmentation seen in incontinentia pigmenti. There is a reduction or complete loss of melanin granules in the basal layer, but there is a less than complete loss of dendritic melanocytes [115].

Rothmund-Thomson syndrome (poikiloderma congenitale) consists of early erythema of the cheeks, later developing into telangiectasia and mottled hyperpigmentation and hypopigmentation. There is dwarfism and hypogonadism. Skin histopathology consists of hydropic degeneration of the basal layer with pigmentary incontinence [116].

Incontinentia pigmenti (Bloch-Sulzberger syndrome) presents in the neonatal period with linear erythematous and vesiculobullous eruptions of the limbs and trunk. The later pigmentary changes do not follow the linear arrangement of the original lesions. Non-cutaneous manifestations include microcephaly, mental retardation, and epilepsy. The vesicobullous lesions are intraepidermal, arising from spongiosis. Large, dyskeratotic cells are seen in the non-spongiotic epidermis. Inheritance is X-linked dominant with male lethality [117].

Patients with Ellis-van Creveld syndrome have short-limbed dwarfism, polydactyly, congenital heart disease, and ectodermal dysplasia. The syndrome is autosomal recessive and has been studied extensively in the Amish [118].

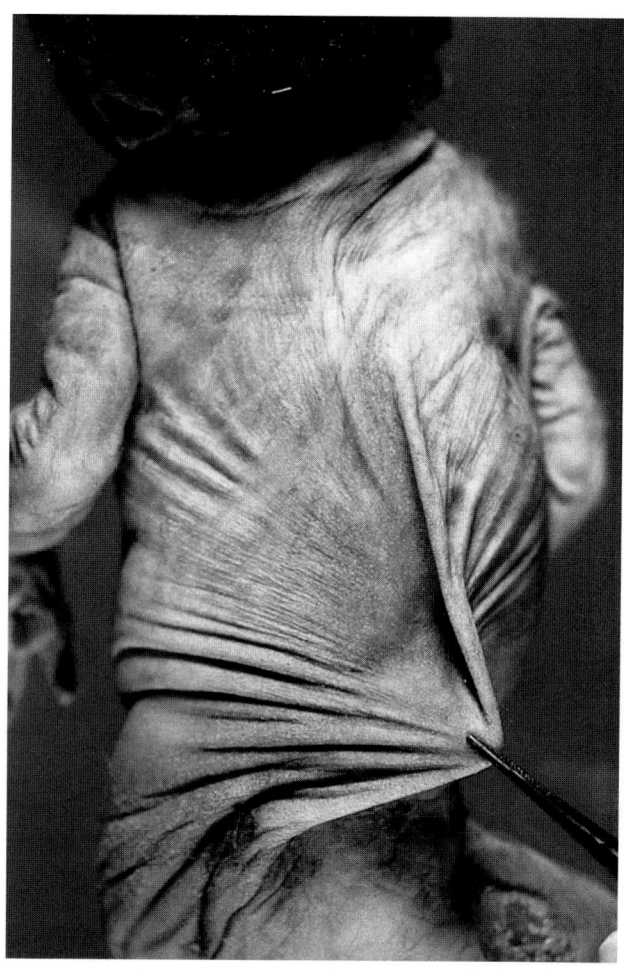

FIGURE 33.18.   *Newborn infant with cutis laxa, dorsal view. After stretching, the skin retracts very slowly.*

SOME MISCELLANEOUS FETAL AND NEONATAL SKIN DISORDERS

Cutis Laxa

Cutis laxa (generalized elastolysis) is very rare (Fig. 33.18). The skin is inelastic (compare with Ehlers-Danlos syndrome), and hangs loosely and pendulously, resulting in a prematurely aged appearance. A severe autosomal recessive type [119] results in a congenital "bloodhound" appearance, and is associated with emphysema, gastrointestinal diverticular disease, rectal prolapse, and hernias. The pathogenesis of the disease is not fully understood, but there is a diminution of elastic fibers in the dermis, and those that are present are thickened at the midportion, and appear granular throughout their length [119]. It has been proposed that these patients lack an elastase inhibitor, but there is no recent work on this topic. In an X-linked recessive form of cutis laxa, there is defective cross-linking of collagen [120]. Abnormalities in lysyl oxidase activity have recently been described [120a].

Neurofibromatosis

This phakomatosis can present clinically in the newborn period. Café au lait spots may or may not be present, and patients usually present with one or more cutaneous neurofibromas [121]. Although prolonged follow-up studies are not available, reports suggest that the lesions may regress in infancy. Congenital fibromatosis is the principal differential diagnosis [122].

Tuberous Sclerosis

Of the various dermatological features of tuberous sclerosis, hypomelanotic macules are the most common lesions present at birth. Biopsy of these lesions may be pivotal in establishing the diagnosis in patients at risk [123]. They are distributed over the entire skin, and do not often show dermatomal or linear patterns that obey the midline. Routine histology is unhelpful, but the intensity of the dopa reaction is reduced in comparison with control skin from the patient.

Aplasia Cutis Congenita

This term signifies localized absence of skin at birth. It must be distinguished from the various forms of EB and from focal dermal hypoplasia. In its fullest form, there is total absence of epidermis and dermis, exposing subcutaneous tissues [124]. Almost any area of the body can be affected, but the most common site is the midline of the vertex of the scalp. Healing can occur, with residual alopecia.

The etiology of aplasia cutis is apparently highly variable [125]. There may be an association between aplasia cutis and the membrane-covered defects seen with neural tube defects [126]. Other cases show impressive pedigrees with multiple family members having lesions in many sites [127]. It also occurs with a number of syndromes, notably trisomy 13 [128], 4p syndrome [129], and Johanson-Blizzard syndrome [130].

It also seems likely that aplasia cutis congenita can result from thromboembolic events related to the intrauterine death of 1 monozygotic twin with fetofetal vascular anastomoses [131].

Subcutaneous Fat Necrosis and Sclerema

These 2 conditions have histological similarities but are quite distinct in their pathogenesis and clinical features. In subcutaneous fat necrosis, discrete nodules and plaques appear in healthy and sick newborns within a few days after birth [132]. The cause is not known, but may not be trauma, as fat necrosis is seen in infants delivered by cesarean section. There may be associated hypercalcemia. The microscopic features are fat necrosis with marked inflammation, foreign-body giant cells, and needle-shaped crystalloid inclusions in viable fat cells (Fig. 33.19).

Sclerema neonatorum is a generalized wax-like hardening of the skin, which feels cold, tight, and indurated. It occurs in sick neonates, the majority of whom die of sepsis [133]. The subcutaneous fat shows zones of increased interlobular fibrous tissue, while fat necrosis and inflammation are rare. However, many adipocytes contain fine, needle-shaped crystals. Features of these 2 diseases are compared in Table 33.5.

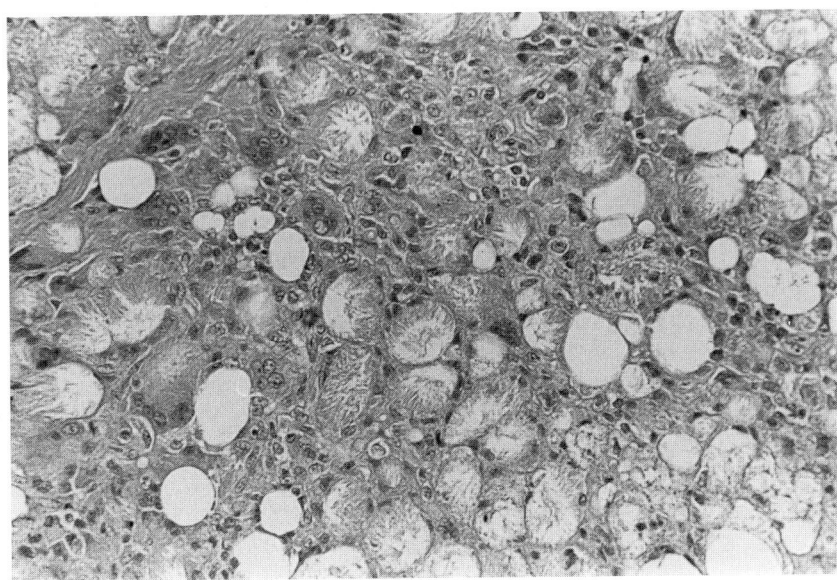

FIGURE 33.19.   *Fat necrosis of the newborn, showing crystals in adipocytes. H&E, ×160.*

Table 33.5.   Comparison of subcutaneous fat necrosis and sclerema

Subcutaneous Fat Necrosis	Sclerema Neonatorum
Healthy newborn infants (majority)	Serious underlying disease (e.g., sepsis, respiratory distress syndrome)
Circumscribed hard nodules	Diffuse, wax-like hardening
Caused by pressure on bony prominences	Hypothermia?; defective fatty acid mobilization?
Fat necrosis; giant cells; inflammation; fatty acid crystals	Edema and thickening of interlobular collagen; fine crystal clefts

Neonatal Lupus Erythematosus and Other Transplacentally Transmitted Maternal Skin Diseases

Neonatal lupus is characterized by erythematous or atrophic skin lesions, sometimes with complete heart block in infants of mothers with serological evidence of systemic lupus erythematosus (SLE). Cutaneous disease usually clears within a few months, but there is evidence that in some patients it recurs later [134].

Neonatal lupus erythematosus (NLE) has been classified into 3 types: 1) erythematous rash or classic discoid lupus without evidence of systemic involvement; 2) skin lesions with evidence of systemic involvement, for example, hepatosplenomegaly had hematological abnormalities; and 3) complete heart block with or without skin and systemic manifestations [135].

Skin lesions are clinically typical of lupus erythematosus, as is the histopathology, which includes telangiectasia, epidermal atrophy, follicular plugging, and liquefaction necrosis of the basal layer [136].

The disease is clearly caused by transplacental transfer of maternal antibodies [137]. Almost 50% of affected neonates have antinuclear antibodies of speckled pattern in high titer. Attention has focused on anti-Ro (SS-A) and anti-La (SS-B) antibodies in NLE [138, 139], which may cause complete heart block and hydrops fetalis.

Neonatal pemphigus vulgaris was found in an infant born to a woman in remission [140].

Of the specific dermatoses of pregnancy, 5% of cases of pemphigoid gestationis affect the neonate with a mild, transient rash [141]. Only 1 case of pruritic urticarial papules and plaques of pregnancy involving mother and infant has been reported [142].

Histiocytic Disorders

The criteria for the diagnosis of neonatal and childhood histiocytic syndromes were reviewed recently [143]. Markers include Birbeck granules, S-100 protein, and OKT6 positivity.

Of the histiocytic proliferative disorders only 4 are of importance in the neonatal period.

1. Acute disseminated Langerhans' cell histiocytosis (Letterer-Siwe disease). The clinicopathological features of this disease are well known to pediatric pathologists through reviews [144, 145].

In a review of a series of 50 patients, 8 neonates had this disease and the distribution of cases was evenly spread (4 each) among the 26 survivors and 24 neonates who died [144]. Of the 8 neonates, 2 had severe skin involvement, and all had some degree of cutaneous histiocytosis (Fig. 33.20). Liver, spleen, lymph nodes, and bone marrow were the other main sites of infiltration. Skin involvement was generally a sign of poor prognosis in this series. Congenital involvement by Langerhans' cell histiocytosis is well recognized [144]; approximately 50% of cases have been fatal.

2. Congenital self-healing histiocytosis (Hashimoto-Pritzker histiocytosis, congenital cutaneous Langerhans' histiocytosis). This variety of Langerhans' cell histiocytosis is limited to the skin, is usually present at birth, and heals to leave minimal scarring within a period of about 3 months [145–147]. Criteria for true Langerhans' cell histiocytosis are fulfilled, as up to 25% of the infiltrative histiocytic cells contain Birbeck granules [146]. However, 40% of the histiocytes also contain lysosomes with paracrystalline bodies and lamellar structures [146]. On purely histological grounds, therefore, the lesion cannot be distinguished from acute disseminated Langerhans' cell histiocytosis, although the clinical picture is of eruptive (i.e., elevated), firm, red-to-brown nodules.

3. Juvenile xanthogranuloma may be present at birth [148]. One or several red-to-yellow nodules up to 1 cm in diameter are the usual pattern, but very large nodules are occasionally seen (Fig. 33.21). The mature lesion contains many typical Touton giant cells admixed with histiocytes, lymphocytes, and eosinophils. Early lesions consist almost entirely of histiocytes, with a few lymphocytes and eosinophils. Birbeck granules are absent [149]. Lesions usually persist, and are frequently excised.

4. Malignant histiocytosis was found in a 5-day-old neonate who developed a maculopapular rash that extended fairly rapidly to cover the trunk and arms [150]. There was evidence of systemic involvement, notably of the bone marrow. Pleomorphic histiocytes were present in the dermal infiltrate, but the bone marrow biopsy specimen showed a dense infiltrate of histiocytes that were morphologically benign, although there was a high mitotic rate. Birbeck granules were absent. Bone marrow cytogenetics showed a diploid line with a reciprocal interautosomal translocation. The infant responded to cytotoxic drug therapy and was well 2 years later.

The monoclonal nature of Langerhans' histiocytosis was proved using X-linked polymorphic restriction fragment-length polymorphism DNA probes [151] in all clinical types of disease.

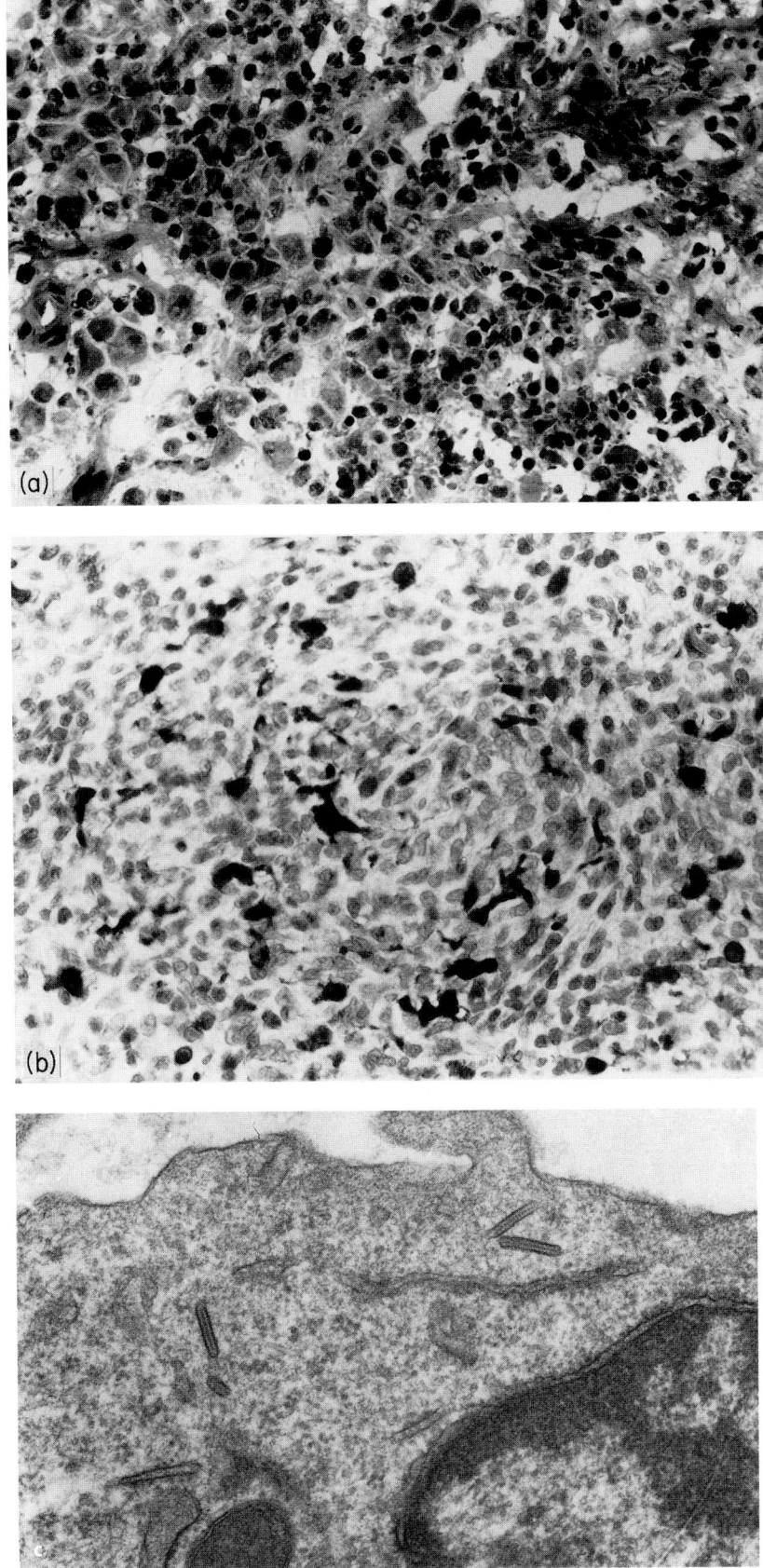

FIGURE 33.20. *(a) Congenital cutaneous Langerhans' cell histiocytosis. H&E, ×67. (b) S-100 protein immunoperoxidase stain in a case of cutaneous Langerhans' cell histiocytosis. H&E, ×67. (c) Birbeck granules demonstrated in histiocyte cytoplasm by electron microscopy.*

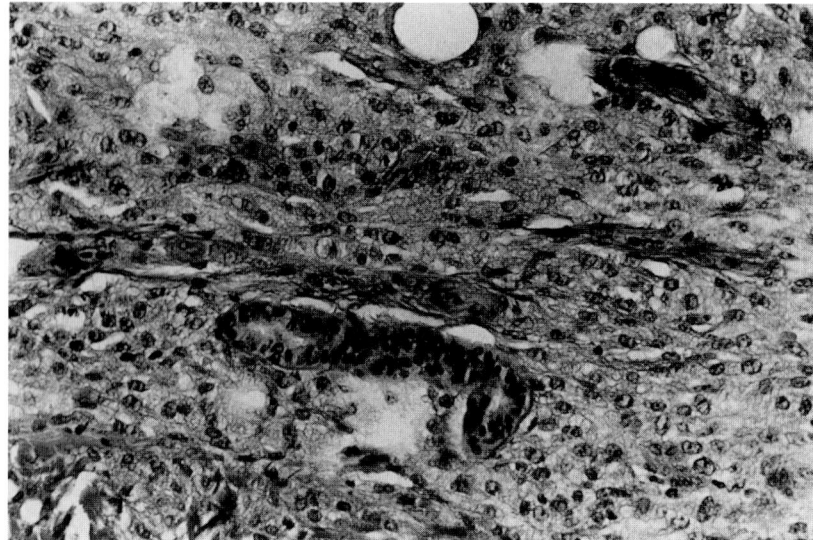

FIGURE 33.21.   *Congenital juvenile xanthogranuloma of the leg. Cellular xanthogranuloma with no Touton giant cells. H&E, ×100.*

IATROGENIC DISEASES

Among the complications of amniocentesis performed during the second trimester for genetic diagnosis is the inadvertent puncture of the fetus. A recent report and review ascertained 36 cases of skin scars from the literature [152]. Eight patients had multiple skin puncture marks [153]. The majority of lesions are found on the extremities, head, and neck. Usually they are depressed scars, resembling dimples, measuring 1–2mm in diameter. In rare patients ileo-cutaneous fistulae occur [154]. The prevalence of skin scarring following second-trimester amniocentesis is estimated at 1–5% [155]. The risk of skin puncture increases with the number of attempted amniocenteses, and the risk of scarring has probably lessened with the use of real-time ultrasound guidance for genetic amniocentesis. The prevalence of skin dimpling is not accurately known for fetuses who have not undergone amniocentesis, and skin dimples do occur as components of some developmental disorders.

Procedures for intrapartum fetal monitoring can also result in iatrogenic skin lesions. Fetal scalp blood sampling has occasionally been complicated by retention of fragments of the pH electrode [156]. Scalp abscesses following fetal scalp blood sampling occur in about 0.5% of fetuses [157]. Scalp electrodes for fetal heart monitoring can also cause ulceration of abscesses [158] that usually develop by about 5 days postpartum. The incidence of such abscesses is 0.1–4.5%, is less with spiral than clip electrodes, and involves a wide variety of aerobic and anaerobic organisms, including streptococci groups A, B, and D, *Escherichia coli*, *Klebsiella pneumoniae*, peptococcus, and *Bacteroides* species. Herpes simplex virus types 1 and 2 were inoculated by fetal scalp electrodes in many cases where the mother showed no overt clinical signs of infection [159].

Scalp lesions from midforceps delivery and vacuum extraction are well recognized. Lacerations and abrasions occur following midforceps delivery [160], although these are of trivial clinical importance.

The chignon of artificial caput is the most common complication of vacuum extraction. Scalp ecchymoses, abrasions, cephalohematoma, and subgaleal and subaponeurotic hemorrhages also can occur [161].

Repeated heel skin puncture for blood sampling in the neonate can leave residua in the form of abscesses and calcaneal chondritis [162]. Calcified nodules may develop in scars from heel skin punctures [163]. They are eventually extruded through the epidermis. These lesions are found most commonly in neonates with birthweights below 1500 grams who needed ventilatory support and had multiple heel sticks. By histology, the lesions are calcified cysts in the superficial dermis, not associated with epidermis.

PRENATAL DIAGNOSIS OF GENODERMATOSES

When the biochemical basis of genodermatosis has been determined, prenatal diagnosis may be feasible on the basis of mutant gene product or by standard methods of DNA analysis such as restriction fragment length polymorphisms from chorionic villus, amniocentesis, or fetal blood samples. In the meantime, prenatal diagnosis is based on fetoscopic skin biopsy and histopathological evaluation [164, 165]. Application is most suitable for EB and the ichthyoses. The disorders that have been diagnosed so far are listed in Table 33.6 [166–173].

NATAL AND NEONATAL TEETH

Deciduous teeth may be present at birth or erupt during the first month of life. Mandibular central incisors most commonly erupt early. The incidence is given as 1 in 2000–3500 births [174]. In some patients without other

Table 33.6.   Prenatal diagnosis of genodermatoses

Reference	Disease	Clinical History	Method	Result
166, 167	Congenital bullous ichthyosiform erythroderma	Mother affected	EM of fetal skin biopsy at 20 weeks' gestation	Abnormal TOP confirmation
168	Junctional EB lethalis	Two previous children affected	EM of fetal skin biopsy at 18 weeks' gestation	Abnormal TOP confirmation
169	Harlequin fetus	One previous infant affected	Light microscopy and EM of fetal skin at 20 weeks' gestation	Abnormal TOP confirmation
170	Recessive EB	One previous infant affected	Light microscopy of fetal skin at 21 weeks' gestation	Abnormal TOP; extensive peeling of fetus
171	Sjögren-Larsson	Two previous children affected	Light microscopy of fetal skin at 23 weeks' gestation	Abnormal confirmed at birth
172	X-Linked ichthyosis	—	Maternal urinary estriol, amniotic fluid DHEA-S	—

EM = electron microscopy; TOP = termination of pregnancy; EB = epidermolysis bullosa; DHEA-S = dehydroepiandrosterone sulfate.

malformations the condition is inherited in an autosomal dominant mode [174]. Syndromes with natal teeth include Hallermann-Streiff syndrome [174], chondroectodermal dysplasia, restrictive dermopathy, and pachyonychia congenita. The subject has been reviewed [175].

PTERYGIA

The topic of redundant skin, including prune belly and pterygia, has been reviewed [176]. Pterygia are webs between adjacent skin areas, usually crossing a joint and causing reduced mobility (Fig. 33.22). The pterygia of the neck in infantile Turner syndrome may be caused by neck immobility secondary to nuchal hygromas that have regressed by birth from a larger size in fetal life. Alternatively, they may be more analogous to prune belly, that is, arising as a result of previous distention. It is also clear that pterygia result from reduced mobility in utero, as by oligohydramnios, bicornuate uterus, twinning, uterine fibroids, and primary neurological and muscular degenerative disorders with onset in utero [177].

RESTRICTIVE DERMOPATHY

In addition to many neuromuscular disorders, abnormally tight skin can cause fetal hypokinesia, with joint contractures, underossified bones, and pulmonary hypoplasia (Fig. 33.23). There may be several distinct autosomal recessive genetic diseases, affecting the dermis or the epidermis [177a–177c]. Histopathologic findings are variable, including disordered increase in dermal collagen and hyperorthokeratosis or hyperparakeratosis.

DISORDERS OF HAIR AND NAILS

Disorders of hair and nails have already been discussed as components of the ectodermal dysplasias. Other disorders are described here.

Abnormal hair color of the forelock is characteristic of Waardenburg syndrome [178]. Other features are a broad,

high nasal bridge, synophrys, heterochromia iridis, and deafness due to malformation of the organ of Corti. There may be patches of vitiligo elsewhere on the body. with characteristic histopathology (i.e., absence of melanocytes).

Generalized hypertrichosis is seen with a number of dis-

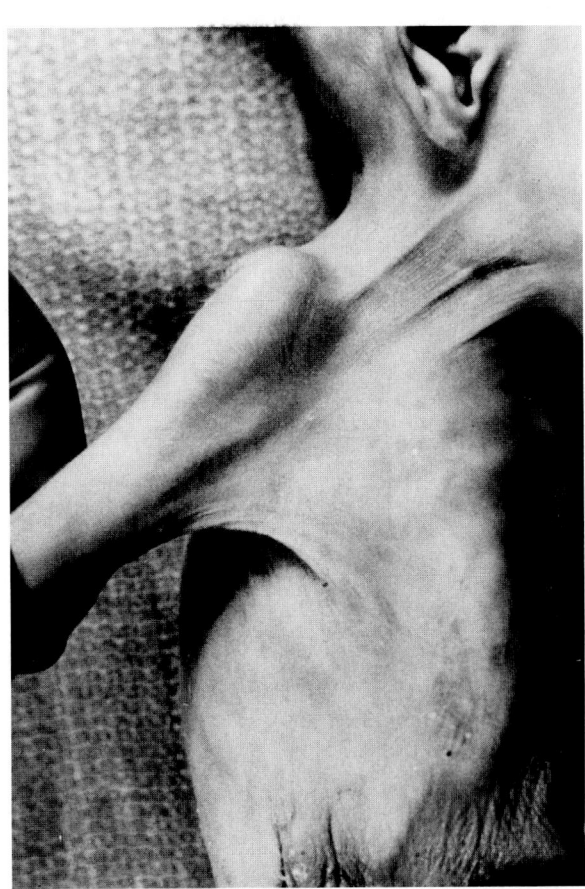

FIGURE 33.22. *Lethal congenital pterygium syndrome. Pterygia are shown in the right axilla and neck. Note the prune belly also.*

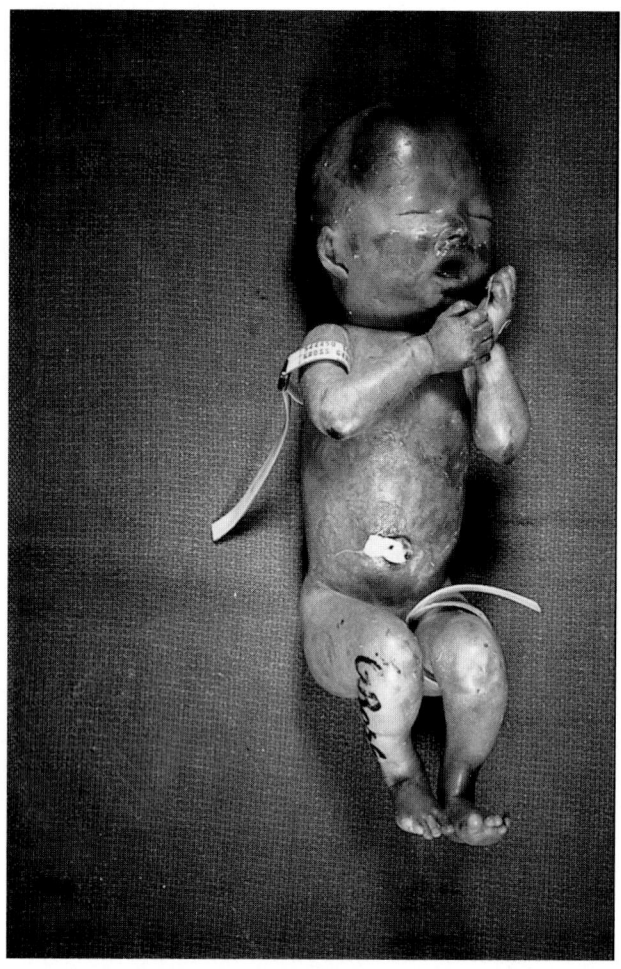

FIGURE 33.23. *Restrictive dermopathy in a newborn. There are flexion contractures, skin slippage, eclabium and thoracic dystrophy.*

orders, including Cornelia de Lange syndrome (in which synophrys is also an important feature) [179] and fetal alcohol syndrome [180].

Abnormalities of the hair shaft may result in increased fragility. Pili torti implies a shaft flattened from side to side, with complete rotation through 180 degrees on the longitudinal axis at irregular intervals [181]. It may cause congenital alopecia, but can also produce a stubble-like appearance because of shaft fracture about 4–5 cm from the scalp. Trichorrhexis nodosa implies node-like swelling with segmental splitting of the hair shaft. In trichorrhexis invaginata (bamboo hair), there is telescope-like invagination of segments of the shaft, causing an effect like a ball-and-socket joint. This anomaly is diagnostic of Netherton syndrome [18]. In Menke disease, both pili torti and trichorrhexis are present. Other features include psychomotor retardation, micrognathia, short stature, unstable body temperature, excessive wormian bones, and low plasma copper and ceruloplasmin levels [182]. In monilethrix, there is alopecia

caused by intermittent shaft constrictions where fractures occur. Mutations have been found in the hair cortex keratin gene hHB6 [182a].

Nail-patella syndrome consists of absent or hypoplastic nails and patellae, renal abnormalities, and heterochromia iridis. It is inherited in an autosomal dominant fashion [183].

Patients with pachyonychia congenita have hypertrophy of the nail bed, oral leukokeratosis, follicular keratosis, and palmoplantar hyperkeratosis, all present at birth. Nail bed biopsy specimens demonstrate hyperkeratosis and dyskeratosis of the matrix. Cutaneous lesions are less diagnostic, with focal parakeratosis and hyperkeratosis. The oral leukokeratosis involves intracellular vacuolization and the absence of prickles in the prickle cell layer [184].

Congenital onychodysplasia consists of anonychia, micronychia, or polyonychia, involving the index fingers bilaterally and never involving the toenails. The nail anomalies are accompanied by generalized hypoplasia of the affected fingers and hypoplasia of the radial digital artery of the index finger. Cases are sporadic, and there are no malformations of other tissues or organs [185].

SOME SELECTED MISCELLANEOUS SKIN DISORDERS AS MARKERS OF SYSTEMIC DISEASE

Immunodeficiency of the Newborn

All forms of immunodeficiency can present with neonatal skin lesions, often candidiasis. The morbilliform rash of graft-versus-host disease may be seen with severe combined immunodeficiency [186]. Patients with Wiscott-Aldrich syndrome usually have severe neonatal eczema [187].

Petechial Hemorrhages in the Newborn

Purpura is one of the principal lesions of the "expanded rubella syndrome" [188]. Where data are available, most cases had platelet counts of less than 90,000 per μL. It is now clear that purpura may be a component of toxoplasmosis and cytomegalic inclusion disease [189, 190].

Congenital amegakaryocytic thrombocytopenia presents with widespread purpura. Erythropoiesis and myelopoiesis are normal, but bone marrow sampling shows an absence of megakaryocytes. Congenital amegakaryocytic thrombocytopenia is found in a number of syndromes, including the thrombocytopenia–absent radius syndrome [191].

Blueberry Muffin Syndrome

This is distinct from thrombocytopenic purpura, although it may coincide with it. In most patients blueberry muffin lesions represent foci of dermal erythropoiesis, causes of which include rubella [188, 192], cytomegalic inclusion disease (see Fig. 17.16) and toxoplasmosis [189]. Blueberry muffin lesions are non-blanching bluish-red macules up to 1 cm in diameter. New lesions seldom appear after the age of 24 hours. They are most commonly found on the head, neck, or trunk. Histologically, there are sharply circumscribed foci of dermal erythropoiesis, although hematopoiesis may occasionally be seen.

Blueberry muffin lesions may also be seen with hematological disorders where there is prenatal or neonatal blood loss or hemolytic anemia. Causes include hereditary spherocytosis [193] and twin transfusion syndrome [194]. Blueberry muffin lesions are not seen with isoimmunization hemolytic anemias, possibly because of the expression of the rhesus blood group antigens in red cell precursors. The skin is a hematopoietic organ in early embryogenesis and up until the middle of the second trimester. Blueberry muffin lesions may represent persistent fetal dermal erythropoiesis.

Blueberry muffin lesions are also seen with congenital metastatic neuroblastoma and stage IVS neuroblastoma. In these cases, the lesions consist of microdeposits of neuroblastoma [195, 196].

Acanthosis Nigricans

This can occur in infancy in at least 2 clinical contexts. A benign infantile familial form is not associated with systemic disease [197]. But it is among the cutaneous features of leprechaunism [198], a syndrome characterized by intrauterine growth retardation, lack of subcutaneous fat, and phallic enlargement. Other cutaneous components of leprechaunism are hypertrichosis, pachyderma, and prominent rugal skin around the orifices.

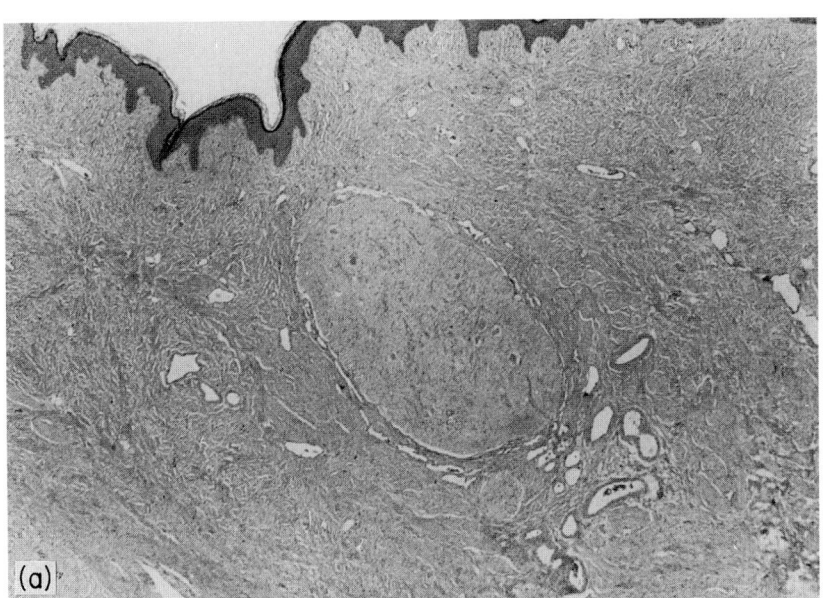

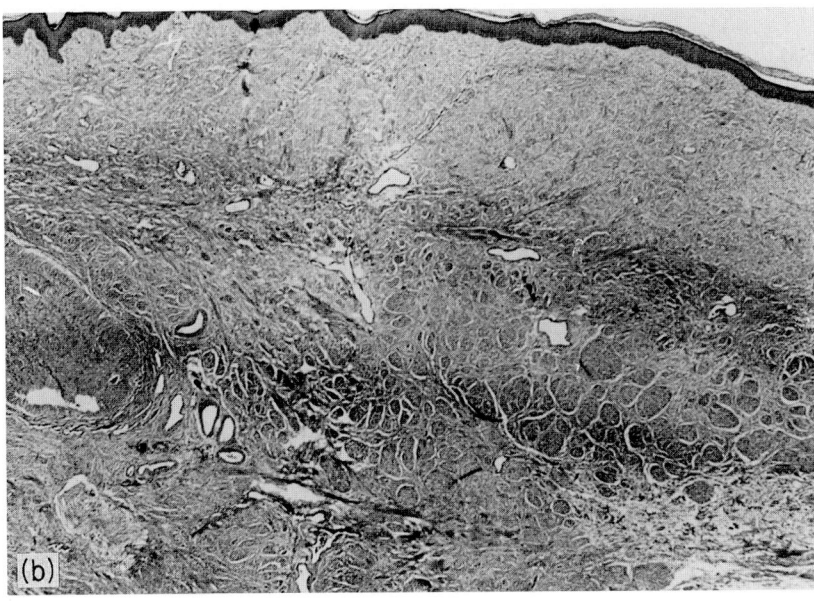

FIGURE 33.24. *A sacrococcygeal cutaneous lesion. (a) There is a superficial focus of tissue resembling spinal cord. H&E, ×100. (b) Bundles of smooth muscle in the reticular dermis resemble Becker's nevus. H&E, ×100.*

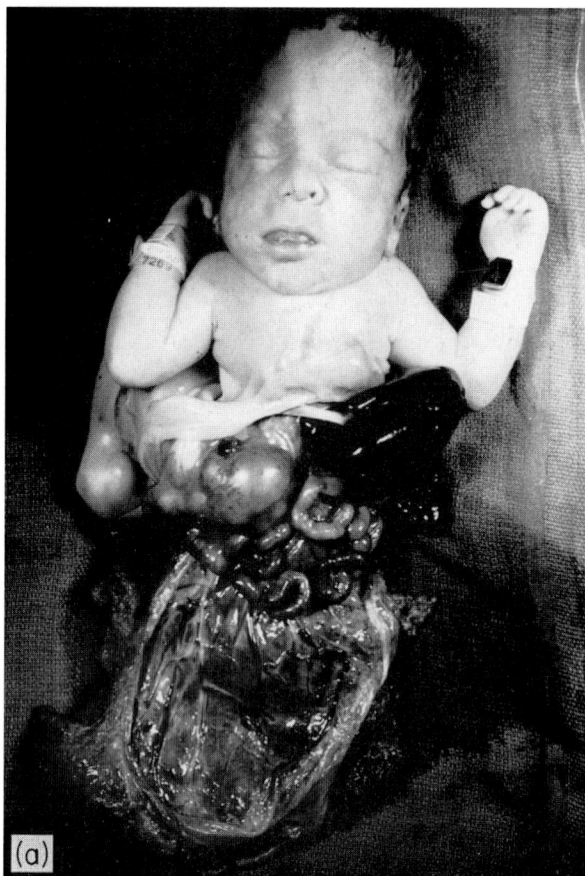
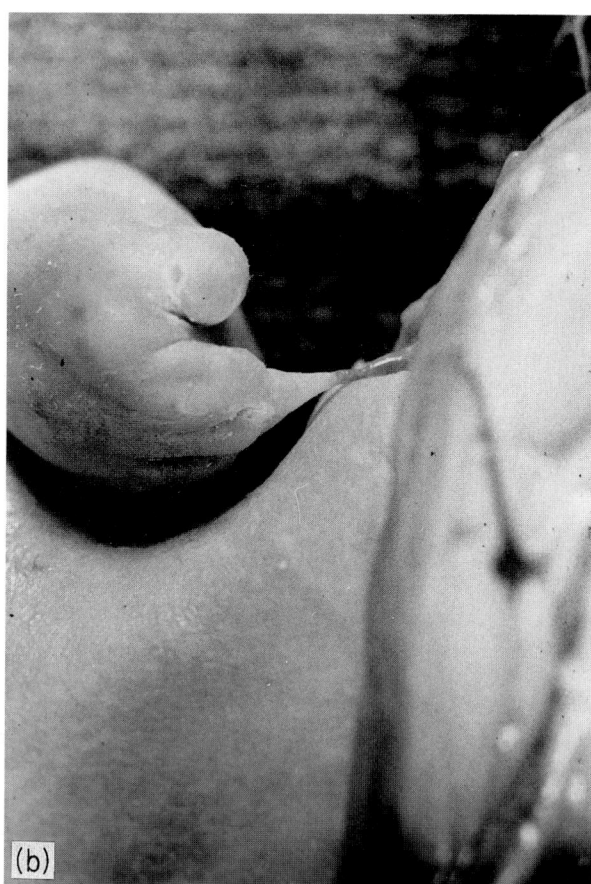

FIGURE 33.25.   *(a) Early amnion rupture–oligohydramnios disrupture (EAROD) diagnosed prenatally by ultrasound. (b) The right foot showed acrosyndactyly/amputation and was attached to the margin of the lateral abdominal wall defect by an amniotic band.*

Sacrococcygeal Cutaneous Lesions

Sacrococcygeal developmental disorders are the subjects of extensive reviews [199, 200]. Skin and subcutaneous lesions encountered in this area include lipomas, epidermal sinus tracts, ependyma-lined sinus tracts, pigmented nevi, sacral dimples, pilonidal sinus tracts, and tail appendages. Many of these lesions are associated with sacrococcygeal teratomas and meningomyeloceles, but they may be the only manifestations of minor degrees of developmental dysplasia in the sacrococcygeal region. Their importance lies in the recognition that lipomas and epidermoid and dermoid cysts may well have connections with intraspinal cysts, while tracts lined by ependyma or meningothelium clearly do have such connections [201] (Fig. 33.24).

Amniotic Band Syndrome

Two principal types of amniotic band syndrome (ABS) are described. In early amnion rupture–oligohydramnios disruption (EAROD) there are widespread disruptions caused by interference with body wall closures (e.g., anterior neu-

ropore, body wall) (Fig. 33.25). The oligohydramnios may result from chronic leakage of amniotic fluid into the chorionic sac, or from the anatomical positioning of the urethral orifice outside the amniotic cavity. Presumably, the amnion rupture occurs early in development, since it appears to interfere with early skin closure events. By contrast, amniotic deformity–adhesion mutilation (ADAM) probably results from later amnion rupture and the defects are less severe. Amputation of limbs or portions thereof are characteristic. Acrosyndactyly also occurs (Fig. 33.26). EAROD and ADAM may coexist in the same patient. Digital amputations may be important in the identification of ABS in patients with extreme degrees of EAROD [202].

Although ABS is usually sporadic, recurrent cases have been reported [203, 204]. Recurrence in sibs and concordance in monozygotic twins could be explained on the basis that at least some cases of ABS are caused by amniotic membrane fragility because the fetus has a heritable connective tissue disorder [205].

Amniotic tags around constriction rings of amputations show disorganized amniotic membrane or vernix granulomas [206] (Fig. 33.27a); the fetal surface of the placenta is denuded of amnion, and shows vernix and squames driven into the chorion [207] (Fig. 33.27b).

Syndactyly

Isolated syndactyly may be found incidentally at autopsy. Six subtypes are described [208]. Syndactyly is also a component of the following syndromes, not all of which are lethal in the perinatal period.

1. Poland syndrome: symbrachydactyly with pectoralis muscle defect
2. The acrocephalosyndactylies (syndactyly with variably cranial synostoses): Apert, Saethre-Chotzen, Pfeiffer, Summit, Herrmann-Opitz, and Waardenburg syndromes

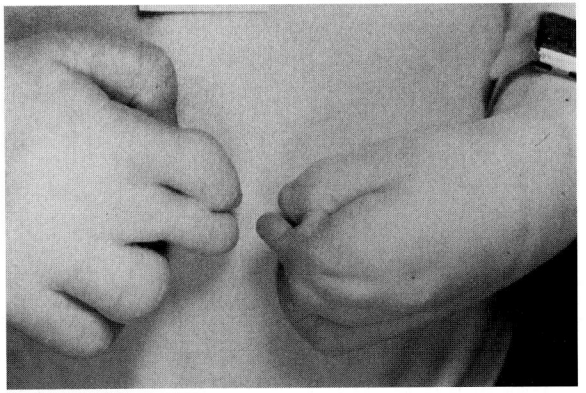

FIGURE 33.26.   *Acrosyndactyly/amputation in a typical case of amniotic deformity–adhesion mutilation (ADAM).*

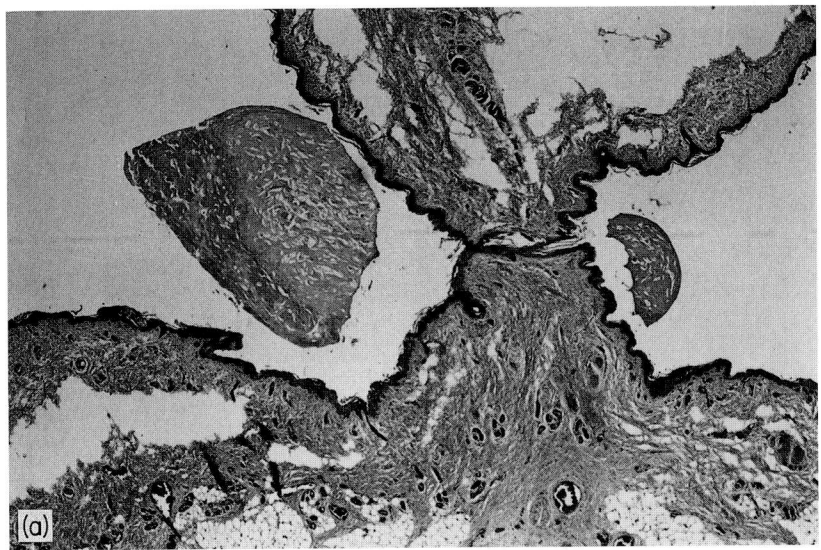

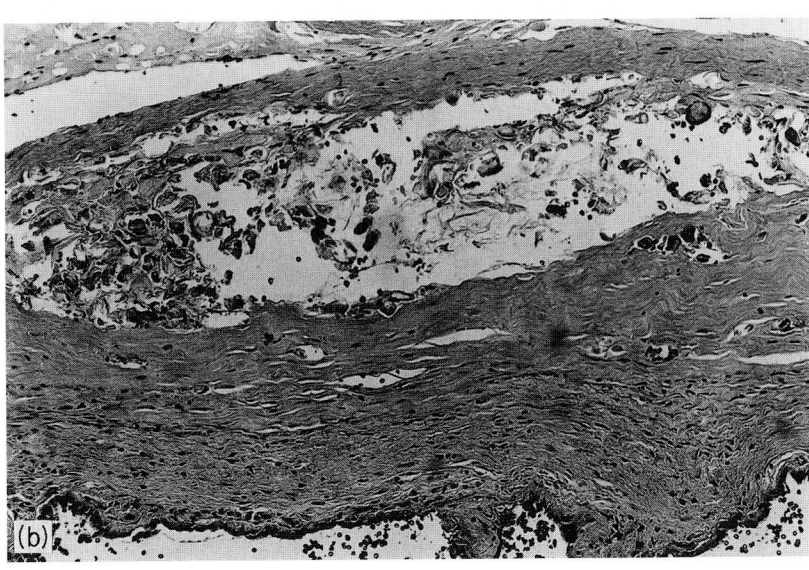

FIGURE 33.27.   *(a) Constricting ring of vernix and chorion around a constriction ring of the upper arm in a patient with EAROD. H&E, ×100. (b) The placenta shows vernix and squames embedded in the chorionic surface. H&E, ×100.*

3. Craniodigital syndrome with mental retardation
4. Oculodentodigital dysplasia
5. The cryptophthalmus syndrome
6. ABS (acrosyndactyly/amputation)
7. Triploidy

Polydactyly

Isolated polydactyly (especially postaxial hexadactyly) is a very common malformation. Major subtypes are preaxial and postaxial polydactyly, and polydactyly of high degree (>6 digits). In syndromes, polydactyly can be an important clue for identification [208]. 1) Postaxial polydactyly occurs in Ellis–van Creveld syndrome, infantile thoracic dystrophy (Jeune's syndrome), Saldino-Noonan type of short ribpolydactyly, Meckel-Gruber syndrome, Bardet-Biedl syndrome, trisomy 13, polydactyly-hydrometrocolpos syndrome, Weyer acrofacial syndrome, Opitz C syndrome, Sugarman syndrome, Biechoud syndrome, Oliver syndrome, and syndromes of cleft palate and postaxial polydactyly. 2) Preaxial polydactyly occurs in acrocephalopolydactyly syndromes (dominant Pfeiffer form, Carpenter, Sakati), Mohr syndrome, Majewski type of short rib (polydactyly), and Towne syndrome.

Skin Dimples

These are found over bone angulations in 3 syndromes: campomelic chondrodysplasia [209], skeletal dysplasia with angulated femora [210], and amyoplasia [211]. They are also found with the following chromosome abnormalities [212]: 4pdel (elbows and knees), trisomy 9p (horizontal chin dimple), and trisomy 9q3 (sacral, elbows).

Sacral dimples are seen in the following disorders: del(4) (pter → p16), dup(9p), del(19q), Bloom, Carpenter, Conradi-Hünermann, Dubowitz, Robinow, and Smith-Lemli-Opitz syndromes.

Lip pits (lower lip) are found in Van der Woude, popliteal web, and oral-facial-digital syndromes.

Nuchal Cystic Hygromas

These are found in a number of disorders, but commonly in 45,X, del(8p), trisomy 21, and Noonan syndromes.

Preauricular Skin Tags

These are found in 4p-syndrome and facio-auriculo-vertebral syndrome.

Synophrys

This is seen with Cornelia de Lange syndrome and also a number of chromosome abnormalities [212].

Scalp Aplasia Cutis

This is a component of del(4p) and trisomy 13 syndromes.

Hirsutism

This occurs with fetal alcohol and hydantoin syndromes, trisomy 3q, Cornelia de Lange syndrome, and trisomy 18.

Single Transverse Palmar Crease

This is an indicator of hypotonia, and therefore occurs with a wide variety of disorders, including fetal alcohol, hydantoin, and trimethadone syndromes; cri du chat syndrome; Cornelia de Lange syndrome; trisomy 21 and 13; triploidy; and 4p-, 18p-, Zellweger and Smith-Lemli-Opitz syndromes.

REFERENCES

1. McLoughlin CB. The importance of mesenchymal factors in the differentiation of chick epidermis. II. Modification of epidermal differentiation by contact with different types of mesenchyme. *J Embryol Exp Morphol* 1961; 9:385–409.
2. Sun TT, Green H. Cultured epithelial cells of cornea, conjunctiva and skin: absence of marked intrinsic divergence of their differentiated states. *Nature* 1977; 269:489–93.
3. Billingham RE, Silvers WK. Studies on the conservation of epidermal specificities of skin and certain mucosas in adult mammals. *J Exp Med* 1967; 125:429–46.
4. Briggaman RA, Wheeler CE. Lamellar ichthyosis: long-term graft studies on congenitally athymic nude mice. *J Invest Dermatol* 1976; 67:567–72.
5. Holbrook KA. The biology of human fetal skin at ages related to prenatal diagnosis. *Pediatr Dermatol* 1983; 1:97–111.
6. Baden HP, Hooker PA. Advances in genetics in dermatology. *Adv Hum Genet* 1982; 12:89–188.
7. Smack DP, Korge BP, James WD. Keratin and keratinization. *J Am Acad Dermatol* 1994; 30:85–102.
8. Steinert PM, Marekov LN, Fraser DB, Parry DAD. Keratin intermediate filament structure. Cross-linking studies yield quantitative information on molecular dimensions and mechanism of assembly. *J Mol Biol* 1993; 230:436–52.
9. Compton JG. Epidermal disease: faulty keratin filaments take their toll. *Nat Genet* 1994; 6:6–7.
10. Williams ML. The ichthyoses—pathogenesis and prenatal diagnosis: a review of recent advances. *Pediatr Dermatol* 1983; 1:1–24.
11. Shapiro LJ, Weiss R, Webster D, France JT. X-Linked ichthyosis due to steroid sulphatase deficiency. *Lancet* 1978; 1:70–2.
12. Yen PH, Allen E, Marsh B, et al. Cloning and expression of steroid sulfatase cDNA and the frequent occurrence of deletion in STS deficiency; implications for X-Y interchange. *Cell* 1987; 49:443–54.
13. Ross JB, Allerdice PW, Shapiro LJ, et al. Familial X-linked ichthyosis, steroid sulphatase deficiency, mental retardation, and nullisomy for Xp223 → pter. *Arch Dermatol* 1985; 121:1524–8.
14. Alperin ES, Shapiro LJ. Characterization of point mutations in patients with X-linked ichthyosis (XLI). *Am J Hum Genet* 1994; 55A:1217.
15. Basler E, Grompe M, Parenti G, Yates J, Ballabio A. Identification of point mutations in the steroid sulfatase gene of three patients with X-linked ichthyosis. *Am J Hum Genet* 1992; 50:483–91.
16. Russell LJ, DiGiovanni JJ, Rogers GT, et al. Mutations in the gene for transglutaminase 1 in autosomal recessive lamellar ichthyosis. *Nat Genet* 1995; 9:279–83.
16a. Laiho E, Ignatius J, Mikkola H, et al. Transglutaminase 1 mutations in autosomal recessive congenital ichthyosis: private and recurrent mutations in an isolated population. *Am J Hum Genet* 1997; 61:529–38.
17. Chiper CC, Korge BP, Markova N, et al. A leucine → proline mutation in the H1 subdomain of keratin 1 causes epidermolytic hyperkeratosis. *Cell* 1992; 70:821–8.
18. Chiper CC, Yang J-M, DiGiovanna JJ, et al. Preferential sites in keratin 10 that are mutated in epidermolytic hyperkeratosis. *Am J Hum Genet* 1994; 54:179–90.
19. Rothnagel JA, Dominey AM, Dempsey LD, et al. Mutations in the rod domains of keratins 1 and 10 in epidermolytic hyperkeratosis. *Science* 1992; 257:1128–30.

20. Cheng J, Snyder AJ, Yu Q-C, et al. The genetic basis of epidermolytic hyperkeratosis: a disorder of differentiation-specific epidermal keratin genes. *Cell* 1992; 70:811–19.

21. McLean WHI, Morley SM, Lane EB, et al. Ichthyosis bullosa of Siemens—a disease involving keratin 2e. *J Invest Dermatol* 1994; 103:277–81.

22. Kremer H, Zeeuwen P, McLean WHI, et al. Ichthyosis bullosa of Siemens is caused by mutations in the keratin 2e gene. *J Invest Dermatol* 1994; 103:286–9.

23. Kanerva L, Karvonen J, Oikarinen A, et al. Ichthyosis hystrix (Curth-Macklin). *Arch Dermatol* 1984; 120:1218–23.

24. Lentz CL, Altman J. Lamellar ichthyosis. The natural clinical course of collodion baby. *Arch Dermatol* 1968; 97:3–13.

25. O'Sherer DM, Metlay LA, Sinkin RA, et al. Congenital ichthyosis with restrictive dermopathy and Gaucher disease: a new syndrome with associated prenatal diagnostic and pathology findings. *Obstet Gynecol* 1993; 81:842–4.

26. Buxman MM, Goodkin PE, Fahrenbach WH, Dimond RL. Harlequin ichthyosis with epidermal lipid abnormality. *Arch Dermatol* 1979; 115:189–93.

27. Baden HP, Kubilus J, Rosenbaum K, Fletcher A. Keratinization in the harlequin fetus. *Arch Dermatol* 1982; 118:14–18.

28. Haftek M, Cambadaro F, Serre G, et al. A longitudinal study of a harlequin infant evolving towards non-bullous congenital ichthyosiform erythroderma (NBCIE). *J Invest Dermatol* 1994; 103:453. Abstract.

29. Lawlor F. Progress of a harlequin fetus to non-bullous ichthyosiform erythroderma. *Pediatrics* 1988; 82:870–3.

30. Viksnins P, Berlin A. Follicular atrophoderma and basal cell carcinomas: the Basex syndrome. *Arch Dermatol* 1977; 113:948–51.

31. Labrisseau A. Rud syndrome: congenital ichthyosis, hypogonadism, mental retardation, retinitis pigmentosa and hypertrophic polyneuropathy. *Neuropediatrics* 1982; 13:95–8.

32. Jurecka W, Aberer E, Mainitz M, Jurgensen O. Keratitis, ichthyosis, and deafness syndrome with glycogen storage. *Arch Dermatol* 1985; 121:799–801.

33. Theile U. Sjögren-Larsson syndrome: oligophrenia-ichthyosis-ditetraplagia. *Hum Genet* 1974; 22:91–118.

34. Caputo R, Vanotti P, Bertani E. Netherton's syndrome in two adult brothers. *Arch Dermatol* 1984; 120:220–1.

35. Davies MG, Marks R, Dykes PJ, Reynolds D. Epidermal abnormalities in Refsum's disease. *Br J Dermatol* 1977; 97:401–6.

36. Silengo MC, Buzzatti I, Silverman FN. Clinical and genetic aspects of Conradi-Hünermann disease. *J Pediatr* 1980; 97:911–7.

37. Lucky AW, McGuire JS. Infantile acropustulosis with eosinophilic pustules. *J Pediatr* 1982; 100:428–9.

38. Marino LY. Toxic erythema present at birth. *Arch Dermatol* 1965; 92:402–3.

39. Ramaswurthy RS, Reveri M, Esterly NB, Fretzin DF, Pildes RS. Transient neonatal pustular melanosis. *J Pediatr* 1976; 88:831–5.

40. Rudolph N, Tariq AA, Reale MR, Goldberg PK, Kozinn PJ. Congenital cutaneous candidiasis. *Arch Dermatol* 1977; 113:1101–3.

41. Delprado WJ, Baird PJ, Russell P. Placental candidiasis: report of three cases with a review of the literature. *Pathology* 1982; 14:191–5.

42. Amon RB, Diamond RL. Toxic epidermal necrolysis: rapid differentiation between staphylococcal- and drug-induced disease. *Arch Dermatol* 1975; 111:1433–7.

43. Honig PJ, Brown D. Congenital herpes simplex virus infection initially resembling epidermolysis bullosa. *J Pediatr* 1982; 101:958–60.

44. Singer DB. Pathology of neonatal herpes simplex virus infection. *Perspect Pediatr Pathol* 1981; 6:243–78.

45. Fine JD, Bauer EA, Briggaman RA, et al. Revised clinical and laboratory criteria for subtypes of inherited epidermolysis bullosa: a consensus report by the Subcommittee in Diagnosis and Classification of the National Epidermolysis Bullosa Registry. *J Am Acad Dermatol* 1991; 24:119–35.

46. Rugg EL, Morley SM, Smith FJD, et al. Missing links: Weber-Cockayne keratin mutations implicate the L12 linker domain in effective cytoskeleton function. *Nat Genet* 1993; 5:294–300.

47. Hovnanian A, Pollack E, Hilal L, et al. A missense mutation in the rod domain of keratin 14 associated with recessive epidermolysis bullosa simplex. *Nat Genet* 1993; 3:327–32.

47a. Smith FJD, Eady RAJ, Leigh IM, et al. Plectin deficiency: hereditary basis for muscular dystrophy with epidermolysis bullosa. *Nat Genet* 1996; 13:450–7.

48. Pulkkinen L, Christiano AM, Airenne T, et al. Mutations in the γ2 chain gene (LAMC2) of kalinin/laminin 5 in the junctional form of epidermolysis bullosa. *Nat Genet* 1994; 6:293–304.

49. Aberdam D, Galliano M-F, Vailly J, et al. Herlitz's junctional epidermolysis bullosa is linked to mutations in the gene (LAMC2) for the γ2 subunit of nicein/kalinin (LAMININ-5). *Nat Genet* 1994; 6:249–304.

49a. Uitto J, Pulkkinen L. Molecular complexity of the cuitaneous basement membrane zone. *Mol Biol Rep* 1996; 23:35–46.

49b. Gatalica B, Pulkkinen L, Li K, et al. Cloning of the human type XVII collagen gene (COLI7A1) and detection of novel mutations in generalized atrophic benign epidermolysis bullosa. *Am J Hum Genet* 1997; 60:352–65.

50. Vidai F, Aberdam D, Miquel C, et al. Integrin β4 mutations with junctional epidermolysis bullosa with pyloric atresia. *Nat Genet* 1995; 10:229–34.

51. Christiano AM, Greenspan DS, Hoffman GG, et al. A missense mutation in type VII collagen in two affected siblings with recessive dystrophic epidermolysis bullosa. *Nat Genet* 1993; 4:62–6.

52. Hilai L, Rochat A, Duquesnoy P, et al. A homozygous insertion-deletion in the type VII collagen gene (COL7A1) in Hallopeau-Siemens dystrophic epidermolysis bullosa. *Nat Genet* 1993; 5:287–93.

53. Dunnill MGS, Richards AJ, Milana G, et al. PCR-SSCP analysis of the type VII collagen gene (COL7A1): detection of a point mutation in five patients. *Am J Hum Genet* 1994; 55:A219.

54. Hovnanian A, Hilal L, Blachot-Bardon C, et al. Recurrent nonsense mutations within the type VII collagen gene in patients with severe recessive dystrophic epidermolysis bullosa. *Am J Hum Genet* 1994; 55:289–96.

55. Johnson WC, Helwig EB. Solitary mastocytosis (urticaria pigmentosa). *Arch Dermatol* 1961; 84:805–15.

56. Fenske NA, Lober CW, Pautler SE. Congenital bullous urticaria pigmentosa. *Arch Dermatol* 1985; 121:115–8.

57. Orkin M, Good RA, Clawson CC, Fisher I, Windhorst DB. Bullous mastocytosis. *Arch Dermatol* 1970; 101:547–64.

58. James MP, Eady RAJ. Familial urticaria pigmentosa with giant mast cell granules. *Arch Dermatol* 1981; 117:713–8.

59. Alper JC, Holmes LB. The incidence and significance of birthmarks in a cohort of 4641 newborns. *Pediatr Dermatol* 1983; 1:58–68.

60. Bolande RP. Neoplasia in early life and its relationships to teratogenesis. *Perspect Pediatr Pathol* 1976; 3:145–83.

61. DiPietro WP, Sweeney EW, Silvers DN. Divided nevi: pigmented and achromatic. *Cutis* 1981; 27:408–9.

62. Hayashi N, Soma Y. A case of epidermal nevi showing a divided form on the fingers. *J Am Acad Dermatol* 1993; 29:281–2.

63. Castilla EE, Dutra MG, Orioli-Parreiras IM. Epidemiology of congenital pigmented nevi: 1. Incidence rates and relative frequencies. *Br J Dermatol* 1981; 104:307–15.

64. Rhodes AR, Wood WC, Sober AJ, Mihm MC. Non-epidermal origin of malignant melanoma associated with giant congenital nevocellular nevus. *Plast Reconstr Surg* 1981; 67:782–90.

65. Reed WB, Becker SW, Nickel WR. Giant pigmented nevi, melanoma, and leptomeningeal melanocytosis. *Arch Dermatol* 1965; 91:100–19.

66. Trozak DJ, Rowland WD, Hu UF. Metastatic malignant melanoma in prepubertal children. *Pediatrics* 1975; 55:191–204.

67. Rhodes AR, Melski JW. Small congenital nevocellular nevi and the risk of cutaneous melanoma. *J Pediatr* 1982; 100:219–4.

68. Solomonn LM. The management of congenital melanocytic nevi. *Arch Dermatol* 1980; 116:1017.

69. Special Symposium. The management of congenital nevocytic nevi. *Pediatr Dermatol* 1984; 2:143–56.

70. Mark GJ, Mihm MC, Liteplo MC, Reed RJ, Clark WJ. Congenital melanocytic nevi of the small and garment type. *Hum Pathol* 1973; 4:395–418.

71. Rhodes AR, Wood WC, Sober AJ, Mihm MC. Nonepidermal origin of malignant melanoma associated with giant congenital nevocellular nevus. *Plast Reconstr Surg* 1981; 67:782–90.

72. Hendrickson MR, Ross JC. Neoplasms arising in congenital giant nevi. Morphologic study of seven cases and a review of the literature. *Am J Surg Pathol* 1981; 5:100–3.

73. Faillace WJ, Okawara S-H, McDonald JV. Neurocutaneous melanosis with extensive cerebral and spinal cord involvement. *J Neurosurg* 1984; 61:782–5.

74. Holaday WJ, Castrow FF. Placental metastasis from a fetal giant pigmented nevus. *Arch Dermatol* 1968; 98:486–8.

75. Marghoob AA, Orlow SJ, Kopf AW. Syndromes associated with melanocytic nevi. *J Am Acad Dermatol* 1993; 29:373–88.

76. Brodsky I, Baren M, Kahn SB, Lewis G, Teelem M. Metastatic malignant melanoma from mother to fetus. *Cancer* 1965; 18:1048–54.

77. Iemoto Y, Kondo Y. Congenital giant cellular blue nevus resulting in dystocia. *Arch Dermatol* 1984; 120:798–9.

78. Nordlund JJ, Lerner AB, Braverman IM, McGuire JS. The multiple lentigines syndrome. *Arch Dermatol* 1973; 107:259–61.

79. Thompson GW, Diehl AC. Partial unilateral lentiginosis. *Arch Dermatol* 1980; 116:356.

80. Kopt AW, Weidman AI. Nevus of Ota. *Arch Dermatol* 1962; 85:195–208.

81. Mishima Y, Mevorah B. Nevus of Ota and nevus of Ito in American blacks. *J Invest Dermatol* 1961; 36:133–54.

82. Chitayat D, Friedman JM, Johnston MM. Hypomelanosis of Ito—a nonspecific marker of somatic mosaicism: report of a case with trisomy 18 mosaicism. *Am J Med Genet* 1990; 35:422–4.

83. Ritter CL, Steele MW, Wehger SL, Cohen BA. Chromosome mosaicism in hypomelanosis of Ito. *Am J Med Genet* 1990; 35:14–17.

84. Flannery DB. Pigmentary dysplasias, hypomelanosis of Ito, and genetic mosaicism. *Am J Med Genet* 1990; 35:18–21.

85. Whitehouse D. Diagnostic value of the café-au-lait spot in children. *Arch Dis Child* 1966; 41:316–9.

86. Hurwitz S, Braveman IM. White spots in tuberous sclerosis. *J Pediatr* 1970; 77:587–94.

87. Rogers M, Poyzer KG. Cutis marmorata telangiectatica congenita. *Arch Dermatol* 1982; 118:895–9.

88. Enjolras O, Riche MC, Merland JJ. Facial port-wine stains and Sturge-Weber syndrome. *Pediatrics* 1985; 76:48–51.

89. Klein JA, Barr RJ. Verrucous hemangioma. *Pediatr Dermatol* 1985; 2:191–3.

90. Elejalde BR, Elejalde MM, Leno J. Nuchal cysts syndromes: etiology, pathogenesis and prenatal diagnosis. *Am J Med Genet* 1985; 21:417–32.

91. Phillips GN, Gordon DH, Martin EC, Haller JO, Casarella W. The Klippel-Trenaunay syndrome: clinical radiologic aspects. *Radiology* 1978; 128:428–34.

92. Lewis RJ, Ketcham AS. Maffucci's syndrome: functional and neoplastic significance. *J Bone Joint Surg* 1973; 55:1465–79.

93. Morris SJ, Kaplan SR, Ballan K. Blue rubber-bleb nevus syndrome. *JAMA* 1978; 239:1887.

94. Stringel G, Mercer S. Giant hemangioma in the newborn and infant. Complications and management. *Clin Pediatr* 1984; 101:582–4.

95. Zonana J, Rimoin DL, David DC. Macrocephaly with multiple lipomas and hemangiomas. *J Pediatr* 1976; 89:600–3.

96. Jessen RT, Thompson S, Smith EB. Cobb syndrome. *Arch Dermatol* 1977; 113:1587–90.

97. Special Symposium. The management of disseminated eruptive hemangiomata in infants. *Pediatr Dermatol* 1984; 1:312–17.

98. Ronan SG, Solomon LM. Benign neonatal eruptive hemangiomatosis in identical twins. *Pediatr Dermatol* 1984; 1:318–21.

99. Hurwitz S. Epidermal nevi and tumors of epidermal origin. *Pediatr Clin North Am* 1983; 30:483–94.

100. Golitz LE, Weston WL. Inflammatory linear verrucous epidermal nevus. Association with epidermal nevus syndrome. *Arch Dermatol* 1979; 115:1208–9.

101. Stosiek N, Ulmer R, von den Driesch P, et al. Chromosomal mosaicism in two patients with epidermal verrucous nevi. *J Am Acad Dermatol* 1994; 30:622–5.

102. Solomon LM, Fretzin DF, DeWald RL. The epidermal nevus syndrome. *Arch Dermatol* 1968; 97:273–85.

103. Domingo J, Helwig EB. Malignant neoplasms associated with nevus sebaceus of Jadassohn. *J Am Acad Dermatol* 1979; 1:546–56.

104. Lovejoy FH, Boyle WE. Linear nevus sebaceous syndrome: report of two cases and a review of the literature. *Pediatrics* 1973; 52:382–7.

105. Engber PB. The nevus comedonicus syndrome. A case report with emphasis on associated internal manifestations. *Int J Dermatol* 1978; 17:745–9.

106. Chapel TA, Tavafoghi V, Mehregan AH, Gagliardi C. Becker's melanosis: an organoid hamartoma. *Cutis* 1981; 27:404–15.

107. Bronson DM, Fretzkin DF, Farrell LN. Congenital pilar and smooth muscle nevus. *J Am Acad Dermatol* 1983; 8:11–4.

108. Nickel WR, Read WB. Tuberous sclerosis. Special reference to the microscopic alterations in the cutaneous hamartomas. *Arch Dermatol* 1962; 85:209–26.

109. Hendricks WM, Limber GK. Nevus lipomatosus cutaneous superficialis. *Cutis* 1982; 29:183–5.

110. Freire-Maia N, Pinheiro M. *Ectodermal Dysplasias: A Clinical and Genetic Study.* New York: Alan R. Liss, 1984.

111. Solomomn LH, Keuer EJ. The ectodermal dysplasias. Problems of classification and some newer syndromes. *Arch Dermatol* 1980; 116:1295–9.

111a. Freire-Maia N, Pinheiro M. Ectodermal dysplasias: a clinical classification and a causal review. *Am J Med Genet* 1994; 53:153–62.

112. Lambert WC, Bilinski DL. Diagnostic pitfalls in anhidrotic ectodermal dysplasia: indications for palmar skin biopsy. *Cutis* 1983; 31:182–7.

112a. Kere J, Srivastava AK, Montenen O, et al. X-linked anhidrotic (hypohidrotic) ectodermal dysplasia is caused by mutation in a novel transmembrane protein. *Nat Genet* 1996; 13:409–16.

113. Kowalski DC, Fenske NA. The focal dermal hypoplasias: report of a kindred and a proposed new classification. *J Am Acad Dermatol* 1992; 27:575–82.

114. Sorrow JM, Hitch JM. Dyskeratosis congenita. First report of its occurrence in a female and a review of the literature. *Arch Dermatol* 1963; 88:340–7.

115. Schwartz MF, Esterly MB, Fretzin DF, Pergament E, Rozenfeld IH. Hypomelanosis of Ito (incontinentia pigmenti achromians): a neurocutaneous syndrome. *J Pediatr* 1979; 90:236–40.

116. Vennos EM, Collins M, James WD. Rothmund-Thomson syndrome: review of the world literature. *J Am Acad Dermatol* 1992; 27:750–62.

117. Carney RG. Incontinentia pigmenti: world statistical analysis. *Arch Dermatol* 1970; 112:535–42.

118. Douglas WF, Schonholtz GJ, Geppert LJ. Chondroectodermal dysplasia (Ellis-van Creveld syndrome). *Am J Dis Child* 1959; 97:473–8.

119. Goltz RW, Hult AM, Goldfarb M, Gorlin RJ. Cutis laxa. *Arch Dermatol* 1965; 92:373–87.

120. Byers PH, Siegel RC, Holbrook KA, et al. X-linked cutis laxa. *N Engl J Med* 1980; 303:61–202.

120a. Khakoo A, Thomas R, Trompeter R, et al. Congenital cutis laxa and lysyl oxidase deficiency. *Clin Genet* 1997; 51:109–14.

121. Eeg-Olofsson O, Lindskog U. Congenital neurofibromatosis. Multiple subcutaneous tumors with spontaneous regression in twins. *Acta Pediatr Scand* 1983; 72:779–80.

122. Roggli VL, Han-Seob K, Hawkins E. Congenital generalized fibromatosis with visceral involvement. A case report. *Cancer* 1980; 45:954–60.

123. Fitzpatrick TB, Szabo G, Hori Y, et al. White leaf-shaped macules. *Arch Dermatol* 1968; 98:1–6.

124. Levin DI, Nolan KS, Esterley NB. Congenital absence of skin. *J Am Acad Dermatol* 1980; 2:203–6.

125. Stephan MJ, Smith DW, Ponzi JW, Alden ER. Origin of scalp vertex aplasia cutis. *J Pediatr* 1982; 101:850–3.

126. Higginbottom MC, Jones KL, James HE, Bruce DA, Schut L. Aplasia cutis congenita: a cutaneous marker of occult spinal dysraphism. *J Pediatr* 1980; 96:687–9.

127. McMurray BR, Martin LW, Dignon PSJ, Fogelson MH. Hereditary aplasia cutis congenita and associated defects. *Clin Pediatr* 1977; 16:610–17.

128. Abuelo D, Feingold M. Scalp defects in trisomy 13. *Clin Pediatr* 1969; 8:416–18.

129. Hirschhorn K, Cooper HL, Firschein IL. Deletion of short arms of chromosome 4 in a child with defects of midline fusion. *Hum Genet* 1965; 1:479–82.

130. Johanson A, Blizzard R. A syndrome of congenital aplasia of the alae nasae, deafness, hypothyroidism, dwarfism, absent permanent teeth and malabsorption. *J Pediatr* 1971; 79:982–7.

131. Mannino FL, Jones KL, Benirschke K. Congenital skin defects and fetus papyraceus. *J Pediatr* 1977; 91:559–64.

132. Katz DA, Huerter C, Bogard P, Braddock SW. Subcutaneous fat necrosis of the newborn. *Arch Dermatol* 1984; 120:1517–8.

133. Kellum RE, Ray TL, Brown GR. Sclerema neonatorum. *Arch Dermatol* 1968; 97:372–80.

134. Jackson R, Gulliver M. Neonatal lupus erythematosus progressing into systemic lupus erythematosus. *Br J Dermatol* 1979; 101:81–6.

135. Rendall JRS, Wilkinson JD. Neonatal lupus erythematosus. *Clin Exp Dermatol* 1978; 3:69–75.

136. Vonderheid EC, Koblenzer PJ, Ming PML, Burgeon CF. Neonatal lupus erythematosus. *Arch Dermatol* 1976; 112:698–705.

137. Miyagawa S, Kitamura W, Yoshioka J, Sakamoto K. Placental transfer of anticytoplasmic antibodies in annular erythema of newborns. *Arch Dermatol* 1981; 117:569–72.

138. Korkij W, Soltani K. Neonatal lupus erythematosus: a review. *Pediatr Dermatol* 1984; 1:189–95.

139. Lee A, Weston WL. New findings in neonatal lupus syndrome. *Am J Dis Child* 1984; 138:233–6.

140. Tope WD, Kamino H, Briggaman RA, Rico MJ, Rose NS. Neonatal pemphigus vulgaris in a child born to a woman in remission. *J Am Acad Dermatol* 1993; 29:480–5.

141. Black MM, Stephens CJM. The specific dermatoses of pregnancy: the British perspective. *Adv Dermatol* 1992; 7:105–26.

142. Uhlin SR. Pruritic urticarial papules and plaques of pregnancy: involvement of the mother and infant. *Arch Dermatol* 1981; 117:238–9.

143. Hansen RC. Childhood histiocytosis syndromes. *Adv Dermatol* 1991; 6:161–97.

144. Nezelof C, Frileux-Herbert F, Cronier-Sachot J. Disseminated histiocytosis X. Analysis of prognostic factors based on a retrospective study of 50 cases. *Cancer* 1979; 44:1824–38.

145. Hashimoto K, Pritzker MS. Electron microscopic study of reticulohis-

tiocytoma. An unusual case of congenital, self-healing reticulohistiocytosis. *Arch Dermatol* 1973; 107:263–70.

146. Bonifazi E, Caputo R, Ceci A, Meneghini C. Congenital self-healing histiocytosis. Clinical, histologic, and ultrastructural study. *Arch Dermatol* 1982; 118:267–72.

147. Kapila PK, Grant-Kels JM, Alfred C, Forouhar F, Capriglione AM. Congenital, spontaneously regressing histiocytosis; a case report and review of the literature. *Pediatr Dermatol* 1985; 2:312–17.

148. Helwig EB, Hackney VC. Juvenile xanthogranuloma (nevoxanthoendothelioma). *Am J Pathol* 1954; 30:625–6.

149. Gonzales-Crussi F, Campbell R. Juvenile xanthogranuloma. Ultrastructural study. *Arch Pathol Lab Med* 1970; 89:65–72.

150. Schouten TJ, Hustinx TWJ, Scheres JHJC, Holland R, de Vaan GAM. Malignant histiocytosis. Clinical and cytogenetic studies in a newborn and a child. *Cancer* 1983; 52:1229–36.

151. Willman CL, Busque L, Griffith BB, et al. Langerhans' cell histiocytosis (histiocytosis X)—a clonal proliferative disease. *N Engl J Med* 1994; 331:154–60.

152. Rainier SS, Rainier BG. Needle puncture scars from midtrimester amniocentesis. *Arch Dermatol* 1984; 120:1360–2.

153. Eply SL, Hanson JW, Cruikshank DP. Fetal injury with mid-trimester diagnostic amniocentesis. *Obstet Gynecol* 1979; 53:77–80.

154. Rickwood AMK. A case of ileal atresia and ileo-cutaneous fistula caused by amniocentesis. *J Pediatr* 1979; 91:312.

155. Finegan JK, Quarrington BJ, Hughes H, et al. Infant outcome following mid-trimester amniocentesis: development and physical status at age six months. *Br J Obstet Gynaecol* 1985; 92:1015–23.

156. Lauerson HN, Miller FC, Paul RH. Continuous intrapartum monitoring of fetal scalp pH. *Am J Obstet Gynecol* 1979; 133:44–50.

157. Balfour HH, Black SH, Bowe ST, James LS. Complications of fetal blood sampling. *Am J Obstet Gynecol* 1970; 107:288–94.

158. Ashkenazi S, Metzker A, Merlob P, Ovadia J, Reisner SH. Scalp changes after fetal monitoring. *Arch Dis Child* 1985; 60:267–9.

159. Goldkrand JW. Intrapartum inoculation of herpes simplex virus by fetal scalp electrode. *Obstet Gynecol* 1982; 59:263–5.

160. Bowes WA, Bowes C. Current role of midforceps operation. *Clin Obstet Gynecol* 1980; 23:549–57.

161. Halme J, Ekbladh L. The vacuum extractor for obstetric delivery. *Clin Obstet Gynecol* 1982; 25:167–75.

162. Blumenfeld TA, Turi GK, Blanc WA. Recommended site and depth of newborn heel skin punctures based on anatomical measurements and histopathology. *Lancet* 1979; 1:230–3.

163. Sell EJ, Hansen RC, Struck-Pierce S. Calcified nodules on the heel: a complication of neonatal intensive care. *J Pediatr* 1980; 96:473–5.

164. Sybert VP, Holbrook KA, Levy M. Prenatal diagnosis of severe dermatologic disease. *Adv Dermatol* 1992; 7:179–209.

165. Elias S, Emerson DS, Simpson JL, Shulman LP, Holbrook KA. Ultrasound guided fetal skin sampling for prenatal diagnosis of genodermatoses. *Obstet Gynecol* 1994; 83:337–41.

166. Golbus MS, Sagebiel RW, Filly RA, Gindhart TD, Hall JG. Prenatal diagnosis of congenital bullous ichthyosiform erythroderma (epidermolytic hyperkeratosis) by fetal skin biopsy. *N Engl J Med* 1980; 302:93–5.

167. Holbrook KA, Dale VA, Sybert VP, Sagebiel RW. Epidermolytic hyperkeratosis: ultrastructure and biochemistry of skin and amniotic cells from affected fetuses and a newborn infant. *J Invest Dermatol* 1983; 80:222–7.

168. Rodeck CH, Eady RAJ, Gosden CM. Prenatal diagnosis of epidermolysis bullosa lethalis. *Lancet* 1980; 1:949–52.

169. Elias S, Mazur M, Sabbagha R, Esterly NB, Simpson JL. Prenatal diagnosis of harlequin fetus. *Clin Genet* 1980; 17:275–80.

170. Anton-Lamprecht I, Rauskolb R, Jovanovic V, et al. Prenatal diagnosis of EB dystrophica Hallopeau-Siemens with electron microscopy of fetal skin. *Lancet* 1981; 2:1077–9.

171. Kousseff BG, Matsuoka LY, Stenn KS, et al. Prenatal diagnosis of Sjögren-Larssen syndrome. *J Pediatr* 1982; 101:998–1001.

172. Braunstein GD, Ziel FH, Allen A, van de Velde R, Wade ME. Prenatal diagnosis of placental steroid sulfatase deficiency. *Am J Obstet Gynecol* 1976; 126:716–19.

173. Elias S, Esterly NB. Prenatal diagnosis of hereditary skin disorders. *Clin Obstet Gynecol* 1981; 24:1069–87.

174. Bodenheff J, Gorlin RJ. Natal and neonatal teeth: folklore and fact. *Pediatrics* 1963; 32:1087–93.

175. Cohen RL. Clinical perspectives on premature tooth eruption and cyst formation in neonates. *Pediatr Dermatol* 1984; 1:301–6.

176. Smith DW. Commentary: redundant skin folds in the infant—their origin and relevance. *J Pediatr* 1979; 94:1021–2.

177. Hall JG, Reed SD, Rosenbaum KN, et al. Limb pterygium syndromes: a review and report of eleven patients. *Am J Med Genet* 1984; 12:377–409.

177a. Lowry RB, Machin GA, Morgan K, et al. Congenital contractures, edema, hyperkeratosis, and intrauterine growth retardation; a fatal syndrome in Hutterite and Mennonite kindreds. *Am J Med Genet* 1985; 22:531–43.

177b. Welsh KM, Smoller BR, Holbrook KA, Johnston K. Restrictive dermopathy. Report of two affected siblings and review of the literature. *Arch Dermatol* 1992; 128:228–31.

177c. Sherer DM, Metlay LA, Mongeon C, et al. Congenital ichthyosis with restrictive dermopathy and Gaucher disease: a new syndrome with associated prenatal diagnostic and pathology findings. *Obstet Gynecol* 1993; 81:842–4.

178. Shah KN, Dalal SJ, Desai MP, et al. White forelock, pigmentary disorder of irides, and long segment Hirschsprung disease: possible variant of Waardenburg syndrome. *J Pediatr* 1981; 99:432–5.

179. Castro-Magana M, Hernandez-Perez E. Cornelia de Lange's syndrome. *Cutis* 1980; 26:59–62.

180. Hanson JW, Jones KL, Smith DW. Hypertrichosis in fetal alcohol syndrome. *JAMA* 1976; 235:1458–60.

181. Book A, Dawber R. *Diseases of the Hair and Scalp*. Oxford: Blackwell Scientific, 1982, pp. 187–96.

182. Ricci MA, Tunnessen WW, Pergolizzi JJ, Hellems MA. Menkes' kinky hair syndrome. *Cutis* 1982; 30:55–7.

182a. Winter H, Rogers MA, Langbein L, et al. Mutations in the hair cortex keratin GHbB cause the inherited hair disease monilethrix. *Nat Genet* 1997; 16:372–4.

183. Silvermann ME, Goodman RM, Cuppage TE. The nail-patella syndrome. Clinical findings and ultrastructural observations in the kidney. *Arch Intern Med* 1967; 120:68–74.

184. Soderquist NA, Reed WB. Pachonychia congenita with epidermal and other congenital dyskeratoses. *Arch Dermatol* 1968; 97:31–3.

185. Baran R, Stroud JD. Congenital onychodysplasia of index fingers. *Arch Dermatol* 1984; 120:243–4.

186. Alain G, Carrier C, Beaumier L, et al. In utero acute graft-versus-host disease in a neonate with severe combined immunodeficiency. *J Am Acad Dermatol* 1993; 29:863–5.

187. Peacocke M, Siminovitch KA. Wiscott-Aldrich syndrome: new molecular and biochemical insights. *J Am Acad Dermatol* 1992; 27:507–19.

188. Bonatvala JE, Horstmann DM, Payne MC, Gluck L. Rubella syndrome and thrombocytopenic purpura in newborn infants. *N Engl J Med* 1965; 273:474–8.

189. Fine J-D, Arndt KA. The TORCH syndrome: a clinical review. *J Am Acad Dermatol* 1985; 12:697–706.

190. Hendricks WM, Hu H-C. Blueberry muffin syndrome: cutaneous erythropoiesis and possible intrauterine viral infection. *Cutis* 1984; 34:549–51.

191. Hall JG, Levin J, Kuhn JP, et al. Thrombocytopenia with absent radius. *Medicine* 1969; 48:411–39.

192. Brough AJ, Jones D, Page RH, Mizukami I. Dermal erythropoiesis in neonatal infant. A manifestation of intrauterine viral disease. *Pediatrics* 1967; 40:627–35.

193. Argyle JC, Zone JJ. Dermal erythropoiesis in a neonate. *Arch Dermatol* 1981; 117:492–94.

194. Schwartz DL, Maniscalco WM, Lane AT, Currao WJ. Twin transfusion syndrome causing cutaneous erythropoiesis. *Pediatrics* 1984; 74:527–9.

195. Shown TE, Durface MF. Blueberry muffin baby: neonatal neuroblastoma with subcutaneous metastases. *J Urol* 1970; 104:193–5.

196. Nguyen TQ, Fisher GB, Tabbarah SO, et al. Metastatic neuroblastoma presenting as skin nodules at birth. *Int J Dermatol* 1988; 28:712–3.

197. Tasjian D, Jarratt M. Familial acanthosis nigricans. *Arch Dermatol* 1984; 120:1351–4.

198. Roth SI, Schedewie HK, Hertzberg VK, et al. Cutaneous manifestations of leprechaunism. *Arch Dermatol* 1981; 117:531–5.

199. Lemire RJ, Beckwith JB. Pathogenesis of congenital tumors and malformations of the sacrococcygeal region. *Teratology* 1982; 25:201–13.

200. Bale PM. Sacrococcygeal developmental abnormalities and tumors in children. *Perspect Pediatr Pathol* 1984; 1:9–56.

201. Harrist TJ, Gang DL, Kleinman GM, Mihm MC, Hendren WH. Unusual sacrococcygeal embryologic malformations with cutaneous manifestations. *Arch Dermatol* 1982; 118:643–8.

202. Higginbottom MC, Jones KL, Hall BD, Smith DW. The amniotic band disruption complex: timing of amniotic rupture and variable spectrum of consequent defects. *J Pediatr* 1979; 95:544–9.

203. Etches PC, Stewart AR, Ives EJ. Familial congenital amputations. *J Pediatr* 1982; 101:448–9.

204. Lubinsky M, Sujansky E, Sanger W, Salyards P, Severn C. Familial amniotic bands. *Am J Med Genet* 1983; 14:81–7.

205. Young ID, Lindenbaum RH, Thompson EM, Pembrey ME. Amniotic bands in connective tissue disorders. *Arch Dis Child* 1985; 60:1061–3.

206. Beyth Y, Perlman M, Ornoy A. Amniogenic bands associated with facial dysplasia and paresis. *J Reprod Med* 1977; 18:83–6.

207. Wang SS, Sanborn JR, Levine AJ, Delp RA. Amniotic rupture, extra-amniotic pregnancy, and vernix granulomata. *Am J Surg Pathol* 1984; 8:117–22.

208. Temtamy SA, McKusick VA. *The Genetics of Hand Malformations*. National Foundation March of Dimes, OAS 14. New York: Alan R. Liss, 1978.

209. Houston CS, Opitz JM, Spranger JW, et al. The camptomelic syndrome: review, report of 17 cases, and follow-up on the currently 17-year old boy first reported by Maroteaux et al in 1971. *Am J Med Genet* 1983; 15:3–28.

210. MacLean RN, Prater WK, Lozzio CB. Skeletal dysplasia with short angulated femora. *Am J Med Genet* 1983; 14:373–80.

211. Hall JG, Reed SD, Driscoll EP. Amyoplasia: a common, sporadic condition with congenital contractures. *Am J Med Genet* 1983; 15:571–90.

212. Schinzel A. *Catalogue of Unbalanced Chromosome Aberrations in Man*. Berlin: de Gruyter, 1984.

Chapter

34

The Hematopoietic System

CALVIN E. OYER DON B. SINGER

DEVELOPMENT OF HEMATOPOIETIC TISSUE

Hematopoiesis begins at 19 days of development in blood islands within the mesenchyme of the yolk sac, chorion, and connecting stalk. These tissues transform into endothelium and hematopoietic stem cells [1]. Within 3 or 4 days, large red blood cells (RBCs) enter the circulation without nuclear expulsion, a process reminiscent of avian erythropoiesis [2]. This first phase of hematopoiesis, the yolk sac phase, is short-lived with rapid subsidence after the 8th developmental week [1]. The second phase, the hepatic phase of hematopoiesis, then predominates. Experimental evidence suggests that a preexisting intact yolk sac is necessary for the subsequent hepatic and myeloid phases of fetal hematopoiesis [3]. Stem cells seed the liver as early as the 4th to 5th weeks of development. One or 2 weeks later, erythroid differentiation is identified in the hepatic sinusoids and these cells continue to proliferate throughout early gestation [2, 4] (Figs. 34.1 and 34.2). The liver remains a major hematopoietic organ throughout fetal life and is not superseded by the marrow until the third trimester [5, 6].

As the liver makes its contribution, non-nucleated erythrocytes appear in the circulation. Based on several studies, the proportion of all circulating erythrocytes that are non-nucleated can be used to estimate the embryonal age [1, 7–10]. If all or almost all erythrocytes are nucleated, the embryo is at the age of 6 completed developmental weeks or less. If almost all are without nuclei, the fetus is older than 9 developmental weeks. The percentage of nucleated erythrocytes progressively decreases during the 7th to 9th developmental weeks (9th to 11th weeks of "gestation" as measured from the last menstrual period). Embryonal and fetal erythrocytes are large, 10–15 μm in diameter (Fig. 34.3), and the mean corpuscular volume (MCV) remains high throughout gestation and the first days of life when values range from 100–115 fL.

Bone marrow stroma first appears in the clavicle during the 7th to 8th developmental weeks. Active hematopoiesis in the bone marrow follows about 3 weeks later [1, 10]. Marrow hematopoiesis gradually increases and all cell lines are represented by 20 developmental weeks [11]. In the third or myeloid phase of hematopoiesis, which occurs in the mid to late third trimester, 30–34 developmental weeks, the marrow becomes the major hematopoietic organ [4] (Figs. 34.4 and 34.5).

Extramedullary hematopoiesis (EMH) is found in the pancreas, thymus, kidneys, lymph nodes, heart, gonads, adrenals, skin, and so on [1]. Such sites can be prominent when abnormally activated. In phylogenesis the earliest sites of hematopoiesis are in many of these same organs [2]. Hematopoiesis may even develop in placental villi during the first trimester of gestation [10, 12]. When dermatitis, pericarditis, or interstitial nephritis is suspected in the fetus or neonate, the cells in question may actually represent EMH.

The spleen, well known as a site of EMH in abnormal conditions in children or adults, is usually listed as a fetal hematopoietic organ [13, 14]. Some immature blood elements are identified in the splenic red pulp as early as the 10th week of development but doubt has been cast on the spleen's role in forming blood cells other than lymphocytes. The spleen contains few granulocytes and megakaryocytes and the splenic myeloid/erythroid ratio is similar to that in fetal blood, suggesting that this organ merely traps circulating immature cells [15].

1143

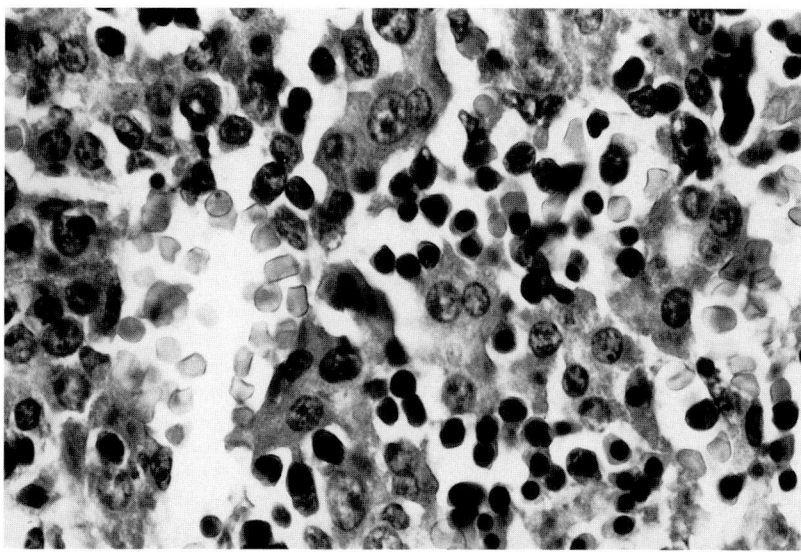

FIGURE 34.1. *Liver from fetus of 12 weeks' gestation with extensive erythropoiesis. H&E, ×820.*

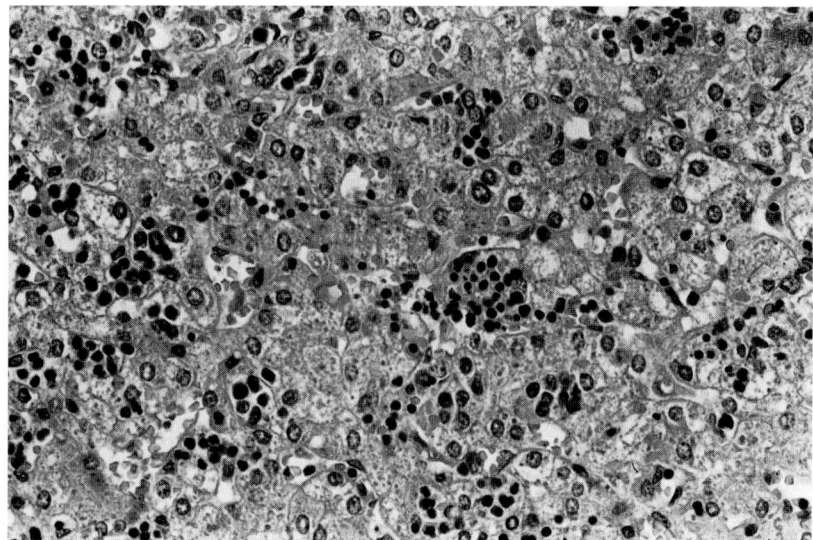

FIGURE 34.2. *Liver from fetus of 28 weeks' gestation with moderate erythropoiesis. H&E, ×490.*

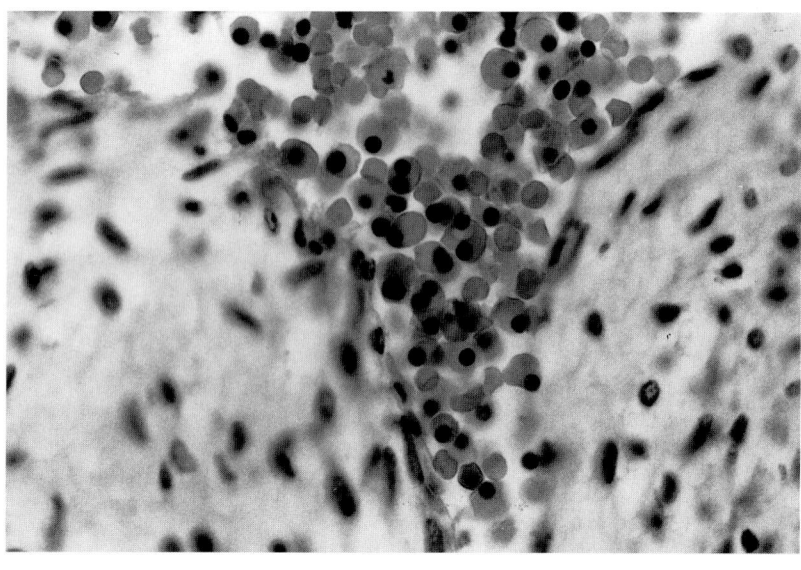

FIGURE 34.3. *Nucleated red blood cells in chorionic vesicle from embryo of 7 weeks' gestation. Note the large size of the red blood cells. H&E, ×820.*

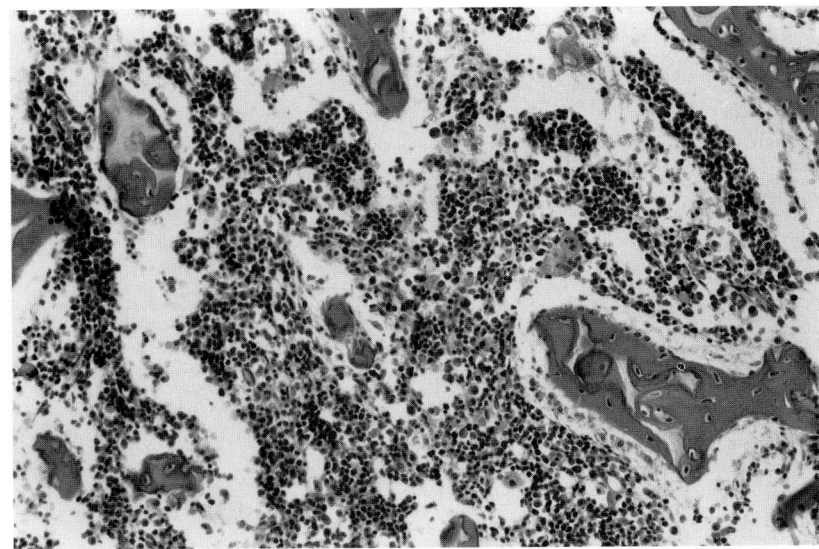

FIGURE 34.4. *Bone marrow from fetus of 28 weeks' gestation with prominent cellularity. H&E, ×205.*

Hematopoietic Stem Cells

Multipotent hematopoietic stem cells give rise to 2 lines of pluripotent hematopoietic stem cells. One line generates all lymphoid cells and the other is parent to more committed stem cells of the erythrocytic, myelomonocytic, and megakaryocytic series [16]. A schema for hematopoiesis is represented in Fig. 34.6 [17, 18].

Fetal blood contains unipotent stem cells (CFU-GM, BFU-E) and pluripotent stem cells (CFU-GEMM) as early as 10 weeks of development [19, 20]. Term neonates have more stem cells in the blood than do adults and extremely premature fetuses have 2 to 4 times as many stem cells as do term infants [3]. For this reason, cord blood may be substituted for marrow when considering transplantation in children with hematological disease, inborn errors of metabolism, or solid tumors [21–23]. The quantity of stem cells

in cord blood may even be adequate for adult recipients and HLA-mismatched recipients of any age but this has yet to be determined [22]. The immunological immaturity of cord blood lymphocytes seems to allow unrelated matched or partially mismatched transplants [24]. Adequate survival of transplanted cord stem cells has been demonstrated in HLA-1 disparate siblings [23]. Stem cells from another source, the liver, have been transplanted in utero in cases of severe immunodeficiency disease and thalassemia major [25].

Erythropoiesis

The earliest committed erythroid is the burst-forming unit (BFU-E) which, in the embryo, requires only erythropoietin for proliferation [26]. When stimulated by erythropoietin, interleukin-3, granulocyte-macrophage colony-stimulating

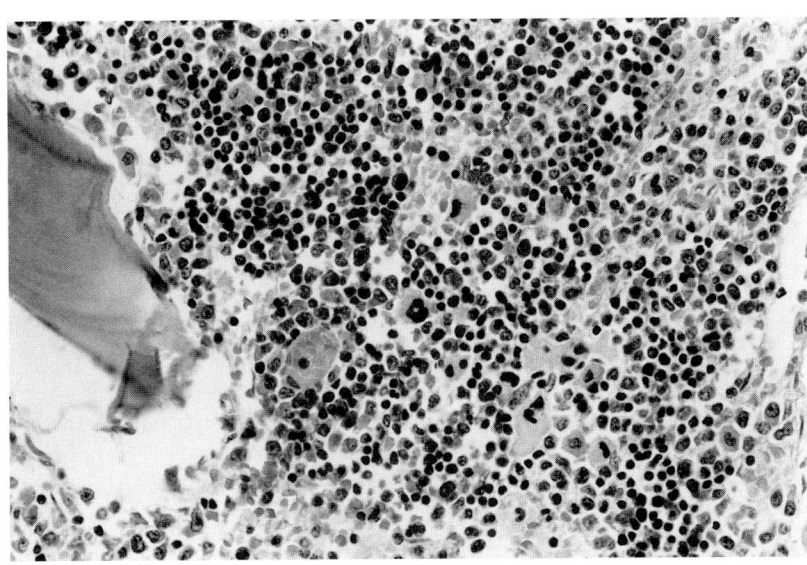

FIGURE 34.5. *Bone marrow from fetus of 28 weeks' gestation, magnified to illustrate varying cellular types. H&E, ×490.*

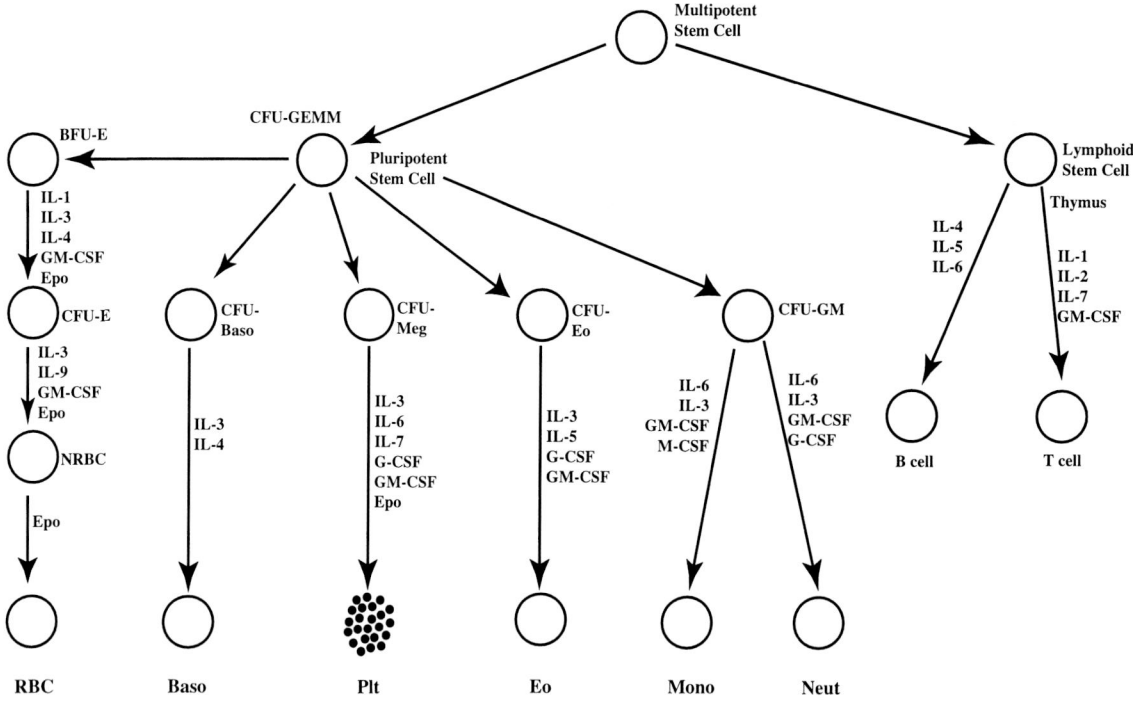

FIGURE 34.6.   *A schema of hematopoiesis and hematopoietic growth factors. The interactions of growth factors are complex. Schema such as this needs frequent re-evaluation as new knowledge is acquired. Baso = basophil; BFU = burst-forming unit; CFU = colony-forming unit; CSF = colony-stimulating factor; Eo = eosinophil; Epo = erythropoietin; G = granulocyte; IL = interleukin; Meg = megakaryocyte; M = macrophage except last M in GEMM = megakaryocyte; Mono = monocyte; Neut = neutrophil; NRBC = nucleated red blood cell; Plt = platelets; RBC = red blood cell. (Adapted from Quesenberry and Lowry [17] and Miller [18].)*

factor (GM-CSF), and other growth factors, BFU-E form colony-forming units (CFU-E).

Erythropoietin

Erythropoietin is produced in the fetal liver where it has both a paracrine effect and an endocrine effect. The relative ratio of volumes of erythroid precursors to hepatic parenchyma is 0.12–0.18 at 21 developmental weeks, falling to about 0.01 at term [27]. This decline is parallel in time to the decline of hepatic erythropoietin levels and the gradual switch to production by the kidney between 23 and 33 developmental weeks [28, 29]. Renal erythropoietin, produced in peritubular cells, has an endocrine effect on CFU-E and BFU-E, which by this time are predominantly located in the bone marrow [30]. Erythropoietin causes both proliferation of erythroblasts and release of reticulocytes into the bloodstream [31]. Erythropoietin production markedly decreases after birth in response to higher oxygen levels compared with those in fetal life. Infants who have congenital heart disease, have respiratory problems, or are otherwise hypoxemic or anemic are capable of increasing erythropoietin production [13, 32]. Maternal pre-eclampsia or diabetes and maternal consumption of alcohol or smoking of tobacco may be associated with increased fetal erythropoietin production [33–36].

Anemia of Prematurity

Because hepatic erythropoietin responds more slowly to anemia and hypoxia than does renal erythropoietin, premature infants whose erythropoietin is predominantly of hepatic origin have a limited ability to compensate for factors such as phlebotomy, hemolysis, and bleeding [29]. This results in "anemia of prematurity" [37]. Human recombinant erythropoietin plus iron is a promising therapy for stable premature infants but the benefits in seriously ill infants are not yet established [37, 38]. A reduction in the need for transfusions has not been clearly demonstrated either [39, 40].

Erythrocytes

Neonatal erythrocytes differ from those of older children and adults in many respects. In premature infants, the life span of RBCs is about 60–80 days but may be as short as 8–10 days [41]. As fetuses approach term gestation, the life span approaches 100 days. A few months after birth, the life span is equal to that of adults, about 120 days. Neonatal RBCs differ from those of adults in that they have weak expression of A and B and Lewis antigens [13]. I antigen is also weakly expressed while i antigen is strong. This relationship is reversed by the age of 18 months [42]. Neonatal RBCs are more susceptible than adult cells to injury from

Table 34.1. Fetal hematological values (mean ± standard deviation)

Week of Gestation	Corrected WBC Count ($\times 10^9$/L)	Normoblast (% WBCs)	Neutrophils (%)	Hemoglobin (gm/dL)	Hematocrit (%)	MCV (fL)	Platelets ($\times 10^9$/L)
18–21	2.57 ± 0.42	45 ± 86	6 ± 4	11.7 ± 1.27	37.3 ± 4.32	131 ± 11	234 ± 57
22–25	3.73 ± 2.17	21 ± 23	6.5 ± 3.5	12.2 ± 1.60	38.6 ± 3.94	125 ± 7.84	247 ± 59
26–29	4.08 ± 0.84	21 ± 67	8.5 ± 4	12.9 ± 1.38	40.9 ± 4.40	118 ± 7.96	242 ± 69
>30	6.40 ± 2.99	17 ± 40	23 ± 15	13.6 ± 2.21	43.5 ± 7.20	114 ± 9.34	232 ± 87

Source: Adapted from Forestier et al [45].
WBC = white blood cell; MCV = mean corpuscular volume.

oxidants; they also consume more oxygen and more readily precipitate denatured hemoglobin intracellularly (Heinz bodies) [13]. The premature infant's reticuloendothelial system removes damaged cells with difficulty, allowing continued circulation of cells with Heinz bodies, Howell-Jolly bodies, or "pocked erythrocytes" [43]. An occasional Howell-Jolly body can be seen in normal neonates, but larger numbers suggest a diagnosis of asplenia.

Circulating nucleated RBCs decrease throughout gestation as does the MCV [42–45] (Table 34.1). In normal term infants, the cord blood contains less than 1 nucleated RBC/100 total nucleated cells. At day 1 of life, 70% of the infants have no nucleated RBCs; by day 8 of life, 99% have no such cells [46]. Infants who are small for gestational age (SGA) have more nucleated RBCs than do those with appropriate weight for age [47]. Term SGA infants also show a high incidence of polycythemia (hematocrit >60%) [48].

The blood smear of the healthy neonate, especially if premature, may demonstrate RBC morphology that would be abnormal at a later age [49]. Changes more frequently seen in the neonate include poikilocytosis, anisocytosis, macrocytes, polychromasia, spherocytes, and RBC fragments.

The total blood volume is 80–85 mL/kg in term and 105 mL/kg in premature infants, with increased plasma contributing the higher value in the latter [50]. Both blood volume and total body mass triple during the last 3 months in utero [51]. Some studies indicated that hemoglobin concentration and hematocrit rise throughout fetal life [52] but others showed no age-related differences from 24 weeks to term [53, 54]. The disparities produce a wide range of reference values for fetal blood.

Because of changes in relative plasma volume, hemoglobin and hematocrit levels are higher in capillary blood than in cord blood. Arterial blood hematocrit equals that in venous blood but both are lower than the hematocrit of capillary blood or venous blood below a tourniquet [55]. The placental vessels contain 50–200 mL of blood and delayed cord clamping can increase the blood volume of the infant by as much as 100 mL, producing a marked effect on hematological measurements [50].

Neonates are born with more RBCs than needed in extrauterine life. After birth, the excess RBCs are rapidly destroyed. After day 3 of life some neonates are unable to process all the free hemoglobin and bilirubin, resulting in jaundice. These processes are more pronounced in the setting of intrauterine growth retardation or when mothers have pregnancy-induced hypertension [56].

Hemoglobin

After reaching a length of 1–2 mm, the developing embryo becomes dependent on an oxygen carrier mechanism, simple diffusion no longer sufficing [57]. Embryonic hemoglobins provide this mechanism. The ε chains are the first globin chains followed shortly by α, γ, and ζ chains [13]. Hemoglobin (Hb) Gower I (either a tetramer of ε or $\zeta_2\varepsilon_2$), Hb Gower II ($\alpha_2\varepsilon_2$), and Hb Portland ($\zeta_2\gamma_2$) are the embryonic hemoglobins [13]. As the site of erythropoiesis shifts to the liver, the production of fetal hemoglobin, Hb F ($\alpha_2\gamma_2$), increases, becoming predominant at about 8 developmental weeks [57]. Hb F comprises about 90% of hemoglobin in the fetus prior to the switch to Hb A and only about 0.5% in the normal adult [58]. Human chromosome 11 contains the information necessary for the switch and the pluripotent stem cell is thought to contain the "developmental clock" for switching [58]. A small quantity of Hb A was detected in a 35 mm embryo but Hb A ($\alpha_2\beta_2$) is not present in significant amounts until the third trimester and does not predominate until 6–8 months after birth [57, 59, 60].

The switches from embryonal to fetal to adult hemoglobin are closely related to gestational age and are not influenced by premature birth [61]. The sites are unrelated to the change in origin of erythropoietin, which gradually shifts from the liver to the kidney, or to the origin of erythrocytes, which changes from the liver to the bone marrow [41]. A cell that produces Hb F can produce Hb A and the proportion of the 2 forms of hemoglobin can vary widely from one cell to the next without regard to acquired fetal disease [31, 41].

The physiological advantage of Hb F is its avidity for oxygen compared with the maternal Hb A. Hb F has less

2,3-diphosphoglycerate (2,3-DPG) than does Hb A and oxygen affinity is inversely related to the amount of 2,3-DPG in the RBC [62]. Thus, oxygen is extracted from the mother's blood in the placental circulation but at the same time Hb F requires special conditions in the fetal tissues in order to release the oxygen. In the normal fetus, these conditions are relative hypoxia and relative acidosis. In abnormal fetuses, these conditions are exaggerated, allowing for greater release of oxygen.

Acute fetal hypoxia has no effect on relative levels of Hb A and Hb F but chronic hypoxia seems to delay the switch to Hb A. The decline of Hb F is delayed in infants who are SGA or are born to diabetic or hypoxemic mothers [18]. Hb F declines more rapidly with rapid cell turnover in conditions such as erythroblastosis fetalis [63]. However, high levels of Hb F persist in β-thalassemia, sickle cell anemia, Fanconi's anemia, and hereditary persistence of Hb F [63].

Iron

Iron is readily transferred from the mother to the fetus. Maternal iron deficiency must be severe before fetal iron deficiency develops. The normal total fetal body iron level is 70–75 mg/kg, of which 50–55 mg/kg is heme iron in erythrocytes, 10 mg/kg is stored iron in various organs, especially the liver, and 7 mg/kg is tissue iron including cytochrome and myoglobin iron [64]. The quantity of heme iron varies with the time of cord clamping at birth. During the first weeks or months of life, decreased erythropoiesis provides a honeymoon period with minimal need for dietary iron. Iron intake becomes important as growth accelerates and erythropoiesis resumes. Premature infants who are born with normal iron concentrations but reduced total body iron are especially prone to develop iron deficiency anemia.

Serum and storage iron is decreased and RBC iron is increased in infants of diabetic mothers, a condition char-acterized by chronic fetal hypoxia [64]. Growth-retarded infants, infants of diabetic mothers, and infants of mothers with pre-eclampsia have reduced cord serum ferritin levels, implying reduced fetal iron stores [65]. In renal agenesis decreased body iron is demonstrated by both chemical analysis and histological evaluation of iron in hepatocytes [66]. Renal agenesis is also associated with chronic fetal hypoxia, growth retardation, and reduced placental blood flow [67, 68].

Myelopoiesis and Megakaryopoiesis

In embryos of 3–5 weeks' developmental age, some granulocytic progenitors can form colonies of granulocytes, erythrocytes, macrophages, and megakaryocytes (CFU-GEMM); others generate mixtures of 2 lineages, for example, erythroid and granulocytic cells (CFU-MIX) [69]. Subsequent progenitors such as CFU-GM are committed to produce granulocytes and macrophages and appear in the fetal liver at 5 weeks of development [69]. In that setting, macrophages are more likely to form than are neutrophils, show more rapid cycling, and have a larger pool size [69]. Other committed progenitors generate eosinophils (CFU-Eo) or megakaryocytes (CFU-MK). Whether basophils are from an exclusively committed progenitor (CFU-Baso) or from a common progenitor with mast cells (CFU-Mast) is uncertain [16].

GM-CSF, granulocyte colony-stimulating factor (G-CSF), macrophage colony-stimulating factor (M-CSF), and interleukin-3, -6, -8, -9, and -11 participate in myelopoiesis [16] (see Fig. 34.6).

Granulocyte precursors are identified in early embryogenesis, but myelopoiesis is not prominent until hematopoiesis is well established in the bone marrow [14]. Monocytes and eosinophils are not seen regularly until the latter half of gestation [14]. In premature fetuses and

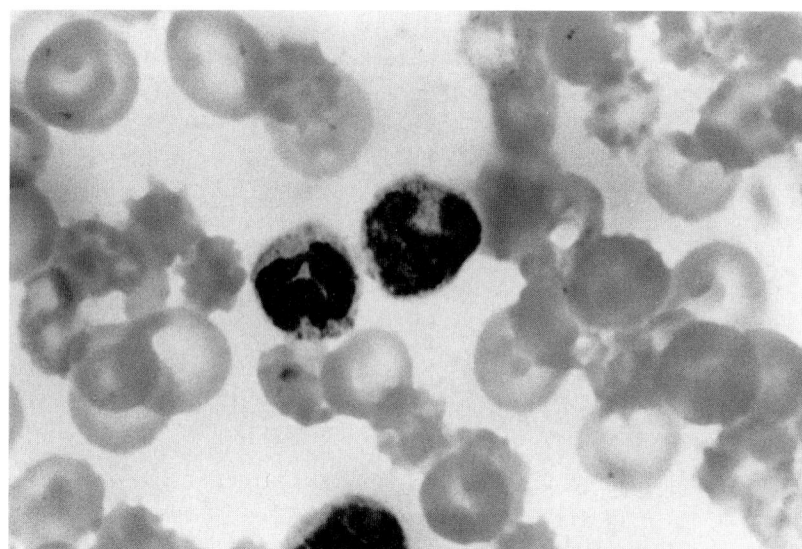

FIGURE 34.7.   *Peripheral blood leukocytes with scanty cytoplasmic granules and thickened nuclear lobules. Wright's stain, ×1480.*

Table 34.2. White blood cell counts

Age (hr)	Percentile	Lymphocytes/ μL	Monocytes/ μL	Eosinophils/ μL
0–60	95	7261	1912	843
	50	4184	600	136
	5	2017	0	0
61–120	95	6623	1740	808
	50	3663	528	176
	5	1915	0	0
120–720	95	9125	1717	839
	50	5616	669	235
	5	2859	97	0

Source: Adapted from Weinberg et al [77].

Table 34.3. Anemia of the fetus and neonate

Anemia of prematurity
Hemorrhage
  Fetofetal (twin-twin transfusion)
  Fetomaternal
  Thrombocytopenia
  Drug-induced coagulopathy
  Hepatic capsular hematomas
Hemolysis
  Alloimmune hemolytic disease
  Drug-induced hemolysis
  Hemoglobinopathies
  Microangiopathic hemolysis
Infections
  Sepsis, bacterial
  Viruses [78]
    Cytomegalovirus
    Rubella
    Parvovirus
  Syphilis [78]
  Toxoplasmosis [78]
Trauma
  Cord rupture
  Needle punctures
  Cephalopelvic disproportion

neonates, granulocytes and lymphocytes may appear large and are sometimes deformed or distorted in smears of peripheral blood. Granules in the neutrophils, eosinophils, and basophils are poorly developed (Fig. 34.7).

Megakaryoblasts appear in the yolk sac at 5 weeks' developmental age and megakaryocytes circulate in the blood of the embryo [1]. Fetal megakaryocytes are small and immature as judged by nuclear/cytoplasmic ratio and nuclear complexity, and do not reach adult size until the age of 1 year [70]. Many megakaryocyte progenitor cells (CFU-MK) and circulating megakaryocytes are present in cord blood [71]. Megakaryocytes are readily identified in the fetal bone marrow (see Fig. 34.5). Thrombopoietin promotes megakaryocyte progenitor expansion and megakaryocyte differentiation [72].

Lymphopoiesis

Stem cell precursors of B and T cells originate in the yolk sac, migrate to the liver, and can be detected there by 8–9 weeks. They then migrate to the bone marrow where neighboring stromal cells promote the growth and differentiation of B cells. B cells with surface immunoglobulins are present in blood, bone marrow, liver, and spleen during the 10th week of development [73]. The capacity to secrete immunoglobulins cannot be demonstrated until about 20 postmenstrual weeks [74].

Stem cell precursors of T cells migrate to the embryonal thymus, with lymphocytes appearing there at 9–10 weeks; some stem cells remain in the marrow and migrate to the thymus in adult life [75]. See Chapter 16 for information regarding the origin and migration of T cells, the role of T and B cells in immunology, and their interactions with one another and with other components of immune reactions.

Fewer T cells and more B cells are present in fetuses of all gestational ages than in older infants, children, and adults. The concentration of helper T cells (OK T4 cells) is equivalent to that of adults but the suppressor T cells (OK T8

cells) are less numerous than in adults through 19–28 weeks' gestation. The ratio of T4 to T8 cells is therefore greater in fetuses and neonates than in adults [52]. Natural killer cells can be detected, especially after induction with interferon [76].

In peripheral blood, lymphocytes decline about the 3rd day of life and reach steady-state values by the age of 1 week (Table 34.2). A reciprocal but earlier rise in neutrophils is noted during the first day of life. Sepsis causes a reduction in the numbers of lymphocytes, eosinophils, and neutrophils during the first 2–3 days of disease. These cell types and the monocyte counts rise as recovery progresses. Babies born to mothers with hypertension have depressed numbers of lymphocytes and neutrophils. Conversely, hemolytic disease due to ABO incompatibility produces an increase in neutrophils and monocytes, as well as in reticulocytes and nucleated RBCs [77].

FETAL AND NEONATAL ANEMIA

The more common causes of anemia in fetuses and neonates are listed in Table 34.3 [78].

Hemolytic Diseases of the Fetus and Newborn

As RBCs are destroyed in the reticuloendothelial tissues, the hemoglobin molecule is split into hematin (iron-containing moiety) and the globin moieties. The iron is extracted and

Table 34.4.   Hyperbilirubinemia in neonates

Blood group incompatibility
Red cell membrane defects
Hemoglobinopathies
Red cell enzyme defects
Extravascular blood, e.g., hematomas
Polycythemia
Increased enterohepatic circulation
  Pyloric stenosis, duodenal atresia, etc.
Metabolic-endocrine disease
  Galactosemia, tyrosinemia, etc.
Biliary atresia
Cystic fibrosis with meconium ileus
Sepsis
Intrauterine infections, e.g., rubella, cytomegalovirus
Hepatitis

Source: From Odel et al [81].

the cyclic tetrapyrole nucleus opens to form biliverdin; this is reduced to bilirubin within phagocytes. Free (unconjugated) bilirubin is bound loosely to albumin in the serum, is carried to the liver, and is incorporated into hepatocytes. Diglucuronide conjugation takes place, and the conjugated bilirubin is carried to the gut and is excreted in the stool. Processing 1 gram of hemoglobin produces 35 mg of bilirubin; when this is diluted in 300 mL of blood, as in a full-term neonate, the liver is presented with 11.7 mg/dL of bilirubin which needs to be conjugated and expelled from the circulation [79]. A small amount of conjugated bilirubin makes its way to the circulation but it is not toxic. Unconjugated bilirubin, on the other hand, is toxic and is capable of crossing cell membranes including the blood–brain barrier [80].

Excessive destruction of fetal RBCs leads to anemia, overloading the reticuloendothelial system with red cell detritus, and the liver with free hemoglobin and unconjugated bilirubin. The anemia can be profound, resulting in acidosis, heart failure, and edema progressing to anasarca in utero (fetal hydrops). Unconjugated bilirubin in large concentrations, whatever the primary cause of the increase, is capable of producing kernicterus. Iron in the excess hemoglobin is converted to hemosiderin. Collectively these are the features of hemolytic diseases of the newborn (HDN). As a corollary, sites of erythropoiesis are hyperplastic. The liver and spleen may be massively enlarged, and nucleated erythrocytes are increased in the circulating blood. Hyperbilirubinemia is often the most striking feature and should be analyzed with attention to the differential diagnoses (Table 34.4) [81].

Immune HDN

Maternal-Fetal Rh Incompatibility   The classic example of HDN occurs when an Rh-negative mother is sensitized by

her fetus's Rh-positive antigen-bearing RBCs. (In this discussion the inclusive "Rh" is used with the understanding that the D antigen is the usual culprit though the less potent Rh antigens can produce disease.) Use of Rh immune globulin, the blocking antibody, has reduced the incidence of this disease to a few percent of its previous incidence.

In the naturally occurring disease, pathogenesis is as follows. Most fetal RBCs reach the maternal circulation at the time of delivery but a few cross the placenta from about 20 weeks of gestation onward [82]. In nearly all cases, the first-born Rh-positive child is unaffected. Each subsequent Rh-positive fetus is at increased risk because the mother is repeatedly sensitized. Some mothers are especially responsive to small numbers of fetal RBCs, which may elicit a large anti-Rh antibody response. In other mothers, weak antibody responses are noted, perhaps because their fetus's RBCs have fewer Rh antigens, or fewer exposed ones, or the mother's own immune response is muted.

Maternal antibodies of IgG type cross from the maternal circulation through the placenta to the fetal circulation where they attach to the fetal RBCs and, with the aid of complement, cause lysis. The IgG subclasses 1 and 3, either of which is capable of fixing complement, induce hemolysis. IgG subclass 2 does not fix complement but may be elevated in cases of incompatibility between mother and fetal RBCs. Because of the latter phenomenon, high titers of maternal antibody specific for fetal blood groups do not necessarily correlate with the severity of disease and may confound interpretation of laboratory tests [83].

Other fetal red cell antigens can cause similar disease but are either less potent immunogens or less frequent than the Rh antigen. These include, in decreasing order of frequency, major blood group antigens A and B (see below), minor blood antigens such as the Rh antigens c and E, Kell, Duffy, Kidd, MS, and so on. Virtually all of the firmly adherent RBC antigens have been implicated in HDN [84].

ABO Fetal-Maternal Blood Group Incompatibility   Among the white population with blood group O, the incidence of maternal-fetal ABO incompatibility is about 1 in 7. Few of these pregnancies result in clinical hemolytic disease in the neonate [85]. ABO incompatibility has essentially the same frequency in blacks as it has in whites but it more frequently causes ABO HDN, possibly due to stronger expression of A and B antigens [86, 87]. Arabs have an incidence of ABO HDN similar to that of blacks and the disease tends to be more severe than in Europeans [87]. The titer of maternal anti-A or anti-B IgG antibodies is not a good indicator of severity since, like the anti-Rh antibodies, much of the IgG may be subclass 2, which does not cause hemolysis [83]. The direct antibody (Coomb's) test of cord blood detects maternal IgG antibodies on the surfaces of the neonate's RBCs. The test result is usually positive with ABO incompatibility but by itself is not an adequate indicator of severity since most of the maternal antibodies may be absorbed onto other fetal cells with A or B antigens. Two useful tests are 1) the antibody-dependent cell-mediated cytotoxicity using exoge-

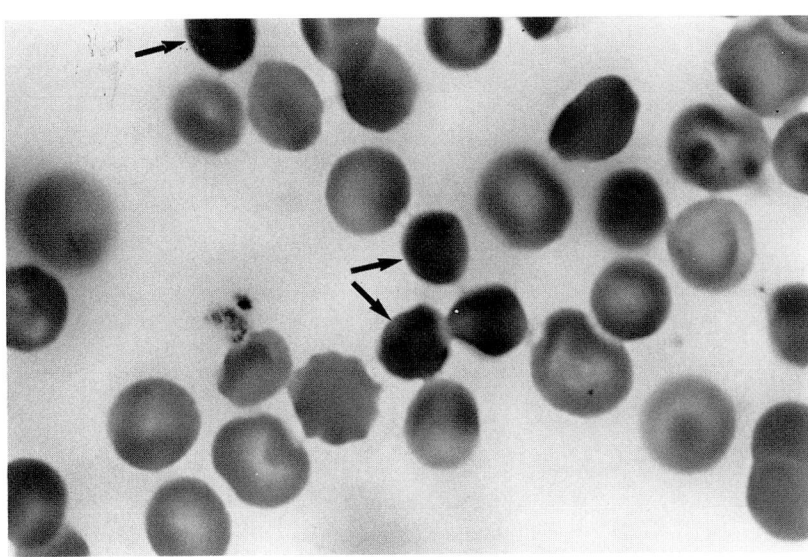

FIGURE 34.8.   *Peripheral red blood cells with several spherocytes (arrows). This is from a baby with ABO-hemolytic disease. Similar numbers of spherocytes may be found in neonates with congenital spherocytosis. Wright's stain, ×1480.*

nous lymphocytes and 2) the density of the A or B antigen on the surfaces of the RBCs. These tests more accurately determine the severity of the disease and suggest which infants may require transfusions or exchange transfusions [83]. In the final analysis ABO HDN is a clinical diagnosis merely supported by laboratory methods. A large number of spherocytes is a clinically useful feature that helps to differentiate ABO incompatibility from other forms of immune hemolytic disease (Fig. 34.8).

Autoantibodies   Though maternal IgG autoantibodies can theoretically cause neonatal anemia, all important neonatal red cell antibodies are alloimmune.

Non-immune HDN

Three main pathogenetic mechanisms are responsible for non-immune hemolytic diseases: 1) abnormalities of hemoglobin synthesis, 2) disorders of the RBC membrane, and 3) disorders of the RBC metabolism.

Hemoglobinopathies   Hb F contains 2 α chains and 2 γ chains. Defects of γ chains [88] and α chains occur in fetuses. Two α-chain genes are located on each of the paired 16 chromosomes. (Genes for β, γ, and δ chains are located in a tightly linked complex on chromosome 11.) When 1 or 2 of the 4 α-chain genes are deleted, no untoward effect is noted but the affected individual becomes a carrier for α-thalassemia. Those with 1 or 2 gene defects show elevated Bart's Hb in cord blood but thereafter can only be definitively diagnosed by molecular techniques. Patients with deletion of 2 genes are asymptomatic or only mildly anemic; however, their RBCs are microcytic and hypochromic. When 3 of the 4 α-chain genes are deleted, the individual suffers from Hb H disease, an anemia of adults with characteristic inclusions in specially stained preparations of RBCs. At birth electrophoresis reveals some Bart's Hb but Hb H, a tetramer of β chains, replaces Bart's Hb as the switch from γ to β chains occurs. If all 4 α-chain genes are deleted, a tetramer

composed of 4 γ chains, Bart's Hb, is substituted and results in the most severe expression of α-thalassemia with fatal hydrops fetalis. This disease is most often found in Southeast Asians in whom α-chain gene deletions are frequent [89]. One or 2 gene defects occur in blacks, but on any given chromosome only 1 gene is missing, thus not allowing for either Hb H or Bart's Hb disease.

Because Hb F has no β chains, it has a protective effect in sickle cell patients. Fetal cells will not sickle even in subjects homozygous for Hb S and sickle cell disease does not develop in early infancy while Hb F persists.

Women with sickle hemoglobin trait can have normal pregnancies and babies despite the prominent sickling phenomenon in the maternal compartment of placentas (Fig. 34.9). Women with homozygous sickle cell disease, or with S-C disease or S-β–thalassemia are at high risk for developing sickle crises, pregnancy-induced hypertension, and urinary tract infections. Fetal deaths are increased by a factor of 10 in women with these abnormal hemoglobins [90].

Unstable hemoglobin variants, most often involving the β chain, cause congenital Heinz body hemolytic anemias but presentation is usually delayed until childhood or adulthood. Hemolysis may be exacerbated by fever. Heinz bodies are detected with supravital staining and are single or multiple granules of denatured globin. Acquired Heinz body hemolytic anemia develops in neonates after oxidative injury [91]. Other causes include pentose phosphate pathway enzyme deficiencies, chronic liver disease, and postsplenectomy states [63].

Membrane Defects in Red Blood Cells   The RBC membrane consists of a network of proteins that maintains the cell's shape and contributes to its ability to deform as it maneuvers through the reticuloendothelial system. Among the proteins involved are the spectrins (α and β), ankyrin, protein 4.1, and actin [92, 93]. Many membrane defects, some poorly defined, produce perinatal hemolytic disease.

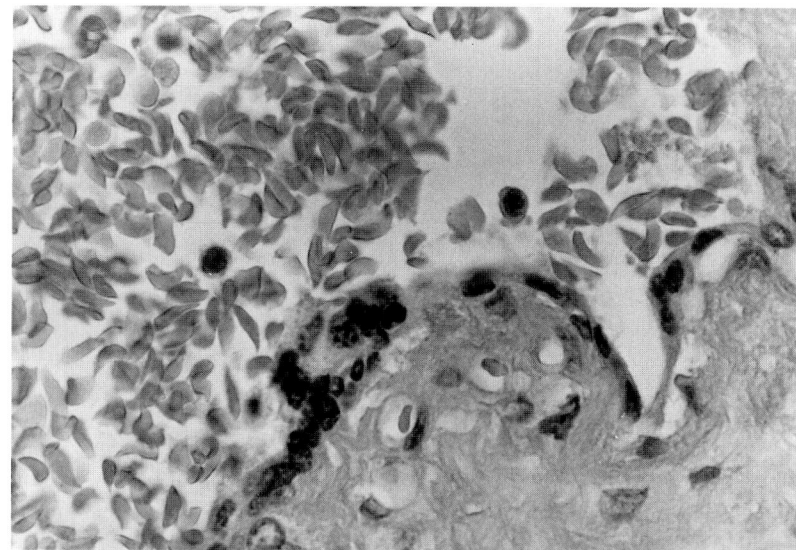

FIGURE 34.9.   *Sickle cells present in intervillous spaces in the placenta. These cells are identified in formalin-fixed placental tissue even when the mother has only sickle trait. H&E, ×592.*

Hereditary spherocytosis (HS) is the most common of these and the most common hemolytic anemia among whites. At least 2 inheritance patterns are known. Among affected families, 75% show an autosomal dominant pattern involving an absent copy of the ankyrin gene on chromosome 8, defects in β-spectrin on chromosome 14, or defects in protein 3 on chromosome 17 [92, 93]. Of the remaining 25% of HS cases, it is uncertain how many are autosomal recessive forms. Neonatal jaundice and anemia develop in 50% of affected babies, although these signs may be delayed for a week or more. The severity of neonatal anemia is not a good predictor of later severity [93]. Spherocytes are demonstrated in the peripheral blood, but may not be numerous until the age of 2 or 3 months. Neonatal HS is sometimes difficult to distinguish from ABO hemolytic disease (see Fig. 34.8). Either condition may have numerous spherocytes and either condition may have increased

osmotic fragility of RBCs. The direct anti-IgG antibody test is negative with HS and serves as a differentiating feature. Examination of first-degree family members for evidence of spherocytes or abnormal osmotic fragility further serves to differentiate the 2 conditions.

Hereditary elliptocytosis (HE) is characterized by cigar-shaped red cells (Fig. 34.10). It is mild or asymptomatic in adults, and is more common in persons of African or Mediterranean ancestry [93]. Genetically and clinically heterogeneous, HE has 2 genes located on chromosome 1, one adjacent to the Rh locus and another near the Duffy locus [92]. A closely related and possibly inseparable disorder is hereditary pyropoikilocytosis (HPP) in which affected neonates, usually of African origin, have severe hemolytic anemia with markedly deformed RBCs. HPP may be merely another form of HE, perhaps the homozygous state. Adult relatives often have typical HE and survivors of HPP

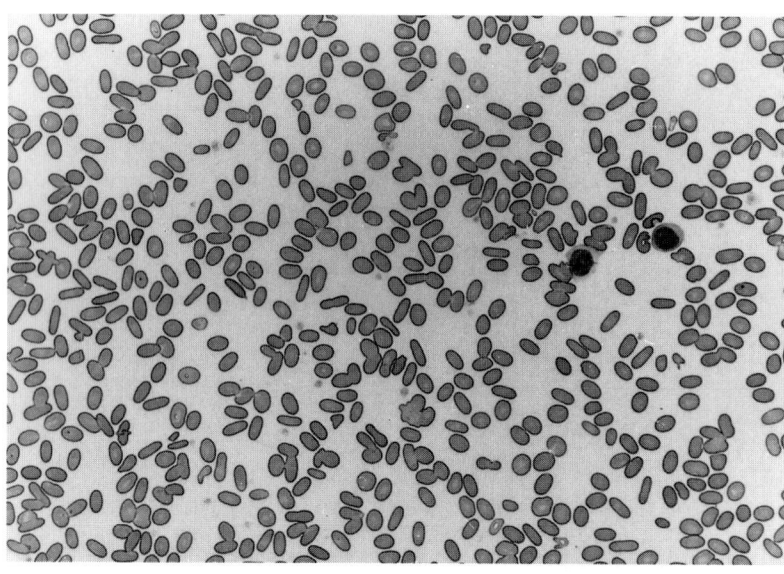

FIGURE 34.10.   *Peripheral red blood cells with elliptocytosis. Though rare, this can produce hemolytic disease in neonates. Wright's stain, ×296.*

have amelioration of disease to a typical HE phenotype [92, 93].

Southeast Asian ovalocytosis is associated with a defect in ankyrin binding and is present in 30% of the population in certain areas where malaria is endemic. It might represent another disorder, along with thalassemia and Hb S, offering resistance to malaria [94].

Vitamin E, an antioxidant, has a complex relationship with infantile anemia. Vitamin E deficiency, especially likely in low-birthweight infants, produces a poorly understood nutritional hemolytic anemia, probably involving membrane proteins in RBCs [92].

Red Cell Enzyme Defects In the Embden-Meyerhof and pentose phosphate pathways of carbohydrate metabolism, fetal and neonatal RBCs may have enzyme deficiencies leading to severe hemolysis and hydrops fetalis. Examples include glucose-6-phosphate dehydrogenase deficiency (manifested after maternal fava bean or sulfisoxazole ingestion), glucose phosphate isomerase deficiency, and deficiencies of hexokinase, pyruvate kinase, phosphofructokinase (PFK), triose phosphate isomerase, and phosphoglycerate kinase [95–99]. Pyruvate kinase deficiency characteristically has scattered burr cells in the peripheral blood (Fig. 34.11).

Disorders of Heme Pathway Metabolism Abnormalities of heme molecules are rarely expressed in the newborn infant. One such disorder is congential erythropoietic porphyria, an autosomal recessive condition with accumulation and hyperexcretion of type I porphyrins. One-third of patients will have symptoms as neonates. Abnormal porphyrin compounds in stool and urine cause an alarming red staining of diapers. Hemolytic anemia and skin eruptions develop in later infancy or childhood [79].

Acquired Hemolytic Disorders

Hemolytic anemia with red cell fragments (schistocytes) and microspherocytes can be secondary to congenital or acquired disorders of the microcirculation (Fig. 34.12). The setting is usually disseminated intravascular coagulopathy (DIC) in which RBCs are sheared as they flow through fibrin strands [100]. Sepsis is likely to be the cause in neonates. Large hemangiomas with localized DIC (Kasabach–Merritt syndrome) can also produce hemolysis in neonates. Infection with parvovirus B19 produces a profound hemolysis in some fetuses.

Pathology of HDN (Erythroblastosis Fetalis)

Whatever the cause in the fetus or newborn, severe hemolytic disease leads to erythroblastosis, fetal anasarca, and intrauterine or early postnatal death. Less severe forms are compatible with neonatal anemia or jaundice. These variations of erythroblastosis fetalis are referred to as hydrops fetalis, congenital anemia of the newborn, and icterus gravis [101]. Erythroblastosis and hydrops develop when the fetal hemoglobin level falls below 7 gm/dL [102]. Heart failure plays a role in the hydrops. The placenta is massive, boggy, and pale. Cytotrophoblast is hyperplastic and the villi appear immature. The heart is enlarged and pale with foci of extramedullary hematopoiesis in the epicardium. Lungs are edematous and adrenal glands are usually enlarged. The liver is greatly enlarged due to congestion and masses of erythropoietic tissue. Although the claim has been made that erythroblastosis before 28 weeks of gestation does not cause enlargement of the liver or spleen, we have seen several cases with these findings in earlier weeks of gestation [46]. The enlarged liver contains excessive iron in hepatocytes and in Kupffer cells. In about 7% of cases, focal hepatic necrosis is found; in about 3% the reticulum in portal zones increases mildly; in 1.4% cirrhosis develops [103]. Precipitated bile pigment forms canalicular bile plugs. Splenic sinusoids are dilated and erythroid colonies and iron deposits are increased (Fig. 34.13). Nucleated erythroid precursors are

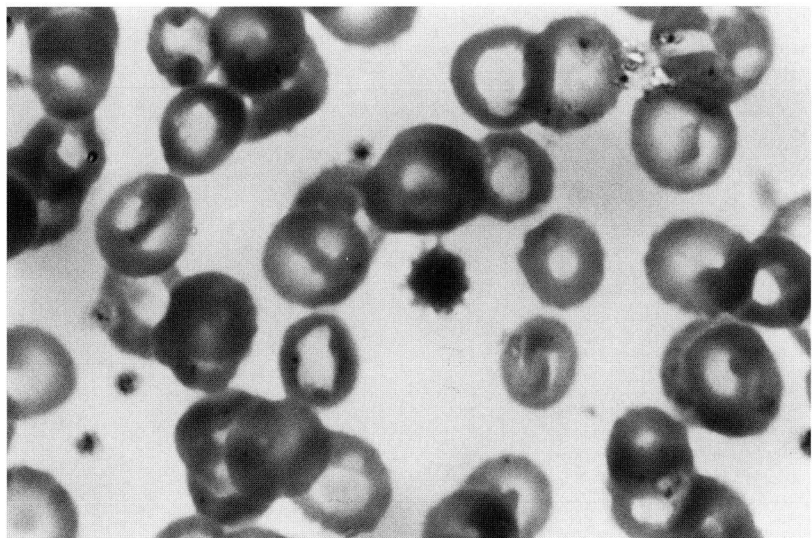

FIGURE 34.11. *Peripheral red blood cells with occasional burr cells, from a neonate with pyruvate kinase deficiency, severe hemolysis, and anemia. Wright's stain, ×1480.*

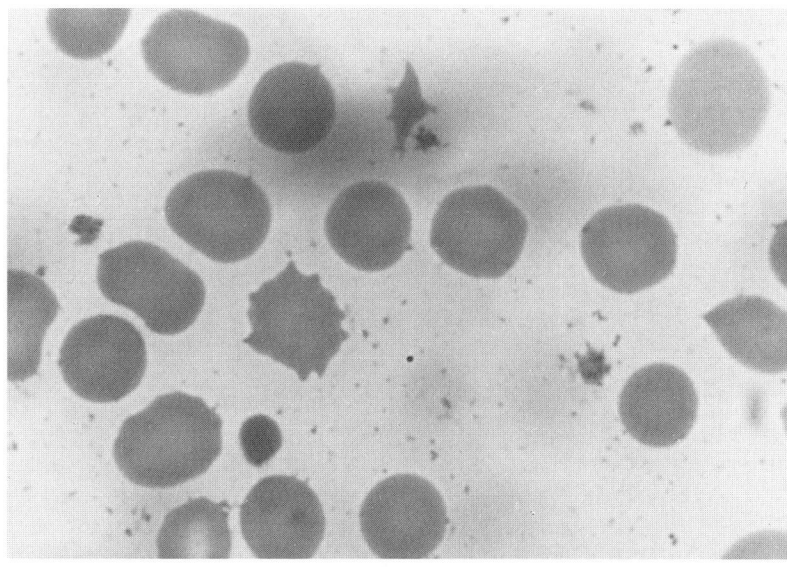

FIGURE 34.12. *Peripheral smear from a neonate with disseminated intravascular coagulation. A red cell fragment and a microspherocyte are seen. Wright's stain, ×1480.*

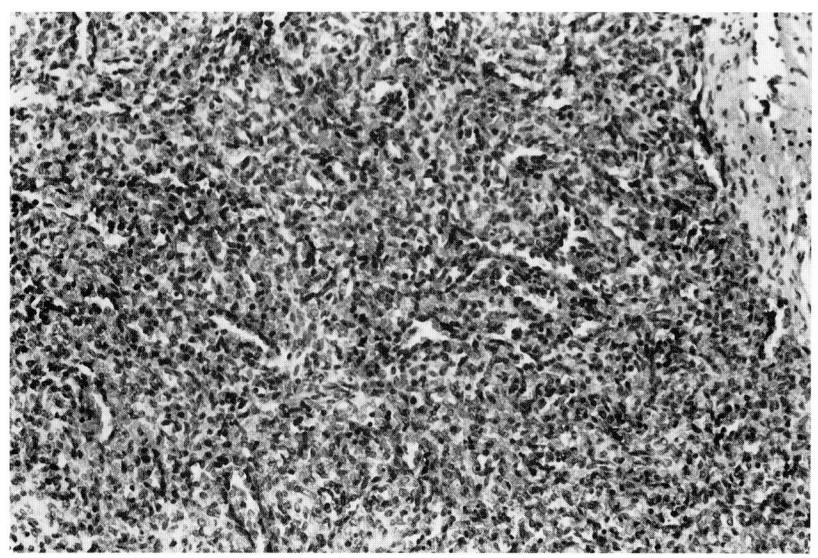

FIGURE 34.13. *Spleen with dilated empty sinusoids, occasional clusters of erythropoiesis, and decreased white pulp. This newborn baby was born at 24 weeks' gestation and had erythroblastosis fetalis. H&E, ×410.*

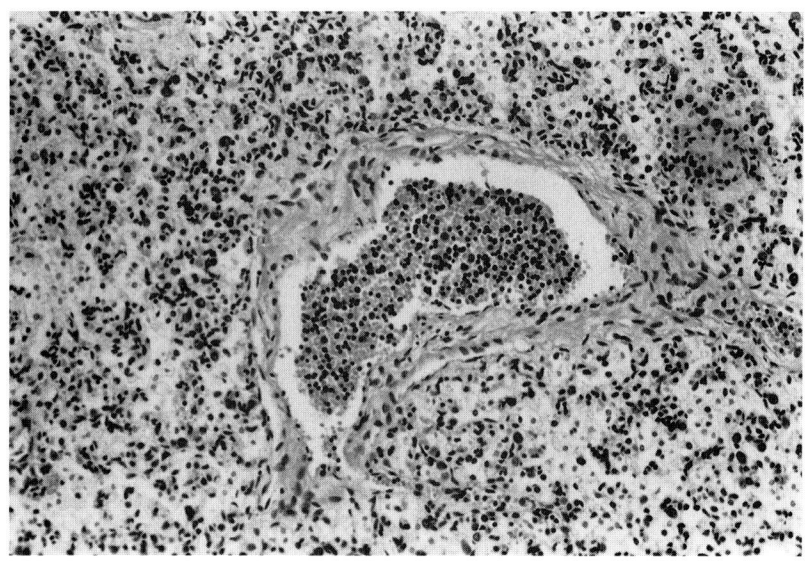

FIGURE 34.14. *Small blood vessel in the autolysed lung of a stillborn fetus with erythroblastosis fetalis, delivered at 28 weeks' gestation. The lumen is filled with nucleated erythroids. H&E, ×410.*

found in the circulating blood, sometimes apparently plugging the lumina of small vessels (Fig. 34.14). Erythropoiesis is especially prominent in the liver, lymph nodes, spleen, thymus, and bone marrow. Almost every organ and tissue in the body, including the dermis, has clusters of erythropoiesis. In fetuses close to term gestation, the breast tissue may appear hemorrhagic, but microscopically will show large masses of erythropoietic elements.

In some cases the thymus may be involuted, lymph nodes inconspicuous, and the spleen small [46]. In our own experience, the spleen is most often enlarged due to congestion and excessive extramedullary erythropoiesis, although the volume of white pulp is reduced (see Fig. 34.13). Splenic rupture is a rare complication. Infants with the most profound anemia may have the largest number of circulating nucleated RBCs but plasma volume may be greatly reduced. Part of the pathogenesis of disease is reduced oxygen-carrying capacity of the antibody-coated RBCs [104]. Some babies develop cutaneous petechiae and purpura and hemorrhages in lungs, brain, meninges, and adrenals. Hypoglycemia is common and, inexplicably, pancreatic islets are increased in both size and number. Radiolucent metaphyseal lines may be seen on radiographs although pathological descriptions are lacking [105]. The number of neutrophils and platelets may be decreased [106].

Jaundice is not usually evident in the first few hours of life. The mother's placental circulation is responsible for clearing the bilirubin from the fetal blood. In severely affected infants or in those born to mothers with liver disease the umbilical cord is stained bright yellow and neonatal skin is visibly jaundiced, if not at birth, then within a few hours [46]. Jaundice may be delayed for several days. As a rule, the earlier the onset of jaundice, the poorer is the prognosis.

When free or unconjugated bilirubin exceeds the binding capacity of the baby's plasma proteins, or when acidosis is severe, bilirubin crosses the blood–brain barrier and is deposited in the cytoplasm of neurons, particularly in the basal ganglia. The toxicity of bilirubin in these cells is poorly understood as is the particular affinity for neurons of the basal ganglia, hippocampus, and cerebellum [107]. Mitochondria are affected [108]. The characteristic yellow or golden deposits are often faint, especially in small premature infants of less than 28 weeks' gestation. Formalin fixation diminishes but does not abolish the intensity of the stain.

Deposits of bilirubin in the brains of term newborns cause classic clinical signs such as opisthotonus, rigidity of limbs, cyanosis, irregular respirations with apneic intervals, frothy blood-tinged mucus, and ultimately circulatory collapse. In untreated infants fever and seizures are frequent and the mortality rate with this clinical picture is 50% [109]. These features are seldom seen today. Serum levels of free, unconjugated bilirubin less than 20 mg/dL are generally considered benign. This "magic" figure, established empirically decades ago in full-term babies, no longer applies since most infants at risk for kernicterus are premature, some of

very low birthweight, with a blood–brain barrier that is more permeable to bilirubin. If the serum unconjugated bilirubin level rapidly rises (i.e., >1 mg/dL/hr), or if the level of serum bilirubin exceeds the binding capacity of the serum albumin, or if acidosis is present, exchange transfusion is the treatment of choice. Survivors of kernicterus may show sensorineural deafness, dyslexia, speech defects, or more severe sequelae such as cerebral palsy with mental retardation, ataxia, or athetosis [110].

Exchange transfusions revolutionized the treatment and outcome of erythroblastosis. The incidence of kernicterus is now much less than it was a few decades ago. In the early experience with exchange transfusion, the routes of delivery of blood were through the sagittal sinus of the skull, the radial artery, the umbilical vein, or the femoral vein [111]. The iatrogenic problems associated with these procedures included electrolyte imbalance, hypervolemia, transient and sometimes fatal cardiac dysrhythmias, infection, hepatic or splenic rupture, focal bowel necrosis, radial artery occlusions, thromboses of the sagittal sinus, and femoral vein and umbilical vein with propagation of thrombi to the liver and with emboli to the lung. The advent of intrauterine blood transfusion (IUT) into the fetal peritoneum in the 1960s was associated with poor results in the hands of most practitioners, but this was better than the utter futility and nearly 100% fetal mortality associated with doing nothing [112–114]. The earlier technique, performed with indirect radiological guidance, resulted in needle puncture wounds to various external and internal body parts, including the eye, brain, and heart. Circulatory overload and shock were common causes of fetal demise. Significant hepatocellular damage was uncommon although serum hepatitis associated with intracerebral hemorrhage was reported after intra-abdominal transfusions in utero [115].

A second revolution in technique is underway with intrauterine ultrasonographically guided cordocentesis and umbilical vein exchange transfusion. When access to the fetal circulation is obtained, the hemoglobin level is determined. The MCV is evaluated to confirm that fetal blood is present. If doubt exists, a Kleihauer-Betke test can be performed. Based on evolving standards, a decision is made regarding transfusion, exchange, or otherwise. These techinques have not replaced amniotic fluid bilirubin concentration for evaluation but have provided more definitive assessment of severity and need for intervention. IUT can be performed as early as 17 weeks' gestation and is usually repeated at 1–3-week intervals until the propitious time for birth arrives [116]. The procedure is not without complications. We have observed a case of florid hepatic giant-cell transformation and cerebral hemorrhage in a baby 16 days old who had 4 intravenous transfusions in utero, 2 of which were exchange transfusions and 2 neonatal exchange transfusions.

Late anemia can complicate Rh disease in untreated patients, patients treated with phototherapy only, or even those treated with exchange transfusions. The latter is less likely if the infant was born at term [117].

Other Causes of Anemia

External Fetal Hemorrhage

Fetuses can bleed into the maternal circulation, into the uterine contents and maternal vagina, or into a fetal sibling in cases of monochorial placentation. Small numbers of fetal RBCs normally enter the maternal circulation but rarely produce significant fetal anemia. In the last trimester fetal erythrocytes are present in the blood of approximately 30% of gravid women but the volume of fetal blood exceeds 0.1 mL in fewer than 6% [118]. Fetal death from fetomaternal hemorrhage (FMH) occurs in about 1 per 1000 births [118]. FMH is associated with trauma, abruptio placentae, amniocentesis, placental tumors, and obstetric manipulations [119, 120]. Chronic FMH may produce fetal or neonatal anemia, edema, and ascites. Placental abnormalities are usually minimal. Nucleated RBCs may be increased in the fetal circulation. Mothers sometimes develop shaking chills and fever, signs of transfusion reaction to incompatible fetal blood. Massive chronic FMH can be successfully treated by repeated IUT [121].

If FMH is suspected the Kleihauer-Betke test is used to detect fetal cells and to differentiate them from adult cells. This test takes advantage of the stability of fetal hemoglobin in acid-eluted preparations as compared with adult hemoglobin. Relative proportions of fetal and maternal cells in maternal blood can be quantitated and the amount of fetal blood in the maternal circulation can be estimated. When Rh incompatibility is present, Du detection or the rosette test are other methods employed to detect fetal cells. Flow cytometry can accurately determine the volume of fetal blood loss [120].

Either the Kleihauer-Betke test or the Apt test, which utilizes the resistance of Hb F to denaturation by alkali, may be used to detect fetal blood in vaginal discharge. The Apt test is also used to test neonatal gastric aspirate, amniotic fluid, or stool but its sensitivity and specificity are low. These tests are of no value when the mother has an elevated Hb F level in her own cells.

In precipitous deliveries or in the setting of a short umbilical cord, the cord may rupture or tear away, usually close to the fetal abdomen, but bleeding usually stops spontaneously. Velamentous cords, while they have delicate vessels unprotected by Wharton's jelly, rarely rupture. Placenta previa, abruptio placentae, and accidental incisions produce significant hemorrhages but rarely produce anemia.

Internal Fetal Hemorrhage

Traumatic fetal hemorrhage is usually confined to the presenting part during labor and delivery. Subgaleal and subaponeurotic hemorrhages may be massive and fatal; nonlethal lesions may lead to significant jaundice as sequestered RBCs are broken down. These lesions usually occur in difficult deliveries or with the use of vacuum extractors.

Enlarged livers or spleens are more easily traumatized than organs of normal size. Bleeding into the adrenal glands, spleen, and kidneys may be associated with difficult breech deliveries. Adrenal hematomas may calcify and be confused with Wolman disease or with neuroblastomas. The increased use of cesarean deliveries has been in part responsible for the reduction of these traumatic lesions. Hypoxia is also associated with fetal hemorrhages and must be considered in the differential diagnoses.

Hepatic subcapsular hematomas are flattened ecchymoses or blebs filled with 0.5 to 5.0 mL of liquid blood. They are single or multiple and are located on all surfaces of the hepatic lobes, even the relatively protected superior (subdiaphragmatic) and inferior surfaces. Most of these remain intact but rupture with hemoperitoneum occurs in about 20% of those who come to autopsy. Blood loss may be minimal, but in some cases fatal hemorrhage develops. Trauma and coagulation disorders were formerly considered predominant causes of hepatic hematomas, but trauma is questionably a true cause [122]. Indeed, stillborn fetuses may have subcapsular hepatic hematomas. Prematurity, thrombocytopenia, mechanical ventilation, sepsis, and manipulations such as chest tube insertion are associated conditions [123, 124]. In our experience, sepsis is the most frequent associated feature. Histologically, the blood accumulates at the interface of hepatic sinusoids and the capsular collagenous structure (Glisson's capsule). A localized stasis of blood expands to form a small pool, lifting the hepatic capsule and dissecting it from its delicate attachments to the parenchyma. Hepatic subcapsular hematomas rupture readily following minimal manipulation.

A neonate with intestinal hemorrhages arising from tortuous, dilated, submucosal vascular channels underlying ulcerated mucosa was reported by Odell et al [125]. Reduced platelet counts were attributed to trapping in the vascular channels; the condition was refractory to platelet transfusions. Though their case was unassociated with similar disease in relatives, the authors suggested that it fell within the spectrum of Osler-Weber-Rendu syndrome (hereditary hemorrhagic telangiectasia), an autosomal dominant disorder in which skin and mucosal lesions can be present at birth but bleeding is usually deferred until later [126–128].

Anemia of Prematurity

In term infants hemoglobin levels range from 14–22 gm/dL in the first few postnatal days and decrease to about 10–12 gm/dL by the age of 8–12 weeks. Premature infants experience an exaggerated version of this "physiologic anemia" with a drop to 7–9 gm/dL at an earlier time, the age of 4–8 weeks [53]. Since fetal hemoglobin releases oxygen less readily than does adult hemoglobin, this degree of anemia can produce severe tachycardia and tachypnea or apnea. Yet, asymptomatic infants with hemoglobin levels as low as 6.5 gm/dL can have adequate oxygenation [129].

POLYCYTHEMIA AND HYPERVISCOSITY

Polycythemia is defined as a hematocrit equal to or greater than 63%, the lowest hematocrit value associated with hyperviscosity [130]. Viscosity is measured by shear rate and expressed as centipoise (cp). Values in the range between 5 and 10 cp are unassociated with symptoms or signs of disease. Polycythemic newborns have values as high as 16 cp when the venous hematocrit is 72% [131]. Premature babies born before 34 weeks of gestation rarely have polycythemia. Newborns with growth retardation, those with asphyxia, newborns with diabetic mothers, recipients in twin transfusion syndrome, newborns with Beckwith-Wiedemann syndrome, or infants who received excess blood from the placenta may have hyperviscosity [130, 132]. Rarely, it is secondary to maternal-fetal transfusion [133]. Babies at sea level are less likely to be polycythemic than are those at high altitude [130]. The source of the blood used to measure hematocrit must be considered; capillary blood and venous blood below a tourniquet have higher hematocrits than does free flowing venous or arterial blood. Polycythemia is not necessary for hyperviscosity. RBCs with decreased deformability and increased plasma protein content (IgM or fibrinogen) may increase the viscosity of blood.

Plethora, cyanosis, tachypnea, jitteriness, seizures, cerebral infarcts, hypoglycemia, and necrotizing enterocolopathy are associated with polycythemia but the majority of polycythemic babies are asymptomatic [134]. When venous hematocrit exceeds 70%, pulmonary vascular resistance increases, cardiac output decreases, and oxygen transport is impaired. Brain, heart, and adrenal glands receive flow preferentially while the skin, gut, and kidneys have diminished flow and may show areas of necrosis [135].

METHEMOGLOBINEMIA

The chief problem with methemoglobinemia is the inability to unload oxygen. Methemoglobinemia may be acquired or congenital, but in either case, the reduction of methemoglobin to hemoglobin is retarded or is counteracted by increased rates of oxidation of the ferrous atom to ferric state. In the most common form of congenital methemoglobinemia, almost always an autosomal recessive condition, deficiency of cytochrome-b_5 reductase is the likely cause. This enzyme enables hemoglobin to be maintained in the reduced form [63]. Activity may be induced or improved by the administration of methylene blue. High doses of methylene blue, which might be injected into amniotic fluid for diagnosis of membrane rupture, can paradoxically induce methemoglobinemia with Heinz body hemolytic anemia due to the oxidant effect of the dye [136, 137]. Methylene blue used in this manner can also cause hemolysis in the fetus [138].

In acquired forms of methemoglobinemia, the enzymic activity is retarded by toxic effects of nitrates, nitrites, aniline dyes, benzocaine, bismuth compounds, carrot juice, and certain local anesthetics given to the mother, or procaine derivatives used for local anesthesia in the infant [139, 140]. The iron in Hb F is more apt to be oxidized than the iron in Hb A, and Bart's Hb is even more easily oxidized [62]. Symptoms may be few but severely affected neonates are cyanotic and may suffer brain damage. RBCs appear normal on smears, but blood in the test tube is distinctly brown, particularly after exposure to air or oxygen [139]. Mild hemolysis may be noted.

Less common congenital forms of methemoglobinemia are due to autosomal dominant inheritance of an amino acid substitution in the β-globin chain. This hemoglobin variant, Hb M, has abnormal oxygen binding and minimal or no hemolysis. Seven such variant Hb M's have been described. Treatment is ineffective but, fortunately, not necessary [63].

DISORDERS OF WHITE BLOOD CELLS

Normal values for leukocytes are presented in Tables 34.1 and 34.2. The published normal ranges for total white blood cell (WBC) and total neutrophil (TN) counts during the first few days of life vary over a wide range [141, 142]. The term neonate's WBC and TN counts are high compared to those in older infants, with normal values at birth between 5 and 30×10^9/L (WBC) and $5–26 \times 10^9$/L (TN) [141–142]. By the age of 12 hours the average value for WBC rises to 22×10^9/L [50]. At 1 week the range for WBC is $5–21 \times 10^9$/L [141]. Premature neonates may have lower normal ranges [142] but this has been disputed [143]. The WBC and TN counts are slightly higher after vaginal delivery than after cesarean section [144].

Neutropenia

The causes of neonatal neutropenia are listed in Table 34.5 [77, 142, 143, 145]. Neutropenia is variously defined as a TN (bands and polymorphonuclear neutrophils) count equal to or less than $1.5–2.0 \times 10^9$/L. It accounts for 5% of admissions to neonatal intensive care units [146]. Bacterial infection is associated in about one-third of the cases and viral infections in a small number, but noninfectious neutropenia accounts for more than half the cases. Low birthweight, respiratory distress, pregnancy-induced hypertension, abruptio placentae, placenta previa, postexchange transfusion, and postoperative state account for many cases. About 1 in 7 such infants is asymptomatic and among those weighing less than 1500 gm, the TN count may be as low as 0.5 $\times 10^9$/L at birth [147]. Bacterial infections are frequently associated with neutropenia in premature infants, and death occurs in about 20% of infants [143].

Vacuoles and toxic granules develop in the cytoplasm of neutrophils but these are of minimal diagnostic value [148]. Granulocytes may be virtually absent in the peripheral blood

Table 34.5.   Neutropenia in the newborn infant

Asphyxia-hypoxia
Pregnancy-induced hypertension
Alloimmune neonatal thrombocytopenia
Schwachman-Diamond syndrome
Reticular dysgenesis
Granulocytopenia with immunodeficiency
Cyclic neutropenia
Benign neutropenia
Hair-cartilage hypoplasia
Autosomal recessive neutropenia

Sources: From Refs 78, 142, 143, 145.

and maturation arrest at the promyelocyte–myelocyte stages is found in the bone marrow [145]. The neutrophil storage pool in the bone marrow, consisting of polymorphonuclear neutrophils, bands, and metamyelocytes, is decreased in as many as 60% of babies with bacterial sepsis but depletion is rarely severe. Neutropenia resolves within 9–36 hours in most patients [146]. Septic newborns with normal or elevated TN counts have a better outcome than do those with neutropenia [149].

Alloimmune neonatal neutropenia is analogous to alloimmune thrombocytopenia and to ABO or Rh incompatibility [142]. The condition is rarely diagnosed but might be more common than realized. Laboratory confirmation is difficult [142, 150]. Neutropenia subsides as maternal IgG is cleared. Plasma exchange and infusion of maternal neutrophils are rarely necessary [142].

Benign congenital neutropenia is almost never symptomatic in the neonate but can be discovered by routine testing. Severe congenital neutropenia (Kostmann syndrome) may present on the first day of life with fatal neonatal infections [149]. The TN count in such patients is less than 0.2×10^9/L [142]. Some cases are familial and show an autosomal recessive pattern of inheritance [142]. Mutations in the gene for G-CSF are involved in the pathogenesis of this disorder and acute myeloid leukemia may develop, either spontaneously or during treatment with G-CSF [151, 152].

The Shwachman–Diamond syndrome is an autosomal recessive condition with dwarfism, metaphyseal chondrodysplasia, exocrine pancreatic insufficiency, diarrhea, eczema, otitis, and pneumonia. While neutropenia is another feature, it is rarely identified in the neonatal period [153]. Hair-cartilage hypoplasia, also an autosomal recessive condition, is found among the Amish people, has associated neutropenia, but is best characterized by the fine hair and short limbs. Cyclic neutropenia cycles about every 21 days so it is not recognized in neonates [142].

Treatment of neutropenia with granulocyte transfusions or with G-CSF or GM-CSF has not been uniformly successful but growth factors may have a useful role in nonimmune neutropenia [29, 154–156]. A definite increase in functioning neutrophils has been demonstrated with administration of G-CSF in Kostmann syndrome [157].

Neutrophilia

Neutrophilia, defined in the adult as a TN count higher than 7.5×10^9/L, is not so readily identified in the neonate. Babies with neutrophilia usually have asphyxia, hypoxia, or infection. Neutrophils in blood smears are large, floppy-appearing, vacuolated, pale blue cells. Granules are fewer than in older children. In small premature infants, the nuclei tend to be round, cleaved, or indented or have thick sausage shapes and with light blue staining of the chromatin with Wright's stain (see Fig. 34.7).

Structural and Functional Abnormalities in Neutrophils

The normal neonate is less responsive to infection than are older patients. Among the neutrophil-related factors are defects in neutrophil adherents, chemotaxis, phagocytosis, and bacterial killing [150]. These defects can be inherited or acquired. Chronic granulomatous disease is a rare genetically heterogeneous syndrome, usually X-linked and manifested in males, caused by failure of the respiratory burst in phagocytes including neutrophils, monocyte/macrophages, and eosinophils [150]. Opsonization, chemotaxis, and ingestion are normal [142]. The disease has genetic defects in any of at least 4 oxidase polypeptides. The most common mutation is in the gene for a 91-kd membrane glycoprotein, the larger subunit of phagocyte-specific cytochrome b [158]. No structural defect identifies the defective phagocyte. The diagnosis is made by demonstrating failure of neutrophils to express a respiratory burst by tests such as nitroblue tetrazolium dye reduction [159–160]. Testing at the molecular level may be necessary for a diagnosis in carriers or affected fetuses [160, 161]. Chronic granulomatous disease may involve neonates with signs including prolonged jaundice and various infections [162, 163]. The disease is more likely to occur late during the first year of life with recurrent, purulent bacterial and fungal infections [150].

Structural abnormalities of neutrophils are rare in neonates. Vacuoles of neutrophils, monocytes, and occasionally lymphocytes (Jordan's anomaly) may be associated with ichthyosis and sulfatase deficiency with adrenal hypoplasia [164]. Such defects as the large granules in the Chediak-Higashi syndrome, the pince-nez neutrophils of the Pelger-Huët anomaly, the increased azurophilic granules in Alder-Reilly anomaly, and the several large cytoplasmic inclusions in monocytes, neutrophils, eosinophils, and basophils in the May-Hegglin anomaly are not usually present in neonates [164, 165].

Eosinophilia

Eosinophilia, defined as an absolute eosinophil count higher than 0.5×10^9/L, may be seen in normal babies at about the age of 1 week. Eosinophilia, in similar numbers and of unknown significance, is frequently observed in premature infants and correlates temporally with an anabolic state [142, 166]. Intravenous lipid administration produces eosinophilia and eosinophilic infiltrates in hepatic tissues. Eosinophils occasionally infiltrate pancreatic islets and thymic medullary stroma in infants of diabetic mothers. Omenn syndrome is a familial reticuloendotheliosis with eosinophilia, small thymus, skin rashes, lymphadenopathy, and hepatomegaly due to histiocytic infiltrates. These and other features may be confused with a graft-versus-host reaction [167–169].

Lymphopenia

Disorders of lymphocytes are most often those associated with decreased numbers (i.e., $<1.0 \times 10^9$/L). Reticular dysgenesis, severe combined immunodeficiency syndromes, and the Nezelof syndrome are sometimes identified in the first month of life, particularly when the family histories are positive. Graft-versus-host disease causes lymphopenia. Another cause of lymphopenia is intestinal lymphangiectasis with lymphocytes sequestered in the abnormal vessels or expelled into the lumen of the bowel.

The graft-versus-host response occurs in infants who have received non-irradiated blood transfusions, including IUTs and rarely spontaneous maternal-fetal transfusions. Lymphoid depletion involves both T and B cells. Thymic hypoplasia, arrest of maturation of Hassall's corpuscles, star-shaped fibrinous deposits in bone marrow, extensive lesions of the skin with hyperkeratosis, apoptosis of lymphocytes, infiltrates of intraepidermal lymphocytes (helper T and suppressor T cells), and localized necrosis of the basement membrane of the epidermis are other features of neonatal graft-versus-host reactions [167, 170, 171].

Congenital Leukemias, Myeloproliferative Disorders, and Myelodysplastic Syndromes

Congenital leukemia is a rare disorder. In our hospital no case of congenital leukemia has been encountered in the last 83,000 births. We have not made the diagnosis in stillborns. It was reported more commonly prior to the 1960s, but since then transient myelopoiesis has been recognized and differentiated, especially in association with Down syndrome, severe erythroblastosis, and infections.

Leukemia in 2 stillborns was reported by Gray et al [172] and another 2 by Las Heras et al [173]. All 4 fetuses were mildly hydropic and showed infiltration of tissues by blasts, myeloblastic in 2 and monoblastic and lymphoblastic in 1 each. The placentas were involved by infiltration in 3 cases and leukemic cells were seen in the vessels of all. There was

no skin infiltration. Of 2 other reports of cases in stillborns, one was subsequently retracted by the author as a reactive phenomenon "in incompatibility situations" [174, 175]. Among congenital leukemias, acute, non-lymphocytic leukemia (ANLL) is more frequent than acute lymphocytic leukemia (ALL), in contrast to the leukemias of older children, and the prognosis is worse for congenital leukemia [142]. Of the ANLLs, acute monocytic leukemia (M5) and acute myelomonocytic leukemia (M4) are the most common but acute megakaryoblastic leukemia (M7), acute erythroblastic leukemia (M6), and acute basophilic leukemia have been reported [142, 176–178]. Skin involvement (leukemia cutis) manifesting as blue, red, or purple nodules is found in about 30% of patients with congenital leukemia and may precede other manifestations [179]. Ocular involvement has been reported [180]. Petechiae, purpura, hepatosplenomegaly, and pallor are often present.

In certain chromosomal disorders there is an increased risk for developing leukemia though it is not usually present at birth. These disorders include Fanconi's anemia, Bloom syndrome, ataxia-telangiectasia, and Down syndrome [181].

The overall increased risk for leukemia in Down syndrome is up to 20 times that for normal individuals with bimodal peaks, one among newborns and the other at 3–6 years. Increased risk extends into adulthood [182]. The distribution of acute leukemia types in Down syndrome is different from that of non-Down syndrome childhood leukemias. In one series of 20 Down syndrome leukemia patients all 14 patients less than 3 years old had M7 leukemia and the older 6 had ALL [183]. The blast cells in 1 ALL patient also expressed myeloid-associated antigens. In M7 leukemia the megakaryoblasts often have a characteristic cytoplasmic projection or bleb (Fig. 34.15).

Myeloproliferative disorders as they are known in the adult are rare in children and evidently non-existent at birth. Chronic myelogenous leukemia comprises 2–5% of childhood leukemias. The adult type has an incidence less than 1 per 100,000 in children less than 2 years old [184]. Juvenile chronic myelogenous leukemia differs from the adult form and presents in the first few yeas of life but not at birth. Transient abnormal myelopoiesis is a myeloproliferative disorder, recognized in utero or at birth, especially in patients with trisomy 21. It must be differentiated from congenital leukemia. Bone marrow assays for CFU-GM show normal cluster/colony ratios and cultures of peripheral leukocytes reveal normal in vitro maturation in transient abnormal myelopoiesis, as opposed to abnormal growth in congenital leukemia [185, 186]. Transient abnormal myelopoiesis has been variously labeled as transient myeloproliferative disorder, transient leukemoid reaction, and "congenital transient leukemia" [187], transient abnormal myelopoiesis, and pseudoleukemia [176, 188]. In our experience transient abnormal myelopoiesis is frequent when trisomy 21 is present. It can occur whether the karyotype is mosaic or non-mosaic and can occur when the phenotype is otherwise normal in spite of the abnormal genotype

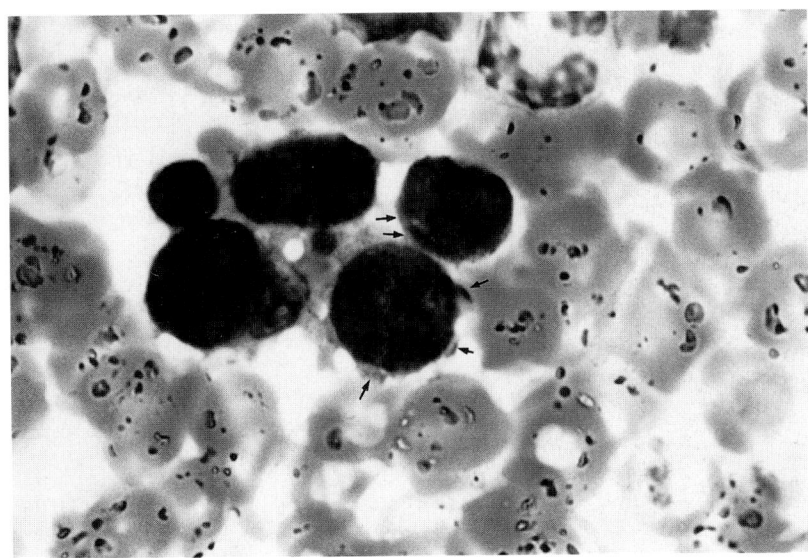

FIGURE 34.15.   *Peripheral blood: megakaryocytic leukemia in a newborn baby with Down syndrome. Note the blebs in the cytoplasm of the small megakaryoblasts (arrows). Wright's stain, ×1480.*

[186, 189–191]. Transient abnormal myelopoiesis may be associated with hydrops in a fetus and has been diagnosed prenatally by cordocentesis in 2 fetuses with Down syndrome; the abnormal myelopoiesis spontaneously remitted in both before the age of 5 weeks [187, 192]. We examined a fetus with hydrops and Down syndrome at 26 weeks' gestation who had many WBC precursors in vessels and extensive myelopoiesis in the epicardium (Fig. 34.16). Aside from EMH, there was no infiltration of tissues.

In either transient abnormal myelopoiesis or congenital leukemia, the peripheral blood count may contain up to 90% blasts with WBC counts higher than 200 × 10⁹/L (Fig. 34.17). No treatment is necessary for resolution of transient abnormal myelopoiesis but the patients are at increased risk for later development of acute leukemia [186].

Myelodysplastic syndromes, often preleukemic in adults, are rare in children [193, 194]. Primary myelodysplasias in children include refractory anemia (RA), refractory anemia with excess blasts (RAEB), RAEB in transformation (RAEBIT), chronic myelomonocytic leukemia (CMML), and infantile monosomy 7 syndrome (M7S) [193, 195]. Congenital myelodysplastic syndrome is extremely rare, with only 4 cases having been recognized before the age of 2 months. These include cases of RA with normal karyotype and RAEBIT with trisomy 21, both treated by bone marrow transplantation, a case of RAEB with abnormal karyotype including trisomy 21 which evolved to fatal erythroleukemia, and a case of RAEB with normal karyotype and survival after chemotherapy [194, 196–198].

The classifications of myelodysplastic syndromes and myeloproliferative disorders in childhood are not well delineated and presently allow much overlap. Entities such as M7S and juvenile chronic myelogenous leukemia are sometimes classified under either group.

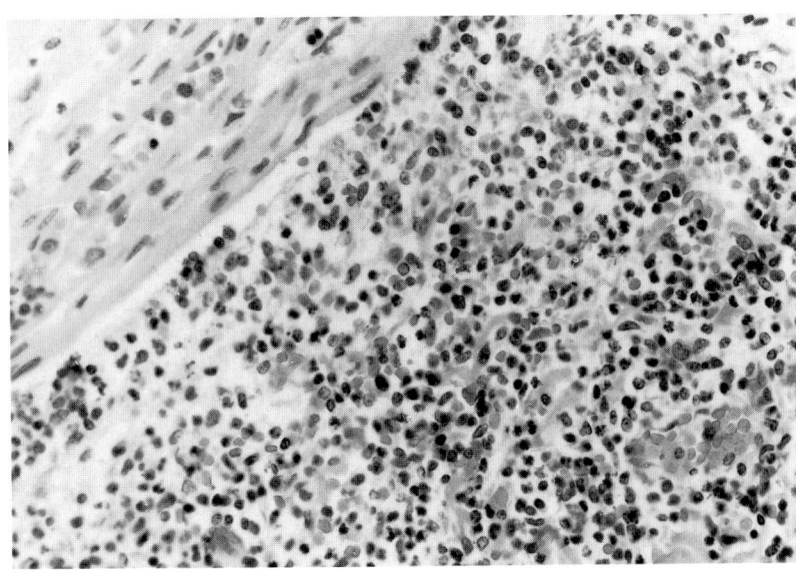

FIGURE 34.16.   *Extensive myelopoiesis in the epicardium of a stillborn with Down syndrome. Increased nucleated blood cells are also seen in the fetal vessels in the myocardium in the upper left corner. H&E, ×296.*

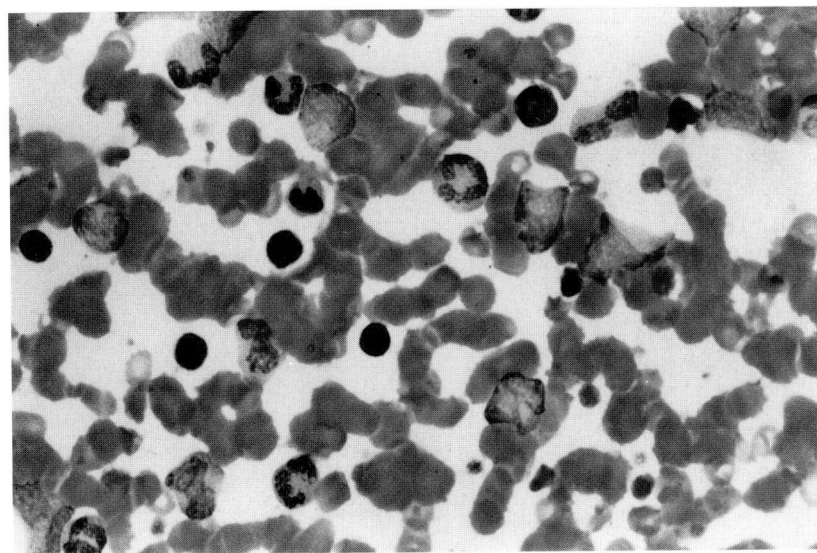

FIGURE 34.17.   *Peripheral blood leukemoid reaction. The white blood cell count was 90,000/μL. Wright's stain, ×450.*

Some patients whose blast cells show monosomy 7 karyotype have clinical features of juvenile chronic myelogenous leukemia [198]. This is an entity with many morphological features akin to chronic monomyelogenous leukemia and many features of M7S, suggesting that in the child these conditions are identical [195, 199]. Monosomy 7 has also been seen in a patient with congenital leukemia [200].

COAGULATION IN THE NEONATE

Normal Development

Both hemostatic and fibrinolytic systems appear by 11–12 weeks' gestation but develop slowly. Between 12 and 24 weeks' gestation most of the coagulation factors are reduced in amount as compared to adult values; for example, the mean fibrinogen level is 90 mg/dL versus 300 mg/dL in adults. Most other factors are 25–50% of adult levels, except for factor V with a mean activity of 75%. At 27–31 weeks' gestation the fibrinogen level has risen to 215 mg/dL and other factors have slowly increased. Prothrombin time (PT) is longer than 20 seconds and the activated partial thromboplastin time (aPTT) is about 100 seconds. The fetus or premature infant of 32–36 weeks has near-adult fibrinogen levels and has PT and aPTT of 18 and 100 seconds, respectively. Factor VIII:C is near adult levels, but factor IX has only about one-third the adult activity. The term infant has adult or near-adult levels of fibrinogen, factor V, von Willebrand's factor, factor VIII:C, and factor XIII. Other factors including factor IX and contact factors are still low. Factors VII and X reach adult levels between 21 and 45 days of postnatal life, factor IX in 3–9 months, and some contact factors within the first 2 weeks or months. The PT is prolonged in premature infants but approaches nearly adult values by term and is at adult values within the first few postnatal days. The aPTT, about 70 seconds at term, takes 2–6 months to reach adult values [201].

Plasminogen levels in term and premature neonates are less than 50% of adult values which are not attained until the baby is 6–7 months old [201]. The levels of tissue plasminogen activators in newborn plasma are elevated to about twice adult levels, probably because of release by endothelial cells during birth [202].

Coagulation Factor Deficiencies

Any of the coagulation factors may be congenitally deficient but acquired defects are much more common. Most of these are vitamin K–dependent proteins: prothrombin (factor II), stable factor or proconvertin (factor VII), plasma thromboplastin compound (PTC) (factor IX), and Stuart-Prower factor (factor X). None of these coagulation factors crosses the placenta; all are synthesized in the fetus. The more common neonatal coagulation disorders are listed in Table 34.6 [203, 204].

Table 34.6.   Coagulation disorders in the neonate

Thrombocytopenia
Disseminated intravascular coagulation
Abnormal platelet function (rare in neonates)
Abnormal coagulation factors
Hemophilia A and B
Afibrinogenemia
Hemorrhagic disease due to reduced factors VII, IX, X
Liver disease
Hemorrhagic shock and encephalopathy [204]

Source: Adapted from Lusher [203].

Hemorrhagic Disease of the Newborn

Vitamin K deficiency or hemorrhagic disease of the newborn was at one time a serious condition with the onset of brisk bleeding or oozing of blood at the age of 3–7 days. Bleeding from the umbilical cord stump, from mucosal surfaces, and into the subcutaneous tissues, the scalp, meninges, lungs, gut, and brain characterizes the condition. The cause is decreased synthesis of the vitamin K–dependent procoagulant proteins, factors II, VII, IX, and X. Though the anticoagulant proteins C and S are also vitamin K–dependent, the net effect of vitamin K deficiency is an increased risk for bleeding. Newborns exposed in utero to the anticonvulsants phenytoin and barbiturates require special consideration because they may have decreased coagulation shortly after delivery, in contrast to presentation on days 2–5 in those with physiological vitamin K deficiency [205].

With prophylactic vitamin K administration, hemorrhagic disease of the newborn should be eliminated but deficiencies of the same procoagulant proteins can arise secondary to severe neonatal liver disease. Factor VII is the most sensitive coagulation factor in that regard [206].

Hemophilia

Hemophilia A and hemophilia B are the most common hereditary bleeding disorders, accounting for about 85% and 15%, respectively, of all cases [207]. Deficiencies for both factor VIII (hemophilia A) and factor IX (hemophilia B) are inherited as X-linked recessive conditions. The spontaneous mutation rate is high so that 20–30% of those afflicted have no family history of the disease [207]. Neonatal bleeding occurs in 35% or more of those with severe deficiency of factor VIII or factor IX and 11% of those with mild deficiency [201]. Severe intracranial bleeding, mostly intracerebral, can be the presenting sign in newborns as young as 1 day [202, 208]. Bleeding from circumcision wounds and large cephalohematomas are strong indications for hemophilia A or hemophilia B although these conditions are rarely fatal. Circumcision in neonates with hemophilia does not always result in hemorrhage. Less than half of those whose eventual diagnosis is severe hemophilia bleed excessively but bleeding becomes almost certain if surgery is performed after the 7th day of life [209]. In severe hemophilia the factor VIII:C or IX level is less than 1% of normal activity. In moderate disease the levels are between 1 and 5%, and in mild disease levels are higher than 5% of normal [207]. von Willebrand's factor and factor VIII–related antigen are present in normal concentrations. With the use of monoclonal antibody and lyophilization, a safe product of factor VIII:C is now in use to treat hemophilia A.

Manifestations of von Willebrand's disease in infancy are rare. Most forms of the disease cannot be diagnosed in the newborn but the most severe form, in which little or no factor VIII or von Willebrand's factor is detectable, can be diagnosed at birth or even prenatally [202, 210].

Hemorrhagic Shock and Encephalopathy

Hemorrhagic shock and encephalopathy comprise a syndrome in infants as early as 6 weeks, with a median age of 15 months [211]. Patients have sudden onset of shock, bleeding, DIC, watery diarrhea, hepatic and renal functional impairment, coma, and convulsions. Petechiae and larger areas of bleeding occur in several organs. Acute renal tubular necrosis, cerebral edema, and pituitary necrosis are common features. Cerebral infarcts may occur [212]. Some observers have been impressed more with hyperthermia than with hemorrhage [213]. Centrilobular necrosis and fatty change may be found in the liver. Plasma levels of α_1-antitrypsin are reduced and trypsin concentrations are increased in older patients. Hepatocytes accumulate α_1-antitrypsin inclusions. In one series of 25 patients, 20 infants and children died and the others were neurologically impaired [204]. Neurologically intact survivors have also been reported [214]. The relationship, if any, of this syndrome to malignant hyperthermia, heat stroke, Reye syndrome, hemolytic-uremic syndrome, and toxic shock syndrome is not yet clear [215].

Platelet Abnormalities

Perinatal Thrombocytopenia

Fetal platelet counts are about $185 \pm 31 \times 10^9$/L at 15 weeks of gestation, gradually increasing to adult levels in cord blood at term [52, 216]. Forestier et al [45] recorded higher platelet counts of $234 \pm 57 \times 10^9$/L at 18–21 weeks of gestation with very little change through more than 30 weeks of gestation. The normal platelet count in neonates at term is essentially the same as that in older children and adults. Neonatal platelet counts less than 150×10^9/L are considered abnormal, but only platelet counts below 100×10^9/L clearly call for investigation [217]. The risk of bleeding is slight even after surgery or trauma, with a platelet count of higher than 80×10^9/L. Spontaneous hemorrhage can occur with a platelet count below 50×10^9/L and especially when counts fall below 20×10^9/L [217]. In infants with low birthweight, thrombocytopenia is associated with an increased frequency and severity of intraventricular hemorrhage [218]. The more common causes of perinatal thrombocytopenia are listed in Table 34.7 [202, 217].

Acquired Thrombocytopenia

Infection is a common cause of thrombocytopenia in the neonate, but thrombocytopenia is a poor marker for sepsis and has a tendency to occur late in the course of the infection [219]. Thrombocytopenia associated with infection is occasionally due to disseminated intravascular clotting, but then it is usually unaccompanied by bleeding [219]. The association between thrombocytopenia and fetal toxoplasmosis, syphilis, or viral infections such as cytomegalovirus infection, rubella, and herpes is well known, and most of those same organisms can be associated with thrombocytopenia in the postnatal period [219]. Premature neonates

Table 34.7. Causes of perinatal thrombocytopenia

Decreased platelet production
 Bone marrow aplasia or hypoplasia
  Thrombocytopenia with absent radii (TAR)
  Fanconi's anemia
  Trisomy syndromes 13, 18, and 21
  Other congenital megakaryocytic hypoplasias
 Bone marrow replacement
  Congenital leukemia or leukemoid reactions
  Disseminated neuroblastoma
  Histiocytosis
  Osteopetrosis
Increased platelet destruction or consumption
 Immune; alloimmune, autoimmune, or maternal drugs
 Disseminated intravascular coagulation
 Kasabach-Merritt syndrome
 Asphyxia, aspiration, respiratory distress syndrome
 Necrotizing enterocolitis
 Congenital hemolytic-uremic/thrombotic thrombocytopenia syndrome
Of mixed or poorly understood etiology
 Perinatal infections, including viral
 Pre-eclampsia
 Hemolytic disease due to Rh incompatibility
 Hyperbilirubinemia, phototherapy
 Total parenteral nutrition
 Wiskott-Aldrich syndrome
 Inborn errors of metabolism

Sources: Adapted from Andrew [202] and Gill [217].

with respiratory distress syndrome, meconium aspiration, sepsis, necrotizing enterocolitis, persistent pulmonary hypertension, umbilical catheters, high serum bilirubin levels, or phototherapy have an increased incidence of thrombocytopenia [201].

Immune Thrombocytopenia

Perinatal alloimmune (isoimmune) thrombocytopenia is analogous to alloimmune hemolytic disease and is caused by maternal antibodies against paternally derived antigens on fetal platelets. The offending antibody is usually formed against the Pl^{A1} antigen by a Pl^{A1}-negative mother [217]. Since Pl^{A1} antigen is lacking in only 2% of the population, the likelihood of a Pl^{A1}-negative mother mating with a man with at least one allele positive for a Pl^{A1} is great. The rarity of Pl^{A1}-negative individuals also makes finding appropriate random donors almost impossible. The diagnosis of perinatal alloimmune thrombocytopenia should be suspected when the fetus or neonate has unexplained thrombocytopenia and the mother has a normal platelet count. Ideal diagnostic work-up includes testing maternal and paternal platelets for Pl^{A1} and Pl^{A2} antigens (establishing homozygosity versus heterozygosity in the father) as well as other antigens such as Bak (HPA-3) and Pen (HPA-4), screening maternal serum for platelet antibodies against panels of

platelets with known antigens, and finally performing a cross-match of paternal platelets with maternal serum. Results will confirm the diagnosis and are important for genetic counseling regarding future pregnancies. Unfortunately, there is no presently available test for rapidly establishing this diagnosis by laboratory means; thus, clinical judgment is required in deciding whether to transfuse maternal platelets into the sick neonate. Additional treatment includes high doses of intravenous immunoglobulin to the mother during pregnancy or to the infant postnatally [220, 221].

Thrombocytopenia in a pregnant woman may have different causes with varying implications for the fetus. Pregnant women should not be considered thrombocytopenic unless the platelet count is 120×10^9/L or less; some women with "gestational thrombocytopenia" suffer no ill effects and their fetuses have no thrombocytopenia [222].

Thrombocytopenia may develop in fetuses of mothers with idiopathic autoimmune thrombocytopenia or that associated with known diseases such as lupus erythematosus. IgG autoantibodies, not discriminatory for maternal or fetal antigens, cross the placenta into the fetal circulation and attack the fetal platelets [202]. Of exposed fetuses, 30–40% have lowered platelet counts but there is poor correlation with the degree of maternal thrombocytopenia or levels of platelet-associated IgG [223]. Even a normal maternal platelet count in a splenectomized mother with idiopathic thrombocytopenic purpura does not ensure normal platelets in her fetus [202]. Neonatal platelet counts less than 50×10^9/L occur in about 12% of babies born to mothers with autoimmune thrombocytopenia [223, 224]. In a study of neonatal thrombocytopenia of all causes, Burrows and Kelton [224] found only 19 (0.12%) of 15,932 infants with cord blood platelet counts less than 50×10^9/L and only 6 infants (0.04%) with counts less than 20×10^9/L. They noted only 3 babies with adverse outcomes, all of which occurred in a setting of neonatal alloimmune thrombocytopenic purpura, suggesting relative benignity of autoimmune thrombocytopenia in the neonate. Among women who had a pre-pregnancy diagnosis of idiopathic thrombocytopenic purpura, Samuels et al [225] found that 18 of 70 who had circulating platelet antibodies delivered babies with platelet counts less than 50×10^9/L and 2 of the 18 affected infants had intracranial hemorrhage, and 1 died. None of the infants born to the 18 mothers with no circulating platelet antibodies had severe thrombocytopenia.

Thrombocytopenia with Absent Radii

Thrombocytopenia with absent radii (TAR) is usually inherited in an autosomal recessive pattern and is associated with periodic leukemoid reactions and eosinophilia. The total leukocyte count often reaches 100,000/μL. Megakaryocytes are reduced in number in the bone marrow [226]. Fatal bleeding can occur in neonates. In survivors, episodes of thrombocytopenia are precipitated by stress, infection, or cows' milk protein. Thrombocytopenia tends to resolve by the age of 1 year [227]. For non-hematological features of TAR, see Chapter 13.

Fanconi's anemia, which also can include skeletal anomalies and thrombocytopenia, is distinguished from TAR by absent thumbs, pancytopenia, and chromosomal breakage. This syndrome rarely has neonatal hematological manifestations [228].

Hemangiomas and Thrombocytopenia

Large hemangiomas and consumptive coagulopathy, usually with severe thrombocytopenia, comprise the Kasabach-Merritt syndrome, with severe neonatal bleeding in approximately 50% of patients [202]. Thrombocytopenia sometimes occurs in newborns whose placentas contain large or numerous chorangiomas and in some, hemangiomas are also present in the fetus [229].

Qualitative Platelet Disorders

The platelets of a normal newborn show decreased and increased aggregation in response to epinephrine and ristocetin, respectively; this poor comparison with adult platelets is unexplained, apparently representing neither a classic storage pool deficiency nor an aspirin-like aggregation defect [202]. Though physiological platelet functional defects have been demonstrated, bleeding times are normal in term and preterm infants and the otherwise normal healthy term neonate does not have a bleeding tendency [201]. Maternal ingestion of aspirin during the few days prior to delivery can be associated with platelet dysfunction and bleeding in both mother and neonate, possibly including intracranial hemorrhage in the latter [201]. The neonatal bleeding tendency might represent the additive effect of physiological platelet dysfunction and aspirin-induced cyclo-oxygenase inhibition [201].

Well-defined platelet disorders of older children and adults, which rarely if ever appear in fetuses and neonates, include defects of platelet adhesion as in the Bernard-Soulier syndrome, defects of secondary aggregation such as the storage pool diseases, or the gray platelet syndrome due to deficiency of α granules. Glanzmann's thrombasthenia, an inherited primary aggregation defect, has been reported in neonates [230].

Thrombocytosis

Excessive numbers of platelets rarely develop in neonates but may be found in babies with asplenia, acute blood loss, myeloproliferative disorders, maternal polydrug use, or congenital neuroblastoma. Some premature infants develop thrombocytosis after the age of 4–6 weeks [202].

Thrombosis in the Neonate

Large venous, aortic, iliac, and cardiac thromboses may develop when indwelling catheters remain for several days [231]. Renal vein thrombosis occurs most frequently in large plethoric fetuses or neonates born to mothers with diabetes or in neonates with congenital nephrotic syndrome [232]. The lesions begin in the small tributary veins of the renal arcuate plexus and propagate toward the larger renal pelvic veins, the main renal vein, and even the inferior vena cava (Fig. 34.18). Pulmonary and systemic emboli may develop, but more often hemorrhagic renal necrosis is the result [233]. Renal vein thrombosis is usually present at birth or within 48 hours [234]. Aortic thromboses occur with regularity among neonates who are catheterized through the umbilical artery and major organ failure may result [231] (see Chap. 3). Spontaneous neonatal aortic thrombosis with extension to the major abdominal branches is rare and seems to be particularly associated with maternal diabetes.

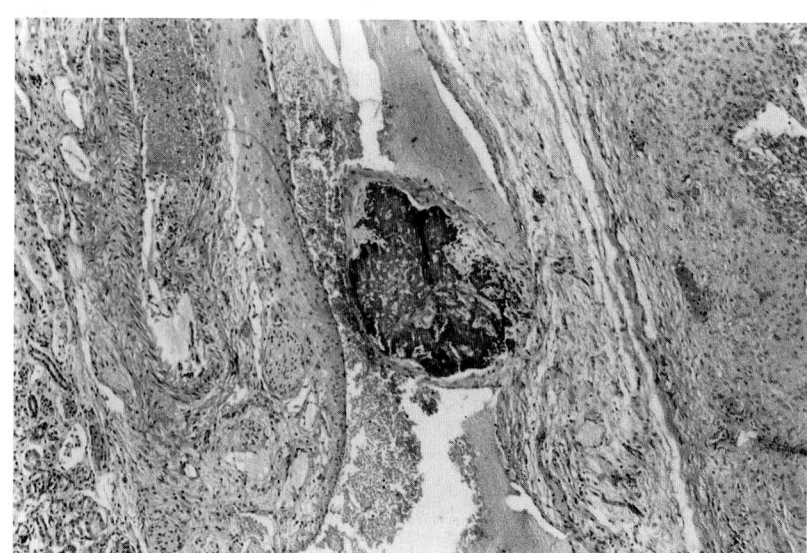

FIGURE 34.18. *Renal vein thrombosis with calcification. H&E, ×125.*

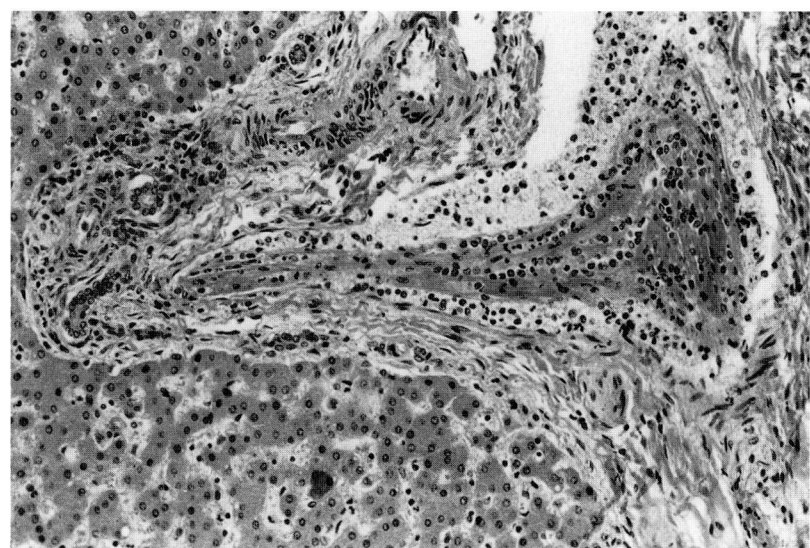

FIGURE 34.19. *Thrombus in the portal vein from a newborn baby who had idiopathic congenital thromboses. Similar lesions were found in the kidney; the brain had extensive encephalomalacia. H&E, ×205.*

Infarcts are found in adrenal glands, kidneys, and intestines [231, 235]. Neonatal thrombosis occurs in arteries or veins in congenital absence or defect of antithrombin III [236], protein C [203, 237–239], or protein S [240], or in idiopathic conditions (Fig. 34.19).

Antithrombin III is synthesized in the liver. Plasma levels in the premature and term neonate are approximately one-third and two-thirds adult levels, respectively [202, 207]. Deficiency, usually inherited in an autosomal recessive pattern, leads to venous thromboses, typically appearing in the second decade of life [241]. Protein C is a vitamin K–dependent protease and its deficiency is transmitted as either an autosomal dominant or an autosomal recessive condition [238, 242]. In the heterozygous state, thrombosis is not usually detected until adolescence, while the homozygous state can lead to severe DIC, purpura fulminans, and central nervous system thromboses in neonates [202]. Aortic, renal, or cerebral arterial and venous thromboses are responsible for the necroses. Blindness can be produced by thrombosis of the ocular vessels. For unexplained reasons, twins are unusually frequent in series of patients with protein C deficiency [238]. Deficiency of protein S occurs in childhood but problems are either extremely rare or nonexistent in the neonate [240].

Capillary thromboses may occur in neonates, particularly with sepsis, trauma, shock, or HDN [243]. Oozing from wounds, purpura, and gastrointestinal tract and urinary tract hemorrhage characterize the typical DIC. Small thrombotic lesions in histological preparations are not easily recognized but favored sites include the lung, kidney, liver, gastrointestinal tract, and spleen. Necroses are most often in the kidney where cortical or medullary necrosis and hemorrhage are noted. In the intestine, necrotizing enterocolopathy may be either a cause or a result of thromboses.

CHROMOSOMAL DISORDERS AND MISCELLANEOUS HEMATOLOGICAL ABNORMALITIES

The WBC count may be lower than normal in trisomy 21 [244]. In trisomy 13, 60–80% of neutrophils have multiple long and thread-like or sessile nuclear excrescences. They should not be confused with the drumstick projections representing X chromosomes [245]. The projections are also seen in eosinophils [245]. The RBCs of neonates with trisomy 13 contain increased Hb F, persistence of embryonal Hb Gower II, and delayed development of Hb A_2 in the rare survivors [246, 247]. Bart's Hb, in amounts up to 1.5%, has been found in the first few days of life in newborn babies with trisomy 13 [248].

Increased phosphofructokinase (PFK) and its type L isoenzyme are seen in trisomy 21. A gene-dose effect related to the localization of the L subunit to chromosome 21 is invoked to explain this finding [249]. PFK is a glycolytic enzyme that interacts with RBC membrane proteins to protect against degradation related to RBC aging. The significance of increased levels is not known but deficiency of PFK can cause a mild hemolytic anemia.

Non-anemic macrocytosis of unknown cause is present in most adults and children with trisomy 21 [244]. Other conditions associated with fetal macrocytosis in the second trimester include triploidy, monosomy X, trisomy 18, and trisomy 13 [250].

PRENATAL DIAGNOSIS OF HEMATOLOGICAL DISORDERS

Techniques used to obtain fetal tissue or blood or trophoblast for prenatal diagnosis include chorionic villus sampling (CVS), amniocentesis, fetal blood sampling (FBS), and

Table 34.8.   Prenatal diagnosis

Disorder	Source	References
Alloimmune thrombocytopenia	T,B,D	254, 255
Autoimmune thrombocytopenia*	B	256
Thrombocytopenia with absent radii (TAR)	B	257–259
Wiskott-Aldrich	T,B,D	260
Hemophilia A and B	T,B,D	18, 261–263
von Willebrand disease	T,B,D	210, 262
Protein C deficiency	T,B,D	18, 264
Antithrombin III deficiency	T,D	265
Chediak-Higashi syndrome	T,B	266, 267
Transient abnormal myelopoiesis in Down syndrome	B	192
Chronic granulomatous disease	T,B,D	18, 161, 262
Thalassemias, α and β	T,B,D	18, 253, 262, 268
Hemoglobins S, C, E	T,B,D	18, 262
RBC enzymes	T,B,D	97, 269
Rh incompatibility	T,B,D	270, 271
Fanconi's anemia	T,B	18
Parvovirus	T,B,D	272, 273

T = tissue; B = blood; D = DNA testing can be performed.
* Available but indications not clear.

fetal biopsy. Many inherited disorders can be diagnosed from DNA analysis of chorionic villi or from cultured amniocytes or fibroblasts. CVS, performed at 9–12 weeks of gestation, allows early diagnosis and offers more tissue than amniocentesis. The latter is usually performed after 16 weeks of gestation, but amniocentesis from 12–15 weeks of gestation is becoming more commonplace. The additional time required for amniocyte culture is a disadvantage of amniocentesis. Fetal biopsy, rarely used at present, can be performed by fetoscopy. Liver, skin, and muscle tissues have been obtained [251]. Fetal cells and trophoblasts can also be extracted from the maternal circulation for use in prenatal diagnosis [252].

Ultrasonography is used to detect early hydrops, for example, in α-thalassemia, other severe hemolytic anemia, or massive FMH.

FBS, also known as percutaneous umbilical blood sampling, done by cordocentesis, is usually performed after 18 weeks of gestation, but has been successfully utilized at 12 weeks of gestation [251, 253]. This technique is particularly suitable when a hematological disorder is suspected. For example, a simple platelet count is useful for a fetus at risk for alloimmune thrombocytopenic purpura. Other tests using fetal blood include measurement of glucose phosphate isomerase in RBCs, hemoglobin electrophoresis and analysis of globin chain synthesis, coagulation testing, chromosome analysis, and DNA analysis. Table 34.8 provides a partial list of hematological disorders amenable to prenatal diagnosis in this rapidly advancing field.

REFERENCES

1. Kelemen E, Calvo W, Fliedner TM. *Atlas of Human Hemopoietic Development.* New York: Springer, 1979, pp. 3–81.
2. Tavassoli M. Embryonic and fetal hemopoiesis: an overview. *Blood Cells* 1991; 1:269–81.
3. Christensen RD. Hematopoiesis in the fetus and neonate. *Pediatr Res* 1989; 26:531–5.
4. Kelemen E, Janossa M, Calvo W, et al. What kind of morphologically recognizable hemopoietic cells do we inject when doing foetal liver infusion in man? *Thymus* 1987; 10:33–44.
5. Erslev AJ. Hemopoietic functions of the liver. In: Arias IM, Jakovy WB, Popper H, Schachter D, Shafritz DA, eds. *The Liver: Biology, and Pathobiology.* 2nd ed. New York: Raven, 1988, pp. 1073–81.
6. Castoldi GL. General aspects of erythropoiesis. In: Zucker-Franklin D, Greaves MF, Grossi CE, Marmont AM, eds. *Atlas of Blood Cells: Function and Pathology.* Philadelphia: Lea & Febiger, 1981, pp. 35–73.
7. Salafia CM, Weigl CA, Foye GJ. Correlation of placental erythrocyte morphology and gestational age. *Pediatr Pathol* 1988; 8:495–502.
8. Thompson EL. Time and rate of loss of nuclei by the red blood cells of human embryos. *Anat Rec* 1951; 111:317–25.
9. Ryerson CS, Sanes S. The age of pregnancy: histologic diagnosis from percentage of erythroblasts in chorionic capillaries. *Arch Pathol* 1934; 17:648–51.
10. Gilmour JR. Normal hemopoiesis in intra-uterine and neonatal life. *J Pathol Bacteriol* 1941; 52:25–54.
11. Chervenick PA, Zucker-Franklin D. In vitro and in vivo hematopoiesis. In: Zucker-Franklin D, Greaves MF, Grossi CE, Marmont AM, eds. *Atlas of Blood Cells: Function and Pathology.* Philadelphia: Lea & Febiger, 1981, pp. 13–31.
12. Alenghat E, Esterly JR. Intravascular hematopoiesis in chorionic villi. *Am J Clin Pathol* 1983; 79:225–7.
13. Oski FA. The erythrocyte and its disorders. In: Nathan DG, Oski FA, eds. *Hematology of Infancy and Childhood.* 4th ed. Philadelphia: WB Saunders, 1993, pp. 18–43.
14. Lukens JN. Blood formation in the embryo, fetus, and newborn. In: Lee GR, Bithell TC, Foerster J, Athens JW, Lukens JN, eds. *Wintrobe's Clinical Hematology.* 9th ed. Philadelphia: Lea & Febiger, 1993, pp. 80–100.
15. Wolf BC, Luevano E, Neiman RS. Evidence to suggest that the human fetal spleen is not a hematopoietic organ. *Am J Clin Pathol* 1983; 80:140–4.
16. Rothstein G. Origin and development of the blood and blood-forming tissues. In: Lee GR, Bithel TC, Foerster J, Athens JW, Lukens JN, eds. *Wintrobe's Clinical Hematology.* 9th ed. Philadelphia: Lea & Febiger, 1993, pp. 41–59.
17. Quesenberry PJ, Lowry PA. The colony-stimulating factors: an overview. *Cancer* 1992; 70(suppl):909–12.
18. Miller DR. Origin and development of blood cells and coagulation factors: maternal-fetal interactions. In: Miller DR, Baehner RL, Miller LP, eds. *Blood Diseases of Infancy and Childhood.* 7th ed. St. Louis: CV Mosby, 1995, pp. 3–29.
19. Hann IM, Bodger MP, Hoffbrand AV. Development of pluripotent hematopoietic progenitor cells in the human fetus. *Blood* 1983; 62:118–23.
20. Linch DC, Knott LJ, Rodeck CH, Huehns ER. Studies of circulating hemopoietic progenitor cells in human fetal blood. *Blood* 1982; 59:976–9.
21. Gluckman E, Broxmeyer HE, Auerbach AD, Friedman HS, Douglas GW. Hematopoietic reconstitution in a patient with Fanconi's anemia by means of umbilical-cord blood from an HLA-identical sibling. *N Engl J Med* 1989; 321:1174–8.
22. Broxmeyer HE, Hangoc G, Cooper S. Clinical and biological aspects of human umbilical cord blood as a source of transplantable hematopoietic stem and progenitor cells. *Bone Marrow Transplant* 1992; 9(suppl):7–10.
23. Wagner JE, Kernan NA, Steinbuch M, Broxmeyer HE, Gluckman E. Allogeneic sibling umbilical-cord-blood transplantation in children with malignant and non-malignant disease. *Lancet* 1995; 346:214–9.
24. Gluckman E, Devergie A, Thierry D, et al. Clinical applications of stem cell transfusion from cord blood and rationale for cord blood banking. *Bone Marrow Transplant* 1992; 9(suppl):114–7.
25. Touraine JL. Rationale and results of in utero transplants of stem cells in humans. *Bone Marrow Transplant* 1992; 10(suppl):121–6.
26. Sieff CA, Nathan DG. The anatomy and physiology of hematopoiesis. In: Nathan DG, Oski FA, eds. *Hematology of Infancy and Childhood.* 4th ed. Philadelphia: WB Saunders, 1993, pp. 156–215.
27. Singer DB. Hepatic erythropoiesis in infants of diabetic mothers: a morphometric study. *Pediatr Pathol* 1986; 5:471–9.

28. Hågå P, Kristiansen S. Role of the kidney in foetal erythropoiesis: erythropoiesis and erythropoietin levels in newborn mice with renal agenesis. *J Embryol Exp Morphol* 1981; 61:165–73.

29. Brown MS. Fetal and neonatal erythropoiesis. In: Stockman JA III, Pochedly C, eds. *Developmental and Neonatal Hematology*. New York: Raven, 1988, pp. 39–56.

30. Groopman JE, Molina J-M, Scadden DT. Hematopoietic growth factors: biology and clinical applications. *N Engl J Med* 1983; 321:1449–59.

31. Bard H, Prosmanne J. Postnatal fetal and adult hemoglobin synthesis in preterm infants weighing less than 1000 grams. *J Clin Invest* 1982; 70:50–52.

32. Moya FR, Grannum PA, Widness JA, et al. Erythropoietin in human fetuses with immune hemolytic anemia and hydrops fetalis. *Obstet Gynecol* 1993; 82:353–8.

33. Ruth V, Widness JA, Clemons G, Raivio KO. Postnatal changes in serum immunoreactive erythropoietin in relation to hypoxia before and after birth. *J Pediatr* 1990; 116:1950–4.

34. Petry CD, Eaton MA, Wobken JD, et al. Iron deficiency of liver, heart, and brain in newborn infants of diabetic mothers. *J Pediatr* 1992; 121:109–14.

35. Halmesmaki E, Teramo KA, Widness JA, Clemons GK, Ylikorkala O. Maternal alcohol abuse is associated with elevated fetal erythropoietin levels. *Obstet Gynecol* 1990; 76:219–22.

36. Varvarigou A, Beratis NG, Makri M, Vagenakis G. Increased levels and positive correlation between erythropoietin and hemoglobin concentrations in newborn children of mothers who are smokers. *J Pediatr* 1994; 124:480–2.

37. Strauss RG. Erythropoietin in the pathogenesis and treatment of neonatal anemia. *Transfusion* 1995; 35:68–73.

38. Strauss RG. Erythropoietin and neonatal anemia. *N Engl J Med* 1994; 330:1227–8.

39. Strauss RG. Red blood cell transfusion practices in the neonate. *Clin Perinatol* 1995; 22:641–55.

40. Shannon K. Recombinant human erythropoietin in neonatal anemia. *Clin Perinatol* 1995; 22:627–40.

41. Mauer AM. *Pediatric Hematology*. New York: McGraw-Hill, 1969, pp. 8ff.

42. Luban NLC. Blood groups and blood component transfusion. In: Miller DR, Baehner RL, Miller LP, eds. *Blood Diseases of Infancy and Childhood*. 7th ed. St. Louis: CV Mosby, 1995, pp. 54–108.

43. Freedman RM, Johnston D, Mahoney MJ, Pearson HA. Brief clinical and laboratory observations: development of splenic reticulo-endothelial function in neonates. *J Pediatr* 1980; 96:466–8.

44. Anderson GW. Studies on the nucleated red cell count in the chorionic capillaries and the cord blood of various ages of pregnancy. *Am J Obstet Gynecol* 1941; 42:1–14.

45. Forestier F, Daffos F, Catherine N, Renard M, Andreux J-P. Deveopmental hematopoiesis in normal human fetal blood. *Blood* 1991; 77:2360–3.

46. Potter EL, Craig JM. *Pathology of the Fetus and the Infant*. Chicago: Year Book Medical, 1975, pp. 654ff.

47. Philip AGS, Tito AM. Increased nucleated red blood cell counts in small for gestational age infants with very low birth weight. *Am J Dis Child* 1989; 143:164–9.

48. Humbert JR, Abelson H, Hathaway WE, Battaglia FC. Polycythemia in small for gestational age infants. *J Pediatr* 1969; 75:812–9.

49. Matsunaga AT, Lubin BH. Hemolytic anemia in the newborn. *Clin Perinatol* 1995; 22:803–28.

50. Miller DR. Normal blood values from birth through adolescence. In: Miller DR, Baehner RL, Miller LP, eds. *Blood Diseases of Infancy and Childhood*. 7th ed. St. Louis: CV Mosby, 1995, pp. 30–53.

51. Pearson HA. Lifespan of the fetal red blood cell. *J Pediatr* 1967; 70:166–71.

52. DeWaele M, Foulon W, Renmans W, et al. Hematologic values and lymphocyte subsets in fetal blood. *Am J Clin Pathol* 1988; 89:742–6.

53. Glader BE. Recognition of anemia and red blood cell disorders during infancy. In: Alter BP, ed. *Perinatal Hematology*. New York: Churchill Livingstone, 1989, pp. 126–64.

54. Zaizov R, Matoth Y. Red cell values on the first post-natal day during the last 16 weeks of gestation. *Am J Hematol* 1976; 1:275–8.

55. Stine MJ, Harris H. Validity of arterial hematocrits in newborns. *Am J Dis Child* 1988; 142:66–7.

56. McIntosh N, Kempson C, Tyler RM. Blood counts in extremely low birthweight infants. *Arch Dis Child* 1988; 63:74–6.

57. Huisman THJ. Human hemoglobin. In: Miller DR, Baehner RL, Miller LP, eds. *Blood Diseases of Infancy and Childhood*. 7th ed. St. Louis: CV Mosby 1995, pp. 385–414.

58. Wood WG, Howes S, Bunch C. Developmental clocks and hemoglobin switching. *Progr Clin Biol Res* 1987; 251:521–9.

59. Kazazian HH, Woodhead AP. Hemoglobin synthesis in the developing fetus. *N Engl J Med* 1973; 289:58–62.

60. Rhondeau SM, Christensen RD, Ross MP, Rothstein G, Simmons MA. Responsiveness to recombinant human erythropoietin to marrow erythroid progenitors from infants with the "anemia of prematurity." *J Pediatr* 1988; 112:935–40.

61. Weatherall DJ, Wood WG, Jones RW, Clegg JB. The developmental genetics of human hemoglobin. *Progr Clin Biol Res* 1985; 191:3–25.

62. Pearson HA. Disorders of hemoglobin synthesis and metabolism. In: Oski FA, Naiman JL, eds. *Hematologic Problems in the Neonate*. 3rd ed. Philadelphia: WB Saunders, 1982, pp. 245–82.

63. Bunn HF. Human hemoglobins: normal and abnormal; methemoglobinemia. In: Nathan DG, Oski FA, eds. *Hematology of Infancy and Childhood*. 4th ed. Philadelphia: WB Saunders, 1993, pp. 698–731.

64. Georgieff MK, Landon MB, Mills MM, et al. Abnormal iron distribution in infants of diabetic mothers: spectrum and maternal antecedence. *J Pediatr* 1990; 117:455–61.

65. Chockilingam UM, Murphy E, Ophoven JC, Weisdorf SA, Georgieff MK. Cord transferrin and ferritin values in newborn infants at risk for prenatal uteroplacental insufficiency and chronic hypoxia. *J Pediatr* 1987; 111:283–6.

66. Georgieff MK, Petry CD, Wobken JD, Oyer CE. Liver and brain iron deficiency in newborn infants with bilateral renal agenesis (Potter's syndrome). *Pediatr Pathol Lab Med* 1996; 16:509–19.

67. Ratten GJ, Beischer NA, Fortune DW. Obsetric complications when the fetus has Potter's syndrome. I. Clinical considerations. *Am J Obstet Gynecol* 1973; 115:890–6.

68. Beischer NA, Ratten GJ, Fortune DW, Macafee J. Obstetric complications when the fetus has Potter's syndrome. II. Fetoplacental function. *Am J Obstet Gynecol* 1973; 116:62–5.

69. Christensen RD. Granulocytopoiesis in the fetus and neonate. *Transf Med Rev* 1990; 4:8–13.

70. Graeve JLA, DeAlarcon PA. Megakaryocytopoiesis in the human fetus. *Arch Dis Child* 1989; 64:481–4.

71. Olson TA, Levine RF, Mazur EM, Wright DG, Salvado AJ. Megakaryocytes and megakaryocyte progenitors in human cord blood. *Am J Pediatr Hematol Oncol* 1992; 14:241–7.

72. Aster RH. What makes platelets go? The cloning of thrombopoietin. *Transfusion* 1995; 35:1–3.

73. Baehner RL. Lymphocytes. In: Miller DR, Baehner RL, Miller LP, eds. *Blood Diseases of Infancy and Childhood*. 6th ed. St. Louis: CV Mosby, 1989, pp. 578–603.

74. Baehner RL, Miller DR. Lymphocytes. In: Miller DR, Baehner RL, Miller LP, eds. *Blood Diseases of Infancy and Childhood*. 7th ed. St. Louis: CV Mosby, 1989, pp. 627–59.

75. McDuffie M, Hayward AR. T-cell development. In: Polin RA, Fox WW, eds. *Fetal and Neonatal Physiology*. Philadelphia: WB Saunders, 1992, pp. 1427–32.

76. Kohl S, Frazier JJ, Greenberg SB, Pickering LK, Loo L-S. Interferon induction of natural killer toxicity in human neonates. *J Pediatr* 1981; 98:379–84.

77. Weinberg AG, Rosenfeld CR, Manroe BL, Browne R. Blood cell counts in health and disease. II. Values for lymphocytes, monocytes, and eosinophils. *J Pediatr* 1985; 106:462–6.

78. Oski FA, Naiman JL. Maternal fetal relationships. In: Oski FA, Naiman JL, eds. *Hematologic Problems in the Newborn*. 3rd ed. Philadelphia: WB Saunders, 1982, pp. 32–55.

79. Oski FA, Naiman JL. Erythroblastosis fetalis. In: Oski FA, Naiman JL, eds. *Hematologic Problems in the Newborn*. 3rd ed. Philadelphia: WB Saunders, 1982, pp. 283–346.

80. Zetterström R. The pathology of kernicterus and cytotoxicity of bilirubin. In: Sass-Korsak A, ed. *Kernicterus*. Toronto: University of Toronto Press, 1961, pp. 135–9.

81. Odel GB, Cukier JO, Maglalang AC. Pathogenesis of neonatal hyperbilirubinemia. In: Young DS, Hicks JM, eds. *The Neonate. Clinical Biochemistry, Physiology and Pathology*. New York: John Wiley, 1976, pp. 271ff.

82. Chown B. Anaemia from bleeding of the fetus into mother's circulation. *Lancet* 1954; 1:1213.

83. Brouwers HAA, Ertbruggen II, Alsbach GPJ, et al. What is the best predictor of the severity of ABO-hemolytic disease in the newborn? *Lancet* 1988; 2:641–4.

84. Bell CA. *A Seminar on Perinatal Blood Banking*. Washington, DC: American Association of Blood Banks, 1978, p. 105.

85. Stern K, Davidsohn I, Buznitsky A. Neonatal serologic diagnosis of hemolytic disease of newborn caused by ABO incompatibility. *J Lab Clin Med* 1957; 50:550–8.

86. Bucher KA, Patterson AM, Elston RC, Jones CA, Kirkman HN Jr. Racial difference in incidence of ABO hemolytic disease. *Am J Public Health* 1976; 66:854–8.

87. Mollison PL, Engelfriet CP, Contreras M. *Blood Transfusion in Clinical Medicine.* 9th ed. Boston: Blackwell Scientific, 1993, p. 585.

88. Kan YW, Forget BG, Nathan DG. Gamma-beta thalassemia: a cause of hemolytic disease of the newborn. *N Engl J Med* 1972; 286:129–32.

89. Hall FW, Lundgrin DB. Screening for alpha-thalassemia in neonates. *Am J Clin Pathol* 1987; 87:389–91.

90. Tuck SM, Studd JWW, White JM. Pregnancy in sickle cell disease in the U.K. *Br J Obstet Gynaecol* 1983; 90:112–7.

91. Ballin A, Brown EJ, Zipursky A. Idiopathic Heinz body hemolytic anemia in newborn infants. *Am J Pediatr Hematol Oncol* 1989; 11:3–7.

92. Becker PS, Lux SE. Disorders of the red cell membrane. In: Nathan DG, Oski FA, eds. *Hematology of Infancy and Childhood.* 4th ed. Philadelphia: WB Saunders, 1993, pp. 529–633.

93. Gallagher PG, Tse WT, Forget BG. Clinical and molecular aspects of disorders of the erythrocyte membrane skeleton. *Semin Perinatol* 1990; 14:351–67.

94. Nagel RL. Red cell cytoskeletal abnormalities—implications for malaria. *N Engl J Med* 1990; 323:1558–60.

95. Mentzer WC Jr, Collier E. Hydrops fetalis associated with erythrocyte G-6-P-D deficiency and maternal ingestion of fava beans and ascorbic acid. *J Pediatr* 1075; 86:565–7.

96. Perkins RP. Hydrops fetalis and stillbirth in a male glucose-6-phosphate dehydrogenase-deficient fetus possibly due to maternal ingestion of sulfisoxazole; a case report. *Am J Obstet Gynecol* 1971; 111:379–81.

97. Whitelaw AGL, Rogers PA, Hopkinson DA, et al. Congenital haemolytic anaemia resulting from glucose phosphate isomerase deficiency: genetics, clinical picture, and prenatal diagnosis. *J Med Genet* 1979; 16:189–96.

98. Ravindranath Y, Paglia DE, Warrier I, et al. Glucose phosphate isomerase deficiency as a cause of hydrops fetalis. *N Engl J Med* 1987; 316:258–61.

99. Matthay KK, Mentzer WC. Erythrocyte enzymopathies in the newborn. *Clin Haematol* 1981; 10:31–55.

100. Kelton JG, Brain MC, Hayward CPM. Destruction of red cells by the vasculature and reticuloendothelial system. In: Nathan DG, Oski FA, eds. *Hematology of Infancy and Childhood.* 4th ed. Philadelphia: WB Saunders, 1993, pp. 511–28.

101. Diamond LK, Blackfan KD, Baty JM. Erythroblastosis fetalis and its association with universal edema of fetus, icterus gravis neonatorum and anemia of the newborn. *J Pediatr* 1932; 1:269–309.

102. Nicolaides KH, Thiliganathan B, Rodeck CH, Mibashan RS. Erythroblastosis and reticulocytosis in anemic fetuses. *Am J Obstet Gynecol* 1988; 159:1063–5.

103. Craig JM. Sequences in the development of cirrhosis of the liver in cases of erythroblastosis fetalis. *Arch Pathol* 1950; 49:665–86.

104. Abrahamov A, Smith CA. Oxygen capacity and affinity of blood from erythroblastotic newborns. *Am J Dis Child* 1959; 97:375.

105. Brenner G, Allen RP. Skeletal changes in erythroblastosis fetalis. *Radiology* 1963; 80:427–30.

106. Chessells JM, Wigglesworth JS. Haemostatic failure in babies with Rhesus isoimmunization. *Arch Dis Child* 1971; 46:38–44.

107. Whitington PF, Gartner LM. Disorders of bilirubin metabolism. In: Nathan DG, Oski FA, eds. *Hematology of Infancy and Childhood.* 4th ed. Philadelphia: WB Saunders, 1993, pp. 74–114.

108. Zipursky A, Chintu C, Brown E, Brown EJ. The quantitation of spherocytes in ABO hemolytic disease. *J Pediatr* 1979; 94:965–7.

109. Oski FA. Kernicterus. In: Taeusch HW, Ballard RA, Avery ME eds. *Diseases of the Newborn.* 6th ed. Philadelphia: WB Saunders, 1991, pp. 760–2.

110. Klemperer MR. Hemolytic anemias: immune defects. In: Miller DR, Baehner RL, Miller LP, eds. *Blood Diseases of Infancy and Childhood.* 7th ed. St. Louis: CV Mosby, 1995, pp. 241–71.

111. Wallerstein H. The management of hemolytic disease of the fetus and newborn infant. *Acta Haematol* 1949; 2:349–68.

112. Frigoletto FD. Management and prevention of erythroblastosis fetalis. *Clin Perinatol* 1974; 3:321–30.

113. Holt EM, Boyd IE, Dewhurst CJ, et al. Intrauterine transfusion: 101 consecutive cases treated at Queen Charlotte's Maternity Hospital. *BMJ* 1973; 3:39–43.

114. Queenan JT. Intrauterine transfusion: a cooperative study. *Am J Obstet Gynecol* 1969; 104:397–405.

115. Mandelbaum B, Brough AJ. Hepatitis following multiple intrauterine transfusions. Report of a case. *Obstet Gynecol* 1967; 30:188–91.

116. Nicolaides KH, Mibashan RS. Fetal red cell isoimmunization. In: Alter BP, ed. *Perinatal Hematology.* New York: Churchill Livingstone, 1989, pp. 108–25.

117. Peterec SM. Management of neonatal Rh disease. *Clin Perinatol* 1995; 22:561–92.

118. Fliegner JRH, Fortune DW, Barrie JU. Occult fetomaternal haemorrhage as a cause of fetal mortality and morbidity. *Aust NZ J Obstet Gynaecol* 1987; 27:158–61.

119. O'Brien JA, Coustan DR, Singer DB, Taylor MA. Prepartum diagnosis of traumatic fetal-maternal hemorrhage. *Am J Perinatol* 1985; 2:214–6.

120. Sebring ES, Polesky HF. Fetomaternal hemorrhage: incidence, risk factors, time of occurrence, and clinical effect. *Transfusion* 1990; 30:344–57.

121. Fischer RL, Kuhlman K, Grover J, Montgomery O, Wapner RJ. Chronic, massive fetomaternal hemorrhage treated with repeated fetal intravascular transfusions. *Am J Obstet Gynecol* 1990; 162:203–4.

122. Andre M, Vert P. Birth injuries. In: Stern L, Vert P, eds. *Neonatal Medicine.* New York: Masson, 1987, pp. 176–91.

123. French CE, Waldstein G. Subcapsular hemorrhage of the liver in the newborn. *Pediatr* 1982; 69:204–8.

124. Ryan CA, Finer NN. Subcapsular hematoma of the liver in infants of very low birth weight. *Can Med Assoc J* 1987; 136:1265–9.

125. Odell JM, Haas JE, Tapper D, Nugent D. Infantile hemorrhagic angiodysplasia. *Pediatr Pathol* 1987; 7:629–36.

126. Schoen FJ. Blood vessels. In: Cotran R, Kumar V, Robbins SL, eds. *Pathologic Basis of Disease.* 5th ed. Philadelphia: WB Saunders, 1994, p. 509.

127. Bussel JB, Corrigan JJ Jr. Platelet and vascular disorders. In: Miller DR, Baehner RL, Miller LP, eds. *Blood Diseases of Infancy and Childhood.* 7th ed. St. Louis: Mosby, 1995, p. 916.

128. Guttmacher AE, Marchuk DA, White RI. Hereditary hemorrhagic telangec-tasia. *N Engl J Med* 1995; 333:918–24.

129. Lachance C, Chessex P, Fouron J-C, Widness JA, Bard H. Myocardial, erythropoietic, and metabolic adaptations to anemia of prematurity. *J Pediatr* 1994; 125:278–82.

130. Oh W. Neonatal polycythemia and hyperviscosity. *Pediatr Clin North Am* 1986; 33:523–30.

131. Oski FA, Naiman JL. Polycythemia and hyperviscosity. In: Oski FA, Naiman JL, eds. *Hematologic Problems in the Newborn.* 3rd ed. Philadelphi: WB Saunders, 1982, pp. 87–96.

132. Saigal S, Usher RH. Symptomatic neonatal plethora. *Biol Neonate* 1977; 32:62–72.

133. Michael AF, Mauer AM. Maternal-fetal transfusion as a cause of plethora in the neonatal period. *Pediatrics* 1961; 28:458–61.

134. Rosenkrantz TS, Oh W. Cerebral blood flow velocity in infants with polycythemia and hyperviscosity. Effects of partial exchange transfusion with plasmanate. *J Pediatr* 1982; 101:94–8.

135. Swetnam SM, Yabek SM, Alverson DC. Hemodynamic consequences of neonatal polycythemia. *J Pediatr* 1987; 110:443–7.

136. Fish WH, Chazen EM. Toxic effects of methylene blue in the fetus. *Am J Dis Child* 1992; 146:1412–3.

137. Sills MR, Zinkham WH. Methylene blue-induced Heinz body hemolytic anemia. *Arch Pediatr Adolesc Med* 1994; 148:306–10.

138. Cowett RW, Hakanson DO, Kocon RW, Oh W. Untoward neonatal effect of intraamniotic administration of methylene blue. *Obstet Gynecol* 1976; 48:74s–5s.

139. Fisch RO, Berglund EB, Bridge AG, et al. Methemoglobinemia in a hospital nursery. A search for causative factors. *JAMA* 1963; 185:760–3.

140. Mandel S. Methemoglobinemia following neonatal circumcision. *JAMA* 1989; 261:702.

141. Dallman PR. Blood and blood forming tissue. In: Rudolph A, ed. *Pediatrics.* 16th ed. New York: Appleton-Century-Crofts, 1977, p. 2111.

142. Glader BE, Zwerdling T. Leukocyte disorders in the newborn. In: Taeusch HW, Ballard RA, Avery ME, eds. *Diseases of the Newborn.* 6th ed. Philadelphia: WB Saunders, 1991, pp. 791–7.

143. Baley JE, Stork EK, Warkentin PI, Shurin SB. Neonatal neutropenia. Clinical manifestations, cause, and outcome. *Am J Dis Child* 1988; 142:1161–6.

144. Hasan R, Inoue S, Banerjee A. Higher white blood cell counts and band forms in newborns delivered vaginally compared with those delivered by cesarean section. *Am J Clin Pathol* 1993; 100:116–8.

145. Miller DR, Freed BA, Lapey JD. Congenital neutropenia. Report of a fatal case in a Negro infant with leukocyte function studies. *Am J Dis Child* 1968; 115:337–46.

146. Engle WA, McGuire WA, Schreiner RL, Yu P-L. Neutrophil storage pool depletion in neonates with sepsis and neutropenia. *J Pediatr* 1988; 113: 747–9.

147. Mouzinho A, Rosenfeld CR, Sanchez PJ, Risser R. Revised reference ranges for circulating neutrophils in very-low-birth-weight neonates. *Pediatrics* 1994; 94:76–82.

148. Liu C-H, Lehan C, Speer ME, Fernbach DJ, Rudolph AJ. Degenerative changes in neutrophils: an indicator of bacterial infection. *Pediatrics* 1984; 74:823–7.

149. Engle WA, Schreiner RL, Baehner RL. Neonatal white blood cell disorders. *Semin Perinatol* 1983; 7:184–200.

150. Curnutte JT. Disorders of granulocyte function and granulopoiesis. In: Nathan DG, Oski FA, eds. *Hematology of Infancy and Childhood.* 4th ed. Philadelphia: WB Saunders, 1993, pp. 904–77.

151. Dong F, Brynes RK, Tidow N, et al. Mutations in the gene for the granulocyte colony-stimulating-factor receptor in patients with acute myeloid leukemia preceded by severe congenital neutropenia. *N Engl J Med* 1995; 333:487–93.

152. Naparstek E. Granulocyte colony-stimulating factor, congenital neutropenia, and acute myeloid leukemia. *N Engl J Med* 1995; 333:516–8.

153. Shwachman H, Diamond LK, Oski FA, Khaw KT. The syndrome of pancreatic insufficiency and bone marrow dysfunction. *J Pediatr* 1964; 65:645–63.

154. Furman WL, Crist WM. Biology and clinical applications of hematopoietins in pediatric practice. *Pediatrics* 1992; 90:716–28.

155. Nemunaitis J. Granulocyte-macrophage-stimulating factor: a review from preclinical development to clinical application. *Transfusion* 1993; 33:70–82.

156. Murray JC, McClain KL, Wearden ME. Using granulocyte colony-stimulating factor for neutropenia during neonatal sepsis. *Arch Pediatr Adolesc Med* 1994; 148:764–6.

157. Bonilla MA, Gillio AP, Ruggiero M, et al. Effects of recombinant human granulocyte colony-stimulating factor on neutropenia in patients with congenital granulocytosis. *N Engl J Med* 1989; 320: 1574–80.

158. Schapiro BL, Newburger PE, Klempner MS, Dinauer MC. Chronic granulomatous disease presenting in a 69-year old man. *N Engl J Med* 1991; 325:1786–90.

159. Yang KD, Hill HR. Neutrophil function disorders: pathophysiology, prevention, and therapy. *J Pediatr* 1991; 119:343–54.

160. Mattia AR. Case records of the Massachusetts General Hospital: case 35-1993. *N Engl J Med* 1993; 329:714–21.

161. Hopkins PJ, Bemiller LS, Curnutte JT. Chronic granulomatous disease: diagnosis and classification at the molecular level. *Clin Lab Med* 1992; 12:277–304.

162. O'Shea PA. Chronic granulomatous disease of childhood. *Perspect Pediatr Pathol* 1982; 7:237–58.

163. Landing BH, Shirkey HS. A syndrome of recurrent infection and infiltration of viscera by pigmented lipid histiocytes. *Pediatrics* 1957; 20:431–8.

164. Stockman JA III. Disorders of leukocytes. In: Oski FA, Naiman JL, eds. *Hematologic Problems in the Newborn.* 3rd ed. Philadelphia: WB Saunders, 1982, pp. 223–44.

165. Oski FA. Hematologic problems. In: Avery GB, ed. *Neonatology.* 2nd ed. Philadelphia: JB Lippincott, 1981, p. 580.

166. Gibson EL, Vaucher Y, Corrigan JJ. Eosinophilia in premature infants: relationship to weight gain. *J Pediatr* 1979; 95:99–101.

167. Jouan H, LeDeist F, Nezelof C. Omenn's syndrome. Pathologic arguments in favor of a graft versus host pathogenesis. A report of nine cases. *Hum Pathol* 1987; 18:1101–8.

168. Omenn GS. Familial reticuloendotheliosis with eosinophilia. *N Engl J Med* 1965; 273:427–32.

169. Hong R, Gilbert EF, Opitz JM. Omenn disease: termination in lymphoma. *Pediatr Pathol* 1985; 3:143–54.

170. Holland PV. Prevention of transfusion-associated graft-vs-host disease. *Arch Pathol Lab Med* 1989; 113;285–8.

171. Darron DA, Bisch AC, Carnahan EA, Zarkowsky HS. Neonatal transfusion practices: results of a national survey. *Lab Med* 1988; 19:814–16.

172. Gray ES, Balch NJ, Kohler H, Thompson WD, Simpson JG. Congenital leukaemia: an unusual cause of stillbirth. *Arch Dis Child* 1986; 61:1001–6.

173. Las Heras J, Leal G, Haust MD. Congenital leukemia with placental involvement: report of a case with ultrastructural study. *Cancer* 1986; 58:2278–81.

174. Bouton MJ, Phillips HJ, Smithells RW, Walker S. Congenital leukaemia with parental consanguinity: case report with chromosome studies. *BMJ* 1961; 2:866–9.

175. Kaufmann HJ, Hess R. Does congenital leukaemia exist? *BMJ* 1962; 1:867–8.

176. Powers LW, Register MK. Down syndrome and acute leukemia: epidemiological and genetic relationships. *Lab Med* 1991; 22:630–6.

177. Allan RR, Wadsworth LD, Kalousek DK, Massing BG. Congenital erythroleukemia: a case report with morphological, immunophenotypic, and cytogenetic findings. *Am J Hematol* 1989; 31:114–21.

178. Kurosawa H, Eguchi M, Sakakibara H, Takahashi H, Furukawa T. Ultra-structural cytochemistry of congenital basophilic leukemia. *Am J Pediatr Hematol Oncol* 1987; 9:27–32.

179. Resnik KS, Brod BB. Leukemia cutis in congenital leukemia. Analysis and review of the world literature with report of an additional case. *Arch Dermatol* 1993; 129:1301–6.

180. Rodgers R, Weiner M, Friedman AH. Ocular involvement in congenital leukemia. *Am J Ophthalmol* 1986; 101:730–2.

181. Miller DR. Hematologic malignancies: leukemia and lymphoma. In: Miller DR, Baehner RL, Miller LP, eds. *Blood Diseases of Infancy and Childhood.* 7th ed. St. Louis: CV Mosby, 1995, pp. 660–804.

182. Fong CT, Brodeur GM. Down's syndrome and leukemia: epidemiology, genetics, cytogenetics and mechanism of leukemogenesis. *Cancer Genet Cytogenet* 1987; 28:55–76.

183. Kojima S, Matsuyama T, Sato T, et al. Down's syndrome and acute leukemia in children: an analysis of phenotype by use of monoclonal antibodies and electron microscopic platelet peroxidase reaction. *Blood* 1990; 76:2348–53.

184. Grier HE, Civin CI. Acute and chronic myeloproliferative disorders and myelodysplasia. In: Nathan DG, Oski FA, eds. *Hematology of Infancy and Childhood.* 4th ed. Philadelphia: WB Saunders, 1993, pp. 1288–318.

185. Jiang C-J, Liang D-C, Tien H-F. Neonatal transient leukaemoid proliferation followed by acute myeloid leukaemia in a phenotypically normal child. *Br J Haematol* 1991; 77:247–8.

186. Liang D-C, Ma S-W, Lu T-H, Lin S-T. Transient myeloproliferative disorder and acute myeloid leukemia: study of six neonatal cases with long-term follow-up. *Leukemia* 1993; 7:1521–4.

187. Donnenfeld AE, Scott SC, Henselder-Kimmel M, Dampier CD. Prenatally diagnosed non-immune hydrops caused by congenital transient leukaemia. *Prenat Diagn* 1994; 14:721–4.

188. Bain B. Down's syndrome—transient abnormal myelopoiesis and acute leukaemia. *Leuk Lymphoma* 1991; 3:309–17.

189. Suda J, Eouchi M, Ozawa T, et al. Platelet peroxidase-positive blast cells in transient myeloproliferative disorder with Down's syndrome. *Br J Haematol* 1988; 68:181–7.

190. Weinberg AG, Schiller G, Windmiller J. Neonatal leukemoid reaction: an isolated manifestation of mosaic trisomy-21. *Am J Dis Child* 1982; 136:310–11.

191. Jones GR, Weaver M, Laug WE. Transient blastemia in phenotypically normal newborns. *Am J Pediatr Hematol Oncol* 1987; 9:153–7.

192. Foucar K, Friedman K, Llewellyn A, et al. Prenatal diagnosis of transient myeloproliferative disorder via percutaneous umbilical blood sampling. *Am J Clin Pathol* 1992; 97:584–90.

193. Jackson GH, Carey PJ, Cant AJ, Bown NP, Reid MM. Myelodysplastic syndromes in children. *Br J Haematol* 1993; 84:185–6.

194. Hasle H, Jacobsen BB, Pedersen NT. Myelodysplastic syndromes in childhood: a population-based study of nine cases. *Br J Haematol* 1992; 81:495–8.

195. Hann IM. Myelodysplastic syndromes. *Arch Dis Child* 1992; 67:962–6.

196. McMullin MF, Chisholm, Hows JW. Congenital myelodysplasia: a newly described disease entity. *Br J Haematol* 1991; 79:340–2.

197. O'Donnell MR, Nademanee AP, Snyder DS, et al. Bone marrow transplantation for myelodysplastic and myeloproliferative disorders. *J Clin Oncol* 1987; 5:1822–6.

198. Brandwein JM, Horsman DE, Eaves AC, et al. Childhood myelodysplasia: suggested classification as myelodysplastic syndromes based on laboratory and clinical findings. *Am J Pediatr Hematol Oncol* 1990; 12:63–70.

199. Baranger L, Baruchel A, Leverger G, Schaison G, Berger R. Monosomy-7 in childhood hemopoietic disorders. *Leukemia* 1990; 4:345–9.

200. Shitara T, Suetake N, Yugami S, et al. A case of congenital leukemia with monosomy 7. *Ann Haematol* 1992; 65:247–7.

201. Stuart MJ. Bleeding in the newborn and pediatric patient. In: Colman RW, Hirsh J, Marder VJ, Salzman EW, eds. *Hemostasis and Thrombosis: Basic Principles and Clinical Practice.* 2nd ed. Philadelphia: JB Lippincott, 1987, pp. 942–57.

202. Andrew M. The hemostatic system in the infant. In: Nathan DG, Oski FA, eds. *Hematology of Infancy and Childhood.* 4th ed. Philadelphia: WB Saunders, 1993, pp. 115–53.

203. Lusher JM. Diseases of coagulation: the fluid phase. In: Nathan DG, Oski FA, eds. *Hematology of Infancy and Childhood.* Philadelphia: WB Saunders, 1987, pp. 1293ff.

204. Levin M, Pincott JR, Hjelm M, et al. Hemorrhagic shock and encephalopathy: clinical, pathologic, and biochemical features. *J Pediatr* 1989; 114: 194–203.

205. Dalessio DJ. Seizure disorders and pregnancy. *N Engl J Med* 1985; 312:559–63.

206. Stockman JA III, Ezekowitz A. Hematologic manifestations of systemic diseases. In: Nathan DG, Oski FA, eds. *Hematology of Infancy and Childhood.* 4th ed. Philadelphia: WB Saunders, 1993, pp. 1834–85.

207. Montgomery RR, Scott JP. Hemostasis: diseases of the fluid phase. In: Nathan DG, Oski FA, eds. *Hematology of Infancy and Childhood.* 4th ed. Philadelphia: WB Saunders, 1993, pp. 1605–50.

208. Yoffe G, Buchanan GR. Intracranial hemorrhage in newborn and young infants with hemophilia. *J Pediatr* 1988; 113:333–6.

209. Smith PS. Congenital coagulation protein deficiencies in the perinatal period. *Semin Perinatol* 1990; 14:384–92.

210. Mibashan RS, Peake IR, Nicolaides KH. Prenatal diagnosis of hemostatic disorders. In: Alter BP, ed. *Perinatal Hematology*. New York: Churchill Livingstone, 1989, pp. 64–107.

211. Bacon CJ, Hall SM. Haemorrhagic shock encephalopathy syndrome in the British Isles. *Arch Dis Child* 1992; 67:985–93.

212. Zureikat GY, Zador I, Aouthmany M, Bhimani S. Cerebral infarct in patients with hemorrhagic shock and encephalopathy syndrome. *Pediatr Radiol* 1990; 20:301–3.

213. Corrigan JJ. The "H" in hemorrhagic shock and encephalopathy syndrome should be 'hyperpyrexia.' *Am J Dis Child* 1990; 144:1077.

214. Bonham JR, Meeds A, Levin M, et al. Complete recovery from hemorrhagic shock and encephalopathy. *J Pediatr* 1992; 120:440–3.

215. Conway EE Jr, Varlotta L, Singer LP, Caspe WB. Hemorrhagic shock and encephalopathy: is it really an entity? *Pediatr Emerg Care* 1990; 6:131–4.

216. Van den Hof MC, Nicolaides KH. Platelet count in normal, small, and anemic fetuses. *Am J Obstet Gynecol* 1990; 162:735–9.

217. Gill FM. Thrombocytopenia in the newborn. *Semin Perinatol* 1983; 7:201–12.

218. Andrew M, Castle V, Saigal S, Carter C, Kelton JG. Clinical impact of neonatal thrombocytopenia. *J Pediatr* 1987; 110;457–64.

219. Klein JO, Marcy SM. Bacterial sepsis and meningitis. In: Remington JS, Klein JO, eds. *Infectious Diseases of the Fetus and Newborn Infant*. 3rd ed. Philadelphia: WB Saunders, 1990, pp. 601–56.

220. Kaplan C, Daffos F, Forestier F, et al. Management of alloimmune thrombocytopenia. Antenatal diagnosis and in utero transfusion of maternal platelets. *Blood* 1988; 72:340–3.

221. Bussel JB, Berkowitz RL, McFarland JG, Lynch L, Chitkara U. Antenatal treatment of neonatal alloimmune thrombocytopenia. *N Engl J Med* 1988; 319:1374–8.

222. Copplestone JA. Asymptomatic thrombocytopenia developing during pregnancy (gestational thrombocytopenia)—a clinical study. *QJM* 1992; 84: 593–601.

223. Kaplan C, Daffos F, Forestier F, et al. Fetla platelet counts in thrombocytopenic pregnancy. *Lancet* 1990; 336:979–82.

224. Burrows RF, Kelton JG. Fetal thrombocytopenia and its relation to maternal thrombocytopenia. *N Engl J Med* 1993; 329:1463–6.

225. Samuels P, Bussel JB, Braitman LE, et al. Estimation of the risk of thrombocytopenia in the offspring of pregnant women with presumed immune thrombocytopenic purpura. *N Engl J Med* 1990; 323:229–35.

226. Homans AC, Cohen JL, Mazur EM. Defective megakaryocytopoiesis in the syndrome of thrombocytopenia with absent radii. *Br J Haematol* 1988; 70:205–10.

227. Hedberg VA, Lipton JM. Thrombocytopenia with absent radii: a review of 100 cases. *Am J Pediatr Hematol Oncol* 1988; 10:51–64.

228. Auerbach AD, Adler B, Chaganti RSK. Prenatal and postnatal diagnosis and carrier detection of Fanconi anemia by a cytogenetic method. *Pediatrics* 1981; 67:128–35.

229. Benirschke K, Kaufmann P. *Pathology of the Human Placenta*. New York: Springer, 1995, p. 713.

230. Zaizov R, Cohen I, Matot HY. Thrombasthenia: a study of two siblings. *Acta Paediatr Scand* 1968; 57:522–6.

231. Schmidt B, Andrew M. Neonatal thrombotic disease: prevention, diagnosis, and treatment. *J Pediatr* 1988; 113:407–10.

232. Alexander F, Campbell WAB. Congenital nephrotic syndrome and renal vein thrombosis in infancy. *J Clin Pathol* 1971; 24:27–40.

233. Oppenheimer EH, Esterly JR. Thrombosis in the newborn. Comparison between infants of diabetic and nondiabetic mothers. *J Pediatr* 1965; 67:549–56.

234. Schmidt B, Andrew M. Neonatal thrombosis: report of a prospective Canadian and international registry. *Pediatrics* 1995; 96:939–43.

235. Haust MD. Maternal diabetes mellitus. Effects on the fetus and placenta. In: Naeye RL, Kissane JM, Kaufman N, eds. *Perinatal Diseases*. Baltimore: Williams & Wilkins, 1981, pp. 201–85.

236. Seguin J, Weatherstone K, Nankervis C. Inherited antithrombin III deficiency in the neonate. *Arch Pediatr Adolesc Med* 1994; 148:389–93.

237. Seligsohn U, Berger A, Abend M, et al. Homozygous protein C deficiency manifested by massive venous thrombosis in the newborn. *N Engl J Med* 1984; 310:559–62.

238. Manco-Johnson M, Hays T, Warady BA, Marlar RA. Severe protein C deficiency in newborn infants. *J Pediatr* 1988; 113:359–63.

239. Matsuda M, Sugo T, Sakata Y, et al. A thrombotic state due to abnormal protein C. *N Engl J Med* 1988; 319:1265–8.

240. O'Sullivan J, Chatuverdi R, Bennett MK, Hunter S. Protein S deficiency: early presentation and pulmonary hypertension. *Arch Dis Child* 1992; 67:960–1.

241. Rick ME. Protein C and protein S; vitamin K-dependent inhibitors of blood coagulation. *JAMA* 1990; 5:701–3.

242. Dusser A, Boyer-Neumann C, Wolf M. Temporary protein C deficiency associated with cerebral arterial thrombosis in childhood. *J Pediatr* 1988; 113:849–51.

243. Oski FA, Naiman JL. Coagulation disorders. In: Oski FA, Naiman JL, eds. *Hematologic Problems in the Newborn*. 3rd ed. Philadelphia: WB Saunders, 1982, pp. 137–74.

244. Akin K. Macrocytosis and leukopenia in Down's syndrome. *JAMA* 1988; 259:842.

245. Lutzner MA, Hecht F. Nuclear anomalies of the neutrophil in a chromosomal triplication: the D₁ (13–15) trisomy syndrome; an electron microscopic study. *Lab Invest* 1966; 15:597–605.

246. Magenis E, Hecht F. Chromosome 13, trisomy 13. In: Buyse ML, ed. *Birth Defects Encyclopedia*. Dover, MA: Center for Birth Defects Information Services, 1990, pp. 368–70.

247. Walzer S, Gerald PS, Breau G, O'Neill D, Diamond LK. Hematologic changes in the D₁ trisomy syndrome. *Pediatrics* 1966; 38:419–29.

248. Huehns ER, Hecht F, Keil JV, Motulsky AG. Development hemoglobin anomalies in a chromosomal triplication: D₁ trisomy syndrome. *Proc Natl Acad Sci USA* 1964; 51:89–97.

249. Miller DR. Hemolytic anemias: metabolic defects. In: Miller DR, Baehner RL, Miller LP, eds. *Blood Diseases of Infancy and Childhood*. 7th ed. St. Louis: CV Mosby, 1995, pp. 316–84.

250. Fisk NM, Tannirandorn Y, Santolaya J, et al. Fetal macrocytosis in association with chromosomal abnormalities. *Obstet Gynecol* 1989; 74:611–6.

251. D'Alton ME, DeCherney AH. Prenatal diagnosis. *N Engl J Med* 1993; 328:114–20.

252. Simpson JL, Elias S. Isolating fetal cells from maternal blood: advances in prenatal diagnosis through molecular technology. *JAMA* 1993; 270: 2357–61.

253. Trapani F DI, Marino M, D'Alcamo E, et al. Prenatal diagnosis of haemoglobin disorders by cardiocentesis at 12 weeks' gestation. *Prenat Diagn* 1991; 11:899–904.

254. Johnson J-AM, McFarland JG, Blanchette VS, Freedman J, Siegel-Bartelt J. Prenatal diagnosis of neonatal alloimmune thrombocytopenia using an allele-specific oligonucleotide probe. *Prenat Diagn* 1993; 13:1037–42.

255. Montemagno R, Soothill PW, Scarcelli M, O'Brien P, Rodeck CH. Detection of alloimmune thrombocytopenia as cause of isolated hydrocephalus by fetal blood sampling. *Lancet* 1994; 343:1300–1.

256. Moishe KJ, Carpenter RJ Jr, Cotton DB, et al. Percutaneous umbilical cord blood sampling in the evaluation of fetal platelet counts in pregnant patients with autoimmune thrombocytopenic purpura. *Obstet Gynecol* 1988; 72:346–50.

257. Donnenfeld AE, Wiseman B, Lavi E, Weiner S. Prenatal diagnosis of thrombocytopenia absent radius syndrome by ultrasound and cardiocentesis. *Prenat Diagn* 1990; 10:29–35.

258. Weinblatt M, Petrikovsky B, Bialer M, Kochen J, Harper R. Prenatal evaluation and in-utero platelet transfusion for thrombocytopenia absent radii syndrome. *Prenat Diagn* 1994; 14:892–6.

259. LaBrune PH, Pons JC, Khalil M, et al. Antinatal thrombocytopenia in three patients with TAR (thrombocytopenia with absent radii) syndrome. *Prenat Diagn* 1993; 13:463–6.

260. Schwartz M, Mibashan RS, Nicolaides KH, et al. First trimester diagnosis of Wiskott-Aldrich syndrome by DNA markers. *Lancet* 1989; 2(8676): 1405.

261. Oberle I, Camerino G, Heilig R, et al. Genetic screening for hemophilia A (classic hemophilia) with a polymorphic DNA probe. *N Engl J Med* 1985; 312:682–6.

262. Romero R, Athanassiadis AP, Inati M. Fetal blood sampling. In: Fleischer AC, Romero R, Manning FA, Jeanty P, James AE Jr, eds. *The Principles and Practice of Ultrasonography in Obstetrics and Gynecology*. 4th ed. Norwalk, CT: Appleton & Lange, 1991, pp. 455–73.

263. Hoyer LW. Hemophilia A. *N Engl J Med* 1994; 330:38–47.

264. Mibashan RS, Millar DS, Rodeck CH, et al. Prenatal diagnosis of hereditary protein C deficiency. *N Engl J Med* 1985; 313:1607.

265. Sharon B. Antithrombin III deficiency. In: Buyse ML, ed. *Birth Defects Encyclopedia*. Dover, MA: Center for Birth Defects Information Services, 1990, pp. 152–4.

266. Diukman R, Tanigawara S, Cowan MJ, Golbus MS. Prenatal diagnosis of Chediak-Higashi syndrome. *Prenat Diagn* 1992; 12:877–85.

267. Durandy A, Breton-Gorius J, Guy-Grand D, Dumez C, Griscelli C. Prenatal diagnosis of syndromes associating albinism and immune deficiencies (Chediak-Higashi syndrome and variant). *Prenat Diagn* 1993; 13:13–20.

268. Antonarakis SE. Medical progress: diagnosis of genetic disorders at the DNA level. *N Engl J Med* 1989; 320:153–62.

269. Beutler E. Glucose-6-phosphate dehydrogenase deficiency. *N Engl J Med* 1991; 324:169–74.

270. Bennett PR, Le Van Kim C, Colin Y, et al. Prenatal determination of fetal RhD type by DNA amplification. *N Engl J Med* 1993; 329:607–10.

271. Brambati B, Anelli MC, Tului L, Columbo G. Fetal RhD typing by DNA amplification in chorionic villus sample. *Lancet* 1994; 344:959–60.

272. Török TJ, Wang Q-Y, Gary GW Jr, et al. Prenatal diagnosis of intrauterine infection with parvovirus B 19 by the polymerase chain reaction technique. *Clin Infect Dis* 1992; 14:149–55.

273. Berry PJ, Gray ES, Porter HJ, Burton PA. Parvovirus infection of the human fetus and newborn. *Semin Diagn Pathol* 1992; 9:4–12.

Note: Page numbers in *italics* refer to illustrations; page numbers followed by t refer to tables.